ICD·10·CM

International Classification of Diseases
10th Revision

Clinical Modification

DISCARDED

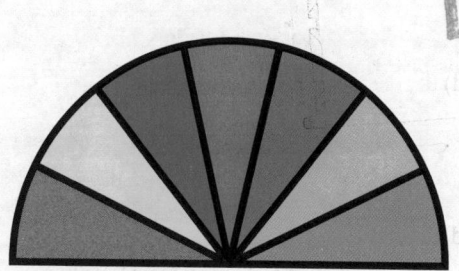

Color Coded

2017

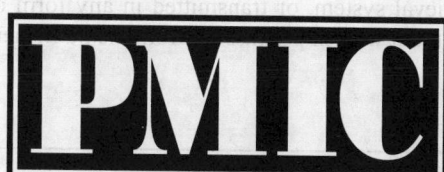

Office, Hospital and Payer Edition

ISBN 978-1-943009-51-0 (Perfect bound)
ISBN 978-1-943009-54-1 (e-Book)

Home Health Edition

ISBN 978-1-943009-79-4 (Perfect bound)
ISBN 978-1-943009-80-0 (e-Book)

Practice Management Information Corporation (PMIC)
4727 Wilshire Boulevard
Los Angeles, California 90010
http://www.pmiconline.com

Copyright 2016 under the Uniform Copyright Convention. All rights reserved. This book is protected by copyright. No part of it may be reproduced, stored in a retrieval system, or transmitted in any form or by any means, electronic mechanical, photocopying, recording, or otherwise, without written permission from the publisher.

Preface

On October 1, 2015, a key element of the data foundation of the United States' health care system underwent a major transformation…the transition from the decades-old Ninth Edition of the International Classification of Diseases (ICD-9) set of diagnosis and inpatient procedure codes to the far more contemporary, vastly larger, and much more detailed Tenth Edition of those code sets—or ICD-10—used by most developed countries throughout the world. The transition had a major impact on any person or entity recording health care information containing a diagnosis and/or inpatient procedure code.

All "covered entities"—as defined by the Health Insurance Portability and Accountability Act of 1996 (HIPAA)—were required to adopt ICD-10 codes for use in all HIPAA transactions with dates of service on or after the October 1, 2015 compliance date. for HIPAA inpatient claims, ICD-10 diagnosis and procedure codes are required for all inpatient stays with discharge dates on or after October 1, 2015.

This edition of ICD-10-CM includes all official codes, descriptions, guidelines, tables and indexes. A new edition is available approximately mid-September of each year. New editions may be purchased from:

Practice Management Information Corporation
4727 Wilshire Boulevard, Suite 300
Los Angeles, CA 90010
1-800-MED-SHOP
http://pmiconline.com

Disclaimer

This publication includes all official ICD-10-CM codes, descriptions, annotations and guidelines. This publication is revised annually so that we may present the most current information possible. Though all of the information is carefully researched and checked for accuracy and completeness, the publisher accepts no responsibility with regard to errors, omissions, misuse or misinterpretation.

Table of Contents

TABLE OF CONTENTS

Introduction to ICD-10-CM

On October 1, 2015, a key element of the data foundation of the United States' health care system underwent a major transformation…the transition from the decades-old Ninth Edition of the International Classification of Diseases (ICD-9) set of diagnosis and inpatient procedure codes to the far more contemporary, vastly larger, and much more detailed Tenth Edition of those code sets—or ICD-10—used by most developed countries throughout the world. The transition had a major impact on any person or entity recording health care information containing a diagnosis and/or inpatient procedure code.

HISTORY OF THE INTERNATIONAL CLASSIFICATION OF DISEASES

For students of medical nomenclature and coding systems, the following history of the International Classification of Diseases excerpted from Wikipedia may be interesting.

HISTORICAL SYNOPSIS

In 1893, a French physician, Jacques Bertillon, introduced the *Bertillon Classification of Causes of Death* at a congress of the International Statistical Institute in Chicago. a number of countries and cities adopted Dr. Bertillon's system, which was based on the principle of distinguishing between general diseases and those localized to a particular organ or anatomical site, as used by the City of Paris for classifying deaths. Subsequent revisions represented a synthesis of English, German and Swiss classifications, expanding from the original 44 titles to 161 titles. in 1898, the American Public Health Association (APHA) recommended that the registrars of Canada, Mexico, and the United States also adopt it. The APHA also recommended revising the system every ten years to ensure the system remained current with medical practice advances. As a result, the first international conference to revise the International Classification of Causes of Death convened in 1900; with revisions occurring every ten years thereafter. At that time the classification system was contained in one book, which included an Alphabetic Index as well as a Tabular List. The book was small compared with current coding texts.

The revisions that followed contained minor changes, until the sixth revision of the classification system. with the sixth revision, the classification system expanded to two volumes. The sixth revision included morbidity and mortality conditions, and its title was modified to reflect the changes: *International Statistical Classification of Diseases, Injuries and Causes of Death (ICD)*. Prior to the sixth revision, responsibility for ICD revisions fell to the Mixed Commission, a group composed of representatives from the International Statistical Institute and the Health Organization of the League of Nations. in 1948, the World Health Organization (WHO) assumed responsibility for preparing and publishing the revisions to the ICD every ten years. WHO sponsored the seventh and eighth revisions in 1957 and 1968, respectively. It later become clear that the established ten-year interval between revisions was too short.

The ICD is currently the most widely used statistical classification system for diseases in the world. International health statistics using this system are available at the WHO Statistical Information System (WHOSIS). in addition, some countries—including Australia, Canada and the United States—have developed their own adaptations of ICD, with more procedure for classification of operative or diagnostic procedures.

HISTORY AND USAGE IN THE UNITED STATES

In the United States, the U.S. Public Health Service published the *International Classification of Diseases, Adapted for Indexing of Hospital Records and Operation Classification (ICDA)*, completed in 1962 and expanding the ICD-7 in a number of areas to more completely meet the indexing needs of hospitals. The U.S. Public Health Service later published the *Eighth Revision, International Classification of Diseases, Adapted for Use in the United States*, commonly referred to as ICDA-8, for official national morbidity and mortality statistics. This was followed by the *ICD, 9th Revision, Clinical Modification*, known as ICD-9-CM, published by the U.S. Department of Health and Human Services and used by hospitals and other healthcare facilities to better describe the clinical picture of the patient. The diagnosis component of ICD-9-CM is completely consistent with ICD-9 codes, and remains the data standard for reporting morbidity. National adaptations of the ICD-10 progressed to incorporate both clinical code (ICD-10-CM) and procedure code (ICD-10-PCS) with the revisions completed in 2003. in 2009, the U.S. Centers for Medicare and Medicaid Services announced that it would begin using ICD-10 on April 1, 2010, with full compliance by all involved parties by 2013.

BRIEF HISTORY OF ICD-10

ICD-10 was first published by the World Health Organization (WHO) in 1992. The National Center for Health Statistics (NCHS), the Federal agency responsible for use of the International Statistical Classification of Diseases and Related Health

Problems, 10th revision (ICD-10) in the United States, has developed a clinical modification of the classification for morbidity purposes. The ICD-10 is used to code and classify mortality data from death certificates, having replaced ICD-9 for this purpose as of January 1, 1999. ICD-10-CM is planned as the replacement for ICD-9-CM, volumes 1 and 2. ICD-10-PCS is the replacement for ICD-9-CM volume 3, Procedures.

ICD-10-CM was developed following a thorough evaluation by a Technical Advisory Panel and extensive additional consultation with physician groups, clinical coders, and others to assure clinical accuracy and utility. Notable improvements in the content and format include: the addition of information relevant to ambulatory and managed care encounters; expanded injury codes; the creation of combination diagnosis/symptom codes to reduce the number of codes needed to fully describe a condition; the addition of a sixth character; incorporation of common 4th and 5th digit subclassifications; laterality; and greater specificity in code assignment. After several delays, ICD-10 was officially implemented on October 1, 2015.

TERMINOLOGY

acute conditions	The medical conditions characterized by sudden onset, severe change, and/or short duration.
additional diagnosis	The secondary diagnosis code used, if available, to provide a more complete picture of the primary diagnosis.
alteration	Modifying the anatomic structure of a body part without affecting the function of the body part
applied mapping	Distillation of a reference mapping to conform to the needs of a particular application (e.g., data quality, research).
approach (5th character)	Defines the technique used to reach the site of the procedure.
backward mapping	mapping that proceeds from a newer code set to an older code set, for example from ICD-10-CM to ICD-9-CM.
bilateral	For bilateral sites, the final character of the codes in the ICD-10-CM indicates laterality. an unspecified side code is also provided should the side not be identified in the medical record. If no bilateral code is provided and the condition is bilateral, assign separate codes for both the left and right side.
body part or region (4th character)	Defines the specific anatomical site where the procedure is performed.
body system (2nd character)	Defines the general physiological system on which the procedure is performed or anatomical region where the procedure is performed.
bypass	Altering the route of passage of the contents of a tubular body part.
category	The three-digit diagnosis code classifications that broadly define each condition (e.g., 250 for diabetes mellitus).
Centers for Disease Control and Prevention (CDC)	A federal health data organization that helps maintain several code sets included in the HIPAA standards, including the ICD-9-CM codes. a division of the Department of Health and Human Services responsible for monitoring, researching and developing public health policies for the prevention of disease, injury and disability and the promotion of healthy behaviors. The National Center for Health Statistics is the part of the CDC that maintains health related statistics including the coordination with World Health Organization (WHO) on use of International Classification of Diseases (ICD) in North America.
Centers for Medicare & Medicaid Services (CMS)	The federal agency that runs the Medicare program. in addition, CMS works with the States to run the Medicaid program. CMS works to make sure that the beneficiaries in these programs are able to get high quality healthcare.
change	Taking out or off a device from a body part and putting back an identical or similar device in or on the same body part without cutting or puncturing the skin or a mucous membrane
character	One of the seven components that comprise an ICD-10-PCS procedure code.

chronic conditions	Medical conditions characterized by long duration, frequent recurrence over a long period of time, and/or slow progression over time.
cluster	in a combination entry, one instance where a code is chosen from each of the choice lists in the target system entry, that when combined satisfies the equivalent meaning of the corresponding code in the source system
combination codes	A single code used to classify any of the following: two diagnoses; a diagnosis with an associated secondary process (manifestation); or a diagnosis with an associated complication.
control	Stopping, or attempting to stop, postprocedural bleeding.
Conventions of ICD-10	The general rules for use of the classification independent of guidelines. These conventions are incorporated within the Index and Tabular of the ICD-10-CM as instructional notes.
creation	Making a new genital structure that does not take over the function of a body part.
crosswalk/mapping	A new test is determined to be similar to an existing test, multiple existing test codes, or a portion of an existing test code. The new test code is then assigned to the related existing local fee schedule amounts and resulting national limitation amount. in some instances, a test may only equate to a portion of a test, and, in those instances, payment at an appropriate percentage of the payment for the existing test is assigned.
Current Procedural Terminology (CPT) Codes	This is the procedural coding system that is currently used in America primarily to report physician professional services. Frequently called "CPT", the Current Procedural Terminology, is a code set, developed in 1966 and maintained by the American Medical Association (AMA), used to describe what healthcare professional services were provided or utilized by healthcare professionals. CPT codes are also known as "Level I" codes. Additional codes to describe use of healthcare facilities and services provided by healthcare professionals are known as "Level II" or "Healthcare Common Procedure Coding System" (HCPCS). Level II codes were developed are maintained by CMS.
destruction	Physical eradication of all or a portion of a body part by the direct use of energy, force or a destructive agent.
detachment	Cutting off all or a portion of the upper or lower extremities.
dilation	Expanding an orifice or the lumen of a tubular body part.
division	Cutting into a body part without draining fluids and/or gases from the body part in order to separate or transect a body part.
drainage	Taking or letting out fluids and/or gases from a body part.
excision	Cutting out or off, without replacement, a portion of a body part.
external (approach)	Procedures performed directly on the skin or mucous membrane and procedures performed indirectly by the application of external force through the skin or mucous membrane.
extirpation	Taking or cutting out solid matter from a body part.
extraction	Pulling or stripping out or off all or a portion of a body part by the use of force.
Federal Register	The "Federal Register" is the official daily publication for rules, proposed rules and notices of federal agencies and organizations, as well as Executive Orders and other Presidential documents.
forward mapping	mapping that proceeds from an older code set to a newer code set, for example from ICD-9-CM Volume 3 to ICD-10-PCS.
fragmentation	Breaking solid matter in a body part into pieces.
GEMs	This reference mapping attempts to include all valid relationships between the codes in the ICD-9-CM diagnosis classification and the ICD-10-CM diagnosis classification.

General Equivalence Map (GEM)	reference mapping that attempts to include all valid relationships between the codes in the ICD-9- CM diagnosis classification and the ICD-10-CM diagnosis classification
Health Insurance Portability & Accountability Act (HIPAA)	A law passed in 1996 which is also sometimes called the "Kassebaum-Kennedy" law. This law expands healthcare coverage for patients who have lost or changed jobs, or have pre-existing conditions. HIPAA does not replace the states' roles as primary regulators of insurance. The HIPAA legislation has the following broad goals, to provide: 1) a way to uniquely identify providers, employers and health plans, 2) a uniform level of protection of health information, known as the "Security Rule," 3) a uniform level of protection of the privacy of health data associated with patients, known as the "Privacy Rule" and 4) a simpler healthcare electronic transaction process by describing standards by which all healthcare administrative entities would use, which is known as the "Transactions and Code Sets Rule".
Healthcare Common Procedure Coding System (HCPCS)	A medical code set that identifies healthcare procedures, equipment, and supplies for claim submission purposes. It has been selected for use in the HIPAA transactions. HCPCS Level I contains numeric CPT codes which are maintained by the AMA. HCPCS Level II contains alphanumeric codes used to identify various items and services that are not included in the CPT medical code set. These are maintained by Health Care Financing Administration (HCFA), Blue Cross and Blue Shield Association (BCBSA), and the Health Insurance Association of America (HIAA). HCPCS Level III contains alphanumeric codes that are assigned by Medicaid state agencies to identify additional items and services not included in levels I or II. These are usually called "local codes", and must have "W", "X", "Y", or "Z" in the first position. HCPCS Procedure Modifier Codes can be used with all three levels, with the WA - ZY range used for locally assigned procedure modifiers.
HIPAA 4010	The original healthcare transactions version of HIPAA (officially known as Version 004010 of the ASC X12 transaction implementation guides) named as part of HIPAA's Electronic Transaction Standards regulation. Version 4010 was required to be used by HIPAA covered healthcare entities by Oct. 16, 2003.
HIPAA 5010	Required by Jan. 1, 2012 to be the new version of the HIPAA healthcare transactions. Officially known as Version 005010 of the ASC X12 transaction Technical Report Type 3. This new version was required as a result of Department of Health and Human Services (HHS) final rules published on Jan. 6, 2009.
ICD-10	The mortality and morbidity classification coding system implemented by WHO in 1993 to replace ICD-9.
ICD-10-CM	The updated version of the clinical modification coding set defined by the National Center for Health Statistics that will replace ICD-9-CM on Oct. 1, 2013.
ICD-10-PCS	The updated procedural coding system defined by CMS that will replace Volume 3 of ICD-9-CM for hospital inpatient services.
ICD-9	The mortality and morbidity classification coding system used prior to ICD-10.
ICD-9-CM	The "clinical modification" to the ICD-9 code used prior to ICD-10-CM in America to report medical diagnoses.
index (to diseases)	The ICD-10-CM is divided into the Alphabetic Index, an alphabetical list of terms and their corresponding code, and the Tabular List, a chronological list of codes divided into chapters based on body system or condition. The Alphabetic Index consists of the following parts: the Index of Diseases and Injury, the Index of External Causes of Injury, the Table of Neoplasms and the Table of Drugs and Chemicals.
insertion	Putting in a nonbiological device that monitors, assists, performs or prevents a physiological function but does not physically take the place of a body part.
inspection	Visually and/or manually exploring a body part.

International Classification of Diseases (ICD)	A medical code set maintained by the World Health Organization (WHO). The primary purpose of this code set is to classify both causes of death or mortality and diseases or morbidity. A U.S. version, known as ICD-CM, "Clinical Modification," is maintained by the NCHS within the CDC to more precisely define ICD use in the U.S.
manifestation codes	Certain conditions have both an underlying etiology and multiple body system manifestations due to the underlying etiology. for such conditions, the ICD-10-CM has a coding convention that requires the underlying condition be sequenced first followed by the manifestation. Wherever such a combination exists, there is a "use additional code" note at the etiology code, and a "code first" note at the manifestation code. These instructional notes indicate the proper sequencing order of the codes, etiology followed by manifestation.
map	Locating the route of passage of electrical impulses and/or locating functional areas in a body part.
medical necessity	Services or supplies that: are proper and needed for the diagnosis or treatment of a medical condition; are provided for the diagnosis, direct care, and treatment of a medical condition; meet the standards of good medical practice in the local area; and are not mainly for the convenience of the patient or doctor.
morbidity	Term refers to the disease rate or number of cases of a particular disease in a given age range, gender, occupation, or other relevant population based grouping.
mortality	Term refers to the death rate reflected by the population in a given region, age range, or other relevant statistical grouping
National Center for Health Statistics (NCHS)	A federal organization within the CDC that collects, analyzes, and distributes healthcare statistics. The NCHS helps maintain the ICD-CM codes.
No Map Flag	attribute in a GEM that when turned on indicates that a code in the source system is not linked to any code in the target system .
occlusion	Completely closing an orifice or the lumen of a tubular body part.
open (approach)	Cutting through the skin or mucous membrane and any other body layers necessary to expose the site of the procedure.
percutaneous (approach)	Entry, by puncture or minor incision, of instrumentation through the skin or mucous membrane and any other body layers necessary to reach the site of the procedure.
percutaneous endoscopic (approach)	Entry, by puncture or minor incision, of instrumentation through the skin or mucous membrane and any other body layers necessary to reach and visualize the site of the procedure.
principle diagnosis	First-listed/primary diagnosis code. The code sequenced first on a medical record defines the primary reason for the encounter as determined at the end of the encounter.
procedure	The complete specification of the ICD-10-PCS seven characters.
reattachment	Putting back in or on all or a portion of a separated body part to its normal location or other suitable location.
release	Freeing a body part from an abnormal physical constraint by cutting or by use of force.
removal	Taking out or off a device from a body part.
repair	Restoring, to the extent possible, a body part to its normal anatomic structure and function.
replacement	Putting in or on biological or synthetic material that physically takes the place and/or function of all or a portion of a body part.
reposition	Moving to its normal location, or other suitable location, all or a portion of a body part.
resection	Cutting out or off, without replacement, all of a body part.

restriction	Partially closing an orifice or the lumen of a tubular body part.
reverse lookup	using a GEM by looking up a target system code to see all the codes in the source system that translate to it.
revision	Correcting, to the extent possible, a portion of a malfunctioning device or the position of a displaced device.
root operation/type (3rd character)	Defines the objective of the procedure.
section (1st character)	Defines the general type of procedure.
sequelae	A late effect is the residual effect (condition produced) after the acute phase of an illness or injury has terminated. There is no time limit on when a late effect code can be used. The residual may be apparent early, such as in cerebral infarction, or it may occur months or years later, such as that due to a previous injury.
signs/symptoms	Codes that describe symptoms and signs, as opposed to diagnoses, are acceptable for reporting purposes when a related definitive diagnosis has not been established (confirmed) by the provider.
source system	code set of origin in the mapping; the set being mapped 'from'
supplement	Putting in or on biological or synthetic material that physically reinforces and/or augments the function of a portion of a body part
Tabular List	It is essential to use both the Alphabetic Index and Tabular List when locating and assigning a code. The Alphabetic Index does not always provide the full code. Selection of the full code, including laterality and any applicable 7th character can only be done in the Tabular List. a dash (-) at the end of an Alphabetic Index entry indicates that additional characters are required. Even if a dash is not included at the Alphabetic Index entry, it is necessary to refer to the Tabular List to verify that no 7th character is required.
target system	destination code set in the mapping; the set being mapped 'to'.
transfer	Moving, without taking out, all or a portion of a body part to another location to take over the function of all or a portion of a body part.
transplantation	Putting in or on all or a portion of a living body part taken from another individual or animal to physically take the place and/or function of all or a portion of a similar body part.
Uniform Hospital Discharge Data Set (UHDDS)	The UHDDS definitions are used by hospitals to report inpatient data elements in a standardized manner. These data elements and their definitions can be found in the July 31, 1985, Federal Register (Vol. 50, No, 147), pp. 31038-40.
value	Individual units defined for each character of ICD-10-PCS and represented by a number or letter.
via natural or artificial opening (approach)	Entry of instrumentation through a natural or artificial external opening to reach the site of the procedure.
via natural or artificial opening endoscopic (approach)	Entry of instrumentation through a natural or artificial external opening to reach and visualize the site of the procedure.
via natural or artificial opening with percutaneous endoscopic assistance (approach)	Entry of instrumentation through a natural or artificial external opening and entry, by puncture or minor incision, of instrumentation through the skin or mucous membrane and any other body layers necessary to aid in the performance of the procedure.
Volume I	The detailed, tabular list of diagnosis codes in the ICD-9-CM manual.
Volume II	The alphabetical index to diseases in the ICD-9-CM diagnosis coding manual.

| Volume III | The ICD-9/ICD-10 list of procedure codes, used in inpatient settings. |
| **World Health Organization (WHO)** | An organization that maintains the International Classification of Diseases (ICD) medical code set. |

ICD-10-CM OVERVIEW

WHAT IS ICD-10-CM?

ICD-10-CM is an acronym for ***International Classification of Diseases, 10th Revision, Clinical Modification***, published under different names since 1900. ICD-10-CM is a statistical classification system that arranges diseases and injuries into groups according to established criteria. Most ICD-9-CM codes are numeric and consist of three seven digits and a description. The codes are revised approximately every 10 years by the World Health Organization and annual updates are published by Center for Medicare and Medicaid Services (CMS).

KEY POINTS REGARDING ICD-10-CM

1. ICD-10-CM codes are three (3) to seven (7) digit alphanumeric codes.

2. ICD-10-CM codes describe illnesses, injuries, signs and symptoms, and procedures.

3. ICD-10-CM codes must be used on all health insurance claims as of October 1, 2014 (subject to extension by CMS).

4. Most ICD-10-CM codes have a specific definition; however, some ICD-10-CM codes have more than one definition.

5. Correct ICD-10-CM coding can make a significant difference in your reimbursement.

6. Accurate ICD-10-CM coding puts you in control of the reimbursement process.

STRUCTURE OF ICD-10-CM COMPARED TO ICD-9-CM

The easiest way to understand the structural difference between ICD-9-CM and ICD-10-CM is with a comparative visual representation of the two coding systems. The illustrations below clearly show the differences in structure and length.

STRUCTURE OF AN ICD-9-CM CODE

414.00   Coronary atherosclerosis of unspecified type of vessel, native or graft

Number or Letter (V/E)	Numbers Only			
1ˢᵗ Digit	**2ⁿᵈ Digit**	**3ʳᵈ Digit**	**4ᵗʰ Digit**	**5ᵗʰ Digit**
4	**1**	**4** .	**0**	**0**
Category			Etiology, anatomic site, manifestation	

Length:	3-5 digits
First character:	Number or Letter (E or V)
Characters 2-5:	Numbers only
Minimum length:	3 characters
Decimal:	After 3ʳᵈ character

STRUCTURE OF AN ICD-10-CM CODE

S32.010A   Wedge compression fracture of first lumbar vertebra, initial encounter for closed fracture

Letter	Number or Letter					
1ST Digit	2nd Digit	3rd Digit	4th Digit	5th Digit	6th Digit	7th Digit
S	**3**	**2** .	**0**	**1**	**0**	**A**
Category			Etiology, anatomic site, severity			Added code extensions for obstetrics, injuries and external causes of injury

Length:	3-7 digits
First character:	Letter only (all letters except U are used)
Character 2:	Number only
Characters 3-7:	Numbers or letter
Decimal:	After 3rd character
Placeholder:	Use of "x" as a dummy placeholder
Letter format:	Letters are case-sensitive

SIMILARITY OF ICD-10-CM TO ICD-9-CM

While there are more codes in the ICD-10-CM coding system than the ICD-9-CM coding system and the coding is a bit more complex, there are many similarities between the two systems. Experienced coders should be able to use the ICD-10-CM system relatively quickly due in part to these similarities.

1. Format – Both ICD-10-CM and ICD-9-CM have a Tabular List and Index.

2. Chapters in the ICD-10-CM Tabular list are structured similarly to ICD-9-CM, with minor exceptions.

    *   A few chapters have been restructured
    *   Sense organs (eye and ear) separated from Nervous System chapter and moved to their own Chapters

3. Index of ICD-10-CM is structured the same as ICD-9-CM.

    *   Alphabetic Index of Diseases and Injuries
    *   Alphabetic Index of External Causes
    *   Table of Neoplasms
    *   Table of Drugs and Chemicals

4. Divided into Alphabetic Index and Tabular List.

    *   Structure and format are the same
    *   Index is alphabetical list of terms and their corresponding codes

5. Alphabetic Index lists main terms in alphabetical order with indented subterms under main terms.

6. The Alphabetic Index is divided into 2 parts: Index to Diseases and Injuries and Index to External Causes.

7. The Tabular List is a chronological list of codes divided into chapters based on body system or condition.

8. The Tabular List is presented in code number order.

9. ICD-10-CM and ICD-9-CM have the same hierarchical structure.

10. Codes are invalid in both ICD-10-CM and ICD-9-CM if they are missing an applicable character.

11. ICD-10-CM and ICD-9-CM codes are looked up the same way.

   - Look up diagnostic terms in Alphabetic Index
   - Then verify code number in Tabular List

12. Many conventions have same meaning in ICD-10-CM and ICD-9-CM.

   - Abbreviations, punctuation, symbols, notes such as "code first" and "use additional code"

13. Nonspecific codes ("unspecified" or "not otherwise specified") are available to use when detailed documentation to support more specific code is not available.

14. ICD-10-CM Official Guidelines for Coding and Reporting accompany and complement ICD-10-CM conventions and instructions.

15. Adherence to the official coding guidelines in all healthcare settings is required under the Health Insurance Portability and Accountability Act.

DIFFERENCES BETWEEN ICD-10-CM AND ICD-9-CM

While there are more similarities than differences between the ICD-10-CM and ICD-9-CM, the differences are significant. Understanding the differences will be the key to a successful transition to the new coding system.

1. All ICD-10-CM codes are alphanumeric (letter and numbers).

   - 1st character is always alpha and alpha characters may appear elsewhere in the code as well

2. ICD-10-CM codes can be up to 7 characters in length.

3. ICD-10-CM codes are more specific than ICD-9-CM codes.

4. ICD-10-CM code titles are more complete (no need to refer back to a category, subcategory, or subclassification level to determine complete meaning of code).

5. Laterality (side of the body affected) has been added to relevant ICD-10-CM codes.

6. ICD-10-CM features an expanded use of combination codes.

   - Certain conditions and associated common symptoms or manifestations
   - Poisonings and associated external cause

7. Injuries grouped by anatomical site rather than type of injury.

8. Codes reflect modern medicine and updated medical terminology.

9. Addition of 7th character

   - Used in certain chapters to provide information about the characteristic of the encounter
   - Must always be used in the 7th character position
   - If a code has an applicable 7th character, the code must be reported with an appropriate 7th character value in order to be valid

Valid 7th Digit Character for Injuries and External Causes

A   Initial encounter
D   Subsequent encounter S Sequela

Note: for aftercare of an injury, assign acute injury code with 7th character "D"

Valid 7th Digit Character for Fractures

A   Initial encounter for closed fracture

B   Initial encounter for open fracture

D   Subsequent encounter for fracture with routine healing

G   Subsequent encounter for fracture with delayed healing

K   Subsequent encounter for fracture with nonunion

P   Subsequent encounter for fracture with malunion

S   Sequela

10. Addition of dummy placeholder "X" is used in certain codes to:

- Allow for future expansion
- Fill out empty characters when a code contains fewer than 6 characters and a 7th character applies

When placeholder character applies, it must be used in order for the code to be considered valid.

11. ICD-10-CM includes two types of Excludes Notes.

- **Excludes 1 Note**

  Indicates that code identified in the note and code where the note appears cannot be reported together because the 2 conditions cannot occur together.

  Examples:

  E10   Type 1 Diabetes mellitus

  Excludes 1: diabetes mellitus due to underlying condition (E08.-)
  drug or chemical induced diabetes mellitus (E09.-)
  gestational diabetes (O24.4-)
  hyperglycemia NOS (R73.9)
  neonatal diabetes mellitus (P70.2)
  type 2 diabetes mellitus (E11.-)

  M21   Other acquired deformities of limbs

  Excludes 1: acquired absence of limb (Z89.-)
  congenital absence of limbs (Q71-Q73)

- **Excludes 2 Note**

  Indicates that condition identified in the note is not part of the condition represented by the code where the note appears, so both codes may be reported together if the patient has both conditions.

Examples:

L89   Pressure ulcer

      Excludes 2: diabetic ulcers (E08.621, E08.622, E09.621, E09.622, E10.621, E10.622, E11.621, E11.622, E13.621, E13.622)
      non-pressure chronic ulcer of skin (L97.-)
      skin infections (L00-L08)
      varicose ulcer (I83.0, I83.2)

I70.2   Atherosclerosis of native arteries of the extremities

      Excludes 2: atherosclerosis of bypass graft of extremities (I70.30-I70.79)

12. ICD-10-CM provides for increased specificity in comparison to ICD-9-CM.

Examples

S72.044G   Nondisplaced fracture of base of neck of right femur, subsequent encounter for closed fracture with delayed healing

I69.351   Sequelae of cerebral infarction, Hemiplegia and hemiparesis following cerebral infarction affecting right dominant side

Z47.81   Encounter for orthopedic aftercare following surgical amputation

Z48.21   Encounter for aftercare following heart transplant

13. ICD-10-CM provides specific codes to identify laterality, i.e. left, right, unspecified. This applies to extremities as well as many organ systems; i.e. eyes, ears, shoulders, arms, hands, hips, legs, feet, lungs, kidneys, ovaries, testicles, etc.

Examples

C50.511   Malignant neoplasm of lower-outer quadrant of <u>right</u> female breast

C50.512   Malignant neoplasm of lower-outer quadrant of <u>left</u> female breast

C50.519   Malignant neoplasm of lower-outer quadrant of <u>unspecified</u> female breast

FORMAT OF ICD-10-CM

The Tabular List (Volume 1)

The ICD-10-CM Tabular List contains categories, subcategories and codes. Characters for categories, subcategories and codes may be either a letter or a number. All categories are 3 characters. a three-character category that has no further subdivision is equivalent to a code. Subcategories are either 4 or 5 characters. Codes may be 3, 4, 5, 6 or 7 characters. That is, each level of subdivision after a category is a subcategory. The final level of subdivision is a code. Codes that have applicable 7th characters are still referred to as codes, not subcategories. a code that has an applicable 7th character is considered invalid without the 7th character.

The Alphabetic Index (Volume 2)

The Alphabetic Index consists of the following parts: the Index of Diseases and Injury, the Index of External Causes of Injury, the Table of Neoplasms and the Table of Drugs and Chemicals.

CONVENTIONS USED IN THE TABULAR LIST

The ICD-10-CM Tabular List (Volume 1) makes use of certain abbreviations, punctuation, symbols, and other conventions that must be clearly understood. The purpose of these conventions is to provide special coding instructions and conserve space. Most of the conventions are defined in the ICD-10-CM Official Guidelines to Coding and Reporting following this chapter. There are sym

SYMBOLS AND COLOR CODING

All PMIC versions of ICD-10-CM include color-coding to alert the user to special coding situations or conditions that require additional attention. The use of color-coding is found in the Tabular List (Volume 1). The color is applied as solid rectangular bars over the codes only so that the descriptions remain clear and legible. The color codes and definitions are printed at the bottom of all right-sided pages of the Tabular List (Volume 1)

Color Coding

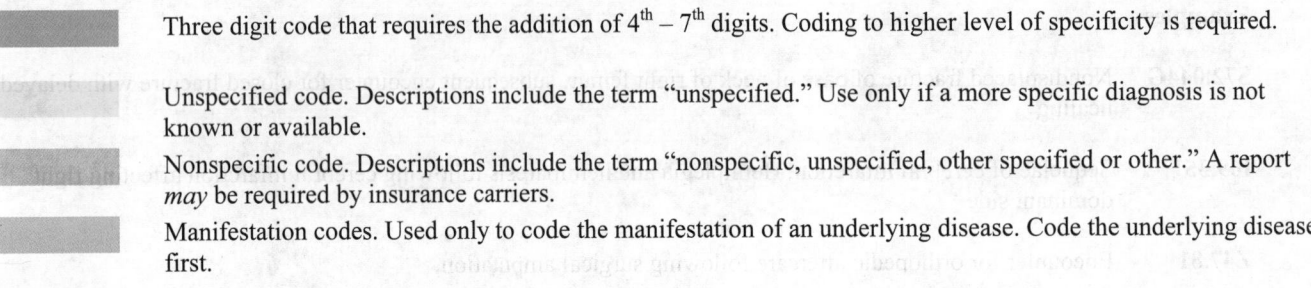

Three digit code that requires the addition of 4th – 7th digits. Coding to higher level of specificity is required.

Unspecified code. Descriptions include the term "unspecified." Use only if a more specific diagnosis is not known or available.

Nonspecific code. Descriptions include the term "nonspecific, unspecified, other specified or other." A report *may* be required by insurance carriers.

Manifestation codes. Used only to code the manifestation of an underlying disease. Code the underlying disease first.

Symbols

● A filled BLACK CIRCLE preceding a code indicates that the code is new to this revision of ICD-9-CM. A symbol key appears on all left-hand pages of the Tabular List, Volume 1.

▲ A filled BLACK TRIANGLE preceding a code indicates that there is a revision to the text of an existing code. A symbol key appears on all left-hand pages of the Tabular List, Volume 1.

⑦ A red circle containing the number 7 preceding a code indicates that a seventh digit is required for coding to the highest level of specificity. The appropriate 7th character is to be added to each code from category. Definitions of valid seventh digits are found under the major category. If a code that requires a 7th character is not 6 characters, a placeholder X must be used to fill in the empty characters.

⊗ A red circle containing the letter P preceding a code indicates that a placeholder character "X" is required for the code to be complete. An example of this is at the poisoning, adverse effect and underdosing codes, categories T36-T50. Where a place holder exists, the X must be used in order for the code to be considered a valid code.

Sex Specific Diagnosis Codes

Some ICD-10-CM codes apply only to female or male patients. Some ICD-10-CM codes include the word "male" or "female" in the diagnosis description, while others are known to apply to female or male because of sex specific terms such as ovary, vagina, prostate, testes, etc. For chapters or sections where all of the diagnosis codes are sex specific, the following alerts appear at the beginning of the section:

NOTE: All Diagnosis Codes In This Section Apply To FEMALE Patients Only

NOTE: All Diagnosis Codes In This Section Apply To MALE Patients Only

Age Specific Diagnosis Codes

Some ICD-10-CM codes apply to patients of general age ranges. These codes are identified by the inclusion of the following terms within the diagnosis description: "adult", "child", "infant", "juvenile", or "newborn".

ICD-10-CM Official Guidelines for Coding and Reporting

The Centers for Medicare and Medicaid Services (CMS) and the National Center for Health Statistics (NCHS), two departments within the U.S. Federal Government's Department of Health and Human Services (DHHS) provide the following guidelines for coding and reporting using the International Classification of Diseases, 10th Revision, Clinical Modification (ICD-10-CM). These guidelines should be used as a companion document to the official version of the ICD-10-CM as published on the NCHS website. The ICD-10-CM is a morbidity classification published by the United States for classifying diagnoses and reason for visits in all health care settings. The ICD-10-CM is based on the ICD-10, the statistical classification of disease published by the World Health Organization (WHO).

These guidelines have been approved by the four organizations that make up the Cooperating Parties for the ICD-10-CM: the American Hospital Association (AHA), the American Health Information Management Association (AHIMA), CMS, and NCHS.

These guidelines are a set of rules that have been developed to accompany and complement the official conventions and instructions provided within the ICD-10-CM itself. The instructions and conventions of the classification take precedence over guidelines. These guidelines are based on the coding and sequencing instructions in the Tabular List and Alphabetic Index of ICD-10-CM, but provide additional instruction. Adherence to these guidelines when assigning ICD-10-CM diagnosis codes is required under the Health Insurance Portability and Accountability Act (HIPAA). The diagnosis codes (Tabular List and Alphabetic Index) have been adopted under HIPAA for all healthcare settings. A joint effort between the healthcare provider and the coder is essential to achieve complete and accurate documentation, code assignment, and reporting of diagnoses and procedures. These guidelines have been developed to assist both the healthcare provider and the coder in identifying those diagnoses that are to be reported. The importance of consistent, complete documentation in the medical record cannot be overemphasized. Without such documentation accurate coding cannot be achieved. The entire record should be reviewed to determine the specific reason for the encounter and the conditions treated.

The term encounter is used for all settings, including hospital admissions. In the context of these guidelines, the term provider is used throughout the guidelines to mean physician or any qualified health care practitioner who is legally accountable for establishing the patient's diagnosis. Only this set of guidelines, approved by the Cooperating Parties, is official.

The guidelines are organized into sections. Section I includes the structure and conventions of the classification and general guidelines that apply to the entire classification, and chapter-specific guidelines that correspond to the chapters as they are arranged in the classification. Section II includes guidelines for selection of principal diagnosis for non-outpatient settings. Section III includes guidelines for reporting additional diagnoses in non-outpatient settings. Section IV is for outpatient coding and reporting. It is necessary to review all sections of the guidelines to fully understand all of the rules and instructions needed to code properly.

SECTION I. CONVENTIONS, GENERAL CODING GUIDELINES AND CHAPTER SPECIFIC GUIDELINES

The conventions, general guidelines and chapter-specific guidelines are applicable to all health care settings unless otherwise indicated. The conventions and instructions of the classification take precedence over guidelines.

A. Conventions for the ICD-10-CM

The conventions for the ICD-10-CM are the general rules for use of the classification independent of the guidelines. These conventions are incorporated within the Alphabetic Index and Tabular List of the ICD-10-CM as instructional notes.

1. The Alphabetic Index and Tabular List

The ICD-10-CM is divided into the Alphabetic Index, an alphabetical list of terms and their corresponding code, and the Tabular List, a structured list of codes divided into chapters based on body system or condition. The Alphabetic Index consists of the following parts: the Index of Diseases and Injury, the Index of External Causes of Injury, the Table of Neoplasms and the Table of Drugs and Chemicals.

See Section I.C2. General guidelines
See Section I.C.19. Adverse effects, poisoning, underdosing and toxic effects

2. **Format and Structure:**

The ICD-10-CM Tabular List contains categories, subcategories and codes. Characters for categories, subcategories and codes may be either a letter or a number. All categories are 3 characters. A three-character category that has no further subdivision is equivalent to a code. Subcategories are either 4 or 5 characters. Codes may be 3, 4, 5, 6 or 7 characters. That is, each level of subdivision after a category is a subcategory. The final level of subdivision is a code. Codes that have applicable 7th characters are still referred to as codes, not subcategories. A code that has an applicable 7th character is considered invalid without the 7th character.

The ICD-10-CM uses an indented format for ease in reference.

3. **Use of codes for reporting purposes**

For reporting purposes only codes are permissible, not categories or subcategories, and any applicable 7th character is required.

4. **Placeholder character**

The ICD-10-CM utilizes a placeholder character "X". The "X" is used as a placeholder at certain codes to allow for future expansion. An example of this is at the poisoning, adverse effect and underdosing codes, categories T36-T50.

Where a placeholder exists, the X must be used in order for the code to be considered a valid code.

5. **7th Characters**

Certain ICD-10-CM categories have applicable 7th characters. The applicable 7th character is required for all codes within the category, or as the notes in the Tabular List instruct. The 7th character must always be the 7th character in the data field. If a code that requires a 7th character is not 6 characters, a placeholder X must be used to fill in the empty characters.

6. **Abbreviations**

   a. **Alphabetic Index abbreviations**

   NEC "Not elsewhere classifiable"

   This abbreviation in the Alphabetic Index represents "other specified." When a specific code is not available for a condition, the Alphabetic Index directs the coder to the "other specified" code in the Tabular List.

   NOS "Not otherwise specified"

   This abbreviation is the equivalent of unspecified.

   b. **Tabular List abbreviations**

   NEC "Not elsewhere classifiable"

   This abbreviation in the Tabular List represents "other specified". When a specific code is not available for a condition, the Tabular List includes an NEC entry under a code to identify the code as the "other specified" code.

   NOS "Not otherwise specified"

This abbreviation is the equivalent of unspecified.

7. **Punctuation**

[ ]   Brackets are used in the Tabular List to enclose synonyms, alternative wording or explanatory phrases. Brackets are used in the Alphabetic Index to identify manifestation codes.

( )   Parentheses are used in both the Alphabetic Index and Tabular List to enclose supplementary words that may be present or absent in the statement of a disease or procedure without affecting the code number to which it is assigned. The terms within the parentheses are referred to as nonessential modifiers. The nonessential modifiers in the Alphabetic Index to Diseases apply to subterms following a main term except when a nonessential modifier and a subentry are mutually exclusive, the subentry takes precedence. For example, in the ICD-10-CM Alphabetic Index under the main term Enteritis, "acute" is a nonessential modifier and "chronic" is a subentry. In this case, the nonessential modifier "acute" does not apply to the subentry "chronic".

:   Colons are used in the Tabular List after an incomplete term which needs one or more of the modifiers following the colon to make it assignable to a given category.

8. **Use of "and".**

See Section I.A.14. Use of the term "And"

9. **Other and Unspecified codes**

a. **"Other" codes**

Codes titled "other" or "other specified" are for use when the information in the medical record provides detail for which a specific code does not exist. Alphabetic Index entries with NEC in the line designate "other" codes in the Tabular List. These Alphabetic Index entries represent specific disease entities for which no specific code exists so the term is included within an "other" code.

b. **"Unspecified" codes**

Codes titled "unspecified" are for use when the information in the medical record is insufficient to assign a more specific code. For those categories for which an unspecified code is not provided, the "other specified" code may represent both other and unspecified.

See Section I.B.18 Use of Signs/Symptom/Unspecified Codes

10. **Includes Notes**

This note appears immediately under a three character code title to further define, or give examples of, the content of the category.

11. **Inclusion terms**

List of terms is included under some codes. These terms are the conditions for which that code is to be used. The terms may be synonyms of the code title, or, in the case of "other specified" codes, the terms are a list of the various conditions assigned to that code. The inclusion terms are not necessarily exhaustive. Additional terms found only in the Alphabetic Index may also be assigned to a code.

12. **Excludes Notes**

The ICD-10-CM has two types of excludes notes. Each type of note has a different definition for use but they are all similar in that they indicate that codes excluded from each other are independent of each other.

a. **Excludes1**

A type 1 Excludes note is a pure excludes note. It means "NOT CODED HERE!" An Excludes1 note indicates that the code excluded should never be used at the same time as the code above the Excludes1 note. An Excludes1 is used when two conditions cannot occur together, such as a congenital form versus an acquired form of the same condition.

An exception to the Excludes1 definition is the circumstance when the two conditions are unrelated to each other. If it is not clear whether the two conditions involving an Excludes1 note are related or not, query the provider. For example, code F45.8, Other somatoform disorders, has an Excludes1 note for "sleep related teeth grinding (G47.63)," because "teeth grinding" is an inclusion term under F45.8.

Only one of these two codes should be assigned for teeth grinding. However psychogenic dysmenorrhea is also an inclusion term under F45.8, and a patient could have both this condition and sleep related teeth grinding. In this case, the two conditions are clearly unrelated to each other, and so it would be appropriate to report F45.8 and G47.63 together.

b. **Excludes2**

A type 2 Excludes note represents "Not included here." An excludes2 note indicates that the condition excluded is not part of the condition represented by the code, but a patient may have both conditions at the same time. When an Excludes2 note appears under a code, it is acceptable to use both the code and the excluded code together, when appropriate.

13. **Etiology/manifestation convention ("code first", "use additional code" and "in diseases classified elsewhere" notes)**

Certain conditions have both an underlying etiology and multiple body system manifestations due to the underlying etiology. For such conditions, the ICD-10-CM has a coding convention that requires the underlying condition be sequenced first, **if** applicable, followed by the manifestation. Wherever such a combination exists, there is a "use additional code" note at the etiology code, and a "code first" note at the manifestation code. These instructional notes indicate the proper sequencing order of the codes, etiology followed by manifestation.

In most cases the manifestation codes will have in the code title, "in diseases classified elsewhere." Codes with this title are a component of the etiology/ manifestation convention. The code title indicates that it is a manifestation code. "In diseases classified elsewhere" codes are never permitted to be used as first-listed or principal diagnosis codes. They must be used in conjunction with an underlying condition code and they must be listed following the underlying condition. See category F02, Dementia in other diseases classified elsewhere, for an example of this convention.

There are manifestation codes that do not have "in diseases classified elsewhere" in the title. For such codes, there is a "use additional code" note at the etiology code and a "code first" note at the manifestation code, and the rules for sequencing apply.

In addition to the notes in the Tabular List, these conditions also have a specific Alphabetic Index entry structure. In the Alphabetic Index both conditions are listed together with the etiology code first followed by the manifestation codes in brackets. The code in brackets is always to be sequenced second.

An example of the etiology/manifestation convention is dementia in Parkinson's disease. In the Alphabetic Index, code G20 is listed first, followed by code F02.80 or F02.81 in brackets. Code G20 represents the underlying etiology, Parkinson's disease, and must be sequenced first, whereas codes F02.80 and F02.81 represent the manifestation of dementia in diseases classified elsewhere, with or without behavioral disturbance.

"Code first" and "Use additional code" notes are also used as sequencing rules in the classification for certain codes that are not part of an etiology/ manifestation combination.

See Section I.B.7. Multiple coding for a single condition.

14. "And"

The word "and" should be interpreted to mean either "and" or "or" when it appears in a title.

For example, cases of "tuberculosis of bones", "tuberculosis of joints" and "tuberculosis of bones and joints" are classified to subcategory A18.0, Tuberculosis of bones and joints.

15. "With"

The word "with" should be interpreted to mean "associated with" or "due to" when it appears in a code title, the Alphabetic Index, or an instructional note in the Tabular List. The classification presumes a causal relationship between the two conditions linked by these terms in the Alphabetic Index or Tabular List.

These conditions should be coded as related even in the absence of provider documentation explicitly linking them, unless the documentation clearly states the conditions are unrelated. For conditions not specifically linked by these relational terms in the classification, provider documentation must link the conditions in order to code them as related.

The word "with" in the Alphabetic Index is sequenced immediately following the main term, not in alphabetical order.

16. "See" and "See Also"

The "see" instruction following a main term in the Alphabetic Index indicates that another term should be referenced. It is necessary to go to the main term referenced with the "see" note to locate the correct code.

A "see also" instruction following a main term in the Alphabetic Index instructs that there is another main term that may also be referenced that may provide additional Alphabetic Index entries that may be useful. It is not necessary to follow the "see also" note when the original main term provides the necessary code.

17. "Code also" note

A "code also" note instructs that two codes may be required to fully describe a condition, but this note does not provide sequencing direction.

18. Default codes

A code listed next to a main term in the ICD-10-CM Alphabetic Index is referred to as a default code. The default code represents that condition that is most commonly associated with the main term, or is the unspecified code for the condition. If a condition is documented in a medical record (for example, appendicitis) without any additional information, such as acute or chronic, the default code should be assigned.

19. Code assignment and Clinical Criteria

The assignment of a diagnosis code is based on the provider's diagnostic statement that the condition exists. The provider's statement that the patient has a particular condition is sufficient. Code assignment is not based on clinical criteria used by the provider to establish the diagnosis.

B. General Coding Guidelines

1. Locating a code in the ICD-10-CM

To select a code in the classification that corresponds to a diagnosis or reason for visit documented in a medical record, first locate the term in the Alphabetic Index, and then verify the code in the Tabular List. Read and be guided by instructional notations that appear in both the Alphabetic Index and the Tabular List.

It is essential to use both the Alphabetic Index and Tabular List when locating and assigning a code. The Alphabetic Index does not always provide the full code. Selection of the full code, including laterality and any applicable 7th character can only be done in the Tabular List. A dash (-) at the end of an Alphabetic Index entry indicates that additional characters are required. Even if a dash is not included at the Alphabetic Index entry, it is necessary to refer to the Tabular List to verify that no 7th character is required.

2. Level of Detail in Coding

Diagnosis codes are to be used and reported at their highest number of characters available.

ICD-10-CM diagnosis codes are composed of codes with 3, 4, 5, 6 or 7 characters. Codes with three characters are included in ICD-10-CM as the heading of a category of codes that may be further subdivided by the use of fourth and/or fifth characters and/or sixth characters, which provide greater detail.

A three-character code is to be used only if it is not further subdivided. A code is invalid if it has not been coded to the full number of characters required for that code, including the 7th character, if applicable.

3. Code or codes from A00.0 through T88.9, Z00-Z99.8

The appropriate code or codes from A00.0 through T88.9, Z00-Z99.8 must be used to identify diagnoses, symptoms, conditions, problems, complaints or other reason(s) for the encounter/visit.

4. Signs and symptoms

Codes that describe symptoms and signs, as opposed to diagnoses, are acceptable for reporting purposes when a related definitive diagnosis has not been established (confirmed) by the provider. Chapter 18 of ICD-10-CM, Symptoms, Signs, and Abnormal Clinical and Laboratory Findings, Not Elsewhere Classified (codes R00.0 - R99) contains many, but not all, codes for symptoms.

See Section I.B.18 Use of Signs/Symptom/Unspecified Codes

5. Conditions that are an integral part of a disease process

Signs and symptoms that are associated routinely with a disease process should not be assigned as additional codes, unless otherwise instructed by the classification.

6. Conditions that are not an integral part of a disease process

Additional signs and symptoms that may not be associated routinely with a disease process should be coded when present.

7. Multiple coding for a single condition

In addition to the etiology/manifestation convention that requires two codes to fully describe a single condition that affects multiple body systems, there are other single conditions that also require more than one code. "Use additional code" notes are found in the Tabular List at codes that are not part of an etiology/manifestation pair where a secondary code is useful to fully describe a condition. The sequencing rule is the same as the etiology/manifestation pair, "use additional code" indicates that a secondary code should be added.

For example, for bacterial infections that are not included in chapter 1, a secondary code from category B95, Streptococcus, Staphylococcus, and Enterococcus, as the cause of diseases classified elsewhere, or B96, Other bacterial agents as the cause of diseases classified elsewhere, may be required to identify the bacterial organism causing the infection. A "use additional code" note will normally be found at the infectious disease code, indicating a need for the organism code to be added as a secondary code.

"Code first" notes are also under certain codes that are not specifically manifestation codes but may be due to an underlying cause. When there is a "code first" note and an underlying condition is present, the underlying condition should be sequenced first.

"Code, if applicable, any causal condition first" notes indicate that this code may be assigned as a principal diagnosis when the causal condition is unknown or not applicable. If a causal condition is known, then the code for that condition should be sequenced as the principal or first-listed diagnosis.

Multiple codes may be needed for sequela, complication codes and obstetric codes to more fully describe a condition. See the specific guidelines for these conditions for further instruction.

8. Acute and Chronic Conditions

If the same condition is described as both acute (subacute) and chronic, and separate subentries exist in the Alphabetic Index at the same indentation level, code both and sequence the acute (subacute) code first.

9. Combination Code

A combination code is a single code used to classify: Two diagnoses, or

A diagnosis with an associated secondary process (manifestation) A diagnosis with an associated complication

Combination codes are identified by referring to subterm entries in the Alphabetic Index and by reading the inclusion and exclusion notes in the Tabular List.

Assign only the combination code when that code fully identifies the diagnostic conditions involved or when the Alphabetic Index so directs. Multiple coding should not be used when the classification provides a combination code that clearly identifies all of the elements documented in the diagnosis. When the combination code lacks necessary specificity in describing the manifestation or complication, an additional code should be used as a secondary code.

10. Sequela (Late Effects)

A sequela is the residual effect (condition produced) after the acute phase of an illness or injury has terminated. There is no time limit on when a sequela code can be used. The residual may be apparent early, such as in cerebral infarction, or it may occur months or years later, such as that due to a previous injury. Examples of sequela include: scar formation resulting from a burn, deviated septum due to a nasal fracture, and infertility due to tubal occlusion from old tuberculosis. Coding of sequela generally requires two codes sequenced in the following order: the condition or nature of the sequela is sequenced first. The sequela code is sequenced second.

An exception to the above guidelines are those instances where the code for the sequela is followed by a manifestation code identified in the Tabular List and title, or the sequela code has been expanded (at the fourth, fifth or sixth character levels) to include the manifestation(s). The code for the acute phase of an illness or injury that led to the sequela is never used with a code for the late effect.

See Section I.C.9. Sequelae of cerebrovascular disease
See Section I.C.15. Sequelae of complication of pregnancy, childbirth and the puerperium
See Section I.C.19. Application of 7th characters for Chapter 19

11. Impending or Threatened Condition

Code any condition described at the time of discharge as "impending" or "threatened" as follows:

If it did occur, code as confirmed diagnosis.

If it did not occur, reference the Alphabetic Index to determine if the condition has a subentry term for "impending" or "threatened" and also reference main term entries for "Impending" and for "Threatened."

If the subterms are listed, assign the given code.

If the subterms are not listed, code the existing underlying condition(s) and not the condition described as impending or threatened.

12. Reporting Same Diagnosis Code More than Once

Each unique ICD-10-CM diagnosis code may be reported only once for an encounter. This applies to bilateral conditions when there are no distinct codes identifying laterality or two different conditions classified to the same ICD-10-CM diagnosis code.

13. Laterality

Some ICD-10-CM codes indicate laterality, specifying whether the condition occurs on the left, right or is bilateral. If no bilateral code is provided and the condition is bilateral, assign separate codes for both the left and right side. If the side is not identified in the medical record, assign the code for the unspecified side.

When a patient has a bilateral condition and each side is treated during separate encounters, assign the "bilateral" code (as the condition still exists on both sides), including for the encounter to treat the first side.

For the second encounter for treatment after one side has previously been treated and the condition no longer exists on that side, assign the appropriate unilateral code for the side where the condition still exists (e.g., cataract surgery performed on each eye in separate encounters). The bilateral code would not be assigned for the subsequent encounter, as the patient no longer has the condition in the previously-treated site. If the treatment on the first side did not completely resolve the condition, then the bilateral code would still be appropriate.

14. Documentation for BMI, *Depth of* Non-pressure ulcers, Pressure Ulcer Stages, Coma Scale, *and NIH Stroke Scale*

For the Body Mass Index (BMI), depth of non-pressure chronic ulcers, pressure ulcer stage, coma scale, and NIH stroke scale (NIHSS) codes, code assignment may be based on medical record documentation from clinicians who are not the patient's provider (i.e., physician or other qualified healthcare practitioner legally accountable for establishing the patient's diagnosis), since this information is typically documented by other clinicians involved in the care of the patient (e.g., a dietitian often documents the BMI, a nurse often documents the pressure ulcer stages, and an emergency medical technician often documents the coma scale). However, the associated diagnosis (such as overweight, obesity, acute stroke, or pressure ulcer) must be documented by the patient's provider. If there is conflicting medical record documentation, either from the same clinician or different clinicians, the patient's attending provider should be queried for clarification.

The BMI, coma scale, and NIHSS codes should only be reported as secondary diagnoses.

15. Syndromes

Follow the Alphabetic Index guidance when coding syndromes. In the absence of Alphabetic Index guidance, assign codes for the documented manifestations of the syndrome. Additional codes for manifestations that are not an integral part of the disease process may also be assigned when the condition does not have a unique code.

16. Documentation of Complications of Care

Code assignment is based on the provider's documentation of the relationship between the condition and the care or procedure, unless otherwise instructed by the classification. The guideline extends to any complications of care, regardless of the chapter the code is located in. It is important to note that not all conditions that occur during or following medical care or surgery are classified as complications. There must be a cause-and-effect relationship between the care provided and the condition, and an indication in the documentation that it is a complication. Query the provider for clarification, if the complication is not clearly documented.

17. Borderline Diagnosis

If the provider documents a "borderline" diagnosis at the time of discharge, the diagnosis is coded as confirmed, unless the classification provides a specific entry (e.g., borderline diabetes). If a borderline condition has a specific index entry in ICD-10-CM, it should be coded as such. Since borderline conditions are not uncertain diagnoses, no distinction is made between the care setting (inpatient versus outpatient). Whenever the documentation is unclear regarding a borderline condition, coders are encouraged to query for clarification.

18. Use of Sign/Symptom/Unspecified Codes

Sign/symptom and "unspecified" codes have acceptable, even necessary, uses. While specific diagnosis codes should be reported when they are supported by the available medical record documentation and clinical knowledge of the patient's health condition, there are instances when signs/symptoms or unspecified codes are the best choices for accurately reflecting the healthcare encounter. Each healthcare encounter should be coded to the level of certainty known for that encounter.

If a definitive diagnosis has not been established by the end of the encounter, it is appropriate to report codes for sign(s) and/or symptom(s) in lieu of a definitive diagnosis. When sufficient clinical information isn't known or available about a particular health condition to assign a more specific code, it is acceptable to report the appropriate "unspecified" code (e.g., a diagnosis of pneumonia has been determined, but not the specific type). Unspecified codes should be reported when they are the codes that most accurately reflect what is known about the patient's condition at the time of that particular encounter. It would be inappropriate to select a specific code that is not supported by the medical record documentation or conduct medically unnecessary diagnostic testing in order to determine a more specific code.

C. Chapter-Specific Coding Guidelines

In addition to general coding guidelines, there are guidelines for specific diagnoses and/or conditions in the classification. Unless otherwise indicated, these guidelines apply to all health care settings. Please refer to Section II for guidelines on the selection of principal diagnosis.

1. Chapter 1: Certain Infectious and Parasitic Diseases (A00-B99)

a. Human Immunodeficiency Virus (HIV) Infections

1) Code only confirmed cases

Code only confirmed cases of HIV infection/illness. This is an exception to the hospital inpatient guideline Section II, H.

In this context, "confirmation" does not require documentation of positive serology or culture for HIV; the provider's diagnostic statement that the patient is HIV positive, or has an HIV-related illness is sufficient.

2) Selection and sequencing of HIV codes

(a) Patient admitted for HIV-related condition

If a patient is admitted for an HIV-related condition, the principal diagnosis should be B20, Human immunodeficiency virus [HIV] disease followed by additional diagnosis codes for all reported HIV-related conditions.

(b) Patient with HIV disease admitted for unrelated condition

If a patient with HIV disease is admitted for an unrelated condition (such as a traumatic injury), the code for the unrelated condition (e.g., the nature of injury code) should be the principal diagnosis.

Other diagnoses would be B20 followed by additional diagnosis codes for all reported HIV-related conditions.

(c) Whether the patient is newly diagnosed

Whether the patient is newly diagnosed or has had previous admissions/encounters for HIV conditions is irrelevant to the sequencing decision.

(d) Asymptomatic human immunodeficiency virus

Z21, Asymptomatic human immunodeficiency virus [HIV] infection status, is to be applied when the patient without any documentation of symptoms is listed as being "HIV positive," "known HIV," "HIV test positive," or similar terminology. Do not use this code if the term "AIDS" is used or if the patient is treated for any HIV-related illness or is described as having any condition(s) resulting from his/her HIV positive status; use B20 in these cases.

(e) Patients with inconclusive HIV serology

Patients with inconclusive HIV serology, but no definitive diagnosis or manifestations of the illness, may be assigned code R75, Inconclusive laboratory evidence of human immunodeficiency virus [HIV].

(f) Previously diagnosed HIV-related illness

Patients with any known prior diagnosis of an HIV-related illness should be coded to B20. Once a patient has developed an HIV-related illness, the patient should always be assigned code B20 on every subsequent admission/encounter. Patients previously diagnosed with any HIV illness (B20) should never be assigned to R75 or Z21, Asymptomatic human immunodeficiency virus [HIV] infection status.

(g) HIV Infection in Pregnancy, Childbirth and the Puerperium

During pregnancy, childbirth or the puerperium, a patient admitted (or presenting for a health care encounter) because of an HIV-related illness should receive a principal diagnosis code of O98.7-, Human immunodeficiency [HIV] disease complicating pregnancy, childbirth and the puerperium, followed by B20 and the code(s) for the HIV-related illness(es). Codes from Chapter 15 always take sequencing priority.

Patients with asymptomatic HIV infection status admitted (or presenting for a health care encounter) during pregnancy, childbirth, or the puerperium should receive codes of O98.7- and Z21.

(h) Encounters for testing for HIV

If a patient is being seen to determine his/her HIV status, use code Z11.4, Encounter for screening for human immunodeficiency virus [HIV]. Use additional codes for any associated high risk behavior.

If a patient with signs or symptoms is being seen for HIV testing, code the signs and symptoms. An additional counseling code Z71.7, Human immunodeficiency virus [HIV] counseling, may be used if counseling is provided during the encounter for the test.

When a patient returns to be informed of his/her HIV test results and the test result is negative, use code Z71.7, Human immunodeficiency virus [HIV] counseling.

If the results are positive, see previous guidelines and assign codes as appropriate.

b. Infectious agents as the cause of diseases classified to other chapters

Certain infections are classified in chapters other than Chapter 1 and no organism is identified as part of the infection code. In these instances, it is necessary to use an additional code from Chapter 1 to identify the organism. A code from category B95, Streptococcus, Staphylococcus, and Enterococcus as the cause of diseases classified to other chapters, B96, Other bacterial agents as the cause of diseases classified to other chapters, or B97, Viral agents as the cause of diseases classified to other chapters, is to be used as an additional code to identify the organism. An instructional note will be found at the infection code advising that an additional organism code is required.

c.   Infections resistant to antibiotics

Many bacterial infections are resistant to current antibiotics. It is necessary to identify all infections documented as antibiotic resistant. Assign a code from category Z16, Resistance to antimicrobial drugs, following the infection code only if the infection code does not identify drug resistance.

d.   Sepsis, Severe Sepsis, and Septic Shock

1)   Coding of Sepsis and Severe Sepsis

(a)   Sepsis

For a diagnosis of sepsis, assign the appropriate code for the underlying systemic infection. If the type of infection or causal organism is not further specified, assign code A41.9, Sepsis, unspecified organism.

A code from subcategory R65.2, Severe sepsis, should not be assigned unless severe sepsis or an associated acute organ dysfunction is documented.

(i)   Negative or inconclusive blood cultures and sepsis

Negative or inconclusive blood cultures do not preclude a diagnosis of sepsis in patients with clinical evidence of the condition; however, the provider should be queried.

(ii)   Urosepsis

The term urosepsis is a nonspecific term. It is not to be considered synonymous with sepsis. It has no default code in the Alphabetic Index. Should a provider use this term, he/she must be queried for clarification.

(iii)   Sepsis with organ dysfunction

If a patient has sepsis and associated acute organ dysfunction or multiple organ dysfunction (MOD), follow the instructions for coding severe sepsis.

(iv)   Acute organ dysfunction that is not clearly associated with the sepsis

If a patient has sepsis and an acute organ dysfunction, but the medical record documentation indicates that the acute organ dysfunction is related to a medical condition other than the sepsis, do not assign a code from subcategory R65.2, Severe sepsis. An acute organ dysfunction must be associated with the sepsis in order to assign the severe sepsis code.

If the documentation is not clear as to whether an acute organ dysfunction is related to the sepsis or another medical condition, query the provider.

(b)   Severe sepsis

The coding of severe sepsis requires a minimum of 2 codes: first a code for the underlying systemic infection, followed by a code from subcategory R65.2, Severe sepsis. If the causal organism is not documented, assign code A41.9, Sepsis, unspecified organism, for the infection. Additional code(s) for the associated acute organ dysfunction are also required.

Due to the complex nature of severe sepsis, some cases may require querying the provider prior to assignment of the codes.

2) **Septic shock**

(a) Septic shock generally refers to circulatory failure associated with severe sepsis, and therefore, it represents a type of acute organ dysfunction.

For cases of septic shock, the code for the systemic infection should be sequenced first, followed by code R65.21, Severe sepsis with septic shock or code T81.12, Postprocedural septic shock. Any additional codes for the other acute organ dysfunctions should also be assigned. As noted in the sequencing instructions in the Tabular List, the code for septic shock cannot be assigned as a principal diagnosis.

3) **Sequencing of severe sepsis**

If severe sepsis is present on admission, and meets the definition of principal diagnosis, the underlying systemic infection should be assigned as principal diagnosis followed by the appropriate code from subcategory R65.2 as required by the sequencing rules in the Tabular List. A code from subcategory R65.2 can never be assigned as a principal diagnosis.

When severe sepsis develops during an encounter (it was not present on admission), the underlying systemic infection and the appropriate code from subcategory R65.2 should be assigned as secondary diagnoses.

Severe sepsis may be present on admission, but the diagnosis may not be confirmed until sometime after admission. If the documentation is not clear whether severe sepsis was present on admission, the provider should be queried.

4) **Sepsis and severe sepsis with a localized infection**

If the reason for admission is both sepsis or severe sepsis and a localized infection, such as pneumonia or cellulitis, a code(s) for the underlying systemic infection should be assigned first and the code for the localized infection should be assigned as a secondary diagnosis. If the patient has severe sepsis, a code from subcategory R65.2 should also be assigned as a secondary diagnosis. If the patient is admitted with a localized infection, such as pneumonia, and sepsis/severe sepsis doesn't develop until after admission, the localized infection should be assigned first, followed by the appropriate sepsis/severe sepsis codes.

5) **Sepsis due to a postprocedural infection**

(a) **Documentation of causal relationship**

As with all postprocedural complications, code assignment is based on the provider's documentation of the relationship between the infection and the procedure.

(b) **Sepsis due to a postprocedural infection**

For such cases, the postprocedural infection code, such as T80.2, Infections following infusion, transfusion, and therapeutic injection, T81.4, Infection following a procedure, T88.0, Infection following immunization, or O86.0, Infection of obstetric surgical wound, should be coded first, followed by the code for the specific infection. If the patient has severe sepsis, the appropriate code

from subcategory R65.2 should also be assigned with the additional code(s) for any acute organ dysfunction.

(c) **Postprocedural infection and postprocedural septic shock**

In cases where a postprocedural infection has occurred and has resulted in severe sepsis the code for the precipitating complication such as code T81.4, Infection following a procedure, or O86.0, Infection of obstetrical surgical wound should be coded first followed by code R65.20, Severe sepsis without septic shock. A code for the systemic infection should also be assigned.

If a postprocedural infection has resulted in postprocedural septic shock, the code for the precipitating complication such as code T81.4, Infection following a procedure, or O86.0, Infection of obstetrical surgical wound should be coded first followed by code T81.12-, Postprocedural septic shock. A code for the systemic infection should also be assigned.

6) **Sepsis and severe sepsis associated with a noninfectious process (condition)**

In some cases a noninfectious process (condition), such as trauma, may lead to an infection which can result in sepsis or severe sepsis. If sepsis or severe sepsis is documented as associated with a noninfectious condition, such as a burn or serious injury, and this condition meets the definition for principal diagnosis, the code for the noninfectious condition should be sequenced first, followed by the code for the resulting infection. If severe sepsis is present, a code from subcategory

R65.2 should also be assigned with any associated organ dysfunction(s) codes. It is not necessary to assign a code from subcategory R65.1, Systemic inflammatory response syndrome (SIRS) of non-infectious origin, for these cases.

If the infection meets the definition of principal diagnosis, it should be sequenced before the non-infectious condition. When both the associated non-infectious condition and the infection meet the definition of principal diagnosis, either may be assigned as principal diagnosis.

Only one code from category R65, Symptoms and signs specifically associated with systemic inflammation and infection, should be assigned. Therefore, when a non-infectious condition leads to an infection resulting in severe sepsis, assign the appropriate code from subcategory R65.2, Severe sepsis. Do not additionally assign a code from subcategory R65.1, Systemic inflammatory response syndrome (SIRS) of non-infectious origin.

See Section I.C.18. SIRS due to non-infectious process

7) **Sepsis and septic shock complicating abortion, pregnancy, childbirth, and the puerperium**

See Section I.C.15. Sepsis and septic shock complicating abortion, pregnancy, childbirth and the puerperium

8) **Newborn sepsis**

See Section I.C.16. f. Bacterial sepsis of Newborn

e. **Methicillin Resistant *Staphylococcus aureus* (MRSA) Conditions**

1) **Selection and sequencing of MRSA codes**

(a) **Combination codes for MRSA infection**

When a patient is diagnosed with an infection that is due to methicillin resistant *Staphylococcus aureus* (MRSA), and that infection has a combination code that includes the causal organism (e.g., sepsis,

pneumonia) assign the appropriate combination code for the condition (e.g., code A41.02, Sepsis due to Methicillin resistant Staphylococcus aureus or code J15.212, Pneumonia due to Methicillin resistant Staphylococcus aureus). Do not assign code B95.62, Methicillin resistant Staphylococcus aureus infection as the cause of diseases classified elsewhere, as an additional code, because the combination code includes the type of infection and the MRSA organism. Do not assign a code from subcategory Z16.11, Resistance to penicillins, as an additional diagnosis.

See Section C.1. for instructions on coding and sequencing of sepsis and severe sepsis.

(b) **Other codes for MRSA infection**

When there is documentation of a current infection (e.g., wound infection, stitch abscess, urinary tract infection) due to MRSA, and that infection does not have a combination code that includes the causal organism, assign the appropriate code to identify the condition along with code B95.62, Methicillin resistant Staphylococcus aureus infection as the cause of diseases classified elsewhere for the MRSA infection. Do not assign a code from subcategory Z16.11, Resistance to penicillins.

(c) **Methicillin susceptible Staphylococcus aureus (MSSA) and MRSA colonization**

The condition or state of being colonized or carrying MSSA or MRSA is called colonization or carriage, while an individual person is described as being colonized or being a carrier. Colonization means that MSSA or MSRA is present on or in the body without necessarily causing illness. A positive MRSA colonization test might be documented by the provider as "MRSA screen positive" or "MRSA nasal swab positive".

Assign code Z22.322, Carrier or suspected carrier of Methicillin resistant Staphylococcus aureus, for patients documented as having MRSA colonization. Assign code Z22.321, Carrier or suspected carrier of Methicillin susceptible Staphylococcus aureus, for patient documented as having MSSA colonization. Colonization is not necessarily indicative of a disease process or as the cause of a specific condition the patient may have unless documented as such by the provider.

(d) **MRSA colonization and infection**

If a patient is documented as having both MRSA colonization and infection during a hospital admission, code Z22.322, Carrier or suspected carrier of Methicillin resistant Staphylococcus aureus, and a code for the MRSA infection may both be assigned.

f.   **Zika virus infections**

1)   **Code only confirmed cases**

Code only a confirmed diagnosis of Zika virus (A92.5, Zika virus disease) as documented by the provider. This is an exception to the hospital inpatient guideline Section II, H.

In this context, "confirmation" does not require documentation of the type of test performed; the physician's diagnostic statement that the condition is confirmed is sufficient. This code should be assigned regardless of the stated mode of transmission.

If the provider documents "suspected", "possible" or "probable" Zika, do not assign code A92.5. Assign a code(s) explaining the reason for encounter (such as fever, rash, or joint pain) or Z20.828, Contact with and (suspected) exposure to other viral communicable diseases.

2.   **Chapter 2: Neoplasms (C00-D49)**

General guidelines

Chapter 2 of the ICD-10-CM contains the codes for most benign and all malignant neoplasms. Certain benign neoplasms, such as prostatic adenomas, may be found in the specific body system chapters. To properly code a neoplasm it is necessary to determine from the record if the neoplasm is benign, in-situ, malignant, or of uncertain histologic behavior. If malignant, any secondary (metastatic) sites should also be determined.

Primary malignant neoplasms overlapping site boundaries

A primary malignant neoplasm that overlaps two or more contiguous (next to each other) sites should be classified to the subcategory/code .8 ('overlapping lesion'), unless the combination is specifically indexed elsewhere. For multiple neoplasms of the same site that are not contiguous such as tumors in different quadrants of the same breast, codes for each site should be assigned.

Malignant neoplasm of ectopic tissue

Malignant neoplasms of ectopic tissue are to be coded to the site of origin mentioned, e.g., ectopic pancreatic malignant neoplasms involving the stomach are coded to pancreas, unspecified (C25.9).

The neoplasm table in the Alphabetic Index should be referenced first. However, if the histological term is documented, that term should be referenced first, rather than going immediately to the Neoplasm Table, in order to determine which column in the Neoplasm Table is appropriate. For example, if the documentation indicates "adenoma," refer to the term in the Alphabetic Index to review the entries under this term and the instructional note to "see also neoplasm, by site, benign." The table provides the proper code based on the type of neoplasm and the site. It is important to select the proper column in the table that corresponds to the type of neoplasm. The Tabular List should then be referenced to verify that the correct code has been selected from the table and that a more specific site code does not exist.

See Section I.C.21. Factors influencing health status and contact with health services, Status, for information regarding Z15.0, codes for genetic susceptibility to cancer.

a.   **Treatment directed at the malignancy**

If the treatment is directed at the malignancy, designate the malignancy as the principal diagnosis.

The only exception to this guideline is if a patient admission/encounter is solely for the administration of chemotherapy, immunotherapy or radiation therapy, assign the appropriate Z51.-- code as the first-listed or principal diagnosis, and the diagnosis or problem for which the service is being performed as a secondary diagnosis.

b.   **Treatment of secondary site**

When a patient is admitted because of a primary neoplasm with metastasis and treatment is directed toward the secondary site only, the secondary neoplasm is designated as the principal diagnosis even though the primary malignancy is still present.

c.   **Coding and sequencing of complications**

Coding and sequencing of complications associated with the malignancies or with the therapy thereof are subject to the following guidelines:

1)   **Anemia associated with malignancy**

When admission/encounter is for management of an anemia associated with the malignancy, and the treatment is only for anemia, the appropriate code for the malignancy is sequenced as the principal or first-listed diagnosis followed by the appropriate code for the anemia (such as code D63.0, Anemia in neoplastic disease).

2) **Anemia associated with chemotherapy, immunotherapy and radiation therapy**

When the admission/encounter is for management of an anemia associated with an adverse effect of the administration of chemotherapy or immunotherapy and the only treatment is for the anemia, the anemia code is sequenced first followed by the appropriate codes for the neoplasm and the adverse effect (T45.1X5, Adverse effect of antineoplastic and immunosuppressive drugs).

When the admission/encounter is for management of an anemia associated with an adverse effect of radiotherapy, the anemia code should be sequenced first, followed by the appropriate neoplasm code and code Y84.2, Radiological procedure and radiotherapy as the cause of abnormal reaction of the patient, or of later complication, without mention of misadventure at the time of the procedure.

3) **Management of dehydration due to the malignancy**

When the admission/encounter is for management of dehydration due to the malignancy and only the dehydration is being treated (intravenous rehydration), the dehydration is sequenced first, followed by the code(s) for the malignancy.

4) **Treatment of a complication resulting from a surgical procedure**

When the admission/encounter is for treatment of a complication resulting from a surgical procedure, designate the complication as the principal or first-listed diagnosis if treatment is directed at resolving the complication.

d. **Primary malignancy previously excised**

When a primary malignancy has been previously excised or eradicated from its site and there is no further treatment directed to that site and there is no evidence of any existing primary malignancy, a code from category Z85, Personal history of malignant neoplasm, should be used to indicate the former site of the malignancy. Any mention of extension, invasion, or metastasis to another site is coded as a secondary malignant neoplasm to that site. The secondary site may be the principal or first-listed with the Z85 code used as a secondary code.

e. **Admissions/Encounters involving chemotherapy, immunotherapy and radiation therapy**

1) **Episode of care involves surgical removal of neoplasm**

When an episode of care involves the surgical removal of a neoplasm, primary or secondary site, followed by adjunct chemotherapy or radiation treatment during the same episode of care, the code for the neoplasm should be assigned as principal or first-listed diagnosis.

2) **Patient admission/encounter solely for administration of chemotherapy, immunotherapy and radiation therapy**

If a patient admission/encounter is solely for the administration of chemotherapy, immunotherapy or radiation therapy assign code Z51.0, Encounter for antineoplastic radiation therapy, or Z51.11, Encounter for antineoplastic chemotherapy, or Z51.12, Encounter for antineoplastic immunotherapy as the first-listed or principal diagnosis. If a patient receives more than one of these therapies during the same admission more than one of these codes may be assigned, in any sequence.

The malignancy for which the therapy is being administered should be assigned as a secondary diagnosis.

3) Patient admitted for radiation therapy, chemotherapy or immunotherapy and develops complications

When a patient is admitted for the purpose of radiotherapy, immunotherapy or chemotherapy and develops complications such as uncontrolled nausea and vomiting or dehydration, the principal or first-listed diagnosis is Z51.0, Encounter for antineoplastic radiation therapy, or Z51.11, Encounter for antineoplastic chemotherapy, or Z51.12, Encounter for antineoplastic immunotherapy followed by any codes for the complications.

f.   Admission/encounter to determine extent of malignancy

When the reason for admission/encounter is to determine the extent of the malignancy, or for a procedure such as paracentesis or thoracentesis, the primary malignancy or appropriate metastatic site is designated as the principal or first-listed diagnosis, even though chemotherapy or radiotherapy is administered.

g.   Symptoms, signs, and abnormal findings listed in Chapter 18 associated with neoplasms

Symptoms, signs, and ill-defined conditions listed in Chapter 18 characteristic of, or associated with, an existing primary or secondary site malignancy cannot be used to replace the malignancy as principal or first-listed diagnosis, regardless of the number of admissions or encounters for treatment and care of the neoplasm.

See section I.C.21. Factors influencing health status and contact with health services, Encounter for prophylactic organ removal.

h.   Admission/encounter for pain control/management

See Section I.C.6. for information on coding admission/encounter for pain control/management.

i.   Malignancy in two or more noncontiguous sites

A patient may have more than one malignant tumor in the same organ. These tumors may represent different primaries or metastatic disease, depending on the site. Should the documentation be unclear, the provider should be queried as to the status of each tumor so that the correct codes can be assigned.

j.   Disseminated malignant neoplasm, unspecified

Code C80.0, Disseminated malignant neoplasm, unspecified, is for use only in those cases where the patient has advanced metastatic disease and no known primary or secondary sites are specified. It should not be used in place of assigning codes for the primary site and all known secondary sites.

k.   Malignant neoplasm without specification of site

Code C80.1, Malignant (primary) neoplasm, unspecified, equates to Cancer, unspecified. This code should only be used when no determination can be made as to the primary site of a malignancy. This code should rarely be used in the inpatient setting.

l.   Sequencing of neoplasm codes

1) Encounter for treatment of primary malignancy

If the reason for the encounter is for treatment of a primary malignancy, assign the malignancy as the principal/first-listed diagnosis. The primary site is to be sequenced first, followed by any metastatic sites.

2) Encounter for treatment of secondary malignancy

When an encounter is for a primary malignancy with metastasis and treatment is directed toward the metastatic (secondary) site(s) only, the metastatic site(s) is designated as the principal/first-listed diagnosis. The primary malignancy is coded as an additional code.

3) Malignant neoplasm in a pregnant patient

When a pregnant woman has a malignant neoplasm, a code from subcategory O9A.1-, Malignant neoplasm complicating pregnancy, childbirth, and the puerperium, should be sequenced first, followed by the appropriate code from Chapter 2 to indicate the type of neoplasm.

4) Encounter for complication associated with a neoplasm

When an encounter is for management of a complication associated with a neoplasm, such as dehydration, and the treatment is only for the complication, the complication is coded first, followed by the appropriate code(s) for the neoplasm.

The exception to this guideline is anemia. When the admission/encounter is for management of an anemia associated with the malignancy, and the treatment is only for anemia, the appropriate code for the malignancy is sequenced as the principal or first-listed diagnosis followed by code D63.0, Anemia in neoplastic disease.

5) Complication from surgical procedure for treatment of a neoplasm

When an encounter is for treatment of a complication resulting from a surgical procedure performed for the treatment of the neoplasm, designate the complication as the principal/first-listed diagnosis. See guideline regarding the coding of a current malignancy versus personal history to determine if the code for the neoplasm should also be assigned.

6) Pathologic fracture due to a neoplasm

When an encounter is for a pathological fracture due to a neoplasm, and the focus of treatment is the fracture, a code from subcategory M84.5, Pathological fracture in neoplastic disease, should be sequenced first, followed by the code for the neoplasm.

If the focus of treatment is the neoplasm with an associated pathological fracture, the neoplasm code should be sequenced first, followed by a code from M84.5 for the pathological fracture.

m. Current malignancy versus personal history of malignancy

When a primary malignancy has been excised but further treatment, such as an additional surgery for the malignancy, radiation therapy or chemotherapy is directed to that site, the primary malignancy code should be used until treatment is completed.

When a primary malignancy has been previously excised or eradicated from its site, there is no further treatment (of the malignancy) directed to that site, and there is no evidence of any existing primary malignancy, a code from category Z85, Personal history of malignant neoplasm, should be used to indicate the former site of the malignancy.

See Section I.C.21. Factors influencing health status and contact with health services, History (of)

n. Leukemia, Multiple Myeloma, and Malignant Plasma Cell Neoplasms in remission versus personal history

The categories for leukemia, and category C90, Multiple myeloma and malignant plasma cell neoplasms, have codes indicating whether or not the leukemia has achieved remission. There are also codes Z85.6, Personal history of leukemia, and Z85.79, Personal history of other malignant neoplasms of lymphoid, hematopoietic and

related tissues. If the documentation is unclear as to whether the leukemia has achieved remission, the provider should be queried.

See Section I.C.21. Factors influencing health status and contact with health services, History (of)

o. **Aftercare following surgery for neoplasm**

See Section I.C.21. Factors influencing health status and contact with health services, Aftercare

p. **Follow-up care for completed treatment of a malignancy**

See Section I.C.21. Factors influencing health status and contact with health services, Follow-up

q. **Prophylactic organ removal for prevention of malignancy**

See Section I.C. 21, Factors influencing health status and contact with health services, Prophylactic organ removal

r. **Malignant neoplasm associated with transplanted organ**

A malignant neoplasm of a transplanted organ should be coded as a transplant complication. Assign first the appropriate code from category T86.-, Complications of transplanted organs and tissue, followed by code C80.2, Malignant neoplasm associated with transplanted organ. Use an additional code for the specific malignancy.

3. **Chapter 3: Disease of the blood and blood-forming organs and certain disorders involving the immune mechanism (D50-D89)**

Reserved for future guideline expansion

4. **Chapter 4: Endocrine, Nutritional, and Metabolic Diseases (E00-E89)**

a. **Diabetes mellitus**

The diabetes mellitus codes are combination codes that include the type of diabetes mellitus, the body system affected, and the complications affecting that body system. As many codes within a particular category

as are necessary to describe all of the complications of the disease may be used. They should be sequenced based on the reason for a particular encounter. Assign as many codes from categories E08 – E13 as needed to identify all of the associated conditions that the patient has.

1) **Type of diabetes**

The age of a patient is not the sole determining factor, though most type 1 diabetics develop the condition before reaching puberty. For this reason type 1 diabetes mellitus is also referred to as juvenile diabetes.

2) **Type of diabetes mellitus not documented**

If the type of diabetes mellitus is not documented in the medical record the default is E11.-, Type 2 diabetes mellitus.

3) **Diabetes mellitus and the use of insulin and oral hypoglycemics**

If the documentation in a medical record does not indicate the type of diabetes but does indicate that the patient uses insulin, code E11, Type 2 diabetes mellitus, should be assigned. Code Z79.4, Long-term (current) use of insulin, or Z79.84, Long term (current) use of oral hypoglycemic drugs, should also be

assigned to indicate that the patient uses insulin or hypoglycemic drugs. Code Z79.4 should not be assigned if insulin is given temporarily to bring a type 2 patient's blood sugar under control during an encounter.

4) Diabetes mellitus in pregnancy and gestational diabetes

See Section I.C.15. Diabetes mellitus in pregnancy.
See Section I.C.15. Gestational (pregnancy induced) diabetes

5) Complications due to insulin pump malfunction

(a) Underdose of insulin due to insulin pump failure

An underdose of insulin due to an insulin pump failure should be assigned to a code from subcategory T85.6, Mechanical complication of other specified internal and external prosthetic devices, implants and grafts, that specifies the type of pump malfunction, as the principal or first-listed code, followed by code T38.3X6-, Underdosing of insulin and oral hypoglycemic [antidiabetic] drugs. Additional codes for the type of diabetes mellitus and any associated complications due to the underdosing should also be assigned.

(b) Overdose of insulin due to insulin pump failure

The principal or first-listed code for an encounter due to an insulin pump malfunction resulting in an overdose of insulin, should also be T85.6-, Mechanical complication of other specified internal and external prosthetic devices, implants and grafts, followed by code T38.3X1-, Poisoning by insulin and oral hypoglycemic [antidiabetic] drugs, accidental (unintentional).

6) Secondary diabetes mellitus

Codes under categories E08, Diabetes mellitus due to underlying condition, E09, Drug or chemical induced diabetes mellitus, and E13, Other specified diabetes mellitus, identify complications/manifestations associated with secondary diabetes mellitus. Secondary diabetes is always caused by another condition or event (e.g., cystic fibrosis, malignant neoplasm of pancreas, pancreatectomy, adverse effect of drug, or poisoning).

(a) Secondary diabetes mellitus and the use of insulin or hypoglycemic drugs

For patients who routinely use insulin or hypoglycemic drugs, code Z79.4, Long-term (current) use of insulin, or Z79.84, Long term (current) use of oral hypoglycemic drugs should also be assigned. Code Z79.4 should not be assigned if insulin is given temporarily to bring a patient's blood sugar under control during an encounter.

(b) Assigning and sequencing secondary diabetes codes and its causes

The sequencing of the secondary diabetes codes in relationship to codes for the cause of the diabetes is based on the Tabular List instructions for categories E08, E09 and E13.

(i) Secondary diabetes mellitus due to pancreatectomy

For postpancreatectomy diabetes mellitus (lack of insulin due to the surgical removal of all or part of the pancreas), assign code E89.1, Postprocedural hypoinsulinemia. Assign a code from category E13 and a code from subcategory Z90.41-, Acquired absence of pancreas, as additional codes.

(ii) Secondary diabetes due to drugs

Secondary diabetes may be caused by an adverse effect of correctly administered medications, poisoning or sequela of poisoning.

See section I.C.19.e for coding of adverse effects and poisoning, and section I.C.20 for external cause code reporting.

5. **Chapter 5: Mental, Behavioral and Neurodevelopmental disorders (F01 – F99)**

    a. **Pain disorders related to psychological factors**

        Assign code F45.41, for pain that is exclusively related to psychological disorders. As indicated by the Excludes 1 note under category G89, a code from category G89 should not be assigned with code F45.41.

        Code F45.42, Pain disorders with related psychological factors, should be used with a code from category G89, Pain, not elsewhere classified, if there is documentation of a psychological component for a patient with acute or chronic pain.

        See Section I.C.6. Pain

    b. **Mental and behavioral disorders due to psychoactive substance use**

        1) **In Remission**

            Selection of codes for "in remission" for categories F10-F19, Mental and behavioral disorders due to psychoactive substance use (categories F10-F19 with -.21) requires the provider's clinical judgment. The appropriate codes for "in remission" are assigned only on the basis of provider documentation (as defined in the Official Guidelines for Coding and Reporting).

        2) **Psychoactive Substance Use, Abuse And Dependence**

            When the provider documentation refers to use, abuse and dependence of the same substance (e.g. alcohol, opioid, cannabis, etc.), only one code should be assigned to identify the pattern of use based on the following hierarchy:

            •   If both use and abuse are documented, assign only the code for abuse

            •   If both abuse and dependence are documented, assign only the code for dependence

            •   If use, abuse and dependence are all documented, assign only the code for dependence

            •   If both use and dependence are documented, assign only the code for dependence.

        3) **Psychoactive Substance Use**

            As with all other diagnoses, the codes for psychoactive substance use (F10.9-, F11.9-, F12.9-, F13.9-, F14.9-, F15.9-, F16.9-) should only be assigned based on provider documentation and when they meet the definition of a reportable diagnosis (see Section III, Reporting Additional Diagnoses). The codes are to be used only when the psychoactive substance use is associated with a mental or behavioral disorder, and such a relationship is documented by the provider.

6. **Chapter 6: Diseases of the Nervous System (G00-G99)**

    a. **Dominant/nondominant side**

        Codes from category G81, Hemiplegia and hemiparesis, and subcategories G83.1, Monoplegia of lower limb, G83.2, Monoplegia of upper limb, and G83.3, Monoplegia, unspecified, identify whether the dominant or nondominant side is affected. Should the affected side be documented, but not specified as dominant or nondominant, and the classification system does not indicate a default, code selection is as follows:

- For ambidextrous patients, the default should be dominant.

- If the left side is affected, the default is non-dominant.

- If the right side is affected, the default is dominant.

b. Pain - Category G89

1) General coding information

Codes in category G89, Pain, not elsewhere classified, may be used in conjunction with codes from other categories and chapters to provide more detail about acute or chronic pain and neoplasm-related pain, unless otherwise indicated below.

If the pain is not specified as acute or chronic, post-thoracotomy, postprocedural, or neoplasm-related, do not assign codes from category G89.

A code from category G89 should not be assigned if the underlying (definitive) diagnosis is known, unless the reason for the encounter is pain control/ management and not management of the underlying condition.

When an admission or encounter is for a procedure aimed at treating the underlying condition (e.g., spinal fusion, kyphoplasty), a code for the underlying condition (e.g., vertebral fracture, spinal stenosis) should be assigned as the principal diagnosis. No code from category G89 should be assigned.

(a) Category G89 Codes as Principal or First-Listed Diagnosis

Category G89 codes are acceptable as principal diagnosis or the first-listed code:

- When pain control or pain management is the reason for the admission/encounter (e.g., a patient with displaced intervertebral disc, nerve impingement and severe back pain presents for injection of steroid into the spinal canal). The underlying cause of the pain should be reported as an additional diagnosis, if known.

- When a patient is admitted for the insertion of a neurostimulator for pain control, assign the appropriate pain code as the principal or first-listed diagnosis. When an admission or encounter is for a procedure aimed at treating the underlying condition and a neurostimulator is inserted for pain control during the same admission/encounter, a code for the underlying condition should be assigned as the principal diagnosis and the appropriate pain code should be assigned as a secondary diagnosis.

(b) Use of Category G89 Codes in Conjunction with Site Specific Pain Codes

(i) Assigning Category G89 and Site-Specific Pain Codes

Codes from category G89 may be used in conjunction with codes that identify the site of pain (including codes from chapter 18) if the category G89 code provides additional information. For example, if the code describes the site of the pain, but does not fully describe whether the pain is acute or chronic, then both codes should be assigned.

(ii) Sequencing of Category G89 Codes with Site-Specific Pain Codes

The sequencing of category G89 codes with site-specific pain codes (including chapter 18 codes), is dependent on the circumstances of the encounter/admission as follows:

- If the encounter is for pain control or pain management, assign the code from category G89 followed by the code identifying the specific site of pain (e.g., encounter for pain management for acute neck pain from trauma is assigned code G89.11, Acute pain due to trauma, followed by code M54.2, Cervicalgia, to identify the site of pain).

- If the encounter is for any other reason except pain control or pain management, and a related definitive diagnosis has not been established (confirmed) by the provider, assign the code for the specific site of pain first, followed by the appropriate code from category G89.

2) **Pain due to devices, implants and grafts**

   See Section I.C.19. Pain due to medical devices

3) **Postoperative Pain**

   The provider's documentation should be used to guide the coding of postoperative pain, as well as *Section III. Reporting Additional Diagnoses* and *Section IV. Diagnostic Coding and Reporting in the Outpatient Setting.*

   The default for post-thoracotomy and other postoperative pain not specified as acute or chronic is the code for the acute form.

   Routine or expected postoperative pain immediately after surgery should not be coded.

   (a) **Postoperative pain not associated with specific postoperative complication**

   Postoperative pain not associated with a specific postoperative complication is assigned to the appropriate postoperative pain code in category G89.

   (b) **Postoperative pain associated with specific postoperative complication**

   Postoperative pain associated with a specific postoperative complication (such as painful wire sutures) is assigned to the appropriate code(s) found in Chapter 19, Injury, poisoning, and certain other consequences of external causes. If appropriate, use additional code(s) from category G89 to identify acute or chronic pain (G89.18 or G89.28).

4) **Chronic pain**

   Chronic pain is classified to subcategory G89.2. There is no time frame defining when pain becomes chronic pain. The provider's documentation should be used to guide use of these codes.

5) **Neoplasm Related Pain**

   Code G89.3 is assigned to pain documented as being related, associated or due to cancer, primary or secondary malignancy, or tumor. This code is assigned regardless of whether the pain is acute or chronic.

   This code may be assigned as the principal or first-listed code when the stated reason for the admission/encounter is documented as pain control/pain management. The underlying neoplasm should be reported as an additional diagnosis.

   When the reason for the admission/encounter is management of the neoplasm and the pain associated with the neoplasm is also documented, code G89.3 may be assigned as an additional diagnosis. It is not necessary to assign an additional code for the site of the pain.

See Section I.C.2 for instructions on the sequencing of neoplasms for all other stated reasons for the admission/encounter (except for pain control/pain management).

6) Chronic pain syndrome

Central pain syndrome (G89.0) and chronic pain syndrome (G89.4) are different than the term "chronic pain," and therefore codes should only be used when the provider has specifically documented this condition.

See Section I.C.5. Pain disorders related to psychological factors

7. Chapter 7: Diseases of the Eye and Adnexa (H00-H59)

a. Glaucoma

1) Assigning Glaucoma Codes

Assign as many codes from category H40, Glaucoma, as needed to identify the type of glaucoma, the affected eye, and the glaucoma stage.

2) Bilateral glaucoma with same type and stage

When a patient has bilateral glaucoma and both eyes are documented as being the same type and stage, and there is a code for bilateral glaucoma, report only the code for the type of glaucoma, bilateral, with the seventh character for the stage.

When a patient has bilateral glaucoma and both eyes are documented as being the same type and stage, and the classification does not provide a code for bilateral glaucoma (i.e. subcategories H40.10, H40.11 and H40.20) report only one code for the type of glaucoma with the appropriate seventh character for the stage.

3) Bilateral glaucoma stage with different types or stages

When a patient has bilateral glaucoma and each eye is documented as having a different type or stage, and the classification distinguishes laterality, assign the appropriate code for each eye rather than the code for bilateral glaucoma.

When a patient has bilateral glaucoma and each eye is documented as having a different type, and the classification does not distinguish laterality (i.e. subcategories H40.10, H40.11 and H40.20), assign one code for each type of glaucoma with the appropriate seventh character for the stage.

When a patient has bilateral glaucoma and each eye is documented as having the same type, but different stage, and the classification does not distinguish laterality (i.e. subcategories H40.10, H40.11 and H40.20), assign a code for

the type of glaucoma for each eye with the seventh character for the specific glaucoma stage documented for each eye.

4) Patient admitted with glaucoma and stage evolves during the admission

If a patient is admitted with glaucoma and the stage progresses during the admission, assign the code for highest stage documented.

5) Indeterminate stage glaucoma

Assignment of the seventh character "4" for "indeterminate stage" should be based on the clinical documentation. The seventh character "4" is used for glaucomas whose stage cannot be clinically

determined. This seventh character should not be confused with the seventh character "0", unspecified, which should be assigned when there is no documentation regarding the stage of the glaucoma.

8. **Chapter 8: Diseases of the Ear and Mastoid Process (H60-H95)**

Reserved for future guideline expansion

9. **Chapter 9: Diseases of the Circulatory System (I00-I99)**

a. **Hypertension**

The classification presumes a causal relationship between hypertension and heart involvement and between hypertension and kidney involvement, as the two conditions are linked by the term "with" in the Alphabetic Index. These conditions should be coded as related even in the absence of provider documentation explicitly linking them, unless the documentation clearly states the conditions are unrelated.

For hypertension and conditions not specifically linked by relational terms such as "with," "associated with" or "due to" in the classification, provider documentation must link the conditions in order to code them as related.

1) **Hypertension with Heart Disease**

Hypertension with heart conditions classified to I50.- or I51.4-I51.9, are assigned to a code from category I11, Hypertensive heart disease. Use an additional code from category I50, Heart failure, to identify the type of heart failure in those patients with heart failure.

The same heart conditions (I50.-, I51.4-I51.9) with hypertension are coded separately if the provider has specifically documented a different cause. Sequence according to the circumstances of the admission/encounter.

2) **Hypertensive Chronic Kidney Disease**

Assign codes from category I12, Hypertensive chronic kidney disease, when both hypertension and a condition classifiable to category N18, Chronic kidney disease (CKD), are present. CKD should not be coded as hypertensive if the physician has specifically documented a different cause.

The appropriate code from category N18 should be used as a secondary code with a code from category I12 to identify the stage of chronic kidney disease.

See Section I.C.14. Chronic kidney disease.

If a patient has hypertensive chronic kidney disease and acute renal failure, an additional code for the acute renal failure is required.

3) **Hypertensive Heart and Chronic Kidney Disease**

Assign codes from combination category I13, Hypertensive heart and chronic kidney disease, when there is hypertension with both heart and kidney involvement. If heart failure is present, assign an additional code from category I50 to identify the type of heart failure.

The appropriate code from category N18, Chronic kidney disease, should be used as a secondary code with a code from category I13 to identify the stage of chronic kidney disease.

See Section I.C.14. Chronic kidney disease.

The codes in category I13, Hypertensive heart and chronic kidney disease, are combination codes that include hypertension, heart disease and chronic kidney disease. The Includes note at I13 specifies that the conditions included at I11 and I12 are included together in I13. If a patient has hypertension, heart disease and chronic kidney disease, then a code from I13 should be used, not individual codes for hypertension, heart disease and chronic kidney disease, or codes from I11 or I12.

For patients with both acute renal failure and chronic kidney disease, an additional code for acute renal failure is required.

4) **Hypertensive Cerebrovascular Disease**

For hypertensive cerebrovascular disease, first assign the appropriate code from categories I60-I69, followed by the appropriate hypertension code.

5) **Hypertensive Retinopathy**

Subcategory H35.0, Background retinopathy and retinal vascular changes, should be used with a code from category I10 – I15, Hypertensive disease to include the systemic hypertension. The sequencing is based on the reason for the encounter.

6) **Hypertension, Secondary**

Secondary hypertension is due to an underlying condition. Two codes are required: one to identify the underlying etiology and one from category I15 to identify the hypertension. Sequencing of codes is determined by the reason for admission/encounter.

7) **Hypertension, Transient**

Assign code R03.0, Elevated blood pressure reading without diagnosis of hypertension, unless patient has an established diagnosis of hypertension. Assign code O13.-, Gestational [pregnancy-induced] hypertension without significant proteinuria, or O14.-, Pre-eclampsia, for transient hypertension of pregnancy.

8) **Hypertension, Controlled**

This diagnostic statement usually refers to an existing state of hypertension under control by therapy. Assign the appropriate code from categories I10-I15, Hypertensive diseases.

9) **Hypertension, Uncontrolled**

Uncontrolled hypertension may refer to untreated hypertension or hypertension not responding to current therapeutic regimen. In either case, assign the appropriate code from categories I10-I15, Hypertensive diseases.

10) **Hypertensive Crisis**

Assign a code from category I16, Hypertensive crisis, for documented hypertensive urgency, hypertensive emergency or unspecified hypertensive crisis. Code also any identified hypertensive disease (I10-I15). The sequencing is based on the reason for the encounter.

b. **Atherosclerotic Coronary Artery Disease and Angina**

ICD-10-CM has combination codes for atherosclerotic heart disease with angina pectoris. The subcategories for these codes are I25.11, Atherosclerotic heart disease of native coronary artery with angina pectoris and I25.7, Atherosclerosis of coronary artery bypass graft(s) and coronary artery of transplanted heart with angina pectoris.

When using one of these combination codes it is not necessary to use an additional code for angina pectoris. A causal relationship can be assumed in a patient with both atherosclerosis and angina pectoris, unless the documentation indicates the angina is due to something other than the atherosclerosis.

If a patient with coronary artery disease is admitted due to an acute myocardial infarction (AMI), the AMI should be sequenced before the coronary artery disease.

See Section I.C.9. Acute myocardial infarction (AMI)

c. **Intraoperative and Postprocedural Cerebrovascular Accident**

Medical record documentation should clearly specify the cause- and-effect relationship between the medical intervention and the cerebrovascular accident in order to assign a code for intraoperative or postprocedural cerebrovascular accident.

Proper code assignment depends on whether it was an infarction or hemorrhage and whether it occurred intraoperatively or postoperatively. If it was a cerebral hemorrhage, code assignment depends on the type of procedure performed.

d. **Sequelae of Cerebrovascular Disease**

1) **Category I69, Sequelae of Cerebrovascular disease**

Category I69 is used to indicate conditions classifiable to categories I60-I67 as the causes of sequela (neurologic deficits), themselves classified elsewhere. These "late effects" include neurologic deficits that persist after initial onset of conditions classifiable to categories I60-I67. The neurologic deficits caused by cerebrovascular disease may be present from the onset or may arise at any time after the onset of the condition classifiable to categories I60-I67.

Codes from category I69, Sequelae of cerebrovascular disease, that specify hemiplegia, hemiparesis and monoplegia identify whether the dominant or nondominant side is affected. Should the affected side be documented, but not specified as dominant or nondominant, and the classification system does not indicate a default, code selection is as follows:

- For ambidextrous patients, the default should be dominant.

- If the left side is affected, the default is non-dominant.

- If the right side is affected, the default is dominant.

2) **Codes from category I69 with codes from I60-I67**

Codes from category I69 may be assigned on a health care record with codes from I60-I67, if the patient has a current cerebrovascular disease and deficits from an old cerebrovascular disease.

3) **Codes from category I69 and Personal history of transient ischemic attack (TIA) and cerebral infarction (Z86.73)**

Codes from category I69 should not be assigned if the patient does not have neurologic deficits.

See Section I.C.21. 4. History (of) for use of personal history codes

e. **Acute myocardial infarction (AMI)**

1) **ST elevation myocardial infarction (STEMI) and non ST elevation myocardial infarction (NSTEMI)**

The ICD-10-CM codes for acute myocardial infarction (AMI) identify the site, such as anterolateral wall or true posterior wall. Subcategories I21.0-I21.2 and code I21.3 are used for ST elevation myocardial infarction (STEMI). Code I21.4, Non-ST elevation (NSTEMI) myocardial infarction, is used for non ST elevation myocardial infarction (NSTEMI) and nontransmural MIs.

If NSTEMI evolves to STEMI, assign the STEMI code. If STEMI converts to NSTEMI due to thrombolytic therapy, it is still coded as STEMI.

For encounters occurring while the myocardial infarction is equal to, or less than, four weeks old, including transfers to another acute setting or a postacute setting, and the myocardial infarction **meets** the definition for "other diagnoses" (see Section III, Reporting Additional Diagnoses), codes from category I21 may continue to be reported. For encounters after the 4 week time frame and the patient is still receiving care related to the myocardial infarction, the appropriate aftercare code should be assigned, rather than a code from category I21. For old or healed myocardial infarctions not requiring further care, code I25.2, Old myocardial infarction, may be assigned.

2) **Acute myocardial infarction, unspecified**

Code I21.3, ST elevation (STEMI) myocardial infarction of unspecified site, is the default for unspecified acute myocardial infarction. If only STEMI or transmural MI without the site is documented, assign code I21.3.

3) **AMI documented as nontransmural or subendocardial but site provided**

If an AMI is documented as nontransmural or subendocardial, but the site is provided, it is still coded as a subendocardial AMI.

See Section I.C.21.3 for information on coding status post administration of tPA in a different facility within the last 24 hours.

4) **Subsequent acute myocardial infarction**

A code from category I22, Subsequent ST elevation (STEMI) and non ST elevation (NSTEMI) myocardial infarction, is to be used when a patient who has suffered an AMI has a new AMI within the 4 week time frame of the initial AMI. A code from category I22 must be used in conjunction with a code from category I21. The sequencing of the I22 and I21 codes depends on the circumstances of the encounter.

10. **Chapter 10: Diseases of the Respiratory System (J00-J99)**

a. **Chronic Obstructive Pulmonary Disease [COPD] and Asthma**

1) **Acute exacerbation of chronic obstructive bronchitis and asthma**

The codes in categories J44 and J45 distinguish between uncomplicated cases and those in acute exacerbation. An acute exacerbation is a worsening or a decompensation of a chronic condition. An acute exacerbation is not equivalent to an infection superimposed on a chronic condition, though an exacerbation may be triggered by an infection.

b. **Acute Respiratory Failure**

1) **Acute respiratory failure as principal diagnosis**

A code from subcategory J96.0, Acute respiratory failure, or subcategory J96.2, Acute and chronic respiratory failure, may be assigned as a principal diagnosis when it is the condition established after study to be chiefly responsible for occasioning the admission to the hospital, and the selection is

supported by the Alphabetic Index and Tabular List. However, chapter-specific coding guidelines (such as obstetrics, poisoning, HIV, newborn) that provide sequencing direction take precedence.

2) Acute respiratory failure as secondary diagnosis

Respiratory failure may be listed as a secondary diagnosis if it occurs after admission, or if it is present on admission, but does not meet the definition of principal diagnosis.

3) Sequencing of acute respiratory failure and another acute condition

When a patient is admitted with respiratory failure and another acute condition, (e.g., myocardial infarction, cerebrovascular accident, aspiration pneumonia), the principal diagnosis will not be the same in every situation. This applies whether the other acute condition is a respiratory or nonrespiratory condition. Selection of the principal diagnosis will be dependent on the circumstances of admission. If both the respiratory failure and the other acute condition are equally responsible for occasioning the admission to the hospital, and there are no chapter-specific sequencing rules, the guideline regarding two or more diagnoses that equally meet the definition for principal diagnosis *(Section II, C.)* may be applied in these situations.

If the documentation is not clear as to whether acute respiratory failure and another condition are equally responsible for occasioning the admission, query the provider for clarification.

c. Influenza due to certain identified influenza viruses

Code only confirmed cases of influenza due to certain identified influenza viruses (category J09), and due to other identified influenza virus (category J10). This is an exception to the hospital inpatient guideline Section II, H. (Uncertain Diagnosis).

In this context, "confirmation" does not require documentation of positive laboratory testing specific for avian or other novel influenza A or other identified influenza virus. However, coding should be based on the provider's diagnostic statement that the patient has avian influenza, or other novel influenza A, for category J09, or has another particular identified strain of influenza, such as H1N1 or H3N2, but not identified as novel or variant, for category J10.

If the provider records "suspected" or "possible" or "probable" avian influenza, or novel influenza, or other identified influenza, then the appropriate influenza code from category J11, Influenza due to unidentified influenza virus, should be assigned. A code from category J09, Influenza due to certain identified influenza viruses, should not be assigned nor should a code from category J10, Influenza due to other identified influenza virus.

d. Ventilator associated Pneumonia

1) Documentation of Ventilator associated Pneumonia

As with all procedural or postprocedural complications, code assignment is based on the provider's documentation of the relationship between the condition and the procedure.

Code J95.851, Ventilator associated pneumonia, should be assigned only when the provider has documented ventilator associated pneumonia (VAP). An additional code to identify the organism (e.g., Pseudomonas aeruginosa, code B96.5) should also be assigned. Do not assign an additional code from categories J12-J18 to identify the type of pneumonia.

Code J95.851 should not be assigned for cases where the patient has pneumonia and is on a mechanical ventilator and the provider has not specifically stated that the pneumonia is ventilator-associated pneumonia. If the documentation is unclear as to whether the patient has a pneumonia that is a complication attributable to the mechanical ventilator, query the provider.

2) **Ventilator associated Pneumonia Develops after Admission**

A patient may be admitted with one type of pneumonia (e.g., code J13, Pneumonia due to Streptococcus pneumonia) and subsequently develop VAP. In this instance, the principal diagnosis would be the appropriate code from categories J12-

J18 for the pneumonia diagnosed at the time of admission. Code J95.851, Ventilator associated pneumonia, would be assigned as an additional diagnosis when the provider has also documented the presence of ventilator associated pneumonia.

11. **Chapter 11: Diseases of the Digestive System (K00-K95)**

Reserved for future guideline expansion

12. **Chapter 12: Diseases of the Skin and Subcutaneous Tissue (L00-L99)**

a. **Pressure ulcer stage codes**

1) **Pressure ulcer stages**

Codes from category L89, Pressure ulcer, identify the site of the pressure ulcer as well as the stage of the ulcer.

The ICD-10-CM classifies pressure ulcer stages based on severity, which is designated by stages 1-4, unspecified stage and unstageable.

Assign as many codes from category L89 as needed to identify all the pressure ulcers the patient has, if applicable.

2) **Unstageable pressure ulcers**

Assignment of the code for unstageable pressure ulcer (L89.--0) should be based on the clinical documentation. These codes are used for pressure ulcers whose stage cannot be clinically determined (e.g., the ulcer is covered by eschar or has been treated with a skin or muscle graft) and pressure ulcers that are documented as deep tissue injury but not documented as due to trauma. This code should not be confused with the codes for unspecified stage (L89.--9). When there is no documentation regarding the stage of the pressure ulcer, assign the appropriate code for unspecified stage (L89.--9).

3) **Documented pressure ulcer stage**

Assignment of the pressure ulcer stage code should be guided by clinical documentation of the stage or documentation of the terms found in the Alphabetic Index. For clinical terms describing the stage that are not found in the Alphabetic Index, and there is no documentation of the stage, the provider should be queried.

4) **Patients admitted with pressure ulcers documented as healed**

No code is assigned if the documentation states that the pressure ulcer is completely healed.

5) **Patients admitted with pressure ulcers documented as healing**

Pressure ulcers described as healing should be assigned the appropriate pressure ulcer stage code based on the documentation in the medical record. If the documentation does not provide information about the stage of the healing pressure ulcer, assign the appropriate code for unspecified stage.

If the documentation is unclear as to whether the patient has a current (new) pressure ulcer or if the patient is being treated for a healing pressure ulcer, query the provider.

For ulcers that were present on admission but healed at the time of discharge, assign the code for the site and stage of the pressure ulcer at the time of admission.

6) Patient admitted with pressure ulcer evolving into another stage during the admission

If a patient is admitted with a pressure ulcer at one stage and it progresses to a higher stage, two separate codes should be assigned: one code for the site and stage of the ulcer on admission and a second code for the same ulcer site and the highest stage reported during the stay.

13. Chapter 13: Diseases of the Musculoskeletal System and Connective Tissue (M00-M99)

a. Site and laterality

Most of the codes within Chapter 13 have site and laterality designations. The site represents the bone, joint or the muscle involved. For some conditions where more than one bone, joint or muscle is usually involved, such as osteoarthritis, there is a "multiple sites" code available. For categories where no multiple site code is provided and more than one bone, joint or muscle is involved, multiple codes should be used to indicate the different sites involved.

1) Bone versus joint

For certain conditions, the bone may be affected at the upper or lower end, (e.g., avascular necrosis of bone, M87, Osteoporosis, M80, M81). Though the portion of the bone affected may be at the joint, the site designation will be the bone, not the joint.

b. Acute traumatic versus chronic or recurrent musculoskeletal conditions

Many musculoskeletal conditions are a result of previous injury or trauma to a site, or are recurrent conditions. Bone, joint or muscle conditions that are the result of a healed injury are usually found in chapter 13. Recurrent bone, joint or muscle conditions are also usually found in chapter 13. Any current, acute injury should be coded to the appropriate injury code from chapter 19. Chronic or recurrent conditions should generally be coded with a code from chapter 13. If it is difficult to determine from the documentation in the record which code is best to describe a condition, query the provider.

c. Coding of Pathologic Fractures

7th character A is for use as long as the patient is receiving active treatment for the fracture. While the patient may be seen by a new or different provider over the course of treatment for a pathological fracture, assignment of the 7th character is based on whether the patient is undergoing active treatment and not whether the provider is seeing the patient for the first time.

7th character D is to be used for encounters after the patient has completed active treatment. The other 7th characters, listed under each subcategory in the Tabular List, are to be used for subsequent encounters for routine care of fractures during the healing and recovery phase as well as treatment of problems associated with the healing, such as malunions, nonunions, and sequelae.

Care for complications of surgical treatment for fracture repairs during the healing or recovery phase should be coded with the appropriate complication codes.

See Section I.C.19. Coding of traumatic fractures.

d. Osteoporosis

Osteoporosis is a systemic condition, meaning that all bones of the musculoskeletal system are affected. Therefore, site is not a component of the codes under category M81, Osteoporosis without current

pathological fracture. The site codes under category M80, Osteoporosis with current pathological fracture, identify the site of the fracture, not the osteoporosis.

1) **Osteoporosis without pathological fracture**

Category M81, Osteoporosis without current pathological fracture, is for use for patients with osteoporosis who do not currently have a pathologic fracture due to the osteoporosis, even if they have had a fracture in the past. For patients with a history of osteoporosis fractures, status code Z87.310, Personal history of (healed) osteoporosis fracture, should follow the code from M81.

2) **Osteoporosis with current pathological fracture**

Category M80, Osteoporosis with current pathological fracture, is for patients who have a current pathologic fracture at the time of an encounter. The codes under M80 identify the site of the fracture. A code from category M80, not a traumatic fracture code, should be used for any patient with known osteoporosis who suffers a fracture, even if the patient had a minor fall or trauma, if that fall or trauma would not usually break a normal, healthy bone.

14. **Chapter 14: Diseases of Genitourinary System (N00-N99)**

a. **Chronic kidney disease**

1) **Stages of chronic kidney disease (CKD)**

The ICD-10-CM classifies CKD based on severity. The severity of CKD is designated by stages 1-5. Stage 2, code N18.2, equates to mild CKD; stage 3, code N18.3, equates to moderate CKD; and stage 4, code N18.4, equates to severe CKD. Code N18.6, End stage renal disease (ESRD), is assigned when the provider has documented end-stage-renal disease (ESRD).

If both a stage of CKD and ESRD are documented, assign code N18.6 only.

2) **Chronic kidney disease and kidney transplant status**

Patients who have undergone kidney transplant may still have some form of chronic kidney disease **(CKD)** because the kidney transplant may not fully restore kidney function. Therefore, the presence of CKD alone does not constitute a transplant complication. Assign the appropriate N18 code for the patient's stage of CKD and code Z94.0, Kidney transplant status. If a transplant complication such as failure or rejection or other transplant complication is documented, see section I.C.19.g for information on coding complications of a kidney transplant. If the documentation is unclear as to whether the patient has a complication of the transplant, query the provider.

3) **Chronic kidney disease with other conditions**

Patients with CKD may also suffer from other serious conditions, most commonly diabetes mellitus and hypertension. The sequencing of the CKD code in relationship to codes for other contributing conditions is based on the conventions in the Tabular List.

See I.C.9. Hypertensive chronic kidney disease.
See I.C.19. Chronic kidney disease and kidney transplant complications.

15. **Chapter 15: Pregnancy, Childbirth, and the Puerperium (O00-O9A)**

a. **General Rules for Obstetric Cases**

1) **Codes from chapter 15 and sequencing priority**

Obstetric cases require codes from chapter 15, codes in the range O00-O9A, Pregnancy, Childbirth, and the Puerperium. Chapter 15 codes have sequencing priority over codes from other chapters. Additional codes from other chapters may be used in conjunction with chapter 15 codes to further specify conditions. Should the provider document that the pregnancy is incidental to the encounter, then code Z33.1, Pregnant state, incidental, should be used in place of any chapter 15 codes. It is the provider's responsibility to state that the condition being treated is not affecting the pregnancy.

2) **Chapter 15 codes used only on the maternal record**

Chapter 15 codes are to be used only on the maternal record, never on the record of the newborn.

3) **Final character for trimester**

The majority of codes in Chapter 15 have a final character indicating the trimester of pregnancy. The timeframes for the trimesters are indicated at the beginning of the chapter. If trimester is not a component of a code, it is because the condition always occurs in a specific trimester, or the concept of trimester of pregnancy is not applicable. Certain codes have characters for only certain trimesters because the condition does not occur in all trimesters, but it may occur in more than just one.

Assignment of the final character for trimester should be based on the provider's documentation of the trimester (or number of weeks) for the current admission/encounter. This applies to the assignment of trimester for pre-existing conditions as well as those that develop during or are due to the pregnancy. The provider's documentation of the number of weeks may be used to assign the appropriate code identifying the trimester.

Whenever delivery occurs during the current admission, and there is an "in childbirth" option for the obstetric complication being coded, the "in childbirth" code should be assigned.

4) **Selection of trimester for inpatient admissions that encompass more than one trimester**

In instances when a patient is admitted to a hospital for complications of pregnancy during one trimester and remains in the hospital into a subsequent trimester, the trimester character for the antepartum complication code should be assigned on the basis of the trimester when the complication developed, not the trimester of the discharge. If the condition developed prior to the current admission/encounter or represents a pre-existing condition, the trimester character for the trimester at the time of the admission/encounter should be assigned.

5) **Unspecified trimester**

Each category that includes codes for trimester has a code for "unspecified trimester." The "unspecified trimester" code should rarely be used, such as when the documentation in the record is insufficient to determine the trimester and it is not possible to obtain clarification.

6) **7th character for Fetus Identification**

Where applicable, a 7th character is to be assigned for certain categories (O31, O32, O33.3 - O33.6, O35, O36, O40, O41, O60.1, O60.2, O64, and O69) to identify the fetus for which the complication code applies.

Assign 7th character "0":

- For single gestations

- When the documentation in the record is insufficient to determine the fetus affected and it is not possible to obtain clarification.

- When it is not possible to clinically determine which fetus is affected.

b. Selection of OB Principal or First-listed Diagnosis

1) Routine outpatient prenatal visits

For routine outpatient prenatal visits when no complications are present, a code from category Z34, Encounter for supervision of normal pregnancy, should be used as the first-listed diagnosis. These codes should not be used in conjunction with chapter 15 codes.

2) *Supervision of High-Risk Pregnancy*

Codes from category O09, Supervision of high-risk pregnancy, are intended for use only during the prenatal period. For complications during the labor or delivery episode as a result of a high-risk pregnancy, assign the applicable complication codes from Chapter 15. If there are no complications during the labor or delivery episode, assign code O80, Encounter for full-term uncomplicated delivery.

For routine prenatal outpatient visits for patients with high-risk pregnancies, a code from category O09, Supervision of high-risk pregnancy, should be used as the first-listed diagnosis. Secondary chapter 15 codes may be used in conjunction with these codes if appropriate.

3) Episodes when no delivery occurs

In episodes when no delivery occurs, the principal diagnosis should correspond to the principal complication of the pregnancy which necessitated the encounter. Should more than one complication exist, all of which are treated or monitored, any of the complications codes may be sequenced first.

4) When a delivery occurs

When an obstetric patient is admitted and delivers during that admission, the condition that prompted the admission should be sequenced as the principal diagnosis. If multiple conditions prompted the admission, sequence the one most related to the delivery as the principal diagnosis. A code for any complication of the delivery should be assigned as an additional diagnosis. In cases of cesarean delivery, if the patient was admitted with a condition that resulted in the performance of a cesarean procedure, that condition should be selected as the principal diagnosis. If the reason for the admission was unrelated to the condition resulting in the cesarean delivery, the condition related to the reason for the admission should be selected as the principal diagnosis.

5) Outcome of delivery

A code from category Z37, Outcome of delivery, should be included on every maternal record when a delivery has occurred. These codes are not to be used on subsequent records or on the newborn record.

c. Pre-existing conditions versus conditions due to the pregnancy

Certain categories in Chapter 15 distinguish between conditions of the mother that existed prior to pregnancy (pre-existing) and those that are a direct result of pregnancy. When assigning codes from Chapter 15, it is important to assess if a condition was pre-existing prior to pregnancy or developed during or due to the pregnancy in order to assign the correct code.

Categories that do not distinguish between pre-existing and pregnancy-related conditions may be used for either. It is acceptable to use codes specifically for the puerperium with codes complicating pregnancy and childbirth if a condition arises postpartum during the delivery encounter.

d. Pre-existing hypertension in pregnancy

Category O10, Pre-existing hypertension complicating pregnancy, childbirth and the puerperium, includes codes for hypertensive heart and hypertensive chronic kidney disease. When assigning one of the O10 codes that includes hypertensive heart disease or hypertensive chronic kidney disease, it is necessary to add a secondary code from the appropriate hypertension category to specify the type of heart failure or chronic kidney disease.

See Section I.C.9. Hypertension.

e.   **Fetal Conditions Affecting the Management of the Mother**

1)   **Codes from categories O35 and O36**

Codes from categories O35, Maternal care for known or suspected fetal abnormality and damage, and O36, Maternal care for other fetal problems, are assigned only when the fetal condition is actually responsible for modifying the management of the mother, i.e., by requiring diagnostic studies, additional observation, special care, or termination of pregnancy. The fact that the fetal condition exists does not justify assigning a code from this series to the mother's record.

2)   **In utero surgery**

In cases when surgery is performed on the fetus, a diagnosis code from category O35, Maternal care for known or suspected fetal abnormality and damage, should be assigned identifying the fetal condition. Assign the appropriate procedure code for the procedure performed.

No code from Chapter 16, the perinatal codes, should be used on the mother's record to identify fetal conditions. Surgery performed in utero on a fetus is still to be coded as an obstetric encounter.

f.   **HIV Infection in Pregnancy, Childbirth and the Puerperium**

During pregnancy, childbirth or the puerperium, a patient admitted because of an HIV-related illness should receive a principal diagnosis from subcategory O98.7-, Human immunodeficiency [HIV] disease complicating pregnancy, childbirth and the puerperium, followed by the code(s) for the HIV-related illness(es).

Patients with asymptomatic HIV infection status admitted during pregnancy, childbirth, or the puerperium should receive codes of O98.7- and Z21, Asymptomatic human immunodeficiency virus [HIV] infection status.

g.   **Diabetes mellitus in pregnancy**

Diabetes mellitus is a significant complicating factor in pregnancy. Pregnant women who are diabetic should be assigned a code from category O24, Diabetes mellitus in pregnancy, childbirth, and the puerperium, first, followed by the appropriate diabetes code(s) (E08-E13) from Chapter 4.

h.   **Long term use of insulin and oral hypoglycemics**

Code Z79.4, Long-term (current) use of insulin, or code Z79.84, Long-term (current) use of oral hypoglycemic drugs, should also be assigned if the diabetes mellitus is being treated with insulin or oral medications. If the patient is treated with both oral medications and insulin, only the code for insulin-controlled should be assigned.

i.   **Gestational (pregnancy induced) diabetes**

Gestational (pregnancy induced) diabetes can occur during the second and third trimester of pregnancy in women who were not diabetic prior to pregnancy. Gestational diabetes can cause complications in the pregnancy similar to those of pre-existing diabetes mellitus. It also puts the woman at greater risk of

developing diabetes after the pregnancy. Codes for gestational diabetes are in subcategory O24.4, Gestational diabetes mellitus. No other code from category O24, Diabetes mellitus in pregnancy, childbirth, and the puerperium, should be used with a code from O24.4.

The codes under subcategory O24.4 include diet controlled, insulin controlled, and controlled by oral hypoglycemic drugs. If a patient with gestational diabetes is treated with both diet and insulin, only the code for insulin-controlled is required. If a patient with gestational diabetes is treated with both diet and oral hypoglycemic medications, only the code for "controlled by oral hypoglycemic drugs" is required. Code Z79.4, Long-term (current) use of insulin or code Z79.84, Long-term (current) use of oral hypoglycemic drugs, should not be assigned with codes from subcategory O24.4.

An abnormal glucose tolerance in pregnancy is assigned a code from subcategory O99.81, Abnormal glucose complicating pregnancy, childbirth, and the puerperium.

j. Sepsis and septic shock complicating abortion, pregnancy, childbirth and the puerperium

When assigning a chapter 15 code for sepsis complicating abortion, pregnancy, childbirth, and the puerperium, a code for the specific type of infection should be assigned as an additional diagnosis. If severe sepsis is present, a code from subcategory R65.2, Severe sepsis, and code(s) for associated organ dysfunction(s) should also be assigned as additional diagnoses.

k. Puerperal sepsis

Code O85, Puerperal sepsis, should be assigned with a secondary code to identify the causal organism (e.g., for a bacterial infection, assign a code from category B95-B96, Bacterial infections in conditions classified elsewhere). A code from category A40, Streptococcal sepsis, or A41, Other sepsis, should not be used for puerperal sepsis. If applicable, use additional codes to identify severe sepsis (R65.2-) and any associated acute organ dysfunction.

l. Alcohol and tobacco use during pregnancy, childbirth and the puerperium

1) Alcohol use during pregnancy, childbirth and the puerperium

Codes under subcategory O99.31, Alcohol use complicating pregnancy, childbirth, and the puerperium, should be assigned for any pregnancy case when a mother uses alcohol during the pregnancy or postpartum. A secondary code from category F10, Alcohol related disorders, should also be assigned to identify manifestations of the alcohol use.

2) Tobacco use during pregnancy, childbirth and the puerperium

Codes under subcategory O99.33, Smoking (tobacco) complicating pregnancy, childbirth, and the puerperium, should be assigned for any pregnancy case when a mother uses any type of tobacco product during the pregnancy or postpartum. A secondary code from category F17, Nicotine dependence, should also be assigned to identify the type of nicotine dependence.

m. Poisoning, toxic effects, adverse effects and underdosing in a pregnant patient

A code from subcategory O9A.2, Injury, poisoning and certain other consequences of external causes complicating pregnancy, childbirth, and the puerperium, should be sequenced first, followed by the appropriate injury, poisoning, toxic effect, adverse effect or underdosing code, and then the additional code(s) that specifies the condition caused by the poisoning, toxic effect, adverse effect or underdosing.

See Section I.C.19. Adverse effects, poisoning, underdosing and toxic effects.

n. Normal Delivery, Code O80

1) Encounter for full term uncomplicated delivery

Code O80 should be assigned when a woman is admitted for a full-term normal delivery and delivers a single, healthy infant without any complications antepartum, during the delivery, or postpartum during the delivery episode. Code O80 is always a principal diagnosis. It is not to be used if any other code from chapter 15 is needed to describe a current complication of the antenatal, delivery, or perinatal period. Additional codes from other chapters may be used with code O80 if they are not related to or are in any way complicating the pregnancy.

2) **Uncomplicated delivery with resolved antepartum complication**

Code O80 may be used if the patient had a complication at some point during the pregnancy, but the complication is not present at the time of the admission for delivery.

3) **Outcome of delivery for O80**

Z37.0, Single live birth, is the only outcome of delivery code appropriate for use with O80.

o. **The Peripartum and Postpartum Periods**

1) **Peripartum and Postpartum periods**

The postpartum period begins immediately after delivery and continues for six weeks following delivery. The peripartum period is defined as the last month of pregnancy to five months postpartum.

2) **Peripartum and postpartum complication**

A postpartum complication is any complication occurring within the six-week period.

3) **Pregnancy-related complications after 6 week period**

Chapter 15 codes may also be used to describe pregnancy-related complications after the peripartum or postpartum period if the provider documents that a condition is pregnancy related.

4) **Admission for routine postpartum care following delivery outside hospital**

When the mother delivers outside the hospital prior to admission and is admitted for routine postpartum care and no complications are noted, code Z39.0, Encounter for care and examination of mother immediately after delivery, should be assigned as the principal diagnosis.

5) **Pregnancy associated cardiomyopathy**

Pregnancy associated cardiomyopathy, code O90.3, is unique in that it may be diagnosed in the third trimester of pregnancy but may continue to progress months after delivery. For this reason, it is referred to as peripartum cardiomyopathy. Code O90.3 is only for use when the cardiomyopathy develops as a result of pregnancy in a woman who did not have pre-existing heart disease.

p. **Code O94, Sequelae of complication of pregnancy, childbirth, and the puerperium**

1) **Code O94**

Code O94, Sequelae of complication of pregnancy, childbirth, and the puerperium, is for use in those cases when an initial complication of a pregnancy develops a sequelae requiring care or treatment at a future date.

2) **After the initial postpartum period**

This code may be used at any time after the initial postpartum period.

3) **Sequencing of Code O94**

This code, like all sequela codes, is to be sequenced following the code describing the sequelae of the complication.

q. *Termination of Pregnancy and Spontaneous abortions*

1) **Abortion with Liveborn Fetus**

When an attempted termination of pregnancy results in a liveborn fetus, assign code Z33.2, Encounter for elective termination of pregnancy and a code from category Z37, Outcome of Delivery.

2) **Retained Products of Conception following an abortion**

Subsequent encounters for retained products of conception following a spontaneous abortion or elective termination of pregnancy are assigned the appropriate code from category O03, Spontaneous abortion, or codes O07.4, Failed attempted termination of pregnancy without complication and Z33.2, Encounter for elective termination of pregnancy. This advice is appropriate even when the patient was discharged previously with a discharge diagnosis of complete abortion.

3) **Complications leading to abortion**

Codes from Chapter 15 may be used as additional codes to identify any documented complications of the pregnancy in conjunction with codes in categories in O07 and O08.

r. **Abuse in a pregnant patient**

For suspected or confirmed cases of abuse of a pregnant patient, a code(s) from subcategories O9A.3, Physical abuse complicating pregnancy, childbirth, and the puerperium, O9A.4, Sexual abuse complicating pregnancy, childbirth, and the puerperium, and O9A.5, Psychological abuse complicating pregnancy, childbirth, and the puerperium, should be sequenced first, followed by the appropriate codes (if applicable) to identify any associated current injury due to physical abuse, sexual abuse, and the perpetrator of abuse.

See Section I.C.19. Adult and child abuse, neglect and other maltreatment.

16. **Chapter 16: Certain Conditions Originating in the Perinatal Period (P00-P96)**

For coding and reporting purposes the perinatal period is defined as before birth through the 28th day following birth. The following guidelines are provided for reporting purposes.

a. **General Perinatal Rules**

1) **Use of Chapter 16 Codes**

Codes in this chapter are never for use on the maternal record. Codes from Chapter 15, the obstetric chapter, are never permitted on the newborn record. Chapter 16 codes may be used throughout the life of the patient if the condition is still present.

2) **Principal Diagnosis for Birth Record**

When coding the birth episode in a newborn record, assign a code from category Z38, Liveborn infants according to place of birth and type of delivery, as the principal diagnosis. A code from category Z38 is assigned only once, to a newborn at the time of birth. If a newborn is transferred to another institution, a code from category Z38 should not be used at the receiving hospital.

A code from category Z38 is used only on the newborn record, not on the mother's record.

3) Use of Codes from other Chapters with Codes from Chapter 16

Codes from other chapters may be used with codes from chapter 16 if the codes from the other chapters provide more specific detail. Codes for signs and symptoms may be assigned when a definitive diagnosis has not been established. If the reason for the encounter is a perinatal condition, the code from chapter 16 should be sequenced first.

4) Use of Chapter 16 Codes after the Perinatal Period

Should a condition originate in the perinatal period, and continue throughout the life of the patient, the perinatal code should continue to be used regardless of the patient's age.

5) Birth process or community acquired conditions

If a newborn has a condition that may be either due to the birth process or community acquired and the documentation does not indicate which it is, the default is due to the birth process and the code from Chapter 16 should be used. If the condition is community-acquired, a code from Chapter 16 should not be assigned.

6) Code all clinically significant conditions

All clinically significant conditions noted on routine newborn examination should be coded. A condition is clinically significant if it requires:

§ clinical evaluation; or

§ therapeutic treatment; or

§ diagnostic procedures; or

§ extended length of hospital stay; or

§ increased nursing care and/or monitoring; or

§ has implications for future health care needs

Note: The perinatal guidelines listed above are the same as the general coding guidelines for "additional diagnoses", except for the final point regarding implications for future health care needs. Codes should be assigned for conditions that have been specified by the provider as having implications for future health care needs.

b. Observation and Evaluation of Newborns for Suspected Conditions not Found

1) Assign a code from category Z05, Observation and evaluation of newborns and infants for suspected conditions ruled out, to identify those instances when a healthy newborn is evaluated for a suspected condition that is determined after study not to be present. Do not use a code from category Z05 when the patient has identified signs or symptoms of a suspected problem; in such cases code the sign or symptom.

2) A code from category Z05 may also be assigned as a principal or first-listed code for readmissions or encounters when the code from category Z38 code no longer applies. Codes from category Z05 are for use only for healthy newborns and infants for which no condition after study is found to be present.

3) Z05 on a birth record

A code from category Z05 is to be used as a secondary code after the code from category Z38, liveborn infants according to place of birth and type of delivery.

c. **Coding Additional Perinatal Diagnoses**

1) **Assigning codes for conditions that require treatment**

Assign codes for conditions that require treatment or further investigation, prolong the length of stay, or require resource utilization.

2) **Codes for conditions specified as having implications for future health care needs**

Assign codes for conditions that have been specified by the provider as having implications for future health care needs.

Note: This guideline should not be used for adult patients.

d. **Prematurity and Fetal Growth Retardation**

Providers utilize different criteria in determining prematurity. A code for prematurity should not be assigned unless it is documented. Assignment of codes in categories P05, Disorders of newborn related to slow fetal growth and fetal malnutrition, and P07, Disorders of newborn related to short gestation and low birth weight, not elsewhere classified, should be based on the recorded birth weight and estimated gestational age. Codes from category P05 should not be assigned with codes from category P07.

When both birth weight and gestational age are available, two codes from category P07 should be assigned, with the code for birth weight sequenced before the code for gestational age.

e. **Low birth weight and immaturity status**

Codes from category P07, Disorders of newborn related to short gestation and low birth weight, not elsewhere classified, are for use for a child or adult who was premature or had a low birth weight as a newborn and this is affecting the patient's current health status.

See Section I.C.21. Factors influencing health status and contact with health services, Status.

f. **Bacterial Sepsis of Newborn**

Category P36, Bacterial sepsis of newborn, includes congenital sepsis. If a perinate is documented as having sepsis without documentation of congenital or community acquired, the default is congenital and a code from category P36 should be assigned. If the P36 code includes the causal organism, an additional code from category B95, Streptococcus, Staphylococcus, and Enterococcus as the cause of diseases classified elsewhere, or B96, Other bacterial agents as the cause of diseases classified elsewhere, should not be assigned. If the P36 code does not include the causal organism, assign an additional code from category B96. If applicable, use additional codes to identify severe sepsis (R65.2-) and any associated acute organ dysfunction.

g. **Stillbirth**

Code P95, Stillbirth, is only for use in institutions that maintain separate records for stillbirths. No other code should be used with P95. Code P95 should not be used on the mother's record.

17. **Chapter 17: Congenital malformations, deformations, and chromosomal abnormalities (Q00-Q99)**

Assign an appropriate code(s) from categories Q00-Q99, Congenital malformations, deformations, and chromosomal abnormalities when a malformation/deformation or chromosomal abnormality is documented. A malformation/deformation/or chromosomal abnormality may be the principal/first-listed diagnosis on a record or a secondary diagnosis.

When a malformation/deformation or chromosomal abnormality does not have a unique code assignment, assign additional code(s) for any manifestations that may be present.

When the code assignment specifically identifies the malformation/deformation or chromosomal abnormality, manifestations that are an inherent component of the anomaly should not be coded separately. Additional codes should be assigned for manifestations that are not an inherent component.

Codes from Chapter 17 may be used throughout the life of the patient. If a congenital malformation or deformity has been corrected, a personal history code should be used to identify the history of the malformation or deformity. Although present at birth, malformation/deformation/or chromosomal abnormality may not be identified until later in life. Whenever the condition is diagnosed by the physician, it is appropriate to assign a code from codes Q00-Q99.For the birth admission, the appropriate code from category Z38, Liveborn infants, according to place of birth and type of delivery, should be sequenced as the principal diagnosis, followed by any congenital anomaly codes, Q00-Q99.

18. **Chapter 18: Symptoms, signs, and abnormal clinical and laboratory findings, not elsewhere classified (R00-R99)**

   Chapter 18 includes symptoms, signs, abnormal results of clinical or other investigative procedures, and ill-defined conditions regarding which no diagnosis classifiable elsewhere is recorded. Signs and symptoms that point to a specific diagnosis have been assigned to a category in other chapters of the classification.

   a. **Use of symptom codes**

   Codes that describe symptoms and signs are acceptable for reporting purposes when a related definitive diagnosis has not been established (confirmed) by the provider.

   b. **Use of a symptom code with a definitive diagnosis code**

   Codes for signs and symptoms may be reported in addition to a related definitive diagnosis when the sign or symptom is not routinely associated with that diagnosis, such as the various signs and symptoms associated with complex syndromes. The definitive diagnosis code should be sequenced before the symptom code.

   Signs or symptoms that are associated routinely with a disease process should not be assigned as additional codes, unless otherwise instructed by the classification.

   c. **Combination codes that include symptoms**

   ICD-10-CM contains a number of combination codes that identify both the definitive diagnosis and common symptoms of that diagnosis. When using one of these combination codes, an additional code should not be assigned for the symptom.

   d. **Repeated falls**

   Code R29.6, Repeated falls, is for use for encounters when a patient has recently fallen and the reason for the fall is being investigated.

   Code Z91.81, History of falling, is for use when a patient has fallen in the past and is at risk for future falls. When appropriate, both codes R29.6 and Z91.81 may be assigned together.

   e. **Coma scale**

   The coma scale codes (R40.2-) can be used in conjunction with traumatic brain injury codes, acute cerebrovascular disease or sequelae of cerebrovascular disease codes. These codes are primarily for use by trauma registries, but they may be used in any setting where this information is collected. The coma scale

may also be used to assess the status of the central nervous system for other non-trauma conditions, such as monitoring patients in the intensive care unit regardless of medical condition. The coma scale codes should be sequenced after the diagnosis code(s).

These codes, one from each subcategory, are needed to complete the scale. The 7th character indicates when the scale was recorded. The 7th character should match for all three codes.

At a minimum, report the initial score documented on presentation at your facility. This may be a score from the emergency medicine technician (EMT) or in the emergency department. If desired, a facility may choose to capture multiple coma scale scores.

Assign code R40.24, Glasgow coma scale, total score, when only the total score is documented in the medical record and not the individual score(s).

f. Functional quadriplegia

Functional quadriplegia (code R53.2) is the lack of ability to use one's limbs or to ambulate due to extreme debility. It is not associated with neurologic deficit or injury, and code R53.2 should not be used for cases of neurologic quadriplegia. It should only be assigned if functional quadriplegia is specifically documented in the medical record.

g. SIRS due to Non-Infectious Process

The systemic inflammatory response syndrome (SIRS) can develop as a result of certain non-infectious disease processes, such as trauma, malignant neoplasm, or pancreatitis. When SIRS is documented with a noninfectious condition, and no subsequent infection is documented, the code for the underlying condition, such as an injury, should be assigned, followed by code R65.10, Systemic inflammatory response syndrome (SIRS) of non-infectious origin without acute organ dysfunction, or code R65.11, Systemic inflammatory response syndrome (SIRS) of non-infectious origin with acute organ dysfunction. If an associated acute organ dysfunction is documented, the appropriate code(s) for the specific type of organ dysfunction(s) should be assigned in addition to code R65.11. If acute organ dysfunction is documented, but it cannot be determined if the acute organ dysfunction is associated with SIRS or due to another condition (e.g., directly due to the trauma), the provider should be queried.

h. Death NOS

Code R99, Ill-defined and unknown cause of mortality, is only for use in the very limited circumstance when a patient who has already died is brought into an emergency department or other healthcare facility and is pronounced dead upon arrival. It does not represent the discharge disposition of death.

i. NIHSS Stroke Scale

The NIH stroke scale (NIHSS) codes (R29.7- -) can be used in conjunction with acute stroke codes (I63) to identify the patient's neurological status and the severity of the stroke. The stroke scale codes should be sequenced after the acute stroke diagnosis code(s).

At a minimum, report the initial score documented. If desired, a facility may choose to capture multiple stroke scale scores.

See Section I.B.14.for information concerning the medical record documentation that may be used for assignment of the NIHSS codes.

19. Chapter 19: Injury, poisoning, and certain other consequences of external causes (S00-T88)

a. Application of 7th Characters in Chapter 19

Most categories in chapter 19 have a 7th character requirement for each applicable code. Most categories in this chapter have three 7th character values (with the exception of fractures): A, initial encounter, D, subsequent encounter and S, sequela. Categories for traumatic fractures have additional 7th character values. While the patient may be seen by a new or different provider over the course of treatment for an injury, assignment of the 7th character is based on whether the patient is undergoing active treatment and not whether the provider is seeing the patient for the first time.

For complication codes, active treatment refers to treatment for the condition described by the code, even though it may be related to an earlier precipitating problem. For example, code T84.50XA, Infection and inflammatory reaction due to unspecified internal joint prosthesis, initial encounter, is used when active treatment is provided for the infection, even though the condition relates to the prosthetic device, implant or graft that was placed at a previous encounter.

7th character "A", initial encounter is used for each encounter where the patient is receiving active treatment for the condition.

7th character "D" subsequent encounter is used for encounters after the patient has completed active treatment of the condition and is receiving routine care for the condition during the healing or recovery phase.

The aftercare Z codes should not be used for aftercare for conditions such as injuries or poisonings, where 7th characters are provided to identify subsequent care. For example, for aftercare of an injury, assign the acute injury code with the 7th character "D" (subsequent encounter).

7th character "S", sequela, is for use for complications or conditions that arise as a direct result of a condition, such as scar formation after a burn. The scars are sequelae of the burn. When using 7th character "S", it is necessary to use both the injury code that precipitated the sequela and the code for the sequela itself. The "S" is added only to the injury code, not the sequela code. The 7th character "S" identifies the injury responsible for the sequela. The specific type of sequela (e.g. scar) is sequenced first, followed by the injury code.

See Section I.B.10 Sequelae, (Late Effects)

b. Coding of Injuries

When coding injuries, assign separate codes for each injury unless a combination code is provided, in which case the combination code is assigned. Code T07, Unspecified multiple injuries should not be assigned in the inpatient setting unless information for a more specific code is not available. Traumatic injury codes (S00-T14.9) are not to be used for normal, healing surgical wounds or to identify complications of surgical wounds.

The code for the most serious injury, as determined by the provider and the focus of treatment, is sequenced first.

1) Superficial injuries

Superficial injuries such as abrasions or contusions are not coded when associated with more severe injuries of the same site.

2) Primary injury with damage to nerves/blood vessels

When a primary injury results in minor damage to peripheral nerves or blood vessels, the primary injury is sequenced first with additional code(s) for injuries to nerves and spinal cord (such as category S04), and/or injury to blood vessels (such as category S15). When the primary injury is to the blood vessels or nerves, that injury should be sequenced first.

c. Coding of Traumatic Fractures

The principles of multiple coding of injuries should be followed in coding fractures. Fractures of specified sites are coded individually by site in accordance with both the provisions within categories S02, S12, S22, S32, S42, S49, S52, S59, S62, S72, S79, S82, S89, S92 and the level of detail furnished by medical record content.

A fracture not indicated as open or closed should be coded to closed. A fracture not indicated whether displaced or not displaced should be coded to displaced.

More specific guidelines are as follows:

1) Initial vs. Subsequent Encounter for Fractures

Traumatic fractures are coded using the appropriate 7th character for initial encounter (A, B, C) for each encounter where the patient is receiving active treatment for the fracture. The appropriate 7th character for initial encounter should also be assigned for a patient who delayed seeking treatment for the fracture or nonunion.

Fractures are coded using the appropriate 7th character for subsequent care for encounters after the patient has completed active treatment of the fracture and is receiving routine care for the fracture during the healing or recovery phase.

Care for complications of surgical treatment for fracture repairs during the healing or recovery phase should be coded with the appropriate complication codes.

Care of complications of fractures, such as malunion and nonunion, should be reported with the appropriate 7th character for subsequent care with nonunion (K, M, N,) or subsequent care with malunion (P, Q, R).

Malunion/nonunion: The appropriate 7th character for initial encounter should also be assigned for a patient who delayed seeking treatment for the fracture or nonunion.

The open fracture designations in the assignment of the 7th character for fractures of the forearm, femur and lower leg, including ankle are based on the Gustilo open fracture classification. When the Gustilo classification type is not specified for an open fracture, the 7th character for open fracture type I or II should be assigned (B, E, H, M, Q).

A code from category M80, not a traumatic fracture code, should be used for any patient with known osteoporosis who suffers a fracture, even if the patient had a minor fall or trauma, if that fall or trauma would not usually break a normal, healthy bone.

See Section I.C.13. Osteoporosis.

The aftercare Z codes should not be used for aftercare for traumatic fractures. For aftercare of a traumatic fracture, assign the acute fracture code with the appropriate 7th character.

2) Multiple fractures sequencing

Multiple fractures are sequenced in accordance with the severity of the fracture.

d. Coding of Burns and Corrosions

The ICD-10-CM makes a distinction between burns and corrosions. The burn codes are for thermal burns, except sunburns, that come from a heat source, such as a fire or hot appliance. The burn codes are also for burns resulting from electricity and radiation. Corrosions are burns due to chemicals. The guidelines are the same for burns and corrosions.

Current burns (T20-T25) are classified by depth, extent and by agent (X code). Burns are classified by depth as first degree (erythema), second degree (blistering), and third degree (full-thickness involvement). Burns of the eye and internal organs (T26-T28) are classified by site, but not by degree.

1) **Sequencing of burn and related condition codes**

Sequence first the code that reflects the highest degree of burn when more than one burn is present.

a. When the reason for the admission or encounter is for treatment of external multiple burns, sequence first the code that reflects the burn of the highest degree.

b. When a patient has both internal and external burns, the circumstances of admission govern the selection of the principal diagnosis or first-listed diagnosis.

c. When a patient is admitted for burn injuries and other related conditions such as smoke inhalation and/or respiratory failure, the circumstances of admission govern the selection of the principal or first-listed diagnosis.

2) **Burns of the same local site**

Classify burns of the same local site (three-character category level, T20-T28) but of different degrees to the subcategory identifying the highest degree recorded in the diagnosis.

3) **Non-healing burns**

Non-healing burns are coded as acute burns.

Necrosis of burned skin should be coded as a non-healed burn.

4) **Infected Burn**

For any documented infected burn site, use an additional code for the infection.

5) **Assign separate codes for each burn site**

When coding burns, assign separate codes for each burn site. Category T30, Burn and corrosion, body region unspecified is extremely vague and should rarely be used.

6) **Burns and Corrosions Classified According to Extent of Body Surface Involved**

Assign codes from category T31, Burns classified according to extent of body surface involved, or T32, Corrosions classified according to extent of body surface involved, when the site of the burn is not specified or when there is a need for additional data. It is advisable to use category T31 as additional coding when needed to provide data for evaluating burn mortality, such as that needed by burn units. It is also advisable to use category T31 as an additional code for reporting purposes when there is mention of a third-degree burn involving 20 percent or more of the body surface.

Categories T31 and T32 are based on the classic "rule of nines" in estimating body surface involved: head and neck are assigned nine percent, each arm nine percent, each leg 18 percent, the anterior trunk 18 percent, posterior trunk 18 percent, and genitalia one percent. Providers may change these percentage assignments where necessary to accommodate infants and children who have proportionately larger heads than adults, and patients who have large buttocks, thighs, or abdomen that involve burns.

7) **Encounters for treatment of sequela of burns**

Encounters for the treatment of the late effects of burns or corrosions (i.e., scars or joint contractures) should be coded with a burn or corrosion code with the 7th character "S" for sequela.

8) **Sequelae with a late effect code and current burn**

When appropriate, both a code for a current burn or corrosion with 7th character "A" or "D" and a burn or corrosion code with 7th character "S" may be assigned on the same record (when both a current burn and sequelae of an old burn exist). Burns and corrosions do not heal at the same rate and a current healing wound may still exist with sequela of a healed burn or corrosion.

See Section I.B.10 Sequela (Late Effects)

9) **Use of an external cause code with burns and corrosions**

An external cause code should be used with burns and corrosions to identify the source and intent of the burn, as well as the place where it occurred.

e. **Adverse Effects, Poisoning, Underdosing and Toxic Effects**

Codes in categories T36-T65 are combination codes that include the substance that was taken as well as the intent. No additional external cause code is required for poisonings, toxic effects, adverse effects and underdosing codes.

1) **Do not code directly from the Table of Drugs**

Do not code directly from the Table of Drugs and Chemicals. Always refer back to the Tabular List.

2) **Use as many codes as necessary to describe**

Use as many codes as necessary to describe completely all drugs, medicinal or biological substances.

3) **If the same code would describe the causative agent**

If the same code would describe the causative agent for more than one adverse reaction, poisoning, toxic effect or underdosing, assign the code only once.

4) **If two or more drugs, medicinal or biological substances**

If two or more drugs, medicinal or biological substances are reported, code each individually unless a combination code is listed in the Table of Drugs and Chemicals.

5) **The occurrence of drug toxicity is classified in ICD-10-CM as follows:**

(a) **Adverse Effect**

When coding an adverse effect of a drug that has been correctly prescribed and properly administered, assign the appropriate code for the nature of the adverse effect followed by the appropriate code for the adverse effect of the drug (T36-T50). The code for the drug should have a 5th or 6th character "5" (for example T36.0X5-) Examples of the nature of an adverse effect are tachycardia, delirium, gastrointestinal hemorrhaging, vomiting, hypokalemia, hepatitis, renal failure, or respiratory failure.

(b) **Poisoning**

When coding a poisoning or reaction to the improper use of a medication (e.g., overdose, wrong substance given or taken in error, wrong route of administration), first assign the appropriate code from categories T36-T50. The poisoning codes have an associated intent as their 5th or 6th

character (accidental, intentional self-harm, assault and undetermined. If the intent of the poisoning is unknown or unspecified, code the intent as accidental intent. The undetermined intent is only for use if the documentation in the record specifies that the intent cannot be determined. Use additional code(s) for all manifestations of poisonings.

If there is also a diagnosis of abuse or dependence of the substance, the abuse or dependence is assigned as an additional code.

Examples of poisoning include:

(i) Error was made in drug prescription Errors made in drug prescription or in the administration of the drug by provider, nurse, patient, or other person.

(ii) Overdose of a drug intentionally taken

If an overdose of a drug was intentionally taken or administered and resulted in drug toxicity, it would be coded as a poisoning.

(iii) Nonprescribed drug taken with correctly prescribed and properly administered drug

If a nonprescribed drug or medicinal agent was taken in combination with a correctly prescribed and properly administered drug, any drug toxicity or other reaction resulting from the interaction of the two drugs would be classified as a poisoning.

(iv) Interaction of drug(s) and alcohol

When a reaction results from the interaction of a drug(s) and alcohol, this would be classified as poisoning.

See Section I.C.4. if poisoning is the result of insulin pump malfunctions.

(c) **Underdosing**

Underdosing refers to taking less of a medication than is prescribed by a provider or a manufacturer's instruction. For underdosing, assign the code from categories T36-T50 (fifth or sixth character "6").

Codes for underdosing should never be assigned as principal or first-listed codes. If a patient has a relapse or exacerbation of the medical condition for which the drug is prescribed because of the reduction in dose, then the medical condition itself should be coded.

Noncompliance (Z91.12-, Z91.13-) or complication of care (Y63.6-Y63.9) codes are to be used with an underdosing code to indicate intent, if known.

(d) **Toxic Effects**

When a harmful substance is ingested or comes in contact with a person, this is classified as a toxic effect. The toxic effect codes are in categories T51-T65.

Toxic effect codes have an associated intent: accidental, intentional self-harm, assault and undetermined.

f. **Adult and child abuse, neglect and other maltreatment**

Sequence first the appropriate code from categories T74.- (Adult and child abuse, neglect and other maltreatment, confirmed) or T76.-(Adult and child abuse, neglect and other maltreatment, suspected) for abuse, neglect and other maltreatment, followed by any accompanying mental health or injury code(s).

If the documentation in the medical record states abuse or neglect it is coded as confirmed (T74.-). It is coded as suspected if it is documented as suspected (T76.-).

For cases of confirmed abuse or neglect an external cause code from the assault section (X92-Y09) should be added to identify the cause of any physical injuries. A perpetrator code (Y07) should be added when the perpetrator of the abuse is known. For suspected cases of abuse or neglect, do not report external cause or perpetrator code.

If a suspected case of abuse, neglect or mistreatment is ruled out during an encounter code Z04.71, Encounter for examination and observation following alleged physical adult abuse, ruled out, or code Z04.72, Encounter for examination and observation following alleged child physical abuse, ruled out, should be used, not a code from T76.

If a suspected case of alleged rape or sexual abuse is ruled out during an encounter code Z04.41, Encounter for examination and observation following alleged adult rape or code Z04.42, Encounter for examination and observation following alleged child rape, should be used, not a code from T76.

See Section I.C.15. Abuse in a pregnant patient.

g. **Complications of care**

1) **General guidelines for complications of care**

(a) **Documentation of complications of care**

See Section I.B.16. for information on documentation of complications of care.

2) **Pain due to medical devices**

Pain associated with devices, implants or grafts left in a surgical site (for example painful hip prosthesis) is assigned to the appropriate code(s) found in Chapter 19, Injury, poisoning, and certain other consequences of external causes. Specific codes for pain due to medical devices are found in the T code section of the ICD-10-CM. Use additional code(s) from category G89 to identify acute or chronic pain due to presence of the device, implant or graft (G89.18 or G89.28).

3) **Transplant complications**

(a) **Transplant complications other than kidney**

Codes under category T86, Complications of transplanted organs and tissues, are for use for both complications and rejection of transplanted organs. A transplant complication code is only assigned if the complication affects the function of the transplanted organ. Two codes are required to fully describe a transplant complication: the appropriate code from category T86 and a secondary code that identifies the complication.

Pre-existing conditions or conditions that develop after the transplant are not coded as complications unless they affect the function of the transplanted organs.

See I.C.21. for transplant organ removal status See I.C.2. for malignant neoplasm associated with transplanted organ.

(b) **Kidney transplant complications**

Patients who have undergone kidney transplant may still have some form of chronic kidney disease (CKD) because the kidney transplant may not fully restore kidney function. Code T86.1- should be assigned for documented complications of a kidney transplant, such as transplant failure or rejection or other transplant complication. Code T86.1- should not be assigned for post kidney transplant patients who have chronic kidney (CKD) unless a transplant complication such as transplant failure or rejection is documented. If the documentation is unclear as to whether the patient has a complication of the transplant, query the provider.

Conditions that affect the function of the transplanted kidney, other than CKD, should be assigned a code from subcategory T86.1, Complications of transplanted organ, Kidney, and a secondary code that identifies the complication.

For patients with CKD following a kidney transplant, but who do not have a complication such as failure or rejection, *see section I.C.14. Chronic kidney disease and kidney transplant status.*

4) Complication codes that include the external cause

As with certain other T codes, some of the complications of care codes have the external cause included in the code. The code includes the nature of the complication as well as the type of procedure that caused the complication. No external cause code indicating the type of procedure is necessary for these codes.

5) Complications of care codes within the body system chapters

Intraoperative and postprocedural complication codes are found within the body system chapters with codes specific to the organs and structures of that body system. These codes should be sequenced first, followed by a code(s) for the specific complication, if applicable.

20. Chapter 20: External Causes of Morbidity (V00-Y99)

The external causes of morbidity codes should never be sequenced as the first-listed or principal diagnosis.

External cause codes are intended to provide data for injury research and evaluation of injury prevention strategies. These codes capture how the injury or health condition happened (cause), the intent (unintentional or accidental; or intentional, such as suicide or assault), the place where the event occurred the activity of the patient at the time of the event, and the person's status (e.g., civilian, military).

There is no national requirement for mandatory ICD-10-CM external cause code reporting. Unless a provider is subject to a state-based external cause code reporting mandate or these codes are required by a particular payer, reporting of ICD-10-CM codes in Chapter 20, External Causes of Morbidity, is not required. In the absence of a mandatory reporting requirement, providers are encouraged to voluntarily report external cause codes, as they provide valuable data for injury research and evaluation of injury prevention strategies.

a. General External Cause Coding Guidelines

1) Used with any code in the range of A00.0-T88.9, Z00-Z99

An external cause code may be used with any code in the range of A00.0-T88.9, Z00-Z99, classification that is a health condition due to an external cause. Though they are most applicable to injuries, they are also valid for use with such things as infections or diseases due to an external source, and other health conditions, such as a heart attack that occurs during strenuous physical activity.

2) External cause code used for length of treatment

Assign the external cause code, with the appropriate 7th character (initial encounter, subsequent encounter or sequela) for each encounter for which the injury or condition is being treated.

Most categories in chapter 20 have a 7th character requirement for each applicable code. Most categories in this chapter have three 7th character values: A, initial encounter, D, subsequent encounter and S, sequela. While the patient may be seen by a new or different provider over the course of treatment for an injury or condition, assignment of the 7th character for external cause should match the 7th character of the code assigned for the associated injury or condition for the encounter.

3) Use the full range of external cause codes

Use the full range of external cause codes to completely describe the cause, the intent, the place of occurrence, and if applicable, the activity of the patient at the time of the event, and the patient's status, for all injuries, and other health conditions due to an external cause.

4) Assign as many external cause codes as necessary

Assign as many external cause codes as necessary to fully explain each cause. If only one external code can be recorded, assign the code most related to the principal diagnosis.

5) The selection of the appropriate external cause code

The selection of the appropriate external cause code is guided by the Alphabetic Index of External Causes and by Inclusion and Exclusion notes in the Tabular List.

6) External cause code can never be a principal diagnosis

An external cause code can never be a principal (first-listed) diagnosis.

7) Combination external cause codes

Certain of the external cause codes are combination codes that identify sequential events that result in an injury, such as a fall which results in striking against an object. The injury may be due to either event or both. The combination external cause code used should correspond to the sequence of events regardless of which caused the most serious injury.

8) No external cause code needed in certain circumstances

No external cause code from Chapter 20 is needed if the external cause and intent are included in a code from another chapter (e.g. T36.0X1- Poisoning by penicillins, accidental (unintentional)).

b. Place of Occurrence Guideline

Codes from category Y92, Place of occurrence of the external cause, are secondary codes for use after other external cause codes to identify the location of the patient at the time of injury or other condition.

Generally, a place of occurrence code is assigned only once, at the initial encounter for treatment. However, in the rare instance that a new injury occurs during hospitalization, an additional place of occurrence code may be assigned. No 7th characters are used for Y92.

Do not use place of occurrence code Y92.9 if the place is not stated or is not applicable.

c. Activity Code

Assign a code from category Y93, Activity code, to describe the activity of the patient at the time the injury or other health condition occurred.

An activity code is used only once, at the initial encounter for treatment. Only one code from Y93 should be recorded on a medical record.

The activity codes are not applicable to poisonings, adverse effects, misadventures or sequela.

Do not assign Y93.9, Unspecified activity, if the activity is not stated.

A code from category Y93 is appropriate for use with external cause and intent codes if identifying the activity provides additional information about the event.

d. Place of Occurrence, Activity, and Status Codes Used with other External Cause Code

When applicable, place of occurrence, activity, and external cause status codes are sequenced after the main external cause code(s). Regardless of the number of external cause codes assigned, generally there should be only one place of occurrence code, one activity code, and one external cause status code assigned to an encounter. However, in the rare instance that a new injury occurs during hospitalization, an additional place of occurrence code may be assigned.

e. If the Reporting Format Limits the Number of External Cause Codes

If the reporting format limits the number of external cause codes that can be used in reporting clinical data, report the code for the cause/intent most related to the principal diagnosis. If the format permits capture of additional external cause codes, the cause/intent, including medical misadventures, of the additional events should be reported rather than the codes for place, activity, or external status.

f. Multiple External Cause Coding Guidelines

More than one external cause code is required to fully describe the external cause of an illness or injury. The assignment of external cause codes should be sequenced in the following priority:

If two or more events cause separate injuries, an external cause code should be assigned for each cause. The first-listed external cause code will be selected in the following order:

External codes for child and adult abuse take priority over all other external cause codes.

See Section I.C.19., Child and Adult abuse guidelines.

External cause codes for terrorism events take priority over all other external cause codes except child and adult abuse.

External cause codes for cataclysmic events take priority over all other external cause codes except child and adult abuse and terrorism.

External cause codes for transport accidents take priority over all other external cause codes except cataclysmic events, child and adult abuse and terrorism.

Activity and external cause status codes are assigned following all causal (intent) external cause codes.

The first-listed external cause code should correspond to the cause of the most serious diagnosis due to an assault, accident, or self-harm, following the order of hierarchy listed above.

g. Child and Adult Abuse Guideline

Adult and child abuse, neglect and maltreatment are classified as assault. Any of the assault codes may be used to indicate the external cause of any injury resulting from the confirmed abuse.

For confirmed cases of abuse, neglect and maltreatment, when the perpetrator is known, a code from Y07, Perpetrator of maltreatment and neglect, should accompany any other assault codes.
See Section I.C.19. Adult and child abuse, neglect and other maltreatment

h. Unknown or Undetermined Intent Guideline

If the intent (accident, self-harm, assault) of the cause of an injury or other condition is unknown or unspecified, code the intent as accidental intent. All transport accident categories assume accidental intent.

1) Use of undetermined intent

External cause codes for events of undetermined intent are only for use if the documentation in the record specifies that the intent cannot be determined.

i. Sequelae (Late Effects) of External Cause Guidelines

1) Sequelae external cause codes

Sequela are reported using the external cause code with the 7th character "S" for sequela. These codes should be used with any report of a late effect or sequela resulting from a previous injury.

See Section I.B.10 Sequela (Late Effects)

2) Sequela external cause code with a related current injury

A sequela external cause code should never be used with a related current nature of injury code.

3) Use of sequela external cause codes for subsequent visits

Use a late effect external cause code for subsequent visits when a late effect of the initial injury is being treated. Do not use a late effect external cause code for subsequent visits for follow-up care (e.g., to assess healing, to receive rehabilitative therapy) of the injury when no late effect of the injury has been documented.

j. Terrorism Guidelines

1) Cause of injury identified by the Federal Government (FBI) as terrorism

When the cause of an injury is identified by the Federal Government (FBI) as terrorism, the first-listed external cause code should be a code from category Y38, Terrorism. The definition of terrorism employed by the FBI is found at the inclusion note at the beginning of category Y38. Use additional code for place of occurrence (Y92.-). More than one Y38 code may be assigned if the injury is the result of more than one mechanism of terrorism.

2) Cause of an injury is suspected to be the result of terrorism

When the cause of an injury is suspected to be the result of terrorism a code from category Y38 should not be assigned. Suspected cases should be classified as assault.

3) Code Y38.9, Terrorism, secondary effects

Assign code Y38.9, Terrorism, secondary effects, for conditions occurring subsequent to the terrorist event. This code should not be assigned for conditions that are due to the initial terrorist act.

It is acceptable to assign code Y38.9 with another code from Y38 if there is an injury due to the initial terrorist event and an injury that is a subsequent result of the terrorist event.

k. External cause status

A code from category Y99, External cause status, should be assigned whenever any other external cause code is assigned for an encounter, including an Activity code, except for the events noted below. Assign a

code from category Y99, External cause status, to indicate the work status of the person at the time the event occurred. The status code indicates whether the event occurred during military activity, whether a non-military person was at work, whether an individual including a student or volunteer was involved in a non-work activity at the time of the causal event.

A code from Y99, External cause status, should be assigned, when applicable, with other external cause codes, such as transport accidents and falls. The external cause status codes are not applicable to poisonings, adverse effects, misadventures or late effects.

Do not assign a code from category Y99 if no other external cause codes (cause, activity) are applicable for the encounter.

An external cause status code is used only once, at the initial encounter for treatment. Only one code from Y99 should be recorded on a medical record.

Do not assign code Y99.9, Unspecified external cause status, if the status is not stated.

21. **Chapter 21: Factors influencing health status and contact with health services (Z00-Z99)**

   Note: The chapter specific guidelines provide additional information about the use of Z codes for specified encounters.

   a. **Use of Z codes in any healthcare setting**

   Z codes are for use in any healthcare setting. Z codes may be used as either a first-listed (principal diagnosis code in the inpatient setting) or secondary code, depending on the circumstances of the encounter. Certain Z codes may only be used as first-listed or principal diagnosis.

   b. **Z Codes indicate a reason for an encounter**

   Z codes are not procedure codes. A corresponding procedure code must accompany a Z code to describe any procedure performed.

   c. **Categories of Z Codes**

   1) **Contact/Exposure**

   Category Z20 indicates contact with, and suspected exposure to, communicable diseases. These codes are for patients who do not show any sign or symptom of a disease but are suspected to have been exposed to it by close personal contact with an infected individual or are in an area where a disease is epidemic.

   Category Z77, Other contact with and (suspected) exposures hazardous to health, indicates contact with and suspected exposures hazardous to health.

   Contact/exposure codes may be used as a first-listed code to explain an encounter for testing, or, more commonly, as a secondary code to identify a potential risk.

   2) **Inoculations and vaccinations**

   Code Z23 is for encounters for inoculations and vaccinations. It indicates that a patient is being seen to receive a prophylactic inoculation against a disease. Procedure codes are required to identify the actual administration of the injection and the type(s) of immunizations given. Code Z23 may be used as a secondary code if the inoculation is given as a routine part of preventive health care, such as a well-baby visit.

3) Status

Status codes indicate that a patient is either a carrier of a disease or has the sequelae or residual of a past disease or condition. This includes such things as the presence of prosthetic or mechanical devices resulting from past treatment. A status code is informative, because the status may affect the course of treatment and its outcome. A status code is distinct from a history code. The history code indicates that the patient no longer has the condition.

A status code should not be used with a diagnosis code from one of the body system chapters, if the diagnosis code includes the information provided by the status code. For example, code Z94.1, Heart transplant status, should not be used with a code from subcategory T86.2, Complications of heart transplant. The status code does not provide additional information. The complication code indicates that the patient is a heart transplant patient.

For encounters for weaning from a mechanical ventilator, assign a code from subcategory J96.1, Chronic respiratory failure, followed by code Z99.11, Dependence on respirator [ventilator] status. The status Z codes/categories are: Z14 Genetic carrier

Genetic carrier status indicates that a person carries a gene, associated with a particular disease, which may be passed to offspring who may develop that disease. The person does not have the disease and is not at risk of developing the disease.

Z15   Genetic susceptibility to disease

Genetic susceptibility indicates that a person has a gene that increases the risk of that person developing the disease.

Codes from category Z15 should not be used as principal or first-listed codes. If the patient has the condition to which he/she is susceptible, and that condition is the reason for the encounter, the code for the current condition should be sequenced first. If the patient is being seen for follow-up after completed treatment for this condition, and the condition no longer exists, a follow-up code should be sequenced first, followed by the appropriate personal history and genetic susceptibility codes. If the purpose of the encounter is genetic counseling associated with procreative management, code Z31.5, Encounter for genetic counseling, should be assigned as the first-listed code, followed by a code from category Z15. Additional codes should be assigned for any applicable family or personal history.

Z16   Resistance to antimicrobial drugs

This code indicates that a patient has a condition that is resistant to antimicrobial drug treatment. Sequence the infection code first.

Z17   Estrogen receptor status

Z18   Retained foreign body fragments

Z19   Hormone sensitivity malignancy status

Z21   Asymptomatic HIV infection status

This code indicates that a patient has tested positive for HIV but has manifested no signs or symptoms of the disease.

Z22   Carrier of infectious disease

Carrier status indicates that a person harbors the specific organisms of a disease without manifest symptoms and is capable of transmitting the infection.

Z28.3   Underimmunization status

Z33.1   Pregnant state, incidental

This code is a secondary code only for use when the pregnancy is in no way complicating the reason for visit. Otherwise, a code from the obstetric chapter is required.

Z66   Do not resuscitate

This code may be used when it is documented by the provider that a patient is on do not resuscitate status at any time during the stay.

Z67   Blood type

Z68   Body mass index (BMI)

As with all other secondary diagnosis codes, the BMI codes should only be assigned when they meet the definition of a reportable diagnosis (see Section III, Reporting Additional Diagnoses).

Z74.01   Bed confinement status

Z76.82   Awaiting organ transplant status

Z78   Other specified health status

Code Z78.1, Physical restraint status, may be used when it is documented by the provider that a patient has been put in restraints during the current encounter. Please note that this code should not be reported when it is documented by the provider that a patient is temporarily restrained during a procedure.

Z79   Long-term (current) drug therapy

Codes from this category indicate a patient's continuous use of a prescribed drug (including such things as aspirin therapy) for the long-term treatment of a condition or for prophylactic use. It is not for use for patients who have addictions to drugs. This subcategory is not for use of medications for detoxification or maintenance programs to prevent withdrawal symptoms in patients with drug dependence (e.g., methadone maintenance for opiate dependence). Assign the appropriate code for the drug dependence instead.

Assign a code from Z79 if the patient is receiving a medication for an extended period as a prophylactic measure (such as for the prevention of deep vein thrombosis) or as treatment of a chronic condition (such as arthritis) or a disease requiring a lengthy course of treatment (such as cancer). Do not assign a code from category Z79 for medication being administered for a brief period of time to treat an acute illness or injury (such as a course of antibiotics to treat acute bronchitis).

Z88   Allergy status to drugs, medicaments and biological substances

Except: Z88.9, Allergy status to unspecified drugs, medicaments and biological substances status

Z89   Acquired absence of limb

Z90   Acquired absence of organs, not elsewhere classified

Z91.0-   Allergy status, other than to drugs and biological substances

Z92.82   Status post administration of tPA (rtPA) in a different facility within the last 24 hours prior to admission to a current facility

Assign code Z92.82, Status post administration of tPA (rtPA) in a different facility within the last 24 hours prior to admission to current facility, as a secondary diagnosis when a patient is received by transfer into a facility and documentation indicates they were administered tissue plasminogen activator (tPA) within the last 24 hours prior to admission to the current facility.

This guideline applies even if the patient is still receiving the tPA at the time they are received into the current facility.

The appropriate code for the condition for which the tPA was administered (such as cerebrovascular disease or myocardial infarction) should be assigned first.

Code Z92.82 is only applicable to the receiving facility record and not to the transferring facility record.

Z93   Artificial opening status

Z94   Transplanted organ and tissue status

Z95   Presence of cardiac and vascular implants and grafts Z96 Presence of other functional implants

Z97   Presence of other devices Z98 Other postprocedural states

Assign code Z98.85, Transplanted organ removal status, to indicate that a transplanted organ has been previously removed. This code should not be assigned for the encounter in which the transplanted organ is removed. The complication necessitating removal of the transplant organ should be assigned for that encounter.

See section I.C19. for information on the coding of organ transplant complications.

Z99   Dependence on enabling machines and devices, not elsewhere classified

Note: Categories Z89-Z90 and Z93-Z99 are for use only if there are no complications or malfunctions of the organ or tissue replaced, the amputation site or the equipment on which the patient is dependent.

4) **History (of)**

There are two types of history Z codes, personal and family. Personal history codes explain a patient's past medical condition that no longer exists and is not receiving any treatment, but that has the potential for recurrence, and therefore may require continued monitoring.

Family history codes are for use when a patient has a family member(s) who has had a particular disease that causes the patient to be at higher risk of also contracting the disease.

Personal history codes may be used in conjunction with follow-up codes and family history codes may be used in conjunction with screening codes to explain the need for a test or procedure. History codes are also acceptable on any medical record regardless of the reason for visit. A history of an illness, even if no longer present, is important information that may alter the type of treatment ordered.

The history Z code categories are:

Z80   Family history of primary malignant neoplasm

Z81	Family history of mental and behavioral disorders
Z82	Family history of certain disabilities and chronic diseases (leading to disablement)
Z83	Family history of other specific disorders
Z84	Family history of other conditions
Z85	Personal history of malignant neoplasm
Z86	Personal history of certain other diseases
Z87	Personal history of other diseases and conditions
Z91.4-	Personal history of psychological trauma, not elsewhere classified
Z91.5	Personal history of self-harm
Z91.8-	Other specified personal risk factors, not elsewhere classified

Exception: Z91.83, Wandering in diseases classified elsewhere

| Z92 | Personal history of medical treatment |

Except: Z92.0, Personal history of contraception

Except: Z92.82, Status post administration of tPA (rtPA) in a different facility within the last 24 hours prior to admission to a current facility

5) Screening

Screening is the testing for disease or disease precursors in seemingly well individuals so that early detection and treatment can be provided for those who test positive for the disease (e.g., screening mammogram).

The testing of a person to rule out or confirm a suspected diagnosis because the patient has some sign or symptom is a diagnostic examination, not a screening. In these cases, the sign or symptom is used to explain the reason for the test.

A screening code may be a first-listed code if the reason for the visit is specifically the screening exam. It may also be used as an additional code if the screening is done during an office visit for other health problems. A screening code is not necessary if the screening is inherent to a routine examination, such as a pap smear done during a routine pelvic examination.

Should a condition be discovered during the screening then the code for the condition may be assigned as an additional diagnosis.

The Z code indicates that a screening exam is planned. A procedure code is required to confirm that the screening was performed.

The screening Z codes/categories:

| Z11 | Encounter for screening for infectious and parasitic diseases |
| Z12 | Encounter for screening for malignant neoplasms |

Z13   Encounter for screening for other diseases and disorders

         Except: Z13.9, Encounter for screening, unspecified

Z36   Encounter for antenatal screening for mother

6) **Observation**

There are three observation Z code categories. They are for use in very limited circumstances when a person is being observed for a suspected condition that is ruled out. The observation codes are not for use if an injury or illness or any signs or symptoms related to the suspected condition are present. In such cases the diagnosis/symptom code is used with the corresponding external cause code.

The observation codes are to be used as principal diagnosis only. The only exception to this is when the principal diagnosis is required to be a code from category Z38, Liveborn infants according to place of birth and type of delivery. Then a code from category Z05, Encounter for observation and evaluation of newborn for suspected diseases and conditions ruled out, is sequenced after the Z38 code. Additional codes may be used in addition to the observation code, but only if they are unrelated to the suspected condition being observed.

Codes from subcategory Z03.7, Encounter for suspected maternal and fetal conditions ruled out, may either be used as a first-listed or as an additional code assignment depending on the case. They are for use in very limited circumstances on a maternal record when an encounter is for a suspected maternal or fetal condition that is ruled out during that encounter (for example, a maternal or fetal condition may be suspected due to an abnormal test result). These codes should not be used when the condition is confirmed. In those cases, the confirmed condition should be coded. In addition, these codes are not for use if an illness or any signs or symptoms related to the suspected condition or problem are present. In such cases the diagnosis/symptom code is used.

Additional codes may be used in addition to the code from subcategory Z03.7, but only if they are unrelated to the suspected condition being evaluated.

Codes from subcategory Z03.7 may not be used for encounters for antenatal screening of mother. *See Section I.C.21. Screening.*

For encounters for suspected fetal condition that are inconclusive following testing and evaluation, assign the appropriate code from category O35, O36, O40 or O41.

The observation Z code categories:

Z03   Encounter for medical observation for suspected diseases and conditions ruled out

Z04   Encounter for examination and observation for other reasons

         Except: Z04.9, Encounter for examination and observation for unspecified reason

Z05   Encounter for observation and evaluation of newborn for suspected diseases and conditions ruled out

7) **Aftercare**

Aftercare visit codes cover situations when the initial treatment of a disease has been performed and the patient requires continued care during the healing or recovery phase, or for the long-term consequences of the disease. The aftercare Z code should not be used if treatment is directed at a current, acute disease. The diagnosis code is to be used in these cases. Exceptions to this rule are codes Z51.0, Encounter for antineoplastic radiation therapy, and codes from subcategory Z51.1, Encounter for antineoplastic chemotherapy and immunotherapy. These codes are to be first-listed, followed by

the diagnosis code when a patient's encounter is solely to receive radiation therapy, chemotherapy, or immunotherapy for the treatment of a neoplasm. If the reason for the encounter is more than one type of antineoplastic therapy, code Z51.0 and a code from subcategory Z51.1 may be assigned together, in which case one of these codes would be reported as a secondary diagnosis.

The aftercare Z codes should also not be used for aftercare for injuries. For aftercare of an injury, assign the acute injury code with the appropriate 7th character (for subsequent encounter).

The aftercare codes are generally first-listed to explain the specific reason for the encounter. An aftercare code may be used as an additional code when some type of aftercare is provided in addition to the reason for admission and no diagnosis code is applicable. An example of this would be the closure of a colostomy during an encounter for treatment of another condition.

Aftercare codes should be used in conjunction with other aftercare codes or diagnosis codes to provide better detail on the specifics of an aftercare encounter visit, unless otherwise directed by the classification. Should a patient receive multiple types of antineoplastic therapy during the same encounter, code Z51.0, Encounter for antineoplastic radiation therapy, and codes from subcategory Z51.1, Encounter for antineoplastic chemotherapy and immunotherapy, may be used together on a record. The sequencing of multiple aftercare codes depends on the circumstances of the encounter.

Certain aftercare Z code categories need a secondary diagnosis code to describe the resolving condition or sequelae. For others, the condition is included in the code title.

Additional Z code aftercare category terms include fitting and adjustment, and attention to artificial openings.

Status Z codes may be used with aftercare Z codes to indicate the nature of the aftercare. For example code Z95.1, Presence of aortocoronary bypass graft, may be used with code Z48.812, Encounter for surgical aftercare following surgery on the circulatory system, to indicate the surgery for which the aftercare is being performed. A status code should not be used when the aftercare code indicates the type of status, such as using Z43.0, Encounter for attention to tracheostomy, with Z93.0, Tracheostomy status.

The aftercare Z category/codes:

Z42   Encounter for plastic and reconstructive surgery following medical procedure or healed injury

Z43   Encounter for attention to artificial openings

Z44   Encounter for fitting and adjustment of external prosthetic device

Z45   Encounter for adjustment and management of implanted device

Z46   Encounter for fitting and adjustment of other devices

Z47   Orthopedic aftercare

Z48   Encounter for other postprocedural aftercare

Z49   Encounter for care involving renal dialysis

Z51   Encounter for other aftercare and medical care

8) **Follow-up**

The follow-up codes are used to explain continuing surveillance following completed treatment of a disease, condition, or injury. They imply that the condition has been fully treated and no longer exists. They should not be confused with aftercare codes, or injury codes with a 7th character for subsequent encounter, that explain ongoing care of a healing condition or its sequelae. Follow-up codes may be used in conjunction with history codes to provide the full picture of the healed condition and its treatment. The follow-up code is sequenced first, followed by the history code.

A follow-up code may be used to explain multiple visits. Should a condition be found to have recurred on the follow-up visit, then the diagnosis code for the condition should be assigned in place of the follow-up code.

The follow-up Z code categories:

Z08   Encounter for follow-up examination after completed treatment for malignant neoplasm

Z09   Encounter for follow-up examination after completed treatment for conditions other than malignant neoplasm

Z39   Encounter for maternal postpartum care and examination

9) Donor

Codes in category Z52, Donors of organs and tissues, are used for living individuals who are donating blood or other body tissue. These codes are only for individuals donating for others, not for self-donations. They are not used to identify cadaveric donations.

10) Counseling

Counseling Z codes are used when a patient or family member receives assistance in the aftermath of an illness or injury, or when support is required in coping with family or social problems. They are not used in conjunction with a diagnosis code when the counseling component of care is considered integral to standard treatment.

The counseling Z codes/categories:

Z30.0-   Encounter for general counseling and advice on contraception

Z31.5   Encounter for genetic counseling

Z31.6-   Encounter for general counseling and advice on procreation

Z32.2   Encounter for childbirth instruction

Z32.3   Encounter for childcare instruction

Z69   Encounter for mental health services for victim and perpetrator of abuse

Z70   Counseling related to sexual attitude, behavior and orientation

Z71   Persons encountering health services for other counseling and medical advice, not elsewhere classified

Z76.81   Expectant mother prebirth pediatrician visit

11) Encounters for Obstetrical and Reproductive Services

See Section I.C.15. Pregnancy, Childbirth, and the Puerperium, for further instruction on the use of these codes.

Z codes for pregnancy are for use in those circumstances when none of the problems or complications included in the codes from the Obstetrics chapter exist (a routine prenatal visit or postpartum care). Codes in category Z34, Encounter for supervision of normal pregnancy, are always first-listed and are not to be used with any other code from the OB chapter.

Codes in category Z3A, Weeks of gestation, may be assigned to provide additional information about the pregnancy. Category Z3A codes should not be assigned for pregnancies with abortive outcomes (categories O00-O08), elective termination of pregnancy (code Z33.32), nor for postpartum conditions, as category Z3A is not applicable to these conditions. The date of the admission should be used to determine weeks of gestation for inpatient admissions that encompass more than one gestational week.

The outcome of delivery, category Z37, should be included on all maternal delivery records. It is always a secondary code. Codes in category Z37 should not be used on the newborn record.

Z codes for family planning (contraceptive) or procreative management and counseling should be included on an obstetric record either during the pregnancy or the postpartum stage, if applicable.

Z codes/categories for obstetrical and reproductive services:

Z30   Encounter for contraceptive management

Z31   Encounter for procreative management

Z32.2   Encounter for childbirth instruction

Z32.3   Encounter for childcare instruction

Z33   Pregnant state

Z34   Encounter for supervision of normal pregnancy

Z36   Encounter for antenatal screening of mother

Z3A   Weeks of gestation

Z37   Outcome of delivery

Z39   Encounter for maternal postpartum care and examination

Z76.81 Expectant mother prebirth pediatrician visit

12) **Newborns and Infants**

See Section I.C.16. Newborn (Perinatal) Guidelines, for further instruction on the use of these codes.

Newborn Z codes/categories:

Z76.1   Encounter for health supervision and care of foundling

Z00.1- Encounter for routine child health examination

Z38   Liveborn infants according to place of birth and type of delivery

13) Routine and administrative examinations

The Z codes allow for the description of encounters for routine examinations, such as, a general check-up, or, examinations for administrative purposes, such as, a pre-employment physical. The codes are not to be used if the examination is for diagnosis of a suspected condition or for treatment purposes. In such cases the diagnosis code is used. During a routine exam, should a diagnosis or condition be discovered, it should be coded as an additional code. Pre-existing and chronic conditions and history codes may also be included as additional codes as long as the examination is for administrative purposes and not focused on any particular condition.

Some of the codes for routine health examinations distinguish between "with" and "without" abnormal findings. Code assignment depends on the information that is known at the time the encounter is being coded. For example, if no abnormal findings were found during the examination, but the encounter is being coded before test results are back, it is acceptable to assign the code for "without abnormal findings." When assigning a code for "with abnormal findings," additional code(s) should be assigned to identify the specific abnormal finding(s).

Pre-operative examination and pre-procedural laboratory examination Z codes are for use only in those situations when a patient is being cleared for a procedure or surgery and no treatment is given.

The Z codes/categories for routine and administrative examinations:

Z00　Encounter for general examination without complaint, suspected or reported diagnosis

Z01　Encounter for other special examination without complaint, suspected or reported diagnosis

Z02　Encounter for administrative examination

　　Except: Z02.9, Encounter for administrative examinations, unspecified

Z32.0-　Encounter for pregnancy test

14) Miscellaneous Z codes

The miscellaneous Z codes capture a number of other health care encounters that do not fall into one of the other categories. Certain of these codes identify the reason for the encounter; others are for use as additional codes that provide useful information on circumstances that may affect a patient's care and treatment.

Prophylactic Organ Removal

For encounters specifically for prophylactic removal of an organ (such as prophylactic removal of breasts due to a genetic susceptibility to cancer or a family history of cancer), the principal or first-listed code should be a code from category Z40, Encounter for prophylactic surgery, followed by the appropriate codes to identify the associated risk factor (such as genetic susceptibility or family history).

If the patient has a malignancy of one site and is having prophylactic removal at another site to prevent either a new primary malignancy or metastatic disease, a code for the malignancy should also be assigned in addition to a code from subcategory Z40.0, Encounter for prophylactic surgery for risk factors related to malignant neoplasms. A Z40.0 code should not be assigned if the patient is having organ removal for treatment of a malignancy, such as the removal of the testes for the treatment of prostate cancer.

Miscellaneous Z codes/categories:

Z28　Immunization not carried out

Except: Z28.3, Underimmunization status

Z29 Encounter for other prophylactic measures

Z40 Encounter for prophylactic surgery

Z41 Encounter for procedures for purposes other than remedying health state

Except: Z41.9, Encounter for procedure for purposes other than remedying health state, unspecified

Z53 Persons encountering health services for specific procedures and treatment, not carried out

Z55 Problems related to education and literacy

Z56 Problems related to employment and unemployment

Z57 Occupational exposure to risk factors

Z58 Problems related to physical environment

Z59 Problems related to housing and economic circumstances

Z60 Problems related to social environment

Z62 Problems related to upbringing

Z63 Other problems related to primary support group, including family circumstances

Z64 Problems related to certain psychosocial circumstances

Z65 Problems related to other psychosocial circumstances

Z72 Problems related to lifestyle

Note: These codes should be assigned only when the documentation specifies that the patient has an associated problem

Z73 Problems related to life management difficulty

Z74 Problems related to care provider dependency

Except: Z74.01, Bed confinement status

Z75 Problems related to medical facilities and other health care

Z76.0 Encounter for issue of repeat prescription

Z76.3 Healthy person accompanying sick person

Z76.4 Other boarder to healthcare facility

Z76.5 Malingerer [conscious simulation]

Z91.1- Patient's noncompliance with medical treatment and regimen

Z91.83   Wandering in diseases classified elsewhere

Z91.89   Other specified personal risk factors, not elsewhere classified

15) Nonspecific Z codes

Certain Z codes are so non-specific, or potentially redundant with other codes in the classification, that there can be little justification for their use in the inpatient setting. Their use in the outpatient setting should be limited to those instances when there is no further documentation to permit more precise coding. Otherwise, any sign or symptom or any other reason for visit that is captured in another code should be used.

Nonspecific Z codes/categories:

Z02.9   Encounter for administrative examinations, unspecified

Z04.9   Encounter for examination and observation for unspecified reason

Z13.9   Encounter for screening, unspecified

Z41.9   Encounter for procedure for purposes other than remedying health state, unspecified

Z52.9   Donor of unspecified organ or tissue

Z86.59   Personal history of other mental and behavioral disorders

Z88.9   Allergy status to unspecified drugs, medicaments and biological substances status

Z92.0   Personal history of contraception

16) Z Codes That May Only be Principal/First-Listed Diagnosis

The following Z codes/categories may only be reported as the principal/first-listed diagnosis, except when there are multiple encounters on the same day and the medical records for the encounters are combined:

Z00   Encounter for general examination without complaint, suspected or reported diagnosis

Except: Z00.6

Z01   Encounter for other special examination without complaint, suspected or reported diagnosis

Z02   Encounter for administrative examination

Z03   Encounter for medical observation for suspected diseases and conditions ruled out

Z04   Encounter for examination and observation for other reasons

Z33.2   Encounter for elective termination of pregnancy

Z31.81   Encounter for male factor infertility in female patient

Z31.83   Encounter for assisted reproductive fertility procedure cycle

Z31.84   Encounter for fertility preservation procedure

Z34   Encounter for supervision of normal pregnancy

Z39   Encounter for maternal postpartum care and examination

Z38   Liveborn infants according to place of birth and type of delivery

Z42   Encounter for plastic and reconstructive surgery following medical procedure or healed injury

Z51.0   Encounter for antineoplastic radiation therapy

Z51.1-   Encounter for antineoplastic chemotherapy and immunotherapy

Z52   Donors of organs and tissues

    Except: Z52.9, Donor of unspecified organ or tissue

Z76.1   Encounter for health supervision and care of foundling

Z76.2   Encounter for health supervision and care of other healthy infant and child

Z99.12   Encounter for respirator [ventilator] dependence during power failure

SECTION II. SELECTION OF PRINCIPAL DIAGNOSIS

The circumstances of inpatient admission always govern the selection of principal diagnosis. The principal diagnosis is defined in the Uniform Hospital Discharge Data Set (UHDDS) as "that condition established after study to be chiefly responsible for occasioning the admission of the patient to the hospital for care."

The UHDDS definitions are used by hospitals to report inpatient data elements in a standardized manner. These data elements and their definitions can be found in the July 31, 1985, Federal Register (Vol. 50, No, 147), pp. 31038-40.

Since that time the application of the UHDDS definitions has been expanded to include all non-outpatient settings (acute care, short term, long term care and psychiatric hospitals; home health agencies; rehab facilities; nursing homes, etc). The UHDDS definitions also apply to hospice services (all levels of care).

In determining principal diagnosis, coding conventions in the ICD-10-CM, the Tabular List and Alphabetic Index take precedence over these official coding guidelines.

(See Section I.A., Conventions for the ICD-10-CM)

The importance of consistent, complete documentation in the medical record cannot be overemphasized. Without such documentation the application of all coding guidelines is a difficult, if not impossible, task.

A. Codes for symptoms, signs, and ill-defined conditions

Codes for symptoms, signs, and ill-defined conditions from Chapter 18 are not to be used as principal diagnosis when a **related definitive diagnosis has been established.**

B. Two or more interrelated conditions, each potentially meeting the definition for principal diagnosis.

When there are two or more interrelated conditions (such as diseases in the same ICD-10-CM chapter or manifestations characteristically associated with a certain disease) potentially meeting the definition of principal diagnosis, either condition may be sequenced first, unless the circumstances of the admission, the therapy provided, the Tabular List, or the Alphabetic Index indicate otherwise.

C. Two or more diagnoses that equally meet the definition for principal diagnosis

In the unusual instance when two or more diagnoses equally meet the criteria for principal diagnosis as determined by the circumstances of admission, diagnostic workup and/or therapy provided, and the Alphabetic Index, Tabular List, or another coding guidelines does not provide sequencing direction, any one of the diagnoses may be sequenced first.

D. Two or more comparative or contrasting conditions

In those rare instances when two or more contrasting or comparative diagnoses are documented as "either/or" (or similar terminology), they are coded as if the diagnoses were confirmed and the diagnoses are sequenced according to the circumstances of the admission. If no further determination can be made as to which diagnosis should be principal, either diagnosis may be sequenced first.

E. A symptom(s) followed by contrasting/comparative diagnoses

Guideline deleted effective October 1, 2014

F. Original treatment plan not carried out

Sequence as the principal diagnosis the condition, which after study occasioned the admission to the hospital, even though treatment may not have been carried out due to unforeseen circumstances.

G. Complications of surgery and other medical care

When the admission is for treatment of a complication resulting from surgery or other medical care, the complication code is sequenced as the principal diagnosis. If the complication is classified to the T80-T88 series and the code lacks the necessary specificity in describing the complication, an additional code for the specific complication should be assigned.

H. Uncertain Diagnosis

If the diagnosis documented at the time of discharge is qualified as "probable", "suspected", "likely", "questionable", "possible", or "still to be ruled out", or other similar terms indicating uncertainty, code the condition as if it existed or was established. The bases for these guidelines are the diagnostic workup, arrangements for further workup or observation, and initial therapeutic approach that correspond most closely with the established diagnosis.

Note: This guideline is applicable only to inpatient admissions to short-term, acute, long-term care and psychiatric hospitals.

I. Admission from Observation Unit

1. Admission Following Medical Observation

When a patient is admitted to an observation unit for a medical condition, which either worsens or does not improve, and is subsequently admitted as an inpatient of the same hospital for this same medical condition, the principal diagnosis would be the medical condition which led to the hospital admission.

2. Admission Following Post-Operative Observation

When a patient is admitted to an observation unit to monitor a condition (or complication) that develops following outpatient surgery, and then is subsequently admitted as an inpatient of the same hospital, hospitals should apply the Uniform Hospital Discharge Data Set (UHDDS) definition of principal diagnosis as "that condition established after study to be chiefly responsible for occasioning the admission of the patient to the hospital for care."

J. Admission from Outpatient Surgery

When a patient receives surgery in the hospital's outpatient surgery department and is subsequently admitted for continuing inpatient care at the same hospital, the following guidelines should be followed in selecting the principal diagnosis for the inpatient admission:

- If the reason for the inpatient admission is a complication, assign the complication as the principal diagnosis.

- If no complication, or other condition, is documented as the reason for the inpatient admission, assign the reason for the outpatient surgery as the principal diagnosis.

- If the reason for the inpatient admission is another condition unrelated to the surgery, assign the unrelated condition as the principal diagnosis.

K. Admissions/Encounters for Rehabilitation

When the purpose for the admission/encounter is rehabilitation, sequence first the code for the condition for which the service is being performed. For example, for an admission/encounter for rehabilitation for right-sided dominant hemiplegia following a cerebrovascular infarction, report code I69.351, Hemiplegia and hemiparesis following cerebral infarction affecting right dominant side, as the first-listed or principal diagnosis.

If the condition for which the rehabilitation service is no longer present, report the appropriate aftercare code as the first-listed or principal diagnosis. For example, if a patient with severe degenerative osteoarthritis of the hip, underwent hip replacement and the current encounter/admission is for rehabilitation, report code Z47.1, Aftercare following joint replacement surgery, as the first-listed or principal diagnosis.

See Section I.C.21.c.7, Factors influencing health states and contact with health services, Aftercare.

SECTION III. REPORTING ADDITIONAL DIAGNOSES

GENERAL RULES FOR OTHER (ADDITIONAL) DIAGNOSES

For reporting purposes the definition for "other diagnoses" is interpreted as additional conditions that affect patient care in terms of requiring:

- clinical evaluation; or therapeutic treatment; or diagnostic procedures; or

- extended length of hospital stay; or increased nursing care and/or monitoring.

The UHDDS item #11-b defines Other Diagnoses as "all conditions that coexist at the time of admission, that develop subsequently, or that affect the treatment received and/or the length of stay. Diagnoses that relate to an earlier episode which have no bearing on the current hospital stay are to be excluded." UHDDS definitions apply to inpatients in acute care, short-term, long term care and psychiatric hospital setting. The UHDDS definitions are used by acute care short-term hospitals to report inpatient data elements in a standardized manner. These data elements and their definitions can be found in the July 31, 1985, Federal Register (Vol. 50, No, 147), pp. 31038-40.

Since that time the application of the UHDDS definitions has been expanded to include all non-outpatient settings (acute care, short term, long term care and psychiatric hospitals; home health agencies; rehab facilities; nursing homes, etc). The UHDDS definitions also apply to hospice services (all levels of care).

The following guidelines are to be applied in designating "other diagnoses" when neither the Alphabetic Index nor the Tabular List in ICD-10-CM provide direction. The listing of the diagnoses in the patient record is the responsibility of the attending provider.

A. Previous conditions

If the provider has included a diagnosis in the final diagnostic statement, such as the discharge summary or the face sheet, it should ordinarily be coded. Some providers include in the diagnostic statement resolved conditions or diagnoses and status-post procedures from previous admission that have no bearing on the current stay. Such conditions are not to be reported and are coded only if required by hospital policy.

However, history codes (categories Z80-Z87) may be used as secondary codes if the historical condition or family history has an impact on current care or influences treatment.

B. Abnormal findings

Abnormal findings (laboratory, x-ray, pathologic, and other diagnostic results) are not coded and reported unless the provider indicates their clinical significance. If the findings are outside the normal range and the attending provider has ordered other tests to evaluate the condition or prescribed treatment, it is appropriate to ask the provider whether the abnormal finding should be added.

Please note: This differs from the coding practices in the outpatient setting for coding encounters for diagnostic tests that have been interpreted by a provider.

C. Uncertain Diagnosis

If the diagnosis documented at the time of discharge is qualified as "probable", "suspected", "likely", "questionable", "possible", or "still to be ruled out" or other similar terms indicating uncertainty, code the condition as if it existed or was established. The bases for these guidelines are the diagnostic workup, arrangements for further workup or observation, and initial therapeutic approach that correspond most closely with the established diagnosis.

Note: This guideline is applicable only to inpatient admissions to short-term, acute, long-term care and psychiatric hospitals.

SECTION IV. DIAGNOSTIC CODING AND REPORTING GUIDELINES FOR OUTPATIENT SERVICES

These coding guidelines for outpatient diagnoses have been approved for use by hospitals/ providers in coding and reporting hospital-based outpatient services and provider-based office visits. Guidelines in Section I, Conventions, general coding guidelines and chapter-specific guidelines, should also be applied for outpatient services and office visits.

Information about the use of certain abbreviations, punctuation, symbols, and other conventions used in the ICD-10-CM Tabular List (code numbers and titles), can be found in Section IA of these guidelines, under "Conventions Used in the Tabular List." Section I.B. contains general guidelines that apply to the entire classification. Section I.C. contains chapter-specific guidelines that correspond to the chapters as they are arranged in the classification. Information about the correct sequence to use in finding a code is also described in Section I.

The terms encounter and visit are often used interchangeably in describing outpatient service contacts and, therefore, appear together in these guidelines without distinguishing one from the other.

Though the conventions and general guidelines apply to all settings, coding guidelines for outpatient and provider reporting of diagnoses will vary in a number of instances from those for inpatient diagnoses, recognizing that:

The Uniform Hospital Discharge Data Set (UHDDS) definition of principal diagnosis does not apply to hospital-based outpatient services and provider-based office visits.

Coding guidelines for inconclusive diagnoses (probable, suspected, rule out, etc.) were developed for inpatient reporting and do not apply to outpatients.

A. Selection of first-listed condition

In the outpatient setting, the term first-listed diagnosis is used in lieu of principal diagnosis.

In determining the first-listed diagnosis the coding conventions of ICD-10-CM, as well as the general and disease specific guidelines take precedence over the outpatient guidelines.

Diagnoses often are not established at the time of the initial encounter/visit. It may take two or more visits before the diagnosis is confirmed.

The most critical rule involves beginning the search for the correct code assignment through the Alphabetic Index. Never begin searching initially in the Tabular List as this will lead to coding errors.

1. Outpatient Surgery

When a patient presents for outpatient surgery (same day surgery), code the reason for the surgery as the first-listed diagnosis (reason for the encounter), even if the surgery is not performed due to a contraindication.

2. Observation Stay

When a patient is admitted for observation for a medical condition, assign a code for the medical condition as the first-listed diagnosis.

When a patient presents for outpatient surgery and develops complications requiring admission to observation, code the reason for the surgery as the first reported diagnosis (reason for the encounter), followed by codes for the complications as secondary diagnoses.

B. Codes from A00.0 through T88.9, Z00-Z99

The appropriate code(s) from A00.0 through T88.9, Z00-Z99 must be used to identify diagnoses, symptoms, conditions, problems, complaints, or other reason(s) for the encounter/visit.

C. Accurate reporting of ICD-10-CM diagnosis codes

For accurate reporting of ICD-10-CM diagnosis codes, the documentation should describe the patient's condition, using terminology which includes specific diagnoses as well as symptoms, problems, or reasons for the encounter. There are ICD-10-CM codes to describe all of these.

D. Codes that describe symptoms and signs

Codes that describe symptoms and signs, as opposed to diagnoses, are acceptable for reporting purposes when a diagnosis has not been established (confirmed) by the provider. Chapter 18 of ICD-10-CM, Symptoms, Signs, and Abnormal Clinical and Laboratory Findings Not Elsewhere Classified (codes R00-R99) contain many, but not all codes for symptoms.

E. Encounters for circumstances other than a disease or injury

ICD-10-CM provides codes to deal with encounters for circumstances other than a disease or injury. The Factors Influencing Health Status and Contact with Health Services codes (Z00-Z99) are provided to deal with occasions when circumstances other than a disease or injury are recorded as diagnosis or problems.

See Section I.C.21. Factors influencing health status and contact with health services.

F. Level of Detail in Coding

1. ICD-10-CM codes with 3, 4, 5, 6 or 7 characters

ICD-10-CM is composed of codes with 3, 4, 5, 6 or 7 characters. Codes with three characters are included in ICD-10-CM as the heading of a category of codes that may be further subdivided by the use of fourth, fifth, sixth or seventh characters to provide greater specificity.

2. Use of full number of characters required for a code

A three-character code is to be used only if it is not further subdivided. A code is invalid if it has not been coded to the full number of characters required for that code, including the 7th character, if applicable.

G. ICD-10-CM code for the diagnosis, condition, problem, or other reason for encounter/visit

List first the ICD-10-CM code for the diagnosis, condition, problem, or other reason for encounter/visit shown in the medical record to be chiefly responsible for the services provided. List additional codes that describe any coexisting conditions. In some cases the first-listed diagnosis may be a symptom when a diagnosis has not been established (confirmed) by the physician.

H. Uncertain diagnosis

Do not code diagnoses documented as "probable", "suspected," "questionable," "rule out," or "working diagnosis" or other similar terms indicating uncertainty. Rather, code the condition(s) to the highest degree of certainty for that encounter/visit, such as symptoms, signs, abnormal test results, or other reason for the visit.

Please note: This differs from the coding practices used by short-term, acute care, long-term care and psychiatric hospitals.

I. Chronic diseases

Chronic diseases treated on an ongoing basis may be coded and reported as many times as the patient receives treatment and care for the condition(s)

J. Code all documented conditions that coexist

Code all documented conditions that coexist at the time of the encounter/visit, and require or affect patient care treatment or management. Do not code conditions that were previously treated and no longer exist. However, history codes (categories Z80-Z87) may be used as secondary codes if the historical condition or family history has an impact on current care or influences treatment.

K. Patients receiving diagnostic services only

For patients receiving diagnostic services only during an encounter/visit, sequence first the diagnosis, condition, problem, or other reason for encounter/visit shown in the medical record to be chiefly responsible for the outpatient services provided during the encounter/visit. Codes for other diagnoses (e.g., chronic conditions) may be sequenced as additional diagnoses.

For encounters for routine laboratory/radiology testing in the absence of any signs, symptoms, or associated diagnosis, assign Z01.89, Encounter for other specified special examinations. If routine testing is performed during the same encounter as a test to evaluate a sign, symptom, or diagnosis, it is appropriate to assign both the Z code and the code describing the reason for the non-routine test.

For outpatient encounters for diagnostic tests that have been interpreted by a physician, and the final report is available at the time of coding, code any confirmed or definitive diagnosis(es) documented in the interpretation. Do not code related signs and symptoms as additional diagnoses.

Please note: This differs from the coding practice in the hospital inpatient setting regarding abnormal findings on test results.

L. Patients receiving therapeutic services only

For patients receiving therapeutic services only during an encounter/visit, sequence first the diagnosis, condition, problem, or other reason for encounter/visit shown in the medical record to be chiefly responsible for the outpatient services provided during the encounter/visit. Codes for other diagnoses (e.g., chronic conditions) may be sequenced as additional diagnoses.

The only exception to this rule is that when the primary reason for the admission/encounter is chemotherapy or radiation therapy, the appropriate Z code for the service is listed first, and the diagnosis or problem for which the service is being performed listed second.

M. Patients receiving preoperative evaluations only

For patients receiving preoperative evaluations only, sequence first a code from subcategory Z01.81, Encounter for pre-procedural examinations, to describe the pre-op consultations. Assign a code for the condition to describe the reason for the surgery as an additional diagnosis. Code also any findings related to the pre-op evaluation.

N. Ambulatory surgery

For ambulatory surgery, code the diagnosis for which the surgery was performed. If the postoperative diagnosis is known to be different from the preoperative diagnosis at the time the diagnosis is confirmed, select the postoperative diagnosis for coding, since it is the most definitive.

O. Routine outpatient prenatal visits

See Section I.C.15. Routine outpatient prenatal visits.

P. Encounters for general medical examinations with abnormal findings

The subcategories for encounters for general medical examinations, Z00.0-, provide codes for with and without abnormal findings. Should a general medical examination result in an abnormal finding, the code for general medical examination with abnormal finding should be assigned as the first-listed diagnosis. An examination with abnormal findings refers to a condition/diagnosis that is newly identified or a change in severity of a chronic condition (such as uncontrolled hypertension, or an acute exacerbation of chronic obstructive pulmonary disease) during a routine physical examination. A secondary code for the abnormal finding should also be coded.

Q. Encounters for routine health screenings

See Section I.C.21. Factors influencing health status and contact with health services, Screening

APPENDIX I

PRESENT ON ADMISSION REPORTING GUIDELINES

INTRODUCTION

These guidelines are to be used as a supplement to the *ICD-10-CM Official Guidelines for Coding and Reporting* to facilitate the assignment of the Present on Admission (POA) indicator for each diagnosis and external cause of injury code reported on claim forms (UB-04 and 837 Institutional).

These guidelines are not intended to replace any guidelines in the main body of the *ICD-10-CM Official Guidelines for Coding and Reporting*. The POA guidelines are not intended to provide guidance on when a condition should be coded, but rather, how to apply the POA indicator to the final set of diagnosis codes that have been assigned in accordance with Sections I, II, and III of the official coding guidelines. Subsequent to the assignment of the ICD-10-CM codes, the POA indicator should then be assigned to those conditions that have been coded.

As stated in the Introduction to the ICD-10-CM Official Guidelines for Coding and Reporting, a joint effort between the healthcare provider and the coder is essential to achieve complete and accurate documentation, code assignment, and reporting of diagnoses and procedures. The importance of consistent, complete documentation in the medical record cannot be overemphasized. Medical record documentation from any provider involved in the care and treatment of the patient may be used to support the determination of whether a condition was present on admission or not. In the context of the official coding guidelines, the term "provider" means a physician or any qualified healthcare practitioner who is legally accountable for establishing the patient's diagnosis.

These guidelines are not a substitute for the provider's clinical judgment as to the determination of whether a condition was/was not present on admission. The provider should be queried regarding issues related to the linking of signs/symptoms, timing of test results, and the timing of findings.

Please see the CDC website for the detailed list of ICD-10-CM codes that do not require the use of a POA indicator (ftp://ftp.cdc.gov/pub/Health_Statistics/NCHS/Publications/ICD10CM/2017/). The conditions on this exempt list represent categories and/or codes for circumstances regarding the healthcare encounter or factors influencing health status that do not represent a current disease or injury or are always present on admission.

General Reporting Requirements

All claims involving inpatient admissions to general acute care hospitals or other facilities that are subject to a law or regulation mandating collection of present on admission information.

Present on admission is defined as present at the time the order for inpatient admission occurs -- conditions that develop during an outpatient encounter, including emergency department, observation, or outpatient surgery, are considered as present on admission.

POA indicator is assigned to principal and secondary diagnoses (as defined in Section II of the Official Guidelines for Coding and Reporting) and the external cause of injury codes.

Issues related to inconsistent, missing, conflicting or unclear documentation must still be resolved by the provider.

If a condition would not be coded and reported based on UHDDS definitions and current official coding guidelines, then the POA indicator would not be reported.

Reporting Options

Y - Yes

N - No

U - Unknown

W - Clinically undetermined

Unreported/Not used – (Exempt from POA reporting)

Reporting Definitions

Y =   present at the time of inpatient admission

N =   not present at the time of inpatient admission

U =   documentation is insufficient to determine if condition is present on admission

W =   provider is unable to clinically determine whether condition was present on admission or not

Timeframe for POA Identification and Documentation

There is no required timeframe as to when a provider (per the definition of "provider" used in these guidelines) must identify or document a condition to be present on admission. In some clinical situations, it may not be possible for a provider to make a definitive diagnosis (or a condition may not be recognized or reported by the patient) for a period of time after admission. In some cases it may be several days before the provider arrives at a definitive diagnosis. This does not mean that the condition was not present on admission. Determination of whether the condition was present on admission or not will be based on the applicable POA guideline as identified in this document, or on the provider's best clinical judgment.

If at the time of code assignment the documentation is unclear as to whether a condition was present on admission or not, it is appropriate to query the provider for clarification.

Assigning the POA Indicator

Condition is on the "Exempt from Reporting" list

Leave the "present on admission" field blank if the condition is on the list of ICD-10-CM codes for which this field is not applicable. This is the only circumstance in which the field may be left blank.

POA Explicitly Documented

Assign Y for any condition the provider explicitly documents as being present on admission.

Assign N for any condition the provider explicitly documents as not present at the time of admission.

Conditions diagnosed prior to inpatient admission

Assign "Y" for conditions that were diagnosed prior to admission (example: hypertension, diabetes mellitus, asthma)

Conditions diagnosed during the admission but clearly present before admission

Assign "Y" for conditions diagnosed during the admission that were clearly present but not diagnosed until after admission occurred.

Diagnoses subsequently confirmed after admission are considered present on admission if at the time of admission they are documented as suspected, possible, rule out, differential diagnosis, or constitute an underlying cause of a symptom that is present at the time of admission.

Condition develops during outpatient encounter prior to inpatient admission

Assign Y for any condition that develops during an outpatient encounter prior to a written order for inpatient admission.

Documentation does not indicate whether condition was present on admission

Assign "U" when the medical record documentation is unclear as to whether the condition was present on admission. "U" should not be routinely assigned and used only in very limited circumstances. Coders are encouraged to query the providers when the documentation is unclear.

Documentation states that it cannot be determined whether the condition was or was not present on admission

Assign "W" when the medical record documentation indicates that it cannot be clinically determined whether or not the condition was present on admission.

Chronic condition with acute exacerbation during the admission

If a single code identifies both the chronic condition and the acute exacerbation, see POA guidelines pertaining to codes that contain multiple clinical concepts.

If a single code only identifies the chronic condition and not the acute exacerbation (e.g., acute exacerbation of chronic leukemia), assign "Y."

Conditions documented as possible, probable, suspected, or rule out at the time of discharge

If the final diagnosis contains a possible, probable, suspected, or rule out diagnosis, and this diagnosis was based on signs, symptoms or clinical findings suspected at the time of inpatient admission, assign "Y."

If the final diagnosis contains a possible, probable, suspected, or rule out diagnosis, and this diagnosis was based on signs, symptoms or clinical findings that were not present on admission, assign "N".

Conditions documented as impending or threatened at the time of discharge

If the final diagnosis contains an impending or threatened diagnosis, and this diagnosis is based on symptoms or clinical findings that were present on admission, assign "Y".

If the final diagnosis contains an impending or threatened diagnosis, and this diagnosis is based on symptoms or clinical findings that were not present on admission, assign "N".

Acute and Chronic Conditions

Assign "Y" for acute conditions that are present at time of admission and N for acute conditions that are not present at time of admission.

Assign "Y" for chronic conditions, even though the condition may not be diagnosed until after admission.

If a single code identifies both an acute and chronic condition, see the POA guidelines for codes that contain multiple clinical concepts.

Codes That Contain Multiple Clinical Concepts

Assign "N" if at least one of the clinical concepts included in the code was not present on admission (e.g., COPD with acute exacerbation and the exacerbation was not present on admission; gastric ulcer that does not start bleeding until after admission; asthma patient develops status asthmaticus after admission).

Assign "Y" if all of the clinical concepts included in the code were present on admission (e.g., duodenal ulcer that perforates prior to admission).

For infection codes that include the causal organism, assign "Y" if the infection (or signs of the infection) **were** present on admission, even though the culture results may not be known until after admission (e.g., patient is admitted with pneumonia and the provider documents Pseudomonas as the causal organism a few days later).

Same Diagnosis Code for Two or More Conditions

When the same ICD-10-CM diagnosis code applies to two or more conditions during the same encounter (e.g. two separate conditions classified to the same ICD-10-CM diagnosis code):

Assign "Y" if all conditions represented by the single ICD-10-CM code were present on admission (e.g. bilateral unspecified age-related cataracts).

Assign "N" if any of the conditions represented by the single ICD-10-CM code was not present on admission (e.g. traumatic secondary and recurrent hemorrhage and seroma is assigned to a single code T79.2, but only one of the conditions was present on admission).

Obstetrical conditions

Whether or not the patient delivers during the current hospitalization does not affect assignment of the POA indicator. The determining factor for POA assignment is whether the pregnancy complication or obstetrical condition described by the code was present at the time of admission or not.

If the pregnancy complication or obstetrical condition was present on admission (e.g., patient admitted in preterm labor), assign "Y".

If the pregnancy complication or obstetrical condition was not present on admission (e.g., 2nd degree laceration during delivery, postpartum hemorrhage that occurred during current hospitalization, fetal distress develops after admission), assign "N".

If the obstetrical code includes more than one diagnosis and any of the diagnoses identified by the code were not present on admission assign "N".

(e.g., Category O11, Pre-existing hypertension with pre-eclampsia)

Perinatal conditions

Newborns are not considered to be admitted until after birth. Therefore, any condition present at birth or that developed in utero is considered present at admission and should be assigned "Y". This includes conditions that occur during delivery (e.g., injury during delivery, meconium aspiration, exposure to streptococcus B in the vaginal canal).

Congenital conditions and anomalies

Assign "Y" for congenital conditions and anomalies except for categories Q00-Q99, Congenital anomalies, which are on the exempt list. Congenital conditions are always considered present on admission.

External cause of injury codes

Assign "Y" for any external cause code representing an external cause of morbidity that occurred prior to inpatient admission (e.g., patient fell out of bed at home, patient fell out of bed in emergency room prior to admission)

Assign "N" for any external cause code representing an external cause of morbidity that occurred during inpatient hospitalization (e.g., patient fell out of hospital bed during hospital stay, patient experienced an adverse reaction to a medication administered after inpatient admission)

Anatomical Illustrations

A fundamental knowledge and understanding of basic human anatomy and physiology is a prerequisite for accurate diagnosis coding. While a comprehensive treatment of anatomy and physiology is beyond the scope of this text, the large scale, full color anatomical illustrations on the following pages are designed to facilitate the procedure coding process for both beginning and experienced coders.

The illustrations provide an anatomical perspective of procedure coding by providing a side-by-side view of the major systems of the human body and a corresponding list of the most common ICD-10-CM categories used to report medical, surgical and diagnostic services performed on the illustrated system.

The ICD-10-CM categories listed on the left facing page of each anatomical illustration are code ranges only and should not be used for coding. These categories are provided as "pointers" to the appropriate section of ICD-10-CM, where the definitive code may be found.

PLATE 1. SKIN AND SUBCUTANEOUS TISSUE – MALE

Viral infections characterized by skin and mucous membrane lesions	**B00-B09**
Bacterial and viral infectious agents	**B95-B97**
Melanoma and other malignant neoplasms of skin	**C43-C44**
Malignant neoplasms of mesothelial and soft tissue	**C45-C49**
Malignant neoplasms of ill-defined, other secondary and unspecified sites	**C76-C80**
In situ neoplasms	**D00-D09**
Benign neoplasms, except benign neuroendocrine tumors	**D10-D36**
Neoplasms of uncertain behavior, polycythemia vera and myelodysplastic syndromes	**D37-D48**
Neoplasms of unspecified behavior	**D49**
Infections of the skin and subcutaneous tissue	**L00-L08**
Bullous disorders	**L10-L14**
Dermatitis and eczema	**L20-L30**
Papulosquamous disorders	**L40-L45**
Urticaria and erythema	**L49-L54**
Radiation-related disorders of the skin and subcutaneous tissue	**L55-L59**
Disorders of skin appendages	**L60-L75**
Intraoperative and postprocedural complications of skin and subcutaneous tissue	**L76**
Other disorders of the skin and subcutaneous tissue	**L80-L99**
Symptoms and signs involving the skin and subcutaneous tissue	**R20-R23**
General symptoms and signs	**R50-R69**
Abnormal findings on diagnostic imaging and in function studies, without diagnosis	**R90-R94**
Burns and corrosions of external body surface, specified by site	**T20-T25**
Burns and corrosions	**T20-T32**
Burns and corrosions of multiple and unspecified body regions	**T30-T32**
Persons encountering health services for examinations	**Z00-Z13**
Encounters for other specific health care	**Z40-Z53**

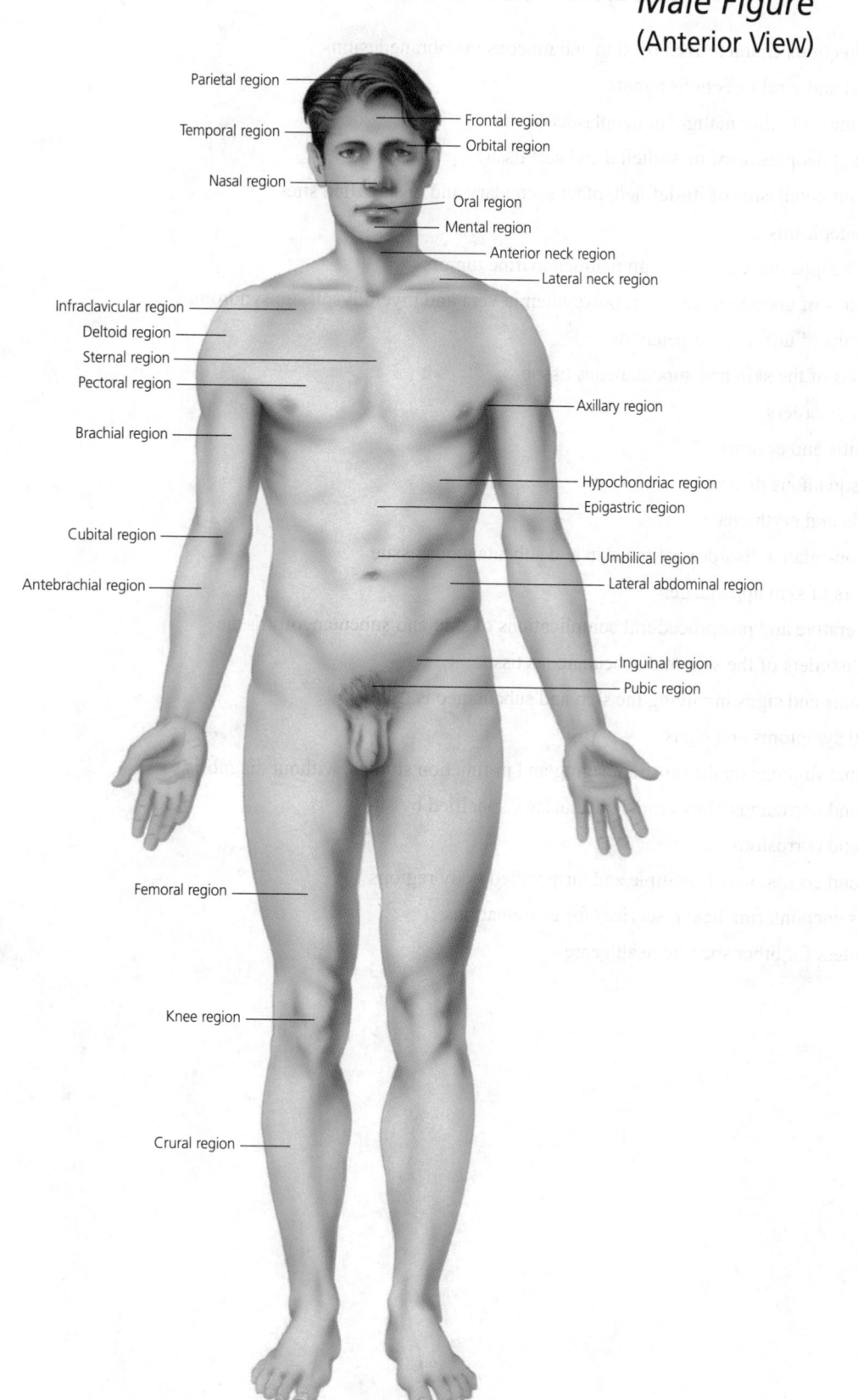

Male Figure
(Anterior View)

Parietal region

Temporal region

Nasal region

Frontal region

Orbital region

Oral region

Mental region

Anterior neck region

Lateral neck region

Infraclavicular region

Deltoid region

Sternal region

Pectoral region

Axillary region

Brachial region

Hypochondriac region

Epigastric region

Cubital region

Umbilical region

Lateral abdominal region

Antebrachial region

Inguinal region

Pubic region

Femoral region

Knee region

Crural region

©Practice Management Information Corp., Los Angeles, CA

PLATE 2. SKIN AND SUBCUTANEOUS TISSUE - FEMALE

Viral infections characterized by skin and mucous membrane lesions	**B00-B09**
Bacterial and viral infectious agents	**B95-B97**
Melanoma and other malignant neoplasms of skin	**C43-C44**
Malignant neoplasms of mesothelial and soft tissue	**C45-C49**
Malignant neoplasms of ill-defined, other secondary and unspecified sites	**C76-C80**
In situ neoplasms	**D00-D09**
Benign neoplasms, except benign neuroendocrine tumors	**D10-D36**
Neoplasms of uncertain behavior, polycythemia vera and myelodysplastic syndromes	**D37-D48**
Neoplasms of unspecified behavior	**D49**
Infections of the skin and subcutaneous tissue	**L00-L08**
Bullous disorders	**L10-L14**
Dermatitis and eczema	**L20-L30**
Papulosquamous disorders	**L40-L45**
Urticaria and erythema	**L49-L54**
Radiation-related disorders of the skin and subcutaneous tissue	**L55-L59**
Disorders of skin appendages	**L60-L75**
Intraoperative and postprocedural complications of skin and subcutaneous tissue	**L76**
Other disorders of the skin and subcutaneous tissue	**L80-L99**
Symptoms and signs involving the skin and subcutaneous tissue	**R20-R23**
General symptoms and signs	**R50-R69**
Abnormal findings on diagnostic imaging and in function studies, without diagnosis	**R90-R94**
Burns and corrosions of external body surface, specified by site	**T20-T25**
Burns and corrosions	**T20-T32**
Burns and corrosions of multiple and unspecified body regions	**T30-T32**
Persons encountering health services for examinations	**Z00-Z13**
Encounters for other specific health care	**Z40-Z53**

Female Figure
(Anterior View)

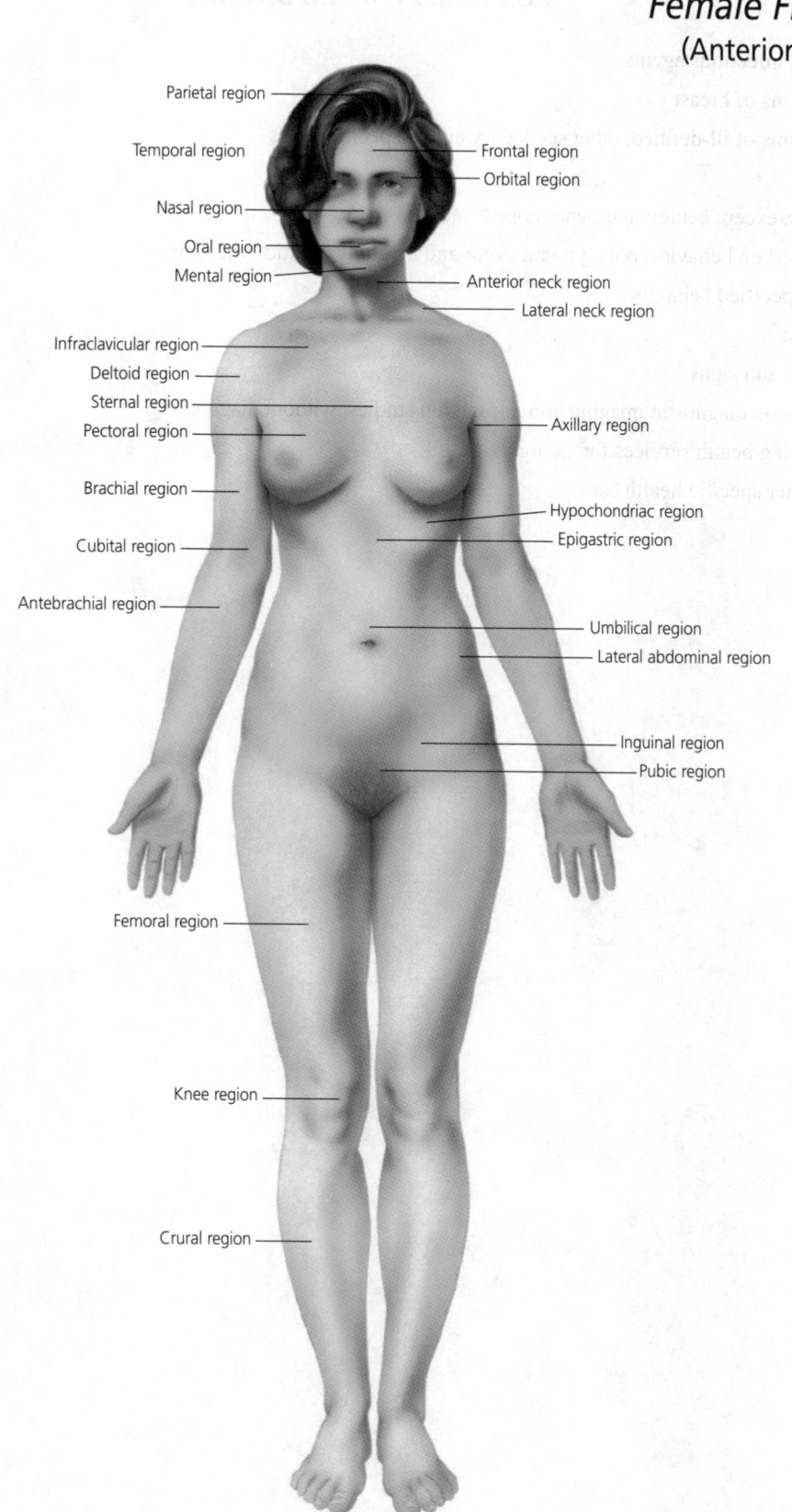

Parietal region

Temporal region

Frontal region

Orbital region

Nasal region

Oral region

Mental region

Anterior neck region

Lateral neck region

Infraclavicular region

Deltoid region

Sternal region

Pectoral region

Axillary region

Brachial region

Hypochondriac region

Cubital region

Epigastric region

Antebrachial region

Umbilical region

Lateral abdominal region

Inguinal region

Pubic region

Femoral region

Knee region

Crural region

©Practice Management Information Corp., Los Angeles, CA

PLATE 3. FEMALE BREAST

Bacterial and viral infectious agents	**B95-B97**
Malignant neoplasms of breast	**C50**
Malignant neoplasms of ill-defined, other secondary and unspecified sites	**C76-C80**
In situ neoplasms	**D00-D09**
Benign neoplasms, except benign neuroendocrine tumors	**D10-D36**
Neoplasms of uncertain behavior, polycythemia vera and myelodysplastic syndromes	**D37-D48**
Neoplasms of unspecified behavior	**D49**
Disorders of breast	**N60-N65**
General symptoms and signs	**R50-R69**
Abnormal findings on diagnostic imaging and in function studies, without diagnosis	**R90-R94**
Persons encountering health services for examinations	**Z00-Z13**
Encounters for other specific health care	**Z40-Z53**

Female Breast

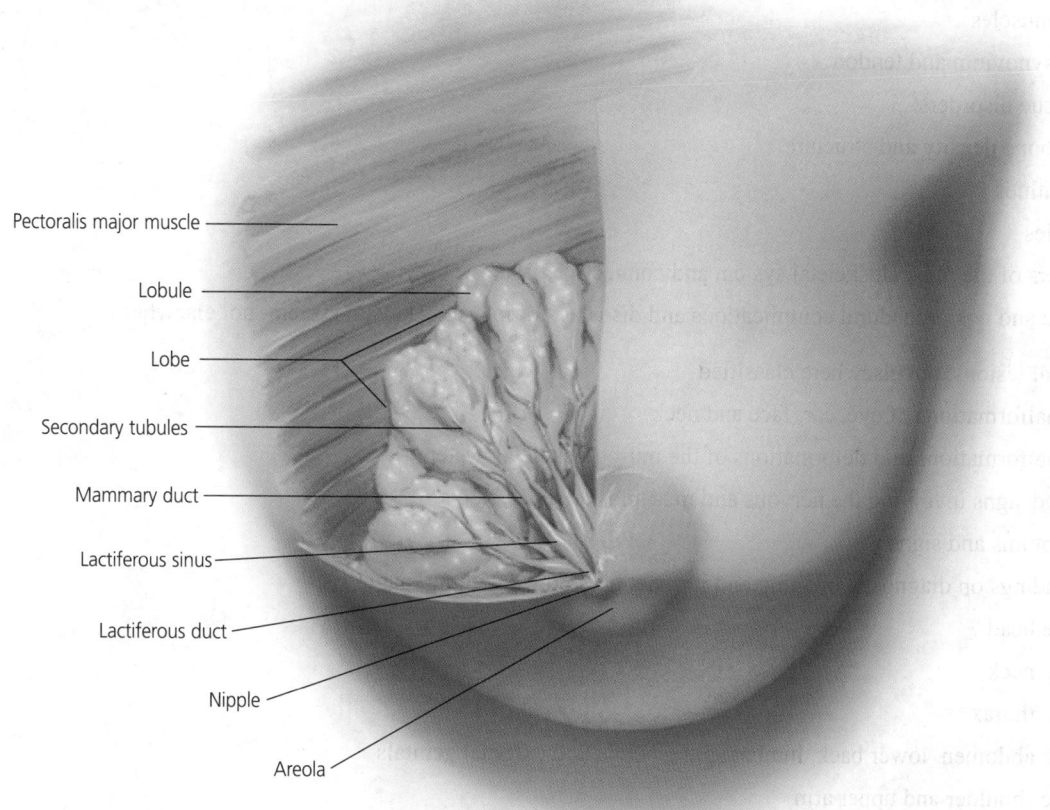

Pectoralis major muscle

Lobule

Lobe

Secondary tubules

Mammary duct

Lactiferous sinus

Lactiferous duct

Nipple

Areola

©Practice Management Information Corp., Los Angeles, CA

PLATE 4. MUSCULAR SYSTEM AND CONNECTIVE TISSUE – ANTERIOR VIEW

Malignant neoplasms of bone and articular cartilage	**C40-C41**
Infectious arthropathies	**M00-M02**
Inflammatory polyarthropathies	**M05-M14**
Osteoarthritis	**M15-M19**
Other joint disorders	**M20-M25**
Dentofacial anomalies [including malocclusion] and other disorders of jaw	**M26-M27**
Systemic connective tissue disorders	**M30-M36**
Deforming dorsopathies	**M40-M43**
Spondylopathies	**M45-M49**
Other dorsopathies	**M50-M54**
Disorders of muscles	**M60-M63**
Disorders of synovium and tendon	**M65-M67**
Other soft tissue disorders	**M70-M79**
Disorders of bone density and structure	**M80-M85**
Other osteopathies	**M86-M90**
Chondropathies	**M91-M94**
Other disorders of the musculoskeletal system and connective tissue	**M95**
Intraoperative and postprocedural complications and disorders of musculoskeletal system, not elsewhere classified	**M96**
Biomechanical lesions, not elsewhere classified	**M99**
Congenital malformations of eye, ear, face and neck	**Q10-Q18**
Congenital malformations and deformations of the musculoskeletal system	**Q65-Q79**
Symptoms and signs involving the nervous and musculoskeletal systems	**R25-R29**
General symptoms and signs	**R50-R69**
Abnormal findings on diagnostic imaging and in function studies, without diagnosis	**R90-R94**
Injuries to the head	**S00-S09**
Injuries to the neck	**S10-S19**
Injuries to the thorax	**S20-S29**
Injuries to the abdomen, lower back, lumbar spine, pelvis and external genitals	**S30-S39**
Injuries to the shoulder and upper arm	**S40-S49**
Injuries to the elbow and forearm	**S50-S59**
Injuries to the wrist, hand and fingers	**S60-S69**
Injuries to the hip and thigh	**S70-S79**
Injuries to the knee and lower leg	**S80-S89**
Injuries to the ankle and foot	**S90-S99**
Injuries involving multiple body regions	**T07**
Certain early complications of trauma	**T79**
Accidents	**V00-X58**
Persons encountering health services for examinations	**Z00-Z13**
Encounters for other specific health care	**Z40-Z53**

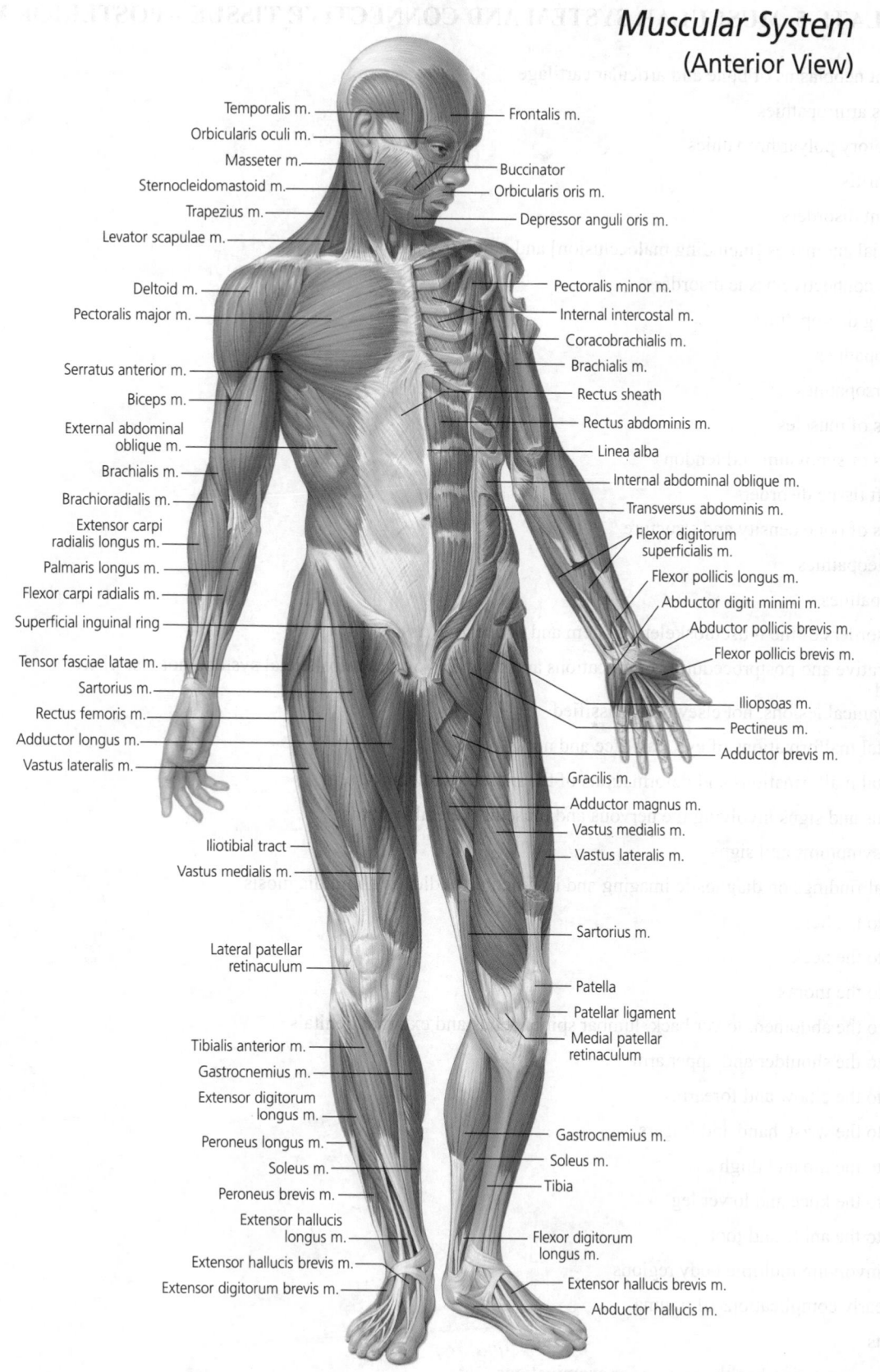

Muscular System
(Anterior View)

Temporalis m.
Orbicularis oculi m.
Masseter m.
Sternocleidomastoid m.
Trapezius m.
Levator scapulae m.

Frontalis m.
Buccinator
Orbicularis oris m.
Depressor anguli oris m.

Deltoid m.
Pectoralis major m.

Serratus anterior m.
Biceps m.
External abdominal oblique m.
Brachialis m.
Brachioradialis m.
Extensor carpi radialis longus m.
Palmaris longus m.
Flexor carpi radialis m.
Superficial inguinal ring
Tensor fasciae latae m.
Sartorius m.
Rectus femoris m.
Adductor longus m.
Vastus lateralis m.

Pectoralis minor m.
Internal intercostal m.
Coracobrachialis m.
Brachialis m.
Rectus sheath
Rectus abdominis m.
Linea alba
Internal abdominal oblique m.
Transversus abdominis m.
Flexor digitorum superficialis m.
Flexor pollicis longus m.
Abductor digiti minimi m.
Abductor pollicis brevis m.
Flexor pollicis brevis m.
Iliopsoas m.
Pectineus m.
Adductor brevis m.
Gracilis m.
Adductor magnus m.
Vastus medialis m.
Vastus lateralis m.

Iliotibial tract
Vastus medialis m.

Sartorius m.

Lateral patellar retinaculum

Patella
Patellar ligament
Medial patellar retinaculum

Tibialis anterior m.
Gastrocnemius m.
Extensor digitorum longus m.
Peroneus longus m.
Soleus m.
Peroneus brevis m.
Extensor hallucis longus m.
Extensor hallucis brevis m.
Extensor digitorum brevis m.

Gastrocnemius m.
Soleus m.
Tibia
Flexor digitorum longus m.
Extensor hallucis brevis m.
Abductor hallucis m.

©Scientific Publishing Ltd., Rolling Meadows, IL

PLATE 5. MUSCULAR SYSTEM AND CONNECTIVE TISSUE – POSTERIOR VIEW

Malignant neoplasms of bone and articular cartilage	**C40-C41**
Infectious arthropathies	**M00-M02**
Inflammatory polyarthropathies	**M05-M14**
Osteoarthritis	**M15-M19**
Other joint disorders	**M20-M25**
Dentofacial anomalies [including malocclusion] and other disorders of jaw	**M26-M27**
Systemic connective tissue disorders	**M30-M36**
Deforming dorsopathies	**M40-M43**
Spondylopathies	**M45-M49**
Other dorsopathies	**M50-M54**
Disorders of muscles	**M60-M63**
Disorders of synovium and tendon	**M65-M67**
Other soft tissue disorders	**M70-M79**
Disorders of bone density and structure	**M80-M85**
Other osteopathies	**M86-M90**
Chondropathies	**M91-M94**
Other disorders of the musculoskeletal system and connective tissue	**M95**
Intraoperative and postprocedural complications and disorders of musculoskeletal system, not elsewhere classified	**M96**
Biomechanical lesions, not elsewhere classified	**M99**
Congenital malformations of eye, ear, face and neck	**Q10-Q18**
Congenital malformations and deformations of the musculoskeletal system	**Q65-Q79**
Symptoms and signs involving the nervous and musculoskeletal systems	**R25-R29**
General symptoms and signs	**R50-R69**
Abnormal findings on diagnostic imaging and in function studies, without diagnosis	**R90-R94**
Injuries to the head	**S00-S09**
Injuries to the neck	**S10-S19**
Injuries to the thorax	**S20-S29**
Injuries to the abdomen, lower back, lumbar spine, pelvis and external genitals	**S30-S39**
Injuries to the shoulder and upper arm	**S40-S49**
Injuries to the elbow and forearm	**S50-S59**
Injuries to the wrist, hand and fingers	**S60-S69**
Injuries to the hip and thigh	**S70-S79**
Injuries to the knee and lower leg	**S80-S89**
Injuries to the ankle and foot	**S90-S99**
Injuries involving multiple body regions	**T07**
Certain early complications of trauma	**T79**
Accidents	**V00-X58**
Persons encountering health services for examinations	**Z00-Z13**
Encounters for other specific health care	**Z40-Z53**

Muscular System
(Posterior View)

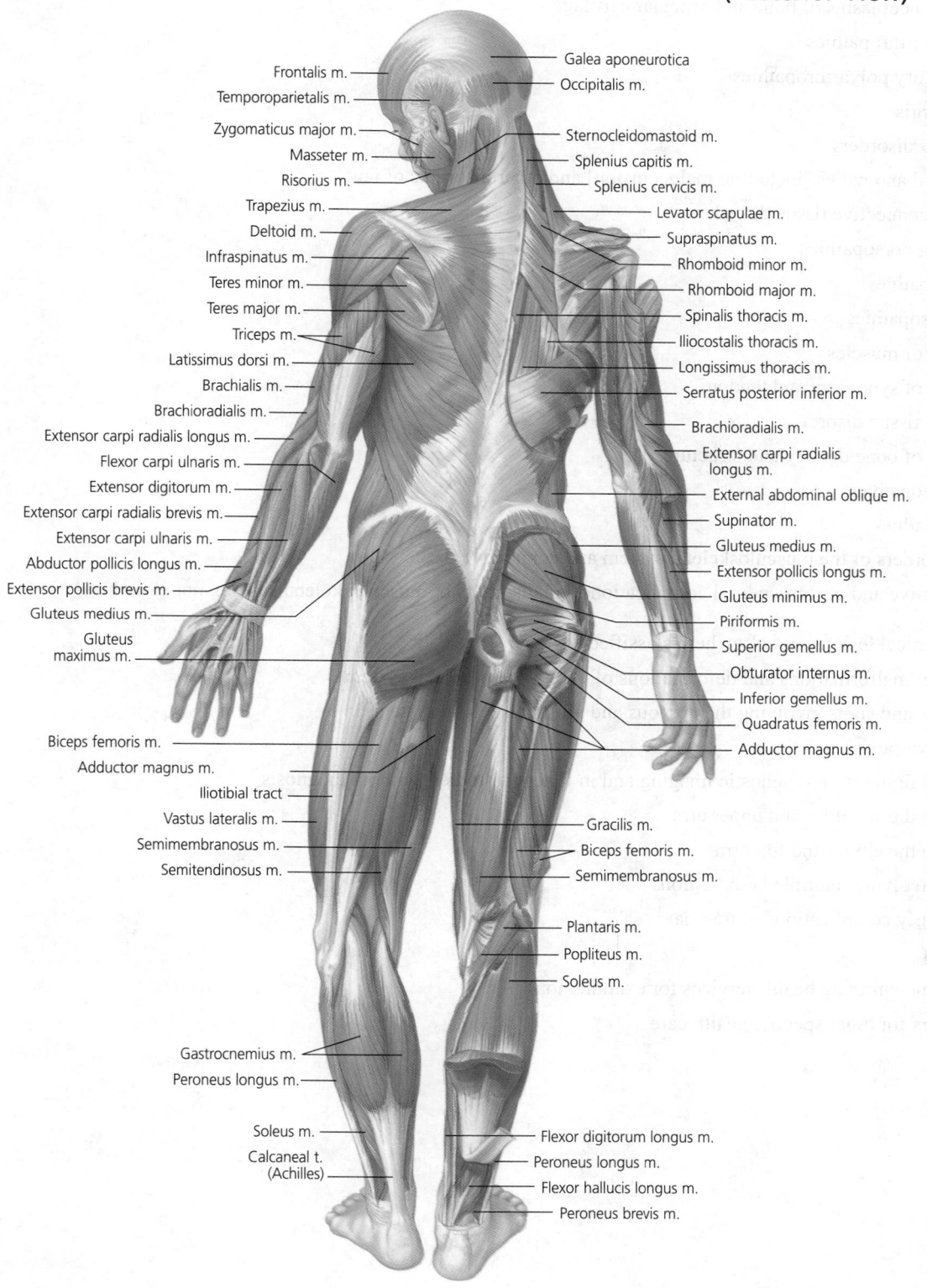

Frontalis m.
Temporoparietalis m.
Zygomaticus major m.
Masseter m.
Risorius m.
Trapezius m.
Deltoid m.
Infraspinatus m.
Teres minor m.
Teres major m.
Triceps m.
Latissimus dorsi m.
Brachialis m.
Brachioradialis m.
Extensor carpi radialis longus m.
Flexor carpi ulnaris m.
Extensor digitorum m.
Extensor carpi radialis brevis m.
Extensor carpi ulnaris m.
Abductor pollicis longus m.
Extensor pollicis brevis m.
Gluteus medius m.
Gluteus maximus m.
Biceps femoris m.
Adductor magnus m.
Iliotibial tract
Vastus lateralis m.
Semimembranosus m.
Semitendinosus m.
Gastrocnemius m.
Peroneus longus m.
Soleus m.
Calcaneal t. (Achilles)

Galea aponeurotica
Occipitalis m.
Sternocleidomastoid m.
Splenius capitis m.
Splenius cervicis m.
Levator scapulae m.
Supraspinatus m.
Rhomboid minor m.
Rhomboid major m.
Spinalis thoracis m.
Iliocostalis thoracis m.
Longissimus thoracis m.
Serratus posterior inferior m.
Brachioradialis m.
Extensor carpi radialis longus m.
External abdominal oblique m.
Supinator m.
Gluteus medius m.
Extensor pollicis longus m.
Gluteus minimus m.
Piriformis m.
Superior gemellus m.
Obturator internus m.
Inferior gemellus m.
Quadratus femoris m.
Adductor magnus m.
Gracilis m.
Biceps femoris m.
Semimembranosus m.
Plantaris m.
Popliteus m.
Soleus m.
Flexor digitorum longus m.
Peroneus longus m.
Flexor hallucis longus m.
Peroneus brevis m.

©Practice Management Information Corp., Los Angeles, CA

PLATE 6. MUSCULAR SYSTEM - SHOULDER AND ELBOW

Malignant neoplasms of bone and articular cartilage	**C40-C41**
Infectious arthropathies	**M00-M02**
Inflammatory polyarthropathies	**M05-M14**
Osteoarthritis	**M15-M19**
Other joint disorders	**M20-M25**
Dentofacial anomalies [including malocclusion] and other disorders of jaw	**M26-M27**
Systemic connective tissue disorders	**M30-M36**
Deforming dorsopathies	**M40-M43**
Spondylopathies	**M45-M49**
Other dorsopathies	**M50-M54**
Disorders of muscles	**M60-M63**
Disorders of synovium and tendon	**M65-M67**
Other soft tissue disorders	**M70-M79**
Disorders of bone density and structure	**M80-M85**
Other osteopathies	**M86-M90**
Chondropathies	**M91-M94**
Other disorders of the musculoskeletal system and connective tissue	**M95**
Intraoperative and postprocedural complications and disorders of musculoskeletal system, not elsewhere classified	**M96**
Biomechanical lesions, not elsewhere classified	**M99**
Congenital malformations and deformations of the musculoskeletal system	**Q65-Q79**
Symptoms and signs involving the nervous and musculoskeletal systems	**R25-R29**
General symptoms and signs	**R50-R69**
Abnormal findings on diagnostic imaging and in function studies, without diagnosis	**R90-R94**
Injuries to the shoulder and upper arm	**S40-S49**
Injuries to the elbow and forearm	**S50-S59**
Injuries involving multiple body regions	**T07**
Certain early complications of trauma	**T79**
Accidents	**V00-X58**
Persons encountering health services for examinations	**Z00-Z13**
Encounters for other specific health care	**Z40-Z53**

Shoulder and Elbow
(Anterior View)

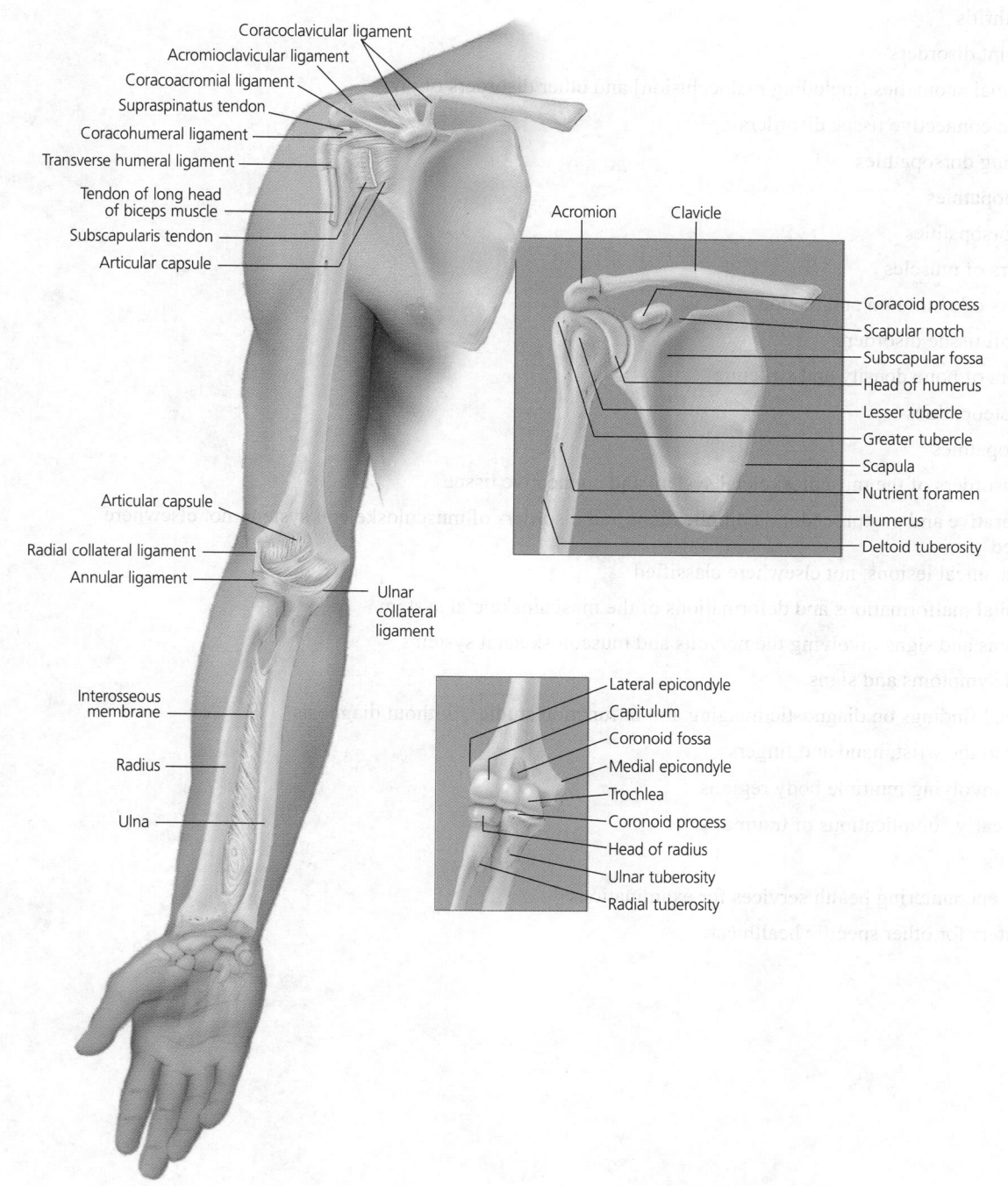

Coracoclavicular ligament
Acromioclavicular ligament
Coracoacromial ligament
Supraspinatus tendon
Coracohumeral ligament
Transverse humeral ligament
Tendon of long head of biceps muscle
Subscapularis tendon
Articular capsule

Acromion
Clavicle

Coracoid process
Scapular notch
Subscapular fossa
Head of humerus
Lesser tubercle
Greater tubercle
Scapula
Nutrient foramen
Humerus
Deltoid tuberosity

Articular capsule
Radial collateral ligament
Annular ligament

Ulnar collateral ligament

Interosseous membrane
Radius
Ulna

Lateral epicondyle
Capitulum
Coronoid fossa
Medial epicondyle
Trochlea
Coronoid process
Head of radius
Ulnar tuberosity
Radial tuberosity

©Scientific Publishing Ltd., Rolling Meadows, IL

PLATE 7. MUSCULAR SYSTEM - HAND AND WRIST

Malignant neoplasms of bone and articular cartilage	**C40-C41**
Infectious arthropathies	**M00-M02**
Inflammatory polyarthropathies	**M05-M14**
Osteoarthritis	**M15-M19**
Other joint disorders	**M20-M25**
Dentofacial anomalies [including malocclusion] and other disorders of jaw	**M26-M27**
Systemic connective tissue disorders	**M30-M36**
Deforming dorsopathies	**M40-M43**
Spondylopathies	**M45-M49**
Other dorsopathies	**M50-M54**
Disorders of muscles	**M60-M63**
Disorders of synovium and tendon	**M65-M67**
Other soft tissue disorders	**M70-M79**
Disorders of bone density and structure	**M80-M85**
Other osteopathies	**M86-M90**
Chondropathies	**M91-M94**
Other disorders of the musculoskeletal system and connective tissue	**M95**
Intraoperative and postprocedural complications and disorders of musculoskeletal system, not elsewhere classified	**M96**
Biomechanical lesions, not elsewhere classified	**M99**
Congenital malformations and deformations of the musculoskeletal system	**Q65-Q79**
Symptoms and signs involving the nervous and musculoskeletal systems	**R25-R29**
General symptoms and signs	**R50-R69**
Abnormal findings on diagnostic imaging and in function studies, without diagnosis	**R90-R94**
Injuries to the wrist, hand and fingers	**S60-S69**
Injuries involving multiple body regions	**T07**
Certain early complications of trauma	**T79**
Accidents	**V00-X58**
Persons encountering health services for examinations	**Z00-Z13**
Encounters for other specific health care	**Z40-Z53**

Hand and Wrist

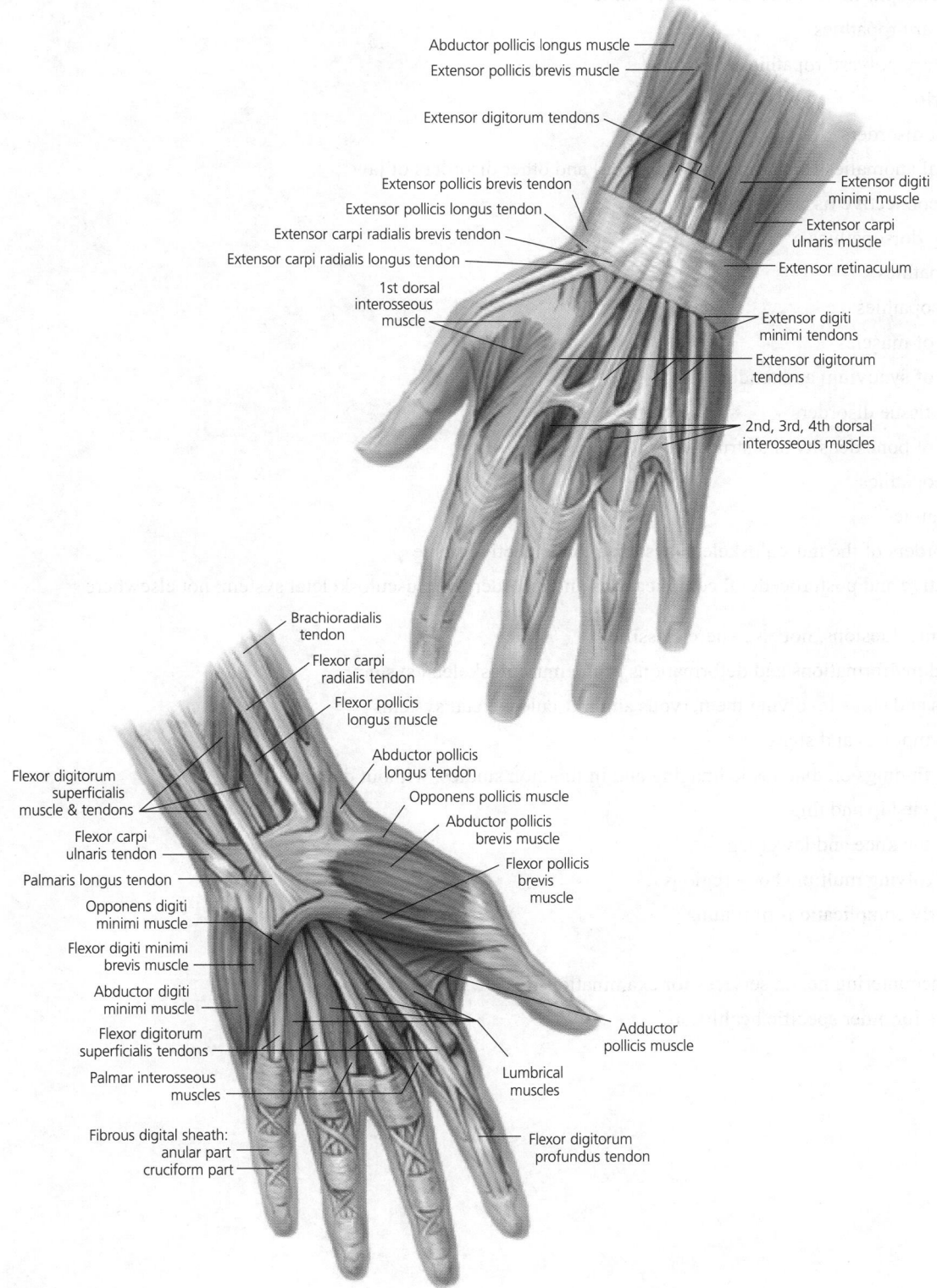

Abductor pollicis longus muscle

Extensor pollicis brevis muscle

Extensor digitorum tendons

Extensor pollicis brevis tendon

Extensor pollicis longus tendon

Extensor carpi radialis brevis tendon

Extensor carpi radialis longus tendon

1st dorsal interosseous muscle

Extensor digiti minimi muscle

Extensor carpi ulnaris muscle

Extensor retinaculum

Extensor digiti minimi tendons

Extensor digitorum tendons

2nd, 3rd, 4th dorsal interosseous muscles

Brachioradialis tendon

Flexor carpi radialis tendon

Flexor pollicis longus muscle

Abductor pollicis longus tendon

Opponens pollicis muscle

Abductor pollicis brevis muscle

Flexor pollicis brevis muscle

Flexor digitorum superficialis muscle & tendons

Flexor carpi ulnaris tendon

Palmaris longus tendon

Opponens digiti minimi muscle

Flexor digiti minimi brevis muscle

Abductor digiti minimi muscle

Flexor digitorum superficialis tendons

Palmar interosseous muscles

Adductor pollicis muscle

Lumbrical muscles

Fibrous digital sheath: anular part cruciform part

Flexor digitorum profundus tendon

©Practice Management Information Corp., Los Angeles, CA

PLATE 8. MUSCULOSKELETAL SYSTEM - HIP AND KNEE

Malignant neoplasms of bone and articular cartilage	**C40-C41**
Infectious arthropathies	**M00-M02**
Inflammatory polyarthropathies	**M05-M14**
Osteoarthritis	**M15-M19**
Other joint disorders	**M20-M25**
Dentofacial anomalies [including malocclusion] and other disorders of jaw	**M26-M27**
Systemic connective tissue disorders	**M30-M36**
Deforming dorsopathies	**M40-M43**
Spondylopathies	**M45-M49**
Other dorsopathies	**M50-M54**
Disorders of muscles	**M60-M63**
Disorders of synovium and tendon	**M65-M67**
Other soft tissue disorders	**M70-M79**
Disorders of bone density and structure	**M80-M85**
Other osteopathies	**M86-M90**
Chondropathies	**M91-M94**
Other disorders of the musculoskeletal system and connective tissue	**M95**
Intraoperative and postprocedural complications and disorders of musculoskeletal system, not elsewhere classified	**M96**
Biomechanical lesions, not elsewhere classified	**M99**
Congenital malformations and deformations of the musculoskeletal system	**Q65-Q79**
Symptoms and signs involving the nervous and musculoskeletal systems	**R25-R29**
General symptoms and signs	**R50-R69**
Abnormal findings on diagnostic imaging and in function studies, without diagnosis	**R90-R94**
Injuries to the hip and thigh	**S70-S79**
Injuries to the knee and lower leg	**S80-S89**
Injuries involving multiple body regions	**T07**
Certain early complications of trauma	**T79**
Accidents	**V00-X58**
Persons encountering health services for examinations	**Z00-Z13**
Encounters for other specific health care	**Z40-Z53**

Hip and Knee
(Anterior View)

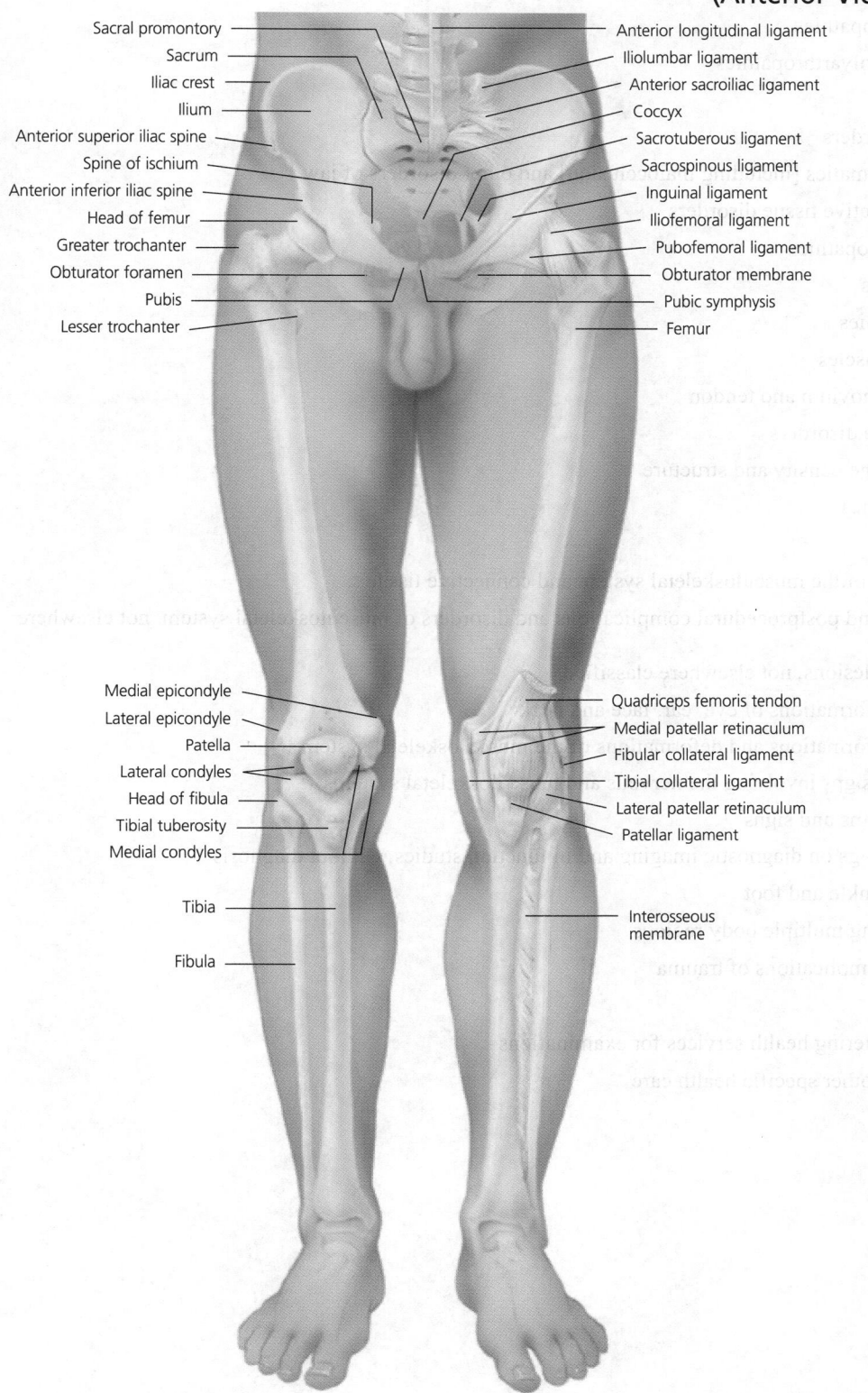

Sacral promontory
Sacrum
Iliac crest
Ilium
Anterior superior iliac spine
Spine of ischium
Anterior inferior iliac spine
Head of femur
Greater trochanter
Obturator foramen
Pubis
Lesser trochanter

Anterior longitudinal ligament
Iliolumbar ligament
Anterior sacroiliac ligament
Coccyx
Sacrotuberous ligament
Sacrospinous ligament
Inguinal ligament
Iliofemoral ligament
Pubofemoral ligament
Obturator membrane
Pubic symphysis
Femur

Medial epicondyle
Lateral epicondyle
Patella
Lateral condyles
Head of fibula
Tibial tuberosity
Medial condyles
Tibia
Fibula

Quadriceps femoris tendon
Medial patellar retinaculum
Fibular collateral ligament
Tibial collateral ligament
Lateral patellar retinaculum
Patellar ligament
Interosseous membrane

©Scientific Publishing Ltd., Rolling Meadows, IL

PLATE 9. MUSCULOSKELETAL SYSTEM – FOOT AND ANKLE

Malignant neoplasms of bone and articular cartilage	**C40-C41**
Infectious arthropathies	**M00-M02**
Inflammatory polyarthropathies	**M05-M14**
Osteoarthritis	**M15-M19**
Other joint disorders	**M20-M25**
Dentofacial anomalies [including malocclusion] and other disorders of jaw	**M26-M27**
Systemic connective tissue disorders	**M30-M36**
Deforming dorsopathies	**M40-M43**
Spondylopathies	**M45-M49**
Other dorsopathies	**M50-M54**
Disorders of muscles	**M60-M63**
Disorders of synovium and tendon	**M65-M67**
Other soft tissue disorders	**M70-M79**
Disorders of bone density and structure	**M80-M85**
Other osteopathies	**M86-M90**
Chondropathies	**M91-M94**
Other disorders of the musculoskeletal system and connective tissue	**M95**
Intraoperative and postprocedural complications and disorders of musculoskeletal system, not elsewhere classified	**M96**
Biomechanical lesions, not elsewhere classified	**M99**
Congenital malformations of eye, ear, face and neck	**Q10-Q18**
Congenital malformations and deformations of the musculoskeletal system	**Q65-Q79**
Symptoms and signs involving the nervous and musculoskeletal systems	**R25-R29**
General symptoms and signs	**R50-R69**
Abnormal findings on diagnostic imaging and in function studies, without diagnosis	**R90-R94**
Injuries to the ankle and foot	**S90-S99**
Injuries involving multiple body regions	**T07**
Certain early complications of trauma	**T79**
Accidents	**V00-X58**
Persons encountering health services for examinations	**Z00-Z13**
Encounters for other specific health care	**Z40-Z53**

Foot and Ankle

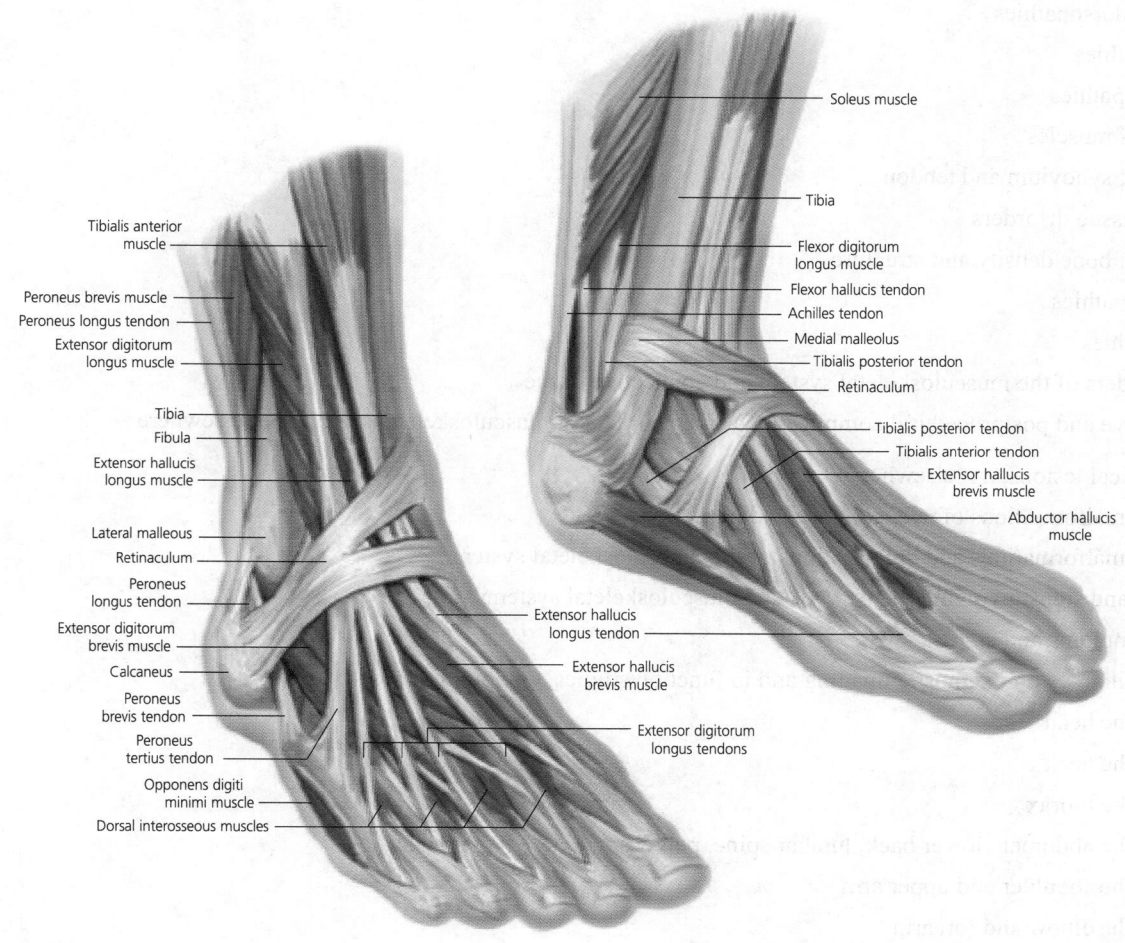

Tibialis anterior muscle

Peroneus brevis muscle
Peroneus longus tendon
Extensor digitorum longus muscle

Tibia
Fibula
Extensor hallucis longus muscle

Lateral malleous
Retinaculum
Peroneus longus tendon
Extensor digitorum brevis muscle
Calcaneus
Peroneus brevis tendon
Peroneus tertius tendon
Opponens digiti minimi muscle
Dorsal interosseous muscles

Extensor hallucis longus tendon
Extensor hallucis brevis muscle
Extensor digitorum longus tendons

Soleus muscle

Tibia
Flexor digitorum longus muscle
Flexor hallucis tendon
Achilles tendon
Medial malleolus
Tibialis posterior tendon
Retinaculum

Tibialis posterior tendon
Tibialis anterior tendon
Extensor hallucis brevis muscle
Abductor hallucis muscle

©Practice Management Information Corp., Los Angeles, CA

PLATE 10. SKELETAL SYSTEM - ANTERIOR VIEW

Malignant neoplasms of bone and articular cartilage	**C40-C41**
Infectious arthropathies	**M00-M02**
Inflammatory polyarthropathies	**M05-M14**
Osteoarthritis	**M15-M19**
Other joint disorders	**M20-M25**
Dentofacial anomalies [including malocclusion] and other disorders of jaw	**M26-M27**
Systemic connective tissue disorders	**M30-M36**
Deforming dorsopathies	**M40-M43**
Spondylopathies	**M45-M49**
Other dorsopathies	**M50-M54**
Disorders of muscles	**M60-M63**
Disorders of synovium and tendon	**M65-M67**
Other soft tissue disorders	**M70-M79**
Disorders of bone density and structure	**M80-M85**
Other osteopathies	**M86-M90**
Chondropathies	**M91-M94**
Other disorders of the musculoskeletal system and connective tissue	**M95**
Intraoperative and postprocedural complications and disorders of musculoskeletal system, not elsewhere classified	**M96**
Biomechanical lesions, not elsewhere classified	**M99**
Congenital malformations of eye, ear, face and neck	**Q10-Q18**
Congenital malformations and deformations of the musculoskeletal system	**Q65-Q79**
Symptoms and signs involving the nervous and musculoskeletal systems	**R25-R29**
General symptoms and signs	**R50-R69**
Abnormal findings on diagnostic imaging and in function studies, without diagnosis	**R90-R94**
Injuries to the head	**S00-S09**
Injuries to the neck	**S10-S19**
Injuries to the thorax	**S20-S29**
Injuries to the abdomen, lower back, lumbar spine, pelvis and external genitals	**S30-S39**
Injuries to the shoulder and upper arm	**S40-S49**
Injuries to the elbow and forearm	**S50-S59**
Injuries to the wrist, hand and fingers	**S60-S69**
Injuries to the hip and thigh	**S70-S79**
Injuries to the knee and lower leg	**S80-S89**
Injuries to the ankle and foot	**S90-S99**
Injuries involving multiple body regions	**T07**
Certain early complications of trauma	**T79**
Accidents	**V00-X58**
Persons encountering health services for examinations	**Z00-Z13**
Encounters for other specific health care	**Z40-Z53**

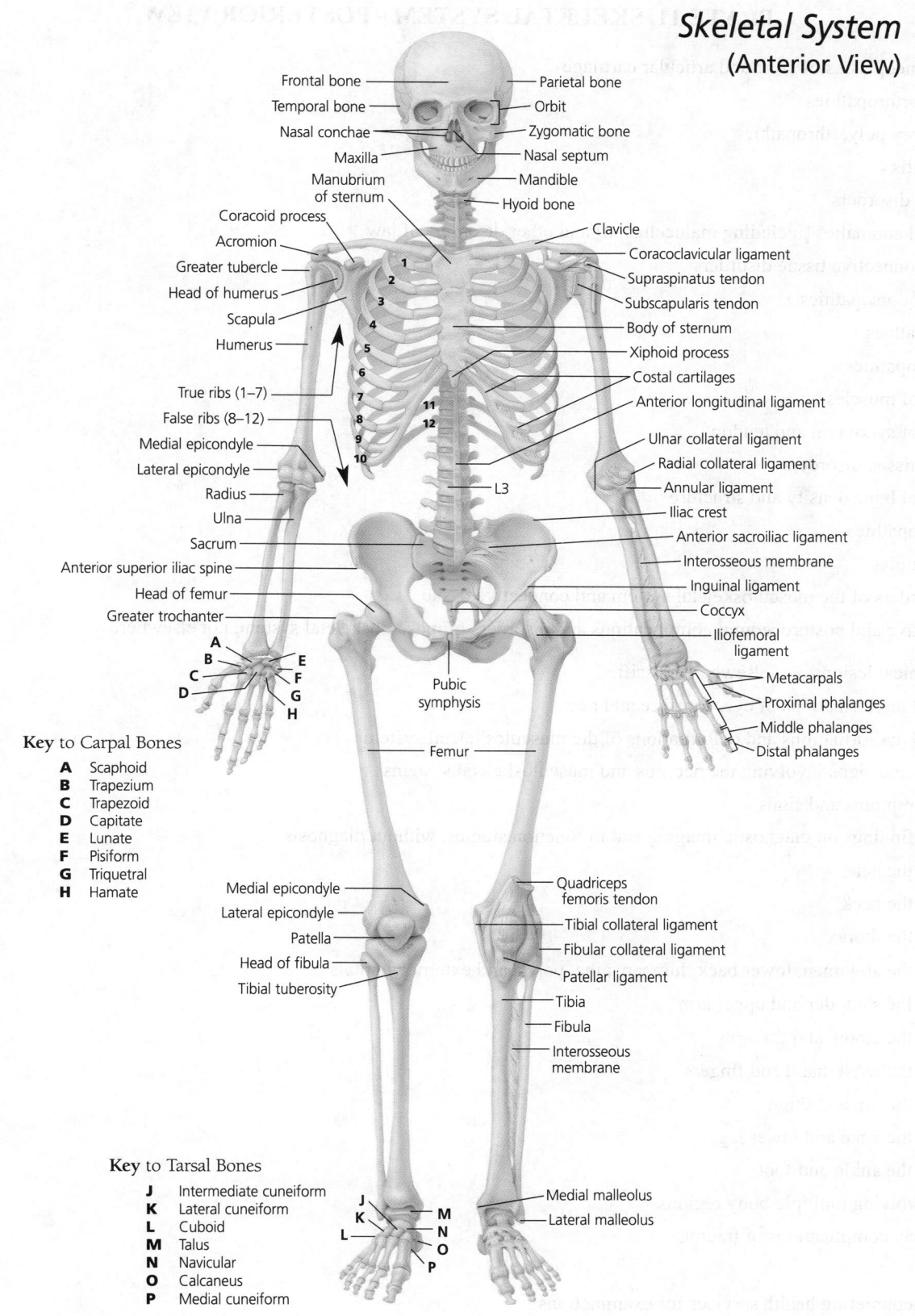

Skeletal System
(Anterior View)

Frontal bone
Temporal bone
Nasal conchae
Maxilla
Manubrium of sternum
Coracoid process
Acromion
Greater tubercle
Head of humerus
Scapula
Humerus
True ribs (1–7)
False ribs (8–12)
Medial epicondyle
Lateral epicondyle
Radius
Ulna
Sacrum
Anterior superior iliac spine
Head of femur
Greater trochanter

Parietal bone
Orbit
Zygomatic bone
Nasal septum
Mandible
Hyoid bone
Clavicle
Coracoclavicular ligament
Supraspinatus tendon
Subscapularis tendon
Body of sternum
Xiphoid process
Costal cartilages
Anterior longitudinal ligament
Ulnar collateral ligament
Radial collateral ligament
Annular ligament
Iliac crest
Anterior sacroiliac ligament
Interosseous membrane
Inguinal ligament
Coccyx
Iliofemoral ligament
Metacarpals
Proximal phalanges
Middle phalanges
Distal phalanges

L3

Pubic symphysis

Femur

Key to Carpal Bones

A Scaphoid
B Trapezium
C Trapezoid
D Capitate
E Lunate
F Pisiform
G Triquetral
H Hamate

Medial epicondyle
Lateral epicondyle
Patella
Head of fibula
Tibial tuberosity

Quadriceps femoris tendon
Tibial collateral ligament
Fibular collateral ligament
Patellar ligament
Tibia
Fibula
Interosseous membrane

Key to Tarsal Bones

J Intermediate cuneiform
K Lateral cuneiform
L Cuboid
M Talus
N Navicular
O Calcaneus
P Medial cuneiform

Medial malleolus
Lateral malleolus

©Scientific Publishing Ltd., Rolling Meadows, IL

PLATE 11. SKELETAL SYSTEM - POSTERIOR VIEW

Malignant neoplasms of bone and articular cartilage	**C40-C41**
Infectious arthropathies	**M00-M02**
Inflammatory polyarthropathies	**M05-M14**
Osteoarthritis	**M15-M19**
Other joint disorders	**M20-M25**
Dentofacial anomalies [including malocclusion] and other disorders of jaw	**M26-M27**
Systemic connective tissue disorders	**M30-M36**
Deforming dorsopathies	**M40-M43**
Spondylopathies	**M45-M49**
Other dorsopathies	**M50-M54**
Disorders of muscles	**M60-M63**
Disorders of synovium and tendon	**M65-M67**
Other soft tissue disorders	**M70-M79**
Disorders of bone density and structure	**M80-M85**
Other osteopathies	**M86-M90**
Chondropathies	**M91-M94**
Other disorders of the musculoskeletal system and connective tissue	**M95**
Intraoperative and postprocedural complications and disorders of musculoskeletal system, not elsewhere classified	**M96**
Biomechanical lesions, not elsewhere classified	**M99**
Congenital malformations of eye, ear, face and neck	**Q10-Q18**
Congenital malformations and deformations of the musculoskeletal system	**Q65-Q79**
Symptoms and signs involving the nervous and musculoskeletal systems	**R25-R29**
General symptoms and signs	**R50-R69**
Abnormal findings on diagnostic imaging and in function studies, without diagnosis	**R90-R94**
Injuries to the head	**S00-S09**
Injuries to the neck	**S10-S19**
Injuries to the thorax	**S20-S29**
Injuries to the abdomen, lower back, lumbar spine, pelvis and external genitals	**S30-S39**
Injuries to the shoulder and upper arm	**S40-S49**
Injuries to the elbow and forearm	**S50-S59**
Injuries to the wrist, hand and fingers	**S60-S69**
Injuries to the hip and thigh	**S70-S79**
Injuries to the knee and lower leg	**S80-S89**
Injuries to the ankle and foot	**S90-S99**
Injuries involving multiple body regions	**T07**
Certain early complications of trauma	**T79**
Accidents	**V00-X58**
Persons encountering health services for examinations	**Z00-Z13**
Encounters for other specific health care	**Z40-Z53**

Skeletal System
(Posterior View)

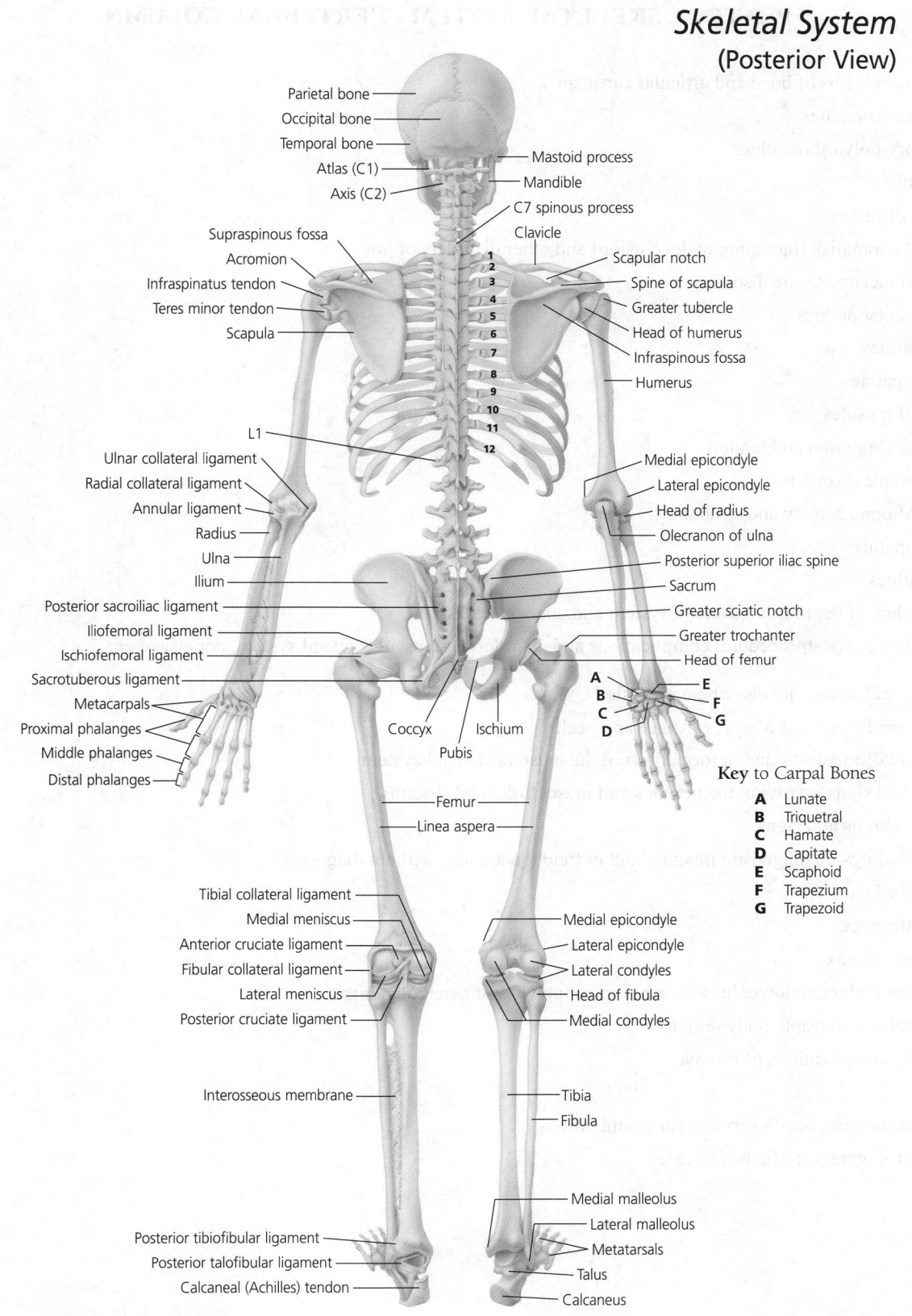

Parietal bone
Occipital bone
Temporal bone
Atlas (C1)
Axis (C2)
Mastoid process
Mandible
C7 spinous process
Clavicle
Supraspinous fossa
Acromion
Infraspinatus tendon
Teres minor tendon
Scapula
Scapular notch
Spine of scapula
Greater tubercle
Head of humerus
Infraspinous fossa
Humerus

1
2
3
4
5
6
7
8
9
10
11
12

L1
Ulnar collateral ligament
Radial collateral ligament
Annular ligament
Radius
Ulna
Ilium
Posterior sacroiliac ligament
Iliofemoral ligament
Ischiofemoral ligament
Sacrotuberous ligament
Metacarpals
Proximal phalanges
Middle phalanges
Distal phalanges

Medial epicondyle
Lateral epicondyle
Head of radius
Olecranon of ulna
Posterior superior iliac spine
Sacrum
Greater sciatic notch
Greater trochanter
Head of femur

A
B
C
D
E
F
G

Coccyx
Ischium
Pubis

Femur
Linea aspera

Tibial collateral ligament
Medial meniscus
Anterior cruciate ligament
Fibular collateral ligament
Lateral meniscus
Posterior cruciate ligament

Medial epicondyle
Lateral epicondyle
Lateral condyles
Head of fibula
Medial condyles

Interosseous membrane

Tibia
Fibula

Key to Carpal Bones

A Lunate
B Triquetral
C Hamate
D Capitate
E Scaphoid
F Trapezium
G Trapezoid

Medial malleolus
Lateral malleolus
Metatarsals
Talus
Calcaneus

Posterior tibiofibular ligament
Posterior talofibular ligament
Calcaneal (Achilles) tendon

©Scientific Publishing Ltd., Rolling Meadows, IL

PLATE 12. SKELETAL SYSTEM - VERTEBRAL COLUMN

Malignant neoplasms of bone and articular cartilage	**C40-C41**
Infectious arthropathies	**M00-M02**
Inflammatory polyarthropathies	**M05-M14**
Osteoarthritis	**M15-M19**
Other joint disorders	**M20-M25**
Dentofacial anomalies [including malocclusion] and other disorders of jaw	**M26-M27**
Systemic connective tissue disorders	**M30-M36**
Deforming dorsopathies	**M40-M43**
Spondylopathies	**M45-M49**
Other dorsopathies	**M50-M54**
Disorders of muscles	**M60-M63**
Disorders of synovium and tendon	**M65-M67**
Other soft tissue disorders	**M70-M79**
Disorders of bone density and structure	**M80-M85**
Other osteopathies	**M86-M90**
Chondropathies	**M91-M94**
Other disorders of the musculoskeletal system and connective tissue	**M95**
Intraoperative and postprocedural complications and disorders of musculoskeletal system, not elsewhere classified	**M96**
Biomechanical lesions, not elsewhere classified	**M99**
Congenital malformations of eye, ear, face and neck	**Q10-Q18**
Congenital malformations and deformations of the musculoskeletal system	**Q65-Q79**
Symptoms and signs involving the nervous and musculoskeletal systems	**R25-R29**
General symptoms and signs	**R50-R69**
Abnormal findings on diagnostic imaging and in function studies, without diagnosis	**R90-R94**
Injuries to the head	**S00-S09**
Injuries to the neck	**S10-S19**
Injuries to the thorax	**S20-S29**
Injuries to the abdomen, lower back, lumbar spine, pelvis and external genitals	**S30-S39**
Injuries involving multiple body regions	**T07**
Certain early complications of trauma	**T79**
Accidents	**V00-X58**
Persons encountering health services for examinations	**Z00-Z13**
Encounters for other specific health care	**Z40-Z53**

Vertebral Column
(Lateral View)

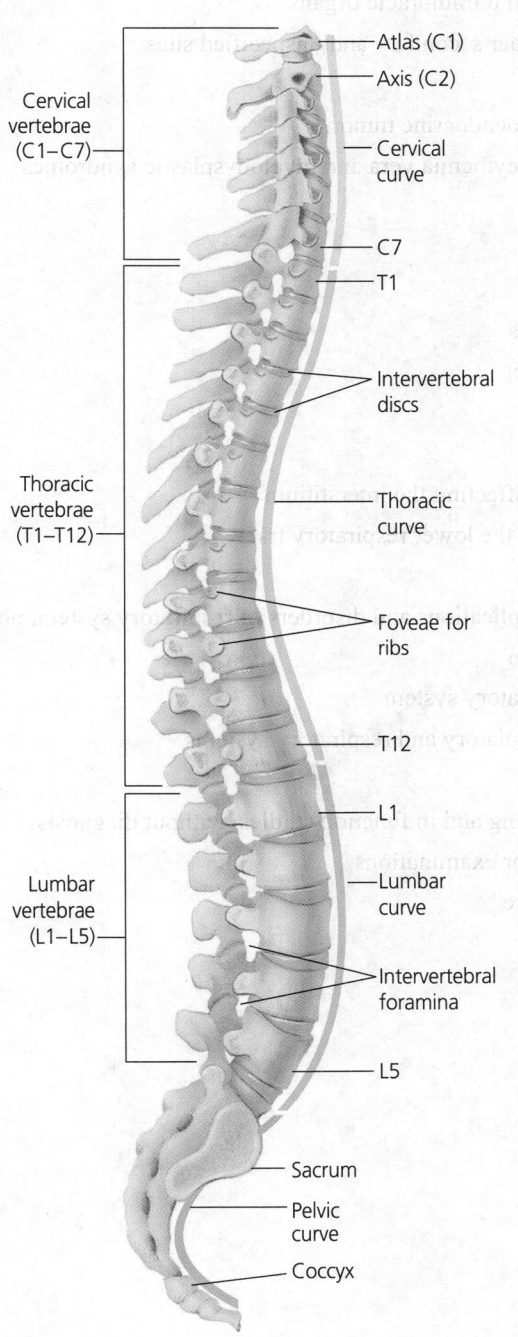

Atlas (C1)

Axis (C2)

Cervical vertebrae (C1–C7)

Cervical curve

C7

T1

Intervertebral discs

Thoracic vertebrae (T1–T12)

Thoracic curve

Foveae for ribs

T12

Lumbar vertebrae (L1–L5)

L1

Lumbar curve

Intervertebral foramina

L5

Sacrum

Pelvic curve

Coccyx

©Scientific Publishing Ltd., Rolling Meadows, IL

PLATE 13. RESPIRATORY SYSTEM

Tuberculosis   **A15-A19**

Bacterial and viral infectious agents   **B95-B97**

Malignant neoplasms of respiratory and intrathoracic organs   **C30-C39**

Malignant neoplasms of ill-defined, other secondary and unspecified sites   **C76-C80**

In situ neoplasms   **D00-D09**

Benign neoplasms, except benign neuroendocrine tumors   **D10-D36**

Neoplasms of uncertain behavior, polycythemia vera and myelodysplastic syndromes   **D37-D48**

Neoplasms of unspecified behavior   **D49**

Acute upper respiratory infections   **J00-J06**

Influenza and pneumonia   **J09-J18**

Other acute lower respiratory infections   **J20-J22**

Other diseases of upper respiratory tract   **J30-J39**

Chronic lower respiratory diseases   **J40-J47**

Lung diseases due to external agents   **J60-J70**

Other respiratory diseases principally affecting the interstitium   **J80-J84**

Suppurative and necrotic conditions of the lower respiratory tract   **J85-J86**

Other diseases of the pleura   **J90-J94**

Intraoperative and postprocedural complications and disorders of respiratory system, not elsewhere classified   **J95**

Other diseases of the respiratory system   **J96-J99**

Congenital malformations of the respiratory system   **Q30-Q34**

Symptoms and signs involving the circulatory and respiratory systems   **R00-R09**

General symptoms and signs   **R50-R69**

Abnormal findings on diagnostic imaging and in function studies, without diagnosis   **R90-R94**

Persons encountering health services for examinations   **Z00-Z13**

Encounters for other specific health care   **Z40-Z53**

Respiratory System

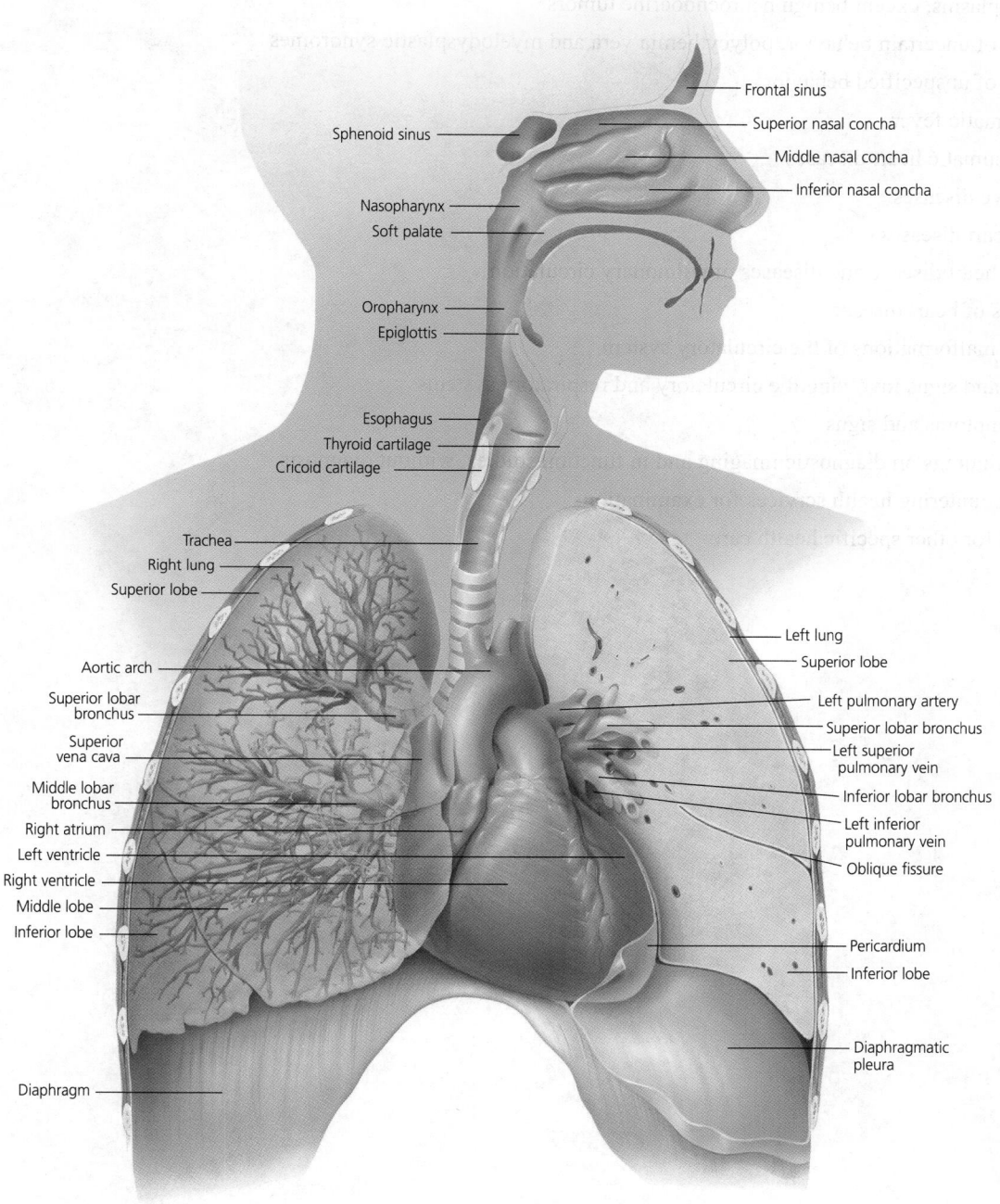

Frontal sinus

Sphenoid sinus

Superior nasal concha

Middle nasal concha

Inferior nasal concha

Nasopharynx

Soft palate

Oropharynx

Epiglottis

Esophagus

Thyroid cartilage

Cricoid cartilage

Trachea

Right lung

Superior lobe

Aortic arch

Superior lobar bronchus

Superior vena cava

Middle lobar bronchus

Right atrium

Left ventricle

Right ventricle

Middle lobe

Inferior lobe

Diaphragm

Left lung

Superior lobe

Left pulmonary artery

Superior lobar bronchus

Left superior pulmonary vein

Inferior lobar bronchus

Left inferior pulmonary vein

Oblique fissure

Pericardium

Inferior lobe

Diaphragmatic pleura

©Scientific Publishing Ltd., Rolling Meadows, IL

PLATE 14. HEART AND PERICARDIUM

Bacterial and viral infectious agents	**B95-B97**
Malignant neoplasms of ill-defined, other secondary and unspecified sites	**C76-C80**
In situ neoplasms	**D00-D09**
Benign neoplasms, except benign neuroendocrine tumors	**D10-D36**
Neoplasms of uncertain behavior, polycythemia vera and myelodysplastic syndromes	**D37-D48**
Neoplasms of unspecified behavior	**D49**
Acute rheumatic fever	**I00-I02**
Chronic rheumatic heart diseases	**I05-I09**
Hypertensive diseases	**I10-I15**
Ischemic heart diseases	**I20-I25**
Pulmonary heart disease and diseases of pulmonary circulation	**I26-I28**
Other forms of heart disease	**I30-I52**
Congenital malformations of the circulatory system	**Q20-Q28**
Symptoms and signs involving the circulatory and respiratory systems	**R00-R09**
General symptoms and signs	**R50-R69**
Abnormal findings on diagnostic imaging and in function studies, without diagnosis	**R90-R94**
Persons encountering health services for examinations	**Z00-Z13**
Encounters for other specific health care	**Z40-Z53**

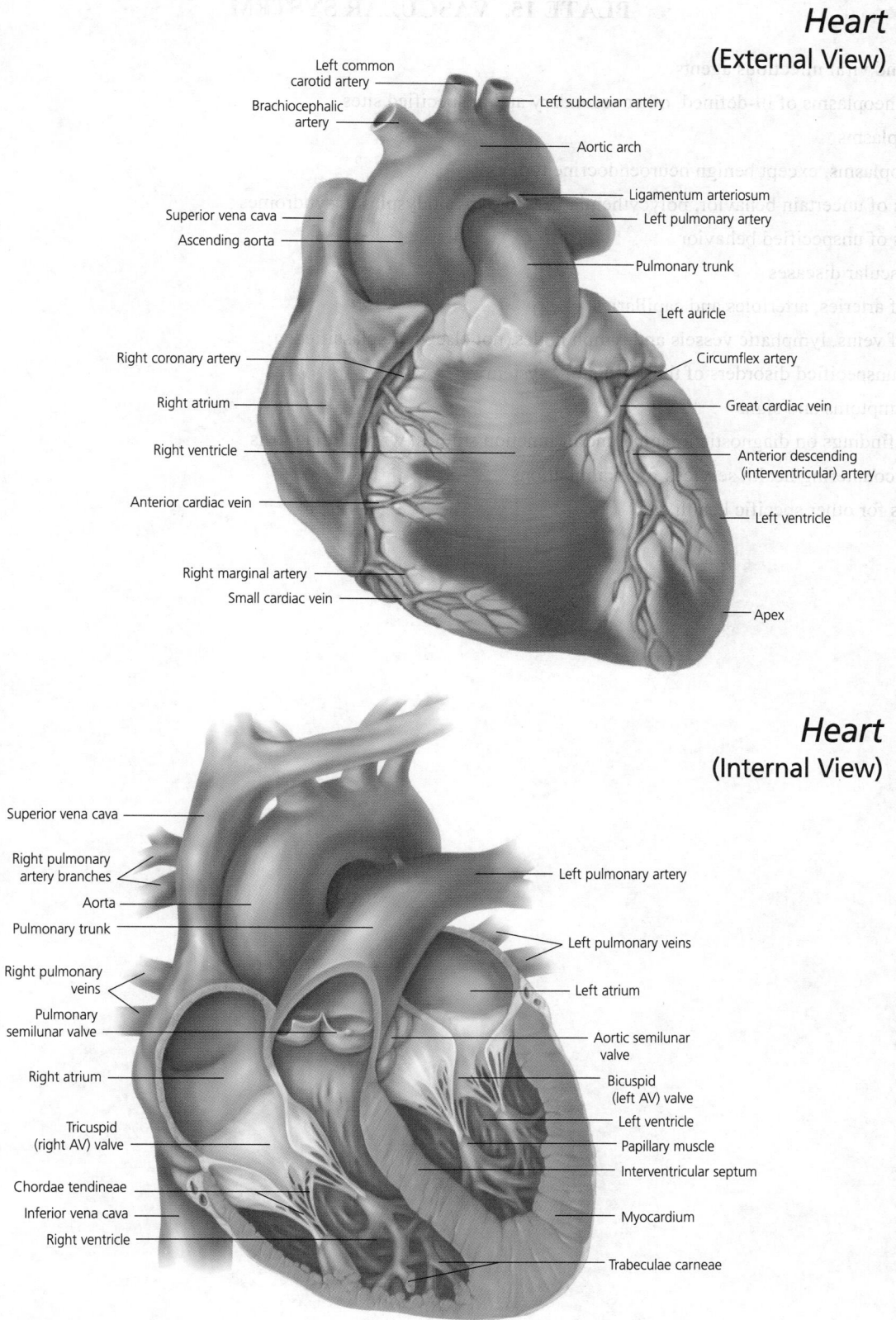

Heart
(External View)

Left common carotid artery

Brachiocephalic artery

Left subclavian artery

Aortic arch

Ligamentum arteriosum

Superior vena cava

Ascending aorta

Left pulmonary artery

Pulmonary trunk

Left auricle

Right coronary artery

Circumflex artery

Right atrium

Great cardiac vein

Right ventricle

Anterior descending (interventricular) artery

Left ventricle

Anterior cardiac vein

Right marginal artery

Small cardiac vein

Apex

Heart
(Internal View)

Superior vena cava

Right pulmonary artery branches

Left pulmonary artery

Aorta

Pulmonary trunk

Left pulmonary veins

Right pulmonary veins

Left atrium

Pulmonary semilunar valve

Aortic semilunar valve

Right atrium

Bicuspid (left AV) valve

Left ventricle

Tricuspid (right AV) valve

Papillary muscle

Interventricular septum

Chordae tendineae

Myocardium

Inferior vena cava

Right ventricle

Trabeculae carneae

©Scientific Publishing Ltd., Rolling Meadows, IL

PLATE 15. VASCULAR SYSTEM

Bacterial and viral infectious agents	**B95-B97**
Malignant neoplasms of ill-defined, other secondary and unspecified sites	**C76-C80**
In situ neoplasms	**D00-D09**
Benign neoplasms, except benign neuroendocrine tumors	**D10-D36**
Neoplasms of uncertain behavior, polycythemia vera and myelodysplastic syndromes	**D37-D48**
Neoplasms of unspecified behavior	**D49**
Cerebrovascular diseases	**I60-I69**
Diseases of arteries, arterioles and capillaries	**I70-I79**
Diseases of veins, lymphatic vessels and lymph nodes, not elsewhere classified	**I80-I89**
Other and unspecified disorders of the circulatory system	**I95-I99**
General symptoms and signs	**R50-R69**
Abnormal findings on diagnostic imaging and in function studies, without diagnosis	**R90-R94**
Persons encountering health services for examinations	**Z00-Z13**
Encounters for other specific health care	**Z40-Z53**

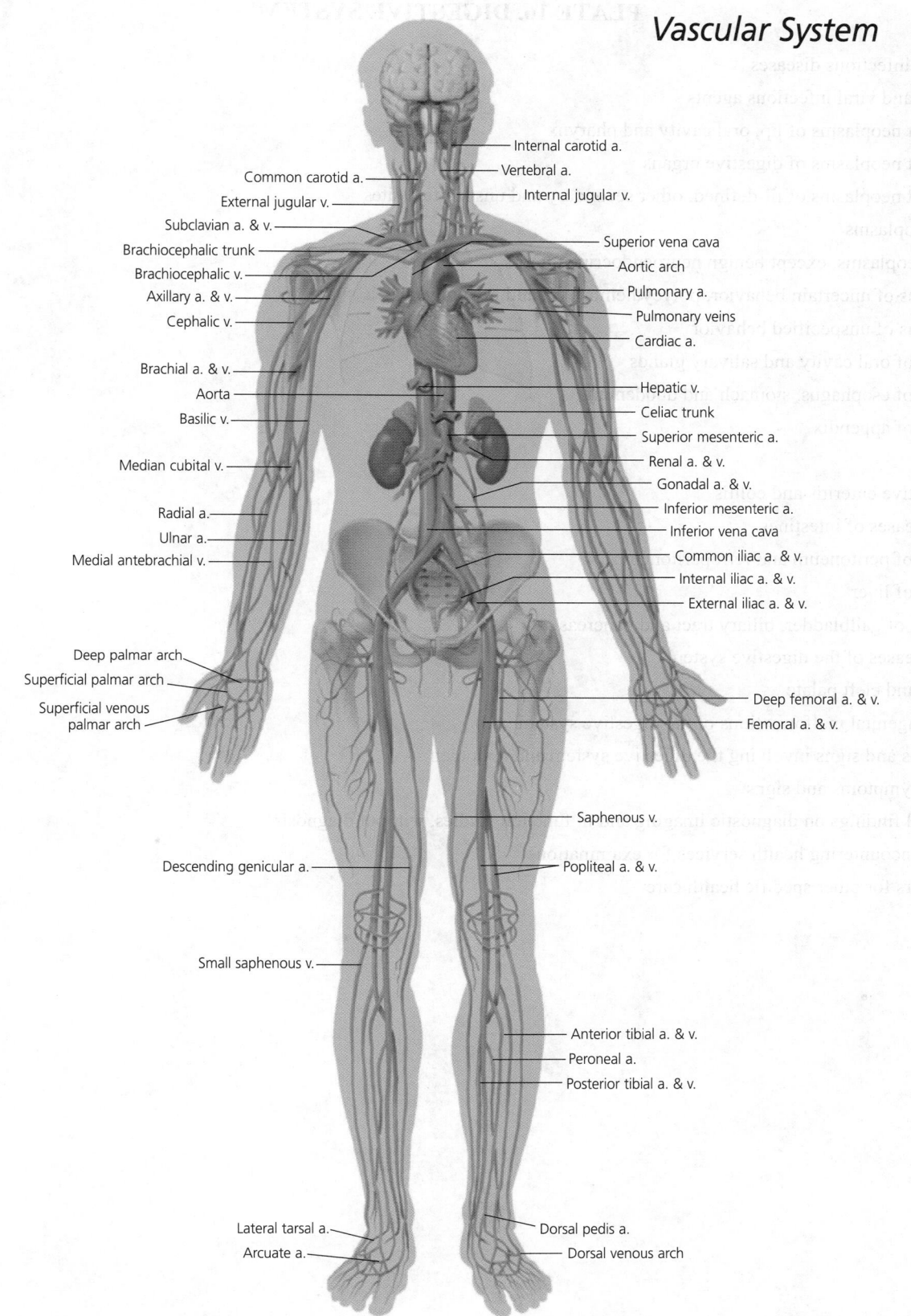

Vascular System

Internal carotid a.

Common carotid a.

Vertebral a.

External jugular v.

Internal jugular v.

Subclavian a. & v.

Brachiocephalic trunk

Superior vena cava

Brachiocephalic v.

Aortic arch

Axillary a. & v.

Pulmonary a.

Cephalic v.

Pulmonary veins

Cardiac a.

Brachial a. & v.

Aorta

Hepatic v.

Basilic v.

Celiac trunk

Superior mesenteric a.

Median cubital v.

Renal a. & v.

Gonadal a. & v.

Radial a.

Inferior mesenteric a.

Ulnar a.

Inferior vena cava

Medial antebrachial v.

Common iliac a. & v.

Internal iliac a. & v.

External iliac a. & v.

Deep palmar arch

Superficial palmar arch

Superficial venous
palmar arch

Deep femoral a. & v.

Femoral a. & v.

Saphenous v.

Descending genicular a.

Popliteal a. & v.

Small saphenous v.

Anterior tibial a. & v.

Peroneal a.

Posterior tibial a. & v.

Lateral tarsal a.

Dorsal pedis a.

Arcuate a.

Dorsal venous arch

©Practice Management Information Corp., Los Angeles, CA

PLATE 16. DIGESTIVE SYSTEM

Intestinal infectious diseases	**A00-A09**
Bacterial and viral infectious agents	**B95-B97**
Malignant neoplasms of lip, oral cavity and pharynx	**C00-C14**
Malignant neoplasms of digestive organs	**C15-C26**
Malignant neoplasms of ill-defined, other secondary and unspecified sites	**C76-C80**
In situ neoplasms	**D00-D09**
Benign neoplasms, except benign neuroendocrine tumors	**D10-D36**
Neoplasms of uncertain behavior, polycythemia vera and myelodysplastic syndromes	**D37-D48**
Neoplasms of unspecified behavior	**D49**
Diseases of oral cavity and salivary glands	**K00-K14**
Diseases of esophagus, stomach and duodenum	**K20-K31**
Diseases of appendix	**K35-K38**
Hernia	**K40-K46**
Noninfective enteritis and colitis	**K50-K52**
Other diseases of intestines	**K55-K64**
Diseases of peritoneum and retroperitoneum	**K65-K68**
Diseases of liver	**K70-K77**
Disorders of gallbladder, biliary tract and pancreas	**K80-K87**
Other diseases of the digestive system	**K90-K95**
Cleft lip and cleft palate	**Q35-Q37**
Other congenital malformations of the digestive system	**Q38-Q45**
Symptoms and signs involving the digestive system and abdomen	**R10-R19**
General symptoms and signs	**R50-R69**
Abnormal findings on diagnostic imaging and in function studies, without diagnosis	**R90-R94**
Persons encountering health services for examinations	**Z00-Z13**
Encounters for other specific health care	**Z40-Z53**

Digestive System

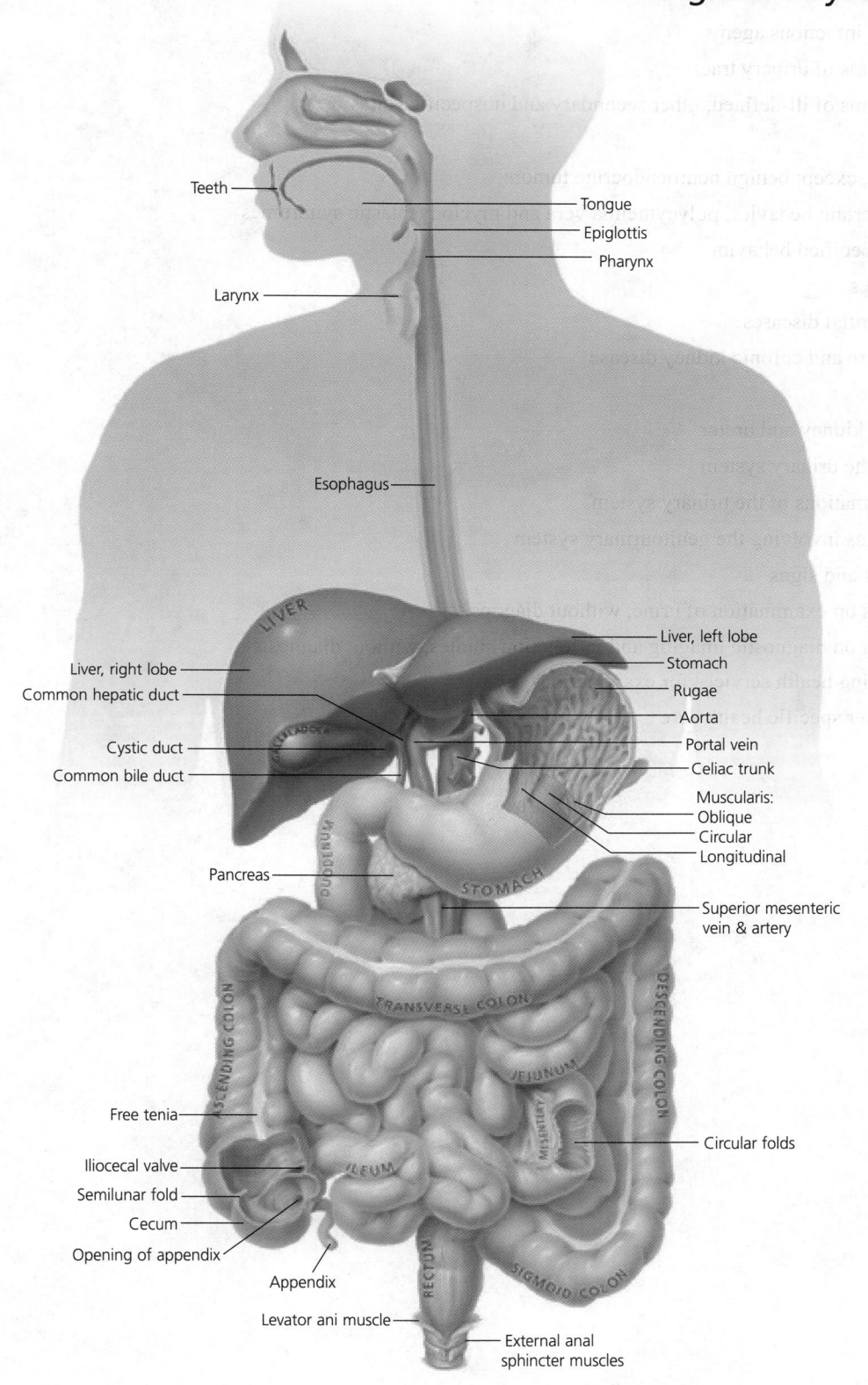

Teeth

Tongue

Epiglottis

Pharynx

Larynx

Esophagus

LIVER

Liver, left lobe

Stomach

Liver, right lobe

Rugae

Common hepatic duct

Aorta

Cystic duct

Portal vein

Common bile duct

Celiac trunk

Muscularis:
Oblique
Circular
Longitudinal

Pancreas

STOMACH

Superior mesenteric
vein & artery

ASCENDING COLON

TRANSVERSE COLON

DESCENDING COLON

JEJUNUM

Free tenia

MESENTERY

Circular folds

Iliocecal valve

ILEUM

Semilunar fold

Cecum

Opening of appendix

Appendix

RECTUM

SIGMOID COLON

Levator ani muscle

External anal
sphincter muscles

©Practice Management Information Corp., Los Angeles, CA

PLATE 17. GENITOURINARY SYSTEM

Bacterial and viral infectious agents	**B95-B97**
Malignant neoplasms of urinary tract	**C64-C68**
Malignant neoplasms of ill-defined, other secondary and unspecified sites	**C76-C80**
In situ neoplasms	**D00-D09**
Benign neoplasms, except benign neuroendocrine tumors	**D10-D36**
Neoplasms of uncertain behavior, polycythemia vera and myelodysplastic syndromes	**D37-D48**
Neoplasms of unspecified behavior	**D49**
Glomerular diseases	**N00-N08**
Renal tubulointerstitial diseases	**N10-N16**
Acute kidney failure and chronic kidney disease	**N17-N19**
Urolithiasis	**N20-N23**
Other disorders of kidney and ureter	**N25-N29**
Other diseases of the urinary system	**N30-N39**
Congenital malformations of the urinary system	**Q60-Q64**
Symptoms and signs involving the genitourinary system	**R30-R39**
General symptoms and signs	**R50-R69**
Abnormal findings on examination of urine, without diagnosis	**R80-R82**
Abnormal findings on diagnostic imaging and in function studies, without diagnosis	**R90-R94**
Persons encountering health services for examinations	**Z00-Z13**
Encounters for other specific health care	**Z40-Z53**

Urinary System

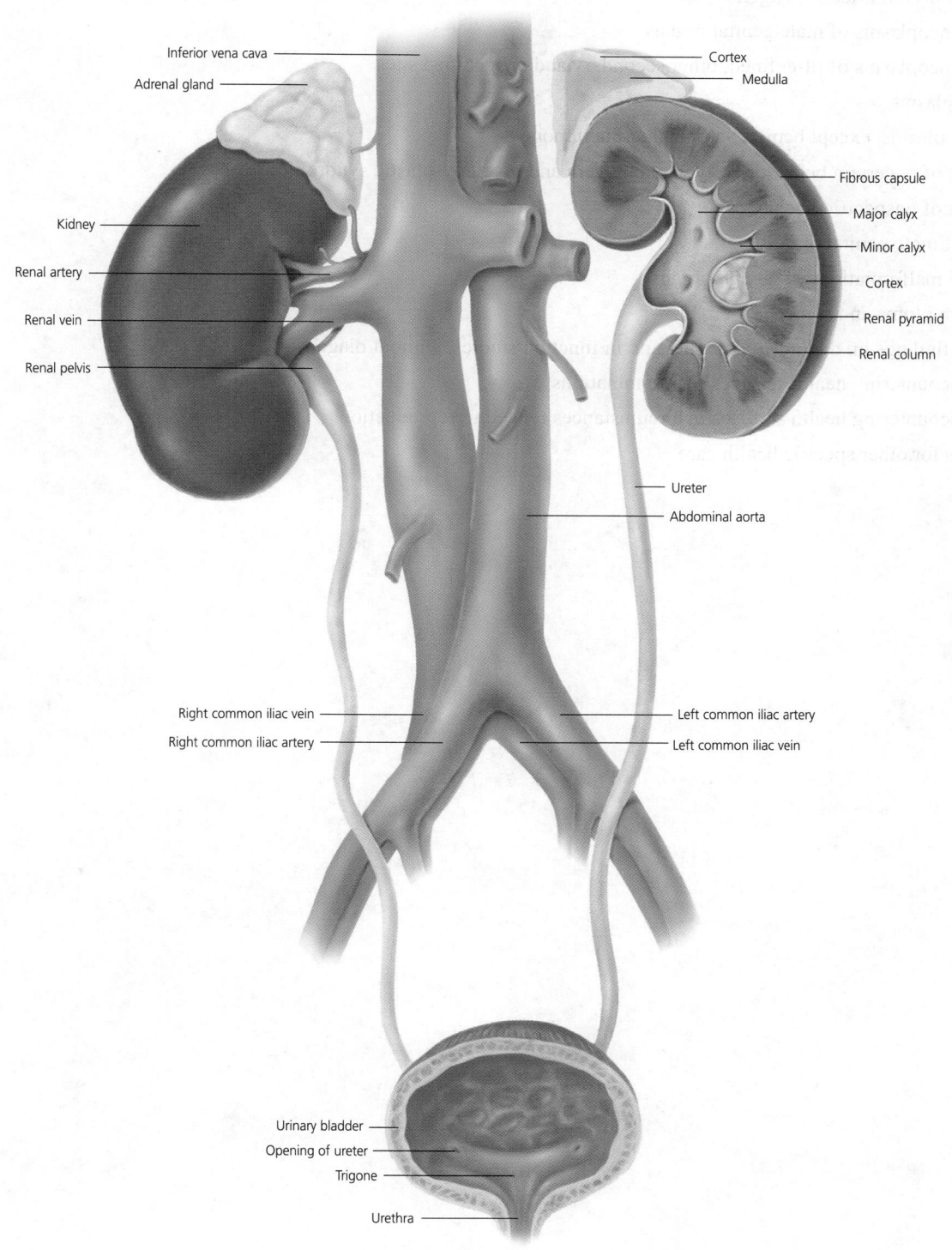

Inferior vena cava

Adrenal gland

Cortex

Medulla

Kidney

Fibrous capsule

Renal artery

Major calyx

Renal vein

Minor calyx

Renal pelvis

Cortex

Renal pyramid

Renal column

Ureter

Abdominal aorta

Right common iliac vein

Left common iliac artery

Right common iliac artery

Left common iliac vein

Urinary bladder

Opening of ureter

Trigone

Urethra

©Practice Management Information Corp., Los Angeles, CA

PLATE 18. MALE REPRODUCTIVE SYSTEM

Infections with a predominantly sexual mode of transmission	**A50-A64**
Bacterial and viral infectious agents	**B95-B97**
Malignant neoplasms of male genital organs	**C60-C63**
Malignant neoplasms of ill-defined, other secondary and unspecified sites	**C76-C80**
In situ neoplasms	**D00-D09**
Benign neoplasms, except benign neuroendocrine tumors	**D10-D36**
Neoplasms of uncertain behavior, polycythemia vera and myelodysplastic syndromes	**D37-D48**
Neoplasms of unspecified behavior	**D49**
Diseases of male genital organs	**N40-N53**
Congenital malformations of genital organs	**Q50-Q56**
General symptoms and signs	**R50-R69**
Abnormal findings on diagnostic imaging and in function studies, without diagnosis	**R90-R94**
Persons encountering health services for examinations	**Z00-Z13**
Persons encountering health services in circumstances related to reproduction	**Z30-Z39**
Encounters for other specific health care	**Z40-Z53**

Male Reproductive System

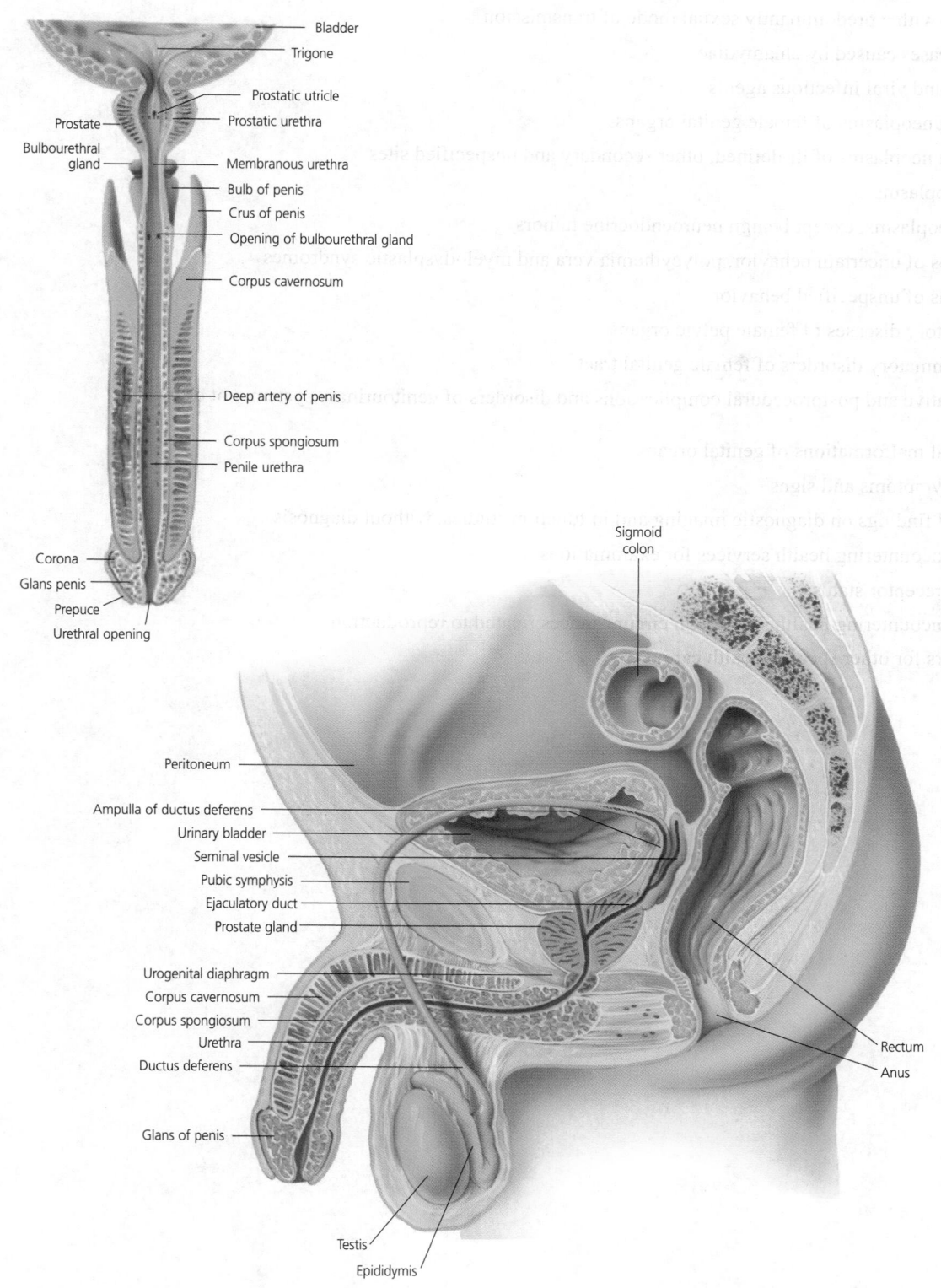

Bladder
Trigone
Prostatic utricle
Prostate
Prostatic urethra
Bulbourethral gland
Membranous urethra
Bulb of penis
Crus of penis
Opening of bulbourethral gland
Corpus cavernosum
Deep artery of penis
Corpus spongiosum
Penile urethra
Corona
Glans penis
Prepuce
Urethral opening

Sigmoid colon

Peritoneum
Ampulla of ductus deferens
Urinary bladder
Seminal vesicle
Pubic symphysis
Ejaculatory duct
Prostate gland
Urogenital diaphragm
Corpus cavernosum
Corpus spongiosum
Urethra
Ductus deferens
Glans of penis
Testis
Epididymis

Rectum
Anus

©Practice Management Information Corp., Los Angeles, CA

PLATE 19. FEMALE REPRODUCTIVE SYSTEM

Infections with a predominantly sexual mode of transmission	**A50-A64**
Other diseases caused by chlamydiae	**A70-A74**
Bacterial and viral infectious agents	**B95-B97**
Malignant neoplasms of female genital organs	**C51-C58**
Malignant neoplasms of ill-defined, other secondary and unspecified sites	**C76-C80**
In situ neoplasms	**D00-D09**
Benign neoplasms, except benign neuroendocrine tumors	**D10-D36**
Neoplasms of uncertain behavior, polycythemia vera and myelodysplastic syndromes	**D37-D48**
Neoplasms of unspecified behavior	**D49**
Inflammatory diseases of female pelvic organs	**N70-N77**
Noninflammatory disorders of female genital tract	**N80-N98**
Intraoperative and postprocedural complications and disorders of genitourinary system, not elsewhere classified	**N99**
Congenital malformations of genital organs	**Q50-Q56**
General symptoms and signs	**R50-R69**
Abnormal findings on diagnostic imaging and in function studies, without diagnosis	**R90-R94**
Persons encountering health services for examinations	**Z00-Z13**
Estrogen receptor status	**Z17**
Persons encountering health services in circumstances related to reproduction	**Z30-Z39**
Encounters for other specific health care	**Z40-Z53**

Female Reproductive System

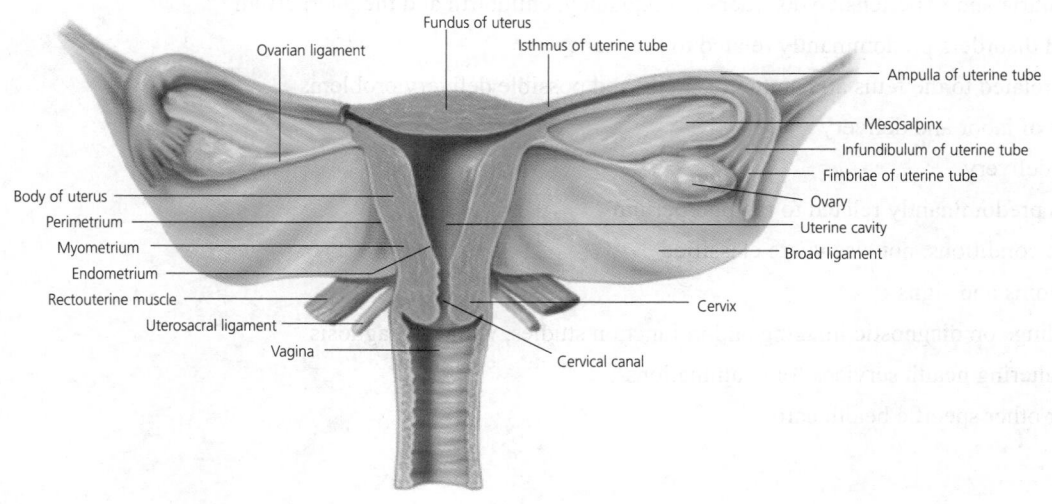

Ovarian ligament
Fundus of uterus
Isthmus of uterine tube
Ampulla of uterine tube
Mesosalpinx
Infundibulum of uterine tube
Fimbriae of uterine tube
Ovary
Body of uterus
Perimetrium
Myometrium
Endometrium
Rectouterine muscle
Uterosacral ligament
Vagina
Uterine cavity
Broad ligament
Cervix
Cervical canal

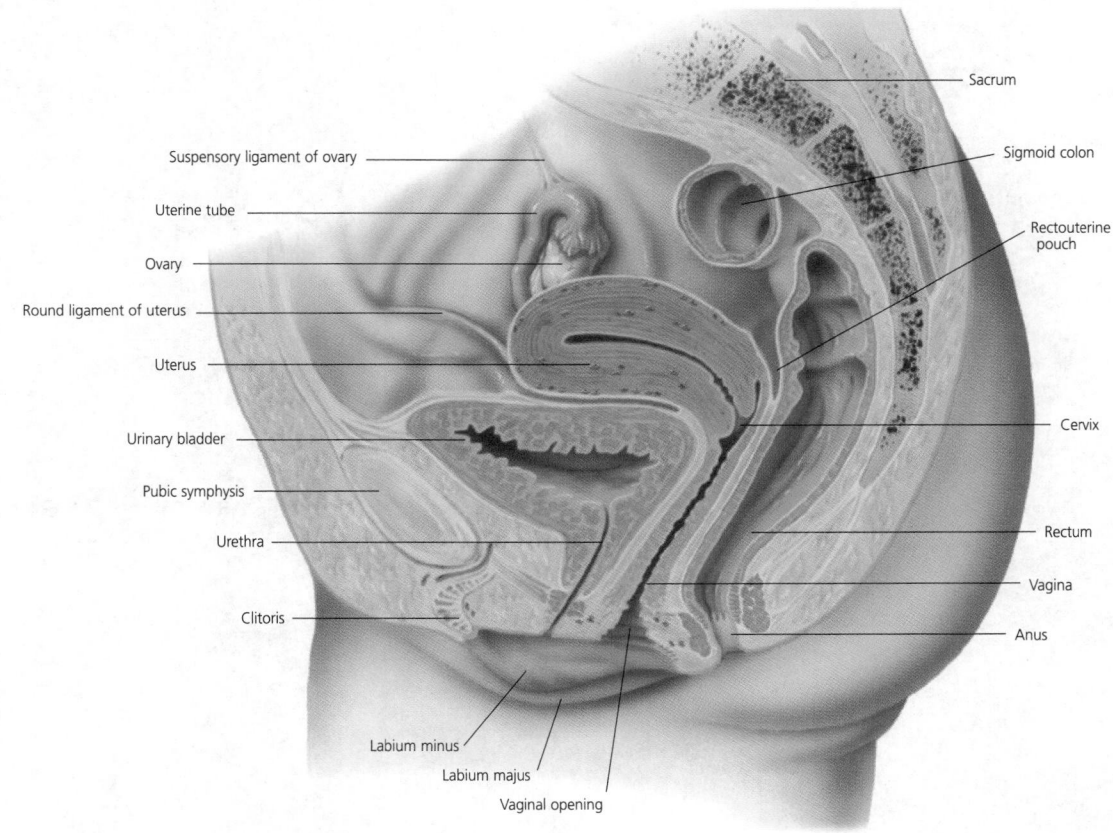

Sacrum
Sigmoid colon
Suspensory ligament of ovary
Uterine tube
Ovary
Round ligament of uterus
Uterus
Urinary bladder
Pubic symphysis
Urethra
Clitoris
Rectouterine pouch
Cervix
Rectum
Vagina
Anus
Labium minus
Labium majus
Vaginal opening

©Practice Management Information Corp., Los Angeles, CA

PLATE 20. PREGNANCY, CHILDBIRTH AND THE PUERPERIUM

Female Reproductive System: Pregnancy
(Lateral View)

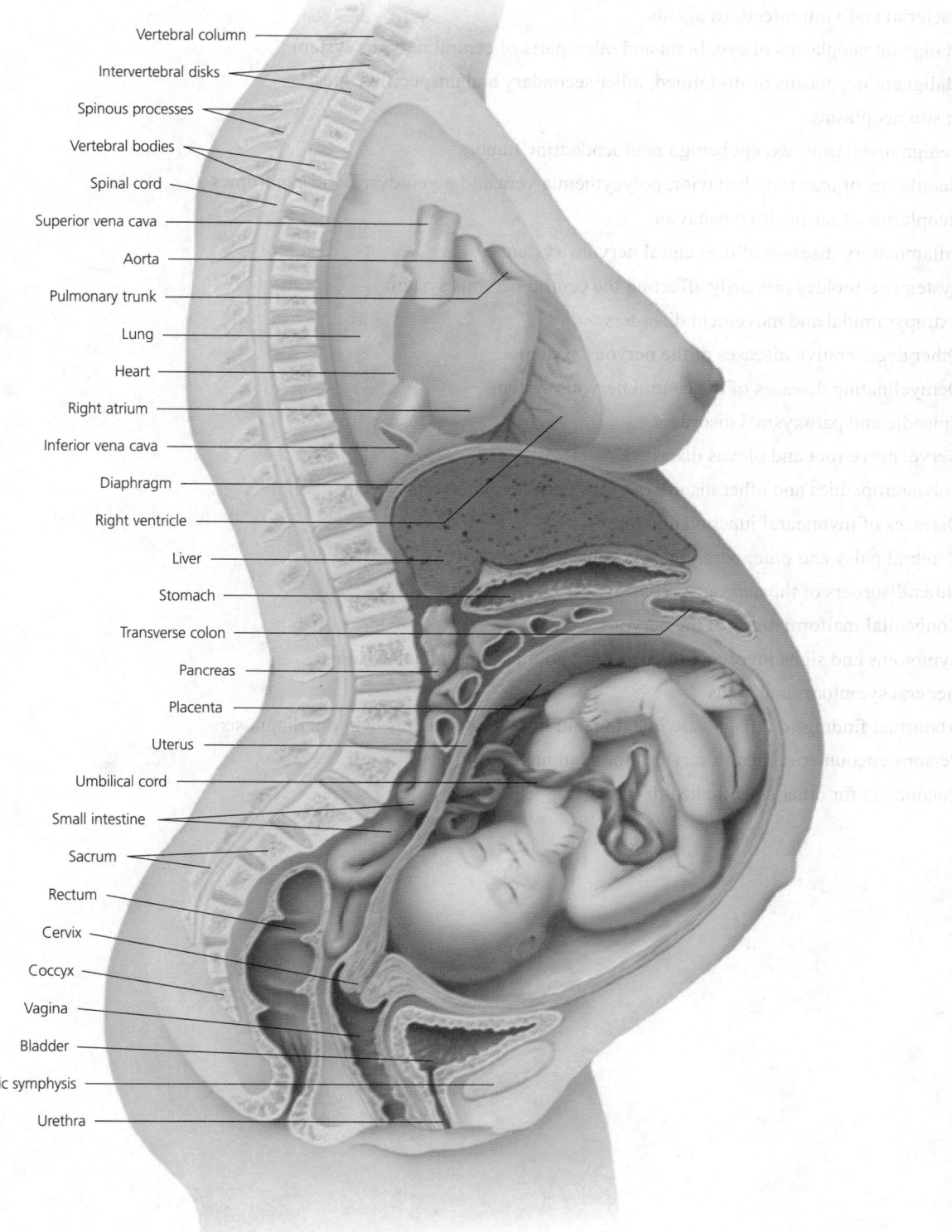

Vertebral column
Intervertebral disks
Spinous processes
Vertebral bodies
Spinal cord
Superior vena cava
Aorta
Pulmonary trunk
Lung
Heart
Right atrium
Inferior vena cava
Diaphragm
Right ventricle
Liver
Stomach
Transverse colon
Pancreas
Placenta
Uterus
Umbilical cord
Small intestine
Sacrum
Rectum
Cervix
Coccyx
Vagina
Bladder
Pubic symphysis
Urethra

©Practice Management Information Corp., Los Angeles, CA

PLATE 21. NERVOUS SYSTEM – BRAIN

Viral and prion infections of the central nervous system	**A80-A89**
Bacterial and viral infectious agents	**B95-B97**
Malignant neoplasms of eye, brain and other parts of central nervous system	**C69-C72**
Malignant neoplasms of ill-defined, other secondary and unspecified sites	**C76-C80**
In situ neoplasms	**D00-D09**
Benign neoplasms, except benign neuroendocrine tumors	**D10-D36**
Neoplasms of uncertain behavior, polycythemia vera and myelodysplastic syndromes	**D37-D48**
Neoplasms of unspecified behavior	**D49**
Inflammatory diseases of the central nervous system	**G00-G09**
Systemic atrophies primarily affecting the central nervous system	**G10-G14**
Extrapyramidal and movement disorders	**G20-G26**
Other degenerative diseases of the nervous system	**G30-G32**
Demyelinating diseases of the central nervous system	**G35-G37**
Episodic and paroxysmal disorders	**G40-G47**
Nerve, nerve root and plexus disorders	**G50-G59**
Polyneuropathies and other disorders of the peripheral nervous system	**G60-G65**
Diseases of myoneural junction and muscle	**G70-G73**
Cerebral palsy and other paralytic syndromes	**G80-G83**
Other disorders of the nervous system	**G89-G99**
Congenital malformations of the nervous system	**Q00-Q07**
Symptoms and signs involving the nervous and musculoskeletal systems	**R25-R29**
General symptoms and signs	**R50-R69**
Abnormal findings on diagnostic imaging and in function studies, without diagnosis	**R90-R94**
Persons encountering health services for examinations	**Z00-Z13**
Encounters for other specific health care	**Z40-Z53**

Brain
(Base View)

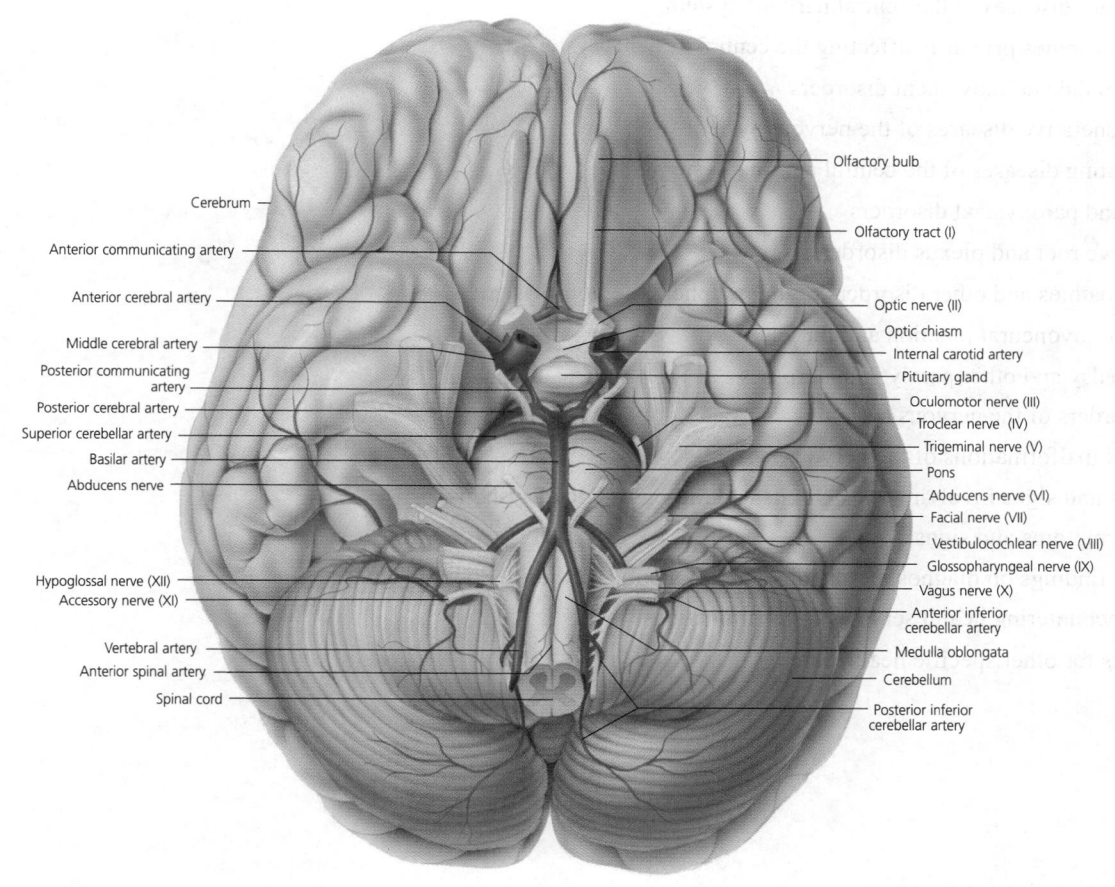

Cerebrum

Anterior communicating artery

Anterior cerebral artery

Middle cerebral artery

Posterior communicating artery

Posterior cerebral artery

Superior cerebellar artery

Basilar artery

Abducens nerve

Hypoglossal nerve (XII)

Accessory nerve (XI)

Vertebral artery

Anterior spinal artery

Spinal cord

Olfactory bulb

Olfactory tract (I)

Optic nerve (II)

Optic chiasm

Internal carotid artery

Pituitary gland

Oculomotor nerve (III)

Troclear nerve (IV)

Trigeminal nerve (V)

Pons

Abducens nerve (VI)

Facial nerve (VII)

Vestibulocochlear nerve (VIII)

Glossopharyngeal nerve (IX)

Vagus nerve (X)

Anterior inferior cerebellar artery

Medulla oblongata

Cerebellum

Posterior inferior cerebellar artery

©Practice Management Information Corp., Los Angeles, CA

PLATE 22. NERVOUS SYSTEM

Viral and prion infections of the central nervous system	**A80-A89**
Bacterial and viral infectious agents	**B95-B97**
Malignant neoplasms of eye, brain and other parts of central nervous system	**C69-C72**
Malignant neoplasms of ill-defined, other secondary and unspecified sites	**C76-C80**
In situ neoplasms	**D00-D09**
Benign neoplasms, except benign neuroendocrine tumors	**D10-D36**
Neoplasms of uncertain behavior, polycythemia vera and myelodysplastic syndromes	**D37-D48**
Neoplasms of unspecified behavior	**D49**
Inflammatory diseases of the central nervous system	**G00-G09**
Systemic atrophies primarily affecting the central nervous system	**G10-G14**
Extrapyramidal and movement disorders	**G20-G26**
Other degenerative diseases of the nervous system	**G30-G32**
Demyelinating diseases of the central nervous system	**G35-G37**
Episodic and paroxysmal disorders	**G40-G47**
Nerve, nerve root and plexus disorders	**G50-G59**
Polyneuropathies and other disorders of the peripheral nervous system	**G60-G65**
Diseases of myoneural junction and muscle	**G70-G73**
Cerebral palsy and other paralytic syndromes	**G80-G83**
Other disorders of the nervous system	**G89-G99**
Congenital malformations of the nervous system	**Q00-Q07**
Symptoms and signs involving the nervous and musculoskeletal systems	**R25-R29**
General symptoms and signs	**R50-R69**
Abnormal findings on diagnostic imaging and in function studies, without diagnosis	**R90-R94**
Persons encountering health services for examinations	**Z00-Z13**
Encounters for other specific health care	**Z40-Z53**

Nervous System

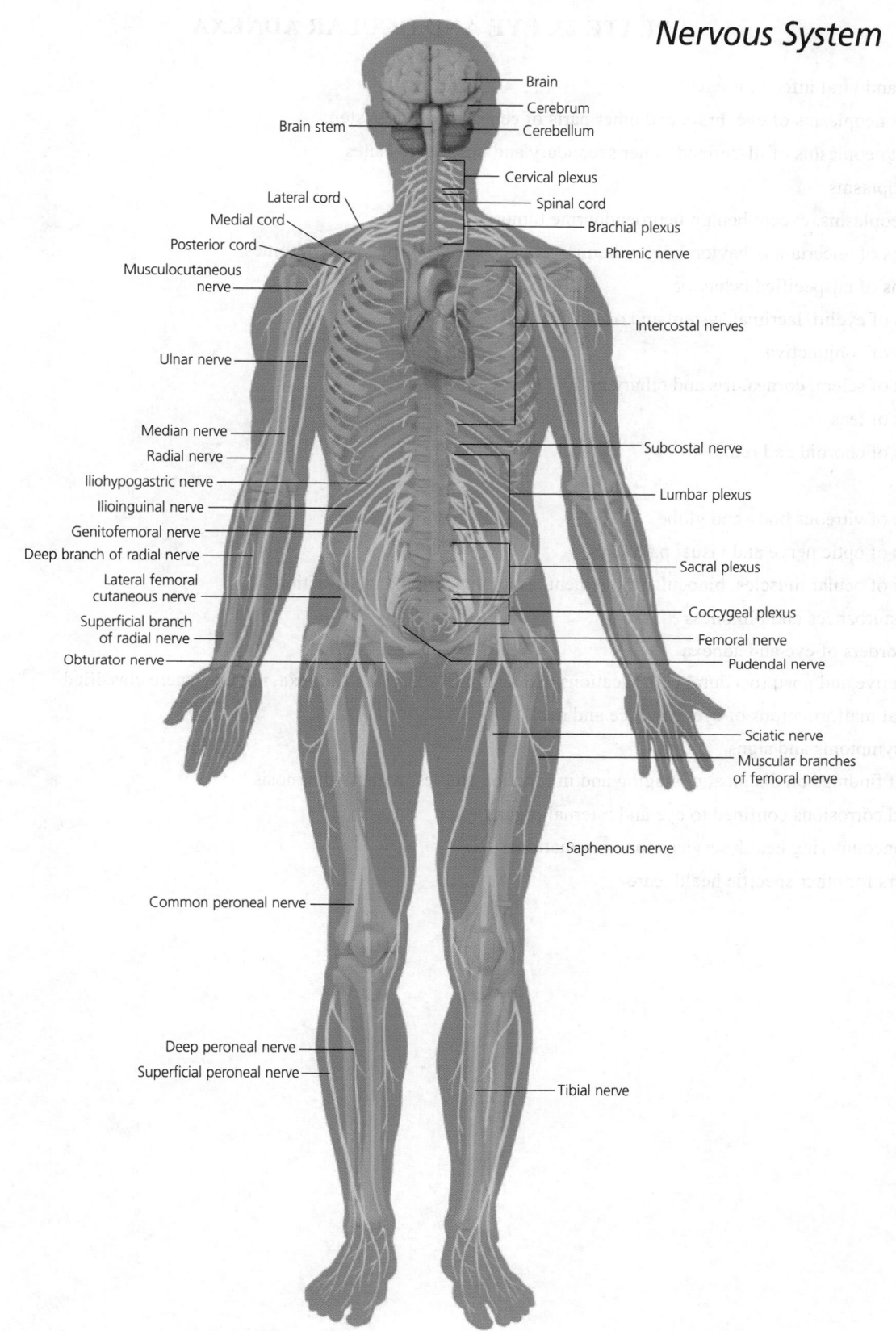

Brain

Cerebrum

Brain stem

Cerebellum

Cervical plexus

Lateral cord

Spinal cord

Medial cord

Brachial plexus

Posterior cord

Phrenic nerve

Musculocutaneous nerve

Intercostal nerves

Ulnar nerve

Median nerve

Subcostal nerve

Radial nerve

Iliohypogastric nerve

Lumbar plexus

Ilioinguinal nerve

Genitofemoral nerve

Deep branch of radial nerve

Sacral plexus

Lateral femoral cutaneous nerve

Coccygeal plexus

Superficial branch of radial nerve

Femoral nerve

Obturator nerve

Pudendal nerve

Sciatic nerve

Muscular branches of femoral nerve

Saphenous nerve

Common peroneal nerve

Deep peroneal nerve

Superficial peroneal nerve

Tibial nerve

©Practice Management Information Corp., Los Angeles, CA

PLATE 23. EYE AND OCULAR ADNEXA

Bacterial and viral infectious agents	**B95-B97**
Malignant neoplasms of eye, brain and other parts of central nervous system	**C69-C72**
Malignant neoplasms of ill-defined, other secondary and unspecified sites	**C76-C80**
In situ neoplasms	**D00-D09**
Benign neoplasms, except benign neuroendocrine tumors	**D10-D36**
Neoplasms of uncertain behavior, polycythemia vera and myelodysplastic syndromes	**D37-D48**
Neoplasms of unspecified behavior	**D49**
Disorders of eyelid, lacrimal system and orbit	**H00-H05**
Disorders of conjunctiva	**H10-H11**
Disorders of sclera, cornea, iris and ciliary body	**H15-H22**
Disorders of lens	**H25-H28**
Disorders of choroid and retina	**H30-H36**
Glaucoma	**H40-H42**
Disorders of vitreous body and globe	**H43-H44**
Disorders of optic nerve and visual pathways	**H46-H47**
Disorders of ocular muscles, binocular movement, accommodation and refraction	**H49-H52**
Visual disturbances and blindness	**H53-H54**
Other disorders of eye and adnexa	**H55-H57**
Intraoperative and postprocedural complications and disorders of eye and adnexa, not elsewhere classified	**H59**
Congenital malformations of eye, ear, face and neck	**Q10-Q18**
General symptoms and signs	**R50-R69**
Abnormal findings on diagnostic imaging and in function studies, without diagnosis	**R90-R94**
Burns and corrosions confined to eye and internal organs	**T26-T28**
Persons encountering health services for examinations	**Z00-Z13**
Encounters for other specific health care	**Z40-Z53**

Right Eye
(Horizontal Section)

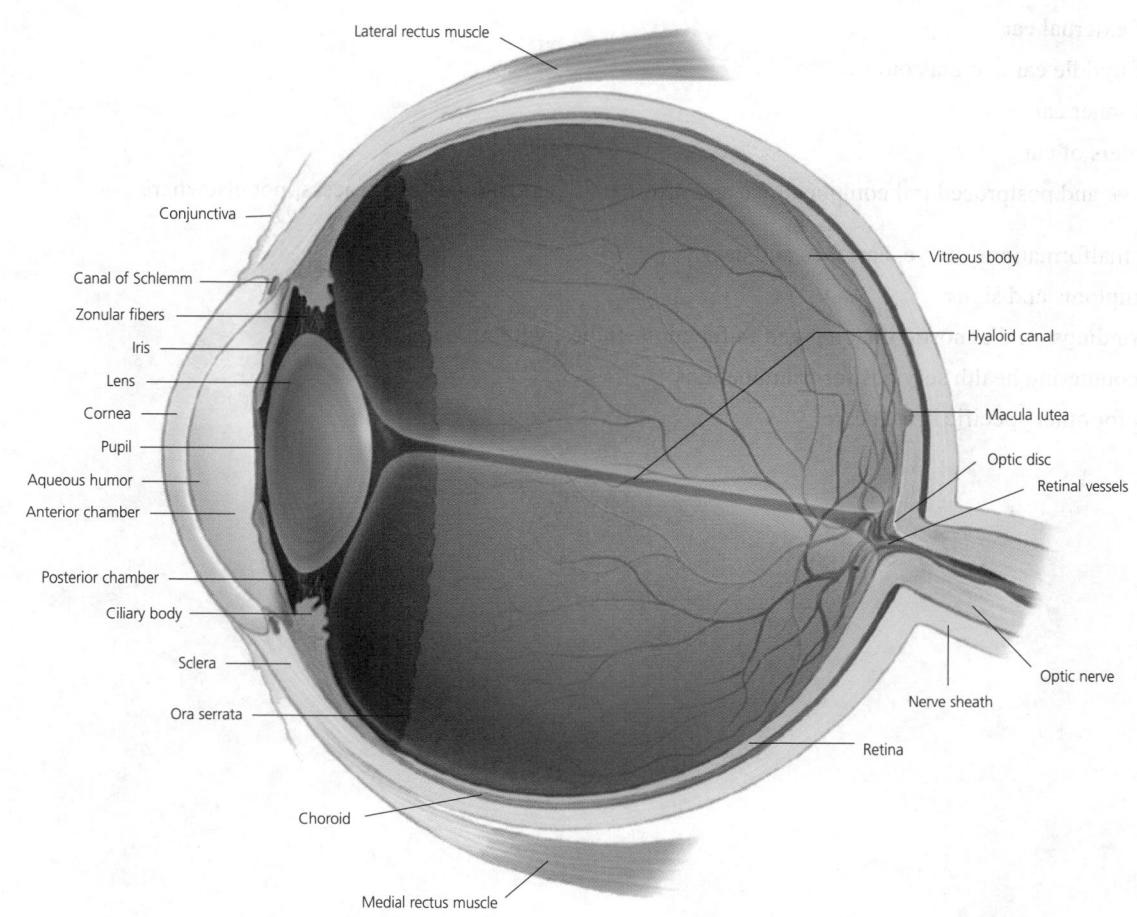

Lateral rectus muscle

Conjunctiva

Canal of Schlemm

Zonular fibers

Iris

Lens

Cornea

Pupil

Aqueous humor

Anterior chamber

Posterior chamber

Ciliary body

Sclera

Ora serrata

Choroid

Medial rectus muscle

Vitreous body

Hyaloid canal

Macula lutea

Optic disc

Retinal vessels

Optic nerve

Nerve sheath

Retina

©Scientific Publishing Ltd., Rolling Meadows, IL

PLATE 24. AUDITORY SYSTEM

Bacterial and viral infectious agents	**B95-B97**
Malignant neoplasms of ill-defined, other secondary and unspecified sites	**C76-C80**
In situ neoplasms	**D00-D09**
Benign neoplasms, except benign neuroendocrine tumors	**D10-D36**
Neoplasms of uncertain behavior, polycythemia vera and myelodysplastic syndromes	**D37-D48**
Neoplasms of unspecified behavior	**D49**
Diseases of external ear	**H60-H62**
Diseases of middle ear and mastoid	**H65-H75**
Diseases of inner ear	**H80-H83**
Other disorders of ear	**H90-H94**
Intraoperative and postprocedural complications and disorders of ear and mastoid process, not elsewhere classified	**H95**
Congenital malformations of eye, ear, face and neck	**Q10-Q18**
General symptoms and signs	**R50-R69**
Abnormal findings on diagnostic imaging and in function studies, without diagnosis	**R90-R94**
Persons encountering health services for examinations	**Z00-Z13**
Encounters for other specific health care	**Z40-Z53**

The Ear

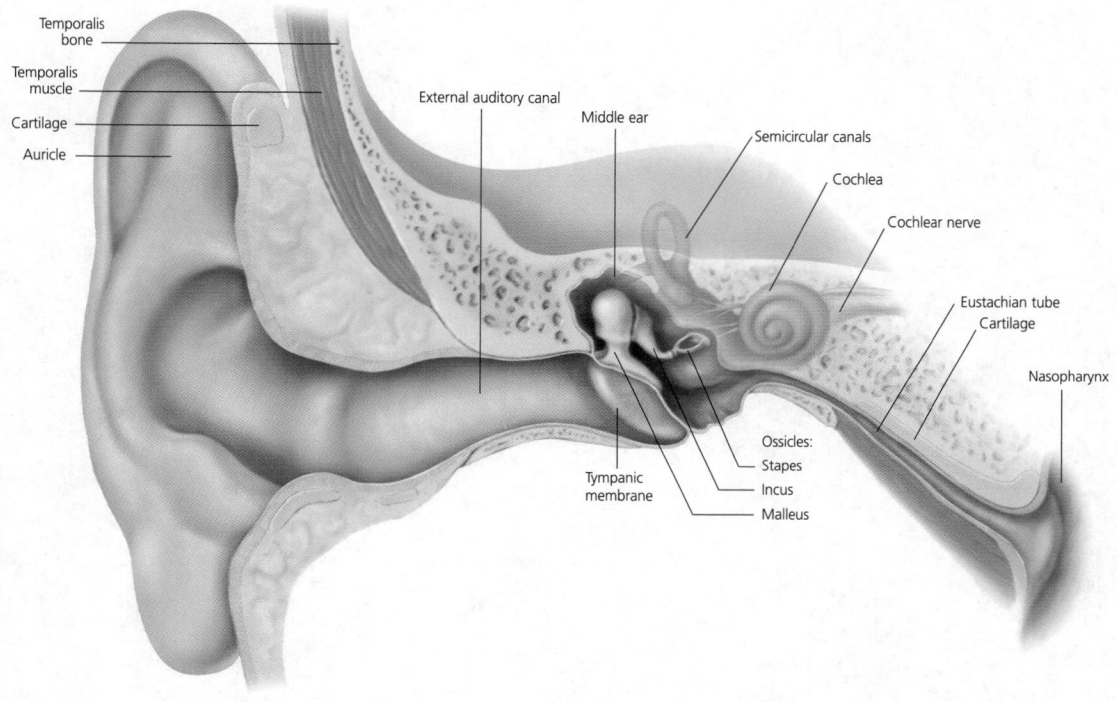

Temporalis bone

Temporalis muscle

Cartilage

Auricle

External auditory canal

Middle ear

Semicircular canals

Cochlea

Cochlear nerve

Eustachian tube

Cartilage

Nasopharynx

Tympanic membrane

Ossicles:
Stapes
Incus
Malleus

©Scientific Publishing Ltd., Rolling Meadows, IL

Chapter 1: Certain Infectious And Parasitic Diseases (A00-B99)

DEFINITIONS

This chapter includes definitions of selected key words, terms and phrases and coding alerts for adding points to the clinical domain, and references to coding late effects where appropriate. An example from this chapter is as follows:

A01 Typhoid and paratyphoid fevers
Definition: Typhoid fever, aka enteric fever, salmonella typhi is an illness caused by the bacterium salmonella enterica serovar typhi.

MULTIPLE CODING FOR A SINGLE CONDITION

In addition to the etiology/manifestation convention that requires two codes to fully describe a single condition that affects multiple body systems, there are other single conditions that also require more than one code. "Use additional code" notes are found in the Tabular List at codes that are not part of an etiology/manifestation pair where a secondary code is useful to fully describe a condition. The sequencing rule is the same as the etiology/manifestation pair, "use additional code" indicates that a secondary code should be added.

For example, for bacterial infections that are not included in chapter 1, a secondary code from category B95, Streptococcus, Staphylococcus, and Enterococcus, as the cause of diseases classified elsewhere, or B96, Other bacterial agents as the cause of diseases classified elsewhere, may be required to identify the bacterial organism causing the infection. A "use additional code" note will normally be found at the infectious disease code, indicating a need for the organism code to be added as a secondary code.

"Code first" notes are also under certain codes that are not specifically manifestation codes but may be due to an underlying cause. When there is a "code first" note and an underlying condition is present, the underlying condition should be sequenced first.

"Code, if applicable, any causal condition first", notes indicate that this code may be assigned as a principal diagnosis when the causal condition is unknown or not applicable. If a causal condition is known, then the code for that condition should be sequenced as the principal or first-listed diagnosis.

Multiple codes may be needed for sequela, complication codes and obstetric codes to more fully describe a condition. See the specific guidelines for these conditions for further instruction.

COMBINATION CODE

A combination code is a single code used to classify: Two diagnoses, or a diagnosis with an associated secondary process (manifestation) A diagnosis with an associated complication

Combination codes are identified by referring to subterm entries in the Alphabetic Index and by reading the inclusion and exclusion notes in the Tabular List.

Assign only the combination code when that code fully identifies the diagnostic conditions involved or when the Alphabetic Index so directs. Multiple coding should not be used when the classification provides a combination code that clearly identifies all of the elements documented in the diagnosis. When the combination code lacks necessary specificity in describing the manifestation or complication, an additional code should be used as a secondary code.

SEQUELA (LATE EFFECTS)

A sequela is the residual effect (condition produced) after the acute phase of an illness or injury has terminated. There is no time limit on when a sequela code can be used. The residual may be apparent early, such as in cerebral infarction, or it may occur months or years later, such as that due to a previous injury. Coding of sequela generally requires two codes sequenced in the following order: The condition or nature of the sequela is sequenced first.

The sequela code is sequenced second.

An exception to the above guidelines are those instances where the code for the sequela is followed by a manifestation code identified in the Tabular List and title, or the sequela code has been expanded (at the fourth, fifth or sixth character levels) to include the manifestation(s). The code for the acute phase of an illness or injury that led to the sequela is never used with a code for the late effect.

HUMAN IMMUNODEFICIENCY VIRUS (HIV) INFECTIONS

1) **Code only confirmed cases**

   Code only confirmed cases of HIV infection/illness. This is an exception to the hospital inpatient guideline Section II, H.

Add 4th-7th digits   Nonspecific code   Unspecified code   Manifestation code   139

In this context, "confirmation" does not require documentation of positive serology or culture for HIV; the provider's diagnostic statement that the patient is HIV positive, or has an HIV-related illness is sufficient.

2) **Selection and sequencing of HIV codes**

(a) **Patient admitted for HIV-related condition**

If a patient is admitted for an HIV-related condition, the principal diagnosis should be B20, Human immunodeficiency virus [HIV] disease followed by additional diagnosis codes for all reported HIV-related conditions.

(b) **Patient with HIV disease admitted for unrelated condition**

If a patient with HIV disease is admitted for an unrelated condition (such as a traumatic injury), the code for the unrelated condition (e.g., the nature of injury code) should be the principal diagnosis. Other diagnoses would be B20 followed by additional diagnosis codes for all reported HIV-related conditions.

(c) **Whether the patient is newly diagnosed**

Whether the patient is newly diagnosed or has had previous admissions/encounters for HIV conditions is irrelevant to the sequencing decision.

(d) **Asymptomatic human immunodeficiency virus**

Z21, Asymptomatic human immunodeficiency virus [HIV] infection status, is to be applied when the patient without any documentation of symptoms is listed as being "HIV positive," "known HIV," "HIV test positive," or similar terminology. Do not use this code if the term "AIDS" is used or if the patient is treated for any HIV-related illness or is described as having any condition(s) resulting from his/her HIV positive status; use B20 in these cases.

(e) **Patients with inconclusive HIV serology**

Patients with inconclusive HIV serology, but no definitive diagnosis or manifestations of the illness, may be assigned code R75, Inconclusive laboratory evidence of human immunodeficiency virus [HIV].

(f) **Previously diagnosed HIV-related illness**

Patients with any known prior diagnosis of an HIV-related illness should be coded to B20. Once a patient has developed an HIV-related illness, the patient should always be assigned code B20 on every subsequent admission/encounter. Patients previously diagnosed with any HIV illness (B20) should never be assigned to R75 or Z21, Asymptomatic human immunodeficiency virus [HIV] infection status.

(g) **HIV Infection in Pregnancy, Childbirth and the Puerperium**

During pregnancy, childbirth or the puerperium, a patient admitted (or presenting for a health care encounter) because of an HIV-related illness should receive a principal diagnosis code of O98.7-, Human immunodeficiency [HIV] disease complicating pregnancy, childbirth and the puerperium, followed by B20 and the code(s) for the HIV-related illness(es). Codes from Chapter 15 always take sequencing priority.

Patients with asymptomatic HIV infection status admitted (or presenting for a health care encounter) during pregnancy, childbirth, or the puerperium should receive codes of O98.7- and Z21.

(h) **Encounters for testing for HIV**

If a patient is being seen to determine his/her HIV status, use code Z11.4, Encounter for screening for human immunodeficiency virus [HIV]. Use additional codes for any associated high risk behavior.

If a patient with signs or symptoms is being seen for HIV testing, code the signs and symptoms. An additional counseling code Z71.7, Human immunodeficiency virus [HIV] counseling, may be used if counseling is provided during the encounter for the test.

When a patient returns to be informed of his/her HIV test results and the test result is negative, use code Z71.7, Human immunodeficiency virus [HIV] counseling.

If the results are positive, see previous guidelines and assign codes as appropriate.

INFECTIOUS AGENTS AS THE CAUSE OF DISEASES CLASSIFIED TO OTHER CHAPTERS

Certain infections are classified in chapters other than Chapter 1 and no organism is identified as part of the infection code. In these instances, it is necessary to use an additional code from Chapter 1 to identify the organism. A code from category B95, Streptococcus, Staphylococcus, and Enterococcus as the cause of diseases classified to other chapters, B96, Other bacterial agents as the cause of diseases classified to other chapters, or B97, Viral agents as the cause of diseases classified to other chapters, is to be used as an additional code to identify the organism. An instructional note will be found at the infection code advising that an additional organism code is required.

INFECTIONS RESISTANT TO ANTIBIOTICS

Many bacterial infections are resistant to current antibiotics. It is necessary to identify all infections documented as antibiotic resistant. Assign a code from category Z16, Resistance to antimicrobial drugs, following the infection code only if the infection code does not identify drug resistance.

SEPSIS, SEVERE SEPSIS, AND SEPTIC SHOCK

1) **Coding of Sepsis and Severe Sepsis**

   (a) **Sepsis**

   For a diagnosis of sepsis, assign the appropriate code for the underlying systemic infection. If the type of infection or causal organism is not further specified, assign code A41.9, Sepsis, unspecified organism.

   A code from subcategory R65.2, Severe sepsis, should not be assigned unless severe sepsis or an associated acute organ dysfunction is documented.

   (i) Negative or inconclusive blood cultures and sepsis

   Negative or inconclusive blood cultures do not preclude a diagnosis of sepsis in patients with clinical evidence of the condition; however, the provider should be queried.

   (ii) Urosepsis

   The term urosepsis is a nonspecific term. It is not to be considered synonymous with sepsis. It has no default code in the Alphabetic Index. Should a provider use this term, he/she must be queried for clarification.

   (iii) Sepsis with organ dysfunction

   If a patient has sepsis and associated acute organ dysfunction or multiple organ dysfunction (MOD), follow the instructions for coding severe sepsis.

   (iv) Acute organ dysfunction that is not clearly associated with the sepsis

   If a patient has sepsis and an acute organ dysfunction, but the medical record documentation indicates that the acute organ dysfunction is related to a medical condition other than the sepsis, do not assign a code from subcategory R65.2, Severe sepsis. An acute organ dysfunction must be associated with the sepsis in order to assign the severe sepsis code.

   If the documentation is not clear as to whether an acute organ dysfunction is related to the sepsis or another medical condition, query the ovider.

   (b) **Severe sepsis**

   The coding of severe sepsis requires a minimum of 2 codes: first a code for the underlying systemic infection, followed by a code from subcategory R65.2, Severe sepsis. If the causal organism is not documented, assign code A41.9, Sepsis, unspecified organism, for the infection. Additional code(s) for the associated acute organ dysfunction are also required.

   Due to the complex nature of severe sepsis, some cases may require querying the provider prior to assignment of the codes.

2) **Septic shock**

   (a) Septic shock generally refers to circulatory failure associated with severe sepsis, and therefore, it represents a type of acute organ dysfunction.

   For cases of septic shock, the code for the systemic infection should be sequenced first, followed by code R65.21, Severe sepsis with septic shock or code T81.12, Postprocedural septic shock. Any additional codes for the other acute organ dysfunctions should also be assigned. As noted in the sequencing instructions in the Tabular List, the code for septic shock cannot be assigned as a principal diagnosis.

3) **Sequencing of severe sepsis**

   If severe sepsis is present on admission, and meets the definition of principal diagnosis, the underlying systemic infection should be assigned as principal diagnosis followed by the appropriate code from subcategory R65.2 as required by the sequencing rules in the Tabular List. A code from subcategory R65.2 can never be assigned as a principal diagnosis.

   When severe sepsis develops during an encounter (it was not present on admission), the underlying systemic infection and the appropriate code from subcategory R65.2 should be assigned as secondary diagnoses.

   Severe sepsis may be present on admission, but the diagnosis may not be confirmed until sometime after admission. If the documentation is not clear whether severe sepsis was present on admission, the provider should be queried.

4) **Sepsis and severe sepsis with a localized infection**

If the reason for admission is both sepsis or severe sepsis and a localized infection, such as pneumonia or cellulitis, a code(s) for the underlying systemic infection should be assigned first and the code for the localized infection should be assigned as a secondary diagnosis. If the patient has severe sepsis, a code from subcategory R65.2 should also be assigned as a secondary diagnosis. If the patient is admitted with a localized infection, such as pneumonia, and sepsis/severe sepsis doesn't develop until after admission, the localized infection should be assigned first, followed by the appropriate sepsis/severe sepsis codes.

5) **Sepsis due to a postprocedural infection**

   (a) **Documentation of causal relationship**

   As with all postprocedural complications, code assignment is based on the provider's documentation of the relationship between the infection and the procedure.

   (b) **Sepsis due to a postprocedural infection**

   For such cases, the postprocedural infection code, such as T80.2, Infections following infusion, transfusion, and therapeutic injection, T81.4, Infection following a procedure, T88.0, Infection following immunization, or O86.0, Infection of obstetric surgical wound, should be coded first, followed by the code for the specific infection. If the patient has severe sepsis, the appropriate code from subcategory R65.2 should also be assigned with the additional code(s) for any acute organ dysfunction.

   (c) **Postprocedural infection and postprocedural septic shock**

   In cases where a postprocedural infection has occurred and has resulted in severe sepsis the code for the precipitating complication such as code T81.4, Infection following a procedure, or O86.0, Infection of obstetrical surgical wound should be coded first followed by code R65.20, Severe sepsis without septic shock. A code for the systemic infection should also be assigned.

   If a postprocedural infection has resulted in postprocedural septic shock, the code for the precipitating complication such as code T81.4, Infection following a procedure, or O86.0, Infection of obstetrical surgical wound should be coded first followed by code T81.12-, Postprocedural septic shock. A code for the systemic infection should also be assigned.

6) **Sepsis and severe sepsis associated with a noninfectious process (condition)**

   In some cases a noninfectious process (condition), such as trauma, may lead to an infection which can result in sepsis or severe sepsis. If sepsis or severe sepsis is documented as associated with a noninfectious condition, such as a burn or serious injury, and this condition meets the definition for principal diagnosis, the code for the noninfectious condition should be sequenced first, followed by the code for the resulting infection. If severe sepsis is present, a code from subcategory

   R65.2 should also be assigned with any associated organ dysfunction(s) codes. It is not necessary to assign a code from subcategory R65.1, Systemic inflammatory response syndrome (SIRS) of non-infectious origin, for these cases.

   If the infection meets the definition of principal diagnosis, it should be sequenced before the non-infectious condition. When both the associated non-infectious condition and the infection meet the definition of principal diagnosis, either may be assigned as principal diagnosis.

   Only one code from category R65, Symptoms and signs specifically associated with systemic inflammation and infection, should be assigned. Therefore, when a non-infectious condition leads to an infection resulting in severe sepsis, assign the appropriate code from subcategory R65.2, Severe sepsis. Do not additionally assign a code from subcategory R65.1, Systemic inflammatory response syndrome (SIRS) of non-infectious origin.

   See Section I.C.18. SIRS due to non-infectious process

7) **Sepsis and septic shock complicating abortion, pregnancy, childbirth, and the puerperium**

   See Section I.C.15. Sepsis and septic shock complicating abortion, pregnancy, childbirth and the puerperium

8) **Newborn sepsis**

   See Section I.C.16. f. Bacterial sepsis of Newborn

METHICILLIN RESISTANT *STAPHYLOCOCCUS AUREUS* (MRSA) CONDITIONS

1) **Selection and sequencing of MRSA codes**

   (a) **Combination codes for MRSA infection**

   When a patient is diagnosed with an infection that is due to methicillin resistant *Staphylococcus aureus* (MRSA), and that infection has a combination code that includes the causal organism (e.g., sepsis, pneumonia) assign the appropriate combination code for the condition (e.g., code A41.02, Sepsis due to Methicillin resistant Staphylococcus aureus or code J15.212, Pneumonia due to Methicillin resistant Staphylococcus aureus). Do not assign code B95.62, Methicillin resistant Staphylococcus aureus infection as the cause of diseases classified elsewhere, as an additional code, because the combination code includes the type of infection and the MRSA organism. Do not assign a code from subcategory Z16.11, Resistance to penicillins, as an additional diagnosis.

   See Section C.1. for instructions on coding and sequencing of sepsis and severe sepsis.

(b) **Other codes for MRSA infection**

When there is documentation of a current infection (e.g., wound infection, stitch abscess, urinary tract infection) due to MRSA, and that infection does not have a combination code that includes the causal organism, assign the appropriate code to identify the condition along with code B95.62, Methicillin resistant Staphylococcus aureus infection as the cause of diseases classified elsewhere for the MRSA infection. Do not assign a code from subcategory Z16.11, Resistance to penicillins.

(c) **Methicillin susceptible Staphylococcus aureus (MSSA) and MRSA colonization**

The condition or state of being colonized or carrying MSSA or MRSA is called colonization or carriage, while an individual person is described as being colonized or being a carrier. Colonization means that MSSA or MSRA is present on or in the body without necessarily causing illness. A positive MRSA colonization test might be documented by the provider as "MRSA screen positive" or "MRSA nasal swab positive".

Assign code Z22.322, Carrier or suspected carrier of Methicillin resistant Staphylococcus aureus, for patients documented as having MRSA colonization. Assign code Z22.321, Carrier or suspected carrier of Methicillin susceptible Staphylococcus aureus, for patient documented as having MSSA colonization. Colonization is not necessarily indicative of a disease process or as the cause of a specific condition the patient may have unless documented as such by the provider.

(d) **MRSA colonization and infection**

If a patient is documented as having both MRSA colonization and infection during a hospital admission, code Z22.322, Carrier or suspected carrier of Methicillin resistant Staphylococcus aureus, and a code for the MRSA infection may both be assigned.

ZIKA VIRUS INFECTIONS

1) Code only confirmed cases

Code only a confirmed diagnosis of Zika virus (A92.5, Zika virus disease) as documented by the provider. This is an exception to the hospital inpatient guideline Section II, H.

In this context, "confirmation" does not require documentation of the type of test performed; the physician's diagnostic statement that the condition is confirmed is sufficient. This code should be assigned regardless of the stated mode of transmission.

If the provider documents "suspected", "possible" or "probable" Zika, do not assign code A92.5. Assign a code(s) explaining the reason for encounter (such as fever, rash, or joint pain) or Z20.828, Contact with and (suspected) exposure to other viral communicable diseases.

● New code   ▲ Revised code   **Excludes1:** Not coded here   **Excludes2:** Not included here   ⊗ Placeholder required   ⑦ 7th digit required

Chapter 1
Certain Infectious and Parasitic Diseases
(A00-B99)

Includes: diseases generally recognized as communicable or transmissible

Use additional code to identify resistance to antimicrobial drugs (Z16.-)

Excludes1: certain localized infections - see body system-related chapters

Excludes2: carrier or suspected carrier of infectious disease (Z22.-)

infectious and parasitic diseases complicating pregnancy, childbirth and the puerperium (O98.-)

infectious and parasitic diseases specific to the perinatal period (P35-P39)

influenza and other acute respiratory infections (J00-J22)

This chapter contains the following blocks:

A00-A09	Intestinal infectious diseases
A15-A19	Tuberculosis
A20-A28	Certain zoonotic bacterial diseases
A30-A49	Other bacterial diseases
A50-A64	Infections with a predominantly sexual mode of transmission
A65-A69	Other spirochetal diseases
A70-A74	Other diseases caused by chlamydiae
A75-A79	Rickettsioses
A80-A89	Viral and prion infections of the central nervous system
A90-A99	Arthropod-borne viral fevers and viral hemorrhagic fevers
B00-B09	Viral infections characterized by skin and mucous membrane lesions
B10	Other human herpesviruses
B15-B19	Viral hepatitis
B20	Human immunodeficiency virus [HIV] disease
B25-B34	Other viral diseases
B35-B49	Mycoses
B50-B64	Protozoal diseases
B65-B83	Helminthiases
B85-B89	Pediculosis, acariasis and other infestations
B90-B94	Sequelae of infectious and parasitic diseases
B95-B97	Bacterial and viral infectious agents
B99	Other infectious diseases

INTESTINAL INFECTIOUS DISEASES (A00-A09)

A00 Cholera

Definition: Cholera, aka asiatic or epidemic cholera, is an infectious gastroenteritis caused by enterotoxin-producing strains of the bacterium vibrio cholerae.

A00.0 Cholera due to Vibrio cholerae 01, biovar cholerae

Classical cholera

A00.1 Cholera due to Vibrio cholerae 01, biovar eltor

Cholera eltor

A00.9 Cholera, unspecified

A01 Typhoid and paratyphoid fevers

A01.0 Typhoid fever

Definition: Typhoid fever, aka enteric fever, salmonella typhi is an illness caused by the bacterium salmonella enterica serovar typhi.

Infection due to Salmonella typhi

A01.00 Typhoid fever, unspecified

A01.01 Typhoid meningitis

A01.02 Typhoid fever with heart involvement

Typhoid endocarditis

Typhoid myocarditis

A01.03 Typhoid pneumonia

A01.04 Typhoid arthritis

A01.05 Typhoid osteomyelitis

A01.09 Typhoid fever with other complications

A01.1 Paratyphoid fever A

A01.2 Paratyphoid fever B

A01.3 Paratyphoid fever C

A01.4 Paratyphoid fever, unspecified

Infection due to Salmonella paratyphi NOS

A02 Other salmonella infections

Definition: Salmonellosis is an infection with salmonella bacteria. Most persons infected with salmonella develop diarrhea, fever, vomiting, and abdominal cramps.

Includes: infection or foodborne intoxication due to any Salmonella species other than S. typhi and S. paratyphi

A02.0 Salmonella enteritis

Salmonellosis

A02.1 Salmonella sepsis

A02.2 Localized salmonella infections

A02.20 Localized salmonella infection, unspecified

A02.21 Salmonella meningitis

A02.22 Salmonella pneumonia

A02.23 Salmonella arthritis

A02.24 Salmonella osteomyelitis

A02.25 Salmonella pyelonephritis

Salmonella tubulo-interstitial nephropathy

A02.29 Salmonella with other localized infection

A02.8 Other specified salmonella infections

A02.9 Salmonella infection, unspecified

A03 Shigellosis

Definition: Shigellosis, aka bacillary dysentery, is a food borne illness caused by infection by bacteria of the genus shigella.

A03.0 Shigellosis due to Shigella dysenteriae

Group A shigellosis [Shiga-Kruse dysentery]

A03.1 Shigellosis due to Shigella flexneri

Group B shigellosis

A03.2 Shigellosis due to Shigella boydii

Group C shigellosis

A03.3 Shigellosis due to Shigella sonnei

Group D shigellosis

A03.8 Other shigellosis

A03.9 Shigellosis, unspecified

Bacillary dysentery NOS

A04 Other bacterial intestinal infections

Excludes1: bacterial foodborne intoxications, NEC (A05.-)

tuberculous enteritis (A18.32)

A04.0 Enteropathogenic Escherichia coli infection

A04.1 Enterotoxigenic Escherichia coli infection

A04.2 Enteroinvasive Escherichia coli infection

A04.3 Enterohemorrhagic Escherichia coli infection

A04.4 Other intestinal Escherichia coli infections

Escherichia coli enteritis NOS

A04.5 **Campylobacter enteritis**

A04.6 **Enteritis due to Yersinia enterocolitica**

Excludes1: extraintestinal yersiniosis (A28.2)

A04.7 **Enterocolitis due to Clostridium difficile**

Foodborne intoxication by Clostridium difficile

Pseudomembraneous colitis

A04.8 **Other specified bacterial intestinal infections**

A04.9 **Bacterial intestinal infection, unspecified**

Bacterial enteritis NOS

A05 **Other bacterial foodborne intoxications, not elsewhere classified**

Excludes1: Clostridium difficile foodborne intoxication and infection (A04.7)

Escherichia coli infection (A04.0-A04.4)

listeriosis (A32.-)

salmonella foodborne intoxication and infection (A02.-)

toxic effect of noxious foodstuffs (T61-T62)

A05.0 **Foodborne staphylococcal intoxication**

A05.1 **Botulism food poisoning**

Botulism NOS

Classical foodborne intoxication due to Clostridium botulinum

Excludes1: infant botulism (A48.51)

wound botulism (A48.52)

A05.2 **Foodborne Clostridium perfringens [Clostridium welchii] intoxication**

Enteritis necroticans

Pig-bel

A05.3 **Foodborne Vibrio parahaemolyticus intoxication**

A05.4 **Foodborne Bacillus cereus intoxication**

A05.5 **Foodborne Vibrio vulnificus intoxication**

A05.8 **Other specified bacterial foodborne intoxications**

A05.9 **Bacterial foodborne intoxication, unspecified**

A06 **Amebiasis**

Definition: Amebiasis is an inflammation of the intestines caused by infection with entamoeba histolytica characterized by frequent, loose stools flecked with blood and mucus.

Includes: infection due to Entamoeba histolytica

Excludes1: Other protozoal intestinal diseases (A07.-)

Excludes2: acanthamebiasis (B60.1-)

Naegleriasis (B60.2)

A06.0 **Acute amebic dysentery**

Acute amebiasis

Intestinal amebiasis NOS

A06.1 **Chronic intestinal amebiasis**

A06.2 **Amebic nondysenteric colitis**

A06.3 **Ameboma of intestine**

Ameboma NOS

A06.4 **Amebic liver abscess**

Hepatic amebiasis

A06.5 **Amebic lung abscess**

Amebic abscess of lung (and liver)

A06.6 **Amebic brain abscess**

Amebic abscess of brain (and liver) (and lung)

A06.7 **Cutaneous amebiasis**

A06.8 **Amebic infection of other sites**

A06.81 **Amebic cystitis**

A06.82 **Other amebic genitourinary infections**

Amebic balanitis

Amebic vesiculitis

Amebic vulvovaginitis

A06.89 **Other amebic infections**

Amebic appendicitis

Amebic splenic abscess

A06.9 **Amebiasis, unspecified**

A07 **Other protozoal intestinal diseases**

Definition: Protozoal intestinal diseases refers to diseases of the intestinal system caused by protozoa, which are single-cell organisms that can only divide within a host organism. Malaria , giardia and toxoplasmosis are examples of diseases caused by protozoa.

A07.0 **Balantidiasis**

Balantidial dysentery

A07.1 **Giardiasis [lambliasis]**

A07.2 **Cryptosporidiosis**

A07.3 **Isosporiasis**

Infection due to Isospora belli and Isospora hominis

Intestinal coccidiosis

Isosporosis

A07.4 **Cyclosporiasis**

A07.8 **Other specified protozoal intestinal diseases**

Intestinal microsporidiosis

Intestinal trichomoniasis

Sarcocystosis

Sarcosporidiosis

A07.9 **Protozoal intestinal disease, unspecified**

Flagellate diarrhea

Protozoal colitis

Protozoal diarrhea

Protozoal dysentery

A08 **Viral and other specified intestinal infections**

Excludes1: influenza with involvement of gastrointestinal tract (J09.X3, J10.2, J11.2)

A08.0 **Rotaviral enteritis**

A08.1 **Acute gastroenteropathy due to Norwalk agent and other small round viruses**

A08.11 **Acute gastroenteropathy due to Norwalk agent**

Acute gastroenteropathy due to Norovirus

Acute gastroenteropathy due to Norwalk-like agent

A08.19 **Acute gastroenteropathy due to other small round viruses**

Acute gastroenteropathy due to small round virus [SRV] NOS

A08.2 **Adenoviral enteritis**

A08.3 **Other viral enteritis**

A08.31 **Calicivirus enteritis**

A08.32 **Astrovirus enteritis**

A08.39 **Other viral enteritis**

Coxsackie virus enteritis

Echovirus enteritis

Enterovirus enteritis NEC

Torovirus enteritis

A08.4   **Viral intestinal infection, unspecified**

Viral enteritis NOS

Viral gastroenteritis NOS

Viral gastroenteropathy NOS

A08.8   **Other specified intestinal infections**

A09   **Infectious gastroenteritis and colitis, unspecified**

Infectious colitis NOS

Infectious enteritis NOS

Infectious gastroenteritis NOS

Excludes1: colitis NOS (K52.9)

diarrhea NOS (R19.7)

enteritis NOS (K52.9)

gastroenteritis NOS (K52.9)

noninfective gastroenteritis and colitis, unspecified (K52.9)

TUBERCULOSIS (A15-A19)

Definition: Tuberculosis is a common and often deadly infectious disease caused by mycobacteria, in humans mainly mycobacterium tuberculosis. Tuberculosis usually attacks the lungs but can also affect the central nervous system, the lymphatic system, the circulatory system, the genitourinary system, the gastrointestinal system, bones, joints, and even the skin.

Includes: infections due to Mycobacterium tuberculosis and Mycobacterium bovis

Excludes1: congenital tuberculosis (P37.0)

nonspecific reaction to test for tuberculosis without active tuberculosis (R76.1-)

pneumoconiosis associated with tuberculosis, any type in A15 (J65)

positive PPD (R76.11)

positive tuberculin skin test without active tuberculosis (R76.11)

sequelae of tuberculosis (B90.-)

silicotuberculosis (J65)

A15   **Respiratory tuberculosis**

A15.0   **Tuberculosis of lung**

Tuberculous bronchiectasis

Tuberculous fibrosis of lung

Tuberculous pneumonia

Tuberculous pneumothorax

A15.4   **Tuberculosis of intrathoracic lymph nodes**

Tuberculosis of hilar lymph nodes

Tuberculosis of mediastinal lymph nodes

Tuberculosis of tracheobronchial lymph nodes

Excludes1: tuberculosis specified as primary (A15.7)

A15.5   **Tuberculosis of larynx, trachea and bronchus**

Tuberculosis of bronchus

Tuberculosis of glottis

Tuberculosis of larynx

Tuberculosis of trachea

A15.6   **Tuberculous pleurisy**

Tuberculosis of pleura

Tuberculous empyema

Excludes1: primary respiratory tuberculosis (A15.7)

A15.7   **Primary respiratory tuberculosis**

A15.8   **Other respiratory tuberculosis**

Mediastinal tuberculosis

Nasopharyngeal tuberculosis

Tuberculosis of nose

Tuberculosis of sinus [any nasal]

A15.9   **Respiratory tuberculosis unspecified**

A17   **Tuberculosis of nervous system**

A17.0   **Tuberculous meningitis**

Tuberculosis of meninges (cerebral)(spinal)

Tuberculous leptomeningitis

Excludes1: tuberculous meningoencephalitis (A17.82)

A17.1   **Meningeal tuberculoma**

Tuberculoma of meninges (cerebral) (spinal)

Excludes2: tuberculoma of brain and spinal cord (A17.81)

A17.8   **Other tuberculosis of nervous system**

A17.81   **Tuberculoma of brain and spinal cord**

Tuberculous abscess of brain and spinal cord

A17.82   **Tuberculous meningoencephalitis**

Tuberculous myelitis

A17.83   **Tuberculous neuritis**

Tuberculous mononeuropathy

A17.89   **Other tuberculosis of nervous system**

Tuberculous polyneuropathy

A17.9   **Tuberculosis of nervous system, unspecified**

A18   **Tuberculosis of other organs**

A18.0   **Tuberculosis of bones and joints**

A18.01   **Tuberculosis of spine**

Pott's disease or curvature of spine

Tuberculous arthritis

Tuberculous osteomyelitis of spine

Tuberculous spondylitis

A18.02   **Tuberculous arthritis of other joints**

Tuberculosis of hip (joint)

Tuberculosis of knee (joint)

A18.03   **Tuberculosis of other bones**

Tuberculous mastoiditis

Tuberculous osteomyelitis

A18.09   **Other musculoskeletal tuberculosis**

Tuberculous myositis

Tuberculous synovitis

Tuberculous tenosynovitis

A18.1   **Tuberculosis of genitourinary system**

A18.10   **Tuberculosis of genitourinary system, unspecified**

A18.11   **Tuberculosis of kidney and ureter**

A18.12   **Tuberculosis of bladder**

A18.13   **Tuberculosis of other urinary organs**

Tuberculous urethritis

A18.14   **Tuberculosis of prostate**

A18.15   **Tuberculosis of other male genital organs**

A18.16   **Tuberculosis of cervix**

A18.17   **Tuberculous female pelvic inflammatory disease**

Tuberculous endometritis

Tuberculous oophoritis and salpingitis

A18.18 **Tuberculosis of other female genital organs**
Tuberculous ulceration of vulva

A18.2 **Tuberculous peripheral lymphadenopathy**
Tuberculous adenitis
Excludes2: tuberculosis of bronchial and mediastinal
lymph nodes (A15.4)
tuberculosis of mesenteric and retroperitoneal
lymph nodes (A18.39)
tuberculous tracheobronchial adenopathy (A15.4)

A18.3 **Tuberculosis of intestines, peritoneum and mesenteric glands**

A18.31 **Tuberculous peritonitis**
Tuberculous ascites

A18.32 **Tuberculous enteritis**
Tuberculosis of anus and rectum
Tuberculosis of intestine (large) (small)

A18.39 **Retroperitoneal tuberculosis**
Tuberculosis of mesenteric glands
Tuberculosis of retroperitoneal (lymph glands)

A18.4 **Tuberculosis of skin and subcutaneous tissue**
Erythema induratum, tuberculous
Lupus excedens
Lupus vulgaris NOS
Lupus vulgaris of eyelid
Scrofuloderma
Tuberculosis of external ear
Excludes2: lupus erythematosus (L93.-)
lupus NOS (M32.9) systemic (M32.-)

A18.5 **Tuberculosis of eye**
Excludes2: lupus vulgaris of eyelid (A18.4)

A18.50 **Tuberculosis of eye, unspecified**

A18.51 **Tuberculous episcleritis**

A18.52 **Tuberculous keratitis**
Tuberculous interstitial keratitis
Tuberculous keratoconjunctivitis (interstitial)
(phlyctenular)

A18.53 **Tuberculous chorioretinitis**

A18.54 **Tuberculous iridocyclitis**

A18.59 **Other tuberculosis of eye**
Tuberculous conjunctivitis

A18.6 **Tuberculosis of (inner) (middle) ear**
Tuberculous otitis media
Excludes2: tuberculosis of external ear (A18.4)
tuberculous mastoiditis (A18.03)

A18.7 **Tuberculosis of adrenal glands**
Tuberculous Addison's disease

A18.8 **Tuberculosis of other specified organs**

A18.81 **Tuberculosis of thyroid gland**

A18.82 **Tuberculosis of other endocrine glands**
Tuberculosis of pituitary gland
Tuberculosis of thymus gland

A18.83 **Tuberculosis of digestive tract organs, not elsewhere classified**
Excludes1: tuberculosis of intestine (A18.32)

A18.84 **Tuberculosis of heart**

Tuberculous cardiomyopathy
Tuberculous endocarditis
Tuberculous myocarditis
Tuberculous pericarditis

A18.85 **Tuberculosis of spleen**

A18.89 **Tuberculosis of other sites**
Tuberculosis of muscle
Tuberculous cerebral arteritis

A19 **Miliary tuberculosis**
Definition: Miliary tuberculosis acute tuberculosis characterized by the appearance of tiny tubercles on one or more organs of the body.
Includes: disseminated tuberculosis
generalized tuberculosis tuberculous polyserositis

A19.0 **Acute miliary tuberculosis of a single specified site**

A19.1 **Acute miliary tuberculosis of multiple sites**

A19.2 **Acute miliary tuberculosis, unspecified**

A19.8 **Other miliary tuberculosis**

A19.9 **Miliary tuberculosis, unspecified**

CERTAIN ZOONOTIC BACTERIAL DISEASES (A20-A28)

A20 **Plague**
Definition: Plague is a deadly infectious disease caused by the enterobacteria yersinia pestis (pasteurella pestis).
Includes: infection due to Yersinia pestis

A20.0 **Bubonic plague**

A20.1 **Cellulocutaneous plague**

A20.2 **Pneumonic plague**

A20.3 **Plague meningitis**

A20.7 **Septicemic plague**

A20.8 **Other forms of plague**
Abortive plague
Asymptomatic plague
Pestis minor

A20.9 **Plague, unspecified**

A21 **Tularemia**
Definition: Tularemia, aka rabbit fever, deer fly fever, O'Hara's fever is a serious infectious disease caused by the bacterium francisella tularensis.
Includes: deer-fly fever
infection due to Francisella tularensis rabbit fever

A21.0 **Ulceroglandular tularemia**

A21.1 **Oculoglandular tularemia**
Ophthalmic tularemia

A21.2 **Pulmonary tularemia**

A21.3 **Gastrointestinal tularemia**
Abdominal tularemia

A21.7 **Generalized tularemia**

A21.8 **Other forms of tularemia**

A21.9 **Tularemia, unspecified**

A22 **Anthrax**
Definition: Anthrax is an acute disease in humans and animals caused by the bacterium bacillus anthracis which is highly lethal in some forms.
Includes: infection due to Bacillus anthracis

A22.0 **Cutaneous anthrax**

Malignant carbuncle

Malignant pustule

A22.1 Pulmonary anthrax

Inhalation anthrax

Ragpicker's disease

Woolsorter's disease

A22.2 Gastrointestinal anthrax

A22.7 Anthrax sepsis

A22.8 Other forms of anthrax

Anthrax meningitis

A22.9 Anthrax, unspecified

A23 Brucellosis

Definition: Brucellosis, aka undulant fever, or malta fever is a highly contagious zoonosis caused by ingestion of unsterilized milk or meat from infected animals, or close contact with their secretions.

Includes: Malta fever

Mediterranean fever undulant fever

A23.0 Brucellosis due to Brucella melitensis

A23.1 Brucellosis due to Brucella abortus

A23.2 Brucellosis due to Brucella suis

A23.3 Brucellosis due to Brucella canis

A23.8 Other brucellosis

A23.9 Brucellosis, unspecified

A24 Glanders and melioidosis

Definition: Glanders is an infectious disease that occurs primarily in horses, mules, and donkeys and other animals such as dogs, cats and goats that can be transmitted to humans. It is caused by infection with the bacterium burkholderia mallei.

A24.0 Glanders

Infection due to Pseudomonas mallei

Malleus

A24.1 Acute and fulminating melioidosis

Melioidosis pneumonia

Melioidosis sepsis

A24.2 Subacute and chronic melioidosis

A24.3 Other melioidosis

A24.9 Melioidosis, unspecified

Infection due to Pseudomonas pseudomallei NOS

Whitmore's disease

A25 Rat-bite fevers

A25.0 Spirillosis

Sodoku

A25.1 Streptobacillosis

Epidemic arthritic erythema

Haverhill fever

Streptobacillary rat-bite fever

A25.9 Rat-bite fever, unspecified

A26 Erysipeloid

A26.0 Cutaneous erysipeloid

Erythema migrans

A26.7 Erysipelothrix sepsis

A26.8 Other forms of erysipeloid

A26.9 Erysipeloid, unspecified

A27 Leptospirosis

A27.0 Leptospirosis icterohemorrhagica

Leptospiral or spirochetal jaundice (hemorrhagic) Weil's disease

A27.8 Other forms of leptospirosis

A27.81 Aseptic meningitis in leptospirosis

A27.89 Other forms of leptospirosis

A27.9 Leptospirosis, unspecified

A28 Other zoonotic bacterial diseases, not elsewhere classified

Definition: Zoonotic refers to other diseases that can be passed from animals, whether wild or domesticated, to humans.

A28.0 Pasteurellosis

A28.1 Cat-scratch disease

Cat-scratch fever

A28.2 Extraintestinal yersiniosis

Excludes1: enteritis due to Yersinia enterocolitica (A04.6)

plague (A20.-)

A28.8 Other specified zoonotic bacterial diseases, not elsewhere classified

A28.9 Zoonotic bacterial disease, unspecified

OTHER BACTERIAL DISEASES (A30-A49)

A30 Leprosy [Hansen's disease]

Definition: Leprosy is an infectious disease characterized by disfiguring skin sores, nerve damage, and progressive debilitation. Leprosy is caused by the organism mycobacterium leprae.

Includes: infection due to Mycobacterium leprae

Excludes1: sequelae of leprosy (B92)

A30.0 Indeterminate leprosy

I leprosy

A30.1 Tuberculoid leprosy

TT leprosy

A30.2 Borderline tuberculoid leprosy

BT leprosy

A30.3 Borderline leprosy

BB leprosy

A30.4 Borderline lepromatous leprosy

BL leprosy

A30.5 Lepromatous leprosy

LL leprosy

A30.8 Other forms of leprosy

A30.9 Leprosy, unspecified

A31 Infection due to other mycobacteria

Excludes2: leprosy (A30.-)

tuberculosis (A15-A19)

A31.0 Pulmonary mycobacterial infection

Infection due to Mycobacterium avium

Infection due to Mycobacterium intracellulare [Battey bacillus]

Infection due to Mycobacterium kansasii

A31.1 Cutaneous mycobacterial infection

Buruli ulcer

Infection due to Mycobacterium marinum

Infection due to Mycobacterium ulcerans

A31.2 Disseminated mycobacterium avium-intracellulare complex (DMAC)

MAC sepsis

A31.8 **Other mycobacterial infections**

A31.9 **Mycobacterial infection, unspecified**

Atypical mycobacterial infection NOS

Mycobacteriosis NOS

A32 **Listeriosis**

Includes: listerial foodborne infection

Excludes1: neonatal (disseminated) listeriosis (P37.2)

A32.0 **Cutaneous listeriosis**

A32.1 **Listerial meningitis and meningoencephalitis**

A32.11 **Listerial meningitis**

A32.12 **Listerial meningoencephalitis**

A32.7 **Listerial sepsis**

A32.8 **Other forms of listeriosis**

A32.81 **Oculoglandular listeriosis**

A32.82 **Listerial endocarditis**

A32.89 **Other forms of listeriosis**

Listerial cerebral arteritis

A32.9 **Listeriosis, unspecified**

A33 **Tetanus neonatorum**

A34 **Obstetrical tetanus**

A35 **Other tetanus**

Tetanus NOS

Excludes1: obstetrical tetanus (A34)

tetanus neonatorum (A33)

A36 **Diphtheria**

Definition: Diphtheria is a highly infectious disease of the upper respiratory tract characterised by a sore throat, fever and causing difficulty in breathing.

A36.0 **Pharyngeal diphtheria**

Diphtheritic membranous angina

Tonsillar diphtheria

A36.1 **Nasopharyngeal diphtheria**

A36.2 **Laryngeal diphtheria**

Diphtheritic laryngotracheitis

A36.3 **Cutaneous diphtheria**

Excludes2: erythrasma (L08.1)

A36.8 **Other diphtheria**

A36.81 **Diphtheritic cardiomyopathy**

Diphtheritic myocarditis

A36.82 **Diphtheritic radiculomyelitis**

A36.83 **Diphtheritic polyneuritis**

A36.84 **Diphtheritic tubulo-interstitial nephropathy**

A36.85 **Diphtheritic cystitis**

A36.86 **Diphtheritic conjunctivitis**

A36.89 **Other diphtheritic complications**

Diphtheritic peritonitis

A36.9 **Diphtheria, unspecified**

A37 **Whooping cough**

Definition: Whooping cough, aka pertussis, is a highly contagious disease caused by bacteria. The most prominent symptom of whooping cough is a distinctive, uncontrollable cough, followed by a sharp, high-pitched intake of air.

A37.0 **Whooping cough due to Bordetella pertussis**

A37.00 **Whooping cough due to Bordetella pertussis without pneumonia**

A37.01 **Whooping cough due to Bordetella pertussis with pneumonia**

A37.1 **Whooping cough due to Bordetella parapertussis**

A37.10 **Whooping cough due to Bordetella parapertussis without pneumonia**

A37.11 **Whooping cough due to Bordetella parapertussis with pneumonia**

A37.8 **Whooping cough due to other Bordetella species**

A37.80 **Whooping cough due to other Bordetella species without pneumonia**

A37.81 **Whooping cough due to other Bordetella species with pneumonia**

A37.9 **Whooping cough, unspecified species**

A37.90 **Whooping cough, unspecified species without pneumonia**

A37.91 **Whooping cough, unspecified species with pneumonia**

A38 **Scarlet fever**

Includes: scarlatina

Excludes2: streptococcal sore throat (J02.0)

A38.0 **Scarlet fever with otitis media**

A38.1 **Scarlet fever with myocarditis**

A38.8 **Scarlet fever with other complications**

A38.9 **Scarlet fever, uncomplicated**

Scarlet fever, NOS

A39 **Meningococcal infection**

A39.0 **Meningococcal meningitis**

A39.1 **Waterhouse-Friderichsen syndrome**

Meningococcal hemorrhagic adrenalitis

Meningococcic adrenal syndrome

A39.2 **Acute meningococcemia**

A39.3 **Chronic meningococcemia**

A39.4 **Meningococcemia, unspecified**

A39.5 **Meningococcal heart disease**

A39.50 **Meningococcal carditis, unspecified**

A39.51 **Meningococcal endocarditis**

A39.52 **Meningococcal myocarditis**

A39.53 **Meningococcal pericarditis**

A39.8 **Other meningococcal infections**

A39.81 **Meningococcal encephalitis**

A39.82 **Meningococcal retrobulbar neuritis**

A39.83 **Meningococcal arthritis**

A39.84 **Postmeningococcal arthritis**

A39.89 **Other meningococcal infections**

Meningococcal conjunctivitis

A39.9 **Meningococcal infection, unspecified**

Meningococcal disease NOS

A40 **Streptococcal sepsis**

Code first postprocedural streptococcal sepsis (T81.4-)

streptococcal sepsis during labor (O75.3)

streptococcal sepsis following abortion or ectopic or molar pregnancy (O03-O07, O08.0)

streptococcal sepsis following immunization (T88.0)

streptococcal sepsis following infusion, transfusion or therapeutic injection (T80.2-)

Excludes1: neonatal (P36.0-P36.1)

puerperal sepsis (O85)

sepsis due to Streptococcus, group D (A41.81)

A40.0 **Sepsis due to streptococcus, group A**

A40.1 **Sepsis due to streptococcus, group B**

A40.3 **Sepsis due to Streptococcus pneumoniae**

Pneumococcal sepsis

A40.8 **Other streptococcal sepsis**

A40.9 **Streptococcal sepsis, unspecified**

A41 **Other sepsis**

Code first postprocedural sepsis (T81.4-)

sepsis during labor (O75.3)

sepsis following abortion, ectopic or molar pregnancy (O03-O07, O08.0)

sepsis following immunization (T88.0)

sepsis following infusion, transfusion or therapeutic injection (T80.2-)

Excludes1: bacteremia NOS (R78.81)

neonatal (P36.-) puerperal sepsis (O85)

streptococcal sepsis (A40.-)

Excludes2: sepsis (due to) (in) actinomycotic (A42.7)

sepsis (due to) (in) anthrax (A22.7)

sepsis (due to) (in) candidal (B37.7)

sepsis (due to) (in) Erysipelothrix (A26.7)

sepsis (due to) (in) extraintestinal yersiniosis (A28.2)

sepsis (due to) (in) gonococcal (A54.86)

sepsis (due to) (in) herpesviral (B00.7)

sepsis (due to) (in) listerial (A32.7)

sepsis (due to) (in) melioidosis (A24.1)

sepsis (due to) (in) meningococcal (A39.2-A39.4)

sepsis (due to) (in) plague (A20.7)

sepsis (due to) (in) tularemia (A21.7)

toxic shock syndrome (A48.3)

A41.0 **Sepsis due to Staphylococcus aureus**

A41.01 **Sepsis due to Methicillin susceptible Staphylococcus aureus**

MSSA sepsis

Staphylococcus aureus sepsis NOS

A41.02 **Sepsis due to Methicillin resistant Staphylococcus aureus**

A41.1 **Sepsis due to other specified staphylococcus**

Coagulase negative staphylococcus sepsis

A41.2 **Sepsis due to unspecified staphylococcus**

A41.3 **Sepsis due to Hemophilus influenzae**

A41.4 **Sepsis due to anaerobes**

Excludes1: gas gangrene (A48.0)

A41.5 **Sepsis due to other Gram-negative organisms**

A41.50 **Gram-negative sepsis, unspecified**

Gram-negative sepsis NOS

A41.51 **Sepsis due to Escherichia coli [E. coli]**

A41.52 **Sepsis due to Pseudomonas**

Pseudomonas aeruginosa

A41.53 **Sepsis due to Serratia**

A41.59 **Other Gram-negative sepsis**

A41.8 **Other specified sepsis**

A41.81 **Sepsis due to Enterococcus**

A41.89 **Other specified sepsis**

A41.9 **Sepsis, unspecified organism**

Septicemia NOS

A42 **Actinomycosis**

Definition: Actinomycosis is an infection primarily caused by the bacterium actinomyces israelii. Infection most often occurs in the face and neck region and is characterized by the presence of a slowly enlarging, hard, red lump.

Excludes1: actinomycetoma (B47.1)

A42.0 **Pulmonary actinomycosis**

A42.1 **Abdominal actinomycosis**

A42.2 **Cervicofacial actinomycosis**

A42.7 **Actinomycotic sepsis**

A42.8 **Other forms of actinomycosis**

A42.81 **Actinomycotic meningitis**

A42.82 **Actinomycotic encephalitis**

A42.89 **Other forms of actinomycosis**

A42.9 **Actinomycosis, unspecified**

A43 **Nocardiosis**

A43.0 **Pulmonary nocardiosis**

A43.1 **Cutaneous nocardiosis**

A43.8 **Other forms of nocardiosis**

A43.9 **Nocardiosis, unspecified**

A44 **Bartonellosis**

A44.0 **Systemic bartonellosis**

Oroya fever

A44.1 **Cutaneous and mucocutaneous bartonellosis**

Verruga peruana

A44.8 **Other forms of bartonellosis**

A44.9 **Bartonellosis, unspecified**

A46 **Erysipelas**

Definition: Erysipelas is an acute febrile disease that is associated with intense often vesicular and edematous local inflammation of the skin and subcutaneous tissues and that is caused by a hemolytic streptococcus.

Excludes1: postpartum or puerperal erysipelas (O86.89)

A48 **Other bacterial diseases, not elsewhere classified**

Excludes1: actinomycetoma (B47.1)

A48.0 **Gas gangrene**

Clostridial cellulitis

Clostridial myonecrosis

A48.1 **Legionnaires' disease**

A48.2 **Nonpneumonic Legionnaires' disease [Pontiac fever]**

A48.3 **Toxic shock syndrome**

Use additional code to identify the organism (B95, B96)

Excludes1: endotoxic shock NOS (R57.8)

sepsis NOS (A41.9)

A48.4 **Brazilian purpuric fever**

Systemic Hemophilus aegyptius infection

A48.5 **Other specified botulism**

Non-foodborne intoxication due to toxins of Clostridium botulinum [C. botulinum]

Excludes1: food poisoning due to toxins of Clostridium botulinum (A05.1)

A48.51 **Infant botulism**

A48.52 **Wound botulism**

Non-foodborne botulism NOS

Use additional code for associated wound

A48.8 **Other specified bacterial diseases**

A49 **Bacterial infection of unspecified site**

Excludes1: bacterial agents as the cause of diseases classified elsewhere (B95-B96)

chlamydial infection NOS (A74.9)

meningococcal infection NOS (A39.9)

rickettsial infection NOS (A79.9)

spirochetal infection NOS (A69.9)

A49.0 **Staphylococcal infection, unspecified site**

A49.01 **Methicillin susceptible Staphylococcus aureus infection, unspecified site**

Methicillin susceptible Staphylococcus aureus (MSSA) infection

Staphylococcus aureus infection NOS

A49.02 **Methicillin resistant Staphylococcus aureus infection, unspecified site**

Methicillin resistant Staphylococcus aureus (MRSA) infection

A49.1 **Streptococcal infection, unspecified site**

A49.2 **Hemophilus influenzae infection, unspecified site**

A49.3 **Mycoplasma infection, unspecified site**

A49.8 **Other bacterial infections of unspecified site**

A49.9 **Bacterial infection, unspecified**

Excludes1: bacteremia NOS (R78.81)

INFECTIONS WITH A PREDOMINANTLY SEXUAL MODE OF TRANSMISSION (A50-A64)

Excludes1: human immunodeficiency virus [HIV] disease (B20)

nonspecific and nongonococcal urethritis (N34.1)

Reiter's disease (M02.3-)

A50 **Congenital syphilis**

Definition: Congenital syphilis is syphilis present in utero and at birth, and occurs when a child is born to a mother with secondary or tertiary syphilis.

A50.0 **Early congenital syphilis, symptomatic**

Any congenital syphilitic condition specified as early or manifest less than two years after birth.

A50.01 **Early congenital syphilitic oculopathy**

A50.02 **Early congenital syphilitic osteochondropathy**

A50.03 **Early congenital syphilitic pharyngitis**

Early congenital syphilitic laryngitis

A50.04 **Early congenital syphilitic pneumonia**

A50.05 **Early congenital syphilitic rhinitis**

A50.06 **Early cutaneous congenital syphilis**

A50.07 **Early mucocutaneous congenital syphilis**

A50.08 **Early visceral congenital syphilis**

A50.09 **Other early congenital syphilis, symptomatic**

A50.1 **Early congenital syphilis, latent**

Congenital syphilis without clinical manifestations, with positive serological reaction and negative

spinal fluid test, less than two years after birth.

A50.2 **Early congenital syphilis, unspecified**

Congenital syphilis NOS less than two years after birth.

A50.3 **Late congenital syphilitic oculopathy**

Excludes1: Hutchinson's triad (A50.53)

A50.30 **Late congenital syphilitic oculopathy, unspecified**

A50.31 **Late congenital syphilitic interstitial keratitis**

A50.32 **Late congenital syphilitic chorioretinitis**

A50.39 **Other late congenital syphilitic oculopathy**

A50.4 **Late congenital neurosyphilis [juvenile neurosyphilis]**

Use additional code to identify any associated mental disorder

Excludes1: Hutchinson's triad (A50.53)

A50.40 **Late congenital neurosyphilis, unspecified**

Juvenile neurosyphilis NOS

A50.41 **Late congenital syphilitic meningitis**

A50.42 **Late congenital syphilitic encephalitis**

A50.43 **Late congenital syphilitic polyneuropathy**

A50.44 **Late congenital syphilitic optic nerve atrophy**

A50.45 **Juvenile general paresis**

Dementia paralytica juvenilis

Juvenile tabetoparetic neurosyphilis

A50.49 **Other late congenital neurosyphilis**

Juvenile tabes dorsalis

A50.5 **Other late congenital syphilis, symptomatic**

Any congenital syphilitic condition specified as late or manifest two years or more after birth.

A50.51 **Clutton's joints**

A50.52 **Hutchinson's teeth**

A50.53 **Hutchinson's triad**

A50.54 **Late congenital cardiovascular syphilis**

A50.55 **Late congenital syphilitic arthropathy**

A50.56 **Late congenital syphilitic osteochondropathy**

A50.57 **Syphilitic saddle nose**

A50.59 **Other late congenital syphilis, symptomatic**

A50.6 **Late congenital syphilis, latent**

Congenital syphilis without clinical manifestations, with positive serological reaction and negative spinal fluid test, two years or more after birth.

A50.7 **Late congenital syphilis, unspecified**

Congenital syphilis NOS two years or more after birth.

A50.9 **Congenital syphilis, unspecified**

A51 **Early syphilis**

Definition: Early syphilis is defined as the stages of syphilis (primary, secondary, and early latent syphilis) that typically occur within the first year after acquisition of the infection.

A51.0 **Primary genital syphilis**

Syphilitic chancre NOS

A51.1 **Primary anal syphilis**

A51.2 **Primary syphilis of other sites**

A51.3 **Secondary syphilis of skin and mucous membranes**

A51.31 **Condyloma latum**

A51.32 **Syphilitic alopecia**

A51.39 **Other secondary syphilis of skin**

Syphilitic leukoderma

Syphilitic mucous patch

Excludes1: late syphilitic leukoderma (A52.79)

A51.4   Other secondary syphilis

A51.41   Secondary syphilitic meningitis

A51.42   Secondary syphilitic female pelvic disease

A51.43   Secondary syphilitic oculopathy

Secondary syphilitic chorioretinitis

Secondary syphilitic iridocyclitis, iritis

Secondary syphilitic uveitis

A51.44   Secondary syphilitic nephritis

A51.45   Secondary syphilitic hepatitis

A51.46   Secondary syphilitic osteopathy

A51.49   Other secondary syphilitic conditions

Secondary syphilitic lymphadenopathy

Secondary syphilitic myositis

A51.5   Early syphilis, latent

Syphilis (acquired) without clinical manifestations, with positive serological reaction and negative spinal fluid test, less than two years after infection.

A51.9   Early syphilis, unspecified

A52   Late syphilis

A52.0   Cardiovascular and cerebrovascular syphilis

Definition: Cardiovascular syphilis refers to the involvement of the cardiovascular system in late syphilis usually resulting in aortitis aneurysm formation, and aortic valvular insufficiency.

A52.00   Cardiovascular syphilis, unspecified

A52.01   Syphilitic aneurysm of aorta

A52.02   Syphilitic aortitis

A52.03   Syphilitic endocarditis

Syphilitic aortic valve incompetence or stenosis

Syphilitic mitral valve stenosis

Syphilitic pulmonary valve regurgitation

A52.04   Syphilitic cerebral arteritis

A52.05   Other cerebrovascular syphilis

Syphilitic cerebral aneurysm (ruptured) (non-ruptured)

Syphilitic cerebral thrombosis

A52.06   Other syphilitic heart involvement

Syphilitic coronary artery disease

Syphilitic myocarditis

Syphilitic pericarditis

A52.09   Other cardiovascular syphilis

A52.1   Symptomatic neurosyphilis

Definition: Neurosyphilis, aka tabes dorsalis, is the slowly progressive degeneration of the spinal cord that occurs in the late (tertiary) phase of syphilis a decade or more after contracting the infection.

A52.10   Symptomatic neurosyphilis, unspecified

A52.11   Tabes dorsalis

Locomotor ataxia (progressive)

Tabetic neurosyphilis

A52.12   Other cerebrospinal syphilis

A52.13   Late syphilitic meningitis

A52.14   Late syphilitic encephalitis

A52.15   Late syphilitic neuropathy

Late syphilitic acoustic neuritis

Late syphilitic optic (nerve) atrophy

Late syphilitic polyneuropathy

Late syphilitic retrobulbar neuritis

A52.16   Charcôt's arthropathy (tabetic)

A52.17   General paresis

Dementia paralytica

A52.19   Other symptomatic neurosyphilis

Syphilitic parkinsonism

A52.2   Asymptomatic neurosyphilis

A52.3   Neurosyphilis, unspecified

Gumma (syphilitic)

Syphilis (late)

Syphiloma

A52.7   Other symptomatic late syphilis

Definition: Late syphilis is defined as involvement of the cardiovascular or central nervous system, or the development of a gumma in any organ, due to infection with treponema pallidum; usually several years to 2-3 decades after the initial infection. Also known as tertiary syphilis.

A52.71   Late syphilitic oculopathy

Late syphilitic chorioretinitis

Late syphilitic episcleritis

A52.72   Syphilis of lung and bronchus

A52.73   Symptomatic late syphilis of other respiratory organs

A52.74   Syphilis of liver and other viscera

Late syphilitic peritonitis

A52.75   Syphilis of kidney and ureter

Syphilitic glomerular disease

A52.76   Other genitourinary symptomatic late syphilis

Late syphilitic female pelvic inflammatory disease

A52.77   Syphilis of bone and joint

A52.78   Syphilis of other musculoskeletal tissue

Late syphilitic bursitis

Syphilis [stage unspecified] of bursa

Syphilis [stage unspecified] of muscle

Syphilis [stage unspecified] of synovium

Syphilis [stage unspecified] of tendon

A52.79   Other symptomatic late syphilis

Late syphilitic leukoderma

Syphilis of adrenal gland

Syphilis of pituitary gland

Syphilis of thyroid gland

Syphilitic splenomegaly

Excludes1: syphilitic leukoderma (secondary) (A51.39)

A52.8   Late syphilis, latent

Syphilis (acquired) without clinical manifestations, with positive serological reaction and negative spinal fluid test, two years or more after infection

A52.9   Late syphilis, unspecified

A53   Other and unspecified syphilis

A53.0 **Latent syphilis, unspecified as early or late**

Latent syphilis NOS

Positive serological reaction for syphilis

A53.9 **Syphilis, unspecified**

Infection due to Treponema pallidum NOS

Syphilis (acquired) NOS

Excludes1: syphilis NOS under two years of age (A50.2)

A54 **Gonococcal infection**

Definition: Gonococcal infection is a sexually transmitted disease caused by gonococcal bacteria that affects the mucous membrane chiefly of the genital and urinary tracts and is characterized by an acute purulent discharge and painful or difficult urination, though women often have no symptoms.

A54.0 **Gonococcal infection of lower genitourinary tract without periurethral or accessory gland abscess**

Excludes1: gonococcal infection with genitourinary gland abscess (A54.1)

gonococcal infection with periurethral abscess (A54.1)

A54.00 **Gonococcal infection of lower genitourinary tract, unspecified**

A54.01 **Gonococcal cystitis and urethritis, unspecified**

A54.02 **Gonococcal vulvovaginitis, unspecified**

A54.03 **Gonococcal cervicitis, unspecified**

A54.09 **Other gonococcal infection of lower genitourinary tract**

A54.1 **Gonococcal infection of lower genitourinary tract with periurethral and accessory gland abscess**

Gonococcal Bartholin's gland abscess

A54.2 **Gonococcal pelviperitonitis and other gonococcal genitourinary infection**

A54.21 **Gonococcal infection of kidney and ureter**

A54.22 **Gonococcal prostatitis**

A54.23 **Gonococcal infection of other male genital organs**

Gonococcal epididymitis

Gonococcal orchitis

A54.24 **Gonococcal female pelvic inflammatory disease**

Gonococcal pelviperitonitis

Excludes1: gonococcal peritonitis (A54.85)

A54.29 **Other gonococcal genitourinary infections**

A54.3 **Gonococcal infection of eye**

A54.30 **Gonococcal infection of eye, unspecified**

A54.31 **Gonococcal conjunctivitis**

Ophthalmia neonatorum due to gonococcus

A54.32 **Gonococcal iridocyclitis**

A54.33 **Gonococcal keratitis**

A54.39 **Other gonococcal eye infection**

Gonococcal endophthalmia

A54.4 **Gonococcal infection of musculoskeletal system**

A54.40 **Gonococcal infection of musculoskeletal system, unspecified**

A54.41 **Gonococcal spondylopathy**

A54.42 **Gonococcal arthritis**

Excludes2: gonococcal infection of spine (A54.41)

A54.43 **Gonococcal osteomyelitis**

Excludes2: gonococcal infection of spine (A54.41)

A54.49 **Gonococcal infection of other musculoskeletal tissue**

Gonococcal bursitis

Gonococcal myositis

Gonococcal synovitis

Gonococcal tenosynovitis

A54.5 **Gonococcal pharyngitis**

A54.6 **Gonococcal infection of anus and rectum**

A54.8 **Other gonococcal infections**

A54.81 **Gonococcal meningitis**

A54.82 **Gonococcal brain abscess**

A54.83 **Gonococcal heart infection**

Gonococcal endocarditis

Gonococcal myocarditis

Gonococcal pericarditis

A54.84 **Gonococcal pneumonia**

A54.85 **Gonococcal peritonitis**

Excludes1: gonococcal pelviperitonitis (A54.24)

A54.86 **Gonococcal sepsis**

A54.89 **Other gonococcal infections**

Gonococcal keratoderma

Gonococcal lymphadenitis

A54.9 **Gonococcal infection, unspecified**

A55 **Chlamydial lymphogranuloma (venereum)**

Climatic or tropical bubo

Durand-Nicolas-Favre disease

Esthiomene

Lymphogranuloma inguinale

A56 **Other sexually transmitted chlamydial diseases**

Includes: sexually transmitted diseases due to Chlamydia trachomatis

Excludes1: neonatal chlamydial conjunctivitis (P39.1)

neonatal chlamydial pneumonia (P23.1)

Excludes2: chlamydial lymphogranuloma (A55)

conditions classified to A74.-

A56.0 **Chlamydial infection of lower genitourinary tract**

A56.00 **Chlamydial infection of lower genitourinary tract, unspecified**

A56.01 **Chlamydial cystitis and urethritis**

A56.02 **Chlamydial vulvovaginitis**

A56.09 **Other chlamydial infection of lower genitourinary tract**

Chlamydial cervicitis

A56.1 **Chlamydial infection of pelviperitoneum and other genitourinary organs**

A56.11 **Chlamydial female pelvic inflammatory disease**

A56.19 **Other chlamydial genitourinary infection**

Chlamydial epididymitis

Chlamydial orchitis

A56.2 **Chlamydial infection of genitourinary tract, unspecified**

A56.3 **Chlamydial infection of anus and rectum**

A56.4 **Chlamydial infection of pharynx**

A56.8 **Sexually transmitted chlamydial infection of other sites**

A57 **Chancroid**

Ulcus molle

A58 **Granuloma inguinale**

Donovanosis

A59 **Trichomoniasis**

Definition: Trichomoniasis is a common sexually transmitted disease caused by the parasite trichomonas vaginalis and infecting the urinary tract or vagina.

Excludes2: intestinal trichomoniasis (A07.8)

A59.0 **Urogenital trichomoniasis**

    A59.00 **Urogenital trichomoniasis, unspecified**

      Fluor (vaginalis) due to Trichomonas

      Leukorrhea (vaginalis) due to Trichomonas

    A59.01 **Trichomonal vulvovaginitis**

    A59.02 **Trichomonal prostatitis**

    A59.03 **Trichomonal cystitis and urethritis**

    A59.09 **Other urogenital trichomoniasis**

      Trichomonas cervicitis

A59.8 **Trichomoniasis of other sites**

A59.9 **Trichomoniasis, unspecified**

A60 **Anogenital herpesviral [herpes simplex] infections**

A60.0 **Herpesviral infection of genitalia and urogenital tract**

    A60.00 **Herpesviral infection of urogenital system, unspecified**

    A60.01 **Herpesviral infection of penis**

    A60.02 **Herpesviral infection of other male genital organs**

    A60.03 **Herpesviral cervicitis**

    A60.04 **Herpesviral vulvovaginitis**

      Herpesviral [herpes simplex] ulceration

      Herpesviral [herpes simplex] vaginitis

      Herpesviral [herpes simplex] vulvitis

    A60.09 **Herpesviral infection of other urogenital tract**

A60.1 **Herpesviral infection of perianal skin and rectum**

A60.9 **Anogenital herpesviral infection, unspecified**

A63 **Other predominantly sexually transmitted diseases, not elsewhere classified**

Excludes2: molluscum contagiosum (B08.1)

papilloma of cervix (D26.0)

A63.0 **Anogenital (venereal) warts**

    Anogenital warts due to (human) papillomavirus [HPV]

    Condyloma acuminatum

A63.8 **Other specified predominantly sexually transmitted diseases**

A64 **Unspecified sexually transmitted disease**

OTHER SPIROCHETAL DISEASES (A65-A69)

Excludes2: leptospirosis (A27.-)

syphilis (A50-A53)

A65 **Nonvenereal syphilis**

Bejel

Endemic syphilis

Njovera

A66 **Yaws**

Definition: Yaws is a contagious tropical disease caused by the spirochete treponema pertenue, characterized by yellowish or reddish tumors, which often resemble currants, strawberries, or raspberries.

Includes: bouba

frambesia (tropica) pian

A66.0 **Initial lesions of yaws**

    Chancre of yaws

    Frambesia, initial or primary

    Initial frambesial ulcer

    Mother yaw

A66.1 **Multiple papillomata and wet crab yaws**

    Frambesioma

    Pianoma

    Plantar or palmar papilloma of yaws

A66.2 **Other early skin lesions of yaws**

    Cutaneous yaws, less than five years after infection

    Early yaws (cutaneous)(macular)(maculopapular) (micropapular)(papular)

    Frambeside of early yaws

A66.3 **Hyperkeratosis of yaws**

    Ghoul hand

    Hyperkeratosis, palmar or plantar (early) (late) due to yaws

    Worm-eaten soles

A66.4 **Gummata and ulcers of yaws**

    Gummatous frambeside

    Nodular late yaws (ulcerated)

A66.5 **Gangosa**

    Rhinopharyngitis mutilans

A66.6 **Bone and joint lesions of yaws**

    Yaws ganglion

    Yaws goundou

    Yaws gumma, bone

    Yaws gummatous osteitis or periostitis

    Yaws hydrarthrosis

    Yaws osteitis

    Yaws periostitis (hypertrophic)

A66.7 **Other manifestations of yaws**

    Juxta-articular nodules of yaws

    Mucosal yaws

A66.8 **Latent yaws**

    Yaws without clinical manifestations, with positive serology

A66.9 **Yaws, unspecified**

A67 **Pinta [carate]**

A67.0 **Primary lesions of pinta**

    Chancre (primary) of pinta

    Papule (primary) of pinta

A67.1 **Intermediate lesions of pinta**

    Erythematous plaques of pinta

    Hyperchromic lesions of pinta

    Hyperkeratosis of pinta

    Pintids

A67.2 **Late lesions of pinta**

Achromic skin lesions of pinta

Cicatricial skin lesions of pinta

Dyschromic skin lesions of pinta

A67.3 Mixed lesions of pinta

Achromic with hyperchromic skin lesions of pinta [carate]

A67.9 Pinta, unspecified

A68 Relapsing fevers

Definition: Relapsing fever is an infection caused by certain bacteria in the genus borrelia. It is a vector-borne disease that is transmitted through louse or soft-bodied tick bites.

Includes: recurrent fever

Excludes2: Lyme disease (A69.2-)

A68.0 Louse-borne relapsing fever

Relapsing fever due to Borrelia recurrentis

A68.1 Tick-borne relapsing fever

Relapsing fever due to any Borrelia species other than Borrelia recurrentis

A68.9 Relapsing fever, unspecified

A69 Other spirochetal infections

A69.0 Necrotizing ulcerative stomatitis

Cancrum oris

Fusospirochetal gangrene Noma

Stomatitis gangrenosa

A69.1 Other Vincent's infections

Fusospirochetal pharyngitis

Necrotizing ulcerative (acute) gingivitis

Necrotizing ulcerative (acute) gingivostomatitis

Spirochetal stomatitis

Trench mouth

Vincent's angina

Vincent's gingivitis

A69.2 Lyme disease

Erythema chronicum migrans due to Borrelia burgdorferi

A69.20 Lyme disease, unspecified

A69.21 Meningitis due to Lyme disease

A69.22 Other neurologic disorders in Lyme disease

Cranial neuritis

Meningoencephalitis

Polyneuropathy

A69.23 Arthritis due to Lyme disease

A69.29 Other conditions associated with Lyme disease

Myopericarditis due to Lyme disease

A69.8 Other specified spirochetal infections

A69.9 Spirochetal infection, unspecified

OTHER DISEASES CAUSED BY CHLAMYDIAE (A70-A74)

Excludes1: sexually transmitted chlamydial diseases (A55-A56)

A70 Chlamydia psittaci infections

Ornithosis

Parrot fever

Psittacosis

A71 Trachoma

Excludes1: sequelae of trachoma (B94.0)

A71.0 Initial stage of trachoma

Trachoma dubium

A71.1 Active stage of trachoma

Granular conjunctivitis (trachomatous)

Trachomatous follicular conjunctivitis

Trachomatous pannus

A71.9 Trachoma, unspecified

A74 Other diseases caused by chlamydiae

Excludes1: neonatal chlamydial conjunctivitis (P39.1)

neonatal chlamydial pneumonia (P23.1)

Reiter's disease (M02.3-)

sexually transmitted chlamydial diseases (A55-A56)

Excludes2: chlamydial pneumonia (J16.0)

A74.0 Chlamydial conjunctivitis

Paratrachoma

A74.8 Other chlamydial diseases

A74.81 Chlamydial peritonitis

A74.89 Other chlamydial diseases

A74.9 Chlamydial infection, unspecified

Chlamydiosis NOS

RICKETTSIOSES (A75-A79)

Definition: Rickettsioses is a disease caused by intracellular bacteria. Examples of rickettsioses include typhus, Rocky Mountain spotted fever, and Rickettsialpox.

A75 Typhus fever

Excludes1: rickettsiosis due to Ehrlichia sennetsu (A79.81)

A75.0 Epidemic louse-borne typhus fever due to Rickettsia prowazekii

Classical typhus (fever)

Epidemic (louse-borne) typhus

A75.1 Recrudescent typhus [Brill's disease]

Brill-Zinsser disease

A75.2 Typhus fever due to Rickettsia typhi

Murine (flea-borne) typhus

A75.3 Typhus fever due to Rickettsia tsutsugamushi

Scrub (mite-borne) typhus

Tsutsugamushi fever

A75.9 Typhus fever, unspecified

Typhus (fever) NOS

A77 Spotted fever [tick-borne rickettsioses]

A77.0 Spotted fever due to Rickettsia rickettsii

Rocky Mountain spotted fever

Sao Paulo fever

A77.1 Spotted fever due to Rickettsia conorii

African tick typhus

Boutonneuse fever

India tick typhus

Kenya tick typhus

Marseilles fever

Mediterranean tick fever

A77.2 Spotted fever due to Rickettsia siberica

North Asian tick fever

Siberian tick typhus

A77.3 Spotted fever due to Rickettsia australis

Queensland tick typhus

A77.4   Ehrlichiosis

Excludes1: Rickettsiosis due to Ehrlichia sennetsu (A79.81)

    A77.40   Ehrlichiosis, unspecified

    A77.41   Ehrlichiosis chafeensis [E. chafeensis]

    A77.49   Other ehrlichiosis

A77.8   Other spotted fevers

A77.9   Spotted fever, unspecified

Tick-borne typhus NOS

A78   Q fever

Infection due to Coxiella burnetii

Nine Mile fever

Quadrilateral fever

A79   Other rickettsioses

A79.0   Trench fever

Quintan fever

Wolhynian fever

A79.1   Rickettsialpox due to Rickettsia akari

Kew Garden fever

Vesicular rickettsiosis

A79.8   Other specified rickettsioses

    A79.81   Rickettsiosis due to Ehrlichia sennetsu

    A79.89   Other specified rickettsioses

A79.9   Rickettsiosis, unspecified

Rickettsial infection NOS

VIRAL AND PRION INFECTIONS OF THE CENTRAL NERVOUS SYSTEM (A80-A89)

Excludes1: postpolio syndrome (G14)

sequelae of poliomyelitis (B91)

sequelae of viral encephalitis (B94.1)

A80   Acute poliomyelitis

A80.0   Acute paralytic poliomyelitis, vaccine-associated

A80.1   Acute paralytic poliomyelitis, wild virus, imported

A80.2   Acute paralytic poliomyelitis, wild virus, indigenous

A80.3   Acute paralytic poliomyelitis, other and unspecified

    A80.30   Acute paralytic poliomyelitis, unspecified

    A80.39   Other acute paralytic poliomyelitis

A80.4   Acute nonparalytic poliomyelitis

A80.9   Acute poliomyelitis, unspecified

A81   Atypical virus infections of central nervous system

Includes: diseases of the central nervous system caused by prions

Use additional code to identify:

dementia with behavioral disturbance (F02.81)

dementia without behavioral disturbance (F02.80)

A81.0   Creutzfeldt-Jakob disease

    A81.00   Creutzfeldt-Jakob disease, unspecified

Jakob-Creutzfeldt disease, unspecified

    A81.01   Variant Creutzfeldt-Jakob disease

vCJD

    A81.09   Other Creutzfeldt-Jakob disease

CJD

Familial Creutzfeldt-Jakob disease

Iatrogenic Creutzfeldt-Jakob disease

Sporadic Creutzfeldt-Jakob disease

Subacute spongiform encephalopathy (with dementia)

A81.1   Subacute sclerosing panencephalitis

Dawson's inclusion body encephalitis

Van Bogaert's sclerosing leukoencephalopathy

A81.2   Progressive multifocal leukoencephalopathy

Multifocal leukoencephalopathy NOS

A81.8   Other atypical virus infections of central nervous system

    A81.81   Kuru

    A81.82   Gerstmann-Sträussler-Scheinker syndrome

GSS syndrome

    A81.83   Fatal familial insomnia

FFI

    A81.89   Other atypical virus infections of central nervous system

A81.9   Atypical virus infection of central nervous system, unspecified

Prion diseases of the central nervous system NOS

A82   Rabies

Definition: Rabies is a viral disease that causes acute encephalitis in warm-blooded animals and people, characterised by abnormal behaviour such as excitement, aggressiveness, and dementia, followed by paralysis and death.

A82.0   Sylvatic rabies

A82.1   Urban rabies

A82.9   Rabies, unspecified

A83   Mosquito-borne viral encephalitis

Includes: mosquito-borne viral meningoencephalitis

Excludes2: Venezuelan equine encephalitis (A92.2)

West Nile fever (A92.3-) West Nile virus (A92.3-)

A83.0   Japanese encephalitis

A83.1   Western equine encephalitis

A83.2   Eastern equine encephalitis

A83.3   St Louis encephalitis

A83.4   Australian encephalitis

Kunjin virus disease

A83.5   California encephalitis

California meningoencephalitis

La Crosse encephalitis

A83.6   Rocio virus disease

A83.8   Other mosquito-borne viral encephalitis

A83.9   Mosquito-borne viral encephalitis, unspecified

A84   Tick-borne viral encephalitis

Includes: tick-borne viral meningoencephalitis

A84.0   Far Eastern tick-borne encephalitis [Russian spring-summer encephalitis]

A84.1   Central European tick-borne encephalitis

A84.8   Other tick-borne viral encephalitis

Louping ill

Powassan virus disease

A84.9   Tick-borne viral encephalitis, unspecified

A85   Other viral encephalitis, not elsewhere classified

Includes: specified viral encephalomyelitis NEC

specified viral meningoencephalitis NEC

Excludes1: benign myalgic encephalomyelitis (G93.3)

encephalitis due to cytomegalovirus (B25.8)

encephalitis due to herpesvirus NEC (B10.0-)

encephalitis due to herpesvirus [herpes simplex] (B00.4)

encephalitis due to measles virus (B05.0)

encephalitis due to mumps virus (B26.2)

encephalitis due to poliomyelitis virus (A80.-)

encephalitis due to zoster (B02.0)

lymphocytic choriomeningitis (A87.2)

A85.0   Enteroviral encephalitis

Enteroviral encephalomyelitis

A85.1   Adenoviral encephalitis

Adenoviral meningoencephalitis

A85.2   Arthropod-borne viral encephalitis, unspecified

Excludes1: West Nile virus with encephalitis (A92.31)

A85.8   Other specified viral encephalitis

Encephalitis lethargica

Von Economo-Cruchet disease

A86   Unspecified viral encephalitis

Viral encephalomyelitis NOS

Viral meningoencephalitis NOS

A87   Viral meningitis

Definition: Meningitis due to enterovirus refers to any of a subgroup of picornaviruses, including polioviruses, coxsackie viruses, and echoviruses, that infect the gastrointestinal tract and often spread to other areas of the body, especially the nervous system

Excludes1: meningitis due to herpesvirus [herpes simplex] (B00.3)

meningitis due to herpesvirus [herpes simplex] (B00.3)

meningitis due to measles virus (B05.1)

meningitis due to mumps virus (B26.1)

meningitis due to poliomyelitis virus (A80.-)

meningitis due to zoster (B02.1)

A87.0   Enteroviral meningitis

Coxsackievirus meningitis

Echovirus meningitis

A87.1   Adenoviral meningitis

A87.2   Lymphocytic choriomeningitis

Lymphocytic meningoencephalitis

A87.8   Other viral meningitis

A87.9   Viral meningitis, unspecified

A88   Other viral infections of central nervous system, not elsewhere classified

Excludes1: viral encephalitis NOS (A86)

viral meningitis NOS (A87.9)

A88.0   Enteroviral exanthematous fever [Boston exanthem]

A88.1   Epidemic vertigo

A88.8   Other specified viral infections of central nervous system

A89   Unspecified viral infection of central nervous system

ARTHROPOD-BORNE VIRAL FEVERS AND VIRAL HEMORRHAGIC FEVERS (A90-A99)

Definition: Hemorrhagic fever is a group of viral infections characterized by fever, chills, headache, malaise, and respiratory or gastrointestinal symptoms, followed by capillary hemorrhages and, in severe infection, by oliguria, kidney failure, hypotension, and possibly death.

A90   Dengue fever [classical dengue]

Excludes1: dengue hemorrhagic fever (A91)

A91   Dengue hemorrhagic fever

A92   Other mosquito-borne viral fevers

Excludes1: Ross River disease (B33.1)

A92.0   Chikungunya virus disease

Chikungunya (hemorrhagic) fever

A92.1   O'nyong-nyong fever

A92.2   Venezuelan equine fever

Venezuelan equine encephalitis

Venezuelan equine encephalomyelitis virus disease

A92.3   West Nile virus infection

West Nile fever

A92.30   West Nile virus infection, unspecified

West Nile fever NOS

West Nile fever without complications

West Nile virus NOS

A92.31   West Nile virus infection with encephalitis

West Nile encephalitis

West Nile encephalomyelitis

A92.32   West Nile virus infection with other neurologic manifestation

Use additional code to specify the neurologic manifestation

A92.39   West Nile virus infection with other complications

Use additional code to specify the other conditions

A92.4   Rift Valley fever

● **A92.5   Zika virus disease**

Zika virus fever

Zika virus infection

Zika NOS

A92.8   Other specified mosquito-borne viral fevers

A92.9   Mosquito-borne viral fever, unspecified

A93   Other arthropod-borne viral fevers, not elsewhere classified

A93.0   Oropouche virus disease

Oropouche fever

A93.1   Sandfly fever

Pappataci fever

Phlebotomus fever

A93.2   Colorado tick fever

A93.8   Other specified arthropod-borne viral fevers

Piry virus disease

Vesicular stomatitis virus disease [Indiana fever]

A94   Unspecified arthropod-borne viral fever

Arboviral fever NOS

Arbovirus infection NOS

A95   Yellow fever

Definition: Yellow fever is an acute systemic (body wide) illness caused by a virus called a flavivirus. In severe cases, the viral infection causes a high fever, bleeding into the skin, and necrosis (death) of cells in the kidney and liver.

A95.0   **Sylvatic yellow fever**

Jungle yellow fever

A95.1   **Urban yellow fever**

A95.9   **Yellow fever, unspecified**

A96   **Arenaviral hemorrhagic fever**

A96.0   **Junin hemorrhagic fever**

Argentinian hemorrhagic fever

A96.1   **Machupo hemorrhagic fever**

Bolivian hemorrhagic fever

A96.2   **Lassa fever**

A96.8   **Other arenaviral hemorrhagic fevers**

A96.9   **Arenaviral hemorrhagic fever, unspecified**

A98   **Other viral hemorrhagic fevers, not elsewhere classified**

Excludes1: chikungunya hemorrhagic fever (A92.0)

dengue hemorrhagic fever (A91)

A98.0   **Crimean-Congo hemorrhagic fever**

Central Asian hemorrhagic fever

A98.1   **Omsk hemorrhagic fever**

A98.2   **Kyasanur Forest disease**

A98.3   **Marburg virus disease**

A98.4   **Ebola virus disease**

A98.5   **Hemorrhagic fever with renal syndrome**

Epidemic hemorrhagic fever

Korean hemorrhagic fever

Russian hemorrhagic fever

Hantaan virus disease

Hantavirus disease with renal manifestations

Nephropathia epidemica

Songo fever

Excludes1: hantavirus (cardio)-pulmonary syndrome (B33.4)

A98.8   **Other specified viral hemorrhagic fevers**

A99   **Unspecified viral hemorrhagic fever**

VIRAL INFECTIONS CHARACTERIZED BY SKIN AND MUCOUS MEMBRANE LESIONS (B00-B09)

B00   **Herpesviral [herpes simplex] infections**

Definition: Herpes simplex is an infection caused by the herpes simplex virus; affects the skin and nervous system; produces small temporary blisters on the skin and mucous membranes.

Excludes1: congenital herpesviral infections (P35.2)

Excludes2: anogenital herpesviral infection (A60.-)

gammaherpesviral mononucleosis (B27.0-)

herpangina (B08.5)

B00.0   **Eczema herpeticum**

Kaposi's varicelliform eruption

B00.1   **Herpesviral vesicular dermatitis**

Herpes simplex facialis

Herpes simplex labialis

Herpes simplex otitis externa

Vesicular dermatitis of ear

Vesicular dermatitis of lip

B00.2   **Herpesviral gingivostomatitis and pharyngotonsillitis**

Herpesviral pharyngitis

B00.3   **Herpesviral meningitis**

B00.4   **Herpesviral encephalitis**

Herpesviral meningoencephalitis

Simian B disease

Excludes1: herpesviral encephalitis due to herpesvirus 6 and 7 (B10.01, B10.09)

non-simplex herpesviral encephalitis (B10.0-)

B00.5   **Herpesviral ocular disease**

B00.50   **Herpesviral ocular disease, unspecified**

B00.51   **Herpesviral iridocyclitis**

Herpesviral iritis

Herpesviral uveitis, anterior

B00.52   **Herpesviral keratitis**

Herpesviral keratoconjunctivitis

B00.53   **Herpesviral conjunctivitis**

B00.59   **Other herpesviral disease of eye**

Herpesviral dermatitis of eyelid

B00.7   **Disseminated herpesviral disease**

Herpesviral sepsis

B00.8   **Other forms of herpesviral infections**

B00.81   **Herpesviral hepatitis**

B00.82   **Herpes simplex myelitis**

B00.89   **Other herpesviral infection**

Herpesviral whitlow

B00.9   **Herpesviral infection, unspecified**

Herpes simplex infection NOS

B01   **Varicella [chickenpox]**

Definition: Chickenpox is an acute contagious disease caused by herpes varicella zoster virus; causes a rash of vesicles on the face and body.

B01.0   **Varicella meningitis**

B01.1   **Varicella encephalitis, myelitis and encephalomyelitis**

Post chickenpox encephalitis, myelitis and encephalomyelitis

B01.11   **Varicella encephalitis and encephalomyelitis**

Post chickenpox encephalitis and encephalomyelitis

B01.12   **Varicella myelitis**

Post chickenpox myelitis

B01.2   **Varicella pneumonia**

B01.8   **Varicella with other complications**

B01.81   **Varicella keratitis**

B01.89   **Other varicella complications**

B01.9   **Varicella without complication**

Varicella NOS

B02   **Zoster [herpes zoster]**

Definition: Herpes zoster is a viral disease characterized by a painful skin rash with blisters in a limited area on one side of the body, often in a stripe.

Includes: shingles

zona

B02.0   **Zoster encephalitis**

Zoster meningoencephalitis

B02.1   **Zoster meningitis**

B02.2   **Zoster with other nervous system involvement**

B02.21   **Postherpetic geniculate ganglionitis**

B02.22   **Postherpetic trigeminal neuralgia**

B02.23   **Postherpetic polyneuropathy**

B02.24   **Postherpetic myelitis**

Herpes zoster myelitis

B02.29   **Other postherpetic nervous system involvement**

Postherpetic radiculopathy

B02.3   **Zoster ocular disease**

B02.30   **Zoster ocular disease, unspecified**

B02.31   **Zoster conjunctivitis**

B02.32   **Zoster iridocyclitis**

B02.33   **Zoster keratitis**

Herpes zoster keratoconjunctivitis

B02.34   **Zoster scleritis**

B02.39   **Other herpes zoster eye disease**

Zoster blepharitis

B02.7   **Disseminated zoster**

B02.8   **Zoster with other complications**

Herpes zoster otitis externa

B02.9   **Zoster without complications**

Zoster NOS

B03   **Smallpox**

Note: In 1980 the 33rd World Health Assembly declared that smallpox had been eradicated.

The classification is maintained for surveillance purposes.

B04   **Monkeypox**

B05   **Measles**

Definition: Measles is a viral infection which causes an illness displaying a characteristic skin rash. Measles is also sometimes called rubeola, 5-day measles, or hard measles.

Includes: morbilli

Excludes1: subacute sclerosing panencephalitis (A81.1)

B05.0   **Measles complicated by encephalitis**

Postmeasles encephalitis

B05.1   **Measles complicated by meningitis**

Postmeasles meningitis

B05.2   **Measles complicated by pneumonia**

Postmeasles pneumonia

B05.3   **Measles complicated by otitis media**

Postmeasles otitis media

B05.4   **Measles with intestinal complications**

B05.8   **Measles with other complications**

B05.81   **Measles keratitis and keratoconjunctivitis**

B05.89   **Other measles complications**

B05.9   **Measles without complication**

Measles NOS

B06   **Rubella [German measles]**

Definition: Rubella is a highly contagious viral disease, aka german measles. The symptoms include swollen glands, joint pain, low fever, and a fine red rash.

Excludes1: congenital rubella (P35.0)

B06.0   **Rubella with neurological complications**

B06.00   **Rubella with neurological complication, unspecified**

B06.01   **Rubella encephalitis**

Rubella meningoencephalitis

B06.02   **Rubella meningitis**

B06.09   **Other neurological complications of rubella**

B06.8   **Rubella with other complications**

B06.81   **Rubella pneumonia**

B06.82   **Rubella arthritis**

B06.89   **Other rubella complications**

B06.9   **Rubella without complication**

Rubella NOS

B07   **Viral warts**

Includes: verruca simplex

verruca vulgaris

viral warts due to human papillomavirus

Excludes2: anogenital (venereal) warts (A63.0)

papilloma of bladder (D41.4)

papilloma of cervix (D26.0)

papilloma larynx (D14.1)

B07.0   **Plantar wart**

Verruca plantaris

B07.8   **Other viral warts**

Common wart

Flat wart

Verruca plana

B07.9   **Viral wart, unspecified**

B08   **Other viral infections characterized by skin and mucous membrane lesions, not elsewhere classified**

Excludes1: vesicular stomatitis virus disease (A93.8)

B08.0   **Other orthopoxvirus infections**

Excludes2: monkeypox (B04)

B08.01   **Cowpox and vaccinia not from vaccine**

B08.010   **Cowpox**

B08.011   **Vaccinia not from vaccine**

Excludes1: vaccinia (from vaccination) (generalized) (T88.1)

B08.02   **ORF virus disease**

Contagious pustular dermatitis

Ecthyma contagiosum

B08.03   **Pseudocowpox [milker's node]**

B08.04   **Paravaccinia, unspecified**

B08.09   **Other orthopoxvirus infections**

Orthopoxvirus infection NOS

B08.1   **Molluscum contagiosum**

B08.2   **Exanthema subitum [sixth disease]**

Roseola infantum

B08.20   **Exanthema subitum [sixth disease], unspecified**

Roseola infantum, unspecified

B08.21   **Exanthema subitum [sixth disease] due to human herpesvirus 6**

Roseola infantum due to human herpesvirus 6

B08.22   **Exanthema subitum [sixth disease] due to human herpesvirus 7**

Roseola infantum due to human herpesvirus 7

B08.3   **Erythema infectiosum [fifth disease]**

B08.4   **Enteroviral vesicular stomatitis with exanthem**

Hand, foot and mouth disease

B08.5   Enteroviral vesicular pharyngitis

Herpangina

B08.6   Parapoxvirus infections

B08.60   Parapoxvirus infection, unspecified

B08.61   Bovine stomatitis

B08.62   Sealpox

B08.69   Other parapoxvirus infections

B08.7   Yatapoxvirus infections

B08.70   Yatapoxvirus infection, unspecified

B08.71   Tanapox virus disease

B08.72   Yaba pox virus disease

Yaba monkey tumor disease

B08.79   Other yatapoxvirus infections

B08.8   Other specified viral infections characterized by skin and mucous membrane lesions

Enteroviral lymphonodular pharyngitis

Foot-and-mouth disease

Poxvirus NEC

B09   Unspecified viral infection characterized by skin and mucous membrane lesions

Viral enanthema NOS

Viral exanthema NOS

OTHER HUMAN HERPESVIRUSES (B10)

Definition: Human herpes viruses, refers to a family of viruses including herpes simplex, varicella zoster, and Epstein-Barr.

B10   Other human herpesviruses

Excludes2: cytomegalovirus (B25.9)

Epstein-Barr virus (B27.0-)

herpes NOS (B00.9)

herpes simplex (B00.-)

herpes zoster (B02.-)

human herpesvirus NOS (B00.-)

human herpesvirus 1 and 2 (B00.-)

human herpesvirus 3 (B01.-, B02.-)

human herpesvirus 4 (B27.0-)

human herpesvirus 5 (B25.-)

varicella (B01.-)

zoster (B02.-)

B10.0   Other human herpesvirus encephalitis

Excludes2: herpes encephalitis NOS (B00.4)

herpes simplex encephalitis (B00.4)

human herpesvirus encephalitis (B00.4)

simian B herpes virus encephalitis (B00.4)

B10.01   Human herpesvirus 6 encephalitis

B10.09   Other human herpesvirus encephalitis

Human herpesvirus 7 encephalitis

B10.8   Other human herpesvirus infection

B10.81   Human herpesvirus 6 infection

B10.82   Human herpesvirus 7 infection

B10.89   Other human herpesvirus infection

Human herpesvirus 8 infection

Kaposi's sarcoma-associated herpesvirus infection

VIRAL HEPATITIS (B15-B19)

Definition: Viral hepatitis is a liver inflammation due to a viral infection. It may present in acute or chronic forms. The most common causes of viral hepatitis are the five unrelated hepatotropic viruses hepatitis A, hepatitis B, hepatitis C, hepatitis D, and hepatitis E.

Excludes1: sequelae of viral hepatitis (B94.2)

Excludes2: cytomegaloviral hepatitis (B25.1)

herpesviral [herpes simplex] hepatitis (B00.81)

B15   Acute hepatitis A

B15.0   Hepatitis A with hepatic coma

B15.9   Hepatitis A without hepatic coma

Hepatitis A (acute)(viral) NOS

B16   Acute hepatitis B

B16.0   Acute hepatitis B with delta-agent with hepatic coma

B16.1   Acute hepatitis B with delta-agent without hepatic coma

B16.2   Acute hepatitis B without delta-agent with hepatic coma

B16.9   Acute hepatitis B without delta-agent and without hepatic coma

Hepatitis B (acute) (viral) NOS

B17   Other acute viral hepatitis

B17.0   Acute delta-(super) infection of hepatitis B carrier

B17.1   Acute hepatitis C

B17.10   Acute hepatitis C without hepatic coma

Acute hepatitis C NOS

B17.11   Acute hepatitis C with hepatic coma

B17.2   Acute hepatitis E

B17.8   Other specified acute viral hepatitis

Hepatitis non-A non-B (acute) (viral) NEC

B17.9   Acute viral hepatitis, unspecified

Acute hepatitis NOS

Acute infectious hepatitis NOS

B18   Chronic viral hepatitis

Includes: Carrier of viral hepatitis

B18.0   Chronic viral hepatitis B with delta-agent

B18.1   Chronic viral hepatitis B without delta-agent

Carrier of viral hepatitis B

Chronic (viral) hepatitis B

B18.2   Chronic viral hepatitis C

Carrier of viral hepatitis C

B18.8   Other chronic viral hepatitis

Carrier of other viral hepatitis

B18.9   Chronic viral hepatitis, unspecified

Carrier of unspecified viral hepatitis

B19   Unspecified viral hepatitis

B19.0   Unspecified viral hepatitis with hepatic coma

B19.1   Unspecified viral hepatitis B

B19.10   Unspecified viral hepatitis B without hepatic coma

Unspecified viral hepatitis B NOS

B19.11   Unspecified viral hepatitis B with hepatic coma

B19.2   Unspecified viral hepatitis C

B19.20   Unspecified viral hepatitis C without hepatic coma

Viral hepatitis C NOS

B19.21   **Unspecified viral hepatitis C with hepatic coma**

B19.9   **Unspecified viral hepatitis without hepatic coma**

Viral hepatitis NOS

HUMAN IMMUNODEFICIENCY VIRUS [HIV] DISEASE (B20)

Definition: Human immunodeficiency virus (HIV) disease is a virus that can lead to acquired immunodeficiency syndrome (AIDS), a condition in humans in which the immune system begins to fail, leading to life-threatening opportunistic infections.

B20   **Human immunodeficiency virus [HIV] disease**

Includes: acquired immune deficiency syndrome [AIDS]

AIDS-related complex [ARC]

HIV infection, symptomatic

Code first Human immunodeficiency virus [HIV] disease complicating pregnancy, childbirth and the puerperium, if applicable (O98.7-)

Use additional code(s) to identify all manifestations of HIV infection

Excludes1: asymptomatic human immunodeficiency virus [HIV] infection status (Z21)

exposure to HIV virus (Z20.6)

inconclusive serologic evidence of HIV (R75)

OTHER VIRAL DISEASES (B25-B34)

B25   **Cytomegaloviral disease**

Excludes1: congenital cytomegalovirus infection (P35.1)

cytomegaloviral mononucleosis (B27.1-)

B25.0   **Cytomegaloviral pneumonitis**

B25.1   **Cytomegaloviral hepatitis**

B25.2   **Cytomegaloviral pancreatitis**

B25.8   **Other cytomegaloviral diseases**

Cytomegaloviral encephalitis

B25.9   **Cytomegaloviral disease, unspecified**

B26   **Mumps**

Includes: epidemic parotitis

infectious parotitis

B26.0   **Mumps orchitis**

B26.1   **Mumps meningitis**

B26.2   **Mumps encephalitis**

B26.3   **Mumps pancreatitis**

B26.8   **Mumps with other complications**

B26.81   **Mumps hepatitis**

B26.82   **Mumps myocarditis**

B26.83   **Mumps nephritis**

B26.84   **Mumps polyneuropathy**

B26.85   **Mumps arthritis**

B26.89   **Other mumps complications**

B26.9   **Mumps without complication**

Mumps NOS

Mumps parotitis NOS

B27   **Infectious mononucleosis**

Definition: Infectious mononucleosis, aka mono, glandular fever, kissing disease is an acute disease characterized by fever and swollen lymph nodes and an abnormal increase of mononuclear leucocytes or monocytes in the bloodstream.

Includes: glandular fever

monocytic angina

Pfeiffer's disease

B27.0   **Gammaherpesviral mononucleosis**

Mononucleosis due to Epstein-Barr virus

B27.00   **Gammaherpesviral mononucleosis without complication**

B27.01   **Gammaherpesviral mononucleosis with polyneuropathy**

B27.02   **Gammaherpesviral mononucleosis with meningitis**

B27.09   **Gammaherpesviral mononucleosis with other complications**

Hepatomegaly in gammaherpesviral mononucleosis

B27.1   **Cytomegaloviral mononucleosis**

B27.10   **Cytomegaloviral mononucleosis without complications**

B27.11   **Cytomegaloviral mononucleosis with polyneuropathy**

B27.12   **Cytomegaloviral mononucleosis with meningitis**

B27.19   **Cytomegaloviral mononucleosis with other complication**

Hepatomegaly in cytomegaloviral mononucleosis

B27.8   **Other infectious mononucleosis**

B27.80   **Other infectious mononucleosis without complication**

B27.81   **Other infectious mononucleosis with polyneuropathy**

B27.82   **Other infectious mononucleosis with meningitis**

B27.89   **Other infectious mononucleosis with other complication**

Hepatomegaly in other infectious mononucleosis

B27.9   **Infectious mononucleosis, unspecified**

B27.90   **Infectious mononucleosis, unspecified without complication**

B27.91   **Infectious mononucleosis, unspecified with polyneuropathy**

B27.92   **Infectious mononucleosis, unspecified with meningitis**

B27.99   **Infectious mononucleosis, unspecified with other complication**

Hepatomegaly in unspecified infectious mononucleosis

B30   **Viral conjunctivitis**

Excludes1: herpesviral [herpes simplex] ocular disease (B00.5)

ocular zoster (B02.3)

B30.0   **Keratoconjunctivitis due to adenovirus**

Epidemic keratoconjunctivitis

Shipyard eye

B30.1   **Conjunctivitis due to adenovirus**

Acute adenoviral follicular conjunctivitis

Swimming-pool conjunctivitis

B30.2   **Viral pharyngoconjunctivitis**

B30.3   **Acute epidemic hemorrhagic conjunctivitis (enteroviral)**

Conjunctivitis due to coxsackievirus 24

Conjunctivitis due to enterovirus 70

Hemorrhagic conjunctivitis (acute)(epidemic)

B30.8   Other viral conjunctivitis

Newcastle conjunctivitis

B30.9   Viral conjunctivitis, unspecified

B33   Other viral diseases, not elsewhere classified

B33.0   Epidemic myalgia

Bornholm disease

B33.1   Ross River disease

Epidemic polyarthritis and exanthema

Ross River fever

B33.2   Viral carditis

Coxsackie (virus) carditis

B33.20   Viral carditis, unspecified

B33.21   Viral endocarditis

B33.22   Viral myocarditis

B33.23   Viral pericarditis

B33.24   Viral cardiomyopathy

B33.3   Retrovirus infections, not elsewhere classified

Retrovirus infection NOS

B33.4   Hantavirus (cardio)-pulmonary syndrome [HPS] [HCPS]

Hantavirus disease with pulmonary manifestations

Sin nombre virus disease

<u>Use additional code</u> to identify any associated acute kidney failure (N17.9)

Excludes1: hantavirus disease with renal manifestations (A98.5)

hemorrhagic fever with renal manifestations (A98.5)

B33.8   Other specified viral diseases

Excludes1: anogenital human papillomavirus infection (A63.0)

viral warts due to human papillomavirus infection (B07)

B34   Viral infection of unspecified site

Excludes1: anogenital human papillomavirus infection (A63.0)

cytomegaloviral disease NOS (B25.9)

herpesvirus [herpes simplex] infection NOS (B00.9)

retrovirus infection NOS (B33.3)

viral agents as the cause of diseases classified elsewhere (B97.-)

viral warts due to human papillomavirus infection (B07)

B34.0   Adenovirus infection, unspecified

B34.1   Enterovirus infection, unspecified

Coxsackievirus infection NOS

Echovirus infection NOS

B34.2   Coronavirus infection, unspecified

Excludes1: pneumonia due to SARS-associated coronavirus (J12.81)

B34.3   Parvovirus infection, unspecified

B34.4   Papovavirus infection, unspecified

B34.8   Other viral infections of unspecified site

B34.9   Viral infection, unspecified

Viremia NOS

MYCOSES (B35-B49)

Excludes2: hypersensitivity pneumonitis due to organic dust (J67.-)

mycosis fungoides (C84.0-)

B35   Dermatophytosis

Definition: Dermatophytosis, aka tinea or ringworm, is a disease that can affect the scalp (tinea capitis), body (tinea corporis), nails (tinea unguium), feet (tinea pedis), groin (tinea cruris), and bearded skin (tinea harbae).

Includes: favus infections due to species of Epidermophyton, Micro-sporum and Trichophyton tinea, any type except those in B36.-

B35.0   Tinea barbae and tinea capitis

Beard ringworm

Kerion

Scalp ringworm

Sycosis, mycotic

B35.1   Tinea unguium

Dermatophytic onychia

Dermatophytosis of nail

Onychomycosis

Ringworm of nails

B35.2   Tinea manuum

Dermatophytosis of hand ringworm

B35.3   Tinea pedis

Athlete's foot

Dermatophytosis of foot ringworm

B35.4   Tinea corporis

Ringworm of the body

B35.5   Tinea imbricata

Tokelau

B35.6   Tinea cruris

Dhobi itch Groin ringworm Jock itch

B35.8   Other dermatophytoses

Disseminated dermatophytosis Granulomatous dermatophytosis

B35.9   Dermatophytosis, unspecified

Ringworm NOS

B36   Other superficial mycoses

B36.0   Pityriasis versicolor Tinea flava

Tinea versicolor

B36.1   Tinea nigra

Keratomycosis nigricans palmaris

Microsporosis nigra

Pityriasis nigra

B36.2   White piedra

Tinea blanca

B36.3   Black piedra

B36.8   Other specified superficial mycoses

B36.9   Superficial mycosis, unspecified

B37   Candidiasis

Definition: Candidiasis is an infection caused by a species of the yeast candida, usually candida albicans. Candidiasis is a common cause of vaginal infections in women.

Includes: candidosis

moniliasis

Excludes1: neonatal candidiasis (P37.5)

B37.0 **Candidal stomatitis**
Oral thrush

B37.1 **Pulmonary candidiasis**
Candidal bronchitis
Candidal pneumonia

B37.2 **Candidiasis of skin and nail**
Candidal onychia
Candidal paronychia
Excludes2: diaper dermatitis (L22)

B37.3 **Candidiasis of vulva and vagina**
Candidal vulvovaginitis
Monilial vulvovaginitis
Vaginal thrush

B37.4 **Candidiasis of other urogenital sites**
    B37.41 **Candidal cystitis and urethritis**
    B37.42 **Candidal balanitis**
    B37.49 **Other urogenital candidiasis**
        Candidal pyelonephritis

B37.5 **Candidal meningitis**

B37.6 **Candidal endocarditis**

B37.7 **Candidal sepsis**
Disseminated candidiasis
Systemic candidiasis

B37.8 **Candidiasis of other sites**
    B37.81 **Candidal esophagitis**
    B37.82 **Candidal enteritis**
        Candidal proctitis
    B37.83 **Candidal cheilitis**
    B37.84 **Candidal otitis externa**
    B37.89 **Other sites of candidiasis**
        Candidal osteomyelitis

B37.9 **Candidiasis, unspecified**
Thrush NOS

B38 **Coccidioidomycosis**

B38.0 **Acute pulmonary coccidioidomycosis**

B38.1 **Chronic pulmonary coccidioidomycosis**

B38.2 **Pulmonary coccidioidomycosis, unspecified**

B38.3 **Cutaneous coccidioidomycosis**

B38.4 **Coccidioidomycosis meningitis**

B38.7 **Disseminated coccidioidomycosis**
Generalized coccidioidomycosis

B38.8 **Other forms of coccidioidomycosis**
    B38.81 **Prostatic coccidioidomycosis**
    B38.89 **Other forms of coccidioidomycosis**

B38.9 **Coccidioidomycosis, unspecified**

B39 **Histoplasmosis**

Definition: Histoplasmosis, aka Darling's disease, is a disease caused by the fungus histoplasma capsulatum. Symptoms vary greatly, but the disease primarily affects the lungs.Histoplasmosis is common among aids patients because of their lowered immune system.

Code first associated AIDS (B20)

Use additional code for any associated manifestations, such as:
endocarditis (I39)
meningitis (G02)

pericarditis (I32)
retinitis (H32)

B39.0 **Acute pulmonary histoplasmosis capsulati**

B39.1 **Chronic pulmonary histoplasmosis capsulati**

B39.2 **Pulmonary histoplasmosis capsulati, unspecified**

B39.3 **Disseminated histoplasmosis capsulati**
Generalized histoplasmosis capsulati

B39.4 **Histoplasmosis capsulati, unspecified**
American histoplasmosis

B39.5 **Histoplasmosis duboisii**
African histoplasmosis

B39.9 **Histoplasmosis, unspecified**

B40 **Blastomycosis**

Definition: Blastomycotic infection, aka North American blastomycosis, blastomycetic dermatitis, and gilchrist's disease, is a fungal infection caused by the organism blastomyces dermatitidis. Endemic to portions of north america, blastomycosis causes clinical symptoms similar to histoplasmosis.

Excludes1: Brazilian blastomycosis (B41.-)
keloidal blastomycosis (B48.0)

B40.0 **Acute pulmonary blastomycosis**

B40.1 **Chronic pulmonary blastomycosis**

B40.2 **Pulmonary blastomycosis, unspecified**

B40.3 **Cutaneous blastomycosis**

B40.7 **Disseminated blastomycosis**
Generalized blastomycosis

B40.8 **Other forms of blastomycosis**
    B40.81 **Blastomycotic meningoencephalitis**
        Meningomyelitis due to blastomycosis
    B40.89 **Other forms of blastomycosis**

B40.9 **Blastomycosis, unspecified**

B41 **Paracoccidioidomycosis**

Includes: Brazilian blastomycosis
Lutz' disease

B41.0 **Pulmonary paracoccidioidomycosis**

B41.7 **Disseminated paracoccidioidomycosis**
Generalized paracoccidioidomycosis

B41.8 **Other forms of paracoccidioidomycosis**

B41.9 **Paracoccidioidomycosis, unspecified**

B42 **Sporotrichosis**

B42.0 **Pulmonary sporotrichosis**

B42.1 **Lymphocutaneous sporotrichosis**

B42.7 **Disseminated sporotrichosis**
Generalized sporotrichosis

B42.8 **Other forms of sporotrichosis**
    B42.81 **Cerebral sporotrichosis**
        Meningitis due to sporotrichosis
    B42.82 **Sporotrichosis arthritis**
    B42.89 **Other forms of sporotrichosis**

B42.9 **Sporotrichosis, unspecified**

B43 **Chromomycosis and pheomycotic abscess**

B43.0 **Cutaneous chromomycosis**
Dermatitis verrucosa

B43.1 **Pheomycotic brain abscess**
Cerebral chromomycosis

B43.2   Subcutaneous pheomycotic abscess and cyst

B43.8   Other forms of chromomycosis

B43.9   Chromomycosis, unspecified

B44   Aspergillosis

Includes: aspergilloma

B44.0   Invasive pulmonary aspergillosis

B44.1   Other pulmonary aspergillosis

B44.2   Tonsillar aspergillosis

B44.7   Disseminated aspergillosis

Generalized aspergillosis

B44.8   Other forms of aspergillosis

B44.81   Allergic bronchopulmonary aspergillosis

B44.89   Other forms of aspergillosis

B44.9   Aspergillosis, unspecified

B45   Cryptococcosis

B45.0   Pulmonary cryptococcosis

B45.1   Cerebral cryptococcosis

Cryptococcal meningitis

Cryptococcosis meningocerebralis

B45.2   Cutaneous cryptococcosis

B45.3   Osseous cryptococcosis

B45.7   Disseminated cryptococcosis

Generalized cryptococcosis

B45.8   Other forms of cryptococcosis

B45.9   Cryptococcosis, unspecified

B46   Zygomycosis

B46.0   Pulmonary mucormycosis

B46.1   Rhinocerebral mucormycosis

B46.2   Gastrointestinal mucormycosis

B46.3   Cutaneous mucormycosis

Subcutaneous mucormycosis

B46.4   Disseminated mucormycosis

Generalized mucormycosis

B46.5   Mucormycosis, unspecified

B46.8   Other zygomycoses

Entomophthoromycosis

B46.9   Zygomycosis, unspecified

Phycomycosis NOS

B47   Mycetoma

B47.0   Eumycetoma

Madura foot, mycotic

Maduromycosis

B47.1   Actinomycetoma

B47.9   Mycetoma, unspecified

Madura foot NOS

B48   Other mycoses, not elsewhere classified

B48.0   Lobomycosis

Keloidal blastomycosis Lobo's disease

B48.1   Rhinosporidiosis

B48.2   Allescheriasis

Infection due to Pseudallescheria boydii

Excludes1: eumycetoma (B47.0)

B48.3   Geotrichosis

Geotrichum stomatitis

B48.4   Penicillosis

B48.8   Other specified mycoses

Adiaspiromycosis

Infection of tissue and organs by Alternaria

Infection of tissue and organs by Drechslera

Infection of tissue and organs by Fusarium

Infection of tissue and organs by saprophytic fungi NEC

B49   Unspecified mycosis

Fungemia NOS

PROTOZOAL DISEASES (B50-B64)

Excludes1: amebiasis (A06.-)

Other protozoal intestinal diseases (A07.-)

B50   Plasmodium falciparum malaria

Includes: mixed infections of Plasmodium falciparum with any other Plasmodium species

B50.0   Plasmodium falciparum malaria with cerebral complications

Cerebral malaria NOS

B50.8   Other severe and complicated Plasmodium falciparum malaria

Severe or complicated Plasmodium falciparum malaria NOS

B50.9   Plasmodium falciparum malaria, unspecified

B51   Plasmodium vivax malaria

Includes: mixed infections of Plasmodium vivax with other Plasmodium species, except Plasmodium falciparum

Excludes1: plasmodium vivax with Plasmodium falciparum (B50.-)

B51.0   Plasmodium vivax malaria with rupture of spleen

B51.8   Plasmodium vivax malaria with other complications

B51.9   Plasmodium vivax malaria without complication

Plasmodium vivax malaria NOS

B52   Plasmodium malariae malaria

Includes: mixed infections of Plasmodium malariae with other Plasmodium species, except Plasmodium falciparum and Plasmodium vivax

Excludes1: Plasmodium falciparum (B50.-)

Plasmodium vivax (B51.-)

B52.0   Plasmodium malariae malaria with nephropathy

B52.8   Plasmodium malariae malaria with other complications

B52.9   Plasmodium malariae malaria without complication

Plasmodium malariae malaria NOS

B53   Other specified malaria

B53.0   Plasmodium ovale malaria

Excludes1: Plasmodium ovale with Plasmodium falciparum (B50.-)

Plasmodium ovale with Plasmodium malariae (B52.-)

Plasmodium ovale with Plasmodium vivax (B51.-)

B53.1   Malaria due to simian plasmodia

Excludes1: Malaria due to simian plasmodia with Plasmodium falciparum (B50.-)

Malaria due to simian plasmodia with Plasmodium malariae (B52.-)

Malaria due to simian plasmodia with Plasmodium ovale (B53.0)

Malaria due to simian plasmodia with Plasmodium vivax (B51.-)

B53.8 **Other malaria, not elsewhere classified**

B54 **Unspecified malaria**

B55 **Leishmaniasis**

B55.0 **Visceral leishmaniasis**
Kala-azar
Post-kala-azar dermal leishmaniasis

B55.1 **Cutaneous leishmaniasis**

B55.2 **Mucocutaneous leishmaniasis**

B55.9 **Leishmaniasis, unspecified**

B56 **African trypanosomiasis**

B56.0 **Gambiense trypanosomiasis**
Infection due to Trypanosoma brucei gambiense
West African sleeping sickness

B56.1 **Rhodesiense trypanosomiasis**
East African sleeping sickness
Infection due to Trypanosoma brucei rhodesiense

B56.9 **African trypanosomiasis, unspecified**
Sleeping sickness NOS

B57 **Chagas' disease**
Includes: American trypanosomiasis
infection due to Trypanosoma cruzi

B57.0 **Acute Chagas' disease with heart involvement**
Acute Chagas' disease with myocarditis

B57.1 **Acute Chagas' disease without heart involvement**
Acute Chagas' disease NOS

B57.2 **Chagas' disease (chronic) with heart involvement**
American trypanosomiasis NOS
Chagas' disease (chronic) NOS
Chagas' disease (chronic) with myocarditis
Trypanosomiasis NOS

B57.3 **Chagas' disease (chronic) with digestive system involvement**

B57.30 **Chagas' disease with digestive system involvement, unspecified**

B57.31 **Megaesophagus in Chagas' disease**

B57.32 **Megacolon in Chagas' disease**

B57.39 **Other digestive system involvement in Chagas' disease**

B57.4 **Chagas' disease (chronic) with nervous system involvement**

B57.40 **Chagas' disease with nervous system involvement, unspecified**

B57.41 **Meningitis in Chagas' disease**

B57.42 **Meningoencephalitis in Chagas' disease**

B57.49 **Other nervous system involvement in Chagas' disease**

B57.5 **Chagas' disease (chronic) with other organ involvement**

B58 **Toxoplasmosis**
Definition: Toxoplasmosis is an infection caused by the parasite named toxoplasma gondii that can invade tissues and damage the brain, especially in a fetus and in a newborn baby. Symptoms include fever, fatigue, headache, swollen lymph glands, and muscle aches and pains.
Includes: infection due to Toxoplasma gondii

Excludes1: congenital toxoplasmosis (P37.1)

B58.0 **Toxoplasma oculopathy**

B58.00 **Toxoplasma oculopathy, unspecified**

B58.01 **Toxoplasma chorioretinitis**

B58.09 **Other toxoplasma oculopathy**
Toxoplasma uveitis

B58.1 **Toxoplasma hepatitis**

B58.2 **Toxoplasma meningoencephalitis**

B58.3 **Pulmonary toxoplasmosis**

B58.8 **Toxoplasmosis with other organ involvement**

B58.81 **Toxoplasma myocarditis**

B58.82 **Toxoplasma myositis**

B58.83 **Toxoplasma tubulo-interstitial nephropathy**
Toxoplasma pyelonephritis

B58.89 **Toxoplasmosis with other organ involvement**

B58.9 **Toxoplasmosis, unspecified**

B59 **Pneumocystosis**
Pneumonia due to Pneumocystis carinii
Pneumonia due to Pneumocystis jiroveci

B60 **Other protozoal diseases, not elsewhere classified**
Excludes1: cryptosporidiosis (A07.2)
intestinal microsporidiosis (A07.8)
isosporiasis (A07.3)

B60.0 **Babesiosis**
Piroplasmosis

B60.1 **Acanthamebiasis**

B60.10 **Acanthamebiasis, unspecified**

B60.11 **Meningoencephalitis due to Acanthamoeba (culbertsoni)**

B60.12 **Conjunctivitis due to Acanthamoeba**

B60.13 **Keratoconjunctivitis due to Acanthamoeba**

B60.19 **Other acanthamebic disease**

B60.2 **Naegleriasis**
Primary amebic meningoencephalitis

B60.8 **Other specified protozoal diseases**
Microsporidiosis

B64 **Unspecified protozoal disease**

HELMINTHIASES (B65-B83)

B65 **Schistosomiasis [bilharziasis]**
Definition: Schistosomiasis [bilharziasis], aka bilharzia, bilharziosis or snail fever, is a parasitic disease caused by several species of fluke of the genus schistosoma. Schistosomiasis often is a chronic illness that can damage internal organs and, in children, impair growth and cognitive development.
Includes: snail fever

B65.0 **Schistosomiasis due to Schistosoma haematobium [urinary schistosomiasis]**

B65.1 **Schistosomiasis due to Schistosoma mansoni [intestinal schistosomiasis]**

B65.2 **Schistosomiasis due to Schistosoma japonicum**
Asiatic schistosomiasis

B65.3 **Cercarial dermatitis**
Swimmer's itch

B65.8 **Other schistosomiasis**

Infection due to Schistosoma intercalatum

Infection due to Schistosoma mattheei

Infection due to Schistosoma mekongi

B65.9   Schistosomiasis, unspecified

B66   Other fluke infections

B66.0   Opisthorchiasis

Infection due to cat liver fluke

Infection due to Opisthorchis (felineus)(viverrini)

B66.1   Clonorchiasis

Chinese liver fluke disease

Infection due to Clonorchis sinensis

Oriental liver fluke disease

B66.2   Dicroceliasis

Infection due to Dicrocoelium dendriticum

Lancet fluke infection

B66.3   Fascioliasis

Infection due to Fasciola gigantica

Infection due to Fasciola hepatica

Infection due to Fasciola indica

Sheep liver fluke disease

B66.4   Paragonimiasis

Infection due to Paragonimus species

Lung fluke disease

Pulmonary distomiasis

B66.5   Fasciolopsiasis

Infection due to Fasciolopsis buski

Intestinal distomiasis

B66.8   Other specified fluke infections

Echinostomiasis

Heterophyiasis

Metagonimiasis Nanophyetiasis Watsoniasis

B66.9   Fluke infection, unspecified

B67   Echinococcosis

Includes: hydatidosis

B67.0   Echinococcus granulosus infection of liver

B67.1   Echinococcus granulosus infection of lung

B67.2   Echinococcus granulosus infection of bone

B67.3   Echinococcus granulosus infection, other and multiple sites

B67.31   Echinococcus granulosus infection, thyroid gland

B67.32   Echinococcus granulosus infection, multiple sites

B67.39   Echinococcus granulosus infection, other sites

B67.4   Echinococcus granulosus infection, unspecified

Dog tapeworm (infection)

B67.5   Echinococcus multilocularis infection of liver

B67.6   Echinococcus multilocularis infection, other and multiple sites

B67.61   Echinococcus multilocularis infection, multiple sites

B67.69   Echinococcus multilocularis infection, other sites

B67.7   Echinococcus multilocularis infection, unspecified

B67.8   Echinococcosis, unspecified, of liver

B67.9   Echinococcosis, other and unspecified

B67.90   Echinococcosis, unspecified

Echinococcosis NOS

B67.99   Other echinococcosis

B68   Taeniasis

Excludes1: cysticercosis (B69.-)

B68.0   Taenia solium taeniasis

Pork tapeworm (infection)

B68.1   Taenia saginata taeniasis

Beef tapeworm (infection)

Infection due to adult tapeworm

Taenia saginata

B68.9   Taeniasis, unspecified

B69   Cysticercosis

Includes: cysticerciasis infection due to larval form of Taenia solium

B69.0   Cysticercosis of central nervous system

B69.1   Cysticercosis of eye

B69.8   Cysticercosis of other sites

B69.81   Myositis in cysticercosis

B69.89   Cysticercosis of other sites

B69.9   Cysticercosis, unspecified

B70   Diphyllobothriasis and sparganosis

B70.0   Diphyllobothriasis

Diphyllobothrium (adult) (latum) (pacificum) infection

Fish tapeworm (infection)

Excludes2: larval diphyllobothriasis (B70.1)

B70.1   Sparganosis

Infection due to Sparganum (mansoni) (proliferum)

Infection due to Spirometra larva

Larval diphyllobothriasis

Spirometrosis

B71   Other cestode infections

B71.0   Hymenolepiasis

Dwarf tapeworm infection

Rat tapeworm (infection)

B71.1   Dipylidiasis

B71.8   Other specified cestode infections

Coenurosis

B71.9   Cestode infection, unspecified

Tapeworm (infection) NOS

B72   Dracunculiasis

Includes: guinea worm infection

infection due to Dracunculus medinensis

B73   Onchocerciasis

Includes: onchocerca volvulus infection

onchocercosis river blindness

B73.0   Onchocerciasis with eye disease

B73.00   Onchocerciasis with eye involvement, unspecified

B73.01   Onchocerciasis with endophthalmitis

B73.02   Onchocerciasis with glaucoma

B73.09   Onchocerciasis with other eye involvement

Infestation of eyelid due to onchocerciasis

B73.1   **Onchocerciasis without eye disease**

B74   **Filariasis**

Excludes2: onchocerciasis (B73)

tropical (pulmonary) eosinophilia NOS (J82)

B74.0   **Filariasis due to Wuchereria bancrofti**

Bancroftian elephantiasis

Bancroftian filariasis

B74.1   **Filariasis due to Brugia malayi**

B74.2   **Filariasis due to Brugia timori**

B74.3   **Loiasis**

Calabar swelling

Eyeworm disease of Africa

Loa Loa infection

B74.4   **Mansonelliasis**

Infection due to Mansonella ozzardi

Infection due to Mansonella perstans

Infection due to Mansonella streptocerca

B74.8   **Other filariases**

Dirofilariasis

B74.9   **Filariasis, unspecified**

B75   **Trichinellosis**

Includes: infection due to Trichinella species

trichiniasis

B76   **Hookworm diseases**

Includes: uncinariasis

B76.0   **Ancylostomiasis**

Infection due to Ancylostoma species

B76.1   **Necatoriasis**

Infection due to Necator americanus

B76.8   **Other hookworm diseases**

B76.9   **Hookworm disease, unspecified**

Cutaneous larva migrans NOS

B77   **Ascariasis**

Includes: ascaridiasis

roundworm infection

B77.0   **Ascariasis with intestinal complications**

B77.8   **Ascariasis with other complications**

B77.81   **Ascariasis pneumonia**

B77.89   **Ascariasis with other complications**

B77.9   **Ascariasis, unspecified**

B78   **Strongyloidiasis**

Excludes1: trichostrongyliasis (B81.2)

B78.0   **Intestinal strongyloidiasis**

B78.1   **Cutaneous strongyloidiasis**

B78.7   **Disseminated strongyloidiasis**

B78.9   **Strongyloidiasis, unspecified**

B79   **Trichuriasis**

Includes: trichocephaliasis

whipworm (disease)(infection)

B80   **Enterobiasis**

Includes: oxyuriasis

pinworm infection threadworm infection

B81   **Other intestinal helminthiases, not elsewhere classified**

Definition: Helminthiases is a disease in which a part of the body

is infested with worms such as pinworm, roundworm or tapeworm.

Excludes1: angiostrongyliasis due to Parastrongylus cantonensis (B83.2)

B81.0   **Anisakiasis**

Infection due to Anisakis larva

B81.1   **Intestinal capillariasis**

Capillariasis NOS

Infection due to Capillaria philippinensis

Excludes2: hepatic capillariasis (B83.8)

B81.2   **Trichostrongyliasis**

B81.3   **Intestinal angiostrongyliasis**

Angiostrongyliasis due to Parastrongylus costaricensis

B81.4   **Mixed intestinal helminthiases**

Infection due to intestinal helminths classified to more than one of the categories B65.0-B81.3 and B81.8

Mixed helminthiasis NOS

B81.8   **Other specified intestinal helminthiases**

Infection due to Oesophagostomum species [esophagostomiasis]

Infection due to Ternidens diminutus [Ternidensiasis]

B82   **Unspecified intestinal parasitism**

B82.0   **Intestinal helminthiasis, unspecified**

B82.9   **Intestinal parasitism, unspecified**

B83   **Other helminthiases**

Excludes1: capillariasis NOS (B81.1)

Excludes2: intestinal capillariasis (B81.1)

B83.0   **Visceral larva migrans**

Toxocariasis

B83.1   **Gnathostomiasis**

Wandering swelling

B83.2   **Angiostrongyliasis due to Parastrongylus cantonensis**

Eosinophilic meningoencephalitis due to Parastrongylus cantonensis

Excludes2: intestinal angiostrongyliasis (B81.3)

B83.3   **Syngamiasis**

Syngamosis

B83.4   **Internal hirudiniasis**

Excludes2: external hirudiniasis (B88.3)

B83.8   **Other specified helminthiases**

Acanthocephaliasis

Gongylonemiasis

Hepatic capillariasis

Metastrongyliasis

Thelaziasis

B83.9   **Helminthiasis, unspecified**

Worms NOS

Excludes1: intestinal helminthiasis NOS (B82.0)

PEDICULOSIS, ACARIASIS AND OTHER INFESTATIONS (B85-B89)

Definition: Pediculosis and phthirus infestation is an infestation with lice (pediculus humanus) or true lice or crab lice (phthirius) resulting in severe itching.

Definition: Acariasis is an infestation with arthropod parasites of the order acarina including the ticks and mites.

B85   **Pediculosis and phthiriasis**

B85.0 **Pediculosis due to Pediculus humanus capitis**

Head-louse infestation

B85.1 **Pediculosis due to Pediculus humanus corporis**

Body-louse infestation

B85.2 **Pediculosis, unspecified**

B85.3 **Phthiriasis**

Infestation by crab-louse

Infestation by Phthirus pubis

B85.4 **Mixed pediculosis and phthiriasis**

Infestation classifiable to more than one of the categories B85.0-B85.3

B86 **Scabies**

Sarcoptic itch

B87 **Myiasis**

Includes: infestation by larva of flies

B87.0 **Cutaneous myiasis**

Creeping myiasis

B87.1 **Wound myiasis**

Traumatic myiasis

B87.2 **Ocular myiasis**

B87.3 **Nasopharyngeal myiasis**

Laryngeal myiasis

B87.4 **Aural myiasis**

B87.8 **Myiasis of other sites**

B87.81 **Genitourinary myiasis**

B87.82 **Intestinal myiasis**

B87.89 **Myiasis of other sites**

B87.9 **Myiasis, unspecified**

B88 **Other infestations**

B88.0 **Other acariasis**

Acarine dermatitis

Dermatitis due to Demodex species

Dermatitis due to Dermanyssus gallinae

Dermatitis due to Liponyssoides sanguineus

Trombiculosis

Excludes2: scabies (B86)

B88.1 **Tungiasis [sandflea infestation]**

B88.2 **Other arthropod infestations**

Scarabiasis

B88.3 **External hirudiniasis**

Leech infestation NOS

Excludes2: internal hirudiniasis (B83.4)

B88.8 **Other specified infestations**

Ichthyoparasitism due to Vandellia cirrhosa

Linguatulosis

Porocephaliasis

B88.9 **Infestation, unspecified**

Infestation (skin) NOS

Infestation by mites NOS

Skin parasites NOS

B89 **Unspecified parasitic disease**

SEQUELAE OF INFECTIOUS AND PARASITIC DISEASES (B90-B94)

Note: Categories B90-B94 are to be used to indicate conditions in categories A00-B89 as the cause of sequelae, which are themselves classified elsewhere. The 'sequelae' include conditions specified as such; they also include residuals of diseases classifiable to the above categories if there is evidence that the disease itself is no longer present. Codes from these categories are not to be used for chronic infections. Code chronic current infections to active infectious disease as appropriate.

Code first condition resulting from (sequela) the infectious or parasitic disease

B90 **Sequelae of tuberculosis**

B90.0 **Sequelae of central nervous system tuberculosis**

B90.1 **Sequelae of genitourinary tuberculosis**

B90.2 **Sequelae of tuberculosis of bones and joints**

B90.8 **Sequelae of tuberculosis of other organs**

Excludes2: sequelae of respiratory tuberculosis (B90.9)

B90.9 **Sequelae of respiratory and unspecified tuberculosis**

Sequelae of tuberculosis NOS

B91 **Sequelae of poliomyelitis**

Excludes1: postpolio syndrome (G14)

B92 **Sequelae of leprosy**

B94 **Sequelae of other and unspecified infectious and parasitic diseases**

B94.0 **Sequelae of trachoma**

B94.1 **Sequelae of viral encephalitis**

B94.2 **Sequelae of viral hepatitis**

B94.8 **Sequelae of other specified infectious and parasitic diseases**

B94.9 **Sequelae of unspecified infectious and parasitic disease**

BACTERIAL AND VIRAL INFECTIOUS AGENTS (B95-B97)

Note: These categories are provided for use as supplementary or additional codes to identify the infectious agent(s) in diseases classified elsewhere.

B95 **Streptococcus, Staphylococcus, and Enterococcus as the cause of diseases classified elsewhere**

B95.0 **Streptococcus, group A, as the cause of diseases classified elsewhere**

B95.1 **Streptococcus, group B, as the cause of diseases classified elsewhere**

B95.2 **Enterococcus as the cause of diseases classified elsewhere**

B95.3 **Streptococcus pneumoniae as the cause of diseases classified elsewhere**

B95.4 **Other streptococcus as the cause of diseases classified elsewhere**

B95.5 **Unspecified streptococcus as the cause of diseases classified elsewhere**

B95.6 **Staphylococcus aureus as the cause of diseases classified elsewhere**

B95.61 **Methicillin susceptible Staphylococcus aureus infection as the cause of diseases classified elsewhere**

Methicillin susceptible Staphylococcus aureus (MSSA) infection as the cause of diseases classified elsewhere

Staphylococcus aureus infection NOS as the cause of diseases classified elsewhere

B95.62 **Methicillin resistant Staphylococcus aureus infection as the cause of diseases classified elsewhere**

Methicillin resistant staphylococcus aureus (MRSA) infection as the cause of diseases classified elsewhere

B95.7 Other staphylococcus as the cause of diseases classified elsewhere

B95.8 Unspecified staphylococcus as the cause of diseases classified elsewhere

B96 Other bacterial agents as the cause of diseases classified elsewhere

B96.0 Mycoplasma pneumoniae [M. pneumoniae] as the cause of diseases classified elsewhere

Pleuro-pneumonia-like-organism [PPLO]

B96.1 Klebsiella pneumoniae [K. pneumoniae] as the cause of diseases classified elsewhere

B96.2 Escherichia coli [E. coli] as the cause of diseases classified elsewhere

B96.20 Unspecified Escherichia coli [E. coli] as the cause of diseases classified elsewhere

Escherichia coli [E. coli] NOS

B96.21 Shiga toxin-producing Escherichia coli [E. coli] (STEC) O157 as the cause of diseases classified elsewhere

E. coli O157:H- (nonmotile) with confirmation of Shiga toxin

E. coli O157 with confirmation of Shiga toxin when H antigen is unknown, or is not H7 O157:H7

Escherichia coli [E. coli] with or without confirmation of Shiga toxin-production

Shiga toxin-producing Escherichia coli [E. coli] O157:H7 with or without confirmation of Shiga toxin-production

STEC O157:H7 with or without confirmation of Shiga toxin-production

B96.22 Other specified Shiga toxin-producing Escherichia coli [E. coli] (STEC) as the cause of diseases classified elsewhere

Non-O157 Shiga toxin-producing Escherichia coli [E. coli]

Non-O157 Shiga toxin-producing Escherichia coli [E. coli] with known O group

B96.23 Unspecified Shiga toxin-producing Escherichia coli [E. coli] (STEC) as the cause of diseases classified elsewhere

Shiga toxin-producing Escherichia coli [E. coli] with unspecified O group STEC NOS

B96.29 Other Escherichia coli [E. coli] as the cause of diseases classified elsewhere

Non-Shiga toxin-producing E. coli

B96.3 Hemophilus influenzae [H. influenzae] as the cause of diseases classified elsewhere

B96.4 Proteus (mirabilis) (morganii) as the cause of diseases classified elsewhere

B96.5 Pseudomonas (aeruginosa) (mallei) (pseudomallei) as the cause of diseases classified elsewhere

B96.6 Bacteroides fragilis [B. fragilis] as the cause of diseases classified elsewhere

B96.7 Clostridium perfringens [C. perfringens] as the cause of diseases classified elsewhere

B96.8 Other specified bacterial agents as the cause of diseases classified elsewhere

B96.81 Helicobacter pylori [H. pylori] as the cause of diseases classified elsewhere

B96.82 Vibrio vulnificus as the cause of diseases classified elsewhere

B96.89 Other specified bacterial agents as the cause of diseases classified elsewhere

B97 Viral agents as the cause of diseases classified elsewhere

B97.0 Adenovirus as the cause of diseases classified elsewhere

B97.1 Enterovirus as the cause of diseases classified elsewhere

B97.10 Unspecified enterovirus as the cause of diseases classified elsewhere

B97.11 Coxsackievirus as the cause of diseases classified elsewhere

B97.12 Echovirus as the cause of diseases classified elsewhere

B97.19 Other enterovirus as the cause of diseases classified elsewhere

B97.2 Coronavirus as the cause of diseases classified elsewhere

B97.21 SARS-associated coronavirus as the cause of diseases classified elsewhere

Excludes1: pneumonia due to SARS-associated coronavirus (J12.81)

B97.29 Other coronavirus as the cause of diseases classified elsewhere

B97.3 Retrovirus as the cause of diseases classified elsewhere

Excludes1: Human immunodeficiency virus [HIV] disease (B20)

B97.30 Unspecified retrovirus as the cause of diseases classified elsewhere

B97.31 Lentivirus as the cause of diseases classified elsewhere

B97.32 Oncovirus as the cause of diseases classified elsewhere

B97.33 Human T-cell lymphotrophic virus, type I [HTLV-I] as the cause of diseases classified elsewhere

B97.34 Human T-cell lymphotrophic virus, type II [HTLV-II] as the cause of diseases classified elsewhere

B97.35 Human immunodeficiency virus, type 2[HIV 2] as the cause of diseases classified elsewhere

B97.39 Other retrovirus as the cause of diseases classified elsewhere

B97.4 Respiratory syncytial virus as the cause of diseases classified elsewhere

B97.5 Reovirus as the cause of diseases classified elsewhere

B97.6 Parvovirus as the cause of diseases classified elsewhere

B97.7 Papillomavirus as the cause of diseases classified elsewhere

B97.8 Other viral agents as the cause of diseases classified elsewhere

B97.81 Human metapneumovirus as the cause of diseases classified elsewhere

B97.89 Other viral agents as the cause of diseases classified elsewhere

OTHER INFECTIOUS DISEASES (B99)

B99 Other and unspecified infectious diseases

B99.8 Other infectious disease

B99.9 Unspecified infectious disease

Chapter 2: Neoplasms (C00-D49)

DEFINITIONS

This chapter includes definitions of selected key words, terms and phrases and coding alerts for adding points to the clinical domain, and references to coding late effects where appropriate. An example from this chapter is as follows:

 C46   Kaposi's sarcoma
    Definition: Kaposi's sarcoma is a form of skin cancer that can involve internal organs. It is most often found in patients with acquired immunodeficiency syndrome (AIDS), and can be fatal.

MULTIPLE CODING FOR A SINGLE CONDITION

In addition to the etiology/manifestation convention that requires two codes to fully describe a single condition that affects multiple body systems, there are other single conditions that also require more than one code. "Use additional code" notes are found in the Tabular List at codes that are not part of an etiology/manifestation pair where a secondary code is useful to fully describe a condition. The sequencing rule is the same as the etiology/manifestation pair, "use additional code" indicates that a secondary code should be added.

For example, for bacterial infections that are not included in chapter 1, a secondary code from category B95, Streptococcus, Staphylococcus, and Enterococcus, as the cause of diseases classified elsewhere, or B96, Other bacterial agents as the cause of diseases classified elsewhere, may be required to identify the bacterial organism causing the infection. A "use additional code" note will normally be found at the infectious disease code, indicating a need for the organism code to be added as a secondary code.

"Code first" notes are also under certain codes that are not specifically manifestation codes but may be due to an underlying cause. When there is a "code first" note and an underlying condition is present, the underlying condition should be sequenced first.

"Code, if applicable, any causal condition first", notes indicate that this code may be assigned as a principal diagnosis when the causal condition is unknown or not applicable. If a causal condition is known, then the code for that condition should be sequenced as the principal or first-listed diagnosis.

Multiple codes may be needed for sequela, complication codes and obstetric codes to more fully describe a condition. See the specific guidelines for these conditions for further instruction.

COMBINATION CODE

A combination code is a single code used to classify: Two diagnoses, or a diagnosis with an associated secondary process (manifestation) A diagnosis with an associated complication

Combination codes are identified by referring to subterm entries in the Alphabetic Index and by reading the inclusion and exclusion notes in the Tabular List.

Assign only the combination code when that code fully identifies the diagnostic conditions involved or when the Alphabetic Index so directs. Multiple coding should not be used when the classification provides a combination code that clearly identifies all of the elements documented in the diagnosis. When the combination code lacks necessary specificity in describing the manifestation or complication, an additional code should be used as a secondary code.

SEQUELA (LATE EFFECTS)

A sequela is the residual effect (condition produced) after the acute phase of an illness or injury has terminated. There is no time limit on when a sequela code can be used. The residual may be apparent early, such as in cerebral infarction, or it may occur months or years later, such as that due to a previous injury. Coding of sequela generally requires two codes sequenced in the following order: The condition or nature of the sequela is sequenced first.

The sequela code is sequenced second.

An exception to the above guidelines are those instances where the code for the sequela is followed by a manifestation code identified in the Tabular List and title, or the sequela code has been expanded (at the fourth, fifth or sixth character levels) to include the manifestation(s). The code for the acute phase of an illness or injury that led to the sequela is never used with a code for the late effect.

GENERAL GUIDELINES

Chapter 2 of the ICD-10-CM contains the codes for most benign and all malignant neoplasms. Certain benign neoplasms, such as prostatic adenomas, may be found in the specific body system chapters. To properly code a neoplasm it is necessary to determine from the record if the neoplasm is benign, in-situ, malignant, or of uncertain histologic behavior. If malignant, any secondary (metastatic) sites should also be determined.

Primary malignant neoplasms overlapping site boundaries

A primary malignant neoplasm that overlaps two or more contiguous (next to each other) sites should be classified to the subcategory/code .8 ('overlapping lesion'), unless the combination is specifically indexed elsewhere. For multiple neoplasms of the same site that are not contiguous such as tumors in different quadrants of the same breast, codes for each site should be assigned.

Malignant neoplasm of ectopic tissue

Malignant neoplasms of ectopic tissue are to be coded to the site of origin mentioned, e.g., ectopic pancreatic malignant neoplasms involving the stomach are coded to pancreas, unspecified (C25.9).

The neoplasm table in the Alphabetic Index should be referenced first. However, if the histological term is documented, that term should be referenced first, rather than going immediately to the Neoplasm Table, in order to determine which column in the Neoplasm Table is appropriate. For example, if the documentation indicates "adenoma," refer to the term in the Alphabetic Index to review the entries under this term and the instructional note to "see also neoplasm, by site, benign." The table provides the proper code based on the type of neoplasm and the site. It is important to select the proper column in the table that corresponds to the type of neoplasm. The Tabular List should then be referenced to verify that the correct code has been selected from the table and that a more specific site code does not exist.

See Section I.C.21. Factors influencing health status and contact with health services, Status, for information regarding Z15.0, codes for genetic susceptibility to cancer.

TREATMENT DIRECTED AT THE MALIGNANCY

If the treatment is directed at the malignancy, designate the malignancy as the principal diagnosis.

The only exception to this guideline is if a patient admission/encounter is solely for the administration of chemotherapy, immunotherapy or radiation therapy, assign the appropriate Z51.-- code as the first-listed or principal diagnosis, and the diagnosis or problem for which the service is being performed as a secondary diagnosis.

TREATMENT OF SECONDARY SITE

When a patient is admitted because of a primary neoplasm with metastasis and treatment is directed toward the secondary site only, the secondary neoplasm is designated as the principal diagnosis even though the primary malignancy is still present.

CODING AND SEQUENCING OF COMPLICATIONS

Coding and sequencing of complications associated with the malignancies or with the therapy thereof are subject to the following guidelines:

1) Anemia associated with malignancy

When admission/encounter is for management of an anemia associated with the malignancy, and the treatment is only for anemia, the appropriate code for the malignancy is sequenced as the principal or first-listed diagnosis followed by the appropriate code for the anemia (such as code D63.0, Anemia in neoplastic disease**).**

2) Anemia associated with chemotherapy, immunotherapy and radiation therapy

When the admission/encounter is for management of an anemia associated with an adverse effect of the administration of chemotherapy or immunotherapy and the only treatment is for the anemia, the anemia code is sequenced first followed by the appropriate codes for the neoplasm and the adverse effect (T45.1X5, Adverse effect of antineoplastic and immunosuppressive drugs).

When the admission/encounter is for management of an anemia associated with an adverse effect of radiotherapy, the anemia code should be sequenced first, followed by the appropriate neoplasm code and code Y84.2, Radiological procedure and radiotherapy as the cause of abnormal reaction of the patient, or of later complication, without mention of misadventure at the time of the procedure.

3) Management of dehydration due to the malignancy

When the admission/encounter is for management of dehydration due to the malignancy and only the dehydration is being treated (intravenous rehydration), the dehydration is sequenced first, followed by the code(s) for the malignancy.

4) Treatment of a complication resulting from a surgical procedure

When the admission/encounter is for treatment of a complication resulting from a surgical procedure, designate the complication as the principal or first-listed diagnosis if treatment is directed at resolving the complication.

PRIMARY MALIGNANCY PREVIOUSLY EXCISED

When a primary malignancy has been previously excised or eradicated from its site and there is no further treatment directed to that site and there is no evidence of any existing primary malignancy, a code from category Z85, Personal history of malignant neoplasm, should be used to indicate the former site of the malignancy. Any mention of extension, invasion, or metastasis to another site is coded as a secondary malignant neoplasm to that site. The secondary site may be the principal or first-listed with the Z85 code used as a secondary code.

ADMISSIONS/ENCOUNTERS INVOLVING CHEMOTHERAPY, IMMUNOTHERAPY AND RADIATION THERAPY

1) Episode of care involves surgical removal of neoplasm

When an episode of care involves the surgical removal of a neoplasm, primary or secondary site, followed by adjunct chemotherapy or radiation treatment during the same episode of care, the code for the neoplasm should be assigned as principal or first-listed diagnosis.

2) Patient admission/encounter solely for administration of chemotherapy, immunotherapy and radiation therapy

If a patient admission/encounter is solely for the administration of chemotherapy, immunotherapy or radiation therapy assign code Z51.0, Encounter for antineoplastic radiation therapy, or Z51.11, Encounter for antineoplastic chemotherapy, or Z51.12, Encounter for antineoplastic immunotherapy as the first-listed or principal diagnosis. If a patient receives more than one of these therapies during the same admission more than one of these codes may be assigned, in any sequence.

The malignancy for which the therapy is being administered should be assigned as a secondary diagnosis.

3) Patient admitted for radiation therapy, chemotherapy or immunotherapy and develops complications

When a patient is admitted for the purpose of radiotherapy, immunotherapy or chemotherapy and develops complications such as uncontrolled nausea and vomiting or dehydration, the principal or first-listed diagnosis is Z51.0, Encounter for antineoplastic radiation therapy, or Z51.11, Encounter for antineoplastic chemotherapy, or Z51.12, Encounter for antineoplastic immunotherapy followed by any codes for the complications.

ADMISSION/ENCOUNTER TO DETERMINE EXTENT OF MALIGNANCY

When the reason for admission/encounter is to determine the extent of the malignancy, or for a procedure such as paracentesis or thoracentesis, the primary malignancy or appropriate metastatic site is designated as the principal or first-listed diagnosis, even though chemotherapy or radiotherapy is administered.

SYMPTOMS, SIGNS, AND ABNORMAL FINDINGS LISTED IN CHAPTER 18 ASSOCIATED WITH NEOPLASMS

Symptoms, signs, and ill-defined conditions listed in Chapter 18 characteristic of, or associated with, an existing primary or secondary site malignancy cannot be used to replace the malignancy as principal or first-listed diagnosis, regardless of the number of admissions or encounters for treatment and care of the neoplasm.

See section I.C.21. Factors influencing health status and contact with health services, Encounter for prophylactic organ removal.

ADMISSION/ENCOUNTER FOR PAIN CONTROL/MANAGEMENT

See Section I.C.6. for information on coding admission/encounter for pain control/management.

MALIGNANCY IN TWO OR MORE NONCONTIGUOUS SITES

A patient may have more than one malignant tumor in the same organ. These tumors may represent different primaries or metastatic disease, depending on the site. Should the documentation be unclear, the provider should be queried as to the status of each tumor so that the correct codes can be assigned.

DISSEMINATED MALIGNANT NEOPLASM, UNSPECIFIED

Code C80.0, Disseminated malignant neoplasm, unspecified, is for use only in those cases where the patient has advanced metastatic disease and no known primary or secondary sites are specified. It should not be used in place of assigning codes for the primary site and all known secondary sites.

MALIGNANT NEOPLASM WITHOUT SPECIFICATION OF SITE

Code C80.1, Malignant (primary) neoplasm, unspecified, equates to Cancer, unspecified. This code should only be used when no determination can be made as to the primary site of a malignancy. This code should rarely be used in the inpatient setting.

SEQUENCING OF NEOPLASM CODES

1) Encounter for treatment of primary malignancy

If the reason for the encounter is for treatment of a primary malignancy, assign the malignancy as the principal/first-listed diagnosis. The primary site is to be sequenced first, followed by any metastatic sites.

2) Encounter for treatment of secondary malignancy

When an encounter is for a primary malignancy with metastasis and treatment is directed toward the metastatic (secondary) site(s) only, the metastatic site(s) is designated as the principal/first-listed diagnosis. The primary malignancy is coded as an additional code.

3) Malignant neoplasm in a pregnant patient

When a pregnant woman has a malignant neoplasm, a code from subcategory O9A.1-, Malignant neoplasm complicating pregnancy, childbirth, and the puerperium, should be sequenced first, followed by the appropriate code from Chapter 2 to indicate the type of neoplasm.

4) **Encounter for complication associated with a neoplasm**

When an encounter is for management of a complication associated with a neoplasm, such as dehydration, and the treatment is only for the complication, the complication is coded first, followed by the appropriate code(s) for the neoplasm.

The exception to this guideline is anemia. When the admission/encounter is for management of an anemia associated with the malignancy, and the treatment is only for anemia, the appropriate code for the malignancy is sequenced as the principal or first-listed diagnosis followed by code D63.0, Anemia in neoplastic disease.

5) **Complication from surgical procedure for treatment of a neoplasm**

When an encounter is for treatment of a complication resulting from a surgical procedure performed for the treatment of the neoplasm, designate the complication as the principal/first-listed diagnosis. See guideline regarding the coding of a current malignancy versus personal history to determine if the code for the neoplasm should also be assigned.

6) **Pathologic fracture due to a neoplasm**

When an encounter is for a pathological fracture due to a neoplasm, and the focus of treatment is the fracture, a code from subcategory M84.5, Pathological fracture in neoplastic disease, should be sequenced first, followed by the code for the neoplasm.

If the focus of treatment is the neoplasm with an associated pathological fracture, the neoplasm code should be sequenced first, followed by a code from M84.5 for the pathological fracture.

CURRENT MALIGNANCY VERSUS PERSONAL HISTORY OF MALIGNANCY

When a primary malignancy has been excised but further treatment, such as an additional surgery for the malignancy, radiation therapy or chemotherapy is directed to that site, the primary malignancy code should be used until treatment is completed.

When a primary malignancy has been previously excised or eradicated from its site, there is no further treatment (of the malignancy) directed to that site, and there is no evidence of any existing primary malignancy, a code from category Z85, Personal history of malignant neoplasm, should be used to indicate the former site of the malignancy.

See Section I.C.21. Factors influencing health status and contact with health services, History (of)

LEUKEMIA, MULTIPLE MYELOMA, AND MALIGNANT PLASMA CELL NEOPLASMS IN REMISSION VERSUS PERSONAL HISTORY

The categories for leukemia, and category C90, Multiple myeloma and malignant plasma cell neoplasms, have codes indicating whether or not the leukemia has achieved remission. There are also codes Z85.6, Personal history of leukemia, and Z85.79, Personal history of other malignant neoplasms of lymphoid, hematopoietic and related tissues. If the documentation is unclear as to whether the leukemia has achieved remission, the provider should be queried.

See Section I.C.21. Factors influencing health status and contact with health services, History (of)

AFTERCARE FOLLOWING SURGERY FOR NEOPLASM

See Section I.C.21. Factors influencing health status and contact with health services, Aftercare

FOLLOW-UP CARE FOR COMPLETED TREATMENT OF A MALIGNANCY

See Section I.C.21. Factors influencing health status and contact with health services, Follow-up

PROPHYLACTIC ORGAN REMOVAL FOR PREVENTION OF MALIGNANCY

See Section I.C. 21, Factors influencing health status and contact with health services, Prophylactic organ removal

MALIGNANT NEOPLASM ASSOCIATED WITH TRANSPLANTED ORGAN

A malignant neoplasm of a transplanted organ should be coded as a transplant complication. Assign first the appropriate code from category T86.-, Complications of transplanted organs and tissue, followed by code C80.2, Malignant neoplasm associated with transplanted organ. Use an additional code for the specific malignancy.

Chapter 2

Neoplasms (C00-D49)

This chapter contains the following blocks:

C00-C14	Malignant neoplasms of lip, oral cavity and pharynx
C15-C26	Malignant neoplasms of digestive organs
C30-C39	Malignant neoplasms of respiratory and intrathoracic organs
C40-C41	Malignant neoplasms of bone and articular cartilage
C43-C44	Melanoma and other Malignant neoplasms of skin
C45-C49	Malignant neoplasms of Mesothelial and soft tissue
C50	Malignant neoplasms of breast
C51-C58	Malignant neoplasms of female genital organs
C60-C63	Malignant neoplasms of Male genital organs
C64-C68	Malignant neoplasms of urinary tract
C69-C72	Malignant neoplasms of eye, brain and other parts of central nervous system
C73-C75	Malignant neoplasms of thyroid and other endocrine glands
C7A	Malignant neuroendocrine tumors
C7B	Secondary neuroendocrine tumors
C76-C80	Malignant neoplasms of ill-defined, other secondary and unspecified sites
C81-C96	Malignant neoplasms of lymphoid, hematopoietic and related tissue
D00-D09	In situ neoplasms
D10-D36	Benign neoplasms, except benign neuroendocrine tumors
D3A	Benign neuroendocrine tumors
D37-D48	Neoplasms of uncertain behavior, polycythemia vera and Myelodysplastic syndromes
D49	Neoplasms of unspecified behavior

Note: Functional activity

All neoplasms are classified in this chapter, whether they are functionally active or not. An additional code from Chapter 4 may be used, to identify functional activity associated with any neoplasm. Morphology [Histology]

Chapter 2 classifies neoplasms primarily by site (topography), with broad groupings for behavior, malignant, in situ, benign, etc. The Table of Neoplasms should be used to identify the correct topography code. In a few cases, such as for malignant melanoma and certain neuroendocrine tumors, the morphology (histologic type) is included in the category and codes.

Primary malignant neoplasms overlapping site boundaries

A primary malignant neoplasm that overlaps two or more contiguous (next to each Other) sites should be classified to the subcategory/code .8 ('overlapping lesion'), unless the combination is specifically indexed elsewhere. For multiple neoplasms of the same site that are not contiguous, such as tumors in different quadrants of the same breast, codes for each site should be assigned.

Malignant neoplasm of ectopic tissue

Malignant neoplasms of ectopic tissue are to be coded to the site mentioned, e.g., ectopic pancreatic malignant neoplasms are coded to pancreas, unspecified (C25.9).

MALIGNANT NEOPLASMS (C00-C96)

Definition: Malignant neoplasm refers to a tumor that tends to grow, invade, and metastasize. The tumor usually has an irregular shape and is composed of poorly differentiated cells. If untreated, it may result in death.

MALIGNANT NEOPLASMS, STATED OR PRESUMED TO BE PRIMARY (OF SPECIFIED SITES), AND CERTAIN SPECIFIED HISTOLOGIES, EXCEPT NEUROENDOCRINE, AND OF LYMPHOID, HEMATOPOIETIC AND RELATED TISSUE

(C00-C75)

MALIGNANT NEOPLASMS OF LIP, ORAL CAVITY AND PHARYNX (C00-C14)

C00 Malignant neoplasm of lip

Use additional code to identify:

alcohol abuse and dependence (F10.-)

history of tobacco dependence (Z87.891)

tobacco dependence (F17.-)

tobacco use (Z72.0)

Excludes1: malignant melanoma of lip (C43.0)

Merkel cell carcinoma of lip (C4A.0)

Other and unspecified malignant neoplasm of skin of lip (C44.0-)

C00.0 Malignant neoplasm of external upper lip

Malignant neoplasm of lipstick area of upper lip

Malignant neoplasm of upper lip NOS

Malignant neoplasm of vermilion border of upper lip

C00.1 Malignant neoplasm of external lower lip

Malignant neoplasm of lower lip NOS

Malignant neoplasm of lipstick area of lower lip

Malignant neoplasm of vermilion border of lower lip

C00.2 Malignant neoplasm of external lip, unspecified

Malignant neoplasm of vermilion border of lip NOS

C00.3 Malignant neoplasm of upper lip, inner aspect

Malignant neoplasm of buccal aspect of upper lip

Malignant neoplasm of frenulum of upper lip

Malignant neoplasm of mucosa of upper lip

Malignant neoplasm of oral aspect of upper lip

C00.4 Malignant neoplasm of lower lip, inner aspect

Malignant neoplasm of buccal aspect of lower lip

Malignant neoplasm of frenulum of lower lip

Malignant neoplasm of mucosa of lower lip

Malignant neoplasm of oral aspect of lower lip

C00.5 Malignant neoplasm of lip, unspecified, inner aspect

Malignant neoplasm of buccal aspect of lip, unspecified

Malignant neoplasm of frenulum of lip, unspecified

Malignant neoplasm of mucosa of lip, unspecified

Malignant neoplasm of oral aspect of lip, unspecified

C00.6 Malignant neoplasm of commissure of lip, unspecified

C00.8 Malignant neoplasm of overlapping sites of lip

C00.9 Malignant neoplasm of lip, unspecified

C01 Malignant neoplasm of base of tongue

Malignant neoplasm of dorsal surface of base of tongue

Malignant neoplasm of fixed part of tongue NOS

Malignant neoplasm of posterior third of tongue

Use additional code to identify:

alcohol abuse and dependence (F10.-)

history of tobacco dependence (Z87.891)

tobacco dependence (F17.-)

tobacco use (Z72.0)

C02 Malignant neoplasm of other and unspecified parts of tongue

Use additional code to identify:

alcohol abuse and dependence (F10.-)

history of tobacco dependence (Z87.891)

tobacco dependence (F17.-)

tobacco use (Z72.0)

C02.0 **Malignant neoplasm of dorsal surface of tongue**

Malignant neoplasm of anterior two-thirds of tongue, dorsal surface

Excludes2: malignant neoplasm of dorsal surface of base of tongue (C01)

C02.1 **Malignant neoplasm of border of tongue**

Malignant neoplasm of tip of tongue

C02.2 **Malignant neoplasm of ventral surface of tongue**

Malignant neoplasm of anterior two-thirds of tongue, ventral surface

Malignant neoplasm of frenulum linguae

C02.3 **Malignant neoplasm of anterior two-thirds of tongue, part unspecified**

Malignant neoplasm of middle third of tongue NOS

Malignant neoplasm of mobile part of tongue NOS

C02.4 **Malignant neoplasm of lingual tonsil**

Excludes2: malignant neoplasm of tonsil NOS (C09.9)

C02.8 **Malignant neoplasm of overlapping sites of tongue**

Malignant neoplasm of two or more contiguous sites of tongue

C02.9 **Malignant neoplasm of tongue, unspecified**

C03 **Malignant neoplasm of gum**

Includes: malignant neoplasm of alveolar (ridge) mucosa

malignant neoplasm of gingiva

Use additional code to identify:

alcohol abuse and dependence (F10.-)

history of tobacco dependence (Z87.891)

tobacco dependence (F17.-)

tobacco use (Z72.0)

Excludes2: malignant odontogenic neoplasms (C41.0-C41.1)

C03.0 **Malignant neoplasm of upper gum**

C03.1 **Malignant neoplasm of lower gum**

C03.9 **Malignant neoplasm of gum, unspecified**

C04 **Malignant neoplasm of floor of mouth**

Use additional code to identify:

alcohol abuse and dependence (F10.-)

history of tobacco dependence (Z87.891)

tobacco dependence (F17.-)

tobacco use (Z72.0)

C04.0 **Malignant neoplasm of anterior floor of mouth**

Malignant neoplasm of anterior to the premolar-canine junction

C04.1 **Malignant neoplasm of lateral floor of mouth**

C04.8 **Malignant neoplasm of overlapping sites of floor of mouth**

C04.9 **Malignant neoplasm of floor of mouth, unspecified**

C05 **Malignant neoplasm of palate**

Use additional code to identify:

alcohol abuse and dependence (F10.-)

history of tobacco dependence (Z87.891)

tobacco dependence (F17.-)

tobacco use (Z72.0)

Excludes1: Kaposi's sarcoma of palate (C46.2)

C05.0 **Malignant neoplasm of hard palate**

C05.1 **Malignant neoplasm of soft palate**

Excludes2: malignant neoplasm of nasopharyngeal surface of soft palate (C11.3)

C05.2 **Malignant neoplasm of uvula**

C05.8 **Malignant neoplasm of overlapping sites of palate**

C05.9 **Malignant neoplasm of palate, unspecified**

Malignant neoplasm of roof of mouth

C06 **Malignant neoplasm of other and unspecified parts of mouth**

Use additional code to identify:

alcohol abuse and dependence (F10.-)

history of tobacco dependence (Z87.891)

tobacco dependence (F17.-)

tobacco use (Z72.0)

C06.0 **Malignant neoplasm of cheek mucosa**

Malignant neoplasm of buccal mucosa NOS

Malignant neoplasm of internal cheek

C06.1 **Malignant neoplasm of vestibule of mouth**

Malignant neoplasm of buccal sulcus (upper) (lower)

Malignant neoplasm of labial sulcus (upper) (lower)

C06.2 **Malignant neoplasm of retromolar area**

C06.8 **Malignant neoplasm of overlapping sites of other and unspecified parts of mouth**

C06.80 **Malignant neoplasm of overlapping sites of unspecified parts of mouth**

C06.89 **Malignant neoplasm of overlapping sites of other parts of mouth**

'book leaf' neoplasm [ventral surface of tongue and floor of mouth]

C06.9 **Malignant neoplasm of mouth, unspecified**

Malignant neoplasm of minor salivary gland, unspecified site

Malignant neoplasm of oral cavity NOS

C07 **Malignant neoplasm of parotid gland**

Use additional code to identify:

alcohol abuse and dependence (F10.-)

exposure to environmental tobacco smoke (Z77.22)

exposure to tobacco smoke in the perinatal period (P96.81)

history of tobacco dependence (Z87.891)

occupational exposure to environmental tobacco smoke (Z57.31)

tobacco dependence (F17.-)

tobacco use (Z72.0)

C08 **Malignant neoplasm of other and unspecified major salivary glands**

Includes: malignant neoplasm of salivary ducts

Use additional code to identify:

alcohol abuse and dependence (F10.-)

exposure to environmental tobacco smoke (Z77.22)

exposure to tobacco smoke in the perinatal period (P96.81)

history of tobacco dependence (Z87.891)

occupational exposure to environmental tobacco smoke (Z57.31)

tobacco dependence (F17.-)

tobacco use (Z72.0)

Excludes1: malignant neoplasms of specified minor salivary glands which are classified according to their anatomical location

Excludes2: malignant neoplasms of minor salivary glands NOS (C06.9)

    malignant neoplasm of parotid gland (C07)

C08.0 **Malignant neoplasm of submandibular gland**

    Malignant neoplasm of submaxillary gland

C08.1 **Malignant neoplasm of sublingual gland**

C08.9 **Malignant neoplasm of major salivary gland, unspecified**

    Malignant neoplasm of salivary gland (major) NOS

C09 **Malignant neoplasm of tonsil**

Use additional code to identify:

alcohol abuse and dependence (F10.-)

exposure to environmental tobacco smoke (Z77.22)

exposure to tobacco smoke in the perinatal period (P96.81)

history of tobacco dependence (Z87.891)

occupational exposure to environmental tobacco smoke (Z57.31)

tobacco dependence (F17.-)

tobacco use (Z72.0)

Excludes2: malignant neoplasm of lingual tonsil (C02.4)

    malignant neoplasm of pharyngeal tonsil (C11.1)

C09.0 **Malignant neoplasm of tonsillar fossa**

C09.1 **Malignant neoplasm of tonsillar pillar (anterior) (posterior)**

C09.8 **Malignant neoplasm of overlapping sites of tonsil**

C09.9 **Malignant neoplasm of tonsil, unspecified**

    Malignant neoplasm of tonsil NOS

    Malignant neoplasm of faucial tonsils

    Malignant neoplasm of palatine tonsils

C10 **Malignant neoplasm of oropharynx**

Use additional code to identify:

alcohol abuse and dependence (F10.-)

exposure to environmental tobacco smoke (Z77.22)

exposure to tobacco smoke in the perinatal period (P96.81)

history of tobacco dependence (Z87.891)

occupational exposure to environmental tobacco smoke (Z57.31)

tobacco dependence (F17.-)

tobacco use (Z72.0)

Excludes2: malignant neoplasm of tonsil (C09.-)

C10.0 **Malignant neoplasm of vallecula**

C10.1 **Malignant neoplasm of anterior surface of epiglottis**

    Malignant neoplasm of epiglottis, free border [margin]

    Malignant neoplasm of glossoepiglottic fold(s)

    Excludes2: malignant neoplasm of epiglottis (suprahyoid portion) NOS (C32.1)

C10.2 **Malignant neoplasm of lateral wall of oropharynx**

C10.3 **Malignant neoplasm of posterior wall of oropharynx**

C10.4 **Malignant neoplasm of branchial cleft**
    Malignant neoplasm of branchial cyst [site of neoplasm]

C10.8 **Malignant neoplasm of overlapping sites of oropharynx**

    Malignant neoplasm of junctional region of oropharynx

C10.9 **Malignant neoplasm of oropharynx, unspecified**

C11 **Malignant neoplasm of nasopharynx**

Use additional code to identify:

exposure to environmental tobacco smoke (Z77.22)

exposure to tobacco smoke in the perinatal period (P96.81)

history of tobacco dependence (Z87.891)

occupational exposure to environmental tobacco smoke (Z57.31)

tobacco dependence (F17.-)

tobacco use (Z72.0)

C11.0 **Malignant neoplasm of superior wall of nasopharynx**

    Malignant neoplasm of roof of nasopharynx

C11.1 **Malignant neoplasm of posterior wall of nasopharynx**

    Malignant neoplasm of adenoid

    Malignant neoplasm of pharyngeal tonsil

C11.2 **Malignant neoplasm of lateral wall of nasopharynx**

    Malignant neoplasm of fossa of Rosenmüller

    Malignant neoplasm of opening of auditory tube

    Malignant neoplasm of pharyngeal recess

C11.3 **Malignant neoplasm of anterior wall of nasopharynx**

    Malignant neoplasm of floor of nasopharynx

    Malignant neoplasm of nasopharyngeal (anterior) (posterior) surface of soft palate

    Malignant neoplasm of posterior margin of nasal choana

    Malignant neoplasm of posterior margin of nasal septum

C11.8 **Malignant neoplasm of overlapping sites of nasopharynx**

C11.9 **Malignant neoplasm of nasopharynx, unspecified**

    Malignant neoplasm of nasopharyngeal wall NOS

C12 **Malignant neoplasm of pyriform sinus**

Malignant neoplasm of pyriform fossa

Use additional code to identify:

exposure to environmental tobacco smoke (Z77.22)

exposure to tobacco smoke in the perinatal period (P96.81)

history of tobacco dependence (Z87.891)

occupational exposure to environmental tobacco smoke (Z57.31)

tobacco dependence (F17.-)

tobacco use (Z72.0)

C13 **Malignant neoplasm of hypopharynx**

Use additional code to identify:

exposure to environmental tobacco smoke (Z77.22)

exposure to tobacco smoke in the perinatal period (P96.81)

history of tobacco dependence (Z87.891)

occupational exposure to environmental tobacco smoke (Z57.31)

tobacco dependence (F17.-)

tobacco use (Z72.0)

Excludes2: malignant neoplasm of pyriform sinus (C12)

C13.0 **Malignant neoplasm of postcricoid region**

C13.1 **Malignant neoplasm of aryepiglottic fold, hypopharyngeal aspect**

    Malignant neoplasm of aryepiglottic fold, marginal zone

    Malignant neoplasm of aryepiglottic fold NOS

    Malignant neoplasm of interarytenoid fold, marginal zone

    Malignant neoplasm of interarytenoid fold NOS

Excludes2: malignant neoplasm of aryepiglottic fold or interarytenoid fold, laryngeal aspect (C32.1)

C13.2 **Malignant neoplasm of posterior wall of hypopharynx**

C13.8 **Malignant neoplasm of overlapping sites of hypopharynx**

C13.9 **Malignant neoplasm of hypopharynx, unspecified**

Malignant neoplasm of hypopharyngeal wall NOS

C14 **Malignant neoplasm of other and ill-defined sites in the lip, oral cavity and pharynx**

Use additional code to identify:

alcohol abuse and dependence (F10.-)

exposure to environmental tobacco smoke (Z77.22)

exposure to tobacco smoke in the perinatal period (P96.81)

history of tobacco dependence (Z87.891)

occupational exposure to environmental tobacco smoke (Z57.31)

tobacco dependence (F17.-)

tobacco use (Z72.0)

Excludes1: malignant neoplasm of oral cavity NOS (C06.9)

C14.0 **Malignant neoplasm of pharynx, unspecified**

C14.2 **Malignant neoplasm of Waldeyer's ring**

C14.8 **Malignant neoplasm of overlapping sites of lip, oral cavity and pharynx**

Primary malignant neoplasm of two or more contiguous sites of lip, oral cavity and pharynx

Excludes1: 'book leaf' neoplasm [ventral surface of tongue and floor of mouth] (C06.89)

MALIGNANT NEOPLASMS OF DIGESTIVE ORGANS (C15-C26)

Excludes1: Kaposi's sarcoma of gastrointestinal sites (C46.4)

Excludes2: gastrointestinal stromal tumors (C49.A-)

C15 **Malignant neoplasm of esophagus**

Use additional code to identify:

alcohol abuse and dependence (F10.-)

C15.3 **Malignant neoplasm of upper third of esophagus**

C15.4 **Malignant neoplasm of middle third of esophagus**

C15.5 **Malignant neoplasm of lower third of esophagus**

Excludes1: malignant neoplasm of cardio-esophageal junction (C16.0)

C15.8 **Malignant neoplasm of overlapping sites of esophagus**

C15.9 **Malignant neoplasm of esophagus, unspecified**

C16 **Malignant neoplasm of stomach**

Use additional code to identify:

alcohol abuse and dependence (F10.-)

Excludes2: malignant carcinoid tumor of the stomach (C7A.092)

C16.0 **Malignant neoplasm of cardia**

Malignant neoplasm of cardiac orifice

Malignant neoplasm of cardio-esophageal junction

Malignant neoplasm of esophagus and stomach

Malignant neoplasm of gastro-esophageal junction

C16.1 **Malignant neoplasm of fundus of stomach**

C16.2 **Malignant neoplasm of body of stomach**

C16.3 **Malignant neoplasm of pyloric antrum**

Malignant neoplasm of gastric antrum

C16.4 **Malignant neoplasm of pylorus**

Malignant neoplasm of prepylorus

Malignant neoplasm of pyloric canal

C16.5 **Malignant neoplasm of lesser curvature of stomach, unspecified**

Malignant neoplasm of lesser curvature of stomach, not classifiable to C16.1-C16.4

C16.6 **Malignant neoplasm of greater curvature of stomach, unspecified**

Malignant neoplasm of greater curvature of stomach, not classifiable to C16.0-C16.4

C16.8 **Malignant neoplasm of overlapping sites of stomach**

C16.9 **Malignant neoplasm of stomach, unspecified**

Gastric cancer NOS

C17 **Malignant neoplasm of small intestine**

Excludes1: malignant carcinoid tumors of the small intestine (C7A.01)

C17.0 **Malignant neoplasm of duodenum**

C17.1 **Malignant neoplasm of jejunum**

C17.2 **Malignant neoplasm of ileum**

Excludes1: malignant neoplasm of ileocecal valve (C18.0)

C17.3 **Meckel's diverticulum, malignant**

Excludes1: Meckel's diverticulum, congenital (Q43.0)

C17.8 **Malignant neoplasm of overlapping sites of small intestine**

C17.9 **Malignant neoplasm of small intestine, unspecified**

C18 **Malignant neoplasm of colon**

Excludes1: malignant carcinoid tumors of the colon (C7A.02-)

C18.0 **Malignant neoplasm of cecum**

Malignant neoplasm of ileocecal valve

C18.1 **Malignant neoplasm of appendix**

C18.2 **Malignant neoplasm of ascending colon**

C18.3 **Malignant neoplasm of hepatic flexure**

C18.4 **Malignant neoplasm of transverse colon**

C18.5 **Malignant neoplasm of splenic flexure**

C18.6 **Malignant neoplasm of descending colon**

C18.7 **Malignant neoplasm of sigmoid colon**

Malignant neoplasm of sigmoid (flexure)

Excludes1: malignant neoplasm of rectosigmoid junction (C19)

C18.8 **Malignant neoplasm of overlapping sites of colon**

C18.9 **Malignant neoplasm of colon, unspecified**

Malignant neoplasm of large intestine NOS

C19 **Malignant neoplasm of rectosigmoid junction**

Malignant neoplasm of colon with rectum

Malignant neoplasm of rectosigmoid (colon)

Excludes1: malignant carcinoid tumors of the colon (C7A.02-)

C20 **Malignant neoplasm of rectum**

Malignant neoplasm of rectal ampulla

Excludes1: malignant carcinoid tumor of the rectum (C7A.026)

C21 **Malignant neoplasm of anus and anal canal**

Excludes2: malignant carcinoid tumors of the colon (C7A.02-)

malignant melanoma of anal margin (C43.51)

malignant melanoma of anal skin (C43.51)

malignant melanoma of perianal skin (C43.51)

Other and unspecified malignant neoplasm of anal margin (C44.500, C44.510, C44.520, C44.590)

Other and unspecified malignant neoplasm of anal skin (C44.500, C44.510, C44.520, C44.590)

Other and unspecified malignant neoplasm of perianal skin (C44.500, C44.510, C44.520, C44.590)

C21.0 **Malignant neoplasm of anus, unspecified**

C21.1 **Malignant neoplasm of anal canal**

Malignant neoplasm of anal sphincter

● New code ▲ Revised code **Excludes1:** Not coded here **Excludes2:** Not included here ⊗ Placeholder required ⑦7th digit required

C21.2 Malignant neoplasm of cloacogenic zone

C21.8 Malignant neoplasm of overlapping sites of rectum, anus and anal canal

Malignant neoplasm of anorectal junction

Malignant neoplasm of anorectum

Primary malignant neoplasm of two or more contiguous sites of rectum, anus and anal canal

C22 Malignant neoplasm of liver and intrahepatic bile ducts

Excludes1: malignant neoplasm of biliary tract NOS (C24.9)

secondary malignant neoplasm of liver and intrahepatic bile duct (C78.7)

Use additional code to identify:

alcohol abuse and dependence (F10.-)

hepatitis B (B16.-, B18.0-B18.1)

hepatitis C (B17.1-, B18.2)

C22.0 Liver cell carcinoma

Hepatocellular carcinoma

Hepatoma

C22.1 Intrahepatic bile duct carcinoma

Cholangiocarcinoma

Excludes1: malignant neoplasm of hepatic duct (C24.0)

C22.2 Hepatoblastoma

C22.3 Angiosarcoma of liver

Kupffer cell sarcoma

C22.4 Other sarcomas of liver

C22.7 Other specified carcinomas of liver

C22.8 Malignant neoplasm of liver, primary, unspecified as to type

C22.9 Malignant neoplasm of liver, not specified as primary or secondary

C23 Malignant neoplasm of gallbladder

C24 Malignant neoplasm of other and unspecified parts of biliary tract

Excludes1: malignant neoplasm of intrahepatic bile duct (C22.1)

C24.0 Malignant neoplasm of extrahepatic bile duct

Malignant neoplasm of biliary duct or passage NOS

Malignant neoplasm of common bile duct

Malignant neoplasm of cystic duct

Malignant neoplasm of hepatic duct

C24.1 Malignant neoplasm of ampulla of Vater

C24.8 Malignant neoplasm of overlapping sites of biliary tract

Malignant neoplasm involving both intrahepatic and extrahepatic bile ducts

Primary malignant neoplasm of two or more contiguous sites of biliary tract

C24.9 Malignant neoplasm of biliary tract, unspecified

C25 Malignant neoplasm of pancreas

Code also exocrine pancreatic insufficiency (K86.81)

Use additional code to identify:

alcohol abuse and dependence (F10.-)

C25.0 Malignant neoplasm of head of pancreas

C25.1 Malignant neoplasm of body of pancreas

C25.2 Malignant neoplasm of tail of pancreas

C25.3 Malignant neoplasm of pancreatic duct

C25.4 Malignant neoplasm of endocrine pancreas

Malignant neoplasm of islets of Langerhans

Use additional code to identify any functional activity.

C25.7 Malignant neoplasm of other parts of pancreas

Malignant neoplasm of neck of pancreas

C25.8 Malignant neoplasm of overlapping sites of pancreas

C25.9 Malignant neoplasm of pancreas, unspecified

C26 Malignant neoplasm of other and ill-defined digestive organs

Excludes1: malignant neoplasm of peritoneum and retroperitoneum (C48.-)

C26.0 Malignant neoplasm of intestinal tract, part unspecified

Malignant neoplasm of intestine NOS

C26.1 Malignant neoplasm of spleen

Excludes1: Hodgkin lymphoma (C81.-)

non-Hodgkin lymphoma (C82-C85)

C26.9 Malignant neoplasm of ill-defined sites within the digestive system

Malignant neoplasm of alimentary canal or tract NOS

Malignant neoplasm of gastrointestinal tract NOS

Excludes1: malignant neoplasm of abdominal NOS (C76.2)

malignant neoplasm of intra-abdominal NOS (C76.2)

MALIGNANT NEOPLASMS OF RESPIRATORY AND INTRATHORACIC ORGANS (C30-C39)

Includes: malignant neoplasm of middle ear

Excludes1: mesothelioma (C45.-)

C30 Malignant neoplasm of nasal cavity and middle ear

C30.0 Malignant neoplasm of nasal cavity

Malignant neoplasm of cartilage of nose

Malignant neoplasm of nasal concha

Malignant neoplasm of internal nose

Malignant neoplasm of septum of nose

Malignant neoplasm of vestibule of nose

Excludes1: malignant neoplasm of nasal bone (C41.0)

malignant neoplasm of nose NOS (C76.0)

malignant neoplasm of olfactory bulb (C72.2-)

malignant neoplasm of posterior margin of nasal septum and choana (C11.3)

malignant melanoma of skin of nose (C43.31)

malignant neoplasm of turbinates (C41.0)

Other and unspecified malignant neoplasm of skin of nose C44.301, C44.311, C44.321, C44.391)

C30.1 Malignant neoplasm of middle ear

Malignant neoplasm of antrum tympanicum

Malignant neoplasm of auditory tube

Malignant neoplasm of eustachian tube

Malignant neoplasm of inner ear

Malignant neoplasm of mastoid air cells

Malignant neoplasm of tympanic cavity

Excludes1: malignant neoplasm of auricular canal (external) (C43.2-,C44.2-)

malignant neoplasm of bone of ear (meatus) (C41.0)

malignant neoplasm of cartilage of ear (C49.0)

malignant melanoma of skin of (external) ear (C43.2-)

Add 4th-7th digits	Nonspecific code	Unspecified code	Manifestation code

Other and unspecified malignant neoplasm of skin of (external) ear (C44.2-)

C31 Malignant neoplasm of accessory sinuses

C31.0 Malignant neoplasm of maxillary sinus

Malignant neoplasm of antrum (Highmore) (maxillary)

C31.1 Malignant neoplasm of ethmoidal sinus

C31.2 Malignant neoplasm of frontal sinus

C31.3 Malignant neoplasm of sphenoid sinus to

C31.8 Malignant neoplasm of overlapping sites of accessory sinuses

C31.9 Malignant neoplasm of accessory sinus, unspecified

C32 Malignant neoplasm of larynx

Use additional code to identify:

alcohol abuse and dependence (F10.-)

exposure to environmental tobacco smoke (Z77.22)

exposure to tobacco smoke in the perinatal period (P96.81)

history of tobacco dependence (Z87.891)

occupational exposure to environmental tobacco smoke (Z57.31)

tobacco dependence (F17.-)

tobacco use (Z72.0)

C32.0 Malignant neoplasm of glottis

Malignant neoplasm of intrinsic larynx

Malignant neoplasm of laryngeal commissure (anterior)(posterior)

Malignant neoplasm of vocal cord (true) NOS

C32.1 Malignant neoplasm of supraglottis

Malignant neoplasm of aryepiglottic fold or interarytenoid fold, laryngeal aspect

Malignant neoplasm of epiglottis (suprahyoid portion) NOS

Malignant neoplasm of extrinsic larynx

Malignant neoplasm of false vocal cord

Malignant neoplasm of posterior (laryngeal) surface of epiglottis

Malignant neoplasm of ventricular bands

Excludes2: malignant neoplasm of anterior surface of epiglottis (C10.1)

malignant neoplasm of aryepiglottic fold or interarytenoid fold, hypopharyngeal aspect (C13.1)

malignant neoplasm of aryepiglottic fold or interarytenoid fold, marginal zone (C13.1)

malignant neoplasm of aryepiglottic fold or interarytenoid fold NOS (C13.1)

C32.2 Malignant neoplasm of subglottis

C32.3 Malignant neoplasm of laryngeal cartilage

C32.8 Malignant neoplasm of overlapping sites of larynx

C32.9 Malignant neoplasm of larynx, unspecified

C33 Malignant neoplasm of trachea

Use additional code to identify:

exposure to environmental tobacco smoke (Z77.22)

exposure to tobacco smoke in the perinatal period (P96.81)

history of tobacco dependence (Z87.891)

occupational exposure to environmental tobacco smoke (Z57.31)

tobacco dependence (F17.-)

tobacco use (Z72.0)

C34 Malignant neoplasm of bronchus and lung

Use additional code to identify:

exposure to environmental tobacco smoke (Z77.22)

exposure to tobacco smoke in the perinatal period (P96.81)

history of tobacco dependence (Z87.891)

occupational exposure to environmental tobacco smoke (Z57.31)

tobacco dependence (F17.-)

tobacco use (Z72.0)

Excludes1: Kaposi's sarcoma of lung (C46.5-)

malignant carcinoid tumor of the bronchus and lung (C7A.090)

C34.0 Malignant neoplasm of main bronchus

Malignant neoplasm of carina

Malignant neoplasm of hilus (of lung)

C34.00 Malignant neoplasm of unspecified main bronchus

C34.01 Malignant neoplasm of right main bronchus

C34.02 Malignant neoplasm of left main bronchus

C34.1 Malignant neoplasm of upper lobe, bronchus or lung

C34.10 Malignant neoplasm of upper lobe, unspecified bronchus or lung

C34.11 Malignant neoplasm of upper lobe, right bronchus or lung

C34.12 Malignant neoplasm of upper lobe, left bronchus or lung

C34.2 Malignant neoplasm of middle lobe, bronchus or lung

C34.3 Malignant neoplasm of lower lobe, bronchus or lung

C34.30 Malignant neoplasm of lower lobe, unspecified bronchus or lung

C34.31 Malignant neoplasm of lower lobe, right bronchus or lung

C34.32 Malignant neoplasm of lower lobe, left bronchus or lung

C34.8 Malignant neoplasm of overlapping sites of bronchus and lung

C34.80 Malignant neoplasm of overlapping sites of unspecified bronchus and lung

C34.81 Malignant neoplasm of overlapping sites of right bronchus and lung

C34.82 Malignant neoplasm of overlapping sites of left bronchus and lung

C34.9 Malignant neoplasm of unspecified part of bronchus or lung

C34.90 Malignant neoplasm of unspecified part of unspecified bronchus or lung

Lung cancer NOS

C34.91 Malignant neoplasm of unspecified part of right bronchus or lung

C34.92 Malignant neoplasm of unspecified part of left bronchus or lung

C37 Malignant neoplasm of thymus

Excludes1: malignant carcinoid tumor of the thymus (C7A.091)

C38 Malignant neoplasm of heart, mediastinum and pleura

Excludes1: mesothelioma (C45.-)

C38.0 Malignant neoplasm of heart

Malignant neoplasm of pericardium

Excludes1: malignant neoplasm of great vessels (C49.3)

● New code ▲ Revised code **Excludes1:** Not coded here **Excludes2:** Not included here ⊗ Placeholder required ⑦7th digit required

C38.1   Malignant neoplasm of anterior mediastinum

C38.2   Malignant neoplasm of posterior mediastinum

C38.3   Malignant neoplasm of mediastinum, part unspecified

C38.4   Malignant neoplasm of pleura

C38.8   Malignant neoplasm of overlapping sites of heart, mediastinum and pleura

C39   Malignant neoplasm of other and ill-defined sites in the respiratory system and intrathoracic organs

Use additional code to identify:

exposure to environmental tobacco smoke (Z77.22)

exposure to tobacco smoke in the perinatal period (P96.81)

history of tobacco dependence (Z87.891)

occupational exposure to environmental tobacco smoke (Z57.31)

tobacco dependence (F17.-)

tobacco use (Z72.0)

Excludes1: intrathoracic malignant neoplasm NOS (C76.1)

thoracic malignant neoplasm NOS (C76.1)

C39.0   Malignant neoplasm of upper respiratory tract, part unspecified

C39.9   Malignant neoplasm of lower respiratory tract, part unspecified

Malignant neoplasm of respiratory tract NOS

MALIGNANT NEOPLASMS OF BONE AND ARTICULAR CARTILAGE (C40-C41)

Includes: malignant neoplasm of cartilage (articular) (joint)

malignant neoplasm of periosteum

Excludes1: malignant neoplasm of bone marrow NOS (C96.9)

malignant neoplasm of synovia (C49.-)

C40   Malignant neoplasm of bone and articular cartilage of limbs

Use additional code to identify major osseous defect, if applicable (M89.7-)

C40.0   Malignant neoplasm of scapula and long bones of upper limb

C40.00   Malignant neoplasm of scapula and long bones of unspecified upper limb

C40.01   Malignant neoplasm of scapula and long bones of right upper limb

C40.02   Malignant neoplasm of scapula and long bones of left upper limb

C40.1   Malignant neoplasm of short bones of upper limb

C40.10   Malignant neoplasm of short bones of unspecified upper limb

C40.11   Malignant neoplasm of short bones of right upper limb

C40.12   Malignant neoplasm of short bones of left upper limb

C40.2   Malignant neoplasm of long bones of lower limb

C40.20   Malignant neoplasm of long bones of unspecified lower limb

C40.21   Malignant neoplasm of long bones of right lower limb

C40.22   Malignant neoplasm of long bones of left lower limb

C40.3   Malignant neoplasm of short bones of lower limb

C40.30   Malignant neoplasm of short bones of unspecified lower limb

C40.31   Malignant neoplasm of short bones of right lower limb

C40.32   Malignant neoplasm of short bones of left lower limb

C40.8   Malignant neoplasm of overlapping sites of bone and articular cartilage of limb

C40.80   Malignant neoplasm of overlapping sites of bone and articular cartilage of unspecified limb

C40.81   Malignant neoplasm of overlapping sites of bone and articular cartilage of right limb

C40.82   Malignant neoplasm of overlapping sites of bone and articular cartilage of left limb

C40.9   Malignant neoplasm of unspecified bones and articular cartilage of limb

C40.90   Malignant neoplasm of unspecified bones and articular cartilage of unspecified limb

C40.91   Malignant neoplasm of unspecified bones and articular cartilage of right limb

C40.92   Malignant neoplasm of unspecified bones and articular cartilage of left limb

C41   Malignant neoplasm of bone and articular cartilage of other and unspecified sites

Excludes1: malignant neoplasm of bones of limbs (C40.-)

malignant neoplasm of cartilage of ear (C49.0)

malignant neoplasm of cartilage of eyelid (C49.0)

malignant neoplasm of cartilage of larynx (C32.3)

malignant neoplasm of cartilage of limbs (C40.-)

malignant neoplasm of cartilage of nose (C30.0)

C41.0   Malignant neoplasm of bones of skull and face

Malignant neoplasm of maxilla (superior)

Malignant neoplasm of orbital bone

Excludes2: carcinoma, any type except intraosseous or odontogenic of:

maxillary sinus (C31.0)

upper jaw (C03.0)

malignant neoplasm of jaw bone (lower) (C41.1)

C41.1   Malignant neoplasm of mandible

Malignant neoplasm of inferior maxilla

Malignant neoplasm of lower jaw bone

Excludes2: carcinoma, any type except intraosseous or odontogenic of:

jaw NOS (C03.9)

lower (C03.1)

malignant neoplasm of upper jaw bone (C41.0)

C41.2   Malignant neoplasm of vertebral column

Excludes1: malignant neoplasm of sacrum and coccyx (C41.4)

C41.3   Malignant neoplasm of ribs, sternum and clavicle

C41.4   Malignant neoplasm of pelvic bones, sacrum and coccyx

C41.9   Malignant neoplasm of bone and articular cartilage, unspecified

MELANOMA AND OTHER MALIGNANT NEOPLASMS OF SKIN (C43-C44)

C43   Malignant melanoma of skin

Excludes1: melanoma in situ (D03.-)

Excludes2: malignant melanoma of skin of genital organs (C51-C52, C60.-, C63.-)

Merkel cell carcinoma (C4A.-)

sites other than skin-code to malignant neoplasm of the site

C43.0 **Malignant melanoma of lip**

Excludes1: malignant neoplasm of vermilion border of lip (C00.0-C00.2)

C43.1 **Malignant melanoma of eyelid, including canthus**

C43.10 **Malignant melanoma of unspecified eyelid, including canthus**

C43.11 **Malignant melanoma of right eyelid, including canthus**

C43.12 **Malignant melanoma of left eyelid, including canthus**

C43.2 **Malignant melanoma of ear and external auricular canal**

C43.20 **Malignant melanoma of unspecified ear and external auricular canal**

C43.21 **Malignant melanoma of right ear and external auricular canal**

C43.22 **Malignant melanoma of left ear and external auricular canal**

C43.3 **Malignant melanoma of other and unspecified parts of face**

C43.30 **Malignant melanoma of unspecified part of face**

C43.31 **Malignant melanoma of nose**

C43.39 **Malignant melanoma of other parts of face**

C43.4 **Malignant melanoma of scalp and neck**

C43.5 **Malignant melanoma of trunk**

Excludes2: malignant neoplasm of anus NOS (C21.0)

malignant neoplasm of scrotum (C63.2)

C43.51 **Malignant melanoma of anal skin**

Malignant melanoma of anal margin

Malignant melanoma of perianal skin

C43.52 **Malignant melanoma of skin of breast**

C43.59 **Malignant melanoma of other part of trunk**

C43.6 **Malignant melanoma of upper limb, including shoulder**

C43.60 **Malignant melanoma of unspecified upper limb, including shoulder**

C43.61 **Malignant melanoma of right upper limb, including shoulder**

C43.62 **Malignant melanoma of left upper limb, including shoulder**

C43.7 **Malignant melanoma of lower limb, including hip**

C43.70 **Malignant melanoma of unspecified lower limb, including hip**

C43.71 **Malignant melanoma of right lower limb, including hip**

C43.72 **Malignant melanoma of left lower limb, including hip**

C43.8 **Malignant melanoma of overlapping sites of skin**

C43.9 **Malignant melanoma of skin, unspecified**

Malignant melanoma of unspecified site of skin

Melanoma (malignant) NOS

C4A **Merkel cell carcinoma**

C4A.0 **Merkel cell carcinoma of lip**

Excludes1: malignant neoplasm of vermilion border of lip (C00.0-C00.2)

C4A.1 **Merkel cell carcinoma of eyelid, including canthus**

C4A.10 **Merkel cell carcinoma of unspecified eyelid, including canthus**

C4A.11 **Merkel cell carcinoma of right eyelid, including canthus**

C4A.12 **Merkel cell carcinoma of left eyelid, including canthus**

C4A.2 **Merkel cell carcinoma of ear and external auricular canal**

C4A.20 **Merkel cell carcinoma of unspecified ear and external auricular canal**

C4A.21 **Merkel cell carcinoma of right ear and external auricular canal**

C4A.22 **Merkel cell carcinoma of left ear and external auricular canal**

C4A.3 **Merkel cell carcinoma of other and unspecified parts of face**

C4A.30 **Merkel cell carcinoma of unspecified part of face**

C4A.31 **Merkel cell carcinoma of nose**

C4A.39 **Merkel cell carcinoma of other parts of face**

C4A.4 **Merkel cell carcinoma of scalp and neck**

C4A.5 **Merkel cell carcinoma of trunk**

Excludes2: malignant neoplasm of anus NOS (C21.0)

malignant neoplasm of scrotum (C63.2)

C4A.51 **Merkel cell carcinoma of anal skin**

Merkel cell carcinoma of anal margin

Merkel cell carcinoma of perianal skin

C4A.52 **Merkel cell carcinoma of skin of breast**

C4A.59 **Merkel cell carcinoma of other part of trunk**

C4A.6 **Merkel cell carcinoma of upper limb, including shoulder**

C4A.60 **Merkel cell carcinoma of unspecified upper limb, including shoulder**

C4A.61 **Merkel cell carcinoma of right upper limb, including shoulder**

C4A.62 **Merkel cell carcinoma of left upper limb, including shoulder**

C4A.7 **Merkel cell carcinoma of lower limb, including hip**

C4A.70 **Merkel cell carcinoma of unspecified lower limb, including hip**

C4A.71 **Merkel cell carcinoma of right lower limb, including hip**

C4A.72 **Merkel cell carcinoma of left lower limb, including hip**

C4A.8 **Merkel cell carcinoma of overlapping sites**

C4A.9 **Merkel cell carcinoma, unspecified**

Merkel cell carcinoma of unspecified site

Merkel cell carcinoma NOS

C44 **Other and unspecified malignant neoplasm of skin**

Includes: malignant neoplasm of sebaceous glands

malignant neoplasm of sweat glands

Excludes1: Kaposi's sarcoma of skin (C46.0)

malignant melanoma of skin (C43.-)

malignant neoplasm of skin of genital organs (C51-C52, C60.-, C63.2)

Merkel cell carcinoma (C4A.-)

C44.0 **Other and unspecified malignant neoplasm of skin of lip**

Excludes1: malignant neoplasm of lip (C00.-)

C44.00 Unspecified malignant neoplasm of skin of lip

C44.01 Basal cell carcinoma of skin of lip

C44.02 Squamous cell carcinoma of skin of lip

C44.09 Other specified malignant neoplasm of skin of lip

C44.1 **Other and unspecified malignant neoplasm of skin of eyelid, including canthus**

Excludes1: connective tissue of eyelid (C49.0)

C44.10 Unspecified malignant neoplasm of skin of eyelid, including canthus

    C44.101 Unspecified malignant neoplasm of skin of unspecified eyelid, including canthus

    C44.102 Unspecified malignant neoplasm of skin of right eyelid, including canthus

    C44.109 Unspecified malignant neoplasm of skin of left eyelid, including canthus

C44.11 Basal cell carcinoma of skin of eyelid, including canthus

    C44.111 Basal cell carcinoma of skin of unspecified eyelid, including canthus

    C44.112 Basal cell carcinoma of skin of right eyelid, including canthus

    C44.119 Basal cell carcinoma of skin of left eyelid, including canthus

C44.12 Squamous cell carcinoma of skin of eyelid, including canthus

    C44.121 Squamous cell carcinoma of skin of unspecified eyelid, including canthus

    C44.122 Squamous cell carcinoma of skin of right eyelid, including canthus

    C44.129 Squamous cell carcinoma of skin of left eyelid, including canthus

C44.19 Other specified malignant neoplasm of skin of eyelid, including canthus

    C44.191 Other specified malignant neoplasm of skin of unspecified eyelid, including canthus

    C44.192 Other specified malignant neoplasm of skin of right eyelid, including canthus

    C44.199 Other specified malignant neoplasm of skin of left eyelid, including canthus

C44.2 **Other and unspecified malignant neoplasm of skin of ear and external auricular canal**

Excludes1: connective tissue of ear (C49.0)

C44.20 Unspecified malignant neoplasm of skin of ear and external auricular canal

    C44.201 Unspecified malignant neoplasm of skin of unspecified ear and external auricular canal

    C44.202 Unspecified malignant neoplasm of skin of right ear and external auricular canal

    C44.209 Unspecified malignant neoplasm of skin of left ear and external auricular canal

C44.21 Basal cell carcinoma of skin of ear and external auricular canal

    C44.211 Basal cell carcinoma of skin of unspecified ear and external auricular canal

    C44.212 Basal cell carcinoma of skin of right ear and external auricular canal

    C44.219 Basal cell carcinoma of skin of left ear and external auricular canal

C44.22 Squamous cell carcinoma of skin of ear and external auricular canal

    C44.221 Squamous cell carcinoma of skin of unspecified ear and external auricular canal

    C44.222 Squamous cell carcinoma of skin of right ear and external auricular canal

    C44.229 Squamous cell carcinoma of skin of left ear and external auricular canal

C44.29 Other specified malignant neoplasm of skin of ear and external auricular canal

    C44.291 Other specified malignant neoplasm of skin of unspecified ear and external auricular canal

    C44.292 Other specified malignant neoplasm of skin of right ear and external auricular canal

    C44.299 Other specified malignant neoplasm of skin of left ear and external auricular canal

C44.3 **Other and unspecified malignant neoplasm of skin of other and unspecified parts of face**

C44.30 Unspecified malignant neoplasm of skin of other and unspecified parts of face

    C44.300 Unspecified malignant neoplasm of skin of unspecified part of face

    C44.301 Unspecified malignant neoplasm of skin of nose

    C44.309 Unspecified malignant neoplasm of skin of other parts of face

C44.31 Basal cell carcinoma of skin of other and unspecified parts of face

    C44.310 Basal cell carcinoma of skin of unspecified parts of face

    C44.311 Basal cell carcinoma of skin of nose

    C44.319 Basal cell carcinoma of skin of other parts of face

C44.32 Squamous cell carcinoma of skin of other and unspecified parts of face

    C44.320 Squamous cell carcinoma of skin of unspecified parts of face

    C44.321 Squamous cell carcinoma of skin of nose

    C44.329 Squamous cell carcinoma of skin of other parts of face

C44.39 Other specified malignant neoplasm of skin of other and unspecified parts of face

    C44.390 Other specified malignant neoplasm of skin of unspecified parts of face

C44.391   **Other specified malignant neoplasm of skin of nose**

C44.399   **Other specified malignant neoplasm of skin of other parts of face**

C44.4   Other and unspecified malignant neoplasm of skin of scalp and neck

C44.40   **Unspecified malignant neoplasm of skin of scalp and neck**

C44.41   **Basal cell carcinoma of skin of scalp and neck**

C44.42   **Squamous cell carcinoma of skin of scalp and neck**

C44.49   **Other specified malignant neoplasm of skin of scalp and neck**

C44.5   Other and unspecified malignant neoplasm of skin of trunk

Excludes1: anus NOS (C21.0)

scrotum (C63.2)

C44.50   **Unspecified malignant neoplasm of skin of trunk**

C44.500   **Unspecified malignant neoplasm of anal skin**

Unspecified malignant neoplasm of anal margin

Unspecified malignant neoplasm of perianal skin

C44.501   **Unspecified malignant neoplasm of skin of breast**

C44.509   **Unspecified malignant neoplasm of skin of other part of trunk**

C44.51   **Basal cell carcinoma of skin of trunk**

C44.510   **Basal cell carcinoma of anal skin**

Basal cell carcinoma of anal margin

Basal cell carcinoma of perianal skin

C44.511   **Basal cell carcinoma of skin of breast**

C44.519   **Basal cell carcinoma of skin of other part of trunk**

C44.52   **Squamous cell carcinoma of skin of trunk**

C44.520   **Squamous cell carcinoma of anal skin**

Squamous cell carcinoma of anal margin

Squamous cell carcinoma of perianal skin

C44.521   **Squamous cell carcinoma of skin of breast**

C44.529   **Squamous cell carcinoma of skin of other part of trunk**

C44.59   **Other specified malignant neoplasm of skin of trunk**

C44.590   **Other specified malignant neoplasm of anal skin**

Other specified malignant neoplasm of anal margin

Other specified malignant neoplasm of perianal skin

C44.591   **Other specified malignant neoplasm of skin of breast**

C44.599   **Other specified malignant neoplasm of skin of other part of trunk**

C44.6   Other and unspecified malignant neoplasm of skin of upper limb, including shoulder

C44.60   **Unspecified malignant neoplasm of skin of upper limb, including shoulder**

C44.601   **Unspecified malignant neoplasm of skin of unspecified upper limb, including shoulder**

C44.602   **Unspecified malignant neoplasm of skin of right upper limb, including shoulder**

C44.609   **Unspecified malignant neoplasm of skin of left upper limb, including shoulder**

C44.61   **Basal cell carcinoma of skin of upper limb, including shoulder**

C44.611   **Basal cell carcinoma of skin of unspecified upper limb, including shoulder**

C44.612   **Basal cell carcinoma of skin of right upper limb, including shoulder**

C44.619   **Basal cell carcinoma of skin of left upper limb, including shoulder**

C44.62   **Squamous cell carcinoma of skin of upper limb, including shoulder**

C44.621   **Squamous cell carcinoma of skin of unspecified upper limb, including shoulder**

C44.622   **Squamous cell carcinoma of skin of right upper limb, including shoulder**

C44.629   **Squamous cell carcinoma of skin of left upper limb, including shoulder**

C44.69   **Other specified malignant neoplasm of skin of upper limb, including shoulder**

C44.691   **Other specified malignant neoplasm of skin of unspecified upper limb, including shoulder**

C44.692   **Other specified malignant neoplasm of skin of right upper limb, including shoulder**

C44.699   **Other specified malignant neoplasm of skin of left upper limb, including shoulder**

C44.7   Other and unspecified malignant neoplasm of skin of lower limb, including hip

C44.70   **Unspecified malignant neoplasm of skin of lower limb, including hip**

C44.701   **Unspecified malignant neoplasm of skin of unspecified lower limb, including hip**

C44.702   **Unspecified malignant neoplasm of skin of right lower limb, including hip**

C44.709   **Unspecified malignant neoplasm of skin of left lower limb, including hip**

C44.71   **Basal cell carcinoma of skin of lower limb, including hip**

C44.711   **Basal cell carcinoma of skin of unspecified lower limb, including hip**

C44.712   **Basal cell carcinoma of skin of right lower limb, including hip**

C44.719　　Basal cell carcinoma of skin of left lower limb, including hip

C44.72　Squamous cell carcinoma of skin of lower limb, including hip

C44.721　　Squamous cell carcinoma of skin of unspecified lower limb, including hip

C44.722　　Squamous cell carcinoma of skin of right lower limb, including hi

C44.729　　Squamous cell carcinoma of skin of left lower limb, including hip

C44.79　Other specified malignant neoplasm of skin of lower limb, including hip

C44.791　　Other specified malignant neoplasm of skin of unspecified lower limb, including hip

C44.792　　Other specified malignant neoplasm of skin of right lower limb, including hip

C44.799　　Other specified malignant neoplasm of skin of left lower limb, including hip

C44.8　Other and unspecified malignant neoplasm of overlapping sites of skin

C44.80　Unspecified malignant neoplasm of overlapping sites of skin

C44.81　Basal cell carcinoma of overlapping sites of skin

C44.82　Squamous cell carcinoma of overlapping sites of skin

C44.89　Other specified malignant neoplasm of overlapping sites of skin

C44.9　Other and unspecified malignant neoplasm of skin, unspecified

C44.90　Unspecified malignant neoplasm of skin, unspecified

Malignant neoplasm of unspecified site of skin

C44.91　Basal cell carcinoma of skin, unspecified

C44.92　Squamous cell carcinoma of skin, unspecified

C44.99　Other specified malignant neoplasm of skin, unspecified

MALIGNANT NEOPLASMS OF MESOTHELIAL AND SOFT TISSUE (C45-C49)

C45　Mesothelioma

C45.0　Mesothelioma of pleura

Excludes1: Other malignant neoplasm of pleura (C38.4)

C45.1　Mesothelioma of peritoneum

Mesothelioma of cul-de-sac

Mesothelioma of mesentery

Mesothelioma of mesocolon

Mesothelioma of omentum

Mesothelioma of peritoneum (parietal) (pelvic)

Excludes1: Other malignant neoplasm of soft tissue of peritoneum (C48.-)

C45.2　Mesothelioma of pericardium

Excludes1: Other malignant neoplasm of pericardium (C38.0)

C45.7　Mesothelioma of other sites

C45.9　Mesothelioma, unspecified

C46　Kaposi's sarcoma

Definition: Kaposi's sarcoma is a form of skin cancer that can involve internal organs. It is most often found in patients with acquired immunodeficiency syndrome (AIDS), and can be fatal.

Code first any human immunodeficiency virus [HIV] disease (B20)

C46.0　Kaposi's sarcoma of skin

C46.1　Kaposi's sarcoma of soft tissue

Kaposi's sarcoma of blood vessel

Kaposi's sarcoma of connective tissue

Kaposi's sarcoma of fascia

Kaposi's sarcoma of ligament

Kaposi's sarcoma of lymphatic(s) NEC

Kaposi's sarcoma of muscle

Excludes2: Kaposi's sarcoma of lymph glands and nodes (C46.3)

C46.2　Kaposi's sarcoma of palate

C46.3　Kaposi's sarcoma of lymph nodes

C46.4　Kaposi's sarcoma of gastrointestinal sites

C46.5　Kaposi's sarcoma of lung

C46.50　Kaposi's sarcoma of unspecified lung

C46.51　Kaposi's sarcoma of right lung

C46.52　Kaposi's sarcoma of left lung

C46.7　Kaposi's sarcoma of other sites

C46.9　Kaposi's sarcoma, unspecified

Kaposi's sarcoma of unspecified site

C47　Malignant neoplasm of peripheral nerves and autonomic nervous system

Includes: malignant neoplasm of sympathetic and parasympathetic nerves and ganglia

Excludes1: Kaposi's sarcoma of soft tissue (C46.1)

C47.0　Malignant neoplasm of peripheral nerves of head, face and neck

Excludes1: malignant neoplasm of peripheral nerves of orbit (C69.6-)

C47.1　Malignant neoplasm of peripheral nerves of upper limb, including shoulder

C47.10　Malignant neoplasm of peripheral nerves of unspecified upper limb, including shoulder

C47.11　Malignant neoplasm of peripheral nerves of right upper limb, including shoulder

C47.12　Malignant neoplasm of peripheral nerves of left upper limb, including shoulder

C47.2　Malignant neoplasm of peripheral nerves of lower limb, including hip

C47.20　Malignant neoplasm of peripheral nerves of unspecified lower limb, including hip

C47.21　Malignant neoplasm of peripheral nerves of right lower limb, including hip

C47.22　Malignant neoplasm of peripheral nerves of left lower limb, including hip

C47.3　Malignant neoplasm of peripheral nerves of thorax

C47.4　Malignant neoplasm of peripheral nerves of abdomen

C47.5　Malignant neoplasm of peripheral nerves of pelvis

C47.6　Malignant neoplasm of peripheral nerves of trunk, unspecified

Malignant neoplasm of peripheral nerves of unspecified part of trunk

C47.8 Malignant neoplasm of overlapping sites of peripheral nerves and autonomic nervous system

C47.9 Malignant neoplasm of peripheral nerves and autonomic nervous system, unspecified

Malignant neoplasm of unspecified site of peripheral nerves and autonomic nervous system

C48 Malignant neoplasm of retroperitoneum and peritoneum

Excludes1: Kaposi's sarcoma of connective tissue (C46.1)

mesothelioma (C45.-)

C48.0 Malignant neoplasm of retroperitoneum

C48.1 Malignant neoplasm of specified parts of peritoneum

Malignant neoplasm of cul-de-sac

Malignant neoplasm of mesentery

Malignant neoplasm of mesocolon

Malignant neoplasm of omentum

Malignant neoplasm of parietal peritoneum

Malignant neoplasm of pelvic peritoneum

C48.2 Malignant neoplasm of peritoneum, unspecified

C48.8 Malignant neoplasm of overlapping sites of retroperitoneum and peritoneum

C49 Malignant neoplasm of other connective and soft tissue

Includes: malignant neoplasm of blood vessel

malignant neoplasm of bursa

malignant neoplasm of cartilage

malignant neoplasm of fascia

malignant neoplasm of fat

malignant neoplasm of ligament, except uterine

malignant neoplasm of lymphatic vessel

malignant neoplasm of muscle

malignant neoplasm of synovia

malignant neoplasm of tendon (sheath)

Excludes1: malignant neoplasm of cartilage (of):

articular (C40-C41)

larynx (C32.3)

nose (C30.0)

malignant neoplasm of connective tissue of breast (C50.-)

Excludes2: Kaposi's sarcoma of soft tissue (C46.1)

malignant neoplasm of heart (C38.0)

malignant neoplasm of peripheral nerves and autonomic nervous system (C47.-)

malignant neoplasm of peritoneum (C48.2)

malignant neoplasm of retroperitoneum (C48.0)

malignant neoplasm of uterine ligament (C57.3)

mesothelioma (C45.-)

C49.0 Malignant neoplasm of connective and soft tissue of head, face and neck

Malignant neoplasm of connective tissue of ear

Malignant neoplasm of connective tissue of eyelid

Excludes1: connective tissue of orbit (C69.6-)

C49.1 Malignant neoplasm of connective and soft tissue of upper limb, including shoulder

C49.10 Malignant neoplasm of connective and soft tissue of unspecified upper limb, including shoulder

C49.11 Malignant neoplasm of connective and soft tissue of right upper limb, including shoulder

C49.12 Malignant neoplasm of connective and soft tissue of left upper limb, including shoulder

C49.2 Malignant neoplasm of connective and soft tissue of lower limb, including hip

C49.20 Malignant neoplasm of connective and soft tissue of unspecified lower limb, including hip

C49.21 Malignant neoplasm of connective and soft tissue of right lower limb, including hip

C49.22 Malignant neoplasm of connective and soft tissue of left lower limb, including hip

C49.3 Malignant neoplasm of connective and soft tissue of thorax

Malignant neoplasm of axilla

Malignant neoplasm of diaphragm

Malignant neoplasm of great vessels

Excludes1: malignant neoplasm of breast (C50.-)

malignant neoplasm of heart (C38.0)

malignant neoplasm of mediastinum (C38.1-C38.3)

malignant neoplasm of thymus (C37)

C49.4 Malignant neoplasm of connective and soft tissue of abdomen

Malignant neoplasm of abdominal wall

Malignant neoplasm of hypochondrium

C49.5 Malignant neoplasm of connective and soft tissue of pelvis

Malignant neoplasm of buttock

Malignant neoplasm of groin

Malignant neoplasm of perineum

C49.6 Malignant neoplasm of connective and soft tissue of trunk, unspecified

Malignant neoplasm of back NOS

C49.8 Malignant neoplasm of overlapping sites of connective and soft tissue

Primary malignant neoplasm of two or more contiguous sites of connective and soft tissue

C49.9 Malignant neoplasm of connective and soft tissue, unspecified

C49.A Gastrointestinal stromal tumor

● **C49.A0** Gastrointestinal stromal tumor, unspecified site

● **C49.A1** Gastrointestinal stromal tumor of esophagus

● **C49.A2** Gastrointestinal stromal tumor of stomach

● **C49.A3** Gastrointestinal stromal tumor of small intestine

● **C49.A4** Gastrointestinal stromal tumor of large intestine

● **C49.A5** Gastrointestinal stromal tumor of rectum

● **C49.A9** Gastrointestinal stromal tumor of other sites

MALIGNANT NEOPLASMS OF BREAST (C50)

C50 Malignant neoplasm of breast

Includes: connective tissue of breast

Paget's disease of breast

Paget's disease of nipple

Use additional code to identify estrogen receptor status (Z17.0, Z17.1)

Excludes1: skin of breast (C44.501, C44.511, C44.521, C44.591)

C50.0 Malignant neoplasm of nipple and areola

    C50.01 Malignant neoplasm of nipple and areola, female

        C50.011 Malignant neoplasm of nipple and areola, right female breast

        C50.012 Malignant neoplasm of nipple and areola, left female breast

        C50.019 Malignant neoplasm of nipple and areola, unspecified female breast

    C50.02 Malignant neoplasm of nipple and areola, male

        C50.021 Malignant neoplasm of nipple and areola, right male breast

        C50.022 Malignant neoplasm of nipple and areola, left male breast

        C50.029 Malignant neoplasm of nipple and areola, unspecified male breast

C50.1 Malignant neoplasm of central portion of breast

    C50.11 Malignant neoplasm of central portion of breast, female

        C50.111 Malignant neoplasm of central portion of right female breast

        C50.112 Malignant neoplasm of central portion of left female breast

        C50.119 Malignant neoplasm of central portion of unspecified female breast

    C50.12 Malignant neoplasm of central portion of breast, male

        C50.121 Malignant neoplasm of central portion of right male breast

        C50.122 Malignant neoplasm of central portion of left male breast

        C50.129 Malignant neoplasm of central portion of unspecified male breast

C50.2 Malignant neoplasm of upper-inner quadrant of breast

    C50.21 Malignant neoplasm of upper-inner quadrant of breast, female

        C50.211 Malignant neoplasm of upper-inner quadrant of right female breast

        C50.212 Malignant neoplasm of upper-inner quadrant of left female breast

        C50.219 Malignant neoplasm of upper-inner quadrant of unspecified female breast

    C50.22 Malignant neoplasm of upper-inner quadrant of breast, male

        C50.221 Malignant neoplasm of upper-inner quadrant of right male breast

        C50.222 Malignant neoplasm of upper-inner quadrant of left male breast

        C50.229 Malignant neoplasm of upper-inner quadrant of unspecified male breast

C50.3 Malignant neoplasm of lower-inner quadrant of breast

    C50.31 Malignant neoplasm of lower-inner quadrant of breast, female

        C50.311 Malignant neoplasm of lower-inner quadrant of right female breast

        C50.312 Malignant neoplasm of lower-inner quadrant of left female breast

        C50.319 Malignant neoplasm of lower-inner quadrant of unspecified female breast

    C50.32 Malignant neoplasm of lower-inner quadrant of breast, male

        C50.321 Malignant neoplasm of lower-inner quadrant of right male breast

        C50.322 Malignant neoplasm of lower-inner quadrant of left male breast

        C50.329 Malignant neoplasm of lower-inner quadrant of unspecified male breast

C50.4 Malignant neoplasm of upper-outer quadrant of breast

    C50.41 Malignant neoplasm of upper-outer quadrant of breast, female

        C50.411 Malignant neoplasm of upper-outer quadrant of right female breast

        C50.412 Malignant neoplasm of upper-outer quadrant of left female breast

        C50.419 Malignant neoplasm of upper-outer quadrant of unspecified female breast

    C50.42 Malignant neoplasm of upper-outer quadrant of breast, male

        C50.421 Malignant neoplasm of upper-outer quadrant of right male breast

        C50.422 Malignant neoplasm of upper-outer quadrant of left male breast

        C50.429 Malignant neoplasm of upper-outer quadrant of unspecified male breast

C50.5 Malignant neoplasm of lower-outer quadrant of breast

    C50.51 Malignant neoplasm of lower-outer quadrant of breast, female

        C50.511 Malignant neoplasm of lower-outer quadrant of right female breast

        C50.512 Malignant neoplasm of lower-outer quadrant of left female breast

        C50.519 Malignant neoplasm of lower-outer quadrant of unspecified female breast

    C50.52 Malignant neoplasm of lower-outer quadrant of breast, male

        C50.521 Malignant neoplasm of lower-outer quadrant of right male breast

        C50.522 Malignant neoplasm of lower-outer quadrant of left male breast

        C50.529 Malignant neoplasm of lower-outer quadrant of unspecified male breast

C50.6 Malignant neoplasm of axillary tail of breast

    C50.61 Malignant neoplasm of axillary tail of breast, female

        C50.611 Malignant neoplasm of axillary tail of right female breast

        C50.612 Malignant neoplasm of axillary tail of left female breast

        C50.619 Malignant neoplasm of axillary tail of unspecified female breast

    C50.62 Malignant neoplasm of axillary tail of breast, male

        C50.621 Malignant neoplasm of axillary tail of right male breast

	C50.622	Malignant neoplasm of axillary tail of left male breast		

C50.622   **Malignant neoplasm of axillary tail of left male breast**

C50.629   **Malignant neoplasm of axillary tail of unspecified male breast**

C50.8   **Malignant neoplasm of overlapping sites of breast**

     C50.81   **Malignant neoplasm of overlapping sites of breast, female**

         C50.811   **Malignant neoplasm of overlapping sites of right female breast**

         C50.812   **Malignant neoplasm of overlapping sites of left female breast**

         C50.819   **Malignant neoplasm of overlapping sites of unspecified female breast**

     C50.82   **Malignant neoplasm of overlapping sites of breast, male**

         C50.821   **Malignant neoplasm of overlapping sites of right male breast**

         C50.822   **Malignant neoplasm of overlapping sites of left male breast**

         C50.829   **Malignant neoplasm of overlapping sites of unspecified male breast**

C50.9   **Malignant neoplasm of breast of unspecified site**

     C50.91   **Malignant neoplasm of breast of unspecified site, female**

         C50.911   **Malignant neoplasm of unspecified site of right female breast**

         C50.912   **Malignant neoplasm of unspecified site of left female breast**

         C50.919   **Malignant neoplasm of unspecified site of unspecified female breast**

     C50.92   **Malignant neoplasm of breast of unspecified site, male**

         C50.921   **Malignant neoplasm of unspecified site of right male breast**

         C50.922   **Malignant neoplasm of unspecified site of left male breast**

         C50.929   **Malignant neoplasm of unspecified site of unspecified male breast**

MALIGNANT NEOPLASMS OF FEMALE GENITAL ORGANS (C51-C58)

> **NOTE: All Diagnosis Codes In This Section Apply To FEMALE Patients Only**

Includes: malignant neoplasm of skin of female genital organs

C51   **Malignant neoplasm of vulva**

     Excludes1: carcinoma in situ of vulva (D07.1)

     C51.0   **Malignant neoplasm of labium majus**

         Malignant neoplasm of Bartholin's [greater vestibular] gland

     C51.1   **Malignant neoplasm of labium minus**

     C51.2   **Malignant neoplasm of clitoris**

     C51.8   **Malignant neoplasm of overlapping sites of vulva**

     C51.9   **Malignant neoplasm of vulva, unspecified**

         Malignant neoplasm of external female genitalia NOS

         Malignant neoplasm of pudendum

C52   **Malignant neoplasm of vagina**

     Excludes1: carcinoma in situ of vagina (D07.2)

C53   **Malignant neoplasm of cervix uteri**

     Excludes1: carcinoma in situ of cervix uteri (D06.-)

C53.0   **Malignant neoplasm of endocervix**

C53.1   **Malignant neoplasm of exocervix**

C53.8   **Malignant neoplasm of overlapping sites of cervix uteri**

C53.9   **Malignant neoplasm of cervix uteri, unspecified**

C54   **Malignant neoplasm of corpus uteri**

     C54.0   **Malignant neoplasm of isthmus uteri**

         Malignant neoplasm of lower uterine segment

     C54.1   **Malignant neoplasm of endometrium**

     C54.2   **Malignant neoplasm of myometrium**

     C54.3   **Malignant neoplasm of fundus uteri**

     C54.8   **Malignant neoplasm of overlapping sites of corpus uteri**

     C54.9   **Malignant neoplasm of corpus uteri, unspecified**

C55   **Malignant neoplasm of uterus, part unspecified**

C56   **Malignant neoplasm of ovary**

     <u>**Use additional code**</u> to identify any functional activity

     C56.1   **Malignant neoplasm of right ovary**

     C56.2   **Malignant neoplasm of left ovary**

     C56.9   **Malignant neoplasm of unspecified ovary**

C57   **Malignant neoplasm of other and unspecified female genital organs**

     C57.0   **Malignant neoplasm of fallopian tube**

         Malignant neoplasm of oviduct

         Malignant neoplasm of uterine tube

         C57.00   **Malignant neoplasm of unspecified fallopian tube**

         C57.01   **Malignant neoplasm of right fallopian tube**

         C57.02   **Malignant neoplasm of left fallopian tube**

     C57.1   **Malignant neoplasm of broad ligament**

         C57.10   **Malignant neoplasm of unspecified broad ligament**

         C57.11   **Malignant neoplasm of right broad ligament**

         C57.12   **Malignant neoplasm of left broad ligament**

     C57.2   **Malignant neoplasm of round ligament**

         C57.20   **Malignant neoplasm of unspecified round ligament**

         C57.21   **Malignant neoplasm of right round ligament**

         C57.22   **Malignant neoplasm of left round ligament**

     C57.3   **Malignant neoplasm of parametrium**

         Malignant neoplasm of uterine ligament NOS

     C57.4   **Malignant neoplasm of uterine adnexa, unspecified**

     C57.7   **Malignant neoplasm of other specified female genital organs**

         Malignant neoplasm of wolffian body or duct

     C57.8   **Malignant neoplasm of overlapping sites of female genital organs**

         Primary malignant neoplasm of two or more contiguous sites of the female genital organs whose point of origin cannot be determined

         Primary tubo-ovarian malignant neoplasm whose point of origin cannot be determined Primary utero-ovarian malignant neoplasm whose point of origin cannot be determined

     C57.9   **Malignant neoplasm of female genital organ, unspecified**

         Malignant neoplasm of female genitourinary tract NOS

C58   **Malignant neoplasm of placenta**

     Includes: choriocarcinoma NOS

chorionepithelioma NOS

Excludes1: chorioadenoma (destruens) (D39.2)

hydatidiform mole NOS (O01.9)

invasive hydatidiform mole (D39.2)

male choriocarcinoma NOS (C62.9-)

malignant hydatidiform mole (D39.2)

MALIGNANT NEOPLASMS OF MALE GENITAL ORGANS (C60-C63)

> NOTE: All Diagnosis Codes In This Section Apply To MALE Patients Only

Includes: malignant neoplasm of skin of male genital organs

C60 **Malignant neoplasm of penis**

C60.0 **Malignant neoplasm of prepuce**

Malignant neoplasm of foreskin

C60.1 **Malignant neoplasm of glans penis**

C60.2 **Malignant neoplasm of body of penis**

Malignant neoplasm of corpus cavernosum

C60.8 **Malignant neoplasm of overlapping sites of penis**

C60.9 **Malignant neoplasm of penis, unspecified**

Malignant neoplasm of skin of penis NOS

C61 **Malignant neoplasm of prostate**

Use additional code to identify:

hormone sensitivity status (Z19.1-Z19.2)

rising PSA following treatment for malignant neoplasm of prostate (R97.21)

Excludes1: malignant neoplasm of seminal vesicle (C63.7)

C62 **Malignant neoplasm of testis**

Use additional code to identify any functional activity

C62.0 **Malignant neoplasm of undescended testis**

Malignant neoplasm of ectopic testis

Malignant neoplasm of retained testis

C62.00 **Malignant neoplasm of unspecified undescended testis**

C62.01 **Malignant neoplasm of undescended right testis**

C62.02 **Malignant neoplasm of undescended left testis**

C62.1 **Malignant neoplasm of descended testis**

Malignant neoplasm of scrotal testis

C62.10 **Malignant neoplasm of unspecified descended testis**

C62.11 **Malignant neoplasm of descended right testis**

C62.12 **Malignant neoplasm of descended left testis**

C62.9 **Malignant neoplasm of testis, unspecified whether descended or undescended**

C62.90 **Malignant neoplasm of unspecified testis, unspecified whether descended or undescended**

Malignant neoplasm of testis NOS

C62.91 **Malignant neoplasm of right testis, unspecified whether descended or undescended**

C62.92 **Malignant neoplasm of left testis, unspecified whether descended or undescended**

C63 **Malignant neoplasm of other and unspecified male genital organs**

C63.0 **Malignant neoplasm of epididymis**

C63.00 **Malignant neoplasm of unspecified epididymis**

C63.01 **Malignant neoplasm of right epididymis**

C63.02 **Malignant neoplasm of left epididymis**

C63.1 **Malignant neoplasm of spermatic cord**

C63.10 **Malignant neoplasm of unspecified spermatic cord**

C63.11 **Malignant neoplasm of right spermatic cord**

C63.12 **Malignant neoplasm of left spermatic cord**

C63.2 **Malignant neoplasm of scrotum**

Malignant neoplasm of skin of scrotum

C63.7 **Malignant neoplasm of other specified male genital organs**

Malignant neoplasm of seminal vesicle

Malignant neoplasm of tunica vaginalis

C63.8 **Malignant neoplasm of overlapping sites of male genital organs**

Primary malignant neoplasm of two or more contiguous sites of male genital organs whose point of origin cannot be determined

C63.9 **Malignant neoplasm of male genital organ, unspecified**

Malignant neoplasm of male genitourinary tract NOS

MALIGNANT NEOPLASMS OF URINARY TRACT (C64-C68)

C64 **Malignant neoplasm of kidney, except renal pelvis**

Excludes1: malignant carcinoid tumor of the kidney (C7A.093)

malignant neoplasm of renal calyces (C65.-)

malignant neoplasm of renal pelvis (C65.-)

C64.1 **Malignant neoplasm of right kidney, except renal pelvis**

C64.2 **Malignant neoplasm of left kidney, except renal pelvis**

C64.9 **Malignant neoplasm of unspecified kidney, except renal pelvis**

C65 **Malignant neoplasm of renal pelvis**

Includes: malignant neoplasm of pelviureteric junction

malignant neoplasm of renal calyces

C65.1 **Malignant neoplasm of right renal pelvis**

C65.2 **Malignant neoplasm of left renal pelvis**

C65.9 **Malignant neoplasm of unspecified renal pelvis**

C66 **Malignant neoplasm of ureter**

Excludes1: malignant neoplasm of ureteric orifice of bladder (C67.6)

C66.1 **Malignant neoplasm of right ureter**

C66.2 **Malignant neoplasm of left ureter**

C66.9 **Malignant neoplasm of unspecified ureter**

C67 **Malignant neoplasm of bladder**

C67.0 **Malignant neoplasm of trigone of bladder**

C67.1 **Malignant neoplasm of dome of bladder**

C67.2 **Malignant neoplasm of lateral wall of bladder**

C67.3 **Malignant neoplasm of anterior wall of bladder**

C67.4 **Malignant neoplasm of posterior wall of bladder**

C67.5 **Malignant neoplasm of bladder neck**

Malignant neoplasm of internal urethral orifice

C67.6 **Malignant neoplasm of ureteric orifice**

C67.7 **Malignant neoplasm of urachus**

C67.8 **Malignant neoplasm of overlapping sites of bladder**

C67.9 **Malignant neoplasm of bladder, unspecified**

C68 **Malignant neoplasm of other and unspecified urinary organs**

Excludes1: malignant neoplasm of female genitourinary tract NOS (C57.9)

malignant neoplasm of male genitourinary tract NOS (C63.9)

C68.0 Malignant neoplasm of urethra

> **Excludes1:** malignant neoplasm of urethral orifice of bladder (C67.5)

C68.1 Malignant neoplasm of paraurethral glands

C68.8 Malignant neoplasm of overlapping sites of urinary organs

> Primary malignant neoplasm of two or more contiguous sites of urinary organs whose point of origin cannot be determined

C68.9 Malignant neoplasm of urinary organ, unspecified

> Malignant neoplasm of urinary system NOS

MALIGNANT NEOPLASMS OF EYE, BRAIN AND OTHER PARTS OF CENTRAL NERVOUS SYSTEM (C69-C72)

C69 Malignant neoplasm of eye and adnexa

> **Excludes1:** malignant neoplasm of connective tissue of eyelid (C49.0)
>
> > malignant neoplasm of eyelid (skin) (C43.1-, C44.1-)
> >
> > malignant neoplasm of optic nerve (C72.3-)

C69.0 Malignant neoplasm of conjunctiva

> **C69.00 Malignant neoplasm of unspecified conjunctiva**
>
> **C69.01 Malignant neoplasm of right conjunctiva**
>
> **C69.02 Malignant neoplasm of left conjunctiva**

C69.1 Malignant neoplasm of cornea

> **C69.10 Malignant neoplasm of unspecified cornea**
>
> **C69.11 Malignant neoplasm of right cornea**
>
> **C69.12 Malignant neoplasm of left cornea**

C69.2 Malignant neoplasm of retina

> **Excludes1:** dark area on retina (D49.81)
>
> > neoplasm of unspecified behavior of retina and choroid (D49.81)
> >
> > retinal freckle (D49.81)
>
> **C69.20 Malignant neoplasm of unspecified retina**
>
> **C69.21 Malignant neoplasm of right retina**
>
> **C69.22 Malignant neoplasm of left retina**

C69.3 Malignant neoplasm of choroid

> **C69.30 Malignant neoplasm of unspecified choroid**
>
> **C69.31 Malignant neoplasm of right choroid**
>
> **C69.32 Malignant neoplasm of left choroid**

C69.4 Malignant neoplasm of ciliary body

> **C69.40 Malignant neoplasm of unspecified ciliary body**
>
> **C69.41 Malignant neoplasm of right ciliary body**
>
> **C69.42 Malignant neoplasm of left ciliary body**

C69.5 Malignant neoplasm of lacrimal gland and duct

> Malignant neoplasm of lacrimal sac
>
> Malignant neoplasm of nasolacrimal duct
>
> **C69.50 Malignant neoplasm of unspecified lacrimal gland and duct**
>
> **C69.51 Malignant neoplasm of right lacrimal gland and duct**
>
> **C69.52 Malignant neoplasm of left lacrimal gland and duct**

C69.6 Malignant neoplasm of orbit

> Malignant neoplasm of connective tissue of orbit
>
> Malignant neoplasm of extraocular muscle
>
> Malignant neoplasm of peripheral nerves of orbit
>
> Malignant neoplasm of retrobulbar tissue
>
> Malignant neoplasm of retro-ocular tissue
>
> **Excludes1:** malignant neoplasm of orbital bone (C41.0)
>
> **C69.60 Malignant neoplasm of unspecified orbit**
>
> **C69.61 Malignant neoplasm of right orbit**
>
> **C69.62 Malignant neoplasm of left orbit**

C69.8 Malignant neoplasm of overlapping sites of eye and adnexa

> **C69.80 Malignant neoplasm of overlapping sites of unspecified eye and adnexa**
>
> **C69.81 Malignant neoplasm of overlapping sites of right eye and adnexa**
>
> **C69.82 Malignant neoplasm of overlapping sites of left eye and adnexa**

C69.9 Malignant neoplasm of unspecified site of eye

> Malignant neoplasm of eyeball
>
> **C69.90 Malignant neoplasm of unspecified site of unspecified eye**
>
> **C69.91 Malignant neoplasm of unspecified site of right eye**
>
> **C69.92 Malignant neoplasm of unspecified site of left eye**

C70 Malignant neoplasm of meninges

C70.0 Malignant neoplasm of cerebral meninges

C70.1 Malignant neoplasm of spinal meninges

C70.9 Malignant neoplasm of meninges, unspecified

C71 Malignant neoplasm of brain

> **Excludes1:** malignant neoplasm of cranial nerves (C72.2-C72.5)
>
> > retrobulbar malignant neoplasm (C69.6-)

C71.0 Malignant neoplasm of cerebrum, except lobes and ventricles

> Malignant neoplasm of supratentorial NOS

C71.1 Malignant neoplasm of frontal lobe

C71.2 Malignant neoplasm of temporal lobe

C71.3 Malignant neoplasm of parietal lobe

C71.4 Malignant neoplasm of occipital lobe

C71.5 Malignant neoplasm of cerebral ventricle

> **Excludes1:** malignant neoplasm of fourth cerebral ventricle (C71.7)

C71.6 Malignant neoplasm of cerebellum

C71.7 Malignant neoplasm of brain stem

> Malignant neoplasm of fourth cerebral ventricle
>
> Infratentorial malignant neoplasm NOS

C71.8 Malignant neoplasm of overlapping sites of brain

C71.9 Malignant neoplasm of brain, unspecified

C72 Malignant neoplasm of spinal cord, cranial nerves and other parts of central nervous system

> **Excludes1:** malignant neoplasm of meninges (C70.-)
>
> > malignant neoplasm of peripheral nerves and autonomic nervous system (C47.-)

C72.0 Malignant neoplasm of spinal cord

C72.1 Malignant neoplasm of cauda equina

C72.2 Malignant neoplasm of olfactory nerve

Malignant neoplasm of olfactory bulb

C72.20 Malignant neoplasm of unspecified olfactory nerve

C72.21 Malignant neoplasm of right olfactory nerve

C72.22 Malignant neoplasm of left olfactory nerve

C72.3 Malignant neoplasm of optic nerve

C72.30 Malignant neoplasm of unspecified optic nerve

C72.31 Malignant neoplasm of right optic nerve

C72.32 Malignant neoplasm of left optic nerve

C72.4 Malignant neoplasm of acoustic nerve

C72.40 Malignant neoplasm of unspecified acoustic nerve

C72.41 Malignant neoplasm of right acoustic nerve

C72.42 Malignant neoplasm of left acoustic nerve

C72.5 Malignant neoplasm of other and unspecified cranial nerves

C72.50 Malignant neoplasm of unspecified cranial nerve

Malignant neoplasm of cranial nerve NOS

C72.59 Malignant neoplasm of other cranial nerves

C72.9 Malignant neoplasm of central nervous system, unspecified

Malignant neoplasm of unspecified site of central nervous system

Malignant neoplasm of nervous system NOS

MALIGNANT NEOPLASMS OF THYROID AND OTHER ENDOCRINE GLANDS (C73-C75)

C73 Malignant neoplasm of thyroid gland

Use additional code to identify any functional activity

C74 Malignant neoplasm of adrenal gland

C74.0 Malignant neoplasm of cortex of adrenal gland

C74.00 Malignant neoplasm of cortex of unspecified adrenal gland

C74.01 Malignant neoplasm of cortex of right adrenal gland

C74.02 Malignant neoplasm of cortex of left adrenal gland

C74.1 Malignant neoplasm of medulla of adrenal gland

C74.10 Malignant neoplasm of medulla of unspecified adrenal gland

C74.11 Malignant neoplasm of medulla of right adrenal gland

C74.12 Malignant neoplasm of medulla of left adrenal gland

C74.9 Malignant neoplasm of unspecified part of adrenal gland

C74.90 Malignant neoplasm of unspecified part of unspecified adrenal gland

C74.91 Malignant neoplasm of unspecified part of right adrenal gland

C74.92 Malignant neoplasm of unspecified part of left adrenal gland

C75 Malignant neoplasm of other endocrine glands and related structures

Excludes1: malignant carcinoid tumors (C7A.0-)

malignant neoplasm of adrenal gland (C74.-)

malignant neoplasm of endocrine pancreas (C25.4)

malignant neoplasm of islets of Langerhans (C25.4)

malignant neoplasm of ovary (C56.-)

malignant neoplasm of testis (C62.-)

malignant neoplasm of thymus (C37)

malignant neoplasm of thyroid gland (C73)

malignant neuroendocrine tumors (C7A.-)

C75.0 Malignant neoplasm of parathyroid gland

C75.1 Malignant neoplasm of pituitary gland

C75.2 Malignant neoplasm of craniopharyngeal duct

C75.3 Malignant neoplasm of pineal gland

C75.4 Malignant neoplasm of carotid body

C75.5 Malignant neoplasm of aortic body and other paraganglia

C75.8 Malignant neoplasm with pluriglandular involvement, unspecified

C75.9 Malignant neoplasm of endocrine gland, unspecified

MALIGNANT NEUROENDOCRINE TUMORS (C7A)

C7A Malignant neuroendocrine tumors

Code also any associated multiple endocrine neoplasia [MEN] syndromes (E31.2-)

Use additional code to identify any associated endocrine syndrome, such as:

carcinoid syndrome (E34.0)

Excludes2: malignant pancreatic islet cell tumors (C25.4)

Merkel cell carcinoma (C4A.-)

C7A.0 Malignant carcinoid tumors

C7A.00 Malignant carcinoid tumor of unspecified site

C7A.01 Malignant carcinoid tumors of the small intestine

C7A.010 Malignant carcinoid tumor of the duodenum

C7A.011 Malignant carcinoid tumor of the jejunum

C7A.012 Malignant carcinoid tumor of the ileum

C7A.019 Malignant carcinoid tumor of the small intestine, unspecified portion

C7A.02 Malignant carcinoid tumors of the appendix, large intestine, and rectum

C7A.020 Malignant carcinoid tumor of the appendix

C7A.021 Malignant carcinoid tumor of the cecum

C7A.022 Malignant carcinoid tumor of the ascending colon

C7A.023 Malignant carcinoid tumor of the transverse colon

C7A.024 Malignant carcinoid tumor of the descending colon

C7A.025 Malignant carcinoid tumor of the sigmoid colon

C7A.026 Malignant carcinoid tumor of the rectum

C7A.029 Malignant carcinoid tumor of the large intestine, unspecified portion

Malignant carcinoid tumor of the colon NOS

C7A.09 **Malignant carcinoid tumors of other sites**

C7A.090 **Malignant carcinoid tumor of the bronchus and lung**

C7A.091 **Malignant carcinoid tumor of the thymus**

C7A.092 **Malignant carcinoid tumor of the stomach**

C7A.093 **Malignant carcinoid tumor of the kidney**

▲C7A.094 **Malignant carcinoid tumor of the foregut, unspecified**

▲C7A.095 **Malignant carcinoid tumor of the midgut, unspecified**

▲C7A.096 **Malignant carcinoid tumor of the hindgut, unspecified**

C7A.098 **Malignant carcinoid tumors of other sites**

C7A.1 **Malignant poorly differentiated neuroendocrine tumors**

Malignant poorly differentiated neuroendocrine tumor NOS

Malignant poorly differentiated neuroendocrine carcinoma, any site

High grade neuroendocrine carcinoma, any site

C7A.8 **Other malignant neuroendocrine tumors**

SECONDARY NEUROENDOCRINE TUMORS (C7B)

C7B **Secondary neuroendocrine tumors**

Use additional code to identify any functional activity

C7B.0 **Secondary carcinoid tumors**

C7B.00 **Secondary carcinoid tumors, unspecified site**

C7B.01 **Secondary carcinoid tumors of distant lymph nodes**

C7B.02 **Secondary carcinoid tumors of liver**

C7B.03 **Secondary carcinoid tumors of bone**

C7B.04 **Secondary carcinoid tumors of peritoneum**

Mesentery metastasis of carcinoid tumor

C7B.09 **Secondary carcinoid tumors of other sites**

C7B.1 **Secondary Merkel cell carcinoma**

Merkel cell carcinoma nodal presentation

Merkel cell carcinoma visceral metastatic presentation

C7B.8 **Other secondary neuroendocrine tumors**

MALIGNANT NEOPLASMS OF ILL-DEFINED, OTHER SECONDARY AND UNSPECIFIED SITES (C76-C80)

C76 **Malignant neoplasm of other and ill-defined sites**

Excludes1: malignant neoplasm of female genitourinary tract NOS (C57.9)

malignant neoplasm of male genitourinary tract NOS (C63.9)

malignant neoplasm of lymphoid, hematopoietic and related tissue (C81-C96)

malignant neoplasm of skin (C44.-)

malignant neoplasm of unspecified site NOS (C80.1)

C76.0 **Malignant neoplasm of head, face and neck**

Malignant neoplasm of cheek NOS

Malignant neoplasm of nose NOS

C76.1 **Malignant neoplasm of thorax**

Intrathoracic malignant neoplasm NOS

Malignant neoplasm of axilla NOS

Thoracic malignant neoplasm NOS

C76.2 **Malignant neoplasm of abdomen**

C76.3 **Malignant neoplasm of pelvis**

Malignant neoplasm of groin NOS

Malignant neoplasm of sites overlapping systems within the pelvis

Rectovaginal (septum) malignant neoplasm

Rectovesical (septum) malignant neoplasm

C76.4 **Malignant neoplasm of upper limb**

C76.40 **Malignant neoplasm of unspecified upper limb**

C76.41 **Malignant neoplasm of right upper limb**

C76.42 **Malignant neoplasm of left upper limb**

C76.5 **Malignant neoplasm of lower limb**

C76.50 **Malignant neoplasm of unspecified lower limb**

C76.51 **Malignant neoplasm of right lower limb**

C76.52 **Malignant neoplasm of left lower limb**

C76.8 **Malignant neoplasm of other specified ill-defined sites**

Malignant neoplasm of overlapping ill-defined sites

C77 **Secondary and unspecified malignant neoplasm of lymph nodes**

Excludes1: malignant neoplasm of lymph nodes, specified as primary (C81-C86, C88, C96.-)

mesentery metastasis of carcinoid tumor (C7B.04)

secondary carcinoid tumors of distant lymph nodes (C7B.01)

C77.0 **Secondary and unspecified malignant neoplasm of lymph nodes of head, face and neck**

Secondary and unspecified malignant neoplasm of supraclavicular lymph nodes

C77.1 **Secondary and unspecified malignant neoplasm of intrathoracic lymph nodes**

C77.2 **Secondary and unspecified malignant neoplasm of intra-abdominal lymph nodes**

C77.3 **Secondary and unspecified malignant neoplasm of axilla and upper limb lymph nodes**

Secondary and unspecified malignant neoplasm of pectoral lymph nodes

C77.4 **Secondary and unspecified malignant neoplasm of inguinal and lower limb lymph nodes**

C77.5 **Secondary and unspecified malignant neoplasm of intrapelvic lymph nodes**

C77.8 **Secondary and unspecified malignant neoplasm of lymph nodes of multiple regions**

C77.9 **Secondary and unspecified malignant neoplasm of lymph node, unspecified**

C78 **Secondary malignant neoplasm of respiratory and digestive organs**

Excludes1: secondary carcinoid tumors of liver (C7B.02)

secondary carcinoid tumors of peritoneum (C7B.04)

Excludes2: lymph node metastases (C77.0)

C78.0 **Secondary malignant neoplasm of lung**

C78.00 **Secondary malignant neoplasm of unspecified lung**

C78.01 **Secondary malignant neoplasm of right lung**

C78.02 **Secondary malignant neoplasm of left lung**

C78.1   Secondary malignant neoplasm of mediastinum

C78.2   Secondary malignant neoplasm of pleura

C78.3   Secondary malignant neoplasm of other and unspecified respiratory organs

     C78.30   Secondary malignant neoplasm of unspecified respiratory organ

     C78.39   Secondary malignant neoplasm of other respiratory organs

C78.4   Secondary malignant neoplasm of small intestine

C78.5   Secondary malignant neoplasm of large intestine and rectum

C78.6   Secondary malignant neoplasm of retroperitoneum and peritoneum

C78.7   Secondary malignant neoplasm of liver and intrahepatic bile duct

C78.8   Secondary malignant neoplasm of other and unspecified digestive organs

     C78.80   Secondary malignant neoplasm of unspecified digestive organ

     C78.89   Secondary malignant neoplasm of other digestive organs

         Code also exocrine pancreatic insufficiency (K86.81)

C79   **Secondary malignant neoplasm of other and unspecified sites**

   Excludes1: secondary carcinoid tumors (C7B.-)

           secondary neuroendocrine tumors (C7B.-)

   Excludes2: lymph node metastases (C77.0)

C79.0   Secondary malignant neoplasm of kidney and renal pelvis

     C79.00   Secondary malignant neoplasm of unspecified kidney and renal pelvis

     C79.01   Secondary malignant neoplasm of right kidney and renal pelvis

     C79.02   Secondary malignant neoplasm of left kidney and renal pelvis

     C79.1   Secondary malignant neoplasm of bladder and other and unspecified urinary organs

     C79.10   Secondary malignant neoplasm of unspecified urinary organs

     C79.11   Secondary malignant neoplasm of bladder

     C79.19   Secondary malignant neoplasm of other urinary organs

C79.2   Secondary malignant neoplasm of skin

     Excludes1: secondary Merkel cell carcinoma (C7B.1)

C79.3   Secondary malignant neoplasm of brain and cerebral meninges

     C79.31   Secondary malignant neoplasm of brain

     C79.32   Secondary malignant neoplasm of cerebral meninges

C79.4   Secondary malignant neoplasm of other and unspecified parts of nervous system

     C79.40   Secondary malignant neoplasm of unspecified part of nervous system

     C79.49   Secondary malignant neoplasm of other parts of nervous system

C79.5   Secondary malignant neoplasm of bone and bone marrow

     Excludes1: secondary carcinoid tumors of bone (C7B.03)

     C79.51   Secondary malignant neoplasm of bone

     C79.52   Secondary malignant neoplasm of bone marrow

C79.6   Secondary malignant neoplasm of ovary

     C79.60   Secondary malignant neoplasm of unspecified ovary

     C79.61   Secondary malignant neoplasm of right ovary

     C79.62   Secondary malignant neoplasm of left ovary

C79.7   Secondary malignant neoplasm of adrenal gland

     C79.70   Secondary malignant neoplasm of unspecified adrenal gland

     C79.71   Secondary malignant neoplasm of right adrenal gland

     C79.72   Secondary malignant neoplasm of left adrenal gland

C79.8   Secondary malignant neoplasm of other specified sites

     C79.81   Secondary malignant neoplasm of breast

     C79.82   Secondary malignant neoplasm of genital organs

     C79.89   Secondary malignant neoplasm of other specified sites

C79.9   Secondary malignant neoplasm of unspecified site

     Metastatic cancer NOS

     Metastatic disease NOS

     Excludes1: carcinomatosis NOS (C80.0)

           generalized cancer NOS (C80.0)

           malignant (primary) neoplasm of unspecified site (C80.1)

C80   **Malignant neoplasm without specification of site**

   Excludes1: malignant carcinoid tumor of unspecified site (C7A.00)

     malignant neoplasm of specified multiple sites- code to each site

C80.0   **Disseminated malignant neoplasm, unspecified**

     Carcinomatosis NOS

     Generalized cancer, unspecified site (primary) (secondary)

     Generalized malignancy, unspecified site (primary) (secondary)

C80.1   **Malignant (primary) neoplasm, unspecified**

     Cancer NOS

     Cancer unspecified site (primary)

     Carcinoma unspecified site (primary)

     Malignancy unspecified site (primary)

     Excludes1: secondary malignant neoplasm of unspecified site (C79.9)

C80.2   **Malignant neoplasm associated with transplanted organ**

     Code first complication of transplanted organ (T86.-)

     Use additional code to identify the specific malignancy

MALIGNANT NEOPLASMS OF LYMPHOID, HEMATOPOIETIC AND RELATED TISSUE (C81-C96)

Excludes2: Kaposi's sarcoma of lymph nodes (C46.3)

   secondary and unspecified neoplasm of lymph nodes (C77.-)

   secondary neoplasm of bone marrow (C79.52)

   secondary neoplasm of spleen (C78.89)

C81   **Hodgkin lymphoma**

   Definition: Hodgkin's disease is a malignant disease of the lymphatic system is characterized by painless enlargement of lymph nodes, the spleen, or other lymphatic tissue. It is sometimes accompanied by symptoms such as fever, weight loss, fatigue and

night sweats.

Excludes1: personal history of Hodgkin lymphoma (Z85.71)

C81.0 Nodular lymphocyte predominant Hodgkin lymphoma

C81.00 Nodular lymphocyte predominant Hodgkin lymphoma, unspecified site

C81.01 Nodular lymphocyte predominant Hodgkin lymphoma, lymph nodes of head, face, and neck

C81.02 Nodular lymphocyte predominant Hodgkin lymphoma, intrathoracic lymph nodes

C81.03 Nodular lymphocyte predominant Hodgkin lymphoma, intra-abdominal lymph nodes

C81.04 Nodular lymphocyte predominant Hodgkin lymphoma, lymph nodes of axilla and upper limb

C81.05 Nodular lymphocyte predominant Hodgkin lymphoma, lymph nodes of inguinal region and lower limb

C81.06 Nodular lymphocyte predominant Hodgkin lymphoma, intrapelvic lymph nodes

C81.07 Nodular lymphocyte predominant Hodgkin lymphoma, spleen

C81.08 Nodular lymphocyte predominant Hodgkin lymphoma, lymph nodes of multiple sites

C81.09 Nodular lymphocyte predominant Hodgkin lymphoma, extranodal and solid organ sites

C81.1 Nodular sclerosis Hodgkin lymphoma

Nodular sclerosis classical Hodgkin lymphoma

▲C81.10 Nodular sclerosis Hodgkin lymphoma, unspecified site

▲C81.11 Nodular sclerosis Hodgkin lymphoma, lymph nodes of head, face, and neck

▲C81.12 Nodular sclerosis Hodgkin lymphoma, intrathoracic lymph nodes

▲C81.13 Nodular sclerosis Hodgkin lymphoma, intra-abdominal lymph nodes

▲C81.14 Nodular sclerosis Hodgkin lymphoma, lymph nodes of axilla and upper limb

▲C81.15 Nodular sclerosis Hodgkin lymphoma, lymph nodes of inguinal region and lower limb

▲C81.16 Nodular sclerosis Hodgkin lymphoma, intrapelvic lymph nodes

▲C81.17 Nodular sclerosis Hodgkin lymphoma, spleen

▲C81.18 Nodular sclerosis Hodgkin lymphoma, lymph nodes of multiple sites

▲C81.19 Nodular sclerosis Hodgkin lymphoma, extranodal and solid organ sites

C81.2 Mixed cellularity Hodgkin lymphoma

Mixed cellularity classical Hodgkin lymphoma

▲C81.20 Mixed cellularity Hodgkin lymphoma, unspecified site

▲C81.21 Mixed cellularity Hodgkin lymphoma, lymph nodes of head, face, and neck

▲C81.22 Mixed cellularity Hodgkin lymphoma, intrathoracic lymph nodes

▲C81.23 Mixed cellularity Hodgkin lymphoma, intra-abdominal lymph nodes

▲C81.24 Mixed cellularity Hodgkin lymphoma, lymph nodes of axilla and upper limb

▲C81.25 Mixed cellularity Hodgkin lymphoma, lymph nodes of inguinal region and lower limb

▲C81.26 Mixed cellularity Hodgkin lymphoma, intrapelvic lymph nodes

▲C81.27 Mixed cellularity Hodgkin lymphoma, spleen

▲C81.28 Mixed cellularity Hodgkin lymphoma, lymph nodes of multiple sites

▲C81.29 Mixed cellularity Hodgkin lymphoma, extranodal and solid organ sites

C81.3 Lymphocyte depleted Hodgkin lymphoma

Lymphocyte depleted classical Hodgkin lymphoma

▲C81.30 Lymphocyte depleted Hodgkin lymphoma, unspecified site

▲C81.31 Lymphocyte depleted Hodgkin lymphoma, lymph nodes of head, face, and neck

▲C81.32 Lymphocyte depleted Hodgkin lymphoma, intrathoracic lymph nodes

▲C81.33 Lymphocyte depleted Hodgkin lymphoma, intra-abdominal lymph nodes

▲C81.34 Lymphocyte depleted Hodgkin lymphoma, lymph nodes of axilla and upper limb

▲C81.35 Lymphocyte depleted Hodgkin lymphoma, lymph nodes of inguinal region and lower limb

▲C81.36 Lymphocyte depleted Hodgkin lymphoma, intrapelvic lymph nodes

▲C81.37 Lymphocyte depleted Hodgkin lymphoma, spleen

▲C81.38 Lymphocyte depleted Hodgkin lymphoma, lymph nodes of multiple sites

▲C81.39 Lymphocyte depleted Hodgkin lymphoma, extranodal and solid organ sites

C81.4 Lymphocyte-rich Hodgkin lymphoma

Lymphocyte-rich classical Hodgkin lymphoma

Excludes1: nodular lymphocyte predominant Hodgkin lymphoma (C81.0-)

▲C81.40 Lymphocyte-rich Hodgkin lymphoma, unspecified site

▲C81.41 Lymphocyte-rich Hodgkin lymphoma, lymph nodes of head, face, and neck

▲C81.42 Lymphocyte-rich Hodgkin lymphoma, intrathoracic lymph nodes

▲C81.43 Lymphocyte-rich Hodgkin lymphoma, intra-abdominal lymph nodes

▲C81.44 Lymphocyte-rich Hodgkin lymphoma, lymph nodes of axilla and upper limb

▲C81.45 Lymphocyte-rich Hodgkin lymphoma, lymph nodes of inguinal region and lower limb

▲C81.46 Lymphocyte-rich Hodgkin lymphoma, intrapelvic lymph nodes

▲C81.47 Lymphocyte-rich Hodgkin lymphoma, spleen

▲C81.48 Lymphocyte-rich Hodgkin lymphoma, lymph nodes of multiple sites

▲C81.49 Lymphocyte-rich Hodgkin lymphoma, extranodal and solid organ sites

C81.7 Other Hodgkin lymphoma

Classical Hodgkin lymphoma NOS

Other classical Hodgkin lymphoma

▲C81.70 Other Hodgkin lymphoma, unspecified site

▲C81.71 Other Hodgkin lymphoma, lymph nodes of head, face, and neck

▲C81.72 Other Hodgkin lymphoma, intrathoracic lymph nodes

▲C81.73 Other Hodgkin lymphoma, intra-abdominal lymph nodes

▲C81.74 Other Hodgkin lymphoma, lymph nodes of axilla and upper limb

▲C81.75 Other Hodgkin lymphoma, lymph nodes of inguinal region and lower limb

▲C81.76 Other Hodgkin lymphoma, intrapelvic lymph nodes

▲C81.77 Other Hodgkin lymphoma, spleen

▲C81.78 Other Hodgkin lymphoma, lymph nodes of multiple sites

▲C81.79 Other Hodgkin lymphoma, extranodal and solid organ sites

C81.9 Hodgkin lymphoma, unspecified

C81.90 Hodgkin lymphoma, unspecified, unspecified site

C81.91 Hodgkin lymphoma, unspecified, lymph nodes of head, face, and neck

C81.92 Hodgkin lymphoma, unspecified, intrathoracic lymph nodes

C81.93 Hodgkin lymphoma, unspecified, intra-abdominal lymph nodes

C81.94 Hodgkin lymphoma, unspecified, lymph nodes of axilla and upper limb

C81.95 Hodgkin lymphoma, unspecified, lymph nodes of inguinal region and lower limb

C81.96 Hodgkin lymphoma, unspecified, intrapelvic lymph nodes

C81.97 Hodgkin lymphoma, unspecified, spleen

C81.98 Hodgkin lymphoma, unspecified, lymph nodes of multiple sites

C81.99 Hodgkin lymphoma, unspecified, extranodal and solid organ sites

C82 **Follicular lymphoma**

Includes: follicular lymphoma with or without diffuse areas

Excludes1: mature T/NK-cell lymphomas (C84.-)

personal history of non-Hodgkin lymphoma (Z85.72)

C82.0 Follicular lymphoma grade I

C82.00 Follicular lymphoma grade I, unspecified site

C82.01 Follicular lymphoma grade I, lymph nodes of head, face, and neck

C82.02 Follicular lymphoma grade I, intrathoracic lymph nodes

C82.03 Follicular lymphoma grade I, intra-abdominal lymph nodes

C82.04 Follicular lymphoma grade I, lymph nodes of axilla and upper limb

C82.05 Follicular lymphoma grade I, lymph nodes of inguinal region and lower limb

C82.06 Follicular lymphoma grade I, intrapelvic lymph nodes

C82.07 Follicular lymphoma grade I, spleen

C82.08 Follicular lymphoma grade I, lymph nodes of multiple sites

C82.09 Follicular lymphoma grade I, extranodal and solid organ sites

C82.1 Follicular lymphoma grade II

C82.10 Follicular lymphoma grade II, unspecified site

C82.11 Follicular lymphoma grade II, lymph nodes of head, face, and neck

C82.12 Follicular lymphoma grade II, intrathoracic lymph nodes

C82.13 Follicular lymphoma grade II, intra-abdominal lymph nodes

C82.14 Follicular lymphoma grade II, lymph nodes of axilla and upper limb

C82.15 Follicular lymphoma grade II, lymph nodes of inguinal region and lower limb

C82.16 Follicular lymphoma grade II, intrapelvic lymph nodes

C82.17 Follicular lymphoma grade II, spleen

C82.18 Follicular lymphoma grade II, lymph nodes of multiple sites

C82.19 Follicular lymphoma grade II, extranodal and solid organ sites

C82.2 Follicular lymphoma grade III, unspecified

C82.20 Follicular lymphoma grade III, unspecified, unspecified site

C82.21 Follicular lymphoma grade III, unspecified, lymph nodes of head, face, and neck

C82.22 Follicular lymphoma grade III, unspecified, intrathoracic lymph nodes

C82.23 Follicular lymphoma grade III, unspecified, intra-abdominal lymph nodes

C82.24 Follicular lymphoma grade III, unspecified, lymph nodes of axilla and upper limb

C82.25 Follicular lymphoma grade III, unspecified, lymph nodes of inguinal region and lower limb

C82.26 Follicular lymphoma grade III, unspecified, intrapelvic lymph nodes

C82.27 Follicular lymphoma grade III, unspecified, spleen

C82.28 Follicular lymphoma grade III, unspecified, lymph nodes of multiple sites

C82.29 Follicular lymphoma grade III, unspecified, extranodal and solid organ sites

C82.3 Follicular lymphoma grade IIIa

C82.30 Follicular lymphoma grade IIIa, unspecified site

C82.31 Follicular lymphoma grade IIIa, lymph nodes of head, face, and neck

C82.32 Follicular lymphoma grade IIIa, intrathoracic lymph nodes

C82.33 Follicular lymphoma grade IIIa, intra-abdominal lymph nodes

C82.34 Follicular lymphoma grade IIIa, lymph nodes of axilla and upper limb

C82.35 Follicular lymphoma grade IIIa, lymph nodes of inguinal region and lower limb

C82.36 Follicular lymphoma grade IIIa, intrapelvic lymph nodes

C82.37 Follicular lymphoma grade IIIa, spleen

C82.38 Follicular lymphoma grade IIIa, lymph nodes of multiple sites

C82.39 Follicular lymphoma grade IIIa, extranodal and solid organ sites

C82.4 Follicular lymphoma grade IIIb

C82.40 Follicular lymphoma grade IIIb, unspecified site

C82.41 Follicular lymphoma grade IIIb, lymph nodes of head, face, and neck

---

C82.42 Follicular lymphoma grade IIIb, intrathoracic lymph nodes

C82.43 Follicular lymphoma grade IIIb, intra-abdominal lymph nodes

C82.44 Follicular lymphoma grade IIIb, lymph nodes of axilla and upper limb

C82.45 Follicular lymphoma grade IIIb, lymph nodes of inguinal region and lower limb

C82.46 Follicular lymphoma grade IIIb, intrapelvic lymph nodes

C82.47 Follicular lymphoma grade IIIb, spleen

C82.48 Follicular lymphoma grade IIIb, lymph nodes of multiple sites

C82.49 Follicular lymphoma grade IIIb, extranodal and solid organ sites

C82.5 Diffuse follicle center lymphoma

C82.50 Diffuse follicle center lymphoma, unspecified site

C82.51 Diffuse follicle center lymphoma, lymph nodes of head, face, and neck

C82.52 Diffuse follicle center lymphoma, intrathoracic lymph nodes

C82.53 Diffuse follicle center lymphoma, intra-abdominal lymph nodes

C82.54 Diffuse follicle center lymphoma, lymph nodes of axilla and upper limb

C82.55 Diffuse follicle center lymphoma, lymph nodes of inguinal region and lower limb

C82.56 Diffuse follicle center lymphoma, intrapelvic lymph nodes

C82.57 Diffuse follicle center lymphoma, spleen

C82.58 Diffuse follicle center lymphoma, lymph nodes of multiple sites

C82.59 Diffuse follicle center lymphoma, extranodal and solid organ sites

C82.6 Cutaneous follicle center lymphoma

C82.60 Cutaneous follicle center lymphoma, unspecified site

C82.61 Cutaneous follicle center lymphoma, lymph nodes of head, face, and neck

C82.62 Cutaneous follicle center lymphoma, intrathoracic lymph nodes

C82.63 Cutaneous follicle center lymphoma, intra-abdominal lymph nodes

C82.64 Cutaneous follicle center lymphoma, lymph nodes of axilla and upper limb

C82.65 Cutaneous follicle center lymphoma, lymph nodes of inguinal region and lower limb

C82.66 Cutaneous follicle center lymphoma, intrapelvic lymph nodes

C82.67 Cutaneous follicle center lymphoma, spleen

C82.68 Cutaneous follicle center lymphoma, lymph nodes of multiple sites

C82.69 Cutaneous follicle center lymphoma, extranodal and solid organ sites

C82.8 Other types of follicular lymphoma

C82.80 Other types of follicular lymphoma, unspecified site

C82.81 Other types of follicular lymphoma, lymph nodes of head, face, and neck

C82.82 Other types of follicular lymphoma, intrathoracic lymph nodes

C82.83 Other types of follicular lymphoma, intra-abdominal lymph nodes

C82.84 Other types of follicular lymphoma, lymph nodes of axilla and upper limb

C82.85 Other types of follicular lymphoma, lymph nodes of inguinal region and lower limb

C82.86 Other types of follicular lymphoma, intrapelvic lymph nodes

C82.87 Other types of follicular lymphoma, spleen

C82.88 Other types of follicular lymphoma, lymph nodes of multiple sites

C82.89 Other types of follicular lymphoma, extranodal and solid organ sites

C82.9 Follicular lymphoma, unspecified

C82.90 Follicular lymphoma, unspecified, unspecified site

C82.91 Follicular lymphoma, unspecified, lymph nodes of head, face, and neck

C82.92 Follicular lymphoma, unspecified, intrathoracic lymph nodes

C82.93 Follicular lymphoma, unspecified, intra-abdominal lymph nodes

C82.94 Follicular lymphoma, unspecified, lymph nodes of axilla and upper limb

C82.95 Follicular lymphoma, unspecified, lymph nodes of inguinal region and lower limb

C82.96 Follicular lymphoma, unspecified, intrapelvic lymph nodes

C82.97 Follicular lymphoma, unspecified, spleen

C82.98 Follicular lymphoma, unspecified, lymph nodes of multiple sites

C82.99 Follicular lymphoma, unspecified, extranodal and solid organ sites

C83 Non-follicular lymphoma

Excludes1: personal history of non-Hodgkin lymphoma (Z85.72)

C83.0 Small cell B-cell lymphoma

Lymphoplasmacytic lymphoma

Nodal marginal zone lymphoma

Non-leukemic variant of B-CLL

Splenic marginal zone lymphoma

Excludes1: chronic lymphocytic leukemia (C91.1)

mature T/NK-cell lymphomas (C84.-)

Waldenström macroglobulinemia (C88.0)

C83.00 Small cell B-cell lymphoma, unspecified site

C83.01 Small cell B-cell lymphoma, lymph nodes of head, face, and neck

C83.02 Small cell B-cell lymphoma, intrathoracic lymph nodes

C83.03 Small cell B-cell lymphoma, intra-abdominal lymph nodes

C83.04 Small cell B-cell lymphoma, lymph nodes of axilla and upper limb

C83.05 Small cell B-cell lymphoma, lymph nodes of inguinal region and lower limb

C83.06 Small cell B-cell lymphoma, intrapelvic lymph nodes

C83.07 Small cell B-cell lymphoma, spleen

C83.08 **Small cell B-cell lymphoma, lymph nodes of multiple sites**

C83.09 **Small cell B-cell lymphoma, extranodal and solid organ sites**

C83.1 **Mantle cell lymphoma**

Centrocytic lymphoma

Malignant lymphomatous polyposis

  C83.10 **Mantle cell lymphoma, unspecified site**

  C83.11 **Mantle cell lymphoma, lymph nodes of head, face, and neck**

  C83.12 **Mantle cell lymphoma, intrathoracic lymph nodes**

  C83.13 **Mantle cell lymphoma, intra-abdominal lymph nodes**

  C83.14 **Mantle cell lymphoma, lymph nodes of axilla and upper limb**

  C83.15 **Mantle cell lymphoma, lymph nodes of inguinal region and lower limb**

  C83.16 **Mantle cell lymphoma, intrapelvic lymph nodes**

  C83.17 **Mantle cell lymphoma, spleen**

  C83.18 **Mantle cell lymphoma, lymph nodes of multiple sites**

  C83.19 **Mantle cell lymphoma, extranodal and solid organ sites**

C83.3 **Diffuse large B-cell lymphoma**

Anaplastic diffuse large B-cell lymphoma

CD30-positive diffuse large B-cell lymphoma

Centroblastic diffuse large B-cell lymphoma

Diffuse large B-cell lymphoma, subtype not specified

Immunoblastic diffuse large B-cell lymphoma

Plasmablastic diffuse large B-cell lymphoma

Diffuse large B-cell lymphoma, subtype not specified

T-cell rich diffuse large B-cell lymphoma

Excludes1: mediastinal (thymic) large B-cell lymphoma (C85.2-)

        mature T/NK-cell lymphomas (C84.-)

  C83.30 **Diffuse large B-cell lymphoma, unspecified site**

  C83.31 **Diffuse large B-cell lymphoma, lymph nodes of head, face, and neck**

  C83.32 **Diffuse large B-cell lymphoma, intrathoracic lymph nodes**

  C83.33 **Diffuse large B-cell lymphoma, intra-abdominal lymph nodes**

  C83.34 **Diffuse large B-cell lymphoma, lymph nodes of axilla and upper limb**

  C83.35 **Diffuse large B-cell lymphoma, lymph nodes of inguinal region and lower limb**

  C83.36 **Diffuse large B-cell lymphoma, intrapelvic lymph nodes**

  C83.37 **Diffuse large B-cell lymphoma, spleen**

  C83.38 **Diffuse large B-cell lymphoma, lymph nodes of multiple sites**

  C83.39 **Diffuse large B-cell lymphoma, extranodal and solid organ sites**

C83.5 **Lymphoblastic (diffuse) lymphoma**

B-precursor lymphoma

Lymphoblastic B-cell lymphoma

Lymphoblastic lymphoma NOS

Lymphoblastic T-cell lymphoma

T-precursor lymphoma

  C83.50 **Lymphoblastic (diffuse) lymphoma, unspecified site**

  C83.51 **Lymphoblastic (diffuse) lymphoma, lymph nodes of head, face, and neck**

  C83.52 **Lymphoblastic (diffuse) lymphoma, intrathoracic lymph nodes**

  C83.53 **Lymphoblastic (diffuse) lymphoma, intra-abdominal lymph nodes**

  C83.54 **Lymphoblastic (diffuse) lymphoma, lymph nodes of axilla and upper limb**

  C83.55 **Lymphoblastic (diffuse) lymphoma, lymph nodes of inguinal region and lower limb**

  C83.56 **Lymphoblastic (diffuse) lymphoma, intrapelvic lymph nodes**

  C83.57 **Lymphoblastic (diffuse) lymphoma, spleen**

  C83.58 **Lymphoblastic (diffuse) lymphoma, lymph nodes of multiple sites**

  C83.59 **Lymphoblastic (diffuse) lymphoma, extranodal and solid organ sites**

C83.7 **Burkitt lymphoma**

Atypical Burkitt lymphoma Burkitt-like lymphoma

Excludes1: mature B-cell leukemia Burkitt type (C91.A-)

  C83.70 **Burkitt lymphoma, unspecified site**

  C83.71 **Burkitt lymphoma, lymph nodes of head, face, and neck**

  C83.72 **Burkitt lymphoma, intrathoracic lymph nodes**

  C83.73 **Burkitt lymphoma, intra-abdominal lymph nodes**

  C83.74 **Burkitt lymphoma, lymph nodes of axilla and upper limb**

  C83.75 **Burkitt lymphoma, lymph nodes of inguinal region and lower limb**

  C83.76 **Burkitt lymphoma, intrapelvic lymph nodes**

  C83.77 **Burkitt lymphoma, spleen**

  C83.78 **Burkitt lymphoma, lymph nodes of multiple sites**

  C83.79 **Burkitt lymphoma, extranodal and solid organ sites**

C83.8 **Other non-follicular lymphoma**

Intravascular large B-cell lymphoma Lymphoid granulomatosis

Primary effusion B-cell lymphoma

Excludes1: mediastinal (thymic) large B-cell lymphoma (C85.2-)

        T-cell rich B-cell lymphoma (C83.3-)

  C83.80 **Other non-follicular lymphoma, unspecified site**

  C83.81 **Other non-follicular lymphoma, lymph nodes of head, face, and neck**

  C83.82 **Other non-follicular lymphoma, intrathoracic lymph nodes**

  C83.83 **Other non-follicular lymphoma, intra-abdominal lymph nodes**

  C83.84 **Other non-follicular lymphoma, lymph nodes of axilla and upper limb**

C83.85 Other non-follicular lymphoma, lymph nodes of inguinal region and lower limb

C83.86 Other non-follicular lymphoma, intrapelvic lymph nodes

C83.87 Other non-follicular lymphoma, spleen

C83.88 Other non-follicular lymphoma, lymph nodes of multiple sites

C83.89 Other non-follicular lymphoma, extranodal and solid organ sites

C83.9 Non-follicular (diffuse) lymphoma, unspecified

   C83.90 Non-follicular (diffuse) lymphoma, unspecified, unspecified site

   C83.91 Non-follicular (diffuse) lymphoma, unspecified, lymph nodes of head, face, and neck

   C83.92 Non-follicular (diffuse) lymphoma, unspecified, intrathoracic lymph nodes

   C83.93 Non-follicular (diffuse) lymphoma, unspecified, intra-abdominal lymph nodes

   C83.94 Non-follicular (diffuse) lymphoma, unspecified, lymph nodes of axilla and upper limb

   C83.95 Non-follicular (diffuse) lymphoma, unspecified, lymph nodes of inguinal region and lower limb

   C83.96 Non-follicular (diffuse) lymphoma, unspecified, intrapelvic lymph nodes

   C83.97 Non-follicular (diffuse) lymphoma, unspecified, spleen

   C83.98 Non-follicular (diffuse) lymphoma, unspecified, lymph nodes of multiple sites

   C83.99 Non-follicular (diffuse) lymphoma, unspecified, extranodal and solid organ sites

C84 **Mature T/NK-cell lymphomas**

   Excludes1: personal history of non-Hodgkin lymphoma (Z85.72)

C84.0 Mycosis fungoides

   Excludes1: peripheral T-cell lymphoma, not classified (C84.4-)

   C84.00 Mycosis fungoides, unspecified site

   C84.01 Mycosis fungoides, lymph nodes of head, face, and neck

   C84.02 Mycosis fungoides, intrathoracic lymph nodes

   C84.03 Mycosis fungoides, intra-abdominal lymph nodes

   C84.04 Mycosis fungoides, lymph nodes of axilla and upper limb

   C84.05 Mycosis fungoides, lymph nodes of inguinal region and lower limb

   C84.06 Mycosis fungoides, intrapelvic lymph nodes

   C84.07 Mycosis fungoides, spleen

   C84.08 Mycosis fungoides, lymph nodes of multiple sites

   C84.09 Mycosis fungoides, extranodal and solid organ sites

C84.1 Sézary disease

   C84.10 Sézary disease, unspecified site

   C84.11 Sézary disease, lymph nodes of head, face, and neck

   C84.12 Sézary disease, intrathoracic lymph nodes

   C84.13 Sézary disease, intra-abdominal lymph nodes

   C84.14 Sézary disease, lymph nodes of axilla and upper limb

   C84.15 Sézary disease, lymph nodes of inguinal region and lower limb

   C84.16 Sézary disease, intrapelvic lymph nodes

   C84.17 Sézary disease, spleen

   C84.18 Sézary disease, lymph nodes of multiple sites

   C84.19 Sézary disease, extranodal and solid organ sites

C84.4 Peripheral T-cell lymphoma, not classified

   Lennert's lymphoma Lymphoepithelioid lymphoma

   Mature T-cell lymphoma, not elsewhere classified

   C84.40 Peripheral T-cell lymphoma, not classified, unspecified site

   C84.41 Peripheral T-cell lymphoma, not classified, lymph nodes of head, face, and neck

   C84.42 Peripheral T-cell lymphoma, not classified, intrathoracic lymph nodes

   C84.43 Peripheral T-cell lymphoma, not classified, intra-abdominal lymph nodes

   C84.44 Peripheral T-cell lymphoma, not classified, lymph nodes of axilla and upper limb

   C84.45 Peripheral T-cell lymphoma, not classified, lymph nodes of inguinal region and lower limb

   C84.46 Peripheral T-cell lymphoma, not classified, intrapelvic lymph nodes

   C84.47 Peripheral T-cell lymphoma, not classified, spleen

   C84.48 Peripheral T-cell lymphoma, not classified, lymph nodes of multiple sites

   C84.49 Peripheral T-cell lymphoma, not classified, extranodal and solid organ sites

C84.6 Anaplastic large cell lymphoma, ALK-positive

   Anaplastic large cell lymphoma, CD30-positive

   C84.60 Anaplastic large cell lymphoma, ALK-positive, unspecified site

   C84.61 Anaplastic large cell lymphoma, ALK-positive, lymph nodes of head, face, and neck

   C84.62 Anaplastic large cell lymphoma, ALK-positive, intrathoracic lymph nodes

   C84.63 Anaplastic large cell lymphoma, ALK-positive, intra-abdominal lymph nodes

   C84.64 Anaplastic large cell lymphoma, ALK-positive, lymph nodes of axilla and upper limb

   C84.65 Anaplastic large cell lymphoma, ALK-positive, lymph nodes of inguinal region and lower limb

   C84.66 Anaplastic large cell lymphoma, ALK-positive, intrapelvic lymph nodes

   C84.67 Anaplastic large cell lymphoma, ALK-positive, spleen

   C84.68 Anaplastic large cell lymphoma, ALK-positive, lymph nodes of multiple sites

   C84.69 Anaplastic large cell lymphoma, ALK-positive, extranodal and solid organ sites

C84.7 Anaplastic large cell lymphoma, ALK-negative

   Excludes1: primary cutaneous CD30-positive T-cell proliferations (C86.6-)

   C84.70 Anaplastic large cell lymphoma, ALK-negative, unspecified site

C84.71 Anaplastic large cell lymphoma, ALK-negative, lymph nodes of head, face, and neck

C84.72 Anaplastic large cell lymphoma, ALK-negative, intrathoracic lymph nodes

C84.73 Anaplastic large cell lymphoma, ALK-negative, intra-abdominal lymph nodes

C84.74 Anaplastic large cell lymphoma, ALK-negative, lymph nodes of axilla and upper limb

C84.75 Anaplastic large cell lymphoma, ALK-negative, lymph nodes of inguinal region and lower limb

C84.76 Anaplastic large cell lymphoma, ALK-negative, intrapelvic lymph nodes

C84.77 Anaplastic large cell lymphoma, ALK-negative, spleen

C84.78 Anaplastic large cell lymphoma, ALK-negative, lymph nodes of multiple sites

C84.79 Anaplastic large cell lymphoma, ALK-negative, extranodal and solid organ sites

C84.A Cutaneous T-cell lymphoma, unspecified

C84.A0 Cutaneous T-cell lymphoma, unspecified, unspecified site

C84.A1 Cutaneous T-cell lymphoma, unspecified lymph nodes of head, face, and neck

C84.A2 Cutaneous T-cell lymphoma, unspecified, intrathoracic lymph nodes

C84.A3 Cutaneous T-cell lymphoma, unspecified, intra-abdominal lymph nodes

C84.A4 Cutaneous T-cell lymphoma, unspecified, lymph nodes of axilla and upper limb

C84.A5 Cutaneous T-cell lymphoma, unspecified, lymph nodes of inguinal region and lower limb

C84.A6 Cutaneous T-cell lymphoma, unspecified, intrapelvic lymph nodes

C84.A7 Cutaneous T-cell lymphoma, unspecified, spleen

C84.A8 Cutaneous T-cell lymphoma, unspecified, lymph nodes of multiple sites

C84.A9 Cutaneous T-cell lymphoma, unspecified, extranodal and solid organ sites

C84.Z Other mature T/NK-cell lymphomas

Note: If T-cell lineage or involvement is mentioned in conjunction with a specific lymphoma, code to the more specific description.

Excludes1: angioimmunoblastic T-cell lymphoma (C86.5)

blastic NK-cell lymphoma (C86.4)

enteropathy-type T-cell lymphoma (C86.2)

extranodal NK-cell lymphoma, nasal type (C86.0)

hepatosplenic T-cell lymphoma (C86.1)

primary cutaneous CD30-positive T-cell proliferations (C86.6)

subcutaneous panniculitis-like T-cell lymphoma (C86.3)

T-cell leukemia (C91.1-)

C84.Z0 Other mature T/NK-cell lymphomas, unspecified site

C84.Z1 Other mature T/NK-cell lymphomas, lymph nodes of head, face, and neck

C84.Z2 Other mature T/NK-cell lymphomas, intrathoracic lymph nodes

C84.Z3 Other mature T/NK-cell lymphomas, intra-abdominal lymph nodes

C84.Z4 Other mature T/NK-cell lymphomas, lymph nodes of axilla and upper limb

C84.Z5 Other mature T/NK-cell lymphomas, lymph nodes of inguinal region and lower limb

C84.Z6 Other mature T/NK-cell lymphomas, intrapelvic lymph nodes

C84.Z7 Other mature T/NK-cell lymphomas, spleen

C84.Z8 Other mature T/NK-cell lymphomas, lymph nodes of multiple sites

C84.Z9 Other mature T/NK-cell lymphomas, extranodal and solid organ sites

C84.9 Mature T/NK-cell lymphomas, unspecified

NK/T cell lymphoma NOS

Excludes1: mature T-cell lymphoma, not elsewhere classified (C84.4-)

C84.90 Mature T/NK-cell lymphomas, unspecified, unspecified site

C84.91 Mature T/NK-cell lymphomas, unspecified, lymph nodes of head, face, and neck

C84.92 Mature T/NK-cell lymphomas, unspecified, intrathoracic lymph nodes

C84.93 Mature T/NK-cell lymphomas, unspecified, intra-abdominal lymph nodes

C84.94 Mature T/NK-cell lymphomas, unspecified, lymph nodes of axilla and upper limb

C84.95 Mature T/NK-cell lymphomas, unspecified, lymph nodes of inguinal region and lower limb

C84.96 Mature T/NK-cell lymphomas, unspecified, intrapelvic lymph nodes

C84.97 Mature T/NK-cell lymphomas, unspecified, spleen

C84.98 Mature T/NK-cell lymphomas, unspecified, lymph nodes of multiple sites

C84.99 Mature T/NK-cell lymphomas, unspecified, extranodal and solid organ sites

C85 Other specified and unspecified types of non-Hodgkin lymphoma

Excludes1: Other specified types of T/NK-cell lymphoma (C86.-)

personal history of non-Hodgkin lymphoma (Z85.72)

C85.1 Unspecified B-cell lymphoma

Note: If B-cell lineage or involvement is mentioned in conjunction with a specific lymphoma, code to the more specific description.

C85.10 Unspecified B-cell lymphoma, unspecified site

C85.11 Unspecified B-cell lymphoma, lymph nodes of head, face, and neck

C85.12 Unspecified B-cell lymphoma, intrathoracic lymph nodes

C85.13 Unspecified B-cell lymphoma, intra-abdominal lymph nodes

C85.14 Unspecified B-cell lymphoma, lymph nodes of axilla and upper limb

C85.15 Unspecified B-cell lymphoma, lymph nodes of inguinal region and lower limb

C85.16 Unspecified B-cell lymphoma, intrapelvic lymph nodes

C85.17 Unspecified B-cell lymphoma, spleen

C85.18   Unspecified B-cell lymphoma, lymph nodes of multiple sites

C85.19   Unspecified B-cell lymphoma, extranodal and solid organ sites

C85.2   Mediastinal (thymic) large B-cell lymphoma

C85.20   Mediastinal (thymic) large B-cell lymphoma, unspecified site

C85.21   Mediastinal (thymic) large B-cell lymphoma, lymph nodes of head, face, and neck

C85.22   Mediastinal (thymic) large B-cell lymphoma, intrathoracic lymph nodes

C85.23   Mediastinal (thymic) large B-cell lymphoma, intra-abdominal lymph nodes

C85.24   Mediastinal (thymic) large B-cell lymphoma, lymph nodes of axilla and upper limb

C85.25   Mediastinal (thymic) large B-cell lymphoma, lymph nodes of inguinal region and lower limb

C85.26   Mediastinal (thymic) large B-cell lymphoma, intrapelvic lymph nodes

C85.27   Mediastinal (thymic) large B-cell lymphoma, spleen

C85.28   Mediastinal (thymic) large B-cell lymphoma, lymph nodes of multiple sites

C85.29   Mediastinal (thymic) large B-cell lymphoma, extranodal and solid organ sites

C85.8   Other specified types of non-Hodgkin lymphoma

C85.80   Other specified types of non-Hodgkin lymphoma, unspecified site

C85.81   Other specified types of non-Hodgkin lymphoma, lymph nodes of head, face, and neck

C85.82   Other specified types of non-Hodgkin lymphoma, intrathoracic lymph nodes

C85.83   Other specified types of non-Hodgkin lymphoma, intra-abdominal lymph nodes

C85.84   Other specified types of non-Hodgkin lymphoma, lymph nodes of axilla and upper limb

C85.85   Other specified types of non-Hodgkin lymphoma, lymph nodes of inguinal region and lower limb

C85.86   Other specified types of non-Hodgkin lymphoma, intrapelvic lymph nodes

C85.87   Other specified types of non-Hodgkin lymphoma, spleen

C85.88   Other specified types of non-Hodgkin lymphoma, lymph nodes of multiple sites

C85.89   Other specified types of non-Hodgkin lymphoma, extranodal and solid organ sites

C85.9   Non-Hodgkin lymphoma, unspecified

Lymphoma NOS

Malignant lymphoma NOS

Non-Hodgkin lymphoma NOS

C85.90   Non-Hodgkin lymphoma, unspecified, unspecified site

C85.91   Non-Hodgkin lymphoma, unspecified, lymph nodes of head, face, and neck

C85.92   Non-Hodgkin lymphoma, unspecified, intrathoracic lymph nodes

C85.93   Non-Hodgkin lymphoma, unspecified, intra-abdominal lymph nodes

C85.94   Non-Hodgkin lymphoma, unspecified, lymph nodes of axilla and upper limb

C85.95   Non-Hodgkin lymphoma, unspecified, lymph nodes of inguinal region and lower limb

C85.96   Non-Hodgkin lymphoma, unspecified, intrapelvic lymph nodes

C85.97   Non-Hodgkin lymphoma, unspecified, spleen

C85.98   Non-Hodgkin lymphoma, unspecified, lymph nodes of multiple sites

C85.99   Non-Hodgkin lymphoma, unspecified, extranodal and solid organ sites

C86   Other specified types of T/NK-cell lymphoma

Excludes1: anaplastic large cell lymphoma, ALK negative (C84.7-)

anaplastic large cell lymphoma, ALK positive (C84.6-)

mature T/NK-cell lymphomas (C84.-)

Other specified types of non-Hodgkin lymphoma (C85.8-)

C86.0   Extranodal NK/T-cell lymphoma, nasal type

C86.1   Hepatosplenic T-cell lymphoma

Alpha-beta and gamma delta types

C86.2   Enteropathy-type (intestinal) T-cell lymphoma

Enteropathy associated T-cell lymphoma

C86.3   Subcutaneous panniculitis-like T-cell lymphoma

C86.4   Blastic NK-cell lymphoma

C86.5   Angioimmunoblastic T-cell lymphoma

Angioimmunoblastic lymphadenopathy with dysproteinemia (AILD)

C86.6   Primary cutaneous CD30-positive T-cell proliferations

Lymphomatoid papulosis

Primary cutaneous anaplastic large cell lymphoma

Primary cutaneous CD30-positive large T-cell lymphoma

C88   Malignant immunoproliferative diseases and certain other B-cell lymphomas

Excludes1: B-cell lymphoma, unspecified (C85.1-)

personal history **of other** malignant neoplasms of lymphoid, hematopoietic and related tissues (Z85.79)

C88.0   Waldenström macroglobulinemia

Lymphoplasmacytic lymphoma with IgM-production

Macroglobulinemia (idiopathic) (primary)

Excludes1: small cell B-cell lymphoma (C83.0)

C88.2   Heavy chain disease

Franklin disease

Gamma heavy chain disease

Mu heavy chain disease

C88.3   Immunoproliferative small intestinal disease

Alpha heavy chain disease

Mediterranean lymphoma

C88.4   Extranodal marginal zone B-cell lymphoma of mucosa-associated lymphoid tissue [MALT-lymphoma]

Lymphoma of skin-associated lymphoid tissue [SALT-lymphoma] Lymphoma of bronchial-associated lymphoid tissue [BALT-lymphoma]

Excludes1: high malignant (diffuse large B-cell) lymphoma (C83.3-)

C88.8   Other malignant immunoproliferative diseases

C88.9   Malignant immunoproliferative disease, unspecified

Immunoproliferative disease NOS

C90   Multiple myeloma and malignant plasma cell neoplasms

Definition: Multiple myeloma and immunoproliferative neoplasms is a cancer in which there is a uncontrolled proliferation and disordered function of cells called plasma cells in the bone marrow., aka a plasma cell neoplasm.

Excludes1: personal history **of other** malignant neoplasms of lymphoid, hematopoietic and related tissues (Z85.79)

C90.0   Multiple myeloma

    Kahler's disease

    Medullary plasmacytoma

    Myelomatosis

    Plasma cell myeloma

    Excludes1: solitary myeloma (C90.3-)

        solitary plasmacytoma (C90.3-)

    C90.00   Multiple myeloma not having achieved remission

        Multiple myeloma with failed remission

        Multiple myeloma NOS

    C90.01   Multiple myeloma in remission

    C90.02   Multiple myeloma in relapse

C90.1   Plasma cell leukemia

    Plasmacytic leukemia

    C90.10   Plasma cell leukemia not having achieved remission

        Plasma cell leukemia with failed remission

        Plasma cell leukemia NOS

    C90.11   Plasma cell leukemia in remission

    C90.12   Plasma cell leukemia in relapse

C90.2   Extramedullary plasmacytoma

    C90.20   Extramedullary plasmacytoma not having achieved remission

        Extramedullary plasmacytoma with failed remission

        Extramedullary plasmacytoma NOS

    C90.21   Extramedullary plasmacytoma in remission

    C90.22   Extramedullary plasmacytoma in relapse

C90.3   Solitary plasmacytoma

    Localized malignant plasma cell tumor NOS

    Plasmacytoma NOS

    Solitary myeloma

    C90.30   Solitary plasmacytoma not having achieved remission

        Solitary plasmacytoma with failed remission

        Solitary plasmacytoma NOS

    C90.31   Solitary plasmacytoma in remission

    C90.32   Solitary plasmacytoma in relapse

C91   Lymphoid leukemia

Excludes1: personal history of leukemia (Z85.6)

C91.0   Acute lymphoblastic leukemia [ALL]

    Note: Code C91.0 should only be used for T-cell and B-cell precursor leukemia

    C91.00   Acute lymphoblastic leukemia not having achieved remission

        Acute lymphoblastic leukemia with failed remission

        Acute lymphoblastic leukemia NOS

    C91.01   Acute lymphoblastic leukemia, in remission

    C91.02   Acute lymphoblastic leukemia, in relapse

C91.1   Chronic lymphocytic leukemia of B-cell type

    Lymphoplasmacytic leukemia

    Richter syndrome

    Excludes1: lymphoplasmacytic lymphoma (C83.0-)

    C91.10   Chronic lymphocytic leukemia of B-cell type not having achieved remission

        Chronic lymphocytic leukemia of B-cell type with failed remission

        Chronic lymphocytic leukemia of B-cell type NOS

    C91.11   Chronic lymphocytic leukemia of B-cell type in remission

    C91.12   Chronic lymphocytic leukemia of B-cell type in relapse

C91.3   Prolymphocytic leukemia of B-cell type

    C91.30   Prolymphocytic leukemia of B-cell type not having achieved remission

        Prolymphocytic leukemia of B-cell type with failed remission

        Prolymphocytic leukemia of B-cell type NOS

    C91.31   Prolymphocytic leukemia of B-cell type, in remission

    C91.32   Prolymphocytic leukemia of B-cell type, in relapse

C91.4   Hairy cell leukemia

    Leukemic reticuloendotheliosis

    C91.40   Hairy cell leukemia not having achieved remission

        Hairy cell leukemia with failed remission

        Hairy cell leukemia NOS

    C91.41   Hairy cell leukemia, in remission

    C91.42   Hairy cell leukemia, in relapse

C91.5   Adult T-cell lymphoma/leukemia (HTLV-1-associated)

    Acute variant of adult T-cell lymphoma/leukemia (HTLV-1-associated)

    Chronic variant of adult T-cell lymphoma/leukemia (HTLV-1-associated)

    Lymphomatoid variant of adult T-cell lymphoma/leukemia (HTLV-1-associated)

    Smouldering variant of adult T-cell lymphoma/leukemia (HTLV-1-associated)

    C91.50   Adult T-cell lymphoma/leukemia (HTLV-1-associated) not having achieved remission

        Adult T-cell lymphoma/leukemia (HTLV-1-associated) with failed remission

        Adult T-cell lymphoma/leukemia (HTLV-1-associated) NOS

    C91.51   Adult T-cell lymphoma/leukemia (HTLV-1-associated), in remission

    C91.52   Adult T-cell lymphoma/leukemia (HTLV-1-associated), in relapse

C91.6   Prolymphocytic leukemia of T-cell type

    C91.60   Prolymphocytic leukemia of T-cell type not having achieved remission

        Prolymphocytic leukemia of T-cell type with failed remission

        Prolymphocytic leukemia of T-cell type NOS

    C91.61   Prolymphocytic leukemia of T-cell type, in remission

C91.62 Prolymphocytic leukemia of T-cell type, in relapse

C91.A Mature B-cell leukemia Burkitt-type

Excludes1: Burkitt lymphoma (C83.7-)

C91.A0 Mature B-cell leukemia Burkitt-type not having achieved remission

Mature B-cell leukemia Burkitt-type with failed remission

Mature B-cell leukemia Burkitt-type NOS

C91.A1 Mature B-cell leukemia Burkitt-type, in remission

C91.A2 Mature B-cell leukemia Burkitt-type, in relapse

C91.Z Other lymphoid leukemia

T-cell large granular lymphocytic leukemia (associated with rheumatoid arthritis)

C91.Z0 Other lymphoid leukemia not having achieved remission

Other lymphoid leukemia with failed remission

Other lymphoid leukemia NOS

C91.Z1 Other lymphoid leukemia, in remission

C91.Z2 Other lymphoid leukemia, in relapse

C91.9 Lymphoid leukemia, unspecified

C91.90 Lymphoid leukemia, unspecified not having achieved remission

Lymphoid leukemia with failed remission

Lymphoid leukemia NOS

C91.91 Lymphoid leukemia, unspecified, in remission

C91.92 Lymphoid leukemia, unspecified, in relapse

C92 Myeloid leukemia

Includes: granulocytic leukemia

myelogenous leukemia

Excludes1: personal history of leukemia (Z85.6)

C92.0 Acute myeloblastic leukemia

Acute myeloblastic leukemia, minimal differentiation

Acute myeloblastic leukemia (with maturation)

Acute myeloblastic leukemia 1/ETO

Acute myeloblastic leukemia M0

Acute myeloblastic leukemia M1

Acute myeloblastic leukemia M2

Acute myeloblastic leukemia with t(8;21)

Acute myeloblastic leukemia (without a FAB classification) NOS

Refractory anemia with excess blasts in transformation [RAEB T]

Excludes1: acute exacerbation of chronic myeloid leukemia (C92.10)

refractory anemia with excess of blasts not in transformation (D46.2-)

C92.00 Acute myeloblastic leukemia, not having achieved remission

Acute myeloblastic leukemia with failed remission

Acute myeloblastic leukemia NOS

C92.01 Acute myeloblastic leukemia, in remission

C92.02 Acute myeloblastic leukemia, in relapse

C92.1 Chronic myeloid leukemia, BCR/ABL-positive

Chronic myelogenous leukemia, Philadelphia chromosome (Ph1) positive

Chronic myelogenous leukemia, t(9;22) (q34;q11)

Chronic myelogenous leukemia with crisis of blast cells

Excludes1: atypical chronic myeloid leukemia BCR/ABL-negative (C92.2-)

chronic myelomonocytic leukemia (C93.1-)

chronic myeloproliferative disease (D47.1)

C92.10 Chronic myeloid leukemia, BCR/ABL-positive, not having achieved remission

Chronic myeloid leukemia, BCR/ABL-positive with failed remission

Chronic myeloid leukemia, BCR/ABL-positive NOS

C92.11 Chronic myeloid leukemia, BCR/ABL-positive, in remission

C92.12 Chronic myeloid leukemia, BCR/ABL-positive, in relapse

C92.2 Atypical chronic myeloid leukemia, BCR/ABL-negative

C92.20 Atypical chronic myeloid leukemia, BCR/ABL-negative, not having achieved remission

Atypical chronic myeloid leukemia, BCR/ABL-negative with failed remission

Atypical chronic myeloid leukemia, BCR/ABL-negative NOS

C92.21 Atypical chronic myeloid leukemia, BCR/ABL-negative, in remission

C92.22 Atypical chronic myeloid leukemia, BCR/ABL-negative, in relapse

C92.3 Myeloid sarcoma

A malignant tumor of immature myeloid cells

Chloroma

Granulocytic sarcoma

C92.30 Myeloid sarcoma, not having achieved remission

Myeloid sarcoma with failed remission

Myeloid sarcoma NOS

C92.31 Myeloid sarcoma, in remission

C92.32 Myeloid sarcoma, in relapse

C92.4 Acute promyelocytic leukemia

AML M3

AML Me with t(15;17) and variants

C92.40 Acute promyelocytic leukemia, not having achieved remission

Acute promyelocytic leukemia with failed remission

Acute promyelocytic leukemia NOS

C92.41 Acute promyelocytic leukemia, in remission

C92.42 Acute promyelocytic leukemia, in relapse

C92.5 Acute myelomonocytic leukemia

AML M4

AML M4 Eo with inv(16) or t(16;16)

C92.50 Acute myelomonocytic leukemia, not having achieved remission

Acute myelomonocytic leukemia with failed remission

Acute myelomonocytic leukemia NOS

C92.51 Acute myelomonocytic leukemia, in remission

C92.52 Acute myelomonocytic leukemia, in relapse

C92.6 Acute myeloid leukemia with 11q23-abnormality

Acute myeloid leukemia with variation of MLL-gene

C92.60 **Acute myeloid leukemia with 11q23-abnormality not having achieved remission**

Acute myeloid leukemia with 11q23-abnormality with failed remission

Acute myeloid leukemia with 11q23-abnormality NOS

C92.61 **Acute myeloid leukemia with 11q23-abnormality in remission**

C92.62 **Acute myeloid leukemia with 11q23-abnormality in relapse**

C92.A Acute myeloid leukemia with multilineage dysplasia

Acute myeloid leukemia with dysplasia of remaining hematopoesis and/or myelodysplastic disease in its history

C92.A0 **Acute myeloid leukemia with multilineage dysplasia, not having achieved remission**

Acute myeloid leukemia with multilineage dysplasia with failed remission

Acute myeloid leukemia with multilineage dysplasia NOS

C92.A1 **Acute myeloid leukemia with multilineage dysplasia, in remission**

C92.A2 **Acute myeloid leukemia with multilineage dysplasia, in relapse**

C92.Z Other myeloid leukemia

C92.Z0 **Other myeloid leukemia not having achieved remission**

Myeloid leukemia NEC with failed remission

Myeloid leukemia NEC

C92.Z1 **Other myeloid leukemia, in remission**

C92.Z2 **Other myeloid leukemia, in relapse**

C92.9 Myeloid leukemia, unspecified

C92.90 **Myeloid leukemia, unspecified, not having achieved remission**

Myeloid leukemia, unspecified with failed remission

Myeloid leukemia, unspecified NOS

C92.91 **Myeloid leukemia, unspecified in remission**

C92.92 **Myeloid leukemia, unspecified in relapse**

C93 Monocytic leukemia

Includes: monocytoid leukemia

Excludes1: personal history of leukemia (Z85.6)

C93.0 Acute monoblastic/monocytic leukemia

AML M5 AML M5a AML M5b

C93.00 **Acute monoblastic/monocytic leukemia, not having achieved remission**

Acute monoblastic/monocytic leukemia with failed remission

Acute monoblastic/monocytic leukemia NOS

C93.01 **Acute monoblastic/monocytic leukemia, in remission**

C93.02 **Acute monoblastic/monocytic leukemia, in relapse**

C93.1 Chronic myelomonocytic leukemia

Chronic monocytic leukemia CMML-1

CMML-2

CMML with eosinophilia

C93.10 **Chronic myelomonocytic leukemia not having achieved remission**

Chronic myelomonocytic leukemia with failed remission

Chronic myelomonocytic leukemia NOS

C93.11 **Chronic myelomonocytic leukemia, in remission**

C93.12 **Chronic myelomonocytic leukemia, in relapse**

C93.3 Juvenile myelomonocytic leukemia

C93.30 **Juvenile myelomonocytic leukemia, not having achieved remission**

Juvenile myelomonocytic leukemia with failed remission Juvenile myelomonocytic leukemia NOS

C93.31 **Juvenile myelomonocytic leukemia, in remission**

C93.32 **Juvenile myelomonocytic leukemia, in relapse**

C93.Z Other monocytic leukemia

C93.Z0 **Other monocytic leukemia, not having achieved remission**

Other monocytic leukemia NOS

C93.Z1 **Other monocytic leukemia, in remission**

C93.Z2 **Other monocytic leukemia, in relapse**

C93.9 Monocytic leukemia, unspecified

C93.90 **Monocytic leukemia, unspecified, not having achieved remission**

Monocytic leukemia, unspecified with failed remission

Monocytic leukemia, unspecified NOS

C93.91 **Monocytic leukemia, unspecified in remission**

C93.92 **Monocytic leukemia, unspecified in relapse**

C94 Other leukemias of specified cell type

Excludes1: leukemic reticuloendotheliosis (C91.4-)

myelodysplastic syndromes (D46.-)

personal history of leukemia (Z85.6)

plasma cell leukemia (C90.1-)

C94.0 Acute erythroid leukemia

Acute myeloid leukemia M6(a)(b)

Erythroleukemia

C94.00 **Acute erythroid leukemia, not having achieved remission**

Acute erythroid leukemia with failed remission

Acute erythroid leukemia NOS

C94.01 **Acute erythroid leukemia, in remission**

C94.02 **Acute erythroid leukemia, in relapse**

C94.2 Acute megakaryoblastic leukemia

Acute myeloid leukemia M7

Acute megakaryocytic leukemia

C94.20 **Acute megakaryoblastic leukemia not having achieved remission**

Acute megakaryoblastic leukemia with failed remission

Acute megakaryoblastic leukemia NOS

C94.21 **Acute megakaryoblastic leukemia, in remission**

C94.22   **Acute megakaryoblastic leukemia, in relapse**

C94.3   **Mast cell leukemia**

C94.30   **Mast cell leukemia not having achieved remission**

Mast cell leukemia with failed remission

Mast cell leukemia NOS

C94.31   **Mast cell leukemia, in remission**

C94.32   **Mast cell leukemia, in relapse**

C94.4   **Acute panmyelosis with myelofibrosis**

Acute myelofibrosis

Excludes1: myelofibrosis NOS (D75.81)

secondary myelofibrosis NOS (D75.81)

C94.40   **Acute panmyelosis with myelofibrosis not having achieved remission**

Acute myelofibrosis NOS

Acute panmyelosis with myelofibrosis with failed remission

Acute panmyelosis NOS

C94.41   **Acute panmyelosis with myelofibrosis, in remission**

C94.42   **Acute panmyelosis with myelofibrosis, in relapse**

C94.6   **Myelodysplastic disease, not classified**

Myeloproliferative disease, not classified

C94.8   **Other specified leukemias**

Aggressive NK-cell leukemia

Acute basophilic leukemia

C94.80   **Other specified leukemias not having achieved remission**

Other specified leukemia with failed remission

Other specified leukemias NOS

C94.81   **Other specified leukemias, in remission**

C94.82   **Other specified leukemias, in relapse**

C95   **Leukemia of unspecified cell type**

Excludes1: personal history of leukemia (Z85.6)

C95.0   **Acute leukemia of unspecified cell type**

Acute bilineal leukemia

Acute mixed lineage leukemia

Biphenotypic acute leukemia

Stem cell leukemia of unclear lineage

Excludes1: acute exacerbation of unspecified chronic leukemia (C95.10)

C95.00   **Acute leukemia of unspecified cell type not having achieved remission**

Acute leukemia of unspecified cell type with failed remission

Acute leukemia NOS

C95.01   **Acute leukemia of unspecified cell type, in remission**

C95.02   **Acute leukemia of unspecified cell type, in relapse**

C95.1   **Chronic leukemia of unspecified cell type**

C95.10   **Chronic leukemia of unspecified cell type not having achieved remission**

Chronic leukemia of unspecified cell type with failed remission

Chronic leukemia NOS

C95.11   **Chronic leukemia of unspecified cell type, in remission**

C95.12   **Chronic leukemia of unspecified cell type, in relapse**

C95.9   **Leukemia, unspecified**

C95.90   **Leukemia, unspecified not having achieved remission**

Leukemia, unspecified with failed remission

Leukemia NOS

C95.91   **Leukemia, unspecified, in remission**

C95.92   **Leukemia, unspecified, in relapse**

C96   **Other and unspecified malignant neoplasms of lymphoid, hematopoietic and related tissue**

Excludes1: personal history **of other** malignant neoplasms of lymphoid, hematopoietic and related tissues (Z85.79)

C96.0   **Multifocal and multisystemic (disseminated) Langerhans-cell histiocytosis**

Histiocytosis X, multisystemic Letterer-Siwe disease

Excludes1: adult pulmonary Langerhans cell histiocytosis J84.82)

multifocal and unisystemic Langerhans-cell histiocytosis (C96.5)

unifocal Langerhans-cell histiocytosis (C96.6)

C96.2   **Malignant mast cell tumor** Aggressive systemic mastocytosis

Mast cell sarcoma

Excludes1: indolent mastocytosis (D47.0)

mast cell leukemia (C94.30)

mastocytosis (congenital) (cutaneous) (Q82.2)

C96.4   **Sarcoma of dendritic cells (accessory cells)**

Follicular dendritic cell sarcoma

Interdigitating dendritic cell sarcoma Langerhans cell sarcoma

C96.5   **Multifocal and unisystemic Langerhans-cell histiocytosis**

Hand-Schüller-Christian disease

Histiocytosis X, multifocal

Excludes1: multifocal and multisystemic (disseminated) Langerhans-cell histiocytosis (C96.0)

unifocal Langerhans-cell histiocytosis (C96.6)

C96.6   **Unifocal Langerhans-cell histiocytosis**

Eosinophilic granuloma

Histiocytosis X, unifocal

Histiocytosis X NOS

Langerhans-cell histiocytosis NOS

Excludes1: multifocal and multisystemic (disseminated) Langerhans-cell histiocytosis (C96.0)

multifocal and unisystemic Langerhans-cell histiocytosis (C96.5)

C96.A   **Histiocytic sarcoma**

Malignant histiocytosis

C96.Z   **Other specified malignant neoplasms of lymphoid, hematopoietic and related tissue**

C96.9   **Malignant neoplasm of lymphoid, hematopoietic and related tissue, unspecified**

IN SITU NEOPLASMS (D00-D09)

Definition: Carcinoma in situ is a cluster of malignant cells that has not yet invaded the deeper epithelial tissue or spread to other parts of the body.

Includes: Bowen's disease

erythroplasia

grade III intraepithelial neoplasia

Queyrat's erythroplasia

D00 **Carcinoma in situ of oral cavity, esophagus and stomach**

Excludes1: melanoma in situ (D03.-)

D00.0 **Carcinoma in situ of lip, oral cavity and pharynx**

Use additional code to identify:

exposure to environmental tobacco smoke (Z77.22)

exposure to tobacco smoke in the perinatal period (P96.81)

history of tobacco dependence (Z87.891)

occupational exposure to environmental tobacco smoke (Z57.31)

tobacco dependence (F17.-)

tobacco use (Z72.0)

Excludes1: carcinoma in situ of aryepiglottic fold or interarytenoid fold, laryngeal aspect (D02.0)

carcinoma in situ of epiglottis NOS (D02.0)

carcinoma in situ of epiglottis suprahyoid portion (D02.0)

carcinoma in situ of skin of lip (D03.0, D04.0)

D00.00 **Carcinoma in situ of oral cavity, unspecified site**

D00.01 **Carcinoma in situ of labial mucosa and vermilion border**

D00.02 **Carcinoma in situ of buccal mucosa**

D00.03 **Carcinoma in situ of gingiva and edentulous alveolar ridge**

D00.04 **Carcinoma in situ of soft palate**

D00.05 **Carcinoma in situ of hard palate**

D00.06 **Carcinoma in situ of floor of mouth**

D00.07 **Carcinoma in situ of tongue**

D00.08 **Carcinoma in situ of pharynx**

Carcinoma in situ of aryepiglottic fold NOS

Carcinoma in situ of hypopharyngeal aspect of aryepiglottic fold

Carcinoma in situ of marginal zone of aryepiglottic fold

D00.1 **Carcinoma in situ of esophagus**

D00.2 **Carcinoma in situ of stomach**

D01 **Carcinoma in situ of other and unspecified digestive organs**

Excludes1: melanoma in situ (D03.-)

D01.0 **Carcinoma in situ of colon**

Excludes1: carcinoma in situ of rectosigmoid junction (D01.1)

D01.1 **Carcinoma in situ of rectosigmoid junction**

D01.2 **Carcinoma in situ of rectum**

D01.3 **Carcinoma in situ of anus and anal canal**

Anal intraepithelial neoplasia III [AIN III]

Severe dysplasia of anus

Excludes1: anal intraepithelial neoplasia I and II [AIN I and AIN II] (K62.82)

carcinoma in situ of anal margin (D04.5)

carcinoma in situ of anal skin (D04.5)

carcinoma in situ of perianal skin (D04.5)

D01.4 **Carcinoma in situ of other and unspecified parts of intestine**

Excludes1: carcinoma in situ of ampulla of Vater (D01.5)

D01.40 **Carcinoma in situ of unspecified part of intestine**

D01.49 **Carcinoma in situ of other parts of intestine**

D01.5 **Carcinoma in situ of liver, gallbladder and bile ducts**

Carcinoma in situ of ampulla of Vater

D01.7 **Carcinoma in situ of other specified digestive organs**

Carcinoma in situ of pancreas

D01.9 **Carcinoma in situ of digestive organ, unspecified**

D02 **Carcinoma in situ of middle ear and respiratory system**

Use additional code to identify:

exposure to environmental tobacco smoke (Z77.22)

exposure to tobacco smoke in the perinatal period (P96.81)

history of tobacco dependence (Z87.891)

occupational exposure to environmental tobacco smoke (Z57.31)

tobacco dependence (F17.-)

tobacco use (Z72.0)

Excludes1: melanoma in situ (D03.-)

D02.0 **Carcinoma in situ of larynx**

Carcinoma in situ of aryepiglottic fold or interarytenoid fold, laryngeal aspect

Carcinoma in situ of epiglottis (suprahyoid portion)

Excludes1: carcinoma in situ of aryepiglottic fold or interarytenoid fold NOS (D00.08)

carcinoma in situ of hypopharyngeal aspect (D00.08)

carcinoma in situ of marginal zone (D00.08)

D02.1 **Carcinoma in situ of trachea**

D02.2 **Carcinoma in situ of bronchus and lung**

D02.20 **Carcinoma in situ of unspecified bronchus and lung**

D02.21 **Carcinoma in situ of right bronchus and lung**

D02.22 **Carcinoma in situ of left bronchus and lung**

D02.3 **Carcinoma in situ of other parts of respiratory system**

Carcinoma in situ of accessory sinuses

Carcinoma in situ of middle ear

Carcinoma in situ of nasal cavities

Excludes1: carcinoma in situ of ear (external) (skin) (D04.2-)

carcinoma in situ of nose NOS D09.8

carcinoma in situ of skin of nose (D04.3)

D02.4 **Carcinoma in situ of respiratory system, unspecified**

D03 **Melanoma in situ**

D03.0 **Melanoma in situ of lip**

D03.1 **Melanoma in situ of eyelid, including canthus**

D03.10 **Melanoma in situ of unspecified eyelid, including canthus**

D03.11 **Melanoma in situ of right eyelid, including canthus**

D03.12 **Melanoma in situ of left eyelid, including canthus**

D03.2 **Melanoma in situ of ear and external auricular canal**

D03.20 **Melanoma in situ of unspecified ear and external auricular canal**

D03.21 Melanoma in situ of right ear and external auricular canal

D03.22 Melanoma in situ of left ear and external auricular canal

D03.3 Melanoma in situ of other and unspecified parts of face

D03.30 Melanoma in situ of unspecified part of face

D03.39 Melanoma in situ of other parts of face

D03.4 Melanoma in situ of scalp and neck

D03.5 Melanoma in situ of trunk

D03.51 Melanoma in situ of anal skin

Melanoma in situ of anal margin

Melanoma in situ of perianal skin

D03.52 Melanoma in situ of breast (skin) (soft tissue)

D03.59 Melanoma in situ of other part of trunk

D03.6 Melanoma in situ of upper limb, including shoulder

D03.60 Melanoma in situ of unspecified upper limb, including shoulder

D03.61 Melanoma in situ of right upper limb, including shoulder

D03.62 Melanoma in situ of left upper limb, including shoulder

D03.7 Melanoma in situ of lower limb, including hip

D03.70 Melanoma in situ of unspecified lower limb, including hip

D03.71 Melanoma in situ of right lower limb, including hip

D03.72 Melanoma in situ of left lower limb, including hip

D03.8 Melanoma in situ of other sites

Melanoma in situ of scrotum

Excludes1: carcinoma in situ of scrotum (D07.61)

D03.9 Melanoma in situ, unspecified

D04 Carcinoma in situ of skin

Excludes1: erythroplasia of Queyrat (penis) NOS (D07.4)

melanoma in situ (D03.-)

D04.0 Carcinoma in situ of skin of lip

Excludes1: carcinoma in situ of vermilion border of lip (D00.01)

D04.1 Carcinoma in situ of skin of eyelid, including canthus

D04.10 Carcinoma in situ of skin of unspecified eyelid, including canthus

D04.11 Carcinoma in situ of skin of right eyelid, including canthus

D04.12 Carcinoma in situ of skin of left eyelid, including canthus

D04.2 Carcinoma in situ of skin of ear and external auricular canal

D04.20 Carcinoma in situ of skin of unspecified ear and external auricular canal

D04.21 Carcinoma in situ of skin of right ear and external auricular canal

D04.22 Carcinoma in situ of skin of left ear and external auricular canal

D04.3 Carcinoma in situ of skin of other and unspecified parts of face

D04.30 Carcinoma in situ of skin of unspecified part of face

D04.39 Carcinoma in situ of skin of other parts of face

D04.4 Carcinoma in situ of skin of scalp and neck

D04.5 Carcinoma in situ of skin of trunk

Carcinoma in situ of anal margin

Carcinoma in situ of anal skin

Carcinoma in situ of perianal skin

Carcinoma in situ of skin of breast

Excludes1: carcinoma in situ of anus NOS (D01.3)

carcinoma in situ of scrotum (D07.61)

carcinoma in situ of skin of genital organs (D07.-)

D04.6 Carcinoma in situ of skin of upper limb, including shoulder

D04.60 Carcinoma in situ of skin of unspecified upper limb, including shoulder

D04.61 Carcinoma in situ of skin of right upper limb, including shoulder

D04.62 Carcinoma in situ of skin of left upper limb, including shoulder

D04.7 Carcinoma in situ of skin of lower limb, including hip

D04.70 Carcinoma in situ of skin of unspecified lower limb, including hip

D04.71 Carcinoma in situ of skin of right lower limb, including hip

D04.72 Carcinoma in situ of skin of left lower limb, including hip

D04.8 Carcinoma in situ of skin of other sites

D04.9 Carcinoma in situ of skin, unspecified

D05 Carcinoma in situ of breast

Excludes1: carcinoma in situ of skin of breast (D04.5)

melanoma in situ of breast (skin) (D03.5)

Paget's disease of breast or nipple (C50.-)

D05.0 Lobular carcinoma in situ of breast

D05.00 Lobular carcinoma in situ of unspecified breast

D05.01 Lobular carcinoma in situ of right breast

D05.02 Lobular carcinoma in situ of left breast

D05.1 Intraductal carcinoma in situ of breast

D05.10 Intraductal carcinoma in situ of unspecified breast

D05.11 Intraductal carcinoma in situ of right breast

D05.12 Intraductal carcinoma in situ of left breast

D05.8 Other specified type of carcinoma in situ of breast

D05.80 Other specified type of carcinoma in situ of unspecified breast

D05.81 Other specified type of carcinoma in situ of right breast

D05.82 Other specified type of carcinoma in situ of left breast

D05.9 Unspecified type of carcinoma in situ of breast

D05.90 Unspecified type of carcinoma in situ of unspecified breast

D05.91 Unspecified type of carcinoma in situ of right breast

D05.92 Unspecified type of carcinoma in situ of left breast

D06 Carcinoma in situ of cervix uteri

Includes: cervical adenocarcinoma in situ

cervical intraepithelial glandular neoplasia

cervical intraepithelial neoplasia III [CIN III]

severe dysplasia of cervix uteri

Excludes1: cervical intraepithelial neoplasia II [CIN II] (N87.1)

cytologic evidence of malignancy of cervix without histologic confirmation (R87.614)

high grade squamous intraepithelial lesion (HGSIL) of cervix (R87.613)

melanoma in situ of cervix (D03.5)

moderate cervical dysplasia (N87.1)

D06.0 **Carcinoma in situ of endocervix**

D06.1 **Carcinoma in situ of exocervix**

D06.7 **Carcinoma in situ of other parts of cervix**

D06.9 **Carcinoma in situ of cervix, unspecified**

D07 **Carcinoma in situ of other and unspecified genital organs**

Excludes1: melanoma in situ of trunk (D03.5)

D07.0 **Carcinoma in situ of endometrium**

D07.1 **Carcinoma in situ of vulva**

Severe dysplasia of vulva

Vulvar intraepithelial neoplasia III [VIN III]

Excludes1: moderate dysplasia of vulva (N90.1)

vulvar intraepithelial neoplasia II [VIN II] (N90.1)

D07.2 **Carcinoma in situ of vagina**

Severe dysplasia of vagina

Vaginal intraepithelial neoplasia III [VAIN III]

Excludes1: moderate dysplasia of vagina (N89.1)

vaginal intraepithelial neoplasia II [VIN II] (N89.1)

D07.3 **Carcinoma in situ of other and unspecified female genital organs**

D07.30 **Carcinoma in situ of unspecified female genital organs**

D07.39 **Carcinoma in situ of other female genital organs**

D07.4 **Carcinoma in situ of penis**

Erythroplasia of Queyrat NOS

D07.5 **Carcinoma in situ of prostate**

Prostatic intraepithelial neoplasia III (PIN III)

Severe dysplasia of prostate

Excludes1: dysplasia (mild) (moderate) of prostate (N42.3-)

prostatic intraepithelial neoplasia II [PIN II] (N42.3-)

D07.6 **Carcinoma in situ of other and unspecified male genital organs**

D07.60 **Carcinoma in situ of unspecified male genital organs**

D07.61 **Carcinoma in situ of scrotum**

D07.69 **Carcinoma in situ of other male genital organs**

D09 **Carcinoma in situ of other and unspecified sites**

Excludes1: melanoma in situ (D03.-)

D09.0 **Carcinoma in situ of bladder**

D09.1 **Carcinoma in situ of other and unspecified urinary organs**

D09.10 **Carcinoma in situ of unspecified urinary organ**

D09.19 **Carcinoma in situ of other urinary organs**

D09.2 **Carcinoma in situ of eye**

Excludes1: carcinoma in situ of skin of eyelid (D04.1-)

D09.20 **Carcinoma in situ of unspecified eye**

D09.21 **Carcinoma in situ of right eye**

D09.22 **Carcinoma in situ of left eye**

D09.3 **Carcinoma in situ of thyroid and other endocrine glands**

Excludes1: carcinoma in situ of endocrine pancreas (D01.7)

carcinoma in situ of ovary (D07.39)

carcinoma in situ of testis (D07.69)

D09.8 **Carcinoma in situ of other specified sites**

D09.9 **Carcinoma in situ, unspecified**

BENIGN NEOPLASMS, EXCEPT BENIGN NEUROENDOCRINE TUMORS (D10-D36)

Definition: A benign neoplasm is a localized tumor that has a fibrous capsule, limited potential for growth, a regular shape, and cells that are well differentiated. A benign neoplasm does not invade surrounding tissue or metastasize to distant sites. Some kinds of benign neoplasms are adenoma, fibroma, hemangioma, and lipoma.

D10 Benign neoplasm of mouth and pharynx

D10 **Benign neoplasm of mouth and pharynx**

D10.0 **Benign neoplasm of lip**

Benign neoplasm of lip (frenulum) (inner aspect) (mucosa) (vermilion border)

Excludes1: benign neoplasm of skin of lip (D22.0, D23.0)

D10.1 **Benign neoplasm of tongue**

Benign neoplasm of lingual tonsil

D10.2 **Benign neoplasm of floor of mouth**

D10.3 **Benign neoplasm of other and unspecified parts of mouth**

D10.30 **Benign neoplasm of unspecified part of mouth**

D10.39 **Benign neoplasm of other parts of mouth**

Benign neoplasm of minor salivary gland NOS

Excludes1: benign odontogenic neoplasms (D16.4-D16.5)

benign neoplasm of mucosa of lip (D10.0)

benign neoplasm of nasopharyngeal surface of soft palate (D10.6)

D10.4 **Benign neoplasm of tonsil**

Benign neoplasm of tonsil (faucial) (palatine)

Excludes1: benign neoplasm of lingual tonsil (D10.1)

benign neoplasm of pharyngeal tonsil (D10.6)

benign neoplasm of tonsillar fossa (D10.5)

benign neoplasm of tonsillar pillars (D10.5)

D10.5 **Benign neoplasm of other parts of oropharynx**

Benign neoplasm of epiglottis, anterior aspect

Benign neoplasm of tonsillar fossa

Benign neoplasm of tonsillar pillars

Benign neoplasm of vallecula

Excludes1: benign neoplasm of epiglottis NOS (D14.1)

benign neoplasm of epiglottis, suprahyoid portion (D14.1)

D10.6 **Benign neoplasm of nasopharynx**

Benign neoplasm of pharyngeal tonsil

Benign neoplasm of posterior margin of septum and choanae

D10.7   **Benign neoplasm of hypopharynx**

D10.9   **Benign neoplasm of pharynx, unspecified**

D11   **Benign neoplasm of major salivary glands**

Excludes1: benign neoplasms of specified minor salivary glands which are classified according to their anatomical location

benign neoplasms of minor salivary glands NOS (D10.39)

D11.0   **Benign neoplasm of parotid gland**

D11.7   **Benign neoplasm of other major salivary glands**

Benign neoplasm of sublingual salivary gland

Benign neoplasm of submandibular salivary gland

D11.9   **Benign neoplasm of major salivary gland, unspecified**

D12   **Benign neoplasm of colon, rectum, anus and anal canal**

Excludes1: benign carcinoid tumors of the large intestine, and rectum (D3A.02-)

D12.0   **Benign neoplasm of cecum**

Benign neoplasm of ileocecal valve

D12.1   **Benign neoplasm of appendix**

Excludes1: benign carcinoid tumor of the appendix (D3A.020)

D12.2   **Benign neoplasm of ascending colon**

D12.3   **Benign neoplasm of transverse colon**

Benign neoplasm of hepatic flexure

Benign neoplasm of splenic flexure

D12.4   **Benign neoplasm of descending colon**

D12.5   **Benign neoplasm of sigmoid colon**

D12.6   **Benign neoplasm of colon, unspecified**

Adenomatosis of colon

Benign neoplasm of large intestine NOS

Polyposis (hereditary) of colon

Excludes1: inflammatory polyp of colon (K51.4-)

polyp of colon NOS (K63.5)

D12.7   **Benign neoplasm of rectosigmoid junction**

D12.8   **Benign neoplasm of rectum**

Excludes1: benign carcinoid tumor of the rectum (D3A.026)

D12.9   **Benign neoplasm of anus and anal canal**

Benign neoplasm of anus NOS

Excludes1: benign neoplasm of anal margin (D22.5, D23.5)

benign neoplasm of anal skin (D22.5, D23.5)

benign neoplasm of perianal skin (D22.5, D23.5)

D13   **Benign neoplasm of other and ill-defined parts of digestive system**

Excludes1: benign stromal tumors of digestive system (D21.4)

D13.0   **Benign neoplasm of esophagus**

D13.1   **Benign neoplasm of stomach**

Excludes1: benign carcinoid tumor of the stomach (D3A.092)

D13.2   **Benign neoplasm of duodenum**

Excludes1: benign carcinoid tumor of the duodenum (D3A.010)

D13.3   **Benign neoplasm of other and unspecified parts of small intestine**

Excludes1: benign carcinoid tumors of the small intestine(D3A.01-)

benign neoplasm of ileocecal valve (D12.0)

D13.30   **Benign neoplasm of unspecified part of small intestine**

D13.39   **Benign neoplasm of other parts of small intestine**

D13.4   **Benign neoplasm of liver**

Benign neoplasm of intrahepatic bile ducts

D13.5   **Benign neoplasm of extrahepatic bile ducts**

D13.6   **Benign neoplasm of pancreas**

Excludes1: benign neoplasm of endocrine pancreas (D13.7)

D13.7   **Benign neoplasm of endocrine pancreas**

Islet cell tumor Benign neoplasm of islets of Langerhans

Use additional code to identify any functional activity.

D13.9   **Benign neoplasm of ill-defined sites within the digestive system**

Benign neoplasm of digestive system NOS

Benign neoplasm of intestine NOS

Benign neoplasm of spleen

D14   **Benign neoplasm of middle ear and respiratory system**

D14.0   **Benign neoplasm of middle ear, nasal cavity and accessory sinuses**

Benign neoplasm of cartilage of nose

Excludes1: benign neoplasm of auricular canal (external) (D22.2-, D23.2-)

benign neoplasm of bone of ear (D16.4)

benign neoplasm of bone of nose (D16.4)

benign neoplasm of cartilage of ear (D21.0)

benign neoplasm of ear (external)(skin) (D22.2-, D23.2-)

benign neoplasm of nose NOS (D36.7)

benign neoplasm of skin of nose (D22.39, D23.39)

benign neoplasm of olfactory bulb (D33.3)

benign neoplasm of posterior margin of septum and choanae (D10.6)

polyp of accessory sinus (J33.8)

polyp of ear (middle) (H74.4)

polyp of nasal (cavity) (J33.-)

D14.1   **Benign neoplasm of larynx**

Adenomatous polyp of larynx

Benign neoplasm of epiglottis (suprahyoid portion)

Excludes1: benign neoplasm of epiglottis, anterior aspect (D10.5)

polyp (nonadenomatous) of vocal cord or larynx (J38.1)

D14.2   **Benign neoplasm of trachea**

D14.3   **Benign neoplasm of bronchus and lung**

Excludes1: benign carcinoid tumor of the bronchus and lung (D3A.090)

D14.30   **Benign neoplasm of unspecified bronchus and lung**

D14.31   **Benign neoplasm of right bronchus and lung**

D14.32   **Benign neoplasm of left bronchus and lung**

D14.4   **Benign neoplasm of respiratory system, unspecified**

D15   **Benign neoplasm of other and unspecified intrathoracic organs**

Excludes1: benign neoplasm of mesothelial tissue (D19.-)

D15.0   **Benign neoplasm of thymus**

Excludes1: benign carcinoid tumor of the thymus (D3A.091)

D15.1   **Benign neoplasm of heart**

Excludes1: benign neoplasm of great vessels (D21.3)

D15.2   **Benign neoplasm of mediastinum**

D15.7   **Benign neoplasm of other specified intrathoracic organs**

D15.9   **Benign neoplasm of intrathoracic organ, unspecified**

D16   **Benign neoplasm of bone and articular cartilage**

Excludes1: benign neoplasm of connective tissue of ear (D21.0)

benign neoplasm of connective tissue of eyelid (D21.0)

benign neoplasm of connective tissue of larynx (D14.1)

benign neoplasm of connective tissue of nose (D14.0)

benign neoplasm of synovia (D21.-)

D16.0   **Benign neoplasm of scapula and long bones of upper limb**

D16.00   **Benign neoplasm of scapula and long bones of unspecified upper limb**

D16.01   **Benign neoplasm of scapula and long bones of right upper limb**

D16.02   **Benign neoplasm of scapula and long bones of left upper limb**

D16.1   **Benign neoplasm of short bones of upper limb**

D16.10   **Benign neoplasm of short bones of unspecified upper limb**

D16.11   **Benign neoplasm of short bones of right upper limb**

D16.12   **Benign neoplasm of short bones of left upper limb**

D16.2   **Benign neoplasm of long bones of lower limb**

D16.20   **Benign neoplasm of long bones of unspecified lower limb**

D16.21   **Benign neoplasm of long bones of right lower limb**

D16.22   **Benign neoplasm of long bones of left lower limb**

D16.3   **Benign neoplasm of short bones of lower limb**

D16.30   **Benign neoplasm of short bones of unspecified lower limb**

D16.31   **Benign neoplasm of short bones of right lower limb**

D16.32   **Benign neoplasm of short bones of left lower limb**

D16.4   **Benign neoplasm of bones of skull and face**

Benign neoplasm of maxilla (superior)

Benign neoplasm of orbital bone

Keratocyst of maxilla

Keratocystic odontogenic tumor of maxilla

Excludes2: benign neoplasm of lower jaw bone (D16.5)

D16.5   **Benign neoplasm of lower jaw bone**

Keratocyst of mandible

Keratocystic odontogenic tumor of mandible

D16.6   **Benign neoplasm of vertebral column**

Excludes1: benign neoplasm of sacrum and coccyx (D16.8)

D16.7   **Benign neoplasm of ribs, sternum and clavicle**

D16.8   **Benign neoplasm of pelvic bones, sacrum and coccyx**

D16.9   **Benign neoplasm of bone and articular cartilage, unspecified**

D17   **Benign lipomatous neoplasm**

D17.0   **Benign lipomatous neoplasm of skin and subcutaneous tissue of head, face and neck**

D17.1   **Benign lipomatous neoplasm of skin and subcutaneous tissue of trunk**

D17.2   **Benign lipomatous neoplasm of skin and subcutaneous tissue of limb**

D17.20   **Benign lipomatous neoplasm of skin and subcutaneous tissue of unspecified limb**

D17.21   **Benign lipomatous neoplasm of skin and subcutaneous tissue of right arm**

D17.22   **Benign lipomatous neoplasm of skin and subcutaneous tissue of left arm**

D17.23   **Benign lipomatous neoplasm of skin and subcutaneous tissue of right leg**

D17.24   **Benign lipomatous neoplasm of skin and subcutaneous tissue of left leg**

D17.3   **Benign lipomatous neoplasm of skin and subcutaneous tissue of other and unspecified sites**

D17.30   **Benign lipomatous neoplasm of skin and subcutaneous tissue of unspecified sites**

D17.39   **Benign lipomatous neoplasm of skin and subcutaneous tissue of other sites**

D17.4   **Benign lipomatous neoplasm of intrathoracic organs**

D17.5   **Benign lipomatous neoplasm of intra-abdominal organs**

Excludes1: benign lipomatous neoplasm of peritoneum and retroperitoneum (D17.79)

D17.6   **Benign lipomatous neoplasm of spermatic cord**

D17.7   **Benign lipomatous neoplasm of other sites**

D17.71   **Benign lipomatous neoplasm of kidney**

D17.72   **Benign lipomatous neoplasm of other genitourinary organ**

D17.79   **Benign lipomatous neoplasm of other sites**

Benign lipomatous neoplasm of peritoneum

Benign lipomatous neoplasm of retroperitoneum

D17.9   **Benign lipomatous neoplasm, unspecified**

Lipoma NOS

D18   **Hemangioma and lymphangioma, any site**

Definition: Hemangioma is a benign skin lesion consisting of dense, usually elevated masses of dilated blood vessels. Lymphangioma is a benign neoplasm characterized by lymph vessel proliferation.

Excludes1: benign neoplasm of glomus jugulare (D35.6)

blue or pigmented nevus (D22.-) nevus NOS (D22.-)

vascular nevus (Q82.5)

D18.0   **Hemangioma**

Angioma NOS

Cavernous nevus

D18.00   **Hemangioma unspecified site**

D18.01   **Hemangioma of skin and subcutaneous tissue**

D18.02   **Hemangioma of intracranial structures**

D18.03   **Hemangioma of intra-abdominal structures**

D18.09   **Hemangioma of other sites**

D18.1   **Lymphangioma, any site**

D19 **Benign neoplasm of mesothelial tissue**

    D19.0   **Benign neoplasm of mesothelial tissue of pleura**

    D19.1   **Benign neoplasm of mesothelial tissue of peritoneum**

    D19.7   **Benign neoplasm of mesothelial tissue of other sites**

    D19.9   **Benign neoplasm of mesothelial tissue, unspecified**

        Benign mesothelioma NOS

D20 **Benign neoplasm of soft tissue of retroperitoneum and peritoneum**

    Excludes1: benign lipomatous neoplasm of peritoneum and retroperitoneum (D17.79)

      benign neoplasm of mesothelial tissue (D19.-)

    D20.0   **Benign neoplasm of soft tissue of retroperitoneum**

    D20.1   **Benign neoplasm of soft tissue of peritoneum**

D21 **Other benign neoplasms of connective and other soft tissue**

    Includes: benign neoplasm of blood vessel

      benign neoplasm of bursa

      benign neoplasm of cartilage

      benign neoplasm of fascia

      benign neoplasm of fat

      benign neoplasm of ligament, except uterine

      benign neoplasm of lymphatic channel

      benign neoplasm of muscle

      benign neoplasm of synovia

      benign neoplasm of tendon (sheath)

      benign stromal tumors

    Excludes1: benign neoplasm of articular cartilage (D16.-)

      benign neoplasm of cartilage of larynx (D14.1)

      benign neoplasm of cartilage of nose (D14.0)

      benign neoplasm of connective tissue of breast (D24.-)

      benign neoplasm of peripheral nerves and autonomic nervous system (D36.1-)

      benign neoplasm of peritoneum (D20.1)

      benign neoplasm of retroperitoneum (D20.0)

      benign neoplasm of uterine ligament, any (D28.2)

      benign neoplasm of vascular tissue (D18.-)

      hemangioma (D18.0-)

      lipomatous neoplasm (D17.-)

      lymphangioma (D18.1)

      uterine leiomyoma (D25.-)

    D21.0   **Benign neoplasm of connective and other soft tissue of head, face and neck**

        Benign neoplasm of connective tissue of ear

        Benign neoplasm of connective tissue of eyelid

        Excludes1: benign neoplasm of connective tissue of orbit (D31.6-)

    D21.1   **Benign neoplasm of connective and other soft tissue of upper limb, including shoulder**

        D21.10   **Benign neoplasm of connective and other soft tissue of unspecified upper limb, including shoulder**

        D21.11   **Benign neoplasm of connective and other soft tissue of right upper limb, including shoulder**

        D21.12   **Benign neoplasm of connective and other soft tissue of left upper limb, including shoulder**

    D21.2   **Benign neoplasm of connective and other soft tissue of lower limb, including hip**

        D21.20   **Benign neoplasm of connective and other soft tissue of unspecified lower limb, including hip**

        D21.21   **Benign neoplasm of connective and other soft tissue of right lower limb, including hip**

        D21.22   **Benign neoplasm of connective and other soft tissue of left lower limb, including hip**

    D21.3   **Benign neoplasm of connective and other soft tissue of thorax**

        Benign neoplasm of axilla

        Benign neoplasm of diaphragm

        Benign neoplasm of great vessels

        Excludes1: benign neoplasm of heart (D15.1)

          benign neoplasm of mediastinum (D15.2)

          benign neoplasm of thymus (D15.0)

    D21.4   **Benign neoplasm of connective and other soft tissue of abdomen**

        Benign stromal tumors of abdomen

    D21.5   **Benign neoplasm of connective and other soft tissue of pelvis**

        Excludes1: benign neoplasm of any uterine ligament (D28.2)

          uterine leiomyoma (D25.-)

    D21.6   **Benign neoplasm of connective and other soft tissue of trunk, unspecified**

        Benign neoplasm of back NOS

    D21.9   **Benign neoplasm of connective and other soft tissue, unspecified**

D22 **Melanocytic nevi**

    Includes: atypical nevus

      blue hairy pigmented nevus NOS

    D22.0   **Melanocytic nevi of lip**

    D22.1   **Melanocytic nevi of eyelid, including canthus**

        D22.10   **Melanocytic nevi of unspecified eyelid, including canthus**

        D22.11   **Melanocytic nevi of right eyelid, including canthus**

        D22.12   **Melanocytic nevi of left eyelid, including canthus**

    D22.2   **Melanocytic nevi of ear and external auricular canal**

        D22.20   **Melanocytic nevi of unspecified ear and external auricular canal**

        D22.21   **Melanocytic nevi of right ear and external auricular canal**

        D22.22   **Melanocytic nevi of left ear and external auricular canal**

    D22.3   **Melanocytic nevi of other and unspecified parts of face**

        D22.30   **Melanocytic nevi of unspecified part of face**

        D22.39   **Melanocytic nevi of other parts of face**

    D22.4   **Melanocytic nevi of scalp and neck**

    D22.5   **Melanocytic nevi of trunk**

        Melanocytic nevi of anal margin

        Melanocytic nevi of anal skin

        Melanocytic nevi of perianal skin

        Melanocytic nevi of skin of breast

    D22.6   **Melanocytic nevi of upper limb, including shoulder**

        D22.60   **Melanocytic nevi of unspecified upper limb, including shoulder**

D22.61   Melanocytic nevi of right upper limb, including shoulder

D22.62   Melanocytic nevi of left upper limb, including shoulder

D22.7   Melanocytic nevi of lower limb, including hip

D22.70   Melanocytic nevi of unspecified lower limb, including hip

D22.71   Melanocytic nevi of right lower limb, including hip

D22.72   Melanocytic nevi of left lower limb, including hip

D22.9   Melanocytic nevi, unspecified

D23   Other benign neoplasms of skin

Includes: benign neoplasm of hair follicles

benign neoplasm of sebaceous glands

benign neoplasm of sweat glands

Excludes1: benign lipomatous neoplasms of skin (D17.0-D17.3)

melanocytic nevi (D22.-)

D23.0   Other benign neoplasm of skin of lip

Excludes1: benign neoplasm of vermilion border of lip (D10.0)

D23.1   Other benign neoplasm of skin of eyelid, including canthus

D23.10   Other benign neoplasm of skin of unspecified eyelid, including canthus

D23.11   Other benign neoplasm of skin of right eyelid, including canthus

D23.12   Other benign neoplasm of skin of left eyelid, including canthus

D23.2   Other benign neoplasm of skin of ear and external auricular canal

D23.20   Other benign neoplasm of skin of unspecified ear and external auricular canal

D23.21   Other benign neoplasm of skin of right ear and external auricular canal

D23.22   Other benign neoplasm of skin of left ear and external auricular canal

D23.3   Other benign neoplasm of skin of other and unspecified parts of face

D23.30   Other benign neoplasm of skin of unspecified part of face

D23.39   Other benign neoplasm of skin of other parts of face

D23.4   Other benign neoplasm of skin of scalp and neck

D23.5   Other benign neoplasm of skin of trunk

Other benign neoplasm of anal margin

Other benign neoplasm of anal skin

Other benign neoplasm of perianal skin

Other benign neoplasm of skin of breast

Excludes1: benign neoplasm of anus NOS (D12.9)

D23.6   Other benign neoplasm of skin of upper limb, including shoulder

D23.60   Other benign neoplasm of skin of unspecified upper limb, including shoulder

D23.61   Other benign neoplasm of skin of right upper limb, including shoulder

D23.62   Other benign neoplasm of skin of left upper limb, including shoulder

D23.7   Other benign neoplasm of skin of lower limb, including hip

D23.70   Other benign neoplasm of skin of unspecified lower limb, including hip

D23.71   Other benign neoplasm of skin of right lower limb, including hip

D23.72   Other benign neoplasm of skin of left lower limb, including hip

D23.9   Other benign neoplasm of skin, unspecified

D24   Benign neoplasm of breast

Includes: benign neoplasm of connective tissue of breast

benign neoplasm of soft parts of breast

fibroadenoma of breast

Excludes2: adenofibrosis of breast (N60.2)

benign cyst of breast (N60.-)

benign mammary dysplasia (N60.-)

benign neoplasm of skin of breast (D22.5, D23.5)

fibrocystic disease of breast (N60.-)

D24.1   Benign neoplasm of right breast

D24.2   Benign neoplasm of left breast

D24.9   Benign neoplasm of unspecified breast

D25   Leiomyoma of uterus

Includes: uterine fibroid

uterine fibromyoma

uterine myoma

D25.0   Submucous leiomyoma of uterus

D25.1   Intramural leiomyoma of uterus

Interstitial leiomyoma of uterus

D25.2   Subserosal leiomyoma of uterus

Subperitoneal leiomyoma of uterus

D25.9   Leiomyoma of uterus, unspecified

D26   Other benign neoplasms of uterus

D26.0   Other benign neoplasm of cervix uteri

D26.1   Other benign neoplasm of corpus uteri

D26.7   Other benign neoplasm of other parts of uterus

D26.9   Other benign neoplasm of uterus, unspecified

D27   Benign neoplasm of ovary

Use additional code to identify any functional activity.

Excludes2: corpus albicans cyst (N83.2-)

corpus luteum cyst (N83.1-)

endometrial cyst (N80.1)

follicular (atretic) cyst (N83.0-)

graafian follicle cyst (N83.0-)

ovarian cyst NEC (N83.2-)

ovarian retention cyst (N83.2-)

D27.0   Benign neoplasm of right ovary

D27.1   Benign neoplasm of left ovary

D27.9   Benign neoplasm of unspecified ovary

D28   Benign neoplasm of other and unspecified female genital organs

Includes: adenomatous polyp

benign neoplasm of skin of female genital organs

benign teratoma

Excludes1: epoophoron cyst (Q50.5)

fimbrial cyst (Q50.4)

Gartner's duct cyst (Q52.4)

parovarian cyst (Q50.5)

D28.0   **Benign neoplasm of vulva**

D28.1   **Benign neoplasm of vagina**

D28.2   **Benign neoplasm of uterine tubes and ligaments**

Benign neoplasm of fallopian tube

Benign neoplasm of uterine ligament (broad) (round)

D28.7   **Benign neoplasm of other specified female genital organs**

D28.9   **Benign neoplasm of female genital organ, unspecified**

D29   **Benign neoplasm of male genital organs**

Includes: benign neoplasm of skin of male genital organs

D29.0   **Benign neoplasm of penis**

D29.1   **Benign neoplasm of prostate**

Excludes1: enlarged prostate (N40.-)

D29.2   **Benign neoplasm of testis**

<u>**Use additional code**</u> to identify any functional activity.

     D29.20   **Benign neoplasm of unspecified testis**

     D29.21   **Benign neoplasm of right testis**

     D29.22   **Benign neoplasm of left testis**

D29.3   **Benign neoplasm of epididymis**

     D29.30   **Benign neoplasm of unspecified epididymis**

     D29.31   **Benign neoplasm of right epididymis**

     D29.32   **Benign neoplasm of left epididymis**

D29.4   **Benign neoplasm of scrotum**

Benign neoplasm of skin of scrotum

D29.8   **Benign neoplasm of other specified male genital organs**

Benign neoplasm of seminal vesicle

Benign neoplasm of spermatic cord

Benign neoplasm of tunica vaginalis

D29.9   **Benign neoplasm of male genital organ, unspecified**

D30   **Benign neoplasm of urinary organs**

D30.0   **Benign neoplasm of kidney**

Excludes1: benign carcinoid tumor of the kidney (D3A.093)

benign neoplasm of renal calyces (D30.1-)

benign neoplasm of renal pelvis (D30.1-)

     D30.00   **Benign neoplasm of unspecified kidney**

     D30.01   **Benign neoplasm of right kidney**

     D30.02   **Benign neoplasm of left kidney**

D30.1   **Benign neoplasm of renal pelvis**

     D30.10   **Benign neoplasm of unspecified renal pelvis**

     D30.11   **Benign neoplasm of right renal pelvis**

     D30.12   **Benign neoplasm of left renal pelvis**

D30.2   **Benign neoplasm of ureter**

Excludes1: benign neoplasm of ureteric orifice of bladder (D30.3)

     D30.20   **Benign neoplasm of unspecified ureter**

     D30.21   **Benign neoplasm of right ureter**

     D30.22   **Benign neoplasm of left ureter**

D30.3   **Benign neoplasm of bladder**

Benign neoplasm of ureteric orifice of bladder

Benign neoplasm of urethral orifice of bladder

D30.4   **Benign neoplasm of urethra**

Excludes1: benign neoplasm of urethral orifice of bladder (D30.3)

D30.8   **Benign neoplasm of other specified urinary organs**

Benign neoplasm of paraurethral glands

D30.9   **Benign neoplasm of urinary organ, unspecified**

Benign neoplasm of urinary system NOS

D31   **Benign neoplasm of eye and adnexa**

Excludes1: benign neoplasm of connective tissue of eyelid (D21.0)

benign neoplasm of optic nerve (D33.3)

benign neoplasm of skin of eyelid (D22.1-, D23.1-)

D31.0   **Benign neoplasm of conjunctiva**

     D31.00   **Benign neoplasm of unspecified conjunctiva**

     D31.01   **Benign neoplasm of right conjunctiva**

     D31.02   **Benign neoplasm of left conjunctiva**

D31.1   **Benign neoplasm of cornea**

     D31.10   **Benign neoplasm of unspecified cornea**

     D31.11   **Benign neoplasm of right cornea**

     D31.12   **Benign neoplasm of left cornea**

D31.2   **Benign neoplasm of retina**

Excludes1: dark area on retina (D49.81)

hemangioma of retina (D49.81)

neoplasm of unspecified behavior of retina and choroid (D49.81)

retinal freckle (D49.81)

     D31.20   **Benign neoplasm of unspecified retina**

     D31.21   **Benign neoplasm of right retina**

     D31.22   **Benign neoplasm of left retina**

D31.3   **Benign neoplasm of choroid**

     D31.30   **Benign neoplasm of unspecified choroid**

     D31.31   **Benign neoplasm of right choroid**

     D31.32   **Benign neoplasm of left choroid**

D31.4   **Benign neoplasm of ciliary body**

     D31.40   **Benign neoplasm of unspecified ciliary body**

     D31.41   **Benign neoplasm of right ciliary body**

     D31.42   **Benign neoplasm of left ciliary body**

D31.5   **Benign neoplasm of lacrimal gland and duct**

Benign neoplasm of lacrimal sac

Benign neoplasm of nasolacrimal duct

     D31.50   **Benign neoplasm of unspecified lacrimal gland and duct**

     D31.51   **Benign neoplasm of right lacrimal gland and duct**

     D31.52   **Benign neoplasm of left lacrimal gland and duct**

D31.6   **Benign neoplasm of unspecified site of orbit**

Benign neoplasm of connective tissue of orbit

Benign neoplasm of extraocular muscle

Benign neoplasm of peripheral nerves of orbit

Benign neoplasm of retrobulbar tissue

Benign neoplasm of retro-ocular tissue

Excludes1: benign neoplasm of orbital bone (D16.4)

     D31.60   **Benign neoplasm of unspecified site of unspecified orbit**

     D31.61   **Benign neoplasm of unspecified site of right orbit**

D31.62 **Benign neoplasm of unspecified site of left orbit**

D31.9 **Benign neoplasm of unspecified part of eye**

Benign neoplasm of eyeball

D31.90 **Benign neoplasm of unspecified part of unspecified eye**

D31.91 **Benign neoplasm of unspecified part of right eye**

D31.92 **Benign neoplasm of unspecified part of left eye**

D32 **Benign neoplasm of meninges**

D32.0 **Benign neoplasm of cerebral meninges**

D32.1 **Benign neoplasm of spinal meninges**

D32.9 **Benign neoplasm of meninges, unspecified**

Meningioma NOS

D33 **Benign neoplasm of brain and other parts of central nervous system**

Excludes1: angioma (D18.0-)

benign neoplasm of meninges (D32.-)

benign neoplasm of peripheral nerves and autonomic nervous system (D36.1-)

hemangioma (D18.0-)

neurofibromatosis (Q85.0-)

retro-ocular benign neoplasm (D31.6-)

D33.0 **Benign neoplasm of brain, supratentorial**

Benign neoplasm of cerebral ventricle

Benign neoplasm of cerebrum

Benign neoplasm of frontal lobe

Benign neoplasm of occipital lobe

Benign neoplasm of parietal lobe

Benign neoplasm of temporal lobe

Excludes1: benign neoplasm of fourth ventricle (D33.1)

D33.1 **Benign neoplasm of brain, infratentorial**

Benign neoplasm of brain stem

Benign neoplasm of cerebellum

Benign neoplasm of fourth ventricle

D33.2 **Benign neoplasm of brain, unspecified**

D33.3 **Benign neoplasm of cranial nerves**

Benign neoplasm of olfactory bulb

D33.4 **Benign neoplasm of spinal cord**

D33.7 **Benign neoplasm of other specified parts of central nervous system**

D33.9 **Benign neoplasm of central nervous system, unspecified**

Benign neoplasm of nervous system (central) NOS

D34 **Benign neoplasm of thyroid gland**

Use additional code to identify any functional activity

D35 **Benign neoplasm of other and unspecified endocrine glands**

Use additional code to identify any functional activity

Excludes1: benign neoplasm of endocrine pancreas (D13.7)

benign neoplasm of ovary (D27.-)

benign neoplasm of testis (D29.2.-)

benign neoplasm of thymus (D15.0)

D35.0 **Benign neoplasm of adrenal gland**

D35.00 **Benign neoplasm of unspecified adrenal gland**

D35.01 **Benign neoplasm of right adrenal gland**

D35.02 **Benign neoplasm of left adrenal gland**

D35.1 **Benign neoplasm of parathyroid gland**

D35.2 **Benign neoplasm of pituitary gland**

D35.3 **Benign neoplasm of craniopharyngeal duct**

D35.4 **Benign neoplasm of pineal gland**

D35.5 **Benign neoplasm of carotid body**

D35.6 **Benign neoplasm of aortic body and other paraganglia**

Benign tumor of glomus jugulare

D35.7 **Benign neoplasm of other specified endocrine glands**

D35.9 **Benign neoplasm of endocrine gland, unspecified**

Benign neoplasm of unspecified endocrine gland

D36 **Benign neoplasm of other and unspecified sites**

D36.0 **Benign neoplasm of lymph nodes**

Excludes1: lymphangioma (D18.1)

D36.1 **Benign neoplasm of peripheral nerves and autonomic nervous system**

Excludes1: benign neoplasm of peripheral nerves of orbit (D31.6-)

neurofibromatosis (Q85.0-)

D36.10 **Benign neoplasm of peripheral nerves and autonomic nervous system, unspecified**

D36.11 **Benign neoplasm of peripheral nerves and autonomic nervous system of face, head, and neck**

D36.12 **Benign neoplasm of peripheral nerves and autonomic nervous system, upper limb, including shoulder**

D36.13 **Benign neoplasm of peripheral nerves and autonomic nervous system of lower limb, including hip**

D36.14 **Benign neoplasm of peripheral nerves and autonomic nervous system of thorax**

D36.15 **Benign neoplasm of peripheral nerves and autonomic nervous system of abdomen**

D36.16 **Benign neoplasm of peripheral nerves and autonomic nervous system of pelvis**

D36.17 **Benign neoplasm of peripheral nerves and autonomic nervous system of trunk, unspecified**

D36.7 **Benign neoplasm of other specified sites**

Benign neoplasm of nose NOS

D36.9 **Benign neoplasm, unspecified site**

BENIGN NEUROENDOCRINE TUMORS (D3A)

Definition: Neuroendocrine tumor is a tumor derived from cells that release a hormone in response to a signal from the nervous system. Examples of neuroendocrine tumors include carcinoid tumors islet cell tumors, medullary thyroid carcinoma, and pheochromocytoma.

D3A **Benign neuroendocrine tumors**

Code also any associated multiple endocrine neoplasia [MEN] syndromes (E31.2-)

Use additional code to identify any associated endocrine syndrome, such as:

carcinoid syndrome (E34.0)

Excludes2: benign pancreatic islet cell tumors (D13.7)

D3A.0 **Benign carcinoid tumors**

D3A.00 **Benign carcinoid tumor of unspecified site**

Carcinoid tumor NOS

D3A.01 **Benign carcinoid tumors of the small intestine**

D3A.010 Benign carcinoid tumor of the duodenum

D3A.011 Benign carcinoid tumor of the jejunum

D3A.012 Benign carcinoid tumor of the ileum

D3A.019 Benign carcinoid tumor of the small intestine, unspecified portion

D3A.020 Benign carcinoid tumor of the appendix

D3A.021 Benign carcinoid tumor of the cecum

D3A.022 Benign carcinoid tumor of the ascending colon

D3A.023 Benign carcinoid tumor of the transverse colon

D3A.024 Benign carcinoid tumor of the descending colon

D3A.025 Benign carcinoid tumor of the sigmoid colon

D3A.026 Benign carcinoid tumor of the rectum

D3A.029 Benign carcinoid tumor of the large intestine, unspecified portion

Benign carcinoid tumor of the colon NOS

D3A.09 Benign carcinoid tumors of other sites

D3A.090 Benign carcinoid tumor of the bronchus and lung

D3A.091 Benign carcinoid tumor of the thymus

D3A.092 Benign carcinoid tumor of the stomach

D3A.093 Benign carcinoid tumor of the kidney

▲**D3A.094** Benign carcinoid tumor of the foregut, unspecified

▲**D3A.095** Benign carcinoid tumor of the midgut, unspecified

▲**D3A.096** Benign carcinoid tumor of the hindgut, unspecified

D3A.098 Benign carcinoid tumors of other sites

D3A.8 Other benign neuroendocrine tumors

Neuroendocrine tumor NOS

NEOPLASMS OF UNCERTAIN BEHAVIOR, POLYCYTHEMIA VERA AND MYELODYSPLASTIC SYNDROMES (D37-D48)

Note: Categories D37-D44, and D48 classify by site neoplasms of uncertain behavior, i.e., histologic confirmation whether the neoplasm is malignant or benign cannot be made.

Excludes1: neoplasms of unspecified behavior (D49.-)

D37 Neoplasm of uncertain behavior of oral cavity and digestive organs

Excludes1: stromal tumors of uncertain behavior of digestive system (D48.1)

D37.0 Neoplasm of uncertain behavior of lip, oral cavity and pharynx

Excludes1: neoplasm of uncertain behavior of aryepiglottic fold or interarytenoid fold, laryngeal aspect (D38.0)

neoplasm of uncertain behavior of epiglottis NOS (D38.0)

neoplasm of uncertain behavior of skin of lip (D48.5)

neoplasm of uncertain behavior of suprahyoid portion of epiglottis (D38.0)

D37.01 Neoplasm of uncertain behavior of lip

Neoplasm of uncertain behavior of vermilion border of lip

D37.02 Neoplasm of uncertain behavior of tongue

D37.03 Neoplasm of uncertain behavior of the major salivary glands

D37.030 Neoplasm of uncertain behavior of the parotid salivary glands

D37.031 Neoplasm of uncertain behavior of the sublingual salivary glands

D37.032 Neoplasm of uncertain behavior of the submandibular salivary glands

D37.039 Neoplasm of uncertain behavior of the major salivary glands, unspecified

D37.04 Neoplasm of uncertain behavior of the minor salivary glands

Neoplasm of uncertain behavior of submucosal salivary glands of lip

Neoplasm of uncertain behavior of submucosal salivary glands of cheek

Neoplasm of uncertain behavior of submucosal salivary glands of hard palate

Neoplasm of uncertain behavior of submucosal salivary glands of soft palate

D37.05 Neoplasm of uncertain behavior of pharynx

Neoplasm of uncertain behavior of aryepiglottic fold of pharynx NOS

Neoplasm of uncertain behavior of hypopharyngeal aspect of aryepiglottic fold of pharynx

Neoplasm of uncertain behavior of marginal zone of aryepiglottic fold of pharynx

D37.09 Neoplasm of uncertain behavior of other specified sites of the oral cavity

D37.1 Neoplasm of uncertain behavior of stomach

D37.2 Neoplasm of uncertain behavior of small intestine

D37.3 Neoplasm of uncertain behavior of appendix

D37.4 Neoplasm of uncertain behavior of colon

D37.5 Neoplasm of uncertain behavior of rectum

Neoplasm of uncertain behavior of rectosigmoid junction

D37.6 Neoplasm of uncertain behavior of liver, gallbladder and bile ducts

Neoplasm of uncertain behavior of ampulla of Vater

D37.8 Neoplasm of uncertain behavior of other specified digestive organs

Neoplasm of uncertain behavior of anal canal

Neoplasm of uncertain behavior of anal sphincter

Neoplasm of uncertain behavior of anus NOS

Neoplasm of uncertain behavior of esophagus

Neoplasm of uncertain behavior of intestine NOS

Neoplasm of uncertain behavior of pancreas

Excludes1: neoplasm of uncertain behavior of anal margin (D48.5)

neoplasm of uncertain behavior of anal skin (D48.5)

neoplasm of uncertain behavior of perianal skin (D48.5)

D37.9 **Neoplasm of uncertain behavior of digestive organ, unspecified**

D38 **Neoplasm of uncertain behavior of middle ear and respiratory and intrathoracic organs**

Excludes1: neoplasm of uncertain behavior of heart (D48.7)

D38.0 **Neoplasm of uncertain behavior of larynx**

Neoplasm of uncertain behavior of aryepiglottic fold or interarytenoid fold, laryngeal aspect

Neoplasm of uncertain behavior of epiglottis (suprahyoid portion)

Excludes1: neoplasm of uncertain behavior of aryepiglottic fold or interarytenoid fold NOS (D37.05)

neoplasm of uncertain behavior of hypopharyngeal aspect of aryepiglottic fold (D37.05)

neoplasm of uncertain behavior of marginal zone of aryepiglottic fold (D37.05)

D38.1 **Neoplasm of uncertain behavior of trachea, bronchus and lung**

D38.2 **Neoplasm of uncertain behavior of pleura**

D38.3 **Neoplasm of uncertain behavior of mediastinum**

D38.4 **Neoplasm of uncertain behavior of thymus**

D38.5 **Neoplasm of uncertain behavior of other respiratory organs**

Neoplasm of uncertain behavior of accessory sinuses

Neoplasm of uncertain behavior of cartilage of nose

Neoplasm of uncertain behavior of middle ear

Neoplasm of uncertain behavior of nasal cavities

Excludes1: neoplasm of uncertain behavior of ear (external) (skin) (D48.5)

neoplasm of uncertain behavior of nose NOS (D48.7)

neoplasm of uncertain behavior of skin of nose (D48.5)

D38.6 **Neoplasm of uncertain behavior of respiratory organ, unspecified**

D39 **Neoplasm of uncertain behavior of female genital organs**

D39.0 **Neoplasm of uncertain behavior of uterus**

D39.1 **Neoplasm of uncertain behavior of ovary**

Use additional code to identify any functional activity.

D39.10 **Neoplasm of uncertain behavior of unspecified ovary**

D39.11 **Neoplasm of uncertain behavior of right ovary**

D39.12 **Neoplasm of uncertain behavior of left ovary**

D39.2 **Neoplasm of uncertain behavior of placenta**

Chorioadenoma destruens

Invasive hydatidiform mole

Malignant hydatidiform mole

Excludes1: hydatidiform mole NOS (O01.9)

D39.8 **Neoplasm of uncertain behavior of other specified female genital organs**

Neoplasm of uncertain behavior of skin of female genital organs

D39.9 **Neoplasm of uncertain behavior of female genital organ, unspecified**

D40 **Neoplasm of uncertain behavior of male genital organs**

D40.0 **Neoplasm of uncertain behavior of prostate**

D40.1 **Neoplasm of uncertain behavior of testis**

D40.10 **Neoplasm of uncertain behavior of unspecified testis**

D40.11 **Neoplasm of uncertain behavior of right testis**

D40.12 **Neoplasm of uncertain behavior of left testis**

D40.8 **Neoplasm of uncertain behavior of other specified male genital organs**

Neoplasm of uncertain behavior of skin of male genital organs

D40.9 **Neoplasm of uncertain behavior of male genital organ, unspecified**

D41 **Neoplasm of uncertain behavior of urinary organs**

D41.0 **Neoplasm of uncertain behavior of kidney**

Excludes1: neoplasm of uncertain behavior of renal pelvis (D41.1-)

D41.00 **Neoplasm of uncertain behavior of unspecified kidney**

D41.01 **Neoplasm of uncertain behavior of right kidney**

D41.02 **Neoplasm of uncertain behavior of left kidney**

D41.1 **Neoplasm of uncertain behavior of renal pelvis**

D41.10 **Neoplasm of uncertain behavior of unspecified renal pelvis**

D41.11 **Neoplasm of uncertain behavior of right renal pelvis**

D41.12 **Neoplasm of uncertain behavior of left renal pelvis**

D41.2 **Neoplasm of uncertain behavior of ureter**

D41.20 **Neoplasm of uncertain behavior of unspecified ureter**

D41.21 **Neoplasm of uncertain behavior of right ureter**

D41.22 **Neoplasm of uncertain behavior of left ureter**

D41.3 **Neoplasm of uncertain behavior of urethra**

D41.4 **Neoplasm of uncertain behavior of bladder**

D41.8 **Neoplasm of uncertain behavior of other specified urinary organs**

D41.9 **Neoplasm of uncertain behavior of unspecified urinary organ**

D42 **Neoplasm of uncertain behavior of meninges**

D42.0 **Neoplasm of uncertain behavior of cerebral meninges**

D42.1 **Neoplasm of uncertain behavior of spinal meninges**

D42.9 **Neoplasm of uncertain behavior of meninges, unspecified**

D43 **Neoplasm of uncertain behavior of brain and central nervous system**

Excludes1: neoplasm of uncertain behavior of peripheral nerves and autonomic nervous system (D48.2)

D43.0 **Neoplasm of uncertain behavior of brain, supratentorial**

Neoplasm of uncertain behavior of cerebral ventricle

Neoplasm of uncertain behavior of cerebrum

Neoplasm of uncertain behavior of frontal lobe

Neoplasm of uncertain behavior of occipital lobe

Neoplasm of uncertain behavior of parietal lobe

Neoplasm of uncertain behavior of temporal lobe

Excludes1: neoplasm of uncertain behavior of fourth ventricle (D43.1)

D43.1 **Neoplasm of uncertain behavior of brain, infratentorial**

Neoplasm of uncertain behavior of brain stem Neoplasm of uncertain behavior of cerebellum Neoplasm of uncertain behavior of fourth ventricle

D43.2 **Neoplasm of uncertain behavior of brain, unspecified**

D43.3 **Neoplasm of uncertain behavior of cranial nerves**

D43.4 **Neoplasm of uncertain behavior of spinal cord**

D43.8 **Neoplasm of uncertain behavior of other specified parts of central nervous system**

D43.9 **Neoplasm of uncertain behavior of central nervous system, unspecified**

Neoplasm of uncertain behavior of nervous system (central) NOS

D44 **Neoplasm of uncertain behavior of endocrine glands**

Excludes1: multiple endocrine adenomatosis (E31.2-)

multiple endocrine neoplasia (E31.2-)

neoplasm of uncertain behavior of endocrine pancreas (D37.8)

neoplasm of uncertain behavior of ovary (D39.1-)

neoplasm of uncertain behavior of testis (D40.1-)

neoplasm of uncertain behavior of thymus (D38.4)

D44.0 **Neoplasm of uncertain behavior of thyroid gland**

D44.1 **Neoplasm of uncertain behavior of adrenal gland**

Use additional code to identify any functional activity.

D44.10 **Neoplasm of uncertain behavior of unspecified adrenal gland**

D44.11 **Neoplasm of uncertain behavior of right adrenal gland**

D44.12 **Neoplasm of uncertain behavior of left adrenal gland**

D44.2 **Neoplasm of uncertain behavior of parathyroid gland**

D44.3 **Neoplasm of uncertain behavior of pituitary gland**

Use additional code to identify any functional activity.

D44.4 **Neoplasm of uncertain behavior of craniopharyngeal duct**

D44.5 **Neoplasm of uncertain behavior of pineal gland**

D44.6 **Neoplasm of uncertain behavior of carotid body**

D44.7 **Neoplasm of uncertain behavior of aortic body and other paraganglia**

D44.9 **Neoplasm of uncertain behavior of unspecified endocrine gland**

D45 **Polycythemia vera**

Excludes1: familial polycythemia (D75.0)

secondary polycythemia (D75.1)

D46 **Myelodysplastic syndromes**

Use additional code for adverse effect, if applicable, to identify drug (T36-T50 with fifth or sixth character 5)

Excludes2: drug-induced aplastic anemia (D61.1)

D46.0 **Refractory anemia without ring sideroblasts, so stated**

Refractory anemia without sideroblasts, without excess of blasts

D46.1 **Refractory anemia with ring sideroblasts**

RARS

D46.2 **Refractory anemia with excess of blasts [RAEB]**

D46.20 **Refractory anemia with excess of blasts, unspecified**

RAEB NOS

D46.21 **Refractory anemia with excess of blasts 1**

RAEB 1

D46.22 **Refractory anemia with excess of blasts 2**

RAEB 2

D46.A **Refractory cytopenia with multilineage dysplasia**

D46.B **Refractory cytopenia with multilineage dysplasia and ring sideroblasts**

RCMD RS

D46.C **Myelodysplastic syndrome with isolated del(5q) chromosomal abnormality**

Myelodysplastic syndrome with 5q deletion 5q minus syndrome NOS

D46.4 **Refractory anemia, unspecified**

D46.Z **Other myelodysplastic syndromes**

Excludes1: chronic myelomonocytic leukemia (C93.1-)

D46.9 **Myelodysplastic syndrome, unspecified**

Myelodysplasia NOS

D47 **Other neoplasms of uncertain behavior of lymphoid, hematopoietic and related tissue**

D47.0 **Histiocytic and mast cell tumors of uncertain behavior** Indolent systemic mastocytosis

Mast cell tumor NOS

Mastocytoma NOS

Excludes1: malignant mast cell tumor (C96.2)

mastocytosis (congenital) (cutaneous) (Q82.2)

D47.1 **Chronic myeloproliferative disease**

Chronic neutrophilic leukemia

Myeloproliferative disease, unspecified

Excludes1: atypical chronic myeloid leukemia BCR/ABL-negative (C92.2-)

chronic myeloid leukemia BCR/ABL-positive (C92.1-)

myelofibrosis NOS (D75.81)

myelophthisic anemia (D61.82)

myelophthisis (D61.82)

secondary myelofibrosis NOS (D75.81)

D47.2 **Monoclonal gammopathy**

Monoclonal gammopathy of undetermined significance [MGUS]

D47.3 **Essential (hemorrhagic) thrombocythemia**

Essential thrombocytosis

Idiopathic hemorrhagic thrombocythemia

D47.4 **Osteomyelofibrosis**

Chronic idiopathic myelofibrosis

Myelofibrosis (idiopathic) (with myeloid metaplasia)

Myelosclerosis (megakaryocytic) with myeloid metaplasia

Secondary myelofibrosis in myeloproliferative disease

Excludes1: acute myelofibrosis (C94.4-)

D47.Z **Other specified neoplasms of uncertain behavior of lymphoid, hematopoietic and related tissue**

D47.Z1 **Post-transplant lymphoproliferative disorder (PTLD)**

Code first complications of transplanted organs and tissue (T86.-)

• **D47.Z2** **Castleman disease**

Code also if applicable human herpesvirus 8 infection (B10.89)

Excludes2: Kaposi's sarcoma (C46-)

D47.Z9 **Other specified neoplasms of uncertain behavior of lymphoid, hematopoietic and related tissue**

Histiocytic tumors of uncertain behavior

D47.9 **Neoplasm of uncertain behavior of lymphoid, hematopoietic and related tissue, unspecified**

Lymphoproliferative disease NOS

D48 **Neoplasm of uncertain behavior of other and unspecified sites**

Excludes1: neurofibromatosis (nonmalignant) (Q85.0-)

D48.0 **Neoplasm of uncertain behavior of bone and articular cartilage**

Excludes1: neoplasm of uncertain behavior of cartilage of ear (D48.1)

neoplasm of uncertain behavior of cartilage of larynx (D38.0)

neoplasm of uncertain behavior of cartilage of nose (D38.5)

neoplasm of uncertain behavior of connective tissue of eyelid (D48.1)

neoplasm of uncertain behavior of synovia (D48.1)

D48.1 **Neoplasm of uncertain behavior of connective and other soft tissue**

Neoplasm of uncertain behavior of connective tissue of ear

Neoplasm of uncertain behavior of connective tissue of eyelid

Stromal tumors of uncertain behavior of digestive system

Excludes1: neoplasm of uncertain behavior of articular cartilage (D48.0)

neoplasm of uncertain behavior of cartilage of larynx (D38.0)

neoplasm of uncertain behavior of cartilage of nose (D38.5)

neoplasm of uncertain behavior of connective tissue of breast (D48.6-)

D48.2 **Neoplasm of uncertain behavior of peripheral nerves and autonomic nervous system**

Excludes1: neoplasm of uncertain behavior of peripheral nerves of orbit (D48.7)

D48.3 **Neoplasm of uncertain behavior of retroperitoneum**

D48.4 **Neoplasm of uncertain behavior of peritoneum**

D48.5 **Neoplasm of uncertain behavior of skin**

Neoplasm of uncertain behavior of anal margin

Neoplasm of uncertain behavior of anal skin

Neoplasm of uncertain behavior of perianal skin

Neoplasm of uncertain behavior of skin of breast

Excludes1: neoplasm of uncertain behavior of anus NOS (D37.8)

neoplasm of uncertain behavior of skin of genital organs (D39.8, D40.8)

neoplasm of uncertain behavior of vermilion border of lip (D37.0)

D48.6 **Neoplasm of uncertain behavior of breast**

Neoplasm of uncertain behavior of connective tissue of breast

Cystosarcoma phyllodes

Excludes1: neoplasm of uncertain behavior of skin of breast (D48.5)

D48.60 **Neoplasm of uncertain behavior of unspecified breast**

D48.61 **Neoplasm of uncertain behavior of right breast**

D48.62 **Neoplasm of uncertain behavior of left breast**

D48.7 **Neoplasm of uncertain behavior of other specified sites**

Neoplasm of uncertain behavior of eye Neoplasm of uncertain behavior of heart

Neoplasm of uncertain behavior of peripheral nerves of orbit

Excludes1: neoplasm of uncertain behavior of connective tissue (D48.1)

neoplasm of uncertain behavior of skin of eyelid (D48.5)

D48.9 **Neoplasm of uncertain behavior, unspecified**

NEOPLASMS OF UNSPECIFIED BEHAVIOR (D49)

D49 **Neoplasms of unspecified behavior Note:**

Category D49 classifies by site neoplasms of unspecified morphology and behavior. The term 'mass', unless otherwise stated, is not to be regarded as a neoplastic growth.

Includes: 'growth' NOS

neoplasm NOS

new growth NOS

tumor NOS

Excludes1: neoplasms of uncertain behavior (D37-D44, D48)

D49.0 **Neoplasm of unspecified behavior of digestive system**

Excludes1: neoplasm of unspecified behavior of margin of anus (D49.2)

neoplasm of unspecified behavior of perianal skin (D49.2)

neoplasm of unspecified behavior of skin of anus (D49.2)

D49.1 **Neoplasm of unspecified behavior of respiratory system**

D49.2 **Neoplasm of unspecified behavior of bone, soft tissue, and skin**

Excludes1: neoplasm of unspecified behavior of anal canal (D49.0)

neoplasm of unspecified behavior of anus NOS (D49.0)

neoplasm of unspecified behavior of bone marrow (D49.89)

neoplasm of unspecified behavior of cartilage of larynx (D49.1)

neoplasm of unspecified behavior of cartilage of nose (D49.1)

neoplasm of unspecified behavior of connective tissue of breast (D49.3)

neoplasm of unspecified behavior of skin of genital organs (D49.59)

neoplasm of unspecified behavior of vermilion border of lip (D49.0)

D49.3 **Neoplasm of unspecified behavior of breast**

Excludes1: neoplasm of unspecified behavior of skin of breast (D49.2)

D49.4 **Neoplasm of unspecified behavior of bladder**

D49.5 Neoplasm of unspecified behavior of other genitourinary organs

    D49.51 Neoplasm of unspecified behavior of kidney

        ●**D49.511** Neoplasm of unspecified behavior of right kidney

        ●**D49.512** Neoplasm of unspecified behavior of left kidney

        ●**D49.519** Neoplasm of unspecified behavior of unspecified kidney

    ●**D49.59** Neoplasm of unspecified behavior of other genitourinary organ

D49.6 Neoplasm of unspecified behavior of brain

    Excludes1: neoplasm of unspecified behavior of cerebral meninges (D49.7)

    neoplasm of unspecified behavior of cranial nerves (D49.7)

D49.7 Neoplasm of unspecified behavior of endocrine glands and other parts of nervous system

    Excludes1: neoplasm of unspecified behavior of peripheral, sympathetic, and parasympathetic nerves and ganglia (D49.2)

D49.8 Neoplasm of unspecified behavior of other specified sites

    Excludes1: neoplasm of unspecified behavior of eyelid (skin) (D49.2)

    neoplasm of unspecified behavior of eyelid cartilage (D49.2)

    neoplasm of unspecified behavior of great vessels (D49.2)

    neoplasm of unspecified behavior of optic nerve (D49.7)

    D49.81 Neoplasm of unspecified behavior of retina and choroid

    Dark area on retina

    Retinal freckle

    D49.89 Neoplasm of unspecified behavior of other specified sites

D49.9 Neoplasm of unspecified behavior of unspecified site

Chapter 3: Diseases Of The Blood And Blood-Forming Organs and Certain Disorders Involving The Immune Mechanism (D50-D89)

DEFINITIONS AND CODING ALERTS

This chapter includes definitions of selected key words, terms and phrases and coding alerts for adding points to the clinical domain, and references to coding late effects where appropriate. An example from this chapter is as follows:

D50 Iron deficiency anemia
Definition: Iron deficiency anemia is a form of anemia due to lack of iron in the diet or to iron loss as a result of chronic bleeding.

MULTIPLE CODING FOR A SINGLE CONDITION

In addition to the etiology/manifestation convention that requires two codes to fully describe a single condition that affects multiple body systems, there are other single conditions that also require more than one code. "Use additional code" notes are found in the Tabular List at codes that are not part of an etiology/manifestation pair where a secondary code is useful to fully describe a condition. The sequencing rule is the same as the etiology/manifestation pair, "use additional code" indicates that a secondary code should be added.

For example, for bacterial infections that are not included in chapter 1, a secondary code from category B95, Streptococcus, Staphylococcus, and Enterococcus, as the cause of diseases classified elsewhere, or B96, Other bacterial agents as the cause of diseases classified elsewhere, may be required to identify the bacterial organism causing the infection. A "use additional code" note will normally be found at the infectious disease code, indicating a need for the organism code to be added as a secondary code.

"Code first" notes are also under certain codes that are not specifically manifestation codes but may be due to an underlying cause. When there is a "code first" note and an underlying condition is present, the underlying condition should be sequenced first.

"Code, if applicable, any causal condition first", notes indicate that this code may be assigned as a principal diagnosis when the causal condition is unknown or not applicable. If a causal condition is known, then the code for that condition should be sequenced as the principal or first-listed diagnosis.

Multiple codes may be needed for sequela, complication codes and obstetric codes to more fully describe a condition. See the specific guidelines for these conditions for further instruction.

COMBINATION CODE

A combination code is a single code used to classify: Two diagnoses, or a diagnosis with an associated secondary process (manifestation) A diagnosis with an associated complication

Combination codes are identified by referring to subterm entries in the Alphabetic Index and by reading the inclusion and exclusion notes in the Tabular List.

Assign only the combination code when that code fully identifies the diagnostic conditions involved or when the Alphabetic Index so directs. Multiple coding should not be used when the classification provides a combination code that clearly identifies all of the elements documented in the diagnosis. When the combination code lacks necessary specificity in describing the manifestation or complication, an additional code should be used as a secondary code.

SEQUELA (LATE EFFECTS)

A sequela is the residual effect (condition produced) after the acute phase of an illness or injury has terminated. There is no time limit on when a sequela code can be used. The residual may be apparent early, such as in cerebral infarction, or it may occur months or years later, such as that due to a previous injury. Coding of sequela generally requires two codes sequenced in the following order: The condition or nature of the sequela is sequenced first.

The sequela code is sequenced second.

An exception to the above guidelines are those instances where the code for the sequela is followed by a manifestation code identified in the Tabular List and title, or the sequela code has been expanded (at the fourth, fifth or sixth character levels) to include the manifestation(s). The code for the acute phase of an illness or injury that led to the sequela is never used with a code for the late effect.

Chapter 3

Diseases of the Blood and Blood-Forming Organs and Certain Disorders Involving the Immune Mechanism (D50-D89)

Excludes2: autoimmune disease (systemic) NOS (M35.9)

certain conditions originating in the perinatal period (P00-P96)

complications of pregnancy, childbirth and the puerperium (O00-O9A)

congenital malformations, deformations and chromosomal abnormalities (Q00-Q99)

endocrine, nutritional and metabolic diseases (E00-E88)

human immunodeficiency virus [HIV] disease (B20)

injury, poisoning and certain other consequences of external causes (S00-T88)

neoplasms (C00-D49)

symptoms, signs and abnormal clinical and laboratory findings, not elsewhere classified (R00-R94)

This chapter contains the following blocks:

D50-D53 Nutritional anemias

D55-D59 Hemolytic anemias

D60-D64 Aplastic and other anemias and other bone marrow failure syndromes

D65-D69 Coagulation defects, purpura and other hemorrhagic conditions

D70-D77 Other disorders of blood and blood-forming organs

D78 Intraoperative and postprocedural complications of the spleen

D80-D89 Certain disorders involving the immune mechanism

NUTRITIONAL ANEMIAS (D50-D53)

D50 **Iron deficiency anemia**

Includes: asiderotic anemia

hypochromic anemia

D50.0 **Iron deficiency anemia secondary to blood loss (chronic)**

Posthemorrhagic anemia (chronic)

Excludes1: acute posthemorrhagic anemia (D62)

congenital anemia from fetal blood loss (P61.3)

D50.1 **Sideropenic dysphagia**

Kelly-Paterson syndrome

Plummer-Vinson syndrome

D50.8 **Other iron deficiency anemias**

Iron deficiency anemia due to inadequate dietary iron intake

D50.9 **Iron deficiency anemia, unspecified**

D51 **Vitamin B12 deficiency anemia**

Excludes1: vitamin B12 deficiency (E53.8)

D51.0 **Vitamin B12 deficiency anemia due to intrinsic factor deficiency**

Addison anemia

Biermer anemia

Pernicious (congenital) anemia

Congenital intrinsic factor deficiency

D51.1 **Vitamin B12 deficiency anemia due to selective vitamin B12 malabsorption with proteinuria**

Imerslund (Gräsbeck) syndrome

Megaloblastic hereditary anemia

D51.2 **Transcobalamin II deficiency**

D51.3 **Other dietary vitamin B12 deficiency anemia**

Vegan anemia

D51.8 **Other vitamin B12 deficiency anemias**

D51.9 **Vitamin B12 deficiency anemia, unspecified**

D52 **Folate deficiency anemia**

Excludes1: folate deficiency without anemia (E53.8)

D52.0 **Dietary folate deficiency anemia**

Nutritional megaloblastic anemia

D52.1 **Drug-induced folate deficiency anemia**

Use additional code for adverse effect, if applicable, to identify drug (T36-T50 with fifth or sixth character 5)

D52.8 **Other folate deficiency anemias**

D52.9 **Folate deficiency anemia, unspecified**

Folic acid deficiency anemia NOS

D53 **Other nutritional anemias**

Includes: megaloblastic anemia unresponsive to vitamin B12 or folate therapy

D53.0 **Protein deficiency anemia**

Amino-acid deficiency anemia

Orotaciduric anemia

Excludes1: Lesch-Nyhan syndrome (E79.1)

D53.1 **Other megaloblastic anemias, not elsewhere classified**

Megaloblastic anemia NOS

Excludes1: Di Guglielmo's disease (C94.0)

D53.2 **Scorbutic anemia**

Excludes1: scurvy (E54)

D53.8 **Other specified nutritional anemias**

Anemia associated with deficiency of copper

Anemia associated with deficiency of molybdenum

Anemia associated with deficiency of zinc

Excludes1: nutritional deficiencies without anemia, such as:

copper deficiency NOS (E61.0)

molybdenum deficiency NOS (E61.5)

zinc deficiency NOS (E60)

D53.9 **Nutritional anemia, unspecified**

Simple chronic anemia

Excludes1: anemia NOS (D64.9)

HEMOLYTIC ANEMIAS (D55-D59)

D55 **Anemia due to enzyme disorders**

Excludes1: drug-induced enzyme deficiency anemia (D59.2)

D55.0 **Anemia due to glucose-6-phosphate dehydrogenase [G6PD] deficiency**

Favism

G6PD deficiency anemia

D55.1 **Anemia due to other disorders of glutathione metabolism**

Anemia (due to) enzyme deficiencies, except G6PD, related to the hexose monophosphate [HMP] shunt pathway

Anemia (due to) hemolytic nonspherocytic (hereditary), type I

D55.2 **Anemia due to disorders of glycolytic enzymes**

Hemolytic nonspherocytic (hereditary) anemia, type II

Hexokinase deficiency anemia

Pyruvate kinase [PK] deficiency anemia

Triose-phosphate isomerase deficiency anemia

Excludes1: disorders of glycolysis not associated with anemia (E74.8)

D55.3 **Anemia due to disorders of nucleotide metabolism**

D55.8 **Other anemias due to enzyme disorders**

D55.9 **Anemia due to enzyme disorder, unspecified**

D56 **Thalassemia**

Excludes1: sickle-cell thalassemia (D57.4-)

D56.0 **Alpha thalassemia**

Alpha thalassemia major

Hemoglobin H Constant Spring

Hemoglobin H disease

Hydrops fetalis due to alpha thalassemia

Severe alpha thalassemia

Triple gene defect alpha thalassemia

Use additional code, if applicable, for hydrops fetalis due to alpha thalassemia (P56.99)

Excludes1: alpha thalassemia trait or minor (D56.3)

asymptomatic alpha thalassemia (D56.3)

hydrops fetalis due to isoimmunization (P56.0)

hydrops fetalis not due to immune hemolysis (P83.2)

D56.1 **Beta thalassemia**

Beta thalassemia major Cooley's anemia

Homozygous beta thalassemia

Severe beta thalassemia

Thalassemia intermedia

Thalassemia major

Excludes1: beta thalassemia minor (D56.3)

beta thalassemia trait (D56.3)

delta-beta thalassemia (D56.2)

hemoglobin E-beta thalassemia (D56.5)

sickle-cell beta thalassemia (D57.4-)

D56.2 **Delta-beta thalassemia**

Homozygous delta-beta thalassemia

Excludes1: delta-beta thalassemia minor (D56.3)

delta-beta thalassemia trait (D56.3)

D56.3 **Thalassemia minor** Alpha thalassemia minor
Alpha thalassemia silent carrier

Alpha thalassemia trait

Beta thalassemia minor Beta thalassemia trait

Delta-beta thalassemia minor

Delta-beta thalassemia trait

Thalassemia trait NOS

Excludes1: alpha thalassemia (D56.0)

beta thalassemia (D56.1)

delta-beta thalassemia (D56.2)

hemoglobin E-beta thalassemia (D56.5)

sickle-cell trait (D57.3)

D56.4 **Hereditary persistence of fetal hemoglobin [HPFH]**

D56.5 **Hemoglobin E-beta thalassemia**

Excludes1: beta thalassemia (D56.1)

beta thalassemia minor (D56.3)

beta thalassemia trait (D56.3)

delta-beta thalassemia (D56.2)

delta-beta thalassemia trait (D56.3)

hemoglobin E disease (D58.2)

Other hemoglobinopathies (D58.2)

sickle-cell beta thalassemia (D57.4-)

D56.8 **Other thalassemias**

Dominant thalassemia

Hemoglobin C thalassemia

Mixed thalassemia

Thalassemia **with other** hemoglobinopathy

Excludes1: hemoglobin C disease (D58.2)

hemoglobin E disease (D58.2)

Other hemoglobinopathies (D58.2)

sickle-cell anemia (D57.-)

sickle-cell thalassemia (D57.4)

D56.9 **Thalassemia, unspecified**

Mediterranean anemia (**with other** hemoglobinopathy)

D57 **Sickle-cell disorders**

Use additional code for any associated fever (R50.81)

Excludes1: Other hemoglobinopathies (D58.-)

D57.0 **Hb-SS disease with crisis**

Sickle-cell disease NOS with crisis

Hb-SS disease with vasoocclusive pain

D57.00 **Hb-SS disease with crisis, unspecified**

D57.01 **Hb-SS disease with acute chest syndrome**

D57.02 **Hb-SS disease with splenic sequestration**

D57.1 **Sickle-cell disease without crisis**

Hb-SS disease without crisis

Sickle-cell anemia NOS

Sickle-cell disease NOS

Sickle-cell disorder NOS

D57.2 **Sickle-cell/Hb-C disease**

Hb-SC disease

Hb-S/Hb-C disease

D57.20 **Sickle-cell/Hb-C disease without crisis**

D57.21 **Sickle-cell/Hb-C disease with crisis**

D57.211 **Sickle-cell/Hb-C disease with acute chest syndrome**

D57.212 **Sickle-cell/Hb-C disease with splenic sequestration**

D57.219 **Sickle-cell/Hb-C disease with crisis, unspecified**

Sickle-cell/Hb-C disease with crisis NOS

D57.3 **Sickle-cell trait**

Hb-S trait

Heterozygous hemoglobin S

D57.4 **Sickle-cell thalassemia**

Sickle-cell beta thalassemia

Thalassemia Hb-S disease

D57.40 Sickle-cell thalassemia without crisis
Microdrepanocytosis
Sickle-cell thalassemia NOS

D57.41 Sickle-cell thalassemia with crisis
Sickle-cell thalassemia with vasoocclusive pain

D57.411 Sickle-cell thalassemia with acute chest syndrome

D57.412 Sickle-cell thalassemia with splenic sequestration

D57.419 Sickle-cell thalassemia with crisis, unspecified
Sickle-cell thalassemia with crisis NOS

D57.8 Other sickle-cell disorders
Hb-SD disease Hb-SE disease

D57.80 Other sickle-cell disorders without crisis

D57.81 Other sickle-cell disorders with crisis

D57.811 Other sickle-cell disorders with acute chest syndrome

D57.812 Other sickle-cell disorders with splenic sequestration

D57.819 Other sickle-cell disorders with crisis, unspecified
Other sickle-cell disorders with crisis NOS

D58 Other hereditary hemolytic anemias
Excludes1: hemolytic anemia of the newborn (P55.-)

D58.0 Hereditary spherocytosis
Acholuric (familial) jaundice
Congenital (spherocytic) hemolytic icterus
Minkowski-Chauffard syndrome

D58.1 Hereditary elliptocytosis
Elliptocytosis (congenital)
Ovalocytosis (congenital) (hereditary)

D58.2 Other hemoglobinopathies
Abnormal hemoglobin NOS
Congenital Heinz body anemia
Hb-C disease
Hb-D disease
Hb-E disease
Hemoglobinopathy NOS
Unstable hemoglobin hemolytic disease
Excludes1: familial polycythemia (D75.0)
Hb-M disease (D74.0)
hemoglobin E-beta thalassemia (D56.5)
hereditary persistence of fetal hemoglobin [HPFH] (D56.4)
high-altitude polycythemia (D75.1)
methemoglobinemia (D74.-)
Other hemoglobinopathies with thalassemia (D56.8)

D58.8 Other specified hereditary hemolytic anemias
Stomatocytosis

D58.9 Hereditary hemolytic anemia, unspecified

D59 Acquired hemolytic anemia

D59.0 Drug-induced autoimmune hemolytic anemia
Use additional code for adverse effect, if applicable, to identify drug (T36-T50 with fifth or sixth character 5)

D59.1 Other autoimmune hemolytic anemias
Autoimmune hemolytic disease (cold type) (warm type)
Chronic cold hemagglutinin disease
Cold agglutinin disease
Cold agglutinin hemoglobinuria
Cold type (secondary) (symptomatic) hemolytic anemia
Warm type (secondary) (symptomatic) hemolytic anemia
Excludes1: Evans syndrome (D69.41)
hemolytic disease of newborn (P55.-)
paroxysmal cold hemoglobinuria (D59.6)

D59.2 Drug-induced nonautoimmune hemolytic anemia
Drug-induced enzyme deficiency anemia
Use additional code for adverse effect, if applicable, to identify drug (T36-T50 with fifth or sixth character 5)

D59.3 Hemolytic-uremic syndrome
Use additional code to identify associated:
E. coli infection (B96.2-)
Pneumococcal pneumonia (J13)
Shigella dysenteriae (A03.9)

D59.4 Other nonautoimmune hemolytic anemias
Mechanical hemolytic anemia
Microangiopathic hemolytic anemia
Toxic hemolytic anemia

D59.5 Paroxysmal nocturnal hemoglobinuria [Marchiafava-Micheli]
Excludes1: hemoglobinuria NOS (R82.3)

D59.6 Hemoglobinuria due to hemolysis from other external causes
Hemoglobinuria from exertion
March hemoglobinuria
Paroxysmal cold hemoglobinuria
Use additional code (Chapter 20) to identify external cause
Excludes1: hemoglobinuria NOS (R82.3)

D59.8 Other acquired hemolytic anemias

D59.9 Acquired hemolytic anemia, unspecified
Idiopathic hemolytic anemia, chronic

APLASTIC AND OTHER ANEMIAS AND OTHER BONE MARROW FAILURE SYNDROMES (D60-D64)

D60 Acquired pure red cell aplasia [erythroblastopenia]
Includes: red cell aplasia (acquired) (adult) (with thymoma)
Excludes1: congenital red cell aplasia (D61.01)

D60.0 Chronic acquired pure red cell aplasia

D60.1 Transient acquired pure red cell aplasia

D60.8 Other acquired pure red cell aplasias

D60.9 Acquired pure red cell aplasia, unspecified

D61 Other aplastic anemias and other bone marrow failure syndromes
Excludes1: neutropenia (D70.-)

D61.0 Constitutional aplastic anemia

D61.01 Constitutional (pure) red blood cell aplasia
Blackfan-Diamond syndrome
Congenital (pure) red cell aplasia
Familial hypoplastic anemia

Primary (pure) red cell aplasia

Red cell (pure) aplasia of infants

> **Excludes1:** acquired red cell aplasia (D60.9)

D61.09 **Other constitutional aplastic anemia**

Fanconi's anemia

Pancytopenia with malformations

D61.1 **Drug-induced aplastic anemia**

Use additional code for adverse effect, if applicable, to identify drug (T36-T50 with fifth or sixth character 5)

D61.2 **Aplastic anemia due to other external agents**

Code first, if applicable, toxic effects of substances chiefly nonmedicinal as to source (T51-T65)

D61.3 **Idiopathic aplastic anemia**

D61.8 **Other specified aplastic anemias and other bone marrow failure syndromes**

D61.81 **Pancytopenia**

> **Excludes1:** pancytopenia (due to) (with) aplastic anemia (D61.9)
>
> pancytopenia (due to) (with) bone marrow infiltration (D61.82)
>
> pancytopenia (due to) (with) congenital (pure) red cell aplasia (D61.01)
>
> pancytopenia (due to) (with) hairy cell leukemia (C91.4-)
>
> pancytopenia (due to) (with) human immunodeficiency virus disease (B20.-)
>
> pancytopenia (due to) (with) leukoerythroblastic anemia (D61.82)
>
> pancytopenia (due to) (with) myeloproliferative disease (D47.1)

> **Excludes2:** pancytopenia (due to) (with) myelodysplastic syndromes (D46.-)

D61.810 **Antineoplastic chemotherapy induced pancytopenia**

> **Excludes2:** aplastic anemia due to antineoplastic chemotherapy (D61.1)

D61.811 **Other drug-induced pancytopenia**

> **Excludes2:** aplastic anemia due to drugs (D61.1)

D61.818 **Other pancytopenia**

D61.82 **Myelophthisis**

Leukoerythroblastic anemia

Myelophthisic anemia

Panmyelophthisis

Code also the underlying disorder, such as:

malignant neoplasm of breast (C50.-)

tuberculosis (A15.-)

> **Excludes1:** idiopathic myelofibrosis (D47.1)
>
> myelofibrosis NOS (D75.81)
>
> myelofibrosis with myeloid metaplasia (D47.4)
>
> primary myelofibrosis (D47.1)
>
> secondary myelofibrosis (D75.81)

D61.89 **Other specified aplastic anemias and other bone marrow failure syndromes**

D61.9 **Aplastic anemia, unspecified**

Hypoplastic anemia NOS

Medullary hypoplasia

D62 **Acute posthemorrhagic anemia**

> **Excludes1:** anemia due to chronic blood loss (D50.0)
>
> blood loss anemia NOS (D50.0)
>
> congenital anemia from fetal blood loss (P61.3)

D63 **Anemia in chronic diseases classified elsewhere**

D63.0 **Anemia in neoplastic disease**

Code first neoplasm (C00-D49)

> **Excludes1:** anemia due to antineoplastic chemotherapy (D64.81)

aplastic anemia due to antineoplastic chemotherapy (D61.1)

D63.1 **Anemia in chronic kidney disease**

Erythropoietin resistant anemia (EPO resistant anemia)

Code first underlying chronic kidney disease (CKD) (N18.-)

D63.8 **Anemia in other chronic diseases classified elsewhere**

Code first underlying disease, such as:

diphyllobothriasis (B70.0)

hookworm disease (B76.0-B76.9)

hypothyroidism (E00.0-E03.9)

malaria (B50.0-B54)

symptomatic late syphilis (A52.79)

tuberculosis (A18.89)

D64 **Other anemias**

> **Excludes1:** refractory anemia (D46.-)
>
> refractory anemia with excess blasts in transformation [RAEB T] (C92.0-)

D64.0 **Hereditary sideroblastic anemia**

Sex-linked hypochromic sideroblastic anemia

D64.1 **Secondary sideroblastic anemia due to disease**

Code first underlying disease

D64.2 **Secondary sideroblastic anemia due to drugs and toxins**

Code first poisoning due to drug or toxin, if applicable (T36-T65 with fifth or sixth character 1-4 or 6)

Use additional code for adverse effect, if applicable, to identify drug (T36-T50 with fifth or sixth character 5)

D64.3 **Other sideroblastic anemias**

Sideroblastic anemia NOS

Pyridoxine-responsive sideroblastic anemia NEC

D64.4 **Congenital dyserythropoietic anemia**

Dyshematopoietic anemia (congenital)

> **Excludes1:** Blackfan-Diamond syndrome (D61.01)
>
> Di Guglielmo's disease (C94.0)

D64.8 **Other specified anemias**

D64.81 **Anemia due to antineoplastic chemotherapy**

Antineoplastic chemotherapy induced anemia

> **Excludes1:** aplastic anemia due to antineoplastic chemotherapy (D61.1)
>
> **Excludes2:** anemia in neoplastic disease (D63.0)

D64.89 **Other specified anemias**

Infantile pseudoleukemia

D64.9 **Anemia, unspecified**

COAGULATION DEFECTS, PURPURA AND OTHER HEMORRHAGIC CONDITIONS (D65-D69)

D65   Disseminated intravascular coagulation [defibrination syndrome]

Afibrinogenemia, acquired

Consumption coagulopathy

Diffuse or disseminated intravascular coagulation [DIC]

Fibrinolytic hemorrhage, acquired

Fibrinolytic purpura

Purpura fulminans

Excludes1: disseminated intravascular coagulation (complicating):

abortion or ectopic or molar pregnancy (O00-O07, O08.1)

in newborn (P60)

pregnancy, childbirth and the puerperium (O45.0, O46.0, O67.0, O72.3)

D66   Hereditary factor VIII deficiency

Classical hemophilia

Deficiency factor VIII (with functional defect)

Hemophilia NOS

Hemophilia A

Excludes1: factor VIII deficiency with vascular defect (D68.0)

D67   Hereditary factor IX deficiency

Christmas disease

Factor IX deficiency (with functional defect)

Hemophilia B

Plasma thromboplastin component [PTC] deficiency

D68   Other coagulation defects

Excludes1: abnormal coagulation profile (R79.1)

coagulation defects complicating abortion or ectopic or molar pregnancy (O00-O07, O08.1)

coagulation defects complicating pregnancy, childbirth and the puerperium (O45.0, O46.0, O67.0, O72.3)

D68.0   Von Willebrand's disease

Angiohemophilia

Factor VIII deficiency with vascular defect

Vascular hemophilia

Excludes1: capillary fragility (hereditary) (D69.8)

factor VIII deficiency NOS (D66)

factor VIII deficiency with functional defect (D66)

D68.1   Hereditary factor XI deficiency

Hemophilia C

Plasma thromboplastin antecedent [PTA] deficiency

Rosenthal's disease

D68.2   Hereditary deficiency of other clotting factors

AC globulin deficiency

Congenital afibrinogenemia

Deficiency of factor I [fibrinogen]

Deficiency of factor II [prothrombin]

Deficiency of factor V [labile]

Deficiency of factor VII [stable]

Deficiency of factor X [Stuart-Prower]

Deficiency of factor XII [Hageman]

Deficiency of factor XIII [fibrin stabilizing]

Dysfibrinogenemia (congenital)

Hypoproconvertinemia

Owren's disease

Proaccelerin deficiency

D68.3   Hemorrhagic disorder due to circulating anticoagulants

D68.31   Hemorrhagic disorder due to intrinsic circulating anticoagulants, antibodies, or inhibitors

D68.311   Acquired hemophilia

Autoimmune hemophilia

Autoimmune inhibitors to clotting factors

Secondary hemophilia

D68.312   Antiphospholipid antibody with hemorrhagic disorder

Lupus anticoagulant (LAC) with hemorrhagic disorder

Systemic lupus erythematosus [SLE] inhibitor with hemorrhagic disorder

Excludes1: antiphospholipid antibody, finding without diagnosis (R76.0)

antiphospholipid antibody syndrome (D68.61)

antiphospholipid antibody with hypercoagulable state (D68.61)

lupus anticoagulant (LAC) finding without diagnosis (R76.0)

lupus anticoagulant (LAC) with hypercoagulable state (D68.62)

systemic lupus erythematosus [SLE] inhibitor finding without diagnosis (R76.0)

systemic lupus erythematosus [SLE] inhibitor with hypercoagulable state (D68.62)

D68.318   Other hemorrhagic disorder due to intrinsic circulating anticoagulants, antibodies, or inhibitors

Antithromboplastinemia

Antithromboplastinogenemia

Hemorrhagic disorder due to intrinsic increase in antithrombin

Hemorrhagic disorder due to intrinsic increase in anti-VIIIa

Hemorrhagic disorder due to intrinsic increase in anti-IXa

Hemorrhagic disorder due to intrinsic increase in anti-XIa

D68.32   Hemorrhagic disorder due to extrinsic circulating anticoagulants

Drug-induced hemorrhagic disorder

Hemorrhagic disorder due to increase in anti-IIa

Hemorrhagic disorder due to increase in anti-Xa

Hyperheparinemia

Use additional code for adverse effect, if applicable, to identify drug (T45.515, T45.525)

D68.4   Acquired coagulation factor deficiency

Deficiency of coagulation factor due to liver disease

Deficiency of coagulation factor due to vitamin K deficiency

Excludes1: vitamin K deficiency of newborn (P53)

D68.5 **Primary thrombophilia**

Primary hypercoagulable states

Excludes1: antiphospholipid syndrome (D68.61)

lupus anticoagulant (D68.62)

secondary activated protein C resistance (D68.69)

secondary antiphospholipid antibody syndrome (D68.69)

secondary lupus anticoagulant with hypercoagulable state (D68.69)

secondary systemic lupus erythematosus [SLE] inhibitor with hypercoagulable state (D68.69)

systemic lupus erythematosus [SLE] inhibitor finding without diagnosis (R76.0)

systemic lupus erythematosus [SLE] inhibitor with hemorrhagic disorder (D68.312)

thrombotic thrombocytopenic purpura (M31.1)

D68.51 **Activated protein C resistance**

Factor V Leiden mutation

D68.52 **Prothrombin gene mutation**

D68.59 **Other primary thrombophilia**

Antithrombin III deficiency

Hypercoagulable state NOS

Primary hypercoagulable state NEC

Primary thrombophilia NEC

Protein C deficiency

Protein S deficiency

Thrombophilia NOS

D68.6 **Other thrombophilia**

Other hypercoagulable states

Excludes1: diffuse or disseminated intravascular coagulation [DIC] (D65)

heparin induced thrombocytopenia (HIT) (D75.82)

hyperhomocysteinemia (E72.11)

D68.61 **Antiphospholipid syndrome**

Anticardiolipin syndrome

Antiphospholipid antibody syndrome

Excludes1: anti-phospholipid antibody, finding without diagnosis (R76.0)

anti-phospholipid antibody with hemorrhagic disorder (D68.312)

lupus anticoagulant syndrome (D68.62)

D68.62 **Lupus anticoagulant syndrome**

Lupus anticoagulant

Presence of systemic lupus erythematosus [SLE] inhibitor

Excludes1: anticardiolipin syndrome (D68.61)

antiphospholipid syndrome (D68.61)

lupus anticoagulant (LAC) finding without diagnosis (R76.0)

lupus anticoagulant (LAC) with hemorrhagic disorder (D68.312)

D68.69 **Other thrombophilia**

Hypercoagulable states NEC

Secondary hypercoagulable state NOS

D68.8 **Other specified coagulation defects**

Excludes1: hemorrhagic disease of newborn (P53)

D68.9 **Coagulation defect, unspecified**

D69 **Purpura and other hemorrhagic conditions**

Excludes1: benign hypergammaglobulinemic purpura (D89.0)

cryoglobulinemic purpura (D89.1)

essential (hemorrhagic) thrombocythemia (D47.3)

hemorrhagic thrombocythemia (D47.3)

purpura fulminans (D65)

thrombotic thrombocytopenic purpura (M31.1)

Waldenström hypergammaglobulinemic purpura (D89.0)

D69.0 **Allergic purpura**

Allergic vasculitis

Nonthrombocytopenic hemorrhagic purpura

Nonthrombocytopenic idiopathic purpura

Purpura anaphylactoid

Purpura Henoch(-Schönlein)

Purpura rheumatica

Vascular purpura

Excludes1: thrombocytopenic hemorrhagic purpura (D69.3)

D69.1 **Qualitative platelet defects**

Bernard-Soulier [giant platelet] syndrome Glanzmann's disease

Grey platelet syndrome

Thromboasthenia (hemorrhagic) (hereditary)

Thrombocytopathy

Excludes1: von Willebrand's disease (D68.0)

D69.2 **Other nonthrombocytopenic purpura**

Purpura NOS

Purpura simplex

Senile purpura

D69.3 **Immune thrombocytopenic purpura**

Hemorrhagic (thrombocytopenic) purpura

Idiopathic thrombocytopenic purpura

Tidal platelet dysgenesis

D69.4 **Other primary thrombocytopenia**

Excludes1: transient neonatal thrombocytopenia (P61.0)

Wiskott-Aldrich syndrome (D82.0)

D69.41 **Evans syndrome**

D69.42 **Congenital and hereditary thrombocytopenia purpura**

Congenital thrombocytopenia

Hereditary thrombocytopenia

Code first congential or hereditary disorder, such as:

thrombocytopenia with absent radius (TAR syndrome) (Q87.2)

D69.49 **Other primary thrombocytopenia**

Megakaryocytic hypoplasia

Primary thrombocytopenia NOS

D69.5 **Secondary thrombocytopenia**

Excludes1: heparin induced thrombocytopenia (HIT) (D75.82)

transient thrombocytopenia of newborn (P61.0)

D69.51 Posttransfusion purpura

Posttransfusion purpura from whole blood (fresh) or blood products PTP

D69.59 Other secondary thrombocytopenia

D69.6 Thrombocytopenia, unspecified

D69.8 Other specified hemorrhagic conditions

Capillary fragility (hereditary)

Vascular pseudohemophilia

D69.9 Hemorrhagic condition, unspecified

OTHER DISORDERS OF BLOOD AND BLOOD-FORMING ORGANS (D70-D77)

D70 Neutropenia

Includes: agranulocytosis

decreased absolute neurophile count (ANC)

Use additional code for any associated:

fever (R50.81)

mucositis (J34.81, K12.3-, K92.81, N76.81)

Excludes1: neutropenic splenomegaly (D73.81)

transient neonatal neutropenia (P61.5)

D70.0 Congenital agranulocytosis

Congenital neutropenia

Infantile genetic agranulocytosis

Kostmann's disease

D70.1 Agranulocytosis secondary to cancer chemotherapy

Code also underlying neoplasm

Use additional code for adverse effect, if applicable, to identify drug (T45.1X5)

D70.2 Other drug-induced agranulocytosis

Use additional code for adverse effect, if applicable, to identify drug (T36-T50 with fifth or sixth character 5)

D70.3 Neutropenia due to infection

D70.4 Cyclic neutropenia

Cyclic hematopoiesis

Periodic neutropenia

D70.8 Other neutropenia

D70.9 Neutropenia, unspecified

D71 Functional disorders of polymorphonuclear neutrophils

Cell membrane receptor complex [CR3] defect

Chronic (childhood) granulomatous disease

Congenital dysphagocytosis

Progressive septic granulomatosis

D72 Other disorders of white blood cells

Definition: White blood cells, aka leukocyte, refers to any of various blood cells that help protect the body from infection and disease. White blood cells include neutrophils, eosinophils, basophils, lymphocytes, and monocytes

Excludes1: basophilia (D72.824)

immunity disorders (D80-D89)

neutropenia (D70)

preleukemia (syndrome) (D46.9)

D72.0 Genetic anomalies of leukocytes

Alder (granulation) (granulocyte) anomaly

Alder syndrome

Hereditary leukocytic hypersegmentation

Hereditary leukocytic hyposegmentation

Hereditary leukomelanopathy

May-Hegglin (granulation) (granulocyte) anomaly

May-Hegglin syndrome

Pelger-Huët (granulation) (granulocyte anomaly

Pelger-Huët syndrome

Excludes1: Chédiak (-Steinbrinck)-Higashi syndrome(E70.330)

D72.1 Eosinophilia

Allergic eosinophilia

Hereditary eosinophilia

Excludes1: Löffler's syndrome (J82)

pulmonary eosinophilia (J82)

D72.8 Other specified disorders of white blood cells

Excludes1: leukemia (C91-C95)

D72.81 Decreased white blood cell count

Excludes1: neutropenia (D70.-)

D72.810 Lymphocytopenia

Decreased lymphocytes

D72.818 Other decreased white blood cell count

Basophilic leukopenia Eosinophilic leukopenia

Monocytopenia

Other decreased leukocytes

Plasmacytopenia

D72.819 Decreased white blood cell count, unspecified

Decreased leukocytes, unspecified

Leukocytopenia, unspecified

Leukopenia

Excludes1: malignant leukopenia (D70.9)

D72.82 Elevated white blood cell count

Excludes1: eosinophilia (D72.1)

D72.820 Lymphocytosis (symptomatic)

Elevated lymphocytes

D72.821 Monocytosis (symptomatic)

Excludes1: infectious mononucleosis (B27.-)

D72.822 Plasmacytosis

D72.823 Leukemoid reaction

Basophilic leukemoid reaction

Leukemoid reaction NOS

Lymphocytic leukemoid reaction

Monocytic leukemoid reaction

Myelocytic leukemoid reaction

Neutrophilic leukemoid reaction

D72.824 Basophilia

D72.825 Bandemia

Bandemia without diagnosis of specific infection

Excludes1: confirmed infection - code to infection

leukemia (C91.-, C92.-, C93.-, C94.-, C95.-)

D72.828 **Other elevated white blood cell count**

D72.829 **Elevated white blood cell count, unspecified**

Elevated leukocytes, unspecified

Leukocytosis, unspecified

D72.89 **Other specified disorders of white blood cells**

Abnormality of white blood cells NEC

D72.9 **Disorder of white blood cells, unspecified**

Abnormal leukocyte differential NOS

D73 Diseases of spleen

D73.0 **Hyposplenism**

Atrophy of spleen

Excludes1: asplenia (congenital) (Q89.01)

postsurgical absence of spleen (Z90.81)

D73.1 **Hypersplenism**

Excludes1: neutropenic splenomegaly (D73.81)

primary splenic neutropenia (D73.81)

splenitis, splenomegaly in late syphilis (A52.79)

splenitis, splenomegaly in tuberculosis (A18.85)

splenomegaly NOS (R16.1)

splenomegaly congenital (Q89.0)

D73.2 **Chronic congestive splenomegaly**

D73.3 **Abscess of spleen**

D73.4 **Cyst of spleen**

D73.5 **Infarction of spleen**

Splenic rupture, nontraumatic

Torsion of spleen

Excludes1: rupture of spleen due to Plasmodium vivax malaria (B51.0)

traumatic rupture of spleen (S36.03-)

D73.8 **Other diseases of spleen**

D73.81 **Neutropenic splenomegaly**

Werner-Schultz disease

D73.89 **Other diseases of spleen**

Fibrosis of spleen NOS

Perisplenitis

Splenitis NOS

D73.9 **Disease of spleen, unspecified**

D74 Methemoglobinemia

D74.0 **Congenital methemoglobinemia**

Congenital NADH-methemoglobin reductase deficiency

Hemoglobin-M [Hb-M] disease

Methemoglobinemia, hereditary

D74.8 **Other methemoglobinemias**

Acquired methemoglobinemia (with sulfhemoglobinemia)

Toxic methemoglobinemia

D74.9 **Methemoglobinemia, unspecified**

D75 Other and unspecified diseases of blood and blood-forming organs

Excludes2: acute lymphadenitis (L04.-)

chronic lymphadenitis (I88.1)

enlarged lymph nodes (R59.-)

hypergammaglobulinemia NOS (D89.2)

lymphadenitis NOS (I88.9)

mesenteric lymphadenitis (acute) (chronic) (I88.0)

D75.0 **Familial erythrocytosis**

Benign polycythemia

Familial polycythemia

Excludes1: hereditary ovalocytosis (D58.1)

D75.1 **Secondary polycythemia**

Acquired polycythemia

Emotional polycythemia

Erythrocytosis NOS

Hypoxemic polycythemia

Nephrogenous polycythemia

Polycythemia due to erythropoietin

Polycythemia due to fall in plasma volume

Polycythemia due to high altitude

Polycythemia due to stress

Polycythemia NOS

Relative polycythemia

Excludes1: polycythemia neonatorum (P61.1)

polycythemia vera (D45)

D75.8 **Other specified diseases of blood and blood-forming organs**

D75.81 **Myelofibrosis**

Myelofibrosis NOS

Secondary myelofibrosis NOS

Code first the underlying disorder, such as:

malignant neoplasm of breast (C50.-)

Use additional code, if applicable, for associated therapy-related myelodysplastic syndrome (D46.-)

Use additional code for adverse effect, if applicable, to identify drug (T45.1X5)

Excludes1: acute myelofibrosis (C94.4-)

idiopathic myelofibrosis (D47.1)

leukoerythroblastic anemia (D61.82)

myelofibrosis with myeloid metaplasia (D47.4)

myelophthisic anemia (D61.82)

myelophthisis (D61.82)

primary myelofibrosis (D47.1)

D75.82 **Heparin induced thrombocytopenia (HIT)**

D75.89 **Other specified diseases of blood and blood-forming organs**

D75.9 **Disease of blood and blood-forming organs, unspecified**

D76 Other specified diseases with participation of lymphoreticular and reticulohistiocytic tissue

Excludes1: (Abt-) Letterer-Siwe disease (C96.0)

eosinophilic granuloma (C96.6)

Hand-Schüller-Christian disease (C96.5)

histiocytic medullary reticulosis (C96.9)

histiocytic sarcoma (C96.A)

histiocytosis X, multifocal (C96.5)

histiocytosis X, unifocal (C96.6)

Langerhans-cell histiocytosis, multifocal (C96.5)

Langerhans-cell histiocytosis NOS (C96.6)

Langerhans-cell histiocytosis, unifocal (C96.6)

leukemic reticuloendotheliosis (C91.4-)

lipomelanotic reticulosis (I89.8)

malignant histiocytosis (C96.A)

malignant reticulosis (C86.0)

nonlipid reticuloendotheliosis (C96.0)

D76.1 **Hemophagocytic lymphohistiocytosis**

Familial hemophagocytic reticulosis

Histiocytoses of mononuclear phagocytes

D76.2 **Hemophagocytic syndrome, infection-associated**

Use additional code to identify infectious agent or disease.

D76.3 **Other histiocytosis syndromes**

Reticulohistiocytoma (giant-cell)

Sinus histiocytosis with massive lymphadenopathy
Xanthogranuloma

D77 **Other disorders of blood and blood-forming organs in diseases classified elsewhere**

Code first underlying disease, such as:

amyloidosis (E85.-)

congenital early syphilis (A50.0)

echinococcosis (B67.0-B67.9)

malaria (B50.0-B54)

schistosomiasis [bilharziasis] (B65.0-B65.9)

vitamin C deficiency (E54)

Excludes1: rupture of spleen due to Plasmodium vivax malaria (B51.0)

splenitis, splenomegaly in late syphilis (A52.79)

splenitis, splenomegaly in tuberculosis (A18.85)

INTRAOPERATIVE AND POSTPROCEDURAL COMPLICATIONS OF THE SPLEEN (D78)

D78 **Intraoperative and postprocedural complications of the spleen**

D78.0 **Intraoperative hemorrhage and hematoma of the spleen complicating a procedure**

Excludes1: intraoperative hemorrhage and hematoma of the spleen due to accidental puncture or laceration during a procedure (D78.1-)

D78.01 **Intraoperative hemorrhage and hematoma of the spleen complicating a procedure on the spleen**

D78.02 **Intraoperative hemorrhage and hematoma of the spleen complicating other procedure**

D78.1 **Accidental puncture and laceration of the spleen during a procedure**

D78.11 **Accidental puncture and laceration of the spleen during a procedure on the spleen**

D78.12 **Accidental puncture and laceration of the spleen during other procedure**

D78.2 **Postprocedural hemorrhage of the spleen following a procedure**

▲**D78.21** **Postprocedural hemorrhage of the spleen following a procedure on the spleen**

▲**D78.22** **Postprocedural hemorrhage of the spleen following other procedure**

D78.3 **Postprocedural hematoma and seroma of the spleen following a procedure**

●**D78.31** **Postprocedural hematoma of the spleen following a procedure on the spleen**

●**D78.32** **Postprocedural hematoma of the spleen following other procedure**

●**D78.33** **Postprocedural seroma of the spleen following a procedure on the spleen**

●**D78.34** **Postprocedural seroma of the spleen following other procedure**

D78.8 **Other intraoperative and postprocedural complications of the spleen**

Use additional code, if applicable, to further specify disorder

D78.81 **Other intraoperative complications of the spleen**

D78.89 **Other postprocedural complications of the spleen**

CERTAIN DISORDERS INVOLVING THE IMMUNE MECHANISM (D80-D89)

Includes: defects in the complement system

immunodeficiency disorders, except human immunodeficiency virus [HIV] disease sarcoidosis

Excludes1: autoimmune disease (systemic) NOS (M35.9)

functional disorders of polymorphonuclear neutrophils (D71)

human immunodeficiency virus [HIV] disease (B20)

D80 **Immunodeficiency with predominantly antibody defects**

D80.0 **Hereditary hypogammaglobulinemia**

Autosomal recessive agammaglobulinemia (Swiss type)

X-linked agammaglobulinemia [Bruton] (with growth hormone deficiency)

D80.1 **Nonfamilial hypogammaglobulinemia**

Agammaglobulinemia with immunoglobulin-bearing B-lymphocytes

Common variable agammaglobulinemia [CVAgamma]

Hypogammaglobulinemia NOS

D80.2 **Selective deficiency of immunoglobulin A [IgA]**

D80.3 **Selective deficiency of immunoglobulin G [IgG] subclasses**

D80.4 **Selective deficiency of immunoglobulin M [IgM]**

D80.5 **Immunodeficiency with increased immunoglobulin M [IgM]**

D80.6 **Antibody deficiency with near-normal immunoglobulins or with hyperimmunoglobulinemia**

D80.7 **Transient hypogammaglobulinemia of infancy**

D80.8 **Other immunodeficiencies with predominantly antibody defects**

Kappa light chain deficiency

D80.9 **Immunodeficiency with predominantly antibody defects, unspecified**

D81 **Combined immunodeficiencies**

Excludes1: autosomal recessive agammaglobulinemia (Swiss type) (D80.0)

D81.0 **Severe combined immunodeficiency [SCID] with reticular dysgenesis**

D81.1 **Severe combined immunodeficiency [SCID] with low T- and B-cell numbers**

D81.2 **Severe combined immunodeficiency [SCID] with low or normal B-cell numbers**

D81.3 **Adenosine deaminase [ADA] deficiency**

D81.4 **Nezelof's syndrome**

D81.5   Purine nucleoside phosphorylase [PNP] deficiency

D81.6   Major histocompatibility complex class I deficiency

      Bare lymphocyte syndrome

D81.7   Major histocompatibility complex class II deficiency

D81.8   Other combined immunodeficiencies

      D81.81   Biotin-dependent carboxylase deficiency

           Multiple carboxylase deficiency

           Excludes1: biotin-dependent carboxylase deficiency due to dietary deficiency of biotin (E53.8)

           D81.810   Biotinidase deficiency

           D81.818   Other biotin-dependent carboxylase deficiency

               Holocarboxylase synthetase deficiency

               Other multiple carboxylase deficiency

           D81.819   Biotin-dependent carboxylase deficiency, unspecified

               Multiple carboxylase deficiency, unspecified

      D81.89   Other combined immunodeficiencies

D81.9   Combined immunodeficiency, unspecified

      Severe combined immunodeficiency disorder [SCID] NOS

D82   Immunodeficiency associated with other major defects

     Excludes1: ataxia telangiectasia [Louis-Bar] (G11.3)

D82.0   Wiskott-Aldrich syndrome

      Immunodeficiency with thrombocytopenia and eczema

D82.1   Di George's syndrome

      Pharyngeal pouch syndrome

      Thymic alymphoplasia

      Thymic aplasia or hypoplasia with immunodeficiency

D82.2   Immunodeficiency with short-limbed stature

D82.3   Immunodeficiency following hereditary defective response to Epstein-Barr virus

      X-linked lymphoproliferative disease

D82.4   Hyperimmunoglobulin E [IgE] syndrome

D82.8   Immunodeficiency associated with other specified major defects

D82.9   Immunodeficiency associated with major defect, unspecified

D83   Common variable immunodeficiency

D83.0   Common variable immunodeficiency with predominant abnormalities of B-cell numbers and function

D83.1   Common variable immunodeficiency with predominant immunoregulatory T-cell disorders

D83.2   Common variable immunodeficiency with autoantibodies to B- or T-cells

D83.8   Other common variable immunodeficiencies

D83.9   Common variable immunodeficiency, unspecified

D84   Other immunodeficiencies

D84.0   Lymphocyte function antigen-1[LFA-1] defect

D84.1   Defects in the complement system

      C1 esterase inhibitor [C1-INH] deficiency

D84.8   Other specified immunodeficiencies

D84.9   Immunodeficiency, unspecified

D86   Sarcoidosis

D86.0   Sarcoidosis of lung

D86.1   Sarcoidosis of lymph nodes

D86.2   Sarcoidosis of lung with sarcoidosis of lymph nodes

D86.3   Sarcoidosis of skin

D86.8   Sarcoidosis of other sites

      D86.81   Sarcoid meningitis

      D86.82   Multiple cranial nerve palsies in sarcoidosis

      D86.83   Sarcoid iridocyclitis

      D86.84   Sarcoid pyelonephritis

           Tubulo-interstitial nephropathy in sarcoidosis

      D86.85   Sarcoid myocarditis

      D86.86   Sarcoid arthropathy

           Polyarthritis in sarcoidosis

      D86.87   Sarcoid myositis

      D86.89   Sarcoidosis of other sites

           Hepatic granuloma

           Uveoparotid fever [Heerfordt]

D86.9   Sarcoidosis, unspecified

D89   Other disorders involving the immune mechanism, not elsewhere classified

     Excludes1: hyperglobulinemia NOS (R77.1)

      monoclonal gammopathy (of undetermined significance) (D47.2)

     Excludes2: transplant failure and rejection (T86.-)

D89.0   Polyclonal hypergammaglobulinemia

      Benign hypergammaglobulinemic purpura

      Polyclonal gammopathy NOS

D89.1   Cryoglobulinemia

      Cryoglobulinemic purpura

      Cryoglobulinemic vasculitis

      Essential cryoglobulinemia

      Idiopathic cryoglobulinemia

      Mixed cryoglobulinemia

      Primary cryoglobulinemia

      Secondary cryoglobulinemia

D89.2   Hypergammaglobulinemia, unspecified

D89.3   Immune reconstitution syndrome

      Immune reconstitution inflammatory syndrome [IRIS]

      <u>Use additional code</u> for adverse effect, if applicable, to identify drug (T36-T50 with fifth or sixth character 5)

D89.4   Mast cell activation syndrome and related disorders

      Excludes1: aggressive systemic mastocytosis (C96.2)

           cutaneous mastocytosis (Q82.2)

           indolent systemic mastocytosis (D47.0)

           malignant mastocytoma (C96.2)

           mast cell leukemia (C94.3-)

           mastocytoma (D47.0)

           systemic mastocytosis associated with a clonal hematologic non-mast cell lineage disease (SM-AHNMD) (D47.0)

      ●D89.40   Mast cell activation, unspecified

           Mast cell activation disorder, unspecified

           Mast cell activation syndrome, NOS

      ●D89.41   Monoclonal mast cell activation syndrome

      ●D89.42   Idiopathic mast cell activation syndrome

•**D89.43** **Secondary mast cell activation**

Secondary mast cell activation syndrome

Code also underlying etiology, if known

•**D89.49** **Other mast cell activation disorder**

Other mast cell activation syndrome

D89.8 **Other specified disorders involving the immune mechanism, not elsewhere classified**

D89.81 **Graft-versus-host disease**

Code first underlying cause, such as:

complications of transplanted organs and tissue (T86.-)

complications of blood transfusion (T80.89)

Use additional code to identify associated manifestations, such as:

desquamative dermatitis (L30.8)

diarrhea (R19.7)

elevated bilirubin (R17)

hair loss (L65.9)

D89.810 **Acute graft-versus-host disease**

D89.811 **Chronic graft-versus-host disease**

D89.812 **Acute on chronic graft-versus-host disease**

D89.813 **Graft-versus-host disease, unspecified**

D89.82 **Autoimmune lymphoproliferative syndrome [ALPS]**

D89.89 **Other specified disorders involving the immune mechanism, not elsewhere classified**

Excludes1: human immunodeficiency virus disease (B20)

D89.9 **Disorder involving the immune mechanism, unspecified**

Immune disease NOS

Chapter 4: Endocrine, Nutritional And Metabolic Diseases (E00-E89)

DEFINITIONS

This chapter includes definitions of selected key words, terms and phrases and coding alerts for adding points to the clinical domain, and references to coding late effects where appropriate. An example from this chapter is as follows:

E20 Hypoparathyroidism

Definition: Parathyroid glands are small endocrine glands in the neck that produce parathyroid hormone. Humans have four parathyroid glands, which are usually located behind the thyroid gland.

MULTIPLE CODING FOR A SINGLE CONDITION

In addition to the etiology/manifestation convention that requires two codes to fully describe a single condition that affects multiple body systems, there are other single conditions that also require more than one code. "Use additional code" notes are found in the Tabular List at codes that are not part of an etiology/manifestation pair where a secondary code is useful to fully describe a condition. The sequencing rule is the same as the etiology/manifestation pair, "use additional code" indicates that a secondary code should be added.

For example, for bacterial infections that are not included in chapter 1, a secondary code from category B95, Streptococcus, Staphylococcus, and Enterococcus, as the cause of diseases classified elsewhere, or B96, Other bacterial agents as the cause of diseases classified elsewhere, may be required to identify the bacterial organism causing the infection. A "use additional code" note will normally be found at the infectious disease code, indicating a need for the organism code to be added as a secondary code.

"Code first" notes are also under certain codes that are not specifically manifestation codes but may be due to an underlying cause. When there is a "code first" note and an underlying condition is present, the underlying condition should be sequenced first.

"Code, if applicable, any causal condition first", notes indicate that this code may be assigned as a principal diagnosis when the causal condition is unknown or not applicable. If a causal condition is known, then the code for that condition should be sequenced as the principal or first-listed diagnosis.

Multiple codes may be needed for sequela, complication codes and obstetric codes to more fully describe a condition. See the specific guidelines for these conditions for further instruction.

COMBINATION CODE

A combination code is a single code used to classify: Two diagnoses, or a diagnosis with an associated secondary process (manifestation) A diagnosis with an associated complication

Combination codes are identified by referring to subterm entries in the Alphabetic Index and by reading the inclusion and exclusion notes in the Tabular List.

Assign only the combination code when that code fully identifies the diagnostic conditions involved or when the Alphabetic Index so directs. Multiple coding should not be used when the classification provides a combination code that clearly identifies all of the elements documented in the diagnosis. When the combination code lacks necessary specificity in describing the manifestation or complication, an additional code should be used as a secondary code.

SEQUELA (LATE EFFECTS)

A sequela is the residual effect (condition produced) after the acute phase of an illness or injury has terminated. There is no time limit on when a sequela code can be used. The residual may be apparent early, such as in cerebral infarction, or it may occur months or years later, such as that due to a previous injury. Coding of sequela generally requires two codes sequenced in the following order: The condition or nature of the sequela is sequenced first.

The sequela code is sequenced second.

An exception to the above guidelines are those instances where the code for the sequela is followed by a manifestation code identified in the Tabular List and title, or the sequela code has been expanded (at the fourth, fifth or sixth character levels) to include the manifestation(s). The code for the acute phase of an illness or injury that led to the sequela is never used with a code for the late effect.

DIABETES MELLITUS

The diabetes mellitus codes are combination codes that include the type of diabetes mellitus, the body system affected, and the complications affecting that body system. As many codes within a particular category

as are necessary to describe all of the complications of the disease may be used. They should be sequenced based on the reason for a particular encounter. Assign as many codes from categories E08 – E13 as needed to identify all of the associated conditions that the patient has.

1) **Type of diabetes**

The age of a patient is not the sole determining factor, though most type 1 diabetics develop the condition before reaching puberty. For this reason type 1 diabetes mellitus is also referred to as juvenile diabetes.

2) **Type of diabetes mellitus not documented**

If the type of diabetes mellitus is not documented in the medical record the default is E11.-, Type 2 diabetes mellitus.

3) **Diabetes mellitus and the use of insulin and oral hypoglycemics**

If the documentation in a medical record does not indicate the type of diabetes but does indicate that the patient uses insulin, code E11, Type 2 diabetes mellitus, should be assigned. Code Z79.4, Long-term (current) use of insulin, or Z79.84, Long term (current) use of oral hypoglycemic drugs, should also be assigned to indicate that the patient uses insulin or hypoglycemic drugs. Code Z79.4 should not be assigned if insulin is given temporarily to bring a type 2 patient's blood sugar under control during an encounter.

4) **Diabetes mellitus in pregnancy and gestational diabetes**

See Section I.C.15. Diabetes mellitus in pregnancy.

See Section I.C.15. Gestational (pregnancy induced) diabetes

5) **Complications due to insulin pump malfunction**

(a) **Underdose of insulin due to insulin pump failure**

An underdose of insulin due to an insulin pump failure should be assigned to a code from subcategory T85.6, Mechanical complication of other specified internal and external prosthetic devices, implants and grafts, that specifies the type of pump malfunction, as the principal or first-listed code, followed by code T38.3X6-, Underdosing of insulin and oral hypoglycemic [antidiabetic] drugs. Additional codes for the type of diabetes mellitus and any associated complications due to the underdosing should also be assigned.

(b) **Overdose of insulin due to insulin pump failure**

The principal or first-listed code for an encounter due to an insulin pump malfunction resulting in an overdose of insulin, should also be T85.6-, Mechanical complication of other specified internal and external prosthetic devices, implants and grafts, followed by code T38.3X1-, Poisoning by insulin and oral hypoglycemic [antidiabetic] drugs, accidental (unintentional).

6) **Secondary diabetes mellitus**

Codes under categories E08, Diabetes mellitus due to underlying condition, E09, Drug or chemical induced diabetes mellitus, and E13, Other specified diabetes mellitus, identify complications/manifestations associated with secondary diabetes mellitus. Secondary diabetes is always caused by another condition or event (e.g., cystic fibrosis, malignant neoplasm of pancreas, pancreatectomy, adverse effect of drug, or poisoning).

(a) **Secondary diabetes mellitus and the use of insulin or hypoglycemic drugs**

For patients who routinely use insulin or hypoglycemic drugs, code Z79.4, Long-term (current) use of insulin, or Z79.84, Long term (current) use of oral hypoglycemic drugs should also be assigned. Code Z79.4 should not be assigned if insulin is given temporarily to bring a patient's blood sugar under control during an encounter.

(b) **Assigning and sequencing secondary diabetes codes and its causes**

The sequencing of the secondary diabetes codes in relationship to codes for the cause of the diabetes is based on the Tabular List instructions for categories E08, E09 and E13.

(i) **Secondary diabetes mellitus due to pancreatectomy**

For postpancreatectomy diabetes mellitus (lack of insulin due to the surgical removal of all or part of the pancreas), assign code E89.1, Postprocedural hypoinsulinemia. Assign a code from category E13 and a code from subcategory Z90.41-, Acquired absence of pancreas, as additional codes.

(ii) **Secondary diabetes due to drugs**

Secondary diabetes may be caused by an adverse effect of correctly administered medications, poisoning or sequela of poisoning.

See section I.C.19.e for coding of adverse effects and poisoning, and section I.C.20 for external cause code reporting.

Chapter 4

Endocrine, Nutritional and Metabolic Diseases (E00-E89)

Note: All neoplasms, whether functionally active or not, are classified in Chapter 2. Appropriate codes in this chapter (i.e. E05.8, E07.0, E16-E31, E34.-) may be used as additional codes to indicate either functional activity by neoplasms and ectopic endocrine tissue or hyperfunction and hypofunction of endocrine glands associated with neoplasms and other conditions classified elsewhere.

Excludes1: transitory endocrine and metabolic disorders specific to newborn (P70-P74)

This chapter contains the following blocks:

E00-E07	Disorders of thyroid gland
E08-E13	Diabetes mellitus
E15-E16	Other disorders of glucose regulation and pancreatic internal secretion
E20-E35	Disorders of other endocrine glands
E36	Intraoperative complications of endocrine system
E40-E46	Malnutrition
E50-E64	Other nutritional deficiencies
E65-E68	Overweight, obesity and other hyperalimentation
E70-E88	Metabolic disorders
E89	Postprocedural endocrine and metabolic complications and disorders, not elsewhere classified

DISORDERS OF THYROID GLAND (E00-E07)

E00 Congenital iodine-deficiency syndrome

Use additional code (F70-F79) to identify associated intellectual disabilities.

Excludes1: subclinical iodine-deficiency hypothyroidism (E02)

E00.0 Congenital iodine-deficiency syndrome, neurological type

Endemic cretinism, neurological type

E00.1 Congenital iodine-deficiency syndrome, myxedematous type

Endemic hypothyroid cretinism

Endemic cretinism, myxedematous type

E00.2 Congenital iodine-deficiency syndrome, mixed type

Endemic cretinism, mixed type

E00.9 Congenital iodine-deficiency syndrome, unspecified

Congenital iodine-deficiency hypothyroidism NOS

Endemic cretinism NOS

E01 Iodine-deficiency related thyroid disorders and allied conditions

Excludes1: congenital iodine-deficiency syndrome (E00.-)

subclinical iodine-deficiency hypothyroidism (E02)

E01.0 Iodine-deficiency related diffuse (endemic) goiter

E01.1 Iodine-deficiency related multinodular (endemic) goiter

Iodine-deficiency related nodular goiter

E01.2 Iodine-deficiency related (endemic) goiter, unspecified

Endemic goiter NOS

E01.8 Other iodine-deficiency related thyroid disorders and allied conditions

Acquired iodine-deficiency hypothyroidism NOS

E02 Subclinical iodine-deficiency hypothyroidism

E03 Other hypothyroidism

Excludes1: iodine-deficiency related hypothyroidism (E00-E02)

postprocedural hypothyroidism (E89.0)

E03.0 Congenital hypothyroidism with diffuse goiter

Congenital parenchymatous goiter (nontoxic)

Congenital goiter (nontoxic) NOS

Excludes1: transitory congenital goiter with normal function (P72.0)

E03.1 Congenital hypothyroidism without goiter

Aplasia of thyroid (with myxedema)

Congenital atrophy of thyroid

Congenital hypothyroidism NOS

E03.2 Hypothyroidism due to medicaments and other exogenous substances

Code first poisoning due to drug or toxin, if applicable (T36-T65 with fifth or sixth character 1-4 or 6)

Use additional code for adverse effect, if applicable, to identify drug (T36-T50 with fifth or sixth character 5)

E03.3 Postinfectious hypothyroidism

E03.4 Atrophy of thyroid (acquired)

Excludes1: congenital atrophy of thyroid (E03.1)

E03.5 Myxedema coma

E03.8 Other specified hypothyroidism

E03.9 Hypothyroidism, unspecified

Myxedema NOS

E04 Other nontoxic goiter

Definition: Nontoxic nodular goiter is a type of simple goiter with enlargement caused by nodules, or lumps, on the thyroid.

Excludes1: congenital goiter (NOS) (diffuse) (parenchymatous) (E03.0)

iodine-deficiency related goiter (E00-E02)

E04.0 Nontoxic diffuse goiter

Diffuse (colloid) nontoxic goiter

Simple nontoxic goiter

E04.1 Nontoxic single thyroid nodule

Colloid nodule (cystic) (thyroid)

Nontoxic uninodular goiter

Thyroid (cystic) nodule NOS

E04.2 Nontoxic multinodular goiter

Cystic goiter NOS

Multinodular (cystic) goiter NOS

E04.8 Other specified nontoxic goiter

E04.9 Nontoxic goiter, unspecified

Goiter NOS

Nodular goiter (nontoxic) NOS

E05 Thyrotoxicosis [hyperthyroidism]

Definition: Thyrotoxicosis with or without goiter is a condition resulting from excessive concentrations of thyroid hormones in the body, as in hyperthyroidism.

Excludes1: chronic thyroiditis with transient thyrotoxicosis (E06.2)

neonatal thyrotoxicosis (P72.1)

E05.0 Thyrotoxicosis with diffuse goiter

Exophthalmic or toxic goiter NOS Graves' disease

Toxic diffuse goiter

E05.00 Thyrotoxicosis with diffuse goiter without thyrotoxic crisis or storm

E05.01 Thyrotoxicosis with diffuse goiter with thyrotoxic crisis or storm

E05.1 **Thyrotoxicosis with toxic single thyroid nodule**

Thyrotoxicosis with toxic uninodular goiter

    E05.10 **Thyrotoxicosis with toxic single thyroid nodule without thyrotoxic crisis or storm**

    E05.11 **Thyrotoxicosis with toxic single thyroid nodule with thyrotoxic crisis or storm**

E05.2 **Thyrotoxicosis with toxic multinodular goiter**

Toxic nodular goiter NOS

    E05.20 **Thyrotoxicosis with toxic multinodular goiter without thyrotoxic crisis or storm**

    E05.21 **Thyrotoxicosis with toxic multinodular goiter with thyrotoxic crisis or storm**

E05.3 **Thyrotoxicosis from ectopic thyroid tissue**

    E05.30 **Thyrotoxicosis from ectopic thyroid tissue without thyrotoxic crisis or storm**

    E05.31 **Thyrotoxicosis from ectopic thyroid tissue with thyrotoxic crisis or storm**

E05.4 **Thyrotoxicosis factitia**

    E05.40 **Thyrotoxicosis factitia without thyrotoxic crisis or storm**

    E05.41 **Thyrotoxicosis factitia with thyrotoxic crisis or storm**

E05.8 **Other thyrotoxicosis**

Overproduction of thyroid-stimulating hormone

    E05.80 **Other thyrotoxicosis without thyrotoxic crisis or storm**

    E05.81 **Other thyrotoxicosis with thyrotoxic crisis or storm**

E05.9 **Thyrotoxicosis, unspecified**

Hyperthyroidism NOS

    E05.90 **Thyrotoxicosis, unspecified without thyrotoxic crisis or storm**

    E05.91 **Thyrotoxicosis, unspecified with thyrotoxic crisis or storm**

E06 **Thyroiditis**

Excludes1: postpartum thyroiditis (O90.5)

E06.0 **Acute thyroiditis**

Abscess of thyroid

Pyogenic thyroiditis

Suppurative thyroiditis

Use additional code (B95-B97) to identify infectious agent.

E06.1 **Subacute thyroiditis**

de Quervain thyroiditis

Giant-cell thyroiditis

Granulomatous thyroiditis

Nonsuppurative thyroiditis

Viral thyroiditis

Excludes1: autoimmune thyroiditis (E06.3)

E06.2 **Chronic thyroiditis with transient thyrotoxicosis**

Excludes1: autoimmune thyroiditis (E06.3)

E06.3 **Autoimmune thyroiditis**

Hashimoto's thyroiditis

Hashitoxicosis (transient)

Lymphadenoid goiter

Lymphocytic thyroiditis

Struma lymphomatosa

E06.4 **Drug-induced thyroiditis**

Use additional code for adverse effect, if applicable, to identify drug (T36-T50 with fifth or sixth character 5)

E06.5 **Other chronic thyroiditis**

Chronic fibrous thyroiditis

Chronic thyroiditis NOS

Ligneous thyroiditis

Riedel thyroiditis

E06.9 **Thyroiditis, unspecified**

E07 **Other disorders of thyroid**

E07.0 **Hypersecretion of calcitonin**

C-cell hyperplasia of thyroid

Hypersecretion of thyrocalcitonin

E07.1 **Dyshormogenetic goiter**

Familial dyshormogenetic goiter

Pendred's syndrome

Excludes1: transitory congenital goiter with normal function (P72.0)

E07.8 **Other specified disorders of thyroid**

    E07.81 **Sick-euthyroid syndrome**

Euthyroid sick-syndrome

    E07.89 **Other specified disorders of thyroid**

Abnormality of thyroid-binding globulin

Hemorrhage of thyroid

Infarction of thyroid

E07.9 **Disorder of thyroid, unspecified**

DIABETES MELLITUS (E08-E13)

Definition: Diabetes mellitus is a condition in which the pancreas no longer produces enough insulin or cells stop responding to the insulin that is produced, so that glucose in the blood cannot be absorbed into the cells of the body. Symptoms include frequent urination, lethargy, excessive thirst, and hunger.

E08 **Diabetes mellitus due to underlying condition**

Code first the underlying condition, such as:

congenital rubella (P35.0)

Cushing's syndrome (E24.-)

cystic fibrosis (E84.-)

malignant neoplasm (C00-C96)

malnutrition (E40-E46)

pancreatitis **and other** diseases of the pancreas (K85-K86.-)

Use additional code to identify control using:

insulin (Z79.4)

oral antidiabetic drugs (Z79.84)

oral hypoglycemic drugs (Z79.84)

Excludes1: drug or chemical induced diabetes mellitus (E09.-)

gestational diabetes (O24.4-)

neonatal diabetes mellitus (P70.2)

postpancreatectomy diabetes mellitus (E13.-)

postprocedural diabetes mellitus (E13.-)

secondary diabetes mellitus NEC (E13.-)

type 1 diabetes mellitus (E10.-)

type 2 diabetes mellitus (E11.-)

E08.0 **Diabetes mellitus due to underlying condition with hyperosmolarity**

E08.00 Diabetes mellitus due to underlying condition with hyperosmolarity without nonketotic hyperglycemic-hyperosmolar coma (NKHHC)

E08.01 Diabetes mellitus due to underlying condition with hyperosmolarity with coma

E08.1 Diabetes mellitus due to underlying condition with ketoacidosis

E08.10 Diabetes mellitus due to underlying condition with ketoacidosis without coma

E08.11 Diabetes mellitus due to underlying condition with ketoacidosis with coma

E08.2 Diabetes mellitus due to underlying condition with kidney complications

E08.21 Diabetes mellitus due to underlying condition with diabetic nephropathy

Diabetes mellitus due to underlying condition with intercapillary glomerulosclerosis

Diabetes mellitus due to underlying condition with intracapillary glomerulonephrosis

Diabetes mellitus due to underlying condition with Kimmelstiel-Wilson disease

E08.22 Diabetes mellitus due to underlying condition with diabetic chronic kidney disease

<u>Use additional code</u> to identify stage of chronic kidney disease (N18.1-N18.6)

E08.29 Diabetes mellitus due to underlying condition with other diabetic kidney complication

Renal tubular degeneration in diabetes mellitus due to underlying condition

E08.3 Diabetes mellitus due to underlying condition with ophthalmic complications

E08.31 Diabetes mellitus due to underlying condition with unspecified diabetic retinopathy

E08.311 Diabetes mellitus due to underlying condition with unspecified diabetic retinopathy with macular edema

E08.319 Diabetes mellitus due to underlying condition with unspecified diabetic retinopathy without macular edema

E08.32 Diabetes mellitus due to underlying condition with mild nonproliferative diabetic retinopathy

Diabetes mellitus due to underlying condition with nonproliferative diabetic retinopathy NOS

One of the following 7th characters is to be assigned to codes in subcategory E08.32 to designate laterality of the disease:

1 - right eye

2 - left eye

3 – bilateral

9 - unspecified eye

● ⑦**E08.321** Diabetes mellitus due to underlying condition with mild nonproliferative diabetic retinopathy with macular edema

● ⑦**E08.329** Diabetes mellitus due to underlying condition with mild nonproliferative diabetic retinopathy without macular edema

E08.33 Diabetes mellitus due to underlying condition with moderate nonproliferative diabetic retinopathy

One of the following 7th characters is to be assigned to codes in subcategory E08.33 to designate laterality of the disease:

1 - right eye

2 - left eye

3 - bilateral

9 - unspecified eye

● ⑦**E08.331** Diabetes mellitus due to underlying condition with moderate nonproliferative diabetic retinopathy with macular edema

● ⑦**E08.339** Diabetes mellitus due to underlying condition with moderate nonproliferative diabetic retinopathy without macular edema

E08.34 Diabetes mellitus due to underlying condition with severe nonproliferative diabetic retinopathy

One of the following 7th characters is to be assigned to codes in subcategory E08.34 to designate laterality of the disease:

1 - right eye

2 - left eye

3 - bilateral

9 - unspecified eye

● ⑦**E08.341** Diabetes mellitus due to underlying condition with severe nonproliferative diabetic retinopathy with macular edema

● ⑦**E08.349** Diabetes mellitus due to underlying condition with severe nonproliferative diabetic retinopathy without macular edema

E08.35 Diabetes mellitus due to underlying condition with proliferative diabetic retinopathy

One of the following 7th characters is to be assigned to codes in subcategory E08.35 to designate laterality of the disease:

1 - right eye

2 - left eye

3 - bilateral

9 - unspecified eye

● ⑦**E08.351** Diabetes mellitus due to underlying condition with proliferative diabetic retinopathy with macular edema

● ⑦**E08.352** Diabetes mellitus due to underlying condition with proliferative diabetic retinopathy with traction retinal detachment involving the macula

● ⑦**E08.353** Diabetes mellitus due to underlying condition with proliferative diabetic retinopathy with traction retinal detachment not involving the macula

● ⑦**E08.354** Diabetes mellitus due to underlying condition with proliferative diabetic retinopathy with combined traction retinal detachment and rhegmatogenous retinal detachment

● ⑦**E08.355** Diabetes mellitus due to underlying condition with stable proliferative diabetic retinopathy

●⑦ **E08.359**   **Diabetes mellitus due to underlying condition with proliferative diabetic retinopathy without macular edema**

E08.36   **Diabetes mellitus due to underlying condition with diabetic cataract**

●⊗⑦ **E08.37**   **Diabetes mellitus due to underlying condition with diabetic macular edema, resolved following treatment**

One of the following 7th characters is to be assigned to code E08.37 to designate laterality of the disease:

1 - right eye

2 - left eye

3 - bilateral

9 - unspecified eye

E08.39   **Diabetes mellitus due to underlying condition with other diabetic ophthalmic complication**

<u>**Use additional code**</u> to identify manifestation, such as:

diabetic glaucoma (H40-H42)

E08.4   **Diabetes mellitus due to underlying condition with neurological complications**

E08.40   **Diabetes mellitus due to underlying condition with diabetic neuropathy, unspecified**

E08.41   **Diabetes mellitus due to underlying condition with diabetic mononeuropathy**

E08.42   **Diabetes mellitus due to underlying condition with diabetic polyneuropathy**

Diabetes mellitus due to underlying condition with diabetic neuralgia

E08.43   **Diabetes mellitus due to underlying condition with diabetic autonomic (poly)neuropathy**

Diabetes mellitus due to underlying condition with diabetic gastroparesis

E08.44   **Diabetes mellitus due to underlying condition with diabetic amyotrophy**

E08.49   **Diabetes mellitus due to underlying condition with other diabetic neurological complication**

E08.5   **Diabetes mellitus due to underlying condition with circulatory complications**

E08.51   **Diabetes mellitus due to underlying condition with diabetic peripheral angiopathy without gangrene**

E08.52   **Diabetes mellitus due to underlying condition with diabetic peripheral angiopathy with gangrene**

Diabetes mellitus due to underlying condition with diabetic gangrene

E08.59   **Diabetes mellitus due to underlying condition with other circulatory complications**

E08.6   **Diabetes mellitus due to underlying condition with other specified complications**

E08.61   **Diabetes mellitus due to underlying condition with diabetic arthropathy**

E08.610   **Diabetes mellitus due to underlying condition with diabetic neuropathic arthropathy**

Diabetes mellitus due to underlying condition with Charcôt's joints

E08.618   **Diabetes mellitus due to underlying condition with other diabetic arthropathy**

E08.62   **Diabetes mellitus due to underlying condition with skin complications**

E08.620   **Diabetes mellitus due to underlying condition with diabetic dermatitis**

Diabetes mellitus due to underlying condition with diabetic necrobiosis lipoidica

E08.621   **Diabetes mellitus due to underlying condition with foot ulcer**

<u>**Use additional code**</u> to identify site of ulcer (L97.4-, L97.5-)

E08.622   **Diabetes mellitus due to underlying condition with other skin ulcer**

<u>**Use additional code**</u> to identify site of ulcer (L97.1-L97.9, L98.41-L98.49)

E08.628   **Diabetes mellitus due to underlying condition with other skin complications**

E08.63   **Diabetes mellitus due to underlying condition with oral complications**

E08.630   **Diabetes mellitus due to underlying condition with periodontal disease**

E08.638   **Diabetes mellitus due to underlying condition with other oral complications**

E08.64   **Diabetes mellitus due to underlying condition with hypoglycemia**

E08.641   **Diabetes mellitus due to underlying condition with hypoglycemia with coma**

E08.649   **Diabetes mellitus due to underlying condition with hypoglycemia without coma**

E08.65   **Diabetes mellitus due to underlying condition with hyperglycemia**

E08.69   **Diabetes mellitus due to underlying condition with other specified complication**

<u>**Use additional code**</u> to identify complication

E08.8   **Diabetes mellitus due to underlying condition with unspecified complications**

E08.9   **Diabetes mellitus due to underlying condition without complications**

E09   **Drug or chemical induced diabetes mellitus**

<u>**Code first**</u> poisoning due to drug or toxin, if applicable (T36-T65 with fifth or sixth character 1-4 or 6)

<u>**Use additional code**</u> for adverse effect, if applicable, to identify drug (T36-T50 with fifth or sixth character 5)

<u>**Use additional code**</u> to identify control using:

insulin (Z79.4)

oral antidiabetic drugs (Z79.84)

oral hypoglycemic drugs (Z79.84)

Excludes1: diabetes mellitus due to underlying condition (E08.-)

gestational diabetes (O24.4-)

neonatal diabetes mellitus (P70.2)

postpancreatectomy diabetes mellitus (E13.-)

postprocedural diabetes mellitus (E13.-)

secondary diabetes mellitus NEC (E13.-)

type 1 diabetes mellitus (E10.-)

type 2 diabetes mellitus (E11.-)

E09.0 **Drug or chemical induced diabetes mellitus with hyperosmolarity**

   E09.00 **Drug or chemical induced diabetes mellitus with hyperosmolarity without nonketotic hyperglycemic-hyperosmolar coma (NKHHC)**

   E09.01 **Drug or chemical induced diabetes mellitus with hyperosmolarity with coma**

E09.1 **Drug or chemical induced diabetes mellitus with ketoacidosis**

   E09.10 **Drug or chemical induced diabetes mellitus with ketoacidosis without coma**

   E09.11 **Drug or chemical induced diabetes mellitus with ketoacidosis with coma**

E09.2 **Drug or chemical induced diabetes mellitus with kidney complications**

   E09.21 **Drug or chemical induced diabetes mellitus with diabetic nephropathy**

   Drug or chemical induced diabetes mellitus with intercapillary glomerulosclerosis

   Drug or chemical induced diabetes mellitus with intracapillary glomerulonephrosis

   Drug or chemical induced diabetes mellitus with Kimmelstiel-Wilson disease

   E09.22 **Drug or chemical induced diabetes mellitus with diabetic chronic kidney disease**

   <u>Use additional code</u> to identify stage of chronic kidney disease (N18.1-N18.6)

   E09.29 **Drug or chemical induced diabetes mellitus with other diabetic kidney complication**

   Drug or chemical induced diabetes mellitus with renal tubular degeneration

E09.3 **Drug or chemical induced diabetes mellitus with ophthalmic complications**

   E09.31 **Drug or chemical induced diabetes mellitus with unspecified diabetic retinopathy**

      E09.311 **Drug or chemical induced diabetes mellitus with unspecified diabetic retinopathy with macular edema**

      E09.319 **Drug or chemical induced diabetes mellitus with unspecified diabetic retinopathywithout macular edema**

   E09.32 **Drug or chemical induced diabetes mellitus with mild nonproliferative diabetic retinopathy**

   Drug or chemical induced diabetes mellitus with nonproliferative diabetic retinopathy NOS

   One of the following 7th characters is to be assigned to codes in subcategory E09.32 to designate laterality of the disease:

   1 - right eye 2 - left eye

   3 - bilateral

   9 - unspecified eye

   ● ⑦**E09.321** **Drug or chemical induced diabetes mellitus with mild nonproliferative diabetic retinopathy with macular edema**

   ● ⑦**E09.329** **Drug or chemical induced diabetes mellitus with mild nonproliferative diabetic retinopathy without macular edema**

E09.33 **Drug or chemical induced diabetes mellitus with moderate nonproliferative diabetic retinopathy**

One of the following 7th characters is to be assigned to codes in subcategory E09.33 to designate laterality of the disease:

1 - right eye

2 - left eye

3 - bilateral

9 - unspecified eye

● ⑦**E09.331** **Drug or chemical induced diabetes mellitus with moderate nonproliferative diabetic retinopathy with macular edema**

● ⑦**E09.339** **Drug or chemical induced diabetes mellitus with moderate nonproliferative diabetic retinopathy without macular edema**

E09.34 **Drug or chemical induced diabetes mellitus with severe nonproliferative diabetic retinopathy**

One of the following 7th characters is to be assigned to codes in subcategory E09.34 to designate laterality of the disease:

1 - right eye

2 - left eye

3 - bilateral

9 - unspecified eye

● ⑦**E09.341** **Drug or chemical induced diabetes mellitus with severe nonproliferative diabetic retinopathy with macular edema**

● ⑦**E09.349** **Drug or chemical induced diabetes mellitus with severe nonproliferative diabetic retinopathy without macular edema**

E09.35 **Drug or chemical induced diabetes mellitus with proliferative diabetic retinopathy**

One of the following 7th characters is to be assigned to codes in subcategory E09.35 to designate laterality of the disease:

1 - right eye

2 - left eye

3 - bilateral

9 - unspecified eye

● ⑦**E09.351** **Drug or chemical induced diabetes mellitus with proliferative diabetic retinopathy with macular edema**

● ⑦**E09.352** **Drug or chemical induced diabetes mellitus with proliferative diabetic retinopathy with traction retinal detachment involving the macula**

● ⑦**E09.353** **Drug or chemical induced diabetes mellitus with proliferative diabetic retinopathy with traction retinal detachment not involving the macula**

● ⑦**E09.354** **Drug or chemical induced diabetes mellitus with proliferative diabetic retinopathy with combined traction retinal detachment and rhegmatogenous retinal detachment**

    Add 4th-7th digits   Nonspecific code   Unspecified code   Manifestation code

●⑦ **E09.355** **Drug or chemical induced diabetes mellitus with stable proliferative diabetic retinopathy**

●⑦ **E09.359** **Drug or chemical induced diabetes mellitus with proliferative diabetic retinopathy without macular edema**

E09.36 **Drug or chemical induced diabetes mellitus with diabetic cataract**

●⊗⑦ **E09.37** **Drug or chemical induced diabetes mellitus with diabetic macular edema, resolved following treatment**

One of the following 7th characters is to be assigned to code E09.37 to designate laterality of the disease:

1 - right eye

2 - left eye

3 - bilateral

9 - unspecified eye

E09.39 **Drug or chemical induced diabetes mellitus with other diabetic ophthalmic complication**

Use additional code to identify manifestation, such as: diabetic glaucoma (H40-H42)

E09.4 **Drug or chemical induced diabetes mellitus with neurological complications**

E09.40 **Drug or chemical induced diabetes mellitus with neurological complications with diabetic neuropathy, unspecified**

E09.41 **Drug or chemical induced diabetes mellitus with neurological complications with diabetic mononeuropathy**

E09.42 **Drug or chemical induced diabetes mellitus with neurological complications with diabetic polyneuropathy**

Drug or chemical induced diabetes mellitus with diabetic neuralgia

E09.43 **Drug or chemical induced diabetes mellitus with neurological complications with diabetic autonomic (poly)neuropathy**

Drug or chemical induced diabetes mellitus with diabetic gastroparesis

E09.44 **Drug or chemical induced diabetes mellitus with neurological complications with diabetic amyotrophy**

E09.49 **Drug or chemical induced diabetes mellitus with neurological complications with other diabetic neurological complication**

E09.5 **Drug or chemical induced diabetes mellitus with circulatory complications**

E09.51 **Drug or chemical induced diabetes mellitus with diabetic peripheral angiopathy without gangrene**

E09.52 **Drug or chemical induced diabetes mellitus with diabetic peripheral angiopathy with gangrene**

Drug or chemical induced diabetes mellitus with diabetic gangrene

E09.59 **Drug or chemical induced diabetes mellitus with other circulatory complications**

E09.6 **Drug or chemical induced diabetes mellitus with other specified complications**

E09.61 **Drug or chemical induced diabetes mellitus with diabetic arthropathy**

E09.610 **Drug or chemical induced diabetes mellitus with diabetic neuropathic arthropathy**

Drug or chemical induced diabetes mellitus with Charcôt's joints

E09.618 **Drug or chemical induced diabetes mellitus with other diabetic arthropathy**

E09.62 **Drug or chemical induced diabetes mellitus with skin complications**

E09.620 **Drug or chemical induced diabetes mellitus with diabetic dermatitis**

Drug or chemical induced diabetes mellitus with diabetic necrobiosis lipoidica

E09.621 **Drug or chemical induced diabetes mellitus with foot ulcer**

Use additional code to identify site of ulcer (L97.4-, L97.5-)

E09.622 **Drug or chemical induced diabetes mellitus with other skin ulcer**

Use additional code to identify site of ulcer (L97.1-L97.9, L98.41-L98.49)

E09.628 **Drug or chemical induced diabetes mellitus with other skin complications**

E09.63 **Drug or chemical induced diabetes mellitus with oral complications**

E09.630 **Drug or chemical induced diabetes mellitus with periodontal disease**

E09.638 **Drug or chemical induced diabetes mellitus with other oral complications**

E09.64 **Drug or chemical induced diabetes mellitus with hypoglycemia**

E09.641 **Drug or chemical induced diabetes mellitus with hypoglycemia with coma**

E09.649 **Drug or chemical induced diabetes mellitus with hypoglycemia without coma**

E09.65 **Drug or chemical induced diabetes mellitus with hyperglycemia**

E09.69 **Drug or chemical induced diabetes mellitus with other specified complication**

Use additional code to identify complication

E09.8 **Drug or chemical induced diabetes mellitus with unspecified complications**

E09.9 **Drug or chemical induced diabetes mellitus without complications**

E10 **Type 1 diabetes mellitus**

Includes: brittle diabetes (mellitus)

diabetes (mellitus) due to autoimmune process

diabetes (mellitus) due to immune mediated pancreatic islet beta-cell destruction idiopathic diabetes (mellitus)

juvenile onset diabetes (mellitus)

ketosis-prone diabetes (mellitus)

Excludes1: diabetes mellitus due to underlying condition (E08.-)

drug or chemical induced diabetes mellitus (E09.-)

gestational diabetes (O24.4-)

hyperglycemia NOS (R73.9)

neonatal diabetes mellitus (P70.2)

postpancreatectomy diabetes mellitus (E13.-)

postprocedural diabetes mellitus (E13.-)

secondary diabetes mellitus NEC (E13.-)

type 2 diabetes mellitus (E11.-)

E10.1 **Type 1 diabetes mellitus with ketoacidosis**

    E10.10 **Type 1diabetes mellitus with ketoacidosis without coma**

    E10.11 **Type 1diabetes mellitus with ketoacidosis with coma**

E10.2 **Type 1 diabetes mellitus with kidney complications**

    E10.21 **Type 1diabetes mellitus with diabetic nephropathy**

    Type 1 diabetes mellitus with intercapillary glomerulosclerosis

    Type 1 diabetes mellitus with intracapillary glomerulonephrosis

    Type 1 diabetes mellitus with Kimmelstiel-Wilson disease

    E10.22 **Type 1diabetes mellitus with diabetic chronic kidney disease**

    <u>Use additional code</u> to identify stage of chronic kidney disease (N18.1-N18.6)

    E10.29 **Type 1diabetes mellitus with other diabetic kidney complication**

    Type 1 diabetes mellitus with renal tubular degeneration

E10.3 **Type 1 Diabetes mellitus with ophthalmic complications**

    E10.31 **Type 1diabetes mellitus with unspecified diabetic retinopathy**

        E10.311 **Type 1 diabetes mellitus with unspecified diabetic retinopathy with macular edema**

        E10.319 **Type 1 diabetes mellitus with unspecified diabetic retinopathy without macular edema**

    E10.32 **Type 1 diabetes mellitus with mild nonproliferative diabetic retinopathy**

    Type 1 diabetes mellitus with nonproliferative diabetic retinopathy NOS

    One of the following 7th characters is to be assigned to codes in subcategory E10.32 to designate laterality of the disease:

    1 - right eye

    2 - left eye

    3 - bilateral

    9 - unspecified eye

    •⑦**E10.321** **Type 1 diabetes mellitus with mild nonproliferative diabetic retinopathy with macular edema**

    •⑦**E10.329** **Type 1 diabetes mellitus with mild nonproliferative diabetic retinopathy without macular edema**

    E10.33 **Type 1 diabetes mellitus with moderate nonproliferative diabetic retinopathy**

    One of the following 7th characters is to be assigned to codes in subcategory E10.33 to designate laterality of the disease:

    1 - right eye

    2 - left eye

3 - bilateral

9 - unspecified eye

•⑦**E10.331** **Type 1 diabetes mellitus with moderate nonproliferative diabetic retinopathy with macular edema**

•⑦**E10.339** **Type 1 diabetes mellitus with moderate nonproliferative diabetic retinopathy without macular edema**

E10.34 **Type 1 diabetes mellitus with severe nonproliferative diabetic retinopathy**

One of the following 7th characters is to be assigned to codes in subcategory E10.34 to designate laterality of the disease:

1 - right eye

2 - left eye

3 - bilateral

9 - unspecified eye

•⑦**E10.341** **Type 1 diabetes mellitus with severe nonproliferative diabetic retinopathy with macular edema**

•⑦**E10.349** **Type 1 diabetes mellitus with severe nonproliferative diabetic retinopathy without macular edema**

E10.35 **Type 1 diabetes mellitus with proliferative diabetic retinopathy**

One of the following 7th characters is to be assigned to codes in subcategory E10.35 to designate laterality of the disease:

1 - right eye

2 - left eye

3 - bilateral

9 - unspecified eye

•⑦**E10.351** **Type 1 diabetes mellitus with proliferative diabetic retinopathy with macular edema**

•⑦**E10.352** **Type 1 diabetes mellitus with proliferative diabetic retinopathy with traction retinal detachment involving the macula**

•⑦**E10.353** **Type 1 diabetes mellitus with proliferative diabetic retinopathy with traction retinal detachment not involving the macula**

•⑦**E10.354** **Type 1 diabetes mellitus with proliferative diabetic retinopathy with combined traction retinal detachment and rhegmatogenous retinal detachment**

•⑦**E10.355** **Type 1 diabetes mellitus with stable proliferative diabetic retinopathy**

•⑦**E10.359** **Type 1 diabetes mellitus with proliferative diabetic retinopathy without macular edema**

⊗⑦**E10.36** **Type 1 diabetes mellitus with diabetic cataract**

•⊗⑦**E10.37** **Type 1 diabetes mellitus with diabetic macular edema, resolved following treatment**

One of the following 7th characters is to be assigned to code E10.37 to designate laterality of the disease:

1 - right eye

2 - left eye

3 - bilateral

9 - unspecified eye

E10.39 **Type 1 diabetes mellitus with other diabetic ophthalmic complication**

<u>Use additional code</u> to identify manifestation, such as:

diabetic glaucoma (H40-H42)

E10.4 **Type 1 diabetes mellitus with neurological complications**

E10.40 **Type 1 diabetes mellitus with diabetic neuropathy, unspecified**

E10.41 **Type 1 diabetes mellitus with diabetic mononeuropathy**

E10.42 **Type 1 diabetes mellitus with diabetic polyneuropathy**

Type 1 diabetes mellitus with diabetic neuralgia

E10.43 **Type 1 diabetes mellitus with diabetic autonomic (poly)neuropathy**

Type 1 diabetes mellitus with diabetic gastroparesis

E10.44 **Type 1 diabetes mellitus with diabetic amyotrophy**

E10.49 **Type 1 diabetes mellitus with other diabetic neurological complication**

E10.5 **Type 1 diabetes mellitus with circulatory complications**

E10.51 **Type 1 diabetes mellitus with diabetic peripheral angiopathy without gangrene**

E10.52 **Type 1 diabetes mellitus with diabetic peripheral angiopathy with gangrene**

Type 1 diabetes mellitus with diabetic gangrene

E10.59 **Type 1 diabetes mellitus with other circulatory complications**

E10.6 **Type 1 diabetes mellitus with other specified complications**

E10.61 **Type 1 diabetes mellitus with diabetic arthropathy**

E10.610 **Type 1 diabetes mellitus with diabetic neuropathic arthropathy**

Type 1 diabetes mellitus with Charcôt's joints

E10.618 **Type 1 diabetes mellitus with other diabetic arthropathy**

E10.62 **Type 1 diabetes mellitus with skin complications**

E10.620 **Type 1 diabetes mellitus with diabetic dermatitis**

Type 1 diabetes mellitus with diabetic necrobiosis lipoidica

E10.621 **Type 1 diabetes mellitus with foot ulcer**

<u>Use additional code</u> to identify site of ulcer (L97.4-, L97.5-)

E10.622 **Type 1 diabetes mellitus with other skin ulcer**

<u>Use additional code</u> to identify site of ulcer (L97.1-L97.9, L98.41-L98.49)

E10.628 **Type 1 diabetes mellitus with other skin complications**

E10.63 **Type 1 diabetes mellitus with oral complications**

E10.630 **Type 1 diabetes mellitus with periodontal disease**

E10.638 **Type 1 diabetes mellitus with other oral complications**

E10.64 **Type 1 diabetes mellitus with hypoglycemia**

E10.641 **Type 1 diabetes mellitus with hypoglycemia with coma**

E10.649 **Type 1 diabetes mellitus with hypoglycemia without coma**

E10.65 **Type 1 diabetes mellitus with hyperglycemia**

E10.69 **Type 1 diabetes mellitus with other specified complication**

<u>Use additional code</u> to identify complication

E10.8 **Type 1 diabetes mellitus with unspecified complications**

E10.9 **Type 1 diabetes mellitus without complications**

E11 **Type 2 diabetes mellitus**

Includes: diabetes (mellitus) due to insulin secretory defect

diabetes NOS

insulin resistant diabetes (mellitus)

<u>Use additional code</u> to identify control using:

insulin (Z79.4)

oral antidiabetic drugs (Z79.84)

oral hypoglycemic drugs (Z79.84)

Excludes1: diabetes mellitus due to underlying condition (E08.-)

drug or chemical induced diabetes mellitus (E09.-)

gestational diabetes (O24.4-)

neonatal diabetes mellitus (P70.2)

postpancreatectomy diabetes mellitus (E13.-)

postprocedural diabetes mellitus (E13.-)

secondary diabetes mellitus NEC (E13.-)

type 1 diabetes mellitus (E10.-)

E11.0 **Type 2 diabetes mellitus with hyperosmolarity**

E11.00 **Type 2 diabetes mellitus with hyperosmolarity without nonketotic hyperglycemic-hyperosmolar coma (NKHHC)**

E11.01 **Type 2 diabetes mellitus with hyperosmolarity with coma**

E11.2 **Type 2 diabetes mellitus with kidney complications**

E11.21 **Type 2 diabetes mellitus with diabetic nephropathy**

Type 2 diabetes mellitus with intercapillary glomerulosclerosis

Type 2 diabetes mellitus with intracapillary glomerulonephrosis

Type 2 diabetes mellitus with Kimmelstiel-Wilson disease

E11.22 **Type 2 diabetes mellitus with diabetic chronic kidney disease**

<u>Use additional code</u> to identify stage of chronic kidney disease (N18.1-N18.6)

E11.29 **Type 2 diabetes mellitus with other diabetic kidney complication**

Type 2 diabetes mellitus with renal tubular degeneration

E11.3 **Type 2 diabetes mellitus with ophthalmic complications**

E11.31 **Type 2 diabetes mellitus with unspecified diabetic retinopathy**

E11.311 **Type 2 diabetes mellitus with unspecified diabetic retinopathy with macular edema**

E11.319 Type 2 diabetes mellitus with unspecified diabetic retinopathy without macular edema

E11.32 Type 2 diabetes mellitus with mild nonproliferative diabetic retinopathy

Type 2 diabetes mellitus with nonproliferative diabetic retinopathy NOS

One of the following 7th characters is to be assigned to codes in subcategory E11.32 to designate laterality of the disease:

1 - right eye

2 - left eye

3 – bilateral

9 - unspecified eye

• ⑦**E11.321** Type 2 diabetes mellitus with mild nonproliferative diabetic retinopathy with macular edema

• ⑦**E11.329** Type 2 diabetes mellitus with mild nonproliferative diabetic retinopathy without macular edema

E11.33 Type 2 diabetes mellitus with moderate nonproliferative diabetic retinopathy

One of the following 7th characters is to be assigned to codes in subcategory E11.33 to designate laterality of the disease:

1 - right eye

2 - left eye

3 - bilateral

9 - unspecified eye

• ⑦**E11.331** Type 2 diabetes mellitus with moderate nonproliferative diabetic retinopathy with macular edema

• ⑦**E11.339** Type 2 diabetes mellitus with moderate nonproliferative diabetic retinopathy without macular edema

E11.34 Type 2 diabetes mellitus with severe nonproliferative diabetic retinopathy

One of the following 7th characters is to be assigned to codes in subcategory E11.34 to designate laterality of the disease:

1 - right eye

2 - left eye

3 - bilateral

9 - unspecified eye

• ⑦**E11.341** Type 2 diabetes mellitus with severe nonproliferative diabetic retinopathy with macular edema

• ⑦**E11.349** Type 2 diabetes mellitus with severe nonproliferative diabetic retinopathy without macular edema

E11.35 Type 2 diabetes mellitus with proliferative diabetic retinopathy

One of the following 7th characters is to be assigned to codes in subcategory E11.35 to designate laterality of the disease:

1 - right eye

2 - left eye

3 - bilateral

9 - unspecified eye

• ⑦**E11.351** Type 2 diabetes mellitus with proliferative diabetic retinopathy with macular edema

• ⑦**E11.352** Type 2 diabetes mellitus with proliferative diabetic retinopathy with traction retinal detachment involving the macula

• ⑦**E11.353** Type 2 diabetes mellitus with proliferative diabetic retinopathy with traction retinal detachment not involving the macula

• ⑦**E11.354** Type 2 diabetes mellitus with proliferative diabetic retinopathy with combined traction retinal detachment and rhegmatogenous retinal detachment

• ⑦**E11.355** Type 2 diabetes mellitus with stable proliferative diabetic retinopathy

• ⑦**E11.359** Type 2 diabetes mellitus with proliferative diabetic retinopathy without macular edema

E11.36 Type 2 diabetes mellitus with diabetic cataract

• ⊗⑦**E11.37** Type 2 diabetes mellitus with diabetic macular edema, resolved following treatment

One of the following 7th characters is to be assigned to code E11.37 to designate laterality of the disease:

1 - right eye

2 - left eye

3 - bilateral

9 - unspecified eye

•**E11.39** Type 2 diabetes mellitus with other diabetic ophthalmic complication

Use additional code to identify manifestation, such as: diabetic glaucoma (H40-H42)

E11.4 Type 2 diabetes mellitus with neurological complications

E11.40 Type 2 diabetes mellitus with diabetic neuropathy, unspecified

E11.41 Type 2 diabetes mellitus with diabetic mononeuropathy

E11.42 Type 2 diabetes mellitus with diabetic polyneuropathy

Type 2 diabetes mellitus with diabetic neuralgia

E11.43 Type 2 diabetes mellitus with diabetic autonomic (poly)neuropathy

Type 2 diabetes mellitus with diabetic gastroparesis

E11.44 Type 2 diabetes mellitus with diabetic amyotrophy

E11.49 Type 2 diabetes mellitus with other diabetic neurological complication

E11.5 Type 2 diabetes mellitus with circulatory complications

E11.51 Type 2 diabetes mellitus with diabetic peripheral angiopathy without gangrene

E11.52 Type 2 diabetes mellitus with diabetic peripheral angiopathy with gangrene

Type 2 diabetes mellitus with diabetic gangrene

E11.59 Type 2 diabetes mellitus with other circulatory complications

E11.6 Type 2 diabetes mellitus with other specified complications

E11.61 Type 2 diabetes mellitus with diabetic arthropathy

    E11.610 Type 2 diabetes mellitus with diabetic neuropathic arthropathy

        Type 2 diabetes mellitus with Charcôt's joints

    E11.618 Type 2 diabetes mellitus with other diabetic arthropathy

E11.62 Type 2 diabetes mellitus with skin complications

    E11.620 Type 2 diabetes mellitus with diabetic dermatitis

        Type 2 diabetes mellitus with diabetic necrobiosis lipoidica

    E11.621 Type 2 diabetes mellitus with foot ulcer

        Use additional code to identify site of ulcer (L97.4-, L97.5-)

    E11.622 Type 2 diabetes mellitus with other skin ulcer

        Use additional code to identify site of ulcer (L97.1-L97.9, L98.41-L98.49)

    E11.628 Type 2 diabetes mellitus with other skin complications

E11.63 Type 2 diabetes mellitus with oral complications

    E11.630 Type 2 diabetes mellitus with periodontal disease

    E11.638 Type 2 diabetes mellitus with other oral complications

E11.64 Type 2 diabetes mellitus with hypoglycemia

    E11.641 Type 2 diabetes mellitus with hypoglycemia with coma

    E11.649 Type 2 diabetes mellitus with hypoglycemia without coma

E11.65 Type 2 diabetes mellitus with hyperglycemia

E11.69 Type 2 diabetes mellitus with other specified complication

    Use additional code to identify complication

E11.8 Type 2 diabetes mellitus with unspecified complications

E11.9 Type 2 diabetes mellitus without complications

E13 Other specified diabetes mellitus

Includes: diabetes mellitus due to genetic defects of beta-cell function

    diabetes mellitus due to genetic defects in insulin action postpancreatectomy diabetes mellitus

    postprocedural diabetes mellitus secondary diabetes mellitus NEC

Use additional code to identify control using:

insulin (Z79.4)

oral antidiabetic drugs (Z79.84)

oral hypoglycemic drugs (Z79.84)

Excludes1: diabetes (mellitus) due to autoimmune process (E10.-)

    diabetes (mellitus) due to immune mediated pancreatic islet beta-cell destruction (E10.-)

    diabetes mellitus due to underlying condition (E08.-)

    drug or chemical induced diabetes mellitus (E09.-)

    gestational diabetes (O24.4-)

    neonatal diabetes mellitus (P70.2)

    type 1 diabetes mellitus (E10.-)

    type 2 diabetes mellitus (E11.-)

E13.0 Other specified diabetes mellitus with hyperosmolarity

    E13.00 Other specified diabetes mellitus with hyperosmolarity without nonketotic hyperglycemic-hyperosmolar coma (NKHHC)

    E13.01 Other specified diabetes mellitus with hyperosmolarity with coma

E13.1 Other specified diabetes mellitus with ketoacidosis

    E13.10 Other specified diabetes mellitus with ketoacidosis without coma

    E13.11 Other specified diabetes mellitus with ketoacidosis with coma

E13.2 Other specified diabetes mellitus with kidney complications

    E13.21 Other specified diabetes mellitus with diabetic nephropathy

        Other specified diabetes mellitus with intercapillary glomerulosclerosis

        Other specified diabetes mellitus with intracapillary glomerulonephrosis

        Other specified diabetes mellitus with Kimmelstiel-Wilson disease

    E13.22 Other specified diabetes mellitus with diabetic chronic kidney disease

        Use additional code to identify stage of chronic kidney disease (N18.1-N18.6)

    E13.29 Other specified diabetes mellitus with other diabetic kidney complication

        Other specified diabetes mellitus with renal tubular degeneration

E13.3 Other specified diabetes mellitus with ophthalmic complications

    E13.31 Other specified diabetes mellitus with unspecified diabetic retinopathy

        E13.311 Other specified diabetes mellitus with unspecified diabetic retinopathy with macular edema

        E13.319 Other specified diabetes mellitus with unspecified diabetic retinopathy without macular edema

    E13.32 Other specified diabetes mellitus with mild nonproliferative diabetic retinopathy

        Other specified diabetes mellitus with nonproliferative diabetic retinopathy NOS

        One of the following 7th characters is to be assigned to codes in subcategory E13.32 to designate laterality of the disease:

        1 - right eye

        2 - left eye

        3 - bilateral

        9 - unspecified eye

        ●⑦ **E13.321** Other specified diabetes mellitus with mild nonproliferative diabetic retinopathy with macular edema

        ●⑦ **E13.329** Other specified diabetes mellitus with mild nonproliferative diabetic retinopathy without macular edema

    E13.33 Other specified diabetes mellitus with moderate nonproliferative diabetic retinopathy

One of the following 7th characters is to be assigned to codes in subcategory E13.33 to designate laterality of the disease:

1 - right eye

2 - left eye

3 - bilateral

9 - unspecified eye

● ⑦ **E13.331**   **Other specified diabetes mellitus with moderate nonproliferative diabetic retinopathy with macular edema**

● ⑦ **E13.339**   **Other specified diabetes mellitus with moderate nonproliferative diabetic retinopathy without macular edema**

E13.34   **Other specified diabetes mellitus with severe nonproliferative diabetic retinopathy**

One of the following 7th characters is to be assigned to codes in subcategory E13.34 to designate laterality of the disease:

1 - right eye

2 - left eye

3 - bilateral

9 - unspecified eye

● ⑦ **E13.341**   **Other specified diabetes mellitus with severe nonproliferative diabetic retinopathy with macular edema**

● ⑦ **E13.349**   **Other specified diabetes mellitus with severe nonproliferative diabetic retinopathy without macular edema**

E13.35   **Other specified diabetes mellitus with proliferative diabetic retinopathy**

One of the following 7th characters is to be assigned to codes in subcategory E13.35 to designate laterality of the disease:

1 - right eye

2 - left eye

3 - bilateral

9 - unspecified eye

● ⑦ **E13.351**   **Other specified diabetes mellitus with proliferative diabetic retinopathy with macular edema**

● ⑦ **E13.352**   **Other specified diabetes mellitus with proliferative diabetic retinopathy with traction retinal detachment involving the macula**

● ⑦ **E13.353**   **Other specified diabetes mellitus with proliferative diabetic retinopathy with traction retinal detachment not involving the macula**

● ⑦ **E13.354**   **Other specified diabetes mellitus with proliferative diabetic retinopathy with combined traction retinal detachment and rhegmatogenous retinal detachment**

● ⑦ **E13.355**   **Other specified diabetes mellitus with stable proliferative diabetic retinopathy**

● ⑦ **E13.359**   **Other specified diabetes mellitus with proliferative diabetic retinopathy without macular edema**

E13.36   **Other specified diabetes mellitus with diabetic cataract**

● ⊗⑦ **E13.37**   **Other specified diabetes mellitus with diabetic macular edema, resolved following treatment**

One of the following 7th characters is to be assigned to code E13.37 to designate laterality of the disease:

1 - right eye

2 - left eye

3 - bilateral

9 - unspecified eye

E13.39   **Other specified diabetes mellitus with other diabetic ophthalmic complication**

<u>Use additional code</u> to identify manifestation, such as:

diabetic glaucoma (H40-H42)

E13.4   **Other specified diabetes mellitus with neurological complications**

E13.40   **Other specified diabetes mellitus with diabetic neuropathy, unspecified**

E13.41   **Other specified diabetes mellitus with diabetic mononeuropathy**

E13.42   **Other specified diabetes mellitus with diabetic polyneuropathy**

Other specified diabetes mellitus with diabetic neuralgia

E13.43   **Other specified diabetes mellitus with diabetic autonomic (poly)neuropathy**

Other specified diabetes mellitus with diabetic gastroparesis

E13.44   **Other specified diabetes mellitus with diabetic amyotrophy**

E13.49   **Other specified diabetes mellitus with other diabetic neurological complication**

E13.5   **Other specified diabetes mellitus with circulatory complications**

E13.51   **Other specified diabetes mellitus with diabetic peripheral angiopathy without gangrene**

E13.52   **Other specified diabetes mellitus with diabetic peripheral angiopathy with gangrene**

Other specified diabetes mellitus with diabetic gangrene

E13.59   **Other specified diabetes mellitus with other circulatory complications**

E13.6   **Other specified diabetes mellitus with other specified complications**

E13.61   **Other specified diabetes mellitus with diabetic arthropathy**

E13.610   **Other specified diabetes mellitus with diabetic neuropathic arthropathy**

Other specified diabetes mellitus with Charcôt's joints

E13.618   **Other specified diabetes mellitus with other diabetic arthropathy**

E13.62   **Other specified diabetes mellitus with skin complications**

E13.620 **Other specified diabetes mellitus with diabetic dermatitis**

Other specified diabetes mellitus with diabetic necrobiosis lipoidica

E13.621 **Other specified diabetes mellitus with foot ulcer**

<u>Use **additional** code</u> to identify site of ulcer (L97.4-, L97.5-)

E13.622 **Other specified diabetes mellitus with other skin ulcer**

<u>Use **additional** code</u> to identify site of ulcer (L97.1-L97.9, L98.41-L98.49)

E13.628 **Other specified diabetes mellitus with other skin complications**

E13.63 **Other specified diabetes mellitus with oral complications**

E13.630 **Other specified diabetes mellitus with periodontal disease**

E13.638 **Other specified diabetes mellitus with other oral complications**

E13.64 **Other specified diabetes mellitus with hypoglycemia**

E13.641 **Other specified diabetes mellitus with hypoglycemia with coma**

E13.649 **Other specified diabetes mellitus with hypoglycemia without coma**

E13.65 **Other specified diabetes mellitus with hyperglycemia**

E13.69 **Other specified diabetes mellitus with other specified complication**

<u>Use **additional** code</u> to identify complication

E13.8 **Other specified diabetes mellitus with unspecified complications**

E13.9 **Other specified diabetes mellitus without complications**

OTHER DISORDERS OF GLUCOSE REGULATION AND PANCREATIC INTERNAL SECRETION (E15-E16)

E15 **Nondiabetic hypoglycemic coma**

Includes: drug-induced insulin coma in nondiabetic

hyperinsulinism with hypoglycemic coma
hypoglycemic coma NOS

E16 **Other disorders of pancreatic internal secretion**

E16.0 **Drug-induced hypoglycemia without coma**

Excludes1: diabetes with hypoglycemia without coma (E09.692)

<u>Use **additional** code</u> for adverse effect, if applicable, to identify drug (T36-T50 with fifth or sixth character 5)

E16.1 **Other hypoglycemia**

Functional hyperinsulinism

Functional nonhyperinsulinemic hypoglycemia

Hyperinsulinism NOS

Hyperplasia of pancreatic islet beta cells NOS

Excludes1: diabetes with hypoglycemia (E08.649, E10.649, E11.649, E13.649)

hypoglycemia in infant of diabetic mother (P70.1)

neonatal hypoglycemia (P70.4)

E16.2 **Hypoglycemia, unspecified**

Definition: Hypoglycemia is the medical term for abnormally low blood sugar usually resulting from excessive insulin or a poor diet.

Excludes1: diabetes with hypoglycemia (E08.649, E10.649, E11.649, E13.649)

E16.3 **Increased secretion of glucagon**

Hyperplasia of pancreatic endocrine cells with glucagon excess

E16.4 **Increased secretion of gastrin**

Hypergastrinemia

Hyperplasia of pancreatic endocrine cells with gastrin excess Zollinger-Ellison syndrome

E16.8 **Other specified disorders of pancreatic internal secretion**

Increased secretion from endocrine pancreas of growth hormone-releasing hormone

Increased secretion from endocrine pancreas of pancreatic polypeptide

Increased secretion from endocrine pancreas of somatostatin

Increased secretion from endocrine pancreas of vasoactive-intestinal polypeptide

E16.9 **Disorder of pancreatic internal secretion, unspecified**

Islet-cell hyperplasia NOS

Pancreatic endocrine cell hyperplasia NOS

DISORDERS OF OTHER ENDOCRINE GLANDS (E20-E35)

Excludes1: galactorrhea (N64.3)

gynecomastia (N62)

E20 **Hypoparathyroidism**

Excludes1: Di George's syndrome (D82.1)

postprocedural hypoparathyroidism (E89.2)

tetany NOS (R29.0)

transitory neonatal hypoparathyroidism (P71.4)

E20.0 **Idiopathic hypoparathyroidism**

E20.1 **Pseudohypoparathyroidism**

E20.8 **Other hypoparathyroidism**

E20.9 **Hypoparathyroidism, unspecified**

Parathyroid tetany

E21 **Hyperparathyroidism and other disorders of parathyroid gland**

Excludes1: adult osteomalacia (M83.-)

ectopic hyperparathyroidism (E34.2)

familial hypocalciuric hypercalcemia (E83.52)

hungry bone syndrome (E83.81)

infantile and juvenile osteomalacia (E55.0)

E21.0 **Primary hyperparathyroidism**

Hyperplasia of parathyroid

Osteitis fibrosa cystica generalisata [von Recklinghausen's disease of bone]

E21.1 **Secondary hyperparathyroidism, not elsewhere classified**

Excludes1: secondary hyperparathyroidism of renal origin (N25.81)

E21.2 **Other hyperparathyroidism**

Tertiary hyperparathyroidism

Excludes1: familial hypocalciuric hypercalcemia (E83.52)

E21.3   **Hyperparathyroidism, unspecified**

E21.4   **Other specified disorders of parathyroid gland**

E21.5   **Disorder of parathyroid gland, unspecified**

E22   **Hyperfunction of pituitary gland**

> **Excludes1:** Cushing's syndrome (E24.-)
>
> Nelson's syndrome (E24.1)
>
> overproduction of ACTH not associated with Cushing's disease (E27.0)
>
> overproduction of pituitary ACTH (E24.0)
>
> overproduction of thyroid-stimulating hormone (E05.8-)

E22.0   **Acromegaly and pituitary gigantism**

Overproduction of growth hormone

> **Excludes1:** constitutional gigantism (E34.4)
>
> constitutional tall stature (E34.4)
>
> increased secretion from endocrine pancreas of growth hormone-releasing hormone (E16.8)

E22.1   **Hyperprolactinemia**

Use additional code for adverse effect, if applicable, to identify drug (T36-T50 with fifth or sixth character 5)

E22.2   **Syndrome of inappropriate secretion of antidiuretic hormone**

E22.8   **Other hyperfunction of pituitary gland**

Central precocious puberty

E22.9   **Hyperfunction of pituitary gland, unspecified**

E23   **Hypofunction and other disorders of the pituitary gland**

> **Includes:** the listed conditions whether the disorder is in the pituitary or the hypothalamus
>
> **Excludes1:** postprocedural hypopituitarism (E89.3)

E23.0   **Hypopituitarism**

Fertile eunuch syndrome

Hypogonadotropic hypogonadism

Idiopathic growth hormone deficiency

Isolated deficiency of gonadotropin

Isolated deficiency of growth hormone

Isolated deficiency of pituitary hormone

Kallmann's syndrome

Lorain-Levi short stature

Necrosis of pituitary gland (postpartum)

Panhypopituitarism

Pituitary cachexia

Pituitary insufficiency NOS

Pituitary short stature

Sheehan's syndrome

Simmonds' disease

E23.1   **Drug-induced hypopituitarism**

Use additional code for adverse effect, if applicable, to identify drug (T36-T50 with fifth or sixth character 5)

E23.2   **Diabetes insipidus**

> **Excludes1:** nephrogenic diabetes insipidus (N25.1)

E23.3   **Hypothalamic dysfunction, not elsewhere classified**

> **Excludes1:** Prader-Willi syndrome (Q87.1)
>
> Russell-Silver syndrome (Q87.1)

E23.6   **Other disorders of pituitary gland**

Abscess of pituitary

Adiposogenital dystrophy

E23.7   **Disorder of pituitary gland, unspecified**

E24   **Cushing's syndrome**

> **Definition:** Cushing's syndrome is a condition due to tumors of the adrenal cortex or the anterior lobe of the pituitary gland.
>
> **Excludes1:** congenital adrenal hyperplasia (E25.0)

E24.0   **Pituitary-dependent Cushing's disease**

Overproduction of pituitary ACTH

Pituitary-dependent hypercorticalism

E24.1   **Nelson's syndrome**

E24.2   **Drug-induced Cushing's syndrome**

Use additional code for adverse effect, if applicable, to identify drug (T36-T50 with fifth or sixth character 5)

E24.3   **Ectopic ACTH syndrome**

E24.4   **Alcohol-induced pseudo-Cushing's syndrome**

E24.8   **Other Cushing's syndrome**

E24.9   **Cushing's syndrome, unspecified**

E25   **Adrenogenital disorders**

> **Includes:** adrenogenital syndromes, virilizing or feminizing, whether acquired or due to adrenal hyperplasia consequent on inborn enzyme defects in hormone synthesis
>
> Female adrenal pseudohermaphroditism
>
> Female heterosexual precocious pseudopuberty
>
> Male isosexual precocious pseudopuberty
>
> Male macrogenitosomia praecox
>
> Male sexual precocity with adrenal hyperplasia
>
> Male virilization (female)
>
> **Excludes1:** indeterminate sex and pseudohermaphroditism (Q56)
>
> chromosomal abnormalities (Q90-Q99)

E25.0   **Congenital adrenogenital disorders associated with enzyme deficiency**

Congenital adrenal hyperplasia 21-Hydroxylase deficiency

Salt-losing congenital adrenal hyperplasia

E25.8   **Other adrenogenital disorders**

Idiopathic adrenogenital disorder

Use additional code for adverse effect, if applicable, to identify drug (T36-T50 with fifth or sixth character 5)

E25.9   **Adrenogenital disorder, unspecified**

Adrenogenital syndrome NOS

E26   **Hyperaldosteronism**

E26.0   **Primary hyperaldosteronism**

E26.01   **Conn's syndrome**

Code also adrenal adenoma (D35.0-)

E26.02   **Glucocorticoid-remediable aldosteronism**

Familial aldosteronism type I

E26.09   **Other primary hyperaldosteronism**

Primary aldosteronism due to adrenal hyperplasia (bilateral)

E26.1   **Secondary hyperaldosteronism**

E26.8   **Other hyperaldosteronism**

E26.81   **Bartter's syndrome**

E26.89   **Other hyperaldosteronism**

E26.9   **Hyperaldosteronism, unspecified**

Aldosteronism NOS

Hyperaldosteronism NOS

E27   **Other disorders of adrenal gland**

E27.0   **Other adrenocortical overactivity**

Overproduction of ACTH, not associated with Cushing's disease

Premature adrenarche

Excludes1: Cushing's syndrome (E24.-)

E27.1   Primary adrenocortical insufficiency

Addison's disease

Autoimmune adrenalitis

Excludes1: Addison only phenotype adrenoleukodystrophy (E71.528)

amyloidosis (E85.-)

tuberculous Addison's disease (A18.7)

Waterhouse-Friderichsen syndrome (A39.1)

E27.2   Addisonian crisis

Adrenal crisis

Adrenocortical crisis

E27.3   Drug-induced adrenocortical insufficiency

Use additional code for adverse effect, if applicable, to identify drug (T36-T50 with fifth or sixth character 5)

E27.4   Other and unspecified adrenocortical insufficiency

Excludes1: adrenoleukodystrophy [Addison-Schilder] (E71.528)

Waterhouse-Friderichsen syndrome (A39.1)

E27.40   Unspecified adrenocortical insufficiency

Adrenocortical insufficiency NOS

Hypoaldosteronism

E27.49   Other adrenocortical insufficiency

Adrenal hemorrhage

Adrenal infarction

E27.5   Adrenomedullary hyperfunction

Adrenomedullary hyperplasia

Catecholamine hypersecretion

E27.8   Other specified disorders of adrenal gland

Abnormality of cortisol-binding globulin

E27.9   Disorder of adrenal gland, unspecified

E28   Ovarian dysfunction

Excludes1: isolated gonadotropin deficiency (E23.0)

postprocedural ovarian failure (E89.4-)

E28.0   Estrogen excess

Use additional code for adverse effect, if applicable, to identify drug (T36-T50 with fifth or sixth character 5)

E28.1   Androgen excess

Hypersecretion of ovarian androgens

Use additional code for adverse effect, if applicable, to identify drug (T36-T50 with fifth or sixth character 5)

E28.2   Polycystic ovarian syndrome

Sclerocystic ovary syndrome

Stein-Leventhal syndrome

E28.3   Primary ovarian failure

Excludes1: pure gonadal dysgenesis (Q99.1)

Turner's syndrome (Q96.-)

E28.31   Premature menopause

E28.310   Symptomatic premature menopause

Symptoms such as flushing, sleeplessness, headache, lack of concentration, associated with premature menopause

E28.319   Asymptomatic premature menopause

Premature menopause NOS

E28.39   Other primary ovarian failure

Decreased estrogen

Resistant ovary syndrome

E28.8   Other ovarian dysfunction

Ovarian hyperfunction NOS

Excludes1: postprocedural ovarian failure (E89.4-)

E28.9   Ovarian dysfunction, unspecified

E29   Testicular dysfunction

Excludes1: androgen insensitivity syndrome (E34.5-)

azoospermia or oligospermia NOS (N46.0-N46.1)

isolated gonadotropin deficiency (E23.0)

Klinefelter's syndrome (Q98.0-Q98.1, Q98.4)

E29.0   Testicular hyperfunction

Hypersecretion of testicular hormones

E29.1   Testicular hypofunction

Defective biosynthesis of testicular androgen NOS

5-delta-Reductase deficiency (with male pseudohermaphroditism)

Testicular hypogonadism NOS

Use additional code for adverse effect, if applicable, to identify drug (T36-T50 with fifth or sixth character 5)

Excludes1: postprocedural testicular hypofunction (E89.5)

E29.8   Other testicular dysfunction

E29.9   Testicular dysfunction, unspecified

E30   Disorders of puberty, not elsewhere classified

E30.0   Delayed puberty

Constitutional delay of puberty

Delayed sexual development

E30.1   Precocious puberty

Precocious menstruation

Excludes1: Albright (-McCune) (-Sternberg) syndrome (Q78.1)

central precocious puberty (E22.8)

congenital adrenal hyperplasia (E25.0)

female heterosexual precocious pseudopuberty (E25.-)

male isosexual precocious pseudopuberty (E25.-)

E30.8   Other disorders of puberty

Premature thelarche

E30.9   Disorder of puberty, unspecified

E31   Polyglandular dysfunction

Excludes1: ataxia telangiectasia [Louis-Bar] (G11.3)

dystrophia myotonica [Steinert] (G71.11)

pseudohypoparathyroidism (E20.1)

E31.0   Autoimmune polyglandular failure

Schmidt's syndrome

E31.1   Polyglandular hyperfunction

Excludes1: multiple endocrine adenomatosis (E31.2-)

multiple endocrine neoplasia (E31.2-)

E31.2   Multiple endocrine neoplasia [MEN] syndromes

Multiple endocrine adenomatosis

Code also any associated malignancies **and other conditions** associated with the syndromes

E31.20 **Multiple endocrine neoplasia [MEN] syndrome, unspecified**

Multiple endocrine adenomatosis NOS

Multiple endocrine neoplasia [MEN] syndrome NOS

E31.21 **Multiple endocrine neoplasia [MEN] type I**

Wermer's syndrome

E31.22 **Multiple endocrine neoplasia [MEN] type IIA**

Sipple's syndrome

E31.23 **Multiple endocrine neoplasia [MEN] type IIB**

E31.8 **Other polyglandular dysfunction**

E31.9 **Polyglandular dysfunction, unspecified**

E32 **Diseases of thymus**

Definition: The thymus is a gland located behind the breastbone that functions in the development of the immune system. The thymus is large in infancy and early childhood but begins to atrophy between ages eight and ten.

Excludes1: aplasia or hypoplasia of thymus with immunodeficiency (D82.1)

myasthenia gravis (G70.0)

E32.0 **Persistent hyperplasia of thymus**

Hypertrophy of thymus

E32.1 **Abscess of thymus**

E32.8 **Other diseases of thymus**

Excludes1: aplasia or hypoplasia with immunodeficiency (D82.1)

thymoma (D15.0)

E32.9 **Disease of thymus, unspecified**

E34 **Other endocrine disorders**

Definition: Endocrine disorders refers to disorders which involve the over-production or under-production of hormone substances from an endocrine gland. Examples include diabetes, hypothyroidism, hyperthyroidism, hyperparathyroidism, Cushing's disease, Cushing's syndrome and acromegaly.

Excludes1: pseudohypoparathyroidism (E20.1)

E34.0 **Carcinoid syndrome**

Note: May be used as an additional code to identify functional activity associated with a carcinoid tumor.

E34.1 **Other hypersecretion of intestinal hormones**

E34.2 **Ectopic hormone secretion, not elsewhere classified**

Excludes1: ectopic ACTH syndrome (E24.3)

E34.3 **Short stature due to endocrine disorder**

Constitutional short stature

Laron-type short stature

Excludes1: achondroplastic short stature (Q77.4)

hypochondroplastic short stature (Q77.4)

nutritional short stature (E45)

pituitary short stature (E23.0)

progeria (E34.8)

renal short stature (N25.0)

Russell-Silver syndrome (Q87.1)

short-limbed stature with immunodeficiency (D82.2)

short stature in specific dysmorphic syndromes - code to syndrome - see Alphabetical Index short stature NOS (R62.52)

E34.4 **Constitutional tall stature**

Constitutional gigantism

E34.5 **Androgen insensitivity syndrome**

E34.50 **Androgen insensitivity syndrome, unspecified**

Androgen insensitivity NOS

E34.51 **Complete androgen insensitivity syndrome**

Complete androgen insensitivity de Quervain syndrome

Goldberg-Maxwell syndrome

E34.52 **Partial androgen insensitivity syndrome**

Partial androgen insensitivity

Reifenstein syndrome

E34.8 **Other specified endocrine disorders**

Pineal gland dysfunction

Progeria

Excludes2: pseudohypoparathyroidism (E20.1)

E34.9 **Endocrine disorder, unspecified**

Endocrine disturbance NOS

Hormone disturbance NOS

E35 **Disorders of endocrine glands in diseases classified elsewhere**

Code first underlying disease, such as:

late congenital syphilis of thymus gland [Dubois disease] (A50.5)

Use additional code , if applicable, to identify:

sequelae of tuberculosis of other organs (B90.8)

Excludes1: Echinococcus granulosus infection of thyroid gland (B67.3)

meningococcal hemorrhagic adrenalitis (A39.1)

syphilis of endocrine gland (A52.79)

tuberculosis of adrenal gland, except calcification (A18.7)

tuberculosis of endocrine gland NEC (A18.82)

tuberculosis of thyroid gland (A18.81)

Waterhouse-Friderichsen syndrome (A39.1)

INTRAOPERATIVE COMPLICATIONS OF ENDOCRINE SYSTEM (E36)

E36 **Intraoperative complications of endocrine system**

Excludes2: postprocedural endocrine and metabolic complications and disorders, not elsewhere classified (E89.-)

E36.0 **Intraoperative hemorrhage and hematoma of an endocrine system organ or structure complicating a procedure**

Excludes1: intraoperative hemorrhage and hematoma of an endocrine system organ or structure due to accidental puncture or laceration during a procedure (E36.1-)

E36.01 **Intraoperative hemorrhage and hematoma of an endocrine system organ or structure complicating an endocrine system procedure**

E36.02 **Intraoperative hemorrhage and hematoma of an endocrine system organ or structure complicating other procedure**

E36.1 **Accidental puncture and laceration of an endocrine system organ or structure during a procedure**

E36.11 **Accidental puncture and laceration of an endocrine system organ or structure during an endocrine system procedure**

E36.12 Accidental puncture and laceration of an endocrine system organ or structure during other procedure

E36.8 Other intraoperative complications of endocrine system

Use additional code, if applicable, to further specify disorder

MALNUTRITION (E40-E46)

Excludes1: intestinal malabsorption (K90.-)

sequelae of protein-calorie malnutrition (E64.0)

Excludes2: nutritional anemias (D50-D53)

starvation (T73.0)

E40 **Kwashiorkor**

Severe malnutrition with nutritional edema with dyspigmentation of skin and hair

Excludes1: marasmic kwashiorkor (E42)

E41 **Nutritional marasmus**

Severe malnutrition with marasmus

Excludes1: marasmic kwashiorkor (E42)

E42 **Marasmic kwashiorkor**

Intermediate form severe protein-calorie malnutrition

Severe protein-calorie malnutrition with signs of both kwashiorkor and marasmus

E43 **Unspecified severe protein-calorie malnutrition**

Starvation edema

E44 **Protein-calorie malnutrition of moderate and mild degree**

E44.0 Moderate protein-calorie malnutrition

E44.1 Mild protein-calorie malnutrition

E45 **Retarded development following protein-calorie malnutrition**

Nutritional short stature

Nutritional stunting

Physical retardation due to malnutrition

E46 **Unspecified protein-calorie malnutrition**

Malnutrition NOS

Protein-calorie imbalance NOS

Excludes1: nutritional deficiency NOS (E63.9)

OTHER NUTRITIONAL DEFICIENCIES (E50-E64)

Excludes2: nutritional anemias (D50-D53)

E50 **Vitamin A deficiency**

Definition: Vitamin A deficiency (VAD) occurs where diets contain insufficient vitamin A for meeting the needs associated with growth and development, physiological functions, and periods of added stress due to illness.

Excludes1: sequelae of vitamin A deficiency (E64.1)

E50.0 Vitamin A deficiency with conjunctival xerosis

E50.1 Vitamin A deficiency with Bitot's spot and conjunctival xerosis

Bitot's spot in the young child

E50.2 Vitamin A deficiency with corneal xerosis

E50.3 Vitamin A deficiency with corneal ulceration and xerosis

E50.4 Vitamin A deficiency with keratomalacia

E50.5 Vitamin A deficiency with night blindness

E50.6 Vitamin A deficiency with xerophthalmic scars of cornea

E50.7 Other ocular manifestations of vitamin A deficiency

Xerophthalmia NOS

E50.8 Other manifestations of vitamin A deficiency

Follicular keratosis Xeroderma

E50.9 Vitamin A deficiency, unspecified

Hypovitaminosis A NOS

E51 **Thiamine deficiency**

Excludes1: sequelae of thiamine deficiency (E64.8)

E51.1 Beriberi

E51.11 Dry beriberi

Beriberi NOS

Beriberi with polyneuropathy

E51.12 Wet beriberi

Beriberi with cardiovascular manifestations

Cardiovascular beriberi

Shoshin disease

E51.2 Wernicke's encephalopathy

E51.8 Other manifestations of thiamine deficiency

E51.9 Thiamine deficiency, unspecified

E52 **Niacin deficiency [pellagra]**

Niacin (-tryptophan) deficiency

Nicotinamide deficiency

Pellagra (alcoholic)

Excludes1: sequelae of niacin deficiency (E64.8)

E53 **Deficiency of other B group vitamins**

Excludes1: sequelae of vitamin B deficiency (E64.8)

E53.0 Riboflavin deficiency

Ariboflavinosis

Vitamin B2 deficiency

E53.1 Pyridoxine deficiency

Vitamin B6 deficiency

Excludes1: pyridoxine-responsive sideroblastic anemia (D64.3)

E53.8 Deficiency of other specified B group vitamins

Biotin deficiency

Cyanocobalamin deficiency

Folate deficiency

Folic acid deficiency

Pantothenic acid deficiency

Vitamin B12 deficiency

Excludes1: folate deficiency anemia (D52.-)

vitamin B12 deficiency anemia (D51.-)

E53.9 Vitamin B deficiency, unspecified

E54 **Ascorbic acid deficiency**

Deficiency of vitamin C

Scurvy

Excludes1: scorbutic anemia (D53.2)

sequelae of vitamin C deficiency (E64.2)

E55 **Vitamin D deficiency**

Excludes1: adult osteomalacia (M83.-)

osteoporosis (M80.-)

sequelae of rickets (E64.3)

E55.0 Rickets, active

Infantile osteomalacia Juvenile osteomalacia

Excludes1: celiac rickets (K90.0)

Crohn's rickets (K50.-)

hereditary vitamin D-dependent rickets (E83.32)

inactive rickets (E64.3)

renal rickets (N25.0)

sequelae of rickets (E64.3)

vitamin D-resistant rickets (E83.31)

E55.9   Vitamin D deficiency, unspecified

Avitaminosis D

E56   Other vitamin deficiencies

Excludes1: sequelae of other vitamin deficiencies (E64.8)

E56.0   Deficiency of vitamin E

E56.1   Deficiency of vitamin K

Excludes1: deficiency of coagulation factor due to vitamin K deficiency (D68.4)

vitamin K deficiency of newborn (P53)

E56.8   Deficiency of other vitamins

E56.9   Vitamin deficiency, unspecified

E58   Dietary calcium deficiency

Excludes1: disorders of calcium metabolism (E83.5-)

sequelae of calcium deficiency (E64.8)

E59   Dietary selenium deficiency

Keshan disease

Excludes1: sequelae of selenium deficiency (E64.8)

E60   Dietary zinc deficiency

E61   Deficiency of other nutrient elements

Use additional code for adverse effect, if applicable, to identify drug (T36-T50 with fifth or sixth character 5)

Excludes1: disorders of mineral metabolism (E83.-)

iodine deficiency related thyroid disorders (E00-E02)

sequelae of malnutrition **and other** nutritional deficiencies (E64.-)

E61.0   Copper deficiency

E61.1   Iron deficiency

Excludes1: iron deficiency anemia (D50.-)

E61.2   Magnesium deficiency

E61.3   Manganese deficiency

E61.4   Chromium deficiency

E61.5   Molybdenum deficiency

E61.6   Vanadium deficiency

E61.7   Deficiency of multiple nutrient elements

E61.8   Deficiency of other specified nutrient elements

E61.9   Deficiency of nutrient element, unspecified

E63   Other nutritional deficiencies

Excludes1: dehydration (E86.0)

failure to thrive, adult (R62.7)

failure to thrive, child (R62.51)

feeding problems in newborn (P92.-)

sequelae of malnutrition **and other** nutritional deficiencies (E64.-)

E63.0   Essential fatty acid [EFA] deficiency

E63.1   Imbalance of constituents of food intake

E63.8   Other specified nutritional deficiencies

E63.9   Nutritional deficiency, unspecified

E64   Sequelae of malnutrition and other nutritional deficiencies

Note: This category is to be used to indicate conditions in categories E43, E44, E46, E50-E63 as the cause of sequelae, which are themselves classified elsewhere. The 'sequelae' include conditions specified as such; they also include the late effects of diseases classifiable to the above categories if the disease itself is no longer present

Code first condition resulting from (sequela) of malnutrition **and other** nutritional deficiencies

E64.0   Sequelae of protein-calorie malnutrition

Excludes2: retarded development following protein-calorie malnutrition (E45)

E64.1   Sequelae of vitamin A deficiency

E64.2   Sequelae of vitamin C deficiency

E64.3   Sequelae of rickets

E64.8   Sequelae of other nutritional deficiencies

E64.9   Sequelae of unspecified nutritional deficiency

OVERWEIGHT, OBESITY AND OTHER HYPERALIMENTATION (E65-E68)

E65   Localized adiposity

Fat pad

E66   Overweight and obesity

Code first obesity complicating pregnancy, childbirth and the puerperium, if applicable (O99.21-)

Use additional code to identify body mass index (BMI), if known (Z68.-)

Excludes1: adiposogenital dystrophy (E23.6)

lipomatosis NOS (E88.2)

lipomatosis dolorosa [Dercum] (E88.2)

Prader-Willi syndrome (Q87.1)

E66.0   Obesity due to excess calories

E66.01   Morbid (severe) obesity due to excess calories

Excludes1: morbid (severe) obesity with alveolar hypoventilation (E66.2)

E66.09   Other obesity due to excess calories

E66.1   Drug-induced obesity

Use additional code for adverse effect, if applicable, to identify drug (T36-T50 with fifth or sixth character 5)

E66.2   Morbid (severe) obesity with alveolar hypoventilation

Obesity hypoventilation syndrome (OHS)

Pickwickian syndrome

E66.3   Overweight

E66.8   Other obesity

E66.9   Obesity, unspecified

Obesity NOS

E67   Other hyperalimentation

Excludes1: hyperalimentation NOS (R63.2)

sequelae of hyperalimentation (E68)

E67.0   Hypervitaminosis A

E67.1   Hypercarotinemia

E67.2   Megavitamin-B6   syndrome

E67.3   Hypervitaminosis D

E67.8   Other specified hyperalimentation

E68   Sequelae of hyperalimentation

Code first condition resulting from (sequela) of hyperalimentation

METABOLIC DISORDERS (E70-E88)

Excludes1: androgen insensitivity syndrome (E34.5-)

congenital adrenal hyperplasia (E25.0)

Ehlers-Danlos syndrome (Q79.6)

hemolytic anemias attributable to enzyme disorders (D55.-)

Marfan's syndrome (Q87.4)

5-alpha-reductase deficiency (E29.1)

E70 Disorders of aromatic amino-acid metabolism

   E70.0 Classical phenylketonuria

   E70.1 Other hyperphenylalaninemias

   E70.2 Disorders of tyrosine metabolism

      Excludes1: transitory tyrosinemia of newborn (P74.5)

      E70.20 Disorder of tyrosine metabolism, unspecified

      E70.21 Tyrosinemia

         Hypertyrosinemia

      E70.29 Other disorders of tyrosine metabolism

         Alkaptonuria

         Ochronosis

   E70.3 Albinism

      E70.30 Albinism, unspecified

      E70.31 Ocular albinism

         E70.310 X-linked ocular albinism

         E70.311 Autosomal recessive ocular albinism

         E70.318 Other ocular albinism

         E70.319 Ocular albinism, unspecified

      E70.32 Oculocutaneous albinism

         Excludes1: Chediak-Higashi syndrome (E70.330)

         Hermansky-Pudlak syndrome (E70.331)

         E70.320 Tyrosinase negative oculocutaneous albinism

            Albinism I

            Oculocutaneous albinism ty-neg

         E70.321 Tyrosinase positive oculocutaneous albinism

            Albinism II

            Oculocutaneous albinism ty-pos

         E70.328 Other oculocutaneous albinism

            Cross syndrome

         E70.329 Oculocutaneous albinism, unspecified

      E70.33 Albinism with hematologic abnormality

         E70.330 Chediak-Higashi syndrome

         E70.331 Hermansky-Pudlak syndrome

         E70.338 Other albinism with hematologic abnormality

         E70.339 Albinism with hematologic abnormality, unspecified

      E70.39 Other specified albinism

         Piebaldism

   E70.4 Disorders of histidine metabolism

      E70.40 Disorders of histidine metabolism, unspecified

      E70.41 Histidinemia

      E70.49 Other disorders of histidine metabolism

   E70.5 Disorders of tryptophan metabolism

   E70.8 Other disorders of aromatic amino-acid metabolism

   E70.9 Disorder of aromatic amino-acid metabolism, unspecified

E71 Disorders of branched-chain amino-acid metabolism and fatty-acid metabolism

   E71.0 Maple-syrup-urine disease

   E71.1 Other disorders of branched-chain amino-acid metabolism

      E71.11 Branched-chain organic acidurias

         E71.110 Isovaleric acidemia

         E71.111 3-methylglutaconic aciduria

         E71.118 Other branched-chain organic acidurias

      E71.12 Disorders of propionate metabolism

         E71.120 Methylmalonic acidemia

         E71.121 Propionic acidemia

         E71.128 Other disorders of propionate metabolism

      E71.19 Other disorders of branched-chain amino-acid metabolism

         Hyperleucine-isoleucinemia

         Hypervalinemia

   E71.2 Disorder of branched-chain amino-acid metabolism, unspecified

   E71.3 Disorders of fatty-acid metabolism

      Excludes1: peroxisomal disorders (E71.5)

         Refsum's disease (G60.1)

         Schilder's disease (G37.0)

      Excludes2: carnitine deficiency due to inborn error of metabolism (E71.42)

      E71.30 Disorder of fatty-acid metabolism, unspecified

      E71.31 Disorders of fatty-acid oxidation

         E71.310 Long chain/very long chain acyl CoA dehydrogenase deficiency

            LCAD

            VLCAD

         E71.311 Medium chain acyl CoA dehydrogenase deficiency

            MCAD

         E71.312 Short chain acyl CoA dehydrogenase deficiency

            SCAD

         E71.313 Glutaric aciduria type II

            Glutaric aciduria type II A

            Glutaric aciduria type II B

            Glutaric aciduria type II C

            Excludes1: glutaric aciduria (type 1) NOS (E72.3)

         E71.314 Muscle carnitine palmitoyltransferase deficiency

         E71.318 Other disorders of fatty-acid oxidation

      E71.32 Disorders of ketone metabolism

      E71.39 Other disorders of fatty-acid metabolism

   E71.4 Disorders of carnitine metabolism

      Excludes1: Muscle carnitine palmitoyltransferase deficiency (E71.314)

E71.40   **Disorder of carnitine metabolism, unspecified**

E71.41   **Primary carnitine deficiency**

E71.42   **Carnitine deficiency due to inborn errors of metabolism**

        Code also associated inborn error or metabolism

E71.43   **Iatrogenic carnitine deficiency**

        Carnitine deficiency due to hemodialysis

        Carnitine deficiency due to Valproic acid therapy

E71.44   **Other secondary carnitine deficiency**

    E71.440   **Ruvalcaba-Myhre-Smith syndrome**

    E71.448   **Other secondary carnitine deficiency**

E71.5   **Peroxisomal disorders**

    Excludes1: Schilder's disease (G37.0)

E71.50   **Peroxisomal disorder, unspecified**

E71.51   **Disorders of peroxisome biogenesis**

        Group 1 peroxisomal disorders

        Excludes1: Refsum's disease (G60.1)

    E71.510   **Zellweger syndrome**

    E71.511   **Neonatal adrenoleukodystrophy**

        Excludes1: X-linked adrenoleukodystrophy (E71.42-)

    E71.518   **Other disorders of peroxisome biogenesis**

E71.52   **X-linked adrenoleukodystrophy**

    E71.520   **Childhood cerebral X-linked adrenoleukodystrophy**

    E71.521   **Adolescent X-linked adrenoleukodystrophy**

    E71.522   **Adrenomyeloneuropathy**

    E71.528   **Other X-linked adrenoleukodystrophy**

        Addison only phenotype adrenoleukodystrophy

        Addison-Schilder adrenoleukodystrophy

    E71.529   **X-linked adrenoleukodystrophy, unspecified type**

E71.53   **Other group 2 peroxisomal disorders**

E71.54   **Other peroxisomal disorders**

    E71.540   **Rhizomelic chondrodysplasia punctata**

        Excludes1: chondrodysplasia punctata NOS (Q77.3)

    E71.541   **Zellweger-like syndrome**

    E71.542   **Other group 3 peroxisomal disorders**

    E71.548   **Other peroxisomal disorders**

E72   **Other disorders of amino-acid metabolism**

    Excludes1: disorders of:

    aromatic amino-acid metabolism (E70.-)

    branched-chain amino-acid metabolism (E71.0-E71.2)

    fatty-acid metabolism (E71.3)

    purine and pyrimidine metabolism (E79.-)

    gout (M1A.-, M10.-)

E72.0   **Disorders of amino-acid transport**

    Excludes1: disorders of tryptophan metabolism (E70.5)

E72.00   **Disorders of amino-acid transport, unspecified**

E72.01   **Cystinuria**

E72.02   **Hartnup's disease**

E72.03   **Lowe's syndrome**

        Use additional code for associated glaucoma (H42)

E72.04   **Cystinosis**

        Fanconi (-de Toni) (-Debré) syndrome with cystinosis

        Excludes1: Fanconi (-de Toni) (-Debré) syndrome without cystinosis (E72.09)

E72.09   **Other disorders of amino-acid transport**

        Fanconi (-de Toni) (-Debré) syndrome, unspecified

E72.1   **Disorders of sulfur-bearing amino-acid metabolism**

    Excludes1: cystinosis (E72.04)

        cystinuria (E72.01)

        transcobalamin II deficiency (D51.2)

E72.10   **Disorders of sulfur-bearing amino-acid metabolism, unspecified**

E72.11   **Homocystinuria**

        Cystathionine synthase deficiency

E72.12   **Methylenetetrahydrofolate reductase deficiency**

E72.19   **Other disorders of sulfur-bearing amino-acid metabolism**

        Cystathioninuria

        Methioninemia

        Sulfite oxidase deficiency

E72.2   **Disorders of urea cycle metabolism**

    Excludes1: disorders of ornithine metabolism (E72.4)

E72.20   **Disorder of urea cycle metabolism, unspecified**

        Hyperammonemia

        Excludes1: hyperammonemia-hyperornithinemia-homocitrullinemia syndrome E72.4

        transient hyperammonemia of newborn (P74.6)

E72.21   **Argininemia**

E72.22   **Arginosuccinic aciduria**

E72.23   **Citrullinemia**

E72.29   **Other disorders of urea cycle metabolism**

E72.3   **Disorders of lysine and hydroxylysine metabolism**

    Glutaric aciduria NOS Glutaric aciduria (type I)

    Hydroxylysinemia

    Hyperlysinemia

    Excludes1: glutaric aciduria type II (E71.313)

    Refsum's disease (G60.1)

    Zellweger syndrome (E71.510)

E72.4   **Disorders of ornithine metabolism**

    Hyperammonemia-Hyperornithinemia-Homocitrullinemia syndrome

    Ornithinemia (types I, II)

    Ornithine transcarbamylase deficiency

    Excludes1: hereditary choroidal dystrophy (H31.2-)

E72.5   **Disorders of glycine metabolism**

E72.50   **Disorder of glycine metabolism, unspecified**

E72.51	**Non-ketotic hyperglycinemia**	
E72.52	**Trimethylaminuria**	
E72.53	**Hyperoxaluria**	
	Oxalosis	
	Oxaluria	

E72.59 **Other disorders of glycine metabolism**

D-glycericacidemia

Hyperhydroxyprolinemia

Hyperprolinemia (types I, II)

Sarcosinemia

E72.8 **Other specified disorders of amino-acid metabolism**

Disorders of beta-amino-acid metabolism

Disorders of gamma-glutamyl cycle

E72.9 **Disorder of amino-acid metabolism, unspecified**

E73 **Lactose intolerance**

E73.0 **Congenital lactase deficiency**

E73.1 **Secondary lactase deficiency**

E73.8 **Other lactose intolerance**

E73.9 **Lactose intolerance, unspecified**

E74 **Other disorders of carbohydrate metabolism**

Excludes1: diabetes mellitus (E08-E13)

hypoglycemia NOS (E16.2)

increased secretion of glucagon (E16.3)

mucopolysaccharidosis (E76.0-E76.3)

E74.0 **Glycogen storage disease**

E74.00 **Glycogen storage disease, unspecified**

E74.01 **von Gierke disease**

Type I glycogen storage disease

E74.02 **Pompe disease**

Cardiac glycogenosis

Type II glycogen storage disease

E74.03 **Cori disease**

Forbes disease

Type III glycogen storage disease

E74.04 **McArdle disease**

Type V glycogen storage disease

E74.09 **Other glycogen storage disease**

Andersen disease

Hers disease

Tauri disease

Glycogen storage disease, types 0, IV, VI-XI

Liver phosphorylase deficiency

Muscle phosphofructokinase deficiency

E74.1 **Disorders of fructose metabolism**

Excludes1: muscle phosphofructokinase deficiency (E74.09)

E74.10 **Disorder of fructose metabolism, unspecified**

E74.11 **Essential fructosuria**

Fructokinase deficiency

E74.12 **Hereditary fructose intolerance**

Fructosemia

E74.19 **Other disorders of fructose metabolism**

Fructose-1, 6-diphosphatase deficiency

E74.2 **Disorders of galactose metabolism**

E74.20 **Disorders of galactose metabolism, unspecified**

E74.21 **Galactosemia**

E74.29 **Other disorders of galactose metabolism**

Galactokinase deficiency

E74.3 **Other disorders of intestinal carbohydrate absorption**

Excludes2: lactose intolerance (E73.-)

E74.31 **Sucrase-isomaltase deficiency**

E74.39 **Other disorders of intestinal carbohydrate absorption**

Disorder of intestinal carbohydrate absorption NOS

Glucose-galactose malabsorption

Sucrase deficiency

E74.4 **Disorders of pyruvate metabolism and gluconeogenesis**

Deficiency of phosphoenolpyruvate carboxykinase

Deficiency of pyruvate carboxylase

Deficiency of pyruvate dehydrogenase

Excludes1: disorders of pyruvate metabolism and gluconeogenesis with anemia (D55.-)

Leigh's syndrome (G31.82)

E74.8 **Other specified disorders of carbohydrate metabolism**

Essential pentosuria

Renal glycosuria

E74.9 **Disorder of carbohydrate metabolism, unspecified**

E75 **Disorders of sphingolipid metabolism and other lipid storage disorders**

Excludes1: mucolipidosis, types I-III (E77.0-E77.1)

Refsum's disease (G60.1)

E75.0 **GM2** **gangliosidosis**

E75.00 **GM2 gangliosidosis, unspecified**

E75.01 **Sandhoff disease**

E75.02 **Tay-Sachs disease**

E75.09 **Other GM2 gangliosidosis**

Adult GM2 gangliosidosis

Juvenile GM2 gangliosidosis

E75.1 **Other and unspecified gangliosidosis**

E75.10 **Unspecified gangliosidosis**

Gangliosidosis NOS

E75.11 **Mucolipidosis IV**

E75.19 **Other gangliosidosis**

GM1 gangliosidosis

GM3 gangliosidosis

E75.2 **Other sphingolipidosis**

Excludes1: adrenoleukodystrophy [Addison-Schilder] (E71.528)

E75.21 **Fabry (-Anderson) disease**

E75.22 **Gaucher disease**

E75.23 **Krabbe disease**

E75.24 **Niemann-Pick disease**

E75.240 **Niemann-Pick disease type A**

E75.241 **Niemann-Pick disease type B**

E75.242 **Niemann-Pick disease type C**

E75.243 **Niemann-Pick disease type D**

E75.248 **Other Niemann-Pick disease**

E75.249 **Niemann-Pick disease, unspecified**

E75.25 **Metachromatic leukodystrophy**

E75.29 **Other sphingolipidosis**

Farber's syndrome

Sulfatase deficiency

Sulfatide lipidosis

E75.3 **Sphingolipidosis, unspecified**

E75.4 **Neuronal ceroid lipofuscinosis**

Batten disease

Bielschowsky-Jansky disease

Kufs disease

Spielmeyer-Vogt disease

E75.5 **Other lipid storage disorders**

Cerebrotendinous cholesterosis [van Bogaert-Scherer-Epstein]

Wolman's disease

E75.6 **Lipid storage disorder, unspecified**

E76 **Disorders of glycosaminoglycan metabolism**

E76.0 **Mucopolysaccharidosis, type I**

E76.01 **Hurler's syndrome**

E76.02 **Hurler-Scheie syndrome**

E76.03 **Scheie's syndrome**

E76.1 **Mucopolysaccharidosis, type II**

Hunter's syndrome

E76.2 **Other mucopolysaccharidoses**

E76.21 **Morquio mucopolysaccharidoses**

E76.210 **Morquio A mucopolysaccharidoses**

Classic Morquio syndrome

Morquio syndrome A

Mucopolysaccharidosis, type IVA

E76.211 **Morquio B mucopolysaccharidoses**

Morquio-like mucopolysaccharidoses

Morquio-like syndrome

Morquio syndrome B

Mucopolysaccharidosis, type IVB

E76.219 **Morquio mucopolysaccharidoses, unspecified**

Morquio syndrome

Mucopolysaccharidosis, type IV

E76.22 **Sanfilippo mucopolysaccharidoses**

Mucopolysaccharidosis, type III (A) (B) (C) (D)

Sanfilippo A syndrome

Sanfilippo B syndrome

Sanfilippo C syndrome

Sanfilippo D syndrome

E76.29 **Other mucopolysaccharidoses**

beta-Glucuronidase deficiency

Maroteaux-Lamy (mild) (severe) syndrome

Mucopolysaccharidosis, types VI, VII

E76.3 **Mucopolysaccharidosis, unspecified**

E76.8 **Other disorders of glucosaminoglycan metabolism**

E76.9 **Glucosaminoglycan metabolism disorder, unspecified**

E77 **Disorders of glycoprotein metabolism**

E77.0 **Defects in post-translational modification of lysosomal enzymes**

Mucolipidosis II [I-cell disease]

Mucolipidosis III [pseudo-Hurler polydystrophy]

E77.1 **Defects in glycoprotein degradation**

Aspartylglucosaminuria

Fucosidosis

Mannosidosis

Sialidosis [mucolipidosis I]

E77.8 **Other disorders of glycoprotein metabolism**

E77.9 **Disorder of glycoprotein metabolism, unspecified**

E78 **Disorders of lipoprotein metabolism and other lipidemias**

Excludes1: sphingolipidosis (E75.0-E75.3)

E78.0 **Pure hypercholesterolemia**

●E78.00 **Pure hypercholesterolemia, unspecified**

Fredrickson's hyperlipoproteinemia, type IIa

Hyperbetalipoproteinemia

Low-density-lipoprotein-type [LDL] hyperlipoproteinemia

●E78.01 **Familial hypercholesterolemia**

E78.1 **Pure hyperglyceridemia**

Elevated fasting triglycerides

Endogenous hyperglyceridemia

Fredrickson's hyperlipoproteinemia, type IV

Hyperlipidemia, group B

Hyperprebetalipoproteinemia

Very-low-density-lipoprotein-type [VLDL] hyperlipoproteinemia

E78.2 **Mixed hyperlipidemia**

Broad- or floating-betalipoproteinemia

Combined hyperlipidemia NOS

Elevated cholesterol with elevated triglycerides NEC

Fredrickson's hyperlipoproteinemia, type IIb or III

Hyperbetalipoproteinemia with prebetalipoproteinemia

Hypercholesteremia with endogenous hyperglyceridemia

Hyperlipidemia, group C

Tubo-eruptive xanthoma Xanthoma tuberosum

Excludes1: cerebrotendinous cholesterosis [van Bogaert-Scherer- Epstein] (E75.5)

familial combined hyperlipidemia (E78.4)

E78.3 **Hyperchylomicronemia**

Chylomicron retention disease

Fredrickson's hyperlipoproteinemia, type I or V

Hyperlipidemia, group D

Mixed hyperglyceridemia

E78.4 **Other hyperlipidemia**

Familial combined hyperlipidemia

E78.5 **Hyperlipidemia, unspecified**

E78.6 **Lipoprotein deficiency**

Abetalipoproteinemia

Depressed HDL cholesterol

High-density lipoprotein deficiency

Hypoalphalipoproteinemia

Hypobetalipoproteinemia (familial)

Lecithin cholesterol acyltransferase deficiency

Tangier disease

E78.7 **Disorders of bile acid and cholesterol metabolism**

Excludes1: Niemann-Pick disease type C (E75.242)

Add 4th-7th digits   Nonspecific code   Unspecified code   Manifestation code

E78.70 Disorder of bile acid and cholesterol metabolism, unspecified

E78.71 Barth syndrome

E78.72 Smith-Lemli-Opitz syndrome

E78.79 Other disorders of bile acid and cholesterol metabolism

E78.8 Other disorders of lipoprotein metabolism

E78.81 Lipoid dermatoarthritis

E78.89 Other lipoprotein metabolism disorders

E78.9 Disorder of lipoprotein metabolism, unspecified

E79 Disorders of purine and pyrimidine metabolism

Excludes1: Ataxia-telangiectasia (Q87.1)

Bloom's syndrome (Q82.8)

Cockayne's syndrome (Q87.1)

calculus of kidney (N20.0)

combined immunodeficiency disorders (D81.-)

Fanconi's anemia (D61.09)

gout (M1A.-, M10.-)

orotaciduric anemia (D53.0)

progeria (E34.8)

Werner's syndrome (E34.8)

xeroderma pigmentosum (Q82.1)

E79.0 Hyperuricemia without signs of inflammatory arthritis and tophaceous disease

Asymptomatic hyperuricemia

E79.1 Lesch-Nyhan syndrome

HGPRT deficiency

E79.2 Myoadenylate deaminase deficiency

E79.8 Other disorders of purine and pyrimidine metabolism

Hereditary xanthinuria

E79.9 Disorder of purine and pyrimidine metabolism, unspecified

E80 Disorders of porphyrin and bilirubin metabolism

Includes: defects of catalase and peroxidase

E80.0 Hereditary erythropoietic porphyria

Congenital erythropoietic porphyria

Erythropoietic protoporphyria

E80.1 Porphyria cutanea tarda

E80.2 Other and unspecified porphyria

E80.20 Unspecified porphyria

Porphyria NOS

E80.21 Acute intermittent (hepatic) porphyria

E80.29 Other porphyria

Hereditary coproporphyria

E80.3 Defects of catalase and peroxidase

Acatalasia [Takahara]

E80.4 Gilbert syndrome

E80.5 Crigler-Najjar syndrome

E80.6 Other disorders of bilirubin metabolism

Dubin-Johnson syndrome

Rotor's syndrome

E80.7 Disorder of bilirubin metabolism, unspecified

E83 Disorders of mineral metabolism

Excludes1: dietary mineral deficiency (E58-E61)

parathyroid disorders (E20-E21)

vitamin D deficiency (E55.-)

E83.0 Disorders of copper metabolism

E83.00 Disorder of copper metabolism, unspecified

E83.01 Wilson's disease

<u>Code also</u> associated Kayser Fleischer ring (H18.04-)

E83.09 Other disorders of copper metabolism

Menkes' (kinky hair) (steely hair) disease

E83.1 Disorders of iron metabolism

Excludes1: iron deficiency anemia (D50.-)

sideroblastic anemia (D64.0-D64.3)

E83.10 Disorder of iron metabolism, unspecified

E83.11 Hemochromatosis

E83.110 Hereditary hemochromatosis

Bronzed diabetes

Pigmentary cirrhosis (of liver)

Primary (hereditary) hemochromatosis

E83.111 Hemochromatosis due to repeated red blood cell transfusions

Iron overload due to repeated red blood cell transfusions

Transfusion (red blood cell) associated hemochromatosis

E83.118 Other hemochromatosis

E83.119 Hemochromatosis, unspecified

E83.19 Other disorders of iron metabolism

<u>Use additional code</u>, if applicable, for idiopathic pulmonary hemosiderosis (J84.03)

E83.2 Disorders of zinc metabolism

Acrodermatitis enteropathica

E83.3 Disorders of phosphorus metabolism and phosphatases

Excludes1: adult osteomalacia (M83.-)

osteoporosis (M80.-)

E83.30 Disorder of phosphorus metabolism, unspecified

E83.31 Familial hypophosphatemia

Vitamin D-resistant osteomalacia

Vitamin D-resistant rickets

Excludes1: vitamin D-deficiency rickets (E55.0)

E83.32 Hereditary vitamin D-dependent rickets (type 1) (type 2)

25-hydroxyvitamin D 1-alpha-hydroxylase deficiency

Pseudovitamin D deficiency

Vitamin D receptor defect

E83.39 Other disorders of phosphorus metabolism

Acid phosphatase deficiency

Hypophosphatasia

E83.4 Disorders of magnesium metabolism

E83.40 Disorders of magnesium metabolism, unspecified

E83.41 Hypermagnesemia

E83.42 Hypomagnesemia

E83.49 Other disorders of magnesium metabolism

E83.5 Disorders of calcium metabolism

Excludes1: chondrocalcinosis (M11.1-M11.2)

● New code ▲ Revised code **Excludes1:** Not coded here **Excludes2:** Not included here ⊗ Placeholder required ⑦ 7th digit required

hungry bone syndrome (E83.81)

hyperparathyroidism (E21.0-E21.3)

E83.50 Unspecified disorder of calcium metabolism

E83.51 Hypocalcemia

E83.52 Hypercalcemia

Familial hypocalciuric hypercalcemia

E83.59 Other disorders of calcium metabolism

Idiopathic hypercalciuria

E83.8 Other disorders of mineral metabolism

E83.81 Hungry bone syndrome

E83.89 Other disorders of mineral metabolism

E83.9 Disorder of mineral metabolism, unspecified

E84 Cystic fibrosis

Includes: mucoviscidosis

Code also exocrine pancreatic insufficiency (K86.81)

E84.0 Cystic fibrosis with pulmonary manifestations

Use additional code to identify any infectious organism present, such as:

Pseudomonas (B96.5)

E84.1 Cystic fibrosis with intestinal manifestations

E84.11 Meconium ileus in cystic fibrosis

Excludes1: meconium ileus not due to cystic fibrosis (P76.0)

E84.19 Cystic fibrosis with other intestinal manifestations

Distal intestinal obstruction syndrome

E84.8 Cystic fibrosis with other manifestations

E84.9 Cystic fibrosis, unspecified

E85 Amyloidosis

Excludes1: Alzheimer's disease (G30.0-)

E85.0 Non-neuropathic heredofamilial amyloidosis

Hereditary amyloid nephropathy

E85.1 Neuropathic heredofamilial amyloidosis

Amyloid polyneuropathy (Portuguese)

E85.2 Heredofamilial amyloidosis, unspecified

E85.3 Secondary systemic amyloidosis

Hemodialysis-associated amyloidosis

E85.4 Organ-limited amyloidosis

Localized amyloidosis

E85.8 Other amyloidosis

E85.9 Amyloidosis, unspecified

E86 Volume depletion

Use additional code(s) for any associated disorders of electrolyte and acid-base balance (E87.-)

Excludes1: dehydration of newborn (P74.1)

hypovolemic shock NOS (R57.1)

postprocedural hypovolemic shock (T81.19)

traumatic hypovolemic shock (T79.4)

E86.0 Dehydration

E86.1 Hypovolemia

Depletion of volume of plasma

E86.9 Volume depletion, unspecified

E87 Other disorders of fluid, electrolyte and acid-base balance

Excludes1: diabetes insipidus (E23.2)

electrolyte imbalance associated with hyperemesis gravidarum (O21.1)

electrolyte imbalance following ectopic or molar pregnancy (O08.5)

familial periodic paralysis (G72.3)

E87.0 Hyperosmolality and hypernatremia

Sodium [Na] excess

Sodium [Na] overload

E87.1 Hypo-osmolality and hyponatremia

Sodium [Na] deficiency

Excludes1: syndrome of inappropriate secretion of antidiuretic hormone (E22.2)

E87.2 Acidosis

Acidosis NOS

Lactic acidosis

Metabolic acidosis

Respiratory acidosis

Excludes1: diabetic acidosis - see categories E08-E10, E13 with ketoacidosis

E87.3 Alkalosis

Alkalosis NOS

Metabolic alkalosis

Respiratory alkalosis

E87.4 Mixed disorder of acid-base balance

E87.5 Hyperkalemia

Potassium [K] excess

Potassium [K] overload

E87.6 Hypokalemia

Potassium [K] deficiency

E87.7 Fluid overload

Excludes1: edema NOS (R60.9)

fluid retention (R60.9)

E87.70 Fluid overload, unspecified

E87.71 Transfusion associated circulatory overload

Fluid overload due to transfusion (blood) (blood components) TACO

E87.79 Other fluid overload

E87.8 Other disorders of electrolyte and fluid balance, not elsewhere classified

Electrolyte imbalance NOS

Hyperchloremia

Hypochloremia

E88 Other and unspecified metabolic disorders

Use additional codes for associated conditions

Excludes1: histiocytosis X (chronic) (C96.6)

E88.0 Disorders of plasma-protein metabolism, not elsewhere classified

Excludes1: disorder of lipoprotein metabolism (E78.-)

monoclonal gammopathy (of undetermined significance) (D47.2)

polyclonal hypergammaglobulinemia (D89.0)

Waldenström macroglobulinemia (C88.0)

E88.01 Alpha-1-antitrypsin deficiency

AAT deficiency

E88.09 Other disorders of plasma-protein metabolism, not elsewhere classified

Bisalbuminemia

E88.1 **Lipodystrophy, not elsewhere classified**

Lipodystrophy NOS

Excludes1: Whipple's disease (K90.81)

E88.2 **Lipomatosis, not elsewhere classified**

Lipomatosis NOS

Lipomatosis (Check) dolorosa [Dercum]

E88.3 **Tumor lysis syndrome**

Tumor lysis syndrome (spontaneous)

Tumor lysis syndrome following antineoplastic drug chemotherapy

Use additional code for adverse effect, if applicable, to identify drug (T45.1X5)

E88.4 **Mitochondrial metabolism disorders**

Excludes1: disorders of pyruvate metabolism (E74.4)

Kearns-Sayre syndrome (H49.81)

Leber's disease (H47.22)

Leigh's encephalopathy (G31.82)

Mitochondrial myopathy, NEC (G71.3)

Reye's syndrome (G93.7)

E88.40 **Mitochondrial metabolism disorder, unspecified**

E88.41 **MELAS syndrome**

Mitochondrial myopathy, encephalopathy, lactic acidosis and stroke-like episodes

E88.42 **MERRF syndrome**

Myoclonic epilepsy associated with ragged-red fibers

Code also progressive myoclonic epilepsy (G40.3-)

E88.49 **Other mitochondrial metabolism disorders**

E88.8 **Other specified metabolic disorders**

E88.81 **Metabolic syndrome**

Dysmetabolic syndrome X

Use additional codes for associated manifestations, such as:

obesity (E66.-)

E88.89 **Other specified metabolic disorders**

Launois-Bensaude adenolipomatosis

Excludes1: adult pulmonary Langerhans cell histiocytosis (J84.82)

E88.9 **Metabolic disorder, unspecified**

POSTPROCEDURAL ENDOCRINE AND METABOLIC COMPLICATIONS AND DISORDERS, NOT ELSEWHERE CLASSIFIED (E89)

E89 **Postprocedural endocrine and metabolic complications and disorders, not elsewhere classified**

Excludes2: intraoperative complications of endocrine system organ or structure (E36.0-, E36.1-, E36.8)

E89.0 **Postprocedural hypothyroidism**

Postirradiation hypothyroidism

Postsurgical hypothyroidism

E89.1 **Postprocedural hypoinsulinemia**

Postpancreatectomy hyperglycemia

Postsurgical hypoinsulinemia

Use additional code, if applicable, to identify:

acquired absence of pancreas (Z90.41-)

diabetes mellitus (postpancreatectomy) (postprocedural) (E13.-)

insulin use (Z79.4)

Excludes1: transient postprocedural hyperglycemia (R73.9)

transient postprocedural hypoglycemia (E16.2)

E89.2 **Postprocedural hypoparathyroidism**

Parathyroprival tetany

E89.3 **Postprocedural hypopituitarism**

Postirradiation hypopituitarism

E89.4 **Postprocedural ovarian failure**

E89.40 **Asymptomatic postprocedural ovarian failure**

Postprocedural ovarian failure NOS

E89.41 **Symptomatic postprocedural ovarian failure**

Symptoms such as flushing, sleeplessness, headache, lack of concentration, associated with postprocedural menopause

E89.5 **Postprocedural testicular hypofunction**

E89.6 **Postprocedural adrenocortical (-medullary) hypofunction**

E89.8 **Other postprocedural endocrine and metabolic complications and disorders**

E89.81 **Postprocedural hemorrhage of an endocrine system organ or structure following a procedure**

▲**E89.810** **Postprocedural hemorrhage of an endocrine system organ or structure following an endocrine system procedure**

▲**E89.811** **Postprocedural hemorrhage of an endocrine system organ or structure following other procedure**

E89.82 **Postprocedural hematoma and seroma of an endocrine system organ or structure**

●**E89.820** **Postprocedural hematoma of an endocrine system organ or structure following an endocrine system procedure**

●**E89.821** **Postprocedural hematoma of an endocrine system organ or structure following other procedure**

●**E89.822** **Postprocedural seroma of an endocrine system organ or structure following an endocrine system procedure**

●**E89.823** **Postprocedural seroma of an endocrine system organ or structure following other procedure**

E89.89 **Other postprocedural endocrine and metabolic complications and disorders**

Use additional code, if applicable, to further specify disorder

Chapter 5: Mental, Behavioral And Neurodevelopmental Disorders (F01-F99)

DEFINITIONS

This chapter includes definitions of selected key words, terms and phrases and coding alerts for adding points to the clinical domain, and references to coding late effects where appropriate. An example from this chapter is as follows:

F02   Dementia in other diseases classified elsewhere
             Definition: Dementia refers to a group of symptoms caused by disorders that affect the brain. It is not a specific disease.

MULTIPLE CODING FOR A SINGLE CONDITION

In addition to the etiology/manifestation convention that requires two codes to fully describe a single condition that affects multiple body systems, there are other single conditions that also require more than one code. "Use additional code" notes are found in the Tabular List at codes that are not part of an etiology/manifestation pair where a secondary code is useful to fully describe a condition. The sequencing rule is the same as the etiology/manifestation pair, "use additional code" indicates that a secondary code should be added.

For example, for bacterial infections that are not included in chapter 1, a secondary code from category B95, Streptococcus, Staphylococcus, and Enterococcus, as the cause of diseases classified elsewhere, or B96, Other bacterial agents as the cause of diseases classified elsewhere, may be required to identify the bacterial organism causing the infection. A "use additional code" note will normally be found at the infectious disease code, indicating a need for the organism code to be added as a secondary code.

 "Code first" notes are also under certain codes that are not specifically manifestation codes but may be due to an underlying cause. When there is a "code first" note and an underlying condition is present, the underlying condition should be sequenced first.

"Code, if applicable, any causal condition first", notes indicate that this code may be assigned as a principal diagnosis when the causal condition is unknown or not applicable. If a causal condition is known, then the code for that condition should be sequenced as the principal or first-listed diagnosis.

Multiple codes may be needed for sequela, complication codes and obstetric codes to more fully describe a condition. See the specific guidelines for these conditions for further instruction.

COMBINATION CODE

A combination code is a single code used to classify: Two diagnoses, or a diagnosis with an associated secondary process (manifestation) A diagnosis with an associated complication

Combination codes are identified by referring to subterm entries in the Alphabetic Index and by reading the inclusion and exclusion notes in the Tabular List.

Assign only the combination code when that code fully identifies the diagnostic conditions involved or when the Alphabetic Index so directs. Multiple coding should not be used when the classification provides a combination code that clearly identifies all of the elements documented in the diagnosis. When the combination code lacks necessary specificity in describing the manifestation or complication, an additional code should be used as a secondary code.

SEQUELA (LATE EFFECTS)

A sequela is the residual effect (condition produced) after the acute phase of an illness or injury has terminated. There is no time limit on when a sequela code can be used. The residual may be apparent early, such as in cerebral infarction, or it may occur months or years later, such as that due to a previous injury. Coding of sequela generally requires two codes sequenced in the following order: The condition or nature of the sequela is sequenced first.

The sequela code is sequenced second.

An exception to the above guidelines are those instances where the code for the sequela is followed by a manifestation code identified in the Tabular List and title, or the sequela code has been expanded (at the fourth, fifth or sixth character levels) to include the manifestation(s). The code for the acute phase of an illness or injury that led to the sequela is never used with a code for the late effect.

PAIN DISORDERS RELATED TO PSYCHOLOGICAL FACTORS

Assign code F45.41, for pain that is exclusively related to psychological disorders. As indicated by the Excludes 1 note under category G89, a code from category G89 should not be assigned with code F45.41.

Code F45.42, Pain disorders with related psychological factors, should be used with a code from category G89, Pain, not elsewhere classified, if there is

F01-F99

documentation of a psychological component for a patient with acute or chronic pain.

See Section I.C.6. Pain

MENTAL AND BEHAVIORAL DISORDERS DUE TO PSYCHOACTIVE SUBSTANCE USE

1)   In Remission

Selection of codes for "in remission" for categories F10-F19, Mental and behavioral disorders due to psychoactive substance use (categories F10-F19 with -.21) requires the provider's clinical judgment. The appropriate codes for "in remission" are assigned only on the basis of provider documentation (as defined in the Official Guidelines for Coding and Reporting).

2)   Psychoactive Substance Use, Abuse And Dependence

When the provider documentation refers to use, abuse and dependence of the same substance (e.g. alcohol, opioid, cannabis, etc.), only one code should be assigned to identify the pattern of use based on the following hierarchy:

- If both use and abuse are documented, assign only the code for abuse

- If both abuse and dependence are documented, assign only the code for dependence

- If use, abuse and dependence are all documented, assign only the code for dependence

- If both use and dependence are documented, assign only the code for dependence.

3)   Psychoactive Substance Use

As with all other diagnoses, the codes for psychoactive substance use (F10.9-, F11.9-, F12.9-, F13.9-, F14.9-, F15.9-, F16.9-) should only be assigned based on provider documentation and when they meet the definition of a reportable diagnosis (see Section III, Reporting Additional Diagnoses). The codes are to be used only when the psychoactive substance use is associated with a mental or behavioral disorder, and such a relationship is documented by the provider.

Chapter 5

Mental, Behavioral and Neurodevelopmental Disorders (F01-F99)

Includes: disorders of psychological development

Excludes2: symptoms, signs and abnormal clinical laboratory findings, not elsewhere classified (R00-R99)

This chapter contains the following blocks:

F01-F09	Mental disorders due to known physiological conditions
F10-F19	Mental and behavioral disorders due to psychoactive substance use
F20-F29	Schizophrenia, schizotypal, delusional, and other non-mood psychotic disorders
F30-F39	Mood [affective] disorders
F40-F48	Anxiety, dissociative, stress-related, somatoform and other nonpsychotic mental disorders
F50-F59	Behavioral syndromes associated with physiological disturbances and physical factors
F60-F69	Disorders of adult personality and behavior
F70-F79	Intellectual disabilities
F80-F89	Pervasive and specific developmental disorders
F90-F98	Behavioral and emotional disorders with onset usually occurring in childhood and adolescence
F99	Unspecified mental disorder

MENTAL DISORDERS DUE TO KNOWN PHYSIOLOGICAL CONDITIONS (F01-F09)

Note: This block comprises a range of mental disorders grouped together on the basis of their having in common a demonstrable etiology in cerebral disease, brain injury, or other insult leading to cerebral dysfunction. The dysfunction may be primary, as in diseases, injuries, and insults that affect the brain directly and selectively; or secondary, as in systemic diseases and disorders that attack the brain only as one of the multiple organs or systems of the body that are involved.

F01 **Vascular dementia**

Vascular dementia as a result of infarction of the brain due to vascular disease, including hypertensive cerebrovascular disease.

Includes: arteriosclerotic dementia

Code first the underlying physiological condition or sequelae of cerebrovascular disease.

F01.5 **Vascular dementia**

F01.50 **Vascular dementia without behavioral disturbance**

Major neurocognitive disorder without behavioral disturbance

F01.51 **Vascular dementia with behavioral disturbance**

Major neurocognitive disorder due to vascular disease, with behavioral disturbance

Major neurocognitive disorder with aggressive behavior

Major neurocognitive disorder with combative behavior

Major neurocognitive disorder with violent behavior

Vascular dementia with aggressive behavior

Vascular dementia with combative behavior

Vascular dementia with violent behavior

Use additional code, if applicable, to identify wandering in vascular dementia (Z91.83)

F02 **Dementia in other diseases classified elsewhere**

Definition: Dementia refers to a group of symptoms caused by disorders that affect the brain. It is not a specific disease.

Includes: Major neurocognitive disorder **in other** diseases classified elsewhere

Code first the underlying physiological condition, such as:

Alzheimer's (G30.-)

cerebral lipidosis (E75.4)

Creutzfeldt-Jakob disease (A81.0-)

dementia with Lewy bodies (G31.83)

dementia with Parkinsonism (G31.83)

epilepsy and recurrent seizures (G40.-)

frontotemporal dementia (G31.09)

hepatolenticular degeneration (E83.0)

human immunodeficiency virus [HIV] disease (B20)

Huntington's disease (G10)

hypercalcemia (E83.52)

hypothyroidism, acquired (E00-E03.-)

intoxications (T36-T65)

Jakob-Creutzfeldt disease (A81.0-)

multiple sclerosis (G35)

neurosyphilis (A52.17)

niacin deficiency [pellagra] (E52)

Parkinson's disease (G20)

Pick's disease (G31.01)

polyarteritis nodosa (M30.0)

prion disease (A81.9)

systemic lupus erythematosus (M32.-)

traumatic brain injury (S06.-)

trypanosomiasis (B56.-, B57.-)

vitamin B deficiency (E53.8)

Excludes2: dementia in alcohol and psychoactive substance disorders (F10-F19, with .17, .27, .97)

vascular dementia (F01.5-)

F02.8 **Dementia in other diseases classified elsewhere**

F02.80 **Dementia in other diseases classified elsewhere without behavioral disturbance**

Dementia **in other** diseases classified elsewhere NOS

Major neurocognitive disorder **in other** diseases classified elsewhere

F02.81 **Dementia in other diseases classified elsewhere with behavioral disturbance**

Dementia **in other** diseases classified elsewhere with aggressive behavior

Dementia **in other** diseases classified elsewhere with combative behavior

Dementia **in other** diseases classified elsewhere with violent behavior

Major neurocognitive disorder **in other** diseases classified elsewhere with aggressive behavior

Major neurocognitive disorder **in other** diseases classified elsewhere with combative behavior

Major neurocognitive disorder **in other** diseases classified elsewhere with violent behavior

Use additional code, if applicable, to identify wandering in dementia in conditions classified elsewhere (Z91.83)

F03 **Unspecified dementia**

Presenile dementia NOS

Presenile psychosis NOS

Primary degenerative dementia NOS

Senile dementia NOS

Senile dementia depressed or paranoid type

Senile psychosis NOS

Excludes1: senility NOS (R41.81)

Excludes2: mild memory disturbance due to known physiological condition (F06.8)

senile dementia with delirium or acute confusional state (F05)

F03.9 **Unspecified dementia**

  F03.90 **Unspecified dementia without behavioral disturbance**

    Dementia NOS

  F03.91 **Unspecified dementia with behavioral disturbance**

    Unspecified dementia with aggressive behavior

    Unspecified dementia with combative behavior

    Unspecified dementia with violent behavior

    Use additional code, if applicable, to identify wandering in unspecified dementia (Z91.83)

F04 **Amnestic disorder due to known physiological condition**

Korsakov's psychosis or syndrome, nonalcoholic

Code first the underlying physiological condition

Excludes1: amnesia NOS (R41.3)

  anterograde amnesia (R41.1)

  dissociative amnesia (F44.0)

  retrograde amnesia (R41.2)

Excludes2: alcohol-induced or unspecified Korsakov's syndrome (F10.26, F10.96)

  Korsakov's syndrome induced by other psychoactive substances (F13.26, F13.96, F19.16, F19.26,F19.96)

F05 **Delirium due to known physiological condition**

Acute or subacute brain syndrome

Acute or subacute confusional state (nonalcoholic)

Acute or subacute infective psychosis

Acute or subacute organic reaction

Acute or subacute psycho-organic syndrome

Delirium of mixed etiology

Delirium superimposed on dementia

Sundowning

  Code first the underlying physiological condition

  Excludes1: delirium NOS (R41.0)

  Excludes2: delirium tremens alcohol-induced or unspecified (F10.231, F10.921)

F06 **Other mental disorders due to known physiological condition**

Includes: mental disorders due to endocrine disorder

  mental disorders due to exogenous hormone

  mental disorders due to exogenous toxic substance

  mental disorders due to primary cerebral disease

  mental disorders due to somatic illness

  mental disorders due to systemic disease affecting the brain

Code first the underlying physiological condition

Excludes1: unspecified dementia (F03)

Excludes2: delirium due to known physiological condition (F05)

  dementia as classified in F01-F02

  Other mental disorders associated with alcohol and other psychoactive substances (F10-F19)

F06.0 **Psychotic disorder with hallucinations due to known physiological condition**

Organic hallucinatory state (nonalcoholic)

Excludes2: hallucinations and perceptual disturbance induced by alcohol and other psychoactive substances (F10-F19 with .151, .251, .951)

  schizophrenia (F20.-)

F06.1 **Catatonic disorder due to known physiological condition**

Catatonia associated with another mental disorder

Catatonia NOS

Excludes1: catatonic stupor (R40.1)

stupor NOS (R40.1)

Excludes2: catatonic schizophrenia (F20.2)

dissociative stupor (F44.2)

F06.2 **Psychotic disorder with delusions due to known physiological condition**

Paranoid and paranoid-hallucinatory organic states

Schizophrenia-like psychosis in epilepsy

Excludes2: alcohol and drug-induced psychotic disorder (F10-F19 with .150, .250, .950)

  brief psychotic disorder (F23)

  delusional disorder (F22)

  schizophrenia (F20.-)

F06.3 **Mood disorder due to known physiological condition**

Excludes2: mood disorders due to alcohol **and other** psychoactive substances (F10-F19 with .14, .24, .94) mood disorders, not due to known physiological condition or unspecified (F30-F39)

  F06.30 **Mood disorder due to known physiological condition, unspecified**

  F06.31 **Mood disorder due to known physiological condition with depressive features**

  F06.32 **Mood disorder due to known physiological condition with major depressive-like episode**

  F06.33 **Mood disorder due to known physiological condition with manic features**

  F06.34 **Mood disorder due to known physiological condition with mixed features**

F06.4 **Anxiety disorder due to known physiological condition**

Excludes2: anxiety disorders due to alcohol and other psychoactive substances (F10-F19 with .180, .280, .980) anxiety disorders, not due to known physiological condition or unspecified (F40.-, F41.-)

F06.8 **Other specified mental disorders due to known physiological condition**

Epileptic psychosis NOS

Organic dissociative disorder

Organic emotionally labile [asthenic] disorder

F07 **Personality and behavioral disorders due to known physiological condition**

Code first the underlying physiological condition

  F07.0 **Personality change due to known physiological condition**

Frontal lobe syndrome

Limbic epilepsy personality syndrome

Lobotomy syndrome

Organic personality disorder

Organic pseudopsychopathic personality

Organic pseudoretarded personality

Postleucotomy syndrome

Code first underlying physiological condition

Excludes1: mild cognitive impairment (G31.84)

postconcussional syndrome (F07.81)

postencephalitic syndrome (F07.89)

signs and symptoms involving emotional state (R45.-)

Excludes2: specific personality disorder (F60.-)

F07.8 **Other personality and behavioral disorders due to known physiological condition**

F07.81 **Postconcussional syndrome**

Postcontusional syndrome (encephalopathy)

Post-traumatic brain syndrome, nonpsychotic

Use additional code to identify associated post-traumatic headache, if applicable (G44.3-)

Excludes1: current concussion (brain) (S06.0-)

postencephalitic syndrome (F07.89)

F07.89 **Other personality and behavioral disorders due to known physiological condition**

Postencephalitic syndrome

Right hemispheric organic affective disorder

F07.9 **Unspecified personality and behavioral disorder due to known physiological condition**

Organic psychosyndrome

F09 **Unspecified mental disorder due to known physiological condition**

Mental disorder NOS due to known physiological condition

Organic brain syndrome NOS

Organic mental disorder NOS

Organic psychosis NOS

Symptomatic psychosis NOS

Code first the underlying physiological condition

Excludes1: psychosis NOS (F29)

MENTAL AND BEHAVIORAL DISORDERS DUE TO PSYCHOACTIVE SUBSTANCE USE (F10-F19)

F10 **Alcohol related disorders**

Definition: Alcohol-induced mental disorders is an alcohol-induced psychological or behavioral pattern that occurs in an individual and is thought to cause distress or disability that is not expected as part of normal development or culture.

Use additional code for blood alcohol level, if applicable (Y90.-)

F10.1 **Alcohol abuse**

Excludes1: alcohol dependence (F10.2-)

alcohol use, unspecified (F10.9-)

F10.10 **Alcohol abuse, uncomplicated**

Alcohol use disorder, mild

F10.12 **Alcohol abuse with intoxication**

F10.120 **Alcohol abuse with intoxication, uncomplicated**

F10.121 **Alcohol abuse with intoxication delirium**

F10.129 **Alcohol abuse with intoxication, unspecified**

F10.14 **Alcohol abuse with alcohol-induced mood disorder**

Alcohol use disorder, mild, with alcohol-induced bipolar or related disorder

Alcohol use disorder, mild, with alcohol-induced depressive disorder

F10.15 **Alcohol abuse with alcohol-induced psychotic disorder**

F10.150 **Alcohol abuse with alcohol-induced psychotic disorder with delusions**

F10.151 **Alcohol abuse with alcohol-induced psychotic disorder with hallucinations**

F10.159 **Alcohol abuse with alcohol-induced psychotic disorder, unspecified**

F10.18 **Alcohol abuse with other alcohol-induced disorders**

F10.180 **Alcohol abuse with alcohol-induced anxiety disorder**

F10.181 **Alcohol abuse with alcohol-induced sexual dysfunction**

F10.182 **Alcohol abuse with alcohol-induced sleep disorder**

F10.188 **Alcohol abuse with other alcohol-induced disorder**

F10.19 **Alcohol abuse with unspecified alcohol-induced disorder**

F10.2 **Alcohol dependence**

Excludes1: alcohol abuse (F10.1-)

alcohol use, unspecified (F10.9-)

Excludes2: toxic effect of alcohol (T51.0-)

F10.20 **Alcohol dependence, uncomplicated**

Alcohol use disorder, moderate

Alcohol use disorder, severe

F10.21 **Alcohol dependence, in remission**

F10.22 **Alcohol dependence with intoxication**

Acute drunkenness (in alcoholism)

Excludes2: alcohol dependence with withdrawal (F10.23-)

F10.220 **Alcohol dependence with intoxication, uncomplicated**

F10.221 **Alcohol dependence with intoxication delirium**

F10.229 **Alcohol dependence with intoxication, unspecified**

F10.23 **Alcohol dependence with withdrawal**

Excludes2: Alcohol dependence with intoxication (F10.22-)

F10.230 **Alcohol dependence with withdrawal, uncomplicated**

F10.231 **Alcohol dependence with withdrawal delirium**

F10.232 **Alcohol dependence with withdrawal with perceptual disturbance**

F10.239 Alcohol dependence with withdrawal, unspecified

F10.24 Alcohol dependence with alcohol-induced mood disorder

Alcohol use disorder, moderate, with alcohol-induced bipolar or related disorder

Alcohol use disorder, moderate, with alcohol-induced depressive disorder

Alcohol use disorder, severe, with alcohol-induced bipolar or related disorder

Alcohol use disorder, severe, with alcohol-induced depressive disorder

F10.25 Alcohol dependence with alcohol-induced psychotic disorder

F10.250 Alcohol dependence with alcohol-induced psychotic disorder with delusions

F10.251 Alcohol dependence with alcohol-induced psychotic disorder with hallucinations

F10.259 Alcohol dependence with alcohol-induced psychotic disorder, unspecified

F10.26 Alcohol dependence with alcohol-induced persisting amnestic disorder

Alcohol use disorder, moderate, with alcohol-induced major neurocognitive disorder, amnestic-confabulatory type

Alcohol use disorder, severe, with alcohol-induced major neurocognitive disorder, amnestic-confabulatory type

F10.27 Alcohol dependence with alcohol-induced persisting dementia

Alcohol use disorder, moderate, with alcohol-induced major neurocognitive disorder, nonamnestic-confabulatory type

Alcohol use disorder, severe, with alcohol-induced major neurocognitive disorder, nonamnestic-confabulatory type

F10.28 Alcohol dependence with other alcohol-induced disorders

F10.280 Alcohol dependence with alcohol-induced anxiety disorder

F10.281 Alcohol dependence with alcohol-induced sexual dysfunction

F10.282 Alcohol dependence with alcohol-induced sleep disorder

F10.288 Alcohol dependence with other alcohol-induced disorder

Alcohol use disorder, moderate, with alcohol-induced mild neurocognitive disorder

Alcohol use disorder, severe, with alcohol-induced mild neurocognitive disorder

F10.29 Alcohol dependence with unspecified alcohol-induced disorder

F10.9 Alcohol use, unspecified

Excludes1: alcohol abuse (F10.1-)

alcohol dependence (F10.2-)

F10.92 Alcohol use, unspecified with intoxication

F10.920 Alcohol use, unspecified with intoxication, uncomplicated

F10.921 Alcohol use, unspecified with intoxication delirium

F10.929 Alcohol use, unspecified with intoxication, unspecified

F10.94 Alcohol use, unspecified with alcohol-induced mood disorder

Alcohol induced bipolar or related disorder, without use disorder

Alcohol induced depressive disorder, without use disorder

F10.95 Alcohol use, unspecified with alcohol-induced psychotic disorder

F10.950 Alcohol use, unspecified with alcohol-induced psychotic disorder with delusions

F10.951 Alcohol use, unspecified with alcohol-induced psychotic disorder with hallucinations

F10.959 Alcohol use, unspecified with alcohol-induced psychotic disorder, unspecified

Alcohol-induced psychotic disorder without use disorder

F10.96 Alcohol use, unspecified with alcohol-induced persisting amnestic disorder

Alcohol-induced major neurocognitive disorder, amnestic-confabulatory type, without use disorder

F10.97 Alcohol use, unspecified with alcohol-induced persisting dementia

Alcohol-induced major neurocognitive disorder, nonamnestic-confabulatory type, without use disorder

F10.98 Alcohol use, unspecified with other alcohol-induced disorders

F10.980 Alcohol use, unspecified with alcohol-induced anxiety disorder

Alcohol induced anxiety disorder, without use disorder

F10.981 Alcohol use, unspecified with alcohol-induced sexual dysfunction

Alcohol induced sexual dysfunction, without use disorder

F10.982 Alcohol use, unspecified with alcohol-induced sleep disorder

Alcohol induced sleep disorder, without use disorder

F10.988 Alcohol use, unspecified with other alcohol-induced disorder

Alcohol induced mild neurocognitive disorder, without use disorder

F10.99 Alcohol use, unspecified with unspecified alcohol-induced disorder

F11 Opioid related disorders

Definition: Opioids are medications that relieve pain. They reduce the intensity of pain signals reaching the brain and affect those brain areas controlling emotion, which diminishes the effects of a painful stimulus. Medications that fall within this class include hydrocodone (e.g., Vicodin), oxycodone (e.g., OxyContin, Percocet), morphine (e.g., Kadian, Avinza), codeine, and related drugs.

F11.1   **Opioid abuse**

     Excludes1: opioid dependence (F11.2-)

     opioid use, unspecified (F11.9-)

     F11.10   **Opioid abuse, uncomplicated**

       Opioid use disorder, mild

     F11.12   **Opioid abuse with intoxication**

       F11.120   **Opioid abuse with intoxication, uncomplicated**

       F11.121   **Opioid abuse with intoxication delirium**

       F11.122   **Opioid abuse with intoxication with perceptual disturbance**

       F11.129   **Opioid abuse with intoxication, unspecified**

     F11.14   **Opioid abuse with opioid-induced mood disorder**

       Opioid use disorder, mild, with opioid-induced depressive disorder

     F11.15   **Opioid abuse with opioid-induced psychotic disorder**

       F11.150   **Opioid abuse with opioid-induced psychotic disorder with delusions**

       F11.151   **Opioid abuse with opioid-induced psychotic disorder with hallucinations**

       F11.159   **Opioid abuse with opioid-induced psychotic disorder, unspecified**

     F11.18   **Opioid abuse with other opioid-induced disorder**

       F11.181   **Opioid abuse with opioid-induced sexual dysfunction**

       F11.182   **Opioid abuse with opioid-induced sleep disorder**

       F11.188   **Opioid abuse with other opioid-induced disorder**

     F11.19   **Opioid abuse with unspecified opioid-induced disorder**

F11.2   **Opioid dependence**

     Excludes1: opioid abuse (F11.1-)

     opioid use, unspecified (F11.9-)

     Excludes2: opioid poisoning (T40.0-T40.2-)

     F11.20   **Opioid dependence, uncomplicated**

       Opioid use disorder, moderate

       Opioid use disorder, severe

     F11.21   **Opioid dependence, in remission**

     F11.22   **Opioid dependence with intoxication**

       Excludes1: opioid dependence with withdrawal (F11.23)

       F11.220   **Opioid dependence with intoxication, uncomplicated**

       F11.221   **Opioid dependence with intoxication delirium**

       F11.222   **Opioid dependence with intoxication with perceptual disturbance**

       F11.229   **Opioid dependence with intoxication, unspecified**

     F11.23   **Opioid dependence with withdrawal**

       Excludes1: opioid dependence with intoxication (F11.22-)

     F11.24   **Opioid dependence with opioid-induced mood disorder**

       Opioid use disorder, moderate, with opioid induced depressive disorder

     F11.25   **Opioid dependence with opioid-induced psychotic disorder**

       F11.250   **Opioid dependence with opioid-induced psychotic disorder with delusions**

       F11.251   **Opioid dependence with opioid-induced psychotic disorder with hallucinations**

       F11.259   **Opioid dependence with opioid-induced psychotic disorder, unspecified**

     F11.28   **Opioid dependence with other opioid-induced disorder**

       F11.281   **Opioid dependence with opioid-induced sexual dysfunction**

       F11.282   **Opioid dependence with opioid-induced sleep disorder**

       F11.288   **Opioid dependence with other opioid-induced disorder**

     F11.29   **Opioid dependence with unspecified opioid-induced disorder**

F11.9   **Opioid use, unspecified**

     Excludes1: opioid abuse (F11.1-)

     opioid dependence (F11.2-)

     F11.90   **Opioid use, unspecified, uncomplicated**

     F11.92   **Opioid use, unspecified with intoxication**

       Excludes1: opioid use, unspecified with withdrawal (F11.93)

       F11.920   **Opioid use, unspecified with intoxication, uncomplicated**

       F11.921   **Opioid use, unspecified with intoxication delirium**

         Opioid-induced delirium

       F11.922   **Opioid use, unspecified with intoxication with perceptual disturbance**

       F11.929   **Opioid use, unspecified with intoxication, unspecified**

     F11.93   **Opioid use, unspecified with withdrawal**

       Excludes1: opioid use, unspecified with intoxication (F11.92-)

     F11.94   **Opioid use, unspecified with opioid-induced mood disorder**

       Opioid induced depressive disorder, without use disorder

     F11.95   **Opioid use, unspecified with opioid-induced psychotic disorder**

       F11.950   **Opioid use, unspecified with opioid-induced psychotic disorder with delusions**

       F11.951   **Opioid use, unspecified with opioid-induced psychotic disorder with hallucinations**

F11.959   Opioid use, unspecified with opioid-induced psychotic disorder, unspecified

F11.98   Opioid use, unspecified with other specified opioid-induced disorder

F11.981   Opioid use, unspecified with opioid-induced sexual dysfunction

Opioid induced sexual dysfunction, without use disorder

F11.982   Opioid use, unspecified with opioid-induced sleep disorder

Opioid induced sleep disorder, without use disorder

F11.988   Opioid use, unspecified with other opioid-induced disorder

Opioid induced anxiety disorder, without use disorder

F11.99   Opioid use, unspecified with unspecified opioid-induced disorder

F12   **Cannabis related disorders**

Includes: marijuana

F12.1   **Cannabis abuse**

Excludes1: cannabis dependence (F12.2-)

cannabis use, unspecified (F12.9-)

F12.10   Cannabis abuse, uncomplicated

Cannabis use disorder, mild

F12.12   Cannabis abuse with intoxication

F12.120   Cannabis abuse with intoxication, uncomplicated

F12.121   Cannabis abuse with intoxication delirium

F12.122   Cannabis abuse with intoxication with perceptual disturbance

F12.129   Cannabis abuse with intoxication, unspecified

F12.15   Cannabis abuse with psychotic disorder

F12.150   Cannabis abuse with psychotic disorder with delusions

F12.151   Cannabis abuse with psychotic disorder with hallucinations

F12.159   Cannabis abuse with psychotic disorder, unspecified

F12.18   Cannabis abuse with other cannabis-induced disorder

F12.180   Cannabis abuse with cannabis-induced anxiety disorder

F12.188   Cannabis abuse with other cannabis-induced disorder

Cannabis use disorder, mild, with cannabis-induced sleep disorder

F12.19   Cannabis abuse with unspecified cannabis-induced disorder

F12.2   **Cannabis dependence**

Excludes1: cannabis abuse (F12.1-)

cannabis use, unspecified (F12.9-)

Excludes2: cannabis poisoning (T40.7-)

F12.20   Cannabis dependence, uncomplicated

Cannabis use disorder, moderate

Cannabis use disorder, severe

F12.21   Cannabis dependence, in remission

F12.22   Cannabis dependence with intoxication

F12.220   Cannabis dependence with intoxication, uncomplicated

F12.221   Cannabis dependence with intoxication delirium

F12.222   Cannabis dependence with intoxication with perceptual disturbance

F12.229   Cannabis dependence with intoxication, unspecified

F12.25   Cannabis dependence with psychotic disorder

F12.250   Cannabis dependence with psychotic disorder with delusions

F12.251   Cannabis dependence with psychotic disorder with hallucinations

F12.259   Cannabis dependence with psychotic disorder, unspecified

F12.28   Cannabis dependence with other cannabis-induced disorder

F12.280   Cannabis dependence with cannabis-induced anxiety disorder

F12.288   Cannabis dependence with other cannabis-induced disorder

Cannabis use disorder, moderate, with cannabis-induced sleep disorder

Cannabis use disorder, severe, with cannabis-induced sleep disorder

Cannabis withdrawal

F12.29   Cannabis dependence with unspecified cannabis-induced disorder

F12.9   **Cannabis use, unspecified**

Excludes1: cannabis abuse (F12.1-)

cannabis dependence (F12.2-)

F12.90   Cannabis use, unspecified, uncomplicated

F12.92   Cannabis use, unspecified with intoxication

F12.920   Cannabis use, unspecified with intoxication, uncomplicated

F12.921   Cannabis use, unspecified with intoxication delirium

F12.922   Cannabis use, unspecified with intoxication with perceptual disturbance

F12.929   Cannabis use, unspecified with intoxication, unspecified

F12.95   Cannabis use, unspecified with psychotic disorder

F12.950   Cannabis use, unspecified with psychotic disorder with delusions

F12.951   Cannabis use, unspecified with psychotic disorder with hallucinations

F12.959   Cannabis use, unspecified with psychotic disorder, unspecified

Cannabis induced psychotic disorder, without use disorder

F12.98   Cannabis use, unspecified with other cannabis-induced disorder

F12.980   Cannabis use, unspecified with anxiety disorder

Cannabis induced anxiety disorder, without use disorder

F12.988 **Cannabis use, unspecified with other cannabis-induced disorder**

Cannabis induced sleep disorder, without use disorder

F12.99 **Cannabis use, unspecified with unspecified cannabis-induced disorder**

F13 **Sedative, hypnotic, or anxiolytic related disorders**

F13.1 **Sedative, hypnotic or anxiolytic-related abuse**

Excludes1: sedative, hypnotic or anxiolytic-related dependence (F13.2-)

sedative, hypnotic, or anxiolytic use, unspecified (F13.9-)

F13.10 **Sedative, hypnotic or anxiolytic abuse, uncomplicated**

Sedative, hypnotic, or anxiolytic use disorder, mild

F13.12 **Sedative, hypnotic or anxiolytic abuse with intoxication**

F13.120 **Sedative, hypnotic or anxiolytic abuse with intoxication, uncomplicated**

F13.121 **Sedative, hypnotic or anxiolytic abuse with intoxication delirium**

F13.129 **Sedative, hypnotic or anxiolytic abuse with intoxication, unspecified**

F13.14 **Sedative, hypnotic or anxiolytic abuse with sedative, hypnotic or anxiolytic-induced mood disorder**

Sedative, hypnotic, or anxiolytic use disorder, mild, with sedative, hypnotic, or anxiolytic induced bipolar or related disorder

Sedative, hypnotic, or anxiolytic use disorder, mild, with sedative, hypnotic, or anxiolytic induced depressive disorder

F13.15 **Sedative, hypnotic or anxiolytic abuse with sedative, hypnotic or anxiolytic-induced psychotic disorder**

F13.150 **Sedative, hypnotic or anxiolytic abuse with sedative, hypnotic or anxiolytic-induced psychotic disorder with delusions**

F13.151 **Sedative, hypnotic or anxiolytic abuse with sedative, hypnotic or anxiolytic-induced psychotic disorder with hallucinations**

F13.159 **Sedative, hypnotic or anxiolytic abuse with sedative, hypnotic or anxiolytic-induced psychotic disorder, unspecified**

F13.18 **Sedative, hypnotic or anxiolytic abuse with other sedative, hypnotic or anxiolytic-induced disorders**

F13.180 **Sedative, hypnotic or anxiolytic abuse with sedative, hypnotic or anxiolytic-induced anxiety disorder**

F13.181 **Sedative, hypnotic or anxiolytic abuse with sedative, hypnotic or anxiolytic-induced sexual dysfunction**

F13.182 **Sedative, hypnotic or anxiolytic abuse with sedative, hypnotic or anxiolytic-induced sleep disorder**

F13.188 **Sedative, hypnotic or anxiolytic abuse with other sedative, hypnotic or anxiolytic-induced disorder**

F13.19 **Sedative, hypnotic or anxiolytic abuse with unspecified sedative, hypnotic or anxiolytic-induced disorder**

F13.2 **Sedative, hypnotic or anxiolytic-related dependence**

Excludes1: sedative, hypnotic or anxiolytic-related abuse (F13.1-)

sedative, hypnotic, or anxiolytic use, unspecified (F13.9-)

Excludes2: sedative, hypnotic, or anxiolytic poisoning (T42.-)

F13.20 **Sedative, hypnotic or anxiolytic dependence, uncomplicated**

F13.21 **Sedative, hypnotic or anxiolytic dependence, in remission**

F13.22 **Sedative, hypnotic or anxiolytic dependence with intoxication**

Excludes1: sedative, hypnotic or anxiolytic dependence with withdrawal (F13.23-)

F13.220 **Sedative, hypnotic or anxiolytic dependence with intoxication, uncomplicated**

F13.221 **Sedative, hypnotic or anxiolytic dependence with intoxication delirium**

F13.229 **Sedative, hypnotic or anxiolytic dependence with intoxication, unspecified**

F13.23 **Sedative, hypnotic or anxiolytic dependence with withdrawal**

Sedative, hypnotic, or anxiolytic use disorder, moderate

Sedative, hypnotic, or anxiolytic use disorder, severe

Excludes1: sedative, hypnotic or anxiolytic dependence with intoxication (F13.22-)

F13.230 **Sedative, hypnotic or anxiolytic dependence with withdrawal, uncomplicated**

F13.231 **Sedative, hypnotic or anxiolytic dependence with withdrawal delirium**

F13.232 **Sedative, hypnotic or anxiolytic dependence with withdrawal with perceptual disturbance**

Sedative, hypnotic, or anxiolytic withdrawal with perceptual disturbances

F13.239 **Sedative, hypnotic or anxiolytic dependence with withdrawal, unspecified**

Sedative, hypnotic, or anxiolytic withdrawal without perceptual disturbances

F13.24 **Sedative, hypnotic or anxiolytic dependence with sedative, hypnotic or anxiolytic-induced mood disorder**

Sedative, hypnotic, or anxiolytic use disorder, moderate, with sedative, hypnotic, or anxiolytic induced bipolar or related disorder

Sedative, hypnotic, or anxiolytic use disorder, moderate, with sedative, hypnotic, or anxiolytic induced depressive disorder

Sedative, hypnotic, or anxiolytic use disorder, severe, with sedative, hypnotic, or anxiolytic-induced bipolar or related disorder

Sedative, hypnotic, or anxiolytic use disorder, severe, with sedative, hypnotic, or anxiolytic induced depressive disorder

F13.25 **Sedative, hypnotic or anxiolytic dependence with sedative, hypnotic or anxiolytic-induced psychotic disorder**

F13.250 **Sedative, hypnotic or anxiolytic dependence with sedative, hypnotic or anxiolytic-induced psychotic disorder with delusions**

F13.251 **Sedative, hypnotic or anxiolytic dependence with sedative, hypnotic or anxiolytic-induced psychotic disorder with hallucinations**

F13.259 **Sedative, hypnotic or anxiolytic dependence with sedative, hypnotic or anxiolytic-induced psychotic disorder, unspecified**

F13.26 **Sedative, hypnotic or anxiolytic dependence with sedative, hypnotic or anxiolytic-induced persisting amnestic disorder**

F13.27 **Sedative, hypnotic or anxiolytic dependence with sedative, hypnotic or anxiolytic-induced persisting dementia**

Sedative, hypnotic, or anxiolytic use disorder, moderate, with sedative, hypnotic, or anxiolytic induced major neurocognitive disorder

Sedative, hypnotic, or anxiolytic use disorder, severe, with sedative, hypnotic, or anxiolytic-induced major neurocognitive disorder

F13.28 **Sedative, hypnotic or anxiolytic dependence with other sedative, hypnotic or anxiolytic-induced disorders**

F13.280 **Sedative, hypnotic or anxiolytic dependence with sedative, hypnotic or anxiolytic-induced anxiety disorder**

F13.281 **Sedative, hypnotic or anxiolytic dependence with sedative, hypnotic or anxiolytic-induced sexual dysfunction**

F13.282 **Sedative, hypnotic or anxiolytic dependence with sedative, hypnotic or anxiolytic-induced sleep disorder**

F13.288 **Sedative, hypnotic or anxiolytic dependence with other sedative, hypnotic or anxiolytic-induced disorder**

Sedative, hypnotic, or anxiolytic use disorder, moderate, with sedative, hypnotic, or anxiolytic induced mild neurocognitive disorder

Sedative, hypnotic, or anxiolytic use disorder, severe, with sedative, hypnotic, or anxiolytic induced mild neurocognitive disorder

F13.29 **Sedative, hypnotic or anxiolytic dependence with unspecified sedative, hypnotic or anxiolytic-induced disorder**

F13.9 **Sedative, hypnotic or anxiolytic-related use, unspecified**

Excludes1: sedative, hypnotic or anxiolytic-related abuse (F13.1-)

sedative, hypnotic or anxiolytic-related dependence (F13.2-)

F13.90 **Sedative, hypnotic, or anxiolytic use, unspecified, uncomplicated**

F13.92 **Sedative, hypnotic or anxiolytic use, unspecified with intoxication**

Excludes1: sedative, hypnotic or anxiolytic use, unspecified with withdrawal (F13.93-)

F13.920 **Sedative, hypnotic or anxiolytic use, unspecified with intoxication, uncomplicated**

F13.921 **Sedative, hypnotic or anxiolytic use, unspecified with intoxication delirium**

Sedative, hypnotic, or anxiolytic-induced delirium

F13.929 **Sedative, hypnotic or anxiolytic use, unspecified with intoxication, unspecified**

F13.93 **Sedative, hypnotic or anxiolytic use, unspecified with withdrawal**

Excludes1: sedative, hypnotic or anxiolytic use, unspecified with intoxication (F13.92-)

F13.930 **Sedative, hypnotic or anxiolytic use, unspecified with withdrawal, uncomplicated**

F13.931 **Sedative, hypnotic or anxiolytic use, unspecified with withdrawal delirium**

F13.932 **Sedative, hypnotic or anxiolytic use, unspecified with withdrawal with perceptual disturbances**

F13.939 **Sedative, hypnotic or anxiolytic use, unspecified with withdrawal, unspecified**

F13.94 **Sedative, hypnotic or anxiolytic use, unspecified with sedative, hypnotic or anxiolytic-induced mood disorder**

Sedative, hypnotic, or anxiolytic-induced bipolar or related disorder, without use disorder

Sedative, hypnotic, or anxiolytic-induced depressive disorder, without use disorder

F13.95 **Sedative, hypnotic or anxiolytic use, unspecified with sedative, hypnotic or anxiolytic-induced psychotic disorder**

F13.950 **Sedative, hypnotic or anxiolytic use, unspecified with sedative, hypnotic or anxiolytic-induced psychotic disorder with delusions**

F13.951 **Sedative, hypnotic or anxiolytic use, unspecified with sedative, hypnotic or anxiolytic-induced psychotic disorder with hallucinations**

F13.959 **Sedative, hypnotic or anxiolytic use, unspecified with sedative, hypnotic or anxiolytic-induced psychotic disorder, unspecified**

Sedative, hypnotic, or anxiolytic induced psychotic disorder, without use disorder

F13.96 **Sedative, hypnotic or anxiolytic use, unspecified with sedative, hypnotic or anxiolytic-induced persisting amnestic disorder**

F13.97 **Sedative, hypnotic or anxiolytic use, unspecified with sedative, hypnotic or anxiolytic-induced persisting dementia**

Sedative, hypnotic, or anxiolytic induced major neurocognitive disorder, without use disorder

F13.98 **Sedative, hypnotic or anxiolytic use, unspecified with other sedative, hypnotic or anxiolytic-induced disorders**

F13.980 **Sedative, hypnotic or anxiolytic use, unspecified with sedative, hypnotic or anxiolytic-induced anxiety disorder**

Sedative, hypnotic, or anxiolytic induced anxiety disorder, without use disorder

F13.981 **Sedative, hypnotic or anxiolytic use, unspecified with sedative, hypnotic or anxiolytic-induced sexual dysfunction**

Sedative, hypnotic, or anxiolytic induced sexual dysfunction disorder, without use disorder

F13.982 **Sedative, hypnotic or anxiolytic use, unspecified with sedative, hypnotic or anxiolytic-induced sleep disorder**

Sedative, hypnotic, or anxiolytic induced sleep disorder, without use disorder

F13.988 **Sedative, hypnotic or anxiolytic use, unspecified with other sedative, hypnotic or anxiolytic-induced disorder**

Sedative, hypnotic, or anxiolytic induced mild neurocognitive disorder

F13.99 **Sedative, hypnotic or anxiolytic use, unspecified with unspecified sedative, hypnotic or anxiolytic-induced disorder**

F14 **Cocaine related disorders**

Excludes2: Other stimulant-related disorders (F15.-)

F14.1 **Cocaine abuse**

Excludes1: cocaine dependence (F14.2-)

cocaine use, unspecified (F14.9-)

F14.10 **Cocaine abuse, uncomplicated**

Cocaine use disorder, mild

F14.12 **Cocaine abuse with intoxication**

F14.120 **Cocaine abuse with intoxication, uncomplicated**

F14.121 **Cocaine abuse with intoxication with delirium**

F14.122 **Cocaine abuse with intoxication with perceptual disturbance**

F14.129 **Cocaine abuse with intoxication, unspecified**

F14.14 **Cocaine abuse with cocaine-induced mood disorder**

Cocaine use disorder, mild, with cocaine-induced bipolar or related disorder

Cocaine use disorder, mild, with cocaine-induced depressive disorder

F14.15 **Cocaine abuse with cocaine-induced psychotic disorder**

F14.150 **Cocaine abuse with cocaine-induced psychotic disorder with delusions**

F14.151 **Cocaine abuse with cocaine-induced psychotic disorder with hallucinations**

F14.159 **Cocaine abuse with cocaine-induced psychotic disorder, unspecified**

F14.18 **Cocaine abuse with other cocaine-induced disorder**

F14.180 **Cocaine abuse with cocaine-induced anxiety disorder**

F14.181 **Cocaine abuse with cocaine-induced sexual dysfunction**

F14.182 **Cocaine abuse with cocaine-induced sleep disorder**

F14.188 **Cocaine abuse with other cocaine-induced disorder**

Cocaine use disorder, mild, with cocaine-induced obsessive compulsive or related disorder

F14.19 **Cocaine abuse with unspecified cocaine-induced disorder**

F14.2 **Cocaine dependence**

Excludes1: cocaine abuse (F14.1-)

cocaine use, unspecified (F14.9-)

Excludes2: cocaine poisoning (T40.5-)

F14.20 **Cocaine dependence, uncomplicated**

Cocaine use disorder, moderate

Cocaine use disorder, severe

F14.21 **Cocaine dependence, in remission**

F14.22 **Cocaine dependence with intoxication**

Excludes1: cocaine dependence with withdrawal (F14.23)

F14.220 **Cocaine dependence with intoxication, uncomplicated**

F14.221 **Cocaine dependence with intoxication delirium**

F14.222 **Cocaine dependence with intoxication with perceptual disturbance**

F14.229 **Cocaine dependence with intoxication, unspecified**

F14.23 **Cocaine dependence with withdrawal**

Excludes1: cocaine dependence with intoxication (F14.22-)

F14.24 **Cocaine dependence with cocaine-induced mood disorder**

Cocaine use disorder, moderate, with cocaine-induced bipolar or related disorder

Cocaine use disorder, moderate, with cocaine-induced depressive disorder

Cocaine use disorder, severe, with cocaine-induced bipolar or related disorder

Cocaine use disorder, severe, with cocaine-induced depressive disorder

F14.25 **Cocaine dependence with cocaine-induced psychotic disorder**

F14.250 **Cocaine dependence with cocaine-induced psychotic disorder with delusions**

F14.251 **Cocaine dependence with cocaine-induced psychotic disorder with hallucinations**

F14.259 **Cocaine dependence with cocaine-induced psychotic disorder, unspecified**

F14.28 **Cocaine dependence with other cocaine-induced disorder**

F14.280 **Cocaine dependence with cocaine-induced anxiety disorder**

F14.281 **Cocaine dependence with cocaine-induced sexual dysfunction**

F14.282 **Cocaine dependence with cocaine-induced sleep disorder**

F14.288 **Cocaine dependence with other cocaine-induced disorder**

Cocaine use disorder, moderate, with cocaine-induced obsessive compulsive or related disorder

Cocaine use disorder, severe, with cocaine-induced obsessive compulsive or related disorder

F14.29 **Cocaine dependence with unspecified cocaine-induced disorder**

F14.9 **Cocaine use, unspecified**

Excludes1: cocaine abuse (F14.1-)
cocaine dependence (F14.2-)

F14.90 **Cocaine use, unspecified, uncomplicated**

F14.92 **Cocaine use, unspecified with intoxication**

F14.920 **Cocaine use, unspecified with intoxication, uncomplicated**

F14.921 **Cocaine use, unspecified with intoxication delirium**

F14.922 **Cocaine use, unspecified with intoxication with perceptual disturbance**

F14.929 **Cocaine use, unspecified with intoxication, unspecified**

F14.94 **Cocaine use, unspecified with cocaine-induced mood disorder**

Cocaine induced bipolar or related disorder, without use disorder

Cocaine induced depressive disorder, without use disorder

F14.95 **Cocaine use, unspecified with cocaine-induced psychotic disorder**

F14.950 **Cocaine use, unspecified with cocaine-induced psychotic disorder with delusions**

F14.951 **Cocaine use, unspecified with cocaine-induced psychotic disorder with hallucinations**

F14.959 **Cocaine use, unspecified with cocaine-induced psychotic disorder, unspecified**

Cocaine induced psychotic disorder, without use disorder

F14.98 **Cocaine use, unspecified with other specified cocaine-induced disorder**

F14.980 **Cocaine use, unspecified with cocaine-induced anxiety disorder**

Cocaine induced anxiety disorder, without use disorder

F14.981 **Cocaine use, unspecified with cocaine-induced sexual dysfunction**

Cocaine induced sexual dysfunction, without use disorder

F14.982 **Cocaine use, unspecified with cocaine-induced sleep disorder**

Cocaine induced sleep disorder, without use disorder

F14.988 **Cocaine use, unspecified with other cocaine-induced disorder**

Cocaine induced obsessive compulsive or related disorder

F14.99 **Cocaine use, unspecified with unspecified cocaine-induced disorder**

F15 **Other stimulant related disorders**

Includes: amphetamine-related disorders
caffeine

Excludes2: cocaine-related disorders (F14.-)

F15.1 **Other stimulant abuse**

Excludes1: Other stimulant dependence (F15.2-)
Other stimulant use, unspecified (F15.9-)

F15.10 **Other stimulant abuse, uncomplicated**

Amphetamine type substance use disorder, mild

Other or unspecified stimulant use disorder, mild

F15.12 **Other stimulant abuse with intoxication**

F15.120 **Other stimulant abuse with intoxication, uncomplicated**

F15.121 **Other stimulant abuse with intoxication delirium**

F15.122 **Other stimulant abuse with intoxication with perceptual disturbance**

Amphetamine or other stimulant use disorder, mild, with amphetamine or other stimulant intoxication, with perceptual disturbances

F15.129 **Other stimulant abuse with intoxication, unspecified**

Amphetamine or other stimulant use disorder, mild, with amphetamine or other stimulant intoxication, without perceptual disturbances

F15.14 **Other stimulant abuse with stimulant-induced mood disorder**

Amphetamine or other stimulant use disorder, mild, with amphetamine or other stimulant induced bipolar or related disorder

Amphetamine or other stimulant use disorder, mild, with amphetamine or other stimulant induced depressive disorder

F15.15 **Other stimulant abuse with stimulant-induced psychotic disorder**

F15.150 **Other stimulant abuse with stimulant-induced psychotic disorder with delusions**

F15.151 **Other stimulant abuse with stimulant-induced psychotic disorder with hallucinations**

F15.159 **Other stimulant abuse with stimulant-induced psychotic disorder, unspecified**

F15.18 **Other stimulant abuse with other stimulant-induced disorder**

F15.180 **Other stimulant abuse with stimulant-induced anxiety disorder**

F15.181 **Other stimulant abuse with stimulant-induced sexual dysfunction**

F15.182 **Other stimulant abuse with stimulant-induced sleep disorder**

F15.188 **Other stimulant abuse with other stimulant-induced disorder**

Amphetamine or other stimulant use disorder, mild, with amphetamine or other stimulant induced obsessive-compulsive or related disorder

F15.19 **Other stimulant abuse with unspecified stimulant-induced disorder**

F15.2 **Other stimulant dependence**

Excludes1: Other stimulant abuse (F15.1-)

Other stimulant use, unspecified (F15.9-)

F15.20 **Other stimulant dependence, uncomplicated**

Amphetamine type substance use disorder, moderate

Amphetamine type substance use disorder, severe

Other or unspecified stimulant use disorder, moderate

Other or unspecified stimulant use disorder, severe

F15.21 **Other stimulant dependence, in remission**

F15.22 **Other stimulant dependence with intoxication**

Excludes1: Other stimulant dependence with withdrawal (F15.23)

F15.220 **Other stimulant dependence with intoxication, uncomplicated**

F15.221 **Other stimulant dependence with intoxication delirium**

F15.222 **Other stimulant dependence with intoxication with perceptual disturbance**

Amphetamine or other stimulant use disorder, moderate, with amphetamine or other stimulant intoxication, with perceptual disturbances

Amphetamine or other stimulant use disorder, severe, with amphetamine or other stimulant intoxication, with perceptual disturbances

F15.229 **Other stimulant dependence with intoxication, unspecified**

Amphetamine **or other** stimulant use disorder, moderate, with amphetamine or other stimulant intoxication, without perceptual disturbances

Amphetamine **or other** stimulant use disorder, severe, with amphetamine **or other** stimulant intoxication, without perceptual disturbances

F15.23 **Other stimulant dependence with withdrawal**

Amphetamine **or other** stimulant withdrawal

Excludes1: Other stimulant dependence with intoxication (F15.22-)

F15.24 **Other stimulant dependence with stimulant-induced mood disorder**

Amphetamine or other stimulant use disorder, moderate, with amphetamine or other stimulant-induced bipolar or related disorder

Amphetamine or other stimulant use disorder, moderate, with amphetamine or other stimulant induced depressive disorder

Amphetamine or other stimulant use disorder, severe, with amphetamine or other stimulant-induced bipolar or related disorder

Amphetamine or other stimulant use disorder, severe, with amphetamine or other stimulant-induced depressive disorder

F15.25 **Other stimulant dependence with stimulant-induced psychotic disorder**

F15.250 **Other stimulant dependence with stimulant-induced psychotic disorder with delusions**

F15.251 **Other stimulant dependence with stimulant-induced psychotic disorder with hallucinations**

F15.259 **Other stimulant dependence with stimulant-induced psychotic disorder, unspecified**

F15.28 **Other stimulant dependence with other stimulant-induced disorder**

F15.280 **Other stimulant dependence with stimulant-induced anxiety disorder**

F15.281 **Other stimulant dependence with stimulant-induced sexual dysfunction**

F15.282 **Other stimulant dependence with stimulant-induced sleep disorder**

F15.288 **Other stimulant dependence with other stimulant-induced disorder**

Amphetamine or other stimulant use disorder, moderate, with amphetamine or other stimulant induced obsessive compulsiveor related disorder

Amphetamine or other stimulant use disorder, severe, with amphetamine or other stimulant induced obsessive compulsiveor related disorder

F15.29 **Other stimulant dependence with unspecified stimulant-induced disorder**

F15.9 **Other stimulant use, unspecified**

Excludes1: Other stimulant abuse (F15.1-)

Other stimulant dependence (F15.2-)

F15.90 **Other stimulant use, unspecified, uncomplicated**

F15.92 **Other stimulant use, unspecified with intoxication**

Excludes1: Other stimulant use, unspecified with withdrawal (F15.93)

Add 4th-7th digits   Nonspecific code   Unspecified code   Manifestation code   271

F15.920 Other stimulant use, unspecified with intoxication, uncomplicated

F15.921 Other stimulant use, unspecified with intoxication delirium

Amphetamine or other stimulant-induced delirium

F15.922 Other stimulant use, unspecified with intoxication with perceptual disturbance

F15.929 Other stimulant use, unspecified with intoxication, unspecified

Caffeine intoxication

F15.93 Other stimulant use, unspecified with withdrawal

Caffeine withdrawal

Excludes1: Other stimulant use, unspecified with intoxication (F15.92-)

F15.94 Other stimulant use, unspecified with stimulant-induced mood disorder

Amphetamine or other stimulant-induced bipolar or related disorder, without use disorder

Amphetamine or other stimulant-induced depressive disorder, without use disorder

F15.95 Other stimulant use, unspecified with stimulant-induced psychotic disorder

F15.950 Other stimulant use, unspecified with stimulant-induced psychotic disorder with delusions

F15.951 Other stimulant use, unspecified with stimulant-induced psychotic disorder with hallucinations

F15.959 Other stimulant use, unspecified with stimulant-induced psychotic disorder, unspecified

Amphetamine or other stimulant-induced induced psychotic disorder, without use disorder

F15.98 Other stimulant use, unspecified with other stimulant-induced disorder

F15.980 Other stimulant use, unspecified with stimulant-induced anxiety disorder

Amphetamine or other stimulant-induced anxiety disorder, without use disorder

Caffeine induced anxiety disorder, without use disorder

F15.981 Other stimulant use, unspecified with stimulant-induced sexual dysfunction

Amphetamine or other stimulant-induced sexual dysfunction, without use disorder

F15.982 Other stimulant use, unspecified with stimulant-induced sleep disorder

Amphetamine or other stimulant-induced sleep disorder, without use disorder

Caffeine induced sleep disorder, without use disorder

F15.988 Other stimulant use, unspecified with other stimulant-induced disorder

Amphetamine or other stimulant-induced obsessive compulsive or related disorder, without use disorder

F15.99 Other stimulant use, unspecified with unspecified stimulant-induced disorder

F16 **Hallucinogen related disorders**

Includes: ecstasy

PCP phencyclidine

F16.1 **Hallucinogen abuse**

Excludes1: hallucinogen dependence (F16.2-)

hallucinogen use, unspecified (F16.9-)

F16.10 Hallucinogen abuse, uncomplicated

Other hallucinogen use disorder, mild

Phencyclidine use disorder, mild

F16.12 Hallucinogen abuse with intoxication

F16.120 Hallucinogen abuse with intoxication, uncomplicated

F16.121 Hallucinogen abuse with intoxication with delirium

F16.122 Hallucinogen abuse with intoxication with perceptual disturbance

F16.129 Hallucinogen abuse with intoxication, unspecified

F16.14 Hallucinogen abuse with hallucinogen-induced mood disorder

Other hallucinogen use disorder, mild, with other hallucinogen induced bipolar or related disorder

Other hallucinogen use disorder, mild, with other hallucinogen induced depressive disorder

Phencyclidine use disorder, mild, with phencyclidine induced bipolar or related disorder

Phencyclidine use disorder, mild, with phencyclidine induced depressive disorder

F16.15 Hallucinogen abuse with hallucinogen-induced psychotic disorder

F16.150 Hallucinogen abuse with hallucinogen-induced psychotic disorder with delusions

F16.151 Hallucinogen abuse with hallucinogen-induced psychotic disorder with hallucinations

F16.159 Hallucinogen abuse with hallucinogen-induced psychotic disorder, unspecified

F16.18 Hallucinogen abuse with other hallucinogen-induced disorder

F16.180 Hallucinogen abuse with hallucinogen-induced anxiety disorder

F16.183 Hallucinogen abuse with hallucinogen persisting perception disorder (flashbacks)

F16.188 Hallucinogen abuse with other hallucinogen-induced disorder

F16.19 Hallucinogen abuse with unspecified hallucinogen-induced disorder

F16.2 **Hallucinogen dependence**

Excludes1: hallucinogen abuse (F16.1-)

hallucinogen use, unspecified (F16.9-)

F16.20 Hallucinogen dependence, uncomplicated

Other hallucinogen use disorder, moderate

Other hallucinogen use disorder, severe

Phencyclidine use disorder, moderate

Phencyclidine use disorder, severe

F16.21 Hallucinogen dependence, in remission

F16.22 Hallucinogen dependence with intoxication

F16.220 Hallucinogen dependence with intoxication, uncomplicated

F16.221 Hallucinogen dependence with intoxication with delirium

F16.229 Hallucinogen dependence with intoxication, unspecified

F16.24 Hallucinogen dependence with hallucinogen-induced mood disorder

Other hallucinogen use disorder, moderate, with other hallucinogen induced bipolar or related disorder

Other hallucinogen use disorder, moderate, with other hallucinogen induced depressive disorder

Other hallucinogen use disorder, severe, with other hallucinogen-induced bipolar or related disorder

Other hallucinogen use disorder, severe, with other hallucinogen-induced depressive disorder

Phencyclidine use disorder, moderate, with phencyclidine induced bipolar or related disorder

Phencyclidine use disorder, moderate, with phencyclidine induced depressive disorder

Phencyclidine use disorder, severe, with phencyclidine induced bipolar or related disorder

Phencyclidine use disorder, severe, with phencyclidine-induced depressive disorder

F16.25 Hallucinogen dependence with hallucinogen-induced psychotic disorder

F16.250 Hallucinogen dependence with hallucinogen-induced psychotic disorder with delusions

F16.251 Hallucinogen dependence with hallucinogen-induced psychotic disorder with hallucinations

F16.259 Hallucinogen dependence with hallucinogen-induced psychotic disorder, unspecified

F16.28 Hallucinogen dependence with other hallucinogen-induced disorder

F16.280 Hallucinogen dependence with hallucinogen-induced anxiety disorder

F16.283 Hallucinogen dependence with hallucinogen persisting perception disorder (flashbacks)

F16.288 Hallucinogen dependence with other hallucinogen-induced disorder

F16.29 Hallucinogen dependence with unspecified hallucinogen-induced disorder

F16.9 Hallucinogen use, unspecified

Excludes1: hallucinogen abuse (F16.1-)

hallucinogen dependence (F16.2-)

F16.90 Hallucinogen use, unspecified, uncomplicated

F16.92 Hallucinogen use, unspecified with intoxication

F16.920 Hallucinogen use, unspecified with intoxication, uncomplicated

F16.921 Hallucinogen use, unspecified with intoxication with delirium

Other hallucinogen intoxication delirium

F16.929 Hallucinogen use, unspecified with intoxication, unspecified

F16.94 Hallucinogen use, unspecified with hallucinogen-induced mood disorder

Other hallucinogen induced bipolar or related disorder, without use disorder

Other hallucinogen induced depressive disorder, without use disorder

Phencyclidine induced bipolar or related disorder, without use disorder

Phencyclidine induced depressive disorder, without use disorder

F16.95 Hallucinogen use, unspecified with hallucinogen-induced psychotic disorder

F16.950 Hallucinogen use, unspecified with hallucinogen-induced psychotic disorder with delusions

F16.951 Hallucinogen use, unspecified with hallucinogen-induced psychotic disorder with hallucinations

F16.959 Hallucinogen use, unspecified with hallucinogen-induced psychotic disorder, unspecified

Other hallucinogen induced psychotic disorder, without use disorder

Phencyclidine induced psychotic disorder, without use disorder

F16.98 Hallucinogen use, unspecified with other specified hallucinogen-induced disorder

F16.980 Hallucinogen use, unspecified with hallucinogen-induced anxiety disorder

Other hallucinogen-induced anxiety disorder, without use disorder

Phencyclidine induced anxiety disorder, without use disorder

F16.983 Hallucinogen use, unspecified with hallucinogen persisting perception disorder (flashbacks)

F16.988 Hallucinogen use, unspecified with other hallucinogen-induced disorder

F16.99 Hallucinogen use, unspecified with unspecified hallucinogen-induced disorder

F17 Nicotine dependence

Excludes1: history of tobacco dependence (Z87.891)

tobacco use NOS (Z72.0)

Excludes2: tobacco use (smoking) during pregnancy, childbirth and the puerperium (O99.33-)

toxic effect of nicotine (T65.2-)

F17.2 Nicotine dependence

F17.20   **Nicotine dependence, unspecified**

    F17.200   **Nicotine dependence, unspecified, uncomplicated**

          Tobacco use disorder, mild

          Tobacco use disorder, moderate

          Tobacco use disorder, severe

    F17.201   **Nicotine dependence, unspecified, in remission**

    F17.203   **Nicotine dependence unspecified, with withdrawal**

          Tobacco withdrawal

    F17.208   **Nicotine dependence, unspecified, with other nicotine-induced disorders**

    F17.209   **Nicotine dependence, unspecified, with unspecified nicotine-induced disorders**

F17.21   **Nicotine dependence, cigarettes**

    F17.210   **Nicotine dependence, cigarettes, uncomplicated**

    F17.211   **Nicotine dependence, cigarettes, in remission**

    F17.213   **Nicotine dependence, cigarettes, with withdrawal**

    F17.218   **Nicotine dependence, cigarettes, with other nicotine-induced disorders**

    F17.219   **Nicotine dependence, cigarettes, with unspecified nicotine-induced disorders**

F17.22   **Nicotine dependence, chewing tobacco**

    F17.220   **Nicotine dependence, chewing tobacco, uncomplicated**

    F17.221   **Nicotine dependence, chewing tobacco, in remission**

    F17.223   **Nicotine dependence, chewing tobacco, with withdrawal**

    F17.228   **Nicotine dependence, chewing tobacco, with other nicotine-induced disorders**

    F17.229   **Nicotine dependence, chewing tobacco, with unspecified nicotine-induced disorders**

F17.29   **Nicotine dependence, other tobacco product**

    F17.290   **Nicotine dependence, other tobacco product, uncomplicated**

    F17.291   **Nicotine dependence, other tobacco product, in remission**

    F17.293   **Nicotine dependence, other tobacco product, with withdrawal**

    F17.298   **Nicotine dependence, other tobacco product, with other nicotine-induced disorders**

    F17.299   **Nicotine dependence, other tobacco product, with unspecified nicotine-induced disorders**

F18   **Inhalant related disorders**

    Includes: volatile solvents

  F18.1 **Inhalant abuse**

    Excludes1: inhalant dependence (F18.2-)

          inhalant use, unspecified (F18.9-)

F18.10   **Inhalant abuse, uncomplicated**

    Inhalant use disorder, mild

F18.12   **Inhalant abuse with intoxication**

    F18.120   **Inhalant abuse with intoxication, uncomplicated**

    F18.121   **Inhalant abuse with intoxication delirium**

    F18.129   **Inhalant abuse with intoxication, unspecified**

F18.14   **Inhalant abuse with inhalant-induced mood disorder**

    Inhalant use disorder, mild, with inhalant induced depressive disorder

F18.15   **Inhalant abuse with inhalant-induced psychotic disorder**

    F18.150   **Inhalant abuse with inhalant-induced psychotic disorder with delusions**

    F18.151   **Inhalant abuse with inhalant-induced psychotic disorder with hallucinations**

    F18.159   **Inhalant abuse with inhalant-induced psychotic disorder, unspecified**

F18.17   **Inhalant abuse with inhalant-induced dementia**

    Inhalant use disorder, mild, with inhalant induced major neurocognitive disorder

F18.18   **Inhalant abuse with other inhalant-induced disorders**

    F18.180   **Inhalant abuse with inhalant-induced anxiety disorder**

    F18.188   **Inhalant abuse with other inhalant-induced disorder**

          Inhalant use disorder, mild, with inhalant induced mild neurocognitive disorder

F18.19   **Inhalant abuse with unspecified inhalant-induced disorder**

F18.2   **Inhalant dependence**

    Excludes1: inhalant abuse (F18.1-)

          inhalant use, unspecified (F18.9-)

F18.20   **Inhalant dependence, uncomplicated**

    Inhalant use disorder, moderate

    Inhalant use disorder, severe

F18.21   **Inhalant dependence, in remission**

F18.22   **Inhalant dependence with intoxication**

    F18.220   **Inhalant dependence with intoxication, uncomplicated**

    F18.221   **Inhalant dependence with intoxication delirium**

    F18.229   **Inhalant dependence with intoxication, unspecified**

F18.24   **Inhalant dependence with inhalant-induced mood disorder**

    Inhalant use disorder, moderate, with inhalant induced depressive disorder

    Inhalant use disorder, severe, with inhalant induced depressive disorder

   ● New code   ▲ Revised code   **Excludes1:** Not coded here   **Excludes2:** Not included here   ⊗ Placeholder required   ⑦7th digit required

MENTAL, BEHAVIORAL AND NEURODEVELOPMENTAL DISORDERS

F18.25 Inhalant dependence with inhalant-induced psychotic disorder

- **F18.250** Inhalant dependence with inhalant-induced psychotic disorder with delusions
- **F18.251** Inhalant dependence with inhalant-induced psychotic disorder with hallucinations
- **F18.259** Inhalant dependence with inhalant-induced psychotic disorder, unspecified

F18.27 Inhalant dependence with inhalant-induced dementia

Inhalant use disorder, moderate, with inhalant induced major neurocognitive disorder

Inhalant use disorder, severe, with inhalant induced major neurocognitive disorder

F18.28 Inhalant dependence with other inhalant-induced disorders

- **F18.280** Inhalant dependence with inhalant-induced anxiety disorder
- **F18.288** Inhalant dependence with other inhalant-induced disorder

Inhalant use disorder, moderate, with inhalant-induced mild neurocognitive disorder

Inhalant use disorder, severe, with inhalant-induced mild neurocognitive disorder

F18.29 Inhalant dependence with unspecified inhalant-induced disorder

F18.9 Inhalant use, unspecified

Excludes1: inhalant abuse (F18.1-)

inhalant dependence (F18.2-)

F18.90 Inhalant use, unspecified, uncomplicated

F18.92 Inhalant use, unspecified with intoxication

- **F18.920** Inhalant use, unspecified with intoxication, uncomplicated
- **F18.921** Inhalant use, unspecified with intoxication with delirium
- **F18.929** Inhalant use, unspecified with intoxication, unspecified

F18.94 Inhalant use, unspecified with inhalant-induced mood disorder

Inhalant induced depressive disorder

F18.95 Inhalant use, unspecified with inhalant-induced psychotic disorder

- **F18.950** Inhalant use, unspecified with inhalant-induced psychotic disorder with delusions
- **F18.951** Inhalant use, unspecified with inhalant-induced psychotic disorder with hallucinations
- **F18.959** Inhalant use, unspecified with inhalant-induced psychotic disorder, unspecified

F18.97 Inhalant use, unspecified with inhalant-induced persisting dementia

Inhalant-induced major neurocognitive disorder

F18.98 Inhalant use, unspecified with other inhalant-induced disorders

- **F18.980** Inhalant use, unspecified with inhalant-induced anxiety disorder
- **F18.988** Inhalant use, unspecified with other inhalant-induced disorder

Inhalant-induced mild neurocognitive disorder

F18.99 Inhalant use, unspecified with unspecified inhalant-induced disorder

F19 Other psychoactive substance related disorders

Includes: polysubstance drug use (indiscriminate drug use)

F19.1 Other psychoactive substance abuse

Excludes1: Other psychoactive substance dependence (F19.2-)

Other psychoactive substance use, unspecified (F19.9-)

F19.10 Other psychoactive substance abuse, uncomplicated

Other (or unknown) substance use disorder, mild

F19.12 Other psychoactive substance abuse with intoxication

- **F19.120** Other psychoactive substance abuse with intoxication, uncomplicated
- **F19.121** Other psychoactive substance abuse with intoxication delirium
- **F19.122** Other psychoactive substance abuse with intoxication with perceptual disturbances
- **F19.129** Other psychoactive substance abuse with intoxication, unspecified

F19.14 Other psychoactive substance abuse with psychoactive substance-induced mood disorder

Other (or unknown) substance use disorder, mild, with other (or unknown) substance-induced bipolar or related disorder

Other (or unknown) substance use disorder, mild, with other (or unknown) substance-induced depressive disorder

F19.15 Other psychoactive substance abuse with psychoactive substance-induced psychotic disorder

- **F19.150** Other psychoactive substance abuse with psychoactive substance-induced psychotic disorder with delusions
- **F19.151** Other psychoactive substance abuse with psychoactive substance-induced psychotic disorder with hallucinations
- **F19.159** Other psychoactive substance abuse with psychoactive substance-induced psychotic disorder, unspecified

F19.16 Other psychoactive substance abuse with psychoactive substance-induced persisting amnestic disorder

F19.17 Other psychoactive substance abuse with psychoactive substance-induced persisting dementia

Other (or unknown) substance use disorder, mild, with other (or unknown) substance-induced major neurocognitive disorder

F19.18   **Other psychoactive substance abuse with other psychoactive substance-induced disorders**

  F19.180   **Other psychoactive substance abuse with psychoactive substance-induced anxiety disorder**

  F19.181   **Other psychoactive substance abuse with psychoactive substance-induced sexual dysfunction**

  F19.182   **Other psychoactive substance abuse with psychoactive substance-induced sleep disorder**

  F19.188   **Other psychoactive substance abuse with other psychoactive substance-induced disorder**

Other (or unknown) substance use disorder, mild, with other (or unknown) substance induced mild neurocognitive disorder

Other (or unknown) substance use disorder, mild, with other (or unknown) substance induced obsessive-compulsive or related disorder

F19.19   **Other psychoactive substance abuse with unspecified psychoactive substance-induced disorder**

F19.2   **Other psychoactive substance dependence**

  Excludes1: Other psychoactive substance abuse (F19.1-)

  Other psychoactive substance use, unspecified (F19.9-)

  F19.20   **Other psychoactive substance dependence, uncomplicated**

Other (or unknown) substance use disorder, moderate **Other** (or unknown) substance use disorder, severe

  F19.21   **Other psychoactive substance dependence, in remission**

  F19.22   **Other psychoactive substance dependence with intoxication**

  Excludes1: Other psychoactive substance dependence with withdrawal (F19.23-)

  F19.220   **Other psychoactive substance dependence with intoxication, uncomplicated**

  F19.221   **Other psychoactive substance dependence with intoxication delirium**

  F9.2122   **Other psychoactive substance dependence with intoxication with perceptual disturbance**

  F19.229   **Other psychoactive substance dependence with intoxication, unspecified**

  F19.23   **Other psychoactive substance dependence with withdrawal**

  Excludes1: Other psychoactive substance dependence with intoxication (F19.22-)

  F19.230   **Other psychoactive substance dependence with withdrawal, uncomplicated**

  F19.231   **Other psychoactive substance dependence with withdrawal delirium**

  F19.232   **Other psychoactive substance dependence with withdrawal with perceptual disturbance**

  F19.239   **Other psychoactive substance dependence with withdrawal, unspecified**

F19.24   **Other psychoactive substance dependence with psychoactive substance-induced mood disorder**

Other (or unknown) substance use disorder, moderate, with other (or unknown) substance induced bipolar or related disorder

Other (or unknown) substance use disorder, moderate, with other (or unknown) substance induced depressive disorder

Other (or unknown) substance use disorder, severe, with other (or unknown) substance induced bipolar or related disorder

Other (or unknown) substance use disorder, severe, with other (or unknown) substance induced depressive disorder

F19.25   **Other psychoactive substance dependence with psychoactive substance-induced psychotic disorder**

  F19.250   **Other psychoactive substance dependence with psychoactive substance-induced psychotic disorder with delusions**

  F19.251   **Other psychoactive substance dependence with psychoactive substance-induced psychotic disorder with hallucinations**

  F19.259   **Other psychoactive substance dependence with psychoactive substance-induced psychotic disorder, unspecified**

F19.26   **Other psychoactive substance dependence with psychoactive substance-induced persisting amnestic disorder**

F19.27   **Other psychoactive substance dependence with psychoactive substance-induced persisting dementia**

Other (or unknown) substance use disorder, moderate, with other (or unknown) substance induced major neurocognitive disorder

Other (or unknown) substance use disorder, severe, with other (or unknown) substance induced major neurocognitive disorder

F19.28   **Other psychoactive substance dependence with other psychoactive substance-induced disorders**

  F19.280   **Other psychoactive substance dependence with psychoactive substance-induced anxiety disorder**

  F19.281   **Other psychoactive substance dependence with psychoactive substance-induced sexual dysfunction**

  F19.282   **Other psychoactive substance dependence with psychoactive substance-induced sleep disorder**

  F19.288   **Other psychoactive substance dependence with other psychoactive substance-induced disorder**

Other (or unknown) substance use disorder, moderate, with other (or unknown) substance induced mild neurocognitive disorder

Other (or unknown) substance use disorder, severe, with other (or unknown) substance induced mild neurocognitive disorder

Other (or unknown) substance use disorder, moderate, with other (or unknown) substance induced obsessive compulsive or related disorder

Other (or unknown) substance use disorder, severe, with other (or unknown) substance induced obsessive-compulsive or related disorder

F19.29 **Other psychoactive substance dependence with unspecified psychoactive substance-induced disorder**

F19.9 **Other psychoactive substance use, unspecified**

Excludes1: Other psychoactive substance abuse (F19.1-)

Other psychoactive substance dependence (F19.2-)

F19.90 **Other psychoactive substance use, unspecified, uncomplicated**

F19.92 **Other psychoactive substance use, unspecified with intoxication**

Excludes1: Other psychoactive substance use, unspecified with withdrawal (F19.93)

F19.920 **Other psychoactive substance use, unspecified with intoxication, uncomplicated**

F19.921 **Other psychoactive substance use, unspecified with intoxication with delirium**

Other (or unknown) substance-induced delirium

F19.922 **Other psychoactive substance use, unspecified with intoxication with perceptual disturbance**

F19.929 **Other psychoactive substance use, unspecified with intoxication, unspecified**

F19.93 **Other psychoactive substance use, unspecified with withdrawal**

Excludes1: Other psychoactive substance use, unspecified with intoxication (F19.92-)

F19.930 **Other psychoactive substance use, unspecified with withdrawal, uncomplicated**

F19.931 **Other psychoactive substance use, unspecified with withdrawal delirium**

F19.932 **Other psychoactive substance use, unspecified with withdrawal with perceptual disturbance**

F19.939 **Other psychoactive substance use, unspecified with withdrawal, unspecified**

F19.94 **Other psychoactive substance use, unspecified with psychoactive substance-induced mood disorder**

Other (or unknown) substance-induced bipolar or related disorder, without use disorder

Other (or unknown) substance-induced depressive disorder, without use disorder

F19.95 **Other psychoactive substance use, unspecified with psychoactive substance-induced psychotic disorder**

F19.950 **Other psychoactive substance use, unspecified with psychoactive substance-induced psychotic disorder with delusions**

F19.951 **Other psychoactive substance use, unspecified with psychoactive substance-induced psychotic disorder with hallucinations**

F19.959 **Other psychoactive substance use, unspecified with psychoactive substance-induced psychotic disorder, unspecified**

Other or unknown substance-induced psychotic disorder, without use disorder

F19.96 **Other psychoactive substance use, unspecified with psychoactive substance-induced persisting amnestic disorder**

F19.97 **Other psychoactive substance use, unspecified with psychoactive substance-induced persisting dementia**

Other (or unknown) substance-induced major neurocognitive disorder, without use disorder

F19.98 **Other psychoactive substance use, unspecified with other psychoactive substance-induced disorders**

F19.980 **Other psychoactive substance use, unspecified with psychoactive substance-induced anxiety disorder**

Other (or unknown) substance-induced anxiety disorder, without use disorder

F19.981 **Other psychoactive substance use, unspecified with psychoactive substance-induced sexual dysfunction**

Other (or unknown) substance-induced sexual dysfunction, without use disorder

F19.982 **Other psychoactive substance use, unspecified with psychoactive substance-induced sleep disorder**

Other (or unknown) substance-induced sleep disorder, without use disorder

F19.988 **Other psychoactive substance use, unspecified with other psychoactive substance-induced disorder**

Other (or unknown) substance-induced mild neurocognitive disorder, without use disorder

Other (or unknown) substance-induced obsessive-compulsive or relateddisorder, without use disorder

F19.99 **Other psychoactive substance use, unspecified with unspecified psychoactive substance-induced disorder**

SCHIZOPHRENIA, SCHIZOTYPAL, DELUSIONAL, AND OTHER NON-MOOD PSYCHOTIC DISORDERS (F20-F29)

F20 **Schizophrenia**

Definition: Schizophrenia is a psychotic disorder marked by severely impaired thinking, emotions, and behaviors. Schizophrenic patients are typically unable to filter sensory stimuli and may have

enhanced perceptions of sounds, colors, and other features of their environment.

Excludes1: brief psychotic disorder (F23)

cyclic schizophrenia (F25.0)

mood [affective] disorders with psychotic symptoms (F30.2, F31.2, F31.5, F31.64, F32.3, F33.3)

schizoaffective disorder (F25.-)

schizophrenic reaction NOS (F23)

Excludes2: schizophrenic reaction in:

alcoholism (F10.15-, F10.25-, F10.95-)

brain disease (F06.2)

epilepsy (F06.2)

psychoactive drug use (F11-F19 with .15, .25, .95)

schizotypal disorder (F21)

F20.0 Paranoid schizophrenia

Paraphrenic schizophrenia

Excludes1: involutional paranoid state (F22)

paranoia (F22)

F20.1 Disorganized schizophrenia

Hebephrenic schizophrenia

Hebephrenia

F20.2 Catatonic schizophrenia

Schizophrenic catalepsy

Schizophrenic catatonia

Schizophrenic flexibilitas cerea

Excludes1: catatonic stupor (R40.1)

F20.3 Undifferentiated schizophrenia

Atypical schizophrenia

Excludes1: acute schizophrenia-like psychotic disorder (F23)

Excludes2: post-schizophrenic depression (F32.89)

F20.5 Residual schizophrenia

Restzustand (schizophrenic)

Schizophrenic residual state

F20.8 Other schizophrenia

F20.81 Schizophreniform disorder

Schizophreniform psychosis NOS

F20.89 Other schizophrenia

Cenesthopathic schizophrenia

Simple schizophrenia

F20.9 Schizophrenia, unspecified

F21 Schizotypal disorder

Borderline schizophrenia

Latent schizophrenia

Latent schizophrenic reaction

Prepsychotic schizophrenia

Prodromal schizophrenia

Pseudoneurotic schizophrenia

Pseudopsychopathic schizophrenia

Schizotypal personality disorder

Excludes2: Asperger's syndrome (F84.5)

schizoid personality disorder (F60.1)

F22 Delusional disorders

Delusional dysmorphophobia

Involutional paranoid state

Paranoia

Paranoia querulans

Paranoid psychosis

Paranoid state

Paraphrenia (late)

Sensitiver Beziehungswahn

Excludes1: mood [affective] disorders with psychotic symptoms (F30.2, F31.2, F31.5, F31.64, F32.3, F33.3)

paranoid schizophrenia (F20.0)

Excludes2: paranoid personality disorder (F60.0)

paranoid psychosis, psychogenic (F23)

paranoid reaction (F23)

F23 Brief psychotic disorder

Paranoid reaction

Psychogenic paranoid psychosis

Excludes2: mood [affective] disorders with psychotic symptoms (F30.2, F31.2, F31.5, F31.64, F32.3, F33.3)

F24 Shared psychotic disorder

Folie à deux

Induced paranoid disorder

Induced psychotic disorder

F25 Schizoaffective disorders

Excludes1: mood [affective] disorders with psychotic symptoms (F30.2, F31.2, F31.5, F31.64, F32.3, F33.3)

schizophrenia (F20.-)

F25.0 Schizoaffective disorder, bipolar type

Cyclic schizophrenia

Schizoaffective disorder, manic type

Schizoaffective disorder, mixed type

Schizoaffective psychosis, bipolar type

Schizophreniform psychosis, manic type

F25.1 Schizoaffective disorder, depressive type

Schizoaffective psychosis, depressive type

Schizophreniform psychosis, depressive type

F25.8 Other schizoaffective disorders

F25.9 Schizoaffective disorder, unspecified

Schizoaffective psychosis NOS

F28 Other psychotic disorder not due to a substance or known physiological condition

Chronic hallucinatory psychosis

F29 Unspecified psychosis not due to a substance or known physiological condition

Psychosis NOS

Excludes1: mental disorder NOS (F99)

unspecified mental disorder due to known physiological condition (F09)

MOOD [AFFECTIVE] DISORDERS (F30-F39)

Definition: A mood disorder, also referred to as an affective disorder, is a condition impacting mood and related functions. In a mood disorder, moods range from extremely low (depressed) to extremely high or irritable (manic).

F30 **Manic episode**

Includes: bipolar disorder, single manic episode

mixed affective episode

Excludes1: bipolar disorder (F31.-)

major depressive disorder, single episode (F32.-)

major depressive disorder, recurrent (F33.-)

F30.1 **Manic episode without psychotic symptoms**

F30.10 **Manic episode without psychotic symptoms, unspecified**

F30.11 **Manic episode without psychotic symptoms, mild**

F30.12 **Manic episode without psychotic symptoms, moderate**

F30.13 **Manic episode, severe, without psychotic symptoms**

F30.2 **Manic episode, severe with psychotic symptoms**

Manic stupor

Mania with mood-congruent psychotic symptoms

Mania with mood-incongruent psychotic symptoms

F30.3 **Manic episode in partial remission**

F30.4 **Manic episode in full remission**

F30.8 **Other manic episodes**

Hypomania

F30.9 **Manic episode, unspecified**

Mania NOS

F31 **Bipolar disorder**

Definition: Bipolar disorder, formerly called manic depression, is a mental illness that brings severe high and low moods and changes in sleep, energy, thinking, and behavior.

Includes: manic-depressive illness

manic-depressive psychosis manic-depressive reaction

Excludes1: bipolar disorder, single manic episode (F30.-)

major depressive disorder, single episode (F32.-)

major depressive disorder, recurrent (F33.-)

Excludes2: cyclothymia (F34.0)

F31.0 **Bipolar disorder, current episode hypomanic**

F31.1 **Bipolar disorder, current episode manic without psychotic features**

F31.10 **Bipolar disorder, current episode manic without psychotic features, unspecified**

F31.11 **Bipolar disorder, current episode manic without psychotic features, mild**

F31.12 **Bipolar disorder, current episode manic without psychotic features, moderate**

F31.13 **Bipolar disorder, current episode manic without psychotic features, severe**

F31.2 **Bipolar disorder, current episode manic severe with psychotic features**

Bipolar disorder, current episode manic with mood-congruent psychotic symptoms

Bipolar disorder, current episode manic with mood-incongruent psychotic symptoms

F31.3 **Bipolar disorder, current episode depressed, mild or moderate severity**

F31.30 **Bipolar disorder, current episode depressed, mild or moderate severity, unspecified**

F31.31 **Bipolar disorder, current episode depressed, mild**

F31.32 **Bipolar disorder, current episode depressed, moderate**

F31.4 **Bipolar disorder, current episode depressed, severe, without psychotic features**

F31.5 **Bipolar disorder, current episode depressed, severe, with psychotic features**

Bipolar disorder, current episode depressed with mood-incongruent psychotic symptoms

Bipolar disorder, current episode depressed with mood-congruent psychotic symptoms

F31.6 **Bipolar disorder, current episode mixed**

F31.60 **Bipolar disorder, current episode mixed, unspecified**

F31.61 **Bipolar disorder, current episode mixed, mild**

F31.62 **Bipolar disorder, current episode mixed, moderate**

F31.63 **Bipolar disorder, current episode mixed, severe, without psychotic features**

F31.64 **Bipolar disorder, current episode mixed, severe, with psychotic features**

Bipolar disorder, current episode mixed with mood-congruent psychotic symptoms

Bipolar disorder, current episode mixed with mood-incongruent psychotic symptoms

F31.7 **Bipolar disorder, currently in remission**

F31.70 **Bipolar disorder, currently in remission, most recent episode unspecified**

F31.71 **Bipolar disorder, in partial remission, most recent episode hypomanic**

F31.72 **Bipolar disorder, in full remission, most recent episode hypomanic**

F31.73 **Bipolar disorder, in partial remission, most recent episode manic**

F31.74 **Bipolar disorder, in full remission, most recent episode manic**

F31.75 **Bipolar disorder, in partial remission, most recent episode depressed**

F31.76 **Bipolar disorder, in full remission, most recent episode depressed**

F31.77 **Bipolar disorder, in partial remission, most recent episode mixed**

F31.78 **Bipolar disorder, in full remission, most recent episode mixed**

F31.8 **Other bipolar disorders**

F31.81 **Bipolar II disorder**

F31.89 **Other bipolar disorder**

Recurrent manic episodes NOS

F31.9 **Bipolar disorder, unspecified**

F32 **Major depressive disorder, single episode**

Includes: single episode of agitated depression

single episode of depressive reaction single episode of major depression

single episode of psychogenic depression single episode of reactive depression single episode of vital depression

Excludes1: bipolar disorder (F31.-)

manic episode (F30.-)

recurrent depressive disorder (F33.-)

Excludes2: adjustment disorder (F43.2)

F32.0 **Major depressive disorder, single episode, mild**

F32.1   Major depressive disorder, single episode, moderate

F32.2   Major depressive disorder, single episode, severe without psychotic features

F32.3   Major depressive disorder, single episode, severe with psychotic features

Single episode of major depression with mood-congruent psychotic symptoms

Single episode of major depression with mood-incongruent psychotic symptoms

Single episode of major depression with psychotic symptoms

Single episode of psychogenic depressive psychosis

Single episode of psychotic depression

Single episode of reactive depressive psychosis

F32.4   Major depressive disorder, single episode, in partial remission

F32.5   Major depressive disorder, single episode, in full remission

F32.8   Other depressive episodes

●F32.81   Premenstrual dysphoric disorder

Excludes1: premenstrual tension syndrome (N94.3)

●F32.89   Other specified depressive episodes

Atypical depression

Post-schizophrenic depression

Single episode of 'masked' depression NOS

F32.9   Major depressive disorder, single episode, unspecified

Depression NOS

Depressive disorder NOS

Major depression NOS

F33   Major depressive disorder, recurrent

Includes: recurrent episodes of depressive reaction

recurrent episodes of endogenous depression recurrent episodes of major depression

recurrent episodes of psychogenic depression recurrent episodes of reactive depression

recurrent episodes of seasonal depressive disorder recurrent episodes of vital depression

Excludes1: bipolar disorder (F31.-)

manic episode (F30.-)

F33.0   Major depressive disorder, recurrent, mild

F33.1   Major depressive disorder, recurrent, moderate

F33.2   Major depressive disorder, recurrent severe without psychotic features

F33.3   Major depressive disorder, recurrent, severe with psychotic symptoms

Endogenous depression with psychotic symptoms

Recurrent severe episodes of major depression with mood-congruent psychotic symptoms

Recurrent severe episodes of major depression with mood-incongruent psychotic symptoms

Recurrent severe episodes of major depression with psychotic symptoms

Recurrent severe episodes of psychogenic depressive psychosis

Recurrent severe episodes of psychotic depression

Recurrent severe episodes of reactive depressive psychosis

F33.4   Major depressive disorder, recurrent, in remission

F33.40   Major depressive disorder, recurrent, in remission, unspecified

F33.41   Major depressive disorder, recurrent, in partial remission

F33.42   Major depressive disorder, recurrent, in full remission

F33.8   Other recurrent depressive disorders

Recurrent brief depressive episodes

F33.9   Major depressive disorder, recurrent, unspecified

Monopolar depression NOS

F34   Persistent mood [affective] disorders

F34.0   Cyclothymic disorder

Affective personality disorder

Cycloid personality

Cyclothymia

Cyclothymic personality

F34.1   Dysthymic disorder

Depressive neurosis

Depressive personality disorder

Dysthymia

Neurotic depression

Persistent anxiety depression

Persistent depressive disorder

Excludes2: anxiety depression (mild or not persistent) (F41.8)

F34.8   Other persistent mood [affective] disorders

●F34.81   Disruptive mood dysregulation disorder

●F34.89   Other specified persistent mood disorders

F34.9   Persistent mood [affective] disorder, unspecified

F39   Unspecified mood [affective] disorder

Affective psychosis NOS

ANXIETY, DISSOCIATIVE, STRESS-RELATED, SOMATOFORM AND OTHER NONPSYCHOTIC MENTAL DISORDERS (F40-F48)

Definition: Anxiety disorders are a group of mental disorders characterized by feelings of anxiety and fear, where anxiety is a worry about future events and fear is a reaction to current events.

F40   Phobic anxiety disorders

F40.0   Agoraphobia

F40.00   Agoraphobia, unspecified

F40.01   Agoraphobia with panic disorder

Panic disorder with agoraphobia

Excludes1: panic disorder without agoraphobia (F41.0)

F40.02   Agoraphobia without panic disorder

F40.1   Social phobias

Anthropophobia

Social anxiety disorder of childhood

Social neurosis

F40.10   Social phobia, unspecified

F40.11   Social phobia, generalized

F40.2   Specific (isolated) phobias

Excludes2: dysmorphophobia (nondelusional) (F45.22)

nosophobia (F45.22)

F40.21   Animal type phobia

F40.210   Arachnophobia

Fear of spiders

F40.218   **Other animal type phobia**

F40.22   **Natural environment type phobia**

F40.220   **Fear of thunderstorms**

F40.228   **Other natural environment type phobia**

F40.23   **Blood, injection, injury type phobia**

F40.230   **Fear of blood**

F40.231   **Fear of injections and transfusions**

F40.232   **Fear of other medical care**

F40.233   **Fear of injury**

F40.24   **Situational type phobia**

F40.240   **Claustrophobia**

F40.241   **Acrophobia**

F40.242   **Fear of bridges**

F40.243   **Fear of flying**

F40.248   **Other situational type phobia**

F40.29   **Other specified phobia**

F40.290   **Androphobia**

Fear of men

F40.291   **Gynephobia**

Fear of women

F40.298   **Other specified phobia**

F40.8   **Other phobic anxiety disorders**

Phobic anxiety disorder of childhood

F40.9   **Phobic anxiety disorder, unspecified**

Phobia NOS

Phobic state NOS

F41   **Other anxiety disorders**

Excludes2: anxiety in:

acute stress reaction (F43.0)

transient adjustment reaction (F43.2)

neurasthenia (F48.8)

psychophysiologic disorders (F45.-)

separation anxiety (F93.0)

F41.0   **Panic disorder [episodic paroxysmal anxiety] without agoraphobia**

Panic attack

Panic state

Excludes1: panic disorder with agoraphobia (F40.01)

F41.1   **Generalized anxiety disorder**

Anxiety neurosis

Anxiety reaction

Anxiety state

Overanxious disorder

Excludes2: neurasthenia (F48.8)

F41.3   **Other mixed anxiety disorders**

F41.8   **Other specified anxiety disorders**

Anxiety depression (mild or not persistent)

Anxiety hysteria

Mixed anxiety and depressive disorder

F41.9   **Anxiety disorder, unspecified**

Anxiety NOS

F42   **Obsessive-compulsive disorder**

Excludes2: obsessive-compulsive personality (disorder) (F60.5)

obsessive-compulsive symptoms occurring in depression (F32-F33)

obsessive-compulsive symptoms occurring in schizophrenia (F20.-)

●F42.2   **Mixed obsessional thoughts and acts**

●F42.3   **Hoarding disorder**

●F42.4   **Excoriation (skin-picking) disorder**

Excludes1: factitial dermatitis (L98.1)

Other specified behavioral and emotional disorders with onset usually occurring in early childhood and adolescence (F98.8)

●F42.8   **Other obsessive-compulsive disorder**

Anancastic neurosis

Obsessive-compulsive neurosis

●F42.9   **Obsessive-compulsive disorder, unspecified**

F43   **Reaction to severe stress, and adjustment disorders**

F43.0   **Acute stress reaction**

Acute crisis reaction

Acute reaction to stress

Combat and operational stress reaction

Combat fatigue

Crisis state

Psychic shock

F43.1   **Post-traumatic stress disorder (PTSD)**

Traumatic neurosis

F43.10   **Post-traumatic stress disorder, unspecified**

F43.11   **Post-traumatic stress disorder, acute**

F43.12   **Post-traumatic stress disorder, chronic**

F43.2   **Adjustment disorders**

Culture shock Grief reaction

Hospitalism in children

Excludes2: separation anxiety disorder of childhood (F93.0)

F43.20   **Adjustment disorder, unspecified**

F43.21   **Adjustment disorder with depressed mood**

F43.22   **Adjustment disorder with anxiety**

F43.23   **Adjustment disorder with mixed anxiety and depressed mood**

F43.24   **Adjustment disorder with disturbance of conduct**

F43.25   **Adjustment disorder with mixed disturbance of emotions and conduct**

F43.29   **Adjustment disorder with other symptoms**

F43.8   **Other reactions to severe stress**

Other specified trauma and stressor-related disorder

F43.9   **Reaction to severe stress, unspecified**

Trauma and stressor-related disorder, NOS

F44   **Dissociative and conversion disorders**

Includes: conversion hysteria

conversion reaction hysteria

hysterical psychosis

Excludes2: malingering [conscious simulation] (Z76.5)

F44.0   **Dissociative amnesia**

Excludes1: amnesia NOS (R41.3)

anterograde amnesia (R41.1)

---

dissociative amnesia with dissociative fugue (F44.1)

retrograde amnesia (R41.2)

Excludes2: alcohol-**or other** psychoactive substance-induced amnestic disorder (F10, F13, F19 with .26, .96)

amnestic disorder due to known physiological condition (F04)

postictal amnesia in epilepsy (G40.-)

F44.1 **Dissociative fugue**

Dissociative amnesia with dissociative fugue

Excludes2: postictal fugue in epilepsy (G40.-)

F44.2 **Dissociative stupor**

Excludes1: catatonic stupor (R40.1)

stupor NOS (R40.1)

Excludes2: catatonic disorder due to known physiological condition (F06.1)

depressive stupor (F32, F33)

manic stupor (F30, F31)

F44.4 **Conversion disorder with motor symptom or deficit**

Dissociative motor disorders

Psychogenic aphonia

Psychogenic dysphonia

F44.5 **Conversion disorder with seizures or convulsions**

Dissociative convulsions

F44.6 **Conversion disorder with sensory symptom or deficit**

Dissociative anesthesia and sensory loss

Psychogenic deafness

F44.7 **Conversion disorder with mixed symptom presentation**

F44.8 **Other dissociative and conversion disorders**

F44.81 **Dissociative identity disorder**

Multiple personality disorder

F44.89 **Other dissociative and conversion disorders**

Ganser's syndrome

Psychogenic confusion

Psychogenic twilight state

Trance and possession disorders

F44.9 **Dissociative and conversion disorder, unspecified**

Dissociative disorder NOS

F45 **Somatoform disorders**

Definition: **Somatoform disorder** is the name for a group of conditions in which the physical pain and symptoms a person feels are related to psychological factors. These symptoms can't be traced to a specific physical cause.

Excludes2: dissociative and conversion disorders (F44.-)

factitious disorders (F68.1-)

hair-plucking (F63.3)

lalling (F80.0)

lisping (F80.0)

malingering [conscious simulation] (Z76.5)

nail-biting (F98.8)

psychological or behavioral factors associated with disorders or diseases classified elsewhere (F54)

sexual dysfunction, not due to a substance or known physiological condition (F52.-)

thumb-sucking (F98.8)

tic disorders (in childhood and adolescence) (F95.-)

Tourette's syndrome (F95.2)

trichotillomania (F63.3)

F45.0 **Somatization disorder**

Briquet's disorder

Multiple psychosomatic disorder

F45.1 **Undifferentiated somatoform disorder**

Somatic symptom disorder

Undifferentiated psychosomatic disorder

F45.2 **Hypochondriacal disorders**

Excludes2: delusional dysmorphophobia (F22)

fixed delusions about bodily functions or shape (F22)

F45.20 **Hypochondriacal disorder, unspecified**

F45.21 **Hypochondriasis**

Hypochondriacal neurosis

Illness anxiety disorder

F45.22 **Body dysmorphic disorder**

Dysmorphophobia (nondelusional)

Nosophobia

F45.29 **Other hypochondriacal disorders**

F45.4 **Pain disorders related to psychological factors**

Excludes1: pain NOS (R52)

F45.41 **Pain disorder exclusively related to psychological factors**

Somatoform pain disorder (persistent)

F45.42 **Pain disorder with related psychological factors**

Code also associated acute or chronic pain (G89.-)

F45.8 **Other somatoform disorders**

Psychogenic dysmenorrhea

Psychogenic dysphagia, including 'globus hystericus'

Psychogenic pruritus

Psychogenic torticollis

Somatoform autonomic dysfunction

Teeth grinding

Excludes1: sleep related teeth grinding (G47.63)

F45.9 **Somatoform disorder, unspecified**

Psychosomatic disorder NOS

F48 **Other nonpsychotic mental disorders**

F48.1 **Depersonalization-derealization syndrome**

F48.2 **Pseudobulbar affect**

Involuntary emotional expression disorder

Code first underlying cause, if known, such as:

amyotrophic lateral sclerosis (G12.21)

multiple sclerosis (G35)

sequelae of cerebrovascular disease (I69.-)

sequelae of traumatic intracranial injury (S06.-)

F48.8 **Other specified nonpsychotic mental disorders**

Dhat syndrome Neurasthenia

Occupational neurosis, including writer's cramp

Psychasthenia

Psychasthenic neurosis

Psychogenic syncope

F48.9 Nonpsychotic mental disorder, unspecified
Neurosis NOS

BEHAVIORAL SYNDROMES ASSOCIATED WITH PHYSIOLOGICAL DISTURBANCES AND PHYSICAL FACTORS (F50-F59)

F50 **Eating disorders**
Excludes1: anorexia NOS (R63.0)
feeding difficulties (R63.3)
polyphagia (R63.2)
Excludes2: feeding disorder in infancy or childhood (F98.2-)

F50.0 **Anorexia nervosa**
Excludes1: loss of appetite (R63.0)
psychogenic loss of appetite (F50.89)

F50.00 **Anorexia nervosa, unspecified**
F50.01 **Anorexia nervosa, restricting type**
F50.02 **Anorexia nervosa, binge eating/purging type**
Excludes1: bulimia nervosa (F50.2)

F50.2 **Bulimia nervosa**
Bulimia NOS
Hyperorexia nervosa
Excludes1: anorexia nervosa, binge eating/purging type (F50.02)

F50.8 **Other eating disorders**
Excludes2: pica of infancy and childhood (F98.3)
●**F50.81** **Binge eating disorder**
●**F50.89** **Other specified eating disorder**
Pica in adults
Psychogenic loss of appetite

F50.9 **Eating disorder, unspecified**
Atypical anorexia nervosa
Atypical bulimia nervosa

F51 **Sleep disorders not due to a substance or known physiological condition**
Excludes2: organic sleep disorders (G47.-)

F51.0 **Insomnia not due to a substance or known physiological condition**
Excludes2: alcohol related insomnia (F10.182, F10.282, F10.982)
drug-related insomnia (F11.182, F11.282, F11.982, F13.182, F13.282, F13.982, F14.182, F14.282, F14.982, F15.182, F15.282, F15.982, F19.182, F19.282, F19.982)
insomnia NOS (G47.0-)
insomnia due to known physiological condition (G47.0-)
organic insomnia (G47.0-)
sleep deprivation (Z72.820)

F51.01 **Primary insomnia**
Idiopathic insomnia
F51.02 **Adjustment insomnia**
F51.03 **Paradoxical insomnia**
F51.04 **Psychophysiologic insomnia**
F51.05 **Insomnia due to other mental disorder**
Code also associated mental disorder
F51.09 **Other insomnia not due to a substance or known physiological condition**

F51.1 **Hypersomnia not due to a substance or known physiological condition**
Excludes2: alcohol related hypersomnia (F10.182, F10.282, F10.982)
drug-related hypersomnia (F11.182, F11.282, F11.982, F13.182, F13.282, F13.982, F14.182,F14.282, F14.982, F15.182, F15.282, F15.982, F19.182, F19.282, F19.982)
hypersomnia NOS (G47.10)
hypersomnia due to known physiological condition (G47.10)
idiopathic hypersomnia (G47.11, G47.12)
narcolepsy (G47.4-)

F51.11 **Primary hypersomnia**
F51.12 **Insufficient sleep syndrome**
Excludes1: sleep deprivation (Z72.820)
F51.13 **Hypersomnia due to other mental disorder**
Code also associated mental disorder
F51.19 **Other hypersomnia not due to a substance or known physiological condition**

F51.3 **Sleepwalking [somnambulism]**
F51.4 **Sleep terrors [night terrors]**
F51.5 **Nightmare disorder**
Dream anxiety disorder
F51.8 **Other sleep disorders not due to a substance or known physiological condition**
F51.9 **Sleep disorder not due to a substance or known physiological condition, unspecified**
Emotional sleep disorder NOS

F52 **Sexual dysfunction not due to a substance or known physiological condition**
Excludes2: Dhat syndrome (F48.8)

F52.0 **Hypoactive sexual desire disorder**
Lack or loss of sexual desire
Sexual anhedonia
Excludes1: decreased libido (R68.82)
F52.1 **Sexual aversion disorder**
Sexual aversion and lack of sexual enjoyment
F52.2 **Sexual arousal disorders**
Failure of genital response
F52.21 **Male erectile disorder**
Psychogenic impotence
Excludes1: impotence of organic origin (N52.-)
impotence NOS (N52.-)
F52.22 **Female sexual arousal disorder**
F52.3 **Orgasmic disorder**
Inhibited orgasm
Psychogenic anorgasmy
F52.31 **Female orgasmic disorder**
F52.32 **Male orgasmic disorder**
Delayed ejaculation
F52.4 **Premature ejaculation**
F52.5 **Vaginismus not due to a substance or known physiological condition**
Psychogenic vaginismus
Excludes2: vaginismus (due to a known physiological condition) (N94.2)

F52.6 **Dyspareunia not due to a substance or known physiological condition**

Genito-pelvic pain penetration disorder

Psychogenic dyspareunia

Excludes2: dyspareunia (due to a known physiological condition) (N94.1-)

F52.8 **Other sexual dysfunction not due to a substance or known physiological condition**

Excessive sexual drive

Nymphomania

Satyriasis

F52.9 **Unspecified sexual dysfunction not due to a substance or known physiological condition**

Sexual dysfunction NOS

F53 **Puerperal psychosis**

Postpartum depression

Excludes1: mood disorders with psychotic features (F30.2, F31.2, F31.5, F31.64, F32.3, F33.3)

postpartum dysphoria (O90.6)

psychosis in schizophrenia, schizotypal, delusional, **and other** psychotic disorders (F20-F29)

F54 **Psychological and behavioral factors associated with disorders or diseases classified elsewhere**

Psychological factors affecting physical conditions

Code first the associated physical disorder, such as:

asthma (J45.-)

dermatitis (L23-L25)

gastric ulcer (K25.-)

mucous colitis (K58.-)

ulcerative colitis (K51.-)

urticaria (L50.-)

Excludes2: tension-type headache (G44.2)

F55 **Abuse of non-psychoactive substances**

Excludes2: abuse of psychoactive substances (F10-F19)

F55.0 **Abuse of antacids**

F55.1 **Abuse of herbal or folk remedies**

F55.2 **Abuse of laxatives**

F55.3 **Abuse of steroids or hormones**

F55.4 **Abuse of vitamins**

F55.8 **Abuse of other non-psychoactive substances**

F59 **Unspecified behavioral syndromes associated with physiological disturbances and physical factors**

Psychogenic physiological dysfunction NOS

DISORDERS OF ADULT PERSONALITY AND BEHAVIOR (F60-F69)

F60 **Specific personality disorders**

F60.0 **Paranoid personality disorder**

Expansive paranoid personality (disorder)

Fanatic personality (disorder)

Querulant personality (disorder)

Paranoid personality (disorder)

Sensitive paranoid personality (disorder)

Excludes2: paranoia (F22)

paranoia querulans (F22)

paranoid psychosis (F22)

paranoid schizophrenia (F20.0)

paranoid state (F22)

F60.1 **Schizoid personality disorder**

Excludes2: Asperger's syndrome (F84.5)

delusional disorder (F22)

schizoid disorder of childhood (F84.5)

schizophrenia (F20.-)

schizotypal disorder (F21)

F60.2 **Antisocial personality disorder**

Amoral personality (disorder)

Asocial personality (disorder)

Dissocial personality disorder

Psychopathic personality (disorder)

Sociopathic personality (disorder)

Excludes1: conduct disorders (F91.-)

Excludes2: borderline personality disorder (F60.3)

F60.3 **Borderline personality disorder**

Aggressive personality (disorder)

Emotionally unstable personality disorder

Explosive personality (disorder)

Excludes2: antisocial personality disorder (F60.2)

F60.4 **Histrionic personality disorder**

Hysterical personality (disorder)

Psychoinfantile personality (disorder)

F60.5 **Obsessive-compulsive personality disorder**

Anankastic personality (disorder)

Compulsive personality (disorder)

Obsessional personality (disorder)

Excludes2: obsessive-compulsive disorder (F42-)

F60.6 **Avoidant personality disorder**

Anxious personality disorder

F60.7 **Dependent personality disorder**

Asthenic personality (disorder)

Inadequate personality (disorder)

Passive personality (disorder)

F60.8 **Other specific personality disorders**

F60.81 **Narcissistic personality disorder**

F60.89 **Other specific personality disorders**

Eccentric personality disorder

'Haltlose' type personality disorder

Immature personality disorder

Passive-aggressive personality disorder

Psychoneurotic personality disorder

Self-defeating personality disorder

F60.9 **Personality disorder, unspecified**

Character disorder NOS

Character neurosis NOS

Pathological personality NOS

F63 **Impulse disorders**

Excludes2: habitual excessive use of alcohol or psychoactive substances (F10-F19)

impulse disorders involving sexual behavior (F65.-)

F63.0 **Pathological gambling**

Compulsive gambling

● New code   ▲ Revised code   **Excludes1:** Not coded here   **Excludes2:** Not included here   ⊗ Placeholder required   ⑦ 7th digit required

Excludes1: gambling and betting NOS (Z72.6)

Excludes2: excessive gambling by manic patients (F30, F31)

gambling in antisocial personality disorder (F60.2)

F63.1 Pyromania

Pathological fire-setting

Excludes2: fire-setting (by) (in):

adult with antisocial personality disorder (F60.2)

alcohol or psychoactive substance intoxication (F10-F19)

conduct disorders (F91.-)

mental disorders due to known physiological condition (F01-F09)

schizophrenia (F20.-)

F63.2 Kleptomania

Pathological stealing

Excludes1: shoplifting as the reason for observation for suspected mental disorder (Z03.8)

Excludes2: depressive disorder with stealing (F31-F33)

stealing due to underlying mental condition-code to mental condition stealing in mental disorders due to known physiological condition (F01-F09)

F63.3 Trichotillomania

Hair plucking

Excludes2: Other stereotyped movement disorder (F98.4)

F63.8 Other impulse disorders

F63.81 Intermittent explosive disorder

F63.89 Other impulse disorders

F63.9 Impulse disorder, unspecified

Impulse control disorder NOS

F64 Gender identity disorders

•F64.0 Transsexualism

Gender identity disorder in adolescence and adulthood

Gender dysphoria in adolescents and adults

▲F64.1 Dual role transvestism

Use additional code to identify sex reassignment status (Z87.890)

Excludes1: gender identity disorder in childhood (F64.2)

Excludes2: fetishistic transvestism (F65.1)

F64.2 Gender identity disorder of childhood

Gender dysphoria in children

Excludes1: gender identity disorder in adolescence and adulthood (F64.0)

Excludes2: sexual maturation disorder (F66)

F64.8 Other gender identity disorders

F64.9 Gender identity disorder, unspecified

Gender-role disorder NOS

F65 Paraphilias

F65.0 Fetishism

F65.1 Transvestic fetishism

Fetishistic transvestism

F65.2 Exhibitionism

F65.3 Voyeurism

F65.4 Pedophilia

F65.5 Sadomasochism

F65.50 Sadomasochism, unspecified

F65.51 Sexual masochism

F65.52 Sexual sadism

F65.8 Other paraphilias

F65.81 Frotteurism

F65.89 Other paraphilias

Necrophilia

F65.9 Paraphilia, unspecified

Sexual deviation NOS

F66 Other sexual disorders

Sexual maturation disorder

Sexual relationship disorder

F68 Other disorders of adult personality and behavior

F68.1 Factitious disorder

Compensation neurosis

Elaboration of physical symptoms for psychological reasons

Hospital hopper syndrome

Münchausen's syndrome

Peregrinating patient

Excludes2: factitial dermatitis (L98.1)

person feigning illness (with obvious motivation) (Z76.5)

F68.10 Factitious disorder, unspecified

F68.11 Factitious disorder with predominantly psychological signs and symptoms

F68.12 Factitious disorder with predominantly physical signs and symptoms

F68.13 Factitious disorder with combined psychological and physical signs and symptoms

F68.8 Other specified disorders of adult personality and behavior

F69 Unspecified disorder of adult personality and behavior

INTELLECTUAL DISABILITIES (F70-F79)

Code first any associated physical or developmental disorders

Excludes1: borderline intellectual functioning, IQ above 70 to 84 (R41.83)

F70 Mild intellectual disabilities

IQ level 50-55 to approximately 70

Mild mental subnormality

F71 Moderate intellectual disabilities

IQ level 35-40 to 50-55

Moderate mental subnormality

F72 Severe intellectual disabilities

IQ 20-25 to 35-40

Severe mental subnormality

F73 Profound intellectual disabilities

IQ level below 20-25 Profound mental subnormality

F78 Other intellectual disabilities

F79 Unspecified intellectual disabilities

Mental deficiency NOS

Mental subnormality NOS

PERVASIVE AND SPECIFIC DEVELOPMENTAL DISORDERS (F80-F89)

F80 Specific developmental disorders of speech and language

F80.0 **Phonological disorder**

Dyslalia

Functional speech articulation disorder

Lalling

Lisping

Phonological developmental disorder

Speech articulation developmental disorder

Speech-sound disorder

Excludes1: speech articulation impairment due to aphasia NOS (R47.01)

speech articulation impairment due to apraxia (R48.2)

Excludes2: speech articulation impairment due to hearing loss (F80.4)

speech articulation impairment due to intellectual disabilities (F70-F79)

speech articulation impairment with expressive language developmental disorder (F80.1)

speech articulation impairment with mixed receptive expressive language developmental disorder (F80.2)

F80.1 **Expressive language disorder**

Developmental dysphasia or aphasia, expressive type

Excludes1: mixed receptive-expressive language disorder (F80.2)

dysphasia and aphasia NOS (R47.-)

Excludes2: acquired aphasia with epilepsy [Landau-Kleffner] (G40.80-)

selective mutism (F94.0)

intellectual disabilities (F70-F79)

pervasive developmental disorders (F84.-)

F80.2 **Mixed receptive-expressive language disorder**

Developmental dysphasia or aphasia, receptive type

Developmental Wernicke's aphasia

Excludes1: central auditory processing disorder (H93.25)

dysphasia or aphasia NOS (R47.-)

expressive language disorder (F80.1)

expressive type dysphasia or aphasia (F80.1)

word deafness (H93.25)

Excludes2: acquired aphasia with epilepsy [Landau-Kleffner] (G40.80-)

pervasive developmental disorders (F84.-)

selective mutism (F94.0)

intellectual disabilities (F70-F79)

F80.4 **Speech and language development delay due to hearing loss**

Code also type of hearing loss (H90.-, H91.-)

F80.8 **Other developmental disorders of speech and language**

F80.81 **Childhood onset fluency disorder**

Cluttering NOS

Stuttering NOS

Excludes1: adult onset fluency disorder (F98.5)

fluency disorder in conditions classified elsewhere (R47.82)

fluency disorder (stuttering) following cerebrovascular disease (I69. with final characters - 23)

●F80.82 **Social pragmatic communication disorder**

Excludes1: Asperger's syndrome (F84.5)

autistic disorder (F84.0)

F80.89 **Other developmental disorders of speech and language**

F80.9 **Developmental disorder of speech and language, unspecified**

Communication disorder NOS

Language disorder NOS

F81 Specific developmental disorders of scholastic skills

F81.0 **Specific reading disorder**

'Backward reading'

Developmental dyslexia

Specific reading retardation

Excludes1: alexia NOS (R48.0)

dyslexia NOS (R48.0)

F81.2 **Mathematics disorder**

Developmental acalculia

Developmental arithmetical disorder

Developmental Gerstmann's syndrome

Excludes1: acalculia NOS (R48.8)

Excludes2: arithmetical difficulties associated with a reading disorder (F81.0)

arithmetical difficulties associated with a spelling disorder (F81.81)

arithmetical difficulties due to inadequate teaching (Z55.8)

F81.8 **Other developmental disorders of scholastic skills**

F81.81 **Disorder of written expression**

Specific spelling disorder

F81.89 **Other developmental disorders of scholastic skills**

F81.9 **Developmental disorder of scholastic skills, unspecified**

Knowledge acquisition disability NOS

Learning disability NOS

Learning disorder NOS

F82 Specific developmental disorder of motor function

Clumsy child syndrome

Developmental coordination disorder

Developmental dyspraxia

Excludes1: abnormalities of gait and mobility (R26.-)

lack of coordination (R27.-)

Excludes2: lack of coordination secondary to intellectual disabilities (F70-F79)

F84 Pervasive developmental disorders

Use additional code to identify any associated medical condition and intellectual disabilities.

F84.0 **Autistic disorder**

Autism spectrum disorder

Infantile autism

Infantile psychosis

Kanner's syndrome

Excludes1: Asperger's syndrome (F84.5)

● New code   ▲ Revised code   **Excludes1:** Not coded here   **Excludes2:** Not included here   ⊗ Placeholder required   ⑦ 7th digit required

F84.2   Rett's syndrome

Excludes1: Asperger's syndrome (F84.5)

Autistic disorder (F84.0)

Other childhood disintegrative disorder (F84.3)

F84.3   Other childhood disintegrative disorder

Dementia infantilis

Disintegrative psychosis

Heller's syndrome

Symbiotic psychosis

Use additional code to identify any associated neurological condition.

Excludes1: Asperger's syndrome (F84.5)

Autistic disorder (F84.0)

Rett's syndrome (F84.2)

F84.5   Asperger's syndrome

Asperger's disorder

Autistic psychopathy

Schizoid disorder of childhood

F84.8   Other pervasive developmental disorders

Overactive disorder associated with intellectual disabilities and stereotyped movements

F84.9   Pervasive developmental disorder, unspecified

Atypical autism

F88   Other disorders of psychological development

Developmental agnosia Global developmental delay

Other specified neurodevelopmental disorder

F89   Unspecified disorder of psychological development

Developmental disorder NOS

Neurodevelopmental disorder NOS

BEHAVIORAL AND EMOTIONAL DISORDERS WITH ONSET USUALLY OCCURRING IN CHILDHOOD AND ADOLESCENCE (F90-F98)

Note: Codes within categories F90-F98 may be used regardless of the age of a patient. These disorders generally have onset within the childhood or adolescent years, but may continue throughout life or not be diagnosed until adulthood

F90   Attention-deficit hyperactivity disorders

Definition: Attention deficit hyperactivity disorder refers to any of a range of behavioral disorders occurring primarily in children, including such symptoms as poor concentration, hyperactivity, and impulsivity.

Includes: attention deficit disorder with hyperactivity

attention deficit syndrome with hyperactivity

Excludes2: anxiety disorders (F40.-, F41.-)

mood [affective] disorders (F30-F39)

pervasive developmental disorders (F84.-)

schizophrenia (F20.-)

F90.0   Attention-deficit hyperactivity disorder, predominantly inattentive type

F90.1   Attention-deficit hyperactivity disorder, predominantly hyperactive type

F90.2   Attention-deficit hyperactivity disorder, combined type

F90.8   Attention-deficit hyperactivity disorder, other type

F90.9   Attention-deficit hyperactivity disorder, unspecified type

Attention-deficit hyperactivity disorder of childhood or adolescence NOS

Attention-deficit hyperactivity disorder NOS

F91   Conduct disorders

Excludes1: antisocial behavior (Z72.81-)

antisocial personality disorder (F60.2)

Excludes2: conduct problems associated with attention-deficit hyperactivity disorder (F90.-)

mood [affective] disorders (F30-F39)

pervasive developmental disorders (F84.-)

schizophrenia (F20.-)

F91.0   Conduct disorder confined to family context

F91.1   Conduct disorder, childhood-onset type

Unsocialized conduct disorder

Conduct disorder, solitary aggressive type

Unsocialized aggressive disorder

F91.2   Conduct disorder, adolescent-onset type

Socialized conduct disorder

Conduct disorder, group type

F91.3   Oppositional defiant disorder

F91.8   Other conduct disorders

Other specified conduct disorder

Other specified disruptive disorder

F91.9   Conduct disorder, unspecified

Behavioral disorder NOS

Conduct disorder NOS

Disruptive behavior disorder NOS

Disruptive disorder NOS

F93   Emotional disorders with onset specific to childhood

F93.0   Separation anxiety disorder of childhood

Excludes2: mood [affective] disorders (F30-F39)

nonpsychotic mental disorders (F40-F48)

phobic anxiety disorder of childhood (F40.8)

social phobia (F40.1)

F93.8   Other childhood emotional disorders

Identity disorder

Excludes2: gender identity disorder of childhood (F64.2)

F93.9   Childhood emotional disorder, unspecified

F94   Disorders of social functioning with onset specific to childhood and adolescence

F94.0   Selective mutism

Elective mutism

Excludes2: pervasive developmental disorders (F84.-)

schizophrenia (F20.-)

specific developmental disorders of speech and language (F80.-)

transient mutism as part of separation anxiety in young children (F93.0)

F94.1   Reactive attachment disorder of childhood

Use additional code to identify any associated failure to thrive or growth retardation

Excludes1: disinhibited attachment disorder of childhood (F94.2)

normal variation in pattern of selective attachment

Excludes2: Asperger's syndrome (F84.5)

---

maltreatment syndromes (T74.-)

sexual or physical abuse in childhood, resulting in psychosocial problems (Z62.81-)

F94.2   Disinhibited attachment disorder of childhood

Affectionless psychopathy

Institutional syndrome

Excludes1: reactive attachment disorder of childhood (F94.1)

Excludes2: Asperger's syndrome (F84.5)

attention-deficit hyperactivity disorders (F90.-)

hospitalism in children (F43.2-)

F94.8   Other childhood disorders of social functioning

F94.9   Childhood disorder of social functioning, unspecified

F95   Tic disorder

F95.0   Transient tic disorder

Provisional tic disorder

F95.1   Chronic motor or vocal tic disorder

F95.2   Tourette's disorder

Combined vocal and multiple motor tic disorder [de la Tourette]

Tourette's syndrome

F95.8   Other tic disorders

F95.9   Tic disorder, unspecified

Tic NOS

F98   Other behavioral and emotional disorders with onset usually occurring in childhood and adolescence

Excludes2: breath-holding spells (R06.89)

gender identity disorder of childhood (F64.2)

Kleine-Levin syndrome (G47.13)

obsessive-compulsive disorder (F42-)

sleep disorders not due to a substance or known physiological condition (F51.-)

F98.0   Enuresis not due to a substance or known physiological condition

Enuresis (primary) (secondary) of nonorganic origin
Functional enuresis

Psychogenic enuresis

Urinary incontinence of nonorganic origin

Excludes1: enuresis NOS (R32)

F98.1   Encopresis not due to a substance or known physiological condition

Functional encopresis

Incontinence of feces of nonorganic origin

Psychogenic encopresis

Use additional code to identify the cause of any coexisting constipation.

Excludes1: encopresis NOS (R15.-)

F98.2   Other feeding disorders of infancy and childhood

Excludes1: feeding difficulties (R63.3)

Excludes2: anorexia nervosa **and other** eating disorders (F50.-)

feeding problems of newborn (P92.-)

pica of infancy or childhood (F98.3)

F98.21   Rumination disorder of infancy

F98.29   Other feeding disorders of infancy and early childhood

F98.3   Pica of infancy and childhood

F98.4   Stereotyped movement disorders

Stereotype/habit disorder

Excludes1: abnormal involuntary movements (R25.-)

Excludes2: compulsions in obsessive-compulsive disorder (F42-)

hair plucking (F63.3)

movement disorders of organic origin (G20-G25)

nail-biting (F98.8)

nose-picking (F98.8)

stereotypies that are part of a broader psychiatric condition (F01-F95)

thumb-sucking (F98.8)

tic disorders (F95.-)

trichotillomania (F63.3)

F98.5   Adult onset fluency disorder

Excludes1: childhood onset fluency disorder (F80.81)

dysphasia (R47.02)

fluency disorder in conditions classified elsewhere (R47.82)

fluency disorder (stuttering)

following cerebrovascular disease (I69. with final characters -23)

tic disorders (F95.-)

F98.8   Other specified behavioral and emotional disorders with onset usually occurring in childhood and adolescence

Excessive masturbation Nail-biting

Nose-picking

Thumb-sucking

F98.9   Unspecified behavioral and emotional disorders with onset usually occurring in childhood and adolescence

UNSPECIFIED MENTAL DISORDER (F99)

F99   Mental disorder, not otherwise specified

Mental illness NOS

Excludes1: unspecified mental disorder due to known physiological condition (F09)

Chapter 6: Diseases Of The Nervous System (G00-G99)

DEFINITIONS

This chapter includes definitions of selected key words, terms and phrases and coding alerts for adding points to the clinical domain, and references to coding late effects where appropriate. An example from this chapter is as follows:

G00   Bacterial meningitis, not elsewhere classified
   Definition: Meningitis is an infectious disease characterized by inflammation of the meninges (the tissues that surround the brain or spinal cord) usually caused by a bacterial infection; symptoms include headache and stiff neck and fever and nausea.

MULTIPLE CODING FOR A SINGLE CONDITION

In addition to the etiology/manifestation convention that requires two codes to fully describe a single condition that affects multiple body systems, there are other single conditions that also require more than one code. "Use additional code" notes are found in the Tabular List at codes that are not part of an etiology/manifestation pair where a secondary code is useful to fully describe a condition. The sequencing rule is the same as the etiology/manifestation pair, "use additional code" indicates that a secondary code should be added.

For example, for bacterial infections that are not included in chapter 1, a secondary code from category B95, Streptococcus, Staphylococcus, and Enterococcus, as the cause of diseases classified elsewhere, or B96, Other bacterial agents as the cause of diseases classified elsewhere, may be required to identify the bacterial organism causing the infection. A "use additional code" note will normally be found at the infectious disease code, indicating a need for the organism code to be added as a secondary code.

"Code first" notes are also under certain codes that are not specifically manifestation codes but may be due to an underlying cause. When there is a "code first" note and an underlying condition is present, the underlying condition should be sequenced first.

"Code, if applicable, any causal condition first", notes indicate that this code may be assigned as a principal diagnosis when the causal condition is unknown or not applicable. If a causal condition is known, then the code for that condition should be sequenced as the principal or first-listed diagnosis.

Multiple codes may be needed for sequela, complication codes and obstetric codes to more fully describe a condition. See the specific guidelines for these conditions for further instruction.

COMBINATION CODE

A combination code is a single code used to classify: Two diagnoses, or a diagnosis with an associated secondary process (manifestation) A diagnosis with an associated complication

Combination codes are identified by referring to subterm entries in the Alphabetic Index and by reading the inclusion and exclusion notes in the Tabular List.

Assign only the combination code when that code fully identifies the diagnostic conditions involved or when the Alphabetic Index so directs. Multiple coding should not be used when the classification provides a combination code that clearly identifies all of the elements documented in the diagnosis. When the combination code lacks necessary specificity in describing the manifestation or complication, an additional code should be used as a secondary code.

SEQUELA (LATE EFFECTS)

A sequela is the residual effect (condition produced) after the acute phase of an illness or injury has terminated. There is no time limit on when a sequela code can be used. The residual may be apparent early, such as in cerebral infarction, or it may occur months or years later, such as that due to a previous injury. Coding of sequela generally requires two codes sequenced in the following order: The condition or nature of the sequela is sequenced first.

The sequela code is sequenced second.

An exception to the above guidelines are those instances where the code for the sequela is followed by a manifestation code identified in the Tabular List and title, or the sequela code has been expanded (at the fourth, fifth or sixth character levels) to include the manifestation(s). The code for the acute phase of an illness or injury that led to the sequela is never used with a code for the late effect.

DOMINANT/NONDOMINANT SIDE

Codes from category G81, Hemiplegia and hemiparesis, and subcategories G83.1, Monoplegia of lower limb, G83.2, Monoplegia of upper limb, and G83.3, Monoplegia, unspecified, identify whether the dominant or nondominant side is affected. Should the affected side be documented, but not specified as dominant or nondominant, and the classification system does not indicate a default, code selection is as follows:

G00-G99

- For ambidextrous patients, the default should be dominant.

- If the left side is affected, the default is non-dominant.

- If the right side is affected, the default is dominant.

PAIN - CATEGORY G89

1) General coding information

Codes in category G89, Pain, not elsewhere classified, may be used in conjunction with codes from other categories and chapters to provide more detail about acute or chronic pain and neoplasm-related pain, unless otherwise indicated below.

If the pain is not specified as acute or chronic, post-thoracotomy, postprocedural, or neoplasm-related, do not assign codes from category G89.

A code from category G89 should not be assigned if the underlying (definitive) diagnosis is known, unless the reason for the encounter is pain control/management and not management of the underlying condition.

When an admission or encounter is for a procedure aimed at treating the underlying condition (e.g., spinal fusion, kyphoplasty), a code for the underlying condition (e.g., vertebral fracture, spinal stenosis) should be assigned as the principal diagnosis. No code from category G89 should be assigned.

(a) Category G89 Codes as Principal or First-Listed Diagnosis

Category G89 codes are acceptable as principal diagnosis or the first-listed code:

- When pain control or pain management is the reason for the admission/encounter (e.g., a patient with displaced intervertebral disc, nerve impingement and severe back pain presents for injection of steroid into the spinal canal). The underlying cause of the pain should be reported as an additional diagnosis, if known.

- When a patient is admitted for the insertion of a neurostimulator for pain control, assign the appropriate pain code as the principal or first-listed diagnosis. When an admission or encounter is for a procedure aimed at treating the underlying condition and a neurostimulator is inserted for pain control during the same admission/encounter, a code for the underlying condition should be assigned as the principal diagnosis and the appropriate pain code should be assigned as a secondary diagnosis.

(b) Use of Category G89 Codes in Conjunction with Site Specific Pain Codes

(i) Assigning Category G89 and Site-Specific Pain Codes

Codes from category G89 may be used in conjunction with codes that identify the site of pain (including codes from chapter 18) if the category G89 code provides additional information. For example, if the code describes the site of the pain, but does not fully describe whether the pain is acute or chronic, then both codes should be assigned.

(ii) Sequencing of Category G89 Codes with Site-Specific Pain Codes

The sequencing of category G89 codes with site-specific pain codes (including chapter 18 codes), is dependent on the circumstances of the encounter/admission as follows:

- If the encounter is for pain control or pain management, assign the code from category G89 followed by the code identifying the specific site of pain (e.g., encounter for pain management for acute neck pain from trauma is assigned code G89.11, Acute pain due to trauma, followed by code M54.2, Cervicalgia, to identify the site of pain).

- If the encounter is for any other reason except pain control or pain management, and a related definitive diagnosis has not been established (confirmed) by the provider, assign the code for the specific site of pain first, followed by the appropriate code from category G89.

2) Pain due to devices, implants and grafts

See Section I.C.19. Pain due to medical devices

3) Postoperative Pain

The provider's documentation should be used to guide the coding of postoperative pain, as well as *Section III. Reporting Additional Diagnoses* and *Section IV. Diagnostic Coding and Reporting in the Outpatient Setting.*

The default for post-thoracotomy and other postoperative pain not specified as acute or chronic is the code for the acute form.

Routine or expected postoperative pain immediately after surgery should not be coded.

(a) Postoperative pain not associated with specific postoperative complication

Postoperative pain not associated with a specific postoperative complication is assigned to the appropriate postoperative pain code in category G89.

(b) **Postoperative pain associated with specific postoperative complication**

Postoperative pain associated with a specific postoperative complication (such as painful wire sutures) is assigned to the appropriate code(s) found in Chapter 19, Injury, poisoning, and certain other consequences of external causes. If appropriate, use additional code(s) from category G89 to identify acute or chronic pain (G89.18 or G89.28).

4) **Chronic pain**

Chronic pain is classified to subcategory G89.2. There is no time frame defining when pain becomes chronic pain. The provider's documentation should be used to guide use of these codes.

5) **Neoplasm Related Pain**

Code G89.3 is assigned to pain documented as being related, associated or due to cancer, primary or secondary malignancy, or tumor. This code is assigned regardless of whether the pain is acute or chronic.

This code may be assigned as the principal or first-listed code when the stated reason for the admission/encounter is documented as pain control/pain management. The underlying neoplasm should be reported as an additional diagnosis.

When the reason for the admission/encounter is management of the neoplasm and the pain associated with the neoplasm is also documented, code G89.3 may be assigned as an additional diagnosis. It is not necessary to assign an additional code for the site of the pain.

See Section I.C.2 for instructions on the sequencing of neoplasms for all other stated reasons for the admission/encounter (except for pain control/pain management).

6) **Chronic pain syndrome**

Central pain syndrome (G89.0) and chronic pain syndrome (G89.4) are different than the term "chronic pain," and therefore codes should only be used when the provider has specifically documented this condition.

See Section I.C.5. Pain disorders related to psychological factors

Chapter 6
Diseases of the Nervous System (G00-G99)

Excludes2: certain conditions originating in the perinatal period (P04-P96)

certain infectious and parasitic diseases (A00-B99)

complications of pregnancy, childbirth and the puerperium (O00-O9A)

congenital malformations, deformations, and chromosomal abnormalities (Q00-Q99)

endocrine, nutritional and metabolic diseases (E00-E88)

injury, poisoning and certain other consequences of external causes (S00-T88)

neoplasms (C00-D49)

symptoms, signs and abnormal clinical and laboratory findings, not elsewhere classified (R00-R94)

This chapter contains the following blocks:

G00-G09	Inflammatory diseases of the central nervous system
G10-G14	Systemic atrophies primarily affecting the central nervous system
G20-G26	Extrapyramidal and movement disorders
G30-G32	Other degenerative diseases of the nervous system
G35-G37	Demyelinating diseases of the central nervous system
G40-G47	Episodic and paroxysmal disorders
G50-G59	Nerve, nerve root and plexus disorders
G60-G65	Polyneuropathies and other disorders of the peripheral nervous system
G70-G73	Diseases of myoneural junction and muscle
G80-G83	Cerebral palsy and other paralytic syndromes
G89-G99	Other disorders of the nervous system

INFLAMMATORY DISEASES OF THE CENTRAL NERVOUS SYSTEM (G00-G09)

G00 **Bacterial meningitis, not elsewhere classified**

Definition: Meningitis is an infectious disease characterized by inflammation of the meninges (the tissues that surround the brain or spinal cord) usually caused by a bacterial infection; symptoms include headache and stiff neck and fever and nausea.

Includes: bacterial arachnoiditis

bacterial leptomeningitis

bacterial meningitis

bacterial pachymeningitis

Excludes1: bacterial:

meningoencephalitis (G04.2)

meningomyelitis (G04.2)

G00.0 **Hemophilus meningitis**

Meningitis due to Hemophilus influenzae

G00.1 **Pneumococcal meningitis**

Meningtitis due to

Streptococcal pneumoniae

G00.2 **Streptococcal meningitis**

Use additional code to further identify organism (B95.0-B95.5)

G00.3 **Staphylococcal meningitis**

Use additional code to further identify organism (B95.61-B95.8)

G00.8 **Other bacterial meningitis**

Meningitis due to Escherichia coli

Meningitis due to Friedländer's bacillus

Meningitis due to Klebsiella

Use additional code to further identify organism (B96.-)

G00.9 **Bacterial meningitis, unspecified**

Meningitis due to gram-negative bacteria, unspecified

Purulent meningitis NOS

Pyogenic meningitis NOS

Suppurative meningitis NOS

G01 **Meningitis in bacterial diseases classified elsewhere**

Code first underlying disease

Excludes1: meningitis (in):

gonococcal (A54.81)

leptospirosis (A27.81)

listeriosis (A32.11)

Lyme disease (A69.21)

meningococcal (A39.0)

neurosyphilis (A52.13)

tuberculosis (A17.0)

meningoencephalitis and meningomyelitis in bacterial diseases classified elsewhere (G05)

G02 **Meningitis in other infectious and parasitic diseases classified elsewhere**

Code first underlying disease, such as:

African trypanosomiasis (B56.-)

poliovirus infection (A80.-)

Excludes1: candidal meningitis (B37.5)

coccidioidomycosis meningitis (B38.4)

cryptococcal meningitis (B45.1)

herpesviral [herpes simplex] meningitis (B00.3)

infectious mononucleosis complicated by meningitis (B27.- with fourth character 2)

measles complicated by meningitis (B05.1)

meningoencephalitis and meningomyelitis in other infectious and parasitic diseases classified elsewhere (G05)

mumps meningitis (B26.1)

rubella meningitis (B06.02)

varicella [chickenpox] meningitis (B01.0)

zoster meningitis (B02.1)

G03 **Meningitis due to other and unspecified causes**

Includes: arachnoiditis NOS

leptomeningitis NOS

meningitis NOS

pachymeningitis NOS

Excludes1: meningoencephalitis (G04.-)

meningomyelitis (G04.-)

G03.0 **Nonpyogenic meningitis**

Aseptic meningitis Nonbacterial meningitis

G03.1 **Chronic meningitis**

G03.2 **Benign recurrent meningitis [Mollaret]**

G03.8 **Meningitis due to other specified causes**

G03.9 **Meningitis, unspecified**

Arachnoiditis (spinal) NOS

G04 **Encephalitis, myelitis and encephalomyelitis**

Definition: Encephalitis is an inflammation of the brain, usually caused by a direct viral infection or a hypersensitivity reaction to a

virus or foreign protein. Myelitis is an inflammation of the spinal column. Encephalomyelitis is an inflammation of the brain and spinal cord.

Includes: acute ascending myelitis

   meningoencephalitis meningomyelitis

Excludes1: encephalopathy NOS (G93.40)

Excludes2: acute transverse myelitis (G37.3-)

   alcoholic encephalopathy (G31.2)

   benign myalgic encephalomyelitis (G93.3)

   multiple sclerosis (G35)

   subacute necrotizing myelitis (G37.4)

   toxic encephalitis (G92)

   toxic encephalopathy (G92)

G04.0   Acute disseminated encephalitis and encephalomyelitis (ADEM)

   Excludes1: acute necrotizing hemorrhagic encephalopathy (G04.3-)

   Other noninfectious acute disseminated encephalomyelitis (noninfectious ADEM) (G04.81)

G04.00   Acute disseminated encephalitis and encephalomyelitis, unspecified

G04.01   Postinfectious acute disseminated encephalitis and encephalomyelitis (postinfectious ADEM)

   Excludes1: post chickenpox encephalitis (B01.1)

   post measles encephalitis (B05.0)

   post measles myelitis (B05.1)

G04.02   Postimmunization acute disseminated encephalitis, myelitis and encephalomyelitis

   Encephalitis, post immunization
   Encephalomyelitis, post immunization

   Use additional code to identify the vaccine (T50.A-, T50.B-, T50.Z-)

G04.1   Tropical spastic paraplegia

G04.2   Bacterial meningoencephalitis and meningomyelitis, not elsewhere classified

G04.3   Acute necrotizing hemorrhagic encephalopathy

   Excludes1: acute disseminated encephalitis and encephalomyelitis (G04.0-)

G04.30   Acute necrotizing hemorrhagic encephalopathy, unspecified

G04.31   Postinfectious acute necrotizing hemorrhagic encephalopathy

G04.32   Postimmunization acute necrotizing hemorrhagic encephalopathy

   Use additional code to identify the vaccine (T50.A-, T50.B-, T50.Z-)

G04.39   Other acute necrotizing hemorrhagic encephalopathy

   Code also underlying etiology, if applicable

G04.8   Other encephalitis, myelitis and encephalomyelitis

   Code also any associated seizure (G40.-, R56.9)

G04.81   Other encephalitis and encephalomyelitis

   Noninfectious acute disseminated encephalomyelitis (noninfectious ADEM)

G04.89   Other myelitis

G04.9   Encephalitis, myelitis and encephalomyelitis, unspecified

G04.90   Encephalitis and encephalomyelitis, unspecified

   Ventriculitis (cerebral) NOS

G04.91   Myelitis, unspecified

G05   Encephalitis, myelitis and encephalomyelitis in diseases classified elsewhere

   Code first underlying disease, such as:

   human immunodeficiency virus [HIV] disease (B20)

   poliovirus (A80.-)

   suppurative otitis media (H66.01-H66.4)

   trichinellosis (B75)

   Excludes1: adenoviral encephalitis, myelitis and encephalomyelitis (A85.1)

   congenital toxoplasmosis encephalitis, myelitis and encephalomyelitis (P37.1)

   cytomegaloviral encephalitis, myelitis and encephalomyelitis (B25.8)

   encephalitis, myelitis and encephalomyelitis (in) measles (B05.0)

   encephalitis, myelitis and encephalomyelitis (in) systemic lupus erythematosus (M32.19)

   enteroviral encephalitis, myelitis and encephalomyelitis (A85.0)

   eosinophilic meningoencephalitis (B83.2)

   herpesviral [herpes simplex] encephalitis, myelitis and encephalomyelitis (B00.4)

   listerial encephalitis, myelitis and encephalomyelitis (A32.12)

   meningococcal encephalitis, myelitis and encephalomyelitis (A39.81)

   mumps encephalitis, myelitis and encephalomyelitis (B26.2)

   postchickenpox encephalitis, myelitis and encephalomyelitis (B01.1-)

   rubella encephalitis, myelitis and encephalomyelitis (B06.01)

   toxoplasmosis encephalitis, myelitis and encephalomyelitis (B58.2)

   zoster encephalitis, myelitis and encephalomyelitis (B02.0)

G05.3   Encephalitis and encephalomyelitis in diseases classified elsewhere

   Meningoencephalitis in diseases classified elsewhere

G05.4   Myelitis in diseases classified elsewhere

   Meningomyelitis in diseases classified elsewhere

G06   Intracranial and intraspinal abscess and granuloma

   Use additional code (B95-B97) to identify infectious agent.

G06.0   Intracranial abscess and granuloma

   Brain [any part] abscess (embolic)

   Cerebellar abscess (embolic)

   Cerebral abscess (embolic)

   Intracranial epidural abscess or granuloma

   Intracranial extradural abscess or granuloma

   Intracranial subdural abscess or granuloma

   Otogenic abscess (embolic)

   Excludes1: tuberculous intracranial abscess and granuloma (A17.81)

G06.1   Intraspinal abscess and granuloma

   Abscess (embolic) of spinal cord [any part]

   Intraspinal epidural abscess or granuloma

   Intraspinal extradural abscess or granuloma

Intraspinal subdural abscess or granuloma

Excludes1: tuberculous intraspinal abscess and granuloma (A17.81)

G06.2 Extradural and subdural abscess, unspecified

G07 Intracranial and intraspinal abscess and granuloma in diseases classified elsewhere

Code first underlying disease, such as:

schistosomiasis granuloma of brain (B65.-)

Excludes1: abscess of brain:

amebic (A06.6)

chromomycotic (B43.1)

gonococcal (A54.82)

tuberculous (A17.81)

tuberculoma of meninges (A17.1)

G08 Intracranial and intraspinal phlebitis and thrombophlebitis

Septic embolism of intracranial or intraspinal venous sinuses and veins

Septic endophlebitis of intracranial or intraspinal venous sinuses and veins

Septic phlebitis of intracranial or intraspinal venous sinuses and veins

Septic thrombophlebitis of intracranial or intraspinal venous sinuses and veins

Septic thrombosis of intracranial or intraspinal venous sinuses and veins

Excludes1: intracranial phlebitis and thrombophlebitis complicating:

abortion, ectopic or molar pregnancy (O00-O07, O08.7)

pregnancy, childbirth and the puerperium (O22.5, O87.3)

nonpyogenic intracranial phlebitis and thrombophlebitis (I67.6)

Excludes2: intracranial phlebitis and thrombophlebitis complicating nonpyogenic intraspinal phlebitis and thrombophlebitis (G95.1)

G09 Sequelae of inflammatory diseases of central nervous system

Note: Category G09 is to be used to indicate conditions whose primary classification is to G00-G08 as the cause of sequelae, themselves classifiable elsewhere. The 'sequelae' include conditions specified as residuals.

Code first condition resulting from (sequela) of inflammatory diseases of central nervous system

SYSTEMIC ATROPHIES PRIMARILY AFFECTING THE CENTRAL NERVOUS SYSTEM (G10-G14)

G10 Huntington's disease

Huntington's chorea

Huntington's dementia

G11 Hereditary ataxia

Excludes2: cerebral palsy (G80.-)

hereditary and idiopathic neuropathy (G60.-)

metabolic disorders (E70-E88)

G11.0 Congenital nonprogressive ataxia

G11.1 Early-onset cerebellar ataxia

Early-onset cerebellar ataxia with essential tremor

Early-onset cerebellar ataxia with myoclonus [Hunt's ataxia]

Early-onset cerebellar ataxia with retained tendon reflexes

Friedreich's ataxia (autosomal recessive)

X-linked recessive spinocerebellar ataxia

G11.2 Late-onset cerebellar ataxia

G11.3 Cerebellar ataxia with defective DNA repair

Ataxia telangiectasia [Louis-Bar]

Excludes2: Cockayne's syndrome (Q87.1)

Other disorders of purine and pyrimidine metabolism (E79.-)

xeroderma pigmentosum (Q82.1)

G11.4 Hereditary spastic paraplegia

G11.8 Other hereditary ataxias

G11.9 Hereditary ataxia, unspecified

Hereditary cerebellar ataxia NOS

Hereditary cerebellar degeneration

Hereditary cerebellar disease

Hereditary cerebellar syndrome

G12 Spinal muscular atrophy and related syndromes

G12.0 Infantile spinal muscular atrophy, type I [Werdnig-Hoffman]

G12.1 Other inherited spinal muscular atrophy

Adult form spinal muscular atrophy

Childhood form, type II spinal muscular atrophy

Distal spinal muscular atrophy

Juvenile form, type III spinal muscular atrophy [Kugelberg-Welander]

Progressive bulbar palsy of childhood [Fazio-Londe]

Scapuloperoneal form spinal muscular atrophy

G12.2 Motor neuron disease

G12.20 Motor neuron disease, unspecified

G12.21 Amyotrophic lateral sclerosis

Progressive spinal muscle atrophy

G12.22 Progressive bulbar palsy

G12.29 Other motor neuron disease

Familial motor neuron disease

Primary lateral sclerosis

G12.8 Other spinal muscular atrophies and related syndromes

G12.9 Spinal muscular atrophy, unspecified

G13 Systemic atrophies primarily affecting central nervous system in diseases classified elsewhere

G13.0 Paraneoplastic neuromyopathy and neuropathy

Carcinomatous neuromyopathy

Sensorial paraneoplastic neuropathy [Denny Brown]

Code first underlying neoplasm (C00-D49)

G13.1 Other systemic atrophy primarily affecting central nervous system in neoplastic disease

Paraneoplastic limbic encephalopathy

Code first underlying neoplasm (C00-D49)

G13.2 Systemic atrophy primarily affecting the central nervous system in myxedema

Code first underlying disease, such as:

hypothyroidism (E03.-)

myxedematous congenital iodine deficiency (E00.1)

G13.8 Systemic atrophy primarily affecting central nervous system in other diseases classified elsewhere

Code first underlying disease

G14 Postpolio syndrome

Includes: postpolio myelitic syndrome

Excludes1: sequelae of poliomyelitis (B91)

EXTRAPYRAMIDAL AND MOVEMENT DISORDERS (G20-G26)

Definition: Extrapyramidal symptoms (EPS) are various movement disorders such as acute dystonic reactions, pseudoparkinsonism, Tardive dyskinesia or akathisia suffered as a result of taking dopamine antagonists, usually antipsychotic (neuroleptic) drugs, which are often used to control psychosis.

G20 Parkinson's disease

Hemiparkinsonism

Idiopathic Parkinsonism or Parkinson's disease

Paralysis agitans

Parkinsonism or Parkinson's disease NOS

Primary Parkinsonism or Parkinson's disease

Excludes1: dementia with Parkinsonism (G31.83)

G21 Secondary parkinsonism

Excludes1: dementia with Parkinsonism (G31.83)

  Huntington's disease (G10)

  Shy-Drager syndrome (G90.3)

  syphilitic Parkinsonism (A52.19)

G21.0 Malignant neuroleptic syndrome

Use additional code for adverse effect, if applicable, to identify drug (T43.3X5, T43.4X5, T43.505, T43.595)

Excludes1: neuroleptic induced parkinsonism (G21.11)

G21.1 Other drug-induced secondary parkinsonism

G21.11 Neuroleptic induced parkinsonism

Use additional code for adverse effect, if applicable, to identify drug (T43.3X5, T43.4X5, T43.505, T43.595)

Excludes1: malignant neuroleptic syndrome (G21.0)

G21.19 Other drug induced secondary parkinsonism

Use additional code for adverse effect, if applicable, to identify drug (T36-T50 with fifth or sixth character 5)

G21.2 Secondary parkinsonism due to other external agents

Code first (T51-T65) to identify external agent

G21.3 Postencephalitic parkinsonism

G21.4 Vascular parkinsonism

G21.8 Other secondary parkinsonism

G21.9 Secondary parkinsonism, unspecified

G23 Other degenerative diseases of basal ganglia

Excludes2: multi-system degeneration of the autonomic nervous system (G90.3)

G23.0 Hallervorden-Spatz disease

Pigmentary pallidal degeneration

G23.1 Progressive supranuclear ophthalmoplegia [Steele-Richardson-Olszewski]

Progressive supranuclear palsy

G23.2 Striatonigral degeneration

G23.8 Other specified degenerative diseases of basal ganglia

Calcification of basal ganglia

G23.9 Degenerative disease of basal ganglia, unspecified

G24 Dystonia

Includes: dyskinesia

Excludes2: athetoid cerebral palsy (G80.3)

G24.0 Drug induced dystonia

Use additional code code for adverse effect, if applicable, to identify drug (T36-T50 with fifth or sixth character 5)

G24.01 Drug induced subacute dyskinesia

Drug induced blepharospasm

Drug induced orofacial dyskinesia

Neuroleptic induced tardive dyskinesia

Tardive dyskinesia

G24.02 Drug induced acute dystonia

Acute dystonic reaction to drugs

Neuroleptic induced acute dystonia

G24.09 Other drug induced dystonia

G24.1 Genetic torsion dystonia

Dystonia deformans progressiva

Dystonia musculorum deformans

Familial torsion dystonia

Idiopathic familial dystonia

Idiopathic (torsion) dystonia NOS (Schwalbe-) Ziehen-Oppenheim disease

G24.2 Idiopathic nonfamilial dystonia

G24.3 Spasmodic torticollis

Excludes1: congenital torticollis (Q68.0)

  hysterical torticollis (F44.4)

  ocular torticollis (R29.891)

  psychogenic torticollis (F45.8)

  torticollis NOS (M43.6)

  traumatic recurrent torticollis (S13.4)

G24.4 Idiopathic orofacial dystonia

Orofacial dyskinesia

Excludes1: drug induced orofacial dyskinesia (G24.01)

G24.5 Blepharospasm

Excludes1: drug induced blepharospasm (G24.01)

G24.8 Other dystonia

Acquired torsion dystonia NOS

G24.9 Dystonia, unspecified

Dyskinesia NOS

G25 Other extrapyramidal and movement disorders

Definition: Extrapyramidal disease is a general term for a number of disorders caused by abnormalities of the basal ganglia or certain brain stem or thalamic nuclei; characterised by motor deficits, loss of postural reflexes, bradykinesia, tremor, rigidity, and various involuntary movements.

Excludes2: sleep related movement disorders (G47.6-)

G25.0 Essential tremor Familial tremor

Excludes1: tremor NOS (R25.1)

G25.1 Drug-induced tremor

Use additional code for adverse effect, if applicable, to identify drug (T36-T50 with fifth or sixth character 5)

G25.2 Other specified forms of tremor

Intention tremor

G25.3 Myoclonus

Drug-induced myoclonus

Palatal myoclonus

Use additional code for adverse effect, if applicable, to identify drug (T36-T50 with fifth or sixth character 5)

Excludes1: facial myokymia (G51.4)

myoclonic epilepsy (G40.-)

G25.4 Drug-induced chorea

Use additional code for adverse effect, if applicable, to identify drug (T36-T50 with fifth or sixth character 5)

G25.5 Other chorea

Chorea NOS

Excludes1: chorea NOS with heart involvement (I02.0)

Huntington's chorea (G10)

rheumatic chorea (I02.-)

Sydenham's chorea (I02.-)

G25.6 Drug induced tics and other tics of organic origin

G25.61 Drug induced tics

Use additional code for adverse effect, if applicable, to identify drug (T36-T50 with fifth or sixth character 5)

G25.69 Other tics of organic origin

Excludes1: habit spasm (F95.9)

tic NOS (F95.9)

Tourette's syndrome (F95.2)

G25.7 Other and unspecified drug induced movement disorders

Use additional code for adverse effect, if applicable, to identify drug (T36-T50 with fifth or sixth character 5)

G25.70 Drug induced movement disorder, unspecified

G25.71 Drug induced akathisia

Drug induced acathisia

Neuroleptic induced acute akathisia

G25.79 Other drug induced movement disorders

G25.8 Other specified extrapyramidal and movement disorders

G25.81 Restless legs syndrome

G25.82 Stiff-man syndrome

G25.83 Benign shuddering attacks

G25.89 Other specified extrapyramidal and movement disorders

G25.9 Extrapyramidal and movement disorder, unspecified

G26 Extrapyramidal and movement disorders in diseases classified elsewhere

Code first underlying disease

OTHER DEGENERATIVE DISEASES OF THE NERVOUS SYSTEM (G30-G32)

G30 Alzheimer's disease

Includes: Alzheimer's dementia senile and presenile forms

Use additional code to identify:

delirium, if applicable (F05)

dementia with behavioral disturbance (F02.81)

dementia without behavioral disturbance (F02.80)

Excludes1: senile degeneration of brain NEC (G31.1)

senile dementia NOS (F03)

senility NOS (R41.81)

G30.0 Alzheimer's disease with early onset

G30.1 Alzheimer's disease with late onset

G30.8 Other Alzheimer's disease

G30.9 Alzheimer's disease, unspecified

G31 Other degenerative diseases of nervous system, not elsewhere classified

Use additional code to identify:

dementia with behavioral disturbance (F02.81)

dementia without behavioral disturbance (F02.80)

Excludes2: Reye's syndrome (G93.7)

G31.0 Frontotemporal dementia

G31.01 Pick's disease

Primary progressive aphasia

Progressive isolated aphasia

G31.09 Other frontotemporal dementia

Frontal dementia

G31.1 Senile degeneration of brain, not elsewhere classified

Excludes1: Alzheimer's disease (G30.-)

senility NOS (R41.81)

G31.2 Degeneration of nervous system due to alcohol

Alcoholic cerebellar ataxia

Alcoholic cerebellar degeneration

Alcoholic cerebral degeneration

Alcoholic encephalopathy

Dysfunction of the autonomic nervous system due to alcohol

Code also associated alcoholism (F10.-)

G31.8 Other specified degenerative diseases of nervous system

G31.81 Alpers disease

Grey-matter degeneration

G31.82 Leigh's disease

Subacute necrotizing encephalopathy

G31.83 Dementia with Lewy bodies

Dementia with Parkinsonism

Lewy body dementia

Lewy body disease

G31.84 Mild cognitive impairment, so stated

Excludes1: age related cognitive decline (R41.81)

altered mental status (R41.82)

cerebral degeneration (G31.9)

change in mental status (R41.82)

cognitive deficits following (sequelae of) cerebral hemorrhage or infarction (I69.01-, I69.11-, I69.21-, I69.31-, I69.81-, I69.91-)

cognitive impairment due to intracranial or head injury (S06.-)

dementia (F01.-, F02.-, F03)

mild memory disturbance (F06.8)

neurologic neglect syndrome (R41.4)

personality change, nonpsychotic (F68.8)

G31.85 Corticobasal degeneration

G31.89 Other specified degenerative diseases of nervous system

G31.9 Degenerative disease of nervous system, unspecified

G32 Other degenerative disorders of nervous system in diseases classified elsewhere

G32.0 Subacute combined degeneration of spinal cord in diseases classified elsewhere

---

Dana-Putnam syndrome

Sclerosis of spinal cord (combined) (dorsolateral) (posterolateral)

Code first underlying disease, such as:

anemia (D51.9)

dietary (D51.3)

pernicious (D51.0)

vitamin B12 deficiency (E53.8)

Excludes1: syphilitic combined degeneration of spinal cord (A52.11)

G32.8 Other specified degenerative disorders of nervous system in diseases classified elsewhere

Code first underlying disease, such as:

amyloidosis cerebral degeneration (E85.-)

cerebral degeneration (due to) hypothyroidism (E00.0-E03.9)

cerebral degeneration (due to) neoplasm (C00-D49)

cerebral degeneration (due to) vitamin B deficiency, except thiamine (E52-E53.-)

Excludes1: superior hemorrhagic polioencephalitis [Wernicke's encephalopathy] (E51.2)

G32.81 Cerebellar ataxia in diseases classified elsewhere

Code first underlying disease, such as:

celiac disease (with gluten ataxia) (K90.0)

cerebellar ataxia (in) neoplastic disease (paraneoplastic cerebellar degeneration) (C00-D49)

non-celiac gluten ataxia (M35.9)

Excludes1: systemic atrophy primarily affecting the central nervous system in alcoholic cerebellar ataxia (G31.2)

systemic atrophy primarily affecting the central nervous system in myxedema (G13.2)

G32.89 Other specified degenerative disorders of nervous system in diseases classified elsewhere

Degenerative encephalopathy in diseases classified elsewhere

DEMYELINATING DISEASES OF THE CENTRAL NERVOUS SYSTEM (G35-G37)

Definition: A demyelinating disease is any condition that results in damage to the protective covering (myelin sheath) that surrounds nerve fibers in your brain and spinal cord. When the myelin sheath is damaged, nerve impulses slow or even stop, causing neurological problems.

G35 Multiple sclerosis

Definition: Multiple sclerosis is a chronic autoimmune disorder affecting movement, sensation, and bodily functions. It is caused by destruction of the myelin insulation covering nerve fibers in the central nervous system.

Disseminated multiple sclerosis Generalized multiple sclerosis

Multiple sclerosis NOS

Multiple sclerosis of brain stem

Multiple sclerosis of cord

G36 Other acute disseminated demyelination

Excludes1: postinfectious encephalitis and encephalomyelitis NOS (G04.01)

G36.0 Neuromyelitis optica [Devic]

Demyelination in optic neuritis

Excludes1: optic neuritis NOS (H46)

G36.1 Acute and subacute hemorrhagic leukoencephalitis [Hurst]

G36.8 Other specified acute disseminated demyelination

G36.9 Acute disseminated demyelination, unspecified

G37 Other demyelinating diseases of central nervous system

Definition: Demyelinating diseases of the central nervous system is any disease of the nervous system in which the myelin sheath of neurons is damaged.

G37.0 Diffuse sclerosis of central nervous system

Periaxial encephalitis

Schilder's disease

Excludes1: X linked adrenoleukodystrophy (E71.52-)

G37.1 Central demyelination of corpus callosum

G37.2 Central pontine myelinolysis

G37.3 Acute transverse myelitis in demyelinating disease of central nervous system

Acute transverse myelitis NOS

Acute transverse myelopathy

Excludes1: multiple sclerosis (G35)

neuromyelitis optica [Devic] (G36.0)

G37.4 Subacute necrotizing myelitis of central nervous system

G37.5 Concentric sclerosis [Balo] of central nervous system

G37.8 Other specified demyelinating diseases of central nervous system

G37.9 Demyelinating disease of central nervous system, unspecified

EPISODIC AND PAROXYSMAL DISORDERS (G40-G47)

G40 Epilepsy and recurrent seizures

Definition: Epilepsy and recurrent seizures is a common chronic neurological disorder characterized by recurrent unprovoked seizures. These seizures are transient signs and/or symptoms of abnormal, excessive or synchronous neuronal activity in the brain.

Note: the following terms are to be considered equivalent to intractable: pharmacoresistant (pharmacologically resistant), treatment resistant, refractory (medically) and poorly controlled

Excludes1: conversion disorder with seizures (F44.5)

convulsions NOS (R56.9)

post traumatic seizures (R56.1)

seizure (convulsive) NOS (R56.9)

seizure of newborn (P90)

Excludes2: hippocampal sclerosis (G93.81)

mesial temporal sclerosis (G93.81)

temporal sclerosis (G93.81)

Todd's paralysis (G83.84)

G40.0 Localization-related (focal) (partial) idiopathic epilepsy and epileptic syndromes with seizures of localized onset

Benign childhood epilepsy with centrotemporal EEG spikes

Childhood epilepsy with occipital EEG paroxysms

Excludes1: adult onset localization-related epilepsy (G40.1-, G40.2-)

G40.00 Localization-related (focal) (partial) idiopathic epilepsy and epileptic syndromes with seizures of localized onset, not intractable

● New code ▲ Revised code **Excludes1:** Not coded here **Excludes2:** Not included here ⊗ Placeholder required ⑦ 7th digit required

Localization-related (focal) (partial) idiopathic epilepsy and epileptic syndromes with seizures of localized onset without intractability

G40.001 **Localization-related (focal) (partial) idiopathic epilepsy and epileptic syndromes with seizures of localized onset, not intractable, with status epilepticus**

G40.009 **Localization-related (focal) (partial) idiopathic epilepsy and epileptic syndromes with seizures of localized onset, not intractable, without status epilepticus**

Localization-related (focal) (partial) idiopathic epilepsy and epileptic syndromes with seizures of localized onset NOS

G40.01 **Localization-related (focal) (partial) idiopathic epilepsy and epileptic syndromes with seizures of localized onset, intractable**

G40.011 **Localization-related (focal) (partial) idiopathic epilepsy and epileptic syndromes with seizures of localized onset, intractable, with status epilepticus**

G40.019 **Localization-related (focal) (partial) idiopathic epilepsy and epileptic syndromes with seizures of localized onset, intractable, without status epilepticus**

G40.1 **Localization-related (focal) (partial) symptomatic epilepsy and epileptic syndromes with simple partial seizures**

Attacks without alteration of consciousness

Epilepsia partialis continua [Kozhevnikof]

Simple partial seizures developing into secondarily generalized seizures

G40.10 **Localization-related (focal) (partial) symptomatic epilepsy and epileptic syndromes with simple partial seizures, not intractable**

Localization-related (focal) (partial) symptomatic epilepsy and epileptic syndromes with simple partial seizures without intractability

G40.101 **Localization-related (focal) (partial) symptomatic epilepsy and epileptic syndromes with simple partial seizures, not intractable, with status epilepticus**

G40.109 **Localization-related (focal) (partial) symptomatic epilepsy and epileptic syndromes with simple partial seizures, not intractable, without status epilepticus**

Localization-related (focal) (partial) symptomatic epilepsy and epileptic syndromes with simple partial seizures NOS

G40.11 **Localization-related (focal) (partial) symptomatic epilepsy and epileptic syndromes with simple partial seizures, intractable**

G40.111 **Localization-related (focal) (partial) symptomatic epilepsy and epileptic syndromes**

with simple partial seizures, intractable, with status epilepticus

G40.119 **Localization-related (focal) (partial) symptomatic epilepsy and epileptic syndromes**

with simple partial seizures, intractable, without status epilepticus

G40.2 **Localization-related (focal) (partial) symptomatic epilepsy and epileptic syndromes with complex partial seizures**

Attacks with alteration of consciousness, often with automatisms

Complex partial seizures developing into secondarily generalized seizures

G40.20 **Localization-related (focal) (partial) symptomatic epilepsy and epileptic syndromes with complex partial seizures, not intractable**

Localization-related (focal) (partial) symptomatic epilepsy and epileptic syndromes with complex partial seizures without intractability

G40.201 **Localization-related (focal) (partial) symptomatic epilepsy and epileptic syndromes with complex partial seizures, not intractable, with status epilepticus**

G40.209 **Localization-related (focal) (partial) symptomatic epilepsy and epileptic syndromes with complex partial seizures, not intractable, without status epilepticus**

Localization-related (focal) (partial) symptomatic epilepsy and epileptic syndromes with complex partial seizures NOS

G40.21 **Localization-related (focal) (partial) symptomatic epilepsy and epileptic syndromes with complex partial seizures, intractable**

G40.211 **Localization-related (focal) (partial) symptomatic epilepsy and epileptic syndromes with complex partial seizures, intractable, with status epilepticus**

G40.219 **Localization-related (focal) (partial) symptomatic epilepsy and epileptic syndromes with complex partial seizures, intractable, without status epilepticus**

G40.3 **Generalized idiopathic epilepsy and epileptic syndromes**

<u>Code also</u> MERRF syndrome, if applicable (E88.42)

G40.30 **Generalized idiopathic epilepsy and epileptic syndromes, not intractable**

Generalized idiopathic epilepsy and epileptic syndromes without intractability

G40.301 **Generalized idiopathic epilepsy and epileptic syndromes, not intractable, with status epilepticus**

G40.309 **Generalized idiopathic epilepsy and epileptic syndromes, not intractable, without status epilepticus**

Generalized idiopathic epilepsy and epileptic syndromes NOS

G40.31 **Generalized idiopathic epilepsy and epileptic syndromes, intractable**

G40.311 Generalized idiopathic epilepsy and epileptic syndromes, intractable, with status epilepticus

G40.319 Generalized idiopathic epilepsy and epileptic syndromes, intractable, without status epilepticus

G40.A Absence epileptic syndrome

Childhood absence epilepsy [pyknolepsy]

Juvenile absence epilepsy

Absence epileptic syndrome, NOS

G40.A0 Absence epileptic syndrome, not intractable

G40.A01 Absence epileptic syndrome, not intractable, with status epilepticus

G40.A09 Absence epileptic syndrome, not intractable, without status epilepticus

G40.A1 Absence epileptic syndrome, intractable

G40.A11 Absence epileptic syndrome, intractable, with status epilepticus

G40.A19 Absence epileptic syndrome, intractable, without status epilepticus

G40.B Juvenile myoclonic epilepsy [impulsive petit mal]

G40.B0 Juvenile myoclonic epilepsy, not intractable

G40.B01 Juvenile myoclonic epilepsy, not intractable, with status epilepticus

G40.B09 Juvenile myoclonic epilepsy, not intractable, without status epilepticus

G40.B1 Juvenile myoclonic epilepsy, intractable

G40.B11 Juvenile myoclonic epilepsy, intractable, with status epilepticus

G40.B19 Juvenile myoclonic epilepsy, intractable, without status epilepticus

G40.4 Other generalized epilepsy and epileptic syndromes

Epilepsy with grand mal seizures on awakening

Epilepsy with myoclonic absences

Epilepsy with myoclonic-astatic seizures

Grand mal seizure NOS

Nonspecific atonic epileptic seizures

Nonspecific clonic epileptic seizures

Nonspecific myoclonic epileptic seizures

Nonspecific tonic epileptic seizures

Nonspecific tonic-clonic epileptic seizures

Symptomatic early myoclonic encephalopathy

G40.40 Other generalized epilepsy and epileptic syndromes, not intractable

Other generalized epilepsy and epileptic syndromes without intractability

Other generalized epilepsy and epileptic syndromes NOS

G40.401 Other generalized epilepsy and epileptic syndromes, not intractable, with status epilepticus

G40.409 Other generalized epilepsy and epileptic syndromes, not intractable, without status epilepticus

G40.41 Other generalized epilepsy and epileptic syndromes, intractable

G40.411 Other generalized epilepsy and epileptic syndromes, intractable, with status epilepticus

G40.419 Other generalized epilepsy and epileptic syndromes, intractable, without status epilepticus

G40.5 Epileptic seizures related to external causes

Epileptic seizures related to alcohol

Epileptic seizures related to drugs

Epileptic seizures related to hormonal changes

Epileptic seizures related to sleep deprivation

Epileptic seizures related to stress

Code also, if applicable, associated epilepsy and recurrent seizures (G40.-)

Use additional code for adverse effect, if applicable, to identify drug (T36-T50 with fifth or sixth character 5)

G40.50 Epileptic seizures related to external causes, not intractable

G40.501 Epileptic seizures related to external causes, not intractable, with status epilepticus

G40.509 Epileptic seizures related to external causes, not intractable, without status epilepticus

Epileptic seizures related to external causes, NOS

G40.8 Other epilepsy and recurrent seizures

Epilepsies and epileptic syndromes undetermined as to whether they are focal or generalized Landau-Kleffner syndrome

G40.80 Other epilepsy

G40.801 Other epilepsy, not intractable, with status epilepticus

Other epilepsy without intractability with status epilepticus

G40.802 Other epilepsy, not intractable, without status epilepticus

Other epilepsy NOS

Other epilepsy without intractability without status epilepticus

G40.803 Other epilepsy, intractable, with status epilepticus

G40.804 Other epilepsy, intractable, without status epilepticus

G40.81 Lennox-Gastaut syndrome

G40.811 Lennox-Gastaut syndrome, not intractable, with status epilepticus

G40.812 Lennox-Gastaut syndrome, not intractable, without status epilepticus

G40.813 Lennox-Gastaut syndrome, intractable, with status epilepticus

G40.814 Lennox-Gastaut syndrome, intractable, without status epilepticus

G40.82 Epileptic spasms

Infantile spasms

Salaam attacks West's syndrome

● New code ▲ Revised code **Excludes1:** Not coded here **Excludes2:** Not included here ⊗ Placeholder required ⑦7th digit required

G40.821 Epileptic spasms, not intractable, with status epilepticus

G40.822 Epileptic spasms, not intractable, without status epilepticus

G40.823 Epileptic spasms, intractable, with status epilepticus

G40.824 Epileptic spasms, intractable, without status epilepticus

G40.89 Other seizures

Excludes1: post traumatic seizures (R56.1)
recurrent seizures NOS (G40.909)
seizure NOS (R56.9)

G40.9 Epilepsy, unspecified

G40.90 Epilepsy, unspecified, not intractable

Epilepsy, unspecified, without intractability

G40.901 Epilepsy, unspecified, not intractable, with status epilepticus

G40.909 Epilepsy, unspecified, not intractable, without status epilepticus

Epilepsy NOS
Epileptic convulsions NOS
Epileptic fits NOS
Epileptic seizures NOS
Recurrent seizures NOS
Seizure disorder NOS

G40.91 Epilepsy, unspecified, intractable

Intractable seizure disorder NOS

G40.911 Epilepsy, unspecified, intractable, with status epilepticus

G40.919 Epilepsy, unspecified, intractable, without status epilepticus

G43 Migraine

Definition: Migraine is a severe, disabling headache, usually affecting only one side of the head, and often accompanied by nausea, vomiting, photophobia and visual disturbances.

Note: the following terms are to be considered equivalent to intractable: pharmacoresistant (pharmacologically resistant), treatment resistant, refractory (medically) and poorly controlled

Use additional code for adverse effect, if applicable, to identify drug (T36-T50 with fifth or sixth character 5)

Excludes1: headache NOS (R51)
lower half migraine (G44.00)

Excludes2: headache syndromes (G44.-)

G43.0 Migraine without aura

Common migraine

Excludes1: chronic migraine without aura (G43.7-)

G43.00 Migraine without aura, not intractable

Migraine without aura without mention of refractory migraine

G43.001 Migraine without aura, not intractable, with status migrainosus

G43.009 Migraine without aura, not intractable, without status migrainosus

Migraine without aura NOS

G43.01 Migraine without aura, intractable

Migraine without aura with refractory migraine

G43.011 Migraine without aura, intractable, with status migrainosus

G43.019 Migraine without aura, intractable, without status migrainosus

G43.1 Migraine with aura

Basilar migraine
Classical migraine
Migraine equivalents
Migraine preceded or accompanied by transient focal neurological phenomena
Migraine triggered seizures
Migraine with acute-onset aura
Migraine with aura without headache (migraine equivalents)
Migraine with prolonged aura
Migraine with typical aura
Retinal migraine

Code also any associated seizure (G40.-, R56.9)

Excludes1: persistent migraine aura (G43.5-, G43.6-)

G43.10 Migraine with aura, not intractable

Migraine with aura without mention of refractory migraine

G43.101 Migraine with aura, not intractable, with status migrainosus

G43.109 Migraine with aura, not intractable, without status migrainosus

Migraine with aura NOS

G43.11 Migraine with aura, intractable

Migraine with aura with refractory migraine

G43.111 Migraine with aura, intractable, with status migrainosus

G43.119 Migraine with aura, intractable, without status migrainosus

G43.4 Hemiplegic migraine

Familial migraine
Sporadic migraine

G43.40 Hemiplegic migraine, not intractable

Hemiplegic migraine without refractory migraine

G43.401 Hemiplegic migraine, not intractable, with status migrainosus

G43.409 Hemiplegic migraine, not intractable, without status migrainosus

Hemiplegic migraine NOS

G43.41 Hemiplegic migraine, intractable

Hemiplegic migraine with refractory migraine

G43.411 Hemiplegic migraine, intractable, with status migrainosus

G43.419 Hemiplegic migraine, intractable, without status migrainosus

G43.5 Persistent migraine aura without cerebral infarction

G43.50 Persistent migraine aura without cerebral infarction, not intractable

Persistent migraine aura without cerebral infarction, without refractory migraine

G43.501 Persistent migraine aura without cerebral infarction, not intractable, with status migrainosus

G43.509 **Persistent migraine aura without cerebral infarction, not intractable, without status migrainosus**

Persistent migraine aura NOS

G43.51 **Persistent migraine aura without cerebral infarction, intractable**

Persistent migraine aura without cerebral infarction, with refractory migraine

G43.511 **Persistent migraine aura without cerebral infarction, intractable, with status migrainosus**

G43.519 **Persistent migraine aura without cerebral infarction, intractable, without status migrainosus**

G43.6 **Persistent migraine aura with cerebral infarction**

<u>Code also</u> the type of cerebral infarction (I63.-)

G43.60 **Persistent migraine aura with cerebral infarction, not intractable**

Persistent migraine aura with cerebral infarction, without refractory migraine

G43.601 **Persistent migraine aura with cerebral infarction, not intractable, with status migrainosus**

G43.609 **Persistent migraine aura with cerebral infarction, not intractable, without status migrainosus**

G43.61 **Persistent migraine aura with cerebral infarction, intractable**

Persistent migraine aura with cerebral infarction, with refractory migraine

G43.611 **Persistent migraine aura with cerebral infarction, intractable, with status migrainosus**

G43.619 **Persistent migraine aura with cerebral infarction, intractable, without status migrainosus**

G43.7 **Chronic migraine without aura**

Transformed migraine

Excludes1: migraine without aura (G43.0-)

G43.70 **Chronic migraine without aura, not intractable**

Chronic migraine without aura, without refractory migraine

G43.701 **Chronic migraine without aura, not intractable, with status migrainosus**

G43.709 **Chronic migraine without aura, not intractable, without status migrainosus**

Chronic migraine without aura NOS

G43.71 **Chronic migraine without aura, intractable**

Chronic migraine without aura, with refractory migraine

G43.711 **Chronic migraine without aura, intractable, with status migrainosus**

G43.719 **Chronic migraine without aura, intractable, without status migrainosus**

G43.A **Cyclical vomiting**

G43.A0 **Cyclical vomiting, not intractable**

Cyclical vomiting, without refractory migraine

G43.A1 **Cyclical vomiting, intractable**

Cyclical vomiting, with refractory migraine

G43.B **Ophthalmoplegic migraine**

G43.B0 **Ophthalmoplegic migraine, not intractable**

Ophthalmoplegic migraine, without refractory migraine

G43.B1 **Ophthalmoplegic migraine, intractable**

Ophthalmoplegic migraine, with refractory migraine

G43.C **Periodic headache syndromes in child or adult**

G43.C0 **Periodic headache syndromes in child or adult, not intractable**

Periodic headache syndromes in child or adult, without refractory migraine

G43.C1 **Periodic headache syndromes in child or adult, intractable**

Periodic headache syndromes in child or adult, with refractory migraine

G43.D **Abdominal migraine**

G43.D0 **Abdominal migraine, not intractable**

Abdominal migraine, without refractory migraine

G43.D1 **Abdominal migraine, intractable**

Abdominal migraine, with refractory migraine

G43.8 **Other migraine**

G43.80 **Other migraine, not intractable**

Other migraine, without refractory migraine

G43.801 **Other migraine, not intractable, with status migrainosus**

G43.809 **Other migraine, not intractable, without status migrainosus**

G43.81 **Other migraine, intractable**

Other migraine, with refractory migraine

G43.811 **Other migraine, intractable, with status migrainosus**

G43.819 **Other migraine, intractable, without status migrainosus**

G43.82 **Menstrual migraine, not intractable**

Menstrual headache, not intractable

Menstrual migraine, without refractory migraine

Menstrually related migraine, not intractable

Pre-menstrual headache, not intractable

Pre-menstrual migraine, not intractable

Pure menstrual migraine, not intractable

<u>Code also</u> associated premenstrual tension syndrome (N94.3)

G43.821 **Menstrual migraine, not intractable, with status migrainosus**

G43.829 **Menstrual migraine, not intractable, without status migrainosus**

Menstrual migraine NOS

G43.83 **Menstrual migraine, intractable**

Menstrual headache, intractable

Menstrual migraine, with refractory migraine

Menstrually related migraine, intractable

Pre-menstrual headache, intractable

Pre-menstrual migraine, intractable

Pure menstrual migraine, intractable

Code also associated premenstrual tension syndrome (N94.3)

> **G43.831** Menstrual migraine, intractable, with status migrainosus
>
> **G43.839** Menstrual migraine, intractable, without status migrainosus

G43.9 Migraine, unspecified

> **G43.90** Migraine, unspecified, not intractable
>
> Migraine, unspecified, without refractory migraine
>
> > **G43.901** Migraine, unspecified, not intractable, with status migrainosus
> >
> > Status migrainosus NOS
> >
> > **G43.909** Migraine, unspecified, not intractable, without status migrainosus
> >
> > Migraine NOS
>
> **G43.91** Migraine, unspecified, intractable
>
> Migraine, unspecified, with refractory migraine
>
> > **G43.911** Migraine, unspecified, intractable, with status migrainosus
> >
> > **G43.919** Migraine, unspecified, intractable, without status migrainosus

G44 Other headache syndromes

Excludes1: headache NOS (R51)

Excludes2: atypical facial pain (G50.1)

headache due to lumbar puncture (G97.1)

migraines (G43.-)

trigeminal neuralgia (G50.0)

G44.0 Cluster headaches and other trigeminal autonomic cephalgias (TAC)

> **G44.00** Cluster headache syndrome, unspecified
>
> Ciliary neuralgia
>
> Cluster headache NOS
>
> Histamine cephalgia
>
> Lower half migraine
>
> Migrainous neuralgia
>
> > **G44.001** Cluster headache syndrome, unspecified, intractable
> >
> > **G44.009** Cluster headache syndrome, unspecified, not intractable
> >
> > Cluster headache syndrome NOS
>
> **G44.01** Episodic cluster headache
>
> > **G44.011** Episodic cluster headache, intractable
> >
> > **G44.019** Episodic cluster headache, not intractable
> >
> > Episodic cluster headache NOS
>
> **G44.02** Chronic cluster headache
>
> > **G44.021** Chronic cluster headache, intractable
> >
> > **G44.029** Chronic cluster headache, not intractable
> >
> > Chronic cluster headache NOS
>
> **G44.03** Episodic paroxysmal hemicrania
>
> Paroxysmal hemicrania NOS
>
> > **G44.031** Episodic paroxysmal hemicrania, intractable

> > **G44.039** Episodic paroxysmal hemicrania, not intractable
> >
> > Episodic paroxysmal hemicrania NOS
>
> **G44.04** Chronic paroxysmal hemicrania
>
> > **G44.041** Chronic paroxysmal hemicrania, intractable
> >
> > **G44.049** Chronic paroxysmal hemicrania, not intractable
> >
> > Chronic paroxysmal hemicrania NOS
>
> **G44.05** Short lasting unilateral neuralgiform headache with conjunctival injection and tearing (SUNCT)
>
> > **G44.051** Short lasting unilateral neuralgiform headache with conjunctival injection and tearing (SUNCT), intractable
> >
> > **G44.059** Short lasting unilateral neuralgiform headache with conjunctival injection and tearing (SUNCT), not intractable
> >
> > Short lasting unilateral neuralgiform headache with conjunctival injection and tearing (SUNCT) NOS
>
> **G44.09** Other trigeminal autonomic cephalgias (TAC)
>
> > **G44.091** Other trigeminal autonomic cephalgias (TAC), intractable
> >
> > **G44.099** Other trigeminal autonomic cephalgias (TAC), not intractable

G44.1 Vascular headache, not elsewhere classified

Excludes2: cluster headache (G44.0)

complicated headache syndromes (G44.5-)

drug-induced headache (G44.4-)

migraine (G43.-)

Other specified headache syndromes (G44.8-)

post-traumatic headache (G44.3-)

tension-type headache (G44.2-)

G44.2 Tension-type headache

> **G44.20** Tension-type headache, unspecified
>
> > **G44.201** Tension-type headache, unspecified, intractable
> >
> > **G44.209** Tension-type headache, unspecified, not intractable
> >
> > Tension headache NOS
>
> **G44.21** Episodic tension-type headache
>
> > **G44.211** Episodic tension-type headache, intractable
> >
> > **G44.219** Episodic tension-type headache, not intractable
> >
> > Episodic tension-type headache NOS
>
> **G44.22** Chronic tension-type headache
>
> > **G44.221** Chronic tension-type headache, intractable
> >
> > **G44.229** Chronic tension-type headache, not intractable
> >
> > Chronic tension-type headache NOS

G44.3 Post-traumatic headache

> **G44.30** Post-traumatic headache, unspecified
>
> > **G44.301** Post-traumatic headache, unspecified, intractable

G44.309 Post-traumatic headache, unspecified, not intractable
Post-traumatic headache NOS

G44.31 Acute post-traumatic headache

G44.311 Acute post-traumatic headache, intractable

G44.319 Acute post-traumatic headache, not intractable
Acute post-traumatic headache NOS

G44.32 Chronic post-traumatic headache

G44.321 Chronic post-traumatic headache, intractable

G44.329 Chronic post-traumatic headache, not intractable
Chronic post-traumatic headache NOS

G44.4 Drug-induced headache, not elsewhere classified
Medication overuse headache
<u>Use additional code</u> for adverse effect, if applicable, to identify drug (T36-T50 with fifth or sixth character 5)

G44.40 Drug-induced headache, not elsewhere classified, not intractable

G44.41 Drug-induced headache, not elsewhere classified, intractable

G44.5 Complicated headache syndromes

G44.51 Hemicrania continua

G44.52 New daily persistent headache (NDPH)

G44.53 Primary thunderclap headache

G44.59 Other complicated headache syndrome

G44.8 Other specified headache syndromes

G44.81 Hypnic headache

G44.82 Headache associated with sexual activity
Orgasmic headache
Preorgasmic headache

G44.83 Primary cough headache

G44.84 Primary exertional headache

G44.85 Primary stabbing headache

G44.89 Other headache syndrome

G45 Transient cerebral ischemic attacks and related syndromes
Definition: Transient cerebral ischemic attack is a brief episode of neurological dysfunction resulting from an interruption in the blood supply to the brain or the eye, sometimes as a precursor to a stroke.
Excludes1: neonatal cerebral ischemia (P91.0)
transient retinal artery occlusion (H34.0-)

G45.0 Vertebro-basilar artery syndrome

G45.1 Carotid artery syndrome (hemispheric)

G45.2 Multiple and bilateral precerebral artery syndromes

G45.3 Amaurosis fugax

G45.4 Transient global amnesia
Excludes1: amnesia NOS (R41.3)

G45.8 Other transient cerebral ischemic attacks and related syndromes

G45.9 Transient cerebral ischemic attack, unspecified
Spasm of cerebral artery TIA
Transient cerebral ischemia NOS

G46 Vascular syndromes of brain in cerebrovascular diseases
<u>Code first</u> underlying cerebrovascular disease (I60-I69)

G46.0 Middle cerebral artery syndrome

G46.1 Anterior cerebral artery syndrome

G46.2 Posterior cerebral artery syndrome

G46.3 Brain stem stroke syndrome
Benedikt syndrome
Claude syndrome
Foville syndrome
Millard-Gubler syndrome
Wallenberg syndrome
Weber syndrome

G46.4 Cerebellar stroke syndrome

G46.5 Pure motor lacunar syndrome

G46.6 Pure sensory lacunar syndrome

G46.7 Other lacunar syndromes

G46.8 Other vascular syndromes of brain in cerebrovascular diseases

G47 Sleep disorders
Excludes2: nightmares (F51.5)
nonorganic sleep disorders (F51.-)
sleep terrors (F51.4)
sleepwalking (F51.3)

G47.0 Insomnia
Excludes2: alcohol related insomnia (F10.182, F10.282, F10.982)
drug-related insomnia (F11.182, F11.282, F11.982, F13.182, F13.282, F13.982, F14.182, F14.282, F14.982, F15.182, F15.282, F15.982, F19.182, F19.282, F19.982)
idiopathic insomnia (F51.01)
insomnia due to a mental disorder (F51.05)
insomnia not due to a substance or known physiological condition (F51.0-)
nonorganic insomnia (F51.0-)
primary insomnia (F51.01)
sleep apnea (G47.3-)

G47.00 Insomnia, unspecified
Insomnia NOS

G47.01 Insomnia due to medical condition
<u>Code also</u> associated medical condition

G47.09 Other insomnia

G47.1 Hypersomnia
Excludes2: alcohol-related hypersomnia (F10.182, F10.282, F10.982)
drug-related hypersomnia (F11.182, F11.282, F11.982, F13.182, F13.282, F13.982, F14.182, F14.282, F14.982, F15.182, F15.282, F15.982, F19.182, F19.282, F19.982)
hypersomnia due to a mental disorder (F51.13)
hypersomnia not due to a substance or known physiological condition (F51.1-)
primary hypersomnia (F51.11)
sleep apnea (G47.3-)

G47.10 Hypersomnia, unspecified
Hypersomnia NOS

G47.11 Idiopathic hypersomnia with long sleep time
Idiopathic hypersomnia NOS

● New code ▲ Revised code **Excludes1:** Not coded here **Excludes2:** Not included here ⊗ Placeholder required ⑦ 7th digit required

G47.12 **Idiopathic hypersomnia without long sleep time**

G47.13 **Recurrent hypersomnia**
Kleine-Levin syndrome
Menstrual related hypersomnia

G47.14 **Hypersomnia due to medical condition**
Code also associated medical condition

G47.19 **Other hypersomnia**

G47.2 **Circadian rhythm sleep disorders**
Disorders of the sleep wake schedule
Inversion of nyctohemeral rhythm
Inversion of sleep rhythm

G47.20 **Circadian rhythm sleep disorder, unspecified type**
Sleep wake schedule disorder NOS

G47.21 **Circadian rhythm sleep disorder, delayed sleep phase type**
Delayed sleep phase syndrome

G47.22 **Circadian rhythm sleep disorder, advanced sleep phase type**

G47.23 **Circadian rhythm sleep disorder, irregular sleep wake type**
Irregular sleep-wake pattern

G47.24 **Circadian rhythm sleep disorder, free running type**

G47.25 **Circadian rhythm sleep disorder, jet lag type**

G47.26 **Circadian rhythm sleep disorder, shift work type**

G47.27 **Circadian rhythm sleep disorder in conditions classified elsewhere**
Code first underlying condition

G47.29 **Other circadian rhythm sleep disorder**

G47.3 **Sleep apnea**
Definition: Sleep apnea is a potentially serious sleep disorder in which breathing repeatedly stops and starts.
Code also any associated underlying condition
Excludes1: apnea NOS (R06.81)
Cheyne-Stokes breathing (R06.3)
pickwickian syndrome (E66.2)
sleep apnea of newborn (P28.3)

G47.30 **Sleep apnea, unspecified**
Sleep apnea NOS

G47.31 **Primary central sleep apnea**

G47.32 **High altitude periodic breathing**

G47.33 **Obstructive sleep apnea (adult) (pediatric)**
Excludes1: obstructive sleep apnea of newborn (P28.3)

G47.34 **Idiopathic sleep related nonobstructive alveolar hypoventilation**
Sleep related hypoxia

G47.35 **Congenital central alveolar hypoventilation syndrome**

G47.36 **Sleep related hypoventilation in conditions classified elsewhere**
Sleep related hypoxemia in conditions classified elsewhere
Code first underlying condition

G47.37 **Central sleep apnea in conditions classified elsewhere**
Code first underlying condition

G47.39 **Other sleep apnea**

G47.4 **Narcolepsy and cataplexy**

G47.41 **Narcolepsy**

G47.411 **Narcolepsy with cataplexy**

G47.419 **Narcolepsy without cataplexy**
Narcolepsy NOS

G47.42 **Narcolepsy in conditions classified elsewhere**
Code first underlying condition

G47.421 **Narcolepsy in conditions classified elsewhere with cataplexy**

G47.429 **Narcolepsy in conditions classified elsewhere without cataplexy**

G47.5 **Parasomnia**
Excludes1: alcohol induced parasomnia (F10.182, F10.282, F10.982)
drug induced parasomnia (F11.182, F11.282, F11.982, F13.182, F13.282, F13.982, F14.182, F14.282, F14.982, F15.182, F15.282, F15.982, F19.182, F19.282, F19.982)
parasomnia not due to a substance or known physiological condition (F51.8)

G47.50 **Parasomnia, unspecified**
Parasomnia NOS

G47.51 **Confusional arousals**

G47.52 **REM sleep behavior disorder**

G47.53 **Recurrent isolated sleep paralysis**

G47.54 **Parasomnia in conditions classified elsewhere**
Code first underlying condition

G47.59 **Other parasomnia**

G47.6 **Sleep related movement disorders**
Excludes2: restless legs syndrome (G25.81)

G47.61 **Periodic limb movement disorder**
Periodic limb movement disorder

G47.62 **Sleep related leg cramps**

G47.63 **Sleep related bruxism**
Excludes1: psychogenic bruxism (F45.8)

G47.69 **Other sleep related movement disorders**

G47.8 **Other sleep disorders**

G47.9 **Sleep disorder, unspecified**
Sleep disorder NOS

NERVE, NERVE ROOT AND PLEXUS DISORDERS (G50-G59)

Excludes1: current traumatic nerve, nerve root and plexus disorders - see Injury, nerve by body region
neuralgia NOS (M79.2)
neuritis NOS (M79.2)
peripheral neuritis in pregnancy (O26.82-)
radiculitis NOS (M54.1-)

G50 **Disorders of trigeminal nerve**
Includes: disorders of 5th cranial nerve

G50.0 **Trigeminal neuralgia**
Syndrome of paroxysmal facial pain
Tic douloureux

G50.1 Atypical facial pain

G50.8 Other disorders of trigeminal nerve

G50.9 Disorder of trigeminal nerve, unspecified

G51 Facial nerve disorders

Definition: Facial nerve disorders refers to a disorder resulting from a weakness of the facial nerve. Bell's palsy is an example of a facial nerve disorder.

Includes: disorders of 7th cranial nerve

G51.0 Bell's palsy

Facial palsy

G51.1 Geniculate ganglionitis

Excludes1: postherpetic geniculate ganglionitis (B02.21)

G51.2 Melkersson's syndrome

Melkersson-Rosenthal syndrome

G51.3 Clonic hemifacial spasm

G51.4 Facial myokymia

G51.8 Other disorders of facial nerve

G51.9 Disorder of facial nerve, unspecified

G52 Disorders of other cranial nerves

Excludes2: disorders of acoustic [8th] nerve (H93.3)

disorders of optic [2nd] nerve (H46, H47.0)

paralytic strabismus due to nerve palsy (H49.0-H49.2)

G52.0 Disorders of olfactory nerve

Disorders of 1st cranial nerve

G52.1 Disorders of glossopharyngeal nerve

Disorder of 9th cranial nerve

Glossopharyngeal neuralgia

G52.2 Disorders of vagus nerve

Disorders of pneumogastric [10th] nerve

G52.3 Disorders of hypoglossal nerve

Disorders of 12th cranial nerve

G52.7 Disorders of multiple cranial nerves

Polyneuritis cranialis

G52.8 Disorders of other specified cranial nerves

G52.9 Cranial nerve disorder, unspecified

G53 Cranial nerve disorders in diseases classified elsewhere

Code first underlying disease, such as:

neoplasm (C00-D49)

Excludes1: multiple cranial nerve palsy in sarcoidosis (D86.82)

multiple cranial nerve palsy in syphilis (A52.15)

postherpetic geniculate ganglionitis (B02.21)

postherpetic trigeminal neuralgia (B02.22)

G54 Nerve root and plexus disorders

Definition: A nerve root is the initial segment of a nerve leaving the central nervous system. Plexus refers to a network of intersecting nerves and blood vessels or of lymphatic vessels. The body contains many plexuses, such as the brachial plexus, the cardiac plexus, the cervical plexus, and the lumbar plexus.

Excludes1: current traumatic nerve root and plexus disorders - see nerve injury by body region

intervertebral disc disorders (M50-M51)

neuralgia or neuritis NOS (M79.2)

neuritis or radiculitis brachial NOS (M54.13)

neuritis or radiculitis lumbar NOS (M54.16)

neuritis or radiculitis lumbosacral NOS (M54.17)

neuritis or radiculitis thoracic NOS (M54.14)

radiculitis NOS (M54.10)

radiculopathy NOS (M54.10)

spondylosis (M47.-)

G54.0 Brachial plexus disorders

Thoracic outlet syndrome

G54.1 Lumbosacral plexus disorders

G54.2 Cervical root disorders, not elsewhere classified

G54.3 Thoracic root disorders, not elsewhere classified

G54.4 Lumbosacral root disorders, not elsewhere classified

G54.5 Neuralgic amyotrophy

Parsonage-Aldren-Turner syndrome

Shoulder-girdle neuritis

Excludes1: neuralgic amyotrophy in diabetes mellitus (E08-E13 with .44)

G54.6 Phantom limb syndrome with pain

G54.7 Phantom limb syndrome without pain

Phantom limb syndrome NOS

G54.8 Other nerve root and plexus disorders

G54.9 Nerve root and plexus disorder, unspecified

G55 Nerve root and plexus compressions in diseases classified elsewhere

Code first underlying disease, such as:

neoplasm (C00-D49)

Excludes1: nerve root compression (due to) (in) ankylosing spondylitis (M45.-)

nerve root compression (due to) (in) dorsopathies (M53.-, M54.-)

nerve root compression (due to) (in) intervertebral disc disorders (M50.1-, M51.1.-)

nerve root compression (due to) (in) spondylopathies (M46.-, M48.-)

nerve root compression (due to) (in) spondylosis (M47.0-M47.2.-)

G56 Mononeuropathies of upper limb

Definition: **Mononeuropathy:** A disorder of a single nerve or nerve trunk. Mononeuropathies may be due to entrapment, compression, stretch injury, ischemia, infection, or inflammation of a nerve.

Excludes1: current traumatic nerve disorder - see nerve injury by body region

G56.0 Carpal tunnel syndrome

G56.00 Carpal tunnel syndrome, unspecified upper limb

G56.01 Carpal tunnel syndrome, right upper limb

G56.02 Carpal tunnel syndrome, left upper limb

●**G56.03 Carpal tunnel syndrome, bilateral upper limbs**

G56.1 Other lesions of median nerve

G56.10 Other lesions of median nerve, unspecified upper limb

G56.11 Other lesions of median nerve, right upper limb

G56.12 Other lesions of median nerve, left upper limb

●**G56.13 Other lesions of median nerve, bilateral upper limbs**

G56.2 Lesion of ulnar nerve

Tardy ulnar nerve palsy

G56.20   Lesion of ulnar nerve, unspecified upper limb

G56.21   Lesion of ulnar nerve, right upper limb

G56.22   Lesion of ulnar nerve, left upper limb

●G56.23   Lesion of ulnar nerve, bilateral upper limbs

G56.3   **Lesion of radial nerve**

G56.30   Lesion of radial nerve, unspecified upper limb

G56.31   Lesion of radial nerve, right upper limb

G56.32   Lesion of radial nerve, left upper limb

●G56.33   Lesion of radial nerve, bilateral upper limbs

G56.4   **Causalgia of upper limb**

Complex regional pain syndrome II of upper limb

Excludes1: complex regional pain syndrome I of lower limb (G90.52-)

complex regional pain syndrome I of upper limb (G90.51-)

complex regional pain syndrome II of lower limb (G57.7-)

reflex sympathetic dystrophy of lower limb (G90.52-)

reflex sympathetic dystrophy of upper limb (G90.51-)

G56.40   Causalgia of unspecified upper limb

G56.41   Causalgia of right upper limb

G56.42   Causalgia of left upper limb

●G56.43   Causalgia of bilateral upper limbs

G56.8   **Other specified mononeuropathies of upper limb**

Interdigital neuroma of upper limb

G56.80   Other specified mononeuropathies of unspecified upper limb

G56.81   Other specified mononeuropathies of right upper limb

G56.82   Other specified mononeuropathies of left upper limb

●G56.83   Other specified mononeuropathies of bilateral upper limbs

G56.9   **Unspecified mononeuropathy of upper limb**

G56.90   Unspecified mononeuropathy of unspecified upper limb

G56.91   Unspecified mononeuropathy of right upper limb

G56.92   Unspecified mononeuropathy of left upper limb

●G56.93   Unspecified mononeuropathy of bilateral upper limbs

G57   **Mononeuropathies of lower limb**

Excludes1: current traumatic nerve disorder - see nerve injury by body region

G57.0   **Lesion of sciatic nerve**

Excludes1: sciatica NOS (M54.3-)

Excludes2: sciatica attributed to intervertebral disc disorder (M51.1.-)

G57.00   Lesion of sciatic nerve, unspecified lower limb

G57.01   Lesion of sciatic nerve, right lower limb

G57.02   Lesion of sciatic nerve, left lower limb

●G57.03   Lesion of sciatic nerve, bilateral lower limbs

G57.1   **Meralgia paresthetica**

Lateral cutaneous nerve of thigh syndrome

G57.10   Meralgia paresthetica, unspecified lower limb

G57.11   Meralgia paresthetica, right lower limb

G57.12   Meralgia paresthetica, left lower limb

●G57.13   Meralgia paresthetica, bilateral lower limbs

G57.2   **Lesion of femoral nerve**

G57.20   Lesion of femoral nerve, unspecified lower limb

G57.21   Lesion of femoral nerve, right lower limb

G57.22   Lesion of femoral nerve, left lower limb

●G57.23   Lesion of femoral nerve, bilateral lower limbs

G57.3   **Lesion of lateral popliteal nerve**

Peroneal nerve palsy

G57.30   Lesion of lateral popliteal nerve, unspecified lower limb

G57.31   Lesion of lateral popliteal nerve, right lower limb

G57.32   Lesion of lateral popliteal nerve, left lower limb

●G57.33   Lesion of lateral popliteal nerve, bilateral lower limbs

G57.4   **Lesion of medial popliteal nerve**

G57.40   Lesion of medial popliteal nerve, unspecified lower limb

G57.41   Lesion of medial popliteal nerve, right lower limb

G57.42   Lesion of medial popliteal nerve, left lower limb

●G57.43   Lesion of medial popliteal nerve, bilateral lower limbs

G57.5   **Tarsal tunnel syndrome**

G57.50   Tarsal tunnel syndrome, unspecified lower limb

G57.51   Tarsal tunnel syndrome, right lower limb

G57.52   Tarsal tunnel syndrome, left lower limb

●G57.53   Tarsal tunnel syndrome, bilateral lower limbs

G57.6   **Lesion of plantar nerve**

Morton's metatarsalgia

G57.60   Lesion of plantar nerve, unspecified lower limb

G57.61   Lesion of plantar nerve, right lower limb

G57.62   Lesion of plantar nerve, left lower limb

●G57.63   Lesion of plantar nerve, bilateral lower limbs

G57.7   **Causalgia of lower limb**

Complex regional pain syndrome II of lower limb

Excludes1: complex regional pain syndrome I of lower limb (G90.52-)

complex regional pain syndrome I of upper limb (G90.51-)

complex regional pain syndrome II of upper limb (G56.4-)

reflex sympathetic dystrophy of lower limb (G90.52-)

reflex sympathetic dystrophy of upper limb (G90.51-)

G57.70   Causalgia of unspecified lower limb

G57.71   Causalgia of right lower limb

G57.72   Causalgia of left lower limb

●G57.73   Causalgia of bilateral lower limbs

G57.8   **Other specified mononeuropathies of lower limb**

Interdigital neuroma of lower limb

G57.80 **Other specified mononeuropathies of unspecified lower limb**

G57.81 **Other specified mononeuropathies of right lower limb**

G57.82 **Other specified mononeuropathies of left lower limb**

•**G57.83** **Other specified mononeuropathies of bilateral lower limbs**

G57.9 **Unspecified mononeuropathy of lower limb**

G57.90 **Unspecified mononeuropathy of unspecified lower limb**

G57.91 **Unspecified mononeuropathy of right lower limb**

G57.92 **Unspecified mononeuropathy of left lower limb**

•**G57.93** **Unspecified mononeuropathy of bilateral lower limbs**

G58 **Other mononeuropathies**

G58.0 **Intercostal neuropathy**

G58.7 **Mononeuritis multiplex**

G58.8 **Other specified mononeuropathies**

G58.9 **Mononeuropathy, unspecified**

G59 **Mononeuropathy in diseases classified elsewhere**

Code first underlying disease

Excludes1: diabetic mononeuropathy (E08-E13 with .41)

syphilitic nerve paralysis (A52.19)

syphilitic neuritis (A52.15)

tuberculous mononeuropathy (A17.83)

POLYNEUROPATHIES AND OTHER DISORDERS OF THE PERIPHERAL NERVOUS SYSTEM (G60-G65)

Definition: Polyneuropathy is damage or disease affecting peripheral nerves (peripheral neuropathy) in roughly the same areas on both sides of the body, featuring weakness, numbness, pins-and-needles and burning pain.

Excludes1: neuralgia NOS (M79.2)

neuritis NOS (M79.2)

peripheral neuritis in pregnancy (O26.82-)

radiculitis NOS (M54.10)

G60 **Hereditary and idiopathic neuropathy**

G60.0 **Hereditary motor and sensory neuropathy**

Charcot-Marie-Tooth disease

Déjérine-Sottas disease

Hereditary motor and sensory neuropathy, types I-IV

Hypertrophic neuropathy of infancy

Peroneal muscular atrophy (axonal type) (hypertrophic type)

Roussy-Levy syndrome

G60.1 **Refsum's disease**

Infantile Refsum disease

G60.2 **Neuropathy in association with hereditary ataxia**

G60.3 **Idiopathic progressive neuropathy**

G60.8 **Other hereditary and idiopathic neuropathies**

Dominantly inherited sensory neuropathy

Morvan's disease

Nelaton's syndrome

Recessively inherited sensory neuropathy

G60.9 **Hereditary and idiopathic neuropathy, unspecified**

G61 **Inflammatory polyneuropathy**

G61.0 **Guillain-Barre syndrome**

Acute (post-)infective polyneuritis

Miller Fisher Syndrome

G61.1 **Serum neuropathy**

Use additional code for adverse effect, if applicable, to identify serum (T50.-)

G61.8 **Other inflammatory polyneuropathies**

G61.81 **Chronic inflammatory demyelinating polyneuritis**

•**G61.82** **Multifocal motor neuropathy**

MMN

G61.89 **Other inflammatory polyneuropathies**

G61.9 **Inflammatory polyneuropathy, unspecified**

G62 **Other and unspecified polyneuropathies**

G62.0 **Drug-induced polyneuropathy**

Use additional code for adverse effect, if applicable, to identify drug (T36-T50 with fifth or sixth character 5)

G62.1 **Alcoholic polyneuropathy**

G62.2 **Polyneuropathy due to other toxic agents**

Code first (T51-T65) to identify toxic agent

G62.8 **Other specified polyneuropathies**

G62.81 **Critical illness polyneuropathy**

Acute motor neuropathy

G62.82 **Radiation-induced polyneuropathy**

Use additional external cause code (W88-W90, X39.0-) to identify cause

G62.89 **Other specified polyneuropathies**

G62.9 **Polyneuropathy, unspecified**

Neuropathy NOS

G63 **Polyneuropathy in diseases classified elsewhere**

Code first underlying disease, such as:

amyloidosis (E85.-)

endocrine disease, except diabetes (E00-E07, E15-E16, E20-E34)

metabolic diseases (E70-E88)

neoplasm (C00-D49)

nutritional deficiency (E40-E64)

Excludes1: polyneuropathy (in):

diabetes mellitus (E08-E13 with .42)

diphtheria (A36.83)

infectious mononucleosis (B27.0-B27.9 with 1)

Lyme disease (A69.22)

mumps (B26.84)

postherpetic (B02.23)

rheumatoid arthritis (M05.33)

scleroderma (M34.83)

systemic lupus erythematosus (M32.19)

G64 **Other disorders of peripheral nervous system**

Disorder of peripheral nervous system NOS

G65 **Sequelae of inflammatory and toxic polyneuropathies**

Code first condition resulting from (sequela) of inflammatory and toxic polyneuropathies

G65.0 **Sequelae of Guillain-Barré syndrome**

G65.1 **Sequelae of other inflammatory polyneuropathy**

G65.2 **Sequelae of toxic polyneuropathy**

DISEASES OF MYONEURAL JUNCTION AND MUSCLE (G70-G73)

G70 **Myasthenia gravis and other myoneural disorders**

Excludes1: botulism (A05.1, A48.51-A48.52)

transient neonatal myasthenia gravis (P94.0)

G70.0 **Myasthenia gravis**

G70.00 **Myasthenia gravis without (acute) exacerbation**

Myasthenia gravis NOS

G70.01 **Myasthenia gravis with (acute) exacerbation**

Myasthenia gravis in crisis

G70.1 **Toxic myoneural disorders**

Code first (T51-T65) to identify toxic agent

G70.2 **Congenital and developmental myasthenia**

G70.8 **Other specified myoneural disorders**

G70.80 **Lambert-Eaton syndrome, unspecified**

Lambert-Eaton syndrome NOS

G70.81 **Lambert-Eaton syndrome in disease classified elsewhere**

Code first underlying disease

Excludes1: Lambert-Eaton syndrome in neoplastic disease (G73.1)

G70.89 **Other specified myoneural disorders**

G70.9 **Myoneural disorder, unspecified**

G71 **Primary disorders of muscles**

Excludes2: arthrogryposis multiplex congenita (Q74.3)

metabolic disorders (E70-E88)

myositis (M60.-)

G71.0 **Muscular dystrophy**

Definition: Muscular dystrophy refers to a group of genetic, hereditary muscle diseases that weaken the muscles that move the human body. Muscular dystrophies are characterized by progressive skeletal muscle weakness, defects in muscle proteins, and the death of muscle cells and tissue.

Autosomal recessive, childhood type, muscular dystrophy resembling Duchenne or Becker muscular dystrophy

Benign [Becker] muscular dystrophy

Benign scapuloperoneal muscular dystrophy with early contractures [Emery-Dreifuss]

Congenital muscular dystrophy NOS

Congenital muscular dystrophy with specific morphological abnormalities of the muscle fiber

Distal muscular dystrophy

Facioscapulohumeral muscular dystrophy

Limb-girdle muscular dystrophy

Ocular muscular dystrophy

Oculopharyngeal muscular dystrophy

Scapuloperoneal muscular dystrophy

Severe [Duchenne] muscular dystrophy

G71.1 **Myotonic disorders**

G71.11 **Myotonic muscular dystrophy**

Dystrophia myotonica [Steinert]

Myotonia atrophica

Myotonic dystrophy

Proximal myotonic myopathy (PROMM)

Steinert disease

G71.12 **Myotonia congenita**

Acetazolamide responsive myotonia congenita

Dominant myotonia congenita [Thomsen disease]

Myotonia levior

Recessive myotonia congenita [Becker disease]

G71.13 **Myotonic chondrodystrophy**

Chondrodystrophic myotonia

Congenital myotonic chondrodystrophy

Schwartz-Jampel disease

G71.14 **Drug induced myotonia**

Use additional code for adverse effect, if applicable, to identify drug (T36-T50 with fifth or sixth

character 5)

G71.19 **Other specified myotonic disorders**

Myotonia fluctuans

Myotonia permanens Neuromyotonia [Isaacs]

Paramyotonia congenita (of von Eulenburg)

Pseudomyotonia

Symptomatic myotonia

G71.2 **Congenital myopathies**

Central core disease

Fiber-type disproportion

Minicore disease

Multicore disease

Myotubular (centronuclear) myopathy Nemaline myopathy

Excludes1: arthrogryposis multiplex congenita (Q74.3)

G71.3 **Mitochondrial myopathy, not elsewhere classified**

Excludes1: Kearns-Sayre syndrome (H49.81)

Leber's disease (H47.21)

Leigh's encephalopathy (G31.82)

mitochondrial metabolism disorders (E88.4.-)

Reye's syndrome (G93.7)

G71.8 **Other primary disorders of muscles**

G71.9 **Primary disorder of muscle, unspecified**

Hereditary myopathy NOS

G72 **Other and unspecified myopathies**

Excludes1: arthrogryposis multiplex congenita (Q74.3)

dermatopolymyositis (M33.-)

ischemic infarction of muscle (M62.2-)

myositis (M60.-)

polymyositis (M33.2.-)

G72.0 **Drug-induced myopathy**

Use additional code for adverse effect, if applicable, to identify drug (T36-T50 with fifth or sixth character 5)

G72.1 **Alcoholic myopathy**

Use additional code to identify alcoholism (F10.-)

G72.2 **Myopathy due to other toxic agents**

Code first (T51-T65) to identify toxic agent

G72.3 **Periodic paralysis**

Familial periodic paralysis

Hyperkalemic periodic paralysis (familial)

Hypokalemic periodic paralysis (familial)

Myotonic periodic paralysis (familial)

Normokalemic paralysis (familial)

Potassium sensitive periodic paralysis

> **Excludes1:** paramyotonia congenita (of von Eulenburg) (G71.19)

G72.4 **Inflammatory and immune myopathies, not elsewhere classified**

G72.41 **Inclusion body myositis [IBM]**

G72.49 **Other inflammatory and immune myopathies, not elsewhere classified**

Inflammatory myopathy NOS

G72.8 **Other specified myopathies**

G72.81 **Critical illness myopathy**

Acute necrotizing myopathy

Acute quadriplegic myopathy

Intensive care (ICU)

myopathy

Myopathy of critical illness

G72.89 **Other specified myopathies**

G72.9 **Myopathy, unspecified**

G73 **Disorders of myoneural junction and muscle in diseases classified elsewhere**

G73.1 **Lambert-Eaton syndrome in neoplastic disease**

Code first underlying neoplasm (C00-D49)

> **Excludes1:** Lambert-Eaton syndrome not associated with neoplasm (G70.80-G70.81)

G73.3 **Myasthenic syndromes in other diseases classified elsewhere**

Code first underlying disease, such as:

neoplasm (C00-D49)

thyrotoxicosis (E05.-)

G73.7 **Myopathy in diseases classified elsewhere**

Code first underlying disease, such as:

hyperparathyroidism (E21.0, E21.3)

hypoparathyroidism (E20.-)

glycogen storage disease (E74.0)

lipid storage disorders (E75.-)

> **Excludes1:** myopathy in:
>
> rheumatoid arthritis (M05.32)
>
> sarcoidosis (D86.87)
>
> scleroderma (M34.82)
>
> sicca syndrome [Sjögren] (M35.03)
>
> systemic lupus erythematosus (M32.19)

CEREBRAL PALSY AND OTHER PARALYTIC SYNDROMES (G80-G83)

Definition: Cerebral palsy is a condition marked by impaired muscle coordination (spastic paralysis) and/or other disabilities, typically caused by damage to the brain before or at birth.

G80 **Cerebral palsy**

> **Excludes1:** hereditary spastic paraplegia (G11.4)

G80.0 **Spastic quadriplegic cerebral palsy**

Congenital spastic paralysis (cerebral)

G80.1 **Spastic diplegic cerebral palsy**

Spastic cerebral palsy NOS

G80.2 **Spastic hemiplegic cerebral palsy**

G80.3 **Athetoid cerebral palsy**

Double athetosis (syndrome)

Dyskinetic cerebral palsy

Dystonic cerebral palsy

Vogt disease

G80.4 **Ataxic cerebral palsy**

G80.8 **Other cerebral palsy**

Mixed cerebral palsy syndromes

G80.9 **Cerebral palsy, unspecified**

Cerebral palsy NOS

G81 **Hemiplegia and hemiparesis**

Definition: Hemiplegia is defined as paralysis or loss of voluntary motion, on one side of the body; may include head and neck, trunk and/or limbs. Hemiparesis is weakness on one side of the body.

Note: This category is to be used only when hemiplegia (complete)(incomplete) is reported without further specification, or is stated to be old or longstanding but of unspecified cause. The category is also for use in multiple coding to identify these types of hemiplegia resulting from any cause.

> **Excludes1:** congenital cerebral palsy (G80.-)

hemiplegia and hemiparesis due to sequela of cerebrovascular disease (I69.05-, I69.15-, I69.25-I69.35-, I69.85-, I69.95-)

G81.0 **Flaccid hemiplegia**

G81.00 **Flaccid hemiplegia affecting unspecified side**

G81.01 **Flaccid hemiplegia affecting right dominant side**

G81.02 **Flaccid hemiplegia affecting left dominant side**

G81.03 **Flaccid hemiplegia affecting right nondominant side**

G81.04 **Flaccid hemiplegia affecting left nondominant side**

G81.1 **Spastic hemiplegia**

G81.10 **Spastic hemiplegia affecting unspecified side**

G81.11 **Spastic hemiplegia affecting right dominant side**

G81.12 **Spastic hemiplegia affecting left dominant side**

G81.13 **Spastic hemiplegia affecting right nondominant side**

G81.14 **Spastic hemiplegia affecting left nondominant side**

G81.9 **Hemiplegia, unspecified**

G81.90 **Hemiplegia, unspecified affecting unspecified side**

G81.91 **Hemiplegia, unspecified affecting right dominant side**

G81.92 **Hemiplegia, unspecified affecting left dominant side**

G81.93 **Hemiplegia, unspecified affecting right nondominant side**

G81.94 **Hemiplegia, unspecified affecting left nondominant side**

G82 **Paraplegia (paraparesis) and quadriplegia (quadriparesis)**

Note: This category is to be used only when the listed conditions are reported without further specification, or are stated to be old or longstanding but of unspecified cause. The category is also for use in multiple coding to identify these conditions resulting from any cause

Excludes1: congenital cerebral palsy (G80.-)

functional quadriplegia (R53.2)

hysterical paralysis (F44.4)

G82.2 Paraplegia

Paralysis of both lower limbs NOS

Paraparesis (lower) NOS

Paraplegia (lower) NOS

G82.20 Paraplegia, unspecified

G82.21 Paraplegia, complete

G82.22 Paraplegia, incomplete

G82.5 Quadriplegia

G82.50 Quadriplegia, unspecified

G82.51 Quadriplegia, C1-C4 complete

G82.52 Quadriplegia, C1-C4 incomplete

G82.53 Quadriplegia, C5-C7 complete

G82.54 Quadriplegia, C5-C7 incomplete

G83 Other paralytic syndromes

Note: This category is to be used only when the listed conditions are reported without further specification, or are stated to be old or longstanding but of unspecified cause. The category is also for use in multiple coding to identify these conditions resulting from any cause.

Includes: paralysis (complete) (incomplete), except as in G80-G82

G83.0 Diplegia of upper limbs

Diplegia (upper)

Paralysis of both upper limbs

G83.1 Monoplegia of lower limb

Paralysis of lower limb

Excludes1: monoplegia of lower limbs due to sequela of cerebrovascular disease (I69.04-, I69.14-, I69.24-, I69.34-, I69.84-, I69.94-)

G83.10 Monoplegia of lower limb affecting unspecified side

G83.11 Monoplegia of lower limb affecting right dominant side

G83.12 Monoplegia of lower limb affecting left dominant side

G83.13 Monoplegia of lower limb affecting right nondominant side

G83.14 Monoplegia of lower limb affecting left nondominant side

G83.2 Monoplegia of upper limb

Paralysis of upper limb

Excludes1: monoplegia of upper limbs due to sequela of cerebrovascular disease (I69.03-, I69.13-, I69.23-, I69.33-, I69.83-, I69.93-)

G83.20 Monoplegia of upper limb affecting unspecified side

G83.21 Monoplegia of upper limb affecting right dominant side

G83.22 Monoplegia of upper limb affecting left dominant side

G83.23 Monoplegia of upper limb affecting right nondominant side

G83.24 Monoplegia of upper limb affecting left nondominant side

G83.3 Monoplegia, unspecified

G83.30 Monoplegia, unspecified affecting unspecified side

G83.31 Monoplegia, unspecified affecting right dominant side

G83.32 Monoplegia, unspecified affecting left dominant side

G83.33 Monoplegia, unspecified affecting right nondominant side

G83.34 Monoplegia, unspecified affecting left nondominant side

G83.4 Cauda equina syndrome

Neurogenic bladder due to cauda equina syndrome

Excludes1: cord bladder NOS (G95.89)

neurogenic bladder NOS (N31.9)

G83.5 Locked-in state

G83.8 Other specified paralytic syndromes

Excludes1: paralytic syndromes due to current spinal cord injury-code to spinal cord injury (S14, S24, S34)

G83.81 Brown-Séquard syndrome

G83.82 Anterior cord syndrome

G83.83 Posterior cord syndrome

G83.84 Todd's paralysis (postepileptic)

G83.89 Other specified paralytic syndromes

G83.9 Paralytic syndrome, unspecified

OTHER DISORDERS OF THE NERVOUS SYSTEM (G89-G99)

G89 Pain, not elsewhere classified

Code also related psychological factors associated with pain (F45.42)

Excludes1: generalized pain NOS (R52)

pain disorders exclusively related to psychological factors (F45.41)

pain NOS (R52)

Excludes2: atypical face pain (G50.1)

headache syndromes (G44.-)

localized pain, unspecified type - code to pain by site, such as: abdomen pain (R10.-)

back pain (M54.9)

breast pain (N64.4)

chest pain (R07.1-R07.9)

ear pain (H92.0-)

eye pain (H57.1)

headache (R51)

joint pain (M25.5-)

limb pain (M79.6-)

lumbar region pain (M54.5)

painful urination (R30.9)

pelvic and perineal pain (R10.2)

shoulder pain (M25.51-)

spine pain (M54.-)

throat pain (R07.0)

tongue pain (K14.6)

tooth pain (K08.8)

renal colic (N23)

migraines (G43.-)

myalgia (M79.1)

pain from prosthetic devices, implants, and grafts (T82.84, T83.84, T84.84, T85.84-)

phantom limb syndrome with pain (G54.6)

vulvar vestibulitis (N94.810)

vulvodynia (N94.81-)

G89.0 Central pain syndrome

Déjérine-Roussy syndrome

Myelopathic pain syndrome

Thalamic pain syndrome (hyperesthetic)

G89.1 Acute pain, not elsewhere classified

    G89.11 Acute pain due to trauma

    G89.12 Acute post-thoracotomy pain

       Post-thoracotomy pain NOS

    G89.18 Other acute postprocedural pain

       Postoperative pain NOS

       Postprocedural pain NOS

G89.2 Chronic pain, not elsewhere classified

    Excludes1: causalgia, lower limb (G57.7-)

       causalgia, upper limb (G56.4-)

       central pain syndrome (G89.0)

       chronic pain syndrome (G89.4)

       complex regional pain syndrome II, lower limb (G57.7-)

       complex regional pain syndrome II, upper limb (G56.4-)

       neoplasm related chronic pain (G89.3)

       reflex sympathetic dystrophy (G90.5-)

    G89.21 Chronic pain due to trauma

    G89.22 Chronic post-thoracotomy pain

    G89.28 Other chronic postprocedural pain

       Other chronic postoperative pain

    G89.29 Other chronic pain

G89.3 Neoplasm related pain (acute) (chronic)

Cancer associated pain

Pain due to malignancy (primary) (secondary)

Tumor associated pain

G89.4 Chronic pain syndrome

Chronic pain associated with significant psychosocial dysfunction

G90 Disorders of autonomic nervous system

Excludes1: dysfunction of the autonomic nervous system due to alcohol (G31.2)

G90.0 Idiopathic peripheral autonomic neuropathy

    G90.01 Carotid sinus syncope

       Carotid sinus syndrome

    G90.09 Other idiopathic peripheral autonomic neuropathy

       Idiopathic peripheral autonomic neuropathy NOS

G90.1 Familial dysautonomia [Riley-Day]

G90.2 Horner's syndrome

Bernard(-Horner) syndrome

Cervical sympathetic dystrophy or paralysis

G90.3 Multi-system degeneration of the autonomic nervous system

Neurogenic orthostatic hypotension [Shy-Drager]

Excludes1: orthostatic hypotension NOS (I95.1)

G90.4 Autonomic dysreflexia

Use additional code to identify the cause, such as:

fecal impaction (K56.41)

pressure ulcer (pressure area) (L89.-)

urinary tract infection (N39.0)

G90.5 Complex regional pain syndrome I (CRPS I)

Reflex sympathetic dystrophy

Excludes1: causalgia of lower limb (G57.7-)

    causalgia of upper limb (G56.4-)

    complex regional pain syndrome II of lower limb (G57.7-)

    complex regional pain syndrome II of upper limb (G56.4-)

    G90.50 Complex regional pain syndrome I, unspecified

    G90.51 Complex regional pain syndrome I of upper limb

       G90.511 Complex regional pain syndrome I of right upper limb

       G90.512 Complex regional pain syndrome I of left upper limb

       G90.513 Complex regional pain syndrome I of upper limb, bilateral

       G90.519 Complex regional pain syndrome I of unspecified upper limb

    G90.52 Complex regional pain syndrome I of lower limb

       G90.521 Complex regional pain syndrome I of right lower limb

       G90.522 Complex regional pain syndrome I of left lower limb

       G90.523 Complex regional pain syndrome I of lower limb, bilateral

       G90.529 Complex regional pain syndrome I of unspecified lower limb

    G90.59 Complex regional pain syndrome I of other specified site

G90.8 Other disorders of autonomic nervous system

G90.9 Disorder of the autonomic nervous system, unspecified

G91 Hydrocephalus

Includes: acquired hydrocephalus

Excludes1: Arnold-Chiari syndrome with hydrocephalus (Q07.-)

congenital hydrocephalus (Q03.-)

spina bifida with hydrocephalus (Q05.-)

G91.0 Communicating hydrocephalus

Secondary normal pressure hydrocephalus

G91.1 Obstructive hydrocephalus

G91.2 (Idiopathic) normal pressure hydrocephalus

Normal pressure hydrocephalus NOS

G91.3 Post-traumatic hydrocephalus, unspecified

G91.4 Hydrocephalus in diseases classified elsewhere

Code first underlying condition, such as:

congenital syphilis (A50.4-)

neoplasm (C00-D49)

Excludes1: hydrocephalus due to congenital toxoplasmosis (P37.1)

G91.8   **Other hydrocephalus**

G91.9   **Hydrocephalus, unspecified**

G92   **Toxic encephalopathy**

Toxic encephalitis

Toxic metabolic encephalopathy

Code first (T51-T65) to identify toxic agent

G93   **Other disorders of brain**

  G93.0   **Cerebral cysts**

    Arachnoid cyst

    Porencephalic cyst, acquired

    Excludes1: acquired periventricular cysts of newborn (P91.1)

        congenital cerebral cysts (Q04.6)

  G93.1   **Anoxic brain damage, not elsewhere classified**

    Excludes1: cerebral anoxia due to anesthesia during labor and delivery (O74.3)

        cerebral anoxia due to anesthesia during the puerperium (O89.2)

        neonatal anoxia (P84)

  G93.2   **Benign intracranial hypertension**

    Excludes1: hypertensive encephalopathy (I67.4)

  G93.3   **Postviral fatigue syndrome**

    Benign myalgic encephalomyelitis

    Excludes1: chronic fatigue syndrome NOS (R53.82)

  G93.4   **Other and unspecified encephalopathy**

    Excludes1: alcoholic encephalopathy (G31.2)

        encephalopathy in diseases classified elsewhere (G94)

        hypertensive encephalopathy (I67.4)

        toxic (metabolic) encephalopathy (G92)

    G93.40   **Encephalopathy, unspecified**

    G93.41   **Metabolic encephalopathy**

      Septic encephalopathy

    G93.49   **Other encephalopathy**

      Encephalopathy NEC

  G93.5   **Compression of brain**

    Arnold-Chiari type 1 compression of brain

    Compression of brain (stem)

    Herniation of brain (stem)

    Excludes1: diffuse traumatic compression of brain (S06.2-)

        focal traumatic compression of brain (S06.3-)

  G93.6   **Cerebral edema**

    Excludes1: cerebral edema due to birth injury (P11.0)

        traumatic cerebral edema (S06.1-)

  G93.7   **Reye's syndrome**

    Code first (T39.0-), if salicylates-induced

  G93.8   **Other specified disorders of brain**

    G93.81   **Temporal sclerosis**

      Hippocampal sclerosis

      Mesial temporal sclerosis

    G93.82   **Brain death**

    G93.89   **Other specified disorders of brain**

      Postradiation encephalopathy

  G93.9   **Disorder of brain, unspecified**

G94   **Other disorders of brain in diseases classified elsewhere**

Code first underlying disease

Excludes1: encephalopathy in congenital syphilis (A50.49)

    encephalopathy in influenza (J09.X9, J10.81, J11.81)

    encephalopathy in syphilis (A52.19)

    hydrocephalus in diseases classified elsewhere (G91.4)

G95   **Other and unspecified diseases of spinal cord**

Excludes2: myelitis (G04.-)

  G95.0   **Syringomyelia and syringobulbia**

  G95.1   **Vascular myelopathies**

    Excludes2: intraspinal phlebitis and thrombophlebitis, except non-pyogenic (G08)

    G95.11   **Acute infarction of spinal cord (embolic) (nonembolic)**

      Anoxia of spinal cord

      Arterial thrombosis of spinal cord

    G95.19   **Other vascular myelopathies**

      Edema of spinal cord

      Hematomyelia

      Nonpyogenic intraspinal phlebitis and thrombophlebitis

      Subacute necrotic myelopathy

  G95.2   **Other and unspecified cord compression**

    G95.20   **Unspecified cord compression**

    G95.29   **Other cord compression**

  G95.8   **Other specified diseases of spinal cord**

    Excludes1: neurogenic bladder NOS (N31.9)

        neurogenic bladder due to cauda equina syndrome (G83.4)

        neuromuscular dysfunction of bladder without spinal cord lesion (N31.-)

    G95.81   **Conus medullaris syndrome**

    G95.89   **Other specified diseases of spinal cord**

      Cord bladder NOS

      Drug-induced myelopathy

      Radiation-induced myelopathy

      Excludes1: myelopathy NOS (G95.9)

  G95.9   **Disease of spinal cord, unspecified**

    Myelopathy NOS

G96   **Other disorders of central nervous system**

  G96.0   **Cerebrospinal fluid leak**

    Excludes1: cerebrospinal fluid leak from spinal puncture (G97.0)

  G96.1   **Disorders of meninges, not elsewhere classified**

    G96.11   **Dural tear**

      Excludes1: accidental puncture or laceration of dura during a procedure (G97.41)

    G96.12   **Meningeal adhesions (cerebral) (spinal)**

    G96.19   **Other disorders of meninges, not elsewhere classified**

  G96.8   **Other specified disorders of central nervous system**

  G96.9   **Disorder of central nervous system, unspecified**

G97   **Intraoperative and postprocedural complications and disorders of nervous system, not elsewhere classified**

Excludes2: intraoperative and postprocedural cerebrovascular infarction (I97.81-, I97.82-)

G97.0 Cerebrospinal fluid leak from spinal puncture

G97.1 Other reaction to spinal and lumbar puncture

Headache due to lumbar puncture

G97.2 Intracranial hypotension following ventricular shunting

G97.3 Intraoperative hemorrhage and hematoma of a nervous system organ or structure complicating a procedure

Excludes1: intraoperative hemorrhage and hematoma of a nervous system organ or structure due to

accidental puncture and laceration during a procedure (G97.4-)

G97.31 Intraoperative hemorrhage and hematoma of a nervous system organ or structure complicating a nervous system procedure

G97.32 Intraoperative hemorrhage and hematoma of a nervous system organ or structure complicating other procedure

G97.4 Accidental puncture and laceration of a nervous system organ or structure during a procedure

G97.41 Accidental puncture or laceration of dura during a procedure Incidental (inadvertent) durotomy

G97.48 Accidental puncture and laceration of other nervous system organ or structure during a nervous system procedure

G97.49 Accidental puncture and laceration of other nervous system organ or structure during other procedure

G97.5 Postprocedural hemorrhage of a nervous system organ or structure following a procedure

▲**G97.51** Postprocedural hemorrhage of a nervous system organ or structure following a nervous system procedure

▲**G97.52** Postprocedural hemorrhage of a nervous system organ or structure following other procedure

G97.6 Postprocedural hematoma and seroma of a nervous system organ or structure following a procedure

●**G97.61** Postprocedural hematoma of a nervous system organ or structure following a nervous system procedure

●**G97.62** Postprocedural hematoma of a nervous system organ or structure following other procedure

●**G97.63** Postprocedural seroma of a nervous system organ or structure following a nervous system procedure

●**G97.64** Postprocedural seroma of a nervous system organ or structure following other procedure

G97.8 Other intraoperative and postprocedural complications and disorders of nervous system

Use additional code to further specify disorder

G97.81 Other intraoperative complications of nervous system

G97.82 Other postprocedural complications and disorders of nervous system

G98 Other disorders of nervous system not elsewhere classified

Includes: nervous system disorder NOS

G98.0 Neurogenic arthritis, not elsewhere classified

Nonsyphilitic neurogenic arthropathy NEC Nonsyphilitic neurogenic spondylopathy NEC

Excludes1: spondylopathy (in):

syringomyelia and syringobulbia (G95.0)

tabes dorsalis (A52.11)

G98.8 Other disorders of nervous system

Nervous system disorder NOS

G99 Other disorders of nervous system in diseases classified elsewhere

G99.0 Autonomic neuropathy in diseases classified elsewhere

Code first underlying disease, such as:

amyloidosis (E85.-)

gout (M1A.-, M10.-)

hyperthyroidism (E05.-)

Excludes1: diabetic autonomic neuropathy (E08-E13 with .43)

G99.2 Myelopathy in diseases classified elsewhere

Code first underlying disease, such as:

neoplasm (C00-D49)

Excludes1: myelopathy in:

intervertebral disease (M50.0-, M51.0-)

spondylosis (M47.0-, M47.1-)

G99.8 Other specified disorders of nervous system in diseases classified elsewhere

Code first underlying disorder, such as:

amyloidosis (E85.-)

avitaminosis (E56.9)

Excludes1: nervous system involvement in:

cysticercosis (B69.0)

rubella (B06.0-)

syphilis (A52.1-)

Chapter 7: Diseases Of The Eye And Adnexa (H00-H59)

DEFINITIONS

This chapter includes definitions of selected key words, terms and phrases and coding alerts for adding points to the clinical domain, and references to coding late effects where appropriate. An example from this chapter is as follows:

H16   **Keratitis**
Definition: Keratitis is an infection or inflammation of the cornea which can be caused by a variety of conditions, including infections, dry eyes, foreign objects, contact lenses, intense light, vitamin a deficiency or allergies.

MULTIPLE CODING FOR A SINGLE CONDITION

In addition to the etiology/manifestation convention that requires two codes to fully describe a single condition that affects multiple body systems, there are other single conditions that also require more than one code. "Use additional code" notes are found in the Tabular List at codes that are not part of an etiology/manifestation pair where a secondary code is useful to fully describe a condition. The sequencing rule is the same as the etiology/manifestation pair, "use additional code" indicates that a secondary code should be added.

For example, for bacterial infections that are not included in chapter 1, a secondary code from category B95, Streptococcus, Staphylococcus, and Enterococcus, as the cause of diseases classified elsewhere, or B96, Other bacterial agents as the cause of diseases classified elsewhere, may be required to identify the bacterial organism causing the infection. A "use additional code" note will normally be found at the infectious disease code, indicating a need for the organism code to be added as a secondary code.

"Code first" notes are also under certain codes that are not specifically manifestation codes but may be due to an underlying cause. When there is a "code first" note and an underlying condition is present, the underlying condition should be sequenced first.

"Code, if applicable, any causal condition first", notes indicate that this code may be assigned as a principal diagnosis when the causal condition is unknown or not applicable. If a causal condition is known, then the code for that condition should be sequenced as the principal or first-listed diagnosis.

Multiple codes may be needed for sequela, complication codes and obstetric codes to more fully describe a condition. See the specific guidelines for these conditions for further instruction.

COMBINATION CODE

A combination code is a single code used to classify: Two diagnoses, or a diagnosis with an associated secondary process (manifestation) A diagnosis with an associated complication

Combination codes are identified by referring to subterm entries in the Alphabetic Index and by reading the inclusion and exclusion notes in the Tabular List.

Assign only the combination code when that code fully identifies the diagnostic conditions involved or when the Alphabetic Index so directs. Multiple coding should not be used when the classification provides a combination code that clearly identifies all of the elements documented in the diagnosis. When the combination code lacks necessary specificity in describing the manifestation or complication, an additional code should be used as a secondary code.

SEQUELA (LATE EFFECTS)

A sequela is the residual effect (condition produced) after the acute phase of an illness or injury has terminated. There is no time limit on when a sequela code can be used. The residual may be apparent early, such as in cerebral infarction, or it may occur months or years later, such as that due to a previous injury. Coding of sequela generally requires two codes sequenced in the following order: The condition or nature of the sequela is sequenced first.

The sequela code is sequenced second.

An exception to the above guidelines are those instances where the code for the sequela is followed by a manifestation code identified in the Tabular List and title, or the sequela code has been expanded (at the fourth, fifth or sixth character levels) to include the manifestation(s). The code for the acute phase of an illness or injury that led to the sequela is never used with a code for the late effect.

GLAUCOMA

1)   **Assigning Glaucoma Codes**

Assign as many codes from category H40, Glaucoma, as needed to identify the type of glaucoma, the affected eye, and the glaucoma stage.

2) **Bilateral glaucoma with same type and stage**

When a patient has bilateral glaucoma and both eyes are documented as being the same type and stage, and there is a code for bilateral glaucoma, report only the code for the type of glaucoma, bilateral, with the seventh character for the stage.

When a patient has bilateral glaucoma and both eyes are documented as being the same type and stage, and the classification does not provide a code for bilateral glaucoma (i.e. subcategories H40.10, H40.11 and H40.20) report only one code for the type of glaucoma with the appropriate seventh character for the stage.

3) **Bilateral glaucoma stage with different types or stages**

When a patient has bilateral glaucoma and each eye is documented as having a different type or stage, and the classification distinguishes laterality, assign the appropriate code for each eye rather than the code for bilateral glaucoma.

When a patient has bilateral glaucoma and each eye is documented as having a different type, and the classification does not distinguish laterality (i.e. subcategories H40.10, H40.11 and H40.20), assign one code for each type of glaucoma with the appropriate seventh character for the stage.

When a patient has bilateral glaucoma and each eye is documented as having the same type, but different stage, and the classification does not distinguish laterality (i.e. subcategories H40.10, H40.11 and H40.20), assign a code for

the type of glaucoma for each eye with the seventh character for the specific glaucoma stage documented for each eye.

4) **Patient admitted with glaucoma and stage evolves during the admission**

If a patient is admitted with glaucoma and the stage progresses during the admission, assign the code for highest stage documented.

5) **Indeterminate stage glaucoma**

Assignment of the seventh character "4" for "indeterminate stage" should be based on the clinical documentation. The seventh character "4" is used for glaucomas whose stage cannot be clinically determined. This seventh character should not be confused with the seventh character "0", unspecified, which should be assigned when there is no documentation regarding the stage of the glaucoma.

Chapter 7

Diseases Of The Eye And Adnexa (H00-H59)

Note: Use an external cause code following the code for the eye condition, if applicable, to identify the cause of the eye condition

Excludes2: certain conditions originating in the perinatal period (P04-P96)

certain infectious and parasitic diseases (A00-B99)

complications of pregnancy, childbirth and the puerperium (O00-O9A)

congenital malformations, deformations, and chromosomal abnormalities (Q00-Q99)

diabetes mellitus related eye conditions (E09.3-, E10.3-, E11.3-, E13.3-)

endocrine, nutritional and metabolic diseases (E00-E88)

injury (trauma) of eye and orbit (S05.-)

injury, poisoning and certain other consequences of external causes (S00-T88)

neoplasms (C00-D49)

symptoms, signs and abnormal clinical and laboratory findings, not elsewhere classified (R00-R94)

syphilis related eye disorders (A50.01, A50.3-, A51.43, A52.71)

This chapter contains the following blocks:

H00-H05	Disorders of eyelid, lacrimal system and orbit
H10-H11	Disorders of conjunctiva
H15-H22	Disorders of sclera, cornea, iris and ciliary body
H25-H28	Disorders of lens
H30-H36	Disorders of choroid and retina
H40-H42	Glaucoma
H43-H44	Disorders of vitreous body and globe
H46-H47	Disorders of optic nerve and visual pathways
H49-H52	Disorders of ocular muscles, binocular movement, accommodation and refraction
H53-H54	Visual disturbances and blindness
H55-H57	Other disorders of eye and adnexa
H59	Intraoperative and postprocedural complications and disorders of eye and adnexa, not elsewhere classified

DISORDERS OF EYELID, LACRIMAL SYSTEM AND ORBIT (H00-H05)

Excludes2: open wound of eyelid (S01.1-)

superficial injury of eyelid (S00.1-, S00.2-)

H00   Hordeolum and chalazion

H00.0   Hordeolum (externum) (internum) of eyelid

H00.01   Hordeolum externum

Hordeolum NOS

Stye

H00.011   Hordeolum externum right upper eyelid

H00.012   Hordeolum externum right lower eyelid

H00.013   Hordeolum externum right eye, unspecified eyelid

H00.014   Hordeolum externum left upper eyelid

H00.015   Hordeolum externum left lower eyelid

H00.016   Hordeolum externum left eye, unspecified eyelid

H00.019   Hordeolum externum unspecified eye, unspecified eyelid

H00.02   Hordeolum internum

Infection of meibomian gland

H00.021   Hordeolum internum right upper eyelid

H00.022   Hordeolum internum right lower eyelid

H00.023   Hordeolum internum right eye, unspecified eyelid

H00.024   Hordeolum internum left upper eyelid

H00.025   Hordeolum internum left lower eyelid

H00.026   Hordeolum internum left eye, unspecified eyelid

H00.029   Hordeolum internum unspecified eye, unspecified eyelid

H00.03   Abscess of eyelid

Furuncle of eyelid

H00.031   Abscess of right upper eyelid

H00.032   Abscess of right lower eyelid

H00.033   Abscess of eyelid right eye, unspecified eyelid

H00.034   Abscess of left upper eyelid

H00.035   Abscess of left lower eyelid

H00.036   Abscess of eyelid left eye, unspecified eyelid

H00.039   Abscess of eyelid unspecified eye, unspecified eyelid

H00.1   Chalazion

Meibomian (gland) cyst

Excludes2: infected meibomian gland (H00.02-)

H00.11   Chalazion right upper eyelid

H00.12   Chalazion right lower eyelid

H00.13   Chalazion right eye, unspecified eyelid

H00.14   Chalazion left upper eyelid

H00.15   Chalazion left lower eyelid

H00.16   Chalazion left eye, unspecified eyelid

H00.19   Chalazion unspecified eye, unspecified eyelid

H01   Other inflammation of eyelid

H01.0   Blepharitis

Excludes1: blepharoconjunctivitis (H10.5-)

H01.00   Unspecified blepharitis

H01.001   Unspecified blepharitis right upper eyelid

H01.002   Unspecified blepharitis right lower eyelid

H01.003   Unspecified blepharitis right eye, unspecified eyelid

H01.004   Unspecified blepharitis left upper eyelid

H01.005   Unspecified blepharitis left lower eyelid

H01.006   Unspecified blepharitis left eye, unspecified eyelid

H01.009   Unspecified blepharitis unspecified eye, unspecified eyelid

H01.01   **Ulcerative blepharitis**

     H01.011   Ulcerative blepharitis right upper eyelid

     H01.012   Ulcerative blepharitis right lower eyelid

     H01.013   Ulcerative blepharitis right eye, unspecified eyelid

     H01.014   Ulcerative blepharitis left upper eyelid

     H01.015   Ulcerative blepharitis left lower eyelid

     H01.016   Ulcerative blepharitis left eye, unspecified eyelid

     H01.019   Ulcerative blepharitis unspecified eye, unspecified eyelid

H01.02   **Squamous blepharitis**

     H01.021   Squamous blepharitis right upper eyelid

     H01.022   Squamous blepharitis right lower eyelid

     H01.023   Squamous blepharitis right eye, unspecified eyelid

     H01.024   Squamous blepharitis left upper eyelid

     H01.025   Squamous blepharitis left lower eyelid

     H01.026   Squamous blepharitis left eye, unspecified eyelid

     H01.029   Squamous blepharitis unspecified eye, unspecified eyelid

H01.1   **Noninfectious dermatoses of eyelid**

H01.11   **Allergic dermatitis of eyelid**

Contact dermatitis of eyelid

     H01.111   Allergic dermatitis of right upper eyelid

     H01.112   Allergic dermatitis of right lower eyelid

     H01.113   Allergic dermatitis of right eye, unspecified eyelid

     H01.114   Allergic dermatitis of left upper eyelid

     H01.115   Allergic dermatitis of left lower eyelid

     H01.116   Allergic dermatitis of left eye, unspecified eyelid

     H01.119   Allergic dermatitis of unspecified eye, unspecified eyelid

H01.12   **Discoid lupus erythematosus of eyelid**

     H01.121   Discoid lupus erythematosus of right upper eyelid

     H01.122   Discoid lupus erythematosus of right lower eyelid

     H01.123   Discoid lupus erythematosus of right eye, unspecified eyelid

     H01.124   Discoid lupus erythematosus of left upper eyelid

     H01.125   Discoid lupus erythematosus of left lower eyelid

     H01.126   Discoid lupus erythematosus of left eye, unspecified eyelid

     H01.129   Discoid lupus erythematosus of unspecified eye, unspecified eyelid

H01.13   **Eczematous dermatitis of eyelid**

     H01.131   Eczematous dermatitis of right upper eyelid

     H01.132   Eczematous dermatitis of right lower eyelid

     H01.133   Eczematous dermatitis of right eye, unspecified eyelid

     H01.134   Eczematous dermatitis of left upper eyelid

     H01.135   Eczematous dermatitis of left lower eyelid

     H01.136   Eczematous dermatitis of left eye, unspecified eyelid

     H01.139   Eczematous dermatitis of unspecified eye, unspecified eyelid

H01.14   **Xeroderma of eyelid**

     H01.141   Xeroderma of right upper eyelid

     H01.142   Xeroderma of right lower eyelid

     H01.143   Xeroderma of right eye, unspecified eyelid

     H01.144   Xeroderma of left upper eyelid

     H01.145   Xeroderma of left lower eyelid

     H01.146   Xeroderma of left eye, unspecified eyelid

     H01.149   Xeroderma of unspecified eye, unspecified eyelid

H01.8   **Other specified inflammations of eyelid**

H01.9   **Unspecified inflammation of eyelid**

Inflammation of eyelid NOS

H02   **Other disorders of eyelid**

Excludes1: congenital malformations of eyelid (Q10.0-Q10.3)

H02.0   **Entropion and trichiasis of eyelid**

H02.00   **Unspecified entropion of eyelid**

     H02.001   Unspecified entropion of right upper eyelid

     H02.002   Unspecified entropion of right lower eyelid

     H02.003   Unspecified entropion of right eye, unspecified eyelid

     H02.004   Unspecified entropion of left upper eyelid

     H02.005   Unspecified entropion of left lower eyelid

     H02.006   Unspecified entropion of left eye, unspecified eyelid

     H02.009   Unspecified entropion of unspecified eye, unspecified eyelid

H02.01   **Cicatricial entropion of eyelid**

     H02.011   Cicatricial entropion of right upper eyelid

     H02.012   Cicatricial entropion of right lower eyelid

     H02.013   Cicatricial entropion of right eye, unspecified eyelid

H02.014 Cicatricial entropion of left upper eyelid

H02.015 Cicatricial entropion of left lower eyelid

H02.016 Cicatricial entropion of left eye, unspecified eyelid

H02.019 Cicatricial entropion of unspecified eye, unspecified eyelid

H02.02 Mechanical entropion of eyelid

H02.021 Mechanical entropion of right upper eyelid

H02.022 Mechanical entropion of right lower eyelid

H02.023 Mechanical entropion of right eye, unspecified eyelid

H02.024 Mechanical entropion of left upper eyelid

H02.025 Mechanical entropion of left lower eyelid

H02.026 Mechanical entropion of left eye, unspecified eyelid

H02.029 Mechanical entropion of unspecified eye, unspecified eyelid

H02.03 Senile entropion of eyelid

H02.031 Senile entropion of right upper eyelid

H02.032 Senile entropion of right lower eyelid

H02.033 Senile entropion of right eye, unspecified eyelid

H02.034 Senile entropion of left upper eyelid

H02.035 Senile entropion of left lower eyelid

H02.036 Senile entropion of left eye, unspecified eyelid

H02.039 Senile entropion of unspecified eye, unspecified eyelid

H02.04 Spastic entropion of eyelid

H02.041 Spastic entropion of right upper eyelid

H02.042 Spastic entropion of right lower eyelid

H02.043 Spastic entropion of right eye, unspecified eyelid

H02.044 Spastic entropion of left upper eyelid

H02.045 Spastic entropion of left lower eyelid

H02.046 Spastic entropion of left eye, unspecified eyelid

H02.049 Spastic entropion of unspecified eye, unspecified eyelid

H02.05 Trichiasis without entropian

H02.051 Trichiasis without entropian right upper eyelid

H02.052 Trichiasis without entropian right lower eyelid

H02.053 Trichiasis without entropian right eye, unspecified eyelid

H02.054 Trichiasis without entropian left upper eyelid

H02.055 Trichiasis without entropian left lower eyelid

H02.056 Trichiasis without entropian left eye, unspecified eyelid

H02.059 Trichiasis without entropian unspecified eye, unspecified eyelid

H02.1 Ectropion of eyelid

H02.10 Unspecified ectropion of eyelid

H02.101 Unspecified ectropion of right upper eyelid

H02.102 Unspecified ectropion of right lower eyelid

H02.103 Unspecified ectropion of right eye, unspecified eyelid

H02.104 Unspecified ectropion of left upper eyelid

H02.105 Unspecified ectropion of left lower eyelid

H02.106 Unspecified ectropion of left eye, unspecified eyelid

H02.109 Unspecified ectropion of unspecified eye, unspecified eyelid

H02.11 Cicatricial ectropion of eyelid

H02.111 Cicatricial ectropion of right upper eyelid

H02.112 Cicatricial ectropion of right lower eyelid

H02.113 Cicatricial ectropion of right eye, unspecified eyelid

H02.114 Cicatricial ectropion of left upper eyelid

H02.115 Cicatricial ectropion of left lower eyelid

H02.116 Cicatricial ectropion of left eye, unspecified eyelid

H02.119 Cicatricial ectropion of unspecified eye, unspecified eyelid

H02.12 Mechanical ectropion of eyelid

H02.121 Mechanical ectropion of right upper eyelid

H02.122 Mechanical ectropion of right lower eyelid

H02.123 Mechanical ectropion of right eye, unspecified eyelid

H02.124 Mechanical ectropion of left upper eyelid

H02.125 Mechanical ectropion of left lower eyelid

H02.126 Mechanical ectropion of left eye, unspecified eyelid

H02.129 Mechanical ectropion of unspecified eye, unspecified eyelid

H02.13 Senile ectropion of eyelid

H02.131 Senile ectropion of right upper eyelid

H02.132 Senile ectropion of right lower eyelid

H02.133 Senile ectropion of right eye, unspecified eyelid

H02.134 Senile ectropion of left upper eyelid

Add 4th-7th digits   Nonspecific code   Unspecified code   Manifestation code   319

H02.135 Senile ectropion of left lower eyelid

H02.136 Senile ectropion of left eye, unspecified eyelid

H02.139 Senile ectropion of unspecified eye, unspecified eyelid

H02.14 Spastic ectropion of eyelid

H02.141 Spastic ectropion of right upper eyelid

H02.142 Spastic ectropion of right lower eyelid

H02.143 Spastic ectropion of right eye, unspecified eyelid

H02.144 Spastic ectropion of left upper eyelid

H02.145 Spastic ectropion of left lower eyelid

H02.146 Spastic ectropion of left eye, unspecified eyelid

H02.149 Spastic ectropion of unspecified eye, unspecified eyelid

H02.2 Lagophthalmos

H02.20 Unspecified lagophthalmos

H02.201 Unspecified lagophthalmos right upper eyelid

H02.202 Unspecified lagophthalmos right lower eyelid

H02.203 Unspecified lagophthalmos right eye, unspecified eyelid

H02.204 Unspecified lagophthalmos left upper eyelid

H02.205 Unspecified lagophthalmos left lower eyelid

H02.206 Unspecified lagophthalmos left eye, unspecified eyelid

H02.209 Unspecified lagophthalmos unspecified eye, unspecified eyelid

H02.21 Cicatricial lagophthalmos

H02.211 Cicatricial lagophthalmos right upper eyelid

H02.212 Cicatricial lagophthalmos right lower eyelid

H02.213 Cicatricial lagophthalmos right eye, unspecified eyelid

H02.214 Cicatricial lagophthalmos left upper eyelid

H02.215 Cicatricial lagophthalmos left lower eyelid

H02.216 Cicatricial lagophthalmos left eye, unspecified eyelid

H02.219 Cicatricial lagophthalmos unspecified eye, unspecified eyelid

H02.22 Mechanical lagophthalmos

H02.221 Mechanical lagophthalmos right upper eyelid

H02.222 Mechanical lagophthalmos right lower eyelid

H02.223 Mechanical lagophthalmos right eye, unspecified eyelid

H02.224 Mechanical lagophthalmos left upper eyelid

H02.225 Mechanical lagophthalmos left lower eyelid

H02.226 Mechanical lagophthalmos left eye, unspecified eyelid

H02.229 Mechanical lagophthalmos unspecified eye, unspecified eyelid

H02.23 Paralytic lagophthalmos

H02.231 Paralytic lagophthalmos right upper eyelid

H02.232 Paralytic lagophthalmos right lower eyelid

H02.233 Paralytic lagophthalmos right eye, unspecified eyelid

H02.234 Paralytic lagophthalmos left upper eyelid

H02.235 Paralytic lagophthalmos left lower eyelid

H02.236 Paralytic lagophthalmos left eye, unspecified eyelid

H02.239 Paralytic lagophthalmos unspecified eye, unspecified eyelid

H02.3 Blepharochalasis

Pseudoptosis

H02.30 Blepharochalasis unspecified eye, unspecified eyelid

H02.31 Blepharochalasis right upper eyelid

H02.32 Blepharochalasis right lower eyelid

H02.33 Blepharochalasis right eye, unspecified eyelid

H02.34 Blepharochalasis left upper eyelid

H02.35 Blepharochalasis left lower eyelid

H02.36 Blepharochalasis left eye, unspecified eyelid

H02.4 Ptosis of eyelid

H02.40 Unspecified ptosis of eyelid

H02.401 Unspecified ptosis of right eyelid

H02.402 Unspecified ptosis of left eyelid

H02.403 Unspecified ptosis of bilateral eyelids

H02.409 Unspecified ptosis of unspecified eyelid

H02.41 Mechanical ptosis of eyelid

H02.411 Mechanical ptosis of right eyelid

H02.412 Mechanical ptosis of left eyelid

H02.413 Mechanical ptosis of bilateral eyelids

H02.419 Mechanical ptosis of unspecified eyelid

H02.42 Myogenic ptosis of eyelid

H02.421 Myogenic ptosis of right eyelid

H02.422 Myogenic ptosis of left eyelid

H02.423 Myogenic ptosis of bilateral eyelids

H02.429 Myogenic ptosis of unspecified eyelid

H02.43 Paralytic ptosis of eyelid

Neurogenic ptosis of eyelid

H02.431 Paralytic ptosis of right eyelid

H02.432 Paralytic ptosis of left eyelid

H02.433 Paralytic ptosis of bilateral eyelids

H02.439 Paralytic ptosis unspecified eyelid

H02.5 **Other disorders affecting eyelid function**
Excludes2: blepharospasm (G24.5)
organic tic (G25.69)
psychogenic tic (F95.-)

H02.51 **Abnormal innervation syndrome**
H02.511 **Abnormal innervation syndrome right upper eyelid**
H02.512 **Abnormal innervation syndrome right lower eyelid**
H02.513 **Abnormal innervation syndrome right eye, unspecified eyelid**
H02.514 **Abnormal innervation syndrome left upper eyelid**
H02.515 **Abnormal innervation syndrome left lower eyelid**
H02.516 **Abnormal innervation syndrome left eye, unspecified eyelid**
H02.519 **Abnormal innervation syndrome unspecified eye, unspecified eyelid**

H02.52 **Blepharophimosis**
Ankyloblepharon
H02.521 **Blepharophimosis right upper eyelid**
H02.522 **Blepharophimosis right lower eyelid**
H02.523 **Blepharophimosis right eye, unspecified eyelid**
H02.524 **Blepharophimosis left upper eyelid**
H02.525 **Blepharophimosis left lower eyelid**
H02.526 **Blepharophimosis left eye, unspecified eyelid**
H02.529 **Blepharophimosis unspecified eye, unspecified lid**

H02.53 **Eyelid retraction**
Eyelid lag
H02.531 **Eyelid retraction right upper eyelid**
H02.532 **Eyelid retraction right lower eyelid**
H02.533 **Eyelid retraction right eye, unspecified eyelid**
H02.534 **Eyelid retraction left upper eyelid**
H02.535 **Eyelid retraction left lower eyelid**
H02.536 **Eyelid retraction left eye, unspecified eyelid**
H02.539 **Eyelid retraction unspecified eye, unspecified lid**

H02.59 **Other disorders affecting eyelid function**
Deficient blink reflex
Sensory disorders

H02.6 **Xanthelasma of eyelid**
H02.60 **Xanthelasma of unspecified eye, unspecified eyelid**
H02.61 **Xanthelasma of right upper eyelid**
H02.62 **Xanthelasma of right lower eyelid**
H02.63 **Xanthelasma of right eye, unspecified eyelid**
H02.64 **Xanthelasma of left upper eyelid**
H02.65 **Xanthelasma of left lower eyelid**
H02.66 **Xanthelasma of left eye, unspecified eyelid**

H02.7 **Other and unspecified degenerative disorders of eyelid and periocular area**

H02.70 **Unspecified degenerative disorders of eyelid and periocular area**

H02.71 **Chloasma of eyelid and periocular area**
Dyspigmentation of eyelid
Hyperpigmentation of eyelid
H02.711 **Chloasma of right upper eyelid and periocular area**
H02.712 **Chloasma of right lower eyelid and periocular area**
H02.713 **Chloasma of right eye, unspecified eyelid and periocular area**
H02.714 **Chloasma of left upper eyelid and periocular area**
H02.715 **Chloasma of left lower eyelid and periocular area**
H02.716 **Chloasma of left eye, unspecified eyelid and periocular area**
H02.719 **Chloasma of unspecified eye, unspecified eyelid and periocular area**

H02.72 **Madarosis of eyelid and periocular area**
Hypotrichosis of eyelid
H02.721 **Madarosis of right upper eyelid and periocular area**
H02.722 **Madarosis of right lower eyelid and periocular area**
H02.723 **Madarosis of right eye, unspecified eyelid and periocular area**
H02.724 **Madarosis of left upper eyelid and periocular area**
H02.725 **Madarosis of left lower eyelid and periocular area**
H02.726 **Madarosis of left eye, unspecified eyelid and periocular area**
H02.729 **Madarosis of unspecified eye, unspecified eyelid and periocular area**

H02.73 **Vitiligo of eyelid and periocular area**
Hypopigmentation of eyelid
H02.731 **Vitiligo of right upper eyelid and periocular area**
H02.732 **Vitiligo of right lower eyelid and periocular area**
H02.733 **Vitiligo of right eye, unspecified eyelid and periocular area**
H02.734 **Vitiligo of left upper eyelid and periocular area**
H02.735 **Vitiligo of left lower eyelid and periocular area**
H02.736 **Vitiligo of left eye, unspecified eyelid and periocular area**
H02.739 **Vitiligo of unspecified eye, unspecified eyelid and periocular area**

H02.79 **Other degenerative disorders of eyelid and periocular area**

H02.8 **Other specified disorders of eyelid**
H02.81 **Retained foreign body in eyelid**
Use additional code to identify the type of retained foreign body (Z18.-)

Excludes1: laceration of eyelid with foreign body (S01.12-)

retained intraocular foreign body (H44.6-, H44.7-)

superficial foreign body of eyelid and periocular area (S00.25-)

H02.811 **Retained foreign body in right upper eyelid**

H02.812 **Retained foreign body in right lower eyelid**

H02.813 **Retained foreign body in right eye, unspecified eyelid**

H02.814 **Retained foreign body in left upper eyelid**

H02.815 **Retained foreign body in left lower eyelid**

H02.816 **Retained foreign body in left eye, unspecified eyelid**

H02.819 **Retained foreign body in unspecified eye, unspecified eyelid**

H02.82 **Cysts of eyelid**

Sebaceous cyst of eyelid

H02.821 **Cysts of right upper eyelid**
H02.822 **Cysts of right lower eyelid**
H02.823 **Cysts of right eye, unspecified eyelid**
H02.824 **Cysts of left upper eyelid**
H02.825 **Cysts of left lower eyelid**
H02.826 **Cysts of left eye, unspecified eyelid**
H02.829 **Cysts of unspecified eye, unspecified eyelid**

H02.83 **Dermatochalasis of eyelid**

H02.831 **Dermatochalasis of right upper eyelid**
H02.832 **Dermatochalasis of right lower eyelid**
H02.833 **Dermatochalasis of right eye, unspecified eyelid**
H02.834 **Dermatochalasis of left upper eyelid**
H02.835 **Dermatochalasis of left lower eyelid**
H02.836 **Dermatochalasis of left eye, unspecified eyelid**
H02.839 **Dermatochalasis of unspecified eye, unspecified eyelid**

H02.84 **Edema of eyelid**

Hyperemia of eyelid

H02.841 **Edema of right upper eyelid**
H02.842 **Edema of right lower eyelid**
H02.843 **Edema of right eye, unspecified eyelid**
H02.844 **Edema of left upper eyelid**
H02.845 **Edema of left lower eyelid**
H02.846 **Edema of left eye, unspecified eyelid**
H02.849 **Edema of unspecified eye, unspecified eyelid**

H02.85 **Elephantiasis of eyelid**

H02.851 **Elephantiasis of right upper eyelid**
H02.852 **Elephantiasis of right lower eyelid**

H02.853 **Elephantiasis of right eye, unspecified eyelid**
H02.854 **Elephantiasis of left upper eyelid**
H02.855 **Elephantiasis of left lower eyelid**
H02.856 **Elephantiasis of left eye, unspecified eyelid**
H02.859 **Elephantiasis of unspecified eye, unspecified eyelid**

H02.86 **Hypertrichosis of eyelid**

H02.861 **Hypertrichosis of right upper eyelid**
H02.862 **Hypertrichosis of right lower eyelid**
H02.863 **Hypertrichosis of right eye, unspecified eyelid**
H02.864 **Hypertrichosis of left upper eyelid**
H02.865 **Hypertrichosis of left lower eyelid**
H02.866 **Hypertrichosis of left eye, unspecified eyelid**
H02.869 **Hypertrichosis of unspecified eye, unspecified eyelid**

H02.87 **Vascular anomalies of eyelid**

H02.871 **Vascular anomalies of right upper eyelid**
H02.872 **Vascular anomalies of right lower eyelid**
H02.873 **Vascular anomalies of right eye, unspecified eyelid**
H02.874 **Vascular anomalies of left upper eyelid**
H02.875 **Vascular anomalies of left lower eyelid**
H02.876 **Vascular anomalies of left eye, unspecified eyelid**
H02.879 **Vascular anomalies of unspecified eye, unspecified eyelid**

H02.89 **Other specified disorders of eyelid**

Hemorrhage of eyelid

H02.9 **Unspecified disorder of eyelid**

Disorder of eyelid NOS

H04 **Disorders of lacrimal system**

Excludes1: congenital malformations of lacrimal system (Q10.4-Q10.6)

H04.0 **Dacryoadenitis**

H04.00 **Unspecified dacryoadenitis**

H04.001 **Unspecified dacryoadenitis, right lacrimal gland**
H04.002 **Unspecified dacryoadenitis, left lacrimal gland**
H04.003 **Unspecified dacryoadenitis, bilateral lacrimal glands**
H04.009 **Unspecified dacryoadenitis, unspecified lacrimal gland**

H04.01 **Acute dacryoadenitis**

H04.011 **Acute dacryoadenitis, right lacrimal gland**
H04.012 **Acute dacryoadenitis, left lacrimal gland**
H04.013 **Acute dacryoadenitis, bilateral lacrimal glands**

H04.019　Acute dacryoadenitis, unspecified lacrimal gland

H04.02　Chronic dacryoadenitis

H04.021　Chronic dacryoadenitis, right lacrimal gland

H04.022　Chronic dacryoadenitis, left lacrimal gland

H04.023　Chronic dacryoadenitis, bilateral lacrimal gland

H04.029　Chronic dacryoadenitis, unspecified lacrimal gland

H04.03　Chronic enlargement of lacrimal gland

H04.031　Chronic enlargement of right lacrimal gland

H04.032　Chronic enlargement of left lacrimal gland

H04.033　Chronic enlargement of bilateral lacrimal glands

H04.039　Chronic enlargement of unspecified lacrimal gland

H04.1　Other disorders of lacrimal gland

H04.11　Dacryops

H04.111　Dacryops of right lacrimal gland

H04.112　Dacryops of left lacrimal gland

H04.113　Dacryops of bilateral lacrimal glands

H04.119　Dacryops of unspecified lacrimal gland

H04.12　Dry eye syndrome

Tear film insufficiency, NOS

H04.121　Dry eye syndrome of right lacrimal gland

H04.122　Dry eye syndrome of left lacrimal gland

H04.123　Dry eye syndrome of bilateral lacrimal glands

H04.129　Dry eye syndrome of unspecified lacrimal gland

H04.13　Lacrimal cyst

Lacrimal cystic degeneration

H04.131　Lacrimal cyst, right lacrimal gland

H04.132　Lacrimal cyst, left lacrimal gland

H04.133　Lacrimal cyst, bilateral lacrimal glands

H04.139　Lacrimal cyst, unspecified lacrimal gland

H04.14　Primary lacrimal gland atrophy

H04.141　Primary lacrimal gland atrophy, right lacrimal gland

H04.142　Primary lacrimal gland atrophy, left lacrimal gland

H04.143　Primary lacrimal gland atrophy, bilateral lacrimal glands

H04.149　Primary lacrimal gland atrophy, unspecified lacrimal gland

H04.15　Secondary lacrimal gland atrophy

H04.151　Secondary lacrimal gland atrophy, right lacrimal gland

H04.152　Secondary lacrimal gland atrophy, left lacrimal gland

H04.153　Secondary lacrimal gland atrophy, bilateral lacrimal glands

H04.159　Secondary lacrimal gland atrophy, unspecified lacrimal gland

H04.16　Lacrimal gland dislocation

H04.161　Lacrimal gland dislocation, right lacrimal gland

H04.162　Lacrimal gland dislocation, left lacrimal gland

H04.163　Lacrimal gland dislocation, bilateral lacrimal glands

H04.169　Lacrimal gland dislocation, unspecified lacrimal gland

H04.19　Other specified disorders of lacrimal gland

H04.2　Epiphora

H04.20　Unspecified epiphora

H04.201　Unspecified epiphora, right lacrimal gland

H04.202　Unspecified epiphora, left lacrimal gland

H04.203　Unspecified epiphora, bilateral lacrimal glands

H04.209　Unspecified epiphora, unspecified lacrimal gland

H04.21　Epiphora due to excess lacrimation

H04.211　Epiphora due to excess lacrimation, right lacrimal gland

H04.212　Epiphora due to excess lacrimation, left lacrimal gland

H04.213　Epiphora due to excess lacrimation, bilateral lacrimal glands

H04.219　Epiphora due to excess lacrimation, unspecified lacrimal gland

H04.22　Epiphora due to insufficient drainage

H04.221　Epiphora due to insufficient drainage, right lacrimal gland

H04.222　Epiphora due to insufficient drainage, left lacrimal gland

H04.223　Epiphora due to insufficient drainage, bilateral lacrimal glands

H04.229　Epiphora due to insufficient drainage, unspecified lacrimal gland

H04.3　Acute and unspecified inflammation of lacrimal passages

Excludes1: neonatal dacryocystitis (P39.1)

H04.30　Unspecified dacryocystitis

H04.301　Unspecified dacryocystitis of right lacrimal passage

H04.302　Unspecified dacryocystitis of left lacrimal passage

H04.303　Unspecified dacryocystitis of bilateral lacrimal passages

H04.309　Unspecified dacryocystitis of unspecified lacrimal passage

H04.31　Phlegmonous dacryocystitis

H04.311　Phlegmonous dacryocystitis of right lacrimal passage

H04.312 Phlegmonous dacryocystitis of left lacrimal passage	**H04.519** Dacryolith of unspecified lacrimal passage
H04.313 Phlegmonous dacryocystitis of bilateral lacrimal passages	**H04.52** Eversion of lacrimal punctum
	H04.521 Eversion of right lacrimal punctum
H04.319 Phlegmonous dacryocystitis of unspecified lacrimal passage	**H04.522** Eversion of left lacrimal punctum
H04.32 Acute dacryocystitis	**H04.523** Eversion of bilateral lacrimal punctum
Acute dacryopericystitis	**H04.529** Eversion of unspecified lacrimal punctum

H04.32 Acute dacryocystitis
Acute dacryopericystitis

  H04.321 Acute dacryocystitis of right lacrimal passage

  H04.322 Acute dacryocystitis of left lacrimal passage

  H04.323 Acute dacryocystitis of bilateral lacrimal passages

  H04.329 Acute dacryocystitis of unspecified lacrimal passage

 H04.33 Acute lacrimal canaliculitis

  H04.331 Acute lacrimal canaliculitis of right lacrimal passage

  H04.332 Acute lacrimal canaliculitis of left lacrimal passage

  H04.333 Acute lacrimal canaliculitis of bilateral lacrimal passages

  H04.339 Acute lacrimal canaliculitis of unspecified lacrimal passage

H04.4 Chronic inflammation of lacrimal passages

 H04.41 Chronic dacryocystitis

  H04.411 Chronic dacryocystitis of right lacrimal passage

  H04.412 Chronic dacryocystitis of left lacrimal passage

  H04.413 Chronic dacryocystitis of bilateral lacrimal passages

  H04.419 Chronic dacryocystitis of unspecified lacrimal passage

 H04.42 Chronic lacrimal canaliculitis

  H04.421 Chronic lacrimal canaliculitis of right lacrimal passage

  H04.422 Chronic lacrimal canaliculitis of left lacrimal passage

  H04.423 Chronic lacrimal canaliculitis of bilateral lacrimal passages

  H04.429 Chronic lacrimal canaliculitis of unspecified lacrimal passage

 H04.43 Chronic lacrimal mucocele

  H04.431 Chronic lacrimal mucocele of right lacrimal passage

  H04.432 Chronic lacrimal mucocele of left lacrimal passage

  H04.433 Chronic lacrimal mucocele of bilateral lacrimal passages

  H04.439 Chronic lacrimal mucocele of unspecified lacrimal passage

H04.5 Stenosis and insufficiency of lacrimal passages

 H04.51 Dacryolith

  H04.511 Dacryolith of right lacrimal passage

  H04.512 Dacryolith of left lacrimal passage

  H04.513 Dacryolith of bilateral lacrimal passages

  H04.519 Dacryolith of unspecified lacrimal passage

 H04.52 Eversion of lacrimal punctum

  H04.521 Eversion of right lacrimal punctum

  H04.522 Eversion of left lacrimal punctum

  H04.523 Eversion of bilateral lacrimal punctum

  H04.529 Eversion of unspecified lacrimal punctum

 H04.53 Neonatal obstruction of nasolacrimal duct

  Excludes1: congenital stenosis and stricture of lacrimal duct (Q10.5)

  H04.531 Neonatal obstruction of right nasolacrimal duct

  H04.532 Neonatal obstruction of left nasolacrimal duct

  H04.533 Neonatal obstruction of bilateral nasolacrimal duct

  H04.539 Neonatal obstruction of unspecified nasolacrimal duct

 H04.54 Stenosis of lacrimal canaliculi

  H04.541 Stenosis of right lacrimal canaliculi

  H04.542 Stenosis of left lacrimal canaliculi

  H04.543 Stenosis of bilateral lacrimal canaliculi

  H04.549 Stenosis of unspecified lacrimal canaliculi

 H04.55 Acquired stenosis of nasolacrimal duct

  H04.551 Acquired stenosis of right nasolacrimal duct

  H04.552 Acquired stenosis of left nasolacrimal duct

  H04.553 Acquired stenosis of bilateral nasolacrimal duct

  H04.559 Acquired stenosis of unspecified nasolacrimal duct

 H04.56 Stenosis of lacrimal punctum

  H04.561 Stenosis of right lacrimal punctum

  H04.562 Stenosis of left lacrimal punctum

  H04.563 Stenosis of bilateral lacrimal punctum

  H04.569 Stenosis of unspecified lacrimal punctum

 H04.57 Stenosis of lacrimal sac

  H04.571 Stenosis of right lacrimal sac

  H04.572 Stenosis of left lacrimal sac

  H04.573 Stenosis of bilateral lacrimal sac

  H04.579 Stenosis of unspecified lacrimal sac

H04.6 Other changes of lacrimal passages

 H04.61 Lacrimal fistula

  H04.611 Lacrimal fistula right lacrimal passage

  H04.612 Lacrimal fistula left lacrimal passage

  H04.613 Lacrimal fistula bilateral lacrimal passages

  H04.619 Lacrimal fistula unspecified lacrimal passage

 H04.69 Other changes of lacrimal passages

H04.8 **Other disorders of lacrimal system**

H04.81 **Granuloma of lacrimal passages**

H04.811 **Granuloma of right lacrimal passage**

H04.812 **Granuloma of left lacrimal passage**

H04.813 **Granuloma of bilateral lacrimal passages**

H04.819 **Granuloma of unspecified lacrimal passage**

H04.89 **Other disorders of lacrimal system**

H04.9 **Disorder of lacrimal system, unspecified**

H05 **Disorders of orbit**

Excludes1: congenital malformation of orbit (Q10.7)

H05.0 **Acute inflammation of orbit**

H05.00 **Unspecified acute inflammation of orbit**

H05.01 **Cellulitis of orbit**

Abscess of orbit

H05.011 **Cellulitis of right orbit**

H05.012 **Cellulitis of left orbit**

H05.013 **Cellulitis of bilateral orbits**

H05.019 **Cellulitis of unspecified orbit**

H05.02 **Osteomyelitis of orbit**

H05.021 **Osteomyelitis of right orbit**

H05.022 **Osteomyelitis of left orbit**

H05.023 **Osteomyelitis of bilateral orbits**

H05.029 **Osteomyelitis of unspecified orbit**

H05.03 **Periostitis of orbit**

H05.031 **Periostitis of right orbit**

H05.032 **Periostitis of left orbit**

H05.033 **Periostitis of bilateral orbits**

H05.039 **Periostitis of unspecified orbit**

H05.04 **Tenonitis of orbit**

H05.041 **Tenonitis of right orbit**

H05.042 **Tenonitis of left orbit**

H05.043 **Tenonitis of bilateral orbits**

H05.049 **Tenonitis of unspecified orbit**

H05.1 **Chronic inflammatory disorders of orbit**

H05.10 **Unspecified chronic inflammatory disorders of orbit**

H05.11 **Granuloma of orbit**

Pseudotumor (inflammatory) of orbit

H05.111 **Granuloma of right orbit**

H05.112 **Granuloma of left orbit**

H05.113 **Granuloma of bilateral orbits**

H05.119 **Granuloma of unspecified orbit**

H05.12 **Orbital myositis**

H05.121 **Orbital myositis, right orbit**

H05.122 **Orbital myositis, left orbit**

H05.123 **Orbital myositis, bilateral**

H05.129 **Orbital myositis, unspecified orbit**

H05.2 **Exophthalmic conditions**

H05.20 **Unspecified exophthalmos**

H05.21 **Displacement (lateral) of globe**

H05.211 **Displacement (lateral) of globe, right eye**

H05.212 **Displacement (lateral) of globe, left eye**

H05.213 **Displacement (lateral) of globe, bilateral**

H05.219 **Displacement (lateral) of globe, unspecified eye**

H05.22 **Edema of orbit**

Orbital congestion

H05.221 **Edema of right orbit**

H05.222 **Edema of left orbit**

H05.223 **Edema of bilateral orbit**

H05.229 **Edema of unspecified orbit**

H05.23 **Hemorrhage of orbit**

H05.231 **Hemorrhage of right orbit**

H05.232 **Hemorrhage of left orbit**

H05.233 **Hemorrhage of bilateral orbit**

H05.239 **Hemorrhage of unspecified orbit**

H05.24 **Constant exophthalmos**

H05.241 **Constant exophthalmos, right eye**

H05.242 **Constant exophthalmos, left eye**

H05.243 **Constant exophthalmos, bilateral**

H05.249 **Constant exophthalmos, unspecified eye**

H05.25 **Intermittent exophthalmos**

H05.251 **Intermittent exophthalmos, right eye**

H05.252 **Intermittent exophthalmos, left eye**

H05.253 **Intermittent exophthalmos, bilateral**

H05.259 **Intermittent exophthalmos, unspecified eye**

H05.26 **Pulsating exophthalmos**

H05.261 **Pulsating exophthalmos, right eye**

H05.262 **Pulsating exophthalmos, left eye**

H05.263 **Pulsating exophthalmos, bilateral**

H05.269 **Pulsating exophthalmos, unspecified eye**

H05.3 **Deformity of orbit**

Excludes1: congenital deformity of orbit (Q10.7)
hypertelorism (Q75.2)

H05.30 **Unspecified deformity of orbit**

H05.31 **Atrophy of orbit**

H05.311 **Atrophy of right orbit**

H05.312 **Atrophy of left orbit**

H05.313 **Atrophy of bilateral orbit**

H05.319 **Atrophy of unspecified orbit**

H05.32 **Deformity of orbit due to bone disease**

<u>Code also</u> associated bone disease

H05.321 **Deformity of right orbit due to bone disease**

H05.322 **Deformity of left orbit due to bone disease**

H05.323 **Deformity of bilateral orbits due to bone disease**

H05.329 **Deformity of unspecified orbit due to bone disease**

H05.33 **Deformity of orbit due to trauma or surgery**

	Add 4th-7th digits	Nonspecific code	Unspecified code	Manifestation code

H05.331   **Deformity of right orbit due to trauma or surgery**

H05.332   **Deformity of left orbit due to trauma or surgery**

H05.333   **Deformity of bilateral orbits due to trauma or surgery**

H05.339   **Deformity of unspecified orbit due to trauma or surgery**

H05.34   **Enlargement of orbit**

    H05.341   **Enlargement of right orbit**

    H05.342   **Enlargement of left orbit**

    H05.343   **Enlargement of bilateral orbits**

    H05.349   **Enlargement of unspecified orbit**

H05.35   **Exostosis of orbit**

    H05.351   **Exostosis of right orbit**

    H05.352   **Exostosis of left orbit**

    H05.353   **Exostosis of bilateral orbits**

    H05.359   **Exostosis of unspecified orbit**

H05.4   Enophthalmos

H05.40   **Unspecified enophthalmos**

    H05.401   **Unspecified enophthalmos, right eye**

    H05.402   **Unspecified enophthalmos, left eye**

    H05.403   **Unspecified enophthalmos, bilateral**

    H05.409   **Unspecified enophthalmos, unspecified eye**

H05.41   **Enophthalmos due to atrophy of orbital tissue**

    H05.411   **Enophthalmos due to atrophy of orbital tissue, right eye**

    H05.412   **Enophthalmos due to atrophy of orbital tissue, left eye**

    H05.413   **Enophthalmos due to atrophy of orbital tissue, bilateral**

    H05.419   **Enophthalmos due to atrophy of orbital tissue, unspecified eye**

H05.42   **Enophthalmos due to trauma or surgery**

    H05.421   **Enophthalmos due to trauma or surgery, right eye**

    H05.422   **Enophthalmos due to trauma or surgery, left eye**

    H05.423   **Enophthalmos due to trauma or surgery, bilateral**

    H05.429   **Enophthalmos due to trauma or surgery, unspecified eye**

H05.5   Retained (old) foreign body following penetrating wound of orbit

Retrobulbar foreign body

Use additional code to identify the type of retained foreign body (Z18.-)

Excludes1: current penetrating wound of orbit (S05.4-)

Excludes2: retained foreign body of eyelid (H02.81-)

retained intraocular foreign body (H44.6-, H44.7-)

H05.50   **Retained (old) foreign body following penetrating wound of unspecified orbit**

H05.51   **Retained (old) foreign body following penetrating wound of right orbit**

H05.52   **Retained (old) foreign body following penetrating wound of left orbit**

H05.53   **Retained (old) foreign body following penetrating wound of bilateral orbits**

H05.8   Other disorders of orbit

H05.81   **Cyst of orbit**

Encephalocele of orbit

    H05.811   **Cyst of right orbit**

    H05.812   **Cyst of left orbit**

    H05.813   **Cyst of bilateral orbits**

    H05.819   **Cyst of unspecified orbit**

H05.82   **Myopathy of extraocular muscles**

    H05.821   **Myopathy of extraocular muscles, right orbit**

    H05.822   **Myopathy of extraocular muscles, left orbit**

    H05.823   **Myopathy of extraocular muscles, bilateral**

    H05.829   **Myopathy of extraocular muscles, unspecified orbit**

H05.89   **Other disorders of orbit**

H05.9   Unspecified disorder of orbit

DISORDERS OF CONJUNCTIVA (H10-H11)

Definition: Disorders of conjunctiva are disorders of the mucous membrane that lines the inner surface of the eyelid and the exposed surface of the eyeball.

H10   Conjunctivitis

Excludes1: keratoconjunctivitis (H16.2-)

H10.0   Mucopurulent conjunctivitis

H10.01   **Acute follicular conjunctivitis**

    H10.011   **Acute follicular conjunctivitis, right eye**

    H10.012   **Acute follicular conjunctivitis, left eye**

    H10.013   **Acute follicular conjunctivitis, bilateral**

    H10.019   **Acute follicular conjunctivitis, unspecified eye**

H10.02   **Other mucopurulent conjunctivitis**

    H10.021   **Other mucopurulent conjunctivitis, right eye**

    H10.022   **Other mucopurulent conjunctivitis, left eye**

    H10.023   **Other mucopurulent conjunctivitis, bilateral**

    H10.029   **Other mucopurulent conjunctivitis, unspecified eye**

H10.1   Acute atopic conjunctivitis

Acute papillary conjunctivitis

H10.10   **Acute atopic conjunctivitis, unspecified eye**

H10.11   **Acute atopic conjunctivitis, right eye**

H10.12   **Acute atopic conjunctivitis, left eye**

H10.13   **Acute atopic conjunctivitis, bilateral**

H10.2   Other acute conjunctivitis

H10.21   **Acute toxic conjunctivitis**

Acute chemical conjunctivitis

Code first (T51-T65) to identify chemical and intent

Excludes1: burn and corrosion of eye and adnexa (T26.-)

    H10.211   **Acute toxic conjunctivitis, right eye**

    H10.212   **Acute toxic conjunctivitis, left eye**

    H10.213   **Acute toxic conjunctivitis, bilateral**

    H10.219   **Acute toxic conjunctivitis, unspecified eye**

  H10.22 **Pseudomembranous conjunctivitis**

    H10.221   **Pseudomembranous conjunctivitis, right eye**

    H10.222   **Pseudomembranous conjunctivitis, left eye**

    H10.223   **Pseudomembranous conjunctivitis, bilateral**

    H10.229   **Pseudomembranous conjunctivitis, unspecified eye**

  H10.23 **Serous conjunctivitis, except viral**

    Excludes1: viral conjunctivitis (B30.-)

    H10.231   **Serous conjunctivitis, except viral, right eye**

    H10.232   **Serous conjunctivitis, except viral, left eye**

    H10.233   **Serous conjunctivitis, except viral, bilateral**

    H10.239   **Serous conjunctivitis, except viral, unspecified eye**

H10.3 **Unspecified acute conjunctivitis**

  Excludes1: ophthalmia neonatorum NOS (P39.1)

  H10.30 **Unspecified acute conjunctivitis, unspecified eye**

  H10.31 **Unspecified acute conjunctivitis, right eye**

  H10.32 **Unspecified acute conjunctivitis, left eye**

  H10.33 **Unspecified acute conjunctivitis, bilateral**

H10.4 **Chronic conjunctivitis**

  H10.40 **Unspecified chronic conjunctivitis**

    H10.401   **Unspecified chronic conjunctivitis, right eye**

    H10.402   **Unspecified chronic conjunctivitis, left eye**

    H10.403   **Unspecified chronic conjunctivitis, bilateral**

    H10.409   **Unspecified chronic conjunctivitis, unspecified eye**

  H10.41 **Chronic giant papillary conjunctivitis**

    H10.411   **Chronic giant papillary conjunctivitis, right eye**

    H10.412   **Chronic giant papillary conjunctivitis, left eye**

    H10.413   **Chronic giant papillary conjunctivitis, bilateral**

    H10.419   **Chronic giant papillary conjunctivitis, unspecified eye**

  H10.42 **Simple chronic conjunctivitis**

    H10.421   **Simple chronic conjunctivitis, right eye**

    H10.422   **Simple chronic conjunctivitis, left eye**

    H10.423   **Simple chronic conjunctivitis, bilateral**

    H10.429   **Simple chronic conjunctivitis, unspecified eye**

  H10.43 **Chronic follicular conjunctivitis**

    H10.431   **Chronic follicular conjunctivitis, right eye**

    H10.432   **Chronic follicular conjunctivitis, left eye**

    H10.433   **Chronic follicular conjunctivitis, bilateral**

    H10.439   **Chronic follicular conjunctivitis, unspecified eye**

  H10.44 **Vernal conjunctivitis**

    Excludes1: vernal keratoconjunctivitis with limbar and corneal involvement (H16.26-)

  H10.45 **Other chronic allergic conjunctivitis**

H10.5 **Blepharoconjunctivitis**

  H10.50 **Unspecified blepharoconjunctivitis**

    H10.501   **Unspecified blepharoconjunctivitis, right eye**

    H10.502   **Unspecified blepharoconjunctivitis, left eye**

    H10.503   **Unspecified blepharoconjunctivitis, bilateral**

    H10.509   **Unspecified blepharoconjunctivitis, unspecified eye**

  H10.51 **Ligneous conjunctivitis**

    H10.511   **Ligneous conjunctivitis, right eye**

    H10.512   **Ligneous conjunctivitis, left eye**

    H10.513   **Ligneous conjunctivitis, bilateral**

    H10.519   **Ligneous conjunctivitis, unspecified eye**

  H10.52 **Angular blepharoconjunctivitis**

    H10.521   **Angular blepharoconjunctivitis, right eye**

    H10.522   **Angular blepharoconjunctivitis, left eye**

    H10.523   **Angular blepharoconjunctivitis, bilateral**

    H10.529   **Angular blepharoconjunctivitis, unspecified eye**

  H10.53 **Contact blepharoconjunctivitis**

    H10.531   **Contact blepharoconjunctivitis, right eye**

    H10.532   **Contact blepharoconjunctivitis, left eye**

    H10.533   **Contact blepharoconjunctivitis, bilateral**

    H10.539   **Contact blepharoconjunctivitis, unspecified eye**

H10.8 **Other conjunctivitis**

  H10.81 **Pingueculitis**

    Excludes1: pinguecula (H11.15-)

    H10.811   **Pingueculitis, right eye**

    H10.812   **Pingueculitis, left eye**

    H10.813   **Pingueculitis, bilateral**

    H10.819   **Pingueculitis, unspecified eye**

  H10.89 **Other conjunctivitis**

H10.9 **Unspecified conjunctivitis**

H11 **Other disorders of conjunctiva**

  Excludes1: keratoconjunctivitis (H16.2-)

H11.0   Pterygium of eye

Excludes1: pseudopterygium (H11.81-)

    H11.00   Unspecified pterygium of eye

        H11.001   Unspecified pterygium of right eye

        H11.002   Unspecified pterygium of left eye

        H11.003   Unspecified pterygium of eye, bilateral

        H11.009   Unspecified pterygium of unspecified eye

    H11.01   Amyloid pterygium

        H11.011   Amyloid pterygium of right eye

        H11.012   Amyloid pterygium of left eye

        H11.013   Amyloid pterygium of eye, bilateral

        H11.019   Amyloid pterygium of unspecified eye

    H11.02   Central pterygium of eye

        H11.021   Central pterygium of right eye

        H11.022   Central pterygium of left eye

        H11.023   Central pterygium of eye, bilateral

        H11.029   Central pterygium of unspecified eye

    H11.03   Double pterygium of eye

        H11.031   Double pterygium of right eye

        H11.032   Double pterygium of left eye

        H11.033   Double pterygium of eye, bilateral

        H11.039   Double pterygium of unspecified eye

    H11.04   Peripheral pterygium of eye, stationary

        H11.041   Peripheral pterygium, stationary, right eye

        H11.042   Peripheral pterygium, stationary, left eye

        H11.043   Peripheral pterygium, stationary, bilateral

        H11.049   Peripheral pterygium, stationary, unspecified eye

    H11.05   Peripheral pterygium of eye, progressive

        H11.051   Peripheral pterygium, progressive, right eye

        H11.052   Peripheral pterygium, progressive, left eye

        H11.053   Peripheral pterygium, progressive, bilateral

        H11.059   Peripheral pterygium, progressive, unspecified eye

    H11.06   Recurrent pterygium of eye

        H11.061   Recurrent pterygium of right eye

        H11.062   Recurrent pterygium of left eye

        H11.063   Recurrent pterygium of eye, bilateral

        H11.069   Recurrent pterygium of unspecified eye

H11.1   Conjunctival degenerations and deposits

Excludes2: pseudopterygium (H11.81)

    H11.10   Unspecified conjunctival degenerations

    H11.11   Conjunctival deposits

        H11.111   Conjunctival deposits, right eye

        H11.112   Conjunctival deposits, left eye

        H11.113   Conjunctival deposits, bilateral

        H11.119   Conjunctival deposits, unspecified eye

    H11.12   Conjunctival concretions

        H11.121   Conjunctival concretions, right eye

        H11.122   Conjunctival concretions, left eye

        H11.123   Conjunctival concretions, bilateral

        H11.129   Conjunctival concretions, unspecified eye

    H11.13   Conjunctival pigmentations

    Conjunctival argyrosis [argyria]

        H11.131   Conjunctival pigmentations, right eye

        H11.132   Conjunctival pigmentations, left eye

        H11.133   Conjunctival pigmentations, bilateral

        H11.139   Conjunctival pigmentations, unspecified eye

    H11.14   Conjunctival xerosis, unspecified

    Excludes1: xerosis of conjunctiva due to vitamin A deficiency (E50.0, E50.1)

        H11.141   Conjunctival xerosis, unspecified, right eye

        H11.142   Conjunctival xerosis, unspecified, left eye

        H11.143   Conjunctival xerosis, unspecified, bilateral

        H11.149   Conjunctival xerosis, unspecified, unspecified eye

    H11.15   Pinguecula

    Excludes1: pingueculitis (H10.81-)

        H11.151   Pinguecula, right eye

        H11.152   Pinguecula, left eye

        H11.153   Pinguecula, bilateral

        H11.159   Pinguecula, unspecified eye

H11.2   Conjunctival scars

    H11.21   Conjunctival adhesions and strands (localized)

        H11.211   Conjunctival adhesions and strands (localized), right eye

        H11.212   Conjunctival adhesions and strands (localized), left eye

        H11.213   Conjunctival adhesions and strands (localized), bilateral

        H11.219   Conjunctival adhesions and strands (localized), unspecified eye

    H11.22   Conjunctival granuloma

        H11.221   Conjunctival granuloma, right eye

        H11.222   Conjunctival granuloma, left eye

        H11.223   Conjunctival granuloma, bilateral

        H11.229   Conjunctival granuloma, unspecified

    H11.23   Symblepharon

        H11.231   Symblepharon, right eye

        H11.232   Symblepharon, left eye

        H11.233   Symblepharon, bilateral

        H11.239   Symblepharon, unspecified eye

● New code   ▲ Revised code   Excludes1: Not coded here   Excludes2: Not included here   ⊗ Placeholder required   ⑦7th digit required

H11.24 Scarring of conjunctiva

    H11.241 Scarring of conjunctiva, right eye

    H11.242 Scarring of conjunctiva, left eye

    H11.243 Scarring of conjunctiva, bilateral

    H11.249 Scarring of conjunctiva, unspecified eye

H11.3 Conjunctival hemorrhage

Subconjunctival hemorrhage

    H11.30 Conjunctival hemorrhage, unspecified eye

    H11.31 Conjunctival hemorrhage, right eye

    H11.32 Conjunctival hemorrhage, left eye

    H11.33 Conjunctival hemorrhage, bilateral

H11.4 Other conjunctival vascular disorders and cysts

    H11.41 Vascular abnormalities of conjunctiva

    Conjunctival aneurysm

        H11.411 Vascular abnormalities of conjunctiva, right eye

        H11.412 Vascular abnormalities of conjunctiva, left eye

        H11.413 Vascular abnormalities of conjunctiva, bilateral

        H11.419 Vascular abnormalities of conjunctiva, unspecified eye

    H11.42 Conjunctival edema

        H11.421 Conjunctival edema, right eye

        H11.422 Conjunctival edema, left eye

        H11.423 Conjunctival edema, bilateral

        H11.429 Conjunctival edema, unspecified eye

    H11.43 Conjunctival hyperemia

        H11.431 Conjunctival hyperemia, right eye

        H11.432 Conjunctival hyperemia, left eye

        H11.433 Conjunctival hyperemia, bilateral

        H11.439 Conjunctival hyperemia, unspecified eye

    H11.44 Conjunctival cysts

        H11.441 Conjunctival cysts, right eye

        H11.442 Conjunctival cysts, left eye

        H11.443 Conjunctival cysts, bilateral

        H11.449 Conjunctival cysts, unspecified eye

H11.8 Other specified disorders of conjunctiva

    H11.81 Pseudopterygium of conjunctiva

        H11.811 Pseudopterygium of conjunctiva, right eye

        H11.812 Pseudopterygium of conjunctiva, left eye

        H11.813 Pseudopterygium of conjunctiva, bilateral

        H11.819 Pseudopterygium of conjunctiva, unspecified eye

    H11.82 Conjunctivochalasis

        H11.821 Conjunctivochalasis, right eye

        H11.822 Conjunctivochalasis, left eye

        H11.823 Conjunctivochalasis, bilateral

        H11.829 Conjunctivochalasis, unspecified eye

    H11.89 Other specified disorders of conjunctiva

H11.9 Unspecified disorder of conjunctiva

DISORDERS OF SCLERA, CORNEA, IRIS AND CILIARY BODY (H15-H22)

H15 Disorders of sclera

    H15.0 Scleritis

        H15.00 Unspecified scleritis

            H15.001 Unspecified scleritis, right eye

            H15.002 Unspecified scleritis, left eye

            H15.003 Unspecified scleritis, bilateral

            H15.009 Unspecified scleritis, unspecified eye

        H15.01 Anterior scleritis

            H15.011 Anterior scleritis, right eye

            H15.012 Anterior scleritis, left eye

            H15.013 Anterior scleritis, bilateral

            H15.019 Anterior scleritis, unspecified eye

        H15.02 Brawny scleritis

            H15.021 Brawny scleritis, right eye

            H15.022 Brawny scleritis, left eye

            H15.023 Brawny scleritis, bilateral

            H15.029 Brawny scleritis, unspecified eye

        H15.03 Posterior scleritis

        Sclerotenonitis

            H15.031 Posterior scleritis, right eye

            H15.032 Posterior scleritis, left eye

            H15.033 Posterior scleritis, bilateral

            H15.039 Posterior scleritis, unspecified eye

        H15.04 Scleritis with corneal involvement

            H15.041 Scleritis with corneal involvement, right eye

            H15.042 Scleritis with corneal involvement, left eye

            H15.043 Scleritis with corneal involvement, bilateral

            H15.049 Scleritis with corneal involvement, unspecified eye

        H15.05 Scleromalacia perforans

            H15.051 Scleromalacia perforans, right eye

            H15.052 Scleromalacia perforans, left eye

            H15.053 Scleromalacia perforans, bilateral

            H15.059 Scleromalacia perforans, unspecified eye

        H15.09 Other scleritis

        Scleral abscess

            H15.091 Other scleritis, right eye

            H15.092 Other scleritis, left eye

            H15.093 Other scleritis, bilateral

            H15.099 Other scleritis, unspecified eye

    H15.1 Episcleritis

        H15.10 Unspecified episcleritis

            H15.101 Unspecified episcleritis, right eye

            H15.102 Unspecified episcleritis, left eye

            H15.103 Unspecified episcleritis, bilateral

            H15.109 Unspecified episcleritis, unspecified eye

        H15.11 Episcleritis periodica fugax

H15.111 **Episcleritis periodica fugax, right eye**

H15.112 **Episcleritis periodica fugax, left eye**

H15.113 **Episcleritis periodica fugax, bilateral**

H15.119 **Episcleritis periodica fugax, unspecified eye**

H15.12 **Nodular episcleritis**

H15.121 **Nodular episcleritis, right eye**

H15.122 **Nodular episcleritis, left eye**

H15.123 **Nodular episcleritis, bilateral**

H15.129 **Nodular episcleritis, unspecified eye**

H15.8 **Other disorders of sclera**

Excludes2: blue sclera (Q13.5)

degenerative myopia (H44.2-)

H15.81 **Equatorial staphyloma**

H15.811 **Equatorial staphyloma, right eye**

H15.812 **Equatorial staphyloma, left eye**

H15.813 **Equatorial staphyloma, bilateral**

H15.819 **Equatorial staphyloma, unspecified eye**

H15.82 **Localized anterior staphyloma**

H15.821 **Localized anterior staphyloma, right eye**

H15.822 **Localized anterior staphyloma, left eye**

H15.823 **Localized anterior staphyloma, bilateral**

H15.829 **Localized anterior staphyloma, unspecified eye**

H15.83 **Staphyloma posticum**

H15.831 **Staphyloma posticum, right eye**

H15.832 **Staphyloma posticum, left eye**

H15.833 **Staphyloma posticum, bilateral**

H15.839 **Staphyloma posticum, unspecified eye**

H15.84 **Scleral ectasia**

H15.841 **Scleral ectasia, right eye**

H15.842 **Scleral ectasia, left eye**

H15.843 **Scleral ectasia, bilateral**

H15.849 **Scleral ectasia, unspecified eye**

H15.85 **Ring staphyloma**

H15.851 **Ring staphyloma, right eye**

H15.852 **Ring staphyloma, left eye**

H15.853 **Ring staphyloma, bilateral**

H15.859 **Ring staphyloma, unspecified eye**

H15.89 **Other disorders of sclera**

H15.9 **Unspecified disorder of sclera**

H16 **Keratitis**

Definition: Keratitis is an infection or inflammation of the cornea which can be caused by a variety of conditions, including infections, dry eyes, foreign objects, contact lenses, intense light, vitamin a deficiency or allergies.

H16.0 **Corneal ulcer**

H16.00 **Unspecified corneal ulcer**

H16.001 **Unspecified corneal ulcer, right eye**

H16.002 **Unspecified corneal ulcer, left eye**

H16.003 **Unspecified corneal ulcer, bilateral**

H16.009 **Unspecified corneal ulcer, unspecified eye**

H16.01 **Central corneal ulcer**

H16.011 **Central corneal ulcer, right eye**

H16.012 **Central corneal ulcer, left eye**

H16.013 **Central corneal ulcer, bilateral**

H16.019 **Central corneal ulcer, unspecified eye**

H16.02 **Ring corneal ulcer**

H16.021 **Ring corneal ulcer, right eye**

H16.022 **Ring corneal ulcer, left eye**

H16.023 **Ring corneal ulcer, bilateral**

H16.029 **Ring corneal ulcer, unspecified eye**

H16.03 **Corneal ulcer with hypopyon**

H16.031 **Corneal ulcer with hypopyon, right eye**

H16.032 **Corneal ulcer with hypopyon, left eye**

H16.033 **Corneal ulcer with hypopyon, bilateral**

H16.039 **Corneal ulcer with hypopyon, unspecified eye**

H16.04 **Marginal corneal ulcer**

H16.041 **Marginal corneal ulcer, right eye**

H16.042 **Marginal corneal ulcer, left eye**

H16.043 **Marginal corneal ulcer, bilateral**

H16.049 **Marginal corneal ulcer, unspecified eye**

H16.05 **Mooren's corneal ulcer**

H16.051 **Mooren's corneal ulcer, right eye**

H16.052 **Mooren's corneal ulcer, left eye**

H16.053 **Mooren's corneal ulcer, bilateral**

H16.059 **Mooren's corneal ulcer, unspecified eye**

H16.06 **Mycotic corneal ulcer**

H16.061 **Mycotic corneal ulcer, right eye**

H16.062 **Mycotic corneal ulcer, left eye**

H16.063 **Mycotic corneal ulcer, bilateral**

H16.069 **Mycotic corneal ulcer, unspecified eye**

H16.07 **Perforated corneal ulcer**

H16.071 **Perforated corneal ulcer, right eye**

H16.072 **Perforated corneal ulcer, left eye**

H16.073 **Perforated corneal ulcer, bilateral**

H16.079 **Perforated corneal ulcer, unspecified eye**

H16.1 **Other and unspecified superficial keratitis without conjunctivitis**

H16.10 **Unspecified superficial keratitis**

H16.101 **Unspecified superficial keratitis, right eye**

H16.102 **Unspecified superficial keratitis, left eye**

H16.103 **Unspecified superficial keratitis, bilateral**

● New code ▲ Revised code **Excludes1:** Not coded here **Excludes2:** Not included here ⊗ Placeholder required ⑦7ᵗʰ digit required

H16.109　Unspecified superficial keratitis, unspecified eye

H16.11　Macular keratitis

Areolar keratitis

Nummular keratitis \

Stellate keratitis \

Striate keratitis

H16.111　Macular keratitis, right eye

H16.112　Macular keratitis, left eye

H16.113　Macular keratitis, bilateral

H16.119　Macular keratitis, unspecified eye

H16.12　Filamentary keratitis

H16.121　Filamentary keratitis, right eye

H16.122　Filamentary keratitis, left eye

H16.123　Filamentary keratitis, bilateral

H16.129　Filamentary keratitis, unspecified eye

H16.13　Photokeratitis

Snow blindness Welders keratitis

H16.131　Photokeratitis, right eye

H16.132　Photokeratitis, left eye

H16.133　Photokeratitis, bilateral

H16.139　Photokeratitis, unspecified eye

H16.14　Punctate keratitis

H16.141　Punctate keratitis, right eye

H16.142　Punctate keratitis, left eye

H16.143　Punctate keratitis, bilateral

H16.149　Punctate keratitis, unspecified eye

H16.2　Keratoconjunctivitis

H16.20　Unspecified keratoconjunctivitis

Superficial keratitis with conjunctivitis NOS

H16.201　Unspecified keratoconjunctivitis, right eye

H16.202　Unspecified keratoconjunctivitis, left eye

H16.203　Unspecified keratoconjunctivitis, bilateral

H16.209　Unspecified keratoconjunctivitis, unspecified eye

H16.21　Exposure keratoconjunctivitis

H16.211　Exposure keratoconjunctivitis, right eye

H16.212　Exposure keratoconjunctivitis, left eye

H16.213　Exposure keratoconjunctivitis, bilateral

H16.219　Exposure keratoconjunctivitis, unspecified eye

H16.22　Keratoconjunctivitis sicca, not specified as Sjögren's

Excludes1: Sjögren's syndrome (M35.01)

H16.221　Keratoconjunctivitis sicca, not specified as Sjögren's, right eye

H16.222　Keratoconjunctivitis sicca, not specified as Sjögren's, left eye

H16.223　Keratoconjunctivitis sicca, not specified as Sjögren's, bilateral

H16.229　Keratoconjunctivitis sicca, not specified as Sjögren's, unspecified eye

H16.23　Neurotrophic keratoconjunctivitis

H16.231　Neurotrophic keratoconjunctivitis, right eye

H16.232　Neurotrophic keratoconjunctivitis, left eye

H16.233　Neurotrophic keratoconjunctivitis, bilateral

H16.239　Neurotrophic keratoconjunctivitis, unspecified eye

H16.24　Ophthalmia nodosa

H16.241　Ophthalmia nodosa, right eye

H16.242　Ophthalmia nodosa, left eye

H16.243　Ophthalmia nodosa, bilateral

H16.249　Ophthalmia nodosa, unspecified eye

H16.25　Phlyctenular keratoconjunctivitis

H16.251　Phlyctenular keratoconjunctivitis, right eye

H16.252　Phlyctenular keratoconjunctivitis, left eye

H16.253　Phlyctenular keratoconjunctivitis, bilateral

H16.259　Phlyctenular keratoconjunctivitis, unspecified eye

H16.26　Vernal keratoconjunctivitis, with limbar and corneal involvement

Excludes1: vernal conjunctivitis without limbar and corneal involvement (H10.44)

H16.261　Vernal keratoconjunctivitis, with limbar and corneal involvement, right eye

H16.262　Vernal keratoconjunctivitis, with limbar and corneal involvement, left eye

H16.263　Vernal keratoconjunctivitis, with limbar and corneal involvement, bilateral

H16.269　Vernal keratoconjunctivitis, with limbar and corneal involvement, unspecified eye

H16.29　Other keratoconjunctivitis

H16.291　Other keratoconjunctivitis, right eye

H16.292　Other keratoconjunctivitis, left eye

H16.293　Other keratoconjunctivitis, bilateral

H16.299　Other keratoconjunctivitis, unspecified eye

H16.3　Interstitial and deep keratitis

H16.30　Unspecified interstitial keratitis

H16.301　Unspecified interstitial keratitis, right eye

H16.302　Unspecified interstitial keratitis, left eye

H16.303　Unspecified interstitial keratitis, bilateral

H16.309　Unspecified interstitial keratitis, unspecified eye

H16.31　Corneal abscess

H16.311   Corneal abscess, right eye

H16.312   Corneal abscess, left eye

H16.313   Corneal abscess, bilateral

H16.319   Corneal abscess, unspecified eye

H16.32   **Diffuse interstitial keratitis**

Cogan's syndrome

H16.321   Diffuse interstitial keratitis, right eye

H16.322   Diffuse interstitial keratitis, left eye

H16.323   Diffuse interstitial keratitis, bilateral

H16.329   Diffuse interstitial keratitis, unspecified eye

H16.33   **Sclerosing keratitis**

H16.331   Sclerosing keratitis, right eye

H16.332   Sclerosing keratitis, left eye

H16.333   Sclerosing keratitis, bilateral

H16.339   Sclerosing keratitis, unspecified eye

H16.39   **Other interstitial and deep keratitis**

H16.391   Other interstitial and deep keratitis, right eye

H16.392   Other interstitial and deep keratitis, left eye

H16.393   Other interstitial and deep keratitis, bilateral

H16.399   Other interstitial and deep keratitis, unspecified eye

H16.4   **Corneal neovascularization**

H16.40   **Unspecified corneal neovascularization**

H16.401   Unspecified corneal neovascularization, right eye

H16.402   Unspecified corneal neovascularization, left eye

H16.403   Unspecified corneal neovascularization, bilateral

H16.409   Unspecified corneal neovascularization, unspecified eye

H16.41   **Ghost vessels (corneal)**

H16.411   Ghost vessels (corneal), right eye

H16.412   Ghost vessels (corneal), left eye

H16.413   Ghost vessels (corneal), bilateral

H16.419   Ghost vessels (corneal), unspecified eye

H16.42   **Pannus (corneal)**

H16.421   Pannus (corneal), right eye

H16.422   Pannus (corneal), left eye

H16.423   Pannus (corneal), bilateral

H16.429   Pannus (corneal), unspecified eye

H16.43   **Localized vascularization of cornea**

H16.431   Localized vascularization of cornea, right eye

H16.432   Localized vascularization of cornea, left eye

H16.433   Localized vascularization of cornea, bilateral

H16.439   Localized vascularization of cornea, unspecified eye

H16.44   **Deep vascularization of cornea**

H16.441   Deep vascularization of cornea, right eye

H16.442   Deep vascularization of cornea, left eye

H16.443   Deep vascularization of cornea, bilateral

H16.449   Deep vascularization of cornea, unspecified eye

H16.8   **Other keratitis**

H16.9   **Unspecified keratitis**

H17   **Corneal scars and opacities**

H17.0   **Adherent leukoma**

H17.00   Adherent leukoma, unspecified eye

H17.01   Adherent leukoma, right eye

H17.02   Adherent leukoma, left eye

H17.03   Adherent leukoma, bilateral

H17.1   **Central corneal opacity**

Definition: Corneal opacity is a cloudy spot in the cornea, which is normally transparent. Causes include corneal scar tissue and infection.

H17.10   Central corneal opacity, unspecified eye

H17.11   Central corneal opacity, right eye

H17.12   Central corneal opacity, left eye

H17.13   Central corneal opacity, bilateral

H17.8   **Other corneal scars and opacities**

H17.81   Minor opacity of cornea

Corneal nebula

H17.811   Minor opacity of cornea, right eye

H17.812   Minor opacity of cornea, left eye

H17.813   Minor opacity of cornea, bilateral

H17.819   Minor opacity of cornea, unspecified eye

H17.82   Peripheral opacity of cornea

H17.821   Peripheral opacity of cornea, right eye

H17.822   Peripheral opacity of cornea, left eye

H17.823   Peripheral opacity of cornea, bilateral

H17.829   Peripheral opacity of cornea, unspecified eye

H17.89   Other corneal scars and opacities

H17.9   **Unspecified corneal scar and opacity**

H18   **Other disorders of cornea**

H18.0   **Corneal pigmentations and deposits**

H18.00   Unspecified corneal deposit

H18.001   Unspecified corneal deposit, right eye

H18.002   Unspecified corneal deposit, left eye

H18.003   Unspecified corneal deposit, bilateral

H18.009   Unspecified corneal deposit, unspecified eye

H18.01   Anterior corneal pigmentations

Staehli's line

H18.011   Anterior corneal pigmentations, right eye

H18.012   **Anterior corneal pigmentations, left eye**

H18.013   **Anterior corneal pigmentations, bilateral**

H18.019   **Anterior corneal pigmentations, unspecified eye**

H18.02   **Argentous corneal deposits**

H18.021   **Argentous corneal deposits, right eye**

H18.022   **Argentous corneal deposits, left eye**

H18.023   **Argentous corneal deposits, bilateral**

H18.029   **Argentous corneal deposits, unspecified eye**

H18.03   **Corneal deposits in metabolic disorders**

<u>Code also</u> associated metabolic disorder

H18.031   **Corneal deposits in metabolic disorders, right eye**

H18.032   **Corneal deposits in metabolic disorders, left eye**

H18.033   **Corneal deposits in metabolic disorders, bilateral**

H18.039   **Corneal deposits in metabolic disorders, unspecified eye**

H18.04   **Kayser-Fleischer ring**

<u>Code also</u> associated Wilson's disease (E83.01)

H18.041   **Kayser-Fleischer ring, right eye**

H18.042   **Kayser-Fleischer ring, left eye**

H18.043   **Kayser-Fleischer ring, bilateral**

H18.049   **Kayser-Fleischer ring, unspecified eye**

H18.05   **Posterior corneal pigmentations**

Krukenberg's spindle

H18.051   **Posterior corneal pigmentations, right eye**

H18.052   **Posterior corneal pigmentations, left eye**

H18.053   **Posterior corneal pigmentations, bilateral**

H18.059   **Posterior corneal pigmentations, unspecified eye**

H18.06   **Stromal corneal pigmentations**

Hematocornea

H18.061   **Stromal corneal pigmentations, right eye**

H18.062   **Stromal corneal pigmentations, left eye**

H18.063   **Stromal corneal pigmentations, bilateral**

H18.069   **Stromal corneal pigmentations, unspecified eye**

H18.1   **Bullous keratopathy**

H18.10   **Bullous keratopathy, unspecified eye**

H18.11   **Bullous keratopathy, right eye**

H18.12   **Bullous keratopathy, left eye**

H18.13   **Bullous keratopathy, bilateral**

H18.2   **Other and unspecified corneal edema**

H18.20   **Unspecified corneal edema**

H18.21   **Corneal edema secondary to contact lens**

Excludes2: Other corneal disorders due to contact lens (H18.82-)

H18.211   **Corneal edema secondary to contact lens, right eye**

H18.212   **Corneal edema secondary to contact lens, left eye**

H18.213   **Corneal edema secondary to contact lens, bilateral**

H18.219   **Corneal edema secondary to contact lens, unspecified eye**

H18.22   **Idiopathic corneal edema**

H18.221   **Idiopathic corneal edema, right eye**

H18.222   **Idiopathic corneal edema, left eye**

H18.223   **Idiopathic corneal edema, bilateral**

H18.229   **Idiopathic corneal edema, unspecified eye**

H18.23   **Secondary corneal edema**

H18.231   **Secondary corneal edema, right eye**

H18.232   **Secondary corneal edema, left eye**

H18.233   **Secondary corneal edema, bilateral**

H18.239   **Secondary corneal edema, unspecified eye**

H18.3   **Changes of corneal membranes**

H18.30   **Unspecified corneal membrane change**

H18.31   **Folds and rupture in Bowman's membrane**

H18.311   **Folds and rupture in Bowman's membrane, right eye**

H18.312   **Folds and rupture in Bowman's membrane, left eye**

H18.313   **Folds and rupture in Bowman's membrane, bilateral**

H18.319   **Folds and rupture in Bowman's membrane, unspecified eye**

H18.32   **Folds in Descemet's membrane**

H18.321   **Folds in Descemet's membrane, right eye**

H18.322   **Folds in Descemet's membrane, left eye**

H18.323   **Folds in Descemet's membrane, bilateral**

H18.329   **Folds in Descemet's membrane, unspecified eye**

H18.33   **Rupture in Descemet's membrane**

H18.331   **Rupture in Descemet's membrane, right eye**

H18.332   **Rupture in Descemet's membrane, left eye**

H18.333   **Rupture in Descemet's membrane, bilateral**

H18.339   **Rupture in Descemet's membrane, unspecified eye**

H18.4   **Corneal degeneration**

Excludes1: Mooren's ulcer (H16.0-)

recurrent erosion of cornea (H18.83-)

H18.40   **Unspecified corneal degeneration**

H18.41   **Arcus senilis**

Senile corneal changes

H18.411   Arcus senilis, right eye

H18.412   Arcus senilis, left eye

H18.413   Arcus senilis, bilateral

H18.419   Arcus senilis, unspecified eye

H18.42   **Band keratopathy**

H18.421   Band keratopathy, right eye

H18.422   Band keratopathy, left eye

H18.423   Band keratopathy, bilateral

H18.429   Band keratopathy, unspecified eye

H18.43   **Other calcerous corneal degeneration**

H18.44   **Keratomalacia**

Excludes1: keratomalacia due to vitamin A deficiency (E50.4)

H18.441   Keratomalacia, right eye

H18.442   Keratomalacia, left eye

H18.443   Keratomalacia, bilateral

H18.449   Keratomalacia, unspecified eye

H18.45   **Nodular corneal degeneration**

H18.451   Nodular corneal degeneration, right eye

H18.452   Nodular corneal degeneration, left eye

H18.453   Nodular corneal degeneration, bilateral

H18.459   Nodular corneal degeneration, unspecified eye

H18.46   **Peripheral corneal degeneration**

H18.461   Peripheral corneal degeneration, right eye

H18.462   Peripheral corneal degeneration, left eye

H18.463   Peripheral corneal degeneration, bilateral

H18.469   Peripheral corneal degeneration, unspecified eye

H18.49   **Other corneal degeneration**

H18.5   **Hereditary corneal dystrophies**

H18.50   **Unspecified hereditary corneal dystrophies**

H18.51   **Endothelial corneal dystrophy**

Fuchs' dystrophy

H18.52   **Epithelial (juvenile) corneal dystrophy**

H18.53   **Granular corneal dystrophy**

H18.54   **Lattice corneal dystrophy**

H18.55   **Macular corneal dystrophy**

H18.59   **Other hereditary corneal dystrophies**

H18.6   **Keratoconus**

H18.60   **Keratoconus, unspecified**

H18.601   Keratoconus, unspecified, right eye

H18.602   Keratoconus, unspecified, left eye

H18.603   Keratoconus, unspecified, bilateral

H18.609   Keratoconus, unspecified, unspecified eye

H18.61   **Keratoconus, stable**

H18.611   Keratoconus, stable, right eye

H18.612   Keratoconus, stable, left eye

H18.613   Keratoconus, stable, bilateral

H18.619   Keratoconus, stable, unspecified eye

H18.62   **Keratoconus, unstable**

Acute hydrops

H18.621   Keratoconus, unstable, right eye

H18.622   Keratoconus, unstable, left eye

H18.623   Keratoconus, unstable, bilateral

H18.629   Keratoconus, unstable, unspecified eye

H18.7   **Other and unspecified corneal deformities**

Excludes1: congenital malformations of cornea (Q13.3-Q13.4)

H18.70   **Unspecified corneal deformity**

H18.71   **Corneal ectasia**

H18.711   Corneal ectasia, right eye

H18.712   Corneal ectasia, left eye

H18.713   Corneal ectasia, bilateral

H18.719   Corneal ectasia, unspecified eye

H18.72   **Corneal staphyloma**

H18.721   Corneal staphyloma, right eye

H18.722   Corneal staphyloma, left eye

H18.723   Corneal staphyloma, bilateral

H18.729   Corneal staphyloma, unspecified eye

H18.73   **Descemetocele**

H18.731   Descemetocele, right eye

H18.732   Descemetocele, left eye

H18.733   Descemetocele, bilateral

H18.739   Descemetocele, unspecified eye

H18.79   **Other corneal deformities**

H18.791   Other corneal deformities, right eye

H18.792   Other corneal deformities, left eye

H18.793   Other corneal deformities, bilateral

H18.799   Other corneal deformities, unspecified eye

H18.8   **Other specified disorders of cornea**

H18.81   **Anesthesia and hypoesthesia of cornea**

H18.811   Anesthesia and hypoesthesia of cornea, right eye

H18.812   Anesthesia and hypoesthesia of cornea, left eye

H18.813   Anesthesia and hypoesthesia of cornea, bilateral

H18.819   Anesthesia and hypoesthesia of cornea, unspecified eye

H18.82   **Corneal disorder due to contact lens**

Excludes2: corneal edema due to contact lens (H18.21-)

H18.821   Corneal disorder due to contact lens, right eye

H18.822   Corneal disorder due to contact lens, left eye

H18.823   Corneal disorder due to contact lens, bilateral

H18.829   Corneal disorder due to contact lens, unspecified eye

H18.83   **Recurrent erosion of cornea**

H18.831 Recurrent erosion of cornea, right eye

H18.832 Recurrent erosion of cornea, left eye

H18.833 Recurrent erosion of cornea, bilateral

H18.839 Recurrent erosion of cornea, unspecified eye

H18.89 Other specified disorders of cornea

H18.891 Other specified disorders of cornea, right eye

H18.892 Other specified disorders of cornea, left eye

H18.893 Other specified disorders of cornea, bilateral

H18.899 Other specified disorders of cornea, unspecified eye

H18.9 Unspecified disorder of cornea

H20 Iridocyclitis

H20.0 Acute and subacute iridocyclitis

Acute anterior uveitis

Acute cyclitis

Acute iritis

Subacute anterior uveitis

Subacute cyclitis

Subacute iritis

Excludes1: iridocyclitis, iritis, uveitis (due to) (in) diabetes mellitus (E08-E13 with .39)

iridocyclitis, iritis, uveitis (due to) (in) diphtheria (A36.89)

iridocyclitis, iritis, uveitis (due to) (in) gonococcal (A54.32)

iridocyclitis, iritis, uveitis (due to) (in) herpes (simplex) (B00.51)

iridocyclitis, iritis, uveitis (due to) (in) herpes zoster (B02.32)

iridocyclitis, iritis, uveitis (due to) (in) late congenital syphilis (A50.39)

iridocyclitis, iritis, uveitis (due to) (in) late syphilis (A52.71)

iridocyclitis, iritis, uveitis (due to) (in) sarcoidosis (D86.83)

iridocyclitis, iritis, uveitis (due to) (in) syphilis (A51.43)

iridocyclitis, iritis, uveitis (due to) (in) toxoplasmosis (B58.09)

iridocyclitis, iritis, uveitis (due to) (in) tuberculosis (A18.54)

H20.00 Unspecified acute and subacute iridocyclitis

H20.01 Primary iridocyclitis

H20.011 Primary iridocyclitis, right eye

H20.012 Primary iridocyclitis, left eye

H20.013 Primary iridocyclitis, bilateral

H20.019 Primary iridocyclitis, unspecified eye

H20.02 Recurrent acute iridocyclitis

H20.021 Recurrent acute iridocyclitis, right eye

H20.022 Recurrent acute iridocyclitis, left eye

H20.023 Recurrent acute iridocyclitis, bilateral

H20.029 Recurrent acute iridocyclitis, unspecified eye

H20.03 Secondary infectious iridocyclitis

H20.031 Secondary infectious iridocyclitis, right eye

H20.032 Secondary infectious iridocyclitis, left eye

H20.033 Secondary infectious iridocyclitis, bilateral

H20.039 Secondary infectious iridocyclitis, unspecified eye

H20.04 Secondary noninfectious iridocyclitis

H20.041 Secondary noninfectious iridocyclitis, right eye

H20.042 Secondary noninfectious iridocyclitis, left eye

H20.043 Secondary noninfectious iridocyclitis, bilateral

H20.049 Secondary noninfectious iridocyclitis, unspecified eye

H20.05 Hypopyon

H20.051 Hypopyon, right eye

H20.052 Hypopyon, left eye

H20.053 Hypopyon, bilateral

H20.059 Hypopyon, unspecified eye

H20.1 Chronic iridocyclitis

Use additional code for any associated cataract (H26.21-)

Excludes2: posterior cyclitis (H30.2-)

H20.10 Chronic iridocyclitis, unspecified eye

H20.11 Chronic iridocyclitis, right eye

H20.12 Chronic iridocyclitis, left eye

H20.13 Chronic iridocyclitis, bilateral

H20.2 Lens-induced iridocyclitis

H20.20 Lens-induced iridocyclitis, unspecified eye

H20.21 Lens-induced iridocyclitis, right eye

H20.22 Lens-induced iridocyclitis, left eye

H20.23 Lens-induced iridocyclitis, bilateral

H20.8 Other iridocyclitis

Excludes2: glaucomatocyclitis crises (H40.4-)

posterior cyclitis (H30.2-) sympathetic uveitis (H44.13-)

H20.81 Fuchs' heterochromic cyclitis

H20.811 Fuchs' heterochromic cyclitis, right eye

H20.812 Fuchs' heterochromic cyclitis, left eye

H20.813 Fuchs' heterochromic cyclitis, bilateral

H20.819 Fuchs' heterochromic cyclitis, unspecified eye

H20.82 Vogt-Koyanagi syndrome

H20.821 Vogt-Koyanagi syndrome, right eye

H20.822 Vogt-Koyanagi syndrome, left eye

H20.823 Vogt-Koyanagi syndrome, bilateral

H20.829 Vogt-Koyanagi syndrome, unspecified eye

H20.9　Unspecified iridocyclitis
　　　　Uveitis NOS

H21　Other disorders of iris and ciliary body
　　Excludes2: sympathetic uveitis (H44.1-)

H21.0　Hyphema
　　　　Excludes1: traumatic hyphema (S05.1-)
　　H21.00　Hyphema, unspecified eye
　　H21.01　Hyphema, right eye
　　H21.02　Hyphema, left eye
　　H21.03　Hyphema, bilateral

H21.1　Other vascular disorders of iris and ciliary body
　　　　Neovascularization of iris or ciliary body
　　　　Rubeosis iridis
　　　　Rubeosis of iris
　　H21.1X　Other vascular disorders of iris and ciliary body
　　　　H21.1X1　Other vascular disorders of iris and ciliary body, right eye
　　　　H21.1X2　Other vascular disorders of iris and ciliary body, left eye
　　　　H21.1X3　Other vascular disorders of iris and ciliary body, bilateral
　　　　H21.1X9　Other vascular disorders of iris and ciliary body, unspecified eye

H21.2　Degeneration of iris and ciliary body
　　H21.21　Degeneration of chamber angle
　　　　H21.211　Degeneration of chamber angle, right eye
　　　　H21.212　Degeneration of chamber angle, left eye
　　　　H21.213　Degeneration of chamber angle, bilateral
　　　　H21.219　Degeneration of chamber angle, unspecified eye
　　H21.22　Degeneration of ciliary body
　　　　H21.221　Degeneration of ciliary body, right eye
　　　　H21.222　Degeneration of ciliary body, left eye
　　　　H21.223　Degeneration of ciliary body, bilateral
　　　　H21.229　Degeneration of ciliary body, unspecified eye
　　H21.23　Degeneration of iris (pigmentary)
　　　　Translucency of iris
　　　　H21.231　Degeneration of iris (pigmentary), right eye
　　　　H21.232　Degeneration of iris (pigmentary), left eye
　　　　H21.233　Degeneration of iris (pigmentary), bilateral
　　　　H21.239　Degeneration of iris (pigmentary), unspecified eye
　　H21.24　Degeneration of pupillary margin
　　　　H21.241　Degeneration of pupillary margin, right eye
　　　　H21.242　Degeneration of pupillary margin, left eye

H21.243　Degeneration of pupillary margin, bilateral
H21.249　Degeneration of pupillary margin, unspecified eye

H21.25　Iridoschisis
　　H21.251　Iridoschisis, right eye
　　H21.252　Iridoschisis, left eye
　　H21.253　Iridoschisis, bilateral
　　H21.259　Iridoschisis, unspecified eye

H21.26　Iris atrophy (essential) (progressive)
　　H21.261　Iris atrophy (essential) (progressive), right eye
　　H21.262　Iris atrophy (essential) (progressive), left eye
　　H21.263　Iris atrophy (essential) (progressive), bilateral
　　H21.269　Iris atrophy (essential) (progressive), unspecified eye

H21.27　Miotic pupillary cyst
　　H21.271　Miotic pupillary cyst, right eye
　　H21.272　Miotic pupillary cyst, left eye
　　H21.273　Miotic pupillary cyst, bilateral
　　H21.279　Miotic pupillary cyst, unspecified eye

H21.29　Other iris atrophy

H21.3　Cyst of iris, ciliary body and anterior chamber
　　　　Excludes2: miotic pupillary cyst (H21.27-)
　　H21.30　Idiopathic cysts of iris, ciliary body or anterior chamber
　　　　Cyst of iris, ciliary body or anterior chamber NOS
　　　　H21.301　Idiopathic cysts of iris, ciliary body or anterior chamber, right eye
　　　　H21.302　Idiopathic cysts of iris, ciliary body or anterior chamber, left eye
　　　　H21.303　Idiopathic cysts of iris, ciliary body or anterior chamber, bilateral
　　　　H21.309　Idiopathic cysts of iris, ciliary body or anterior chamber, unspecified eye
　　H21.31　Exudative cysts of iris or anterior chamber
　　　　H21.311　Exudative cysts of iris or anterior chamber, right eye
　　　　H21.312　Exudative cysts of iris or anterior chamber, left eye
　　　　H21.313　Exudative cysts of iris or anterior chamber, bilateral
　　　　H21.319　Exudative cysts of iris or anterior chamber, unspecified eye
　　H21.32　Implantation cysts of iris, ciliary body or anterior chamber
　　　　H21.321　Implantation cysts of iris, ciliary body or anterior chamber, right eye
　　　　H21.322　Implantation cysts of iris, ciliary body or anterior chamber, left eye
　　　　H21.323　Implantation cysts of iris, ciliary body or anterior chamber, bilateral
　　　　H21.329　Implantation cysts of iris, ciliary body or anterior chamber, unspecified eye

H21.33 **Parasitic cyst of iris, ciliary body or anterior chamber**

    H21.331 **Parasitic cyst of iris, ciliary body or anterior chamber, right eye**

    H21.332 **Parasitic cyst of iris, ciliary body or anterior chamber, left eye**

    H21.333 **Parasitic cyst of iris, ciliary body or anterior chamber, bilateral**

    H21.339 **Parasitic cyst of iris, ciliary body or anterior chamber, unspecified eye**

H21.34 **Primary cyst of pars plana**

    H21.341 **Primary cyst of pars plana, right eye**

    H21.342 **Primary cyst of pars plana, left eye**

    H21.343 **Primary cyst of pars plana, bilateral**

    H21.349 **Primary cyst of pars plana, unspecified eye**

H21.35 **Exudative cyst of pars plana**

    H21.351 **Exudative cyst of pars plana, right eye**

    H21.352 **Exudative cyst of pars plana, left eye**

    H21.353 **Exudative cyst of pars plana, bilateral**

    H21.359 **Exudative cyst of pars plana, unspecified eye**

H21.4 **Pupillary membranes**

Iris bombé

Pupillary occlusion

Pupillary seclusion

Excludes1: congenital pupillary membranes (Q13.8)

H21.40 **Pupillary membranes, unspecified eye**

H21.41 **Pupillary membranes, right eye**

H21.42 **Pupillary membranes, left eye**

H21.43 **Pupillary membranes, bilateral**

H21.5 **Other and unspecified adhesions and disruptions of iris and ciliary body**

Excludes1: corectopia (Q13.2)

H21.50 **Unspecified adhesions of iris**

Synechia (iris) NOS

    H21.501 **Unspecified adhesions of iris, right eye**

    H21.502 **Unspecified adhesions of iris, left eye**

    H21.503 **Unspecified adhesions of iris, bilateral**

    H21.509 **Unspecified adhesions of iris and ciliary body, unspecified eye**

H21.51 **Anterior synechiae (iris)**

    H21.511 **Anterior synechiae (iris), right eye**

    H21.512 **Anterior synechiae (iris), left eye**

    H21.513 **Anterior synechiae (iris), bilateral**

    H21.519 **Anterior synechiae (iris), unspecified eye**

H21.52 **Goniosynechiae**

    H21.521 **Goniosynechiae, right eye**

    H21.522 **Goniosynechiae, left eye**

    H21.523 **Goniosynechiae, bilateral**

    H21.529 **Goniosynechiae, unspecified eye**

H21.53 **Iridodialysis**

    H21.531 **Iridodialysis, right eye**

    H21.532 **Iridodialysis, left eye**

    H21.533 **Iridodialysis, bilateral**

    H21.539 **Iridodialysis, unspecified eye**

H21.54 **Posterior synechiae (iris)**

    H21.541 **Posterior synechiae (iris), right eye**

    H21.542 **Posterior synechiae (iris), left eye**

    H21.543 **Posterior synechiae (iris), bilateral**

    H21.549 **Posterior synechiae (iris), unspecified eye**

H21.55 **Recession of chamber angle**

    H21.551 **Recession of chamber angle, right eye**

    H21.552 **Recession of chamber angle, left eye**

    H21.553 **Recession of chamber angle, bilateral**

    H21.559 **Recession of chamber angle, unspecified eye**

H21.56 **Pupillary abnormalities**

Deformed pupil

Ectopic pupil

Rupture of sphincter, pupil

Excludes1: congenital deformity of pupil (Q13.2-)

    H21.561 **Pupillary abnormality, right eye**

    H21.562 **Pupillary abnormality, left eye**

    H21.563 **Pupillary abnormality, bilateral**

    H21.569 **Pupillary abnormality, unspecified eye**

H21.8 **Other specified disorders of iris and ciliary body**

H21.81 **Floppy iris syndrome**

Intraoperative floppy iris syndrome (IFIS)

Use additional code for adverse effect, if applicable, to identify drug (T36-T50 with fifth or sixth character 5)

H21.82 **Plateau iris syndrome (post-iridectomy) (postprocedural)**

H21.89 **Other specified disorders of iris and ciliary body**

H21.9 **Unspecified disorder of iris and ciliary body**

H22 **Disorders of iris and ciliary body in diseases classified elsewhere**

Code first underlying disease, such as:

gout (M1A.-, M10.-)

leprosy (A30.-)

parasitic disease (B89)

DISORDERS OF LENS (H25-H28)

H25 **Age-related cataract**

Definition: A cataract is a clouding that develops in the crystalline lens of the eye or in its envelope, varying in degree from slight to complete opacity and obstructing the passage of light.

Senile cataract

Excludes2: capsular glaucoma with pseudoexfoliation of lens (H40.1-)

H25.0 **Age-related incipient cataract**

H25.01 **Cortical age-related cataract**

    H25.011 **Cortical age-related cataract, right eye**

    H25.012 **Cortical age-related cataract, left eye**

    H25.013 **Cortical age-related cataract, bilateral**

    H25.019 **Cortical age-related cataract, unspecified eye**

H25.03 **Anterior subcapsular polar age-related cataract**

    H25.031 **Anterior subcapsular polar age-related cataract, right eye**

    H25.032 **Anterior subcapsular polar age-related cataract, left eye**

    H25.033 **Anterior subcapsular polar age-related cataract, bilateral**

    H25.039 **Anterior subcapsular polar age-related cataract, unspecified eye**

H25.04 **Posterior subcapsular polar age-related cataract**

    H25.041 **Posterior subcapsular polar age-related cataract, right eye**

    H25.042 **Posterior subcapsular polar age-related cataract, left eye**

    H25.043 **Posterior subcapsular polar age-related cataract, bilateral**

    H25.049 **Posterior subcapsular polar age-related cataract, unspecified eye**

H25.09 **Other age-related incipient cataract**

Coronary age-related cataract

Punctate age-related cataract

Water clefts

    H25.091 **Other age-related incipient cataract, right eye**

    H25.092 **Other age-related incipient cataract, left eye**

    H25.093 **Other age-related incipient cataract, bilateral**

    H25.099 **Other age-related incipient cataract, unspecified eye**

H25.1 **Age-related nuclear cataract**

Cataracta brunescens Nuclear sclerosis cataract

H25.10 **Age-related nuclear cataract, unspecified eye**

H25.11 **Age-related nuclear cataract, right eye**

H25.12 **Age-related nuclear cataract, left eye**

H25.13 **Age-related nuclear cataract, bilateral**

H25.2 **Age-related cataract, morgagnian type**

Age-related hypermature cataract

H25.20 **Age-related cataract, morgagnian type, unspecified eye**

H25.21 **Age-related cataract, morgagnian type, right eye**

H25.22 **Age-related cataract, morgagnian type, left eye**

H25.23 **Age-related cataract, morgagnian type, bilateral**

H25.8 **Other age-related cataract**

H25.81 **Combined forms of age-related cataract**

    H25.811 **Combined forms of age-related cataract, right eye**

    H25.812 **Combined forms of age-related cataract, left eye**

    H25.813 **Combined forms of age-related cataract, bilateral**

    H25.819 **Combined forms of age-related cataract, unspecified eye**

H25.89 **Other age-related cataract**

H25.9 **Unspecified age-related cataract**

H26 **Other cataract**

Excludes1: congenital cataract (Q12.0)

H26.0 **Infantile and juvenile cataract**

H26.00 **Unspecified infantile and juvenile cataract**

    H26.001 **Unspecified infantile and juvenile cataract, right eye**

    H26.002 **Unspecified infantile and juvenile cataract, left eye**

    H26.003 **Unspecified infantile and juvenile cataract, bilateral**

    H26.009 **Unspecified infantile and juvenile cataract, unspecified eye**

H26.01 **Infantile and juvenile cortical, lamellar, or zonular cataract**

    H26.011 **Infantile and juvenile cortical, lamellar, or zonular cataract, right eye**

    H26.012 **Infantile and juvenile cortical, lamellar, or zonular cataract, left eye**

    H26.013 **Infantile and juvenile cortical, lamellar, or zonular cataract, bilateral**

    H26.019 **Infantile and juvenile cortical, lamellar, or zonular cataract, unspecified eye**

H26.03 **Infantile and juvenile nuclear cataract**

    H26.031 **Infantile and juvenile nuclear cataract, right eye**

    H26.032 **Infantile and juvenile nuclear cataract, left eye**

    H26.033 **Infantile and juvenile nuclear cataract, bilateral**

    H26.039 **Infantile and juvenile nuclear cataract, unspecified eye**

H26.04 **Anterior subcapsular polar infantile and juvenile cataract**

    H26.041 **Anterior subcapsular polar infantile and juvenile cataract, right eye**

    H26.042 **Anterior subcapsular polar infantile and juvenile cataract, left eye**

    H26.043 **Anterior subcapsular polar infantile and juvenile cataract, bilateral**

    H26.049 **Anterior subcapsular polar infantile and juvenile cataract, unspecified eye**

H26.05 **Posterior subcapsular polar infantile and juvenile cataract**

    H26.051 **Posterior subcapsular polar infantile and juvenile cataract, right eye**

● New code   ▲ Revised code   **Excludes1:** Not coded here   **Excludes2:** Not included here   ⊗ Placeholder required   ⑦ 7th digit required

H26.052   **Posterior subcapsular polar infantile and juvenile cataract, left eye**

H26.053   **Posterior subcapsular polar infantile and juvenile cataract, bilateral**

H26.059   **Posterior subcapsular polar infantile and juvenile cataract, unspecified eye**

H26.06   **Combined forms of infantile and juvenile cataract**

H26.061   **Combined forms of infantile and juvenile cataract, right eye**

H26.062   **Combined forms of infantile and juvenile cataract, left eye**

H26.063   **Combined forms of infantile and juvenile cataract, bilateral**

H26.069   **Combined forms of infantile and juvenile cataract, unspecified eye**

H26.09   **Other infantile and juvenile cataract**

H26.1   Traumatic cataract

<u>Use additional code</u> (Chapter 20) to identify external cause

H26.10   **Unspecified traumatic cataract**

H26.101   **Unspecified traumatic cataract, right eye**

H26.102   **Unspecified traumatic cataract, left eye**

H26.103   **Unspecified traumatic cataract, bilateral**

H26.109   **Unspecified traumatic cataract, unspecified eye**

H26.11   **Localized traumatic opacities**

H26.111   **Localized traumatic opacities, right eye**

H26.112   **Localized traumatic opacities, left eye**

H26.113   **Localized traumatic opacities, bilateral**

H26.119   **Localized traumatic opacities, unspecified eye**

H26.12   **Partially resolved traumatic cataract**

H26.121   **Partially resolved traumatic cataract, right eye**

H26.122   **Partially resolved traumatic cataract, left eye**

H26.123   **Partially resolved traumatic cataract, bilateral**

H26.129   **Partially resolved traumatic cataract, unspecified eye**

H26.13   **Total traumatic cataract**

H26.131   **Total traumatic cataract, right eye**

H26.132   **Total traumatic cataract, left eye**

H26.133   **Total traumatic cataract, bilateral**

H26.139   **Total traumatic cataract, unspecified eye**

H26.2   Complicated cataract

H26.20   **Unspecified complicated cataract**

Cataracta complicata NOS

H26.21   **Cataract with neovascularization**

<u>Code also</u> associated condition, such as:

    chronic iridocyclitis (H20.1-)

H26.211   **Cataract with neovascularization, right eye**

H26.212   **Cataract with neovascularization, left eye**

H26.213   **Cataract with neovascularization, bilateral**

H26.219   **Cataract with neovascularization, unspecified eye**

H26.22   **Cataract secondary to ocular disorders (degenerative) (inflammatory)**

<u>Code also</u> associated ocular disorder

H26.221   **Cataract secondary to ocular disorders (degenerative) (inflammatory), right eye**

H26.222   **Cataract secondary to ocular disorders (degenerative) (inflammatory), left eye**

H26.223   **Cataract secondary to ocular disorders (degenerative) (inflammatory), bilateral**

H26.229   **Cataract secondary to ocular disorders (degenerative) (inflammatory), unspecified eye**

H26.23   **Glaucomatous flecks (subcapsular)**

<u>Code first</u> underlying glaucoma (H40-H42)

H26.231   **Glaucomatous flecks (subcapsular), right eye**

H26.232   **Glaucomatous flecks (subcapsular), left eye**

H26.233   **Glaucomatous flecks (subcapsular), bilateral**

H26.239   **Glaucomatous flecks (subcapsular), unspecified eye**

H26.3   Drug-induced cataract

Toxic cataract

<u>Use additional code</u> for adverse effect, if applicable, to identify drug (T36-T50 with fifth or sixth character 5)

H26.30   **Drug-induced cataract, unspecified eye**

H26.31   **Drug-induced cataract, right eye**

H26.32   **Drug-induced cataract, left eye**

H26.33   **Drug-induced cataract, bilateral**

H26.4   Secondary cataract

H26.40   **Unspecified secondary cataract**

H26.41   **Soemmering's ring**

H26.411   **Soemmering's ring, right eye**

H26.412   **Soemmering's ring, left eye**

H26.413   **Soemmering's ring, bilateral**

H26.419   **Soemmering's ring, unspecified eye**

H26.49   **Other secondary cataract**

H26.491   **Other secondary cataract, right eye**

H26.492   **Other secondary cataract, left eye**

H26.493   **Other secondary cataract, bilateral**

H26.499   **Other secondary cataract, unspecified eye**

H26.8   Other specified cataract

H26.9   Unspecified cataract

H27 **Other disorders of lens**

Excludes1: congenital lens malformations (Q12.-)

mechanical complications of intraocular lens implant (T85.2)

pseudophakia (Z96.1)

H27.0 **Aphakia**

Acquired absence of lens

Acquired aphakia

Aphakia due to trauma

Excludes1: cataract extraction status (Z98.4-)

congenital absence of lens (Q12.3)

congenital aphakia (Q12.3)

H27.00 **Aphakia, unspecified eye**

H27.01 **Aphakia, right eye**

H27.02 **Aphakia, left eye**

H27.03 **Aphakia, bilateral**

H27.1 **Dislocation of lens**

H27.10 **Unspecified dislocation of lens**

H27.11 **Subluxation of lens**

H27.111 **Subluxation of lens, right eye**

H27.112 **Subluxation of lens, left eye**

H27.113 **Subluxation of lens, bilateral**

H27.119 **Subluxation of lens, unspecified eye**

H27.12 **Anterior dislocation of lens**

H27.121 **Anterior dislocation of lens, right eye**

H27.122 **Anterior dislocation of lens, left eye**

H27.123 **Anterior dislocation of lens, bilateral**

H27.129 **Anterior dislocation of lens, unspecified eye**

H27.13 **Posterior dislocation of lens**

H27.131 **Posterior dislocation of lens, right eye**

H27.132 **Posterior dislocation of lens, left eye**

H27.133 **Posterior dislocation of lens, bilateral**

H27.139 **Posterior dislocation of lens, unspecified eye**

H27.8 **Other specified disorders of lens**

H27.9 **Unspecified disorder of lens**

H28 **Cataract in diseases classified elsewhere**

Code first underlying disease, such as:

hypoparathyroidism (E20.-)

myotonia (G71.1-)

myxedema (E03.-)

protein-calorie malnutrition (E40-E46)

Excludes1: cataract in diabetes mellitus (E08.36, E09.36, E10.36, E11.36, E13.36)

DISORDERS OF CHOROID AND RETINA (H30-H36)

H30 **Chorioretinal inflammation**

H30.0 **Focal chorioretinal inflammation**

Focal chorioretinitis

Focal choroiditis

Focal retinitis

Focal retinochoroiditis

H30.00 **Unspecified focal chorioretinal inflammation**

Focal chorioretinitis NOS

Focal choroiditis NOS

Focal retinitis NOS

Focal retinochoroiditis NOS

H30.001 **Unspecified focal chorioretinal inflammation, right eye**

H30.002 **Unspecified focal chorioretinal inflammation, left eye**

H30.003 **Unspecified focal chorioretinal inflammation, bilateral**

H30.009 **Unspecified focal chorioretinal inflammation, unspecified eye**

H30.01 **Focal chorioretinal inflammation, juxtapapillary**

H30.011 **Focal chorioretinal inflammation, juxtapapillary, right eye**

H30.012 **Focal chorioretinal inflammation, juxtapapillary, left eye**

H30.013 **Focal chorioretinal inflammation, juxtapapillary, bilateral**

H30.019 **Focal chorioretinal inflammation, juxtapapillary, unspecified eye**

H30.02 **Focal chorioretinal inflammation of posterior pole**

H30.021 **Focal chorioretinal inflammation of posterior pole, right eye**

H30.022 **Focal chorioretinal inflammation of posterior pole, left eye**

H30.023 **Focal chorioretinal inflammation of posterior pole, bilateral**

H30.029 **Focal chorioretinal inflammation of posterior pole, unspecified eye**

H30.03 **Focal chorioretinal inflammation, peripheral**

H30.031 **Focal chorioretinal inflammation, peripheral, right eye**

H30.032 **Focal chorioretinal inflammation, peripheral, left eye**

H30.033 **Focal chorioretinal inflammation, peripheral, bilateral**

H30.039 **Focal chorioretinal inflammation, peripheral, unspecified eye**

H30.04 **Focal chorioretinal inflammation, macular or paramacular**

H30.041 **Focal chorioretinal inflammation, macular or paramacular, right eye**

H30.042 **Focal chorioretinal inflammation, macular or paramacular, left eye**

H30.043 **Focal chorioretinal inflammation, macular or paramacular, bilateral**

H30.049 **Focal chorioretinal inflammation, macular or paramacular, unspecified eye**

H30.1 **Disseminated chorioretinal inflammation**

Disseminated chorioretinitis

Disseminated choroiditis

Disseminated retinitis

Disseminated retinochoroiditis

Excludes2: exudative retinopathy (H35.02-)

● New code ▲ Revised code **Excludes1:** Not coded here **Excludes2:** Not included here ⊗ Placeholder required ⑦ 7th digit required

H30.10 **Unspecified disseminated chorioretinal inflammation**

Disseminated chorioretinitis NOS

Disseminated choroiditis NOS

Disseminated retinitis NOS

Disseminated retinochoroiditis NOS

    H30.101 **Unspecified disseminated chorioretinal inflammation, right eye**

    H30.102 **Unspecified disseminated chorioretinal inflammation, left eye**

    H30.103 **Unspecified disseminated chorioretinal inflammation, bilateral**

    H30.109 **Unspecified disseminated chorioretinal inflammation, unspecified eye**

H30.11 **Disseminated chorioretinal inflammation of posterior pole**

    H30.111 **Disseminated chorioretinal inflammation of posterior pole, right eye**

    H30.112 **Disseminated chorioretinal inflammation of posterior pole, left eye**

    H30.113 **Disseminated chorioretinal inflammation of posterior pole, bilateral**

    H30.119 **Disseminated chorioretinal inflammation of posterior pole, unspecified eye**

H30.12 **Disseminated chorioretinal inflammation, peripheral**

    H30.121 **Disseminated chorioretinal inflammation, peripheral right eye**

    H30.122 **Disseminated chorioretinal inflammation, peripheral, left eye**

    H30.123 **Disseminated chorioretinal inflammation, peripheral, bilateral**

    H30.129 **Disseminated chorioretinal inflammation, peripheral, unspecified eye**

H30.13 **Disseminated chorioretinal inflammation, generalized**

    H30.131 **Disseminated chorioretinal inflammation, generalized, right eye**

    H30.132 **Disseminated chorioretinal inflammation, generalized, left eye**

    H30.133 **Disseminated chorioretinal inflammation, generalized, bilateral**

    H30.139 **Disseminated chorioretinal inflammation, generalized, unspecified eye**

H30.14 **Acute posterior multifocal placoid pigment epitheliopathy**

    H30.141 **Acute posterior multifocal placoid pigment epitheliopathy, right eye**

    H30.142 **Acute posterior multifocal placoid pigment epitheliopathy, left eye**

    H30.143 **Acute posterior multifocal placoid pigment epitheliopathy, bilateral**

    H30.149 **Acute posterior multifocal placoid pigment epitheliopathy, unspecified eye**

H30.2 **Posterior cyclitis**

Pars planitis

  H30.20 **Posterior cyclitis, unspecified eye**

  H30.21 **Posterior cyclitis, right eye**

  H30.22 **Posterior cyclitis, left eye**

  H30.23 **Posterior cyclitis, bilateral**

H30.8 **Other chorioretinal inflammations**

  H30.81 **Harada's disease**

    H30.811 **Harada's disease, right eye**

    H30.812 **Harada's disease, left eye**

    H30.813 **Harada's disease, bilateral**

    H30.819 **Harada's disease, unspecified eye**

  H30.89 **Other chorioretinal inflammations**

    H30.891 **Other chorioretinal inflammations, right eye**

    H30.892 **Other chorioretinal inflammations, left eye**

    H30.893 **Other chorioretinal inflammations, bilateral**

    H30.899 **Other chorioretinal inflammations, unspecified eye**

H30.9 **Unspecified chorioretinal inflammation**

Chorioretinitis NOS

Choroiditis NOS Neuroretinitis NOS

Retinitis NOS

Retinochoroiditis NOS

  H30.90 **Unspecified chorioretinal inflammation, unspecified eye**

  H30.91 **Unspecified chorioretinal inflammation, right eye**

  H30.92 **Unspecified chorioretinal inflammation, left eye**

  H30.93 **Unspecified chorioretinal inflammation, bilateral**

H31 **Other disorders of choroid**

H31.0 **Chorioretinal scars**

Excludes2: postsurgical chorioretinal scars (H59.81-)

  H31.00 **Unspecified chorioretinal scars**

    H31.001 **Unspecified chorioretinal scars, right eye**

    H31.002 **Unspecified chorioretinal scars, left eye**

    H31.003 **Unspecified chorioretinal scars, bilateral**

    H31.009 **Unspecified chorioretinal scars, unspecified eye**

  H31.01 **Macula scars of posterior pole (postinflammatory) (post-traumatic)**

Excludes1: postprocedural chorioretinal scar (H59.81-)

    H31.011 **Macula scars of posterior pole (postinflammatory) (post-traumatic), right eye**

    H31.012 **Macula scars of posterior pole (postinflammatory) (post-traumatic), left eye**

H31.013   **Macula scars of posterior pole (postinflammatory) (post-traumatic), bilateral**

H31.019   **Macula scars of posterior pole (postinflammatory) (post-traumatic), unspecified eye**

H31.02   **Solar retinopathy**

    H31.021   **Solar retinopathy, right eye**

    H31.022   **Solar retinopathy, left eye**

    H31.023   **Solar retinopathy, bilateral**

    H31.029   **Solar retinopathy, unspecified eye**

H31.09   **Other chorioretinal scars**

    H31.091   **Other chorioretinal scars, right eye**

    H31.092   **Other chorioretinal scars, left eye**

    H31.093   **Other chorioretinal scars, bilateral**

    H31.099   **Other chorioretinal scars, unspecified eye**

H31.1   Choroidal degeneration

> **Excludes2:**   angioid streaks of macula (H35.33)

H31.10   **Unspecified choroidal degeneration**

Choroidal sclerosis NOS

    H31.101   **Choroidal degeneration, unspecified, right eye**

    H31.102   **Choroidal degeneration, unspecified, left eye**

    H31.103   **Choroidal degeneration, unspecified, bilateral**

    H31.109   **Choroidal degeneration, unspecified, unspecified eye**

H31.11   **Age-related choroidal atrophy**

    H31.111   **Age-related choroidal atrophy, right eye**

    H31.112   **Age-related choroidal atrophy, left eye**

    H31.113   **Age-related choroidal atrophy, bilateral**

    H31.119   **Age-related choroidal atrophy, unspecified eye**

H31.12   **Diffuse secondary atrophy of choroid**

    H31.121   **Diffuse secondary atrophy of choroid, right eye**

    H31.122   **Diffuse secondary atrophy of choroid, left eye**

    H31.123   **Diffuse secondary atrophy of choroid, bilateral**

    H31.129   **Diffuse secondary atrophy of choroid, unspecified eye**

H31.2   Hereditary choroidal dystrophy

> **Excludes2:**   hyperornithinemia (E72.4)
>
>   ornithinemia (E72.4)

H31.20   **Hereditary choroidal dystrophy, unspecified**

H31.21   **Choroideremia**

H31.22   **Choroidal dystrophy (central areolar) (generalized) (peripapillary)**

H31.23   **Gyrate atrophy, choroid**

H31.29   **Other hereditary choroidal dystrophy**

H31.3   Choroidal hemorrhage and rupture

H31.30   **Unspecified choroidal hemorrhage**

    H31.301   **Unspecified choroidal hemorrhage, right eye**

    H31.302   **Unspecified choroidal hemorrhage, left eye**

    H31.303   **Unspecified choroidal hemorrhage, bilateral**

    H31.309   **Unspecified choroidal hemorrhage, unspecified eye**

H31.31   **Expulsive choroidal hemorrhage**

    H31.311   **Expulsive choroidal hemorrhage, right eye**

    H31.312   **Expulsive choroidal hemorrhage, left eye**

    H31.313   **Expulsive choroidal hemorrhage, bilateral**

    H31.319   **Expulsive choroidal hemorrhage, unspecified eye**

H31.32   **Choroidal rupture**

    H31.321   **Choroidal rupture, right eye**

    H31.322   **Choroidal rupture, left eye**

    H31.323   **Choroidal rupture, bilateral**

    H31.329   **Choroidal rupture, unspecified eye**

H31.4   Choroidal detachment

H31.40   **Unspecified choroidal detachment**

    H31.401   **Unspecified choroidal detachment, right eye**

    H31.402   **Unspecified choroidal detachment, left eye**

    H31.403   **Unspecified choroidal detachment, bilateral**

    H31.409   **Unspecified choroidal detachment, unspecified eye**

H31.41   **Hemorrhagic choroidal detachment**

    H31.411   **Hemorrhagic choroidal detachment, right eye**

    H31.412   **Hemorrhagic choroidal detachment, left eye**

    H31.413   **Hemorrhagic choroidal detachment, bilateral**

    H31.419   **Hemorrhagic choroidal detachment, unspecified eye**

H31.42   **Serous choroidal detachment**

    H31.421   **Serous choroidal detachment, right eye**

    H31.422   **Serous choroidal detachment, left eye**

    H31.423   **Serous choroidal detachment, bilateral**

    H31.429   **Serous choroidal detachment, unspecified eye**

H31.8   Other specified disorders of choroid

H31.9   Unspecified disorder of choroid

H32   Chorioretinal disorders in diseases classified elsewhere

Code first underlying disease, such as:

congenital toxoplasmosis (P37.1)

histoplasmosis (B39.-)

leprosy (A30.-)

> **Excludes1:**   chorioretinitis (in):
>
>   toxoplasmosis (acquired) (B58.01)

tuberculosis (A18.53)

H33   Retinal detachments and breaks

Definition: Retinal detachment is a disorder of the eye in which the retina peels away from its underlying layer of support tissue.

Excludes1: detachment of retinal pigment epithelium (H35.72-, H35.73-)

H33.0   Retinal detachment with retinal break

Rhegmatogenous retinal detachment

Excludes1: serous retinal detachment (without retinal break) (H33.2-)

H33.00   Unspecified retinal detachment with retinal break

H33.001   Unspecified retinal detachment with retinal break, right eye

H33.002   Unspecified retinal detachment with retinal break, left eye

H33.003   Unspecified retinal detachment with retinal break, bilateral

H33.009   Unspecified retinal detachment with retinal break, unspecified eye

H33.01   Retinal detachment with single break

H33.011   Retinal detachment with single break, right eye

H33.012   Retinal detachment with single break, left eye

H33.013   Retinal detachment with single break, bilateral

H33.019   Retinal detachment with single break, unspecified eye

H33.02   Retinal detachment with multiple breaks

H33.021   Retinal detachment with multiple breaks, right eye

H33.022   Retinal detachment with multiple breaks, left eye

H33.023   Retinal detachment with multiple breaks, bilateral

H33.029   Retinal detachment with multiple breaks, unspecified eye

H33.03   Retinal detachment with giant retinal tear

H33.031   Retinal detachment with giant retinal tear, right eye

H33.032   Retinal detachment with giant retinal tear, left eye

H33.033   Retinal detachment with giant retinal tear, bilateral

H33.039   Retinal detachment with giant retinal tear, unspecified eye

H33.04   Retinal detachment with retinal dialysis

H33.041   Retinal detachment with retinal dialysis, right eye

H33.042   Retinal detachment with retinal dialysis, left eye

H33.043   Retinal detachment with retinal dialysis, bilateral

H33.049   Retinal detachment with retinal dialysis, unspecified eye

H33.05   Total retinal detachment

H33.051   Total retinal detachment, right eye

H33.052   Total retinal detachment, left eye

H33.053   Total retinal detachment, bilateral

H33.059   Total retinal detachment, unspecified eye

H33.1   Retinoschisis and retinal cysts

Excludes1: congenital retinoschisis (Q14.1)

microcystoid degeneration of retina (H35.42-)

H33.10   Unspecified retinoschisis

H33.101   Unspecified retinoschisis, right eye

H33.102   Unspecified retinoschisis, left eye

H33.103   Unspecified retinoschisis, bilateral

H33.109   Unspecified retinoschisis, unspecified eye

H33.11   Cyst of ora serrata

H33.111   Cyst of ora serrata, right eye

H33.112   Cyst of ora serrata, left eye

H33.113   Cyst of ora serrata, bilateral

H33.119   Cyst of ora serrata, unspecified eye

H33.12   Parasitic cyst of retina

H33.121   Parasitic cyst of retina, right eye

H33.122   Parasitic cyst of retina, left eye

H33.123   Parasitic cyst of retina, bilateral

H33.129   Parasitic cyst of retina, unspecified eye

H33.19   Other retinoschisis and retinal cysts

Pseudocyst of retina

H33.191   Other retinoschisis and retinal cysts, right eye

H33.192   Other retinoschisis and retinal cysts, left eye

H33.193   Other retinoschisis and retinal cysts, bilateral

H33.199   Other retinoschisis and retinal cysts, unspecified eye

H33.2   Serous retinal detachment

Retinal detachment NOS

Retinal detachment without retinal break

Excludes1: central serous chorioretinopathy (H35.71-)

H33.20   Serous retinal detachment, unspecified eye

H33.21   Serous retinal detachment, right eye

H33.22   Serous retinal detachment, left eye

H33.23   Serous retinal detachment, bilateral

H33.3   Retinal breaks without detachment

Excludes1: chorioretinal scars after surgery for detachment (H59.81-)

peripheral retinal degeneration without break (H35.4-)

H33.30   Unspecified retinal break

H33.301   Unspecified retinal break, right eye

H33.302   Unspecified retinal break, left eye

H33.303   Unspecified retinal break, bilateral

H33.309   Unspecified retinal break, unspecified eye

H33.31   Horseshoe tear of retina without detachment

Operculum of retina without detachment

H33.311   Horseshoe tear of retina without detachment, right eye

H33.312   Horseshoe tear of retina without detachment, left eye

	H33.313	Horseshoe tear of retina without detachment, bilateral	H34.233	Retinal artery branch occlusion, bilateral
	H33.319	Horseshoe tear of retina without detachment, unspecified eye	H34.239	Retinal artery branch occlusion, unspecified eye

H33.32 **Round hole of retina without detachment**

H33.321 **Round hole, right eye**

H33.322 **Round hole, left eye**

H33.323 **Round hole, bilateral**

H33.329 **Round hole, unspecified eye**

H33.33 **Multiple defects of retina without detachment**

H33.331 **Multiple defects of retina without detachment, right eye**

H33.332 **Multiple defects of retina without detachment, left eye**

H33.333 **Multiple defects of retina without detachment, bilateral**

H33.339 **Multiple defects of retina without detachment, unspecified eye**

H33.4 **Traction detachment of retina**

Proliferative vitreo-retinopathy with retinal detachment

H33.40 **Traction detachment of retina, unspecified eye**

H33.41 **Traction detachment of retina, right eye**

H33.42 **Traction detachment of retina, left eye**

H33.43 **Traction detachment of retina, bilateral**

H33.8 **Other retinal detachments**

H34 Retinal vascular occlusions

Excludes1: amaurosis fugax (G45.3)

H34.0 **Transient retinal artery occlusion**

H34.00 **Transient retinal artery occlusion, unspecified eye**

H34.01 **Transient retinal artery occlusion, right eye**

H34.02 **Transient retinal artery occlusion, left eye**

H34.03 **Transient retinal artery occlusion, bilateral**

H34.1 **Central retinal artery occlusion**

H34.10 **Central retinal artery occlusion, unspecified eye**

H34.11 **Central retinal artery occlusion, right eye**

H34.12 **Central retinal artery occlusion, left eye**

H34.13 **Central retinal artery occlusion, bilateral**

H34.2 **Other retinal artery occlusions**

H34.21 **Partial retinal artery occlusion**

Hollenhorst's plaque

Retinal microembolism

H34.211 **Partial retinal artery occlusion, right eye**

H34.212 **Partial retinal artery occlusion, left eye**

H34.213 **Partial retinal artery occlusion, bilateral**

H34.219 **Partial retinal artery occlusion, unspecified eye**

H34.23 **Retinal artery branch occlusion**

H34.231 **Retinal artery branch occlusion, right eye**

H34.232 **Retinal artery branch occlusion, left eye**

H34.8 **Other retinal vascular occlusions**

H34.81 **Central retinal vein occlusion**

One of the following 7th characters is to be assigned to codes in subcategory H34.81 to designate the severity of the occlusion:

0 - with macular edema

1 - with retinal neovascularization

2 – stable Old central retinal vein occlusion

●⑦H34.811 **Central retinal vein occlusion, right eye**

●⑦H34.812 **Central retinal vein occlusion, left eye**

●⑦H34.813 **Central retinal vein occlusion, bilateral**

●⑦H34.819 **Central retinal vein occlusion, unspecified eye**

H34.82 **Venous engorgement**

Incipient retinal vein occlusion

Partial retinal vein occlusion

H34.821 **Venous engorgement, right eye**

H34.822 **Venous engorgement, left eye**

H34.823 **Venous engorgement, bilateral**

H34.829 **Venous engorgement, unspecified eye**

H34.83 **Tributary (branch) retinal vein occlusion**

One of the following 7th characters is to be assigned to codes in subcategory H34.83 to designate the severity of the occlusion:

0 - with macular edema

1 - with retinal neovascularization

2 – stable Old tributary (branch) retinal vein occlusion

●⑦H34.831 **Tributary (branch) retinal vein occlusion, right eye**

●⑦H34.832 **Tributary (branch) retinal vein occlusion, left eye**

●⑦H34.833 **Tributary (branch) retinal vein occlusion, bilateral**

●⑦H34.839 **Tributary (branch) retinal vein occlusion, unspecified eye**

H34.9 **Unspecified retinal vascular occlusion**

H35 Other retinal disorders

Excludes2: diabetic retinal disorders (E08.311-E08.359, E09.311-E09.359, E10.311-E10.359, E11.311-E11.359, E13.311-E13.359)

H35.0 **Background retinopathy and retinal vascular changes**

Code also any associated hypertension (I10.-)

H35.00 **Unspecified background retinopathy**

H35.01 **Changes in retinal vascular appearance**

Retinal vascular sheathing

H35.011 **Changes in retinal vascular appearance, right eye**

H35.012 **Changes in retinal vascular appearance, left eye**

H35.013 **Changes in retinal vascular appearance, bilateral**

H35.019   **Changes in retinal vascular appearance, unspecified eye**

H35.02   **Exudative retinopathy**

Coats retinopathy

    H35.021   **Exudative retinopathy, right eye**

    H35.022   **Exudative retinopathy, left eye**

    H35.023   **Exudative retinopathy, bilateral**

    H35.029   **Exudative retinopathy, unspecified eye**

H35.03   **Hypertensive retinopathy**

    •H35.031   **Hypertensive retinopathy, right eye**

    H35.032   **Hypertensive retinopathy, left eye**

    H35.033   **Hypertensive retinopathy, bilateral**

    H35.039   **Hypertensive retinopathy, unspecified eye**

H35.04   **Retinal micro-aneurysms, unspecified**

    H35.041   **Retinal micro-aneurysms, unspecified, right eye**

    H35.042   **Retinal micro-aneurysms, unspecified, left eye**

    H35.043   **Retinal micro-aneurysms, unspecified, bilateral**

    H35.049   **Retinal micro-aneurysms, unspecified, unspecified eye**

H35.05   **Retinal neovascularization, unspecified**

    H35.051   **Retinal neovascularization, unspecified, right eye**

    H35.052   **Retinal neovascularization, unspecified, left eye**

    H35.053   **Retinal neovascularization, unspecified, bilateral**

    H35.059   **Retinal neovascularization, unspecified, unspecified eye**

H35.06   **Retinal vasculitis**

Eales disease

Retinal perivasculitis

    H35.061   **Retinal vasculitis, right eye**

    H35.062   **Retinal vasculitis, left eye**

    H35.063   **Retinal vasculitis, bilateral**

    H35.069   **Retinal vasculitis, unspecified eye**

H35.07   **Retinal telangiectasis**

    H35.071   **Retinal telangiectasis, right eye**

    H35.072   **Retinal telangiectasis, left eye**

    H35.073   **Retinal telangiectasis, bilateral**

    H35.079   **Retinal telangiectasis, unspecified eye**

H35.09   **Other intraretinal microvascular abnormalities**

Retinal varices

H35.1   **Retinopathy of prematurity**

H35.10   **Retinopathy of prematurity, unspecified**

Retinopathy of prematurity NOS

    H35.101   **Retinopathy of prematurity, unspecified, right eye**

    H35.102   **Retinopathy of prematurity, unspecified, left eye**

    H35.103   **Retinopathy of prematurity, unspecified, bilateral**

H35.109   **Retinopathy of prematurity, unspecified, unspecified eye**

H35.11   **Retinopathy of prematurity, stage 0**

    H35.111   **Retinopathy of prematurity, stage 0, right eye**

    H35.112   **Retinopathy of prematurity, stage 0, left eye**

    H35.113   **Retinopathy of prematurity, stage 0, bilateral**

    H35.119   **Retinopathy of prematurity, stage 0, unspecified eye**

H35.12   **Retinopathy of prematurity, stage 1**

    H35.121   **Retinopathy of prematurity, stage 1, right eye**

    H35.122   **Retinopathy of prematurity, stage 1, left eye**

    H35.123   **Retinopathy of prematurity, stage 1, bilateral**

    H35.129   **Retinopathy of prematurity, stage 1, unspecified eye**

H35.13   **Retinopathy of prematurity, stage 2**

    H35.131   **Retinopathy of prematurity, stage 2, right eye**

    H35.132   **Retinopathy of prematurity, stage 2, left eye**

    H35.133   **Retinopathy of prematurity, stage 2, bilateral**

    H35.139   **Retinopathy of prematurity, stage 2, unspecified eye**

H35.14   **Retinopathy of prematurity, stage 3**

    H35.141   **Retinopathy of prematurity, stage 3, right eye**

    H35.142   **Retinopathy of prematurity, stage 3, left eye**

    H35.143   **Retinopathy of prematurity, stage 3, bilateral**

    H35.149   **Retinopathy of prematurity, stage 3, unspecified eye**

H35.15   **Retinopathy of prematurity, stage 4**

    H35.151   **Retinopathy of prematurity, stage 4, right eye**

    H35.152   **Retinopathy of prematurity, stage 4, left eye**

    H35.153   **Retinopathy of prematurity, stage 4, bilateral**

    H35.159   **Retinopathy of prematurity, stage 4, unspecified eye**

H35.16   **Retinopathy of prematurity, stage 5**

    H35.161   **Retinopathy of prematurity, stage 5, right eye**

    H35.162   **Retinopathy of prematurity, stage 5, left eye**

    H35.163   **Retinopathy of prematurity, stage 5, bilateral**

    H35.169   **Retinopathy of prematurity, stage 5, unspecified eye**

H35.17   **Retrolental fibroplasia**

    H35.171   **Retrolental fibroplasia, right eye**

    H35.172   **Retrolental fibroplasia, left eye**

    H35.173   **Retrolental fibroplasia, bilateral**

Add 4th-7th digits   Nonspecific code   Unspecified code   Manifestation code

H35.179 **Retrolental fibroplasia, unspecified eye**

H35.2 **Other non-diabetic proliferative retinopathy**

Proliferative vitreo-retinopathy

Excludes1: proliferative vitreo-retinopathy with retinal detachment (H33.4-)

H35.20 **Other non-diabetic proliferative retinopathy, unspecified eye**

H35.21 **Other non-diabetic proliferative retinopathy, right eye**

H35.22 **Other non-diabetic proliferative retinopathy, left eye**

H35.23 **Other non-diabetic proliferative retinopathy, bilateral**

H35.3 **Degeneration of macula and posterior pole**

H35.30 **Unspecified macular degeneration**

Age-related macular degeneration

H35.31 **Nonexudative age-related macular degeneration**

Atrophic age-related macular degeneration

Dry age-related macular degeneration

One of the following 7th characters is to be assigned to codes in subcategory H35.31 to designate the stage of the disease:

0 - stage unspecified

1 - early dry stage

2 - intermediate dry stage

3 - advanced atrophic without subfoveal involvement advanced dry stage

4 - advanced atrophic with subfoveal involvement

● ⑦ H35.311 **Nonexudative age-related macular degeneration, right eye**

● ⑦ H35.312 **Nonexudative age-related macular degeneration, left eye**

● ⑦ H35.313 **Nonexudative age-related macular degeneration, bilateral**

● ⑦ H35.319 **Nonexudative age-related macular degeneration, unspecified eye**

H35.32 **Exudative age-related macular degeneration**

Wet age-related macular degeneration

One of the following 7th characters is to be assigned to codes in subcategory H35.32 to designate the stage of the disease:

0 - stage unspecified

1 - with active choroidal neovascularization

2 - with inactive choroidal neovascularization with involuted or regressed neovascularization

3 - with inactive scar

● ⑦ H35.321 **Exudative age-related macular degeneration, right eye**

● ⑦ H35.322 **Exudative age-related macular degeneration, left eye**

● ⑦ H35.323 **Exudative age-related macular degeneration, bilateral**

● ⑦ H35.329 **Exudative age-related macular degeneration, unspecified eye**

H35.33 **Angioid streaks of macula**

H35.34 **Macular cyst, hole, or pseudohole**

H35.341 **Macular cyst, hole, or pseudohole, right eye**

H35.342 **Macular cyst, hole, or pseudohole, left eye**

H35.343 **Macular cyst, hole, or pseudohole, bilateral**

H35.349 **Macular cyst, hole, or pseudohole, unspecified eye**

H35.35 **Cystoid macular degeneration**

Excludes1: cystoid macular edema following cataract surgery (H59.03-)

H35.351 **Cystoid macular degeneration, right eye**

H35.352 **Cystoid macular degeneration, left eye**

H35.353 **Cystoid macular degeneration, bilateral**

H35.359 **Cystoid macular degeneration, unspecified eye**

H35.36 **Drusen (degenerative) of macula**

H35.361 **Drusen (degenerative) of macula, right eye**

H35.362 **Drusen (degenerative) of macula, left eye**

H35.363 **Drusen (degenerative) of macula, bilateral**

H35.369 **Drusen (degenerative) of macula, unspecified eye**

H35.37 **Puckering of macula**

H35.371 **Puckering of macula, right eye**

H35.372 **Puckering of macula, left eye**

H35.373 **Puckering of macula, bilateral**

H35.379 **Puckering of macula, unspecified eye**

H35.38 **Toxic maculopathy**

Code first poisoning due to drug or toxin, if applicable (T36-T65 with fifth or sixth character 1-4 or 6)

Use additional code for adverse effect, if applicable, to identify drug (T36-T50 with fifth or sixth character 5)

H35.381 **Toxic maculopathy, right eye**

H35.382 **Toxic maculopathy, left eye**

H35.383 **Toxic maculopathy, bilateral**

H35.389 **Toxic maculopathy, unspecified eye**

H35.4 **Peripheral retinal degeneration**

Excludes1: hereditary retinal degeneration (dystrophy) (H35.5-)

peripheral retinal degeneration with retinal break (H33.3-)

H35.40 **Unspecified peripheral retinal degeneration**

H35.41 **Lattice degeneration of retina**

Palisade degeneration of retina

H35.411 **Lattice degeneration of retina, right eye**

H35.412 **Lattice degeneration of retina, left eye**

H35.413 **Lattice degeneration of retina, bilateral**

H35.419 Lattice degeneration of retina, unspecified eye

H35.42 Microcystoid degeneration of retina

H35.421 Microcystoid degeneration of retina, right eye

H35.422 Microcystoid degeneration of retina, left eye

H35.423 Microcystoid degeneration of retina, bilateral

H35.429 Microcystoid degeneration of retina, unspecified eye

H35.43 Paving stone degeneration of retina

H35.431 Paving stone degeneration of retina, right eye

H35.432 Paving stone degeneration of retina, left eye

H35.433 Paving stone degeneration of retina, bilateral

H35.439 Paving stone degeneration of retina, unspecified eye

H35.44 Age-related reticular degeneration of retina

H35.441 Age-related reticular degeneration of retina, right eye

H35.442 Age-related reticular degeneration of retina, left eye

H35.443 Age-related reticular degeneration of retina, bilateral

H35.449 Age-related reticular degeneration of retina, unspecified eye

H35.45 Secondary pigmentary degeneration

H35.451 Secondary pigmentary degeneration, right eye

H35.452 Secondary pigmentary degeneration, left eye

H35.453 Secondary pigmentary degeneration, bilateral

H35.459 Secondary pigmentary degeneration, unspecified eye

H35.46 Secondary vitreoretinal degeneration

H35.461 Secondary vitreoretinal degeneration, right eye

H35.462 Secondary vitreoretinal degeneration, left eye

H35.463 Secondary vitreoretinal degeneration, bilateral

H35.469 Secondary vitreoretinal degeneration, unspecified eye

H35.5 Hereditary retinal dystrophy

Excludes1: dystrophies primarily involving Bruch's membrane (H31.1-)

H35.50 Unspecified hereditary retinal dystrophy

H35.51 Vitreoretinal dystrophy

H35.52 Pigmentary retinal dystrophy

Albipunctate retinal dystrophy

Retinitis pigmentosa

Tapetoretinal dystrophy

H35.53 Other dystrophies primarily involving the sensory retina

Stargardt's disease

H35.54 Dystrophies primarily involving the retinal pigment epithelium

Vitelliform retinal dystrophy

H35.6 Retinal hemorrhage

H35.60 Retinal hemorrhage, unspecified eye

H35.61 Retinal hemorrhage, right eye

H35.62 Retinal hemorrhage, left eye

H35.63 Retinal hemorrhage, bilateral

H35.7 Separation of retinal layers

Excludes1: retinal detachment (serous) (H33.2-)

rhegmatogenous retinal detachment (H33.0-)

H35.70 Unspecified separation of retinal layers

H35.71 Central serous chorioretinopathy

H35.711 Central serous chorioretinopathy, right eye

H35.712 Central serous chorioretinopathy, left eye

H35.713 Central serous chorioretinopathy, bilateral

H35.719 Central serous chorioretinopathy, unspecified eye

H35.72 Serous detachment of retinal pigment epithelium

H35.721 Serous detachment of retinal pigment epithelium, right eye

H35.722 Serous detachment of retinal pigment epithelium, left eye

H35.723 Serous detachment of retinal pigment epithelium, bilateral

H35.729 Serous detachment of retinal pigment epithelium, unspecified eye

H35.73 Hemorrhagic detachment of retinal pigment epithelium

H35.731 Hemorrhagic detachment of retinal pigment epithelium, right eye

H35.732 Hemorrhagic detachment of retinal pigment epithelium, left eye

H35.733 Hemorrhagic detachment of retinal pigment epithelium, bilateral

H35.739 Hemorrhagic detachment of retinal pigment epithelium, unspecified eye

H35.8 Other specified retinal disorders

Excludes2: retinal hemorrhage (H35.6-)

H35.81 Retinal edema

Retinal cotton wool spots

H35.82 Retinal ischemia

H35.89 Other specified retinal disorders

H35.9 Unspecified retinal disorder

H36 Retinal disorders in diseases classified elsewhere

Code first underlying disease, such as:

lipid storage disorders (E75.-)

sickle-cell disorders (D57.-)

Excludes1: arteriosclerotic retinopathy (H35.0-)

diabetic retinopathy (E08.3-, E09.3-, E10.3-, E11.3-, E13.3-)

GLAUCOMA (H40-H42)

Definition: Glaucoma is a group of eye diseases characterized by

damage to the optic nerve usually due to excessively high intraocular pressure.

H40   Glaucoma

Excludes1: absolute glaucoma (H44.51-)

congenital glaucoma (Q15.0)

traumatic glaucoma due to birth injury (P15.3)

H40.0   Glaucoma suspect

H40.00   Preglaucoma, unspecified

H40.001   Preglaucoma, unspecified, right eye

H40.002   Preglaucoma, unspecified, left eye

H40.003   Preglaucoma, unspecified, bilateral

H40.009   Preglaucoma, unspecified, unspecified eye

H40.01   Open angle with borderline findings, low risk

Open angle, low risk

H40.011   Open angle with borderline findings, low risk, right eye

H40.012   Open angle with borderline findings, low risk, left eye

H40.013   Open angle with borderline findings, low risk, bilateral

H40.019   Open angle with borderline findings, low risk, unspecified eye

H40.02   Open angle with borderline findings, high risk

Open angle, high risk

H40.021   Open angle with borderline findings, high risk, right eye

H40.022   Open angle with borderline findings, high risk, left eye

H40.023   Open angle with borderline findings, high risk, bilateral

H40.029   Open angle with borderline findings, high risk, unspecified eye

H40.03   Anatomical narrow angle

Primary angle closure suspect

H40.031   Anatomical narrow angle, right eye

H40.032   Anatomical narrow angle, left eye

H40.033   Anatomical narrow angle, bilateral

H40.039   Anatomical narrow angle, unspecified eye

H40.04   Steroid responder

H40.041   Steroid responder, right eye

H40.042   Steroid responder, left eye

H40.043   Steroid responder, bilateral

H40.049   Steroid responder, unspecified eye

H40.05   Ocular hypertension

H40.051   Ocular hypertension, right eye

H40.052   Ocular hypertension, left eye

H40.053   Ocular hypertension, bilateral

H40.059   Ocular hypertension, unspecified eye

H40.06   Primary angle closure without glaucoma damage

H40.061   Primary angle closure without glaucoma damage, right eye

H40.062   Primary angle closure without glaucoma damage, left eye

H40.063   Primary angle closure without glaucoma damage, bilateral

H40.069   Primary angle closure without glaucoma damage, unspecified eye

H40.1   Open-angle glaucoma

⊗⑦**H40.10   Unspecified open-angle glaucoma**

One of the following 7th characters is to be assigned to code H40.10 to designate the stage of glaucoma

0 - stage unspecified

1 - mild stage

2 - moderate stage

3 - severe stage

4 - indeterminate stage

H40.11   Primary open-angle glaucoma

Chronic simple glaucoma

One of the following 7th characters is to be assigned to each code in subcategory H40.11 to designate the stage of glaucoma

0 - stage unspecified

1 - mild stage

2 - moderate stage

3 - severe stage

4 - indeterminate stage

●⑦**H40.111   Primary open-angle glaucoma, right eye**

●⑦**H40.112   Primary open-angle glaucoma, left eye**

●⑦**H40.113   Primary open-angle glaucoma, bilateral**

●⑦**H40.119   Primary open-angle glaucoma, unspecified eye**

H40.12   Low-tension glaucoma

One of the following 7th characters is to be assigned to each code in subcategory H40.12 to designate the stage of glaucoma

0 - stage unspecified

1 - mild stage

2 - moderate stage

3 - severe stage

4 - indeterminate stage

⑦**H40.121   Low-tension glaucoma, right eye**

⑦**H40.122   Low-tension glaucoma, left eye**

⑦**H40.123   Low-tension glaucoma, bilateral**

⑦**H40.129   Low-tension glaucoma, unspecified eye**

H40.13   Pigmentary glaucoma

One of the following 7th characters is to be assigned to each code in subcategory H40.13 to designate the stage of glaucoma

0 - stage unspecified

1 - mild stage

2 - moderate stage

3 - severe stage

4 - indeterminate stage

⑦**H40.131   Pigmentary glaucoma, right eye**

⑦**H40.132   Pigmentary glaucoma, left eye**

⑦**H40.133** **Pigmentary glaucoma, bilateral**

⑦**H40.139** **Pigmentary glaucoma, unspecified eye**

H40.14 **Capsular glaucoma with pseudoexfoliation of lens**

One of the following 7th characters is to be assigned to each code in subcategory H40.14 to designate the stage of glaucoma

0 - stage unspecified

1 - mild stage

2 - moderate stage

3 - severe stage

4 - indeterminate stage

⑦**H40.141** **Capsular glaucoma with pseudoexfoliation of lens, right eye**

⑦**H40.142** **Capsular glaucoma with pseudoexfoliation of lens, left eye**

⑦**H40.143** **Capsular glaucoma with pseudoexfoliation of lens, bilateral**

⑦**H40.149** **Capsular glaucoma with pseudoexfoliation of lens, unspecified eye**

H40.15 **Residual stage of open-angle glaucoma**

H40.151 **Residual stage of open-angle glaucoma, right eye**

H40.152 **Residual stage of open-angle glaucoma, left eye**

H40.153 **Residual stage of open-angle glaucoma, bilateral**

H40.159 **Residual stage of open-angle glaucoma, unspecified eye**

H40.2 **Primary angle-closure glaucoma**

Excludes1: aqueous misdirection (H40.83-)

malignant glaucoma (H40.83-)

⊗⑦**H40.20** **Unspecified primary angle-closure glaucoma**

One of the following 7th characters is to be assigned to code H40.20 to designate the stage of glaucoma

0 - stage unspecified

1 - mild stage

2 - moderate stage

3 - severe stage

4 - indeterminate stage

H40.21 **Acute angle-closure glaucoma**

Acute angle-closure glaucoma attack

Acute angle-closure glaucoma crisis

H40.212 **Acute angle-closure glaucoma, left eye**

H40.213 **Acute angle-closure glaucoma, bilateral**

H40.219 **Acute angle-closure glaucoma, unspecified eye**

H40.22 **Chronic angle-closure glaucoma**

Chronic primary angle closure glaucoma

One of the following 7th characters is to be assigned to each code in subcategory H40.22 to designate the stage of glaucoma

0 - stage unspecified

1 - mild stage

2 - moderate stage

3 - severe stage

4 - indeterminate stage

⑦**H40.221** **Chronic angle-closure glaucoma, right eye**

⑦**H40.222** **Chronic angle-closure glaucoma, left eye**

⑦**H40.223** **Chronic angle-closure glaucoma, bilateral**

⑦**H40.229** **Chronic angle-closure glaucoma, unspecified eye**

H40.23 **Intermittent angle-closure glaucoma**

H40.231 **Intermittent angle-closure glaucoma, right eye**

H40.232 **Intermittent angle-closure glaucoma, left eye**

H40.233 **Intermittent angle-closure glaucoma, bilateral**

H40.239 **Intermittent angle-closure glaucoma, unspecified eye**

H40.24 **Residual stage of angle-closure glaucoma**

H40.241 **Residual stage of angle-closure glaucoma, right eye**

H40.242 **Residual stage of angle-closure glaucoma, left eye**

H40.243 **Residual stage of angle-closure glaucoma, bilateral**

H40.249 **Residual stage of angle-closure glaucoma, unspecified eye**

H40.3 **Glaucoma secondary to eye trauma**

Code also underlying condition

One of the following 7th characters is to be assigned to each code in subcategory H40.3 to designate the stage of glaucoma

0 - stage unspecified

1 - mild stage

2 - moderate stage

3 - severe stage

4 - indeterminate stage

⊗⑦**H40.30** **Glaucoma secondary to eye trauma, unspecified eye**

⊗⑦**H40.31** **Glaucoma secondary to eye trauma, right eye**

⊗⑦**H40.32** **Glaucoma secondary to eye trauma, left eye**

⊗⑦**H40.33** **Glaucoma secondary to eye trauma, bilateral**

H40.4 **Glaucoma secondary to eye inflammation**

Code also underlying condition

One of the following 7th characters is to be assigned to each code in subcategory H40.4 to designate the stage of glaucoma

0 - stage unspecified

1 - mild stage

2 - moderate stage

3 - severe stage

4 - indeterminate stage

⊗⑦**H40.40** **Glaucoma secondary to eye inflammation, unspecified eye**

⊗⑦**H40.41** **Glaucoma secondary to eye inflammation, right eye**

⊗⑦H40.42   Glaucoma secondary to eye inflammation, left eye

⊗⑦H40.43   Glaucoma secondary to eye inflammation, bilateral

H40.5   **Glaucoma secondary to other eye disorders**

<u>Code also</u> underlying eye disorder

One of the following 7th characters is to be assigned to each code in subcategory H40.5 to designate the stage of glaucoma

0 - stage unspecified

1 - mild stage

2 - moderate stage

3 - severe stage

4 - indeterminate stage

⊗⑦**H40.50**   **Glaucoma secondary to other eye disorders, unspecified eye**

⊗⑦**H40.51**   **Glaucoma secondary to other eye disorders, right eye**

⊗⑦**H40.52**   **Glaucoma secondary to other eye disorders, left eye**

⊗⑦**H40.53**   **Glaucoma secondary to other eye disorders, bilateral**

H40.6   **Glaucoma secondary to drugs**

<u>Use additional code</u> for adverse effect, if applicable, to identify drug (T36-T50 with fifth or sixth character 5)

One of the following 7th characters is to be assigned to each code in subcategory H40.6 to designate the stage of glaucoma

0 - stage unspecified

1 - mild stage

2 - moderate stage

3 - severe stage

4 - indeterminate stage

⊗⑦**H40.60**   Glaucoma secondary to drugs, unspecified eye

⊗⑦**H40.61**   Glaucoma secondary to drugs, right eye

⊗⑦**H40.62**   Glaucoma secondary to drugs, left eye

⊗⑦**H40.63**   Glaucoma secondary to drugs, bilateral

H40.8   **Other glaucoma**

H40.81   **Glaucoma with increased episcleral venous pressure**

H40.811   **Glaucoma with increased episcleral venous pressure, right eye**

H40.812   **Glaucoma with increased episcleral venous pressure, left eye**

H40.813   **Glaucoma with increased episcleral venous pressure, bilateral**

H40.819   **Glaucoma with increased episcleral venous pressure, unspecified eye**

H40.82   **Hypersecretion glaucoma**

H40.821   Hypersecretion glaucoma, right eye

H40.822   Hypersecretion glaucoma, left eye

H40.823   Hypersecretion glaucoma, bilateral

H40.829   Hypersecretion glaucoma, unspecified eye

H40.83   **Aqueous misdirection**

Malignant glaucoma

H40.831   **Aqueous misdirection, right eye**

H40.832   **Aqueous misdirection, left eye**

H40.833   **Aqueous misdirection, bilateral**

H40.839   **Aqueous misdirection, unspecified eye**

H40.89   **Other specified glaucoma**

H40.9   **Unspecified glaucoma**

H42   **Glaucoma in diseases classified elsewhere**

<u>Code first</u> underlying condition, such as:

amyloidosis (E85.-)

aniridia (Q13.1)

Lowe's syndrome (E72.03)

Reiger's anomaly (Q13.81)

specified metabolic disorder (E70-E88)

Excludes1: glaucoma (in) onchocerciasis (B73.02)

glaucoma (in) syphilis (A52.71)

glaucoma (in) tuberculous (A18.59)

Excludes2: glaucoma (in) diabetes mellitus (E08.39, E09.39, E10.39, E11.39, E13.39)

DISORDERS OF VITREOUS BODY AND GLOBE (H43-H44)

H43   **Disorders of vitreous body**

H43.0   **Vitreous prolapse**

Excludes1: vitreous syndrome following cataract surgery (H59.0-)

traumatic vitreous prolapse (S05.2-)

H43.00   **Vitreous prolapse, unspecified eye**

H43.01   **Vitreous prolapse, right eye**

H43.02   **Vitreous prolapse, left eye**

H43.03   **Vitreous prolapse, bilateral**

H43.1   **Vitreous hemorrhage**

H43.10   **Vitreous hemorrhage, unspecified eye**

H43.11   **Vitreous hemorrhage, right eye**

H43.12   **Vitreous hemorrhage, left eye**

H43.13   **Vitreous hemorrhage, bilateral**

H43.2   **Crystalline deposits in vitreous body**

H43.20   **Crystalline deposits in vitreous body, unspecified eye**

H43.21   **Crystalline deposits in vitreous body, right eye**

H43.22   **Crystalline deposits in vitreous body, left eye**

H43.23   **Crystalline deposits in vitreous body, bilateral**

H43.3   **Other vitreous opacities**

H43.31   **Vitreous membranes and strands**

H43.311   **Vitreous membranes and strands, right eye**

H43.312   **Vitreous membranes and strands, left eye**

H43.313   **Vitreous membranes and strands, bilateral**

H43.319   **Vitreous membranes and strands, unspecified eye**

H43.39   **Other vitreous opacities**

Vitreous floaters

H43.391   **Other vitreous opacities, right eye**

H43.392   **Other vitreous opacities, left eye**

H43.393   **Other vitreous opacities, bilateral**

H43.399   **Other vitreous opacities, unspecified eye**

H43.8 **Other disorders of vitreous body**

Excludes1: proliferative vitreo-retinopathy with retinal detachment (H33.4-)

Excludes2: vitreous abscess (H44.02-)

H43.81 **Vitreous degeneration**

Vitreous detachment

H43.811 **Vitreous degeneration, right eye**

H43.812 **Vitreous degeneration, left eye**

H43.813 **Vitreous degeneration, bilateral**

H43.819 **Vitreous degeneration, unspecified eye**

H43.82 **Vitreomacular adhesion**

Vitreomacular traction

H43.821 **Vitreomacular adhesion, right eye**

H43.822 **Vitreomacular adhesion, left eye**

H43.823 **Vitreomacular adhesion, bilateral**

H43.829 **Vitreomacular adhesion, unspecified eye**

H43.89 **Other disorders of vitreous body**

H43.9 **Unspecified disorder of vitreous body**

H44 **Disorders of globe**

Includes: disorders affecting multiple structures of eye

H44.0 **Purulent endophthalmitis**

Use additional code to identify organism

Excludes1: bleb associated endophthalmitis (H59.4-)

H44.00 **Unspecified purulent endophthalmitis**

H44.001 **Unspecified purulent endophthalmitis, right eye**

H44.002 **Unspecified purulent endophthalmitis, left eye**

H44.003 **Unspecified purulent endophthalmitis, bilateral**

H44.009 **Unspecified purulent endophthalmitis, unspecified eye**

H44.01 **Panophthalmitis (acute)**

H44.011 **Panophthalmitis (acute), right eye**

H44.012 **Panophthalmitis (acute), left eye**

H44.013 **Panophthalmitis (acute), bilateral**

H44.019 **Panophthalmitis (acute), unspecified eye**

H44.02 **Vitreous abscess (chronic)**

H44.021 **Vitreous abscess (chronic), right eye**

H44.022 **Vitreous abscess (chronic), left eye**

H44.023 **Vitreous abscess (chronic), bilateral**

H44.029 **Vitreous abscess (chronic), unspecified eye**

H44.1 **Other endophthalmitis**

Excludes1: bleb associated endophthalmitis (H59.4-)

Excludes2: ophthalmia nodosa (H16.2-)

H44.11 **Panuveitis**

H44.111 **Panuveitis, right eye**

H44.112 **Panuveitis, left eye**

H44.113 **Panuveitis, bilateral**

H44.119 **Panuveitis, unspecified eye**

H44.12 **Parasitic endophthalmitis, unspecified**

H44.121 **Parasitic endophthalmitis, unspecified, right eye**

H44.122 **Parasitic endophthalmitis, unspecified, left eye**

H44.123 **Parasitic endophthalmitis, unspecified, bilateral**

H44.129 **Parasitic endophthalmitis, unspecified, unspecified eye**

H44.13 **Sympathetic uveitis**

H44.131 **Sympathetic uveitis, right eye**

H44.132 **Sympathetic uveitis, left eye**

H44.133 **Sympathetic uveitis, bilateral**

H44.139 **Sympathetic uveitis, unspecified eye**

H44.19 **Other endophthalmitis**

H44.2 **Degenerative myopia**

Malignant myopia

H44.20 **Degenerative myopia, unspecified eye**

H44.21 **Degenerative myopia, right eye**

H44.22 **Degenerative myopia, left eye**

H44.23 **Degenerative myopia, bilateral**

H44.3 **Other and unspecified degenerative disorders of globe**

H44.30 **Unspecified degenerative disorder of globe**

H44.31 **Chalcosis**

H44.311 **Chalcosis, right eye**

H44.312 **Chalcosis, left eye**

H44.313 **Chalcosis, bilateral**

H44.319 **Chalcosis, unspecified eye**

H44.32 **Siderosis of eye**

H44.321 **Siderosis of eye, right eye**

H44.322 **Siderosis of eye, left eye**

H44.323 **Siderosis of eye, bilateral**

H44.329 **Siderosis of eye, unspecified eye**

H44.39 **Other degenerative disorders of globe**

H44.391 **Other degenerative disorders of globe, right eye**

H44.392 **Other degenerative disorders of globe, left eye**

H44.393 **Other degenerative disorders of globe, bilateral**

H44.399 **Other degenerative disorders of globe, unspecified eye**

H44.4 **Hypotony of eye**

H44.40 **Unspecified hypotony of eye**

H44.41 **Flat anterior chamber hypotony of eye**

H44.411 **Flat anterior chamber hypotony of right eye**

H44.412 **Flat anterior chamber hypotony of left eye**

H44.413 **Flat anterior chamber hypotony of eye, bilateral**

H44.419 **Flat anterior chamber hypotony of unspecified eye**

H44.42 **Hypotony of eye due to ocular fistula**

H44.421 **Hypotony of right eye due to ocular fistula**

H44.422 **Hypotony of left eye due to ocular fistula**

H44.423 **Hypotony of eye due to ocular fistula, bilateral**

H44.429 **Hypotony of unspecified eye due to ocular fistula**

H44.43 **Hypotony of eye due to other ocular disorders**

H44.431 **Hypotony of eye due to other ocular disorders, right eye**

H44.432 **Hypotony of eye due to other ocular disorders, left eye**

H44.433 **Hypotony of eye due to other ocular disorders, bilateral**

H44.439 **Hypotony of eye due to other ocular disorders, unspecified eye**

H44.44 **Primary hypotony of eye**

H44.441 **Primary hypotony of right eye**

H44.442 **Primary hypotony of left eye**

H44.443 **Primary hypotony of eye, bilateral**

H44.449 **Primary hypotony of unspecified eye**

H44.5 **Degenerated conditions of globe**

H44.50 **Unspecified degenerated conditions of globe**

H44.51 **Absolute glaucoma**

H44.511 **Absolute glaucoma, right eye**

H44.512 **Absolute glaucoma, left eye**

H44.513 **Absolute glaucoma, bilateral**

H44.519 **Absolute glaucoma, unspecified eye**

H44.52 **Atrophy of globe**

Phthisis bulbi

H44.521 **Atrophy of globe, right eye**

H44.522 **Atrophy of globe, left eye**

H44.523 **Atrophy of globe, bilateral**

H44.529 **Atrophy of globe, unspecified eye**

H44.53 **Leucocoria**

H44.531 **Leucocoria, right eye**

H44.532 **Leucocoria, left eye**

H44.533 **Leucocoria, bilateral**

H44.539 **Leucocoria, unspecified eye**

H44.6 **Retained (old) intraocular foreign body, magnetic**

Use additional code to identify magnetic foreign body (Z18.11)

Excludes1: current intraocular foreign body (S05.-)

Excludes2: retained foreign body in eyelid (H02.81-)

retained (old) foreign body following penetrating wound of orbit (H05.5-)

retained (old) intraocular foreign body, nonmagnetic (H44.7-)

H44.60 **Unspecified retained (old) intraocular foreign body, magnetic**

H44.601 **Unspecified retained (old) intraocular foreign body, magnetic, right eye**

H44.602 **Unspecified retained (old) intraocular foreign body, magnetic, left eye**

H44.603 **Unspecified retained (old) intraocular foreign body, magnetic, bilateral**

H44.609 **Unspecified retained (old) intraocular foreign body, magnetic, unspecified eye**

H44.61 **Retained (old) magnetic foreign body in anterior chamber**

H44.611 **Retained (old) magnetic foreign body in anterior chamber, right eye**

H44.612 **Retained (old) magnetic foreign body in anterior chamber, left eye**

H44.613 **Retained (old) magnetic foreign body in anterior chamber, bilateral**

H44.619 **Retained (old) magnetic foreign body in anterior chamber, unspecified eye**

H44.62 **Retained (old) magnetic foreign body in iris or ciliary body**

H44.621 **Retained (old) magnetic foreign body in iris or ciliary body, right eye**

H44.622 **Retained (old) magnetic foreign body in iris or ciliary body, left eye**

H44.623 **Retained (old) magnetic foreign body in iris or ciliary body, bilateral**

H44.629 **Retained (old) magnetic foreign body in iris or ciliary body, unspecified eye**

H44.63 **Retained (old) magnetic foreign body in lens**

H44.631 **Retained (old) magnetic foreign body in lens, right eye**

H44.632 **Retained (old) magnetic foreign body in lens, left eye**

H44.633 **Retained (old) magnetic foreign body in lens, bilateral**

H44.639 **Retained (old) magnetic foreign body in lens, unspecified eye**

H44.64 **Retained (old) magnetic foreign body in posterior wall of globe**

H44.641 **Retained (old) magnetic foreign body in posterior wall of globe, right eye**

H44.642 **Retained (old) magnetic foreign body in posterior wall of globe, left eye**

H44.643 **Retained (old) magnetic foreign body in posterior wall of globe, bilateral**

H44.649 **Retained (old) magnetic foreign body in posterior wall of globe, unspecified eye**

H44.65 **Retained (old) magnetic foreign body in vitreous body**

H44.651 **Retained (old) magnetic foreign body in vitreous body, right eye**

H44.652 **Retained (old) magnetic foreign body in vitreous body, left eye**

H44.653 **Retained (old) magnetic foreign body in vitreous body, bilateral**

H44.659 **Retained (old) magnetic foreign body in vitreous body, unspecified eye**

H44.69 **Retained (old) intraocular foreign body, magnetic, in other or multiple sites**

H44.691 Retained (old) intraocular foreign body, magnetic, in other or multiple sites, right eye

H44.692 Retained (old) intraocular foreign body, magnetic, in other or multiple sites, left eye

H44.693 Retained (old) intraocular foreign body, magnetic, in other or multiple sites, bilateral

H44.699 Retained (old) intraocular foreign body, magnetic, in other or multiple sites, unspecified eye

H44.7 Retained (old) intraocular foreign body, nonmagnetic

Use additional code to identify nonmagnetic foreign body (Z18.01-Z18.10, Z18.12, Z18.2-Z18.9)

Excludes1: current intraocular foreign body (S05.-)

Excludes2: retained foreign body in eyelid (H02.81-)

retained (old) foreign body following penetrating wound of orbit (H05.5-)

retained (old) intraocular foreign body, magnetic (H44.6-)

H44.70 Unspecified retained (old) intraocular foreign body, nonmagnetic

H44.701 Unspecified retained (old) intraocular foreign body, nonmagnetic, right eye

H44.702 Unspecified retained (old) intraocular foreign body, nonmagnetic, left eye

H44.703 Unspecified retained (old) intraocular foreign body, nonmagnetic, bilateral

H44.709 Unspecified retained (old) intraocular foreign body, nonmagnetic, unspecified eye

Retained (old) intraocular foreign body NOS

H44.71 Retained (nonmagnetic) (old) foreign body in anterior chamber

H44.711 Retained (nonmagnetic) (old) foreign body in anterior chamber, right eye

H44.712 Retained (nonmagnetic) (old) foreign body in anterior chamber, left eye

H44.713 Retained (nonmagnetic) (old) foreign body in anterior chamber, bilateral

H44.719 Retained (nonmagnetic) (old) foreign body in anterior chamber, unspecified eye

H44.72 Retained (nonmagnetic) (old) foreign body in iris or ciliary body

H44.721 Retained (nonmagnetic) (old) foreign body in iris or ciliary body, right eye

H44.722 Retained (nonmagnetic) (old) foreign body in iris or ciliary body, left eye

H44.723 Retained (nonmagnetic) (old) foreign body in iris or ciliary body, bilateral

H44.729 Retained (nonmagnetic) (old) foreign body in iris or ciliary body, unspecified eye

H44.73 Retained (nonmagnetic) (old) foreign body in lens

H44.731 Retained (nonmagnetic) (old) foreign body in lens, right eye

H44.732 Retained (nonmagnetic) (old) foreign body in lens, left eye

H44.733 Retained (nonmagnetic) (old) foreign body in lens, bilateral

H44.739 Retained (nonmagnetic) (old) foreign body in lens, unspecified eye

H44.74 Retained (nonmagnetic) (old) foreign body in posterior wall of globe

H44.741 Retained (nonmagnetic) (old) foreign body in posterior wall of globe, right eye

H44.742 Retained (nonmagnetic) (old) foreign body in posterior wall of globe, left eye

H44.743 Retained (nonmagnetic) (old) foreign body in posterior wall of globe, bilateral

H44.749 Retained (nonmagnetic) (old) foreign body in posterior wall of globe, unspecified eye

H44.75 Retained (nonmagnetic) (old) foreign body in vitreous body

H44.751 Retained (nonmagnetic) (old) foreign body in vitreous body, right eye

H44.752 Retained (nonmagnetic) (old) foreign body in vitreous body, left eye

H44.753 Retained (nonmagnetic) (old) foreign body in vitreous body, bilateral

H44.759 Retained (nonmagnetic) (old) foreign body in vitreous body, unspecified eye

H44.79 Retained (old) intraocular foreign body, nonmagnetic, in other or multiple sites

H44.791 Retained (old) intraocular foreign body, nonmagnetic, in other or multiple sites, right eye

H44.792 Retained (old) intraocular foreign body, nonmagnetic, in other or multiple sites, left eye

H44.793 Retained (old) intraocular foreign body, nonmagnetic, in other or multiple sites, bilateral

H44.799 Retained (old) intraocular foreign body, nonmagnetic, in other or multiple sites, unspecified eye

H44.8 Other disorders of globe

H44.81 Hemophthalmos

H44.811 Hemophthalmos, right eye

H44.812 Hemophthalmos, left eye

H44.813 Hemophthalmos, bilateral

H44.819 Hemophthalmos, unspecified eye

H44.82 Luxation of globe

H44.821　Luxation of globe, right eye

H44.822　Luxation of globe, left eye

H44.823　Luxation of globe, bilateral

H44.829　Luxation of globe, unspecified eye

H44.89　Other disorders of globe

H44.9　Unspecified disorder of globe

DISORDERS OF OPTIC NERVE AND VISUAL PATHWAYS (H46-H47)

H46　Optic neuritis

Excludes2: ischemic optic neuropathy (H47.01-)

neuromyelitis optica [Devic] (G36.0)

H46.0　Optic papillitis

H46.00　Optic papillitis, unspecified eye

H46.01　Optic papillitis, right eye

H46.02　Optic papillitis, left eye

H46.03　Optic papillitis, bilateral

H46.1　Retrobulbar neuritis

Retrobulbar neuritis NOS

Excludes1: syphilitic retrobulbar neuritis (A52.15)

H46.10　Retrobulbar neuritis, unspecified eye

H46.11　Retrobulbar neuritis, right eye

H46.12　Retrobulbar neuritis, left eye

H46.13　Retrobulbar neuritis, bilateral

H46.2　Nutritional optic neuropathy

H46.3　Toxic optic neuropathy

Code first (T51-T65) to identify cause

H46.8　Other optic neuritis

H46.9　Unspecified optic neuritis

H47　Other disorders of optic [2nd] nerve and visual pathways

H47.0　Disorders of optic nerve, not elsewhere classified

H47.01　Ischemic optic neuropathy

H47.011　Ischemic optic neuropathy, right eye

H47.012　Ischemic optic neuropathy, left eye

H47.013　Ischemic optic neuropathy, bilateral

H47.019　Ischemic optic neuropathy, unspecified eye

H47.02　Hemorrhage in optic nerve sheath

H47.021　Hemorrhage in optic nerve sheath, right eye

H47.022　Hemorrhage in optic nerve sheath, left eye

H47.023　Hemorrhage in optic nerve sheath, bilateral

H47.029　Hemorrhage in optic nerve sheath, unspecified eye

H47.03　Optic nerve hypoplasia

H47.031　Optic nerve hypoplasia, right eye

H47.032　Optic nerve hypoplasia, left eye

H47.033　Optic nerve hypoplasia, bilateral

H47.039　Optic nerve hypoplasia, unspecified eye

H47.09　Other disorders of optic nerve, not elsewhere classified

Compression of optic nerve

H47.091　Other disorders of optic nerve, not elsewhere classified, right eye

H47.092　Other disorders of optic nerve, not elsewhere classified, left eye

H47.093　Other disorders of optic nerve, not elsewhere classified, bilateral

H47.099　Other disorders of optic nerve, not elsewhere classified, unspecified eye

H47.1　Papilledema

H47.10　Unspecified papilledema

H47.11　Papilledema associated with increased intracranial pressure

H47.12　Papilledema associated with decreased ocular pressure

H47.13　Papilledema associated with retinal disorder

H47.14　Foster-Kennedy syndrome

H47.141　Foster-Kennedy syndrome, right eye

H47.142　Foster-Kennedy syndrome, left eye

H47.143　Foster-Kennedy syndrome, bilateral

H47.149　Foster-Kennedy syndrome, unspecified eye

H47.2　Optic atrophy

H47.20　Unspecified optic atrophy

H47.21　Primary optic atrophy

H47.211　Primary optic atrophy, right eye

H47.212　Primary optic atrophy, left eye

H47.213　Primary optic atrophy, bilateral

H47.219　Primary optic atrophy, unspecified eye

H47.22　Hereditary optic atrophy

Leber's optic atrophy

H47.23　Glaucomatous optic atrophy

H47.231　Glaucomatous optic atrophy, right eye

H47.232　Glaucomatous optic atrophy, left eye

H47.233　Glaucomatous optic atrophy, bilateral

H47.239　Glaucomatous optic atrophy, unspecified eye

H47.29　Other optic atrophy

Temporal pallor of optic disc

H47.291　Other optic atrophy, right eye

H47.292　Other optic atrophy, left eye

H47.293　Other optic atrophy, bilateral

H47.299　Other optic atrophy, unspecified eye

H47.3　Other disorders of optic disc

H47.31　Coloboma of optic disc

H47.311　Coloboma of optic disc, right eye

H47.312　Coloboma of optic disc, left eye

H47.313　Coloboma of optic disc, bilateral

H47.319　Coloboma of optic disc, unspecified eye

H47.32　Drusen of optic disc

H47.321　Drusen of optic disc, right eye

H47.322 **Drusen of optic disc, left eye**

H47.323 **Drusen of optic disc, bilateral**

H47.329 **Drusen of optic disc, unspecified eye**

H47.33 **Pseudopapilledema of optic disc**

H47.331 **Pseudopapilledema of optic disc, right eye**

H47.332 **Pseudopapilledema of optic disc, left eye**

H47.333 **Pseudopapilledema of optic disc, bilateral**

H47.339 **Pseudopapilledema of optic disc, unspecified eye**

H47.39 **Other disorders of optic disc**

H47.391 **Other disorders of optic disc, right eye**

H47.392 **Other disorders of optic disc, left eye**

H47.393 **Other disorders of optic disc, bilateral**

H47.399 **Other disorders of optic disc, unspecified eye**

H47.4 **Disorders of optic chiasm**

Code also underlying condition

H47.41 **Disorders of optic chiasm in (due to) inflammatory disorders**

H47.42 **Disorders of optic chiasm in (due to) neoplasm**

H47.43 **Disorders of optic chiasm in (due to) vascular disorders**

H47.49 **Disorders of optic chiasm in (due to) other disorders**

H47.5 **Disorders of other visual pathways**

Disorders of optic tracts, geniculate nuclei and optic radiations

Code also underlying condition

H47.51 **Disorders of visual pathways in (due to) inflammatory disorders**

H47.511 **Disorders of visual pathways in (due to) inflammatory disorders, right side**

H47.512 **Disorders of visual pathways in (due to) inflammatory disorders, left side**

H47.519 **Disorders of visual pathways in (due to) inflammatory disorders, unspecified side**

H47.52 **Disorders of visual pathways in (due to) neoplasm**

H47.521 **Disorders of visual pathways in (due to) neoplasm, right side**

H47.522 **Disorders of visual pathways in (due to) neoplasm, left side**

H47.529 **Disorders of visual pathways in (due to) neoplasm, unspecified side**

H47.53 **Disorders of visual pathways in (due to) vascular disorders**

H47.531 **Disorders of visual pathways in (due to) vascular disorders, right side**

H47.532 **Disorders of visual pathways in (due to) vascular disorders, left side**

H47.539 **Disorders of visual pathways in (due to) vascular disorders, unspecified side**

H47.6 **Disorders of visual cortex**

Code also underlying condition

Excludes1: injury to visual cortex S04.04

H47.61 **Cortical blindness**

H47.611 **Cortical blindness, right side of brain**

H47.612 **Cortical blindness, left side of brain**

H47.619 **Cortical blindness, unspecified side of brain**

H47.62 **Disorders of visual cortex in (due to) inflammatory disorders**

H47.621 **Disorders of visual cortex in (due to) inflammatory disorders, right side of brain**

H47.622 **Disorders of visual cortex in (due to) inflammatory disorders, left side of brain**

H47.629 **Disorders of visual cortex in (due to) inflammatory disorders, unspecified side of brain**

H47.63 **Disorders of visual cortex in (due to) neoplasm**

H47.631 **Disorders of visual cortex in (due to) neoplasm, right side of brain**

H47.632 **Disorders of visual cortex in (due to) neoplasm, left side of brain**

H47.639 **Disorders of visual cortex in (due to) neoplasm, unspecified side of brain**

H47.64 **Disorders of visual cortex in (due to) vascular disorders**

H47.641 **Disorders of visual cortex in (due to) vascular disorders, right side of brain**

H47.642 **Disorders of visual cortex in (due to) vascular disorders, left side of brain**

H47.649 **Disorders of visual cortex in (due to) vascular disorders, unspecified side of brain**

H47.9 **Unspecified disorder of visual pathways**

DISORDERS OF OCULAR MUSCLES, BINOCULAR MOVEMENT, ACCOMMODATION AND REFRACTION (H49-H52)

Definition: Refraction is the ability of the eye to bend light so that an image is focused on the retina. Accommodation is the automatic adjustment in focal length of the natural lens of the eye.

Excludes2: nystagmus **and other** irregular eye movements (H55)

H49 **Paralytic strabismus**

Definition: Strabismus, aka crossed eyes, is a visual defect in which the eyes are misaligned and point in different directions. Strabismus usually occurs in childhood but can occur later in life.

Excludes2: internal ophthalmoplegia (H52.51-)

internuclear ophthalmoplegia (H51.2-)

progressive supranuclear ophthalmoplegia (G23.1)

H49.0 **Third [oculomotor] nerve palsy**

H49.00 **Third [oculomotor] nerve palsy, unspecified eye**

H49.01   Third [oculomotor] nerve palsy, right eye

H49.02   Third [oculomotor] nerve palsy, left eye

H49.03   Third [oculomotor] nerve palsy, bilateral

H49.1   Fourth [trochlear] nerve palsy

H49.10   Fourth [trochlear] nerve palsy, unspecified eye

H49.11   Fourth [trochlear] nerve palsy, right eye

H49.12   Fourth [trochlear] nerve palsy, left eye

H49.13   Fourth [trochlear] nerve palsy, bilateral

H49.2   Sixth [abducent] nerve palsy

H49.20   Sixth [abducent] nerve palsy, unspecified eye

H49.21   Sixth [abducent] nerve palsy, right eye

H49.22   Sixth [abducent] nerve palsy, left eye

H49.23   Sixth [abducent] nerve palsy, bilateral

H49.3   Total (external) ophthalmoplegia

H49.30   Total (external) ophthalmoplegia, unspecified eye

H49.31   Total (external) ophthalmoplegia, right eye

H49.32   Total (external) ophthalmoplegia, left eye

H49.33   Total (external) ophthalmoplegia, bilateral

H49.4   Progressive external ophthalmoplegia

Excludes1: Kearns-Sayre syndrome (H49.81-)

H49.40   Progressive external ophthalmoplegia, unspecified eye

H49.41   Progressive external ophthalmoplegia, right eye

H49.42   Progressive external ophthalmoplegia, left eye

H49.43   Progressive external ophthalmoplegia, bilateral

H49.8   Other paralytic strabismus

H49.81   Kearns-Sayre syndrome

Progressive external ophthalmoplegia with pigmentary retinopathy

Use additional code for other manifestation, such as: heart block (I45.9)

H49.811   Kearns-Sayre syndrome, right eye

H49.812   Kearns-Sayre syndrome, left eye

H49.813   Kearns-Sayre syndrome, bilateral

H49.819   Kearns-Sayre syndrome, unspecified eye

H49.88   Other paralytic strabismus

External ophthalmoplegia NOS

H49.881   Other paralytic strabismus, right eye

H49.882   Other paralytic strabismus, left eye

H49.883   Other paralytic strabismus, bilateral

H49.889   Other paralytic strabismus, unspecified eye

H49.9   Unspecified paralytic strabismus

H50   **Other strabismus**

H50.0   Esotropia

Convergent concomitant strabismus

Excludes1: intermittent esotropia (H50.31-, H50.32)

H50.00   Unspecified esotropia

H50.01   Monocular esotropia

H50.011   Monocular esotropia, right eye

H50.012   Monocular esotropia, left eye

H50.02   Monocular esotropia with A pattern

H50.021   Monocular esotropia with A pattern, right eye

H50.022   Monocular esotropia with A pattern, left eye

H50.03   Monocular esotropia with V pattern

H50.031   Monocular esotropia with V pattern, right eye

H50.032   Monocular esotropia with V pattern, left eye

H50.04   Monocular esotropia with other noncomitancies

H50.041   Monocular esotropia with other noncomitancies, right eye

H50.042   Monocular esotropia with other noncomitancies, left eye

H50.05   Alternating esotropia

H50.06   Alternating esotropia with A pattern

H50.07   Alternating esotropia with V pattern

H50.08   Alternating esotropia with other noncomitancies

H50.1   Exotropia

Divergent concomitant strabismus

Excludes1: intermittent exotropia (H50.33-, H50.34)

H50.10   Unspecified exotropia

H50.11   Monocular exotropia

H50.111   Monocular exotropia, right eye

H50.112   Monocular exotropia, left eye

H50.12   Monocular exotropia with A pattern

H50.121   Monocular exotropia with A pattern, right eye

H50.122   Monocular exotropia with A pattern, left eye

H50.13   Monocular exotropia with V pattern

H50.131   Monocular exotropia with V pattern, right eye

H50.132   Monocular exotropia with V pattern, left eye

H50.14   Monocular exotropia with other noncomitancies

H50.141   Monocular exotropia with other noncomitancies, right eye

H50.142   Monocular exotropia with other noncomitancies, left eye

H50.15   Alternating exotropia

H50.16   Alternating exotropia with A pattern

H50.17   Alternating exotropia with V pattern

H50.18   Alternating exotropia with other noncomitancies

H50.2   Vertical strabismus

Hypertropia

H50.21   Vertical strabismus, right eye

H50.22   Vertical strabismus, left eye

H50.3   Intermittent heterotropia

H50.30   Unspecified intermittent heterotropia

H50.31   Intermittent monocular esotropia

H50.311 Intermittent monocular esotropia, right eye

H50.312 Intermittent monocular esotropia, left eye

H50.32 Intermittent alternating esotropia

H50.33 Intermittent monocular exotropia

H50.331 Intermittent monocular exotropia, right eye

H50.332 Intermittent monocular exotropia, left eye

H50.34 Intermittent alternating exotropia

H50.4 Other and unspecified heterotropia

H50.40 Unspecified heterotropia

H50.41 Cyclotropia

H50.411 Cyclotropia, right eye

H50.412 Cyclotropia, left eye

H50.42 Monofixation syndrome

H50.43 Accommodative component in esotropia

H50.5 Heterophoria

H50.50 Unspecified heterophoria

H50.51 Esophoria

H50.52 Exophoria

H50.53 Vertical heterophoria

H50.54 Cyclophoria

H50.55 Alternating heterophoria

H50.6 Mechanical strabismus

H50.60 Mechanical strabismus, unspecified

H50.61 Brown's sheath syndrome

H50.611 Brown's sheath syndrome, right eye

H50.612 Brown's sheath syndrome, left eye

H50.69 Other mechanical strabismus

Strabismus due to adhesions

Traumatic limitation of duction of eye muscle

H50.8 Other specified strabismus

H50.81 Duane's syndrome

H50.811 Duane's syndrome, right eye

H50.812 Duane's syndrome, left eye

H50.89 Other specified strabismus

H50.9 Unspecified strabismus

H51 Other disorders of binocular movement

H51.0 Palsy (spasm) of conjugate gaze

H51.1 Convergence insufficiency and excess

H51.11 Convergence insufficiency

H51.12 Convergence excess

H51.2 Internuclear ophthalmoplegia

H51.20 Internuclear ophthalmoplegia, unspecified eye

H51.21 Internuclear ophthalmoplegia, right eye

H51.22 Internuclear ophthalmoplegia, left eye

H51.23 Internuclear ophthalmoplegia, bilateral

H51.8 Other specified disorders of binocular movement

H51.9 Unspecified disorder of binocular movement

H52 Disorders of refraction and accommodation

H52.0 Hypermetropia

H52.00 Hypermetropia, unspecified eye

H52.01 Hypermetropia, right eye

H52.02 Hypermetropia, left eye

H52.03 Hypermetropia, bilateral

H52.1 Myopia

Excludes1: degenerative myopia (H44.2-)

H52.10 Myopia, unspecified eye

H52.11 Myopia, right eye

H52.12 Myopia, left eye

H52.13 Myopia, bilateral

H52.2 Astigmatism

H52.20 Unspecified astigmatism

H52.201 Unspecified astigmatism, right eye

H52.202 Unspecified astigmatism, left eye

H52.203 Unspecified astigmatism, bilateral

H52.209 Unspecified astigmatism, unspecified eye

H52.21 Irregular astigmatism

H52.211 Irregular astigmatism, right eye

H52.212 Irregular astigmatism, left eye

H52.213 Irregular astigmatism, bilateral

H52.219 Irregular astigmatism, unspecified eye

H52.22 Regular astigmatism

H52.221 Regular astigmatism, right eye

H52.222 Regular astigmatism, left eye

H52.223 Regular astigmatism, bilateral

H52.229 Regular astigmatism, unspecified eye

H52.3 Anisometropia and aniseikonia

H52.31 Anisometropia

H52.32 Aniseikonia

H52.4 Presbyopia

H52.5 Disorders of accommodation

H52.51 Internal ophthalmoplegia (complete) (total)

H52.511 Internal ophthalmoplegia (complete) (total), right eye

H52.512 Internal ophthalmoplegia (complete) (total), left eye

H52.513 Internal ophthalmoplegia (complete) (total), bilateral

H52.519 Internal ophthalmoplegia (complete) (total), unspecified eye

H52.52 Paresis of accommodation

H52.521 Paresis of accommodation, right eye

H52.522 Paresis of accommodation, left eye

H52.523 Paresis of accommodation, bilateral

H52.529 Paresis of accommodation, unspecified eye

H52.53 Spasm of accommodation

H52.531 Spasm of accommodation, right eye

H52.532 Spasm of accommodation, left eye

H52.533 Spasm of accommodation, bilateral

H52.539 Spasm of accommodation, unspecified eye

H52.6 Other disorders of refraction

H52.7 Unspecified disorder of refraction

Add 4th-7th digits   Nonspecific code   Unspecified code   Manifestation code   357

VISUAL DISTURBANCES AND BLINDNESS (H53-H54)

H53   **Visual disturbances**

    H53.0 **Amblyopia ex anopsia**

        Excludes1: amblyopia due to vitamin A deficiency (E50.5)

        H53.00 **Unspecified amblyopia**

            H53.001 **Unspecified amblyopia, right eye**

            H53.002 **Unspecified amblyopia, left eye**

            H53.003 **Unspecified amblyopia, bilateral**

            H53.009 **Unspecified amblyopia, unspecified eye**

        H53.01 **Deprivation amblyopia**

            H53.011 **Deprivation amblyopia, right eye**

            H53.012 **Deprivation amblyopia, left eye**

            H53.013 **Deprivation amblyopia, bilateral**

            H53.019 **Deprivation amblyopia, unspecified eye**

        H53.02 **Refractive amblyopia**

            H53.021 **Refractive amblyopia, right eye**

            H53.022 **Refractive amblyopia, left eye**

            H53.023 **Refractive amblyopia, bilateral**

            H53.029 **Refractive amblyopia, unspecified eye**

        H53.03 **Strabismic amblyopia**

            Excludes1: strabismus (H50.-)

            H53.031 **Strabismic amblyopia, right eye**

            H53.032 **Strabismic amblyopia, left eye**

            H53.033 **Strabismic amblyopia, bilateral**

            H53.039 **Strabismic amblyopia, unspecified eye**

        H53.04 **Amblyopia suspect**

            ●H53.041 **Amblyopia suspect, right eye**

            ●H53.042 **Amblyopia suspect, left eye**

            ●H53.043 **Amblyopia suspect, bilateral**

            ●H53.049 **Amblyopia suspect, unspecified eye**

    H53.1 **Subjective visual disturbances**

        subjective visual disturbances due to vitamin A deficiency (E50.5)

        visual hallucinations (R44.1)

        H53.10 **Unspecified subjective visual disturbances**

        H53.11 **Day blindness**

            Hemeralopia

        H53.12 **Transient visual loss**

            Scintillating scotoma amaurosis fugax (G45.3-)

            transient retinal artery occlusion (H34.0-)

            H53.121 **Transient visual loss, right eye**

            H53.122 **Transient visual loss, left eye**

            H53.123 **Transient visual loss, bilateral**

            H53.129 **Transient visual loss, unspecified eye**

        H53.13 **Sudden visual loss**

            H53.131 **Sudden visual loss, right eye**

            H53.132 **Sudden visual loss, left eye**

            H53.133 **Sudden visual loss, bilateral**

            H53.139 **Sudden visual loss, unspecified eye**

        H53.14 **Visual discomfort**

            Asthenopia

            Photophobia

            H53.141 **Visual discomfort, right eye**

            H53.142 **Visual discomfort, left eye**

            H53.143 **Visual discomfort, bilateral**

            H53.149 **Visual discomfort, unspecified**

        H53.15 **Visual distortions of shape and size**

            Metamorphopsia

        H53.16 **Psychophysical visual disturbances**

        H53.19 **Other subjective visual disturbances**

            Visual halos

    H53.2 **Diplopia**

        Double vision

    H53.3 **Other and unspecified disorders of binocular vision**

        H53.30 **Unspecified disorder of binocular vision**

        H53.31 **Abnormal retinal correspondence**

        H53.32 **Fusion with defective stereopsis**

        H53.33 **Simultaneous visual perception without fusion**

        H53.34 **Suppression of binocular vision**

    H53.4 **Visual field defects**

        H53.40 **Unspecified visual field defects**

        H53.41 **Scotoma involving central area**

            Central scotoma

            H53.411 **Scotoma involving central area, right eye**

            H53.412 **Scotoma involving central area, left eye**

            H53.413 **Scotoma involving central area, bilateral**

            H53.419 **Scotoma involving central area, unspecified eye**

        H53.42 **Scotoma of blind spot area**

            Enlarged blind spot

            H53.421 **Scotoma of blind spot area, right eye**

            H53.422 **Scotoma of blind spot area, left eye**

            H53.423 **Scotoma of blind spot area, bilateral**

            H53.429 **Scotoma of blind spot area, unspecified eye**

        H53.43 **Sector or arcuate defects**

            Arcuate scotoma

            Bjerrum scotoma

            H53.431 **Sector or arcuate defects, right eye**

            H53.432 **Sector or arcuate defects, left eye**

            H53.433 **Sector or arcuate defects, bilateral**

            H53.439 **Sector or arcuate defects, unspecified eye**

        H53.45 **Other localized visual field defect**

            Peripheral visual field defect

            Ring scotoma NOS

            Scotoma NOS

            H53.451 **Other localized visual field defect, right eye**

            H53.452 **Other localized visual field defect, left eye**

H53.453 Other localized visual field defect, bilateral

H53.459 Other localized visual field defect, unspecified eye

H53.46 Homonymous bilateral field defects

Homonymous hemianopia

Homonymous hemianopsia

Quadrant anopia

Quadrant anopsia

H53.461 Homonymous bilateral field defects, right side

H53.462 Homonymous bilateral field defects, left side

H53.469 Homonymous bilateral field defects, unspecified side

Homonymous bilateral field defects NOS

H53.47 Heteronymous bilateral field defects

Heteronymous hemianop(s)ia

H53.48 Generalized contraction of visual field

H53.481 Generalized contraction of visual field, right eye

H53.482 Generalized contraction of visual field, left eye

H53.483 Generalized contraction of visual field, bilateral

H53.489 Generalized contraction of visual field, unspecified eye

H53.5 Color vision deficiencies

Color blindness

Excludes2: day blindness (H53.11)

H53.50 Unspecified color vision deficiencies

Color blindness NOS

H53.51 Achromatopsia

H53.52 Acquired color vision deficiency

H53.53 Deuteranomaly

Deuteranopia

H53.54 Protanomaly

Protanopia

H53.55 Tritanomaly

Tritanopia

H53.59 Other color vision deficiencies

H53.6 Night blindness

Excludes1: night blindness due to vitamin A deficiency (E50.5)

H53.60 Unspecified night blindness

H53.61 Abnormal dark adaptation curve

H53.62 Acquired night blindness

H53.63 Congenital night blindness

H53.69 Other night blindness

H53.7 Vision sensitivity deficiencies

H53.71 Glare sensitivity

H53.72 Impaired contrast sensitivity

H53.8 Other visual disturbances

H53.9 Unspecified visual disturbance

H54 Blindness and low vision

Note: For definition of visual impairment categories see table below

Code first any associated underlying cause of the blindness

Excludes1: amaurosis fugax (G45.3)

H54.0 Blindness, both eyes

Visual impairment categories 3, 4, 5 in both eyes.

H54.1 Blindness, one eye, low vision other eye

Visual impairment categories 3, 4, 5 in one eye, with categories 1 or 2 in **the other** eye.

H54.10 Blindness, one eye, low vision other eye, unspecified eyes

H54.11 Blindness, right eye, low vision left eye

H54.12 Blindness, left eye, low vision right eye

H54.2 Low vision, both eyes

Visual impairment categories 1 or 2 in both eyes.

H54.3 Unqualified visual loss, both eyes

Visual impairment category 9 in both eyes.

H54.4 Blindness, one eye

Visual impairment categories 3, 4, 5 in one eye [normal vision in other eye]

H54.40 Blindness, one eye, unspecified eye

H54.41 Blindness, right eye, normal vision left eye

H54.42 Blindness, left eye, normal vision right eye

H54.5 Low vision, one eye

Visual impairment categories 1 or 2 in one eye [normal vision in other eye].

H54.50 Low vision, one eye, unspecified eye

H54.51 Low vision, right eye, normal vision left eye

H54.52 Low vision, left eye, normal vision right eye

H54.6 Unqualified visual loss, one eye

Visual impairment category 9 in one eye [normal vision in other eye].

H54.60 Unqualified visual loss, one eye, unspecified

H54.61 Unqualified visual loss, right eye, normal vision left eye

H54.62 Unqualified visual loss, left eye, normal vision right eye

H54.7 Unspecified visual loss

Visual impairment category 9 NOS

H54.8 Legal blindness, as defined in USA

Blindness NOS according to USA definition

Excludes1: legal blindness with specification of impairment level (H54.0-H54.7)

Note: The table below gives a classification of severity of visual impairment recommended by a WHO Study Group on the Prevention of Blindness, Geneva, 6-10 November 1972.

The term 'low vision' in category H54 comprises categories 1 and 2 of the table, the term 'blindness' categories 3, 4 and 5, and the term 'unqualified visual loss' category 9.

If the extent of the visual field is taken into account, patients with a field no greater than 10 but greater than 5 around central fixation should be placed in category 3 and patients with a field no greater than 5 around central fixation should be placed in category 4, even if the central acuity is not impaired. (Document 508 compliance requires all cells in the following table to be filled.)

Category of visual impairment	Visual acuity with best possible correction	
	Maximum less than:	Minimum equal to or

		better than:
-	6/18	6/60
3/10(0.3)	1/10(0.1)	-
20/70	20/200	-
-	6/60	3/60
1/10(0.1)	1/20(0.05	-
20/200	20/400	-
-	3/60	1/60(finger counting at one meter)
1/200(0.05)	1/50(0.02)	-
20/400	5/300(20/1200)	-
-	1/60(finger counting at one meter)	Light perception
1/50(0.02)	-	-
5/300	-	-
-	No light perception	-
-	Undetermined or unspecified	-

OTHER DISORDERS OF EYE AND ADNEXA (H55-H57)

H55 **Nystagmus and other irregular eye movements**

    H55.0 **Nystagmus**

        H55.00 **Unspecified nystagmus**

        H55.01 **Congenital nystagmus**

        H55.02 **Latent nystagmus**

        H55.03 **Visual deprivation nystagmus**

        H55.04 **Dissociated nystagmus**

        H55.09 **Other forms of nystagmus**

    H55.8 **Other irregular eye movements**

        H55.81 **Saccadic eye movements**

        H55.89 **Other irregular eye movements**

H57 **Other disorders of eye and adnexa**

    H57.0 **Anomalies of pupillary function**

        H57.00 **Unspecified anomaly of pupillary function**

        H57.01 **Argyll Robertson pupil, atypical**

          Excludes1: syphilitic Argyll Robertson pupil (A52.19)

        H57.02 **Anisocoria**

        H57.03 **Miosis**

        H57.04 **Mydriasis**

        H57.05 **Tonic pupil**

          H57.051 **Tonic pupil, right eye**

          H57.052 **Tonic pupil, left eye**

          H57.053 **Tonic pupil, bilateral**

          H57.059 **Tonic pupil, unspecified eye**

        H57.09 **Other anomalies of pupillary function**

    H57.1 **Ocular pain**

        H57.10 **Ocular pain, unspecified eye**

        H57.11 **Ocular pain, right eye**

        H57.12 **Ocular pain, left eye**

        H57.13 **Ocular pain, bilateral**

H57.8 **Other specified disorders of eye and adnexa**

H57.9 **Unspecified disorder of eye and adnexa**

INTRAOPERATIVE AND POSTPROCEDURAL COMPLICATIONS AND DISORDERS OF EYE AND ADNEXA, NOT ELSEWHERE CLASSIFIED (H59)

H59 **Intraoperative and postprocedural complications and disorders of eye and adnexa, not elsewhere classified**

    Excludes1: mechanical complication of intraocular lens (T85.2)

    mechanical complication **of other** ocular prosthetic devices, implants and grafts (T85.3)

    pseudophakia (Z96.1)

    secondary cataracts (H26.4-)

    H59.0 **Disorders of the eye following cataract surgery**

        H59.01 **Keratopathy (bullous aphakic) following cataract surgery**

          Vitreal corneal syndrome

          Vitreous (touch) syndrome

          H59.011 **Keratopathy (bullous aphakic) following cataract surgery, right eye**

          H59.012 **Keratopathy (bullous aphakic) following cataract surgery, left eye**

          H59.013 **Keratopathy (bullous aphakic) following cataract surgery, bilateral**

          H59.019 **Keratopathy (bullous aphakic) following cataract surgery, unspecified eye**

        H59.02 **Cataract (lens) fragments in eye following cataract surgery**

          H59.021 **Cataract (lens) fragments in eye following cataract surgery, right eye**

          H59.022 **Cataract (lens) fragments in eye following cataract surgery, left eye**

          H59.023 **Cataract (lens) fragments in eye following cataract surgery, bilateral**

          H59.029 **Cataract (lens) fragments in eye following cataract surgery, unspecified eye**

        H59.03 **Cystoid macular edema following cataract surgery**

          H59.031 **Cystoid macular edema following cataract surgery, right eye**

          H59.032 **Cystoid macular edema following cataract surgery, left eye**

          H59.033 **Cystoid macular edema following cataract surgery, bilateral**

          H59.039 **Cystoid macular edema following cataract surgery, unspecified eye**

        H59.09 **Other disorders of the eye following cataract surgery**

          H59.091 **Other disorders of the right eye following cataract surgery**

          H59.092 **Other disorders of the left eye following cataract surgery**

          H59.093 **Other disorders of the eye following cataract surgery, bilateral**

          H59.099 **Other disorders of unspecified eye following cataract surgery**

    H59.1 **Intraoperative hemorrhage and hematoma of eye and adnexa complicating a procedure**

Excludes1: intraoperative hemorrhage and hematoma of eye and adnexa due to accidental puncture or laceration during a procedure (H59.2-)

H59.11 **Intraoperative hemorrhage and hematoma of eye and adnexa complicating an ophthalmic procedure**

H59.111 **Intraoperative hemorrhage and hematoma of right eye and adnexa complicating an ophthalmic procedure**

H59.112 **Intraoperative hemorrhage and hematoma of left eye and adnexa complicating an ophthalmic procedure**

H59.113 **Intraoperative hemorrhage and hematoma of eye and adnexa complicating an ophthalmic procedure, bilateral**

H59.119 **Intraoperative hemorrhage and hematoma of unspecified eye and adnexa complicating an ophthalmic procedure**

H59.12 **Intraoperative hemorrhage and hematoma of eye and adnexa complicating other procedure**

H59.121 **Intraoperative hemorrhage and hematoma of right eye and adnexa complicating other procedure**

H59.122 **Intraoperative hemorrhage and hematoma of left eye and adnexa complicating other procedure**

H59.123 **Intraoperative hemorrhage and hematoma of eye and adnexa complicating other procedure, bilateral**

H59.129 **Intraoperative hemorrhage and hematoma of unspecified eye and adnexa complicating other procedure**

H59.2 **Accidental puncture and laceration of eye and adnexa during a procedure**

H59.21 **Accidental puncture and laceration of eye and adnexa during an ophthalmic procedure**

H59.211 **Accidental puncture and laceration of right eye and adnexa during an ophthalmic procedure**

H59.212 **Accidental puncture and laceration of left eye and adnexa during an ophthalmic procedure**

H59.213 **Accidental puncture and laceration of eye and adnexa during an ophthalmic procedure, bilateral**

H59.219 **Accidental puncture and laceration of unspecified eye and adnexa during an ophthalmic procedure**

H59.22 **Accidental puncture and laceration of eye and adnexa during other procedure**

H59.221 **Accidental puncture and laceration of right eye and adnexa during other procedure**

H59.222 **Accidental puncture and laceration of left eye and adnexa during other procedure**

H59.223 **Accidental puncture and laceration of eye and adnexa during other procedure, bilateral**

H59.229 **Accidental puncture and laceration of unspecified eye and adnexa during other procedure**

H59.3 **Postprocedural hemorrhage, hematoma, and seroma of eye and adnexa following a procedure**

H59.31 **Postprocedural hemorrhage of eye and adnexa following an ophthalmic procedure**

▲H59.311 **Postprocedural hemorrhage of right eye and adnexa following an ophthalmic procedure**

▲H59.312 **Postprocedural hemorrhage of left eye and adnexa following an ophthalmic procedure**

▲H59.313 **Postprocedural hemorrhage of eye and adnexa following an ophthalmic procedure, bilateral**

▲H59.319 **Postprocedural hemorrhage of unspecified eye and adnexa following an ophthalmic procedure**

H59.32 **Postprocedural hemorrhage of eye and adnexa following other procedure**

▲H59.321 **Postprocedural hemorrhage of right eye and adnexa following other procedure**

▲H59.322 **Postprocedural hemorrhage of left eye and adnexa following other procedure**

▲H59.323 **Postprocedural hemorrhage of eye and adnexa following other procedure, bilateral**

▲H59.329 **Postprocedural hemorrhage of unspecified eye and adnexa following other procedure**

H59.33 **Postprocedural hematoma of eye and adnexa following an ophthalmic procedure**

•H59.331 **Postprocedural hematoma of right eye and adnexa following an ophthalmic procedure**

•H59.332 **Postprocedural hematoma of left eye and adnexa following an ophthalmic procedure**

•H59.333 **Postprocedural hematoma of eye and adnexa following an ophthalmic procedure, bilateral**

•H59.339 **Postprocedural hematoma of unspecified eye and adnexa following an ophthalmic procedure**

H59.34 **Postprocedural hematoma of eye and adnexa following other procedure**

•H59.341 **Postprocedural hematoma of right eye and adnexa following other procedure**

•H59.342 **Postprocedural hematoma of left eye and adnexa following other procedure**

•H59.343 **Postprocedural hematoma of eye and adnexa following other procedure, bilateral**

•H59.349 **Postprocedural hematoma of unspecified eye and adnexa following other procedure**

H59.35 **Postprocedural seroma of eye and adnexa following an ophthalmic procedure**

- **H59.351** Postprocedural seroma of right eye and adnexa following an ophthalmic procedure
- **H59.352** Postprocedural seroma of left eye and adnexa following an ophthalmic procedure
- **H59.353** Postprocedural seroma of eye and adnexa following an ophthalmic procedure, bilateral
- **H59.359** Postprocedural seroma of unspecified eye and adnexa following an ophthalmic procedure

H59.36 **Postprocedural seroma of eye and adnexa following other procedure**

- **H59.361** Postprocedural seroma of right eye and adnexa following other procedure
- **H59.362** Postprocedural seroma of left eye and adnexa following other procedure
- **H59.363** Postprocedural seroma of eye and adnexa following other procedure, bilateral
- **H59.369** Postprocedural seroma of unspecified eye and adnexa following other procedure

H59.4 **Inflammation (infection) of postprocedural bleb**

Postprocedural blebitis

Excludes1: filtering (vitreous) bleb after glaucoma surgery status (Z98.83)

H59.40 **Inflammation (infection) of postprocedural bleb, unspecified**

H59.41 **Inflammation (infection) of postprocedural bleb, stage 1**

H59.42 **Inflammation (infection) of postprocedural bleb, stage 2**

H59.43 **Inflammation (infection) of postprocedural bleb, stage 3**

Bleb endophthalmitis

H59.8 **Other intraoperative and postprocedural complications and disorders of eye and adnexa, not elsewhere classified**

H59.81 **Chorioretinal scars after surgery for detachment**

H59.811 Chorioretinal scars after surgery for detachment, right eye

H59.812 Chorioretinal scars after surgery for detachment, left eye

H59.813 Chorioretinal scars after surgery for detachment, bilateral

H59.819 Chorioretinal scars after surgery for detachment, unspecified eye

H59.88 **Other intraoperative complications of eye and adnexa, not elsewhere classified**

H59.89 **Other postprocedural complications and disorders of eye and adnexa, not elsewhere classified**

Chapter 8: Diseases Of The Ear And Mastoid Process (H60-H95)

DEFINITIONS

This chapter includes definitions of selected key words, terms and phrases and coding alerts for adding points to the clinical domain, and references to coding late effects where appropriate. An example from this chapter is as follows:

H65 Nonsuppurative otitis media
Definition: Nonsuppurative otitis media and eustachian tube disorders, otitis media is an inflammation of the middle ear without the formation or discharge of pus.

MULTIPLE CODING FOR A SINGLE CONDITION

In addition to the etiology/manifestation convention that requires two codes to fully describe a single condition that affects multiple body systems, there are other single conditions that also require more than one code. "Use additional code" notes are found in the Tabular List at codes that are not part of an etiology/manifestation pair where a secondary code is useful to fully describe a condition. The sequencing rule is the same as the etiology/manifestation pair, "use additional code" indicates that a secondary code should be added.

For example, for bacterial infections that are not included in chapter 1, a secondary code from category B95, Streptococcus, Staphylococcus, and Enterococcus, as the cause of diseases classified elsewhere, or B96, Other bacterial agents as the cause of diseases classified elsewhere, may be required to identify the bacterial organism causing the infection. A "use additional code" note will normally be found at the infectious disease code, indicating a need for the organism code to be added as a secondary code.

 "Code first" notes are also under certain codes that are not specifically manifestation codes but may be due to an underlying cause. When there is a "code first" note and an underlying condition is present, the underlying condition should be sequenced first.

"Code, if applicable, any causal condition first", notes indicate that this code may be assigned as a principal diagnosis when the causal condition is unknown or not applicable. If a causal condition is known, then the code for that condition should be sequenced as the principal or first-listed diagnosis.

Multiple codes may be needed for sequela, complication codes and obstetric codes to more fully describe a condition. See the specific guidelines for these conditions for further instruction.

COMBINATION CODE

A combination code is a single code used to classify: Two diagnoses, or a diagnosis with an associated secondary process (manifestation) A diagnosis with an associated complication

Combination codes are identified by referring to subterm entries in the Alphabetic Index and by reading the inclusion and exclusion notes in the Tabular List.

Assign only the combination code when that code fully identifies the diagnostic conditions involved or when the Alphabetic Index so directs. Multiple coding should not be used when the classification provides a combination code that clearly identifies all of the elements documented in the diagnosis. When the combination code lacks necessary specificity in describing the manifestation or complication, an additional code should be used as a secondary code.

SEQUELA (LATE EFFECTS)

A sequela is the residual effect (condition produced) after the acute phase of an illness or injury has terminated. There is no time limit on when a sequela code can be used. The residual may be apparent early, such as in cerebral infarction, or it may occur months or years later, such as that due to a previous injury. Coding of sequela generally requires two codes sequenced in the following order: The condition or nature of the sequela is sequenced first.

The sequela code is sequenced second.

An exception to the above guidelines are those instances where the code for the sequela is followed by a manifestation code identified in the Tabular List and title, or the sequela code has been expanded (at the fourth, fifth or sixth character levels) to include the manifestation(s). The code for the acute phase of an illness or injury that led to the sequela is never used with a code for the late effect.

Chapter 8

Diseases Of The Ear And Mastoid Process (H60-H95)

Note: Use an external cause code following the code for the ear condition, if applicable, to identify the cause of the ear condition

Excludes2: certain conditions originating in the perinatal period (P04-P96)

certain infectious and parasitic diseases (A00-B99)

complications of pregnancy, childbirth and the puerperium (O00-O9A)

congenital malformations, deformations and chromosomal abnormalities (Q00-Q99)

endocrine, nutritional and metabolic diseases (E00-E88)

injury, poisoning and certain other consequences of external causes (S00-T88)

neoplasms (C00-D49)

symptoms, signs and abnormal clinical and laboratory findings, not elsewhere classified (R00-R94)

This chapter contains the following blocks:

H60-H62	Diseases of external ear
H65-H75	Diseases of middle ear and mastoid
H80-H83	Diseases of inner ear
H90-H94	Other disorders of ear
H95	Intraoperative and postprocedural complications and disorders of ear and mastoid process, not elsewhere classified

DISEASES OF EXTERNAL EAR (H60-H62)

H60   Otitis externa

H60.0   Abscess of external ear

Boil of external ear

Carbuncle of auricle or external auditory canal

Furuncle of external ear

H60.00   Abscess of external ear, unspecified ear

H60.01   Abscess of right external ear

H60.02   Abscess of left external ear

H60.03   Abscess of external ear, bilateral

H60.1   Cellulitis of external ear

Cellulitis of auricle

Cellulitis of external auditory canal

H60.10   Cellulitis of external ear, unspecified ear

H60.11   Cellulitis of right external ear

H60.12   Cellulitis of left external ear

H60.13   Cellulitis of external ear, bilateral

H60.2   Malignant otitis externa

H60.20   Malignant otitis externa, unspecified ear

H60.21   Malignant otitis externa, right ear

H60.22   Malignant otitis externa, left ear

H60.23   Malignant otitis externa, bilateral

H60.3   Other infective otitis externa

H60.31   Diffuse otitis externa

H60.311   Diffuse otitis externa, right ear

H60.312   Diffuse otitis externa, left ear

H60.313   Diffuse otitis externa, bilateral

H60.319   Diffuse otitis externa, unspecified ear

H60.32   Hemorrhagic otitis externa

H60.321   Hemorrhagic otitis externa, right ear

H60.322   Hemorrhagic otitis externa, left ear

H60.323   Hemorrhagic otitis externa, bilateral

H60.329   Hemorrhagic otitis externa, unspecified ear

H60.33   Swimmer's ear

H60.331   Swimmer's ear, right ear

H60.332   Swimmer's ear, left ear

H60.333   Swimmer's ear, bilateral

H60.339   Swimmer's ear, unspecified ear

H60.39   Other infective otitis externa

H60.391   Other infective otitis externa, right ear

H60.392   Other infective otitis externa, left ear

H60.393   Other infective otitis externa, bilateral

H60.399   Other infective otitis externa, unspecified ear

H60.4   Cholesteatoma of external ear

Keratosis obturans of external ear (canal)

Excludes2: cholesteatoma of middle ear (H71.-)

recurrent cholesteatoma of postmastoidectomy cavity (H95.0-)

H60.40   Cholesteatoma of external ear, unspecified ear

H60.41   Cholesteatoma of right external ear

H60.42   Cholesteatoma of left external ear

H60.43   Cholesteatoma of external ear, bilateral

H60.5   Acute noninfective otitis externa

H60.50   Unspecified acute noninfective otitis externa

Acute otitis externa NOS

H60.501   Unspecified acute noninfective otitis externa, right ear

H60.502   Unspecified acute noninfective otitis externa, left ear

H60.503   Unspecified acute noninfective otitis externa, bilateral

H60.509   Unspecified acute noninfective otitis externa, unspecified ear

H60.51   Acute actinic otitis externa

H60.511   Acute actinic otitis externa, right ear

H60.512   Acute actinic otitis externa, left ear

H60.513   Acute actinic otitis externa, bilateral

H60.519   Acute actinic otitis externa, unspecified ear

H60.52   Acute chemical otitis externa

H60.521   Acute chemical otitis externa, right ear

H60.522   Acute chemical otitis externa, left ear

H60.523   Acute chemical otitis externa, bilateral

H60.529   Acute chemical otitis externa, unspecified ear

H60.53   Acute contact otitis externa

    H60.531   Acute contact otitis externa, right ear

    H60.532   Acute contact otitis externa, left ear

    H60.533   Acute contact otitis externa, bilateral

    H60.539   Acute contact otitis externa, unspecified ear

H60.54   Acute eczematoid otitis externa

    H60.541   Acute eczematoid otitis externa, right ear

    H60.542   Acute eczematoid otitis externa, left ear

    H60.543   Acute eczematoid otitis externa, bilateral

    H60.549   Acute eczematoid otitis externa, unspecified ear

H60.55   Acute reactive otitis externa

    H60.551   Acute reactive otitis externa, right ear

    H60.552   Acute reactive otitis externa, left ear

    H60.553   Acute reactive otitis externa, bilateral

    H60.559   Acute reactive otitis externa, unspecified ear

H60.59   Other noninfective acute otitis externa

    H60.591   Other noninfective acute otitis externa, right ear

    H60.592   Other noninfective acute otitis externa, left ear

    H60.593   Other noninfective acute otitis externa, bilateral

    H60.599   Other noninfective acute otitis externa, unspecified ear

H60.6   Unspecified chronic otitis externa

    H60.60   Unspecified chronic otitis externa, unspecified ear

    H60.61   Unspecified chronic otitis externa, right ear

    H60.62   Unspecified chronic otitis externa, left ear

    H60.63   Unspecified chronic otitis externa, bilateral

H60.8   Other otitis externa

    H60.8X   Other otitis externa

        H60.8X1   Other otitis externa, right ear

        H60.8X2   Other otitis externa, left ear

        H60.8X3   Other otitis externa, bilateral

        H60.8X9   Other otitis externa, unspecified ear

H60.9   Unspecified otitis externa

    H60.90   Unspecified otitis externa, unspecified ear

    H60.91   Unspecified otitis externa, right ear

    H60.92   Unspecified otitis externa, left ear

    H60.93   Unspecified otitis externa, bilateral

H61   Other disorders of external ear

H61.0   Chondritis and perichondritis of external ear

    Chondrodermatitis nodularis chronica helicis

    Perichondritis of auricle

    Perichondritis of pinna

    H61.00   Unspecified perichondritis of external ear

        H61.001   Unspecified perichondritis of right external ear

        H61.002   Unspecified perichondritis of left external ear

        H61.003   Unspecified perichondritis of external ear, bilateral

        H61.009   Unspecified perichondritis of external ear, unspecified ear

    H61.01   Acute perichondritis of external ear

        H61.011   Acute perichondritis of right external ear

        H61.012   Acute perichondritis of left external ear

        H61.013   Acute perichondritis of external ear, bilateral

        H61.019   Acute perichondritis of external ear, unspecified ear

    H61.02   Chronic perichondritis of external ear

        H61.021   Chronic perichondritis of right external ear

        H61.022   Chronic perichondritis of left external ear

        H61.023   Chronic perichondritis of external ear, bilateral

        H61.029   Chronic perichondritis of external ear, unspecified ear

    H61.03   Chondritis of external ear

        Chondritis of auricle

        Chondritis of pinna

        H61.031   Chondritis of right external ear

        H61.032   Chondritis of left external ear

        H61.033   Chondritis of external ear, bilateral

        H61.039   Chondritis of external ear, unspecified ear

H61.1   Noninfective disorders of pinna

    Excludes2: cauliflower ear (M95.1-)

        gouty tophi of ear (M1A.-)

    H61.10   Unspecified noninfective disorders of pinna

    Disorder of pinna NOS

        H61.101   Unspecified noninfective disorders of pinna, right ear

        H61.102   Unspecified noninfective disorders of pinna, left ear

        H61.103   Unspecified noninfective disorders of pinna, bilateral

        H61.109   Unspecified noninfective disorders of pinna, unspecified ear

    H61.11   Acquired deformity of pinna

    Acquired deformity of auricle

    Excludes2: cauliflower ear (M95.1-)

        H61.111   Acquired deformity of pinna, right ear

        H61.112   Acquired deformity of pinna, left ear

        H61.113   Acquired deformity of pinna, bilateral

        H61.119   Acquired deformity of pinna, unspecified ear

    H61.12   Hematoma of pinna

● New code   ▲ Revised code   **Excludes1:** Not coded here   **Excludes2:** Not included here   ⊗ Placeholder required   ⑦7th digit required

Hematoma of auricle

H61.121 Hematoma of pinna, right ear

H61.122 Hematoma of pinna, left ear

H61.123 Hematoma of pinna, bilateral

H61.129 Hematoma of pinna, unspecified ear

H61.19 Other noninfective disorders of pinna

H61.191 Noninfective disorders of pinna, right ear

H61.192 Noninfective disorders of pinna, left ear

H61.193 Noninfective disorders of pinna, bilateral

H61.199 Noninfective disorders of pinna, unspecified ear

H61.2 Impacted cerumen

Wax in ear

H61.20 Impacted cerumen, unspecified ear

H61.21 Impacted cerumen, right ear

H61.22 Impacted cerumen, left ear

H61.23 Impacted cerumen, bilateral

H61.3 Acquired stenosis of external ear canal

Collapse of external ear canal

Excludes1: postprocedural stenosis of external ear canal (H95.81-)

H61.30 Acquired stenosis of external ear canal, unspecified

H61.301 Acquired stenosis of right external ear canal, unspecified

H61.302 Acquired stenosis of left external ear canal, unspecified

H61.303 Acquired stenosis of external ear canal, unspecified, bilateral

H61.309 Acquired stenosis of external ear canal, unspecified, unspecified ear

H61.31 Acquired stenosis of external ear canal secondary to trauma

H61.311 Acquired stenosis of right external ear canal secondary to trauma

H61.312 Acquired stenosis of left external ear canal secondary to trauma

H61.313 Acquired stenosis of external ear canal secondary to trauma, bilateral

H61.319 Acquired stenosis of external ear canal secondary to trauma, unspecified ear

H61.32 Acquired stenosis of external ear canal secondary to inflammation and infection

H61.321 Acquired stenosis of right external ear canal secondary to inflammation and infection

H61.322 Acquired stenosis of left external ear canal secondary to inflammation and infection

H61.323 Acquired stenosis of external ear canal secondary to inflammation and infection, bilateral

H61.329 Acquired stenosis of external ear canal secondary to inflammation and infection, unspecified ear

H61.39 Other acquired stenosis of external ear canal

H61.391 Other acquired stenosis of right external ear canal

H61.392 Other acquired stenosis of left external ear canal

H61.393 Other acquired stenosis of external ear canal, bilateral

H61.399 Other acquired stenosis of external ear canal, unspecified ear

H61.8 Other specified disorders of external ear

H61.81 Exostosis of external canal

H61.811 Exostosis of right external canal

H61.812 Exostosis of left external canal

H61.813 Exostosis of external canal, bilateral

H61.819 Exostosis of external canal, unspecified ear

H61.89 Other specified disorders of external ear

H61.891 Other specified disorders of right external ear

H61.892 Other specified disorders of left external ear

H61.893 Other specified disorders of external ear, bilateral

H61.899 Other specified disorders of external ear, unspecified ear

H61.9 Disorder of external ear, unspecified

H61.90 Disorder of external ear, unspecified, unspecified ear

H61.91 Disorder of right external ear, unspecified

H61.92 Disorder of left external ear, unspecified

H61.93 Disorder of external ear, unspecified, bilateral

H62 Disorders of external ear in diseases classified elsewhere

H62.4 Otitis externa in other diseases classified elsewhere

Code first underlying disease, such as:

erysipelas (A46)

impetigo (L01.0)

Excludes1: otitis externa (in):

candidiasis (B37.84)

herpes viral [herpes simplex] (B00.1)

herpes zoster (B02.8)

H62.40 Otitis externa in other diseases classified elsewhere, unspecified ear

H62.41 Otitis externa in other diseases classified elsewhere, right ear

H62.42 Otitis externa in other diseases classified elsewhere, left ear

H62.43 Otitis externa in other diseases classified elsewhere, bilateral

H62.8 Other disorders of external ear in diseases classified elsewhere

Code first underlying disease, such as:

gout (M1A.-, M10.-)

H62.8X Other disorders of external ear in diseases classified elsewhere

H62.8X1 Other disorders of right external ear in diseases classified elsewhere

H62.8X2 Other disorders of left external ear in diseases classified elsewhere

H62.8X3 Other disorders of external ear in diseases classified elsewhere, bilateral

H62.8X9 Other disorders of external ear in diseases classified elsewhere, unspecified ear

DISEASES OF MIDDLE EAR AND MASTOID (H65-H75)

H65 Nonsuppurative otitis media

Definition: Nonsuppurative otitis media and eustachian tube disorders, otitis media is an inflammation of the middle ear without the formation or discharge of pus.

Includes: nonsuppurative otitis media with myringitis

Use additional code for any associated perforated tympanic membrane (H72.-)

Use additional code to identify:

exposure to environmental tobacco smoke (Z77.22)

exposure to tobacco smoke in the perinatal period (P96.81)

history of tobacco dependence (Z87.891)

occupational exposure to environmental tobacco smoke (Z57.31)

tobacco dependence (F17.-)

tobacco use (Z72.0)

H65.0 Acute serous otitis media

Acute and subacute secretory otitis

H65.00 Acute serous otitis media, unspecified ear

H65.01 Acute serous otitis media, right ear

H65.02 Acute serous otitis media, left ear

H65.03 Acute serous otitis media, bilateral

H65.04 Acute serous otitis media, recurrent, right ear

H65.05 Acute serous otitis media, recurrent, left ear

H65.06 Acute serous otitis media, recurrent, bilateral

H65.07 Acute serous otitis media, recurrent, unspecified ear

H65.1 Other acute nonsuppurative otitis media

Excludes1: otitic barotrauma (T70.0)

otitis media (acute) NOS (H66.9)

H65.11 Acute and subacute allergic otitis media (mucoid) (sanguinous) (serous)

H65.111 Acute and subacute allergic otitis media (mucoid) (sanguinous) (serous), right ear

H65.112 Acute and subacute allergic otitis media (mucoid) (sanguinous) (serous), left ear

H65.113 Acute and subacute allergic otitis media (mucoid) (sanguinous) (serous), bilateral

H65.114 Acute and subacute allergic otitis media (mucoid) (sanguinous) (serous), recurrent, right ear

H65.115 Acute and subacute allergic otitis media (mucoid) (sanguinous) (serous), recurrent, left ear

H65.116 Acute and subacute allergic otitis media (mucoid) (sanguinous) (serous), recurrent, bilateral

H65.117 Acute and subacute allergic otitis media (mucoid) (sanguinous) (serous), recurrent, unspecified ear

H65.119 Acute and subacute allergic otitis media (mucoid) (sanguinous) (serous), unspecified ear

H65.19 Other acute nonsuppurative otitis media

Acute and subacute mucoid otitis media

Acute and subacute nonsuppurative otitis media NOS

Acute and subacute sanguinous otitis media

Acute and subacute seromucinous otitis media

H65.191 Other acute nonsuppurative otitis media, right ear

H65.192 Other acute nonsuppurative otitis media, left ear

H65.193 Other acute nonsuppurative otitis media, bilateral

H65.194 Other acute nonsuppurative otitis media, recurrent, right ear

H65.195 Other acute nonsuppurative otitis media, recurrent, left ear

H65.196 Other acute nonsuppurative otitis media, recurrent, bilateral

H65.197 Other acute nonsuppurative otitis media recurrent, unspecified ear

H65.199 Other acute nonsuppurative otitis media, unspecified ear

H65.2 Chronic serous otitis media

Chronic tubotympanal catarrh

H65.20 Chronic serous otitis media, unspecified ear

H65.21 Chronic serous otitis media, right ear

H65.22 Chronic serous otitis media, left ear

H65.23 Chronic serous otitis media, bilateral

H65.3 Chronic mucoid otitis media

Chronic mucinous otitis media

Chronic secretory otitis media

Chronic transudative otitis media Glue ear

Excludes1: adhesive middle ear disease (H74.1)

H65.30 Chronic mucoid otitis media, unspecified ear

H65.31 Chronic mucoid otitis media, right ear

H65.32 Chronic mucoid otitis media, left ear

H65.33 Chronic mucoid otitis media, bilateral

H65.4 Other chronic nonsuppurative otitis media

H65.41 Chronic allergic otitis media

H65.411 Chronic allergic otitis media, right ear

H65.412 Chronic allergic otitis media, left ear

H65.413 Chronic allergic otitis media, bilateral

H65.419 Chronic allergic otitis media, unspecified ear

H65.49 Other chronic nonsuppurative otitis media

Chronic exudative otitis media

Chronic nonsuppurative otitis media NOS

Chronic otitis media with effusion (nonpurulent)

Chronic seromucinous otitis media

H65.491 Other chronic nonsuppurative otitis media, right ear

● New code ▲ Revised code **Excludes1:** Not coded here **Excludes2:** Not included here ⊗ Placeholder required ⑦7th digit required

H65.492	Other chronic nonsuppurative otitis media, left ear
H65.493	Other chronic nonsuppurative otitis media, bilateral
H65.499	Other chronic nonsuppurative otitis media, unspecified ear

H65.9 Unspecified nonsuppurative otitis media

Allergic otitis media NOS

Catarrhal otitis media NOS

Exudative otitis media NOS

Mucoid otitis media NOS

Otitis media with effusion (nonpurulent) NOS

Secretory otitis media NOS

Seromucinous otitis media NOS

Serous otitis media NOS

Transudative otitis media NOS

H65.90	Unspecified nonsuppurative otitis media, unspecified ear
H65.91	Unspecified nonsuppurative otitis media, right ear
H65.92	Unspecified nonsuppurative otitis media, left ear
H65.93	Unspecified nonsuppurative otitis media, bilateral

H66 Suppurative and unspecified otitis media

Definition: Suppurative and unspecified otitis media is an inflammation of the middle ear including the formation or discharge of pus.

Includes: suppurative and unspecified otitis media with myringitis

Use additional code to identify:

exposure to environmental tobacco smoke (Z77.22)

exposure to tobacco smoke in the perinatal period (P96.81)

history of tobacco dependence (Z87.891)

occupational exposure to environmental tobacco smoke (Z57.31)

tobacco dependence (F17.-)

tobacco use (Z72.0)

H66.0 Acute suppurative otitis media

H66.00	Acute suppurative otitis media without spontaneous rupture of ear drum
H66.001	Acute suppurative otitis media without spontaneous rupture of ear drum, right ear
H66.002	Acute suppurative otitis media without spontaneous rupture of ear drum, left ear
H66.003	Acute suppurative otitis media without spontaneous rupture of ear drum, bilateral
H66.004	Acute suppurative otitis media without spontaneous rupture of ear drum, recurrent, right ear
H66.005	Acute suppurative otitis media without spontaneous rupture of ear drum, recurrent, left ear
H66.006	Acute suppurative otitis media without spontaneous rupture of ear drum, recurrent, bilateral
H66.007	Acute suppurative otitis media without spontaneous rupture of ear drum, recurrent, unspecified ear

H66.009	Acute suppurative otitis media without spontaneous rupture of ear drum, unspecified ear
H66.01	Acute suppurative otitis media with spontaneous rupture of ear drum
H66.011	Acute suppurative otitis media with spontaneous rupture of ear drum, right ear
H66.012	Acute suppurative otitis media with spontaneous rupture of ear drum, left ear
H66.013	Acute suppurative otitis media with spontaneous rupture of ear drum, bilateral
H66.014	Acute suppurative otitis media with spontaneous rupture of ear drum, recurrent, right ear
H66.015	Acute suppurative otitis media with spontaneous rupture of ear drum, recurrent, left ear
H66.016	Acute suppurative otitis media with spontaneous rupture of ear drum, recurrent, bilateral
H66.017	Acute suppurative otitis media with spontaneous rupture of ear drum, recurrent, unspecified ear
H66.019	Acute suppurative otitis media with spontaneous rupture of ear drum, unspecified ear

H66.1 Chronic tubotympanic suppurative otitis media

Benign chronic suppurative otitis media

Chronic tubotympanic disease

Use additional code for any associated perforated tympanic membrane (H72.-)

H66.10	Chronic tubotympanic suppurative otitis media, unspecified
H66.11	Chronic tubotympanic suppurative otitis media, right ear
H66.12	Chronic tubotympanic suppurative otitis media, left ear
H66.13	Chronic tubotympanic suppurative otitis media, bilateral

H66.2 Chronic atticoantral suppurative otitis media

Chronic atticoantral disease

Use additional code for any associated perforated tympanic membrane (H72.-)

H66.20	Chronic atticoantral suppurative otitis media, unspecified ear
H66.21	Chronic atticoantral suppurative otitis media, right ear
H66.22	Chronic atticoantral suppurative otitis media, left ear
H66.23	Chronic atticoantral suppurative otitis media, bilateral

H66.3 Other chronic suppurative otitis media

Chronic suppurative otitis media NOS

Use additional code for any associated perforated tympanic membrane (H72.-)

Excludes1: tuberculous otitis media (A18.6)

| H66.3X | Other chronic suppurative otitis media |
| H66.3X1 | Other chronic suppurative otitis media, right ear |

H66.3X2 **Other chronic suppurative otitis media, left ear**

H66.3X3 **Other chronic suppurative otitis media, bilateral**

H66.3X9 **Other chronic suppurative otitis media, unspecified ear**

H66.4 **Suppurative otitis media, unspecified**

Purulent otitis media NOS

Use additional code for any associated perforated tympanic membrane (H72.-)

H66.40 **Suppurative otitis media, unspecified, unspecified ear**

H66.41 **Suppurative otitis media, unspecified, right ear**

H66.42 **Suppurative otitis media, unspecified, left ear**

H66.43 **Suppurative otitis media, unspecified, bilateral**

H66.9 **Otitis media, unspecified**

Otitis media NOS

Acute otitis media NOS

Chronic otitis media NOS

Use additional code for any associated perforated tympanic membrane (H72.-)

H66.90 **Otitis media, unspecified, unspecified ear**

H66.91 **Otitis media, unspecified, right ear**

H66.92 **Otitis media, unspecified, left ear**

H66.93 **Otitis media, unspecified, bilateral**

H67 **Otitis media in diseases classified elsewhere**

Code first underlying disease, such as:

viral disease NEC (B00-B34)

Use additional code for any associated perforated tympanic membrane (H72.-)

Excludes1: otitis media in:

influenza (J09.X9, J10.83, J11.83)

measles (B05.3)

scarlet fever (A38.0)

tuberculosis (A18.6)

H67.1 **Otitis media in diseases classified elsewhere, right ear**

H67.2 **Otitis media in diseases classified elsewhere, left ear**

H67.3 **Otitis media in diseases classified elsewhere, bilateral**

H67.9 **Otitis media in diseases classified elsewhere, unspecified ear**

H68 **Eustachian salpingitis and obstruction**

H68.0 **Eustachian salpingitis**

H68.00 **Unspecified Eustachian salpingitis**

H68.001 **Unspecified Eustachian salpingitis, right ear**

H68.002 **Unspecified Eustachian salpingitis, left ear**

H68.003 **Unspecified Eustachian salpingitis, bilateral**

H68.009 **Unspecified Eustachian salpingitis, unspecified ear**

H68.01 **Acute Eustachian salpingitis**

H68.011 **Acute Eustachian salpingitis, right ear**

H68.012 **Acute Eustachian salpingitis, left ear**

H68.013 **Acute Eustachian salpingitis, bilateral**

H68.019 **Acute Eustachian salpingitis, unspecified ear**

H68.02 **Chronic Eustachian salpingitis**

H68.021 **Chronic Eustachian salpingitis, right ear**

H68.022 **Chronic Eustachian salpingitis, left ear**

H68.023 **Chronic Eustachian salpingitis, bilateral**

H68.029 **Chronic Eustachian salpingitis, unspecified ear**

H68.1 **Obstruction of Eustachian tube**

Stenosis of Eustachian tube

Stricture of Eustachian tube

H68.10 **Unspecified obstruction of Eustachian tube**

H68.101 **Unspecified obstruction of Eustachian tube, right ear**

H68.102 **Unspecified obstruction of Eustachian tube, left ear**

H68.103 **Unspecified obstruction of Eustachian tube, bilateral**

H68.109 **Unspecified obstruction of Eustachian tube, unspecified ear**

H68.11 **Osseous obstruction of Eustachian tube**

H68.111 **Osseous obstruction of Eustachian tube, right ear**

H68.112 **Osseous obstruction of Eustachian tube, left ear**

H68.113 **Osseous obstruction of Eustachian tube, bilateral**

H68.119 **Osseous obstruction of Eustachian tube, unspecified ear**

H68.12 **Intrinsic cartilagenous obstruction of Eustachian tube**

H68.121 **Intrinsic cartilagenous obstruction of Eustachian tube, right ear**

H68.122 **Intrinsic cartilagenous obstruction of Eustachian tube, left ear**

H68.123 **Intrinsic cartilagenous obstruction of Eustachian tube, bilateral**

H68.129 **Intrinsic cartilagenous obstruction of Eustachian tube, unspecified ear**

H68.13 **Extrinsic cartilagenous obstruction of Eustachian tube**

Compression of Eustachian tube

H68.131 **Extrinsic cartilagenous obstruction of Eustachian tube, right ear**

H68.132 **Extrinsic cartilagenous obstruction of Eustachian tube, left ear**

H68.133 **Extrinsic cartilagenous obstruction of Eustachian tube, bilateral**

H68.139 **Extrinsic cartilagenous obstruction of Eustachian tube, unspecified ear**

H69 **Other and unspecified disorders of Eustachian tube**

H69.0 **Patulous Eustachian tube**

H69.00 **Patulous Eustachian tube, unspecified ear**

H69.01 **Patulous Eustachian tube, right ear**

H69.02 **Patulous Eustachian tube, left ear**

● New code   ▲ Revised code   Excludes1: Not coded here   Excludes2: Not included here   ⊗ Placeholder required   ⑦7th digit required

H69.03 Patulous Eustachian tube, bilateral

H69.8 Other specified disorders of Eustachian tube

H69.80 Other specified disorders of Eustachian tube, unspecified ear

H69.81 Other specified disorders of Eustachian tube, right ear

H69.82 Other specified disorders of Eustachian tube, left ear

H69.83 Other specified disorders of Eustachian tube, bilateral

H69.9 Unspecified Eustachian tube disorder

H69.90 Unspecified Eustachian tube disorder, unspecified ear

H69.91 Unspecified Eustachian tube disorder, right ear

H69.92 Unspecified Eustachian tube disorder, left ear

H69.93 Unspecified Eustachian tube disorder, bilateral

H70 Mastoiditis and related conditions

Definition: Mastoiditis is an infection of the spaces within the mastoid bone. It is almost always associated with otitis media, an infection of the middle ear. In the most serious cases, the bone itself becomes infected.

H70.0 Acute mastoiditis

Abscess of mastoid Empyema of mastoid

H70.00 Acute mastoiditis without complications

H70.001 Acute mastoiditis without complications, right ear

H70.002 Acute mastoiditis without complications, left ear

H70.003 Acute mastoiditis without complications, bilateral

H70.009 Acute mastoiditis without complications, unspecified ear

H70.01 Subperiosteal abscess of mastoid

H70.011 Subperiosteal abscess of mastoid, right ear

H70.012 Subperiosteal abscess of mastoid, left ear

H70.013 Subperiosteal abscess of mastoid, bilateral

H70.019 Subperiosteal abscess of mastoid, unspecified ear

H70.09 Acute mastoiditis with other complications

H70.091 Acute mastoiditis with other complications, right ear

H70.092 Acute mastoiditis with other complications, left ear

H70.093 Acute mastoiditis with other complications, bilateral

H70.099 Acute mastoiditis with other complications, unspecified ear

H70.1 Chronic mastoiditis

Caries of mastoid

Fistula of mastoid

Excludes1: tuberculous mastoiditis (A18.03)

H70.10 Chronic mastoiditis, unspecified ear

H70.11 Chronic mastoiditis, right ear

H70.12 Chronic mastoiditis, left ear

H70.13 Chronic mastoiditis, bilateral

H70.2 Petrositis

Inflammation of petrous bone

H70.20 Unspecified petrositis

H70.201 Unspecified petrositis, right ear

H70.202 Unspecified petrositis, left ear

H70.203 Unspecified petrositis, bilateral

H70.209 Unspecified petrositis, unspecified ear

H70.21 Acute petrositis

H70.211 Acute petrositis, right ear

H70.212 Acute petrositis, left ear

H70.213 Acute petrositis, bilateral

H70.219 Acute petrositis, unspecified ear

H70.22 Chronic petrositis

H70.221 Chronic petrositis, right ear

H70.222 Chronic petrositis, left ear

H70.223 Chronic petrositis, bilateral

H70.229 Chronic petrositis, unspecified ear

H70.8 Other mastoiditis and related conditions

Excludes1: preauricular sinus and cyst (Q18.1)

sinus, fistula, and cyst of branchial cleft (Q18.0)

H70.81 Postauricular fistula

H70.811 Postauricular fistula, right ear

H70.812 Postauricular fistula, left ear

H70.813 Postauricular fistula, bilateral

H70.819 Postauricular fistula, unspecified ear

H70.89 Other mastoiditis and related conditions

H70.891 Other mastoiditis and related conditions, right ear

H70.892 Other mastoiditis and related conditions, left ear

H70.893 Other mastoiditis and related conditions, bilateral

H70.899 Other mastoiditis and related conditions, unspecified ear

H70.9 Unspecified mastoiditis

H70.90 Unspecified mastoiditis, unspecified ear

H70.91 Unspecified mastoiditis, right ear

H70.92 Unspecified mastoiditis, left ear

H70.93 Unspecified mastoiditis, bilateral

H71 Cholesteatoma of middle ear

Excludes2: cholesteatoma of external ear (H60.4-)

recurrent cholesteatoma of postmastoidectomy cavity (H95.0-)

H71.0 Cholesteatoma of attic

H71.00 Cholesteatoma of attic, unspecified ear

H71.01 Cholesteatoma of attic, right ear

H71.02 Cholesteatoma of attic, left ear

H71.03 Cholesteatoma of attic, bilateral

H71.1 Cholesteatoma of tympanum

H71.10 Cholesteatoma of tympanum, unspecified ear

H71.11 Cholesteatoma of tympanum, right ear

H71.12 Cholesteatoma of tympanum, left ear

H71.13 Cholesteatoma of tympanum, bilateral

H71.2 **Cholesteatoma of mastoid**

    H71.20 **Cholesteatoma of mastoid, unspecified ear**

    H71.21 **Cholesteatoma of mastoid, right ear**

    H71.22 **Cholesteatoma of mastoid, left ear**

    H71.23 **Cholesteatoma of mastoid, bilateral**

H71.3 **Diffuse cholesteatosis**

    H71.30 **Diffuse cholesteatosis, unspecified ear**

    H71.31 **Diffuse cholesteatosis, right ear**

    H71.32 **Diffuse cholesteatosis, left ear**

    H71.33 **Diffuse cholesteatosis, bilateral**

H71.9 **Unspecified cholesteatoma**

    H71.90 **Unspecified cholesteatoma, unspecified ear**

    H71.91 **Unspecified cholesteatoma, right ear**

    H71.92 **Unspecified cholesteatoma, left ear**

    H71.93 **Unspecified cholesteatoma, bilateral**

H72 **Perforation of tympanic membrane**

Includes: persistent post-traumatic perforation of ear drum

    postinflammatory perforation of ear drum

Code first any associated otitis media (H65.-, H66.1-, H66.2-, H66.3-, H66.4-, H66.9-, H67.-)

Excludes1: acute suppurative otitis media with rupture of the tympanic membrane (H66.01-)

    traumatic rupture of ear drum (S09.2-)

H72.0 **Central perforation of tympanic membrane**

    H72.00 **Central perforation of tympanic membrane, unspecified ear**

    H72.01 **Central perforation of tympanic membrane, right ear**

    H72.02 **Central perforation of tympanic membrane, left ear**

    H72.03 **Central perforation of tympanic membrane, bilateral**

H72.1 **Attic perforation of tympanic membrane**

    Perforation of pars flaccida

    H72.10 **Attic perforation of tympanic membrane, unspecified ear**

    H72.11 **Attic perforation of tympanic membrane, right ear**

    H72.12 **Attic perforation of tympanic membrane, left ear**

    H72.13 **Attic perforation of tympanic membrane, bilateral**

H72.2 **Other marginal perforations of tympanic membrane**

    H72.2X **Other marginal perforations of tympanic membrane**

        H72.2X1 **Other marginal perforations of tympanic membrane, right ear**

        H72.2X2 **Other marginal perforations of tympanic membrane, left ear**

        H72.2X3 **Other marginal perforations of tympanic membrane, bilateral**

        H72.2X9 **Other marginal perforations of tympanic membrane, unspecified ear**

H72.8 **Other perforations of tympanic membrane**

    H72.81 **Multiple perforations of tympanic membrane**

        H72.811 **Multiple perforations of tympanic membrane, right ear**

        H72.812 **Multiple perforations of tympanic membrane, left ear**

        H72.813 **Multiple perforations of tympanic membrane, bilateral**

        H72.819 **Multiple perforations of tympanic membrane, unspecified ear**

    H72.82 **Total perforations of tympanic membrane**

        H72.821 **Total perforations of tympanic membrane, right ear**

        H72.822 **Total perforations of tympanic membrane, left ear**

        H72.823 **Total perforations of tympanic membrane, bilateral**

        H72.829 **Total perforations of tympanic membrane, unspecified ear**

H72.9 **Unspecified perforation of tympanic membrane**

    H72.90 **Unspecified perforation of tympanic membrane, unspecified ear**

    H72.91 **Unspecified perforation of tympanic membrane, right ear**

    H72.92 **Unspecified perforation of tympanic membrane, left ear**

    H72.93 **Unspecified perforation of tympanic membrane, bilateral**

H73 **Other disorders of tympanic membrane**

H73.0 **Acute myringitis**

    Excludes1: acute myringitis with otitis media (H65, H66)

    H73.00 **Unspecified acute myringitis**

        Acute tympanitis NOS

        H73.001 **Acute myringitis, right ear**

        H73.002 **Acute myringitis, left ear**

        H73.003 **Acute myringitis, bilateral**

        H73.009 **Acute myringitis, unspecified ear**

    H73.01 **Bullous myringitis**

        H73.011 **Bullous myringitis, right ear**

        H73.012 **Bullous myringitis, left ear**

        H73.013 **Bullous myringitis, bilateral**

        H73.019 **Bullous myringitis, unspecified ear**

    H73.09 **Other acute myringitis**

        H73.091 **Other acute myringitis, right ear**

        H73.092 **Other acute myringitis, left ear**

        H73.093 **Other acute myringitis, bilateral**

        H73.099 **Other acute myringitis, unspecified ear**

H73.1 **Chronic myringitis**

    Chronic tympanitis

    Excludes1: chronic myringitis with otitis media (H65, H66)

    H73.10 **Chronic myringitis, unspecified ear**

    H73.11 **Chronic myringitis, right ear**

    H73.12 **Chronic myringitis, left ear**

    H73.13 **Chronic myringitis, bilateral**

H73.2 **Unspecified myringitis**

    H73.20 **Unspecified myringitis, unspecified ear**

    H73.21 **Unspecified myringitis, right ear**

    H73.22 **Unspecified myringitis, left ear**

    H73.23 **Unspecified myringitis, bilateral**

H73.8 Other specified disorders of tympanic membrane

    H73.81 Atrophic flaccid tympanic membrane

        H73.811 Atrophic flaccid tympanic membrane, right ear

        H73.812 Atrophic flaccid tympanic membrane, left ear

        H73.813 Atrophic flaccid tympanic membrane, bilateral

        H73.819 Atrophic flaccid tympanic membrane, unspecified ear

    H73.82 Atrophic nonflaccid tympanic membrane

        H73.821 Atrophic nonflaccid tympanic membrane, right ear

        H73.822 Atrophic nonflaccid tympanic membrane, left ear

        H73.823 Atrophic nonflaccid tympanic membrane, bilateral

        H73.829 Atrophic nonflaccid tympanic membrane, unspecified ear

    H73.89 Other specified disorders of tympanic membrane

        H73.891 Other specified disorders of tympanic membrane, right ear

        H73.892 Other specified disorders of tympanic membrane, left ear

        H73.893 Other specified disorders of tympanic membrane, bilateral

        H73.899 Other specified disorders of tympanic membrane, unspecified ear

H73.9 Unspecified disorder of tympanic membrane

    H73.90 Unspecified disorder of tympanic membrane, unspecified ear

    H73.91 Unspecified disorder of tympanic membrane, right ear

    H73.92 Unspecified disorder of tympanic membrane, left ear

    H73.93 Unspecified disorder of tympanic membrane, bilateral

H74 OTHER DISORDERS OF MIDDLE EAR MASTOID

Definition: The middle ear is the space between the eardrum and the inner ear that contains the three auditory ossicles, which convey vibrations through the oval window to the cochlea. The mastoid is the bone located directly behind the external ear.

Excludes2: mastoiditis (H70.-)

H74.0 Tympanosclerosis

    H74.01 Tympanosclerosis, right ear

    H74.02 Tympanosclerosis, left ear

    H74.03 Tympanosclerosis, bilateral

    H74.09 Tympanosclerosis, unspecified ear

H74.1 Adhesive middle ear disease

    Adhesive otitis

    Excludes1: glue ear (H65.3-)

    H74.11 Adhesive right middle ear disease

    H74.12 Adhesive left middle ear disease

    H74.13 Adhesive middle ear disease, bilateral

    H74.19 Adhesive middle ear disease, unspecified ear

H74.2 Discontinuity and dislocation of ear ossicles

    H74.20 Discontinuity and dislocation of ear ossicles, unspecified ear

    H74.21 Discontinuity and dislocation of right ear ossicles

    H74.22 Discontinuity and dislocation of left ear ossicles

    H74.23 Discontinuity and dislocation of ear ossicles, bilateral

H74.3 Other acquired abnormalities of ear ossicles

    H74.31 Ankylosis of ear ossicles

        H74.311 Ankylosis of ear ossicles, right ear

        H74.312 Ankylosis of ear ossicles, left ear

        H74.313 Ankylosis of ear ossicles, bilateral

        H74.319 Ankylosis of ear ossicles, unspecified ear

    H74.32 Partial loss of ear ossicles

        H74.321 Partial loss of ear ossicles, right ear

        H74.322 Partial loss of ear ossicles, left ear

        H74.323 Partial loss of ear ossicles, bilateral

        H74.329 Partial loss of ear ossicles, unspecified ear

    H74.39 Other acquired abnormalities of ear ossicles

        H74.391 Other acquired abnormalities of right ear ossicles

        H74.392 Other acquired abnormalities of left ear ossicles

        H74.393 Other acquired abnormalities of ear ossicles, bilateral

        H74.399 Other acquired abnormalities of ear ossicles, unspecified ear

H74.4 Polyp of middle ear

    H74.40 Polyp of middle ear, unspecified ear

    H74.41 Polyp of right middle ear

    H74.42 Polyp of left middle ear

    H74.43 Polyp of middle ear, bilateral

H74.8 Other specified disorders of middle ear and mastoid

    H74.8X Other specified disorders of middle ear and mastoid

        H74.8X1 Other specified disorders of right middle ear and mastoid

        H74.8X2 Other specified disorders of left middle ear and mastoid

        H74.8X3 Other specified disorders of middle ear and mastoid, bilateral

        H74.8X9 Other specified disorders of middle ear and mastoid, unspecified ear

H74.9 Unspecified disorder of middle ear and mastoid

    H74.90 Unspecified disorder of middle ear and mastoid, unspecified ear

    H74.91 Unspecified disorder of right middle ear and mastoid

    H74.92 Unspecified disorder of left middle ear and mastoid

    H74.93 Unspecified disorder of middle ear and mastoid, bilateral

H75 OTHER DISORDERS OF MIDDLE EAR AND MASTOID IN DISEASES CLASSIFIED ELSEWHERE

Code first underlying disease

H75.0 **Mastoiditis in infectious and parasitic diseases classified elsewhere**

Excludes1: mastoiditis (in):

syphilis (A52.77)

tuberculosis (A18.03)

    H75.00 **Mastoiditis in infectious and parasitic diseases classified elsewhere, unspecified ear**

    H75.01 **Mastoiditis in infectious and parasitic diseases classified elsewhere, right ear**

    H75.02 **Mastoiditis in infectious and parasitic diseases classified elsewhere, left ear**

    H75.03 **Mastoiditis in infectious and parasitic diseases classified elsewhere, bilateral**

H75.8 **Other specified disorders of middle ear and mastoid in diseases classified elsewhere**

    H75.80 **Other specified disorders of middle ear and mastoid in diseases classified elsewhere, unspecified ear**

    H75.81 **Other specified disorders of right middle ear and mastoid in diseases classified elsewhere**

    H75.82 **Other specified disorders of left middle ear and mastoid in diseases classified elsewhere**

    H75.83 **Other specified disorders of middle ear and mastoid in diseases classified elsewhere, bilateral**

DISEASES OF INNER EAR (H80-H83)

H80 **Otosclerosis**

Includes: Otospongiosis

H80.0 **Otosclerosis involving oval window, nonobliterative**

    H80.00 **Otosclerosis involving oval window, nonobliterative, unspecified ear**

    H80.01 **Otosclerosis involving oval window, nonobliterative, right ear**

    H80.02 **Otosclerosis involving oval window, nonobliterative, left ear**

    H80.03 **Otosclerosis involving oval window, nonobliterative, bilateral**

H80.1 **Otosclerosis involving oval window, obliterative**

    H80.10 **Otosclerosis involving oval window, obliterative, unspecified ear**

    H80.11 **Otosclerosis involving oval window, obliterative, right ear**

    H80.12 **Otosclerosis involving oval window, obliterative, left ear**

    H80.13 **Otosclerosis involving oval window, obliterative, bilateral**

H80.2 **Cochlear otosclerosis**

Otosclerosis involving otic capsule

Otosclerosis involving round window

    H80.20 **Cochlear otosclerosis, unspecified ear**

    H80.21 **Cochlear otosclerosis, right ear**

    H80.22 **Cochlear otosclerosis, left ear**

    H80.23 **Cochlear otosclerosis, bilateral**

H80.8 **Other otosclerosis**

    H80.80 **Other otosclerosis, unspecified ear**

    H80.81 **Other otosclerosis, right ear**

    H80.82 **Other otosclerosis, left ear**

    H80.83 **Other otosclerosis, bilateral**

H80.9 **Unspecified otosclerosis**

    H80.90 **Unspecified otosclerosis, unspecified ear**

    H80.91 **Unspecified otosclerosis, right ear**

    H80.92 **Unspecified otosclerosis, left ear**

    H80.93 **Unspecified otosclerosis, bilateral**

H81 **Disorders of vestibular function**

Excludes1: epidemic vertigo (A88.1)

vertigo NOS (R42)

H81.0 **Ménière's disease**

Labyrinthine hydrops

Ménière's syndrome or vertigo

    H81.01 **Ménière's disease, right ear**

    H81.02 **Ménière's disease, left ear**

    H81.03 **Ménière's disease, bilateral**

    H81.09 **Ménière's disease, unspecified ear**

H81.1 **Benign paroxysmal vertigo**

    H81.10 **Benign paroxysmal vertigo, unspecified ear**

    H81.11 **Benign paroxysmal vertigo, right ear**

    H81.12 **Benign paroxysmal vertigo, left ear**

    H81.13 **Benign paroxysmal vertigo, bilateral**

H81.2 **Vestibular neuronitis**

    H81.20 **Vestibular neuronitis, unspecified ear**

    H81.21 **Vestibular neuronitis, right ear**

    H81.22 **Vestibular neuronitis, left ear**

    H81.23 **Vestibular neuronitis, bilateral**

H81.3 **Other peripheral vertigo**

    H81.31 **Aural vertigo**

        H81.311 **Aural vertigo, right ear**

        H81.312 **Aural vertigo, left ear**

        H81.313 **Aural vertigo, bilateral**

        H81.319 **Aural vertigo, unspecified ear**

    H81.39 **Other peripheral vertigo**

Lermoyez' syndrome

Otogenic vertigo

Peripheral vertigo NOS

        H81.391 **Other peripheral vertigo, right ear**

        H81.392 **Other peripheral vertigo, left ear**

        H81.393 **Other peripheral vertigo, bilateral**

        H81.399 **Other peripheral vertigo, unspecified ear**

H81.4 **Vertigo of central origin**

Central positional nystagmus

    H81.41 **Vertigo of central origin, right ear**

    H81.42 **Vertigo of central origin, left ear**

    H81.43 **Vertigo of central origin, bilateral**

    H81.49 **Vertigo of central origin, unspecified ear**

H81.8 **Other disorders of vestibular function**

    H81.8X **Other disorders of vestibular function**

        H81.8X1 **Other disorders of vestibular function, right ear**

        H81.8X2 **Other disorders of vestibular function, left ear**

        H81.8X3 **Other disorders of vestibular function, bilateral**

H81.8X9 Other disorders of vestibular function, unspecified ear

H81.9 Unspecified disorder of vestibular function

Vertiginous syndrome NOS

H81.90 Unspecified disorder of vestibular function, unspecified ear

H81.91 Unspecified disorder of vestibular function, right ear

H81.92 Unspecified disorder of vestibular function, left ear

H81.93 Unspecified disorder of vestibular function, bilateral

H82 **Vertiginous syndromes in diseases classified elsewhere**

Code first underlying disease

Excludes1: epidemic vertigo (A88.1)

H82.1 Vertiginous syndromes in diseases classified elsewhere, right ear

H82.2 Vertiginous syndromes in diseases classified elsewhere, left ear

H82.3 Vertiginous syndromes in diseases classified elsewhere, bilateral

H82.9 Vertiginous syndromes in diseases classified elsewhere, unspecified ear

H83 **Other diseases of inner ear**

H83.0 Labyrinthitis

H83.01 Labyrinthitis, right ear

H83.02 Labyrinthitis, left ear

H83.03 Labyrinthitis, bilateral

H83.09 Labyrinthitis, unspecified ear

H83.1 Labyrinthine fistula

H83.11 Labyrinthine fistula, right ear

H83.12 Labyrinthine fistula, left ear

H83.13 Labyrinthine fistula, bilateral

H83.19 Labyrinthine fistula, unspecified ear

H83.2 Labyrinthine dysfunction

Labyrinthine hypersensitivity

Labyrinthine hypofunction

Labyrinthine loss of function

H83.2X Labyrinthine dysfunction

H83.2X1 Labyrinthine dysfunction, right ear

H83.2X2 Labyrinthine dysfunction, left ear

H83.2X3 Labyrinthine dysfunction, bilateral

H83.2X9 Labyrinthine dysfunction, unspecified ear

H83.3 Noise effects on inner ear

Acoustic trauma of inner ear

Noise-induced hearing loss of inner ear

H83.3X Noise effects on inner ear

H83.3X1 Noise effects on right inner ear

H83.3X2 Noise effects on left inner ear

H83.3X3 Noise effects on inner ear, bilateral

H83.3X9 Noise effects on inner ear, unspecified ear

H83.8 Other specified diseases of inner ear

H83.8X Other specified diseases of inner ear

H83.8X1 Other specified diseases of right inner ear

H83.8X2 Other specified diseases of left inner ear

H83.8X3 Other specified diseases of inner ear, bilateral

H83.8X9 Other specified diseases of inner ear, unspecified ear

H83.9 Unspecified disease of inner ear

H83.90 Unspecified disease of inner ear, unspecified ear

H83.91 Unspecified disease of right inner ear

H83.92 Unspecified disease of left inner ear

H83.93 Unspecified disease of inner ear, bilateral

OTHER DISORDERS OF EAR (H90-H94)

H90 **Conductive and sensorineural hearing loss**

Excludes1: deaf nonspeaking NEC (H91.3)

deafness NOS (H91.9-)

hearing loss NOS (H91.9-)

noise-induced hearing loss (H83.3-)

ototoxic hearing loss (H91.0-)

sudden (idiopathic) hearing loss (H91.2-)

H90.0 Conductive hearing loss, bilateral

H90.1 Conductive hearing loss, unilateral with unrestricted hearing on the contralateral side

H90.11 Conductive hearing loss, unilateral, right ear, with unrestricted hearing on the contralateral side

H90.12 Conductive hearing loss, unilateral, left ear, with unrestricted hearing on the contralateral side

H90.2 Conductive hearing loss, unspecified

Conductive deafness NOS

H90.3 Sensorineural hearing loss, bilateral

H90.4 Sensorineural hearing loss, unilateral with unrestricted hearing on the contralateral side

H90.41 Sensorineural hearing loss, unilateral, right ear, with unrestricted hearing on the contralateral side

H90.42 Sensorineural hearing loss, unilateral, left ear, with unrestricted hearing on the contralateral side

H90.5 Unspecified sensorineural hearing loss

Central hearing loss NOS

Congenital deafness NOS

Neural hearing loss NOS

Perceptive hearing loss NOS

Sensorineural deafness NOS

Sensory hearing loss NOS

Excludes1: abnormal auditory perception (H93.2-)

psychogenic deafness (F44.6)

H90.6 Mixed conductive and sensorineural hearing loss, bilateral

H90.7 Mixed conductive and sensorineural hearing loss, unilateral with unrestricted hearing on the contralateral side

H90.71 Mixed conductive and sensorineural hearing loss, unilateral, right ear, with unrestricted hearing on the contralateral side

Add 4th-7th digits   Nonspecific code   Unspecified code   Manifestation code

H90.72 Mixed conductive and sensorineural hearing loss, unilateral, left ear, with unrestricted hearing on the contralateral side

H90.8 Mixed conductive and sensorineural hearing loss, unspecified

H90.A Conductive and sensorineural hearing loss with restricted hearing on the contralateral side

   H90.A1 Conductive hearing loss, unilateral, with restricted hearing on the contralateral side

      ●**H90.A11** Conductive hearing loss, unilateral, right ear with restricted hearing on the contralateral side

      ●**H90.A12** Conductive hearing loss, unilateral, left ear with restricted hearing on the contralateral side

   H90.A2 Sensorineural hearing loss, unilateral, with restricted hearing on the contralateral side

      ●**H90.A21** Sensorineural hearing loss, unilateral, right ear, with restricted hearing on the contralateral side

      ●**H90.A22** Sensorineural hearing loss, unilateral, left ear, with restricted hearing on the contralateral side

   H90.A3 Mixed conductive and sensorineural hearing loss, unilateral with restricted hearing on the contralateral side

      ●**H90.A31** Mixed conductive and sensorineural hearing loss, unilateral, right ear with restricted hearing on the contralateral side

      ●**H90.A32** Mixed conductive and sensorineural hearing loss, unilateral, left ear with restricted hearing on the contralateral side

H91 **Other and unspecified hearing loss**

Excludes1: abnormal auditory perception (H93.2-)

   hearing loss as classified in H90.-

   impacted cerumen (H61.2-)

   noise-induced hearing loss (H83.3-)

   psychogenic deafness (F44.6)

   transient ischemic deafness (H93.01-)

H91.0 **Ototoxic hearing loss**

Code first poisoning due to drug or toxin, if applicable (T36-T65 with fifth or sixth character 1-4 or 6)

Use additional code for adverse effect, if applicable, to identify drug (T36-T50 with fifth or sixth character 5)

   H91.01 Ototoxic hearing loss, right ear

   H91.02 Ototoxic hearing loss, left ear

   H91.03 Ototoxic hearing loss, bilateral

   H91.09 Ototoxic hearing loss, unspecified ear

H91.1 **Presbycusis**

Presbyacusia

   H91.10 Presbycusis, unspecified ear

   H91.11 Presbycusis, right ear

   H91.12 Presbycusis, left ear

   H91.13 Presbycusis, bilateral

H91.2 **Sudden idiopathic hearing loss**

Sudden hearing loss NOS

   H91.20 Sudden idiopathic hearing loss, unspecified ear

   H91.21 Sudden idiopathic hearing loss, right ear

   H91.22 Sudden idiopathic hearing loss, left ear

   H91.23 Sudden idiopathic hearing loss, bilateral

H91.3 Deaf nonspeaking, not elsewhere classified

H91.8 Other specified hearing loss

   H91.8X Other specified hearing loss

      H91.8X1 Other specified hearing loss, right ear

      H91.8X2 Other specified hearing loss, left ear

      H91.8X3 Other specified hearing loss, bilateral

      H91.8X9 Other specified hearing loss, unspecified ear

H91.9 **Unspecified hearing loss**

Deafness NOS

High frequency deafness

Low frequency deafness

   H91.90 Unspecified hearing loss, unspecified ear

   H91.91 Unspecified hearing loss, right ear

   H91.92 Unspecified hearing loss, left ear

   H91.93 Unspecified hearing loss, bilateral

H92 **Otalgia and effusion of ear**

H92.0 **Otalgia**

   H92.01 Otalgia, right ear

   H92.02 Otalgia, left ear

   H92.03 Otalgia, bilateral

   H92.09 Otalgia, unspecified ear

H92.1 **Otorrhea**

Excludes1: leakage of cerebrospinal fluid through ear (G96.0)

   H92.10 Otorrhea, unspecified ear

   H92.11 Otorrhea, right ear

   H92.12 Otorrhea, left ear

   H92.13 Otorrhea, bilateral

H92.2 **Otorrhagia**

Excludes1: traumatic otorrhagia - code to injury

   H92.20 Otorrhagia, unspecified ear

   H92.21 Otorrhagia, right ear

   H92.22 Otorrhagia, left ear

   H92.23 Otorrhagia, bilateral

H93 **Other disorders of ear, not elsewhere classified**

H93.0 **Degenerative and vascular disorders of ear**

Excludes1: presbycusis (H91.1)

   H93.01 Transient ischemic deafness

      H93.011 Transient ischemic deafness, right ear

      H93.012 Transient ischemic deafness, left ear

      H93.013 Transient ischemic deafness, bilateral

      H93.019 Transient ischemic deafness, unspecified ear

   H93.09 Unspecified degenerative and vascular disorders of ear

      H93.091 Unspecified degenerative and vascular disorders of right ear

● New code ▲ Revised code **Excludes1:** Not coded here **Excludes2:** Not included here ⊗ Placeholder required ⑦7th digit required

H93.092 Unspecified degenerative and vascular disorders of left ear

H93.093 Unspecified degenerative and vascular disorders of ear, bilateral

H93.099 Unspecified degenerative and vascular disorders of unspecified ear

H93.1 Tinnitus

H93.11 Tinnitus, right ear

H93.12 Tinnitus, left ear

H93.13 Tinnitus, bilateral

H93.19 Tinnitus, unspecified ear

H93.A Pulsatile tinnitus

●H93.A1 Pulsatile tinnitus, right ear

●H93.A2 Pulsatile tinnitus, left ear

●H93.A3 Pulsatile tinnitus, bilateral

●H93.A9 Pulsatile tinnitus, unspecified ear

H93.2 Other abnormal auditory perceptions

Excludes2: auditory hallucinations (R44.0)

H93.21 Auditory recruitment

H93.211 Auditory recruitment, right ear

H93.212 Auditory recruitment, left ear

H93.213 Auditory recruitment, bilateral

H93.219 Auditory recruitment, unspecified ear

H93.22 Diplacusis

H93.221 Diplacusis, right ear

H93.222 Diplacusis, left ear

H93.223 Diplacusis, bilateral

H93.229 Diplacusis, unspecified ear

H93.23 Hyperacusis

H93.231 Hyperacusis, right ear

H93.232 Hyperacusis, left ear

H93.233 Hyperacusis, bilateral

H93.239 Hyperacusis, unspecified ear

H93.24 Temporary auditory threshold shift

H93.241 Temporary auditory threshold shift, right ear

H93.242 Temporary auditory threshold shift, left ear

H93.243 Temporary auditory threshold shift, bilateral

H93.249 Temporary auditory threshold shift, unspecified ear

H93.25 Central auditory processing disorder

Congenital auditory imperception Word deafness

Excludes1: mixed receptive-expressive language disorder (F80.2)

H93.29 Other abnormal auditory perceptions

H93.291 Other abnormal auditory perceptions, right ear

H93.292 Other abnormal auditory perceptions, left ear

H93.293 Other abnormal auditory perceptions, bilateral

H93.299 Other abnormal auditory perceptions, unspecified ear

H93.3 Disorders of acoustic nerve

Disorder of 8th cranial nerve

Excludes1: acoustic neuroma (D33.3)

syphilitic acoustic neuritis (A52.15)

H93.3X Disorders of acoustic nerve

H93.3X1 Disorders of right acoustic nerve

H93.3X2 Disorders of left acoustic nerve

H93.3X3 Disorders of bilateral acoustic nerves

H93.3X9 Disorders of unspecified acoustic nerve

H93.8 Other specified disorders of ear

H93.8X Other specified disorders of ear

H93.8X1 Other specified disorders of right ear

H93.8X2 Other specified disorders of left ear

H93.8X3 Other specified disorders of ear, bilateral

H93.8X9 Other specified disorders of ear, unspecified ear

H93.9 Unspecified disorder of ear

H93.90 Unspecified disorder of ear, unspecified ear

H93.91 Unspecified disorder of right ear

H93.92 Unspecified disorder of left ear

H93.93 Unspecified disorder of ear, bilateral

H94 Other disorders of ear in diseases classified elsewhere

H94.0 Acoustic neuritis in infectious and parasitic diseases classified elsewhere

Code first underlying disease, such as:

parasitic disease (B65-B89)

Excludes1: acoustic neuritis (in):

herpes zoster (B02.29)

syphilis (A52.15)

H94.00 Acoustic neuritis in infectious and parasitic diseases classified elsewhere, unspecified ear

H94.01 Acoustic neuritis in infectious and parasitic diseases classified elsewhere, right ear

H94.02 Acoustic neuritis in infectious and parasitic diseases classified elsewhere, left ear

H94.03 Acoustic neuritis in infectious and parasitic diseases classified elsewhere, bilateral

H94.8 Other specified disorders of ear in diseases classified elsewhere

Code first underlying disease, such as:

congenital syphilis (A50.0)

Excludes1: aural myiasis (B87.4)

syphilitic labyrinthitis (A52.79)

H94.80 Other specified disorders of ear in diseases classified elsewhere, unspecified ear

H94.81 Other specified disorders of right ear in diseases classified elsewhere

H94.82 Other specified disorders of left ear in diseases classified elsewhere

H94.83 Other specified disorders of ear in diseases classified elsewhere, bilateral

INTRAOPERATIVE AND POSTPROCEDURAL COMPLICATIONS AND DISORDERS OF EAR AND MASTOID PROCESS, NOT ELSEWHERE CLASSIFIED (H95)

H95 Intraoperative and postprocedural complications and disorders of ear and mastoid process, not elsewhere classified

H95.0 Recurrent cholesteatoma of postmastoidectomy cavity

H95.00 Recurrent cholesteatoma of postmastoidectomy cavity, unspecified ear

H95.01 Recurrent cholesteatoma of postmastoidectomy cavity, right ear

H95.02 Recurrent cholesteatoma of postmastoidectomy cavity, left ear

H95.03 Recurrent cholesteatoma of postmastoidectomy cavity, bilateral ears

H95.1 Other disorders of ear and mastoid process following mastoidectomy

H95.11 Chronic inflammation of postmastoidectomy cavity

H95.111 Chronic inflammation of postmastoidectomy cavity, right ear

H95.112 Chronic inflammation of postmastoidectomy cavity, left ear

H95.113 Chronic inflammation of postmastoidectomy cavity, bilateral ears

H95.119 Chronic inflammation of postmastoidectomy cavity, unspecified ear

H95.12 Granulation of postmastoidectomy cavity

H95.121 Granulation of postmastoidectomy cavity, right ear

H95.122 Granulation of postmastoidectomy cavity, left ear

H95.123 Granulation of postmastoidectomy cavity, bilateral ears

H95.129 Granulation of postmastoidectomy cavity, unspecified ear

H95.13 Mucosal cyst of postmastoidectomy cavity

H95.131 Mucosal cyst of postmastoidectomy cavity, right ear

H95.132 Mucosal cyst of postmastoidectomy cavity, left ear

H95.133 Mucosal cyst of postmastoidectomy cavity, bilateral ears

H95.139 Mucosal cyst of postmastoidectomy cavity, unspecified ear

H95.19 Other disorders following mastoidectomy

H95.191 Other disorders following mastoidectomy, right ear

H95.192 Other disorders following mastoidectomy, left ear

H95.193 Other disorders following mastoidectomy, bilateral ears

H95.199 Other disorders following mastoidectomy, unspecified ear

H95.2 Intraoperative hemorrhage and hematoma of ear and mastoid process complicating a procedure

Excludes1: intraoperative hemorrhage and hematoma of ear and mastoid process due to accidental puncture or laceration during a procedure (H95.3-)

H95.21 Intraoperative hemorrhage and hematoma of ear and mastoid process complicating a procedure on the ear and mastoid process

H95.22 Intraoperative hemorrhage and hematoma of ear and mastoid process complicating other procedure

H95.3 Accidental puncture and laceration of ear and mastoid process during a procedure

H95.31 Accidental puncture and laceration of the ear and mastoid process during a procedure on the ear and mastoid process

H95.32 Accidental puncture and laceration of the ear and mastoid process during other procedure

H95.4 Postprocedural hemorrhage of ear and mastoid process following a procedure

▲H95.41 Postprocedural hemorrhage of ear and mastoid process following a procedure on the ear and mastoid process

▲H95.42 Postprocedural hemorrhage of ear and mastoid process following other procedure

H95.5 Postprocedural hematoma and seroma of ear and mastoid process following a procedure

●H95.51 Postprocedural hematoma of ear and mastoid process following a procedure on the ear and mastoid process

●H95.52 Postprocedural hematoma of ear and mastoid process following other procedure

●H95.53 Postprocedural seroma of ear and mastoid process following a procedure on the ear and mastoid process

●H95.54 Postprocedural seroma of ear and mastoid process following other procedure

H95.8 Other intraoperative and postprocedural complications and disorders of the ear and mastoid process, not elsewhere classified

Excludes2: postprocedural complications and disorders following mastoidectomy (H95.0-, H95.1-)

H95.81 Postprocedural stenosis of external ear canal

H95.811 Postprocedural stenosis of right external ear canal

H95.812 Postprocedural stenosis of left external ear canal

H95.813 Postprocedural stenosis of external ear canal, bilateral

H95.819 Postprocedural stenosis of unspecified external ear canal

H95.88 Other intraoperative complications and disorders of the ear and mastoid process, not elsewhere classified

Use additional code, if applicable, to further specify disorder

H95.89 Other postprocedural complications and disorders of the ear and mastoid process, not elsewhere classified

Use additional code, if applicable, to further specify disorder

Chapter 9: Diseases Of The Circulatory System (I00-I99)

DEFINITIONS

This chapter includes definitions of selected key words, terms and phrases and coding alerts for adding points to the clinical domain, and references to coding late effects where appropriate. An example from this chapter is as follows:

I12   Hypertensive chronic kidney disease
　　　　Definition: Hypertensive chronic kidney disease, refers to diseases of the kidney caused by high blood pressure.

MULTIPLE CODING FOR A SINGLE CONDITION

In addition to the etiology/manifestation convention that requires two codes to fully describe a single condition that affects multiple body systems, there are other single conditions that also require more than one code. "Use additional code" notes are found in the Tabular List at codes that are not part of an etiology/manifestation pair where a secondary code is useful to fully describe a condition. The sequencing rule is the same as the etiology/manifestation pair, "use additional code" indicates that a secondary code should be added.

For example, for bacterial infections that are not included in chapter 1, a secondary code from category B95, Streptococcus, Staphylococcus, and Enterococcus, as the cause of diseases classified elsewhere, or B96, Other bacterial agents as the cause of diseases classified elsewhere, may be required to identify the bacterial organism causing the infection. A "use additional code" note will normally be found at the infectious disease code, indicating a need for the organism code to be added as a secondary code.

 "Code first" notes are also under certain codes that are not specifically manifestation codes but may be due to an underlying cause. When there is a "code first" note and an underlying condition is present, the underlying condition should be sequenced first.

"Code, if applicable, any causal condition first", notes indicate that this code may be assigned as a principal diagnosis when the causal condition is unknown or not applicable. If a causal condition is known, then the code for that condition should be sequenced as the principal or first-listed diagnosis.

Multiple codes may be needed for sequela, complication codes and obstetric codes to more fully describe a condition. See the specific guidelines for these conditions for further instruction.

COMBINATION CODE

A combination code is a single code used to classify: Two diagnoses, or a diagnosis with an associated secondary process (manifestation) A diagnosis with an associated complication

Combination codes are identified by referring to subterm entries in the Alphabetic Index and by reading the inclusion and exclusion notes in the Tabular List.

Assign only the combination code when that code fully identifies the diagnostic conditions involved or when the Alphabetic Index so directs. Multiple coding should not be used when the classification provides a combination code that clearly identifies all of the elements documented in the diagnosis. When the combination code lacks necessary specificity in describing the manifestation or complication, an additional code should be used as a secondary code.

SEQUELA (LATE EFFECTS)

A sequela is the residual effect (condition produced) after the acute phase of an illness or injury has terminated. There is no time limit on when a sequela code can be used. The residual may be apparent early, such as in cerebral infarction, or it may occur months or years later, such as that due to a previous injury. Coding of sequela generally requires two codes sequenced in the following order: The condition or nature of the sequela is sequenced first.

The sequela code is sequenced second.

An exception to the above guidelines are those instances where the code for the sequela is followed by a manifestation code identified in the Tabular List and title, or the sequela code has been expanded (at the fourth, fifth or sixth character levels) to include the manifestation(s). The code for the acute phase of an illness or injury that led to the sequela is never used with a code for the late effect.

HYPERTENSION

The classification presumes a causal relationship between hypertension and heart involvement and between hypertension and kidney involvement, as the two conditions are linked by the term "with" in the Alphabetic Index. These conditions should be coded as related even in the absence of provider documentation explicitly linking them, unless the documentation clearly states the conditions are unrelated.

For hypertension and conditions not specifically linked by relational terms such as "with," "associated with" or "due to" in the classification, provider documentation must link the conditions in order to code them as related.

1)   **Hypertension with Heart Disease**

Hypertension with heart conditions classified to I50.- or I51.4-I51.9, are assigned to a code from category I11, Hypertensive heart disease. Use an additional code from category I50, Heart failure, to identify the type of heart failure in those patients with heart failure.

The same heart conditions (I50.-, I51.4-I51.9) with hypertension are coded separately if the provider has specifically documented a different cause. Sequence according to the circumstances of the admission/encounter.

2) **Hypertensive Chronic Kidney Disease**

Assign codes from category I12, Hypertensive chronic kidney disease, when both hypertension and a condition classifiable to category N18, Chronic kidney disease (CKD), are present. CKD should not be coded as hypertensive if the physician has specifically documented a different cause.

The appropriate code from category N18 should be used as a secondary code with a code from category I12 to identify the stage of chronic kidney disease.

See Section I.C.14. Chronic kidney disease.

If a patient has hypertensive chronic kidney disease and acute renal failure, an additional code for the acute renal failure is required.

3) **Hypertensive Heart and Chronic Kidney Disease**

Assign codes from combination category I13, Hypertensive heart and chronic kidney disease, when there is hypertension with both heart and kidney involvement. If heart failure is present, assign an additional code from category I50 to identify the type of heart failure.

The appropriate code from category N18, Chronic kidney disease, should be used as a secondary code with a code from category I13 to identify the stage of chronic kidney disease.

See Section I.C.14. Chronic kidney disease.

The codes in category I13, Hypertensive heart and chronic kidney disease, are combination codes that include hypertension, heart disease and chronic kidney disease. The Includes note at I13 specifies that the conditions included at I11 and I12 are included together in I13. If a patient has hypertension, heart disease and chronic kidney disease, then a code from I13 should be used, not individual codes for hypertension, heart disease and chronic kidney disease, or codes from I11 or I12.

For patients with both acute renal failure and chronic kidney disease, an additional code for acute renal failure is required.

4) **Hypertensive Cerebrovascular Disease**

For hypertensive cerebrovascular disease, first assign the appropriate code from categories I60-I69, followed by the appropriate hypertension code.

5) **Hypertensive Retinopathy**

Subcategory H35.0, Background retinopathy and retinal vascular changes, should be used with a code from category I10 – I15, Hypertensive disease to include the systemic hypertension. The sequencing is based on the reason for the encounter.

6) **Hypertension, Secondary**

Secondary hypertension is due to an underlying condition. Two codes are required: one to identify the underlying etiology and one from category I15 to identify the hypertension. Sequencing of codes is determined by the reason for admission/encounter.

7) **Hypertension, Transient**

Assign code R03.0, Elevated blood pressure reading without diagnosis of hypertension, unless patient has an established diagnosis of hypertension. Assign code O13.-, Gestational [pregnancy-induced] hypertension without significant proteinuria, or O14.-, Pre-eclampsia, for transient hypertension of pregnancy.

8) **Hypertension, Controlled**

This diagnostic statement usually refers to an existing state of hypertension under control by therapy. Assign the appropriate code from categories I10-I15, Hypertensive diseases.

9) **Hypertension, Uncontrolled**

Uncontrolled hypertension may refer to untreated hypertension or hypertension not responding to current therapeutic regimen. In either case, assign the appropriate code from categories I10-I15, Hypertensive diseases.

10) **Hypertensive Crisis**

Assign a code from category I16, Hypertensive crisis, for documented hypertensive urgency, hypertensive emergency or unspecified hypertensive crisis. Code also any identified hypertensive disease (I10-I15). The sequencing is based on the reason for the encounter.

ATHEROSCLEROTIC CORONARY ARTERY DISEASE AND ANGINA

ICD-10-CM has combination codes for atherosclerotic heart disease with angina pectoris. The subcategories for these codes are I25.11, Atherosclerotic heart disease of native coronary artery with angina pectoris and I25.7, Atherosclerosis of coronary artery bypass graft(s) and coronary artery of transplanted heart with angina pectoris.

When using one of these combination codes it is not necessary to use an additional code for angina pectoris. A causal relationship can be assumed in a patient with both atherosclerosis and angina pectoris, unless the documentation indicates the angina is due to something other than the atherosclerosis.

If a patient with coronary artery disease is admitted due to an acute myocardial infarction (AMI), the AMI should be sequenced before the coronary artery disease.

See Section I.C.9. Acute myocardial infarction (AMI)

INTRAOPERATIVE AND POSTPROCEDURAL CEREBROVASCULAR ACCIDENT

Medical record documentation should clearly specify the cause- and-effect relationship between the medical intervention and the cerebrovascular accident in order to assign a code for intraoperative or postprocedural cerebrovascular accident.

Proper code assignment depends on whether it was an infarction or hemorrhage and whether it occurred intraoperatively or postoperatively. If it was a cerebral hemorrhage, code assignment depends on the type of procedure performed.

SEQUELAE OF CEREBROVASCULAR DISEASE

1) **Category I69, Sequelae of Cerebrovascular disease**

Category I69 is used to indicate conditions classifiable to categories I60-I67 as the causes of sequela (neurologic deficits), themselves classified elsewhere. These "late effects" include neurologic deficits that persist after initial onset of conditions classifiable to categories I60-I67. The neurologic deficits caused by cerebrovascular disease may be present from the onset or may arise at any time after the onset of the condition classifiable to categories I60-I67.

Codes from category I69, Sequelae of cerebrovascular disease, that specify hemiplegia, hemiparesis and monoplegia identify whether the dominant or nondominant side is affected. Should the affected side be documented, but not specified as dominant or nondominant, and the classification system does not indicate a default, code selection is as follows:

- For ambidextrous patients, the default should be dominant.

- If the left side is affected, the default is non-dominant.

- If the right side is affected, the default is dominant.

2) **Codes from category I69 with codes from I60-I67**

Codes from category I69 may be assigned on a health care record with codes from I60-I67, if the patient has a current cerebrovascular disease and deficits from an old cerebrovascular disease.

3) **Codes from category I69 and Personal history of transient ischemic attack (TIA) and cerebral infarction (Z86.73)**

Codes from category I69 should not be assigned if the patient does not have neurologic deficits.

See Section I.C.21. 4. History (of) for use of personal history codes

ACUTE MYOCARDIAL INFARCTION (AMI)

1) **ST elevation myocardial infarction (STEMI) and non ST elevation myocardial infarction (NSTEMI)**

The ICD-10-CM codes for acute myocardial infarction (AMI) identify the site, such as anterolateral wall or true posterior wall. Subcategories I21.0-I21.2 and code I21.3 are used for ST elevation myocardial infarction (STEMI). Code I21.4, Non-ST elevation (NSTEMI) myocardial infarction, is used for non ST elevation myocardial infarction (NSTEMI) and nontransmural MIs.

If NSTEMI evolves to STEMI, assign the STEMI code. If STEMI converts to NSTEMI due to thrombolytic therapy, it is still coded as STEMI.

For encounters occurring while the myocardial infarction is equal to, or less than, four weeks old, including transfers to another acute setting or a postacute setting, and the myocardial infarction **meets** the definition for "other diagnoses" (see Section III, Reporting Additional Diagnoses), codes from category I21 may continue to be reported. For encounters after the 4 week time frame and the patient is still receiving care related to the myocardial infarction, the appropriate aftercare code should be assigned, rather than a code from category I21. For old or healed myocardial infarctions not requiring further care, code I25.2, Old myocardial infarction, may be assigned.

2) **Acute myocardial infarction, unspecified**

Code I21.3, ST elevation (STEMI) myocardial infarction of unspecified site, is the default for unspecified acute myocardial infarction. If only STEMI or transmural MI without the site is documented, assign code I21.3.

3) AMI documented as nontransmural or subendocardial but site provided

If an AMI is documented as nontransmural or subendocardial, but the site is provided, it is still coded as a subendocardial AMI.

See Section I.C.21.3 for information on coding status post administration of tPA in a different facility within the last 24 hours.

4) Subsequent acute myocardial infarction

A code from category I22, Subsequent ST elevation (STEMI) and non ST elevation (NSTEMI) myocardial infarction, is to be used when a patient who has suffered an AMI has a new AMI within the 4 week time frame of the initial AMI. A code from category I22 must be used in conjunction with a code from category I21. The sequencing of the I22 and I21 codes depends on the circumstances of the encounter.

● New code ▲ Revised code **Excludes1:** Not coded here **Excludes2:** Not included here ⊗ Placeholder required ⑦ 7ᵗʰ digit required

Chapter 9

Diseases Of The Circulatory System (I00-I99)

Excludes2: certain conditions originating in the perinatal period (P04-P96)

certain infectious and parasitic diseases (A00-B99)

complications of pregnancy, childbirth and the puerperium (O00-O9A)

congenital malformations, deformations, and chromosomal abnormalities (Q00-Q99)

endocrine, nutritional and metabolic diseases (E00-E88)

injury, poisoning and certain other consequences of external causes (S00-T88)

neoplasms (C00-D49)

symptoms, signs and abnormal clinical and laboratory findings, not elsewhere classified (R00-R94)

systemic connective tissue disorders (M30-M36)

transient cerebral ischemic attacks and related syndromes (G45.-)

This chapter contains the following blocks:

I00-I02	Acute rheumatic fever
I05-I09	Chronic rheumatic heart diseases
I10-I16	Hypertensive diseases
I20-I25	Ischemic heart diseases
I26-I28	Pulmonary heart disease and diseases of pulmonary circulation
I30-I52	Other forms of heart disease
I60-I69	Cerebrovascular diseases
I70-I79	Diseases of arteries, arterioles and capillaries
I80-I89	Diseases of veins, lymphatic vessels and lymph nodes, not elsewhere classified
I95-I99	Other and unspecified disorders of the circulatory system

ACUTE RHEUMATIC FEVER (I00-I02)

I00 **Rheumatic fever without heart involvement**

Includes: arthritis, rheumatic, acute or subacute

Excludes1: rheumatic fever with heart involvement (I01.0 -I01.9)

I01 **Rheumatic fever with heart involvement**

Excludes1: chronic diseases of rheumatic origin (I05-I09) unless rheumatic fever is also present or there is evidence of reactivation or activity of the rheumatic process.

I01.0 **Acute rheumatic pericarditis**

Any condition in I00 with pericarditis

Rheumatic pericarditis (acute)

Excludes1: acute pericarditis not specified as rheumatic (I30.-)

I01.1 **Acute rheumatic endocarditis**

Any condition in I00 with endocarditis or valvulitis

Acute rheumatic valvulitis

I01.2 **Acute rheumatic myocarditis**

Any condition in I00 with myocarditis

I01.8 **Other acute rheumatic heart disease**

Any condition in I00 **with other** or multiple types of heart involvement

Acute rheumatic pancarditis

I01.9 **Acute rheumatic heart disease, unspecified**

Any condition in I00 with unspecified type of heart involvement

Rheumatic carditis, acute

Rheumatic heart disease, active or acute

I02 **Rheumatic chorea**

Includes: Sydenham's chorea

Excludes1: chorea NOS (G25.5)

Huntington's chorea (G10)

I02.0 **Rheumatic chorea with heart involvement**

Chorea NOS with heart involvement

Rheumatic chorea with heart involvement of any type classifiable under I01.-

I02.9 **Rheumatic chorea without heart involvement**

Rheumatic chorea NOS

CHRONIC RHEUMATIC HEART DISEASES (I05-I09)

Definition: Rheumatic heart disease refers to a thickening and stenosis of one or more of the heart valves and often requires surgery to repair or replace the involved valve(s).

I05 **Rheumatic mitral valve diseases**

Includes: conditions classifiable to both I05.0 and I05.2-I05.9, whether specified as rheumatic or not

Excludes1: mitral valve disease specified as nonrheumatic (I34.-)

mitral valve disease with aortic and/or tricuspid valve involvement (I08.-)

I05.0 **Rheumatic mitral stenosis**

Mitral (valve) obstruction (rheumatic)

I05.1 **Rheumatic mitral insufficiency**

Rheumatic mitral incompetence

Rheumatic mitral regurgitation

Excludes1: mitral insufficiency not specified as rheumatic (I34.0)

I05.2 **Rheumatic mitral stenosis with insufficiency**

Rheumatic mitral stenosis with incompetence or regurgitation

I05.8 **Other rheumatic mitral valve diseases**

Rheumatic mitral (valve) failure

I05.9 **Rheumatic mitral valve disease, unspecified**

Rheumatic mitral (valve) disorder (chronic) NOS

I06 **Rheumatic aortic valve diseases**

Excludes1: aortic valve disease not specified as rheumatic (I35.-)

aortic valve disease with mitral and/or tricuspid valve involvement (I08.-)

I06.0 **Rheumatic aortic stenosis**

Rheumatic aortic (valve) obstruction

I06.1 **Rheumatic aortic insufficiency**

Rheumatic aortic incompetence

Rheumatic aortic regurgitation

I06.2 **Rheumatic aortic stenosis with insufficiency**

Rheumatic aortic stenosis with incompetence or regurgitation

I06.8 **Other rheumatic aortic valve diseases**

I06.9 **Rheumatic aortic valve disease, unspecified**

Rheumatic aortic (valve) disease NOS

I07 **Rheumatic tricuspid valve diseases**

Includes: rheumatic tricuspid valve diseases specified as rheumatic or unspecified

Excludes1: tricuspid valve disease specified as nonrheumatic (I36.-)

tricuspid valve disease with aortic and/or mitral valve involvement (I08.-)

I07.0   **Rheumatic tricuspid stenosis**

Tricuspid (valve) stenosis (rheumatic)

I07.1   **Rheumatic tricuspid insufficiency**

Tricuspid (valve) insufficiency (rheumatic)

I07.2   **Rheumatic tricuspid stenosis and insufficiency**

I07.8   **Other rheumatic tricuspid valve diseases**

I07.9   **Rheumatic tricuspid valve disease, unspecified**

Rheumatic tricuspid valve disorder NOS

I08   **Multiple valve diseases**

Includes: multiple valve diseases specified as rheumatic or unspecified

Excludes1: endocarditis, valve unspecified (I38)

multiple valve disease specified a nonrheumatic (I34.-, I35.-, I36.-, I37.-, I38.-, Q22.-, Q23.-, Q24.8-)

rheumatic valve disease NOS (I09.1)

I08.0   **Rheumatic disorders of both mitral and aortic valves**

Involvement of both mitral and aortic valves specified as rheumatic or unspecified

I08.1   **Rheumatic disorders of both mitral and tricuspid valves**

I08.2   **Rheumatic disorders of both aortic and tricuspid valves**

I08.3   **Combined rheumatic disorders of mitral, aortic and tricuspid valves**

I08.8   **Other rheumatic multiple valve diseases**

I08.9   **Rheumatic multiple valve disease, unspecified**

I09   **Other rheumatic heart diseases**

I09.0   **Rheumatic myocarditis**

Excludes1: myocarditis not specified as rheumatic (I51.4)

I09.1   **Rheumatic diseases of endocardium, valve unspecified**

Rheumatic endocarditis (chronic)

Rheumatic valvulitis (chronic)

Excludes1: endocarditis, valve unspecified (I38)

I09.2   **Chronic rheumatic pericarditis**

Adherent pericardium, rheumatic

Chronic rheumatic mediastinopericarditis

Chronic rheumatic myopericarditis

Excludes1: chronic pericarditis not specified as rheumatic (I31.-)

I09.8   **Other specified rheumatic heart diseases**

     I09.81   **Rheumatic heart failure**

        Use additional code to identify type of heart ailure (I50.-)

     I09.89   **Other specified rheumatic heart diseases**

        Rheumatic disease of pulmonary valve

I09.9   **Rheumatic heart disease, unspecified**

Rheumatic carditis

Excludes1: rheumatoid carditis (M05.31)

HYPERTENSIVE DISEASES (I10-I16)

Definition: Hypertensive heart disease refers to heart disease caused by high blood pressure, especially localised high blood pressure.

Use additional code to identify:

exposure to environmental tobacco smoke (Z77.22)

history of tobacco dependence (Z87.891)

occupational exposure to environmental tobacco smoke (Z57.31)

tobacco dependence (F17.-)

tobacco use (Z72.0)

Excludes1: neonatal hypertension (P29.2)

primary pulmonary hypertension (I27.0)

Excludes2: hypertensive disease complicating pregnancy, childbirth and the puerperium (O10-O11, O13-O16)

I10   **Essential (primary) hypertension**

Includes: high blood pressure

hypertension (arterial) (benign) (essential) (malignant) (primary) (systemic)

Excludes1: hypertensive disease complicating pregnancy, childbirth and the puerperium (O10-O11, O13-O16)

Excludes2: essential (primary) hypertension involving vessels of brain (I60-I69)

essential (primary) hypertension involving vessels of eye (H35.0-)

I11   **Hypertensive heart disease**

Includes: any condition in I51.4-I51.9 due to hypertension

I11.0   **Hypertensive heart disease with heart failure**

Hypertensive heart failure

Use additional code to identify type of heart failure (I50.-)

I11.9   **Hypertensive heart disease without heart failure**

Hypertensive heart disease NOS

I12   **Hypertensive chronic kidney disease**

Includes: any condition in N18 and N26 - due to hypertension

arteriosclerosis of kidney

arteriosclerotic nephritis (chronic) (interstitial) hypertensive nephropathy

nephrosclerosis

Excludes1: hypertension due to kidney disease (I15.0, I15.1)

renovascular hypertension (I15.0) secondary hypertension (I15.-)

Excludes2: acute kidney failure (N17.-)

I12.0   **Hypertensive chronic kidney disease with stage 5 chronic kidney disease or end stage renal disease**

Use additional code to identify the stage of chronic kidney disease (N18.5, N18.6)

I12.9   **Hypertensive chronic kidney disease with stage 1through stage 4 chronic kidney disease, or unspecified chronic kidney disease**

Hypertensive chronic kidney disease NOS Hypertensive renal disease NOS

Use additional code to identify the stage of chronic kidney disease (N18.1-N18.4, N18.9)

I13   **Hypertensive heart and chronic kidney disease**

Includes: any condition in I11.- with any condition in I12.-

cardiorenal disease cardiovascular renal disease

I13.0   **Hypertensive heart and chronic kidney disease with heart failure and stage 1through stage 4chronic kidney disease, or unspecified chronic kidney disease**

Use additional code to identify type of heart failure (I50.-)

Use additional code to identify stage of chronic kidney disease (N18.1-N18.4, N18.9)

I13.1   **Hypertensive heart and chronic kidney disease without heart failure**

     I13.10   **Hypertensive heart and chronic kidney disease without heart failure, with stage 1through stage 4chronic kidney disease, or unspecified chronic kidney disease**

Hypertensive heart disease and hypertensive chronic kidney disease NOS

Use additional code to identify the stage of chronic kidney disease (N18.1-N18.4, N18.9)

I13.11 **Hypertensive heart and chronic kidney disease without heart failure, with stage 5 chronic kidney disease, or end stage renal disease**

Use additional code to identify the stage of chronic kidney disease (N18.5, N18.6)

I13.2 **Hypertensive heart and chronic kidney disease with heart failure and with stage 5 chronic kidney disease, or end stage renal disease**

Use additional code to identify type of heart failure (I50.-)

Use additional code to identify the stage of chronic kidney disease (N18.5, N18.6)

I15 **Secondary hypertension**

Definition: Secondary hypertension is a type of hypertension caused by an identifiable underlying secondary cause.

Code also underlying condition

Excludes1: postprocedural hypertension (I97.3)

Excludes2: secondary hypertension involving vessels of brain (I60-I69)

secondary hypertension involving vessels of eye (H35.0-)

I15.0 **Renovascular hypertension**

I15.1 **Hypertension secondary to other renal disorders**

I15.2 **Hypertension secondary to endocrine disorders**

I15.8 **Other secondary hypertension**

I15.9 **Secondary hypertension, unspecified**

I16 **Hypertensive crisis**

Code also any identified hypertensive disease (I10-I15)

•**I16.0** **Hypertensive urgency**

•**I16.1** **Hypertensive emergency**

•**I16.9** **Hypertensive crisis, unspecified**

ISCHEMIC HEART DISEASES (I20-I25)

Definition: Ischemic heart disease is a condition caused by a reduced amount of blood supplying the heart muscle. It can be caused by cholesterol and other lipids building up on the inner walls of arteries that supply the heart, forming a thick plaque that can reduce the amount of blood carrying nutrients and oxygen to heart tissue.

Use additional code to identify presence of hypertension (I10-I16)

I20 **Angina pectoris**

Use additional code to identify:

exposure to environmental tobacco smoke (Z77.22)

history of tobacco dependence (Z87.891)

occupational exposure to environmental tobacco smoke (Z57.31)

tobacco dependence (F17.-)

tobacco use (Z72.0)

Excludes1: angina pectoris with atherosclerotic heart disease of native coronary arteries (I25.1-)

atherosclerosis of coronary artery bypass graft(s) and coronary artery of transplanted heart with angina pectoris (I25.7-)

postinfarction angina (I23.7)

I20.0 **Unstable angina**

Accelerated angina

Crescendo angina

De novo effort angina

Intermediate coronary syndrome

Preinfarction syndrome

Worsening effort angina

I20.1 **Angina pectoris with documented spasm**

Angiospastic angina

Prinzmetal angina

Spasm-induced angina

Variant angina

I20.8 **Other forms of angina pectoris**

Angina equivalent

Angina of effort

Coronary slow flow syndrome

Stenocardia

Stable angina

Use additional code(s) for symptoms associated with angina equivalent

I20.9 **Angina pectoris, unspecified**

Angina NOS

Anginal syndrome

Cardiac angina

Ischemic chest pain

I21 **ST elevation (STEMI) and non-ST elevation (NSTEMI) myocardial infarction**

Definition: Myocardial infarction, commonly known as a heart attack, occurs when the blood supply to part of the heart is interrupted causing some heart cells to die.

Includes: cardiac infarction

coronary (artery) embolism

coronary (artery) occlusion

coronary (artery) rupture

coronary (artery) thrombosis

infarction of heart, myocardium, or ventricle

myocardial infarction specified as acute or with a stated duration of 4 weeks (28 days) or less from onset

Use additional code, if applicable, to identify:

exposure to environmental tobacco smoke (Z77.22)

history of tobacco dependence (Z87.891)

occupational exposure to environmental tobacco smoke (Z57.31)

status post administration of tPA (rtPA) in a different facility within the last 24 hours prior to admission to current facility (Z92.82)

tobacco dependence (F17.-)

tobacco use (Z72.0)

Excludes2: old myocardial infarction (I25.2)

postmyocardial infarction syndrome (I24.1)

subsequent myocardial infarction (I22.-)

I21.0 **ST elevation (STEMI) myocardial infarction of anterior wall**

I21.01 **ST elevation (STEMI) myocardial infarction involving left main coronary artery**

I21.02 **ST elevation (STEMI) myocardial infarction involving left anterior descending coronary artery**

ST elevation (STEMI) myocardial infarction involving diagonal coronary artery

I21.09 **ST elevation (STEMI) myocardial infarction involving other coronary artery of anterior wall**

Acute transmural myocardial infarction of anterior wall

Anteroapical transmural (Q wave) infarction (acute)

Anterolateral transmural (Q wave) infarction (acute)

Anteroseptal transmural (Q wave) infarction (acute)

Transmural (Q wave) infarction (acute) (of) anterior (wall) NOS

I21.1 ST elevation (STEMI) myocardial infarction of inferior wall

I21.11 ST elevation (STEMI) myocardial infarction involving right coronary artery

Inferoposterior transmural (Q wave) infarction (acute)

I21.19 ST elevation (STEMI) myocardial infarction involving other coronary artery of inferior wall

Acute transmural myocardial infarction of inferior wall

Inferolateral transmural (Q wave) infarction (acute)

Transmural (Q wave) infarction (acute) (of) diaphragmatic wall

Transmural (Q wave) infarction (acute) (of) inferior (wall) NOS

Excludes2: ST elevation (STEMI) myocardial infarction involving left circumflex coronary artery (I21.21)

I21.2 ST elevation (STEMI) myocardial infarction of other sites

I21.21 ST elevation (STEMI) myocardial infarction involving left circumflex coronary artery

ST elevation (STEMI) myocardial infarction involving oblique marginal coronary artery

I21.29 ST elevation (STEMI) myocardial infarction involving other sites

Acute transmural myocardial infarction **of other** sites

Apical-lateral transmural (Q wave) infarction (acute)

Basal-lateral transmural (Q wave) infarction (acute)

High lateral transmural (Q wave) infarction (acute)

Lateral (wall) NOS transmural (Q wave) infarction (acute)

Posterior (true) transmural (Q wave) infarction (acute)

Posterobasal transmural (Q wave) infarction (acute)

Posterolateral transmural (Q wave) infarction (acute)

Posteroseptal transmural (Q wave) infarction (acute)

Septal transmural (Q wave) infarction (acute) NOS

I21.3 ST elevation (STEMI) myocardial infarction of unspecified site

Acute transmural myocardial infarction of unspecified site

Myocardial infarction (acute) NOS

Transmural (Q wave) myocardial infarction NOS

I21.4 Non-ST elevation (NSTEMI) myocardial infarction

Acute subendocardial myocardial infarction

Non-Q wave myocardial infarction NOS

Nontransmural myocardial infarction NOS

I22 Subsequent ST elevation (STEMI) and non-ST elevation (NSTEMI) myocardial infarction

Includes: acute myocardial infarction occurring within four weeks (28 days) of a previous acute myocardial infarction, regardless of site cardiac infarction

coronary (artery) embolism coronary (artery) occlusion

coronary (artery) rupture coronary (artery) thrombosis

infarction of heart, myocardium, or ventricle recurrent myocardial infarction

reinfarction of myocardium

rupture of heart, myocardium, or ventricle

Use additional code, if applicable, to identify:

exposure to environmental tobacco smoke (Z77.22)

history of tobacco dependence (Z87.891)

occupational exposure to environmental tobacco smoke (Z57.31)

status post administration of tPA (rtPA) in a different facility within the last 24 hours prior to admission to current facility (Z92.82)

tobacco dependence (F17.-)

tobacco use (Z72.0)

I22.0 Subsequent ST elevation (STEMI) myocardial infarction of anterior wall

Subsequent acute transmural myocardial infarction of anterior wall

Subsequent transmural (Q wave) infarction (acute)(of) anterior (wall) NOS

Subsequent anteroapical transmural (Q wave) infarction (acute)

Subsequent anterolateral transmural (Q wave) infarction (acute)

Subsequent anteroseptal transmural (Q wave) infarction (acute)

I22.1 Subsequent ST elevation (STEMI) myocardial infarction of inferior wall

Subsequent acute transmural myocardial infarction of inferior wall

Subsequent transmural (Q wave) infarction (acute)(of) diaphragmatic wall

Subsequent transmural (Q wave) infarction (acute)(of) inferior (wall) NOS

Subsequent inferolateral transmural (Q wave) infarction (acute)

Subsequent inferoposterior transmural (Q wave) infarction (acute)

I22.2 Subsequent non-ST elevation (NSTEMI) myocardial infarction

Subsequent acute subendocardial myocardial infarction

Subsequent non-Q wave myocardial infarction NOS

Subsequent nontransmural myocardial infarction NOS

I22.8 Subsequent ST elevation (STEMI) myocardial infarction of other sites

Subsequent acute transmural myocardial infarction **of other** sites

Subsequent apical-lateral transmural (Q wave) myocardial infarction (acute)

Subsequent basal-lateral transmural (Q wave) myocardial infarction (acute)

Subsequent high lateral transmural (Q wave) myocardial infarction (acute)

Subsequent transmural (Q wave) myocardial infarction (acute)(of) lateral (wall) NOS

Subsequent posterior (true)transmural (Q wave) myocardial infarction (acute)

Subsequent posterobasal transmural (Q wave) myocardial infarction (acute)

Subsequent posterolateral transmural (Q wave) myocardial infarction (acute)

Subsequent posteroseptal transmural (Q wave) myocardial infarction (acute)

Subsequent septal NOS transmural (Q wave) myocardial infarction (acute)

I22.9 Subsequent ST elevation (STEMI) myocardial infarction of unspecified site

Subsequent acute myocardial infarction of unspecified site

Subsequent myocardial infarction (acute) NOS

I23 Certain current complications following ST elevation (STEMI) and non-ST elevation (NSTEMI) myocardial infarction (within the 28 day period)

I23.0 Hemopericardium as current complication following acute myocardial infarction

Excludes1: hemopericardium not specified as current complication following acute myocardial infarction (I31.2)

I23.1 Atrial septal defect as current complication following acute myocardial infarction

Excludes1: acquired atrial septal defect not specified as current complication following acute myocardial infarction (I51.0)

I23.2 Ventricular septal defect as current complication following acute myocardial infarction

Excludes1: acquired ventricular septal defect not specified as current complication following acute myocardial infarction (I51.0)

I23.3 Rupture of cardiac wall without hemopericardium as current complication following acute myocardial infarction

I23.4 Rupture of chordae tendineae as current complication following acute myocardial infarction

Excludes1: rupture of chordae tendineae not specified as current complication following acute myocardial infarction (I51.1)

I23.5 Rupture of papillary muscle as current complication following acute myocardial infarction

Excludes1: rupture of papillary muscle not specified as current complication following acute myocardial infarction (I51.2)

I23.6 Thrombosis of atrium, auricular appendage, and ventricle as current complications following acute myocardial infarction

Excludes1: thrombosis of atrium, auricular appendage, and ventricle not specified as current complication following acute myocardial infarction (I51.3)

I23.7 Postinfarction angina

I23.8 Other current complications following acute myocardial infarction

I24 Other acute ischemic heart diseases

Excludes1: angina pectoris (I20.-)

transient myocardial ischemia in newborn (P29.4)

I24.0 Acute coronary thrombosis not resulting in myocardial infarction

Acute coronary (artery) (vein) embolism not resulting in myocardial infarction

Acute coronary (artery) (vein) occlusion not resulting in myocardial infarction

Acute coronary (artery) (vein) thromboembolism not resulting in myocardial infarction

Excludes1: atherosclerotic heart disease (I25.1-)

I24.1 Dressler's syndrome

Postmyocardial infarction syndrome

Excludes1: postinfarction angina (I23.7)

I24.8 Other forms of acute ischemic heart disease

I24.9 Acute ischemic heart disease, unspecified

Excludes1: ischemic heart disease (chronic) NOS (I25.9)

I25 Chronic ischemic heart disease

Use additional code to identify:

chronic total occlusion of coronary artery (I25.82)

exposure to environmental tobacco smoke (Z77.22)

history of tobacco dependence (Z87.891)

occupational exposure to environmental tobacco smoke (Z57.31)

tobacco dependence (F17.-)

tobacco use (Z72.0)

I25.1 Atherosclerotic heart disease of native coronary artery

Atherosclerotic cardiovascular disease

Coronary (artery) atheroma

Coronary (artery) atherosclerosis

Coronary (artery) disease

Coronary (artery) sclerosis

Use additional code, if applicable, to identify:

coronary atherosclerosis due to calcified coronary lesion (I25.84)

coronary atherosclerosis due to lipid rich plaque (I25.83)

Excludes2: atheroembolism (I75.-)

atherosclerosis of coronary artery bypass graft(s) and transplanted heart (I25.7-)

I25.10 Atherosclerotic heart disease of native coronary artery without angina pectoris

Atherosclerotic heart disease NOS

I25.11 Atherosclerotic heart disease of native coronary artery with angina pectoris

I25.110 Atherosclerotic heart disease of native coronary artery with unstable angina pectoris

Excludes1: unstable angina without atherosclerotic heart disease (I20.0)

I25.111 Atherosclerotic heart disease of native coronary artery with angina pectoris with documented spasm

Excludes1: angina pectoris with documented spasm without atherosclerotic heart disease (I20.1)

I25.118 Atherosclerotic heart disease of native coronary artery with other forms of angina pectoris

Excludes1: Other forms of angina pectoris without atherosclerotic heart disease (I20.8)

I25.119　**Atherosclerotic heart disease of native coronary artery with unspecified angina pectoris**

Atherosclerotic heart disease with angina NOS

Atherosclerotic heart disease with ischemic chest pain

Excludes1: unspecified angina pectoris without atherosclerotic heart disease (I20.9)

I25.2　**Old myocardial infarction**

Definition: Old myocardial infarction refers to an old occlusion or blockage of arteries supplying the muscles of the heart, resulting in injury or necrosis of the heart muscle.

Healed myocardial infarction

Past myocardial infarction diagnosed by ECG **or other** investigation, but currently presenting no symptoms

I25.3　**Aneurysm of heart**

Mural aneurysm

Ventricular aneurysm

I25.4　**Coronary artery aneurysm and dissection**

I25.41　**Coronary artery aneurysm**

Coronary arteriovenous fistula, acquired

Excludes1: congenital coronary (artery) aneurysm (Q24.5)

I25.42　**Coronary artery dissection**

I25.5　**Ischemic cardiomyopathy**

Excludes2: coronary atherosclerosis (I25.1-, I25.7-)

I25.6　**Silent myocardial ischemia**

I25.7　**Atherosclerosis of coronary artery bypass graft(s) and coronary artery of transplanted heart with angina pectoris**

Use additional code, if applicable, to identify:

coronary atherosclerosis due to calcified coronary lesion (I25.84)

coronary atherosclerosis due to lipid rich plaque (I25.83)

Excludes1: atherosclerosis of bypass graft(s) of transplanted heart without angina pectoris (I25.812)

atherosclerosis of coronary artery bypass graft(s) without angina pectoris (I25.810)

atherosclerosis of native coronary artery of transplanted heart without angina pectoris (I25.811)

embolism or thrombus of coronary artery bypass graft(s) (T82.8-)

I25.70　**Atherosclerosis of coronary artery bypass graft(s), unspecified, with angina pectoris**

I25.700　**Atherosclerosis of coronary artery bypass graft(s), unspecified, with unstable angina pectoris**

Excludes1: unstable angina pectoris without atherosclerosis of coronary artery bypass graft (I20.0)

I25.701　**Atherosclerosis of coronary artery bypass graft(s), unspecified, with angina pectoris with documented spasm**

Excludes1: angina pectoris with documented spasm without atherosclerosis of coronary artery bypass graft (I20.1)

I25.708　**Atherosclerosis of coronary artery bypass graft(s), unspecified, with other forms of angina pectoris**

Excludes1: Other forms of angina pectoris without atherosclerosis of coronary artery bypass graft (I20.8)

I25.709　**Atherosclerosis of coronary artery bypass graft(s), unspecified, with unspecified angina pectoris**

Excludes1: unspecified angina pectoris without atherosclerosis of coronary artery bypass graft (I20.9)

I25.71　**Atherosclerosis of autologous vein coronary artery bypass graft(s) with angina pectoris**

I25.710　**Atherosclerosis of autologous vein coronary artery bypass graft(s) with unstable angina pectoris**

Excludes1: unstable angina without atherosclerosis of autologous vein coronary artery bypass graft(s) (I20.0)

I25.711　**Atherosclerosis of autologous vein coronary artery bypass graft(s) with angina pectoris with documented spasm**

Excludes1: angina pectoris with documented spasm without atherosclerosis of autologous vein coronary artery bypass graft(s) (I20.1)

I25.718　**Atherosclerosis of autologous vein coronary artery bypass graft(s) with other forms of angina pectoris**

Excludes1: Other forms of angina pectoris without atherosclerosis of autologous vein coronary artery bypass graft(s) (I20.8)

I25.719　**Atherosclerosis of autologous vein coronary artery bypass graft(s) with unspecified angina pectoris**

Excludes1: unspecified angina pectoris without atherosclerosis of autologous vein coronary artery bypass graft(s) (I20.9)

I25.72　**Atherosclerosis of autologous artery coronary artery bypass graft(s) with angina pectoris**

Atherosclerosis of internal mammary artery graft with angina pectoris

I25.720　**Atherosclerosis of autologous artery coronary artery bypass graft(s) with unstable angina pectoris**

Excludes1: unstable angina without atherosclerosis of autologous artery coronary artery bypass graft(s) (I20.0)

I25.721　**Atherosclerosis of autologous artery coronary artery bypass graft(s) with angina pectoris with documented spasm**

Excludes1: angina pectoris with documented spasm without atherosclerosis of autologous artery coronary artery bypass graft(s) (I20.1)

I25.728 **Atherosclerosis of autologous artery coronary artery bypass graft(s) with other forms of angina pectoris**

Excludes1: Other forms of angina pectoris without atherosclerosis of autologous artery coronary artery bypass graft(s) (I20.8)

I25.729 **Atherosclerosis of autologous artery coronary artery bypass graft(s) with unspecified angina pectoris**

Excludes1: unspecified angina pectoris without atherosclerosis of autologous artery coronary artery bypass graft(s) (I20.9)

I25.73 **Atherosclerosis of nonautologous biological coronary artery bypass graft(s) with angina pectoris**

I25.730 **Atherosclerosis of nonautologous biological coronary artery bypass graft(s) with unstable angina pectoris**

Excludes1: unstable angina without atherosclerosis of nonautologous biological coronary artery bypass graft(s) (I20.0)

I25.731 **Atherosclerosis of nonautologous biological coronary artery bypass graft(s) with angina pectoris with documented spasm**

Excludes1: angina pectoris with documented spasm without atherosclerosis of nonautologous biological coronary artery bypass graft(s) (I20.1)

I25.738 **Atherosclerosis of nonautologous biological coronary artery bypass graft(s) with other forms of angina pectoris**

Excludes1: Other forms of angina pectoris without atherosclerosis of nonautologous biological coronary artery bypass graft(s) (I20.8)

I25.739 **Atherosclerosis of nonautologous biological coronary artery bypass graft(s) with unspecified angina pectoris**

Excludes1: unspecified angina pectoris without atherosclerosis of nonautologous biological coronary artery bypass graft(s) (I20.9)

I25.75 **Atherosclerosis of native coronary artery of transplanted heart with angina pectoris**

Excludes1: atherosclerosis of native coronary artery of transplanted heart without angina pectoris (I25.811)

I25.750 **Atherosclerosis of native coronary artery of transplanted heart with unstable angina**

I25.751 **Atherosclerosis of native coronary artery of transplanted heart with angina pectoris with documented spasm**

I25.758 **Atherosclerosis of native coronary artery of transplanted heart with other forms of angina pectoris**

I25.759 **Atherosclerosis of native coronary artery of transplanted heart with unspecified angina pectoris**

I25.76 **Atherosclerosis of bypass graft of coronary artery of transplanted heart with angina pectoris**

Excludes1: atherosclerosis of bypass graft of coronary artery of transplanted heart without angina pectoris (I25.812)

I25.760 **Atherosclerosis of bypass graft of coronary artery of transplanted heart with unstable angina**

I25.761 **Atherosclerosis of bypass graft of coronary artery of transplanted heart with angina pectoris with documented spasm**

I25.768 **Atherosclerosis of bypass graft of coronary artery of transplanted heart with other forms of angina pectoris**

I25.769 **Atherosclerosis of bypass graft of coronary artery of transplanted heart with unspecified angina pectoris**

I25.79 **Atherosclerosis of other coronary artery bypass graft(s) with angina pectoris**

I25.790 **Atherosclerosis of other coronary artery bypass graft(s) with unstable angina pectoris**

Excludes1: unstable angina without atherosclerosis of other coronary artery bypass graft(s) (I20.0)

I25.791 **Atherosclerosis of other coronary artery bypass graft(s) with angina pectoris with documented spasm**

Excludes1: angina pectoris with documented spasm without atherosclerosis of other coronary artery bypass graft(s) (I20.1)

I25.798 **Atherosclerosis of other coronary artery bypass graft(s) with other forms of angina pectoris**

Excludes1: Other forms of angina pectoris without atherosclerosis of other coronary artery bypass graft(s) (I20.8)

I25.799 **Atherosclerosis of other coronary artery bypass graft(s) with unspecified angina pectoris**

Excludes1: unspecified angina pectoris without atherosclerosis of other coronary artery bypass graft(s) (I20.9)

I25.8 **Other forms of chronic ischemic heart disease**

I25.81 **Atherosclerosis of other coronary vessels without angina pectoris**

Use additional code, if applicable, to identify:

coronary atherosclerosis due to calcified coronary lesion (I25.84)

coronary atherosclerosis due to lipid rich plaque (I25.83)

Excludes1: atherosclerotic heart disease of native coronary artery without angina pectoris (I25.10)

I25.810   **Atherosclerosis of coronary artery bypass graft(s) without angina pectoris**

Atherosclerosis of coronary artery bypass graft NOS

Excludes1: atherosclerosis of coronary bypass graft(s) with angina pectoris (I25.70-I25.73-,I25.79-)

I25.811   **Atherosclerosis of native coronary artery of transplanted heart without angina pectoris**

Atherosclerosis of native coronary artery of transplanted heart NOS

Excludes1: atherosclerosis of native coronary artery of transplanted heart with angina pectoris (I25.75-)

I25.812   **Atherosclerosis of bypass graft of coronary artery of transplanted heart without angina pectoris**

Atherosclerosis of bypass graft of transplanted heart NOS

Excludes1: atherosclerosis of bypass graft of transplanted heart with angina pectoris (I25.76)

I25.82   **Chronic total occlusion of coronary artery**

Complete occlusion of coronary artery

Total occlusion of coronary artery

Code first coronary atherosclerosis (I25.1-, I25.7-, I25.81-)

Excludes1: acute coronary occlusion with myocardial infarction (I21.-, I22.-)

acute coronary occlusion without myocardial infarction (I24.0)

I25.83   **Coronary atherosclerosis due to lipid rich plaque**

Code first coronary atherosclerosis (I25.1-, I25.7-, I25.81-)

I25.84   **Coronary atherosclerosis due to calcified coronary lesion**

Coronary atherosclerosis due to severely calcified coronary lesion

Code first coronary atherosclerosis (I25.1-, I25.7-, I25.81-)

I25.89   **Other forms of chronic ischemic heart disease**

I25.9   **Chronic ischemic heart disease, unspecified**

Ischemic heart disease (chronic) NOS

PULMONARY HEART DISEASE AND DISEASES OF PULMONARY CIRCULATION (I26-I28)

Definition: Pulmonary heart disease is the enlargement and eventual failure of the right ventricle of the heart due to disorders of the lungs or their blood vessels or chest wall abnormalities.

Definition: Pulmonary circulation is the circulation of blood through the lungs for the purpose of oxygenation and the release of carbon dioxide. Also known as lesser circulation.

I26   **Pulmonary embolism**

Includes: pulmonary (acute) (artery)(vein) infarction

pulmonary (acute) (artery)(vein) thromboembolism
pulmonary (acute) (artery)(vein) thrombosis

Excludes2: chronic pulmonary embolism (I27.82)

personal history of pulmonary embolism (Z86.711)

pulmonary embolism complicating abortion, ectopic or molar pregnancy (O00-O07, O08.2)

pulmonary embolism complicating pregnancy, childbirth and the puerperium (O88.-)

pulmonary embolism due to trauma (T79.0, T79.1)

pulmonary embolism due to complications of surgical and medical care (T80.0, T81.7-, T82.8-)

septic (non-pulmonary) arterial embolism (I76)

I26.0   **Pulmonary embolism with acute cor pulmonale**

I26.01   **Septic pulmonary embolism with acute cor pulmonale**

Code first underlying infection

I26.02   **Saddle embolus of pulmonary artery with acute cor pulmonale**

I26.09   **Other pulmonary embolism with acute cor pulmonale**

Acute cor pulmonale NOS

I26.9   **Pulmonary embolism without acute cor pulmonale**

I26.90   **Septic pulmonary embolism without acute cor pulmonale**

Code first underlying infection

I26.92   **Saddle embolus of pulmonary artery without acute cor pulmonale**

I26.99   **Other pulmonary embolism without acute cor pulmonale**

Acute pulmonary embolism NOS

Pulmonary embolism NOS

I27   **Other pulmonary heart diseases**

I27.0   **Primary pulmonary hypertension**

Excludes1: pulmonary hypertension NOS (I27.2)

secondary pulmonary hypertension (I27.2)

I27.1   **Kyphoscoliotic heart disease**

I27.2   **Other secondary pulmonary hypertension**

Pulmonary hypertension NOS

Code also associated underlying condition

I27.8   **Other specified pulmonary heart diseases**

I27.81   **Cor pulmonale (chronic)**

Cor pulmonale NOS

Excludes1: acute cor pulmonale (I26.0-)

I27.82   **Chronic pulmonary embolism**

Use additional code, if applicable, for associated long-term (current) use of anticoagulants (Z79.01)

Excludes1: personal history of pulmonary embolism (Z86.711)

I27.89   **Other specified pulmonary heart diseases**

Eisenmenger's complex

Eisenmenger's syndrome

Excludes1: Eisenmenger's defect (Q21.8)

I27.9   **Pulmonary heart disease, unspecified**

Chronic cardiopulmonary disease

I28   **Other diseases of pulmonary vessels**

I28.0   **Arteriovenous fistula of pulmonary vessels**

Excludes1: congenital arteriovenous fistula (Q25.72)

I28.1   **Aneurysm of pulmonary artery**

Excludes1: congenital aneurysm (Q25.79)

congenital arteriovenous aneurysm (Q25.72)

I28.8 Other diseases of pulmonary vessels

Pulmonary arteritis

Pulmonary endarteritis

Rupture of pulmonary vessels

Stenosis of pulmonary vessels

Stricture of pulmonary vessels

I28.9 Disease of pulmonary vessels, unspecified

OTHER FORMS OF HEART DISEASE (I30-I52)

I30 Acute pericarditis

Definition: Pericarditis is an inflammation of the two layers of the thin, sac-like membrane that surrounds the heart.

Includes: acute mediastinopericarditis

acute myopericarditis

acute pericardial effusion

acute pleuropericarditis

acute pneumopericarditis

Excludes1: Dressler's syndrome (I24.1)

rheumatic pericarditis (acute) (I01.0)

I30.0 Acute nonspecific idiopathic pericarditis

I30.1 Infective pericarditis

Pneumococcal pericarditis

Pneumopyopericardium

Purulent pericarditis

Pyopericarditis

Pyopericardium

Pyopneumopericardium

Staphylococcal pericarditis

Streptococcal pericarditis

Suppurative pericarditis

Viral pericarditis

Use additional code (B95-B97) to identify infectious agent

I30.8 Other forms of acute pericarditis

I30.9 Acute pericarditis, unspecified

I31 Other diseases of pericardium

Excludes1: diseases of pericardium specified as rheumatic (I09.2)

postcardiotomy syndrome (I97.0)

traumatic injury to pericardium (S26.-)

I31.0 Chronic adhesive pericarditis

Accretio cordis

Adherent pericardium

Adhesive mediastinopericarditis

I31.1 Chronic constrictive pericarditis

Concretio cordis

Pericardial calcification

I31.2 Hemopericardium, not elsewhere classified

Excludes1: hemopericardium as current complication following acute myocardial infarction (I23.0)

I31.3 Pericardial effusion (noninflammatory)

Chylopericardium

Excludes1: acute pericardial effusion (I30.9)

I31.4 Cardiac tamponade

Code first underlying cause

I31.8 Other specified diseases of pericardium

Epicardial plaques

Focal pericardial adhesions

I31.9 Disease of pericardium, unspecified

Pericarditis (chronic) NOS

I32 Pericarditis in diseases classified elsewhere

Code first underlying disease

Excludes1: pericarditis (in):

coxsackie (virus) (B33.23)

gonococcal (A54.83)

meningococcal (A39.53)

rheumatoid (arthritis) (M05.31)

syphilitic (A52.06)

systemic lupus erythematosus (M32.12)

tuberculosis (A18.84)

I33 Acute and subacute endocarditis

Definition: Endocarditis is an infection of the lining of the heart chambers and heart valves that is caused by bacteria, fungi, or other infectious substances.

Excludes1: acute rheumatic endocarditis (I01.1)

endocarditis NOS (I38)

I33.0 Acute and subacute infective endocarditis

Bacterial endocarditis (acute) (subacute)

Infective endocarditis (acute) (subacute) NOS

Endocarditis lenta (acute) (subacute)

Malignant endocarditis (acute) (subacute)

Purulent endocarditis (acute) (subacute)

Septic endocarditis (acute) (subacute)

Ulcerative endocarditis (acute) (subacute)

Vegetative endocarditis (acute) (subacute)

Use additional code (B95-B97) to identify infectious agent

I33.9 Acute and subacute endocarditis, unspecified

Acute endocarditis NOS

Acute myoendocarditis NOS

Acute periendocarditis NOS

Subacute endocarditis NOS

Subacute myoendocarditis NOS

Subacute periendocarditis NOS

I34 Nonrheumatic mitral valve disorders

Excludes1: mitral valve disease (I05.9)

mitral valve failure (I05.8)

mitral valve stenosis (I05.0)

mitral valve disorder of unspecified cause with diseases of aortic and/or tricuspid valve(s) (I08.-)

mitral valve disorder of unspecified cause with mitral stenosis or obstruction (I05.0)

mitral valve disorder specified as congenital (Q23.2, Q23.3)

mitral valve disorder specified as rheumatic (I05.-)

I34.0 Nonrheumatic mitral (valve) insufficiency

Nonrheumatic mitral (valve) incompetence NOS

Nonrheumatic mitral (valve) regurgitation NOS

I34.1 Nonrheumatic mitral (valve) prolapse

Floppy nonrheumatic mitral valve syndrome

Excludes1: Marfan's syndrome (Q87.4-)

I34.2 Nonrheumatic mitral (valve) stenosis

I34.8   **Other nonrheumatic mitral valve disorders**

I34.9   **Nonrheumatic mitral valve disorder, unspecified**

I35   **Nonrheumatic aortic valve disorders**

Excludes1: aortic valve disorder of unspecified cause but with diseases of mitral and/or tricuspid valve(s) (I08.-)

aortic valve disorder specified as congenital (Q23.0, Q23.1)

aortic valve disorder specified as rheumatic (I06.-)

hypertrophic subaortic stenosis (I42.1)

I35.0   **Nonrheumatic aortic (valve) stenosis**

I35.1   **Nonrheumatic aortic (valve) insufficiency**

Nonrheumatic aortic (valve) incompetence NOS

Nonrheumatic aortic (valve) regurgitation NOS

I35.2   **Nonrheumatic aortic (valve) stenosis with insufficiency**

I35.8   **Other nonrheumatic aortic valve disorders**

I35.9   **Nonrheumatic aortic valve disorder, unspecified**

I36   **Nonrheumatic tricuspid valve disorders**

Excludes1: tricuspid valve disorders of unspecified cause (I07.-)

tricuspid valve disorders specified as congenital (Q22.4, Q22.8, Q22.9)

tricuspid valve disorders specified as rheumatic (I07.-)

tricuspid valve disorders with aortic and/or mitral valve involvement (I08.-)

I36.0   **Nonrheumatic tricuspid (valve) stenosis**

I36.1   **Nonrheumatic tricuspid (valve) insufficiency**

Nonrheumatic tricuspid (valve) incompetence

Nonrheumatic tricuspid (valve) regurgitation

I36.2   **Nonrheumatic tricuspid (valve) stenosis with insufficiency**

I36.8   **Other nonrheumatic tricuspid valve disorders**

I36.9   **Nonrheumatic tricuspid valve disorder, unspecified**

I37   **Nonrheumatic pulmonary valve disorders**

Excludes1: pulmonary valve disorder specified as congenital (Q22.1, Q22.2, Q22.3)

pulmonary valve disorder specified as rheumatic (I09.89)

I37.0   **Nonrheumatic pulmonary valve stenosis**

I37.1   **Nonrheumatic pulmonary valve insufficiency**

Nonrheumatic pulmonary valve incompetence

Nonrheumatic pulmonary valve regurgitation

I37.2   **Nonrheumatic pulmonary valve stenosis with insufficiency**

I37.8   **Other nonrheumatic pulmonary valve disorders**

I37.9   **Nonrheumatic pulmonary valve disorder, unspecified**

I38   **Endocarditis, valve unspecified**

Includes: endocarditis (chronic) NOS

valvular incompetence NOS

valvular insufficiency NOS

valvular regurgitation NOS

valvular stenosis NOS

valvulitis (chronic) NOS

Excludes1: congenital insufficiency of cardiac valve NOS (Q24.8)

congenital stenosis of cardiac valve NOS (Q24.8)

endocardial fibroelastosis (I42.4)

endocarditis specified as rheumatic (I09.1)

I39   **Endocarditis and heart valve disorders in diseases classified elsewhere**

Code first underlying disease, such as:

Q fever (A78)

Excludes1: endocardial involvement in:

candidiasis (B37.6) gonococcal infection (A54.83)

Libman-Sacks disease (M32.11)

listerosis (A32.82)

meningococcal infection (A39.51)

rheumatoid arthritis (M05.31)

syphilis (A52.03)

tuberculosis (A18.84)

typhoid fever (A01.02)

I40   **Acute myocarditis**

Includes: subacute myocarditis

Excludes1: acute rheumatic myocarditis (I01.2)

I40.0   **Infective myocarditis**

Septic myocarditis

Use additional code (B95-B97) to identify infectious agent

I40.1   **Isolated myocarditis**

Fiedler's myocarditis

Giant cell myocarditis

Idiopathic myocarditis

I40.8   **Other acute myocarditis**

I40.9   **Acute myocarditis, unspecified**

I41   **Myocarditis in diseases classified elsewhere**

Code first underlying disease, such as:

typhus (A75.0-A75.9)

Excludes1: myocarditis (in):

Chagas' disease (chronic) (B57.2)

acute (B57.0)

coxsackie (virus) infection (B33.22)

diphtheritic (A36.81)

gonococcal (A54.83)

influenzal (J09.X9, J10.82, J11.82)

meningococcal (A39.52)

mumps (B26.82)

rheumatoid arthritis (M05.31)

sarcoid (D86.85)

syphilis (A52.06)

toxoplasmosis (B58.81)

tuberculous (A18.84)

I42   **Cardiomyopathy**

Definition: Cardiomyopathy is a weakening of the heart muscle or a change in heart muscle structure. It is often associated with inadequate heart pumping or other heart function problems.

Includes: myocardiopathy

Code first pre-existing cardiomyopathy complicating pregnancy and puerperium (O99.4)

Excludes2: ischemic cardiomyopathy (I25.5)

peripartum cardiomyopathy (O90.3)

ventricular hypertrophy (I51.7)

I42.0   **Dilated cardiomyopathy**

Congestive cardiomyopathy

I42.1   **Obstructive hypertrophic cardiomyopathy**

Hypertrophic subaortic stenosis (idiopathic)

I42.2   **Other hypertrophic cardiomyopathy**

Nonobstructive hypertrophic cardiomyopathy

I42.3   **Endomyocardial (eosinophilic) disease**

Endomyocardial (tropical) fibrosis

Löffler's endocarditis

I42.4   **Endocardial fibroelastosis**

Congenital cardiomyopathy

Elastomyofibrosis

I42.5   **Other restrictive cardiomyopathy**

Constrictive cardiomyopathy NOS

I42.6   **Alcoholic cardiomyopathy**

<u>Code also</u> presence of alcoholism (F10.-)

I42.7   **Cardiomyopathy due to drug and external agent**

<u>Code first</u> poisoning due to drug or toxin, if applicable (T36-T65 with fifth or sixth character 1-4 or 6)

<u>Use additional code</u> for adverse effect, if applicable, to identify drug (T36-T50 with fifth or sixth character 5)

I42.8   **Other cardiomyopathies**

I42.9   **Cardiomyopathy, unspecified**

Cardiomyopathy (primary) (secondary) NOS

I43   **Cardiomyopathy in diseases classified elsewhere**

<u>Code first</u> underlying disease, such as:

amyloidosis (E85.-)

glycogen storage disease (E74.0) gout (M10.0-)

thyrotoxicosis (E05.0-E05.9-)

Excludes1: cardiomyopathy (in):

     coxsackie (virus) (B33.24)

     diphtheria (A36.81)

     sarcoidosis (D86.85)

     tuberculosis (A18.84)

I44   **Atrioventricular and left bundle-branch block**

I44.0   **Atrioventricular block, first degree**

I44.1   **Atrioventricular block, second degree**

Atrioventricular block, type I and II

Möbitz block block, type I and II

Second degree block, type I and II

Wenckebach's block

I44.2   **Atrioventricular block, complete**

Complete heart block NOS

Third degree block

I44.3   **Other and unspecified atrioventricular block**

Atrioventricular block NOS

   I44.30   **Unspecified atrioventricular block**

   I44.39   **Other atrioventricular block**

I44.4   **Left anterior fascicular block**

I44.5   **Left posterior fascicular block**

I44.6   **Other and unspecified fascicular block**

   I44.60   **Unspecified fascicular block**

     Left bundle-branch hemiblock NOS

   I44.69   **Other fascicular block**

I44.7   **Left bundle-branch block, unspecified**

I45   **Other conduction disorders**

I45.0   **Right fascicular block**

I45.1   **Other and unspecified right bundle-branch block**

   I45.10   **Unspecified right bundle-branch block**

     Right bundle-branch block NOS

   I45.19   **Other right bundle-branch block**

I45.2   **Bifascicular block**

I45.3   **Trifascicular block**

I45.4   **Nonspecific intraventricular block**

Bundle-branch block NOS

I45.5   **Other specified heart block**

Sinoatrial block

Sinoauricular block

   Excludes1: heart block NOS (I45.9)

I45.6   **Pre-excitation syndrome**

Accelerated atrioventricular conduction

Accessory atrioventricular conduction

Anomalous atrioventricular excitation

Lown-Ganong-Levine syndrome

Pre-excitation atrioventricular conduction

Wolff-Parkinson-White syndrome

I45.8   **Other specified conduction disorders**

   I45.81   **Long QT syndrome**

   I45.89   **Other specified conduction disorders**

     Atrioventricular [AV] dissociation

     Interference dissociation

     Isorhythmic dissociation

     Nonparoxysmal AV nodal tachycardia

I45.9   **Conduction disorder, unspecified**

Heart block NOS

Stokes-Adams syndrome

I46   **Cardiac arrest**

Excludes1: cardiogenic shock (R57.0)

I46.2   **Cardiac arrest due to underlying cardiac condition**

<u>Code first</u> underlying cardiac condition

I46.8   **Cardiac arrest due to other underlying condition**

<u>Code first</u> underlying condition

I46.9   **Cardiac arrest, cause unspecified**

I47   **Paroxysmal tachycardia**

<u>Code first</u> tachycardia complicating:

abortion or ectopic or molar pregnancy (O00-O07, O08.8)

obstetric surgery and procedures (O75.4)

Excludes1: tachycardia NOS (R00.0)

   sinoauricular tachycardia NOS (R00.0)

   sinus [sinusal] tachycardia NOS (R00.0)

I47.0   **Re-entry ventricular arrhythmia**

I47.1   **Supraventricular tachycardia**

Atrial (paroxysmal) tachycardia

Atrioventricular [AV] (paroxysmal) tachycardia

Atrioventricular re-entrant (nodal) tachycardia [AVNRT] [AVRT]

Junctional (paroxysmal) tachycardia

Nodal (paroxysmal) tachycardia

I47.2   **Ventricular tachycardia**

I47.9   **Paroxysmal tachycardia, unspecified**

Bouveret (-Hoffman) syndrome

I48   **Atrial fibrillation and flutter**

I48.0   **Paroxysmal atrial fibrillation**

I48.1   **Persistent atrial fibrillation**

I48.2   **Chronic atrial fibrillation**

Permanent atrial fibrillation

I48.3   **Typical atrial flutter**

Type I atrial flutter

I48.4   **Atypical atrial flutter**

Type II atrial flutter

I48.9   **Unspecified atrial fibrillation and atrial flutter**

I48.91   **Unspecified atrial fibrillation**

I48.92   **Unspecified atrial flutter**

I49   **Other cardiac arrhythmias**

Code first cardiac arrhythmia complicating:

abortion or ectopic or molar pregnancy (O00-O07, O08.8)

obstetric surgery and procedures (O75.4)

Excludes1: bradycardia NOS (R00.1)

neonatal dysrhythmia (P29.1-)

sinoatrial bradycardia (R00.1)

sinus bradycardia (R00.1)

vagal bradycardia (R00.1)

I49.0   **Ventricular fibrillation and flutter**

I49.01   **Ventricular fibrillation**

I49.02   **Ventricular flutter**

I49.1   **Atrial premature depolarization**

Atrial premature beats

I49.2   **Junctional premature depolarization**

I49.3   **Ventricular premature depolarization**

I49.4   **Other and unspecified premature depolarization**

I49.40   **Unspecified premature depolarization**

Premature beats NOS

I49.49   **Other premature depolarization**

Ectopic beats

Extrasystoles

Extrasystolic arrhythmias

Premature contractions

I49.5   **Sick sinus syndrome**

Tachycardia-bradycardia syndrome

I49.8   **Other specified cardiac arrhythmias**

Coronary sinus rhythm disorder

Ectopic rhythm disorder

Nodal rhythm disorder

I49.9   **Cardiac arrhythmia, unspecified**

Arrhythmia (cardiac) NOS

I50   **Heart failure**

Definition: Heart failure is a condition where there is ineffective pumping of the heart leading to an accumulation of fluid in the lungs. Typical symptoms include shortness of breath with exertion, difficulty breathing when lying flat and leg or ankle swelling.

Code first heart failure complicating abortion or ectopic or molar pregnancy (O00-O07, O08.8)

heart failure due to hypertension (I11.0)

heart failure due to hypertension with chronic kidney disease (I13.-)

heart failure following surgery (I97.13-)

obstetric surgery and procedures (O75.4)

rheumatic heart failure (I09.81)

Excludes1: neonatal cardiac failure (P29.0)

Excludes2: cardiac arrest (I46.-)

I50.1   **Left ventricular failure**

Cardiac asthma

Edema of lung with heart disease NOS

Edema of lung with heart failure

Left heart failure

Pulmonary edema with heart disease NOS

Pulmonary edema with heart failure

Excludes1: edema of lung without heart disease or heart failure (J81.-)

pulmonary edema without heart disease or failure (J81.-)

I50.2   **Systolic (congestive) heart failure**

Excludes1: combined systolic (congestive) and diastolic (congestive) heart failure (I50.4-)

I50.20   **Unspecified systolic (congestive) heart failure**

I50.21   **Acute systolic (congestive) heart failure**

I50.22   **Chronic systolic (congestive) heart failure**

I50.23   **Acute on chronic systolic (congestive) heart failure**

I50.3   **Diastolic (congestive) heart failure**

Excludes1: combined systolic (congestive) and diastolic (congestive) heart failure (I50.4-)

I50.30   **Unspecified diastolic (congestive) heart failure**

I50.31   **Acute diastolic (congestive) heart failure**

I50.32   **Chronic diastolic (congestive) heart failure**

I50.33   **Acute on chronic diastolic (congestive) heart failure**

I50.4   **Combined systolic (congestive) and diastolic (congestive) heart failure**

I50.40   **Unspecified combined systolic (congestive) and diastolic (congestive) heart failure**

I50.41   **Acute combined systolic (congestive) and diastolic (congestive) heart failure**

I50.42   **Chronic combined systolic (congestive) and diastolic (congestive) heart failure**

I50.43   **Acute on chronic combined systolic (congestive) and diastolic (congestive) heart failure**

I50.9   **Heart failure, unspecified**

Biventricular (heart) failure NOS

Cardiac, heart or myocardial failure NOS

Congestive heart disease

Congestive heart failure NOS

Right ventricular failure (secondary to left heart failure)

Excludes2: fluid overload (E87.70)

I51   **Complications and ill-defined descriptions of heart disease**

Excludes1: any condition in I51.4-I51.9 due to hypertension (I11.-)

any condition in I51.4-I51.9 due to hypertension and chronic kidney disease (I13.-)

heart disease specified as rheumatic (I00-I09)

I51.0   **Cardiac septal defect, acquired**

Acquired septal atrial defect (old)

Acquired septal auricular defect (old)

Acquired septal ventricular defect (old)

Excludes1: cardiac septal defect as current complication following acute myocardial infarction (I23.1, I23.2)

I51.1   Rupture of chordae tendineae, not elsewhere classified

Excludes1: rupture of chordae tendineae as current complication following acute myocardial infarction (I23.4)

I51.2   Rupture of papillary muscle, not elsewhere classified

Excludes1: rupture of papillary muscle as current complication following acute myocardial infarction (I23.5)

I51.3   Intracardiac thrombosis, not elsewhere classified

Apical thrombosis (old)

Atrial thrombosis (old)

Auricular thrombosis (old)

Mural thrombosis (old)

Ventricular thrombosis (old)

Excludes1: intracardiac thrombosis as current complication following acute myocardial infarction (I23.6)

I51.4   Myocarditis, unspecified

Chronic (interstitial) myocarditis

Myocardial fibrosis

Myocarditis NOS

Excludes1: acute or subacute myocarditis (I40.-)

I51.5   Myocardial degeneration

Fatty degeneration of heart or myocardium

Myocardial disease

Senile degeneration of heart or myocardium

I51.7   Cardiomegaly

Cardiac dilatation

Cardiac hypertrophy

Ventricular dilatation

I51.8   Other ill-defined heart diseases

I51.81   Takotsubo syndrome

Reversible left ventricular dysfunction following sudden emotional stress

Stress induced cardiomyopathy

Takotsubo cardiomyopathy

Transient left ventricular apical ballooning syndrome

I51.89   Other ill-defined heart diseases

Carditis (acute)(chronic)

Pancarditis (acute)(chronic)

I51.9   Heart disease, unspecified

I52   Other heart disorders in diseases classified elsewhere

Code first underlying disease, such as:

congenital syphilis (A50.5)

mucopolysaccharidosis (E76.3)

schistosomiasis (B65.0-B65.9)

Excludes1: heart disease (in):

gonococcal infection (A54.83)

meningococcal infection (A39.50)

rheumatoid arthritis (M05.31)

syphilis (A52.06)

CEREBROVASCULAR DISEASES (I60-I69)

Use additional code to identify presence of:

alcohol abuse and dependence (F10.-)

exposure to environmental tobacco smoke (Z77.22)

history of tobacco dependence (Z87.891) hypertension (I10-I15)

occupational exposure to environmental tobacco smoke (Z57.31)

tobacco dependence (F17.-)

tobacco use (Z72.0)

Excludes1: transient cerebral ischemic attacks and related syndromes (G45.-)

traumatic intracranial hemorrhage (S06.-)

I60   Nontraumatic subarachnoid hemorrhage

Definition: Subarachnoid hemorrhage refers to bleeding within the head into the space between two membranes that surround the brain.

Includes: ruptured cerebral aneurysm

Excludes1: syphilitic ruptured cerebral aneurysm (A52.05)

Excludes2: sequelae of subarachnoid hemorrhage (I69.0-)

I60.0   Nontraumatic subarachnoid hemorrhage from carotid siphon and bifurcation

I60.00   Nontraumatic subarachnoid hemorrhage from unspecified carotid siphon and bifurcation

I60.01   Nontraumatic subarachnoid hemorrhage from right carotid siphon and bifurcation

I60.02   Nontraumatic subarachnoid hemorrhage from left carotid siphon and bifurcation

I60.1   Nontraumatic subarachnoid hemorrhage from middle cerebral artery

I60.10   Nontraumatic subarachnoid hemorrhage from unspecified middle cerebral artery

I60.11   Nontraumatic subarachnoid hemorrhage from right middle cerebral artery

I60.12   Nontraumatic subarachnoid hemorrhage from left middle cerebral artery

•I60.2   Nontraumatic subarachnoid hemorrhage from anterior communicating artery

I60.3   Nontraumatic subarachnoid hemorrhage from posterior communicating artery

I60.30   Nontraumatic subarachnoid hemorrhage from unspecified posterior communicating artery

I60.31   Nontraumatic subarachnoid hemorrhage from right posterior communicating artery

I60.32   Nontraumatic subarachnoid hemorrhage from left posterior communicating artery

I60.4   Nontraumatic subarachnoid hemorrhage from basilar artery

I60.5   Nontraumatic subarachnoid hemorrhage from vertebral artery

I60.50   Nontraumatic subarachnoid hemorrhage from unspecified vertebral artery

I60.51   Nontraumatic subarachnoid hemorrhage from right vertebral artery

I60.52   Nontraumatic subarachnoid hemorrhage from left vertebral artery

I60.6   Nontraumatic subarachnoid hemorrhage from other intracranial arteries

I60.7   Nontraumatic subarachnoid hemorrhage from unspecified intracranial artery

Ruptured (congenital) berry aneurysm

Ruptured (congenital) cerebral aneurysm

Subarachnoid hemorrhage (nontraumatic) from cerebral artery NOS

Subarachnoid hemorrhage (nontraumatic) from communicating artery NOS

Excludes1: berry aneurysm, nonruptured (I67.1)

I60.8   **Other nontraumatic subarachnoid hemorrhage**
   Meningeal hemorrhage
   Rupture of cerebral arteriovenous malformation

I60.9   **Nontraumatic subarachnoid hemorrhage, unspecified**

I61   **Nontraumatic intracerebral hemorrhage**

   Definition: Intracerebral hemorrhage is a medical condition indicated by the rupturing of a blood vessel in the brain and the subsequent bleeding into the tissues of the brain.

   Excludes2: sequelae of intracerebral hemorrhage (I69.1-)

I61.0   **Nontraumatic intracerebral hemorrhage in hemisphere, subcortical**
   Deep intracerebral hemorrhage (nontraumatic)

I61.1   **Nontraumatic intracerebral hemorrhage in hemisphere, cortical**
   Cerebral lobe hemorrhage (nontraumatic)
   Superficial intracerebral hemorrhage (nontraumatic)

I61.2   **Nontraumatic intracerebral hemorrhage in hemisphere, unspecified**

I61.3   **Nontraumatic intracerebral hemorrhage in brain stem**

I61.4   **Nontraumatic intracerebral hemorrhage in cerebellum**

I61.5   **Nontraumatic intracerebral hemorrhage, intraventricular**

I61.6   **Nontraumatic intracerebral hemorrhage, multiple localized**

I61.8   **Other nontraumatic intracerebral hemorrhage**

I61.9   **Nontraumatic intracerebral hemorrhage, unspecified**

I62   **Other and unspecified nontraumatic intracranial hemorrhage**

   Definition: Intracranial hemorrhage is bleeding in the brain caused by the breaking (rupture) of a blood vessel in the head.

   Excludes2: sequelae of intracranial hemorrhage (I69.2)

I62.0   **Nontraumatic subdural hemorrhage**

   I62.00   **Nontraumatic subdural hemorrhage, unspecified**

   I62.01   **Nontraumatic acute subdural hemorrhage**

   I62.02   **Nontraumatic subacute subdural hemorrhage**

   I62.03   **Nontraumatic chronic subdural hemorrhage**

I62.1   **Nontraumatic extradural hemorrhage**
   Nontraumatic epidural hemorrhage

I62.9   **Nontraumatic intracranial hemorrhage, unspecified**

I63   **Cerebral infarction**

   Includes: occlusion and stenosis of cerebral and precerebral arteries, resulting in cerebral infarction

   Use additional code, if applicable, to identify status post administration of tPA (rtPA) in a different facility within the last 24 hours prior to admission to current facility (Z92.82)

   Use additional code, if known, to indicate National Institutes of Health Stroke Scale (NIHSS) score (R29.7-)

   Excludes2: sequelae of cerebral infarction (I69.3-)

I63.0   **Cerebral infarction due to thrombosis of precerebral arteries**

   I63.00   **Cerebral infarction due to thrombosis of unspecified precerebral artery**

   I63.01   **Cerebral infarction due to thrombosis of vertebral artery**

      I63.011   **Cerebral infarction due to thrombosis of right vertebral artery**

      I63.012   **Cerebral infarction due to thrombosis of left vertebral artery**

      ●**I63.013**   **Cerebral infarction due to thrombosis of bilateral vertebral arteries**

      I63.019   **Cerebral infarction due to thrombosis of unspecified vertebral artery**

   I63.02   **Cerebral infarction due to thrombosis of basilar artery**

   I63.03   **Cerebral infarction due to thrombosis of carotid artery**

      I63.031   **Cerebral infarction due to thrombosis of right carotid artery**

      I63.032   **Cerebral infarction due to thrombosis of left carotid artery**

      ●**I63.033**   **Cerebral infarction due to thrombosis of bilateral carotid arteries**

      I63.039   **Cerebral infarction due to thrombosis of unspecified carotid artery**

   I63.09   **Cerebral infarction due to thrombosis of other precerebral artery**

I63.1   **Cerebral infarction due to embolism of precerebral arteries**

   I63.10   **Cerebral infarction due to embolism of unspecified precerebral artery**

   I63.11   **Cerebral infarction due to embolism of vertebral artery**

      I63.111   **Cerebral infarction due to embolism of right vertebral artery**

      I63.112   **Cerebral infarction due to embolism of left vertebral artery**

      ●**I63.113**   **Cerebral infarction due to embolism of bilateral vertebral arteries**

      I63.119   **Cerebral infarction due to embolism of unspecified vertebral artery**

   I63.12   **Cerebral infarction due to embolism of basilar artery**

   I63.13   **Cerebral infarction due to embolism of carotid artery**

      I63.131   **Cerebral infarction due to embolism of right carotid artery**

      I63.132   **Cerebral infarction due to embolism of left carotid artery**

      ●**I63.133**   **Cerebral infarction due to embolism of bilateral carotid arteries**

      I63.139   **Cerebral infarction due to embolism of unspecified carotid artery**

   I63.19   **Cerebral infarction due to embolism of other precerebral artery**

I63.2   **Cerebral infarction due to unspecified occlusion or stenosis of precerebral arteries**

   I63.20   **Cerebral infarction due to unspecified occlusion or stenosis of unspecified precerebral arteries**

   I63.21   **Cerebral infarction due to unspecified occlusion or stenosis of vertebral arteries**

● New code   ▲ Revised code   **Excludes1:** Not coded here   **Excludes2:** Not included here   ⊗ Placeholder required   ⑦ 7th digit required

I63.211   Cerebral infarction due to unspecified occlusion or stenosis of right vertebral arteries

I63.212   Cerebral infarction due to unspecified occlusion or stenosis of left vertebral arteries

• I63.213   Cerebral infarction due to unspecified occlusion or stenosis of bilateral vertebral arteries

I63.219   Cerebral infarction due to unspecified occlusion or stenosis of unspecified vertebral arteries

I63.22   Cerebral infarction due to unspecified occlusion or stenosis of basilar arteries

I63.23   Cerebral infarction due to unspecified occlusion or stenosis of carotid arteries

I63.231   Cerebral infarction due to unspecified occlusion or stenosis of right carotid arteries

I63.232   Cerebral infarction due to unspecified occlusion or stenosis of left carotid arteries

• I63.233   Cerebral infarction due to unspecified occlusion or stenosis of bilateral carotid arteries

I63.239   Cerebral infarction due to unspecified occlusion or stenosis of unspecified carotid arteries

I63.29   Cerebral infarction due to unspecified occlusion or stenosis of other precerebral arteries

I63.3   Cerebral infarction due to thrombosis of cerebral arteries

I63.30   Cerebral infarction due to thrombosis of unspecified cerebral artery

I63.31   Cerebral infarction due to thrombosis of middle cerebral artery

I63.311   Cerebral infarction due to thrombosis of right middle cerebral artery

I63.312   Cerebral infarction due to thrombosis of left middle cerebral artery

• I63.313   Cerebral infarction due to thrombosis of bilateral middle cerebral arteries

I63.319   Cerebral infarction due to thrombosis of unspecified middle cerebral artery

I63.32   Cerebral infarction due to thrombosis of anterior cerebral artery

I63.321   Cerebral infarction due to thrombosis of right anterior cerebral artery

I63.322   Cerebral infarction due to thrombosis of left anterior cerebral artery

• I63.323   Cerebral infarction due to thrombosis of bilateral anterior arteries

I63.329   Cerebral infarction due to thrombosis of unspecified anterior cerebral artery

I63.33   Cerebral infarction due to thrombosis of posterior cerebral artery

I63.331   Cerebral infarction due to thrombosis of right posterior cerebral artery

I63.332   Cerebral infarction due to thrombosis of left posterior cerebral artery

• I63.333   Cerebral infarction to thrombosis of bilateral posterior arteries

I63.339   Cerebral infarction due to thrombosis of unspecified posterior cerebral artery

I63.34   Cerebral infarction due to thrombosis of cerebellar artery

I63.341   Cerebral infarction due to thrombosis of right cerebellar artery

I63.342   Cerebral infarction due to thrombosis of left cerebellar artery

• I63.343   Cerebral infarction to thrombosis of bilateral cerebellar arteries

I63.349   Cerebral infarction due to thrombosis of unspecified cerebellar artery

I63.39   Cerebral infarction due to thrombosis of other cerebral artery

I63.4   Cerebral infarction due to embolism of cerebral arteries

I63.40   Cerebral infarction due to embolism of unspecified cerebral artery

I63.41   Cerebral infarction due to embolism of middle cerebral artery

I63.411   Cerebral infarction due to embolism of right middle cerebral artery

I63.412   Cerebral infarction due to embolism of left middle cerebral artery

• I63.413   Cerebral infarction due to embolism of bilateral middle cerebral arteries

I63.419   Cerebral infarction due to embolism of unspecified middle cerebral artery

I63.42   Cerebral infarction due to embolism of anterior cerebral artery

I63.421   Cerebral infarction due to embolism of right anterior cerebral artery

I63.422   Cerebral infarction due to embolism of left anterior cerebral artery

• I63.423   Cerebral infarction due to embolism of bilateral anterior cerebral arteries

I63.429   Cerebral infarction due to embolism of unspecified anterior cerebral artery

I63.43   Cerebral infarction due to embolism of posterior cerebral artery

I63.431 Cerebral infarction due to embolism of right posterior cerebral artery

I63.432 Cerebral infarction due to embolism of left posterior cerebral artery

•I63.433 Cerebral infarction due to embolism of bilateral posterior cerebral arteries

I63.439 Cerebral infarction due to embolism of unspecified posterior cerebral artery

I63.44 Cerebral infarction due to embolism of cerebellar artery

I63.441 Cerebral infarction due to embolism of right cerebellar artery

I63.442 Cerebral infarction due to embolism of left cerebellar artery

•I63.443 Cerebral infarction due to embolism of bilateral cerebellar arteries

I63.449 Cerebral infarction due to embolism of unspecified cerebellar artery

I63.49 Cerebral infarction due to embolism of other cerebral artery

I63.5 Cerebral infarction due to unspecified occlusion or stenosis of cerebral arteries

I63.50 Cerebral infarction due to unspecified occlusion or stenosis of unspecified cerebral artery

I63.51 Cerebral infarction due to unspecified occlusion or stenosis of middle cerebral artery

I63.511 Cerebral infarction due to unspecified occlusion or stenosis of right middle cerebral artery

I63.512 Cerebral infarction due to unspecified occlusion or stenosis of left middle cerebral artery

•I63.513 Cerebral infarction due to unspecified occlusion or stenosis of bilateral middle arteries

I63.519 Cerebral infarction due to unspecified occlusion or stenosis of unspecified middle cerebral artery

I63.52 Cerebral infarction due to unspecified occlusion or stenosis of anterior cerebral artery

I63.521 Cerebral infarction due to unspecified occlusion or stenosis of right anterior cerebral artery

I63.522 Cerebral infarction due to unspecified occlusion or stenosis of left anterior cerebral artery

•I63.523 Cerebral infarction due to unspecified occlusion or stenosis of bilateral anterior arteries

I63.529 Cerebral infarction due to unspecified occlusion or stenosis of unspecified anterior cerebral artery

I63.53 Cerebral infarction due to unspecified occlusion or stenosis of posterior cerebral artery

I63.531 Cerebral infarction due to unspecified occlusion or stenosis of right posterior cerebral artery

I63.532 Cerebral infarction due to unspecified occlusion or stenosis of left posterior cerebral artery

•I63.533 Cerebral infarction due to unspecified occlusion or stenosis of bilateral posterior arteries

I63.539 Cerebral infarction due to unspecified occlusion or stenosis of unspecified posterior cerebral artery

I63.54 Cerebral infarction due to unspecified occlusion or stenosis of cerebellar artery

I63.541 Cerebral infarction due to unspecified occlusion or stenosis of right cerebellar artery

I63.542 Cerebral infarction due to unspecified occlusion or stenosis of left cerebellar artery

•I63.543 Cerebral infarction due to unspecified occlusion or stenosis of bilateral cerebellar arteries

I63.549 Cerebral infarction due to unspecified occlusion or stenosis of unspecified cerebellar artery

I63.59 Cerebral infarction due to unspecified occlusion or stenosis of other cerebral artery

I63.6 Cerebral infarction due to cerebral venous thrombosis, nonpyogenic

I63.8 Other cerebral infarction

I63.9 Cerebral infarction, unspecified

Stroke NOS

I65 **Occlusion and stenosis of precerebral arteries, not resulting in cerebral infarction**

Includes: embolism of precerebral artery

narrowing of precerebral artery

obstruction (complete) (partial) of precerebral artery

thrombosis of precerebral artery

Excludes1: insufficiency, NOS, of precerebral artery (G45.-)

insufficiency of precerebral arteries causing cerebral infarction (I63.0-I63.2)

I65.0 Occlusion and stenosis of vertebral artery

I65.01 Occlusion and stenosis of right vertebral artery

I65.02 Occlusion and stenosis of left vertebral artery

I65.03 Occlusion and stenosis of bilateral vertebral arteries

I65.09 Occlusion and stenosis of unspecified vertebral artery

I65.1 Occlusion and stenosis of basilar artery

I65.2 Occlusion and stenosis of carotid artery

I65.21 Occlusion and stenosis of right carotid artery

I65.22 Occlusion and stenosis of left carotid artery

I65.23 Occlusion and stenosis of bilateral carotid arteries

I65.29 Occlusion and stenosis of unspecified carotid artery

I65.8 Occlusion and stenosis of other precerebral arteries

I65.9   **Occlusion and stenosis of unspecified precerebral artery**
Occlusion and stenosis of precerebral artery NOS

I66   **Occlusion and stenosis of cerebral arteries, not resulting in cerebral infarction**
Includes: embolism of cerebral artery
narrowing of cerebral artery
obstruction (complete) (partial) of cerebral artery
thrombosis of cerebral artery
Excludes1: Occlusion and stenosis of cerebral artery causing cerebral infarction (I63.3-I63.5)

I66.0   **Occlusion and stenosis of middle cerebral artery**
I66.01   **Occlusion and stenosis of right middle cerebral artery**
I66.02   **Occlusion and stenosis of left middle cerebral artery**
I66.03   **Occlusion and stenosis of bilateral middle cerebral arteries**
I66.09   **Occlusion and stenosis of unspecified middle cerebral artery**

I66.1   **Occlusion and stenosis of anterior cerebral artery**
I66.11   **Occlusion and stenosis of right anterior cerebral artery**
I66.12   **Occlusion and stenosis of left anterior cerebral artery**
I66.13   **Occlusion and stenosis of bilateral anterior cerebral arteries**
I66.19   **Occlusion and stenosis of unspecified anterior cerebral artery**

I66.2   **Occlusion and stenosis of posterior cerebral artery**
I66.21   **Occlusion and stenosis of right posterior cerebral artery**
I66.22   **Occlusion and stenosis of left posterior cerebral artery**
I66.23   **Occlusion and stenosis of bilateral posterior cerebral arteries**
I66.29   **Occlusion and stenosis of unspecified posterior cerebral artery**

I66.3   **Occlusion and stenosis of cerebellar arteries**
I66.8   **Occlusion and stenosis of other cerebral arteries**
Occlusion and stenosis of perforating arteries
I66.9   **Occlusion and stenosis of unspecified cerebral artery**

I67   **Other cerebrovascular diseases**
Excludes2: sequelae of the listed conditions (I69.8)
I67.0   **Dissection of cerebral arteries, nonruptured**
Excludes1: ruptured cerebral arteries (I60.7)
I67.1   **Cerebral aneurysm, nonruptured**
Cerebral aneurysm NOS
Cerebral arteriovenous fistula, acquired
Internal carotid artery aneurysm, intracranial portion
Internal carotid artery aneurysm, NOS
Excludes1: congenital cerebral aneurysm, nonruptured (Q28.-)
ruptured cerebral aneurysm (I60.7)
I67.2   **Cerebral atherosclerosis**
Atheroma of cerebral and precerebral arteries
I67.3   **Progressive vascular leukoencephalopathy**
Binswanger's disease
I67.4   **Hypertensive encephalopathy**

I67.5   **Moyamoya disease**
I67.6   **Nonpyogenic thrombosis of intracranial venous system**
Nonpyogenic thrombosis of cerebral vein
Nonpyogenic thrombosis of intracranial venous sinus
Excludes1: nonpyogenic thrombosis of intracranial venous system causing infarction (I63.6)
I67.7   **Cerebral arteritis, not elsewhere classified**
Granulomatous angiitis of the nervous system
Excludes1: allergic granulomatous angiitis (M30.1)
I67.8   **Other specified cerebrovascular diseases**
I67.81   **Acute cerebrovascular insufficiency**
Acute cerebrovascular insufficiency unspecified as to location or reversibility
I67.82   **Cerebral ischemia**
Chronic cerebral ischemia
I67.83   **Posterior reversible encephalopathy syndrome**
PRES
I67.84   **Cerebral vasospasm and vasoconstriction**
I67.841   **Reversible cerebrovascular vasoconstriction syndrome**
Call-Fleming syndrome
Code first underlying condition, if applicable, such as eclampsia (O15.00-O15.9)
I67.848   **Other cerebrovascular vasospasm and vasoconstriction**
I67.89   **Other cerebrovascular disease**
I67.9   **Cerebrovascular disease, unspecified**

I68   **Cerebrovascular disorders in diseases classified elsewhere**
I68.0   **Cerebral amyloid angiopathy**
Code first underlying amyloidosis (E85.-)
I68.2   **Cerebral arteritis in other diseases classified elsewhere**
Code first underlying disease
Excludes1: cerebral arteritis (in):
listerosis (A32.89)
systemic lupus erythematosus (M32.19)
syphilis (A52.04)
tuberculosis (A18.89)
I68.8   **Other cerebrovascular disorders in diseases classified elsewhere**
Code first underlying disease
Excludes1: syphilitic cerebral aneurysm (A52.05)

I69   **Sequelae of cerebrovascular disease**
Note: Category I69 is to be used to indicate conditions in I60-I67 as the cause of sequelae. The 'sequelae' include conditions specified as such or as residuals which may occur at any time after the onset of the causal condition
Excludes1: personal history of cerebral infarction without residual deficit (Z86.73)
personal history of prolonged reversible ischemic neurologic deficit (PRIND) (Z86.73)
personal history of reversible ischemic neurologcial deficit (RIND) (Z86.73)
sequelae of traumatic intracranial injury (S06.-)
transient ischemic attack (TIA) (G45.9)
I69.0   **Sequelae of nontraumatic subarachnoid hemorrhage**
I69.00   **Unspecified sequelae of nontraumatic subarachnoid hemorrhage**

I69.01 **Cognitive deficits following nontraumatic subarachnoid hemorrhage**

•I69.010 **Attention and concentration deficit following nontraumatic subarachnoid hemorrhage**

•I69.011 **Memory deficit following nontraumatic subarachnoid hemorrhage**

•I69.012 **Visuospatial deficit and spatial neglect following nontraumatic subarachnoid hemorrhage**

•I69.013 **Psychomotor deficit following nontraumatic subarachnoid hemorrhage**

•I69.014 **Frontal lobe and executive function deficit following nontraumatic subarachnoid hemorrhage**

•I69.015 **Cognitive social or emotional deficit following nontraumatic subarachnoid hemorrhage**

•I69.018 **Other symptoms and signs involving cognitive functions following nontraumatic subarachnoid hemorrhage**

•I69.019 **Unspecified symptoms and signs involving cognitive functions following nontraumatic subarachnoid hemorrhage**

I69.02 **Speech and language deficits following nontraumatic subarachnoid hemorrhage**

I69.020 **Aphasia following nontraumatic subarachnoid hemorrhage**

I69.021 **Dysphasia following nontraumatic subarachnoid hemorrhage**

I69.022 **Dysarthria following nontraumatic subarachnoid hemorrhage**

I69.023 **Fluency disorder following nontraumatic subarachnoid hemorrhage**

Stuttering following nontraumatic subarachnoid hemorrhage

I69.028 **Other speech and language deficits following nontraumatic subarachnoid hemorrhage**

I69.03 **Monoplegia of upper limb following nontraumatic subarachnoid hemorrhage**

I69.031 **Monoplegia of upper limb following nontraumatic subarachnoid hemorrhage affecting right dominant side**

I69.032 **Monoplegia of upper limb following nontraumatic subarachnoid hemorrhage affecting left dominant side**

I69.033 **Monoplegia of upper limb following nontraumatic subarachnoid hemorrhage affecting right non-dominant side**

I69.034 **Monoplegia of upper limb following nontraumatic subarachnoid hemorrhage affecting left non-dominant side**

I69.039 **Monoplegia of upper limb following nontraumatic subarachnoid**

hemorrhage affecting unspecified side

I69.04 **Monoplegia of lower limb following nontraumatic subarachnoid hemorrhage**

I69.041 **Monoplegia of lower limb following nontraumatic subarachnoid hemorrhage affecting right dominant side**

I69.042 **Monoplegia of lower limb following nontraumatic subarachnoid hemorrhage affecting left dominant side**

I69.043 **Monoplegia of lower limb following nontraumatic subarachnoid hemorrhage affecting right non-dominant side**

I69.044 **Monoplegia of lower limb following nontraumatic subarachnoid hemorrhage affecting left non-dominant side**

I69.049 **Monoplegia of lower limb following nontraumatic subarachnoid hemorrhage affecting unspecified side**

I69.05 **Hemiplegia and hemiparesis following nontraumatic subarachnoid hemorrhage**

I69.051 **Hemiplegia and hemiparesis following nontraumatic subarachnoid hemorrhage affecting right dominant side**

I69.052 **Hemiplegia and hemiparesis following nontraumatic subarachnoid hemorrhage affecting left dominant side**

I69.053 **Hemiplegia and hemiparesis following nontraumatic subarachnoid hemorrhage affecting right non-dominant side**

I69.054 **Hemiplegia and hemiparesis following nontraumatic subarachnoid hemorrhage affecting left non-dominant side**

I69.059 **Hemiplegia and hemiparesis following nontraumatic subarachnoid hemorrhage affecting unspecified side**

I69.06 **Other paralytic syndrome following nontraumatic subarachnoid hemorrhage**

Use additional code to identify type of paralytic syndrome, such as:

locked-in state (G83.5)

quadriplegia (G82.5-)

Excludes1: hemiplegia/hemiparesis following nontraumatic subarachnoid hemorrhage (I69.05-)

monoplegia of lower limb following nontraumatic subarachnoid hemorrhage (I69.04-)

monoplegia of upper limb following nontraumatic subarachnoid hemorrhage (I69.03-)

I69.061 **Other paralytic syndrome following nontraumatic subarachnoid hemorrhage affecting right dominant side**

I69.062 Other paralytic syndrome following nontraumatic subarachnoid hemorrhage affecting left dominant side

I69.063 Other paralytic syndrome following nontraumatic subarachnoid hemorrhage affecting right non-dominant side

I69.064 Other paralytic syndrome following nontraumatic subarachnoid hemorrhage affecting left non-dominant side

I69.065 Other paralytic syndrome following nontraumatic subarachnoid hemorrhage, bilateral

I69.069 Other paralytic syndrome following nontraumatic subarachnoid hemorrhage affecting unspecified side

I69.09 Other sequelae of nontraumatic subarachnoid hemorrhage

I69.090 Apraxia following nontraumatic subarachnoid hemorrhage

I69.091 Dysphagia following nontraumatic subarachnoid hemorrhage

Use additional code to identify the type of dysphagia, if known (R13.1-)

I69.092 Facial weakness following nontraumatic subarachnoid hemorrhage

Facial droop following nontraumatic subarachnoid hemorrhage

I69.093 Ataxia following nontraumatic subarachnoid hemorrhage

I69.098 Other sequelae following nontraumatic subarachnoid hemorrhage

Alterations of sensation following nontraumatic subarachnoid hemorrhage

Disturbance of vision following nontraumatic subarachnoid hemorrhage

Use additional code to identify the sequelae

I69.1 Sequelae of nontraumatic intracerebral hemorrhage

I69.10 Unspecified sequelae of nontraumatic intracerebral hemorrhage

I69.11 Cognitive deficits following nontraumatic intracerebral hemorrhage

•**I69.110** Attention and concentration deficit following nontraumatic intracerebral hemorrhage

•**I69.111** Memory deficit following nontraumatic intracerebral hemorrhage

•**I69.112** Visuospatial deficit and spatial neglect following nontraumatic intracerebral hemorrhage

•**I69.113** Psychomotor deficit following nontraumatic intracerebral hemorrhage

•**I69.114** Frontal lobe and executive function deficit following nontraumatic intracerebral hemorrhage

•**I69.115** Cognitive social or emotional deficit following nontraumatic intracerebral hemorrhage

•**I69.118** Other symptoms and signs involving cognitive functions following nontraumatic intracerebral hemorrhage

•**I69.119** Unspecified symptoms and signs involving cognitive functions following nontraumatic intracerebral hemorrhage

I69.12 Speech and language deficits following nontraumatic intracerebral hemorrhage

I69.120 Aphasia following nontraumatic intracerebral hemorrhage

I69.121 Dysphasia following nontraumatic intracerebral hemorrhage

I69.122 Dysarthria following nontraumatic intracerebral hemorrhage

I69.123 Fluency disorder following nontraumatic intracerebral hemorrhage

Stuttering following nontraumatic intracerebral hemorrhage

I69.128 Other speech and language deficits following nontraumatic intracerebral hemorrhage

I69.13 Monoplegia of upper limb following nontraumatic intracerebral hemorrhage

I69.131 Monoplegia of upper limb following nontraumatic intracerebral hemorrhage affecting right dominant side

I69.132 Monoplegia of upper limb following nontraumatic intracerebral hemorrhage affecting left dominant side

I69.133 Monoplegia of upper limb following nontraumatic intracerebral hemorrhage affecting right non-dominant side

I69.134 Monoplegia of upper limb following nontraumatic intracerebral hemorrhage affecting left non-dominant side

I69.139 Monoplegia of upper limb following nontraumatic intracerebral hemorrhage affecting unspecified side

I69.14 Monoplegia of lower limb following nontraumatic intracerebral hemorrhage

I69.141 Monoplegia of lower limb following nontraumatic intracerebral hemorrhage affecting right dominant side

I69.142 Monoplegia of lower limb following nontraumatic intracerebral hemorrhage affecting left dominant side

I69.143 Monoplegia of lower limb following nontraumatic intracerebral hemorrhage

hemorrhage affecting right non-dominant side

I69.144 **Monoplegia of lower limb following nontraumatic intracerebral hemorrhage affecting left non-dominant side**

I69.149 **Monoplegia of lower limb following nontraumatic intracerebral hemorrhage affecting unspecified side**

I69.15 **Hemiplegia and hemiparesis following nontraumatic intracerebral hemorrhage**

I69.151 **Hemiplegia and hemiparesis following nontraumatic intracerebral hemorrhage affecting right dominant side**

I69.152 **Hemiplegia and hemiparesis following nontraumatic intracerebral hemorrhage affecting left dominant side**

I69.153 **Hemiplegia and hemiparesis following nontraumatic intracerebral hemorrhage affecting right non-dominant side**

I69.154 **Hemiplegia and hemiparesis following nontraumatic intracerebral hemorrhage affecting left non-dominant side**

I69.159 **Hemiplegia and hemiparesis following nontraumatic intracerebral hemorrhage affecting unspecified side**

I69.16 **Other paralytic syndrome following nontraumatic intracerebral hemorrhage**

Use additional code to identify type of paralytic syndrome, such as:

locked-in state (G83.5)

quadriplegia (G82.5-)

Excludes1: hemiplegia/hemiparesis following nontraumatic intracerebral hemorrhage (I69.15-)

monoplegia of lower limb following nontraumatic intracerebral hemorrhage (I69.14-)

monoplegia of upper limb following nontraumatic intracerebral hemorrhage (I69.13-)

I69.161 **Other paralytic syndrome following nontraumatic intracerebral hemorrhage affecting right dominant side**

I69.162 **Other paralytic syndrome following nontraumatic intracerebral hemorrhage affecting left dominant side**

I69.163 **Other paralytic syndrome following nontraumatic intracerebral hemorrhage affecting right non-dominant side**

I69.164 **Other paralytic syndrome following nontraumatic intracerebral hemorrhage affecting left non-dominant side**

I69.165 **Other paralytic syndrome following nontraumatic intracerebral hemorrhage, bilateral**

I69.169 **Other paralytic syndrome following nontraumatic intracerebral hemorrhage affecting unspecified side**

I69.19 **Other sequelae of nontraumatic intracerebral hemorrhage**

I69.190 **Apraxia following nontraumatic intracerebral hemorrhage**

I69.191 **Dysphagia following nontraumatic intracerebral hemorrhage**

Use additional code to identify the type of dysphagia, if known (R13.1-)

I69.192 **Facial weakness following nontraumatic intracerebral hemorrhage**

Facial droop following nontraumatic intracerebral hemorrhage

I69.193 **Ataxia following nontraumatic intracerebral hemorrhage**

I69.198 **Other sequelae of nontraumatic intracerebral hemorrhage**

Alteration of sensations following nontraumatic intracerebral hemorrhage

Disturbance of vision following nontraumatic intracerebral hemorrhage

Use additional code to identify the sequelae

I69.2 **Sequelae of other nontraumatic intracranial hemorrhage**

I69.20 **Unspecified sequelae of other nontraumatic intracranial hemorrhage**

I69.21 **Cognitive deficits following other nontraumatic intracranial hemorrhage**

● **I69.210** **Attention and concentration deficit following other nontraumatic intracranial hemorrhage**

● **I69.211** **Memory deficit following other nontraumatic intracranial hemorrhage**

● **I69.212** **Visuospatial deficit and spatial neglect following other nontraumatic intracranial hemorrhage**

● **I69.213** **Psychomotor deficit following other nontraumatic intracranial hemorrhage**

● **I69.214** **Frontal lobe and executive function deficit following other nontraumatic intracranial hemorrhage**

● **I69.215** **Cognitive social or emotional deficit following other nontraumatic intracranial hemorrhage**

● **I69.218** **Other symptoms and signs involving cognitive functions following other nontraumatic intracranial hemorrhage**

● **I69.219** **Unspecified symptoms and signs involving cognitive functions following other nontraumatic intracranial hemorrhage**

I69.22 **Speech and language deficits following other nontraumatic intracranial hemorrhage**

I69.220   **Aphasia following other nontraumatic intracranial hemorrhage**

I69.221   **Dysphasia following other nontraumatic intracranial hemorrhage**

I69.222   **Dysarthria following other nontraumatic intracranial hemorrhage**

I69.223   **Fluency disorder following other nontraumatic intracranial hemorrhage**

Stuttering following other nontraumatic intracranial hemorrhage

I69.228   **Other speech and language deficits following other nontraumatic intracranial hemorrhage**

I69.23   **Monoplegia of upper limb following other nontraumatic intracranial hemorrhage**

I69.231   **Monoplegia of upper limb following other nontraumatic intracranial hemorrhage affecting right dominant side**

I69.232   **Monoplegia of upper limb following other nontraumatic intracranial hemorrhage affecting left dominant side**

I69.233   **Monoplegia of upper limb following other nontraumatic intracranial hemorrhage affecting right non-dominant side**

I69.234   **Monoplegia of upper limb following other nontraumatic intracranial hemorrhage affecting left non-dominant side**

I69.239   **Monoplegia of upper limb following other nontraumatic intracranial hemorrhage affecting unspecified side**

I69.24   **Monoplegia of lower limb following other nontraumatic intracranial hemorrhage**

I69.241   **Monoplegia of lower limb following other nontraumatic intracranial hemorrhage affecting right dominant side**

I69.242   **Monoplegia of lower limb following other nontraumatic intracranial hemorrhage affecting left dominant side**

I69.243   **Monoplegia of lower limb following other nontraumatic intracranial hemorrhage affecting right non-dominant side**

I69.244   **Monoplegia of lower limb following other nontraumatic intracranial hemorrhage affecting left non-dominant side**

I69.249   **Monoplegia of lower limb following other nontraumatic intracranial hemorrhage affecting unspecified side**

I69.25   **Hemiplegia and hemiparesis following other nontraumatic intracranial hemorrhage**

I69.251   **Hemiplegia and hemiparesis following other nontraumatic intracranial hemorrhage affecting right dominant side**

I69.252   **Hemiplegia and hemiparesis following other nontraumatic intracranial hemorrhage affecting left dominant side**

I69.253   **Hemiplegia and hemiparesis following other nontraumatic intracranial hemorrhage affecting right non-dominant side**

I69.254   **Hemiplegia and hemiparesis following other nontraumatic intracranial hemorrhage affecting left non-dominant side**

I69.259   **Hemiplegia and hemiparesis following other nontraumatic intracranial hemorrhage affecting unspecified side**

I69.26   **Other paralytic syndrome following other nontraumatic intracranial hemorrhage**

<u>Use additional code</u> to identify type of paralytic syndrome, such as:

locked-in state (G83.5)

quadriplegia (G82.5-)

Excludes1: hemiplegia/hemiparesis following other nontraumatic intracranial hemorrhage (I69.25-)

monoplegia of lower limb following other nontraumatic intracranial hemorrhage (I69.24-)

monoplegia of upper limb following other nontraumatic intracranial hemorrhage (I69.23-)

I69.261   **Other paralytic syndrome following other nontraumatic intracranial hemorrhage affecting right dominant side**

I69.262   **Other paralytic syndrome following other nontraumatic intracranial hemorrhage affecting left dominant side**

I69.263   **Other paralytic syndrome following other nontraumatic intracranial hemorrhage affecting right non-dominant side**

I69.264   **Other paralytic syndrome following other nontraumatic intracranial hemorrhage affecting left non-dominant side**

I69.265   **Other paralytic syndrome following other nontraumatic intracranial hemorrhage, bilateral**

I69.269   **Other paralytic syndrome following other nontraumatic intracranial hemorrhage affecting unspecified side**

I69.29   **Other sequelae of other nontraumatic intracranial hemorrhage**

I69.290   **Apraxia following other nontraumatic intracranial hemorrhage**

I69.291   **Dysphagia following other nontraumatic intracranial hemorrhage**

Use additional code to identify the type of dysphagia, if known (R13.1-)

I69.292 **Facial weakness following other nontraumatic intracranial hemorrhage**

Facial droop following other nontraumatic intracranial hemorrhage

I69.293 **Ataxia following other nontraumatic intracranial hemorrhage**

I69.298 **Other sequelae of other nontraumatic intracranial hemorrhage**

Alteration of sensation following other nontraumatic intracranial hemorrhage

Disturbance of vision following other nontraumatic intracranial hemorrhage

Use additional code to identify the sequelae

I69.3 **Sequelae of cerebral infarction**

Sequelae of stroke NOS

I69.30 **Unspecified sequelae of cerebral infarction**

I69.31 **Cognitive deficits following cerebral infarction**

- **I69.310** **Attention and concentration deficit following cerebral infarction**

- **I69.311** **Memory deficit following cerebral infarction**

- **I69.312** **Visuospatial deficit and spatial neglect following cerebral infarction**

- **I69.313** **Psychomotor deficit following cerebral infarction**

- **I69.314** **Frontal lobe and executive function deficit following cerebral infarction**

- **I69.315** **Cognitive social or emotional deficit following cerebral infarction**

- **I69.318** **Other symptoms and signs involving cognitive functions following cerebral infarction**

- **I69.319** **Unspecified symptoms and signs involving cognitive functions following cerebral infarction**

I69.32 **Speech and language deficits following cerebral infarction**

I69.320 **Aphasia following cerebral infarction**

I69.321 **Dysphasia following cerebral infarction**

I69.322 **Dysarthria following cerebral infarction**

I69.323 **Fluency disorder following cerebral infarction**

Stuttering following cerebral infarction

I69.328 **Other speech and language deficits following cerebral infarction**

I69.33 **Monoplegia of upper limb following cerebral infarction**

I69.331 **Monoplegia of upper limb following cerebral infarction affecting right dominant side**

I69.332 **Monoplegia of upper limb following cerebral infarction affecting left dominant side**

I69.333 **Monoplegia of upper limb following cerebral infarction affecting right non-dominant side**

I69.334 **Monoplegia of upper limb following cerebral infarction affecting left non-dominant side**

I69.339 **Monoplegia of upper limb following cerebral infarction affecting unspecified side**

I69.34 **Monoplegia of lower limb following cerebral infarction**

I69.341 **Monoplegia of lower limb following cerebral infarction affecting right dominant side**

I69.342 **Monoplegia of lower limb following cerebral infarction affecting left dominant side**

I69.343 **Monoplegia of lower limb following cerebral infarction affecting right non-dominant side**

I69.344 **Monoplegia of lower limb following cerebral infarction affecting left non-dominant side**

I69.349 **Monoplegia of lower limb following cerebral infarction affecting unspecified side**

I69.35 **Hemiplegia and hemiparesis following cerebral infarction**

I69.351 **Hemiplegia and hemiparesis following cerebral infarction affecting right dominant side**

I69.352 **Hemiplegia and hemiparesis following cerebral infarction affecting left dominant side**

I69.353 **Hemiplegia and hemiparesis following cerebral infarction affecting right non-dominant side**

I69.354 **Hemiplegia and hemiparesis following cerebral infarction affecting left non-dominant side**

I69.359 **Hemiplegia and hemiparesis following cerebral infarction affecting unspecified side**

I69.36 **Other paralytic syndrome following cerebral infarction**

Use additional code to identify type of paralytic syndrome, such as:

locked-in state (G83.5)

quadriplegia (G82.5-)

Excludes1: hemiplegia/hemiparesis following cerebral infarction (I69.35-)

monoplegia of lower limb following cerebral infarction (I69.34-)

monoplegia of upper limb following cerebral infarction (I69.33-)

I69.361 **Other paralytic syndrome following cerebral infarction affecting right dominant side**

● New code ▲ Revised code **Excludes1:** Not coded here **Excludes2:** Not included here ⊗ Placeholder required ⑦7th digit required

I69.362   **Other paralytic syndrome following cerebral infarction affecting left dominant side**

I69.363   **Other paralytic syndrome following cerebral infarction affecting right non-dominant side**

I69.364   **Other paralytic syndrome following cerebral infarction affecting left non-dominant side**

I69.365   **Other paralytic syndrome following cerebral infarction, bilateral**

I69.369   **Other paralytic syndrome following cerebral infarction affecting unspecified side**

I69.39   **Other sequelae of cerebral infarction**

I69.390   **Apraxia following cerebral infarction**

I69.391   **Dysphagia following cerebral infarction**

> **Use additional code** to identify the type of dysphagia, if known (R13.1-)

I69.392   **Facial weakness following cerebral infarction**

> Facial droop following cerebral infarction

I69.393   **Ataxia following cerebral infarction**

I69.398   **Other sequelae of cerebral infarction**

> Alteration of sensation following cerebral infarction
>
> Disturbance of vision following cerebral infarction
>
> **Use additional code** to identify the sequelae

I69.8   **Sequelae of other cerebrovascular diseases**

> **Excludes1:** sequelae of traumatic intracranial injury (S06.-)

I69.80   **Unspecified sequelae of other cerebrovascular disease**

I69.81   **Cognitive deficits following other cerebrovascular disease**

●**I69.810**   **Attention and concentration deficit following other cerebrovascular disease**

●**I69.811**   **Memory deficit following other cerebrovascular disease**

●**I69.812**   **Visuospatial deficit and spatial neglect following other cerebrovascular disease**

●**I69.813**   **Psychomotor deficit following other cerebrovascular disease**

●**I69.814**   **Frontal lobe and executive function deficit following other cerebrovascular disease**

●**I69.815**   **Cognitive social or emotional deficit following other cerebrovascular disease**

●**I69.818**   **Other symptoms and signs involving cognitive functions following other cerebrovascular disease**

●**I69.819**   **Unspecified symptoms and signs involving cognitive functions following other cerebrovascular disease**

I69.82   **Speech and language deficits following other cerebrovascular disease**

I69.820   **Aphasia following other cerebrovascular disease**

I69.821   **Dysphasia following other cerebrovascular disease**

I69.822   **Dysarthria following other cerebrovascular disease**

I69.823   **Fluency disorder following other cerebrovascular disease**

> Stuttering following other cerebrovascular disease

I69.828   **Other speech and language deficits following other cerebrovascular disease**

I69.83   **Monoplegia of upper limb following other cerebrovascular disease**

I69.831   **Monoplegia of upper limb following other cerebrovascular disease affecting right dominant side**

I69.832   **Monoplegia of upper limb following other cerebrovascular disease affecting left dominant side**

I69.833   **Monoplegia of upper limb following other cerebrovascular disease affecting right non-dominant side**

I69.834   **Monoplegia of upper limb following other cerebrovascular disease affecting left non-dominant side**

I69.839   **Monoplegia of upper limb following other cerebrovascular disease affecting unspecified side**

I69.84   **Monoplegia of lower limb following other cerebrovascular disease**

I69.841   **Monoplegia of lower limb following other cerebrovascular disease affecting right dominant side**

I69.842   **Monoplegia of lower limb following other cerebrovascular disease affecting left dominant side**

I69.843   **Monoplegia of lower limb following other cerebrovascular disease affecting right non-dominant side**

I69.844   **Monoplegia of lower limb following other cerebrovascular disease affecting left non-dominant side**

I69.849   **Monoplegia of lower limb following other cerebrovascular disease affecting unspecified side**

I69.85   **Hemiplegia and hemiparesis following other cerebrovascular disease**

I69.851   **Hemiplegia and hemiparesis following other cerebrovascular disease affecting right dominant side**

I69.852   **Hemiplegia and hemiparesis following other cerebrovascular disease affecting left dominant side**

I69.853   **Hemiplegia and hemiparesis following other cerebrovascular**

disease affecting right non-dominant side

I69.854 Hemiplegia and hemiparesis following other cerebrovascular disease affecting left non-dominant side

I69.859 Hemiplegia and hemiparesis following other cerebrovascular disease affecting unspecified side

I69.86 Other paralytic syndrome following other cerebrovascular disease

Use additional code to identify type of paralytic syndrome, such as:

locked-in state (G83.5)

quadriplegia (G82.5-)

Excludes1: hemiplegia/hemiparesis following other cerebrovascular disease (I69.85-)

monoplegia of lower limb following other cerebrovascular disease

(I69.84-)

monoplegia of upper limb following other cerebrovascular disease

(I69.83-)

I69.861 Other paralytic syndrome following other cerebrovascular disease affecting right dominant side

I69.862 Other paralytic syndrome following other cerebrovascular disease affecting left dominant side

I69.863 Other paralytic syndrome following other cerebrovascular disease affecting right non-dominant side

I69.864 Other paralytic syndrome following other cerebrovascular disease affecting left non-dominant side

I69.865 Other paralytic syndrome following other cerebrovascular disease, bilateral

I69.869 Other paralytic syndrome following other cerebrovascular disease affecting unspecified side

I69.89 Other sequelae of other cerebrovascular disease

I69.890 Apraxia following other cerebrovascular disease

I69.891 Dysphagia following other cerebrovascular disease

Use additional code to identify the type of dysphagia, if known (R13.1-)

I69.892 Facial weakness following other cerebrovascular disease

Facial droop following other cerebrovascular disease

I69.893 Ataxia following other cerebrovascular disease

I69.898 Other sequelae of other cerebrovascular disease

Alteration of sensation following other cerebrovascular disease

Disturbance of vision following other cerebrovascular disease

Use additional code to identify the sequelae

I69.9 Sequelae of unspecified cerebrovascular diseases

Excludes1: sequelae of stroke (I69.3)

sequelae of traumatic intracranial injury (S06.-)

I69.90 Unspecified sequelae of unspecified cerebrovascular disease

I69.91 Cognitive deficits following unspecified cerebrovascular disease

●**I69.910** Attention and concentration deficit following unspecified cerebrovascular disease

●**I69.911** Memory deficit following unspecified cerebrovascular disease

●**I69.912** Visuospatial deficit and spatial neglect following unspecified cerebrovascular disease

●**I69.913** Psychomotor deficit following unspecified cerebrovascular disease

●**I69.914** Frontal lobe and executive function deficit following unspecified cerebrovascular disease

●**I69.915** Cognitive social or emotional deficit following unspecified cerebrovascular disease

●**I69.918** Other symptoms and signs involving cognitive functions following unspecified cerebrovascular disease

●**I69.919** Unspecified symptoms and signs involving cognitive functions following unspecified cerebrovascular disease

I69.92 Speech and language deficits following unspecified cerebrovascular disease

I69.920 Aphasia following unspecified cerebrovascular disease

I69.921 Dysphasia following unspecified cerebrovascular disease

I69.922 Dysarthria following unspecified cerebrovascular disease

I69.923 Fluency disorder following unspecified cerebrovascular disease

Stuttering following unspecified cerebrovascular disease

I69.928 Other speech and language deficits following unspecified cerebrovascular disease

I69.93 Monoplegia of upper limb following unspecified cerebrovascular disease

I69.931 Monoplegia of upper limb following unspecified cerebrovascular disease affecting right dominant side

I69.932 Monoplegia of upper limb following unspecified cerebrovascular disease affecting left dominant side

I69.933 Monoplegia of upper limb following unspecified cerebrovascular disease affecting right non-dominant side

I69.934 Monoplegia of upper limb following unspecified cerebrovascular disease affecting left non-dominant side

● New code ▲ Revised code Excludes1: Not coded here Excludes2: Not included here ⊗ Placeholder required ⑦7th digit required

I69.939 Monoplegia of upper limb following unspecified cerebrovascular disease affecting unspecified side

I69.94 Monoplegia of lower limb following unspecified cerebrovascular disease

I69.941 Monoplegia of lower limb following unspecified cerebrovascular disease affecting right dominant side

I69.942 Monoplegia of lower limb following unspecified cerebrovascular disease affecting left dominant side

I69.943 Monoplegia of lower limb following unspecified cerebrovascular disease affecting right non-dominant side

I69.944 Monoplegia of lower limb following unspecified cerebrovascular disease affecting left non-dominant side

I69.949 Monoplegia of lower limb following unspecified cerebrovascular disease affecting unspecified side

I69.95 Hemiplegia and hemiparesis following unspecified cerebrovascular disease

I69.951 Hemiplegia and hemiparesis following unspecified cerebrovascular disease affecting right dominant side

I69.952 Hemiplegia and hemiparesis following unspecified cerebrovascular disease affecting left dominant side

I69.953 Hemiplegia and hemiparesis following unspecified cerebrovascular disease affecting right non-dominant side

I69.954 Hemiplegia and hemiparesis following unspecified cerebrovascular disease affecting left non-dominant side

I69.959 Hemiplegia and hemiparesis following unspecified cerebrovascular disease affecting unspecified side

I69.96 Other paralytic syndrome following unspecified cerebrovascular disease

Use additional code to identify type of paralytic syndrome, such as:

locked-in state (G83.5)

quadriplegia (G82.5-)

Excludes1: hemiplegia/hemiparesis following unspecified cerebrovascular disease (I69.95-)

monoplegia of lower limb following unspecified cerebrovascular disease (I69.94-)

monoplegia of upper limb following unspecified cerebrovascular disease (I69.93-)

I69.961 Other paralytic syndrome following unspecified cerebrovascular disease affecting right dominant side

I69.962 Other paralytic syndrome following unspecified cerebrovascular disease affecting left dominant side

I69.963 Other paralytic syndrome following unspecified cerebrovascular disease affecting right non-dominant side

I69.964 Other paralytic syndrome following unspecified cerebrovascular disease affecting left non-dominant side

I69.965 Other paralytic syndrome following unspecified cerebrovascular disease, bilateral

I69.969 Other paralytic syndrome following unspecified cerebrovascular disease affecting unspecified side

I69.99 Other sequelae of unspecified cerebrovascular disease

I69.990 Apraxia following unspecified cerebrovascular disease

I69.991 Dysphagia following unspecified cerebrovascular disease

Use additional code to identify the type of dysphagia, if known (R13.1-)

I69.992 Facial weakness following unspecified cerebrovascular disease

Facial droop following unspecified cerebrovascular disease

I69.993 Ataxia following unspecified cerebrovascular disease

I69.998 Other sequelae following unspecified cerebrovascular disease

Alteration in sensation following unspecified cerebrovascular disease

Disturbance of vision following unspecified cerebrovascular disease

Use additional code to identify the sequelae

DISEASES OF ARTERIES, ARTERIOLES AND CAPILLARIES (I70-I79)

I70 **Atherosclerosis**

Definition: Atherosclerosis is a condition in which an artery wall thickens as the result of a build up of fatty materials such as cholesterol. It is a syndrome affecting arterial blood vessels.

Includes: arteriolosclerosis

arterial degeneration arteriosclerosis

arteriosclerotic vascular disease

arteriovascular degeneration atheroma

endarteritis deformans or obliterans

senile arteritis

senile endarteritis vascular degeneration

Use additional code to identify:

exposure to environmental tobacco smoke (Z77.22) history of tobacco dependence (Z87.891)

occupational exposure to environmental tobacco smoke (Z57.31) tobacco dependence (F17.-)

tobacco use (Z72.0)

Excludes2: arteriosclerotic cardiovascular disease (I25.1-)

arteriosclerotic heart disease (I25.1-)

atheroembolism (I75.-)

cerebral atherosclerosis (I67.2)

coronary atherosclerosis (I25.1-)

mesenteric atherosclerosis (K55.1)

precerebral atherosclerosis (I67.2)

primary pulmonary atherosclerosis (I27.0)

I70.0   Atherosclerosis of aorta

I70.1   Atherosclerosis of renal artery

Goldblatt's kidney

Excludes2: atherosclerosis of renal arterioles (I12.-)

I70.2   Atherosclerosis of native arteries of the extremities

Mönckeberg's (medial) sclerosis

Use additional code, if applicable, to identify chronic total occlusion of artery of extremity (I70.92)

Excludes2: atherosclerosis of bypass graft of extremities (I70.30-I70.79)

I70.20   Unspecified atherosclerosis of native arteries of extremities

I70.201   Unspecified atherosclerosis of native arteries of extremities, right leg

I70.202   Unspecified atherosclerosis of native arteries of extremities, left leg

I70.203   Unspecified atherosclerosis of native arteries of extremities, bilateral legs

I70.208   Unspecified atherosclerosis of native arteries of extremities, other extremity

I70.209   Unspecified atherosclerosis of native arteries of extremities, unspecified extremity

I70.21   Atherosclerosis of native arteries of extremities with intermittent claudication

I70.211   Atherosclerosis of native arteries of extremities with intermittent claudication, right leg

I70.212   Atherosclerosis of native arteries of extremities with intermittent claudication, left leg

I70.213   Atherosclerosis of native arteries of extremities with intermittent claudication, bilateral legs

I70.218   Atherosclerosis of native arteries of extremities with intermittent claudication, other extremity

I70.219   Atherosclerosis of native arteries of extremities with intermittent claudication, unspecified extremity

I70.22   Atherosclerosis of native arteries of extremities with rest pain

Includes: any condition classifiable to I70.21-

I70.221   Atherosclerosis of native arteries of extremities with rest pain, right leg

I70.222   Atherosclerosis of native arteries of extremities with rest pain, left leg

I70.223   Atherosclerosis of native arteries of extremities with rest pain, bilateral legs

I70.228   Atherosclerosis of native arteries of extremities with rest pain, other extremity

I70.229   Atherosclerosis of native arteries of extremities with rest pain, unspecified extremity

I70.23   Atherosclerosis of native arteries of right leg with ulceration

Includes: any condition classifiable to I70.211 and I70.221

Use additional code to identify severity of ulcer (L97.-)

I70.231   Atherosclerosis of native arteries of right leg with ulceration of thigh

I70.232   Atherosclerosis of native arteries of right leg with ulceration of calf

I70.233   Atherosclerosis of native arteries of right leg with ulceration of ankle

I70.234   Atherosclerosis of native arteries of right leg with ulceration of heel and midfoot

Atherosclerosis of native arteries of right leg with ulceration of plantar surface of midfoot

I70.235   Atherosclerosis of native arteries of right leg with ulceration of other part of foot

Atherosclerosis of native arteries of right leg extremities with ulceration of toe

I70.238   Atherosclerosis of native arteries of right leg with ulceration of other part of lower right leg

I70.239   Atherosclerosis of native arteries of right leg with ulceration of unspecified site

I70.24   Atherosclerosis of native arteries of left leg with ulceration

Includes: any condition classifiable to I70.212 and I70.222

Use additional code to identify severity of ulcer (L97.-)

I70.241   Atherosclerosis of native arteries of left leg with ulceration of thigh

I70.242   Atherosclerosis of native arteries of left leg with ulceration of calf

I70.243   Atherosclerosis of native arteries of left leg with ulceration of ankle

I70.244   Atherosclerosis of native arteries of left leg with ulceration of heel and midfoot

Atherosclerosis of native arteries of left leg with ulceration of plantar surface of midfoot

I70.245   Atherosclerosis of native arteries of left leg with ulceration of other part of foot

Atherosclerosis of native arteries of left leg extremities with ulceration of toe

I70.248   Atherosclerosis of native arteries of left leg with ulceration of other part of lower left leg

I70.249   Atherosclerosis of native arteries of left leg with ulceration of unspecified site

I70.25   Atherosclerosis of native arteries of other extremities with ulceration

Includes: any condition classifiable to I70.218 and I70.228

● New code   ▲ Revised code   **Excludes1:** Not coded here   **Excludes2:** Not included here   ⊗ Placeholder required   ⑦7th digit required

Use additional code to identify the severity of the ulcer (L98.49-)

I70.26 **Atherosclerosis of native arteries of extremities with gangrene**

Includes: any condition classifiable to I70.21-, I70.22-, I70.23-, I70.24-, and I70.25-

Use additional code to identify the severity of any ulcer (L97.-, L98.49-), if applicable

  I70.261 **Atherosclerosis of native arteries of extremities with gangrene, right leg**

  I70.262 **Atherosclerosis of native arteries of extremities with gangrene, left leg**

  I70.263 **Atherosclerosis of native arteries of extremities with gangrene, bilateral legs**

  I70.268 **Atherosclerosis of native arteries of extremities with gangrene, other extremity**

  I70.269 **Atherosclerosis of native arteries of extremities with gangrene, unspecified extremity**

I70.29 **Other atherosclerosis of native arteries of extremities**

  I70.291 **Other atherosclerosis of native arteries of extremities, right leg**

  I70.292 **Other atherosclerosis of native arteries of extremities, left leg**

  I70.293 **Other atherosclerosis of native arteries of extremities, bilateral legs**

  I70.298 **Other atherosclerosis of native arteries of extremities, other extremity**

  I70.299 **Other atherosclerosis of native arteries of extremities, unspecified extremity**

I70.3 **Atherosclerosis of unspecified type of bypass graft(s) of the extremities**

Use additional code, if applicable, to identify chronic total occlusion of artery of extremity (I70.92)

Excludes1: embolism or thrombus of bypass graft(s) of extremities (T82.8-)

I70.30 **Unspecified atherosclerosis of unspecified type of bypass graft(s) of the extremities**

  I70.301 **Unspecified atherosclerosis of unspecified type of bypass graft(s) of the extremities, right leg**

  I70.302 **Unspecified atherosclerosis of unspecified type of bypass graft(s) of the extremities, left leg**

  I70.303 **Unspecified atherosclerosis of unspecified type of bypass graft(s) of the extremities, bilateral legs**

  I70.308 **Unspecified atherosclerosis of unspecified type of bypass graft(s) of the extremities, other extremity**

  I70.309 **Unspecified atherosclerosis of unspecified type of bypass graft(s) of the extremities, unspecified extremity**

I70.31 **Atherosclerosis of unspecified type of bypass graft(s) of the extremities with intermittent claudication**

  I70.311 **Atherosclerosis of unspecified type of bypass graft(s) of the extremities with intermittent claudication, right leg**

  I70.312 **Atherosclerosis of unspecified type of bypass graft(s) of the extremities with intermittent claudication, left leg**

  I70.313 **Atherosclerosis of unspecified type of bypass graft(s) of the extremities with intermittent claudication, bilateral legs**

  I70.318 **Atherosclerosis of unspecified type of bypass graft(s) of the extremities with intermittent claudication, other extremity**

  I70.319 **Atherosclerosis of unspecified type of bypass graft(s) of the extremities with intermittent claudication, unspecified extremity**

I70.32 **Atherosclerosis of unspecified type of bypass graft(s) of the extremities with rest pain**

Includes: any condition classifiable to I70.31-

  I70.321 **Atherosclerosis of unspecified type of bypass graft(s) of the extremities with rest pain, right leg**

  I70.322 **Atherosclerosis of unspecified type of bypass graft(s) of the extremities with rest pain, left leg**

  I70.323 **Atherosclerosis of unspecified type of bypass graft(s) of the extremities with rest pain, bilateral legs**

  I70.328 **Atherosclerosis of unspecified type of bypass graft(s) of the extremities with rest pain, other extremity**

  I70.329 **Atherosclerosis of unspecified type of bypass graft(s) of the extremities with rest pain, unspecified extremity**

I70.33 **Atherosclerosis of unspecified type of bypass graft(s) of the right leg with ulceration**

Includes: any condition classifiable to I70.311 and I70.321

Use additional code to identify severity of ulcer (L97.-)

  I70.331 **Atherosclerosis of unspecified type of bypass graft(s) of the right leg with ulceration of thigh**

  I70.332 **Atherosclerosis of unspecified type of bypass graft(s) of the right leg with ulceration of calf**

  I70.333 **Atherosclerosis of unspecified type of bypass graft(s) of the right leg with ulceration of ankle**

  I70.334 **Atherosclerosis of unspecified type of bypass graft(s) of the right leg with ulceration of heel and midfoot**

    Atherosclerosis of unspecified type of bypass graft(s) of right leg with ulceration of plantar surface of midfoot

  I70.335 **Atherosclerosis of unspecified type of bypass graft(s) of the right leg with ulceration of other part of foot**

Atherosclerosis of unspecified type of bypass graft(s) of the right leg with ulceration of toe

I70.338 Atherosclerosis of unspecified type of bypass graft(s) of the right leg with ulceration of other part of lower leg

I70.339 Atherosclerosis of unspecified type of bypass graft(s) of the right leg with ulceration of unspecified site

I70.34 Atherosclerosis of unspecified type of bypass graft(s) of the left leg with ulceration

Includes: any condition classifiable to I70.312 and I70.322

Use additional code to identify severity of ulcer (L97.-)

I70.341 Atherosclerosis of unspecified type of bypass graft(s) of the left leg with ulceration of thigh

I70.342 Atherosclerosis of unspecified type of bypass graft(s) of the left leg with ulceration of calf

I70.343 Atherosclerosis of unspecified type of bypass graft(s) of the left leg with ulceration of ankle

I70.344 Atherosclerosis of unspecified type of bypass graft(s) of the left leg with ulceration of heel and midfoot

Atherosclerosis of unspecified type of bypass graft(s) of left leg with ulceration of plantar surface of midfoot

I70.345 Atherosclerosis of unspecified type of bypass graft(s) of the left leg with ulceration of other part of foot

Atherosclerosis of unspecified type of bypass graft(s) of the left leg with ulceration of toe

I70.348 Atherosclerosis of unspecified type of bypass graft(s) of the left leg with ulceration of other part of lower leg

I70.349 Atherosclerosis of unspecified type of bypass graft(s) of the left leg with ulceration of unspecified site

I70.35 Atherosclerosis of unspecified type of bypass graft(s) of other extremity with ulceration

Includes: any condition classifiable to I70.318 and I70.328

Use additional code to identify severity of ulcer (L98.49-)

I70.36 Atherosclerosis of unspecified type of bypass graft(s) of the extremities with gangrene

Includes: any condition classifiable to I70.31-, I70.32-, I70.33-, I70.34-, I70.35

Use additional code to identify the severity of any ulcer (L97.-, L98.49-), if applicable

I70.361 Atherosclerosis of unspecified type of bypass graft(s) of the extremities with gangrene, right leg

I70.362 Atherosclerosis of unspecified type of bypass graft(s) of the extremities with gangrene, left leg

I70.363 Atherosclerosis of unspecified type of bypass graft(s) of the extremities with gangrene, bilateral legs

I70.368 Atherosclerosis of unspecified type of bypass graft(s) of the extremities with gangrene, other extremity

I70.369 Atherosclerosis of unspecified type of bypass graft(s) of the extremities with gangrene, unspecified extremity

I70.39 Other atherosclerosis of unspecified type of bypass graft(s) of the extremities

I70.391 Other atherosclerosis of unspecified type of bypass graft(s) of the extremities, right leg

I70.392 Other atherosclerosis of unspecified type of bypass graft(s) of the extremities, left leg

I70.393 Other atherosclerosis of unspecified type of bypass graft(s) of the extremities, bilateral legs

I70.398 Other atherosclerosis of unspecified type of bypass graft(s) of the extremities, other extremity

I70.399 Other atherosclerosis of unspecified type of bypass graft(s) of the extremities, unspecified extremity

I70.4 Atherosclerosis of autologous vein bypass graft(s) of the extremities

Use additional code, if applicable, to identify chronic total occlusion of artery of extremity (I70.92)

I70.40 Unspecified atherosclerosis of autologous vein bypass graft(s) of the extremities

I70.401 Unspecified atherosclerosis of autologous vein bypass graft(s) of the extremities, right leg

I70.402 Unspecified atherosclerosis of autologous vein bypass graft(s) of the extremities, left leg

I70.403 Unspecified atherosclerosis of autologous vein bypass graft(s) of the extremities, bilateral legs

I70.408 Unspecified atherosclerosis of autologous vein bypass graft(s) of the extremities, other extremity

I70.409 Unspecified atherosclerosis of autologous vein bypass graft(s) of the extremities, unspecified extremity

I70.41 Atherosclerosis of autologous vein bypass graft(s) of the extremities with intermittent claudication

I70.411 Atherosclerosis of autologous vein bypass graft(s) of the extremities with intermittent claudication, right leg

I70.412 Atherosclerosis of autologous vein bypass graft(s) of the extremities with intermittent claudication, left leg

I70.413 Atherosclerosis of autologous vein bypass graft(s) of the extremities with intermittent claudication, bilateral legs

I70.418   **Atherosclerosis of autologous vein bypass graft(s) of the extremities with intermittent claudication, other extremity**

I70.419   **Atherosclerosis of autologous vein bypass graft(s) of the extremities with intermittent claudication, unspecified extremity**

I70.42   **Atherosclerosis of autologous vein bypass graft(s) of the extremities with rest pain**

Includes: any condition classifiable to I70.41-

I70.421   **Atherosclerosis of autologous vein bypass graft(s) of the extremities with rest pain, right leg**

I70.422   **Atherosclerosis of autologous vein bypass graft(s) of the extremities with rest pain, left leg**

I70.423   **Atherosclerosis of autologous vein bypass graft(s) of the extremities with rest pain, bilateral legs**

I70.428   **Atherosclerosis of autologous vein bypass graft(s) of the extremities with rest pain, other extremity**

I70.429   **Atherosclerosis of autologous vein bypass graft(s) of the extremities with rest pain, unspecified extremity**

I70.43   **Atherosclerosis of autologous vein bypass graft(s) of the right leg with ulceration**

Includes: any condition classifiable to I70.411 and I70.421

Use additional code to identify severity of ulcer (L97.-)

I70.431   **Atherosclerosis of autologous vein bypass graft(s) of the right leg with ulceration of thigh**

I70.432   **Atherosclerosis of autologous vein bypass graft(s) of the right leg with ulceration of calf**

I70.433   **Atherosclerosis of autologous vein bypass graft(s) of the right leg with ulceration of ankle**

I70.434   **Atherosclerosis of autologous vein bypass graft(s) of the right leg with ulceration of heel and midfoot**

Atherosclerosis of autologous vein bypass graft(s) of right leg with ulceration of plantar surface of midfoot

I70.435   **Atherosclerosis of autologous vein bypass graft(s) of the right leg with ulceration of other part of foot**

Atherosclerosis of autologous vein bypass graft(s) of right leg with ulceration of toe

I70.438   **Atherosclerosis of autologous vein bypass graft(s) of the right leg with ulceration of other part of lower leg**

I70.439   **Atherosclerosis of autologous vein bypass graft(s) of the right leg with ulceration of unspecified site**

I70.44   **Atherosclerosis of autologous vein bypass graft(s) of the left leg with ulceration**

Includes: any condition classifiable to I70.412 and I70.422

Use additional code to identify severity of ulcer (L97.-)

I70.441   **Atherosclerosis of autologous vein bypass graft(s) of the left leg with ulceration of thigh**

I70.442   **Atherosclerosis of autologous vein bypass graft(s) of the left leg with ulceration of calf**

I70.443   **Atherosclerosis of autologous vein bypass graft(s) of the left leg with ulceration of ankle**

I70.444   **Atherosclerosis of autologous vein bypass graft(s) of the left leg with ulceration of heel and midfoot**

Atherosclerosis of autologous vein bypass graft(s) of left leg with ulceration of plantar surface of midfoot

I70.445   **Atherosclerosis of autologous vein bypass graft(s) of the left leg with ulceration of other part of foot**

Atherosclerosis of autologous vein bypass graft(s) of left leg with ulceration of toe

I70.448   **Atherosclerosis of autologous vein bypass graft(s) of the left leg with ulceration of other part of lower leg**

I70.449   **Atherosclerosis of autologous vein bypass graft(s) of the left leg with ulceration of unspecified site**

I70.45   **Atherosclerosis of autologous vein bypass graft(s) of other extremity with ulceration**

Includes: any condition classifiable to I70.418, I70.428, and I70.438

Use additional code to identify severity of ulcer (L98.49)

I70.46   **Atherosclerosis of autologous vein bypass graft(s) of the extremities with gangrene**

Includes: any condition classifiable to I70.41-, I70.42-, and I70.43-, I70.44-, I70.45

Use additional code to identify the severity of any ulcer (L97.-, L98.49-), if applicable

I70.461   **Atherosclerosis of autologous vein bypass graft(s) of the extremities with gangrene, right leg**

I70.462   **Atherosclerosis of autologous vein bypass graft(s) of the extremities with gangrene, left leg**

I70.463   **Atherosclerosis of autologous vein bypass graft(s) of the extremities with gangrene, bilateral legs**

I70.468   **Atherosclerosis of autologous vein bypass graft(s) of the extremities with gangrene, other extremity**

I70.469   **Atherosclerosis of autologous vein bypass graft(s) of the extremities with gangrene, unspecified extremity**

I70.49   **Other atherosclerosis of autologous vein bypass graft(s) of the extremities**

I70.491 Other atherosclerosis of autologous vein bypass graft(s) of the extremities, right leg

I70.492 Other atherosclerosis of autologous vein bypass graft(s) of the extremities, left leg

I70.493 Other atherosclerosis of autologous vein bypass graft(s) of the extremities, bilateral legs

I70.498 Other atherosclerosis of autologous vein bypass graft(s) of the extremities, other extremity

I70.499 Other atherosclerosis of autologous vein bypass graft(s) of the extremities, unspecified extremity

I70.5 Atherosclerosis of nonautologous biological bypass graft(s) of the extremities

Use additional code, if applicable, to identify chronic total occlusion of artery of extremity (I70.92)

I70.50 Unspecified atherosclerosis of nonautologous biological bypass graft(s) of the extremities

I70.501 Unspecified atherosclerosis of nonautologous biological bypass graft(s) of the extremities, right leg

I70.502 Unspecified atherosclerosis of nonautologous biological bypass graft(s) of the extremities, left leg

I70.503 Unspecified atherosclerosis of nonautologous biological bypass graft(s) of the extremities, bilateral legs

I70.508 Unspecified atherosclerosis of nonautologous biological bypass graft(s) of the extremities, other extremity

I70.509 Unspecified atherosclerosis of nonautologous biological bypass graft(s) of the extremities, unspecified extremity

I70.51 Atherosclerosis of nonautologous biological bypass graft(s) of the extremities intermittent claudication

I70.511 Atherosclerosis of nonautologous biological bypass graft(s) of the extremities with intermittent claudication, right leg

I70.512 Atherosclerosis of nonautologous biological bypass graft(s) of the extremities with intermittent claudication, left leg

I70.513 Atherosclerosis of nonautologous biological bypass graft(s) of the extremities with intermittent claudication, bilateral legs

I70.518 Atherosclerosis of nonautologous biological bypass graft(s) of the extremities with intermittent claudication, other extremity

I70.519 Atherosclerosis of nonautologous biological bypass graft(s) of the extremities with intermittent claudication, unspecified extremity

I70.52 Atherosclerosis of nonautologous biological bypass graft(s) of the extremities with rest pain

Includes: any condition classifiable to I70.51-

I70.521 Atherosclerosis of nonautologous biological bypass graft(s) of the extremities with rest pain, right leg

I70.522 Atherosclerosis of nonautologous biological bypass graft(s) of the extremities with rest pain, left leg

I70.523 Atherosclerosis of nonautologous biological bypass graft(s) of the extremities with rest pain, bilateral legs

I70.528 Atherosclerosis of nonautologous biological bypass graft(s) of the extremities with rest pain, other extremity

I70.529 Atherosclerosis of nonautologous biological bypass graft(s) of the extremities with rest pain, unspecified extremity

I70.53 Atherosclerosis of nonautologous biological bypass graft(s) of the right leg with ulceration

Includes: any condition classifiable to I70.511 and I70.521

Use additional code to identify severity of ulcer (L97.-)

I70.531 Atherosclerosis of nonautologous biological bypass graft(s) of the right leg with ulceration of thigh

I70.532 Atherosclerosis of nonautologous biological bypass graft(s) of the right leg with ulceration of calf

I70.533 Atherosclerosis of nonautologous biological bypass graft(s) of the right leg with ulceration of ankle

I70.534 Atherosclerosis of nonautologous biological bypass graft(s) of the right leg with ulceration of heel and midfoot

Atherosclerosis of nonautologous biological bypass graft(s) of right leg with ulceration of plantar surface of midfoot

I70.535 Atherosclerosis of nonautologous biological bypass graft(s) of the right leg with ulceration of other part of foot

Atherosclerosis of nonautologous biological bypass graft(s) of the right leg with ulceration of toe

I70.538 Atherosclerosis of nonautologous biological bypass graft(s) of the right leg with ulceration of other part of lower leg

I70.539 Atherosclerosis of nonautologous biological bypass graft(s) of the right leg with ulceration of unspecified site

I70.54 Atherosclerosis of nonautologous biological bypass graft(s) of the left leg with ulceration

Includes: any condition classifiable to I70.512 and I70.522

Use additional code to identify severity of ulcer (L97.-)

● New code ▲ Revised code **Excludes1:** Not coded here **Excludes2:** Not included here ⊗ Placeholder required ⑦ 7th digit required

I70.541 Atherosclerosis of nonautologous biological bypass graft(s) of the left leg with ulceration of thigh

I70.542 Atherosclerosis of nonautologous biological bypass graft(s) of the left leg with ulceration of calf

I70.543 Atherosclerosis of nonautologous biological bypass graft(s) of the left leg with ulceration of ankle

I70.544 Atherosclerosis of nonautologous biological bypass graft(s) of the left leg with ulceration of heel and midfoot

Atherosclerosis of nonautologous biological bypass graft(s) of left leg with ulceration of plantar surface of midfoot

I70.545 Atherosclerosis of nonautologous biological bypass graft(s) of the left leg with ulceration of other part of foot

Atherosclerosis of nonautologous biological bypass graft(s) of the left leg with ulceration of toe

I70.548 Atherosclerosis of nonautologous biological bypass graft(s) of the left leg with ulceration of other part of lower leg

I70.549 Atherosclerosis of nonautologous biological bypass graft(s) of the left leg with ulceration of unspecified site

I70.55 Atherosclerosis of nonautologous biological bypass graft(s) of other extremity with ulceration

Includes: any condition classifiable to I70.518, I70.528, and I70.538

Use additional code to identify severity of ulcer (L98.49)

I70.56 Atherosclerosis of nonautologous biological bypass graft(s) of the extremities with gangrene

Includes: any condition classifiable to I70.51-, I70.52-, and I70.53-, I70.54-, I70.55

Use additional code to identify the severity of any ulcer (L97.-, L98.49-), if applicable

I70.561 Atherosclerosis of nonautologous biological bypass graft(s) of the extremities with gangrene, right leg

I70.562 Atherosclerosis of nonautologous biological bypass graft(s) of the extremities with gangrene, left leg

I70.563 Atherosclerosis of nonautologous biological bypass graft(s) of the extremities with gangrene, bilateral legs

I70.568 Atherosclerosis of nonautologous biological bypass graft(s) of the extremities with gangrene, other extremity

I70.569 Atherosclerosis of nonautologous biological bypass graft(s) of the extremities with gangrene, unspecified extremity

I70.59 Other atherosclerosis of nonautologous biological bypass graft(s) of the extremities

I70.591 Other atherosclerosis of nonautologous biological bypass graft(s) of the extremities, right leg

I70.592 Other atherosclerosis of nonautologous biological bypass graft(s) of the extremities, left leg

I70.593 Other atherosclerosis of nonautologous biological bypass graft(s) of the extremities, bilateral legs

I70.598 Other atherosclerosis of nonautologous biological bypass graft(s) of the extremities, other extremity

I70.599 Other atherosclerosis of nonautologous biological bypass graft(s) of the extremities, unspecified extremity

I70.6 Atherosclerosis of nonbiological bypass graft(s) of the extremities

Use additional code, if applicable, to identify chronic total occlusion of artery of extremity (I70.92)

I70.60 Unspecified atherosclerosis of nonbiological bypass graft(s) of the extremities

I70.601 Unspecified atherosclerosis of nonbiological bypass graft(s) of the extremities, right leg

I70.602 Unspecified atherosclerosis of nonbiological bypass graft(s) of the extremities, left leg

I70.603 Unspecified atherosclerosis of nonbiological bypass graft(s) of the extremities, bilateral legs

I70.608 Unspecified atherosclerosis of nonbiological bypass graft(s) of the extremities, other extremity

I70.609 Unspecified atherosclerosis of nonbiological bypass graft(s) of the extremities, unspecified extremity

I70.61 Atherosclerosis of nonbiological bypass graft(s) of the extremities with intermittent claudication

I70.611 Atherosclerosis of nonbiological bypass graft(s) of the extremities with intermittent claudication, right leg

I70.612 Atherosclerosis of nonbiological bypass graft(s) of the extremities with intermittent claudication, left leg

I70.613 Atherosclerosis of nonbiological bypass graft(s) of the extremities with intermittent claudication, bilateral legs

I70.618 Atherosclerosis of nonbiological bypass graft(s) of the extremities with intermittent claudication, other extremity

I70.619 Atherosclerosis of nonbiological bypass graft(s) of the extremities with intermittent claudication, unspecified extremity

I70.62 **Atherosclerosis of nonbiological bypass graft(s) of the extremities with rest pain**

Includes: any condition classifiable to I70.61-

I70.621 **Atherosclerosis of nonbiological bypass graft(s) of the extremities with rest pain, right leg**

I70.622 **Atherosclerosis of nonbiological bypass graft(s) of the extremities with rest pain, left leg**

I70.623 **Atherosclerosis of nonbiological bypass graft(s) of the extremities with rest pain, bilateral legs**

I70.628 **Atherosclerosis of nonbiological bypass graft(s) of the extremities with rest pain, other extremity**

I70.629 **Atherosclerosis of nonbiological bypass graft(s) of the extremities with rest pain, unspecified extremity**

I70.63 **Atherosclerosis of nonbiological bypass graft(s) of the right leg with ulceration**

Includes: any condition classifiable to I70.611 and I70.621

Use additional code to identify severity of ulcer (L97.-)

I70.631 **Atherosclerosis of nonbiological bypass graft(s) of the right leg with ulceration of thigh**

I70.632 **Atherosclerosis of nonbiological bypass graft(s) of the right leg with ulceration of calf**

I70.633 **Atherosclerosis of nonbiological bypass graft(s) of the right leg with ulceration of ankle**

I70.634 **Atherosclerosis of nonbiological bypass graft(s) of the right leg with ulceration of heel and midfoot**

Atherosclerosis of nonbiological bypass graft(s) of right leg with ulceration of plantar surface of midfoot

I70.635 **Atherosclerosis of nonbiological bypass graft(s) of the right leg with ulceration of other part of foot**

Atherosclerosis of nonbiological bypass graft(s) of the right leg with ulceration of toe

I70.638 **Atherosclerosis of nonbiological bypass graft(s) of the right leg with ulceration of other part of lower leg**

I70.639 **Atherosclerosis of nonbiological bypass graft(s) of the right leg with ulceration of unspecified site**

I70.64 **Atherosclerosis of nonbiological bypass graft(s) of the left leg with ulceration**

Includes: any condition classifiable to I70.612 and I70.622

Use additional code to identify severity of ulcer (L97.-)

I70.641 **Atherosclerosis of nonbiological bypass graft(s) of the left leg with ulceration of thigh**

I70.642 **Atherosclerosis of nonbiological bypass graft(s) of the left leg with ulceration of calf**

I70.643 **Atherosclerosis of nonbiological bypass graft(s) of the left leg with ulceration of ankle**

I70.644 **Atherosclerosis of nonbiological bypass graft(s) of the left leg with ulceration of heel and midfoot**

Atherosclerosis of nonbiological bypass graft(s) of left leg with ulceration of plantar surface of midfoot

I70.645 **Atherosclerosis of nonbiological bypass graft(s) of the left leg with ulceration of other part of foot**

Atherosclerosis of nonbiological bypass graft(s) of the left leg with ulceration of toe

I70.648 **Atherosclerosis of nonbiological bypass graft(s) of the left leg with ulceration of other part of lower leg**

I70.649 **Atherosclerosis of nonbiological bypass graft(s) of the left leg with ulceration of unspecified site**

I70.65 **Atherosclerosis of nonbiological bypass graft(s) of other extremity with ulceration**

Includes: any condition classifiable to I70.618 and I70.628

Use additional code to identify severity of ulcer (L98.49)

I70.66 **Atherosclerosis of nonbiological bypass graft(s) of the extremities with gangrene**

Includes: any condition classifiable to I70.61-, I70.62-, I70.63-, I70.64-, I70.65

Use additional code to identify the severity of any ulcer (L97.-, L98.49-), if applicable

I70.661 **Atherosclerosis of nonbiological bypass graft(s) of the extremities with gangrene, right leg**

I70.662 **Atherosclerosis of nonbiological bypass graft(s) of the extremities with gangrene, left leg**

I70.663 **Atherosclerosis of nonbiological bypass graft(s) of the extremities with gangrene, bilateral legs**

I70.668 **Atherosclerosis of nonbiological bypass graft(s) of the extremities with gangrene, other extremity**

I70.669 **Atherosclerosis of nonbiological bypass graft(s) of the extremities with gangrene, unspecified extremity**

I70.69 **Other atherosclerosis of nonbiological bypass graft(s) of the extremities**

I70.691 **Other atherosclerosis of nonbiological bypass graft(s) of the extremities, right leg**

I70.692 **Other atherosclerosis of nonbiological bypass graft(s) of the extremities, left leg**

I70.693 **Other atherosclerosis of nonbiological bypass graft(s) of the extremities, bilateral legs**

I70.698 Other atherosclerosis of nonbiological bypass graft(s) of the extremities, other extremity

I70.699 Other atherosclerosis of nonbiological bypass graft(s) of the extremities, unspecified extremity

I70.7 Atherosclerosis of other type of bypass graft(s) of the extremities

Use additional code, if applicable, to identify chronic total occlusion of artery of extremity (I70.92)

I70.70 Unspecified atherosclerosis of other type of bypass graft(s) of the extremities

I70.701 Unspecified atherosclerosis of other type of bypass graft(s) of the extremities, right leg

I70.702 Unspecified atherosclerosis of other type of bypass graft(s) of the extremities, left leg

I70.703 Unspecified atherosclerosis of other type of bypass graft(s) of the extremities, bilateral legs

I70.708 Unspecified atherosclerosis of other type of bypass graft(s) of the extremities, other extremity

I70.709 Unspecified atherosclerosis of other type of bypass graft(s) of the extremities, unspecified extremity

I70.71 Atherosclerosis of other type of bypass graft(s) of the extremities with intermittent claudication

I70.711 Atherosclerosis of other type of bypass graft(s) of the extremities with intermittent claudication, right leg

I70.712 Atherosclerosis of other type of bypass graft(s) of the extremities with intermittent claudication, left leg

I70.713 Atherosclerosis of other type of bypass graft(s) of the extremities with intermittent claudication, bilateral legs

I70.718 Atherosclerosis of other type of bypass graft(s) of the extremities with intermittent claudication, other extremity

I70.719 Atherosclerosis of other type of bypass graft(s) of the extremities with intermittent claudication, unspecified extremity

I70.72 Atherosclerosis of other type of bypass graft(s) of the extremities with rest pain

Includes: any condition classifiable to I70.71-

I70.721 Atherosclerosis of other type of bypass graft(s) of the extremities with rest pain, right leg

I70.722 Atherosclerosis of other type of bypass graft(s) of the extremities with rest pain, left leg

I70.723 Atherosclerosis of other type of bypass graft(s) of the extremities with rest pain, bilateral legs

I70.728 Atherosclerosis of other type of bypass graft(s) of the extremities with rest pain, other extremity

I70.729 Atherosclerosis of other type of bypass graft(s) of the extremities with rest pain, unspecified extremity

I70.73 Atherosclerosis of other type of bypass graft(s) of the right leg with ulceration

Includes: any condition classifiable to I70.711 and I70.721

Use additional code to identify severity of ulcer (L97.-)

I70.731 Atherosclerosis of other type of bypass graft(s) of the right leg with ulceration of thigh

I70.732 Atherosclerosis of other type of bypass graft(s) of the right leg with ulceration of calf

I70.733 Atherosclerosis of other type of bypass graft(s) of the right leg with ulceration of ankle

I70.734 Atherosclerosis of other type of bypass graft(s) of the right leg with ulceration of heel and midfoot

Atherosclerosis of other type of bypass graft(s) of right leg with ulceration of plantar surface of midfoot

I70.735 Atherosclerosis of other type of bypass graft(s) of the right leg with ulceration of other part of foot

Atherosclerosis of other type of bypass graft(s) of right leg with ulceration of toe

I70.738 Atherosclerosis of other type of bypass graft(s) of the right leg with ulceration of other part of lower leg

I70.739 Atherosclerosis of other type of bypass graft(s) of the right leg with ulceration of unspecified site

I70.74 Atherosclerosis of other type of bypass graft(s) of the left leg with ulceration

Includes: any condition classifiable to I70.712 and I70.722

Use additional code to identify severity of ulcer (L97.-)

I70.741 Atherosclerosis of other type of bypass graft(s) of the left leg with ulceration of thigh

I70.742 Atherosclerosis of other type of bypass graft(s) of the left leg with ulceration of calf

I70.743 Atherosclerosis of other type of bypass graft(s) of the left leg with ulceration of ankle

I70.744 Atherosclerosis of other type of bypass graft(s) of the left leg with ulceration of heel and midfoot

Atherosclerosis of other type of bypass graft(s) of left leg with ulceration of plantar surface of midfoot

I70.745 **Atherosclerosis of other type of bypass graft(s) of the left leg with ulceration of other part of foot**

Atherosclerosis of other type of bypass graft(s) of left leg with ulceration of toe

I70.748 **Atherosclerosis of other type of bypass graft(s) of the left leg with ulceration of other part of lower leg**

I70.749 **Atherosclerosis of other type of bypass graft(s) of the left leg with ulceration of unspecified site**

I70.75 **Atherosclerosis of other type of bypass graft(s) of other extremity with ulceration**

Includes: any condition classifiable to I70.718 and I70.728

Use additional code to identify severity of ulcer (L98.49)

I70.76 **Atherosclerosis of other type of bypass graft(s) of the extremities with gangrene**

Includes: any condition classifiable to I70.71-, I70.72-, I70.73-, I70.74-, I70.75

Use additional code to identify the severity of any ulcer (L97.-, L98.49-), if applicable

I70.761 **Atherosclerosis of other type of bypass graft(s) of the extremities with gangrene, right leg**

I70.762 **Atherosclerosis of other type of bypass graft(s) of the extremities with gangrene, left leg**

I70.763 **Atherosclerosis of other type of bypass graft(s) of the extremities with gangrene, bilateral legs**

I70.768 **Atherosclerosis of other type of bypass graft(s) of the extremities with gangrene, other extremity**

I70.769 **Atherosclerosis of other type of bypass graft(s) of the extremities with gangrene, unspecified extremity**

I70.79 **Other atherosclerosis of other type of bypass graft(s) of the extremities**

I70.791 **Other atherosclerosis of other type of bypass graft(s) of the extremities, right leg**

I70.792 **Other atherosclerosis of other type of bypass graft(s) of the extremities, left leg**

I70.793 **Other atherosclerosis of other type of bypass graft(s) of the extremities, bilateral legs**

I70.798 **Other atherosclerosis of other type of bypass graft(s) of the extremities, other extremity**

I70.799 **Other atherosclerosis of other type of bypass graft(s) of the extremities, unspecified extremity**

I70.8 **Atherosclerosis of other arteries**

I70.9 **Other and unspecified atherosclerosis**

I70.90 **Unspecified atherosclerosis**

I70.91 **Generalized atherosclerosis**

I70.92 **Chronic total occlusion of artery of the extremities**

Complete occlusion of artery of the extremities

Total occlusion of artery of the extremities

Code first atherosclerosis of arteries of the extremities (I70.2-, I70.3-, I70.4-, I70.5-, I70.6-, I70.7-)

I71 **Aortic aneurysm and dissection**

Definition: Aortic aneurysm and dissection is a localized, abnormal and persistent dilation of a section of the aorta. This usually results from a weakness in the vessel wall. If severe enough, rupture of the aorta with severe hemorrhage is a potential hazard.

Excludes1: aortic ectasia (I77.81-)

syphilitic aortic aneurysm (A52.01)

traumatic aortic aneurysm (S25.09, S35.09)

I71.0 **Dissection of aorta**

I71.00 **Dissection of unspecified site of aorta**

I71.01 **Dissection of thoracic aorta**

I71.02 **Dissection of abdominal aorta**

I71.03 **Dissection of thoracoabdominal aorta**

I71.1 **Thoracic aortic aneurysm, ruptured**

I71.2 **Thoracic aortic aneurysm, without rupture**

I71.3 **Abdominal aortic aneurysm, ruptured**

I71.4 **Abdominal aortic aneurysm, without rupture**

I71.5 **Thoracoabdominal aortic aneurysm, ruptured**

I71.6 **Thoracoabdominal aortic aneurysm, without rupture**

I71.8 **Aortic aneurysm of unspecified site, ruptured**

Rupture of aorta NOS

I71.9 **Aortic aneurysm of unspecified site, without rupture**

Aneurysm of aorta

Dilatation of aorta

Hyaline necrosis of aorta

I72 **Other aneurysm**

Includes: aneurysm (cirsoid) (false) (ruptured)

Excludes2: acquired aneurysm (I77.0)

aneurysm (of) aorta (I71.-)

aneurysm (of) arteriovenous NOS (Q27.3-)

carotid artery dissection (I77.71)

cerebral (nonruptured) aneurysm (I67.1)

coronary aneurysm (I25.4)

coronary artery dissection (I25.42)

dissection of artery NEC (I77.79)

dissection of precerebral artery, congenital (nonruptured) (Q28.1)

heart aneurysm (I25.3)

iliac artery dissection (I77.72)

pulmonary artery aneurysm (I28.1)

renal artery dissection (I77.73)

retinal aneurysm (H35.0)

ruptured cerebral aneurysm (I60.7)

varicose aneurysm (I77.0)

vertebral artery dissection (I77.74)

I72.0 **Aneurysm of carotid artery**

Aneurysm of common carotid artery

Aneurysm of external carotid artery

Aneurysm of internal carotid artery, extracranial portion

● New code ▲ Revised code **Excludes1:** Not coded here **Excludes2:** Not included here ⊗ Placeholder required ⑦7th digit required

Excludes1: aneurysm of internal carotid artery, intracranial portion (I67.1)

aneurysm of internal carotid artery NOS (I67.1)

I72.1   **Aneurysm of artery of upper extremity**

I72.2   **Aneurysm of renal artery**

I72.3   **Aneurysm of iliac artery**

I72.4   **Aneurysm of artery of lower extremity**

•**I72.5**   **Aneurysm of other precerebral arteries**

Aneurysm of basilar artery (trunk)

Excludes2: aneurysm of carotid artery (I72.0)

aneurysm of vertebral artery (I72.6)

dissection of carotid artery (I77.71)

dissection of other precerebral arteries (I77.75)

dissection of vertebral artery (I77.74)

•**I72.6**   **Aneurysm of vertebral artery**

Excludes2: dissection of vertebral artery (I77.74)

I72.8   **Aneurysm of other specified arteries**

I72.9   **Aneurysm of unspecified site**

I73   **Other peripheral vascular diseases**

Excludes2: chilblains (T69.1)

frostbite (T33-T34)

immersion hand or foot (T69.0-)

spasm of cerebral artery (G45.9)

I73.0   **Raynaud's syndrome**

Raynaud's disease

Raynaud's phenomenon (secondary)

I73.00   **Raynaud's syndrome without gangrene**

I73.01   **Raynaud's syndrome with gangrene**

I73.1   **Thromboangiitis obliterans [Buerger's disease]**

I73.8   **Other specified peripheral vascular diseases**

Excludes1: diabetic (peripheral) angiopathy (E08-E13 with .51-.52)

I73.81   **Erythromelalgia**

I73.89   **Other specified peripheral vascular diseases**

Acrocyanosis

Erythrocyanosis

Simple acroparesthesia [Schultze's type]

Vasomotor acroparesthesia [Nothnagel's type]

I73.9   **Peripheral vascular disease, unspecified**

Intermittent claudication

Peripheral angiopathy NOS

Spasm of artery

Excludes1: atherosclerosis of the extremities (I70.2--I70.7-)

I74   **Arterial embolism and thrombosis**

Definition: An embolism is a sudden interruption in arterial blood flow to an organ or body extremity. The blockage is caused by a blood clot or foreign object. A Thrombosis is the formation or presence of a thrombus (a clot of coagulated blood) in a blood

Includes: embolic infarction

embolic occlusion thrombotic infarction thrombotic occlusion

Code first embolism and thrombosis complicating abortion or ectopic or molar pregnancy (O00-O07, O08.2)

embolism and thrombosis complicating pregnancy, childbirth and the puerperium (O88.-)

Excludes2: atheroembolism (I75.-)

basilar embolism and thrombosis (I63.0-I63.2, I65.1)

carotid embolism and thrombosis (I63.0-I63.2, I65.2)

cerebral embolism and thrombosis (I63.3-I63.5, I66.-)

coronary embolism and thrombosis (I21-I25)

mesenteric embolism and thrombosis (K55.0-)

ophthalmic embolism and thrombosis (H34.-)

precerebral embolism and thrombosis NOS (I63.0-I63.2, I65.9)

pulmonary embolism and thrombosis (I26.-)

renal embolism and thrombosis (N28.0)

retinal embolism and thrombosis (H34.-)

septic embolism and thrombosis (I76)

vertebral embolism and thrombosis (I63.0-I63.2, I65.0)

I74.0   **Embolism and thrombosis of abdominal aorta**

I74.01   **Saddle embolus of abdominal aorta**

I74.09   **Other arterial embolism and thrombosis of abdominal aorta**

Aortic bifurcation syndrome

Aortoiliac obstruction

Leriche's syndrome

I74.1   **Embolism and thrombosis of other and unspecified parts of aorta**

I74.10   **Embolism and thrombosis of unspecified parts of aorta**

I74.11   **Embolism and thrombosis of thoracic aorta**

I74.19   **Embolism and thrombosis of other parts of aorta**

I74.2   **Embolism and thrombosis of arteries of the upper extremities**

I74.3   **Embolism and thrombosis of arteries of the lower extremities**

I74.4   **Embolism and thrombosis of arteries of extremities, unspecified**

Peripheral arterial embolism NOS

I74.5   **Embolism and thrombosis of iliac artery**

I74.8   **Embolism and thrombosis of other arteries**

I74.9   **Embolism and thrombosis of unspecified artery**

I75   **Atheroembolism**

Includes: atherothrombotic microembolism

cholesterol embolism

I75.0   **Atheroembolism of extremities**

I75.01   **Atheroembolism of upper extremity**

I75.011   **Atheroembolism of right upper extremity**

I75.012   **Atheroembolism of left upper extremity**

I75.013   **Atheroembolism of bilateral upper extremities**

I75.019   **Atheroembolism of unspecified upper extremity**

I75.02   **Atheroembolism of lower extremity**

I75.021   **Atheroembolism of right lower extremity**

I75.022   **Atheroembolism of left lower extremity**

I75.023   **Atheroembolism of bilateral lower extremities**

I75.029   Atheroembolism of unspecified lower extremity

I75.8   Atheroembolism of other sites

     I75.81   Atheroembolism of kidney

       Use additional code for any associated acute kidney failure and chronic kidney disease (N17.-, N18.-)

     I75.89   Atheroembolism of other site

I76   Septic arterial embolism

Code first underlying infection, such as:

infective endocarditis (I33.0)

lung abscess (J85.-)

Use additional code to identify the site of the embolism (I74.-)

Excludes2: septic pulmonary embolism (I26.01, I26.90)

I77   Other disorders of arteries and arterioles

Excludes2: collagen (vascular) diseases (M30-M36)

       hypersensitivity angiitis (M31.0)

       pulmonary artery (I28.-)

I77.0   Arteriovenous fistula, acquired

Aneurysmal varix

Arteriovenous aneurysm, acquired

Excludes1: arteriovenous aneurysm NOS (Q27.3-)

       presence of arteriovenous shunt (fistula) for dialysis (Z99.2)

       traumatic - see injury of blood vessel by body region

Excludes2: cerebral (I67.1)

       coronary (I25.4)

I77.1   Stricture of artery

Narrowing of artery

I77.2   Rupture of artery

Erosion of artery

Fistula of artery

Ulcer of artery

Excludes1: traumatic rupture of artery - see injury of blood vessel by body region

I77.3   Arterial fibromuscular dysplasia

Fibromuscular hyperplasia (of) carotid artery

Fibromuscular hyperplasia (of) renal artery

I77.4   Celiac artery compression syndrome

I77.5   Necrosis of artery

I77.6   Arteritis, unspecified

Aortitis NOS

Endarteritis NOS

Excludes1: arteritis or endarteritis:

       aortic arch (M31.4)

       cerebral NEC (I67.7)

       coronary (I25.89)

       deformans (I70.-)

       giant cell (M31.5., M31.6)

       obliterans (I70.-)

       senile (I70.-)

I77.7   Other arterial dissection

Excludes2: dissection of aorta (I71.0-)

       dissection of coronary artery (I25.42)

● **I77.70**   Dissection of unspecified artery

I77.71   Dissection of carotid artery

I77.72   Dissection of iliac artery

I77.73   Dissection of renal artery

I77.74   Dissection of vertebral artery

       Excludes2: aneurysm of vertebral artery (I72.6)

● **I77.75**   Dissection of other precerebral arteries

       Dissection of basilar artery (trunk)

       Excludes2: aneurysm of carotid artery (I72.0)

             aneurysm of other precerebral arteries (I72.5)

             aneurysm of vertebral artery (I72.6)

             dissection of carotid artery (I77.71)

             dissection of vertebral artery (I77.74)

● **I77.76**   Dissection of artery of upper extremity

● **I77.77**   Dissection of artery of lower extremity

I77.79   Dissection of other specified artery

I77.8   Other specified disorders of arteries and arterioles

     I77.81   Aortic ectasia

       Ectasis aorta

       Excludes1: aortic aneurysm and dissection (I71.0-)

       I77.810   Thoracic aortic ectasia

       I77.811   Abdominal aortic ectasia

       I77.812   Thoracoabdominal aortic ectasia

       I77.819   Aortic ectasia, unspecified site

     I77.89   Other specified disorders of arteries and arterioles

I77.9   Disorder of arteries and arterioles, unspecified

I78   Diseases of capillaries

I78.0   Hereditary hemorrhagic telangiectasia

Rendu-Osler-Weber disease

I78.1   Nevus, non-neoplastic

Araneus nevus

Senile nevus

Spider nevus

Stellar nevus

Excludes1: nevus NOS (D22.-)

       vascular NOS (Q82.5)

Excludes2: blue nevus (D22.-)

       flammeus nevus (Q82.5)

       hairy nevus (D22.-)

       melanocytic nevus (D22.-)

       pigmented nevus (D22.-)

       portwine nevus (Q82.5)

       sanguineous nevus (Q82.5)

       strawberry nevus (Q82.5)

       verrucous nevus (Q82.5)

I78.8   Other diseases of capillaries

I78.9   Disease of capillaries, unspecified

I79   Disorders of arteries, arterioles and capillaries in diseases classified elsewhere

I79.0   Aneurysm of aorta in diseases classified elsewhere

Code first underlying disease

Excludes1: syphilitic aneurysm (A52.01)

   ● New code   ▲ Revised code   **Excludes1:** Not coded here   **Excludes2:** Not included here   ⊗ Placeholder required   ⑦7ᵗʰ digit required

I79.1 **Aortitis in diseases classified elsewhere**

Code first underlying disease

Excludes1: syphilitic aortitis (A52.02)

I79.8 **Other disorders of arteries, arterioles and capillaries in diseases classified elsewhere**

Code first underlying disease, such as:

amyloidosis (E85.-)

Excludes1: diabetic (peripheral) angiopathy (E08-E13 with .51-.52)

syphilitic endarteritis (A52.09)

tuberculous endarteritis (A18.89)

DISEASES OF VEINS, LYMPHATIC VESSELS AND LYMPH NODES, NOT ELSEWHERE CLASSIFIED (I80-I89)

I80 **Phlebitis and thrombophlebitis**

Includes: endophlebitis

inflammation, vein periphlebitis suppurative phlebitis

Code first phlebitis and thrombophlebitis complicating abortion, ectopic or molar pregnancy (O00-O07, O08.7)

phlebitis and thrombophlebitis complicating pregnancy, childbirth and the puerperium (O22.-, O87.-)

Excludes1: venous embolism and thrombosis of lower extremities (I82.4-, I82.5-, I82.81-)

I80.0 **Phlebitis and thrombophlebitis of superficial vessels of lower extremities**

Phlebitis and thrombophlebitis of femoropopliteal vein

I80.00 **Phlebitis and thrombophlebitis of superficial vessels of unspecified lower extremity**

I80.01 **Phlebitis and thrombophlebitis of superficial vessels of right lower extremity**

I80.02 **Phlebitis and thrombophlebitis of superficial vessels of left lower extremity**

I80.03 **Phlebitis and thrombophlebitis of superficial vessels of lower extremities, bilateral**

I80.1 **Phlebitis and thrombophlebitis of femoral vein**

I80.10 **Phlebitis and thrombophlebitis of unspecified femoral vein**

I80.11 **Phlebitis and thrombophlebitis of right femoral vein**

I80.12 **Phlebitis and thrombophlebitis of left femoral vein**

I80.13 **Phlebitis and thrombophlebitis of femoral vein, bilateral**

I80.2 **Phlebitis and thrombophlebitis of other and unspecified deep vessels of lower extremities**

I80.20 **Phlebitis and thrombophlebitis of unspecified deep vessels of lower extremities**

I80.201 **Phlebitis and thrombophlebitis of unspecified deep vessels of right lower extremity**

I80.202 **Phlebitis and thrombophlebitis of unspecified deep vessels of left lower extremity**

I80.203 **Phlebitis and thrombophlebitis of unspecified deep vessels of lower extremities, bilateral**

I80.209 **Phlebitis and thrombophlebitis of unspecified deep vessels of unspecified lower extremity**

I80.21 **Phlebitis and thrombophlebitis of iliac vein**

I80.211 **Phlebitis and thrombophlebitis of right iliac vein**

I80.212 **Phlebitis and thrombophlebitis of left iliac vein**

I80.213 **Phlebitis and thrombophlebitis of iliac vein, bilateral**

I80.219 **Phlebitis and thrombophlebitis of unspecified iliac vein**

I80.22 **Phlebitis and thrombophlebitis of popliteal vein**

I80.221 **Phlebitis and thrombophlebitis of right popliteal vein**

I80.222 **Phlebitis and thrombophlebitis of left popliteal vein**

I80.223 **Phlebitis and thrombophlebitis of popliteal vein, bilateral**

I80.229 **Phlebitis and thrombophlebitis of unspecified popliteal vein**

I80.23 **Phlebitis and thrombophlebitis of tibial vein**

I80.231 **Phlebitis and thrombophlebitis of right tibial vein**

I80.232 **Phlebitis and thrombophlebitis of left tibial vein**

I80.233 **Phlebitis and thrombophlebitis of tibial vein, bilateral**

I80.239 **Phlebitis and thrombophlebitis of unspecified tibial vein**

I80.29 **Phlebitis and thrombophlebitis of other deep vessels of lower extremities**

I80.291 **Phlebitis and thrombophlebitis of other deep vessels of right lower extremity**

I80.292 **Phlebitis and thrombophlebitis of other deep vessels of left lower extremity**

I80.293 **Phlebitis and thrombophlebitis of other deep vessels of lower extremity, bilateral**

I80.299 **Phlebitis and thrombophlebitis of other deep vessels of unspecified lower extremity**

I80.3 **Phlebitis and thrombophlebitis of lower extremities, unspecified**

I80.8 **Phlebitis and thrombophlebitis of other sites**

I80.9 **Phlebitis and thrombophlebitis of unspecified site**

I81 **Portal vein thrombosis**

Portal (vein) obstruction

Excludes2: hepatic vein thrombosis (I82.0)

phlebitis of portal vein (K75.1)

I82 **Other venous embolism and thrombosis**

Definition: Venous embolism and thrombosis is a mass of clotted blood or other material moved by the blood from one vein and forced into a smaller one.

Code first venous embolism and thrombosis complicating:

abortion, ectopic or molar pregnancy (O00-O07, O08.7)

pregnancy, childbirth and the puerperium (O22.-, O87.-)

Excludes2: venous embolism and thrombosis (of):

cerebral (I63.6, I67.6)

coronary (I21-I25)

intracranial and intraspinal, septic or NOS (G08)

intracranial, nonpyogenic (I67.6)

intraspinal, nonpyogenic (G95.1)

mesenteric (K55.0-)

portal (I81)

pulmonary (I26.-)

I82.0   Budd-Chiari syndrome

Hepatic vein thrombosis

I82.1   Thrombophlebitis migrans

I82.2   Embolism and thrombosis of vena cava and other thoracic veins

  I82.21   Embolism and thrombosis of superior vena cava

    I82.210   Acute embolism and thrombosis of superior vena cava

      Embolism and thrombosis of superior vena cava NOS

    I82.211   Chronic embolism and thrombosis of superior vena cava

  I82.22   Embolism and thrombosis of inferior vena cava

    I82.220   Acute embolism and thrombosis of inferior vena cava

      Embolism and thrombosis of inferior vena cava NOS

    I82.221   Chronic embolism and thrombosis of inferior vena cava

  I82.29   Embolism and thrombosis of other thoracic veins

    Embolism and thrombosis of brachiocephalic (innominate) vein

    I82.290   Acute embolism and thrombosis of other thoracic veins

    I82.291   Chronic embolism and thrombosis of other thoracic veins

I82.3   Embolism and thrombosis of renal vein

I82.4   Acute embolism and thrombosis of deep veins of lower extremity

  I82.40   Acute embolism and thrombosis of unspecified deep veins of lower extremity

    Deep vein thrombosis NOS

    DVT NOS

    Excludes1: acute embolism and thrombosis of unspecified deep veins of distal lower extremity (I82.4Z-)

    acute embolism and thrombosis of unspecified deep veins of proximal lower extremity (I82.4Y-)

    I82.401   Acute embolism and thrombosis of unspecified deep veins of right lower extremity

    I82.402   Acute embolism and thrombosis of unspecified deep veins of left lower extremity

    I82.403   Acute embolism and thrombosis of unspecified deep veins of lower extremity, bilateral

    I82.409   Acute embolism and thrombosis of unspecified deep veins of unspecified lower extremity

I82.41   Acute embolism and thrombosis of femoral vein

  I82.411   Acute embolism and thrombosis of right femoral vein

  I82.412   Acute embolism and thrombosis of left femoral vein

  I82.413   Acute embolism and thrombosis of femoral vein, bilateral

  I82.419   Acute embolism and thrombosis of unspecified femoral vein

I82.42   Acute embolism and thrombosis of iliac vein

  I82.421   Acute embolism and thrombosis of right iliac vein

  I82.422   Acute embolism and thrombosis of left iliac vein

  I82.423   Acute embolism and thrombosis of iliac vein, bilateral

  I82.429   Acute embolism and thrombosis of unspecified iliac vein

I82.43   Acute embolism and thrombosis of popliteal vein

  I82.431   Acute embolism and thrombosis of right popliteal vein

  I82.432   Acute embolism and thrombosis of left popliteal vein

  I82.433   Acute embolism and thrombosis of popliteal vein, bilateral

  I82.439   Acute embolism and thrombosis of unspecified popliteal vein

I82.44   Acute embolism and thrombosis of tibial vein

  I82.441   Acute embolism and thrombosis of right tibial vein

  I82.442   Acute embolism and thrombosis of left tibial vein

  I82.443   Acute embolism and thrombosis of tibial vein, bilateral

  I82.449   Acute embolism and thrombosis of unspecified tibial vein

I82.49   Acute embolism and thrombosis of other specified deep vein of lower extremity

  I82.491   Acute embolism and thrombosis of other specified deep vein of right lower extremity

  I82.492   Acute embolism and thrombosis of other specified deep vein of left lower extremity

  I82.493   Acute embolism and thrombosis of other specified deep vein of lower extremity, bilateral

  I82.499   Acute embolism and thrombosis of other specified deep vein of unspecified lower extremity

I82.4Y   Acute embolism and thrombosis of unspecified deep veins of proximal lower extremity

  Acute embolism and thrombosis of deep vein of thigh NOS

  Acute embolism and thrombosis of deep vein of upper leg NOS

  I82.4Y1   Acute embolism and thrombosis of unspecified deep veins of right proximal lower extremity

   ● New code   ▲ Revised code   **Excludes1:** Not coded here   **Excludes2:** Not included here   ⊗ Placeholder required   ⑦7th digit required

I82.4Y2 Acute embolism and thrombosis of unspecified deep veins of left proximal lower extremity

I82.4Y3 Acute embolism and thrombosis of unspecified deep veins of proximal lower extremity, bilateral

I82.4Y9 Acute embolism and thrombosis of unspecified deep veins of unspecified proximal lower extremity

I82.4Z Acute embolism and thrombosis of unspecified deep veins of distal lower extremity

Acute embolism and thrombosis of deep vein of calf NOS

Acute embolism and thrombosis of deep vein of lower leg NOS

I82.4Z1 Acute embolism and thrombosis of unspecified deep veins of right distal lower extremity

I82.4Z2 Acute embolism and thrombosis of unspecified deep veins of left distal lower extremity

I82.4Z3 Acute embolism and thrombosis of unspecified deep veins of distal lower extremity, bilateral

I82.4Z9 Acute embolism and thrombosis of unspecified deep veins of unspecified distal lower extremity

I82.5 Chronic embolism and thrombosis of deep veins of lower extremity

Use additional code, if applicable, for associated long-term (current) use of anticoagulants (Z79.01)

Excludes1: personal history of venous embolism and thrombosis (Z86.718)

I82.50 Chronic embolism and thrombosis of unspecified deep veins of lower extremity

Excludes1: chronic embolism and thrombosis of unspecified deep veins of distal lower extremity (I82.5Z-)

chronic embolism and thrombosis of unspecified deep veins of proximal lower extremity (I82.5Y-)

I82.501 Chronic embolism and thrombosis of unspecified deep veins of right lower extremity

I82.502 Chronic embolism and thrombosis of unspecified deep veins of left lower extremity

I82.503 Chronic embolism and thrombosis of unspecified deep veins of lower extremity, bilateral

I82.509 Chronic embolism and thrombosis of unspecified deep veins of unspecified lower extremity

I82.51 Chronic embolism and thrombosis of femoral vein

I82.511 Chronic embolism and thrombosis of right femoral vein

I82.512 Chronic embolism and thrombosis of left femoral vein

I82.513 Chronic embolism and thrombosis of femoral vein, bilateral

I82.519 Chronic embolism and thrombosis of unspecified femoral vein

I82.52 Chronic embolism and thrombosis of iliac vein

I82.521 Chronic embolism and thrombosis of right iliac vein

I82.522 Chronic embolism and thrombosis of left iliac vein

I82.523 Chronic embolism and thrombosis of iliac vein, bilateral

I82.529 Chronic embolism and thrombosis of unspecified iliac vein

I82.53 Chronic embolism and thrombosis of popliteal vein

I82.531 Chronic embolism and thrombosis of right popliteal vein

I82.532 Chronic embolism and thrombosis of left popliteal vein

I82.533 Chronic embolism and thrombosis of popliteal vein, bilateral

I82.539 Chronic embolism and thrombosis of unspecified popliteal vein

I82.54 Chronic embolism and thrombosis of tibial vein

I82.541 Chronic embolism and thrombosis of right tibial vein

I82.542 Chronic embolism and thrombosis of left tibial vein

I82.543 Chronic embolism and thrombosis of tibial vein, bilateral

I82.549 Chronic embolism and thrombosis of unspecified tibial vein

I82.59 Chronic embolism and thrombosis of other specified deep vein of lower extremity

I82.591 Chronic embolism and thrombosis of other specified deep vein of right lower extremity

I82.592 Chronic embolism and thrombosis of other specified deep vein of left lower extremity

I82.593 Chronic embolism and thrombosis of other specified deep vein of lower extremity, bilateral

I82.599 Chronic embolism and thrombosis of other specified deep vein of unspecified lower extremity

I82.5Y Chronic embolism and thrombosis of unspecified deep veins of proximal lower extremity

Chronic embolism and thrombosis of deep veins of thigh NOS

Chronic embolism and thrombosis of deep veins of upper leg NOS

I82.5Y1 Chronic embolism and thrombosis of unspecified deep veins of right proximal lower extremity

I82.5Y2 Chronic embolism and thrombosis of unspecified deep veins of left proximal lower extremity

I82.5Y3 Chronic embolism and thrombosis of unspecified deep veins of proximal lower extremity, bilateral

I82.5Y9 Chronic embolism and thrombosis of unspecified deep veins of unspecified proximal lower extremity

I82.5Z Chronic embolism and thrombosis of unspecified deep veins of distal lower extremity

Chronic embolism and thrombosis of deep veins of calf NOS

Chronic embolism and thrombosis of deep veins of lower leg NOS

I82.5Z1 Chronic embolism and thrombosis of unspecified deep veins of right distal lower extremity

I82.5Z2 Chronic embolism and thrombosis of unspecified deep veins of left distal lower extremity

I82.5Z3 Chronic embolism and thrombosis of unspecified deep veins of distal lower extremity, bilateral

I82.5Z9 Chronic embolism and thrombosis of unspecified deep veins of unspecified distal lower extremity

I82.6 Acute embolism and thrombosis of veins of upper extremity

I82.60 Acute embolism and thrombosis of unspecified veins of upper extremity

I82.601 Acute embolism and thrombosis of unspecified veins of right upper extremity

I82.602 Acute embolism and thrombosis of unspecified veins of left upper extremity

I82.603 Acute embolism and thrombosis of unspecified veins of upper extremity, bilateral

I82.609 Acute embolism and thrombosis of unspecified veins of unspecified upper extremity

I82.61 Acute embolism and thrombosis of superficial veins of upper extremity

Acute embolism and thrombosis of antecubital vein

Acute embolism and thrombosis of basilic vein

Acute embolism and thrombosis of cephalic vein

I82.611 Acute embolism and thrombosis of superficial veins of right upper extremity

I82.612 Acute embolism and thrombosis of superficial veins of left upper extremity

I82.613 Acute embolism and thrombosis of superficial veins of upper extremity, bilateral

I82.619 Acute embolism and thrombosis of superficial veins of unspecified upper extremity

I82.62 Acute embolism and thrombosis of deep veins of upper extremity

Acute embolism and thrombosis of brachial vein

Acute embolism and thrombosis of radial vein

Acute embolism and thrombosis of ulnar vein

I82.621 Acute embolism and thrombosis of deep veins of right upper extremity

I82.622 Acute embolism and thrombosis of deep veins of left upper extremity

I82.623 Acute embolism and thrombosis of deep veins of upper extremity, bilateral

I82.629 Acute embolism and thrombosis of deep veins of unspecified upper extremity

I82.7 Chronic embolism and thrombosis of veins of upper extremity

Use additional code, if applicable, for associated long-term (current) use of anticoagulants (Z79.01)

Excludes1: personal history of venous embolism and thrombosis (Z86.718)

I82.70 Chronic embolism and thrombosis of unspecified veins of upper extremity

I82.701 Chronic embolism and thrombosis of unspecified veins of right upper extremity

I82.702 Chronic embolism and thrombosis of unspecified veins of left upper extremity

I82.703 Chronic embolism and thrombosis of unspecified veins of upper extremity, bilateral

I82.709 Chronic embolism and thrombosis of unspecified veins of unspecified upper extremity

I82.71 Chronic embolism and thrombosis of superficial veins of upper extremity

Chronic embolism and thrombosis of antecubital vein

Chronic embolism and thrombosis of basilic vein

Chronic embolism and thrombosis of cephalic vein

I82.711 Chronic embolism and thrombosis of superficial veins of right upper extremity

I82.712 Chronic embolism and thrombosis of superficial veins of left upper extremity

I82.713 Chronic embolism and thrombosis of superficial veins of upper extremity, bilateral

I82.719 Chronic embolism and thrombosis of superficial veins of unspecified upper extremity

I82.72 Chronic embolism and thrombosis of deep veins of upper extremity

Chronic embolism and thrombosis of brachial vein

Chronic embolism and thrombosis of radial vein

Chronic embolism and thrombosis of ulnar vein

I82.721 Chronic embolism and thrombosis of deep veins of right upper extremity

I82.722 Chronic embolism and thrombosis of deep veins of left upper extremity

I82.723 Chronic embolism and thrombosis of deep veins of upper extremity, bilateral

● New code   ▲ Revised code   **Excludes1:** Not coded here   **Excludes2:** Not included here   ⊗ Placeholder required   ⑦7th digit required

I82.729 Chronic embolism and thrombosis of deep veins of unspecified upper extremity

I82.A Embolism and thrombosis of axillary vein

I82.A1 Acute embolism and thrombosis of axillary vein

I82.A11 Acute embolism and thrombosis of right axillary vein

I82.A12 Acute embolism and thrombosis of left axillary vein

I82.A13 Acute embolism and thrombosis of axillary vein, bilateral

I82.A19 Acute embolism and thrombosis of unspecified axillary vein

I82.A2 Chronic embolism and thrombosis of axillary vein

I82.A21 Chronic embolism and thrombosis of right axillary vein

I82.A22 Chronic embolism and thrombosis of left axillary vein

I82.A23 Chronic embolism and thrombosis of axillary vein, bilateral

I82.A29 Chronic embolism and thrombosis of unspecified axillary vein

I82.B Embolism and thrombosis of subclavian vein

I82.B1 Acute embolism and thrombosis of subclavian vein

I82.B11 Acute embolism and thrombosis of right subclavian vein

I82.B12 Acute embolism and thrombosis of left subclavian vein

I82.B13 Acute embolism and thrombosis of subclavian vein, bilateral

I82.B19 Acute embolism and thrombosis of unspecified subclavian vein

I82.B2 Chronic embolism and thrombosis of subclavian vein

I82.B21 Chronic embolism and thrombosis of right subclavian vein

I82.B22 Chronic embolism and thrombosis of left subclavian vein

I82.B23 Chronic embolism and thrombosis of subclavian vein, bilateral

I82.B29 Chronic embolism and thrombosis of unspecified subclavian vein

I82.C Embolism and thrombosis of internal jugular vein

I82.C1 Acute embolism and thrombosis of internal jugular vein

I82.C11 Acute embolism and thrombosis of right internal jugular vein

I82.C12 Acute embolism and thrombosis of left internal jugular vein

I82.C13 Acute embolism and thrombosis of internal jugular vein, bilateral

I82.C19 Acute embolism and thrombosis of unspecified internal jugular vein

I82.C2 Chronic embolism and thrombosis of internal jugular vein

I82.C21 Chronic embolism and thrombosis of right internal jugular vein

I82.C22 Chronic embolism and thrombosis of left internal jugular vein

I82.C23 Chronic embolism and thrombosis of internal jugular vein, bilateral

I82.C29 Chronic embolism and thrombosis of unspecified internal jugular vein

I82.8 Embolism and thrombosis of other specified veins

Use additional code, if applicable, for associated long-term (current) use of anticoagulants (Z79.01)

I82.81 Embolism and thrombosis of superficial veins of lower extremities

Embolism and thrombosis of saphenous vein (greater) (lesser)

I82.811 Embolism and thrombosis of superficial veins of right lower extremities

I82.812 Embolism and thrombosis of superficial veins of left lower extremities

I82.813 Embolism and thrombosis of superficial veins of lower extremities, bilateral

I82.819 Embolism and thrombosis of superficial veins of unspecified lower extremities

I82.89 Embolism and thrombosis of other specified veins

I82.890 Acute embolism and thrombosis of other specified veins

I82.891 Chronic embolism and thrombosis of other specified veins

I82.9 Embolism and thrombosis of unspecified vein

I82.90 Acute embolism and thrombosis of unspecified vein

Embolism of vein NOS

Thrombosis (vein) NOS

I82.91 Chronic embolism and thrombosis of unspecified vein

I83 Varicose veins of lower extremities

Definition: Varicose veins are dilated (widened) tortuous (twisting) veins, usually involving a superficial vein in the leg, often associated with incompetency of the valves in the vein

Excludes1: varicose veins complicating pregnancy (O22.0-)

varicose veins complicating the puerperium (O87.4)

I83.0 Varicose veins of lower extremities with ulcer

Use additional code to identify severity of ulcer (L97.-)

I83.00 Varicose veins of unspecified lower extremity with ulcer

I83.001 Varicose veins of unspecified lower extremity with ulcer of thigh

I83.002 Varicose veins of unspecified lower extremity with ulcer of calf

I83.003 Varicose veins of unspecified lower extremity with ulcer of ankle

I83.004 Varicose veins of unspecified lower extremity with ulcer of heel and midfoot

Varicose veins of unspecified lower extremity with ulcer of plantar surface of midfoot

---

Add 4th-7th digits   Nonspecific code   Unspecified code   Manifestation code   423

I83.005   **Varicose veins of unspecified lower extremity with ulcer other part of foot**

Varicose veins of unspecified lower extremity with ulcer of toe

I83.008   **Varicose veins of unspecified lower extremity with ulcer other part of lower leg**

I83.009   **Varicose veins of unspecified lower extremity with ulcer of unspecified site**

I83.01   **Varicose veins of right lower extremity with ulcer**

I83.011   **Varicose veins of right lower extremity with ulcer of thigh**

I83.012   **Varicose veins of right lower extremity with ulcer of calf**

I83.013   **Varicose veins of right lower extremity with ulcer of ankle**

I83.014   **Varicose veins of right lower extremity with ulcer of heel and midfoot**

Varicose veins of right lower extremity with ulcer of plantar surface of midfoot

I83.015   **Varicose veins of right lower extremity with ulcer other part of foot**

Varicose veins of right lower extremity with ulcer of toe

I83.018   **Varicose veins of right lower extremity with ulcer other part of lower leg**

I83.019   **Varicose veins of right lower extremity with ulcer of unspecified site**

I83.02   **Varicose veins of left lower extremity with ulcer**

I83.021   **Varicose veins of left lower extremity with ulcer of thigh**

I83.022   **Varicose veins of left lower extremity with ulcer of calf**

I83.023   **Varicose veins of left lower extremity with ulcer of ankle**

I83.024   **Varicose veins of left lower extremity with ulcer of heel and midfoot**

Varicose veins of left lower extremity with ulcer of plantar surface of midfoot

I83.025   **Varicose veins of left lower extremity with ulcer other part of foot**

Varicose veins of left lower extremity with ulcer of toe

I83.028   **Varicose veins of left lower extremity with ulcer other part of lower leg**

I83.029   **Varicose veins of left lower extremity with ulcer of unspecified site**

I83.1   **Varicose veins of lower extremities with inflammation**

I83.10   **Varicose veins of unspecified lower extremity with inflammation**

I83.11   **Varicose veins of right lower extremity with inflammation**

I83.12   **Varicose veins of left lower extremity with inflammation**

I83.2   **Varicose veins of lower extremities with both ulcer and inflammation**

Use additional code to identify severity of ulcer (L97.-)

I83.20   **Varicose veins of unspecified lower extremity with both ulcer and inflammation**

I83.201   **Varicose veins of unspecified lower extremity with both ulcer of thigh and inflammation**

I83.202   **Varicose veins of unspecified lower extremity with both ulcer of calf and inflammation**

I83.203   **Varicose veins of unspecified lower extremity with both ulcer of ankle and inflammation**

I83.204   **Varicose veins of unspecified lower extremity with both ulcer of heel and midfoot and inflammation**

Varicose veins of unspecified lower extremity with both ulcer of plantar surface of midfoot and inflammation

I83.205   **Varicose veins of unspecified lower extremity with both ulcer other part of foot and inflammation**

Varicose veins of unspecified lower extremity with both ulcer of toe and inflammation

I83.208   **Varicose veins of unspecified lower extremity with both ulcer of other part of lower extremity and inflammation**

I83.209   **Varicose veins of unspecified lower extremity with both ulcer of unspecified site and inflammation**

I83.21   **Varicose veins of right lower extremity with both ulcer and inflammation**

I83.211   **Varicose veins of right lower extremity with both ulcer of thigh and inflammation**

I83.212   **Varicose veins of right lower extremity with both ulcer of calf and inflammation**

I83.213   **Varicose veins of right lower extremity with both ulcer of ankle and inflammation**

I83.214   **Varicose veins of right lower extremity with both ulcer of heel and midfoot and inflammation**

Varicose veins of right lower extremity with both ulcer of plantar surface of midfoot and inflammation

I83.215   **Varicose veins of right lower extremity with both ulcer other part of foot and inflammation**

Varicose veins of right lower extremity with both ulcer of toe and inflammation

I83.218   **Varicose veins of right lower extremity with both ulcer of other**

part of lower extremity and inflammation

I83.219   Varicose veins of right lower extremity with both ulcer of unspecified site and inflammation

I83.22   Varicose veins of left lower extremity with both ulcer and inflammation

I83.221   Varicose veins of left lower extremity with both ulcer of thigh and inflammation

I83.222   Varicose veins of left lower extremity with both ulcer of calf and inflammation

I83.223   Varicose veins of left lower extremity with both ulcer of ankle and inflammation

I83.224   Varicose veins of left lower extremity with both ulcer of heel and midfoot and inflammation

Varicose veins of left lower extremity with bothulcer of plantar surface of midfoot and inflammation

I83.225   Varicose veins of left lower extremity with both ulcer other part of foot and inflammation

Varicose veins of left lower extremity with both ulcer of toe and inflammation

I83.228   Varicose veins of left lower extremity with both ulcer of other part of lower extremity and inflammation

I83.229   Varicose veins of left lower extremity with both ulcer of unspecified site and inflammation

I83.8   Varicose veins of lower extremities with other complications

I83.81   Varicose veins of lower extremities with pain

I83.811   Varicose veins of right lower extremities with pain

I83.812   Varicose veins of left lower extremities with pain

I83.813   Varicose veins of bilateral lower extremities with pain

I83.819   Varicose veins of unspecified lower extremities with pain

I83.89   Varicose veins of lower extremities with other complications

Varicose veins of lower extremities with edema

Varicose veins of lower extremities with swelling

I83.891   Varicose veins of right lower extremities with other complications

I83.892   Varicose veins of left lower extremities with other complications

I83.893   Varicose veins of bilateral lower extremities with other complications

I83.899   Varicose veins of unspecified lower extremities with other complications

I83.9   Asymptomatic varicose veins of lower extremities

Phlebectasia of lower extremities

Varicose veins of lower extremities

Varix of lower extremities

I83.90   Asymptomatic varicose veins of unspecified lower extremity

Varicose veins NOS

I83.91   Asymptomatic varicose veins of right lower extremity

I83.92   Asymptomatic varicose veins of left lower extremity

I83.93   Asymptomatic varicose veins of bilateral lower extremities

I85   **Esophageal varices**

Use additional code to identify:

alcohol abuse and dependence (F10.-)

I85.0   Esophageal varices

Idiopathic esophageal varices

Primary esophageal varices

I85.00   Esophageal varices without bleeding

Esophageal varices NOS

I85.01   Esophageal varices with bleeding

I85.1   Secondary esophageal varices

Esophageal varices secondary to alcoholic liver disease

Esophageal varices secondary to cirrhosis of liver

Esophageal varices secondary to schistosomiasis

Esophageal varices secondary to toxic liver disease

Code first underlying disease

I85.10   Secondary esophageal varices without bleeding

I85.11   Secondary esophageal varices with bleeding

I86   **Varicose veins of other sites**

Excludes1: varicose veins of unspecified site (I83.9-)

Excludes2: retinal varices (H35.0-)

I86.0   Sublingual varices

I86.1   Scrotal varices

Varicocele

I86.2   Pelvic varices

I86.3   Vulval varices

Excludes1: vulval varices complicating childbirth and the puerperium (O87.8)

vulval varices complicating pregnancy (O22.1-)

I86.4   Gastric varices

I86.8   Varicose veins of other specified sites

Varicose ulcer of nasal septum

I87   **Other disorders of veins**

I87.0   Postthrombotic syndrome

Chronic venous hypertension due to deep vein thrombosis

Postphlebitic syndrome

Excludes1: chronic venous hypertension without deep vein thrombosis (I87.3-)

I87.00   Postthrombotic syndrome without complications

Asymptomatic Postthrombotic syndrome

I87.001   Postthrombotic syndrome without complications of right lower extremity

I87.002   Postthrombotic syndrome without complications of left lower extremity

---

I87.003   **Postthrombotic syndrome without complications of bilateral lower extremity**

I87.009   **Postthrombotic syndrome without complications of unspecified extremity**

Postthrombotic syndrome NOS

I87.01   **Postthrombotic syndrome with ulcer**

<u>Use additional code</u> to specify site and severity of ulcer (L97.-)

I87.011   **Postthrombotic syndrome with ulcer of right lower extremity**

I87.012   **Postthrombotic syndrome with ulcer of left lower extremity**

I87.013   **Postthrombotic syndrome with ulcer of bilateral lower extremity**

I87.019   **Postthrombotic syndrome with ulcer of unspecified lower extremity**

I87.02   **Postthrombotic syndrome with inflammation**

I87.021   **Postthrombotic syndrome with inflammation of right lower extremity**

I87.022   **Postthrombotic syndrome with inflammation of left lower extremity**

I87.023   **Postthrombotic syndrome with inflammation of bilateral lower extremity**

I87.029   **Postthrombotic syndrome with inflammation of unspecified lower extremity**

I87.03   **Postthrombotic syndrome with ulcer and inflammation**

<u>Use additional code</u> to specify site and severity of ulcer (L97.-)

I87.031   **Postthrombotic syndrome with ulcer and inflammation of right lower extremity**

I87.032   **Postthrombotic syndrome with ulcer and inflammation of left lower extremity**

I87.033   **Postthrombotic syndrome with ulcer and inflammation of bilateral lower extremity**

I87.039   **Postthrombotic syndrome with ulcer and inflammation of unspecified lower extremity**

I87.09   **Postthrombotic syndrome with other complications**

I87.091   **Postthrombotic syndrome with other complications of right lower extremity**

I87.092   **Postthrombotic syndrome with other complications of left lower extremity**

I87.093   **Postthrombotic syndrome with other complications of bilateral lower extremity**

I87.099   **Postthrombotic syndrome with other complications of unspecified lower extremity**

I87.1   **Compression of vein**

Stricture of vein

Vena cava syndrome (inferior) (superior)

Excludes2: compression of pulmonary vein (I28.8)

I87.2   **Venous insufficiency (chronic) (peripheral)**

Stasis dermatitis

Excludes1: stasis dermatitis with varicose veins of lower extremities (I83.1-, I83.2-)

I87.3   **Chronic venous hypertension (idiopathic)**

Stasis edema

Excludes1: chronic venous hypertension due to deep vein thrombosis (I87.0-)

varicose veins of lower extremities (I83.-)

I87.30   **Chronic venous hypertension (idiopathic) without complications**

Asymptomatic chronic venous hypertension (idiopathic)

I87.301   **Chronic venous hypertension (idiopathic) without complications of right lower extremity**

I87.302   **Chronic venous hypertension (idiopathic) without complications of left lower extremity**

I87.303   **Chronic venous hypertension (idiopathic) without complications of bilateral lower extremity**

I87.309   **Chronic venous hypertension (idiopathic) without complications of unspecified lower extremity**

Chronic venous hypertension NOS

I87.31   **Chronic venous hypertension (idiopathic) with ulcer**

<u>Use additional code</u> to specify site and severity of ulcer (L97.-)

I87.311   **Chronic venous hypertension (idiopathic) with ulcer of right lower extremity**

I87.312   **Chronic venous hypertension (idiopathic) with ulcer of left lower extremity**

I87.313   **Chronic venous hypertension (idiopathic) with ulcer of bilateral lower extremity**

I87.319   **Chronic venous hypertension (idiopathic) with ulcer of unspecified lower extremity**

I87.32   **Chronic venous hypertension (idiopathic) with inflammation**

I87.321   **Chronic venous hypertension (idiopathic) with inflammation of right lower extremity**

I87.322   **Chronic venous hypertension (idiopathic) with inflammation of left lower extremity**

I87.323   **Chronic venous hypertension (idiopathic) with inflammation of bilateral lower extremity**

I87.329   **Chronic venous hypertension (idiopathic) with inflammation of unspecified lower extremity**

I87.33   **Chronic venous hypertension (idiopathic) with ulcer and inflammation**

<u>Use additional code</u> to specify site and severity of ulcer (L97.-)

I87.331 Chronic venous hypertension (idiopathic) with ulcer and inflammation of right lower extremity

I87.332 Chronic venous hypertension (idiopathic) with ulcer and inflammation of left lower extremity

I87.333 Chronic venous hypertension (idiopathic) with ulcer and inflammation of bilateral lower extremity

I87.339 Chronic venous hypertension (idiopathic) with ulcer and inflammation of unspecified lower extremity

I87.39 Chronic venous hypertension (idiopathic) with other complications

I87.391 Chronic venous hypertension (idiopathic) with other complications of right lower extremity

I87.392 Chronic venous hypertension (idiopathic) with other complications of left lower extremity

I87.393 Chronic venous hypertension (idiopathic) with other complications of bilateral lower extremity

I87.399 Chronic venous hypertension (idiopathic) with other complications of unspecified lower extremity

I87.8 Other specified disorders of veins

Phlebosclerosis

Venofibrosis

I87.9 Disorder of vein, unspecified

I88 Nonspecific lymphadenitis

Excludes1: acute lymphadenitis, except mesenteric (L04.-)

enlarged lymph nodes NOS (R59.-)

human immunodeficiency virus [HIV] disease resulting in generalized lymphadenopathy (B20)

I88.0 Nonspecific mesenteric lymphadenitis

Mesenteric lymphadenitis (acute)(chronic)

I88.1 Chronic lymphadenitis, except mesenteric

Adenitis

Lymphadenitis

I88.8 Other nonspecific lymphadenitis

I88.9 Nonspecific lymphadenitis, unspecified

Lymphadenitis NOS

I89 Other noninfective disorders of lymphatic vessels and lymph nodes

Excludes1: chylocele, tunica vaginalis (nonfilarial) NOS (N50.89)

enlarged lymph nodes NOS (R59.-)

filarial chylocele (B74.-)

hereditary lymphedema (Q82.0)

I89.0 Lymphedema, not elsewhere classified

Elephantiasis (nonfilarial) NOS

Lymphangiectasis

Obliteration, lymphatic vessel

Praecox lymphedema

Secondary lymphedema

Excludes1: postmastectomy lymphedema (I97.2)

I89.1 Lymphangitis

Chronic lymphangitis

Lymphangitis NOS

Subacute lymphangitis

Excludes1: acute lymphangitis (L03.-)

I89.8 Other specified noninfective disorders of lymphatic vessels and lymph nodes

Chylocele (nonfilarial)

Chylous ascites

Chylous cyst

Lipomelanotic reticulosis

Lymph node or vessel fistula

Lymph node or vessel infarction

Lymph node or vessel rupture

I89.9 Noninfective disorder of lymphatic vessels and lymph nodes, unspecified

Disease of lymphatic vessels NOS

OTHER AND UNSPECIFIED DISORDERS OF THE CIRCULATORY SYSTEM (I95-I99)

I95 Hypotension

Excludes1: cardiovascular collapse (R57.9)

maternal hypotension syndrome (O26.5-)

nonspecific low blood pressure reading NOS (R03.1)

I95.0 Idiopathic hypotension

I95.1 Orthostatic hypotension

Hypotension, postural

Excludes1: neurogenic orthostatic hypotension [Shy-Drager] (G90.3)

orthostatic hypotension due to drugs (I95.2)

I95.2 Hypotension due to drugs

Orthostatic hypotension due to drugs

Use additional code for adverse effect, if applicable, to identify drug (T36-T50 with fifth or sixth character 5)

I95.3 Hypotension of hemodialysis

Intra-dialytic hypotension

I95.8 Other hypotension

I95.81 Postprocedural hypotension

I95.89 Other hypotension

Chronic hypotension

I95.9 Hypotension, unspecified

I96 Gangrene, not elsewhere classified

Gangrenous cellulitis

Excludes1: gangrene in atherosclerosis of native arteries of the extremities (I70.26)

gangrene in diabetes mellitus (E08-E13 with .52)

gangrene in hernia (K40.1, K40.4, K41.1, K41.4, K42.1, K43.1-, K44.1, K45.1, K46.1)

gangrene in other peripheral vascular diseases (I73.-)

gangrene of certain specified sites - see Alphabetical Index gas gangrene (A48.0)

pyoderma gangrenosum (L88)

I97 **Intraoperative and postprocedural complications and disorders of circulatory system, not elsewhere classified**

Excludes2: postprocedural shock (T81.1-)

I97.0 **Postcardiotomy syndrome**

I97.1 **Other postprocedural cardiac functional disturbances**

Excludes2: acute pulmonary insufficiency following thoracic surgery (J95.1)

intraoperative cardiac functional disturbances (I97.7-)

I97.11 **Postprocedural cardiac insufficiency**

I97.110 **Postprocedural cardiac insufficiency following cardiac surgery**

I97.111 **Postprocedural cardiac insufficiency following other surgery**

I97.12 **Postprocedural cardiac arrest**

I97.120 **Postprocedural cardiac arrest following cardiac surgery**

I97.121 **Postprocedural cardiac arrest following other surgery**

I97.13 **Postprocedural heart failure**

Use additional code to identify the heart failure (I50.-)

I97.130 **Postprocedural heart failure following cardiac surgery**

I97.131 **Postprocedural heart failure following other surgery**

I97.19 **Other postprocedural cardiac functional disturbances**

Use additional code, if applicable, to further specify disorder

I97.190 **Other postprocedural cardiac functional disturbances following cardiac surgery**

I97.191 **Other postprocedural cardiac functional disturbances following other surgery**

I97.2 **Postmastectomy lymphedema syndrome**

Elephantiasis due to mastectomy

Obliteration of lymphatic vessels

I97.3 **Postprocedural hypertension**

I97.4 **Intraoperative hemorrhage and hematoma of a circulatory system organ or structure complicating a procedure**

Excludes1: intraoperative hemorrhage and hematoma of a circulatory system organ or structure due to

accidental puncture and laceration during a procedure (I97.5-)

Excludes2: intraoperative cerebrovascular hemorrhage complicating a procedure (G97.3-)

I97.41 **Intraoperative hemorrhage and hematoma of a circulatory system organ or structure complicating a circulatory system procedure**

I97.410 **Intraoperative hemorrhage and hematoma of a circulatory system organ or structure complicating a cardiac catheterization**

I97.411 **Intraoperative hemorrhage and hematoma of a circulatory system**

organ or structure complicating a cardiac bypass

I97.418 **Intraoperative hemorrhage and hematoma of a circulatory system organ or structure complicating other circulatory system procedure**

I97.42 **Intraoperative hemorrhage and hematoma of a circulatory system organ or structure complicating other procedure**

I97.5 **Accidental puncture and laceration of a circulatory system organ or structure during a procedure**

Excludes2: accidental puncture and laceration of brain during a procedure (G97.4-)

I97.51 **Accidental puncture and laceration of a circulatory system organ or structure during a circulatory system procedure**

I97.52 **Accidental puncture and laceration of a circulatory system organ or structure during other procedure**

I97.6 **Postprocedural hemorrhage, hematoma and seroma of a circulatory system organ or structure following a procedure**

Excludes2: postprocedural cerebrovascular hemorrhage complicating a procedure (G97.5-)

I97.61 **Postprocedural hemorrhage of a circulatory system organ or structure following a circulatory system procedure**

▲I97.610 **Postprocedural hemorrhage of a circulatory system organ or structure following a cardiac catheterization**

▲I97.611 **Postprocedural hemorrhage of a circulatory system organ or structure following cardiac bypass**

▲I97.618 **Postprocedural hemorrhage of a circulatory system organ or structure following other circulatory system procedure**

I97.62 **Postprocedural hemorrhage, hematoma and seroma of a circulatory system organ or structure following other procedure**

●I97.620 **Postprocedural hemorrhage of a circulatory system organ or structure following other procedure**

●I97.621 **Postprocedural hematoma of a circulatory system organ or structure following other procedure**

●I97.622 **Postprocedural seroma of a circulatory system organ or structure following other procedure**

I97.63 **Postprocedural hematoma of a circulatory system organ or structure following a circulatory system procedure**

●I97.630 **Postprocedural hematoma of a circulatory system organ or structure following a cardiac catheterization**

●I97.631 **Postprocedural hematoma of a circulatory system organ or structure following cardiac bypass**

●I97.638 **Postprocedural hematoma of a circulatory system organ or structure following other circulatory system procedure**

I97.64   **Postprocedural seroma of a circulatory system organ or structure following a circulatory system procedure**

- I97.640 **Postprocedural seroma of a circulatory system organ or structure following a cardiac catheterization**
- I97.641 **Postprocedural seroma of a circulatory system organ or structure following cardiac bypass**
- I97.648 **Postprocedural seroma of a circulatory system organ or structure following other circulatory system procedure**

I97.7 **Intraoperative cardiac functional disturbances**

Excludes2: acute pulmonary insufficiency following thoracic surgery (J95.1)

postprocedural cardiac functional disturbances (I97.1-)

I97.71 **Intraoperative cardiac arrest**

I97.710 **Intraoperative cardiac arrest during cardiac surgery**

I97.711 **Intraoperative cardiac arrest during other surgery**

I97.79 **Other intraoperative cardiac functional disturbances**

Use additional code, if applicable, to further specify disorder

I97.790 **Other intraoperative cardiac functional disturbances during cardiac surgery**

I97.791 **Other intraoperative cardiac functional disturbances during other surgery**

I97.8 **Other intraoperative and postprocedural complications and disorders of the circulatory system, not elsewhere classified**

Use additional code, if applicable, to further specify disorder

I97.81 **Intraoperative cerebrovascular infarction**

I97.810 **Intraoperative cerebrovascular infarction during cardiac surgery**

I97.811 **Intraoperative cerebrovascular infarction during other surgery**

I97.82 **Postprocedural cerebrovascular infarction**

▲I97.820 **Postprocedural cerebrovascular infarction following cardiac surgery**

▲I97.821 **Postprocedural cerebrovascular infarction following other surgery**

I97.88 **Other intraoperative complications of the circulatory system, not elsewhere classified**

I97.89 **Other postprocedural complications and disorders of the circulatory system, not elsewhere classified**

I99 **Other and unspecified disorders of circulatory system**

I99.8 **Other disorder of circulatory system**

I99.9 **Unspecified disorder of circulatory system**

● New code ▲ Revised code **Excludes1:** Not coded here **Excludes2:** Not included here ⊗ Placeholder required ⑦ 7ᵗʰ digit required

Chapter 10: Diseases Of The Respiratory System (J00-J99)

DEFINITIONS

This chapter includes definitions of selected key words, terms and phrases and coding alerts for adding points to the clinical domain, and references to coding late effects where appropriate. An example from this chapter is as follows:

J01   Acute sinusitis
    Definition: Sinusitis is an infection of the small, air-filled cavities inside the cheekbones and forehead.

MULTIPLE CODING FOR A SINGLE CONDITION

In addition to the etiology/manifestation convention that requires two codes to fully describe a single condition that affects multiple body systems, there are other single conditions that also require more than one code. "Use additional code" notes are found in the Tabular List at codes that are not part of an etiology/manifestation pair where a secondary code is useful to fully describe a condition. The sequencing rule is the same as the etiology/manifestation pair, "use additional code" indicates that a secondary code should be added.

For example, for bacterial infections that are not included in chapter 1, a secondary code from category B95, Streptococcus, Staphylococcus, and Enterococcus, as the cause of diseases classified elsewhere, or B96, Other bacterial agents as the cause of diseases classified elsewhere, may be required to identify the bacterial organism causing the infection. A "use additional code" note will normally be found at the infectious disease code, indicating a need for the organism code to be added as a secondary code.

"Code first" notes are also under certain codes that are not specifically manifestation codes but may be due to an underlying cause. When there is a "code first" note and an underlying condition is present, the underlying condition should be sequenced first.

"Code, if applicable, any causal condition first", notes indicate that this code may be assigned as a principal diagnosis when the causal condition is unknown or not applicable. If a causal condition is known, then the code for that condition should be sequenced as the principal or first-listed diagnosis.

Multiple codes may be needed for sequela, complication codes and obstetric codes to more fully describe a condition. See the specific guidelines for these conditions for further instruction.

COMBINATION CODE

A combination code is a single code used to classify: Two diagnoses, or a diagnosis with an associated secondary process (manifestation) A diagnosis with an associated complication

Combination codes are identified by referring to subterm entries in the Alphabetic Index and by reading the inclusion and exclusion notes in the Tabular List.

Assign only the combination code when that code fully identifies the diagnostic conditions involved or when the Alphabetic Index so directs. Multiple coding should not be used when the classification provides a combination code that clearly identifies all of the elements documented in the diagnosis. When the combination code lacks necessary specificity in describing the manifestation or complication, an additional code should be used as a secondary code.

SEQUELA (LATE EFFECTS)

A sequela is the residual effect (condition produced) after the acute phase of an illness or injury has terminated. There is no time limit on when a sequela code can be used. The residual may be apparent early, such as in cerebral infarction, or it may occur months or years later, such as that due to a previous injury. Coding of sequela generally requires two codes sequenced in the following order: The condition or nature of the sequela is sequenced first.

The sequela code is sequenced second.

An exception to the above guidelines are those instances where the code for the sequela is followed by a manifestation code identified in the Tabular List and title, or the sequela code has been expanded (at the fourth, fifth or sixth character levels) to include the manifestation(s). The code for the acute phase of an illness or injury that led to the sequela is never used with a code for the late effect.

CHRONIC OBSTRUCTIVE PULMONARY DISEASE [COPD] AND ASTHMA

1) **Acute exacerbation of chronic obstructive bronchitis and asthma**

    The codes in categories J44 and J45 distinguish between uncomplicated cases and those in acute exacerbation. An acute exacerbation is a worsening or a decompensation of a chronic condition. An acute exacerbation is not equivalent to an infection superimposed on a chronic condition, though an exacerbation may be triggered by an infection.

ACUTE RESPIRATORY FAILURE

1) **Acute respiratory failure as principal diagnosis**

A code from subcategory J96.0, Acute respiratory failure, or subcategory J96.2, Acute and chronic respiratory failure, may be assigned as a principal diagnosis when it is the condition established after study to be chiefly responsible for occasioning the admission to the hospital, and the selection is supported by the Alphabetic Index and Tabular List. However, chapter-specific coding guidelines (such as obstetrics, poisoning, HIV, newborn) that provide sequencing direction take precedence.

2) Acute respiratory failure as secondary diagnosis

Respiratory failure may be listed as a secondary diagnosis if it occurs after admission, or if it is present on admission, but does not meet the definition of principal diagnosis.

3) Sequencing of acute respiratory failure and another acute condition

When a patient is admitted with respiratory failure and another acute condition, (e.g., myocardial infarction, cerebrovascular accident, aspiration pneumonia), the principal diagnosis will not be the same in every situation. This applies whether the other acute condition is a respiratory or nonrespiratory condition. Selection of the principal diagnosis will be dependent on the circumstances of admission. If both the respiratory failure and the other acute condition are equally responsible for occasioning the admission to the hospital, and there are no chapter-specific sequencing rules, the guideline regarding two or more diagnoses that equally meet the definition for principal diagnosis *(Section II, C.)* may be applied in these situations.

If the documentation is not clear as to whether acute respiratory failure and another condition are equally responsible for occasioning the admission, query the provider for clarification.

INFLUENZA DUE TO CERTAIN IDENTIFIED INFLUENZA VIRUSES

Code only confirmed cases of influenza due to certain identified influenza viruses (category J09), and due to other identified influenza virus (category J10). This is an exception to the hospital inpatient guideline Section II, H. (Uncertain Diagnosis).

In this context, "confirmation" does not require documentation of positive laboratory testing specific for avian or other novel influenza A or other identified influenza virus. However, coding should be based on the provider's diagnostic statement that the patient has avian influenza, or other novel influenza A, for category J09, or has another particular identified strain of influenza, such as H1N1 or H3N2, but not identified as novel or variant, for category J10.

If the provider records "suspected" or "possible" or "probable" avian influenza, or novel influenza, or other identified influenza, then the appropriate influenza code from category J11, Influenza due to unidentified influenza virus, should be assigned. A code from category J09, Influenza due to certain identified influenza viruses, should not be assigned nor should a code from category J10, Influenza due to other identified influenza virus.

VENTILATOR ASSOCIATED PNEUMONIA

1) Documentation of Ventilator associated Pneumonia

As with all procedural or postprocedural complications, code assignment is based on the provider's documentation of the relationship between the condition and the procedure.

Code J95.851, Ventilator associated pneumonia, should be assigned only when the provider has documented ventilator associated pneumonia (VAP). An additional code to identify the organism (e.g., Pseudomonas aeruginosa, code B96.5) should also be assigned. Do not assign an additional code from categories J12-J18 to identify the type of pneumonia.

Code J95.851 should not be assigned for cases where the patient has pneumonia and is on a mechanical ventilator and the provider has not specifically stated that the pneumonia is ventilator-associated pneumonia. If the documentation is unclear as to whether the patient has a pneumonia that is a complication attributable to the mechanical ventilator, query the provider.

2) Ventilator associated Pneumonia Develops after Admission

A patient may be admitted with one type of pneumonia (e.g., code J13, Pneumonia due to Streptococcus pneumonia) and subsequently develop VAP. In this instance, the principal diagnosis would be the appropriate code from categories J12-

J18 for the pneumonia diagnosed at the time of admission. Code J95.851, Ventilator associated pneumonia, would be assigned as an additional diagnosis when the provider has also documented the presence of ventilator associated pneumonia.

Chapter 10

Diseases Of The Respiratory System (J00-J99)

Note: When a respiratory condition is described as occurring in more than one site and is not specifically indexed, it should be classified to the lower anatomic site (e.g. tracheobronchitis to bronchitis in J40).

Use additional code, where applicable, to identify:

exposure to environmental tobacco smoke (Z77.22)

exposure to tobacco smoke in the perinatal period (P96.81)

history of tobacco dependence (Z87.891)

occupational exposure to environmental tobacco smoke (Z57.31)

tobacco dependence (F17.-)

tobacco use (Z72.0)

Excludes2: certain conditions originating in the perinatal period (P04-P96)

certain infectious and parasitic diseases (A00-B99)

complications of pregnancy, childbirth and the puerperium (O00-O9A)

congenital malformations, deformations and chromosomal abnormalities (Q00-Q99)

endocrine, nutritional and metabolic diseases (E00-E88)

injury, poisoning and certain other consequences of external causes (S00-T88) neoplasms (C00-D49)

smoke inhalation (T59.81-)

symptoms, signs and abnormal clinical and laboratory findings, not elsewhere classified (R00-R94)

This chapter contains the following blocks:

J00-J06	Acute upper respiratory infections
J09-J18	Influenza and pneumonia
J20-J22	Other acute lower respiratory infections
J30-J39	Other diseases of upper respiratory tract
J40-J47	Chronic lower respiratory diseases
J60-J70	Lung diseases due to external agents
J80-J84	Other respiratory diseases principally affecting the interstitium
J85-J86	Suppurative and necrotic conditions of the lower respiratory tract
J90-J94	Other diseases of the pleura
J95	Intraoperative and postprocedural complications and disorders of respiratory system, not elsewhere classified
J96-J99	Other diseases of the respiratory system

ACUTE UPPER RESPIRATORY INFECTIONS (J00-J06)

Excludes1: chronic obstructive pulmonary disease with acute lower respiratory infection (J44.0)

influenza virus **with other** respiratory manifestations (J09.X2, J10.1, J11.1)

J00   **Acute nasopharyngitis [common cold]**

Acute rhinitis

Coryza (acute)

Infective nasopharyngitis NOS

Infective rhinitis

Nasal catarrh, acute Nasopharyngitis NOS

Excludes1: acute pharyngitis (J02.-)

acute sore throat NOS (J02.9)

pharyngitis NOS (J02.9)

rhinitis NOS (J31.0)

sore throat NOS (J02.9)

Excludes2: allergic rhinitis (J30.1-J30.9)

chronic pharyngitis (J31.2)

chronic rhinitis (J31.0)

chronic sore throat (J31.2)

nasopharyngitis, chronic (J31.1)

vasomotor rhinitis (J30.0)

J01   **Acute sinusitis**

Includes: acute abscess of sinus

acute empyema of sinus

acute infection of sinus

acute inflammation of sinus

acute suppuration of sinus

Use additional code (B95-B97) to identify infectious agent.

Excludes1: sinusitis NOS (J32.9)

Excludes2: chronic sinusitis (J32.0-J32.8)

J01.0   **Acute maxillary sinusitis**

Acute antritis

   J01.00   **Acute maxillary sinusitis, unspecified**

   J01.01   **Acute recurrent maxillary sinusitis**

J01.1   **Acute frontal sinusitis**

   J01.10   **Acute frontal sinusitis, unspecified**

   J01.11   **Acute recurrent frontal sinusitis**

J01.2   **Acute ethmoidal sinusitis**

   J01.20   **Acute ethmoidal sinusitis, unspecified**

   J01.21   **Acute recurrent ethmoidal sinusitis**

J01.3   **Acute sphenoidal sinusitis**

   J01.30   **Acute sphenoidal sinusitis, unspecified**

   J01.31   **Acute recurrent sphenoidal sinusitis**

J01.4   **Acute pansinusitis**

   J01.40   **Acute pansinusitis, unspecified**

   J01.41   **Acute recurrent pansinusitis**

J01.8   **Other acute sinusitis**

   J01.80   **Other acute sinusitis**

   Acute sinusitis involving more than one sinus but not pansinusitis

   J01.81   **Other acute recurrent sinusitis**

   Acute recurrent sinusitis involving more than one sinus but not pansinusitis

J01.9   **Acute sinusitis, unspecified**

   J01.90   **Acute sinusitis, unspecified**

   J01.91   **Acute recurrent sinusitis, unspecified**

J02   **Acute pharyngitis**

Includes: acute sore throat

Excludes1: acute laryngopharyngitis (J06.0)

peritonsillar abscess (J36)

pharyngeal abscess (J39.1)

retropharyngeal abscess (J39.0)

Excludes2: chronic pharyngitis (J31.2)

J02.0   **Streptococcal pharyngitis**

Septic pharyngitis

Streptococcal sore throat

Excludes2: scarlet fever (A38.-)

J02.8 **Acute pharyngitis due to other specified organisms**

Use additional code (B95-B97) to identify infectious agent

Excludes1: acute pharyngitis due to coxsackie virus (B08.5)

acute pharyngitis due to gonococcus (A54.5)

acute pharyngitis due to herpes [simplex] virus (B00.2)

acute pharyngitis due to infectious mononucleosis (B27.-)

enteroviral vesicular pharyngitis (B08.5)

J02.9 **Acute pharyngitis, unspecified**

Gangrenous pharyngitis (acute)

Infective pharyngitis (acute) NOS

Pharyngitis (acute) NOS

Sore throat (acute) NOS

Suppurative pharyngitis (acute)

Ulcerative pharyngitis (acute)

J03 **Acute tonsillitis**

Excludes1: acute sore throat (J02.-)

hypertrophy of tonsils (J35.1)

peritonsillar abscess (J36)

sore throat NOS (J02.9)

streptococcal sore throat (J02.0)

Excludes2: chronic tonsillitis (J35.0)

J03.0 **Streptococcal tonsillitis**

J03.00 **Acute streptococcal tonsillitis, unspecified**

J03.01 **Acute recurrent streptococcal tonsillitis**

J03.8 **Acute tonsillitis due to other specified organisms**

Use additional code (B95-B97) to identify infectious agent.

Excludes1: diphtheritic tonsillitis (A36.0)

herpesviral pharyngotonsillitis (B00.2)

streptococcal tonsillitis (J03.0)

tuberculous tonsillitis (A15.8)

Vincent's tonsillitis (A69.1)

J03.80 **Acute tonsillitis due to other specified organisms**

J03.81 **Acute recurrent tonsillitis due to other specified organisms**

J03.9 **Acute tonsillitis, unspecified**

Follicular tonsillitis (acute) Gangrenous tonsillitis (acute)

Infective tonsillitis (acute)

Tonsillitis (acute) NOS

Ulcerative tonsillitis (acute)

J03.90 **Acute tonsillitis, unspecified**

J03.91 **Acute recurrent tonsillitis, unspecified**

J04 **Acute laryngitis and tracheitis**

Use additional code (B95-B97) to identify infectious agent.

Excludes1: acute obstructive laryngitis [croup] and epiglottitis (J05.-)

Excludes2: laryngismus (stridulus) (J38.5)

J04.0 **Acute laryngitis**

Edematous laryngitis (acute)

Laryngitis (acute) NOS

Subglottic laryngitis (acute)

Suppurative laryngitis (acute)

Ulcerative laryngitis (acute)

Excludes1: acute obstructive laryngitis (J05.0)

Excludes2: chronic laryngitis (J37.0)

J04.1 **Acute tracheitis**

Acute viral tracheitis

Catarrhal tracheitis (acute)

Tracheitis (acute) NOS

Excludes2: chronic tracheitis (J42)

J04.10 **Acute tracheitis without obstruction**

J04.11 **Acute tracheitis with obstruction**

J04.2 **Acute laryngotracheitis**

Laryngotracheitis NOS

Tracheitis (acute) with laryngitis (acute)

Excludes1: acute obstructive laryngotracheitis (J05.0)

Excludes2: chronic laryngotracheitis (J37.1)

J04.3 **Supraglottitis, unspecified**

J04.30 **Supraglottitis, unspecified, without obstruction**

J04.31 **Supraglottitis, unspecified, with obstruction**

J05 **Acute obstructive laryngitis [croup] and epiglottitis**

Use additional code (B95-B97) to identify infectious agent.

J05.0 **Acute obstructive laryngitis [croup]**

Obstructive laryngitis (acute) NOS

Obstructive laryngotracheitis NOS

J05.1 **Acute epiglottitis**

Excludes2: epiglottitis, chronic (J37.0)

J05.10 **Acute epiglottitis without obstruction**

Epiglottitis NOS

J05.11 **Acute epiglottitis with obstruction**

J06 **Acute upper respiratory infections of multiple and unspecified sites**

Excludes1: acute respiratory infection NOS (J22)

streptococcal pharyngitis (J02.0)

J06.0 **Acute laryngopharyngitis**

J06.9 **Acute upper respiratory infection, unspecified**

Upper respiratory disease, acute

Upper respiratory infection NOS

INFLUENZA AND PNEUMONIA (J09-J18)

Excludes2: allergic or eosinophilic pneumonia (J82)

aspiration pneumonia NOS (J69.0)

meconium pneumonia (P24.01)

neonatal aspiration pneumonia (P24.-)

pneumonia due to solids and liquids (J69.-)

congenital pneumonia (P23.9)

lipid pneumonia (J69.1)

rheumatic pneumonia (I00)

ventilator associated pneumonia (J95.851)

J09 **Influenza due to certain identified influenza viruses**

Excludes1: influenza due to other identified influenza virus (J10.-)

influenza due to unidentified influenza virus (J11.-)

seasonal influenza due to other identified influenza virus (J10.-)

seasonal influenza due to unidentified influenza virus (J11.-)

J09.X **Influenza due to identified novel influenza A virus**

Avian influenza

Bird influenza

Influenza A/H5N1

Influenza **of** other animal origin, not bird or swine

Swine influenza virus (viruses that normally cause infections in pigs)

J09.X1 **Influenza due to identified novel influenza A virus with pneumonia**

Code also, if applicable, associated:

lung abscess (J85.1)

Other specified type of pneumonia

J09.X2 **Influenza due to identified novel influenza A virus with other respiratory manifestations**

Influenza due to identified novel influenza A virus NOS

Influenza due to identified novel influenza A virus with laryngitis

Influenza due to identified novel influenza A virus with pharyngitis

Influenza due to identified novel influenza A virus with upper respiratory symptoms

Use additional code, if applicable, for associated:

pleural effusion (J91.8)

sinusitis (J01.-)

J09.X3 **Influenza due to identified novel influenza A virus with gastrointestinal manifestations**

Influenza due to identified novel influenza A virus gastroenteritis

Excludes1: 'intestinal flu' [viral gastroenteritis] (A08.-)

J09.X9 **Influenza due to identified novel influenza A virus with other manifestations**

Influenza due to identified novel influenza A virus with encephalopathy

Influenza due to identified novel influenza A virus with myocarditis

Influenza due to identified novel influenza A virus with otitis media

Use additional code to identify manifestation

J10 **Influenza due to other identified influenza virus**

Excludes1: influenza due to avian influenza virus (J09.X-)

influenza due to swine flu (J09.X-)

influenza due to unidentifed influenza virus (J11.-)

J10.0 **Influenza due to other identified influenza virus with pneumonia**

Code also associated lung abscess, if applicable (J85.1)

J10.00 **Influenza due to other identified influenza virus with unspecified type of pneumonia**

J10.01 **Influenza due to other identified influenza virus with the same other identified influenza virus pneumonia**

J10.08 **Influenza due to other identified influenza virus with other specified pneumonia**

Code also other specified type of pneumonia

J10.1 **Influenza due to other identified influenza virus with other respiratory manifestations**

Influenza due **to other** identified influenza virus NOS

Influenza due **to** other identified influenza virus with laryngitis

Influenza due to other identified influenza virus with pharyngitis

Influenza due to other identified influenza virus with upper respiratory symptoms

Use additional code for associated pleural effusion, if applicable (J91.8)

Use additional code for associated sinusitis, if applicable (J01.-)

J10.2 **Influenza due to other identified influenza virus with gastrointestinal manifestations**

Influenza due **to other** identified influenza virus gastroenteritis

Excludes1: 'intestinal flu' [viral gastroenteritis] (A08.-)

J10.8 **Influenza due to other identified influenza virus with other manifestations**

J10.81 **Influenza due to other identified influenza virus with encephalopathy**

J10.82 **Influenza due to other identified influenza virus with myocarditis**

J10.83 **Influenza due to other identified influenza virus with otitis media**

Use additional code for any associated perforated tympanic membrane (H72.-)

J10.89 **Influenza due to other identified influenza virus with other manifestations**

Use additional code to identify the manifestations

J11 **Influenza due to unidentified influenza virus**

J11.0 **Influenza due to unidentified influenza virus with pneumonia**

Code also associated lung abscess, if applicable (J85.1)

J11.00 **Influenza due to unidentified influenza virus with unspecified type of pneumonia**

Influenza with pneumonia NOS

J11.08 **Influenza due to unidentified influenza virus with specified pneumonia**

Code also other specified type of pneumonia

J11.1 **Influenza due to unidentified influenza virus with other respiratory manifestations**

Influenza NOS

Influenzal laryngitis NOS

Influenzal pharyngitis NOS

Influenza with upper respiratory symptoms NOS

Use additional code for associated pleural effusion, if applicable (J91.8)

Use additional code for associated sinusitis, if applicable (J01.-)

J11.2 **Influenza due to unidentified influenza virus with gastrointestinal manifestations**

Influenza gastroenteritis NOS

Excludes1: 'intestinal flu' [viral gastroenteritis] (A08.-)

J11.8 **Influenza due to unidentified influenza virus with other manifestations**

J11.81 **Influenza due to unidentified influenza virus with encephalopathy**

Influenzal encephalopathy NOS

J11.82   Influenza due to unidentified influenza virus with myocarditis

Influenzal myocarditis NOS

J11.83   Influenza due to unidentified influenza virus with otitis media

Influenzal otitis media NOS

Use additional code for any associated perforated tympanic membrane (H72.-)

J11.89   Influenza due to unidentified influenza virus with other manifestations

Use additional codes to identify the manifestations

J12   Viral pneumonia, not elsewhere classified

Includes: bronchopneumonia due to viruses other than influenza viruses

Code first associated influenza, if applicable (J09.X1, J10.0-, J11.0-)

Code also associated abscess, if applicable (J85.1)

Excludes1: aspiration pneumonia due to anesthesia during labor and delivery (O74.0)

aspiration pneumonia due to anesthesia during pregnancy (O29)

aspiration pneumonia due to anesthesia during puerperium (O89.0)

aspiration pneumonia due to solids and liquids (J69.-)

aspiration pneumonia NOS (J69.0)

congenital pneumonia (P23.0)

congenital rubella pneumonitis (P35.0)

interstitial pneumonia NOS (J84.9)

lipid pneumonia (J69.1)

neonatal aspiration pneumonia (P24.-)

J12.0   Adenoviral pneumonia

J12.1   Respiratory syncytial virus pneumonia

J12.2   Parainfluenza virus pneumonia

J12.3   Human metapneumovirus pneumonia

J12.8   Other viral pneumonia

J12.81   Pneumonia due to SARS-associated coronavirus

Severe acute respiratory syndrome NOS

J12.89   Other viral pneumonia

J12.9   Viral pneumonia, unspecified

J13   Pneumonia due to Streptococcus pneumoniae

Bronchopneumonia due to S. pneumoniae

Code first associated influenza, if applicable (J09.X1, J10.0-, J11.0-)

Code also associated abscess, if applicable (J85.1)

Excludes1: congenital pneumonia due to S. pneumoniae (P23.6)

lobar pneumonia, unspecified organism (J18.1)

pneumonia due **to other** streptococci (J15.3-J15.4)

J14   Pneumonia due to Hemophilus influenzae

Bronchopneumonia due to H. influenzae

Code first associated influenza, if applicable (J09.X1, J10.0-, J11.0-)

Code also associated abscess, if applicable (J85.1)

Excludes1: congenital pneumonia due to H. influenzae (P23.6)

J15   Bacterial pneumonia, not elsewhere classified

Includes: bronchopneumonia due to bacteria other than S. pneumoniae and H. influenzae

Code first associated influenza, if applicable (J09.X1, J10.0-, J11.0-)

Code also associated abscess, if applicable (J85.1)

Excludes1: chlamydial pneumonia (J16.0)

congenital pneumonia (P23.-)

Legionnaires' disease (A48.1)

spirochetal pneumonia (A69.8)

J15.0   Pneumonia due to Klebsiella pneumoniae

J15.1   Pneumonia due to Pseudomonas

J15.2   Pneumonia due to staphylococcus

J15.20   Pneumonia due to staphylococcus, unspecified

J15.21   Pneumonia due to staphylococcus aureus

J15.211   Pneumonia due to Methicillin susceptible Staphylococcus aureus

MSSA pneumonia

Pneumonia due to Staphylococcus aureus NOS

J15.212   Pneumonia due to Methicillin resistant Staphylococcus aureus

J15.29   Pneumonia due to other staphylococcus

J15.3   Pneumonia due to streptococcus, group B

J15.4   Pneumonia due to other streptococci

Excludes1: pneumonia due to streptococcus, group B (J15.3)

pneumonia due to Streptococcus pneumoniae (J13)

J15.5   Pneumonia due to Escherichia coli

J15.6   Pneumonia due to other aerobic Gram-negative bacteria

Pneumonia due to Serratia marcescens

J15.7   Pneumonia due to Mycoplasma pneumoniae

J15.8   Pneumonia due to other specified bacteria

J15.9   Unspecified bacterial pneumonia

Pneumonia due to gram-positive bacteria

J16   Pneumonia due to other infectious organisms, not elsewhere classified

Code first associated influenza, if applicable (J09.X1, J10.0-, J11.0-)

Code also associated abscess, if applicable (J85.1)

Excludes1: congenital pneumonia (P23.-)

ornithosis (A70)

pneumocystosis (B59)

pneumonia NOS (J18.9)

J16.0   Chlamydial pneumonia

J16.8   Pneumonia due to other specified infectious organisms

J17   Pneumonia in diseases classified elsewhere

Code first underlying disease, such as:

Q fever (A78) rheumatic fever (I00)

schistosomiasis (B65.0-B65.9)

Excludes1: candidial pneumonia (B37.1)

chlamydial pneumonia (J16.0)

gonorrheal pneumonia (A54.84)

histoplasmosis pneumonia (B39.0-B39.2)

measles pneumonia (B05.2)

nocardiosis pneumonia (A43.0)

pneumocystosis (B59)

pneumonia due to Pneumocystis carinii (B59)

pneumonia due to Pneumocystis jiroveci (B59)

pneumonia in actinomycosis (A42.0)

pneumonia in anthrax (A22.1)

pneumonia in ascariasis (B77.81)

pneumonia in aspergillosis (B44.0-B44.1)

pneumonia in coccidioidomycosis (B38.0-B38.2)

pneumonia in cytomegalovirus disease (B25.0)

pneumonia in toxoplasmosis (B58.3)

rubella pneumonia (B06.81)

salmonella pneumonia (A02.22)

spirochetal infection NEC with pneumonia (A69.8)

tularemia pneumonia (A21.2)

typhoid fever with pneumonia (A01.03)

varicella pneumonia (B01.2)

whooping cough with pneumonia (A37 with fifth-character 1)

J18   Pneumonia, unspecified organism

Code first associated influenza, if applicable (J09.X1, J10.0-, J11.0-)

Excludes1: abscess of lung with pneumonia (J85.1)

aspiration pneumonia due to anesthesia during labor and delivery (O74.0)

aspiration pneumonia due to anesthesia during pregnancy (O29)

aspiration pneumonia due to anesthesia during puerperium (O89.0)

aspiration pneumonia due to solids and liquids (J69.-)

aspiration pneumonia NOS (J69.0)

congenital pneumonia (P23.0)

drug-induced interstitial lung disorder (J70.2-J70.4)

interstitial pneumonia NOS (J84.9)

lipid pneumonia (J69.1)

neonatal aspiration pneumonia (P24.-)

pneumonitis due to external agents (J67-J70)

pneumonitis due to fumes and vapors (J68.0)

usual interstitial pneumonia (J84.17)

J18.0   Bronchopneumonia, unspecified organism

Definition: Bronchopneumonia is a pneumonia characterized by acute inflammation of the walls of the bronchioles

Excludes1: hypostatic bronchopneumonia (J18.2)

lipid pneumonia (J69.1)

Excludes2: acute bronchiolitis (J21.-)

chronic bronchiolitis (J44.9)

J18.1   Lobar pneumonia, unspecified organism

J18.2   Hypostatic pneumonia, unspecified organism

Hypostatic bronchopneumonia

Passive pneumonia

J18.8   Other pneumonia, unspecified organism

J18.9   Pneumonia, unspecified organism

OTHER ACUTE LOWER RESPIRATORY INFECTIONS (J20-J22)

Excludes2: chronic obstructive pulmonary disease with acute lower respiratory infection (J44.0)

J20   Acute bronchitis

Includes: acute and subacute bronchitis (with) bronchospasm

acute and subacute bronchitis (with) tracheitis

acute and subacute bronchitis (with) tracheobronchitis,

acute acute and subacute fibrinous bronchitis

acute and subacute membranous bronchitis acute and subacute purulent bronchitis acute and subacute septic bronchitis

Excludes1: bronchitis NOS (J40)

tracheobronchitis NOS (J40)

Excludes2: acute bronchitis with bronchiectasis (J47.0)

acute bronchitis with chronic obstructive asthma (J44.0)

acute bronchitis with chronic obstructive pulmonary disease (J44.0)

allergic bronchitis NOS (J45.909-)

bronchitis due to chemicals, fumes and vapors (J68.0)

chronic bronchitis NOS (J42)

chronic mucopurulent bronchitis (J41.1)

chronic obstructive bronchitis (J44.-)

chronic obstructive tracheobronchitis (J44.-)

chronic simple bronchitis (J41.0)

chronic tracheobronchitis (J42)

J20.0   Acute bronchitis due to Mycoplasma pneumoniae

J20.1   Acute bronchitis due to Hemophilus influenzae

J20.2   Acute bronchitis due to streptococcus

J20.3   Acute bronchitis due to coxsackievirus

J20.4   Acute bronchitis due to parainfluenza virus

J20.5   Acute bronchitis due to respiratory syncytial virus

J20.6   Acute bronchitis due to rhinovirus

J20.7   Acute bronchitis due to echovirus

J20.8   Acute bronchitis due to other specified organisms

J20.9   Acute bronchitis, unspecified

J21   Acute bronchiolitis

Includes: acute bronchiolitis with bronchospasm

Excludes2: respiratory bronchiolitis interstitial lung disease (J84.115)

J21.0   Acute bronchiolitis due to respiratory syncytial virus

J21.1   Acute bronchiolitis due to human metapneumovirus

J21.8   Acute bronchiolitis due to other specified organisms

J21.9   Acute bronchiolitis, unspecified

Bronchiolitis (acute)

Excludes1: chronic bronchiolitis (J44.-)

J22   Unspecified acute lower respiratory infection

Acute (lower) respiratory (tract) infection NOS

Excludes1: upper respiratory infection (acute) (J06.9)

OTHER DISEASES OF UPPER RESPIRATORY TRACT (J30-J39)

J30   Vasomotor and allergic rhinitis

Includes: spasmodic rhinorrhea

Excludes1: allergic rhinitis with asthma (bronchial) (J45.909)

rhinitis NOS (J31.0)

J30.0   Vasomotor rhinitis

J30.1   Allergic rhinitis due to pollen

Definition: Allergic rhinitis refers to a group of symptoms similar to those of a cold such as runny nose and sore throat, caused by an allergic reaction to an allergen such as dust, plant pollens or animal dander.

Allergy NOS due to pollen

Hay fever

Pollinosis

J30.2   Other seasonal allergic rhinitis

J30.5   Allergic rhinitis due to food

J30.8   Other allergic rhinitis

J30.81   Allergic rhinitis due to animal (cat) (dog) hair and dander

J30.89   Other allergic rhinitis

Perennial allergic rhinitis

J30.9   Allergic rhinitis, unspecified

J31   Chronic rhinitis, nasopharyngitis and pharyngitis

Use additional code to identify:

exposure to environmental tobacco smoke (Z77.22)

exposure to tobacco smoke in the perinatal period (P96.81)

history of tobacco dependence (Z87.891)

occupational exposure to environmental tobacco smoke (Z57.31)

tobacco dependence (F17.-)

tobacco use (Z72.0)

J31.0   Chronic rhinitis

Atrophic rhinitis (chronic)

Granulomatous rhinitis (chronic)

Hypertrophic rhinitis (chronic)

Obstructive rhinitis (chronic)

Ozena

Purulent rhinitis (chronic)

Rhinitis (chronic) NOS

Ulcerative rhinitis (chronic)

Excludes1: allergic rhinitis (J30.1-J30.9)

vasomotor rhinitis (J30.0)

J31.1   Chronic nasopharyngitis

Excludes2: acute nasopharyngitis (J00)

J31.2   Chronic pharyngitis

Chronic sore throat

Atrophic pharyngitis (chronic)

Granular pharyngitis (chronic)

Hypertrophic pharyngitis (chronic)

Excludes2: acute pharyngitis (J02.9)

J32   Chronic sinusitis

Includes: sinus abscess

sinus empyema

sinus infection

sinus suppuration

Use additional code to identify:

exposure to environmental tobacco smoke (Z77.22)

exposure to tobacco smoke in the perinatal period (P96.81)

history of tobacco dependence (Z87.891)

infectious agent (B95-B97)

occupational exposure to environmental tobacco smoke (Z57.31)

tobacco dependence (F17.-)

tobacco use (Z72.0)

Excludes2: acute sinusitis (J01.-)

J32.0   Chronic maxillary sinusitis

Antritis (chronic)

Maxillary sinusitis NOS

J32.1   Chronic frontal sinusitis

Frontal sinusitis NOS

J32.2   Chronic ethmoidal sinusitis

Ethmoidal sinusitis NOS

Excludes1: Woakes' ethmoiditis (J33.1)

J32.3   Chronic sphenoidal sinusitis

Sphenoidal sinusitis NOS

J32.4   Chronic pansinusitis

Pansinusitis NOS

J32.8   Other chronic sinusitis

Sinusitis (chronic) involving more than one sinus but not pansinusitis

J32.9   Chronic sinusitis, unspecified

Sinusitis (chronic) NOS

J33   Nasal polyp

Use additional code to identify:

exposure to environmental tobacco smoke (Z77.22)

exposure to tobacco smoke in the perinatal period (P96.81)

history of tobacco dependence (Z87.891)

occupational exposure to environmental tobacco smoke (Z57.31)

tobacco dependence (F17.-)

tobacco use (Z72.0)

Excludes1: adenomatous polyps (D14.0)

J33.0   Polyp of nasal cavity

Choanal polyp Nasopharyngeal polyp

J33.1   Polypoid sinus degeneration

Woakes' syndrome or ethmoiditis

J33.8   Other polyp of sinus

Accessory polyp of sinus

Ethmoidal polyp of sinus

Maxillary polyp of sinus \

Sphenoidal polyp of sinus

J33.9   Nasal polyp, unspecified

J34   Other and unspecified disorders of nose and nasal sinuses

Excludes2: varicose ulcer of nasal septum (I86.8)

J34.0   Abscess, furuncle and carbuncle of nose

Cellulitis of nose

Necrosis of nose

Ulceration of nose

J34.1   Cyst and mucocele of nose and nasal sinus

J34.2   Deviated nasal septum

Deflection or deviation of septum (nasal) (acquired)

Excludes1: congenital deviated nasal septum (Q67.4)

J34.3   Hypertrophy of nasal turbinates

J34.8   Other specified disorders of nose and nasal sinuses

J34.81   Nasal mucositis (ulcerative)

Code also type of associated therapy, such as:

antineoplastic and immunosuppressive drugs (T45.1X-)

radiological procedure and radiotherapy (Y84.2)

Excludes2: gastrointestinal mucositis (ulcerative) (K92.81)

mucositis (ulcerative) of vagina and vulva (N76.81)

oral mucositis (ulcerative) (K12.3-)

J34.89   **Other specified disorders of nose and nasal sinuses**

Perforation of nasal septum NOS

Rhinolith

J34.9   **Unspecified disorder of nose and nasal sinuses**

J35   **Chronic diseases of tonsils and adenoids**

Use additional code to identify:

exposure to environmental tobacco smoke (Z77.22)

exposure to tobacco smoke in the perinatal period (P96.81)

history of tobacco dependence (Z87.891)

occupational exposure to environmental tobacco smoke (Z57.31)

tobacco dependence (F17.-)

tobacco use (Z72.0)

J35.0   **Chronic tonsillitis and adenoiditis**

Excludes2: acute tonsillitis (J03.-)

J35.01   **Chronic tonsillitis**

J35.02   **Chronic adenoiditis**

J35.03   **Chronic tonsillitis and adenoiditis**

J35.1   **Hypertrophy of tonsils**

Enlargement of tonsils

Excludes1: hypertrophy of tonsils with tonsillitis (J35.0-)

J35.2   **Hypertrophy of adenoids**

Enlargement of adenoids

Excludes1: hypertrophy of adenoids with adenoiditis (J35.0-)

J35.3   **Hypertrophy of tonsils with hypertrophy of adenoids**

Excludes1: hypertrophy of tonsils and adenoids with tonsillitis and adenoiditis (J35.03)

J35.8   **Other chronic diseases of tonsils and adenoids**

Adenoid vegetations

Amygdalolith

Calculus, tonsil

Cicatrix of tonsil (and adenoid)

Tonsillar tag

Ulcer of tonsil

J35.9   **Chronic disease of tonsils and adenoids, unspecified**

Disease (chronic) of tonsils and adenoids NOS

J36   **Peritonsillar abscess**

Definition: A Peritonsillar abscess is an abscess forming in acute tonsillitis around one or both tonsils.

Includes: abscess of tonsil

peritonsillar cellulitis quinsy

Use additional code (B95-B97) to identify infectious agent.

Excludes1: acute tonsillitis (J03.-)

chronic tonsillitis (J35.0)

retropharyngeal abscess (J39.0)

tonsillitis NOS (J03.9-)

J37   **Chronic laryngitis and laryngotracheitis**

Use additional code to identify:

exposure to environmental tobacco smoke (Z77.22)

exposure to tobacco smoke in the perinatal period (P96.81)

history of tobacco dependence (Z87.891)

infectious agent (B95-B97)

occupational exposure to environmental tobacco smoke (Z57.31)

tobacco dependence (F17.-)

tobacco use (Z72.0)

J37.0   **Chronic laryngitis**

Catarrhal laryngitis

Hypertrophic laryngitis

Sicca laryngitis

Excludes2: acute laryngitis (J04.0)

obstructive (acute) laryngitis (J05.0)

J37.1   **Chronic laryngotracheitis**

Laryngitis, chronic, with tracheitis (chronic)

Tracheitis, chronic, with laryngitis

Excludes1: chronic tracheitis (J42)

Excludes2: acute laryngotracheitis (J04.2)

acute tracheitis (J04.1)

J38   **Diseases of vocal cords and larynx, not elsewhere classified**

Use additional code to identify:

exposure to environmental tobacco smoke (Z77.22)

exposure to tobacco smoke in the perinatal period (P96.81)

history of tobacco dependence (Z87.891)

occupational exposure to environmental tobacco smoke (Z57.31)

tobacco dependence (F17.-)

tobacco use (Z72.0)

Excludes1: congenital laryngeal stridor (P28.89)

obstructive laryngitis (acute) (J05.0)

postprocedural subglottic stenosis (J95.5)

stridor (R06.1)

ulcerative laryngitis (J04.0)

J38.0   **Paralysis of vocal cords and larynx**

Laryngoplegia

Paralysis of glottis

J38.00   **Paralysis of vocal cords and larynx, unspecified**

J38.01   **Paralysis of vocal cords and larynx, unilateral**

J38.02   **Paralysis of vocal cords and larynx, bilateral**

J38.1   **Polyp of vocal cord and larynx**

Excludes1: adenomatous polyps (D14.1)

J38.2   **Nodules of vocal cords**

Chorditis (fibrinous)(nodosa)(tuberosa)

Singer's nodes

Teacher's nodes

J38.3   **Other diseases of vocal cords**

Abscess of vocal cords

Cellulitis of vocal cords

Granuloma of vocal cords

Leukokeratosis of vocal cords

Leukoplakia of vocal cords

J38.4   **Edema of larynx**

Edema (of) glottis

Subglottic edema

Supraglottic edema

Excludes1: acute obstructive laryngitis [croup] (J05.0)

edematous laryngitis (J04.0)

J38.5 **Laryngeal spasm**

Laryngismus (stridulus)

J38.6 **Stenosis of larynx**

J38.7 **Other diseases of larynx**

Abscess of larynx

Cellulitis of larynx

Disease of larynx NOS

Necrosis of larynx

Pachyderma of larynx

Perichondritis of larynx

Ulcer of larynx

J39 **Other diseases of upper respiratory tract**

Excludes1: acute respiratory infection NOS (J22)

acute upper respiratory infection (J06.9)

upper respiratory inflammation due to chemicals, gases, fumes or vapors (J68.2)

J39.0 **Retropharyngeal and parapharyngeal abscess**

Peripharyngeal abscess

Excludes1: peritonsillar abscess (J36)

J39.1 **Other abscess of pharynx**

Cellulitis of pharynx Nasopharyngeal abscess

J39.2 **Other diseases of pharynx**

Cyst of pharynx

Edema of pharynx

Excludes2: chronic pharyngitis (J31.2)

ulcerative pharyngitis (J02.9)

J39.3 **Upper respiratory tract hypersensitivity reaction, site unspecified**

Excludes1: hypersensitivity reaction of upper respiratory tract, such as:

extrinsic allergic alveolitis (J67.9)

pneumoconiosis (J60-J67.9)

J39.8 **Other specified diseases of upper respiratory tract**

J39.9 **Disease of upper respiratory tract, unspecified**

CHRONIC LOWER RESPIRATORY DISEASES (J40-J47)

Excludes1: bronchitis due to chemicals, gases, fumes and vapors (J68.0)

Excludes2: cystic fibrosis (E84.-)

J40 **Bronchitis, not specified as acute or chronic**

Bronchitis NOS

Bronchitis with tracheitis NOS

Catarrhal bronchitis

Tracheobronchitis NOS

Use additional code to identify:

exposure to environmental tobacco smoke (Z77.22)

exposure to tobacco smoke in the perinatal period (P96.81)

history of tobacco dependence (Z87.891)

occupational exposure to environmental tobacco smoke (Z57.31)

tobacco dependence (F17.-)

tobacco use (Z72.0)

Excludes1: acute bronchitis (J20.-)

allergic bronchitis NOS (J45.909-)

asthmatic bronchitis NOS (J45.9-)

bronchitis due to chemicals, gases, fumes and vapors (J68.0)

J41 **Simple and mucopurulent chronic bronchitis**

Use additional code to identify:

exposure to environmental tobacco smoke (Z77.22)

exposure to tobacco smoke in the perinatal period (P96.81)

history of tobacco dependence (Z87.891)

occupational exposure to environmental tobacco smoke (Z57.31)

tobacco dependence (F17.-)

tobacco use (Z72.0)

Excludes1: chronic bronchitis NOS (J42)

chronic obstructive bronchitis (J44.-)

J41.0 **Simple chronic bronchitis**

J41.1 **Mucopurulent chronic bronchitis**

J41.8 **Mixed simple and mucopurulent chronic bronchitis**

J42 **Unspecified chronic bronchitis**

Chronic bronchitis NOS

Chronic tracheitis

Chronic tracheobronchitis

Use additional code to identify:

exposure to environmental tobacco smoke (Z77.22)

exposure to tobacco smoke in the perinatal period (P96.81)

history of tobacco dependence (Z87.891)

occupational exposure to environmental tobacco smoke (Z57.31)

tobacco dependence (F17.-)

tobacco use (Z72.0)

Excludes1: chronic asthmatic bronchitis (J44.-)

chronic bronchitis with airways obstruction (J44.-)

chronic emphysematous bronchitis (J44.-)

chronic obstructive pulmonary disease NOS (J44.9)

simple and mucopurulent chronic bronchitis (J41.-)

J43 **Emphysema**

Definition: Emphysema is a chronic respiratory disease where there is over-inflation of the air sacs (alveoli) in the lungs, causing a decrease in lung function, and often, breathlessness.

Use additional code to identify:

exposure to environmental tobacco smoke (Z77.22)

history of tobacco dependence (Z87.891)

occupational exposure to environmental tobacco smoke (Z57.31)

tobacco dependence (F17.-)

tobacco use (Z72.0)

Excludes1: compensatory emphysema (J98.3)

emphysema due to inhalation of chemicals, gases, fumes or vapors (J68.4)

emphysema with chronic (obstructive) bronchitis (J44.-)

emphysematous (obstructive) bronchitis (J44.-)

interstitial emphysema (J98.2)

mediastinal emphysema (J98.2)

neonatal interstitial emphysema (P25.0)

surgical (subcutaneous) emphysema (T81.82)

traumatic subcutaneous emphysema (T79.7)

J43.0   **Unilateral pulmonary emphysema [MacLeod's syndrome]**

Swyer-James syndrome

Unilateral emphysema

Unilateral hyperlucent lung

Unilateral pulmonary artery functional hypoplasia

Unilateral transparency of lung

J43.1   **Panlobular emphysema**

Panacinar emphysema

J43.2   **Centrilobular emphysema**

J43.8   **Other emphysema**

J43.9   **Emphysema, unspecified**

Bullous emphysema (lung)(pulmonary)

Emphysema (lung)(pulmonary) NOS

Emphysematous bleb

Vesicular emphysema (lung)(pulmonary)

J44   **Other chronic obstructive pulmonary disease**

Includes: asthma with chronic obstructive pulmonary disease

chronic asthmatic (obstructive) bronchitis

chronic bronchitis with airways obstruction

chronic bronchitis with emphysema

chronic emphysematous bronchitis

chronic obstructive asthma

chronic obstructive bronchitis

chronic obstructive tracheobronchitis

Code also type of asthma, if applicable (J45.-)

Use additional code to identify:

exposure to environmental tobacco smoke (Z77.22) history of tobacco dependence (Z87.891)

occupational exposure to environmental tobacco smoke (Z57.31) tobacco dependence (F17.-)

tobacco use (Z72.0)

Excludes1: bronchiectasis (J47.-)

chronic bronchitis NOS (J42)

chronic simple and mucopurulent bronchitis (J41.-)

chronic tracheitis (J42)

chronic tracheobronchitis (J42)

emphysema without chronic bronchitis (J43.-)

Excludes2: lung diseases due to external agents (J60-J70)

J44.0   **Chronic obstructive pulmonary disease with acute lower respiratory infection**

Use additional code to identify the infection

J44.1   **Chronic obstructive pulmonary disease with (acute) exacerbation**

Decompensated COPD

Decompensated COPD with (acute) exacerbation

Excludes2: chronic obstructive pulmonary disease [COPD] with acute bronchitis (J44.0)

J44.9   **Chronic obstructive pulmonary disease, unspecified**

Chronic obstructive airway disease NOS

Chronic obstructive lung disease NOS

J45   **Asthma**

Includes: allergic (predominantly) asthma

allergic bronchitis NOS

allergic rhinitis with asthma

atopic asthma

extrinsic allergic asthma

hay fever with asthma

idiosyncratic asthma

intrinsic nonallergic asthma

nonallergic asthma

Use additional code to identify:

exposure to environmental tobacco smoke (Z77.22)

exposure to tobacco smoke in the perinatal period (P96.81)

history of tobacco dependence (Z87.891)

occupational exposure to environmental tobacco smoke (Z57.31)

tobacco dependence (F17.-)

tobacco use (Z72.0)

Excludes1: detergent asthma (J69.8)

eosinophilic asthma (J82)

lung diseases due to external agents (J60-J70)

miner's asthma (J60)

wheezing NOS (R06.2)

wood asthma (J67.8)

Excludes2: asthma with chronic obstructive pulmonary disease (J44.9)

chronic asthmatic (obstructive) bronchitis (J44.9)

chronic obstructive asthma (J44.9)

J45.2   **Mild intermittent asthma**

J45.20   **Mild intermittent asthma, uncomplicated**

Mild intermittent asthma NOS

J45.21   **Mild intermittent asthma with (acute) exacerbation**

J45.22   **Mild intermittent asthma with status asthmaticus**

J45.3   **Mild persistent asthma**

J45.30   **Mild persistent asthma, uncomplicated**

Mild persistent asthma NOS

J45.31   **Mild persistent asthma with (acute) exacerbation**

J45.32   **Mild persistent asthma with status asthmaticus**

J45.4   **Moderate persistent asthma**

J45.40   **Moderate persistent asthma, uncomplicated**

Moderate persistent asthma NOS

J45.41   **Moderate persistent asthma with (acute) exacerbation**

J45.42   **Moderate persistent asthma with status asthmaticus**

J45.5   **Severe persistent asthma**

J45.50   **Severe persistent asthma, uncomplicated**

Severe persistent asthma NOS

J45.51   **Severe persistent asthma with (acute) exacerbation**

J45.52   **Severe persistent asthma with status asthmaticus**

J45.9   **Other and unspecified asthma**

J45.90   **Unspecified asthma**

Asthmatic bronchitis NOS

Childhood asthma NOS

Late onset asthma

J45.901 Unspecified asthma with (acute) exacerbation

J45.902 Unspecified asthma with status asthmaticus

J45.909 Unspecified asthma, uncomplicated

Asthma NOS

J45.99 Other asthma

J45.990 Exercise induced bronchospasm

J45.991 Cough variant asthma

J45.998 Other asthma

J47 **Bronchiectasis**

Definition: Bronchiectasis is a condition characterized by abnormal dilatation of the bronchi (airways) and excessive mucus production. The mucus accumulation may obstruct the bronchi. Is often associated with repeated bronchial infections.

Includes: bronchiolectasis

Use additional code to identify:

exposure to environmental tobacco smoke (Z77.22)

exposure to tobacco smoke in the perinatal period (P96.81)

history of tobacco dependence (Z87.891)

occupational exposure to environmental tobacco smoke (Z57.31)

tobacco dependence (F17.-)

tobacco use (Z72.0)

Excludes1: congenital bronchiectasis (Q33.4)

tuberculous bronchiectasis (current disease) (A15.0)

J47.0 **Bronchiectasis with acute lower respiratory infection**

Bronchiectasis with acute bronchitis

Use additional code to identify the infection

J47.1 **Bronchiectasis with (acute) exacerbation**

J47.9 **Bronchiectasis, uncomplicated**

Bronchiectasis NOS

LUNG DISEASES DUE TO EXTERNAL AGENTS (J60-J70)

Excludes2: asthma (J45.-)

malignant neoplasm of bronchus and lung (C34.-)

J60 **Coalworker's pneumoconiosis**

Anthracosilicosis

Anthracosis

Black lung disease

Coalworker's lung

Excludes1: coalworker pneumoconiosis with tuberculosis, any type in A15 (J65)

J61 **Pneumoconiosis due to asbestos and other mineral fibers**

Asbestosis

Excludes1: pleural plaque with asbestosis (J92.0)

pneumoconiosis with tuberculosis, any type in A15 (J65)

J62 **Pneumoconiosis due to dust containing silica**

Includes: silicotic fibrosis (massive) of lung

Excludes1: pneumoconiosis with tuberculosis, any type in A15 (J65)

J62.0 **Pneumoconiosis due to talc dust**

J62.8 **Pneumoconiosis due to other dust containing silica**

Silicosis NOS

J63 **Pneumoconiosis due to other inorganic dusts**

Excludes1: pneumoconiosis with tuberculosis, any type in A15 (J65)

J63.0 **Aluminosis (of lung)**

J63.1 **Bauxite fibrosis (of lung)**

J63.2 **Berylliosis**

J63.3 **Graphite fibrosis (of lung)**

J63.4 **Siderosis**

J63.5 **Stannosis**

J63.6 **Pneumoconiosis due to other specified inorganic dusts**

J64 **Unspecified pneumoconiosis**

Excludes1: pneumonoconiosis with tuberculosis, any type in A15 (J65)

J65 **Pneumoconiosis associated with tuberculosis**

Any condition in J60-J64 with tuberculosis, any type in A15

Silicotuberculosis

J66 **Airway disease due to specific organic dust**

Excludes2: allergic alveolitis (J67.-)

asbestosis (J61)

bagassosis (J67.1)

farmer's lung (J67.0)

hypersensitivity pneumonitis due to organic dust (J67.-)

reactive airways dysfunction syndrome (J68.3)

J66.0 **Byssinosis**

Airway disease due to cotton dust

J66.1 **Flax-dressers' disease**

J66.2 **Cannabinosis**

J66.8 **Airway disease due to other specific organic dusts**

J67 **Hypersensitivity pneumonitis due to organic dust**

Includes: allergic alveolitis and pneumonitis due to inhaled organic dust and particles of fungal, actinomycetic **or other** origin

Excludes1: pneumonitis due to inhalation of chemicals, gases, fumes or vapors (J68.0)

J67.0 **Farmer's lung**

Harvester's lung

Haymaker's lung

Moldy hay disease

J67.1 **Bagassosis**

Bagasse disease

Bagasse pneumonitis

J67.2 **Bird fancier's lung**

Budgerigar fancier's disease or lung

Pigeon fancier's disease or lung

J67.3 **Suberosis**

Corkhandler's disease or lung

Corkworker's disease or lung

J67.4 **Maltworker's lung**

Alveolitis due to Aspergillus clavatus

J67.5 **Mushroom-worker's lung**

J67.6 **Maple-bark-stripper's lung**

Alveolitis due to

Cryptostroma corticale

Cryptostromosis

J67.7 **Air conditioner and humidifier lung**

Allergic alveolitis due to fungal, thermophilic actinomycetes **and other** organisms growing in ventilation [air conditioning] systems

J67.8 **Hypersensitivity pneumonitis due to other organic dusts**

Cheese-washer's lung

Coffee-worker's lung

Fish-meal worker's lung

Furrier's lung

Sequoiosis

J67.9 Hypersensitivity pneumonitis due to unspecified organic dust

Allergic alveolitis (extrinsic) NOS

Hypersensitivity pneumonitis NOS

J68 Respiratory conditions due to inhalation of chemicals, gases, fumes and vapors

Code first (T51-T65) to identify cause

Use additional code to identify associated respiratory conditions, such as:

acute respiratory failure (J96.0-)

J68.0 Bronchitis and pneumonitis due to chemicals, gases, fumes and vapors

Chemical bronchitis (acute)

J68.1 Pulmonary edema due to chemicals, gases, fumes and vapors

Chemical pulmonary edema (acute) (chronic)

Excludes1: pulmonary edema (acute) (chronic) NOS (J81.-)

J68.2 Upper respiratory inflammation due to chemicals, gases, fumes and vapors, not elsewhere classified

J68.3 Other acute and subacute respiratory conditions due to chemicals, gases, fumes and vapors

Reactive airways dysfunction syndrome

J68.4 Chronic respiratory conditions due to chemicals, gases, fumes and vapors

Emphysema (diffuse) (chronic) due to inhalation of chemicals, gases, fumes and vapors

Obliterative bronchiolitis (chronic) (subacute) due to inhalation of chemicals, gases, fumes and vapors

Pulmonary fibrosis (chronic) due to inhalation of chemicals, gases, fumes and vapors

Excludes1: chronic pulmonary edema due to chemicals, gases, fumes and vapors (J68.1)

J68.8 Other respiratory conditions due to chemicals, gases, fumes and vapors

J68.9 Unspecified respiratory condition due to chemicals, gases, fumes and vapors

J69 Pneumonitis due to solids and liquids

Excludes1: neonatal aspiration syndromes (P24.-)

postprocedural pneumonitis (J95.4)

J69.0 Pneumonitis due to inhalation of food and vomit

Aspiration pneumonia NOS

Aspiration pneumonia (due to) food (regurgitated)

Aspiration pneumonia (due to) gastric secretions

Aspiration pneumonia (due to) milk

Aspiration pneumonia (due to) vomit

Code also any associated foreign body in respiratory tract (T17.-)

Excludes1: chemical pneumonitis due to anesthesia (J95.4)

obstetric aspiration pneumonitis (O74.0)

J69.1 Pneumonitis due to inhalation of oils and essences

Exogenous lipoid pneumonia

Lipid pneumonia NOS

Code first (T51-T65) to identify substance

Excludes1: endogenous lipoid pneumonia (J84.89)

J69.8 Pneumonitis due to inhalation of other solids and liquids

Pneumonitis due to aspiration of blood

Pneumonitis due to aspiration of detergent

Code first (T51-T65) to identify substance

J70 Respiratory conditions due to other external agents

J70.0 Acute pulmonary manifestations due to radiation

Radiation pneumonitis

Use additional code (W88-W90, X39.0-) to identify the external cause

J70.1 Chronic and other pulmonary manifestations due to radiation

Fibrosis of lung following radiation

Use additional code (W88-W90, X39.0-) to identify the external cause

J70.2 Acute drug-induced interstitial lung disorders

Use additional code for adverse effect, if applicable, to identify drug (T36-T50 with fifth or sixth character 5)

Excludes1: interstitial pneumonia NOS (J84.9)

lymphoid interstitial pneumonia (J84.2)

J70.3 Chronic drug-induced interstitial lung disorders

Use additional code for adverse effect, if applicable, to identify drug (T36-T50 with fifth or sixth character 5)

Excludes1: interstitial pneumonia NOS (J84.9)

lymphoid interstitial pneumonia (J84.2)

J70.4 Drug-induced interstitial lung disorders, unspecified

Use additional code for adverse effect, if applicable, to identify drug (T36-T50 with fifth or sixth character 5)

Excludes1: interstitial pneumonia NOS (J84.9)

lymphoid interstitial pneumonia (J84.2)

J70.5 Respiratory conditions due to smoke inhalation

Smoke inhalation NOS

Excludes1: smoke inhalation due to chemicals, gases, fumes and vapors (J68.9)

J70.8 Respiratory conditions due to other specified external agents

Code first (T51-T65) to identify the external agent

J70.9 Respiratory conditions due to unspecified external agent

Code first (T51-T65) to identify the external agent

OTHER RESPIRATORY DISEASES PRINCIPALLY AFFECTING THE INTERSTITIUM (J80-J84)

J80 Acute respiratory distress syndrome

Acute respiratory distress syndrome in adult or child

Adult hyaline membrane disease

Excludes1: respiratory distress syndrome in newborn (perinatal) (P22.0)

J81 Pulmonary edema

Use additional code to identify:

exposure to environmental tobacco smoke (Z77.22)

history of tobacco dependence (Z87.891)

occupational exposure to environmental tobacco smoke (Z57.31)

tobacco dependence (F17.-)

tobacco use (Z72.0)

Excludes1: chemical (acute) pulmonary edema (J68.1)

hypostatic pneumonia (J18.2)

passive pneumonia (J18.2)

pulmonary edema due to external agents (J60-J70)

pulmonary edema with heart disease NOS (I50.1)

pulmonary edema with heart failure (I50.1)

J81.0   Acute pulmonary edema

Acute edema of lung

J81.1   Chronic pulmonary edema

Pulmonary congestion (chronic) (passive)

Pulmonary edema NOS

J82   Pulmonary eosinophilia, not elsewhere classified

Allergic pneumonia

Eosinophilic asthma

Eosinophilic pneumonia

Löffler's pneumonia

Tropical (pulmonary) eosinophilia NOS

Excludes1: pulmonary eosinophilia due to aspergillosis (B44.-)

pulmonary eosinophilia due to drugs (J70.2-J70.4)

pulmonary eosinophilia due to specified parasitic

infection (B50-B83)

pulmonary eosinophilia due to systemic connective tissue

disorders (M30-M36)

pulmonary infiltrate NOS (R91.8)

J84   Other interstitial pulmonary diseases

Excludes1: drug-induced interstitial lung disorders (J70.2-J70.4)

interstitial emphysema (J98.2)

lung diseases due to external agents (J60-J70)

J84.0   Alveolar and parieto-alveolar conditions

J84.01   Alveolar proteinosis

J84.02   Pulmonary alveolar microlithiasis

J84.03   Idiopathic pulmonary hemosiderosis

Essential brown induration of lung

Code first underlying disease, such as:

disorders of iron metabolism (E83.1-)

Excludes1: acute idiopathic pulmonary

hemorrhage in infants [AIPHI] (R04.81)

J84.09   Other alveolar and parieto-alveolar conditions

J84.1   Other interstitial pulmonary diseases with fibrosis

Excludes1: pulmonary fibrosis (chronic) due to inhalation

of chemicals, gases, fumes or vapors (J68.4)

pulmonary fibrosis (chronic) following radiation

(J70.1)

J84.10   Pulmonary fibrosis, unspecified

Definition: Pulmonary fibrosis is a condition

characterized by deposition of fibrous tissue in

the lung. It decreases lung compliance and results

in a restrictive ventilatory defect as seen in

pulmonary function testing.

Capillary fibrosis of lung

Cirrhosis of lung (chronic) NOS

Fibrosis of lung (atrophic) (chronic) (confluent)

(massive) (perialveolar) (peribronchial) NOS

Induration of lung (chronic) NOS

Postinflammatory pulmonary fibrosis

J84.11   Idiopathic interstitial pneumonia

Excludes1: lymphoid interstitial pneumonia

(J84.2)

pneumocystis pneumonia (B59)

J84.111   Idiopathic interstitial pneumonia, not otherwise specified

J84.112   Idiopathic pulmonary fibrosis

Cryptogenic fibrosing alveolitis

Idiopathic fibrosing alveolitis

J84.113   Idiopathic non-specific interstitial pneumonitis

Excludes1: non-specific interstitial

pneumonia NOS, or due to known

underlying cause (J84.89)

J84.114   Acute interstitial pneumonitis

Hamman-Rich syndrome

Excludes1: pneumocystis pneumonia

(B59)

J84.115   Respiratory bronchiolitis interstitial lung disease

J84.116   Cryptogenic organizing pneumonia

Excludes1: organizing pneumonia

NOS, or due to known underlying

cause (J84.89)

J84.117   Desquamative interstitial pneumonia

J84.17   Other interstitial pulmonary diseases with fibrosis in diseases classified elsewhere

Interstitial pneumonia (nonspecific) (usual) due

to collagen vascular disease

Interstitial pneumonia (nonspecific) (usual) in

diseases classified elsewhere

Organizing pneumonia due to collagen vascular

disease

Organizing pneumonia in diseases classified

elsewhere

Code first underlying disease, such as:

progressive systemic sclerosis (M34.0)

rheumatoid arthritis (M05.00-M06.9)

systemic lupus erythematosis (M32.0-M32.9)

J84.2   Lymphoid interstitial pneumonia

Lymphoid interstitial pneumonitis

J84.8   Other specified interstitial pulmonary diseases

Excludes1: exogenous lipoid pneumonia (J69.1)

unspecified lipoid pneumonia (J69.1)

J84.81   Lymphangioleiomyomatosis

Lymphangiomyomatosis

J84.82   Adult pulmonary Langerhans cell histiocytosis

Adult PLCH

J84.83   Surfactant mutations of the lung

J84.84   Other interstitial lung diseases of childhood

J84.841   Neuroendocrine cell hyperplasia of infancy

J84.842   Pulmonary interstitial glycogenosis

J84.843   Alveolar capillary dysplasia with vein misalignment

J84.848   Other interstitial lung diseases of childhood

J84.89   Other specified interstitial pulmonary diseases

Endogenous lipoid pneumonia

Interstitial pneumonitis

Non-specific interstitial pneumonitis NOS

Organizing pneumonia NOS

Code first, if applicable:

poisoning due to drug or toxin (T51-T65 with fifth or sixth character to indicate intent), for toxic pneumonopathy

underlying cause of pneumonopathy, if known

Use additional code, for adverse effect, to identify drug (T36-T50 with fifth or sixth character 5), if drug-induced

Excludes1: cryptogenic organizing pneumonia (J84.116)

idiopathic non-specific interstitial pneumonitis (J84.113)

lipoid pneumonia, exogenous or unspecified (J69.1)

lymphoid interstitial pneumonia (J84.2)

J84.9 Interstitial pulmonary disease, unspecified

Interstitial pneumonia NOS

SUPPURATIVE AND NECROTIC CONDITIONS OF THE LOWER RESPIRATORY TRACT (J85-J86)

J85 Abscess of lung and mediastinum

Use additional code (B95-B97) to identify infectious agent.

J85.0 Gangrene and necrosis of lung

J85.1 Abscess of lung with pneumonia

Code also the type of pneumonia

J85.2 Abscess of lung without pneumonia

Abscess of lung NOS

J85.3 Abscess of mediastinum

J86 Pyothorax

Use additional code (B95-B97) to identify infectious agent.

Excludes1: abscess of lung (J85.-)

pyothorax due to tuberculosis (A15.6)

J86.0 Pyothorax with fistula

Bronchocutaneous fistula

Bronchopleural fistula

Hepatopleural fistula

Mediastinal fistula

Pleural fistula

Thoracic fistula

Any condition classifiable to J86.9 with fistula

J86.9 Pyothorax without fistula

Abscess of pleura

Abscess of thorax

Empyema (chest) (lung) (pleura)

Fibrinopurulent pleurisy

Purulent pleurisy

Pyopneumothorax

Septic pleurisy

Seropurulent pleurisy

Suppurative pleurisy

OTHER DISEASES OF THE PLEURA (J90-J94)

J90 Pleural effusion, not elsewhere classified

Definition: Pleurisy is an inflammation of the membrane that surrounds and protects the lungs (the pleura). Inflammation occurs when an infection or damaging agent irritates the pleural surface.

Encysted pleurisy

Pleural effusion NOS

Pleurisy with effusion (exudative) (serous)

Excludes1: chylous (pleural) effusion (J94.0)

malignant pleural effusion (J91.0))

pleurisy NOS (R09.1)

tuberculous pleural effusion (A15.6)

J91 Pleural effusion in conditions classified elsewhere

Excludes2: pleural effusion in heart failure (I50.-)

pleural effusion in systemic lupus erythematosus (M32.13)

J91.0 Malignant pleural effusion

Code first underlying neoplasm

J91.8 Pleural effusion in other conditions classified elsewhere

Code first underlying disease, such as:

filariasis (B74.0-B74.9)

influenza (J09.X2, J10.1, J11.1)

J92 Pleural plaque

Includes: pleural thickening

J92.0 Pleural plaque with presence of asbestos

J92.9 Pleural plaque without asbestos

Pleural plaque NOS

J93 Pneumothorax and air leak

Excludes1: congenital or perinatal pneumothorax (P25.1)

postprocedural air leak (J95.812)

postprocedural pneumothorax (J95.811)

traumatic pneumothorax (S27.0)

tuberculous (current disease)

pneumothorax (A15.-)

pyopneumothorax (J86.-)

J93.0 Spontaneous tension pneumothorax

J93.1 Other spontaneous pneumothorax

J93.11 Primary spontaneous pneumothorax

J93.12 Secondary spontaneous pneumothorax

Code first underlying condition, such as:

catamenial pneumothorax due to endometriosis (N80.8)

cystic fibrosis (E84.-)

eosinophilic pneumonia (J82)

lymphangioleiomyomatosis (J84.81)

malignant neoplasm of bronchus and lung (C34.-)

Marfan's syndrome (Q87.4)

pneumonia due to Pneumocystis carinii (B59)

secondary malignant neoplasm of lung (C78.0-)

spontaneous rupture of the esophagus (K22.3)

J93.8 Other pneumothorax and air leak

J93.81 Chronic pneumothorax

J93.82 Other air leak

Persistent air leak

J93.83 Other pneumothorax

Acute pneumothorax

Spontaneous pneumothorax NOS

J93.9 **Pneumothorax, unspecified**

Pneumothorax NOS

J94 **Other pleural conditions**

Excludes1: pleurisy NOS (R09.1)

traumatic hemopneumothorax (S27.2)

traumatic hemothorax (S27.1)

tuberculous pleural conditions (current disease) (A15.-)

J94.0 **Chylous effusion**

Chyliform effusion

J94.1 **Fibrothorax**

J94.2 **Hemothorax**

Hemopneumothorax

J94.8 **Other specified pleural conditions**

Hydropneumothorax

Hydrothorax

J94.9 **Pleural condition, unspecified**

INTRAOPERATIVE AND POSTPROCEDURAL COMPLICATIONS AND DISORDERS OF RESPIRATORY SYSTEM, NOT ELSEWHERE CLASSIFIED (J95)

J95 **Intraoperative and postprocedural complications and disorders of respiratory system, not elsewhere classified**

Excludes2: aspiration pneumonia (J69.-)

emphysema (subcutaneous) resulting from a procedure (T81.82)

hypostatic pneumonia (J18.2)

pulmonary manifestations due to radiation (J70.0-J70.1)

J95.0 **Tracheostomy complications**

J95.00 **Unspecified tracheostomy complication**

J95.01 **Hemorrhage from tracheostomy stoma**

J95.02 **Infection of tracheostomy stoma**

Use additional code to identify type of infection, such as:

cellulitis of neck (L03.8)

sepsis (A40, A41.-)

J95.03 **Malfunction of tracheostomy stoma**

Mechanical complication of tracheostomy stoma

Obstruction of tracheostomy airway

Tracheal stenosis due to tracheostomy

J95.04 **Tracheo-esophageal fistula following tracheostomy**

J95.09 **Other tracheostomy complication**

J95.1 **Acute pulmonary insufficiency following thoracic surgery**

Excludes2: Functional disturbances following cardiac surgery (I97.0, I97.1-)

J95.2 **Acute pulmonary insufficiency following nonthoracic surgery**

Excludes2: Functional disturbances following cardiac surgery (I97.0, I97.1-)

J95.3 **Chronic pulmonary insufficiency following surgery**

Excludes2: Functional disturbances following cardiac surgery (I97.0, I97.1-)

J95.4 **Chemical pneumonitis due to anesthesia**

Mendelson's syndrome

Postprocedural aspiration pneumonia

Use additional code for adverse effect, if applicable, to identify drug (T41.- with fifth or sixth character 5)

Excludes1: aspiration pneumonitis due to anesthesia complicating labor and delivery (O74.0)

aspiration pneumonitis due to anesthesia complicating pregnancy (O29)

aspiration pneumonitis due to anesthesia complicating the puerperium (O89.01)

J95.5 **Postprocedural subglottic stenosis**

J95.6 **Intraoperative hemorrhage and hematoma of a respiratory system organ or structure complicating a procedure**

Excludes1: intraoperative hemorrhage and hematoma of a respiratory system organ or structure due to

accidental puncture and laceration during procedure (J95.7-)

J95.61 **Intraoperative hemorrhage and hematoma of a respiratory system organ or structure complicating a respiratory system procedure**

J95.62 **Intraoperative hemorrhage and hematoma of a respiratory system organ or structure complicating other procedure**

J95.7 **Accidental puncture and laceration of a respiratory system organ or structure during a procedure**

Excludes2: postprocedural pneumothorax (J95.811)

J95.71 **Accidental puncture and laceration of a respiratory system organ or structure during a respiratory system procedure**

J95.72 **Accidental puncture and laceration of a respiratory system organ or structure during other procedure**

J95.8 **Other intraoperative and postprocedural complications and disorders of respiratory system, not elsewhere classified**

J95.81 **Postprocedural pneumothorax and air leak**

J95.811 **Postprocedural pneumothorax**

J95.812 **Postprocedural air leak**

J95.82 **Postprocedural respiratory failure**

Excludes1: Respiratory failure in other conditions (J96.-)

J95.821 **Acute postprocedural respiratory failure**

Postprocedural respiratory failure NOS

J95.822 **Acute and chronic postprocedural respiratory failure**

J95.83 **Postprocedural hemorrhage of a respiratory system organ or structure following a procedure**

▲**J95.830** **Postprocedural hemorrhage of a respiratory system organ or structure following a respiratory system procedure**

▲**J95.831** **Postprocedural hemorrhage of a respiratory system organ or structure following other procedure**

J95.84 **Transfusion-related acute lung injury (TRALI)**

J95.85 **Complication of respirator [ventilator]**

J95.850 **Mechanical complication of respirator** Excludes1: encounter for

respirator [ventilator] dependence during power failure (Z99.12)

J95.851 Ventilator associated pneumonia

Ventilator associated pneumonitis

Use additional code to identify the organism, if known (B95.-, B96.-, B97.-)

Excludes1: ventilator lung in newborn (P27.8)

J95.859 Other complication of respirator [ventilator]

J95.86 Postprocedural hematoma and seroma of a respiratory system organ or structure following a procedure

●**J95.860 Postprocedural hematoma of a respiratory system organ or structure following a respiratory system procedure**

●**J95.861 Postprocedural hematoma of a respiratory system organ or structure following other procedure**

●**J95.862 Postprocedural seroma of a respiratory system organ or structure following a respiratory system procedure**

●**J95.863 Postprocedural seroma of a respiratory system organ or structure following other procedure**

J95.88 Other intraoperative complications of respiratory system, not elsewhere classified

J95.89 Other postprocedural complications and disorders of respiratory system, not elsewhere classified

Use additional code to identify disorder, such as:

aspiration pneumonia (J69.-)

bacterial or viral pneumonia (J12-J18)

Excludes2: acute pulmonary insufficiency following thoracic surgery (J95.1)

postprocedural subglottic stenosis (J95.5)

OTHER DISEASES OF THE RESPIRATORY SYSTEM (J96-J99)

J96 Respiratory failure, not elsewhere classified

Excludes1: acute respiratory distress syndrome (J80)

cardiorespiratory failure (R09.2)

newborn respiratory distress syndrome (P22.0)

postprocedural respiratory failure (J95.82-)

respiratory arrest (R09.2)

respiratory arrest of newborn (P28.81)

respiratory failure of newborn (P28.5)

J96.0 Acute respiratory failure

J96.00 Acute respiratory failure, unspecified whether with hypoxia or hypercapnia

J96.01 Acute respiratory failure with hypoxia

J96.02 Acute respiratory failure with hypercapnia

J96.1 Chronic respiratory failure

J96.10 Chronic respiratory failure, unspecified whether with hypoxia or hypercapnia

J96.11 Chronic respiratory failure with hypoxia

J96.12 Chronic respiratory failure with hypercapnia

J96.2 Acute and chronic respiratory failure

Acute on chronic respiratory failure

J96.20 Acute and chronic respiratory failure, unspecified whether with hypoxia or hypercapnia

J96.21 Acute and chronic respiratory failure with hypoxia

J96.22 Acute and chronic respiratory failure with hypercapnia

J96.9 Respiratory failure, unspecified

J96.90 Respiratory failure, unspecified, unspecified whether with hypoxia or hypercapnia

J96.91 Respiratory failure, unspecified with hypoxia

J96.92 Respiratory failure, unspecified with hypercapnia

J98 Other respiratory disorders

Use additional code to identify:

exposure to environmental tobacco smoke (Z77.22)

exposure to tobacco smoke in the perinatal period (P96.81)

history of tobacco dependence (Z87.891)

occupational exposure to environmental tobacco smoke (Z57.31)

tobacco dependence (F17.-)

tobacco use (Z72.0)

Excludes1: newborn apnea (P28.4)

newborn sleep apnea (P28.3)

Excludes2: apnea NOS (R06.81)

sleep apnea (G47.3-)

J98.0 Diseases of bronchus, not elsewhere classified

J98.01 Acute bronchospasm

Excludes1: acute bronchiolitis with bronchospasm (J21.-)

acute bronchitis with bronchospasm (J20.-)

asthma (J45.-)

exercise induced bronchospasm (J45.990)

J98.09 Other diseases of bronchus, not elsewhere classified

Broncholithiasis

Calcification of bronchus

Stenosis of bronchus

Tracheobronchial collapse

Tracheobronchial dyskinesia

Ulcer of bronchus

J98.1 Pulmonary collapse

Excludes1: therapeutic collapse of lung status (Z98.3)

J98.11 Atelectasis

Excludes1: newborn atelectasis

tuberculous atelectasis (current disease) (A15)

J98.19 Other pulmonary collapse

J98.2 Interstitial emphysema

Mediastinal emphysema

Excludes1: emphysema NOS (J43.9)

emphysema in newborn (P25.0)

surgical emphysema (subcutaneous) (T81.82)

traumatic subcutaneous emphysema (T79.7)

J98.3 **Compensatory emphysema**

J98.4 **Other disorders of lung**

Calcification of lung

Cystic lung disease (acquired)

Lung disease NOS

Pulmolithiasis

Excludes1: acute interstitial pneumonitis (J84.114)

pulmonary insufficiency following surgery (J95.1-J95.2)

J98.5 **Diseases of mediastinum, not elsewhere classified**

Excludes2: abscess of mediastinum (J85.3)

• **J98.51** **Mediastinitis**

Code first underlying condition, if applicable, such as postoperative mediastinitis (T81.-)

• **J98.59** **Other diseases of mediastinum, not elsewhere classified**

Fibrosis of mediastinum

Hernia of mediastinum

Retraction of mediastinum

J98.6 **Disorders of diaphragm**

Diaphragmatitis

Paralysis of diaphragm

Relaxation of diaphragm

Excludes1: congenital malformation of diaphragm NEC (Q79.1)

congenital diaphragmatic hernia (Q79.0)

Excludes2: diaphragmatic hernia (K44.-)

J98.8 **Other specified respiratory disorders**

J98.9 **Respiratory disorder, unspecified**

Respiratory disease (chronic) NOS

J99 **Respiratory disorders in diseases classified elsewhere**

Code first underlying disease, such as:

amyloidosis (E85.-)

ankylosing spondylitis (M45)

congenital syphilis (A50.5)

cryoglobulinemia (D89.1)

early congenital syphilis (A50.0)

schistosomiasis (B65.0-B65.9)

Excludes1: respiratory disorders in:

amebiasis (A06.5)

blastomycosis (B40.0-B40.2)

candidiasis (B37.1)

coccidioidomycosis (B38.0-B38.2)

cystic fibrosis with pulmonary manifestations (E84.0)

dermatomyositis (M33.01, M33.11)

histoplasmosis (B39.0-B39.2)

late syphilis (A52.72, A52.73)

polymyositis (M33.21)

sicca syndrome (M35.02)

systemic lupus erythematosus (M32.13)

systemic sclerosis (M34.81)

Wegener's granulomatosis (M31.30-M31.31)

● New code   ▲ Revised code   **Excludes1:** Not coded here   **Excludes2:** Not included here   ⊗ Placeholder required   ⑦ 7ᵗʰ digit required

Chapter 11: Diseases Of The Digestive System (K00-K95)

DEFINITIONS

This chapter includes definitions of selected key words, terms and phrases and coding alerts for adding points to the clinical domain, and references to coding late effects where appropriate. An example from this chapter is as follows:

K04   Diseases of pulp and periapical tissues
        Definition: Pulp is the part in the center of a tooth made up of living soft tissue and cells called odontoblasts.

MULTIPLE CODING FOR A SINGLE CONDITION

In addition to the etiology/manifestation convention that requires two codes to fully describe a single condition that affects multiple body systems, there are other single conditions that also require more than one code. "Use additional code" notes are found in the Tabular List at codes that are not part of an etiology/manifestation pair where a secondary code is useful to fully describe a condition. The sequencing rule is the same as the etiology/manifestation pair, "use additional code" indicates that a secondary code should be added.

For example, for bacterial infections that are not included in chapter 1, a secondary code from category B95, Streptococcus, Staphylococcus, and Enterococcus, as the cause of diseases classified elsewhere, or B96, Other bacterial agents as the cause of diseases classified elsewhere, may be required to identify the bacterial organism causing the infection. A "use additional code" note will normally be found at the infectious disease code, indicating a need for the organism code to be added as a secondary code.

"Code first" notes are also under certain codes that are not specifically manifestation codes but may be due to an underlying cause. When there is a "code first" note and an underlying condition is present, the underlying condition should be sequenced first.

"Code, if applicable, any causal condition first", notes indicate that this code may be assigned as a principal diagnosis when the causal condition is unknown or not applicable. If a causal condition is known, then the code for that condition should be sequenced as the principal or first-listed diagnosis.

Multiple codes may be needed for sequela, complication codes and obstetric codes to more fully describe a condition. See the specific guidelines for these conditions for further instruction.

COMBINATION CODE

A combination code is a single code used to classify: Two diagnoses, or a diagnosis with an associated secondary process (manifestation) A diagnosis with an associated complication

Combination codes are identified by referring to subterm entries in the Alphabetic Index and by reading the inclusion and exclusion notes in the Tabular List.

Assign only the combination code when that code fully identifies the diagnostic conditions involved or when the Alphabetic Index so directs. Multiple coding should not be used when the classification provides a combination code that clearly identifies all of the elements documented in the diagnosis. When the combination code lacks necessary specificity in describing the manifestation or complication, an additional code should be used as a secondary code.

SEQUELA (LATE EFFECTS)

A sequela is the residual effect (condition produced) after the acute phase of an illness or injury has terminated. There is no time limit on when a sequela code can be used. The residual may be apparent early, such as in cerebral infarction, or it may occur months or years later, such as that due to a previous injury. Coding of sequela generally requires two codes sequenced in the following order: The condition or nature of the sequela is sequenced first.

The sequela code is sequenced second.

An exception to the above guidelines are those instances where the code for the sequela is followed by a manifestation code identified in the Tabular List and title, or the sequela code has been expanded (at the fourth, fifth or sixth character levels) to include the manifestation(s). The code for the acute phase of an illness or injury that led to the sequela is never used with a code for the late effect.

Chapter 11

Diseases Of The Digestive System (K00-K95)

Excludes2: certain conditions originating in the perinatal period (P04-P96)

certain infectious and parasitic diseases (A00-B99)

complications of pregnancy, childbirth and the puerperium (O00-O9A)

congenital malformations, deformations and chromosomal abnormalities (Q00-Q99)

endocrine, nutritional and metabolic diseases (E00-E88)

injury, poisoning and certain other consequences of external causes (S00-T88)

neoplasms (C00-D49)

symptoms, signs and abnormal clinical and laboratory findings, not elsewhere classified (R00-R94)

This chapter contains the following blocks:

K00-K14	Diseases of oral cavity and salivary glands
K20-K31	Diseases of esophagus, stomach and duodenum
K35-K38	Diseases of appendix
K40-K46	Hernia
K50-K52	Noninfective enteritis and colitis
K55-K64	Other diseases of intestines
K65-K68	Diseases of peritoneum and retroperitoneum
K70-K77	Diseases of liver
K80-K87	Disorders of gallbladder, biliary tract and pancreas
K90-K95	Other diseases of the digestive system

DISEASES OF ORAL CAVITY AND SALIVARY GLANDS (K00-K14)

K00 Disorders of tooth development and eruption

Excludes2: embedded and impacted teeth (K01.-)

K00.0 Anodontia

Hypodontia

Oligodontia

Excludes1: acquired absence of teeth (K08.1-)

K00.1 Supernumerary teeth

Distomolar Fourth molar

Mesiodens Paramolar

Supplementary teeth

Excludes2: supernumerary roots (K00.2)

K00.2 Abnormalities of size and form of teeth

Concrescence of teeth

Fusion of teeth

Gemination of teeth

Dens evaginatus

Dens in dente

Dens invaginatus

Enamel pearls

Macrodontia

Microdontia

Peg-shaped [conical] teeth

Supernumerary roots

Taurodontism

Tuberculum paramolare

Excludes1: abnormalities of teeth due to congenital syphilis (A50.5)

tuberculum Carabelli, which is regarded as a normal variation and should not be coded

K00.3 Mottled teeth

Dental fluorosis

Mottling of enamel

Nonfluoride enamel opacities

Excludes2: deposits [accretions] on teeth (K03.6)

K00.4 Disturbances in tooth formation

Aplasia and hypoplasia of cementum

Dilaceration of tooth

Enamel hypoplasia (neonatal) (postnatal) (prenatal)

Regional odontodysplasia

Turner's tooth

Excludes1: Hutchinson's teeth and mulberry molars in congenital syphilis (A50.5)

Excludes2: mottled teeth (K00.3)

K00.5 Hereditary disturbances in tooth structure, not elsewhere classified

Amelogenesis imperfecta

Dentinogenesis imperfecta

Odontogenesis imperfecta

Dentinal dysplasia

Shell teeth

K00.6 Disturbances in tooth eruption

Dentia praecox Natal tooth Neonatal tooth

Premature eruption of tooth

Premature shedding of primary [deciduous] tooth

Prenatal teeth

Retained [persistent] primary tooth

Excludes2: embedded and impacted teeth (K01.-)

K00.7 Teething syndrome

K00.8 Other disorders of tooth development

Color changes during tooth formation

Intrinsic staining of teeth NOS

Excludes2: posteruptive color changes (K03.7)

K00.9 Disorder of tooth development, unspecified

Disorder of odontogenesis NOS

K01 Embedded and impacted teeth

Excludes1: abnormal position of fully erupted teeth (M26.3-)

K01.0 Embedded teeth

K01.1 Impacted teeth

K02 Dental caries

Includes: caries of dentine

dental cavities

early childhood caries

pre-eruptive caries

recurrent caries (dentino enamel junction) (enamel) (to the pulp) tooth decay

K02.3 Arrested dental caries

Arrested coronal and root caries

K02.5 Dental caries on pit and fissure surface

Dental caries on chewing surface of tooth

K02.51 **Dental caries on pit and fissure surface limited to enamel**

White spot lesions [initial caries] on pit and fissure surface of tooth

K02.52 **Dental caries on pit and fissure surface penetrating into dentin**

Primary dental caries, cervical origin

K02.53 **Dental caries on pit and fissure surface penetrating into pulp**

K02.6 **Dental caries on smooth surface**

K02.61 **Dental caries on smooth surface limited to enamel**

White spot lesions [initial caries] on smooth surface of tooth

K02.62 **Dental caries on smooth surface penetrating into dentin**

K02.63 **Dental caries on smooth surface penetrating into pulp**

K02.7 **Dental root caries**

K02.9 **Dental caries, unspecified**

K03 **Other diseases of hard tissues of teeth**

Excludes2: bruxism (F45.8)

dental caries (K02.-)

teeth-grinding NOS (F45.8)

K03.0 **Excessive attrition of teeth**

Approximal wear of teeth

Occlusal wear of teeth

K03.1 **Abrasion of teeth**

Dentifrice abrasion of teeth

Habitual abrasion of teeth

Occupational abrasion of teeth

Ritual abrasion of teeth

Traditional abrasion of teeth Wedge defect NOS

K03.2 **Erosion of teeth**

Erosion of teeth due to diet

Erosion of teeth due to drugs and medicaments

Erosion of teeth due to persistent vomiting

Erosion of teeth NOS

Idiopathic erosion of teeth

Occupational erosion of teeth

K03.3 **Pathological resorption of teeth**

Internal granuloma of pulp

Resorption of teeth (external)

K03.4 **Hypercementosis**

Cementation hyperplasia

K03.5 **Ankylosis of teeth**

K03.6 **Deposits [accretions] on teeth**

Betel deposits [accretions] on teeth

Black deposits [accretions] on teeth

Extrinsic staining of teeth NOS

Green deposits [accretions] on teeth

Materia alba deposits [accretions] on teeth

Orange deposits [accretions] on teeth

Staining of teeth NOS

Subgingival dental calculus

Supragingival dental calculus

Tobacco deposits [accretions] on teeth

K03.7 **Posteruptive color changes of dental hard tissues**

Excludes2: deposits [accretions] on teeth (K03.6)

K03.8 **Other specified diseases of hard tissues of teeth**

K03.81 **Cracked tooth**

Excludes1: asymptomatic craze lines in enamel - omit code

broken or fractured tooth due to trauma (S02.5)

K03.89 **Other specified diseases of hard tissues of teeth**

K03.9 **Disease of hard tissues of teeth, unspecified**

K04 **Diseases of pulp and periapical tissues**

Definition: Pulp is the part in the center of a tooth made up of living soft tissue and cells called odontoblasts.

K04.0 **Pulpitis**

Acute pulpitis

Chronic (hyperplastic) (ulcerative) pulpitis

●**K04.01** **Reversible pulpitis**

●**K04.02** **Irreversible pulpitis**

K04.1 **Necrosis of pulp**

Pulpal gangrene

K04.2 **Pulp degeneration**

Denticles

Pulpal calcifications

Pulpal stones

K04.3 **Abnormal hard tissue formation in pulp**

Secondary or irregular dentine

K04.4 **Acute apical periodontitis of pulpal origin**

Acute apical periodontitis NOS

Excludes1: acute periodontitis (K05.2-)

K04.5 **Chronic apical periodontitis**

Apical or periapical granuloma

Apical periodontitis NOS

Excludes1: chronic periodontitis (K05.3-)

K04.6 **Periapical abscess with sinus**

Dental abscess with sinus

Dentoalveolar abscess with sinus

K04.7 **Periapical abscess without sinus**

Dental abscess without sinus

Dentoalveolar abscess without sinus

Periapical abscess without sinus

K04.8 **Radicular cyst**

Apical (periodontal) cyst

Periapical cyst

Residual radicular cyst

Excludes2: lateral periodontal cyst (K09.0)

K04.9 **Other and unspecified diseases of pulp and periapical tissues**

K04.90 **Unspecified diseases of pulp and periapical tissues**

K04.99 **Other diseases of pulp and periapical tissues**

K05 **Gingivitis and periodontal diseases**

Use additional code to identify:

alcohol abuse and dependence (F10.-)

exposure to environmental tobacco smoke (Z77.22)

● New code   ▲ Revised code   Excludes1: Not coded here   Excludes2: Not included here   ⊗ Placeholder required   ⑦ 7th digit required

exposure to tobacco smoke in the perinatal period (P96.81)

history of tobacco dependence (Z87.891)

occupational exposure to environmental tobacco smoke (Z57.31)

tobacco dependence (F17.-)

tobacco use (Z72.0)

K05.0   Acute gingivitis

    Excludes1: acute necrotizing ulcerative gingivitis (A69.1)

    herpesviral [herpes simplex] gingivostomatitis (B00.2)

K05.00   Acute gingivitis, plaque induced

    Acute gingivitis NOS

    Plaque induced gingival disease

K05.01   Acute gingivitis, non-plaque induced

K05.1   Chronic gingivitis

    Desquamative gingivitis (chronic)

    Gingivitis (chronic) NOS

    Hyperplastic gingivitis (chronic)

    Pregnancy associated gingivitis

    Simple marginal gingivitis (chronic)

    Ulcerative gingivitis (chronic)

    Code first, if applicable, diseases of the digestive system complicating pregnancy (O99.61-)

K05.10   Chronic gingivitis, plaque induced

    Chronic gingivitis NOS Gingivitis NOS

K05.11   Chronic gingivitis, non-plaque induced

K05.2   Aggressive periodontitis

    Acute pericoronitis

    Excludes1: acute apical periodontitis (K04.4)

    periapical abscess (K04.7)

    periapical abscess with sinus (K04.6)

K05.20   Aggressive periodontitis, unspecified

K05.21   Aggressive periodontitis, localized

    Periodontal abscess

- **K05.211   Aggressive periodontitis, localized, slight**
- **K05.212   Aggressive periodontitis, localized, moderate**
- **K05.213   Aggressive periodontitis, localized, severe**
- **K05.219   Aggressive periodontitis, localized, unspecified severity**

K05.22   Aggressive periodontitis, generalized

- **K05.221   Aggressive periodontitis, generalized, slight**
- **K05.222   Aggressive periodontitis, generalized, moderate**
- **K05.223   Aggressive periodontitis, generalized, severe**
- **K05.229   Aggressive periodontitis, generalized, unspecified severity**

K05.3   Chronic periodontitis

    Chronic pericoronitis

    Complex periodontitis

    Periodontitis NOS

    Simplex periodontitis

    Excludes1: chronic apical periodontitis (K04.5)

K05.30   Chronic periodontitis, unspecified

K05.31   Chronic periodontitis, localized

- **K05.311   Chronic periodontitis, localized, slight**
- **K05.312   Chronic periodontitis, localized, moderate**
- **K05.313   Chronic periodontitis, localized, severe**
- **K05.319   Chronic periodontitis, localized, unspecified severity**

K05.32   Chronic periodontitis, generalized

- **K05.321   Chronic periodontitis, generalized, slight**
- **K05.322   Chronic periodontitis, generalized, moderate**
- **K05.323   Chronic periodontitis, generalized, severe**
- **K05.329   Chronic periodontitis, generalized, unspecified severity**

K05.4   Periodontosis

    Juvenile periodontosis

K05.5   Other periodontal diseases

    Combined periodontic-endodontic lesion

    Narrow gingival width (of periodontal soft tissue)

    Excludes2: leukoplakia of gingiva (K13.21)

K05.6   Periodontal disease, unspecified

K06   Other disorders of gingiva and edentulous alveolar ridge

    Excludes2: acute gingivitis (K05.0)

    atrophy of edentulous alveolar ridge (K08.2)

    chronic gingivitis (K05.1)

    gingivitis NOS (K05.1)

K06.0   Gingival recession

    Gingival recession (generalized) (localized) (postinfective) (postprocedural)

K06.1   Gingival enlargement

    Gingival fibromatosis

K06.2   Gingival and edentulous alveolar ridge lesions associated with trauma

    Irritative hyperplasia of edentulous ridge [denture hyperplasia]

    Use additional code (Chapter 20) to identify external cause or denture status (Z97.2)

- **K06.3   Horizontal alveolar bone loss**

K06.8   Other specified disorders of gingiva and edentulous alveolar ridge

    Fibrous epulis

    Flabby alveolar ridge

    Giant cell epulis

    Peripheral giant cell granuloma of gingiva

    Pyogenic granuloma of gingiva

    Vertical ridge deficiency

    Excludes2: gingival cyst (K09.0)

K06.9   Disorder of gingiva and edentulous alveolar ridge, unspecified

K08   Other disorders of teeth and supporting structures

    Excludes2: dentofacial anomalies [including malocclusion] (M26.-)

    disorders of jaw (M27.-)

K08.0 **Exfoliation of teeth due to systemic causes**

Code also underlying systemic condition

K08.1 **Complete loss of teeth**

Acquired loss of teeth, complete

Excludes1: congenital absence of teeth (K00.0)

exfoliation of teeth due to systemic causes (K08.0)

partial loss of teeth (K08.4-)

K08.10 **Complete loss of teeth, unspecified cause**

K08.101 **Complete loss of teeth, unspecified cause, class I**

K08.102 **Complete loss of teeth, unspecified cause, class II**

K08.103 **Complete loss of teeth, unspecified cause, class III**

K08.104 **Complete loss of teeth, unspecified cause, class IV**

K08.109 **Complete loss of teeth, unspecified cause, unspecified class**

Edentulism NOS

K08.11 **Complete loss of teeth due to trauma**

K08.111 **Complete loss of teeth due to trauma, class I**

K08.112 **Complete loss of teeth due to trauma, class II**

K08.113 **Complete loss of teeth due to trauma, class III**

K08.114 **Complete loss of teeth due to trauma, class IV**

K08.119 **Complete loss of teeth due to trauma, unspecified class**

K08.12 **Complete loss of teeth due to periodontal diseases**

K08.121 **Complete loss of teeth due to periodontal diseases, class I**

K08.122 **Complete loss of teeth due to periodontal diseases, class II**

K08.123 **Complete loss of teeth due to periodontal diseases, class III**

K08.124 **Complete loss of teeth due to periodontal diseases, class IV**

K08.129 **Complete loss of teeth due to periodontal diseases, unspecified class**

K08.13 **Complete loss of teeth due to caries**

K08.131 **Complete loss of teeth due to caries, class I**

K08.132 **Complete loss of teeth due to caries, class II**

K08.133 **Complete loss of teeth due to caries, class III**

K08.134 **Complete loss of teeth due to caries, class IV**

K08.139 **Complete loss of teeth due to caries, unspecified class**

K08.19 **Complete loss of teeth due to other specified cause**

K08.191 **Complete loss of teeth due to other specified cause, class I**

K08.192 **Complete loss of teeth due to other specified cause, class II**

K08.193 **Complete loss of teeth due to other specified cause, class III**

K08.194 **Complete loss of teeth due to other specified cause, class IV**

K08.199 **Complete loss of teeth due to other specified cause, unspecified class**

K08.2 **Atrophy of edentulous alveolar ridge**

K08.20 **Unspecified atrophy of edentulous alveolar ridge**

Atrophy of the mandible NOS

Atrophy of the maxilla NOS

K08.21 **Minimal atrophy of the mandible**

Minimal atrophy of the edentulous mandible

K08.22 **Moderate atrophy of the mandible**

Moderate atrophy of the edentulous mandible

K08.23 **Severe atrophy of the mandible**

Severe atrophy of the edentulous mandible

K08.24 **Minimal atrophy of maxilla**

Minimal atrophy of the edentulous maxilla

K08.25 **Moderate atrophy of the maxilla**

Moderate atrophy of the edentulous maxilla

K08.26 **Severe atrophy of the maxilla**

Severe atrophy of the edentulous maxilla

K08.3 **Retained dental root**

K08.4 **Partial loss of teeth**

Acquired loss of teeth, partial

Excludes1: complete loss of teeth (K08.1-)

congenital absence of teeth (K00.0)

Excludes2: exfoliation of teeth due to systemic causes (K08.0)

K08.40 **Partial loss of teeth, unspecified cause**

K08.401 **Partial loss of teeth, unspecified cause, class I**

K08.402 **Partial loss of teeth, unspecified cause, class II**

K08.403 **Partial loss of teeth, unspecified cause, class III**

K08.404 **Partial loss of teeth, unspecified cause, class IV**

K08.409 **Partial loss of teeth, unspecified cause, unspecified class**

Tooth extraction status NOS

K08.41 **Partial loss of teeth due to trauma**

K08.411 **Partial loss of teeth due to trauma, class I**

K08.412 **Partial loss of teeth due to trauma, class II**

K08.413 **Partial loss of teeth due to trauma, class III**

K08.414 **Partial loss of teeth due to trauma, class IV**

K08.419 **Partial loss of teeth due to trauma, unspecified class**

K08.42 **Partial loss of teeth due to periodontal diseases**

K08.421 **Partial loss of teeth due to periodontal diseases, class I**

● New code ▲ Revised code **Excludes1:** Not coded here **Excludes2:** Not included here ⊗ Placeholder required ⑦7th digit required

K08.422 **Partial loss of teeth due to periodontal diseases, class II**

K08.423 **Partial loss of teeth due to periodontal diseases, class III**

K08.424 **Partial loss of teeth due to periodontal diseases, class IV**

K08.429 **Partial loss of teeth due to periodontal diseases, unspecified class**

K08.43 **Partial loss of teeth due to caries**

K08.431 **Partial loss of teeth due to caries, class I**

K08.432 **Partial loss of teeth due to caries, class II**

K08.433 **Partial loss of teeth due to caries, class III**

K08.434 **Partial loss of teeth due to caries, class IV**

K08.439 **Partial loss of teeth due to caries, unspecified class**

K08.49 **Partial loss of teeth due to other specified cause**

K08.491 **Partial loss of teeth due to other specified cause, class I**

K08.492 **Partial loss of teeth due to other specified cause, class II**

K08.493 **Partial loss of teeth due to other specified cause, class III**

K08.494 **Partial loss of teeth due to other specified cause, class IV**

K08.499 **Partial loss of teeth due to other specified cause, unspecified class**

K08.5 **Unsatisfactory restoration of tooth**

Defective bridge, crown, filling

Defective dental restoration

Excludes1: dental restoration status (Z98.811)

Excludes2: endosseous dental implant failure (M27.6-)

unsatisfactory endodontic treatment (M27.5-)

K08.50 **Unsatisfactory restoration of tooth, unspecified**

Defective dental restoration NOS

K08.51 **Open restoration margins of tooth**

Dental restoration failure of marginal integrity

Open margin on tooth restoration

Poor gingival margin to tooth restoration

K08.52 **Unrepairable overhanging of dental restorative materials**

Overhanging of tooth restoration

K08.53 **Fractured dental restorative material**

Excludes1: cracked tooth (K03.81)

traumatic fracture of tooth (S02.5)

K08.530 **Fractured dental restorative material without loss of material**

K08.531 **Fractured dental restorative material with loss of material**

K08.539 **Fractured dental restorative material, unspecified**

K08.54 **Contour of existing restoration of tooth biologically incompatible with oral health**

Dental restoration failure of periodontal anatomical integrity

Unacceptable contours of existing restoration of tooth

Unacceptable morphology of existing restoration of tooth

K08.55 **Allergy to existing dental restorative material**

Use additional code to identify the specific type of allergy

K08.56 **Poor aesthetic of existing restoration of tooth**

Dental restoration aesthetically inadequate or displeasing

K08.59 **Other unsatisfactory restoration of tooth**

Other defective dental restoration

K08.8 **Other specified disorders of teeth and supporting structures**

●K08.81 **Primary occlusal trauma**

●K08.82 **Secondary occlusal trauma**

●K08.89 **Other specified disorders of teeth and supporting structures**

Enlargement of alveolar ridge NOS

Insufficient anatomic crown height

Insufficient clinical crown length

Irregular alveolar process

Toothache NOS

K08.9 **Disorder of teeth and supporting structures, unspecified**

K09 **Cysts of oral region, not elsewhere classified**

Includes: lesions showing histological features both of aneurysmal cyst and of another fibro-osseous lesion

Excludes2: cysts of jaw (M27.0-, M27.4-)

radicular cyst (K04.8)

K09.0 **Developmental odontogenic cysts**

Dentigerous cyst

Eruption cyst

Follicular cyst

Gingival cyst

Lateral periodontal cyst

Primordial cyst

Excludes2: keratocysts (D16.4, D16.5)

odontogenic keratocystic tumors (D16.4, D16.5)

K09.1 **Developmental (nonodontogenic) cysts of oral region**

Cyst (of) incisive canal

Cyst (of) palatine of papilla Globulomaxillary cyst

Median palatal cyst Nasoalveolar cyst Nasolabial cyst Nasopalatine duct cyst

K09.8 **Other cysts of oral region, not elsewhere classified**

Dermoid cyst

Epidermoid cyst

Lymphoepithelial cyst

Epstein's pearl

K09.9 **Cyst of oral region, unspecified**

K11 **Diseases of salivary glands**

Definition: The salivary gland is a gland that secretes saliva, especially any of three pairs of large glands, the parotid, submaxillary, and sublingual, whose secretions enter the mouth and mingle in saliva.

Use additional code to identify:

alcohol abuse and dependence (F10.-)

exposure to environmental tobacco smoke (Z77.22)

exposure to tobacco smoke in the perinatal period (P96.81)

history of tobacco dependence (Z87.891)

occupational exposure to environmental tobacco smoke (Z57.31)
tobacco dependence (F17.-)

tobacco use (Z72.0)

K11.0   Atrophy of salivary gland

K11.1   Hypertrophy of salivary gland

K11.2   Sialoadenitis

Parotitis

Excludes1: epidemic parotitis (B26.-)

          mumps (B26.-)

          uveoparotid fever [Heerfordt] (D86.89)

K11.20   Sialoadenitis, unspecified

K11.21   Acute sialoadenitis

Excludes1: acute recurrent sialoadenitis (K11.22)

K11.22   Acute recurrent sialoadenitis

K11.23   Chronic sialoadenitis

K11.3   Abscess of salivary gland

K11.4   Fistula of salivary gland

Excludes1: congenital fistula of salivary gland (Q38.4)

K11.5   Sialolithiasis

Calculus of salivary gland or duct

Stone of salivary gland or duct

K11.6   Mucocele of salivary gland

Mucous extravasation cyst of salivary gland

Mucous retention cyst of salivary gland

Ranula

K11.7   Disturbances of salivary secretion

Hypoptyalism

Ptyalism

Xerostomia

Excludes2: dry mouth NOS (R68.2)

K11.8   Other diseases of salivary glands

Benign lymphoepithelial lesion of salivary gland

Mikulicz' disease

Necrotizing sialometaplasia

Sialectasia

Stenosis of salivary duct

Stricture of salivary duct

Excludes1: sicca syndrome [Sjögren] (M35.0-)

K11.9   Disease of salivary gland, unspecified

Sialoadenopathy NOS

K12   Stomatitis and related lesions

Use additional code to identify:

alcohol abuse and dependence (F10.-)

exposure to environmental tobacco smoke (Z77.22)

exposure to tobacco smoke in the perinatal period (P96.81)

history of tobacco dependence (Z87.891)

occupational exposure to environmental tobacco smoke (Z57.31)

tobacco dependence (F17.-)

tobacco use (Z72.0)

Excludes1: cancrum oris (A69.0)

cheilitis (K13.0)

gangrenous stomatitis (A69.0)

herpesviral [herpes simplex] gingivostomatitis (B00.2)

noma (A69.0)

K12.0   Recurrent oral aphthae

Aphthous stomatitis (major) (minor)

Bednar's aphthae

Periadenitis mucosa necrotica recurrens

Recurrent aphthous ulcer

Stomatitis herpetiformis

K12.1   Other forms of stomatitis

Stomatitis NOS

Denture stomatitis

Ulcerative stomatitis

Vesicular stomatitis

Excludes1: acute necrotizing ulcerative stomatitis (A69.1)

          Vincent's stomatitis (A69.1)

K12.2   Cellulitis and abscess of mouth

Cellulitis of mouth (floor)

Submandibular abscess

Excludes2: abscess of salivary gland (K11.3)

          abscess of tongue (K14.0)

          periapical abscess (K04.6-K04.7)

          periodontal abscess (K05.21)

          peritonsillar abscess (J36)

K12.3   Oral mucositis (ulcerative)

Mucositis (oral) (oropharyneal)

Excludes2: gastrointestinal mucositis (ulcerative) (K92.81)

          mucositis (ulcerative) of vagina and vulva (N76.81)

          nasal mucositis (ulcerative) (J34.81)

K12.30   Oral mucositis (ulcerative), unspecified

K12.31   Oral mucositis (ulcerative) due to antineoplastic therapy

Use additional code for adverse effect, if applicable, to identify antineoplastic and immunosuppressive drugs (T45.1X5)

Use additional code for other antineoplastic therapy, such as:

radiological procedure and radiotherapy (Y84.2)

K12.32   Oral mucositis (ulcerative) due to other drugs

Use additional code for adverse effect, if applicable, to identify drug (T36-T50 with fifth or sixth character 5)

K12.33   Oral mucositis (ulcerative) due to radiation

Use additional external cause code (W88-W90, X39.0-) to identify cause

K12.39   Other oral mucositis (ulcerative)

Viral oral mucositis (ulcerative)

K13   Other diseases of lip and oral mucosa

Includes: epithelial disturbances of tongue

Use additional code to identify:

alcohol abuse and dependence (F10.-)

exposure to environmental tobacco smoke (Z77.22)

exposure to tobacco smoke in the perinatal period (P96.81)

history of tobacco dependence (Z87.891)

occupational exposure to environmental tobacco smoke (Z57.31)

tobacco dependence (F17.-)

tobacco use (Z72.0)

Excludes2: certain disorders of gingiva and edentulous alveolar ridge (K05-K06)

    cysts of oral region (K09.-)

    diseases of tongue (K14.-)

    stomatitis and related lesions (K12.-)

K13.0   **Diseases of lips**

    Abscess of lips

    Angular cheilitis

    Cellulitis of lips

    Cheilitis NOS

    Cheilodynia

    Cheilosis

    Exfoliative cheilitis

    Fistula of lips

    Glandular cheilitis

    Hypertrophy of lips

    Perlèche NEC

    Excludes1: ariboflavinosis (E53.0)

        cheilitis due to radiation-related disorders (L55-L59)

        congenital fistula of lips (Q38.0)

        congenital hypertrophy of lips (Q18.6)

        Perlèche due to candidiasis (B37.83)

        Perlèche due to riboflavin deficiency (E53.0)

K13.1   **Cheek and lip biting**

K13.2   **Leukoplakia and other disturbances of oral epithelium, including tongue**

    Excludes1: carcinoma in situ of oral epithelium (D00.0-)

        hairy leukoplakia (K13.3)

    K13.21   **Leukoplakia of oral mucosa, including tongue**

        Leukokeratosis of oral mucosa

        Leukoplakia of gingiva, lips, tongue

        Excludes1: hairy leukoplakia (K13.3)

        leukokeratosis nicotina palati (K13.24)

    K13.22   **Minimal keratinized residual ridge mucosa**

        Minimal keratinization of alveolar ridge mucosa

    K13.23   **Excessive keratinized residual ridge mucosa**

        Excessive keratinization of alveolar ridge mucosa

    K13.24   **Leukokeratosis nicotina palati**

        Smoker's palate

    K13.29   **Other disturbances of oral epithelium, including tongue**

        Erythroplakia of mouth or tongue

        Focal epithelial hyperplasia of mouth or tongue

        Leukoedema of mouth or tongue

        Other oral epithelium disturbances

K13.3   **Hairy leukoplakia**

K13.4   **Granuloma and granuloma-like lesions of oral mucosa**

    Eosinophilic granuloma Granuloma pyogenicum

    Verrucous xanthoma

K13.5   **Oral submucous fibrosis**

    Submucous fibrosis of tongue

K13.6   **Irritative hyperplasia of oral mucosa**

    Excludes2: irritative hyperplasia of edentulous ridge [denture hyperplasia] (K06.2)

K13.7   **Other and unspecified lesions of oral mucosa**

    K13.70   **Unspecified lesions of oral mucosa**

    K13.79   **Other lesions of oral mucosa**

    Focal oral mucinosis

K14   **Diseases of tongue**

Use additional code to identify:

alcohol abuse and dependence (F10.-)

exposure to environmental tobacco smoke (Z77.22)

history of tobacco dependence (Z87.891)

occupational exposure to environmental tobacco smoke (Z57.31)

tobacco dependence (F17.-)

tobacco use (Z72.0)

Excludes2: erythroplakia (K13.29)

    focal epithelial hyperplasia (K13.29)

    leukedema of tongue (K13.29)

    leukoplakia of tongue (K13.21)

    hairy leukoplakia (K13.3)

    macroglossia (congenital) (Q38.2)

    submucous fibrosis of tongue (K13.5)

K14.0   **Glossitis**

    Abscess of tongue

    Ulceration (traumatic) of tongue

    Excludes1: atrophic glossitis (K14.4)

K14.1   **Geographic tongue**

    Benign migratory glossitis Glossitis areata exfoliativa

K14.2   **Median rhomboid glossitis**

K14.3   **Hypertrophy of tongue papillae**

    Black hairy tongue

    Coated tongue

    Hypertrophy of foliate papillae

    Lingua villosa nigra

K14.4   **Atrophy of tongue papillae**

    Atrophic glossitis

K14.5   **Plicated tongue**

    Fissured tongue

    Furrowed tongue

    Scrotal tongue

    Excludes1: fissured tongue, congenital (Q38.3)

K14.6   **Glossodynia**

    Glossopyrosis

    Painful tongue

K14.8   **Other diseases of tongue**

    Atrophy of tongue

    Crenated tongue

    Enlargement of tongue

    Glossocele

    Glossoptosis

    Hypertrophy of tongue

K14.9   **Disease of tongue, unspecified**

    Glossopathy NOS

DISEASES OF ESOPHAGUS, STOMACH AND DUODENUM (K20-K31)

Excludes2: hiatus hernia (K44.-)

K20   Esophagitis

Use additional code to identify:

alcohol abuse and dependence (F10.-)

Excludes1: erosion of esophagus (K22.1-)

esophagitis with gastro-esophageal reflux disease (K21.0)

reflux esophagitis (K21.0)

ulcerative esophagitis (K22.1-)

Excludes2: eosinophilic gastritis or gastroenteritis (K52.81)

K20.0   Eosinophilic esophagitis

K20.8   Other esophagitis

Abscess of esophagus

K20.9   Esophagitis, unspecified

Esophagitis NOS

K21   Gastro-esophageal reflux disease

Excludes1: newborn esophageal reflux (P78.83)

K21.0   Gastro-esophageal reflux disease with esophagitis

Reflux esophagitis

K21.9   Gastro-esophageal reflux disease without esophagitis

Esophageal reflux NOS

K22   Other diseases of esophagus

Excludes2: esophageal varices (I85.-)

K22.0   Achalasia of cardia

Achalasia NOS

Cardiospasm

Excludes1: congenital cardiospasm (Q39.5)

K22.1   Ulcer of esophagus

Barrett's ulcer

Erosion of esophagus

Fungal ulcer of esophagus

Peptic ulcer of esophagus

Ulcer of esophagus due to ingestion of chemicals

Ulcer of esophagus due to ingestion of drugs and medicaments

Ulcerative esophagitis

Code first poisoning due to drug or toxin, if applicable (T36-T65 with fifth or sixth character 1-4 or 6)

Use additional code for adverse effect, if applicable, to identify drug (T36-T50 with fifth or sixth character 5)

Excludes1: Barrett's esophagus (K22.7-)

K22.10   Ulcer of esophagus without bleeding

Ulcer of esophagus NOS

K22.11   Ulcer of esophagus with bleeding

Excludes2: bleeding esophageal varices (I85.01, I85.11)

K22.2   Esophageal obstruction

Compression of esophagus

Constriction of esophagus

Stenosis of esophagus

Stricture of esophagus

Excludes1: congenital stenosis or stricture of esophagus (Q39.3)

K22.3   Perforation of esophagus

Rupture of esophagus

Excludes1: traumatic perforation of (thoracic) esophagus (S27.8-)

K22.4   Dyskinesia of esophagus

Corkscrew esophagus

Diffuse esophageal spasm

Spasm of esophagus

Excludes1: cardiospasm (K22.0)

K22.5   Diverticulum of esophagus, acquired

Esophageal pouch, acquired

Excludes1: diverticulum of esophagus (congenital) (Q39.6)

K22.6   Gastro-esophageal laceration-hemorrhage syndrome

Mallory-Weiss syndrome

K22.7   Barrett's esophagus

Barrett's disease

Barrett's syndrome

Excludes1: Barrett's ulcer (K22.1)

malignant neoplasm of esophagus (C15.-)

K22.70   Barrett's esophagus without dysplasia

Barrett's esophagus NOS

K22.71   Barrett's esophagus with dysplasia

K22.710   Barrett's esophagus with low grade dysplasia

K22.711   Barrett's esophagus with high grade dysplasia

K22.719   Barrett's esophagus with dysplasia, unspecified

K22.8   Other specified diseases of esophagus

Hemorrhage of esophagus NOS

Excludes2: esophageal varices (I85.-)

Paterson-Kelly syndrome (D50.1)

K22.9   Disease of esophagus, unspecified

K23   Disorders of esophagus in diseases classified elsewhere

Code first underlying disease, such as:

congenital syphilis (A50.5)

Excludes1: late syphilis (A52.79)

megaesophagus due to Chagas' disease (B57.31)

tuberculosis (A18.83)

K25   Gastric ulcer

Definition: A Gastric ulcer is a hole in the lining of the stomach corroded by the acidic digestive juices which are secreted by the stomach cells.

Includes: erosion (acute) of stomach

pylorus ulcer (peptic) stomach ulcer (peptic)

Use additional code to identify:

alcohol abuse and dependence (F10.-)

Excludes1: acute gastritis (K29.0-)

peptic ulcer NOS (K27.-)

K25.0   Acute gastric ulcer with hemorrhage

K25.1   Acute gastric ulcer with perforation

K25.2   Acute gastric ulcer with both hemorrhage and perforation

K25.3   Acute gastric ulcer without hemorrhage or perforation

K25.4   Chronic or unspecified gastric ulcer with hemorrhage

K25.5   Chronic or unspecified gastric ulcer with perforation

K25.6 Chronic or unspecified gastric ulcer with both hemorrhage and perforation

K25.7 Chronic gastric ulcer without hemorrhage or perforation

K25.9 Gastric ulcer, unspecified as acute or chronic, without hemorrhage or perforation

K26 **Duodenal ulcer**

Definition: A Duodenal ulcer is a ulcer in the lining of the first part of the small intestine (duodenum).

Includes: erosion (acute) of duodenum

duodenum ulcer (peptic)

postpyloric ulcer (peptic)

Use additional code to identify:

alcohol abuse and dependence (F10.-)

Excludes1: peptic ulcer NOS (K27.-)

K26.0 Acute duodenal ulcer with hemorrhage

K26.1 Acute duodenal ulcer with perforation

K26.2 Acute duodenal ulcer with both hemorrhage and perforation

K26.3 Acute duodenal ulcer without hemorrhage or perforation

K26.4 Chronic or unspecified duodenal ulcer with hemorrhage

K26.5 Chronic or unspecified duodenal ulcer with perforation

K26.6 Chronic or unspecified duodenal ulcer with both hemorrhage and perforation

K26.7 Chronic duodenal ulcer without hemorrhage or perforation

K26.9 Duodenal ulcer, unspecified as acute or chronic, without hemorrhage or perforation

K27 **Peptic ulcer, site unspecified**

Definition: A Peptic ulcer is an ulcer of the mucous membrane lining of the alimentary tract

Includes: gastroduodenal ulcer NOS

peptic ulcer NOS

Use additional code to identify:

alcohol abuse and dependence (F10.-)

Excludes1: peptic ulcer of newborn (P78.82)

K27.0 Acute peptic ulcer, site unspecified, with hemorrhage

K27.1 Acute peptic ulcer, site unspecified, with perforation

K27.2 Acute peptic ulcer, site unspecified, with both hemorrhage and perforation

K27.3 Acute peptic ulcer, site unspecified, without hemorrhage or perforation

K27.4 Chronic or unspecified peptic ulcer, site unspecified, with hemorrhage

K27.5 Chronic or unspecified peptic ulcer, site unspecified, with perforation

K27.6 Chronic or unspecified peptic ulcer, site unspecified, with both hemorrhage and perforation

K27.7 Chronic peptic ulcer, site unspecified, without hemorrhage or perforation

K27.9 Peptic ulcer, site unspecified, unspecified as acute or chronic, without hemorrhage or perforation

K28 **Gastrojejunal ulcer**

Definition: A gastrojejunal ulcer is an ulcer that forms in the area between the stomach and the part of the small intestine known as the jejunum.

Includes: anastomotic ulcer (peptic) or erosion

gastrocolic ulcer (peptic) or erosion

gastrointestinal ulcer (peptic) or erosion

gastrojejunal ulcer (peptic) or erosion

jejunal ulcer (peptic) or erosion

marginal ulcer (peptic) or erosion

stomal ulcer (peptic) or erosion

Use additional code to identify:

alcohol abuse and dependence (F10.-)

Excludes1: primary ulcer of small intestine (K63.3)

K28.0 Acute gastrojejunal ulcer with hemorrhage

K28.1 Acute gastrojejunal ulcer with perforation

K28.2 Acute gastrojejunal ulcer with both hemorrhage and perforation

K28.3 Acute gastrojejunal ulcer without hemorrhage or perforation

K28.4 Chronic or unspecified gastrojejunal ulcer with hemorrhage

K28.5 Chronic or unspecified gastrojejunal ulcer with perforation

K28.6 Chronic or unspecified gastrojejunal ulcer with both hemorrhage and perforation

K28.7 Chronic gastrojejunal ulcer without hemorrhage or perforation

K28.9 Gastrojejunal ulcer, unspecified as acute or chronic, without hemorrhage or perforation

K29 **Gastritis and duodenitis**

Excludes1: eosinophilic gastritis or gastroenteritis (K52.81)

Zollinger-Ellison syndrome (E16.4)

K29.0 Acute gastritis

Use additional code to identify:

alcohol abuse and dependence (F10.-)

Excludes1: erosion (acute) of stomach (K25.-)

K29.00 Acute gastritis without bleeding

K29.01 Acute gastritis with bleeding

K29.2 Alcoholic gastritis

Use additional code to identify:

alcohol abuse and dependence (F10.-)

K29.20 Alcoholic gastritis without bleeding

K29.21 Alcoholic gastritis with bleeding

K29.3 Chronic superficial gastritis

K29.30 Chronic superficial gastritis without bleeding

K29.31 Chronic superficial gastritis with bleeding

K29.4 Chronic atrophic gastritis

Gastric atrophy

K29.40 Chronic atrophic gastritis without bleeding

K29.41 Chronic atrophic gastritis with bleeding

K29.5 Unspecified chronic gastritis

Chronic antral gastritis

Chronic fundal gastritis

K29.50 Unspecified chronic gastritis without bleeding

K29.51 Unspecified chronic gastritis with bleeding

K29.6 Other gastritis

Giant hypertrophic gastritis Granulomatous gastritis

Ménétrier's disease

K29.60 Other gastritis without bleeding

K29.61 Other gastritis with bleeding

Add 4th-7th digits   Nonspecific code   Unspecified code   Manifestation code   459

K29.7 **Gastritis, unspecified**

    K29.70 **Gastritis, unspecified, without bleeding**

    K29.71 **Gastritis, unspecified, with bleeding**

K29.8 **Duodenitis**

    K29.80 **Duodenitis without bleeding**

    K29.81 **Duodenitis with bleeding**

K29.9 **Gastroduodenitis, unspecified**

    K29.90 **Gastroduodenitis, unspecified, without bleeding**

    K29.91 **Gastroduodenitis, unspecified, with bleeding**

K30 Functional dyspepsia

Indigestion

Excludes1: dyspepsia NOS (R10.13)

    heartburn (R12)

    nervous dyspepsia (F45.8)

    neurotic dyspepsia (F45.8)

    psychogenic dyspepsia (F45.8)

K31 Other diseases of stomach and duodenum

Includes: functional disorders of stomach

Excludes2: diabetic gastroparesis (E08.43, E09.43, E10.43, E11.43, E13.43)

    diverticulum of duodenum (K57.00-K57.13)

K31.0 **Acute dilatation of stomach**

Acute distention of stomach

K31.1 **Adult hypertrophic pyloric stenosis**

Pyloric stenosis NOS

Excludes1: congenital or infantile pyloric stenosis (Q40.0)

K31.2 **Hourglass stricture and stenosis of stomach**

Excludes1: congenital hourglass stomach (Q40.2)

    hourglass contraction of stomach (K31.89)

K31.3 **Pylorospasm, not elsewhere classified**

Excludes1: congenital or infantile pylorospasm (Q40.0)

    neurotic pylorospasm (F45.8)

    psychogenic pylorospasm (F45.8)

K31.4 **Gastric diverticulum**

Excludes1: congenital diverticulum of stomach (Q40.2)

K31.5 **Obstruction of duodenum**

Constriction of duodenum

Duodenal ileus (chronic)

Stenosis of duodenum

Stricture of duodenum

Volvulus of duodenum

Excludes1: congenital stenosis of duodenum (Q41.0)

K31.6 **Fistula of stomach and duodenum**

Gastrocolic fistula

Gastrojejunocolic fistula

K31.7 **Polyp of stomach and duodenum**

Excludes1: adenomatous polyp of stomach (D13.1)

K31.8 **Other specified diseases of stomach and duodenum**

    K31.81 **Angiodysplasia of stomach and duodenum**

        K31.811 **Angiodysplasia of stomach and duodenum with bleeding**

        K31.819 **Angiodysplasia of stomach and duodenum without bleeding**

        Angiodysplasia of stomach and duodenum NOS

    K31.82 **Dieulafoy lesion (hemorrhagic) of stomach and duodenum**

        Excludes2: Dieulafoy lesion of intestine (K63.81)

    K31.83 **Achlorhydria**

    K31.84 **Gastroparesis**

        Gastroparalysis

        Code first underlying disease, if known, such as:

        anorexia nervosa (F50.0-)

        diabetes mellitus (E08.43, E09.43, E10.43, E11.43, E13.43)

        scleroderma (M34.-)

    K31.89 **Other diseases of stomach and duodenum**

K31.9 **Disease of stomach and duodenum, unspecified**

DISEASES OF APPENDIX (K35-K38)

K35 Acute appendicitis

K35.2 **Acute appendicitis with generalized peritonitis**

Appendicitis (acute) with generalized (diffuse) peritonitis following rupture or perforation of appendix

Perforated appendix NOS

Ruptured appendix NOS

K35.3 **Acute appendicitis with localized peritonitis**

Acute appendicitis with or without perforation or rupture with peritonitis NOS

Acute appendicitis with or without perforation or rupture with localized peritonitis

Acute appendicitis with peritoneal abscess

K35.8 **Other and unspecified acute appendicitis**

    K35.80 **Unspecified acute appendicitis**

        Acute appendicitis NOS

        Acute appendicitis without (localized) (generalized) peritonitis

    K35.89 **Other acute appendicitis**

K36 Other appendicitis

Chronic appendicitis

Recurrent appendicitis

K37 Unspecified appendicitis

Excludes1: -unspecified appendicitis with peritonitis (K35.2-K35.3)

K38 Other diseases of appendix

K38.0 **Hyperplasia of appendix**

K38.1 **Appendicular concretions**

Fecalith of appendix

Stercolith of appendix

K38.2 **Diverticulum of appendix**

K38.3 **Fistula of appendix**

K38.8 **Other specified diseases of appendix**

Intussusception of appendix

K38.9 **Disease of appendix, unspecified**

HERNIA (K40-K46)

Note: Hernia with both gangrene and obstruction is classified to hernia with gangrene.

Includes: acquired hernia

    congenital [except diaphragmatic or hiatus] hernia

recurrent hernia

K40 **Inguinal hernia**

Includes: bubonocele

direct inguinal hernia

double inguinal hernia

indirect inguinal hernia

inguinal hernia NOS

oblique inguinal hernia

scrotal hernia

K40.0 **Bilateral inguinal hernia, with obstruction, without gangrene**

Inguinal hernia (bilateral) causing obstruction without gangrene

Incarcerated inguinal hernia (bilateral) without gangrene

Irreducible inguinal hernia (bilateral) without gangrene

Strangulated inguinal hernia (bilateral) without gangrene

K40.00 **Bilateral inguinal hernia, with obstruction, without gangrene, not specified as recurrent**

Bilateral inguinal hernia, with obstruction, without gangrene NOS

K40.01 **Bilateral inguinal hernia, with obstruction, without gangrene, recurrent**

K40.1 **Bilateral inguinal hernia, with gangrene**

K40.10 **Bilateral inguinal hernia, with gangrene, not specified as recurrent**

Bilateral inguinal hernia, with gangrene NOS

K40.11 **Bilateral inguinal hernia, with gangrene, recurrent**

K40.2 **Bilateral inguinal hernia, without obstruction or gangrene**

K40.20 **Bilateral inguinal hernia, without obstruction or gangrene, not specified as recurrent**

Bilateral inguinal hernia NOS

K40.21 **Bilateral inguinal hernia, without obstruction or gangrene, recurrent**

K40.3 **Unilateral inguinal hernia, with obstruction, without gangrene**

Inguinal hernia (unilateral) causing obstruction without gangrene

Incarcerated inguinal hernia (unilateral) without gangrene

Irreducible inguinal hernia (unilateral) without gangrene

Strangulated inguinal hernia (unilateral) without gangrene

K40.30 **Unilateral inguinal hernia, with obstruction, without gangrene, not specified as recurrent**

Inguinal hernia, with obstruction NOS

Unilateral inguinal hernia, with obstruction, without gangrene NOS

K40.31 **Unilateral inguinal hernia, with obstruction, without gangrene, recurrent**

K40.4 **Unilateral inguinal hernia, with gangrene**

K40.40 **Unilateral inguinal hernia, with gangrene, not specified as recurrent**

Inguinal hernia with gangrene NOS

Unilateral inguinal hernia with gangrene NOS

K40.41 **Unilateral inguinal hernia, with gangrene, recurrent**

K40.9 **Unilateral inguinal hernia, without obstruction or gangrene**

K40.90 **Unilateral inguinal hernia, without obstruction or gangrene, not specified as recurrent**

Inguinal hernia NOS

Unilateral inguinal hernia NOS

K40.91 **Unilateral inguinal hernia, without obstruction or gangrene, recurrent**

K41 **Femoral hernia**

K41.0 **Bilateral femoral hernia, with obstruction, without gangrene**

Femoral hernia (bilateral) causing obstruction, without gangrene

Incarcerated femoral hernia (bilateral), without gangrene

Irreducible femoral hernia (bilateral), without gangrene

Strangulated femoral hernia (bilateral), without gangrene

K41.00 **Bilateral femoral hernia, with obstruction, without gangrene, not specified as recurrent**

Bilateral femoral hernia, with obstruction, without gangrene NOS

K41.01 **Bilateral femoral hernia, with obstruction, without gangrene, recurrent**

K41.1 **Bilateral femoral hernia, with gangrene**

K41.10 **Bilateral femoral hernia, with gangrene, not specified as recurrent**

Bilateral femoral hernia, with gangrene NOS

K41.11 **Bilateral femoral hernia, with gangrene, recurrent**

K41.2 **Bilateral femoral hernia, without obstruction or gangrene**

K41.20 **Bilateral femoral hernia, without obstruction or gangrene, not specified as recurrent**

Bilateral femoral hernia NOS

K41.21 **Bilateral femoral hernia, without obstruction or gangrene, recurrent**

K41.3 **Unilateral femoral hernia, with obstruction, without gangrene**

Femoral hernia (unilateral) causing obstruction, without gangrene

Incarcerated femoral hernia (unilateral), without gangrene

Irreducible femoral hernia (unilateral), without gangrene

Strangulated femoral hernia (unilateral), without gangrene

K41.30 **Unilateral femoral hernia, with obstruction, without gangrene, not specified as recurrent**

Femoral hernia, with obstruction NOS

Unilateral femoral hernia, with obstruction NOS

K41.31 **Unilateral femoral hernia, with obstruction, without gangrene, recurrent**

K41.4 **Unilateral femoral hernia, with gangrene**

K41.40 **Unilateral femoral hernia, with gangrene, not specified as recurrent**

Femoral hernia, with gangrene NOS

Unilateral femoral hernia, with gangrene NOS

K41.41 **Unilateral femoral hernia, with gangrene, recurrent**

K41.9 **Unilateral femoral hernia, without obstruction or gangrene**

K41.90 **Unilateral femoral hernia, without obstruction or gangrene, not specified as recurrent**

Femoral hernia NOS

Unilateral femoral hernia NOS

K41.91   **Unilateral femoral hernia, without obstruction or gangrene, recurrent**

K42   **Umbilical hernia**

Includes: paraumbilical hernia

Excludes1: omphalocele (Q79.2)

K42.0   **Umbilical hernia with obstruction, without gangrene**

Umbilical hernia causing obstruction, without gangrene

Incarcerated umbilical hernia, without gangrene

Irreducible umbilical hernia, without gangrene

Strangulated umbilical hernia, without gangrene

K42.1   **Umbilical hernia with gangrene**

Gangrenous umbilical hernia

K42.9   **Umbilical hernia without obstruction or gangrene**

Umbilical hernia NOS

K43   **Ventral hernia**

K43.0   **Incisional hernia with obstruction, without gangrene**

Incisional hernia causing obstruction, without gangrene

Incarcerated incisional hernia, without gangrene

Irreducible incisional hernia, without gangrene

Strangulated incisional hernia, without gangrene

K43.1   **Incisional hernia with gangrene**

Gangrenous incisional hernia

K43.2   **Incisional hernia without obstruction or gangrene**

Incisional hernia NOS

K43.3   **Parastomal hernia with obstruction, without gangrene**

Incarcerated parastomal hernia, without gangrene

Irreducible parastomal hernia, without gangrene

Parastomal hernia causing obstruction, without gangrene

Strangulated parastomal hernia, without gangrene

K43.4   **Parastomal hernia with gangrene**

Gangrenous parastomal hernia

K43.5   **Parastomal hernia without obstruction or gangrene**

Parastomal hernia NOS

K43.6   **Other and unspecified ventral hernia with obstruction, without gangrene**

Epigastric hernia causing obstruction, without gangrene

Hypogastric hernia causing obstruction, without gangrene

Incarcerated epigastric hernia without gangrene

Incarcerated hypogastric hernia without gangrene

Incarcerated midline hernia without gangrene

Incarcerated spigelian hernia without gangrene

Incarcerated subxiphoid hernia without gangrene

Irreducible epigastric hernia without gangrene

Irreducible hypogastric hernia without gangrene

Irreducible midline hernia without gangrene

Irreducible spigelian hernia without gangrene

Irreducible subxiphoid hernia without gangrene

Midline hernia causing obstruction, without gangrene

Spigelian hernia causing obstruction, without gangrene

Strangulated epigastric hernia without gangrene

Strangulated hypogastric hernia without gangrene

Strangulated midline hernia without gangrene

Strangulated spigelian hernia without gangrene

Strangulated subxiphoid hernia without gangrene

Subxiphoid hernia causing obstruction, without gangrene

K43.7   **Other and unspecified ventral hernia with gangrene**

Any condition listed under K43.6 specified as gangrenous

K43.9   **Ventral hernia without obstruction or gangrene**

Epigastric hernia

Ventral hernia NOS

K44   **Diaphragmatic hernia**

Includes: hiatus hernia (esophageal) (sliding)

paraesophageal hernia

Excludes1: congenital diaphragmatic hernia (Q79.0)

congenital hiatus hernia (Q40.1)

K44.0   **Diaphragmatic hernia with obstruction, without gangrene**

Diaphragmatic hernia causing obstruction

Incarcerated diaphragmatic hernia

Irreducible diaphragmatic hernia

Strangulated diaphragmatic hernia

K44.1   **Diaphragmatic hernia with gangrene**

Gangrenous diaphragmatic hernia

K44.9   **Diaphragmatic hernia without obstruction or gangrene**

Diaphragmatic hernia NOS

K45   **Other abdominal hernia**

Includes: abdominal hernia, specified site NEC

lumbar hernia

obturator hernia

pudendal hernia

retroperitoneal hernia

sciatic hernia

K45.0   **Other specified abdominal hernia with obstruction, without gangrene**

Other specified abdominal hernia causing obstruction

Other specified incarcerated abdominal hernia

Other specified irreducible abdominal hernia

Other specified strangulated abdominal hernia

K45.1   **Other specified abdominal hernia with gangrene**

Any condition listed under K45 specified as gangrenous

K45.8   **Other specified abdominal hernia without obstruction or gangrene**

K46   **Unspecified abdominal hernia**

Includes: enterocele

epiplocele hernia NOS

interstitial hernia

intestinal hernia

intra-abdominal hernia

Excludes1: vaginal enterocele (N81.5)

K46.0   **Unspecified abdominal hernia with obstruction, without gangrene**

Unspecified abdominal hernia causing obstruction

Unspecified incarcerated abdominal hernia

Unspecified irreducible abdominal hernia

Unspecified strangulated abdominal hernia

K46.1   **Unspecified abdominal hernia with gangrene**

Any condition listed under K46 specified as gangrenous

K46.9 Unspecified abdominal hernia without obstruction or gangrene

Abdominal hernia NOS

NONINFECTIVE ENTERITIS AND COLITIS (K50-K52)

Includes: noninfective inflammatory bowel disease

Excludes1: irritable bowel syndrome (K58.-)

megacolon (K59.3-)

K50 Crohn's disease [regional enteritis]

Includes: granulomatous enteritis

Use additional code to identify manifestations, such as:

pyoderma gangrenosum (L88)

Excludes1: ulcerative colitis (K51.-)

K50.0 Crohn's disease of small intestine

Crohn's disease [regional enteritis] of duodenum

Crohn's disease [regional enteritis] of ileum

Crohn's disease [regional enteritis] of jejunum

Regional ileitis

Terminal ileitis

Excludes1: Crohn's disease of both small and large intestine (K50.8-)

K50.00 Crohn's disease of small intestine without complications

K50.01 Crohn's disease of small intestine with complications

K50.011 Crohn's disease of small intestine with rectal bleeding

K50.012 Crohn's disease of small intestine with intestinal obstruction

K50.013 Crohn's disease of small intestine with fistula

K50.014 Crohn's disease of small intestine with abscess

K50.018 Crohn's disease of small intestine with other complication

K50.019 Crohn's disease of small intestine with unspecified complications

K50.1 Crohn's disease of large intestine

Crohn's disease [regional enteritis] of colon

Crohn's disease [regional enteritis] of large bowel

Crohn's disease [regional enteritis] of rectum

Granulomatous colitis

Regional colitis

Excludes1: Crohn's disease of both small and large intestine (K50.8)

K50.10 Crohn's disease of large intestine without complications

K50.11 Crohn's disease of large intestine with complications

K50.111 Crohn's disease of large intestine with rectal bleeding

K50.112 Crohn's disease of large intestine with intestinal obstruction

K50.113 Crohn's disease of large intestine with fistula

K50.114 Crohn's disease of large intestine with abscess

K50.118 Crohn's disease of large intestine with other complication

K50.119 Crohn's disease of large intestine with unspecified complications

K50.8 Crohn's disease of both small and large intestine

K50.80 Crohn's disease of both small and large intestine without complications

K50.81 Crohn's disease of both small and large intestine with complications

K50.811 Crohn's disease of both small and large intestine with rectal bleeding

K50.812 Crohn's disease of both small and large intestine with intestinal obstruction

K50.813 Crohn's disease of both small and large intestine with fistula

K50.814 Crohn's disease of both small and large intestine with abscess

K50.818 Crohn's disease of both small and large intestine with other complication

K50.819 Crohn's disease of both small and large intestine with unspecified complications

K50.9 Crohn's disease, unspecified

K50.90 Crohn's disease, unspecified, without complications

Crohn's disease NOS

Regional enteritis NOS

K50.91 Crohn's disease, unspecified, with complications

K50.911 Crohn's disease, unspecified, with rectal bleeding

K50.912 Crohn's disease, unspecified, with intestinal obstruction

K50.913 Crohn's disease, unspecified, with fistula

K50.914 Crohn's disease, unspecified, with abscess

K50.918 Crohn's disease, unspecified, with other complication

K50.919 Crohn's disease, unspecified, with unspecified complications

K51 Ulcerative colitis

Definition: Ulcerative colitis ulcerative colitis is a form of inflammatory bowel disease (ibd). It causes swelling, ulcerations, and loss of function of the large intestine.

Use additional code to identify manifestations, such as:

pyoderma gangrenosum (L88)

Excludes1: Crohn's disease [regional enteritis] (K50.-)

K51.0 Ulcerative (chronic) pancolitis

Backwash ileitis

K51.00 Ulcerative (chronic) pancolitis without complications

Ulcerative (chronic) pancolitis NOS

K51.01 Ulcerative (chronic) pancolitis with complications

K51.011 Ulcerative (chronic) pancolitis with rectal bleeding

K51.012   Ulcerative (chronic) pancolitis with intestinal obstruction

K51.013   Ulcerative (chronic) pancolitis with fistula

K51.014   Ulcerative (chronic) pancolitis with abscess

K51.018   Ulcerative (chronic) pancolitis with other complication

K51.019   Ulcerative (chronic) pancolitis with unspecified complications

K51.2   **Ulcerative (chronic) proctitis**

    K51.20   Ulcerative (chronic) proctitis without complications

        Ulcerative (chronic) proctitis NOS

    K51.21   Ulcerative (chronic) proctitis with complications

K51.211   Ulcerative (chronic) proctitis with rectal bleeding

K51.212   Ulcerative (chronic) proctitis with intestinal obstruction

K51.213   Ulcerative (chronic) proctitis with fistula

K51.214   Ulcerative (chronic) proctitis with abscess

K51.218   Ulcerative (chronic) proctitis with other complication

K51.219   Ulcerative (chronic) proctitis with unspecified complications

K51.3   **Ulcerative (chronic) rectosigmoiditis**

    K51.30   Ulcerative (chronic) rectosigmoiditis without complications

        Ulcerative (chronic) rectosigmoiditis NOS

    K51.31   Ulcerative (chronic) rectosigmoiditis with complications

K51.311   Ulcerative (chronic) rectosigmoiditis with rectal bleeding

K51.312   Ulcerative (chronic) rectosigmoiditis with intestinal obstruction

K51.313   Ulcerative (chronic) rectosigmoiditis with fistula

K51.314   Ulcerative (chronic) rectosigmoiditis with abscess

K51.318   Ulcerative (chronic) rectosigmoiditis with other complication

K51.319   Ulcerative (chronic) rectosigmoiditis with unspecified complications

K51.4   **Inflammatory polyps of colon**

    Excludes1: adenomatous polyp of colon (D12.6)

        polyposis of colon (D12.6) polyps of colon NOS (K63.5)

    K51.40   Inflammatory polyps of colon without complications

        Inflammatory polyps of colon NOS

    K51.41   Inflammatory polyps of colon with complications

K51.411   Inflammatory polyps of colon with rectal bleeding

K51.412   Inflammatory polyps of colon with intestinal obstruction

K51.413   Inflammatory polyps of colon with fistula

K51.414   Inflammatory polyps of colon with abscess

K51.418   Inflammatory polyps of colon with other complication

K51.419   Inflammatory polyps of colon with unspecified complications

K51.5   **Left sided colitis**

    Left hemicolitis

    K51.50   Left sided colitis without complications

    Left sided colitis NOS

    K51.51   Left sided colitis with complications

K51.511   Left sided colitis with rectal bleeding

K51.512   Left sided colitis with intestinal obstruction

K51.513   Left sided colitis with fistula

K51.514   Left sided colitis with abscess

K51.518   Left sided colitis with other complication

K51.519   Left sided colitis with unspecified complications

K51.8   **Other ulcerative colitis**

    K51.80   Other ulcerative colitis without complications

    K51.81   Other ulcerative colitis with complications

K51.811   Other ulcerative colitis with rectal bleeding

K51.812   Other ulcerative colitis with intestinal obstruction

K51.813   Other ulcerative colitis with fistula

K51.814   Other ulcerative colitis with abscess

K51.818   Other ulcerative colitis with other complication

K51.819   Other ulcerative colitis with unspecified complications

K51.9   **Ulcerative colitis, unspecified**

    K51.90   Ulcerative colitis, unspecified, without complications

    K51.91   Ulcerative colitis, unspecified, with complications

K51.911   Ulcerative colitis, unspecified with rectal bleeding

K51.912   Ulcerative colitis, unspecified with intestinal obstruction

K51.913   Ulcerative colitis, unspecified with fistula

K51.914   Ulcerative colitis, unspecified with abscess

K51.918   Ulcerative colitis, unspecified with other complication

K51.919   Ulcerative colitis, unspecified with unspecified complications

K52   **Other and unspecified noninfective gastroenteritis and colitis**

K52.0   **Gastroenteritis and colitis due to radiation**

K52.1   **Toxic gastroenteritis and colitis**

    Drug-induced gastroenteritis and colitis

<u>Code first</u> (T51-T65) to identify toxic agent

<u>Use additional code</u> for adverse effect, if applicable, to identify drug (T36-T50 with fifth or sixth character 5)

K52.2 Allergic and dietetic gastroenteritis and colitis

Food hypersensitivity gastroenteritis or colitis

<u>Use additional code</u> to identify type of food allergy (Z91.01-, Z91.02-)

Excludes2: allergic eosinophilic colitis (K52.82)

allergic eosinophilic esophagitis (K20.0)

allergic eosinophilic gastritis (K52.81)

allergic eosinophilic gastroenteritis (K52.81)

food protein-induced proctocolitis (K52.82)

- **K52.21 Food protein-induced enterocolitis syndrome**

    <u>Use additional code</u> for hypovolemic shock, if present (R57.1)

- **K52.22 Food protein-induced enteropathy**

- **K52.29 Other allergic and dietetic gastroenteritis and colitis**

    Food hypersensitivity gastroenteritis or colitis

    Immediate gastrointestinal hypersensitivity

- **K52.3 Indeterminate colitis**

    Colonic inflammatory bowel disease unclassified (IBDU)

    Excludes1: unspecified colitis (K52.9)

K52.8 Other specified noninfective gastroenteritis and colitis

K52.81 Eosinophilic gastritis or gastroenteritis

Eosinophilic enteritis

Excludes2: eosinophilic esophagitis (K20.0)

K52.82 Eosinophilic colitis

Allergic proctocolitis

Food-induced eosinophilic proctocolitis

Food protein-induced proctocolitis

Milk protein-induced proctocolitis

K52.83 Microscopic colitis

- **K52.831 Collagenous colitis**

- **K52.832 Lymphocytic colitis**

- **K52.838 Other microscopic colitis**

- **K52.839 Microscopic colitis, unspecified**

K52.89 Other specified noninfective gastroenteritis and colitis

K52.9 Noninfective gastroenteritis and colitis, unspecified

Colitis NOS

Enteritis NOS

Gastroenteritis NOS

Ileitis NOS

Jejunitis NOS

Sigmoiditis NOS

Excludes1: diarrhea NOS (R19.7)

functional diarrhea (K59.1)

infectious gastroenteritis and colitis NOS (A09)

neonatal diarrhea (noninfective) (P78.3)

psychogenic diarrhea (F45.8)

OTHER DISEASES OF INTESTINES (K55-K64)

K55 Vascular disorders of intestine

Excludes1: necrotizing enterocolitis of newborn (P77.-)

K55.0 Acute vascular disorders of intestine

Infarction of appendices epiploicae

Mesenteric (artery) (vein) embolism

Mesenteric (artery) (vein) infarction

Mesenteric (artery) (vein) thrombosis

K55.01 Acute (reversible) ischemia of small intestine

- **K55.011 Focal (segmental) acute (reversible) ischemia of small intestine**

- **K55.012 Diffuse acute (reversible) ischemia of small intestine**

- **K55.019 Acute (reversible) ischemia of small intestine, extent unspecified**

K55.02 Acute infarction of small intestine

Gangrene of small intestine

Necrosis of small intestine

- **K55.021 Focal (segmental) acute infarction of small intestine**

- **K55.022 Diffuse acute infarction of small intestine**

- **K55.029 Acute infarction of small intestine, extent unspecified**

K55.03 Acute (reversible) ischemia of large intestine

Acute fulminant ischemic colitis

Subacute ischemic colitis

- **K55.031 Focal (segmental) acute (reversible) ischemia of large intestine**

- **K55.032 Diffuse acute (reversible) ischemia of large intestine**

- **K55.039 Acute (reversible) ischemia of large intestine, extent unspecified**

K55.04 Acute infarction of large intestine

Gangrene of large intestine

Necrosis of large intestine

- **K55.041 Focal (segmental) acute infarction of large intestine**

- **K55.042 Diffuse acute infarction of large intestine**

- **K55.049 Acute infarction of large intestine, extent unspecified**

K55.05 Acute (reversible) ischemia of intestine, part unspecified

- **K55.051 Focal (segmental) acute (reversible) ischemia of intestine, part unspecified**

- **K55.052 Diffuse acute (reversible) ischemia of intestine, part unspecified**

- **K55.059 Acute (reversible) ischemia of intestine, part and extent unspecified**

K55.06 Acute infarction of intestine, part unspecified

Acute intestinal infarction

Gangrene of intestine

Necrosis of intestine

- **K55.061 Focal (segmental) acute infarction of intestine, part unspecified**

- **K55.062 Diffuse acute infarction of intestine, part unspecified**

- **K55.069 Acute infarction of intestine, part and extent unspecified**

Add 4th-7th digits   Nonspecific code   Unspecified code   Manifestation code   465

K55.1   Chronic vascular disorders of intestine

Chronic ischemic colitis

Chronic ischemic enteritis

Chronic ischemic enterocolitis

Ischemic stricture of intestine

Mesenteric atherosclerosis

Mesenteric vascular insufficiency

K55.2   Angiodysplasia of colon

    K55.20   Angiodysplasia of colon without hemorrhage

    K55.21   Angiodysplasia of colon with hemorrhage

K55.3   Necrotizing enterocolitis

    Excludes1: necrotizing enterocolitis of newborn (P77.-)

    Excludes2: necrotizing enterocolitis due to Clostridium difficile (A04.7)

    ●**K55.30   Necrotizing enterocolitis, unspecified**

      Necrotizing enterocolitis, NOS

    ●**K55.31   Stage 1 necrotizing enterocolitis**

      Necrotizing enterocolitis without pneumatosis, without perforation

    ●**K55.32   Stage 2 necrotizing enterocolitis**

      Necrotizing enterocolitis with pneumatosis, without perforation

    ●**K55.33   Stage 3 necrotizing enterocolitis**

      Necrotizing enterocolitis with perforation

      Necrotizing enterocolitis with pneumatosis and perforation

K55.8   Other vascular disorders of intestine

K55.9   Vascular disorder of intestine, unspecified

Ischemic colitis Ischemic enteritis

Ischemic enterocolitis

K56   Paralytic ileus and intestinal obstruction without hernia

Excludes1: congenital stricture or stenosis of intestine (Q41-Q42)

cystic fibrosis with meconium ileus (E84.11)

ischemic stricture of intestine (K55.1)

meconium ileus NOS (P76.0)

neonatal intestinal obstructions classifiable to P76.- obstruction of duodenum (K31.5)

postprocedural intestinal obstruction (K91.3)

stenosis of anus or rectum (K62.4)

intestinal obstruction with hernia (K40-K46)

K56.0   Paralytic ileus

Paralysis of bowel

Paralysis of colon

Paralysis of intestine

Excludes1: gallstone ileus (K56.3)

ileus NOS (K56.7)

obstructive ileus NOS (K56.69)

K56.1   Intussusception

Intussusception or invagination of bowel

Intussusception or invagination of colon

Intussusception or invagination of intestine

Intussusception or invagination of rectum

Excludes2: intussusception of appendix (K38.8)

K56.2   Volvulus

Strangulation of colon or intestine

Torsion of colon or intestine

Twist of colon or intestine

Excludes2: volvulus of duodenum (K31.5)

K56.3   Gallstone ileus

Obstruction of intestine by gallstone

K56.4   Other impaction of intestine

    K56.41   Fecal impaction

      Excludes1: constipation (K59.0-)

            incomplete defecation (R15.0)

    K56.49   Other impaction of intestine

K56.5   Intestinal adhesions [bands] with obstruction (postprocedural) (postinfection)

Abdominal hernia due to adhesions with obstruction

Peritoneal adhesions [bands] with intestinal obstruction (postprocedural) (postinfection)

K56.6   Other and unspecified intestinal obstruction

    K56.60   Unspecified intestinal obstruction

      Intestinal obstruction NOS

      Excludes1: intestinal obstruction due to specified condition-code to condition

    K56.69   Other intestinal obstruction

      Enterostenosis NOS

      Obstructive ileus NOS

      Occlusion of colon or intestine NOS

      Stenosis of colon or intestine NOS

      Stricture of colon or intestine NOS

      Excludes1: intestinal obstruction due to specified condition-code to condition

K56.7   Ileus, unspecified

Excludes1: obstructive ileus (K56.69)

K57   Diverticular disease of intestine

Definition: Diverticulitis is a common digestive disease which involves the formation of pouches (diverticula) within the bowel wall. This process is known as diverticulosis, and typically occurs within the large intestine, or colon, although it can occasionally occur in the small intestine as well. Diverticulitis results when one of these diverticula becomes inflamed.

Excludes1: congenital diverticulum of intestine (Q43.8)

Meckel's diverticulum (Q43.0)

Excludes2: diverticulum of appendix (K38.2)

K57.0   Diverticulitis of small intestine with perforation and abscess

Diverticulitis of small intestine with peritonitis

Excludes1: diverticulitis of both small and large intestine with perforation and abscess (K57.4-)

    K57.00   Diverticulitis of small intestine with perforation and abscess without bleeding

    K57.01   Diverticulitis of small intestine with perforation and abscess with bleeding

K57.1   Diverticular disease of small intestine without perforation or abscess

Excludes1: diverticular disease of both small and large intestine without perforation or abscess (K57.5-)

    K57.10   Diverticulosis of small intestine without perforation or abscess without bleeding

      Diverticular disease of small intestine NOS

    K57.11   Diverticulosis of small intestine without perforation or abscess with bleeding

K57.12 Diverticulitis of small intestine without perforation or abscess without bleeding

K57.13 Diverticulitis of small intestine without perforation or abscess with bleeding

K57.2 Diverticulitis of large intestine with perforation and abscess

Diverticulitis of colon with peritonitis

Excludes1: diverticulitis of both small and large intestine with perforation and abscess (K57.4-)

K57.20 Diverticulitis of large intestine with perforation and abscess without bleeding

K57.21 Diverticulitis of large intestine with perforation and abscess with bleeding

K57.3 Diverticular disease of large intestine without perforation or abscess

Excludes1: diverticular disease of both small and large intestine without perforation or abscess (K57.5-)

K57.30 Diverticulosis of large intestine without perforation or abscess without bleeding

Diverticular disease of colon NOS

K57.31 Diverticulosis of large intestine without perforation or abscess with bleeding

K57.32 Diverticulitis of large intestine without perforation or abscess without bleeding

K57.33 Diverticulitis of large intestine without perforation or abscess with bleeding

K57.4 Diverticulitis of both small and large intestine with perforation and abscess

Diverticulitis of both small and large intestine with peritonitis

K57.40 Diverticulitis of both small and large intestine with perforation and abscess without bleeding

K57.41 Diverticulitis of both small and large intestine with perforation and abscess with bleeding

K57.5 Diverticular disease of both small and large intestine without perforation or abscess

K57.50 Diverticulosis of both small and large intestine without perforation or abscess without bleeding

Diverticular disease of both small and large intestine NOS

K57.51 Diverticulosis of both small and large intestine without perforation or abscess with bleeding

K57.52 Diverticulitis of both small and large intestine without perforation or abscess without bleeding

K57.53 Diverticulitis of both small and large intestine without perforation or abscess with bleeding

K57.8 Diverticulitis of intestine, part unspecified, with perforation and abscess

Diverticulitis of intestine NOS with peritonitis

K57.80 Diverticulitis of intestine, part unspecified, with perforation and abscess without bleeding

K57.81 Diverticulitis of intestine, part unspecified, with perforation and abscess with bleeding

K57.9 Diverticular disease of intestine, part unspecified, without perforation or abscess

K57.90 Diverticulosis of intestine, part unspecified, without perforation or abscess without bleeding

Diverticular disease of intestine NOS

K57.91 Diverticulosis of intestine, part unspecified, without perforation or abscess with bleeding

K57.92 Diverticulitis of intestine, part unspecified, without perforation or abscess without bleeding

K57.93 Diverticulitis of intestine, part unspecified, without perforation or abscess with bleeding

K58 Irritable bowel syndrome

Includes: irritable colon

spastic colon

K58.0 Irritable bowel syndrome with diarrhea

●**K58.1** Irritable bowel syndrome with constipation

●**K58.2** Mixed irritable bowel syndrome

●**K58.8** Other irritable bowel syndrome

K58.9 Irritable bowel syndrome without diarrhea

Irritable bowel syndrome NOS

K59 Other functional intestinal disorders

Excludes1: change in bowel habit NOS (R19.4)

intestinal malabsorption (K90.-)

psychogenic intestinal disorders (F45.8)

Excludes2: functional disorders of stomach (K31.-)

K59.0 Constipation

Use additional code for adverse effect, if applicable, to identify drug (T36-T50 with fifth or sixth character 5)

Excludes1: fecal impaction (K56.41)

incomplete defecation (R15.0)

K59.00 Constipation, unspecified

K59.01 Slow transit constipation

K59.02 Outlet dysfunction constipation

●**K59.03** Drug induced constipation

Use additional code for adverse effect, if applicable, to identify drug (T36-T50 with fifth or sixth character 5

●**K59.04** Chronic idiopathic constipation

Functional constipation

K59.09 Other constipation

Chronic constipation

K59.1 Functional diarrhea

Excludes1: diarrhea NOS (R19.7)

irritable bowel syndrome with diarrhea (K58.0)

K59.2 Neurogenic bowel, not elsewhere classified

K59.3 Megacolon, not elsewhere classified

Dilatation of colon

Code first, if applicable (T51-T65) to identify toxic agent

Excludes1: congenital megacolon (aganglionic) (Q43.1)

megacolon (due to) (in) Chagas' disease (B57.32)

megacolon (due to) (in) Clostridium difficile (A04.7)

megacolon (due to) (in) Hirschsprung's disease (Q43.1)

●**K59.31** Toxic megacolon

●**K59.39** Other megacolon

Megacolon NOS

K59.4 Anal spasm

Proctalgia fugax

K59.8 Other specified functional intestinal disorders

Atony of colon

Pseudo-obstruction (acute) (chronic) of intestine

K59.9 Functional intestinal disorder, unspecified

K60 Fissure and fistula of anal and rectal regions

Excludes1: fissure and fistula of anal and rectal regions with abscess or cellulitis (K61.-)

Excludes2: anal sphincter tear (healed) (nontraumatic) (old) (K62.81)

K60.0 Acute anal fissure

K60.1 Chronic anal fissure

K60.2 Anal fissure, unspecified

K60.3 Anal fistula

K60.4 Rectal fistula

Fistula of rectum to skin

Excludes1: rectovaginal fistula (N82.3)

vesicorectal fistual (N32.1)

K60.5 Anorectal fistula

K61 Abscess of anal and rectal regions

Includes: abscess of anal and rectal regions

cellulitis of anal and rectal regions

K61.0 Anal abscess

Perianal abscess

Excludes1: intrasphincteric abscess (K61.4)

K61.1 Rectal abscess

Perirectal abscess

Excludes1: ischiorectal abscess (K61.3)

K61.2 Anorectal abscess

K61.3 Ischiorectal abscess

Abscess of ischiorectal fossa

K61.4 Intrasphincteric abscess

K62 Other diseases of anus and rectum

Includes: anal canal

Excludes2: colostomy and enterostomy malfunction (K94.0-, K94.1-)

fecal incontinence (R15.-)

hemorrhoids (K64.-)

K62.0 Anal polyp

K62.1 Rectal polyp

Excludes1: adenomatous polyp (D12.8)

K62.2 Anal prolapse

Prolapse of anal canal

K62.3 Rectal prolapse

Prolapse of rectal mucosa

K62.4 Stenosis of anus and rectum

Stricture of anus (sphincter)

K62.5 Hemorrhage of anus and rectum

Excludes1: gastrointestinal bleeding NOS (K92.2)

melena (K92.1)

neonatal rectal hemorrhage (P54.2)

K62.6 Ulcer of anus and rectum

Solitary ulcer of anus and rectum

Stercoral ulcer of anus and rectum

Excludes1: fissure and fistula of anus and rectum (K60.-)

ulcerative colitis (K51.-)

K62.7 Radiation proctitis

Use additional code to identify the type of radiation (W90.-)

K62.8 Other specified diseases of anus and rectum

Excludes2: ulcerative proctitis (K51.2)

K62.81 Anal sphincter tear (healed) (nontraumatic) (old)

Tear of anus, nontraumatic

Use additional code for any associated fecal incontinence (R15.-)

Excludes2: anal fissure (K60.-)

anal sphincter tear (healed) (old) complicating delivery (O34.7-)

traumatic tear of anal sphincter (S31.831)

K62.82 Dysplasia of anus

Anal intraepithelial neoplasia I and II (AIN I and II) (histologically confirmed)

Dysplasia of anus NOS

Mild and moderate dysplasia of anus (histologically confirmed)

Excludes1: abnormal results from anal cytologic examination without histologic confirmation (R85.61-)

anal intraepithelial neoplasia III (D01.3)

carcinoma in situ of anus (D01.3)

HGSIL of anus (R85.613)

severe dysplasia of anus (D01.3)

K62.89 Other specified diseases of anus and rectum

Proctitis NOS

Use additional code for any associated fecal incontinence (R15.-)

K62.9 Disease of anus and rectum, unspecified

K63 Other diseases of intestine

K63.0 Abscess of intestine

Excludes1: abscess of intestine with Crohn's disease (K50.014, K50.114, K50.814, K50.914,)

abscess of intestine with diverticular disease (K57.0, K57.2, K57.4, K57.8)

abscess of intestine with ulcerative colitis (K51.014, K51.214, K51.314, K51.414, K51.514, K51.814, K51.914)

Excludes2: abscess of anal and rectal regions (K61.-)

abscess of appendix (K35.3)

K63.1 Perforation of intestine (nontraumatic)

Perforation (nontraumatic) of rectum

Excludes1: perforation (nontraumatic) of duodenum (K26.-)

perforation (nontraumatic) of intestine with diverticular disease (K57.0, K57.2, K57.4, K57.8)

Excludes2: perforation (nontraumatic) of appendix (K35.2, K35.3)

K63.2 Fistula of intestine

Excludes1: fistula of duodenum (K31.6)

fistula of intestine with Crohn's disease (K50.013, K50.113, K50.813, K50.913,)

fistula of intestine with ulcerative colitis (K51.013, K51.213, K51.313, K51.413, K51.513, K51.813, K51.913)

Excludes2: fistula of anal and rectal regions (K60.-)

fistula of appendix (K38.3)

intestinal-genital fistula, female (N82.2-N82.4)

vesicointestinal fistula (N32.1)

K63.3 Ulcer of intestine

Primary ulcer of small intestine

Excludes1: duodenal ulcer (K26.-)

gastrointestinal ulcer (K28.-)

gastrojejunal ulcer (K28.-)

jejunal ulcer (K28.-)

peptic ulcer, site unspecified (K27.-)

ulcer of intestine with perforation (K63.1)

ulcer of anus or rectum (K62.6)

ulcerative colitis (K51.-)

K63.4 Enteroptosis

K63.5 Polyp of colon

Excludes1: adenomatous polyp of colon (D12.6)

inflammatory polyp of colon (K51.4-)

polyposis of colon (D12.6)

K63.8 Other specified diseases of intestine

K63.81 Dieulafoy lesion of intestine

Excludes2: Dieulafoy lesion of stomach and duodenum (K31.82)

K63.89 Other specified diseases of intestine

K63.9 Disease of intestine, unspecified

K64 Hemorrhoids and perianal venous thrombosis

Includes: piles

Excludes1: hemorrhoids complicating childbirth and the puerperium (O87.2)

hemorrhoids complicating pregnancy (O22.4)

K64.0 First degree hemorrhoids

Grade/stage I hemorrhoids

Hemorrhoids (bleeding) without prolapse outside of anal canal

K64.1 Second degree hemorrhoids

Grade/stage II hemorrhoids

Hemorrhoids (bleeding) that prolapse with straining, but retract spontaneously

K64.2 Third degree hemorrhoids

Grade/stage III hemorrhoids

Hemorrhoids (bleeding) that prolapse with straining and require manual replacement back inside anal canal

K64.3 Fourth degree hemorrhoids

Grade/stage IV hemorrhoids

Hemorrhoids (bleeding) with prolapsed tissue that cannot be manually replaced

K64.4 Residual hemorrhoidal skin tags

External hemorrhoids, NOS

Skin tags of anus

K64.5 Perianal venous thrombosis

External hemorrhoids with thrombosis

Perianal hematoma

Thrombosed hemorrhoids NOS

K64.8 Other hemorrhoids

Internal hemorrhoids, without mention of degree

Prolapsed hemorrhoids, degree not specified

K64.9 Unspecified hemorrhoids

Hemorrhoids (bleeding) NOS

Hemorrhoids (bleeding) without mention of degree

DISEASES OF PERITONEUM AND RETROPERITONEUM (K65-K68)

K65 Peritonitis

Definition: Peritonitis is an inflammation of the membrane which lines the inside of the abdomen and all of the internal organs.

Use additional code (B95-B97), to identify infectious agent

Excludes1: acute appendicitis with generalized peritonitis (K35.2)

aseptic peritonitis (T81.6)

benign paroxysmal peritonitis (E85.0)

chemical peritonitis (T81.6)

diverticulitis of both small and large intestine with peritonitis (K57.4-)

diverticulitis of colon with peritonitis (K57.2-)

diverticulitis of intestine, NOS, with peritonitis (K57.8-)

diverticulitis of small intestine with peritonitis (K57.0-)

gonococcal peritonitis (A54.85)

neonatal peritonitis (P78.0-P78.1)

pelvic peritonitis, female (N73.3-N73.5)

periodic familial peritonitis (E85.0)

peritonitis due to talc **or other** foreign substance (T81.6)

peritonitis in chlamydia (A74.81)

peritonitis in diphtheria (A36.89)

peritonitis in syphilis (late) (A52.74)

peritonitis in tuberculosis (A18.31)

peritonitis with or following abortion or ectopic or molar pregnancy (O00-O07, O08.0)

peritonitis with or following appendicitis (K35.-)

peritonitis with or following diverticular disease of intestine (K57.-)

puerperal peritonitis (O85)

retroperitoneal infections (K68.-)

K65.0 Generalized (acute) peritonitis

Pelvic peritonitis (acute), male

Subphrenic peritonitis (acute)

Suppurative peritonitis (acute)

K65.1 Peritoneal abscess

Abdominopelvic abscess

Abscess (of) omentum

Abscess (of) peritoneum

Mesenteric abscess

Retrocecal abscess

Subdiaphragmatic abscess

Subhepatic abscess

Subphrenic abscess

K65.2 Spontaneous bacterial peritonitis

Excludes1: bacterial peritonitis NOS (K65.9)

K65.3 Choleperitonitis

Peritonitis due to bile

Add 4th-7th digits   Nonspecific code   Unspecified code   Manifestation code   469

K65.4 **Sclerosing mesenteritis**

Fat necrosis of peritoneum (Idiopathic) sclerosing mesenteric fibrosis

Mesenteric lipodystrophy

Mesenteric panniculitis

Retractile mesenteritis

K65.8 **Other peritonitis**

Chronic proliferative peritonitis

Peritonitis due to urine

K65.9 **Peritonitis, unspecified**

Bacterial peritonitis NOS

K66 **Other disorders of peritoneum**

Excludes2: ascites (R18.-)

peritoneal effusion (chronic) (R18.8)

K66.0 **Peritoneal adhesions (postprocedural) (postinfection)**

Adhesions (of) abdominal (wall)

Adhesions (of) diaphragm

Adhesions (of) intestine

Adhesions (of) male pelvis

Adhesions (of) omentum

Adhesions (of) stomach

Adhesive bands

Mesenteric adhesions

Excludes1: female pelvic adhesions [bands] (N73.6)

peritoneal adhesions with intestinal obstruction (K56.5)

K66.1 **Hemoperitoneum**

Excludes1: traumatic hemoperitoneum (S36.8-)

K66.8 **Other specified disorders of peritoneum**

K66.9 **Disorder of peritoneum, unspecified**

K67 **Disorders of peritoneum in infectious diseases classified elsewhere**

Code first underlying disease, such as :

congenital syphilis (A50.0)

helminthiasis (B65.0 -B83.9)

Excludes1: peritonitis in chlamydia (A74.81)

peritonitis in diphtheria (A36.89)

peritonitis in gonococcal (A54.85)

peritonitis in syphilis (late) (A52.74)

peritonitis in tuberculosis (A18.31)

K68 **Disorders of retroperitoneum**

K68.1 **Retroperitoneal abscess**

K68.11 **Postprocedural retroperitoneal abscess**

K68.12 **Psoas muscle abscess**

K68.19 **Other retroperitoneal abscess**

K68.9 **Other disorders of retroperitoneum**

DISEASES OF LIVER (K70-K77)

Excludes1: jaundice NOS (R17)

Excludes2: hemochromatosis (E83.11-)

Reye's syndrome (G93.7)

viral hepatitis (B15-B19)

Wilson's disease (E83.0)

K70 **Alcoholic liver disease**

Use additional code to identify:

alcohol abuse and dependence (F10.-)

K70.0 **Alcoholic fatty liver**

K70.1 **Alcoholic hepatitis**

K70.10 **Alcoholic hepatitis without ascites**

K70.11 **Alcoholic hepatitis with ascites**

K70.2 **Alcoholic fibrosis and sclerosis of liver**

K70.3 **Alcoholic cirrhosis of liver**

Alcoholic cirrhosis NOS

K70.30 **Alcoholic cirrhosis of liver without ascites**

K70.31 **Alcoholic cirrhosis of liver with ascites**

K70.4 **Alcoholic hepatic failure**

Acute alcoholic hepatic failure

Alcoholic hepatic failure NOS

Chronic alcoholic hepatic failure

Subacute alcoholic hepatic failure

K70.40 **Alcoholic hepatic failure without coma**

K70.41 **Alcoholic hepatic failure with coma**

K70.9 **Alcoholic liver disease, unspecified**

K71 **Toxic liver disease**

Includes: drug-induced idiosyncratic (unpredictable) liver disease

drug-induced toxic (predictable) liver disease

Code first poisoning due to drug or toxin, if applicable (T36-T65 with fifth or sixth character 1-4 or 6)

Use additional code for adverse effect, if applicable, to identify drug (T36-T50 with fifth or sixth character 5)

Excludes2: alcoholic liver disease (K70.-)

Budd-Chiari syndrome (I82.0)

K71.0 **Toxic liver disease with cholestasis**

Cholestasis with hepatocyte injury 'Pure' cholestasis

K71.1 **Toxic liver disease with hepatic necrosis**

Hepatic failure (acute) (chronic) due to drugs

K71.10 **Toxic liver disease with hepatic necrosis, without coma**

K71.11 **Toxic liver disease with hepatic necrosis, with coma**

K71.2 **Toxic liver disease with acute hepatitis**

K71.3 **Toxic liver disease with chronic persistent hepatitis**

K71.4 **Toxic liver disease with chronic lobular hepatitis**

K71.5 **Toxic liver disease with chronic active hepatitis**

Toxic liver disease with lupoid hepatitis

K71.50 **Toxic liver disease with chronic active hepatitis without ascites**

K71.51 **Toxic liver disease with chronic active hepatitis with ascites**

K71.6 **Toxic liver disease with hepatitis, not elsewhere classified**

K71.7 **Toxic liver disease with fibrosis and cirrhosis of liver**

K71.8 **Toxic liver disease with other disorders of liver**

Toxic liver disease with focal nodular hyperplasia

Toxic liver disease with hepatic granulomas

Toxic liver disease with peliosis hepatis

Toxic liver disease with veno-occlusive disease of liver

K71.9 **Toxic liver disease, unspecified**

K72 **Hepatic failure, not elsewhere classified**

Includes: fulminant hepatitis NEC, with hepatic failure

hepatic encephalopathy NOS

liver (cell) necrosis with hepatic failure

malignant hepatitis NEC, with hepatic failure yellow liver atrophy or dystrophy

Excludes1: alcoholic hepatic failure (K70.4)

hepatic failure with toxic liver disease (K71.1-)

icterus of newborn (P55-P59)

postprocedural hepatic failure (K91.82)

Excludes2: hepatic failure complicating abortion or ectopic or molar pregnancy (O00-O07, O08.8)

hepatic failure complicating pregnancy, childbirth and the puerperium (O26.6-)

viral hepatitis with hepatic coma (B15-B19)

K72.0 **Acute and subacute hepatic failure**

Acute non-viral hepatitis NOS

K72.00 **Acute and subacute hepatic failure without coma**

K72.01 **Acute and subacute hepatic failure with coma**

K72.1 **Chronic hepatic failure**

K72.10 **Chronic hepatic failure without coma**

K72.11 **Chronic hepatic failure with coma**

K72.9 **Hepatic failure, unspecified**

K72.90 **Hepatic failure, unspecified without coma**

K72.91 **Hepatic failure, unspecified with coma**

Hepatic coma NOS

K73 **Chronic hepatitis, not elsewhere classified**

Excludes1: alcoholic hepatitis (chronic) (K70.1-)

drug-induced hepatitis (chronic) (K71.-)

granulomatous hepatitis (chronic) NEC (K75.3)

reactive, nonspecific hepatitis (chronic) (K75.2)

viral hepatitis (chronic) (B15-B19)

K73.0 **Chronic persistent hepatitis, not elsewhere classified**

K73.1 **Chronic lobular hepatitis, not elsewhere classified**

K73.2 **Chronic active hepatitis, not elsewhere classified**

K73.8 **Other chronic hepatitis, not elsewhere classified**

K73.9 **Chronic hepatitis, unspecified**

K74 **Fibrosis and cirrhosis of liver**

Definition: Cirrhosis is the chronic scarring of the liver, leading to loss of normal liver function.

Code also, if applicable, viral hepatitis (acute) (chronic) (B15-B19)

Excludes1: alcoholic cirrhosis (of liver) (K70.3)

alcoholic fibrosis of liver (K70.2)

cardiac sclerosis of liver (K76.1)

cirrhosis (of liver) with toxic liver disease (K71.7)

congenital cirrhosis (of liver) (P78.81)

pigmentary cirrhosis (of liver) (E83.110)

K74.0 **Hepatic fibrosis**

K74.1 **Hepatic sclerosis**

K74.2 **Hepatic fibrosis with hepatic sclerosis**

K74.3 **Primary biliary cirrhosis**

Chronic nonsuppurative destructive cholangitis

K74.4 **Secondary biliary cirrhosis**

K74.5 **Biliary cirrhosis, unspecified**

K74.6 **Other and unspecified cirrhosis of liver**

K74.60 **Unspecified cirrhosis of liver**

Cirrhosis (of liver) NOS

K74.69 **Other cirrhosis of liver**

Cryptogenic cirrhosis (of liver)

Macronodular cirrhosis (of liver)

Micronodular cirrhosis (of liver)

Mixed type cirrhosis (of liver)

Portal cirrhosis (of liver)

Postnecrotic cirrhosis (of liver)

K75 **Other inflammatory liver diseases**

Excludes2: toxic liver disease (K71.-)

K75.0 **Abscess of liver**

Cholangitic hepatic abscess

Hematogenic hepatic abscess

Hepatic abscess NOS

Lymphogenic hepatic abscess

Pylephlebitic hepatic abscess

Excludes1: amebic liver abscess (A06.4)

cholangitis without liver abscess (K83.0)

pylephlebitis without liver abscess (K75.1)

Excludes2: acute or subacute hepatitis NOS (B17.9)

acute or subacute non-viral hepatitis (K72.0)

chronic hepatitis NEC (K73.8)

K75.1 **Phlebitis of portal vein**

Pylephlebitis

Excludes1: pylephlebitic liver abscess (K75.0)

K75.2 **Nonspecific reactive hepatitis**

Excludes1: acute or subacute hepatitis (K72.0-)

chronic hepatitis NEC (K73.-)

viral hepatitis (B15-B19)

K75.3 **Granulomatous hepatitis, not elsewhere classified**

Excludes1: acute or subacute hepatitis (K72.0-)

chronic hepatitis NEC (K73.-)

viral hepatitis (B15-B19)

K75.4 **Autoimmune hepatitis**

Lupoid hepatitis NEC

K75.8 **Other specified inflammatory liver diseases**

K75.81 **Nonalcoholic steatohepatitis (NASH)**

K75.89 **Other specified inflammatory liver diseases**

K75.9 **Inflammatory liver disease, unspecified**

Hepatitis NOS

Excludes1: acute or subacute hepatitis (K72.0-)

chronic hepatitis NEC (K73.-)

viral hepatitis (B15-B19)

K76 **Other diseases of liver**

Excludes2: alcoholic liver disease (K70.-)

amyloid degeneration of liver (E85.-)

cystic disease of liver (congenital) (Q44.6)

hepatic vein thrombosis (I82.0)

hepatomegaly NOS (R16.0)

pigmentary cirrhosis (of liver) (E83.110)

portal vein thrombosis (I81)

toxic liver disease (K71.-)

K76.0 **Fatty (change of) liver, not elsewhere classified**

Nonalcoholic fatty liver disease (NAFLD)

Excludes1: nonalcoholic steatohepatitis (NASH) (K75.81)

K76.1 Chronic passive congestion of liver

Cardiac cirrhosis

Cardiac sclerosis

K76.2 Central hemorrhagic necrosis of liver

Excludes1: liver necrosis with hepatic failure (K72.-)

K76.3 Infarction of liver

K76.4 Peliosis hepatis

Hepatic angiomatosis

K76.5 Hepatic veno-occlusive disease

Excludes1: Budd-Chiari syndrome (I82.0)

K76.6 Portal hypertension

Use additional code for any associated complications, such as:

portal hypertensive gastropathy (K31.89)

K76.7 Hepatorenal syndrome

Excludes1: hepatorenal syndrome following labor and delivery (O90.4)

postprocedural hepatorenal syndrome (K91.83)

K76.8 Other specified diseases of liver

K76.81 Hepatopulmonary syndrome

Code first underlying liver disease, such as:

alcoholic cirrhosis of liver (K70.3-)

cirrhosis of liver without mention of alcohol (K74.6-)

K76.89 Other specified diseases of liver

Cyst (simple) of liver

Focal nodular hyperplasia of liver

Hepatoptosis

K76.9 Liver disease, unspecified

K77 Liver disorders in diseases classified elsewhere

Code first underlying disease, such as:

amyloidosis (E85.-)

congenital syphilis (A50.0, A50.5)

congenital toxoplasmosis (P37.1)

schistosomiasis (B65.0-B65.9)

Excludes1: alcoholic hepatitis (K70.1-)

alcoholic liver disease (K70.-)

cytomegaloviral hepatitis (B25.1)

herpesviral [herpes simplex] hepatitis (B00.81)

infectious mononucleosis with liver disease (B27.0-B27.9 with .9)

mumps hepatitis (B26.81)

sarcoidosis with liver disease (D86.89)

secondary syphilis with liver disease (A51.45)

syphilis (late) with liver disease (A52.74)

toxoplasmosis (acquired) hepatitis (B58.1)

tuberculosis with liver disease (A18.83)

DISORDERS OF GALLBLADDER, BILIARY TRACT AND PANCREAS (K80-K87)

K80 Cholelithiasis

Excludes1: retained cholelithiasis following cholecystectomy (K91.86)

K80.0 Calculus of gallbladder with acute cholecystitis

Any condition listed in K80.2 with acute cholecystitis

K80.00 Calculus of gallbladder with acute cholecystitis without obstruction

K80.01 Calculus of gallbladder with acute cholecystitis with obstruction

K80.1 Calculus of gallbladder with other cholecystitis

K80.10 Calculus of gallbladder with chronic cholecystitis without obstruction

Cholelithiasis with cholecystitis NOS

K80.11 Calculus of gallbladder with chronic cholecystitis with obstruction

K80.12 Calculus of gallbladder with acute and chronic cholecystitis without obstruction

K80.13 Calculus of gallbladder with acute and chronic cholecystitis with obstruction

K80.18 Calculus of gallbladder with other cholecystitis without obstruction

K80.19 Calculus of gallbladder with other cholecystitis with obstruction

K80.2 Calculus of gallbladder without cholecystitis

Cholecystolithiasis without cholecystitis

Cholelithiasis (without cholecystitis)

Colic (recurrent) of gallbladder (without cholecystitis)

Gallstone (impacted) of cystic duct (without cholecystitis)

Gallstone (impacted) of gallbladder (without cholecystitis)

K80.20 Calculus of gallbladder without cholecystitis without obstruction

K80.21 Calculus of gallbladder without cholecystitis with obstruction

K80.3 Calculus of bile duct with cholangitis

Any condition listed in K80.5 with cholangitis

K80.30 Calculus of bile duct with cholangitis, unspecified, without obstruction

K80.31 Calculus of bile duct with cholangitis, unspecified, with obstruction

K80.32 Calculus of bile duct with acute cholangitis without obstruction

K80.33 Calculus of bile duct with acute cholangitis with obstruction

K80.34 Calculus of bile duct with chronic cholangitis without obstruction

K80.35 Calculus of bile duct with chronic cholangitis with obstruction

K80.36 Calculus of bile duct with acute and chronic cholangitis without obstruction

K80.37 Calculus of bile duct with acute and chronic cholangitis with obstruction

K80.4 Calculus of bile duct with cholecystitis

Any condition listed in K80.5 with cholecystitis (with cholangitis)

K80.40 Calculus of bile duct with cholecystitis, unspecified, without obstruction

K80.41 Calculus of bile duct with cholecystitis, unspecified, with obstruction

K80.42 Calculus of bile duct with acute cholecystitis without obstruction

K80.43 Calculus of bile duct with acute cholecystitis with obstruction

K80.44 **Calculus of bile duct with chronic cholecystitis without obstruction**

K80.45 **Calculus of bile duct with chronic cholecystitis with obstruction**

K80.46 **Calculus of bile duct with acute and chronic cholecystitis without obstruction**

K80.47 **Calculus of bile duct with acute and chronic cholecystitis with obstruction**

K80.5 **Calculus of bile duct without cholangitis or cholecystitis**

Choledocholithiasis (without cholangitis or cholecystitis)

Gallstone (impacted) of bile duct NOS (without cholangitis or cholecystitis)

Gallstone (impacted) of common duct (without cholangitis or cholecystitis)

Gallstone (impacted) of hepatic duct (without cholangitis or cholecystitis)

Hepatic cholelithiasis (without cholangitis or cholecystitis)

Hepatic colic (recurrent) (without cholangitis or cholecystitis)

K80.50 **Calculus of bile duct without cholangitis or cholecystitis without obstruction**

K80.51 **Calculus of bile duct without cholangitis or cholecystitis with obstruction**

K80.6 **Calculus of gallbladder and bile duct with cholecystitis**

K80.60 **Calculus of gallbladder and bile duct with cholecystitis, unspecified, without obstruction**

K80.61 **Calculus of gallbladder and bile duct with cholecystitis, unspecified, with obstruction**

K80.62 **Calculus of gallbladder and bile duct with acute cholecystitis without obstruction**

K80.63 **Calculus of gallbladder and bile duct with acute cholecystitis with obstruction**

K80.64 **Calculus of gallbladder and bile duct with chronic cholecystitis without obstruction**

K80.65 **Calculus of gallbladder and bile duct with chronic cholecystitis with obstruction**

K80.66 **Calculus of gallbladder and bile duct with acute and chronic cholecystitis without obstruction**

K80.67 **Calculus of gallbladder and bile duct with acute and chronic cholecystitis with obstruction**

K80.7 **Calculus of gallbladder and bile duct without cholecystitis**

K80.70 **Calculus of gallbladder and bile duct without cholecystitis without obstruction**

K80.71 **Calculus of gallbladder and bile duct without cholecystitis with obstruction**

K80.8 **Other cholelithiasis**

K80.80 **Other cholelithiasis without obstruction**

K80.81 **Other cholelithiasis with obstruction**

K81 **Cholecystitis**

Excludes1: cholecystitis with cholelithiasis (K80.-)

K81.0 **Acute cholecystitis**

Abscess of gallbladder

Angiocholecystitis

Emphysematous (acute) cholecystitis

Empyema of gallbladder

Gangrene of gallbladder

Gangrenous cholecystitis

Suppurative cholecystitis

K81.1 **Chronic cholecystitis**

K81.2 **Acute cholecystitis with chronic cholecystitis**

K81.9 **Cholecystitis, unspecified**

K82 **Other diseases of gallbladder**

Excludes1: nonvisualization of gallbladder (R93.2)

postcholecystectomy syndrome (K91.5)

K82.0 **Obstruction of gallbladder**

Occlusion of cystic duct or gallbladder without cholelithiasis

Stenosis of cystic duct or gallbladder without cholelithiasis

Stricture of cystic duct or gallbladder without cholelithiasis

Excludes1: obstruction of gallbladder with cholelithiasis (K80.-)

K82.1 **Hydrops of gallbladder**

Mucocele of gallbladder

K82.2 **Perforation of gallbladder**

Rupture of cystic duct or gallbladder

K82.3 **Fistula of gallbladder**

Cholecystocolic fistula

Cholecystoduodenal fistula

K82.4 **Cholesterolosis of gallbladder**

Strawberry gallbladder

Excludes1: cholesterolosis of gallbladder with cholecystitis (K81.-)

cholesterolosis of gallbladder with cholelithiasis (K80.-)

K82.8 **Other specified diseases of gallbladder**

Adhesions of cystic duct or gallbladder

Atrophy of cystic duct or gallbladder

Cyst of cystic duct or gallbladder

Dyskinesia of cystic duct or gallbladder

Hypertrophy of cystic duct or gallbladder

Nonfunctioning of cystic duct or gallbladder

Ulcer of cystic duct or gallbladder

K82.9 **Disease of gallbladder, unspecified**

K83 **Other diseases of biliary tract**

Excludes1: postcholecystectomy syndrome (K91.5)

Excludes2: conditions involving the gallbladder (K81-K82)

conditions involving the cystic duct (K81-K82)

K83.0 **Cholangitis**

Ascending cholangitis

Cholangitis NOS

Primary cholangitis

Recurrent cholangitis

Sclerosing cholangitis

Secondary cholangitis

Stenosing cholangitis

Suppurative cholangitis

Excludes1: cholangitic liver abscess (K75.0)

cholangitis with choledocholithiasis (K80.3-, K80.4-)

chronic nonsuppurative destructive cholangitis (K74.3)

K83.1 **Obstruction of bile duct**

Occlusion of bile duct without cholelithiasis

Stenosis of bile duct without cholelithiasis

Stricture of bile duct without cholelithiasis

Excludes1: congenital obstruction of bile duct (Q44.3)

obstruction of bile duct with cholelithiasis (K80.-)

K83.2 Perforation of bile duct

Rupture of bile duct

K83.3 Fistula of bile duct

Choledochoduodenal fistula

K83.4 Spasm of sphincter of Oddi

K83.5 Biliary cyst

K83.8 Other specified diseases of biliary tract

Adhesions of biliary tract

Atrophy of biliary tract

Hypertrophy of biliary tract

Ulcer of biliary tract

K83.9 Disease of biliary tract, unspecified

K85 Acute pancreatitis

Includes: acute (recurrent) pancreatitis

subacute pancreatitis

K85.0 Idiopathic acute pancreatitis

- **K85.00 Idiopathic acute pancreatitis without necrosis or infection**

- **K85.01 Idiopathic acute pancreatitis with uninfected necrosis**

- **K85.02 Idiopathic acute pancreatitis with infected necrosis**

K85.1 Biliary acute pancreatitis

Gallstone pancreatitis

- **K85.10 Biliary acute pancreatitis without necrosis or infection**

- **K85.11 Biliary acute pancreatitis with uninfected necrosis**

- **K85.12 Biliary acute pancreatitis with infected necrosis**

K85.2 Alcohol induced acute pancreatitis

Excludes2: alcohol induced chronic pancreatitis (K86.0)

- **K85.20 Alcohol induced acute pancreatitis without necrosis or infection**

- **K85.21 Alcohol induced acute pancreatitis with uninfected necrosis**

- **K85.22 Alcohol induced acute pancreatitis with infected necrosis**

K85.3 Drug induced acute pancreatitis

Use additional code for adverse effect, if applicable, to identify drug (T36-T50 with fifth or sixth character 5)

Use additional code to identify drug abuse and dependence (F11.-F17.-)

- **K85.30 Drug induced acute pancreatitis without necrosis or infection**

- **K85.31 Drug induced acute pancreatitis with uninfected necrosis**

- **K85.32 Drug induced acute pancreatitis with infected necrosis**

K85.8 Other acute pancreatitis

- **K85.80 Other acute pancreatitis without necrosis or infection**

- **K85.81 Other acute pancreatitis with uninfected necrosis**

- **K85.82 Other acute pancreatitis with infected necrosis**

K85.9 Acute pancreatitis, unspecified

Pancreatitis NOS

- **K85.90 Acute pancreatitis without necrosis or infection, unspecified**

- **K85.91 Acute pancreatitis with uninfected necrosis, unspecified**

- **K85.92 Acute pancreatitis with infected necrosis, unspecified**

K86 Other diseases of pancreas

Excludes2: fibrocystic disease of pancreas (E84.-)

islet cell tumor (of pancreas) (D13.7)

pancreatic steatorrhea (K90.3)

K86.0 Alcohol-induced chronic pancreatitis

Use additional code to identify:

alcohol abuse and dependence (F10.-)

Code also exocrine pancreatic insufficiency (K86.81)

Excludes2: alcohol induced acute pancreatitis (K85.2-)

K86.1 Other chronic pancreatitis

Chronic pancreatitis NOS

Infectious chronic pancreatitis

Recurrent chronic pancreatitis

Relapsing chronic pancreatitis

Code also exocrine pancreatic insufficiency (K86.81)

K86.2 Cyst of pancreas

K86.3 Pseudocyst of pancreas

K86.8 Other specified diseases of pancreas

- **K86.81 Exocrine pancreatic insufficiency**

- **K86.89 Other specified diseases of pancreas**

Aseptic pancreatic necrosis, unrelated to acute pancreatitis

Atrophy of pancreas

Calculus of pancreas

Cirrhosis of pancreas

Fibrosis of pancreas

Pancreatic fat necrosis, unrelated to acute pancreatitis

Pancreatic infantilism

Pancreatic necrosis NOS, unrelated to acute pancreatitis

K86.9 Disease of pancreas, unspecified

K87 Disorders of gallbladder, biliary tract and pancreas in diseases classified elsewhere

Code first underlying disease

Excludes1: cytomegaloviral pancreatitis(B25.2)

mumps pancreatitis (B26.3)

syphilitic gallbladder (A52.74)

syphilitic pancreas (A52.74)

tuberculosis of gallbladder (A18.83)

tuberculosis of pancreas (A18.83)

OTHER DISEASES OF THE DIGESTIVE SYSTEM (K90-K95)

K90 Intestinal malabsorption

Definition: Intestinal malabsorption is a state arising from

abnormality in digestion or absorption of food nutrients across the gastrointestinal(GI) tract.

Excludes1: intestinal malabsorption following gastrointestinal surgery (K91.2)

K90.0 Celiac disease

Celiac disease with steatorrhea Gluten-sensitive enteropathy Nontropical sprue

Use additional code for associated disorders including:

dermatitis herpetiformis (L13.0)

gluten ataxia (G32.81)

Code also exocrine pancreatic insufficiency (K86.81)

K90.1 Tropical sprue

Sprue NOS

Tropical steatorrhea

K90.2 Blind loop syndrome, not elsewhere classified

Blind loop syndrome NOS

Excludes1: congenital blind loop syndrome (Q43.8)

postsurgical blind loop syndrome (K91.2)

K90.3 Pancreatic steatorrhea

K90.4 Other malabsorption due to intolerance

Excludes2: gluten-sensitive enteropathy (K90.0)

lactose intolerance (E73.-)

● **K90.41 Non-celiac gluten sensitivity**

Gluten sensitivity NOS

Non-celiac gluten sensitive enteropathy

● **K90.49 Malabsorption due to intolerance, not elsewhere classified**

Malabsorption due to intolerance to carbohydrate

Malabsorption due to intolerance to fat

Malabsorption due to intolerance to protein

Malabsorption due to intolerance to starch

K90.8 Other intestinal malabsorption

K90.81 Whipple's disease

K90.89 Other intestinal malabsorption

K90.9 Intestinal malabsorption, unspecified

K91 Intraoperative and postprocedural complications and disorders of digestive system, not elsewhere classified

Excludes2: complications of artificial opening of digestive system (K94.-)

complications of bariatric procedures (K95.-)

gastrojejunal ulcer (K28.-)

postprocedural (radiation) retroperitoneal abscess (K68.11)

radiation colitis (K52.0)

radiation gastroenteritis (K52.0)

radiation proctitis (K62.7)

K91.0 Vomiting following gastrointestinal surgery

K91.1 Postgastric surgery syndromes

Dumping syndrome

Postgastrectomy syndrome

Postvagotomy syndrome

K91.2 Postsurgical malabsorption, not elsewhere classified

Postsurgical blind loop syndrome

Excludes1: malabsorption osteomalacia in adults (M83.2)

malabsorption osteoporosis, postsurgical (M80.8-, M81.8)

K91.3 Postprocedural intestinal obstruction

K91.5 Postcholecystectomy syndrome

K91.6 Intraoperative hemorrhage and hematoma of a digestive system organ or structure complicating a procedure

Excludes1: intraoperative hemorrhage and hematoma of a digestive system organ or structure due to accidental puncture and laceration during a procedure (K91.7-)

▲**K91.61 Intraoperative hemorrhage and hematoma of a digestive system organ or structure complicating a digestive system procedure**

K91.62 Intraoperative hemorrhage and hematoma of a digestive system organ or structure complicating other procedure

K91.7 Accidental puncture and laceration of a digestive system organ or structure during a procedure

K91.71 Accidental puncture and laceration of a digestive system organ or structure during a digestive system procedure

K91.72 Accidental puncture and laceration of a digestive system organ or structure during other procedure

K91.8 Other intraoperative and postprocedural complications and disorders of digestive system

K91.81 Other intraoperative complications of digestive system

K91.82 Postprocedural hepatic failure

K91.83 Postprocedural hepatorenal syndrome

K91.84 Postprocedural hemorrhage of a digestive system organ or structure following a procedure

▲**K91.840 Postprocedural hemorrhage of a digestive system organ or structure following a digestive system procedure**

▲**K91.841 Postprocedural hemorrhage of a digestive system organ or structure following other procedure**

K91.85 Complications of intestinal pouch

K91.850 Pouchitis

Inflammation of internal ileoanal pouch

K91.858 Other complications of intestinal pouch

K91.86 Retained cholelithiasis following cholecystectomy

K91.87 Postprocedural hematoma and seroma of a digestive system organ or structure following a procedure

● **K91.870 Postprocedural hematoma of a digestive system organ or structure following a digestive system procedure**

● **K91.871 Postprocedural hematoma of a digestive system organ or structure following other procedure**

● **K91.872 Postprocedural seroma of a digestive system organ or structure following a digestive system procedure**

● **K91.873 Postprocedural seroma of a digestive system organ or structure following other procedure**

K91.89 **Other postprocedural complications and disorders of digestive system**

Use additional code, if applicable, to further specify disorder

Excludes2: postprocedural retroperitoneal abscess (K68.11)

K92 **Other diseases of digestive system**

Excludes1: neonatal gastrointestinal hemorrhage (P54.0-P54.3)

K92.0 **Hematemesis**

K92.1 **Melena**

Excludes1: occult blood in feces (R19.5)

K92.2 **Gastrointestinal hemorrhage, unspecified**

Gastric hemorrhage NOS

Intestinal hemorrhage NOS

Excludes1: acute hemorrhagic gastritis (K29.01)

hemorrhage of anus and rectum (K62.5)

angiodysplasia of stomach with hemorrhage (K31.811)

diverticular disease with hemorrhage (K57.-)

gastritis and duodenitis with hemorrhage (K29.-)

peptic ulcer with hemorrhage (K25-K28)

K92.8 **Other specified diseases of the digestive system**

K92.81 **Gastrointestinal mucositis (ulcerative)**

Code also type of associated therapy, such as:

antineoplastic and immunosuppressive drugs (T45.1X-)

radiological procedure and radiotherapy (Y84.2)

Excludes2: mucositis (ulcerative) of vagina and vulva (N76.81)

nasal mucositis (ulcerative) (J34.81)

oral mucositis (ulcerative) (K12.3-)

K92.89 **Other specified diseases of the digestive system**

K92.9 **Disease of digestive system, unspecified**

K94 **Complications of artificial openings of the digestive system**

K94.0 **Colostomy complications**

K94.00 **Colostomy complication, unspecified**

K94.01 **Colostomy hemorrhage**

K94.02 **Colostomy infection**

Use additional code to specify type of infection, such as:

cellulitis of abdominal wall (L03.311) sepsis (A40.-, A41.-)

K94.03 **Colostomy malfunction**

Mechanical complication of colostomy

K94.09 **Other complications of colostomy**

K94.1 **Enterostomy complications**

K94.10 **Enterostomy complication, unspecified**

K94.11 **Enterostomy hemorrhage**

K94.12 **Enterostomy infection**

Use additional code to specify type of infection, such as:

cellulitis of abdominal wall (L03.311) sepsis (A40.-, A41.-)

K94.13 **Enterostomy malfunction**

Mechanical complication of enterostomy

K94.19 **Other complications of enterostomy**

K94.2 **Gastrostomy complications**

K94.20 **Gastrostomy complication, unspecified**

K94.21 **Gastrostomy hemorrhage**

K94.22 **Gastrostomy infection**

Use additional code to specify type of infection, such as:

cellulitis of abdominal wall (L03.311)

sepsis (A40.-, A41.-)

K94.23 **Gastrostomy malfunction**

Mechanical complication of gastrostomy

K94.29 **Other complications of gastrostomy**

K94.3 **Esophagostomy complications**

K94.30 **Esophagostomy complications, unspecified**

K94.31 **Esophagostomy hemorrhage**

K94.32 **Esophagostomy infection**

Use additional code to identify the infection

K94.33 **Esophagostomy malfunction**

Mechanical complication of esophagostomy

K94.39 **Other complications of esophagostomy**

K95 **Complications of bariatric procedures**

K95.0 **Complications of gastric band procedure**

K95.01 **Infection due to gastric band procedure**

Use additional code to specify type of infection or organism, such as:

bacterial and viral infectious agents (B95.-, B96.-)

cellulitis of abdominal wall (L03.311)

sepsis (A40.-, A41.-)

K95.09 **Other complications of gastric band procedure**

Use additional code, if applicable, to further specify complication

K95.8 **Complications of other bariatric procedure**

Excludes1: complications of gastric band surgery (K95.0-)

K95.81 **Infection due to other bariatric procedure**

Use additional code to specify type of infection or organism, such as:

bacterial and viral infectious agents (B95.-, B96.-)

cellulitis of abdominal wall (L03.311)

sepsis (A40.-, A41.-)

K95.89 **Other complications of other bariatric procedure**

Use additional code, if applicable, to further specify complication

● New code   ▲ Revised code   Excludes1: Not coded here   Excludes2: Not included here   ⊗ Placeholder required   ⑦ 7th digit required

Chapter 12: Diseases Of The Skin And Subcutaneous Tissue (L00-L99)

DEFINITIONS

This chapter includes definitions of selected key words, terms and phrases and coding alerts for adding points to the clinical domain, and references to coding late effects where appropriate. An example from this chapter is as follows:

L49 Exfoliation due to erythematous conditions according to extent of body surface involved
Definition: Erythematous conditions refers to conditions causing diffuse or patchy redness of skin.

MULTIPLE CODING FOR A SINGLE CONDITION

In addition to the etiology/manifestation convention that requires two codes to fully describe a single condition that affects multiple body systems, there are other single conditions that also require more than one code. "Use additional code" notes are found in the Tabular List at codes that are not part of an etiology/manifestation pair where a secondary code is useful to fully describe a condition. The sequencing rule is the same as the etiology/manifestation pair, "use additional code" indicates that a secondary code should be added.

For example, for bacterial infections that are not included in chapter 1, a secondary code from category B95, Streptococcus, Staphylococcus, and Enterococcus, as the cause of diseases classified elsewhere, or B96, Other bacterial agents as the cause of diseases classified elsewhere, may be required to identify the bacterial organism causing the infection. A "use additional code" note will normally be found at the infectious disease code, indicating a need for the organism code to be added as a secondary code.

"Code first" notes are also under certain codes that are not specifically manifestation codes but may be due to an underlying cause. When there is a "code first" note and an underlying condition is present, the underlying condition should be sequenced first.

"Code, if applicable, any causal condition first", notes indicate that this code may be assigned as a principal diagnosis when the causal condition is unknown or not applicable. If a causal condition is known, then the code for that condition should be sequenced as the principal or first-listed diagnosis.

Multiple codes may be needed for sequela, complication codes and obstetric codes to more fully describe a condition. See the specific guidelines for these conditions for further instruction.

COMBINATION CODE

A combination code is a single code used to classify: Two diagnoses, or a diagnosis with an associated secondary process (manifestation) A diagnosis with an associated complication

Combination codes are identified by referring to subterm entries in the Alphabetic Index and by reading the inclusion and exclusion notes in the Tabular List.

Assign only the combination code when that code fully identifies the diagnostic conditions involved or when the Alphabetic Index so directs. Multiple coding should not be used when the classification provides a combination code that clearly identifies all of the elements documented in the diagnosis. When the combination code lacks necessary specificity in describing the manifestation or complication, an additional code should be used as a secondary code.

SEQUELA (LATE EFFECTS)

A sequela is the residual effect (condition produced) after the acute phase of an illness or injury has terminated. There is no time limit on when a sequela code can be used. The residual may be apparent early, such as in cerebral infarction, or it may occur months or years later, such as that due to a previous injury. Coding of sequela generally requires two codes sequenced in the following order: The condition or nature of the sequela is sequenced first.

The sequela code is sequenced second.

An exception to the above guidelines are those instances where the code for the sequela is followed by a manifestation code identified in the Tabular List and title, or the sequela code has been expanded (at the fourth, fifth or sixth character levels) to include the manifestation(s). The code for the acute phase of an illness or injury that led to the sequela is never used with a code for the late effect.

PRESSURE ULCER STAGE CODES

1) Pressure ulcer stages

Codes from category L89, Pressure ulcer, identify the site of the pressure ulcer as well as the stage of the ulcer.

The ICD-10-CM classifies pressure ulcer stages based on severity, which is designated by stages 1-4, unspecified stage and unstageable.

Assign as many codes from category L89 as needed to identify all the pressure ulcers the patient has, if applicable.

2) **Unstageable pressure ulcers**

Assignment of the code for unstageable pressure ulcer (L89.--0) should be based on the clinical documentation. These codes are used for pressure ulcers whose stage cannot be clinically determined (e.g., the ulcer is covered by eschar or has been treated with a skin or muscle graft) and pressure ulcers that are documented as deep tissue injury but not documented as due to trauma. This code should not be confused with the codes for unspecified stage (L89.--9). When there is no documentation regarding the stage of the pressure ulcer, assign the appropriate code for unspecified stage (L89.--9).

3) **Documented pressure ulcer stage**

Assignment of the pressure ulcer stage code should be guided by clinical documentation of the stage or documentation of the terms found in the Alphabetic Index. For clinical terms describing the stage that are not found in the Alphabetic Index, and there is no documentation of the stage, the provider should be queried.

4) **Patients admitted with pressure ulcers documented as healed**

No code is assigned if the documentation states that the pressure ulcer is completely healed.

5) **Patients admitted with pressure ulcers documented as healing**

Pressure ulcers described as healing should be assigned the appropriate pressure ulcer stage code based on the documentation in the medical record. If the documentation does not provide information about the stage of the healing pressure ulcer, assign the appropriate code for unspecified stage.

If the documentation is unclear as to whether the patient has a current (new) pressure ulcer or if the patient is being treated for a healing pressure ulcer, query the provider.

For ulcers that were present on admission but healed at the time of discharge, assign the code for the site and stage of the pressure ulcer at the time of admission.

6) **Patient admitted with pressure ulcer evolving into another stage during the admission**

If a patient is admitted with a pressure ulcer at one stage and it progresses to a higher stage, two separate codes should be assigned: one code for the site and stage of the ulcer on admission and a second code for the same ulcer site and the highest stage reported during the stay.

● New code   ▲ Revised code   **Excludes1:** Not coded here   **Excludes2:** Not included here   ⊗ Placeholder required   ⑦ 7ᵗʰ digit required

Chapter 12

Diseases Of The Skin And Subcutaneous Tissue (L00-L99)

Excludes2: certain conditions originating in the perinatal period (P04-P96)

certain infectious and parasitic diseases (A00-B99)

complications of pregnancy, childbirth and the puerperium (O00-O9A)

congenital malformations, deformations, and chromosomal abnormalities (Q00-Q99)

endocrine, nutritional and metabolic diseases (E00-E88)

lipomelanotic reticulosis (I89.8)

neoplasms (C00-D49)

symptoms, signs and abnormal clinical and laboratory findings, not elsewhere classified (R00-R94)

systemic connective tissue disorders (M30-M36)

viral warts (B07.-)

This chapter contains the following blocks:

L00-L08	Infections of the skin and subcutaneous tissue
L10-L14	Bullous disorders
L20-L30	Dermatitis and eczema
L40-L45	Papulosquamous disorders
L49-L54	Urticaria and erythema
L55-L59	Radiation-related disorders of the skin and subcutaneous tissue
L60-L75	Disorders of skin appendages
L76	Intraoperative and postprocedural complications of skin and subcutaneous tissue
L80-L99	Other disorders of the skin and subcutaneous tissue

INFECTIONS OF THE SKIN AND SUBCUTANEOUS TISSUE (L00-L08)

Use additional code (B95-B97) to identify infectious agent.

Excludes2: hordeolum (H00.0)

infective dermatitis (L30.3)

local infections of skin classified in Chapter 1

lupus panniculitis (L93.2)

panniculitis NOS (M79.3)

panniculitis of neck and back (M54.0-)

Perlèche NOS (K13.0)

Perlèche due to candidiasis (B37.0)

Perlèche due to riboflavin deficiency (E53.0)

pyogenic granuloma (L98.0)

relapsing panniculitis [Weber-Christian] (M35.6)

viral warts (B07.-)

zoster (B02.-)

L00   Staphylococcal scalded skin syndrome

Ritter's disease

Use additional code to identify percentage of skin exfoliation (L49.-)

Excludes1: bullous impetigo (L01.03)

pemphigus neonatorum (L01.03)

toxic epidermal necrolysis [Lyell] (L51.2)

L01   Impetigo

Excludes1: impetigo herpetiformis (L40.1)

L01.0   Impetigo

Impetigo contagiosa Impetigo vulgaris

L01.00   Impetigo, unspecified

Impetigo NOS

L01.01   Non-bullous impetigo

L01.02   Bockhart's impetigo

Impetigo follicularis

Perifolliculitis NOS

Superficial pustular perifolliculitis

L01.03   Bullous impetigo

Impetigo neonatorum

Pemphigus neonatorum

L01.09   Other impetigo

Ulcerative impetigo

L01.1   Impetiginization of other dermatoses

L02   Cutaneous abscess, furuncle and carbuncle

Definition: A carbuncle is an abscess larger than a boil, usually with one or more openings draining pus onto the skin. It is usually caused by bacterial infection, most commonly staphylococcus aureus. A furuncle is a skin disease caused by the infection of hair follicles, resulting in the localized accumulation of pus and dead tissue.

Use additional code to identify organism (B95-B96)

Excludes2: abscess of anus and rectal regions (K61.-)

abscess of female genital organs (external) (N76.4)

abscess of male genital organs (external) (N48.2, N49.-)

L02.0   Cutaneous abscess, furuncle and carbuncle of face

Excludes2: abscess of ear, external (H60.0)

abscess of eyelid (H00.0)

abscess of head [any part, except face] (L02.8)

abscess of lacrimal gland (H04.0)

abscess of lacrimal passages (H04.3)

abscess of mouth (K12.2)

abscess of nose (J34.0)

abscess of orbit (H05.0)

submandibular abscess (K12.2)

L02.01   Cutaneous abscess of face

L02.02   Furuncle of face

Boil of face

Folliculitis of face

L02.03   Carbuncle of face

L02.1   Cutaneous abscess, furuncle and carbuncle of neck

L02.11   Cutaneous abscess of neck

L02.12   Furuncle of neck

Boil of neck

Folliculitis of neck

L02.13   Carbuncle of neck

L02.2   Cutaneous abscess, furuncle and carbuncle of trunk

Excludes1: non-newborn omphalitis (L08.82)

omphalitis of newborn (P38.-)

Excludes2: abscess of breast (N61.1)

abscess of buttocks (L02.3)

abscess of female external genital organs (N76.4)

▓ Add 4th-7th digits	▓ Nonspecific code	▓ Unspecified code	▓ Manifestation code

abscess of male external genital organs (N48.2, N49.-)

abscess of hip (L02.4)

L02.21 **Cutaneous abscess of trunk**

L02.211 **Cutaneous abscess of abdominal wall**

L02.212 **Cutaneous abscess of back [any part, except buttock]**

L02.213 **Cutaneous abscess of chest wall**

L02.214 **Cutaneous abscess of groin**

L02.215 **Cutaneous abscess of perineum**

L02.216 **Cutaneous abscess of umbilicus**

L02.219 **Cutaneous abscess of trunk, unspecified**

L02.22 **Furuncle of trunk**

Boil of trunk

Folliculitis of trunk

L02.221 **Furuncle of abdominal wall**

L02.222 **Furuncle of back [any part, except buttock]**

L02.223 **Furuncle of chest wall**

L02.224 **Furuncle of groin**

L02.225 **Furuncle of perineum**

L02.226 **Furuncle of umbilicus**

L02.229 **Furuncle of trunk, unspecified**

L02.23 **Carbuncle of trunk**

L02.231 **Carbuncle of abdominal wall**

L02.232 **Carbuncle of back [any part, except buttock]**

L02.233 **Carbuncle of chest wall**

L02.234 **Carbuncle of groin**

L02.235 **Carbuncle of perineum**

L02.236 **Carbuncle of umbilicus**

L02.239 **Carbuncle of trunk, unspecified**

L02.3 **Cutaneous abscess, furuncle and carbuncle of buttock**

Excludes1: pilonidal cyst with abscess (L05.01)

L02.31 **Cutaneous abscess of buttock**

Cutaneous abscess of gluteal region

L02.32 **Furuncle of buttock**

Boil of buttock

Folliculitis of buttock

Furuncle of gluteal region

L02.33 **Carbuncle of buttock**

Carbuncle of gluteal region

L02.4 **Cutaneous abscess, furuncle and carbuncle of limb**

Excludes2: Cutaneous abscess, furuncle and carbuncle of groin (L02.214, L02.224, L02.234)

Cutaneous abscess, furuncle and carbuncle of hand (L02.5-)

Cutaneous abscess, furuncle and carbuncle of foot (L02.6-)

L02.41 **Cutaneous abscess of limb**

L02.411 **Cutaneous abscess of right axilla**

L02.412 **Cutaneous abscess of left axilla**

L02.413 **Cutaneous abscess of right upper limb**

L02.414 **Cutaneous abscess of left upper limb**

L02.415 **Cutaneous abscess of right lower limb**

L02.416 **Cutaneous abscess of left lower limb**

L02.419 **Cutaneous abscess of limb, unspecified**

L02.42 **Furuncle of limb**

Boil of limb

Folliculitis of limb

L02.421 **Furuncle of right axilla**

L02.422 **Furuncle of left axilla**

L02.423 **Furuncle of right upper limb**

L02.424 **Furuncle of left upper limb**

L02.425 **Furuncle of right lower limb**

L02.426 **Furuncle of left lower limb**

L02.429 **Furuncle of limb, unspecified**

L02.43 **Carbuncle of limb**

L02.431 **Carbuncle of right axilla**

L02.432 **Carbuncle of left axilla**

L02.433 **Carbuncle of right upper limb**

L02.434 **Carbuncle of left upper limb**

L02.435 **Carbuncle of right lower limb**

L02.436 **Carbuncle of left lower limb**

L02.439 **Carbuncle of limb, unspecified**

L02.5 **Cutaneous abscess, furuncle and carbuncle of hand**

L02.51 **Cutaneous abscess of hand**

L02.511 **Cutaneous abscess of right hand**

L02.512 **Cutaneous abscess of left hand**

L02.519 **Cutaneous abscess of unspecified hand**

L02.52 **Furuncle hand**

Boil of hand

Folliculitis of hand

L02.521 **Furuncle right hand**

L02.522 **Furuncle left hand**

L02.529 **Furuncle unspecified hand**

L02.53 **Carbuncle of hand**

L02.531 **Carbuncle of right hand**

L02.532 **Carbuncle of left hand**

L02.539 **Carbuncle of unspecified hand**

L02.6 **Cutaneous abscess, furuncle and carbuncle of foot**

L02.61 **Cutaneous abscess of foot**

L02.611 **Cutaneous abscess of right foot**

L02.612 **Cutaneous abscess of left foot**

L02.619 **Cutaneous abscess of unspecified foot**

L02.62 **Furuncle of foot**

Boil of foot

Folliculitis of foot

L02.621 **Furuncle of right foot**

L02.622 **Furuncle of left foot**

L02.629 **Furuncle of unspecified foot**

L02.63 **Carbuncle of foot**

L02.631 **Carbuncle of right foot**

L02.632   **Carbuncle of left foot**

L02.639   **Carbuncle of unspecified foot**

L02.8   **Cutaneous abscess, furuncle and carbuncle of other sites**

     L02.81   **Cutaneous abscess of other sites**

         L02.811   **Cutaneous abscess of head [any part, except face]**

         L02.818   **Cutaneous abscess of other sites**

     L02.82   **Furuncle of other sites**

        Boil **of other** sites

        Folliculitis **of other** sites

         L02.821   **Furuncle of head [any part, except face]**

         L02.828   **Furuncle of other sites**

     L02.83   **Carbuncle of other sites**

         L02.831   **Carbuncle of head [any part, except face]**

         L02.838   **Carbuncle of other sites**

L02.9   **Cutaneous abscess, furuncle and carbuncle, unspecified**

     L02.91   **Cutaneous abscess, unspecified**

     L02.92   **Furuncle, unspecified**

        Boil NOS

        Furunculosis NOS

     L02.93   **Carbuncle, unspecified**

L03   **Cellulitis and acute lymphangitis**

     Excludes2: cellulitis of anal and rectal region (K61.-)

        cellulitis of external auditory canal (H60.1)

        cellulitis of eyelid (H00.0)

        cellulitis of female external genital organs (N76.4)

        cellulitis of lacrimal apparatus (H04.3)

        cellulitis of male external genital organs (N48.2, N49.-)

        cellulitis of mouth (K12.2)

        cellulitis of nose (J34.0)

        eosinophilic cellulitis [Wells] (L98.3)

        febrile neutrophilic dermatosis [Sweet] (L98.2)

        lymphangitis (chronic) (subacute) (I89.1)

L03.0   **Cellulitis and acute lymphangitis of finger and toe**

     Infection of nail

     Onychia

     Paronychia

     Perionychia

     L03.01   **Cellulitis of finger**

        Felon Whitlow

        Excludes1: herpetic whitlow (B00.89)

         L03.011   **Cellulitis of right finger**

         L03.012   **Cellulitis of left finger**

         L03.019   **Cellulitis of unspecified finger**

     L03.02   **Acute lymphangitis of finger**

        Hangnail with lymphangitis of finger

         L03.021   **Acute lymphangitis of right finger**

         L03.022   **Acute lymphangitis of left finger**

         L03.029   **Acute lymphangitis of unspecified finger**

     L03.03   **Cellulitis of toe**

         L03.031   **Cellulitis of right toe**

         L03.032   **Cellulitis of left toe**

         L03.039   **Cellulitis of unspecified toe**

     L03.04   **Acute lymphangitis of toe**

        Hangnail with lymphangitis of toe

         L03.041   **Acute lymphangitis of right toe**

         L03.042   **Acute lymphangitis of left toe**

         L03.049   **Acute lymphangitis of unspecified toe**

L03.1   **Cellulitis and acute lymphangitis of other parts of limb**

     L03.11   **Cellulitis of other parts of limb**

        Excludes2: cellulitis of fingers (L03.01-)

           cellulitis of toes (L03.03-)

           groin (L03.314)

         L03.111   **Cellulitis of right axilla**

         L03.112   **Cellulitis of left axilla**

         L03.113   **Cellulitis of right upper limb**

         L03.114   **Cellulitis of left upper limb**

         L03.115   **Cellulitis of right lower limb**

         L03.116   **Cellulitis of left lower limb**

         L03.119   **Cellulitis of unspecified part of limb**

     L03.12   **Acute lymphangitis of other parts of limb**

        Excludes2: acute lymphangitis of fingers (L03.2-)

           acute lymphangitis of toes (L03.04-)

           acute lymphangitis of groin (L03.324)

         L03.121   **Acute lymphangitis of right axilla**

         L03.122   **Acute lymphangitis of left axilla**

         L03.123   **Acute lymphangitis of right upper limb**

         L03.124   **Acute lymphangitis of left upper limb**

         L03.125   **Acute lymphangitis of right lower limb**

         L03.126   **Acute lymphangitis of left lower limb**

         L03.129   **Acute lymphangitis of unspecified part of limb**

L03.2   **Cellulitis and acute lymphangitis of face and neck**

     L03.21   **Cellulitis and acute lymphangitis of face**

         L03.211   **Cellulitis of face**

           Excludes2: abscess of orbit (H05.01-)

             cellulitis of ear (H60.1-)

             cellulitis of eyelid (H00.0-)

             cellulitis of head (L03.81)

             cellulitis of lacrimal apparatus (H04.3)

             cellulitis of lip (K13.0)

             cellulitis of mouth (K12.2)

             cellulitis of nose (internal) (J34.0)

             cellulitis of orbit (H05.01-)

             cellulitis of scalp (L03.81)

         L03.212   **Acute lymphangitis of face**

         ●**L03.213**   **Periorbital cellulitis**

Preseptal cellulitis

L03.22   **Cellulitis and acute lymphangitis of neck**

    L03.221   **Cellulitis of neck**

    L03.222   **Acute lymphangitis of neck**

L03.3   **Cellulitis and acute lymphangitis of trunk**

   L03.31   **Cellulitis of trunk**

     Excludes2: cellulitis of anal and rectal regions (K61.-)

        cellulitis of breast NOS (N61.0)

        cellulitis of female external genital organs (N76.4)

        cellulitis of male external genital organs (N48.2, N49.-)

        omphalitis of newborn (P38.-)

        puerperal cellulitis of breast (O91.2)

    L03.311   **Cellulitis of abdominal wall**

      Excludes2: cellulitis of umbilicus (L03.316)

          cellulitis of groin (L03.314)

    L03.312   **Cellulitis of back [any part except buttock]**

    L03.313   **Cellulitis of chest wall**

    L03.314   **Cellulitis of groin**

    L03.315   **Cellulitis of perineum**

    L03.316   **Cellulitis of umbilicus**

    L03.317   **Cellulitis of buttock**

    L03.319   **Cellulitis of trunk, unspecified**

   L03.32   **Acute lymphangitis of trunk**

    L03.321   **Acute lymphangitis of abdominal wall**

    L03.322   **Acute lymphangitis of back [any part except buttock]**

    L03.323   **Acute lymphangitis of chest wall**

    L03.324   **Acute lymphangitis of groin**

    L03.325   **Acute lymphangitis of perineum**

    L03.326   **Acute lymphangitis of umbilicus**

    L03.327   **Acute lymphangitis of buttock**

    L03.329   **Acute lymphangitis of trunk, unspecified**

L03.8   **Cellulitis and acute lymphangitis of other sites**

   L03.81   **Cellulitis of other sites**

    L03.811   **Cellulitis of head [any part, except face]**

        Cellulitis of scalp

      Excludes2: cellulitis of face (L03.211)

    L03.818   **Cellulitis of other sites**

   L03.89   **Acute lymphangitis of other sites**

    L03.891   **Acute lymphangitis of head [any part, except face]**

    L03.898   **Acute lymphangitis of other sites**

L03.9   **Cellulitis and acute lymphangitis, unspecified**

   L03.90   **Cellulitis, unspecified**

   L03.91   **Acute lymphangitis, unspecified**

     Excludes1: lymphangitis NOS (I89.1)

L04   **Acute lymphadenitis**

Definition: Lymphadenitis is an inflammation of a lymph node. It is often a complication of a bacterial infection of a wound, although it can also be caused by viruses or other disease agents.

Includes: abscess (acute) of lymph nodes, except mesenteric

    acute lymphadenitis, except mesenteric

Excludes1: chronic or subacute lymphadenitis, except mesenteric (I88.1)

    enlarged lymph nodes (R59.-)

    human immunodeficiency virus [HIV] disease resulting in generalized lymphadenopathy (B20)

    lymphadenitis NOS (I88.9)

    nonspecific mesenteric lymphadenitis (I88.0)

L04.0   **Acute lymphadenitis of face, head and neck**

L04.1   **Acute lymphadenitis of trunk**

L04.2   **Acute lymphadenitis of upper limb**

    Acute lymphadenitis of axilla

    Acute lymphadenitis of shoulder

L04.3   **Acute lymphadenitis of lower limb**

    Acute lymphadenitis of hip

    Excludes2: acute lymphadenitis of groin (L04.1)

L04.8   **Acute lymphadenitis of other sites**

L04.9   **Acute lymphadenitis, unspecified**

L05   **Pilonidal cyst and sinus**

L05.0   **Pilonidal cyst and sinus with abscess**

   L05.01   **Pilonidal cyst with abscess**

    Pilonidal abscess

    Pilonidal dimple with abscess

    Postanal dimple with abscess

    Excludes2: congenital sacral dimple (Q82.6)

          parasacral dimple (Q82.6)

   L05.02   **Pilonidal sinus with abscess**

    Coccygeal fistula with abscess

    Coccygeal sinus with abscess

    Pilonidal fistula with abscess

L05.9   **Pilonidal cyst and sinus without abscess**

   L05.91   **Pilonidal cyst without abscess**

    Pilonidal dimple

    Postanal dimple

    Pilonidal cyst NOS

    Excludes2: congenital sacral dimple (Q82.6)

          parasacral dimple (Q82.6)

   L05.92   **Pilonidal sinus without abscess**

    Coccygeal fistula

    Coccygeal sinus without abscess

    Pilonidal fistula

L08   **Other local infections of skin and subcutaneous tissue**

L08.0   **Pyoderma**

    Dermatitis gangrenosa

    Purulent dermatitis

    Septic dermatitis

    Suppurative dermatitis

    Excludes1: pyoderma gangrenosum (L88)

          pyoderma vegetans (L08.81)

L08.1   **Erythrasma**

L08.8 **Other specified local infections of the skin and subcutaneous tissue**

    L08.81 **Pyoderma vegetans**

      Excludes1: pyoderma gangrenosum (L88)

                pyoderma NOS (L08.0)

    L08.82 **Omphalitis not of newborn**

      Excludes1: omphalitis of newborn (P38.-)

    L08.89 **Other specified local infections of the skin and subcutaneous tissue**

L08.9 **Local infection of the skin and subcutaneous tissue, unspecified**

BULLOUS DISORDERS (L10-L14)

Excludes1: benign familial pemphigus [Hailey-Hailey] (Q82.8)

staphylococcal scalded skin syndrome (L00)

toxic epidermal necrolysis [Lyell] (L51.2)

L10 **Pemphigus**

    Excludes1: pemphigus neonatorum (L01.03)

L10.0 **Pemphigus vulgaris**

L10.1 **Pemphigus vegetans**

L10.2 **Pemphigus foliaceous**

L10.3 **Brazilian pemphigus [fogo selvagem]**

L10.4 **Pemphigus erythematosus**

    Senear-Usher syndrome

L10.5 **Drug-induced pemphigus**

    Use additional code for adverse effect, if applicable, to identify drug (T36-T50 with fifth or sixth character 5)

L10.8 **Other pemphigus**

    L10.81 **Paraneoplastic pemphigus**

    L10.89 **Other pemphigus**

L10.9 **Pemphigus, unspecified**

L11 **Other acantholytic disorders**

L11.0 **Acquired keratosis follicularis**

    Excludes1: keratosis follicularis (congenital) [Darier-White] (Q82.8)

L11.1 **Transient acantholytic dermatosis [Grover]**

L11.8 **Other specified acantholytic disorders**

L11.9 **Acantholytic disorder, unspecified**

L12 **Pemphigoid**

    Excludes1: herpes gestationis (O26.4-)

                impetigo herpetiformis (L40.1)

L12.0 **Bullous pemphigoid**

L12.1 **Cicatricial pemphigoid**

    Benign mucous membrane pemphigoid

L12.2 **Chronic bullous disease of childhood**

    Juvenile dermatitis herpetiformis

L12.3 **Acquired epidermolysis bullosa**

    Excludes1: epidermolysis bullosa (congenital) (Q81.-)

    L12.30 **Acquired epidermolysis bullosa, unspecified**

    L12.31 **Epidermolysis bullosa due to drug**

      Use additional code for adverse effect, if applicable, to identify drug (T36-T50 with fifth or sixth character 5)

    L12.35 **Other acquired epidermolysis bullosa**

L12.8 **Other pemphigoid**

L12.9 **Pemphigoid, unspecified**

L13 **Other bullous disorders**

L13.0 **Dermatitis herpetiformis**

    Duhring's disease

    Hydroa herpetiformis

    Excludes1: juvenile dermatitis herpetiformis (L12.2)

                senile dermatitis herpetiformis (L12.0)

L13.1 **Subcorneal pustular dermatitis**

    Sneddon-Wilkinson disease

L13.8 **Other specified bullous disorders**

L13.9 **Bullous disorder, unspecified**

L14 **Bullous disorders in diseases classified elsewhere**

    Code first underlying disease

DERMATITIS AND ECZEMA (L20-L30)

Note: In this block the terms dermatitis and eczema are used synonymously and interchangeably.

Excludes2: chronic (childhood) granulomatous disease (D71)

dermatitis gangrenosa (L08.0)

dermatitis herpetiformis (L13.0)

dry skin dermatitis (L85.3)

factitial dermatitis (L98.1)

perioral dermatitis (L71.0)

radiation-related disorders of the skin and subcutaneous tissue (L55-L59)

stasis dermatitis (I87.2)

L20 **Atopic dermatitis**

    Definition: Atopic dermatitis and related conditions, aka eczema, is a chronic, recurring inflammatory skin disorder that usually first appears in babies or very young children and may last through adulthood. Eczema causes the skin to itch and develop a red, scaly, patchy rash.

L20.0 **Besnier's prurigo**

L20.8 **Other atopic dermatitis**

    Excludes2: circumscribed neurodermatitis (L28.0)

    L20.81 **Atopic neurodermatitis**

      Diffuse neurodermatitis

    L20.82 **Flexural eczema**

    L20.83 **Infantile (acute) (chronic) eczema**

    L20.84 **Intrinsic (allergic) eczema**

    L20.89 **Other atopic dermatitis**

L20.9 **Atopic dermatitis, unspecified**

L21 **Seborrheic dermatitis**

    Excludes2: infective dermatitis (L30.3)

                seborrheic keratosis (L82.-)

L21.0 **Seborrhea capitis**

    Cradle cap

L21.1 **Seborrheic infantile dermatitis**

L21.8 **Other seborrheic dermatitis**

L21.9 **Seborrheic dermatitis, unspecified**

    Seborrhea NOS

L22 **Diaper dermatitis**

    Diaper erythema

    Diaper rash

    Psoriasiform diaper rash

L23 **Allergic contact dermatitis**

    Excludes1: allergy NOS (T78.40)

contact dermatitis NOS (L25.9)

dermatitis NOS (L30.9)

Excludes2: dermatitis due to substances taken internally (L27.-)

dermatitis of eyelid (H01.1-)

diaper dermatitis (L22)

eczema of external ear (H60.5-)

irritant contact dermatitis (L24.-)

perioral dermatitis (L71.0)

radiation-related disorders of the skin and subcutaneous tissue (L55-L59)

L23.0   Allergic contact dermatitis due to metals

Allergic contact dermatitis due to chromium

Allergic contact dermatitis due to nickel

L23.1   Allergic contact dermatitis due to adhesives

L23.2   Allergic contact dermatitis due to cosmetics

L23.3   Allergic contact dermatitis due to drugs in contact with skin

Use additional code for adverse effect, if applicable, to identify drug (T36-T50 with fifth or sixth character 5)

Excludes2: dermatitis due to ingested drugs and medicaments (L27.0-L27.1)

L23.4   Allergic contact dermatitis due to dyes

L23.5   Allergic contact dermatitis due to other chemical products

Allergic contact dermatitis due to cement

Allergic contact dermatitis due to insecticide

Allergic contact dermatitis due to plastic

Allergic contact dermatitis due to rubber

L23.6   Allergic contact dermatitis due to food in contact with the skin

Excludes2: dermatitis due to ingested food (L27.2)

L23.7   Allergic contact dermatitis due to plants, except food

Excludes2: allergy NOS due to pollen (J30.1)

L23.8   Allergic contact dermatitis due to other agents

L23.81   Allergic contact dermatitis due to animal (cat) (dog) dander

Allergic contact dermatitis due to animal (cat) (dog) hair

L23.89   Allergic contact dermatitis due to other agents

L23.9   Allergic contact dermatitis, unspecified cause

Allergic contact eczema NOS

L24   Irritant contact dermatitis

Excludes1: allergy NOS (T78.40)

contact dermatitis NOS (L25.9)

dermatitis NOS (L30.9)

Excludes2: allergic contact dermatitis (L23.-)

dermatitis due to substances taken internally (L27.-)

dermatitis of eyelid (H01.1-)

diaper dermatitis (L22)

eczema of external ear (H60.5-)

perioral dermatitis (L71.0)

radiation-related disorders of the skin and subcutaneous tissue (L55-L59)

L24.0   Irritant contact dermatitis due to detergents

L24.1   Irritant contact dermatitis due to oils and greases

L24.2   Irritant contact dermatitis due to solvents

Irritant contact dermatitis due to chlorocompound

Irritant contact dermatitis due to cyclohexane

Irritant contact dermatitis due to ester

Irritant contact dermatitis due to glycol

Irritant contact dermatitis due to hydrocarbon

Irritant contact dermatitis due to ketone

L24.3   Irritant contact dermatitis due to cosmetics

L24.4   Irritant contact dermatitis due to drugs in contact with skin

Use additional code for adverse effect, if applicable, to identify drug (T36-T50 with fifth or sixth character 5)

L24.5   Irritant contact dermatitis due to other chemical products

Irritant contact dermatitis due to cement

Irritant contact dermatitis due to insecticide

Irritant contact dermatitis due to plastic

Irritant contact dermatitis due to rubber

L24.6   Irritant contact dermatitis due to food in contact with skin

Excludes2: dermatitis due to ingested food (L27.2)

L24.7   Irritant contact dermatitis due to plants, except food

Excludes2: allergy NOS to pollen (J30.1)

L24.8   Irritant contact dermatitis due to other agents

L24.81   Irritant contact dermatitis due to metals

Irritant contact dermatitis due to chromium

Irritant contact dermatitis due to nickel

L24.89   Irritant contact dermatitis due to other agents

Irritant contact dermatitis due to dyes

L24.9   Irritant contact dermatitis, unspecified cause

Irritant contact eczema NOS

L25   Unspecified contact dermatitis

Excludes1: allergic contact dermatitis (L23.-)

allergy NOS (T78.40)

dermatitis NOS (L30.9)

irritant contact dermatitis (L24.-)

Excludes2: dermatitis due to ingested substances (L27.-)

dermatitis of eyelid (H01.1-)

eczema of external ear (H60.5-)

perioral dermatitis (L71.0)

radiation-related disorders of the skin and subcutaneous tissue (L55-L59)

L25.0   Unspecified contact dermatitis due to cosmetics

L25.1   Unspecified contact dermatitis due to drugs in contact with skin

Use additional code for adverse effect, if applicable, to identify drug (T36-T50 with fifth or sixth character 5)

Excludes2: dermatitis due to ingested drugs and medicaments (L27.0-L27.1)

L25.2   Unspecified contact dermatitis due to dyes

L25.3   Unspecified contact dermatitis due to other chemical products

Unspecified contact dermatitis due to cement

Unspecified contact dermatitis due to insecticide

L25.4   Unspecified contact dermatitis due to food in contact with skin

Excludes2: dermatitis due to ingested food (L27.2)

● New code   ▲ Revised code   **Excludes1:** Not coded here   **Excludes2:** Not included here   ⊗ Placeholder required   ⑦ 7th digit required

L25.5 **Unspecified contact dermatitis due to plants, except food**

    Excludes1: nettle rash (L50.9)

    Excludes2: allergy NOS due to pollen (J30.1)

L25.8 **Unspecified contact dermatitis due to other agents**

L25.9 **Unspecified contact dermatitis, unspecified cause**

    Contact dermatitis (occupational) NOS

    Contact eczema (occupational) NOS

L26 **Exfoliative dermatitis**

    Hebra's pityriasis

    Excludes1: Ritter's disease (L00)

L27 **Dermatitis due to substances taken internally**

    Excludes1: allergy NOS (T78.40)

    Excludes2: adverse food reaction, except dermatitis (T78.0-T78.1)

    contact dermatitis (L23-L25)

    drug photoallergic response (L56.1)

    drug phototoxic response (L56.0)

    urticaria (L50.-)

L27.0 **Generalized skin eruption due to drugs and medicaments taken internally**

    Use additional code for adverse effect, if applicable, to identify drug (T36-T50 with fifth or sixth character 5)

L27.1 **Localized skin eruption due to drugs and medicaments taken internally**

    Use additional code for adverse effect, if applicable, to identify drug (T36-T50 with fifth or sixth character 5)

L27.2 **Dermatitis due to ingested food**

    Excludes2: dermatitis due to food in contact with skin (L23.6, L24.6, L25.4)

L27.8 **Dermatitis due to other substances taken internally**

L27.9 **Dermatitis due to unspecified substance taken internally**

L28 **Lichen simplex chronicus and prurigo**

L28.0 **Lichen simplex chronicus**

    Circumscribed neurodermatitis

    Lichen NOS

L28.1 **Prurigo nodularis**

L28.2 **Other prurigo**

    Prurigo NOS

    Prurigo Hebra

    Prurigo mitis

    Urticaria papulosa

L29 **Pruritus**

    Excludes1: neurotic excoriation (L98.1)

            psychogenic pruritus (F45.8)

L29.0 **Pruritus ani**

L29.1 **Pruritus scroti**

L29.2 **Pruritus vulvae**

L29.3 **Anogenital pruritus, unspecified**

L29.8 **Other pruritus**

L29.9 **Pruritus, unspecified**

    Itch NOS

L30 **Other and unspecified dermatitis**

    Excludes2: contact dermatitis (L23-L25)

    dry skin dermatitis (L85.3)

    small plaque parapsoriasis (L41.3)

    stasis dermatitis (I87.2)

L30.0 **Nummular dermatitis**

L30.1 **Dyshidrosis [pompholyx]**

L30.2 **Cutaneous autosensitization**

    Candidid [levurid]

    Dermatophytid Eczematid

L30.3 **Infective dermatitis**

    Infectious eczematoid dermatitis

L30.4 **Erythema intertrigo**

L30.5 **Pityriasis alba**

L30.8 **Other specified dermatitis**

L30.9 **Dermatitis, unspecified**

    Eczema NOS

PAPULOSQUAMOUS DISORDERS (L40-L45)

L40 **Psoriasis**

L40.0 **Psoriasis vulgaris**

    Nummular psoriasis

    Plaque psoriasis

L40.1 **Generalized pustular psoriasis**

    Impetigo herpetiformis

    Von Zumbusch's disease

L40.2 **Acrodermatitis continua**

L40.3 **Pustulosis palmaris et plantaris**

L40.4 **Guttate psoriasis**

L40.5 **Arthropathic psoriasis**

    L40.50 **Arthropathic psoriasis, unspecified**

    L40.51 **Distal interphalangeal psoriatic arthropathy**

    L40.52 **Psoriatic arthritis mutilans**

    L40.53 **Psoriatic spondylitis**

    L40.54 **Psoriatic juvenile arthropathy**

    L40.59 **Other psoriatic arthropathy**

L40.8 **Other psoriasis**

    Flexural psoriasis

L40.9 **Psoriasis, unspecified**

L41 **Parapsoriasis**

    Excludes1: poikiloderma vasculare atrophicans (L94.5)

L41.0 **Pityriasis lichenoides et varioliformis acuta**

    Mucha-Habermann disease

L41.1 **Pityriasis lichenoides chronica**

L41.3 **Small plaque parapsoriasis**

L41.4 **Large plaque parapsoriasis**

L41.5 **Retiform parapsoriasis**

L41.8 **Other parapsoriasis**

L41.9 **Parapsoriasis, unspecified**

L42 **Pityriasis rosea**

L43 **Lichen planus**

    Excludes1: lichen planopilaris (L66.1)

L43.0 **Hypertrophic lichen planus**

L43.1 **Bullous lichen planus**

L43.2 **Lichenoid drug reaction**

    Use additional code for adverse effect, if applicable, to identify drug (T36-T50 with fifth or sixth character 5)

L43.3 **Subacute (active) lichen planus**

Lichen planus tropicus

L43.8   **Other lichen planus**

L43.9   **Lichen planus, unspecified**

L44   **Other papulosquamous disorders**

L44.0   **Pityriasis rubra pilaris**

L44.1   **Lichen nitidus**

L44.2   **Lichen striatus**

L44.3   **Lichen ruber moniliformis**

L44.4   **Infantile papular acrodermatitis [Gianotti-Crosti]**

L44.8   **Other specified papulosquamous disorders**

L44.9   **Papulosquamous disorder, unspecified**

L45   **Papulosquamous disorders in diseases classified elsewhere**

<u>**Code first**</u> underlying disease.

URTICARIA AND ERYTHEMA (L49-L54)

Excludes1: Lyme disease (A69.2-)

rosacea (L71.-)

L49   **Exfoliation due to erythematous conditions according to extent of body surface involved**

<u>**Code first**</u> erythematous condition causing exfoliation, such as:

Ritter's disease (L00)

(Staphylococcal) scalded skin syndrom (L00)

Stevens-Johnson syndrome (L51.1)

Stevens-Johnson syndrome-toxic epidermal necrolysis overlap syndrome (L51.3)

Toxic epidermal necrolysis (L51.2)

L49.0   **Exfoliation due to erythematous condition involving less than 10 percent of body surface**

Exfoliation due to erythematous condition NOS

L49.1   **Exfoliation due to erythematous condition involving 10-19 percent of body surface**

L49.2   **Exfoliation due to erythematous condition involving 20-29 percent of body surface**

L49.3   **Exfoliation due to erythematous condition involving 30-39 percent of body surface**

L49.4   **Exfoliation due to erythematous condition involving 40-49 percent of body surface**

L49.5   **Exfoliation due to erythematous condition involving 50-59 percent of body surface**

L49.6   **Exfoliation due to erythematous condition involving 60-69 percent of body surface**

L49.7   **Exfoliation due to erythematous condition involving 70-79 percent of body surface**

L49.8   **Exfoliation due to erythematous condition involving 80-89 percent of body surface**

L49.9   **Exfoliation due to erythematous condition involving 90 or more percent of body surface**

L50   **Urticaria**

Excludes1: allergic contact dermatitis (L23.-)

angioneurotic edema (T78.3)

giant urticaria (T78.3)

hereditary angio-edema (D84.1)

Quincke's edema (T78.3)

serum urticaria (T80.6-)

solar urticaria (L56.3)

urticaria neonatorum (P83.8)

urticaria papulosa (L28.2)

urticaria pigmentosa (Q82.2)

L50.0   **Allergic urticaria**

L50.1   **Idiopathic urticaria**

L50.2   **Urticaria due to cold and heat**

Excludes2: familial cold urticaria (M04.2)

L50.3   **Dermatographic urticaria**

L50.4   **Vibratory urticaria**

L50.5   **Cholinergic urticaria**

L50.6   **Contact urticaria**

L50.8   **Other urticaria**

Chronic urticaria

Recurrent periodic urticaria

L50.9   **Urticaria, unspecified**

L51   **Erythema multiforme**

<u>**Use additional code**</u> for adverse effect, if applicable, to identify drug (T36-T50 with fifth or sixth character 5)

<u>**Use additional code**</u> to identify associated manifestations, such as:

arthropathy associated with dermatological disorders (M14.8-)

conjunctival edema (H11.42)

conjunctivitis (H10.22-)

corneal scars and opacities (H17.-)

corneal ulcer (H16.0-)

edema of eyelid (H02.84)

inflammation of eyelid (H01.8)

keratoconjunctivitis sicca (H16.22-)

mechanical lagophthalmos (H02.22-)

stomatitis (K12.-)

symblepharon (H11.23-)

<u>**Use additional code**</u> to identify percentage of skin exfoliation (L49.-)

Excludes1: staphylococcal scalded skin syndrome (L00)

Ritter's disease (L00)

L51.0   **Nonbullous erythema multiforme**

L51.1   **Stevens-Johnson syndrome**

L51.2   **Toxic epidermal necrolysis [Lyell]**

L51.3   **Stevens-Johnson syndrome-toxic epidermal necrolysis overlap syndrome**

SJS-TEN overlap syndrome

L51.8   **Other erythema multiforme**

L51.9   **Erythema multiforme, unspecified**

Erythema iris

Erythema multiforme major NOS

Erythema multiforme minor NOS

Herpes iris

L52   **Erythema nodosum**

Excludes1: tuberculous erythema nodosum (A18.4)

L53   **Other erythematous conditions**

Excludes1: erythema ab igne (L59.0)

erythema due to external agents in contact with skin (L23-L25)

erythema intertrigo (L30.4)

L53.0   **Toxic erythema**

<u>**Code first**</u> poisoning due to drug or toxin, if applicable (T36-T65 with fifth or sixth character 1-4 or 6)

Use additional code for adverse effect, if applicable, to identify drug (T36-T50 with fifth or sixth character 5)

Excludes1: neonatal erythema toxicum (P83.1)

L53.1 **Erythema annulare centrifugum**

L53.2 **Erythema marginatum**

L53.3 **Other chronic figurate erythema**

L53.8 **Other specified erythematous conditions**

L53.9 **Erythematous condition, unspecified**

Erythema NOS

Erythroderma NOS

L54 **Erythema in diseases classified elsewhere**

Code first underlying disease.

RADIATION-RELATED DISORDERS OF THE SKIN AND SUBCUTANEOUS TISSUE (L55-L59)

L55 **Sunburn**

L55.0 **Sunburn of first degree**

L55.1 **Sunburn of second degree**

L55.2 **Sunburn of third degree**

L55.9 **Sunburn, unspecified**

L56 **Other acute skin changes due to ultraviolet radiation**

Use additional code to identify the source of the ultraviolet radiation (W89, X32)

L56.0 **Drug phototoxic response**

Use additional code for adverse effect, if applicable, to identify drug (T36-T50 with fifth or sixth character 5)

L56.1 **Drug photoallergic response**

Use additional code for adverse effect, if applicable, to identify drug (T36-T50 with fifth or sixth character 5)

L56.2 **Photocontact dermatitis [berloque dermatitis]**

L56.3 **Solar urticaria**

L56.4 **Polymorphous light eruption**

L56.5 **Disseminated superficial actinic porokeratosis (DSAP)**

L56.8 **Other specified acute skin changes due to ultraviolet radiation**

L56.9 **Acute skin change due to ultraviolet radiation, unspecified**

L57 **Skin changes due to chronic exposure to nonionizing radiation**

Use additional code to identify the source of the ultraviolet radiation (W89, X32)

L57.0 **Actinic keratosis**

Keratosis NOS

Senile keratosis

Solar keratosis

L57.1 **Actinic reticuloid**

L57.2 **Cutis rhomboidalis nuchae**

L57.3 **Poikiloderma of Civatte**

L57.4 **Cutis laxa senilis**

Elastosis senilis

L57.5 **Actinic granuloma**

L57.8 **Other skin changes due to chronic exposure to nonionizing radiation**

Farmer's skin

Sailor's skin

Solar dermatitis

L57.9 **Skin changes due to chronic exposure to nonionizing radiation, unspecified**

L58 **Radiodermatitis**

Use additional code to identify the source of the radiation (W88, W90)

L58.0 **Acute radiodermatitis**

L58.1 **Chronic radiodermatitis**

L58.9 **Radiodermatitis, unspecified**

L59 **Other disorders of skin and subcutaneous tissue related to radiation**

L59.0 **Erythema ab igne [dermatitis ab igne]**

L59.8 **Other specified disorders of the skin and subcutaneous tissue related to radiation**

L59.9 **Disorder of the skin and subcutaneous tissue related to radiation, unspecified**

DISORDERS OF SKIN APPENDAGES (L60-L75)

Excludes1: congenital malformations of integument (Q84.-)

L60 **Nail disorders**

Excludes2: clubbing of nails (R68.3)

onychia and paronychia (L03.0-)

L60.0 **Ingrowing nail**

L60.1 **Onycholysis**

L60.2 **Onychogryphosis**

L60.3 **Nail dystrophy**

L60.4 **Beau's lines**

L60.5 **Yellow nail syndrome**

L60.8 **Other nail disorders**

L60.9 **Nail disorder, unspecified**

L62 **Nail disorders in diseases classified elsewhere**

Code first underlying disease, such as:

pachydermoperiostosis (M89.4-)

L63 **Alopecia areata**

L63.0 **Alopecia (capitis) totalis**

L63.1 **Alopecia universalis**

L63.2 **Ophiasis**

L63.8 **Other alopecia areata**

L63.9 **Alopecia areata, unspecified**

L64 **Androgenic alopecia**

Includes: male-pattern baldness

L64.0 **Drug-induced androgenic alopecia**

Use additional code for adverse effect, if applicable, to identify drug (T36-T50 with fifth or sixth character 5)

L64.8 **Other androgenic alopecia**

L64.9 **Androgenic alopecia, unspecified**

L65 **Other nonscarring hair loss**

Use additional code for adverse effect, if applicable, to identify drug (T36-T50 with fifth or sixth character 5)

Excludes1: trichotillomania (F63.3)

L65.0 **Telogen effluvium**

L65.1 **Anagen effluvium**

L65.2 **Alopecia mucinosa**

L65.8 **Other specified nonscarring hair loss**

L65.9 **Nonscarring hair loss, unspecified**

Alopecia NOS

L66 **Cicatricial alopecia [scarring hair loss]**

L66.0   **Pseudopelade**

L66.1   **Lichen planopilaris**

     Follicular lichen planus

L66.2   **Folliculitis decalvans**

L66.3   **Perifolliculitis capitis abscedens**

L66.4   **Folliculitis ulerythematosa reticulata**

L66.8   **Other cicatricial alopecia**

L66.9   **Cicatricial alopecia, unspecified**

L67   **Hair color and hair shaft abnormalities**

     Excludes1: monilethrix (Q84.1)

         pili annulati (Q84.1)

         telogen effluvium (L65.0)

L67.0   **Trichorrhexis nodosa**

L67.1   **Variations in hair color** Canities

     Greyness, hair (premature)

     Heterochromia of hair

     Poliosis circumscripta, acquired

     Poliosis NOS

L67.8   **Other hair color and hair shaft abnormalities**

     Fragilitas crinium

L67.9   **Hair color and hair shaft abnormality, unspecified**

L68   **Hypertrichosis**

     Includes: excess hair

     Excludes1: congenital hypertrichosis (Q84.2)

         persistent lanugo (Q84.2)

L68.0   **Hirsutism**

L68.1   **Acquired hypertrichosis lanuginosa**

L68.2   **Localized hypertrichosis**

L68.3   **Polytrichia**

L68.8   **Other hypertrichosis**

L68.9   **Hypertrichosis, unspecified**

L70   **Acne**

     Excludes2: acne keloid (L73.0)

L70.0   **Acne vulgaris**

L70.1   **Acne conglobata**

L70.2   **Acne varioliformis**

     Acne necrotica miliaris

L70.3   **Acne tropica**

L70.4   **Infantile acne**

▲**L70.5**   **Acné excoriée**

     Acné excoriée des jeunes filles

     Picker's acne

L70.8   **Other acne**

L70.9   **Acne, unspecified**

L71   **Rosacea**

     Use additional code for adverse effect, if applicable, to identify drug (T36-T50 with fifth or sixth character 5)

L71.0   **Perioral dermatitis**

L71.1   **Rhinophyma**

L71.8   **Other rosacea**

L71.9   **Rosacea, unspecified**

L72   **Follicular cysts of skin and subcutaneous tissue**

L72.0   **Epidermal cyst**

L72.1   **Pilar and trichodermal cyst**

L72.11   **Pilar cyst**

L72.12   **Trichodermal cyst**

     Trichilemmal (proliferating) cyst

L72.2   **Steatocystoma multiplex**

L72.3   **Sebaceous cyst**

     Excludes2: pilar cyst (L72.11)

         trichilemmal (proliferating) cyst (L72.12)

L72.8   **Other follicular cysts of the skin and subcutaneous tissue**

L72.9   **Follicular cyst of the skin and subcutaneous tissue, unspecified**

L73   **Other follicular disorders**

L73.0   **Acne keloid**

L73.1   **Pseudofolliculitis barbae**

L73.2   **Hidradenitis suppurativa**

L73.8   **Other specified follicular disorders**

     Sycosis barbae

L73.9   **Follicular disorder, unspecified**

L74   **Eccrine sweat disorders**

     Excludes2: generalized hyperhidrosis (R61)

L74.0   **Miliaria rubra**

L74.1   **Miliaria crystallina**

L74.2   **Miliaria profunda**

     Miliaria tropicalis

L74.3   **Miliaria, unspecified**

L74.4   **Anhidrosis**

     Hypohidrosis

L74.5   **Focal hyperhidrosis**

     L74.51   **Primary focal hyperhidrosis**

         L74.510   **Primary focal hyperhidrosis, axilla**

         L74.511   **Primary focal hyperhidrosis, face**

         L74.512   **Primary focal hyperhidrosis, palms**

         L74.513   **Primary focal hyperhidrosis, soles**

         L74.519   **Primary focal hyperhidrosis, unspecified**

     L74.52   **Secondary focal hyperhidrosis**

         Frey's syndrome

L74.8   **Other eccrine sweat disorders**

L74.9   **Eccrine sweat disorder, unspecified**

     Sweat gland disorder NOS

L75   **Apocrine sweat disorders**

     Excludes1: dyshidrosis (L30.1)

         hidradenitis suppurativa (L73.2)

L75.0   **Bromhidrosis**

L75.1   **Chromhidrosis**

L75.2   **Apocrine miliaria**

     Fox-Fordyce disease

L75.8   **Other apocrine sweat disorders**

L75.9   **Apocrine sweat disorder, unspecified**

INTRAOPERATIVE AND POSTPROCEDURAL COMPLICATIONS OF SKIN AND SUBCUTANEOUS TISSUE (L76)

L76   **Intraoperative and postprocedural complications of skin and subcutaneous tissue**

L76.0 **Intraoperative hemorrhage and hematoma of skin and subcutaneous tissue complicating a procedure**

Excludes1: intraoperative hemorrhage and hematoma of skin and subcutaneous tissue due to accidental puncture and laceration during a procedure (L76.1-)

L76.01 **Intraoperative hemorrhage and hematoma of skin and subcutaneous tissue complicating a dermatologic procedure**

L76.02 **Intraoperative hemorrhage and hematoma of skin and subcutaneous tissue complicating other procedure**

L76.1 **Accidental puncture and laceration of skin and subcutaneous tissue during a procedure**

L76.11 **Accidental puncture and laceration of skin and subcutaneous tissue during a dermatologic procedure**

L76.12 **Accidental puncture and laceration of skin and subcutaneous tissue during other procedure**

L76.2 **Postprocedural hemorrhage of skin and subcutaneous tissue following a procedure**

▲**L76.21** **Postprocedural hemorrhage of skin and subcutaneous tissue following a dermatologic procedure**

▲**L76.22** **Postprocedural hemorrhage of skin and subcutaneous tissue following other procedure**

L76.3 **Postprocedural hematoma and seroma of skin and subcutaneous tissue following a procedure**

●**L76.31** **Postprocedural hematoma of skin and subcutaneous tissue following a dermatologic procedure**

●**L76.32** **Postprocedural hematoma of skin and subcutaneous tissue following other procedure**

●**L76.33** **Postprocedural seroma of skin and subcutaneous tissue following a dermatologic procedure**

●**L76.34** **Postprocedural seroma of skin and subcutaneous tissue following other procedure**

L76.8 **Other intraoperative and postprocedural complications of skin and subcutaneous tissue**

Use additional code, if applicable, to further specify disorder

L76.81 **Other intraoperative complications of skin and subcutaneous tissue**

L76.82 **Other postprocedural complications of skin and subcutaneous tissue**

OTHER DISORDERS OF THE SKIN AND SUBCUTANEOUS TISSUE (L80-L99)

L80 **Vitiligo**

Excludes2: vitiligo of eyelids (H02.73-)

vitiligo of vulva (N90.89)

L81 **Other disorders of pigmentation**

Excludes1: birthmark NOS (Q82.5)

Peutz-Jeghers syndrome (Q85.8)

Excludes2: nevus - see Alphabetical Index

L81.0 **Postinflammatory hyperpigmentation**

L81.1 **Chloasma**

L81.2 **Freckles**

L81.3 **Café au lait spots**

L81.4 **Other melanin hyperpigmentation**

Lentigo

L81.5 **Leukoderma, not elsewhere classified**

L81.6 **Other disorders of diminished melanin formation**

L81.7 **Pigmented purpuric dermatosis**

Angioma serpiginosum

L81.8 **Other specified disorders of pigmentation**

Iron pigmentation

Tattoo pigmentation

L81.9 **Disorder of pigmentation, unspecified**

L82 **Seborrheic keratosis**

Includes: basal cell papilloma

dermatosis papulosa nigra

Leser-Trélat disease

Excludes2: seborrheic dermatitis (L21.-)

L82.0 **Inflamed seborrheic keratosis**

L82.1 **Other seborrheic keratosis**

Seborrheic keratosis NOS

L83 **Acanthosis nigricans**

Confluent and reticulated papillomatosis

L84 **Corns and callosities**

Callus Clavus

L85 **Other epidermal thickening**

Excludes2: hypertrophic disorders of the skin (L91.-)

L85.0 **Acquired ichthyosis**

Excludes1: congenital ichthyosis (Q80.-)

L85.1 **Acquired keratosis [keratoderma] palmaris et plantaris**

Excludes1: inherited keratosis palmaris et plantaris (Q82.8)

L85.2 **Keratosis punctata (palmaris et plantaris)**

L85.3 **Xerosis cutis**

Dry skin dermatitis

L85.8 **Other specified epidermal thickening**

Cutaneous horn

L85.9 **Epidermal thickening, unspecified**

L86 **Keratoderma in diseases classified elsewhere**

Code first underlying disease, such as:

Reiter's disease (M02.3-)

Excludes1: gonococcal keratoderma (A54.89)

gonococcal keratosis (A54.89)

keratoderma due to vitamin A deficiency (E50.8)

keratosis due to vitamin A deficiency (E50.8)

xeroderma due to vitamin A deficiency (E50.8)

L87 **Transepidermal elimination disorders**

Excludes1: granuloma annulare (perforating) (L92.0)

L87.0 **Keratosis follicularis et parafollicularis in cutem penetrans**

Kyrle disease

Hyperkeratosis follicularis penetrans

L87.1 **Reactive perforating collagenosis**

L87.2 **Elastosis perforans serpiginosa**

L87.8 **Other transepidermal elimination disorders**

L87.9 **Transepidermal elimination disorder, unspecified**

L88 **Pyoderma gangrenosum**

Phagedenic pyoderma

Excludes1: dermatitis gangrenosa (L08.0)

L89 **Pressure ulcer**

Includes: bed sore

decubitus ulcer

plaster ulcer

pressure area

pressure sore

Code first any associated gangrene (I96)

Excludes2: decubitus (trophic) ulcer of cervix (uteri) (N86)

diabetic ulcers (E08.621, E08.622, E09.621, E09.622, E10.621, E10.622, E11.621, E11.622, E13.621, E13.622)

non-pressure chronic ulcer of skin (L97.-)

skin infections (L00-L08)

varicose ulcer (I83.0, I83.2)

L89.0 **Pressure ulcer of elbow**

L89.00 **Pressure ulcer of unspecified elbow**

L89.000 **Pressure ulcer of unspecified elbow, unstageable**

L89.001 **Pressure ulcer of unspecified elbow, stage 1**

Healing pressure ulcer of unspecified elbow, stage 1

Pressure pre-ulcer skin changes limited to persistent focal edema, unspecified elbow

L89.002 **Pressure ulcer of unspecified elbow, stage 2**

Healing pressure ulcer of unspecified elbow, stage 2

Pressure ulcer with abrasion, blister, partial thickness skin loss involving epidermis and/or dermis, unspecified elbow

L89.003 **Pressure ulcer of unspecified elbow, stage 3**

Healing pressure ulcer of unspecified elbow, stage 3

Pressure ulcer with full thickness skin loss involving damage or necrosis of subcutaneous tissue, unspecified elbow

L89.004 **Pressure ulcer of unspecified elbow, stage 4**

Healing pressure ulcer of unspecified elbow, stage 4

Pressure ulcer with necrosis of soft tissues through to underlying muscle, tendon, or bone, unspecified elbow

L89.009 **Pressure ulcer of unspecified elbow, unspecified stage**

Healing pressure ulcer of elbow NOS

Healing pressure ulcer of unspecified elbow, unspecified stage

L89.01 **Pressure ulcer of right elbow**

L89.010 **Pressure ulcer of right elbow, unstageable**

L89.011 **Pressure ulcer of right elbow, stage 1**

Healing pressure ulcer of right elbow, stage 1

Pressure pre-ulcer skin changes limited to persistent focal edema, right elbow

L89.012 **Pressure ulcer of right elbow, stage 2**

Healing pressure ulcer of right elbow, stage 2

Pressure ulcer with abrasion, blister, partial thickness skin loss involving epidermis and/or dermis, right elbow

L89.013 **Pressure ulcer of right elbow, stage 3**

Healing pressure ulcer of right elbow, stage 3

Pressure ulcer with full thickness skin loss involving damage or necrosis of subcutaneous tissue, right elbow

L89.014 **Pressure ulcer of right elbow, stage 4**

Healing pressure ulcer of right elbow, stage 4

Pressure ulcer with necrosis of soft tissues through to underlying muscle, tendon, or bone, right elbow

L89.019 **Pressure ulcer of right elbow, unspecified stage**

Healing pressure right of elbow NOS

Healing pressure ulcer of unspecified elbow, unspecified stage

L89.02 **Pressure ulcer of left elbow**

L89.020 **Pressure ulcer of left elbow, unstageable**

L89.021 **Pressure ulcer of left elbow, stage 1**

Healing pressure ulcer of left elbow, stage 1

Pressure pre-ulcer skin changes limited to persistent focal edema, left elbow

L89.022 **Pressure ulcer of left elbow, stage 2**

Healing pressure ulcer of left elbow, stage 2

Pressure ulcer with abrasion, blister, partial thickness skin loss involving epidermis and/or dermis, left elbow

L89.023 **Pressure ulcer of left elbow, stage 3**

Healing pressure ulcer of left elbow, stage 3

Pressure ulcer with full thickness skin loss involving damage or necrosis of subcutaneous tissue, left elbow

L89.024 **Pressure ulcer of left elbow, stage 4**

Healing pressure ulcer of left elbow, stage 4

Pressure ulcer with necrosis of soft tissues through to underlying muscle, tendon, or bone, left elbow

L89.029 **Pressure ulcer of left elbow, unspecified stage**

Healing pressure ulcer of left of elbow NOS

● New code ▲ Revised code **Excludes1:** Not coded here **Excludes2:** Not included here ⊗ Placeholder required ⑦7th digit required

Healing pressure ulcer of unspecified elbow, unspecified stage

L89.1 **Pressure ulcer of back**

L89.10 **Pressure ulcer of unspecified part of back**

L89.100 **Pressure ulcer of unspecified part of back, unstageable**

L89.101 **Pressure ulcer of unspecified part of back, stage 1**

Healing pressure ulcer of unspecified part of back, stage 1

Pressure pre-ulcer skin changes limited to persistent focal edema, unspecified part of back

L89.102 **Pressure ulcer of unspecified part of back, stage 2**

Healing pressure ulcer of unspecified part of back, stage 2

Pressure ulcer with abrasion, blister, partial thickness skin loss involving epidermis and/or dermis, unspecified part of back

L89.103 **Pressure ulcer of unspecified part of back, stage 3**

Healing pressure ulcer of unspecified part of back, stage 3

Pressure ulcer with full thickness skin loss involving damage or necrosis of subcutaneous tissue, unspecified part of back

L89.104 **Pressure ulcer of unspecified part of back, stage 4**

Healing pressure ulcer of unspecified part of back, stage 4

Pressure ulcer with necrosis of soft tissues through to underlying muscle, tendon, or bone, unspecified part of back

L89.109 **Pressure ulcer of unspecified part of back, unspecified stage**

Healing pressure ulcer of unspecified part of back NOS

Healing pressure ulcer of unspecified part of back, unspecified stage

L89.11 **Pressure ulcer of right upper back**

Pressure ulcer of right shoulder blade

L89.110 **Pressure ulcer of right upper back, unstageable**

L89.111 **Pressure ulcer of right upper back, stage 1**

Healing pressure ulcer of right upper back, stage 1

Pressure pre-ulcer skin changes limited to persistent focal edema, right upper back

L89.112 **Pressure ulcer of right upper back, stage 2**

Healing pressure ulcer of right upper back, stage 2

Pressure ulcer with abrasion, blister, partial thickness skin loss involving epidermis and/or dermis, right upper back

L89.113 **Pressure ulcer of right upper back, stage 3**

Healing pressure ulcer of right upper back, stage 3

Pressure ulcer with full thickness skin loss involving damage or necrosis of subcutaneous tissue, right upper back

L89.114 **Pressure ulcer of right upper back, stage 4**

Healing pressure ulcer of right upper back, stage 4

Pressure ulcer with necrosis of soft tissues through to underlying muscle, tendon, or bone, right upper back

L89.119 **Pressure ulcer of right upper back, unspecified stage**

Healing pressure ulcer of right upper back NOS

Healing pressure ulcer of right upper back, unspecified stage

L89.12 **Pressure ulcer of left upper back**

Pressure ulcer of left shoulder blade

L89.120 **Pressure ulcer of left upper back, unstageable**

L89.121 **Pressure ulcer of left upper back, stage 1**

Healing pressure ulcer of left upper back, stage 1

Pressure pre-ulcer skin changes limited to persistent focal edema, left upper back

L89.122 **Pressure ulcer of left upper back, stage 2**

Healing pressure ulcer of left upper back, stage 2

Pressure ulcer with abrasion, blister, partial thickness skin loss involving epidermis and/or dermis, left upper back

L89.123 **Pressure ulcer of left upper back, stage 3**

Healing pressure ulcer of left upper back, stage 3

Pressure ulcer with full thickness skin loss involving damage or necrosis of subcutaneous tissue, left upper back

L89.124 **Pressure ulcer of left upper back, stage 4**

Healing pressure ulcer of left upper back, stage 4

Pressure ulcer with necrosis of soft tissues through to underlying muscle, tendon, or bone, left upper back

L89.129 **Pressure ulcer of left upper back, unspecified stage**

Healing pressure ulcer of left upper back NOS

Healing pressure ulcer of left upper back, unspecified stage

L89.13 **Pressure ulcer of right lower back**

L89.130 **Pressure ulcer of right lower back, unstageable**

L89.131 **Pressure ulcer of right lower back, stage 1**

Healing pressure ulcer of right lower back, stage 1

Pressure pre-ulcer skin changes limited to persistent focal edema, right lower back

L89.132 **Pressure ulcer of right lower back, stage 2**

Healing pressure ulcer of right lower back, stage 2

Pressure ulcer with abrasion, blister, partial thickness skin loss involving epidermis and/or dermis, right lower back

L89.133 **Pressure ulcer of right lower back, stage 3**

Healing pressure ulcer of right lower back, stage 3

Pressure ulcer with full thickness skin loss involving damage or necrosis of subcutaneous tissue, right lower back

L89.134 **Pressure ulcer of right lower back, stage 4**

Healing pressure ulcer of right lower back, stage 4

Pressure ulcer with necrosis of soft tissues through to underlying muscle, tendon, or bone, right lower back

L89.139 **Pressure ulcer of right lower back, unspecified stage**

Healing pressure ulcer of right lower back NOS

Healing pressure ulcer of right lower back, unspecified stage

L89.14 **Pressure ulcer of left lower back**

L89.140 **Pressure ulcer of left lower back, unstageable**

L89.141 **Pressure ulcer of left lower back, stage 1**

Healing pressure ulcer of left lower back, stage 1

Pressure pre-ulcer skin changes limited to persistent focal edema, left lower back

L89.142 **Pressure ulcer of left lower back, stage 2**

Healing pressure ulcer of left lower back, stage 2

Pressure ulcer with abrasion, blister, partial thickness skin loss involving epidermis and/or dermis, left lower back

L89.143 **Pressure ulcer of left lower back, stage 3**

Healing pressure ulcer of left lower back, stage 3

Pressure ulcer with full thickness skin loss involving damage or necrosis of subcutaneous tissue, left lower back

L89.144 **Pressure ulcer of left lower back, stage 4**

Healing pressure ulcer of left lower back, stage 4

Pressure ulcer with necrosis of soft tissues through to underlying muscle, tendon, or bone, left lower back

L89.149 **Pressure ulcer of left lower back, unspecified stage**

Healing pressure ulcer of left lower back NOS

Healing pressure ulcer of left lower back, unspecified stage

L89.15 **Pressure ulcer of sacral region**

Pressure ulcer of coccyx

Pressure ulcer of tailbone

L89.150 **Pressure ulcer of sacral region, unstageable**

L89.151 **Pressure ulcer of sacral region, stage 1**

Healing pressure ulcer of sacral region, stage 1

Pressure pre-ulcer skin changes limited to persistent focal edema, sacral region

L89.152 **Pressure ulcer of sacral region, stage 2**

Healing pressure ulcer of sacral region, stage 2

Pressure ulcer with abrasion, blister, partial thickness skin loss involving epidermis and/or dermis, sacral region

L89.153 **Pressure ulcer of sacral region, stage 3**

Healing pressure ulcer of sacral region, stage 3

Pressure ulcer with full thickness skin loss involving damage or necrosis of subcutaneous tissue, sacral region

L89.154 **Pressure ulcer of sacral region, stage 4**

Healing pressure ulcer of sacral region, stage 4

Pressure ulcer with necrosis of soft tissues through to underlying muscle, tendon, or bone, sacral region

L89.159 **Pressure ulcer of sacral region, unspecified stage**

Healing pressure ulcer of sacral region NOS

Healing pressure ulcer of sacral region, unspecified stage

L89.2 **Pressure ulcer of hip**

L89.20 **Pressure ulcer of unspecified hip**

L89.200 **Pressure ulcer of unspecified hip, unstageable**

L89.201 **Pressure ulcer of unspecified hip, stage 1**

Healing pressure ulcer of unspecified hip back, stage 1

Pressure pre-ulcer skin changes limited to persistent focal edema, unspecified hip

● New code ▲ Revised code **Excludes1:** Not coded here **Excludes2:** Not included here ⊗ Placeholder required ⑦ 7th digit required

L89.202 Pressure ulcer of unspecified hip, stage 2

Healing pressure ulcer of unspecified hip, stage 2

Pressure ulcer with abrasion, blister, partial thickness skin loss involving epidermis and/or dermis, unspecified hip

L89.203 Pressure ulcer of unspecified hip, stage 3

Healing pressure ulcer of unspecified hip, stage 3

Pressure ulcer with full thickness skin loss involving damage or necrosis of subcutaneous tissue, unspecified hip

L89.204 Pressure ulcer of unspecified hip, stage 4

Healing pressure ulcer of unspecified hip, stage 4

Pressure ulcer with necrosis of soft tissues through to underlying muscle, tendon, or bone, unspecified hip

L89.209 Pressure ulcer of unspecified hip, unspecified stage

Healing pressure ulcer of unspecified hip NOS

Healing pressure ulcer of unspecified hip, unspecified stage

L89.21 Pressure ulcer of right hip

L89.210 Pressure ulcer of right hip, unstageable

L89.211 Pressure ulcer of right hip, stage 1

Healing pressure ulcer of right hip back, stage 1

Pressure pre-ulcer skin changes limited to persistent focal edema, right hip

L89.212 Pressure ulcer of right hip, stage 2

Healing pressure ulcer of right hip, stage 2

Pressure ulcer with abrasion, blister, partial thickness skin loss involving epidermis and/or dermis, right hip

L89.213 Pressure ulcer of right hip, stage 3

Healing pressure ulcer of right hip, stage 3

Pressure ulcer with full thickness skin loss involving damage or necrosis of subcutaneous tissue, right hip

L89.214 Pressure ulcer of right hip, stage 4

Healing pressure ulcer of right hip, stage 4

Pressure ulcer with necrosis of soft tissues through to underlying muscle, tendon, or bone, right hip

L89.219 Pressure ulcer of right hip, unspecified stage

Healing pressure ulcer of right hip NOS

Healing pressure ulcer of right hip, unspecified stage

L89.22 Pressure ulcer of left hip

L89.220 Pressure ulcer of left hip, unstageable

L89.221 Pressure ulcer of left hip, stage 1

Healing pressure ulcer of left hip back, stage 1

Pressure pre-ulcer skin changes limited to persistent focal edema, left hip

L89.222 Pressure ulcer of left hip, stage 2

Healing pressure ulcer of left hip, stage 2

Pressure ulcer with abrasion, blister, partial thickness skin loss involving epidermis and/or dermis, left hip

L89.223 Pressure ulcer of left hip, stage 3

Healing pressure ulcer of left hip, stage 3

Pressure ulcer with full thickness skin loss involving damage or necrosis of subcutaneous tissue, left hip

L89.224 Pressure ulcer of left hip, stage 4

Healing pressure ulcer of left hip, stage 4

Pressure ulcer with necrosis of soft tissues through to underlying muscle, tendon, or bone, left hip

L89.229 Pressure ulcer of left hip, unspecified stage

Healing pressure ulcer of left hip NOS

Healing pressure ulcer of left hip, unspecified stage

L89.3 Pressure ulcer of buttock

L89.30 Pressure ulcer of unspecified buttock

L89.300 Pressure ulcer of unspecified buttock, unstageable

L89.301 Pressure ulcer of unspecified buttock, stage 1

Healing pressure ulcer of unspecified buttock, stage 1

Pressure pre-ulcer skin changes limited to persistent focal edema, unspecified buttock

L89.302 Pressure ulcer of unspecified buttock, stage 2

Healing pressure ulcer of unspecified buttock, stage 2

Pressure ulcer with abrasion, blister, partial thickness skin loss involving epidermis and/or dermis, unspecified buttock

L89.303 Pressure ulcer of unspecified buttock, stage 3

Healing pressure ulcer of unspecified buttock, stage 3

Pressure ulcer with full thickness skin loss involving damage or necrosis of subcutaneous tissue, unspecified buttock

L89.304 Pressure ulcer of unspecified buttock, stage 4

Healing pressure ulcer of unspecified buttock, stage 4

Pressure ulcer with necrosis of soft tissues through to underlying muscle, tendon, or bone, unspecified buttock

L89.309 **Pressure ulcer of unspecified buttock, unspecified stage**

Healing pressure ulcer of unspecified buttock NOS

Healing pressure ulcer of unspecified buttock, unspecified stage

L89.31 **Pressure ulcer of right buttock**

L89.310 **Pressure ulcer of right buttock, unstageable**

L89.311 **Pressure ulcer of right buttock, stage 1**

Healing pressure ulcer of right buttock, stage 1

Pressure pre-ulcer skin changes limited to persistent focal edema, right buttock

L89.312 **Pressure ulcer of right buttock, stage 2**

Healing pressure ulcer of right buttock, stage 2

Pressure ulcer with abrasion, blister, partial thickness skin loss involving epidermis and/or dermis, right buttock

L89.313 **Pressure ulcer of right buttock, stage 3**

Healing pressure ulcer of right buttock, stage 3

Pressure ulcer with full thickness skin loss involving damage or necrosis of subcutaneous tissue, right buttock

L89.314 **Pressure ulcer of right buttock, stage 4**

Healing pressure ulcer of right buttock, stage 4

Pressure ulcer with necrosis of soft tissues through to underlying muscle, tendon, or bone, right buttock

L89.319 **Pressure ulcer of right buttock, unspecified stage**

Healing pressure ulcer of right buttock NOS

Healing pressure ulcer of right buttock, unspecified stage

L89.32 **Pressure ulcer of left buttock**

L89.320 **Pressure ulcer of left buttock, unstageable**

L89.321 **Pressure ulcer of left buttock, stage 1**

Healing pressure ulcer of left buttock, stage 1

Pressure pre-ulcer skin changes limited to persistent focal edema, left buttock

L89.322 **Pressure ulcer of left buttock, stage 2**

Healing pressure ulcer of left buttock, stage 2

Pressure ulcer with abrasion, blister, partial thickness skin loss involving epidermis and/or dermis, left buttock

L89.323 **Pressure ulcer of left buttock, stage 3**

Healing pressure ulcer of left buttock, stage 3

Pressure ulcer with full thickness skin loss involving damage or necrosis of subcutaneous tissue, left buttock

L89.324 **Pressure ulcer of left buttock, stage 4**

Healing pressure ulcer of left buttock, stage 4

Pressure ulcer with necrosis of soft tissues through to underlying muscle, tendon, or bone, left buttock

L89.329 **Pressure ulcer of left buttock, unspecified stage**

Healing pressure ulcer of left buttock NOS

Healing pressure ulcer of left buttock, unspecified stage

L89.4 **Pressure ulcer of contiguous site of back, buttock and hip**

L89.40 **Pressure ulcer of contiguous site of back, buttock and hip, unspecified stage**

Healing pressure ulcer of contiguous site of back, buttock and hip NOS

Healing pressure ulcer of contiguous site of back, buttock and hip, unspecified stage

L89.41 **Pressure ulcer of contiguous site of back, buttock and hip, stage 1**

Healing pressure ulcer of contiguous site of back, buttock and hip, stage 1

Pressure pre-ulcer skin changes limited to persistent focal edema, contiguous site of back, buttock and hip

L89.42 **Pressure ulcer of contiguous site of back, buttock and hip, stage 2**

Healing pressure ulcer of contiguous site of back, buttock and hip, stage 2

Pressure ulcer with abrasion, blister, partial thickness skin loss involving epidermis and/or dermis, contiguous site of back, buttock and hip

L89.43 **Pressure ulcer of contiguous site of back, buttock and hip, stage 3**

Healing pressure ulcer of contiguous site of back, buttock and hip, stage 3

Pressure ulcer with full thickness skin loss involving damage or necrosis of subcutaneous tissue, contiguous site of back, buttock and hip

L89.44 **Pressure ulcer of contiguous site of back, buttock and hip, stage 4**

Healing pressure ulcer of contiguous site of back, buttock and hip, stage 4

Pressure ulcer with necrosis of soft tissues through to underlying muscle, tendon, or bone, contiguous site of back, buttock and hip

L89.45 **Pressure ulcer of contiguous site of back, buttock and hip, unstageable**

L89.5 **Pressure ulcer of ankle**

L89.50 **Pressure ulcer of unspecified ankle**

L89.500 **Pressure ulcer of unspecified ankle, unstageable**

L89.501 **Pressure ulcer of unspecified ankle, stage 1**

Healing pressure ulcer of unspecified ankle, stage 1

Pressure pre-ulcer skin changes limited to persistent focal edema, unspecified ankle

L89.502 **Pressure ulcer of unspecified ankle, stage 2**

Healing pressure ulcer of unspecified ankle, stage 2

Pressure ulcer with abrasion, blister, partial thickness skin loss involving epidermis and/or dermis, unspecified ankle

L89.503 **Pressure ulcer of unspecified ankle, stage 3**

Healing pressure ulcer of unspecified ankle, stage 3

Pressure ulcer with full thickness skin loss involving damage or necrosis of subcutaneous tissue, unspecified ankle

L89.504 **Pressure ulcer of unspecified ankle, stage 4**

Healing pressure ulcer of unspecified ankle, stage 4

Pressure ulcer with necrosis of soft tissues through to underlying muscle, tendon, or bone, unspecified ankle

L89.509 **Pressure ulcer of unspecified ankle, unspecified stage**

Healing pressure ulcer of unspecified ankle NOS

Healing pressure ulcer of unspecified ankle, unspecified stage

L89.51 **Pressure ulcer of right ankle**

L89.510 **Pressure ulcer of right ankle, unstageable**

L89.511 **Pressure ulcer of right ankle, stage 1**

Healing pressure ulcer of right ankle, stage 1

Pressure pre-ulcer skin changes limited to persistent focal edema, right ankle

L89.512 **Pressure ulcer of right ankle, stage 2**

Healing pressure ulcer of right ankle, stage 2

Pressure ulcer with abrasion, blister, partial thickness skin loss involving epidermis and/or dermis, right ankle

L89.513 **Pressure ulcer of right ankle, stage 3**

Healing pressure ulcer of right ankle, stage 3

Pressure ulcer with full thickness skin loss involving damage or necrosis of subcutaneous tissue, right ankle

L89.514 **Pressure ulcer of right ankle, stage 4**

Healing pressure ulcer of right ankle, stage 4

Pressure ulcer with necrosis of soft tissues through to underlying muscle, tendon, or bone, right ankle

L89.519 **Pressure ulcer of right ankle, unspecified stage**

Healing pressure ulcer of right ankle NOS

Healing pressure ulcer of right ankle, unspecified stage

L89.52 **Pressure ulcer of left ankle**

L89.520 **Pressure ulcer of left ankle, unstageable**

L89.521 **Pressure ulcer of left ankle, stage 1**

Healing pressure ulcer of left ankle, stage 1

Pressure pre-ulcer skin changes limited to persistent focal edema, left ankle

L89.522 **Pressure ulcer of left ankle, stage 2**

Healing pressure ulcer of left ankle, stage 2

Pressure ulcer with abrasion, blister, partial thickness skin loss involving epidermis and/or dermis, left ankle

L89.523 **Pressure ulcer of left ankle, stage 3**

Healing pressure ulcer of left ankle, stage 3

Pressure ulcer with full thickness skin loss involving damage or necrosis of subcutaneous tissue, left ankle

L89.524 **Pressure ulcer of left ankle, stage 4**

Healing pressure ulcer of left ankle, stage 4

Pressure ulcer with necrosis of soft tissues through to underlying muscle, tendon, or bone, left ankle

L89.529 **Pressure ulcer of left ankle, unspecified stage**

Healing pressure ulcer of left ankle NOS

Healing pressure ulcer of left ankle, unspecified stage

L89.6 **Pressure ulcer of heel**

L89.60 **Pressure ulcer of unspecified heel**

L89.600 **Pressure ulcer of unspecified heel, unstageable**

L89.601 **Pressure ulcer of unspecified heel, stage 1**

Healing pressure ulcer of unspecified heel, stage 1

Pressure pre-ulcer skin changes limited to persistent focal edema, unspecified heel

L89.602 **Pressure ulcer of unspecified heel, stage 2**

Healing pressure ulcer of unspecified heel, stage 2

| | Add 4th-7th digits | | Nonspecific code | | Unspecified code | | Manifestation code | 495 |

Pressure ulcer with abrasion, blister, partial thickness skin loss involving epidermis and/or dermis, unspecified heel

L89.603 Pressure ulcer of unspecified heel, stage 3

Healing pressure ulcer of unspecified heel, stage 3

Pressure ulcer with full thickness skin loss involving damage or necrosis of subcutaneous tissue, unspecified heel

L89.604 Pressure ulcer of unspecified heel, stage 4

Healing pressure ulcer of unspecified heel, stage 4

Pressure ulcer with necrosis of soft tissues through to underlying muscle, tendon, or bone, unspecified heel

L89.609 Pressure ulcer of unspecified heel, unspecified stage

Healing pressure ulcer of unspecified heel NOS

Healing pressure ulcer of unspecified heel, unspecified stage

L89.61 Pressure ulcer of right heel

L89.610 Pressure ulcer of right heel, unstageable

L89.611 Pressure ulcer of right heel, stage 1

Healing pressure ulcer of right heel, stage 1

Pressure pre-ulcer skin changes limited to persistent focal edema, right heel

L89.612 Pressure ulcer of right heel, stage 2

Healing pressure ulcer of right heel, stage 2

Pressure ulcer with abrasion, blister, partial thickness skin loss involving epidermis and/or dermis, right heel

L89.613 Pressure ulcer of right heel, stage 3

Healing pressure ulcer of right heel, stage 3

Pressure ulcer with full thickness skin loss involving damage or necrosis of subcutaneous tissue, right heel

L89.614 Pressure ulcer of right heel, stage 4

Healing pressure ulcer of right heel, stage 4

Pressure ulcer with necrosis of soft tissues through to underlying muscle, tendon, or bone, right heel

L89.619 Pressure ulcer of right heel, unspecified stage

Healing pressure ulcer of right heel NOS

Healing pressure ulcer of unspecified heel, right stage

L89.62 Pressure ulcer of left heel

L89.620 Pressure ulcer of left heel, unstageable

L89.621 Pressure ulcer of left heel, stage 1

Healing pressure ulcer of left heel, stage 1

Pressure pre-ulcer skin changes limited to persistent focal edema, left heel

L89.622 Pressure ulcer of left heel, stage 2

Healing pressure ulcer of left heel, stage 2

Pressure ulcer with abrasion, blister, partial thickness skin loss involving epidermis and/or dermis, left heel

L89.623 Pressure ulcer of left heel, stage 3

Healing pressure ulcer of left heel, stage 3

Pressure ulcer with full thickness skin loss involving damage or necrosis of subcutaneous tissue, left heel

L89.624 Pressure ulcer of left heel, stage 4

Healing pressure ulcer of left heel, stage 4

Pressure ulcer with necrosis of soft tissues through to underlying muscle, tendon, or bone, left heel

L89.629 Pressure ulcer of left heel, unspecified stage

Healing pressure ulcer of left heel NOS

Healing pressure ulcer of left heel, unspecified stage

L89.8 Pressure ulcer of other site

L89.81 Pressure ulcer of head

Pressure ulcer of face

L89.810 Pressure ulcer of head, unstageable

L89.811 Pressure ulcer of head, stage 1

Healing pressure ulcer of head, stage 1

Pressure pre-ulcer skin changes limited to persistent focal edema, head

L89.812 Pressure ulcer of head, stage 2

Healing pressure ulcer of head, stage 2

Pressure ulcer with abrasion, blister, partial thickness skin loss involving epidermis and/or dermis, head

L89.813 Pressure ulcer of head, stage 3

Healing pressure ulcer of head, stage 3

Pressure ulcer with full thickness skin loss involving damage or necrosis of subcutaneous tissue, head

L89.814 Pressure ulcer of head, stage 4

Healing pressure ulcer of head, stage 4

Pressure ulcer with necrosis of soft tissues through to underlying muscle, tendon, or bone, head

L89.819 Pressure ulcer of head, unspecified stage

Healing pressure ulcer of head NOS

Healing pressure ulcer of head, unspecified stage

L89.89 Pressure ulcer of other site

L89.890 Pressure ulcer of other site, unstageable

● New code ▲ Revised code **Excludes1:** Not coded here **Excludes2:** Not included here ⊗ Placeholder required ⑦ 7th digit required

L89.891   **Pressure ulcer of other site, stage 1**

Healing pressure ulcer **of other** site, stage 1

Pressure pre-ulcer skin changes limited to persistent focal edema, **other** site

L89.892   **Pressure ulcer of other site, stage 2**

Healing pressure ulcer **of other** site, stage 2

Pressure ulcer with abrasion, blister, partial thickness skin loss involving epidermis and/or dermis, **other** site

L89.893   **Pressure ulcer of other site, stage 3**

Healing pressure ulcer **of other** site, stage 3

Pressure ulcer with full thickness skin loss involving damage or necrosis of subcutaneous tissue, **other** site

L89.894   **Pressure ulcer of other site, stage 4**

Healing pressure ulcer **of other** site, stage 4

Pressure ulcer with necrosis of soft tissues through to underlying muscle, tendon, or bone, **other** site

L89.899   **Pressure ulcer of other site, unspecified stage**

Healing pressure ulcer **of other** site NOS

Healing pressure ulcer **of other** site, unspecified stage

L89.9   **Pressure ulcer of unspecified site**

L89.90   **Pressure ulcer of unspecified site, unspecified stage**

Healing pressure ulcer of unspecified site NOS

Healing pressure ulcer of unspecified site, unspecified stage

L89.91   **Pressure ulcer of unspecified site, stage 1**

Healing pressure ulcer of unspecified site, stage 1

Pressure pre-ulcer skin changes limited to persistent focal edema, unspecified site

L89.92   **Pressure ulcer of unspecified site, stage 2**

Healing pressure ulcer of unspecified site, stage 2

Pressure ulcer with abrasion, blister, partial thickness skin loss involving epidermis and/or dermis, unspecified site

L89.93   **Pressure ulcer of unspecified site, stage 3**

Healing pressure ulcer of unspecified site, stage 3

Pressure ulcer with full thickness skin loss involving damage or necrosis of subcutaneous tissue, unspecified site

L89.94   **Pressure ulcer of unspecified site, stage 4**

Healing pressure ulcer of unspecified site, stage 4

Pressure ulcer with necrosis of soft tissues through to underlying muscle, tendon, or bone, unspecified site

L89.95   **Pressure ulcer of unspecified site, unstageable**

L90   **Atrophic disorders of skin**

L90.0   **Lichen sclerosus et atrophicus**

Excludes2: lichen sclerosus of external female genital organs (N90.4)

lichen sclerosus of external male genital organs (N48.0)

L90.1   **Anetoderma of Schweninger-Buzzi**

L90.2   **Anetoderma of Jadassohn-Pellizzari**

L90.3   **Atrophoderma of Pasini and Pierini**

L90.4   **Acrodermatitis chronica atrophicans**

L90.5   **Scar conditions and fibrosis of skin**

Adherent scar (skin)

Cicatrix

Disfigurement of skin due to scar

Fibrosis of skin NOS

Scar NOS

Excludes2: hypertrophic scar (L91.0)

keloid scar (L91.0)

L90.6   **Striae atrophicae**

L90.8   **Other atrophic disorders of skin**

L90.9   **Atrophic disorder of skin, unspecified**

L91   **Hypertrophic disorders of skin**

L91.0   **Hypertrophic scar**

Keloid

Keloid scar

Excludes2: acne keloid (L73.0)

scar NOS (L90.5)

L91.8   **Other hypertrophic disorders of the skin**

L91.9   **Hypertrophic disorder of the skin, unspecified**

L92   **Granulomatous disorders of skin and subcutaneous tissue**

Excludes2: actinic granuloma (L57.5)

L92.0   **Granuloma annulare**

Perforating granuloma annulare

L92.1   **Necrobiosis lipoidica, not elsewhere classified**

Excludes1: necrobiosis lipoidica associated with diabetes mellitus (E08-E13 with .620)

L92.2   **Granuloma faciale [eosinophilic granuloma of skin]**

L92.3   **Foreign body granuloma of the skin and subcutaneous tissue**

Use additional code to identify the type of retained foreign body (Z18.-)

L92.8   **Other granulomatous disorders of the skin and subcutaneous tissue**

L92.9   **Granulomatous disorder of the skin and subcutaneous tissue, unspecified**

L93   **Lupus erythematosus**

Use additional code for adverse effect, if applicable, to identify drug (T36-T50 with fifth or sixth character 5)

Excludes1: lupus exedens (A18.4)

lupus vulgaris (A18.4)

scleroderma (M34.-)

systemic lupus erythematosus (M32.-)

L93.0   **Discoid lupus erythematosus**

Lupus erythematosus NOS

L93.1   **Subacute cutaneous lupus erythematosus**

L93.2   **Other local lupus erythematosus**

Lupus erythematosus profundus

Lupus panniculitis

L94   **Other localized connective tissue disorders**

Excludes1: systemic connective tissue disorders (M30-M36)

L94.0 **Localized scleroderma [morphea]**
Circumscribed scleroderma

L94.1 **Linear scleroderma**
En coup de sabre lesion

L94.2 **Calcinosis cutis**

L94.3 **Sclerodactyly**

L94.4 **Gottron's papules**

L94.5 **Poikiloderma vasculare atrophicans**

L94.6 **Ainhum**

L94.8 **Other specified localized connective tissue disorders**

L94.9 **Localized connective tissue disorder, unspecified**

L95 **Vasculitis limited to skin, not elsewhere classified**
Excludes1: angioma serpiginosum (L81.7)
Henoch(-Schönlein) purpura (D69.0)
hypersensitivity angiitis (M31.0)
lupus panniculitis (L93.2)
panniculitis NOS (M79.3)
panniculitis of neck and back (M54.0-)
polyarteritis nodosa (M30.0)
relapsing panniculitis (M35.6)
rheumatoid vasculitis (M05.2)
serum sickness (T80.6-)
urticaria (L50.-)
Wegener's granulomatosis (M31.3-)

L95.0 **Livedoid vasculitis**
Atrophie blanche (en plaque)

L95.1 **Erythema elevatum diutinum**

L95.8 **Other vasculitis limited to the skin**

L95.9 **Vasculitis limited to the skin, unspecified**

L97 **Non-pressure chronic ulcer of lower limb, not elsewhere classified**
Includes: chronic ulcer of skin of lower limb NOS
non-healing ulcer of skin non-infected sinus of skin trophic ulcer NOS
tropical ulcer NOS
ulcer of skin of lower limb NOS

Code first any associated underlying condition, such as:
any associated gangrene (I96)
atherosclerosis of the lower extremities (I70.23-, I70.24-, I70.33-, I70.34-, I70.43-, I70.44-, I70.53-, I70.54-, I70.63-, I70.64-, I70.73-, I70.74-)
chronic venous hypertension (I87.31-, I87.33-)
diabetic ulcers (E08.621, E08.622, E09.621, E09.622, E10.621, E10.622, E11.621, E11.622, E13.621, E13.622)
postphlebitic syndrome (I87.01-, I87.03-)
postthrombotic syndrome (I87.01-, I87.03-)
varicose ulcer (I83.0-, I83.2-)
Excludes2: pressure ulcer (pressure area) (L89.-)
skin infections (L00-L08)
specific infections classified to A00-B99

L97.1 **Non-pressure chronic ulcer of thigh**

L97.10 **Non-pressure chronic ulcer of unspecified thigh**

L97.101 **Non-pressure chronic ulcer of unspecified thigh limited to breakdown of skin**

L97.102 **Non-pressure chronic ulcer of unspecified thigh with fat layer exposed**

L97.103 **Non-pressure chronic ulcer of unspecified thigh with necrosis of muscle**

L97.104 **Non-pressure chronic ulcer of unspecified thigh with necrosis of bone**

L97.109 **Non-pressure chronic ulcer of unspecified thigh with unspecified severity**

L97.11 **Non-pressure chronic ulcer of right thigh**

L97.111 **Non-pressure chronic ulcer of right thigh limited to breakdown of skin**

L97.112 **Non-pressure chronic ulcer of right thigh with fat layer exposed**

L97.113 **Non-pressure chronic ulcer of right thigh with necrosis of muscle**

L97.114 **Non-pressure chronic ulcer of right thigh with necrosis of bone**

L97.119 **Non-pressure chronic ulcer of right thigh with unspecified severity**

L97.12 **Non-pressure chronic ulcer of left thigh**

L97.121 **Non-pressure chronic ulcer of left thigh limited to breakdown of skin**

L97.122 **Non-pressure chronic ulcer of left thigh with fat layer exposed**

L97.123 **Non-pressure chronic ulcer of left thigh with necrosis of muscle**

L97.124 **Non-pressure chronic ulcer of left thigh with necrosis of bone**

L97.129 **Non-pressure chronic ulcer of left thigh with unspecified severity**

L97.2 **Non-pressure chronic ulcer of calf**

L97.20 **Non-pressure chronic ulcer of unspecified calf**

L97.201 **Non-pressure chronic ulcer of unspecified calf limited to breakdown of skin**

L97.202 **Non-pressure chronic ulcer of unspecified calf with fat layer exposed**

L97.203 **Non-pressure chronic ulcer of unspecified calf with necrosis of muscle**

L97.204 **Non-pressure chronic ulcer of unspecified calf with necrosis of bone**

L97.209 **Non-pressure chronic ulcer of unspecified calf with unspecified severity**

L97.21 **Non-pressure chronic ulcer of right calf**

L97.211 **Non-pressure chronic ulcer of right calf limited to breakdown of skin**

L97.212 **Non-pressure chronic ulcer of right calf with fat layer exposed**

L97.213 **Non-pressure chronic ulcer of right calf with necrosis of muscle**

L97.214 **Non-pressure chronic ulcer of right calf with necrosis of bone**

L97.219 **Non-pressure chronic ulcer of right calf with unspecified severity**

● New code ▲ Revised code **Excludes1:** Not coded here **Excludes2:** Not included here ⊗ Placeholder required ⑦7th digit required

L97.22   Non-pressure chronic ulcer of left calf

     L97.221   Non-pressure chronic ulcer of left calf limited to breakdown of skin

     L97.222   Non-pressure chronic ulcer of left calf with fat layer exposed

     L97.223   Non-pressure chronic ulcer of left calf with necrosis of muscle

     L97.224   Non-pressure chronic ulcer of left calf with necrosis of bone

     L97.229   Non-pressure chronic ulcer of left calf with unspecified severity

L97.3   **Non-pressure chronic ulcer of ankle**

   L97.30   Non-pressure chronic ulcer of unspecified ankle

     L97.301   Non-pressure chronic ulcer of unspecified ankle limited to breakdown of skin

     L97.302   Non-pressure chronic ulcer of unspecified ankle with fat layer exposed

     L97.303   Non-pressure chronic ulcer of unspecified ankle with necrosis of muscle

     L97.304   Non-pressure chronic ulcer of unspecified ankle with necrosis of bone

     L97.309   Non-pressure chronic ulcer of unspecified ankle with unspecified severity

   L97.31   Non-pressure chronic ulcer of right ankle

     L97.311   Non-pressure chronic ulcer of right ankle limited to breakdown of skin

     L97.312   Non-pressure chronic ulcer of right ankle with fat layer exposed

     L97.313   Non-pressure chronic ulcer of right ankle with necrosis of muscle

     L97.314   Non-pressure chronic ulcer of right ankle with necrosis of bone

     L97.319   Non-pressure chronic ulcer of right ankle with unspecified severity

   L97.32   Non-pressure chronic ulcer of left ankle

     L97.321   Non-pressure chronic ulcer of left ankle limited to breakdown of skin

     L97.322   Non-pressure chronic ulcer of left ankle with fat layer exposed

     L97.323   Non-pressure chronic ulcer of left ankle with necrosis of muscle

     L97.324   Non-pressure chronic ulcer of left ankle with necrosis of bone

     L97.329   Non-pressure chronic ulcer of left ankle with unspecified severity

L97.4   **Non-pressure chronic ulcer of heel and midfoot**

Non-pressure chronic ulcer of plantar surface of midfoot

   L97.40   Non-pressure chronic ulcer of unspecified heel and midfoot

     L97.401   Non-pressure chronic ulcer of unspecified heel and midfoot limited to breakdown of skin

     L97.402   Non-pressure chronic ulcer of unspecified heel and midfoot with fat layer exposed

     L97.403   Non-pressure chronic ulcer of unspecified heel and midfoot with necrosis of muscle

     L97.404   Non-pressure chronic ulcer of unspecified heel and midfoot with necrosis of bone

     L97.409   Non-pressure chronic ulcer of unspecified heel and midfoot with unspecified severity

   L97.41   Non-pressure chronic ulcer of right heel and midfoot

     L97.411   Non-pressure chronic ulcer of right heel and midfoot limited to breakdown of skin

     L97.412   Non-pressure chronic ulcer of right heel and midfoot with fat layer exposed

     L97.413   Non-pressure chronic ulcer of right heel and midfoot with necrosis of muscle

     L97.414   Non-pressure chronic ulcer of right heel and midfoot with necrosis of bone

     L97.419   Non-pressure chronic ulcer of right heel and midfoot with unspecified severity

   L97.42   Non-pressure chronic ulcer of left heel and midfoot

     L97.421   Non-pressure chronic ulcer of left heel and midfoot limited to breakdown of skin

     L97.422   Non-pressure chronic ulcer of left heel and midfoot with fat layer exposed

     L97.423   Non-pressure chronic ulcer of left heel and midfoot with necrosis of muscle

     L97.424   Non-pressure chronic ulcer of left heel and midfoot with necrosis of bone

     L97.429   Non-pressure chronic ulcer of left heel and midfoot with unspecified severity

L97.5   **Non-pressure chronic ulcer of other part of foot**

Non-pressure chronic ulcer of toe

   L97.50   Non-pressure chronic ulcer of other part of unspecified foot

     L97.501   Non-pressure chronic ulcer of other part of unspecified foot limited to breakdown of skin

     L97.502   Non-pressure chronic ulcer of other part of unspecified foot with fat layer exposed

     L97.503   Non-pressure chronic ulcer of other part of unspecified foot with necrosis of muscle

     L97.504   Non-pressure chronic ulcer of other part of unspecified foot with necrosis of bone

     L97.509   Non-pressure chronic ulcer of other part of unspecified foot with unspecified severity

   L97.51   Non-pressure chronic ulcer of other part of right foot

L97.511 Non-pressure chronic ulcer of other part of right foot limited to breakdown of skin

L97.512 Non-pressure chronic ulcer of other part of right foot with fat layer exposed

L97.513 Non-pressure chronic ulcer of other part of right foot with necrosis of muscle

L97.514 Non-pressure chronic ulcer of other part of right foot with necrosis of bone

L97.519 Non-pressure chronic ulcer of other part of right foot with unspecified severity

L97.52 Non-pressure chronic ulcer of other part of left foot

L97.521 Non-pressure chronic ulcer of other part of left foot limited to breakdown of skin

L97.522 Non-pressure chronic ulcer of other part of left foot with fat layer exposed

L97.523 Non-pressure chronic ulcer of other part of left foot with necrosis of muscle

L97.524 Non-pressure chronic ulcer of other part of left foot with necrosis of bone

L97.529 Non-pressure chronic ulcer of other part of left foot with unspecified severity

L97.8 Non-pressure chronic ulcer of other part of lower leg

L97.80 Non-pressure chronic ulcer of other part of unspecified lower leg

L97.801 Non-pressure chronic ulcer of other part of unspecified lower leg limited to breakdown of skin

L97.802 Non-pressure chronic ulcer of other part of unspecified lower leg with fat layer exposed

L97.803 Non-pressure chronic ulcer of other part of unspecified lower leg with necrosis of muscle

L97.804 Non-pressure chronic ulcer of other part of unspecified lower leg with necrosis of bone

L97.809 Non-pressure chronic ulcer of other part of unspecified lower leg with unspecified severity

L97.81 Non-pressure chronic ulcer of other part of right lower leg

L97.811 Non-pressure chronic ulcer of other part of right lower leg limited to breakdown of skin

L97.812 Non-pressure chronic ulcer of other part of right lower leg with fat layer exposed

L97.813 Non-pressure chronic ulcer of other part of right lower leg with necrosis of muscle

L97.814 Non-pressure chronic ulcer of other part of right lower leg with necrosis of bone

L97.819 Non-pressure chronic ulcer of other part of right lower leg with unspecified severity

L97.82 Non-pressure chronic ulcer of other part of left lower leg

L97.821 Non-pressure chronic ulcer of other part of left lower leg limited to breakdown of skin

L97.822 Non-pressure chronic ulcer of other part of left lower leg with fat layer exposed

L97.823 Non-pressure chronic ulcer of other part of left lower leg with necrosis of muscle

L97.824 Non-pressure chronic ulcer of other part of left lower leg with necrosis of bone

L97.829 Non-pressure chronic ulcer of other part of left lower leg with unspecified severity

L97.9 Non-pressure chronic ulcer of unspecified part of lower leg

L97.90 Non-pressure chronic ulcer of unspecified part of unspecified lower leg

L97.901 Non-pressure chronic ulcer of unspecified part of unspecified lower leg limited to breakdown of skin

L97.902 Non-pressure chronic ulcer of unspecified part of unspecified lower leg with fat layer exposed

L97.903 Non-pressure chronic ulcer of unspecified part of unspecified lower leg with necrosis of muscle

L97.904 Non-pressure chronic ulcer of unspecified part of unspecified lower leg with necrosis of bone

L97.909 Non-pressure chronic ulcer of unspecified part of unspecified lower leg with unspecified severity

L97.91 Non-pressure chronic ulcer of unspecified part of right lower leg

L97.911 Non-pressure chronic ulcer of unspecified part of right lower leg limited to breakdown of skin

L97.912 Non-pressure chronic ulcer of unspecified part of right lower leg with fat layer exposed

L97.913 Non-pressure chronic ulcer of unspecified part of right lower leg with necrosis of muscle

L97.914 Non-pressure chronic ulcer of unspecified part of right lower leg with necrosis of bone

L97.919 Non-pressure chronic ulcer of unspecified part of right lower leg with unspecified severity

L97.92 Non-pressure chronic ulcer of unspecified part of left lower leg

L97.921 Non-pressure chronic ulcer of unspecified part of left lower leg limited to breakdown of skin

● New code   ▲ Revised code   **Excludes1:** Not coded here   **Excludes2:** Not included here   ⊗ Placeholder required   ⑦ 7th digit required

L97.922 Non-pressure chronic ulcer of unspecified part of left lower leg with fat layer exposed

L97.923 Non-pressure chronic ulcer of unspecified part of left lower leg with necrosis of muscle

L97.924 Non-pressure chronic ulcer of unspecified part of left lower leg with necrosis of bone

L97.929 Non-pressure chronic ulcer of unspecified part of left lower leg with unspecified severity

L98 Other disorders of skin and subcutaneous tissue, not elsewhere classified

L98.0 Pyogenic granuloma

Excludes2: pyogenic granuloma of gingiva (K06.8)

pyogenic granuloma of maxillary alveolar ridge (K04.5)

pyogenic granuloma of oral mucosa (K13.4)

L98.1 Factitial dermatitis

Neurotic excoriation

Excludes1: Excoriation (skin-picking) disorder (F42.4)

L98.2 Febrile neutrophilic dermatosis [Sweet]

L98.3 Eosinophilic cellulitis [Wells]

L98.4 Non-pressure chronic ulcer of skin, not elsewhere classified

Chronic ulcer of skin NOS

Tropical ulcer NOS

Ulcer of skin NOS

Excludes2: pressure ulcer (pressure area) (L89.-)

gangrene (I96)

skin infections (L00-L08)

specific infections classified to A00-B99

ulcer of lower limb NEC (L97.-)

varicose ulcer (I83.0-I82.2)

L98.41 Non-pressure chronic ulcer of buttock

L98.411 Non-pressure chronic ulcer of buttock limited to breakdown of skin

L98.412 Non-pressure chronic ulcer of buttock with fat layer exposed

L98.413 Non-pressure chronic ulcer of buttock with necrosis of muscle

L98.414 Non-pressure chronic ulcer of buttock with necrosis of bone

L98.419 Non-pressure chronic ulcer of buttock with unspecified severity

L98.42 Non-pressure chronic ulcer of back

L98.421 Non-pressure chronic ulcer of back limited to breakdown of skin

L98.422 Non-pressure chronic ulcer of back with fat layer exposed

L98.423 Non-pressure chronic ulcer of back with necrosis of muscle

L98.424 Non-pressure chronic ulcer of back with necrosis of bone

L98.429 Non-pressure chronic ulcer of back with unspecified severity

L98.49 Non-pressure chronic ulcer of skin of other sites

Non-pressure chronic ulcer of skin NOS

L98.491 Non-pressure chronic ulcer of skin of other sites limited to breakdown of skin

L98.492 Non-pressure chronic ulcer of skin of other sites with fat layer exposed

L98.493 Non-pressure chronic ulcer of skin of other sites with necrosis of muscle

L98.494 Non-pressure chronic ulcer of skin of other sites with necrosis of bone

L98.499 Non-pressure chronic ulcer of skin of other sites with unspecified severity

L98.5 Mucinosis of the skin

Focal mucinosis

Lichen myxedematosus

Reticular erythematous mucinosis

Excludes1: focal oral mucinosis (K13.79)

myxedema (E03.9)

L98.6 Other infiltrative disorders of the skin and subcutaneous tissue

Excludes1: hyalinosis cutis et mucosae (E78.89)

•**L98.7** Excessive and redundant skin and subcutaneous tissue

Loose or sagging skin following bariatric surgery weight loss

Loose or sagging skin following dietary weight loss

Loose or sagging skin, NOS

Excludes2: acquired excess or redundant skin of eyelid (H02.3-)

congenital excess or redundant skin of eyelid (Q10.3)

skin changes due to chronic exposure to nonionizing radiation (L57.-)

L98.8 Other specified disorders of the skin and subcutaneous tissue

L98.9 Disorder of the skin and subcutaneous tissue, unspecified

L99 Other disorders of skin and subcutaneous tissue in diseases classified elsewhere

Code first underlying disease, such as:

amyloidosis (E85.-)

Excludes1: skin disorders in diabetes (E08-E13 with .62)

skin disorders in gonorrhea (A54.89)

skin disorders in syphilis (A51.31, A52.79)

● New code　▲ Revised code　Excludes1: Not coded here　Excludes2: Not included here　⊗ Placeholder required　⑦7th digit required

Chapter 13: Diseases Of The Musculoskeletal System And Connective Tissue (M00-M99)

DEFINITIONS

This chapter includes definitions of selected key words, terms and phrases and coding alerts for adding points to the clinical domain, and references to coding late effects where appropriate. An example from this chapter is as follows:

M05   Rheumatoid arthritis with rheumatoid factor
        Definition: Rheumatoid arthritis is a chronic, systemic inflammatory disorder that may affect many tissues and organs, but principally attacks the joints producing a inflammatory synovitis that often progresses to destruction of the articular cartilage and ankylosis of the joints.

MULTIPLE CODING FOR A SINGLE CONDITION

In addition to the etiology/manifestation convention that requires two codes to fully describe a single condition that affects multiple body systems, there are other single conditions that also require more than one code. "Use additional code" notes are found in the Tabular List at codes that are not part of an etiology/manifestation pair where a secondary code is useful to fully describe a condition. The sequencing rule is the same as the etiology/manifestation pair, "use additional code" indicates that a secondary code should be added.

For example, for bacterial infections that are not included in chapter 1, a secondary code from category B95, Streptococcus, Staphylococcus, and Enterococcus, as the cause of diseases classified elsewhere, or B96, Other bacterial agents as the cause of diseases classified elsewhere, may be required to identify the bacterial organism causing the infection. A "use additional code" note will normally be found at the infectious disease code, indicating a need for the organism code to be added as a secondary code.

"Code first" notes are also under certain codes that are not specifically manifestation codes but may be due to an underlying cause. When there is a "code first" note and an underlying condition is present, the underlying condition should be sequenced first.

"Code, if applicable, any causal condition first", notes indicate that this code may be assigned as a principal diagnosis when the causal condition is unknown or not applicable. If a causal condition is known, then the code for that condition should be sequenced as the principal or first-listed diagnosis.

Multiple codes may be needed for sequela, complication codes and obstetric codes to more fully describe a condition. See the specific guidelines for these conditions for further instruction.

COMBINATION CODE

A combination code is a single code used to classify: Two diagnoses, or a diagnosis with an associated secondary process (manifestation) A diagnosis with an associated complication

Combination codes are identified by referring to subterm entries in the Alphabetic Index and by reading the inclusion and exclusion notes in the Tabular List.

Assign only the combination code when that code fully identifies the diagnostic conditions involved or when the Alphabetic Index so directs. Multiple coding should not be used when the classification provides a combination code that clearly identifies all of the elements documented in the diagnosis. When the combination code lacks necessary specificity in describing the manifestation or complication, an additional code should be used as a secondary code.

SEQUELA (LATE EFFECTS)

A sequela is the residual effect (condition produced) after the acute phase of an illness or injury has terminated. There is no time limit on when a sequela code can be used. The residual may be apparent early, such as in cerebral infarction, or it may occur months or years later, such as that due to a previous injury. Coding of sequela generally requires two codes sequenced in the following order: The condition or nature of the sequela is sequenced first.

The sequela code is sequenced second.

An exception to the above guidelines are those instances where the code for the sequela is followed by a manifestation code identified in the Tabular List and title, or the sequela code has been expanded (at the fourth, fifth or sixth character levels) to include the manifestation(s). The code for the acute phase of an illness or injury that led to the sequela is never used with a code for the late effect.

SITE AND LATERALITY

Most of the codes within Chapter 13 have site and laterality designations. The site represents the bone, joint or the muscle involved. For some conditions where more than one bone, joint or muscle is usually involved, such as osteoarthritis, there is a "multiple sites" code available. For categories where no multiple site code is provided and more than one bone, joint or muscle is involved, multiple codes should be used to indicate the different sites involved.

1)   Bone versus joint

For certain conditions, the bone may be affected at the upper or lower end, (e.g., avascular necrosis of bone, M87, Osteoporosis, M80, M81). Though the portion of the bone affected may be at the joint, the site designation will be the bone, not the joint.

ACUTE TRAUMATIC VERSUS CHRONIC OR RECURRENT MUSCULOSKELETAL CONDITIONS

Many musculoskeletal conditions are a result of previous injury or trauma to a site, or are recurrent conditions. Bone, joint or muscle conditions that are the result of a healed injury are usually found in chapter 13. Recurrent bone, joint or muscle conditions are also usually found in chapter 13. Any current, acute injury should be coded to the appropriate injury code from chapter 19. Chronic or recurrent conditions should generally be coded with a code from chapter 13. If it is difficult to determine from the documentation in the record which code is best to describe a condition, query the provider.

CODING OF PATHOLOGIC FRACTURES

7th character A is for use as long as the patient is receiving active treatment for the fracture. While the patient may be seen by a new or different provider over the course of treatment for a pathological fracture, assignment of the 7th character is based on whether the patient is undergoing active treatment and not whether the provider is seeing the patient for the first time.

7th character D is to be used for encounters after the patient has completed active treatment. The other 7th characters, listed under each subcategory in the Tabular List, are to be used for subsequent encounters for routine care of fractures during the healing and recovery phase as well as treatment of problems associated with the healing, such as malunions, nonunions, and sequelae.

Care for complications of surgical treatment for fracture repairs during the healing or recovery phase should be coded with the appropriate complication codes.

See Section I.C.19. Coding of traumatic fractures.

OSTEOPOROSIS

Osteoporosis is a systemic condition, meaning that all bones of the musculoskeletal system are affected. Therefore, site is not a component of the codes under category M81, Osteoporosis without current pathological fracture. The site codes under category M80, Osteoporosis with current pathological fracture, identify the site of the fracture, not the osteoporosis.

1) **Osteoporosis without pathological fracture**

    Category M81, Osteoporosis without current pathological fracture, is for use for patients with osteoporosis who do not currently have a pathologic fracture due to the osteoporosis, even if they have had a fracture in the past. For patients with a history of osteoporosis fractures, status code Z87.310, Personal history of (healed) osteoporosis fracture, should follow the code from M81.

2) **Osteoporosis with current pathological fracture**

    Category M80, Osteoporosis with current pathological fracture, is for patients who have a current pathologic fracture at the time of an encounter. The codes under M80 identify the site of the fracture. A code from category M80, not a traumatic fracture code, should be used for any patient with known osteoporosis who suffers a fracture, even if the patient had a minor fall or trauma, if that fall or trauma would not usually break a normal, healthy bone.

● New code   ▲ Revised code   **Excludes1:** Not coded here   **Excludes2:** Not included here   ⊗ Placeholder required   ⑦7ᵗʰ digit required

Chapter 13

Diseases Of The Musculoskeletal System And Connective Tissue (M00-M99)

Note: Use an external cause code following the code for the musculoskeletal condition, if applicable, to identify the cause of the musculoskeletal condition

Excludes2: arthropathic psoriasis (L40.5-)

certain conditions originating in the perinatal period (P04-P96)

certain infectious and parasitic diseases (A00-B99)

compartment syndrome (traumatic) (T79.A-)

complications of pregnancy, childbirth and the puerperium (O00-O9A)

congenital malformations, deformations, and chromosomal abnormalities (Q00-Q99)

endocrine, nutritional and metabolic diseases (E00-E88)

injury, poisoning and certain other consequences of external causes (S00-T88)

neoplasms (C00-D49)

symptoms, signs and abnormal clinical and laboratory findings, not elsewhere classified (R00-R94)

This chapter contains the following blocks:

M00-M02	Infectious arthropathies
M04	Autoinflammatory syndromes
M05-M14	Inflammatory polyarthropathies
M15-M19	Osteoarthritis
M20-M25	Other joint disorders
M26-M27	Dentofacial anomalies [including malocclusion] and other disorders of jaw
M30-M36	Systemic connective tissue disorders
M40-M43	Deforming dorsopathies
M45-M49	Spondylopathies
M50-M54	Other dorsopathies
M60-M63	Disorders of muscles
M65-M67	Disorders of synovium and tendon
M70-M79	Other soft tissue disorders
M80-M85	Disorders of bone density and structure
M86-M90	Other osteopathies
M91-M94	Chondropathies
M95	Other disorders of the musculoskeletal system and connective tissue
M96	Intraoperative and postprocedural complications and disorders of musculoskeletal system, not elsewhere classified
M97	Periprosthetic fracture around internal prosthetic joint
M99	Biomechanical lesions, not elsewhere classified

ARTHROPATHIES (M00-M25)

Includes: Disorders affecting predominantly peripheral (limb) joints

INFECTIOUS ARTHROPATHIES (M00-M02)

Note: This block comprises arthropathies due to microbiological agents. Distinction is made between the following types of etiological relationship:

a) direct infection of joint, where organisms invade synovial tissue and microbial antigen is present in the joint; b) indirect infection, which may be of two types: a reactive arthropathy, where microbial infection of the body is established but neither organisms nor antigens can be identified in the joint, and a postinfective arthropathy, where microbial antigen is

present but recovery of an organism is inconstant and evidence of local multiplication is lacking.

M00 Pyogenic arthritis

    M00.0 Staphylococcal arthritis and polyarthritis

        Use additional code (B95.61-B95.8) to identify bacterial agent

        Excludes2: infection and inflammatory reaction due to internal joint prosthesis (T84.5-)

        M00.00 Staphylococcal arthritis, unspecified joint

        M00.01 Staphylococcal arthritis, shoulder

            M00.011 Staphylococcal arthritis, right shoulder

            M00.012 Staphylococcal arthritis, left shoulder

            M00.019 Staphylococcal arthritis, unspecified shoulder

        M00.02 Staphylococcal arthritis, elbow

            M00.021 Staphylococcal arthritis, right elbow

            M00.022 Staphylococcal arthritis, left elbow

            M00.029 Staphylococcal arthritis, unspecified elbow

        M00.03 Staphylococcal arthritis, wrist

        Staphylococcal arthritis of carpal bones

            M00.031 Staphylococcal arthritis, right wrist

            M00.032 Staphylococcal arthritis, left wrist

            M00.039 Staphylococcal arthritis, unspecified wrist

        M00.04 Staphylococcal arthritis, hand

        Staphylococcal arthritis of metacarpus and phalanges

            M00.041 Staphylococcal arthritis, right hand

            M00.042 Staphylococcal arthritis, left hand

            M00.049 Staphylococcal arthritis, unspecified hand

        M00.05 Staphylococcal arthritis, hip

            M00.051 Staphylococcal arthritis, right hip

            M00.052 Staphylococcal arthritis, left hip

            M00.059 Staphylococcal arthritis, unspecified hip

        M00.06 Staphylococcal arthritis, knee

            M00.061 Staphylococcal arthritis, right knee

            M00.062 Staphylococcal arthritis, left knee

            M00.069 Staphylococcal arthritis, unspecified knee

        M00.07 Staphylococcal arthritis, ankle and foot

        Staphylococcal arthritis, tarsus, metatarsus and phalanges

            M00.071 Staphylococcal arthritis, right ankle and foot

            M00.072 Staphylococcal arthritis, left ankle and foot

            M00.079 Staphylococcal arthritis, unspecified ankle and foot

        M00.08 Staphylococcal arthritis, vertebrae

        M00.09 Staphylococcal polyarthritis

    M00.1 Pneumococcal arthritis and polyarthritis

        M00.10 Pneumococcal arthritis, unspecified joint

M00.11   Pneumococcal arthritis, shoulder

    M00.111   Pneumococcal arthritis, right shoulder

    M00.112   Pneumococcal arthritis, left shoulder

    M00.119   Pneumococcal arthritis, unspecified shoulder

M00.12   Pneumococcal arthritis, elbow

    M00.121   Pneumococcal arthritis, right elbow

    M00.122   Pneumococcal arthritis, left elbow

    M00.129   Pneumococcal arthritis, unspecified elbow

M00.13   Pneumococcal arthritis, wrist

    Pneumococcal arthritis of carpal bones

    M00.131   Pneumococcal arthritis, right wrist

    M00.132   Pneumococcal arthritis, left wrist

    M00.139   Pneumococcal arthritis, unspecified wrist

M00.14   Pneumococcal arthritis, hand

    Pneumococcal arthritis of metacarpus and phalanges

    M00.141   Pneumococcal arthritis, right hand

    M00.142   Pneumococcal arthritis, left hand

    M00.149   Pneumococcal arthritis, unspecified hand

M00.15   Pneumococcal arthritis, hip

    M00.151   Pneumococcal arthritis, right hip

    M00.152   Pneumococcal arthritis, left hip

    M00.159   Pneumococcal arthritis, unspecified hip

M00.16   Pneumococcal arthritis, knee

    M00.161   Pneumococcal arthritis, right knee

    M00.162   Pneumococcal arthritis, left knee

    M00.169   Pneumococcal arthritis, unspecified knee

M00.17   Pneumococcal arthritis, ankle and foot

    Pneumococcal arthritis, tarsus, metatarsus and phalanges

    M00.171   Pneumococcal arthritis, right ankle and foot

    M00.172   Pneumococcal arthritis, left ankle and foot

    M00.179   Pneumococcal arthritis, unspecified ankle and foot

M00.18   Pneumococcal arthritis, vertebrae

M00.19   Pneumococcal polyarthritis

M00.2   Other streptococcal arthritis and polyarthritis

    <u>Use additional code</u> (B95.0-B95.2, B95.4-B95.5) to identify bacterial agent

M00.20   Other streptococcal arthritis, unspecified joint

M00.21   Other streptococcal arthritis, shoulder

    M00.211   Other streptococcal arthritis, right shoulder

    M00.212   Other streptococcal arthritis, left shoulder

    M00.219   Other streptococcal arthritis, unspecified shoulder

M00.22   Other streptococcal arthritis, elbow

    M00.221   Other streptococcal arthritis, right elbow

    M00.222   Other streptococcal arthritis, left elbow

    M00.229   Other streptococcal arthritis, unspecified elbow

M00.23   Other streptococcal arthritis, wrist

    Other streptococcal arthritis of carpal bones

    M00.231   Other streptococcal arthritis, right wrist

    M00.232   Other streptococcal arthritis, left wrist

    M00.239   Other streptococcal arthritis, unspecified wrist

M00.24   Other streptococcal arthritis, hand

    Other streptococcal arthritis metacarpus and phalanges

    M00.241   Other streptococcal arthritis, right hand

    M00.242   Other streptococcal arthritis, left hand

    M00.249   Other streptococcal arthritis, unspecified hand

M00.25   Other streptococcal arthritis, hip

    M00.251   Other streptococcal arthritis, right hip

    M00.252   Other streptococcal arthritis, left hip

    M00.259   Other streptococcal arthritis, unspecified hip

M00.26   Other streptococcal arthritis, knee

    M00.261   Other streptococcal arthritis, right knee

    M00.262   Other streptococcal arthritis, left knee

    M00.269   Other streptococcal arthritis, unspecified knee

M00.27   Other streptococcal arthritis, ankle and foot

    Other streptococcal arthritis, tarsus, metatarsus and phalanges

    M00.271   Other streptococcal arthritis, right ankle and foot

    M00.272   Other streptococcal arthritis, left ankle and foot

    M00.279   Other streptococcal arthritis, unspecified ankle and foot

M00.28   Other streptococcal arthritis, vertebrae

M00.29   Other streptococcal polyarthritis

M00.8   Arthritis and polyarthritis due to other bacteria

    <u>Use additional code</u> (B96) to identify bacteria

M00.80   Arthritis due to other bacteria, unspecified joint

M00.81   Arthritis due to other bacteria, shoulder

    M00.811   Arthritis due to other bacteria, right shoulder

    M00.812   Arthritis due to other bacteria, left shoulder

    M00.819   Arthritis due to other bacteria, unspecified shoulder

M00.82   Arthritis due to other bacteria, elbow

● New code   ▲ Revised code   **Excludes1:** Not coded here   **Excludes2:** Not included here   ⊗ Placeholder required   ⑦7th digit required

M00.821 **Arthritis due to other bacteria, right elbow**

M00.822 **Arthritis due to other bacteria, left elbow**

M00.829 **Arthritis due to other bacteria, unspecified elbow**

M00.83 **Arthritis due to other bacteria, wrist**

Arthritis due to other bacteria, carpal bones

M00.831 **Arthritis due to other bacteria, right wrist**

M00.832 **Arthritis due to other bacteria, left wrist**

M00.839 **Arthritis due to other bacteria, unspecified wrist**

M00.84 **Arthritis due to other bacteria, hand**

Arthritis due to other bacteria, metacarpus and phalanges

M00.841 **Arthritis due to other bacteria, right hand**

M00.842 **Arthritis due to other bacteria, left hand**

M00.849 **Arthritis due to other bacteria, unspecified hand**

M00.85 **Arthritis due to other bacteria, hip**

M00.851 **Arthritis due to other bacteria, right hip**

M00.852 **Arthritis due to other bacteria, left hip**

M00.859 **Arthritis due to other bacteria, unspecified hip**

M00.86 **Arthritis due to other bacteria, knee**

M00.861 **Arthritis due to other bacteria, right knee**

M00.862 **Arthritis due to other bacteria, left knee**

M00.869 **Arthritis due to other bacteria, unspecified knee**

M00.87 **Arthritis due to other bacteria, ankle and foot**

Arthritis due to other bacteria, tarsus, metatarsus, and phalanges

M00.871 **Arthritis due to other bacteria, right ankle and foot**

M00.872 **Arthritis due to other bacteria, left ankle and foot**

M00.879 **Arthritis due to other bacteria, unspecified ankle and foot**

M00.88 **Arthritis due to other bacteria, vertebrae**

M00.89 **Polyarthritis due to other bacteria**

M00.9 **Pyogenic arthritis, unspecified**

Infective arthritis NOS

M01 **Direct infections of joint in infectious and parasitic diseases classified elsewhere**

Code first underlying disease, such as:

leprosy [Hansen's disease] (A30.-)

mycoses (B35-B49)

O'nyong-nyong fever (A92.1)

paratyphoid fever (A01.1-A01.4)

Excludes1: arthropathy in Lyme disease (A69.23)

gonococcal arthritis (A54.42)

meningococcal arthritis (A39.83)

mumps arthritis (B26.85)

postinfective arthropathy (M02.-)

postmeningococcal arthritis (A39.84)

reactive arthritis (M02.3)

rubella arthritis (B06.82)

sarcoidosis arthritis (D86.86)

typhoid fever arthritis (A01.04)

tuberculosis arthritis (A18.01-A18.02)

M01.X **Direct infection of joint in infectious and parasitic diseases classified elsewhere**

M01.X0 **Direct infection of unspecified joint in infectious and parasitic diseases classified elsewhere**

M01.X1 **Direct infection of shoulder joint in infectious and parasitic diseases classified elsewhere**

M01.X11 **Direct infection of right shoulder in infectious and parasitic diseases classified elsewhere**

M01.X12 **Direct infection of left shoulder in infectious and parasitic diseases classified elsewhere**

M01.X19 **Direct infection of unspecified shoulder in infectious and parasitic diseases classified elsewhere**

M01.X2 **Direct infection of elbow in infectious and parasitic diseases classified elsewhere**

M01.X21 **Direct infection of right elbow in infectious and parasitic diseases classified elsewhere**

M01.X22 **Direct infection of left elbow in infectious and parasitic diseases classified elsewhere**

M01.X29 **Direct infection of unspecified elbow in infectious and parasitic diseases classified elsewhere**

M01.X3 **Direct infection of wrist in infectious and parasitic diseases classified elsewhere**

Direct infection of carpal bones in infectious and parasitic diseases classified elsewhere

M01.X31 **Direct infection of right wrist in infectious and parasitic diseases classified elsewhere**

M01.X32 **Direct infection of left wrist in infectious and parasitic diseases classified elsewhere**

M01.X39 **Direct infection of unspecified wrist in infectious and parasitic diseases classified elsewhere**

M01.X4 **Direct infection of hand in infectious and parasitic diseases classified elsewhere**

Direct infection of metacarpus and phalanges in infectious and parasitic diseases classified elsewhere

M01.X41 **Direct infection of right hand in infectious and parasitic diseases classified elsewhere**

M01.X42 **Direct infection of left hand in infectious and parasitic diseases classified elsewhere**

M01.X49   Direct infection of unspecified hand in infectious and parasitic diseases classified elsewhere

M01.X5   **Direct infection of hip in infectious and parasitic diseases classified elsewhere**

M01.X51   Direct infection of right hip in infectious and parasitic diseases classified elsewhere

M01.X52   Direct infection of left hip in infectious and parasitic diseases classified elsewhere

M01.X59   Direct infection of unspecified hip in infectious and parasitic diseases classified elsewhere

M01.X6   **Direct infection of knee in infectious and parasitic diseases classified elsewhere**

M01.X61   Direct infection of right knee in infectious and parasitic diseases classified elsewhere

M01.X62   Direct infection of left knee in infectious and parasitic diseases classified elsewhere

M01.X69   Direct infection of unspecified knee in infectious and parasitic diseases classified elsewhere

M01.X7   **Direct infection of ankle and foot in infectious and parasitic diseases classified elsewhere**

Direct infection of tarsus, metatarsus and phalanges in infectious and parasitic diseases classified elsewhere

M01.X71   Direct infection of right ankle and foot in infectious and parasitic diseases classified elsewhere

M01.X72   Direct infection of left ankle and foot in infectious and parasitic diseases classified elsewhere

M01.X79   Direct infection of unspecified ankle and foot in infectious and parasitic diseases

classified elsewhere

M01.X8   **Direct infection of vertebrae in infectious and parasitic diseases classified elsewhere**

M01.X9   **Direct infection of multiple joints in infectious and parasitic diseases classified elsewhere**

M02   **Postinfective and reactive arthropathies**

Code first underlying disease, such as:

congenital syphilis [Clutton's joints] (A50.5) enteritis due to Yersinia enterocolitica (A04.6)

infective endocarditis (I33.0)

viral hepatitis (B15-B19)

Excludes1: Behçet's disease (M35.2)

direct infections of joint in infectious and parasitic diseases classified elsewhere (M01.-)

postmeningococcal arthritis (A39.84)

mumps arthritis (B26.85)

rubella arthritis (B06.82)

syphilis arthritis (late) (A52.77)

rheumatic fever (I00)

tabetic arthropathy [Charcôt's] (A52.16)

M02.0   **Arthropathy following intestinal bypass**

M02.00   Arthropathy following intestinal bypass, unspecified site

M02.01   Arthropathy following intestinal bypass, shoulder

M02.011   Arthropathy following intestinal bypass, right shoulder

M02.012   Arthropathy following intestinal bypass, left shoulder

M02.019   Arthropathy following intestinal bypass, unspecified shoulder

M02.02   Arthropathy following intestinal bypass, elbow

M02.021   Arthropathy following intestinal bypass, right elbow

M02.022   Arthropathy following intestinal bypass, left elbow

M02.029   Arthropathy following intestinal bypass, unspecified elbow

M02.03   Arthropathy following intestinal bypass, wrist

Arthropathy following intestinal bypass, carpal bones

M02.031   Arthropathy following intestinal bypass, right wrist

M02.032   Arthropathy following intestinal bypass, left wrist

M02.039   Arthropathy following intestinal bypass, unspecified wrist

M02.04   Arthropathy following intestinal bypass, hand

Arthropathy following intestinal bypass, metacarpals and phalanges

M02.041   Arthropathy following intestinal bypass, right hand

M02.042   Arthropathy following intestinal bypass, left hand

M02.049   Arthropathy following intestinal bypass, unspecified hand

M02.05   Arthropathy following intestinal bypass, hip

M02.051   Arthropathy following intestinal bypass, right hip

M02.052   Arthropathy following intestinal bypass, left hip

M02.059   Arthropathy following intestinal bypass, unspecified hip

M02.06   Arthropathy following intestinal bypass, knee

M02.061   Arthropathy following intestinal bypass, right knee

M02.062   Arthropathy following intestinal bypass, left knee

M02.069   Arthropathy following intestinal bypass, unspecified knee

M02.07   Arthropathy following intestinal bypass, ankle and foot

Arthropathy following intestinal bypass, tarsus, metatarsus and phalanges

M02.071   Arthropathy following intestinal bypass, right ankle and foot

M02.072   Arthropathy following intestinal bypass, left ankle and foot

M02.079   Arthropathy following intestinal bypass, unspecified ankle and foot

M02.08   Arthropathy following intestinal bypass, vertebrae

M02.09 Arthropathy following intestinal bypass, multiple sites

M02.1 Postdysenteric arthropathy

  M02.10 Postdysenteric arthropathy, unspecified site

  M02.11 Postdysenteric arthropathy, shoulder

    M02.111 Postdysenteric arthropathy, right shoulder

    M02.112 Postdysenteric arthropathy, left shoulder

    M02.119 Postdysenteric arthropathy, unspecified shoulder

  M02.12 Postdysenteric arthropathy, elbow

    M02.121 Postdysenteric arthropathy, right elbow

    M02.122 Postdysenteric arthropathy, left elbow

    M02.129 Postdysenteric arthropathy, unspecified elbow

  M02.13 Postdysenteric arthropathy, wrist

    Postdysenteric arthropathy, carpal bones

    M02.131 Postdysenteric arthropathy, right wrist

    M02.132 Postdysenteric arthropathy, left wrist

    M02.139 Postdysenteric arthropathy, unspecified wrist

  M02.14 Postdysenteric arthropathy, hand

    Postdysenteric arthropathy, metacarpus and phalanges

    M02.141 Postdysenteric arthropathy, right hand

    M02.142 Postdysenteric arthropathy, left hand

    M02.149 Postdysenteric arthropathy, unspecified hand

  M02.15 Postdysenteric arthropathy, hip

    M02.151 Postdysenteric arthropathy, right hip

    M02.152 Postdysenteric arthropathy, left hip

    M02.159 Postdysenteric arthropathy, unspecified hip

  M02.16 Postdysenteric arthropathy, knee

    M02.161 Postdysenteric arthropathy, right knee

    M02.162 Postdysenteric arthropathy, left knee

    M02.169 Postdysenteric arthropathy, unspecified knee

  M02.17 Postdysenteric arthropathy, ankle and foot

    Postdysenteric arthropathy, tarsus, metatarsus and phalanges

    M02.171 Postdysenteric arthropathy, right ankle and foot

    M02.172 Postdysenteric arthropathy, left ankle and foot

    M02.179 Postdysenteric arthropathy, unspecified ankle and foot

  M02.18 Postdysenteric arthropathy, vertebrae

  M02.19 Postdysenteric arthropathy, multiple sites

M02.2 Postimmunization arthropathy

  M02.20 Postimmunization arthropathy, unspecified site

  M02.21 Postimmunization arthropathy, shoulder

    M02.211 Postimmunization arthropathy, right shoulder

    M02.212 Postimmunization arthropathy, left shoulder

    M02.219 Postimmunization arthropathy, unspecified shoulder

  M02.22 Postimmunization arthropathy, elbow

    M02.221 Postimmunization arthropathy, right elbow

    M02.222 Postimmunization arthropathy, left elbow

    M02.229 Postimmunization arthropathy, unspecified elbow

  M02.23 Postimmunization arthropathy, wrist

    Postimmunization arthropathy, carpal bones

    M02.231 Postimmunization arthropathy, right wrist

    M02.232 Postimmunization arthropathy, left wrist

    M02.239 Postimmunization arthropathy, unspecified wrist

  M02.24 Postimmunization arthropathy, hand

    Postimmunization arthropathy, metacarpus and phalanges

    M02.241 Postimmunization arthropathy, right hand

    M02.242 Postimmunization arthropathy, left hand

    M02.249 Postimmunization arthropathy, unspecified hand

  M02.25 Postimmunization arthropathy, hip

    M02.251 Postimmunization arthropathy, right hip

    M02.252 Postimmunization arthropathy, left hip

    M02.259 Postimmunization arthropathy, unspecified hip

  M02.26 Postimmunization arthropathy, knee

    M02.261 Postimmunization arthropathy, right knee

    M02.262 Postimmunization arthropathy, left knee

    M02.269 Postimmunization arthropathy, unspecified knee

  M02.27 Postimmunization arthropathy, ankle and foot

    Postimmunization arthropathy, tarsus, metatarsus and phalanges

    M02.271 Postimmunization arthropathy, right ankle and foot

    M02.272 Postimmunization arthropathy, left ankle and foot

    M02.279 Postimmunization arthropathy, unspecified ankle and foot

  M02.28 Postimmunization arthropathy, vertebrae

  M02.29 Postimmunization arthropathy, multiple sites

M02.3 Reiter's disease

Reactive arthritis

M02.30 Reiter's disease, unspecified site

M02.31 Reiter's disease, shoulder

　　　M02.311 Reiter's disease, right shoulder

　　　M02.312 Reiter's disease, left shoulder

　　　M02.319 Reiter's disease, unspecified shoulder

M02.32 Reiter's disease, elbow

　　　M02.321 Reiter's disease, right elbow

　　　M02.322 Reiter's disease, left elbow

　　　M02.329 Reiter's disease, unspecified elbow

M02.33 Reiter's disease, wrist

　　Reiter's disease, carpal bones

　　　M02.331 Reiter's disease, right wrist

　　　M02.332 Reiter's disease, left wrist

　　　M02.339 Reiter's disease, unspecified wrist

M02.34 Reiter's disease, hand

　　Reiter's disease, metacarpus and phalanges

　　　M02.341 Reiter's disease, right hand

　　　M02.342 Reiter's disease, left hand

　　　M02.349 Reiter's disease, unspecified hand

M02.35 Reiter's disease, hip

　　　M02.351 Reiter's disease, right hip

　　　M02.352 Reiter's disease, left hip

　　　M02.359 Reiter's disease, unspecified hip

M02.36 Reiter's disease, knee

　　　M02.361 Reiter's disease, right knee

　　　M02.362 Reiter's disease, left knee

　　　M02.369 Reiter's disease, unspecified knee

M02.37 Reiter's disease, ankle and foot

　　Reiter's disease, tarsus, metatarsus and phalanges

　　　M02.371 Reiter's disease, right ankle and foot

　　　M02.372 Reiter's disease, left ankle and foot

　　　M02.379 Reiter's disease, unspecified ankle and foot

M02.38 Reiter's disease, vertebrae

M02.39 Reiter's disease, multiple sites

M02.8 Other reactive arthropathies

M02.80 Other reactive arthropathies, unspecified site

M02.81 Other reactive arthropathies, shoulder

　　　M02.811 Other reactive arthropathies, right shoulder

　　　M02.812 Other reactive arthropathies, left shoulder

　　　M02.819 Other reactive arthropathies, unspecified shoulder

M02.82 Other reactive arthropathies, elbow

　　　M02.821 Other reactive arthropathies, right elbow

　　　M02.822 Other reactive arthropathies, left elbow

　　　M02.829 Other reactive arthropathies, unspecified elbow

M02.83 Other reactive arthropathies, wrist

　　Other reactive arthropathies, carpal bones

　　　M02.831 Other reactive arthropathies, right wrist

　　　M02.832 Other reactive arthropathies, left wrist

　　　M02.839 Other reactive arthropathies, unspecified wrist

M02.84 Other reactive arthropathies, hand

　　Other reactive arthropathies, metacarpus and phalanges

　　　M02.841 Other reactive arthropathies, right hand

　　　M02.842 Other reactive arthropathies, left hand

　　　M02.849 Other reactive arthropathies, unspecified hand

M02.85 Other reactive arthropathies, hip

　　　M02.851 Other reactive arthropathies, right hip

　　　M02.852 Other reactive arthropathies, left hip

　　　M02.859 Other reactive arthropathies, unspecified hip

M02.86 Other reactive arthropathies, knee

　　　M02.861 Other reactive arthropathies, right knee

　　　M02.862 Other reactive arthropathies, left knee

　　　M02.869 Other reactive arthropathies, unspecified knee

M02.87 Other reactive arthropathies, ankle and foot

　　Other reactive arthropathies, tarsus, metatarsus and phalanges

　　　M02.871 Other reactive arthropathies, right ankle and foot

　　　M02.872 Other reactive arthropathies, left ankle and foot

　　　M02.879 Other reactive arthropathies, unspecified ankle and foot

M02.88 Other reactive arthropathies, vertebrae

M02.89 Other reactive arthropathies, multiple sites

M02.9 Reactive arthropathy, unspecified

AUTOINFLAMMATORY SYNDROMES (M04)

M04 **Autoinflammatory syndromes**

　　Excludes2: Crohn's disease (K50.-)

●**M04.1** **Periodic fever syndromes**

　　Familial Mediterranean fever

　　Hyperimmunoglobin D syndrome

　　Mevalonate kinase deficiency

　　Tumor necrosis factor receptor associated periodic syndrome [TRAPS]

●**M04.2** **Cryopyrin-associated periodic syndromes**

　　Chronic infantile neurological, cutaneous and articular syndrome [CINCA]

　　Familial cold autoinflammatory syndrome

　　Familial cold urticaria

　　Muckle-Wells syndrome

　　Neonatal onset multisystemic inflammatory disorder [NOMID]

• **M04.8** **Other autoinflammatory syndromes**

Blau syndrome

Deficiency of interleukin 1 receptor antagonist [DIRA]

Majeed syndrome

Periodic fever, aphthous stomatitis, pharyngitis, and adenopathy syndrome [PFAPA]

Pyogenic arthritis, pyoderma gangrenosum, and acne syndrome [PAPA]

• **M04.9** **Autoinflammatory syndrome, unspecified**

INFLAMMATORY POLYARTHROPATHIES (M05-M14)

M05 **Rheumatoid arthritis with rheumatoid factor**

Definition: Rheumatoid arthritis is a chronic, systemic inflammatory disorder that may affect many tissues and organs, but principally attacks the joints producing a inflammatory synovitis that often progresses to destruction of the articular cartilage and ankylosis of the joints.

Excludes1: rheumatic fever (I00)

juvenile rheumatoid arthritis (M08.-)

rheumatoid arthritis of spine (M45.-)

M05.0 **Felty's syndrome**

Rheumatoid arthritis with splenoadenomegaly and leukopenia

M05.00 **Felty's syndrome, unspecified site**

M05.01 **Felty's syndrome, shoulder**

M05.011 **Felty's syndrome, right shoulder**

M05.012 **Felty's syndrome, left shoulder**

M05.019 **Felty's syndrome, unspecified shoulder**

M05.02 **Felty's syndrome, elbow**

M05.021 **Felty's syndrome, right elbow**

M05.022 **Felty's syndrome, left elbow**

M05.029 **Felty's syndrome, unspecified elbow**

M05.03 **Felty's syndrome, wrist**

Felty's syndrome, carpal bones

M05.031 **Felty's syndrome, right wrist**

M05.032 **Felty's syndrome, left wrist**

M05.039 **Felty's syndrome, unspecified wrist**

M05.04 **Felty's syndrome, hand**

Felty's syndrome, metacarpus and phalanges

M05.041 **Felty's syndrome, right hand**

M05.042 **Felty's syndrome, left hand**

M05.049 **Felty's syndrome, unspecified hand**

M05.05 **Felty's syndrome, hip**

M05.051 **Felty's syndrome, right hip**

M05.052 **Felty's syndrome, left hip**

M05.059 **Felty's syndrome, unspecified hip**

M05.06 **Felty's syndrome, knee**

M05.061 **Felty's syndrome, right knee**

M05.062 **Felty's syndrome, left knee**

M05.069 **Felty's syndrome, unspecified knee**

M05.07 **Felty's syndrome, ankle and foot**

Felty's syndrome, tarsus, metatarsus and phalanges

M05.071 **Felty's syndrome, right ankle and foot**

M05.072 **Felty's syndrome, left ankle and foot**

M05.079 **Felty's syndrome, unspecified ankle and foot**

M05.09 **Felty's syndrome, multiple sites**

M05.1 **Rheumatoid lung disease with rheumatoid arthritis**

M05.10 **Rheumatoid lung disease with rheumatoid arthritis of unspecified site**

M05.11 **Rheumatoid lung disease with rheumatoid arthritis of shoulder**

M05.111 **Rheumatoid lung disease with rheumatoid arthritis of right shoulder**

M05.112 **Rheumatoid lung disease with rheumatoid arthritis of left shoulder**

M05.119 **Rheumatoid lung disease with rheumatoid arthritis of unspecified shoulder**

M05.12 **Rheumatoid lung disease with rheumatoid arthritis of elbow**

M05.121 **Rheumatoid lung disease with rheumatoid arthritis of right elbow**

M05.122 **Rheumatoid lung disease with rheumatoid arthritis of left elbow**

M05.129 **Rheumatoid lung disease with rheumatoid arthritis of unspecified elbow**

M05.13 **Rheumatoid lung disease with rheumatoid arthritis of wrist**

Rheumatoid lung disease with rheumatoid arthritis, carpal bones

M05.131 **Rheumatoid lung disease with rheumatoid arthritis of right wrist**

M05.132 **Rheumatoid lung disease with rheumatoid arthritis of left wrist**

M05.139 **Rheumatoid lung disease with rheumatoid arthritis of unspecified wrist**

M05.14 **Rheumatoid lung disease with rheumatoid arthritis of hand**

Rheumatoid lung disease with rheumatoid arthritis, metacarpus and phalanges

M05.141 **Rheumatoid lung disease with rheumatoid arthritis of right hand**

M05.142 **Rheumatoid lung disease with rheumatoid arthritis of left hand**

M05.149 **Rheumatoid lung disease with rheumatoid arthritis of unspecified hand**

M05.15 **Rheumatoid lung disease with rheumatoid arthritis of hip**

M05.151 **Rheumatoid lung disease with rheumatoid arthritis of right hip**

M05.152 **Rheumatoid lung disease with rheumatoid arthritis of left hip**

M05.159 **Rheumatoid lung disease with rheumatoid arthritis of unspecified hip**

M05.16 **Rheumatoid lung disease with rheumatoid arthritis of knee**

M05.161 **Rheumatoid lung disease with rheumatoid arthritis of right knee**

M05.162   Rheumatoid lung disease with rheumatoid arthritis of left knee

M05.169   Rheumatoid lung disease with rheumatoid arthritis of unspecified knee

M05.17   Rheumatoid lung disease with rheumatoid arthritis of ankle and foot

Rheumatoid lung disease with rheumatoid arthritis, tarsus, metatarsus and phalanges

M05.171   Rheumatoid lung disease with rheumatoid arthritis of right ankle and foot

M05.172   Rheumatoid lung disease with rheumatoid arthritis of left ankle and foot

M05.179   Rheumatoid lung disease with rheumatoid arthritis of unspecified ankle and foot

M05.19   Rheumatoid lung disease with rheumatoid arthritis of multiple sites

M05.2   Rheumatoid vasculitis with rheumatoid arthritis

M05.20   Rheumatoid vasculitis with rheumatoid arthritis of unspecified site

M05.21   Rheumatoid vasculitis with rheumatoid arthritis of shoulder

M05.211   Rheumatoid vasculitis with rheumatoid arthritis of right shoulder

M05.212   Rheumatoid vasculitis with rheumatoid arthritis of left shoulder

M05.219   Rheumatoid vasculitis with rheumatoid arthritis of unspecified shoulder

M05.22   Rheumatoid vasculitis with rheumatoid arthritis of elbow

M05.221   Rheumatoid vasculitis with rheumatoid arthritis of right elbow

M05.222   Rheumatoid vasculitis with rheumatoid arthritis of left elbow

M05.229   Rheumatoid vasculitis with rheumatoid arthritis of unspecified elbow

M05.23   Rheumatoid vasculitis with rheumatoid arthritis of wrist

Rheumatoid vasculitis with rheumatoid arthritis, carpal bones

M05.231   Rheumatoid vasculitis with rheumatoid arthritis of right wrist

M05.232   Rheumatoid vasculitis with rheumatoid arthritis of left wrist

M05.239   Rheumatoid vasculitis with rheumatoid arthritis of unspecified wrist

M05.24   Rheumatoid vasculitis with rheumatoid arthritis of hand

Rheumatoid vasculitis with rheumatoid arthritis, metacarpus and phalanges

M05.241   Rheumatoid vasculitis with rheumatoid arthritis of right hand

M05.242   Rheumatoid vasculitis with rheumatoid arthritis of left hand

M05.249   Rheumatoid vasculitis with rheumatoid arthritis of unspecified hand

M05.25   Rheumatoid vasculitis with rheumatoid arthritis of hip

M05.251   Rheumatoid vasculitis with rheumatoid arthritis of right hip

M05.252   Rheumatoid vasculitis with rheumatoid arthritis of left hip

M05.259   Rheumatoid vasculitis with rheumatoid arthritis of unspecified hip

M05.26   Rheumatoid vasculitis with rheumatoid arthritis of knee

M05.261   Rheumatoid vasculitis with rheumatoid arthritis of right knee

M05.262   Rheumatoid vasculitis with rheumatoid arthritis of left knee

M05.269   Rheumatoid vasculitis with rheumatoid arthritis of unspecified knee

M05.27   Rheumatoid vasculitis with rheumatoid arthritis of ankle and foot

Rheumatoid vasculitis with rheumatoid arthritis, tarsus, metatarsus and phalanges

M05.271   Rheumatoid vasculitis with rheumatoid arthritis of right ankle and foot

M05.272   Rheumatoid vasculitis with rheumatoid arthritis of left ankle and foot

M05.279   Rheumatoid vasculitis with rheumatoid arthritis of unspecified ankle and foot

M05.29   Rheumatoid vasculitis with rheumatoid arthritis of multiple sites

M05.3   Rheumatoid heart disease with rheumatoid arthritis

Rheumatoid carditis

Rheumatoid endocarditis

Rheumatoid myocarditis

Rheumatoid pericarditis

M05.30   Rheumatoid heart disease with rheumatoid arthritis of unspecified site

M05.31   Rheumatoid heart disease with rheumatoid arthritis of shoulder

M05.311   Rheumatoid heart disease with rheumatoid arthritis of right shoulder

M05.312   Rheumatoid heart disease with rheumatoid arthritis of left shoulder

M05.319   Rheumatoid heart disease with rheumatoid arthritis of unspecified shoulder

M05.32   Rheumatoid heart disease with rheumatoid arthritis of elbow

M05.321   Rheumatoid heart disease with rheumatoid arthritis of right elbow

M05.322   Rheumatoid heart disease with rheumatoid arthritis of left elbow

M05.329   Rheumatoid heart disease with rheumatoid arthritis of unspecified elbow

M05.33   **Rheumatoid heart disease with rheumatoid arthritis of wrist**

Rheumatoid heart disease with rheumatoid arthritis, carpal bones

   M05.331   **Rheumatoid heart disease with rheumatoid arthritis of right wrist**

   M05.332   **Rheumatoid heart disease with rheumatoid arthritis of left wrist**

   M05.339   **Rheumatoid heart disease with rheumatoid arthritis of unspecified wrist**

M05.34   **Rheumatoid heart disease with rheumatoid arthritis of hand**

Rheumatoid heart disease with rheumatoid arthritis, metacarpus and phalanges

   M05.341   **Rheumatoid heart disease with rheumatoid arthritis of right hand**

   M05.342   **Rheumatoid heart disease with rheumatoid arthritis of left hand**

   M05.349   **Rheumatoid heart disease with rheumatoid arthritis of unspecified hand**

M05.35   **Rheumatoid heart disease with rheumatoid arthritis of hip**

   M05.351   **Rheumatoid heart disease with rheumatoid arthritis of right hip**

   M05.352   **Rheumatoid heart disease with rheumatoid arthritis of left hip**

   M05.359   **Rheumatoid heart disease with rheumatoid arthritis of unspecified hip**

M05.36   **Rheumatoid heart disease with rheumatoid arthritis of knee**

   M05.361   **Rheumatoid heart disease with rheumatoid arthritis of right knee**

   M05.362   **Rheumatoid heart disease with rheumatoid arthritis of left knee**

   M05.369   **Rheumatoid heart disease with rheumatoid arthritis of unspecified knee**

M05.37   **Rheumatoid heart disease with rheumatoid arthritis of ankle and foot**

Rheumatoid heart disease with rheumatoid arthritis, tarsus, metatarsus and phalanges

   M05.371   **Rheumatoid heart disease with rheumatoid arthritis of right ankle and foot**

   M05.372   **Rheumatoid heart disease with rheumatoid arthritis of left ankle and foot**

   M05.379   **Rheumatoid heart disease with rheumatoid arthritis of unspecified ankle and foot**

M05.39   **Rheumatoid heart disease with rheumatoid arthritis of multiple sites**

M05.4   **Rheumatoid myopathy with rheumatoid arthritis**

M05.40   **Rheumatoid myopathy with rheumatoid arthritis of unspecified site**

M05.41   **Rheumatoid myopathy with rheumatoid arthritis of shoulder**

   M05.411   **Rheumatoid myopathy with rheumatoid arthritis of right shoulder**

   M05.412   **Rheumatoid myopathy with rheumatoid arthritis of left shoulder**

   M05.419   **Rheumatoid myopathy with rheumatoid arthritis of unspecified shoulder**

M05.42   **Rheumatoid myopathy with rheumatoid arthritis of elbow**

   M05.421   **Rheumatoid myopathy with rheumatoid arthritis of right elbow**

   M05.422   **Rheumatoid myopathy with rheumatoid arthritis of left elbow**

   M05.429   **Rheumatoid myopathy with rheumatoid arthritis of unspecified elbow**

M05.43   **Rheumatoid myopathy with rheumatoid arthritis of wrist**

Rheumatoid myopathy with rheumatoid arthritis, carpal bones

   M05.431   **Rheumatoid myopathy with rheumatoid arthritis of right wrist**

   M05.432   **Rheumatoid myopathy with rheumatoid arthritis of left wrist**

   M05.439   **Rheumatoid myopathy with rheumatoid arthritis of unspecified wrist**

M05.44   **Rheumatoid myopathy with rheumatoid arthritis of hand**

Rheumatoid myopathy with rheumatoid arthritis, metacarpus and phalanges

   M05.441   **Rheumatoid myopathy with rheumatoid arthritis of right hand**

   M05.442   **Rheumatoid myopathy with rheumatoid arthritis of left hand**

   M05.449   **Rheumatoid myopathy with rheumatoid arthritis of unspecified hand**

M05.45   **Rheumatoid myopathy with rheumatoid arthritis of hip**

   M05.451   **Rheumatoid myopathy with rheumatoid arthritis of right hip**

   M05.452   **Rheumatoid myopathy with rheumatoid arthritis of left hip**

   M05.459   **Rheumatoid myopathy with rheumatoid arthritis of unspecified hip**

M05.46   **Rheumatoid myopathy with rheumatoid arthritis of knee**

   M05.461   **Rheumatoid myopathy with rheumatoid arthritis of right knee**

   M05.462   **Rheumatoid myopathy with rheumatoid arthritis of left knee**

   M05.469   **Rheumatoid myopathy with rheumatoid arthritis of unspecified knee**

M05.47   **Rheumatoid myopathy with rheumatoid arthritis of ankle and foot**

Rheumatoid myopathy with rheumatoid arthritis, tarsus, metatarsus and phalanges

M05.471 Rheumatoid myopathy with rheumatoid arthritis of right ankle and foot

M05.472 Rheumatoid myopathy with rheumatoid arthritis of left ankle and foot

M05.479 Rheumatoid myopathy with rheumatoid arthritis of unspecified ankle and foot

M05.49 Rheumatoid myopathy with rheumatoid arthritis of multiple sites

M05.5 Rheumatoid polyneuropathy with rheumatoid arthritis

M05.50 Rheumatoid polyneuropathy with rheumatoid arthritis of unspecified site

M05.51 Rheumatoid polyneuropathy with rheumatoid arthritis of shoulder

M05.511 Rheumatoid polyneuropathy with rheumatoid arthritis of right shoulder

M05.512 Rheumatoid polyneuropathy with rheumatoid arthritis of left shoulder

M05.519 Rheumatoid polyneuropathy with rheumatoid arthritis of unspecified shoulder

M05.52 Rheumatoid polyneuropathy with rheumatoid arthritis of elbow

M05.521 Rheumatoid polyneuropathy with rheumatoid arthritis of right elbow

M05.522 Rheumatoid polyneuropathy with rheumatoid arthritis of left elbow

M05.529 Rheumatoid polyneuropathy with rheumatoid arthritis of unspecified elbow

M05.53 Rheumatoid polyneuropathy with rheumatoid arthritis of wrist

Rheumatoid polyneuropathy with rheumatoid arthritis, carpal bones

M05.531 Rheumatoid polyneuropathy with rheumatoid arthritis of right wrist

M05.532 Rheumatoid polyneuropathy with rheumatoid arthritis of left wrist

M05.539 Rheumatoid polyneuropathy with rheumatoid arthritis of unspecified wrist

M05.54 Rheumatoid polyneuropathy with rheumatoid arthritis of hand

Rheumatoid polyneuropathy with rheumatoid arthritis, metacarpus and phalanges

M05.541 Rheumatoid polyneuropathy with rheumatoid arthritis of right hand

M05.542 Rheumatoid polyneuropathy with rheumatoid arthritis of left hand

M05.549 Rheumatoid polyneuropathy with rheumatoid arthritis of unspecified hand

M05.55 Rheumatoid polyneuropathy with rheumatoid arthritis of hip

M05.551 Rheumatoid polyneuropathy with rheumatoid arthritis of right hip

M05.552 Rheumatoid polyneuropathy with rheumatoid arthritis of left hip

M05.559 Rheumatoid polyneuropathy with rheumatoid arthritis of unspecified hip

M05.56 Rheumatoid polyneuropathy with rheumatoid arthritis of knee

M05.561 Rheumatoid polyneuropathy with rheumatoid arthritis of right knee

M05.562 Rheumatoid polyneuropathy with rheumatoid arthritis of left knee

M05.569 Rheumatoid polyneuropathy with rheumatoid arthritis of unspecified knee

M05.57 Rheumatoid polyneuropathy with rheumatoid arthritis of ankle and foot

Rheumatoid polyneuropathy with rheumatoid arthritis, tarsus, metatarsus and phalanges

M05.571 Rheumatoid polyneuropathy with rheumatoid arthritis of right ankle and foot

M05.572 Rheumatoid polyneuropathy with rheumatoid arthritis of left ankle and foot

M05.579 Rheumatoid polyneuropathy with rheumatoid arthritis of unspecified ankle and foot

M05.59 Rheumatoid polyneuropathy with rheumatoid arthritis of multiple sites

M05.6 Rheumatoid arthritis with involvement of other organs and systems

M05.60 Rheumatoid arthritis of unspecified site with involvement of other organs and systems

M05.61 Rheumatoid arthritis of shoulder with involvement of other organs and systems

M05.611 Rheumatoid arthritis of right shoulder with involvement of other organs and systems

M05.612 Rheumatoid arthritis of left shoulder with involvement of other organs and systems

M05.619 Rheumatoid arthritis of unspecified shoulder with involvement of other organs and systems

M05.62 Rheumatoid arthritis of elbow with involvement of other organs and systems

M05.621 Rheumatoid arthritis of right elbow with involvement of other organs and systems

M05.622 Rheumatoid arthritis of left elbow with involvement of other organs and systems

M05.629 Rheumatoid arthritis of unspecified elbow with involvement of other organs and systems

M05.63 Rheumatoid arthritis of wrist with involvement of other organs and systems

Rheumatoid arthritis of carpal bones with involvement of other organs and systems

M05.631 Rheumatoid arthritis of right wrist with involvement of other organs and systems

M05.632 Rheumatoid arthritis of left wrist with involvement of other organs and systems

● New code   ▲ Revised code   **Excludes1:** Not coded here   **Excludes2:** Not included here   ⊗ Placeholder required   ⑦7th digit required

M05.639 Rheumatoid arthritis of unspecified wrist with involvement of other organs and systems

M05.64 Rheumatoid arthritis of hand with involvement of other organs and systems

Rheumatoid arthritis of metacarpus and phalanges with involvement of other organs and systems

M05.641 Rheumatoid arthritis of right hand with involvement of other organs and systems

M05.642 Rheumatoid arthritis of left hand with involvement of other organs and systems

M05.649 Rheumatoid arthritis of unspecified hand with involvement of other organs and systems

M05.65 Rheumatoid arthritis of hip with involvement of other organs and systems

M05.651 Rheumatoid arthritis of right hip with involvement of other organs and systems

M05.652 Rheumatoid arthritis of left hip with involvement of other organs and systems

M05.659 Rheumatoid arthritis of unspecified hip with involvement of other organs and systems

M05.66 Rheumatoid arthritis of knee with involvement of other organs and systems

M05.661 Rheumatoid arthritis of right knee with involvement of other organs and systems

M05.662 Rheumatoid arthritis of left knee with involvement of other organs and systems

M05.669 Rheumatoid arthritis of unspecified knee with involvement of other organs and systems

M05.67 Rheumatoid arthritis of ankle and foot with involvement of other organs and systems

Rheumatoid arthritis of tarsus, metatarsus and phalanges with involvement of other organs and systems

M05.671 Rheumatoid arthritis of right ankle and foot with involvement of other organs and systems

M05.672 Rheumatoid arthritis of left ankle and foot with involvement of other organs and systems

M05.679 Rheumatoid arthritis of unspecified ankle and foot with involvement of other organs and systems

M05.69 Rheumatoid arthritis of multiple sites with involvement of other organs and systems

M05.7 Rheumatoid arthritis with rheumatoid factor without organ or systems involvement

M05.70 Rheumatoid arthritis with rheumatoid factor of unspecified site without organ or systems involvement

M05.71 Rheumatoid arthritis with rheumatoid factor of shoulder without organ or systems involvement

M05.711 Rheumatoid arthritis with rheumatoid factor of right shoulder without organ or systems involvement

M05.712 Rheumatoid arthritis with rheumatoid factor of left shoulder without organ or systems involvement

M05.719 Rheumatoid arthritis with rheumatoid factor of unspecified shoulder without organ or systems involvement

M05.72 Rheumatoid arthritis with rheumatoid factor of elbow without organ or systems involvement

M05.721 Rheumatoid arthritis with rheumatoid factor of right elbow without organ or systems involvement

M05.722 Rheumatoid arthritis with rheumatoid factor of left elbow without organ or systems involvement

M05.729 Rheumatoid arthritis with rheumatoid factor of unspecified elbow without organ or systems involvement

M05.73 Rheumatoid arthritis with rheumatoid factor of wrist without organ or systems involvement

M05.731 Rheumatoid arthritis with rheumatoid factor of right wrist without organ or systems involvement

M05.732 Rheumatoid arthritis with rheumatoid factor of left wrist without organ or systems involvement

M05.739 Rheumatoid arthritis with rheumatoid factor of unspecified wrist without organ or systems involvement

M05.74 Rheumatoid arthritis with rheumatoid factor of hand without organ or systems involvement

M05.741 Rheumatoid arthritis with rheumatoid factor of right hand without organ or systems involvement

M05.742 Rheumatoid arthritis with rheumatoid factor of left hand without organ or systems involvement

M05.749 Rheumatoid arthritis with rheumatoid factor of unspecified hand without organ or systems involvement

M05.75 Rheumatoid arthritis with rheumatoid factor of hip without organ or systems involvement

M05.751 Rheumatoid arthritis with rheumatoid factor of right hip without organ or systems involvement

M05.752 Rheumatoid arthritis with rheumatoid factor of left hip without organ or systems involvement

M05.759 Rheumatoid arthritis with rheumatoid factor of unspecified hip without organ or systems involvement

M05.76 Rheumatoid arthritis with rheumatoid factor of knee without organ or systems involvement

M05.761 Rheumatoid arthritis with rheumatoid factor of right knee without organ or systems involvement

M05.762 Rheumatoid arthritis with rheumatoid factor of left knee without organ or systems involvement

M05.769 Rheumatoid arthritis with rheumatoid factor of unspecified knee without organ or systems involvement

M05.77 Rheumatoid arthritis with rheumatoid factor of ankle and foot without organ or systems involvement

M05.771 Rheumatoid arthritis with rheumatoid factor of right ankle and foot without organ or systems involvement

M05.772 Rheumatoid arthritis with rheumatoid factor of left ankle and foot without organ or systems involvement

M05.779 Rheumatoid arthritis with rheumatoid factor of unspecified ankle and foot without organ or systems involvement

M05.79 Rheumatoid arthritis with rheumatoid factor of multiple sites without organ or systems involvement

M05.8 Other rheumatoid arthritis with rheumatoid factor

M05.80 Other rheumatoid arthritis with rheumatoid factor of unspecified site

M05.81 Other rheumatoid arthritis with rheumatoid factor of shoulder

M05.811 Other rheumatoid arthritis with rheumatoid factor of right shoulder

M05.812 Other rheumatoid arthritis with rheumatoid factor of left shoulder

M05.819 Other rheumatoid arthritis with rheumatoid factor of unspecified shoulder

M05.82 Other rheumatoid arthritis with rheumatoid factor of elbow

M05.821 Other rheumatoid arthritis with rheumatoid factor of right elbow

M05.822 Other rheumatoid arthritis with rheumatoid factor of left elbow

M05.829 Other rheumatoid arthritis with rheumatoid factor of unspecified elbow

M05.83 Other rheumatoid arthritis with rheumatoid factor of wrist

M05.831 Other rheumatoid arthritis with rheumatoid factor of right wrist

M05.832 Other rheumatoid arthritis with rheumatoid factor of left wrist

M05.839 Other rheumatoid arthritis with rheumatoid factor of unspecified wrist

M05.84 Other rheumatoid arthritis with rheumatoid factor of hand

M05.841 Other rheumatoid arthritis with rheumatoid factor of right hand

M05.842 Other rheumatoid arthritis with rheumatoid factor of left hand

M05.849 Other rheumatoid arthritis with rheumatoid factor of unspecified hand

M05.85 Other rheumatoid arthritis with rheumatoid factor of hip

M05.851 Other rheumatoid arthritis with rheumatoid factor of right hip

M05.852 Other rheumatoid arthritis with rheumatoid factor of left hip

M05.859 Other rheumatoid arthritis with rheumatoid factor of unspecified hip

M05.86 Other rheumatoid arthritis with rheumatoid factor of knee

M05.861 Other rheumatoid arthritis with rheumatoid factor of right knee

M05.862 Other rheumatoid arthritis with rheumatoid factor of left knee

M05.869 Other rheumatoid arthritis with rheumatoid factor of unspecified knee

M05.87 Other rheumatoid arthritis with rheumatoid factor of ankle and foot

M05.871 Other rheumatoid arthritis with rheumatoid factor of right ankle and foot

M05.872 Other rheumatoid arthritis with rheumatoid factor of left ankle and foot

M05.879 Other rheumatoid arthritis with rheumatoid factor of unspecified ankle and foot

M05.89 Other rheumatoid arthritis with rheumatoid factor of multiple sites

M05.9 Rheumatoid arthritis with rheumatoid factor, unspecified

M06 Other rheumatoid arthritis

M06.0 Rheumatoid arthritis without rheumatoid factor

M06.00 Rheumatoid arthritis without rheumatoid factor, unspecified site

M06.01 Rheumatoid arthritis without rheumatoid factor, shoulder

M06.011 Rheumatoid arthritis without rheumatoid factor, right shoulder

M06.012 Rheumatoid arthritis without rheumatoid factor, left shoulder

M06.019 Rheumatoid arthritis without rheumatoid factor, unspecified shoulder

M06.02 Rheumatoid arthritis without rheumatoid factor, elbow

M06.021 Rheumatoid arthritis without rheumatoid factor, right elbow

● New code   ▲ Revised code   **Excludes1:** Not coded here   **Excludes2:** Not included here   ⊗ Placeholder required   ⑦ 7th digit required

M06.022   Rheumatoid arthritis without rheumatoid factor, left elbow

M06.029   Rheumatoid arthritis without rheumatoid factor, unspecified elbow

M06.03   Rheumatoid arthritis without rheumatoid factor, wrist

M06.031   Rheumatoid arthritis without rheumatoid factor, right wrist

M06.032   Rheumatoid arthritis without rheumatoid factor, left wrist

M06.039   Rheumatoid arthritis without rheumatoid factor, unspecified wrist

M06.04   Rheumatoid arthritis without rheumatoid factor, hand

M06.041   Rheumatoid arthritis without rheumatoid factor, right hand

M06.042   Rheumatoid arthritis without rheumatoid factor, left hand

M06.049   Rheumatoid arthritis without rheumatoid factor, unspecified hand

M06.05   Rheumatoid arthritis without rheumatoid factor, hip

M06.051   Rheumatoid arthritis without rheumatoid factor, right hip

M06.052   Rheumatoid arthritis without rheumatoid factor, left hip

M06.059   Rheumatoid arthritis without rheumatoid factor, unspecified hip

M06.06   Rheumatoid arthritis without rheumatoid factor, knee

M06.061   Rheumatoid arthritis without rheumatoid factor, right knee

M06.062   Rheumatoid arthritis without rheumatoid factor, left knee

M06.069   Rheumatoid arthritis without rheumatoid factor, unspecified knee

M06.07   Rheumatoid arthritis without rheumatoid factor, ankle and foot

M06.071   Rheumatoid arthritis without rheumatoid factor, right ankle and foot

M06.072   Rheumatoid arthritis without rheumatoid factor, left ankle and foot

M06.079   Rheumatoid arthritis without rheumatoid factor, unspecified ankle and foot

M06.08   Rheumatoid arthritis without rheumatoid factor, vertebrae

M06.09   Rheumatoid arthritis without rheumatoid factor, multiple sites

M06.1   Adult-onset Still's disease

Excludes1: Still's disease NOS (M08.2-)

M06.2   Rheumatoid bursitis

M06.20   Rheumatoid bursitis, unspecified site

M06.21   Rheumatoid bursitis, shoulder

M06.211   Rheumatoid bursitis, right shoulder

M06.212   Rheumatoid bursitis, left shoulder

M06.219   Rheumatoid bursitis, unspecified shoulder

M06.22   Rheumatoid bursitis, elbow

M06.221   Rheumatoid bursitis, right elbow

M06.222   Rheumatoid bursitis, left elbow

M06.229   Rheumatoid bursitis, unspecified elbow

M06.23   Rheumatoid bursitis, wrist

M06.231   Rheumatoid bursitis, right wrist

M06.232   Rheumatoid bursitis, left wrist

M06.239   Rheumatoid bursitis, unspecified wrist

M06.24   Rheumatoid bursitis, hand

M06.241   Rheumatoid bursitis, right hand

M06.242   Rheumatoid bursitis, left hand

M06.249   Rheumatoid bursitis, unspecified hand

M06.25   Rheumatoid bursitis, hip

M06.251   Rheumatoid bursitis, right hip

M06.252   Rheumatoid bursitis, left hip

M06.259   Rheumatoid bursitis, unspecified hip

M06.26   Rheumatoid bursitis, knee

M06.261   Rheumatoid bursitis, right knee

M06.262   Rheumatoid bursitis, left knee

M06.269   Rheumatoid bursitis, unspecified knee

M06.27   Rheumatoid bursitis, ankle and foot

M06.271   Rheumatoid bursitis, right ankle and foot

M06.272   Rheumatoid bursitis, left ankle and foot

M06.279   Rheumatoid bursitis, unspecified ankle and foot

M06.28   Rheumatoid bursitis, vertebrae

M06.29   Rheumatoid bursitis, multiple sites

M06.3   Rheumatoid nodule

M06.30   Rheumatoid nodule, unspecified site

M06.31   Rheumatoid nodule, shoulder

M06.311   Rheumatoid nodule, right shoulder

M06.312   Rheumatoid nodule, left shoulder

M06.319   Rheumatoid nodule, unspecified shoulder

M06.32   Rheumatoid nodule, elbow

M06.321   Rheumatoid nodule, right elbow

M06.322   Rheumatoid nodule, left elbow

M06.329   Rheumatoid nodule, unspecified elbow

M06.33   Rheumatoid nodule, wrist

M06.331   Rheumatoid nodule, right wrist

M06.332   Rheumatoid nodule, left wrist

M06.339   Rheumatoid nodule, unspecified wrist

M06.34   Rheumatoid nodule, hand

M06.341   Rheumatoid nodule, right hand

M06.342   Rheumatoid nodule, left hand

M06.349 Rheumatoid nodule, unspecified hand

M06.35 Rheumatoid nodule, hip

M06.351 Rheumatoid nodule, right hip

M06.352 Rheumatoid nodule, left hip

M06.359 Rheumatoid nodule, unspecified hip

M06.36 Rheumatoid nodule, knee

M06.361 Rheumatoid nodule, right knee

M06.362 Rheumatoid nodule, left knee

M06.369 Rheumatoid nodule, unspecified knee

M06.37 Rheumatoid nodule, ankle and foot

M06.371 Rheumatoid nodule, right ankle and foot

M06.372 Rheumatoid nodule, left ankle and foot

M06.379 Rheumatoid nodule, unspecified ankle and foot

M06.38 Rheumatoid nodule, vertebrae

M06.39 Rheumatoid nodule, multiple sites

M06.4 Inflammatory polyarthropathy

Excludes1: polyarthritis NOS (M13.0)

M06.8 Other specified rheumatoid arthritis

M06.80 Other specified rheumatoid arthritis, unspecified site

M06.81 Other specified rheumatoid arthritis, shoulder

M06.811 Other specified rheumatoid arthritis, right shoulder

M06.812 Other specified rheumatoid arthritis, left shoulder

M06.819 Other specified rheumatoid arthritis, unspecified shoulder

M06.82 Other specified rheumatoid arthritis, elbow

M06.821 Other specified rheumatoid arthritis, right elbow

M06.822 Other specified rheumatoid arthritis, left elbow

M06.829 Other specified rheumatoid arthritis, unspecified elbow

M06.83 Other specified rheumatoid arthritis, wrist

M06.831 Other specified rheumatoid arthritis, right wrist

M06.832 Other specified rheumatoid arthritis, left wrist

M06.839 Other specified rheumatoid arthritis, unspecified wrist

M06.84 Other specified rheumatoid arthritis, hand

M06.841 Other specified rheumatoid arthritis, right hand

M06.842 Other specified rheumatoid arthritis, left hand

M06.849 Other specified rheumatoid arthritis, unspecified hand

M06.85 Other specified rheumatoid arthritis, hip

M06.851 Other specified rheumatoid arthritis, right hip

M06.852 Other specified rheumatoid arthritis, left hip

M06.859 Other specified rheumatoid arthritis, unspecified hip

M06.86 Other specified rheumatoid arthritis, knee

M06.861 Other specified rheumatoid arthritis, right knee

M06.862 Other specified rheumatoid arthritis, left knee

M06.869 Other specified rheumatoid arthritis, unspecified knee

M06.87 Other specified rheumatoid arthritis, ankle and foot

M06.871 Other specified rheumatoid arthritis, right ankle and foot

M06.872 Other specified rheumatoid arthritis, left ankle and foot

M06.879 Other specified rheumatoid arthritis, unspecified ankle and foot

M06.88 Other specified rheumatoid arthritis, vertebrae

M06.89 Other specified rheumatoid arthritis, multiple sites

M06.9 Rheumatoid arthritis, unspecified

M07 Enteropathic arthropathies

Code also associated enteropathy, such as:

regional enteritis [Crohn's disease] (K50.-)

ulcerative colitis (K51.-)

Excludes1: psoriatic arthropathies (L40.5-)

M07.6 Enteropathic arthropathies

M07.60 Enteropathic arthropathies, unspecified site

M07.61 Enteropathic arthropathies, shoulder

M07.611 Enteropathic arthropathies, right shoulder

M07.612 Enteropathic arthropathies, left shoulder

M07.619 Enteropathic arthropathies, unspecified shoulder

M07.62 Enteropathic arthropathies, elbow

M07.621 Enteropathic arthropathies, right elbow

M07.622 Enteropathic arthropathies, left elbow

M07.629 Enteropathic arthropathies, unspecified elbow

M07.63 Enteropathic arthropathies, wrist

M07.631 Enteropathic arthropathies, right wrist

M07.632 Enteropathic arthropathies, left wrist

M07.639 Enteropathic arthropathies, unspecified wrist

M07.64 Enteropathic arthropathies, hand

M07.641 Enteropathic arthropathies, right hand

M07.642 Enteropathic arthropathies, left hand

M07.649 Enteropathic arthropathies, unspecified hand

M07.65 Enteropathic arthropathies, hip

M07.651   Enteropathic arthropathies, right hip

M07.652   Enteropathic arthropathies, left hip

M07.659   Enteropathic arthropathies, unspecified hip

M07.66   Enteropathic arthropathies, knee

M07.661   Enteropathic arthropathies, right knee

M07.662   Enteropathic arthropathies, left knee

M07.669   Enteropathic arthropathies, unspecified knee

M07.67   Enteropathic arthropathies, ankle and foot

M07.671   Enteropathic arthropathies, right ankle and foot

M07.672   Enteropathic arthropathies, left ankle and foot

M07.679   Enteropathic arthropathies, unspecified ankle and foot

M07.68   Enteropathic arthropathies, vertebrae

M07.69   Enteropathic arthropathies, multiple sites

M08   **Juvenile arthritis**

Code also any associated underlying condition, such as:

regional enteritis [Crohn's disease] (K50.-)

ulcerative colitis (K51.-)

Excludes1: arthropathy in Whipple's disease (M14.8)

Felty's syndrome (M05.0)

juvenile dermatomyositis (M33.0-)

psoriatic juvenile arthropathy (L40.54)

M08.0   **Unspecified juvenile rheumatoid arthritis**

Juvenile rheumatoid arthritis with or without rheumatoid factor

M08.00   Unspecified juvenile rheumatoid arthritis of unspecified site

M08.01   Unspecified juvenile rheumatoid arthritis, shoulder

M08.011   Unspecified juvenile rheumatoid arthritis, right shoulder

M08.012   Unspecified juvenile rheumatoid arthritis, left shoulder

M08.019   Unspecified juvenile rheumatoid arthritis, unspecified shoulder

M08.02   Unspecified juvenile rheumatoid arthritis of elbow

M08.021   Unspecified juvenile rheumatoid arthritis, right elbow

M08.022   Unspecified juvenile rheumatoid arthritis, left elbow

M08.029   Unspecified juvenile rheumatoid arthritis, unspecified elbow

M08.03   Unspecified juvenile rheumatoid arthritis, wrist

M08.031   Unspecified juvenile rheumatoid arthritis, right wrist

M08.032   Unspecified juvenile rheumatoid arthritis, left wrist

M08.039   Unspecified juvenile rheumatoid arthritis, unspecified wrist

M08.04   Unspecified juvenile rheumatoid arthritis, hand

M08.041   Unspecified juvenile rheumatoid arthritis, right hand

M08.042   Unspecified juvenile rheumatoid arthritis, left hand

M08.049   Unspecified juvenile rheumatoid arthritis, unspecified hand

M08.05   Unspecified juvenile rheumatoid arthritis, hip

M08.051   Unspecified juvenile rheumatoid arthritis, right hip

M08.052   Unspecified juvenile rheumatoid arthritis, left hip

M08.059   Unspecified juvenile rheumatoid arthritis, unspecified hip

M08.06   Unspecified juvenile rheumatoid arthritis, knee

M08.061   Unspecified juvenile rheumatoid arthritis, right knee

M08.062   Unspecified juvenile rheumatoid arthritis, left knee

M08.069   Unspecified juvenile rheumatoid arthritis, unspecified knee

M08.07   Unspecified juvenile rheumatoid arthritis, ankle and foot

M08.071   Unspecified juvenile rheumatoid arthritis, right ankle and foot

M08.072   Unspecified juvenile rheumatoid arthritis, left ankle and foot

M08.079   Unspecified juvenile rheumatoid arthritis, unspecified ankle and foot

M08.08   Unspecified juvenile rheumatoid arthritis, vertebrae

M08.09   Unspecified juvenile rheumatoid arthritis, multiple sites

M08.1   **Juvenile ankylosing spondylitis**

Excludes1: ankylosing spondylitis in adults (M45.0-)

M08.2   **Juvenile rheumatoid arthritis with systemic onset**

Still's disease NOS

Excludes1: adult-onset Still's disease (M06.1-)

M08.20   Juvenile rheumatoid arthritis with systemic onset, unspecified site

M08.21   Juvenile rheumatoid arthritis with systemic onset, shoulder

M08.211   Juvenile rheumatoid arthritis with systemic onset, right shoulder

M08.212   Juvenile rheumatoid arthritis with systemic onset, left shoulder

M08.219   Juvenile rheumatoid arthritis with systemic onset, unspecified shoulder

M08.22   Juvenile rheumatoid arthritis with systemic onset, elbow

M08.221   Juvenile rheumatoid arthritis with systemic onset, right elbow

M08.222   Juvenile rheumatoid arthritis with systemic onset, left elbow

M08.229   Juvenile rheumatoid arthritis with systemic onset, unspecified elbow

M08.23   Juvenile rheumatoid arthritis with systemic onset, wrist

M08.231 Juvenile rheumatoid arthritis with systemic onset, right wrist

M08.232 Juvenile rheumatoid arthritis with systemic onset, left wrist

M08.239 Juvenile rheumatoid arthritis with systemic onset, unspecified wrist

M08.24 Juvenile rheumatoid arthritis with systemic onset, hand

M08.241 Juvenile rheumatoid arthritis with systemic onset, right hand

M08.242 Juvenile rheumatoid arthritis with systemic onset, left hand

M08.249 Juvenile rheumatoid arthritis with systemic onset, unspecified hand

M08.25 Juvenile rheumatoid arthritis with systemic onset, hip

M08.251 Juvenile rheumatoid arthritis with systemic onset, right hip

M08.252 Juvenile rheumatoid arthritis with systemic onset, left hip

M08.259 Juvenile rheumatoid arthritis with systemic onset, unspecified hip

M08.26 Juvenile rheumatoid arthritis with systemic onset, knee

M08.261 Juvenile rheumatoid arthritis with systemic onset, right knee

M08.262 Juvenile rheumatoid arthritis with systemic onset, left knee

M08.269 Juvenile rheumatoid arthritis with systemic onset, unspecified knee

M08.27 Juvenile rheumatoid arthritis with systemic onset, ankle and foot

M08.271 Juvenile rheumatoid arthritis with systemic onset, right ankle and foot

M08.272 Juvenile rheumatoid arthritis with systemic onset, left ankle and foot

M08.279 Juvenile rheumatoid arthritis with systemic onset, unspecified ankle and foot

M08.28 Juvenile rheumatoid arthritis with systemic onset, vertebrae

M08.29 Juvenile rheumatoid arthritis with systemic onset, multiple sites

M08.3 Juvenile rheumatoid polyarthritis (seronegative)

M08.4 Pauciarticular juvenile rheumatoid arthritis

M08.40 Pauciarticular juvenile rheumatoid arthritis, unspecified site

M08.41 Pauciarticular juvenile rheumatoid arthritis, shoulder

M08.411 Pauciarticular juvenile rheumatoid arthritis, right shoulder

M08.412 Pauciarticular juvenile rheumatoid arthritis, left shoulder

M08.419 Pauciarticular juvenile rheumatoid arthritis, unspecified shoulder

M08.42 Pauciarticular juvenile rheumatoid arthritis, elbow

M08.421 Pauciarticular juvenile rheumatoid arthritis, right elbow

M08.422 Pauciarticular juvenile rheumatoid arthritis, left elbow

M08.429 Pauciarticular juvenile rheumatoid arthritis, unspecified elbow

M08.43 Pauciarticular juvenile rheumatoid arthritis, wrist

M08.431 Pauciarticular juvenile rheumatoid arthritis, right wrist

M08.432 Pauciarticular juvenile rheumatoid arthritis, left wrist

M08.439 Pauciarticular juvenile rheumatoid arthritis, unspecified wrist

M08.44 Pauciarticular juvenile rheumatoid arthritis, hand

M08.441 Pauciarticular juvenile rheumatoid arthritis, right hand

M08.442 Pauciarticular juvenile rheumatoid arthritis, left hand

M08.449 Pauciarticular juvenile rheumatoid arthritis, unspecified hand

M08.45 Pauciarticular juvenile rheumatoid arthritis, hip

M08.451 Pauciarticular juvenile rheumatoid arthritis, right hip

M08.452 Pauciarticular juvenile rheumatoid arthritis, left hip

M08.459 Pauciarticular juvenile rheumatoid arthritis, unspecified hip

M08.46 Pauciarticular juvenile rheumatoid arthritis, knee

M08.461 Pauciarticular juvenile rheumatoid arthritis, right knee

M08.462 Pauciarticular juvenile rheumatoid arthritis, left knee

M08.469 Pauciarticular juvenile rheumatoid arthritis, unspecified knee

M08.47 Pauciarticular juvenile rheumatoid arthritis, ankle and foot

M08.471 Pauciarticular juvenile rheumatoid arthritis, right ankle and foot

M08.472 Pauciarticular juvenile rheumatoid arthritis, left ankle and foot

M08.479 Pauciarticular juvenile rheumatoid arthritis, unspecified ankle and foot

M08.48 Pauciarticular juvenile rheumatoid arthritis, vertebrae

M08.8 Other juvenile arthritis

M08.80 Other juvenile arthritis, unspecified site

M08.81 Other juvenile arthritis, shoulder

M08.811 Other juvenile arthritis, right shoulder

M08.812 Other juvenile arthritis, left shoulder

M08.819 Other juvenile arthritis, unspecified shoulder

M08.82 Other juvenile arthritis, elbow

M08.821 Other juvenile arthritis, right elbow

M08.822 Other juvenile arthritis, left elbow

M08.829 Other juvenile arthritis, unspecified elbow

M08.83 Other juvenile arthritis, wrist

M08.831 Other juvenile arthritis, right wrist

● New code ▲ Revised code **Excludes1:** Not coded here **Excludes2:** Not included here ⊗ Placeholder required ⑦ 7th digit required

M08.832 Other juvenile arthritis, left wrist

M08.839 Other juvenile arthritis, unspecified wrist

M08.84 Other juvenile arthritis, hand

M08.841 Other juvenile arthritis, right hand

M08.842 Other juvenile arthritis, left hand

M08.849 Other juvenile arthritis, unspecified hand

M08.85 Other juvenile arthritis, hip

M08.851 Other juvenile arthritis, right hip

M08.852 Other juvenile arthritis, left hip

M08.859 Other juvenile arthritis, unspecified hip

M08.86 Other juvenile arthritis, knee

M08.861 Other juvenile arthritis, right knee

M08.862 Other juvenile arthritis, left knee

M08.869 Other juvenile arthritis, unspecified knee

M08.87 Other juvenile arthritis, ankle and foot

M08.871 Other juvenile arthritis, right ankle and foot

M08.872 Other juvenile arthritis, left ankle and foot

M08.879 Other juvenile arthritis, unspecified ankle and foot

M08.88 Other juvenile arthritis, other specified site

Other juvenile arthritis, vertebrae

M08.89 Other juvenile arthritis, multiple sites

M08.9 Juvenile arthritis, unspecified

Excludes1: juvenile rheumatoid arthritis, unspecified (M08.0-)

M08.90 Juvenile arthritis, unspecified, unspecified site

M08.91 Juvenile arthritis, unspecified, shoulder

M08.911 Juvenile arthritis, unspecified, right shoulder

M08.912 Juvenile arthritis, unspecified, left shoulder

M08.919 Juvenile arthritis, unspecified, unspecified shoulder

M08.92 Juvenile arthritis, unspecified, elbow

M08.921 Juvenile arthritis, unspecified, right elbow

M08.922 Juvenile arthritis, unspecified, left elbow

M08.929 Juvenile arthritis, unspecified, unspecified elbow

M08.93 Juvenile arthritis, unspecified, wrist

M08.931 Juvenile arthritis, unspecified, right wrist

M08.932 Juvenile arthritis, unspecified, left wrist

M08.939 Juvenile arthritis, unspecified, unspecified wrist

M08.94 Juvenile arthritis, unspecified, hand

M08.941 Juvenile arthritis, unspecified, right hand

M08.942 Juvenile arthritis, unspecified, left hand

M08.949 Juvenile arthritis, unspecified, unspecified hand

M08.95 Juvenile arthritis, unspecified, hip

M08.951 Juvenile arthritis, unspecified, right hip

M08.952 Juvenile arthritis, unspecified, left hip

M08.959 Juvenile arthritis, unspecified, unspecified hip

M08.96 Juvenile arthritis, unspecified, knee

M08.961 Juvenile arthritis, unspecified, right knee

M08.962 Juvenile arthritis, unspecified, left knee

M08.969 Juvenile arthritis, unspecified, unspecified knee

M08.97 Juvenile arthritis, unspecified, ankle and foot

M08.971 Juvenile arthritis, unspecified, right ankle and foot

M08.972 Juvenile arthritis, unspecified, left ankle and foot

M08.979 Juvenile arthritis, unspecified, unspecified ankle and foot

M08.98 Juvenile arthritis, unspecified, vertebrae

M08.99 Juvenile arthritis, unspecified, multiple sites

M1A Chronic gout

Use additional code to identify:

Autonomic neuropathy in diseases classified elsewhere (G99.0)

Calculus of urinary tract in diseases classified elsewhere (N22)

Cardiomyopathy in diseases classified elsewhere (I43)

Disorders of external ear in diseases classified elsewhere (H61.1-, H62.8-)

Disorders of iris and ciliary body in diseases classified elsewhere (H22)

Glomerular disorders in diseases classified elsewhere (N08)

Excludes1: gout NOS (M10.-)

Excludes2: acute gout (M10.-)

The appropriate 7th character is to be added to each code from category M1A

0 - without tophus (tophi)

1 - with tophus (tophi)

M1A.0 Idiopathic chronic gout

Chronic gouty bursitis

Primary chronic gout

⊗⑦M1A.00 Idiopathic chronic gout, unspecified site

M1A.01 Idiopathic chronic gout, shoulder

⑦M1A.011 Idiopathic chronic gout, right shoulder

⑦M1A.012 Idiopathic chronic gout, left shoulder

⑦M1A.019 Idiopathic chronic gout, unspecified shoulder

M1A.02 Idiopathic chronic gout, elbow

⑦M1A.021 Idiopathic chronic gout, right elbow

⑦M1A.022 Idiopathic chronic gout, left elbow

⑦M1A.029 Idiopathic chronic gout, unspecified elbow

M1A.03 Idiopathic chronic gout, wrist

⑦M1A.031 Idiopathic chronic gout, right wrist

⑦M1A.032 Idiopathic chronic gout, left wrist

⑦M1A.039 Idiopathic chronic gout, unspecified wrist

M1A.04 Idiopathic chronic gout, hand

⑦M1A.041 Idiopathic chronic gout, right hand

⑦M1A.042 Idiopathic chronic gout, left hand

⑦M1A.049 Idiopathic chronic gout, unspecified hand

M1A.05 Idiopathic chronic gout, hip

⑦M1A.051 Idiopathic chronic gout, right hip

⑦M1A.052 Idiopathic chronic gout, left hip

⑦M1A.059 Idiopathic chronic gout, unspecified hip

M1A.06 Idiopathic chronic gout, knee

⑦M1A.061 Idiopathic chronic gout, right knee

⑦M1A.062 Idiopathic chronic gout, left knee

⑦M1A.069 Idiopathic chronic gout, unspecified knee

M1A.07 Idiopathic chronic gout, ankle and foot

⑦M1A.071 Idiopathic chronic gout, right ankle and foot

⑦M1A.072 Idiopathic chronic gout, left ankle and foot

⑦M1A.079 Idiopathic chronic gout, unspecified ankle and foot

⊗⑦M1A.08 Idiopathic chronic gout, vertebrae

⊗⑦M1A.09 Idiopathic chronic gout, multiple sites

M1A.1 Lead-induced chronic gout

Code first toxic effects of lead and its compounds (T56.0-)

⊗⑦M1A.10 Lead-induced chronic gout, unspecified site

M1A.11 Lead-induced chronic gout, shoulder

⑦M1A.111 Lead-induced chronic gout, right shoulder

⑦M1A.112 Lead-induced chronic gout, left shoulder

⑦M1A.119 Lead-induced chronic gout, unspecified shoulder

M1A.12 Lead-induced chronic gout, elbow

⑦M1A.121 Lead-induced chronic gout, right elbow

⑦M1A.122 Lead-induced chronic gout, left elbow

⑦M1A.129 Lead-induced chronic gout, unspecified elbow

M1A.13 Lead-induced chronic gout, wrist

⑦M1A.131 Lead-induced chronic gout, right wrist

⑦M1A.132 Lead-induced chronic gout, left wrist

⑦M1A.139 Lead-induced chronic gout, unspecified wrist

M1A.14 Lead-induced chronic gout, hand

⑦M1A.141 Lead-induced chronic gout, right hand

⑦M1A.142 Lead-induced chronic gout, left hand

⑦M1A.149 Lead-induced chronic gout, unspecified hand

M1A.15 Lead-induced chronic gout, hip

⑦M1A.151 Lead-induced chronic gout, right hip

⑦M1A.152 Lead-induced chronic gout, left hip

⑦M1A.159 Lead-induced chronic gout, unspecified hip

M1A.16 Lead-induced chronic gout, knee

⑦M1A.161 Lead-induced chronic gout, right knee

⑦M1A.162 Lead-induced chronic gout, left knee

⑦M1A.169 Lead-induced chronic gout, unspecified knee

M1A.17 Lead-induced chronic gout, ankle and foot

⑦M1A.171 Lead-induced chronic gout, right ankle and foot

⑦M1A.172 Lead-induced chronic gout, left ankle and foot

⑦M1A.179 Lead-induced chronic gout, unspecified ankle and foot

⊗⑦M1A.18 Lead-induced chronic gout, vertebrae

⊗⑦M1A.19 Lead-induced chronic gout, multiple sites

M1A.2 Drug-induced chronic gout

Use additional code for adverse effect, if applicable, to identify drug (T36-T50 with fifth or sixth character 5)

⊗⑦M1A.20 Drug-induced chronic gout, unspecified site

M1A.21 Drug-induced chronic gout, shoulder

⑦M1A.211 Drug-induced chronic gout, right shoulder

⑦M1A.212 Drug-induced chronic gout, left shoulder

⑦M1A.219 Drug-induced chronic gout, unspecified shoulder

M1A.22 Drug-induced chronic gout, elbow

⑦M1A.221 Drug-induced chronic gout, right elbow

⑦M1A.222 Drug-induced chronic gout, left elbow

⑦M1A.229 Drug-induced chronic gout, unspecified elbow

M1A.23 Drug-induced chronic gout, wrist

⑦M1A.231 Drug-induced chronic gout, right wrist

⑦M1A.232 Drug-induced chronic gout, left wrist

⑦M1A.239 Drug-induced chronic gout, unspecified wrist

M1A.24 Drug-induced chronic gout, hand

⑦M1A.241 Drug-induced chronic gout, right hand

⑦M1A.242 Drug-induced chronic gout, left hand

⑦M1A.249 Drug-induced chronic gout, unspecified hand

M1A.25 Drug-induced chronic gout, hip

⑦M1A.251 Drug-induced chronic gout, right hip

⑦M1A.252 Drug-induced chronic gout, left hip

⑦M1A.259 Drug-induced chronic gout, unspecified hip

M1A.26 Drug-induced chronic gout, knee

⑦M1A.261 Drug-induced chronic gout, right knee

⑦M1A.262 Drug-induced chronic gout, left knee

⑦M1A.269 Drug-induced chronic gout, unspecified knee

M1A.27 Drug-induced chronic gout, ankle and foot

⑦M1A.271 Drug-induced chronic gout, right ankle and foot

⑦M1A.272 Drug-induced chronic gout, left ankle and foot

⑦M1A.279 Drug-induced chronic gout, unspecified ankle and foot

⊗⑦M1A.28 Drug-induced chronic gout, vertebrae

⊗⑦M1A.29 Drug-induced chronic gout, multiple sites

M1A.3 Chronic gout due to renal impairment

Code first associated renal disease

⊗⑦M1A.30 Chronic gout due to renal impairment, unspecified site

M1A.31 Chronic gout due to renal impairment, shoulder

⑦M1A.311 Chronic gout due to renal impairment, right shoulder

⑦M1A.312 Chronic gout due to renal impairment, left shoulder

⑦M1A.319 Chronic gout due to renal impairment, unspecified shoulder

M1A.32 Chronic gout due to renal impairment, elbow

⑦M1A.321 Chronic gout due to renal impairment, right elbow

⑦M1A.322 Chronic gout due to renal impairment, left elbow

⑦M1A.329 Chronic gout due to renal impairment, unspecified elbow

M1A.33 Chronic gout due to renal impairment, wrist

⑦M1A.331 Chronic gout due to renal impairment, right wrist

⑦M1A.332 Chronic gout due to renal impairment, left wrist

⑦M1A.339 Chronic gout due to renal impairment, unspecified wrist

M1A.34 Chronic gout due to renal impairment, hand

⑦M1A.341 Chronic gout due to renal impairment, right hand

⑦M1A.342 Chronic gout due to renal impairment, left hand

⑦M1A.349 Chronic gout due to renal impairment, unspecified hand

M1A.35 Chronic gout due to renal impairment, hip

⑦M1A.351 Chronic gout due to renal impairment, right hip

⑦M1A.352 Chronic gout due to renal impairment, left hip

⑦M1A.359 Chronic gout due to renal impairment, unspecified hip

M1A.36 Chronic gout due to renal impairment, knee

⑦M1A.361 Chronic gout due to renal impairment, right knee

⑦M1A.362 Chronic gout due to renal impairment, left knee

⑦M1A.369 Chronic gout due to renal impairment, unspecified knee

M1A.37 Chronic gout due to renal impairment, ankle and foot

⑦M1A.371 Chronic gout due to renal impairment, right ankle and foot

⑦M1A.372 Chronic gout due to renal impairment, left ankle and foot

⑦M1A.379 Chronic gout due to renal impairment, unspecified ankle and foot

⊗⑦M1A.38 Chronic gout due to renal impairment, vertebrae

⊗⑦M1A.39 Chronic gout due to renal impairment, multiple sites

M1A.4 Other secondary chronic gout

Code first associated condition

⊗M1A.40 Other secondary chronic gout, unspecified site

M1A.41 Other secondary chronic gout, shoulder

⑦M1A.411 Other secondary chronic gout, right shoulder

⑦M1A.412 Other secondary chronic gout, left shoulder

⑦M1A.419 Other secondary chronic gout, unspecified shoulder

M1A.42 Other secondary chronic gout, elbow

⑦M1A.421 Other secondary chronic gout, right elbow

⑦M1A.422 Other secondary chronic gout, left elbow

⑦M1A.429 Other secondary chronic gout, unspecified elbow

M1A.43 Other secondary chronic gout, wrist

⑦M1A.431 Other secondary chronic gout, right wrist

⑦M1A.432 Other secondary chronic gout, left wrist

⑦M1A.439 Other secondary chronic gout, unspecified wrist

M1A.44 Other secondary chronic gout, hand

⑦M1A.441 Other secondary chronic gout, right hand

⑦M1A.442 Other secondary chronic gout, left hand

⑦M1A.449 Other secondary chronic gout, unspecified hand

M1A.45 Other secondary chronic gout, hip

⑦M1A.451 Other secondary chronic gout, right hip

⑦M1A.452 Other secondary chronic gout, left hip

⑦M1A.459 Other secondary chronic gout, unspecified hip

M1A.46 Other secondary chronic gout, knee

⑦M1A.461 Other secondary chronic gout, right knee

⑦ **M1A.462** Other secondary chronic gout, left knee

⑦ **M1A.469** Other secondary chronic gout, unspecified knee

M1A.47 Other secondary chronic gout, ankle and foot

⑦ **M1A.471** Other secondary chronic gout, right ankle and foot

⑦ **M1A.472** Other secondary chronic gout, left ankle and foot

⑦ **M1A.479** Other secondary chronic gout, unspecified ankle and foot

⊗⑦**M1A.48** Other secondary chronic gout, vertebrae

⊗⑦**M1A.49** Other secondary chronic gout, multiple sites

⊗⑦**M1A.9** Chronic gout, unspecified

M10 **Gout**

Acute gout

Gout attack

Gout flare

Podagra

Use additional code to identify:

Autonomic neuropathy in diseases classified elsewhere (G99.0)

Calculus of urinary tract in diseases classified elsewhere (N22)

Cardiomyopathy in diseases classified elsewhere (I43)

Disorders of external ear in diseases classified elsewhere (H61.1-, H62.8-)

Disorders of iris and ciliary body in diseases classified elsewhere (H22)

Glomerular disorders in diseases classified elsewhere (N08)

Excludes2: chronic gout (M1A.-)

M10.0 **Idiopathic gout**

Gouty bursitis

Primary gout

M10.00 Idiopathic gout, unspecified site

M10.01 Idiopathic gout, shoulder

M10.011 Idiopathic gout, right shoulder

M10.012 Idiopathic gout, left shoulder

M10.019 Idiopathic gout, unspecified shoulder

M10.02 Idiopathic gout, elbow

M10.021 Idiopathic gout, right elbow

M10.022 Idiopathic gout, left elbow

M10.029 Idiopathic gout, unspecified elbow

M10.03 Idiopathic gout, wrist

M10.031 Idiopathic gout, right wrist

M10.032 Idiopathic gout, left wrist

M10.039 Idiopathic gout, unspecified wrist

M10.04 Idiopathic gout, hand

M10.041 Idiopathic gout, right hand

M10.042 Idiopathic gout, left hand

M10.049 Idiopathic gout, unspecified hand

M10.05 Idiopathic gout, hip

M10.051 Idiopathic gout, right hip

M10.052 Idiopathic gout, left hip

M10.059 Idiopathic gout, unspecified hip

M10.06 Idiopathic gout, knee

M10.061 Idiopathic gout, right knee

M10.062 Idiopathic gout, left knee

M10.069 Idiopathic gout, unspecified knee

M10.07 Idiopathic gout, ankle and foot

M10.071 Idiopathic gout, right ankle and foot

M10.072 Idiopathic gout, left ankle and foot

M10.079 Idiopathic gout, unspecified ankle and foot

M10.08 Idiopathic gout, vertebrae

M10.09 Idiopathic gout, multiple sites

M10.1 **Lead-induced gout**

Code first toxic effects of lead and its compounds (T56.0-)

M10.10 Lead-induced gout, unspecified site

M10.11 Lead-induced gout, shoulder

M10.111 Lead-induced gout, right shoulder

M10.112 Lead-induced gout, left shoulder

M10.119 Lead-induced gout, unspecified shoulder

M10.12 Lead-induced gout, elbow

M10.121 Lead-induced gout, right elbow

M10.122 Lead-induced gout, left elbow

M10.129 Lead-induced gout, unspecified elbow

M10.13 Lead-induced gout, wrist

M10.131 Lead-induced gout, right wrist

M10.132 Lead-induced gout, left wrist

M10.139 Lead-induced gout, unspecified wrist

M10.14 Lead-induced gout, hand

M10.141 Lead-induced gout, right hand

M10.142 Lead-induced gout, left hand

M10.149 Lead-induced gout, unspecified hand

M10.15 Lead-induced gout, hip

M10.151 Lead-induced gout, right hip

M10.152 Lead-induced gout, left hip

M10.159 Lead-induced gout, unspecified hip

M10.16 Lead-induced gout, knee

M10.161 Lead-induced gout, right knee

M10.162 Lead-induced gout, left knee

M10.169 Lead-induced gout, unspecified knee

M10.17 Lead-induced gout, ankle and foot

M10.171 Lead-induced gout, right ankle and foot

M10.172 Lead-induced gout, left ankle and foot

M10.179 Lead-induced gout, unspecified ankle and foot

M10.18 Lead-induced gout, vertebrae

M10.19 Lead-induced gout, multiple sites

M10.2 **Drug-induced gout**

Use additional code for adverse effect, if applicable, to identify drug (T36-T50 with fifth or sixth character 5)

M10.20 Drug-induced gout, unspecified site

M10.21 Drug-induced gout, shoulder

M10.211 Drug-induced gout, right shoulder

M10.212   Drug-induced gout, left shoulder

M10.219   Drug-induced gout, unspecified shoulder

M10.22   Drug-induced gout, elbow

M10.221   Drug-induced gout, right elbow

M10.222   Drug-induced gout, left elbow

M10.229   Drug-induced gout, unspecified elbow

M10.23   Drug-induced gout, wrist

M10.231   Drug-induced gout, right wrist

M10.232   Drug-induced gout, left wrist

M10.239   Drug-induced gout, unspecified wrist

M10.24   Drug-induced gout, hand

M10.241   Drug-induced gout, right hand

M10.242   Drug-induced gout, left hand

M10.249   Drug-induced gout, unspecified hand

M10.25   Drug-induced gout, hip

M10.251   Drug-induced gout, right hip

M10.252   Drug-induced gout, left hip

M10.259   Drug-induced gout, unspecified hip

M10.26   Drug-induced gout, knee

M10.261   Drug-induced gout, right knee

M10.262   Drug-induced gout, left knee

M10.269   Drug-induced gout, unspecified knee

M10.27   Drug-induced gout, ankle and foot

M10.271   Drug-induced gout, right ankle and foot

M10.272   Drug-induced gout, left ankle and foot

M10.279   Drug-induced gout, unspecified ankle and foot

M10.28   Drug-induced gout, vertebrae

M10.29   Drug-induced gout, multiple sites

M10.3   Gout due to renal impairment

Code first associated renal disease

M10.30   Gout due to renal impairment, unspecified site

M10.31   Gout due to renal impairment, shoulder

M10.311   Gout due to renal impairment, right shoulder

M10.312   Gout due to renal impairment, left shoulder

M10.319   Gout due to renal impairment, unspecified shoulder

M10.32   Gout due to renal impairment, elbow

M10.321   Gout due to renal impairment, right elbow

M10.322   Gout due to renal impairment, left elbow

M10.329   Gout due to renal impairment, unspecified elbow

M10.33   Gout due to renal impairment, wrist

M10.331   Gout due to renal impairment, right wrist

M10.332   Gout due to renal impairment, left wrist

M10.339   Gout due to renal impairment, unspecified wrist

M10.34   Gout due to renal impairment, hand

M10.341   Gout due to renal impairment, right hand

M10.342   Gout due to renal impairment, left hand

M10.349   Gout due to renal impairment, unspecified hand

M10.35   Gout due to renal impairment, hip

M10.351   Gout due to renal impairment, right hip

M10.352   Gout due to renal impairment, left hip

M10.359   Gout due to renal impairment, unspecified hip

M10.36   Gout due to renal impairment, knee

M10.361   Gout due to renal impairment, right knee

M10.362   Gout due to renal impairment, left knee

M10.369   Gout due to renal impairment, unspecified knee

M10.37   Gout due to renal impairment, ankle and foot

M10.371   Gout due to renal impairment, right ankle and foot

M10.372   Gout due to renal impairment, left ankle and foot

M10.379   Gout due to renal impairment, unspecified ankle and foot

M10.38   Gout due to renal impairment, vertebrae

M10.39   Gout due to renal impairment, multiple sites

M10.4   Other secondary gout

Code first associated condition

M10.40   Other secondary gout, unspecified site

M10.41   Other secondary gout, shoulder

M10.411   Other secondary gout, right shoulder

M10.412   Other secondary gout, left shoulder

M10.419   Other secondary gout, unspecified shoulder

M10.42   Other secondary gout, elbow

M10.421   Other secondary gout, right elbow

M10.422   Other secondary gout, left elbow

M10.429   Other secondary gout, unspecified elbow

M10.43   Other secondary gout, wrist

M10.431   Other secondary gout, right wrist

M10.432   Other secondary gout, left wrist

M10.439   Other secondary gout, unspecified wrist

M10.44   Other secondary gout, hand

M10.441   Other secondary gout, right hand

M10.442   Other secondary gout, left hand

M10.449   Other secondary gout, unspecified hand

M10.45   Other secondary gout, hip

M10.451   Other secondary gout, right hip

M10.452   Other secondary gout, left hip

M10.459   Other secondary gout, unspecified hip

M10.46   Other secondary gout, knee

 M10.461   Other secondary gout, right knee

 M10.462   Other secondary gout, left knee

 M10.469   Other secondary gout, unspecified knee

M10.47   Other secondary gout, ankle and foot

 M10.471   Other secondary gout, right ankle and foot

 M10.472   Other secondary gout, left ankle and foot

 M10.479   Other secondary gout, unspecified ankle and foot

M10.48   Other secondary gout, vertebrae

M10.49   Other secondary gout, multiple sites

M10.9   **Gout, unspecified**

Gout NOS

M11   **Other crystal arthropathies**

Definition: Crystal arthropathies refers to a type of arthropathy characterized by accumulation of crystals in joints.

M11.0   **Hydroxyapatite deposition disease**

M11.00   **Hydroxyapatite deposition disease, unspecified site**

M11.01   **Hydroxyapatite deposition disease, shoulder**

 M11.011   Hydroxyapatite deposition disease, right shoulder

 M11.012   Hydroxyapatite deposition disease, left shoulder

 M11.019   Hydroxyapatite deposition disease, unspecified shoulder

M11.02   **Hydroxyapatite deposition disease, elbow**

 M11.021   Hydroxyapatite deposition disease, right elbow

 M11.022   Hydroxyapatite deposition disease, left elbow

 M11.029   Hydroxyapatite deposition disease, unspecified elbow

M11.03   **Hydroxyapatite deposition disease, wrist**

 M11.031   Hydroxyapatite deposition disease, right wrist

 M11.032   Hydroxyapatite deposition disease, left wrist

 M11.039   Hydroxyapatite deposition disease, unspecified wrist

M11.04   **Hydroxyapatite deposition disease, hand**

 M11.041   Hydroxyapatite deposition disease, right hand

 M11.042   Hydroxyapatite deposition disease, left hand

 M11.049   Hydroxyapatite deposition disease, unspecified hand

M11.05   **Hydroxyapatite deposition disease, hip**

 M11.051   Hydroxyapatite deposition disease, right hip

 M11.052   Hydroxyapatite deposition disease, left hip

M11.059   Hydroxyapatite deposition disease, unspecified hip

M11.06   **Hydroxyapatite deposition disease, knee**

 M11.061   Hydroxyapatite deposition disease, right knee

 M11.062   Hydroxyapatite deposition disease, left knee

 M11.069   Hydroxyapatite deposition disease, unspecified knee

M11.07   **Hydroxyapatite deposition disease, ankle and foot**

 M11.071   Hydroxyapatite deposition disease, right ankle and foot

 M11.072   Hydroxyapatite deposition disease, left ankle and foot

 M11.079   Hydroxyapatite deposition disease, unspecified ankle and foot

M11.08   **Hydroxyapatite deposition disease, vertebrae**

M11.09   **Hydroxyapatite deposition disease, multiple sites**

M11.1   **Familial chondrocalcinosis**

M11.10   **Familial chondrocalcinosis, unspecified site**

M11.11   **Familial chondrocalcinosis, shoulder**

 M11.111   Familial chondrocalcinosis, right shoulder

 M11.112   Familial chondrocalcinosis, left shoulder

 M11.119   Familial chondrocalcinosis, unspecified shoulder

M11.12   **Familial chondrocalcinosis, elbow**

 M11.121   Familial chondrocalcinosis, right elbow

 M11.122   Familial chondrocalcinosis, left elbow

 M11.129   Familial chondrocalcinosis, unspecified elbow

M11.13   **Familial chondrocalcinosis, wrist**

 M11.131   Familial chondrocalcinosis, right wrist

 M11.132   Familial chondrocalcinosis, left wrist

 M11.139   Familial chondrocalcinosis, unspecified wrist

M11.14   **Familial chondrocalcinosis, hand**

 M11.141   Familial chondrocalcinosis, right hand

 M11.142   Familial chondrocalcinosis, left hand

 M11.149   Familial chondrocalcinosis, unspecified hand

M11.15   **Familial chondrocalcinosis, hip**

 M11.151   Familial chondrocalcinosis, right hip

 M11.152   Familial chondrocalcinosis, left hip

 M11.159   Familial chondrocalcinosis, unspecified hip

M11.16   **Familial chondrocalcinosis, knee**

 M11.161   Familial chondrocalcinosis, right knee

M11.162 Familial chondrocalcinosis, left knee

M11.169 Familial chondrocalcinosis, unspecified knee

M11.17 Familial chondrocalcinosis, ankle and foot

M11.171 Familial chondrocalcinosis, right ankle and foot

M11.172 Familial chondrocalcinosis, left ankle and foot

M11.179 Familial chondrocalcinosis, unspecified ankle and foot

M11.18 Familial chondrocalcinosis, vertebrae

M11.19 Familial chondrocalcinosis, multiple sites

M11.2 Other chondrocalcinosis

Chondrocalcinosis NOS

M11.20 Other chondrocalcinosis, unspecified site

M11.21 Other chondrocalcinosis, shoulder

M11.211 Other chondrocalcinosis, right shoulder

M11.212 Other chondrocalcinosis, left shoulder

M11.219 Other chondrocalcinosis, unspecified shoulder

M11.22 Other chondrocalcinosis, elbow

M11.221 Other chondrocalcinosis, right elbow

M11.222 Other chondrocalcinosis, left elbow

M11.229 Other chondrocalcinosis, unspecified elbow

M11.23 Other chondrocalcinosis, wrist

M11.231 Other chondrocalcinosis, right wrist

M11.232 Other chondrocalcinosis, left wrist

M11.239 Other chondrocalcinosis, unspecified wrist

M11.24 Other chondrocalcinosis, hand

M11.241 Other chondrocalcinosis, right hand

M11.242 Other chondrocalcinosis, left hand

M11.249 Other chondrocalcinosis, unspecified hand

M11.25 Other chondrocalcinosis, hip

M11.251 Other chondrocalcinosis, right hip

M11.252 Other chondrocalcinosis, left hip

M11.259 Other chondrocalcinosis, unspecified hip

M11.26 Other chondrocalcinosis, knee

M11.261 Other chondrocalcinosis, right knee

M11.262 Other chondrocalcinosis, left knee

M11.269 Other chondrocalcinosis, unspecified knee

M11.27 Other chondrocalcinosis, ankle and foot

M11.271 Other chondrocalcinosis, right ankle and foot

M11.272 Other chondrocalcinosis, left ankle and foot

M11.279 Other chondrocalcinosis, unspecified ankle and foot

M11.28 Other chondrocalcinosis, vertebrae

M11.29 Other chondrocalcinosis, multiple sites

M11.8 Other specified crystal arthropathies

M11.80 Other specified crystal arthropathies, unspecified site

M11.81 Other specified crystal arthropathies, shoulder

M11.811 Other specified crystal arthropathies, right shoulder

M11.812 Other specified crystal arthropathies, left shoulder

M11.819 Other specified crystal arthropathies, unspecified shoulder

M11.82 Other specified crystal arthropathies, elbow

M11.821 Other specified crystal arthropathies, right elbow

M11.822 Other specified crystal arthropathies, left elbow

M11.829 Other specified crystal arthropathies, unspecified elbow

M11.83 Other specified crystal arthropathies, wrist

M11.831 Other specified crystal arthropathies, right wrist

M11.832 Other specified crystal arthropathies, left wrist

M11.839 Other specified crystal arthropathies, unspecified wrist

M11.84 Other specified crystal arthropathies, hand

M11.841 Other specified crystal arthropathies, right hand

M11.842 Other specified crystal arthropathies, left hand

M11.849 Other specified crystal arthropathies, unspecified hand

M11.85 Other specified crystal arthropathies, hip

M11.851 Other specified crystal arthropathies, right hip

M11.852 Other specified crystal arthropathies, left hip

M11.859 Other specified crystal arthropathies, unspecified hip

M11.86 Other specified crystal arthropathies, knee

M11.861 Other specified crystal arthropathies, right knee

M11.862 Other specified crystal arthropathies, left knee

M11.869 Other specified crystal arthropathies, unspecified knee

M11.87 Other specified crystal arthropathies, ankle and foot

M11.871 Other specified crystal arthropathies, right ankle and foot

M11.872 Other specified crystal arthropathies, left ankle and foot

M11.879 Other specified crystal arthropathies, unspecified ankle and foot

M11.88 Other specified crystal arthropathies, vertebrae

M11.89 Other specified crystal arthropathies, multiple sites

M11.9 Crystal arthropathy, unspecified

M12 Other and unspecified arthropathy

Excludes1: arthrosis (M15-M19)

cricoarytenoid arthropathy (J38.7)

M12.0 **Chronic postrheumatic arthropathy [Jaccoud]**

    M12.00   Chronic postrheumatic arthropathy [Jaccoud], unspecified site

    M12.01   Chronic postrheumatic arthropathy [Jaccoud], shoulder

        M12.011   Chronic postrheumatic arthropathy [Jaccoud], right shoulder

        M12.012   Chronic postrheumatic arthropathy [Jaccoud], left shoulder

        M12.019   Chronic postrheumatic arthropathy [Jaccoud], unspecified shoulder

    M12.02   Chronic postrheumatic arthropathy [Jaccoud], elbow

        M12.021   Chronic postrheumatic arthropathy [Jaccoud], right elbow

        M12.022   Chronic postrheumatic arthropathy [Jaccoud], left elbow

        M12.029   Chronic postrheumatic arthropathy [Jaccoud], unspecified elbow

    M12.03   Chronic postrheumatic arthropathy [Jaccoud], wrist

        M12.031   Chronic postrheumatic arthropathy [Jaccoud], right wrist

        M12.032   Chronic postrheumatic arthropathy [Jaccoud], left wrist

        M12.039   Chronic postrheumatic arthropathy [Jaccoud], unspecified wrist

    M12.04   Chronic postrheumatic arthropathy [Jaccoud], hand

        M12.041   Chronic postrheumatic arthropathy [Jaccoud], right hand

        M12.042   Chronic postrheumatic arthropathy [Jaccoud], left hand

        M12.049   Chronic postrheumatic arthropathy [Jaccoud], unspecified hand

    M12.05   Chronic postrheumatic arthropathy [Jaccoud], hip

        M12.051   Chronic postrheumatic arthropathy [Jaccoud], right hip

        M12.052   Chronic postrheumatic arthropathy [Jaccoud], left hip

        M12.059   Chronic postrheumatic arthropathy [Jaccoud], unspecified hip

    M12.06   Chronic postrheumatic arthropathy [Jaccoud], knee

        M12.061   Chronic postrheumatic arthropathy [Jaccoud], right knee

        M12.062   Chronic postrheumatic arthropathy [Jaccoud], left knee

        M12.069   Chronic postrheumatic arthropathy [Jaccoud], unspecified knee

    M12.07   Chronic postrheumatic arthropathy [Jaccoud], ankle and foot

        M12.071   Chronic postrheumatic arthropathy [Jaccoud], right ankle and foot

        M12.072   Chronic postrheumatic arthropathy [Jaccoud], left ankle and foot

        M12.079   Chronic postrheumatic arthropathy [Jaccoud], unspecified ankle and foot

    M12.08   Chronic postrheumatic arthropathy [Jaccoud], other specified site

        Chronic postrheumatic arthropathy [Jaccoud], vertebrae

    M12.09   Chronic postrheumatic arthropathy [Jaccoud], multiple sites

M12.1 **Kaschin-Beck disease**

    Osteochondroarthrosis deformans endemica

    M12.10   Kaschin-Beck disease, unspecified site

    M12.11   Kaschin-Beck disease, shoulder

        M12.111   Kaschin-Beck disease, right shoulder

        M12.112   Kaschin-Beck disease, left shoulder

        M12.119   Kaschin-Beck disease, unspecified shoulder

    M12.12   Kaschin-Beck disease, elbow

        M12.121   Kaschin-Beck disease, right elbow

        M12.122   Kaschin-Beck disease, left elbow

        M12.129   Kaschin-Beck disease, unspecified elbow

    M12.13   Kaschin-Beck disease, wrist

        M12.131   Kaschin-Beck disease, right wrist

        M12.132   Kaschin-Beck disease, left wrist

        M12.139   Kaschin-Beck disease, unspecified wrist

    M12.14   Kaschin-Beck disease, hand

        M12.141   Kaschin-Beck disease, right hand

        M12.142   Kaschin-Beck disease, left hand

        M12.149   Kaschin-Beck disease, unspecified hand

    M12.15   Kaschin-Beck disease, hip

        M12.151   Kaschin-Beck disease, right hip

        M12.152   Kaschin-Beck disease, left hip

        M12.159   Kaschin-Beck disease, unspecified hip

    M12.16   Kaschin-Beck disease, knee

        M12.161   Kaschin-Beck disease, right knee

        M12.162   Kaschin-Beck disease, left knee

        M12.169   Kaschin-Beck disease, unspecified knee

    M12.17   Kaschin-Beck disease, ankle and foot

        M12.171   Kaschin-Beck disease, right ankle and foot

        M12.172   Kaschin-Beck disease, left ankle and foot

        M12.179   Kaschin-Beck disease, unspecified ankle and foot

    M12.18   Kaschin-Beck disease, vertebrae

    M12.19   Kaschin-Beck disease, multiple sites

M12.2 **Villonodular synovitis (pigmented)**

    M12.20   Villonodular synovitis (pigmented), unspecified site

    M12.21   Villonodular synovitis (pigmented), shoulder

        M12.211   Villonodular synovitis (pigmented), right shoulder

  ● New code   ▲ Revised code   **Excludes1:** Not coded here   **Excludes2:** Not included here   ⊗ Placeholder required   ⑦ 7th digit required

M12.212 Villonodular synovitis (pigmented), left shoulder

M12.219 Villonodular synovitis (pigmented), unspecified shoulder

M12.22 Villonodular synovitis (pigmented), elbow

M12.221 Villonodular synovitis (pigmented), right elbow

M12.222 Villonodular synovitis (pigmented), left elbow

M12.229 Villonodular synovitis (pigmented), unspecified elbow

M12.23 Villonodular synovitis (pigmented), wrist

M12.231 Villonodular synovitis (pigmented), right wrist

M12.232 Villonodular synovitis (pigmented), left wrist

M12.239 Villonodular synovitis (pigmented), unspecified wrist

M12.24 Villonodular synovitis (pigmented), hand

M12.241 Villonodular synovitis (pigmented), right hand

M12.242 Villonodular synovitis (pigmented), left hand

M12.249 Villonodular synovitis (pigmented), unspecified hand

M12.25 Villonodular synovitis (pigmented), hip

M12.251 Villonodular synovitis (pigmented), right hip

M12.252 Villonodular synovitis (pigmented), left hip

M12.259 Villonodular synovitis (pigmented), unspecified hip

M12.26 Villonodular synovitis (pigmented), knee

M12.261 Villonodular synovitis (pigmented), right knee

M12.262 Villonodular synovitis (pigmented), left knee

M12.269 Villonodular synovitis (pigmented), unspecified knee

M12.27 Villonodular synovitis (pigmented), ankle and foot

M12.271 Villonodular synovitis (pigmented), right ankle and foot

M12.272 Villonodular synovitis (pigmented), left ankle and foot

M12.279 Villonodular synovitis (pigmented), unspecified ankle and foot

M12.28 Villonodular synovitis (pigmented), other specified site

Villonodular synovitis (pigmented), vertebrae

M12.29 Villonodular synovitis (pigmented), multiple sites

M12.3 Palindromic rheumatism

M12.30 Palindromic rheumatism, unspecified site

M12.31 Palindromic rheumatism, shoulder

M12.311 Palindromic rheumatism, right shoulder

M12.312 Palindromic rheumatism, left shoulder

M12.319 Palindromic rheumatism, unspecified shoulder

M12.32 Palindromic rheumatism, elbow

M12.321 Palindromic rheumatism, right elbow

M12.322 Palindromic rheumatism, left elbow

M12.329 Palindromic rheumatism, unspecified elbow

M12.33 Palindromic rheumatism, wrist

M12.331 Palindromic rheumatism, right wrist

M12.332 Palindromic rheumatism, left wrist

M12.339 Palindromic rheumatism, unspecified wrist

M12.34 Palindromic rheumatism, hand

M12.341 Palindromic rheumatism, right hand

M12.342 Palindromic rheumatism, left hand

M12.349 Palindromic rheumatism, unspecified hand

M12.35 Palindromic rheumatism, hip

M12.351 Palindromic rheumatism, right hip

M12.352 Palindromic rheumatism, left hip

M12.359 Palindromic rheumatism, unspecified hip

M12.36 Palindromic rheumatism, knee

M12.361 Palindromic rheumatism, right knee

M12.362 Palindromic rheumatism, left knee

M12.369 Palindromic rheumatism, unspecified knee

M12.37 Palindromic rheumatism, ankle and foot

M12.371 Palindromic rheumatism, right ankle and foot

M12.372 Palindromic rheumatism, left ankle and foot

M12.379 Palindromic rheumatism, unspecified ankle and foot

M12.38 Palindromic rheumatism, other specified site

Palindromic rheumatism, vertebrae

M12.39 Palindromic rheumatism, multiple sites

M12.4 Intermittent hydrarthrosis

M12.40 Intermittent hydrarthrosis, unspecified site

M12.41 Intermittent hydrarthrosis, shoulder

M12.411 Intermittent hydrarthrosis, right shoulder

M12.412 Intermittent hydrarthrosis, left shoulder

M12.419 Intermittent hydrarthrosis, unspecified shoulder

M12.42 Intermittent hydrarthrosis, elbow

M12.421 Intermittent hydrarthrosis, right elbow

M12.422 Intermittent hydrarthrosis, left elbow

M12.429 Intermittent hydrarthrosis, unspecified elbow

M12.43 Intermittent hydrarthrosis, wrist

M12.431 Intermittent hydrarthrosis, right wrist

M12.432 Intermittent hydrarthrosis, left wrist

M12.439 Intermittent hydrarthrosis, unspecified wrist

M12.44 Intermittent hydrarthrosis, hand

M12.441 Intermittent hydrarthrosis, right hand

M12.442 Intermittent hydrarthrosis, left hand

M12.449 Intermittent hydrarthrosis, unspecified hand

M12.45 Intermittent hydrarthrosis, hip

M12.451 Intermittent hydrarthrosis, right hip

M12.452 Intermittent hydrarthrosis, left hip

M12.459 Intermittent hydrarthrosis, unspecified hip

M12.46 Intermittent hydrarthrosis, knee

M12.461 Intermittent hydrarthrosis, right knee

M12.462 Intermittent hydrarthrosis, left knee

M12.469 Intermittent hydrarthrosis, unspecified knee

M12.47 Intermittent hydrarthrosis, ankle and foot

M12.471 Intermittent hydrarthrosis, right ankle and foot

M12.472 Intermittent hydrarthrosis, left ankle and foot

M12.479 Intermittent hydrarthrosis, unspecified ankle and foot

M12.48 Intermittent hydrarthrosis, other site

M12.49 Intermittent hydrarthrosis, multiple sites

M12.5 **Traumatic arthropathy**

Excludes1: current injury-see Alphabetic Index

post-traumatic osteoarthritis of first carpometacarpal joint (M18.2-M18.3)

post-traumatic osteoarthritis of hip (M16.4-M16.5)

post-traumatic osteoarthritis of knee (M17.2-M17.3)

post-traumatic osteoarthritis NOS (M19.1-)

post-traumatic osteoarthritis **of other** single joints (M19.1-)

M12.50 Traumatic arthropathy, unspecified site

M12.51 Traumatic arthropathy, shoulder

M12.511 Traumatic arthropathy, right shoulder

M12.512 Traumatic arthropathy, left shoulder

M12.519 Traumatic arthropathy, unspecified shoulder

M12.52 Traumatic arthropathy, elbow

M12.521 Traumatic arthropathy, right elbow

M12.522 Traumatic arthropathy, left elbow

M12.529 Traumatic arthropathy, unspecified elbow

M12.53 Traumatic arthropathy, wrist

M12.531 Traumatic arthropathy, right wrist

M12.532 Traumatic arthropathy, left wrist

M12.539 Traumatic arthropathy, unspecified wrist

M12.54 Traumatic arthropathy, hand

M12.541 Traumatic arthropathy, right hand

M12.542 Traumatic arthropathy, left hand

M12.549 Traumatic arthropathy, unspecified hand

M12.55 Traumatic arthropathy, hip

M12.551 Traumatic arthropathy, right hip

M12.552 Traumatic arthropathy, left hip

M12.559 Traumatic arthropathy, unspecified hip

M12.56 Traumatic arthropathy, knee

M12.561 Traumatic arthropathy, right knee

M12.562 Traumatic arthropathy, left knee

M12.569 Traumatic arthropathy, unspecified knee

M12.57 Traumatic arthropathy, ankle and foot

M12.571 Traumatic arthropathy, right ankle and foot

M12.572 Traumatic arthropathy, left ankle and foot

M12.579 Traumatic arthropathy, unspecified ankle and foot

M12.58 Traumatic arthropathy, other specified site

Traumatic arthropathy, vertebrae

M12.59 Traumatic arthropathy, multiple sites

M12.8 **Other specific arthropathies, not elsewhere classified**

Transient arthropathy

M12.80 Other specific arthropathies, not elsewhere classified, unspecified site

M12.81 Other specific arthropathies, not elsewhere classified, shoulder

M12.811 Other specific arthropathies, not elsewhere classified, right shoulder

M12.812 Other specific arthropathies, not elsewhere classified, left shoulder

M12.819 Other specific arthropathies, not elsewhere classified, unspecified shoulder

M12.82 Other specific arthropathies, not elsewhere classified, elbow

M12.821 Other specific arthropathies, not elsewhere classified, right elbow

M12.822 Other specific arthropathies, not elsewhere classified, left elbow

M12.829 Other specific arthropathies, not elsewhere classified, unspecified elbow

M12.83 Other specific arthropathies, not elsewhere classified, wrist

M12.831 Other specific arthropathies, not elsewhere classified, right wrist

M12.832 Other specific arthropathies, not elsewhere classified, left wrist

M12.839 Other specific arthropathies, not elsewhere classified, unspecified wrist

● New code ▲ Revised code Excludes1: Not coded here Excludes2: Not included here ⊗ Placeholder required ⑦ 7th digit required

M12.84 Other specific arthropathies, not elsewhere classified, hand

    M12.841 Other specific arthropathies, not elsewhere classified, right hand

    M12.842 Other specific arthropathies, not elsewhere classified, left hand

    M12.849 Other specific arthropathies, not elsewhere classified, unspecified hand

M12.85 Other specific arthropathies, not elsewhere classified, hip

    M12.851 Other specific arthropathies, not elsewhere classified, right hip

    M12.852 Other specific arthropathies, not elsewhere classified, left hip

    M12.859 Other specific arthropathies, not elsewhere classified, unspecified hip

M12.86 Other specific arthropathies, not elsewhere classified, knee

    M12.861 Other specific arthropathies, not elsewhere classified, right knee

    M12.862 Other specific arthropathies, not elsewhere classified, left knee

    M12.869 Other specific arthropathies, not elsewhere classified, unspecified knee

M12.87 Other specific arthropathies, not elsewhere classified, ankle and foot

    M12.871 Other specific arthropathies, not elsewhere classified, right ankle and foot

    M12.872 Other specific arthropathies, not elsewhere classified, left ankle and foot

    M12.879 Other specific arthropathies, not elsewhere classified, unspecified ankle and foot

M12.88 Other specific arthropathies, not elsewhere classified, other specified site

Other specific arthropathies, not elsewhere classified, vertebrae

M12.89 Other specific arthropathies, not elsewhere classified, multiple sites

M12.9 Arthropathy, unspecified

M13 Other arthritis

Excludes1: arthrosis (M15-M19)

osteoarthritis (M15-M19)

M13.0 Polyarthritis, unspecified

M13.1 Monoarthritis, not elsewhere classified

M13.10 Monoarthritis, not elsewhere classified, unspecified site

M13.11 Monoarthritis, not elsewhere classified, shoulder

    M13.111 Monoarthritis, not elsewhere classified, right shoulder

    M13.112 Monoarthritis, not elsewhere classified, left shoulder

    M13.119 Monoarthritis, not elsewhere classified, unspecified shoulder

M13.12 Monoarthritis, not elsewhere classified, elbow

    M13.121 Monoarthritis, not elsewhere classified, right elbow

    M13.122 Monoarthritis, not elsewhere classified, left elbow

    M13.129 Monoarthritis, not elsewhere classified, unspecified elbow

M13.13 Monoarthritis, not elsewhere classified, wrist

    M13.131 Monoarthritis, not elsewhere classified, right wrist

    M13.132 Monoarthritis, not elsewhere classified, left wrist

    M13.139 Monoarthritis, not elsewhere classified, unspecified wrist

M13.14 Monoarthritis, not elsewhere classified, hand

    M13.141 Monoarthritis, not elsewhere classified, right hand

    M13.142 Monoarthritis, not elsewhere classified, left hand

    M13.149 Monoarthritis, not elsewhere classified, unspecified hand

M13.15 Monoarthritis, not elsewhere classified, hip

    M13.151 Monoarthritis, not elsewhere classified, right hip

    M13.152 Monoarthritis, not elsewhere classified, left hip

    M13.159 Monoarthritis, not elsewhere classified, unspecified hip

M13.16 Monoarthritis, not elsewhere classified, knee

    M13.161 Monoarthritis, not elsewhere classified, right knee

    M13.162 Monoarthritis, not elsewhere classified, left knee

    M13.169 Monoarthritis, not elsewhere classified, unspecified knee

M13.17 Monoarthritis, not elsewhere classified, ankle and foot

    M13.171 Monoarthritis, not elsewhere classified, right ankle and foot

    M13.172 Monoarthritis, not elsewhere classified, left ankle and foot

    M13.179 Monoarthritis, not elsewhere classified, unspecified ankle and foot

M13.8 Other specified arthritis

Allergic arthritis

Excludes1: osteoarthritis (M15-M19)

M13.80 Other specified arthritis, unspecified site

M13.81 Other specified arthritis, shoulder

    M13.811 Other specified arthritis, right shoulder

    M13.812 Other specified arthritis, left shoulder

    M13.819 Other specified arthritis, unspecified shoulder

M13.82 Other specified arthritis, elbow

    M13.821 Other specified arthritis, right elbow

    M13.822 Other specified arthritis, left elbow

    M13.829 Other specified arthritis, unspecified elbow

M13.83 Other specified arthritis, wrist

> **M13.831 Other specified arthritis, right wrist**
>
> **M13.832 Other specified arthritis, left wrist**
>
> **M13.839 Other specified arthritis, unspecified wrist**

M13.84 Other specified arthritis, hand

> **M13.841 Other specified arthritis, right hand**
>
> **M13.842 Other specified arthritis, left hand**
>
> **M13.849 Other specified arthritis, unspecified hand**

M13.85 Other specified arthritis, hip

> **M13.851 Other specified arthritis, right hip**
>
> **M13.852 Other specified arthritis, left hip**
>
> **M13.859 Other specified arthritis, unspecified hip**

M13.86 Other specified arthritis, knee

> **M13.861 Other specified arthritis, right knee**
>
> **M13.862 Other specified arthritis, left knee**
>
> **M13.869 Other specified arthritis, unspecified knee**

M13.87 Other specified arthritis, ankle and foot

> **M13.871 Other specified arthritis, right ankle and foot**
>
> **M13.872 Other specified arthritis, left ankle and foot**
>
> **M13.879 Other specified arthritis, unspecified ankle and foot**

M13.88 Other specified arthritis, other site

M13.89 Other specified arthritis, multiple sites

M14 Arthropathies in other diseases classified elsewhere

> **Excludes1:** arthropathy in:
>
> diabetes mellitus (E08-E13 with .61-)
>
> hematological disorders (M36.2-M36.3)
>
> hypersensitivity reactions (M36.4)
>
> neoplastic disease (M36.1)
>
> neurosyphillis (A52.16)
>
> sarcoidosis (D86.86)
>
> enteropathic arthropathies (M07.-)
>
> juvenile psoriatic arthropathy (L40.54)
>
> lipoid dermatoarthritis (E78.81)

M14.6 Charcôt's joint

> Neuropathic arthropathy
>
> **Excludes1:** Charcôt's joint in diabetes mellitus (E08-E13 with .610)
>
> Charcôt's joint in tabes dorsalis (A52.16)

M14.60 Charcôt's joint, unspecified site

M14.61 Charcôt's joint, shoulder

> **M14.611 Charcôt's joint, right shoulder**
>
> **M14.612 Charcôt's joint, left shoulder**
>
> **M14.619 Charcôt's joint, unspecified shoulder**

M14.62 Charcôt's joint, elbow

> **M14.621 Charcôt's joint, right elbow**
>
> **M14.622 Charcôt's joint, left elbow**
>
> **M14.629 Charcôt's joint, unspecified elbow**

M14.63 Charcôt's joint, wrist

> **M14.631 Charcôt's joint, right wrist**
>
> **M14.632 Charcôt's joint, left wrist**
>
> **M14.639 Charcôt's joint, unspecified wrist**

M14.64 Charcôt's joint, hand

> **M14.641 Charcôt's joint, right hand**
>
> **M14.642 Charcôt's joint, left hand**
>
> **M14.649 Charcôt's joint, unspecified hand**

M14.65 Charcôt's joint, hip

> **M14.651 Charcôt's joint, right hip**
>
> **M14.652 Charcôt's joint, left hip**
>
> **M14.659 Charcôt's joint, unspecified hip**

M14.66 Charcôt's joint, knee

> **M14.661 Charcôt's joint, right knee**
>
> **M14.662 Charcôt's joint, left knee**
>
> **M14.669 Charcôt's joint, unspecified knee**

M14.67 Charcôt's joint, ankle and foot

> **M14.671 Charcôt's joint, right ankle and foot**
>
> **M14.672 Charcôt's joint, left ankle and foot**
>
> **M14.679 Charcôt's joint, unspecified ankle and foot**

M14.68 Charcôt's joint, vertebrae

M14.69 Charcôt's joint, multiple sites

M14.8 Arthropathies in other specified diseases classified elsewhere

> **Code first** underlying disease, such as:
>
> amyloidosis (E85.-)
>
> erythema multiforme (L51.-)
>
> erythema nodosum (L52)
>
> hemochromatosis (E83.11-)
>
> hyperparathyroidism (E21.-)
>
> hypothyroidism (E00-E03)
>
> sickle-cell disorders (D57.-)
>
> thyrotoxicosis [hyperthyroidism] (E05.-)
>
> Whipple's disease (K90.81)

M14.80 Arthropathies in other specified diseases classified elsewhere, unspecified site

M14.81 Arthropathies in other specified diseases classified elsewhere, shoulder

> **M14.811 Arthropathies in other specified diseases classified elsewhere, right shoulder**
>
> **M14.812 Arthropathies in other specified diseases classified elsewhere, left shoulder**
>
> **M14.819 Arthropathies in other specified diseases classified elsewhere, unspecified shoulder**

M14.82 Arthropathies in other specified diseases classified elsewhere, elbow

> **M14.821 Arthropathies in other specified diseases classified elsewhere, right elbow**
>
> **M14.822 Arthropathies in other specified diseases classified elsewhere, left elbow**
>
> **M14.829 Arthropathies in other specified diseases classified elsewhere, unspecified elbow**

● New code ▲ Revised code **Excludes1:** Not coded here **Excludes2:** Not included here ⊗ Placeholder required ⑦ 7th digit required

M14.83 Arthropathies in other specified diseases classified elsewhere, wrist

    M14.831 Arthropathies in other specified diseases classified elsewhere, right wrist

    M14.832 Arthropathies in other specified diseases classified elsewhere, left wrist

    M14.839 Arthropathies in other specified diseases classified elsewhere, unspecified wrist

M14.84 Arthropathies in other specified diseases classified elsewhere, hand

    M14.841 Arthropathies in other specified diseases classified elsewhere, right hand

    M14.842 Arthropathies in other specified diseases classified elsewhere, left hand

    M14.849 Arthropathies in other specified diseases classified elsewhere, unspecified hand

M14.85 Arthropathies in other specified diseases classified elsewhere, hip

    M14.851 Arthropathies in other specified diseases classified elsewhere, right hip

    M14.852 Arthropathies in other specified diseases classified elsewhere, left hip

    M14.859 Arthropathies in other specified diseases classified elsewhere, unspecified hip

M14.86 Arthropathies in other specified diseases classified elsewhere, knee

    M14.861 Arthropathies in other specified diseases classified elsewhere, right knee

    M14.862 Arthropathies in other specified diseases classified elsewhere, left knee

    M14.869 Arthropathies in other specified diseases classified elsewhere, unspecified knee

M14.87 Arthropathies in other specified diseases classified elsewhere, ankle and foot

    M14.871 Arthropathies in other specified diseases classified elsewhere, right ankle and foot

    M14.872 Arthropathies in other specified diseases classified elsewhere, left ankle and foot

    M14.879 Arthropathies in other specified diseases classified elsewhere, unspecified ankle and foot

M14.88 Arthropathies in other specified diseases classified elsewhere, vertebrae

M14.89 Arthropathies in other specified diseases classified elsewhere, multiple sites

OSTEOARTHRITIS (M15-M19)

Definition: Osteoarthritis (OA), which is also known as osteoarthrosis or degenerative joint disease (DJD), is a progressivedisorder of the joints caused by gradual loss of cartilage a nd resulting in the development of bony spurs and cysts at the margins of the joints.

Excludes2: osteoarthritis of spine (M47.-)

M15 Polyosteoarthritis

Includes: arthritis of multiple sites

Excludes1: bilateral involvement of single joint (M16-M19)

M15.0 Primary generalized (osteo)arthritis

M15.1 Heberden's nodes (with arthropathy)

    Interphalangeal distal osteoarthritis

M15.2 Bouchard's nodes (with arthropathy)

    Juxtaphalangeal distal osteoarthritis

M15.3 Secondary multiple arthritis

    Post-traumatic polyosteoarthritis

M15.4 Erosive (osteo)arthritis

M15.8 Other polyosteoarthritis

M15.9 Polyosteoarthritis, unspecified

    Generalized osteoarthritis NOS

M16 Osteoarthritis of hip

M16.0 Bilateral primary osteoarthritis of hip

M16.1 Unilateral primary osteoarthritis of hip

    Primary osteoarthritis of hip NOS

    M16.10 Unilateral primary osteoarthritis, unspecified hip

    M16.11 Unilateral primary osteoarthritis, right hip

    M16.12 Unilateral primary osteoarthritis, left hip

M16.2 Bilateral osteoarthritis resulting from hip dysplasia

M16.3 Unilateral osteoarthritis resulting from hip dysplasia

    Dysplastic osteoarthritis of hip NOS

    M16.30 Unilateral osteoarthritis resulting from hip dysplasia, unspecified hip

    M16.31 Unilateral osteoarthritis resulting from hip dysplasia, right hip

    M16.32 Unilateral osteoarthritis resulting from hip dysplasia, left hip

M16.4 Bilateral post-traumatic osteoarthritis of hip

M16.5 Unilateral post-traumatic osteoarthritis of hip

    Post-traumatic osteoarthritis of hip NOS

    M16.50 Unilateral post-traumatic osteoarthritis, unspecified hip

    M16.51 Unilateral post-traumatic osteoarthritis, right hip

    M16.52 Unilateral post-traumatic osteoarthritis, left hip

M16.6 Other bilateral secondary osteoarthritis of hip

M16.7 Other unilateral secondary osteoarthritis of hip

    Secondary osteoarthritis of hip NOS

M16.9 Osteoarthritis of hip, unspecified

M17 Osteoarthritis of knee

M17.0 Bilateral primary osteoarthritis of knee

M17.1 Unilateral primary osteoarthritis of knee

    Primary osteoarthritis of knee NOS

    M17.10 Unilateral primary osteoarthritis, unspecified knee

    M17.11 Unilateral primary osteoarthritis, right knee

    M17.12 Unilateral primary osteoarthritis, left knee

M17.2 Bilateral post-traumatic osteoarthritis of knee

M17.3 **Unilateral post-traumatic osteoarthritis of knee**

Post-traumatic osteoarthritis of knee NOS

M17.30 **Unilateral post-traumatic osteoarthritis, unspecified knee**

M17.31 **Unilateral post-traumatic osteoarthritis, right knee**

M17.32 **Unilateral post-traumatic osteoarthritis, left knee**

M17.4 **Other bilateral secondary osteoarthritis of knee**

M17.5 **Other unilateral secondary osteoarthritis of knee**

Secondary osteoarthritis of knee NOS

M17.9 **Osteoarthritis of knee, unspecified**

M18 **Osteoarthritis of first carpometacarpal joint**

M18.0 **Bilateral primary osteoarthritis of first carpometacarpal joints**

M18.1 **Unilateral primary osteoarthritis of first carpometacarpal joint**

Primary osteoarthritis of first carpometacarpal joint NOS

M18.10 **Unilateral primary osteoarthritis of first carpometacarpal joint, unspecified hand**

M18.11 **Unilateral primary osteoarthritis of first carpometacarpal joint, right hand**

M18.12 **Unilateral primary osteoarthritis of first carpometacarpal joint, left hand**

M18.2 **Bilateral post-traumatic osteoarthritis of first carpometacarpal joints**

M18.3 **Unilateral post-traumatic osteoarthritis of first carpometacarpal joint**

Post-traumatic osteoarthritis of first carpometacarpal joint NOS

M18.30 **Unilateral post-traumatic osteoarthritis of first carpometacarpal joint, unspecified hand**

M18.31 **Unilateral post-traumatic osteoarthritis of first carpometacarpal joint, right hand**

M18.32 **Unilateral post-traumatic osteoarthritis of first carpometacarpal joint, left hand**

M18.4 **Other bilateral secondary osteoarthritis of first carpometacarpal joints**

M18.5 **Other unilateral secondary osteoarthritis of first carpometacarpal joint**

Secondary osteoarthritis of first carpometacarpal joint NOS

M18.50 **Other unilateral secondary osteoarthritis of first carpometacarpal joint, unspecified hand**

M18.51 **Other unilateral secondary osteoarthritis of first carpometacarpal joint, right hand**

M18.52 **Other unilateral secondary osteoarthritis of first carpometacarpal joint, left hand**

M18.9 **Osteoarthritis of first carpometacarpal joint, unspecified**

M19 **Other and unspecified osteoarthritis**

Excludes1: polyarthritis (M15.-)

Excludes2: arthrosis of spine (M47.-)

hallux rigidus (M20.2)

osteoarthritis of spine (M47.-)

M19.0 **Primary osteoarthritis of other joints**

M19.01 **Primary osteoarthritis, shoulder**

M19.011 **Primary osteoarthritis, right shoulder**

M19.012 **Primary osteoarthritis, left shoulder**

M19.019 **Primary osteoarthritis, unspecified shoulder**

M19.02 **Primary osteoarthritis, elbow**

M19.021 **Primary osteoarthritis, right elbow**

M19.022 **Primary osteoarthritis, left elbow**

M19.029 **Primary osteoarthritis, unspecified elbow**

M19.03 **Primary osteoarthritis, wrist**

M19.031 **Primary osteoarthritis, right wrist**

M19.032 **Primary osteoarthritis, left wrist**

M19.039 **Primary osteoarthritis, unspecified wrist**

M19.04 **Primary osteoarthritis, hand**

Excludes2: primary osteoarthritis of first carpometacarpal joint (M18.0-, M18.1-)

M19.041 **Primary osteoarthritis, right hand**

M19.042 **Primary osteoarthritis, left hand**

M19.049 **Primary osteoarthritis, unspecified hand**

M19.07 **Primary osteoarthritis ankle and foot**

M19.071 **Primary osteoarthritis, right ankle and foot**

M19.072 **Primary osteoarthritis, left ankle and foot**

M19.079 **Primary osteoarthritis, unspecified ankle and foot**

M19.1 **Post-traumatic osteoarthritis of other joints**

M19.11 **Post-traumatic osteoarthritis, shoulder**

M19.111 **Post-traumatic osteoarthritis, right shoulder**

M19.112 **Post-traumatic osteoarthritis, left shoulder**

M19.119 **Post-traumatic osteoarthritis, unspecified shoulder**

M19.12 **Post-traumatic osteoarthritis, elbow**

M19.121 **Post-traumatic osteoarthritis, right elbow**

M19.122 **Post-traumatic osteoarthritis, left elbow**

M19.129 **Post-traumatic osteoarthritis, unspecified elbow**

M19.13 **Post-traumatic osteoarthritis, wrist**

M19.131 **Post-traumatic osteoarthritis, right wrist**

M19.132 **Post-traumatic osteoarthritis, left wrist**

M19.139 **Post-traumatic osteoarthritis, unspecified wrist**

M19.14 **Post-traumatic osteoarthritis, hand**

Excludes2: post-traumatic osteoarthritis of first carpometacarpal joint (M18.2-, M18.3-)

M19.141 **Post-traumatic osteoarthritis, right hand**

M19.142 **Post-traumatic osteoarthritis, left hand**

M19.149 **Post-traumatic osteoarthritis, unspecified hand**

M19.17 **Post-traumatic osteoarthritis, ankle and foot**

M19.171 Post-traumatic osteoarthritis, right ankle and foot

M19.172 Post-traumatic osteoarthritis, left ankle and foot

M19.179 Post-traumatic osteoarthritis, unspecified ankle and foot

M19.2 Secondary osteoarthritis of other joints

  M19.21 Secondary osteoarthritis, shoulder

    M19.211 Secondary osteoarthritis, right shoulder

    M19.212 Secondary osteoarthritis, left shoulder

    M19.219 Secondary osteoarthritis, unspecified shoulder

  M19.22 Secondary osteoarthritis, elbow

    M19.221 Secondary osteoarthritis, right elbow

    M19.222 Secondary osteoarthritis, left elbow

    M19.229 Secondary osteoarthritis, unspecified elbow

  M19.23 Secondary osteoarthritis, wrist

    M19.231 Secondary osteoarthritis, right wrist

    M19.232 Secondary osteoarthritis, left wrist

    M19.239 Secondary osteoarthritis, unspecified wrist

  M19.24 Secondary osteoarthritis, hand

    M19.241 Secondary osteoarthritis, right hand

    M19.242 Secondary osteoarthritis, left hand

    M19.249 Secondary osteoarthritis, unspecified hand

  M19.27 Secondary osteoarthritis, ankle and foot

    M19.271 Secondary osteoarthritis, right ankle and foot

    M19.272 Secondary osteoarthritis, left ankle and foot

    M19.279 Secondary osteoarthritis, unspecified ankle and foot

M19.9 Osteoarthritis, unspecified site

  M19.90 Unspecified osteoarthritis, unspecified site

    Arthrosis NOS

    Arthritis NOS

    Osteoarthritis NOS

  M19.91 Primary osteoarthritis, unspecified site

    Primary osteoarthritis NOS

  M19.92 Post-traumatic osteoarthritis, unspecified site

    Post-traumatic osteoarthritis NOS

  M19.93 Secondary osteoarthritis, unspecified site

    Secondary osteoarthritis NOS

OTHER JOINT DISORDERS (M20-M25)

Excludes2: joints of the spine (M40-M54)

M20 Acquired deformities of fingers and toes

  Excludes1: acquired absence of fingers and toes (Z89.-)

    congenital absence of fingers and toes (Q71.3-, Q72.3-)

    congenital deformities and malformations of fingers and toes (Q66.-, Q68-Q70, Q74.-)

  M20.0 Deformity of finger(s)

    Excludes1: clubbing of fingers (R68.3)

      palmar fascial fibromatosis [Dupuytren] (M72.0)

      trigger finger (M65.3)

    M20.00 Unspecified deformity of finger(s)

      M20.001 Unspecified deformity of right finger(s)

      M20.002 Unspecified deformity of left finger(s)

      M20.009 Unspecified deformity of unspecified finger(s)

    M20.01 Mallet finger

      M20.011 Mallet finger of right finger(s)

      M20.012 Mallet finger of left finger(s)

      M20.019 Mallet finger of unspecified finger(s)

    M20.02 Boutonnière deformity

      M20.021 Boutonnière deformity of right finger(s)

      M20.022 Boutonnière deformity of left finger(s)

      M20.029 Boutonnière deformity of unspecified finger(s)

    M20.03 Swan-neck deformity

      M20.031 Swan-neck deformity of right finger(s)

      M20.032 Swan-neck deformity of left finger(s)

      M20.039 Swan-neck deformity of unspecified finger(s)

    M20.09 Other deformity of finger(s)

      M20.091 Other deformity of right finger(s)

      M20.092 Other deformity of left finger(s)

      M20.099 Other deformity of finger(s), unspecified finger(s)

  M20.1 Hallux valgus (acquired)

    Excludes2: bunion (M21.6-)

    M20.10 Hallux valgus (acquired), unspecified foot

    M20.11 Hallux valgus (acquired), right foot

    M20.12 Hallux valgus (acquired), left foot

  M20.2 Hallux rigidus

    M20.20 Hallux rigidus, unspecified foot

    M20.21 Hallux rigidus, right foot

    M20.22 Hallux rigidus, left foot

  M20.3 Hallux varus (acquired)

    M20.30 Hallux varus (acquired), unspecified foot

    M20.31 Hallux varus (acquired), right foot

    M20.32 Hallux varus (acquired), left foot

  M20.4 Other hammer toe(s) (acquired)

    M20.40 Other hammer toe(s) (acquired), unspecified foot

    M20.41 Other hammer toe(s) (acquired), right foot

    M20.42 Other hammer toe(s) (acquired), left foot

  M20.5 Other deformities of toe(s) (acquired)

    M20.5X Other deformities of toe(s) (acquired)

      M20.5X1 Other deformities of toe(s) (acquired), right foot

---

▨ Add 4th-7th digits	▨ Nonspecific code	▨ Unspecified code	▨ Manifestation code

M20.5X2 Other deformities of toe(s) (acquired), left foot

M20.5X9 Other deformities of toe(s) (acquired), unspecified foot

M20.6 Acquired deformities of toe(s), unspecified

    M20.60 Acquired deformities of toe(s), unspecified, unspecified foot

    M20.61 Acquired deformities of toe(s), unspecified, right foot

    M20.62 Acquired deformities of toe(s), unspecified, left foot

M21 **Other acquired deformities of limbs**

    Excludes1: acquired absence of limb (Z89.-)

    congenital absence of limbs (Q71-Q73)

    congenital deformities and malformations of limbs (Q65-Q66, Q68-Q74)

    Excludes2: acquired deformities of fingers or toes (M20.-)

    coxa plana (M91.2)

M21.0 Valgus deformity, not elsewhere classified

    Excludes1: metatarsus valgus (Q66.6)

    talipes calcaneovalgus (Q66.4)

    M21.00 Valgus deformity, not elsewhere classified, unspecified site

    M21.02 Valgus deformity, not elsewhere classified, elbow

    Cubitus valgus

        M21.021 Valgus deformity, not elsewhere classified, right elbow

        M21.022 Valgus deformity, not elsewhere classified, left elbow

        M21.029 Valgus deformity, not elsewhere classified, unspecified elbow

    M21.05 Valgus deformity, not elsewhere classified, hip

        M21.051 Valgus deformity, not elsewhere classified, right hip

        M21.052 Valgus deformity, not elsewhere classified, left hip

        M21.059 Valgus deformity, not elsewhere classified, unspecified hip

    M21.06 Valgus deformity, not elsewhere classified, knee

    Genu valgum

    Knock knee

        M21.061 Valgus deformity, not elsewhere classified, right knee

        M21.062 Valgus deformity, not elsewhere classified, left knee

        M21.069 Valgus deformity, not elsewhere classified, unspecified knee

    M21.07 Valgus deformity, not elsewhere classified, ankle

        M21.071 Valgus deformity, not elsewhere classified, right ankle

        M21.072 Valgus deformity, not elsewhere classified, left ankle

        M21.079 Valgus deformity, not elsewhere classified, unspecified ankle

M21.1 Varus deformity, not elsewhere classified

    Excludes1: metatarsus varus (Q66.22)

tibia vara (M92.5)

    M21.10 Varus deformity, not elsewhere classified, unspecified site

    M21.12 Varus deformity, not elsewhere classified, elbow

    Cubitus varus, elbow

        M21.121 Varus deformity, not elsewhere classified, right elbow

        M21.122 Varus deformity, not elsewhere classified, left elbow

        M21.129 Varus deformity, not elsewhere classified, unspecified elbow

    M21.15 Varus deformity, not elsewhere classified, hip

        M21.151 Varus deformity, not elsewhere classified, right hip

        M21.152 Varus deformity, not elsewhere classified, left hip

        M21.159 Varus deformity, not elsewhere classified, unspecified

    M21.16 Varus deformity, not elsewhere classified, knee

    Bow leg Genu varum

        M21.161 Varus deformity, not elsewhere classified, right knee

        M21.162 Varus deformity, not elsewhere classified, left knee

        M21.169 Varus deformity, not elsewhere classified, unspecified knee

    M21.17 Varus deformity, not elsewhere classified, ankle

        M21.171 Varus deformity, not elsewhere classified, right ankle

        M21.172 Varus deformity, not elsewhere classified, left ankle

        M21.179 Varus deformity, not elsewhere classified, unspecified ankle

M21.2 **Flexion deformity**

    M21.20 Flexion deformity, unspecified site

    M21.21 Flexion deformity, shoulder

        M21.211 Flexion deformity, right shoulder

        M21.212 Flexion deformity, left shoulder

        M21.219 Flexion deformity, unspecified shoulder

    M21.22 Flexion deformity, elbow

        M21.221 Flexion deformity, right elbow

        M21.222 Flexion deformity, left elbow

        M21.229 Flexion deformity, unspecified elbow

    M21.23 Flexion deformity, wrist

        M21.231 Flexion deformity, right wrist

        M21.232 Flexion deformity, left wrist

        M21.239 Flexion deformity, unspecified wrist

    M21.24 Flexion deformity, finger joints

        M21.241 Flexion deformity, right finger joints

        M21.242 Flexion deformity, left finger joints

        M21.249 Flexion deformity, unspecified finger joints

    M21.25 Flexion deformity, hip

● New code   ▲ Revised code   **Excludes1:** Not coded here   **Excludes2:** Not included here   ⊗ Placeholder required   ⑦ 7th digit required

M21.251 Flexion deformity, right hip

M21.252 Flexion deformity, left hip

M21.259 Flexion deformity, unspecified hip

M21.26 Flexion deformity, knee

M21.261 Flexion deformity, right knee

M21.262 Flexion deformity, left knee

M21.269 Flexion deformity, unspecified knee

M21.27 Flexion deformity, ankle and toes

M21.271 Flexion deformity, right ankle and toes

M21.272 Flexion deformity, left ankle and toes

M21.279 Flexion deformity, unspecified ankle and toes

M21.3 Wrist or foot drop (acquired)

M21.33 Wrist drop (acquired)

M21.331 Wrist drop, right wrist

M21.332 Wrist drop, left wrist

M21.339 Wrist drop, unspecified wrist

M21.37 Foot drop (acquired)

M21.371 Foot drop, right foot

M21.372 Foot drop, left foot

M21.379 Foot drop, unspecified foot

M21.4 Flat foot [pes planus] (acquired)

Excludes1: congenital pes planus (Q66.5-)

M21.40 Flat foot [pes planus] (acquired), unspecified foot

M21.41 Flat foot [pes planus] (acquired), right foot

M21.42 Flat foot [pes planus] (acquired), left foot

M21.5 Acquired clawhand, clubhand, clawfoot and clubfoot

Excludes1: clubfoot, not specified as acquired (Q66.89)

M21.51 Acquired clawhand

M21.511 Acquired clawhand, right hand

M21.512 Acquired clawhand, left hand

M21.519 Acquired clawhand, unspecified hand

M21.52 Acquired clubhand

M21.521 Acquired clubhand, right hand

M21.522 Acquired clubhand, left hand

M21.529 Acquired clubhand, unspecified hand

M21.53 Acquired clawfoot

M21.531 Acquired clawfoot, right foot

M21.532 Acquired clawfoot, left foot

M21.539 Acquired clawfoot, unspecified foot

M21.54 Acquired clubfoot

M21.541 Acquired clubfoot, right foot

M21.542 Acquired clubfoot, left foot

M21.549 Acquired clubfoot, unspecified foot

M21.6 Other acquired deformities of foot

Excludes2: deformities of toe (acquired) (M20.1-M20.6-)

M21.61 Bunion

•M21.611 Bunion of right foot

•M21.612 Bunion of left foot

•M21.619 Bunion of unspecified foot

M21.62 Bunionette

•M21.621 Bunionette of right foot

•M21.622 Bunionette of left foot

•M21.629 Bunionette of unspecified foot

M21.6X Other acquired deformities of foot

M21.6X1 Other acquired deformities of right foot

M21.6X2 Other acquired deformities of left foot

M21.6X9 Other acquired deformities of unspecified foot

M21.7 Unequal limb length (acquired)

Note: The site used should correspond to the shorter limb

M21.70 Unequal limb length (acquired), unspecified site

M21.72 Unequal limb length (acquired), humerus

M21.721 Unequal limb length (acquired), right humerus

M21.722 Unequal limb length (acquired), left humerus

M21.729 Unequal limb length (acquired), unspecified humerus

M21.73 Unequal limb length (acquired), ulna and radius

M21.731 Unequal limb length (acquired), right ulna

M21.732 Unequal limb length (acquired), left ulna

M21.733 Unequal limb length (acquired), right radius

M21.734 Unequal limb length (acquired), left radius

M21.739 Unequal limb length (acquired), unspecified ulna and radius

M21.75 Unequal limb length (acquired), femur

M21.751 Unequal limb length (acquired), right femur

M21.752 Unequal limb length (acquired), left femur

M21.759 Unequal limb length (acquired), unspecified femur

M21.76 Unequal limb length (acquired), tibia and fibula

M21.761 Unequal limb length (acquired), right tibia

M21.762 Unequal limb length (acquired), left tibia

M21.763 Unequal limb length (acquired), right fibula

M21.764 Unequal limb length (acquired), left fibula

M21.769 Unequal limb length (acquired), unspecified tibia and fibula

M21.8 Other specified acquired deformities of limbs

Excludes2: coxa plana (M91.2)

M21.80 Other specified acquired deformities of unspecified limb

M21.82 Other specified acquired deformities of upper arm

M21.821   Other specified acquired deformities of right upper arm

M21.822   Other specified acquired deformities of left upper arm

M21.829   Other specified acquired deformities of unspecified upper arm

M21.83   Other specified acquired deformities of forearm

M21.831   Other specified acquired deformities of right forearm

M21.832   Other specified acquired deformities of left forearm

M21.839   Other specified acquired deformities of unspecified forearm

M21.85   Other specified acquired deformities of thigh

M21.851   Other specified acquired deformities of right thigh

M21.852   Other specified acquired deformities of left thigh

M21.859   Other specified acquired deformities of unspecified thigh

M21.86   Other specified acquired deformities of lower leg

M21.861   Other specified acquired deformities of right lower leg

M21.862   Other specified acquired deformities of left lower leg

M21.869   Other specified acquired deformities of unspecified lower leg

M21.9   Unspecified acquired deformity of limb and hand

M21.90   Unspecified acquired deformity of unspecified limb

M21.92   Unspecified acquired deformity of upper arm

M21.921   Unspecified acquired deformity of right upper arm

M21.922   Unspecified acquired deformity of left upper arm

M21.929   Unspecified acquired deformity of unspecified upper arm

M21.93   Unspecified acquired deformity of forearm

M21.931   Unspecified acquired deformity of right forearm

M21.932   Unspecified acquired deformity of left forearm

M21.939   Unspecified acquired deformity of unspecified forearm

M21.94   Unspecified acquired deformity of hand

M21.941   Unspecified acquired deformity of hand, right hand

M21.942   Unspecified acquired deformity of hand, left hand

M21.949   Unspecified acquired deformity of hand, unspecified hand

M21.95   Unspecified acquired deformity of thigh

M21.951   Unspecified acquired deformity of right thigh

M21.952   Unspecified acquired deformity of left thigh

M21.959   Unspecified acquired deformity of unspecified thigh

M21.96   Unspecified acquired deformity of lower leg

M21.961   Unspecified acquired deformity of right lower leg

M21.962   Unspecified acquired deformity of left lower leg

M21.969   Unspecified acquired deformity of unspecified lower leg

M22   **Disorder of patella**

Excludes1: traumatic dislocation of patella (S83.0-)

M22.0   Recurrent dislocation of patella

M22.00   Recurrent dislocation of patella, unspecified knee

M22.01   Recurrent dislocation of patella, right knee

M22.02   Recurrent dislocation of patella, left knee

M22.1   Recurrent subluxation of patella

Incomplete dislocation of patella

M22.10   Recurrent subluxation of patella, unspecified knee

M22.11   Recurrent subluxation of patella, right knee

M22.12   Recurrent subluxation of patella, left knee

M22.2   Patellofemoral disorders

M22.2X   Patellofemoral disorders

M22.2X1   Patellofemoral disorders, right knee

M22.2X2   Patellofemoral disorders, left knee

M22.2X9   Patellofemoral disorders, unspecified knee

M22.3   Other derangements of patella

M22.3X   Other derangements of patella

M22.3X1   Other derangements of patella, right knee

M22.3X2   Other derangements of patella, left knee

M22.3X9   Other derangements of patella, unspecified knee

M22.4   Chondromalacia patellae

M22.40   Chondromalacia patellae, unspecified knee

M22.41   Chondromalacia patellae, right knee

M22.42   Chondromalacia patellae, left knee

M22.8   Other disorders of patella

M22.8X   Other disorders of patella

M22.8X1   Other disorders of patella, right knee

M22.8X2   Other disorders of patella, left knee

M22.8X9   Other disorders of patella, unspecified knee

M22.9   Unspecified disorder of patella

M22.90   Unspecified disorder of patella, unspecified knee

M22.91   Unspecified disorder of patella, right knee

M22.92   Unspecified disorder of patella, left knee

M23   **Internal derangement of knee**

Definition: Internal derangement of knee is a term that describes internal damage to the knee joint, generally caused by trauma. It is a nonspecific term that usually must be further refined by history, physical exam, x-rays, and frequently mri studies.

Excludes1: ankylosis (M24.66)

current injury - see injury of knee and lower leg (S80-S89)

  ● New code   ▲ Revised code   Excludes1: Not coded here   Excludes2: Not included here   ⊗ Placeholder required   ⑦ 7th digit required

deformity of knee (M21.-)

osteochondritis dissecans (M93.2)

recurrent dislocation or subluxation of joints (M24.4)

recurrent dislocation or subluxation of patella (M22.0-M22.1)

M23.0   Cystic meniscus

    M23.00   Cystic meniscus, unspecified meniscus

        Cystic meniscus, unspecified lateral meniscus

        Cystic meniscus, unspecified medial meniscus

        M23.000   Cystic meniscus, unspecified lateral meniscus, right knee

        M23.001   Cystic meniscus, unspecified lateral meniscus, left knee

        M23.002   Cystic meniscus, unspecified lateral meniscus, unspecified knee

        M23.003   Cystic meniscus, unspecified medial meniscus, right knee

        M23.004   Cystic meniscus, unspecified medial meniscus, left knee

        M23.005   Cystic meniscus, unspecified medial meniscus, unspecified knee

        M23.006   Cystic meniscus, unspecified meniscus, right knee

        M23.007   Cystic meniscus, unspecified meniscus, left knee

        M23.009   Cystic meniscus, unspecified meniscus, unspecified knee

    M23.01   Cystic meniscus, anterior horn of medial meniscus

        M23.011   Cystic meniscus, anterior horn of medial meniscus, right knee

        M23.012   Cystic meniscus, anterior horn of medial meniscus, left knee

        M23.019   Cystic meniscus, anterior horn of medial meniscus, unspecified knee

    M23.02   Cystic meniscus, posterior horn of medial meniscus

        M23.021   Cystic meniscus, posterior horn of medial meniscus, right knee

        M23.022   Cystic meniscus, posterior horn of medial meniscus, left knee

        M23.029   Cystic meniscus, posterior horn of medial meniscus, unspecified knee

    M23.03   Cystic meniscus, other medial meniscus

        M23.031   Cystic meniscus, other medial meniscus, right knee

        M23.032   Cystic meniscus, other medial meniscus, left knee

        M23.039   Cystic meniscus, other medial meniscus, unspecified knee

    M23.04   Cystic meniscus, anterior horn of lateral meniscus

        M23.041   Cystic meniscus, anterior horn of lateral meniscus, right knee

        M23.042   Cystic meniscus, anterior horn of lateral meniscus, left knee

        M23.049   Cystic meniscus, anterior horn of lateral meniscus, unspecified knee

    M23.05   Cystic meniscus, posterior horn of lateral meniscus

        M23.051   Cystic meniscus, posterior horn of lateral meniscus, right knee

        M23.052   Cystic meniscus, posterior horn of lateral meniscus, left knee

        M23.059   Cystic meniscus, posterior horn of lateral meniscus, unspecified knee

    M23.06   Cystic meniscus, other lateral meniscus

        M23.061   Cystic meniscus, other lateral meniscus, right knee

        M23.062   Cystic meniscus, other lateral meniscus, left knee

        M23.069   Cystic meniscus, other lateral meniscus, unspecified knee

M23.2   Derangement of meniscus due to old tear or injury

    Old bucket-handle tear

    M23.20   Derangement of unspecified meniscus due to old tear or injury

        Derangement of unspecified lateral meniscus due to old tear or injury

        Derangement of unspecified medial meniscus due to old tear or injury

        M23.200   Derangement of unspecified lateral meniscus due to old tear or injury, right knee

        M23.201   Derangement of unspecified lateral meniscus due to old tear or injury, left knee

        M23.202   Derangement of unspecified lateral meniscus due to old tear or injury, unspecified knee

        M23.203   Derangement of unspecified medial meniscus due to old tear or injury, right knee

        M23.204   Derangement of unspecified medial meniscus due to old tear or injury, left knee

        M23.205   Derangement of unspecified medial meniscus due to old tear or injury, unspecified knee

        M23.206   Derangement of unspecified meniscus due to old tear or injury, right knee

        M23.207   Derangement of unspecified meniscus due to old tear or injury, left knee

        M23.209   Derangement of unspecified meniscus due to old tear or injury, unspecified knee

    M23.21   Derangement of anterior horn of medial meniscus due to old tear or injury

        M23.211   Derangement of anterior horn of medial meniscus due to old tear or injury, right knee

        M23.212   Derangement of anterior horn of medial meniscus due to old tear or injury, left knee

        M23.219   Derangement of anterior horn of medial meniscus due to old tear or injury, unspecified knee

    M23.22   Derangement of posterior horn of medial meniscus due to old tear or injury

M23.221 Derangement of posterior horn of medial meniscus due to old tear or injury, right knee

M23.222 Derangement of posterior horn of medial meniscus due to old tear or injury, left knee

M23.229 Derangement of posterior horn of medial meniscus due to old tear or injury, unspecified knee

M23.23 Derangement of other medial meniscus due to old tear or injury

M23.231 Derangement of other medial meniscus due to old tear or injury, right knee

M23.232 Derangement of other medial meniscus due to old tear or injury, left knee

M23.239 Derangement of other medial meniscus due to old tear or injury, unspecified knee

M23.24 Derangement of anterior horn of lateral meniscus due to old tear or injury

M23.241 Derangement of anterior horn of lateral meniscus due to old tear or injury, right knee

M23.242 Derangement of anterior horn of lateral meniscus due to old tear or injury, left knee

M23.249 Derangement of anterior horn of lateral meniscus due to old tear or injury, unspecified knee

M23.25 Derangement of posterior horn of lateral meniscus due to old tear or injury

M23.251 Derangement of posterior horn of lateral meniscus due to old tear or injury, right knee

M23.252 Derangement of posterior horn of lateral meniscus due to old tear or injury, left knee

M23.259 Derangement of posterior horn of lateral meniscus due to old tear or injury, unspecified knee

M23.26 Derangement of other lateral meniscus due to old tear or injury

M23.261 Derangement of other lateral meniscus due to old tear or injury, right knee

M23.262 Derangement of other lateral meniscus due to old tear or injury, left knee

M23.269 Derangement of other lateral meniscus due to old tear or injury, unspecified knee

M23.3 Other meniscus derangements

Degenerate meniscus

Detached meniscus

Retained meniscus

M23.30 Other meniscus derangements, unspecified meniscus

Other meniscus derangements, unspecified lateral meniscus

Other meniscus derangements, unspecified medial meniscus

M23.300 Other meniscus derangements, unspecified lateral meniscus, right knee

M23.301 Other meniscus derangements, unspecified lateral meniscus, left knee

M23.302 Other meniscus derangements, unspecified lateral meniscus, unspecified knee

M23.303 Other meniscus derangements, unspecified medial meniscus, right knee

M23.304 Other meniscus derangements, unspecified medial meniscus, left knee

M23.305 Other meniscus derangements, unspecified medial meniscus, unspecified knee

M23.306 Other meniscus derangements, unspecified meniscus, right knee

M23.307 Other meniscus derangements, unspecified meniscus, left knee

M23.309 Other meniscus derangements, unspecified meniscus, unspecified knee

M23.31 Other meniscus derangements, anterior horn of medial meniscus

M23.311 Other meniscus derangements, anterior horn of medial meniscus, right knee

M23.312 Other meniscus derangements, anterior horn of medial meniscus, left knee

M23.319 Other meniscus derangements, anterior horn of medial meniscus, unspecified knee

M23.32 Other meniscus derangements, posterior horn of medial meniscus

M23.321 Other meniscus derangements, posterior horn of medial meniscus, right knee

M23.322 Other meniscus derangements, posterior horn of medial meniscus, left knee

M23.329 Other meniscus derangements, posterior horn of medial meniscus, unspecified knee

M23.33 Other meniscus derangements, other medial meniscus

M23.331 Other meniscus derangements, other medial meniscus, right knee

M23.332 Other meniscus derangements, other medial meniscus, left knee

M23.339 Other meniscus derangements, other medial meniscus, unspecified knee

M23.34 Other meniscus derangements, anterior horn of lateral meniscus

M23.341 Other meniscus derangements, anterior horn of lateral meniscus, right knee

M23.342 Other meniscus derangements, anterior horn of lateral meniscus, left knee

● New code ▲ Revised code **Excludes1:** Not coded here **Excludes2:** Not included here ⊗ Placeholder required ⑦ 7th digit required

M23.349 Other meniscus derangements, anterior horn of lateral meniscus, unspecified knee

M23.35 Other meniscus derangements, posterior horn of lateral meniscus

   M23.351 Other meniscus derangements, posterior horn of lateral meniscus, right knee

   M23.352 Other meniscus derangements, posterior horn of lateral meniscus, left knee

   M23.359 Other meniscus derangements, posterior horn of lateral meniscus, unspecified knee

M23.36 Other meniscus derangements, other lateral meniscus

   M23.361 Other meniscus derangements, other lateral meniscus, right knee

   M23.362 Other meniscus derangements, other lateral meniscus, left knee

   M23.369 Other meniscus derangements, other lateral meniscus, unspecified knee

M23.4 Loose body in knee

   M23.40 Loose body in knee, unspecified knee

   M23.41 Loose body in knee, right knee

   M23.42 Loose body in knee, left knee

M23.5 Chronic instability of knee

   M23.50 Chronic instability of knee, unspecified knee

   M23.51 Chronic instability of knee, right knee

   M23.52 Chronic instability of knee, left knee

M23.6 Other spontaneous disruption of ligament(s) of knee

   M23.60 Other spontaneous disruption of unspecified ligament of knee

     M23.601 Other spontaneous disruption of unspecified ligament of right knee

     M23.602 Other spontaneous disruption of unspecified ligament of left knee

     M23.609 Other spontaneous disruption of unspecified ligament of unspecified knee

   M23.61 Other spontaneous disruption of anterior cruciate ligament of knee

     M23.611 Other spontaneous disruption of anterior cruciate ligament of right knee

     M23.612 Other spontaneous disruption of anterior cruciate ligament of left knee

     M23.619 Other spontaneous disruption of anterior cruciate ligament of unspecified knee

   M23.62 Other spontaneous disruption of posterior cruciate ligament of knee

     M23.621 Other spontaneous disruption of posterior cruciate ligament of right knee

     M23.622 Other spontaneous disruption of posterior cruciate ligament of left knee

     M23.629 Other spontaneous disruption of posterior cruciate ligament of unspecified knee

   M23.63 Other spontaneous disruption of medial collateral ligament of knee

     M23.631 Other spontaneous disruption of medial collateral ligament of right knee

     M23.632 Other spontaneous disruption of medial collateral ligament of left knee

     M23.639 Other spontaneous disruption of medial collateral ligament of unspecified knee

   M23.64 Other spontaneous disruption of lateral collateral ligament of knee

     M23.641 Other spontaneous disruption of lateral collateral ligament of right knee

     M23.642 Other spontaneous disruption of lateral collateral ligament of left knee

     M23.649 Other spontaneous disruption of lateral collateral ligament of unspecified knee

   M23.67 Other spontaneous disruption of capsular ligament of knee

     M23.671 Other spontaneous disruption of capsular ligament of right knee

     M23.672 Other spontaneous disruption of capsular ligament of left knee

     M23.679 Other spontaneous disruption of capsular ligament of unspecified knee

M23.8 Other internal derangements of knee

Laxity of ligament of knee

Snapping knee

   M23.8X Other internal derangements of knee

     M23.8X1 Other internal derangements of right knee

     M23.8X2 Other internal derangements of left knee

     M23.8X9 Other internal derangements of unspecified knee

M23.9 Unspecified internal derangement of knee

   M23.90 Unspecified internal derangement of unspecified knee

   M23.91 Unspecified internal derangement of right knee

   M23.92 Unspecified internal derangement of left knee

M24 Other specific joint derangements

Excludes1: current injury - see injury of joint by body region

Excludes2: ganglion (M67.4)

snapping knee (M23.8-)

temporomandibular joint disorders (M26.6-)

M24.0 Loose body in joint

Excludes2: loose body in knee (M23.4)

   M24.00 Loose body in unspecified joint

   M24.01 Loose body in shoulder

     M24.011 Loose body in right shoulder

M24.012   Loose body in left shoulder

M24.019   Loose body in unspecified shoulder

M24.02   Loose body in elbow

     M24.021   Loose body in right elbow

     M24.022   Loose body in left elbow

     M24.029   Loose body in unspecified elbow

M24.03   Loose body in wrist

     M24.031   Loose body in right wrist

     M24.032   Loose body in left wrist

     M24.039   Loose body in unspecified wrist

M24.04   Loose body in finger joints

     M24.041   Loose body in right finger joint(s)

     M24.042   Loose body in left finger joint(s)

     M24.049   Loose body in unspecified finger joint(s)

M24.05   Loose body in hip

     M24.051   Loose body in right hip

     M24.052   Loose body in left hip

     M24.059   Loose body in unspecified hip

M24.07   Loose body in ankle and toe joints

     M24.071   Loose body in right ankle

     M24.072   Loose body in left ankle

     M24.073   Loose body in unspecified ankle

     M24.074   Loose body in right toe joint(s)

     M24.075   Loose body in left toe joint(s)

     M24.076   Loose body in unspecified toe joints

M24.08   Loose body, other site

M24.1   **Other articular cartilage disorders**

   Excludes2: chondrocalcinosis (M11.1, M11.2-)

     internal derangement of knee (M23.-)

     metastatic calcification (E83.5)

     ochronosis (E70.2)

M24.10   Other articular cartilage disorders, unspecified site

M24.11   Other articular cartilage disorders, shoulder

     M24.111   Other articular cartilage disorders, right shoulder

     M24.112   Other articular cartilage disorders, left shoulder

     M24.119   Other articular cartilage disorders, unspecified shoulder

M24.12   Other articular cartilage disorders, elbow

     M24.121   Other articular cartilage disorders, right elbow

     M24.122   Other articular cartilage disorders, left elbow

     M24.129   Other articular cartilage disorders, unspecified elbow

M24.13   Other articular cartilage disorders, wrist

     M24.131   Other articular cartilage disorders, right wrist

     M24.132   Other articular cartilage disorders, left wrist

     M24.139   Other articular cartilage disorders, unspecified wrist

M24.14   Other articular cartilage disorders, hand

     M24.141   Other articular cartilage disorders, right hand

     M24.142   Other articular cartilage disorders, left hand

     M24.149   Other articular cartilage disorders, unspecified hand

M24.15   Other articular cartilage disorders, hip

     M24.151   Other articular cartilage disorders, right hip

     M24.152   Other articular cartilage disorders, left hip

     M24.159   Other articular cartilage disorders, unspecified hip

M24.17   Other articular cartilage disorders, ankle and foot

     M24.171   Other articular cartilage disorders, right ankle

     M24.172   Other articular cartilage disorders, left ankle

     M24.173   Other articular cartilage disorders, unspecified ankle

     M24.174   Other articular cartilage disorders, right foot

     M24.175   Other articular cartilage disorders, left foot

     M24.176   Other articular cartilage disorders, unspecified foot

M24.2   **Disorder of ligament**

Instability secondary to old ligament injury

Ligamentous laxity NOS

   Excludes1: familial ligamentous laxity (M35.7)

   Excludes2: internal derangement of knee (M23.5-M23.89)

M24.20   Disorder of ligament, unspecified site

M24.21   Disorder of ligament, shoulder

     M24.211   Disorder of ligament, right shoulder

     M24.212   Disorder of ligament, left shoulder

     M24.219   Disorder of ligament, unspecified shoulder

M24.22   Disorder of ligament, elbow

     M24.221   Disorder of ligament, right elbow

     M24.222   Disorder of ligament, left elbow

     M24.229   Disorder of ligament, unspecified elbow

M24.23   Disorder of ligament, wrist

     M24.231   Disorder of ligament, right wrist

     M24.232   Disorder of ligament, left wrist

     M24.239   Disorder of ligament, unspecified wrist

M24.24   Disorder of ligament, hand

     M24.241   Disorder of ligament, right hand

     M24.242   Disorder of ligament, left hand

     M24.249   Disorder of ligament, unspecified hand

M24.25   Disorder of ligament, hip

     M24.251   Disorder of ligament, right hip

     M24.252   Disorder of ligament, left hip

     M24.259   Disorder of ligament, unspecified hip

M24.27   Disorder of ligament, ankle and foot

    M24.271   Disorder of ligament, right ankle

    M24.272   Disorder of ligament, left ankle

    M24.273   Disorder of ligament, unspecified ankle

    M24.274   Disorder of ligament, right foot

    M24.275   Disorder of ligament, left foot

    M24.276   Disorder of ligament, unspecified foot

M24.28   Disorder of ligament, vertebrae

M24.3   Pathological dislocation of joint, not elsewhere classified

Excludes1: congenital dislocation or displacement of joint- see congenital malformations and deformations of the musculoskeletal system (Q65-Q79)

current injury - see injury of joints and ligaments by body region

recurrent dislocation of joint (M24.4-)

M24.30   Pathological dislocation of unspecified joint, not elsewhere classified

M24.31   Pathological dislocation of shoulder, not elsewhere classified

    M24.311   Pathological dislocation of right shoulder, not elsewhere classified

    M24.312   Pathological dislocation of left shoulder, not elsewhere classified

    M24.319   Pathological dislocation of unspecified shoulder, not elsewhere classified

M24.32   Pathological dislocation of elbow, not elsewhere classified

    M24.321   Pathological dislocation of right elbow, not elsewhere classified

    M24.322   Pathological dislocation of left elbow, not elsewhere classified

    M24.329   Pathological dislocation of unspecified elbow, not elsewhere classified

M24.33   Pathological dislocation of wrist, not elsewhere classified

    M24.331   Pathological dislocation of right wrist, not elsewhere classified

    M24.332   Pathological dislocation of left wrist, not elsewhere classified

    M24.339   Pathological dislocation of unspecified wrist, not elsewhere classified

M24.34   Pathological dislocation of hand, not elsewhere classified

    M24.341   Pathological dislocation of right hand, not elsewhere classified

    M24.342   Pathological dislocation of left hand, not elsewhere classified

    M24.349   Pathological dislocation of unspecified hand, not elsewhere classified

M24.35   Pathological dislocation of hip, not elsewhere classified

    M24.351   Pathological dislocation of right hip, not elsewhere classified

    M24.352   Pathological dislocation of left hip, not elsewhere classified

    M24.359   Pathological dislocation of unspecified hip, not elsewhere classified

M24.36   Pathological dislocation of knee, not elsewhere classified

    M24.361   Pathological dislocation of right knee, not elsewhere classified

    M24.362   Pathological dislocation of left knee, not elsewhere classified

    M24.369   Pathological dislocation of unspecified knee, not elsewhere classified

M24.37   Pathological dislocation of ankle and foot, not elsewhere classified

    M24.371   Pathological dislocation of right ankle, not elsewhere classified

    M24.372   Pathological dislocation of left ankle, not elsewhere classified

    M24.373   Pathological dislocation of unspecified ankle, not elsewhere classified

    M24.374   Pathological dislocation of right foot, not elsewhere classified

    M24.375   Pathological dislocation of left foot, not elsewhere classified

    M24.376   Pathological dislocation of unspecified foot, not elsewhere classified

M24.4   Recurrent dislocation of joint

Recurrent subluxation of joint

Excludes2: recurrent dislocation of patella (M22.0-M22.1)

recurrent vertebral dislocation (M43.3-, M43.4, M43.5-)

M24.40   Recurrent dislocation, unspecified joint

M24.41   Recurrent dislocation, shoulder

    M24.411   Recurrent dislocation, right shoulder

    M24.412   Recurrent dislocation, left shoulder

    M24.419   Recurrent dislocation, unspecified shoulder

M24.42   Recurrent dislocation, elbow

    M24.421   Recurrent dislocation, right elbow

    M24.422   Recurrent dislocation, left elbow

    M24.429   Recurrent dislocation, unspecified elbow

M24.43   Recurrent dislocation, wrist

    M24.431   Recurrent dislocation, right wrist

    M24.432   Recurrent dislocation, left wrist

    M24.439   Recurrent dislocation, unspecified wrist

M24.44   Recurrent dislocation, hand and finger(s)

    M24.441   Recurrent dislocation, right hand

    M24.442   Recurrent dislocation, left hand

    M24.443   Recurrent dislocation, unspecified hand

    M24.444   Recurrent dislocation, right finger

    M24.445   Recurrent dislocation, left finger

    M24.446   Recurrent dislocation, unspecified finger

M24.45　Recurrent dislocation, hip
　　　　M24.451　Recurrent dislocation, right hip
　　　　M24.452　Recurrent dislocation, left hip
　　　　M24.459　Recurrent dislocation, unspecified hip
M24.46　Recurrent dislocation, knee
　　　　M24.461　Recurrent dislocation, right knee
　　　　M24.462　Recurrent dislocation, left knee
　　　　M24.469　Recurrent dislocation, unspecified knee
M24.47　Recurrent dislocation, ankle, foot and toes
　　　　M24.471　Recurrent dislocation, right ankle
　　　　M24.472　Recurrent dislocation, left ankle
　　　　M24.473　Recurrent dislocation, unspecified ankle
　　　　M24.474　Recurrent dislocation, right foot
　　　　M24.475　Recurrent dislocation, left foot
　　　　M24.476　Recurrent dislocation, unspecified foot
　　　　M24.477　Recurrent dislocation, right toe(s)
　　　　M24.478　Recurrent dislocation, left toe(s)
　　　　M24.479　Recurrent dislocation, unspecified toe(s)

M24.5　Contracture of joint
　　Excludes1: contracture of muscle without contracture of joint (M62.4-)
　　　contracture of tendon (sheath) without contracture of joint (M62.4-)
　　　Dupuytren's contracture (M72.0)
　　Excludes2: acquired deformities of limbs (M20-M21)
　　M24.50　Contracture, unspecified joint
　　M24.51　Contracture, shoulder
　　　　M24.511　Contracture, right shoulder
　　　　M24.512　Contracture, left shoulder
　　　　M24.519　Contracture, unspecified shoulder
　　M24.52　Contracture, elbow
　　　　M24.521　Contracture, right elbow
　　　　M24.522　Contracture, left elbow
　　　　M24.529　Contracture, unspecified elbow
　　M24.53　Contracture, wrist
　　　　M24.531　Contracture, right wrist
　　　　M24.532　Contracture, left wrist
　　　　M24.539　Contracture, unspecified wrist
　　M24.54　Contracture, hand
　　　　M24.541　Contracture, right hand
　　　　M24.542　Contracture, left hand
　　　　M24.549　Contracture, unspecified hand
　　M24.55　Contracture, hip
　　　　M24.551　Contracture, right hip
　　　　M24.552　Contracture, left hip
　　　　M24.559　Contracture, unspecified hip
　　M24.56　Contracture, knee
　　　　M24.561　Contracture, right knee
　　　　M24.562　Contracture, left knee
　　　　M24.569　Contracture, unspecified knee

M24.57　Contracture, ankle and foot
　　　　M24.571　Contracture, right ankle
　　　　M24.572　Contracture, left ankle
　　　　M24.573　Contracture, unspecified ankle
　　　　M24.574　Contracture, right foot
　　　　M24.575　Contracture, left foot
　　　　M24.576　Contracture, unspecified foot

M24.6　Ankylosis of joint
　　Excludes1: stiffness of joint without ankylosis (M25.6-)
　　Excludes2: spine (M43.2-)
　　M24.60　Ankylosis, unspecified joint
　　M24.61　Ankylosis, shoulder
　　　　M24.611　Ankylosis, right shoulder
　　　　M24.612　Ankylosis, left shoulder
　　　　M24.619　Ankylosis, unspecified shoulder
　　M24.62　Ankylosis, elbow
　　　　M24.621　Ankylosis, right elbow
　　　　M24.622　Ankylosis, left elbow
　　　　M24.629　Ankylosis, unspecified elbow
　　M24.63　Ankylosis, wrist
　　　　M24.631　Ankylosis, right wrist
　　　　M24.632　Ankylosis, left wrist
　　　　M24.639　Ankylosis, unspecified wrist
　　M24.64　Ankylosis, hand
　　　　M24.641　Ankylosis, right hand
　　　　M24.642　Ankylosis, left hand
　　　　M24.649　Ankylosis, unspecified hand
　　M24.65　Ankylosis, hip
　　　　M24.651　Ankylosis, right hip
　　　　M24.652　Ankylosis, left hip
　　　　M24.659　Ankylosis, unspecified hip
　　M24.66　Ankylosis, knee
　　　　M24.661　Ankylosis, right knee
　　　　M24.662　Ankylosis, left knee
　　　　M24.669　Ankylosis, unspecified knee
　　M24.67　Ankylosis, ankle and foot
　　　　M24.671　Ankylosis, right ankle
　　　　M24.672　Ankylosis, left ankle
　　　　M24.673　Ankylosis, unspecified ankle
　　　　M24.674　Ankylosis, right foot
　　　　M24.675　Ankylosis, left foot
　　　　M24.676　Ankylosis, unspecified foot

M24.7　Protrusio acetabuli

M24.8　Other specific joint derangements, not elsewhere classified
　　Excludes2: iliotibial band syndrome (M76.3)
　　M24.80　Other specific joint derangements of unspecified joint, not elsewhere classified
　　M24.81　Other specific joint derangements of shoulder, not elsewhere classified
　　　　M24.811　Other specific joint derangements of right shoulder, not elsewhere classified

M24.812 Other specific joint derangements of left shoulder, not elsewhere classified

M24.819 Other specific joint derangements of unspecified shoulder, not elsewhere classified

M24.82 Other specific joint derangements of elbow, not elsewhere classified

M24.821 Other specific joint derangements of right elbow, not elsewhere classified

M24.822 Other specific joint derangements of left elbow, not elsewhere classified

M24.829 Other specific joint derangements of unspecified elbow, not elsewhere classified

M24.83 Other specific joint derangements of wrist, not elsewhere classified

M24.831 Other specific joint derangements of right wrist, not elsewhere classified

M24.832 Other specific joint derangements of left wrist, not elsewhere classified

M24.839 Other specific joint derangements of unspecified wrist, not elsewhere classified

M24.84 Other specific joint derangements of hand, not elsewhere classified

M24.841 Other specific joint derangements of right hand, not elsewhere classified

M24.842 Other specific joint derangements of left hand, not elsewhere classified

M24.849 Other specific joint derangements of unspecified hand, not elsewhere classified

M24.85 Other specific joint derangements of hip, not elsewhere classified

Irritable hip

M24.851 Other specific joint derangements of right hip, not elsewhere classified

M24.852 Other specific joint derangements of left hip, not elsewhere classified

M24.859 Other specific joint derangements of unspecified hip, not elsewhere classified

M24.87 Other specific joint derangements of ankle and foot, not elsewhere classified

M24.871 Other specific joint derangements of right ankle, not elsewhere classified

M24.872 Other specific joint derangements of left ankle, not elsewhere classified

M24.873 Other specific joint derangements of unspecified ankle, not elsewhere classified

M24.874 Other specific joint derangements of right foot, not elsewhere classified

M24.875 Other specific joint derangements left foot, not elsewhere classified

M24.876 Other specific joint derangements of unspecified foot, not elsewhere classified

M24.9 Joint derangement, unspecified

M25 Other joint disorder, not elsewhere classified

Excludes2: abnormality of gait and mobility (R26.-)

acquired deformities of limb (M20-M21)

calcification of bursa (M71.4-)

calcification of shoulder (joint) (M75.3)

calcification of tendon (M65.2-)

difficulty in walking (R26.2)

temporomandibular joint disorder (M26.6-)

M25.0 Hemarthrosis

Excludes1: current injury - see injury of joint by body region

hemophilic arthropathy (M36.2)

M25.00 Hemarthrosis, unspecified joint

M25.01 Hemarthrosis, shoulder

M25.011 Hemarthrosis, right shoulder

M25.012 Hemarthrosis, left shoulder

M25.019 Hemarthrosis, unspecified shoulder

M25.02 Hemarthrosis, elbow

M25.021 Hemarthrosis, right elbow

M25.022 Hemarthrosis, left elbow

M25.029 Hemarthrosis, unspecified elbow

M25.03 Hemarthrosis, wrist

M25.031 Hemarthrosis, right wrist

M25.032 Hemarthrosis, left wrist

M25.039 Hemarthrosis, unspecified wrist

M25.04 Hemarthrosis, hand

M25.041 Hemarthrosis, right hand

M25.042 Hemarthrosis, left hand

M25.049 Hemarthrosis, unspecified hand

M25.05 Hemarthrosis, hip

M25.051 Hemarthrosis, right hip

M25.052 Hemarthrosis, left hip

M25.059 Hemarthrosis, unspecified hip

M25.06 Hemarthrosis, knee

M25.061 Hemarthrosis, right knee

M25.062 Hemarthrosis, left knee

M25.069 Hemarthrosis, unspecified knee

M25.07 Hemarthrosis, ankle and foot

M25.071 Hemarthrosis, right ankle

M25.072 Hemarthrosis, left ankle

M25.073 Hemarthrosis, unspecified ankle

M25.074 Hemarthrosis, right foot

M25.075 Hemarthrosis, left foot

M25.076 Hemarthrosis, unspecified foot

M25.08 Hemarthrosis, other specified site

Hemarthrosis, vertebrae

M25.1 Fistula of joint

M25.10 Fistula, unspecified joint

M25.11 Fistula, shoulder

M25.111 Fistula, right shoulder

M25.112 Fistula, left shoulder

M25.119 Fistula, unspecified shoulder

M25.12 Fistula, elbow

   M25.121 Fistula, right elbow

   M25.122 Fistula, left elbow

   M25.129 Fistula, unspecified elbow

M25.13 Fistula, wrist

   M25.131 Fistula, right wrist

   M25.132 Fistula, left wrist

   M25.139 Fistula, unspecified wrist

M25.14 Fistula, hand

   M25.141 Fistula, right hand

   M25.142 Fistula, left hand

   M25.149 Fistula, unspecified hand

M25.15 Fistula, hip

   M25.151 Fistula, right hip

   M25.152 Fistula, left hip

   M25.159 Fistula, unspecified hip

M25.16 Fistula, knee

   M25.161 Fistula, right knee

   M25.162 Fistula, left knee

   M25.169 Fistula, unspecified knee

M25.17 Fistula, ankle and foot

   M25.171 Fistula, right ankle

   M25.172 Fistula, left ankle

   M25.173 Fistula, unspecified ankle

   M25.174 Fistula, right foot

   M25.175 Fistula, left foot

   M25.176 Fistula, unspecified foot

M25.18 Fistula, other specified site

   Fistula, vertebrae

M25.2 Flail joint

M25.20 Flail joint, unspecified joint

M25.21 Flail joint, shoulder

   M25.211 Flail joint, right shoulder

   M25.212 Flail joint, left shoulder

   M25.219 Flail joint, unspecified shoulder

M25.22 Flail joint, elbow

   M25.221 Flail joint, right elbow

   M25.222 Flail joint, left elbow

   M25.229 Flail joint, unspecified elbow

M25.23 Flail joint, wrist

   M25.231 Flail joint, right wrist

   M25.232 Flail joint, left wrist

   M25.239 Flail joint, unspecified wrist

M25.24 Flail joint, hand

   M25.241 Flail joint, right hand

   M25.242 Flail joint, left hand

   M25.249 Flail joint, unspecified hand

M25.25 Flail joint, hip

   M25.251 Flail joint, right hip

   M25.252 Flail joint, left hip

   M25.259 Flail joint, unspecified hip

M25.26 Flail joint, knee

   M25.261 Flail joint, right knee

   M25.262 Flail joint, left knee

   M25.269 Flail joint, unspecified knee

M25.27 Flail joint, ankle and foot

   M25.271 Flail joint, right ankle and foot

   M25.272 Flail joint, left ankle and foot

   M25.279 Flail joint, unspecified ankle and foot

M25.28 Flail joint, other site

M25.3 Other instability of joint

Excludes1: instability of joint secondary to old ligament injury (M24.2-)

   instability of joint secondary to removal of joint prosthesis (M96.8-)

Excludes2: spinal instabilities (M53.2-)

M25.30 Other instability, unspecified joint

M25.31 Other instability, shoulder

   M25.311 Other instability, right shoulder

   M25.312 Other instability, left shoulder

   M25.319 Other instability, unspecified shoulder

M25.32 Other instability, elbow

   M25.321 Other instability, right elbow

   M25.322 Other instability, left elbow

   M25.329 Other instability, unspecified elbow

M25.33 Other instability, wrist

   M25.331 Other instability, right wrist

   M25.332 Other instability, left wrist

   M25.339 Other instability, unspecified wrist

M25.34 Other instability, hand

   M25.341 Other instability, right hand

   M25.342 Other instability, left hand

   M25.349 Other instability, unspecified hand

M25.35 Other instability, hip

   M25.351 Other instability, right hip

   M25.352 Other instability, left hip

   M25.359 Other instability, unspecified hip

M25.36 Other instability, knee

   M25.361 Other instability, right knee

   M25.362 Other instability, left knee

   M25.369 Other instability, unspecified knee

M25.37 Other instability, ankle and foot

   M25.371 Other instability, right ankle

   M25.372 Other instability, left ankle

   M25.373 Other instability, unspecified ankle

   M25.374 Other instability, right foot

   M25.375 Other instability, left foot

   M25.376 Other instability, unspecified foot

M25.4 Effusion of joint

Excludes1: hydrarthrosis in yaws (A66.6)

   intermittent hydrarthrosis (M12.4-)

   Other infective (teno)synovitis (M65.1-)

M25.40 Effusion, unspecified joint

M25.41 Effusion, shoulder

   M25.411 Effusion, right shoulder

   M25.412 Effusion, left shoulder

M25.419　Effusion, unspecified shoulder

M25.42　Effusion, elbow
- M25.421　Effusion, right elbow
- M25.422　Effusion, left elbow
- M25.429　Effusion, unspecified elbow

M25.43　Effusion, wrist
- M25.431　Effusion, right wrist
- M25.432　Effusion, left wrist
- M25.439　Effusion, unspecified wrist

M25.44　Effusion, hand
- M25.441　Effusion, right hand
- M25.442　Effusion, left hand
- M25.449　Effusion, unspecified hand

M25.45　Effusion, hip
- M25.451　Effusion, right hip
- M25.452　Effusion, left hip
- M25.459　Effusion, unspecified hip

M25.46　Effusion, knee
- M25.461　Effusion, right knee
- M25.462　Effusion, left knee
- M25.469　Effusion, unspecified knee

M25.47　Effusion, ankle and foot
- M25.471　Effusion, right ankle
- M25.472　Effusion, left ankle
- M25.473　Effusion, unspecified ankle
- M25.474　Effusion, right foot
- M25.475　Effusion, left foot
- M25.476　Effusion, unspecified foot

M25.48　Effusion, other site

M25.5　Pain in joint

Excludes2: pain in hand (M79.64-)
　　　　　pain in fingers (M79.64-)
　　　　　pain in foot (M79.67-)
　　　　　pain in limb (M79.6-)
　　　　　pain in toes (M79.67-)

M25.50　Pain in unspecified joint

M25.51　Pain in shoulder
- M25.511　Pain in right shoulder
- M25.512　Pain in left shoulder
- M25.519　Pain in unspecified shoulder

M25.52　Pain in elbow
- M25.521　Pain in right elbow
- M25.522　Pain in left elbow
- M25.529　Pain in unspecified elbow

M25.53　Pain in wrist
- M25.531　Pain in right wrist
- M25.532　Pain in left wrist
- M25.539　Pain in unspecified wrist

M25.54　Pain in joints of hand
- ●M25.541　Pain in joints of right hand
- ●M25.542　Pain in joints of left hand
- ●M25.549　Pain in joints of unspecified hand
　　　　　Pain in joints of hand NOS

M25.55　Pain in hip

M25.551　Pain in right hip
M25.552　Pain in left hip
M25.559　Pain in unspecified hip

M25.56　Pain in knee
- M25.561　Pain in right knee
- M25.562　Pain in left knee
- M25.569　Pain in unspecified knee

M25.57　Pain in ankle and joints of foot
- M25.571　Pain in right ankle and joints of right foot
- M25.572　Pain in left ankle and joints of left foot
- M25.579　Pain in unspecified ankle and joints of unspecified foot

M25.6　Stiffness of joint, not elsewhere classified

Excludes1: ankylosis of joint (M24.6-)
　　　　　contracture of joint (M24.5-)

M25.60　Stiffness of unspecified joint, not elsewhere classified

M25.61　Stiffness of shoulder, not elsewhere classified
- M25.611　Stiffness of right shoulder, not elsewhere classified
- M25.612　Stiffness of left shoulder, not elsewhere classified
- M25.619　Stiffness of unspecified shoulder, not elsewhere classified

M25.62　Stiffness of elbow, not elsewhere classified
- M25.621　Stiffness of right elbow, not elsewhere classified
- M25.622　Stiffness of left elbow, not elsewhere classified
- M25.629　Stiffness of unspecified elbow, not elsewhere classified

M25.63　Stiffness of wrist, not elsewhere classified
- M25.631　Stiffness of right wrist, not elsewhere classified
- M25.632　Stiffness of left wrist, not elsewhere classified
- M25.639　Stiffness of unspecified wrist, not elsewhere classified

M25.64　Stiffness of hand, not elsewhere classified
- M25.641　Stiffness of right hand, not elsewhere classified
- M25.642　Stiffness of left hand, not elsewhere classified
- M25.649　Stiffness of unspecified hand, not elsewhere classified

M25.65　Stiffness of hip, not elsewhere classified
- M25.651　Stiffness of right hip, not elsewhere classified
- M25.652　Stiffness of left hip, not elsewhere classified
- M25.659　Stiffness of unspecified hip, not elsewhere classified

M25.66　Stiffness of knee, not elsewhere classified
- M25.661　Stiffness of right knee, not elsewhere classified
- M25.662　Stiffness of left knee, not elsewhere classified

M25.669	Stiffness of unspecified knee, not elsewhere classified	
M25.67	Stiffness of ankle and foot, not elsewhere classified	
M25.671	Stiffness of right ankle, not elsewhere classified	
M25.672	Stiffness of left ankle, not elsewhere classified	
M25.673	Stiffness of unspecified ankle, not elsewhere classified	
M25.674	Stiffness of right foot, not elsewhere classified	
M25.675	Stiffness of left foot, not elsewhere classified	
M25.676	Stiffness of unspecified foot, not elsewhere classified	

M25.7 Osteophyte

M25.70 Osteophyte, unspecified joint

M25.71 Osteophyte, shoulder

    M25.711 Osteophyte, right shoulder

    M25.712 Osteophyte, left shoulder

    M25.719 Osteophyte, unspecified shoulder

M25.72 Osteophyte, elbow

    M25.721 Osteophyte, right elbow

    M25.722 Osteophyte, left elbow

    M25.729 Osteophyte, unspecified elbow

M25.73 Osteophyte, wrist

    M25.731 Osteophyte, right wrist

    M25.732 Osteophyte, left wrist

    M25.739 Osteophyte, unspecified wrist

M25.74 Osteophyte, hand

    M25.741 Osteophyte, right hand

    M25.742 Osteophyte, left hand

    M25.749 Osteophyte, unspecified hand

M25.75 Osteophyte, hip

    M25.751 Osteophyte, right hip

    M25.752 Osteophyte, left hip

    M25.759 Osteophyte, unspecified hip

M25.76 Osteophyte, knee

    M25.761 Osteophyte, right knee

    M25.762 Osteophyte, left knee

    M25.769 Osteophyte, unspecified knee

M25.77 Osteophyte, ankle and foot

    M25.771 Osteophyte, right ankle

    M25.772 Osteophyte, left ankle

    M25.773 Osteophyte, unspecified ankle

    M25.774 Osteophyte, right foot

    M25.775 Osteophyte, left foot

    M25.776 Osteophyte, unspecified foot

M25.78 Osteophyte, vertebrae

M25.8 Other specified joint disorders

M25.80 Other specified joint disorders, unspecified joint

M25.81 Other specified joint disorders, shoulder

    M25.811 Other specified joint disorders, right shoulder

    M25.812 Other specified joint disorders, left shoulder

    M25.819 Other specified joint disorders, unspecified shoulder

M25.82 Other specified joint disorders, elbow

    M25.821 Other specified joint disorders, right elbow

    M25.822 Other specified joint disorders, left elbow

    M25.829 Other specified joint disorders, unspecified elbow

M25.83 Other specified joint disorders, wrist

    M25.831 Other specified joint disorders, right wrist

    M25.832 Other specified joint disorders, left wrist

    M25.839 Other specified joint disorders, unspecified wrist

M25.84 Other specified joint disorders, hand

    M25.841 Other specified joint disorders, right hand

    M25.842 Other specified joint disorders, left hand

    M25.849 Other specified joint disorders, unspecified hand

M25.85 Other specified joint disorders, hip

    M25.851 Other specified joint disorders, right hip

    M25.852 Other specified joint disorders, left hip

    M25.859 Other specified joint disorders, unspecified hip

M25.86 Other specified joint disorders, knee

    M25.861 Other specified joint disorders, right knee

    M25.862 Other specified joint disorders, left knee

    M25.869 Other specified joint disorders, unspecified knee

M25.87 Other specified joint disorders, ankle and foot

    M25.871 Other specified joint disorders, right ankle and foot

    M25.872 Other specified joint disorders, left ankle and foot

    M25.879 Other specified joint disorders, unspecified ankle and foot

M25.9 Joint disorder, unspecified

DENTOFACIAL ANOMALIES [INCLUDING MALOCCLUSION] AND OTHER DISORDERS OF JAW (M26-M27)

Excludes1: hemifacial atrophy or hypertrophy (Q67.4)

    unilateral condylar hyperplasia or hypoplasia (M27.8)

M26 Dentofacial anomalies [including malocclusion]

M26.0 Major anomalies of jaw size

    Excludes1: acromegaly (E22.0)

    Robin's syndrome (Q87.0)

    M26.00 Unspecified anomaly of jaw size

    M26.01 Maxillary hyperplasia

    M26.02 Maxillary hypoplasia

M26.03   Mandibular hyperplasia

M26.04   Mandibular hypoplasia

M26.05   Macrogenia

M26.06   Microgenia

M26.07   Excessive tuberosity of jaw

    Entire maxillary tuberosity

M26.09   Other specified anomalies of jaw size

M26.1   Anomalies of jaw-cranial base relationship

M26.10   Unspecified anomaly of jaw-cranial base relationship

M26.11   Maxillary asymmetry

M26.12   Other jaw asymmetry

M26.19   Other specified anomalies of jaw-cranial base relationship

M26.2   Anomalies of dental arch relationship

M26.20   Unspecified anomaly of dental arch relationship

M26.21   Malocclusion, Angle's class

  M26.211   Malocclusion, Angle's class I

    Neutro-occlusion

  M26.212   Malocclusion, Angle's class II

    Disto-occlusion Division I

    Disto-occlusion Division II

  M26.213   Malocclusion, Angle's class III

    Mesio-occlusion

  M26.219   Malocclusion, Angle's class, unspecified

M26.22   Open occlusal relationship

  M26.220   Open anterior occlusal relationship

    Anterior openbite

  M26.221   Open posterior occlusal relationship

    Posterior openbite

M26.23   Excessive horizontal overlap

    Excessive horizontal overjet

M26.24   Reverse articulation

    Crossbite (anterior) (posterior)

M26.25   Anomalies of interarch distance

M26.29   Other anomalies of dental arch relationship

    Midline deviation of dental arch

    Overbite (excessive) deep

    Overbite (excessive) horizontal

    Overbite (excessive) vertical

    Posterior lingual occlusion of mandibular teeth

M26.3   Anomalies of tooth position of fully erupted tooth or teeth

  Excludes2: embedded and impacted teeth (K01.-)

M26.30   Unspecified anomaly of tooth position of fully erupted tooth or teeth

    Abnormal spacing of fully erupted tooth or teeth NOS

    Displacement of fully erupted tooth or teeth NOS

    Transposition of fully erupted tooth or teeth NOS

M26.31   Crowding of fully erupted teeth

M26.32   Excessive spacing of fully erupted teeth

    Diastema of fully erupted tooth or teeth NOS

M26.33   Horizontal displacement of fully erupted tooth or teeth

    Tipped tooth or teeth

    Tipping of fully erupted tooth

M26.34   Vertical displacement of fully erupted tooth or teeth

    Extruded tooth

    Infraeruption of tooth or teeth

    Supraeruption of tooth or teeth

M26.35   Rotation of fully erupted tooth or teeth

M26.36   Insufficient interocclusal distance of fully erupted teeth (ridge)

    Lack of adequate intermaxillary vertical dimension of fully erupted teeth

M26.37   Excessive interocclusal distance of fully erupted teeth

    Excessive intermaxillary vertical dimension of fully erupted teeth

    Loss of occlusal vertical dimension of fully erupted teeth

M26.39   Other anomalies of tooth position of fully erupted tooth or teeth

M26.4   Malocclusion, unspecified

M26.5   Dentofacial functional abnormalities

  Excludes1: bruxism (F45.8)

    teeth-grinding NOS (F45.8)

M26.50   Dentofacial functional abnormalities, unspecified

M26.51   Abnormal jaw closure

M26.52   Limited mandibular range of motion

M26.53   Deviation in opening and closing of the mandible

M26.54   Insufficient anterior guidance

    Insufficient anterior occlusal guidance

M26.55   Centric occlusion maximum intercuspation discrepancy

  Excludes1: centric occlusion NOS (M26.59)

M26.56   Non-working side interference

    Balancing side interference

M26.57   Lack of posterior occlusal support

M26.59   Other dentofacial functional abnormalities

    Centric occlusion (of teeth) NOS

    Malocclusion due to abnormal swallowing

    Malocclusion due to mouth breathing

    Malocclusion due to tongue, lip or finger habits

M26.6   Temporomandibular joint disorders

  Excludes2: current temporomandibular joint dislocation (S03.0)

    current temporomandibular joint sprain (S03.4)

M26.60   Temporomandibular joint disorder, unspecified

  ●M26.601   Right temporomandibular joint disorder, unspecified

  ●M26.602   Left temporomandibular joint disorder, unspecified

  ●M26.603   Bilateral temporomandibular joint disorder, unspecified

●**M26.609** **Unspecified temporomandibular joint disorder, unspecified side**

Temporomandibular joint disorder NOS

M26.61 **Adhesions and ankylosis of temporomandibular joint**

●**M26.611** **Adhesions and ankylosis of right temporomandibular joint**

●**M26.612** **Adhesions and ankylosis of left temporomandibular joint**

●**M26.613** **Adhesions and ankylosis of bilateral temporomandibular joint**

●**M26.619** **Adhesions and ankylosis of temporomandibular joint, unspecified side**

M26.62 **Arthralgia of temporomandibular joint**

●**M26.621** **Arthralgia of right temporomandibular joint**

●**M26.622** **Arthralgia of left temporomandibular joint**

●**M26.623** **Arthralgia of bilateral temporomandibular joint**

●**M26.629** **Arthralgia of temporomandibular joint, unspecified side**

M26.63 **Articular disc disorder of temporomandibular joint**

●**M26.631** **Articular disc disorder of right temporomandibular joint**

●**M26.632** **Articular disc disorder of left temporomandibular joint**

●**M26.633** **Articular disc disorder of bilateral temporomandibular joint**

●**M26.639** **Articular disc disorder of temporomandibular joint, unspecified side**

M26.69 **Other specified disorders of temporomandibular joint**

M26.7 **Dental alveolar anomalies**

M26.70 **Unspecified alveolar anomaly**

M26.71 **Alveolar maxillary hyperplasia**

M26.72 **Alveolar mandibular hyperplasia**

M26.73 **Alveolar maxillary hypoplasia**

M26.74 **Alveolar mandibular hypoplasia**

M26.79 **Other specified alveolar anomalies**

M26.8 **Other dentofacial anomalies**

M26.81 **Anterior soft tissue impingement**

Anterior soft tissue impingement on teeth

M26.82 **Posterior soft tissue impingement**

Posterior soft tissue impingement on teeth

M26.89 **Other dentofacial anomalies**

M26.9 **Dentofacial anomaly, unspecified**

M27 **Other diseases of jaws**

M27.0 **Developmental disorders of jaws**

Latent bone cyst of jaw

Stafne's cyst

Torus mandibularis

Torus palatinus

M27.1 **Giant cell granuloma, central**

Giant cell granuloma NOS

Excludes1: peripheral giant cell granuloma (K06.8)

M27.2 **Inflammatory conditions of jaws**

Osteitis of jaw(s)

Osteomyelitis (neonatal) jaw(s)

Osteoradionecrosis jaw(s)

Periostitis jaw(s)

Sequestrum of jaw bone

Use additional code (W88-W90, X39.0) to identify radiation, if radiation-induced

Excludes2: osteonecrosis of jaw due to drug (M87.180)

M27.3 **Alveolitis of jaws**

Alveolar osteitis

Dry socket

M27.4 **Other and unspecified cysts of jaw**

Excludes1: cysts of oral region (K09.-)

latent bone cyst of jaw (M27.0)

Stafne's cyst (M27.0)

M27.40 **Unspecified cyst of jaw**

Cyst of jaw NOS

M27.49 **Other cysts of jaw**

Aneurysmal cyst of jaw

Hemorrhagic cyst of jaw

Traumatic cyst of jaw

M27.5 **Periradicular pathology associated with previous endodontic treatment**

M27.51 **Perforation of root canal space due to endodontic treatment**

M27.52 **Endodontic overfill**

M27.53 **Endodontic underfill**

M27.59 **Other periradicular pathology associated with previous endodontic treatment**

M27.6 **Endosseous dental implant failure**

M27.61 **Osseointegration failure of dental implant**

Hemorrhagic complications of dental implant placement

Iatrogenic osseointegration failure of dental implant

Osseointegration failure of dental implant due to complications of systemic disease

Osseointegration failure of dental implant due to poor bone quality

Pre-integration failure of dental implant NOS

Pre-osseointegration failure of dental implant

M27.62 **Post-osseointegration biological failure of dental implant**

Failure of dental implant due to lack of attached gingiva

Failure of dental implant due to occlusal trauma (caused by poor prosthetic design)

Failure of dental implant due to parafunctional habits

Failure of dental implant due to periodontal infection (peri-implantitis)

Failure of dental implant due to poor oral hygiene

Iatrogenic post-osseointegration failure of dental implant

Post-osseointegration failure of dental implant due to complications of systemic disease

M27.63 Post-osseointegration mechanical failure of dental implant

Failure of dental prosthesis causing loss of dental implant

Fracture of dental implant

Excludes2: cracked tooth (K03.81)

fractured dental restorative material with loss of material (K08.531)

fractured dental restorative material without loss of material (K08.530)

fractured tooth (S02.5)

M27.69 Other endosseous dental implant failure

Dental implant failure NOS

M27.8 Other specified diseases of jaws

Cherubism

Exostosis

Fibrous dysplasia

Unilateral condylar hyperplasia

Unilateral condylar hypoplasia

Excludes1: jaw pain (R68.84)

M27.9 Disease of jaws, unspecified

SYSTEMIC CONNECTIVE TISSUE DISORDERS (M30-M36)

Includes: autoimmune disease NOS

collagen (vascular) disease NOS

systemic autoimmune disease systemic collagen (vascular) disease

Excludes1: autoimmune disease, single organ or single cell-type -code to relevant condition category

M30 Polyarteritis nodosa and related conditions

Excludes1: microscopic polyarteritis (M31.7)

M30.0 Polyarteritis nodosa

M30.1 Polyarteritis with lung involvement [Churg-Strauss]

Allergic granulomatous angiitis

M30.2 Juvenile polyarteritis

M30.3 Mucocutaneous lymph node syndrome [Kawasaki]

M30.8 Other conditions related to polyarteritis nodosa

Polyangiitis overlap syndrome

M31 Other necrotizing vasculopathies

M31.0 Hypersensitivity angiitis

Goodpasture's syndrome

M31.1 Thrombotic microangiopathy

Thrombotic thrombocytopenic purpura

M31.2 Lethal midline granuloma

M31.3 Wegener's granulomatosis

Necrotizing respiratory granulomatosis

M31.30 Wegener's granulomatosis without renal involvement

Wegener's granulomatosis NOS

M31.31 Wegener's granulomatosis with renal involvement

M31.4 Aortic arch syndrome [Takayasu]

M31.5 Giant cell arteritis with polymyalgia rheumatica

M31.6 Other giant cell arteritis

M31.7 Microscopic polyangiitis

Microscopic polyarteritis

Excludes1: polyarteritis nodosa (M30.0)

M31.8 Other specified necrotizing vasculopathies

Hypocomplementemic vasculitis

Septic vasculitis

M31.9 Necrotizing vasculopathy, unspecified

M32 Systemic lupus erythematosus (SLE)

Excludes1: lupus erythematosus (discoid) (NOS) (L93.0)

M32.0 Drug-induced systemic lupus erythematosus

Use additional code for adverse effect, if applicable, to identify drug (T36-T50 with fifth or sixth character 5)

M32.1 Systemic lupus erythematosus with organ or system involvement

M32.10 Systemic lupus erythematosus, organ or system involvement unspecified

M32.11 Endocarditis in systemic lupus erythematosus

Libman-Sacks disease

M32.12 Pericarditis in systemic lupus erythematosus

Lupus pericarditis

M32.13 Lung involvement in systemic lupus erythematosus

Pleural effusion due to systemic lupus erythematosus

M32.14 Glomerular disease in systemic lupus erythematosus

Lupus renal disease NOS

M32.15 Tubulo-interstitial nephropathy in systemic lupus erythematosus

M32.19 Other organ or system involvement in systemic lupus erythematosus

M32.8 Other forms of systemic lupus erythematosus

M32.9 Systemic lupus erythematosus, unspecified

SLE NOS

Systemic lupus erythematosus NOS

Systemic lupus erythematosus without organ involvement

M33 Dermatopolymyositis

M33.0 Juvenile dermatopolymyositis

M33.00 Juvenile dermatopolymyositis, organ involvement unspecified

M33.01 Juvenile dermatopolymyositis with respiratory involvement

M33.02 Juvenile dermatopolymyositis with myopathy

M33.09 Juvenile dermatopolymyositis with other organ involvement

M33.1 Other dermatopolymyositis

M33.10 Other dermatopolymyositis, organ involvement unspecified

M33.11 Other dermatopolymyositis with respiratory involvement

M33.12 Other dermatopolymyositis with myopathy

M33.19 Other dermatopolymyositis with other organ involvement

M33.2 Polymyositis

M33.20 Polymyositis, organ involvement unspecified

M33.21 Polymyositis with respiratory involvement

M33.22 Polymyositis with myopathy

M33.29 Polymyositis with other organ involvement

M33.9 Dermatopolymyositis, unspecified

    M33.90 Dermatopolymyositis, unspecified, organ involvement unspecified

    M33.91 Dermatopolymyositis, unspecified with respiratory involvement

    M33.92 Dermatopolymyositis, unspecified with myopathy

    M33.99 Dermatopolymyositis, unspecified with other organ involvement

M34 Systemic sclerosis [scleroderma]

    Excludes1: circumscribed scleroderma (L94.0)

    neonatal scleroderma (P83.8)

M34.0 Progressive systemic sclerosis

M34.1 CR(E)ST syndrome

    Combination of calcinosis, Raynaud's phenomenon, esophageal dysfunction, sclerodactyly, telangiectasia

M34.2 Systemic sclerosis induced by drug and chemical

    Code first poisoning due to drug or toxin, if applicable (T36-T65 with fifth or sixth character 1-4 or 6)

    Use additional code for adverse effect, if applicable, to identify drug (T36-T50 with fifth or sixth character 5)

M34.8 Other forms of systemic sclerosis

    M34.81 Systemic sclerosis with lung involvement

    M34.82 Systemic sclerosis with myopathy

    M34.83 Systemic sclerosis with polyneuropathy

    M34.89 Other systemic sclerosis

M34.9 Systemic sclerosis, unspecified

M35 Other systemic involvement of connective tissue

    Excludes1: reactive perforating collagenosis (L87.1)

M35.0 Sicca syndrome [Sjögren]

    M35.00 Sicca syndrome, unspecified

    M35.01 Sicca syndrome with keratoconjunctivitis

    M35.02 Sicca syndrome with lung involvement

    M35.03 Sicca syndrome with myopathy

    M35.04 Sicca syndrome with tubulo-interstitial nephropathy

        Renal tubular acidosis in sicca syndrome

    M35.09 Sicca syndrome with other organ involvement

M35.1 Other overlap syndromes

    Mixed connective tissue disease

    Excludes1: polyangiitis overlap syndrome (M30.8)

M35.2 Behçet's disease

M35.3 Polymyalgia rheumatica

    Definition: Polymyalgia rheumatica is a rheumatic disorder that is associated with moderate to severe muscle pain and stiffness in the neck, shoulder and hip areas.

    Excludes1: polymyalgia rheumatica with giant cell arteritis (M31.5)

M35.4 Diffuse (eosinophilic) fasciitis

M35.5 Multifocal fibrosclerosis

M35.6 Relapsing panniculitis [Weber-Christian]

    Excludes1: lupus panniculitis (L93.2)

    panniculitis NOS (M79.3-)

M35.7 Hypermobility syndrome

    Familial ligamentous laxity

    Excludes1: Ehlers-Danlos syndrome (Q79.6)

    ligamentous laxity, NOS (M24.2-)

M35.8 Other specified systemic involvement of connective tissue

M35.9 Systemic involvement of connective tissue, unspecified

    Autoimmune disease (systemic) NOS

    Collagen (vascular) disease NOS

M36 Systemic disorders of connective tissue in diseases classified elsewhere

    Excludes2: arthropathies in diseases classified elsewhere (M14.-)

M36.0 Dermato(poly)myositis in neoplastic disease

    Code first underlying neoplasm (C00-D49)

M36.1 Arthropathy in neoplastic disease

    Code first underlying neoplasm, such as:

        leukemia (C91-C95)

        malignant histiocytosis (C96.A)

        multiple myeloma (C90.0)

M36.2 Hemophilic arthropathy

    Hemarthrosis in hemophilic arthropathy

    Code first underlying disease, such as:

        factor VIII deficiency (D66)

        with vascular defect (D68.0)

        factor IX deficiency (D67)

        hemophilia (classical) (D66)

        hemophilia B (D67)

        hemophilia C (D68.1)

M36.3 Arthropathy in other blood disorders

M36.4 Arthropathy in hypersensitivity reactions classified elsewhere

    Code first underlying disease, such as:

        Henoch (-Schönlein) purpura (D69.0)

        serum sickness (T80.6-)

M36.8 Systemic disorders of connective tissue in other diseases classified elsewhere

    Code first underlying disease, such as:

        alkaptonuria (E70.2)

        hypogammaglobulinemia (D80.-)

        ochronosis (E70.2)

DORSOPATHIES (M40-M54)

Deforming dorsopathies (M40-M43)

M40 Kyphosis and lordosis

    Excludes1: congenital kyphosis and lordosis (Q76.4)

    kyphoscoliosis (M41.-)

    postprocedural kyphosis and lordosis (M96.-)

M40.0 Postural kyphosis

    Excludes1: osteochondrosis of spine (M42.-)

    M40.00 Postural kyphosis, site unspecified

    M40.03 Postural kyphosis, cervicothoracic region

    M40.04 Postural kyphosis, thoracic region

    M40.05 Postural kyphosis, thoracolumbar region

M40.1 Other secondary kyphosis

    M40.10 Other secondary kyphosis, site unspecified

    M40.12 Other secondary kyphosis, cervical region

M40.13 Other secondary kyphosis, cervicothoracic region

M40.14 Other secondary kyphosis, thoracic region

M40.15 Other secondary kyphosis, thoracolumbar region

M40.2 Other and unspecified kyphosis

M40.20 Unspecified kyphosis

M40.202 Unspecified kyphosis, cervical region

M40.203 Unspecified kyphosis, cervicothoracic region

M40.204 Unspecified kyphosis, thoracic region

M40.205 Unspecified kyphosis, thoracolumbar region

M40.209 Unspecified kyphosis, site unspecified

M40.29 Other kyphosis

M40.292 Other kyphosis, cervical region

M40.293 Other kyphosis, cervicothoracic region

M40.294 Other kyphosis, thoracic region

M40.295 Other kyphosis, thoracolumbar region

M40.299 Other kyphosis, site unspecified

M40.3 Flatback syndrome

M40.30 Flatback syndrome, site unspecified

M40.35 Flatback syndrome, thoracolumbar region

M40.36 Flatback syndrome, lumbar region

M40.37 Flatback syndrome, lumbosacral region

M40.4 Postural lordosis

Acquired lordosis

M40.40 Postural lordosis, site unspecified

M40.45 Postural lordosis, thoracolumbar region

M40.46 Postural lordosis, lumbar region

M40.47 Postural lordosis, lumbosacral region

M40.5 Lordosis, unspecified

M40.50 Lordosis, unspecified, site unspecified

M40.55 Lordosis, unspecified, thoracolumbar region

M40.56 Lordosis, unspecified, lumbar region

M40.57 Lordosis, unspecified, lumbosacral region

M41 Scoliosis

Includes: kyphoscoliosis

Excludes1: congenital scoliosis NOS (Q67.5)

congenital scoliosis due to bony malformation (Q76.3)

postural congenital scoliosis (Q67.5)

kyphoscoliotic heart disease (I27.1)

postprocedural scoliosis (M96.-)

M41.0 Infantile idiopathic scoliosis

M41.00 Infantile idiopathic scoliosis, site unspecified

M41.02 Infantile idiopathic scoliosis, cervical region

M41.03 Infantile idiopathic scoliosis, cervicothoracic region

M41.04 Infantile idiopathic scoliosis, thoracic region

M41.05 Infantile idiopathic scoliosis, thoracolumbar region

M41.06 Infantile idiopathic scoliosis, lumbar region

M41.07 Infantile idiopathic scoliosis, lumbosacral region

M41.08 Infantile idiopathic scoliosis, sacral and sacrococcygeal region

M41.1 Juvenile and adolescent idiopathic scoliosis

M41.11 Juvenile idiopathic scoliosis

M41.112 Juvenile idiopathic scoliosis, cervical region

M41.113 Juvenile idiopathic scoliosis, cervicothoracic region

M41.114 Juvenile idiopathic scoliosis, thoracic region

M41.115 Juvenile idiopathic scoliosis, thoracolumbar region

M41.116 Juvenile idiopathic scoliosis, lumbar region

M41.117 Juvenile idiopathic scoliosis, lumbosacral region

M41.119 Juvenile idiopathic scoliosis, site unspecified

M41.12 Adolescent scoliosis

M41.122 Adolescent idiopathic scoliosis, cervical region

M41.123 Adolescent idiopathic scoliosis, cervicothoracic region

M41.124 Adolescent idiopathic scoliosis, thoracic region

M41.125 Adolescent idiopathic scoliosis, thoracolumbar region

M41.126 Adolescent idiopathic scoliosis, lumbar region

M41.127 Adolescent idiopathic scoliosis, lumbosacral region

M41.129 Adolescent idiopathic scoliosis, site unspecified

M41.2 Other idiopathic scoliosis

M41.20 Other idiopathic scoliosis, site unspecified

M41.22 Other idiopathic scoliosis, cervical region

M41.23 Other idiopathic scoliosis, cervicothoracic region

M41.24 Other idiopathic scoliosis, thoracic region

M41.25 Other idiopathic scoliosis, thoracolumbar region

M41.26 Other idiopathic scoliosis, lumbar region

M41.27 Other idiopathic scoliosis, lumbosacral region

M41.3 Thoracogenic scoliosis

M41.30 Thoracogenic scoliosis, site unspecified

M41.34 Thoracogenic scoliosis, thoracic region

M41.35 Thoracogenic scoliosis, thoracolumbar region

M41.4 Neuromuscular scoliosis

Scoliosis secondary to cerebral palsy, Friedreich's ataxia, poliomyelitis **and other** neuromuscular disorders

Code also underlying condition

M41.40 Neuromuscular scoliosis, site unspecified

M41.41 Neuromuscular scoliosis, occipito-atlanto-axial region

M41.42 Neuromuscular scoliosis, cervical region

M41.43 Neuromuscular scoliosis, cervicothoracic region

M41.44 Neuromuscular scoliosis, thoracic region

M41.45 Neuromuscular scoliosis, thoracolumbar region

M41.46 Neuromuscular scoliosis, lumbar region

M41.47 Neuromuscular scoliosis, lumbosacral region

M41.5 Other secondary scoliosis

  M41.50 Other secondary scoliosis, site unspecified

  M41.52 Other secondary scoliosis, cervical region

  M41.53 Other secondary scoliosis, cervicothoracic region

  M41.54 Other secondary scoliosis, thoracic region

  M41.55 Other secondary scoliosis, thoracolumbar region

  M41.56 Other secondary scoliosis, lumbar region

  M41.57 Other secondary scoliosis, lumbosacral region

M41.8 Other forms of scoliosis

  M41.80 Other forms of scoliosis, site unspecified

  M41.82 Other forms of scoliosis, cervical region

  M41.83 Other forms of scoliosis, cervicothoracic region

  M41.84 Other forms of scoliosis, thoracic region

  M41.85 Other forms of scoliosis, thoracolumbar region

  M41.86 Other forms of scoliosis, lumbar region

  M41.87 Other forms of scoliosis, lumbosacral region

M41.9 Scoliosis, unspecified

M42 Spinal osteochondrosis

M42.0 Juvenile osteochondrosis of spine

Calvé's disease

Scheuermann's disease

Excludes1: postural kyphosis (M40.0)

  M42.00 Juvenile osteochondrosis of spine, site unspecified

  M42.01 Juvenile osteochondrosis of spine, occipito-atlanto-axial region

  M42.02 Juvenile osteochondrosis of spine, cervical region

  M42.03 Juvenile osteochondrosis of spine, cervicothoracic region

  M42.04 Juvenile osteochondrosis of spine, thoracic region

  M42.05 Juvenile osteochondrosis of spine, thoracolumbar region

  M42.06 Juvenile osteochondrosis of spine, lumbar region

  M42.07 Juvenile osteochondrosis of spine, lumbosacral region

  M42.08 Juvenile osteochondrosis of spine, sacral and sacrococcygeal region

  M42.09 Juvenile osteochondrosis of spine, multiple sites in spine

M42.1 Adult osteochondrosis of spine

  M42.10 Adult osteochondrosis of spine, site unspecified

  M42.11 Adult osteochondrosis of spine, occipito-atlanto-axial region

  M42.12 Adult osteochondrosis of spine, cervical region

  M42.13 Adult osteochondrosis of spine, cervicothoracic region

M42.14 Adult osteochondrosis of spine, thoracic region

M42.15 Adult osteochondrosis of spine, thoracolumbar region

M42.16 Adult osteochondrosis of spine, lumbar region

M42.17 Adult osteochondrosis of spine, lumbosacral region

M42.18 Adult osteochondrosis of spine, sacral and sacrococcygeal region

M42.19 Adult osteochondrosis of spine, multiple sites in spine

M42.9 Spinal osteochondrosis, unspecified

M43 Other deforming dorsopathies

Excludes1: congenital spondylolysis and spondylolisthesis (Q76.2)

hemivertebra (Q76.3-Q76.4)

Klippel-Feil syndrome (Q76.1)

lumbarization and sacralization (Q76.4)

platyspondylisis (Q76.4)

spina bifida occulta (Q76.0)

spinal curvature in osteoporosis (M80.-)

spinal curvature in

Paget's disease of bone [osteitis deformans] (M88.-)

M43.0 Spondylolysis

Excludes1: congenital spondylolysis (Q76.2)

spondylolisthesis (M43.1)

  M43.00 Spondylolysis, site unspecified

  M43.01 Spondylolysis, occipito-atlanto-axial region

  M43.02 Spondylolysis, cervical region

  M43.03 Spondylolysis, cervicothoracic region

  M43.04 Spondylolysis, thoracic region

  M43.05 Spondylolysis, thoracolumbar region

  M43.06 Spondylolysis, lumbar region

  M43.07 Spondylolysis, lumbosacral region

  M43.08 Spondylolysis, sacral and sacrococcygeal region

  M43.09 Spondylolysis, multiple sites in spine

M43.1 Spondylolisthesis

Excludes1: acute traumatic of lumbosacral region (S33.1)

acute traumatic of **sites other** than lumbosacral-code to Fracture, vertebra, by region congenital spondylolisthesis (Q76.2)

  M43.10 Spondylolisthesis, site unspecified

  M43.11 Spondylolisthesis, occipito-atlanto-axial region

  M43.12 Spondylolisthesis, cervical region

  M43.13 Spondylolisthesis, cervicothoracic region

  M43.14 Spondylolisthesis, thoracic region

  M43.15 Spondylolisthesis, thoracolumbar region

  M43.16 Spondylolisthesis, lumbar region

  M43.17 Spondylolisthesis, lumbosacral region

  M43.18 Spondylolisthesis, sacral and sacrococcygeal region

  M43.19 Spondylolisthesis, multiple sites in spine

M43.2 Fusion of spine

Ankylosis of spinal joint

Excludes1: ankylosing spondylitis (M45.0-)

congenital fusion of spine (Q76.4)

Excludes2: arthrodesis status (Z98.1)

pseudoarthrosis after fusion or arthrodesis (M96.0)

M43.20 Fusion of spine, site unspecified

M43.21 Fusion of spine, occipito-atlanto-axial region

M43.22 Fusion of spine, cervical region

M43.23 Fusion of spine, cervicothoracic region

M43.24 Fusion of spine, thoracic region

M43.25 Fusion of spine, thoracolumbar region

M43.26 Fusion of spine, lumbar region

M43.27 Fusion of spine, lumbosacral region

M43.28 Fusion of spine, sacral and sacrococcygeal region

M43.3 Recurrent atlantoaxial dislocation with myelopathy

M43.4 Other recurrent atlantoaxial dislocation

M43.5 Other recurrent vertebral dislocation

Excludes1: biomechanical lesions NEC (M99.-)

M43.5X Other recurrent vertebral dislocation

M43.5X2 Other recurrent vertebral dislocation, cervical region

M43.5X3 Other recurrent vertebral dislocation, cervicothoracic region

M43.5X4 Other recurrent vertebral dislocation, thoracic region

M43.5X5 Other recurrent vertebral dislocation, thoracolumbar region

M43.5X6 Other recurrent vertebral dislocation, lumbar region

M43.5X7 Other recurrent vertebral dislocation, lumbosacral region

M43.5X8 Other recurrent vertebral dislocation, sacral and sacrococcygeal region

M43.5X9 Other recurrent vertebral dislocation, site unspecified

M43.6 Torticollis

Excludes1: congenital (sternomastoid) torticollis (Q68.0)

current injury - see Injury, of spine, by body region

ocular torticollis (R29.891)

psychogenic torticollis (F45.8)

spasmodic torticollis (G24.3)

torticollis due to birth injury (P15.2)

M43.8 Other specified deforming dorsopathies

Excludes2: kyphosis and lordosis (M40.-)

scoliosis (M41.-)

M43.8X Other specified deforming dorsopathies

M43.8X1 Other specified deforming dorsopathies, occipito-atlanto-axial region

M43.8X2 Other specified deforming dorsopathies, cervical region

M43.8X3 Other specified deforming dorsopathies, cervicothoracic region

M43.8X4 Other specified deforming dorsopathies, thoracic region

M43.8X5 Other specified deforming dorsopathies, thoracolumbar region

M43.8X6 Other specified deforming dorsopathies, lumbar region

M43.8X7 Other specified deforming dorsopathies, lumbosacral region

M43.8X8 Other specified deforming dorsopathies, sacral and sacrococcygeal region

M43.8X9 Other specified deforming dorsopathies, site unspecified

M43.9 Deforming dorsopathy, unspecified

Curvature of spine NOS

SPONDYLOPATHIES (M45-M49)

M45 Ankylosing spondylitis

Definition: Ankylosing spondylitis is a long-term disease that causes inflammation of the joints between the spinal bones and the joints between the spine and the pelvis. It eventually causes the affected spinal bones to join together.

Rheumatoid arthritis of spine

Excludes1: arthropathy in Reiter's disease (M02.3-)

juvenile (ankylosing) spondylitis (M08.1)

Excludes2: Behçet's disease (M35.2)

M45.0 Ankylosing spondylitis of multiple sites in spine

M45.1 Ankylosing spondylitis of occipito-atlanto-axial region

M45.2 Ankylosing spondylitis of cervical region

M45.3 Ankylosing spondylitis of cervicothoracic region

M45.4 Ankylosing spondylitis of thoracic region

M45.5 Ankylosing spondylitis of thoracolumbar region

M45.6 Ankylosing spondylitis lumbar region

M45.7 Ankylosing spondylitis of lumbosacral region

M45.8 Ankylosing spondylitis sacral and sacrococcygeal region

M45.9 Ankylosing spondylitis of unspecified sites in spine

M46 Other inflammatory spondylopathies

M46.0 Spinal enthesopathy

Definition: Enthesopathies are disorders of peripheral ligamentous or muscular attachments, abnormalities in the zones of attachment, for ligaments and tendons to bone.

Disorder of ligamentous or muscular attachments of spine

M46.00 Spinal enthesopathy, site unspecified

M46.01 Spinal enthesopathy, occipito-atlanto-axial region

M46.02 Spinal enthesopathy, cervical region

M46.03 Spinal enthesopathy, cervicothoracic region

M46.04 Spinal enthesopathy, thoracic region

M46.05 Spinal enthesopathy, thoracolumbar region

M46.06 Spinal enthesopathy, lumbar region

M46.07 Spinal enthesopathy, lumbosacral region

M46.08 Spinal enthesopathy, sacral and sacrococcygeal region

M46.09 Spinal enthesopathy, multiple sites in spine

M46.1 Sacroiliitis, not elsewhere classified

M46.2 Osteomyelitis of vertebra

Definition: Osteomyelitis is an inflammation of bone and bone marrow (usually caused by bacterial infection).

M46.20 Osteomyelitis of vertebra, site unspecified

M46.21 Osteomyelitis of vertebra, occipito-atlanto-axial region

M46.22 Osteomyelitis of vertebra, cervical region

M46.23 Osteomyelitis of vertebra, cervicothoracic region

M46.24 Osteomyelitis of vertebra, thoracic region

M46.25 Osteomyelitis of vertebra, thoracolumbar region

M46.26 Osteomyelitis of vertebra, lumbar region

M46.27 Osteomyelitis of vertebra, lumbosacral region

M46.28 Osteomyelitis of vertebra, sacral and sacrococcygeal region

M46.3 Infection of intervertebral disc (pyogenic)

Use additional code (B95-B97) to identify infectious agent.

M46.30 Infection of intervertebral disc (pyogenic), site unspecified

M46.31 Infection of intervertebral disc (pyogenic), occipito-atlanto-axial region

M46.32 Infection of intervertebral disc (pyogenic), cervical region

M46.33 Infection of intervertebral disc (pyogenic), cervicothoracic region

M46.34 Infection of intervertebral disc (pyogenic), thoracic region

M46.35 Infection of intervertebral disc (pyogenic), thoracolumbar region

M46.36 Infection of intervertebral disc (pyogenic), lumbar region

M46.37 Infection of intervertebral disc (pyogenic), lumbosacral region

M46.38 Infection of intervertebral disc (pyogenic), sacral and sacrococcygeal region

M46.39 Infection of intervertebral disc (pyogenic), multiple sites in spine

M46.4 Discitis, unspecified

M46.40 Discitis, unspecified, site unspecified

M46.41 Discitis, unspecified, occipito-atlanto-axial region

M46.42 Discitis, unspecified, cervical region

M46.43 Discitis, unspecified, cervicothoracic region

M46.44 Discitis, unspecified, thoracic region

M46.45 Discitis, unspecified, thoracolumbar region

M46.46 Discitis, unspecified, lumbar region

M46.47 Discitis, unspecified, lumbosacral region

M46.48 Discitis, unspecified, sacral and sacrococcygeal region

M46.49 Discitis, unspecified, multiple sites in spine

M46.5 Other infective spondylopathies

M46.50 Other infective spondylopathies, site unspecified

M46.51 Other infective spondylopathies, occipito-atlanto-axial region

M46.52 Other infective spondylopathies, cervical region

M46.53 Other infective spondylopathies, cervicothoracic region

M46.54 Other infective spondylopathies, thoracic region

M46.55 Other infective spondylopathies, thoracolumbar region

M46.56 Other infective spondylopathies, lumbar region

M46.57 Other infective spondylopathies, lumbosacral region

M46.58 Other infective spondylopathies, sacral and sacrococcygeal region

M46.59 Other infective spondylopathies, multiple sites in spine

M46.8 Other specified inflammatory spondylopathies

M46.80 Other specified inflammatory spondylopathies, site unspecified

M46.81 Other specified inflammatory spondylopathies, occipito-atlanto-axial region

M46.82 Other specified inflammatory spondylopathies, cervical region

M46.83 Other specified inflammatory spondylopathies, cervicothoracic region

M46.84 Other specified inflammatory spondylopathies, thoracic region

M46.85 Other specified inflammatory spondylopathies, thoracolumbar region

M46.86 Other specified inflammatory spondylopathies, lumbar region

M46.87 Other specified inflammatory spondylopathies, lumbosacral region

M46.88 Other specified inflammatory spondylopathies, sacral and sacrococcygeal region

M46.89 Other specified inflammatory spondylopathies, multiple sites in spine

M46.9 Unspecified inflammatory spondylopathy

M46.90 Unspecified inflammatory spondylopathy, site unspecified

M46.91 Unspecified inflammatory spondylopathy, occipito-atlanto-axial region

M46.92 Unspecified inflammatory spondylopathy, cervical region

M46.93 Unspecified inflammatory spondylopathy, cervicothoracic region

M46.94 Unspecified inflammatory spondylopathy, thoracic region

M46.95 Unspecified inflammatory spondylopathy, thoracolumbar region

M46.96 Unspecified inflammatory spondylopathy, lumbar region

M46.97 Unspecified inflammatory spondylopathy, lumbosacral region

M46.98 Unspecified inflammatory spondylopathy, sacral and sacrococcygeal region

M46.99 Unspecified inflammatory spondylopathy, multiple sites in spine

M47 Spondylosis

Definition: Spondylosis is degenerative arthritis (osteoarthritis) of the spinal vertebra and related tissue.

Includes: arthrosis or osteoarthritis of spine
degeneration of facet joints

M47.0 Anterior spinal and vertebral artery compression syndromes

M47.01 Anterior spinal artery compression syndromes

M47.011 Anterior spinal artery compression syndromes, occipito-atlanto-axial region

● New code ▲ Revised code Excludes1: Not coded here Excludes2: Not included here ⊗ Placeholder required ⑦ 7th digit required

M47.012   **Anterior spinal artery compression syndromes, cervical region**

M47.013   **Anterior spinal artery compression syndromes, cervicothoracic region**

M47.014   **Anterior spinal artery compression syndromes, thoracic region**

M47.015   **Anterior spinal artery compression syndromes, thoracolumbar region**

M47.016   **Anterior spinal artery compression syndromes, lumbar region**

M47.019   **Anterior spinal artery compression syndromes, site unspecified**

M47.02   **Vertebral artery compression syndromes**

M47.021   **Vertebral artery compression syndromes, occipito-atlanto-axial region**

M47.022   **Vertebral artery compression syndromes, cervical region**

M47.029   **Vertebral artery compression syndromes, site unspecified**

M47.1   **Other spondylosis with myelopathy**

Spondylogenic compression of spinal cord

Excludes1: vertebral subluxation (M43.3-M43.59)

M47.10   **Other spondylosis with myelopathy, site unspecified**

M47.11   **Other spondylosis with myelopathy, occipito-atlanto-axial region**

M47.12   **Other spondylosis with myelopathy, cervical region**

M47.13   **Other spondylosis with myelopathy, cervicothoracic region**

M47.14   **Other spondylosis with myelopathy, thoracic region**

M47.15   **Other spondylosis with myelopathy, thoracolumbar region**

M47.16   **Other spondylosis with myelopathy, lumbar region**

M47.2   **Other spondylosis with radiculopathy**

M47.20   **Other spondylosis with radiculopathy, site unspecified**

M47.21   **Other spondylosis with radiculopathy, occipito-atlanto-axial region**

M47.22   **Other spondylosis with radiculopathy, cervical region**

M47.23   **Other spondylosis with radiculopathy, cervicothoracic region**

M47.24   **Other spondylosis with radiculopathy, thoracic region**

M47.25   **Other spondylosis with radiculopathy, thoracolumbar region**

M47.26   **Other spondylosis with radiculopathy, lumbar region**

M47.27   **Other spondylosis with radiculopathy, lumbosacral region**

M47.28   **Other spondylosis with radiculopathy, sacral and sacrococcygeal region**

M47.8   **Other spondylosis**

M47.81   **Spondylosis without myelopathy or radiculopathy**

M47.811   **Spondylosis without myelopathy or radiculopathy, occipito-atlanto-axial region**

M47.812   **Spondylosis without myelopathy or radiculopathy, cervical region**

M47.813   **Spondylosis without myelopathy or radiculopathy, cervicothoracic region**

M47.814   **Spondylosis without myelopathy or radiculopathy, thoracic region**

M47.815   **Spondylosis without myelopathy or radiculopathy, thoracolumbar region**

M47.816   **Spondylosis without myelopathy or radiculopathy, lumbar region**

M47.817   **Spondylosis without myelopathy or radiculopathy, lumbosacral region**

M47.818   **Spondylosis without myelopathy or radiculopathy, sacral and sacrococcygeal region**

M47.819   **Spondylosis without myelopathy or radiculopathy, site unspecified**

M47.89   **Other spondylosis**

M47.891   **Other spondylosis, occipito-atlanto-axial region**

M47.892   **Other spondylosis, cervical region**

M47.893   **Other spondylosis, cervicothoracic region**

M47.894   **Other spondylosis, thoracic region**

M47.895   **Other spondylosis, thoracolumbar region**

M47.896   **Other spondylosis, lumbar region**

M47.897   **Other spondylosis, lumbosacral region**

M47.898   **Other spondylosis, sacral and sacrococcygeal region**

M47.899   **Other spondylosis, site unspecified**

M47.9   **Spondylosis, unspecified**

M48   **Other spondylopathies**

M48.0   **Spinal stenosis**

Caudal stenosis

M48.00   **Spinal stenosis, site unspecified**

M48.01   **Spinal stenosis, occipito-atlanto-axial region**

M48.02   **Spinal stenosis, cervical region**

M48.03   **Spinal stenosis, cervicothoracic region**

M48.04   **Spinal stenosis, thoracic region**

M48.05   **Spinal stenosis, thoracolumbar region**

M48.06   **Spinal stenosis, lumbar region**

M48.07   **Spinal stenosis, lumbosacral region**

M48.08   **Spinal stenosis, sacral and sacrococcygeal region**

M48.1   **Ankylosing hyperostosis [Forestier]**

Diffuse idiopathic skeletal hyperostosis [DISH]

M48.10   **Ankylosing hyperostosis [Forestier], site unspecified**

M48.11   **Ankylosing hyperostosis [Forestier], occipito-atlanto-axial region**

M48.12   **Ankylosing hyperostosis [Forestier], cervical region**

M48.13 Ankylosing hyperostosis [Forestier], cervicothoracic region

M48.14 Ankylosing hyperostosis [Forestier], thoracic region

M48.15 Ankylosing hyperostosis [Forestier], thoracolumbar region

M48.16 Ankylosing hyperostosis [Forestier], lumbar region

M48.17 Ankylosing hyperostosis [Forestier], lumbosacral region

M48.18 Ankylosing hyperostosis [Forestier], sacral and sacrococcygeal region

M48.19 Ankylosing hyperostosis [Forestier], multiple sites in spine

M48.2 Kissing spine

M48.20 Kissing spine, site unspecified

M48.21 Kissing spine, occipito-atlanto-axial region

M48.22 Kissing spine, cervical region

M48.23 Kissing spine, cervicothoracic region

M48.24 Kissing spine, thoracic region

M48.25 Kissing spine, thoracolumbar region

M48.26 Kissing spine, lumbar region

M48.27 Kissing spine, lumbosacral region

M48.3 Traumatic spondylopathy

M48.30 Traumatic spondylopathy, site unspecified

M48.31 Traumatic spondylopathy, occipito-atlanto-axial region

M48.32 Traumatic spondylopathy, cervical region

M48.33 Traumatic spondylopathy, cervicothoracic region

M48.34 Traumatic spondylopathy, thoracic region

M48.35 Traumatic spondylopathy, thoracolumbar region

M48.36 Traumatic spondylopathy, lumbar region

M48.37 Traumatic spondylopathy, lumbosacral region

M48.38 Traumatic spondylopathy, sacral and sacrococcygeal region

M48.4 Fatigue fracture of vertebra

Stress fracture of vertebra

Excludes1: pathological fracture NOS (M84.4-)

pathological fracture of vertebra due to neoplasm (M84.58)

pathological fracture of vertebra due to **other** diagnosis (M84.68)

pathological fracture of vertebra due to osteoporosis (M80.-)

traumatic fracture of vertebrae (S12.0-S12.3-, S22.0-, S32.0-)

The appropriate 7th character is to be added to each code from subcategory M48.4:

A - initial encounter for fracture

D - subsequent encounter for fracture with routine healing

G - subsequent encounter for fracture with delayed healing

S - sequela of fracture

⊗⑦**M48.40** Fatigue fracture of vertebra, site unspecified

⊗⑦**M48.41** Fatigue fracture of vertebra, occipito-atlanto-axial region

⊗⑦**M48.42** Fatigue fracture of vertebra, cervical region

⊗⑦**M48.43** Fatigue fracture of vertebra, cervicothoracic region

⊗⑦**M48.44** Fatigue fracture of vertebra, thoracic region

⊗⑦**M48.45** Fatigue fracture of vertebra, thoracolumbar region

⊗⑦**M48.46** Fatigue fracture of vertebra, lumbar region

⊗⑦**M48.47** Fatigue fracture of vertebra, lumbosacral region

⊗⑦**M48.48** Fatigue fracture of vertebra, sacral and sacrococcygeal region

M48.5 Collapsed vertebra, not elsewhere classified

Collapsed vertebra NOS

Compression fracture of vertebra NOS

Wedging of vertebra NOS

Excludes1: current injury - see Injury of spine, by body region

fatigue fracture of vertebra (M48.4)

pathological fracture of vertebra due to neoplasm (M84.58)

pathological fracture of vertebra due to **other** diagnosis (M84.68)

pathological fracture of vertebra due to osteoporosis (M80.-)

pathological fracture NOS (M84.4-)

stress fracture of vertebra (M48.4-)

traumatic fracture of vertebra (S12.-, S22.-, S32.-)

The appropriate 7th character is to be added to each code from subcategory M48.5:

A - initial encounter for fracture

D - subsequent encounter for fracture with routine healing

G - subsequent encounter for fracture with delayed healing

S - sequela of fracture

⊗⑦**M48.50** Collapsed vertebra, not elsewhere classified, site unspecified

⊗⑦**M48.51** Collapsed vertebra, not elsewhere classified, occipito-atlanto-axial region

⊗⑦**M48.52** Collapsed vertebra, not elsewhere classified, cervical region

⊗⑦**M48.53** Collapsed vertebra, not elsewhere classified, cervicothoracic region

⊗⑦**M48.54** Collapsed vertebra, not elsewhere classified, thoracic region

⊗⑦**M48.55** Collapsed vertebra, not elsewhere classified, thoracolumbar region

⊗⑦**M48.56** Collapsed vertebra, not elsewhere classified, lumbar region

⊗⑦**M48.57** Collapsed vertebra, not elsewhere classified, lumbosacral region

⊗⑦**M48.58** Collapsed vertebra, not elsewhere classified, sacral and sacrococcygeal region

M48.8 Other specified spondylopathies

Ossification of posterior longitudinal ligament

M48.8X Other specified spondylopathies

M48.8X1 Other specified spondylopathies, occipito-atlanto-axial region

M48.8X2 Other specified spondylopathies, cervical region

M48.8X3 Other specified spondylopathies, cervicothoracic region

M48.8X4 Other specified spondylopathies, thoracic region

M48.8X5 Other specified spondylopathies, thoracolumbar region

M48.8X6 Other specified spondylopathies, lumbar region

M48.8X7 Other specified spondylopathies, lumbosacral region

M48.8X8 Other specified spondylopathies, sacral and sacrococcygeal region

M48.8X9 Other specified spondylopathies, site unspecified

M48.9 Spondylopathy, unspecified

M49 Spondylopathies in diseases classified elsewhere

Includes: curvature of spine in diseases classified elsewhere

deformity of spine in diseases classified elsewhere

kyphosis in diseases classified elsewhere

scoliosis in diseases classified elsewhere

spondylopathy in diseases classified elsewhere

Code first underlying disease, such as:

brucellosis (A23.-)

Charcot-Marie-Tooth disease (G60.0)

enterobacterial infections (A01-A04)

osteitis fibrosa cystica (E21.0)

Excludes1: curvature of spine in tuberculosis [Pott's] (A18.01)

enteropathic arthropathies (M07.-)

gonococcal spondylitis (A54.41)

neuropathic [tabes dorsalis] spondylitis (A52.11)

neuropathic spondylopathy in syringomyelia (G95.0)

neuropathic spondylopathy in tabes dorsalis (A52.11)

nonsyphilitic neuropathic spondylopathy NEC (G98.0)

spondylitis in syphilis (acquired) (A52.77)

tuberculous spondylitis (A18.01)

typhoid fever spondylitis (A01.05)

M49.8 Spondylopathy in diseases classified elsewhere

M49.80 Spondylopathy in diseases classified elsewhere, site unspecified

M49.81 Spondylopathy in diseases classified elsewhere, occipito-atlanto-axial region

M49.82 Spondylopathy in diseases classified elsewhere, cervical region

M49.83 Spondylopathy in diseases classified elsewhere, cervicothoracic region

M49.84 Spondylopathy in diseases classified elsewhere, thoracic region

M49.85 Spondylopathy in diseases classified elsewhere, thoracolumbar region

M49.86 Spondylopathy in diseases classified elsewhere, lumbar region

M49.87 Spondylopathy in diseases classified elsewhere, lumbosacral region

M49.88 Spondylopathy in diseases classified elsewhere, sacral and sacrococcygeal region

M49.89 Spondylopathy in diseases classified elsewhere, multiple sites in spine

OTHER DORSOPATHIES (M50-M54)

Excludes1: current injury - see injury of spine by body region

discitis NOS (M46.4-)

M50 Cervical disc disorders

Note: code to the most superior level of disorder

Includes: cervicothoracic disc disorders with cervicalgia

cervicothoracic disc disorders

M50.0 Cervical disc disorder with myelopathy

M50.00 Cervical disc disorder with myelopathy, unspecified cervical region

M50.01 Cervical disc disorder with myelopathy, high cervical region

C2-C3 disc disorder with myelopathy

C3-C4 disc disorder with myelopathy

M50.02 Cervical disc disorder with myelopathy, mid-cervical region

●**M50.020** Cervical disc disorder with myelopathy, mid-cervical region, unspecified level

●**M50.021** Cervical disc disorder at C4-C5 evel with myelopathy

C4-C5 disc disorder with myelopathy

●**M50.022** Cervical disc disorder at C5-C6 level with myelopathy

C5-C6 disc disorder with myelopathy

●**M50.023** Cervical disc disorder at C6-C7 level with myelopathy

C6-C7 disc disorder with myelopathy

M50.03 Cervical disc disorder with myelopathy, cervicothoracic region

C7-T1 disc disorder with myelopathy

M50.1 Cervical disc disorder with radiculopathy

Excludes2: brachial radiculitis NOS (M54.13)

M50.10 Cervical disc disorder with radiculopathy, unspecified cervical region

M50.11 Cervical disc disorder with radiculopathy, high cervical region

C2-C3 disc disorder with radiculopathy

C3 radiculopathy due to disc disorder

C3-C4 disc disorder with radiculopathy

C4 radiculopathy due to disc disorder

M50.12 Cervical disc disorder with radiculopathy, mid-cervical region

●**M50.120** Mid-cervical disc disorder, unspecified

●**M50.121** Cervical disc disorder at C4-C5 level with radiculopathy

C4-C5 disc disorder with radiculopathy

C5 radiculopathy due to disc disorder

●**M50.122** Cervical disc disorder at C5-C6 level with radiculopathy

C5-C6 disc disorder with radiculopathy

C6 radiculopathy due to disc disorder

●**M50.123** Cervical disc disorder at C6-C7 level with radiculopathy

C6-C7 disc disorder with radiculopathy

C7 radiculopathy due to disc disorder

M50.13   Cervical disc disorder with radiculopathy, cervicothoracic region

C7-T1 disc disorder with radiculopathy

C8 radiculopathy due to disc disorder

M50.2   Other cervical disc displacement

M50.20   Other cervical disc displacement, unspecified cervical region

M50.21   Other cervical disc displacement, high cervical region

Other C2-C3 cervical disc displacement

Other C3-C4 cervical disc displacement

M50.22   Other cervical disc displacement, mid-cervical region

●**M50.220   Other cervical disc displacement, mid-cervical region, unspecified level**

●**M50.221   Other cervical disc displacement at C4-C5 level**

Other C4-C5 cervical disc displacement

●**M50.222   Other cervical disc displacement at C5-C6 level**

Other C5-C6 cervical disc displacement

●**M50.223   Other cervical disc displacement at C6-C7 level**

Other C6-C7 cervical disc displacement

M50.23   Other cervical disc displacement, cervicothoracic region

Other C7-T1 cervical disc displacement

M50.3   Other cervical disc degeneration

M50.30   Other cervical disc degeneration, unspecified cervical region

M50.31   Other cervical disc degeneration, high cervical region

Other C2-C3 cervical disc degeneration

Other C3-C4 cervical disc degeneration

M50.32   Other cervical disc degeneration, mid-cervical region

●**M50.320   Other cervical disc degeneration, mid-cervical region, unspecified level**

●**M50.321   Other cervical disc degeneration at C4-C5 level**

Other C4-C5 cervical disc degeneration

●**M50.322   Other cervical disc degeneration at C5-C6 level**

Other C5-C6 cervical disc degeneration

●**M50.323   Other cervical disc degeneration at C6-C7 level**

Other C6-C7 cervical disc degeneration

M50.33   Other cervical disc degeneration, cervicothoracic region

Other C7-T1 cervical disc degeneration

M50.8   Other cervical disc disorders

M50.80   Other cervical disc disorders, unspecified cervical region

M50.81   Other cervical disc disorders, high cervical region

Other C2-C3 cervical disc disorders

Other C3-C4 cervical disc disorders

M50.82   Other cervical disc disorders, mid-cervical region

●**M50.820   Other cervical disc disorders, mid-cervical region, unspecified level**

●**M50.821   Other cervical disc disorders at C4-C5 level**

Other C4-C5 cervical disc disorders

●**M50.822   Other cervical disc disorders at C5-C6 level**

Other C5-C6 cervical disc disorders

●**M50.823   Other cervical disc disorders at C6-C7 level**

Other C6-C7 cervical disc disorders

M50.83   Other cervical disc disorders, cervicothoracic region

Other C7-T1 cervical disc disorders

M50.9   Cervical disc disorder, unspecified

M50.90   Cervical disc disorder, unspecified, unspecified cervical region

M50.91   Cervical disc disorder, unspecified, high cervical region

C2-C3 cervical disc disorder, unspecified

C3-C4 cervical disc disorder, unspecified

M50.92   Cervical disc disorder, unspecified, mid-cervical region

●**M50.920   Unspecified cervical disc disorder, mid-cervical region, unspecified level**

●**M50.921   Unspecified cervical disc disorder at C4-C5 level**

Unspecified C4-C5 cervical disc disorder

●**M50.922   Unspecified cervical disc disorder at C5-C6 level**

Unspecified C5-C6 cervical disc disorder

●**M50.923   Unspecified cervical disc disorder at C6-C7 level**

Unspecified C6-C7 cervical disc disorder

M50.93   Cervical disc disorder, unspecified, cervicothoracic region

C7-T1 cervical disc disorder, unspecified

M51   Thoracic, thoracolumbar, and lumbosacral intervertebral disc disorders

Definition: Intervertebral disc disorders result from a protrusion or herniation of one of the gel-like cushions (discs) that separate the vertebrae of the spine.

Excludes2: cervical and cervicothoracic disc disorders (M50.-)

sacral and sacrococcygeal disorders (M53.3)

M51.0   Thoracic, thoracolumbar and lumbosacral intervertebral disc disorders with myelopathy

M51.04 Intervertebral disc disorders with myelopathy, thoracic region

M51.05 Intervertebral disc disorders with myelopathy, thoracolumbar region

M51.06 Intervertebral disc disorders with myelopathy, lumbar region

M51.1 Thoracic, thoracolumbar and lumbosacral intervertebral disc disorders with radiculopathy

Sciatica due to intervertebral disc disorder

Excludes1: lumbar radiculitis NOS (M54.16)

sciatica NOS (M54.3)

M51.14 Intervertebral disc disorders with radiculopathy, thoracic region

M51.15 Intervertebral disc disorders with radiculopathy, thoracolumbar region

M51.16 Intervertebral disc disorders with radiculopathy, lumbar region

M51.17 Intervertebral disc disorders with radiculopathy, lumbosacral region

M51.2 Other thoracic, thoracolumbar and lumbosacral intervertebral disc displacement

Lumbago due to displacement of intervertebral disc

M51.24 Other intervertebral disc displacement, thoracic region

M51.25 Other intervertebral disc displacement, thoracolumbar region

M51.26 Other intervertebral disc displacement, lumbar region

M51.27 Other intervertebral disc displacement, lumbosacral region

M51.3 Other thoracic, thoracolumbar and lumbosacral intervertebral disc degeneration

M51.34 Other intervertebral disc degeneration, thoracic region

M51.35 Other intervertebral disc degeneration, thoracolumbar region

M51.36 Other intervertebral disc degeneration, lumbar region

M51.37 Other intervertebral disc degeneration, lumbosacral region

M51.4 Schmorl's nodes

M51.44 Schmorl's nodes, thoracic region

M51.45 Schmorl's nodes, thoracolumbar region

M51.46 Schmorl's nodes, lumbar region

M51.47 Schmorl's nodes, lumbosacral region

M51.8 Other thoracic, thoracolumbar and lumbosacral intervertebral disc disorders

M51.84 Other intervertebral disc disorders, thoracic region

M51.85 Other intervertebral disc disorders, thoracolumbar region

M51.86 Other intervertebral disc disorders, lumbar region

M51.87 Other intervertebral disc disorders, lumbosacral region

M51.9 Unspecified thoracic, thoracolumbar and lumbosacral intervertebral disc disorder

M53 Other and unspecified dorsopathies, not elsewhere classified

M53.0 Cervicocranial syndrome

Posterior cervical sympathetic syndrome

M53.1 Cervicobrachial syndrome

Excludes2: cervical disc disorder (M50.-)

thoracic outlet syndrome (G54.0)

M53.2 Spinal instabilities

M53.2X Spinal instabilities

M53.2X1 Spinal instabilities, occipito-atlanto-axial region

M53.2X2 Spinal instabilities, cervical region

M53.2X3 Spinal instabilities, cervicothoracic region

M53.2X4 Spinal instabilities, thoracic region

M53.2X5 Spinal instabilities, thoracolumbar region

M53.2X6 Spinal instabilities, lumbar region

M53.2X7 Spinal instabilities, lumbosacral region

M53.2X8 Spinal instabilities, sacral and sacrococcygeal region

M53.2X9 Spinal instabilities, site unspecified

M53.3 Sacrococcygeal disorders, not elsewhere classified

Coccygodynia

M53.8 Other specified dorsopathies

M53.80 Other specified dorsopathies, site unspecified

M53.81 Other specified dorsopathies, occipito-atlanto-axial region

M53.82 Other specified dorsopathies, cervical region

M53.83 Other specified dorsopathies, cervicothoracic region

M53.84 Other specified dorsopathies, thoracic region

M53.85 Other specified dorsopathies, thoracolumbar region

M53.86 Other specified dorsopathies, lumbar region

M53.87 Other specified dorsopathies, lumbosacral region

M53.88 Other specified dorsopathies, sacral and sacrococcygeal region

M53.9 Dorsopathy, unspecified

M54 Dorsalgia

Excludes1: psychogenic dorsalgia (F45.41)

M54.0 Panniculitis affecting regions of neck and back

Excludes1: lupus panniculitis (L93.2)

panniculitis NOS (M79.3)

relapsing [Weber-Christian] panniculitis (M35.6)

M54.00 Panniculitis affecting regions of neck and back, site unspecified

M54.01 Panniculitis affecting regions of neck and back, occipito-atlanto-axial region

M54.02 Panniculitis affecting regions of neck and back, cervical region

M54.03 Panniculitis affecting regions of neck and back, cervicothoracic region

M54.04 Panniculitis affecting regions of neck and back, thoracic region

M54.05 Panniculitis affecting regions of neck and back, thoracolumbar region

M54.06 Panniculitis affecting regions of neck and back, lumbar region

M54.07 **Panniculitis affecting regions of neck and back, lumbosacral region**

M54.08 **Panniculitis affecting regions of neck and back, sacral and sacrococcygeal region**

M54.09 **Panniculitis affecting regions, neck and back, multiple sites in spine**

M54.1 **Radiculopathy**

Brachial neuritis or radiculitis NOS

Lumbar neuritis or radiculitis NOS

Lumbosacral neuritis or radiculitis NOS

Thoracic neuritis or radiculitis NOS

Radiculitis NOS

Excludes1: neuralgia and neuritis NOS (M79.2)

radiculopathy with cervical disc disorder (M50.1)

radiculopathy with lumbar **and other** intervertebral disc disorder (M51.1-)

radiculopathy with spondylosis (M47.2-)

M54.10 **Radiculopathy, site unspecified**

M54.11 **Radiculopathy, occipito-atlanto-axial region**

M54.12 **Radiculopathy, cervical region**

M54.13 **Radiculopathy, cervicothoracic region**

M54.14 **Radiculopathy, thoracic region**

M54.15 **Radiculopathy, thoracolumbar region**

M54.16 **Radiculopathy, lumbar region**

M54.17 **Radiculopathy, lumbosacral region**

M54.18 **Radiculopathy, sacral and sacrococcygeal region**

M54.2 **Cervicalgia**

Excludes1: cervicalgia due to intervertebral cervical disc disorder (M50.-)

M54.3 **Sciatica**

Excludes1: lesion of sciatic nerve (G57.0)

sciatica due to intervertebral disc disorder (M51.1-)

sciatica with lumbago (M54.4-)

M54.30 **Sciatica, unspecified side**

M54.31 **Sciatica, right side**

M54.32 **Sciatica, left side**

M54.4 **Lumbago with sciatica**

Excludes1: lumbago with sciatica due to intervertebral disc disorder (M51.1-)

M54.40 **Lumbago with sciatica, unspecified side**

M54.41 **Lumbago with sciatica, right side**

M54.42 **Lumbago with sciatica, left side**

M54.5 **Low back pain**

Loin pain

Lumbago NOS

Excludes1: low back strain (S39.012)

lumbago due to intervertebral disc displacement (M51.2-)

lumbago with sciatica (M54.4-)

M54.6 **Pain in thoracic spine**

Excludes1: pain in thoracic spine due to intervertebral disc disorder (M51.-)

M54.8 **Other dorsalgia**

Excludes1: dorsalgia in thoracic region (M54.6)

low back pain (M54.5)

M54.81 **Occipital neuralgia**

M54.89 **Other dorsalgia**

M54.9 **Dorsalgia, unspecified**

Backache NOS

Back pain NOS

SOFT TISSUE DISORDERS (M60-M79)

DISORDERS OF MUSCLES (M60-M63)

Excludes1: dermatopolymyositis (M33.-)

muscular dystrophies and myopathies (G71-G72)

myopathy in amyloidosis (E85.-)

myopathy in polyarteritis nodosa (M30.0)

myopathy in rheumatoid arthritis (M05.32)

myopathy in scleroderma (M34.-)

myopathy in Sjögren's syndrome (M35.03)

myopathy in systemic lupus erythematosus (M32.-)

M60 **Myositis**

Excludes2: inclusion body myositis [IBM] (G72.41)

M60.0 **Infective myositis**

Tropical pyomyositis

Use additional code (B95-B97) to identify infectious agent

M60.00 **Infective myositis, unspecified site**

M60.000 **Infective myositis, unspecified right arm**

Infective myositis, right upper limb NOS

M60.001 **Infective myositis, unspecified left arm**

Infective myositis, left upper limb NOS

M60.002 **Infective myositis, unspecified arm**

Infective myositis, upper limb NOS

M60.003 **Infective myositis, unspecified right leg**

Infective myositis, right lower limb NOS

M60.004 **Infective myositis, unspecified left leg**

Infective myositis, left lower limb NOS

M60.005 **Infective myositis, unspecified leg**

Infective myositis, lower limb NOS

M60.009 **Infective myositis, unspecified site**

M60.01 **Infective myositis, shoulder**

M60.011 **Infective myositis, right shoulder**

M60.012 **Infective myositis, left shoulder**

M60.019 **Infective myositis, unspecified shoulder**

M60.02 **Infective myositis, upper arm**

M60.021 **Infective myositis, right upper arm**

M60.022 **Infective myositis, left upper arm**

M60.029 **Infective myositis, unspecified upper arm**

M60.03 **Infective myositis, forearm**

M60.031 **Infective myositis, right forearm**

M60.032 Infective myosis, left forearm

M60.039 Infective myositis, unspecified forearm

M60.04 Infective myositis, hand and fingers

    M60.041 Infective myositis, right hand

    M60.042 Infective myositis, left hand

    M60.043 Infective myositis, unspecified hand

    M60.044 Infective myositis, right finger(s)

    M60.045 Infective myositis, left finger(s)

    M60.046 Infective myositis, unspecified finger(s)

M60.05 Infective myositis, thigh

    M60.051 Infective myositis, right thigh

    M60.052 Infective myositis, left thigh

    M60.059 Infective myositis, unspecified thigh

M60.06 Infective myositis, lower leg

    M60.061 Infective myositis, right lower leg

    M60.062 Infective myositis, left lower leg

    M60.069 Infective myositis, unspecified lower leg

M60.07 Infective myositis, ankle, foot and toes

    M60.070 Infective myositis, right ankle

    M60.071 Infective myositis, left ankle

    M60.072 Infective myositis, unspecified ankle

    M60.073 Infective myositis, right foot

    M60.074 Infective myositis, left foot

    M60.075 Infective myositis, unspecified foot

    M60.076 Infective myositis, right toe(s)

    M60.077 Infective myositis, left toe(s)

    M60.078 Infective myositis, unspecified toe(s)

M60.08 Infective myositis, other site

M60.09 Infective myositis, multiple sites

M60.1 Interstitial myositis

M60.10 Interstitial myositis of unspecified site

M60.11 Interstitial myositis, shoulder

    M60.111 Interstitial myositis, right shoulder

    M60.112 Interstitial myositis, left shoulder

    M60.119 Interstitial myositis, unspecified shoulder

M60.12 Interstitial myositis, upper arm

    M60.121 Interstitial myositis, right upper arm

    M60.122 Interstitial myositis, left upper arm

    M60.129 Interstitial myositis, unspecified upper arm

M60.13 Interstitial myositis, forearm

    M60.131 Interstitial myositis, right forearm

    M60.132 Interstitial myositis, left forearm

    M60.139 Interstitial myositis, unspecified forearm

M60.14 Interstitial myositis, hand

    M60.141 Interstitial myositis, right hand

    M60.142 Interstitial myositis, left hand

    M60.149 Interstitial myositis, unspecified hand

M60.15 Interstitial myositis, thigh

M60.151 Interstitial myositis, right thigh

M60.152 Interstitial myositis, left thigh

M60.159 Interstitial myositis, unspecified thigh

M60.16 Interstitial myositis, lower leg

    M60.161 Interstitial myositis, right lower leg

    M60.162 Interstitial myositis, left lower leg

    M60.169 Interstitial myositis, unspecified lower leg

M60.17 Interstitial myositis, ankle and foot

    M60.171 Interstitial myositis, right ankle and foot

    M60.172 Interstitial myositis, left ankle and foot

    M60.179 Interstitial myositis, unspecified ankle and foot

M60.18 Interstitial myositis, other site

M60.19 Interstitial myositis, multiple sites

M60.2 Foreign body granuloma of soft tissue, not elsewhere classified

Use additional code to identify the type of retained foreign body (Z18.-)

Excludes1: foreign body granuloma of skin and subcutaneous tissue (L92.3)

M60.20 Foreign body granuloma of soft tissue, not elsewhere classified, unspecified site

M60.21 Foreign body granuloma of soft tissue, not elsewhere classified, shoulder

    M60.211 Foreign body granuloma of soft tissue, not elsewhere classified, right shoulder

    M60.212 Foreign body granuloma of soft tissue, not elsewhere classified, left shoulder

    M60.219 Foreign body granuloma of soft tissue, not elsewhere classified, unspecified shoulder

M60.22 Foreign body granuloma of soft tissue, not elsewhere classified, upper arm

    M60.221 Foreign body granuloma of soft tissue, not elsewhere classified, right upper arm

    M60.222 Foreign body granuloma of soft tissue, not elsewhere classified, left upper arm

    M60.229 Foreign body granuloma of soft tissue, not elsewhere classified, unspecified upper arm

M60.23 Foreign body granuloma of soft tissue, not elsewhere classified, forearm

    M60.231 Foreign body granuloma of soft tissue, not elsewhere classified, right forearm

    M60.232 Foreign body granuloma of soft tissue, not elsewhere classified, left forearm

    M60.239 Foreign body granuloma of soft tissue, not elsewhere classified, unspecified forearm

M60.24 Foreign body granuloma of soft tissue, not elsewhere classified, hand

M60.241 Foreign body granuloma of soft tissue, not elsewhere classified, right hand

M60.242 Foreign body granuloma of soft tissue, not elsewhere classified, left hand

M60.249 Foreign body granuloma of soft tissue, not elsewhere classified, unspecified hand

M60.25 Foreign body granuloma of soft tissue, not elsewhere classified, thigh

M60.251 Foreign body granuloma of soft tissue, not elsewhere classified, right thigh

M60.252 Foreign body granuloma of soft tissue, not elsewhere classified, left thigh

M60.259 Foreign body granuloma of soft tissue, not elsewhere classified, unspecified thigh

M60.26 Foreign body granuloma of soft tissue, not elsewhere classified, lower leg

M60.261 Foreign body granuloma of soft tissue, not elsewhere classified, right lower leg

M60.262 Foreign body granuloma of soft tissue, not elsewhere classified, left lower leg

M60.269 Foreign body granuloma of soft tissue, not elsewhere classified, unspecified lower leg

M60.27 Foreign body granuloma of soft tissue, not elsewhere classified, ankle and foot

M60.271 Foreign body granuloma of soft tissue, not elsewhere classified, right ankle and foot

M60.272 Foreign body granuloma of soft tissue, not elsewhere classified, left ankle and foot

M60.279 Foreign body granuloma of soft tissue, not elsewhere classified, unspecified ankle and foot

M60.28 Foreign body granuloma of soft tissue, not elsewhere classified, other site

M60.8 Other myositis

M60.80 Other myositis, unspecified site

M60.81 Other myositis shoulder

M60.811 Other myositis, right shoulder

M60.812 Other myositis, left shoulder

M60.819 Other myositis, unspecified shoulder

M60.82 Other myositis, upper arm

M60.821 Other myositis, right upper arm

M60.822 Other myositis, left upper arm

M60.829 Other myositis, unspecified upper arm

M60.83 Other myositis, forearm

M60.831 Other myositis, right forearm

M60.832 Other myositis, left forearm

M60.839 Other myositis, unspecified forearm

M60.84 Other myositis, hand

M60.841 Other myositis, right hand

M60.842 Other myositis, left hand

M60.849 Other myositis, unspecified hand

M60.85 Other myositis, thigh

M60.851 Other myositis, right thigh

M60.852 Other myositis, left thigh

M60.859 Other myositis, unspecified thigh

M60.86 Other myositis, lower leg

M60.861 Other myositis, right lower leg

M60.862 Other myositis, left lower leg

M60.869 Other myositis, unspecified lower leg

M60.87 Other myositis, ankle and foot

M60.871 Other myositis, right ankle and foot

M60.872 Other myositis, left ankle and foot

M60.879 Other myositis, unspecified ankle and foot

M60.88 Other myositis, other site

M60.89 Other myositis, multiple sites

M60.9 Myositis, unspecified

M61 Calcification and ossification of muscle

M61.0 Myositis ossificans traumatica

M61.00 Myositis ossificans traumatica, unspecified site

M61.01 Myositis ossificans traumatica, shoulder

M61.011 Myositis ossificans traumatica, right shoulder

M61.012 Myositis ossificans traumatica, left shoulder

M61.019 Myositis ossificans traumatica, unspecified shoulder

M61.02 Myositis ossificans traumatica, upper arm

M61.021 Myositis ossificans traumatica, right upper arm

M61.022 Myositis ossificans traumatica, left upper arm

M61.029 Myositis ossificans traumatica, unspecified upper arm

M61.03 Myositis ossificans traumatica, forearm

M61.031 Myositis ossificans traumatica, right forearm

M61.032 Myositis ossificans traumatica, left forearm

M61.039 Myositis ossificans traumatica, unspecified forearm

M61.04 Myositis ossificans traumatica, hand

M61.041 Myositis ossificans traumatica, right hand

M61.042 Myositis ossificans traumatica, left hand

M61.049 Myositis ossificans traumatica, unspecified hand

M61.05 Myositis ossificans traumatica, thigh

M61.051 Myositis ossificans traumatica, right thigh

M61.052 Myositis ossificans traumatica, left thigh

M61.059 Myositis ossificans traumatica, unspecified thigh

● New code ▲ Revised code **Excludes1:** Not coded here **Excludes2:** Not included here ⊗ Placeholder required ⑦ 7th digit required

M61.06 Myositis ossificans traumatica, lower leg

    M61.061 Myositis ossificans traumatica, right lower leg

    M61.062 Myositis ossificans traumatica, left lower leg

    M61.069 Myositis ossificans traumatica, unspecified lower leg

M61.07 Myositis ossificans traumatica, ankle and foot

    M61.071 Myositis ossificans traumatica, right ankle and foot

    M61.072 Myositis ossificans traumatica, left ankle and foot

    M61.079 Myositis ossificans traumatica, unspecified ankle and foot

M61.08 Myositis ossificans traumatica, other site

M61.09 Myositis ossificans traumatica, multiple sites

M61.1 **Myositis ossificans progressiva**

Fibrodysplasia ossificans progressiva

M61.10 Myositis ossificans progressiva, unspecified site

M61.11 Myositis ossificans progressiva, shoulder

    M61.111 Myositis ossificans progressiva, right shoulder

    M61.112 Myositis ossificans progressiva, left shoulder

    M61.119 Myositis ossificans progressiva, unspecified shoulder

M61.12 Myositis ossificans progressiva, upper arm

    M61.121 Myositis ossificans progressiva, right upper arm

    M61.122 Myositis ossificans progressiva, left upper arm

    M61.129 Myositis ossificans progressiva, unspecified arm

M61.13 Myositis ossificans progressiva, forearm

    M61.131 Myositis ossificans progressiva, right forearm

    M61.132 Myositis ossificans progressiva, left forearm

    M61.139 Myositis ossificans progressiva, unspecified forearm

M61.14 Myositis ossificans progressiva, hand and finger(s)

    M61.141 Myositis ossificans progressiva, right hand

    M61.142 Myositis ossificans progressiva, left hand

    M61.143 Myositis ossificans progressiva, unspecified hand

    M61.144 Myositis ossificans progressiva, right finger(s)

    M61.145 Myositis ossificans progressiva, left finger(s)

    M61.146 Myositis ossificans progressiva, unspecified finger(s)

M61.15 Myositis ossificans progressiva, thigh

    M61.151 Myositis ossificans progressiva, right thigh

    M61.152 Myositis ossificans progressiva, left thigh

    M61.159 Myositis ossificans progressiva, unspecified thigh

M61.16 Myositis ossificans progressiva, lower leg

    M61.161 Myositis ossificans progressiva, right lower leg

    M61.162 Myositis ossificans progressiva, left lower leg

    M61.169 Myositis ossificans progressiva, unspecified lower leg

M61.17 Myositis ossificans progressiva, ankle, foot and toe(s)

    M61.171 Myositis ossificans progressiva, right ankle

    M61.172 Myositis ossificans progressiva, left ankle

    M61.173 Myositis ossificans progressiva, unspecified ankle

    M61.174 Myositis ossificans progressiva, right foot

    M61.175 Myositis ossificans progressiva, left foot

    M61.176 Myositis ossificans progressiva, unspecified foot

    M61.177 Myositis ossificans progressiva, right toe(s)

    M61.178 Myositis ossificans progressiva, left toe(s)

    M61.179 Myositis ossificans progressiva, unspecified toe(s)

M61.18 Myositis ossificans progressiva, other site

M61.19 Myositis ossificans progressiva, multiple sites

M61.2 **Paralytic calcification and ossification of muscle**

Myositis ossificans associated with quadriplegia or paraplegia

M61.20 Paralytic calcification and ossification of muscle, unspecified site

M61.21 Paralytic calcification and ossification of muscle, shoulder

    M61.211 Paralytic calcification and ossification of muscle, right shoulder

    M61.212 Paralytic calcification and ossification of muscle, left shoulder

    M61.219 Paralytic calcification and ossification of muscle, unspecified shoulder

M61.22 Paralytic calcification and ossification of muscle, upper arm

    M61.221 Paralytic calcification and ossification of muscle, right upper arm

    M61.222 Paralytic calcification and ossification of muscle, left upper arm

    M61.229 Paralytic calcification and ossification of muscle, unspecified upper arm

M61.23 Paralytic calcification and ossification of muscle, forearm

    M61.231 Paralytic calcification and ossification of muscle, right forearm

M61.232   Paralytic calcification and ossification of muscle, left forearm

M61.239   Paralytic calcification and ossification of muscle, unspecified forearm

M61.24 Paralytic calcification and ossification of muscle, hand

    M61.241   Paralytic calcification and ossification of muscle, right hand

    M61.242   Paralytic calcification and ossification of muscle, left hand

    M61.249   Paralytic calcification and ossification of muscle, unspecified hand

M61.25 Paralytic calcification and ossification of muscle, thigh

    M61.251   Paralytic calcification and ossification of muscle, right thigh

    M61.252   Paralytic calcification and ossification of muscle, left thigh

    M61.259   Paralytic calcification and ossification of muscle, unspecified thigh

M61.26 Paralytic calcification and ossification of muscle, lower leg

    M61.261   Paralytic calcification and ossification of muscle, right lower leg

    M61.262   Paralytic calcification and ossification of muscle, left lower leg

    M61.269   Paralytic calcification and ossification of muscle, unspecified lower leg

M61.27 Paralytic calcification and ossification of muscle, ankle and foot

    M61.271   Paralytic calcification and ossification of muscle, right ankle and foot

    M61.272   Paralytic calcification and ossification of muscle, left ankle and foot

    M61.279   Paralytic calcification and ossification of muscle, unspecified ankle and foot

M61.28 Paralytic calcification and ossification of muscle, other site

M61.29 Paralytic calcification and ossification of muscle, multiple sites

M61.3 Calcification and ossification of muscles associated with burns

Myositis ossificans associated with burns

M61.30 Calcification and ossification of muscles associated with burns, unspecified site

M61.31 Calcification and ossification of muscles associated with burns, shoulder

    M61.311   Calcification and ossification of muscles associated with burns, right shoulder

    M61.312   Calcification and ossification of muscles associated with burns, left shoulder

M61.319   Calcification and ossification of muscles associated with burns, unspecified shoulder

M61.32 Calcification and ossification of muscles associated with burns, upper arm

    M61.321   Calcification and ossification of muscles associated with burns, right upper arm

    M61.322   Calcification and ossification of muscles associated with burns, left upper arm

    M61.329   Calcification and ossification of muscles associated with burns, unspecified upper arm

M61.33 Calcification and ossification of muscles associated with burns, forearm

    M61.331   Calcification and ossification of muscles associated with burns, right forearm

    M61.332   Calcification and ossification of muscles associated with burns, left forearm

    M61.339   Calcification and ossification of muscles associated with burns, unspecified forearm

M61.34 Calcification and ossification of muscles associated with burns, hand

    M61.341   Calcification and ossification of muscles associated with burns, right hand

    M61.342   Calcification and ossification of muscles associated with burns, left hand

    M61.349   Calcification and ossification of muscles associated with burns, unspecified hand

M61.35 Calcification and ossification of muscles associated with burns, thigh

    M61.351   Calcification and ossification of muscles associated with burns, right thigh

    M61.352   Calcification and ossification of muscles associated with burns, left thigh

    M61.359   Calcification and ossification of muscles associated with burns, unspecified thigh

M61.36 Calcification and ossification of muscles associated with burns, lower leg

    M61.361   Calcification and ossification of muscles associated with burns, right lower leg

    M61.362   Calcification and ossification of muscles associated with burns, left lower leg

    M61.369   Calcification and ossification of muscles associated with burns, unspecified lower leg

M61.37 Calcification and ossification of muscles associated with burns, ankle and foot

    M61.371   Calcification and ossification of muscles associated with burns, right ankle and foot

M61.372   Calcification and ossification of muscles associated with burns, left ankle and foot

M61.379   Calcification and ossification of muscles associated with burns, unspecified ankle and foot

M61.38   Calcification and ossification of muscles associated with burns, other site

M61.39   Calcification and ossification of muscles associated with burns, multiple sites

M61.4   Other calcification of muscle

> **Excludes1:** calcific tendinitis NOS (M65.2-)
>
> calcific tendinitis of shoulder (M75.3)

M61.40   Other calcification of muscle, unspecified site

M61.41   Other calcification of muscle, shoulder

M61.411   Other calcification of muscle, right shoulder

M61.412   Other calcification of muscle, left shoulder

M61.419   Other calcification of muscle, unspecified shoulder

M61.42   Other calcification of muscle, upper arm

M61.421   Other calcification of muscle, right upper arm

M61.422   Other calcification of muscle, left upper arm

M61.429   Other calcification of muscle, unspecified upper arm

M61.43   Other calcification of muscle, forearm

M61.431   Other calcification of muscle, right forearm

M61.432   Other calcification of muscle, left forearm

M61.439   Other calcification of muscle, unspecified forearm

M61.44   Other calcification of muscle, hand

M61.441   Other calcification of muscle, right hand

M61.442   Other calcification of muscle, left hand

M61.449   Other calcification of muscle, unspecified hand

M61.45   Other calcification of muscle, thigh

M61.451   Other calcification of muscle, right thigh

M61.452   Other calcification of muscle, left thigh

M61.459   Other calcification of muscle, unspecified thigh

M61.46   Other calcification of muscle, lower leg

M61.461   Other calcification of muscle, right lower leg

M61.462   Other calcification of muscle, left lower leg

M61.469   Other calcification of muscle, unspecified lower leg

M61.47   Other calcification of muscle, ankle and foot

M61.471   Other calcification of muscle, right ankle and foot

M61.472   Other calcification of muscle, left ankle and foot

M61.479   Other calcification of muscle, unspecified ankle and foot

M61.48   Other calcification of muscle, other site

M61.49   Other calcification of muscle, multiple sites

M61.5   Other ossification of muscle

M61.50   Other ossification of muscle, unspecified site

M61.51   Other ossification of muscle, shoulder

M61.511   Other ossification of muscle, right shoulder

M61.512   Other ossification of muscle, left shoulder

M61.519   Other ossification of muscle, unspecified shoulder

M61.52   Other ossification of muscle, upper arm

M61.521   Other ossification of muscle, right upper arm

M61.522   Other ossification of muscle, left upper arm

M61.529   Other ossification of muscle, unspecified upper arm

M61.53   Other ossification of muscle, forearm

M61.531   Other ossification of muscle, right forearm

M61.532   Other ossification of muscle, left forearm

M61.539   Other ossification of muscle, unspecified forearm

M61.54   Other ossification of muscle, hand

M61.541   Other ossification of muscle, right hand

M61.542   Other ossification of muscle, left hand

M61.549   Other ossification of muscle, unspecified hand

M61.55   Other ossification of muscle, thigh

M61.551   Other ossification of muscle, right thigh

M61.552   Other ossification of muscle, left thigh

M61.559   Other ossification of muscle, unspecified thigh

M61.56   Other ossification of muscle, lower leg

M61.561   Other ossification of muscle, right lower leg

M61.562   Other ossification of muscle, left lower leg

M61.569   Other ossification of muscle, unspecified lower leg

M61.57   Other ossification of muscle, ankle and foot

M61.571   Other ossification of muscle, right ankle and foot

M61.572   Other ossification of muscle, left ankle and foot

M61.579   Other ossification of muscle, unspecified ankle and foot

M61.58   Other ossification of muscle, other site

M61.59   Other ossification of muscle, multiple sites

M61.9 Calcification and ossification of muscle, unspecified

M62 Other disorders of muscle

> **Excludes1:** alcoholic myopathy (G72.1)
>
> cramp and spasm (R25.2)
>
> drug-induced myopathy (G72.0)
>
> myalgia (M79.1)
>
> stiff-man syndrome (G25.82)
>
> **Excludes2:** nontraumatic hematoma of muscle (M79.81)

M62.0 Separation of muscle (nontraumatic)

Diastasis of muscle

> **Excludes1:** diastasis recti complicating pregnancy, labor and delivery (O71.8)

traumatic separation of muscle- see strain of muscle by body region

M62.00 Separation of muscle (nontraumatic), unspecified site

M62.01 Separation of muscle (nontraumatic), shoulder

M62.011 Separation of muscle (nontraumatic), right shoulder

M62.012 Separation of muscle (nontraumatic), left shoulder

M62.019 Separation of muscle (nontraumatic), unspecified shoulder

M62.02 Separation of muscle (nontraumatic), upper arm

M62.021 Separation of muscle (nontraumatic), right upper arm

M62.022 Separation of muscle (nontraumatic), left upper arm

M62.029 Separation of muscle (nontraumatic), unspecified upper arm

M62.03 Separation of muscle (nontraumatic), forearm

M62.031 Separation of muscle (nontraumatic), right forearm

M62.032 Separation of muscle (nontraumatic), left forearm

M62.039 Separation of muscle (nontraumatic), unspecified forearm

M62.04 Separation of muscle (nontraumatic), hand

M62.041 Separation of muscle (nontraumatic), right hand

M62.042 Separation of muscle (nontraumatic), left hand

M62.049 Separation of muscle (nontraumatic), unspecified hand

M62.05 Separation of muscle (nontraumatic), thigh

M62.051 Separation of muscle (nontraumatic), right thigh

M62.052 Separation of muscle (nontraumatic), left thigh

M62.059 Separation of muscle (nontraumatic), unspecified thigh

M62.06 Separation of muscle (nontraumatic), lower leg

M62.061 Separation of muscle (nontraumatic), right lower leg

M62.062 Separation of muscle (nontraumatic), left lower leg

M62.069 Separation of muscle (nontraumatic), unspecified lower leg

M62.07 Separation of muscle (nontraumatic), ankle and foot

M62.071 Separation of muscle (nontraumatic), right ankle and foot

M62.072 Separation of muscle (nontraumatic), left ankle and foot

M62.079 Separation of muscle (nontraumatic), unspecified ankle and foot

M62.08 Separation of muscle (nontraumatic), other site

M62.1 Other rupture of muscle (nontraumatic)

> **Excludes1:** traumatic rupture of muscle - see strain of muscle by body region
>
> **Excludes2:** rupture of tendon (M66.-)

M62.10 Other rupture of muscle (nontraumatic), unspecified site

M62.11 Other rupture of muscle (nontraumatic), shoulder

M62.111 Other rupture of muscle (nontraumatic), right shoulder

M62.112 Other rupture of muscle (nontraumatic), left shoulder

M62.119 Other rupture of muscle (nontraumatic), unspecified shoulder

M62.12 Other rupture of muscle (nontraumatic), upper arm

M62.121 Other rupture of muscle (nontraumatic), right upper arm

M62.122 Other rupture of muscle (nontraumatic), left upper arm

M62.129 Other rupture of muscle (nontraumatic), unspecified upper arm

M62.13 Other rupture of muscle (nontraumatic), forearm

M62.131 Other rupture of muscle (nontraumatic), right forearm

M62.132 Other rupture of muscle (nontraumatic), left forearm

M62.139 Other rupture of muscle (nontraumatic), unspecified forearm

M62.14 Other rupture of muscle (nontraumatic), hand

M62.141 Other rupture of muscle (nontraumatic), right hand

M62.142 Other rupture of muscle (nontraumatic), left hand

M62.149 Other rupture of muscle (nontraumatic), unspecified hand

M62.15 Other rupture of muscle (nontraumatic), thigh

M62.151 Other rupture of muscle (nontraumatic), right thigh

M62.152 Other rupture of muscle (nontraumatic), left thigh

● New code   ▲ Revised code   **Excludes1:** Not coded here   **Excludes2:** Not included here   ⊗ Placeholder required   ⑦7th digit required

M62.159 Other rupture of muscle (nontraumatic), unspecified thigh

M62.16 Other rupture of muscle (nontraumatic), lower leg

  M62.161 Other rupture of muscle (nontraumatic), right lower leg

  M62.162 Other rupture of muscle (nontraumatic), left lower leg

  M62.169 Other rupture of muscle (nontraumatic), unspecified lower leg

M62.17 Other rupture of muscle (nontraumatic), ankle and foot

  M62.171 Other rupture of muscle (nontraumatic), right ankle and foot

  M62.172 Other rupture of muscle (nontraumatic), left ankle and foot

  M62.179 Other rupture of muscle (nontraumatic), unspecified ankle and foot

M62.18 Other rupture of muscle (nontraumatic), other site

M62.2 Nontraumatic ischemic infarction of muscle

  Excludes1: compartment syndrome (traumatic) (T79.A-)

  nontraumatic compartment syndrome (M79.A-)

  traumatic ischemia of muscle (T79.6)

  rhabdomyolysis (M62.82)

  Volkmann's ischemic contracture (T79.6)

M62.20 Nontraumatic ischemic infarction of muscle, unspecified site

M62.21 Nontraumatic ischemic infarction of muscle, shoulder

  M62.211 Nontraumatic ischemic infarction of muscle, right shoulder

  M62.212 Nontraumatic ischemic infarction of muscle, left shoulder

  M62.219 Nontraumatic ischemic infarction of muscle, unspecified shoulder

M62.22 Nontraumatic ischemic infarction of muscle, upper arm

  M62.221 Nontraumatic ischemic infarction of muscle, right upper arm

  M62.222 Nontraumatic ischemic infarction of muscle, left upper arm

  M62.229 Nontraumatic ischemic infarction of muscle, unspecified upper arm

M62.23 Nontraumatic ischemic infarction of muscle, forearm

  M62.231 Nontraumatic ischemic infarction of muscle, right forearm

  M62.232 Nontraumatic ischemic infarction of muscle, left forearm

  M62.239 Nontraumatic ischemic infarction of muscle, unspecified forearm

M62.24 Nontraumatic ischemic infarction of muscle, hand

  M62.241 Nontraumatic ischemic infarction of muscle, right hand

  M62.242 Nontraumatic ischemic infarction of muscle, left hand

M62.249 Nontraumatic ischemic infarction of muscle, unspecified hand

M62.25 Nontraumatic ischemic infarction of muscle, thigh

  M62.251 Nontraumatic ischemic infarction of muscle, right thigh

  M62.252 Nontraumatic ischemic infarction of muscle, left thigh

  M62.259 Nontraumatic ischemic infarction of muscle, unspecified thigh

M62.26 Nontraumatic ischemic infarction of muscle, lower leg

  M62.261 Nontraumatic ischemic infarction of muscle, right lower leg

  M62.262 Nontraumatic ischemic infarction of muscle, left lower leg

  M62.269 Nontraumatic ischemic infarction of muscle, unspecified lower leg

M62.27 Nontraumatic ischemic infarction of muscle, ankle and foot

  M62.271 Nontraumatic ischemic infarction of muscle, right ankle and foot

  M62.272 Nontraumatic ischemic infarction of muscle, left ankle and foot

  M62.279 Nontraumatic ischemic infarction of muscle, unspecified ankle and foot

M62.28 Nontraumatic ischemic infarction of muscle, other site

M62.3 Immobility syndrome (paraplegic)

M62.4 Contracture of muscle

  Contracture of tendon (sheath)

  Excludes1: contracture of joint (M24.5-)

M62.40 Contracture of muscle, unspecified site

M62.41 Contracture of muscle, shoulder

  M62.411 Contracture of muscle, right shoulder

  M62.412 Contracture of muscle, left shoulder

  M62.419 Contracture of muscle, unspecified shoulder

M62.42 Contracture of muscle, upper arm

  M62.421 Contracture of muscle, right upper arm

  M62.422 Contracture of muscle, left upper arm

  M62.429 Contracture of muscle, unspecified upper arm

M62.43 Contracture of muscle, forearm

  M62.431 Contracture of muscle, right forearm

  M62.432 Contracture of muscle, left forearm

  M62.439 Contracture of muscle, unspecified forearm

M62.44 Contracture of muscle, hand

  M62.441 Contracture of muscle, right hand

  M62.442 Contracture of muscle, left hand

  M62.449 Contracture of muscle, unspecified hand

M62.45 Contracture of muscle, thigh

  M62.451 Contracture of muscle, right thigh

M62.452 Contracture of muscle, left thigh

M62.459 Contracture of muscle, unspecified thigh

M62.46 Contracture of muscle, lower leg

M62.461 Contracture of muscle, right lower leg

M62.462 Contracture of muscle, left lower leg

M62.469 Contracture of muscle, unspecified lower leg

M62.47 Contracture of muscle, ankle and foot

M62.471 Contracture of muscle, right ankle and foot

M62.472 Contracture of muscle, left ankle and foot

M62.479 Contracture of muscle, unspecified ankle and foot

M62.48 Contracture of muscle, other site

M62.49 Contracture of muscle, multiple sites

M62.5 Muscle wasting and atrophy, not elsewhere classified

Disuse atrophy NEC

Excludes1: neuralgic amyotrophy (G54.5)

progressive muscular atrophy (G12.29)

sarcopenia (M62.84)

Excludes2: pelvic muscle wasting (N81.84)

M62.50 Muscle wasting and atrophy, not elsewhere classified, unspecified site

M62.51 Muscle wasting and atrophy, not elsewhere classified, shoulder

M62.511 Muscle wasting and atrophy, not elsewhere classified, right shoulder

M62.512 Muscle wasting and atrophy, not elsewhere classified, left shoulder

M62.519 Muscle wasting and atrophy, not elsewhere classified, unspecified shoulder

M62.52 Muscle wasting and atrophy, not elsewhere classified, upper arm

M62.521 Muscle wasting and atrophy, not elsewhere classified, right upper arm

M62.522 Muscle wasting and atrophy, not elsewhere classified, left upper arm

M62.529 Muscle wasting and atrophy, not elsewhere classified, unspecified upper arm

M62.53 Muscle wasting and atrophy, not elsewhere classified, forearm

M62.531 Muscle wasting and atrophy, not elsewhere classified, right forearm

M62.532 Muscle wasting and atrophy, not elsewhere classified, left forearm

M62.539 Muscle wasting and atrophy, not elsewhere classified, unspecified forearm

M62.54 Muscle wasting and atrophy, not elsewhere classified, hand

M62.541 Muscle wasting and atrophy, not elsewhere classified, right hand

M62.542 Muscle wasting and atrophy, not elsewhere classified, left hand

M62.549 Muscle wasting and atrophy, not elsewhere classified, unspecified hand

M62.55 Muscle wasting and atrophy, not elsewhere classified, thigh

M62.551 Muscle wasting and atrophy, not elsewhere classified, right thigh

M62.552 Muscle wasting and atrophy, not elsewhere classified, left thigh

M62.559 Muscle wasting and atrophy, not elsewhere classified, unspecified thigh

M62.56 Muscle wasting and atrophy, not elsewhere classified, lower leg

M62.561 Muscle wasting and atrophy, not elsewhere classified, right lower leg

M62.562 Muscle wasting and atrophy, not elsewhere classified, left lower leg

M62.569 Muscle wasting and atrophy, not elsewhere classified, unspecified lower leg

M62.57 Muscle wasting and atrophy, not elsewhere classified, ankle and foot

M62.571 Muscle wasting and atrophy, not elsewhere classified, right ankle and foot

M62.572 Muscle wasting and atrophy, not elsewhere classified, left ankle and foot

M62.579 Muscle wasting and atrophy, not elsewhere classified, unspecified ankle and foot

M62.58 Muscle wasting and atrophy, not elsewhere classified, other site

M62.59 Muscle wasting and atrophy, not elsewhere classified, multiple sites

M62.8 Other specified disorders of muscle

Excludes2: nontraumatic hematoma of muscle (M79.81)

M62.81 Muscle weakness (generalized)

Excludes1: muscle weakness in sarcopenia (M62.84)

M62.82 Rhabdomyolysis

Excludes1: traumatic rhabdomyolysis (T79.6)

M62.83 Muscle spasm

M62.830 Muscle spasm of back

M62.831 Muscle spasm of calf

Charley-horse

M62.838 Other muscle spasm

● **M62.84** Sarcopenia

Age-related sarcopenia

Code first underlying disease, if applicable, such as:

disorders of myoneural junction and muscle disease in diseases classified elsewhere (G73.-)

Other and unspecified myopathies (G72.-)

primary disorders of muscles (G71.-)

M62.89 Other specified disorders of muscle

Muscle (sheath) hernia

● New code ▲ Revised code **Excludes1:** Not coded here **Excludes2:** Not included here ⊗ Placeholder required ⑦7ᵗʰ digit required

M62.9 Disorder of muscle, unspecified

M63 Disorders of muscle in diseases classified elsewhere

Code first underlying disease, such as:

leprosy (A30.-)

neoplasm (C49.-, C79.89, D21.-, D48.1)

schistosomiasis (B65.-)

trichinellosis (B75)

Excludes1: myopathy in cysticercosis (B69.81)

myopathy in endocrine diseases (G73.7)

myopathy in metabolic diseases (G73.7)

myopathy in sarcoidosis (D86.87)

myopathy in secondary syphilis (A51.49)

myopathy in syphilis (late) (A52.78)

myopathy in toxoplasmosis (B58.82)

myopathy in tuberculosis (A18.09)

M63.8 Disorders of muscle in diseases classified elsewhere

M63.80 Disorders of muscle in diseases classified elsewhere, unspecified site

M63.81 Disorders of muscle in diseases classified elsewhere, shoulder

M63.811 Disorders of muscle in diseases classified elsewhere, right shoulder

M63.812 Disorders of muscle in diseases classified elsewhere, left shoulder

M63.819 Disorders of muscle in diseases classified elsewhere, unspecified shoulder

M63.82 Disorders of muscle in diseases classified elsewhere, upper arm

M63.821 Disorders of muscle in diseases classified elsewhere, right upper arm

M63.822 Disorders of muscle in diseases classified elsewhere, left upper arm

M63.829 Disorders of muscle in diseases classified elsewhere, unspecified upper arm

M63.83 Disorders of muscle in diseases classified elsewhere, forearm

M63.831 Disorders of muscle in diseases classified elsewhere, right forearm

M63.832 Disorders of muscle in diseases classified elsewhere, left forearm

M63.839 Disorders of muscle in diseases classified elsewhere, unspecified forearm

M63.84 Disorders of muscle in diseases classified elsewhere, hand

M63.841 Disorders of muscle in diseases classified elsewhere, right hand

M63.842 Disorders of muscle in diseases classified elsewhere, left hand

M63.849 Disorders of muscle in diseases classified elsewhere, unspecified hand

M63.85 Disorders of muscle in diseases classified elsewhere, thigh

M63.851 Disorders of muscle in diseases classified elsewhere, right thigh

M63.852 Disorders of muscle in diseases classified elsewhere, left thigh

M63.859 Disorders of muscle in diseases classified elsewhere, unspecified thigh

M63.86 Disorders of muscle in diseases classified elsewhere, lower leg

M63.861 Disorders of muscle in diseases classified elsewhere, right lower leg

M63.862 Disorders of muscle in diseases classified elsewhere, left lower leg

M63.869 Disorders of muscle in diseases classified elsewhere, unspecified lower leg

M63.87 Disorders of muscle in diseases classified elsewhere, ankle and foot

M63.871 Disorders of muscle in diseases classified elsewhere, right ankle and foot

M63.872 Disorders of muscle in diseases classified elsewhere, left ankle and foot

M63.879 Disorders of muscle in diseases classified elsewhere, unspecified ankle and foot

M63.88 Disorders of muscle in diseases classified elsewhere, other site

M63.89 Disorders of muscle in diseases classified elsewhere, multiple sites

DISORDERS OF SYNOVIUM AND TENDON (M65-M67)

M65 Synovitis and tenosynovitis

Excludes1: chronic crepitant synovitis of hand and wrist (M70.0-)

current injury - see injury of ligament or tendon by body region soft tissue disorders related to use, overuse and pressure (M70.-)

M65.0 Abscess of tendon sheath

Use additional code (B95-B96) to identify bacterial agent.

M65.00 Abscess of tendon sheath, unspecified site

M65.01 Abscess of tendon sheath, shoulder

M65.011 Abscess of tendon sheath, right shoulder

M65.012 Abscess of tendon sheath, left shoulder

M65.019 Abscess of tendon sheath, unspecified shoulder

M65.02 Abscess of tendon sheath, upper arm

M65.021 Abscess of tendon sheath, right upper arm

M65.022 Abscess of tendon sheath, left upper arm

M65.029 Abscess of tendon sheath, unspecified upper arm

M65.03 Abscess of tendon sheath, forearm

M65.031 Abscess of tendon sheath, right forearm

M65.032 Abscess of tendon sheath, left forearm

M65.039 Abscess of tendon sheath, unspecified forearm

M65.04 Abscess of tendon sheath, hand

M65.041 Abscess of tendon sheath, right hand

M65.042 Abscess of tendon sheath, left hand

M65.049 Abscess of tendon sheath, unspecified hand

M65.05 Abscess of tendon sheath, thigh

M65.051 Abscess of tendon sheath, right thigh

M65.052 Abscess of tendon sheath, left thigh

M65.059 Abscess of tendon sheath, unspecified thigh

M65.06 Abscess of tendon sheath, lower leg

M65.061 Abscess of tendon sheath, right lower leg

M65.062 Abscess of tendon sheath, left lower leg

M65.069 Abscess of tendon sheath, unspecified lower leg

M65.07 Abscess of tendon sheath, ankle and foot

M65.071 Abscess of tendon sheath, right ankle and foot

M65.072 Abscess of tendon sheath, left ankle and foot

M65.079 Abscess of tendon sheath, unspecified ankle and foot

M65.08 Abscess of tendon sheath, other site

M65.1 Other infective (teno)synovitis

M65.10 Other infective (teno)synovitis, unspecified site

M65.11 Other infective (teno)synovitis, shoulder

M65.111 Other infective (teno)synovitis, right shoulder

M65.112 Other infective (teno)synovitis, left shoulder

M65.119 Other infective (teno)synovitis, unspecified shoulder

M65.12 Other infective (teno)synovitis, elbow

M65.121 Other infective (teno)synovitis, right elbow

M65.122 Other infective (teno)synovitis, left elbow

M65.129 Other infective (teno)synovitis, unspecified elbow

M65.13 Other infective (teno)synovitis, wrist

M65.131 Other infective (teno)synovitis, right wrist

M65.132 Other infective (teno)synovitis, left wrist

M65.139 Other infective (teno)synovitis, unspecified wrist

M65.14 Other infective (teno)synovitis, hand

M65.141 Other infective (teno)synovitis, right hand

M65.142 Other infective (teno)synovitis, left hand

M65.149 Other infective (teno)synovitis, unspecified hand

M65.15 Other infective (teno)synovitis, hip

M65.151 Other infective (teno)synovitis, right hip

M65.152 Other infective (teno)synovitis, left hip

M65.159 Other infective (teno)synovitis, unspecified hip

M65.16 Other infective (teno)synovitis, knee

M65.161 Other infective (teno)synovitis, right knee

M65.162 Other infective (teno)synovitis, left knee

M65.169 Other infective (teno)synovitis, unspecified knee

M65.17 Other infective (teno)synovitis, ankle and foot

M65.171 Other infective (teno)synovitis, right ankle and foot

M65.172 Other infective (teno)synovitis, left ankle and foot

M65.179 Other infective (teno)synovitis, unspecified ankle and foot

M65.18 Other infective (teno)synovitis, other site

M65.19 Other infective (teno)synovitis, multiple sites

M65.2 Calcific tendinitis

Excludes1: tendinitis as classified in M75-M77

calcified tendinitis of shoulder (M75.3)

M65.20 Calcific tendinitis, unspecified site

M65.22 Calcific tendinitis, upper arm

M65.221 Calcific tendinitis, right upper arm

M65.222 Calcific tendinitis, left upper arm

M65.229 Calcific tendinitis, unspecified upper arm

M65.23 Calcific tendinitis, forearm

M65.231 Calcific tendinitis, right forearm

M65.232 Calcific tendinitis, left forearm

M65.239 Calcific tendinitis, unspecified forearm

M65.24 Calcific tendinitis, hand

M65.241 Calcific tendinitis, right hand

M65.242 Calcific tendinitis, left hand

M65.249 Calcific tendinitis, unspecified hand

M65.25 Calcific tendinitis, thigh

M65.251 Calcific tendinitis, right thigh

M65.252 Calcific tendinitis, left thigh

M65.259 Calcific tendinitis, unspecified thigh

M65.26 Calcific tendinitis, lower leg

M65.261 Calcific tendinitis, right lower leg

M65.262 Calcific tendinitis, left lower leg

M65.269 Calcific tendinitis, unspecified lower leg

M65.27 Calcific tendinitis, ankle and foot

M65.271 Calcific tendinitis, right ankle and foot

M65.272 Calcific tendinitis, left ankle and foot

M65.279 Calcific tendinitis, unspecified ankle and foot

M65.28 Calcific tendinitis, other site

M65.29 Calcific tendinitis, multiple sites

M65.3 Trigger finger

Nodular tendinous disease

M65.30   **Trigger finger, unspecified finger**

M65.31   **Trigger thumb**

     M65.311   **Trigger thumb, right thumb**

     M65.312   **Trigger thumb, left thumb**

     M65.319   **Trigger thumb, unspecified thumb**

M65.32   **Trigger finger, index finger**

     M65.321   **Trigger finger, right index finger**

     M65.322   **Trigger finger, left index finger**

     M65.329   **Trigger finger, unspecified index finger**

M65.33   **Trigger finger, middle finger**

     M65.331   **Trigger finger, right middle finger**

     M65.332   **Trigger finger, left middle finger**

     M65.339   **Trigger finger, unspecified middle finger**

M65.34   **Trigger finger, ring finger**

     M65.341   **Trigger finger, right ring finger**

     M65.342   **Trigger finger, left ring finger**

     M65.349   **Trigger finger, unspecified ring finger**

M65.35   **Trigger finger, little finger**

     M65.351   **Trigger finger, right little finger**

     M65.352   **Trigger finger, left little finger**

     M65.359   **Trigger finger, unspecified little finger**

M65.4   **Radial styloid tenosynovitis [de Quervain]**

M65.8   **Other synovitis and tenosynovitis**

   M65.80   **Other synovitis and tenosynovitis, unspecified site**

   M65.81   **Other synovitis and tenosynovitis, shoulder**

     M65.811   **Other synovitis and tenosynovitis, right shoulder**

     M65.812   **Other synovitis and tenosynovitis, left shoulder**

     M65.819   **Other synovitis and tenosynovitis, unspecified shoulder**

   M65.82   **Other synovitis and tenosynovitis, upper arm**

     M65.821   **Other synovitis and tenosynovitis, right upper arm**

     M65.822   **Other synovitis and tenosynovitis, left upper arm**

     M65.829   **Other synovitis and tenosynovitis, unspecified upper arm**

   M65.83   **Other synovitis and tenosynovitis, forearm**

     M65.831   **Other synovitis and tenosynovitis, right forearm**

     M65.832   **Other synovitis and tenosynovitis, left forearm**

     M65.839   **Other synovitis and tenosynovitis, unspecified forearm**

   M65.84   **Other synovitis and tenosynovitis, hand**

     M65.841   **Other synovitis and tenosynovitis, right hand**

     M65.842   **Other synovitis and tenosynovitis, left hand**

     M65.849   **Other synovitis and tenosynovitis, unspecified hand**

   M65.85   **Other synovitis and tenosynovitis, thigh**

     M65.851   **Other synovitis and tenosynovitis, right thigh**

     M65.852   **Other synovitis and tenosynovitis, left thigh**

     M65.859   **Other synovitis and tenosynovitis, unspecified thigh**

   M65.86   **Other synovitis and tenosynovitis, lower leg**

     M65.861   **Other synovitis and tenosynovitis, right lower leg**

     M65.862   **Other synovitis and tenosynovitis, left lower leg**

     M65.869   **Other synovitis and tenosynovitis, unspecified lower leg**

   M65.87   **Other synovitis and tenosynovitis, ankle and foot**

     M65.871   **Other synovitis and tenosynovitis, right ankle and foot**

     M65.872   **Other synovitis and tenosynovitis, left ankle and foot**

     M65.879   **Other synovitis and tenosynovitis, unspecified ankle and foot**

   M65.88   **Other synovitis and tenosynovitis, other site**

   M65.89   **Other synovitis and tenosynovitis, multiple sites**

M65.9   **Synovitis and tenosynovitis, unspecified**

M66   **Spontaneous rupture of synovium and tendon**

   Includes: rupture that occurs when a normal force is applied to tissues that are inferred to have less than normal strength

   Excludes2: rotator cuff syndrome (M75.1-)

   rupture where an abnormal force is applied to normal tissue - see injury of tendon by body region

M66.0   **Rupture of popliteal cyst**

M66.1   **Rupture of synovium**

   Rupture of synovial cyst

   Excludes2: rupture of popliteal cyst (M66.0)

   M66.10   **Rupture of synovium, unspecified joint**

   M66.11   **Rupture of synovium, shoulder**

     M66.111   **Rupture of synovium, right shoulder**

     M66.112   **Rupture of synovium, left shoulder**

     M66.119   **Rupture of synovium, unspecified shoulder**

   M66.12   **Rupture of synovium, elbow**

     M66.121   **Rupture of synovium, right elbow**

     M66.122   **Rupture of synovium, left elbow**

     M66.129   **Rupture of synovium, unspecified elbow**

   M66.13   **Rupture of synovium, wrist**

     M66.131   **Rupture of synovium, right wrist**

     M66.132   **Rupture of synovium, left wrist**

     M66.139   **Rupture of synovium, unspecified wrist**

   M66.14   **Rupture of synovium, hand and fingers**

     M66.141   **Rupture of synovium, right hand**

     M66.142   **Rupture of synovium, left hand**

     M66.143   **Rupture of synovium, unspecified hand**

M66.144   Rupture of synovium, right finger(s)

M66.145   Rupture of synovium, left finger(s)

M66.146   Rupture of synovium, unspecified finger(s)

M66.15   **Rupture of synovium, hip**

M66.151   Rupture of synovium, right hip

M66.152   Rupture of synovium, left hip

M66.159   Rupture of synovium, unspecified hip

M66.17   **Rupture of synovium, ankle, foot and toes**

M66.171   Rupture of synovium, right ankle

M66.172   Rupture of synovium, left ankle

M66.173   Rupture of synovium, unspecified ankle

M66.174   Rupture of synovium, right foot

M66.175   Rupture of synovium, left foot

M66.176   Rupture of synovium, unspecified foot

M66.177   Rupture of synovium, right toe(s)

M66.178   Rupture of synovium, left toe(s)

M66.179   Rupture of synovium, unspecified toe(s)

M66.18   **Rupture of synovium, other site**

M66.2   **Spontaneous rupture of extensor tendons**

M66.20   **Spontaneous rupture of extensor tendons, unspecified site**

M66.21   **Spontaneous rupture of extensor tendons, shoulder**

M66.211   Spontaneous rupture of extensor tendons, right shoulder

M66.212   Spontaneous rupture of extensor tendons, left shoulder

M66.219   Spontaneous rupture of extensor tendons, unspecified shoulder

M66.22   **Spontaneous rupture of extensor tendons, upper arm**

M66.221   Spontaneous rupture of extensor tendons, right upper arm

M66.222   Spontaneous rupture of extensor tendons, left upper arm

M66.229   Spontaneous rupture of extensor tendons, unspecified upper arm

M66.23   **Spontaneous rupture of extensor tendons, forearm**

M66.231   Spontaneous rupture of extensor tendons, right forearm

M66.232   Spontaneous rupture of extensor tendons, left forearm

M66.239   Spontaneous rupture of extensor tendons, unspecified forearm

M66.24   **Spontaneous rupture of extensor tendons, hand**

M66.241   Spontaneous rupture of extensor tendons, right hand

M66.242   Spontaneous rupture of extensor tendons, left hand

M66.249   Spontaneous rupture of extensor tendons, unspecified hand

M66.25   **Spontaneous rupture of extensor tendons, thigh**

M66.251   Spontaneous rupture of extensor tendons, right thigh

M66.252   Spontaneous rupture of extensor tendons, left thigh

M66.259   Spontaneous rupture of extensor tendons, unspecified thigh

M66.26   **Spontaneous rupture of extensor tendons, lower leg**

M66.261   Spontaneous rupture of extensor tendons, right lower leg

M66.262   Spontaneous rupture of extensor tendons, left lower leg

M66.269   Spontaneous rupture of extensor tendons, unspecified lower leg

M66.27   **Spontaneous rupture of extensor tendons, ankle and foot**

M66.271   Spontaneous rupture of extensor tendons, right ankle and foot

M66.272   Spontaneous rupture of extensor tendons, left ankle and foot

M66.279   Spontaneous rupture of extensor tendons, unspecified ankle and foot

M66.28   **Spontaneous rupture of extensor tendons, other site**

M66.29   **Spontaneous rupture of extensor tendons, multiple sites**

M66.3   **Spontaneous rupture of flexor tendons**

M66.30   **Spontaneous rupture of flexor tendons, unspecified site**

M66.31   **Spontaneous rupture of flexor tendons, shoulder**

M66.311   Spontaneous rupture of flexor tendons, right shoulder

M66.312   Spontaneous rupture of flexor tendons, left shoulder

M66.319   Spontaneous rupture of flexor tendons, unspecified shoulder

M66.32   **Spontaneous rupture of flexor tendons, upper arm**

M66.321   Spontaneous rupture of flexor tendons, right upper arm

M66.322   Spontaneous rupture of flexor tendons, left upper arm

M66.329   Spontaneous rupture of flexor tendons, unspecified upper arm

M66.33   **Spontaneous rupture of flexor tendons, forearm**

M66.331   Spontaneous rupture of flexor tendons, right forearm

M66.332   Spontaneous rupture of flexor tendons, left forearm

M66.339   Spontaneous rupture of flexor tendons, unspecified forearm

M66.34   **Spontaneous rupture of flexor tendons, hand**

M66.341   Spontaneous rupture of flexor tendons, right hand

M66.342   Spontaneous rupture of flexor tendons, left hand

  ● New code   ▲ Revised code   **Excludes1:** Not coded here   **Excludes2:** Not included here   ⊗ Placeholder required   ⑦ 7th digit required

M66.349 Spontaneous rupture of flexor tendons, unspecified hand

M66.35 Spontaneous rupture of flexor tendons, thigh

M66.351 Spontaneous rupture of flexor tendons, right thigh

M66.352 Spontaneous rupture of flexor tendons, left thigh

M66.359 Spontaneous rupture of flexor tendons, unspecified thigh

M66.36 Spontaneous rupture of flexor tendons, lower leg

M66.361 Spontaneous rupture of flexor tendons, right lower leg

M66.362 Spontaneous rupture of flexor tendons, left lower leg

M66.369 Spontaneous rupture of flexor tendons, unspecified lower leg

M66.37 Spontaneous rupture of flexor tendons, ankle and foot

M66.371 Spontaneous rupture of flexor tendons, right ankle and foot

M66.372 Spontaneous rupture of flexor tendons, left ankle and foot

M66.379 Spontaneous rupture of flexor tendons, unspecified ankle and foot

M66.38 Spontaneous rupture of flexor tendons, other site

M66.39 Spontaneous rupture of flexor tendons, multiple sites

M66.8 Spontaneous rupture of other tendons

M66.80 Spontaneous rupture of other tendons, unspecified site

M66.81 Spontaneous rupture of other tendons, shoulder

M66.811 Spontaneous rupture of other tendons, right shoulder

M66.812 Spontaneous rupture of other tendons, left shoulder

M66.819 Spontaneous rupture of other tendons, unspecified shoulder

M66.82 Spontaneous rupture of other tendons, upper arm

M66.821 Spontaneous rupture of other tendons, right upper arm

M66.822 Spontaneous rupture of other tendons, left upper arm

M66.829 Spontaneous rupture of other tendons, unspecified upper arm

M66.83 Spontaneous rupture of other tendons, forearm

M66.831 Spontaneous rupture of other tendons, right forearm

M66.832 Spontaneous rupture of other tendons, left forearm

M66.839 Spontaneous rupture of other tendons, unspecified forearm

M66.84 Spontaneous rupture of other tendons, hand

M66.841 Spontaneous rupture of other tendons, right hand

M66.842 Spontaneous rupture of other tendons, left hand

M66.849 Spontaneous rupture of other tendons, unspecified hand

M66.85 Spontaneous rupture of other tendons, thigh

M66.851 Spontaneous rupture of other tendons, right thigh

M66.852 Spontaneous rupture of other tendons, left thigh

M66.859 Spontaneous rupture of other tendons, unspecified thigh

M66.86 Spontaneous rupture of other tendons, lower leg

M66.861 Spontaneous rupture of other tendons, right lower leg

M66.862 Spontaneous rupture of other tendons, left lower leg

M66.869 Spontaneous rupture of other tendons, unspecified lower leg

M66.87 Spontaneous rupture of other tendons, ankle and foot

M66.871 Spontaneous rupture of other tendons, right ankle and foot

M66.872 Spontaneous rupture of other tendons, left ankle and foot

M66.879 Spontaneous rupture of other tendons, unspecified ankle and foot

M66.88 Spontaneous rupture of other tendons, other

M66.89 Spontaneous rupture of other tendons, multiple sites

M66.9 Spontaneous rupture of unspecified tendon

Rupture at musculotendinous junction, nontraumatic

M67 Other disorders of synovium and tendon

Excludes1: palmar fascial fibromatosis [Dupuytren] (M72.0)

tendinitis NOS (M77.9-)

xanthomatosis localized to tendons (E78.2)

M67.0 Short Achilles tendon (acquired)

M67.00 Short Achilles tendon (acquired), unspecified ankle

M67.01 Short Achilles tendon (acquired), right ankle

M67.02 Short Achilles tendon (acquired), left ankle

M67.2 Synovial hypertrophy, not elsewhere classified

Excludes1: villonodular synovitis (pigmented) (M12.2-)

M67.20 Synovial hypertrophy, not elsewhere classified, unspecified site

M67.21 Synovial hypertrophy, not elsewhere classified, shoulder

M67.211 Synovial hypertrophy, not elsewhere classified, right shoulder

M67.212 Synovial hypertrophy, not elsewhere classified, left shoulder

M67.219 Synovial hypertrophy, not elsewhere classified, unspecified shoulder

M67.22 Synovial hypertrophy, not elsewhere classified, upper arm

M67.221 Synovial hypertrophy, not elsewhere classified, right upper arm

M67.222 Synovial hypertrophy, not elsewhere classified, left upper arm

M67.229   Synovial hypertrophy, not elsewhere classified, unspecified upper arm

M67.23   Synovial hypertrophy, not elsewhere classified, forearm

    M67.231   Synovial hypertrophy, not elsewhere classified, right forearm

    M67.232   Synovial hypertrophy, not elsewhere classified, left forearm

    M67.239   Synovial hypertrophy, not elsewhere classified, unspecified forearm

M67.24   Synovial hypertrophy, not elsewhere classified, hand

    M67.241   Synovial hypertrophy, not elsewhere classified, right hand

    M67.242   Synovial hypertrophy, not elsewhere classified, left hand

    M67.249   Synovial hypertrophy, not elsewhere classified, unspecified hand

M67.25   Synovial hypertrophy, not elsewhere classified, thigh

    M67.251   Synovial hypertrophy, not elsewhere classified, right thigh

    M67.252   Synovial hypertrophy, not elsewhere classified, left thigh

    M67.259   Synovial hypertrophy, not elsewhere classified, unspecified thigh

M67.26   Synovial hypertrophy, not elsewhere classified, lower leg

    M67.261   Synovial hypertrophy, not elsewhere classified, right lower leg

    M67.262   Synovial hypertrophy, not elsewhere classified, left lower leg

    M67.269   Synovial hypertrophy, not elsewhere classified, unspecified lower leg

M67.27   Synovial hypertrophy, not elsewhere classified, ankle and foot

    M67.271   Synovial hypertrophy, not elsewhere classified, right ankle and foot

    M67.272   Synovial hypertrophy, not elsewhere classified, left ankle and foot

    M67.279   Synovial hypertrophy, not elsewhere classified, unspecified ankle and foot

M67.28   Synovial hypertrophy, not elsewhere classified, other site

M67.29   Synovial hypertrophy, not elsewhere classified, multiple sites

M67.3   Transient synovitis

Toxic synovitis

Excludes1: palindromic rheumatism (M12.3-)

M67.30   Transient synovitis, unspecified site

M67.31   Transient synovitis, shoulder

    M67.311   Transient synovitis, right shoulder

    M67.312   Transient synovitis, left shoulder

    M67.319   Transient synovitis, unspecified shoulder

M67.32   Transient synovitis, elbow

    M67.321   Transient synovitis, right elbow

    M67.322   Transient synovitis, left elbow

    M67.329   Transient synovitis, unspecified elbow

M67.33   Transient synovitis, wrist

    M67.331   Transient synovitis, right wrist

    M67.332   Transient synovitis, left wrist

    M67.339   Transient synovitis, unspecified wrist

M67.34   Transient synovitis, hand

    M67.341   Transient synovitis, right hand

    M67.342   Transient synovitis, left hand

    M67.349   Transient synovitis, unspecified hand

M67.35   Transient synovitis, hip

    M67.351   Transient synovitis, right hip

    M67.352   Transient synovitis, left hip

    M67.359   Transient synovitis, unspecified hip

M67.36   Transient synovitis, knee

    M67.361   Transient synovitis, right knee

    M67.362   Transient synovitis, left knee

    M67.369   Transient synovitis, unspecified knee

M67.37   Transient synovitis, ankle and foot

    M67.371   Transient synovitis, right ankle and foot

    M67.372   Transient synovitis, left ankle and foot

    M67.379   Transient synovitis, unspecified ankle and foot

M67.38   Transient synovitis, other site

M67.39   Transient synovitis, multiple sites

M67.4   Ganglion

Ganglion of joint or tendon (sheath)

Excludes1: ganglion in yaws (A66.6)

Excludes2: cyst of bursa (M71.2-M71.3)

cyst of synovium (M71.2-M71.3)

M67.40   Ganglion, unspecified site

M67.41   Ganglion, shoulder

    M67.411   Ganglion, right shoulder

    M67.412   Ganglion, left shoulder

    M67.419   Ganglion, unspecified shoulder

M67.42   Ganglion, elbow

    M67.421   Ganglion, right elbow

    M67.422   Ganglion, left elbow

    M67.429   Ganglion, unspecified elbow

M67.43   Ganglion, wrist

    M67.431   Ganglion, right wrist

    M67.432   Ganglion, left wrist

    M67.439   Ganglion, unspecified wrist

M67.44   Ganglion, hand

    M67.441   Ganglion, right hand

    M67.442   Ganglion, left hand

M67.449   Ganglion, unspecified hand

M67.45   Ganglion, hip

    M67.451   Ganglion, right hip

    M67.452   Ganglion, left hip

    M67.459   Ganglion, unspecified hip

M67.46   Ganglion, knee

    M67.461   Ganglion, right knee

    M67.462   Ganglion, left knee

    M67.469   Ganglion, unspecified knee

M67.47   Ganglion, ankle and foot

    M67.471   Ganglion, right ankle and foot

    M67.472   Ganglion, left ankle and foot

    M67.479   Ganglion, unspecified ankle and foot

M67.48   Ganglion, other site

M67.49   Ganglion, multiple sites

M67.5   Plica syndrome

    Plica knee

M67.50   Plica syndrome, unspecified knee

M67.51   Plica syndrome, right knee

M67.52   Plica syndrome, left knee

M67.8   Other specified disorders of synovium and tendon

M67.80   Other specified disorders of synovium and tendon, unspecified site

M67.81   Other specified disorders of synovium and tendon, shoulder

    M67.811   Other specified disorders of synovium, right shoulder

    M67.812   Other specified disorders of synovium, left shoulder

    M67.813   Other specified disorders of tendon, right shoulder

    M67.814   Other specified disorders of tendon, left shoulder

    M67.819   Other specified disorders of synovium and tendon, unspecified shoulder

M67.82   Other specified disorders of synovium and tendon, elbow

    M67.821   Other specified disorders of synovium, right elbow

    M67.822   Other specified disorders of synovium, left elbow

    M67.823   Other specified disorders of tendon, right elbow

    M67.824   Other specified disorders of tendon, left elbow

    M67.829   Other specified disorders of synovium and tendon, unspecified elbow

M67.83   Other specified disorders of synovium and tendon, wrist

    M67.831   Other specified disorders of synovium, right wrist

    M67.832   Other specified disorders of synovium, left wrist

    M67.833   Other specified disorders of tendon, right wrist

    M67.834   Other specified disorders of tendon, left wrist

    M67.839   Other specified disorders of synovium and tendon, unspecified forearm

M67.84   Other specified disorders of synovium and tendon, hand

    M67.841   Other specified disorders of synovium, right hand

    M67.842   Other specified disorders of synovium, left hand

    M67.843   Other specified disorders of tendon, right hand

    M67.844   Other specified disorders of tendon, left hand

    M67.849   Other specified disorders of synovium and tendon, unspecified hand

M67.85   Other specified disorders of synovium and tendon, hip

    M67.851   Other specified disorders of synovium, right hip

    M67.852   Other specified disorders of synovium, left hip

    M67.853   Other specified disorders of tendon, right hip

    M67.854   Other specified disorders of tendon, left hip

    M67.859   Other specified disorders of synovium and tendon, unspecified hip

M67.86   Other specified disorders of synovium and tendon, knee

    M67.861   Other specified disorders of synovium, right knee

    M67.862   Other specified disorders of synovium, left knee

    M67.863   Other specified disorders of tendon, right knee

    M67.864   Other specified disorders of tendon, left knee

    M67.869   Other specified disorders of synovium and tendon, unspecified knee

M67.87   Other specified disorders of synovium and tendon, ankle and foot

    M67.871   Other specified disorders of synovium, right ankle and foot

    M67.872   Other specified disorders of synovium, left ankle and foot

    M67.873   Other specified disorders of tendon, right ankle and foot

    M67.874   Other specified disorders of tendon, left ankle and foot

    M67.879   Other specified disorders of synovium and tendon, unspecified ankle and foot

M67.88   Other specified disorders of synovium and tendon, other site

M67.89   Other specified disorders of synovium and tendon, multiple sites

M67.9   Unspecified disorder of synovium and tendon

M67.90 Unspecified disorder of synovium and tendon, unspecified site

M67.91 Unspecified disorder of synovium and tendon, shoulder

    M67.911 Unspecified disorder of synovium and tendon, right shoulder

    M67.912 Unspecified disorder of synovium and tendon, left shoulder

    M67.919 Unspecified disorder of synovium and tendon, unspecified shoulder

M67.92 Unspecified disorder of synovium and tendon, upper arm

    M67.921 Unspecified disorder of synovium and tendon, right upper arm

    M67.922 Unspecified disorder of synovium and tendon, left upper arm

    M67.929 Unspecified disorder of synovium and tendon, unspecified upper arm

M67.93 Unspecified disorder of synovium and tendon, forearm

    M67.931 Unspecified disorder of synovium and tendon, right forearm

    M67.932 Unspecified disorder of synovium and tendon, left forearm

    M67.939 Unspecified disorder of synovium and tendon, unspecified forearm

M67.94 Unspecified disorder of synovium and tendon, hand

    M67.941 Unspecified disorder of synovium and tendon, right hand

    M67.942 Unspecified disorder of synovium and tendon, left hand

    M67.949 Unspecified disorder of synovium and tendon, unspecified hand

M67.95 Unspecified disorder of synovium and tendon, thigh

    M67.951 Unspecified disorder of synovium and tendon, right thigh

    M67.952 Unspecified disorder of synovium and tendon, left thigh

    M67.959 Unspecified disorder of synovium and tendon, unspecified thigh

M67.96 Unspecified disorder of synovium and tendon, lower leg

    M67.961 Unspecified disorder of synovium and tendon, right lower leg

    M67.962 Unspecified disorder of synovium and tendon, left lower leg

    M67.969 Unspecified disorder of synovium and tendon, unspecified lower leg

M67.97 Unspecified disorder of synovium and tendon, ankle and foot

    M67.971 Unspecified disorder of synovium and tendon, right ankle and foot

    M67.972 Unspecified disorder of synovium and tendon, left ankle and foot

    M67.979 Unspecified disorder of synovium and tendon, unspecified ankle and foot

M67.98 Unspecified disorder of synovium and tendon, other site

M67.99 Unspecified disorder of synovium and tendon, multiple sites

OTHER SOFT TISSUE DISORDERS (M70-M79)

M70 **Soft tissue disorders related to use, overuse and pressure**

Includes: soft tissue disorders of occupational origin

Use additional external cause code to identify activity causing disorder (Y93.-)

Excludes1: bursitis NOS (M71.9-)

Excludes2: bursitis of shoulder (M75.5)

    enthesopathies (M76-M77)

    pressure ulcer (pressure area) (L89.-)

M70.0 **Crepitant synovitis (acute) (chronic) of hand and wrist**

    M70.03 Crepitant synovitis (acute) (chronic), wrist

        M70.031 Crepitant synovitis (acute) (chronic), right wrist

        M70.032 Crepitant synovitis (acute) (chronic), left wrist

        M70.039 Crepitant synovitis (acute) (chronic), unspecified wrist

    M70.04 Crepitant synovitis (acute) (chronic), hand

        M70.041 Crepitant synovitis (acute) (chronic), right hand

        M70.042 Crepitant synovitis (acute) (chronic), left hand

        M70.049 Crepitant synovitis (acute) (chronic), unspecified hand

M70.1 **Bursitis of hand**

    M70.10 Bursitis, unspecified hand

    M70.11 Bursitis, right hand

    M70.12 Bursitis, left hand

M70.2 **Olecranon bursitis**

    M70.20 Olecranon bursitis, unspecified elbow

    M70.21 Olecranon bursitis, right elbow

    M70.22 Olecranon bursitis, left elbow

M70.3 **Other bursitis of elbow**

    M70.30 Other bursitis of elbow, unspecified elbow

    M70.31 Other bursitis of elbow, right elbow

    M70.32 Other bursitis of elbow, left elbow

M70.4 **Prepatellar bursitis**

    M70.40 Prepatellar bursitis, unspecified knee

    M70.41 Prepatellar bursitis, right knee

    M70.42 Prepatellar bursitis, left knee

M70.5 **Other bursitis of knee**

    M70.50 Other bursitis of knee, unspecified knee

    M70.51 Other bursitis of knee, right knee

    M70.52 Other bursitis of knee, left knee

M70.6 **Trochanteric bursitis**

Trochanteric tendinitis

    M70.60 Trochanteric bursitis, unspecified hip

    M70.61 Trochanteric bursitis, right hip

    M70.62 Trochanteric bursitis, left hip

M70.7 **Other bursitis of hip**

Ischial bursitis

    M70.70 Other bursitis of hip, unspecified hip

    M70.71 Other bursitis of hip, right hip

M70.72 Other bursitis of hip, left hip

M70.8 Other soft tissue disorders related to use, overuse and pressure

    M70.80 Other soft tissue disorders related to use, overuse and pressure of unspecified site

    M70.81 Other soft tissue disorders related to use, overuse and pressure of shoulder

        M70.811 Other soft tissue disorders related to use, overuse and pressure, right shoulder

        M70.812 Other soft tissue disorders related to use, overuse and pressure, left shoulder

        M70.819 Other soft tissue disorders related to use, overuse and pressure, unspecified shoulder

    M70.82 Other soft tissue disorders related to use, overuse and pressure of upper arm

        M70.821 Other soft tissue disorders related to use, overuse and pressure, right upper arm

        M70.822 Other soft tissue disorders related to use, overuse and pressure, left upper arm

        M70.829 Other soft tissue disorders related to use, overuse and pressure, unspecified upper arms

    M70.83 Other soft tissue disorders related to use, overuse and pressure of forearm

        M70.831 Other soft tissue disorders related to use, overuse and pressure, right forearm

        M70.832 Other soft tissue disorders related to use, overuse and pressure, left forearm

        M70.839 Other soft tissue disorders related to use, overuse and pressure, unspecified forearm

    M70.84 Other soft tissue disorders related to use, overuse and pressure of hand

        M70.841 Other soft tissue disorders related to use, overuse and pressure, right hand

        M70.842 Other soft tissue disorders related to use, overuse and pressure, left hand

        M70.849 Other soft tissue disorders related to use, overuse and pressure, unspecified hand

    M70.85 Other soft tissue disorders related to use, overuse and pressure of thigh

        M70.851 Other soft tissue disorders related to use, overuse and pressure, right thigh

        M70.852 Other soft tissue disorders related to use, overuse and pressure, left thigh

        M70.859 Other soft tissue disorders related to use, overuse and pressure, unspecified thigh

    M70.86 Other soft tissue disorders related to use, overuse and pressure lower leg

        M70.861 Other soft tissue disorders related to use, overuse and pressure, right lower leg

        M70.862 Other soft tissue disorders related to use, overuse and pressure, left lower leg

        M70.869 Other soft tissue disorders related to use, overuse and pressure, unspecified leg

    M70.87 Other soft tissue disorders related to use, overuse and pressure of ankle and foot

        M70.871 Other soft tissue disorders related to use, overuse and pressure, right ankle and foot

        M70.872 Other soft tissue disorders related to use, overuse and pressure, left ankle and foot

        M70.879 Other soft tissue disorders related to use, overuse and pressure, unspecified ankle and foot

    M70.88 Other soft tissue disorders related to use, overuse and pressure other site

    M70.89 Other soft tissue disorders related to use, overuse and pressure multiple sites

M70.9 Unspecified soft tissue disorder related to use, overuse and pressure

    M70.90 Unspecified soft tissue disorder related to use, overuse and pressure of unspecified site

    M70.91 Unspecified soft tissue disorder related to use, overuse and pressure of shoulder

        M70.911 Unspecified soft tissue disorder related to use, overuse and pressure, right shoulder

        M70.912 Unspecified soft tissue disorder related to use, overuse and pressure, left shoulder

        M70.919 Unspecified soft tissue disorder related to use, overuse and pressure, unspecified shoulder

    M70.92 Unspecified soft tissue disorder related to use, overuse and pressure of upper arm

        M70.921 Unspecified soft tissue disorder related to use, overuse and pressure, right upper arm

        M70.922 Unspecified soft tissue disorder related to use, overuse and pressure, left upper arm

        M70.929 Unspecified soft tissue disorder related to use, overuse and pressure, unspecified upper arm

    M70.93 Unspecified soft tissue disorder related to use, overuse and pressure of forearm

        M70.931 Unspecified soft tissue disorder related to use, overuse and pressure, right forearm

        M70.932 Unspecified soft tissue disorder related to use, overuse and pressure, left forearm

        M70.939 Unspecified soft tissue disorder related to use, overuse and pressure, unspecified forearm

    M70.94 Unspecified soft tissue disorder related to use, overuse and pressure of hand

M70.941 **Unspecified soft tissue disorder related to use, overuse and pressure, right hand**

M70.942 **Unspecified soft tissue disorder related to use, overuse and pressure, left hand**

M70.949 **Unspecified soft tissue disorder related to use, overuse and pressure, unspecified hand**

M70.95 **Unspecified soft tissue disorder related to use, overuse and pressure of thigh**

M70.951 **Unspecified soft tissue disorder related to use, overuse and pressure, right thigh**

M70.952 **Unspecified soft tissue disorder related to use, overuse and pressure, left thigh**

M70.959 **Unspecified soft tissue disorder related to use, overuse and pressure, unspecified thigh**

M70.96 **Unspecified soft tissue disorder related to use, overuse and pressure lower leg**

M70.961 **Unspecified soft tissue disorder related to use, overuse and pressure, right lower leg**

M70.962 **Unspecified soft tissue disorder related to use, overuse and pressure, left lower leg**

M70.969 **Unspecified soft tissue disorder related to use, overuse and pressure, unspecified lower leg**

M70.97 **Unspecified soft tissue disorder related to use, overuse and pressure of ankle and foot**

M70.971 **Unspecified soft tissue disorder related to use, overuse and pressure, right ankle and foot**

M70.972 **Unspecified soft tissue disorder related to use, overuse and pressure, left ankle and foot**

M70.979 **Unspecified soft tissue disorder related to use, overuse and pressure, unspecified ankle and foot**

M70.98 **Unspecified soft tissue disorder related to use, overuse and pressure other**

M70.99 **Unspecified soft tissue disorder related to use, overuse and pressure multiple sites**

M71 **Other bursopathies**

Excludes1: bunion (M20.1)

bursitis related to use, overuse or pressure (M70.-)

enthesopathies (M76-M77)

M71.0 **Abscess of bursa**

Use additional code (B95.-, B96.-) to identify causative organism

M71.00 **Abscess of bursa, unspecified site**

M71.01 **Abscess of bursa, shoulder**

M71.011 **Abscess of bursa, right shoulder**

M71.012 **Abscess of bursa, left shoulder**

M71.019 **Abscess of bursa, unspecified shoulder**

M71.02 **Abscess of bursa, elbow**

M71.021 **Abscess of bursa, right elbow**

M71.022 **Abscess of bursa, left elbow**

M71.029 **Abscess of bursa, unspecified elbow**

M71.03 **Abscess of bursa, wrist**

M71.031 **Abscess of bursa, right wrist**

M71.032 **Abscess of bursa, left wrist**

M71.039 **Abscess of bursa, unspecified wrist**

M71.04 **Abscess of bursa, hand**

M71.041 **Abscess of bursa, right hand**

M71.042 **Abscess of bursa, left hand**

M71.049 **Abscess of bursa, unspecified hand**

M71.05 **Abscess of bursa, hip**

M71.051 **Abscess of bursa, right hip**

M71.052 **Abscess of bursa, left hip**

M71.059 **Abscess of bursa, unspecified hip**

M71.06 **Abscess of bursa, knee**

M71.061 **Abscess of bursa, right knee**

M71.062 **Abscess of bursa, left knee**

M71.069 **Abscess of bursa, unspecified knee**

M71.07 **Abscess of bursa, ankle and foot**

M71.071 **Abscess of bursa, right ankle and foot**

M71.072 **Abscess of bursa, left ankle and foot**

M71.079 **Abscess of bursa, unspecified ankle and foot**

M71.08 **Abscess of bursa, other site**

M71.09 **Abscess of bursa, multiple sites**

M71.1 **Other infective bursitis**

Use additional code (B95.-, B96.-) to identify causative organism

M71.10 **Other infective bursitis, unspecified site**

M71.11 **Other infective bursitis, shoulder**

M71.111 **Other infective bursitis, right shoulder**

M71.112 **Other infective bursitis, left shoulder**

M71.119 **Other infective bursitis, unspecified shoulder**

M71.12 **Other infective bursitis, elbow**

M71.121 **Other infective bursitis, right elbow**

M71.122 **Other infective bursitis, left elbow**

M71.129 **Other infective bursitis, unspecified elbow**

M71.13 **Other infective bursitis, wrist**

M71.131 **Other infective bursitis, right wrist**

M71.132 **Other infective bursitis, left wrist**

M71.139 **Other infective bursitis, unspecified wrist**

M71.14 **Other infective bursitis, hand**

M71.141 **Other infective bursitis, right hand**

M71.142 **Other infective bursitis, left hand**

M71.149 **Other infective bursitis, unspecified hand**

M71.15 **Other infective bursitis, hip**

M71.151 **Other infective bursitis, right hip**

M71.152 **Other infective bursitis, left hip**

M71.159 Other infective bursitis, unspecified hip

M71.16 Other infective bursitis, knee

    M71.161 Other infective bursitis, right knee

    M71.162 Other infective bursitis, left knee

    M71.169 Other infective bursitis, unspecified knee

M71.17 Other infective bursitis, ankle and foot

    M71.171 Other infective bursitis, right ankle and foot

    M71.172 Other infective bursitis, left ankle and foot

    M71.179 Other infective bursitis, unspecified ankle and foot

M71.18 Other infective bursitis, other site

M71.19 Other infective bursitis, multiple sites

M71.2 **Synovial cyst of popliteal space [Baker]**

  Excludes1: synovial cyst of popliteal space with rupture (M66.0)

M71.20 Synovial cyst of popliteal space [Baker], unspecified knee

M71.21 Synovial cyst of popliteal space [Baker], right knee

M71.22 Synovial cyst of popliteal space [Baker], left knee

M71.3 **Other bursal cyst**

Synovial cyst NOS

  Excludes1: synovial cyst with rupture (M66.1-)

M71.30 Other bursal cyst, unspecified site

M71.31 Other bursal cyst, shoulder

    M71.311 Other bursal cyst, right shoulder

    M71.312 Other bursal cyst, left shoulder

    M71.319 Other bursal cyst, unspecified shoulder

M71.32 Other bursal cyst, elbow

    M71.321 Other bursal cyst, right elbow

    M71.322 Other bursal cyst, left elbow

    M71.329 Other bursal cyst, unspecified elbow

M71.33 Other bursal cyst, wrist

    M71.331 Other bursal cyst, right wrist

    M71.332 Other bursal cyst, left wrist

    M71.339 Other bursal cyst, unspecified wrist

M71.34 Other bursal cyst, hand

    M71.341 Other bursal cyst, right hand

    M71.342 Other bursal cyst, left hand

    M71.349 Other bursal cyst, unspecified hand

M71.35 Other bursal cyst, hip

    M71.351 Other bursal cyst, right hip

    M71.352 Other bursal cyst, left hip

    M71.359 Other bursal cyst, unspecified hip

M71.37 Other bursal cyst, ankle and foot

    M71.371 Other bursal cyst, right ankle and foot

    M71.372 Other bursal cyst, left ankle and foot

M71.379 Other bursal cyst, unspecified ankle and foot

M71.38 Other bursal cyst, other site

M71.39 Other bursal cyst, multiple sites

M71.4 **Calcium deposit in bursa**

  Excludes2: calcium deposit in bursa of shoulder (M75.3)

M71.40 Calcium deposit in bursa, unspecified site

M71.42 Calcium deposit in bursa, elbow

    M71.421 Calcium deposit in bursa, right elbow

    M71.422 Calcium deposit in bursa, left elbow

    M71.429 Calcium deposit in bursa, unspecified elbow

M71.43 Calcium deposit in bursa, wrist

    M71.431 Calcium deposit in bursa, right wrist

    M71.432 Calcium deposit in bursa, left wrist

    M71.439 Calcium deposit in bursa, unspecified wrist

M71.44 Calcium deposit in bursa, hand

    M71.441 Calcium deposit in bursa, right hand

    M71.442 Calcium deposit in bursa, left hand

    M71.449 Calcium deposit in bursa, unspecified hand

M71.45 Calcium deposit in bursa, hip

    M71.451 Calcium deposit in bursa, right hip

    M71.452 Calcium deposit in bursa, left hip

    M71.459 Calcium deposit in bursa, unspecified hip

M71.46 Calcium deposit in bursa, knee

    M71.461 Calcium deposit in bursa, right knee

    M71.462 Calcium deposit in bursa, left knee

    M71.469 Calcium deposit in bursa, unspecified knee

M71.47 Calcium deposit in bursa, ankle and foot

    M71.471 Calcium deposit in bursa, right ankle and foot

    M71.472 Calcium deposit in bursa, left ankle and foot

    M71.479 Calcium deposit in bursa, unspecified ankle and foot

M71.48 Calcium deposit in bursa, other site

M71.49 Calcium deposit in bursa, multiple sites

M71.5 **Other bursitis, not elsewhere classified**

  Excludes1: bursitis NOS (M71.9-)

  Excludes2: bursitis of shoulder (M75.5)

  bursitis of tibial collateral [Pellegrini-Stieda] (M76.4-)

M71.50 Other bursitis, not elsewhere classified, unspecified site

M71.52 Other bursitis, not elsewhere classified, elbow

    M71.521 Other bursitis, not elsewhere classified, right elbow

    M71.522 Other bursitis, not elsewhere classified, left elbow

M71.529 Other bursitis, not elsewhere classified, unspecified elbow

M71.53 Other bursitis, not elsewhere classified, wrist

M71.531 Other bursitis, not elsewhere classified, right wrist

M71.532 Other bursitis, not elsewhere classified, left wrist

M71.539 Other bursitis, not elsewhere classified, unspecified wrist

M71.54 Other bursitis, not elsewhere classified, hand

M71.541 Other bursitis, not elsewhere classified, right hand

M71.542 Other bursitis, not elsewhere classified, left hand

M71.549 Other bursitis, not elsewhere classified, unspecified hand

M71.55 Other bursitis, not elsewhere classified, hip

M71.551 Other bursitis, not elsewhere classified, right hip

M71.552 Other bursitis, not elsewhere classified, left hip

M71.559 Other bursitis, not elsewhere classified, unspecified hip

M71.56 Other bursitis, not elsewhere classified, knee

M71.561 Other bursitis, not elsewhere classified, right knee

M71.562 Other bursitis, not elsewhere classified, left knee

M71.569 Other bursitis, not elsewhere classified, unspecified knee

M71.57 Other bursitis, not elsewhere classified, ankle and foot

M71.571 Other bursitis, not elsewhere classified, right ankle and foot

M71.572 Other bursitis, not elsewhere classified, left ankle and foot

M71.579 Other bursitis, not elsewhere classified, unspecified ankle and foot

M71.58 Other bursitis, not elsewhere classified, other site

M71.8 Other specified bursopathies

M71.80 Other specified bursopathies, unspecified site

M71.81 Other specified bursopathies, shoulder

M71.811 Other specified bursopathies, right shoulder

M71.812 Other specified bursopathies, left shoulder

M71.819 Other specified bursopathies, unspecified shoulder

M71.82 Other specified bursopathies, elbow

M71.821 Other specified bursopathies, right elbow

M71.822 Other specified bursopathies, left elbow

M71.829 Other specified bursopathies, unspecified elbow

M71.83 Other specified bursopathies, wrist

M71.831 Other specified bursopathies, right wrist

M71.832 Other specified bursopathies, left wrist

M71.839 Other specified bursopathies, unspecified wrist

M71.84 Other specified bursopathies, hand

M71.841 Other specified bursopathies, right hand

M71.842 Other specified bursopathies, left hand

M71.849 Other specified bursopathies, unspecified hand

M71.85 Other specified bursopathies, hip

M71.851 Other specified bursopathies, right hip

M71.852 Other specified bursopathies, left hip

M71.859 Other specified bursopathies, unspecified hip

M71.86 Other specified bursopathies, knee

M71.861 Other specified bursopathies, right knee

M71.862 Other specified bursopathies, left knee

M71.869 Other specified bursopathies, unspecified knee

M71.87 Other specified bursopathies, ankle and foot

M71.871 Other specified bursopathies, right ankle and foot

M71.872 Other specified bursopathies, left ankle and foot

M71.879 Other specified bursopathies, unspecified ankle and foot

M71.88 Other specified bursopathies, other site

M71.89 Other specified bursopathies, multiple sites

M71.9 Bursopathy, unspecified

Bursitis NOS

M72 **Fibroblastic disorders**

Excludes2: retroperitoneal fibromatosis (D48.3)

M72.0 Palmar fascial fibromatosis [Dupuytren]

M72.1 Knuckle pads

M72.2 Plantar fascial fibromatosis

Plantar fasciitis

M72.4 Pseudosarcomatous fibromatosis

Nodular fasciitis

M72.6 Necrotizing fasciitis

Use additional code (B95.-, B96.-) to identify causative organism

M72.8 Other fibroblastic disorders

Abscess of fascia

Fasciitis NEC

Other infective fasciitis

Use additional code to (B95.-, B96.-) identify causative organism

Excludes1: diffuse (eosinophilic) fasciitis (M35.4)

necrotizing fasciitis (M72.6)

nodular fasciitis (M72.4)

perirenal fasciitis NOS (N13.5)

perirenal fasciitis with infection (N13.6)

plantar fasciitis (M72.2)

M72.9 Fibroblastic disorder, unspecified

Fasciitis NOS

Fibromatosis NOS

M75 Shoulder lesions

Excludes2: shoulder-hand syndrome (M89.0-)

M75.0 Adhesive capsulitis of shoulder

Frozen shoulder

Periarthritis of shoulder

M75.00 Adhesive capsulitis of unspecified shoulder

M75.01 Adhesive capsulitis of right shoulder

M75.02 Adhesive capsulitis of left shoulder

M75.1 Rotator cuff tear or rupture, not specified as traumatic

Rotator cuff syndrome

Supraspinatus tear or rupture, not specified as traumatic

Supraspinatus syndrome

Excludes1: tear of rotator cuff, traumatic (S46.01-)

M75.10 Unspecified rotator cuff tear or rupture, not specified as traumatic

M75.100 Unspecified rotator cuff tear or rupture of unspecified shoulder, not specified as traumatic

M75.101 Unspecified rotator cuff tear or rupture of right shoulder, not specified as traumatic

M75.102 Unspecified rotator cuff tear or rupture of left shoulder, not specified as traumatic

M75.11 Incomplete rotator cuff tear or rupture not specified as traumatic

M75.110 Incomplete rotator cuff tear or rupture of unspecified shoulder, not specified as traumatic

M75.111 Incomplete rotator cuff tear or rupture of right shoulder, not specified as traumatic

M75.112 Incomplete rotator cuff tear or rupture of left shoulder, not specified as traumatic

M75.12 Complete rotator cuff tear or rupture not specified as traumatic

M75.120 Complete rotator cuff tear or rupture of unspecified shoulder, not specified as traumatic

M75.121 Complete rotator cuff tear or rupture of right shoulder, not specified as traumatic

M75.122 Complete rotator cuff tear or rupture of left shoulder, not specified as traumatic

M75.2 Bicipital tendinitis

M75.20 Bicipital tendinitis, unspecified shoulder

M75.21 Bicipital tendinitis, right shoulder

M75.22 Bicipital tendinitis, left shoulder

M75.3 Calcific tendinitis of shoulder

Calcified bursa of shoulder

M75.30 Calcific tendinitis of unspecified shoulder

M75.31 Calcific tendinitis of right shoulder

M75.32 Calcific tendinitis of left shoulder

M75.4 Impingement syndrome of shoulder

M75.40 Impingement syndrome of unspecified shoulder

M75.41 Impingement syndrome of right shoulder

M75.42 Impingement syndrome of left shoulder

M75.5 Bursitis of shoulder

M75.50 Bursitis of unspecified shoulder

M75.51 Bursitis of right shoulder

M75.52 Bursitis of left shoulder

M75.8 Other shoulder lesions

M75.80 Other shoulder lesions, unspecified shoulder

M75.81 Other shoulder lesions, right shoulder

M75.82 Other shoulder lesions, left shoulder

M75.9 Shoulder lesion, unspecified

M75.90 Shoulder lesion, unspecified, unspecified shoulder

M75.91 Shoulder lesion, unspecified, right shoulder

M75.92 Shoulder lesion, unspecified, left shoulder

M76 Enthesopathies, lower limb, excluding foot

Excludes2: bursitis due to use, overuse and pressure (M70.-)

enthesopathies of ankle and foot (M77.5-)

M76.0 Gluteal tendinitis

M76.00 Gluteal tendinitis, unspecified hip

M76.01 Gluteal tendinitis, right hip

M76.02 Gluteal tendinitis, left hip

M76.1 Psoas tendinitis

M76.10 Psoas tendinitis, unspecified hip

M76.11 Psoas tendinitis, right hip

M76.12 Psoas tendinitis, left hip

M76.2 Iliac crest spur

M76.20 Iliac crest spur, unspecified hip

M76.21 Iliac crest spur, right hip

M76.22 Iliac crest spur, left hip

M76.3 Iliotibial band syndrome

M76.30 Iliotibial band syndrome, unspecified leg

M76.31 Iliotibial band syndrome, right leg

M76.32 Iliotibial band syndrome, left leg

M76.4 Tibial collateral bursitis [Pellegrini-Stieda]

M76.40 Tibial collateral bursitis [Pellegrini-Stieda], unspecified leg

M76.41 Tibial collateral bursitis [Pellegrini-Stieda], right leg

M76.42 Tibial collateral bursitis [Pellegrini-Stieda], left leg

M76.5 Patellar tendinitis

M76.50 Patellar tendinitis, unspecified knee

M76.51 Patellar tendinitis, right knee

M76.52 Patellar tendinitis, left knee

M76.6 Achilles tendinitis

Achilles bursitis

M76.60 Achilles tendinitis, unspecified leg

M76.61 Achilles tendinitis, right leg

M76.62 Achilles tendinitis, left leg

M76.7 Peroneal tendinitis

M76.70 Peroneal tendinitis, unspecified leg

Add 4th-7th digits　　Nonspecific code　　Unspecified code　　Manifestation code　　583

M76.71 Peroneal tendinitis, right leg

M76.72 Peroneal tendinitis, left leg

M76.8 Other specified enthesopathies of lower limb, excluding foot

    M76.81 Anterior tibial syndrome

        M76.811 Anterior tibial syndrome, right leg

        M76.812 Anterior tibial syndrome, left leg

        M76.819 Anterior tibial syndrome, unspecified leg

    M76.82 Posterior tibial tendinitis

        M76.821 Posterior tibial tendinitis, right leg

        M76.822 Posterior tibial tendinitis, left leg

        M76.829 Posterior tibial tendinitis, unspecified leg

    M76.89 Other specified enthesopathies of lower limb, excluding foot

        M76.891 Other specified enthesopathies of right lower limb, excluding foot

        M76.892 Other specified enthesopathies of left lower limb, excluding foot

        M76.899 Other specified enthesopathies of unspecified lower limb, excluding foot

M76.9 Unspecified enthesopathy, lower limb, excluding foot

M77 Other enthesopathies

Excludes1: bursitis NOS (M71.9-)

Excludes2: bursitis due to use, overuse and pressure (M70.-)

    osteophyte (M25.7)

    spinal enthesopathy (M46.0-)

M77.0 Medial epicondylitis

    M77.00 Medial epicondylitis, unspecified elbow

    M77.01 Medial epicondylitis, right elbow

    M77.02 Medial epicondylitis, left elbow

M77.1 Lateral epicondylitis

    Tennis elbow

    M77.10 Lateral epicondylitis, unspecified elbow

    M77.11 Lateral epicondylitis, right elbow

    M77.12 Lateral epicondylitis, left elbow

M77.2 Periarthritis of wrist

    M77.20 Periarthritis, unspecified wrist

    M77.21 Periarthritis, right wrist

    M77.22 Periarthritis, left wrist

M77.3 Calcaneal spur

    M77.30 Calcaneal spur, unspecified foot

    M77.31 Calcaneal spur, right foot

    M77.32 Calcaneal spur, left foot

M77.4 Metatarsalgia

    Excludes1: Morton's metatarsalgia (G57.6)

    M77.40 Metatarsalgia, unspecified foot

    M77.41 Metatarsalgia, right foot

    M77.42 Metatarsalgia, left foot

M77.5 Other enthesopathy of foot

    M77.50 Other enthesopathy of unspecified foot

    M77.51 Other enthesopathy of right foot

    M77.52 Other enthesopathy of left foot

M77.8 Other enthesopathies, not elsewhere classified

M77.9 Enthesopathy, unspecified

    Bone spur NOS

    Capsulitis NOS

    Periarthritis NOS

    Tendinitis NOS

M79 Other and unspecified soft tissue disorders, not elsewhere classified

Excludes1: psychogenic rheumatism (F45.8)

    soft tissue pain, psychogenic (F45.41)

M79.0 Rheumatism, unspecified

    Definition: Rheumatism refers to 1) any painful disorder of the joints or muscles or connective tissues or 2) a chronic autoimmune disease with inflammation of the joints and marked deformities.

    Excludes1: fibromyalgia (M79.7)

        palindromic rheumatism (M12.3-)

M79.1 Myalgia

    Myofascial pain syndrome

    Excludes1: fibromyalgia (M79.7)

        myositis (M60.-)

M79.2 Neuralgia and neuritis, unspecified

    Excludes1: brachial radiculitis NOS (M54.1)

        lumbosacral radiculitis NOS (M54.1)

        mononeuropathies (G56-G58)

        radiculitis NOS (M54.1)

        sciatica (M54.3-M54.4)

M79.3 Panniculitis, unspecified

    Excludes1: lupus panniculitis (L93.2)

        neck and back panniculitis (M54.0-)

        relapsing [Weber-Christian] panniculitis (M35.6)

M79.4 Hypertrophy of (infrapatellar) fat pad

M79.5 Residual foreign body in soft tissue

    Excludes1: foreign body granuloma of skin and subcutaneous tissue (L92.3)

        foreign body granuloma of soft tissue (M60.2-)

M79.6 Pain in limb, hand, foot, fingers and toes

    Excludes2: pain in joint (M25.5-)

    M79.60 Pain in limb, unspecified

        M79.601 Pain in right arm

            Pain in right upper limb NOS

        M79.602 Pain in left arm

            Pain in left upper limb NOS

        M79.603 Pain in arm, unspecified

            Pain in upper limb NOS

        M79.604 Pain in right leg

            Pain in right lower limb NOS

        M79.605 Pain in left leg

            Pain in left lower limb NOS

        M79.606 Pain in leg, unspecified

            Pain in lower limb NOS

        M79.609 Pain in unspecified limb

            Pain in limb NOS

    M79.62 Pain in upper arm

        Pain in axillary region

        M79.621 Pain in right upper arm

M79.622   Pain in left upper arm

M79.629   Pain in unspecified upper arm

M79.63   **Pain in forearm**

M79.631   Pain in right forearm

M79.632   Pain in left forearm

M79.639   Pain in unspecified forearm

M79.64   **Pain in hand and fingers**

M79.641   Pain in right hand

M79.642   Pain in left hand

M79.643   Pain in unspecified hand

M79.644   Pain in right finger(s)

M79.645   Pain in left finger(s)

M79.646   Pain in unspecified finger(s)

M79.65   **Pain in thigh**

M79.651   Pain in right thigh

M79.652   Pain in left thigh

M79.659   Pain in unspecified thigh

M79.66   **Pain in lower leg**

M79.661   Pain in right lower leg

M79.662   Pain in left lower leg

M79.669   Pain in unspecified lower leg

M79.67   **Pain in foot and toes**

M79.671   Pain in right foot

M79.672   Pain in left foot

M79.673   Pain in unspecified foot

M79.674   Pain in right toe(s)

M79.675   Pain in left toe(s)

M79.676   Pain in unspecified toe(s)

M79.7   **Fibromyalgia**

Fibromyositis

Fibrositis

Myofibrositis

M79.A   **Nontraumatic compartment syndrome**

Code first, if applicable, associated postprocedural complication

Excludes1: compartment syndrome NOS (T79.A-)

fibromyalgia (M79.7)

nontraumatic ischemic infarction of muscle (M62.2-)

traumatic compartment syndrome (T79.A-)

M79.A1   **Nontraumatic compartment syndrome of upper extremity**

Nontraumatic compartment syndrome of shoulder, arm, forearm, wrist, hand, and fingers

M79.A11   **Nontraumatic compartment syndrome of right upper extremity**

M79.A12   **Nontraumatic compartment syndrome of left upper extremity**

M79.A19   **Nontraumatic compartment syndrome of unspecified upper extremity**

M79.A2   **Nontraumatic compartment syndrome of lower extremity**

Nontraumatic compartment syndrome of hip, buttock, thigh, leg, foot, and toes

M79.A21   **Nontraumatic compartment syndrome of right lower extremity**

M79.A22   **Nontraumatic compartment syndrome of left lower extremity**

M79.A29   **Nontraumatic compartment syndrome of unspecified lower extremity**

M79.A3   **Nontraumatic compartment syndrome of abdomen**

M79.A9   **Nontraumatic compartment syndrome of other sites**

M79.8   **Other specified soft tissue disorders**

M79.81   **Nontraumatic hematoma of soft tissue**

Nontraumatic hematoma of muscle

Nontraumatic seroma of muscle and soft tissue

M79.89   **Other specified soft tissue disorders**

Polyalgia

M79.9   **Soft tissue disorder, unspecified**

OSTEOPATHIES AND CHONDROPATHIES (M80-M94)

DISORDERS OF BONE DENSITY AND STRUCTURE (M80-M85)

M80   **Osteoporosis with current pathological fracture**

Includes: osteoporosis with current fragility fracture

Use additional code to identify major osseous defect, if applicable (M89.7-)

Excludes1: collapsed vertebra NOS (M48.5)

pathological fracture NOS (M84.4)

wedging of vertebra NOS (M48.5)

Excludes2: personal history of (healed) osteoporosis fracture (Z87.310)

The appropriate 7th character is to be added to each code from category M80:

A - initial encounter for fracture

D - subsequent encounter for fracture with routine healing

G - subsequent encounter for fracture with delayed healing

K - subsequent encounter for fracture with nonunion

P - subsequent encounter for fracture with malunion

S - sequela

M80.0   **Age-related osteoporosis with current pathological fracture**

Involutional osteoporosis with current pathological fracture

Osteoporosis NOS with current pathological fracture

Postmenopausal osteoporosis with current pathological fracture

Senile osteoporosis with current pathological fracture

⊗⑦**M80.00**   **Age-related osteoporosis with current pathological fracture, unspecified site**

M80.01   **Age-related osteoporosis with current pathological fracture, shoulder**

⑦**M80.011**   **Age-related osteoporosis with current pathological fracture, right shoulder**

⑦**M80.012**   **Age-related osteoporosis with current pathological fracture, left shoulder**

⑦**M80.019**   **Age-related osteoporosis with current pathological fracture, unspecified shoulder**

M80.02   **Age-related osteoporosis with current pathological fracture, humerus**

⑦ **M80.021** Age-related osteoporosis with current pathological fracture, right humerus

⑦ **M80.022** Age-related osteoporosis with current pathological fracture, left humerus

⑦ **M80.029** Age-related osteoporosis with current pathological fracture, unspecified humerus

M80.03 Age-related osteoporosis with current pathological fracture, forearm

Age-related osteoporosis with current pathological fracture of wrist

⑦ **M80.031** Age-related osteoporosis with current pathological fracture, right forearm

⑦ **M80.032** Age-related osteoporosis with current pathological fracture, left forearm

⑦ **M80.039** Age-related osteoporosis with current pathological fracture, unspecified forearm

M80.04 Age-related osteoporosis with current pathological fracture, hand

⑦ **M80.041** Age-related osteoporosis with current pathological fracture, right hand

⑦ **M80.042** Age-related osteoporosis with current pathological fracture, left hand

⑦ **M80.049** Age-related osteoporosis with current pathological fracture, unspecified hand

M80.05 Age-related osteoporosis with current pathological fracture, femur

Age-related osteoporosis with current pathological fracture of hip

⑦ **M80.051** Age-related osteoporosis with current pathological fracture, right femur

⑦ **M80.052** Age-related osteoporosis with current pathological fracture, left femur

⑦ **M80.059** Age-related osteoporosis with current pathological fracture, unspecified femur

M80.06 Age-related osteoporosis with current pathological fracture, lower leg

⑦ **M80.061** Age-related osteoporosis with current pathological fracture, right lower leg

⑦ **M80.062** Age-related osteoporosis with current pathological fracture, left lower leg

⑦ **M80.069** Age-related osteoporosis with current pathological fracture, unspecified lower leg

M80.07 Age-related osteoporosis with current pathological fracture, ankle and foot

⑦ **M80.071** Age-related osteoporosis with current pathological fracture, right ankle and foot

⑦ **M80.072** Age-related osteoporosis with current pathological fracture, left ankle and foot

⑦ **M80.079** Age-related osteoporosis with current pathological fracture, unspecified ankle and foot

⊗⑦ **M80.08** Age-related osteoporosis with current pathological fracture, vertebra(e)

M80.8 Other osteoporosis with current pathological fracture

Drug-induced osteoporosis with current pathological fracture

Idiopathic osteoporosis with current pathological fracture

Osteoporosis of disuse with current pathological fracture

Postoophorectomy osteoporosis with current pathological fracture

Postsurgical malabsorption osteoporosis with current pathological fracture

Post-traumatic osteoporosis with current pathological fracture

<u>Use additional code</u> for adverse effect, if applicable, to identify drug (T36-T50 with fifth or sixth character 5)

⊗⑦ **M80.80** Other osteoporosis with current pathological fracture, unspecified site

M80.81 Other osteoporosis with pathological fracture, shoulder

⑦ **M80.811** Other osteoporosis with current pathological fracture, right shoulder

⑦ **M80.812** Other osteoporosis with current pathological fracture, left shoulder

⑦ **M80.819** Other osteoporosis with current pathological fracture, unspecified shoulder

M80.82 Other osteoporosis with current pathological fracture, humerus

⑦ **M80.821** Other osteoporosis with current pathological fracture, right humerus

⑦ **M80.822** Other osteoporosis with current pathological fracture, left humerus

⑦ **M80.829** Other osteoporosis with current pathological fracture, unspecified humerus

M80.83 Other osteoporosis with current pathological fracture, forearm

Other osteoporosis with current pathological fracture of wrist

⑦ **M80.831** Other osteoporosis with current pathological fracture, right forearm

⑦ **M80.832** Other osteoporosis with current pathological fracture, left forearm

⑦ **M80.839** Other osteoporosis with current pathological fracture, unspecified forearm

M80.84 Other osteoporosis with current pathological fracture, hand

⑦ **M80.841** Other osteoporosis with current pathological fracture, right hand

⑦ **M80.842** Other osteoporosis with current pathological fracture, left hand

• New code ▲ Revised code **Excludes1:** Not coded here **Excludes2:** Not included here ⊗ Placeholder required ⑦ 7th digit required

⑦**M80.849** Other osteoporosis with current pathological fracture, unspecified hand

M80.85 Other osteoporosis with current pathological fracture, femur

Other osteoporosis with current pathological fracture of hip

⑦**M80.851** Other osteoporosis with current pathological fracture, right femur

⑦**M80.852** Other osteoporosis with current pathological fracture, left femur

⑦**M80.859** Other osteoporosis with current pathological fracture, unspecified femur

M80.86 Other osteoporosis with current pathological fracture, lower leg

⑦**M80.861** Other osteoporosis with current pathological fracture, right lower leg

⑦**M80.862** Other osteoporosis with current pathological fracture, left lower leg

⑦**M80.869** Other osteoporosis with current pathological fracture, unspecified lower leg

M80.87 Other osteoporosis with current pathological fracture, ankle and foot

⑦**M80.871** Other osteoporosis with current pathological fracture, right ankle and foot

⑦**M80.872** Other osteoporosis with current pathological fracture, left ankle and foot

⑦**M80.879** Other osteoporosis with current pathological fracture, unspecified ankle and foot

⊗⑦**M80.88** Other osteoporosis with current pathological fracture, vertebra(e)

M81 **Osteoporosis without current pathological fracture**

Use additional code to identify:

major osseous defect, if applicable (M89.7-)

personal history of (healed) osteoporosis fracture, if applicable (Z87.310)

Excludes1: osteoporosis with current pathological fracture (M80.-)

Sudeck's atrophy (M89.0)

M81.0 **Age-related osteoporosis without current pathological fracture**

Involutional osteoporosis without current pathological fracture

Osteoporosis NOS

Postmenopausal osteoporosis without current pathological fracture

Senile osteoporosis without current pathological fracture

M81.6 **Localized osteoporosis [Lequesne]**

Excludes1: Sudeck's atrophy (M89.0)

M81.8 **Other osteoporosis without current pathological fracture**

Drug-induced osteoporosis without current pathological fracture

Idiopathic osteoporosis without current pathological fracture

Osteoporosis of disuse without current pathological fracture

Postoophorectomy osteoporosis without current pathological fracture

Postsurgical malabsorption osteoporosis without current pathological fracture

Post-traumatic osteoporosis without current pathological fracture

Use additional code for adverse effect, if applicable, to identify drug (T36-T50 with fifth or sixth character 5)

M83 **Adult osteomalacia**

Excludes1: infantile and juvenile osteomalacia (E55.0)

renal osteodystrophy (N25.0)

rickets (active) (E55.0)

rickets (active) sequelae (E64.3)

vitamin D-resistant osteomalacia (E83.3)

vitamin D-resistant rickets (active) (E83.3)

M83.0 **Puerperal osteomalacia**

M83.1 **Senile osteomalacia**

M83.2 **Adult osteomalacia due to malabsorption**

Postsurgical malabsorption osteomalacia in adults

M83.3 **Adult osteomalacia due to malnutrition**

M83.4 **Aluminum bone disease**

M83.5 **Other drug-induced osteomalacia in adults**

Use additional code for adverse effect, if applicable, to identify drug (T36-T50 with fifth or sixth character 5)

M83.8 **Other adult osteomalacia**

M83.9 **Adult osteomalacia, unspecified**

M84 **Disorder of continuity of bone**

Excludes2: traumatic fracture of bone-see fracture, by site

M84.3 **Stress fracture**

Fatigue fracture

March fracture

Stress fracture NOS

Stress reaction

Use additional external cause code(s) to identify the cause of the stress fracture

Excludes1: pathological fracture NOS (M84.4.-)

pathological fracture due to osteoporosis (M80.-)

traumatic fracture (S12.-, S22.-, S32.-, S42.-, S52.-, S62.-, S72.-, S82.-, S92.-)

Excludes2: personal history of (healed) stress (fatigue) fracture (Z87.312)

stress fracture of vertebra (M48.4-)

The appropriate 7th character is to be added to each code from subcategory M84.3:

A - initial encounter for fracture

D - subsequent encounter for fracture with routine healing

G - subsequent encounter for fracture with delayed healing

K - subsequent encounter for fracture with nonunion

P - subsequent encounter for fracture with malunion S - sequela

⊗⑦**M84.30** Stress fracture, unspecified site

M84.31 Stress fracture, shoulder

⑦**M84.311** Stress fracture, right shoulder

⑦**M84.312** Stress fracture, left shoulder

⑦ **M84.319**   **Stress fracture, unspecified shoulder**

M84.32   **Stress fracture, humerus**

⑦ **M84.321**   **Stress fracture, right humerus**

⑦ **M84.322**   **Stress fracture, left humerus**

⑦ **M84.329**   **Stress fracture, unspecified humerus**

M84.33   **Stress fracture, ulna and radius**

⑦ **M84.331**   **Stress fracture, right ulna**

⑦ **M84.332**   **Stress fracture, left ulna**

⑦ **M84.333**   **Stress fracture, right radius**

⑦ **M84.334**   **Stress fracture, left radius**

⑦ **M84.339**   **Stress fracture, unspecified ulna and radius**

M84.34   **Stress fracture, hand and fingers**

⑦ **M84.341**   **Stress fracture, right hand**

⑦ **M84.342**   **Stress fracture, left hand**

⑦ **M84.343**   **Stress fracture, unspecified hand**

⑦ **M84.344**   **Stress fracture, right finger(s)**

⑦ **M84.345**   **Stress fracture, left finger(s)**

⑦ **M84.346**   **Stress fracture, unspecified finger(s)**

M84.35   **Stress fracture, pelvis and femur**

Stress fracture, hip

⑦ **M84.350**   **Stress fracture, pelvis**

⑦ **M84.351**   **Stress fracture, right femur**

⑦ **M84.352**   **Stress fracture, left femur**

⑦ **M84.353**   **Stress fracture, unspecified femur**

⑦ **M84.359**   **Stress fracture, hip, unspecified**

M84.36   **Stress fracture, tibia and fibula**

⑦ **M84.361**   **Stress fracture, right tibia**

⑦ **M84.362**   **Stress fracture, left tibia**

⑦ **M84.363**   **Stress fracture, right fibula**

⑦ **M84.364**   **Stress fracture, left fibula**

⑦ **M84.369**   **Stress fracture, unspecified tibia and fibula**

M84.37   **Stress fracture, ankle, foot and toes**

⑦ **M84.371**   **Stress fracture, right ankle**

⑦ **M84.372**   **Stress fracture, left ankle**

⑦ **M84.373**   **Stress fracture, unspecified ankle**

⑦ **M84.374**   **Stress fracture, right foot**

⑦ **M84.375**   **Stress fracture, left foot**

⑦ **M84.376**   **Stress fracture, unspecified foot**

⑦ **M84.377**   **Stress fracture, right toe(s)**

⑦ **M84.378**   **Stress fracture, left toe(s)**

⑦ **M84.379**   **Stress fracture, unspecified toe(s)**

⊗⑦ **M84.38**   **Stress fracture, other site**

Excludes2: stress fracture of vertebra (M48.4-)

M84.4   **Pathological fracture, not elsewhere classified**

Chronic fracture

Pathological fracture NOS

Excludes1: collapsed vertebra NEC (M48.5)

pathological fracture in neoplastic disease (M84.5-)

pathological fracture in osteoporosis (M80.-)

pathological fracture **in other** disease (M84.6-)

stress fracture (M84.3-)

traumatic fracture (S12.-, S22.-, S32.-, S42.-, S52.-, S62.-, S72.-, S82.-, S92.-)

Excludes2: personal history of (healed) pathological fracture (Z87.311)

The appropriate 7th character is to be added to each code from subcategory M84.4:

A - initial encounter for fracture

D - subsequent encounter for fracture with routine healing

G - subsequent encounter for fracture with delayed healing

K - subsequent encounter for fracture with nonunion

P - subsequent encounter for fracture with malunion

S - sequela

⊗⑦ **M84.40**   **Pathological fracture, unspecified site**

M84.41   **Pathological fracture, shoulder**

⑦ **M84.411**   **Pathological fracture, right shoulder**

⑦ **M84.412**   **Pathological fracture, left shoulder**

⑦ **M84.419**   **Pathological fracture, unspecified shoulder**

M84.42   **Pathological fracture, humerus**

⑦ **M84.421**   **Pathological fracture, right humerus**

⑦ **M84.422**   **Pathological fracture, left humerus**

⑦ **M84.429**   **Pathological fracture, unspecified humerus**

M84.43   **Pathological fracture, ulna and radius**

⑦ **M84.431**   **Pathological fracture, right ulna**

⑦ **M84.432**   **Pathological fracture, left ulna**

⑦ **M84.433**   **Pathological fracture, right radius**

⑦ **M84.434**   **Pathological fracture, left radius**

⑦ **M84.439**   **Pathological fracture, unspecified ulna and radius**

M84.44   **Pathological fracture, hand and fingers**

⑦ **M84.441**   **Pathological fracture, right hand**

⑦ **M84.442**   **Pathological fracture, left hand**

⑦ **M84.443**   **Pathological fracture, unspecified hand**

⑦ **M84.444**   **Pathological fracture, right finger(s)**

⑦ **M84.445**   **Pathological fracture, left finger(s)**

⑦ **M84.446**   **Pathological fracture, unspecified finger(s)**

M84.45   **Pathological fracture, femur and pelvis**

⑦ **M84.451**   **Pathological fracture, right femur**

⑦ **M84.452**   **Pathological fracture, left femur**

⑦ **M84.453**   **Pathological fracture, unspecified femur**

⑦ **M84.454**   **Pathological fracture, pelvis**

⑦ **M84.459**   **Pathological fracture, hip, unspecified**

M84.46   **Pathological fracture, tibia and fibula**

⑦ **M84.461**   **Pathological fracture, right tibia**

⑦ **M84.462**   **Pathological fracture, left tibia**

⑦ **M84.463**   **Pathological fracture, right fibula**

⑦ **M84.464**   **Pathological fracture, left fibula**

⑦ **M84.469**   **Pathological fracture, unspecified tibia and fibula**

M84.47 Pathological fracture, ankle, foot and toes

⑦M84.471 Pathological fracture, right ankle

⑦M84.472 Pathological fracture, left ankle

⑦M84.473 Pathological fracture, unspecified ankle

⑦M84.474 Pathological fracture, right foot

⑦M84.475 Pathological fracture, left foot

⑦M84.476 Pathological fracture, unspecified foot

⑦M84.477 Pathological fracture, right toe(s)

⑦M84.478 Pathological fracture, left toe(s)

⑦M84.479 Pathological fracture, unspecified toe(s)

⊗⑦M84.48 Pathological fracture, other site

M84.5 Pathological fracture in neoplastic disease

Code also underlying neoplasm

The appropriate 7th character is to be added to each code from subcategory M84.5:

A - initial encounter for fracture

D - subsequent encounter for fracture with routine healing

G - subsequent encounter for fracture with delayed healing

K - subsequent encounter for fracture with nonunion

P - subsequent encounter for fracture with malunion

S - sequela

⊗⑦M84.50 Pathological fracture in neoplastic disease, unspecified site

M84.51 Pathological fracture in neoplastic disease, shoulder

⑦M84.511 Pathological fracture in neoplastic disease, right shoulder

⑦M84.512 Pathological fracture in neoplastic disease, left shoulder

⑦M84.519 Pathological fracture in neoplastic disease, unspecified shoulder

M84.52 Pathological fracture in neoplastic disease, humerus

⑦M84.521 Pathological fracture in neoplastic disease, right humerus

⑦M84.522 Pathological fracture in neoplastic disease, left humerus

⑦M84.529 Pathological fracture in neoplastic disease, unspecified humerus

M84.53 Pathological fracture in neoplastic disease, ulna and radius

⑦M84.531 Pathological fracture in neoplastic disease, right ulna

⑦M84.532 Pathological fracture in neoplastic disease, left ulna

⑦M84.533 Pathological fracture in neoplastic disease, right radius

⑦M84.534 Pathological fracture in neoplastic disease, left radius

⑦M84.539 Pathological fracture in neoplastic disease, unspecified ulna and radius

M84.54 Pathological fracture in neoplastic disease, hand

⑦M84.541 Pathological fracture in neoplastic disease, right hand

⑦M84.542 Pathological fracture in neoplastic disease, left hand

⑦M84.549 Pathological fracture in neoplastic disease, unspecified hand

M84.55 Pathological fracture in neoplastic disease, pelvis and femur

⑦M84.550 Pathological fracture in neoplastic disease, pelvis

⑦M84.551 Pathological fracture in neoplastic disease, right femur

⑦M84.552 Pathological fracture in neoplastic disease, left femur

⑦M84.553 Pathological fracture in neoplastic disease, unspecified femur

⑦M84.559 Pathological fracture in neoplastic disease, hip, unspecified

M84.56 Pathological fracture in neoplastic disease, tibia and fibula

⑦M84.561 Pathological fracture in neoplastic disease, right tibia

⑦M84.562 Pathological fracture in neoplastic disease, left tibia

⑦M84.563 Pathological fracture in neoplastic disease, right fibula

⑦M84.564 Pathological fracture in neoplastic disease, left fibula

⑦M84.569 Pathological fracture in neoplastic disease, unspecified tibia and fibula

M84.57 Pathological fracture in neoplastic disease, ankle and foot

⑦M84.571 Pathological fracture in neoplastic disease, right ankle

⑦M84.572 Pathological fracture in neoplastic disease, left ankle

⑦M84.573 Pathological fracture in neoplastic disease, unspecified ankle

⑦M84.574 Pathological fracture in neoplastic disease, right foot

⑦M84.575 Pathological fracture in neoplastic disease, left foot

⑦M84.576 Pathological fracture in neoplastic disease, unspecified foot

⊗⑦M84.58 Pathological fracture in neoplastic disease, other specified site

Pathological fracture in neoplastic disease, vertebrae

M84.6 Pathological fracture in other disease

Code also underlying condition

Excludes1: pathological fracture in osteoporosis (M80.-)

The appropriate 7th character is to be added to each code from subcategory M84.6:

A - initial encounter for fracture

D - subsequent encounter for fracture with routine healing

G - subsequent encounter for fracture with delayed healing

K - subsequent encounter for fracture with nonunion

P - subsequent encounter for fracture with malunion

S - sequela

⊗⑦M84.60 Pathological fracture in other disease, unspecified site

M84.61 Pathological fracture in other disease, shoulder

⑦ **M84.611** Pathological fracture in other disease, right shoulder

⑦ **M84.612** Pathological fracture in other disease, left shoulder

⑦ **M84.619** Pathological fracture in other disease, unspecified shoulder

M84.62 Pathological fracture in other disease, humerus

⑦ **M84.621** Pathological fracture in other disease, right humerus

⑦ **M84.622** Pathological fracture in other disease, left humerus

⑦ **M84.629** Pathological fracture in other disease, unspecified humerus

M84.63 Pathological fracture in other disease, ulna and radius

⑦ **M84.631** Pathological fracture in other disease, right ulna

⑦ **M84.632** Pathological fracture in other disease, left ulna

⑦ **M84.633** Pathological fracture in other disease, right radius

⑦ **M84.634** Pathological fracture in other disease, left radius

⑦ **M84.639** Pathological fracture in other disease, unspecified ulna and radius

M84.64 Pathological fracture in other disease, hand

⑦ **M84.641** Pathological fracture in other disease, right hand

⑦ **M84.642** Pathological fracture in other disease, left hand

⑦ **M84.649** Pathological fracture in other disease, unspecified hand

M84.65 Pathological fracture in other disease, pelvis and femur

⑦ **M84.650** Pathological fracture in other disease, pelvis

⑦ **M84.651** Pathological fracture in other disease, right femur

⑦ **M84.652** Pathological fracture in other disease, left femur

⑦ **M84.653** Pathological fracture in other disease, unspecified femur

⑦ **M84.659** Pathological fracture in other disease, hip, unspecified

M84.66 Pathological fracture in other disease, tibia and fibula

⑦ **M84.661** Pathological fracture in other disease, right tibia

⑦ **M84.662** Pathological fracture in other disease, left tibia

⑦ **M84.663** Pathological fracture in other disease, right fibula

⑦ **M84.664** Pathological fracture in other disease, left fibula

⑦ **M84.669** Pathological fracture in other disease, unspecified tibia and fibula

M84.67 Pathological fracture in other disease, ankle and foot

⑦ **M84.671** Pathological fracture in other disease, right ankle

⑦ **M84.672** Pathological fracture in other disease, left ankle

⑦ **M84.673** Pathological fracture in other disease, unspecified ankle

⑦ **M84.674** Pathological fracture in other disease, right foot

⑦ **M84.675** Pathological fracture in other disease, left foot

⑦ **M84.676** Pathological fracture in other disease, unspecified foot

⊗⑦ **M84.68** Pathological fracture in other disease, other site

M84.7 Nontraumatic fracture, not elsewhere classified

M84.75 Atypical femoral fracture

The appropriate 7th character is to be added to each code from M84.75:

A - initial encounter for fracture

D - subsequent encounter for fracture with routine healing

G - subsequent encounter for fracture with delayed healing

K - subsequent encounter for fracture with nonunion

P - subsequent encounter for fracture with malunion

S - sequela

●⑦ **M84.750** Atypical femoral fracture, unspecified

●⑦ **M84.751** Incomplete atypical femoral fracture, right leg

●⑦ **M84.752** Incomplete atypical femoral fracture, left leg

●⑦ **M84.753** Incomplete atypical femoral fracture, unspecified leg

●⑦ **M84.754** Complete transverse atypical femoral fracture, right leg

●⑦ **M84.755** Complete transverse atypical femoral fracture, left leg

●⑦ **M84.756** Complete transverse atypical femoral fracture, unspecified leg

●⑦ **M84.757** Complete oblique atypical femoral fracture, right leg

●⑦ **M84.758** Complete oblique atypical femoral fracture, left leg

●⑦ **M84.759** Complete oblique atypical femoral fracture, unspecified leg

M84.8 Other disorders of continuity of bone

⊗⑦ **M84.80** Other disorders of continuity of bone, unspecified site

M84.81 Other disorders of continuity of bone, shoulder

⑦ **M84.811** Other disorders of continuity of bone, right shoulder

⑦ **M84.812** Other disorders of continuity of bone, left shoulder

⑦ **M84.819** Other disorders of continuity of bone, unspecified shoulder

M84.82 Other disorders of continuity of bone, humerus

⑦**M84.821** Other disorders of continuity of bone, right humerus

⑦**M84.822** Other disorders of continuity of bone, left humerus

⑦**M84.829** Other disorders of continuity of bone, unspecified humerus

M84.83 Other disorders of continuity of bone, ulna and radius

⑦**M84.831** Other disorders of continuity of bone, right ulna

⑦**M84.832** Other disorders of continuity of bone, left ulna

⑦**M84.833** Other disorders of continuity of bone, right radius

⑦**M84.834** Other disorders of continuity of bone, left radius

⑦**M84.839** Other disorders of continuity of bone, unspecified ulna and radius

M84.84 Other disorders of continuity of bone, hand

⑦**M84.841** Other disorders of continuity of bone, right hand

⑦**M84.842** Other disorders of continuity of bone, left hand

⑦**M84.849** Other disorders of continuity of bone, unspecified hand

M84.85 Other disorders of continuity of bone, pelvic region and thigh

⑦**M84.851** Other disorders of continuity of bone, right pelvic region and thigh

⑦**M84.852** Other disorders of continuity of bone, left pelvic region and thigh

⑦**M84.859** Other disorders of continuity of bone, unspecified pelvic region and thigh

M84.86 Other disorders of continuity of bone, tibia and fibula

⑦**M84.861** Other disorders of continuity of bone, right tibia

⑦**M84.862** Other disorders of continuity of bone, left tibia

⑦**M84.863** Other disorders of continuity of bone, right fibula

⑦**M84.864** Other disorders of continuity of bone, left fibula

⑦**M84.869** Other disorders of continuity of bone, unspecified tibia and fibula

M84.87 Other disorders of continuity of bone, ankle and foot

⑦**M84.871** Other disorders of continuity of bone, right ankle and foot

⑦**M84.872** Other disorders of continuity of bone, left ankle and foot

⑦**M84.879** Other disorders of continuity of bone, unspecified ankle and foot

⊗⑦**M84.88** Other disorders of continuity of bone, other site

⊗⑦**M84.9** Disorder of continuity of bone, unspecified

M85 Other disorders of bone density and structure

Excludes1: osteogenesis imperfecta (Q78.0)

osteopetrosis (Q78.2)

osteopoikilosis (Q78.8)

polyostotic fibrous dysplasia (Q78.1)

M85.0 Fibrous dysplasia (monostotic)

Excludes2: fibrous dysplasia of jaw (M27.8)

M85.00 Fibrous dysplasia (monostotic), unspecified site

M85.01 Fibrous dysplasia (monostotic), shoulder

M85.011 Fibrous dysplasia (monostotic), right shoulder

M85.012 Fibrous dysplasia (monostotic), left shoulder

M85.019 Fibrous dysplasia (monostotic), unspecified shoulder

M85.02 Fibrous dysplasia (monostotic), upper arm

M85.021 Fibrous dysplasia (monostotic), right upper arm

M85.022 Fibrous dysplasia (monostotic), left upper arm

M85.029 Fibrous dysplasia (monostotic), unspecified upper arm

M85.03 Fibrous dysplasia (monostotic), forearm

M85.031 Fibrous dysplasia (monostotic), right forearm

M85.032 Fibrous dysplasia (monostotic), left forearm

M85.039 Fibrous dysplasia (monostotic), unspecified forearm

M85.04 Fibrous dysplasia (monostotic), hand

M85.041 Fibrous dysplasia (monostotic), right hand

M85.042 Fibrous dysplasia (monostotic), left hand

M85.049 Fibrous dysplasia (monostotic), unspecified hand

M85.05 Fibrous dysplasia (monostotic), thigh

M85.051 Fibrous dysplasia (monostotic), right thigh

M85.052 Fibrous dysplasia (monostotic), left thigh

M85.059 Fibrous dysplasia (monostotic), unspecified thigh

M85.06 Fibrous dysplasia (monostotic), lower leg

M85.061 Fibrous dysplasia (monostotic), right lower leg

M85.062 Fibrous dysplasia (monostotic), left lower leg

M85.069 Fibrous dysplasia (monostotic), unspecified lower leg

M85.07 Fibrous dysplasia (monostotic), ankle and foot

M85.071 Fibrous dysplasia (monostotic), right ankle and foot

M85.072 Fibrous dysplasia (monostotic), left ankle and foot

M85.079 Fibrous dysplasia (monostotic), unspecified ankle and foot

M85.08 Fibrous dysplasia (monostotic), other site

M85.09 Fibrous dysplasia (monostotic), multiple sites

M85.1 Skeletal fluorosis

M85.10 Skeletal fluorosis, unspecified site

M85.11 Skeletal fluorosis, shoulder

Add 4th-7th digits   Nonspecific code   Unspecified code   Manifestation code   591

M85.111   Skeletal fluorosis, right shoulder

M85.112   Skeletal fluorosis, left shoulder

M85.119   Skeletal fluorosis, unspecified shoulder

M85.12   Skeletal fluorosis, upper arm

M85.121   Skeletal fluorosis, right upper arm

M85.122   Skeletal fluorosis, left upper arm

M85.129   Skeletal fluorosis, unspecified upper arm

M85.13   Skeletal fluorosis, forearm

M85.131   Skeletal fluorosis, right forearm

M85.132   Skeletal fluorosis, left forearm

M85.139   Skeletal fluorosis, unspecified forearm

M85.14   Skeletal fluorosis, hand

M85.141   Skeletal fluorosis, right hand

M85.142   Skeletal fluorosis, left hand

M85.149   Skeletal fluorosis, unspecified hand

M85.15   Skeletal fluorosis, thigh

M85.151   Skeletal fluorosis, right thigh

M85.152   Skeletal fluorosis, left thigh

M85.159   Skeletal fluorosis, unspecified thigh

M85.16   Skeletal fluorosis, lower leg

M85.161   Skeletal fluorosis, right lower leg

M85.162   Skeletal fluorosis, left lower leg

M85.169   Skeletal fluorosis, unspecified lower leg

M85.17   Skeletal fluorosis, ankle and foot

M85.171   Skeletal fluorosis, right ankle and foot

M85.172   Skeletal fluorosis, left ankle and foot

M85.179   Skeletal fluorosis, unspecified ankle and foot

M85.18   Skeletal fluorosis, other site

M85.19   Skeletal fluorosis, multiple sites

M85.2   **Hyperostosis of skull**

M85.3   **Osteitis condensans**

M85.30   Osteitis condensans, unspecified site

M85.31   Osteitis condensans, shoulder

M85.311   Osteitis condensans, right shoulder

M85.312   Osteitis condensans, left shoulder

M85.319   Osteitis condensans, unspecified shoulder

M85.32   Osteitis condensans, upper arm

M85.321   Osteitis condensans, right upper arm

M85.322   Osteitis condensans, left upper arm

M85.329   Osteitis condensans, unspecified upper arm

M85.33   Osteitis condensans, forearm

M85.331   Osteitis condensans, right forearm

M85.332   Osteitis condensans, left forearm

M85.339   Osteitis condensans, unspecified forearm

M85.34   Osteitis condensans, hand

M85.341   Osteitis condensans, right hand

M85.342   Osteitis condensans, left hand

M85.349   Osteitis condensans, unspecified hand

M85.35   Osteitis condensans, thigh

M85.351   Osteitis condensans, right thigh

M85.352   Osteitis condensans, left thigh

M85.359   Osteitis condensans, unspecified thigh

M85.36   Osteitis condensans, lower leg

M85.361   Osteitis condensans, right lower leg

M85.362   Osteitis condensans, left lower leg

M85.369   Osteitis condensans, unspecified lower leg

M85.37   Osteitis condensans, ankle and foot

M85.371   Osteitis condensans, right ankle and foot

M85.372   Osteitis condensans, left ankle and foot

M85.379   Osteitis condensans, unspecified ankle and foot

M85.38   Osteitis condensans, other site

M85.39   Osteitis condensans, multiple sites

M85.4   **Solitary bone cyst**

Excludes2: solitary cyst of jaw (M27.4)

M85.40   Solitary bone cyst, unspecified site

M85.41   Solitary bone cyst, shoulder

M85.411   Solitary bone cyst, right shoulder

M85.412   Solitary bone cyst, left shoulder

M85.419   Solitary bone cyst, unspecified shoulder

M85.42   Solitary bone cyst, humerus

M85.421   Solitary bone cyst, right humerus

M85.422   Solitary bone cyst, left humerus

M85.429   Solitary bone cyst, unspecified humerus

M85.43   Solitary bone cyst, ulna and radius

M85.431   Solitary bone cyst, right ulna and radius

M85.432   Solitary bone cyst, left ulna and radius

M85.439   Solitary bone cyst, unspecified ulna and radius

M85.44   Solitary bone cyst, hand

M85.441   Solitary bone cyst, right hand

M85.442   Solitary bone cyst, left hand

M85.449   Solitary bone cyst, unspecified hand

M85.45   Solitary bone cyst, pelvis

M85.451   Solitary bone cyst, right pelvis

M85.452   Solitary bone cyst, left pelvis

M85.459   Solitary bone cyst, unspecified pelvis

M85.46   Solitary bone cyst, tibia and fibula

M85.461   Solitary bone cyst, right tibia and fibula

M85.462   Solitary bone cyst, left tibia and fibula

● New code   ▲ Revised code   **Excludes1:** Not coded here   **Excludes2:** Not included here   ⊗ Placeholder required   ⑦7th digit required

M85.469 Solitary bone cyst, unspecified tibia and fibula

M85.47 Solitary bone cyst, ankle and foot

M85.471 Solitary bone cyst, right ankle and foot

M85.472 Solitary bone cyst, left ankle and foot

M85.479 Solitary bone cyst, unspecified ankle and foot

M85.48 Solitary bone cyst, other site

M85.5 Aneurysmal bone cyst

Excludes2: aneurysmal cyst of jaw (M27.4)

M85.50 Aneurysmal bone cyst, unspecified site

M85.51 Aneurysmal bone cyst, shoulder

M85.511 Aneurysmal bone cyst, right shoulder

M85.512 Aneurysmal bone cyst, left shoulder

M85.519 Aneurysmal bone cyst, unspecified shoulder

M85.52 Aneurysmal bone cyst, upper arm

M85.521 Aneurysmal bone cyst, right upper arm

M85.522 Aneurysmal bone cyst, left upper arm

M85.529 Aneurysmal bone cyst, unspecified upper arm

M85.53 Aneurysmal bone cyst, forearm

M85.531 Aneurysmal bone cyst, right forearm

M85.532 Aneurysmal bone cyst, left forearm

M85.539 Aneurysmal bone cyst, unspecified forearm

M85.54 Aneurysmal bone cyst, hand

M85.541 Aneurysmal bone cyst, right hand

M85.542 Aneurysmal bone cyst, left hand

M85.549 Aneurysmal bone cyst, unspecified hand

M85.55 Aneurysmal bone cyst, thigh

M85.551 Aneurysmal bone cyst, right thigh

M85.552 Aneurysmal bone cyst, left thigh

M85.559 Aneurysmal bone cyst, unspecified thigh

M85.56 Aneurysmal bone cyst, lower leg

M85.561 Aneurysmal bone cyst, right lower leg

M85.562 Aneurysmal bone cyst, left lower leg

M85.569 Aneurysmal bone cyst, unspecified lower leg

M85.57 Aneurysmal bone cyst, ankle and foot

M85.571 Aneurysmal bone cyst, right ankle and foot

M85.572 Aneurysmal bone cyst, left ankle and foot

M85.579 Aneurysmal bone cyst, unspecified ankle and foot

M85.58 Aneurysmal bone cyst, other site

M85.59 Aneurysmal bone cyst, multiple sites

M85.6 Other cyst of bone

Excludes1: cyst of jaw NEC (M27.4)

osteitis fibrosa cystica generalisata [von Recklinghausen's disease of bone] (E21.0)

M85.60 Other cyst of bone, unspecified site

M85.61 Other cyst of bone, shoulder

M85.611 Other cyst of bone, right shoulder

M85.612 Other cyst of bone, left shoulder

M85.619 Other cyst of bone, unspecified shoulder

M85.62 Other cyst of bone, upper arm

M85.621 Other cyst of bone, right upper arm

M85.622 Other cyst of bone, left upper arm

M85.629 Other cyst of bone, unspecified upper arm

M85.63 Other cyst of bone, forearm

M85.631 Other cyst of bone, right forearm

M85.632 Other cyst of bone, left forearm

M85.639 Other cyst of bone, unspecified forearm

M85.64 Other cyst of bone, hand

M85.641 Other cyst of bone, right hand

M85.642 Other cyst of bone, left hand

M85.649 Other cyst of bone, unspecified hand

M85.65 Other cyst of bone, thigh

M85.651 Other cyst of bone, right thigh

M85.652 Other cyst of bone, left thigh

M85.659 Other cyst of bone, unspecified thigh

M85.66 Other cyst of bone, lower leg

M85.661 Other cyst of bone, right lower leg

M85.662 Other cyst of bone, left lower leg

M85.669 Other cyst of bone, unspecified lower leg

M85.67 Other cyst of bone, ankle and foot

M85.671 Other cyst of bone, right ankle and foot

M85.672 Other cyst of bone, left ankle and foot

M85.679 Other cyst of bone, unspecified ankle and foot

M85.68 Other cyst of bone, other site

M85.69 Other cyst of bone, multiple sites

M85.8 Other specified disorders of bone density and structure

Hyperostosis of bones, except skull

Osteosclerosis, acquired

Excludes1: diffuse idiopathic skeletal hyperostosis [DISH] (M48.1)

osteosclerosis congenita (Q77.4)

osteosclerosis fragilitas (generalista) (Q78.2)

osteosclerosis myelofibrosis (D75.81)

M85.80 Other specified disorders of bone density and structure, unspecified site

M85.81 Other specified disorders of bone density and structure, shoulder

M85.811 Other specified disorders of bone density and structure, right shoulder

M85.812 Other specified disorders of bone density and structure, left shoulder

M85.819 Other specified disorders of bone density and structure, unspecified shoulder

M85.82 Other specified disorders of bone density and structure, upper arm

M85.821 Other specified disorders of bone density and structure, right upper arm

M85.822 Other specified disorders of bone density and structure, left upper arm

M85.829 Other specified disorders of bone density and structure, unspecified upper arm

M85.83 Other specified disorders of bone density and structure, forearm

M85.831 Other specified disorders of bone density and structure, right forearm

M85.832 Other specified disorders of bone density and structure, left forearm

M85.839 Other specified disorders of bone density and structure, unspecified forearm

M85.84 Other specified disorders of bone density and structure, hand

M85.841 Other specified disorders of bone density and structure, right hand

M85.842 Other specified disorders of bone density and structure, left hand

M85.849 Other specified disorders of bone density and structure, unspecified hand

M85.85 Other specified disorders of bone density and structure, thigh

M85.851 Other specified disorders of bone density and structure, right thigh

M85.852 Other specified disorders of bone density and structure, left thigh

M85.859 Other specified disorders of bone density and structure, unspecified thigh

M85.86 Other specified disorders of bone density and structure, lower leg

M85.861 Other specified disorders of bone density and structure, right lower leg

M85.862 Other specified disorders of bone density and structure, left lower leg

M85.869 Other specified disorders of bone density and structure, unspecified lower leg

M85.87 Other specified disorders of bone density and structure, ankle and foot

M85.871 Other specified disorders of bone density and structure, right ankle and foot

M85.872 Other specified disorders of bone density and structure, left ankle and foot

M85.879 Other specified disorders of bone density and structure, unspecified ankle and foot

M85.88 Other specified disorders of bone density and structure, other site

M85.89 Other specified disorders of bone density and structure, multiple sites

M85.9 Disorder of bone density and structure, unspecified

OTHER OSTEOPATHIES (M86-M90)

Excludes1: postprocedural osteopathies (M96.-)

M86 Osteomyelitis

Use additional code (B95-B97) to identify infectious agent

Use additional code to identify major osseous defect, if applicable (M89.7-)

Excludes1: osteomyelitis due to:

echinococcus (B67.2)

gonococcus (A54.43)

salmonella (A02.24)

Excludes2: ostemyelitis of:

orbit (H05.0-)

petrous bone (H70.2-)

vertebra (M46.2-)

M86.0 Acute hematogenous osteomyelitis

M86.00 Acute hematogenous osteomyelitis, unspecified site

M86.01 Acute hematogenous osteomyelitis, shoulder

M86.011 Acute hematogenous osteomyelitis, right shoulder

M86.012 Acute hematogenous osteomyelitis, left shoulder

M86.019 Acute hematogenous osteomyelitis, unspecified shoulder

M86.02 Acute hematogenous osteomyelitis, humerus

M86.021 Acute hematogenous osteomyelitis, right humerus

M86.022 Acute hematogenous osteomyelitis, left humerus

M86.029 Acute hematogenous osteomyelitis, unspecified humerus

M86.03 Acute hematogenous osteomyelitis, radius and ulna

M86.031 Acute hematogenous osteomyelitis, right radius and ulna

M86.032 Acute hematogenous osteomyelitis, left radius and ulna

M86.039 Acute hematogenous osteomyelitis, unspecified radius and ulna

M86.04 Acute hematogenous osteomyelitis, hand

M86.041 Acute hematogenous osteomyelitis, right hand

M86.042 Acute hematogenous osteomyelitis, left hand

M86.049 Acute hematogenous osteomyelitis, unspecified hand

M86.05 Acute hematogenous osteomyelitis, femur

M86.051 Acute hematogenous osteomyelitis, right femur

M86.052 Acute hematogenous osteomyelitis, left femur

M86.059 Acute hematogenous osteomyelitis, unspecified femur

M86.06 Acute hematogenous osteomyelitis, tibia and fibula

M86.061 Acute hematogenous osteomyelitis, right tibia and fibula

M86.062 Acute hematogenous osteomyelitis, left tibia and fibula

M86.069 Acute hematogenous osteomyelitis, unspecified tibia and fibula

M86.07 Acute hematogenous osteomyelitis, ankle and foot

M86.071 Acute hematogenous osteomyelitis, right ankle and foot

M86.072 Acute hematogenous osteomyelitis, left ankle and foot

M86.079 Acute hematogenous osteomyelitis, unspecified ankle and foot

M86.08 Acute hematogenous osteomyelitis, other sites

M86.09 Acute hematogenous osteomyelitis, multiple sites

M86.1 Other acute osteomyelitis

M86.10 Other acute osteomyelitis, unspecified site

M86.11 Other acute osteomyelitis, shoulder

M86.111 Other acute osteomyelitis, right shoulder

M86.112 Other acute osteomyelitis, left shoulder

M86.119 Other acute osteomyelitis, unspecified shoulder

M86.12 Other acute osteomyelitis, humerus

M86.121 Other acute osteomyelitis, right humerus

M86.122 Other acute osteomyelitis, left humerus

M86.129 Other acute osteomyelitis, unspecified humerus

M86.13 Other acute osteomyelitis, radius and ulna

M86.131 Other acute osteomyelitis, right radius and ulna

M86.132 Other acute osteomyelitis, left radius and ulna

M86.139 Other acute osteomyelitis, unspecified radius and ulna

M86.14 Other acute osteomyelitis, hand

M86.141 Other acute osteomyelitis, right hand

M86.142 Other acute osteomyelitis, left hand

M86.149 Other acute osteomyelitis, unspecified hand

M86.15 Other acute osteomyelitis, femur

M86.151 Other acute osteomyelitis, right femur

M86.152 Other acute osteomyelitis, left femur

M86.159 Other acute osteomyelitis, unspecified femur

M86.16 Other acute osteomyelitis, tibia and fibula

M86.161 Other acute osteomyelitis, right tibia and fibula

M86.162 Other acute osteomyelitis, left tibia and fibula

M86.169 Other acute osteomyelitis, unspecified tibia and fibula

M86.17 Other acute osteomyelitis, ankle and foot

M86.171 Other acute osteomyelitis, right ankle and foot

M86.172 Other acute osteomyelitis, left ankle and foot

M86.179 Other acute osteomyelitis, unspecified ankle and foot

M86.18 Other acute osteomyelitis, other site

M86.19 Other acute osteomyelitis, multiple sites

M86.2 Subacute osteomyelitis

M86.20 Subacute osteomyelitis, unspecified site

M86.21 Subacute osteomyelitis, shoulder

M86.211 Subacute osteomyelitis, right shoulder

M86.212 Subacute osteomyelitis, left shoulder

M86.219 Subacute osteomyelitis, unspecified shoulder

M86.22 Subacute osteomyelitis, humerus

M86.221 Subacute osteomyelitis, right humerus

M86.222 Subacute osteomyelitis, left humerus

M86.229 Subacute osteomyelitis, unspecified humerus

M86.23 Subacute osteomyelitis, radius and ulna

M86.231 Subacute osteomyelitis, right radius and ulna

M86.232 Subacute osteomyelitis, left radius and ulna

M86.239 Subacute osteomyelitis, unspecified radius and ulna

M86.24 Subacute osteomyelitis, hand

M86.241 Subacute osteomyelitis, right hand

M86.242 Subacute osteomyelitis, left hand

M86.249 Subacute osteomyelitis, unspecified hand

M86.25 Subacute osteomyelitis, femur

M86.251 Subacute osteomyelitis, right femur

M86.252 Subacute osteomyelitis, left femur

M86.259 Subacute osteomyelitis, unspecified femur

M86.26 Subacute osteomyelitis, tibia and fibula

M86.261 Subacute osteomyelitis, right tibia and fibula

M86.262 Subacute osteomyelitis, left tibia and fibula

M86.269 Subacute osteomyelitis, unspecified tibia and fibula

M86.27 Subacute osteomyelitis, ankle and foot

M86.271 Subacute osteomyelitis, right ankle and foot

M86.272 Subacute osteomyelitis, left ankle and foot

M86.279 Subacute osteomyelitis, unspecified ankle and foot

M86.28 Subacute osteomyelitis, other site

M86.29 Subacute osteomyelitis, multiple sites

M86.3 Chronic multifocal osteomyelitis

M86.30 Chronic multifocal osteomyelitis, unspecified site

M86.31 Chronic multifocal osteomyelitis, shoulder

M86.311 Chronic multifocal osteomyelitis, right shoulder

M86.312 Chronic multifocal osteomyelitis, left shoulder

M86.319 Chronic multifocal osteomyelitis, unspecified shoulder

M86.32 Chronic multifocal osteomyelitis, humerus

M86.321 Chronic multifocal osteomyelitis, right humerus

M86.322 Chronic multifocal osteomyelitis, left humerus

M86.329 Chronic multifocal osteomyelitis, unspecified humerus

M86.33 Chronic multifocal osteomyelitis, radius and ulna

M86.331 Chronic multifocal osteomyelitis, right radius and ulna

M86.332 Chronic multifocal osteomyelitis, left radius and ulna

M86.339 Chronic multifocal osteomyelitis, unspecified radius and ulna

M86.34 Chronic multifocal osteomyelitis, hand

M86.341 Chronic multifocal osteomyelitis, right hand

M86.342 Chronic multifocal osteomyelitis, left hand

M86.349 Chronic multifocal osteomyelitis, unspecified hand

M86.35 Chronic multifocal osteomyelitis, femur

M86.351 Chronic multifocal osteomyelitis, right femur

M86.352 Chronic multifocal osteomyelitis, left femur

M86.359 Chronic multifocal osteomyelitis, unspecified femur

M86.36 Chronic multifocal osteomyelitis, tibia and fibula

M86.361 Chronic multifocal osteomyelitis, right tibia and fibula

M86.362 Chronic multifocal osteomyelitis, left tibia and fibula

M86.369 Chronic multifocal osteomyelitis, unspecified tibia and fibula

M86.37 Chronic multifocal osteomyelitis, ankle and foot

M86.371 Chronic multifocal osteomyelitis, right ankle and foot

M86.372 Chronic multifocal osteomyelitis, left ankle and foot

M86.379 Chronic multifocal osteomyelitis, unspecified ankle and foot

M86.38 Chronic multifocal osteomyelitis, other site

M86.39 Chronic multifocal osteomyelitis, multiple sites

M86.4 Chronic osteomyelitis with draining sinus

M86.40 Chronic osteomyelitis with draining sinus, unspecified site

M86.41 Chronic osteomyelitis with draining sinus, shoulder

M86.411 Chronic osteomyelitis with draining sinus, right shoulder

M86.412 Chronic osteomyelitis with draining sinus, left shoulder

M86.419 Chronic osteomyelitis with draining sinus, unspecified shoulder

M86.42 Chronic osteomyelitis with draining sinus, humerus

M86.421 Chronic osteomyelitis with draining sinus, right humerus

M86.422 Chronic osteomyelitis with draining sinus, left humerus

M86.429 Chronic osteomyelitis with draining sinus, unspecified humerus

M86.43 Chronic osteomyelitis with draining sinus, radius and ulna

M86.431 Chronic osteomyelitis with draining sinus, right radius and ulna

M86.432 Chronic osteomyelitis with draining sinus, left radius and ulna

M86.439 Chronic osteomyelitis with draining sinus, unspecified radius and ulna

M86.44 Chronic osteomyelitis with draining sinus, hand

M86.441 Chronic osteomyelitis with draining sinus, right hand

M86.442 Chronic osteomyelitis with draining sinus, left hand

M86.449 Chronic osteomyelitis with draining sinus, unspecified hand

M86.45 Chronic osteomyelitis with draining sinus, femur

M86.451 Chronic osteomyelitis with draining sinus, right femur

M86.452 Chronic osteomyelitis with draining sinus, left femur

M86.459 Chronic osteomyelitis with draining sinus, unspecified femur

M86.46 Chronic osteomyelitis with draining sinus, tibia and fibula

M86.461 Chronic osteomyelitis with draining sinus, right tibia and fibula

M86.462 Chronic osteomyelitis with draining sinus, left tibia and fibula

M86.469 Chronic osteomyelitis with draining sinus, unspecified tibia and fibula

M86.47 Chronic osteomyelitis with draining sinus, ankle and foot

M86.471 Chronic osteomyelitis with draining sinus, right ankle and foot

● New code   ▲ Revised code   **Excludes1:** Not coded here   **Excludes2:** Not included here   ⊗ Placeholder required   ⑦7th digit required

M86.472 Chronic osteomyelitis with draining sinus, left ankle and foot

M86.479 Chronic osteomyelitis with draining sinus, unspecified ankle and foot

M86.48 Chronic osteomyelitis with draining sinus, other site

M86.49 Chronic osteomyelitis with draining sinus, multiple sites

M86.5 Other chronic hematogenous osteomyelitis

M86.50 Other chronic hematogenous osteomyelitis, unspecified site

M86.51 Other chronic hematogenous osteomyelitis, shoulder

M86.511 Other chronic hematogenous osteomyelitis, right shoulder

M86.512 Other chronic hematogenous osteomyelitis, left shoulder

M86.519 Other chronic hematogenous osteomyelitis, unspecified shoulder

M86.52 Other chronic hematogenous osteomyelitis, humerus

M86.521 Other chronic hematogenous osteomyelitis, right humerus

M86.522 Other chronic hematogenous osteomyelitis, left humerus

M86.529 Other chronic hematogenous osteomyelitis, unspecified humerus

M86.53 Other chronic hematogenous osteomyelitis, radius and ulna

M86.531 Other chronic hematogenous osteomyelitis, right radius and ulna

M86.532 Other chronic hematogenous osteomyelitis, left radius and ulna

M86.539 Other chronic hematogenous osteomyelitis, unspecified radius and ulna

M86.54 Other chronic hematogenous osteomyelitis, hand

M86.541 Other chronic hematogenous osteomyelitis, right hand

M86.542 Other chronic hematogenous osteomyelitis, left hand

M86.549 Other chronic hematogenous osteomyelitis, unspecified hand

M86.55 Other chronic hematogenous osteomyelitis, femur

M86.551 Other chronic hematogenous osteomyelitis, right femur

M86.552 Other chronic hematogenous osteomyelitis, left femur

M86.559 Other chronic hematogenous osteomyelitis, unspecified femur

M86.56 Other chronic hematogenous osteomyelitis, tibia and fibula

M86.561 Other chronic hematogenous osteomyelitis, right tibia and fibula

M86.562 Other chronic hematogenous osteomyelitis, left tibia and fibula

M86.569 Other chronic hematogenous osteomyelitis, unspecified tibia and fibula

M86.57 Other chronic hematogenous osteomyelitis, ankle and foot

M86.571 Other chronic hematogenous osteomyelitis, right ankle and foot

M86.572 Other chronic hematogenous osteomyelitis, left ankle and foot

M86.579 Other chronic hematogenous osteomyelitis, unspecified ankle and foot

M86.58 Other chronic hematogenous osteomyelitis, other site

M86.59 Other chronic hematogenous osteomyelitis, multiple sites

M86.6 Other chronic osteomyelitis

M86.60 Other chronic osteomyelitis, unspecified site

M86.61 Other chronic osteomyelitis, shoulder

M86.611 Other chronic osteomyelitis, right shoulder

M86.612 Other chronic osteomyelitis, left shoulder

M86.619 Other chronic osteomyelitis, unspecified shoulder

M86.62 Other chronic osteomyelitis, humerus

M86.621 Other chronic osteomyelitis, right humerus

M86.622 Other chronic osteomyelitis, left humerus

M86.629 Other chronic osteomyelitis, unspecified humerus

M86.63 Other chronic osteomyelitis, radius and ulna

M86.631 Other chronic osteomyelitis, right radius and ulna

M86.632 Other chronic osteomyelitis, left radius and ulna

M86.639 Other chronic osteomyelitis, unspecified radius and ulna

M86.64 Other chronic osteomyelitis, hand

M86.641 Other chronic osteomyelitis, right hand

M86.642 Other chronic osteomyelitis, left hand

M86.649 Other chronic osteomyelitis, unspecified hand

M86.65 Other chronic osteomyelitis, thigh

M86.651 Other chronic osteomyelitis, right thigh

M86.652 Other chronic osteomyelitis, left thigh

M86.659 Other chronic osteomyelitis, unspecified thigh

M86.66 Other chronic osteomyelitis, tibia and fibula

M86.661 Other chronic osteomyelitis, right tibia and fibula

M86.662 Other chronic osteomyelitis, left tibia and fibula

M86.669 Other chronic osteomyelitis, unspecified tibia and fibula

M86.67 Other chronic osteomyelitis, ankle and foot

M86.671 Other chronic osteomyelitis, right ankle and foot

Add 4th-7th digits   Nonspecific code   Unspecified code   Manifestation code

M86.672   Other chronic osteomyelitis, left ankle and foot

M86.679   Other chronic osteomyelitis, unspecified ankle and foot

M86.68   Other chronic osteomyelitis, other site

M86.69   Other chronic osteomyelitis, multiple sites

M86.8   Other osteomyelitis

Brodie's abscess

M86.8X   Other osteomyelitis

M86.8X0   Other osteomyelitis, multiple sites

M86.8X1   Other osteomyelitis, shoulder

M86.8X2   Other osteomyelitis, upper arm

M86.8X3   Other osteomyelitis, forearm

M86.8X4   Other osteomyelitis, hand

M86.8X5   Other osteomyelitis, thigh

M86.8X6   Other osteomyelitis, lower leg

M86.8X7   Other osteomyelitis, ankle and foot

M86.8X8   Other osteomyelitis, other site

M86.8X9   Other osteomyelitis, unspecified sites

M86.9   Osteomyelitis, unspecified

Infection of bone NOS

Periostitis without osteomyelitis

M87   Osteonecrosis

Includes: avascular necrosis of bone

Use additional code to identify major osseous defect, if applicable (M89.7-)

Excludes1: juvenile osteonecrosis (M91-M92)

osteochondropathies (M90-M93)

M87.0   Idiopathic aseptic necrosis of bone

M87.00   Idiopathic aseptic necrosis of unspecified bone

M87.01   Idiopathic aseptic necrosis of shoulder

Idiopathic aseptic necrosis of clavicle and scapula

M87.011   Idiopathic aseptic necrosis of right shoulder

M87.012   Idiopathic aseptic necrosis of left shoulder

M87.019   Idiopathic aseptic necrosis of unspecified shoulder

M87.02   Idiopathic aseptic necrosis of humerus

M87.021   Idiopathic aseptic necrosis of right humerus

M87.022   Idiopathic aseptic necrosis of left humerus

M87.029   Idiopathic aseptic necrosis of unspecified humerus

M87.03   Idiopathic aseptic necrosis of radius, ulna and carpus

M87.031   Idiopathic aseptic necrosis of right radius

M87.032   Idiopathic aseptic necrosis of left radius

M87.033   Idiopathic aseptic necrosis of unspecified radius

M87.034   Idiopathic aseptic necrosis of right ulna

M87.035   Idiopathic aseptic necrosis of left ulna

M87.036   Idiopathic aseptic necrosis of unspecified ulna

M87.037   Idiopathic aseptic necrosis of right carpus

M87.038   Idiopathic aseptic necrosis of left carpus

M87.039   Idiopathic aseptic necrosis of unspecified carpus

M87.04   Idiopathic aseptic necrosis of hand and fingers

Idiopathic aseptic necrosis of metacarpals and phalanges of hands

M87.041   Idiopathic aseptic necrosis of right hand

M87.042   Idiopathic aseptic necrosis of left hand

M87.043   Idiopathic aseptic necrosis of unspecified hand

M87.044   Idiopathic aseptic necrosis of right finger(s)

M87.045   Idiopathic aseptic necrosis of left finger(s)

M87.046   Idiopathic aseptic necrosis of unspecified finger(s)

M87.05   Idiopathic aseptic necrosis of pelvis and femur

M87.050   Idiopathic aseptic necrosis of pelvis

M87.051   Idiopathic aseptic necrosis of right femur

M87.052   Idiopathic aseptic necrosis of left femur

M87.059   Idiopathic aseptic necrosis of unspecified femur

Idiopathic aseptic necrosis of hip NOS

M87.06   Idiopathic aseptic necrosis of tibia and fibula

M87.061   Idiopathic aseptic necrosis of right tibia

M87.062   Idiopathic aseptic necrosis of left tibia

M87.063   Idiopathic aseptic necrosis of unspecified tibia

M87.064   Idiopathic aseptic necrosis of right fibula

M87.065   Idiopathic aseptic necrosis of left fibula

M87.066   Idiopathic aseptic necrosis of unspecified fibula

M87.07   Idiopathic aseptic necrosis of ankle, foot and toes

Idiopathic aseptic necrosis of metatarsus, tarsus, and phalanges of toes

M87.071   Idiopathic aseptic necrosis of right ankle

M87.072   Idiopathic aseptic necrosis of left ankle

M87.073   Idiopathic aseptic necrosis of unspecified ankle

M87.074   Idiopathic aseptic necrosis of right foot

M87.075   Idiopathic aseptic necrosis of left foot

M87.076   Idiopathic aseptic necrosis of unspecified foot

M87.077   Idiopathic aseptic necrosis of right toe(s)

M87.078   Idiopathic aseptic necrosis of left toe(s)

M87.079   Idiopathic aseptic necrosis of unspecified toe(s)

M87.08   Idiopathic aseptic necrosis of bone, other site

M87.09   Idiopathic aseptic necrosis of bone, multiple sites

M87.1   **Osteonecrosis due to drugs**

Use additional code for adverse effect, if applicable, to identify drug (T36-T50 with fifth or sixth character 5)

M87.10   Osteonecrosis due to drugs, unspecified bone

M87.11   Osteonecrosis due to drugs, shoulder

M87.111   Osteonecrosis due to drugs, right shoulder

M87.112   Osteonecrosis due to drugs, left shoulder

M87.119   Osteonecrosis due to drugs, unspecified shoulder

M87.12   Osteonecrosis due to drugs, humerus

M87.121   Osteonecrosis due to drugs, right humerus

M87.122   Osteonecrosis due to drugs, left humerus

M87.129   Osteonecrosis due to drugs, unspecified humerus

M87.13   Osteonecrosis due to drugs of radius, ulna and carpus

M87.131   Osteonecrosis due to drugs of right radius

M87.132   Osteonecrosis due to drugs of left radius

M87.133   Osteonecrosis due to drugs of unspecified radius

M87.134   Osteonecrosis due to drugs of right ulna

M87.135   Osteonecrosis due to drugs of left ulna

M87.136   Osteonecrosis due to drugs of unspecified ulna

M87.137   Osteonecrosis due to drugs of right carpus

M87.138   Osteonecrosis due to drugs of left carpus

M87.139   Osteonecrosis due to drugs of unspecified carpus

M87.14   Osteonecrosis due to drugs, hand and fingers

M87.141   Osteonecrosis due to drugs, right hand

M87.142   Osteonecrosis due to drugs, left hand

M87.143   Osteonecrosis due to drugs, unspecified hand

M87.144   Osteonecrosis due to drugs, right finger(s)

M87.145   Osteonecrosis due to drugs, left finger(s)

M87.146   Osteonecrosis due to drugs, unspecified finger(s)

M87.15   Osteonecrosis due to drugs, pelvis and femur

M87.150   Osteonecrosis due to drugs, pelvis

M87.151   Osteonecrosis due to drugs, right femur

M87.152   Osteonecrosis due to drugs, left femur

M87.159   Osteonecrosis due to drugs, unspecified femur

M87.16   Osteonecrosis due to drugs, tibia and fibula

M87.161   Osteonecrosis due to drugs, right tibia

M87.162   Osteonecrosis due to drugs, left tibia

M87.163   Osteonecrosis due to drugs, unspecified tibia

M87.164   Osteonecrosis due to drugs, right fibula

M87.165   Osteonecrosis due to drugs, left fibula

M87.166   Osteonecrosis due to drugs, unspecified fibula

M87.17   Osteonecrosis due to drugs, ankle, foot and toes

M87.171   Osteonecrosis due to drugs, right ankle

M87.172   Osteonecrosis due to drugs, left ankle

M87.173   Osteonecrosis due to drugs, unspecified ankle

M87.174   Osteonecrosis due to drugs, right foot

M87.175   Osteonecrosis due to drugs, left foot

M87.176   Osteonecrosis due to drugs, unspecified foot

M87.177   Osteonecrosis due to drugs, right toe(s)

M87.178   Osteonecrosis due to drugs, left toe(s)

M87.179   Osteonecrosis due to drugs, unspecified toe(s)

M87.18   Osteonecrosis due to drugs, other site

M87.180   Osteonecrosis due to drugs, jaw

M87.188   Osteonecrosis due to drugs, other site

M87.19   Osteonecrosis due to drugs, multiple sites

M87.2   **Osteonecrosis due to previous trauma**

M87.20   Osteonecrosis due to previous trauma, unspecified bone

M87.21   Osteonecrosis due to previous trauma, shoulder

M87.211   Osteonecrosis due to previous trauma, right shoulder

M87.212   Osteonecrosis due to previous trauma, left shoulder

M87.219   Osteonecrosis due to previous trauma, unspecified shoulder

M87.22   Osteonecrosis due to previous trauma, humerus

M87.221   Osteonecrosis due to previous trauma, right humerus

M87.222 Osteonecrosis due to previous trauma, left humerus

M87.229 Osteonecrosis due to previous trauma, unspecified humerus

M87.23 Osteonecrosis due to previous trauma of radius, ulna and carpus

M87.231 Osteonecrosis due to previous trauma of right radius

M87.232 Osteonecrosis due to previous trauma of left radius

M87.233 Osteonecrosis due to previous trauma of unspecified radius

M87.234 Osteonecrosis due to previous trauma of right ulna

M87.235 Osteonecrosis due to previous trauma of left ulna

M87.236 Osteonecrosis due to previous trauma of unspecified ulna

M87.237 Osteonecrosis due to previous trauma of right carpus

M87.238 Osteonecrosis due to previous trauma of left carpus

M87.239 Osteonecrosis due to previous trauma of unspecified carpus

M87.24 Osteonecrosis due to previous trauma, hand and fingers

M87.241 Osteonecrosis due to previous trauma, right hand

M87.242 Osteonecrosis due to previous trauma, left hand

M87.243 Osteonecrosis due to previous trauma, unspecified hand

M87.244 Osteonecrosis due to previous trauma, right finger(s)

M87.245 Osteonecrosis due to previous trauma, left finger(s)

M87.246 Osteonecrosis due to previous trauma, unspecified finger(s)

M87.25 Osteonecrosis due to previous trauma, pelvis and femur

M87.250 Osteonecrosis due to previous trauma, pelvis

M87.251 Osteonecrosis due to previous trauma, right femur

M87.252 Osteonecrosis due to previous trauma, left femur

M87.256 Osteonecrosis due to previous trauma, unspecified femur

M87.26 Osteonecrosis due to previous trauma, tibia and fibula

M87.261 Osteonecrosis due to previous trauma, right tibia

M87.262 Osteonecrosis due to previous trauma, left tibia

M87.263 Osteonecrosis due to previous trauma, unspecified tibia

M87.264 Osteonecrosis due to previous trauma, right fibula

M87.265 Osteonecrosis due to previous trauma, left fibula

M87.266 Osteonecrosis due to previous trauma, unspecified fibula

M87.27 Osteonecrosis due to previous trauma, ankle, foot and toes

M87.271 Osteonecrosis due to previous trauma, right ankle

M87.272 Osteonecrosis due to previous trauma, left ankle

M87.273 Osteonecrosis due to previous trauma, unspecified ankle

M87.274 Osteonecrosis due to previous trauma, right foot

M87.275 Osteonecrosis due to previous trauma, left foot

M87.276 Osteonecrosis due to previous trauma, unspecified foot

M87.277 Osteonecrosis due to previous trauma, right toe(s)

M87.278 Osteonecrosis due to previous trauma, left toe(s)

M87.279 Osteonecrosis due to previous trauma, unspecified toe(s)

M87.28 Osteonecrosis due to previous trauma, other site

M87.29 Osteonecrosis due to previous trauma, multiple sites

M87.3 Other secondary osteonecrosis

M87.30 Other secondary osteonecrosis, unspecified bone

M87.31 Other secondary osteonecrosis, shoulder

M87.311 Other secondary osteonecrosis, right shoulder

M87.312 Other secondary osteonecrosis, left shoulder

M87.319 Other secondary osteonecrosis, unspecified shoulder

M87.32 Other secondary osteonecrosis, humerus

M87.321 Other secondary osteonecrosis, right humerus

M87.322 Other secondary osteonecrosis, left humerus

M87.329 Other secondary osteonecrosis, unspecified humerus

M87.33 Other secondary osteonecrosis of radius, ulna and carpus

M87.331 Other secondary osteonecrosis of right radius

M87.332 Other secondary osteonecrosis of left radius

M87.333 Other secondary osteonecrosis of unspecified radius

M87.334 Other secondary osteonecrosis of right ulna

M87.335 Other secondary osteonecrosis of left ulna

M87.336 Other secondary osteonecrosis of unspecified ulna

M87.337 Other secondary osteonecrosis of right carpus

M87.338 Other secondary osteonecrosis of left carpus

● New code ▲ Revised code **Excludes1:** Not coded here **Excludes2:** Not included here ⊗ Placeholder required ⑦7th digit required

M87.339   Other secondary osteonecrosis of unspecified carpus

M87.34   Other secondary osteonecrosis, hand and fingers

M87.341   Other secondary osteonecrosis, right hand

M87.342   Other secondary osteonecrosis, left hand

M87.343   Other secondary osteonecrosis, unspecified hand

M87.344   Other secondary osteonecrosis, right finger(s)

M87.345   Other secondary osteonecrosis, left finger(s)

M87.346   Other secondary osteonecrosis, unspecified finger(s)

M87.35   Other secondary osteonecrosis, pelvis and femur

M87.350   Other secondary osteonecrosis, pelvis

M87.351   Other secondary osteonecrosis, right femur

M87.352   Other secondary osteonecrosis, left femur

M87.353   Other secondary osteonecrosis, unspecified femur

M87.36   Other secondary osteonecrosis, tibia and fibula

M87.361   Other secondary osteonecrosis, right tibia

M87.362   Other secondary osteonecrosis, left tibia

M87.363   Other secondary osteonecrosis, unspecified tibia

M87.364   Other secondary osteonecrosis, right fibula

M87.365   Other secondary osteonecrosis, left fibula

M87.366   Other secondary osteonecrosis, unspecified fibula

M87.37   Other secondary osteonecrosis, ankle and foot

M87.371   Other secondary osteonecrosis, right ankle

M87.372   Other secondary osteonecrosis, left ankle

M87.373   Other secondary osteonecrosis, unspecified ankle

M87.374   Other secondary osteonecrosis, right foot

M87.375   Other secondary osteonecrosis, left foot

M87.376   Other secondary osteonecrosis, unspecified foot

M87.377   Other secondary osteonecrosis, right toe(s)

M87.378   Other secondary osteonecrosis, left toe(s)

M87.379   Other secondary osteonecrosis, unspecified toe(s)

M87.38   Other secondary osteonecrosis, other site

M87.39   Other secondary osteonecrosis, multiple sites

M87.8   Other osteonecrosis

M87.80   Other osteonecrosis, unspecified bone

M87.81   Other osteonecrosis, shoulder

M87.811   Other osteonecrosis, right shoulder

M87.812   Other osteonecrosis, left shoulder

M87.819   Other osteonecrosis, unspecified shoulder

M87.82   Other osteonecrosis, humerus

M87.821   Other osteonecrosis, right humerus

M87.822   Other osteonecrosis, left humerus

M87.829   Other osteonecrosis, unspecified humerus

M87.83   Other osteonecrosis of radius, ulna and carpus

M87.831   Other osteonecrosis of right radius

M87.832   Other osteonecrosis of left radius

M87.833   Other osteonecrosis of unspecified radius

M87.834   Other osteonecrosis of right ulna

M87.835   Other osteonecrosis of left ulna

M87.836   Other osteonecrosis of unspecified ulna

M87.837   Other osteonecrosis of right carpus

M87.838   Other osteonecrosis of left carpus

M87.839   Other osteonecrosis of unspecified carpus

M87.84   Other osteonecrosis, hand and fingers

M87.841   Other osteonecrosis, right hand

M87.842   Other osteonecrosis, left hand

M87.843   Other osteonecrosis, unspecified hand

M87.844   Other osteonecrosis, right finger(s)

M87.845   Other osteonecrosis, left finger(s)

M87.849   Other osteonecrosis, unspecified finger(s)

M87.85   Other osteonecrosis, pelvis and femur

M87.850   Other osteonecrosis, pelvis

M87.851   Other osteonecrosis, right femur

M87.852   Other osteonecrosis, left femur

M87.859   Other osteonecrosis, unspecified femur

M87.86   Other osteonecrosis, tibia and fibula

M87.861   Other osteonecrosis, right tibia

M87.862   Other osteonecrosis, left tibia

M87.863   Other osteonecrosis, unspecified tibia

M87.864   Other osteonecrosis, right fibula

M87.865   Other osteonecrosis, left fibula

M87.869   Other osteonecrosis, unspecified fibula

M87.87   Other osteonecrosis, ankle, foot and toes

M87.871   Other osteonecrosis, right ankle

M87.872   Other osteonecrosis, left ankle

M87.873   Other osteonecrosis, unspecified ankle

M87.874   Other osteonecrosis, right foot

M87.875   Other osteonecrosis, left foot

M87.876 **Other osteonecrosis, unspecified foot**

M87.877 **Other osteonecrosis, right toe(s)**

M87.878 **Other osteonecrosis, left toe(s)**

M87.879 **Other osteonecrosis, unspecified toe(s)**

M87.88 **Other osteonecrosis, other site**

M87.89 **Other osteonecrosis, multiple sites**

M87.9 **Osteonecrosis, unspecified**

Necrosis of bone NOS

M88 **Osteitis deformans [Paget's disease of bone]**

Definition: Osteitis deformans, aka paget's disease, is a disease of bone occurring in the middle aged and elderly; excessive bone destruction sometimes leading to bone pain and fractures and skeletal deformities.

Excludes1: osteitis deformans in neoplastic disease (M90.6)

M88.0 **Osteitis deformans of skull**

M88.1 **Osteitis deformans of vertebrae**

M88.8 **Osteitis deformans of other bones**

M88.81 **Osteitis deformans of shoulder**

M88.811 **Osteitis deformans of right shoulder**

M88.812 **Osteitis deformans of left shoulder**

M88.819 **Osteitis deformans of unspecified shoulder**

M88.82 **Osteitis deformans of upper arm**

M88.821 **Osteitis deformans of right upper arm**

M88.822 **Osteitis deformans of left upper arm**

M88.829 **Osteitis deformans of unspecified upper arm**

M88.83 **Osteitis deformans of forearm**

M88.831 **Osteitis deformans of right forearm**

M88.832 **Osteitis deformans of left forearm**

M88.839 **Osteitis deformans of unspecified forearm**

M88.84 **Osteitis deformans of hand**

M88.841 **Osteitis deformans of right hand**

M88.842 **Osteitis deformans of left hand**

M88.849 **Osteitis deformans of unspecified hand**

M88.85 **Osteitis deformans of thigh**

M88.851 **Osteitis deformans of right thigh**

M88.852 **Osteitis deformans of left thigh**

M88.859 **Osteitis deformans of unspecified thigh**

M88.86 **Osteitis deformans of lower leg**

M88.861 **Osteitis deformans of right lower leg**

M88.862 **Osteitis deformans of left lower leg**

M88.869 **Osteitis deformans of unspecified lower leg**

M88.87 **Osteitis deformans of ankle and foot**

M88.871 **Osteitis deformans of right ankle and foot**

M88.872 **Osteitis deformans of left ankle and foot**

M88.879 **Osteitis deformans of unspecified ankle and foot**

M88.88 **Osteitis deformans of other bones**

Excludes2: osteitis deformans of skull (M88.0)

osteitis deformans of vertebrae (M88.1)

M88.89 **Osteitis deformans of multiple sites**

M88.9 **Osteitis deformans of unspecified bone**

M89 **Other disorders of bone**

M89.0 **Algoneurodystrophy**

Shoulder-hand syndrome

Sudeck's atrophy

Excludes1: causalgia, lower limb (G57.7-)

causalgia, upper limb (G56.4-)

complex regional pain syndrome II, lower limb (G57.7-)

complex regional pain syndrome II, upper limb (G56.4-)

reflex sympathetic dystrophy (G90.5-)

M89.00 **Algoneurodystrophy, unspecified site**

M89.01 **Algoneurodystrophy, shoulder**

M89.011 **Algoneurodystrophy, right shoulder**

M89.012 **Algoneurodystrophy, left shoulder**

M89.019 **Algoneurodystrophy, unspecified shoulder**

M89.02 **Algoneurodystrophy, upper arm**

M89.021 **Algoneurodystrophy, right upper arm**

M89.022 **Algoneurodystrophy, left upper arm**

M89.029 **Algoneurodystrophy, unspecified upper arm**

M89.03 **Algoneurodystrophy, forearm**

M89.031 **Algoneurodystrophy, right forearm**

M89.032 **Algoneurodystrophy, left forearm**

M89.039 **Algoneurodystrophy, unspecified forearm**

M89.04 **Algoneurodystrophy, hand**

M89.041 **Algoneurodystrophy, right hand**

M89.042 **Algoneurodystrophy, left hand**

M89.049 **Algoneurodystrophy, unspecified hand**

M89.05 **Algoneurodystrophy, thigh**

M89.051 **Algoneurodystrophy, right thigh**

M89.052 **Algoneurodystrophy, left thigh**

M89.059 **Algoneurodystrophy, unspecified thigh**

M89.06 **Algoneurodystrophy, lower leg**

M89.061 **Algoneurodystrophy, right lower leg**

M89.062 **Algoneurodystrophy, left lower leg**

M89.069 **Algoneurodystrophy, unspecified lower leg**

M89.07 **Algoneurodystrophy, ankle and foot**

M89.071 **Algoneurodystrophy, right ankle and foot**

M89.072 **Algoneurodystrophy, left ankle and foot**

• New code   ▲ Revised code   **Excludes1:** Not coded here   **Excludes2:** Not included here   ⊗ Placeholder required   ⑦7th digit required

M89.079 Algoneurodystrophy, unspecified ankle and foot

M89.08 Algoneurodystrophy, other site

M89.09 Algoneurodystrophy, multiple sites

M89.1 **Physeal arrest**
Arrest of growth plate
Epiphyseal arrest
Growth plate arrest

M89.12 **Physeal arrest, humerus**

M89.121 Complete physeal arrest, right proximal humerus

M89.122 Complete physeal arrest, left proximal humerus

M89.123 Partial physeal arrest, right proximal humerus

M89.124 Partial physeal arrest, left proximal humerus

M89.125 Complete physeal arrest, right distal humerus

M89.126 Complete physeal arrest, left distal humerus

M89.127 Partial physeal arrest, right distal humerus

M89.128 Partial physeal arrest, left distal humerus

M89.129 Physeal arrest, humerus, unspecified

M89.13 **Physeal arrest, forearm**

M89.131 Complete physeal arrest, right distal radius

M89.132 Complete physeal arrest, left distal radius

M89.133 Partial physeal arrest, right distal radius

M89.134 Partial physeal arrest, left distal radius

M89.138 Other physeal arrest of forearm

M89.139 Physeal arrest, forearm, unspecified

M89.15 **Physeal arrest, femur**

M89.151 Complete physeal arrest, right proximal femur

M89.152 Complete physeal arrest, left proximal femur

M89.153 Partial physeal arrest, right proximal femur

M89.154 Partial physeal arrest, left proximal femur

M89.155 Complete physeal arrest, right distal femur

M89.156 Complete physeal arrest, left distal femur

M89.157 Partial physeal arrest, right distal femur

M89.158 Partial physeal arrest, left distal femur

M89.159 Physeal arrest, femur, unspecified

M89.16 **Physeal arrest, lower leg**

M89.160 Complete physeal arrest, right proximal tibia

M89.161 Complete physeal arrest, left proximal tibia

M89.162 Partial physeal arrest, right proximal tibia

M89.163 Partial physeal arrest, left proximal tibia

M89.164 Complete physeal arrest, right distal tibia

M89.165 Complete physeal arrest, left distal tibia

M89.166 Partial physeal arrest, right distal tibia

M89.167 Partial physeal arrest, left distal tibia

M89.168 Other physeal arrest of lower leg

M89.169 Physeal arrest, lower leg, unspecified

M89.18 **Physeal arrest, other site**

M89.2 **Other disorders of bone development and growth**

M89.20 Other disorders of bone development and growth, unspecified site

M89.21 Other disorders of bone development and growth, shoulder

M89.211 Other disorders of bone development and growth, right shoulder

M89.212 Other disorders of bone development and growth, left shoulder

M89.219 Other disorders of bone development and growth, unspecified shoulder

M89.22 Other disorders of bone development and growth, humerus

M89.221 Other disorders of bone development and growth, right humerus

M89.222 Other disorders of bone development and growth, left humerus

M89.229 Other disorders of bone development and growth, unspecified humerus

M89.23 Other disorders of bone development and growth, ulna and radius

M89.231 Other disorders of bone development and growth, right ulna

M89.232 Other disorders of bone development and growth, left ulna

M89.233 Other disorders of bone development and growth, right radius

M89.234 Other disorders of bone development and growth, left radius

M89.239 Other disorders of bone development and growth, unspecified ulna and radius

M89.24 Other disorders of bone development and growth, hand

M89.241 Other disorders of bone development and growth, right hand

M89.242 Other disorders of bone development and growth, left hand

M89.249 Other disorders of bone development and growth, unspecified hand

M89.25 Other disorders of bone development and growth, femur

M89.251 Other disorders of bone development and growth, right femur

M89.252 Other disorders of bone development and growth, left femur

M89.259 Other disorders of bone development and growth, unspecified femur

M89.26 Other disorders of bone development and growth, tibia and fibula

M89.261 Other disorders of bone development and growth, right tibia

M89.262 Other disorders of bone development and growth, left tibia

M89.263 Other disorders of bone development and growth, right fibula

M89.264 Other disorders of bone development and growth, left fibula

M89.269 Other disorders of bone development and growth, unspecified lower leg

M89.27 Other disorders of bone development and growth, ankle and foot

M89.271 Other disorders of bone development and growth, right ankle and foot

M89.272 Other disorders of bone development and growth, left ankle and foot

M89.279 Other disorders of bone development and growth, unspecified ankle and foot

M89.28 Other disorders of bone development and growth, other site

M89.29 Other disorders of bone development and growth, multiple sites

M89.3 **Hypertrophy of bone**

M89.30 Hypertrophy of bone, unspecified site

M89.31 Hypertrophy of bone, shoulder

M89.311 Hypertrophy of bone, right shoulder

M89.312 Hypertrophy of bone, left shoulder

M89.319 Hypertrophy of bone, unspecified shoulder

M89.32 Hypertrophy of bone, humerus

M89.321 Hypertrophy of bone, right humerus

M89.322 Hypertrophy of bone, left humerus

M89.329 Hypertrophy of bone, unspecified humerus

M89.33 Hypertrophy of bone, ulna and radius

M89.331 Hypertrophy of bone, right ulna

M89.332 Hypertrophy of bone, left ulna

M89.333 Hypertrophy of bone, right radius

M89.334 Hypertrophy of bone, left radius

M89.339 Hypertrophy of bone, unspecified ulna and radius

M89.34 Hypertrophy of bone, hand

M89.341 Hypertrophy of bone, right hand

M89.342 Hypertrophy of bone, left hand

M89.349 Hypertrophy of bone, unspecified hand

M89.35 Hypertrophy of bone, femur

M89.351 Hypertrophy of bone, right femur

M89.352 Hypertrophy of bone, left femur

M89.359 Hypertrophy of bone, unspecified femur

M89.36 Hypertrophy of bone, tibia and fibula

M89.361 Hypertrophy of bone, right tibia

M89.362 Hypertrophy of bone, left tibia

M89.363 Hypertrophy of bone, right fibula

M89.364 Hypertrophy of bone, left fibula

M89.369 Hypertrophy of bone, unspecified tibia and fibula

M89.37 Hypertrophy of bone, ankle and foot

M89.371 Hypertrophy of bone, right ankle and foot

M89.372 Hypertrophy of bone, left ankle and foot

M89.379 Hypertrophy of bone, unspecified ankle and foot

M89.38 Hypertrophy of bone, other site

M89.39 Hypertrophy of bone, multiple sites

M89.4 **Other hypertrophic osteoarthropathy**

Marie-Bamberger disease

Pachydermoperiostosis

M89.40 Other hypertrophic osteoarthropathy, unspecified site

M89.41 Other hypertrophic osteoarthropathy, shoulder

M89.411 Other hypertrophic osteoarthropathy, right shoulder

M89.412 Other hypertrophic osteoarthropathy, left shoulder

M89.419 Other hypertrophic osteoarthropathy, unspecified shoulder

M89.42 Other hypertrophic osteoarthropathy, upper arm

M89.421 Other hypertrophic osteoarthropathy, right upper arm

M89.422 Other hypertrophic osteoarthropathy, left upper arm

M89.429 Other hypertrophic osteoarthropathy, unspecified upper arm

M89.43 Other hypertrophic osteoarthropathy, forearm

M89.431 Other hypertrophic osteoarthropathy, right forearm

M89.432 Other hypertrophic osteoarthropathy, left forearm

M89.439 Other hypertrophic osteoarthropathy, unspecified forearm

M89.44 Other hypertrophic osteoarthropathy, hand

M89.441 Other hypertrophic osteoarthropathy, right hand

M89.442 Other hypertrophic osteoarthropathy, left hand

M89.449 Other hypertrophic osteoarthropathy, unspecified hand

M89.45 Other hypertrophic osteoarthropathy, thigh

M89.451 Other hypertrophic osteoarthropathy, right thigh

M89.452 Other hypertrophic osteoarthropathy, left thigh

M89.459 Other hypertrophic osteoarthropathy, unspecified thigh

M89.46 Other hypertrophic osteoarthropathy, lower leg

M89.461 Other hypertrophic osteoarthropathy, right lower leg

M89.462 Other hypertrophic osteoarthropathy, left lower leg

M89.469 Other hypertrophic osteoarthropathy, unspecified lower leg

M89.47 Other hypertrophic osteoarthropathy, ankle and foot

M89.471 Other hypertrophic osteoarthropathy, right ankle and foot

M89.472 Other hypertrophic osteoarthropathy, left ankle and foot

M89.479 Other hypertrophic osteoarthropathy, unspecified ankle and foot

M89.48 Other hypertrophic osteoarthropathy, other site

M89.49 Other hypertrophic osteoarthropathy, multiple sites

M89.5 Osteolysis

Use additional code to identify major osseous defect, if applicable (M89.7-)

Excludes2: periprosthetic osteolysis of internal prosthetic joint (T84.05-)

M89.50 Osteolysis, unspecified site

M89.51 Osteolysis, shoulder

M89.511 Osteolysis, right shoulder

M89.512 Osteolysis, left shoulder

M89.519 Osteolysis, unspecified shoulder

M89.52 Osteolysis, upper arm

M89.521 Osteolysis, right upper arm

M89.522 Osteolysis, left upper arm

M89.529 Osteolysis, unspecified upper arm

M89.53 Osteolysis, forearm

M89.531 Osteolysis, right forearm

M89.532 Osteolysis, left forearm

M89.539 Osteolysis, unspecified forearm

M89.54 Osteolysis, hand

M89.541 Osteolysis, right hand

M89.542 Osteolysis, left hand

M89.549 Osteolysis, unspecified hand

M89.55 Osteolysis, thigh

M89.551 Osteolysis, right thigh

M89.552 Osteolysis, left thigh

M89.559 Osteolysis, unspecified thigh

M89.56 Osteolysis, lower leg

M89.561 Osteolysis, right lower leg

M89.562 Osteolysis, left lower leg

M89.569 Osteolysis, unspecified lower leg

M89.57 Osteolysis, ankle and foot

M89.571 Osteolysis, right ankle and foot

M89.572 Osteolysis, left ankle and foot

M89.579 Osteolysis, unspecified ankle and foot

M89.58 Osteolysis, other site

M89.59 Osteolysis, multiple sites

M89.6 Osteopathy after poliomyelitis

Use additional code (B91) to identify previous poliomyelitis

Excludes1: postpolio syndrome (G14)

M89.60 Osteopathy after poliomyelitis, unspecified site

M89.61 Osteopathy after poliomyelitis, shoulder

M89.611 Osteopathy after poliomyelitis, right shoulder

M89.612 Osteopathy after poliomyelitis, left shoulder

M89.619 Osteopathy after poliomyelitis, unspecified shoulder

M89.62 Osteopathy after poliomyelitis, upper arm

M89.621 Osteopathy after poliomyelitis, right upper arm

M89.622 Osteopathy after poliomyelitis, left upper arm

M89.629 Osteopathy after poliomyelitis, unspecified upper arm

M89.63 Osteopathy after poliomyelitis, forearm

M89.631 Osteopathy after poliomyelitis, right forearm

M89.632 Osteopathy after poliomyelitis, left forearm

M89.639 Osteopathy after poliomyelitis, unspecified forearm

M89.64 Osteopathy after poliomyelitis, hand

M89.641 Osteopathy after poliomyelitis, right hand

M89.642 Osteopathy after poliomyelitis, left hand

M89.649 Osteopathy after poliomyelitis, unspecified hand

M89.65 Osteopathy after poliomyelitis, thigh

M89.651 Osteopathy after poliomyelitis, right thigh

M89.652 Osteopathy after poliomyelitis, left thigh

M89.659 Osteopathy after poliomyelitis, unspecified thigh

M89.66 Osteopathy after poliomyelitis, lower leg

   M89.661 Osteopathy after poliomyelitis, right lower leg

   M89.662 Osteopathy after poliomyelitis, left lower leg

   M89.669 Osteopathy after poliomyelitis, unspecified lower leg

M89.67 Osteopathy after poliomyelitis, ankle and foot

   M89.671 Osteopathy after poliomyelitis, right ankle and foot

   M89.672 Osteopathy after poliomyelitis, left ankle and foot

   M89.679 Osteopathy after poliomyelitis, unspecified ankle and foot

M89.68 Osteopathy after poliomyelitis, other site

M89.69 Osteopathy after poliomyelitis, multiple sites

M89.7 **Major osseous defect**

  <u>Code first</u> underlying disease, if known, such as:

     aseptic necrosis of bone (M87.-)

     malignant neoplasm of bone (C40.-)

     osteolysis (M89.5)

     osteomyelitis (M86.-)

     osteonecrosis (M87.-)

     osteoporosis (M80.-, M81.-)

     periprosthetic osteolysis (T84.05-)

M89.70 Major osseous defect, unspecified site

M89.71 Major osseous defect, shoulder region

  Major osseous defect clavicle or scapula

   M89.711 Major osseous defect, right shoulder region

   M89.712 Major osseous defect, left shoulder region

   M89.719 Major osseous defect, unspecified shoulder region

M89.72 Major osseous defect, humerus

   M89.721 Major osseous defect, right humerus

   M89.722 Major osseous defect, left humerus

   M89.729 Major osseous defect, unspecified humerus

M89.73 Major osseous defect, forearm

  Major osseous defect of radius and ulna

   M89.731 Major osseous defect, right forearm

   M89.732 Major osseous defect, left forearm

   M89.739 Major osseous defect, unspecified forearm

M89.74 Major osseous defect, hand

  Major osseous defect of carpus, fingers, metacarpus

   M89.741 Major osseous defect, right hand

   M89.742 Major osseous defect, left hand

   M89.749 Major osseous defect, unspecified hand

M89.75 Major osseous defect, pelvic region and thigh

  Major osseous defect of femur and pelvis

   M89.751 Major osseous defect, right pelvic region and thigh

   M89.752 Major osseous defect, left pelvic region and thigh

   M89.759 Major osseous defect, unspecified pelvic region and thigh

M89.76 Major osseous defect, lower leg

  Major osseous defect of fibula and tibia

   M89.761 Major osseous defect, right lower leg

   M89.762 Major osseous defect, left lower leg

   M89.769 Major osseous defect, unspecified lower leg

M89.77 Major osseous defect, ankle and foot

  Major osseous defect of metatarsus, tarsus, toes

   M89.771 Major osseous defect, right ankle and foot

   M89.772 Major osseous defect, left ankle and foot

   M89.779 Major osseous defect, unspecified ankle and foot

M89.78 Major osseous defect, other site

M89.79 Major osseous defect, multiple sites

M89.8 **Other specified disorders of bone**

  Infantile cortical hyperostoses

  Post-traumatic subperiosteal ossification

M89.8X Other specified disorders of bone

   M89.8X0 Other specified disorders of bone, multiple sites

   M89.8X1 Other specified disorders of bone, shoulder

   M89.8X2 Other specified disorders of bone, upper arm

   M89.8X3 Other specified disorders of bone, forearm

   M89.8X4 Other specified disorders of bone, hand

   M89.8X5 Other specified disorders of bone, thigh

   M89.8X6 Other specified disorders of bone, lower leg

   M89.8X7 Other specified disorders of bone, ankle and foot

   M89.8X8 Other specified disorders of bone, other site

   M89.8X9 Other specified disorders of bone, unspecified site

M89.9 **Disorder of bone, unspecified**

M90 **Osteopathies in diseases classified elsewhere**

  Excludes1: osteochondritis, osteomyelitis, and osteopathy (in):

     cryptococcosis (B45.3)

     diabetes mellitus (E08-E13 with .69-)

     gonococcal (A54.43)

     neurogenic syphilis (A52.11)

     renal osteodystrophy (N25.0)

     salmonellosis (A02.24)

     secondary syphilis (A51.46)

     syphilis (late) (A52.77)

M90.5 **Osteonecrosis in diseases classified elsewhere**

  <u>Code first</u> underlying disease, such as:

caisson disease (T70.3)

hemoglobinopathy (D50-D64)

M90.50 Osteonecrosis in diseases classified elsewhere, unspecified site

M90.51 Osteonecrosis in diseases classified elsewhere, shoulder

M90.511 Osteonecrosis in diseases classified elsewhere, right shoulder

M90.512 Osteonecrosis in diseases classified elsewhere, left shoulder

M90.519 Osteonecrosis in diseases classified elsewhere, unspecified shoulder

M90.52 Osteonecrosis in diseases classified elsewhere, upper arm

M90.521 Osteonecrosis in diseases classified elsewhere, right upper arm

M90.522 Osteonecrosis in diseases classified elsewhere, left upper arm

M90.529 Osteonecrosis in diseases classified elsewhere, unspecified upper arm

M90.53 Osteonecrosis in diseases classified elsewhere, forearm

M90.531 Osteonecrosis in diseases classified elsewhere, right forearm

M90.532 Osteonecrosis in diseases classified elsewhere, left forearm

M90.539 Osteonecrosis in diseases classified elsewhere, unspecified forearm

M90.54 Osteonecrosis in diseases classified elsewhere, hand

M90.541 Osteonecrosis in diseases classified elsewhere, right hand

M90.542 Osteonecrosis in diseases classified elsewhere, left hand

M90.549 Osteonecrosis in diseases classified elsewhere, unspecified hand

M90.55 Osteonecrosis in diseases classified elsewhere, thigh

M90.551 Osteonecrosis in diseases classified elsewhere, right thigh

M90.552 Osteonecrosis in diseases classified elsewhere, left thigh

M90.559 Osteonecrosis in diseases classified elsewhere, unspecified thigh

M90.56 Osteonecrosis in diseases classified elsewhere, lower leg

M90.561 Osteonecrosis in diseases classified elsewhere, right lower leg

M90.562 Osteonecrosis in diseases classified elsewhere, left lower leg

M90.569 Osteonecrosis in diseases classified elsewhere, unspecified lower leg

M90.57 Osteonecrosis in diseases classified elsewhere, ankle and foot

M90.571 Osteonecrosis in diseases classified elsewhere, right ankle and foot

M90.572 Osteonecrosis in diseases classified elsewhere, left ankle and foot

M90.579 Osteonecrosis in diseases classified elsewhere, unspecified ankle and foot

M90.58 Osteonecrosis in diseases classified elsewhere, other site

M90.59 Osteonecrosis in diseases classified elsewhere, multiple sites

M90.6 Osteitis deformans in neoplastic diseases

Osteitis deformans in malignant neoplasm of bone

<u>Code first</u> the neoplasm (C40.-, C41.-)

Excludes1: osteitis deformans [Paget's disease of bone] (M88.-)

M90.60 Osteitis deformans in neoplastic diseases, unspecified site

M90.61 Osteitis deformans in neoplastic diseases, shoulder

M90.611 Osteitis deformans in neoplastic diseases, right shoulder

M90.612 Osteitis deformans in neoplastic diseases, left shoulder

M90.619 Osteitis deformans in neoplastic diseases, unspecified shoulder

M90.62 Osteitis deformans in neoplastic diseases, upper arm

M90.621 Osteitis deformans in neoplastic diseases, right upper arm

M90.622 Osteitis deformans in neoplastic diseases, left upper arm

M90.629 Osteitis deformans in neoplastic diseases, unspecified upper arm

M90.63 Osteitis deformans in neoplastic diseases, forearm

M90.631 Osteitis deformans in neoplastic diseases, right forearm

M90.632 Osteitis deformans in neoplastic diseases, left forearm

M90.639 Osteitis deformans in neoplastic diseases, unspecified forearm

M90.64 Osteitis deformans in neoplastic diseases, hand

M90.641 Osteitis deformans in neoplastic diseases, right hand

M90.642 Osteitis deformans in neoplastic diseases, left hand

M90.649 Osteitis deformans in neoplastic diseases, unspecified hand

M90.65 Osteitis deformans in neoplastic diseases, thigh

M90.651 Osteitis deformans in neoplastic diseases, right thigh

M90.652 Osteitis deformans in neoplastic diseases, left thigh

M90.659 Osteitis deformans in neoplastic diseases, unspecified thigh

M90.66 Osteitis deformans in neoplastic diseases, lower leg

M90.661 Osteitis deformans in neoplastic diseases, right lower leg

M90.662 Osteitis deformans in neoplastic diseases, left lower leg

M90.669 Osteitis deformans in neoplastic diseases, unspecified lower leg

M90.67 Osteitis deformans in neoplastic diseases, ankle and foot

M90.671 Osteitis deformans in neoplastic diseases, right ankle and foot

M90.672　Osteitis deformans in neoplastic diseases, left ankle and foot

M90.679　Osteitis deformans in neoplastic diseases, unspecified ankle and foot

M90.68　Osteitis deformans in neoplastic diseases, other site

M90.69　Osteitis deformans in neoplastic diseases, multiple sites

M90.8　Osteopathy in diseases classified elsewhere

<u>Code first</u> underlying disease, such as:

rickets (E55.0)

vitamin-D-resistant rickets (E83.3)

M90.80　Osteopathy in diseases classified elsewhere, unspecified site

M90.81　Osteopathy in diseases classified elsewhere, shoulder

M90.811　Osteopathy in diseases classified elsewhere, right shoulder

M90.812　Osteopathy in diseases classified elsewhere, left shoulder

M90.819　Osteopathy in diseases classified elsewhere, unspecified shoulder

M90.82　Osteopathy in diseases classified elsewhere, upper arm

M90.821　Osteopathy in diseases classified elsewhere, right upper arm

M90.822　Osteopathy in diseases classified elsewhere, left upper arm

M90.829　Osteopathy in diseases classified elsewhere, unspecified upper arm

M90.83　Osteopathy in diseases classified elsewhere, forearm

M90.831　Osteopathy in diseases classified elsewhere, right forearm

M90.832　Osteopathy in diseases classified elsewhere, left forearm

M90.839　Osteopathy in diseases classified elsewhere, unspecified forearm

M90.84　Osteopathy in diseases classified elsewhere, hand

M90.841　Osteopathy in diseases classified elsewhere, right hand

M90.842　Osteopathy in diseases classified elsewhere, left hand

M90.849　Osteopathy in diseases classified elsewhere, unspecified hand

M90.85　Osteopathy in diseases classified elsewhere, thigh

M90.851　Osteopathy in diseases classified elsewhere, right thigh

M90.852　Osteopathy in diseases classified elsewhere, left thigh

M90.859　Osteopathy in diseases classified elsewhere, unspecified thigh

M90.86　Osteopathy in diseases classified elsewhere, lower leg

M90.861　Osteopathy in diseases classified elsewhere, right lower leg

M90.862　Osteopathy in diseases classified elsewhere, left lower leg

M90.869　Osteopathy in diseases classified elsewhere, unspecified lower leg

M90.87　Osteopathy in diseases classified elsewhere, ankle and foot

M90.871　Osteopathy in diseases classified elsewhere, right ankle and foot

M90.872　Osteopathy in diseases classified elsewhere, left ankle and foot

M90.879　Osteopathy in diseases classified elsewhere, unspecified ankle and foot

M90.88　Osteopathy in diseases classified elsewhere, other site

M90.89　Osteopathy in diseases classified elsewhere, multiple sites

CHONDROPATHIES (M91-M94)

Excludes1: postprocedural chondropathies (M96.-)

M91　Juvenile osteochondrosis of hip and pelvis

Excludes1: slipped upper femoral epiphysis (nontraumatic) (M93.0)

M91.0　Juvenile osteochondrosis of pelvis

Osteochondrosis (juvenile) of acetabulum

Osteochondrosis (juvenile) of iliac crest [Buchanan]

Osteochondrosis (juvenile) of ischiopubic synchondrosis [van Neck]

Osteochondrosis (juvenile) of symphysis pubis [Pierson]

M91.1　Juvenile osteochondrosis of head of femur [Legg-Calvé-Perthes]

M91.10　Juvenile osteochondrosis of head of femur [Legg-Calvé-Perthes], unspecified leg

M91.11　Juvenile osteochondrosis of head of femur [Legg-Calvé-Perthes], right leg

M91.12　Juvenile osteochondrosis of head of femur [Legg-Calvé-Perthes], left leg

M91.2　Coxa plana

Hip deformity due to previous juvenile osteochondrosis

M91.20　Coxa plana, unspecified hip

M91.21　Coxa plana, right hip

M91.22　Coxa plana, left hip

M91.3　Pseudocoxalgia

M91.30　Pseudocoxalgia, unspecified hip

M91.31　Pseudocoxalgia, right hip

M91.32　Pseudocoxalgia, left hip

M91.4　Coxa magna

M91.40　Coxa magna, unspecified hip

M91.41　Coxa magna, right hip

M91.42　Coxa magna, left hip

M91.8　Other juvenile osteochondrosis of hip and pelvis

Juvenile osteochondrosis after reduction of congenital dislocation of hip

M91.80　Other juvenile osteochondrosis of hip and pelvis, unspecified leg

M91.81　Other juvenile osteochondrosis of hip and pelvis, right leg

M91.82　Other juvenile osteochondrosis of hip and pelvis, left leg

M91.9　Juvenile osteochondrosis of hip and pelvis, unspecified

---

　● New code　▲ Revised code　**Excludes1:** Not coded here　**Excludes2:** Not included here　⊗ Placeholder required　⑦7th digit required

M91.90 Juvenile osteochondrosis of hip and pelvis, unspecified, unspecified leg

M91.91 Juvenile osteochondrosis of hip and pelvis, unspecified, right leg

M91.92 Juvenile osteochondrosis of hip and pelvis, unspecified, left leg

M92 **Other juvenile osteochondrosis**

M92.0 **Juvenile osteochondrosis of humerus**

Osteochondrosis (juvenile) of capitulum of humerus [Panner]

Osteochondrosis (juvenile) of head of humerus [Haas]

M92.00 Juvenile osteochondrosis of humerus, unspecified arm

M92.01 Juvenile osteochondrosis of humerus, right arm

M92.02 Juvenile osteochondrosis of humerus, left arm

M92.1 **Juvenile osteochondrosis of radius and ulna**

Osteochondrosis (juvenile) of lower ulna [Burns]

Osteochondrosis (juvenile) of radial head [Brailsford]

M92.10 Juvenile osteochondrosis of radius and ulna, unspecified arm

M92.11 Juvenile osteochondrosis of radius and ulna, right arm

M92.12 Juvenile osteochondrosis of radius and ulna, left arm

M92.2 **Juvenile osteochondrosis, hand**

M92.20 Unspecified juvenile osteochondrosis, hand

M92.201 Unspecified juvenile osteochondrosis, right hand

M92.202 Unspecified juvenile osteochondrosis, left hand

M92.209 Unspecified juvenile osteochondrosis, unspecified hand

M92.21 Osteochondrosis (juvenile) of carpal lunate [Kienböck]

M92.211 Osteochondrosis (juvenile) of carpal lunate [Kienböck], right hand

M92.212 Osteochondrosis (juvenile) of carpal lunate [Kienböck], left hand

M92.219 Osteochondrosis (juvenile) of carpal lunate [Kienböck], unspecified hand

M92.22 Osteochondrosis (juvenile) of metacarpal heads [Mauclaire]

M92.221 Osteochondrosis (juvenile) of metacarpal heads [Mauclaire], right hand

M92.222 Osteochondrosis (juvenile) of metacarpal heads [Mauclaire], left hand

M92.229 Osteochondrosis (juvenile) of metacarpal heads [Mauclaire], unspecified hand

M92.29 Other juvenile osteochondrosis, hand

M92.291 Other juvenile osteochondrosis, right hand

M92.292 Other juvenile osteochondrosis, left hand

M92.299 Other juvenile osteochondrosis, unspecified hand

M92.3 **Other juvenile osteochondrosis, upper limb**

M92.30 Other juvenile osteochondrosis, unspecified upper limb

M92.31 Other juvenile osteochondrosis, right upper limb

M92.32 Other juvenile osteochondrosis, left upper limb

M92.4 **Juvenile osteochondrosis of patella**

Osteochondrosis (juvenile) of primary patellar center [Köhler]

Osteochondrosis (juvenile) of secondary patellar centre [Sinding Larsen]

M92.40 Juvenile osteochondrosis of patella, unspecified knee

M92.41 Juvenile osteochondrosis of patella, right knee

M92.42 Juvenile osteochondrosis of patella, left knee

M92.5 **Juvenile osteochondrosis of tibia and fibula**

Osteochondrosis (juvenile) of proximal tibia [Blount]

Osteochondrosis (juvenile) of tibial tubercle [Osgood-Schlatter]

Tibia vara

M92.50 Juvenile osteochondrosis of tibia and fibula, unspecified leg

M92.51 Juvenile osteochondrosis of tibia and fibula, right leg

M92.52 Juvenile osteochondrosis of tibia and fibula, left leg

M92.6 **Juvenile osteochondrosis of tarsus**

Osteochondrosis (juvenile) of calcaneum [Sever]

Osteochondrosis (juvenile) of os tibiale externum [Haglund]

Osteochondrosis (juvenile) of talus [Diaz]

Osteochondrosis (juvenile) of tarsal navicular [Köhler]

M92.60 Juvenile osteochondrosis of tarsus, unspecified ankle

M92.61 Juvenile osteochondrosis of tarsus, right ankle

M92.62 Juvenile osteochondrosis of tarsus, left ankle

M92.7 **Juvenile osteochondrosis of metatarsus**

Osteochondrosis (juvenile) of fifth metatarsus [Iselin]

Osteochondrosis (juvenile) of second metatarsus [Freiberg]

M92.70 Juvenile osteochondrosis of metatarsus, unspecified foot

M92.71 Juvenile osteochondrosis of metatarsus, right foot

M92.72 Juvenile osteochondrosis of metatarsus, left foot

M92.8 **Other specified juvenile osteochondrosis**

Calcaneal apophysitis

M92.9 **Juvenile osteochondrosis, unspecified**

Juvenile apophysitis NOS

Juvenile epiphysitis NOS

Juvenile osteochondritis NOS

Juvenile osteochondrosis NOS

M93 **Other osteochondropathies**

Excludes2: osteochondrosis of spine (M42.-)

M93.0 **Slipped upper femoral epiphysis (nontraumatic)**

Use additional code for associated chondrolysis (M94.3)

M93.00 Unspecified slipped upper femoral epiphysis (nontraumatic)

M93.001   **Unspecified slipped upper femoral epiphysis (nontraumatic), right hip**

M93.002   **Unspecified slipped upper femoral epiphysis (nontraumatic), left hip**

M93.003   **Unspecified slipped upper femoral epiphysis (nontraumatic), unspecified hip**

M93.01   **Acute slipped upper femoral epiphysis (nontraumatic)**

M93.011   **Acute slipped upper femoral epiphysis (nontraumatic), right hip**

M93.012   **Acute slipped upper femoral epiphysis (nontraumatic), left hip**

M93.013   **Acute slipped upper femoral epiphysis (nontraumatic), unspecified hip**

M93.02   **Chronic slipped upper femoral epiphysis (nontraumatic)**

M93.021   **Chronic slipped upper femoral epiphysis (nontraumatic), right hip**

M93.022   **Chronic slipped upper femoral epiphysis (nontraumatic), left hip**

M93.023   **Chronic slipped upper femoral epiphysis (nontraumatic), unspecified hip**

M93.03   **Acute on chronic slipped upper femoral epiphysis (nontraumatic)**

M93.031   **Acute on chronic slipped upper femoral epiphysis (nontraumatic), right hip**

M93.032   **Acute on chronic slipped upper femoral epiphysis (nontraumatic), left hip**

M93.033   **Acute on chronic slipped upper femoral epiphysis (nontraumatic), unspecified hip**

M93.1   **Kienböck's disease of adults**

Adult osteochondrosis of carpal lunates

M93.2   **Osteochondritis dissecans**

M93.20   **Osteochondritis dissecans of unspecified site**

M93.21   **Osteochondritis dissecans of shoulder**

M93.211   **Osteochondritis dissecans, right shoulder**

M93.212   **Osteochondritis dissecans, left shoulder**

M93.219   **Osteochondritis dissecans, unspecified shoulder**

M93.22   **Osteochondritis dissecans of elbow**

M93.221   **Osteochondritis dissecans, right elbow**

M93.222   **Osteochondritis dissecans, left elbow**

M93.229   **Osteochondritis dissecans, unspecified elbow**

M93.23   **Osteochondritis dissecans of wrist**

M93.231   **Osteochondritis dissecans, right wrist**

M93.232   **Osteochondritis dissecans, left wrist**

M93.239   **Osteochondritis dissecans, unspecified wrist**

M93.24   **Osteochondritis dissecans of joints of hand**

M93.241   **Osteochondritis dissecans, joints of right hand**

M93.242   **Osteochondritis dissecans, joints of left hand**

M93.249   **Osteochondritis dissecans, joints of unspecified hand**

M93.25   **Osteochondritis dissecans of hip**

M93.251   **Osteochondritis dissecans, right hip**

M93.252   **Osteochondritis dissecans, left hip**

M93.259   **Osteochondritis dissecans, unspecified hip**

M93.26   **Osteochondritis dissecans knee**

M93.261   **Osteochondritis dissecans, right knee**

M93.262   **Osteochondritis dissecans, left knee**

M93.269   **Osteochondritis dissecans, unspecified knee**

M93.27   **Osteochondritis dissecans of ankle and joints of foot**

M93.271   **Osteochondritis dissecans, right ankle and joints of right foot**

M93.272   **Osteochondritis dissecans, left ankle and joints of left foot**

M93.279   **Osteochondritis dissecans, unspecified ankle and joints of foot**

M93.28   **Osteochondritis dissecans other site**

M93.29   **Osteochondritis dissecans multiple sites**

M93.8   **Other specified osteochondropathies**

M93.80   **Other specified osteochondropathies of unspecified site**

M93.81   **Other specified osteochondropathies of shoulder**

M93.811   **Other specified osteochondropathies, right shoulder**

M93.812   **Other specified osteochondropathies, left shoulder**

M93.819   **Other specified osteochondropathies, unspecified shoulder**

M93.82   **Other specified osteochondropathies of upper arm**

M93.821   **Other specified osteochondropathies, right upper arm**

M93.822   **Other specified osteochondropathies, left upper arm**

M93.829   **Other specified osteochondropathies, unspecified upper arm**

M93.83   **Other specified osteochondropathies of forearm**

M93.831   **Other specified osteochondropathies, right forearm**

M93.832   **Other specified osteochondropathies, left forearm**

M93.839   **Other specified osteochondropathies, unspecified forearm**

M93.84   **Other specified osteochondropathies of hand**

M93.841   **Other specified osteochondropathies, right hand**

M93.842 Other specified osteochondropathies, left hand

M93.849 Other specified osteochondropathies, unspecified hand

M93.85 Other specified osteochondropathies of thigh

M93.851 Other specified osteochondropathies, right thigh

M93.852 Other specified osteochondropathies, left thigh

M93.859 Other specified osteochondropathies, unspecified thigh

M93.86 Other specified osteochondropathies lower leg

M93.861 Other specified osteochondropathies, right lower leg

M93.862 Other specified osteochondropathies, left lower leg

M93.869 Other specified osteochondropathies, unspecified lower leg

M93.87 Other specified osteochondropathies of ankle and foot

M93.871 Other specified osteochondropathies, right ankle and foot

M93.872 Other specified osteochondropathies, left ankle and foot

M93.879 Other specified osteochondropathies, unspecified ankle and foot

M93.88 Other specified osteochondropathies other

M93.89 Other specified osteochondropathies multiple sites

M93.9 Osteochondropathy, unspecified

Apophysitis NOS

Epiphysitis NOS

Osteochondritis NOS

Osteochondrosis NOS

M93.90 Osteochondropathy, unspecified of unspecified site

M93.91 Osteochondropathy, unspecified of shoulder

M93.911 Osteochondropathy, unspecified, right shoulder

M93.912 Osteochondropathy, unspecified, left shoulder

M93.919 Osteochondropathy, unspecified, unspecified shoulder

M93.92 Osteochondropathy, unspecified of upper arm

M93.921 Osteochondropathy, unspecified, right upper arm

M93.922 Osteochondropathy, unspecified, left upper arm

M93.929 Osteochondropathy, unspecified, unspecified upper arm

M93.93 Osteochondropathy, unspecified of forearm

M93.931 Osteochondropathy, unspecified, right forearm

M93.932 Osteochondropathy, unspecified, left forearm

M93.939 Osteochondropathy, unspecified, unspecified forearm

M93.94 Osteochondropathy, unspecified of hand

M93.941 Osteochondropathy, unspecified, right hand

M93.942 Osteochondropathy, unspecified, left hand

M93.949 Osteochondropathy, unspecified, unspecified hand

M93.95 Osteochondropathy, unspecified of thigh

M93.951 Osteochondropathy, unspecified, right thigh

M93.952 Osteochondropathy, unspecified, left thigh

M93.959 Osteochondropathy, unspecified, unspecified thigh

M93.96 Osteochondropathy, unspecified lower leg

M93.961 Osteochondropathy, unspecified, right lower leg

M93.962 Osteochondropathy, unspecified, left lower leg

M93.969 Osteochondropathy, unspecified, unspecified lower leg

M93.97 Osteochondropathy, unspecified of ankle and foot

M93.971 Osteochondropathy, unspecified, right ankle and foot

M93.972 Osteochondropathy, unspecified, left ankle and foot

M93.979 Osteochondropathy, unspecified, unspecified ankle and foot

M93.98 Osteochondropathy, unspecified other

M93.99 Osteochondropathy, unspecified multiple sites

M94 Other disorders of cartilage

M94.0 Chondrocostal junction syndrome [Tietze]

Costochondritis

M94.1 Relapsing polychondritis

M94.2 Chondromalacia

Excludes1: chondromalacia patellae (M22.4)

M94.20 Chondromalacia, unspecified site

M94.21 Chondromalacia, shoulder

M94.211 Chondromalacia, right shoulder

M94.212 Chondromalacia, left shoulder

M94.219 Chondromalacia, unspecified shoulder

M94.22 Chondromalacia, elbow

M94.221 Chondromalacia, right elbow

M94.222 Chondromalacia, left elbow

M94.229 Chondromalacia, unspecified elbow

M94.23 Chondromalacia, wrist

M94.231 Chondromalacia, right wrist

M94.232 Chondromalacia, left wrist

M94.239 Chondromalacia, unspecified wrist

M94.24 Chondromalacia, joints of hand

M94.241 Chondromalacia, joints of right hand

M94.242 Chondromalacia, joints of left hand

M94.249 Chondromalacia, joints of unspecified hand

M94.25 Chondromalacia, hip

M94.251 Chondromalacia, right hip

M94.252 Chondromalacia, left hip

M94.259 Chondromalacia, unspecified hip

M94.26 Chondromalacia, knee

M94.261 Chondromalacia, right knee

M94.262 Chondromalacia, left knee

M94.269 Chondromalacia, unspecified knee

M94.27 Chondromalacia, ankle and joints of foot

M94.271 Chondromalacia, right ankle and joints of right foot

M94.272 Chondromalacia, left ankle and joints of left foot

M94.279 Chondromalacia, unspecified ankle and joints of foot

M94.28 Chondromalacia, other site

M94.29 Chondromalacia, multiple sites

M94.3 Chondrolysis

Code first any associated slipped upper femoral epiphysis (nontraumatic) (M93.0-)

M94.35 Chondrolysis, hip

M94.351 Chondrolysis, right hip

M94.352 Chondrolysis, left hip

M94.359 Chondrolysis, unspecified hip

M94.8 Other specified disorders of cartilage

M94.8X Other specified disorders of cartilage

M94.8X0 Other specified disorders of cartilage, multiple sites

M94.8X1 Other specified disorders of cartilage, shoulder

M94.8X2 Other specified disorders of cartilage, upper arm

M94.8X3 Other specified disorders of cartilage, forearm

M94.8X4 Other specified disorders of cartilage, hand

M94.8X5 Other specified disorders of cartilage, thigh

M94.8X6 Other specified disorders of cartilage, lower leg

M94.8X7 Other specified disorders of cartilage, ankle and foot

M94.8X8 Other specified disorders of cartilage, other site

M94.8X9 Other specified disorders of cartilage, unspecified sites

M94.9 Disorder of cartilage, unspecified

OTHER DISORDERS OF THE MUSCULOSKELETAL SYSTEM AND CONNECTIVE TISSUE (M95)

M95 Other acquired deformities of musculoskeletal system and connective tissue

Excludes2: acquired absence of limbs and organs (Z89-Z90)

acquired deformities of limbs (M20-M21)

congenital malformations and deformations of the musculoskeletal system (Q65-Q79)

deforming dorsopathies (M40-M43)

dentofacial anomalies [including malocclusion] (M26.-)

postprocedural musculoskeletal disorders (M96.-)

M95.0 Acquired deformity of nose

Excludes2: deviated nasal septum (J34.2)

M95.1 Cauliflower ear

Excludes2: Other acquired deformities of ear (H61.1)

M95.10 Cauliflower ear, unspecified ear

M95.11 Cauliflower ear, right ear

M95.12 Cauliflower ear, left ear

M95.2 Other acquired deformity of head

M95.3 Acquired deformity of neck

M95.4 Acquired deformity of chest and rib

M95.5 Acquired deformity of pelvis

Excludes1: maternal care for known or suspected disproportion (O33.-)

M95.8 Other specified acquired deformities of musculoskeletal system

M95.9 Acquired deformity of musculoskeletal system, unspecified

INTRAOPERATIVE AND POSTPROCEDURAL COMPLICATIONS AND DISORDERS OF MUSCULOSKELETAL SYSTEM, NOT ELSEWHERE CLASSIFIED (M96)

M96 Intraoperative and postprocedural complications and disorders of musculoskeletal system, not elsewhere classified

Excludes2: arthropathy following intestinal bypass (M02.0-)

complications of internal orthopedic prosthetic devices, implants and grafts (T84.-)

disorders associated with osteoporosis (M80)

periprosthetic fracture around internal prosthetic joint (M97.-)

presence of functional implants **and other** devices (Z96-Z97)

M96.0 Pseudarthrosis after fusion or arthrodesis

M96.1 Postlaminectomy syndrome, not elsewhere classified

M96.2 Postradiation kyphosis

M96.3 Postlaminectomy kyphosis

M96.4 Postsurgical lordosis

M96.5 Postradiation scoliosis

M96.6 Fracture of bone following insertion of orthopedic implant, joint prosthesis, or bone plate

Intraoperative fracture of bone during insertion of orthopedic implant, joint prosthesis, or bone plate

Excludes2: complication of internal orthopedic devices, implants or grafts (T84.-)

M96.62 Fracture of humerus following insertion of orthopedic implant, joint prosthesis, or bone plate

M96.621 Fracture of humerus following insertion of orthopedic implant, joint prosthesis, or bone plate, right arm

M96.622 Fracture of humerus following insertion of orthopedic implant, joint prosthesis, or bone plate, left arm

M96.629 Fracture of humerus following insertion of orthopedic implant,

● New code ▲ Revised code Excludes1: Not coded here Excludes2: Not included here ⊗ Placeholder required ⑦7th digit required

joint prosthesis, or bone plate,
nspecified arm

M96.63 **Fracture of radius or ulna following insertion of orthopedic implant, joint prosthesis, or bone plate**

M96.631 Fracture of radius or ulna following insertion of orthopedic implant, joint prosthesis, or bone plate, right arm

M96.632 Fracture of radius or ulna following insertion of orthopedic implant, joint prosthesis, or bone plate, left arm

M96.639 Fracture of radius or ulna following insertion of orthopedic implant, joint prosthesis, or bone plate, unspecified arm

M96.65 **Fracture of pelvis following insertion of orthopedic implant, joint prosthesis, or bone plate**

M96.66 **Fracture of femur following insertion of orthopedic implant, joint prosthesis, or bone plate**

M96.661 Fracture of femur following insertion of orthopedic implant, joint prosthesis, or bone plate, right leg

M96.662 Fracture of femur following insertion of orthopedic implant, joint prosthesis, or bone plate, left leg

M96.669 Fracture of femur following insertion of orthopedic implant, joint prosthesis, or bone plate, unspecified leg

M96.67 **Fracture of tibia or fibula following insertion of orthopedic implant, joint prosthesis, or bone plate**

M96.671 Fracture of tibia or fibula following insertion of orthopedic implant, joint prosthesis, or bone plate, right leg

M96.672 Fracture of tibia or fibula following insertion of orthopedic implant, joint prosthesis, or bone plate, left leg

M96.679 Fracture of tibia or fibula following insertion of orthopedic implant, joint prosthesis, or bone plate, unspecified leg

M96.69 **Fracture of other bone following insertion of orthopedic implant, joint prosthesis, or bone plate**

M96.8 **Other intraoperative and postprocedural complications and disorders of musculoskeletal system, not elsewhere classified**

M96.81 **Intraoperative hemorrhage and hematoma of a musculoskeletal structure complicating a procedure**

Excludes1: intraoperative hemorrhage and hematoma of a musculoskeletal structure due to accidental puncture and laceration during a procedure (M96.82-)

M96.810 Intraoperative hemorrhage and hematoma of a musculoskeletal structure complicating a musculoskeletal system procedure

M96.811 Intraoperative hemorrhage and hematoma of a musculoskeletal structure complicating other procedure

M96.82 **Accidental puncture and laceration of a musculoskeletal structure during a procedure**

M96.820 Accidental puncture and laceration of a musculoskeletal structure during a musculoskeletal system procedure

M96.821 Accidental puncture and laceration of a musculoskeletal structure during other procedure

M96.83 **Postprocedural hemorrhage of a musculoskeletal structure following a procedure**

▲M96.830 Postprocedural hemorrhage of a musculoskeletal structure following a musculoskeletal system procedure

▲M96.831 Postprocedural hemorrhage of a musculoskeletal structure following other procedure

M96.84 **Postprocedural hematoma and seroma of a musculoskeletal structure following a procedure**

●M96.840 Postprocedural hematoma of a musculoskeletal structure following a musculoskeletal system procedure

●M96.841 Postprocedural hematoma of a musculoskeletal structure following other procedure

●M96.842 Postprocedural seroma of a musculoskeletal structure following a musculoskeletal system procedure

●M96.843 Postprocedural seroma of a musculoskeletal structure following other procedure

M96.89 **Other intraoperative and postprocedural complications and disorders of the musculoskeletal system**

Instability of joint secondary to removal of joint prosthesis

Use additional code, if applicable, to further specify disorder

PERIPROSTHETIC FRACTURE AROUND INTERNAL PROSTHETIC JOINT (M97)

M97 **Periprosthetic fracture around internal prosthetic joint**

Excludes2: fracture of bone following insertion of orthopedic implant, joint prosthesis or bone plate (M96.6-)

breakage (fracture) of prosthetic joint (T84.01-)

The appropriate 7th character is to be added to each code from category M97

A - initial encounter

D - subsequent encounter

S - sequela

M97.0 **Periprosthetic fracture around internal prosthetic hip joint**

●⊗⑦M97.01 Periprosthetic fracture around internal prosthetic right hip joint

- ⊗⑦M97.02 **Periprosthetic fracture around internal prosthetic left hip joint**

M97.1 **Periprosthetic fracture around internal prosthetic knee joint**

- ⊗⑦M97.11 **Periprosthetic fracture around internal prosthetic right knee joint**

- ⊗⑦M97.12 **Periprosthetic fracture around internal prosthetic left knee joint**

M97.2 **Periprosthetic fracture around internal prosthetic ankle joint**

- ⊗⑦M97.21 **Periprosthetic fracture around internal prosthetic right ankle joint**

- ⊗⑦M97.22 **Periprosthetic fracture around internal prosthetic left ankle joint**

M97.3 **Periprosthetic fracture around internal prosthetic shoulder joint**

- ⊗⑦M97.31 **Periprosthetic fracture around internal prosthetic right shoulder joint**

- ⊗⑦M97.32 **Periprosthetic fracture around internal prosthetic left shoulder joint**

M97.4 **Periprosthetic fracture around internal prosthetic elbow joint**

- ⊗⑦M97.41 **Periprosthetic fracture around internal prosthetic right elbow joint**

- ⊗⑦M97.42 **Periprosthetic fracture around internal prosthetic left elbow joint**

- ⊗⑦M97.8 **Periprosthetic fracture around other internal prosthetic joint**

  Periprosthetic fracture around internal prosthetic finger joint

  Periprosthetic fracture around internal prosthetic spinal joint

  Periprosthetic fracture around internal prosthetic toe joint

  Periprosthetic fracture around internal prosthetic wrist joint

  <u>Use additional code</u> to identify the joint (Z96.6-)

- ⊗⑦M97.9 **Periprosthetic fracture around unspecified internal prosthetic joint**

BIOMECHANICAL LESIONS, NOT ELSEWHERE CLASSIFIED (M99)

M99 **Biomechanical lesions, not elsewhere classified**

Note: This category should not be used if the condition can be classified elsewhere.

M99.0 **Segmental and somatic dysfunction**

M99.00 **Segmental and somatic dysfunction of head region**

M99.01 **Segmental and somatic dysfunction of cervical region**

M99.02 **Segmental and somatic dysfunction of thoracic region**

M99.03 **Segmental and somatic dysfunction of lumbar region**

M99.04 **Segmental and somatic dysfunction of sacral region**

M99.05 **Segmental and somatic dysfunction of pelvic region**

M99.06 **Segmental and somatic dysfunction of lower extremity**

M99.07 **Segmental and somatic dysfunction of upper extremity**

M99.08 **Segmental and somatic dysfunction of rib cage**

M99.09 **Segmental and somatic dysfunction of abdomen and other regions**

M99.1 **Subluxation complex (vertebral)**

M99.10 **Subluxation complex (vertebral) of head region**

M99.11 **Subluxation complex (vertebral) of cervical region**

M99.12 **Subluxation complex (vertebral) of thoracic region**

M99.13 **Subluxation complex (vertebral) of lumbar region**

M99.14 **Subluxation complex (vertebral) of sacral region**

M99.15 **Subluxation complex (vertebral) of pelvic region**

M99.16 **Subluxation complex (vertebral) of lower extremity**

M99.17 **Subluxation complex (vertebral) of upper extremity**

M99.18 **Subluxation complex (vertebral) of rib cage**

M99.19 **Subluxation complex (vertebral) of abdomen and other regions**

M99.2 **Subluxation stenosis of neural canal**

M99.20 **Subluxation stenosis of neural canal of head region**

M99.21 **Subluxation stenosis of neural canal of cervical region**

M99.22 **Subluxation stenosis of neural canal of thoracic region**

M99.23 **Subluxation stenosis of neural canal of lumbar region**

M99.24 **Subluxation stenosis of neural canal of sacral region**

M99.25 **Subluxation stenosis of neural canal of pelvic region**

M99.26 **Subluxation stenosis of neural canal of lower extremity**

M99.27 **Subluxation stenosis of neural canal of upper extremity**

M99.28 **Subluxation stenosis of neural canal of rib cage**

M99.29 **Subluxation stenosis of neural canal of abdomen and other regions**

M99.3 **Osseous stenosis of neural canal**

M99.30 **Osseous stenosis of neural canal of head region**

M99.31 **Osseous stenosis of neural canal of cervical region**

M99.32 **Osseous stenosis of neural canal of thoracic region**

M99.33 **Osseous stenosis of neural canal of lumbar region**

M99.34 **Osseous stenosis of neural canal of sacral region**

M99.35 **Osseous stenosis of neural canal of pelvic region**

M99.36 **Osseous stenosis of neural canal of lower extremity**

M99.37 **Osseous stenosis of neural canal of upper extremity**

● New code ▲ Revised code **Excludes1:** Not coded here **Excludes2:** Not included here ⊗ Placeholder required ⑦7th digit required

M99.38 Osseous stenosis of neural canal of rib cage

M99.39 Osseous stenosis of neural canal of abdomen and other regions

M99.4 Connective tissue stenosis of neural canal

M99.40 Connective tissue stenosis of neural canal of head region

M99.41 Connective tissue stenosis of neural canal of cervical region

M99.42 Connective tissue stenosis of neural canal of thoracic region

M99.43 Connective tissue stenosis of neural canal of lumbar region

M99.44 Connective tissue stenosis of neural canal of sacral region

M99.45 Connective tissue stenosis of neural canal of pelvic region

M99.46 Connective tissue stenosis of neural canal of lower extremity

M99.47 Connective tissue stenosis of neural canal of upper extremity

M99.48 Connective tissue stenosis of neural canal of rib cage

M99.49 Connective tissue stenosis of neural canal of abdomen and other regions

M99.5 Intervertebral disc stenosis of neural canal

M99.50 Intervertebral disc stenosis of neural canal of head region

M99.51 Intervertebral disc stenosis of neural canal of cervical region

M99.52 Intervertebral disc stenosis of neural canal of thoracic region

M99.53 Intervertebral disc stenosis of neural canal of lumbar region

M99.54 Intervertebral disc stenosis of neural canal of sacral region

M99.55 Intervertebral disc stenosis of neural canal of pelvic region

M99.56 Intervertebral disc stenosis of neural canal of lower extremity

M99.57 Intervertebral disc stenosis of neural canal of upper extremity

M99.58 Intervertebral disc stenosis of neural canal of rib cage

M99.59 Intervertebral disc stenosis of neural canal of abdomen and other regions

M99.6 Osseous and subluxation stenosis of intervertebral foramina

M99.60 Osseous and subluxation stenosis of intervertebral foramina of head region

M99.61 Osseous and subluxation stenosis of intervertebral foramina of cervical region

M99.62 Osseous and subluxation stenosis of intervertebral foramina of thoracic region

M99.63 Osseous and subluxation stenosis of intervertebral foramina of lumbar region

M99.64 Osseous and subluxation stenosis of intervertebral foramina of sacral region

M99.65 Osseous and subluxation stenosis of intervertebral foramina of pelvic region

M99.66 Osseous and subluxation stenosis of intervertebral foramina of lower extremity

M99.67 Osseous and subluxation stenosis of intervertebral foramina of upper extremity

M99.68 Osseous and subluxation stenosis of intervertebral foramina of rib cage

M99.69 Osseous and subluxation stenosis of intervertebral foramina of abdomen and other regions

M99.7 Connective tissue and disc stenosis of intervertebral foramina

M99.70 Connective tissue and disc stenosis of intervertebral foramina of head region

M99.71 Connective tissue and disc stenosis of intervertebral foramina of cervical region

M99.72 Connective tissue and disc stenosis of intervertebral foramina of thoracic region

M99.73 Connective tissue and disc stenosis of intervertebral foramina of lumbar region

M99.74 Connective tissue and disc stenosis of intervertebral foramina of sacral region

M99.75 Connective tissue and disc stenosis of intervertebral foramina of pelvic region

M99.76 Connective tissue and disc stenosis of intervertebral foramina of lower extremity

M99.77 Connective tissue and disc stenosis of intervertebral foramina of upper extremity

M99.78 Connective tissue and disc stenosis of intervertebral foramina of rib cage

M99.79 Connective tissue and disc stenosis of intervertebral foramina of abdomen and other regions

M99.8 Other biomechanical lesions

M99.80 Other biomechanical lesions of head region

M99.81 Other biomechanical lesions of cervical region

M99.82 Other biomechanical lesions of thoracic region

M99.83 Other biomechanical lesions of lumbar region

M99.84 Other biomechanical lesions of sacral region

M99.85 Other biomechanical lesions of pelvic region

M99.86 Other biomechanical lesions of lower extremity

M99.87 Other biomechanical lesions of upper extremity

M99.88 Other biomechanical lesions of rib cage

M99.89 Other biomechanical lesions of abdomen and other regions

M99.9 Biomechanical lesion, unspecified

Chapter 14: Diseases Of The Genitourinary System (N00-N99)

DEFINITIONS

This chapter includes definitions of selected key words, terms and phrases and coding alerts for adding points to the clinical domain, and references to coding late effects where appropriate. An example from this chapter is as follows:

N03   Chronic nephritic syndrome
   Definition: Nephritic syndrome is a collection of signs associated with disorders affecting the kidneys, more specifically glomerular disorders.

MULTIPLE CODING FOR A SINGLE CONDITION

In addition to the etiology/manifestation convention that requires two codes to fully describe a single condition that affects multiple body systems, there are other single conditions that also require more than one code. "Use additional code" notes are found in the Tabular List at codes that are not part of an etiology/manifestation pair where a secondary code is useful to fully describe a condition. The sequencing rule is the same as the etiology/manifestation pair, "use additional code" indicates that a secondary code should be added.

For example, for bacterial infections that are not included in chapter 1, a secondary code from category B95, Streptococcus, Staphylococcus, and Enterococcus, as the cause of diseases classified elsewhere, or B96, Other bacterial agents as the cause of diseases classified elsewhere, may be required to identify the bacterial organism causing the infection. A "use additional code" note will normally be found at the infectious disease code, indicating a need for the organism code to be added as a secondary code.

"Code first" notes are also under certain codes that are not specifically manifestation codes but may be due to an underlying cause. When there is a "code first" note and an underlying condition is present, the underlying condition should be sequenced first.

"Code, if applicable, any causal condition first", notes indicate that this code may be assigned as a principal diagnosis when the causal condition is unknown or not applicable. If a causal condition is known, then the code for that condition should be sequenced as the principal or first-listed diagnosis.

Multiple codes may be needed for sequela, complication codes and obstetric codes to more fully describe a condition. See the specific guidelines for these conditions for further instruction.

COMBINATION CODE

A combination code is a single code used to classify: Two diagnoses, or a diagnosis with an associated secondary process (manifestation) A diagnosis with an associated complication

Combination codes are identified by referring to subterm entries in the Alphabetic Index and by reading the inclusion and exclusion notes in the Tabular List.

Assign only the combination code when that code fully identifies the diagnostic conditions involved or when the Alphabetic Index so directs. Multiple coding should not be used when the classification provides a combination code that clearly identifies all of the elements documented in the diagnosis. When the combination code lacks necessary specificity in describing the manifestation or complication, an additional code should be used as a secondary code.

SEQUELA (LATE EFFECTS)

A sequela is the residual effect (condition produced) after the acute phase of an illness or injury has terminated. There is no time limit on when a sequela code can be used. The residual may be apparent early, such as in cerebral infarction, or it may occur months or years later, such as that due to a previous injury. Coding of sequela generally requires two codes sequenced in the following order: The condition or nature of the sequela is sequenced first.

The sequela code is sequenced second.

An exception to the above guidelines are those instances where the code for the sequela is followed by a manifestation code identified in the Tabular List and title, or the sequela code has been expanded (at the fourth, fifth or sixth character levels) to include the manifestation(s). The code for the acute phase of an illness or injury that led to the sequela is never used with a code for the late effect.

CHRONIC KIDNEY DISEASE

1) **Stages of chronic kidney disease (CKD)**

   The ICD-10-CM classifies CKD based on severity. The severity of CKD is designated by stages 1-5. Stage 2, code N18.2, equates to mild CKD; stage 3, code N18.3, equates to moderate CKD; and stage 4, code N18.4, equates to severe CKD. Code N18.6, End stage renal disease (ESRD), is assigned when the provider has documented end-stage-renal disease (ESRD).

   If both a stage of CKD and ESRD are documented, assign code N18.6 only.

2) **Chronic kidney disease and kidney transplant status**

   Patients who have undergone kidney transplant may still have some form of chronic kidney disease (CKD) because the kidney transplant may not fully restore kidney function. Therefore, the presence of CKD alone does not constitute a transplant complication. Assign the appropriate N18 code for the

Add 4th-7th digits   Nonspecific code   Unspecified code   Manifestation code   617

patient's stage of CKD and code Z94.0, Kidney transplant status. If a transplant complication such as failure or rejection or other transplant complication is documented, see section I.C.19.g for information on coding complications of a kidney transplant. If the documentation is unclear as to whether the patient has a complication of the transplant, query the provider.

3) Chronic kidney disease with other conditions

Patients with CKD may also suffer from other serious conditions, most commonly diabetes mellitus and hypertension. The sequencing of the CKD code in relationship to codes for other contributing conditions is based on the conventions in the Tabular List.

See I.C.9. Hypertensive chronic kidney disease.
See I.C.19. Chronic kidney disease and kidney transplant complications.

Chapter 14

Diseases Of The Genitourinary System (N00-N99)

Excludes2: certain conditions originating in the perinatal period (P04-P96)

certain infectious and parasitic diseases (A00-B99)

complications of pregnancy, childbirth and the puerperium (O00-O9A)

congenital malformations, deformations and chromosomal abnormalities (Q00-Q99)

endocrine, nutritional and metabolic diseases (E00-E88)

injury, poisoning and certain other consequences of external causes (S00-T88)

neoplasms (C00-D49)

symptoms, signs and abnormal clinical and laboratory findings, not elsewhere classified (R00-R94)

This chapter contains the following blocks: N00-N08 Glomerular diseases

N10-N16	Renal tubulo-interstitial diseases
N17-N19	Acute kidney failure and chronic kidney disease
N20-N23	Urolithiasis
N25-N29	Other disorders of kidney and ureter
N30-N39	Other diseases of the urinary system
N40-N53	Diseases of male genital organs
N60-N65	Disorders of breast
N70-N77	Inflammatory diseases of female pelvic organs
N80-N98	Noninflammatory disorders of female genital tract
N99	Intraoperative and postprocedural complications and disorders of genitourinary system, not elsewhere classified

GLOMERULAR DISEASES (N00-N08)

Definition: Glomerulonephritis is a form of nephritis with inflammation of the capillary loops in the renal glomeruli. The acute form is characterized by proteinuria, edema, hematuria, renal failure, and hypertension, sometimes preceded by tonsillitis or febrile pharyngitis.

Code also any associated kidney failure (N17-N19).

Excludes1: hypertensive chronic kidney disease (I12.-)

N00   Acute nephritic syndrome

Includes: acute glomerular disease

acute glomerulonephritis acute nephritis

Excludes1: acute tubulo-interstitial nephritis (N10)

nephritic syndrome NOS (N05.-)

N00.0   Acute nephritic syndrome with minor glomerular abnormality

Acute nephritic syndrome with minimal change lesion

N00.1   Acute nephritic syndrome with focal and segmental glomerular lesions

Acute nephritic syndrome with focal and segmental hyalinosis

Acute nephritic syndrome with focal and segmental sclerosis

Acute nephritic syndrome with focal glomerulonephritis

N00.2   Acute nephritic syndrome with diffuse membranous glomerulonephritis

N00.3   Acute nephritic syndrome with diffuse mesangial proliferative glomerulonephritis

N00.4   Acute nephritic syndrome with diffuse endocapillary proliferative glomerulonephritis

N00.5   Acute nephritic syndrome with diffuse mesangiocapillary glomerulonephritis

Acute nephritic syndrome with membranoproliferative glomerulonephritis, types 1 and 3, or NOS

N00.6   Acute nephritic syndrome with dense deposit disease

Acute nephritic syndrome with membranoproliferative glomerulonephritis, type 2

N00.7   Acute nephritic syndrome with diffuse crescentic glomerulonephritis

Acute nephritic syndrome with extracapillary glomerulonephritis

N00.8   Acute nephritic syndrome with other morphologic changes

Acute nephritic syndrome with proliferative glomerulonephritis NOS

N00.9   Acute nephritic syndrome with unspecified morphologic changes

N01   Rapidly progressive nephritic syndrome

Includes: rapidly progressive glomerular disease

rapidly progressive glomerulonephritis rapidly progressive nephritis

Excludes1: nephritic syndrome NOS (N05.-)

N01.0   Rapidly progressive nephritic syndrome with minor glomerular abnormality

Rapidly progressive nephritic syndrome with minimal change lesion

N01.1   Rapidly progressive nephritic syndrome with focal and segmental glomerular lesions

Rapidly progressive nephritic syndrome with focal and segmental hyalinosis

Rapidly progressive nephritic syndrome with focal and segmental sclerosis

Rapidly progressive nephritic syndrome with focal glomerulonephritis

N01.2   Rapidly progressive nephritic syndrome with diffuse membranous glomerulonephritis

N01.3   Rapidly progressive nephritic syndrome with diffuse mesangial proliferative glomerulonephritis

N01.4   Rapidly progressive nephritic syndrome with diffuse endocapillary proliferative glomerulonephritis

N01.5   Rapidly progressive nephritic syndrome with diffuse mesangiocapillary glomerulonephritis

Rapidly progressive nephritic syndrome with membranoproliferative glomerulonephritis, types 1 and 3, or NOS

N01.6   Rapidly progressive nephritic syndrome with dense deposit disease

Rapidly progressive nephritic syndrome with membranoproliferative glomerulonephritis, type 2

N01.7   Rapidly progressive nephritic syndrome with diffuse crescentic glomerulonephritis

Rapidly progressive nephritic syndrome with extracapillary glomerulonephritis

N01.8   Rapidly progressive nephritic syndrome with other morphologic changes

Rapidly progressive nephritic syndrome with proliferative glomerulonephritis NOS

N01.9   Rapidly progressive nephritic syndrome with unspecified morphologic changes

N02   Recurrent and persistent hematuria

Excludes1: acute cystitis with hematuria (N30.01)

hematuria NOS (R31.9)

hematuria not associated with specified morphologic lesions (R31.-)

N02.0   Recurrent and persistent hematuria with minor glomerular abnormality

Recurrent and persistent hematuria with minimal change lesion

N02.1   Recurrent and persistent hematuria with focal and segmental glomerular lesions

Recurrent and persistent hematuria with focal and segmental hyalinosis

Recurrent and persistent hematuria with focal and segmental sclerosis

Recurrent and persistent hematuria with focal glomerulonephritis

N02.2   Recurrent and persistent hematuria with diffuse membranous glomerulonephritis

N02.3   Recurrent and persistent hematuria with diffuse mesangial proliferative glomerulonephritis

N02.4   Recurrent and persistent hematuria with diffuse endocapillary proliferative glomerulonephritis

N02.5   Recurrent and persistent hematuria with diffuse mesangiocapillary glomerulonephritis

Recurrent and persistent hematuria with membranoproliferative glomerulonephritis, types 1 and 3, or NOS

N02.6   Recurrent and persistent hematuria with dense deposit disease

Recurrent and persistent hematuria with membranoproliferative glomerulonephritis, type 2

N02.7   Recurrent and persistent hematuria with diffuse crescentic glomerulonephritis

Recurrent and persistent hematuria with extracapillary glomerulonephritis

N02.8   Recurrent and persistent hematuria with other morphologic changes

Recurrent and persistent hematuria with proliferative glomerulonephritis NOS

N02.9   Recurrent and persistent hematuria with unspecified morphologic changes

N03   Chronic nephritic syndrome

Definition: Nephritic syndrome is a collection of signs associated with disorders affecting the kidneys, more specifically glomerular disorders.

Includes: chronic glomerular disease

chronic glomerulonephritis chronic nephritis

Excludes1: chronic tubulo-interstitial nephritis (N11.-)

diffuse sclerosing glomerulonephritis (N05.8-)

nephritic syndrome NOS (N05.-)

N03.0   Chronic nephritic syndrome with minor glomerular abnormality

Chronic nephritic syndrome with minimal change lesion

N03.1   Chronic nephritic syndrome with focal and segmental glomerular lesions

Chronic nephritic syndrome with focal and segmental hyalinosis

Chronic nephritic syndrome with focal and segmental sclerosis

Chronic nephritic syndrome with focal glomerulonephritis

N03.2   Chronic nephritic syndrome with diffuse membranous glomerulonephritis

N03.3   Chronic nephritic syndrome with diffuse mesangial proliferative glomerulonephritis

N03.4   Chronic nephritic syndrome with diffuse endocapillary proliferative glomerulonephritis

N03.5   Chronic nephritic syndrome with diffuse mesangiocapillary glomerulonephritis

Chronic nephritic syndrome with membranoproliferative glomerulonephritis, types 1 and 3, or NOS

N03.6   Chronic nephritic syndrome with dense deposit disease

Chronic nephritic syndrome with membranoproliferative glomerulonephritis, type 2

N03.7   Chronic nephritic syndrome with diffuse crescentic glomerulonephritis

Chronic nephritic syndrome with extracapillary glomerulonephritis

N03.8   Chronic nephritic syndrome with other morphologic changes

Chronic nephritic syndrome with proliferative glomerulonephritis NOS

N03.9   Chronic nephritic syndrome with unspecified morphologic changes

N04   Nephrotic syndrome

Definition: Nephrotic syndrome is a collection of symptoms which occur because the glomeruli (tiny blood vessels) in the kidney become leaky. This allows protein, normally never passed out in the urine, to leave the body in large amounts.

Includes: congenital nephrotic syndrome

lipoid nephrosis

N04.0   Nephrotic syndrome with minor glomerular abnormality

Nephrotic syndrome with minimal change lesion

N04.1   Nephrotic syndrome with focal and segmental glomerular lesions

Nephrotic syndrome with focal and segmental hyalinosis

Nephrotic syndrome with focal and segmental sclerosis

Nephrotic syndrome with focal glomerulonephritis

N04.2   Nephrotic syndrome with diffuse membranous glomerulonephritis

N04.3   Nephrotic syndrome with diffuse mesangial proliferative glomerulonephritis

N04.4   Nephrotic syndrome with diffuse endocapillary proliferative glomerulonephritis

N04.5   Nephrotic syndrome with diffuse mesangiocapillary glomerulonephritis

Nephrotic syndrome with membranoproliferative glomerulonephritis, types 1 and 3, or NOS

N04.6   Nephrotic syndrome with dense deposit disease

Nephrotic syndrome with membranoproliferative glomerulonephritis, type 2

N04.7   Nephrotic syndrome with diffuse crescentic glomerulonephritis

Nephrotic syndrome with extracapillary glomerulonephritis

N04.8   Nephrotic syndrome with other morphologic changes

Nephrotic syndrome with proliferative glomerulonephritis NOS

N04.9   Nephrotic syndrome with unspecified morphologic changes

N05   Unspecified nephritic syndrome

Includes: glomerular disease NOS

glomerulonephritis NOS nephritis NOS

nephropathy NOS and renal disease NOS with morphological lesion specified in .0-.8

Excludes1: nephropathy NOS with no stated morphological lesion (N28.9)

renal disease NOS with no stated morphological lesion (N28.9)

tubulo-interstitial nephritis NOS (N12)

N05.0 Unspecified nephritic syndrome with minor glomerular abnormality

Unspecified nephritic syndrome with minimal change lesion

N05.1 Unspecified nephritic syndrome with focal and segmental glomerular lesions

Unspecified nephritic syndrome with focal and segmental hyalinosis

Unspecified nephritic syndrome with focal and segmental sclerosis

Unspecified nephritic syndrome with focal glomerulonephritis

N05.2 Unspecified nephritic syndrome with diffuse membranous glomerulonephritis

N05.3 Unspecified nephritic syndrome with diffuse mesangial proliferative glomerulonephritis

N05.4 Unspecified nephritic syndrome with diffuse endocapillary proliferative glomerulonephritis

N05.5 Unspecified nephritic syndrome with diffuse mesangiocapillary glomerulonephritis

Unspecified nephritic syndrome with membranoproliferative glomerulonephritis, types 1 and 3, or NOS

N05.6 Unspecified nephritic syndrome with dense deposit disease

Unspecified nephritic syndrome with membranoproliferative glomerulonephritis, type 2

N05.7 Unspecified nephritic syndrome with diffuse crescentic glomerulonephritis

Unspecified nephritic syndrome with extracapillary glomerulonephritis

N05.8 Unspecified nephritic syndrome with other morphologic changes

Unspecified nephritic syndrome with proliferative glomerulonephritis NOS

N05.9 Unspecified nephritic syndrome with unspecified morphologic changes

N06 Isolated proteinuria with specified morphological lesion

Excludes1: Proteinuria not associated with specific morphologic lesions (R80.0)

N06.0 Isolated proteinuria with minor glomerular abnormality

Isolated proteinuria with minimal change lesion

N06.1 Isolated proteinuria with focal and segmental glomerular lesions

Isolated proteinuria with focal and segmental hyalinosis

Isolated proteinuria with focal and segmental sclerosis

Isolated proteinuria with focal glomerulonephritis

N06.2 Isolated proteinuria with diffuse membranous glomerulonephritis

N06.3 Isolated proteinuria with diffuse mesangial proliferative glomerulonephritis

N06.4 Isolated proteinuria with diffuse endocapillary proliferative glomerulonephritis

N06.5 Isolated proteinuria with diffuse mesangiocapillary glomerulonephritis

Isolated proteinuria with membranoproliferative glomerulonephritis, types 1 and 3, or NOS

N06.6 Isolated proteinuria with dense deposit disease

Isolated proteinuria with membranoproliferative glomerulonephritis, type 2

N06.7 Isolated proteinuria with diffuse crescentic glomerulonephritis

Isolated proteinuria with extracapillary glomerulonephritis

N06.8 Isolated proteinuria with other morphologic lesion

Isolated proteinuria with proliferative glomerulonephritis NOS

N06.9 Isolated proteinuria with unspecified morphologic lesion

N07 Hereditary nephropathy, not elsewhere classified

Excludes2: Alport's syndrome (Q87.81-)

hereditary amyloid nephropathy (E85.-)

nail patella syndrome (Q87.2)

non-neuropathic heredofamilial amyloidosis (E85.-)

N07.0 Hereditary nephropathy, not elsewhere classified with minor glomerular abnormality

Hereditary nephropathy, not elsewhere classified with minimal change lesion

N07.1 Hereditary nephropathy, not elsewhere classified with focal and segmental glomerular lesions

Hereditary nephropathy, not elsewhere classified with focal and segmental hyalinosis

Hereditary nephropathy, not elsewhere classified with focal and segmental sclerosis

Hereditary nephropathy, not elsewhere classified with focal glomerulonephritis

N07.2 Hereditary nephropathy, not elsewhere classified with diffuse membranous glomerulonephritis

N07.3 Hereditary nephropathy, not elsewhere classified with diffuse mesangial proliferative glomerulonephritis

N07.4 Hereditary nephropathy, not elsewhere classified with diffuse endocapillary proliferative glomerulonephritis

N07.5 Hereditary nephropathy, not elsewhere classified with diffuse mesangiocapillary glomerulonephritis

Hereditary nephropathy, not elsewhere classified with membranoproliferative glomerulonephritis, types 1 and 3, or NOS

N07.6 Hereditary nephropathy, not elsewhere classified with dense deposit disease

Hereditary nephropathy, not elsewhere classified with membranoproliferative glomerulonephritis, type 2

N07.7 Hereditary nephropathy, not elsewhere classified with diffuse crescentic glomerulonephritis

Hereditary nephropathy, not elsewhere classified with extracapillary glomerulonephritis

N07.8 Hereditary nephropathy, not elsewhere classified with other morphologic lesions

Hereditary nephropathy, not elsewhere classified with proliferative glomerulonephritis NOS

N07.9 Hereditary nephropathy, not elsewhere classified with unspecified morphologic lesions

N08 Glomerular disorders in diseases classified elsewhere

Glomerulonephritis Nephritis Nephropathy

<u>Code first</u> underlying disease, such as:

amyloidosis (E85.-)

congenital syphilis (A50.5)

cryoglobulinemia (D89.1)

disseminated intravascular coagulation (D65)

gout (M1A.-, M10.-)

microscopic polyangiitis (M31.7)

multiple myeloma (C90.0-)

sepsis (A40.0-A41.9)

sickle-cell disease (D57.0-D57.8)

Excludes1: glomerulonephritis, nephritis and nephropathy (in):

antiglomerular basement membrane disease (M31.0)

diabetes (E08-E13 with .21)

gonococcal (A54.21)

Goodpasture's syndrome (M31.0)

hemolytic-uremic syndrome (D59.3)

lupus (M32.14)

mumps (B26.83)

syphilis (A52.75)

systemic lupus erythematosus (M32.14)

Wegener's granulomatosis (M31.31)

pyelonephritis in diseases classified elsewhere (N16)

renal tubulo-interstitial disorders classified elsewhere (N16)

RENAL TUBULO-INTERSTITIAL DISEASES (N10-N16)

Includes: pyelonephritis

Excludes1: pyeloureteritis cystica (N28.85)

▲N10 Acute pyelonephritis

Acute infectious interstitial nephritis

Acute pyelitis

Acute tubulo-interstitial nephritis

Hemoglobin nephrosis

Myoglobin nephrosis

<u>Use additional code</u> (B95-B97), to identify infectious agent.

N11 Chronic tubulo-interstitial nephritis

Includes: chronic infectious interstitial nephritis

chronic pyelitis chronic pyelonephritis

<u>Use additional code</u> (B95-B97), to identify infectious agent.

N11.0 Nonobstructive reflux-associated chronic pyelonephritis

Pyelonephritis (chronic) associated with (vesicoureteral) reflux

Excludes1: vesicoureteral reflux NOS (N13.70)

N11.1 Chronic obstructive pyelonephritis

Pyelonephritis (chronic) associated with anomaly of pelviureteric junction

Pyelonephritis (chronic) associated with anomaly of pyeloureteric junction

Pyelonephritis (chronic) associated with crossing of vessel

Pyelonephritis (chronic) associated with kinking of ureter

Pyelonephritis (chronic) associated with obstruction of ureter

Pyelonephritis (chronic) associated with stricture of pelviureteric junction

Pyelonephritis (chronic) associated with stricture of ureter

Excludes1: calculous pyelonephritis (N20.9)

obstructive uropathy (N13.-)

N11.8 Other chronic tubulo-interstitial nephritis

Nonobstructive chronic pyelonephritis NOS

N11.9 Chronic tubulo-interstitial nephritis, unspecified

Chronic interstitial nephritis NOS

Chronic pyelitis NOS

Chronic pyelonephritis NOS

N12 Tubulo-interstitial nephritis, not specified as acute or chronic

Interstitial nephritis NOS

Pyelitis NOS

Pyelonephritis NOS

Excludes1: calculous pyelonephritis (N20.9)

N13 Obstructive and reflux uropathy

Excludes2: calculus of kidney and ureter without hydronephrosis (N20.-)

congenital obstructive defects of renal pelvis and ureter (Q62.0-Q62.3)

hydronephrosis with ureteropelvic junction obstruction (Q62.1)

obstructive pyelonephritis (N11.1)

•N13.0 Hydronephrosis with ureteropelvic junction obstruction

Definition: Hydronephrosis is a condition that occurs as a result of urine accumulation in the upper urinary tract. This usually occurs from a blockage somewhere along the urinary tract.

Hydronephrosis due to acquired occlusion of ureteropelvic junction

Excludes2: Hydronephrosis with ureteropelvic junction obstruction due to calculus (N13.2)

N13.1 Hydronephrosis with ureteral stricture, not elsewhere classified

Excludes1: Hydronephrosis with ureteral stricture with infection (N13.6)

N13.2 Hydronephrosis with renal and ureteral calculous obstruction

Excludes1: Hydronephrosis with renal and ureteral calculous obstruction with infection (N13.6)

N13.3 Other and unspecified hydronephrosis

Excludes1: hydronephrosis with infection (N13.6)

N13.30 Unspecified hydronephrosis

N13.39 Other hydronephrosis

N13.4 Hydroureter

Excludes1: congenital hydroureter (Q62.3-)

hydroureter with infection (N13.6)

vesicoureteral-reflux with hydroureter (N13.73-)

N13.5 Crossing vessel and stricture of ureter without hydronephrosis

Kinking and stricture of ureter without hydronephrosis

Excludes1: Crossing vessel and stricture of ureter without hydronephrosis with infection (N13.6)

N13.6 Pyonephrosis

Conditions in N13.0-N13.5 with infection

Obstructive uropathy with infection

> **Use additional code** (B95-B97), to identify infectious agent.

N13.7 Vesicoureteral-reflux

> **Excludes1:** reflux-associated pyelonephritis (N11.0)

N13.70 Vesicoureteral-reflux, unspecified

> Vesicoureteral-reflux NOS

N13.71 Vesicoureteral-reflux without reflux nephropathy

N13.72 Vesicoureteral-reflux with reflux nephropathy without hydroureter

N13.721 Vesicoureteral-reflux with reflux nephropathy without hydroureter, unilateral

N13.722 Vesicoureteral-reflux with reflux nephropathy without hydroureter, bilateral

N13.729 Vesicoureteral-reflux with reflux nephropathy without hydroureter, unspecified

N13.731 Vesicoureteral-reflux with reflux nephropathy with hydroureter, unilateral

N13.732 Vesicoureteral-reflux with reflux nephropathy with hydroureter, bilateral

N13.739 Vesicoureteral-reflux with reflux nephropathy with hydroureter, unspecified

N13.8 Other obstructive and reflux uropathy

> Urinary tract obstruction due to specified cause

> **Code first**, if applicable, any causal condition, such as:
> enlarged prostate (N40.1)

N13.9 Obstructive and reflux uropathy, unspecified

> Urinary tract obstruction NOS

N14 Drug- and heavy-metal-induced tubulo-interstitial and tubular conditions

> **Code first** poisoning due to drug or toxin, if applicable (T36-T65 with fifth or sixth character 1-4 or 6)

> **Use additional code** for adverse effect, if applicable, to identify drug (T36-T50 with fifth or sixth character 5)

N14.0 Analgesic nephropathy

N14.1 Nephropathy induced by other drugs, medicaments and biological substances

N14.2 Nephropathy induced by unspecified drug, medicament or biological substance

N14.3 Nephropathy induced by heavy metals

N14.4 Toxic nephropathy, not elsewhere classified

N15 Other renal tubulo-interstitial diseases

N15.0 Balkan nephropathy

> Balkan endemic nephropathy

N15.1 Renal and perinephric abscess

N15.8 Other specified renal tubulo-interstitial diseases

N15.9 Renal tubulo-interstitial disease, unspecified

> Infection of kidney NOS

> **Excludes1:** urinary tract infection NOS (N39.0)

N16 Renal tubulo-interstitial disorders in diseases classified elsewhere

> Pyelonephritis

Tubulo-interstitial nephritis

> **Code first** underlying disease, such as:
> brucellosis (A23.0-A23.9)
> cryoglobulinemia (D89.1)
> glycogen storage disease (E74.0)
> leukemia (C91-C95)
> lymphoma (C81.0-C85.9, C96.0-C96.9)
> multiple myeloma (C90.0-)
> sepsis (A40.0-A41.9)
> Wilson's disease (E83.0)

> **Excludes1:** diphtheritic pyelonephritis and tubulo-interstitial nephritis (A36.84)
> pyelonephritis and tubulo-interstitial nephritis in candidiasis (B37.49)
> pyelonephritis and tubulo-interstitial nephritis in cystinosis (E72.04)
> pyelonephritis and tubulo-interstitial nephritis in salmonella infection (A02.25)
> pyelonephritis and tubulo-interstitial nephritis in sarcoidosis (D86.84)
> pyelonephritis and tubulo-interstitial nephritis in sicca syndrome [Sjogren's] (M35.04)
> pyelonephritis and tubulo-interstitial nephritis in systemic lupus erythematosus (M32.15)
> pyelonephritis and tubulo-interstitial nephritis in toxoplasmosis (B58.83)
> renal tubular degeneration in diabetes (E08-E13 with .29)
> syphilitic pyelonephritis and tubulo-interstitial nephritis (A52.75)

ACUTE KIDNEY FAILURE AND CHRONIC KIDNEY DISEASE (N17-N19)

> **Excludes2:** congenital renal failure (P96.0)
> drug- and heavy-metal-induced tubulo-interstitial and tubular conditions (N14.-) extrarenal uremia (R39.2)
> hemolytic-uremic syndrome (D59.3) hepatorenal syndrome (K76.7)
> postpartum hepatorenal syndrome (O90.4) posttraumatic renal failure (T79.5) prerenal uremia (R39.2)
> renal failure complicating abortion or ectopic or molar pregnancy (O00-O07, O08.4) renal failure following labor and delivery (O90.4)
> renal failure postprocedural (N99.0)

N17 Acute kidney failure

> **Code also** associated underlying condition

> **Excludes1:** posttraumatic renal failure (T79.5)

N17.0 Acute kidney failure with tubular necrosis

> Acute tubular necrosis
> Renal tubular necrosis
> Tubular necrosis NOS

N17.1 Acute kidney failure with acute cortical necrosis

> Acute cortical necrosis
> Cortical necrosis NOS
> Renal cortical necrosis

N17.2 Acute kidney failure with medullary necrosis

> Medullary [papillary] necrosis NOS
> Acute medullary [papillary] necrosis
> Renal medullary [papillary] necrosis

N17.8   **Other acute kidney failure**

N17.9   **Acute kidney failure, unspecified**

    Acute kidney injury (nontraumatic)

    Excludes2: traumatic kidney injury (S37.0-)

N18   **Chronic kidney disease (CKD)**

    Definition: Chronic kidney disease (CKD), aka chronic renal disease, is a progressive loss of renal function over a period of months or years.

    Code first any associated:

    diabetic chronic kidney disease (E08.22, E09.22, E10.22, E11.22, E13.22)

    hypertensive chronic kidney disease (I12.-, I13.-)

    Use additional code to identify kidney transplant status, if applicable, (Z94.0)

N18.1   **Chronic kidney disease, stage 1**

N18.2   **Chronic kidney disease, stage 2 (mild)**

N18.3   **Chronic kidney disease, stage 3 (moderate)**

N18.4   **Chronic kidney disease, stage 4 (severe)**

N18.5   **Chronic kidney disease, stage 5**

    Excludes1: chronic kidney disease, stage 5 requiring chronic dialysis (N18.6)

N18.6   **End stage renal disease**

    Chronic kidney disease requiring chronic dialysis

    Use additional code to identify dialysis status (Z99.2)

N18.9   **Chronic kidney disease, unspecified**

    Chronic renal disease

    Chronic renal failure NOS

    Chronic renal insufficiency

    Chronic uremia

N19   **Unspecified kidney failure**

    Uremia NOS

    Excludes1: acute kidney failure (N17.-)

    chronic kidney disease (N18.-)

    chronic uremia (N18.9)

    extrarenal uremia (R39.2)

    prerenal uremia (R39.2)

    renal insufficiency (acute) (N28.9)

    uremia of newborn (P96.0)

UROLITHIASIS (N20-N23)

N20   **Calculus of kidney and ureter**

    Calculous pyelonephritis

    Excludes1: nephrocalcinosis (E83.5)

    that with hydronephrosis (N13.2)

N20.0   **Calculus of kidney**

    Nephrolithiasis NOS

    Renal calculus

    Renal stone

    Staghorn calculus

    Stone in kidney

N20.1   **Calculus of ureter**

    Ureteric stone

N20.2   **Calculus of kidney with calculus of ureter**

N20.9   **Urinary calculus, unspecified**

N21   **Calculus of lower urinary tract**

    Includes: calculus of lower urinary tract with cystitis and urethritis

N21.0   **Calculus in bladder**

    Calculus in diverticulum of bladder

    Urinary bladder stone

    Excludes2: staghorn calculus (N20.0)

N21.1   **Calculus in urethra**

    Excludes2: calculus of prostate (N42.0)

N21.8   **Other lower urinary tract calculus**

N21.9   **Calculus of lower urinary tract, unspecified**

    Excludes1: calculus of urinary tract NOS (N20.9)

N22   **Calculus of urinary tract in diseases classified elsewhere**

    Code first underlying disease, such as:

    gout (M1A.-, M10.-)

    schistosomiasis (B65.0-B65.9)

N23   **Unspecified renal colic**

OTHER DISORDERS OF KIDNEY AND URETER (N25-N29)

Excludes2: disorders of kidney and ureter with urolithiasis (N20-N23)

N25   **Disorders resulting from impaired renal tubular function**

    Excludes1: metabolic disorders classifiable to E70-E88

N25.0   **Renal osteodystrophy**

    Azotemic osteodystrophy

    Phosphate-losing tubular disorders

    Renal rickets

    Renal short stature

N25.1   **Nephrogenic diabetes insipidus**

    Excludes1: diabetes insipidus NOS (E23.2)

N25.8   **Other disorders resulting from impaired renal tubular function**

    N25.81   **Secondary hyperparathyroidism of renal origin**

        Excludes1: secondary hyperparathyroidism, non-renal (E21.1)

    N25.89   **Other disorders resulting from impaired renal tubular function**

        Hypokalemic nephropathy

        Lightwood-Albright syndrome

        Renal tubular acidosis NOS

N25.9   **Disorder resulting from impaired renal tubular function, unspecified**

N26   **Unspecified contracted kidney**

    Excludes1: contracted kidney due to hypertension (I12.-)

    diffuse sclerosing glomerulonephritis (N05.8.-)

    hypertensive nephrosclerosis (arteriolar) (arteriosclerotic) (I12.-)

    small kidney of unknown cause (N27.-)

N26.1   **Atrophy of kidney (terminal)**

N26.2   **Page kidney**

N26.9   **Renal sclerosis, unspecified**

N27   **Small kidney of unknown cause**

    Includes: oligonephronia

N27.0   **Small kidney, unilateral**

N27.1   **Small kidney, bilateral**

N27.9   **Small kidney, unspecified**

N28   **Other disorders of kidney and ureter, not elsewhere classified**

N28.0   Ischemia and infarction of kidney

Renal artery embolism

Renal artery obstruction

Renal artery occlusion

Renal artery thrombosis

Renal infarct

Excludes1: atherosclerosis of renal artery (extrarenal part) (I70.1)

congenital stenosis of renal artery (Q27.1)

Goldblatt's kidney (I70.1)

N28.1   Cyst of kidney, acquired

Cyst (multiple)(solitary) of kidney, acquired

Excludes1: cystic kidney disease (congenital) (Q61.-)

N28.8   Other specified disorders of kidney and ureter

Excludes1: hydroureter (N13.4)

ureteric stricture with hydronephrosis (N13.1)

ureteric stricture without hydronephrosis (N13.5)

N28.81   Hypertrophy of kidney

N28.82   Megaloureter

N28.83   Nephroptosis

N28.84   Pyelitis cystica

N28.85   Pyeloureteritis cystica

N28.86   Ureteritis cystica

N28.89   Other specified disorders of kidney and ureter

N28.9   Disorder of kidney and ureter, unspecified

Nephropathy NOS

Renal disease (acute) NOS

Renal insufficiency (acute)

Excludes1: chronic renal insufficiency (N18.9)

unspecified nephritic syndrome (N05.-)

N29   Other disorders of kidney and ureter in diseases classified elsewhere

Code first underlying disease, such as:

amyloidosis (E85.-)

nephrocalcinosis (E83.5)

schistosomiasis (B65.0-B65.9)

Excludes1: disorders of kidney and ureter in:

cystinosis (E72.0)

gonorrhea (A54.21)

syphilis (A52.75)

tuberculosis (A18.11)

OTHER DISEASES OF THE URINARY SYSTEM (N30-N39)

Excludes1: urinary infection (complicating):

abortion or ectopic or molar pregnancy (O00-O07, O08.8)

pregnancy, childbirth and the puerperium (O23.-, O75.3, O86.2-)

N30   Cystitis

Use additional code to identify infectious agent (B95-B97)

Excludes1: prostatocystitis (N41.3)

N30.0   Acute cystitis

Excludes1: irradiation cystitis (N30.4-)

trigonitis (N30.3-)

N30.00   Acute cystitis without hematuria

N30.01   Acute cystitis with hematuria

N30.1   Interstitial cystitis (chronic)

N30.10   Interstitial cystitis (chronic) without hematuria

N30.11   Interstitial cystitis (chronic) with hematuria

N30.2   Other chronic cystitis

N30.20   Other chronic cystitis without hematuria

N30.21   Other chronic cystitis with hematuria

N30.3   Trigonitis

Urethrotrigonitis

N30.30   Trigonitis without hematuria

N30.31   Trigonitis with hematuria

N30.4   Irradiation cystitis

N30.40   Irradiation cystitis without hematuria

N30.41   Irradiation cystitis with hematuria

N30.8   Other cystitis

Abscess of bladder

N30.80   Other cystitis without hematuria

N30.81   Other cystitis with hematuria

N30.9   Cystitis, unspecified

N30.90   Cystitis, unspecified without hematuria

N30.91   Cystitis, unspecified with hematuria

N31   Neuromuscular dysfunction of bladder, not elsewhere classified

Use additional code to identify any associated urinary incontinence (N39.3-N39.4-)

Excludes1: cord bladder NOS (G95.89)

neurogenic bladder due to cauda equina syndrome (G83.4)

neuromuscular dysfunction due to spinal cord lesion (G95.89)

N31.0   Uninhibited neuropathic bladder, not elsewhere classified

N31.1   Reflex neuropathic bladder, not elsewhere classified

N31.2   Flaccid neuropathic bladder, not elsewhere classified

Atonic (motor) (sensory) neuropathic bladder

Autonomous neuropathic bladder

Nonreflex neuropathic bladder

N31.8   Other neuromuscular dysfunction of bladder

N31.9   Neuromuscular dysfunction of bladder, unspecified

Neurogenic bladder dysfunction NOS

N32   Other disorders of bladder

Excludes2: calculus of bladder (N21.0)

cystocele (N81.1-)

hernia or prolapse of bladder, female (N81.1-)

N32.0   Bladder-neck obstruction

Bladder-neck stenosis (acquired)

Excludes1: congenital bladder-neck obstruction (Q64.3-)

N32.1   Vesicointestinal fistula

Vesicorectal fistula

N32.2   Vesical fistula, not elsewhere classified

Excludes1: fistula between bladder and female genital tract (N82.0-N82.1)

N32.3   Diverticulum of bladder

Excludes1: congenital diverticulum of bladder (Q64.6)

diverticulitis of bladder (N30.8-)

N32.8   Other specified disorders of bladder

N32.81   Overactive bladder

Detrusor muscle hyperactivity

Excludes1: frequent urination due to specified bladder condition- code to condition

N32.89 **Other specified disorders of bladder**

Bladder hemorrhage

Bladder hypertrophy

Calcified bladder

Contracted bladder

N32.9 **Bladder disorder, unspecified**

N33 **Bladder disorders in diseases classified elsewhere**

Code first underlying disease, such as:

schistosomiasis (B65.0-B65.9)

Excludes1: bladder disorder in syphilis (A52.76)

bladder disorder in tuberculosis (A18.12)

candidal cystitis (B37.41)

chlamydial cystitis (A56.01)

cystitis in gonorrhea (A54.01)

cystitis in neurogenic bladder (N31.-)

diphtheritic cystitis (A36.85)

syphilitic cystitis (A52.76)

trichomonal cystitis (A59.03)

N34 **Urethritis and urethral syndrome**

Use additional code (B95-B97), to identify infectious agent.

Excludes2: Reiter's disease (M02.3-)

urethritis in diseases with a predominantly sexual mode of transmission (A50-A64)

urethrotrigonitis (N30.3-)

N34.0 **Urethral abscess**

Abscess (of) Cowper's gland

Abscess (of) Littré's gland

Abscess (of) urethral (gland)

Periurethral abscess

Excludes1: urethral caruncle (N36.2)

N34.1 **Nonspecific urethritis**

Nongonococcal urethritis Nonvenereal urethritis

N34.2 **Other urethritis**

Meatitis, urethral

Postmenopausal urethritis

Ulcer of urethra (meatus)

Urethritis NOS

N34.3 **Urethral syndrome, unspecified**

N35 **Urethral stricture**

Excludes1: congenital urethral stricture (Q64.3-)

postprocedural urethral stricture (N99.1-)

N35.0 **Post-traumatic urethral stricture**

Urethral stricture due to injury

Excludes1: postprocedural urethral stricture (N99.1-)

N35.01 **Post-traumatic urethral stricture, male**

N35.010 **Post-traumatic urethral stricture, male, meatal**

N35.011 **Post-traumatic bulbous urethral stricture**

N35.012 **Post-traumatic membranous urethral stricture**

N35.013 **Post-traumatic anterior urethral stricture**

N35.014 **Post-traumatic urethral stricture, male, unspecified**

N35.02 **Post-traumatic urethral stricture, female**

N35.021 **Urethral stricture due to childbirth**

N35.028 **Other post-traumatic urethral stricture, female**

N35.1 **Postinfective urethral stricture, not elsewhere classified**

Excludes1: urethral stricture associated with schistosomiasis (B65.-, N29)

gonococcal urethral stricture (A54.01)

syphilitic urethral stricture (A52.76)

N35.11 **Postinfective urethral stricture, not elsewhere classified, male**

N35.111 **Postinfective urethral stricture, not elsewhere classified, male, meatal**

N35.112 **Postinfective bulbous urethral stricture, not elsewhere classified**

N35.113 **Postinfective membranous urethral stricture, not elsewhere classified**

N35.114 **Postinfective anterior urethral stricture, not elsewhere classified**

N35.119 **Postinfective urethral stricture, not elsewhere classified, male, unspecified**

N35.12 **Postinfective urethral stricture, not elsewhere classified, female**

N35.8 **Other urethral stricture**

Excludes1: postprocedural urethral stricture (N99.1-)

N35.9 **Urethral stricture, unspecified**

N36 **Other disorders of urethra**

N36.0 **Urethral fistula**

Urethroperineal fistula

Urethrorectal fistula

Urinary fistula NOS

Excludes1: urethroscrotal fistula (N50.89)

urethrovaginal fistula (N82.1)

urethrovesicovaginal fistula (N82.1)

N36.1 **Urethral diverticulum**

N36.2 **Urethral caruncle**

N36.4 **Urethral functional and muscular disorders**

Use additional code to identify associated urinary stress incontinence (N39.3)

N36.41 **Hypermobility of urethra**

N36.42 **Intrinsic sphincter deficiency (ISD)**

N36.43 **Combined hypermobility of urethra and intrinsic sphincter deficiency**

N36.44 **Muscular disorders of urethra**

Bladder sphincter dyssynergy

N36.5 **Urethral false passage**

N36.8 **Other specified disorders of urethra**

Excludes1: congenital urethrocele (Q64.7)

female urethrocele (N81.0)

N36.9 **Urethral disorder, unspecified**

N37 **Urethral disorders in diseases classified elsewhere**

Code first underlying disease

Excludes1: urethritis (in):

candidal infection (B37.41)

chlamydial (A56.01)

gonorrhea (A54.01)

syphilis (A52.76)

trichomonal infection (A59.03)

tuberculosis (A18.13)

N39 **Other disorders of urinary system**

Excludes2: hematuria NOS (R31.-)

recurrent or persistent hematuria (N02.-)

recurrent or persistent hematuria with specified morphological lesion (N02.-)

proteinuria NOS (R80.-)

N39.0 **Urinary tract infection, site not specified**

Use additional code (B95-B97), to identify infectious agent.

Excludes1: candidiasis of urinary tract (B37.4-)

neonatal urinary tract infection (P39.3)

urinary tract infection of specified site, such as: cystitis (N30.-)

urethritis (N34.-)

N39.3 **Stress incontinence (female) (male)**

Code also any associated overactive bladder (N32.81)

Excludes1: mixed incontinence (N39.46)

N39.4 **Other specified urinary incontinence**

Code also any associated overactive bladder (N32.81)

Excludes1: enuresis NOS (R32)

functional urinary incontinence (R39.81)

urinary incontinence associated with cognitive impairment (R39.81)

urinary incontinence NOS (R32)

urinary incontinence of nonorganic origin (F98.0)

N39.41 **Urge incontinence**

Excludes1: mixed incontinence (N39.46)

N39.42 **Incontinence without sensory awareness**

Insensible (urinary) incontinence

N39.43 **Post-void dribbling**

N39.44 **Nocturnal enuresis**

N39.45 **Continuous leakage**

N39.46 **Mixed incontinence**

Urge and stress incontinence

N39.49 **Other specified urinary incontinence**

N39.490 **Overflow incontinence**

●**N39.491** **Coital incontinence**

●**N39.492** **Postural (urinary) incontinence**

N39.498 **Other specified urinary incontinence**

Reflex incontinence

Total incontinence

N39.8 **Other specified disorders of urinary system**

N39.9 **Disorder of urinary system, unspecified**

DISEASES OF MALE GENITAL ORGANS (N40-N53)

> NOTE: All Diagnosis Codes In This Section Apply To MALE Patients Only

N40 **Benign prostatic hyperplasia**

Includes: adenofibromatous hypertrophy of prostate

benign hypertrophy of the prostate

benign prostatic hypertrophy

BPH

enlarged prostate nodular prostate

polyp of prostate

Excludes1: benign neoplasms of prostate (adenoma, benign) (fibroadenoma) (fibroma) (myoma) (D29.1)

Excludes2: malignant neoplasm of prostate (C61)

▲**N40.0** **Benign prostatic hyperplasia without lower urinary tract symptoms**

Enlarged prostate without LUTS

Enlarged prostate NOS

▲**N40.1** **Benign prostatic hyperplasia with lower urinary tract symptoms**

Enlarged prostate with LUTS

Use additional code for associated symptoms, when specified:

incomplete bladder emptying (R39.14)

nocturia (R35.1)

straining on urination (R39.16)

urinary frequency (R35.0)

urinary hesitancy (R39.11)

urinary incontinence (N39.4-)

urinary obstruction (N13.8)

urinary retention (R33.8)

urinary urgency (R39.15)

weak urinary stream (R39.12)

N40.2 **Nodular prostate without lower urinary tract symptoms**

Nodular prostate without LUTS

N40.3 **Nodular prostate with lower urinary tract symptoms**

Use additional code for associated symptoms, when specified:

incomplete bladder emptying (R39.14)

nocturia (R35.1)

straining on urination (R39.16)

urinary frequency (R35.0)

urinary hesitancy (R39.11)

urinary incontinence (N39.4-)

urinary obstruction (N13.8)

urinary retention (R33.8)

urinary urgency (R39.15)

weak urinary stream (R39.12)

N41 **Inflammatory diseases of prostate**

Use additional code (B95-B97), to identify infectious agent.

N41.0 **Acute prostatitis**

N41.1 **Chronic prostatitis**

N41.2 **Abscess of prostate**

N41.3 **Prostatocystitis**

N41.4 **Granulomatous prostatitis**

N41.8 **Other inflammatory diseases of prostate**

N41.9 Inflammatory disease of prostate, unspecified

Prostatitis NOS

N42 Other and unspecified disorders of prostate

N42.0 Calculus of prostate

Prostatic stone

N42.1 Congestion and hemorrhage of prostate

Excludes1: enlarged prostate (N40.-)

hematuria (R31.-)

hyperplasia of prostate (N40.-)

inflammatory diseases of prostate (N41.-)

N42.3 Dysplasia of prostate

● **N42.30** Unspecified dysplasia of prostate

● **N42.31** Prostatic intraepithelial neoplasia

PIN

Prostatic intraepithelial neoplasia I (PIN I)

Prostatic intraepithelial neoplasia II (PIN II)

Excludes1: prostatic intraepithelial neoplasia III (PIN III) (D07.5)

● **N42.32** Atypical small acinar proliferation of prostate

● **N42.39** Other dysplasia of prostate

N42.8 Other specified disorders of prostate

N42.81 Prostatodynia syndrome

Painful prostate syndrome

N42.82 Prostatosis syndrome

N42.83 Cyst of prostate

N42.89 Other specified disorders of prostate

N42.9 Disorder of prostate, unspecified

N43 Hydrocele and spermatocele

Definition: A Hydrocele is a painless swelling of the scrotum, caused by a collection of fluid around the testicle; commonly occurs in middle-aged men.

Includes: hydrocele of spermatic cord, testis or tunica vaginalis

Excludes1: congenital hydrocele (P83.5)

N43.0 Encysted hydrocele

N43.1 Infected hydrocele

Use additional code (B95-B97), to identify infectious agent

N43.2 Other hydrocele

N43.3 Hydrocele, unspecified

N43.4 Spermatocele of epididymis

Spermatic cyst

N43.40 Spermatocele of epididymis, unspecified

N43.41 Spermatocele of epididymis, single

N43.42 Spermatocele of epididymis, multiple

N44 Noninflammatory disorders of testis

N44.0 Torsion of testis

N44.00 Torsion of testis, unspecified

N44.01 Extravaginal torsion of spermatic cord

N44.02 Intravaginal torsion of spermatic cord

Torsion of spermatic cord NOS

N44.03 Torsion of appendix testis

N44.04 Torsion of appendix epididymis

N44.1 Cyst of tunica albuginea testis

N44.2 Benign cyst of testis

N44.8 Other noninflammatory disorders of the testis

N45 Orchitis and epididymitis

Definition: Orchitis is the inflammation and swelling of the testes as a result of infection or physical injury. Epididymitis is an inflammation of the epididymis which is located along the posterior aspect of the testicle.

Use additional code (B95-B97), to identify infectious agent.

N45.1 Epididymitis

N45.2 Orchitis

N45.3 Epididymo-orchitis

N45.4 Abscess of epididymis or testis

N46 Male infertility

Excludes1: vasectomy status (Z98.52)

N46.0 Azoospermia

Absolute male infertility

Male infertility due to germinal (cell) aplasia

Male infertility due to spermatogenic arrest (complete)

N46.01 Organic azoospermia

Azoospermia NOS

N46.02 Azoospermia due to extratesticular causes

Code also associated cause

N46.021 Azoospermia due to drug therapy

N46.022 Azoospermia due to infection

N46.023 Azoospermia due to obstruction of efferent ducts

N46.024 Azoospermia due to radiation

N46.025 Azoospermia due to systemic disease

N46.029 Azoospermia due to other extratesticular causes

N46.1 Oligospermia

Male infertility due to germinal cell desquamation

Male infertility due to hypospermatogenesis

Male infertility due to incomplete spermatogenic arrest

N46.11 Organic oligospermia

Oligospermia NOS

N46.12 Oligospermia due to extratesticular causes

Code also associated cause

N46.121 Oligospermia due to drug therapy

N46.122 Oligospermia due to infection

N46.123 Oligospermia due to obstruction of efferent ducts

N46.124 Oligospermia due to radiation

N46.125 Oligospermia due to systemic disease

N46.129 Oligospermia due to other extratesticular causes

N46.8 Other male infertility

N46.9 Male infertility, unspecified

N47 Disorders of prepuce

N47.0 Adherent prepuce, newborn

N47.1 Phimosis

N47.2 Paraphimosis

N47.3 Deficient foreskin

N47.4 Benign cyst of prepuce

N47.5 Adhesions of prepuce and glans penis

N47.6 Balanoposthitis

Use additional code (B95-B97), to identify infectious agent.

Excludes1: balanitis (N48.1)

N47.7 **Other inflammatory diseases of prepuce**

Use additional code (B95-B97), to identify infectious agent.

N47.8 **Other disorders of prepuce**

N48 **Other disorders of penis**

N48.0 **Leukoplakia of penis**

Balanitis xerotica obliterans

Kraurosis of penis

Lichen sclerosus of external male genital organs

Excludes1: carcinoma in situ of penis (D07.4)

N48.1 **Balanitis**

Use additional code (B95-B97), to identify infectious agent

Excludes1: amebic balanitis (A06.8)

balanitis xerotica obliterans (N48.0)

candidal balanitis (B37.42)

gonococcal balanitis (A54.23)

herpesviral [herpes simplex] balanitis (A60.01)

N48.2 **Other inflammatory disorders of penis**

Use additional code (B95-B97), to identify infectious agent.

Excludes1: balanitis (N48.1)

balanitis xerotica obliterans (N48.0)

balanoposthitis (N47.6)

N48.21 **Abscess of corpus cavernosum and penis**

N48.22 **Cellulitis of corpus cavernosum and penis**

N48.29 **Other inflammatory disorders of penis**

N48.3 **Priapism**

Painful erection

Code first underlying cause

N48.30 **Priapism, unspecified**

N48.31 **Priapism due to trauma**

N48.32 **Priapism due to disease classified elsewhere**

N48.33 **Priapism, drug-induced**

N48.39 **Other priapism**

N48.5 **Ulcer of penis**

N48.6 **Induration penis plastica**

Peyronie's disease

Plastic induration of penis

N48.8 **Other specified disorders of penis**

N48.81 **Thrombosis of superficial vein of penis**

N48.82 **Acquired torsion of penis**

Acquired torsion of penis NOS

Excludes1: congenital torsion of penis (Q55.63)

N48.83 **Acquired buried penis**

Excludes1: congenital hidden penis (Q55.64)

N48.89 **Other specified disorders of penis**

N48.9 **Disorder of penis, unspecified**

N49 **Inflammatory disorders of male genital organs, not elsewhere classified**

Use additional code (B95-B97), to identify infectious agent

Excludes1: inflammation of penis (N48.1, N48.2-)

orchitis and epididymitis (N45.-)

N49.0 **Inflammatory disorders of seminal vesicle**

Vesiculitis NOS

N49.1 **Inflammatory disorders of spermatic cord, tunica vaginalis and vas deferens**

Vasitis

N49.2 **Inflammatory disorders of scrotum**

N49.3 **Fournier gangrene**

N49.8 **Inflammatory disorders of other specified male genital organs**

Inflammation of multiple sites in male genital organs

N49.9 **Inflammatory disorder of unspecified male genital organ**

Abscess of unspecified male genital organ

Boil of unspecified male genital organ

Carbuncle of unspecified male genital organ

Cellulitis of unspecified male genital organ

N50 **Other and unspecified disorders of male genital organs**

Excludes2: torsion of testis (N44.0-)

N50.0 **Atrophy of testis**

N50.1 **Vascular disorders of male genital organs**

Hematocele, NOS, of male genital organs

Hemorrhage of male genital organs

Thrombosis of male genital organs

N50.3 **Cyst of epididymis**

N50.8 **Other specified disorders of male genital organs**

N50.81 **Testicular pain**

•**N50.811** **Right testicular pain**

•**N50.812** **Left testicular pain**

•**N50.819** **Testicular pain, unspecified**

•**N50.82** **Scrotal pain**

•**N50.89** **Other specified disorders of the male genital organs**

Atrophy of scrotum, seminal vesicle, spermatic cord, tunica vaginalis and vas deferens

Chylocele, tunica vaginalis (nonfilarial) NOS

Edema of scrotum, seminal vesicle, spermatic cord, tunica vaginalis and vas deferens

Hypertrophy of scrotum, seminal vesicle, spermatic cord, tunica vaginalis and vas deferens

Stricture of spermatic cord, tunica vaginalis, and vas deferens

Ulcer of scrotum, seminal vesicle, spermatic cord, testis, tunica vaginalis and vas deferens

Urethroscrotal fistula

N50.9 **Disorder of male genital organs, unspecified**

N51 **Disorders of male genital organs in diseases classified elsewhere**

Code first underlying disease, such as:

filariasis (B74.0-B74.9)

Excludes1: amebic balanitis (A06.8)

candidal balanitis (B37.42)

gonococcal balanitis (A54.23)

gonococcal prostatitis (A54.22)

herpesviral [herpes simplex] balanitis (A60.01)

trichomonal prostatitis (A59.02)

tuberculous prostatitis (A18.14)

N52 **Male erectile dysfunction**

> **Excludes1:** psychogenic impotence (F52.21)

N52.0 **Vasculogenic erectile dysfunction**

> **N52.01** **Erectile dysfunction due to arterial insufficiency**
>
> **N52.02** **Corporo-venous occlusive erectile dysfunction**
>
> **N52.03** **Combined arterial insufficiency and corporo-venous occlusive erectile dysfunction**

N52.1 **Erectile dysfunction due to diseases classified elsewhere**

> <u>Code first</u> underlying disease

N52.2 **Drug-induced erectile dysfunction**

N52.3 **Postprocedural erectile dysfunction**

> **N52.31** **Erectile dysfunction following radical prostatectomy**
>
> **N52.32** **Erectile dysfunction following radical cystectomy**
>
> **N52.33** **Erectile dysfunction following urethral surgery**
>
> **N52.34** **Erectile dysfunction following simple prostatectomy**
>
> ●**N52.35** **Erectile dysfunction following radiation therapy**
>
> ●**N52.36** **Erectile dysfunction following interstitial seed therapy**
>
> ●**N52.37** **Erectile dysfunction following prostate ablative therapy**
>
> > Erectile dysfunction following cry**Other**apy
> >
> > Erectile dysfunction follow**ing other** prostate ablative therapies
> >
> > Erectile dysfunction following ultrasound ablative therapies
>
> ▲**N52.39** **Other and unspecified postprocedural erectile dysfunction**

N52.8 **Other male erectile dysfunction**

N52.9 **Male erectile dysfunction, unspecified**

> Impotence NOS

N53 **Other male sexual dysfunction**

> **Excludes1:** psychogenic sexual dysfunction (F52.-)

N53.1 **Ejaculatory dysfunction**

> **Excludes1:** premature ejaculation (F52.4)
>
> **N53.11** **Retarded ejaculation**
>
> **N53.12** **Painful ejaculation**
>
> **N53.13** **Anejaculatory orgasm**
>
> **N53.14** **Retrograde ejaculation**
>
> **N53.19** **Other ejaculatory dysfunction**
>
> > Ejaculatory dysfunction NOS

N53.8 **Other male sexual dysfunction**

N53.9 **Unspecified male sexual dysfunction**

DISORDERS OF BREAST (N60-N65)

Excludes1: disorders of breast associated with childbirth (O91-O92)

N60 **Benign mammary dysplasia**

> **Definition:** Mammary dysplasia is a common condition marked by benign (noncancerous) changes in breast tissue. These changes may include irregular lumps or cysts, breast discomfort, sensitive nipples, and itching.
>
> **Includes:** fibrocystic mastopathy

N60.0 **Solitary cyst of breast**

> Cyst of breast
>
> **N60.01** **Solitary cyst of right breast**
>
> **N60.02** **Solitary cyst of left breast**
>
> **N60.09** **Solitary cyst of unspecified breast**

N60.1 **Diffuse cystic mastopathy**

> Cystic breast
>
> Fibrocystic disease of breast
>
> **Excludes1:** diffuse cystic mastopathy with epithelial proliferation (N60.3-)
>
> **N60.11** **Diffuse cystic mastopathy of right breast**
>
> **N60.12** **Diffuse cystic mastopathy of left breast**
>
> **N60.19** **Diffuse cystic mastopathy of unspecified breast**

N60.2 **Fibroadenosis of breast**

> Adenofibrosis of breast
>
> **Excludes2:** fibroadenoma of breast (D24.-)
>
> **N60.21** **Fibroadenosis of right breast**
>
> **N60.22** **Fibroadenosis of left breast**
>
> **N60.29** **Fibroadenosis of unspecified breast**

N60.3 **Fibrosclerosis of breast**

> Cystic mastopathy with epithelial proliferation
>
> **N60.31** **Fibrosclerosis of right breast**
>
> **N60.32** **Fibrosclerosis of left breast**
>
> **N60.39** **Fibrosclerosis of unspecified breast**

N60.4 **Mammary duct ectasia**

> **N60.41** **Mammary duct ectasia of right breast**
>
> **N60.42** **Mammary duct ectasia of left breast**
>
> **N60.49** **Mammary duct ectasia of unspecified breast**

N60.8 **Other benign mammary dysplasias**

> **N60.81** **Other benign mammary dysplasias of right breast**
>
> **N60.82** **Other benign mammary dysplasias of left breast**
>
> **N60.89** **Other benign mammary dysplasias of unspecified breast**

N60.9 **Unspecified benign mammary dysplasia**

> **N60.91** **Unspecified benign mammary dysplasia of right breast**
>
> **N60.92** **Unspecified benign mammary dysplasia of left breast**
>
> **N60.99** **Unspecified benign mammary dysplasia of unspecified breast**

N61 **Inflammatory disorders of breast**

> **Excludes1:** inflammatory carcinoma of breast (C50.9)
>
> inflammatory disorder of breast associated with childbirth (O91.-)
>
> neonatal infective mastitis (P39.0)
>
> thrombophlebitis of breast [Mondor's disease] (I80.8)

●**N61.0** **Mastitis without abscess**

> Infective mastitis (acute) (nonpuerperal) (subacute)
>
> Mastitis (acute) (nonpuerperal) (subacute) NOS
>
> Cellulitis (acute) (nonpuerperal) (subacute) of breast NOS
>
> Cellulitis (acute) (nonpuerperal) (subacute) of nipple NOS

●**N61.1** **Abscess of the breast and nipple**

> Abscess (acute) (chronic) (nonpuerperal) of areola

● New code ▲ Revised code **Excludes1:** Not coded here **Excludes2:** Not included here ⊗ Placeholder required ⑦ 7th digit required

Abscess (acute) (chronic) (nonpuerperal) of breast

Carbuncle of breast

Mastitis with abscess

N62   Hypertrophy of breast

Gynecomastia

Hypertrophy of breast NOS

Massive pubertal hypertrophy of breast

Excludes1: breast engorgement of newborn (P83.4)

disproportion of reconstructed breast (N65.1)

N63   Unspecified lump in breast

Nodule(s) NOS in breast

N64   Other disorders of breast

Excludes2: mechanical complication of breast prosthesis and implant (T85.4-)

N64.0   Fissure and fistula of nipple

N64.1   Fat necrosis of breast

Fat necrosis (segmental) of breast

Code first breast necrosis due to breast graft (T85.898)

N64.2   Atrophy of breast

N64.3   Galactorrhea not associated with childbirth

N64.4   Mastodynia

N64.5   Other signs and symptoms in breast

Excludes2: abnormal findings on diagnostic imaging of breast (R92.-)

N64.51   Induration of breast

N64.52   Nipple discharge

Excludes1: abnormal findings in nipple discharge (R89.-)

N64.53   Retraction of nipple

N64.59   Other signs and symptoms in breast

N64.8   Other specified disorders of breast

N64.81   Ptosis of breast

Excludes1: ptosis of native breast in relation to reconstructed breast (N65.1)

N64.82   Hypoplasia of breast

Micromastia

Excludes1: congenital absence of breast (Q83.0)

hypoplasia of native breast in relation to reconstructed breast (N65.1)

N64.89   Other specified disorders of breast

Galactocele

Subinvolution of breast (postlactational)

N64.9   Disorder of breast, unspecified

N65   Deformity and disproportion of reconstructed breast

N65.0   Deformity of reconstructed breast

Contour irregularity in reconstructed breast

Excess tissue in reconstructed breast

Misshapen reconstructed breast

N65.1   Disproportion of reconstructed breast

Breast asymmetry between native breast and reconstructed breast

Disproportion between native breast and reconstructed breast

INFLAMMATORY DISEASES OF FEMALE PELVIC ORGANS (N70-N77)

> NOTE: All Diagnosis Codes In This Section Apply To FEMALE Patients Only

Excludes1: inflammatory diseases of female pelvic organs complicating:

abortion or ectopic or molar pregnancy (O00-O07, O08.0)

pregnancy, childbirth and the puerperium (O23.-, O75.3, O85, O86.-)

N70   Salpingitis and oophoritis

Includes: abscess (of) fallopian tube

abscess (of) ovary pyosalpinx salpingo-oophoritis

tubo-ovarian abscess

tubo-ovarian inflammatory disease

Use additional code (B95-B97), to identify infectious agent

Excludes1: gonococcal infection (A54.24)

tuberculous infection (A18.17)

N70.0   Acute salpingitis and oophoritis

N70.01   Acute salpingitis

N70.02   Acute oophoritis

N70.03   Acute salpingitis and oophoritis

N70.1   Chronic salpingitis and oophoritis

Hydrosalpinx

N70.11   Chronic salpingitis

N70.12   Chronic oophoritis

N70.13   Chronic salpingitis and oophoritis

N70.9   Salpingitis and oophoritis, unspecified

N70.91   Salpingitis, unspecified

N70.92   Oophoritis, unspecified

N70.93   Salpingitis and oophoritis, unspecified

N71   Inflammatory disease of uterus, except cervix

Includes: endo (myo) metritis

metritis myometritis pyometra uterine abscess

Use additional code (B95-B97), to identify infectious agent

Excludes1: hyperplastic endometritis (N85.0-)

infection of uterus following delivery (O85, O86.-)

N71.0   Acute inflammatory disease of uterus

N71.1   Chronic inflammatory disease of uterus

N71.9   Inflammatory disease of uterus, unspecified

N72   Inflammatory disease of cervix uteri

Includes: cervicitis (with or without erosion or ectropion)

endocervicitis (with or without erosion or ectropion)

exocervicitis (with or without erosion or ectropion)

Use additional code (B95-B97), to identify infectious agent

Excludes1: erosion and ectropion of cervix without cervicitis (N86)

N73   Other female pelvic inflammatory diseases

Use additional code (B95-B97), to identify infectious agent.

N73.0   Acute parametritis and pelvic cellulitis

Abscess of broad ligament

Abscess of parametrium

Pelvic cellulitis, female

N73.1   Chronic parametritis and pelvic cellulitis

Any condition in N73.0 specified as chronic

Excludes1: tuberculous parametritis and pelvic cellultis (A18.17)

N73.2 **Unspecified parametritis and pelvic cellulitis**

Any condition in N73.0 unspecified whether acute or chronic

N73.3 **Female acute pelvic peritonitis**

N73.4 **Female chronic pelvic peritonitis**

Excludes1: tuberculous pelvic (female) peritonitis (A18.17)

N73.5 **Female pelvic peritonitis, unspecified**

N73.6 **Female pelvic peritoneal adhesions (postinfective)**

Excludes2: postprocedural pelvic peritoneal adhesions (N99.4)

N73.8 **Other specified female pelvic inflammatory diseases**

N73.9 **Female pelvic inflammatory disease, unspecified**

Female pelvic infection or inflammation NOS

N74 **Female pelvic inflammatory disorders in diseases classified elsewhere**

Code first underlying disease

Excludes1: chlamydial cervicitis (A56.02)

chlamydial pelvic inflammatory disease (A56.11)

gonococcal cervicitis (A54.03)

gonococcal pelvic inflammatory disease (A54.24)

herpesviral [herpes simplex] cervicitis (A60.03)

herpesviral [herpes simplex] pelvic inflammatory disease (A60.09)

syphilitic cervicitis (A52.76)

syphilitic pelvic inflammatory disease (A52.76)

trichomonal cervicitis (A59.09)

tuberculous cervicitis (A18.16)

tuberculous pelvic inflammatory disease (A18.17)

N75 **Diseases of Bartholin's gland**

N75.0 **Cyst of Bartholin's gland**

N75.1 **Abscess of Bartholin's gland**

N75.8 **Other diseases of Bartholin's gland**

Bartholinitis

N75.9 **Disease of Bartholin's gland, unspecified**

N76 **Other inflammation of vagina and vulva**

Use additional code (B95-B97), to identify infectious agent

Excludes2: senile (atrophic) vaginitis (N95.2)

vulvar vestibulitis (N94.810)

N76.0 **Acute vaginitis**

Acute vulvovaginitis

Vaginitis NOS

Vulvovaginitis NOS

N76.1 **Subacute and chronic vaginitis**

Chronic vulvovaginitis

Subacute vulvovaginitis

N76.2 **Acute vulvitis**

Vulvitis NOS

N76.3 **Subacute and chronic vulvitis**

N76.4 **Abscess of vulva**

Furuncle of vulva

N76.5 **Ulceration of vagina**

N76.6 **Ulceration of vulva**

N76.8 **Other specified inflammation of vagina and vulva**

N76.81 **Mucositis (ulcerative) of vagina and vulva**

Code also type of associated therapy, such as:

antineoplastic and immunosuppressive drugs (T45.1X-)

radiological procedure and radiotherapy (Y84.2)

Excludes2: gastrointestinal mucositis (ulcerative) (K92.81)

nasal mucositis (ulcerative) (J34.81)

oral mucositis (ulcerative) (K12.3-)

N76.89 **Other specified inflammation of vagina and vulva**

N77 **Vulvovaginal ulceration and inflammation in diseases classified elsewhere**

N77.0 **Ulceration of vulva in diseases classified elsewhere**

Code first underlying disease, such as:

Behçet's disease (M35.2)

Excludes1: ulceration of vulva in gonococcal infection (A54.02)

ulceration of vulva in herpesviral [herpes simplex] infection (A60.04)

ulceration of vulva in syphilis (A51.0)

ulceration of vulva in tuberculosis (A18.18)

N77.1 **Vaginitis, vulvitis and vulvovaginitis in diseases classified elsewhere**

Code first underlying disease, such as:

pinworm (B80)

Excludes1: candidal vulvovaginitis (B37.3)

chlamydial vulvovaginitis (A56.02)

gonococcal vulvovaginitis (A54.02)

herpesviral [herpes simplex] vulvovaginitis (A60.04)

trichomonal vulvovaginitis (A59.01)

tuberculous vulvovaginitis (A18.18)

vulvovaginitis in early syphilis (A51.0)

vulvovaginitis in late syphilis (A52.76)

NONINFLAMMATORY DISORDERS OF FEMALE GENITAL TRACT (N80-N98)

N80 **Endometriosis**

Definition: Endometriosis is a condition where tissue that normally lines the uterus grows in other areas of the body. This can cause pain, irregular menstrual bleeding, and infertility for some women.

N80.0 **Endometriosis of uterus**

Adenomyosis

Excludes1: stromal endometriosis (D39.0)

N80.1 **Endometriosis of ovary**

N80.2 **Endometriosis of fallopian tube**

N80.3 **Endometriosis of pelvic peritoneum**

N80.4 **Endometriosis of rectovaginal septum and vagina**

N80.5 **Endometriosis of intestine**

N80.6 **Endometriosis in cutaneous scar**

N80.8 **Other endometriosis**

N80.9 **Endometriosis, unspecified**

N81 **Female genital prolapse**

Definition: Genital prolapse is a condition in which the vaginal wall or uterus descend below their normal positions; part of the bladder or rectum may protrude from the vagina.

● New code   ▲ Revised code   Excludes1: Not coded here   Excludes2: Not included here   ⊗ Placeholder required   ⑦7th digit required

Excludes1: genital prolapse complicating pregnancy, labor or delivery (O34.5-)

prolapse and hernia of ovary and fallopian tube (N83.4-)

prolapse of vaginal vault after hysterectomy (N99.3)

N81.0   Urethrocele

    Excludes1: urethrocele with cystocele (N81.1-)

    urethrocele with prolapse of uterus (N81.2-N81.4)

N81.1   Cystocele

    Cystocele with urethrocele

    Cystourethrocele

    Excludes1: cystocele with prolapse of uterus (N81.2-N81.4)

    N81.10   Cystocele, unspecified

        Prolapse of (anterior) vaginal wall NOS

    N81.11   Cystocele, midline

    N81.12   Cystocele, lateral

        Paravaginal cystocele

N81.2   Incomplete uterovaginal prolapse

    First degree uterine prolapse

    Prolapse of cervix NOS

    Second degree uterine prolapse

    Excludes1: cervical stump prolaspe (N81.85)

N81.3   Complete uterovaginal prolapse

    Procidentia (uteri) NOS

    Third degree uterine prolapse

N81.4   Uterovaginal prolapse, unspecified

    Prolapse of uterus NOS

N81.5   Vaginal enterocele

    Excludes1: enterocele with prolapse of uterus (N81.2-N81.4)

N81.6   Rectocele

    Prolapse of posterior vaginal wall

    Use additional code for any associated fecal incontinence, if applicable (R15.-)

    Excludes2: perineocele (N81.81)

        rectal prolapse (K62.3)

        rectocele with prolapse of uterus (N81.2-N81.4)

N81.8   Other female genital prolapse

    N81.81   Perineocele

    N81.82   Incompetence or weakening of pubocervical tissue

    N81.83   Incompetence or weakening of rectovaginal tissue

    N81.84   Pelvic muscle wasting

        Disuse atrophy of pelvic muscles and anal sphincter

    N81.85   Cervical stump prolapse

    N81.89   Other female genital prolapse

        Deficient perineum

        Old laceration of muscles of pelvic floor

N81.9   Female genital prolapse, unspecified

N82   Fistulae involving female genital tract

Definition: A fistula involving female genital tract is a fistula that has formed in the wall of the vagina. A vaginal fistula may open into the urinary tract, the rectum, the colon, or the small bowel.

Excludes1: vesicointestinal fistulae (N32.1)

N82.0   Vesicovaginal fistula

N82.1   Other female urinary-genital tract fistulae

    Cervicovesical fistula

    Ureterovaginal fistula

    Urethrovaginal fistula

    Uteroureteric fistula

    Uterovesical fistula

N82.2   Fistula of vagina to small intestine

N82.3   Fistula of vagina to large intestine

    Rectovaginal fistula

N82.4   Other female intestinal-genital tract fistulae

    Intestinouterine fistula

N82.5   Female genital tract-skin fistulae

    Uterus to abdominal wall fistula

    Vaginoperineal fistula

N82.8   Other female genital tract fistulae

N82.9   Female genital tract fistula, unspecified

N83   Noninflammatory disorders of ovary, fallopian tube and broad ligament

Excludes2: hydrosalpinx (N70.1-)

N83.0   Follicular cyst of ovary

    Cyst of graafian follicle

    Hemorrhagic follicular cyst (of ovary)

    ●**N83.00   Follicular cyst of ovary, unspecified side**

    ●**N83.01   Follicular cyst of right ovary**

    ●**N83.02   Follicular cyst of left ovary**

N83.1   Corpus luteum cyst

    Hemorrhagic corpus luteum cyst

    ●**N83.10   Corpus luteum cyst of ovary, unspecified side**

    ●**N83.11   Corpus luteum cyst of right ovary**

    ●**N83.12   Corpus luteum cyst of left ovary**

N83.2   Other and unspecified ovarian cysts

    Excludes1: developmental ovarian cyst (Q50.1)

        neoplastic ovarian cyst (D27.-)

        polycystic ovarian syndrome (E28.2)

        Stein-Leventhal syndrome (E28.2)

    N83.20   Unspecified ovarian cysts

        ●**N83.201   Unspecified ovarian cyst, right side**

        ●**N83.202   Unspecified ovarian cyst, left side**

        ●**N83.209   Unspecified ovarian cyst, unspecified side**

            Ovarian cyst, NOS

    N83.29   Other ovarian cysts

        Retention cyst of ovary

    Simple cyst of ovary

        ●**N83.291   Other ovarian cyst, right side**

        ●**N83.292   Other ovarian cyst, left side**

        ●**N83.299   Other ovarian cyst, unspecified side**

N83.3   Acquired atrophy of ovary and fallopian tube

    N83.31   Acquired atrophy of ovary

        ●**N83.311   Acquired atrophy of right ovary**

        ●**N83.312   Acquired atrophy of left ovary**

        ●**N83.319   Acquired atrophy of ovary, unspecified side**

            Acquired atrophy of ovary, NOS

N83.32   Acquired atrophy of fallopian tube

  ●N83.321   Acquired atrophy of right fallopian tube

  ●N83.322   Acquired atrophy of left fallopian tube

  ●N83.329   Acquired atrophy of fallopian tube, unspecified side

      Acquired atrophy of fallopian tube, NOS

N83.33   Acquired atrophy of ovary and fallopian tube

  ●N83.331   Acquired atrophy of right ovary and fallopian tube

  ●N83.332   Acquired atrophy of left ovary and fallopian tube

  ●N83.339   Acquired atrophy of ovary and fallopian tube, unspecified side

      Acquired atrophy of ovary and fallopian tube, NOS

N83.4   Prolapse and hernia of ovary and fallopian tube

  ●N83.40   Prolapse and hernia of ovary and fallopian tube, unspecified side

      Prolapse and hernia of ovary and fallopian tube, NOS

  ●N83.41   Prolapse and hernia of right ovary and fallopian tube

  ●N83.42   Prolapse and hernia of left ovary and fallopian tube

N83.5   Torsion of ovary, ovarian pedicle and fallopian tube

  Torsion of accessory tube

N83.51   Torsion of ovary and ovarian pedicle

  ●N83.511   Torsion of right ovary and ovarian pedicle

  ●N83.512   Torsion of left ovary and ovarian pedicle

  ●N83.519   Torsion of ovary and ovarian pedicle, unspecified side

      Torsion of ovary and ovarian pedicle, NOS

N83.52   Torsion of fallopian tube

  Torsion of hydatid of Morgagni

  ●N83.521   Torsion of right fallopian tube

  ●N83.522   Torsion of left fallopian tube

  ●N83.529   Torsion of fallopian tube, unspecified side

      Torsion of fallopian tube, NOS

N83.53   Torsion of ovary, ovarian pedicle and fallopian tube

N83.6   Hematosalpinx

  Excludes1: hematosalpinx (with) (in):

      hematocolpos (N89.7)

      hematometra (N85.7)

      tubal pregnancy (O00.1-)

N83.7   Hematoma of broad ligament

N83.8   Other noninflammatory disorders of ovary, fallopian tube and broad ligament

  Broad ligament laceration syndrome [Allen-Masters]

N83.9   Noninflammatory disorder of ovary, fallopian tube and broad ligament, unspecified

N84   Polyp of female genital tract

Excludes1: adenomatous polyp (D28.-)

  placental polyp (O90.89)

N84.0   Polyp of corpus uteri

  Polyp of endometrium

  Polyp of uterus NOS

  Excludes1: polypoid endometrial hyperplasia (N85.0-)

N84.1   Polyp of cervix uteri

  Mucous polyp of cervix

N84.2   Polyp of vagina

N84.3   Polyp of vulva

  Polyp of labia

N84.8   Polyp of other parts of female genital tract

N84.9   Polyp of female genital tract, unspecified

N85   Other noninflammatory disorders of uterus, except cervix

Excludes1: endometriosis (N80.-)

  inflammatory diseases of uterus (N71.-)

  noninflammatory disorders of cervix, except malposition (N86-N88)

  polyp of corpus uteri (N84.0)

  uterine prolapse (N81.-)

N85.0   Endometrial hyperplasia

N85.00   Endometrial hyperplasia, unspecified

  Hyperplasia (adenomatous) (cystic) (glandular) of endometrium

  Hyperplastic endometritis

N85.01   Benign endometrial hyperplasia

  Endometrial hyperplasia (complex) (simple) without atypia

N85.02   Endometrial intraepithelial neoplasia [EIN]

  Endometrial hyperplasia with atypia

  Excludes1: malignant neoplasm of endometrium (with endometrial intraepithelial neoplasia [EIN]) (C54.1)

N85.2   Hypertrophy of uterus

  Bulky or enlarged uterus

  Excludes1: puerperal hypertrophy of uterus (O90.89)

N85.3   Subinvolution of uterus

  Excludes1: puerperal subinvolution of uterus (O90.89)

N85.4   Malposition of uterus

  Anteversion of uterus

  Retroflexion of uterus

  Retroversion of uterus

  Excludes1: malposition of uterus complicating pregnancy, labor or delivery (O34.5-, O65.5)

N85.5   Inversion of uterus

  Excludes1: current obstetric trauma (O71.2)

      postpartum inversion of uterus (O71.2)

N85.6   Intrauterine synechiae

N85.7   Hematometra

  Hematosalpinx with hematometra

  Excludes1: hematometra with hematocolpos (N89.7)

N85.8   Other specified noninflammatory disorders of uterus

  Atrophy of uterus, acquired

  Fibrosis of uterus NOS

N85.9   Noninflammatory disorder of uterus, unspecified

Disorder of uterus NOS

N86   Erosion and ectropion of cervix uteri

Decubitus (trophic) ulcer of cervix

Eversion of cervix

Excludes1: erosion and ectropion of cervix with cervicitis (N72)

N87   Dysplasia of cervix uteri

Excludes1: abnormal results from cervical cytologic examination without histologic confirmation (R87.61-)

carcinoma in situ of cervix uteri (D06.-)

cervical intraepithelial neoplasia III [CIN III] (D06.-)

HGSIL of cervix (R87.613)

severe dysplasia of cervix uteri (D06.-)

N87.0   Mild cervical dysplasia

Cervical intraepithelial neoplasia I [CIN I]

N87.1   Moderate cervical dysplasia

Cervical intraepithelial neoplasia II [CIN II]

N87.9   Dysplasia of cervix uteri, unspecified

Anaplasia of cervix

Cervical atypism

Cervical dysplasia NOS

N88   Other noninflammatory disorders of cervix uteri

Excludes2: inflammatory disease of cervix (N72)

polyp of cervix (N84.1)

N88.0   Leukoplakia of cervix uteri

N88.1   Old laceration of cervix uteri

Adhesions of cervix

Excludes1: current obstetric trauma (O71.3)

N88.2   Stricture and stenosis of cervix uteri

Excludes1: stricture and stenosis of cervix uteri complicating labor (O65.5)

N88.3   Incompetence of cervix uteri

Investigation and management of (suspected) cervical incompetence in a nonpregnant woman

Excludes1: cervical incompetence complicating pregnancy (O34.3-)

N88.4   Hypertrophic elongation of cervix uteri

N88.8   Other specified noninflammatory disorders of cervix uteri

Excludes1: current obstetric trauma (O71.3)

N88.9   Noninflammatory disorder of cervix uteri, unspecified

N89   Other noninflammatory disorders of vagina

Excludes1: abnormal results from vaginal cytologic examination without histologic confirmation (R87.62-)

carcinoma in situ of vagina (D07.2)

HGSIL of vagina (R87.623)

inflammation of vagina (N76.-)

senile (atrophic) vaginitis (N95.2)

severe dysplasia of vagina (D07.2)

trichomonal leukorrhea (A59.00)

vaginal intraepithelial neoplasia [VAIN], grade III (D07.2)

N89.0   Mild vaginal dysplasia

Vaginal intraepithelial neoplasia [VAIN], grade I

N89.1   Moderate vaginal dysplasia

Vaginal intraepithelial neoplasia [VAIN], grade II

N89.3   Dysplasia of vagina, unspecified

N89.4   Leukoplakia of vagina

N89.5   Stricture and atresia of vagina

Vaginal adhesions

Vaginal stenosis

Excludes1: congenital atresia or stricture (Q52.4)

postprocedural adhesions of vagina (N99.2)

N89.6   Tight hymenal ring

Rigid hymen

Tight introitus

Excludes1: imperforate hymen (Q52.3)

N89.7   Hematocolpos

Hematocolpos with hematometra or hematosalpinx

N89.8   Other specified noninflammatory disorders of vagina

Leukorrhea NOS

Old vaginal laceration

Pessary ulcer of vagina

Excludes1: current obstetric trauma (O70.-, O71.4, O71.7-O71.8)

old laceration involving muscles of pelvic floor (N81.8)

N89.9   Noninflammatory disorder of vagina, unspecified

N90   Other noninflammatory disorders of vulva and perineum

Excludes1: anogenital (venereal) warts (A63.0)

carcinoma in situ of vulva (D07.1)

condyloma acuminatum (A63.0)

current obstetric trauma (O70.-, O71.7-O71.8)

inflammation of vulva (N76.-)

severe dysplasia of vulva (D07.1)

vulvar intraepithelial neoplasm III [VIN III] (D07.1)

N90.0   Mild vulvar dysplasia

Vulvar intraepithelial neoplasia [VIN], grade I

N90.1   Moderate vulvar dysplasia

Vulvar intraepithelial neoplasia [VIN], grade II

N90.3   Dysplasia of vulva, unspecified

N90.4   Leukoplakia of vulva

Dystrophy of vulva

Kraurosis of vulva

Lichen sclerosus of external female genital organs

N90.5   Atrophy of vulva

Stenosis of vulva

N90.6   Hypertrophy of vulva

●**N90.60   Unspecified hypertrophy of vulva**

Unspecified hypertrophy of labia

●**N90.61   Childhood asymmetric labium majus enlargement**

CALME

●**N90.69   Other specified hypertrophy of vulva**

Other specified hypertrophy of labia

N90.7   Vulvar cyst

N90.8   Other specified noninflammatory disorders of vulva and perineum

N90.81   Female genital mutilation status

Female genital cutting status

N90.810 **Female genital mutilation status, unspecified**

Female genital cutting status, unspecified

Female genital mutilation status NOS

N90.811 **Female genital mutilation Type I status**

Clitorectomy status

Female genital cutting Type I status

N90.812 **Female genital mutilation Type II status**

Clitorectomy with excision of labia minora status

Female genital cutting Type II status

N90.813 **Female genital mutilation Type III status**

Female genital cutting Type III status

Infibulation status

N90.818 **Other female genital mutilation status**

Female genital cutting Type IV status

Female genital mutilation Type IV status

Other female genital cutting status

N90.89 **Other specified noninflammatory disorders of vulva and perineum**

Adhesions of vulva

Hypertrophy of clitoris

N90.9 **Noninflammatory disorder of vulva and perineum, unspecified**

N91 **Absent, scanty and rare menstruation**

Excludes1: ovarian dysfunction (E28.-)

N91.0 **Primary amenorrhea**

N91.1 **Secondary amenorrhea**

N91.2 **Amenorrhea, unspecified**

N91.3 **Primary oligomenorrhea**

N91.4 **Secondary oligomenorrhea**

N91.5 **Oligomenorrhea, unspecified**

Hypomenorrhea NOS

N92 **Excessive, frequent and irregular menstruation**

Excludes1: postmenopausal bleeding (N95.0)

precocious puberty (menstruation) (E30.1)

N92.0 **Excessive and frequent menstruation with regular cycle**

Heavy periods NOS

Menorrhagia NOS

Polymenorrhea

N92.1 **Excessive and frequent menstruation with irregular cycle**

Irregular intermenstrual bleeding

Irregular, shortened intervals between menstrual bleeding

Menometrorrhagia

Metrorrhagia

N92.2 **Excessive menstruation at puberty**

Excessive bleeding associated with onset of menstrual periods

Pubertal menorrhagia

Puberty bleeding

N92.3 **Ovulation bleeding**

Regular intermenstrual bleeding

N92.4 **Excessive bleeding in the premenopausal period**

Climacteric menorrhagia or metrorrhagia

Menopausal menorrhagia or metrorrhagia

Preclimacteric menorrhagia or metrorrhagia

Premenopausal menorrhagia or metrorrhagia

N92.5 **Other specified irregular menstruation**

N92.6 **Irregular menstruation, unspecified**

Irregular bleeding NOS

Irregular periods NOS

Excludes1: irregular menstruation with:

lengthened intervals or scanty bleeding (N91.3-N91.5)

shortened intervals or excessive bleeding (N92.1)

N93 **Other abnormal uterine and vaginal bleeding**

Excludes1: neonatal vaginal hemorrhage (P54.6)

precocious puberty (menstruation) (E30.1)

pseudomenses (P54.6)

N93.0 **Postcoital and contact bleeding**

•N93.1 **Pre-pubertal vaginal bleeding**

N93.8 **Other specified abnormal uterine and vaginal bleeding**

Dysfunctional or functional uterine or vaginal bleeding NOS

N93.9 **Abnormal uterine and vaginal bleeding, unspecified**

N94 **Pain and other conditions associated with female genital organs and menstrual cycle**

N94.0 **Mittelschmerz**

N94.1 **Dyspareunia**

Excludes1: psychogenic dyspareunia (F52.6)

•N94.10 **Unspecified dyspareunia**

•N94.11 **Superficial (introital) dyspareunia**

•N94.12 **Deep dyspareunia**

•N94.19 **Other specified dyspareunia**

N94.2 **Vaginismus**

Excludes1: psychogenic vaginismus (F52.5)

N94.3 **Premenstrual tension syndrome**

Premenstrual dysphoric disorder

Code also associated menstrual migraine (G43.82-, G43.83-)

Excludes1: Premenstrual dysphoric disorder (F32.81)

N94.4 **Primary dysmenorrhea**

N94.5 **Secondary dysmenorrhea**

N94.6 **Dysmenorrhea, unspecified**

Excludes1: psychogenic dysmenorrhea (F45.8)

N94.8 **Other specified conditions associated with female genital organs and menstrual cycle**

N94.81 **Vulvodynia**

N94.810 **Vulvar vestibulitis**

N94.818 **Other vulvodynia**

N94.819 **Vulvodynia, unspecified**

Vulvodynia NOS

N94.89 **Other specified conditions associated with female genital organs and menstrual cycle**

N94.9 **Unspecified condition associated with female genital organs and menstrual cycle**

N95 **Menopausal and other perimenopausal disorders**

Menopausal **and other** perimenopausal disorders due to naturally occurring (age-related) menopause and perimenopause

Excludes1: excessive bleeding in the premenopausal period (N92.4)

menopausal and perimenopausal disorders due to artificial or premature menopause (E89.4-, E28.31-)

premature menopause (E28.31-)

Excludes2: postmenopausal osteoporosis (M81.0-)

postmenopausal osteoporosis with current pathological fracture (M80.0-)

postmenopausal urethritis (N34.2)

N95.0 **Postmenopausal bleeding**

N95.1 **Menopausal and female climacteric states**

Symptoms such as flushing, sleeplessness, headache, lack of concentration, associated with natural (age-related) menopause

Use additional code for associated symptoms

Excludes1: asymptomatic menopausal state (Z78.0)

symptoms associated with artificial menopause (E89.41)

symptoms associated with premature menopause (E28.310)

N95.2 **Postmenopausal atrophic vaginitis**

Senile (atrophic) vaginitis

N95.8 **Other specified menopausal and perimenopausal disorders**

N95.9 **Unspecified menopausal and perimenopausal disorder**

N96 **Recurrent pregnancy loss**

Investigation or care in a nonpregnant woman with history of recurrent pregnancy loss

Excludes1: recurrent pregancy loss with current pregnancy (O26.2-)

N97 **Female infertility**

Includes: inability to achieve a pregnancy

sterility, female NOS

Excludes1: female infertility associated with:

hypopituitarism (E23.0)

Stein-Leventhal syndrome (E28.2)

Excludes2: incompetence of cervix uteri (N88.3)

N97.0 **Female infertility associated with anovulation**

N97.1 **Female infertility of tubal origin**

Female infertility associated with congenital anomaly of tube female infertility due to tubal block

Female infertility due to tubal occlusion female infertility due to tubal stenosis

N97.2 **Female infertility of uterine origin**

Female infertility associated with congenital anomaly of uterus female infertility due to nonimplantation of ovum

N97.8 **Female infertility of other origin**

N97.9 **Female infertility, unspecified**

N98 **Complications associated with artificial fertilization**

N98.0 **Infection associated with artificial insemination**

N98.1 **Hyperstimulation of ovaries**

Hyperstimulation of ovaries NOS

Hyperstimulation of ovaries associated with induced ovulation

N98.2 **Complications of attempted introduction of fertilized ovum following in vitro fertilization**

N98.3 **Complications of attempted introduction of embryo in embryo transfer**

N98.8 **Other complications associated with artificial fertilization**

N98.9 **Complication associated with artificial fertilization, unspecified**

INTRAOPERATIVE AND POSTPROCEDURAL COMPLICATIONS AND DISORDERS OF GENITOURINARY SYSTEM, NOT ELSEWHERE CLASSIFIED (N99)

N99 **Intraoperative and postprocedural complications and disorders of genitourinary system, not elsewhere classified**

Excludes2: irradiation cystitis (N30.4-)

postoophorectomy osteoporosis with current pathological fracture (M80.8-)

postoophorectomy osteoporosis without current pathological fracture (M81.8)

N99.0 **Postprocedural (acute) (chronic) kidney failure**

Use additional code to type of kidney disease

N99.1 **Postprocedural urethral stricture**

Postcatheterization urethral stricture

N99.11 **Postprocedural urethral stricture, male**

N99.110 **Postprocedural urethral stricture, male, meatal**

N99.111 **Postprocedural bulbous urethral stricture**

N99.112 **Postprocedural membranous urethral stricture**

▲**N99.113** **Postprocedural anterior bulbous urethral stricture**

N99.114 **Postprocedural urethral stricture, male, unspecified**

•**N99.115** **Postprocedural fossa navicularis urethral stricture**

N99.12 **Postprocedural urethral stricture, female**

N99.2 **Postprocedural adhesions of vagina**

N99.3 **Prolapse of vaginal vault after hysterectomy**

N99.4 **Postprocedural pelvic peritoneal adhesions**

Excludes2: pelvic peritoneal adhesions NOS (N73.6)

postinfective pelvic peritoneal adhesions (N73.6)

N99.5 **Complications of stoma of urinary tract**

Excludes2: mechanical complication of urinary catheter (T83.0-)

N99.51 **Complication of cystostomy**

N99.510 **Cystostomy hemorrhage**

N99.511 **Cystostomy infection**

N99.512 **Cystostomy malfunction**

N99.518 **Other cystostomy complication**

N99.52 **Complication of incontinent external stoma of urinary tract**

▲**N99.520** **Hemorrhage of incontinent external stoma of urinary tract**

▲**N99.521** **Infection of incontinent external stoma of urinary tract**

▲**N99.522** **Malfunction of incontinent external stoma of urinary tract**

● N99.523   Herniation of incontinent stoma of urinary tract

● N99.524   Stenosis of incontinent stoma of urinary tract

▲ N99.528   Other complication of incontinent external stoma of urinary tract

N99.53   Complication of continent stoma of urinary tract

▲ N99.530   Hemorrhage of continent stoma of urinary tract

▲ N99.531   Infection of continent stoma of urinary tract

▲ N99.532   Malfunction of continent stoma of urinary tract

● N99.533   Herniation of continent stoma of urinary tract

● N99.534   Stenosis of continent stoma of urinary tract

▲ N99.538   Other complication of continent stoma of urinary tract

N99.6   Intraoperative hemorrhage and hematoma of a genitourinary system organ or structure complicating a procedure

> **Excludes1:** intraoperative hemorrhage and hematoma of a genitourinary system organ or structure due to accidental puncture or laceration during a procedure (N99.7-)

N99.61   Intraoperative hemorrhage and hematoma of a genitourinary system organ or structure complicating a genitourinary system procedure

N99.62   Intraoperative hemorrhage and hematoma of a genitourinary system organ or structure complicating other procedure

N99.7   Accidental puncture and laceration of a genitourinary system organ or structure during a procedure

N99.71   Accidental puncture and laceration of a genitourinary system organ or structure during a genitourinary system procedure

N99.72   Accidental puncture and laceration of a genitourinary system organ or structure during other procedure

N99.8   Other intraoperative and postprocedural complications and disorders of genitourinary system

N99.81   Other intraoperative complications of genitourinary system

N99.82   Postprocedural hemorrhage of a genitourinary system organ or structure following a procedure

▲ N99.820   Postprocedural hemorrhage of a genitourinary system organ or structure following a genitourinary system procedure

▲ N99.821   Postprocedural hemorrhage of a genitourinary system organ or structure following other procedure

N99.83   Residual ovary syndrome

N99.84   Postprocedural hematoma and seroma of a genitourinary system organ or structure following a procedure

● N99.840   Postprocedural hematoma of a genitourinary system organ or structure following a genitourinary system procedure

● N99.841   Postprocedural hematoma of a genitourinary system organ or structure following other procedure

● N99.842   Postprocedural seroma of a genitourinary system organ or structure following a genitourinary system procedure

● N99.843   Postprocedural seroma of a genitourinary system organ or structure following other procedure

N99.89   Other postprocedural complications and disorders of genitourinary system

---

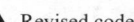 New code   Revised code   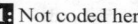 **Excludes1:** Not coded here   **Excludes2:** Not included here   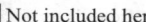 ⊗ Placeholder required   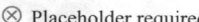 ⑦ 7th digit required

Chapter 15: Pregnancy, Childbirth And The Puerperium (O00-O9A)

DEFINITIONS

This chapter includes definitions of selected key words, terms and phrases and coding alerts for adding points to the clinical domain, and references to coding late effects where appropriate. An example from this chapter is as follows:

O03 Spontaneous abortion
Definition: *Spontaneous abortion* refers to the loss of pregnancy before 20 weeks of gestation without outside intervention.

MULTIPLE CODING FOR A SINGLE CONDITION

In addition to the etiology/manifestation convention that requires two codes to fully describe a single condition that affects multiple body systems, there are other single conditions that also require more than one code. "Use additional code" notes are found in the Tabular List at codes that are not part of an etiology/manifestation pair where a secondary code is useful to fully describe a condition. The sequencing rule is the same as the etiology/manifestation pair, "use additional code" indicates that a secondary code should be added.

For example, for bacterial infections that are not included in chapter 1, a secondary code from category B95, Streptococcus, Staphylococcus, and Enterococcus, as the cause of diseases classified elsewhere, or B96, Other bacterial agents as the cause of diseases classified elsewhere, may be required to identify the bacterial organism causing the infection. A "use additional code" note will normally be found at the infectious disease code, indicating a need for the organism code to be added as a secondary code.

"Code first" notes are also under certain codes that are not specifically manifestation codes but may be due to an underlying cause. When there is a "code first" note and an underlying condition is present, the underlying condition should be sequenced first.

"Code, if applicable, any causal condition first", notes indicate that this code may be assigned as a principal diagnosis when the causal condition is unknown or not applicable. If a causal condition is known, then the code for that condition should be sequenced as the principal or first-listed diagnosis.

Multiple codes may be needed for sequela, complication codes and obstetric codes to more fully describe a condition. See the specific guidelines for these conditions for further instruction.

COMBINATION CODE

A combination code is a single code used to classify: Two diagnoses, or a diagnosis with an associated secondary process (manifestation) A diagnosis with an associated complication

Combination codes are identified by referring to subterm entries in the Alphabetic Index and by reading the inclusion and exclusion notes in the Tabular List.

Assign only the combination code when that code fully identifies the diagnostic conditions involved or when the Alphabetic Index so directs. Multiple coding should not be used when the classification provides a combination code that clearly identifies all of the elements documented in the diagnosis. When the combination code lacks necessary specificity in describing the manifestation or complication, an additional code should be used as a secondary code.

SEQUELA (LATE EFFECTS)

A sequela is the residual effect (condition produced) after the acute phase of an illness or injury has terminated. There is no time limit on when a sequela code can be used. The residual may be apparent early, such as in cerebral infarction, or it may occur months or years later, such as that due to a previous injury. Coding of sequela generally requires two codes sequenced in the following order: The condition or nature of the sequela is sequenced first.

The sequela code is sequenced second.

An exception to the above guidelines are those instances where the code for the sequela is followed by a manifestation code identified in the Tabular List and title, or the sequela code has been expanded (at the fourth, fifth or sixth character levels) to include the manifestation(s). The code for the acute phase of an illness or injury that led to the sequela is never used with a code for the late effect.

GENERAL RULES FOR OBSTETRIC CASES

1) **Codes from chapter 15 and sequencing priority**

   Obstetric cases require codes from chapter 15, codes in the range O00-O9A, Pregnancy, Childbirth, and the Puerperium. Chapter 15 codes have sequencing priority over codes from other chapters. Additional codes from other chapters may be used in conjunction with chapter 15 codes to further specify conditions. Should the provider document that the pregnancy is incidental to the encounter, then code Z33.1, Pregnant state, incidental, should be used in place of any chapter 15 codes. It is the provider's responsibility to state that the condition being treated is not affecting the pregnancy.

2) **Chapter 15 codes used only on the maternal record**

   Chapter 15 codes are to be used only on the maternal record, never on the record of the newborn.

3) **Final character for trimester**

The majority of codes in Chapter 15 have a final character indicating the trimester of pregnancy. The timeframes for the trimesters are indicated at the beginning of the chapter. If trimester is not a component of a code, it is because the condition always occurs in a specific trimester, or the concept of trimester of pregnancy is not applicable. Certain codes have characters for only certain trimesters because the condition does not occur in all trimesters, but it may occur in more than just one.

Assignment of the final character for trimester should be based on the provider's documentation of the trimester (or number of weeks) for the current admission/encounter. This applies to the assignment of trimester for pre-existing conditions as well as those that develop during or are due to the pregnancy. The provider's documentation of the number of weeks may be used to assign the appropriate code identifying the trimester.

Whenever delivery occurs during the current admission, and there is an "in childbirth" option for the obstetric complication being coded, the "in childbirth" code should be assigned.

4)   Selection of trimester for inpatient admissions that encompass more than one trimester

In instances when a patient is admitted to a hospital for complications of pregnancy during one trimester and remains in the hospital into a subsequent trimester, the trimester character for the antepartum complication code should be assigned on the basis of the trimester when the complication developed, not the trimester of the discharge. If the condition developed prior to the current admission/encounter or represents a pre-existing condition, the trimester character for the trimester at the time of the admission/encounter should be assigned.

5)   Unspecified trimester

Each category that includes codes for trimester has a code for "unspecified trimester." The "unspecified trimester" code should rarely be used, such as when the documentation in the record is insufficient to determine the trimester and it is not possible to obtain clarification.

6)   7th character for Fetus Identification

Where applicable, a 7th character is to be assigned for certain categories (O31, O32, O33.3 - O33.6, O35, O36, O40, O41, O60.1, O60.2, O64, and O69) to identify the fetus for which the complication code applies.

Assign 7th character "0":

- For single gestations

- When the documentation in the record is insufficient to determine the fetus affected and it is not possible to obtain clarification.

- When it is not possible to clinically determine which fetus is affected.

SELECTION OF OB PRINCIPAL OR FIRST-LISTED DIAGNOSIS

1)   Routine outpatient prenatal visits

For routine outpatient prenatal visits when no complications are present, a code from category Z34, Encounter for supervision of normal pregnancy, should be used as the first-listed diagnosis. These codes should not be used in conjunction with chapter 15 codes.

2)   Supervision of High-Risk Pregnancy

Codes from category O09, Supervision of high-risk pregnancy, are intended for use only during the prenatal period. For complications during the labor or delivery episode as a result of a high-risk pregnancy, assign the applicable complication codes from Chapter 15. If there are no complications during the labor or delivery episode, assign code O80, Encounter for full-term uncomplicated delivery.

For routine prenatal outpatient visits for patients with high-risk pregnancies, a code from category O09, Supervision of high-risk pregnancy, should be used as the first-listed diagnosis. Secondary chapter 15 codes may be used in conjunction with these codes if appropriate.

3)   Episodes when no delivery occurs

In episodes when no delivery occurs, the principal diagnosis should correspond to the principal complication of the pregnancy which necessitated the encounter. Should more than one complication exist, all of which are treated or monitored, any of the complications codes may be sequenced first.

4)   When a delivery occurs

When an obstetric patient is admitted and delivers during that admission, the condition that prompted the admission should be sequenced as the principal diagnosis. If multiple conditions prompted the admission, sequence the one most related to the delivery as the principal diagnosis. A code for any complication of the delivery should be assigned as an additional diagnosis. In cases of cesarean delivery, if the patient was admitted with a condition that resulted in the performance of a cesarean procedure, that condition should be selected as the principal diagnosis. If the reason for the admission was unrelated to the condition resulting in the cesarean delivery, the condition related to the reason for the admission should be selected as the principal diagnosis.

5)   Outcome of delivery

A code from category Z37, Outcome of delivery, should be included on every maternal record when a delivery has occurred. These codes are not to be used on subsequent records or on the newborn record.

PRE-EXISTING CONDITIONS VERSUS CONDITIONS DUE TO THE PREGNANCY

Certain categories in Chapter 15 distinguish between conditions of the mother that existed prior to pregnancy (pre-existing) and those that are a direct result of pregnancy. When assigning codes from Chapter 15, it is important to assess if a condition was pre-existing prior to pregnancy or developed during or due to the pregnancy in order to assign the correct code.

Categories that do not distinguish between pre-existing and pregnancy-related conditions may be used for either. It is acceptable to use codes specifically for the puerperium with codes complicating pregnancy and childbirth if a condition arises postpartum during the delivery encounter.

PRE-EXISTING HYPERTENSION IN PREGNANCY

Category O10, Pre-existing hypertension complicating pregnancy, childbirth and the puerperium, includes codes for hypertensive heart and hypertensive chronic kidney disease. When assigning one of the O10 codes that includes hypertensive heart disease or hypertensive chronic kidney disease, it is necessary to add a secondary code from the appropriate hypertension category to specify the type of heart failure or chronic kidney disease.

See Section I.C.9. Hypertension.

FETAL CONDITIONS AFFECTING THE MANAGEMENT OF THE MOTHER

1) **Codes from categories O35 and O36**

   Codes from categories O35, Maternal care for known or suspected fetal abnormality and damage, and O36, Maternal care for other fetal problems, are assigned only when the fetal condition is actually responsible for modifying the management of the mother, i.e., by requiring diagnostic studies, additional observation, special care, or termination of pregnancy. The fact that the fetal condition exists does not justify assigning a code from this series to the mother's record.

2) **In utero surgery**

   In cases when surgery is performed on the fetus, a diagnosis code from category O35, Maternal care for known or suspected fetal abnormality and damage, should be assigned identifying the fetal condition. Assign the appropriate procedure code for the procedure performed.

   No code from Chapter 16, the perinatal codes, should be used on the mother's record to identify fetal conditions. Surgery performed in utero on a fetus is still to be coded as an obstetric encounter.

HIV INFECTION IN PREGNANCY, CHILDBIRTH AND THE PUERPERIUM

During pregnancy, childbirth or the puerperium, a patient admitted because of an HIV-related illness should receive a principal diagnosis from subcategory O98.7-, Human immunodeficiency [HIV] disease complicating pregnancy, childbirth and the puerperium, followed by the code(s) for the HIV-related illness(es).

Patients with asymptomatic HIV infection status admitted during pregnancy, childbirth, or the puerperium should receive codes of O98.7- and Z21, Asymptomatic human immunodeficiency virus [HIV] infection status.

DIABETES MELLITUS IN PREGNANCY

Diabetes mellitus is a significant complicating factor in pregnancy. Pregnant women who are diabetic should be assigned a code from category O24, Diabetes mellitus in pregnancy, childbirth, and the puerperium, first, followed by the appropriate diabetes code(s) (E08-E13) from Chapter 4.

LONG TERM USE OF INSULIN AND ORAL HYPOGLYCEMICS

Code Z79.4, Long-term (current) use of insulin, or code Z79.84, Long-term (current) use of oral hypoglycemic drugs, should also be assigned if the diabetes mellitus is being treated with insulin or oral medications. If the patient is treated with both oral medications and insulin, only the code for insulin-controlled should be assigned.

GESTATIONAL (PREGNANCY INDUCED) DIABETES

Gestational (pregnancy induced) diabetes can occur during the second and third trimester of pregnancy in women who were not diabetic prior to pregnancy. Gestational diabetes can cause complications in the pregnancy similar to those of pre-existing diabetes mellitus. It also puts the woman at greater risk of developing diabetes after the pregnancy. Codes for gestational diabetes are in subcategory O24.4, Gestational diabetes mellitus. No other code from category O24, Diabetes mellitus in pregnancy, childbirth, and the puerperium, should be used with a code from O24.4.

The codes under subcategory O24.4 include diet controlled, insulin controlled, and controlled by oral hypoglycemic drugs. If a patient with gestational diabetes is treated with both diet and insulin, only the code for insulin-controlled is required. If a patient with gestational diabetes is treated with both diet and oral hypoglycemic medications, only the code for "controlled by oral hypoglycemic drugs" is required. Code Z79.4, Long-term (current) use of insulin or code Z79.84, Long-term (current) use of oral hypoglycemic drugs, should not be assigned with codes from subcategory O24.4. An abnormal glucose tolerance in pregnancy is assigned a code from subcategory O99.81, Abnormal glucose complicating pregnancy, childbirth, and the puerperium.

SEPSIS AND SEPTIC SHOCK COMPLICATING ABORTION, PREGNANCY, CHILDBIRTH AND THE PUERPERIUM

When assigning a chapter 15 code for sepsis complicating abortion, pregnancy, childbirth, and the puerperium, a code for the specific type of infection should be assigned as an additional diagnosis. If severe sepsis is present, a code from subcategory R65.2, Severe sepsis, and code(s) for associated organ dysfunction(s) should also be assigned as additional diagnoses.

PUERPERAL SEPSIS

Code O85, Puerperal sepsis, should be assigned with a secondary code to identify the causal organism (e.g., for a bacterial infection, assign a code from category B95-B96, Bacterial infections in conditions classified elsewhere). A code from category A40, Streptococcal sepsis, or A41, Other sepsis, should not be used for puerperal sepsis. If applicable, use additional codes to identify severe sepsis (R65.2-) and any associated acute organ dysfunction.

ALCOHOL AND TOBACCO USE DURING PREGNANCY, CHILDBIRTH AND THE PUERPERIUM

1) Alcohol use during pregnancy, childbirth and the puerperium

Codes under subcategory O99.31, Alcohol use complicating pregnancy, childbirth, and the puerperium, should be assigned for any pregnancy case when a mother uses alcohol during the pregnancy or postpartum. A secondary code from category F10, Alcohol related disorders, should also be assigned to identify manifestations of the alcohol use.

2) Tobacco use during pregnancy, childbirth and the puerperium

Codes under subcategory O99.33, Smoking (tobacco) complicating pregnancy, childbirth, and the puerperium, should be assigned for any pregnancy case when a mother uses any type of tobacco product during the pregnancy or postpartum. A secondary code from category F17, Nicotine dependence, should also be assigned to identify the type of nicotine dependence.

POISONING, TOXIC EFFECTS, ADVERSE EFFECTS AND UNDERDOSING IN A PREGNANT PATIENT

A code from subcategory O9A.2, Injury, poisoning and certain other consequences of external causes complicating pregnancy, childbirth, and the puerperium, should be sequenced first, followed by the appropriate injury, poisoning, toxic effect, adverse effect or underdosing code, and then the additional code(s) that specifies the condition caused by the poisoning, toxic effect, adverse effect or underdosing.

See Section I.C.19. Adverse effects, poisoning, underdosing and toxic effects.

NORMAL DELIVERY, CODE O80

1) Encounter for full term uncomplicated delivery

Code O80 should be assigned when a woman is admitted for a full-term normal delivery and delivers a single, healthy infant without any complications antepartum, during the delivery, or postpartum during the delivery episode. Code O80 is always a principal diagnosis. It is not to be used if any other code from chapter 15 is needed to describe a current complication of the antenatal, delivery, or perinatal period. Additional codes from other chapters may be used with code O80 if they are not related to or are in any way complicating the pregnancy.

2) Uncomplicated delivery with resolved antepartum complication

Code O80 may be used if the patient had a complication at some point during the pregnancy, but the complication is not present at the time of the admission for delivery.

3) Outcome of delivery for O80

Z37.0, Single live birth, is the only outcome of delivery code appropriate for use with O80.

THE PERIPARTUM AND POSTPARTUM PERIODS

1) Peripartum and Postpartum periods

The postpartum period begins immediately after delivery and continues for six weeks following delivery. The peripartum period is defined as the last month of pregnancy to five months postpartum.

2) Peripartum and postpartum complication

A postpartum complication is any complication occurring within the six-week period.

3) Pregnancy-related complications after 6 week period

Chapter 15 codes may also be used to describe pregnancy-related complications after the peripartum or postpartum period if the provider documents that a condition is pregnancy related.

4) Admission for routine postpartum care following delivery outside hospital

When the mother delivers outside the hospital prior to admission and is admitted for routine postpartum care and no complications are noted, code Z39.0, Encounter for care and examination of mother immediately after delivery, should be assigned as the principal diagnosis.

5)   Pregnancy associated cardiomyopathy

Pregnancy associated cardiomyopathy, code O90.3, is unique in that it may be diagnosed in the third trimester of pregnancy but may continue to progress months after delivery. For this reason, it is referred to as peripartum cardiomyopathy. Code O90.3 is only for use when the cardiomyopathy develops as a result of pregnancy in a woman who did not have pre-existing heart disease.

CODE O94, SEQUELAE OF COMPLICATION OF PREGNANCY, CHILDBIRTH, AND THE PUERPERIUM

1)   Code O94

Code O94, Sequelae of complication of pregnancy, childbirth, and the puerperium, is for use in those cases when an initial complication of a pregnancy develops a sequelae requiring care or treatment at a future date.

2)   After the initial postpartum period

This code may be used at any time after the initial postpartum period.

3)   Sequencing of Code O94

This code, like all sequela codes, is to be sequenced following the code describing the sequelae of the complication.

TERMINATION OF PREGNANCY AND SPONTANEOUS ABORTIONS

1)   Abortion with Liveborn Fetus

When an attempted termination of pregnancy results in a liveborn fetus, assign code Z33.2, Encounter for elective termination of pregnancy and a code from category Z37, Outcome of Delivery.

2)   Retained Products of Conception following an abortion

Subsequent encounters for retained products of conception following a spontaneous abortion or elective termination of pregnancy are assigned the appropriate code from category O03, Spontaneous abortion, or codes O07.4, Failed attempted termination of pregnancy without complication and Z33.2, Encounter for elective termination of pregnancy. This advice is appropriate even when the patient was discharged previously with a discharge diagnosis of complete abortion.

3)   Complications leading to abortion

Codes from Chapter 15 may be used as additional codes to identify any documented complications of the pregnancy in conjunction with codes in categories in O07 and O08.

ABUSE IN A PREGNANT PATIENT

For suspected or confirmed cases of abuse of a pregnant patient, a code(s) from subcategories O9A.3, Physical abuse complicating pregnancy, childbirth, and the puerperium, O9A.4, Sexual abuse complicating pregnancy, childbirth, and the puerperium, and O9A.5, Psychological abuse complicating pregnancy, childbirth, and the puerperium, should be sequenced first, followed by the appropriate codes (if applicable) to identify any associated current injury due to physical abuse, sexual abuse, and the perpetrator of abuse.

See Section I.C.19. Adult and child abuse, neglect and other maltreatment.

Chapter 15

Pregnancy, Childbirth And The Puerperium (O00-O9A)

NOTE: All Diagnosis Codes In This Chapter Apply To FEMALE Patients Only

NOTE: CODES FROM THIS CHAPTER ARE FOR USE ONLY ON MATERNAL RECORDS, NEVER ON NEWBORN RECORDS

Codes from this chapter are for use for conditions related to or aggravated by the pregnancy, childbirth, or by the puerperium (maternal causes or obstetric causes) trimesters are counted from the first day of the last menstrual period. They are defined as follows:

1st trimester- less than 14 weeks 0 days

2nd trimester- 14 weeks 0 days to less than 28 weeks 0 days

3rd trimester- 28 weeks 0 days until delivery

Use additional code from category Z3A, Weeks of gestation, to identify the specific week of the pregnancy, if known.

Excludes1: supervision of normal pregnancy (Z34.-)

Excludes2: mental and behavioral disorders associated with the puerperium (F53)

obstetrical tetanus (A34)

postpartum necrosis of pituitary gland (E23.0)

puerperal osteomalacia (M83.0)

This chapter contains the following blocks:

O00-O08	Pregnancy with abortive outcome
O09	Supervision of high risk pregnancy
O10-O16	Edema, proteinuria and hypertensive disorders in pregnancy, childbirth and the puerperium
O20-O29	Other maternal disorders predominantly related to pregnancy
O30-O48	Maternal care related to the fetus and amniotic cavity and possible delivery problems
O60-O77	Complications of labor and delivery
O80-O82	Encounter for delivery
O85-O92	Complications predominantly related to the puerperium
O94-O9A	Other obstetric conditions, not elsewhere classified

PREGNANCY WITH ABORTIVE OUTCOME (O00-O08)

Excludes1: continuing pregnancy in multiple gestation after abortion of one fetus or more (O31.1-, O31.3-)

O00 Ectopic pregnancy

Includes: ruptured ectopic pregnancy

Use additional code from category O08 to identify any associated complication

O00.0 Abdominal pregnancy

Excludes1: maternal care for viable fetus in abdominal pregnancy (O36.7-)

● **O00.00 Abdominal pregnancy without intrauterine pregnancy**

Abdominal pregnancy NOS

● **O00.01 Abdominal pregnancy with intrauterine pregnancy**

O00.1 Tubal pregnancy

Fallopian pregnancy

Rupture of (fallopian) tube due to pregnancy

Tubal abortion

● **O00.10 Tubal pregnancy without intrauterine pregnancy**

Tubal pregnancy NOS

● **O00.11 Tubal pregnancy with intrauterine pregnancy**

O00.2 Ovarian pregnancy

● **O00.20 Ovarian pregnancy without intrauterine pregnancy**

Ovarian pregnancy NOS

● **O00.21 Ovarian pregnancy with intrauterine pregnancy**

O00.8 Other ectopic pregnancy

Definition: Ectopic pregnancy occurs with the implantation and subsequent development of a fertilized ovum outside the uterus, as in a fallopian tube.

Cervical pregnancy

Cornual pregnancy

Intraligamentous pregnancy

Mural pregnancy

● **O00.80 Other ectopic pregnancy without intrauterine pregnancy**

Other ectopic pregnancy NOS

● **O00.81 Other ectopic pregnancy with intrauterine pregnancy**

O00.9 Ectopic pregnancy, unspecified

● **O00.90 Unspecified ectopic pregnancy without intrauterine pregnancy**

Ectopic pregnancy NOS

● **O00.91 Unspecified ectopic pregnancy with intrauterine pregnancy**

O01 Hydatidiform mole

Definition: A Hydatidiform mole is a rare mass or growth that forms inside the uterus at the beginning of a pregnancy. It is a type of gestational trophoblastic disease (GTD).

Use additional code from category O08 to identify any associated complication.

Excludes1: chorioadenoma (destruens) (D39.2)

malignant hydatidiform mole (D39.2)

O01.0 Classical hydatidiform mole

Complete hydatidiform mole

O01.1 Incomplete and partial hydatidiform mole

O01.9 Hydatidiform mole, unspecified

Trophoblastic disease NOS

Vesicular mole NOS

O02 Other abnormal products of conception

Use additional code from category O08 to identify any associated complication.

Excludes1: papyraceous fetus (O31.0-)

O02.0 Blighted ovum and nonhydatidiform mole

Carneous mole

Fleshy mole

Intrauterine mole NOS

Molar pregnancy NEC

Pathological ovum

O02.1 Missed abortion

Definition: A missed abortion is an abortion in which the fetus dies but is retained within the uterus for two months or longer.

Early fetal death, before completion of 20 weeks of gestation, with retention of dead fetus

Excludes1: failed induced abortion (O07.-)

fetal death (intrauterine) (late) (O36.4)

missed abortion with blighted ovum (O02.0)

missed abortion with hydatidiform mole (O01.-)

missed abortion with nonhydatidiform (O02.0)

missed abortion with other abnormal products of conception (O02.8-)

missed delivery (O36.4)

stillbirth (P95)

O02.8 Other specified abnormal products of conception

Excludes1: abnormal products of conception with blighted ovum (O02.0)

abnormal products of conception with hydatidiform mole (O01.-)

abnormal products of conception with nonhydatidiform mole (O02.0)

O02.81 Inappropriate change in quantitative human chorionic gonadotropin (hCG) in early pregnancy

Biochemical pregnancy

Chemical pregnancy

Inappropriate level of quantitative human chorionic gonadotropin (hCG) for gestational age in early pregnancy

O02.89 Other abnormal products of conception

O02.9 Abnormal product of conception, unspecified

O03 Spontaneous abortion

Definition: Spontaneous abortion refers to the loss of pregnancy before 20 weeks of gestation without outside intervention.

Note: Incomplete abortion includes retained products of conception following spontaneous abortion

Includes: miscarriage

O03.0 Genital tract and pelvic infection following incomplete spontaneous abortion

Endometritis following incomplete spontaneous abortion

Oophoritis following incomplete spontaneous abortion

Parametritis following incomplete spontaneous abortion

Pelvic peritonitis following incomplete spontaneous abortion

Salpingitis following incomplete spontaneous abortion

Salpingo-oophoritis following incomplete spontaneous abortion

Excludes1: sepsis following incomplete spontaneous abortion (O03.37)

urinary tract infection following incomplete spontaneous abortion (O03.38)

O03.1 Delayed or excessive hemorrhage following incomplete spontaneous abortion

Afibrinogenemia following incomplete spontaneous abortion

Defibrination syndrome following incomplete spontaneous abortion

Hemolysis following incomplete spontaneous abortion

Intravascular coagulation following incomplete spontaneous abortion

O03.2 Embolism following incomplete spontaneous abortion

Air embolism following incomplete spontaneous abortion

Amniotic fluid embolism following incomplete spontaneous abortion

Blood-clot embolism following incomplete spontaneous abortion

Embolism NOS following incomplete spontaneous abortion

Fat embolism following incomplete spontaneous abortion

Pulmonary embolism following incomplete spontaneous abortion

Pyemic embolism following incomplete spontaneous abortion

Septic or septicopyemic embolism following incomplete spontaneous abortion

Soap embolism following incomplete spontaneous abortion

O03.3 Other and unspecified complications following incomplete spontaneous abortion

O03.30 Unspecified complication following incomplete spontaneous abortion

O03.31 Shock following incomplete spontaneous abortion

Circulatory collapse following incomplete spontaneous abortion

Shock (postprocedural) following incomplete spontaneous abortion

Excludes1: shock due to infection following incomplete spontaneous abortion (O03.37)

O03.32 Renal failure following incomplete spontaneous abortion

Kidney failure (acute) following incomplete spontaneous abortion

Oliguria following incomplete spontaneous abortion

Renal shutdown following incomplete spontaneous abortion

Renal tubular necrosis following incomplete spontaneous abortion

Uremia following incomplete spontaneous abortion

O03.33 Metabolic disorder following incomplete spontaneous abortion

O03.34 Damage to pelvic organs following incomplete spontaneous abortion

Laceration, perforation, tear or chemical damage of bladder following incomplete spontaneous abortion

Laceration, perforation, tear or chemical damage of bowel following incomplete spontaneous abortion

Laceration, perforation, tear or chemical damage of broad ligament following incomplete spontaneous abortion

Laceration, perforation, tear or chemical damage of cervix following incomplete spontaneous abortion

Laceration, perforation, tear or chemical damage of periurethral tissue following incomplete spontaneous abortion

Laceration, perforation, tear or chemical damage of uterus following incomplete spontaneous abortion

Laceration, perforation, tear or chemical damage of vagina following incomplete spontaneous abortion

● New code ▲ Revised code Excludes1: Not coded here Excludes2: Not included here ⊗ Placeholder required ⑦7th digit required

O03.35 Other venous complications following incomplete spontaneous abortion

O03.36 Cardiac arrest following incomplete spontaneous abortion

O03.37 Sepsis following incomplete spontaneous abortion

Use additional code to identify infectious agent (B95-B97)

Use additional code to identify severe sepsis, if applicable (R65.2-)

Excludes1: septic or septicopyemic embolism following incomplete spontaneous abortion (O03.2)

O03.38 Urinary tract infection following incomplete spontaneous abortion

Cystitis following incomplete spontaneous abortion

O03.39 Incomplete spontaneous abortion with other complications

O03.4 Incomplete spontaneous abortion without complication

O03.5 Genital tract and pelvic infection following complete or unspecified spontaneous abortion

Endometritis following complete or unspecified spontaneous abortion

Oophoritis following complete or unspecified spontaneous abortion

Parametritis following complete or unspecified spontaneous abortion

Pelvic peritonitis following complete or unspecified spontaneous abortion

Salpingitis following complete or unspecified spontaneous abortion

Salpingo-oophoritis following complete or unspecified spontaneous abortion

Excludes1: sepsis following complete or unspecified spontaneous abortion (O03.87)

urinary tract infection following complete or unspecified spontaneous abortion (O03.88)

O03.6 Delayed or excessive hemorrhage following complete or unspecified spontaneous abortion

Afibrinogenemia following complete or unspecified spontaneous abortion

Defibrination syndrome following complete or unspecified spontaneous abortion

Hemolysis following complete or unspecified spontaneous abortion

Intravascular coagulation following complete or unspecified spontaneous abortion

O03.7 Embolism following complete or unspecified spontaneous abortion

Air embolism following complete or unspecified spontaneous abortion

Amniotic fluid embolism following complete or unspecified spontaneous abortion

Blood-clot embolism following complete or unspecified spontaneous abortion

Embolism NOS following complete or unspecified spontaneous abortion

Fat embolism following complete or unspecified spontaneous abortion

Pulmonary embolism following complete or unspecified spontaneous abortion

Pyemic embolism following complete or unspecified spontaneous abortion

Septic or septicopyemic embolism following complete or unspecified spontaneous abortion

Soap embolism following complete or unspecified spontaneous abortion

O03.8 Other and unspecified complications following complete or unspecified spontaneous abortion

O03.80 Unspecified complication following complete or unspecified spontaneous abortion

O03.81 Shock following complete or unspecified spontaneous abortion

Circulatory collapse following complete or unspecified spontaneous abortion

Shock (postprocedural) following complete or unspecified spontaneous abortion

Excludes1: shock due to infection following complete or unspecified spontaneous abortion (O03.87)

O03.82 Renal failure following complete or unspecified spontaneous abortion

Kidney failure (acute) following complete or unspecified spontaneous abortion

Oliguria following complete or unspecified spontaneous abortion

Renal shutdown following complete or unspecified spontaneous abortion

Renal tubular necrosis following complete or unspecified spontaneous abortion

Uremia following complete or unspecified spontaneous abortion

O03.83 Metabolic disorder following complete or unspecified spontaneous abortion

O03.84 Damage to pelvic organs following complete or unspecified spontaneous abortion

Laceration, perforation, tear or chemical damage of bladder following complete or unspecified spontaneous abortion

Laceration, perforation, tear or chemical damage of bowel following complete or unspecified spontaneous abortion

Laceration, perforation, tear or chemical damage of broad ligament following complete or unspecified spontaneous abortion

Laceration, perforation, tear or chemical damage of cervix following complete or unspecified spontaneous abortion

Laceration, perforation, tear or chemical damage of periurethral tissue following complete or unspecified spontaneous abortion

Laceration, perforation, tear or chemical damage of uterus following complete or unspecified spontaneous abortion

Laceration, perforation, tear or chemical damage of vagina following complete or unspecified spontaneous abortion

O03.85 Other venous complications following complete or unspecified spontaneous abortion

O03.86 Cardiac arrest following complete or unspecified spontaneous abortion

O03.87 **Sepsis following complete or unspecified spontaneous abortion**

Use additional code to identify infectious agent (B95-B97)

Use additional code to identify severe sepsis, if applicable (R65.2-)

Excludes1: septic or septicopyemic embolism following complete or unspecified spontaneous abortion (O03.7)

O03.88 **Urinary tract infection following complete or unspecified spontaneous abortion**

Cystitis following complete or unspecified spontaneous abortion

O03.89 **Complete or unspecified spontaneous abortion with other complications**

O03.9 **Complete or unspecified spontaneous abortion without complication**

Miscarriage NOS

Spontaneous abortion NOS

O04 **Complications following (induced) termination of pregnancy**

Includes: complications following (induced) termination of pregnancy

Excludes1: encounter for elective termination of pregnancy, uncomplicated (Z33.2)

failed attempted termination of pregnancy (O07.-)

O04.5 **Genital tract and pelvic infection following (induced) termination of pregnancy**

Endometritis following (induced) termination of pregnancy

Oophoritis following (induced) termination of pregnancy

Parametritis following (induced) termination of pregnancy

Pelvic peritonitis following (induced) termination of pregnancy

Salpingitis following (induced) termination of pregnancy

Salpingo-oophoritis following (induced) termination of pregnancy

Excludes1: sepsis following (induced) termination of pregnancy (O04.87)

urinary tract infection following (induced) termination of pregnancy (O04.88)

O04.6 **Delayed or excessive hemorrhage following (induced) termination of pregnancy**

Afibrinogenemia following (induced) termination of pregnancy

Defibrination syndrome following (induced) termination of pregnancy

Hemolysis following (induced) termination of pregnancy

Intravascular coagulation following (induced) termination of pregnancy

O04.7 **Embolism following (induced) termination of pregnancy**

Air embolism following (induced) termination of pregnancy

Amniotic fluid embolism following (induced) termination of pregnancy

Blood-clot embolism following (induced) termination of pregnancy

Embolism NOS following (induced) termination of pregnancy

Fat embolism following (induced) termination of pregnancy

Pulmonary embolism following (induced) termination of pregnancy

Pyemic embolism following (induced) termination of pregnancy

Septic or septicopyemic embolism following (induced) termination of pregnancy

Soap embolism following (induced) termination of pregnancy

O04.8 **(Induced) termination of pregnancy with other and unspecified complications**

O04.80 **(Induced) termination of pregnancy with unspecified complications**

O04.81 **Shock following (induced) termination of pregnancy**

Circulatory collapse following (induced) termination of pregnancy

Shock (postprocedural) following (induced) termination of pregnancy

Excludes1: shock due to infection following (induced) termination of pregnancy (O04.87)

O04.82 **Renal failure following (induced) termination of pregnancy**

Kidney failure (acute) following (induced) termination of pregnancy

Oliguria following (induced) termination of pregnancy

Renal shutdown following (induced) termination of pregnancy

Renal tubular necrosis following (induced) termination of pregnancy

Uremia following (induced) termination of pregnancy

O04.83 **Metabolic disorder following (induced) termination of pregnancy**

O04.84 **Damage to pelvic organs following (induced) termination of pregnancy**

Laceration, perforation, tear or chemical damage of bladder following (induced) termination of pregnancy

Laceration, perforation, tear or chemical damage of bowel following (induced) termination of pregnancy

Laceration, perforation, tear or chemical damage of broad ligament following (induced) termination of pregnancy

Laceration, perforation, tear or chemical damage of cervix following (induced) termination of pregnancy

Laceration, perforation, tear or chemical damage of periurethral tissue following (induced) termination of pregnancy

Laceration, perforation, tear or chemical damage of uterus following (induced) termination of pregnancy

Laceration, perforation, tear or chemical damage of vagina following (induced) termination of pregnancy

O04.85 **Other venous complications following (induced) termination of pregnancy**

O04.86 **Cardiac arrest following (induced) termination of pregnancy**

● New code   ▲ Revised code   **Excludes1:** Not coded here   **Excludes2:** Not included here   ⊗ Placeholder required   ⑦7th digit required

O04.87 Sepsis following (induced) termination of pregnancy

Use additional code to identify infectious agent (B95-B97)

Use additional code to identify severe sepsis, if applicable (R65.2-)

Excludes1: septic or septicopyemic embolism following (induced) termination of pregnancy (O04.7)

O04.88 Urinary tract infection following (induced) termination of pregnancy

Cystitis following (induced) termination of pregnancy

O04.89 (Induced) termination of pregnancy with other complications

O07 Failed attempted termination of pregnancy

Includes: failure of attempted induction of termination of pregnancy

incomplete elective abortion

Excludes1: incomplete spontaneous abortion (O03.0-)

O07.0 Genital tract and pelvic infection following failed attempted termination of pregnancy

Endometritis following failed attempted termination of pregnancy

Oophoritis following failed attempted termination of pregnancy

Parametritis following failed attempted termination of pregnancy

Pelvic peritonitis following failed attempted termination of pregnancy

Salpingitis following failed attempted termination of pregnancy

Salpingo-oophoritis following failed attempted termination of pregnancy

Excludes1: sepsis following failed attempted termination of pregnancy (O07.37)

urinary tract infection following failed attempted termination of pregnancy (O07.38)

O07.1 Delayed or excessive hemorrhage following failed attempted termination of pregnancy

Afibrinogenemia following failed attempted termination of pregnancy

Defibrination syndrome following failed attempted termination of pregnancy

Hemolysis following failed attempted termination of pregnancy

Intravascular coagulation following failed attempted termination of pregnancy

O07.2 Embolism following failed attempted termination of pregnancy

Air embolism following failed attempted termination of pregnancy

Amniotic fluid embolism following failed attempted termination of pregnancy

Blood-clot embolism following failed attempted termination of pregnancy

Embolism NOS following failed attempted termination of pregnancy

Fat embolism following failed attempted termination of pregnancy

Pulmonary embolism following failed attempted termination of pregnancy

Pyemic embolism following failed attempted termination of pregnancy

Septic or septicopyemic embolism following failed attempted termination of pregnancy

Soap embolism following failed attempted termination of pregnancy

O07.3 Failed attempted termination of pregnancy with other and unspecified complications

O07.30 Failed attempted termination of pregnancy with unspecified complications

O07.31 Shock following failed attempted termination of pregnancy

Circulatory collapse following failed attempted termination of pregnancy

Shock (postprocedural) following failed attempted termination of pregnancy

Excludes1: shock due to infection following failed attempted termination of pregnancy (O07.37)

O07.32 Renal failure following failed attempted termination of pregnancy

Kidney failure (acute) following failed attempted termination of pregnancy

Oliguria following failed attempted termination of pregnancy

Renal shutdown following failed attempted termination of pregnancy

Renal tubular necrosis following failed attempted termination of pregnancy

Uremia following failed attempted termination of pregnancy

O07.33 Metabolic disorder following failed attempted termination of pregnancy

O07.34 Damage to pelvic organs following failed attempted termination of pregnancy

Laceration, perforation, tear or chemical damage of bladder following failed attempted termination of pregnancy

Laceration, perforation, tear or chemical damage of bowel following failed attempted termination of pregnancy

Laceration, perforation, tear or chemical damage of broad ligament following failed attempted termination of pregnancy

Laceration, perforation, tear or chemical damage of cervix following failed attempted termination of pregnancy

Laceration, perforation, tear or chemical damage of periurethral tissue following failed attempted termination of pregnancy

Laceration, perforation, tear or chemical damage of uterus following failed attempted termination of pregnancy

Laceration, perforation, tear or chemical damage of vagina following failed attempted termination of pregnancy

O07.35 Other venous complications following failed attempted termination of pregnancy

O07.36 Cardiac arrest following failed attempted termination of pregnancy

O07.37 Sepsis following failed attempted termination of pregnancy

Use additional code (B95-B97), to identify infectious agent

Use additional code (R65.2-) to identify severe sepsis, if applicable

Excludes1: septic or septicopyemic embolism following failed attempted termination of pregnancy (O07.2)

O07.38 Urinary tract infection following failed attempted termination of pregnancy

Cystitis following failed attempted termination of pregnancy

O07.39 Failed attempted termination of pregnancy with other complications

O07.4 Failed attempted termination of pregnancy without complication

O08 Complications following ectopic and molar pregnancy

This category is for use with categories O00-O02 to identify any associated complications

O08.0 Genital tract and pelvic infection following ectopic and molar pregnancy

Endometritis following ectopic and molar pregnancy

Oophoritis following ectopic and molar pregnancy

Parametritis following ectopic and molar pregnancy

Pelvic peritonitis following ectopic and molar pregnancy

Salpingitis following ectopic and molar pregnancy

Salpingo-oophoritis following ectopic and molar pregnancy

Excludes1: sepsis following ectopic and molar pregnancy (O08.82)

urinary tract infection (O08.83)

O08.1 Delayed or excessive hemorrhage following ectopic and molar pregnancy

Afibrinogenemia following ectopic and molar pregnancy

Defibrination syndrome following ectopic and molar pregnancy

Hemolysis following ectopic and molar pregnancy

Intravascular coagulation following ectopic and molar pregnancy

Excludes1: delayed or excessive hemorrhage due to incomplete abortion (O03.1)

O08.2 Embolism following ectopic and molar pregnancy

Air embolism following ectopic and molar pregnancy

Amniotic fluid embolism following ectopic and molar pregnancy

Blood-clot embolism following ectopic and molar pregnancy

Embolism NOS following ectopic and molar pregnancy

Fat embolism following ectopic and molar pregnancy

Pulmonary embolism following ectopic and molar pregnancy

Pyemic embolism following ectopic and molar pregnancy

Septic or septicopyemic embolism following ectopic and molar pregnancy

Soap embolism following ectopic and molar pregnancy

O08.3 Shock following ectopic and molar pregnancy

Circulatory collapse following ectopic and molar pregnancy

Shock (postprocedural) following ectopic and molar pregnancy

Excludes1: shock due to infection following ectopic and molar pregnancy (O08.82)

O08.4 Renal failure following ectopic and molar pregnancy

Kidney failure (acute) following ectopic and molar pregnancy

Oliguria following ectopic and molar pregnancy

Renal shutdown following ectopic and molar pregnancy

Renal tubular necrosis following ectopic and molar pregnancy

Uremia following ectopic and molar pregnancy

O08.5 Metabolic disorders following an ectopic and molar pregnancy

O08.6 Damage to pelvic organs and tissues following an ectopic and molar pregnancy

Laceration, perforation, tear or chemical damage of bladder following an ectopic and molar pregnancy

Laceration, perforation, tear or chemical damage of bowel following an ectopic and molar pregnancy

Laceration, perforation, tear or chemical damage of broad ligament following an ectopic and molar pregnancy

Laceration, perforation, tear or chemical damage of cervix following an ectopic and molar pregnancy

Laceration, perforation, tear or chemical damage of periurethral tissue following an ectopic and molar pregnancy

Laceration, perforation, tear or chemical damage of uterus following an ectopic and molar pregnancy

Laceration, perforation, tear or chemical damage of vagina following an ectopic and molar pregnancy

O08.7 Other venous complications following an ectopic and molar pregnancy

O08.8 Other complications following an ectopic and molar pregnancy

O08.81 Cardiac arrest following an ectopic and molar pregnancy

O08.82 Sepsis following ectopic and molar pregnancy

Use additional code (B95-B97), to identify infectious agent

Use additional code (R65.2-) to identify severe sepsis, if applicable

Excludes1: septic or septicopyemic embolism following ectopic and molar pregnancy (O08.2)

O08.83 Urinary tract infection following an ectopic and molar pregnancy

Cystitis following an ectopic and molar pregnancy

O08.89 Other complications following an ectopic and molar pregnancy

O08.9 Unspecified complication following an ectopic and molar pregnancy

SUPERVISION OF HIGH RISK PREGNANCY (O09)

O09 Supervision of high risk pregnancy

O09.0 Supervision of pregnancy with history of infertility

O09.00 Supervision of pregnancy with history of infertility, unspecified trimester

O09.01 Supervision of pregnancy with history of infertility, first trimester

● New code ▲ Revised code Excludes1: Not coded here Excludes2: Not included here ⊗ Placeholder required ⑦7th digit required

PREGNANCY, CHILDBIRTH AND THE PUERPERIUM

O09.02 Supervision of pregnancy with history of infertility, second trimester

O09.03 Supervision of pregnancy with history of infertility, third trimester

O09.1 Supervision of pregnancy with history of ectopic pregnancy

▲O09.10 Supervision of pregnancy with history of ectopic pregnancy, unspecified trimester

▲O09.11 Supervision of pregnancy with history of ectopic pregnancy, first trimester

▲O09.12 Supervision of pregnancy with history of ectopic pregnancy, second trimester

▲O09.13 Supervision of pregnancy with history of ectopic pregnancy, third trimester

O09.A Supervision of pregnancy with history of molar pregnancy

•O09.A0 Supervision of pregnancy with history of molar pregnancy, unspecified trimester

•O09.A1 Supervision of pregnancy with history of molar pregnancy, first trimester

•O09.A2 Supervision of pregnancy with history of molar pregnancy, second trimester

•O09.A3 Supervision of pregnancy with history of molar pregnancy, third trimester

O09.2 Supervision of pregnancy with other poor reproductive or obstetric history

Excludes2: pregnancy care for patient with history of recurrent pregnancy loss (O26.2-)

O09.21 Supervision of pregnancy with history of pre-term labor

O09.211 Supervision of pregnancy with history of pre-term labor, first trimester

O09.212 Supervision of pregnancy with history of pre-term labor, second trimester

O09.213 Supervision of pregnancy with history of pre-term labor, third trimester

O09.219 Supervision of pregnancy with history of pre-term labor, unspecified trimester

O09.29 Supervision of pregnancy with other poor reproductive or obstetric history

Supervision of pregnancy with history of neonatal death

Supervision of pregnancy with history of stillbirth

O09.291 Supervision of pregnancy with other poor reproductive or obstetric history, first trimester

O09.292 Supervision of pregnancy with other poor reproductive or obstetric history, second trimester

O09.293 Supervision of pregnancy with other poor reproductive or obstetric history, third trimester

O09.299 Supervision of pregnancy with other poor reproductive or obstetric history, unspecified trimester

O09.3 Supervision of pregnancy with insufficient antenatal care

Supervision of concealed pregnancy

Supervision of hidden pregnancy

O09.30 Supervision of pregnancy with insufficient antenatal care, unspecified trimester

O09.31 Supervision of pregnancy with insufficient antenatal care, first trimester

O09.32 Supervision of pregnancy with insufficient antenatal care, second trimester

O09.33 Supervision of pregnancy with insufficient antenatal care, third trimester

O09.4 Supervision of pregnancy with grand multiparity

O09.40 Supervision of pregnancy with grand multiparity, unspecified trimester

O09.41 Supervision of pregnancy with grand multiparity, first trimester

O09.42 Supervision of pregnancy with grand multiparity, second trimester

O09.43 Supervision of pregnancy with grand multiparity, third trimester

O09.5 Supervision of elderly primigravida and multigravida

Pregnancy for a female 35 years and older at expected date of delivery

O09.51 Supervision of elderly primigravida

O09.511 Supervision of elderly primigravida, first trimester

O09.512 Supervision of elderly primigravida, second trimester

O09.513 Supervision of elderly primigravida, third trimester

O09.519 Supervision of elderly primigravida, unspecified trimester

O09.52 Supervision of elderly multigravida

O09.521 Supervision of elderly multigravida, first trimester

O09.522 Supervision of elderly multigravida, second trimester

O09.523 Supervision of elderly multigravida, third trimester

O09.529 Supervision of elderly multigravida, unspecified trimester

O09.6 Supervision of young primigravida and multigravida

Supervision of pregnancy for a female less than 16 years old at expected date of delivery

O09.61 Supervision of young primigravida

O09.611 Supervision of young primigravida, first trimester

O09.612 Supervision of young primigravida, second trimester

O09.613 Supervision of young primigravida, third trimester

O09.619 Supervision of young primigravida, unspecified trimester

O09.62 Supervision of young multigravida

O09.621 Supervision of young multigravida, first trimester

O09.622 Supervision of young multigravida, second trimester

O09.623 Supervision of young multigravida, third trimester

O09.629 Supervision of young multigravida, unspecified trimester

O09.7 **Supervision of high risk pregnancy due to social problems**

O09.70 Supervision of high risk pregnancy due to social problems, unspecified trimester

O09.71 Supervision of high risk pregnancy due to social problems, first trimester

O09.72 Supervision of high risk pregnancy due to social problems, second trimester

O09.73 Supervision of high risk pregnancy due to social problems, third trimester

O09.8 **Supervision of other high risk pregnancies**

O09.81 Supervision of pregnancy resulting from assisted reproductive technology

Supervision of pregnancy resulting from in-vitro fertilization

Excludes2: gestational carrier status (Z33.3)

O09.811 Supervision of pregnancy resulting from assisted reproductive technology, first trimester

O09.812 Supervision of pregnancy resulting from assisted reproductive technology, second trimester

O09.813 Supervision of pregnancy resulting from assisted reproductive technology, third trimester

O09.819 Supervision of pregnancy resulting from assisted reproductive technology, unspecified trimester

O09.82 Supervision of pregnancy with history of in utero procedure during previous pregnancy

O09.821 Supervision of pregnancy with history of in utero procedure during previous pregnancy, first trimester

O09.822 Supervision of pregnancy with history of in utero procedure during previous pregnancy, second trimester

O09.823 Supervision of pregnancy with history of in utero procedure during previous pregnancy, third trimester

O09.829 Supervision of pregnancy with history of in utero procedure during previous pregnancy, unspecified trimester

Excludes1: supervision of pregnancy affected by in utero procedure during current pregnancy (O35.7)

O09.89 **Supervision of other high risk pregnancies**

O09.891 Supervision of other high risk pregnancies, first trimester

O09.892 Supervision of other high risk pregnancies, second trimester

O09.893 Supervision of other high risk pregnancies, third trimester

O09.899 Supervision of other high risk pregnancies, unspecified trimester

O09.9 **Supervision of high risk pregnancy, unspecified**

O09.90 Supervision of high risk pregnancy, unspecified, unspecified trimester

O09.91 Supervision of high risk pregnancy, unspecified, first trimester

O09.92 Supervision of high risk pregnancy, unspecified, second trimester

O09.93 Supervision of high risk pregnancy, unspecified, third trimester

EDEMA, PROTEINURIA AND HYPERTENSIVE DISORDERS IN PREGNANCY, CHILDBIRTH AND THE PUERPERIUM (O10-O16)

O10 **Pre-existing hypertension complicating pregnancy, childbirth and the puerperium**

Includes: pre-existing hypertension with pre-existing proteinuria complicating pregnancy, childbirth and the puerperium

Excludes2: pre-existing hypertension with superimposed pre-eclampsia complicating pregnancy, childbirth and the puerperium (O11.-)

O10.0 **Pre-existing essential hypertension complicating pregnancy, childbirth and the puerperium**

Any condition in I10 specified as a reason for obstetric care during pregnancy, childbirth or the puerperium

O10.01 Pre-existing essential hypertension complicating pregnancy

O10.011 Pre-existing essential hypertension complicating pregnancy, first trimester

O10.012 Pre-existing essential hypertension complicating pregnancy, second trimester

O10.013 Pre-existing essential hypertension complicating pregnancy, third trimester

O10.019 Pre-existing essential hypertension complicating pregnancy, unspecified trimester

O10.02 Pre-existing essential hypertension complicating childbirth

O10.03 Pre-existing essential hypertension complicating the puerperium

O10.1 **Pre-existing hypertensive heart disease complicating pregnancy, childbirth and the puerperium**

Any condition in I11 specified as a reason for obstetric care during pregnancy, childbirth or the puerperium

Use additional code from I11 to identify the type of hypertensive heart disease

O10.11 Pre-existing hypertensive heart disease complicating pregnancy

O10.111 Pre-existing hypertensive heart disease complicating pregnancy, first trimester

O10.112 Pre-existing hypertensive heart disease complicating pregnancy, second trimester

O10.113 Pre-existing hypertensive heart disease complicating pregnancy, third trimester

O10.119 Pre-existing hypertensive heart disease complicating pregnancy, unspecified trimester

O10.12 Pre-existing hypertensive heart disease complicating childbirth

O10.13 Pre-existing hypertensive heart disease complicating the puerperium

O10.2 **Pre-existing hypertensive chronic kidney disease complicating pregnancy, childbirth and the puerperium**

Any condition in I12 specified as a reason for obstetric care during pregnancy, childbirth or the puerperium

Use additional code from I12 to identify the type of hypertensive chronic kidney disease

O10.21 **Pre-existing hypertensive chronic kidney disease complicating pregnancy**

O10.211 **Pre-existing hypertensive chronic kidney disease complicating pregnancy, first trimester**

O10.212 **Pre-existing hypertensive chronic kidney disease complicating pregnancy, second trimester**

O10.213 **Pre-existing hypertensive chronic kidney disease complicating pregnancy, third trimester**

O10.219 **Pre-existing hypertensive chronic kidney disease complicating pregnancy, unspecified trimester**

O10.22 **Pre-existing hypertensive chronic kidney disease complicating childbirth**

O10.23 **Pre-existing hypertensive chronic kidney disease complicating the puerperium**

O10.3 **Pre-existing hypertensive heart and chronic kidney disease complicating pregnancy, childbirth and the puerperium**

Any condition in I13 specified as a reason for obstetric care during pregnancy, childbirth or the puerperium

Use additional code from I13 to identify the type of hypertensive heart and chronic kidney disease

O10.31 **Pre-existing hypertensive heart and chronic kidney disease complicating pregnancy**

O10.311 **Pre-existing hypertensive heart and chronic kidney disease complicating pregnancy, first trimester**

O10.312 **Pre-existing hypertensive heart and chronic kidney disease complicating pregnancy, second trimester**

O10.313 **Pre-existing hypertensive heart and chronic kidney disease complicating pregnancy, third trimester**

O10.319 **Pre-existing hypertensive heart and chronic kidney disease complicating pregnancy, unspecified trimester**

O10.32 **Pre-existing hypertensive heart and chronic kidney disease complicating childbirth**

O10.33 **Pre-existing hypertensive heart and chronic kidney disease complicating the puerperium**

O10.4 **Pre-existing secondary hypertension complicating pregnancy, childbirth and the puerperium**

Any condition in I15 specified as a reason for obstetric care during pregnancy, childbirth or the puerperium

Use additional code from I15 to identify the type of secondary hypertension

O10.41 **Pre-existing secondary hypertension complicating pregnancy**

O10.411 **Pre-existing secondary hypertension complicating pregnancy, first trimester**

O10.412 **Pre-existing secondary hypertension complicating pregnancy, second trimester**

O10.413 **Pre-existing secondary hypertension complicating pregnancy, third trimester**

O10.419 **Pre-existing secondary hypertension complicating pregnancy, unspecified trimester**

O10.42 **Pre-existing secondary hypertension complicating childbirth**

O10.43 **Pre-existing secondary hypertension complicating the puerperium**

O10.9 **Unspecified pre-existing hypertension complicating pregnancy, childbirth and the puerperium**

O10.91 **Unspecified pre-existing hypertension complicating pregnancy**

O10.911 **Unspecified pre-existing hypertension complicating pregnancy, first trimester**

O10.912 **Unspecified pre-existing hypertension complicating pregnancy, second trimester**

O10.913 **Unspecified pre-existing hypertension complicating pregnancy, third trimester**

O10.919 **Unspecified pre-existing hypertension complicating pregnancy, unspecified trimester**

O10.92 **Unspecified pre-existing hypertension complicating childbirth**

O10.93 **Unspecified pre-existing hypertension complicating the puerperium**

O11 **Pre-existing hypertension with pre-eclampsia**

Includes: conditions in O10 complicated by pre-eclampsia

pre-eclampsia superimposed pre-existing hypertension

Use additional code from O10 to identify the type of hypertension

O11.1 **Pre-existing hypertension with pre-eclampsia, first trimester**

O11.2 **Pre-existing hypertension with pre-eclampsia, second trimester**

O11.3 **Pre-existing hypertension with pre-eclampsia, third trimester**

●**O11.4** **Pre-existing hypertension with pre-eclampsia, complicating childbirth**

●**O11.5** **Pre-existing hypertension with pre-eclampsia, complicating the puerperium**

O11.9 **Pre-existing hypertension with pre-eclampsia, unspecified trimester**

O12 **Gestational [pregnancy-induced] edema and proteinuria without hypertension**

O12.0 **Gestational edema**

O12.00 **Gestational edema, unspecified trimester**

O12.01 **Gestational edema, first trimester**

O12.02 **Gestational edema, second trimester**

O12.03 **Gestational edema, third trimester**

●**O12.04** **Gestational edema, complicating childbirth**

●**O12.05** **Gestational edema, complicating the puerperium**

O12.1 **Gestational proteinuria**

O12.10 **Gestational proteinuria, unspecified trimester**

O12.11 **Gestational proteinuria, first trimester**

O12.12 **Gestational proteinuria, second trimester**

O12.13　Gestational proteinuria, third trimester

●O12.14　Gestational proteinuria, complicating childbirth

●O12.15　Gestational proteinuria, complicating the puerperium

O12.2　Gestational edema with proteinuria

O12.20　Gestational edema with proteinuria, unspecified trimester

O12.21　Gestational edema with proteinuria, first trimester

O12.22　Gestational edema with proteinuria, second trimester

O12.23　Gestational edema with proteinuria, third trimester

●O12.24　Gestational edema with proteinuria, complicating childbirth

●O12.25　Gestational edema with proteinuria, complicating the puerperium

O13　Gestational [pregnancy-induced] hypertension without significant proteinuria

Includes: gestational hypertension NOS

transient hypertension of pregnancy

O13.1　Gestational [pregnancy-induced] hypertension without significant proteinuria, first trimester

O13.2　Gestational [pregnancy-induced] hypertension without significant proteinuria, second trimester

O13.3　Gestational [pregnancy-induced] hypertension without significant proteinuria, third trimester

●O13.4　Gestational [pregnancy-induced] hypertension without significant proteinuria, complicating childbirth

●O13.5　Gestational [pregnancy-induced] hypertension without significant proteinuria, complicating the puerperium

O13.9　Gestational [pregnancy-induced] hypertension without significant proteinuria, unspecified trimester

O14　Pre-eclampsia

Excludes1: pre-existing hypertension with pre-eclampsia (O11)

O14.0　Mild to moderate pre-eclampsia

O14.00　Mild to moderate pre-eclampsia, unspecified trimester

O14.02　Mild to moderate pre-eclampsia, second trimester

O14.03　Mild to moderate pre-eclampsia, third trimester

●O14.04　Mild to moderate pre-eclampsia, complicating childbirth

●O14.05　Mild to moderate pre-eclampsia, complicating the puerperium

O14.1　Severe pre-eclampsia

Excludes1: HELLP syndrome (O14.2-)

O14.10　Severe pre-eclampsia, unspecified trimester

O14.12　Severe pre-eclampsia, second trimester

O14.13　Severe pre-eclampsia, third trimester

●O14.14　Severe pre-eclampsia complicating childbirth

●O14.15　Severe pre-eclampsia, complicating the puerperium

O14.2　HELLP syndrome

Severe pre-eclampsia with hemolysis, elevated liver enzymes and low platelet count (HELLP)

O14.20　HELLP syndrome (HELLP), unspecified trimester

O14.22　HELLP syndrome (HELLP), second trimester

O14.23　HELLP syndrome (HELLP), third trimester

●O14.24　HELLP syndrome, complicating childbirth

●O14.25　HELLP syndrome, complicating the puerperium

O14.9　Unspecified pre-eclampsia

O14.90　Unspecified pre-eclampsia, unspecified trimester

O14.92　Unspecified pre-eclampsia, second trimester

O14.93　Unspecified pre-eclampsia, third trimester

●O14.94　Unspecified pre-eclampsia, complicating childbirth

●O14.95　Unspecified pre-eclampsia, complicating the puerperium

O15　Eclampsia

Includes: convulsions following conditions in O10-O14 and O16

O15.0　Eclampsia complicating pregnancy

▲O15.00　Eclampsia complicating pregnancy, unspecified trimester

▲O15.02　Eclampsia complicating pregnancy, second trimester

▲O15.03　Eclampsia complicating pregnancy, third trimester

▲O15.1　Eclampsia complicating labor

▲O15.2　Eclampsia complicating the puerperium

O15.9　Eclampsia, unspecified as to time period

Eclampsia NOS

O16　Unspecified maternal hypertension

O16.1　Unspecified maternal hypertension, first trimester

O16.2　Unspecified maternal hypertension, second trimester

O16.3　Unspecified maternal hypertension, third trimester

●O16.4　Unspecified maternal hypertension, complicating childbirth

●O16.5　Unspecified maternal hypertension, complicating the puerperium

O16.9　Unspecified maternal hypertension, unspecified trimester

OTHER MATERNAL DISORDERS PREDOMINANTLY RELATED TO PREGNANCY (O20-O29)

Excludes2: maternal care related to the fetus and amniotic cavity and possible delivery problems (O30-O48)

maternal diseases classifiable elsewhere but complicating pregnancy, labor and delivery, and the puerperium (O98-O99)

O20　Hemorrhage in early pregnancy

Includes: hemorrhage before completion of 20 weeks gestation

Excludes1: pregnancy with abortive outcome (O00-O08)

O20.0　Threatened abortion

Hemorrhage specified as due to threatened abortion

O20.8　Other hemorrhage in early pregnancy

O20.9　Hemorrhage in early pregnancy, unspecified

O21　Excessive vomiting in pregnancy

O21.0　Mild hyperemesis gravidarum

Hyperemesis gravidarum, mild or unspecified, starting before the end of the 20th week of gestation

O21.1   Hyperemesis gravidarum with metabolic disturbance

Hyperemesis gravidarum, starting before the end of the 20th week of gestation, with metabolic disturbance such as carbohydrate depletion

Hyperemesis gravidarum, starting before the end of the 20th week of gestation, with metabolic disturbance such as dehydration

Hyperemesis gravidarum, starting before the end of the 20th week of gestation, with metabolic disturbance such as electrolyte imbalance

O21.2   Late vomiting of pregnancy

Excessive vomiting starting after 20 completed weeks of gestation

O21.8   Other vomiting complicating pregnancy

Vomiting due to diseases classified elsewhere, complicating pregnancy

<u>Use additional code</u>, to identify cause.

O21.9   Vomiting of pregnancy, unspecified

O22   Venous complications and hemorrhoids in pregnancy

Excludes1: venous complications of:

abortion NOS (O03.9)

ectopic or molar pregnancy (O08.7)

failed attempted abortion (O07.35)

induced abortion (O04.85)

spontaneous abortion (O03.89)

Excludes2: obstetric pulmonary embolism (O88.-)

venous complications and hemorrhoids of childbirth and the puerperium (O87.-)

O22.0   Varicose veins of lower extremity in pregnancy

Varicose veins NOS in pregnancy

O22.00   Varicose veins of lower extremity in pregnancy, unspecified trimester

O22.01   Varicose veins of lower extremity in pregnancy, first trimester

O22.02   Varicose veins of lower extremity in pregnancy, second trimester

O22.03   Varicose veins of lower extremity in pregnancy, third trimester

O22.1   Genital varices in pregnancy

Perineal varices in pregnancy

Vaginal varices in pregnancy

Vulval varices in pregnancy

O22.10   Genital varices in pregnancy, unspecified trimester

O22.11   Genital varices in pregnancy, first trimester

O22.12   Genital varices in pregnancy, second trimester

O22.13   Genital varices in pregnancy, third trimester

O22.2   Superficial thrombophlebitis in pregnancy

Phlebitis in pregnancy NOS

Thrombophlebitis of legs in pregnancy

Thrombosis in pregnancy NOS

<u>Use additional code</u> to identify the superficial thrombophlebitis (I80.0-)

O22.20   Superficial thrombophlebitis in pregnancy, unspecified trimester

O22.21   Superficial thrombophlebitis in pregnancy, first trimester

O22.22   Superficial thrombophlebitis in pregnancy, second trimester

O22.23   Superficial thrombophlebitis in pregnancy, third trimester

O22.3   Deep phlebothrombosis in pregnancy

Deep vein thrombosis, antepartum

<u>Use additional code</u> to identify the deep vein thrombosis (I82.4-, I82.5-, I82.62-. I82.72-)

<u>Use additional code</u>, if applicable, for associated long-term (current) use of anticoagulants (Z79.01)

O22.30   Deep phlebothrombosis in pregnancy, unspecified trimester

O22.31   Deep phlebothrombosis in pregnancy, first trimester

O22.32   Deep phlebothrombosis in pregnancy, second trimester

O22.33   Deep phlebothrombosis in pregnancy, third trimester

O22.4   Hemorrhoids in pregnancy

O22.40   Hemorrhoids in pregnancy, unspecified trimester

O22.41   Hemorrhoids in pregnancy, first trimester

O22.42   Hemorrhoids in pregnancy, second trimester

O22.43   Hemorrhoids in pregnancy, third trimester

O22.5   Cerebral venous thrombosis in pregnancy

Cerebrovenous sinus thrombosis in pregnancy

O22.50   Cerebral venous thrombosis in pregnancy, unspecified trimester

O22.51   Cerebral venous thrombosis in pregnancy, first trimester

O22.52   Cerebral venous thrombosis in pregnancy, second trimester

O22.53   Cerebral venous thrombosis in pregnancy, third trimester

O22.8   Other venous complications in pregnancy

O22.8X   Other venous complications in pregnancy

O22.8X1   Other venous complications in pregnancy, first trimester

O22.8X2   Other venous complications in pregnancy, second trimester

O22.8X3   Other venous complications in pregnancy, third trimester

O22.8X9   Other venous complications in pregnancy, unspecified trimester

O22.9   Venous complication in pregnancy, unspecified

Gestational phlebitis NOS

Gestational phlebopathy NOS

Gestational thrombosis NOS

O22.90   Venous complication in pregnancy, unspecified, unspecified trimester

O22.91   Venous complication in pregnancy, unspecified, first trimester

O22.92   Venous complication in pregnancy, unspecified, second trimester

O22.93   Venous complication in pregnancy, unspecified, third trimester

O23   Infections of genitourinary tract in pregnancy

<u>Use additional code</u> to identify organism (B95.-, B96.-)

▨ Add 4th-7th digits	▨ Nonspecific code	▨ Unspecified code	▨ Manifestation code

Excludes2: gonococcal infections complicating pregnancy, childbirth and the puerperium (O98.2)

infections with a predominantly sexual mode of transmission NOS complicating pregnancy, childbirth and the puerperium (O98.3)

syphilis complicating pregnancy, childbirth and the puerperium (O98.1)

tuberculosis of genitourinary system complicating pregnancy, childbirth and the puerperium (O98.0)

venereal disease NOS complicating pregnancy, childbirth and the puerperium (O98.3)

O23.0 Infections of kidney in pregnancy
Pyelonephritis in pregnancy

O23.00 Infections of kidney in pregnancy, unspecified trimester

O23.01 Infections of kidney in pregnancy, first trimester

O23.02 Infections of kidney in pregnancy, second trimester

O23.03 Infections of kidney in pregnancy, third trimester

O23.1 Infections of bladder in pregnancy

O23.10 Infections of bladder in pregnancy, unspecified trimester

O23.11 Infections of bladder in pregnancy, first trimester

O23.12 Infections of bladder in pregnancy, second trimester

O23.13 Infections of bladder in pregnancy, third trimester

O23.2 Infections of urethra in pregnancy

O23.20 Infections of urethra in pregnancy, unspecified trimester

O23.21 Infections of urethra in pregnancy, first trimester

O23.22 Infections of urethra in pregnancy, second trimester

O23.23 Infections of urethra in pregnancy, third trimester

O23.3 Infections of other parts of urinary tract in pregnancy

O23.30 Infections of other parts of urinary tract in pregnancy, unspecified trimester

O23.31 Infections of other parts of urinary tract in pregnancy, first trimester

O23.32 Infections of other parts of urinary tract in pregnancy, second trimester

O23.33 Infections of other parts of urinary tract in pregnancy, third trimester

O23.4 Unspecified infection of urinary tract in pregnancy

O23.40 Unspecified infection of urinary tract in pregnancy, unspecified trimester

O23.41 Unspecified infection of urinary tract in pregnancy, first trimester

O23.42 Unspecified infection of urinary tract in pregnancy, second trimester

O23.43 Unspecified infection of urinary tract in pregnancy, third trimester

O23.5 Infections of the genital tract in pregnancy

O23.51 Infection of cervix in pregnancy

O23.511 Infections of cervix in pregnancy, first trimester

O23.512 Infections of cervix in pregnancy, second trimester

O23.513 Infections of cervix in pregnancy, third trimester

O23.519 Infections of cervix in pregnancy, unspecified trimester

O23.52 Salpingo-oophoritis in pregnancy
Oophoritis in pregnancy
Salpingitis in pregnancy

O23.521 Salpingo-oophoritis in pregnancy, first trimester

O23.522 Salpingo-oophoritis in pregnancy, second trimester

O23.523 Salpingo-oophoritis in pregnancy, third trimester

O23.529 Salpingo-oophoritis in pregnancy, unspecified trimester

O23.59 Infection of other part of genital tract in pregnancy

O23.591 Infection of other part of genital tract in pregnancy, first trimester

O23.592 Infection of other part of genital tract in pregnancy, second trimester

O23.593 Infection of other part of genital tract in pregnancy, third trimester

O23.599 Infection of other part of genital tract in pregnancy, unspecified trimester

O23.9 Unspecified genitourinary tract infection in pregnancy
Genitourinary tract infection in pregnancy NOS

O23.90 Unspecified genitourinary tract infection in pregnancy, unspecified trimester

O23.91 Unspecified genitourinary tract infection in pregnancy, first trimester

O23.92 Unspecified genitourinary tract infection in pregnancy, second trimester

O23.93 Unspecified genitourinary tract infection in pregnancy, third trimester

O24 Diabetes mellitus in pregnancy, childbirth, and the puerperium

O24.0 Pre-existing type 1 diabetes mellitus, in pregnancy, childbirth and the puerperium
Juvenile onset diabetes mellitus, in pregnancy, childbirth and the puerperium
Ketosis-prone diabetes mellitus in pregnancy, childbirth and the puerperium

Use additional code from category E10 to further identify any manifestations

O24.01 Pre-existing type 1 Diabetes mellitus, in pregnancy

▲**O24.011** Pre-existing type 1 diabetes mellitus, in pregnancy, first trimester

▲**O24.012** Pre-existing type 1 diabetes mellitus, in pregnancy, second trimester

▲**O24.013** Pre-existing type 1 diabetes mellitus, in pregnancy, third trimester

● New code ▲ Revised code **Excludes1:** Not coded here **Excludes2:** Not included here ⊗ Placeholder required ⑦7th digit required

▲O24.019 Pre-existing type 1 diabetes mellitus, in pregnancy, unspecified trimester

▲O24.02 Pre-existing type 1 diabetes mellitus, in childbirth

▲O24.03 Pre-existing type 1 diabetes mellitus, in the puerperium

O24.1 Pre-existing type 2 diabetes mellitus, in pregnancy, childbirth and the puerperium

Insulin-resistant diabetes mellitus in pregnancy, childbirth and the puerperium

<u>Use additional code</u> (for):

from category E11 to further identify any manifestations long-term (current) use of insulin (Z79.4)

O24.11 Pre-existing type 2 diabetes mellitus, in pregnancy

▲O24.111 Pre-existing type 2 diabetes mellitus, in pregnancy, first trimester

▲O24.112 Pre-existing type 2 diabetes mellitus, in pregnancy, second trimester

▲O24.113 Pre-existing type 2 diabetes mellitus, in pregnancy, third trimester

▲O24.119 Pre-existing type 2 diabetes mellitus, in pregnancy, unspecified trimester

▲O24.12 Pre-existing type 2 diabetes mellitus, in childbirth

▲O24.13 Pre-existing type 2 diabetes mellitus, in the puerperium

O24.3 Unspecified pre-existing diabetes mellitus in pregnancy, childbirth and the puerperium

<u>Use additional code</u> (for):

from category E11 to further identify any manifestation long-term (current) use of insulin (Z79.4)

O24.31 Unspecified pre-existing diabetes mellitus in pregnancy

O24.311 Unspecified pre-existing diabetes mellitus in pregnancy, first trimester

O24.312 Unspecified pre-existing diabetes mellitus in pregnancy, second trimester

O24.313 Unspecified pre-existing diabetes mellitus in pregnancy, third trimester

O24.319 Unspecified pre-existing diabetes mellitus in pregnancy, unspecified trimester

O24.32 Unspecified pre-existing diabetes mellitus in childbirth

O24.33 Unspecified pre-existing diabetes mellitus in the puerperium

O24.4 Gestational diabetes mellitus

Diabetes mellitus arising in pregnancy

Gestational diabetes mellitus NOS

O24.41 Gestational diabetes mellitus in pregnancy

O24.410 Gestational diabetes mellitus in pregnancy, diet controlled

O24.414 Gestational diabetes mellitus in pregnancy, insulin controlled

●O24.415 Gestational diabetes mellitus in pregnancy, controlled by oral hypoglycemic drugs

Gestational diabetes mellitus in pregnancy, controlled by oral antidiabetic drugs

O24.419 Gestational diabetes mellitus in pregnancy, unspecified control

O24.42 Gestational diabetes mellitus in childbirth

O24.420 Gestational diabetes mellitus in childbirth, diet controlled

O24.424 Gestational diabetes mellitus in childbirth, insulin controlled

●O24.425 Gestational diabetes mellitus in childbirth, controlled by oral hypoglycemic drugs

Gestational diabetes mellitus in childbirth, controlled by oral antidiabetic drugs

O24.429 Gestational diabetes mellitus in childbirth, unspecified control

O24.43 Gestational diabetes mellitus in the puerperium

O24.430 Gestational diabetes mellitus in the puerperium, diet controlled

O24.434 Gestational diabetes mellitus in the puerperium, insulin controlled

●O24.435 Gestational diabetes mellitus in puerperium, controlled by oral hypoglycemic drugs

Gestational diabetes mellitus in puerperium, controlled by oral antidiabetic drugs

O24.439 Gestational diabetes mellitus in the puerperium, unspecified control

O24.8 Other pre-existing diabetes mellitus in pregnancy, childbirth, and the puerperium

<u>Use additional code</u> (for):

from categories E08, E09 and E13 to further identify any manifestation long-term (current) use of insulin (Z79.4)

O24.81 Other pre-existing diabetes mellitus in pregnancy

O24.811 Other pre-existing diabetes mellitus in pregnancy, first trimester

O24.812 Other pre-existing diabetes mellitus in pregnancy, second trimester

O24.813 Other pre-existing diabetes mellitus in pregnancy, third trimester

O24.819 Other pre-existing diabetes mellitus in pregnancy, unspecified trimester

O24.82 Other pre-existing diabetes mellitus in childbirth

O24.83 Other pre-existing diabetes mellitus in the puerperium

O24.9 Unspecified diabetes mellitus in pregnancy, childbirth and the puerperium

<u>Use additional code</u> for long-term (current) use of insulin (Z79.4)

O24.91 Unspecified diabetes mellitus in pregnancy

O24.911 Unspecified diabetes mellitus in pregnancy, first trimester

O24.912 Unspecified diabetes mellitus in pregnancy, second trimester

O24.913 Unspecified diabetes mellitus in pregnancy, third trimester

O24.919 Unspecified diabetes mellitus in pregnancy, unspecified trimester

O24.92 Unspecified diabetes mellitus in childbirth

O24.93 Unspecified diabetes mellitus in the puerperium

O25 Malnutrition in pregnancy, childbirth and the puerperium

O25.1 Malnutrition in pregnancy

O25.10 Malnutrition in pregnancy, unspecified trimester

O25.11 Malnutrition in pregnancy, first trimester

O25.12 Malnutrition in pregnancy, second trimester

O25.13 Malnutrition in pregnancy, third trimester

O25.2 Malnutrition in childbirth

O25.3 Malnutrition in the puerperium

O26 Maternal care for other conditions predominantly related to pregnancy

O26.0 Excessive weight gain in pregnancy

Excludes2: gestational edema (O12.0, O12.2)

O26.00 Excessive weight gain in pregnancy, unspecified trimester

O26.01 Excessive weight gain in pregnancy, first trimester

O26.02 Excessive weight gain in pregnancy, second trimester

O26.03 Excessive weight gain in pregnancy, third trimester

O26.1 Low weight gain in pregnancy

O26.10 Low weight gain in pregnancy, unspecified trimester

O26.11 Low weight gain in pregnancy, first trimester

O26.12 Low weight gain in pregnancy, second trimester

O26.13 Low weight gain in pregnancy, third trimester

O26.2 Pregnancy care for patient with recurrent pregnancy loss

O26.20 Pregnancy care for patient with recurrent pregnancy loss, unspecified trimester

O26.21 Pregnancy care for patient with recurrent pregnancy loss, first trimester

O26.22 Pregnancy care for patient with recurrent pregnancy loss, second trimester

O26.23 Pregnancy care for patient with recurrent pregnancy loss, third trimester

O26.3 Retained intrauterine contraceptive device in pregnancy

O26.30 Retained intrauterine contraceptive device in pregnancy, unspecified trimester

O26.31 Retained intrauterine contraceptive device in pregnancy, first trimester

O26.32 Retained intrauterine contraceptive device in pregnancy, second trimester

O26.33 Retained intrauterine contraceptive device in pregnancy, third trimester

O26.4 Herpes gestationis

O26.40 Herpes gestationis, unspecified trimester

O26.41 Herpes gestationis, first trimester

O26.42 Herpes gestationis, second trimester

O26.43 Herpes gestationis, third trimester

O26.5 Maternal hypotension syndrome

Supine hypotensive syndrome

O26.50 Maternal hypotension syndrome, unspecified trimester

O26.51 Maternal hypotension syndrome, first trimester

O26.52 Maternal hypotension syndrome, second trimester

O26.53 Maternal hypotension syndrome, third trimester

O26.6 Liver and biliary tract disorders in pregnancy, childbirth and the puerperium

Use additional code to identify the specific disorder

Excludes2: hepatorenal syndrome following labor and delivery (O90.4)

O26.61 Liver and biliary tract disorders in pregnancy

O26.611 Liver and biliary tract disorders in pregnancy, first trimester

O26.612 Liver and biliary tract disorders in pregnancy, second trimester

O26.613 Liver and biliary tract disorders in pregnancy, third trimester

O26.619 Liver and biliary tract disorders in pregnancy, unspecified trimester

O26.62 Liver and biliary tract disorders in childbirth

O26.63 Liver and biliary tract disorders in the puerperium

O26.7 Subluxation of symphysis (pubis) in pregnancy, childbirth and the puerperium

Excludes1: traumatic separation of symphysis (pubis) during childbirth (O71.6)

O26.71 Subluxation of symphysis (pubis) in pregnancy

O26.711 Subluxation of symphysis (pubis) in pregnancy, first trimester

O26.712 Subluxation of symphysis (pubis) in pregnancy, second trimester

O26.713 Subluxation of symphysis (pubis) in pregnancy, third trimester

O26.719 Subluxation of symphysis (pubis) in pregnancy, unspecified trimester

O26.72 Subluxation of symphysis (pubis) in childbirth

O26.73 Subluxation of symphysis (pubis) in the puerperium

O26.8 Other specified pregnancy related conditions

O26.81 Pregnancy related exhaustion and fatigue

O26.811 Pregnancy related exhaustion and fatigue, first trimester

O26.812 Pregnancy related exhaustion and fatigue, second trimester

O26.813 Pregnancy related exhaustion and fatigue, third trimester

O26.819 Pregnancy related exhaustion and fatigue, unspecified trimester

O26.82 Pregnancy related peripheral neuritis

● New code   ▲ Revised code   Excludes1: Not coded here   Excludes2: Not included here   ⊗ Placeholder required   ⑦7th digit required

O26.821 **Pregnancy related peripheral neuritis, first trimester**

O26.822 **Pregnancy related peripheral neuritis, second trimester**

O26.823 **Pregnancy related peripheral neuritis, third trimester**

O26.829 **Pregnancy related peripheral neuritis, unspecified trimester**

O26.83 **Pregnancy related renal disease**

Use additional code to identify the specific disorder

O26.831 **Pregnancy related renal disease, first trimester**

O26.832 **Pregnancy related renal disease, second trimester**

O26.833 **Pregnancy related renal disease, third trimester**

O26.839 **Pregnancy related renal disease, unspecified trimester**

O26.84 **Uterine size-date discrepancy complicating pregnancy**

Excludes1: encounter for suspected problem with fetal growth ruled out (Z03.74)

O26.841 **Uterine size-date discrepancy, first trimester**

O26.842 **Uterine size-date discrepancy, second trimester**

O26.843 **Uterine size-date discrepancy, third trimester**

O26.849 **Uterine size-date discrepancy, unspecified trimester**

O26.85 **Spotting complicating pregnancy**

O26.851 **Spotting complicating pregnancy, first trimester**

O26.852 **Spotting complicating pregnancy, second trimester**

O26.853 **Spotting complicating pregnancy, third trimester**

O26.859 **Spotting complicating pregnancy, unspecified trimester**

O26.86 **Pruritic urticarial papules and plaques of pregnancy (PUPPP)**

Polymorphic eruption of pregnancy

O26.87 **Cervical shortening**

Excludes1: encounter for suspected cervical shortening ruled out (Z03.75)

O26.872 **Cervical shortening, second trimester**

O26.873 **Cervical shortening, third trimester**

O26.879 **Cervical shortening, unspecified trimester**

O26.89 **Other specified pregnancy related conditions**

O26.891 **Other specified pregnancy related conditions, first trimester**

O26.892 **Other specified pregnancy related conditions, second trimester**

O26.893 **Other specified pregnancy related conditions, third trimester**

O26.899 **Other specified pregnancy related conditions, unspecified trimester**

O26.9 **Pregnancy related conditions, unspecified**

O26.90 **Pregnancy related conditions, unspecified, unspecified trimester**

O26.91 **Pregnancy related conditions, unspecified, first trimester**

O26.92 **Pregnancy related conditions, unspecified, second trimester**

O26.93 **Pregnancy related conditions, unspecified, third trimester**

O28 **Abnormal findings on antenatal screening of mother**

Excludes1: diagnostic findings classified elsewhere - see Alphabetical Index

O28.0 **Abnormal hematological finding on antenatal screening of mother**

O28.1 **Abnormal biochemical finding on antenatal screening of mother**

O28.2 **Abnormal cytological finding on antenatal screening of mother**

O28.3 **Abnormal ultrasonic finding on antenatal screening of mother**

O28.4 **Abnormal radiological finding on antenatal screening of mother**

O28.5 **Abnormal chromosomal and genetic finding on antenatal screening of mother**

O28.8 **Other abnormal findings on antenatal screening of mother**

O28.9 **Unspecified abnormal findings on antenatal screening of mother**

O29 **Complications of anesthesia during pregnancy**

Includes: maternal complications arising from the administration of a general, regional or local anesthetic, analgesic or other sedation during pregnancy

Use additional code, if necessary, to identify the complication

Excludes2: complications of anesthesia during labor and delivery (O74.-)

complications of anesthesia during the puerperium (O89.-)

O29.0 **Pulmonary complications of anesthesia during pregnancy**

O29.01 **Aspiration pneumonitis due to anesthesia during pregnancy**

Inhalation of stomach contents or secretions NOS due to anesthesia during pregnancy

Mendelson's syndrome due to anesthesia during pregnancy

O29.011 **Aspiration pneumonitis due to anesthesia during pregnancy, first trimester**

O29.012 **Aspiration pneumonitis due to anesthesia during pregnancy, second trimester**

O29.013 **Aspiration pneumonitis due to anesthesia during pregnancy, third trimester**

O29.019 **Aspiration pneumonitis due to anesthesia during pregnancy, unspecified trimester**

O29.02 **Pressure collapse of lung due to anesthesia during pregnancy**

O29.021 **Pressure collapse of lung due to anesthesia during pregnancy, first trimester**

O29.022 **Pressure collapse of lung due to anesthesia during pregnancy, second trimester**

O29.023 **Pressure collapse of lung due to anesthesia during pregnancy, third trimester**

O29.029 **Pressure collapse of lung due to anesthesia during pregnancy, unspecified trimester**

O29.09 **Other pulmonary complications of anesthesia during pregnancy**

O29.091 **Other pulmonary complications of anesthesia during pregnancy, first trimester**

O29.092 **Other pulmonary complications of anesthesia during pregnancy, second trimester**

O29.093 **Other pulmonary complications of anesthesia during pregnancy, third trimester**

O29.099 **Other pulmonary complications of anesthesia during pregnancy, unspecified trimester**

O29.1 **Cardiac complications of anesthesia during pregnancy**

O29.11 **Cardiac arrest due to anesthesia during pregnancy**

O29.111 **Cardiac arrest due to anesthesia during pregnancy, first trimester**

O29.112 **Cardiac arrest due to anesthesia during pregnancy, second trimester**

O29.113 **Cardiac arrest due to anesthesia during pregnancy, third trimester**

O29.119 **Cardiac arrest due to anesthesia during pregnancy, unspecified trimester**

O29.12 **Cardiac failure due to anesthesia during pregnancy**

O29.121 **Cardiac failure due to anesthesia during pregnancy, first trimester**

O29.122 **Cardiac failure due to anesthesia during pregnancy, second trimester**

O29.123 **Cardiac failure due to anesthesia during pregnancy, third trimester**

O29.129 **Cardiac failure due to anesthesia during pregnancy, unspecified trimester**

O29.19 **Other cardiac complications of anesthesia during pregnancy**

O29.191 **Other cardiac complications of anesthesia during pregnancy, first trimester**

O29.192 **Other cardiac complications of anesthesia during pregnancy, second trimester**

O29.193 **Other cardiac complications of anesthesia during pregnancy, third trimester**

O29.199 **Other cardiac complications of anesthesia during pregnancy, unspecified trimester**

O29.2 **Central nervous system complications of anesthesia during pregnancy**

O29.21 **Cerebral anoxia due to anesthesia during pregnancy**

O29.211 **Cerebral anoxia due to anesthesia during pregnancy, first trimester**

O29.212 **Cerebral anoxia due to anesthesia during pregnancy, second trimester**

O29.213 **Cerebral anoxia due to anesthesia during pregnancy, third trimester**

O29.219 **Cerebral anoxia due to anesthesia during pregnancy, unspecified trimester**

O29.29 **Other central nervous system complications of anesthesia during pregnancy**

O29.291 **Other central nervous system complications of anesthesia during pregnancy, first trimester**

O29.292 **Other central nervous system complications of anesthesia during pregnancy, second trimester**

O29.293 **Other central nervous system complications of anesthesia during pregnancy, third trimester**

O29.299 **Other central nervous system complications of anesthesia during pregnancy, unspecified trimester**

O29.3 **Toxic reaction to local anesthesia during pregnancy**

O29.3X **Toxic reaction to local anesthesia during pregnancy**

O29.3X1 **Toxic reaction to local anesthesia during pregnancy, first trimester**

O29.3X2 **Toxic reaction to local anesthesia during pregnancy, second trimester**

O29.3X3 **Toxic reaction to local anesthesia during pregnancy, third trimester**

O29.3X9 **Toxic reaction to local anesthesia during pregnancy, unspecified trimester**

O29.4 **Spinal and epidural anesthesia induced headache during pregnancy**

O29.40 **Spinal and epidural anesthesia induced headache during pregnancy, unspecified trimester**

O29.41 **Spinal and epidural anesthesia induced headache during pregnancy, first trimester**

O29.42 **Spinal and epidural anesthesia induced headache during pregnancy, second trimester**

O29.43 **Spinal and epidural anesthesia induced headache during pregnancy, third trimester**

O29.5 **Other complications of spinal and epidural anesthesia during pregnancy**

O29.5X **Other complications of spinal and epidural anesthesia during pregnancy**

O29.5X1 **Other complications of spinal and epidural anesthesia during pregnancy, first trimester**

O29.5X2 **Other complications of spinal and epidural anesthesia during pregnancy, second trimester**

O29.5X3 **Other complications of spinal and epidural anesthesia during pregnancy, third trimester**

● New code ▲ Revised code **Excludes1:** Not coded here **Excludes2:** Not included here ⊗ Placeholder required ⑦ 7th digit required

O29.5X9 Other complications of spinal and epidural anesthesia during pregnancy, unspecified trimester

O29.6 Failed or difficult intubation for anesthesia during pregnancy

O29.60 Failed or difficult intubation for anesthesia during pregnancy, unspecified trimester

O29.61 Failed or difficult intubation for anesthesia during pregnancy, first trimester

O29.62 Failed or difficult intubation for anesthesia during pregnancy, second trimester

O29.63 Failed or difficult intubation for anesthesia during pregnancy, third trimester

O29.8 Other complications of anesthesia during pregnancy

O29.8X Other complications of anesthesia during pregnancy

O29.8X1 Other complications of anesthesia during pregnancy, first trimester

O29.8X2 Other complications of anesthesia during pregnancy, second trimester

O29.8X3 Other complications of anesthesia during pregnancy, third trimester

O29.8X9 Other complications of anesthesia during pregnancy, unspecified trimester

O29.9 Unspecified complication of anesthesia during pregnancy

O29.90 Unspecified complication of anesthesia during pregnancy, unspecified trimester

O29.91 Unspecified complication of anesthesia during pregnancy, first trimester

O29.92 Unspecified complication of anesthesia during pregnancy, second trimester

O29.93 Unspecified complication of anesthesia during pregnancy, third trimester

MATERNAL CARE RELATED TO THE FETUS AND AMNIOTIC CAVITY AND POSSIBLE DELIVERY PROBLEMS (O30-O48)

O30 Multiple gestation

Code also any complications specific to multiple gestation

O30.0 Twin pregnancy

O30.00 Twin pregnancy, unspecified number of placenta and unspecified number of amniotic sacs

O30.001 Twin pregnancy, unspecified number of placenta and unspecified number of amniotic sacs, first trimester

O30.002 Twin pregnancy, unspecified number of placenta and unspecified number of amniotic sacs, second trimester

O30.003 Twin pregnancy, unspecified number of placenta and unspecified number of amniotic sacs, third trimester

O30.009 Twin pregnancy, unspecified number of placenta and unspecified number of amniotic sacs, unspecified trimester

O30.01 Twin pregnancy, monochorionic/ monoamniotic

Twin pregnancy, one placenta, one amniotic sac

Excludes1: conjoined twins (O30.02-)

O30.011 Twin pregnancy, monochorionic/monoamniotic, first trimester

O30.012 Twin pregnancy, monochorionic/monoamniotic, second trimester

O30.013 Twin pregnancy, monochorionic/monoamniotic, third trimester

O30.019 Twin pregnancy, monochorionic/monoamniotic, unspecified trimester

O30.02 Conjoined twin pregnancy

O30.021 Conjoined twin pregnancy, first trimester

O30.022 Conjoined twin pregnancy, second trimester

O30.023 Conjoined twin pregnancy, third trimester

O30.029 Conjoined twin pregnancy, unspecified trimester

O30.03 Twin pregnancy, monochorionic/ diamniotic
Twin pregnancy, one placenta, two amniotic sacs

O30.031 Twin pregnancy, monochorionic/diamniotic, first trimester

O30.032 Twin pregnancy, monochorionic/diamniotic, second trimester

O30.033 Twin pregnancy, monochorionic/diamniotic, third trimester

O30.039 Twin pregnancy, monochorionic/diamniotic, unspecified trimester

O30.04 Twin pregnancy, dichorionic/diamniotic Twin pregnancy, two placentae, two amniotic sacs

O30.041 Twin pregnancy, dichorionic/diamniotic, first trimester

O30.042 Twin pregnancy, dichorionic/diamniotic, second trimester

O30.043 Twin pregnancy, dichorionic/diamniotic, third trimester

O30.049 Twin pregnancy, dichorionic/diamniotic, unspecified trimester

O30.09 Twin pregnancy, unable to determine number of placenta and number of amniotic sacs

O30.091 Twin pregnancy, unable to determine number of placenta and number of amniotic sacs, first trimester

O30.092 Twin pregnancy, unable to determine number of placenta and number of amniotic sacs, second trimester

O30.093 Twin pregnancy, unable to determine number of placenta and number of amniotic sacs, third trimester

---

Add 4th-7th digits   Nonspecific code   Unspecified code   Manifestation code   661

O30.099   Twin pregnancy, unable to determine number of placenta and number of amniotic sacs, unspecified trimester

O30.1   Triplet pregnancy

O30.10   Triplet pregnancy, unspecified number of placenta and unspecified number of amniotic sacs

O30.101   Triplet pregnancy, unspecified number of placenta and unspecified number of amniotic sacs, first trimester

O30.102   Triplet pregnancy, unspecified number of placenta and unspecified number of amniotic sacs, second trimester

O30.103   Triplet pregnancy, unspecified number of placenta and unspecified number of amniotic sacs, third trimester

O30.109   Triplet pregnancy, unspecified number of placenta and unspecified number of amniotic sacs, unspecified trimester

O30.11   Triplet pregnancy with two or more monochorionic fetuses

O30.111   Triplet pregnancy with two or more monochorionic fetuses, first trimester

O30.112   Triplet pregnancy with two or more monochorionic fetuses, second trimester

O30.113   Triplet pregnancy with two or more monochorionic fetuses, third trimester

O30.119   Triplet pregnancy with two or more monochorionic fetuses, unspecified trimester

O30.12   Triplet pregnancy with two or more monoamniotic fetuses

O30.121   Triplet pregnancy with two or more monoamniotic fetuses, first trimester

O30.122   Triplet pregnancy with two or more monoamniotic fetuses, second trimester

O30.123   Triplet pregnancy with two or more monoamniotic fetuses, third trimester

O30.129   Triplet pregnancy with two or more monoamniotic fetuses, unspecified trimester

O30.19   Triplet pregnancy, unable to determine number of placenta and number of amniotic sacs

O30.191   Triplet pregnancy, unable to determine number of placenta and number of amniotic sacs, first trimester

O30.192   Triplet pregnancy, unable to determine number of placenta and number of amniotic sacs, second trimester

O30.193   Triplet pregnancy, unable to determine number of placenta and

number of amniotic sacs, third trimester

O30.199   Triplet pregnancy, unable to determine number of placenta and number of amniotic sacs, unspecified trimester

O30.2   Quadruplet pregnancy

O30.20   Quadruplet pregnancy, unspecified number of placenta and unspecified number of amniotic sacs

O30.201   Quadruplet pregnancy, unspecified number of placenta and unspecified number of amniotic sacs, first trimester

O30.202   Quadruplet pregnancy, unspecified number of placenta and unspecified number of amniotic sacs, second trimester

O30.203   Quadruplet pregnancy, unspecified number of placenta and unspecified number of amniotic sacs, third trimester

O30.209   Quadruplet pregnancy, unspecified number of placenta and unspecified number of amniotic sacs, unspecified trimester

O30.21   Quadruplet pregnancy with two or more monochorionic fetuses

O30.211   Quadruplet pregnancy with two or more monochorionic fetuses, first trimester

O30.212   Quadruplet pregnancy with two or more monochorionic fetuses, second trimester

O30.213   Quadruplet pregnancy with two or more monochorionic fetuses, third trimester

O30.219   Quadruplet pregnancy with two or more monochorionic fetuses, unspecified trimester

O30.22   Quadruplet pregnancy with two or more monoamniotic fetuses

O30.221   Quadruplet pregnancy with two or more monoamniotic fetuses, first trimester

O30.222   Quadruplet pregnancy with two or more monoamniotic fetuses, second trimester

O30.223   Quadruplet pregnancy with two or more monoamniotic fetuses, third trimester

O30.229   Quadruplet pregnancy with two or more monoamniotic fetuses, unspecified trimester

O30.29   Quadruplet pregnancy, unable to determine number of placenta and number of amniotic sacs

O30.291   Quadruplet pregnancy, unable to determine number of placenta and number of amniotic sacs, first trimester

O30.292   Quadruplet pregnancy, unable to determine number of placenta and number of amniotic sacs, second trimester

  ● New code   ▲ Revised code   **Excludes1:** Not coded here   **Excludes2:** Not included here   ⊗ Placeholder required   ⑦7th digit required

O30.293   Quadruplet pregnancy, unable to determine number of placenta and number of amniotic sacs, third trimester

O30.299   Quadruplet pregnancy, unable to determine number of placenta and number of amniotic sacs, unspecified trimester

O30.8   **Other specified multiple gestation**

Multiple gestation pregnancy greater then quadruplets

O30.80   **Other specified multiple gestation, unspecified number of placenta and unspecified number of amniotic sacs**

O30.801   Other specified multiple gestation, unspecified number of placenta and unspecified number of amniotic sacs, first trimester

O30.802   Other specified multiple gestation, unspecified number of placenta and unspecified number of amniotic sacs, second trimester

O30.803   Other specified multiple gestation, unspecified number of placenta and unspecified number of amniotic sacs, third trimester

O30.809   Other specified multiple gestation, unspecified number of placenta and unspecified number of amniotic sacs, unspecified trimester

O30.81   **Other specified multiple gestation with two or more monochorionic fetuses**

O30.811   Other specified multiple gestation with two or more monochorionic fetuses, first trimester

O30.812   Other specified multiple gestation with two or more monochorionic fetuses, second trimester

O30.813   Other specified multiple gestation with two or more monochorionic fetuses, third trimester

O30.819   Other specified multiple gestation with two or more monochorionic fetuses, unspecified trimester

O30.82   **Other specified multiple gestation with two or more monoamniotic fetuses**

O30.821   Other specified multiple gestation with two or more monoamniotic fetuses, first trimester

O30.822   Other specified multiple gestation with two or more monoamniotic fetuses, second trimester

O30.823   Other specified multiple gestation with two or more monoamniotic fetuses, third trimester

O30.829   Other specified multiple gestation with two or more monoamniotic fetuses, unspecified trimester

O30.89   **Other specified multiple gestation, unable to determine number of placenta and number of amniotic sacs**

O30.891   Other specified multiple gestation, unable to determine number of placenta and number of amniotic sacs, first trimester

O30.892   Other specified multiple gestation, unable to determine number of placenta and number of amniotic sacs, second trimester

O30.893   Other specified multiple gestation, unable to determine number of placenta and number of amniotic sacs, third trimester

O30.899   Other specified multiple gestation, unable to determine number of placenta and number of amniotic sacs, unspecified trimester

O30.9   **Multiple gestation, unspecified**

Multiple pregnancy NOS

O30.90   Multiple gestation, unspecified, unspecified trimester

O30.91   Multiple gestation, unspecified, first trimester

O30.92   Multiple gestation, unspecified, second trimester

O30.93   Multiple gestation, unspecified, third trimester

O31   **Complications specific to multiple gestation**

Excludes2: delayed delivery of second twin, triplet, etc. (O63.2)

malpresentation of one fetus or more (O32.9)

placental transfusion syndromes (O43.0-)

One of the following 7th characters is to be assigned to each code under category O31. 7th character 0 is for single gestations and multiple gestations where the fetus is unspecified. 7th characters 1 through 9 are for cases of multiple gestations to identify the fetus for which the code applies. The appropriate code from category O30, Multiple gestation, must also be assigned when assigning a code from category O31 that has a 7th character of 1 through 9.

0 - not applicable or unspecified

1 - fetus 1

2 - fetus 2

3 - fetus 3

4 - fetus 4

5 - fetus 5

9 - Other fetus

O31.0   **Papyraceous fetus**

Fetus compressus

⊗⑦O31.00   Papyraceous fetus, unspecified trimester

⊗⑦O31.01   Papyraceous fetus, first trimester

⊗⑦O31.02   Papyraceous fetus, second trimester

⊗⑦O31.03   Papyraceous fetus, third trimester

O31.1   **Continuing pregnancy after spontaneous abortion of one fetus or more**

⊗⑦O31.10   Continuing pregnancy after spontaneous abortion of one fetus or more, unspecified trimester

⊗⑦O31.11   Continuing pregnancy after spontaneous abortion of one fetus or more, first trimester

⊗⑦O31.12   Continuing pregnancy after spontaneous abortion of one fetus or more, second trimester

⊗⑦O31.13   Continuing pregnancy after spontaneous abortion of one fetus or more, third trimester

O31.2   **Continuing pregnancy after intrauterine death of one fetus or more**

⊗⑦O31.20   Continuing pregnancy after intrauterine death of one fetus or more, unspecified trimester

⊗⑦**O31.21** **Continuing pregnancy after intrauterine death of one fetus or more, first trimester**

⊗⑦**O31.22** **Continuing pregnancy after intrauterine death of one fetus or more, second trimester**

⊗⑦**O31.23** **Continuing pregnancy after intrauterine death of one fetus or more, third trimester**

O31.3 **Continuing pregnancy after elective fetal reduction of one fetus or more**

Continuing pregnancy after selective termination of one fetus or more

⊗⑦**O31.30** **Continuing pregnancy after elective fetal reduction of one fetus or more, unspecified trimester**

⊗⑦**O31.31** **Continuing pregnancy after elective fetal reduction of one fetus or more, first trimester**

⊗⑦**O31.32** **Continuing pregnancy after elective fetal reduction of one fetus or more, second trimester**

⊗⑦**O31.33** **Continuing pregnancy after elective fetal reduction of one fetus or more, third trimester**

O31.8 **Other complications specific to multiple gestation**

O31.8X **Other complications specific to multiple gestation**

⑦**O31.8X1** **Other complications specific to multiple gestation, first trimester**

⑦**O31.8X2** **Other complications specific to multiple gestation, second trimester**

⑦**O31.8X3** **Other complications specific to multiple gestation, third trimester**

⑦**O31.8X9** **Other complications specific to multiple gestation, unspecified trimester**

O32 **Maternal care for malpresentation of fetus**

Includes: the listed conditions as a reason for observation, hospitalization **or other** obstetric care of the mother, or for cesarean delivery before onset of labor

Excludes1: malpresentation of fetus with obstructed labor (O64.-)

One of the following 7th characters is to be assigned to each code under category O32. 7th character 0 is for single gestations and multiple gestations where the fetus is unspecified. 7th characters 1 through 9 are for cases of multiple gestations to identify the fetus for which the code applies. The appropriate code from category O30, Multiple gestation, must also be assigned when assigning a code from category O32 that has a 7th character of 1 through 9.

0 - not applicable or unspecified

1 - fetus 1

2 - fetus 2

3 - fetus 3

4 - fetus 4

5 - fetus 5

9 - Other fetus

⊗⑦**O32.0** **Maternal care for unstable lie**

⊗⑦**O32.1** **Maternal care for breech presentation**

Maternal care for buttocks presentation

Maternal care for complete breech

Maternal care for frank breech

Excludes1: footling presentation (O32.8)

incomplete breech (O32.8)

⊗⑦**O32.2** **Maternal care for transverse and oblique lie**

Maternal care for oblique presentation

Maternal care for transverse presentation

⊗⑦**O32.3** **Maternal care for face, brow and chin presentation**

⊗⑦**O32.4** **Maternal care for high head at term**

Maternal care for failure of head to enter pelvic brim

⊗⑦**O32.6** **Maternal care for compound presentation**

⊗⑦**O32.8** **Maternal care for other malpresentation of fetus**

Maternal care for footling presentation

Maternal care for incomplete breech

⊗⑦**O32.9** **Maternal care for malpresentation of fetus, unspecified**

O33 **Maternal care for disproportion**

Includes: the listed conditions as a reason for observation, hospitalization **or other** obstetric care of the mother, or for cesarean delivery before onset of labor

Excludes1: disproportion with obstructed labor (O65-O66)

O33.0 **Maternal care for disproportion due to deformity of maternal pelvic bones**

Maternal care for disproportion due to pelvic deformity causing disproportion NOS

O33.1 **Maternal care for disproportion due to generally contracted pelvis**

Maternal care for disproportion due to contracted pelvis NOS causing disproportion

O33.2 **Maternal care for disproportion due to inlet contraction of pelvis**

Maternal care for disproportion due to inlet contraction (pelvis) causing disproportion

⊗⑦**O33.3** **Maternal care for disproportion due to outlet contraction of pelvis**

Maternal care for disproportion due to mid-cavity contraction (pelvis)

Maternal care for disproportion due to outlet contraction (pelvis)

One of the following 7th characters is to be assigned to code O33.3. 7th character 0 is for single gestations and multiple gestations where the fetus is unspecified. 7th characters 1 through 9 are for cases of multiple gestations to identify the fetus for which the code applies. The appropriate code from category O30, Multiple gestation, must also be assigned when assigning code O33.3 with a 7th character of 1 through 9.

0 - not applicable or unspecified

1 - fetus 1

2 - fetus 2

3 - fetus 3

4 - fetus 4

5 - fetus 5

9 - Other fetus

⊗⑦**O33.4** **Maternal care for disproportion of mixed maternal and fetal origin**

One of the following 7th characters is to be assigned to code O33.4. 7th character 0 is for single gestations and multiple gestations where the fetus is unspecified. 7th characters 1 through 9 are for cases of multiple gestations to identify the fetus for which the code applies. The appropriate code from category O30,

Multiple gestation, must also be assigned when assigning code O33.4 with a 7th character of 1 through 9.

0 - not applicable or unspecified

1 - fetus 1

2 - fetus 2

● New code ▲ Revised code **Excludes1:** Not coded here **Excludes2:** Not included here ⊗ Placeholder required ⑦ 7th digit required

3 - fetus 3

4 - fetus 4

5 - fetus 5

9 - Other fetus

⊗⑦**O33.5** **Maternal care for disproportion due to unusually large fetus**

Maternal care for disproportion due to disproportion of fetal origin with normally formed fetus

Maternal care for disproportion due to fetal disproportion NOS

One of the following 7th characters is to be assigned to code O33.5. 7th character 0 is for single gestations and multiple gestations where the fetus is unspecified. 7th characters 1 through 9 are for cases of multiple gestations to identify the fetus for which the code applies. The appropriate code from category O30,

Multiple gestation, must also be assigned when assigning code O33.5 with a 7th character of 1 through 9.

0 - not applicable or unspecified

1 - fetus 1

2 - fetus 2

3 - fetus 3

4 - fetus 4

5 - fetus 5

9 - Other fetus

⊗⑦**O33.6** **Maternal care for disproportion due to hydrocephalic fetus**

One of the following 7th characters is to be assigned to code O33.6. 7th character 0 is for single gestations and multiple gestations where the fetus is unspecified. 7th characters 1 through 9 are for cases of multiple gestations to identify the fetus for which the code applies. The appropriate code from category O30,

Multiple gestation, must also be assigned when assigning code O33.6 with a 7th character of 1 through 9.

0 - not applicable or unspecified

1 - fetus 1

2 - fetus 2

3 - fetus 3

4 - fetus 4

5 - fetus 5

9 - Other fetus

●⊗⑦**O33.7** **Maternal care for disproportion due to other fetal deformities**

Maternal care for disproportion due to fetal ascites

Maternal care for disproportion due to fetal hydrops

Maternal care for disproportion due to fetal meningomyelocele

Maternal care for disproportion due to fetal sacral teratoma

Maternal care for disproportion due to fetal tumor

One of the following 7th characters is to be assigned to code O33.7. 7th character 0 is for single gestations and multiple gestations where the fetus is unspecified. 7th characters 1 through 9 are for cases of multiple gestations to identify the fetus for which the code applies. The appropriate code from category O30,

Multiple gestation, must also be assigned when assigning code O33.7 with a 7th character of 1 through 9.

0 - not applicable or unspecified

1 - fetus 1

2 - fetus 2

3 - fetus 3

4 - fetus 4

5 - fetus 5

9 - Other fetus

Excludes1: obstructed labor due **to other** fetal deformities (O66.3)

O33.8 **Maternal care for disproportion of other origin**

O33.9 **Maternal care for disproportion, unspecified**

Maternal care for disproportion due to cephalopelvic disproportion NOS

Maternal care for disproportion due to fetopelvic disproportion NOS

O34 **Maternal care for abnormality of pelvic organs**

Includes: the listed conditions as a reason for hospitalization **or other** obstetric care of the mother, or for cesarean

delivery before onset of labor

Code first any associated obstructed labor (O65.5)

Use additional code for specific condition

O34.0 **Maternal care for congenital malformation of uterus**

Maternal care for double uterus

Maternal care for uterus bicornis

O34.00 **Maternal care for unspecified congenital malformation of uterus, unspecified trimester**

O34.01 **Maternal care for unspecified congenital malformation of uterus, first trimester**

O34.02 **Maternal care for unspecified congenital malformation of uterus, second trimester**

O34.03 **Maternal care for unspecified congenital malformation of uterus, third trimester**

O34.1 **Maternal care for benign tumor of corpus uteri**

Excludes2: maternal care for benign tumor of cervix (O34.4-)

maternal care for malignant neoplasm of uterus (O9A.1-)

O34.10 **Maternal care for benign tumor of corpus uteri, unspecified trimester**

O34.11 **Maternal care for benign tumor of corpus uteri, first trimester**

O34.12 **Maternal care for benign tumor of corpus uteri, second trimester**

O34.13 **Maternal care for benign tumor of corpus uteri, third trimester**

O34.2 **Maternal care due to uterine scar from previous surgery**

O34.21 **Maternal care for scar from previous cesarean delivery**

●**O34.211** **Maternal care for low transverse scar from previous cesarean delivery**

●**O34.212** **Maternal care for vertical scar from previous cesarean delivery**

Maternal care for classical scar from previous cesarean delivery

●**O34.219** **Maternal care for unspecified type scar from previous cesarean delivery**

O34.29 **Maternal care due to uterine scar from other previous surgery**

Maternal care due to uterine scar **from other** transmural uterine incision

O34.3 Maternal care for cervical incompetence

Maternal care for cerclage with or without cervical incompetence

Maternal care for Shirodkar suture with or without cervical incompetence

O34.30 Maternal care for cervical incompetence, unspecified trimester

O34.31 Maternal care for cervical incompetence, first trimester

O34.32 Maternal care for cervical incompetence, second trimester

O34.33 Maternal care for cervical incompetence, third trimester

O34.4 Maternal care for other abnormalities of cervix

O34.40 Maternal care for other abnormalities of cervix, unspecified trimester

O34.41 Maternal care for other abnormalities of cervix, first trimester

O34.42 Maternal care for other abnormalities of cervix, second trimester

O34.43 Maternal care for other abnormalities of cervix, third trimester

O34.5 Maternal care for other abnormalities of gravid uterus

O34.51 Maternal care for incarceration of gravid uterus

O34.511 Maternal care for incarceration of gravid uterus, first trimester

O34.512 Maternal care for incarceration of gravid uterus, second trimester

O34.513 Maternal care for incarceration of gravid uterus, third trimester

O34.519 Maternal care for incarceration of gravid uterus, unspecified trimester

O34.52 Maternal care for prolapse of gravid uterus

O34.521 Maternal care for prolapse of gravid uterus, first trimester

O34.522 Maternal care for prolapse of gravid uterus, second trimester

O34.523 Maternal care for prolapse of gravid uterus, third trimester

O34.529 Maternal care for prolapse of gravid uterus, unspecified trimester

O34.53 Maternal care for retroversion of gravid uterus

O34.531 Maternal care for retroversion of gravid uterus, first trimester

O34.532 Maternal care for retroversion of gravid uterus, second trimester

O34.533 Maternal care for retroversion of gravid uterus, third trimester

O34.539 Maternal care for retroversion of gravid uterus, unspecified trimester

O34.59 Maternal care for other abnormalities of gravid uterus

O34.591 Maternal care for other abnormalities of gravid uterus, first trimester

O34.592 Maternal care for other abnormalities of gravid uterus, second trimester

O34.593 Maternal care for other abnormalities of gravid uterus, third trimester

O34.599 Maternal care for other abnormalities of gravid uterus, unspecified trimester

O34.6 Maternal care for abnormality of vagina

Excludes2: maternal care for vaginal varices in pregnancy (O22.1-)

O34.60 Maternal care for abnormality of vagina, unspecified trimester

O34.61 Maternal care for abnormality of vagina, first trimester

O34.62 Maternal care for abnormality of vagina, second trimester

O34.63 Maternal care for abnormality of vagina, third trimester

O34.7 Maternal care for abnormality of vulva and perineum

Excludes2: maternal care for perineal and vulval varices in pregnancy (O22.1-)

O34.70 Maternal care for abnormality of vulva and perineum, unspecified trimester

O34.71 Maternal care for abnormality of vulva and perineum, first trimester

O34.72 Maternal care for abnormality of vulva and perineum, second trimester

O34.73 Maternal care for abnormality of vulva and perineum, third trimester

O34.8 Maternal care for other abnormalities of pelvic organs

O34.80 Maternal care for other abnormalities of pelvic organs, unspecified trimester

O34.81 Maternal care for other abnormalities of pelvic organs, first trimester

O34.82 Maternal care for other abnormalities of pelvic organs, second trimester

O34.83 Maternal care for other abnormalities of pelvic organs, third trimester

O34.9 Maternal care for abnormality of pelvic organ, unspecified

O34.90 Maternal care for abnormality of pelvic organ, unspecified, unspecified trimester

O34.91 Maternal care for abnormality of pelvic organ, unspecified, first trimester

O34.92 Maternal care for abnormality of pelvic organ, unspecified, second trimester

O34.93 Maternal care for abnormality of pelvic organ, unspecified, third trimester

O35 Maternal care for known or suspected fetal abnormality and damage

Includes: the listed conditions in the fetus as a reason for hospitalization **or other** obstetric care to the mother, or for termination of pregnancy

Code also any associated maternal condition

Excludes1: encounter for suspected maternal and fetal conditions ruled out (Z03.7-)

One of the following 7th characters is to be assigned to each code under category O35. 7th character 0 is for single gestations and multiple gestations where the fetus is unspecified. 7th characters 1

● New code   ▲ Revised code   **Excludes1:** Not coded here   **Excludes2:** Not included here   ⊗ Placeholder required   ⑦7ᵗʰ digit required

through 9 are for cases of multiple gestations to identify the fetus for which the code applies. The appropriate code from category O30,

Multiple gestation, must also be assigned when assigning a code from category O35 that has a 7th character of 1 through 9.

0 - not applicable or unspecified

1 - fetus 1

2 - fetus 2

3 - fetus 3

4 - fetus 4

5 - fetus 5

9 - Other fetus

⊗⑦**O35.0 Maternal care for (suspected) central nervous system malformation in fetus**

Maternal care for fetal anencephaly

Maternal care for fetal hydrocephalus

Maternal care for fetal spina bifida

Excludes2: chromosomal abnormality in fetus (O35.1)

⊗⑦**O35.1 Maternal care for (suspected) chromosomal abnormality in fetus**

⊗⑦**O35.2 Maternal care for (suspected) hereditary disease in fetus**

Excludes2: chromosomal abnormality in fetus (O35.1)

⊗⑦**O35.3 Maternal care for (suspected) damage to fetus from viral disease in mother**

Maternal care for damage to fetus from maternal cytomegalovirus infection

Maternal care for damage to fetus from maternal rubella

⊗⑦**O35.4 Maternal care for (suspected) damage to fetus from alcohol**

⊗⑦**O35.5 Maternal care for (suspected) damage to fetus by drugs**

Maternal care for damage to fetus from drug addiction

⊗⑦**O35.6 Maternal care for (suspected) damage to fetus by radiation**

⊗⑦**O35.7 Maternal care for (suspected) damage to fetus by other medical procedures**

Maternal care for damage to fetus by amniocentesis

Maternal care for damage to fetus by biopsy procedures

Maternal care for damage to fetus by hematological investigation

Maternal care for damage to fetus by intrauterine contraceptive device

Maternal care for damage to fetus by intrauterine surgery

⊗⑦**O35.8 Maternal care for other (suspected) fetal abnormality and damage**

Maternal care for damage to fetus from maternal listeriosis

Maternal care for damage to fetus from maternal toxoplasmosis

⊗⑦**O35.9 Maternal care for (suspected) fetal abnormality and damage, unspecified**

O36 Maternal care for other fetal problems

Includes: the listed conditions in the fetus as a reason for `hospitalization **or other** obstetric care of the mother, or for termination of pregnancy

Excludes1: encounter for suspected maternal and fetal conditions ruled out (Z03.7-)

placental transfusion syndromes (O43.0-)

Excludes2: labor and delivery complicated by fetal stress (O77.-)

One of the following 7th characters is to be assigned to each code under category O36. 7th character 0 is for single gestations and multiple gestations where the fetus is unspecified. 7th characters 1 through 9 are for cases of multiple gestations to identify the fetus for which the code applies. The appropriate code from category O30,

Multiple gestation, must also be assigned when assigning a code from category O36 that has a 7th character of 1 through 9.

0 - not applicable or unspecified

1 - fetus 1

2 - fetus 2

3 - fetus 3

4 - fetus 4

5 - fetus 5

9 - Other fetus

O36.0 Maternal care for rhesus isoimmunization

Maternal care for Rh incompatibility (with hydrops fetalis)

O36.01 Maternal care for anti-D [Rh] antibodies

⑦**O36.011 Maternal care for anti-D [Rh] antibodies, first trimester**

⑦**O36.012 Maternal care for anti-D [Rh] antibodies, second trimester**

⑦**O36.013 Maternal care for anti-D [Rh] antibodies, third trimester**

⑦**O36.019 Maternal care for anti-D [Rh] antibodies, unspecified trimester**

O36.09 Maternal care for other rhesus isoimmunization

⑦**O36.091 Maternal care for other rhesus isoimmunization, first trimester**

⑦**O36.092 Maternal care for other rhesus isoimmunization, second trimester**

⑦**O36.093 Maternal care for other rhesus isoimmunization, third trimester**

⑦**O36.099 Maternal care for other rhesus isoimmunization, unspecified trimester**

O36.1 Maternal care for other isoimmunization

Maternal care for ABO isoimmunization

O36.11 Maternal care for Anti-A sensitization

Maternal care for isoimmunization NOS (with hydrops fetalis)

⑦**O36.111 Maternal care for Anti-A sensitization, first trimester**

⑦**O36.112 Maternal care for Anti-A sensitization, second trimester**

⑦**O36.113 Maternal care for Anti-A sensitization, third trimester**

⑦**O36.119 Maternal care for Anti-A sensitization, unspecified trimester**

O36.19 Maternal care for other isoimmunization

Maternal care for Anti-B sensitization

⑦**O36.191 Maternal care for other isoimmunization, first trimester**

⑦**O36.192 Maternal care for other isoimmunization, second trimester**

⑦**O36.193 Maternal care for other isoimmunization, third trimester**

⑦ O36.199   **Maternal care for other isoimmunization, unspecified trimester**

O36.2   **Maternal care for hydrops fetalis**

Maternal care for hydrops fetalis NOS

Maternal care for hydrops fetalis not associated with isoimmunization

Excludes1: hydrops fetalis associated with ABO isoimmunization (O36.1-)

hydrops fetalis associated with rhesus isoimmunization (O36.0-)

⊗⑦ O36.20   **Maternal care for hydrops fetalis, unspecified trimester**

⊗⑦ O36.21   **Maternal care for hydrops fetalis, first trimester**

⊗⑦ O36.22   **Maternal care for hydrops fetalis, second trimester**

⊗⑦ O36.23   **Maternal care for hydrops fetalis, third trimester**

⊗⑦ O36.4   **Maternal care for intrauterine death**

Maternal care for intrauterine fetal death NOS

Maternal care for intrauterine fetal death after completion of 20 weeks of gestation

Maternal care for late fetal death

Maternal care for missed delivery

Excludes1: missed abortion (O02.1)

stillbirth (P95)

O36.5   **Maternal care for known or suspected poor fetal growth**

O36.51   **Maternal care for known or suspected placental insufficiency**

⑦ O36.511   **Maternal care for known or suspected placental insufficiency, first trimester**

⑦ O36.512   **Maternal care for known or suspected placental insufficiency, second trimester**

⑦ O36.513   **Maternal care for known or suspected placental insufficiency, third trimester**

⑦ O36.519   **Maternal care for known or suspected placental insufficiency, unspecified trimester**

O36.59   **Maternal care for other known or suspected poor fetal growth**

Maternal care for known or suspected light-for-dates NOS

Maternal care for known or suspected small-for-dates NOS

⑦ O36.591   **Maternal care for other known or suspected poor fetal growth, first trimester**

⑦ O36.592   **Maternal care for other known or suspected poor fetal growth, second trimester**

⑦ O36.593   **Maternal care for other known or suspected poor fetal growth, third trimester**

⑦ O36.599   **Maternal care for other known or suspected poor fetal growth, unspecified trimester**

O36.6   **Maternal care for excessive fetal growth**

Maternal care for known or suspected large-for-dates

⊗⑦ O36.60   **Maternal care for excessive fetal growth, unspecified trimester**

⊗⑦ O36.61   **Maternal care for excessive fetal growth, first trimester**

⊗⑦ O36.62   **Maternal care for excessive fetal growth, second trimester**

⊗⑦ O36.63   **Maternal care for excessive fetal growth, third trimester**

O36.7   **Maternal care for viable fetus in abdominal pregnancy**

⊗⑦ O36.70   **Maternal care for viable fetus in abdominal pregnancy, unspecified trimester**

⊗⑦ O36.71   **Maternal care for viable fetus in abdominal pregnancy, first trimester**

⊗⑦ O36.72   **Maternal care for viable fetus in abdominal pregnancy, second trimester**

⊗⑦ O36.73   **Maternal care for viable fetus in abdominal pregnancy, third trimester**

O36.8   **Maternal care for other specified fetal problems**

⊗⑦ O36.80   **Pregnancy with inconclusive fetal viability**

Encounter to determine fetal viability of pregnancy

O36.81   **Decreased fetal movements**

⑦ O36.812   **Decreased fetal movements, second trimester**

⑦ O36.813   **Decreased fetal movements, third trimester**

⑦ O36.819   **Decreased fetal movements, unspecified trimester**

O36.82   **Fetal anemia and thrombocytopenia**

⑦ O36.821   **Fetal anemia and thrombocytopenia, first trimester**

⑦ O36.822   **Fetal anemia and thrombocytopenia, second trimester**

⑦ O36.823   **Fetal anemia and thrombocytopenia, third trimester**

⑦ O36.829   **Fetal anemia and thrombocytopenia, unspecified trimester**

O36.89   **Maternal care for other specified fetal problems**

⑦ O36.891   **Maternal care for other specified fetal problems, first trimester**

⑦ O36.892   **Maternal care for other specified fetal problems, second trimester**

⑦ O36.893   **Maternal care for other specified fetal problems, third trimester**

⑦ O36.899   **Maternal care for other specified fetal problems, unspecified trimester**

O36.9   **Maternal care for fetal problem, unspecified**

⊗⑦ O36.90   **Maternal care for fetal problem, unspecified, unspecified trimester**

⊗⑦ O36.91   **Maternal care for fetal problem, unspecified, first trimester**

⊗⑦ O36.92   **Maternal care for fetal problem, unspecified, second trimester**

⊗⑦ O36.93   **Maternal care for fetal problem, unspecified, third trimester**

   ● New code   ▲ Revised code   **Excludes1:** Not coded here   **Excludes2:** Not included here   ⊗ Placeholder required   ⑦ 7ᵗʰ digit required

O40 Polyhydramnios

Definition: Polyhydramnios is a condition that exists when there is too much amniotic fluid in the uterus.

Includes: hydramnios

Excludes1: encounter for suspected maternal and fetal conditions ruled out (Z03.7-)

One of the following 7th characters is to be assigned to each code under category O40. 7th character 0 is for single gestations and multiple gestations where the fetus is unspecified. 7th characters 1 through 9 are for cases of multiple gestations to identify the fetus for which the code applies. The appropriate code from category O30,

Multiple gestation, must also be assigned when assigning a code from category O40 that has a 7th character of 1 through 9.

0 - not applicable or unspecified

1 - fetus 1

2 - fetus 2

3 - fetus 3

4 - fetus 4

5 - fetus 5

9 - Other fetus

⊗⑦ **O40.1 Polyhydramnios, first trimester**

⊗⑦ **O40.2 Polyhydramnios, second trimester**

⊗⑦ **O40.3 Polyhydramnios, third trimester**

⊗⑦ **O40.9 Polyhydramnios, unspecified trimester**

O41 Other disorders of amniotic fluid and membranes

Excludes1: encounter for suspected maternal and fetal conditions ruled out (Z03.7-)

One of the following 7th characters is to be assigned to each code under category O41. 7th character 0 is for single gestations and multiple gestations where the fetus is unspecified. 7th characters 1 through 9 are for cases of multiple gestations to identify the fetus for which the code applies. The appropriate code from category O30,

Multiple gestation, must also be assigned when assigning a code from category O41 that has a 7th character of 1 through 9.

0 - not applicable or unspecified

1 - fetus 1

2 - fetus 2

3 - fetus 3

4 - fetus 4

5 - fetus 5

9 - Other fetus

O41.0 Oligohydramnios

Oligohydramnios without rupture of membranes

⊗⑦ **O41.00 Oligohydramnios, unspecified trimester**

⊗⑦ **O41.01 Oligohydramnios, first trimester**

⊗⑦ **O41.02 Oligohydramnios, second trimester**

⊗⑦ **O41.03 Oligohydramnios, third trimester**

O41.1 Infection of amniotic sac and membranes

O41.10 Infection of amniotic sac and membranes, unspecified

⑦ **O41.101 Infection of amniotic sac and membranes, unspecified, first trimester**

⑦ **O41.102 Infection of amniotic sac and membranes, unspecified, second trimester**

⑦ **O41.103 Infection of amniotic sac and membranes, unspecified, third trimester**

⑦ **O41.109 Infection of amniotic sac and membranes, unspecified, unspecified trimester**

O41.12 Chorioamnionitis

⑦ **O41.121 Chorioamnionitis, first trimester**

⑦ **O41.122 Chorioamnionitis, second trimester**

⑦ **O41.123 Chorioamnionitis, third trimester**

⑦ **O41.129 Chorioamnionitis, unspecified trimester**

O41.14 Placentitis

⑦ **O41.141 Placentitis, first trimester**

⑦ **O41.142 Placentitis, second trimester**

⑦ **O41.143 Placentitis, third trimester**

⑦ **O41.149 Placentitis, unspecified trimester**

O41.8 Other specified disorders of amniotic fluid and membranes

O41.8X Other specified disorders of amniotic fluid and membranes

⑦ **O41.8X1 Other specified disorders of amniotic fluid and membranes, first trimester**

⑦ **O41.8X2 Other specified disorders of amniotic fluid and membranes, second trimester**

⑦ **O41.8X3 Other specified disorders of amniotic fluid and membranes, third trimester**

⑦ **O41.8X9 Other specified disorders of amniotic fluid and membranes, unspecified trimester**

O41.9 Disorder of amniotic fluid and membranes, unspecified

⊗⑦ **O41.90 Disorder of amniotic fluid and membranes, unspecified, unspecified trimester**

⊗⑦ **O41.91 Disorder of amniotic fluid and membranes, unspecified, first trimester**

⊗⑦ **O41.92 Disorder of amniotic fluid and membranes, unspecified, second trimester**

⊗⑦ **O41.93 Disorder of amniotic fluid and membranes, unspecified, third trimester**

O42 Premature rupture of membranes

O42.0 Premature rupture of membranes, onset of labor within 24 hours of rupture

O42.00 Premature rupture of membranes, onset of labor within 24 hours of rupture, unspecified weeks of gestation

O42.01 Preterm premature rupture of membranes, onset of labor within 24 hours of rupture

Premature rupture of membranes before 37 completed weeks of gestation

O42.011 Preterm premature rupture of membranes, onset of labor within 24 hours of rupture, first trimester

O42.012 Preterm premature rupture of membranes, onset of labor within 24 hours of rupture, second trimester

O42.013 Preterm premature rupture of membranes, onset of labor within 24 hours of rupture, third trimester

O42.019 Preterm premature rupture of membranes, onset of labor within 24 hours of rupture, unspecified trimester

O42.02 Full-term premature rupture of membranes, onset of labor within 24 hours of rupture

Premature rupture of membranes at or after 37 completed weeks of gestation, onset of labor within 24 hours of rupture

O42.1 Premature rupture of membranes, onset of labor more than 24 hours following rupture

O42.10 Premature rupture of membranes, onset of labor more than 24 hours following rupture, unspecified weeks of gestation

O42.11 Preterm premature rupture of membranes, onset of labor more than 24 hours following rupture

Premature rupture of membranes before 37 completed weeks of gestation

O42.111 Preterm premature rupture of membranes, onset of labor more than 24 hours following rupture, first trimester

O42.112 Preterm premature rupture of membranes, onset of labor more than 24 hours following rupture, second trimester

O42.113 Preterm premature rupture of membranes, onset of labor more than 24 hours following rupture, third trimester

O42.119 Preterm premature rupture of membranes, onset of labor more than 24 hours following rupture, unspecified trimester

O42.12 Full-term premature rupture of membranes, onset of labor more than 24 hours following rupture

Premature rupture of membranes at or after 37 completed weeks of gestation, onset of labor more than 24 hours following rupture

O42.9 Premature rupture of membranes, unspecified as to length of time between rupture and onset of labor

O42.90 Premature rupture of membranes, unspecified as to length of time between rupture and onset of labor, unspecified weeks of gestation

O42.91 Preterm premature rupture of membranes, unspecified as to length of time between rupture and onset of labor

Premature rupture of membranes before 37 completed weeks of gestation

O42.911 Preterm premature rupture of membranes, unspecified as to length of time between rupture and onset of labor, first trimester

O42.912 Preterm premature rupture of membranes, unspecified as to length of time between rupture and onset of labor, second trimester

O42.913 Preterm premature rupture of membranes, unspecified as to length

of time between rupture and onset of labor, third trimester

O42.919 Preterm premature rupture of membranes, unspecified as to length of time between rupture and onset of labor, unspecified trimester

O42.92 Full-term premature rupture of membranes, unspecified as to length of time between rupture and onset of labor

Premature rupture of membranes at or after 37 completed weeks of gestation, unspecified as to length of time between rupture and onset of labor

O43 Placental disorders

Excludes2: maternal care for poor fetal growth due to placental insufficiency (O36.5-)

placenta previa (O44.-)

placental polyp (O90.89)

placentitis (O41.14-)

premature separation of placenta [abruptio placentae] (O45.-)

O43.0 Placental transfusion syndromes

O43.01 Fetomaternal placental transfusion syndrome

Maternofetal placental transfusion syndrome

O43.011 Fetomaternal placental transfusion syndrome, first trimester

O43.012 Fetomaternal placental transfusion syndrome, second trimester

O43.013 Fetomaternal placental transfusion syndrome, third trimester

O43.019 Fetomaternal placental transfusion syndrome, unspecified trimester

O43.02 Fetus-to-fetus placental transfusion syndrome

O43.021 Fetus-to-fetus placental transfusion syndrome, first trimester

O43.022 Fetus-to-fetus placental transfusion syndrome, second trimester

O43.023 Fetus-to-fetus placental transfusion syndrome, third trimester

O43.029 Fetus-to-fetus placental transfusion syndrome, unspecified trimester

O43.1 Malformation of placenta

O43.10 Malformation of placenta, unspecified

Abnormal placenta NOS

O43.101 Malformation of placenta, unspecified, first trimester

O43.102 Malformation of placenta, unspecified, second trimester

O43.103 Malformation of placenta, unspecified, third trimester

O43.109 Malformation of placenta, unspecified, unspecified trimester

O43.11 Circumvallate placenta

O43.111 Circumvallate placenta, first trimester

O43.112 Circumvallate placenta, second trimester

O43.113 Circumvallate placenta, third trimester

O43.119 Circumvallate placenta, unspecified trimester

O43.12 Velamentous insertion of umbilical cord

    O43.121 Velamentous insertion of umbilical cord, first trimester

    O43.122 Velamentous insertion of umbilical cord, second trimester

    O43.123 Velamentous insertion of umbilical cord, third trimester

    O43.129 Velamentous insertion of umbilical cord, unspecified trimester

O43.19 Other malformation of placenta

    O43.191 Other malformation of placenta, first trimester

    O43.192 Other malformation of placenta, second trimester

    O43.193 Other malformation of placenta, third trimester

    O43.199 Other malformation of placenta, unspecified trimester

O43.2 Morbidly adherent placenta

Code also associated third stage postpartum hemorrhage, if applicable (O72.0)

Excludes1: retained placenta (O73.-)

O43.21 Placenta accreta

    O43.211 Placenta accreta, first trimester

    O43.212 Placenta accreta, second trimester

    O43.213 Placenta accreta, third trimester

    O43.219 Placenta accreta, unspecified trimester

O43.22 Placenta increta

    O43.221 Placenta increta, first trimester

    O43.222 Placenta increta, second trimester

    O43.223 Placenta increta, third trimester

    O43.229 Placenta increta, unspecified trimester

O43.23 Placenta percreta

    O43.231 Placenta percreta, first trimester

    O43.232 Placenta percreta, second trimester

    O43.233 Placenta percreta, third trimester

    O43.239 Placenta percreta, unspecified trimester

O43.8 Other placental disorders

O43.81 Placental infarction

    O43.811 Placental infarction, first trimester

    O43.812 Placental infarction, second trimester

    O43.813 Placental infarction, third trimester

    O43.819 Placental infarction, unspecified trimester

O43.89 Other placental disorders

Placental dysfunction

    O43.891 Other placental disorders, first trimester

    O43.892 Other placental disorders, second trimester

    O43.893 Other placental disorders, third trimester

    O43.899 Other placental disorders, unspecified trimester

O43.9 Unspecified placental disorder

O43.90 Unspecified placental disorder, unspecified trimester

O43.91 Unspecified placental disorder, first trimester

O43.92 Unspecified placental disorder, second trimester

O43.93 Unspecified placental disorder, third trimester

O44 Placenta previa

O44.0 Complete placenta previa NOS or without hemorrhage

Placenta previa NOS

▲O44.00 Complete placenta previa NOS or without hemorrhage, unspecified trimester

▲O44.01 Complete placenta previa NOS or without hemorrhage, first trimester

▲O44.02 Complete placenta previa NOS or without hemorrhage, second trimester

▲O44.03 Complete placenta previa NOS or without hemorrhage, third trimester

O44.1 Complete placenta previa with hemorrhage

Excludes1: labor and delivery complicated by hemorrhage from vasa previa (O69.4)

▲O44.10 Complete placenta previa with hemorrhage, unspecified trimester

▲O44.11 Complete placenta previa with hemorrhage, first trimester

▲O44.12 Complete placenta previa with hemorrhage, second trimester

▲O44.13 Complete placenta previa with hemorrhage, third trimester

O44.2 Partial placenta previa without hemorrhage

Marginal placenta previa, NOS or without hemorrhage

●O44.20 Partial placenta previa NOS or without hemorrhage, unspecified trimester

●O44.21 Partial placenta previa NOS or without hemorrhage, first trimester

●O44.22 Partial placenta previa NOS or without hemorrhage, second trimester

●O44.23 Partial placenta previa NOS or without hemorrhage, third trimester

O44.3 Partial placenta previa with hemorrhage

Marginal placenta previa with hemorrhage

●O44.30 Partial placenta previa with hemorrhage, unspecified trimester

●O44.31 Partial placenta previa with hemorrhage, first trimester

●O44.32 Partial placenta previa with hemorrhage, second trimester

●O44.33 Partial placenta previa with hemorrhage, third trimester

O44.4 Low lying placenta NOS or without hemorrhage

Low implantation of placenta NOS or without hemorrhage

●O44.40 Low lying placenta NOS or without hemorrhage, unspecified trimester

●O44.41 Low lying placenta NOS or without hemorrhage, first trimester

●O44.42 Low lying placenta NOS or without hemorrhage, second trimester

●O44.43 Low lying placenta NOS or without hemorrhage, third trimester

O44.5   Low lying placenta with hemorrhage

Low implantation of placenta with hemorrhage

•**O44.50   Low lying placenta with hemorrhage, unspecified trimester**

•**O44.51   Low lying placenta with hemorrhage, first trimester**

•**O44.52   Low lying placenta with hemorrhage, second trimester**

•**O44.53   Low lying placenta with hemorrhage, third trimester**

O45   Premature separation of placenta [abruptio placentae]

O45.0   Premature separation of placenta with coagulation defect

O45.00   Premature separation of placenta with coagulation defect, unspecified

O45.001   Premature separation of placenta with coagulation defect, unspecified, first trimester

O45.002   Premature separation of placenta with coagulation defect, unspecified, second trimester

O45.003   Premature separation of placenta with coagulation defect, unspecified, third trimester

O45.009   Premature separation of placenta with coagulation defect, unspecified, unspecified trimester

O45.01   Premature separation of placenta with afibrinogenemia

Premature separation of placenta with hypofibrinogenemia

O45.011   Premature separation of placenta with afibrinogenemia, first trimester

O45.012   Premature separation of placenta with afibrinogenemia, second trimester

O45.013   Premature separation of placenta with afibrinogenemia, third trimester

O45.019   Premature separation of placenta with afibrinogenemia, unspecified trimester

O45.02   Premature separation of placenta with disseminated intravascular coagulation

O45.021   Premature separation of placenta with disseminated intravascular coagulation, first trimester

O45.022   Premature separation of placenta with disseminated intravascular coagulation, second trimester

O45.023   Premature separation of placenta with disseminated intravascular coagulation, third trimester

O45.029   Premature separation of placenta with disseminated intravascular coagulation, unspecified trimester

O45.09   Premature separation of placenta with other coagulation defect

O45.091   Premature separation of placenta with other coagulation defect, first trimester

O45.092   Premature separation of placenta with other coagulation defect, second trimester

O45.093   Premature separation of placenta with other coagulation defect, third trimester

O45.099   Premature separation of placenta with other coagulation defect, unspecified trimester

O45.8   Other premature separation of placenta

O45.8X   Other premature separation of placenta

O45.8X1   Other premature separation of placenta, first trimester

O45.8X2   Other premature separation of placenta, second trimester

O45.8X3   Other premature separation of placenta, third trimester

O45.8X9   Other premature separation of placenta, unspecified trimester

O45.9   Premature separation of placenta, unspecified

Abruptio placentae NOS

O45.90   Premature separation of placenta, unspecified, unspecified trimester

O45.91   Premature separation of placenta, unspecified, first trimester

O45.92   Premature separation of placenta, unspecified, second trimester

O45.93   Premature separation of placenta, unspecified, third trimester

O46   Antepartum hemorrhage, not elsewhere classified

Excludes1: hemorrhage in early pregnancy (O20.-)

intrapartum hemorrhage NEC (O67.-) placenta previa (O44.-)

premature separation of placenta [abruptio placentae] (O45.-)

O46.0   Antepartum hemorrhage with coagulation defect

O46.00   Antepartum hemorrhage with coagulation defect, unspecified

O46.001   Antepartum hemorrhage with coagulation defect, unspecified, first trimester

O46.002   Antepartum hemorrhage with coagulation defect, unspecified, second trimester

O46.003   Antepartum hemorrhage with coagulation defect, unspecified, third trimester

O46.009   Antepartum hemorrhage with coagulation defect, unspecified, unspecified trimester

O46.01   Antepartum hemorrhage with afibrinogenemia

Antepartum hemorrhage with hypofibrinogenemia

O46.011   Antepartum hemorrhage with afibrinogenemia, first trimester

O46.012   Antepartum hemorrhage with afibrinogenemia, second trimester

O46.013   Antepartum hemorrhage with afibrinogenemia, third trimester

• New code   ▲ Revised code   **Excludes1:** Not coded here   **Excludes2:** Not included here   ⊗ Placeholder required   ⑦ 7th digit required

O46.019 Antepartum hemorrhage with afibrinogenemia, unspecified trimester

O46.02 Antepartum hemorrhage with disseminated intravascular coagulation

O46.021 Antepartum hemorrhage with disseminated intravascular coagulation, first trimester

O46.022 Antepartum hemorrhage with disseminated intravascular coagulation, second trimester

O46.023 Antepartum hemorrhage with disseminated intravascular coagulation, third trimester

O46.029 Antepartum hemorrhage with disseminated intravascular coagulation, unspecified trimester

O46.09 Antepartum hemorrhage with other coagulation defect

O46.091 Antepartum hemorrhage with other coagulation defect, first trimester

O46.092 Antepartum hemorrhage with other coagulation defect, second trimester

O46.093 Antepartum hemorrhage with other coagulation defect, third trimester

O46.099 Antepartum hemorrhage with other coagulation defect, unspecified trimester

O46.8 Other antepartum hemorrhage

O46.8X Other antepartum hemorrhage

O46.8X1 Other antepartum hemorrhage, first trimester

O46.8X2 Other antepartum hemorrhage, second trimester

O46.8X3 Other antepartum hemorrhage, third trimester

O46.8X9 Other antepartum hemorrhage, unspecified trimester

O46.9 Antepartum hemorrhage, unspecified

O46.90 Antepartum hemorrhage, unspecified, unspecified trimester

O46.91 Antepartum hemorrhage, unspecified, first trimester

O46.92 Antepartum hemorrhage, unspecified, second trimester

O46.93 Antepartum hemorrhage, unspecified, third trimester

O47 False labor

Includes: Braxton Hicks contractions

threatened labor

Excludes1: preterm labor (O60.-)

O47.0 False labor before 37completed weeks of gestation

O47.00 False labor before 37 completed weeks of gestation, unspecified trimester

O47.02 False labor before 37 completed weeks of gestation, second trimester

O47.03 False labor before 37 completed weeks of gestation, third trimester

O47.1 False labor at or after 37completed weeks of gestation

O47.9 False labor, unspecified

O48 Late pregnancy

O48.0 Post-term pregnancy

Pregnancy over 40 completed weeks to 42 completed weeks gestation

O48.1 Prolonged pregnancy

Pregnancy which has advanced beyond 42 completed weeks gestation

COMPLICATIONS OF LABOR AND DELIVERY (O60-O77)

O60 Preterm labor Includes: onset (spontaneous) of labor before 37 completed weeks of gestation

Excludes1: false labor (O47.0-)

threatened labor NOS (O47.0-)

O60.0 Preterm labor without delivery

O60.00 Preterm labor without delivery, unspecified trimester

O60.02 Preterm labor without delivery, second trimester

O60.03 Preterm labor without delivery, third trimester

O60.1 Preterm labor with preterm delivery

One of the following 7th characters is to be assigned to each code under subcategory O60.1. 7th character 0 is for single gestations and multiple gestations where the fetus is unspecified. 7th characters 1 through 9 are for cases of multiple gestations to identify the fetus for which the code applies. The appropriate code from category O30, Multiple gestation, must also be assigned when assigning a code from subcategory O60.1 that has a 7th character of 1 through 9.

0 - not applicable or unspecified

1 - fetus 1

2 - fetus 2

3 - fetus 3

4 - fetus 4

5 - fetus 5

9 - Other fetus

⊗⑦O60.10 Preterm labor with preterm delivery, unspecified trimester

Preterm labor with delivery NOS

⊗⑦O60.12 Preterm labor second trimester with preterm delivery second trimester

⊗⑦O60.13 Preterm labor second trimester with preterm delivery third trimester

⊗⑦O60.14 Preterm labor third trimester with preterm delivery third trimester

O60.2 Term delivery with preterm labor

One of the following 7th characters is to be assigned to each code under subcategory O60.2. 7th character 0 is for single gestations and multiple gestations where the fetus is unspecified. 7th characters 1 through 9 are for cases of multiple gestations to identify the fetus for which the code applies. The appropriate code from category O30, Multiple gestation, must also be assigned when assigning a code from subcategory O60.2 that has a 7th character of 1 through 9.

0 - not applicable or unspecified

1 - fetus 1

2 - fetus 2

3 - fetus 3

4 - fetus 4

5 - fetus 5

9 - Other fetus

⊗⑦**O60.20**   **Term delivery with preterm labor, unspecified trimester**

⊗⑦**O60.22**   **Term delivery with preterm labor, second trimester**

⊗⑦**O60.23**   **Term delivery with preterm labor, third trimester**

O61   **Failed induction of labor**

O61.0   **Failed medical induction of labor**

Failed induction (of labor) by oxytocin

Failed induction (of labor) by prostaglandins

O61.1   **Failed instrumental induction of labor**

Failed mechanical induction (of labor)

Failed surgical induction (of labor)

O61.8   **Other failed induction of labor**

O61.9   **Failed induction of labor, unspecified**

O62   **Abnormalities of forces of labor**

O62.0   **Primary inadequate contractions**

Failure of cervical dilatation

Primary hypotonic uterine dysfunction

Uterine inertia during latent phase of labor

O62.1   **Secondary uterine inertia**

Arrested active phase of labor

Secondary hypotonic uterine dysfunction

O62.2   **Other uterine inertia**

Atony of uterus without hemorrhage

Atony of uterus NOS

Desultory labor

Hypotonic uterine dysfunction NOS

Irregular labor

Poor contractions

Slow slope active phase of labor

Uterine inertia NOS

Excludes1: atony of uterus with hemorrhage (postpartum) (O72.1)

postpartum atony of uterus without hemorrhage (O75.89)

O62.3   **Precipitate labor**

O62.4   **Hypertonic, incoordinate, and prolonged uterine contractions**

Cervical spasm

Contraction ring dystocia

Dyscoordinate labor hour-glass contraction of uterus

Hypertonic uterine dysfunction

Incoordinate uterine action

Tetanic contractions

Uterine dystocia NOS

Uterine spasm

Excludes1: dystocia (fetal) (maternal) NOS (O66.9)

O62.8   **Other abnormalities of forces of labor**

O62.9   **Abnormality of forces of labor, unspecified**

O63   **Long labor**

O63.0   **Prolonged first stage (of labor)**

O63.1   **Prolonged second stage (of labor)**

O63.2   **Delayed delivery of second twin, triplet, etc.**

O63.9   **Long labor, unspecified**

Prolonged labor NOS

O64   **Obstructed labor due to malposition and malpresentation of fetus**

Definition: Malposition and malpresentation of fetus refers to presentation of the fetal parts in inappropriate positions for the easiest passage through the cervix, e.g. Retention of the head, breech presentation.

One of the following 7th characters is to be assigned to each code under category O64. 7th character 0 is for single gestations and multiple gestations where the fetus is unspecified. 7th characters 1 through 9 are for cases of multiple gestations to identify the fetus for which the code applies. The appropriate code from category O30, Multiple gestation, must also be assigned when assigning a code from category O64 that has a 7th character of 1 through 9.

0 - not applicable or unspecified

1 - fetus 1

2 - fetus 2

3 - fetus 3

4 - fetus 4

5 - fetus 5

9 - Other fetus

⊗⑦**O64.0**   **Obstructed labor due to incomplete rotation of fetal head**

Deep transverse arrest

Obstructed labor due to persistent occipitoiliac (position)

Obstructed labor due to persistent occipitoposterior (position)

Obstructed labor due to persistent occipitosacral (position)

Obstructed labor due to persistent occipitotransverse (position)

⊗⑦**O64.1**   **Obstructed labor due to breech presentation**

Obstructed labor due to buttocks presentation

Obstructed labor due to complete breech presentation

Obstructed labor due to frank breech presentation

⊗⑦**O64.2**   **Obstructed labor due to face presentation**

Obstructed labor due to chin presentation

⊗⑦**O64.3**   **Obstructed labor due to brow presentation**

⊗⑦**O64.4**   **Obstructed labor due to shoulder presentation**

Prolapsed arm

Excludes1: impacted shoulders (O66.0)

shoulder dystocia (O66.0)

⊗⑦**O64.5**   **Obstructed labor due to compound presentation**

⊗⑦**O64.8**   **Obstructed labor due to other malposition and malpresentation**

Obstructed labor due to footling presentation

Obstructed labor due to incomplete breech presentation

⊗⑦**O64.9**   **Obstructed labor due to malposition and malpresentation, unspecified**

O65   **Obstructed labor due to maternal pelvic abnormality**

O65.0   **Obstructed labor due to deformed pelvis**

O65.1   **Obstructed labor due to generally contracted pelvis**

O65.2   **Obstructed labor due to pelvic inlet contraction**

O65.3   **Obstructed labor due to pelvic outlet and mid-cavity contraction**

● New code   ▲ Revised code   **Excludes1:** Not coded here   **Excludes2:** Not included here   ⊗ Placeholder required   ⑦ 7th digit required

O65.4 **Obstructed labor due to fetopelvic disproportion, unspecified**

> **Excludes1:** dystocia due to abnormality of fetus (O66.2-O66.3)

O65.5 **Obstructed labor due to abnormality of maternal pelvic organs**

> Obstructed labor due to conditions listed in O34.-
>
> **Use additional code** to identify abnormality of pelvic organs O34.-

O65.8 **Obstructed labor due to other maternal pelvic abnormalities**

O65.9 **Obstructed labor due to maternal pelvic abnormality, unspecified**

O66 **Other obstructed labor**

O66.0 **Obstructed labor due to shoulder dystocia**

> Impacted shoulders

O66.1 **Obstructed labor due to locked twins**

O66.2 **Obstructed labor due to unusually large fetus**

O66.3 **Obstructed labor due to other abnormalities of fetus**

> Dystocia due to fetal ascites
>
> Dystocia due to fetal hydrops
>
> Dystocia due to fetal meningomyelocele
>
> Dystocia due to fetal sacral teratoma
>
> Dystocia due to fetal tumor
>
> Dystocia due to hydrocephalic fetus
>
> **Use additional code** to identify cause of obstruction

O66.4 **Failed trial of labor O66.40 Failed trial of labor, unspecified**

> **O66.40** **Failed trial of labor, unspecified**
>
> **O66.41** **Failed attempted vaginal birth after previous cesarean delivery**
>
> > **Code first** rupture of uterus, if applicable (O71.0-O71.1)

O66.5 **Attempted application of vacuum extractor and forceps**

> Attempted application of vacuum or forceps, with subsequent delivery by forceps or cesarean delivery

O66.6 **Obstructed labor due to other multiple fetuses**

O66.8 **Other specified obstructed labor**

> **Use additional code** to identify cause of obstruction

O66.9 **Obstructed labor, unspecified**

> Dystocia NOS
>
> Fetal dystocia NOS
>
> Maternal dystocia NOS

O67 **Labor and delivery complicated by intrapartum hemorrhage, not elsewhere classified**

> **Excludes1:** antepartum hemorrhage NEC (O46.-)
>
> placenta previa (O44.-)
>
> premature separation of placenta [abruptio placentae] (O45.-)
>
> **Excludes2:** postpartum hemorrhage (O72.-)

O67.0 **Intrapartum hemorrhage with coagulation defect**

> Intrapartum hemorrhage (excessive) associated with afibrinogenemia
>
> Intrapartum hemorrhage (excessive) associated with disseminated intravascular coagulation
>
> Intrapartum hemorrhage (excessive) associated with hyperfibrinolysis

Intrapartum hemorrhage (excessive) associated with hypofibrinogenemia

O67.8 **Other intrapartum hemorrhage**

> Excessive intrapartum hemorrhage

O67.9 **Intrapartum hemorrhage, unspecified**

O68 **Labor and delivery complicated by abnormality of fetal acid-base balance**

> Fetal acidemia complicating labor and delivery
>
> Fetal acidosis complicating labor and delivery
>
> Fetal alkalosis complicating labor and delivery
>
> Fetal metabolic acidemia complicating labor and delivery
>
> **Excludes1:** fetal stress NOS (O77.9)
>
> labor and delivery complicated by electrocardiographic evidence of fetal stress (O77.8)
>
> labor and delivery complicated by ultrasonic evidence of fetal stress (O77.8)
>
> **Excludes2:** abnormality in fetal heart rate or rhythm (O76)
>
> labor and delivery complicated by meconium in amniotic fluid (O77.0)

O69 **Labor and delivery complicated by umbilical cord complications**

> One of the following 7th characters is to be assigned to each code under category O69. 7th character 0 is for single gestations and multiple gestations where the fetus is unspecified. 7th characters 1 through 9 are for cases of multiple gestations to identify the fetus for which the code applies. The appropriate code from category O30, Multiple gestation, must also be assigned when assigning a code from category O69 that has a 7th character of 1 through 9.
>
> 0 - not applicable or unspecified
>
> 1 - fetus 1
>
> 2 - fetus 2
>
> 3 - fetus 3
>
> 4 - fetus 4
>
> 5 - fetus 5
>
> 9 - Other fetus

⊗⑦O69.0 **Labor and delivery complicated by prolapse of cord**

⊗⑦O69.1 **Labor and delivery complicated by cord around neck, with compression**

> **Excludes1:** labor and delivery complicated by cord around neck, without compression (O69.81)

⊗⑦O69.2 **Labor and delivery complicated by other cord entanglement, with compression**

> Labor and delivery complicated by compression of cord NOS
>
> Labor and delivery complicated by entanglement of cords of twins in monoamniotic sac
>
> Labor and delivery complicated by knot in cord
>
> **Excludes1:** labor and delivery complicated by other cord entanglement, without compression (O69.82)

⊗⑦O69.3 **Labor and delivery complicated by short cord**

⊗⑦O69.4 **Labor and delivery complicated by vasa previa**

> Labor and delivery complicated by hemorrhage from vasa previa

⊗⑦O69.5 **Labor and delivery complicated by vascular lesion of cord**

> Labor and delivery complicated by cord bruising
>
> Labor and delivery complicated by cord hematoma
>
> Labor and delivery complicated by thrombosis of umbilical vessels

O69.8 **Labor and delivery complicated by other cord complications**

⊗⑦**O69.81** **Labor and delivery complicated by cord around neck, without compression**

⊗⑦**O69.82** **Labor and delivery complicated by other cord entanglement, without compression**

⊗⑦**O69.89** **Labor and delivery complicated by other cord complications**

⊗⑦**O69.9** **Labor and delivery complicated by cord complication, unspecified**

O70 **Perineal laceration during delivery**

Includes: episiotomy extended by laceration

Excludes1: obstetric high vaginal laceration alone (O71.4)

O70.0 **First degree perineal laceration during delivery**

Perineal laceration, rupture or tear involving fourchette during delivery

Perineal laceration, rupture or tear involving labia during delivery

Perineal laceration, rupture or tear involving skin during delivery

Perineal laceration, rupture or tear involving vagina during delivery

Perineal laceration, rupture or tear involving vulva during delivery

Slight perineal laceration, rupture or tear during delivery

O70.1 **Second degree perineal laceration during delivery**

Perineal laceration, rupture or tear during delivery as in O70.0, also involving pelvic floor

Perineal laceration, rupture or tear during delivery as in O70.0, also involving perineal muscles

Perineal laceration, rupture or tear during delivery as in O70.0, also involving vaginal muscles

Excludes1: perineal laceration involving anal sphincter (O70.2)

O70.2 **Third degree perineal laceration during delivery**

Perineal laceration, rupture or tear during delivery as in O70.1, also involving anal sphincter

Perineal laceration, rupture or tear during delivery as in O70.1, also involving rectovaginal septum

Perineal laceration, rupture or tear during delivery as in O70.1, also involving sphincter NOS

Excludes1: anal sphincter tear during delivery without third degree perineal laceration (O70.4)

perineal laceration involving anal or rectal mucosa (O70.3)

●**O70.20** **Third degree perineal laceration during delivery, unspecified**

●**O70.21** **Third degree perineal laceration during delivery, IIIa**

Third degree perineal laceration during delivery with less than 50% of external anal sphincter (EAS) thickness torn

●**O70.22** **Third degree perineal laceration during delivery, IIIb**

Third degree perineal laceration during delivery with more than 50% external anal sphincter (EAS) thickness torn

●**O70.23** **Third degree perineal laceration during delivery, IIIc**

Third degree perineal laceration during delivery with both external anal sphincter (EAS) and internal anal sphincter (IAS) torn

O70.3 **Fourth degree perineal laceration during delivery**

Perineal laceration, rupture or tear during delivery as in O70.2, also involving anal mucosa

Perineal laceration, rupture or tear during delivery as in O70.2, also involving rectal mucosa

O70.4 **Anal sphincter tear complicating delivery, not associated with third degree laceration**

Excludes1: anal sphincter tear with third degree perineal laceration (O70.2)

O70.9 **Perineal laceration during delivery, unspecified**

O71 **Other obstetric trauma**

Includes: obstetric damage from instruments

O71.0 **Rupture of uterus (spontaneous) before onset of labor**

Excludes1: disruption of (current) cesarean delivery wound (O90.0)

laceration of uterus, NEC (O71.81)

O71.00 **Rupture of uterus before onset of labor, unspecified trimester**

O71.02 **Rupture of uterus before onset of labor, second trimester**

O71.03 **Rupture of uterus before onset of labor, third trimester**

O71.1 **Rupture of uterus during labor**

Rupture of uterus not stated as occurring before onset of labor

Excludes1: disruption of cesarean delivery wound (O90.0)

laceration of uterus, NEC (O71.81)

O71.2 **Postpartum inversion of uterus**

O71.3 **Obstetric laceration of cervix**

Annular detachment of cervix

O71.4 **Obstetric high vaginal laceration alone**

Laceration of vaginal wall without perineal laceration

Excludes1: obstetric high vaginal laceration with perineal laceration (O70.-)

O71.5 **Other obstetric injury to pelvic organs**

Obstetric injury to bladder

Obstetric injury to urethra

Excludes2: obstetric periurethral trauma (O71.82)

O71.6 **Obstetric damage to pelvic joints and ligaments**

Obstetric avulsion of inner symphyseal cartilage

Obstetric damage to coccyx

Obstetric traumatic separation of symphysis (pubis)

O71.7 **Obstetric hematoma of pelvis**

Obstetric hematoma of perineum

Obstetric hematoma of vagina

Obstetric hematoma of vulva

O71.8 **Other specified obstetric trauma**

O71.81 **Laceration of uterus, not elsewhere classified**

O71.82 **Other specified trauma to perineum and vulva**

Obstetric periurethral trauma

O71.89 **Other specified obstetric trauma**

O71.9 **Obstetric trauma, unspecified**

O72 **Postpartum hemorrhage**

Includes: hemorrhage after delivery of fetus or infant

● New code   ▲ Revised code   **Excludes1:** Not coded here   **Excludes2:** Not included here   ⊗ Placeholder required   ⑦ 7th digit required

O72.0 **Third-stage hemorrhage**

Hemorrhage associated with retained, trapped or adherent placenta

Retained placenta NOS

<u>Code also</u> type of adherent placenta (O43.2-)

O72.1 **Other immediate postpartum hemorrhage**

Hemorrhage following delivery of placenta

Postpartum hemorrhage (atonic) NOS

Uterine atony with hemorrhage

Excludes1: uterine atony NOS (O62.2)

uterine atony without hemorrhage (O62.2)

postpartum atony of uterus without hemorrhage (O75.89)

O72.2 **Delayed and secondary postpartum hemorrhage**

Hemorrhage associated with retained portions of placenta or membranes after the first 24 hours following delivery of placenta

Retained products of conception NOS, following delivery

O72.3 **Postpartum coagulation defects**

Postpartum afibrinogenemia

Postpartum fibrinolysis

O73 **Retained placenta and membranes, without hemorrhage**

Excludes1: placenta accreta (O43.21-)

placenta increta (O43.22-)

placenta percreta (O43.23-)

O73.0 **Retained placenta without hemorrhage**

Adherent placenta, without hemorrhage

Trapped placenta without hemorrhage

O73.1 **Retained portions of placenta and membranes, without hemorrhage**

Retained products of conception following delivery, without hemorrhage

O74 **Complications of anesthesia during labor and delivery**

Includes: maternal complications arising from the administration of a general, regional or local anesthetic, analgesic **or other** sedation during labor and delivery

<u>Use additional code</u>, if applicable, to identify specific complication

O74.0 **Aspiration pneumonitis due to anesthesia during labor and delivery**

Inhalation of stomach contents or secretions NOS due to anesthesia during labor and delivery

Mendelson's syndrome due to anesthesia during labor and delivery

O74.1 **Other pulmonary complications of anesthesia during labor and delivery**

O74.2 **Cardiac complications of anesthesia during labor and delivery**

O74.3 **Central nervous system complications of anesthesia during labor and delivery**

O74.4 **Toxic reaction to local anesthesia during labor and delivery**

O74.5 **Spinal and epidural anesthesia-induced headache during labor and delivery**

O74.6 **Other complications of spinal and epidural anesthesia during labor and delivery**

O74.7 **Failed or difficult intubation for anesthesia during labor and delivery**

O74.8 **Other complications of anesthesia during labor and delivery**

O74.9 **Complication of anesthesia during labor and delivery, unspecified**

O75 **Other complications of labor and delivery, not elsewhere classified**

Excludes2: puerperal (postpartum) infection (O86.-)

puerperal (postpartum) sepsis (O85)

O75.0 **Maternal distress during labor and delivery**

O75.1 **Shock during or following labor and delivery**

Obstetric shock following labor and delivery

O75.2 **Pyrexia during labor, not elsewhere classified**

O75.3 **Other infection during labor** Sepsis during labor <u>Use additional code</u> (B95-B97), to identify infectious agent

O75.4 **Other complications of obstetric surgery and procedures**

Cardiac arrest following obstetric surgery or procedures

Cardiac failure following obstetric surgery or procedures

Cerebral anoxia following obstetric surgery or procedures

Pulmonary edema following obstetric surgery or procedures

<u>Use additional code</u> to identify specific complication

Excludes2: complications of anesthesia during labor and delivery (O74.-)

disruption of obstetrical (surgical) wound (O90.0-O90.1)

hematoma of obstetrical (surgical) wound (O90.2)

infection of obstetrical (surgical) wound (O86.0)

O75.5 **Delayed delivery after artificial rupture of membranes**

O75.8 **Other specified complications of labor and delivery**

O75.81 **Maternal exhaustion complicating labor and delivery**

O75.82 **Onset (spontaneous) of labor after 37 completed weeks of gestation but before 39 completed weeks gestation, with delivery by (planned) cesarean section**

Delivery by (planned) cesarean section occurring after 37 completed weeks of gestation but before 39 completed weeks gestation due to (spontaneous) onset of labor

<u>Code first</u> to specify reason for planned cesarean section such as:

cephalopelvic disproportion (normally formed fetus) (O33.9)

previous cesarean delivery (O34.21)

O75.89 **Other specified complications of labor and delivery**

O75.9 **Complication of labor and delivery, unspecified**

O76 **Abnormality in fetal heart rate and rhythm complicating labor and delivery**

Depressed fetal heart rate tones complicating labor and delivery

Fetal bradycardia complicating labor and delivery

Fetal heart rate decelerations complicating labor and delivery

Fetal heart rate irregularity complicating labor and delivery

Fetal heart rate abnormal variability complicating labor and delivery

Fetal tachycardia complicating labor and delivery

Non-reassuring fetal heart rate or rhythm complicating labor and delivery

Excludes1: fetal stress NOS (O77.9)

labor and delivery complicated by electrocardiographic evidence of fetal stress (O77.8)

labor and delivery complicated by ultrasonic evidence of fetal stress (O77.8)

Excludes2: fetal metabolic acidemia (O68)

Other fetal stress (O77.0-O77.1)

O77   Other fetal stress complicating labor and delivery

O77.0   Labor and delivery complicated by meconium in amniotic fluid

O77.1   Fetal stress in labor or delivery due to drug administration

O77.8   Labor and delivery complicated by other evidence of fetal stress

Labor and delivery complicated by electrocardiographic evidence of fetal stress

Labor and delivery complicated by ultrasonic evidence of fetal stress

Excludes1: abnormality of fetal acid-base balance (O68)

abnormality in fetal heart rate or rhythm (O76)

fetal metabolic acidemia (O68)

O77.9   Labor and delivery complicated by fetal stress, unspecified

Excludes1: abnormality of fetal acid-base balance (O68)

abnormality in fetal heart rate or rhythm (O76)

fetal metabolic acidemia (O68)

ENCOUNTER FOR DELIVERY (O80-O82)

O80   Encounter for full-term uncomplicated delivery

Delivery requiring minimal or no assistance, with or without episiotomy, without fetal manipulation [e.g., rotation version] or instrumentation [forceps] of a spontaneous, cephalic, vaginal, full-term, single, live-born infant. This code is for use as a single diagnosis code and is not to be used with any other code from chapter 15.

Use additional code to indicate outcome of delivery (Z37.0)

O82   Encounter for cesarean delivery without indication

Use additional code to indicate outcome of delivery (Z37.0)

COMPLICATIONS PREDOMINANTLY RELATED TO THE PUERPERIUM (O85-O92)

Excludes2: mental and behavioral disorders associated with the puerperium (F53)

obstetrical tetanus (A34)

puerperal osteomalacia (M83.0)

O85   Puerperal sepsis

Postpartum sepsis

Puerperal peritonitis

Puerperal pyemia

Use additional code (B95-B97), to identify infectious agent

Use additional code (R65.2-) to identify severe sepsis, if applicable

Excludes1: fever of unknown origin following delivery (O86.4)

genital tract infection following delivery (O86.1-)

obstetric pyemic and septic embolism (O88.3-)

puerperal septic thrombophlebitis (O86.81)

urinary tract infection following delivery (O86.2-)

Excludes2: sepsis during labor (O75.3)

O86   Other puerperal infections

Use additional code (B95-B97), to identify infectious agent

Excludes2: infection during labor (O75.3)

obstetrical tetanus (A34)

O86.0   Infection of obstetric surgical wound

Infected cesarean delivery wound following delivery

Infected perineal repair following delivery

O86.1   Other infection of genital tract following delivery

O86.11   Cervicitis following delivery

O86.12   Endometritis following delivery

O86.13   Vaginitis following delivery

O86.19   Other infection of genital tract following delivery

O86.2   Urinary tract infection following delivery

O86.20   Urinary tract infection following delivery, unspecified

Puerperal urinary tract infection NOS

O86.21   Infection of kidney following delivery

O86.22   Infection of bladder following delivery

Infection of urethra following delivery

O86.29   Other urinary tract infection following delivery

O86.4   Pyrexia of unknown origin following delivery

Puerperal infection NOS following delivery

Puerperal pyrexia NOS following delivery

Excludes2: pyrexia during labor (O75.2)

O86.8   Other specified puerperal infections

O86.81   Puerperal septic thrombophlebitis

O86.89   Other specified puerperal infections

O87   Venous complications and hemorrhoids in the puerperium

Includes: venous complications in labor, delivery and the puerperium

Excludes2: obstetric embolism (O88.-)

puerperal septic thrombophlebitis (O86.81)

venous complications in pregnancy (O22.-)

O87.0   Superficial thrombophlebitis in the puerperium

Puerperal phlebitis NOS

Puerperal thrombosis NOS

O87.1   Deep phlebothrombosis in the puerperium

Deep vein thrombosis, postpartum

Pelvic thrombophlebitis, postpartum

Use additional code to identify the deep vein thrombosis (I82.4-, I82.5-, I82.62-. I82.72-)

Use additional code, if applicable, for associated long-term (current) use of anticoagulants (Z79.01)

O87.2   Hemorrhoids in the puerperium

O87.3   Cerebral venous thrombosis in the puerperium

Cerebrovenous sinus thrombosis in the puerperium

O87.4   Varicose veins of lower extremity in the puerperium

O87.8   Other venous complications in the puerperium

Genital varices in the puerperium

O87.9   Venous complication in the puerperium, unspecified

Puerperal phlebopathy NOS

O88   Obstetric embolism

● New code   ▲ Revised code   **Excludes1:** Not coded here   **Excludes2:** Not included here   ⊗ Placeholder required   ⑦ 7th digit required

Excludes1: embolism complicating abortion NOS (O03.2)

embolism complicating ectopic or molar pregnancy (O08.2)

embolism complicating failed attempted abortion (O07.2)

embolism complicating induced abortion (O04.7)

embolism complicating spontaneous abortion (O03.2, O03.7)

O88.0   Obstetric air embolism

    O88.01   Obstetric air embolism in pregnancy

        O88.011   Air embolism in pregnancy, first trimester

        O88.012   Air embolism in pregnancy, second trimester

        O88.013   Air embolism in pregnancy, third trimester

        O88.019   Air embolism in pregnancy, unspecified trimester

    O88.02   Air embolism in childbirth

    O88.03   Air embolism in the puerperium

O88.1   Amniotic fluid embolism

Anaphylactoid syndrome in pregnancy

    O88.11   Amniotic fluid embolism in pregnancy

        O88.111   Amniotic fluid embolism in pregnancy, first trimester

        O88.112   Amniotic fluid embolism in pregnancy, second trimester

        O88.113   Amniotic fluid embolism in pregnancy, third trimester

        O88.119   Amniotic fluid embolism in pregnancy, unspecified trimester

    O88.12   Amniotic fluid embolism in childbirth

    O88.13   Amniotic fluid embolism in the puerperium

O88.2   Obstetric thromboembolism

    O88.21   Thromboembolism in pregnancy

Obstetric (pulmonary) embolism NOS

        O88.211   Thromboembolism in pregnancy, first trimester

        O88.212   Thromboembolism in pregnancy, second trimester

        O88.213   Thromboembolism in pregnancy, third trimester

        O88.219   Thromboembolism in pregnancy, unspecified trimester

    O88.22   Thromboembolism in childbirth

    O88.23   Thromboembolism in the puerperium

Puerperal (pulmonary) embolism NOS

O88.3   Obstetric pyemic and septic embolism

    O88.31   Pyemic and septic embolism in pregnancy

        O88.311   Pyemic and septic embolism in pregnancy, first trimester

        O88.312   Pyemic and septic embolism in pregnancy, second trimester

        O88.313   Pyemic and septic embolism in pregnancy, third trimester

        O88.319   Pyemic and septic embolism in pregnancy, unspecified trimester

    O88.32   Pyemic and septic embolism in childbirth

    O88.33   Pyemic and septic embolism in the puerperium

O88.8   Other obstetric embolism

Obstetric fat embolism

    O88.81   Other embolism in pregnancy

        O88.811   Other embolism in pregnancy, first trimester

        O88.812   Other embolism in pregnancy, second trimester

        O88.813   Other embolism in pregnancy, third trimester

        O88.819   Other embolism in pregnancy, unspecified trimester

    O88.82   Other embolism in childbirth

    O88.83   Other embolism in the puerperium

O89   Complications of anesthesia during the puerperium

Includes: maternal complications arising from the administration of a general, regional or local anesthetic, analgesic **or other** sedation during the puerperium

Use additional code, if applicable, to identify specific complication

O89.0   Pulmonary complications of anesthesia during the puerperium

    O89.01   Aspiration pneumonitis due to anesthesia during the puerperium

Inhalation of stomach contents or secretions NOS due to anesthesia during the puerperium

Mendelson's syndrome due to anesthesia during the puerperium

    O89.09   Other pulmonary complications of anesthesia during the puerperium

O89.1   Cardiac complications of anesthesia during the puerperium

O89.2   Central nervous system complications of anesthesia during the puerperium

O89.3   Toxic reaction to local anesthesia during the puerperium

O89.4   Spinal and epidural anesthesia-induced headache during the puerperium

O89.5   Other complications of spinal and epidural anesthesia during the puerperium

O89.6   Failed or difficult intubation for anesthesia during the puerperium

O89.8   Other complications of anesthesia during the puerperium

O89.9   Complication of anesthesia during the puerperium, unspecified

O90   Complications of the puerperium, not elsewhere classified

O90.0   Disruption of cesarean delivery wound

Dehiscence of cesarean delivery wound

Excludes1: rupture of uterus (spontaneous) before onset of labor (O71.0-)

rupture of uterus during labor (O71.1)

O90.1   Disruption of perineal obstetric wound

Disruption of wound of episiotomy

Disruption of wound of perineal laceration

Secondary perineal tear

O90.2   Hematoma of obstetric wound

O90.3   Peripartum cardiomyopathy

Conditions in I42.- arising during pregnancy and the puerperium

Excludes1: pre-existing heart disease complicating pregnancy and the puerperium (O99.4-)

O90.4 **Postpartum acute kidney failure**

Hepatorenal syndrome following labor and delivery

O90.5 **Postpartum thyroiditis**

O90.6 **Postpartum mood disturbance**

Postpartum blues

Postpartum dysphoria

Postpartum sadness

Excludes1: postpartum depression (F53)

puerperal psychosis (F53)

O90.8 **Other complications of the puerperium, not elsewhere classified**

O90.81 **Anemia of the puerperium**

Postpartum anemia NOS

Excludes1: pre-existing anemia complicating the puerperium (O99.03)

O90.89 **Other complications of the puerperium, not elsewhere classified**

Placental polyp

O90.9 **Complication of the puerperium, unspecified**

O91 **Infections of breast associated with pregnancy, the puerperium and lactation**

Use additional code to identify infection

O91.0 **Infection of nipple associated with pregnancy, the puerperium and lactation**

O91.01 **Infection of nipple associated with pregnancy**

Gestational abscess of nipple

O91.011 **Infection of nipple associated with pregnancy, first trimester**

O91.012 **Infection of nipple associated with pregnancy, second trimester**

O91.013 **Infection of nipple associated with pregnancy, third trimester**

O91.019 **Infection of nipple associated with pregnancy, unspecified trimester**

O91.02 **Infection of nipple associated with the puerperium**

Puerperal abscess of nipple

O91.03 **Infection of nipple associated with lactation**

Abscess of nipple associated with lactation

O91.1 **Abscess of breast associated with pregnancy, the puerperium and lactation**

O91.11 **Abscess of breast associated with pregnancy**

Gestational mammary abscess

Gestational purulent mastitis

Gestational subareolar abscess

O91.111 **Abscess of breast associated with pregnancy, first trimester**

O91.112 **Abscess of breast associated with pregnancy, second trimester**

O91.113 **Abscess of breast associated with pregnancy, third trimester**

O91.119 **Abscess of breast associated with pregnancy, unspecified trimester**

O91.12 **Abscess of breast associated with the puerperium**

Puerperal mammary abscess

Puerperal purulent mastitis

Puerperal subareolar abscess

O91.13 **Abscess of breast associated with lactation**

Mammary abscess associated with lactation

Purulent mastitis associated with lactation

Subareolar abscess associated with lactation

O91.2 **Nonpurulent mastitis associated with pregnancy, the puerperium and lactation**

O91.21 **Nonpurulent mastitis associated with pregnancy**

Gestational interstitial mastitis

Gestational lymphangitis of breast

Gestational mastitis NOS

Gestational parenchymatous mastitis

O91.211 **Nonpurulent mastitis associated with pregnancy, first trimester**

O91.212 **Nonpurulent mastitis associated with pregnancy, second trimester**

O91.213 **Nonpurulent mastitis associated with pregnancy, third trimester**

O91.219 **Nonpurulent mastitis associated with pregnancy, unspecified trimester**

O91.22 **Nonpurulent mastitis associated with the puerperium**

Puerperal interstitial mastitis

Puerperal lymphangitis of breast

Puerperal mastitis NOS

Puerperal parenchymatous mastitis

O91.23 **Nonpurulent mastitis associated with lactation**

Interstitial mastitis associated with lactation

Lymphangitis of breast associated with lactation

Mastitis NOS associated with lactation

Parenchymatous mastitis associated with lactation

O92 **Other disorders of breast and disorders of lactation associated with pregnancy and the puerperium**

O92.0 **Retracted nipple associated with pregnancy, the puerperium, and lactation**

O92.01 **Retracted nipple associated with pregnancy**

O92.011 **Retracted nipple associated with pregnancy, first trimester**

O92.012 **Retracted nipple associated with pregnancy, second trimester**

O92.013 **Retracted nipple associated with pregnancy, third trimester**

O92.019 **Retracted nipple associated with pregnancy, unspecified trimester**

O92.02 **Retracted nipple associated with the puerperium**

O92.03 **Retracted nipple associated with lactation**

O92.1 **Cracked nipple associated with pregnancy, the puerperium, and lactation**

Fissure of nipple, gestational or puerperal

O92.11 **Cracked nipple associated with pregnancy**

O92.111 **Cracked nipple associated with pregnancy, first trimester**

● New code   ▲ Revised code   Excludes1: Not coded here   Excludes2: Not included here   ⊗ Placeholder required   ⑦7th digit required

O92.112 **Cracked nipple associated with pregnancy, second trimester**

O92.113 **Cracked nipple associated with pregnancy, third trimester**

O92.119 **Cracked nipple associated with pregnancy, unspecified trimester**

O92.12 **Cracked nipple associated with the puerperium**

O92.13 **Cracked nipple associated with lactation**

O92.2 **Other and unspecified disorders of breast associated with pregnancy and the puerperium**

O92.20 **Unspecified disorder of breast associated with pregnancy and the puerperium**

O92.29 **Other disorders of breast associated with pregnancy and the puerperium**

O92.3 **Agalactia**

Primary agalactia

Excludes1: Elective agalactia (O92.5)

Secondary agalactia (O92.5)

Therapeutic agalactia (O92.5)

O92.4 **Hypogalactia**

O92.5 **Suppressed lactation**

Elective agalactia

Secondary agalactia

Therapeutic agalactia

Excludes1: primary agalactia (O92.3)

O92.6 **Galactorrhea**

O92.7 **Other and unspecified disorders of lactation**

O92.70 **Unspecified disorders of lactation**

O92.79 **Other disorders of lactation**

Puerperal galactocele

OTHER OBSTETRIC CONDITIONS, NOT ELSEWHERE CLASSIFIED (O94-O9A)

O94 **Sequelae of complication of pregnancy, childbirth, and the puerperium**

Note: This category is to be used to indicate conditions in O00-O77.-, O85-O94 and O98-O9A.- as the cause of late effects. The sequelae include conditions specified as such, or as late effects, which may occur at any time after the puerperium

Code first condition resulting from (sequela) of complication of pregnancy, childbirth, and the puerperium

O98 **Maternal infectious and parasitic diseases classifiable elsewhere but complicating pregnancy, childbirth and the puerperium**

Includes: the listed conditions when complicating the pregnant state, when aggravated by the pregnancy, or as a reason for obstetric care

Use additional code (Chapter 1), to identify specific infectious or parasitic disease

Excludes2: herpes gestationis (O26.4-)

infectious carrier state (O99.82-, O99.83-)

obstetrical tetanus (A34)

puerperal infection (O86.-)

puerperal sepsis (O85)

when the reason for maternal care is that the disease is known or suspected to have affected the fetus (O35-O36)

O98.0 **Tuberculosis complicating pregnancy, childbirth and the puerperium**

Conditions in A15-A19

O98.01 **Tuberculosis complicating pregnancy**

O98.011 **Tuberculosis complicating pregnancy, first trimester**

O98.012 **Tuberculosis complicating pregnancy, second trimester**

O98.013 **Tuberculosis complicating pregnancy, third trimester**

O98.019 **Tuberculosis complicating pregnancy, unspecified trimester**

O98.02 **Tuberculosis complicating childbirth**

O98.03 **Tuberculosis complicating the puerperium**

O98.1 **Syphilis complicating pregnancy, childbirth and the puerperium**

Conditions in A50-A53

O98.11 **Syphilis complicating pregnancy**

O98.111 **Syphilis complicating pregnancy, first trimester**

O98.112 **Syphilis complicating pregnancy, second trimester**

O98.113 **Syphilis complicating pregnancy, third trimester**

O98.119 **Syphilis complicating pregnancy, unspecified trimester**

O98.12 **Syphilis complicating childbirth**

O98.13 **Syphilis complicating the puerperium**

O98.2 **Gonorrhea complicating pregnancy, childbirth and the puerperium**

Conditions in A54.-

O98.21 **Gonorrhea complicating pregnancy**

O98.211 **Gonorrhea complicating pregnancy, first trimester**

O98.212 **Gonorrhea complicating pregnancy, second trimester**

O98.213 **Gonorrhea complicating pregnancy, third trimester**

O98.219 **Gonorrhea complicating pregnancy, unspecified trimester**

O98.22 **Gonorrhea complicating childbirth**

O98.23 **Gonorrhea complicating the puerperium**

O98.3 **Other infections with a predominantly sexual mode of transmission complicating pregnancy, childbirth and the puerperium** Conditions in A55-A64

O98.31 **Other infections with a predominantly sexual mode of transmission complicating pregnancy**

O98.311 **Other infections with a predominantly sexual mode of transmission complicating pregnancy, first trimester**

O98.312 **Other infections with a predominantly sexual mode of transmission complicating pregnancy, second trimester**

O98.313 **Other infections with a predominantly sexual mode of transmission complicating pregnancy, third trimester**

O98.319 **Other infections with a predominantly sexual mode of transmission complicating pregnancy, unspecified trimester**

O98.32   Other infections with a predominantly sexual mode of transmission complicating childbirth

O98.33   Other infections with a predominantly sexual mode of transmission complicating the puerperium

O98.4   **Viral hepatitis complicating pregnancy, childbirth and the puerperium**

Conditions in B15-B19

O98.41   Viral hepatitis complicating pregnancy

    O98.411   Viral hepatitis complicating pregnancy, first trimester

    O98.412   Viral hepatitis complicating pregnancy, second trimester

    O98.413   Viral hepatitis complicating pregnancy, third trimester

    O98.419   Viral hepatitis complicating pregnancy, unspecified trimester

O98.42   Viral hepatitis complicating childbirth

O98.43   Viral hepatitis complicating the puerperium

O98.5   **Other viral diseases complicating pregnancy, childbirth and the puerperium**

Conditions in A80-B09, B25-B34, R87.81-, R87.82-

Excludes1: human immunodeficiency virus [HIV] disease complicating pregnancy, childbirth and the puerperium (O98.7-)

O98.51   Other viral diseases complicating pregnancy

    O98.511   Other viral diseases complicating pregnancy, first trimester

    O98.512   Other viral diseases complicating pregnancy, second trimester

    O98.513   Other viral diseases complicating pregnancy, third trimester

    O98.519   Other viral diseases complicating pregnancy, unspecified trimester

O98.52   Other viral diseases complicating childbirth

O98.53   Other viral diseases complicating the puerperium

O98.6   **Protozoal diseases complicating pregnancy, childbirth and the puerperium**

Conditions in B50-B64

O98.61   Protozoal diseases complicating pregnancy

    O98.611   Protozoal diseases complicating pregnancy, first trimester

    O98.612   Protozoal diseases complicating pregnancy, second trimester

    O98.613   Protozoal diseases complicating pregnancy, third trimester

    O98.619   Protozoal diseases complicating pregnancy, unspecified trimester

O98.62   Protozoal diseases complicating childbirth

O98.63   Protozoal diseases complicating the puerperium

O98.7   **Human immunodeficiency virus [HIV] disease complicating pregnancy, childbirth and the puerperium**

Use additional code to identify the type of HIV disease:

Acquired immune deficiency syndrome (AIDS) (B20)

Asymptomatic HIV status (Z21)

HIV positive NOS (Z21)

Symptomatic HIV disease (B20)

O98.71   Human immunodeficiency virus [HIV] disease complicating pregnancy

    O98.711   Human immunodeficiency virus [HIV] disease complicating pregnancy, first trimester

    O98.712   Human immunodeficiency virus [HIV] disease complicating pregnancy, second trimester

    O98.713   Human immunodeficiency virus [HIV] disease complicating pregnancy, third trimester

    O98.719   Human immunodeficiency virus [HIV] disease complicating pregnancy, unspecified trimester

O98.72   Human immunodeficiency virus [HIV] disease complicating childbirth

O98.73   Human immunodeficiency virus [HIV] disease complicating the puerperium

O98.8   **Other maternal infectious and parasitic diseases complicating pregnancy, childbirth and the puerperium**

O98.81   Other maternal infectious and parasitic diseases complicating pregnancy

    O98.811   Other maternal infectious and parasitic diseases complicating pregnancy, first trimester

    O98.812   Other maternal infectious and parasitic diseases complicating pregnancy, second trimester

    O98.813   Other maternal infectious and parasitic diseases complicating pregnancy, third trimester

    O98.819   Other maternal infectious and parasitic diseases complicating pregnancy, unspecified trimester

O98.82   Other maternal infectious and parasitic diseases complicating childbirth

O98.83   Other maternal infectious and parasitic diseases complicating the puerperium

O98.9   **Unspecified maternal infectious and parasitic disease complicating pregnancy, childbirth and the puerperium**

O98.91   Unspecified maternal infectious and parasitic disease complicating pregnancy

    O98.911   Unspecified maternal infectious and parasitic disease complicating pregnancy, first trimester

    O98.912   Unspecified maternal infectious and parasitic disease complicating pregnancy, second trimester

    O98.913   Unspecified maternal infectious and parasitic disease complicating pregnancy, third trimester

    O98.919   Unspecified maternal infectious and parasitic disease complicating pregnancy, unspecified trimester

O98.92   Unspecified maternal infectious and parasitic disease complicating childbirth

O98.93   Unspecified maternal infectious and parasitic disease complicating the puerperium

O99   **Other maternal diseases classifiable elsewhere but complicating pregnancy, childbirth and the puerperium**

Includes: conditions which complicate the pregnant state, are aggravated by the pregnancy or are a main reason for obstetric care

Use additional code to identify specific condition

  ● New code   ▲ Revised code   **Excludes1:** Not coded here   **Excludes2:** Not included here   ⊗ Placeholder required   ⑦ 7th digit required

Excludes2: when the reason for maternal care is that the condition is known or suspected to have affected the fetus (O35-O36)

O99.0 **Anemia complicating pregnancy, childbirth and the puerperium**

Conditions in D50-D64

Excludes1: anemia arising in the puerperium (O90.81)

postpartum anemia NOS (O90.81)

O99.01 **Anemia complicating pregnancy**

O99.011 **Anemia complicating pregnancy, first trimester**

O99.012 **Anemia complicating pregnancy, second trimester**

O99.013 **Anemia complicating pregnancy, third trimester**

O99.019 **Anemia complicating pregnancy, unspecified trimester**

O99.02 **Anemia complicating childbirth**

O99.03 **Anemia complicating the puerperium**

Excludes1: postpartum anemia not pre-existing prior to delivery (O90.81)

O99.1 **Other diseases of the blood and blood-forming organs and certain disorders involving the immune mechanism complicating pregnancy, childbirth and the puerperium**

Conditions in D65-D89

Excludes2: hemorrhage with coagulation defects (O45.-, O46.0-, O67.0, O72.3)

O99.11 **Other diseases of the blood and blood-forming organs and certain disorders involving the immune mechanism complicating pregnancy**

O99.111 **Other diseases of the blood and blood-forming organs and certain disorders involving the immune mechanism complicating pregnancy, first trimester**

O99.112 **Other diseases of the blood and blood-forming organs and certain disorders involving the immune mechanism complicating pregnancy, second trimester**

O99.113 **Other diseases of the blood and blood-forming organs and certain disorders involving the immune mechanism complicating pregnancy, third trimester**

O99.119 **Other diseases of the blood and blood-forming organs and certain disorders involving the immune mechanism complicating pregnancy, unspecified trimester**

O99.12 **Other diseases of the blood and blood-forming organs and certain disorders involving the immune mechanism complicating childbirth**

O99.13 **Other diseases of the blood and blood-forming organs and certain disorders involving the immune mechanism complicating the puerperium**

O99.2 **Endocrine, nutritional and metabolic diseases complicating pregnancy, childbirth and the puerperium**

Conditions in E00-E88

Excludes2: diabetes mellitus (O24.-)

malnutrition (O25.-)

postpartum thyroiditis (O90.5)

O99.21 **Obesity complicating pregnancy, childbirth, and the puerperium**

Use additional code to identify the type of obesity (E66.-)

O99.210 **Obesity complicating pregnancy, unspecified trimester**

O99.211 **Obesity complicating pregnancy, first trimester**

O99.212 **Obesity complicating pregnancy, second trimester**

O99.213 **Obesity complicating pregnancy, third trimester**

O99.214 **Obesity complicating childbirth**

O99.215 **Obesity complicating the puerperium**

O99.28 **Other endocrine, nutritional and metabolic diseases complicating pregnancy, childbirth and the puerperium**

O99.280 **Endocrine, nutritional and metabolic diseases complicating pregnancy, unspecified trimester**

O99.281 **Endocrine, nutritional and metabolic diseases complicating pregnancy, first trimester**

O99.282 **Endocrine, nutritional and metabolic diseases complicating pregnancy, second trimester**

O99.283 **Endocrine, nutritional and metabolic diseases complicating pregnancy, third trimester**

O99.284 **Endocrine, nutritional and metabolic diseases complicating childbirth**

O99.285 **Endocrine, nutritional and metabolic diseases complicating the puerperium**

O99.3 **Mental disorders and diseases of the nervous system complicating pregnancy, childbirth and the puerperium**

O99.31 **Alcohol use complicating pregnancy, childbirth, and the puerperium**

Use additional code(s) from F10 to identify manifestations of the alcohol use

O99.310 **Alcohol use complicating pregnancy, unspecified trimester**

O99.311 **Alcohol use complicating pregnancy, first trimester**

O99.312 **Alcohol use complicating pregnancy, second trimester**

O99.313 **Alcohol use complicating pregnancy, third trimester**

O99.314 **Alcohol use complicating childbirth**

O99.315 **Alcohol use complicating the puerperium**

O99.32 **Drug use complicating pregnancy, childbirth, and the puerperium**

Use additional code(s) from F11-F16 and F18-F19 to identify manifestations of the drug use

O99.320 **Drug use complicating pregnancy, unspecified trimester**

O99.321 **Drug use complicating pregnancy, first trimester**

O99.322 Drug use complicating pregnancy, second trimester

O99.323 Drug use complicating pregnancy, third trimester

O99.324 Drug use complicating childbirth

O99.325 Drug use complicating the puerperium

O99.33 Tobacco use disorder complicating pregnancy, childbirth, and the puerperium

Smoking complicating pregnancy, childbirth, and the puerperium

<u>Use additional code</u> from category F17 to identify type of tobacco nicotine dependence

O99.330 Smoking (tobacco) complicating pregnancy, unspecified trimester

O99.331 Smoking (tobacco) complicating pregnancy, first trimester

O99.332 Smoking (tobacco) complicating pregnancy, second trimester

O99.333 Smoking (tobacco) complicating pregnancy, third trimester

O99.334 Smoking (tobacco) complicating childbirth

O99.335 Smoking (tobacco) complicating the puerperium

O99.34 Other mental disorders complicating pregnancy, childbirth, and the puerperium

Conditions in F01-F09 and F20-F99

Excludes2: postpartum mood disturbance (O90.6)

postnatal psychosis (F53)

puerperal psychosis (F53)

O99.340 Other mental disorders complicating pregnancy, unspecified trimester

O99.341 Other mental disorders complicating pregnancy, first trimester

O99.342 Other mental disorders complicating pregnancy, second trimester

O99.343 Other mental disorders complicating pregnancy, third trimester

O99.344 Other mental disorders complicating childbirth

O99.345 Other mental disorders complicating the puerperium

O99.35 Diseases of the nervous system complicating pregnancy, childbirth, and the puerperium

Conditions in G00-G99

Excludes2: pregnancy related peripheral neuritis (O26.8-)

O99.350 Diseases of the nervous system complicating pregnancy, unspecified trimester

O99.351 Diseases of the nervous system complicating pregnancy, first trimester

O99.352 Diseases of the nervous system complicating pregnancy, second trimester

O99.353 Diseases of the nervous system complicating pregnancy, third trimester

O99.354 Diseases of the nervous system complicating childbirth

O99.355 Diseases of the nervous system complicating the puerperium

O99.4 Diseases of the circulatory system complicating pregnancy, childbirth and the puerperium

Conditions in I00-I99

Excludes1: peripartum cardiomyopathy (O90.3)

Excludes2: hypertensive disorders (O10-O16)

obstetric embolism (O88.-)

venous complications and cerebrovenous sinus thrombosis in labor, childbirth and the puerperium (O87.-)

venous complications and cerebrovenous sinus thrombosis in pregnancy (O22.-)

O99.41 Diseases of the circulatory system complicating pregnancy

O99.411 Diseases of the circulatory system complicating pregnancy, first trimester

O99.412 Diseases of the circulatory system complicating pregnancy, second trimester

O99.413 Diseases of the circulatory system complicating pregnancy, third trimester

O99.419 Diseases of the circulatory system complicating pregnancy, unspecified trimester

O99.42 Diseases of the circulatory system complicating childbirth

O99.43 Diseases of the circulatory system complicating the puerperium

O99.5 Diseases of the respiratory system complicating pregnancy, childbirth and the puerperium

Conditions in J00-J99

O99.51 Diseases of the respiratory system complicating pregnancy

O99.511 Diseases of the respiratory system complicating pregnancy, first trimester

O99.512 Diseases of the respiratory system complicating pregnancy, second trimester

O99.513 Diseases of the respiratory system complicating pregnancy, third trimester

O99.519 Diseases of the respiratory system complicating pregnancy, unspecified trimester

O99.52 Diseases of the respiratory system complicating childbirth

O99.53 Diseases of the respiratory system complicating the puerperium

O99.6 Diseases of the digestive system complicating pregnancy, childbirth and the puerperium

Conditions in K00-K93

Excludes2: hemorrhoids in pregnancy (O22.4-)

liver and biliary tract disorders in pregnancy, childbirth and the puerperium (O26.6-)

O99.61 **Diseases of the digestive system complicating pregnancy**

    O99.611 **Diseases of the digestive system complicating pregnancy, first trimester**

    O99.612 **Diseases of the digestive system complicating pregnancy, second trimester**

    O99.613 **Diseases of the digestive system complicating pregnancy, third trimester**

    O99.619 **Diseases of the digestive system complicating pregnancy, unspecified trimester**

O99.62 **Diseases of the digestive system complicating childbirth**

O99.63 **Diseases of the digestive system complicating the puerperium**

O99.7 **Diseases of the skin and subcutaneous tissue complicating pregnancy, childbirth and the puerperium**

Conditions in L00-L99

Excludes2: herpes gestationis (O26.4)

pruritic urticarial papules and plaques of pregnancy (PUPPP) (O26.86)

O99.71 **Diseases of the skin and subcutaneous tissue complicating pregnancy**

    O99.711 **Diseases of the skin and subcutaneous tissue complicating pregnancy, first trimester**

    O99.712 **Diseases of the skin and subcutaneous tissue complicating pregnancy, second trimester**

    O99.713 **Diseases of the skin and subcutaneous tissue complicating pregnancy, third trimester**

    O99.719 **Diseases of the skin and subcutaneous tissue complicating pregnancy, unspecified trimester**

O99.72 **Diseases of the skin and subcutaneous tissue complicating childbirth**

O99.73 **Diseases of the skin and subcutaneous tissue complicating the puerperium**

O99.8 **Other specified diseases and conditions complicating pregnancy, childbirth and the puerperium**

Conditions in D00-D48, H00-H95, M00-N99, and Q00-Q99

Use additional code to identify condition

Excludes2: genitourinary infections in pregnancy (O23.-)

infection of genitourinary tract following delivery (O86.1-O86.3)

malignant neoplasm complicating pregnancy, childbirth and the puerperium (O9A.1-)

maternal care for known or suspected abnormality of maternal pelvic organs (O34.-)

postpartum acute kidney failure (O90.4)

traumatic injuries in pregnancy (O9A.2-)

O99.81 **Abnormal glucose complicating pregnancy, childbirth and the puerperium**

    Excludes1: gestational diabetes (O24.4-)

    O99.810 **Abnormal glucose complicating pregnancy**

    O99.814 **Abnormal glucose complicating childbirth**

    O99.815 **Abnormal glucose complicating the puerperium**

O99.82 **Streptococcus B carrier state complicating pregnancy, childbirth and the puerperium**

    Excludes1: Carrier of streptococcus group B (GBS) in a nonpregnant woman (Z22.330)

    O99.820 **Streptococcus B carrier state complicating pregnancy**

    O99.824 **Streptococcus B carrier state complicating childbirth**

    O99.825 **Streptococcus B carrier state complicating the puerperium**

O99.83 **Other infection carrier state complicating pregnancy, childbirth and the puerperium**

Use additional code to identify the carrier state (Z22.-)

    O99.830 **Other infection carrier state complicating pregnancy**

    O99.834 **Other infection carrier state complicating childbirth**

    O99.835 **Other infection carrier state complicating the puerperium**

O99.84 **Bariatric surgery status complicating pregnancy, childbirth and the puerperium**

Gastric banding status complicating pregnancy, childbirth and the puerperium

Gastric bypass status for obesity complicating pregnancy, childbirth and the puerperium

Obesity surgery status complicating pregnancy, childbirth and the puerperium

    O99.840 **Bariatric surgery status complicating pregnancy, unspecified trimester**

    O99.841 **Bariatric surgery status complicating pregnancy, first trimester**

    O99.842 **Bariatric surgery status complicating pregnancy, second trimester**

    O99.843 **Bariatric surgery status complicating pregnancy, third trimester**

    O99.844 **Bariatric surgery status complicating childbirth**

    O99.845 **Bariatric surgery status complicating the puerperium**

O99.89 **Other specified diseases and conditions complicating pregnancy, childbirth and the puerperium**

O9A **Maternal malignant neoplasms, traumatic injuries and abuse classifiable elsewhere but complicating pregnancy, childbirth and the puerperium**

O9A.1 **Malignant neoplasm complicating pregnancy, childbirth and the puerperium**

Conditions in C00-C96

Use additional code to identify neoplasm

Excludes2: maternal care for benign tumor of corpus uteri (O34.1-)

maternal care for benign tumor of cervix (O34.4-)

O9A.11 Malignant neoplasm complicating pregnancy

    O9A.111 Malignant neoplasm complicating pregnancy, first trimester

    O9A.112 Malignant neoplasm complicating pregnancy, second trimester

    O9A.113 Malignant neoplasm complicating pregnancy, third trimester

    O9A.119 Malignant neoplasm complicating pregnancy, unspecified trimester

O9A.12 Malignant neoplasm complicating childbirth

O9A.13 Malignant neoplasm complicating the puerperium

O9A.2 Injury, poisoning and certain other consequences of external causes complicating pregnancy, childbirth and the puerperium

Conditions in S00-T88, except T74 and T76

Use additional code(s) to identify the injury or poisoning

Excludes2: physical, sexual and psychological abuse complicating pregnancy, childbirth and the puerperium (O9A.3-, O9A.4-, O9A.5-)

O9A.21 Injury, poisoning and certain other consequences of external causes complicating pregnancy

    O9A.211 Injury, poisoning and certain other consequences of external causes complicating pregnancy, first trimester

    O9A.212 Injury, poisoning and certain other consequences of external causes complicating pregnancy, second trimester

    O9A.213 Injury, poisoning and certain other consequences of external causes complicating pregnancy, third trimester

    O9A.219 Injury, poisoning and certain other consequences of external causes complicating pregnancy, unspecified trimester

O9A.22 Injury, poisoning and certain other consequences of external causes complicating childbirth

O9A.23 Injury, poisoning and certain other consequences of external causes complicating the puerperium

O9A.3 Physical abuse complicating pregnancy, childbirth and the puerperium

Conditions in T74.11 or T76.11

Use additional code (if applicable):

to identify any associated current injury due to physical abuse to identify the perpetrator of abuse (Y07.-)

Excludes2: sexual abuse complicating pregnancy, childbirth and the puerperium (O9A.4)

O9A.31 Physical abuse complicating pregnancy

    O9A.311 Physical abuse complicating pregnancy, first trimester

    O9A.312 Physical abuse complicating pregnancy, second trimester

    O9A.313 Physical abuse complicating pregnancy, third trimester

    O9A.319 Physical abuse complicating pregnancy, unspecified trimester

O9A.32 Physical abuse complicating childbirth

O9A.33 Physical abuse complicating the puerperium

O9A.4 Sexual abuse complicating pregnancy, childbirth and the puerperium

Conditions in T74.21 or T76.21

Use additional code (if applicable):

to identify any associated current injury due to sexual abuse to identify the perpetrator of abuse (Y07.-)

O9A.41 Sexual abuse complicating pregnancy

    O9A.411 Sexual abuse complicating pregnancy, first trimester

    O9A.412 Sexual abuse complicating pregnancy, second trimester

    O9A.413 Sexual abuse complicating pregnancy, third trimester

    O9A.419 Sexual abuse complicating pregnancy, unspecified trimester

O9A.42 Sexual abuse complicating childbirth

O9A.43 Sexual abuse complicating the puerperium

O9A.5 Psychological abuse complicating pregnancy, childbirth and the puerperium

Conditions in T74.31 or T76.31

Use additional code to identify the perpetrator of abuse (Y07.-)

O9A.51 Psychological abuse complicating pregnancy

    O9A.511 Psychological abuse complicating pregnancy, first trimester

    O9A.512 Psychological abuse complicating pregnancy, second trimester

    O9A.513 Psychological abuse complicating pregnancy, third trimester

    O9A.519 Psychological abuse complicating pregnancy, unspecified trimester

O9A.52 Psychological abuse complicating childbirth

O9A.53 Psychological abuse complicating the puerperium

● New code   ▲ Revised code   **Excludes1:** Not coded here   **Excludes2:** Not included here   ⊗ Placeholder required   ⑦ 7th digit required

Chapter 16: Certain Conditions Originating In The Perinatal Period (P00-P96)

DEFINITIONS

This chapter includes definitions of selected key words, terms and phrases and coding alerts for adding points to the clinical domain, and references to coding late effects where appropriate. An example from this chapter is as follows:

P36   Bacterial sepsis of newborn
         Definition: Neonatal sepsis is a blood infection that occurs in an infant younger than 90 days old. Early-onset sepsis is seen in the first week of life.

MULTIPLE CODING FOR A SINGLE CONDITION

In addition to the etiology/manifestation convention that requires two codes to fully describe a single condition that affects multiple body systems, there are other single conditions that also require more than one code. "Use additional code" notes are found in the Tabular List at codes that are not part of an etiology/manifestation pair where a secondary code is useful to fully describe a condition. The sequencing rule is the same as the etiology/manifestation pair, "use additional code" indicates that a secondary code should be added.

For example, for bacterial infections that are not included in chapter 1, a secondary code from category B95, Streptococcus, Staphylococcus, and Enterococcus, as the cause of diseases classified elsewhere, or B96, Other bacterial agents as the cause of diseases classified elsewhere, may be required to identify the bacterial organism causing the infection. A "use additional code" note will normally be found at the infectious disease code, indicating a need for the organism code to be added as a secondary code.

"**Code first**" notes are also under certain codes that are not specifically manifestation codes but may be due to an underlying cause. When there is a "**Code first**" note and an underlying condition is present, the underlying condition should be sequenced first.

"Code, if applicable, any causal condition first", notes indicate that this code may be assigned as a principal diagnosis when the causal condition is unknown or not applicable. If a causal condition is known, then the code for that condition should be sequenced as the principal or first-listed diagnosis.

Multiple codes may be needed for sequela, complication codes and obstetric codes to more fully describe a condition. See the specific guidelines for these conditions for further instruction.

COMBINATION CODE

A combination code is a single code used to classify: Two diagnoses, or a diagnosis with an associated secondary process (manifestation) A diagnosis with an associated complication

Combination codes are identified by referring to subterm entries in the Alphabetic Index and by reading the inclusion and exclusion notes in the Tabular List.

Assign only the combination code when that code fully identifies the diagnostic conditions involved or when the Alphabetic Index so directs. Multiple coding should not be used when the classification provides a combination code that clearly identifies all of the elements documented in the diagnosis. When the combination code lacks necessary specificity in describing the manifestation or complication, an additional code should be used as a secondary code.

SEQUELA (LATE EFFECTS)

A sequela is the residual effect (condition produced) after the acute phase of an illness or injury has terminated. There is no time limit on when a sequela code can be used. The residual may be apparent early, such as in cerebral infarction, or it may occur months or years later, such as that due to a previous injury. Coding of sequela generally requires two codes sequenced in the following order: The condition or nature of the sequela is sequenced first.

The sequela code is sequenced second.

An exception to the above guidelines are those instances where the code for the sequela is followed by a manifestation code identified in the Tabular List and title, or the sequela code has been expanded (at the fourth, fifth or sixth character levels) to include the manifestation(s). The code for the acute phase of an illness or injury that led to the sequela is never used with a code for the late effect.

GENERAL PERINATAL RULES

1)   **Use of Chapter 16 Codes**

      Codes in this chapter are <u>never</u> for use on the maternal record. Codes from Chapter 15, the obstetric chapter, are never permitted on the newborn record. Chapter 16 codes may be used throughout the life of the patient if the condition is still present.

2) Principal Diagnosis for Birth Record

When coding the birth episode in a newborn record, assign a code from category Z38, Liveborn infants according to place of birth and type of delivery, as the principal diagnosis. A code from category Z38 is assigned only once, to a newborn at the time of birth. If a newborn is transferred to another institution, a code from category Z38 should not be used at the receiving hospital.

A code from category Z38 is used only on the newborn record, not on the mother's record.

3) Use of Codes from other Chapters with Codes from Chapter 16

Codes from other chapters may be used with codes from chapter 16 if the codes from the other chapters provide more specific detail. Codes for signs and symptoms may be assigned when a definitive diagnosis has not been established. If the reason for the encounter is a perinatal condition, the code from chapter 16 should be sequenced first.

4) Use of Chapter 16 Codes after the Perinatal Period

Should a condition originate in the perinatal period, and continue throughout the life of the patient, the perinatal code should continue to be used regardless of the patient's age.

5) Birth process or community acquired conditions

If a newborn has a condition that may be either due to the birth process or community acquired and the documentation does not indicate which it is, the default is due to the birth process and the code from Chapter 16 should be used. If the condition is community-acquired, a code from Chapter 16 should not be assigned.

6) Code all clinically significant conditions

All clinically significant conditions noted on routine newborn examination should be coded. A condition is clinically significant if it requires:

§ clinical evaluation; or

§ therapeutic treatment; or

§ diagnostic procedures; or

§ extended length of hospital stay; or

§ increased nursing care and/or monitoring; or

§ has implications for future health care needs

Note: The perinatal guidelines listed above are the same as the general coding guidelines for "additional diagnoses", except for the final point regarding implications for future health care needs. Codes should be assigned for conditions that have been specified by the provider as having implications for future health care needs.

OBSERVATION AND EVALUATION OF NEWBORNS FOR SUSPECTED CONDITIONS NOT FOUND

1) Assign a code from category Z05, Observation and evaluation of newborns and infants for suspected conditions ruled out, to identify those instances when a healthy newborn is evaluated for a suspected condition that is determined after study not to be present. Do not use a code from category Z05 when the patient has identified signs or symptoms of a suspected problem; in such cases code the sign or symptom.

2) A code from category Z05 may also be assigned as a principal or first-listed code for readmissions or encounters when the code from category Z38 code no longer applies. Codes from category Z05 are for use only for healthy newborns and infants for which no condition after study is found to be present.

3) Z05 on a birth record

A code from category Z05 is to be used as a secondary code after the code from category Z38, liveborn infants according to place of birth and type of delivery.

CODING ADDITIONAL PERINATAL DIAGNOSES

1) Assigning codes for conditions that require treatment

Assign codes for conditions that require treatment or further investigation, prolong the length of stay, or require resource utilization.

2) Codes for conditions specified as having implications for future health care needs

Assign codes for conditions that have been specified by the provider as having implications for future health care needs.

Note: This guideline should not be used for adult patients.

PREMATURITY AND FETAL GROWTH RETARDATION

Providers utilize different criteria in determining prematurity. A code for prematurity should not be assigned unless it is documented. Assignment of codes in categories P05, Disorders of newborn related to slow fetal growth and fetal malnutrition, and P07, Disorders of newborn related to short gestation and low birth weight, not elsewhere classified, should be based on the recorded birth weight and estimated gestational age. Codes from category P05 should not be assigned with codes from category P07.

When both birth weight and gestational age are available, two codes from category P07 should be assigned, with the code for birth weight sequenced before the code for gestational age.

LOW BIRTH WEIGHT AND IMMATURITY STATUS

Codes from category P07, Disorders of newborn related to short gestation and low birth weight, not elsewhere classified, are for use for a child or adult who was premature or had a low birth weight as a newborn and this is affecting the patient's current health status.

See Section I.C.21. Factors influencing health status and contact with health services, Status.

BACTERIAL SEPSIS OF NEWBORN

Category P36, Bacterial sepsis of newborn, includes congenital sepsis. If a perinate is documented as having sepsis without documentation of congenital or community acquired, the default is congenital and a code from category P36 should be assigned. If the P36 code includes the causal organism, an additional code from category B95, Streptococcus, Staphylococcus, and Enterococcus as the cause of diseases classified elsewhere, or B96, Other bacterial agents as the cause of diseases classified elsewhere, should not be assigned. If the P36 code does not include the causal organism, assign an additional code from category B96. If applicable, use additional codes to identify severe sepsis (R65.2-) and any associated acute organ dysfunction.

STILLBIRTH

Code P95, Stillbirth, is only for use in institutions that maintain separate records for stillbirths. No other code should be used with P95. Code P95 should not be used on the mother's record.

Chapter 16

Certain Conditions Originating In The Perinatal Period (P00-P96)

NOTE: CODES FROM THIS CHAPTER ARE FOR USE ON NEWBORN RECORDS ONLY, NEVER ON MATERNAL RECORDS

Includes: conditions that have their origin in the fetal or perinatal period (before birth through the first 28 days after birth) even if morbidity occurs later

Excludes2: congenital malformations, deformations and chromosomal abnormalities (Q00-Q99)

endocrine, nutritional and metabolic diseases (E00-E88)

injury, poisoning and certain other consequences of external causes (S00-T88)

neoplasms (C00-D49)

tetanus neonatorum (A33)

This chapter contains the following blocks:

P00-P04	Newborn affected by maternal factors and by complications of pregnancy, labor, and delivery
P05-P08	Disorders of newborn related to length of gestation and fetal growth
P09	Abnormal findings on neonatal screening
P10-P15	Birth trauma
P19-P29	Respiratory and cardiovascular disorders specific to the perinatal period
P35-P39	Infections specific to the perinatal period
P50-P61	Hemorrhagic and hematological disorders of newborn
P70-P74	Transitory endocrine and metabolic disorders specific to newborn
P76-P78	Digestive system disorders of newborn
P80-P83	Conditions involving the integument and temperature regulation of newborn
P84	Other problems with newborn
P90-P96	Other disorders originating in the perinatal period

NEWBORN AFFECTED BY MATERNAL FACTORS AND BY COMPLICATIONS OF PREGNANCY, LABOR, AND DELIVERY (P00-P04)

Note: These codes are for use when the listed maternal conditions are specified as the cause of confirmed morbidity or potential morbidity which have their origin in the perinatal period (before birth through the first 28 days after birth).

P00 **Newborn affected by maternal conditions that may be unrelated to present pregnancy**

Code first any current condition in newborn

Excludes2: encounter for observation of newborn for suspected diseases and conditions ruled out (Z05.-)

newborn affected by maternal complications of pregnancy (P01.-)

newborn affected by maternal endocrine and metabolic disorders (P70-P74)

newborn affected by noxious substances transmitted via placenta or breast milk (P04.-)

▲P00.0 **Newborn affected by maternal hypertensive disorders**

Newborn affected by maternal conditions classifiable to O10-O11, O13-O16

▲P00.1 **Newborn affected by maternal renal and urinary tract diseases**

Newborn affected by maternal conditions classifiable to N00-N39

▲P00.2 **Newborn affected by maternal infectious and parasitic diseases**

Newborn affected by maternal infectious disease classifiable to A00-B99, J09 and J10

Excludes1: infections specific to the perinatal period (P35-P39)

maternal genital tract or other localized infections (P00.8)

▲P00.3 **Newborn affected by other maternal circulatory and respiratory diseases**

Newborn affected by maternal conditions classifiable to I00-I99, J00-J99, Q20-Q34 and not included in P00.0, P00.2

▲P00.4 **Newborn affected by maternal nutritional disorders**

Newborn affected by maternal disorders classifiable to E40-E64

Maternal malnutrition NOS

▲P00.5 **Newborn affected by maternal injury**

Newborn affected by maternal conditions classifiable to O9A.2-

▲P00.6 **Newborn affected by surgical procedure on mother**

Newborn affected by amniocentesis

Excludes1: Cesarean delivery for present delivery (P03.4)

damage to placenta from amniocentesis, Cesarean delivery or surgical induction (P02.1)

previous surgery to uterus or pelvic organs (P03.89)

Excludes2: newborn affected by complication of (fetal) intrauterine procedure (P96.5)

▲P00.7 **Newborn affected by other medical procedures on mother, not elsewhere classified**

Newborn affected by radiation to mother

Excludes1: damage to placenta from amniocentesis, cesarean delivery or surgical induction (P02.1)

newborn affected by other complications of labor and delivery (P03.-)

P00.8 **Newborn affected by other maternal conditions**

▲P00.81 **Newborn affected by periodontal disease in mother**

▲P00.89 **Newborn affected by other maternal conditions**

Newborn affected by conditions classifiable to T80-T88

Newborn affected by maternal genital tract or other localized infections

Newborn affected by maternal systemic lupus erythematosus

▲P00.9 **Newborn affected by unspecified maternal condition**

P01 **Newborn affected by maternal complications of pregnancy**

Code first any current condition in newborn

Excludes2: encounter for observation of newborn for suspected diseases and conditions ruled out (Z05.-)

▲P01.0 **Newborn affected by incompetent cervix**

▲P01.1 **Newborn affected by premature rupture of membranes**

▲P01.2 **Newborn affected by oligohydramnios**

Excludes1: oligohydramnios due to premature rupture of membranes (P01.1)

▲P01.3 **Newborn affected by polyhydramnios**

Newborn affected by hydramnios

▲P01.4 **Newborn affected by ectopic pregnancy**

Newborn affected by abdominal pregnancy

▲P01.5 **Newborn affected by multiple pregnancy**

Newborn affected by triplet (pregnancy)

Newborn affected by twin (pregnancy)

▲P01.6 **Newborn affected by maternal death**

▲P01.7 **Newborn affected by malpresentation before labor**

Newborn affected by breech presentation before labor

Newborn affected by external version before labor

Newborn affected by face presentation before labor

Newborn affected by transverse lie before labor

Newborn affected by unstable lie before labor

▲P01.8 **Newborn affected by other maternal complications of pregnancy**

▲P01.9 **Newborn affected by maternal complication of pregnancy, unspecified**

P02 **Newborn affected by complications of placenta, cord and membranes**

Code first any current condition in newborn

Excludes2: encounter for observation of newborn for suspected diseases and conditions ruled out (Z05.-)

▲P02.0 **Newborn affected by placenta previa**

▲P02.1 **Newborn affected by other forms of placental separation and hemorrhage**

Newborn affected by abruptio placenta

Newborn affected by accidental hemorrhage

Newborn affected by antepartum hemorrhage

Newborn affected by damage to placenta from amniocentesis, cesarean delivery or surgical induction

Newborn affected by maternal blood loss

Newborn affected by premature separation of placenta

P02.2 **Newborn affected by other and unspecified morphological and functional abnormalities of placenta**

▲P02.20 **Newborn affected by unspecified morphological and functional abnormalities of placenta**

▲P02.29 **Newborn affected by other morphological and functional abnormalities of placenta**

Newborn affected by placental dysfunction

Newborn affected by placental infarction

Newborn affected by placental insufficiency

▲P02.3 **Newborn affected by placental transfusion syndromes**

Newborn affected by placental and cord abnormalities resulting in twin-to-twin **or other** transplacental transfusion

▲P02.4 **Newborn affected by prolapsed cord**

▲P02.5 **Newborn affected by other compression of umbilical cord**

Newborn affected by umbilical cord (tightly) around neck

Newborn affected by entanglement of umbilical cord

Newborn affected by knot in umbilical cord

P02.6 **Newborn affected by other and unspecified conditions of umbilical cord**

▲P02.60 **Newborn affected by unspecified conditions of umbilical cord**

▲P02.69 **Newborn affected by other conditions of umbilical cord**

Newborn affected by short umbilical cord

Newborn affected by vasa previa

Excludes1: newborn affected by single umbilical artery (Q27.0)

▲P02.7 **Newborn affected by chorioamnionitis**

Newborn affected by amnionitis

Newborn affected by membranitis

Newborn affected by placentitis

▲P02.8 **Newborn affected by other abnormalities of membranes**

▲P02.9 **Newborn affected by abnormality of membranes, unspecified**

P03 **Newborn affected by other complications of labor and delivery**

Code first any current condition in newborn

Excludes2: encounter for observation of newborn for suspected diseases and conditions ruled out (Z05.-)

▲P03.0 **Newborn affected by breech delivery and extraction**

▲P03.1 **Newborn affected by other malpresentation, malposition and disproportion during labor and delivery**

Newborn affected by contracted pelvis

Newborn affected by conditions classifiable to O64-O66

Newborn affected by persistent occipitoposterior

Newborn affected by transverse lie

▲P03.2 **Newborn affected by forceps delivery**

▲P03.3 **Newborn affected by delivery by vacuum extractor [ventouse]**

▲P03.4 **Newborn affected by Cesarean delivery**

▲P03.5 **Newborn affected by precipitate delivery**

Newborn affected by rapid second stage

▲P03.6 **Newborn affected by abnormal uterine contractions**

Newborn affected by conditions classifiable to O62.-, except O62.3

Newborn affected by hypertonic labor

Newborn affected by uterine inertia

P03.8 **Newborn affected by other specified complications of labor and delivery**

P03.81 **Newborn affected by abnormality in fetal (intrauterine) heart rate or rhythm**

Excludes1: neonatal cardiac dysrhythmia (P29.1-)

▲P03.810 **Newborn affected by abnormality in fetal (intrauterine) heart rate or rhythm before the onset of labor**

▲P03.811 **Newborn affected by abnormality in fetal (intrauterine) heart rate or rhythm during labor**

▲P03.819 **Newborn affected by abnormality in fetal (intrauterine) heart rate or rhythm, unspecified as to time of onset**

P03.82 **Meconium passage during delivery**

Excludes1: meconium aspiration (P24.00, P24.01)

meconium staining (P96.83)

▲P03.89 **Newborn affected by other specified complications of labor and delivery**

● New code ▲ Revised code **Excludes1:** Not coded here **Excludes2:** Not included here ⊗ Placeholder required ⑦7th digit required

Newborn affected by abnormality of maternal soft tissues

Newborn affected by conditions classifiable to O60-O75 and by procedures used in labor and delivery not included in P02.- and P03.0-P03.6

Newborn affected by induction of labor

▲**P03.9   Newborn affected by complication of labor and delivery, unspecified**

P04   Newborn affected by noxious substances transmitted via placenta or breast milk

Includes: nonteratogenic effects of substances transmitted via placenta

Excludes2: congenital malformations (Q00-Q99)

encounter for observation of newborn for suspected diseases and conditions ruled out (Z05.-)

neonatal jaundice from excessive hemolysis due to drugs or toxins transmitted from mother (P58.4)

newborn in contact with and (suspected) exposures hazardous to health not transmitted via placenta or breast milk (Z77.-)

▲**P04.0   Newborn affected by maternal anesthesia and analgesia in pregnancy, labor and delivery**

Newborn affected by reactions and intoxications from maternal opiates and tranquilizers administered during labor and delivery

▲**P04.1   Newborn affected by other maternal medication**

Newborn affected by cancer chemotherapy

Newborn affected by cytotoxic drugs

Excludes1: dysmorphism due to warfarin (Q86.2)

fetal hydantoin syndrome (Q86.1)

maternal use of drugs of addiction (P04.4-)

▲**P04.2   Newborn affected by maternal use of tobacco**

Newborn affected by exposure in utero to tobacco smoke

Excludes2: newborn exposure to environmental tobacco smoke (P96.81)

▲**P04.3   Newborn affected by maternal use of alcohol**

Excludes1: fetal alcohol syndrome (Q86.0)

P04.4   Newborn affected by maternal use of drugs of addiction

▲**P04.41   Newborn affected by maternal use of cocaine**

'Crack baby'

▲**P04.49   Newborn affected by maternal use of other drugs of addiction**

Excludes2: newborn affected by maternal anesthesia and analgesia (P04.0)

withdrawal symptoms from maternal use of drugs of addiction (P96.1)

▲**P04.5   Newborn affected by maternal use of nutritional chemical substances**

▲**P04.6   Newborn affected by maternal exposure to environmental chemical substances**

▲**P04.8   Newborn affected by other maternal noxious substances**

▲**P04.9   Newborn affected by maternal noxious substance, unspecified**

DISORDERS OF NEWBORN RELATED TO LENGTH OF GESTATION AND FETAL GROWTH (P05-P08)

P05   Disorders of newborn related to slow fetal growth and fetal malnutrition

P05.0   Newborn light for gestational age

Newborn light-for-dates

Weight below but length above 10th percentile for gestational age

P05.00   Newborn light for gestational age, unspecified weight

P05.01   Newborn light for gestational age, less than 500 grams

P05.02   Newborn light for gestational age, 500-749 grams

P05.03   Newborn light for gestational age, 750-999 grams

P05.04   Newborn light for gestational age, 1000-1249 grams

P05.05   Newborn light for gestational age, 1250-1499 grams

P05.06   Newborn light for gestational age, 1500-1749 grams

P05.07   Newborn light for gestational age, 1750-1999 grams

P05.08   Newborn light for gestational age, 2000-2499 grams

●**P05.09   Newborn light for gestational age, 2500 grams and over**

Newborn light for gestational age, **other**

P05.1   Newborn small for gestational age

Newborn small-and-light-for-dates

Newborn small-for-dates

Weight and length below 10th percentile for gestational age

P05.10   Newborn small for gestational age, unspecified weight

P05.11   Newborn small for gestational age, less than 500 grams

P05.12   Newborn small for gestational age, 500-749 grams

P05.13   Newborn small for gestational age, 750-999 grams

P05.14   Newborn small for gestational age, 1000-1249 grams

P05.15   Newborn small for gestational age, 1250-1499 grams

P05.16   Newborn small for gestational age, 1500-1749 grams

P05.17   Newborn small for gestational age, 1750-1999 grams

P05.18   Newborn small for gestational age, 2000-2499 grams

●**P05.19   Newborn small for gestational age, other**

Newborn small for gestational age, 2500 grams and over

P05.2   Newborn affected by fetal (intrauterine) malnutrition not light or small for gestational age

Infant, not light or small for gestational age, showing signs of fetal malnutrition, such as dry, peeling skin and loss of subcutaneous tissue

Excludes1: newborn affected by fetal malnutrition with light for gestational age (P05.0-)

newborn affected by fetal malnutrition with small for gestational age (P05.1-)

P05.9   Newborn affected by slow intrauterine growth, unspecified

Newborn affected by fetal growth retardation NOS

P07 **Disorders of newborn related to short gestation and low birth weight, not elsewhere classified**

Note: When both birth weight and gestational age of the newborn are available, both should be coded with birth weight sequenced before gestational age

Includes: the listed conditions, without further specification, as the cause of morbidity or additional care, in newborn

P07.0 **Extremely low birth weight newborn**

Newborn birth weight 999 g. or less

Excludes1: low birth weight due to slow fetal growth and fetal malnutrition (P05.-)

P07.00 **Extremely low birth weight newborn, unspecified weight**

P07.01 **Extremely low birth weight newborn, less than 500 grams**

P07.02 **Extremely low birth weight newborn, 500-749 grams**

P07.03 **Extremely low birth weight newborn, 750-999 grams**

P07.1 **Other low birth weight newborn**

Newborn birth weight 1000-2499 g.

Excludes1: low birth weight due to slow fetal growth and fetal malnutrition (P05.-)

P07.10 **Other low birth weight newborn, unspecified weight**

P07.14 **Other low birth weight newborn, 1000-1249 grams**

P07.15 **Other low birth weight newborn, 1250-1499 grams**

P07.16 **Other low birth weight newborn, 1500-1749 grams**

P07.17 **Other low birth weight newborn, 1750-1999 grams**

P07.18 **Other low birth weight newborn, 2000-2499 grams**

P07.2 **Extreme immaturity of newborn**

Less than 28 completed weeks (less than 196 completed days) of gestation.

P07.20 **Extreme immaturity of newborn, unspecified weeks of gestation**

Gestational age less than 28 completed weeks NOS

P07.21 **Extreme immaturity of newborn, gestational age less than 23 completed weeks**

Extreme immaturity of newborn, gestational age less than 23 weeks, 0 days

P07.22 **Extreme immaturity of newborn, gestational age 23 completed weeks**

Extreme immaturity of newborn, gestational age 23 weeks, 0 days through 23 weeks, 6 days

P07.23 **Extreme immaturity of newborn, gestational age 24completed weeks**

Extreme immaturity of newborn, gestational age 24 weeks, 0 days through 24 weeks, 6 days

P07.24 **Extreme immaturity of newborn, gestational age 25completed weeks**

Extreme immaturity of newborn, gestational age 25 weeks, 0 days through 25 weeks, 6 days

P07.25 **Extreme immaturity of newborn, gestational age 26completed weeks**

Extreme immaturity of newborn, gestational age 26 weeks, 0 days through 26 weeks, 6 days

P07.26 **Extreme immaturity of newborn, gestational age 27completed weeks**

Extreme immaturity of newborn, gestational age 27 weeks, 0 days through 27 weeks, 6 days

P07.3 **Preterm [premature] newborn [Other]**

28 completed weeks or more but less than 37 completed weeks (196 completed days but less than 259 completed days) of gestation.

Prematurity NOS

P07.30 **Preterm newborn, unspecified weeks of gestation**

P07.31 **Preterm newborn, gestational age 28 completed weeks**

Preterm newborn, gestational age 28 weeks, 0 days through 28 weeks, 6 days

P07.32 **Preterm newborn, gestational age 29 completed weeks**

Preterm newborn, gestational age 29 weeks, 0 days through 29 weeks, 6 days

P07.33 **Preterm newborn, gestational age 30 completed weeks**

Preterm newborn, gestational age 30 weeks, 0 days through 30 weeks, 6 days

P07.34 **Preterm newborn, gestational age 31 completed weeks**

Preterm newborn, gestational age 31 weeks, 0 days through 31 weeks, 6 days

P07.35 **Preterm newborn, gestational age 32 completed weeks**

Preterm newborn, gestational age 32 weeks, 0 days through 32 weeks, 6 days

P07.36 **Preterm newborn, gestational age 33 completed weeks**

Preterm newborn, gestational age 33 weeks, 0 days through 33 weeks, 6 days

P07.37 **Preterm newborn, gestational age 34 completed weeks**

Preterm newborn, gestational age 34 weeks, 0 days through 34 weeks, 6 days

P07.38 **Preterm newborn, gestational age 35 completed weeks**

Preterm newborn, gestational age 35 weeks, 0 days through 35 weeks, 6 days

P07.39 **Preterm newborn, gestational age 36 completed weeks**

Preterm newborn, gestational age 36 weeks, 0 days through 36 weeks, 6 days

P08 **Disorders of newborn related to long gestation and high birth weight**

Note: When both birth weight and gestational age of the newborn are available, priority of assignment should be given to birth weight

Includes: the listed conditions, without further specification, as causes of morbidity or additional care, in newborn

P08.0 **Exceptionally large newborn baby**

Usually implies a birth weight of 4500 g. or more

Excludes1: syndrome of infant of diabetic mother (P70.1)

syndrome of infant of mother with gestational diabetes (P70.0)

P08.1 **Other heavy for gestational age newborn**

Other newborn heavy- or large-for-dates regardless of period of gestation Usually implies a birth weight of 4000 g. to 4499 g.

Excludes1: newborn with a birth weight of 4500 or more (P08.0)

syndrome of infant of diabetic mother (P70.1)

syndrome of infant of mother with gestational diabetes (P70.0).

P08.2   Late newborn, not heavy for gestational age

P08.21   Post-term newborn

Newborn with gestation period over 40 completed weeks to 42 completed weeks

P08.22   Prolonged gestation of newborn

Newborn with gestation period over 42 completed weeks (294 days or more), not heavy- or large-for-dates.

Postmaturity NOS

ABNORMAL FINDINGS ON NEONATAL SCREENING (P09)

P09   Abnormal findings on neonatal screening

Use additional code to identify signs, symptoms and conditions associated with the screening

Excludes2: nonspecific serologic evidence of human immunodeficiency virus [HIV] (R75)

BIRTH TRAUMA (P10-P15)

Definition: Birth trauma refers to: 1) a physical injury sustained by an infant during birth; or 2) the psychological shock said to be experienced by an infant during birth.

P10   Intracranial laceration and hemorrhage due to birth injury

Excludes1: intracranial hemorrhage of newborn NOS (P52.9)

intracranial hemorrhage of newborn due to anoxia or hypoxia (P52.-)

nontraumatic intracranial hemorrhage of newborn (P52.-)

P10.0   Subdural hemorrhage due to birth injury

Subdural hematoma (localized) due to birth injury

Excludes1: subdural hemorrhage accompanying tentorial tear (P10.4)

P10.1   Cerebral hemorrhage due to birth injury

P10.2   Intraventricular hemorrhage due to birth injury

P10.3   Subarachnoid hemorrhage due to birth injury

P10.4   Tentorial tear due to birth injury

P10.8   Other intracranial lacerations and hemorrhages due to birth injury

P10.9   Unspecified intracranial laceration and hemorrhage due to birth injury

P11   Other birth injuries to central nervous system

P11.0   Cerebral edema due to birth injury

P11.1   Other specified brain damage due to birth injury

P11.2   Unspecified brain damage due to birth injury

P11.3   Birth injury to facial nerve

Facial palsy due to birth injury

P11.4   Birth injury to other cranial nerves

P11.5   Birth injury to spine and spinal cord

Fracture of spine due to birth injury

P11.9   Birth injury to central nervous system, unspecified

P12   Birth injury to scalp

P12.0   Cephalhematoma due to birth injury

P12.1   Chignon (from vacuum extraction) due to birth injury

P12.2   Epicranial subaponeurotic hemorrhage due to birth injury

Subgaleal hemorrhage

P12.3   Bruising of scalp due to birth injury

P12.4   Injury of scalp of newborn due to monitoring equipment

Sampling incision of scalp of newborn

Scalp clip (electrode) injury of newborn

P12.8   Other birth injuries to scalp

P12.81   Caput succedaneum

P12.89   Other birth injuries to scalp

P12.9   Birth injury to scalp, unspecified

P13   Birth injury to skeleton

Excludes2: birth injury to spine (P11.5)

P13.0   Fracture of skull due to birth injury

P13.1   Other birth injuries to skull

Excludes1: cephalhematoma (P12.0)

P13.2   Birth injury to femur

P13.3   Birth injury to other long bones

P13.4   Fracture of clavicle due to birth injury

P13.8   Birth injuries to other parts of skeleton

P13.9   Birth injury to skeleton, unspecified

P14   Birth injury to peripheral nervous system

P14.0   Erb's paralysis due to birth injury

P14.1   Klumpke's paralysis due to birth injury

P14.2   Phrenic nerve paralysis due to birth injury

P14.3   Other brachial plexus birth injuries

P14.8   Birth injuries to other parts of peripheral nervous system

P14.9   Birth injury to peripheral nervous system, unspecified

P15   Other birth injuries

P15.0   Birth injury to liver

Rupture of liver due to birth injury

P15.1   Birth injury to spleen

Rupture of spleen due to birth injury

P15.2   Sternomastoid injury due to birth injury

P15.3   Birth injury to eye

Subconjunctival hemorrhage due to birth injury

Traumatic glaucoma due to birth injury

P15.4   Birth injury to face

Facial congestion due to birth injury

P15.5   Birth injury to external genitalia

P15.6   Subcutaneous fat necrosis due to birth injury

P15.8   Other specified birth injuries

P15.9   Birth injury, unspecified

RESPIRATORY AND CARDIOVASCULAR DISORDERS SPECIFIC TO THE PERINATAL PERIOD (P19-P29)

P19   Metabolic acidemia in newborn

Includes: metabolic acidemia in newborn

P19.0   Metabolic acidemia in newborn first noted before onset of labor

P19.1   Metabolic acidemia in newborn first noted during labor

P19.2   Metabolic acidemia noted at birth

P19.9   Metabolic acidemia, unspecified

| | Add 4th-7th digits | | Nonspecific code | | Unspecified code | | Manifestation code | 695 |

P22 Respiratory distress of newborn

Excludes1: respiratory arrest of newborn (P28.81)

respiratory failure of newborn NOS (P28.5)

P22.0 Respiratory distress syndrome of newborn

Definition: Respiratory distress syndrome (RDS), formerly known as hyaline membrane disease, is a syndrome of respiratory difficulty in newborn infants caused by a deficiency of a molecule called surfactant.

Cardiorespiratory distress syndrome of newborn

Hyaline membrane disease

Idiopathic respiratory distress syndrome [IRDS or RDS] of newborn

Pulmonary hypoperfusion syndrome

Respiratory distress syndrome, type I

P22.1 Transient tachypnea of newborn

Idiopathic tachypnea of newborn

Respiratory distress syndrome, type II

Wet lung syndrome

P22.8 Other respiratory distress of newborn

P22.9 Respiratory distress of newborn, unspecified

P23 Congenital pneumonia

Includes: infective pneumonia acquired in utero or during birth

Excludes1: neonatal pneumonia resulting from aspiration (P24.-)

P23.0 Congenital pneumonia due to viral agent

Use additional code (B97) to identify organism

Excludes1: congenital rubella pneumonitis (P35.0)

P23.1 Congenital pneumonia due to Chlamydia

P23.2 Congenital pneumonia due to staphylococcus

P23.3 Congenital pneumonia due to streptococcus, group B

P23.4 Congenital pneumonia due to Escherichia coli

P23.5 Congenital pneumonia due to Pseudomonas

P23.6 Congenital pneumonia due to other bacterial agents

Congenital pneumonia due to Hemophilus influenzae

Congenital pneumonia due to Klebsiella pneumoniae

Congenital pneumonia due to Mycoplasma

Congenital pneumonia due to Streptococcus, except group B

Use additional code (B95-B96) to identify organism

P23.8 Congenital pneumonia due to other organisms

P23.9 Congenital pneumonia, unspecified

P24 Neonatal aspiration

Includes: aspiration in utero and during delivery

P24.0 Meconium aspiration

Excludes1: meconium passage (without aspiration) during delivery (P03.82)

meconium staining (P96.83)

P24.00 Meconium aspiration without respiratory symptoms

Meconium aspiration NOS

P24.01 Meconium aspiration with respiratory symptoms

Meconium aspiration pneumonia

Meconium aspiration pneumonitis

Meconium aspiration syndrome NOS

Use additional code to identify any secondary pulmonary hypertension, if applicable (I27.2)

P24.1 Neonatal aspiration of (clear) amniotic fluid and mucus

Neonatal aspiration of liquor (amnii)

P24.10 Neonatal aspiration of (clear) amniotic fluid and mucus without respiratory symptoms

Neonatal aspiration of amniotic fluid and mucus NOS

P24.11 Neonatal aspiration of (clear) amniotic fluid and mucus with respiratory symptoms

Neonatal aspiration of amniotic fluid and mucus with pneumonia

Neonatal aspiration of amniotic fluid and mucus with pneumonitis

Use additional code to identify any secondary pulmonary hypertension, if applicable (I27.2)

P24.2 Neonatal aspiration of blood

P24.20 Neonatal aspiration of blood without respiratory symptoms

Neonatal aspiration of blood NOS

P24.21 Neonatal aspiration of blood with respiratory symptoms

Neonatal aspiration of blood with pneumonia

Neonatal aspiration of blood with pneumonitis

Use additional code to identify any secondary pulmonary hypertension, if applicable (I27.2)

P24.3 Neonatal aspiration of milk and regurgitated food

Neonatal aspiration of stomach contents

P24.30 Neonatal aspiration of milk and regurgitated food without respiratory symptoms

Neonatal aspiration of milk and regurgitated food NOS

P24.31 Neonatal aspiration of milk and regurgitated food with respiratory symptoms

Neonatal aspiration of milk and regurgitated food with pneumonia

Neonatal aspiration of milk and regurgitated food with pneumonitis

Use additional code to identify any secondary pulmonary hypertension, if applicable (I27.2)

P24.8 Other neonatal aspiration

P24.80 Other neonatal aspiration without respiratory symptoms

Neonatal aspiration NEC

P24.81 Other neonatal aspiration with respiratory symptoms

Neonatal aspiration pneumonia NEC

Neonatal aspiration with pneumonitis NEC

Neonatal aspiration with pneumonia NOS

Neonatal aspiration with pneumonitis NOS

Use additional code to identify any secondary pulmonary hypertension, if applicable (I27.2)

P24.9 Neonatal aspiration, unspecified

P25 Interstitial emphysema and related conditions originating in the perinatal period

P25.0 Interstitial emphysema originating in the perinatal period

P25.1 Pneumothorax originating in the perinatal period

P25.2 Pneumomediastinum originating in the perinatal period

P25.3 Pneumopericardium originating in the perinatal period

P25.8 Other conditions related to interstitial emphysema originating in the perinatal period

P26 Pulmonary hemorrhage originating in the perinatal period

Excludes1: acute idiopathic hemorrhage in infants over 28 days old (R04.81)

P26.0 Tracheobronchial hemorrhage originating in the perinatal period

P26.1 Massive pulmonary hemorrhage originating in the perinatal period

P26.8 Other pulmonary hemorrhages originating in the perinatal period

P26.9 Unspecified pulmonary hemorrhage originating in the perinatal period

P27 Chronic respiratory disease originating in the perinatal period

Excludes1: respiratory distress of newborn (P22.0-P22.9)

P27.0 Wilson-Mikity syndrome

Pulmonary dysmaturity

P27.1 Bronchopulmonary dysplasia originating in the perinatal period

P27.8 Other chronic respiratory diseases originating in the perinatal period

Congenital pulmonary fibrosis

Ventilator lung in newborn

P27.9 Unspecified chronic respiratory disease originating in the perinatal period

P28 Other respiratory conditions originating in the perinatal period

Excludes1: congenital malformations of the respiratory system (Q30-Q34)

P28.0 Primary atelectasis of newborn

Primary failure to expand terminal respiratory units

Pulmonary hypoplasia associated with short gestation

Pulmonary immaturity NOS

P28.1 Other and unspecified atelectasis of newborn

P28.10 Unspecified atelectasis of newborn

Atelectasis of newborn NOS

P28.11 Resorption atelectasis without respiratory distress syndrome

Excludes1: resorption atelectasis with respiratory distress syndrome (P22.0)

P28.19 Other atelectasis of newborn

Partial atelectasis of newborn

Secondary atelectasis of newborn

P28.2 Cyanotic attacks of newborn

Excludes1: apnea of newborn (P28.3-P28.4)

P28.3 Primary sleep apnea of newborn

Central sleep apnea of newborn

Obstructive sleep apnea of newborn

Sleep apnea of newborn NOS

P28.4 Other apnea of newborn

Apnea of prematurity

Obstructive apnea of newborn

Excludes1: obstructive sleep apnea of newborn (P28.3)

P28.5 Respiratory failure of newborn

Excludes1: respiratory arrest of newborn (P28.81)

respiratory distress of newborn (P22.0-)

P28.8 Other specified respiratory conditions of newborn

P28.81 Respiratory arrest of newborn

P28.89 Other specified respiratory conditions of newborn

Congenital laryngeal stridor

Sniffles in newborn

Snuffles in newborn

Excludes1: early congenital syphilitic rhinitis (A50.05)

P28.9 Respiratory condition of newborn, unspecified

Respiratory depression in newborn

P29 Cardiovascular disorders originating in the perinatal period

Excludes1: congenital malformations of the circulatory system (Q20-Q28)

P29.0 Neonatal cardiac failure

P29.1 Neonatal cardiac dysrhythmia

P29.11 Neonatal tachycardia

P29.12 Neonatal bradycardia

P29.2 Neonatal hypertension

P29.3 Persistent fetal circulation

Delayed closure of ductus arteriosus (Persistent)

pulmonary hypertension of newborn

P29.4 Transient myocardial ischemia in newborn

P29.8 Other cardiovascular disorders originating in the perinatal period

P29.81 Cardiac arrest of newborn

P29.89 Other cardiovascular disorders originating in the perinatal period

P29.9 Cardiovascular disorder originating in the perinatal period, unspecified

INFECTIONS SPECIFIC TO THE PERINATAL PERIOD (P35-P39)

Infections acquired in utero, during birth via the umbilicus, or during the first 28 days after birth

Excludes2: asymptomatic human immunodeficiency virus [HIV] infection status (Z21)

congenital gonococcal infection (A54.-)

congenital pneumonia (P23.-)

congenital syphilis (A50.-)

human immunodeficiency virus [HIV] disease (B20)

infant botulism (A48.51)

infectious diseases not specific to the perinatal period (A00-B99, J09, J10.-)

intestinal infectious disease (A00-A09)

laboratory evidence of human immunodeficiency virus [HIV] (R75)

tetanus neonatorum (A33)

P35 Congenital viral diseases

Includes: infections acquired in utero or during birth

P35.0 Congenital rubella syndrome

Congenital rubella pneumonitis

P35.1 Congenital cytomegalovirus infection

P35.2 Congenital herpesviral [herpes simplex] infection

P35.3 Congenital viral hepatitis

P35.8 Other congenital viral diseases

Congenital varicella [chickenpox]

P35.9 Congenital viral disease, unspecified

P36 Bacterial sepsis of newborn

Definition: Neonatal sepsis is a blood infection that occurs in an

infant younger than 90 days old. Early-onset sepsis is seen in the first week of life. Late-onset sepsis occurs between days 8 and 89.

Includes: congenital sepsis

Use additional code(s), if applicable, to identify severe sepsis (R652-) and associated acute organ dysfunction(s)

P36.0   Sepsis of newborn due to streptococcus, group B

P36.1   Sepsis of newborn due to other and unspecified streptococci

   P36.10   Sepsis of newborn due to unspecified streptococci

   P36.19   Sepsis of newborn due to other streptococci

P36.2   Sepsis of newborn due to Staphylococcus aureus

P36.3   Sepsis of newborn due to other and unspecified staphylococci

   P36.30   Sepsis of newborn due to unspecified staphylococci

   P36.39   Sepsis of newborn due to other staphylococci

P36.4   Sepsis of newborn due to Escherichia coli

P36.5   Sepsis of newborn due to anaerobes

P36.8   Other bacterial sepsis of newborn

   Use additional code from category B96 to identify organism

P36.9   Bacterial sepsis of newborn, unspecified

P37   Other congenital infectious and parasitic diseases

   Excludes2: congenital syphilis (A50.-)

      infectious neonatal diarrhea (A00-A09)

      necrotizing enterocolitis in newborn (P77.-)

      noninfectious neonatal diarrhea (P78.3)

      ophthalmia neonatorum due to gonococcus (A54.31)

      tetanus neonatorum (A33)

P37.0   Congenital tuberculosis

P37.1   Congenital toxoplasmosis

   Hydrocephalus due to congenital toxoplasmosis

P37.2   Neonatal (disseminated) listeriosis

P37.3   Congenital falciparum malaria

P37.4   Other congenital malaria

P37.5   Neonatal candidiasis

P37.8   Other specified congenital infectious and parasitic diseases

P37.9   Congenital infectious or parasitic disease, unspecified

P38   Omphalitis of newborn

   Definition: Omphalitis is the medical term for inflammation of the umbilical cord stump in the neonatal newborn period, most commonly attributed to a bacterial infection.

   Excludes1: omphalitis not of newborn (L08.82)

      tetanus omphalitis (A33)

      umbilical hemorrhage of newborn (P51.-)

P38.1   Omphalitis with mild hemorrhage

P38.9   Omphalitis without hemorrhage

   Omphalitis of newborn NOS

P39   Other infections specific to the perinatal period

   Use additional code to identify organism or specific infection

P39.0   Neonatal infective mastitis

   Excludes1: breast engorgement of newborn (P83.4)

      noninfective mastitis of newborn (P83.4)

P39.1   Neonatal conjunctivitis and dacryocystitis

Neonatal chlamydial conjunctivitis

Ophthalmia neonatorum NOS

Excludes1: gonococcal conjunctivitis (A54.31)

P39.2   Intra-amniotic infection affecting newborn, not elsewhere classified

P39.3   Neonatal urinary tract infection

P39.4   Neonatal skin infection

Neonatal pyoderma

Excludes1: pemphigus neonatorum (L00)

      staphylococcal scalded skin syndrome (L00)

P39.8   Other specified infections specific to the perinatal period

P39.9   Infection specific to the perinatal period, unspecified

HEMORRHAGIC AND HEMATOLOGICAL DISORDERS OF NEWBORN (P50-P61)

Excludes1: congenital stenosis and stricture of bile ducts (Q44.3)

   Crigler-Najjar syndrome (E80.5)

   Dubin-Johnson syndrome (E80.6)

   Gilbert syndrome (E80.4)

   hereditary hemolytic anemias (D55-D58)

P50   Newborn affected by intrauterine (fetal) blood loss

   Excludes1: congenital anemia from intrauterine (fetal) blood loss (P61.3)

P50.0   Newborn affected by intrauterine (fetal) blood loss from vasa previa

P50.1   Newborn affected by intrauterine (fetal) blood loss from ruptured cord

P50.2   Newborn affected by intrauterine (fetal) blood loss from placenta

P50.3   Newborn affected by hemorrhage into co-twin

P50.4   Newborn affected by hemorrhage into maternal circulation

P50.5   Newborn affected by intrauterine (fetal) blood loss from cut end of co-twin's cord

P50.8   Newborn affected by other intrauterine (fetal) blood loss

P50.9   Newborn affected by intrauterine (fetal) blood loss, unspecified

Newborn affected by fetal hemorrhage NOS

P51   Umbilical hemorrhage of newborn

   Excludes1: omphalitis with mild hemorrhage (P38.1)

      umbilical hemorrhage from cut end of co-twins cord (P50.5)

P51.0   Massive umbilical hemorrhage of newborn

P51.8   Other umbilical hemorrhages of newborn

Slipped umbilical ligature NOS

P51.9   Umbilical hemorrhage of newborn, unspecified

P52   Intracranial nontraumatic hemorrhage of newborn

   Includes: intracranial hemorrhage due to anoxia or hypoxia

   Excludes1: intracranial hemorrhage due to birth injury (P10.-)

      intracranial hemorrhage due **to other** injury (S06.-)

P52.0   Intraventricular (nontraumatic) hemorrhage, grade 1, of newborn

Subependymal hemorrhage (without intraventricular extension)

Bleeding into germinal matrix

P52.1 **Intraventricular (nontraumatic) hemorrhage, grade 2, of newborn**

Subependymal hemorrhage with intraventricular extension

Bleeding into ventricle

P52.2 **Intraventricular (nontraumatic) hemorrhage, grade 3 and grade 4, of newborn**

P52.21 **Intraventricular (nontraumatic) hemorrhage, grade 3, of newborn**

Subependymal hemorrhage with intraventricular extension with enlargement of ventricle

P52.22 **Intraventricular (nontraumatic) hemorrhage, grade 4, of newborn**

Bleeding into cerebral cortex

Subependymal hemorrhage with intracerebral extension

P52.3 **Unspecified intraventricular (nontraumatic) hemorrhage of newborn**

P52.4 **Intracerebral (nontraumatic) hemorrhage of newborn**

P52.5 **Subarachnoid (nontraumatic) hemorrhage of newborn**

P52.6 **Cerebellar (nontraumatic) and posterior fossa hemorrhage of newborn**

P52.8 **Other intracranial (nontraumatic) hemorrhages of newborn**

P52.9 **Intracranial (nontraumatic) hemorrhage of newborn, unspecified**

P53 **Hemorrhagic disease of newborn**

Vitamin K deficiency of newborn

P54 **Other neonatal hemorrhages**

Excludes1: newborn affected by (intrauterine) blood loss (P50.-)

pulmonary hemorrhage originating in the perinatal period (P26.-)

P54.0 **Neonatal hematemesis**

Excludes1: neonatal hematemesis due to swallowed maternal blood (P78.2)

P54.1 **Neonatal melena**

Excludes1: neonatal melena due to swallowed maternal blood (P78.2)

P54.2 **Neonatal rectal hemorrhage**

P54.3 **Other neonatal gastrointestinal hemorrhage**

P54.4 **Neonatal adrenal hemorrhage**

P54.5 **Neonatal cutaneous hemorrhage**

Neonatal bruising

Neonatal ecchymoses

Neonatal petechiae

Neonatal superficial hematomata

Excludes2: bruising of scalp due to birth injury (P12.3)

cephalhematoma due to birth injury (P12.0)

P54.6 **Neonatal vaginal hemorrhage**

Neonatal pseudomenses

P54.8 **Other specified neonatal hemorrhages**

P54.9 **Neonatal hemorrhage, unspecified**

P55 **Hemolytic disease of newborn**

P55.0 **Rh isoimmunization of newborn**

P55.1 **ABO isoimmunization of newborn**

P55.8 **Other hemolytic diseases of newborn**

P55.9 **Hemolytic disease of newborn, unspecified**

P56 **Hydrops fetalis due to hemolytic disease**

Excludes1: hydrops fetalis NOS (P83.2)

P56.0 **Hydrops fetalis due to isoimmunization**

P56.9 **Hydrops fetalis due to other and unspecified hemolytic disease**

P56.90 **Hydrops fetalis due to unspecified hemolytic disease**

P56.99 **Hydrops fetalis due to other hemolytic disease**

P57 **Kernicterus**

Definition: Kernicterus is a disorder that is due to severe jaundice in the newborn, with deposition of the pigment bilirubin in the brain that causes damage to the brain, potentially leading to athetoid cerebral palsy, hearing loss, vision problems, or mental retardation.

P57.0 **Kernicterus due to isoimmunization**

P57.8 **Other specified kernicterus**

Excludes1: Crigler-Najjar syndrome (E80.5)

P57.9 **Kernicterus, unspecified**

P58 **Neonatal jaundice due to other excessive hemolysis**

Excludes1: jaundice due to isoimmunization (P55-P57)

P58.0 **Neonatal jaundice due to bruising**

P58.1 **Neonatal jaundice due to bleeding**

P58.2 **Neonatal jaundice due to infection**

P58.3 **Neonatal jaundice due to polycythemia**

P58.4 **Neonatal jaundice due to drugs or toxins transmitted from mother or given to newborn**

Code first poisoning due to drug or toxin, if applicable (T36-T65 with fifth or sixth character 1-4 or 6)

Use additional code for adverse effect, if applicable, to identify drug (T36-T50 with fifth or sixth character 5)

P58.41 **Neonatal jaundice due to drugs or toxins transmitted from mother**

P58.42 **Neonatal jaundice due to drugs or toxins given to newborn**

P58.5 **Neonatal jaundice due to swallowed maternal blood**

P58.8 **Neonatal jaundice due to other specified excessive hemolysis**

P58.9 **Neonatal jaundice due to excessive hemolysis, unspecified**

P59 **Neonatal jaundice from other and unspecified causes**

Excludes1: jaundice due to inborn errors of metabolism (E70-E88)

kernicterus (P57.-)

P59.0 **Neonatal jaundice associated with preterm delivery**

Hyperbilirubinemia of prematurity

Jaundice due to delayed conjugation associated with preterm delivery

P59.1 **Inspissated bile syndrome**

P59.2 **Neonatal jaundice from other and unspecified hepatocellular damage**

Excludes1: congenital viral hepatitis (P35.3)

P59.20 **Neonatal jaundice from unspecified hepatocellular damage**

P59.29 **Neonatal jaundice from other hepatocellular damage**

Neonatal giant cell hepatitis

Neonatal (idiopathic) hepatitis

P59.3 **Neonatal jaundice from breast milk inhibitor**

P59.8 **Neonatal jaundice from other specified causes**

P59.9 **Neonatal jaundice, unspecified**

Neonatal physiological jaundice (intense)(prolonged) NOS

P60 **Disseminated intravascular coagulation of newborn**

Defibrination syndrome of newborn

P61 **Other perinatal hematological disorders**

Excludes1: transient hypogammaglobulinemia of infancy (D80.7)

P61.0 **Transient neonatal thrombocytopenia**

Neonatal thrombocytopenia due to exchange transfusion

Neonatal thrombocytopenia due to idiopathic maternal thrombocytopenia

Neonatal thrombocytopenia due to isoimmunization

P61.1 **Polycythemia neonatorum**

P61.2 **Anemia of prematurity**

P61.3 **Congenital anemia from fetal blood loss**

P61.4 **Other congenital anemias, not elsewhere classified**

Congenital anemia NOS

P61.5 **Transient neonatal neutropenia**

Excludes1: congenital neutropenia (nontransient) (D70.0)

P61.6 **Other transient neonatal disorders of coagulation**

P61.8 **Other specified perinatal hematological disorders**

P61.9 **Perinatal hematological disorder, unspecified**

TRANSITORY ENDOCRINE AND METABOLIC DISORDERS SPECIFIC TO NEWBORN (P70-P74)

Includes: transitory endocrine and metabolic disturbances caused by the infant's response to maternal endocrine and metabolic factors, or its adjustment to extrauterine environment

P70 **Transitory disorders of carbohydrate metabolism specific to newborn**

P70.0 **Syndrome of infant of mother with gestational diabetes**

Newborn (with hypoglycemia) affected by maternal gestational diabetes

Excludes1: newborn (with hypoglycemia) affected by maternal (pre-existing) diabetes mellitus (P70.1)

syndrome of infant of a diabetic mother (P70.1)

P70.1 **Syndrome of infant of a diabetic mother**

Newborn (with hypoglycemia) affected by maternal (pre-existing) diabetes mellitus

Excludes1: newborn (with hypoglycemia) affected by maternal gestational diabetes (P70.0)

syndrome of infant of mother with gestational diabetes (P70.0)

P70.2 **Neonatal diabetes mellitus**

P70.3 **Iatrogenic neonatal hypoglycemia**

P70.4 **Other neonatal hypoglycemia**

Transitory neonatal hypoglycemia

P70.8 **Other transitory disorders of carbohydrate metabolism of newborn**

P70.9 **Transitory disorder of carbohydrate metabolism of newborn, unspecified**

P71 **Transitory neonatal disorders of calcium and magnesium metabolism**

P71.0 **Cow's milk hypocalcemia in newborn**

P71.1 **Other neonatal hypocalcemia**

Excludes1: neonatal hypoparathyroidism (P71.4)

P71.2 **Neonatal hypomagnesemia**

P71.3 **Neonatal tetany without calcium or magnesium deficiency**

Neonatal tetany NOS

P71.4 **Transitory neonatal hypoparathyroidism**

P71.8 **Other transitory neonatal disorders of calcium and magnesium metabolism**

P71.9 **Transitory neonatal disorder of calcium and magnesium metabolism, unspecified**

P72 **Other transitory neonatal endocrine disorders**

Excludes1: congenital hypothyroidism with or without goiter (E03.0-E03.1)

dyshormogenetic goiter (E07.1)

Pendred's syndrome (E07.1)

P72.0 **Neonatal goiter, not elsewhere classified**

Transitory congenital goiter with normal functioning

P72.1 **Transitory neonatal hyperthyroidism**

Neonatal thyrotoxicosis

P72.2 **Other transitory neonatal disorders of thyroid function, not elsewhere classified**

Transitory neonatal hypothyroidism

P72.8 **Other specified transitory neonatal endocrine disorders**

P72.9 **Transitory neonatal endocrine disorder, unspecified**

P74 **Other transitory neonatal electrolyte and metabolic disturbances**

P74.0 **Late metabolic acidosis of newborn**

Excludes1: (fetal) metabolic acidosis of newborn (P19)

P74.1 **Dehydration of newborn**

P74.2 **Disturbances of sodium balance of newborn**

P74.3 **Disturbances of potassium balance of newborn**

P74.4 **Other transitory electrolyte disturbances of newborn**

P74.5 **Transitory tyrosinemia of newborn**

P74.6 **Transitory hyperammonemia of newborn**

P74.8 **Other transitory metabolic disturbances of newborn**

Amino-acid metabolic disorders described as transitory

P74.9 **Transitory metabolic disturbance of newborn, unspecified**

DIGESTIVE SYSTEM DISORDERS OF NEWBORN (P76-P78)

P76 **Other intestinal obstruction of newborn**

P76.0 **Meconium plug syndrome**

Meconium ileus NOS

Excludes1: meconium ileus in cystic fibrosis (E84.11)

P76.1 **Transitory ileus of newborn**

Excludes1: Hirschsprung's disease (Q43.1)

P76.2 **Intestinal obstruction due to inspissated milk**

P76.8 **Other specified intestinal obstruction of newborn**

Excludes1: intestinal obstruction classifiable to K56.-

P76.9 **Intestinal obstruction of newborn, unspecified**

P77 **Necrotizing enterocolitis of newborn**

P77.1 **Stage 1 necrotizing enterocolitis in newborn**

Necrotizing enterocolitis without pneumatosis, without perforation

P77.2 **Stage 2 necrotizing enterocolitis in newborn**

Necrotizing enterocolitis with pneumatosis, without perforation

P77.3 **Stage 3 necrotizing enterocolitis in newborn**

Necrotizing enterocolitis with perforation

Necrotizing enterocolitis with pneumatosis and perforation

P77.9   **Necrotizing enterocolitis in newborn, unspecified**

Necrotizing enterocolitis in newborn, NOS

P78   **Other perinatal digestive system disorders**

Excludes1: cystic fibrosis (E84.0-E84.9)

neonatal gastrointestinal hemorrhages (P54.0-P54.3)

P78.0   **Perinatal intestinal perforation**

Meconium peritonitis

P78.1   **Other neonatal peritonitis**

Neonatal peritonitis NOS

P78.2   **Neonatal hematemesis and melena due to swallowed maternal blood**

P78.3   **Noninfective neonatal diarrhea**

Neonatal diarrhea NOS

P78.8   **Other specified perinatal digestive system disorders**

P78.81   **Congenital cirrhosis (of liver)**

P78.82   **Peptic ulcer of newborn**

P78.83   **Newborn esophageal reflux**

Neonatal esophageal reflux

P78.89   **Other specified perinatal digestive system disorders**

P78.9   **Perinatal digestive system disorder, unspecified**

CONDITIONS INVOLVING THE INTEGUMENT AND TEMPERATURE REGULATION OF NEWBORN (P80-P83)

P80   **Hypothermia of newborn**

P80.0   **Cold injury syndrome**

Severe and usually chronic hypothermia associated with a pink flushed appearance, edema and neurological and biochemical abnormalities.

Excludes1: mild hypothermia of newborn (P80.8)

P80.8   **Other hypothermia of newborn**

Mild hypothermia of newborn

P80.9   **Hypothermia of newborn, unspecified**

P81   **Other disturbances of temperature regulation of newborn**

P81.0   **Environmental hyperthermia of newborn**

P81.8   **Other specified disturbances of temperature regulation of newborn**

P81.9   **Disturbance of temperature regulation of newborn, unspecified**

Fever of newborn NOS

P83   **Other conditions of integument specific to newborn**

Excludes1: congenital malformations of skin and integument (Q80-Q84)

hydrops fetalis due to hemolytic disease (P56.-)

neonatal skin infection (P39.4)

staphylococcal scalded skin syndrome (L00)

Excludes2: cradle cap (L21.0)

diaper [napkin] dermatitis (L22)

P83.0   **Sclerema neonatorum**

P83.1   **Neonatal erythema toxicum**

P83.2   **Hydrops fetalis not due to hemolytic disease**

Hydrops fetalis NOS

P83.3   **Other and unspecified edema specific to newborn**

P83.30   **Unspecified edema specific to newborn**

P83.39   **Other edema specific to newborn**

P83.4   **Breast engorgement of newborn**

Noninfective mastitis of newborn

P83.5   **Congenital hydrocele**

P83.6   **Umbilical polyp of newborn**

P83.8   **Other specified conditions of integument specific to newborn**

Bronze baby syndrome

Neonatal scleroderma

Urticaria neonatorum

P83.9   **Condition of the integument specific to newborn, unspecified**

OTHER PROBLEMS WITH NEWBORN (P84)

P84   **Other problems with newborn**

Acidemia of newborn

Acidosis of newborn

Anoxia of newborn NOS

Asphyxia of newborn NOS

Hypercapnia of newborn

Hypoxemia of newborn

Hypoxia of newborn NOS

Mixed metabolic and respiratory acidosis of newborn

Excludes1: intracranial hemorrhage due to anoxia or hypoxia (P52.-)

hypoxic ischemic encephalopathy [HIE] (P91.6-)

late metabolic acidosis of newborn (P74.0)

OTHER DISORDERS ORIGINATING IN THE PERINATAL PERIOD (P90-P96)

P90   **Convulsions of newborn**

Excludes1: benign myoclonic epilepsy in infancy (G40.3-)

benign neonatal convulsions (familial) (G40.3-)

P91   **Other disturbances of cerebral status of newborn**

P91.0   **Neonatal cerebral ischemia**

P91.1   **Acquired periventricular cysts of newborn**

P91.2   **Neonatal cerebral leukomalacia**

Periventricular leukomalacia

P91.3   **Neonatal cerebral irritability**

P91.4   **Neonatal cerebral depression**

P91.5   **Neonatal coma**

P91.6   **Hypoxic ischemic encephalopathy [HIE]**

P91.60   **Hypoxic ischemic encephalopathy [HIE], unspecified**

P91.61   **Mild hypoxic ischemic encephalopathy [HIE]**

P91.62   **Moderate hypoxic ischemic encephalopathy [HIE]**

P91.63   **Severe hypoxic ischemic encephalopathy [HIE]**

P91.8   **Other specified disturbances of cerebral status of newborn**

P91.9   **Disturbance of cerebral status of newborn, unspecified**

P92   **Feeding problems of newborn**

Excludes1: feeding problems in child over 28 days old (R63.3)

P92.0   **Vomiting of newborn**

Excludes1: vomiting of child over 28 days old (R11.-)

P92.01   **Bilious vomiting of newborn**

Excludes1: bilious vomiting in child over 28 days old (R11.14)

P92.09 **Other vomiting of newborn**

Excludes1: regurgitation of food in newborn (P92.1)

P92.1 **Regurgitation and rumination of newborn**

P92.2 **Slow feeding of newborn**

P92.3 **Underfeeding of newborn**

P92.4 **Overfeeding of newborn**

P92.5 **Neonatal difficulty in feeding at breast**

P92.6 **Failure to thrive in newborn**

Excludes1: failure to thrive in child over 28 days old (R62.51)

P92.8 **Other feeding problems of newborn**

P92.9 **Feeding problem of newborn, unspecified**

P93 **Reactions and intoxications due to drugs administered to newborn**

Includes: reactions and intoxications due to drugs administered to fetus affecting newborn

Excludes1: jaundice due to drugs or toxins transmitted from mother or given to newborn (P58.4-)

reactions and intoxications from maternal opiates, tranquilizers **and other** medication (P04.0-P04.1, P04.4)

withdrawal symptoms from maternal use of drugs of addiction (P96.1)

withdrawal symptoms from therapeutic use of drugs in newborn (P96.2)

P93.0 **Grey baby syndrome**

Grey syndrome from chloramphenicol administration in newborn

P93.8 **Other reactions and intoxications due to drugs administered to newborn**

Use additional code for adverse effect, if applicable, to identify drug (T36-T50 with fifth or sixth character 5)

P94 **Disorders of muscle tone of newborn**

P94.0 **Transient neonatal myasthenia gravis**

Excludes1: myasthenia gravis (G70.0)

P94.1 **Congenital hypertonia**

P94.2 **Congenital hypotonia**

Floppy baby syndrome, unspecified

P94.8 **Other disorders of muscle tone of newborn**

P94.9 **Disorder of muscle tone of newborn, unspecified**

P95 **Stillbirth**

Deadborn fetus NOS

Fetal death of unspecified cause

Stillbirth NOS

Excludes1: maternal care for intrauterine death (O36.4)

missed abortion (O02.1)

outcome of delivery, stillbirth (Z37.1, Z37.3, Z37.4, Z37.7)

P96 **Other conditions originating in the perinatal period**

P96.0 **Congenital renal failure**

Uremia of newborn

P96.1 **Neonatal withdrawal symptoms from maternal use of drugs of addiction**

Drug withdrawal syndrome in infant of dependent mother

Neonatal abstinence syndrome

Excludes1: reactions and intoxications from maternal opiates and tranquilizers administered during labor and delivery (P04.0)

P96.2 **Withdrawal symptoms from therapeutic use of drugs in newborn**

P96.3 **Wide cranial sutures of newborn**

Neonatal craniotabes

P96.5 **Complication to newborn due to (fetal) intrauterine procedure**

Excludes2: newborn affected by amniocentesis (P00.6)

P96.8 **Other specified conditions originating in the perinatal period**

P96.81 **Exposure to (parental) (environmental) tobacco smoke in the perinatal period**

Excludes2: newborn affected by in utero exposure to tobacco (P04.2)

exposure to environmental tobacco smoke after the perinatal period (Z77.22)

P96.82 **Delayed separation of umbilical cord**

P96.83 **Meconium staining**

Excludes1: meconium aspiration (P24.00, P24.01)

meconium passage during delivery (P03.82)

P96.89 **Other specified conditions originating in the perinatal period**

Use additional code to specify condition

P96.9 **Condition originating in the perinatal period, unspecified**

Congenital debility NOS

• New code ▲ Revised code **Excludes1:** Not coded here **Excludes2:** Not included here ⊗ Placeholder required ⑦7th digit required

Chapter 17: Congenital Malformations, Deformations And Chromosomal Abnormalities (Q00-Q99)

DEFINITIONS

This chapter includes definitions of selected key words, terms and phrases and coding alerts for adding points to the clinical domain, and references to coding late effects where appropriate. An example from this chapter is as follows:

Q11   Anophthalmos, microphthalmos and macrophthalmos
      Definition: Anophthalmos is the absence of one or both eyes. Both the globe and the ocular tissue are missing from the orbit.

MULTIPLE CODING FOR A SINGLE CONDITION

In addition to the etiology/manifestation convention that requires two codes to fully describe a single condition that affects multiple body systems, there are other single conditions that also require more than one code. "Use additional code" notes are found in the Tabular List at codes that are not part of an etiology/manifestation pair where a secondary code is useful to fully describe a condition. The sequencing rule is the same as the etiology/manifestation pair, "use additional code" indicates that a secondary code should be added.

For example, for bacterial infections that are not included in chapter 1, a secondary code from category B95, Streptococcus, Staphylococcus, and Enterococcus, as the cause of diseases classified elsewhere, or B96, Other bacterial agents as the cause of diseases classified elsewhere, may be required to identify the bacterial organism causing the infection. A "use additional code" note will normally be found at the infectious disease code, indicating a need for the organism code to be added as a secondary code.

"Code first" notes are also under certain codes that are not specifically manifestation codes but may be due to an underlying cause. When there is a "code first" note and an underlying condition is present, the underlying condition should be sequenced first.

"Code, if applicable, any causal condition first", notes indicate that this code may be assigned as a principal diagnosis when the causal condition is unknown or not applicable. If a causal condition is known, then the code for that condition should be sequenced as the principal or first-listed diagnosis.

Multiple codes may be needed for sequela, complication codes and obstetric codes to more fully describe a condition. See the specific guidelines for these conditions for further instruction.

COMBINATION CODE

A combination code is a single code used to classify: Two diagnoses, or a diagnosis with an associated secondary process (manifestation) A diagnosis with an associated complication

Combination codes are identified by referring to subterm entries in the Alphabetic Index and by reading the inclusion and exclusion notes in the Tabular List.

Assign only the combination code when that code fully identifies the diagnostic conditions involved or when the Alphabetic Index so directs. Multiple coding should not be used when the classification provides a combination code that clearly identifies all of the elements documented in the diagnosis. When the combination code lacks necessary specificity in describing the manifestation or complication, an additional code should be used as a secondary code.

SEQUELA (LATE EFFECTS)

A sequela is the residual effect (condition produced) after the acute phase of an illness or injury has terminated. There is no time limit on when a sequela code can be used. The residual may be apparent early, such as in cerebral infarction, or it may occur months or years later, such as that due to a previous injury. Coding of sequela generally requires two codes sequenced in the following order: The condition or nature of the sequela is sequenced first.

The sequela code is sequenced second.

An exception to the above guidelines are those instances where the code for the sequela is followed by a manifestation code identified in the Tabular List and title, or the sequela code has been expanded (at the fourth, fifth or sixth character levels) to include the manifestation(s). The code for the acute phase of an illness or injury that led to the sequela is never used with a code for the late effect.

Assign an appropriate code(s) from categories Q00-Q99, Congenital malformations, deformations, and chromosomal abnormalities when a malformation/deformation or chromosomal abnormality is documented. A malformation/deformation/or chromosomal abnormality may be the principal/first-listed diagnosis on a record or a secondary diagnosis.

Q00-Q99

When a malformation/deformation or chromosomal abnormality does not have a unique code assignment, assign additional code(s) for any manifestations that may be present.

When the code assignment specifically identifies the malformation/deformation or chromosomal abnormality, manifestations that are an inherent component of the anomaly should not be coded separately. Additional codes should be assigned for manifestations that are not an inherent component.

Codes from Chapter 17 may be used throughout the life of the patient. If a congenital malformation or deformity has been corrected, a personal history code should be used to identify the history of the malformation or deformity. Although present at birth, malformation/deformation/or chromosomal abnormality may not be identified until later in life. Whenever the condition is diagnosed by the physician, it is appropriate to assign a code from codes Q00-Q99. For the birth admission, the appropriate code from category Z38, Liveborn infants, according to place of birth and type of delivery, should be sequenced as the principal diagnosis, followed by any congenital anomaly codes, Q00-Q99.

Chapter 17

Congenital Malformations, Deformations And Chromosomal Abnormalities (Q00-Q99)

Note: Codes from this chapter are not for use on maternal or fetal records

Excludes2: inborn errors of metabolism (E70-E88)

This chapter contains the following blocks:

Q00-Q07	Congenital malformations of the nervous system
Q10-Q18	Congenital malformations of eye, ear, face and neck
Q20-Q28	Congenital malformations of the circulatory system
Q30-Q34	Congenital malformations of the respiratory system
Q35-Q37	Cleft lip and cleft palate
Q38-Q45	Other congenital malformations of the digestive system
Q50-Q56	Congenital malformations of genital organs
Q60-Q64	Congenital malformations of the urinary system
Q65-Q79	Congenital malformations and deformations of the musculoskeletal system
Q80-Q89	Other congenital malformations
Q90-Q99	Chromosomal abnormalities, not elsewhere classified

CONGENITAL MALFORMATIONS OF THE NERVOUS SYSTEM (Q00-Q07)

Q00 **Anencephaly and similar malformations**

Definition: Anencephaly is the absence of a major portion of the brain, skull, and scalp that occurs during embryonic development.

Q00.0 **Anencephaly**

Acephaly

Acrania

Amyelencephaly

Hemianencephaly

Hemicephaly

Q00.1 **Craniorachischisis**

Q00.2 **Iniencephaly**

Q01 **Encephalocele**

Includes: Arnold-Chiari syndrome, type III

encephalocystocele

encephalomyelocele

hydroencephalocele

hydromeningocele, cranial meningocele, cerebral meningoencephalocele

Excludes1: Meckel-Gruber syndrome (Q61.9)

Q01.0 **Frontal encephalocele**

Q01.1 **Nasofrontal encephalocele**

Q01.2 **Occipital encephalocele**

Q01.8 **Encephalocele of other sites**

Q01.9 **Encephalocele, unspecified**

Q02 **Microcephaly**

Includes: hydromicrocephaly

micrencephalon

Excludes1: Meckel-Gruber syndrome (Q61.9)

Q03 **Congenital hydrocephalus**

Includes: hydrocephalus in newborn

Excludes1: Arnold-Chiari syndrome, type II (Q07.0-)

acquired hydrocephalus (G91.-)

hydrocephalus due to congenital toxoplasmosis (P37.1)

hydrocephalus with spina bifida (Q05.0-Q05.4)

Q03.0 **Malformations of aqueduct of Sylvius**

Anomaly of aqueduct of Sylvius

Obstruction of aqueduct of Sylvius, congenital

Stenosis of aqueduct of Sylvius

Q03.1 **Atresia of foramina of Magendie and Luschka**

Dandy-Walker syndrome

Q03.8 **Other congenital hydrocephalus**

Q03.9 **Congenital hydrocephalus, unspecified**

Q04 **Other congenital malformations of brain**

Excludes1: cyclopia (Q87.0)

macrocephaly (Q75.3)

Q04.0 **Congenital malformations of corpus callosum**

Agenesis of corpus callosum

Q04.1 **Arhinencephaly**

Q04.2 **Holoprosencephaly**

Q04.3 **Other reduction deformities of brain**

Absence of part of brain

Agenesis of part of brain

Agyria

Aplasia of part of brain

Hydranencephaly

Hypoplasia of part of brain

Lissencephaly

Microgyria

Pachygyria

Excludes1: congenital malformations of corpus callosum (Q04.0)

Q04.4 **Septo-optic dysplasia of brain**

Q04.5 **Megalencephaly**

Q04.6 **Congenital cerebral cysts**

Porencephaly

Schizencephaly

Excludes1: acquired porencephalic cyst (G93.0)

Q04.8 **Other specified congenital malformations of brain**

Arnold-Chiari syndrome, type IV

Macrogyria

Q04.9 **Congenital malformation of brain, unspecified**

Congenital anomaly NOS of brain

Congenital deformity NOS of brain

Congenital disease or lesion NOS of brain

Multiple anomalies NOS of brain, congenital

Q05 **Spina bifida**

Definition: Spina bifida is a serious birth abnormality in which the spinal cord is malformed and lacks its usual protective skeletal and soft tissue coverings.

Includes: hydromeningocele (spinal)

meningocele (spinal)

meningomyelocele

myelocele

myelomeningocele

rachischisis

spina bifida (aperta)(cystica)

syringomyelocele

Use additional code for any associated paraplegia (paraparesis) (G82.2-)

Excludes1: Arnold-Chiari syndrome, type II (Q07.0-)

spina bifida occulta (Q76.0)

Q05.0   **Cervical spina bifida with hydrocephalus**

Q05.1   **Thoracic spina bifida with hydrocephalus**

Dorsal spina bifida with hydrocephalus

Thoracolumbar spina bifida with hydrocephalus

Q05.2   **Lumbar spina bifida with hydrocephalus**

Lumbosacral spina bifida with hydrocephalus

Q05.3   **Sacral spina bifida with hydrocephalus**

Q05.4   **Unspecified spina bifida with hydrocephalus**

Q05.5   **Cervical spina bifida without hydrocephalus**

Q05.6   **Thoracic spina bifida without hydrocephalus**

Dorsal spina bifida NOS

Thoracolumbar spina bifida NOS

Q05.7   **Lumbar spina bifida without hydrocephalus**

Lumbosacral spina bifida NOS

Q05.8   **Sacral spina bifida without hydrocephalus**

Q05.9   **Spina bifida, unspecified**

Q06   **Other congenital malformations of spinal cord**

Q06.0   **Amyelia**

Q06.1   **Hypoplasia and dysplasia of spinal cord**

Atelomyelia

Myelatelia

Myelodysplasia of spinal cord

Q06.2   **Diastematomyelia**

Q06.3   **Other congenital cauda equina malformations**

Q06.4   **Hydromyelia**

Hydrorachis

Q06.8   **Other specified congenital malformations of spinal cord**

Q06.9   **Congenital malformation of spinal cord, unspecified**

Congenital anomaly NOS of spinal cord

Congenital deformity NOS of spinal cord

Congenital disease or lesion NOS of spinal cord

Q07   **Other congenital malformations of nervous system**

Excludes2: congenital central alveolar hypoventilation syndrome (G47.35)

familial dysautonomia [Riley-Day] (G90.1)

neurofibromatosis (nonmalignant) (Q85.0-)

Q07.0   **Arnold-Chiari syndrome**

Arnold-Chiari syndrome, type II

Excludes1: Arnold-Chiari syndrome, type III (Q01.-)

Arnold-Chiari syndrome, type IV (Q04.8)

Q07.00   **Arnold-Chiari syndrome without spina bifida or hydrocephalus**

Q07.01   **Arnold-Chiari syndrome with spina bifida**

Q07.02   **Arnold-Chiari syndrome with hydrocephalus**

Q07.03   **Arnold-Chiari syndrome with spina bifida and hydrocephalus**

Q07.8   **Other specified congenital malformations of nervous system**

Agenesis of nerve

Displacement of brachial plexus Jaw-winking syndrome

Marcus Gunn's syndrome

Q07.9   **Congenital malformation of nervous system, unspecified**

Congenital anomaly NOS of nervous system

Congenital deformity NOS of nervous system

Congenital disease or lesion NOS of nervous system

CONGENITAL MALFORMATIONS OF EYE, EAR, FACE AND NECK (Q10-Q18)

Excludes2: cleft lip and cleft palate (Q35-Q37)

congenital malformation of cervical spine (Q05.0, Q05.5, Q67.5, Q76.0-Q76.4)

congenital malformation of larynx (Q31.-)

congenital malformation of lip NEC (Q38.0)

congenital malformation of nose (Q30.-)

congenital malformation of parathyroid gland (Q89.2)

congenital malformation of thyroid gland (Q89.2)

Q10   **Congenital malformations of eyelid, lacrimal apparatus and orbit**

Excludes1: cryptophthalmos NOS (Q11.2)

cryptophthalmos syndrome (Q87.0)

Q10.0   **Congenital ptosis**

Q10.1   **Congenital ectropion**

Q10.2   **Congenital entropion**

Q10.3   **Other congenital malformations of eyelid**

Ablepharon

Blepharophimosis, congenital

Coloboma of eyelid

Congenital absence or agenesis of cilia

Congenital absence or agenesis of eyelid

Congenital accessory eyelid

Congenital accessory eye muscle

Congenital malformation of eyelid NOS

Q10.4   **Absence and agenesis of lacrimal apparatus**

Congenital absence of punctum lacrimale

Q10.5   **Congenital stenosis and stricture of lacrimal duct**

Q10.6   **Other congenital malformations of lacrimal apparatus**

Congenital malformation of lacrimal apparatus NOS

Q10.7   **Congenital malformation of orbit**

Q11   **Anophthalmos, microphthalmos and macrophthalmos**

Q11.0   **Cystic eyeball**

Q11.1   **Other anophthalmos**

Anophthalmos NOS

Agenesis of eye

Aplasia of eye

Q11.2   **Microphthalmos**

Cryptophthalmos NOS

Dysplasia of eye

Hypoplasia of eye

Rudimentary eye

Excludes1: cryptophthalmos syndrome (Q87.0)

Q11.3   **Macrophthalmos**

Excludes1: macrophthalmos in congenital glaucoma (Q15.0)

Q12   **Congenital lens malformations**

● New code   ▲ Revised code   **Excludes1:** Not coded here   **Excludes2:** Not included here   ⊗ Placeholder required   ⑦7th digit required

Q12.0   **Congenital cataract**

Q12.1   **Congenital displaced lens**

Q12.2   **Coloboma of lens**

Q12.3   **Congenital aphakia**

Q12.4   **Spherophakia**

Q12.8   **Other congenital lens malformations**

Microphakia

Q12.9   **Congenital lens malformation, unspecified**

Q13   **Congenital malformations of anterior segment of eye**

Q13.0   **Coloboma of iris**

Coloboma NOS

Q13.1   **Absence of iris**

Aniridia

<u>**Use additional code**</u> for associated glaucoma (H42)

Q13.2   **Other congenital malformations of iris**

Anisocoria, congenital

Atresia of pupil

Congenital malformation of iris NOS

Corectopia

Q13.3   **Congenital corneal opacity**

Q13.4   **Other congenital corneal malformations**

Congenital malformation of cornea NOS

Microcornea

Peter's anomaly

Q13.5   **Blue sclera**

Q13.8   **Other congenital malformations of anterior segment of eye**

Q13.81   **Rieger's anomaly**

<u>**Use additional code**</u> for associated glaucoma (H42)

Q13.89   **Other congenital malformations of anterior segment of eye**

Q13.9   **Congenital malformation of anterior segment of eye, unspecified**

Q14   **Congenital malformations of posterior segment of eye**

Excludes2: optic nerve hypoplasia (H47.03-)

Q14.0   **Congenital malformation of vitreous humor**

Congenital vitreous opacity

Q14.1   **Congenital malformation of retina**

Congenital retinal aneurysm

Q14.2   **Congenital malformation of optic disc**

Coloboma of optic disc

Q14.3   **Congenital malformation of choroid**

Q14.8   **Other congenital malformations of posterior segment of eye**

Coloboma of the fundus

Q14.9   **Congenital malformation of posterior segment of eye, unspecified**

Q15   **Other congenital malformations of eye**

Excludes1: congenital nystagmus (H55.01)

ocular albinism (E70.31-)

optic nerve hypoplasia (H47.03-)

retinitis pigmentosa (H35.52)

Q15.0   **Congenital glaucoma**

Axenfeld's anomaly

Buphthalmos Glaucoma of childhood Glaucoma of newborn Hydrophthalmos

Keratoglobus, congenital, with glaucoma

Macrocornea with glaucoma

Macrophthalmos in congenital glaucoma

Megalocornea with glaucoma

Q15.8   **Other specified congenital malformations of eye**

Q15.9   **Congenital malformation of eye, unspecified**

Congenital anomaly of eye

Congenital deformity of eye

Q16   **Congenital malformations of ear causing impairment of hearing**

Excludes1: congenital deafness (H90.-)

Q16.0   **Congenital absence of (ear) auricle**

Q16.1   **Congenital absence, atresia and stricture of auditory canal (external)**

Congenital atresia or stricture of osseous meatus

Q16.2   **Absence of eustachian tube**

Q16.3   **Congenital malformation of ear ossicles**

Congenital fusion of ear ossicles

Q16.4   **Other congenital malformations of middle ear**

Congenital malformation of middle ear NOS

Q16.5   **Congenital malformation of inner ear**

Congenital anomaly of membranous labyrinth

Congenital anomaly of organ of Corti

Q16.9   **Congenital malformation of ear causing impairment of hearing, unspecified**

Congenital absence of ear NOS

Q17   **Other congenital malformations of ear**

Excludes1: congenital malformations of ear with impairment of hearing (Q16.0-Q16.9)

preauricular sinus (Q18.1)

Q17.0   **Accessory auricle**

Accessory tragus

Polyotia

Preauricular appendage or tag

Supernumerary ear

Supernumerary lobule

Q17.1   **Macrotia**

Q17.2   **Microtia**

Q17.3   **Other misshapen ear**

Pointed ear

Q17.4   **Misplaced ear**

Low-set ears

Excludes1: cervical auricle (Q18.2)

Q17.5   **Prominent ear**

Bat ear

Q17.8   **Other specified congenital malformations of ear**

Congenital absence of lobe of ear

Q17.9   **Congenital malformation of ear, unspecified**

Congenital anomaly of ear NOS

Q18   **Other congenital malformations of face and neck**

Excludes1: cleft lip and cleft palate (Q35-Q37)

conditions classified to Q67.0-Q67.4

congenital malformations of skull and face bones (Q75.-)

cyclopia (Q87.0)

dentofacial anomalies [including malocclusion] (M26.-)

malformation syndromes affecting facial appearance (Q87.0)

persistent thyroglossal duct (Q89.2)

Q18.0   Sinus, fistula and cyst of branchial cleft Branchial vestige

Q18.1   Preauricular sinus and cyst

Fistula of auricle, congenital

Cervicoaural fistula

Q18.2   Other branchial cleft malformations

Branchial cleft malformation NOS

Cervical auricle

Otocephaly

Q18.3   Webbing of neck

Pterygium colli

Q18.4   Macrostomia

Q18.5   Microstomia

Q18.6   Macrocheilia

Hypertrophy of lip, congenital

Q18.7   Microcheilia

Q18.8   Other specified congenital malformations of face and neck

Medial cyst of face and neck

Medial fistula of face and neck

Medial sinus of face and neck

Q18.9   Congenital malformation of face and neck, unspecified

Congenital anomaly NOS of face and neck

CONGENITAL MALFORMATIONS OF THE CIRCULATORY SYSTEM (Q20-Q28)

Q20   Congenital malformations of cardiac chambers and connections

Excludes1: dextrocardia with situs inversus (Q89.3)

mirror-image atrial arrangement with situs inversus (Q89.3)

Q20.0   Common arterial trunk

Persistent truncus arteriosus

Excludes1: aortic septal defect (Q21.4)

Q20.1   Double outlet right ventricle

Taussig-Bing syndrome

Q20.2   Double outlet left ventricle

Q20.3   Discordant ventriculoarterial connection

Dextrotransposition of aorta

Transposition of great vessels (complete)

Q20.4   Double inlet ventricle

Common ventricle

Cor triloculare biatriatum

Single ventricle

Q20.5   Discordant atrioventricular connection

Corrected transposition

Levotransposition

Ventricular inversion

Q20.6   Isomerism of atrial appendages

Isomerism of atrial appendages with asplenia or polysplenia

Q20.8   Other congenital malformations of cardiac chambers and connections

Cor binoculare

Q20.9   Congenital malformation of cardiac chambers and connections, unspecified

Q21   Congenital malformations of cardiac septa

Excludes1: acquired cardiac septal defect (I51.0)

Q21.0   Ventricular septal defect

Roger's disease

Q21.1   Atrial septal defect

Coronary sinus defect

Patent or persistent foramen ovale

Patent or persistent ostium secundum defect (type II)

Patent or persistent sinus venosus defect

Q21.2   Atrioventricular septal defect

Common atrioventricular canal

Endocardial cushion defect

Ostium primum atrial septal defect (type I)

Q21.3   Tetralogy of Fallot

Definition: Tetralogy of Fallot, which is one of the most common congenital heart disorders, comprises right ventricular (RV) outflow tract obstruction (RVOTO) (infundibular stenosis), ventricular septal defect (VSD), aorta dextroposition, and RV hypertrophy.

Ventricular septal defect with pulmonary stenosis or atresia, dextroposition of aorta and hypertrophy of right ventricle.

Q21.4   Aortopulmonary septal defect

Aortic septal defect

Aortopulmonary window

Q21.8   Other congenital malformations of cardiac septa

Eisenmenger's defect

Pentalogy of Fallot

Excludes1: Eisenmenger's complex (I27.8)

Eisenmenger's syndrome (I27.8)

Q21.9   Congenital malformation of cardiac septum, unspecified

Septal (heart) defect NOS

Q22   Congenital malformations of pulmonary and tricuspid valves

Q22.0   Pulmonary valve atresia

Q22.1   Congenital pulmonary valve stenosis

Q22.2   Congenital pulmonary valve insufficiency

Congenital pulmonary valve regurgitation

Q22.3   Other congenital malformations of pulmonary valve

Congenital malformation of pulmonary valve NOS

Supernumerary cusps of pulmonary valve

Q22.4   Congenital tricuspid stenosis

Congenital tricuspid atresia

Q22.5   Ebstein's anomaly

Q22.6   Hypoplastic right heart syndrome

Q22.8   Other congenital malformations of tricuspid valve

Q22.9   Congenital malformation of tricuspid valve, unspecified

Q23   Congenital malformations of aortic and mitral valves

Q23.0   Congenital stenosis of aortic valve

Congenital aortic atresia

Congenital aortic stenosis NOS

Excludes1: congenital stenosis of aortic valve in hypoplastic left heart syndrome (Q23.4)

congenital subaortic stenosis (Q24.4)

supravalvular aortic stenosis (congenital) (Q25.3)

Q23.1 Congenital insufficiency of aortic valve

Bicuspid aortic valve

Congenital aortic insufficiency

Q23.2 Congenital mitral stenosis

Congenital mitral atresia

Q23.3 Congenital mitral insufficiency

Q23.4 Hypoplastic left heart syndrome

Q23.8 Other congenital malformations of aortic and mitral valves

Q23.9 Congenital malformation of aortic and mitral valves, unspecified

Q24 Other congenital malformations of heart

Excludes1: endocardial fibroelastosis (I42.4)

Q24.0 Dextrocardia

Excludes1: dextrocardia with situs inversus (Q89.3)

isomerism of atrial appendages (with asplenia or polysplenia) (Q20.6)

mirror-image atrial arrangement with situs inversus (Q89.3)

Q24.1 Levocardia

Q24.2 Cor triatriatum

Q24.3 Pulmonary infundibular stenosis

Subvalvular pulmonic stenosis

Q24.4 Congenital subaortic stenosis

Q24.5 Malformation of coronary vessels

Congenital coronary (artery) aneurysm

Q24.6 Congenital heart block

Q24.8 Other specified congenital malformations of heart

Congenital diverticulum of left ventricle

Congenital malformation of myocardium

Congenital malformation of pericardium

Malposition of heart

Uhl's disease

Q24.9 Congenital malformation of heart, unspecified

Congenital anomaly of heart

Congenital disease of heart

Q25 Congenital malformations of great arteries

Q25.0 Patent ductus arteriosus

Patent ductus

Botallo

Persistent ductus arteriosus

Q25.1 Coarctation of aorta

Coarctation of aorta (preductal) (postductal)

Stenosis of aorta

Q25.2 Atresia of aorta

●**Q25.21 Interruption of aortic arch**

Atresia of aortic arch

●**Q25.29 Other atresia of aorta**

Atresia of aorta

Q25.3 Supravalvular aortic stenosis

Excludes1: congenital aortic stenosis NOS (Q23.0)

congenital stenosis of aortic valve (Q23.0)

Q25.4 Other congenital malformations of aorta

Excludes1: hypoplasia of aorta in hypoplastic left heart syndrome (Q23.4)

●**Q25.40 Congenital malformation of aorta unspecified**

●**Q25.41 Absence and aplasia of aorta**

●**Q25.42 Hypoplasia of aorta**

●**Q25.43 Congenital aneurysm of aorta**

Congenital aneurysm of aortic root

Congenital aneurysm of aortic sinus

●**Q25.44 Congenital dilation of aorta**

●**Q25.45 Double aortic arch**

Vascular ring of aorta

●**Q25.46 Tortuous aortic arch**

Persistent convolutions of aortic arch

●**Q25.47 Right aortic arch**

Persistent right aortic arch

●**Q25.48 Anomalous origin of subclavian artery**

●**Q25.49 Other congenital malformations of aorta**

Q25.5 Atresia of pulmonary artery

Q25.6 Stenosis of pulmonary artery

Supravalvular pulmonary stenosis

Q25.7 Other congenital malformations of pulmonary artery

Q25.71 Coarctation of pulmonary artery

Q25.72 Congenital pulmonary arteriovenous malformation

Congenital pulmonary arteriovenous aneurysm

Q25.79 Other congenital malformations of pulmonary artery

Aberrant pulmonary artery

Agenesis of pulmonary artery

Congenital aneurysm of pulmonary artery

Congenital anomaly of pulmonary artery

Hypoplasia of pulmonary artery

Q25.8 Other congenital malformations of other great arteries

Q25.9 Congenital malformation of great arteries, unspecified

Q26 Congenital malformations of great veins

Q26.0 Congenital stenosis of vena cava

Congenital stenosis of vena cava (inferior)(superior)

Q26.1 Persistent left superior vena cava

Q26.2 Total anomalous pulmonary venous connection

Total anomalous pulmonary venous return [TAPVR], subdiaphragmatic

Total anomalous pulmonary venous return [TAPVR], supradiaphragmatic

Q26.3 Partial anomalous pulmonary venous connection

Partial anomalous pulmonary venous return

Q26.4 Anomalous pulmonary venous connection, unspecified

Q26.5 Anomalous portal venous connection

Q26.6 Portal vein-hepatic artery fistula

Q26.8 Other congenital malformations of great veins

Absence of vena cava (inferior) (superior)

Azygos continuation of inferior vena cava

Persistent left posterior cardinal vein

Scimitar syndrome

Q26.9 **Congenital malformation of great vein, unspecified**
Congenital anomaly of vena cava (inferior) (superior) NOS

Q27 **Other congenital malformations of peripheral vascular system**
Excludes2: anomalies of cerebral and precerebral vessels (Q28.0-Q28.3)
anomalies of coronary vessels (Q24.5)
anomalies of pulmonary artery (Q25.5-Q25.7)
congenital retinal aneurysm (Q14.1)
hemangioma and lymphangioma (D18.-)

Q27.0 **Congenital absence and hypoplasia of umbilical artery**
Single umbilical artery

Q27.1 **Congenital renal artery stenosis**

Q27.2 **Other congenital malformations of renal artery**
Congenital malformation of renal artery NOS
Multiple renal arteries

Q27.3 **Arteriovenous malformation (peripheral)**
Arteriovenous aneurysm
Excludes1: acquired arteriovenous aneurysm (I77.0)
Excludes2: arteriovenous malformation of cerebral vessels (Q28.2)
arteriovenous malformation of precerebral vessels (Q28.0)

Q27.30 **Arteriovenous malformation, site unspecified**

Q27.31 **Arteriovenous malformation of vessel of upper limb**

Q27.32 **Arteriovenous malformation of vessel of lower limb**

Q27.33 **Arteriovenous malformation of digestive system vessel**

Q27.34 **Arteriovenous malformation of renal vessel**

Q27.39 **Arteriovenous malformation, other site**

Q27.4 **Congenital phlebectasia**

Q27.8 **Other specified congenital malformations of peripheral vascular system**
Absence of peripheral vascular system
Atresia of peripheral vascular system
Congenital aneurysm (peripheral)
Congenital stricture, artery
Congenital varix
Excludes1: arteriovenous malformation (Q27.3-)

Q27.9 **Congenital malformation of peripheral vascular system, unspecified**
Anomaly of artery or vein NOS

Q28 **Other congenital malformations of circulatory system**
Excludes1: congenital aneurysm NOS (Q27.8)
congenital coronary aneurysm (Q24.5)
ruptured cerebral arteriovenous malformation (I60.8)
ruptured malformation of precerebral vessels (I72.0)
Excludes2: congenital peripheral aneurysm (Q27.8)
congenital pulmonary aneurysm (Q25.79)
congenital retinal aneurysm (Q14.1)

Q28.0 **Arteriovenous malformation of precerebral vessels**
Congenital arteriovenous precerebral aneurysm (nonruptured)

Q28.1 **Other malformations of precerebral vessels**
Congenital malformation of precerebral vessels NOS

Congenital precerebral aneurysm (nonruptured)

Q28.2 **Arteriovenous malformation of cerebral vessels**
Arteriovenous malformation of brain NOS
Congenital arteriovenous cerebral aneurysm (nonruptured)

Q28.3 **Other malformations of cerebral vessels**
Congenital cerebral aneurysm (nonruptured)
Congenital malformation of cerebral vessels NOS
Developmental venous anomaly

Q28.8 **Other specified congenital malformations of circulatory system**
Congenital aneurysm, specified site NEC
Spinal vessel anomaly

Q28.9 **Congenital malformation of circulatory system, unspecified**

CONGENITAL MALFORMATIONS OF THE RESPIRATORY SYSTEM (Q30-Q34)

Q30 **Congenital malformations of nose**
Excludes1: congenital deviation of nasal septum (Q67.4)

Q30.0 **Choanal atresia**
Atresia of nares (anterior) (posterior)
Congenital stenosis of nares (anterior) (posterior)

Q30.1 **Agenesis and underdevelopment of nose**
Congenital absent of nose

Q30.2 **Fissured, notched and cleft nose**

Q30.3 **Congenital perforated nasal septum**

Q30.8 **Other congenital malformations of nose**
Accessory nose
Congenital anomaly of nasal sinus wall

Q30.9 **Congenital malformation of nose, unspecified**

Q31 **Congenital malformations of larynx**
Excludes1: congenital laryngeal stridor NOS (P28.89)

Q31.0 **Web of larynx**
Glottic web of larynx
Subglottic web of larynx
Web of larynx NOS

Q31.1 **Congenital subglottic stenosis**

Q31.2 **Laryngeal hypoplasia**

Q31.3 **Laryngocele**

Q31.5 **Congenital laryngomalacia**

Q31.8 **Other congenital malformations of larynx**
Absence of larynx
Agenesis of larynx
Atresia of larynx
Congenital cleft thyroid cartilage
Congenital fissure of epiglottis
Congenital stenosis of larynx NEC
Posterior cleft of cricoid cartilage

Q31.9 **Congenital malformation of larynx, unspecified**

Q32 **Congenital malformations of trachea and bronchus**
Excludes1: congenital bronchiectasis (Q33.4)

Q32.0 **Congenital tracheomalacia**

Q32.1 **Other congenital malformations of trachea**
Atresia of trachea

Congenital anomaly of tracheal cartilage

Congenital dilatation of trachea

Congenital malformation of trachea

Congenital stenosis of trachea

Congenital tracheocele

Q32.2 Congenital bronchomalacia

Q32.3 Congenital stenosis of bronchus

Q32.4 Other congenital malformations of bronchus

Absence of bronchus

Agenesis of bronchus

Atresia of bronchus

Congenital diverticulum of bronchus

Congenital malformation of bronchus NOS

Q33 Congenital malformations of lung

Q33.0 Congenital cystic lung

Congenital cystic lung disease

Congenital honeycomb lung

Congenital polycystic lung disease

Excludes1: cystic fibrosis (E84.0)

cystic lung disease, acquired or unspecified (J98.4)

Q33.1 Accessory lobe of lung

Azygos lobe (fissured), lung

Q33.2 Sequestration of lung

Q33.3 Agenesis of lung

Congenital absence of lung (lobe)

Q33.4 Congenital bronchiectasis

Q33.5 Ectopic tissue in lung

Q33.6 Congenital hypoplasia and dysplasia of lung

Excludes1: pulmonary hypoplasia associated with short gestation (P28.0)

Q33.8 Other congenital malformations of lung

Q33.9 Congenital malformation of lung, unspecified

Q34 Other congenital malformations of respiratory system

Excludes2: congenital central alveolar hypoventilation syndrome (G47.35)

Q34.0 Anomaly of pleura

Q34.1 Congenital cyst of mediastinum

Q34.8 Other specified congenital malformations of respiratory system

Atresia of nasopharynx

Q34.9 Congenital malformation of respiratory system, unspecified

Congenital absence of respiratory system

Congenital anomaly of respiratory system NOS

CLEFT LIP AND CLEFT PALATE (Q35-Q37)

Definition: Cleft lip is a congenital deformity characterized by a vertical cleft or pair of clefts in the upper lip, with or without involvement of the palate. Cleft palate is a congenital fissure in the roof of the mouth, resulting from incomplete fusion of the palate during embryonic development.

Use additional code to identify associated malformation of the nose (Q30.2)

Excludes1: Robin's syndrome (Q87.0)

Q35 Cleft palate

Includes: fissure of palate

palatoschisis

Excludes1: cleft palate with cleft lip (Q37.-)

Q35.1 Cleft hard palate

Q35.3 Cleft soft palate

Q35.5 Cleft hard palate with cleft soft palate

Q35.7 Cleft uvula

Q35.9 Cleft palate, unspecified

Cleft palate NOS

Q36 Cleft lip

Includes: cheiloschisis

congenital fissure of lip harelip

labium leporinum

Excludes1: cleft lip with cleft palate (Q37.-)

Q36.0 Cleft lip, bilateral

Q36.1 Cleft lip, median

Q36.9 Cleft lip, unilateral

Cleft lip NOS

Q37 Cleft palate with cleft lip

Includes: cheilopalatoschisis

Q37.0 Cleft hard palate with bilateral cleft lip

Q37.1 Cleft hard palate with unilateral cleft lip

Cleft hard palate with cleft lip NOS

Q37.2 Cleft soft palate with bilateral cleft lip

Q37.3 Cleft soft palate with unilateral cleft lip

Cleft soft palate with cleft lip NOS

Q37.4 Cleft hard and soft palate with bilateral cleft lip

Q37.5 Cleft hard and soft palate with unilateral cleft lip

Cleft hard and soft palate with cleft lip NOS

Q37.8 Unspecified cleft palate with bilateral cleft lip

Q37.9 Unspecified cleft palate with unilateral cleft lip

Cleft palate with cleft lip NOS

OTHER CONGENITAL MALFORMATIONS OF THE DIGESTIVE SYSTEM (Q38-Q45)

Q38 Other congenital malformations of tongue, mouth and pharynx

Excludes1: dentofacial anomalies (M26.-)

macrostomia (Q18.4) microstomia (Q18.5)

Q38.0 Congenital malformations of lips, not elsewhere classified

Congenital fistula of lip

Congenital malformation of lip NOS

Van der Woude's syndrome

Excludes1: cleft lip (Q36.-)

cleft lip with cleft palate (Q37.-)

macrocheilia (Q18.6) microcheilia (Q18.7)

Q38.1 Ankyloglossia

Tongue tie

Q38.2 Macroglossia

Congenital hypertrophy of tongue

Q38.3 Other congenital malformations of tongue

Aglossia

Bifid tongue

Congenital adhesion of tongue

Congenital fissure of tongue

Congenital malformation of tongue NOS

Double tongue

Hypoglossia

Hypoplasia of tongue

Microglossia

Q38.4 **Congenital malformations of salivary glands and ducts**

Atresia of salivary glands and ducts

Congenital absence of salivary glands and ducts

Congenital accessory salivary glands and ducts

Congenital fistula of salivary gland

Q38.5 **Congenital malformations of palate, not elsewhere classified**

Congenital absence of uvula

Congenital malformation of palate NOS

Congenital high arched palate

Excludes1: cleft palate (Q35.-)

cleft palate with cleft lip (Q37.-)

Q38.6 **Other congenital malformations of mouth**

Congenital malformation of mouth NOS

Q38.7 **Congenital pharyngeal pouch**

Congenital diverticulum of pharynx

Excludes1: pharyngeal pouch syndrome (D82.1)

Q38.8 **Other congenital malformations of pharynx**

Congenital malformation of pharynx NOS

Imperforate pharynx

Q39 **Congenital malformations of esophagus**

Q39.0 **Atresia of esophagus without fistula**

Atresia of esophagus NOS

Q39.1 **Atresia of esophagus with tracheo-esophageal fistula**

Atresia of esophagus with broncho-esophageal fistula

Q39.2 **Congenital tracheo-esophageal fistula without atresia**

Congenital tracheo-esophageal fistula NOS

Q39.3 **Congenital stenosis and stricture of esophagus**

Q39.4 **Esophageal web**

Q39.5 **Congenital dilatation of esophagus**

Congenital cardiospasm

Q39.6 **Congenital diverticulum of esophagus**

Congenital esophageal pouch

Q39.8 **Other congenital malformations of esophagus**

Congenital absence of esophagus

Congenital displacement of esophagus

Congenital duplication of esophagus

Q39.9 **Congenital malformation of esophagus, unspecified**

Q40 **Other congenital malformations of upper alimentary tract**

Q40.0 **Congenital hypertrophic pyloric stenosis**

Congenital or infantile constriction

Congenital or infantile hypertrophy

Congenital or infantile spasm

Congenital or infantile stenosis

Congenital or infantile stricture

Q40.1 **Congenital hiatus hernia**

Congenital displacement of cardia through esophageal hiatus

Excludes1: congenital diaphragmatic hernia (Q79.0)

Q40.2 **Other specified congenital malformations of stomach**

Congenital displacement of stomach

Congenital diverticulum of stomach

Congenital hourglass stomach

Congenital duplication of stomach

Megalogastria

Microgastria

Q40.3 **Congenital malformation of stomach, unspecified**

Q40.8 **Other specified congenital malformations of upper alimentary tract**

Q40.9 **Congenital malformation of upper alimentary tract, unspecified**

Congenital anomaly of upper alimentary tract

Congenital deformity of upper alimentary tract

Q41 **Congenital absence, atresia and stenosis of small intestine**

Includes: congenital obstruction, occlusion or stricture of small intestine or intestine NOS

Excludes1: cystic fibrosis with intestinal manifestation (E84.11)

meconium ileus NOS (without cystic fibrosis) (P76.0)

Q41.0 **Congenital absence, atresia and stenosis of duodenum**

Q41.1 **Congenital absence, atresia and stenosis of jejunum**

Apple peel syndrome

Imperforate jejunum

Q41.2 **Congenital absence, atresia and stenosis of ileum**

Q41.8 **Congenital absence, atresia and stenosis of other specified parts of small intestine**

Q41.9 **Congenital absence, atresia and stenosis of small intestine, part unspecified**

Congenital absence, atresia and stenosis of intestine NOS

Q42 **Congenital absence, atresia and stenosis of large intestine**

Includes: congenital obstruction, occlusion and stricture of large intestine

Q42.0 **Congenital absence, atresia and stenosis of rectum with fistula**

Q42.1 **Congenital absence, atresia and stenosis of rectum without fistula**

Imperforate rectum

Q42.2 **Congenital absence, atresia and stenosis of anus with fistula**

Q42.3 **Congenital absence, atresia and stenosis of anus without fistula**

Imperforate anus

Q42.8 **Congenital absence, atresia and stenosis of other parts of large intestine**

Q42.9 **Congenital absence, atresia and stenosis of large intestine, part unspecified**

Q43 **Other congenital malformations of intestine**

Q43.0 **Meckel's diverticulum (displaced) (hypertrophic)**

Persistent omphalomesenteric duct

Persistent vitelline duct

Q43.1 **Hirschsprung's disease**

Aganglionosis

Congenital (aganglionic) megacolon

Q43.2 **Other congenital functional disorders of colon**

Congenital dilatation of colon

Q43.3 **Congenital malformations of intestinal fixation**

Congenital omental, anomalous adhesions [bands]

● New code ▲ Revised code Excludes1: Not coded here Excludes2: Not included here ⊗ Placeholder required ⑦7th digit required

Congenital peritoneal adhesions [bands]

Incomplete rotation of cecum and colon

Insufficient rotation of cecum and colon

Jackson's membrane

Malrotation of colon

Rotation failure of cecum and colon

Universal mesentery

Q43.4 Duplication of intestine

Q43.5 Ectopic anus

Q43.6 Congenital fistula of rectum and anus

Excludes1: congenital fistula of anus with absence, atresia and stenosis (Q42.2)

congenital fistula of rectum with absence, atresia and stenosis (Q42.0)

congenital rectovaginal fistula (Q52.2)

congenital urethrorectal fistula (Q64.73)

pilonidal fistula or sinus (L05.-)

Q43.7 Persistent cloaca

Cloaca NOS

Q43.8 Other specified congenital malformations of intestine

Congenital blind loop syndrome

Congenital diverticulitis, colon

Congenital diverticulum, intestine

Dolichocolon

Megaloappendix

Megaloduodenum

Microcolon

Transposition of appendix

Transposition of colon

Transposition of intestine

Q43.9 Congenital malformation of intestine, unspecified

Q44 Congenital malformations of gallbladder, bile ducts and liver

Q44.0 Agenesis, aplasia and hypoplasia of gallbladder

Congenital absence of gallbladder

Q44.1 Other congenital malformations of gallbladder

Congenital malformation of gallbladder NOS

Intrahepatic gallbladder

Q44.2 Atresia of bile ducts

Q44.3 Congenital stenosis and stricture of bile ducts

Q44.4 Choledochal cyst

Q44.5 Other congenital malformations of bile ducts

Accessory hepatic duct

Biliary duct duplication

Congenital malformation of bile duct NOS

Cystic duct duplication

Q44.6 Cystic disease of liver

Fibrocystic disease of liver

Q44.7 Other congenital malformations of liver

Accessory liver

Alagille's syndrome

Congenital absence of liver

Congenital hepatomegaly

Congenital malformation of liver NOS

Q45 Other congenital malformations of digestive system

Excludes2: congenital diaphragmatic hernia (Q79.0)

congenital hiatus hernia (Q40.1)

Q45.0 Agenesis, aplasia and hypoplasia of pancreas

Congenital absence of pancreas

Q45.1 Annular pancreas

Q45.2 Congenital pancreatic cyst

Q45.3 Other congenital malformations of pancreas and pancreatic duct

Accessory pancreas

Congenital malformation of pancreas or pancreatic duct NOS

Excludes1: congenital diabetes mellitus (E10.-)

cystic fibrosis (E84.0-E84.9)

fibrocystic disease of pancreas (E84.-)

neonatal diabetes mellitus (P70.2)

Q45.8 Other specified congenital malformations of digestive system

Absence (complete) (partial) of alimentary tract NOS

Duplication of digestive system

Malposition, congenital of digestive system

Q45.9 Congenital malformation of digestive system, unspecified

Congenital anomaly of digestive system

Congenital deformity of digestive system

CONGENITAL MALFORMATIONS OF GENITAL ORGANS (Q50-Q56)

Excludes1: androgen insensitivity syndrome (E34.5-)

syndromes associated with anomalies in the number and form of chromosomes (Q90-Q99)

Q50 Congenital malformations of ovaries, fallopian tubes and broad ligaments

Q50.0 Congenital absence of ovary

Excludes1: Turner's syndrome (Q96.-)

Q50.01 Congenital absence of ovary, unilateral

Q50.02 Congenital absence of ovary, bilateral

Q50.1 Developmental ovarian cyst

Q50.2 Congenital torsion of ovary

Q50.3 Other congenital malformations of ovary

Q50.31 Accessory ovary

Q50.32 Ovarian streak

46, XX with streak gonads

Q50.39 Other congenital malformation of ovary

Congenital malformation of ovary NOS

Q50.4 Embryonic cyst of fallopian tube

Fimbrial cyst

Q50.5 Embryonic cyst of broad ligament

Epoophoron cyst

Parovarian cyst

Q50.6 Other congenital malformations of fallopian tube and broad ligament

Absence of fallopian tube and broad ligament

Accessory fallopian tube and broad ligament

Atresia of fallopian tube and broad ligament

Congenital malformation of fallopian tube or broad ligament NOS

Add 4th-7th digits	Nonspecific code	Unspecified code	Manifestation code

Q51 Congenital malformations of uterus and cervix

Q51.0 Agenesis and aplasia of uterus

Congenital absence of uterus

Q51.1 Doubling of uterus with doubling of cervix and vagina

Q51.10 Doubling of uterus with doubling of cervix and vagina without obstruction

Doubling of uterus with doubling of cervix and vagina NOS

Q51.11 Doubling of uterus with doubling of cervix and vagina with obstruction

Q51.2 Other doubling of uterus

Doubling of uterus NOS

Septate uterus, complete or partial

Q51.3 Bicornate uterus

Bicornate uterus, complete or partial

Q51.4 Unicornate uterus

Unicornate uterus with or without a separate uterine horn

Uterus with only one functioning horn

Q51.5 Agenesis and aplasia of cervix

Congenital absence of cervix

Q51.6 Embryonic cyst of cervix

Q51.7 Congenital fistulae between uterus and digestive and urinary tracts

Q51.8 Other congenital malformations of uterus and cervix

Q51.81 Other congenital malformations of uterus

Q51.810 Arcuate uterus

Arcuatus uterus

Q51.811 Hypoplasia of uterus

Q51.818 Other congenital malformations of uterus

Müllerian anomaly of uterus NEC

Q51.82 Other congenital malformations of cervix

Q51.820 Cervical duplication

Q51.821 Hypoplasia of cervix

Q51.828 Other congenital malformations of cervix

Q51.9 Congenital malformation of uterus and cervix, unspecified

Q52 Other congenital malformations of female genitalia

Q52.0 Congenital absence of vagina

Vaginal agenesis, total or partial

Q52.1 Doubling of vagina

Excludes1: doubling of vagina with doubling of uterus and cervix (Q51.1-)

Q52.10 Doubling of vagina, unspecified

Septate vagina NOS

Q52.11 Transverse vaginal septum

Q52.12 Longitudinal vaginal septum

•Q52.120 Longitudinal vaginal septum, nonobstructing

•Q52.121 Longitudinal vaginal septum, obstructing, right side

•Q52.122 Longitudinal vaginal septum, obstructing, left side

•Q52.123 Longitudinal vaginal septum, microperforate, right side

•Q52.124 Longitudinal vaginal septum, microperforate, left side

•**Q52.129** Other and unspecified longitudinal vaginal septum

Q52.2 Congenital rectovaginal fistula

Excludes1: cloaca (Q43.7)

Q52.3 Imperforate hymen

Q52.4 Other congenital malformations of vagina

Canal of Nuck cyst, congenital

Congenital malformation of vagina NOS

Embryonic vaginal cyst

Gartner's duct cyst

Q52.5 Fusion of labia

Q52.6 Congenital malformation of clitoris

Q52.7 Other and unspecified congenital malformations of vulva

Q52.70 Unspecified congenital malformations of vulva

Congenital malformation of vulva NOS

Q52.71 Congenital absence of vulva

Q52.79 Other congenital malformations of vulva

Congenital cyst of vulva

Q52.8 Other specified congenital malformations of female genitalia

Q52.9 Congenital malformation of female genitalia, unspecified

Q53 Undescended and ectopic testicle

Q53.0 Ectopic testis

Q53.00 Ectopic testis, unspecified

Q53.01 Ectopic testis, unilateral

Q53.02 Ectopic testes, bilateral

Q53.1 Undescended testicle, unilateral

Q53.10 Unspecified undescended testicle, unilateral

Q53.11 Abdominal testis, unilateral

Q53.12 Ectopic perineal testis, unilateral

Q53.2 Undescended testicle, bilateral

Q53.20 Undescended testicle, unspecified, bilateral

Q53.21 Abdominal testis, bilateral

Q53.22 Ectopic perineal testis, bilateral

Q53.9 Undescended testicle, unspecified

Cryptorchism NOS

Q54 Hypospadias

Excludes1: epispadias (Q64.0)

Q54.0 Hypospadias, balanic

Hypospadias, coronal

Hypospadias, glandular

Q54.1 Hypospadias, penile

Q54.2 Hypospadias, penoscrotal

Q54.3 Hypospadias, perineal

Q54.4 Congenital chordee

Chordee without hypospadias

Q54.8 Other hypospadias

Hypospadias with intersex state

Q54.9 Hypospadias, unspecified

Q55 Other congenital malformations of male genital organs

Excludes1: congenital hydrocele (P83.5)

hypospadias (Q54.-)

Q55.0   **Absence and aplasia of testis**

Monorchism

Q55.1   **Hypoplasia of testis and scrotum**

Fusion of testes

Q55.2   **Other and unspecified congenital malformations of testis and scrotum**

    Q55.20   **Unspecified congenital malformations of testis and scrotum**

        Congenital malformation of testis or scrotum NOS

    Q55.21   **Polyorchism**

    Q55.22   **Retractile testis**

    Q55.23   **Scrotal transposition**

    Q55.29   **Other congenital malformations of testis and scrotum**

Q55.3   **Atresia of vas deferens**

Code first any associated cystic fibrosis (E84.-)

Q55.4   **Other congenital malformations of vas deferens, epididymis, seminal vesicles and prostate**

Absence or aplasia of prostate

Absence or aplasia of spermatic cord

Congenital malformation of vas deferens, epididymis, seminal vesicles or prostate NOS

Q55.5   **Congenital absence and aplasia of penis**

Q55.6   **Other congenital malformations of penis**

    Q55.61   **Curvature of penis (lateral)**

    Q55.62   **Hypoplasia of penis**

        Micropenis

    Q55.63   **Congenital torsion of penis**

        Excludes1: acquired torsion of penis (N48.82)

    Q55.64   **Hidden penis**

        Buried penis

        Concealed penis

        Excludes1: acquired buried penis (N48.83)

    Q55.69   **Other congenital malformation of penis**

        Congenital malformation of penis NOS

Q55.7   **Congenital vasocutaneous fistula**

Q55.8   **Other specified congenital malformations of male genital organs**

Q55.9   **Congenital malformation of male genital organ, unspecified**

Congenital anomaly of male genital organ

Congenital deformity of male genital organ

Q56   **Indeterminate sex and pseudohermaphroditism**

Excludes1: 46,XX true hermaphrodite (Q99.1)

androgen insensitivity syndrome (E34.5-)

chimera 46,XX/46,XY true hermaphrodite (Q99.0)

female pseudohermaphroditism with adrenocortical disorder (E25.-)

pseudohermaphroditism with specified chromosomal anomaly (Q96-Q99)

pure gonadal dysgenesis (Q99.1)

Q56.0   **Hermaphroditism, not elsewhere classified**

Ovotestis

Q56.1   **Male pseudohermaphroditism, not elsewhere classified**

46, XY with streak gonads

Male pseudohermaphroditism NOS

Q56.2   **Female pseudohermaphroditism, not elsewhere classified**

Female pseudohermaphroditism NOS

Q56.3   **Pseudohermaphroditism, unspecified**

Q56.4   **Indeterminate sex, unspecified**

Ambiguous genitalia

CONGENITAL MALFORMATIONS OF THE URINARY SYSTEM (Q60-Q64)

Q60   **Renal agenesis and other reduction defects of kidney**

Includes: congenital absence of kidney

        congenital atrophy of kidney infantile atrophy of kidney

Q60.0   **Renal agenesis, unilateral**

Q60.1   **Renal agenesis, bilateral**

Q60.2   **Renal agenesis, unspecified**

Q60.3   **Renal hypoplasia, unilateral**

Q60.4   **Renal hypoplasia, bilateral**

Q60.5   **Renal hypoplasia, unspecified**

Q60.6   **Potter's syndrome**

Q61   **Cystic kidney disease**

Excludes1: acquired cyst of kidney (N28.1)

        Potter's syndrome (Q60.6)

Q61.0   **Congenital renal cyst**

    Q61.00   **Congenital renal cyst, unspecified**

        Cyst of kidney NOS (congenital)

    Q61.01   **Congenital single renal cyst**

    Q61.02   **Congenital multiple renal cysts**

Q61.1   **Polycystic kidney, infantile type**

Polycystic kidney, autosomal recessive

    Q61.11   **Cystic dilatation of collecting ducts**

    Q61.19   **Other polycystic kidney, infantile type**

Q61.2   **Polycystic kidney, adult type**

Polycystic kidney, autosomal dominant

Q61.3   **Polycystic kidney, unspecified**

Q61.4   **Renal dysplasia**

Multicystic dysplastic kidney

Multicystic kidney (development)

Multicystic kidney disease

Multicystic renal dysplasia

Excludes1: polycystic kidney disease (Q61.11-Q61.3)

Q61.5   **Medullary cystic kidney**

Nephronopthisis

Sponge kidney NOS

Q61.8   **Other cystic kidney diseases**

Fibrocystic kidney

Fibrocystic renal degeneration or disease

Q61.9   **Cystic kidney disease, unspecified**

Meckel-Gruber syndrome

Q62   **Congenital obstructive defects of renal pelvis and congenital malformations of ureter**

Q62.0   **Congenital hydronephrosis**

Q62.1   **Congenital occlusion of ureter**

Atresia and stenosis of ureter

    Q62.10   **Congenital occlusion of ureter, unspecified**

Q62.11　Congenital occlusion of ureteropelvic junction

Q62.12　Congenital occlusion of ureterovesical orifice

Q62.2　Congenital megaureter

Congenital dilatation of ureter

Q62.3　Other obstructive defects of renal pelvis and ureter

Q62.31　Congenital ureterocele, orthotopic

Q62.32　Cecoureterocele

Ectopic ureterocele

Q62.39　Other obstructive defects of renal pelvis and ureter

Ureteropelvic junction obstruction NOS

Q62.4　Agenesis of ureter

Congenital absence ureter

Q62.5　Duplication of ureter

Accessory ureter

Double ureter

Q62.6　Malposition of ureter

Q62.60　Malposition of ureter, unspecified

Q62.61　Deviation of ureter

Q62.62　Displacement of ureter

Q62.63　Anomalous implantation of ureter

Ectopia of ureter

Ectopic ureter

Q62.69　Other malposition of ureter

Q62.7　Congenital vesico-uretero-renal reflux

Q62.8　Other congenital malformations of ureter

Anomaly of ureter NOS

Q63　Other congenital malformations of kidney

Excludes1: congenital nephrotic syndrome (N04.-)

Q63.0　Accessory kidney

Q63.1　Lobulated, fused and horseshoe kidney

Q63.2　Ectopic kidney

Congenital displaced kidney

Malrotation of kidney

Q63.3　Hyperplastic and giant kidney

Compensatory hypertrophy of kidney

Q63.8　Other specified congenital malformations of kidney

Congenital renal calculi

Q63.9　Congenital malformation of kidney, unspecified

Q64　Other congenital malformations of urinary system

Q64.0　Epispadias

Excludes1: hypospadias (Q54.-)

Q64.1　Exstrophy of urinary bladder

Q64.10　Exstrophy of urinary bladder, unspecified

Ectopia vesicae

Q64.11　Supravesical fissure of urinary bladder

Q64.12　Cloacal extrophy of urinary bladder

Q64.19　Other exstrophy of urinary bladder

Extroversion of bladder

Q64.2　Congenital posterior urethral valves

Q64.3　Other atresia and stenosis of urethra and bladder neck

Q64.31　Congenital bladder neck obstruction

Congenital obstruction of vesicourethral orifice

Q64.32　Congenital stricture of urethra

Q64.33　Congenital stricture of urinary meatus

Q64.39　Other atresia and stenosis of urethra and bladder neck

Atresia and stenosis of urethra and bladder neck NOS

Q64.4　Malformation of urachus

Cyst of urachus

Patent urachus

Prolapse of urachus

Q64.5　Congenital absence of bladder and urethra

Q64.6　Congenital diverticulum of bladder

Q64.7　Other and unspecified congenital malformations of bladder and urethra

Excludes1: congenital prolapse of bladder (mucosa) (Q79.4)

Q64.70　Unspecified congenital malformation of bladder and urethra

Malformation of bladder or urethra NOS

Q64.71　Congenital prolapse of urethra

Q64.72　Congenital prolapse of urinary meatus

Q64.73　Congenital urethrorectal fistula

Q64.74　Double urethra

Q64.75　Double urinary meatus

Q64.79　Other congenital malformations of bladder and urethra

Q64.8　Other specified congenital malformations of urinary system

Q64.9　Congenital malformation of urinary system, unspecified

Congenital anomaly NOS of urinary system

Congenital deformity NOS of urinary system

CONGENITAL MALFORMATIONS AND DEFORMATIONS OF THE MUSCULOSKELETAL SYSTEM (Q65-Q79)

Q65　Congenital deformities of hip

Excludes1: clicking hip (R29.4)

Q65.0　Congenital dislocation of hip, unilateral

Q65.00　Congenital dislocation of unspecified hip, unilateral

Q65.01　Congenital dislocation of right hip, unilateral

Q65.02　Congenital dislocation of left hip, unilateral

Q65.1　Congenital dislocation of hip, bilateral

Q65.2　Congenital dislocation of hip, unspecified

Q65.3　Congenital partial dislocation of hip, unilateral

Q65.30　Congenital partial dislocation of unspecified hip, unilateral

Q65.31　Congenital partial dislocation of right hip, unilateral

Q65.32　Congenital partial dislocation of left hip, unilateral

Q65.4　Congenital partial dislocation of hip, bilateral

Q65.5　Congenital partial dislocation of hip, unspecified

Q65.6　Congenital unstable hip

Congenital dislocatable hip

Q65.8　Other congenital deformities of hip

Q65.81　Congenital coxa valga

Q65.82　Congenital coxa vara

Q65.89　Other specified congenital deformities of hip

Anteversion of femoral neck

Congenital acetabular dysplasia

Q65.9   Congenital deformity of hip, unspecified

Q66   Congenital deformities of feet

Excludes1: reduction defects of feet (Q72.-)

valgus deformities (acquired) (M21.0-)

varus deformities (acquired) (M21.1-)

Q66.0   Congenital talipes equinovarus

Q66.1   Congenital talipes calcaneovarus

Q66.2   Congenital metatarsus (primus) varus

    Q66.21   Congenital metatarsus primus varus

    Q66.22   Congenital metatarsus adductus

        Congenital metatarsus varus

Q66.3   Other congenital varus deformities of feet

Hallux varus, congenital

Q66.4   Congenital talipes calcaneovalgus

Q66.5   Congenital pes planus

Congenital flat foot

Congenital rigid flat foot

Congenital spastic (everted) flat foot

    Excludes1: pes planus, acquired (M21.4)

    Q66.50   Congenital pes planus, unspecified foot

    Q66.51   Congenital pes planus, right foot

    Q66.52   Congenital pes planus, left foot

Q66.6   Other congenital valgus deformities of feet

Congenital metatarsus valgus

Q66.7   Congenital pes cavus

Q66.8   Other congenital deformities of feet

    Q66.80   Congenital vertical talus deformity, unspecified foot

    Q66.81   Congenital vertical talus deformity, right foot

    Q66.82   Congenital vertical talus deformity, left foot

    Q66.89   Other specified congenital deformities of feet

        Congenital asymmetric talipes

        Congenital clubfoot NOS

        Congenital talipes NOS

        Congenital tarsal coalition

        Hammer toe, congenital

Q66.9   Congenital deformity of feet, unspecified

Q67   Congenital musculoskeletal deformities of head, face, spine and chest

Excludes1: congenital malformation syndromes classified to Q87.-

Potter's syndrome (Q60.6)

Q67.0   Congenital facial asymmetry

Q67.1   Congenital compression facies

Q67.2   Dolichocephaly

Q67.3   Plagiocephaly

Q67.4   Other congenital deformities of skull, face and jaw

Congenital depressions in skull

Congenital hemifacial atrophy or hypertrophy

Deviation of nasal septum, congenital

Squashed or bent nose, congenital

    Excludes1: dentofacial anomalies [including malocclusion] (M26.-)

        syphilitic saddle nose (A50.5)

Q67.5   Congenital deformity of spine

Congenital postural scoliosis

Congenital scoliosis NOS

    Excludes1: infantile idiopathic scoliosis (M41.0)

        scoliosis due to congenital bony malformation (Q76.3)

Q67.6   Pectus excavatum

Congenital funnel chest

Q67.7   Pectus carinatum

Congenital pigeon chest

Q67.8   Other congenital deformities of chest

Congenital deformity of chest wall NOS

Q68   Other congenital musculoskeletal deformities

Excludes1: reduction defects of limb(s) (Q71-Q73)

Excludes2: congenital myotonic chondrodystrophy (G71.13)

Q68.0   Congenital deformity of sternocleidomastoid muscle

Congenital contracture of sternocleidomastoid (muscle)

Congenital (sternomastoid) torticollis

Sternomastoid tumor (congenital)

Q68.1   Congenital deformity of finger(s) and hand

Congenital clubfinger

Spade-like hand (congenital)

Q68.2   Congenital deformity of knee

Congenital dislocation of knee

Congenital genu recurvatum

Q68.3   Congenital bowing of femur

    Excludes1: anteversion of femur (neck) (Q65.89)

Q68.4   Congenital bowing of tibia and fibula

Q68.5   Congenital bowing of long bones of leg, unspecified

Q68.6   Discoid meniscus

Q68.8   Other specified congenital musculoskeletal deformities

Congenital deformity of clavicle

Congenital deformity of elbow

Congenital deformity of forearm

Congenital deformity of scapula

Congenital deformity of wrist

Congenital dislocation of elbow

Congenital dislocation of shoulder

Congenital dislocation of wrist

Q69   Polydactyly

Q69.0   Accessory finger(s)

Q69.1   Accessory thumb(s)

Q69.2   Accessory toe(s)

Accessory hallux

Q69.9   Polydactyly, unspecified

Supernumerary digit(s) NOS

Q70   Syndactyly

Q70.0   Fused fingers

Complex syndactyly of fingers with synostosis

    Q70.00   Fused fingers, unspecified hand

    Q70.01   Fused fingers, right hand

    Q70.02   Fused fingers, left hand

    Q70.03   Fused fingers, bilateral

Q70.1   Webbed fingers

Simple syndactyly of fingers without synostosis

Q70.10   **Webbed fingers, unspecified hand**

Q70.11   **Webbed fingers, right hand**

Q70.12   **Webbed fingers, left hand**

Q70.13   **Webbed fingers, bilateral**

Q70.2   **Fused toes**

Complex syndactyly of toes with synostosis

Q70.20   **Fused toes, unspecified foot**

Q70.21   **Fused toes, right foot**

Q70.22   **Fused toes, left foot**

Q70.23   **Fused toes, bilateral**

Q70.3   **Webbed toes**

Simple syndactyly of toes without synostosis

Q70.30   **Webbed toes, unspecified foot**

Q70.31   **Webbed toes, right foot**

Q70.32   **Webbed toes, left foot**

Q70.33   **Webbed toes, bilateral**

Q70.4   **Polysyndactyly, unspecified**

Excludes1: specified syndactyly of hand and feet - code to specified conditions (Q70.0- -Q70.3-)

Q70.9   **Syndactyly, unspecified**

Symphalangy NOS

Q71   **Reduction defects of upper limb**

Q71.0   **Congenital complete absence of upper limb**

Q71.00   **Congenital complete absence of unspecified upper limb**

Q71.01   **Congenital complete absence of right upper limb**

Q71.02   **Congenital complete absence of left upper limb**

Q71.03   **Congenital complete absence of upper limb, bilateral**

Q71.1   **Congenital absence of upper arm and forearm with hand present**

Q71.10   **Congenital absence of unspecified upper arm and forearm with hand present**

Q71.11   **Congenital absence of right upper arm and forearm with hand present**

Q71.12   **Congenital absence of left upper arm and forearm with hand present**

Q71.13   **Congenital absence of upper arm and forearm with hand present, bilateral**

Q71.2   **Congenital absence of both forearm and hand**

Q71.20   **Congenital absence of both forearm and hand, unspecified upper limb**

Q71.21   **Congenital absence of both forearm and hand, right upper limb**

Q71.22   **Congenital absence of both forearm and hand, left upper limb**

Q71.23   **Congenital absence of both forearm and hand, bilateral**

Q71.3   **Congenital absence of hand and finger**

Q71.30   **Congenital absence of unspecified hand and finger**

Q71.31   **Congenital absence of right hand and finger**

Q71.32   **Congenital absence of left hand and finger**

Q71.33   **Congenital absence of hand and finger, bilateral**

Q71.4   **Longitudinal reduction defect of radius**

Clubhand (congenital)

Radial clubhand

Q71.40   **Longitudinal reduction defect of unspecified radius**

Q71.41   **Longitudinal reduction defect of right radius**

Q71.42   **Longitudinal reduction defect of left radius**

Q71.43   **Longitudinal reduction defect of radius, bilateral**

Q71.5   **Longitudinal reduction defect of ulna**

Q71.50   **Longitudinal reduction defect of unspecified ulna**

Q71.51   **Longitudinal reduction defect of right ulna**

Q71.52   **Longitudinal reduction defect of left ulna**

Q71.53   **Longitudinal reduction defect of ulna, bilateral**

Q71.6   **Lobster-claw hand**

Q71.60   **Lobster-claw hand, unspecified hand**

Q71.61   **Lobster-claw right hand**

Q71.62   **Lobster-claw left hand**

Q71.63   **Lobster-claw hand, bilateral**

Q71.8   **Other reduction defects of upper limb**

Q71.81   **Congenital shortening of upper limb**

Q71.811   **Congenital shortening of right upper limb**

Q71.812   **Congenital shortening of left upper limb**

Q71.813   **Congenital shortening of upper limb, bilateral**

Q71.819   **Congenital shortening of unspecified upper limb**

Q71.89   **Other reduction defects of upper limb**

Q71.891   **Other reduction defects of right upper limb**

Q71.892   **Other reduction defects of left upper limb**

Q71.893   **Other reduction defects of upper limb, bilateral**

Q71.899   **Other reduction defects of unspecified upper limb**

Q71.9   **Unspecified reduction defect of upper limb**

Q71.90   **Unspecified reduction defect of unspecified upper limb**

Q71.91   **Unspecified reduction defect of right upper limb**

Q71.92   **Unspecified reduction defect of left upper limb**

Q71.93   **Unspecified reduction defect of upper limb, bilateral**

Q72   **Reduction defects of lower limb**

Q72.0   **Congenital complete absence of lower limb**

Q72.00   **Congenital complete absence of unspecified lower limb**

Q72.01   **Congenital complete absence of right lower limb**

Q72.02   **Congenital complete absence of left lower limb**

Q72.03   **Congenital complete absence of lower limb, bilateral**

Q72.1   **Congenital absence of thigh and lower leg with foot present**

    Q72.10   Congenital absence of unspecified thigh and lower leg with foot present

    Q72.11   Congenital absence of right thigh and lower leg with foot present

    Q72.12   Congenital absence of left thigh and lower leg with foot present

    Q72.13   Congenital absence of thigh and lower leg with foot present, bilateral

Q72.2   **Congenital absence of both lower leg and foot**

    Q72.20   Congenital absence of both lower leg and foot, unspecified lower limb

    Q72.21   Congenital absence of both lower leg and foot, right lower limb

    Q72.22   Congenital absence of both lower leg and foot, left lower limb

    Q72.23   Congenital absence of both lower leg and foot, bilateral

Q72.3   **Congenital absence of foot and toe(s)**

    Q72.30   Congenital absence of unspecified foot and toe(s)

    Q72.31   Congenital absence of right foot and toe(s)

    Q72.32   Congenital absence of left foot and toe(s)

    Q72.33   Congenital absence of foot and toe(s), bilateral

Q72.4   **Longitudinal reduction defect of femur**

Proximal femoral focal deficiency

    Q72.40   Longitudinal reduction defect of unspecified femur

    Q72.41   Longitudinal reduction defect of right femur

    Q72.42   Longitudinal reduction defect of left femur

    Q72.43   Longitudinal reduction defect of femur, bilateral

Q72.5   **Longitudinal reduction defect of tibia**

    Q72.50   Longitudinal reduction defect of unspecified tibia

    Q72.51   Longitudinal reduction defect of right tibia

    Q72.52   Longitudinal reduction defect of left tibia

    Q72.53   Longitudinal reduction defect of tibia, bilateral

Q72.6   **Longitudinal reduction defect of fibula**

    Q72.60   Longitudinal reduction defect of unspecified fibula

    Q72.61   Longitudinal reduction defect of right fibula

    Q72.62   Longitudinal reduction defect of left fibula

    Q72.63   Longitudinal reduction defect of fibula, bilateral

Q72.7   **Split foot**

    Q72.70   Split foot, unspecified lower limb

    Q72.71   Split foot, right lower limb

    Q72.72   Split foot, left lower limb

    Q72.73   Split foot, bilateral

Q72.8   **Other reduction defects of lower limb**

    Q72.81   Congenital shortening of lower limb

      Q72.811   Congenital shortening of right lower limb

      Q72.812   Congenital shortening of left lower limb

      Q72.813   Congenital shortening of lower limb, bilateral

      Q72.819   Congenital shortening of unspecified lower limb

    Q72.89   Other reduction defects of lower limb

      Q72.891   Other reduction defects of right lower limb

      Q72.892   Other reduction defects of left lower limb

      Q72.893   Other reduction defects of lower limb, bilateral

      Q72.899   Other reduction defects of unspecified lower limb

Q72.9   **Unspecified reduction defect of lower limb**

    Q72.90   Unspecified reduction defect of unspecified lower limb

    Q72.91   Unspecified reduction defect of right lower limb

    Q72.92   Unspecified reduction defect of left lower limb

    Q72.93   Unspecified reduction defect of lower limb, bilateral

Q73   **Reduction defects of unspecified limb**

Q73.0   **Congenital absence of unspecified limb(s)**

Amelia NOS

Q73.1   **Phocomelia, unspecified limb(s)**

Phocomelia NOS

Q73.8   **Other reduction defects of unspecified limb(s)**

Longitudinal reduction deformity of unspecified limb(s)

Ectromelia of limb NOS

Hemimelia of limb NOS

Reduction defect of limb NOS

Q74   **Other congenital malformations of limb(s)**

Excludes1: polydactyly (Q69.-)

    reduction defect of limb (Q71-Q73)

    syndactyly (Q70.-)

Q74.0   **Other congenital malformations of upper limb(s), including shoulder girdle**

Accessory carpal bones

Cleidocranial dysostosis

Congenital pseudarthrosis of clavicle

Macrodactylia (fingers)

Madelung's deformity

Radioulnar synostosis

Sprengel's deformity

Triphalangeal thumb

Q74.1   **Congenital malformation of knee**

Congenital absence of patella

Congenital dislocation of patella

Congenital genu valgum

Congenital genu varum

Rudimentary patella

Excludes1: congenital dislocation of knee (Q68.2)

    congenital genu recurvatum (Q68.2)

    nail patella syndrome (Q87.2)

Q74.2   **Other congenital malformations of lower limb(s), including pelvic girdle**

Congenital fusion of sacroiliac joint

Congenital malformation of ankle joint

Congenital malformation of sacroiliac joint

Excludes1: anteversion of femur (neck) (Q65.89)

Q74.3 **Arthrogryposis multiplex congenita**

Q74.8 **Other specified congenital malformations of limb(s)**

Q74.9 **Unspecified congenital malformation of limb(s)**

Congenital anomaly of limb(s) NOS

Q75 **Other congenital malformations of skull and face bones**

Excludes1: congenital malformation of face NOS (Q18.-)

congenital malformation syndromes classified to Q87.-

dentofacial anomalies [including malocclusion] (M26.-)

musculoskeletal deformities of head and face (Q67.0-Q67.4)

skull defects associated with congenital anomalies of brain such as: anencephaly (Q00.0)

encephalocele (Q01.-)

hydrocephalus (Q03.-)

microcephaly (Q02)

Q75.0 **Craniosynostosis**

Acrocephaly

Imperfect fusion of skull

Oxycephaly

Trigonocephaly

Q75.1 **Craniofacial dysostosis**

Crouzon's disease

Q75.2 **Hypertelorism**

Q75.3 **Macrocephaly**

Q75.4 **Mandibulofacial dysostosis**

Franceschetti syndrome

Treacher Collins syndrome

Q75.5 **Oculomandibular dysostosis**

Q75.8 **Other specified congenital malformations of skull and face bones**

Absence of skull bone, congenital

Congenital deformity of forehead

Platybasia

Q75.9 **Congenital malformation of skull and face bones, unspecified**

Congenital anomaly of face bones NOS

Congenital anomaly of skull NOS

Q76 **Congenital malformations of spine and bony thorax**

Excludes1: congenital musculoskeletal deformities of spine and chest (Q67.5-Q67.8)

Q76.0 **Spina bifida occulta**

Excludes1: meningocele (spinal) (Q05.-)

spina bifida (aperta) (cystica) (Q05.-)

Q76.1 **Klippel-Feil syndrome**

Cervical fusion syndrome

Q76.2 **Congenital spondylolisthesis**

Congenital spondylolysis

Excludes1: spondylolisthesis (acquired) (M43.1-)

spondylolysis (acquired) (M43.0-)

Q76.3 **Congenital scoliosis due to congenital bony malformation**

Hemivertebra fusion or failure of segmentation with scoliosis

Q76.4 **Other congenital malformations of spine, not associated with scoliosis**

Q76.41 **Congenital kyphosis**

Q76.411 **Congenital kyphosis, occipito-atlanto-axial region**

Q76.412 **Congenital kyphosis, cervical region**

Q76.413 **Congenital kyphosis, cervicothoracic region**

Q76.414 **Congenital kyphosis, thoracic region**

Q76.415 **Congenital kyphosis, thoracolumbar region**

Q76.419 **Congenital kyphosis, unspecified region**

Q76.42 **Congenital lordosis**

Q76.425 **Congenital lordosis, thoracolumbar region**

Q76.426 **Congenital lordosis, lumbar region**

Q76.427 **Congenital lordosis, lumbosacral region**

Q76.428 **Congenital lordosis, sacral and sacrococcygeal region**

Q76.429 **Congenital lordosis, unspecified region**

Q76.49 **Other congenital malformations of spine, not associated with scoliosis**

Congenital absence of vertebra NOS

Congenital fusion of spine NOS

Congenital malformation of lumbosacral (joint) (region) NOS

Congenital malformation of spine NOS

Hemivertebra NOS

Malformation of spine NOS

Platyspondylisis NOS

Supernumerary vertebra NOS

Q76.5 **Cervical rib**

Supernumerary rib in cervical region

Q76.6 **Other congenital malformations of ribs**

Accessory rib

Congenital absence of rib

Congenital fusion of ribs

Congenital malformation of ribs NOS

Excludes1: short rib syndrome (Q77.2)

Q76.7 **Congenital malformation of sternum**

Congenital absence of sternum

Sternum bifidum

Q76.8 **Other congenital malformations of bony thorax**

Q76.9 **Congenital malformation of bony thorax, unspecified**

Q77 **Osteochondrodysplasia with defects of growth of tubular bones and spine**

Excludes1: mucopolysaccharidosis (E76.0-E76.3)

Excludes2: congenital myotonic chondrodystrophy (G71.13)

Q77.0 **Achondrogenesis**

Hypochondrogenesis

Q77.1 **Thanatophoric short stature**

● New code   ▲ Revised code   **Excludes1:** Not coded here   **Excludes2:** Not included here   ⊗ Placeholder required   ⑦7th digit required

Q77.2 **Short rib syndrome**
Asphyxiating thoracic dysplasia [Jeune]

Q77.3 **Chondrodysplasia punctata**
Excludes1: Rhizomelic chondrodysplasia punctata (E71.43)

Q77.4 **Achondroplasia**
Hypochondroplasia
Osteosclerosis congenita

Q77.5 **Diastrophic dysplasia**

Q77.6 **Chondroectodermal dysplasia**
Ellis-van Creveld syndrome

Q77.7 **Spondyloepiphyseal dysplasia**

Q77.8 **Other osteochondrodysplasia with defects of growth of tubular bones and spine**

Q77.9 **Osteochondrodysplasia with defects of growth of tubular bones and spine, unspecified**

Q78 **Other osteochondrodysplasias**
Excludes2: congenital myotonic chondrodystrophy (G71.13)

Q78.0 **Osteogenesis imperfecta**
Fragilitas ossium
Osteopsathyrosis

Q78.1 **Polyostotic fibrous dysplasia**
Albright(-McCune)(-Sternberg) syndrome

Q78.2 **Osteopetrosis**
Albers-Schönberg syndrome
Osteosclerosis NOS

Q78.3 **Progressive diaphyseal dysplasia**
Camurati-Engelmann syndrome

Q78.4 **Enchondromatosis**
Maffucci's syndrome
Ollier's disease

Q78.5 **Metaphyseal dysplasia**
Pyle's syndrome

Q78.6 **Multiple congenital exostoses**
Diaphyseal aclasis

Q78.8 **Other specified osteochondrodysplasias**
Osteopoikilosis

Q78.9 **Osteochondrodysplasia, unspecified**
Chondrodystrophy NOS
Osteodystrophy NOS

Q79 **Congenital malformations of musculoskeletal system, not elsewhere classified**
Excludes2: congenital (sternomastoid) torticollis (Q68.0)

Q79.0 **Congenital diaphragmatic hernia**
Excludes1: congenital hiatus hernia (Q40.1)

Q79.1 **Other congenital malformations of diaphragm**
Absence of diaphragm
Congenital malformation of diaphragm NOS
Eventration of diaphragm

Q79.2 **Exomphalos**
Omphalocele
Excludes1: umbilical hernia (K42.-)

Q79.3 **Gastroschisis**

Q79.4 **Prune belly syndrome**
Congenital prolapse of bladder mucosa

Eagle-Barrett syndrome

Q79.5 **Other congenital malformations of abdominal wall**
Excludes1: umbilical hernia (K42.-)

Q79.51 **Congenital hernia of bladder**

Q79.59 **Other congenital malformations of abdominal wall**

Q79.6 **Ehlers-Danlos syndrome**

Q79.8 **Other congenital malformations of musculoskeletal system**
Absence of muscle
Absence of tendon
Accessory muscle
Amyotrophia congenita
Congenital constricting bands
Congenital shortening of tendon
Poland syndrome

Q79.9 **Congenital malformation of musculoskeletal system, unspecified**
Congenital anomaly of musculoskeletal system NOS
Congenital deformity of musculoskeletal system NOS

OTHER CONGENITAL MALFORMATIONS (Q80-Q89)

Q80 **Congenital ichthyosis**
Excludes1: Refsum's disease (G60.1)

Q80.0 **Ichthyosis vulgaris**

Q80.1 **X-linked ichthyosis**

Q80.2 **Lamellar ichthyosis**
Collodion baby

Q80.3 **Congenital bullous ichthyosiform erythroderma**

Q80.4 **Harlequin fetus**

Q80.8 **Other congenital ichthyosis**

Q80.9 **Congenital ichthyosis, unspecified**

Q81 **Epidermolysis bullosa**

Q81.0 **Epidermolysis bullosa simplex**
Excludes1: Cockayne's syndrome (Q87.1)

Q81.1 **Epidermolysis bullosa letalis**
Herlitz' syndrome

Q81.2 **Epidermolysis bullosa dystrophica**

Q81.8 **Other epidermolysis bullosa**

Q81.9 **Epidermolysis bullosa, unspecified**

Q82 **Other congenital malformations of skin**
Excludes1: acrodermatitis enteropathica (E83.2)
congenital erythropoietic porphyria (E80.0)
pilonidal cyst or sinus (L05.-)
Sturge-Weber (-Dimitri) syndrome (Q85.8)

Q82.0 **Hereditary lymphedema**

Q82.1 **Xeroderma pigmentosum**

Q82.2 **Mastocytosis**
Urticaria pigmentosa
Excludes1: malignant mastocytosis (C96.2)

Q82.3 **Incontinentia pigmenti**

Q82.4 **Ectodermal dysplasia (anhidrotic)**
Excludes1: Ellis-van Creveld syndrome (Q77.6)

Q82.5 **Congenital non-neoplastic nevus**
Birthmark NOS

Flammeus Nevus

Portwine Nevus

Sanguineous Nevus

Strawberry Nevus

Vascular Nevus NOS

Verrucous Nevus

Excludes2: Café au lait spots (L81.3)

lentigo (L81.4) nevus NOS (D22.-)

araneus nevus (I78.1)

melanocytic nevus (D22.-)

pigmented nevus (D22.-)

spider nevus (I78.1)

stellar nevus (I78.1)

•Q82.6   **Congenital sacral dimple**

Parasacral dimple

Excludes2: pilonidal cyst with abscess (L05.01)

pilonidal cyst without abscess (L05.91)

Q82.8   **Other specified congenital malformations of skin**

Abnormal palmar creases

Accessory skin tags

Benign familial pemphigus [Hailey-Hailey]

Congenital poikiloderma

Cutis laxa (hyperelastica)

Dermatoglyphic anomalies

Inherited keratosis palmaris et plantaris

Keratosis follicularis [Darier-White]

Excludes1: Ehlers-Danlos syndrome (Q79.6)

Q82.9   **Congenital malformation of skin, unspecified**

Q83   **Congenital malformations of breast**

Excludes2: absence of pectoral muscle (Q79.8)

hypoplasia of breast (N64.82)

micromastia (N64.82)

Q83.0   **Congenital absence of breast with absent nipple**

Q83.1   **Accessory breast**

Supernumerary breast

Q83.2   **Absent nipple**

Q83.3   **Accessory nipple**

Supernumerary nipple

Q83.8   **Other congenital malformations of breast**

Q83.9   **Congenital malformation of breast, unspecified**

Q84   **Other congenital malformations of integument**

Q84.0   **Congenital alopecia**

Congenital atrichosis

Q84.1   **Congenital morphological disturbances of hair, not elsewhere classified**

Beaded hair

Monilethrix

Pili annulati

Excludes1: Menkes' kinky hair syndrome (E83.0)

Q84.2   **Other congenital malformations of hair**

Congenital hypertrichosis

Congenital malformation of hair NOS

Persistent lanugo

Q84.3   **Anonychia**

Excludes1: nail patella syndrome (Q87.2)

Q84.4   **Congenital leukonychia**

Q84.5   **Enlarged and hypertrophic nails**

Congenital onychauxis

Pachyonychia

Q84.6   **Other congenital malformations of nails**

Congenital clubnail

Congenital koilonychia

Congenital malformation of nail NOS

Q84.8   **Other specified congenital malformations of integument**

Aplasia cutis congenita

Q84.9   **Congenital malformation of integument, unspecified**

Congenital anomaly of integument NOS

Congenital deformity of integument NOS

Q85   **Phakomatoses, not elsewhere classified**

Excludes1: ataxia telangiectasia [Louis-Bar] (G11.3)

familial dysautonomia [Riley-Day] (G90.1)

Q85.0   **Neurofibromatosis (nonmalignant)**

Q85.00   **Neurofibromatosis, unspecified**

Q85.01   **Neurofibromatosis, type 1**

Von Recklinghausen disease

Q85.02   **Neurofibromatosis, type 2**

Acoustic neurofibromatosis

Q85.03   **Schwannomatosis**

Q85.09   **Other neurofibromatosis**

Q85.1   **Tuberous sclerosis**

Bourneville's disease

Epiloia

Q85.8   **Other phakomatoses, not elsewhere classified**

Peutz-Jeghers Syndrome

Sturge-Weber(-Dimitri) syndrome von Hippel-Lindau syndrome

Excludes1: Meckel-Gruber syndrome (Q61.9)

Q85.9   **Phakomatosis, unspecified**

Hamartosis NOS

Q86   **Congenital malformation syndromes due to known exogenous causes, not elsewhere classified**

Excludes2: iodine-deficiency-related hypothyroidism (E00-E02)

nonteratogenic effects of substances transmitted via placenta or breast milk (P04.-)

Q86.0   **Fetal alcohol syndrome (dysmorphic)**

Q86.1   **Fetal hydantoin syndrome**

Meadow's syndrome

Q86.2   **Dysmorphism due to warfarin**

Q86.8   **Other congenital malformation syndromes due to known exogenous causes**

Q87   **Other specified congenital malformation syndromes affecting multiple systems**

Use additional code(s) to identify all associated manifestations

Q87.0   **Congenital malformation syndromes predominantly affecting facial appearance**

Acrocephalopolysyndactyly

Acrocephalosyndactyly [Apert]

Cryptophthalmos syndrome

Cyclopia

Goldenhar syndrome

Moebius syndrome

Oro-facial-digital syndrome

Robin syndrome

Whistling face

Q87.1 **Congenital malformation syndromes predominantly associated with short stature**

Aarskog syndrome

Cockayne syndrome

De Lange syndrome

Dubowitz syndrome Noonan syndrome

Prader-Willi syndrome

Robinow-Silverman-Smith syndrome

Russell-Silver syndrome

Seckel syndrome

Excludes1: Ellis-van Creveld syndrome (Q77.6)

Smith-Lemli-Opitz syndrome (E78.72)

Q87.2 **Congenital malformation syndromes predominantly involving limbs**

Holt-Oram syndrome

Klippel-Trenaunay-Weber syndrome Nail patella syndrome

Rubinstein-Taybi syndrome

Sirenomelia syndrome

Thrombocytopenia with absent radius [TAR] syndrome

VATER syndrome

Q87.3 **Congenital malformation syndromes involving early overgrowth**

Beckwith-Wiedemann syndrome

Sotos syndrome

Weaver syndrome

Q87.4 **Marfan's syndrome**

Q87.40 **Marfan's syndrome, unspecified**

Q87.41 **Marfan's syndrome with cardiovascular manifestations**

Q87.410 **Marfan's syndrome with aortic dilation**

Q87.418 **Marfan's syndrome with other cardiovascular manifestations**

Q87.42 **Marfan's syndrome with ocular manifestations**

Q87.43 **Marfan's syndrome with skeletal manifestation**

Q87.5 **Other congenital malformation syndromes with other skeletal changes**

Q87.8 **Other specified congenital malformation syndromes, not elsewhere classified**

Excludes1: Zellweger syndrome (E71.510)

Q87.81 **Alport syndrome**

Use additional code to identify stage of chronic kidney disease (N18.1-N18.6)

• **Q87.82** **Arterial tortuosity syndrome**

Q87.89 **Other specified congenital malformation syndromes, not elsewhere classified**

Laurence-Moon (-Bardet)-Biedl syndrome

Q89 **Other congenital malformations, not elsewhere classified**

Q89.0 **Congenital absence and malformations of spleen**

Excludes1: isomerism of atrial appendages (with asplenia or polysplenia) (Q20.6)

Q89.01 **Asplenia (congenital)**

Q89.09 **Congenital malformations of spleen**

Congenital splenomegaly

Q89.1 **Congenital malformations of adrenal gland**

Excludes1: adrenogenital disorders (E25.-)

congenital adrenal hyperplasia (E25.0)

Q89.2 **Congenital malformations of other endocrine glands**

Congenital malformation of parathyroid or thyroid gland

Persistent thyroglossal duct

Thyroglossal cyst

Excludes1: congenital goiter (E03.0)

congenital hypothyroidism (E03.1)

Q89.3 **Situs inversus**

Dextrocardia with situs inversus

Mirror-image atrial arrangement with situs inversus

Situs inversus or transversus abdominalis

Situs inversus or transversus thoracis

Transposition of abdominal viscera

Transposition of thoracic viscera

Excludes1: dextrocardia NOS (Q24.0)

Q89.4 **Conjoined twins**

Craniopagus

Dicephaly

Pygopagus

Thoracopagus

Q89.7 **Multiple congenital malformations, not elsewhere classified**

Multiple congenital anomalies NOS

Multiple congenital deformities NOS

Excludes1: congenital malformation syndromes affecting multiple systems (Q87.-)

Q89.8 **Other specified congenital malformations**

Use additional code(s) to identify all associated manifestations

Q89.9 **Congenital malformation, unspecified**

Congenital anomaly NOS

Congenital deformity NOS

CHROMOSOMAL ABNORMALITIES, NOT ELSEWHERE CLASSIFIED (Q90-Q99)

Excludes2: mitochondrial metabolic disorders (E88.4-)

Q90 **Down syndrome**

Use additional code(s) to identify any associated physical conditions and degree of intellectual disabilities (F70-F79)

Q90.0 **Trisomy 21, nonmosaicism (meiotic nondisjunction)**

Q90.1 **Trisomy 21, mosaicism (mitotic nondisjunction)**

Q90.2 **Trisomy 21, translocation**

Q90.9 **Down syndrome, unspecified**

Trisomy 21 NOS

Q91 **Trisomy 18 and Trisomy 13**

Q91.0 **Trisomy 18, nonmosaicism (meiotic nondisjunction)**

Q91.1 **Trisomy 18, mosaicism (mitotic nondisjunction)**

Q91.2 **Trisomy 18, translocation**

Q91.3 **Trisomy 18, unspecified**

Q91.4 **Trisomy 13, nonmosaicism (meiotic nondisjunction)**

Q91.5   **Trisomy 13, mosaicism (mitotic nondisjunction)**

Q91.6   **Trisomy 13, translocation**

Q91.7   **Trisomy 13, unspecified**

Q92   **Other trisomies and partial trisomies of the autosomes, not elsewhere classified**

Includes: unbalanced translocations and insertions

Excludes1: trisomies of chromosomes 13, 18, 21 (Q90-Q91)

Q92.0   **Whole chromosome trisomy, nonmosaicism (meiotic nondisjunction)**

Q92.1   **Whole chromosome trisomy, mosaicism (mitotic nondisjunction)**

Q92.2   **Partial trisomy**

Less than whole arm duplicated Whole arm or more duplicated

Excludes1: partial trisomy due to unbalanced translocation (Q92.5)

Q92.5   **Duplications with other complex rearrangements**

Partial trisomy due to unbalanced translocations

Code also any associated deletions due to unbalanced translocations, inversions and insertions (Q93.7)

Q92.6   **Marker chromosomes**

Trisomies due to dicentrics

Trisomies due to extra rings

Trisomies due to isochromosomes

Individual with marker heterochromatin

Q92.61   **Marker chromosomes in normal individual**

Q92.62   **Marker chromosomes in abnormal individual**

Q92.7   **Triploidy and polyploidy**

Q92.8   **Other specified trisomies and partial trisomies of autosomes**

Duplications identified by fluorescence in situ hybridization (FISH)

Duplications identified by in situ hybridization (ISH)

Duplications seen only at prometaphase

Q92.9   **Trisomy and partial trisomy of autosomes, unspecified**

Q93   **Monosomies and deletions from the autosomes, not elsewhere classified**

Q93.0   **Whole chromosome monosomy, nonmosaicism (meiotic nondisjunction)**

Q93.1   **Whole chromosome monosomy, mosaicism (mitotic nondisjunction)**

Q93.2   **Chromosome replaced with ring, dicentric or isochromosome**

Q93.3   **Deletion of short arm of chromosome 4**

Wolff-Hirschorn syndrome

Q93.4   **Deletion of short arm of chromosome 5**

Cri-du-chat syndrome

Q93.5   **Other deletions of part of a chromosome**

Angelman syndrome

Q93.7   **Deletions with other complex rearrangements**

Deletions due to unbalanced translocations, inversions and insertions

Code also any associated duplications due to unbalanced translocations, inversions and insertions (Q92.5)

Q93.8   **Other deletions from the autosomes**

Q93.81   **Velo-cardio-facial syndrome**

Deletion 22q11.2

Q93.88   **Other microdeletions**

Miller-Dieker syndrome

Smith-Magenis syndrome

Q93.89   **Other deletions from the autosomes**

Deletions identified by fluorescence in situ hybridization (FISH)

Deletions identified by in situ hybridization (ISH)

Deletions seen only at prometaphase

Q93.9   **Deletion from autosomes, unspecified**

Q95   **Balanced rearrangements and structural markers, not elsewhere classified**

Includes: Robertsonian and balanced reciprocal translocations and insertions

Q95.0   **Balanced translocation and insertion in normal individual**

Q95.1   **Chromosome inversion in normal individual**

Q95.2   **Balanced autosomal rearrangement in abnormal individual**

Q95.3   **Balanced sex/autosomal rearrangement in abnormal individual**

Q95.5   **Individual with autosomal fragile site**

Q95.8   **Other balanced rearrangements and structural markers**

Q95.9   **Balanced rearrangement and structural marker, unspecified**

Q96   **Turner's syndrome**

Excludes1: Noonan syndrome (Q87.1)

Q96.0   **Karyotype 45, X**

Q96.1   **Karyotype 46, X iso (Xq)**

Karyotype 46, isochromosome Xq

Q96.2   **Karyotype 46, X with abnormal sex chromosome, except iso (Xq)**

Karyotype 46, X with abnormal sex chromosome, except isochromosome Xq

Q96.3   **Mosaicism, 45, X/46, XX or XY**

Q96.4   **Mosaicism, 45, X/Other cell line(s) with abnormal sex chromosome**

Q96.8   **Other variants of Turner's syndrome**

Q96.9   **Turner's syndrome, unspecified**

Q97   **Other sex chromosome abnormalities, female phenotype, not elsewhere classified**

Excludes1: Turner's syndrome (Q96.-)

Q97.0   **Karyotype 47, XXX**

Q97.1   **Female with more than three X chromosomes**

Q97.2   **Mosaicism, lines with various numbers of X chromosomes**

Q97.3   **Female with 46, XY karyotype**

Q97.8   **Other specified sex chromosome abnormalities, female phenotype**

Q97.9   **Sex chromosome abnormality, female phenotype, unspecified**

Q98   **Other sex chromosome abnormalities, male phenotype, not elsewhere classified**

Q98.0   **Klinefelter syndrome karyotype 47, XXY**

Q98.1   **Klinefelter syndrome, male with more than two X chromosomes**

Q98.3   **Other male with 46, XX karyotype**

Q98.4   **Klinefelter syndrome, unspecified**

● New code   ▲ Revised code   **Excludes1:** Not coded here   **Excludes2:** Not included here   ⊗ Placeholder required   ⑦7th digit required

Q98.5   **Karyotype 47, XYY**

Q98.6   **Male with structurally abnormal sex chromosome**

Q98.7   **Male with sex chromosome mosaicism**

Q98.8   **Other specified sex chromosome abnormalities, male phenotype**

Q98.9   **Sex chromosome abnormality, male phenotype, unspecified**

Q99   **Other chromosome abnormalities, not elsewhere classified**

Q99.0   **Chimera 46, XX/46, XY**

     Chimera 46, XX/46, XY true hermaphrodite

Q99.1   **46, XX true hermaphrodite**

     46, XX with streak gonads

     46, XY with streak gonads

     Pure gonadal dysgenesis

Q99.2   **Fragile X chromosome**

     Fragile X syndrome

Q99.8   **Other specified chromosome abnormalities**

Q99.9   **Chromosomal abnormality, unspecified**

● New code ▲ Revised code **Excludes1:** Not coded here **Excludes2:** Not included here ⊗ Placeholder required ⑦ 7th digit required

Chapter 18: Symptoms, Signs And Abnormal Clinical And Laboratory Findings, Not Elsewhere Classified (R00-R99)

DEFINITIONS

This chapter includes definitions of selected key words, terms and phrases and coding alerts for adding points to the clinical domain, and references to coding late effects where appropriate. An example from this chapter is as follows:

R16 Hepatomegaly and splenomegaly, not elsewhere classified
Definition: Hepatomegaly refers to abnormal enlargement of the liver. Splenomegaly refers to abnormal enlargement of the spleen.

MULTIPLE CODING FOR A SINGLE CONDITION

In addition to the etiology/manifestation convention that requires two codes to fully describe a single condition that affects multiple body systems, there are other single conditions that also require more than one code. "Use additional code" notes are found in the Tabular List at codes that are not part of an etiology/manifestation pair where a secondary code is useful to fully describe a condition. The sequencing rule is the same as the etiology/manifestation pair, "use additional code" indicates that a secondary code should be added.

For example, for bacterial infections that are not included in chapter 1, a secondary code from category B95, Streptococcus, Staphylococcus, and Enterococcus, as the cause of diseases classified elsewhere, or B96, Other bacterial agents as the cause of diseases classified elsewhere, may be required to identify the bacterial organism causing the infection. A "use additional code" note will normally be found at the infectious disease code, indicating a need for the organism code to be added as a secondary code.

"Code first" notes are also under certain codes that are not specifically manifestation codes but may be due to an underlying cause. When there is a "code first" note and an underlying condition is present, the underlying condition should be sequenced first.

"Code, if applicable, any causal condition first", notes indicate that this code may be assigned as a principal diagnosis when the causal condition is unknown or not applicable. If a causal condition is known, then the code for that condition should be sequenced as the principal or first-listed diagnosis.

Multiple codes may be needed for sequela, complication codes and obstetric codes to more fully describe a condition. See the specific guidelines for these conditions for further instruction.

COMBINATION CODE

A combination code is a single code used to classify: Two diagnoses, or a diagnosis with an associated secondary process (manifestation) A diagnosis with an associated complication

Combination codes are identified by referring to subterm entries in the Alphabetic Index and by reading the inclusion and exclusion notes in the Tabular List.

Assign only the combination code when that code fully identifies the diagnostic conditions involved or when the Alphabetic Index so directs. Multiple coding should not be used when the classification provides a combination code that clearly identifies all of the elements documented in the diagnosis. When the combination code lacks necessary specificity in describing the manifestation or complication, an additional code should be used as a secondary code.

SEQUELA (LATE EFFECTS)

A sequela is the residual effect (condition produced) after the acute phase of an illness or injury has terminated. There is no time limit on when a sequela code can be used. The residual may be apparent early, such as in cerebral infarction, or it may occur months or years later, such as that due to a previous injury. Coding of sequela generally requires two codes sequenced in the following order: The condition or nature of the sequela is sequenced first.

The sequela code is sequenced second.

An exception to the above guidelines are those instances where the code for the sequela is followed by a manifestation code identified in the Tabular List and title, or the sequela code has been expanded (at the fourth, fifth or sixth character levels) to include the manifestation(s). The code for the acute phase of an illness or injury that led to the sequela is never used with a code for the late effect.

Chapter 18 includes symptoms, signs, abnormal results of clinical or other investigative procedures, and ill-defined conditions regarding which no diagnosis classifiable elsewhere is recorded. Signs and symptoms that point to a specific diagnosis have been assigned to a category in other chapters of the classification.

USE OF SYMPTOM CODES

Codes that describe symptoms and signs are acceptable for reporting purposes when a related definitive diagnosis has not been established (confirmed) by the provider.

USE OF A SYMPTOM CODE WITH A DEFINITIVE DIAGNOSIS CODE

Codes for signs and symptoms may be reported in addition to a related definitive diagnosis when the sign or symptom is not routinely associated with that diagnosis, such as the various signs and symptoms associated with complex syndromes. The definitive diagnosis code should be sequenced before the symptom code.

Signs or symptoms that are associated routinely with a disease process should not be assigned as additional codes, unless otherwise instructed by the classification.

COMBINATION CODES THAT INCLUDE SYMPTOMS

ICD-10-CM contains a number of combination codes that identify both the definitive diagnosis and common symptoms of that diagnosis. When using one of these combination codes, an additional code should not be assigned for the symptom.

REPEATED FALLS

Code R29.6, Repeated falls, is for use for encounters when a patient has recently fallen and the reason for the fall is being investigated.

Code Z91.81, History of falling, is for use when a patient has fallen in the past and is at risk for future falls. When appropriate, both codes R29.6 and Z91.81 may be assigned together.

COMA SCALE

The coma scale codes (R40.2-) can be used in conjunction with traumatic brain injury codes, acute cerebrovascular disease or sequelae of cerebrovascular disease codes. These codes are primarily for use by trauma registries, but they may be used in any setting where this information is collected. The coma scale may also be used to assess the status of the central nervous system for other non-trauma conditions, such as monitoring patients in the intensive care unit regardless of medical condition. The coma scale codes should be sequenced after the diagnosis code(s).

These codes, one from each subcategory, are needed to complete the scale. The 7th character indicates when the scale was recorded. The 7th character should match for all three codes.

At a minimum, report the initial score documented on presentation at your facility. This may be a score from the emergency medicine technician (EMT) or in the emergency department. If desired, a facility may choose to capture multiple coma scale scores.

Assign code R40.24, Glasgow coma scale, total score, when only the total score is documented in the medical record and not the individual score(s).

FUNCTIONAL QUADRIPLEGIA

Functional quadriplegia (code R53.2) is the lack of ability to use one's limbs or to ambulate due to extreme debility. It is not associated with neurologic deficit or injury, and code R53.2 should not be used for cases of neurologic quadriplegia. It should only be assigned if functional quadriplegia is specifically documented in the medical record.

SIRS DUE TO NON-INFECTIOUS PROCESS

The systemic inflammatory response syndrome (SIRS) can develop as a result of certain non-infectious disease processes, such as trauma, malignant neoplasm, or pancreatitis. When SIRS is documented with a noninfectious condition, and no subsequent infection is documented, the code for the underlying condition, such as an injury, should be assigned, followed by code R65.10, Systemic inflammatory response syndrome (SIRS) of non-infectious origin without acute organ dysfunction, or code R65.11, Systemic inflammatory response syndrome (SIRS) of non-infectious origin with acute organ dysfunction. If an associated acute organ dysfunction is documented, the appropriate code(s) for the specific type of organ dysfunction(s) should be assigned in addition to code R65.11. If acute organ dysfunction is documented, but it cannot be determined if the acute organ dysfunction is associated with SIRS or due to another condition (e.g., directly due to the trauma), the provider should be queried.

DEATH NOS

Code R99, Ill-defined and unknown cause of mortality, is only for use in the very limited circumstance when a patient who has already died is brought into an emergency department or other healthcare facility and is pronounced dead upon arrival. It does not represent the discharge disposition of death.

NIHSS STROKE SCALE

The NIH stroke scale (NIHSS) codes (R29.7- -) can be used in conjunction with acute stroke codes (I63) to identify the patient's neurological status and the severity of the stroke. The stroke scale codes should be sequenced after the acute stroke diagnosis code(s).

At a minimum, report the initial score documented. If desired, a facility may choose to capture multiple stroke scale scores.

See Section I.B.14.for information concerning the medical record documentation that may be used for assignment of the NIHSS codes.

Chapter 18

Symptoms, Signs And Abnormal Clinical And Laboratory Findings, Not Elsewhere Classified (R00-R99)

Note: This chapter includes symptoms, signs, abnormal results of clinical or other investigative procedures, and ill-defined conditions regarding which no diagnosis classifiable elsewhere is recorded.

Signs and symptoms that point rather definitely to a given diagnosis have been assigned to a category in other chapters of the classification. In general, categories in this chapter include the less well-defined conditions and symptoms that, without the necessary study of the case to establish a final diagnosis, point perhaps equally to two or more diseases or to two or more systems of the body. Practically all categories in the chapter could be designated 'not otherwise specified', 'unknown etiology' or 'transient'. The Alphabetical Index should be consulted to determine which symptoms and signs are to be allocated here and which to other chapters. The residual subcategories, numbered .8, are generally provided for other relevant symptoms that cannot be allocated elsewhere in the classification.

The conditions and signs or symptoms included in categories R00-R94 consist of: (a) cases for which no more specific diagnosis can be made even after all the facts bearing on the case have been investigated; (b) signs or symptoms existing at the time of initial encounter that proved to be transient and whose causes could not be determined; (c) provisional diagnosis in a patient who failed to return for further investigation or care; (d) cases referred elsewhere for investigation or treatment before the diagnosis was made; (e) cases in which a more precise diagnosis was not available for any other reason; (f) certain symptoms, for which supplementary information is provided, that represent important problems in medical care in their own right.

Excludes2: abnormal findings on antenatal screening of mother (O28.-)

certain conditions originating in the perinatal period (P04-P96)

signs and symptoms classified in the body system chapters signs and symptoms of breast (N63, N64.5)

This chapter contains the following blocks:

R00-R09	Symptoms and signs involving the circulatory and respiratory systems
R10-R19	Symptoms and signs involving the digestive system and abdomen
R20-R23	Symptoms and signs involving the skin and subcutaneous tissue
R25-R29	Symptoms and signs involving the nervous and musculoskeletal systems
R30-R39	Symptoms and signs involving the genitourinary system
R40-R46	Symptoms and signs involving cognition, perception, emotional state and behavior
R47-R49	Symptoms and signs involving speech and voice
R50-R69	General symptoms and signs
R70-R79	Abnormal findings on examination of blood, without diagnosis
R80-R82	Abnormal findings on examination of urine, without diagnosis
R83-R89	Abnormal findings on examination of other body fluids, substances and tissues, without diagnosis
R90-R94	Abnormal findings on diagnostic imaging and in function studies, without diagnosis
R97	Abnormal tumor markers
R99	Ill-defined and unknown cause of mortality

SYMPTOMS AND SIGNS INVOLVING THE CIRCULATORY AND RESPIRATORY SYSTEMS (R00-R09)

R00   **Abnormalities of heart beat**

Excludes1: abnormalities originating in the perinatal period (P29.1-)

Excludes2: specified arrhythmias (I47-I49)

R00.0   **Tachycardia, unspecified**

Rapid heart beat

Sinoauricular tachycardia NOS

Sinus [sinusal] tachycardia NOS

Excludes1: neonatal tachycardia (P29.11)

paroxysmal tachycardia (I47.-)

R00.1   **Bradycardia, unspecified**

Sinoatrial bradycardia

Sinus bradycardia

Slow heart beat

Vagal bradycardia

Use additional code for adverse effect, if applicable, to identify drug (T36-T50 with fifth or sixth character 5)

Excludes1: neonatal bradycardia (P29.12)

R00.2   **Palpitations**

Awareness of heart beat

R00.8   **Other abnormalities of heart beat**

R00.9   **Unspecified abnormalities of heart beat**

R01   **Cardiac murmurs and other cardiac sounds**

Excludes1: cardiac murmurs and sounds originating in the perinatal period (P29.8)

R01.0   **Benign and innocent cardiac murmurs**

Functional cardiac murmur

R01.1   **Cardiac murmur, unspecified**

Cardiac bruit NOS

Heart murmur NOS

Systolic murmur NOS

R01.2   **Other cardiac sounds**

Cardiac dullness, increased or decreased

Precordial friction

R03   **Abnormal blood-pressure reading, without diagnosis**

R03.0   **Elevated blood-pressure reading, without diagnosis of hypertension**

Note: This category is to be used to record an episode of elevated blood pressure in a patient in whom no formal diagnosis of hypertension has been made, or as an isolated incidental finding.

R03.1   **Nonspecific low blood-pressure reading**

Excludes1: hypotension (I95.-)

maternal hypotension syndrome (O26.5-)

neurogenic orthostatic hypotension (G90.3)

R04   **Hemorrhage from respiratory passages**

R04.0   **Epistaxis**

Hemorrhage from nose Nosebleed

R04.1   **Hemorrhage from throat**

Excludes2: hemoptysis (R04.2)

R04.2   **Hemoptysis**

Blood-stained sputum

Cough with hemorrhage

R04.8   **Hemorrhage from other sites in respiratory passages**

R04.81   **Acute idiopathic pulmonary hemorrhage in infants**

AIPHI

Acute idiopathic hemorrhage in infants over 28 days old

Excludes1: perinatal pulmonary hemorrhage (P26.-)

von Willebrand's disease (D68.0)

R04.89 **Hemorrhage from other sites in respiratory passages**

Pulmonary hemorrhage NOS

R04.9 **Hemorrhage from respiratory passages, unspecified**

R05 **Cough**

Excludes1: cough with hemorrhage (R04.2)

smoker's cough (J41.0)

R06 **Abnormalities of breathing**

Excludes1: acute respiratory distress syndrome (J80)

respiratory arrest (R09.2)

respiratory arrest of newborn (P28.81)

respiratory distress syndrome of newborn (P22.-)

respiratory failure (J96.-)

respiratory failure of newborn (P28.5)

R06.0 **Dyspnea**

Excludes1: tachypnea NOS (R06.82)

transient tachypnea of newborn (P22.1)

R06.00 **Dyspnea, unspecified**

R06.01 **Orthopnea**

R06.02 **Shortness of breath**

R06.09 **Other forms of dyspnea**

R06.1 **Stridor **

Excludes1: congenital laryngeal stridor (P28.89)

laryngismus (stridulus) (J38.5)

R06.2 **Wheezing**

Excludes1: Asthma (J45.-)

R06.3 **Periodic breathing**

Cheyne-Stokes breathing

R06.4 **Hyperventilation**

Excludes1: psychogenic hyperventilation (F45.8)

R06.5 **Mouth breathing**

Excludes2: dry mouth NOS (R68.2)

R06.6 **Hiccough**

Excludes1: psychogenic hiccough (F45.8)

R06.7 **Sneezing**

R06.8 **Other abnormalities of breathing**

R06.81 **Apnea, not elsewhere classified**

Apnea NOS

Excludes1: apnea (of) newborn (P28.4)

sleep apnea (G47.3-)

sleep apnea of newborn (primary) (P28.3)

R06.82 **Tachypnea, not elsewhere classified**

Tachypnea NOS

Excludes1: transitory tachypnea of newborn (P22.1)

R06.83 **Snoring**

R06.89 **Other abnormalities of breathing**

Breath-holding (spells)

Sighing

R06.9 **Unspecified abnormalities of breathing**

R07 **Pain in throat and chest**

Excludes1: epidemic myalgia (B33.0)

Excludes2: jaw pain R68.84

pain in breast (N64.4)

R07.0 **Pain in throat**

Excludes1: chronic sore throat (J31.2)

sore throat (acute) NOS (J02.9)

Excludes2: dysphagia (R13.1-)

pain in neck (M54.2)

R07.1 **Chest pain on breathing**

Painful respiration

R07.2 **Precordial pain**

R07.8 **Other chest pain**

R07.81 **Pleurodynia**

Pleurodynia NOS

Excludes1: epidemic pleurodynia (B33.0)

R07.82 **Intercostal pain**

R07.89 **Other chest pain**

Anterior chest-wall pain NOS

R07.9 **Chest pain, unspecified**

R09 **Other symptoms and signs involving the circulatory and respiratory system**

Excludes1: acute respiratory distress syndrome (J80)

respiratory arrest of newborn (P28.81)

respiratory distress syndrome of newborn (P22.0)

respiratory failure (J96.-)

respiratory failure of newborn (P28.5)

R09.0 **Asphyxia and hypoxemia**

Excludes1: asphyxia due to carbon monoxide (T58.-)

asphyxia due to foreign body in respiratory tract (T17.-)

birth (intrauterine) asphyxia (P84)

hypercapnia (R06.4)

hyperventilation (R06.4) traumatic asphyxia (T71.-)

R09.01 **Asphyxia**

R09.02 **Hypoxemia**

R09.1 **Pleurisy**

Excludes1: pleurisy with effusion (J90)

R09.2 **Respiratory arrest**

Cardiorespiratory failure

Excludes1: cardiac arrest (I46.-)

respiratory arrest of newborn (P28.81)

respiratory distress of newborn (P22.0)

respiratory failure (J96.-)

respiratory failure of newborn (P28.5)

respiratory insufficiency (R06.89)

respiratory insufficiency of newborn (P28.5)

R09.3 **Abnormal sputum**

Abnormal amount of sputum

Abnormal color of sputum

Abnormal odor of sputum

Excessive sputum

Excludes1: blood-stained sputum (R04.2)

R09.8 **Other specified symptoms and signs involving the circulatory and respiratory systems**

R09.81 **Nasal congestion**

R09.82 **Postnasal drip**

R09.89 **Other specified symptoms and signs involving the circulatory and respiratory systems**

Bruit (arterial)

Abnormal chest percussion

Feeling of foreign body in throat

Friction sounds in chest

Chest tympany Choking sensation

Rales

Weak pulse

Excludes2: foreign body in throat (T17.2-)

wheezing (R06.2)

SYMPTOMS AND SIGNS INVOLVING THE DIGESTIVE SYSTEM AND ABDOMEN (R10-R19)

Excludes2: congenital or infantile pylorospasm (Q40.0)

gastrointestinal hemorrhage (K92.0-K92.2)

intestinal obstruction (K56.-)

newborn gastrointestinal hemorrhage (P54.0-P54.3)

newborn intestinal obstruction (P76.-)

pylorospasm (K31.3)

signs and symptoms involving the urinary system (R30-R39)

symptoms referable to female genital organs (N94.-)

symptoms referable to male genital organs (N48-N50)

R10 **Abdominal and pelvic pain**

Excludes1: renal colic (N23)

Excludes2: dorsalgia (M54.-)

flatulence and related conditions (R14.-)

R10.0 **Acute abdomen**

Severe abdominal pain (generalized) (with abdominal rigidity)

Excludes1: abdominal rigidity NOS (R19.3)

generalized abdominal pain NOS (R10.84)

localized abdominal pain (R10.1-R10.3-)

R10.1 **Pain localized to upper abdomen**

R10.10 **Upper abdominal pain, unspecified**

R10.11 **Right upper quadrant pain**

R10.12 **Left upper quadrant pain**

R10.13 **Epigastric pain**

Dyspepsia

Excludes1: functional dyspepsia (K30)

R10.2 **Pelvic and perineal pain**

Excludes1: vulvodynia (N94.81)

R10.3 **Pain localized to other parts of lower abdomen**

R10.30 **Lower abdominal pain, unspecified**

R10.31 **Right lower quadrant pain**

R10.32 **Left lower quadrant pain**

R10.33 **Periumbilical pain**

R10.8 **Other abdominal pain**

R10.81 **Abdominal tenderness**

Abdominal tenderness NOS

R10.811 **Right upper quadrant abdominal tenderness**

R10.812 **Left upper quadrant abdominal tenderness**

R10.813 **Right lower quadrant abdominal tenderness**

R10.814 **Left lower quadrant abdominal tenderness**

R10.815 **Periumbilic abdominal tenderness**

R10.816 **Epigastric abdominal tenderness**

R10.817 **Generalized abdominal tenderness**

R10.819 **Abdominal tenderness, unspecified site**

R10.82 **Rebound abdominal tenderness**

R10.821 **Right upper quadrant rebound abdominal tenderness**

R10.822 **Left upper quadrant rebound abdominal tenderness**

R10.823 **Right lower quadrant rebound abdominal tenderness**

R10.824 **Left lower quadrant rebound abdominal tenderness**

R10.825 **Periumbilic rebound abdominal tenderness**

R10.826 **Epigastric rebound abdominal tenderness**

R10.827 **Generalized rebound abdominal tenderness**

R10.829 **Rebound abdominal tenderness, unspecified site**

R10.83 **Colic**

Colic NOS

Infantile colic

Excludes1: colic in adult and child over 12 months old (R10.84)

R10.84 **Generalized abdominal pain**

Excludes1: generalized abdominal pain associated with acute abdomen (R10.0)

R10.9 **Unspecified abdominal pain**

R11 **Nausea and vomiting**

Excludes1: cyclical vomiting associated with migraine (G43.A-)

excessive vomiting in pregnancy (O21.-)

hematemesis (K92.0)

neonatal hematemesis (P54.0)

newborn vomiting (P92.0-)

psychogenic vomiting (F50.89)

vomiting associated with bulimia nervosa (F50.2)

vomiting following gastrointestinal surgery (K91.0)

R11.0 **Nausea**

Nausea NOS

Nausea without vomiting

R11.1 **Vomiting**

R11.10 **Vomiting, unspecified**

Vomiting NOS

R11.11 **Vomiting without nausea**

R11.12 **Projectile vomiting**

R11.13 **Vomiting of fecal matter**

R11.14 **Bilious vomiting**

Bilious emesis

R11.2 Nausea with vomiting, unspecified

Persistent nausea with vomiting NOS

R12 Heartburn

Excludes1: dyspepsia NOS (R10.13)

functional dyspepsia (K30)

R13 Aphagia and dysphagia

R13.0 Aphagia

Inability to swallow

Excludes1: psychogenic aphagia (F50.9)

R13.1 Dysphagia

Code first, if applicable, dysphagia following cerebrovascular disease (I69. with final characters -91)

Excludes1: psychogenic dysphagia (F45.8)

R13.10 Dysphagia, unspecified

Difficulty in swallowing NOS

R13.11 Dysphagia, oral phase

R13.12 Dysphagia, oropharyngeal phase

R13.13 Dysphagia, pharyngeal phase

R13.14 Dysphagia, pharyngoesophageal phase

R13.19 Other dysphagia

Cervical dysphagia Neurogenic dysphagia

R14 Flatulence and related conditions

Excludes1: psychogenic aerophagy (F45.8)

R14.0 Abdominal distension (gaseous)

Bloating

Tympanites (abdominal) (intestinal)

R14.1 Gas pain

R14.2 Eructation

R14.3 Flatulence

R15 Fecal incontinence

Includes: encopresis NOS

Excludes1: fecal incontinence of nonorganic origin (F98.1)

R15.0 Incomplete defecation

Excludes1: constipation (K59.0-)

fecal impaction (K56.41)

R15.1 Fecal smearing

Fecal soiling

R15.2 Fecal urgency

R15.9 Full incontinence of feces

Fecal incontinence NOS

R16 Hepatomegaly and splenomegaly, not elsewhere classified

Definition: Cleft lip is a congenital deformity characterized by a vertical cleft or pair of clefts in the upper lip, with or without involvement of the palate. Cleft palate is a congenital fissure in the roof of the mouth, resulting from incomplete fusion of the palate during embryonic development.

R16.0 Hepatomegaly, not elsewhere classified

Hepatomegaly NOS

R16.1 Splenomegaly, not elsewhere classified

Splenomegaly NOS

R16.2 Hepatomegaly with splenomegaly, not elsewhere classified

Hepatosplenomegaly NOS

R17 Unspecified jaundice

Excludes1: neonatal jaundice (P55, P57-P59)

R18 Ascites

Includes: fluid in peritoneal cavity

Excludes1: ascites in alcoholic cirrhosis (K70.31)

ascites in alcoholic hepatitis (K70.11)

ascites in toxic liver disease with chronic active hepatitis (K71.51)

R18.0 Malignant ascites

Code first malignancy, such as:

malignant neoplasm of ovary (C56.-)

secondary malignant neoplasm of retroperitoneum and peritoneum (C78.6)

R18.8 Other ascites

Ascites NOS

Peritoneal effusion (chronic)

R19 Other symptoms and signs involving the digestive system and abdomen

Excludes1: acute abdomen (R10.0)

R19.0 Intra-abdominal and pelvic swelling, mass and lump

Excludes1: abdominal distension (gaseous) (R14.-)

ascites (R18.-)

R19.00 Intra-abdominal and pelvic swelling, mass and lump, unspecified site

R19.01 Right upper quadrant abdominal swelling, mass and lump

R19.02 Left upper quadrant abdominal swelling, mass and lump

R19.03 Right lower quadrant abdominal swelling, mass and lump

R19.04 Left lower quadrant abdominal swelling, mass and lump

R19.05 Periumbilic swelling, mass or lump

Diffuse or generalized umbilical swelling or mass

R19.06 Epigastric swelling, mass or lump

R19.07 Generalized intra-abdominal and pelvic swelling, mass and lump

Diffuse or generalized intra-abdominal swelling or mass NOS

Diffuse or generalized pelvic swelling or mass NOS

R19.09 Other intra-abdominal and pelvic swelling, mass and lump

R19.1 Abnormal bowel sounds

R19.11 Absent bowel sounds

R19.12 Hyperactive bowel sounds

R19.15 Other abnormal bowel sounds

Abnormal bowel sounds NOS

R19.2 Visible peristalsis

Definition: Peristalsis is the involuntary constriction and relaxation of the muscles of the intestine or another canal, creating wavelike movements that push the contents of the canal forward.

Hyperperistalsis

R19.3 Abdominal rigidity

Excludes1: abdominal rigidity with severe abdominal pain (R10.0)

R19.30 Abdominal rigidity, unspecified site

R19.31 Right upper quadrant abdominal rigidity

● New code ▲ Revised code **Excludes1:** Not coded here **Excludes2:** Not included here ⊗ Placeholder required ⑦ 7th digit required

R19.32　Left upper quadrant abdominal rigidity

R19.33　Right lower quadrant abdominal rigidity

R19.34　Left lower quadrant abdominal rigidity

R19.35　Periumbilic abdominal rigidity

R19.36　Epigastric abdominal rigidity

R19.37　Generalized abdominal rigidity

R19.4　Change in bowel habit

Excludes1: constipation (K59.0-)

functional diarrhea (K59.1)

R19.5　Other fecal abnormalities

Abnormal stool color

Bulky stools

Mucus in stools

Occult blood in feces

Occult blood in stools

Excludes1: melena (K92.1)

neonatal melena (P54.1)

R19.6　Halitosis

R19.7　Diarrhea, unspecified

Diarrhea NOS

Excludes1: functional diarrhea (K59.1)

neonatal diarrhea (P78.3) psychogenic diarrhea (F45.8)

R19.8　Other specified symptoms and signs involving the digestive system and abdomen

SYMPTOMS AND SIGNS INVOLVING THE SKIN AND SUBCUTANEOUS TISSUE (R20-R23)

Excludes2: symptoms relating to breast (N64.4-N64.5)

R20　Disturbances of skin sensation

Excludes1: dissociative anesthesia and sensory loss (F44.6)

psychogenic disturbances (F45.8)

R20.0　Anesthesia of skin

R20.1　Hypoesthesia of skin

R20.2　Paresthesia of skin

Formication

Pins and needles

Tingling skin

Excludes1: acroparesthesia (I73.8)

R20.3　Hyperesthesia

R20.8　Other disturbances of skin sensation

R20.9　Unspecified disturbances of skin sensation

R21　Rash and other nonspecific skin eruption

Includes: rash NOS

Excludes1: specified type of rash- code to condition

vesicular eruption (R23.8)

R22　Localized swelling, mass and lump of skin and subcutaneous tissue

Includes: subcutaneous nodules (localized)(superficial)

Excludes1: abnormal findings on diagnostic imaging (R90-R93)

edema (R60.-)

enlarged lymph nodes (R59.-) \

localized adiposity (E65)

swelling of joint (M25.4-)

R22.0　Localized swelling, mass and lump, head

R22.1　Localized swelling, mass and lump, neck

R22.2　Localized swelling, mass and lump, trunk

Excludes1: intra-abdominal or pelvic mass and lump (R19.0-)

intra-abdominal or pelvic swelling (R19.0-)

Excludes2: breast mass and lump (N63)

R22.3　Localized swelling, mass and lump, upper limb

R22.30　Localized swelling, mass and lump, unspecified upper limb

R22.31　Localized swelling, mass and lump, right upper limb

R22.32　Localized swelling, mass and lump, left upper limb

R22.33　Localized swelling, mass and lump, upper limb, bilateral

R22.4　Localized swelling, mass and lump, lower limb

R22.40　Localized swelling, mass and lump, unspecified lower limb

R22.41　Localized swelling, mass and lump, right lower limb

R22.42　Localized swelling, mass and lump, left lower limb

R22.43　Localized swelling, mass and lump, lower limb, bilateral

R22.9　Localized swelling, mass and lump, unspecified

R23　Other skin changes

R23.0　Cyanosis

Excludes1: acrocyanosis (I73.8)

cyanotic attacks of newborn (P28.2)

R23.1　Pallor Clammy skin

R23.2　Flushing

Excessive blushing

Code first, if applicable, menopausal and female climacteric states (N95.1)

R23.3　Spontaneous ecchymoses

Petechiae

Excludes1: ecchymoses of newborn (P54.5)

purpura (D69.-)

R23.4　Changes in skin texture

Desquamation of skin

Induration of skin

Scaling of skin

Excludes1: epidermal thickening NOS (L85.9)

R23.8　Other skin changes

R23.9　Unspecified skin changes

SYMPTOMS AND SIGNS INVOLVING THE NERVOUS AND MUSCULOSKELETAL SYSTEMS (R25-R29)

R25　Abnormal involuntary movements

Excludes1: specific movement disorders (G20-G26)

stereotyped movement disorders (F98.4)

tic disorders (F95.-)

R25.0　Abnormal head movements

R25.1　Tremor, unspecified

Excludes1: chorea NOS (G25.5)

essential tremor (G25.0)

hysterical tremor (F44.4)

| Add 4th-7th digits | Nonspecific code | Unspecified code | Manifestation code |

intention tremor (G25.2)

R25.2 Cramp and spasm

Excludes2: carpopedal spasm (R29.0)

charley-horse (M62.831)

infantile spasms (G40.4-)

muscle spasm of back (M62.830)

muscle spasm of calf (M62.831)

R25.3 Fasciculation

Twitching NOS

R25.8 Other abnormal involuntary movements

R25.9 Unspecified abnormal involuntary movements

R26 Abnormalities of gait and mobility

Excludes1: ataxia NOS (R27.0)

hereditary ataxia (G11.-)

locomotor (syphilitic) ataxia (A52.11)

immobility syndrome (paraplegic) (M62.3)

R26.0 Ataxic gait

Staggering gait

R26.1 Paralytic gait

Spastic gait

R26.2 Difficulty in walking, not elsewhere classified

Excludes1: falling (R29.6)

unsteadiness on feet (R26.81)

R26.8 Other abnormalities of gait and mobility

R26.81 Unsteadiness on feet

R26.89 Other abnormalities of gait and mobility

R26.9 Unspecified abnormalities of gait and mobility

R27 Other lack of coordination

Excludes1: ataxic gait (R26.0)

hereditary ataxia (G11.-)

vertigo NOS (R42)

R27.0 Ataxia, unspecified

Excludes1: ataxia following cerebrovascular disease (I69. with final characters -93)

R27.8 Other lack of coordination

R27.9 Unspecified lack of coordination

R29 Other symptoms and signs involving the nervous and musculoskeletal systems

R29.0 Tetany Carpopedal spasm

Excludes1: hysterical tetany (F44.5)

neonatal tetany (P71.3)

parathyroid tetany (E20.9)

post-thyroidectomy tetany (E89.2)

R29.1 Meningismus

R29.2 Abnormal reflex

Excludes2: abnormal pupillary reflex (H57.0)

hyperactive gag reflex (J39.2)

vasovagal reaction or syncope (R55)

R29.3 Abnormal posture

R29.4 Clicking hip

Excludes1: congenital deformities of hip (Q65.-)

R29.5 Transient paralysis

Code first any associated spinal cord injury (S14.0, S14.1-, S24.0, S24.1-, S34.0-, S34.1-)

Excludes1: transient ischemic attack (G45.9)

R29.6 Repeated falls

Falling

Tendency to fall

Excludes2: at risk for falling (Z91.81)

history of falling (Z91.81)

R29.7 National Institutes of Health Stroke Scale (NIHSS) score

Code first the type of cerebral infarction (I63-)

R29.70 NIHSS score 0-9

•**R29.700 NIHSS score 0**

•**R29.701 NIHSS score 1**

•**R29.702 NIHSS score 2**

•**R29.703 NIHSS score 3**

•**R29.704 NIHSS score 4**

•**R29.705 NIHSS score 5**

•**R29.706 NIHSS score 6**

•**R29.707 NIHSS score 7**

•**R29.708 NIHSS score 8**

•**R29.709 NIHSS score 9**

R29.71 NIHSS score 10-19

•**R29.710 NIHSS score 10**

•**R29.711 NIHSS score 11**

•**R29.712 NIHSS score 12**

•**R29.713 NIHSS score 13**

•**R29.714 NIHSS score 14**

•**R29.715 NIHSS score 15**

•**R29.716 NIHSS score 16**

•**R29.717 NIHSS score 17**

•**R29.718 NIHSS score 18**

•**R29.719 NIHSS score 19**

R29.72 NIHSS score 20-29

•**R29.720 NIHSS score 20**

•**R29.721 NIHSS score 21**

•**R29.722 NIHSS score 22**

•**R29.723 NIHSS score 23**

•**R29.724 NIHSS score 24**

•**R29.725 NIHSS score 25**

•**R29.726 NIHSS score 26**

•**R29.727 NIHSS score 27**

•**R29.728 NIHSS score 28**

•**R29.729 NIHSS score 29**

R29.73 NIHSS score 30-39

•**R29.730 NIHSS score 30**

•**R29.731 NIHSS score 31**

•**R29.732 NIHSS score 32**

•**R29.733 NIHSS score 33**

•**R29.734 NIHSS score 34**

•**R29.735 NIHSS score 35**

•**R29.736 NIHSS score 36**

•**R29.737 NIHSS score 37**

•**R29.738 NIHSS score 38**

•**R29.739 NIHSS score 39**

R29.74 NIHSS score 40-42

- •R29.740 **NIHSS score 40**
- •R29.741 **NIHSS score 41**
- •R29.742 **NIHSS score 42**

R29.8 **Other symptoms and signs involving the nervous and musculoskeletal systems**

  R29.81 **Other symptoms and signs involving the nervous system**

    R29.810 **Facial weakness**

    Facial droop

    Excludes1: Bell's palsy (G51.0)

    facial weakness following cerebrovascular disease (I69. with final characters -92)

    R29.818 **Other symptoms and signs involving the nervous system**

  R29.89 **Other symptoms and signs involving the musculoskeletal system**

    Excludes2: pain in limb (M79.6-)

    R29.890 **Loss of height**

    Excludes1: osteoporosis (M80-M81)

    R29.891 **Ocular torticollis**

    Excludes1: congenital (sternomastoid) torticollis Q68.0

    psychogenic torticollis (F45.8)

    spasmodic torticollis (G24.3)

    torticollis due to birth injury (P15.8)

    torticollis NOS M43.6

    R29.898 **Other symptoms and signs involving the musculoskeletal system**

R29.9 **Unspecified symptoms and signs involving the nervous and musculoskeletal systems**

  R29.90 **Unspecified symptoms and signs involving the nervous system**

  R29.91 **Unspecified symptoms and signs involving the musculoskeletal system**

SYMPTOMS AND SIGNS INVOLVING THE GENITOURINARY SYSTEM (R30-R39)

R30 **Pain associated with micturition**

Excludes1: psychogenic pain associated with micturition (F45.8)

R30.0 **Dysuria**

Strangury

R30.1 **Vesical tenesmus**

R30.9 **Painful micturition, unspecified**

Painful urination NOS

R31 **Hematuria**

Excludes1: hematuria included with underlying conditions, such as:

acute cystitis with hematuria (N30.01)

recurrent and persistent hematuria in glomerular diseases (N02.-)

R31.0 **Gross hematuria**

R31.1 **Benign essential microscopic hematuria**

R31.2 **Other microscopic hematuria**

  •R31.21 **Asymptomatic microscopic hematuria**

  AMH

  •R31.29 **Other microscopic hematuria**

R31.9 **Hematuria, unspecified**

R32 **Unspecified urinary incontinence**

Enuresis NOS

Excludes1: functional urinary incontinence (R39.81)

nonorganic enuresis (F98.0)

stress incontinence and other specified urinary incontinence (N39.3-N39.4-)

urinary incontinence associated with cognitive impairment (R39.81)

R33 **Retention of urine**

Excludes1: psychogenic retention of urine (F45.8)

R33.0 **Drug induced retention of urine**

Use additional code for adverse effect, if applicable, to identify drug (T36-T50 with fifth or sixth character 5)

R33.8 **Other retention of urine**

Code first, if applicable, any causal condition, such as: enlarged prostate (N40.1)

R33.9 **Retention of urine, unspecified**

R34 **Anuria and oliguria**

Excludes1: anuria and oliguria complicating abortion or ectopic or molar pregnancy (O00-O07, O08.4)

anuria and oliguria complicating pregnancy (O26.83-)

anuria and oliguria complicating the puerperium (O90.4)

R35 **Polyuria**

Code first, if applicable, any causal condition, such as: enlarged prostate (N40.1)

Excludes1: psychogenic polyuria (F45.8)

R35.0 **Frequency of micturition**

R35.1 **Nocturia**

R35.8 **Other polyuria**

Polyuria NOS

R36 **Urethral discharge**

R36.0 **Urethral discharge without blood**

R36.1 **Hematospermia**

R36.9 **Urethral discharge, unspecified**

Penile discharge NOS

Urethrorrhea

R37 **Sexual dysfunction, unspecified**

R39 **Other and unspecified symptoms and signs involving the genitourinary system**

R39.0 **Extravasation of urine**

R39.1 **Other difficulties with micturition**

Code first, if applicable, any causal condition, such as: enlarged prostate (N40.1)

R39.11 **Hesitancy of micturition**

R39.12 **Poor urinary stream**

Weak urinary steam

R39.13 **Splitting of urinary stream**

R39.14 **Feeling of incomplete bladder emptying**

R39.15 **Urgency of urination**

Excludes1: urge incontinence (N39.41, N39.46)

R39.16 **Straining to void**

R39.19 **Other difficulties with micturition**

  •R39.191 **Need to immediately re-void**

  •R39.192 **Position dependent micturition**

●**R39.198**   **Other difficulties with micturition**

R39.2   **Extrarenal uremia**

Prerenal uremia

Excludes1: uremia NOS (N19)

R39.8   **Other symptoms and signs involving the genitourinary system**

R39.81   **Functional urinary incontinence**

Urinary incontinence due to cognitive impairment, or severe physical disability or immobility

Excludes1: stress incontinence **and other** specified urinary incontinence (N39.3-N39.4-)

urinary incontinence NOS (R32)

●**R39.82**   **Chronic bladder pain**

R39.89   **Other symptoms and signs involving the genitourinary system**

R39.9   **Unspecified symptoms and signs involving the genitourinary system**

SYMPTOMS AND SIGNS INVOLVING COGNITION, PERCEPTION, EMOTIONAL STATE AND BEHAVIOR (R40-R46)

Excludes2: symptoms and signs constituting part of a pattern of mental disorder (F01-F99)

R40   **Somnolence, stupor and coma**

Definition: Somnolence (or "drowsiness") is a state of near-sleep, a strong desire for sleep, or sleeping for unusually long periods (cf. hypersomnia).

Excludes1: neonatal coma (P91.5)

somnolence, stupor and coma in diabetes (E08-E13)

somnolence, stupor and coma in hepatic failure (K72.-)

somnolence, stupor and coma in hypoglycemia (nondiabetic) (E15)

R40.0   **Somnolence**

Drowsiness

Excludes1: coma (R40.2-)

R40.1   **Stupor** Catatonic stupor

Semicoma

Excludes1: catatonic schizophrenia (F20.2)

coma (R40.2-)

depressive stupor (F31-F33)

dissociative stupor (F44.2)

manic stupor (F30.2)

R40.2   **Coma**

Code first any associated:

fracture of skull (S02.-)

intracranial injury (S06.-)

Note: One code from each subcategory, R40.21-R40.23, is required to complete the coma scale

R40.20   **Unspecified coma**

Coma NOS

Unconsciousness NOS

R40.21   **Coma scale, eyes open**

The following appropriate 7th character is to be added to subcategory R40.21-:

0 - unspecified time

1 - in the field [EMT or ambulance]

2 - at arrival to emergency department

3 - at hospital admission

4 - 24 hours or more after hospital admission

⑦**R40.211**   **Coma scale, eyes open, never**

⑦**R40.212**   **Coma scale, eyes open, to pain**

⑦**R40.213**   **Coma scale, eyes open, to sound**

⑦**R40.214**   **Coma scale, eyes open, spontaneous**

R40.22   **Coma scale, best verbal response**

The following appropriate 7th character is to be added to subcategory R40.22-:

0 - unspecified time

1 - in the field [EMT or ambulance]

2 - at arrival to emergency department

3 - at hospital admission

4 - 24 hours or more after hospital admission

⑦**R40.221**   **Coma scale, best verbal response, none**

⑦**R40.222**   **Coma scale, best verbal response, incomprehensible words**

⑦**R40.223**   **Coma scale, best verbal response, inappropriate words**

⑦**R40.224**   **Coma scale, best verbal response, confused conversation**

⑦**R40.225**   **Coma scale, best verbal response, oriented**

R40.23   **Coma scale, best motor response**

The following appropriate 7th character is to be added to subcategory R40.23-:

0 - unspecified time

1 - in the field [EMT or ambulance]

2 - at arrival to emergency department

3 - at hospital admission

4 - 24 hours or more after hospital admission

⑦**R40.231**   **Coma scale, best motor response, none**

⑦**R40.232**   **Coma scale, best motor response, extension**

⑦**R40.233**   **Coma scale, best motor response, abnormal**

⑦**R40.234**   **Coma scale, best motor response, flexion withdrawal**

⑦**R40.235**   **Coma scale, best motor response, localizes pain**

⑦**R40.236**   **Coma scale, best motor response, obeys commands**

R40.24   **Glasgow coma scale, total score**

Note: Assign a code from subcategory R40.24, when only the total coma score is documented

The following appropriate 7th character is to be added to subcategory R40.24-:

0 - unspecified time

1 - in the field [EMT or ambulance]

2 - at arrival to emergency department

3 - at hospital admission

4 - 24 hours or more after hospital admission

●⑦**R40.241**   **Glasgow coma scale score 13-15**

●⑦**R40.242**   **Glasgow coma scale score 9-12**

●⑦**R40.243**   **Glasgow coma scale score 3-8**

● ⑦ **R40.244**   **Other coma, without documented Glasgow coma scale score, or with partial score reported**

R40.3   **Persistent vegetative state**

R40.4   **Transient alteration of awareness**

R41   **Other symptoms and signs involving cognitive functions and awareness**

   Excludes1: dissociative [conversion] disorders (F44.-)

     mild cognitive impairment, so stated (G31.84)

R41.0   **Disorientation, unspecified**

   Confusion NOS

   Delirium NOS

R41.1   **Anterograde amnesia**

R41.2   **Retrograde amnesia**

R41.3   **Other amnesia**

   Amnesia NOS

   Memory loss NOS

   Excludes1: amnestic disorder due to known physiologic condition (F04)

     amnestic syndrome due to psychoactive substance use (F10-F19 with 5th character .6)

     mild memory disturbance due to known physiological condition (F06.8)

     transient global amnesia (G45.4)

R41.4   **Neurologic neglect syndrome**

   Asomatognosia

   Hemi-akinesia

   Hemi-inattention

   Hemispatial neglect

   Left-sided neglect

   Sensory neglect

   Visuospatial neglect

   Excludes1: visuospatial deficit (R41.842)

R41.8   **Other symptoms and signs involving cognitive functions and awareness**

   R41.81   **Age-related cognitive decline**

     Senility NOS

   R41.82   **Altered mental status, unspecified**

     Change in mental status NOS

     Excludes1: altered level of consciousness (R40.-)

     altered mental status due to known condition - code to condition delirium NOS (R41.0)

   R41.83   **Borderline intellectual functioning**

     IQ level 71 to 84

     Excludes1: intellectual disabilities (F70-F79)

   R41.84   **Other specified cognitive deficit**

     Excludes1: cognitive deficits as sequelae of cerebrovascular disease (I69.01-, I69.11-, I69.21-, I69.31-, I69.81-, I69.91-)

     R41.840   **Attention and concentration deficit**

       Excludes1: attention-deficit hyperactivity disorders (F90.-)

     R41.841   **Cognitive communication deficit**

     R41.842   **Visuospatial deficit**

     R41.843   **Psychomotor deficit**

     R41.844   **Frontal lobe and executive function deficit**

   R41.89   **Other symptoms and signs involving cognitive functions and awareness**

     Anosognosia

R41.9   **Unspecified symptoms and signs involving cognitive functions and awareness**

R42   **Dizziness and giddiness**

   Light-headedness

   Vertigo NOS

   Excludes1: vertiginous syndromes (H81.-)

     vertigo from infrasound (T75.23)

R43   **Disturbances of smell and taste**

R43.0   **Anosmia**

R43.1   **Parosmia**

R43.2   **Parageusia**

R43.8   **Other disturbances of smell and taste**

   Mixed disturbance of smell and taste

R43.9   **Unspecified disturbances of smell and taste**

R44   **Other symptoms and signs involving general sensations and perceptions**

   Excludes1: alcoholic hallucinations (F1.5)

     hallucinations in drug psychosis (F11-F19 with .5)

     hallucinations in mood disorders with psychotic symptoms (F30.2, F31.5, F32.3, F33.3)

     hallucinations in schizophrenia, schizotypal and delusional disorders (F20-F29)

   Excludes2: disturbances of skin sensation (R20.-)

R44.0   **Auditory hallucinations**

R44.1   **Visual hallucinations**

R44.2   **Other hallucinations**

R44.3   **Hallucinations, unspecified**

R44.8   **Other symptoms and signs involving general sensations and perceptions**

R44.9   **Unspecified symptoms and signs involving general sensations and perceptions**

R45   **Symptoms and signs involving emotional state**

R45.0   **Nervousness**

   Nervous tension

R45.1   **Restlessness and agitation**

R45.2   **Unhappiness**

R45.3   **Demoralization and apathy**

   Excludes1: anhedonia (R45.84)

R45.4   **Irritability and anger**

R45.5   **Hostility**

R45.6   **Violent behavior**

R45.7   **State of emotional shock and stress, unspecified**

R45.8   **Other symptoms and signs involving emotional state**

   R45.81   **Low self-esteem**

   R45.82   **Worries**

   R45.83   **Excessive crying of child, adolescent or adult**

     Excludes1: excessive crying of infant (baby) R68.11

   R45.84   **Anhedonia**

   R45.85   **Homicidal and suicidal ideations**

     Excludes1: suicide attempt (T14.91)

     R45.850   **Homicidal ideations**

     R45.851   **Suicidal ideations**

R45.86   **Emotional lability**

R45.87   **Impulsiveness**

R45.89   **Other symptoms and signs involving emotional state**

R46   **Symptoms and signs involving appearance and behavior**

Excludes1: appearance and behavior in schizophrenia, schizotypal and delusional disorders (F20-F29)

mental and behavioral disorders (F01-F99)

R46.0   **Very low level of personal hygiene**

R46.1   **Bizarre personal appearance**

R46.2   **Strange and inexplicable behavior**

R46.3   **Overactivity**

R46.4   **Slowness and poor responsiveness**

Excludes1: stupor (R40.1)

R46.5   **Suspiciousness and marked evasiveness**

R46.6   **Undue concern and preoccupation with stressful events**

R46.7   **Verbosity and circumstantial detail obscuring reason for contact**

R46.8   **Other symptoms and signs involving appearance and behavior**

R46.81   **Obsessive-compulsive behavior** **Excludes1:** obsessive-compulsive disorder (F42-)

R46.89   **Other symptoms and signs involving appearance and behavior**

SYMPTOMS AND SIGNS INVOLVING SPEECH AND VOICE (R47-R49)

R47   **Speech disturbances, not elsewhere classified**

Excludes1: autism (F84.0)

cluttering (F80.81)

specific developmental disorders of speech and language (F80.-)

stuttering (F80.81)

R47.0   **Dysphasia and aphasia**

R47.01   **Aphasia**

Excludes1: aphasia following cerebrovascular disease (I69. with final characters -20)

progressive isolated aphasia (G31.01)

R47.02   **Dysphasia**

Excludes1: dysphasia following cerebrovascular disease (I69. with final characters -21)

R47.1   **Dysarthria and anarthria**

Excludes1: dysarthria following cerebrovascular disease (I69. with final characters -22)

R47.8   **Other speech disturbances**

Excludes1: dysarthria following cerebrovascular disease (I69. with final characters -28)

R47.81   **Slurred speech**

R47.82   **Fluency disorder in conditions classified elsewhere**

Stuttering in conditions classified elsewhere

Code first underlying disease or condition, such as:

Parkinson's disease (G20)

Excludes1: adult onset fluency disorder (F98.5)

childhood onset fluency disorder (F80.81)

fluency disorder (stuttering) following cerebrovascular disease (I69. with final characters -23)

R47.89   **Other speech disturbances**

R47.9   **Unspecified speech disturbances**

R48   **Dyslexia and other symbolic dysfunctions, not elsewhere classified**

Definition: Dyslexia is a general term for disorders that involve difficulty in learning to read or interpret words, letters, and other symbols, but that do not affect general intelligence.

Excludes1: specific developmental disorders of scholastic skills (F81.-)

R48.0   **Dyslexia and alexia**

R48.1   **Agnosia**

Astereognosia (astereognosis)

Autotopagnosia

Excludes1: visual object agnosia (R48.3)

R48.2   **Apraxia**

Excludes1: apraxia following cerebrovascular disease (I69. with final characters -90)

R48.3   **Visual agnosia**

Prosopagnosia

Simultanagnosia (asimultagnosia)

R48.8   **Other symbolic dysfunctions**

Acalculia

Agraphia

R48.9   **Unspecified symbolic dysfunctions**

R49   **Voice and resonance disorders**

Excludes1: psychogenic voice and resonance disorders (F44.4)

R49.0   **Dysphonia**

Hoarseness

R49.1   **Aphonia**

Loss of voice

R49.2   **Hypernasality and hyponasality**

R49.21   **Hypernasality**

R49.22   **Hyponasality**

R49.8   **Other voice and resonance disorders**

R49.9   **Unspecified voice and resonance disorder**

Change in voice NOS Resonance disorder NOS

GENERAL SYMPTOMS AND SIGNS (R50-R69)

R50   **Fever of other and unknown origin**

Excludes1: chills without fever (R68.83)

febrile convulsions (R56.0-)

fever of unknown origin during labor (O75.2) fever of unknown origin in newborn (P81.9)

hypothermia due to illness (R68.0)

malignant hyperthermia due to anesthesia (T88.3) puerperal pyrexia NOS (O86.4)

R50.2   **Drug induced fever**

Use additional code for adverse effect, if applicable, to identify drug (T36-T50 with fifth or sixth character 5)

Excludes1: postvaccination (postimmunization) fever (R50.83)

R50.8   **Other specified fever**

R50.81   **Fever presenting with conditions classified elsewhere**

Code first underlying condition when associated fever is present, such as with:

leukemia (C91-C95)

neutropenia (D70.-)

sickle-cell disease (D57.-)

R50.82   Postprocedural fever

Excludes1: postprocedural infection (T81.4-)

posttransfusion fever (R50.84)

postvaccination (postimmunization) fever (R50.83)

R50.83   Postvaccination fever

Postimmunization fever

R50.84   Febrile nonhemolytic transfusion reaction

FNHTR Posttransfusion fever

R50.9   Fever, unspecified

Fever NOS

Fever of unknown origin [FUO]

Fever with chills

Fever with rigors

Hyperpyrexia NOS

Persistent fever

Pyrexia NOS

R51   Headache

Facial pain NOS

Excludes1: atypical face pain (G50.1)

migraine **and other** headache syndromes (G43-G44)

trigeminal neuralgia (G50.0)

R52   Pain, unspecified

Acute pain NOS

Generalized pain NOS

Pain NOS

Excludes1: acute and chronic pain, not elsewhere classified (G89.-)

localized pain, unspecified type - code to pain by site, such as: abdomen pain (R10.-)

back pain (M54.9)

breast pain (N64.4)

chest pain (R07.1-R07.9)

ear pain (H92.0-)

eye pain (H57.1)

headache (R51)

joint pain (M25.5-)

limb pain (M79.6-)

lumbar region pain (M54.5)

pelvic and perineal pain (R10.2)

shoulder pain (M25.51-)

spine pain (M54.-)

throat pain (R07.0)

tongue pain (K14.6)

tooth pain (K08.8)

renal colic (N23)

pain disorders exclusively related to psychological factors (F45.41)

R53   Malaise and fatigue

R53.0   Neoplastic (malignant) related fatigue

Code first associated neoplasm

R53.1   Weakness

Asthenia NOS

Excludes1: age-related weakness (R54)

muscle weakness (M62.8-)

sarcopenia (M62.84)

senile asthenia (R54)

R53.2   Functional quadriplegia

Complete immobility due to severe physical disability or frailty

Excludes1: frailty NOS (R54)

hysterical paralysis (F44.4)

immobility syndrome (M62.3)

neurologic quadriplegia (G82.5-)

quadriplegia (G82.50)

R53.8   Other malaise and fatigue

Excludes1: combat exhaustion and fatigue (F43.0)

congenital debility (P96.9)

exhaustion and fatigue due to depressive episode (F32.-)

exhaustion and fatigue due to excessive exertion (T73.3)

exhaustion and fatigue due to exposure (T73.2)

exhaustion and fatigue due to heat (T67.-)

exhaustion and fatigue due to pregnancy (O26.8-)

exhaustion and fatigue due to recurrent depressive episode (F33)

exhaustion and fatigue due to senile debility (R54)

R53.81   Other malaise

Chronic debility

Debility NOS

General physical deterioration

Malaise NOS

Nervous debility

Excludes1: age-related physical debility (R54)

R53.82   Chronic fatigue, unspecified

Chronic fatigue syndrome NOS

Excludes1: postviral fatigue syndrome (G93.3)

R53.83   Other fatigue

Fatigue NOS

Lack of energy

Lethargy

Tiredness

R54   Age-related physical debility

Frailty

Old age

Senescence

Senile asthenia

Senile debility

Excludes1: age-related cognitive decline (R41.81)

sarcopenia (M62.84)

senile psychosis (F03)

senility NOS (R41.81)

R55   Syncope and collapse

Blackout

Add 4th-7th digits   Nonspecific code   Unspecified code   Manifestation code   739

Fainting

Vasovagal attack

Excludes1: cardiogenic shock (R57.0)

carotid sinus syncope (G90.01) heat syncope (T67.1)

neurocirculatory asthenia (F45.8)

neurogenic orthostatic hypotension (G90.3)

orthostatic hypotension (I95.1)

postprocedural shock (T81.1-)

psychogenic syncope (F48.8)

shock NOS (R57.9)

shock complicating or following abortion or ectopic or molar pregnancy (O00-O07, O08.3)

shock complicating or following labor and delivery (O75.1)

Stokes-Adams attack (I45.9)

unconsciousness NOS (R40.2-)

R56 Convulsions, not elsewhere classified

Excludes1: dissociative convulsions and seizures (F44.5)

epileptic convulsions and seizures (G40.-)

newborn convulsions and seizures (P90)

R56.0 Febrile convulsions

R56.00 Simple febrile convulsions

Febrile convulsion NOS

Febrile seizure NOS

R56.01 Complex febrile convulsions

Atypical febrile seizure

Complex febrile seizure

Complicated febrile seizure

Excludes1: status epilepticus (G40.901)

R56.1 Post traumatic seizures

Excludes1: post traumatic epilepsy (G40.-)

R56.9 Unspecified convulsions

Convulsion disorder

Fit NOS

Recurrent convulsions

Seizure(s) (convulsive) NOS

R57 Shock, not elsewhere classified

Excludes1: anaphylactic shock NOS (T78.2)

anaphylactic reaction or shock due to adverse food reaction (T78.0-)

anaphylactic shock due to adverse effect of correct drug or medicament properly administered (T88.6)

anaphylactic shock due to serum (T80.5-)

anesthetic shock (T88.3)

electric shock (T75.4)

obstetric shock (O75.1)

postprocedural shock (T81.1-)

psychic shock (F43.0)

septic shock (R65.21)

shock complicating or following ectopic or molar pregnancy (O00-O07, O08.3)

shock due to lightning (T75.01)

traumatic shock (T79.4)

toxic shock syndrome (A48.3)

R57.0 Cardiogenic shock

R57.1 Hypovolemic shock

R57.8 Other shock

R57.9 Shock, unspecified

Failure of peripheral circulation NOS

R58 Hemorrhage, not elsewhere classified

Hemorrhage NOS

Excludes1: hemorrhage included with underlying conditions, such as:

acute duodenal ulcer with hemorrhage (K26.0)

acute gastritis with bleeding (K29.01)

ulcerative enterocolitis with rectal bleeding (K51.01)

R59 Enlarged lymph nodes

Includes: swollen glands

Excludes1: lymphadenitis NOS (I88.9)

acute lymphadenitis (L04.-)

chronic lymphadenitis (I88.1)

mesenteric (acute) (chronic) lymphadenitis (I88.0)

R59.0 Localized enlarged lymph nodes

R59.1 Generalized enlarged lymph nodes

Lymphadenopathy NOS

R59.9 Enlarged lymph nodes, unspecified

R60 Edema, not elsewhere classified

Excludes1: angioneurotic edema (T78.3)

ascites (R18.-)

cerebral edema (G93.6)

cerebral edema due to birth injury (P11.0)

edema of larynx (J38.4)

edema of nasopharynx (J39.2)

edema of pharynx (J39.2)

gestational edema (O12.0-)

hereditary edema (Q82.0)

hydrops fetalis NOS (P83.2)

hydrothorax (J94.8)

nutritional edema (E40-E46)

hydrops fetalis NOS (P83.2)

newborn edema (P83.3)

pulmonary edema (J81.-)

R60.0 Localized edema

R60.1 Generalized edema

R60.9 Edema, unspecified

Fluid retention NOS

R61 Generalized hyperhidrosis

Excessive sweating Night sweats

Secondary hyperhidrosis

Code first, if applicable, menopausal and female climacteric states (N95.1)

Excludes1: focal (primary) (secondary) hyperhidrosis (L74.5-)

Frey's syndrome (L74.52)

localized (primary) (secondary) hyperhidrosis (L74.5-)

R62 Lack of expected normal physiological development in childhood and adults

Excludes1: delayed puberty (E30.0)

gonadal dysgenesis (Q99.1)

hypopituitarism (E23.0)

R62.0 Delayed milestone in childhood

Delayed attainment of expected physiological developmental stage

Late talker

Late walker

R62.5 **Other and unspecified lack of expected normal physiological development in childhood**

Excludes1: HIV disease resulting in failure to thrive (B20)

physical retardation due to malnutrition (E45)

R62.50 **Unspecified lack of expected normal physiological development in childhood**

Infantilism NOS

R62.51 **Failure to thrive (child)**

Failure to gain weight

Excludes1: failure to thrive in child under 28 days old (P92.6)

R62.52 **Short stature (child)**

Lack of growth

Physical retardation

Short stature NOS

Excludes1: short stature due to endocrine disorder (E34.3)

R62.59 **Other lack of expected normal physiological development in childhood**

R62.7 **Adult failure to thrive**

R63 **Symptoms and signs concerning food and fluid intake**

Excludes1: bulimia NOS (F50.2)

eating disorders of nonorganic origin (F50.-)

malnutrition (E40-E46)

R63.0 **Anorexia**

Loss of appetite

Excludes1: anorexia nervosa (F50.0-)

loss of appetite of nonorganic origin (F50.89)

R63.1 **Polydipsia**

Excessive thirst

R63.2 **Polyphagia**

Excessive eating

Hyperalimentation NOS

R63.3 **Feeding difficulties**

Feeding problem (elderly) (infant) NOS

Excludes1: feeding problems of newborn (P92.-)

infant feeding disorder of nonorganic origin (F98.2-)

R63.4 **Abnormal weight loss**

R63.5 **Abnormal weight gain**

Excludes1: excessive weight gain in pregnancy (O26.0-)

obesity (E66.-)

R63.6 **Underweight**

Use additional code to identify body mass index (BMI), if known (Z68.-)

Excludes1: abnormal weight loss (R63.4)

anorexia nervosa (F50.0-)

malnutrition (E40-E46)

R63.8 **Other symptoms and signs concerning food and fluid intake**

R64 **Cachexia**

Wasting syndrome

Code first underlying condition, if known

Excludes1: abnormal weight loss (R63.4)

nutritional marasmus (E41)

R65 **Symptoms and signs specifically associated with systemic inflammation and infection**

R65.1 **Systemic inflammatory response syndrome (SIRS) of non-infectious origin**

Code first underlying condition, such as:

heatstroke (T67.0)

injury and trauma (S00-T88)

Excludes1: sepsis- code to infection

severe sepsis (R65.2)

R65.10 **Systemic inflammatory response syndrome (SIRS) of non-infectious origin without acute organ dysfunction**

Systemic inflammatory response syndrome (SIRS) NOS

R65.11 **Systemic inflammatory response syndrome (SIRS) of non-infectious origin with acute organ dysfunction**

Use additional code to identify specific acute organ dysfunction, such as:

acute kidney failure (N17.-)

acute respiratory failure (J96.0-)

critical illness myopathy (G72.81)

critical illness polyneuropathy (G62.81)

disseminated intravascular coagulopathy [DIC] (D65)

encephalopathy (metabolic) (septic) (G93.41)

hepatic failure (K72.0-)

R65.2 **Severe sepsis**

Infection with associated acute organ dysfunction

Sepsis with acute organ dysfunction

Sepsis with multiple organ dysfunction

Systemic inflammatory response syndrome due to infectious process with acute organ dysfunction

Code first underlying infection, such as:

infection following a procedure (T81.4-)

infections following infusion, transfusion and therapeutic injection (T80.2-)

puerperal sepsis (O85)

sepsis following complete or unspecified spontaneous abortion (O03.87)

sepsis following ectopic and molar pregnancy (O08.82)

sepsis following incomplete spontaneous abortion (O03.37)

sepsis following (induced) termination of pregnancy (O04.87)

sepsis NOS (A41.9)

Use additional code to identify specific acute organ dysfunction, such as:

acute kidney failure (N17.-)

acute respiratory failure (J96.0-)

critical illness myopathy (G72.81)

critical illness polyneuropathy (G62.81)

disseminated intravascular coagulopathy [DIC] (D65)

encephalopathy (metabolic) (septic) (G93.41)

hepatic failure (K72.0-)

R65.20   Severe sepsis without septic shock

Severe sepsis NOS

R65.21   Severe sepsis with septic shock

R68   Other general symptoms and signs

R68.0   Hypothermia, not associated with low environmental temperature

Excludes1: hypothermia NOS (accidental) (T68)

hypothermia due to anesthesia (T88.51)

hypothermia due to low environmental temperature (T68)

newborn hypothermia (P80.-)

R68.1   Nonspecific symptoms peculiar to infancy

Excludes1: colic, infantile (R10.83)

neonatal cerebral irritability (P91.3)

teething syndrome (K00.7)

R68.11   Excessive crying of infant (baby)

Excludes1: excessive crying of child, adolescent, or adult (R45.83)

R68.12   Fussy infant (baby)

Irritable infant

R68.13   Apparent life threatening event in infant (ALTE)

Apparent life threatening event in newborn

Code first confirmed diagnosis, if known

Use additional code(s) for associated signs and symptoms if no confirmed diagnosis established, or if signs and symptoms are not associated routinely with confirmed diagnosis, or provide additional information for cause of ALTE

R68.19   Other nonspecific symptoms peculiar to infancy

R68.2   Dry mouth, unspecified

Excludes1: dry mouth due to dehydration (E86.0)

dry mouth due to sicca syndrome [Sjögren] (M35.0-)

salivary gland hyposecretion (K11.7)

R68.3   Clubbing of fingers

Clubbing of nails

Excludes1: congenital clubfinger (Q68.1)

R68.8   Other general symptoms and signs

R68.81   Early satiety

R68.82   Decreased libido

Decreased sexual desire

R68.83   Chills (without fever)

Chills NOS

Excludes1: chills with fever (R50.9)

R68.84   Jaw pain

Mandibular pain

Maxilla pain

Excludes1: temporomandibular joint arthralgia (M26.62-)

R68.89   Other general symptoms and signs

R69   Illness, unspecified

Unknown and unspecified cases of morbidity

ABNORMAL FINDINGS ON EXAMINATION OF BLOOD, WITHOUT DIAGNOSIS (R70-R79)

Excludes2: abnormal findings on antenatal screening of mother (O28.-)

abnormalities of lipids (E78.-)

abnormalities of platelets and thrombocytes (D69.-)

abnormalities of white blood cells classified elsewhere (D70-D72)

coagulation hemorrhagic disorders (D65-D68)

diagnostic abnormal findings classified elsewhere - see Alphabetical Index hemorrhagic and hematological disorders of newborn (P50-P61)

R70   Elevated erythrocyte sedimentation rate and abnormality of plasma viscosity

R70.0   Elevated erythrocyte sedimentation rate

R70.1   Abnormal plasma viscosity

R71   Abnormality of red blood cells

Excludes1: anemias (D50-D64)

anemia of premature infant (P61.2)

benign (familial) polycythemia (D75.0)

congenital anemias (P61.2-P61.4)

newborn anemia due to isoimmunization (P55.-)

polycythemia neonatorum (P61.1)

polycythemia NOS (D75.1)

polycythemia vera (D45) secondary polycythemia (D75.1)

R71.0   Precipitous drop in hematocrit

Drop (precipitous) in hemoglobin

Drop in hematocrit

R71.8   Other abnormality of red blood cells

Abnormal red-cell morphology NOS

Abnormal red-cell volume NOS

Anisocytosis

Poikilocytosis

R73   Elevated blood glucose level

Excludes1: diabetes mellitus (E08-E13)

diabetes mellitus in pregnancy, childbirth and the puerperium (O24.-)

neonatal disorders (P70.0-P70.2)

postsurgical hypoinsulinemia (E89.1)

R73.0   Abnormal glucose

Excludes1: abnormal glucose in pregnancy (O99.81-)

diabetes mellitus (E08-E13)

dysmetabolic syndrome X (E88.81)

gestational diabetes (O24.4-)

glycosuria (R81)

hypoglycemia (E16.2)

R73.01   Impaired fasting glucose

Elevated fasting glucose

R73.02   Impaired glucose tolerance (oral)

Elevated glucose tolerance

●**R73.03   Prediabetes**

Latent diabetes

R73.09   Other abnormal glucose

Abnormal glucose NOS

Abnormal non-fasting glucose tolerance

R73.9   Hyperglycemia, unspecified

R74   Abnormal serum enzyme levels

● New code   ▲ Revised code   Excludes1: Not coded here   Excludes2: Not included here   ⊗ Placeholder required   ⑦7th digit required

R74.0   **Nonspecific elevation of levels of transaminase and lactic acid dehydrogenase [LDH]**

R74.8   **Abnormal levels of other serum enzymes**

Abnormal level of acid phosphatase

Abnormal level of alkaline phosphatase

Abnormal level of amylase

Abnormal level of lipase [triacylglycerol lipase]

R74.9   **Abnormal serum enzyme level, unspecified**

R75   **Inconclusive laboratory evidence of human immunodeficiency virus [HIV]**

Nonconclusive HIV-test finding in infants

Excludes1: asymptomatic human immunodeficiency virus [HIV] infection status (Z21)

human immunodeficiency virus [HIV] disease (B20)

R76   **Other abnormal immunological findings in serum**

R76.0   **Raised antibody titer**

Excludes1: isoimmunization in pregnancy (O36.0-O36.1)

isoimmunization affecting newborn (P55.-)

R76.1   **Nonspecific reaction to test for tuberculosis**

R76.11   **Nonspecific reaction to tuberculin skin test without active tuberculosis**

Abnormal result of Mantoux test

PPD positive

Tuberculin (skin test) positive

Tuberculin (skin test) reactor

Excludes1: nonspecific reaction to cell mediated immunity measurement of gamma interferon antigen response without active tuberculosis (R76.12)

R76.12   **Nonspecific reaction to cell mediated immunity measurement of gamma interferon antigen response without active tuberculosis**

Nonspecific reaction to QuantiFERON-TB test (QFT) without active tuberculosis

Excludes1: nonspecific reaction to tuberculin skin test without active tuberculosis (R76.11)

positive tuberculin skin test (R76.11)

R76.8   **Other specified abnormal immunological findings in serum**

Raised level of immunoglobulins NOS

R76.9   **Abnormal immunological finding in serum, unspecified**

R77   **Other abnormalities of plasma proteins**

Excludes1: disorders of plasma-protein metabolism (E88.0)

R77.0   **Abnormality of albumin**

R77.1   **Abnormality of globulin**

Hyperglobulinemia NOS

R77.2   **Abnormality of alphafetoprotein**

R77.8   **Other specified abnormalities of plasma proteins**

R77.9   **Abnormality of plasma protein, unspecified**

R78   **Findings of drugs and other substances, not normally found in blood**

Use additional code to identify the any retained foreign body, if applicable (Z18.-)

Excludes1: mental or behavioral disorders due to psychoactive substance use (F10-F19)

R78.0   **Finding of alcohol in blood**

Use additional external cause code (Y90.-), for detail regarding alcohol level.

R78.1   **Finding of opiate drug in blood**

R78.2   **Finding of cocaine in blood**

R78.3   **Finding of hallucinogen in blood**

R78.4   **Finding of other drugs of addictive potential in blood**

R78.5   **Finding of other psychotropic drug in blood**

R78.6   **Finding of steroid agent in blood**

R78.7   **Finding of abnormal level of heavy metals in blood**

R78.71   **Abnormal lead level in blood**

Excludes1: lead poisoning (T56.0-)

R78.79   **Finding of abnormal level of heavy metals in blood**

R78.8   **Finding of other specified substances, not normally found in blood**

R78.81   **Bacteremia**

Excludes1: sepsis-code to specified infection

R78.89   **Finding of other specified substances, not normally found in blood**

Finding of abnormal level of lithium in blood

R78.9   **Finding of unspecified substance, not normally found in blood**

R79   **Other abnormal findings of blood chemistry**

Use additional code to identify any retained foreign body, if applicable (Z18.-)

Excludes1: abnormality of fluid, electrolyte or acid-base balance (E86-E87)

asymptomatic hyperuricemia (E79.0)

hyperglycemia NOS (R73.9) hypoglycemia NOS (E16.2)

neonatal hypoglycemia (P70.3-P70.4)

specific findings indicating disorder of amino-acid metabolism (E70-E72)

specific findings indicating disorder of carbohydrate metabolism (E73-E74)

specific findings indicating disorder of lipid metabolism (E75.-)

R79.0   **Abnormal level of blood mineral**

Abnormal blood level of cobalt

Abnormal blood level of copper

Abnormal blood level of iron

Abnormal blood level of magnesium

Abnormal blood level of mineral NEC

Abnormal blood level of zinc

Excludes1: abnormal level of lithium (R78.89)

disorders of mineral metabolism (E83.-)

neonatal hypomagnesemia (P71.2)

nutritional mineral deficiency (E58-E61)

R79.1   **Abnormal coagulation profile**

Abnormal or prolonged bleeding time

Abnormal or prolonged coagulation time

Abnormal or prolonged partial thromboplastin time [PTT]

Abnormal or prolonged prothrombin time [PT]

Excludes1: coagulation defects (D68.-)

R79.8   **Other specified abnormal findings of blood chemistry**

R79.81   **Abnormal blood-gas level**

R79.82   **Elevated C-reactive protein (CRP)**

R79.89   **Other specified abnormal findings of blood chemistry**

R79.9 Abnormal finding of blood chemistry, unspecified

ABNORMAL FINDINGS ON EXAMINATION OF URINE, WITHOUT DIAGNOSIS (R80-R82)

Excludes1: abnormal findings on antenatal screening of mother (O28.-)

diagnostic abnormal findings classified elsewhere - see Alphabetical Index specific findings indicating disorder of amino-acid metabolism (E70-E72) specific findings indicating disorder of carbohydrate metabolism (E73-E74)

R80 Proteinuria

Excludes1: gestational proteinuria (O12.1-)

R80.0 Isolated proteinuria

Idiopathic proteinuria

Excludes1: isolated proteinuria with specific morphological lesion (N06.-)

R80.1 Persistent proteinuria, unspecified

R80.2 Orthostatic proteinuria, unspecified

Postural proteinuria

R80.3 Bence Jones proteinuria

R80.8 Other proteinuria

R80.9 Proteinuria, unspecified

Albuminuria NOS

R81 Glycosuria

Excludes1: renal glycosuria (E74.8)

R82 Other and unspecified abnormal findings in urine

Includes: chromoabnormalities in urine

Use additional code to identify any retained foreign body, if applicable (Z18.-)

Excludes2: hematuria (R31.-)

R82.0 Chyluria

Excludes1: filarial chyluria (B74.-)

R82.1 Myoglobinuria

R82.2 Biliuria

R82.3 Hemoglobinuria

Excludes1: hemoglobinuria due to hemolysis from external causes NEC (D59.6)

hemoglobinuria due to paroxysmal nocturnal [Marchiafava-Micheli] (D59.5)

R82.4 Acetonuria

Ketonuria

R82.5 Elevated urine levels of drugs, medicaments and biological substances

Elevated urine levels of catecholamines

Elevated urine levels of indoleacetic acid

Elevated urine levels of 17-ketosteroids

Elevated urine levels of steroids

R82.6 Abnormal urine levels of substances chiefly nonmedicinal as to source

Abnormal urine level of heavy metals

R82.7 Abnormal findings on microbiological examination of urine

Excludes1: colonization status (Z22.-)

●**R82.71** Bacteriuria

●**R82.79** Other abnormal findings on microbiological examination of urine

Positive culture findings of urine

R82.8 Abnormal findings on cytological and histological examination of urine

R82.9 Other and unspecified abnormal findings in urine

R82.90 Unspecified abnormal findings in urine

R82.91 Other chromoabnormalities of urine

Chromoconversion (dipstick)

Idiopathic dipstick converts positive for blood with no cellular forms in sediment

Excludes1: hemoglobinuria (R82.3)

myoglobinuria (R82.1)

R82.99 Other abnormal findings in urine

Cells and casts in urine

Crystalluria

Melanuria

ABNORMAL FINDINGS ON EXAMINATION OF OTHER BODY FLUIDS, SUBSTANCES AND TISSUES, WITHOUT DIAGNOSIS (R83-R89)

Excludes1: abnormal findings on antenatal screening of mother (O28.-)

diagnostic abnormal findings classified elsewhere - see Alphabetical Index

Excludes2: abnormal findings on examination of blood, without diagnosis (R70-R79)

abnormal findings on examination of urine, without diagnosis (R80-R82)

abnormal tumor markers (R97.-)

R83 Abnormal findings in cerebrospinal fluid

R83.0 Abnormal level of enzymes in cerebrospinal fluid

R83.1 Abnormal level of hormones in cerebrospinal fluid

R83.2 Abnormal level of other drugs, medicaments and biological substances in cerebrospinal fluid

R83.3 Abnormal level of substances chiefly nonmedicinal as to source in cerebrospinal fluid

R83.4 Abnormal immunological findings in cerebrospinal fluid

R83.5 Abnormal microbiological findings in cerebrospinal fluid

Positive culture findings in cerebrospinal fluid

Excludes1: colonization status (Z22.-)

R83.6 Abnormal cytological findings in cerebrospinal fluid

R83.8 Other abnormal findings in cerebrospinal fluid

Abnormal chromosomal findings in cerebrospinal fluid

R83.9 Unspecified abnormal finding in cerebrospinal fluid

R84 Abnormal findings in specimens from respiratory organs and thorax

Includes: abnormal findings in bronchial washings

abnormal findings in nasal secretions

abnormal findings in pleural fluid

abnormal findings in sputum

abnormal findings in throat scrapings

Excludes1: blood-stained sputum (R04.2)

R84.0 Abnormal level of enzymes in specimens from respiratory organs and thorax

R84.1 Abnormal level of hormones in specimens from respiratory organs and thorax

R84.2 Abnormal level of other drugs, medicaments and biological substances in specimens from respiratory organs and thorax

● New code   ▲ Revised code   Excludes1: Not coded here   Excludes2: Not included here   ⊗ Placeholder required   ⑦7th digit required

R84.3　Abnormal level of substances chiefly nonmedicinal as to source in specimens from respiratory organs and thorax

R84.4　Abnormal immunological findings in specimens from respiratory organs and thorax

R84.5　Abnormal microbiological findings in specimens from respiratory organs and thorax

Positive culture findings in specimens from respiratory organs and thorax

Excludes1: colonization status (Z22.-)

R84.6　Abnormal cytological findings in specimens from respiratory organs and thorax

R84.7　Abnormal histological findings in specimens from respiratory organs and thorax

R84.8　Other abnormal findings in specimens from respiratory organs and thorax

Abnormal chromosomal findings in specimens from respiratory organs and thorax

R84.9　Unspecified abnormal finding in specimens from respiratory organs and thorax

R85　Abnormal findings in specimens from digestive organs and abdominal cavity

Includes: abnormal findings in peritoneal fluid

abnormal findings in saliva

Excludes1: cloudy peritoneal dialysis effluent (R88.0)

fecal abnormalities (R19.5)

R85.0　Abnormal level of enzymes in specimens from digestive organs and abdominal cavity

R85.1　Abnormal level of hormones in specimens from digestive organs and abdominal cavity

R85.2　Abnormal level of other drugs, medicaments and biological substances in specimens from digestive organs and abdominal cavity

R85.3　Abnormal level of substances chiefly nonmedicinal as to source in specimens from digestive organs and abdominal cavity

R85.4　Abnormal immunological findings in specimens from digestive organs and abdominal cavity

R85.5　Abnormal microbiological findings in specimens from digestive organs and abdominal cavity

Positive culture findings in specimens from digestive organs and abdominal cavity

Excludes1: colonization status (Z22.-)

R85.6　Abnormal cytological findings in specimens from digestive organs and abdominal cavity

R85.61　Abnormal cytologic smear of anus

Excludes1: abnormal cytological findings in specimens from other digestive organs and abdominal cavity (R85.69)

carcinoma in situ of anus (histologically confirmed) (D01.3)

anal intraepithelial neoplasia I [AIN I] (K62.82)

anal intraepithelial neoplasia II [AIN II] (K62.82)

anal intraepithelial neoplasia III [AIN III] (D01.3)

dysplasia (mild) (moderate) of anus (histologically confirmed) (K62.82)

severe dysplasia of anus (histologically confirmed) (D01.3)

Excludes2: anal high risk human papillomavirus (HPV) DNA test positive (R85.81)

anal low risk human papillomavirus (HPV) DNA test positive (R85.82)

R85.610　Atypical squamous cells of undetermined significance on cytologic smear of anus (ASC-US)

R85.611　Atypical squamous cells cannot exclude high grade squamous intraepithelial lesion on cytologic smear of anus (ASC-H)

R85.612　Low grade squamous intraepithelial lesion on cytologic smear of anus (LGSIL)

R85.613　High grade squamous intraepithelial lesion on cytologic smear of anus (HGSIL)

R85.614　Cytologic evidence of malignancy on smear of anus

R85.615　Unsatisfactory cytologic smear of anus

Inadequate sample of cytologic smear of anus

R85.616　Satisfactory anal smear but lacking transformation zone

R85.618　Other abnormal cytological findings on specimens from anus

R85.619　Unspecified abnormal cytological findings in specimens from anus

Abnormal anal cytology NOS

Atypical glandular cells of anus NOS

R85.69　Abnormal cytological findings in specimens from other digestive organs and abdominal cavity

R85.7　Abnormal histological findings in specimens from digestive organs and abdominal cavity

R85.8　Other abnormal findings in specimens from digestive organs and abdominal cavity

R85.81　Anal high risk human papillomavirus (HPV) DNA test positive

Excludes1: anogenital warts due to human papillomavirus (HPV) (A63.0)

condyloma acuminatum (A63.0)

R85.82　Anal low risk human papillomavirus (HPV) DNA test positive

Use additional code for associated human papillomavirus (B97.7)

R85.89　Other abnormal findings in specimens from digestive organs and abdominal cavity

Abnormal chromosomal findings in specimens from digestive organs and abdominal cavity

R85.9　Unspecified abnormal finding in specimens from digestive organs and abdominal cavity

R86　Abnormal findings in specimens from male genital organs

Includes: abnormal findings in prostatic secretions

abnormal findings in semen, seminal fluid

abnormal spermatozoa

Excludes1: azoospermia (N46.0-)

oligospermia (N46.1-)

R86.0　Abnormal level of enzymes in specimens from male genital organs

R86.1　Abnormal level of hormones in specimens from male genital organs

R86.2 Abnormal level of other drugs, medicaments and biological substances in specimens from male genital organs

R86.3 Abnormal level of substances chiefly nonmedicinal as to source in specimens from male genital organs

R86.4 Abnormal immunological findings in specimens from male genital organs

R86.5 Abnormal microbiological findings in specimens from male genital organs

Positive culture findings in specimens from male genital organs

Excludes1: colonization status (Z22.-)

R86.6 Abnormal cytological findings in specimens from male genital organs

R86.7 Abnormal histological findings in specimens from male genital organs

R86.8 Other abnormal findings in specimens from male genital organs

Abnormal chromosomal findings in specimens from male genital organs

R86.9 Unspecified abnormal finding in specimens from male genital organs

R87 Abnormal findings in specimens from female genital organs

Includes: abnormal findings in secretion and smears from cervix uteri

abnormal findings in secretion and smears from vagina

abnormal findings in secretion and smears from vulva

R87.0 Abnormal level of enzymes in specimens from female genital organs

R87.1 Abnormal level of hormones in specimens from female genital organs

R87.2 Abnormal level of other drugs, medicaments and biological substances in specimens from female genital organs

R87.3 Abnormal level of substances chiefly nonmedicinal as to source in specimens from female genital organs

R87.4 Abnormal immunological findings in specimens from female genital organs

R87.5 Abnormal microbiological findings in specimens from female genital organs

Positive culture findings in specimens from female genital organs

Excludes1: colonization status (Z22.-)

R87.6 Abnormal cytological findings in specimens from female genital organs

R87.61 Abnormal cytological findings in specimens from cervix uteri

Excludes1: abnormal cytological findings in specimens from other female genital organs (R87.69)

abnormal cytological findings in specimens from vagina (R87.62-)

carcinoma in situ of cervix uteri (histologically confirmed) (D06.-)

cervical intraepithelial neoplasia I [CIN I] (N87.0)

cervical intraepithelial neoplasia II [CIN II] (N87.1)

cervical intraepithelial neoplasia III [CIN III] (D06.-)

dysplasia (mild) (moderate) of cervix uteri (histologically confirmed) (N87.-)

severe dysplasia of cervix uteri (histologically confirmed) (D06.-)

Excludes2: cervical high risk human papillomavirus (HPV) DNA test positive (R87.810)

cervical low risk human papillomavirus (HPV) DNA test positive (R87.820)

R87.610 Atypical squamous cells of undetermined significance on cytologic smear of cervix (ASC-US)

R87.611 Atypical squamous cells cannot exclude high grade squamous intraepithelial lesion on cytologic smear of cervix (ASC-H)

R87.612 Low grade squamous intraepithelial lesion on cytologic smear of cervix (LGSIL)

R87.613 High grade squamous intraepithelial lesion on cytologic smear of cervix (HGSIL)

R87.614 Cytologic evidence of malignancy on smear of cervix

R87.615 Unsatisfactory cytologic smear of cervix

Inadequate sample of cytologic smear of cervix

R87.616 Satisfactory cervical smear but lacking transformation zone

R87.618 Other abnormal cytological findings on specimens from cervix uteri

R87.619 Unspecified abnormal cytological findings in specimens from cervix uteri

Abnormal cervical cytology NOS

Abnormal Papanicolaou smear of cervix NOS

Abnormal thin preparation smear of cervix NOS

Atypical endocervial cells of cervix NOS

Atypical endometrial cells of cervix NOS

Atypical glandular cells of cervix NOS

R87.62 Abnormal cytological findings in specimens from vagina

Use additional code to identify acquired absence of uterus and cervix, if applicable (Z90.71-)

Excludes1: abnormal cytological findings in specimens from cervix uteri (R87.61-)

abnormal cytological findings in specimens from other female genital organs (R87.69)

carcinoma in situ of vagina (histologically confirmed) (D07.2)

vaginal intraepithelial neoplasia I [VAIN I] (N89.0)

vaginal intraepithelial neoplasia II [VAIN II] (N89.1)

vaginal intraepithelial neoplasia III [VAIN III] (D07.2)

dysplasia (mild) (moderate) of vagina (histologically confirmed) (N89.-)

severe dysplasia of vagina (histologically confirmed) (D07.2)

Excludes2: vaginal high risk human papillomavirus (HPV) DNA test positive (R87.811)

vaginal low risk human papillomavirus (HPV) DNA test positive (R87.821)

R87.620 Atypical squamous cells of undetermined significance on cytologic smear of vagina (ASC-US)

R87.621 Atypical squamous cells cannot exclude high grade squamous intraepithelial lesion on cytologic smear of vagina (ASC-H)

R87.622 Low grade squamous intraepithelial lesion on cytologic smear of vagina (LGSIL)

R87.623 High grade squamous intraepithelial lesion on cytologic smear of vagina (HGSIL)

R87.624 Cytologic evidence of malignancy on smear of vagina

R87.625 Unsatisfactory cytologic smear of vagina

Inadequate sample of cytologic smear of vagina

R87.628 Other abnormal cytological findings on specimens from vagina

R87.629 Unspecified abnormal cytological findings in specimens from vagina

Abnormal Papanicolaou smear of vagina NOS

Abnormal thin preparation smear of vagina NOS

Abnormal vaginal cytology NOS

Atypical endocervical cells of vagina NOS

Atypical endometrial cells of vagina NOS

Atypical glandular cells of vagina NOS

R87.69 Abnormal cytological findings in specimens from other female genital organs

Abnormal cytological findings in specimens from female genital organs NOS

Excludes1: dysplasia of vulva (histologically confirmed) (N90.0-N90.3)

R87.7 Abnormal histological findings in specimens from female genital organs

Excludes1: carcinoma in situ (histologically confirmed) of female genital organs (D06-D07.3)

cervical intraepithelial neoplasia I [CIN I] (N87.0)

cervical intraepithelial neoplasia II [CIN II] (N87.1)

cervical intraepithelial neoplasia III [CIN III] (D06.-)

dysplasia (mild) (moderate) of cervix uteri (histologically confirmed) (N87.-)

dysplasia (mild) (moderate) of vagina (histologically confirmed) (N89.-)

vaginal intraepithelial neoplasia I [VAIN I] (N89.0)

vaginal intraepithelial neoplasia II [VAIN II] (N89.1)

vaginal intraepithelial neoplasia III [VAIN III] (D07.2)

severe dysplasia of cervix uteri (histologically confirmed) (D06.-)

severe dysplasia of vagina (histologically confirmed) (D07.2)

R87.8 Other abnormal findings in specimens from female genital organs

R87.81 High risk human papillomavirus (HPV) DNA test positive from female genital organs

Excludes1: anogenital warts due to human papillomavirus (HPV) (A63.0)

condyloma acuminatum (A63.0)

R87.810 Cervical high risk human papillomavirus (HPV) DNA test positive

R87.811 Vaginal high risk human papillomavirus (HPV) DNA test positive

R87.82 Low risk human papillomavirus (HPV) DNA test positive from female genital organs

Use additional code for associated human papillomavirus (B97.7)

R87.820 Cervical low risk human papillomavirus (HPV) DNA test positive

R87.821 Vaginal low risk human papillomavirus (HPV) DNA test positive

R87.89 Other abnormal findings in specimens from female genital organs

Abnormal chromosomal findings in specimens from female genital organs

R87.9 Unspecified abnormal finding in specimens from female genital organs

R88 Abnormal findings in other body fluids and substances

R88.0 Cloudy (hemodialysis) (peritoneal) dialysis effluent

R88.8 Abnormal findings in other body fluids and substances

R89 Abnormal findings in specimens from other organs, systems and tissues

Includes: abnormal findings in nipple discharge

abnormal findings in synovial fluid abnormal findings in wound secretions

R89.0 Abnormal level of enzymes in specimens from other organs, systems and tissues

R89.1 Abnormal level of hormones in specimens from other organs, systems and tissues

R89.2 Abnormal level of other drugs, medicaments and biological substances in specimens from other organs, systems and tissues

R89.3 Abnormal level of substances chiefly nonmedicinal as to source in specimens from other organs, systems and tissues

R89.4 Abnormal immunological findings in specimens from other organs, systems and tissues

R89.5 Abnormal microbiological findings in specimens from other organs, systems and tissues

Positive culture findings in specimens **from other** organs, systems and tissues

> **Excludes1:** colonization status (Z22.-)

R89.6 **Abnormal cytological findings in specimens from other organs, systems and tissues**

R89.7 **Abnormal histological findings in specimens from other organs, systems and tissues**

R89.8 **Other abnormal findings in specimens from other organs, systems and tissues**

Abnormal chromosomal findings in specimens **from other** organs, systems and tissues

R89.9 **Unspecified abnormal finding in specimens from other organs, systems and tissues**

ABNORMAL FINDINGS ON DIAGNOSTIC IMAGING AND IN FUNCTION STUDIES, WITHOUT DIAGNOSIS (R90-R94)

Includes: nonspecific abnormal findings on diagnostic imaging by computerized axial tomography [CAT scan]

nonspecific abnormal findings on diagnostic imaging by magnetic resonance imaging [MRI][NMR]

nonspecific abnormal findings on diagnostic imaging by positron emission tomography [PET scan]

nonspecific abnormal findings on diagnostic imaging by thermography

nonspecific abnormal findings on diagnostic imaging by ultrasound [echogram]

nonspecific abnormal findings on diagnostic imaging by X-ray examination

> **Excludes1:** abnormal findings on antenatal screening of mother (O28.-)

diagnostic abnormal findings classified elsewhere - see Alphabetical Index

R90 **Abnormal findings on diagnostic imaging of central nervous system**

R90.0 **Intracranial space-occupying lesion found on diagnostic imaging of central nervous system**

R90.8 **Other abnormal findings on diagnostic imaging of central nervous system**

R90.81 **Abnormal echoencephalogram**

R90.82 **White matter disease, unspecified**

R90.89 **Other abnormal findings on diagnostic imaging of central nervous system**

Other cerebrovascular abnormality found on diagnostic imaging of central nervous system

R91 **Abnormal findings on diagnostic imaging of lung**

R91.1 **Solitary pulmonary nodule**

Coin lesion lung

Solitary pulmonary nodule, subsegmental branch of the bronchial tree

R91.8 **Other nonspecific abnormal finding of lung field**

Lung mass NOS found on diagnostic imaging of lung

Pulmonary infiltrate NOS

Shadow, lung

R92 **Abnormal and inconclusive findings on diagnostic imaging of breast**

R92.0 **Mammographic microcalcification found on diagnostic imaging of breast**

> **Excludes2:** mammographic calcification (calculus) found on diagnostic imaging of breast (R92.1)

R92.1 **Mammographic calcification found on diagnostic imaging of breast**

Mammographic calculus found on diagnostic imaging of breast

R92.2 **Inconclusive mammogram**

Dense breasts NOS

Inconclusive mammogram NEC

Inconclusive mammography due to dense breasts

Inconclusive mammography NEC

R92.8 **Other abnormal and inconclusive findings on diagnostic imaging of breast**

R93 **Abnormal findings on diagnostic imaging of other body structures**

R93.0 **Abnormal findings on diagnostic imaging of skull and head, not elsewhere classified**

> **Excludes1:** intracranial space-occupying lesion found on diagnostic imaging (R90.0)

R93.1 **Abnormal findings on diagnostic imaging of heart and coronary circulation**

Abnormal echocardiogram NOS

Abnormal heart shadow

R93.2 **Abnormal findings on diagnostic imaging of liver and biliary tract**

Nonvisualization of gallbladder

R93.3 **Abnormal findings on diagnostic imaging of other parts of digestive tract**

R93.4 **Abnormal findings on diagnostic imaging of urinary organs**

> **Excludes2:** hypertrophy of kidney (N28.81)

● **R93.41** **Abnormal radiologic findings on diagnostic imaging of renal pelvis, ureter, or bladder**

Filling defect of bladder found on diagnostic imaging

Filling defect of renal pelvis found on diagnostic imaging

Filling defect of ureter found on diagnostic imaging

R93.42 **Abnormal radiologic findings on diagnostic imaging of kidney**

● **R93.421** **Abnormal radiologic findings on diagnostic imaging of right kidney**

● **R93.422** **Abnormal radiologic findings on diagnostic imaging of left kidney**

● **R93.429** **Abnormal radiologic findings on diagnostic imaging of unspecified kidney**

R93.49 **Abnormal radiologic findings on diagnostic imaging of other urinary organs**

R93.5 **Abnormal findings on diagnostic imaging of other abdominal regions, including retroperitoneum**

R93.6 **Abnormal findings on diagnostic imaging of limbs**

> **Excludes2:** abnormal finding in skin and subcutaneous tissue (R93.8)

R93.7 **Abnormal findings on diagnostic imaging of other parts of musculoskeletal system**

> **Excludes2:** abnormal findings on diagnostic imaging of skull (R93.0)

R93.8 **Abnormal findings on diagnostic imaging of other specified body structures**

Abnormal finding by radioisotope localization of placenta

● New code ▲ Revised code **Excludes1:** Not coded here **Excludes2:** Not included here ⊗ Placeholder required ⑦ 7th digit required

Abnormal radiological finding in skin and subcutaneous tissue

Mediastinal shift

R93.9 Diagnostic imaging inconclusive due to excess body fat of patient

R94 Abnormal results of function studies

Includes: abnormal results of radionuclide [radioisotope] uptake studies

abnormal results of scintigraphy

R94.0 Abnormal results of function studies of central nervous system

R94.01 Abnormal electroencephalogram [EEG]

R94.02 Abnormal brain scan

R94.09 Abnormal results of other function studies of central nervous system

R94.1 Abnormal results of function studies of peripheral nervous system and special senses

R94.11 Abnormal results of function studies of eye

R94.110 Abnormal electro-oculogram [EOG]

R94.111 Abnormal electroretinogram [ERG]

Abnormal retinal function study

R94.112 Abnormal visually evoked potential [VEP]

R94.113 Abnormal oculomotor study

R94.118 Abnormal results of other function studies of eye

R94.12 Abnormal results of function studies of ear and other special senses

R94.120 Abnormal auditory function study

R94.121 Abnormal vestibular function study

R94.128 Abnormal results of other function studies of ear and other special senses

R94.13 Abnormal results of function studies of peripheral nervous system

R94.130 Abnormal response to nerve stimulation, unspecified

R94.131 Abnormal electromyogram [EMG]

Excludes1: electromyogram of eye (R94.113)

R94.138 Abnormal results of other function studies of peripheral nervous system

R94.2 Abnormal results of pulmonary function studies

Reduced ventilatory capacity Reduced vital capacity

R94.3 Abnormal results of cardiovascular function studies

R94.30 Abnormal result of cardiovascular function study, unspecified

R94.31 Abnormal electrocardiogram [ECG] [EKG]

Excludes1: long QT syndrome (I45.81)

R94.39 Abnormal result of other cardiovascular function study

Abnormal electrophysiological intracardiac studies

Abnormal phonocardiogram

Abnormal vectorcardiogram

R94.4 Abnormal results of kidney function studies

Abnormal renal function test

R94.5 Abnormal results of liver function studies

R94.6 Abnormal results of thyroid function studies

R94.7 Abnormal results of other endocrine function studies

Excludes2: abnormal glucose (R73.0-)

R94.8 Abnormal results of function studies of other organs and systems

Abnormal basal metabolic rate [BMR]

Abnormal bladder function test

Abnormal splenic function test

ABNORMAL TUMOR MARKERS (R97)

Definition: A tumor marker is a biomarker found in the blood, urine, or body tissues that can be elevated in cancer, among other tissue types. There are many different **tumor** markers, each indicative of a particular disease process, and they are used in oncology to help detect the presence of cancer.

R97 Abnormal tumor markers

Elevated tumor associated antigens [TAA]

Elevated tumor specific antigens [TSA]

R97.0 Elevated carcinoembryonic antigen [CEA]

R97.1 Elevated cancer antigen 125 [CA 125]

R97.2 Elevated prostate specific antigen [PSA]

● **R97.20 Elevated prostate specific antigen [PSA]**

● **R97.21 Rising PSA following treatment for malignant neoplasm of prostate**

R97.8 Other abnormal tumor markers

ILL-DEFINED AND UNKNOWN CAUSE OF MORTALITY (R99)

R99 Ill-defined and unknown cause of mortality

Death (unexplained) NOS

Unspecified cause of mortality

Chapter 19: Injury, Poisoning And Certain Other Consequences Of External Causes (S00-T88)

DEFINITIONS

This chapter includes definitions of selected key words, terms and phrases and coding alerts for adding points to the clinical domain, and references to coding late effects where appropriate. An example from this chapter is as follows:

S05.7   Avulsion of eye
            Traumatic enucleation
            Definition: An avulsion is an injury in which a body structure is forcibly detached from its normal point of insertion by either trauma or surgery (from the Latin *avellere*, meaning "to tear off"). The term most commonly refers to a surface trauma where all layers of the skin have been torn away, exposing the underlying structures (i.e., subcutaneous tissue, muscle, tendons, or bone).

MULTIPLE CODING FOR A SINGLE CONDITION

In addition to the etiology/manifestation convention that requires two codes to fully describe a single condition that affects multiple body systems, there are other single conditions that also require more than one code. "Use additional code" notes are found in the Tabular List at codes that are not part of an etiology/manifestation pair where a secondary code is useful to fully describe a condition. The sequencing rule is the same as the etiology/manifestation pair, "use additional code" indicates that a secondary code should be added.

For example, for bacterial infections that are not included in chapter 1, a secondary code from category B95, Streptococcus, Staphylococcus, and Enterococcus, as the cause of diseases classified elsewhere, or B96, Other bacterial agents as the cause of diseases classified elsewhere, may be required to identify the bacterial organism causing the infection. A "use additional code" note will normally be found at the infectious disease code, indicating a need for the organism code to be added as a secondary code.

"**Code first**" notes are also under certain codes that are not specifically manifestation codes but may be due to an underlying cause. When there is a "**Code first**" note and an underlying condition is present, the underlying condition should be sequenced first.

"Code, if applicable, any causal condition first", notes indicate that this code may be assigned as a principal diagnosis when the causal condition is unknown or not applicable. If a causal condition is known, then the code for that condition should be sequenced as the principal or first-listed diagnosis.

Multiple codes may be needed for sequela, complication codes and obstetric codes to more fully describe a condition. See the specific guidelines for these conditions for further instruction.

COMBINATION CODE

A combination code is a single code used to classify: Two diagnoses, or a diagnosis with an associated secondary process (manifestation) A diagnosis with an associated complication

Combination codes are identified by referring to subterm entries in the Alphabetic Index and by reading the inclusion and exclusion notes in the Tabular List.

Assign only the combination code when that code fully identifies the diagnostic conditions involved or when the Alphabetic Index so directs. Multiple coding should not be used when the classification provides a combination code that clearly identifies all of the elements documented in the diagnosis. When the combination code lacks necessary specificity in describing the manifestation or complication, an additional code should be used as a secondary code.

SEQUELA (LATE EFFECTS)

A sequela is the residual effect (condition produced) after the acute phase of an illness or injury has terminated. There is no time limit on when a sequela code can be used. The residual may be apparent early, such as in cerebral infarction, or it may occur months or years later, such as that due to a previous injury. Coding of sequela generally requires two codes sequenced in the following order: The condition or nature of the sequela is sequenced first.

The sequela code is sequenced second.

An exception to the above guidelines are those instances where the code for the sequela is followed by a manifestation code identified in the Tabular List and title, or the sequela code has been expanded (at the fourth, fifth or sixth character levels) to include the manifestation(s). The code for the acute phase of an illness or injury that led to the sequela is never used with a code for the late effect.

APPLICATION OF 7TH CHARACTERS IN CHAPTER 19

Most categories in chapter 19 have a 7th character requirement for each applicable code. Most categories in this chapter have three 7th character values (with the exception of fractures): A, initial encounter, D, subsequent encounter and S, sequela. Categories for traumatic fractures have additional 7th character values. While the patient may be seen by a new or different provider over the course of treatment for an injury, assignment of the 7th character is based on whether the patient is undergoing active treatment and not whether the provider is seeing the patient for the first time.

For complication codes, active treatment refers to treatment for the condition described by the code, even though it may be related to an earlier precipitating problem. For example, code T84.50XA, Infection and inflammatory reaction due to unspecified internal joint prosthesis, initial encounter, is used when

S00-T88

active treatment is provided for the infection, even though the condition relates to the prosthetic device, implant or graft that was placed at a previous encounter.

7th character "A", initial encounter is used for each encounter where the patient is receiving active treatment for the condition.

7th character "D" subsequent encounter is used for encounters after the patient has completed active treatment of the condition and is receiving routine care for the condition during the healing or recovery phase.

The aftercare Z codes should not be used for aftercare for conditions such as injuries or poisonings, where 7th characters are provided to identify subsequent care. For example, for aftercare of an injury, assign the acute injury code with the 7th character "D" (subsequent encounter).

7th character "S", sequela, is for use for complications or conditions that arise as a direct result of a condition, such as scar formation after a burn. The scars are sequelae of the burn. When using 7th character "S", it is necessary to use both the injury code that precipitated the sequela and the code for the sequela itself. The "S" is added only to the injury code, not the sequela code. The 7th character "S" identifies the injury responsible for the sequela. The specific type of sequela (e.g. scar) is sequenced first, followed by the injury code.

See Section I.B.10 Sequelae, (Late Effects)

CODING OF INJURIES

When coding injuries, assign separate codes for each injury unless a combination code is provided, in which case the combination code is assigned. Code T07, Unspecified multiple injuries should not be assigned in the inpatient setting unless information for a more specific code is not available. Traumatic injury codes (S00-T14.9) are not to be used for normal, healing surgical wounds or to identify complications of surgical wounds.

The code for the most serious injury, as determined by the provider and the focus of treatment, is sequenced first.

1) **Superficial injuries**

   Superficial injuries such as abrasions or contusions are not coded when associated with more severe injuries of the same site.

2) **Primary injury with damage to nerves/blood vessels**

   When a primary injury results in minor damage to peripheral nerves or blood vessels, the primary injury is sequenced first with additional code(s) for injuries to nerves and spinal cord (such as category S04), and/or injury to blood vessels (such as category S15). When the primary injury is to the blood vessels or nerves, that injury should be sequenced first.

CODING OF TRAUMATIC FRACTURES

The principles of multiple coding of injuries should be followed in coding fractures. Fractures of specified sites are coded individually by site in accordance with both the provisions within categories S02, S12, S22, S32, S42, S49, S52, S59, S62, S72, S79, S82, S89, S92 and the level of detail furnished by medical record content.

A fracture not indicated as open or closed should be coded to closed. A fracture not indicated whether displaced or not displaced should be coded to displaced.

More specific guidelines are as follows:

1) **Initial vs. Subsequent Encounter for Fractures**

   Traumatic fractures are coded using the appropriate 7th character for initial encounter (A, B, C) for each encounter where the patient is receiving active treatment for the fracture. The appropriate 7th character for initial encounter should also be assigned for a patient who delayed seeking treatment for the fracture or nonunion.

   Fractures are coded using the appropriate 7th character for subsequent care for encounters after the patient has completed active treatment of the fracture and is receiving routine care for the fracture during the healing or recovery phase.

   Care for complications of surgical treatment for fracture repairs during the healing or recovery phase should be coded with the appropriate complication codes.

   Care of complications of fractures, such as malunion and nonunion, should be reported with the appropriate 7th character for subsequent care with nonunion (K, M, N,) or subsequent care with malunion (P, Q, R).

   Malunion/nonunion: The appropriate 7th character for initial encounter should also be assigned for a patient who delayed seeking treatment for the fracture or nonunion.

   The open fracture designations in the assignment of the 7th character for fractures of the forearm, femur and lower leg, including ankle are based on the Gustilo open fracture classification. When the Gustilo classification type is not specified for an open fracture, the 7th character for open fracture type I or II should be assigned (B, E, H, M, Q).

   A code from category M80, not a traumatic fracture code, should be used for any patient with known osteoporosis who suffers a fracture, even if the patient had a minor fall or trauma, if that fall or trauma would not usually break a normal, healthy bone.

See Section I.C.13. Osteoporosis.

The aftercare Z codes should not be used for aftercare for traumatic fractures. For aftercare of a traumatic fracture, assign the acute fracture code with the appropriate 7th character.

2)   Multiple fractures sequencing

Multiple fractures are sequenced in accordance with the severity of the fracture.

CODING OF BURNS AND CORROSIONS

The ICD-10-CM makes a distinction between burns and corrosions. The burn codes are for thermal burns, except sunburns, that come from a heat source, such as a fire or hot appliance. The burn codes are also for burns resulting from electricity and radiation. Corrosions are burns due to chemicals. The guidelines are the same for burns and corrosions.

Current burns (T20-T25) are classified by depth, extent and by agent (X code). Burns are classified by depth as first degree (erythema), second degree (blistering), and third degree (full-thickness involvement). Burns of the eye and internal organs (T26-T28) are classified by site, but not by degree.

1)   Sequencing of burn and related condition codes

Sequence first the code that reflects the highest degree of burn when more than one burn is present.

a.   When the reason for the admission or encounter is for treatment of external multiple burns, sequence first the code that reflects the burn of the highest degree.

b.   When a patient has both internal and external burns, the circumstances of admission govern the selection of the principal diagnosis or first-listed diagnosis.

c.   When a patient is admitted for burn injuries and other related conditions such as smoke inhalation and/or respiratory failure, the circumstances of admission govern the selection of the principal or first-listed diagnosis.

2)   Burns of the same local site

Classify burns of the same local site (three-character category level, T20-T28) but of different degrees to the subcategory identifying the highest degree recorded in the diagnosis.

3)   Non-healing burns

Non-healing burns are coded as acute burns.

Necrosis of burned skin should be coded as a non-healed burn.

4)   Infected Burn

For any documented infected burn site, use an additional code for the infection.

5)   Assign separate codes for each burn site

When coding burns, assign separate codes for each burn site. Category T30, Burn and corrosion, body region unspecified is extremely vague and should rarely be used.

6)   Burns and Corrosions Classified According to Extent of Body Surface Involved

Assign codes from category T31, Burns classified according to extent of body surface involved, or T32, Corrosions classified according to extent of body surface involved, when the site of the burn is not specified or when there is a need for additional data. It is advisable to use category T31 as additional coding when needed to provide data for evaluating burn mortality, such as that needed by burn units. It is also advisable to use category T31 as an additional code for reporting purposes when there is mention of a third-degree burn involving 20 percent or more of the body surface.

Categories T31 and T32 are based on the classic "rule of nines" in estimating body surface involved: head and neck are assigned nine percent, each arm nine percent, each leg 18 percent, the anterior trunk 18 percent, posterior trunk 18 percent, and genitalia one percent. Providers may change these percentage assignments where necessary to accommodate infants and children who have proportionately larger heads than adults, and patients who have large buttocks, thighs, or abdomen that involve burns.

7)   Encounters for treatment of sequela of burns

Encounters for the treatment of the late effects of burns or corrosions (i.e., scars or joint contractures) should be coded with a burn or corrosion code with the 7th character "S" for sequela.

8)   Sequelae with a late effect code and current burn

When appropriate, both a code for a current burn or corrosion with 7th character "A" or "D" and a burn or corrosion code with 7th character "S" may be assigned on the same record (when both a current burn and sequelae of an old burn exist). Burns and corrosions do not heal at the same rate and a current healing wound may still exist with sequela of a healed burn or corrosion.

See Section I.B.10 Sequela (Late Effects)

9) **Use of an external cause code with burns and corrosions**

An external cause code should be used with burns and corrosions to identify the source and intent of the burn, as well as the place where it occurred.

ADVERSE EFFECTS, POISONING, UNDERDOSING AND TOXIC EFFECTS

Codes in categories T36-T65 are combination codes that include the substance that was taken as well as the intent. No additional external cause code is required for poisonings, toxic effects, adverse effects and underdosing codes.

1) **Do not code directly from the Table of Drugs**

Do not code directly from the Table of Drugs and Chemicals. Always refer back to the Tabular List.

2) **Use as many codes as necessary to describe**

Use as many codes as necessary to describe completely all drugs, medicinal or biological substances.

3) **If the same code would describe the causative agent**

If the same code would describe the causative agent for more than one adverse reaction, poisoning, toxic effect or underdosing, assign the code only once.

4) **If two or more drugs, medicinal or biological substances**

If two or more drugs, medicinal or biological substances are reported, code each individually unless a combination code is listed in the Table of Drugs and Chemicals.

5) **The occurrence of drug toxicity is classified in ICD-10-CM as follows:**

(a) **Adverse Effect**

When coding an adverse effect of a drug that has been correctly prescribed and properly administered, assign the appropriate code for the nature of the adverse effect followed by the appropriate code for the adverse effect of the drug (T36-T50). The code for the drug should have a 5th or 6th character "5" (for example T36.0X5-) Examples of the nature of an adverse effect are tachycardia, delirium, gastrointestinal hemorrhaging, vomiting, hypokalemia, hepatitis, renal failure, or respiratory failure.

(b) **Poisoning**

When coding a poisoning or reaction to the improper use of a medication (e.g., overdose, wrong substance given or taken in error, wrong route of administration), first assign the appropriate code from categories T36-T50. The poisoning codes have an associated intent as their 5th or 6th character (accidental, intentional self-harm, assault and undetermined. If the intent of the poisoning is unknown or unspecified, code the intent as accidental intent. The undetermined intent is only for use if the documentation in the record specifies that the intent cannot be determined. Use additional code(s) for all manifestations of poisonings.

If there is also a diagnosis of abuse or dependence of the substance, the abuse or dependence is assigned as an additional code.

Examples of poisoning include:

(i) Error was made in drug prescription Errors made in drug prescription or in the administration of the drug by provider, nurse, patient, or other person.

(ii) Overdose of a drug intentionally taken

If an overdose of a drug was intentionally taken or administered and resulted in drug toxicity, it would be coded as a poisoning.

(iii) Nonprescribed drug taken with correctly prescribed and properly administered drug

If a nonprescribed drug or medicinal agent was taken in combination with a correctly prescribed and properly administered drug, any drug toxicity or other reaction resulting from the interaction of the two drugs would be classified as a poisoning.

(iv) Interaction of drug(s) and alcohol

When a reaction results from the interaction of a drug(s) and alcohol, this would be classified as poisoning.

See Section I.C.4. if poisoning is the result of insulin pump malfunctions.

● New code   ▲ Revised code   **Excludes1:** Not coded here   **Excludes2:** Not included here   ⊗ Placeholder required   ⑦7th digit required

(c)   **Underdosing**

Underdosing refers to taking less of a medication than is prescribed by a provider or a manufacturer's instruction. For underdosing, assign the code from categories T36-T50 (fifth or sixth character "6").

Codes for underdosing should never be assigned as principal or first-listed codes. If a patient has a relapse or exacerbation of the medical condition for which the drug is prescribed because of the reduction in dose, then the medical condition itself should be coded.

Noncompliance (Z91.12-, Z91.13-) or complication of care (Y63.6-Y63.9) codes are to be used with an underdosing code to indicate intent, if known.

(d)   **Toxic Effects**

When a harmful substance is ingested or comes in contact with a person, this is classified as a toxic effect. The toxic effect codes are in categories T51-T65.

Toxic effect codes have an associated intent: accidental, intentional self-harm, assault and undetermined.

ADULT AND CHILD ABUSE, NEGLECT AND OTHER MALTREATMENT

Sequence first the appropriate code from categories T74.- (Adult and child abuse, neglect and other maltreatment, confirmed) or T76.-(Adult and child abuse, neglect and other maltreatment, suspected) for abuse, neglect and other maltreatment, followed by any accompanying mental health or injury code(s).

If the documentation in the medical record states abuse or neglect it is coded as confirmed (T74.-). It is coded as suspected if it is documented as suspected (T76.-).

For cases of confirmed abuse or neglect an external cause code from the assault section (X92-**Y09**) should be added to identify the cause of any physical injuries. A perpetrator code (Y07) should be added when the perpetrator of the abuse is known. For suspected cases of abuse or neglect, do not report external cause or perpetrator code.

If a suspected case of abuse, neglect or mistreatment is ruled out during an encounter code Z04.71, Encounter for examination and observation following alleged physical adult abuse, ruled out, or code Z04.72, Encounter for examination and observation following alleged child physical abuse, ruled out, should be used, not a code from T76.

If a suspected case of alleged rape or sexual abuse is ruled out during an encounter code Z04.41, Encounter for examination and observation following alleged **adult rape** or code Z04.42, Encounter for examination and observation following alleged **child** rape, should be used, not a code from T76.

See Section I.C.15. Abuse in a pregnant patient.

COMPLICATIONS OF CARE

1)   **General guidelines for complications of care**

(a)   **Documentation of complications of care**

See Section I.B.16. for information on documentation of complications of care.

2)   **Pain due to medical devices**

Pain associated with devices, implants or grafts left in a surgical site (for example painful hip prosthesis) is assigned to the appropriate code(s) found in Chapter 19, Injury, poisoning, and certain other consequences of external causes. Specific codes for pain due to medical devices are found in the T code section of the ICD-10-CM. Use additional code(s) from category G89 to identify acute or chronic pain due to presence of the device, implant or graft (G89.18 or G89.28).

3)   **Transplant complications**

(a)   **Transplant complications other than kidney**

Codes under category T86, Complications of transplanted organs and tissues, are for use for both complications and rejection of transplanted organs. A transplant complication code is only assigned if the complication affects the function of the transplanted organ. Two codes are required to fully describe a transplant complication: the appropriate code from category T86 and a secondary code that identifies the complication.

Pre-existing conditions or conditions that develop after the transplant are not coded as complications unless they affect the function of the transplanted organs.

See I.C.21. for transplant organ removal status See I.C.2. for malignant neoplasm associated with transplanted organ.

(b)   **Kidney transplant complications**

Patients who have undergone kidney transplant may still have some form of chronic kidney disease (CKD) because the kidney transplant may not fully restore kidney function. Code T86.1- should be assigned for documented complications of a kidney transplant, such as transplant failure or

rejection or other transplant complication. Code T86.1- should not be assigned for post kidney transplant patients who have chronic kidney (CKD) unless a transplant complication such as transplant failure or rejection is documented. If the documentation is unclear as to whether the patient has a complication of the transplant, query the provider.

Conditions that affect the function of the transplanted kidney, other than CKD, should be assigned a code from subcategory T86.1, Complications of transplanted organ, Kidney, and a secondary code that identifies the complication.

For patients with CKD following a kidney transplant, but who do not have a complication such as failure or rejection, *see section I.C.14. Chronic kidney disease and kidney transplant status.*

4) **Complication codes that include the external cause**

As with certain other T codes, some of the complications of care codes have the external cause included in the code. The code includes the nature of the complication as well as the type of procedure that caused the complication. No external cause code indicating the type of procedure is necessary for these codes.

5) **Complications of care codes within the body system chapters**

Intraoperative and postprocedural complication codes are found within the body system chapters with codes specific to the organs and structures of that body system. These codes should be sequenced first, followed by a code(s) for the specific complication, if applicable.

● New code ▲ Revised code **Excludes1:** Not coded here **Excludes2:** Not included here ⊗ Placeholder required ⑦ 7th digit required

Chapter 19

Injury, Poisoning And Certain Other Consequences Of External Causes (S00-T88)

Note: Use secondary code(s) from Chapter 20, External causes of morbidity, to indicate cause of injury. Codes within the T section that include the external cause do not require an additional external cause code

<u>**Use additional code**</u> to identify any retained foreign body, if applicable (Z18.-)

Excludes1: birth trauma (P10-P15)

　　　　　obstetric trauma (O70-O71)

This chapter contains the following blocks:

S00-S09	Injuries to the head
S10-S19	Injuries to the neck
S20-S29	Injuries to the thorax
S30-S39	Injuries to the abdomen, lower back, lumbar spine, pelvis and external genitals
S40-S49	Injuries to the shoulder and upper arm
S50-S59	Injuries to the elbow and forearm
S60-S69	Injuries to the wrist, hand and fingers
S70-S79	Injuries to the hip and thigh
S80-S89	Injuries to the knee and lower leg
S90-S99	Injuries to the ankle and foot
T07	Injuries involving multiple body regions
T14	Injury of unspecified body region
T15-T19	Effects of foreign body entering through natural orifice
T20-T32	Burns and corrosions
T20-T25	Burns and corrosions of external body surface, specified by site
T26-T28	Burns and corrosions confined to eye and internal organs
T30-T32	Burns and corrosions of multiple and unspecified body regions
T33-T34	Frostbite
T36-T50	Poisoning by, adverse effect of and underdosing of drugs, medicaments and biological substances
T51-T65	Toxic effects of substances chiefly nonmedicinal as to source
T66-T78	Other and unspecified effects of external causes
T79	Certain early complications of trauma
T80-T88	Complications of surgical and medical care, not elsewhere classified

Note: The chapter uses the S-section for coding different types of injuries related to single body regions and the T-section to cover injuries to unspecified body regions as well as poisoning and certain other consequences of external causes.

INJURIES TO THE HEAD (S00-S09)

Includes: injuries of ear

　　　　injuries of eye

　　　　injuries of face [any part] injuries of gum

　　　　injuries of jaw injuries of oral cavity injuries of palate

　　　　injuries of periocular area injuries of scalp

　　　　injuries of temporomandibular joint area injuries of tongue

　　　　injuries of tooth

<u>**Code also**</u> for any associated infection

Excludes2: burns and corrosions (T20-T32)

　　　　　effects of foreign body in ear (T16)

effects of foreign body in larynx (T17.3)

effects of foreign body in mouth NOS (T18.0)

effects of foreign body in nose (T17.0-T17.1)

effects of foreign body in pharynx (T17.2)

effects of foreign body on external eye (T15.-)

frostbite (T33-T34)

insect bite or sting, venomous (T63.4)

S00 **Superficial injury of head**

Excludes1: diffuse cerebral contusion (S06.2-)

　　　　　focal cerebral contusion (S06.3-)

　　　　　injury of eye and orbit (S05.-)

　　　　　open wound of head (S01.-)

The appropriate 7th character is to be added to each code from category S00

A - initial encounter

D - subsequent encounter

S - sequela

S00.0　**Superficial injury of scalp**

　　⊗⑦**S00.00**　**Unspecified superficial injury of scalp**

　　⊗⑦**S00.01**　**Abrasion of scalp**

　　⊗⑦**S00.02**　**Blister (nonthermal) of scalp**

　　⊗⑦**S00.03**　**Contusion of scalp**

　　　　Bruise of scalp

　　　　Hematoma of scalp

　　⊗⑦**S00.04**　**External constriction of part of scalp**

　　⊗⑦**S00.05**　**Superficial foreign body of scalp**

　　　　Splinter in the scalp

　　⊗⑦**S00.06**　**Insect bite (nonvenomous) of scalp**

　　⊗⑦**S00.07**　**Other superficial bite of scalp**

　　　　Excludes1: open bite of scalp (S01.05)

S00.1　**Contusion of eyelid and periocular area**

　　　Black eye

　　　Excludes2: contusion of eyeball and orbital tissues (S05.1)

　　⊗⑦**S00.10**　**Contusion of unspecified eyelid and periocular area**

　　⊗⑦**S00.11**　**Contusion of right eyelid and periocular area**

　　⊗⑦**S00.12**　**Contusion of left eyelid and periocular area**

S00.2　**Other and unspecified superficial injuries of eyelid and periocular area**

　　　Excludes2: superficial injury of conjunctiva and cornea (S05.0-)

　　S00.20　**Unspecified superficial injury of eyelid and periocular area**

　　　　⑦**S00.201**　**Unspecified superficial injury of right eyelid and periocular area**

　　　　⑦**S00.202**　**Unspecified superficial injury of left eyelid and periocular area**

　　　　⑦**S00.209**　**Unspecified superficial injury of unspecified eyelid and periocular area**

　　S00.21　**Abrasion of eyelid and periocular area**

　　　　⑦**S00.211**　**Abrasion of right eyelid and periocular area**

　　　　⑦**S00.212**　**Abrasion of left eyelid and periocular area**

⑦S00.219   **Abrasion of unspecified eyelid and periocular area**

S00.22   **Blister (nonthermal) of eyelid and periocular area**

⑦S00.221   **Blister (nonthermal) of right eyelid and periocular area**

⑦S00.222   **Blister (nonthermal) of left eyelid and periocular area**

⑦S00.229   **Blister (nonthermal) of unspecified eyelid and periocular area**

S00.24   **External constriction of eyelid and periocular area**

⑦S00.241   **External constriction of right eyelid and periocular area**

⑦S00.242   **External constriction of left eyelid and periocular area**

⑦S00.249   **External constriction of unspecified eyelid and periocular area**

S00.25   **Superficial foreign body of eyelid and periocular area**

Splinter of eyelid and periocular area

Excludes2: retained foreign body in eyelid (H02.81-)

⑦S00.251   **Superficial foreign body of right eyelid and periocular area**

⑦S00.252   **Superficial foreign body of left eyelid and periocular area**

⑦S00.259   **Superficial foreign body of unspecified eyelid and periocular area**

S00.26   **Insect bite (nonvenomous) of eyelid and periocular area**

⑦S00.261   **Insect bite (nonvenomous) of right eyelid and periocular area**

⑦S00.262   **Insect bite (nonvenomous) of left eyelid and periocular area**

⑦S00.269   **Insect bite (nonvenomous) of unspecified eyelid and periocular area**

S00.27   **Other superficial bite of eyelid and periocular area**

Excludes1: open bite of eyelid and periocular area (S01.15)

⑦S00.271   **Other superficial bite of right eyelid and periocular area**

⑦S00.272   **Other superficial bite of left eyelid and periocular area**

⑦S00.279   **Other superficial bite of unspecified eyelid and periocular area**

S00.3   **Superficial injury of nose**

⊗⑦S00.30   **Unspecified superficial injury of nose**

⊗⑦S00.31   **Abrasion of nose**

⊗⑦S00.32   **Blister (nonthermal) of nose**

⊗⑦S00.33   **Contusion of nose**

Bruise of nose

Hematoma of nose

⊗⑦S00.34   **External constriction of nose**

⊗⑦S00.35   **Superficial foreign body of nose**

Splinter in the nose

⊗⑦S00.36   **Insect bite (nonvenomous) of nose**

⊗⑦S00.37   **Other superficial bite of nose**

Excludes1: open bite of nose (S01.25)

S00.4   **Superficial injury of ear**

S00.40   **Unspecified superficial injury of ear**

⑦S00.401   **Unspecified superficial injury of right ear**

⑦S00.402   **Unspecified superficial injury of left ear**

⑦S00.409   **Unspecified superficial injury of unspecified ear**

S00.41   **Abrasion of ear**

⑦S00.411   **Abrasion of right ear**

⑦S00.412   **Abrasion of left ear**

⑦S00.419   **Abrasion of unspecified ear**

S00.42   **Blister (nonthermal) of ear**

⑦S00.421   **Blister (nonthermal) of right ear**

⑦S00.422   **Blister (nonthermal) of left ear**

⑦S00.429   **Blister (nonthermal) of unspecified ear**

S00.43   **Contusion of ear**

Bruise of ear

Hematoma of ear

⑦S00.431   **Contusion of right ear**

⑦S00.432   **Contusion of left ear**

⑦S00.439   **Contusion of unspecified ear**

S00.44   **External constriction of ear**

⑦S00.441   **External constriction of right ear**

⑦S00.442   **External constriction of left ear**

⑦S00.449   **External constriction of unspecified ear**

S00.45   **Superficial foreign body of ear**

Splinter in the ear

⑦S00.451   **Superficial foreign body of right ear**

⑦S00.452   **Superficial foreign body of left ear**

⑦S00.459   **Superficial foreign body of unspecified ear**

S00.46   **Insect bite (nonvenomous) of ear**

⑦S00.461   **Insect bite (nonvenomous) of right ear**

⑦S00.462   **Insect bite (nonvenomous) of left ear**

⑦S00.469   **Insect bite (nonvenomous) of unspecified ear**

S00.47   **Other superficial bite of ear**

Excludes1: open bite of ear (S01.35)

⑦S00.471   **Other superficial bite of right ear**

⑦S00.472   **Other superficial bite of left ear**

⑦S00.479   **Other superficial bite of unspecified ear**

S00.5   **Superficial injury of lip and oral cavity**

S00.50   **Unspecified superficial injury of lip and oral cavity**

⑦S00.501   **Unspecified superficial injury of lip**

⑦S00.502   **Unspecified superficial injury of oral cavity**

S00.51   **Abrasion of lip and oral cavity**

⑦S00.511   **Abrasion of lip**

● New code   ▲ Revised code   Excludes1: Not coded here   Excludes2: Not included here   ⊗ Placeholder required   ⑦7th digit required

⑦**S00.512**   **Abrasion of oral cavity**

S00.52   **Blister (nonthermal) of lip and oral cavity**

⑦**S00.521**   **Blister (nonthermal) of lip**

⑦**S00.522**   **Blister (nonthermal) of oral cavity**

S00.53   **Contusion of lip and oral cavity**

⑦**S00.531**   **Contusion of lip**

Bruise of lip

Hematoma of oral cavity

⑦**S00.532**   **Contusion of oral cavity**

Bruise of lip

Hematoma of oral cavity

S00.54   **External constriction of lip and oral cavity**

⑦**S00.541**   **External constriction of lip**

⑦**S00.542**   **External constriction of oral cavity**

S00.55   **Superficial foreign body of lip and oral cavity**

⑦**S00.551**   **Superficial foreign body of lip**

Splinter of lip and oral cavity

⑦**S00.552**   **Superficial foreign body of oral cavity**

Splinter of lip and oral cavity

S00.56   **Insect bite (nonvenomous) of lip and oral cavity**

⑦**S00.561**   **Insect bite (nonvenomous) of lip**

⑦**S00.562**   **Insect bite (nonvenomous) of oral cavity**

S00.57   **Other superficial bite of lip and oral cavity**

⑦**S00.571**   **Other superficial bite of lip**

Excludes1: open bite of lip (S01.551)

⑦**S00.572**   **Other superficial bite of oral cavity**

Excludes1: open bite of oral cavity (S01.552)

S00.8   **Superficial injury of other parts of head**

Superficial injuries of face [any part]

⊗⑦**S00.80**   **Unspecified superficial injury of other part of head**

⊗⑦**S00.81**   **Abrasion of other part of head**

⊗⑦**S00.82**   **Blister (nonthermal) of other part of head**

⊗⑦**S00.83**   **Contusion of other part of head**

Bruise of other part of head

Hematoma of other part of head

⊗⑦**S00.84**   **External constriction of other part of head**

⊗⑦**S00.85**   **Superficial foreign body of other part of head**

Splinter in other part of head

⊗⑦**S00.86**   **Insect bite (nonvenomous) of other part of head**

⊗⑦**S00.87**   **Other superficial bite of other part of head**

Excludes1: open bite of other part of head (S01.85)

S00.9   **Superficial injury of unspecified part of head**

⊗⑦**S00.90**   **Unspecified superficial injury of unspecified part of head**

⊗⑦**S00.91**   **Abrasion of unspecified part of head**

⊗⑦**S00.92**   **Blister (nonthermal) of unspecified part of head**

⊗⑦**S00.93**   **Contusion of unspecified part of head**

Bruise of head

Hematoma of head

⊗**S00.94**   **External constriction of unspecified part of head**

⊗**S00.95**   **Superficial foreign body of unspecified part of head**

Splinter of head

⊗**S00.96**   **Insect bite (nonvenomous) of unspecified part of head**

⊗**S00.97**   **Other superficial bite of unspecified part of head**

Excludes1: open bite of head (S01.95)

S01   **Open wound of head**

Code also any associated:

injury of cranial nerve (S04.-)

injury of muscle and tendon of head (S09.1-)

intracranial injury (S06.-)

wound infection

Excludes1: open skull fracture (S02.- with 7th character B)

Excludes2: injury of eye and orbit (S05.-)

traumatic amputation of part of head (S08.-)

The appropriate 7th character is to be added to each code from category S01

A - initial encounter

D - subsequent encounter

S - sequela

S01.0   **Open wound of scalp**

Excludes1: avulsion of scalp (S08.0)

⊗⑦**S01.00**   **Unspecified open wound of scalp**

⊗⑦**S01.01**   **Laceration without foreign body of scalp**

⊗⑦**S01.02**   **Laceration with foreign body of scalp**

⊗⑦**S01.03**   **Puncture wound without foreign body of scalp**

⊗⑦**S01.04**   **Puncture wound with foreign body of scalp**

⊗⑦**S01.05**   **Open bite of scalp**

Bite of scalp NOS

Excludes1: superficial bite of scalp (S00.06, S00.07-)

S01.1   **Open wound of eyelid and periocular area**

Open wound of eyelid and periocular area with or without involvement of lacrimal passages

S01.10   **Unspecified open wound of eyelid and periocular area**

⑦**S01.101**   **Unspecified open wound of right eyelid and periocular area**

⑦**S01.102**   **Unspecified open wound of left eyelid and periocular area**

⑦**S01.109**   **Unspecified open wound of unspecified eyelid and periocular area**

S01.11   **Laceration without foreign body of eyelid and periocular area**

⑦**S01.111**   **Laceration without foreign body of right eyelid and periocular area**

⑦**S01.112**   **Laceration without foreign body of left eyelid and periocular area**

⑦**S01.119**   **Laceration without foreign body of unspecified eyelid and periocular area**

S01.12   Laceration with foreign body of eyelid and periocular area

⑦S01.121   Laceration with foreign body of right eyelid and periocular area

⑦S01.122   Laceration with foreign body of left eyelid and periocular area

⑦S01.129   Laceration with foreign body of unspecified eyelid and periocular area

S01.13   Puncture wound without foreign body of eyelid and periocular area

⑦S01.131   Puncture wound without foreign body of right eyelid and periocular area

⑦S01.132   Puncture wound without foreign body of left eyelid and periocular area

⑦S01.139   Puncture wound without foreign body of unspecified eyelid and periocular area

S01.14   Puncture wound with foreign body of eyelid and periocular area

⑦S01.141   Puncture wound with foreign body of right eyelid and periocular area

⑦S01.142   Puncture wound with foreign body of left eyelid and periocular area

⑦S01.149   Puncture wound with foreign body of unspecified eyelid and periocular area

S01.15   Open bite of eyelid and periocular area

Bite of eyelid and periocular area NOS

Excludes1: superficial bite of eyelid and periocular area (S00.26, S00.27)

⑦S01.151   Open bite of right eyelid and periocular area

⑦S01.152   Open bite of left eyelid and periocular area

⑦S01.159   Open bite of unspecified eyelid and periocular area

S01.2   Open wound of nose

⊗⑦S01.20   Unspecified open wound of nose

⊗⑦S01.21   Laceration without foreign body of nose

⊗⑦S01.22   Laceration with foreign body of nose

⊗⑦S01.23   Puncture wound without foreign body of nose

⊗⑦S01.24   Puncture wound with foreign body of nose

⊗⑦S01.25   Open bite of nose

Bite of nose NOS

Excludes1: superficial bite of nose (S00.36, S00.37)

S01.3   Open wound of ear

S01.30   Unspecified open wound of ear

⑦S01.301   Unspecified open wound of right ear

⑦S01.302   Unspecified open wound of left ear

⑦S01.309   Unspecified open wound of unspecified ear

S01.31   Laceration without foreign body of ear

⑦S01.311   Laceration without foreign body of right ear

⑦S01.312   Laceration without foreign body of left ear

⑦S01.319   Laceration without foreign body of unspecified ear

S01.32   Laceration with foreign body of ear

⑦S01.321   Laceration with foreign body of right ear

⑦S01.322   Laceration with foreign body of left ear

⑦S01.329   Laceration with foreign body of unspecified ear

S01.33   Puncture wound without foreign body of ear

⑦S01.331   Puncture wound without foreign body of right ear

⑦S01.332   Puncture wound without foreign body of left ear

⑦S01.339   Puncture wound without foreign body of unspecified ear

S01.34   Puncture wound with foreign body of ear

⑦S01.341   Puncture wound with foreign body of right ear

⑦S01.342   Puncture wound with foreign body of left ear

⑦S01.349   Puncture wound with foreign body of unspecified ear

S01.35   Open bite of ear

Bite of ear NOS

Excludes1: superficial bite of ear (S00.46, S00.47)

⑦S01.351   Open bite of right ear

⑦S01.352   Open bite of left ear

⑦S01.359   Open bite of unspecified ear

S01.4   Open wound of cheek and temporomandibular area

S01.40   Unspecified open wound of cheek and temporomandibular area

⑦S01.401   Unspecified open wound of right cheek and temporomandibular area

⑦S01.402   Unspecified open wound of left cheek and temporomandibular area

⑦S01.409   Unspecified open wound of unspecified cheek and temporomandibular area

S01.41   Laceration without foreign body of cheek and temporomandibular area

⑦S01.411   Laceration without foreign body of right cheek and temporomandibular area

⑦S01.412   Laceration without foreign body of left cheek and temporomandibular area

⑦S01.419   Laceration without foreign body of unspecified cheek and temporomandibular area

S01.42   Laceration with foreign body of cheek and temporomandibular area

⑦S01.421   Laceration with foreign body of right cheek and temporomandibular area

⑦S01.422   Laceration with foreign body of left cheek and temporomandibular area

● New code   ▲ Revised code   **Excludes1:** Not coded here   **Excludes2:** Not included here   ⊗ Placeholder required   ⑦7th digit required

⑦**S01.429** **Laceration with foreign body of unspecified cheek and temporomandibular area**

S01.43 **Puncture wound without foreign body of cheek and temporomandibular area**

⑦**S01.431** **Puncture wound without foreign body of right cheek and temporomandibular area**

⑦**S01.432** **Puncture wound without foreign body of left cheek and temporomandibular area**

⑦**S01.439** **Puncture wound without foreign body of unspecified cheek and temporomandibular area**

S01.44 **Puncture wound with foreign body of cheek and temporomandibular area**

⑦**S01.441** **Puncture wound with foreign body of right cheek and temporomandibular area**

⑦**S01.442** **Puncture wound with foreign body of left cheek and temporomandibular area**

⑦**S01.449** **Puncture wound with foreign body of unspecified cheek and temporomandibular area**

S01.45 **Open bite of cheek and temporomandibular area**

Bite of cheek and temporomandibular area NOS

Excludes2: superficial bite of cheek and temporomandibular area (S00.86, S00.87)

⑦**S01.451** **Open bite of right cheek and temporomandibular area**

⑦**S01.452** **Open bite of left cheek and temporomandibular area**

⑦**S01.459** **Open bite of unspecified cheek and temporomandibular area**

S01.5 **Open wound of lip and oral cavity**

Excludes2: tooth dislocation (S03.2)

tooth fracture (S02.5)

S01.50 **Unspecified open wound of lip and oral cavity**

⑦**S01.501** **Unspecified open wound of lip**

⑦**S01.502** **Unspecified open wound of oral cavity**

S01.51 **Laceration of lip and oral cavity without foreign body**

⑦**S01.511** **Laceration without foreign body of lip**

⑦**S01.512** **Laceration without foreign body of oral cavity**

S01.52 **Laceration of lip and oral cavity with foreign body**

⑦**S01.521** **Laceration with foreign body of lip**

⑦**S01.522** **Laceration with foreign body of oral cavity**

S01.53 **Puncture wound of lip and oral cavity without foreign body**

⑦**S01.531** **Puncture wound without foreign body of lip**

⑦**S01.532** **Puncture wound without foreign body of oral cavity**

S01.54 **Puncture wound of lip and oral cavity with foreign body**

⑦**S01.541** **Puncture wound with foreign body of lip**

⑦**S01.542** **Puncture wound with foreign body of oral cavity**

S01.55 **Open bite of lip and oral cavity**

⑦**S01.551** **Open bite of lip**

Bite of lip NOS

Excludes1: superficial bite of lip (S00.571)

⑦**S01.552** **Open bite of oral cavity**

Bite of oral cavity NOS

Excludes1: superficial bite of oral cavity (S00.572)

S01.8 **Open wound of other parts of head**

⊗⑦**S01.80** **Unspecified open wound of other part of head**

⊗⑦**S01.81** **Laceration without foreign body of other part of head**

⊗⑦**S01.82** **Laceration with foreign body of other part of head**

⊗⑦**S01.83** **Puncture wound without foreign body of other part of head**

⊗⑦**S01.84** **Puncture wound with foreign body of other part of head**

⊗⑦**S01.85** **Open bite of other part of head**

Bite **of other** part of head NOS

Excludes1: superficial bite **of other** part of head (S00.85)

S01.9 **Open wound of unspecified part of head**

⊗⑦**S01.90** **Unspecified open wound of unspecified part of head**

⊗⑦**S01.91** **Laceration without foreign body of unspecified part of head**

⊗⑦**S01.92** **Laceration with foreign body of unspecified part of head**

⊗⑦**S01.93** **Puncture wound without foreign body of unspecified part of head**

⊗⑦**S01.94** **Puncture wound with foreign body of unspecified part of head**

⊗⑦**S01.95** **Open bite of unspecified part of head**

Bite of head NOS

Excludes1: superficial bite of head NOS (S00.97)

S02 **Fracture of skull and facial bones**

Note: A fracture not indicated as open or closed should be coded to closed

Code also any associated intracranial injury (S06.-)

The appropriate 7th character is to be added to each code from category S02

A - initial encounter for closed fracture

B - initial encounter for open fracture

D - subsequent encounter for fracture with routine healing

G - subsequent encounter for fracture with delayed healing

K - subsequent encounter for fracture with nonunion

S - sequela

⊗⑦**S02.0** **Fracture of vault of skull**

Fracture of frontal bone

Fracture of parietal bone

S02.1 **Fracture of base of skull**

Excludes1: orbit NOS (S02.8)

Excludes2: orbital floor (S02.3-)

    S02.10 **Unspecified fracture of base of skull**

      ●⑦**S02.101** **Fracture of base of skull, right side**

      ●⑦**S02.102** **Fracture of base of skull, left side**

      ●⑦**S02.109** **Fracture of base of skull, unspecified side**

    S02.11 **Fracture of occiput**

      ▲⑦**S02.110** **Type I occipital condyle fracture, unspecified side**

      ▲⑦**S02.111** **Type II occipital condyle fracture, unspecified side**

      ▲⑦**S02.112** **Type III occipital condyle fracture, unspecified side**

      ⑦**S02.113** **Unspecified occipital condyle fracture**

      ▲⑦**S02.118** **Other fracture of occiput, unspecified side**

      ⑦**S02.119** **Unspecified fracture of occiput**

      ●⑦**S02.11A** **Type I occipital condyle fracture, right side**

      ●⑦**S02.11B** **Type I occipital condyle fracture, left side**

      ●⑦**S02.11C** **Type II occipital condyle fracture, right side**

      ●⑦**S02.11D** **Type II occipital condyle fracture, left side**

      ●⑦**S02.11E** **Type III occipital condyle fracture, right side**

      ●⑦**S02.11F** **Type III occipital condyle fracture, left side**

      ●**S02.11G** **Other fracture of occiput, right side**

      ●**S02.11H** **Other fracture of occiput, left side**

    ⊗⑦**S02.19** **Other fracture of base of skull**

      Fracture of anterior fossa of base of skull

      Fracture of ethmoid sinus

      Fracture of frontal sinus

      Fracture of middle fossa of base of skull

      Fracture of orbital roof

      Fracture of posterior fossa of base of skull

      Fracture of sphenoid

      Fracture of temporal bone

⊗⑦**S02.2** **Fracture of nasal bones**

S02.3 **Fracture of orbital floor**

Excludes1: orbit NOS (S02.8)

Excludes2: orbital roof (S02.1-)

  ●⊗⑦**S02.30** **Fracture of orbital floor, unspecified side**

  ●⊗⑦**S02.31** **Fracture of orbital floor, right side**

  ●⊗⑦**S02.32** **Fracture of orbital floor, left side**

S02.4 **Fracture of malar, maxillary and zygoma bones**

  Fracture of superior maxilla

  Fracture of upper jaw (bone)

  Fracture of zygomatic process of temporal bone

    S02.40 **Fracture of malar, maxillary and zygoma bones, unspecified**

      ●⑦**S02.400** **Malar fracture, unspecified side**

      ●⑦**S02.401** **Maxillary fracture, unspecified side**

      ●⑦**S02.402** **Zygomatic fracture, unspecified side**

      ●⑦**S02.40A** **Malar fracture, right side**

      ●⑦**S02.40B** **Malar fracture, left side**

      ●⑦**S02.40C** **Maxillary fracture, right side**

      ●⑦**S02.40D** **Maxillary fracture, left side**

      ●⑦**S02.40E** **Zygomatic fracture, right side**

      ●⑦**S02.40F** **Zygomatic fracture, left side**

    S02.41 **LeFort fracture**

      ⑦**S02.411** **LeFort I fracture**

      ⑦**S02.412** **LeFort II fracture**

      ⑦**S02.413** **LeFort III fracture**

  ⊗⑦**S02.42** **Fracture of alveolus of maxilla**

⊗⑦**S02.5** **Fracture of tooth (traumatic)**

  Broken tooth

  Excludes1: cracked tooth (nontraumatic) (K03.81)

S02.6 **Fracture of mandible**

  Fracture of lower jaw (bone)

    S02.60 **Fracture of mandible, unspecified**

      ▲⑦**S02.600** **Fracture of unspecified part of body of mandible, unspecified side**

      ●⑦**S02.601** **Fracture of unspecified part of body of right mandible**

      ●⑦**S02.602** **Fracture of unspecified part of body of left mandible**

      ⑦**S02.609** **Fracture of mandible, unspecified**

    S02.61 **Fracture of condylar process of mandible**

      ●⑦**S02.610** **Fracture of condylar process of mandible, unspecified side**

      ●⑦**S02.611** **Fracture of condylar process of right mandible**

      ●⑦**S02.612** **Fracture of condylar process of left mandible**

    S02.62 **Fracture of subcondylar process of mandible**

      ●⑦**S02.620** **Fracture of subcondylar process of mandible, unspecified side**

      ●⑦**S02.621** **Fracture of subcondylar process of right mandible**

      ●⑦**S02.622** **Fracture of subcondylar process of left mandible**

    S02.63 **Fracture of coronoid process of mandible**

      ●⑦**S02.630** **Fracture of coronoid process of mandible, unspecified side**

      ●⑦**S02.631** **Fracture of coronoid process of right mandible**

      ●⑦**S02.632** **Fracture of coronoid process of left mandible**

    S02.64 **Fracture of ramus of mandible**

      ●⑦**S02.640** **Fracture of ramus of mandible, unspecified side**

      ●⑦**S02.641** **Fracture of ramus of right mandible**

      ●⑦**S02.642** **Fracture of ramus of left mandible**

    S02.65 **Fracture of angle of mandible**

      ●⑦**S02.650** **Fracture of angle of mandible, unspecified side**

   ● New code   ▲ Revised code   **Excludes1:** Not coded here   **Excludes2:** Not included here   ⊗ Placeholder required   ⑦7th digit required

- ⑦S02.651   **Fracture of angle of right mandible**
- ⑦S02.652   **Fracture of angle of left mandible**

⊗⑦**S02.66**   **Fracture of symphysis of mandible**

S02.67   **Fracture of alveolus of mandible**

- ⑦**S02.670**   **Fracture of alveolus of mandible, unspecified side**
- ⑦**S02.671**   **Fracture of alveolus of right mandible**
- ⑦**S02.672**   **Fracture of alveolus of left mandible**

⊗⑦**S02.69**   **Fracture of mandible of other specified site**

S02.8   **Fractures of other specified skull and facial bones**

Fracture of orbit NOS

Fracture of palate

Excludes1: fracture of orbital floor (S02.3-)

fracture of orbital roof (S02.1-)

- ⊗⑦**S02.80**   **Fracture of other specified skull and facial bones, unspecified side**
- ⊗⑦**S02.81**   **Fracture of other specified skull and facial bones, right side**
- ⊗⑦**S02.82**   **Fracture of other specified skull and facial bones, left side**

S02.9   **Fracture of unspecified skull and facial bones**

⊗⑦**S02.91**   **Unspecified fracture of skull**

⊗⑦**S02.92**   **Unspecified fracture of facial bones**

S03   **Dislocation and sprain of joints and ligaments of head**

Includes: avulsion of joint (capsule) or ligament of head

laceration of cartilage, joint (capsule) or ligament of head

sprain of cartilage, joint (capsule) or ligament of head

traumatic hemarthrosis of joint or ligament of head

traumatic rupture of joint or ligament of head

traumatic subluxation of joint or ligament of head

traumatic tear of joint or ligament of head

Code also any associated open wound

Excludes2: Strain of muscle or tendon of head (S09.1)

The appropriate 7th character is to be added to each code from category S03

A - initial encounter

D - subsequent encounter

S - sequela

S03.0   **Dislocation of jaw**

Dislocation of jaw (cartilage) (meniscus)

Dislocation of mandible

Dislocation of temporomandibular (joint)

- ⊗⑦**S03.00**   **Dislocation of jaw, unspecified side**
- ⊗⑦**S03.01**   **Dislocation of jaw, right side**
- ⊗⑦**S03.02**   **Dislocation of jaw, left side**
- ⊗⑦**S03.03**   **Dislocation of jaw, bilateral**

⊗⑦**S03.1**   **Dislocation of septal cartilage of nose**

⊗⑦**S03.2**   **Dislocation of tooth**

S03.4   **Sprain of jaw**

Sprain of temporomandibular (joint) (ligament)

- ⊗⑦**S03.40**   **Sprain of jaw, unspecified side**
- ⊗⑦**S03.41**   **Sprain of jaw, right side**
- ⊗⑦**S03.42**   **Sprain of jaw, left side**
- ⊗⑦**S03.43**   **Sprain of jaw, bilateral**

⊗⑦**S03.8**   **Sprain of joints and ligaments of other parts of head**

⊗⑦**S03.9**   **Sprain of joints and ligaments of unspecified parts of head**

S04   **Injury of cranial nerve**

The selection of side should be based on the side of the body being affected

Code first any associated intracranial injury (S06.-)

Code also any associated:

open wound of head (S01.-) skull fracture (S02.-)

The appropriate 7th character is to be added to each code from category S04

A - initial encounter

D - subsequent encounter

S - sequela

S04.0   **Injury of optic nerve and pathways**

Use additional code to identify any visual field defect or blindness (H53.4-, H54)

S04.01   **Injury of optic nerve**

Injury of 2nd cranial nerve

⑦**S04.011**   **Injury of optic nerve, right eye**

⑦**S04.012**   **Injury of optic nerve, left eye**

⑦**S04.019**   **Injury of optic nerve, unspecified eye**

Injury of optic nerve NOS

⊗⑦**S04.02**   **Injury of optic chiasm**

S04.03   **Injury of optic tract and pathways**

Injury of optic radiation

⑦**S04.031**   **Injury of optic tract and pathways, right eye**

⑦**S04.032**   **Injury of optic tract and pathways, left eye**

⑦**S04.039**   **Injury of optic tract and pathways, unspecified eye**

Injury of optic tract and pathways NOS

S04.04   **Injury of visual cortex**

⑦**S04.041**   **Injury of visual cortex, right eye**

⑦**S04.042**   **Injury of visual cortex, left eye**

⑦**S04.049**   **Injury of visual cortex, unspecified eye**

Injury of visual cortex NOS

S04.1   **Injury of oculomotor nerve**

Injury of 3rd cranial nerve

⊗⑦**S04.10**   **Injury of oculomotor nerve, unspecified side**

⊗⑦**S04.11**   **Injury of oculomotor nerve, right side**

⊗⑦**S04.12**   **Injury of oculomotor nerve, left side**

S04.2   **Injury of trochlear nerve**

Injury of 4th cranial nerve

⊗⑦**S04.20**   **Injury of trochlear nerve, unspecified side**

⊗⑦**S04.21**   **Injury of trochlear nerve, right side**

⊗⑦**S04.22**   **Injury of trochlear nerve, left side**

S04.3   **Injury of trigeminal nerve**

Injury of 5th cranial nerve

⊗⑦**S04.30**   **Injury of trigeminal nerve, unspecified side**

⊗⑦**S04.31**   **Injury of trigeminal nerve, right side**

⊗⑦**S04.32**   **Injury of trigeminal nerve, left side**

S04.4   **Injury of abducent nerve**

	Add 4th-7th digits		Nonspecific code		Unspecified code		Manifestation code

Injury of 6th cranial nerve

⊗⑦**S04.40**　**Injury of abducent nerve, unspecified side**

⊗⑦**S04.41**　**Injury of abducent nerve, right side**

⊗⑦**S04.42**　**Injury of abducent nerve, left side**

S04.5　**Injury of facial nerve**

Injury of 7th cranial nerve

⊗⑦**S04.50**　**Injury of facial nerve, unspecified side**

⊗⑦**S04.51**　**Injury of facial nerve, right side**

⊗⑦**S04.52**　**Injury of facial nerve, left side**

S04.6　**Injury of acoustic nerve**

Injury of auditory nerve Injury of 8th cranial nerve

⊗⑦**S04.60**　**Injury of acoustic nerve, unspecified side**

⊗⑦**S04.61**　**Injury of acoustic nerve, right side**

⊗⑦**S04.62**　**Injury of acoustic nerve, left side**

S04.7　**Injury of accessory nerve**

Injury of 11th cranial nerve

⊗⑦**S04.70**　**Injury of accessory nerve, unspecified side**

⊗⑦**S04.71**　**Injury of accessory nerve, right side**

⊗⑦**S04.72**　**Injury of accessory nerve, left side**

S04.8　**Injury of other cranial nerves**

　　S04.81　**Injury of olfactory [1st] nerve**

⑦　S04.811　**Injury of olfactory [1st] nerve, right side**

⑦　S04.812　**Injury of olfactory [1st] nerve, left side**

⑦　S04.819　**Injury of olfactory [1st] nerve, unspecified side**

　　S04.89　**Injury of other cranial nerves**

Injury of vagus [10th] nerve

⑦　S04.891　**Injury of other cranial nerves, right side**

⑦　S04.892　**Injury of other cranial nerves, left side**

⑦　S04.899　**Injury of other cranial nerves, unspecified side**

⊗⑦**S04.9**　**Injury of unspecified cranial nerve**

S05　**Injury of eye and orbit**

Includes: open wound of eye and orbit

Excludes2: 2nd cranial [optic] nerve injury (S04.0-)

3rd cranial [oculomotor] nerve injury (S04.1-)

open wound of eyelid and periocular area (S01.1-)

orbital bone fracture (S02.1-, S02.3-, S02.8-)

superficial injury of eyelid (S00.1-S00.2)

The appropriate 7th character is to be added to each code from category S05

A - initial encounter

D - subsequent encounter

S - sequela

S05.0　**Injury of conjunctiva and corneal abrasion without foreign body**

Excludes1: foreign body in conjunctival sac (T15.1)

foreign body in cornea (T15.0)

⊗⑦**S05.00**　**Injury of conjunctiva and corneal abrasion without foreign body, unspecified eye**

⊗⑦**S05.01**　**Injury of conjunctiva and corneal abrasion without foreign body, right eye**

⊗⑦**S05.02**　**Injury of conjunctiva and corneal abrasion without foreign body, left eye**

S05.1　**Contusion of eyeball and orbital tissues**

Traumatic hyphema

Excludes2: black eye NOS (S00.1)

contusion of eyelid and periocular area (S00.1)

⊗⑦**S05.10**　**Contusion of eyeball and orbital tissues, unspecified eye**

⊗⑦**S05.11**　**Contusion of eyeball and orbital tissues, right eye**

⊗⑦**S05.12**　**Contusion of eyeball and orbital tissues, left eye**

S05.2　**Ocular laceration and rupture with prolapse or loss of intraocular tissue**

⊗⑦**S05.20**　**Ocular laceration and rupture with prolapse or loss of intraocular tissue, unspecified eye**

⊗⑦**S05.21**　**Ocular laceration and rupture with prolapse or loss of intraocular tissue, right eye**

⊗⑦**S05.22**　**Ocular laceration and rupture with prolapse or loss of intraocular tissue, left eye**

S05.3　**Ocular laceration without prolapse or loss of intraocular tissue**

Laceration of eye NOS

⊗⑦**S05.30**　**Ocular laceration without prolapse or loss of intraocular tissue, unspecified eye**

⊗⑦**S05.31**　**Ocular laceration without prolapse or loss of intraocular tissue, right eye**

⊗⑦**S05.32**　**Ocular laceration without prolapse or loss of intraocular tissue, left eye**

S05.4　**Penetrating wound of orbit with or without foreign body**

Excludes2: retained (old) foreign body following penetrating wound in orbit (H05.5-)

⊗⑦**S05.40**　**Penetrating wound of orbit with or without foreign body, unspecified eye**

⊗⑦**S05.41**　**Penetrating wound of orbit with or without foreign body, right eye**

⊗⑦**S05.42**　**Penetrating wound of orbit with or without foreign body, left eye**

S05.5　**Penetrating wound with foreign body of eyeball**

Excludes2: retained (old) intraocular foreign body (H44.6-, H44.7)

⊗⑦**S05.50**　**Penetrating wound with foreign body of unspecified eyeball**

⊗⑦**S05.51**　**Penetrating wound with foreign body of right eyeball**

⊗⑦**S05.52**　**Penetrating wound with foreign body of left eyeball**

S05.6　**Penetrating wound without foreign body of eyeball**

Ocular penetration NOS

⊗⑦**S05.60**　**Penetrating wound without foreign body of unspecified eyeball**

⊗⑦**S05.61**　**Penetrating wound without foreign body of right eyeball**

⊗⑦**S05.62**　**Penetrating wound without foreign body of left eyeball**

S05.7　**Avulsion of eye**

Definition: An avulsion is an injury in which a body structure is forcibly detached from its normal point of insertion by either trauma or surgery.

Traumatic enucleation

　● New code　▲ Revised code　**Excludes1:** Not coded here　**Excludes2:** Not included here　⊗ Placeholder required　⑦ 7th digit required

⊗⑦**S05.70** Avulsion of unspecified eye

⊗⑦**S05.71** Avulsion of right eye

⊗⑦**S05.72** Avulsion of left eye

S05.8 Other injuries of eye and orbit

Lacrimal duct injury

S05.8X Other injuries of eye and orbit

⑦**S05.8X1** Other injuries of right eye and orbit

⑦**S05.8X2** Other injuries of left eye and orbit

⑦**S05.8X9** Other injuries of unspecified eye and orbit

S05.9 Unspecified injury of eye and orbit

Injury of eye NOS

⊗⑦**S05.90** Unspecified injury of unspecified eye and orbit

⊗⑦**S05.91** Unspecified injury of right eye and orbit

⊗⑦**S05.92** Unspecified injury of left eye and orbit

S06 **Intracranial injury**

Includes: traumatic brain injury

Code also any associated:

open wound of head (S01.-)

skull fracture (S02.-)

Excludes1: head injury NOS (S09.90)

The appropriate 7th character is to be added to each code from category S06

A - initial encounter

D - subsequent encounter

S - sequela

S06.0 **Concussion**

Commotio cerebri

Excludes1: concussion with other intracranial injuries classified in subcategories S06.1- to S06.6- , S06.81- and S06.82- code to specified intracranial injury

S06.0X Concussion

⑦**S06.0X0** Concussion without loss of consciousness

⑦**S06.0X1** Concussion with loss of consciousness of 30 minutes or less

⑦**S06.0X9** Concussion with loss of consciousness of unspecified duration

Concussion NOS

S06.1 **Traumatic cerebral edema**

Diffuse traumatic cerebral edema

Focal traumatic cerebral edema

S06.1X Traumatic cerebral edema

⑦**S06.1X0** Traumatic cerebral edema without loss of consciousness

⑦**S06.1X1** Traumatic cerebral edema with loss of consciousness of 30 minutes or less

⑦**S06.1X2** Traumatic cerebral edema with loss of consciousness of 31 minutes to 59 minutes

⑦**S06.1X3** Traumatic cerebral edema with loss of consciousness of 1hour to 5 hours 59 minutes

⑦**S06.1X4** Traumatic cerebral edema with loss of consciousness of 6 hours to 24 hours

⑦**S06.1X5** Traumatic cerebral edema with loss of consciousness greater than 24 hours with return to pre-existing conscious level

⑦**S06.1X6** Traumatic cerebral edema with loss of consciousness greater than 24 hours without return to pre-existing conscious level with patient surviving

⑦**S06.1X7** Traumatic cerebral edema with loss of consciousness of any duration with death due to brain injury prior to regaining consciousness

⑦**S06.1X8** Traumatic cerebral edema with loss of consciousness of any duration with death due to other cause prior to regaining consciousness

⑦**S06.1X9** Traumatic cerebral edema with loss of consciousness of unspecified duration

Traumatic cerebral edema NOS

S06.2 **Diffuse traumatic brain injury**

Diffuse axonal brain injury

Excludes1: traumatic diffuse cerebral edema (S06.1X-)

S06.2X Diffuse traumatic brain injury

⑦**S06.2X0** Diffuse traumatic brain injury without loss of consciousness

⑦**S06.2X1** Diffuse traumatic brain injury with loss of consciousness of 30 minutes or less

⑦**S06.2X2** Diffuse traumatic brain injury with loss of consciousness of 31 minutes to 59 minutes

⑦**S06.2X3** Diffuse traumatic brain injury with loss of consciousness of 1 hour to 5 hours 59 minutes

⑦**S06.2X4** Diffuse traumatic brain injury with loss of consciousness of 6 hours to 24 hours

⑦**S06.2X5** Diffuse traumatic brain injury with loss of consciousness greater than 24 hours with return to pre-existing conscious levels

⑦**S06.2X6** Diffuse traumatic brain injury with loss of consciousness greater than 24 hours without return to pre-existing conscious level with patient surviving

⑦**S06.2X7** Diffuse traumatic brain injury with loss of consciousness of any duration with death due to brain injury prior to regaining consciousness

⑦**S06.2X8** Diffuse traumatic brain injury with loss of consciousness of any duration with death due to other cause prior to regaining consciousness

⑦**S06.2X9** Diffuse traumatic brain injury with loss of consciousness of unspecified duration

Diffuse traumatic brain injury NOS

S06.3 **Focal traumatic brain injury**

Excludes1: any condition classifiable to S06.4-S06.6

focal cerebral edema (S06.1)

S06.30   Unspecified focal traumatic brain injury

⑦ S06.300   Unspecified focal traumatic brain injury without loss of consciousness

⑦ S06.301   Unspecified focal traumatic brain injury with loss of consciousness of 30 minutes or less

⑦ S06.302   Unspecified focal traumatic brain injury with loss of consciousness of 31 minutes to 59 minutes

⑦ S06.303   Unspecified focal traumatic brain injury with loss of consciousness of 1 hour to 5 hours 59 minutes

⑦ S06.304   Unspecified focal traumatic brain injury with loss of consciousness of 6 hours to 24 hours

⑦ S06.305   Unspecified focal traumatic brain injury with loss of consciousness greater than 24 hours with return to pre-existing conscious level

⑦ S06.306   Unspecified focal traumatic brain injury with loss of consciousness greater than 24 hours without return to pre-existing conscious level with patient surviving

⑦ S06.307   Unspecified focal traumatic brain injury with loss of consciousness of any duration with death due to brain injury prior to regaining consciousness

⑦ S06.308   Unspecified focal traumatic brain injury with loss of consciousness of any duration with death due to other cause prior to regaining consciousness

⑦ S06.309   Unspecified focal traumatic brain injury with loss of consciousness of unspecified duration

Unspecified focal traumatic brain injury NOS

S06.31   Contusion and laceration of right cerebrum

⑦ S06.310   Contusion and laceration of right cerebrum without loss of consciousness

⑦ S06.311   Contusion and laceration of right cerebrum with loss of consciousness of 30 minutes or less

⑦ S06.312   Contusion and laceration of right cerebrum with loss of consciousness of 31 minutes to 59 minutes

⑦ S06.313   Contusion and laceration of right cerebrum with loss of consciousness of 1 hour to 5 hours 59 minutes

⑦ S06.314   Contusion and laceration of right cerebrum with loss of consciousness of 6 hours to 24 hours

⑦ S06.315   Contusion and laceration of right cerebrum with loss of consciousness greater than 24 hours with return to pre-existing conscious level

⑦ S06.316   Contusion and laceration of right cerebrum with loss of consciousness greater than 24 hours without return to pre-existing conscious level with patient surviving

⑦ S06.317   Contusion and laceration of right cerebrum with loss of consciousness of any duration with death due to brain injury prior to regaining consciousness

⑦ S06.318   Contusion and laceration of right cerebrum with loss of consciousness of any duration with death due to other cause prior to regaining consciousness

⑦ S06.319   Contusion and laceration of right cerebrum with loss of consciousness of unspecified duration

Contusion and laceration of right cerebrum NOS

S06.32   Contusion and laceration of left cerebrum

⑦ S06.320   Contusion and laceration of left cerebrum without loss of consciousness

⑦ S06.321   Contusion and laceration of left cerebrum with loss of consciousness of 30 minutes or less

⑦ S06.322   Contusion and laceration of left cerebrum with loss of consciousness of 31 minutes to 59 minutes

⑦ S06.323   Contusion and laceration of left cerebrum with loss of consciousness of 1 hour to 5 hours 59 minutes

⑦ S06.324   Contusion and laceration of left cerebrum with loss of consciousness of 6 hours to 24 hours

⑦ S06.325   Contusion and laceration of left cerebrum with loss of consciousness greater than 24 hours with return to pre-existing conscious level

⑦ S06.326   Contusion and laceration of left cerebrum with loss of consciousness greater than 24 hours without return to pre-existing conscious level with patient surviving

⑦ S06.327   Contusion and laceration of left cerebrum with loss of consciousness of any duration with death due to brain injury prior to regaining consciousness

⑦ S06.328   Contusion and laceration of left cerebrum with loss of consciousness of any duration with death due to other cause prior to regaining consciousness

⑦ S06.329   Contusion and laceration of left cerebrum with loss of consciousness of unspecified duration

Contusion and laceration of left cerebrum NOS

S06.33   Contusion and laceration of cerebrum, unspecified

⑦ S06.330   Contusion and laceration of cerebrum, unspecified, without loss of consciousness

⑦ S06.331   Contusion and laceration of cerebrum, unspecified, with loss of consciousness of 30 minutes or less

⑦ S06.332   Contusion and laceration of cerebrum, unspecified, with loss of

consciousness of 31 minutes to 59 minutes

⑦S06.333 **Contusion and laceration of cerebrum, unspecified, with loss of consciousness of 1 hour to 5 hours 59 minutes**

⑦S06.334 **Contusion and laceration of cerebrum, unspecified, with loss of consciousness of 6 hours to 24 hours**

⑦S06.335 **Contusion and laceration of cerebrum, unspecified, with loss of consciousness greater than 24 hours with return to pre-existing conscious level**

⑦S06.336 **Contusion and laceration of cerebrum, unspecified, with loss of consciousness greater than 24 hours without return to pre-existing conscious level with patient surviving**

⑦S06.337 **Contusion and laceration of cerebrum, unspecified, with loss of consciousness of any duration with death due to brain injury prior to regaining consciousness**

⑦S06.338 **Contusion and laceration of cerebrum, unspecified, with loss of consciousness of any duration with death due to other cause prior to regaining consciousness**

⑦S06.339 **Contusion and laceration of cerebrum, unspecified, with loss of consciousness of unspecified duration**

Contusion and laceration of cerebrum NOS

S06.34 **Traumatic hemorrhage of right cerebrum**

Traumatic intracerebral hemorrhage and hematoma of right cerebrum

⑦S06.340 **Traumatic hemorrhage of right cerebrum without loss of consciousness**

⑦S06.341 **Traumatic hemorrhage of right cerebrum with loss of consciousness of 30 minutes or less**

⑦S06.342 **Traumatic hemorrhage of right cerebrum with loss of consciousness of 31 minutes to 59 minutes**

⑦S06.343 **Traumatic hemorrhage of right cerebrum with loss of consciousness of 1 hours to 5 hours 59 minutes**

⑦S06.344 **Traumatic hemorrhage of right cerebrum with loss of consciousness of 6 hours to 24 hours**

⑦S06.345 **Traumatic hemorrhage of right cerebrum with loss of consciousness greater than 24 hours with return to pre-existing conscious level**

⑦S06.346 **Traumatic hemorrhage of right cerebrum with loss of consciousness greater than 24 hours without return to pre-existing conscious level with patient surviving**

⑦S06.347 **Traumatic hemorrhage of right cerebrum with loss of consciousness**

of any duration with death due to brain injury prior to regaining consciousness

⑦S06.348 **Traumatic hemorrhage of right cerebrum with loss of consciousness of any duration with death due to other cause prior to regaining consciousness**

⑦S06.349 **Traumatic hemorrhage of right cerebrum with loss of consciousness of unspecified duration**

Traumatic hemorrhage of right cerebrum NOS

S06.35 **Traumatic hemorrhage of left cerebrum**

Traumatic intracerebral hemorrhage and hematoma of left cerebrum

⑦S06.350 **Traumatic hemorrhage of left cerebrum without loss of consciousness**

⑦S06.351 **Traumatic hemorrhage of left cerebrum with loss of consciousness of 30 minutes or less**

⑦S06.352 **Traumatic hemorrhage of left cerebrum with loss of consciousness of 31 minutes to 59 minutes**

⑦S06.353 **Traumatic hemorrhage of left cerebrum with loss of consciousness of 1 hours to 5 hours 59 minutes**

⑦S06.354 **Traumatic hemorrhage of left cerebrum with loss of consciousness of 6 hours to 24 hours**

⑦S06.355 **Traumatic hemorrhage of left cerebrum with loss of consciousness greater than 24 hours with return to pre-existing conscious level**

⑦S06.356 **Traumatic hemorrhage of left cerebrum with loss of consciousness greater than 24 hours without return to pre-existing conscious level with patient surviving**

⑦S06.357 **Traumatic hemorrhage of left cerebrum with loss of consciousness of any duration with death due to brain injury prior to regaining consciousness**

⑦S06.358 **Traumatic hemorrhage of left cerebrum with loss of consciousness of any duration with death due to other cause prior to regaining consciousness**

⑦S06.359 **Traumatic hemorrhage of left cerebrum with loss of consciousness of unspecified duration**

Traumatic hemorrhage of left cerebrum NOS

S06.36 **Traumatic hemorrhage of cerebrum, unspecified**

Traumatic intracerebral hemorrhage and hematoma, unspecified

⑦S06.360 **Traumatic hemorrhage of cerebrum, unspecified, without loss of consciousness**

⑦S06.361 **Traumatic hemorrhage of cerebrum, unspecified, with loss of consciousness of 30 minutes or less**

⑦ **S06.362** **Traumatic hemorrhage of cerebrum, unspecified, with loss of consciousness of 31 minutes to 59 minutes**

⑦ **S06.363** **Traumatic hemorrhage of cerebrum, unspecified, with loss of consciousness of 1 hours to 5 hours 59 minutes**

⑦ **S06.364** **Traumatic hemorrhage of cerebrum, unspecified, with loss of consciousness of 6 hours to 24 hours**

⑦ **S06.365** **Traumatic hemorrhage of cerebrum, unspecified, with loss of consciousness greater than 24 hours with return to pre-existing conscious level**

⑦ **S06.366** **Traumatic hemorrhage of cerebrum, unspecified, with loss of consciousness greater than 24 hours without return to pre-existing conscious level with patient surviving**

⑦ **S06.367** **Traumatic hemorrhage of cerebrum, unspecified, with loss of consciousness of any duration with death due to brain injury prior to regaining consciousness**

⑦ **S06.368** **Traumatic hemorrhage of cerebrum, unspecified, with loss of consciousness of any duration with death due to other cause prior to regaining consciousness**

⑦ **S06.369** **Traumatic hemorrhage of cerebrum, unspecified, with loss of consciousness of unspecified duration**

Traumatic hemorrhage of cerebrum NOS

S06.37 **Contusion, laceration, and hemorrhage of cerebellum**

⑦ **S06.370** **Contusion, laceration, and hemorrhage of cerebellum without loss of consciousness**

⑦ **S06.371** **Contusion, laceration, and hemorrhage of cerebellum with loss of consciousness of 30 minutes or less**

⑦ **S06.372** **Contusion, laceration, and hemorrhage of cerebellum with loss of consciousness of 31 minutes to 59 minutes**

⑦ **S06.373** **Contusion, laceration, and hemorrhage of cerebellum with loss of consciousness of 1 hour to 5 hours 59 minutes**

⑦ **S06.374** **Contusion, laceration, and hemorrhage of cerebellum with loss of consciousness of 6 hours to 24 hours**

⑦ **S06.375** **Contusion, laceration, and hemorrhage of cerebellum with loss of consciousness greater than 24 hours with return to pre-existing conscious level**

⑦ **S06.376** **Contusion, laceration, and hemorrhage of cerebellum with loss of consciousness greater than 24 hours without return to pre-existing conscious level with patient surviving**

⑦ **S06.377** **Contusion, laceration, and hemorrhage of cerebellum with loss of consciousness of any duration with death due to brain injury prior to regaining consciousness**

⑦ **S06.378** **Contusion, laceration, and hemorrhage of cerebellum with loss of consciousness of any duration with death due to other cause prior to regaining consciousness**

⑦ **S06.379** **Contusion, laceration, and hemorrhage of cerebellum with loss of consciousness of unspecified duration**

Contusion, laceration, and hemorrhage of cerebellum NOS

S06.38 **Contusion, laceration, and hemorrhage of brainstem**

⑦ **S06.380** **Contusion, laceration, and hemorrhage of brainstem without loss of consciousness**

⑦ **S06.381** **Contusion, laceration, and hemorrhage of brainstem with loss of consciousness of 30 minutes or less**

⑦ **S06.382** **Contusion, laceration, and hemorrhage of brainstem with loss of consciousness of 31 minutes to 59 minutes**

⑦ **S06.383** **Contusion, laceration, and hemorrhage of brainstem with loss of consciousness of 1 hour to 5 hours 59 minutes**

⑦ **S06.384** **Contusion, laceration, and hemorrhage of brainstem with loss of consciousness of 6 hours to 24 hours**

⑦ **S06.385** **Contusion, laceration, and hemorrhage of brainstem with loss of consciousness greater than 24 hours with return to pre-existing conscious level**

⑦ **S06.386** **Contusion, laceration, and hemorrhage of brainstem with loss of consciousness greater than 24 hours without return to pre-existing conscious level with patient surviving**

⑦ **S06.387** **Contusion, laceration, and hemorrhage of brainstem with loss of consciousness of any duration with death due to brain injury prior to regaining consciousness**

⑦ **S06.388** **Contusion, laceration, and hemorrhage of brainstem with loss of consciousness of any duration with death due to other cause prior to regaining consciousness**

⑦ **S06.389** **Contusion, laceration, and hemorrhage of brainstem with loss of consciousness of unspecified duration**

● New code ▲ Revised code **Excludes1:** Not coded here **Excludes2:** Not included here ⊗ Placeholder required ⑦ 7th digit required

upper ventrical cavities — thoracic cavity - chest cavity. midportion is mediastinum.
↳ lateral subdivisions of thoracic cavity are R/L pleural cavities

lower vent. cavities — - include abdominal & pelvic cavities.

abdominopelvic (no physical partition)

- diaphragm separates thoracic from abdominopelvic

- upper abdominopelvic regions- right hypochondriac region, left hr, & epigastric lie across abdomen at level of 9th rib cages

RUQ	LUQ superior
RLQ	LLQ inferior

R. Hypochondriac	epigastric	L Hypochondriac
R Lumbar	Umbilical	L Lumbar (Flank)
R. iliac (inguinal)	Hypogastric (pubic)	L. iliac (inguinal)

Contusion, laceration, and hemorrhage of brainstem NOS

S06.4   Epidural hemorrhage

Extradural hemorrhage NOS

Extradural hemorrhage (traumatic)

S06.4X   Epidural hemorrhage

⑦**S06.4X0**   Epidural hemorrhage without loss of consciousness

⑦**S06.4X1**   Epidural hemorrhage with loss of consciousness of 30 minutes or less

⑦**S06.4X2**   Epidural hemorrhage with loss of consciousness of 31 minutes to 59 minutes

⑦**S06.4X3**   Epidural hemorrhage with loss of consciousness of 1 hour to 5 hours 59 minutes

⑦**S06.4X4**   Epidural hemorrhage with loss of consciousness of 6 hours to 24 hours

⑦**S06.4X5**   Epidural hemorrhage with loss of consciousness greater than 24 hours with return to pre-existing conscious level

⑦**S06.4X6**   Epidural hemorrhage with loss of consciousness greater than 24 hours without return to pre-existing conscious level with patient surviving

⑦**S06.4X7**   Epidural hemorrhage with loss of consciousness of any duration with death due to brain injury prior to regaining consciousness

⑦**S06.4X8**   Epidural hemorrhage with loss of consciousness of any duration with death due to other causes prior to regaining consciousness

⑦**S06.4X9**   Epidural hemorrhage with loss of consciousness of unspecified duration

Epidural hemorrhage NOS

S06.5   Traumatic subdural hemorrhage

S06.5X   Traumatic subdural hemorrhage

⑦**S06.5X0**   Traumatic subdural hemorrhage without loss of consciousness

⑦**S06.5X1**   Traumatic subdural hemorrhage with loss of consciousness of 30 minutes or less

⑦**S06.5X2**   Traumatic subdural hemorrhage with loss of consciousness of 31 minutes to 59 minutes

⑦**S06.5X3**   Traumatic subdural hemorrhage with loss of consciousness of 1 hour to 5 hours 59 minutes

⑦**S06.5X4**   Traumatic subdural hemorrhage with loss of consciousness of 6 hours to 24 hours

⑦**S06.5X5**   Traumatic subdural hemorrhage with loss of consciousness greater than 24 hours with return to pre-existing conscious level

⑦**S06.5X6**   Traumatic subdural hemorrhage with loss of consciousness greater than 24 hours without return to

pre-existing conscious level with patient surviving

⑦**S06.5X7**   Traumatic subdural hemorrhage with loss of consciousness of any duration with death due to brain injury before regaining consciousness

⑦**S06.5X8**   Traumatic subdural hemorrhage with loss of consciousness of any duration with death due to other cause before regaining consciousness

⑦**S06.5X9**   Traumatic subdural hemorrhage with loss of consciousness of unspecified duration

Traumatic subdural hemorrhage NOS

S06.6   Traumatic subarachnoid hemorrhage

S06.6X   Traumatic subarachnoid hemorrhage

⑦**S06.6X0**   Traumatic subarachnoid hemorrhage without loss of consciousness

⑦**S06.6X1**   Traumatic subarachnoid hemorrhage with loss of consciousness of 30 minutes or less

⑦**S06.6X2**   Traumatic subarachnoid hemorrhage with loss of consciousness of 31 minutes to 59 minutes

⑦**S06.6X3**   Traumatic subarachnoid hemorrhage with loss of consciousness of 1 hour to 5 hours 59 minutes

⑦**S06.6X4**   Traumatic subarachnoid hemorrhage with loss of consciousness of 6 hours to 24 hours

⑦**S06.6X5**   Traumatic subarachnoid hemorrhage with loss of consciousness greater than 24 hours with return to pre-existing conscious level

⑦**S06.6X6**   Traumatic subarachnoid hemorrhage with loss of consciousness greater than 24 hours without return to pre-existing conscious level with patient

⑦**S06.6X7**   Traumatic subarachnoid hemorrhage with loss of consciousness of any duration with death due to brain injury prior to regaining consciousness

⑦**S06.6X8**   Traumatic subarachnoid hemorrhage with loss of consciousness of any duration with death due to other cause prior to regaining consciousness

⑦**S06.6X9**   Traumatic subarachnoid hemorrhage with loss of consciousness of unspecified duration

Traumatic subarachnoid hemorrhage NOS

S06.8   Other specified intracranial injuries

S06.81   Injury of right internal carotid artery, intracranial portion, not elsewhere classified

⑦ S06.810 **Injury of right internal carotid artery, intracranial portion, not elsewhere classified without loss of consciousness**

⑦ S06.811 **Injury of right internal carotid artery, intracranial portion, not elsewhere classified with loss of consciousness of 30 minutes or less**

⑦ S06.812 **Injury of right internal carotid artery, intracranial portion, not elsewhere classified with loss of consciousness of 31 minutes to 59 minutes**

⑦ S06.813 **Injury of right internal carotid artery, intracranial portion, not elsewhere classified with loss of consciousness of 1 hour to 5 hours 59 minutes**

⑦ S06.814 **Injury of right internal carotid artery, intracranial portion, not elsewhere classified with loss of consciousness of 6 hours to 24 hours**

⑦ S06.815 **Injury of right internal carotid artery, intracranial portion, not elsewhere classified with loss of consciousness greater than 24 hours with return to pre-existing conscious level**

⑦ S06.816 **Injury of right internal carotid artery, intracranial portion, not elsewhere classified with loss of consciousness greater than 24 hours without return to pre-existing conscious level with patient surviving**

⑦ S06.817 **Injury of right internal carotid artery, intracranial portion, not elsewhere classified with loss of consciousness of any duration with death due to brain injury prior to regaining consciousness**

⑦ S06.818 **Injury of right internal carotid artery, intracranial portion, not elsewhere classified with loss of consciousness of any duration with death due to other cause prior to regaining consciousness**

⑦ S06.819 **Injury of right internal carotid artery, intracranial portion, not elsewhere classified with loss of consciousness of unspecified duration**

Injury of right internal carotid artery, intracranial portion, not elsewhere classified NOS

S06.82 **Injury of left internal carotid artery, intracranial portion, not elsewhere classified**

⑦ S06.820 **Injury of left internal carotid artery, intracranial portion, not elsewhere classified without loss of consciousness**

⑦ S06.821 **Injury of left internal carotid artery, intracranial portion, not elsewhere classified with loss of consciousness of 30 minutes or less**

⑦ S06.822 **Injury of left internal carotid artery, intracranial portion, not elsewhere classified with loss of consciousness of 31 minutes to 59 minutes**

⑦ S06.823 **Injury of left internal carotid artery, intracranial portion, not elsewhere classified with loss of consciousness of 1 hour to 5 hours 59 minutes**

⑦ S06.824 **Injury of left internal carotid artery, intracranial portion, not elsewhere classified with loss of consciousness of 6 hours to 24 hours**

⑦ S06.825 **Injury of left internal carotid artery, intracranial portion, not elsewhere classified with loss of consciousness greater than 24 hours with return to pre-existing conscious level**

⑦ S06.826 **Injury of left internal carotid artery, intracranial portion, not elsewhere classified with loss of consciousness greater than 24 hours without return to pre-existing conscious level with patient surviving**

⑦ S06.827 **Injury of left internal carotid artery, intracranial portion, not elsewhere classified with loss of consciousness of any duration with death due to brain injury prior to regaining consciousness**

⑦ S06.828 **Injury of left internal carotid artery, intracranial portion, not elsewhere classified with loss of consciousness of any duration with death due to other cause prior to regaining consciousness**

⑦ S06.829 **Injury of left internal carotid artery, intracranial portion, not elsewhere classified with loss of consciousness of unspecified duration**

Injury of left internal carotid artery, intracranial portion, not elsewhere classified NOS

S06.89 **Other specified intracranial injury**

Excludes1: concussion (S06.0X-)

⑦ S06.890 **Other specified intracranial injury without loss of consciousness**

⑦ S06.891 **Other specified intracranial injury with loss of consciousness of 30 minutes or less**

⑦ S06.892 **Other specified intracranial injury with loss of consciousness of 31 minutes to 59 minutes**

⑦ S06.893 **Other specified intracranial injury with loss of consciousness of 1 hour to 5 hours 59 minutes**

⑦ S06.894 **Other specified intracranial injury with loss of consciousness of 6 hours to 24 hours**

⑦ S06.895 **Other specified intracranial injury with loss of consciousness greater than 24 hours with return to pre-existing conscious level**

⑦**S06.896**   **Other specified intracranial injury with loss of consciousness greater than 24 hours without return to pre-existing conscious level with patient surviving**

⑦**S06.897**   **Other specified intracranial injury with loss of consciousness of any duration with death due to brain injury prior to regaining consciousness**

⑦**S06.898**   **Other specified intracranial injury with loss of consciousness of any duration with death due to other cause prior to regaining consciousness**

⑦**S06.899**   **Other specified intracranial injury with loss of consciousness of unspecified duration**

S06.9   **Unspecified intracranial injury**

Brain injury NOS

Head injury NOS with loss of consciousness

Traumatic brain injury NOS

Excludes1: conditions classifiable to S06.0- to S06.8-code to specified intracranial injury

head injury NOS (S09.90)

S06.9X   **Unspecified intracranial injury**

⑦**S06.9X0**   **Unspecified intracranial injury without loss of consciousness**

⑦**S06.9X1**   **Unspecified intracranial injury with loss of consciousness of 30 minutes or less**

⑦**S06.9X2**   **Unspecified intracranial injury with loss of consciousness of 31 minutes to 59 minutes**

⑦**S06.9X3**   **Unspecified intracranial injury with loss of consciousness of 1 hour to 5 hours 59 minutes**

⑦**S06.9X4**   **Unspecified intracranial injury with loss of consciousness of 6 hours to 24 hours**

⑦**S06.9X5**   **Unspecified intracranial injury with loss of consciousness greater than 24 hours with return to pre-existing conscious level**

⑦**S06.9X6**   **Unspecified intracranial injury with loss of consciousness greater than 24 hours without return to pre-existing conscious level with patient surviving**

⑦**S06.9X7**   **Unspecified intracranial injury with loss of consciousness of any duration with death due to brain injury prior to regaining consciousness**

⑦**S06.9X8**   **Unspecified intracranial injury with loss of consciousness of any duration with death due to other cause prior to regaining consciousness**

⑦**S06.9X9**   **Unspecified intracranial injury with loss of consciousness of unspecified duration**

S07   **Crushing injury of head**

Use additional code for all associated injuries, such as:

intracranial injuries (S06.-)

skull fractures (S02.-)

The appropriate 7th character is to be added to each code from category S07

A - initial encounter

D - subsequent encounter

S - sequela

⊗⑦**S07.0**   **Crushing injury of face**

⊗⑦**S07.1**   **Crushing injury of skull**

⊗⑦**S07.8**   **Crushing injury of other parts of head**

⊗⑦**S07.9**   **Crushing injury of head, part unspecified**

S08   **Avulsion and traumatic amputation of part of head**

An amputation not identified as partial or complete should be coded to complete

The appropriate 7th character is to be added to each code from category S08

A - initial encounter

D - subsequent encounter

S - sequela

⊗⑦**S08.0**   **Avulsion of scalp**

S08.1   **Traumatic amputation of ear**

S08.11   **Complete traumatic amputation of ear**

⑦**S08.111**   **Complete traumatic amputation of right ear**

⑦**S08.112**   **Complete traumatic amputation of left ear**

⑦**S08.119**   **Complete traumatic amputation of unspecified ear**

S08.12   **Partial traumatic amputation of ear**

⑦**S08.121**   **Partial traumatic amputation of right ear**

⑦**S08.122**   **Partial traumatic amputation of left ear**

⑦**S08.129**   **Partial traumatic amputation of unspecified ear**

S08.8   **Traumatic amputation of other parts of head**

S08.81   **Traumatic amputation of nose**

⑦**S08.811**   **Complete traumatic amputation of nose**

⑦**S08.812**   **Partial traumatic amputation of nose**

⊗⑦**S08.89**   **Traumatic amputation of other parts of head**

S09   **Other and unspecified injuries of head**

The appropriate 7th character is to be added to each code from category S09

A - initial encounter

D - subsequent encounter

S - sequela

⊗⑦**S09.0**   **Injury of blood vessels of head, not elsewhere classified**

Excludes1: injury of cerebral blood vessels (S06.-)

injury of precerebral blood vessels (S15.-)

S09.1   **Injury of muscle and tendon of head**

Code also any associated open wound (S01.-)

Excludes2: sprain to joints and ligament of head (S03.9)

⊗⑦**S09.10**   **Unspecified injury of muscle and tendon of head**

Injury of muscle and tendon of head NOS

⊗⑦S09.11   **Strain of muscle and tendon of head**

⊗⑦S09.12   **Laceration of muscle and tendon of head**

⊗⑦S09.19   **Other specified injury of muscle and tendon of head**

S09.2   **Traumatic rupture of ear drum**

Excludes1: traumatic rupture of ear drum due to blast injury (S09.31-)

⊗⑦S09.20   **Traumatic rupture of unspecified ear drum**

⊗⑦S09.21   **Traumatic rupture of right ear drum**

⊗⑦S09.22   **Traumatic rupture of left ear drum**

S09.3   **Other specified and unspecified injury of middle and inner ear**

Excludes1: injury to ear NOS (S09.91-)

Excludes2: injury to external ear (S00.4-, S01.3-, S08.1-)

S09.30   **Unspecified injury of middle and inner ear**

⑦ S09.301   **Unspecified injury of right middle and inner ear**

⑦ S09.302   **Unspecified injury of left middle and inner ear**

⑦ S09.309   **Unspecified injury of unspecified middle and inner ear**

S09.31   **Primary blast injury of ear**

Blast injury of ear NOS

⑦ S09.311   **Primary blast injury of right ear**

⑦ S09.312   **Primary blast injury of left ear**

⑦ S09.313   **Primary blast injury of ear, bilateral**

⑦ S09.319   **Primary blast injury of unspecified ear**

S09.39   **Other specified injury of middle and inner ear**

Secondary blast injury to ear

⑦ S09.391   **Other specified injury of right middle and inner ear**

⑦ S09.392   **Other specified injury of left middle and inner ear**

⑦ S09.399   **Other specified injury of unspecified middle and inner ear**

⊗⑦S09.8   **Other specified injuries of head**

S09.9   **Unspecified injury of face and head**

⊗⑦S09.90   **Unspecified injury of head**

Head injury NOS

Excludes1: brain injury NOS (S06.9-)

head injury NOS with loss of consciousness (S06.9-)

intracranial injury NOS (S06.9-)

⊗⑦S09.91   **Unspecified injury of ear**

Injury of ear NOS

⊗⑦S09.92   **Unspecified injury of nose**

Injury of nose NOS

⊗⑦S09.93   **Unspecified injury of face**

Injury of face NOS

INJURIES TO THE NECK (S10-S19)

Includes: injuries of nape

injuries of supraclavicular region injuries of throat

Excludes2: burns and corrosions (T20-T32)

effects of foreign body in esophagus (T18.1)

effects of foreign body in larynx (T17.3)

effects of foreign body in pharynx (T17.2)

effects of foreign body in trachea (T17.4)

frostbite (T33-T34)

insect bite or sting, venomous (T63.4)

S10   **Superficial injury of neck**

The appropriate 7th character is to be added to each code from category S10

A - initial encounter

D - subsequent encounter

S - sequela

⊗⑦S10.0   **Contusion of throat**

Contusion of cervical esophagus

Contusion of larynx

Contusion of pharynx

Contusion of trachea

S10.1   **Other and unspecified superficial injuries of throat**

⊗⑦S10.10   **Unspecified superficial injuries of throat**

⊗⑦S10.11   **Abrasion of throat**

⊗⑦S10.12   **Blister (nonthermal) of throat**

⊗⑦S10.14   **External constriction of part of throat**

⊗⑦S10.15   **Superficial foreign body of throat**

Splinter in the throat

⊗⑦S10.16   **Insect bite (nonvenomous) of throat**

⊗⑦S10.17   **Other superficial bite of throat**

Excludes1: open bite of throat (S11.85)

S10.8   **Superficial injury of other specified parts of neck**

⊗⑦S10.80   **Unspecified superficial injury of other specified part of neck**

⊗⑦S10.81   **Abrasion of other specified part of neck**

⊗⑦S10.82   **Blister (nonthermal) of other specified part of neck**

⊗⑦S10.83   **Contusion of other specified part of neck**

⊗⑦S10.84   **External constriction of other specified part of neck**

⊗⑦S10.85   **Superficial foreign body of other specified part of neck**

Splinter in other specified part of neck

⊗⑦S10.86   **Insect bite of other specified part of neck**

⊗⑦S10.87   **Other superficial bite of other specified part of neck**

Excludes1: open bite of other specified parts of neck (S11.85)

S10.9   **Superficial injury of unspecified part of neck**

⊗⑦S10.90   **Unspecified superficial injury of unspecified part of neck**

⊗⑦S10.91   **Abrasion of unspecified part of neck**

⊗⑦S10.92   **Blister (nonthermal) of unspecified part of neck**

⊗⑦S10.93   **Contusion of unspecified part of neck**

⊗⑦S10.94   **External constriction of unspecified part of neck**

⊗⑦S10.95   **Superficial foreign body of unspecified part of neck**

⊗⑦S10.96   **Insect bite of unspecified part of neck**

⊗⑦S10.97   **Other superficial bite of unspecified part of neck**

● New code   ▲ Revised code   **Excludes1:** Not coded here   **Excludes2:** Not included here   ⊗ Placeholder required   ⑦ 7th digit required

S11   **Open wound of neck**

Code also any associated:

spinal cord injury (S14.0, S14.1-)

wound infection

Excludes2: open fracture of vertebra (S12.- with 7th character B)

The appropriate 7th character is to be added to each code from category S11

A - initial encounter

D - subsequent encounter

S - sequela

S11.0   **Open wound of larynx and trachea**

    S11.01   **Open wound of larynx**

      Excludes2: open wound of vocal cord (S11.03)

      ⑦S11.011   Laceration without foreign body of larynx

      ⑦S11.012   Laceration with foreign body of larynx

      ⑦S11.013   Puncture wound without foreign body of larynx

      ⑦S11.014   Puncture wound with foreign body of larynx

      ⑦S11.015   Open bite of larynx

        Bite of larynx NOS

      ⑦S11.019   Unspecified open wound of larynx

    S11.02   **Open wound of trachea**

      Open wound of cervical trachea

      Open wound of trachea NOS

      Excludes2: open wound of thoracic trachea (S27.5-)

      ⑦S11.021   Laceration without foreign body of trachea

      ⑦S11.022   Laceration with foreign body of trachea

      ⑦S11.023   Puncture wound without foreign body of trachea

      ⑦S11.024   Puncture wound with foreign body of trachea

      ⑦S11.025   Open bite of trachea

        Bite of trachea NOS

      ⑦S11.029   Unspecified open wound of trachea

    S11.03   **Open wound of vocal cord**

      ⑦S11.031   Laceration without foreign body of vocal cord

      ⑦S11.032   Laceration with foreign body of vocal cord

      ⑦S11.033   Puncture wound without foreign body of vocal cord

      ⑦S11.034   Puncture wound with foreign body of vocal cord

      ⑦S11.035   Open bite of vocal cord

        Bite of vocal cord NOS

      ⑦S11.039   Unspecified open wound of vocal cord

    S11.1   **Open wound of thyroid gland**

      ⊗⑦S11.10   Unspecified open wound of thyroid gland

      ⊗⑦S11.11   Laceration without foreign body of thyroid gland

      ⊗⑦S11.12   Laceration with foreign body of thyroid gland

      ⊗⑦S11.13   Puncture wound without foreign body of thyroid gland

      ⊗⑦S11.14   Puncture wound with foreign body of thyroid gland

      ⊗⑦S11.15   Open bite of thyroid gland

        Bite of thyroid gland NOS

    S11.2   **Open wound of pharynx and cervical esophagus**

      Excludes1: open wound of esophagus NOS (S27.8-)

      ⊗⑦S11.20   Unspecified open wound of pharynx and cervical esophagus

      ⊗⑦S11.21   Laceration without foreign body of pharynx and cervical esophagus

      ⊗⑦S11.22   Laceration with foreign body of pharynx and cervical esophagus

      ⊗⑦S11.23   Puncture wound without foreign body of pharynx and cervical esophagus

      ⊗⑦S11.24   Puncture wound with foreign body of pharynx and cervical esophagus

      ⊗⑦S11.25   Open bite of pharynx and cervical esophagus

        Bite of pharynx and cervical esophagus NOS

    S11.8   **Open wound of other specified parts of neck**

      ⊗⑦S11.80   Unspecified open wound of other specified part of neck

      ⊗⑦S11.81   Laceration without foreign body of other specified part of neck

      ⊗⑦S11.82   Laceration with foreign body of other specified part of neck

      ⊗⑦S11.83   Puncture wound without foreign body of other specified part of neck

      ⊗⑦S11.84   Puncture wound with foreign body of other specified part of neck

      ⊗⑦S11.85   Open bite of other specified part of neck

        Bite of other specified part of neck NOS

      Excludes1: superficial bite of other specified part of neck (S10.87)

      ⊗⑦S11.89   Other open wound of other specified part of neck

    S11.9   **Open wound of unspecified part of neck**

      ⊗⑦S11.90   Unspecified open wound of unspecified part of neck

      ⊗⑦S11.91   Laceration without foreign body of unspecified part of neck

      ⊗⑦S11.92   Laceration with foreign body of unspecified part of neck

      ⊗⑦S11.93   Puncture wound without foreign body of unspecified part of neck

      ⊗⑦S11.94   Puncture wound with foreign body of unspecified part of neck

      ⊗⑦S11.95   Open bite of unspecified part of neck

        Bite of neck NOS

      Excludes1: superficial bite of neck (S10.97)

S12   **Fracture of cervical vertebra and other parts of neck**

Note: A fracture not indicated as displaced or nondisplaced should be coded to displaced

A fracture not indicated as open or closed should be coded to closed

Includes: fracture of cervical neural arch

    fracture of cervical spine

    fracture of cervical spinous process

    fracture of cervical transverse process

fracture of cervical vertebral arch fracture of neck

Code first any associated cervical spinal cord injury (S14.0, S14.1-)

The appropriate 7th character is to be added to all codes from subcategories S12.0-S12.6

A - initial encounter for closed fracture

B - initial encounter for open fracture

D - subsequent encounter for fracture with routine healing

G - subsequent encounter for fracture with delayed healing

K - subsequent encounter for fracture with nonunion

S - sequela

S12.0   Fracture of first cervical vertebra
   Atlas

  S12.00 Unspecified fracture of first cervical vertebra

    ⑦ **S12.000 Unspecified displaced fracture of first cervical vertebra**

    ⑦ **S12.001 Unspecified nondisplaced fracture of first cervical vertebra**

  ⊗⑦ **S12.01 Stable burst fracture of first cervical vertebra**

  ⊗⑦ **S12.02 Unstable burst fracture of first cervical vertebra**

  S12.03 Posterior arch fracture of first cervical vertebra

    ⑦ **S12.030 Displaced posterior arch fracture of first cervical vertebra**

    ⑦ **S12.031 Nondisplaced posterior arch fracture of first cervical vertebra**

  S12.04 Lateral mass fracture of first cervical vertebra

    ⑦ **S12.040 Displaced lateral mass fracture of first cervical vertebra**

    ⑦ **S12.041 Nondisplaced lateral mass fracture of first cervical vertebra**

  S12.09 Other fracture of first cervical vertebra

    ⑦ **S12.090 Other displaced fracture of first cervical vertebra**

    ⑦ **S12.091 Other nondisplaced fracture of first cervical vertebra**

S12.1   Fracture of second cervical vertebra
   Axis

  S12.10 Unspecified fracture of second cervical vertebra

    ⑦ **S12.100 Unspecified displaced fracture of second cervical vertebra**

    ⑦ **S12.101 Unspecified nondisplaced fracture of second cervical vertebra**

  S12.11 Type II dens fracture

    ⑦ **S12.110 Anterior displaced Type II dens fracture**

    ⑦ **S12.111 Posterior displaced Type II dens fracture**

    ⑦ **S12.112 Nondisplaced Type II dens fracture**

  S12.12 Other dens fracture

    ⑦ **S12.120 Other displaced dens fracture**

    ⑦ **S12.121 Other nondisplaced dens fracture**

  S12.13 Unspecified traumatic spondylolisthesis of second cervical vertebra

    ⑦ **S12.130 Unspecified traumatic displaced spondylolisthesis of second cervical vertebra**

    ⑦ **S12.131 Unspecified traumatic nondisplaced spondylolisthesis of second cervical vertebra**

  ⊗⑦ **S12.14 Type III traumatic spondylolisthesis of second cervical vertebra**

  S12.15 Other traumatic spondylolisthesis of second cervical vertebra

    ⑦ **S12.150 Other traumatic displaced spondylolisthesis of second cervical vertebra**

    ⑦ **S12.151 Other traumatic nondisplaced spondylolisthesis of second cervical vertebra**

  S12.19 Other fracture of second cervical vertebra

    ⑦ **S12.190 Other displaced fracture of second cervical vertebra**

    ⑦ **S12.191 Other nondisplaced fracture of second cervical vertebra**

S12.2   Fracture of third cervical vertebra

  S12.20 Unspecified fracture of third cervical vertebra

    ⑦ **S12.200 Unspecified displaced fracture of third cervical vertebra**

    ⑦ **S12.201 Unspecified nondisplaced fracture of third cervical vertebra**

  S12.23 Unspecified traumatic spondylolisthesis of third cervical vertebra

    ⑦ **S12.230 Unspecified traumatic displaced spondylolisthesis of third cervical vertebra**

    ⑦ **S12.231 Unspecified traumatic nondisplaced spondylolisthesis of third cervical vertebra**

  ⊗⑦ **S12.24 Type III traumatic spondylolisthesis of third cervical vertebra**

  S12.25 Other traumatic spondylolisthesis of third cervical vertebra

    ⑦ **S12.250 Other traumatic displaced spondylolisthesis of third cervical vertebra**

    ⑦ **S12.251 Other traumatic nondisplaced spondylolisthesis of third cervical vertebra**

  S12.29 Other fracture of third cervical vertebra

    ⑦ **S12.290 Other displaced fracture of third cervical vertebra**

    ⑦ **S12.291 Other nondisplaced fracture of third cervical vertebra**

S12.3   Fracture of fourth cervical vertebra

  S12.30 Unspecified fracture of fourth cervical vertebra

    ⑦ **S12.300 Unspecified displaced fracture of fourth cervical vertebra**

    ⑦ **S12.301 Unspecified nondisplaced fracture of fourth cervical vertebra**

  S12.33 Unspecified traumatic spondylolisthesis of fourth cervical vertebra

    ⑦ **S12.330 Unspecified traumatic displaced spondylolisthesis of fourth cervical vertebra**

    ⑦ **S12.331 Unspecified traumatic nondisplaced spondylolisthesis of fourth cervical vertebra**

⊗⑦S12.34 Type III traumatic spondylolisthesis of fourth cervical vertebra

S12.35 Other traumatic spondylolisthesis of fourth cervical vertebra

⑦S12.350 Other traumatic displaced spondylolisthesis of fourth cervical vertebra

⑦S12.351 Other traumatic nondisplaced spondylolisthesis of fourth cervical vertebra

S12.39 Other fracture of fourth cervical vertebra

⑦S12.390 Other displaced fracture of fourth cervical vertebra

⑦S12.391 Other nondisplaced fracture of fourth cervical vertebra

S12.4 Fracture of fifth cervical vertebra

S12.40 Unspecified fracture of fifth cervical vertebra

⑦S12.400 Unspecified displaced fracture of fifth cervical vertebra

⑦S12.401 Unspecified nondisplaced fracture of fifth cervical vertebra

S12.43 Unspecified traumatic spondylolisthesis of fifth cervical vertebra

⑦S12.430 Unspecified traumatic displaced spondylolisthesis of fifth cervical vertebra

⑦S12.431 Unspecified traumatic nondisplaced spondylolisthesis of fifth cervical vertebra

⊗⑦S12.44 Type III traumatic spondylolisthesis of fifth cervical vertebra

S12.45 Other traumatic spondylolisthesis of fifth cervical vertebra

⑦S12.450 Other traumatic displaced spondylolisthesis of fifth cervical vertebra

⑦S12.451 Other traumatic nondisplaced spondylolisthesis of fifth cervical vertebra

S12.49 Other fracture of fifth cervical vertebra

⑦S12.490 Other displaced fracture of fifth cervical vertebra

⑦S12.491 Other nondisplaced fracture of fifth cervical vertebra

S12.5 Fracture of sixth cervical vertebra

S12.50 Unspecified fracture of sixth cervical vertebra

⑦S12.500 Unspecified displaced fracture of sixth cervical vertebra

⑦S12.501 Unspecified nondisplaced fracture of sixth cervical vertebra

S12.53 Unspecified traumatic spondylolisthesis of sixth cervical vertebra

⑦S12.530 Unspecified traumatic displaced spondylolisthesis of sixth cervical vertebra

⑦S12.531 Unspecified traumatic nondisplaced spondylolisthesis of sixth cervical vertebra

⊗⑦S12.54 Type III traumatic spondylolisthesis of sixth cervical vertebra

S12.55 Other traumatic spondylolisthesis of sixth cervical vertebra

⑦S12.550 Other traumatic displaced spondylolisthesis of sixth cervical vertebra

⑦S12.551 Other traumatic nondisplaced spondylolisthesis of sixth cervical vertebra

S12.59 Other fracture of sixth cervical vertebra

⑦S12.590 Other displaced fracture of sixth cervical vertebra

⑦S12.591 Other nondisplaced fracture of sixth cervical vertebra

S12.6 Fracture of seventh cervical vertebra

S12.60 Unspecified fracture of seventh cervical vertebra

⑦S12.600 Unspecified displaced fracture of seventh cervical vertebra

⑦S12.601 Unspecified nondisplaced fracture of seventh cervical vertebra

S12.63 Unspecified traumatic spondylolisthesis of seventh cervical vertebra

⑦S12.630 Unspecified traumatic displaced spondylolisthesis of seventh cervical vertebra

⑦S12.631 Unspecified traumatic nondisplaced spondylolisthesis of seventh cervical vertebra

⑦S12.64 Type III traumatic spondylolisthesis of seventh cervical vertebra

S12.65 Other traumatic spondylolisthesis of seventh cervical vertebra

⑦S12.650 Other traumatic displaced spondylolisthesis of seventh cervical vertebra

⑦S12.651 Other traumatic nondisplaced spondylolisthesis of seventh cervical vertebra

S12.69 Other fracture of seventh cervical vertebra

⑦S12.690 Other displaced fracture of seventh cervical vertebra

⑦S12.691 Other nondisplaced fracture of seventh cervical vertebra

⊗⑦S12.8 Fracture of other parts of neck

Hyoid bone

Larynx

Thyroid cartilage

Trachea

The appropriate 7th character is to be added to code S12.8

A - initial encounter

D - subsequent encounter

S - sequela

⊗⑦S12.9 Fracture of neck, unspecified

Fracture of neck NOS

Fracture of cervical spine NOS

Fracture of cervical vertebra NOS

The appropriate 7th character is to be added to code S12.9

A - initial encounter

D - subsequent encounter

S - sequela

S13 Dislocation and sprain of joints and ligaments at neck level

Includes: avulsion of joint or ligament at neck level

laceration of cartilage, joint or ligament at neck level

sprain of cartilage, joint or ligament at neck level

traumatic hemarthrosis of joint or ligament at neck level

traumatic rupture of joint or ligament at neck level

traumatic subluxation of joint or ligament at neck level

traumatic tear of joint or ligament at neck level

Code also any associated open wound

Excludes2: strain of muscle or tendon at neck level (S16.1)

The appropriate 7th character is to be added to each code from category S13

A - initial encounter

D - subsequent encounter

S - sequela

⊗⑦**S13.0   Traumatic rupture of cervical intervertebral disc**

Excludes1: rupture or displacement (nontraumatic) of cervical intervertebral disc NOS (M50.-)

S13.1   Subluxation and dislocation of cervical vertebrae

Definition: Subluxation is a condition that occurs when a joint begins to dislocate. Instead of the joint surfaces completely losing contact, a subluxation can be considered a "partial dislocation." A subluxation can be the result of a trauma or acute injury. In these cases, the injury can be quite painful. Subluxations can also occur as a result of loose joints.

Code also any associated:

open wound of neck (S11.-)

spinal cord injury (S14.1-)

Excludes2: fracture of cervical vertebrae (S12.0-S12.3-)

S13.10   Subluxation and dislocation of unspecified cervical vertebrae

⑦**S13.100   Subluxation of unspecified cervical vertebrae**

⑦**S13.101   Dislocation of unspecified cervical vertebrae**

S13.11   Subluxation and dislocation of C0/C1 cervical vertebrae

Subluxation and dislocation of atlantooccipital joint

Subluxation and dislocation of atloidooccipital joint

Subluxation and dislocation of occipitoatloid joint

⑦**S13.110   Subluxation of C0/C1 cervical vertebrae**

⑦**S13.111   Dislocation of C0/C1 cervical vertebrae**

S13.12   Subluxation and dislocation of C1/C2 cervical vertebrae

Subluxation and dislocation of atlantoaxial joint

⑦**S13.120   Subluxation of C1/C2 cervical vertebrae**

⑦**S13.121   Dislocation of C1/C2 cervical vertebrae**

S13.13   Subluxation and dislocation of C2/C3 cervical vertebrae

⑦**S13.130   Subluxation of C2/C3 cervical vertebrae**

⑦**S13.131   Dislocation of C2/C3 cervical vertebrae**

S13.14   Subluxation and dislocation of C3/C4 cervical vertebrae

⑦**S13.140   Subluxation of C3/C4 cervical vertebrae**

⑦**S13.141   Dislocation of C3/C4 cervical vertebrae**

S13.15   Subluxation and dislocation of C4/C5 cervical vertebrae

⑦**S13.150   Subluxation of C4/C5 cervical vertebrae**

⑦**S13.151   Dislocation of C4/C5 cervical vertebrae**

S13.16   Subluxation and dislocation of C5/C6 cervical vertebrae

⑦**S13.160   Subluxation of C5/C6 cervical vertebrae**

⑦**S13.161   Dislocation of C5/C6 cervical vertebrae**

S13.17   Subluxation and dislocation of C6/C7 cervical vertebrae

⑦**S13.170   Subluxation of C6/C7 cervical vertebrae**

⑦**S13.171   Dislocation of C6/C7 cervical vertebrae**

S13.18   Subluxation and dislocation of C7/T1 cervical vertebrae

⑦**S13.180   Subluxation of C7/T1 cervical vertebrae**

⑦**S13.181   Dislocation of C7/T1 cervical vertebrae**

S13.2   Dislocation of other and unspecified parts of neck

⊗⑦**S13.20   Dislocation of unspecified parts of neck**

⊗⑦**S13.29   Dislocation of other parts of neck**

⊗⑦**S13.4   Sprain of ligaments of cervical spine**

Sprain of anterior longitudinal (ligament), cervical

Sprain of atlanto-axial (joints)

Sprain of atlanto-occipital (joints)

Whiplash injury of cervical spine

⊗⑦**S13.5   Sprain of thyroid region**

Sprain of cricoarytenoid (joint) (ligament)

Sprain of cricothyroid (joint) (ligament)

Sprain of thyroid cartilage

⊗⑦**S13.8   Sprain of joints and ligaments of other parts of neck**

⊗⑦**S13.9   Sprain of joints and ligaments of unspecified parts of neck**

S14   Injury of nerves and spinal cord at neck level

Note: Code to highest level of cervical cord injury

Code also any associated:

fracture of cervical vertebra (S12.0--S12.6.-)

open wound of neck (S11.-)

transient paralysis (R29.5)

The appropriate 7th character is to be added to each code from category S14

A - initial encounter

D - subsequent encounter

S - sequela

⊗⑦**S14.0** **Concussion and edema of cervical spinal cord**

S14.1 **Other and unspecified injuries of cervical spinal cord**

    S14.10 **Unspecified injury of cervical spinal cord**

      ⑦**S14.101** **Unspecified injury at C1 level of cervical spinal cord**

      ⑦**S14.102** **Unspecified injury at C2 level of cervical spinal cord**

      ⑦**S14.103** **Unspecified injury at C3 level of cervical spinal cord**

      ⑦**S14.104** **Unspecified injury at C4 level of cervical spinal cord**

      ⑦**S14.105** **Unspecified injury at C5 level of cervical spinal cord**

      ⑦**S14.106** **Unspecified injury at C6 level of cervical spinal cord**

      ⑦**S14.107** **Unspecified injury at C7 level of cervical spinal cord**

      ⑦**S14.108** **Unspecified injury at C8 level of cervical spinal cord**

      ⑦**S14.109** **Unspecified injury at unspecified level of cervical spinal cord**

           Injury of cervical spinal cord NOS

    S14.11 **Complete lesion of cervical spinal cord**

      ⑦**S14.111** **Complete lesion at C1 level of cervical spinal cord**

      ⑦**S14.112** **Complete lesion at C2 level of cervical spinal cord**

      ⑦**S14.113** **Complete lesion at C3 level of cervical spinal cord**

      ⑦**S14.114** **Complete lesion at C4 level of cervical spinal cord**

      ⑦**S14.115** **Complete lesion at C5 level of cervical spinal cord**

      ⑦**S14.116** **Complete lesion at C6 level of cervical spinal cord**

      ⑦**S14.117** **Complete lesion at C7 level of cervical spinal cord**

      ⑦**S14.118** **Complete lesion at C8 level of cervical spinal cord**

      ⑦**S14.119** **Complete lesion at unspecified level of cervical spinal cord**

    S14.12 **Central cord syndrome of cervical spinal cord**

      ⑦**S14.121** **Central cord syndrome at C1 level of cervical spinal cord**

      ⑦**S14.122** **Central cord syndrome at C2 level of cervical spinal cord**

      ⑦**S14.123** **Central cord syndrome at C3 level of cervical spinal cord**

      ⑦**S14.124** **Central cord syndrome at C4 level of cervical spinal cord**

      ⑦**S14.125** **Central cord syndrome at C5 level of cervical spinal cord**

      ⑦**S14.126** **Central cord syndrome at C6 level of cervical spinal cord**

      ⑦**S14.127** **Central cord syndrome at C7 level of cervical spinal cord**

      ⑦**S14.128** **Central cord syndrome at C8 level of cervical spinal cord**

      ⑦**S14.129** **Central cord syndrome at unspecified level of cervical spinal cord**

S14.13 **Anterior cord syndrome of cervical spinal cord**

      ⑦**S14.131** **Anterior cord syndrome at C1 level of cervical spinal cord**

      ⑦**S14.132** **Anterior cord syndrome at C2 level of cervical spinal cord**

      ⑦**S14.133** **Anterior cord syndrome at C3 level of cervical spinal cord**

      ⑦**S14.134** **Anterior cord syndrome at C4 level of cervical spinal cord**

      ⑦**S14.135** **Anterior cord syndrome at C5 level of cervical spinal cord**

      ⑦**S14.136** **Anterior cord syndrome at C6 level of cervical spinal cord**

      ⑦**S14.137** **Anterior cord syndrome at C7 level of cervical spinal cord**

      ⑦**S14.138** **Anterior cord syndrome at C8 level of cervical spinal cord**

      ⑦**S14.139** **Anterior cord syndrome at unspecified level of cervical spinal cord**

S14.14 **Brown-Séquard syndrome of cervical spinal cord**

      ⑦**S14.141** **Brown-Séquard syndrome at C1 level of cervical spinal cord**

      ⑦**S14.142** **Brown-Séquard syndrome at C2 level of cervical spinal cord**

      ⑦**S14.143** **Brown-Séquard syndrome at C3 level of cervical spinal cord**

      ⑦**S14.144** **Brown-Séquard syndrome at C4 level of cervical spinal cord**

      ⑦**S14.145** **Brown-Séquard syndrome at C5 level of cervical spinal cord**

      ⑦**S14.146** **Brown-Séquard syndrome at C6 level of cervical spinal cord**

      ⑦**S14.147** **Brown-Séquard syndrome at C7 level of cervical spinal cord**

      ⑦**S14.148** **Brown-Séquard syndrome at C8 level of cervical spinal cord**

      ⑦**S14.149** **Brown-Séquard syndrome at unspecified level of cervical spinal cord**

S14.15 **Other incomplete lesions of cervical spinal cord**

           Incomplete lesion of cervical spinal cord NOS

           Posterior cord syndrome of cervical spinal cord

      ⑦**S14.151** **Other incomplete lesion at C1 level of cervical spinal cord**

      ⑦**S14.152** **Other incomplete lesion at C2 level of cervical spinal cord**

      ⑦**S14.153** **Other incomplete lesion at C3 level of cervical spinal cord**

      ⑦**S14.154** **Other incomplete lesion at C4 level of cervical spinal cord**

      ⑦**S14.155** **Other incomplete lesion at C5 level of cervical spinal cord**

      ⑦**S14.156** **Other incomplete lesion at C6 level of cervical spinal cord**

      ⑦**S14.157** **Other incomplete lesion at C7 level of cervical spinal cord**

⑦ S14.158   **Other incomplete lesion at C8 level of cervical spinal cord**

⑦ S14.159   **Other incomplete lesion at unspecified level of cervical spinal cord**

⊗⑦ **S14.2**   **Injury of nerve root of cervical spine**

⊗⑦ **S14.3**   **Injury of brachial plexus**

⊗⑦ **S14.4**   **Injury of peripheral nerves of neck**

⊗⑦ **S14.5**   **Injury of cervical sympathetic nerves**

⊗⑦ **S14.8**   **Injury of other specified nerves of neck**

⊗⑦ **S14.9**   **Injury of unspecified nerves of neck**

S15   **Injury of blood vessels at neck level**

     Code also any associated open wound (S11.-)

     The appropriate 7th character is to be added to each code from category S15

     A - initial encounter

     D - subsequent encounter

     S - sequela

     S15.0   **Injury of carotid artery of neck**

       Injury of carotid artery (common) (external) (internal, extracranial portion)

       Injury of carotid artery NOS

       Excludes1: injury of internal carotid artery, intracranial portion (S06.8)

       S15.00   **Unspecified injury of carotid artery**

         ⑦ S15.001   **Unspecified injury of right carotid artery**

         ⑦ S15.002   **Unspecified injury of left carotid artery**

         ⑦ S15.009   **Unspecified injury of unspecified carotid artery**

       S15.01   **Minor laceration of carotid artery**

         Incomplete transection of carotid artery

         Laceration of carotid artery NOS

         Superficial laceration of carotid artery

         ⑦ S15.011   **Minor laceration of right carotid artery**

         ⑦ S15.012   **Minor laceration of left carotid artery**

         ⑦ S15.019   **Minor laceration of unspecified carotid artery**

       S15.02   **Major laceration of carotid artery**

         Complete transection of carotid artery

         Traumatic rupture of carotid artery

         ⑦ S15.021   **Major laceration of right carotid artery**

         ⑦ S15.022   **Major laceration of left carotid artery**

         ⑦ S15.029   **Major laceration of unspecified carotid artery**

       S15.09   **Other specified injury of carotid artery**

         ⑦ S15.091   **Other specified injury of right carotid artery**

         ⑦ S15.092   **Other specified injury of left carotid artery**

         ⑦ S15.099   **Other specified injury of unspecified carotid artery**

     S15.1   **Injury of vertebral artery**

     S15.10   **Unspecified injury of vertebral artery**

       ⑦ S15.101   **Unspecified injury of right vertebral artery**

       ⑦ S15.102   **Unspecified injury of left vertebral artery**

       ⑦ S15.109   **Unspecified injury of unspecified vertebral artery**

     S15.11   **Minor laceration of vertebral artery**

       Incomplete transection of vertebral artery

       Laceration of vertebral artery NOS

       Superficial laceration of vertebral artery

       ⑦ S15.111   **Minor laceration of right vertebral artery**

       ⑦ S15.112   **Minor laceration of left vertebral artery**

       ⑦ S15.119   **Minor laceration of unspecified vertebral artery**

     S15.12   **Major laceration of vertebral artery**

       Complete transection of vertebral artery

       Traumatic rupture of vertebral artery

       ⑦ S15.121   **Major laceration of right vertebral artery**

       ⑦ S15.122   **Major laceration of left vertebral artery**

       ⑦ S15.129   **Major laceration of unspecified vertebral artery**

     S15.19   **Other specified injury of vertebral artery**

       ⑦ S15.191   **Other specified injury of right vertebral artery**

       ⑦ S15.192   **Other specified injury of left vertebral artery**

       ⑦ S15.199   **Other specified injury of unspecified vertebral artery**

     S15.2   **Injury of external jugular vein**

     S15.20   **Unspecified injury of external jugular vein**

       ⑦ S15.201   **Unspecified injury of right external jugular vein**

       ⑦ S15.202   **Unspecified injury of left external jugular vein**

       ⑦ S15.209   **Unspecified injury of unspecified external jugular vein**

     S15.21   **Minor laceration of external jugular vein**

       Incomplete transection of external jugular vein

       Laceration of external jugular vein NOS

       Superficial laceration of external jugular vein

       ⑦ S15.211   **Minor laceration of right external jugular vein**

       ⑦ S15.212   **Minor laceration of left external jugular vein**

       ⑦ S15.219   **Minor laceration of unspecified external jugular vein**

     S15.22   **Major laceration of external jugular vein**

       Complete transection of external jugular vein

       Traumatic rupture of external jugular vein

       ⑦ S15.221   **Major laceration of right external jugular vein**

       ⑦ S15.222   **Major laceration of left external jugular vein**

   ● New code   ▲ Revised code   **Excludes1:** Not coded here   **Excludes2:** Not included here   ⊗ Placeholder required   ⑦ 7th digit required

⑦S15.229   Major laceration of unspecified external jugular vein

S15.29   Other specified injury of external jugular vein

⑦S15.291   Other specified injury of right external jugular vein

⑦S15.292   Other specified injury of left external jugular vein

⑦S15.299   Other specified injury of unspecified external jugular vein

S15.3   Injury of internal jugular vein

S15.30   Unspecified injury of internal jugular vein

⑦S15.301   Unspecified injury of right internal jugular vein

⑦S15.302   Unspecified injury of left internal jugular vein

⑦S15.309   Unspecified injury of unspecified internal jugular vein

S15.31   Minor laceration of internal jugular vein

Incomplete transection of internal jugular vein

Laceration of internal jugular vein NOS

Superficial laceration of internal jugular vein

⑦S15.311   Minor laceration of right internal jugular vein

⑦S15.312   Minor laceration of left internal jugular vein

⑦S15.319   Minor laceration of unspecified internal jugular vein

⑦S15.32   Major laceration of internal jugular vein

Complete transection of internal jugular vein

Traumatic rupture of internal jugular vein

⑦S15.321   Major laceration of right internal jugular vein

⑦S15.322   Major laceration of left internal jugular vein

⑦S15.329   Major laceration of unspecified internal jugular vein

⑦S15.39   Other specified injury of internal jugular vein

⑦S15.391   Other specified injury of right internal jugular vein

⑦S15.392   Other specified injury of left internal jugular vein

⑦S15.399   Other specified injury of unspecified internal jugular vein

⊗⑦S15.8   Injury of other specified blood vessels at neck level

⊗⑦S15.9   Injury of unspecified blood vessel at neck level

S16   Injury of muscle, fascia and tendon at neck level

Code also any associated open wound (S11.-)

Excludes2: sprain of joint or ligament at neck level (S13.9)

The appropriate 7th character is to be added to each code from category S16

A - initial encounter

D - subsequent encounter

S - sequela

⊗⑦S16.1   Strain of muscle, fascia and tendon at neck level

⊗⑦S16.2   Laceration of muscle, fascia and tendon at neck level

⊗⑦S16.8   Other specified injury of muscle, fascia and tendon at neck level

⊗⑦S16.9   Unspecified injury of muscle, fascia and tendon at neck level

S17   Crushing injury of neck

Use additional code for all associated injuries, such as:

injury of blood vessels (S15.-)

open wound of neck (S11.-)

spinal cord injury (S14.0, S14.1-)

vertebral fracture (S12.0--S12.3-)

The appropriate 7th character is to be added to each code from category S17

A - initial encounter

D - subsequent encounter

S - sequela

⊗⑦S17.0   Crushing injury of larynx and trachea

⊗⑦S17.8   Crushing injury of other specified parts of neck

⊗⑦S17.9   Crushing injury of neck, part unspecified

S19   Other specified and unspecified injuries of neck

The appropriate 7th character is to be added to each code from category S19

A - initial encounter

D - subsequent encounter

S - sequela

S19.8   Other specified injuries of neck

⊗⑦S19.80   Other specified injuries of unspecified part of neck

⊗⑦S19.81   Other specified injuries of larynx

⊗⑦S19.82   Other specified injuries of cervical trachea

Excludes2: Other specified injury of thoracic trachea (S27.5-)

⊗⑦S19.83   Other specified injuries of vocal cord

⊗⑦S19.84   Other specified injuries of thyroid gland

⊗⑦S19.85   Other specified injuries of pharynx and cervical esophagus

⊗⑦S19.89   Other specified injuries of other specified part of neck

⊗⑦S19.9   Unspecified injury of neck

INJURIES TO THE THORAX (S20-S29)

Includes: injuries of breast

injuries of chest (wall)

injuries of interscapular area

Excludes2: burns and corrosions (T20-T32)

effects of foreign body in bronchus (T17.5)

effects of foreign body in esophagus (T18.1)

effects of foreign body in lung (T17.8)

effects of foreign body in trachea (T17.4)

frostbite (T33-T34)

injuries of axilla injuries of clavicle

injuries of scapular region injuries of shoulder insect bite or sting, venomous (T63.4)

S20   Superficial injury of thorax

The appropriate 7th character is to be added to each code from category S20

A - initial encounter

D - subsequent encounter

S - sequela

S20.0 Contusion of breast
⊗⑦**S20.00 Contusion of breast, unspecified breast**
⊗⑦**S20.01 Contusion of right breast**
⊗⑦**S20.02 Contusion of left breast**
S20.1 Other and unspecified superficial injuries of breast
  S20.10 Unspecified superficial injuries of breast
    ⑦**S20.101 Unspecified superficial injuries of breast, right breast**
    ⑦**S20.102 Unspecified superficial injuries of breast, left breast**
    ⑦**S20.109 Unspecified superficial injuries of breast, unspecified breast**
  S20.11 Abrasion of breast
    ⑦**S20.111 Abrasion of breast, right breast**
    ⑦**S20.112 Abrasion of breast, left breast**
    ⑦**S20.119 Abrasion of breast, unspecified breast**
  S20.12 Blister (nonthermal) of breast
    ⑦**S20.121 Blister (nonthermal) of breast, right breast**
    ⑦**S20.122 Blister (nonthermal) of breast, left breast**
    ⑦**S20.129 Blister (nonthermal) of breast, unspecified breast**
  S20.14 External constriction of part of breast
    ⑦**S20.141 External constriction of part of breast, right breast**
    ⑦**S20.142 External constriction of part of breast, left breast**
    ⑦**S20.149 External constriction of part of breast, unspecified breast**
  S20.15 ⑦ Superficial foreign body of breast
    Splinter in the breast
    ⑦**S20.151 Superficial foreign body of breast, right breast**
    ⑦**S20.152 Superficial foreign body of breast, left breast**
    ⑦**S20.159 Superficial foreign body of breast, unspecified breast**
  S20.16 Insect bite (nonvenomous) of breast
    ⑦**S20.161 Insect bite (nonvenomous) of breast, right breast**
    ⑦**S20.162 Insect bite (nonvenomous) of breast, left breast**
    ⑦**S20.169 Insect bite (nonvenomous) of breast, unspecified breast**
  S20.17 Other superficial bite of breast
    Excludes1: open bite of breast (S21.05-)
    ⑦**S20.171 Other superficial bite of breast, right breast**
    ⑦**S20.172 Other superficial bite of breast, left breast**
    ⑦**S20.179 Other superficial bite of breast, unspecified breast**
S20.2 Contusion of thorax
  ⊗⑦**S20.20 Contusion of thorax, unspecified**
  S20.21 Contusion of front wall of thorax
    ⑦**S20.211 Contusion of right front wall of thorax**

⑦**S20.212 Contusion of left front wall of thorax**
⑦**S20.219 Contusion of unspecified front wall of thorax**
  S20.22 Contusion of back wall of thorax
    ⑦**S20.221 Contusion of right back wall of thorax**
    ⑦**S20.222 Contusion of left back wall of thorax**
    ⑦**S20.229 Contusion of unspecified back wall of thorax**
S20.3 Other and unspecified superficial injuries of front wall of thorax
  S20.30 Unspecified superficial injuries of front wall of thorax
    ⑦**S20.301 Unspecified superficial injuries of right front wall of thorax**
    ⑦**S20.302 Unspecified superficial injuries of left front wall of thorax**
    ⑦**S20.309 Unspecified superficial injuries of unspecified front wall of thorax**
  S20.31 Abrasion of front wall of thorax
    ⑦**S20.311 Abrasion of right front wall of thorax**
    ⑦**S20.312 Abrasion of left front wall of thorax**
    ⑦**S20.319 Abrasion of unspecified front wall of thorax**
  S20.32 Blister (nonthermal) of front wall of thorax
    ⑦**S20.321 Blister (nonthermal) of right front wall of thorax**
    ⑦**S20.322 Blister (nonthermal) of left front wall of thorax**
    ⑦**S20.329 Blister (nonthermal) of unspecified front wall of thorax**
  S20.34 External constriction of front wall of thorax
    ⑦**S20.341 External constriction of right front wall of thorax**
    ⑦**S20.342 External constriction of left front wall of thorax**
    ⑦**S20.349 External constriction of unspecified front wall of thorax**
  S20.35 Superficial foreign body of front wall of thorax
    Splinter in front wall of thorax
    ⑦**S20.351 ⑦ Superficial foreign body of right front wall of thorax**
    ⑦**S20.352 ⑦ Superficial foreign body of left front wall of thorax**
    ⑦**S20.359 ⑦ Superficial foreign body of unspecified front wall of thorax**
  S20.36 Insect bite (nonvenomous) of front wall of thorax
    ⑦**S20.361 Insect bite (nonvenomous) of right front wall of thorax**
    ⑦**S20.362 Insect bite (nonvenomous) of left front wall of thorax**
    ⑦**S20.369 Insect bite (nonvenomous) of unspecified front wall of thorax**
  S20.37 Other superficial bite of front wall of thorax

● New code ▲ Revised code **Excludes1:** Not coded here **Excludes2:** Not included here ⊗ Placeholder required ⑦ 7ᵗʰ digit required

Excludes1: open bite of front wall of thorax (S21.14)

⑦**S20.371** Other superficial bite of right front wall of thorax

⑦**S20.372** Other superficial bite of left front wall of thorax

⑦**S20.379** Other superficial bite of unspecified front wall of thorax

S20.4 Other and unspecified superficial injuries of back wall of thorax

S20.40 Unspecified superficial injuries of back wall of thorax

⑦**S20.401** Unspecified superficial injuries of right back wall of thorax

⑦**S20.402** Unspecified superficial injuries of left back wall of thorax

⑦**S20.409** Unspecified superficial injuries of unspecified back wall of thorax

S20.41 Abrasion of back wall of thorax

⑦**S20.411** Abrasion of right back wall of thorax

⑦**S20.412** Abrasion of left back wall of thorax

⑦**S20.419** Abrasion of unspecified back wall of thorax

S20.42 Blister (nonthermal) of back wall of thorax

⑦**S20.421** Blister (nonthermal) of right back wall of thorax

⑦**S20.422** Blister (nonthermal) of left back wall of thorax

⑦**S20.429** Blister (nonthermal) of unspecified back wall of thorax

S20.44 External constriction of back wall of thorax

⑦**S20.441** External constriction of right back wall of thorax

⑦**S20.442** External constriction of left back wall of thorax

⑦**S20.449** External constriction of unspecified back wall of thorax

S20.45 Superficial foreign body of back wall of thorax

Splinter of back wall of thorax

⑦**S20.451** Superficial foreign body of right back wall of thorax

⑦**S20.452** Superficial foreign body of left back wall of thorax

⑦**S20.459** Superficial foreign body of unspecified back wall of thorax

S20.46 Insect bite (nonvenomous) of back wall of thorax

⑦**S20.461** Insect bite (nonvenomous) of right back wall of thorax

⑦**S20.462** Insect bite (nonvenomous) of left back wall of thorax

⑦**S20.469** Insect bite (nonvenomous) of unspecified back wall of thorax

S20.47 Other superficial bite of back wall of thorax

Excludes1: open bite of back wall of thorax (S21.24)

⑦**S20.471** Other superficial bite of right back wall of thorax

⑦**S20.472** Other superficial bite of left back wall of thorax

⑦**S20.479** Other superficial bite of unspecified back wall of thorax

S20.9 Superficial injury of unspecified parts of thorax

Excludes1: contusion of thorax NOS (S20.20)

⊗⑦**S20.90** Unspecified superficial injury of unspecified parts of thorax

Superficial injury of thoracic wall NOS

⊗⑦**S20.91** Abrasion of unspecified parts of thorax

⊗⑦**S20.92** Blister (nonthermal) of unspecified parts of thorax

⊗⑦**S20.94** External constriction of unspecified parts of thorax

⊗⑦**S20.95** Superficial foreign body of unspecified parts of thorax

Splinter in thorax NOS

⊗⑦**S20.96** Insect bite (nonvenomous) of unspecified parts of thorax

⊗⑦**S20.97** Other superficial bite of unspecified parts of thorax

Excludes1: open bite of thorax NOS (S21.95)

S21 Open wound of thorax

<u>Code also</u> any associated injury, such as:

injury of heart (S26.-)

injury of intrathoracic organs (S27.-)

rib fracture (S22.3-, S22.4-)

spinal cord injury (S24.0-, S24.1-)

traumatic hemopneumothorax (S27.3)

traumatic hemothorax (S27.1)

traumatic pneumothorax (S27.0) wound infection

Excludes1: traumatic amputation (partial) of thorax (S28.1)

The appropriate 7th character is to be added to each code from category S21

A - initial encounter

D - subsequent encounter

S - sequela

S21.0 Open wound of breast

S21.00 Unspecified open wound of breast

⑦**S21.001** Unspecified open wound of right breast

⑦**S21.002** Unspecified open wound of left breast

⑦**S21.009** Unspecified open wound of unspecified breast

S21.01 Laceration without foreign body of breast

⑦**S21.011** Laceration without foreign body of right breast

⑦**S21.012** Laceration without foreign body of left breast

⑦**S21.019** Laceration without foreign body of unspecified breast

S21.02 Laceration with foreign body of breast

⑦**S21.021** Laceration with foreign body of right breast

⑦**S21.022** Laceration with foreign body of left breast

⑦ **S21.029**   Laceration with foreign body of unspecified breast

S21.03   Puncture wound without foreign body of breast

     ⑦ **S21.031**   Puncture wound without foreign body of right breast

     ⑦ **S21.032**   Puncture wound without foreign body of left breast

     ⑦ **S21.039**   Puncture wound without foreign body of unspecified breast

S21.04   Puncture wound with foreign body of breast

     ⑦ **S21.041**   Puncture wound with foreign body of right breast

     ⑦ **S21.042**   Puncture wound with foreign body of left breast

     ⑦ **S21.049**   Puncture wound with foreign body of unspecified breast

S21.05   Open bite of breast

Bite of breast NOS

Excludes1: superficial bite of breast (S20.17)

     ⑦ **S21.051**   **Open bite of right breast**

     ⑦ **S21.052**   **Open bite of left breast**

     ⑦ **S21.059**   **Open bite of unspecified breast**

S21.1   **Open wound of front wall of thorax without penetration into thoracic cavity**

Open wound of chest without penetration into thoracic cavity

   S21.10   Unspecified open wound of front wall of thorax without penetration into thoracic cavity

     ⑦ **S21.101**   Unspecified open wound of right front wall of thorax without penetration into thoracic cavity

     ⑦ **S21.102**   Unspecified open wound of left front wall of thorax without penetration into thoracic cavity

     ⑦ **S21.109**   Unspecified open wound of unspecified front wall of thorax without penetration into thoracic cavity

   S21.11   Laceration without foreign body of front wall of thorax without penetration into thoracic cavity

     ⑦ **S21.111**   Laceration without foreign body of right front wall of thorax without penetration into thoracic cavity

     ⑦ **S21.112**   Laceration without foreign body of left front wall of thorax without penetration into thoracic cavity

     ⑦ **S21.119**   Laceration without foreign body of unspecified front wall of thorax without penetration into thoracic cavity

   S21.12   Laceration with foreign body of front wall of thorax without penetration into thoracic cavity

     ⑦ **S21.121**   Laceration with foreign body of right front wall of thorax without penetration into thoracic cavity

     ⑦ **S21.122**   Laceration with foreign body of left front wall of thorax without penetration into thoracic cavity

⑦ **S21.129**   Laceration with foreign body of unspecified front wall of thorax without penetration into thoracic cavity

S21.13   Puncture wound without foreign body of front wall of thorax without penetration into thoracic cavity

     ⑦ **S21.131**   Puncture wound without foreign body of right front wall of thorax without penetration into thoracic cavity

     ⑦ **S21.132**   Puncture wound without foreign body of left front wall of thorax without penetration into thoracic cavity

     ⑦ **S21.139**   Puncture wound without foreign body of unspecified front wall of thorax without penetration into thoracic cavity

S21.14   Puncture wound with foreign body of front wall of thorax without penetration into thoracic cavity

     ⑦ **S21.141**   Puncture wound with foreign body of right front wall of thorax without penetration into thoracic cavity

     ⑦ **S21.142**   Puncture wound with foreign body of left front wall of thorax without penetration into thoracic cavity

     ⑦ **S21.149**   Puncture wound with foreign body of unspecified front wall of thorax without penetration into thoracic cavity

S21.15   Open bite of front wall of thorax without penetration into thoracic cavity

Bite of front wall of thorax NOS

Excludes1: superficial bite of front wall of thorax (S20.37)

     ⑦ **S21.151**   Open bite of right front wall of thorax without penetration into thoracic cavity

     ⑦ **S21.152**   Open bite of left front wall of thorax without penetration into thoracic cavity

     ⑦ **S21.159**   Open bite of unspecified front wall of thorax without penetration into thoracic cavity

S21.2   **Open wound of back wall of thorax without penetration into thoracic cavity**

   S21.20   Unspecified open wound of back wall of thorax without penetration into thoracic cavity

     ⑦ **S21.201**   Unspecified open wound of right back wall of thorax without penetration into thoracic cavity

     ⑦ **S21.202**   Unspecified open wound of left back wall of thorax without penetration into thoracic cavity

     ⑦ **S21.209**   Unspecified open wound of unspecified back wall of thorax without penetration into thoracic cavity

   S21.21   Laceration without foreign body of back wall of thorax without penetration into thoracic cavity

   ● New code   ▲ Revised code   **Excludes1:** Not coded here   **Excludes2:** Not included here   ⊗ Placeholder required   ⑦ 7ᵗʰ digit required

⑦S21.211   Laceration without foreign body of right back wall of thorax without penetration into thoracic cavity

⑦S21.212   Laceration without foreign body of left back wall of thorax without penetration into thoracic cavity

⑦S21.219   Laceration without foreign body of unspecified back wall of thorax without penetration into thoracic cavity

S21.22   **Laceration with foreign body of back wall of thorax without penetration into thoracic cavity**

⑦S21.221   Laceration with foreign body of right back wall of thorax without penetration into thoracic cavity

⑦S21.222   Laceration with foreign body of left back wall of thorax without penetration into thoracic cavity

⑦S21.229   Laceration with foreign body of unspecified back wall of thorax without penetration into thoracic cavity

S21.23   **Puncture wound without foreign body of back wall of thorax without penetration into thoracic cavity**

⑦S21.231   Puncture wound without foreign body of right back wall of thorax without penetration into thoracic cavity

⑦S21.232   Puncture wound without foreign body of left back wall of thorax without penetration into thoracic cavity

⑦S21.239   Puncture wound without foreign body of unspecified back wall of thorax without penetration into thoracic cavity

S21.24   **Puncture wound with foreign body of back wall of thorax without penetration into thoracic cavity**

⑦S21.241   Puncture wound with foreign body of right back wall of thorax without penetration into thoracic cavity

⑦S21.242   Puncture wound with foreign body of left back wall of thorax without penetration into thoracic cavity

⑦S21.249   Puncture wound with foreign body of unspecified back wall of thorax without penetration into thoracic cavity

S21.25   **Open bite of back wall of thorax without penetration into thoracic cavity**

Bite of back wall of thorax NOS

Excludes1: superficial bite of back wall of thorax (S20.47)

⑦S21.251   Open bite of right back wall of thorax without penetration into thoracic cavity

⑦S21.252   Open bite of left back wall of thorax without penetration into thoracic cavity

⑦S21.259   Open bite of unspecified back wall of thorax without penetration into thoracic cavity

S21.3   **Open wound of front wall of thorax with penetration into thoracic cavity**

Open wound of chest with penetration into thoracic cavity

S21.30   **Unspecified open wound of front wall of thorax with penetration into thoracic cavity**

⑦S21.301   Unspecified open wound of right front wall of thorax with penetration into thoracic cavity

⑦S21.302   Unspecified open wound of left front wall of thorax with penetration into thoracic cavity

⑦S21.309   Unspecified open wound of unspecified front wall of thorax with penetration into thoracic cavity

S21.31   **Laceration without foreign body of front wall of thorax with penetration into thoracic cavity**

⑦S21.311   Laceration without foreign body of right front wall of thorax with penetration into thoracic cavity

⑦S21.312   Laceration without foreign body of left front wall of thorax with penetration into thoracic cavity

⑦S21.319   Laceration without foreign body of unspecified front wall of thorax with penetration into thoracic cavity

S21.32   **Laceration with foreign body of front wall of thorax with penetration into thoracic cavity**

⑦S21.321   Laceration with foreign body of right front wall of thorax with penetration into thoracic cavity

⑦S21.322   Laceration with foreign body of left front wall of thorax with penetration into thoracic cavity

⑦S21.329   Laceration with foreign body of unspecified front wall of thorax with penetration into thoracic cavity

S21.33   **Puncture wound without foreign body of front wall of thorax with penetration into thoracic cavity**

⑦S21.331   Puncture wound without foreign body of right front wall of thorax with penetration into thoracic cavity

⑦S21.332   Puncture wound without foreign body of left front wall of thorax with penetration into thoracic cavity

⑦S21.339   Puncture wound without foreign body of unspecified front wall of thorax with penetration into thoracic cavity

S21.34   **Puncture wound with foreign body of front wall of thorax with penetration into thoracic cavity**

⑦S21.341   Puncture wound with foreign body of right front wall of thorax with penetration into thoracic cavity

⑦S21.342   Puncture wound with foreign body of left front wall of thorax with penetration into thoracic cavity

⑦S21.349   **Puncture wound with foreign body of unspecified front wall of thorax with penetration into thoracic cavity**

S21.35   **Open bite of front wall of thorax with penetration into thoracic cavity**

Excludes1: superficial bite of front wall of thorax (S20.37)

⑦S21.351   **Open bite of right front wall of thorax with penetration into thoracic cavity**

⑦S21.352   **Open bite of left front wall of thorax with penetration into thoracic cavity**

⑦S21.359   **Open bite of unspecified front wall of thorax with penetration into thoracic cavity**

S21.4   **Open wound of back wall of thorax with penetration into thoracic cavity**

S21.40   **Unspecified open wound of back wall of thorax with penetration into thoracic cavity**

⑦S21.401   **Unspecified open wound of right back wall of thorax with penetration into thoracic cavity**

⑦S21.402   **Unspecified open wound of left back wall of thorax with penetration into thoracic cavity**

⑦S21.409   **Unspecified open wound of unspecified back wall of thorax with penetration into thoracic cavity**

S21.41   **Laceration without foreign body of back wall of thorax with penetration into thoracic cavity**

⑦S21.411   **Laceration without foreign body of right back wall of thorax with penetration into thoracic cavity**

⑦S21.412   **Laceration without foreign body of left back wall of thorax with penetration into thoracic cavity**

⑦S21.419   **Laceration without foreign body of unspecified back wall of thorax with penetration into thoracic cavity**

S21.42   **Laceration with foreign body of back wall of thorax with penetration into thoracic cavity**

⑦S21.421   **Laceration with foreign body of right back wall of thorax with penetration into thoracic cavity**

⑦S21.422   **Laceration with foreign body of left back wall of thorax with penetration into thoracic cavity**

⑦S21.429   **Laceration with foreign body of unspecified back wall of thorax with penetration into thoracic cavity**

S21.43   **Puncture wound without foreign body of back wall of thorax with penetration into thoracic cavity**

⑦S21.431   **Puncture wound without foreign body of right back wall of thorax with penetration into thoracic cavity**

⑦S21.432   **Puncture wound without foreign body of left back wall of thorax with penetration into thoracic cavity**

⑦S21.439   **Puncture wound without foreign body of unspecified back wall of**

thorax with penetration into thoracic cavity

S21.44   **Puncture wound with foreign body of back wall of thorax with penetration into thoracic cavity**

⑦S21.441   **Puncture wound with foreign body of right back wall of thorax with penetration into thoracic cavity**

⑦S21.442   **Puncture wound with foreign body of left back wall of thorax with penetration into thoracic cavity**

⑦S21.449   **Puncture wound with foreign body of unspecified back wall of thorax with penetration into thoracic cavity**

S21.45   **Open bite of back wall of thorax with penetration into thoracic cavity**

Bite of back wall of thorax NOS

Excludes1: superficial bite of back wall of thorax (S20.47)

⑦S21.451   **Open bite of right back wall of thorax with penetration into thoracic cavity**

⑦S21.452   **Open bite of left back wall of thorax with penetration into thoracic cavity**

⑦S21.459   **Open bite of unspecified back wall of thorax with penetration into thoracic cavity**

S21.9   **Open wound of unspecified part of thorax**

Open wound of thoracic wall NOS

⊗⑦S21.90   **Unspecified open wound of unspecified part of thorax**

⊗⑦S21.91   **Laceration without foreign body of unspecified part of thorax**

⊗⑦S21.92   **Laceration with foreign body of unspecified part of thorax**

⊗⑦S21.93   **Puncture wound without foreign body of unspecified part of thorax**

⊗⑦S21.94   **Puncture wound with foreign body of unspecified part of thorax**

⊗⑦S21.95   **Open bite of unspecified part of thorax**

Excludes1: superficial bite of thorax (S20.97)

S22 **Fracture of rib(s), sternum and thoracic spine**

Note: A fracture not indicated as displaced or nondisplaced should be coded to displaced

A fracture not indicated as open or closed should be coded to closed

Includes: fracture of thoracic neural arch

      fracture of thoracic spinous process

      fracture of thoracic transverse process

      fracture of thoracic vertebra

      fracture of thoracic vertebral arch

Code first any associated:

injury of intrathoracic organ (S27.-)

spinal cord injury (S24.0-, S24.1-)

Excludes1: transection of thorax (S28.1)

Excludes2: fracture of clavicle (S42.0-)

      fracture of scapula (S42.1-)

The appropriate 7th character is to be added to each code from category S22

   ● New code   ▲ Revised code   **Excludes1:** Not coded here   **Excludes2:** Not included here   ⊗ Placeholder required   ⑦7ᵗʰ digit required

A - initial encounter for closed fracture

B - initial encounter for open fracture

D - subsequent encounter for fracture with routine healing

G - subsequent encounter for fracture with delayed healing

K - subsequent encounter for fracture with nonunion

S - sequela

S22.0   Fracture of thoracic vertebra

    S22.00   Fracture of unspecified thoracic vertebra

        ⑦S22.000   **Wedge compression fracture of unspecified thoracic vertebra**

        ⑦S22.001   **Stable burst fracture of unspecified thoracic vertebra**

        ⑦S22.002   **Unstable burst fracture of unspecified thoracic vertebra**

        ⑦S22.008   **Other fracture of unspecified thoracic vertebra**

        ⑦S22.009   **Unspecified fracture of unspecified thoracic vertebra**

    S22.01   Fracture of first thoracic vertebra

        ⑦S22.010   **Wedge compression fracture of first thoracic vertebra**

        ⑦S22.011   **Stable burst fracture of first thoracic vertebra**

        ⑦S22.012   **Unstable burst fracture of first thoracic vertebra**

        ⑦S22.018   **Other fracture of first thoracic vertebra**

        ⑦S22.019   **Unspecified fracture of first thoracic vertebra**

    S22.02   Fracture of second thoracic vertebra

        ⑦S22.020   **Wedge compression fracture of second thoracic vertebra**

        ⑦S22.021   **Stable burst fracture of second thoracic vertebra**

        ⑦S22.022   **Unstable burst fracture of second thoracic vertebra**

        ⑦S22.028   **Other fracture of second thoracic vertebra**

        ⑦S22.029   **Unspecified fracture of second thoracic vertebra**

    S22.03   Fracture of third thoracic vertebra

        ⑦S22.030   **Wedge compression fracture of third thoracic vertebra**

        ⑦S22.031   **Stable burst fracture of third thoracic vertebra**

        ⑦S22.032   **Unstable burst fracture of third thoracic vertebra**

        ⑦S22.038   **Other fracture of third thoracic vertebra**

        ⑦S22.039   **Unspecified fracture of third thoracic vertebra**

    S22.04   Fracture of fourth thoracic vertebra

        ⑦S22.040   **Wedge compression fracture of fourth thoracic vertebra**

        ⑦S22.041   **Stable burst fracture of fourth thoracic vertebra**

        ⑦S22.042   **Unstable burst fracture of fourth thoracic vertebra**

        ⑦S22.048   **Other fracture of fourth thoracic vertebra**

        ⑦S22.049   **Unspecified fracture of fourth thoracic vertebra**

    S22.05   Fracture of T5-T6 vertebra

        ⑦S22.050   **Wedge compression fracture of T5-T6 vertebra**

        ⑦S22.051   **Stable burst fracture of T5-T6 vertebra**

        ⑦S22.052   **Unstable burst fracture of T5-T6 vertebra**

        ⑦S22.058   **Other fracture of T5-T6 vertebra**

        ⑦S22.059   **Unspecified fracture of T5-T6 vertebra**

    S22.06   Fracture of T7-T8 vertebra

        ⑦S22.060   **Wedge compression fracture of T7-T8 vertebra**

        ⑦S22.061   **Stable burst fracture of T7-T8 vertebra**

        ⑦S22.062   **Unstable burst fracture of T7-T8 vertebra**

        ⑦S22.068   **Other fracture of T7-T8 thoracic vertebra**

        ⑦S22.069   **Unspecified fracture of T7-T8 vertebra**

    S22.07   Fracture of T9-T10 vertebra

        ⑦S22.070   **Wedge compression fracture of T9-T10 vertebra**

        ⑦S22.071   **Stable burst fracture of T9-T10 vertebra**

        ⑦S22.072   **Unstable burst fracture of T9-T10 vertebra**

        ⑦S22.078   **Other fracture of T9-T10 vertebra**

        ⑦S22.079   **Unspecified fracture of T9-T10 vertebra**

    S22.08   Fracture of T11-T12 vertebra

        ⑦S22.080   **Wedge compression fracture of T11-T12 vertebra**

        ⑦S22.081   **Stable burst fracture of T11-T12 vertebra**

        ⑦S22.082   **Unstable burst fracture of T11-T12 vertebra**

        ⑦S22.088   **Other fracture of T11-T12 vertebra**

        ⑦S22.089   **Unspecified fracture of T11-T12 vertebra**

S22.2   Fracture of sternum

    ⊗⑦S22.20   **Unspecified fracture of sternum**

    ⊗⑦S22.21   **Fracture of manubrium**

    ⊗⑦S22.22   **Fracture of body of sternum**

    ⊗⑦S22.23   **Sternal manubrial dissociation**

    ⊗⑦S22.24   **Fracture of xiphoid process**

S22.3   Fracture of one rib

    ⊗⑦S22.31   **Fracture of one rib, right side**

    ⊗⑦S22.32   **Fracture of one rib, left side**

    ⊗⑦S22.39   **Fracture of one rib, unspecified side**

S22.4   Multiple fractures of ribs

    Fractures of two or more ribs

    Excludes1: flail chest (S22.5-)

    ⊗⑦S22.41   **Multiple fractures of ribs, right side**

    ⊗⑦S22.42   **Multiple fractures of ribs, left side**

▨ Add 4th-7th digits	▨ Nonspecific code	▨ Unspecified code	▨ Manifestation code

⊗⑦**S22.43** **Multiple fractures of ribs, bilateral**

⊗⑦**S22.49** **Multiple fractures of ribs, unspecified side**

⊗⑦**S22.5** **Flail chest**

⊗⑦**S22.9** **Fracture of bony thorax, part unspecified**

S23 **Dislocation and sprain of joints and ligaments of thorax**

Includes: avulsion of joint or ligament of thorax

laceration of cartilage, joint or ligament of thorax

sprain of cartilage, joint or ligament of thorax

traumatic hemarthrosis of joint or ligament of thorax

traumatic rupture of joint or ligament of thorax

traumatic subluxation of joint or ligament of thorax

traumatic tear of joint or ligament of thorax

Code also any associated open wound

Excludes2: dislocation, sprain of sternoclavicular joint (S43.2, S43.6)

strain of muscle or tendon of thorax (S29.01-)

The appropriate 7th character is to be added to each code from category S23

A - initial encounter

D - subsequent encounter

S - sequela

⊗⑦**S23.0** **Traumatic rupture of thoracic intervertebral disc**

Excludes1: rupture or displacement (nontraumatic) of thoracic intervertebral disc NOS (M51.- with fifth character 4)

S23.1 **Subluxation and dislocation of thoracic vertebra**

Code also any associated

open wound of thorax (S21.-)

spinal cord injury (S24.0-, S24.1-)

Excludes2: fracture of thoracic vertebrae (S22.0-)

S23.10 **Subluxation and dislocation of unspecified thoracic vertebra**

⑦**S23.100** **Subluxation of unspecified thoracic vertebra**

⑦**S23.101** **Dislocation of unspecified thoracic vertebra**

S23.11 **Subluxation and dislocation of T1/T2 thoracic vertebra**

⑦**S23.110** **Subluxation of T1/T2 thoracic vertebra**

⑦**S23.111** **Dislocation of T1/T2 thoracic vertebra**

S23.12 **Subluxation and dislocation of T2/T3-T3/T4 thoracic vertebra**

⑦**S23.120** **Subluxation of T2/T3 thoracic vertebra**

⑦**S23.121** **Dislocation of T2/T3 thoracic vertebra**

⑦**S23.122** **Subluxation of T3/T4 thoracic vertebra**

⑦**S23.123** **Dislocation of T3/T4 thoracic vertebra**

S23.13 **Subluxation and dislocation of T4/T5-T5/T6 thoracic vertebra**

⑦**S23.130** **Subluxation of T4/T5 thoracic vertebra**

⑦**S23.131** **Dislocation of T4/T5 thoracic vertebra**

⑦**S23.132** **Subluxation of T5/T6 thoracic vertebra**

⑦**S23.133** **Dislocation of T5/T6 thoracic vertebra**

S23.14 **Subluxation and dislocation of T6/T7-T7/T8 thoracic vertebra**

⑦**S23.140** **Subluxation of T6/T7 thoracic vertebra**

⑦**S23.141** **Dislocation of T6/T7 thoracic vertebra**

⑦**S23.142** **Subluxation of T7/T8 thoracic vertebra**

⑦**S23.143** **Dislocation of T7/T8thoracic vertebra**

S23.15 **Subluxation and dislocation of T8/T9-T9/T10 thoracic vertebra**

⑦**S23.150** **Subluxation of T8/T9thoracic vertebra**

⑦**S23.151** **Dislocation of T8/T9thoracic vertebra**

⑦**S23.152** **Subluxation of T9/T10thoracic vertebra**

⑦**S23.153** **Dislocation of T9/T10thoracic vertebra**

S23.16 **Subluxation and dislocation of T10/T11-T11/T12 thoracic vertebra**

⑦**S23.160** **Subluxation of T10/T11thoracic vertebra**

⑦**S23.161** **Dislocation of T10/T11thoracic vertebra**

⑦**S23.162** **Subluxation of T11/T12thoracic vertebra**

⑦**S23.163** **Dislocation of T11/T12thoracic vertebra**

S23.17 **Subluxation and dislocation of T12/L1 thoracic vertebra**

⑦**S23.170** **Subluxation of T12/L1 thoracic vertebra**

⑦**S23.171** **Dislocation of T12/L1 thoracic vertebra**

S23.2 **Dislocation of other and unspecified parts of thorax**

⊗⑦**S23.20** **Dislocation of unspecified part of thorax**

⊗⑦**S23.29** **Dislocation of other parts of thorax**

⊗⑦**S23.3** **Sprain of ligaments of thoracic spine**

S23.4 **Sprain of ribs and sternum**

⊗⑦**S23.41** **Sprain of ribs**

S23.42 **Sprain of sternum**

⑦**S23.420** **Sprain of sternoclavicular (joint) (ligament)**

⑦**S23.421** **Sprain of chondrosternal joint**

⑦**S23.428** **Other sprain of sternum**

⑦**S23.429** **Unspecified sprain of sternum**

⊗⑦**S23.8** **Sprain of other specified parts of thorax**

⊗⑦**S23.9** **Sprain of unspecified parts of thorax**

S24 **Injury of nerves and spinal cord at thorax level**

Note: Code to highest level of thoracic spinal cord injury

Injuries to the spinal cord (S24.0 and S24.1) refer to the cord level and not bone level injury, and can affect nerve roots at and below the level given.

● New code ▲ Revised code **Excludes1:** Not coded here **Excludes2:** Not included here ⊗ Placeholder required ⑦7th digit required

Code also any associated:

fracture of thoracic vertebra (S22.0-)

open wound of thorax (S21.-)

transient paralysis (R29.5)

Excludes2: injury of brachial plexus (S14.3)

The appropriate 7th character is to be added to each code from category S24

A - initial encounter

D - subsequent encounter

S - sequela

⊗⑦**S24.0   Concussion and edema of thoracic spinal cord**

S24.1   Other and unspecified injuries of thoracic spinal cord

 S24.10   Unspecified injury of thoracic spinal cord

  ⑦**S24.101   Unspecified injury at T1 level of thoracic spinal cord**

  ⑦**S24.102   Unspecified injury at T2-T6 level of thoracic spinal cord**

  ⑦**S24.103   Unspecified injury at T7-T10 level of thoracic spinal cord**

  ⑦**S24.104   Unspecified injury at T11-T12 level of thoracic spinal cord**

  ⑦**S24.109   Unspecified injury at unspecified level of thoracic spinal cord**

   Injury of thoracic spinal cord NOS

 S24.11   Complete lesion of thoracic spinal cord

  ⑦**S24.111   Complete lesion at T1 level of thoracic spinal cord**

  ⑦**S24.112   Complete lesion at T2-T6 level of thoracic spinal cord**

  ⑦**S24.113   Complete lesion at T7-T10 level of thoracic spinal cord**

  ⑦**S24.114   Complete lesion at T11-T12 level of thoracic spinal cord**

  ⑦**S24.119   Complete lesion at unspecified level of thoracic spinal cord**

 S24.13   Anterior cord syndrome of thoracic spinal cord

  ⑦**S24.131   Anterior cord syndrome at T1 level of thoracic spinal cord**

  ⑦**S24.132   Anterior cord syndrome at T2-T6 level of thoracic spinal cord**

  ⑦**S24.133   Anterior cord syndrome at T7-T10 level of thoracic spinal cord**

  ⑦**S24.134   Anterior cord syndrome at T11-T12 level of thoracic spinal cord**

  ⑦**S24.139   Anterior cord syndrome at unspecified level of thoracic spinal cord**

 S24.14   Brown-Séquard syndrome of thoracic spinal cord

  ⑦**S24.141   Brown-Séquard syndrome at T1 level of thoracic spinal cord**

  ⑦**S24.142   Brown-Séquard syndrome at T2-T6 level of thoracic spinal cord**

  ⑦**S24.143   Brown-Séquard syndrome at T7-T10 level of thoracic spinal cord**

  ⑦**S24.144   Brown-Séquard syndrome at T11-T12 level of thoracic spinal cord**

  ⑦**S24.149   Brown-Séquard syndrome at unspecified level of thoracic spinal cord**

 S24.15   Other incomplete lesions of thoracic spinal cord

  Incomplete lesion of thoracic spinal cord NOS

  Posterior cord syndrome of thoracic spinal cord

  ⑦**S24.151   Other incomplete lesion at T1 level of thoracic spinal cord**

  ⑦**S24.152   Other incomplete lesion at T2-T6 level of thoracic spinal cord**

  ⑦**S24.153   Other incomplete lesion at T7-T10 level of thoracic spinal cord**

  ⑦**S24.154   Other incomplete lesion at T11-T12 level of thoracic spinal cord**

  ⑦**S24.159   Other incomplete lesion at unspecified level of thoracic spinal cord**

⊗⑦**S24.2   Injury of nerve root of thoracic spine**

⊗⑦**S24.3   Injury of peripheral nerves of thorax**

⊗⑦**S24.4   Injury of thoracic sympathetic nervous system**

 Injury of cardiac plexus

 Injury of esophageal plexus

 Injury of pulmonary plexus

 Injury of stellate ganglion

 Injury of thoracic sympathetic ganglion

⊗⑦**S24.8   Injury of other specified nerves of thorax**

⊗⑦**S24.9   Injury of unspecified nerve of thorax**

S25   Injury of blood vessels of thorax

Code also any associated open wound (S21.-)

The appropriate 7th character is to be added to each code from category S25

A - initial encounter

D - subsequent encounter

S - sequela

S25.0   Injury of thoracic aorta

 Injury of aorta NOS

 ⊗⑦**S25.00   Unspecified injury of thoracic aorta**

 ⊗⑦**S25.01   Minor laceration of thoracic aorta**

  Incomplete transection of thoracic aorta

  Laceration of thoracic aorta NOS

  Superficial laceration of thoracic aorta

 ⊗⑦**S25.02   Major laceration of thoracic aorta**

  Complete transection of thoracic aorta

  Traumatic rupture of thoracic aorta

 ⊗⑦**S25.09   Other specified injury of thoracic aorta**

S25.1   Injury of innominate or subclavian artery

 S25.10   Unspecified injury of innominate or subclavian artery

  ⑦**S25.101   Unspecified injury of right innominate or subclavian artery injury of left innominate or subclavian artery**

  ⑦**S25.109   Unspecified injury of unspecified innominate or subclavian artery**

 S25.11   Minor laceration of innominate or subclavian artery

Incomplete transection of innominate or subclavian artery

Laceration of innominate or subclavian artery NOS

Superficial laceration of innominate or subclavian artery

⑦S25.111 **Minor laceration of right innominate or subclavian artery**

⑦S25.112 **Minor laceration of left innominate or subclavian artery**

⑦S25.119 **Minor laceration of unspecified innominate or subclavian artery**

S25.12 **Major laceration of innominate or subclavian artery**

Complete transection of innominate or subclavian artery

Traumatic rupture of innominate or subclavian artery

⑦S25.121 **Major laceration of right innominate or subclavian artery**

⑦S25.122 **Major laceration of left innominate or subclavian artery**

⑦S25.129 **Major laceration of unspecified innominate or subclavian artery**

S25.19 **Other specified injury of innominate or subclavian artery**

⑦S25.191 **Other specified injury of right innominate or subclavian artery**

⑦S25.192 **Other specified injury of left innominate or subclavian artery**

⑦S25.199 **Other specified injury of unspecified innominate or subclavian artery**

S25.2 **Injury of superior vena cava**

Injury of vena cava NOS

⊗⑦S25.20 **Unspecified injury of superior vena cava**

⊗⑦S25.21 **Minor laceration of superior vena cava**

Incomplete transection of superior vena cava

Laceration of superior vena cava NOS

Superficial laceration of superior vena cava

⊗⑦S25.22 **Major laceration of superior vena cava**

Complete transection of superior vena cava

Traumatic rupture of superior vena cava

⊗⑦S25.29 **Other specified injury of superior vena cava**

S25.3 **Injury of innominate or subclavian vein**

S25.30 **Unspecified injury of innominate or subclavian vein**

⑦S25.301 **Unspecified injury of right innominate or subclavian vein**

⑦S25.302 **Unspecified injury of left innominate or subclavian vein**

⑦S25.309 **Unspecified injury of unspecified innominate or subclavian vein**

S25.31 **Minor laceration of innominate or subclavian vein**

Incomplete transection of innominate or subclavian vein

Laceration of innominate or subclavian vein NOS

Superficial laceration of innominate or subclavian vein

⑦S25.311 **Minor laceration of right innominate or subclavian vein**

⑦S25.312 **Minor laceration of left innominate or subclavian vein**

⑦S25.319 **Minor laceration of unspecified innominate or subclavian vein**

S25.32 **Major laceration of innominate or subclavian vein**

Complete transection of innominate or subclavian vein

Traumatic rupture of innominate or subclavian vein

⑦S25.321 **Major laceration of right innominate or subclavian vein**

⑦S25.322 **Major laceration of left innominate or subclavian vein**

⑦S25.329 **Major laceration of unspecified innominate or subclavian vein**

S25.39 **Other specified injury of innominate or subclavian vein**

⑦S25.391 **Other specified injury of right innominate or subclavian vein**

⑦S25.392 **Other specified injury of left innominate or subclavian vein**

⑦S25.399 **Other specified injury of unspecified innominate or subclavian vein**

S25.4 **Injury of pulmonary blood vessels**

S25.40 **Unspecified injury of pulmonary blood vessels**

⑦S25.401 **Unspecified injury of right pulmonary blood vessels**

⑦S25.402 **Unspecified injury of left pulmonary blood vessels**

⑦S25.409 **Unspecified injury of unspecified pulmonary blood vessels**

S25.41 **Minor laceration of pulmonary blood vessels**

Incomplete transection of pulmonary blood vessels

Laceration of pulmonary blood vessels NOS

Superficial laceration of pulmonary blood vessels

⑦S25.411 **Minor laceration of right pulmonary blood vessels**

⑦S25.412 **Minor laceration of left pulmonary blood vessels**

⑦S25.419 **Minor laceration of unspecified pulmonary blood vessels**

S25.42 **Major laceration of pulmonary blood vessels**

Complete transection of pulmonary blood vessels

Traumatic rupture of pulmonary blood vessels

⑦S25.421 **Major laceration of right pulmonary blood vessels**

⑦S25.422 **Major laceration of left pulmonary blood vessels**

⑦S25.429 **Major laceration of unspecified pulmonary blood vessels**

S25.49 **Other specified injury of pulmonary blood vessels**

⑦S25.491 **Other specified injury of right pulmonary blood vessels**

● New code   ▲ Revised code   **Excludes1:** Not coded here   **Excludes2:** Not included here   ⊗ Placeholder required   ⑦ 7th digit required

⑦**S25.492** **Other specified injury of left pulmonary blood vessels**

⑦**S25.499** **Other specified injury of unspecified pulmonary blood vessels**

S25.5 **Injury of intercostal blood vessels**

    S25.50 **Unspecified injury of intercostal blood vessels**

      ⑦**S25.501** **Unspecified injury of intercostal blood vessels, right side**

      ⑦**S25.502** **Unspecified injury of intercostal blood vessels, left side**

      ⑦**S25.509** **Unspecified injury of intercostal blood vessels, unspecified side**

    S25.51 **Laceration of intercostal blood vessels**

      ⑦**S25.511** **Laceration of intercostal blood vessels, right side**

      ⑦**S25.512** **Laceration of intercostal blood vessels, left side**

      ⑦**S25.519** **Laceration of intercostal blood vessels, unspecified side**

    S25.59 **Other specified injury of intercostal blood vessels**

      ⑦**S25.591** **Other specified injury of intercostal blood vessels, right side**

      ⑦**S25.592** **Other specified injury of intercostal blood vessels, left side**

      ⑦**S25.599** **Other specified injury of intercostal blood vessels, unspecified side**

S25.8 **Injury of other blood vessels of thorax**

    Injury of azygos vein

    Injury of mammary artery or vein

    S25.80 **Unspecified injury of other blood vessels of thorax**

      ⑦**S25.801** **Unspecified injury of other blood vessels of thorax, right side**

      ⑦**S25.802** **Unspecified injury of other blood vessels of thorax, left side**

      ⑦**S25.809** **Unspecified injury of other blood vessels of thorax, unspecified side**

    S25.81 **Laceration of other blood vessels of thorax**

      ⑦**S25.811** **Laceration of other blood vessels of thorax, right side**

      ⑦**S25.812** **Laceration of other blood vessels of thorax, left side**

      ⑦**S25.819** **Laceration of other blood vessels of thorax, unspecified side**

    S25.89 **Other specified injury of other blood vessels of thorax**

      ⑦**S25.891** **Other specified injury of other blood vessels of thorax, right side**

      ⑦**S25.892** **Other specified injury of other blood vessels of thorax, left side**

      ⑦**S25.899** **Other specified injury of other blood vessels of thorax, unspecified side**

S25.9 **Injury of unspecified blood vessel of thorax**

    S25.90 **Unspecified injury of unspecified blood vessel of thorax**

      ⑦**S25.90** **Unspecified injury of unspecified blood vessel of thorax**

      ⑦**S25.91** **Laceration of unspecified blood vessel of thorax**

⑦**S25.99** **Other specified injury of unspecified blood vessel of thorax**

S26 **Injury of heart**

Code also any associated:

open wound of thorax (S21.-)

traumatic hemopneumothorax (S27.2)

traumatic hemothorax (S27.1)

traumatic pneumothorax (S27.0)

The appropriate 7th character is to be added to each code from category S26

A - initial encounter

D - subsequent encounter

S - sequela

S26.0 **Injury of heart with hemopericardium**

    ⊗⑦**S26.00** **Unspecified injury of heart with hemopericardium**

    ⊗⑦**S26.01** **Contusion of heart with hemopericardium**

    S26.02 **Laceration of heart with hemopericardium**

      ⑦**S26.020** **Mild laceration of heart with hemopericardium**

          Laceration of heart without penetration of heart chamber

      ⑦**S26.021** **Moderate laceration of heart with hemopericardium**

          Laceration of heart with penetration of heart chamber

      ⑦**S26.022** **Major laceration of heart with hemopericardium**

          Laceration of heart with penetration of multiple heart chambers

    ⊗⑦**S26.09** **Other injury of heart with hemopericardium**

S26.1 **Injury of heart without hemopericardium**

    ⊗⑦**S26.10** **Unspecified injury of heart without hemopericardium**

    ⊗⑦**S26.11** **Contusion of heart without hemopericardium**

    ⊗⑦**S26.12** **Laceration of heart without hemopericardium**

    ⊗⑦**S26.19** **Other injury of heart without hemopericardium**

S26.9 **Injury of heart, unspecified with or without hemopericardium**

    ⊗⑦**S26.90** **Unspecified injury of heart, unspecified with or without hemopericardium**

    ⊗⑦**S26.91** **Contusion of heart, unspecified with or without hemopericardium**

    ⊗⑦**S26.92** **Laceration of heart, unspecified with or without hemopericardium**

      Laceration of heart NOS

    ⊗⑦**S26.99** **Other injury of heart, unspecified with or without hemopericardium**

S27 **Injury of other and unspecified intrathoracic organs**

Code also any associated open wound of thorax (S21.-)

Excludes2: injury of cervical esophagus (S10-S19)

    injury of trachea (cervical) (S10-S19)

The appropriate 7th character is to be added to each code from category S27

A - initial encounter

D - subsequent encounter

S - sequela

⊗⑦**S27.0** **Traumatic pneumothorax**

    Excludes1: spontaneous pneumothorax (J93.-)

⊗⑦**S27.1** **Traumatic hemothorax**

⊗⑦**S27.2** **Traumatic hemopneumothorax**

⊗⑦**S27.3** **Other and unspecified injuries of lung**

    S27.30 **Unspecified injury of lung**

      ⑦**S27.301** **Unspecified injury of lung, unilateral**

      ⑦**S27.302** **Unspecified injury of lung, bilateral**

      ⑦**S27.309** **Unspecified injury of lung, unspecified**

    S27.31 **Primary blast injury of lung**

      Blast injury of lung NOS

      ⑦**S27.311** **Primary blast injury of lung, unilateral**

      ⑦**S27.312** **Primary blast injury of lung, bilateral**

      ⑦**S27.319** **Primary blast injury of lung, unspecified**

    S27.32 **Contusion of lung**

      ⑦**S27.321** **Contusion of lung, unilateral**

      ⑦**S27.322** **Contusion of lung, bilateral**

      ⑦**S27.329** **Contusion of lung, unspecified**

    S27.33 **Laceration of lung**

      ⑦**S27.331** **Laceration of lung, unilateral**

      ⑦**S27.332** **Laceration of lung, bilateral**

      ⑦**S27.339** **Laceration of lung, unspecified**

    S27.39 **Other injuries of lung**

      Secondary blast injury of lung

      ⑦**S27.391** **Other injuries of lung, unilateral**

      ⑦**S27.392** **Other injuries of lung, bilateral**

      ⑦**S27.399** **Other injuries of lung, unspecified**

S27.4 **Injury of bronchus**

    S27.40 **Unspecified injury of bronchus**

      ⑦**S27.401** **Unspecified injury of bronchus, unilateral**

      ⑦**S27.402** **Unspecified injury of bronchus, bilateral**

      ⑦**S27.409** **Unspecified injury of bronchus, unspecified**

    S27.41 **Primary blast injury of bronchus**

      Blast injury of bronchus NOS

      ⑦**S27.411** **Primary blast injury of bronchus, unilateral**

      ⑦**S27.412** **Primary blast injury of bronchus, bilateral**

      ⑦**S27.419** **Primary blast injury of bronchus, unspecified**

    S27.42 **Contusion of bronchus**

      ⑦**S27.421** **Contusion of bronchus, unilateral**

      ⑦**S27.422** **Contusion of bronchus, bilateral**

      ⑦**S27.429** **Contusion of bronchus, unspecified**

    S27.43 **Laceration of bronchus**

      ⑦**S27.431** **Laceration of bronchus, unilateral**

      ⑦**S27.432** **Laceration of bronchus, bilateral**

      ⑦**S27.439** **Laceration of bronchus, unspecified**

    S27.49 **Other injury of bronchus**

      Secondary blast injury of bronchus

      ⑦**S27.491** **Other injury of bronchus, unilateral**

      ⑦**S27.492** **Other injury of bronchus, bilateral**

      ⑦**S27.499** **Other injury of bronchus, unspecified**

S27.5 **Injury of thoracic trachea**

    ⊗⑦**S27.50** **Unspecified injury of thoracic trachea**

    ⊗⑦**S27.51** **Primary blast injury of thoracic trachea**

      Blast injury of thoracic trachea NOS

    ⊗⑦**S27.52** **Contusion of thoracic trachea**

    ⊗⑦**S27.53** **Laceration of thoracic trachea**

    ⊗⑦**S27.59** **Other injury of thoracic trachea**

      Secondary blast injury of thoracic trachea

S27.6 **Injury of pleura**

    ⊗⑦**S27.60** **Unspecified injury of pleura**

    ⊗⑦**S27.63** **Laceration of pleura**

    ⊗⑦**S27.69** **Other injury of pleura**

S27.8 **Injury of other specified intrathoracic organs**

    S27.80 **Injury of diaphragm**

      ⑦**S27.802** **Contusion of diaphragm**

      ⑦**S27.803** **Laceration of diaphragm**

      ⑦**S27.808** **Other injury of diaphragm**

      ⑦**S27.809** **Unspecified injury of diaphragm**

    S27.81 **Injury of esophagus (thoracic part)**

      ⑦**S27.812** **Contusion of esophagus (thoracic part)**

      ⑦**S27.813** **Laceration of esophagus (thoracic part)**

      ⑦**S27.818** **Other injury of esophagus (thoracic part)**

      ⑦**S27.819** **Unspecified injury of esophagus (thoracic part)**

    S27.89 **Injury of other specified intrathoracic organs**

      Injury of lymphatic thoracic duct

      Injury of thymus gland

      ⑦**S27.892** **Contusion of other specified intrathoracic organs**

      ⑦**S27.893** **Laceration of other specified intrathoracic organs**

      ⑦**S27.898** **Other injury of other specified intrathoracic organs**

      ⑦**S27.899** **Unspecified injury of other specified intrathoracic organs**

⊗⑦**S27.9** **Injury of unspecified intrathoracic organ**

S28 **Crushing injury of thorax, and traumatic amputation of part of thorax**

The appropriate 7th character is to be added to each code from category S28

A - initial encounter

D - subsequent encounter

S - sequela

⊗⑦**S28.0** **Crushed chest**

    Use additional code for all associated injuries

    Excludes1: flail chest (S22.5)

⊗⑦**S28.1** **Traumatic amputation (partial) of part of thorax, except breast**

● New code   ▲ Revised code   **Excludes1:** Not coded here   **Excludes2:** Not included here   ⊗ Placeholder required   ⑦ 7th digit required

S28.2   **Traumatic amputation of breast**

    S28.21   **Complete traumatic amputation of breast**

        Traumatic amputation of breast NOS

        ⑦ **S28.211**   **Complete traumatic amputation of right breast**

        ⑦ **S28.212**   **Complete traumatic amputation of left breast**

        ⑦ **S28.219**   **Complete traumatic amputation of unspecified breast**

    S28.22   **Partial traumatic amputation of breast**

        ⑦ **S28.221**   **Partial traumatic amputation of right breast**

        ⑦ **S28.222**   **Partial traumatic amputation of left breast**

        ⑦ **S28.229**   **Partial traumatic amputation of unspecified breast**

S29   **Other and unspecified injuries of thorax**

Code also any associated open wound (S21.-)

The appropriate 7th character is to be added to each code from category S29

A - initial encounter

D - subsequent encounter

S - sequela

S29.0   **Injury of muscle and tendon at thorax level**

    S29.00   **Unspecified injury of muscle and tendon of thorax**

        ⑦ **S29.001**   **Unspecified injury of muscle and tendon of front wall of thorax**

        ⑦ **S29.002**   **Unspecified injury of muscle and tendon of back wall of thorax**

        ⑦ **S29.009**   **Unspecified injury of muscle and tendon of unspecified wall of thorax**

    S29.01   **Strain of muscle and tendon of thorax**

        ⑦ **S29.011**   **Strain of muscle and tendon of front wall of thorax**

        ⑦ **S29.012**   **Strain of muscle and tendon of back wall of thorax**

        ⑦ **S29.019**   **Strain of muscle and tendon of unspecified wall of thorax**

    S29.02   **Laceration of muscle and tendon of thorax**

        ⑦ **S29.021**   **Laceration of muscle and tendon of front wall of thorax**

        ⑦ **S29.022**   **Laceration of muscle and tendon of back wall of thorax**

        ⑦ **S29.029**   **Laceration of muscle and tendon of unspecified wall of thorax**

    S29.09   **Other injury of muscle and tendon of thorax**

        ⑦ **S29.091**   **Other injury of muscle and tendon of front wall of thorax**

        ⑦ **S29.092**   **Other injury of muscle and tendon of back wall of thorax**

        ⑦ **S29.099**   **Other injury of muscle and tendon of unspecified wall of thorax**

⊗⑦ **S29.8**   **Other specified injuries of thorax**

⊗⑦ **S29.9**   **Unspecified injury of thorax**

INJURIES TO THE ABDOMEN, LOWER BACK, LUMBAR SPINE, PELVIS AND EXTERNAL GENITALS (S30-S39)

Includes: injuries to the abdominal wall

injuries to the anus injuries to the buttock

injuries to the external genitalia injuries to the flank

injuries to the groin

Excludes2: burns and corrosions (T20-T32)

effects of foreign body in anus and rectum (T18.5)

effects of foreign body in genitourinary tract (T19.-)

effects of foreign body in stomach, small intestine and colon (T18.2-T18.4)

frostbite (T33-T34)

insect bite or sting, venomous (T63.4)

S30   **Superficial injury of abdomen, lower back, pelvis and external genitals**

Excludes2: superficial injury of hip (S70.-)

The appropriate 7th character is to be added to each code from category S30

A - initial encounter

D - subsequent encounter

S - sequela

⊗⑦ **S30.0**   **Contusion of lower back and pelvis**

    Contusion of buttock

⊗⑦ **S30.1**   **Contusion of abdominal wall**

    Contusion of flank

    Contusion of groin

S30.2   **Contusion of external genital organs**

    S30.20   **Contusion of unspecified external genital organ**

        ⑦ **S30.201**   **Contusion of unspecified external genital organ, male**

        ⑦ **S30.202**   **Contusion of unspecified external genital organ, female**

    ⊗⑦ **S30.21**   **Contusion of penis**

    ⊗⑦ **S30.22**   **Contusion of scrotum and testes**

    ⊗⑦ **S30.23**   **Contusion of vagina and vulva**

S30.3   **Contusion of anus**

S30.8   **Other superficial injuries of abdomen, lower back, pelvis and external genitals**

    S30.81   **Abrasion of abdomen, lower back, pelvis and external genitals**

        ⑦ **S30.810**   **Abrasion of lower back and pelvis**

        ⑦ **S30.811**   **Abrasion of abdominal wall**

        ⑦ **S30.812**   **Abrasion of penis**

        ⑦ **S30.813**   **Abrasion of scrotum and testes**

        ⑦ **S30.814**   **Abrasion of vagina and vulva**

        ⑦ **S30.815**   **Abrasion of unspecified external genital organs, male**

        ⑦ **S30.816**   **Abrasion of unspecified external genital organs, female**

        ⑦ **S30.817**   **Abrasion of anus**

    S30.82   **Blister (nonthermal) of abdomen, lower back, pelvis and external genitals**

        ⑦ **S30.820**   **Blister (nonthermal) of lower back and pelvis**

        ⑦ **S30.821**   **Blister (nonthermal) of abdominal wall**

        ⑦ **S30.822**   **Blister (nonthermal) of penis**

        ⑦ **S30.823**   **Blister (nonthermal) of scrotum and testes**

⑦S30.824   **Blister (nonthermal) of vagina and vulva**

⑦S30.825   **Blister (nonthermal) of unspecified external genital organs, male**

⑦S30.826   **Blister (nonthermal) of unspecified external genital organs, female**

⑦S30.827   **Blister (nonthermal) of anus**

S30.84   **External constriction of abdomen, lower back, pelvis and external genitals**

⑦S30.840   **External constriction of lower back and pelvis**

⑦S30.841   **External constriction of abdominal wall**

⑦S30.842   **External constriction of penis**

Hair tourniquet syndrome of penis

Use additional cause code to identify the constricting item (W49.0-)

⑦S30.843   **External constriction of scrotum and testes**

⑦S30.844   **External constriction of vagina and vulva**

⑦S30.845   **External constriction of unspecified external genital organs, male**

⑦S30.846   **External constriction of unspecified external genital organs, female**

S30.85   **Superficial foreign body of abdomen, lower back, pelvis and external genitals**

Splinter in the abdomen, lower back, pelvis and external genitals

⑦S30.850   **Superficial foreign body of lower back and pelvis**

⑦S30.851   **Superficial foreign body of abdominal wall**

⑦S30.852   **Superficial foreign body of penis**

⑦S30.853   **Superficial foreign body of scrotum and testes**

⑦S30.854   **Superficial foreign body of vagina and vulva**

⑦S30.855   **Superficial foreign body of unspecified external genital organs, male**

⑦S30.856   **Superficial foreign body of unspecified external genital organs, female**

⑦S30.857   **Superficial foreign body of anus**

S30.86   **Insect bite (nonvenomous) of abdomen, lower back, pelvis and external genitals**

⑦S30.860   **Insect bite (nonvenomous) of lower back and pelvis**

⑦S30.861   **Insect bite (nonvenomous) of abdominal wall**

⑦S30.862   **Insect bite (nonvenomous) of penis**

⑦S30.863   **Insect bite (nonvenomous) of scrotum and testes**

⑦S30.864   **Insect bite (nonvenomous) of vagina and vulva**

⑦S30.865   **Insect bite (nonvenomous) of unspecified external genital organs, male**

⑦S30.866   **Insect bite (nonvenomous) of unspecified external genital organs, female**

⑦S30.867   **Insect bite (nonvenomous) of anus**

S30.87   **Other superficial bite of abdomen, lower back, pelvis and external genitals**

Excludes1: open bite of abdomen, lower back, pelvis and external genitals (S31.05, S31.15, S31.25, S31.35, S31.45, S31.55)

⑦S30.870   **Other superficial bite of lower back and pelvis**

⑦S30.871   **Other superficial bite of abdominal wall**

⑦S30.872   **Other superficial bite of penis**

⑦S30.873   **Other superficial bite of scrotum and testes**

⑦S30.874   **Other superficial bite of vagina and vulva**

⑦S30.875   **Other superficial bite of unspecified external genital organs, male**

⑦S30.876   **Other superficial bite of unspecified external genital organs, female**

⑦S30.877   **Other superficial bite of anus**

S30.9   **Unspecified superficial injury of abdomen, lower back, pelvis and external genitals**

⊗⑦S30.91   **Unspecified superficial injury of lower back and pelvis**

⊗⑦S30.92   **Unspecified superficial injury of abdominal wall**

⊗⑦S30.93   **Unspecified superficial injury of penis**

⊗⑦S30.94   **Unspecified superficial injury of scrotum and testes**

⊗⑦S30.95   **Unspecified superficial injury of vagina and vulva**

⊗⑦S30.96   **Unspecified superficial injury of unspecified external genital organs, male**

⊗⑦S30.97   **Unspecified superficial injury of unspecified external genital organs, female**

⊗⑦S30.98   **Unspecified superficial injury of anus**

S31   **Open wound of abdomen, lower back, pelvis and external genitals**

Code also any associated:

spinal cord injury (S24.0, S24.1-, S34.0-, S34.1-)

wound infection

Excludes1: traumatic amputation of part of abdomen, lower back and pelvis (S38.2-, S38.3)

Excludes2: open wound of hip (S71.00-S71.02)

open fracture of pelvis (S32.1--S32.9 with 7th character B)

The appropriate 7th character is to be added to each code from category S31

A - initial encounter

D - subsequent encounter

S - sequela

S31.0   **Open wound of lower back and pelvis**

S31.00   **Unspecified open wound of lower back and pelvis**

⑦S31.000   **Unspecified open wound of lower back and pelvis without penetration into retroperitoneum**

● New code   ▲ Revised code   **Excludes1:** Not coded here   **Excludes2:** Not included here   ⊗ Placeholder required   ⑦7th digit required

Unspecified open wound of lower back and pelvis NOS

⑦ **S31.001** **Unspecified open wound of lower back and pelvis with penetration into retroperitoneum**

S31.01 **Laceration without foreign body of lower back and pelvis**

⑦ **S31.010** **Laceration without foreign body of lower back and pelvis without penetration into retroperitoneum**

Laceration without foreign body of lower back and pelvis NOS

⑦ **S31.011** **Laceration without foreign body of lower back and pelvis with penetration into retroperitoneum**

S31.02 **Laceration with foreign body of lower back and pelvis**

⑦ **S31.020** **Laceration with foreign body of lower back and pelvis without penetration into retroperitoneum**

Laceration with foreign body of lower back and pelvis NOS

⑦ **S31.021** **Laceration with foreign body of lower back and pelvis with penetration into retroperitoneum**

S31.03 **Puncture wound without foreign body of lower back and pelvis**

⑦ **S31.030** **Puncture wound without foreign body of lower back and pelvis without penetration into retroperitoneum**

Puncture wound without foreign body of lower back and pelvis NOS

⑦ **S31.031** **Puncture wound without foreign body of lower back and pelvis with penetration into retroperitoneum**

S31.04 **Puncture wound with foreign body of lower back and pelvis**

⑦ **S31.040** **Puncture wound with foreign body of lower back and pelvis without penetration into retroperitoneum**

Puncture wound with foreign body of lower back and pelvis NOS

⑦ **S31.041** **Puncture wound with foreign body of lower back and pelvis with penetration into retroperitoneum**

S31.05 **Open bite of lower back and pelvis**

Bite of lower back and pelvis NOS

Excludes1: superficial bite of lower back and pelvis (S30.860, S30.870)

⑦ **S31.050** **Open bite of lower back and pelvis without penetration into retroperitoneum**

Open bite of lower back and pelvis NOS

⑦ **S31.051** **Open bite of lower back and pelvis with penetration into retroperitoneum**

S31.1 **Open wound of abdominal wall without penetration into peritoneal cavity**

Open wound of abdominal wall NOS

Excludes2: open wound of abdominal wall with penetration into peritoneal cavity (S31.6-)

S31.10 **Unspecified open wound of abdominal wall without penetration into peritoneal cavity**

⑦ **S31.100** **Unspecified open wound of abdominal wall, right upper quadrant without penetration into peritoneal cavity**

⑦ **S31.101** **Unspecified open wound of abdominal wall, left upper quadrant without penetration into peritoneal cavity**

⑦ **S31.102** **Unspecified open wound of abdominal wall, epigastric region without penetration into peritoneal cavity**

⑦ **S31.103** **Unspecified open wound of abdominal wall, right lower quadrant without penetration into peritoneal cavity**

⑦ **S31.104** **Unspecified open wound of abdominal wall, left lower quadrant without penetration into peritoneal cavity**

⑦ **S31.105** **Unspecified open wound of abdominal wall, periumbilic region without penetration into peritoneal cavity**

⑦ **S31.109** **Unspecified open wound of abdominal wall, unspecified quadrant without penetration into peritoneal cavity**

Unspecified open wound of abdominal wall NOS

⑦ **S31.11** **Laceration without foreign body of abdominal wall without penetration into peritoneal cavity**

⑦ **S31.110** **Laceration without foreign body of abdominal wall, right upper quadrant without penetration into peritoneal cavity**

⑦ **S31.111** **Laceration without foreign body of abdominal wall, left upper quadrant without penetration into peritoneal cavity**

⑦ **S31.112** **Laceration without foreign body of abdominal wall, epigastric region without penetration into peritoneal cavity**

⑦ **S31.113** **Laceration without foreign body of abdominal wall, right lower quadrant without penetration into peritoneal cavity**

⑦ **S31.114** **Laceration without foreign body of abdominal wall, left lower quadrant without penetration into peritoneal cavity**

⑦ **S31.115** **Laceration without foreign body of abdominal wall, periumbilic region without penetration into peritoneal cavity**

⑦ **S31.119** **Laceration without foreign body of abdominal wall, unspecified quadrant without penetration into peritoneal cavity**

S31.12 **Laceration with foreign body of abdominal wall without penetration into peritoneal cavity**

⑦ **S31.120** Laceration of abdominal wall with foreign body, right upper quadrant without penetration into peritoneal cavity

⑦ **S31.121** Laceration of abdominal wall with foreign body, left upper quadrant without penetration into peritoneal cavity

⑦ **S31.122** Laceration of abdominal wall with foreign body, epigastric region without penetration into peritoneal cavity

⑦ **S31.123** Laceration of abdominal wall with foreign body, right lower quadrant without penetration into peritoneal cavity

⑦ **S31.124** Laceration of abdominal wall with foreign body, left lower quadrant without penetration into peritoneal cavity

⑦ **S31.125** Laceration of abdominal wall with foreign body, periumbilic region without penetration into peritoneal cavity

⑦ **S31.129** Laceration of abdominal wall with foreign body, unspecified quadrant without penetration into peritoneal cavity

S31.13 Puncture wound of abdominal wall without foreign body without penetration into peritoneal cavity

⑦ **S31.130** Puncture wound of abdominal wall without foreign body, right upper quadrant without penetration into peritoneal cavity

⑦ **S31.131** Puncture wound of abdominal wall without foreign body, left upper quadrant without penetration into peritoneal cavity

⑦ **S31.132** Puncture wound of abdominal wall without foreign body, epigastric region without penetration into peritoneal cavity

⑦ **S31.133** Puncture wound of abdominal wall without foreign body, right lower quadrant without penetration into peritoneal cavity

⑦ **S31.134** Puncture wound of abdominal wall without foreign body, left lower quadrant without penetration into peritoneal cavity

⑦ **S31.135** Puncture wound of abdominal wall without foreign body, periumbilic region without penetration into peritoneal cavity

⑦ **S31.139** Puncture wound of abdominal wall without foreign body, unspecified quadrant without penetration into peritoneal cavity

S31.14 Puncture wound of abdominal wall with foreign body without penetration into peritoneal cavity

⑦ **S31.140** Puncture wound of abdominal wall with foreign body, right upper quadrant without penetration into peritoneal cavity

⑦ **S31.141** Puncture wound of abdominal wall with foreign body, left upper quadrant without penetration into peritoneal cavity

⑦ **S31.142** Puncture wound of abdominal wall with foreign body, epigastric region without penetration into peritoneal cavity

⑦ **S31.143** Puncture wound of abdominal wall with foreign body, right lower quadrant without penetration into peritoneal cavity

⑦ **S31.144** Puncture wound of abdominal wall with foreign body, left lower quadrant without penetration into peritoneal cavity

⑦ **S31.145** Puncture wound of abdominal wall with foreign body, periumbilic region without penetration into peritoneal cavity

⑦ **S31.149** Puncture wound of abdominal wall with foreign body, unspecified quadrant without penetration into peritoneal cavity

S31.15 Open bite of abdominal wall without penetration into peritoneal cavity

Bite of abdominal wall NOS

Excludes1: superficial bite of abdominal wall (S30.871)

⑦ **S31.150** Open bite of abdominal wall, right upper quadrant without penetration into peritoneal cavity

⑦ **S31.151** Open bite of abdominal wall, left upper quadrant without penetration into peritoneal cavity

⑦ **S31.152** Open bite of abdominal wall, epigastric region without penetration into peritoneal cavity

⑦ **S31.153** Open bite of abdominal wall, right lower quadrant without penetration into peritoneal cavity

⑦ **S31.154** Open bite of abdominal wall, left lower quadrant without penetration into peritoneal cavity

⑦ **S31.155** Open bite of abdominal wall, periumbilic region without penetration into peritoneal cavity

⑦ **S31.159** Open bite of abdominal wall, unspecified quadrant without penetration into peritoneal cavity

S31.2 Open wound of penis

⊗⑦ **S31.20** Unspecified open wound of penis

⊗⑦ **S31.21** Laceration without foreign body of penis

⊗⑦ **S31.22** Laceration with foreign body of penis

⊗⑦ **S31.23** Puncture wound without foreign body of penis

⊗⑦ **S31.24** Puncture wound with foreign body of penis

⊗⑦ **S31.25** Open bite of penis

Bite of penis NOS

Excludes1: superficial bite of penis (S30.862, S30.872)

S31.3 Open wound of scrotum and testes

⊗⑦ **S31.30** Unspecified open wound of scrotum and testes

● New code ▲ Revised code **Excludes1:** Not coded here **Excludes2:** Not included here ⊗ Placeholder required ⑦7th digit required

⊗⑦**S31.31**   **Laceration without foreign body of scrotum and testes**

⊗⑦**S31.32**   **Laceration with foreign body of scrotum and testes**

⊗⑦**S31.33**   **Puncture wound without foreign body of scrotum and testes**

⊗⑦**S31.34**   **Puncture wound with foreign body of scrotum and testes**

⊗⑦**S31.35**   **Open bite of scrotum and testes**
Bite of scrotum and testes NOS
Excludes1: superficial bite of scrotum and testes (S30.863, S30.873)

S31.4   **Open wound of vagina and vulva**
Excludes1: injury to vagina and vulva during delivery (O70.-, O71.4)

⊗⑦**S31.40**   **Unspecified open wound of vagina and vulva**

⊗⑦**S31.41**   **Laceration without foreign body of vagina and vulva**

⊗⑦**S31.42**   **Laceration with foreign body of vagina and vulva**

⊗⑦**S31.43**   **Puncture wound without foreign body of vagina and vulva**

⊗⑦**S31.44**   **Puncture wound with foreign body of vagina and vulva**

⊗⑦**S31.45**   **Open bite of vagina and vulva**
Bite of vagina and vulva NOS
Excludes1: superficial bite of vagina and vulva (S30.864, S30.874)

S31.5   **Open wound of unspecified external genital organs**
Excludes1: traumatic amputation of external genital organs (S38.21, S38.22)

S31.50   **Unspecified open wound of unspecified external genital organs**

⑦**S31.501**   **Unspecified open wound of unspecified external genital organs, male**

⑦**S31.502**   **Unspecified open wound of unspecified external genital organs, female**

S31.51   **Laceration without foreign body of unspecified external genital organs**

⑦**S31.511**   **Laceration without foreign body of unspecified external genital organs, male**

⑦**S31.512**   **Laceration without foreign body of unspecified external genital organs, female**

S31.52   **Laceration with foreign body of unspecified external genital organs**

⑦**S31.521**   **Laceration with foreign body of unspecified external genital organs, male**

⑦**S31.522**   **Laceration with foreign body of unspecified external genital organs, female**

S31.53   **Puncture wound without foreign body of unspecified external genital organs**

⑦**S31.531**   **Puncture wound without foreign body of unspecified external genital organs, male**

⑦**S31.532**   **Puncture wound without foreign body of unspecified external genital organs, female**

S31.54   **Puncture wound with foreign body of unspecified external genital organs**

⑦**S31.541**   **Puncture wound with foreign body of unspecified external genital organs, male**

⑦**S31.542**   **Puncture wound with foreign body of unspecified external genital organs, female**

S31.55   **Open bite of unspecified external genital organs**
Bite of unspecified external genital organs NOS
Excludes1: superficial bite of unspecified external genital organs (S30.865, S30.866, S30.875, S30.876)

⑦**S31.551**   **Open bite of unspecified external genital organs, male**

⑦**S31.552**   **Open bite of unspecified external genital organs, female**

S31.6   **Open wound of abdominal wall with penetration into peritoneal cavity**

S31.60   **Unspecified open wound of abdominal wall with penetration into peritoneal cavity**

⑦**S31.600**   **Unspecified open wound of abdominal wall, right upper quadrant with penetration into peritoneal cavity**

⑦**S31.601**   **Unspecified open wound of abdominal wall, left upper quadrant with penetration into peritoneal cavity**

⑦**S31.602**   **Unspecified open wound of abdominal wall, epigastric region with penetration into peritoneal cavity**

⑦**S31.603**   **Unspecified open wound of abdominal wall, right lower quadrant with penetration into peritoneal cavity**

⑦**S31.604**   **Unspecified open wound of abdominal wall, left lower quadrant with penetration into peritoneal cavity**

⑦**S31.605**   **Unspecified open wound of abdominal wall, periumbilic region with penetration into peritoneal cavity**

⑦**S31.609**   **Unspecified open wound of abdominal wall, unspecified quadrant with penetration into peritoneal cavity**

S31.61   **Laceration without foreign body of abdominal wall with penetration into peritoneal cavity**

⑦**S31.610**   **Laceration without foreign body of abdominal wall, right upper quadrant with penetration into peritoneal cavity**

⑦**S31.611**   **Laceration without foreign body of abdominal wall, left upper quadrant with penetration into peritoneal cavity**

⑦S31.612 Laceration without foreign body of abdominal wall, epigastric region with penetration into peritoneal cavity

⑦S31.613 Laceration without foreign body of abdominal wall, right lower quadrant with penetration into peritoneal cavity

⑦S31.614 Laceration without foreign body of abdominal wall, left lower quadrant with penetration into peritoneal cavity

⑦S31.615 Laceration without foreign body of abdominal wall, periumbilic region with penetration into peritoneal cavity

⑦S31.619 Laceration without foreign body of abdominal wall, unspecified quadrant with penetration into peritoneal cavity

S31.62 Laceration with foreign body of abdominal wall with penetration into peritoneal cavity

⑦S31.620 Laceration with foreign body of abdominal wall, right upper quadrant with penetration into peritoneal cavity

⑦S31.621 Laceration with foreign body of abdominal wall, left upper quadrant with penetration into peritoneal cavity

⑦S31.622 Laceration with foreign body of abdominal wall, epigastric region with penetration into peritoneal cavity

⑦S31.623 Laceration with foreign body of abdominal wall, right lower quadrant with penetration into peritoneal cavity

⑦S31.624 Laceration with foreign body of abdominal wall, left lower quadrant with penetration into peritoneal cavity

⑦S31.625 Laceration with foreign body of abdominal wall, periumbilic region with penetration into peritoneal cavity

⑦S31.629 Laceration with foreign body of abdominal wall, unspecified quadrant with penetration into peritoneal cavity

S31.63 Puncture wound without foreign body of abdominal wall with penetration into peritoneal cavity

⑦S31.630 Puncture wound without foreign body of abdominal wall, right upper quadrant with penetration into peritoneal cavity

⑦S31.631 Puncture wound without foreign body of abdominal wall, left upper quadrant with penetration into peritoneal cavity

⑦S31.632 Puncture wound without foreign body of abdominal wall, epigastric region with penetration into peritoneal cavity

⑦S31.633 Puncture wound without foreign body of abdominal wall, right lower quadrant with penetration into peritoneal cavity

⑦S31.634 Puncture wound without foreign body of abdominal wall, left lower quadrant with penetration into peritoneal cavity

⑦S31.635 Puncture wound without foreign body of abdominal wall, periumbilic region with penetration into peritoneal cavity

⑦S31.639 Puncture wound without foreign body of abdominal wall, unspecified quadrant with penetration into peritoneal cavity

S31.64 Puncture wound with foreign body of abdominal wall with penetration into peritoneal cavity

⑦S31.640 Puncture wound with foreign body of abdominal wall, right upper quadrant with penetration into peritoneal cavity

⑦S31.641 Puncture wound with foreign body of abdominal wall, left upper quadrant with penetration into peritoneal cavity

⑦S31.642 Puncture wound with foreign body of abdominal wall, epigastric region with penetration into peritoneal cavity

⑦S31.643 Puncture wound with foreign body of abdominal wall, right lower quadrant with penetration into peritoneal cavity

⑦S31.644 Puncture wound with foreign body of abdominal wall, left lower quadrant with penetration into peritoneal cavity

⑦S31.645 Puncture wound with foreign body of abdominal wall, periumbilic region with penetration into peritoneal cavity

⑦S31.649 Puncture wound with foreign body of abdominal wall, unspecified quadrant with penetration into peritoneal cavity

S31.65 Open bite of abdominal wall with penetration into peritoneal cavity

Excludes1: superficial bite of abdominal wall (S30.861, S30.871)

⑦S31.650 Open bite of abdominal wall, right upper quadrant with penetration into peritoneal cavity

⑦S31.651 Open bite of abdominal wall, left upper quadrant with penetration into peritoneal cavity

⑦S31.652 Open bite of abdominal wall, epigastric region with penetration into peritoneal cavity

⑦S31.653 Open bite of abdominal wall, right lower quadrant with penetration into peritoneal cavity

⑦S31.654 **Open bite of abdominal wall, left lower quadrant with penetration into peritoneal cavity**

⑦S31.655 **Open bite of abdominal wall, periumbilic region with penetration into peritoneal cavity**

⑦S31.659 **Open bite of abdominal wall, unspecified quadrant with penetration into peritoneal cavity**

S31.8 **Open wound of other parts of abdomen, lower back and pelvis**

S31.80 **Open wound of unspecified buttock**

⑦S31.801 **Laceration without foreign body of unspecified buttock**

⑦S31.802 **Laceration with foreign body of unspecified buttock**

⑦S31.803 **Puncture wound without foreign body of unspecified buttock**

⑦S31.804 **Puncture wound with foreign body of unspecified buttock**

⑦S31.805 **Open bite of unspecified buttock**
Bite of buttock NOS
Excludes1: superficial bite of buttock (S30.870)

⑦S31.809 **Unspecified open wound of unspecified buttock**

S31.81 **Open wound of right buttock**

⑦S31.811 **Laceration without foreign body of right buttock**

⑦S31.812 **Laceration with foreign body of right buttock**

⑦S31.813 **Puncture wound without foreign body of right buttock**

⑦S31.814 **Puncture wound with foreign body of right buttock**

⑦S31.815 **Open bite of right buttock**
Bite of right buttock NOS
Excludes1: superficial bite of buttock (S30.870)

⑦S31.819 **Unspecified open wound of right buttock**

S31.82 **Open wound of left buttock**

⑦S31.821 **Laceration without foreign body of left buttock**

⑦S31.822 **Laceration with foreign body of left buttock**

⑦S31.823 **Puncture wound without foreign body of left buttock**

⑦S31.824 **Puncture wound with foreign body of left buttock**

⑦S31.825 **Open bite of left buttock**
Bite of left buttock NOS
Excludes1: superficial bite of buttock (S30.870)

⑦S31.829 **Unspecified open wound of left buttock**

⑦S31.83 **Open wound of anus**

⑦S31.831 **Laceration without foreign body of anus**

⑦S31.832 **Laceration with foreign body of anus**

⑦S31.833 **Puncture wound without foreign body of anus**

⑦S31.834 **Puncture wound with foreign body of anus**

⑦S31.835 **Open bite of anus**
Bite of anus NOS
Excludes1: superficial bite of anus (S30.877)

⑦S31.839 **Unspecified open wound of anus**

S32 **Fracture of lumbar spine and pelvis**
Note: A fracture not indicated as displaced or nondisplaced should be coded to displaced
A fracture not indicated as opened or closed should be coded to closed
Includes: fracture of lumbosacral neural arch
fracture of lumbosacral spinous process
fracture of lumbosacral transverse process
fracture of lumbosacral vertebra
fracture of lumbosacral vertebral arch
Code first any associated spinal cord and spinal nerve injury (S34.-)
Excludes1: transection of abdomen (S38.3)
Excludes2: fracture of hip NOS (S72.0-)
The appropriate 7th character is to be added to each code from category S32
A - initial encounter for closed fracture
B - initial encounter for open fracture
D - subsequent encounter for fracture with routine healing
G - subsequent encounter for fracture with delayed healing
K - subsequent encounter for fracture with nonunion
S - sequela

S32.0 **Fracture of lumbar vertebra**
Fracture of lumbar spine NOS

S32.00 **Fracture of unspecified lumbar vertebra**

⑦S32.000 **Wedge compression fracture of unspecified lumbar vertebra**

⑦S32.001 **Stable burst fracture of unspecified lumbar vertebra**

⑦S32.002 **Unstable burst fracture of unspecified lumbar vertebra**

⑦S32.008 **Other fracture of unspecified lumbar vertebra**

⑦S32.009 **Unspecified fracture of unspecified lumbar vertebra**

S32.01 **Fracture of first lumbar vertebra**

⑦S32.010 **Wedge compression fracture of first lumbar vertebra**

⑦S32.011 **Stable burst fracture of first lumbar vertebra**

⑦S32.012 **Unstable burst fracture of first lumbar vertebra**

⑦S32.018 **Other fracture of first lumbar vertebra**

⑦S32.019 **Unspecified fracture of first lumbar vertebra**

S32.02 **Fracture of second lumbar vertebra**

⑦S32.020 **Wedge compression fracture of second lumbar vertebra**

⑦S32.021 **Stable burst fracture of second lumbar vertebra**

⑦S32.022 **Unstable burst fracture of second lumbar vertebra**

⑦S32.028 **Other fracture of second lumbar vertebra**

⑦S32.029 **Unspecified fracture of second lumbar vertebra**

S32.03 **Fracture of third lumbar vertebra**

⑦S32.030 **Wedge compression fracture of third lumbar vertebra**

⑦S32.031 **Stable burst fracture of third lumbar vertebra**

⑦S32.032 **Unstable burst fracture of third lumbar vertebra**

⑦S32.038 **Other fracture of third lumbar vertebra**

⑦S32.039 **Unspecified fracture of third lumbar vertebra**

S32.04 **Fracture of fourth lumbar vertebra**

⑦S32.040 **Wedge compression fracture of fourth lumbar vertebra**

⑦S32.041 **Stable burst fracture of fourth lumbar vertebra**

⑦S32.042 **Unstable burst fracture of fourth lumbar vertebra**

⑦S32.048 **Other fracture of fourth lumbar vertebra**

⑦S32.049 **Unspecified fracture of fourth lumbar vertebra**

S32.05 **Fracture of fifth lumbar vertebra**

⑦S32.050 **Wedge compression fracture of fifth lumbar vertebra**

⑦S32.051 **Stable burst fracture of fifth lumbar vertebra**

⑦S32.052 **Unstable burst fracture of fifth lumbar vertebra**

⑦S32.058 **Other fracture of fifth lumbar vertebra**

⑦S32.059 **Unspecified fracture of fifth lumbar vertebra**

S32.1 **Fracture of sacrum**

For vertical fractures, code to most medial fracture extension

Use two codes if both a vertical and transverse fracture are present

Code also any associated fracture of pelvic ring (S32.8-)

⊗⑦S32.10 **Unspecified fracture of sacrum**

S32.11 **Zone I fracture of sacrum**

Vertical sacral ala fracture of sacrum

⑦S32.110 **Nondisplaced Zone I fracture of sacrum**

⑦S32.111 **Minimally displaced Zone I fracture of sacrum**

⑦S32.112 **Severely displaced Zone I fracture of sacrum**

⑦S32.119 **Unspecified Zone I fracture of sacrum**

S32.12 **Zone II fracture of sacrum**

Vertical foraminal region fracture of sacrum

⑦S32.120 **Nondisplaced Zone II fracture of sacrum**

⑦S32.121 **Minimally displaced Zone II fracture of sacrum**

⑦S32.122 **Severely displaced Zone II fracture of sacrum**

⑦S32.129 **Unspecified Zone II fracture of sacrum**

S32.13 **Zone III fracture of sacrum**

Vertical fracture into spinal canal region of sacrum

⑦S32.130 **Nondisplaced Zone III fracture of sacrum**

⑦S32.131 **Minimally displaced Zone III fracture of sacrum**

⑦S32.132 **Severely displaced Zone III fracture of sacrum**

⑦S32.139 **Unspecified Zone III fracture of sacrum**

S32.14 **Type 1   fracture of sacrum**

Transverse flexion fracture of sacrum without displacement

⊗⑦S32.15 **Type 2 fracture of sacrum**

Transverse flexion fracture of sacrum with posterior displacement

⊗⑦S32.16 **Type 3 fracture of sacrum**

Transverse extension fracture of sacrum with anterior displacement

⊗⑦S32.17 **Type 4 fracture of sacrum**

Transverse segmental comminution of upper sacrum

⊗⑦S32.19 **Other fracture of sacrum**

⊗⑦S32.2 **Fracture of coccyx**

S32.3 **Fracture of ilium**

Excludes1: fracture of ilium with associated disruption of pelvic ring (S32.8-)

S32.30 **Unspecified fracture of ilium**

⑦S32.301 **Unspecified fracture of right ilium**

⑦S32.302 **Unspecified fracture of left ilium**

⑦S32.309 **Unspecified fracture of unspecified ilium**

S32.31 **Avulsion fracture of ilium**

⑦S32.311 **Displaced avulsion fracture of right ilium**

⑦S32.312 **Displaced avulsion fracture of left ilium**

⑦S32.313 **Displaced avulsion fracture of unspecified ilium**

⑦S32.314 **Nondisplaced avulsion fracture of right ilium**

⑦S32.315 **Nondisplaced avulsion fracture of left ilium**

⑦S32.316 **Nondisplaced avulsion fracture of unspecified ilium**

S32.39 **Other fracture of ilium**

⑦S32.391 **Other fracture of right ilium**

⑦S32.392 **Other fracture of left ilium**

● New code   ▲ Revised code   **Excludes1:** Not coded here   **Excludes2:** Not included here   ⊗ Placeholder required   ⑦7th digit required

⑦ **S32.399**   Other fracture of unspecified ilium

S32.4   **Fracture of acetabulum**

Code also any associated fracture of pelvic ring (S32.8-)

S32.40   **Unspecified fracture of acetabulum**

⑦ **S32.401**   Unspecified fracture of right acetabulum

⑦ **S32.402**   Unspecified fracture of left acetabulum

⑦ **S32.409**   Unspecified fracture of unspecified acetabulum

S32.41   **Fracture of anterior wall of acetabulum**

⑦ **S32.411**   Displaced fracture of anterior wall of right acetabulum

⑦ **S32.412**   Displaced fracture of anterior wall of left acetabulum

⑦ **S32.413**   Displaced fracture of anterior wall of unspecified acetabulum

⑦ **S32.414**   Nondisplaced fracture of anterior wall of right acetabulum

⑦ **S32.415**   Nondisplaced fracture of anterior wall of left acetabulum

⑦ **S32.416**   Nondisplaced fracture of anterior wall of unspecified acetabulum

S32.42   **Fracture of posterior wall of acetabulum**

⑦ **S32.421**   Displaced fracture of posterior wall of right acetabulum

⑦ **S32.422**   Displaced fracture of posterior wall of left acetabulum

⑦ **S32.423**   Displaced fracture of posterior wall of unspecified acetabulum

⑦ **S32.424**   Nondisplaced fracture of posterior wall of right acetabulum

⑦ **S32.425**   Nondisplaced fracture of posterior wall of left acetabulum

⑦ **S32.426**   Nondisplaced fracture of posterior wall of unspecified acetabulum

S32.43   **Fracture of anterior column [iliopubic] of acetabulum**

⑦ **S32.431**   Displaced fracture of anterior column [iliopubic] of right acetabulum

⑦ **S32.432**   Displaced fracture of anterior column [iliopubic] of left acetabulum

⑦ **S32.433**   Displaced fracture of anterior column [iliopubic] of unspecified acetabulum

⑦ **S32.434**   Nondisplaced fracture of anterior column [iliopubic] of right acetabulum

⑦ **S32.435**   Nondisplaced fracture of anterior column [iliopubic] of left acetabulum

⑦ **S32.436**   Nondisplaced fracture of anterior column [iliopubic] of unspecified acetabulum

S32.44   **Fracture of posterior column [ilioischial] of acetabulum**

⑦ **S32.441**   Displaced fracture of posterior column [ilioischial] of right acetabulum

⑦ **S32.442**   Displaced fracture of posterior column [ilioischial] of left acetabulum

⑦ **S32.443**   Displaced fracture of posterior column [ilioischial] of unspecified acetabulum

⑦ **S32.444**   Nondisplaced fracture of posterior column [ilioischial] of right acetabulum

⑦ **S32.445**   Nondisplaced fracture of posterior column [ilioischial] of left acetabulum

⑦ **S32.446**   Nondisplaced fracture of posterior column [ilioischial] of unspecified acetabulum

S32.45   **Transverse fracture of acetabulum**

⑦ **S32.451**   Displaced transverse fracture of right acetabulum

⑦ **S32.452**   Displaced transverse fracture of left acetabulum

⑦ **S32.453**   Displaced transverse fracture of unspecified acetabulum

⑦ **S32.454**   Nondisplaced transverse fracture of right acetabulum

⑦ **S32.455**   Nondisplaced transverse fracture of left acetabulum

⑦ **S32.456**   Nondisplaced transverse fracture of unspecified acetabulum

S32.46   **Associated transverse-posterior fracture of acetabulum**

⑦ **S32.461**   Displaced associated transverse-posterior fracture of right acetabulum

⑦ **S32.462**   Displaced associated transverse-posterior fracture of left acetabulum

⑦ **S32.463**   Displaced associated transverse-posterior fracture of unspecified acetabulum

⑦ **S32.464**   Nondisplaced associated transverse-posterior fracture of right acetabulum

⑦ **S32.465**   Nondisplaced associated transverse-posterior fracture of left acetabulum

⑦ **S32.466**   Nondisplaced associated transverse-posterior fracture of unspecified acetabulum

S32.47   **Fracture of medial wall of acetabulum**

⑦ **S32.471**   Displaced fracture of medial wall of right acetabulum

⑦ **S32.472**   Displaced fracture of medial wall of left acetabulum

⑦ **S32.473**   Displaced fracture of medial wall of unspecified acetabulum

⑦ **S32.474**   Nondisplaced fracture of medial wall of right acetabulum

⑦ **S32.475**   Nondisplaced fracture of medial wall of left acetabulum

⑦ **S32.476**   Nondisplaced fracture of medial wall of unspecified acetabulum

S32.48   **Dome fracture of acetabulum**

⑦**S32.481** **Displaced dome fracture of right acetabulum**

⑦**S32.482** **Displaced dome fracture of left acetabulum**

⑦**S32.483** **Displaced dome fracture of unspecified acetabulum**

⑦**S32.484** **Nondisplaced dome fracture of right acetabulum**

⑦**S32.485** **Nondisplaced dome fracture of left acetabulum**

⑦**S32.486** **Nondisplaced dome fracture of unspecified acetabulum**

S32.49 **Other specified fracture of acetabulum**

⑦**S32.491** **Other specified fracture of right acetabulum**

⑦**S32.492** **Other specified fracture of left acetabulum**

⑦**S32.499** **Other specified fracture of unspecified acetabulum**

S32.5 **Fracture of pubis**

Excludes1: fracture of pubis with associated disruption of pelvic ring (S32.8-)

S32.50 **Unspecified fracture of pubis**

⑦**S32.501** **Unspecified fracture of right pubis**

⑦**S32.502** **Unspecified fracture of left pubis**

⑦**S32.509** **Unspecified fracture of unspecified pubis**

S32.51 **Fracture of superior rim of pubis**

⑦**S32.511** **Fracture of superior rim of right pubis**

⑦**S32.512** **Fracture of superior rim of left pubis**

⑦**S32.519** **Fracture of superior rim of unspecified pubis**

S32.59 **Other specified fracture of pubis**

⑦**S32.591** **Other specified fracture of right pubis**

⑦**S32.592** **Other specified fracture of left pubis**

⑦**S32.599** **Other specified fracture of unspecified pubis**

S32.6 **Fracture of ischium**

Excludes1: fracture of ischium with associated disruption of pelvic ring (S32.8-)

S32.60 **Unspecified fracture of ischium**

⑦**S32.601** **Unspecified fracture of right ischium**

⑦**S32.602** **Unspecified fracture of left ischium**

⑦**S32.609** **Unspecified fracture of unspecified ischium**

S32.61 **Avulsion fracture of ischium**

⑦**S32.611** **Displaced avulsion fracture of right ischium**

⑦**S32.612** **Displaced avulsion fracture of left ischium**

⑦**S32.613** **Displaced avulsion fracture of unspecified ischium**

⑦**S32.614** **Nondisplaced avulsion fracture of right ischium**

⑦**S32.615** **Nondisplaced avulsion fracture of left ischium**

⑦**S32.616** **Nondisplaced avulsion fracture of unspecified ischium**

S32.69 **Other specified fracture of ischium**

⑦**S32.691** **Other specified fracture of right ischium**

⑦**S32.692** **Other specified fracture of left ischium**

⑦**S32.699** **Other specified fracture of unspecified ischium**

S32.8 **Fracture of other parts of pelvis**

Code also any associated:

fracture of acetabulum (S32.4-)

sacral fracture (S32.1-)

S32.81 **Multiple fractures of pelvis with disruption of pelvic ring**

Multiple pelvic fractures with disruption of pelvic circle

⑦**S32.810** **Multiple fractures of pelvis with stable disruption of pelvic ring**

⑦**S32.811** **Multiple fractures of pelvis with unstable disruption of pelvic ring**

⊗⑦**S32.82** **Multiple fractures of pelvis without disruption of pelvic ring**

Multiple pelvic fractures without disruption of pelvic circle

⊗⑦**S32.89** **Fracture of other parts of pelvis**

S32.9 **Fracture of unspecified parts of lumbosacral spine and pelvis**

Fracture of lumbosacral spine NOS

Fracture of pelvis NOS

S33 **Dislocation and sprain of joints and ligaments of lumbar spine and pelvis**

Includes: avulsion of joint or ligament of lumbar spine and pelvis

laceration of cartilage, joint or ligament of lumbar spine and pelvis

sprain of cartilage, joint or ligament of lumbar spine and pelvis

traumatic hemarthrosis of joint or ligament of lumbar spine and pelvis

traumatic rupture of joint or ligament of lumbar spine and pelvis

traumatic subluxation of joint or ligament of lumbar spine and pelvis

traumatic tear of joint or ligament of lumbar spine and pelvis

Code also any associated open wound

Excludes1: nontraumatic rupture or displacement of lumbar intervertebral disc NOS (M51.-)

obstetric damage to pelvic joints and ligaments (O71.6)

Excludes2: dislocation and sprain of joints and ligaments of hip (S73.-)

strain of muscle of lower back and pelvis (S39.01-)

The appropriate 7th character is to be added to each code from category S33

A - initial encounter

D - subsequent encounter

S - sequela

⊗⑦**S33.0   Traumatic rupture of lumbar intervertebral disc**

Excludes1: rupture or displacement (nontraumatic) of lumbar intervertebral disc NOS (M51.- with fifth character 6)

S33.1   Subluxation and dislocation of lumbar vertebra

Code also any associated:

open wound of abdomen, lower back and pelvis (S31)

spinal cord injury (S24.0, S24.1-, S34.0-, S34.1-)

Excludes2: fracture of lumbar vertebrae (S32.0-)

S33.10   Subluxation and dislocation of unspecified lumbar vertebra

⑦**S33.100   Subluxation of unspecified lumbar vertebra**

⑦**S33.101   Dislocation of unspecified lumbar vertebra**

S33.11   Subluxation and dislocation of L1/L2 lumbar vertebra

⑦**S33.110   Subluxation of L1/L2 lumbar vertebra**

⑦**S33.111   Dislocation of L1/L2 lumbar vertebra**

S33.12   Subluxation and dislocation of L2/L3 lumbar vertebra

⑦**S33.120   Subluxation of L2/L3 lumbar vertebra**

⑦**S33.121   Dislocation of L2/L3 lumbar vertebra**

S33.13   Subluxation and dislocation of L3/L4 lumbar vertebra

⑦**S33.130   Subluxation of L3/L4 lumbar vertebra**

⑦**S33.131   Dislocation of L3/L4 lumbar vertebra**

⑦**S33.14   Subluxation and dislocation of L4/L5 lumbar vertebra**

⑦**S33.140   Subluxation of L4/L5 lumbar vertebra**

⑦**S33.141   Dislocation of L4/L5 lumbar vertebra**

⊗⑦**S33.2   Dislocation of sacroiliac and sacrococcygeal joint**

S33.3   Dislocation of other and unspecified parts of lumbar spine and pelvis

⊗⑦**S33.30   Dislocation of unspecified parts of lumbar spine and pelvis**

⊗⑦**S33.39   Dislocation of other parts of lumbar spine and pelvis**

⊗⑦**S33.4   Traumatic rupture of symphysis pubis**

⊗⑦**S33.5   Sprain of ligaments of lumbar spine**

⊗⑦**S33.6   Sprain of sacroiliac joint**

⊗⑦**S33.8   Sprain of other parts of lumbar spine and pelvis**

⊗⑦**S33.9   Sprain of unspecified parts of lumbar spine and pelvis**

S34   Injury of lumbar and sacral spinal cord and nerves at abdomen, lower back and pelvis level

Note: Code to highest level of lumbar cord injury

Injuries to the spinal cord (S34.0 and S34.1) refer to the cord level and not bone level injury, and can affect nerve roots at and below the level given.

Code also any associated:

fracture of vertebra (S22.0-, S32.0-)

open wound of abdomen, lower back and pelvis (S31.-)

transient paralysis (R29.5)

The appropriate 7th character is to be added to each code from category S34

A - initial encounter

D - subsequent encounter

S - sequela

S34.0   Concussion and edema of lumbar and sacral spinal cord

⊗⑦**S34.01   Concussion and edema of lumbar spinal cord**

⊗⑦**S34.02   Concussion and edema of sacral spinal cord**

Concussion and edema of conus medullaris

S34.1   Other and unspecified injury of lumbar and sacral spinal cord

S34.10   Unspecified injury to lumbar spinal cord

⑦**S34.101   Unspecified injury to L1 level of lumbar spinal cord**

Unspecified injury to lumbar spinal cord level 1

⑦**S34.102   Unspecified injury to L2 level of lumbar spinal cord**

Unspecified injury to lumbar spinal cord level 2

⑦**S34.103   Unspecified injury to L3 level of lumbar spinal cord**

Unspecified injury to lumbar spinal cord level 3

⑦**S34.104   Unspecified injury to L4 level of lumbar spinal cord**

Unspecified injury to lumbar spinal cord level 4

⑦**S34.105   Unspecified injury to L5 level of lumbar spinal cord**

Unspecified injury to lumbar spinal cord level 5

⑦**S34.109   Unspecified injury to unspecified level of lumbar spinal cord**

S34.11   Complete lesion of lumbar spinal cord

⑦**S34.111   Complete lesion of L1 level of lumbar spinal cord**

Complete lesion of lumbar spinal cord level 1

⑦**S34.112   Complete lesion of L2 level of lumbar spinal cord**

Complete lesion of lumbar spinal cord level 2

⑦**S34.113   Complete lesion of L3 level of lumbar spinal cord**

Complete lesion of lumbar spinal cord level 3

⑦**S34.114   Complete lesion of L4 level of lumbar spinal cord**

Complete lesion of lumbar spinal cord level 4

⑦**S34.115   Complete lesion of L5 level of lumbar spinal cord**

Complete lesion of lumbar spinal cord level 5

⑦**S34.119   Complete lesion of unspecified level of lumbar spinal cord**

S34.12   Incomplete lesion of lumbar spinal cord

⑦S34.121 **Incomplete lesion of L1 level of lumbar spinal cord**

Incomplete lesion of lumbar spinal cord level 1

⑦S34.122 **Incomplete lesion of L2 level of lumbar spinal cord**

Incomplete lesion of lumbar spinal cord level 2

⑦S34.123 **Incomplete lesion of L3 level of lumbar spinal cord**

Incomplete lesion of lumbar spinal cord level 3

⑦S34.124 **Incomplete lesion of L4 level of lumbar spinal cord**

Incomplete lesion of lumbar spinal cord level 4

⑦S34.125 **Incomplete lesion of L5 level of lumbar spinal cord**

Incomplete lesion of lumbar spinal cord level 5

⑦S34.129 **Incomplete lesion of unspecified level of lumbar spinal cord**

S34.13 **Other and unspecified injury to sacral spinal cord**

Other injury to conus medullaris

⑦S34.131 **Complete lesion of sacral spinal cord**

Complete lesion of conus medullaris

⑦S34.132 **Incomplete lesion of sacral spinal cord**

Incomplete lesion of conus medullaris

⑦S34.139 **Unspecified injury to sacral spinal cord**

Unspecified injury of conus medullaris

S34.2 **Injury of nerve root of lumbar and sacral spine**

⊗⑦S34.21 **Injury of nerve root of lumbar spine**

⊗⑦S34.22 **Injury of nerve root of sacral spine**

⊗⑦S34.3 **Injury of cauda equina**

⊗⑦S34.4 **Injury of lumbosacral plexus**

⊗⑦S34.5 **Injury of lumbar, sacral and pelvic sympathetic nerves**

Injury of celiac ganglion or plexus

Injury of hypogastric plexus

Injury of mesenteric plexus (inferior) (superior)

Injury of splanchnic nerve

⊗⑦S34.6 **Injury of peripheral nerve(s) at abdomen, lower back and pelvis level**

⊗⑦S34.8 **Injury of other nerves at abdomen, lower back and pelvis level**

⊗⑦S34.9 **Injury of unspecified nerves at abdomen, lower back and pelvis level**

S35 **Injury of blood vessels at abdomen, lower back and pelvis level**

Code also any associated open wound (S31.-)

The appropriate 7th character is to be added to each code from category S35

A - initial encounter

D - subsequent encounter

S - sequela

S35.0 **Injury of abdominal aorta**

Excludes1: injury of aorta NOS (S25.0)

⊗⑦S35.00 **Unspecified injury of abdominal aorta**

⊗⑦S35.01 **Minor laceration of abdominal aorta**

Incomplete transection of abdominal aorta

Laceration of abdominal aorta NOS

Superficial laceration of abdominal aorta

⊗⑦S35.02 **Major laceration of abdominal aorta**

Complete transection of abdominal aorta

Traumatic rupture of abdominal aorta

⊗⑦S35.09 **Other injury of abdominal aorta**

S35.1 **Injury of inferior vena cava**

Injury of hepatic vein

Excludes1: injury of vena cava NOS (S25.2)

⊗⑦S35.10 **Unspecified injury of inferior vena cava**

⊗⑦S35.11 **Minor laceration of inferior vena cava**

Incomplete transection of inferior vena cava

Laceration of inferior vena cava NOS

Superficial laceration of inferior vena cava

⊗⑦S35.12 **Major laceration of inferior vena cava**

Complete transection of inferior vena cava

Traumatic rupture of inferior vena cava

⊗⑦S35.19 **Other injury of inferior vena cava**

S35.2 **Injury of celiac or mesenteric artery and branches**

S35.21 **Injury of celiac artery**

⑦S35.211 **Minor laceration of celiac artery**

Incomplete transection of celiac artery

Laceration of celiac artery NOS

Superficial laceration of celiac artery

⑦S35.212 **Major laceration of celiac artery**

Complete transection of celiac artery

Traumatic rupture of celiac artery

⑦S35.218 **Other injury of celiac artery**

⑦S35.219 **Unspecified injury of celiac artery**

S35.22 **Injury of superior mesenteric artery**

⑦S35.221 **Minor laceration of superior mesenteric artery**

Incomplete transection of superior mesenteric artery

Laceration of superior mesenteric artery NOS

Superficial laceration of superior mesenteric artery

⑦S35.222 **Major laceration of superior mesenteric artery**

Complete transection of superior mesenteric artery

Traumatic rupture of superior mesenteric artery

⑦S35.228 **Other injury of superior mesenteric artery**

⑦S35.229 **Unspecified injury of superior mesenteric artery**

S35.23 **Injury of inferior mesenteric artery**

⑦S35.231 **Minor laceration of inferior mesenteric artery**

Incomplete transection of inferior mesenteric artery

Laceration of inferior mesenteric artery NOS

Superficial laceration of inferior mesenteric artery

⑦S35.232 **Major laceration of inferior mesenteric artery**

Complete transection of inferior mesenteric artery

Traumatic rupture of inferior mesenteric artery

⑦S35.238 **Other injury of inferior mesenteric artery**

⑦S35.239 **Unspecified injury of inferior mesenteric artery**

S35.29 **Injury of branches of celiac and mesenteric artery**

Injury of gastric artery

Injury of gastroduodenal artery

Injury of hepatic artery

Injury of splenic artery

⑦S35.291 **Minor laceration of branches of celiac and mesenteric artery**

Incomplete transection of branches of celiac and mesenteric artery

Laceration of branches of celiac and mesenteric artery NOS

Superficial laceration of branches of celiac and mesenteric artery

⑦S35.292 **Major laceration of branches of celiac and mesenteric artery**

Complete transection of branches of celiac and mesenteric artery

Traumatic rupture of branches of celiac and mesenteric artery

⑦S35.298 **Other injury of branches of celiac and mesenteric artery**

⑦S35.299 **Unspecified injury of branches of celiac and mesenteric artery**

S35.3 **Injury of portal or splenic vein and branches**

S35.31 **Injury of portal vein**

⑦S35.311 **Laceration of portal vein**

⑦S35.318 **Other specified injury of portal vein**

⑦S35.319 **Unspecified injury of portal vein**

S35.32 **Injury of splenic vein**

⑦S35.321 **Laceration of splenic vein**

⑦S35.328 **Other specified injury of splenic vein**

⑦S35.329 **Unspecified injury of splenic vein**

S35.33 **Injury of superior mesenteric vein**

⑦S35.331 **Laceration of superior mesenteric vein**

⑦S35.338 **Other specified injury of superior mesenteric vein**

⑦S35.339 **Unspecified injury of superior mesenteric vein**

S35.34 **Injury of inferior mesenteric vein**

⑦S35.341 **Laceration of inferior mesenteric vein**

⑦S35.348 **Other specified injury of inferior mesenteric vein**

⑦S35.349 **Unspecified injury of inferior mesenteric vein**

S35.4 **Injury of renal blood vessels**

S35.40 **Unspecified injury of renal blood vessel**

⑦S35.401 **Unspecified injury of right renal artery**

⑦S35.402 **Unspecified injury of left renal artery**

⑦S35.403 **Unspecified injury of unspecified renal artery**

⑦S35.404 **Unspecified injury of right renal vein**

⑦S35.405 **Unspecified injury of left renal vein**

⑦S35.406 **Unspecified injury of unspecified renal vein**

S35.41 **Laceration of renal blood vessel**

⑦S35.411 **Laceration of right renal artery**

⑦S35.412 **Laceration of left renal artery**

⑦S35.413 **Laceration of unspecified renal artery**

⑦S35.414 **Laceration of right renal vein**

⑦S35.415 **Laceration of left renal vein**

⑦S35.416 **Laceration of unspecified renal vein**

S35.49 **Other specified injury of renal blood vessel**

⑦S35.491 **Other specified injury of right renal artery**

⑦S35.492 **Other specified injury of left renal artery**

⑦S35.493 **Other specified injury of unspecified renal artery**

⑦S35.494 **Other specified injury of right renal vein**

⑦S35.495 **Other specified injury of left renal vein**

⑦S35.496 **Other specified injury of unspecified renal vein**

S35.5 **Injury of iliac blood vessels**

⊗⑦S35.50 **Injury of unspecified iliac blood vessel(s)**

S35.51 **Injury of iliac artery or vein**

Injury of hypogastric artery or vein

⑦S35.511 **Injury of right iliac artery**

⑦S35.512 **Injury of left iliac artery**

⑦S35.513 **Injury of unspecified iliac artery**

⑦S35.514 **Injury of right iliac vein**

⑦S35.515 **Injury of left iliac vein**

⑦S35.516 **Injury of unspecified iliac vein**

S35.53 **Injury of uterine artery or vein**

⑦S35.531 **Injury of right uterine artery**

⑦S35.532 **Injury of left uterine artery**

⑦S35.533 **Injury of unspecified uterine artery**

⑦S35.534 **Injury of right uterine vein**

⑦S35.535 **Injury of left uterine vein**

⑦S35.536 **Injury of unspecified uterine vein**

⊗⑦S35.59 **Injury of other iliac blood vessels**

S35.8 **Injury of other blood vessels at abdomen, lower back and pelvis level**

Injury of ovarian artery or vein

    S35.8X **Injury of other blood vessels at abdomen, lower back and pelvis level**

      ⑦**S35.8X1** **Laceration of other blood vessels at abdomen, lower back and pelvis level**

      ⑦**S35.8X8** **Other specified injury of other blood vessels at abdomen, lower back and pelvis level**

      ⑦**S35.8X9** **Unspecified injury of other blood vessels at abdomen, lower back and pelvis level**

S35.9 **Injury of unspecified blood vessel at abdomen, lower back and pelvis level**

    ⊗⑦**S35.90** **Unspecified injury of unspecified blood vessel at abdomen, lower back and pelvis level**

    ⊗⑦**S35.91** **Laceration of unspecified blood vessel at abdomen, lower back and pelvis level**

    ⊗⑦**S35.99** **Other specified injury of unspecified blood vessel at abdomen, lower back and pelvis level**

S36 **Injury of intra-abdominal organs**

<u>Code also</u> any associated open wound (S31.-)

The appropriate 7th character is to be added to each code from category S36

A - initial encounter

D - subsequent encounter

S - sequela

S36.0 **Injury of spleen**

    ⊗⑦**S36.00** **Unspecified injury of spleen**

    S36.02 **Contusion of spleen**

      ⑦**S36.020** **Minor contusion of spleen**

      Contusion of spleen less than 2 cm

      ⑦**S36.021** **Major contusion of spleen**

      Contusion of spleen greater than 2 cm

      ⑦**S36.029** **Unspecified contusion of spleen**

    S36.03 **Laceration of spleen**

      ⑦**S36.030** ⑦**Superficial (capsular) laceration of spleen**

      Laceration of spleen less than 1 cm

      Minor laceration of spleen

      ⑦**S36.031** **Moderate laceration of spleen**

      Laceration of spleen 1 to 3 cm

      ⑦**S36.032** **Major laceration of spleen**

      Avulsion of spleen

      Laceration of spleen greater than 3 cm

      Massive laceration of spleen

      Multiple moderate lacerations of spleen Stellate laceration of spleen

      ⑦**S36.039** **Unspecified laceration of spleen**

    S36.09 **Other injury of spleen**

S36.1 **Injury of liver and gallbladder and bile duct**

    S36.11 **Injury of liver**

      ⑦**S36.112** **Contusion of liver**

      ⑦**S36.113** **Laceration of liver, unspecified degree**

      ⑦**S36.114** **Minor laceration of liver**

Laceration involving capsule only, or, without significant involvement of hepatic parenchyma [i.e., less than 1 cm deep]

      ⑦**S36.115** **Moderate laceration of liver**

Laceration involving parenchyma but without major disruption of parenchyma [i.e., less than 10 cm long and less than 3 cm deep]

      ⑦**S36.116** **Major laceration of liver**

Laceration with significant disruption of hepatic parenchyma [i.e., greater than 10 cm long and 3 cm deep]

Multiple moderate lacerations, with or without hematoma

Stellate laceration of liver

      ⑦**S36.118** **Other injury of liver**

      ⑦**S36.119** **Unspecified injury of liver**

    S36.12 **Injury of gallbladder**

      ⑦**S36.122** **Contusion of gallbladder**

      ⑦**S36.123** **Laceration of gallbladder**

      ⑦**S36.128** **Other injury of gallbladder**

      ⑦**S36.129** **Unspecified injury of gallbladder**

    ⊗⑦**S36.13** **Injury of bile duct**

S36.2 **Injury of pancreas**

    S36.20 **Unspecified injury of pancreas**

      ⑦**S36.200** **Unspecified injury of head of pancreas**

      ⑦**S36.201** **Unspecified injury of body of pancreas**

      ⑦**S36.202** **Unspecified injury of tail of pancreas**

      ⑦**S36.209** **Unspecified injury of unspecified part of pancreas**

    S36.22 **Contusion of pancreas**

      ⑦**S36.220** **Contusion of head of pancreas**

      ⑦**S36.221** **Contusion of body of pancreas**

      ⑦**S36.222** **Contusion of tail of pancreas**

      ⑦**S36.229** **Contusion of unspecified part of pancreas**

    S36.23 **Laceration of pancreas, unspecified degree**

      ⑦**S36.230** **Laceration of head of pancreas, unspecified degree**

      ⑦**S36.231** **Laceration of body of pancreas, unspecified degree**

      ⑦**S36.232** **Laceration of tail of pancreas, unspecified degree**

      ⑦**S36.239** **Laceration of unspecified part of pancreas, unspecified degree**

    S36.24 **Minor laceration of pancreas**

      ⑦**S36.240** **Minor laceration of head of pancreas**

      ⑦**S36.241** **Minor laceration of body of pancreas**

      ⑦**S36.242** **Minor laceration of tail of pancreas**

      ⑦**S36.249** **Minor laceration of unspecified part of pancreas**

    S36.25 **Moderate laceration of pancreas**

⑦S36.250 Moderate laceration of head of pancreas

⑦S36.251 Moderate laceration of body of pancreas

⑦S36.252 Moderate laceration of tail of pancreas

⑦S36.259 Moderate laceration of unspecified part of pancreas

S36.26 Major laceration of pancreas

⑦S36.260 Major laceration of head of pancreas

⑦S36.261 Major laceration of body of pancreas

⑦S36.262 Major laceration of tail of pancreas

⑦S36.269 Major laceration of unspecified part of pancreas

S36.29 Other injury of pancreas

⑦S36.290 Other injury of head of pancreas

⑦S36.291 Other injury of body of pancreas

⑦S36.292 Other injury of tail of pancreas

⑦S36.299 Other injury of unspecified part of pancreas

S36.3 Injury of stomach

⊗⑦S36.30 Unspecified injury of stomach

⊗⑦S36.32 Contusion of stomach

⊗⑦S36.33 Laceration of stomach

⊗⑦S36.39 Other injury of stomach

S36.4 Injury of small intestine

S36.40 Unspecified injury of small intestine

⑦S36.400 Unspecified injury of duodenum

⑦S36.408 Unspecified injury of other part of small intestine

⑦S36.409 Unspecified injury of unspecified part of small intestine

S36.41 Primary blast injury of small intestine

Blast injury of small intestine NOS

⑦S36.410 Primary blast injury of duodenum

⑦S36.418 Primary blast injury of other part of small intestine

⑦S36.419 Primary blast injury of unspecified part of small intestine

S36.42 Contusion of small intestine

⑦S36.420 Contusion of duodenum

⑦S36.428 Contusion of other part of small intestine

⑦S36.429 Contusion of unspecified part of small intestine

S36.43 Laceration of small intestine

⑦S36.430 Laceration of duodenum

⑦S36.438 Laceration of other part of small intestine

⑦S36.439 Laceration of unspecified part of small intestine

S36.49 Other injury of small intestine

⑦S36.490 Other injury of duodenum

⑦S36.498 Other injury of other part of small intestine

⑦S36.499 Other injury of unspecified part of small intestine

S36.5 Injury of colon

Excludes2: injury of rectum (S36.6-)

S36.50 Unspecified injury of colon

⑦S36.500 Unspecified injury of ascending [right] colon

⑦S36.501 Unspecified injury of transverse colon

⑦S36.502 Unspecified injury of descending [left] colon

⑦S36.503 Unspecified injury of sigmoid colon

⑦S36.508 Unspecified injury of other part of colon

⑦S36.509 Unspecified injury of unspecified part of colon

S36.51 Primary blast injury of colon

Blast injury of colon NOS

⑦S36.510 Primary blast injury of ascending [right] colon

⑦S36.511 Primary blast injury of transverse colon

⑦S36.512 Primary blast injury of descending [left] colon

⑦S36.513 Primary blast injury of sigmoid colon

⑦S36.518 Primary blast injury of other part of colon

⑦S36.519 Primary blast injury of unspecified part of colon

S36.52 Contusion of colon

⑦S36.520 Contusion of ascending [right] colon

⑦S36.521 Contusion of transverse colon

⑦S36.522 Contusion of descending [left] colon

⑦S36.523 Contusion of sigmoid colon

⑦S36.528 Contusion of other part of colon

⑦S36.529 Contusion of unspecified part of colon

S36.53 Laceration of colon

⑦S36.530 Laceration of ascending [right] colon

⑦S36.531 Laceration of transverse colon

⑦S36.532 Laceration of descending [left] colon

⑦S36.533 Laceration of sigmoid colon

⑦S36.538 Laceration of other part of colon

⑦S36.539 Laceration of unspecified part of colon

S36.59 Other injury of colon

Secondary blast injury of colon

⑦S36.590 Other injury of ascending [right] colon

⑦S36.591 Other injury of transverse colon

⑦S36.592 Other injury of descending [left] colon

⑦S36.593 Other injury of sigmoid colon

⑦S36.598 Other injury of other part of colon

⑦S36.599 Other injury of unspecified part of colon

S36.6 Injury of rectum

⊗⑦S36.60 Unspecified injury of rectum

⊗⑦S36.61 Primary blast injury of rectum

Blast injury of rectum NOS

⊗⑦S36.62 Contusion of rectum

⊗⑦S36.63 Laceration of rectum

⊗⑦S36.69 Other injury of rectum

Secondary blast injury of rectum

S36.8 Injury of other intra-abdominal organs

⊗⑦S36.81 Injury of peritoneum

S36.89 Injury of other intra-abdominal organs

Injury of retroperitoneum

⑦S36.892 Contusion of other intra-abdominal organs

⑦S36.893 Laceration of other intra-abdominal organs

⑦S36.898 Other injury of other intra-abdominal organs

⑦S36.899 Unspecified injury of other intra-abdominal organs

S36.9 Injury of unspecified intra-abdominal organ

⊗⑦S36.90 Unspecified injury of unspecified intra-abdominal organ

⊗⑦S36.92 Contusion of unspecified intra-abdominal organ

⊗⑦S36.93 Laceration of unspecified intra-abdominal organ

⊗⑦S36.99 Other injury of unspecified intra-abdominal organ

S37 Injury of urinary and pelvic organs

Code also any associated open wound (S31.-)

Excludes1: obstetric trauma to pelvic organs (O71.-)

Excludes2: injury of peritoneum (S36.81)

injury of retroperitoneum (S36.89-)

The appropriate 7th character is to be added to each code from category S37

A - initial encounter

D - subsequent encounter

S - sequela

S37.0 Injury of kidney

Excludes2: acute kidney injury (nontraumatic) (N17.9)

S37.00 Unspecified injury of kidney

⑦S37.001 Unspecified injury of right kidney

⑦S37.002 Unspecified injury of left kidney

⑦S37.009 Unspecified injury of unspecified kidney

S37.01 Minor contusion of kidney

Contusion of kidney less than 2 cm

Contusion of kidney NOS

⑦S37.011 Minor contusion of right kidney

⑦S37.012 Minor contusion of left kidney

⑦S37.019 Minor contusion of unspecified kidney

S37.02 Major contusion of kidney

Contusion of kidney greater than 2 cm

⑦S37.021 Major contusion of right kidney

⑦S37.022 Major contusion of left kidney

⑦S37.029 Major contusion of unspecified kidney

S37.03 Laceration of kidney, unspecified degree

⑦S37.031 Laceration of right kidney, unspecified degree

⑦S37.032 Laceration of left kidney, unspecified degree

⑦S37.039 Laceration of unspecified kidney, unspecified degree

S37.04 Minor laceration of kidney

Laceration of kidney less than 1 cm

⑦S37.041 Minor laceration of right kidney

⑦S37.042 Minor laceration of left kidney

⑦S37.049 Minor laceration of unspecified kidney

S37.05 Moderate laceration of kidney

Laceration of kidney 1 to 3 cm

⑦S37.051 Moderate laceration of right kidney

⑦S37.052 Moderate laceration of left kidney

⑦S37.059 Moderate laceration of unspecified kidney

S37.06 Major laceration of kidney

Avulsion of kidney

Laceration of kidney greater than 3 cm

Massive laceration of kidney

Multiple moderate lacerations of kidney

Stellate laceration of kidney

⑦S37.061 Major laceration of right kidney

⑦S37.062 Major laceration of left kidney

⑦S37.069 Major laceration of unspecified kidney

S37.09 Other injury of kidney

⑦S37.091 Other injury of right kidney

⑦S37.092 Other injury of left kidney

⑦S37.099 Other injury of unspecified kidney

S37.1 Injury of ureter

⊗⑦S37.10 Unspecified injury of ureter

⊗⑦S37.12 Contusion of ureter

⊗⑦S37.13 Laceration of ureter

⊗⑦S37.19 Other injury of ureter

S37.2 Injury of bladder

⊗⑦S37.20 Unspecified injury of bladder

⊗⑦S37.22 Contusion of bladder

⊗⑦S37.23 Laceration of bladder

⊗⑦S37.29 Other injury of bladder

S37.3 Injury of urethra

⊗⑦S37.30 Unspecified injury of urethra

⊗⑦S37.32 Contusion of urethra

⊗⑦S37.33 Laceration of urethra

⊗⑦S37.39 Other injury of urethra

S37.4 Injury of ovary

S37.40 Unspecified injury of ovary

⑦S37.401 Unspecified injury of ovary, unilateral

⑦S37.402   Unspecified injury of ovary, bilateral

⑦S37.409   Unspecified injury of ovary, unspecified

S37.42   Contusion of ovary

⑦S37.421   Contusion of ovary, unilateral

⑦S37.422   Contusion of ovary, bilateral

⑦S37.429   Contusion of ovary, unspecified

S37.43   Laceration of ovary

⑦S37.431   Laceration of ovary, unilateral

⑦S37.432   Laceration of ovary, bilateral

⑦S37.439   Laceration of ovary, unspecified

S37.49   Other injury of ovary

⑦S37.491   Other injury of ovary, unilateral

⑦S37.492   Other injury of ovary, bilateral

⑦S37.499   Other injury of ovary, unspecified

S37.5   Injury of fallopian tube

S37.50   Unspecified injury of fallopian tube

⑦S37.501   Unspecified injury of fallopian tube, unilateral

⑦S37.502   Unspecified injury of fallopian tube, bilateral

⑦S37.509   Unspecified injury of fallopian tube, unspecified

S37.51   Primary blast injury of fallopian tube

Blast injury of fallopian tube NOS

⑦S37.511   Primary blast injury of fallopian tube, unilateral

⑦S37.512   Primary blast injury of fallopian tube, bilateral

⑦S37.519   Primary blast injury of fallopian tube, unspecified

S37.52   Contusion of fallopian tube

⑦S37.521   Contusion of fallopian tube, unilateral

⑦S37.522   Contusion of fallopian tube, bilateral

⑦S37.529   Contusion of fallopian tube, unspecified

S37.53   Laceration of fallopian tube

⑦S37.531   Laceration of fallopian tube, unilateral

⑦S37.532   Laceration of fallopian tube, bilateral

⑦S37.539   Laceration of fallopian tube, unspecified

S37.59   Other injury of fallopian tube

Secondary blast injury of fallopian tube

⑦S37.591   Other injury of fallopian tube, unilateral

⑦S37.592   Other injury of fallopian tube, bilateral

⑦S37.599   Other injury of fallopian tube, unspecified

S37.6   Injury of uterus

Excludes1: injury to gravid uterus (O9A.2-)

injury to uterus during delivery (O71.-)

⊗⑦S37.60   Unspecified injury of uterus

⊗⑦S37.62   Contusion of uterus

⊗⑦S37.63   Laceration of uterus

⊗⑦S37.69   Other injury of uterus

S37.8   Injury of other urinary and pelvic organs

S37.81   Injury of adrenal gland

⑦S37.812   Contusion of adrenal gland

⑦S37.813   Laceration of adrenal gland

⑦S37.818   Other injury of adrenal gland

⑦S37.819   Unspecified injury of adrenal gland

S37.82   Injury of prostate

⑦S37.822   Contusion of prostate

⑦S37.823   Laceration of prostate

⑦S37.828   Other injury of prostate

⑦S37.829   Unspecified injury of prostate

S37.89   Injury of other urinary and pelvic organ

⑦S37.892   Contusion of other urinary and pelvic organ

⑦S37.893   Laceration of other urinary and pelvic organ

⑦S37.898   Other injury of other urinary and pelvic organ

⑦S37.899   Unspecified injury of other urinary and pelvic organ

S37.9   Injury of unspecified urinary and pelvic organ

⊗⑦S37.90   Unspecified injury of unspecified urinary and pelvic organ

⊗⑦S37.92   Contusion of unspecified urinary and pelvic organ

⊗⑦S37.93   Laceration of unspecified urinary and pelvic organ

⊗⑦S37.99   Other injury of unspecified urinary and pelvic organ

S38   Crushing injury and traumatic amputation of abdomen, lower back, pelvis and external genitals

An amputation not identified as partial or complete should be coded to complete

The appropriate 7th character is to be added to each code from category S38

A - initial encounter

D - subsequent encounter

S - sequela

S38.0   Crushing injury of external genital organs

Use additional code for any associated injuries

S38.00   Crushing injury of unspecified external genital organs

⑦S38.001   Crushing injury of unspecified external genital organs, male

⑦S38.002   Crushing injury of unspecified external genital organs, female

⊗⑦S38.01   Crushing injury of penis

⊗⑦S38.02   Crushing injury of scrotum and testis

⊗⑦S38.03   Crushing injury of vulva

S38.1   Crushing injury of abdomen, lower back, and pelvis

Use additional code for all associated injuries, such as:

fracture of thoracic or lumbar spine and pelvis (S22.0-, S32.-)

injury to intra-abdominal organs (S36.-)

injury to urinary and pelvic organs (S37.-)

Add 4th-7th digits   Nonspecific code   Unspecified code   Manifestation code

open wound of abdominal wall (S31.-)

spinal cord injury (S34.0, S34.1-)

Excludes2: crushing injury of external genital organs (S38.0-)

S38.2 Traumatic amputation of external genital organs

S38.21 Traumatic amputation of female external genital organs

Traumatic amputation of clitoris

Traumatic amputation of labium (majus) (minus)

Traumatic amputation of vulva

⑦**S38.211** Complete traumatic amputation of female external genital organs

⑦**S38.212** Partial traumatic amputation of female external genital organs

S38.22 Traumatic amputation of penis

⑦**S38.221** Complete traumatic amputation of penis

⑦**S38.222** Partial traumatic amputation of penis

S38.23 Traumatic amputation of scrotum and testis

⑦**S38.231** Complete traumatic amputation of scrotum and testis

⑦**S38.232** Partial traumatic amputation of scrotum and testis

⊗⑦**S38.3** Transection (partial) of abdomen

S39 Other and unspecified injuries of abdomen, lower back, pelvis and external genitals

Code also any associated open wound (S31.-)

Excludes2: sprain of joints and ligaments of lumbar spine and pelvis (S33.-)

The appropriate 7th character is to be added to each code from category S39

A - initial encounter

D - subsequent encounter

S - sequela

S39.0 Injury of muscle, fascia and tendon of abdomen, lower back and pelvis

S39.00 Unspecified injury of muscle, fascia and tendon of abdomen, lower back and pelvis

⑦**S39.001** Unspecified injury of muscle, fascia and tendon of abdomen

⑦**S39.002** Unspecified injury of muscle, fascia and tendon of lower back

⑦**S39.003** Unspecified injury of muscle, fascia and tendon of pelvis

S39.01 Strain of muscle, fascia and tendon of abdomen, lower back and pelvis

⑦**S39.011** Strain of muscle, fascia and tendon of abdomen

⑦**S39.012** Strain of muscle, fascia and tendon of lower back

⑦**S39.013** Strain of muscle, fascia and tendon of pelvis

S39.02 Laceration of muscle, fascia and tendon of abdomen, lower back and pelvis

⑦**S39.021** Laceration of muscle, fascia and tendon of abdomen

⑦**S39.022** Laceration of muscle, fascia and tendon of lower back

⑦**S39.023** Laceration of muscle, fascia and tendon of pelvis

S39.09 Other injury of muscle, fascia and tendon of abdomen, lower back and pelvis

⑦**S39.091** Other injury of muscle, fascia and tendon of abdomen

⑦**S39.092** Other injury of muscle, fascia and tendon of lower back

⑦**S39.093** Other injury of muscle, fascia and tendon of pelvis

S39.8 Other specified injuries of abdomen, lower back, pelvis and external genitals

⊗⑦**S39.81** Other specified injuries of abdomen

⊗⑦**S39.82** Other specified injuries of lower back

⊗⑦**S39.83** Other specified injuries of pelvis

S39.84 Other specified injuries of external genitals

⑦**S39.840** Fracture of corpus cavernosum penis

⑦**S39.848** Other specified injuries of external genitals

S39.9 Unspecified injury of abdomen, lower back, pelvis and external genitals

⊗⑦**S39.91** Unspecified injury of abdomen

⊗⑦**S39.92** Unspecified injury of lower back

⊗⑦**S39.93** Unspecified injury of pelvis

⊗⑦**S39.94** Unspecified injury of external genitals

INJURIES TO THE SHOULDER AND UPPER ARM (S40-S49)

Includes: injuries of axilla

injuries of scapular region

Excludes2: burns and corrosions (T20-T32)

frostbite (T33-T34)

injuries of elbow (S50-S59)

insect bite or sting, venomous (T63.4)

S40 Superficial injury of shoulder and upper arm

The appropriate 7th character is to be added to each code from category S40

A - initial encounter

D - subsequent encounter

S - sequela

S40.0 Contusion of shoulder and upper arm

S40.01 Contusion of shoulder

⑦**S40.011** Contusion of right shoulder

⑦**S40.012** Contusion of left shoulder

⑦**S40.019** Contusion of unspecified shoulder

S40.02 Contusion of upper arm

⑦**S40.021** Contusion of right upper arm

⑦**S40.022** Contusion of left upper arm

⑦**S40.029** Contusion of unspecified upper arm

S40.2 Other superficial injuries of shoulder

S40.21 Abrasion of shoulder

⑦**S40.211** Abrasion of right shoulder

⑦**S40.212** Abrasion of left shoulder

⑦**S40.219** Abrasion of unspecified shoulder

S40.22 Blister (nonthermal) of shoulder

⑦**S40.221**   **Blister (nonthermal) of right shoulder**

⑦**S40.222**   **Blister (nonthermal) of left shoulder**

⑦**S40.229**   **Blister (nonthermal) of unspecified shoulder**

S40.24   **External constriction of shoulder**

⑦**S40.241**   **External constriction of right shoulder**

⑦**S40.242**   **External constriction of left shoulder**

⑦**S40.249**   **External constriction of unspecified shoulder**

S40.25   **Superficial foreign body of shoulder**

Splinter in the shoulder

⑦**S40.251**   **Superficial foreign body of right shoulder**

⑦**S40.252**   **Superficial foreign body of left shoulder**

⑦**S40.259**   **Superficial foreign body of unspecified shoulder**

S40.26   **Insect bite (nonvenomous) of shoulder**

⑦**S40.261**   **Insect bite (nonvenomous) of right shoulder**

⑦**S40.262**   **Insect bite (nonvenomous) of left shoulder**

⑦**S40.269**   **Insect bite (nonvenomous) of unspecified shoulder**

S40.27   **Other superficial bite of shoulder**

Excludes1: open bite of shoulder (S41.05)

⑦**S40.271**   **Other superficial bite of right shoulder**

⑦**S40.272**   **Other superficial bite of left shoulder**

⑦**S40.279**   **Other superficial bite of unspecified shoulder**

S40.8   **Other superficial injuries of upper arm**

S40.81   **Abrasion of upper arm**

⑦**S40.811**   **Abrasion of right upper arm**

⑦**S40.812**   **Abrasion of left upper arm**

⑦**S40.819**   **Abrasion of unspecified upper arm**

S40.82   **Blister (nonthermal) of upper arm**

⑦**S40.821**   **Blister (nonthermal) of right upper arm**

⑦**S40.822**   **Blister (nonthermal) of left upper arm**

⑦**S40.829**   **Blister (nonthermal) of unspecified upper arm**

S40.84   **External constriction of upper arm**

⑦**S40.841**   **External constriction of right upper arm**

⑦**S40.842**   **External constriction of left upper arm**

⑦**S40.849**   **External constriction of unspecified upper arm**

S40.85   **Superficial foreign body of upper arm**

Splinter in the upper arm

⑦**S40.851**   **Superficial foreign body of right upper arm**

⑦**S40.852**   **Superficial foreign body of left upper arm**

⑦**S40.859**   **Superficial foreign body of unspecified upper arm**

S40.86   **Insect bite (nonvenomous) of upper arm**

⑦**S40.861**   **Insect bite (nonvenomous) of right upper arm**

⑦**S40.862**   **Insect bite (nonvenomous) of left upper arm**

⑦**S40.869**   **Insect bite (nonvenomous) of unspecified upper arm**

S40.87   **Other superficial bite of upper arm**

Excludes1: open bite of upper arm (S41.14)

Excludes2: Other superficial bite of shoulder (S40.27-)

⑦**S40.871**   **Other superficial bite of right upper arm**

⑦**S40.872**   **Other superficial bite of left upper arm**

⑦**S40.879**   **Other superficial bite of unspecified upper arm**

S40.9   **Unspecified superficial injury of shoulder and upper arm**

S40.91   **Unspecified superficial injury of shoulder**

⑦**S40.911**   **Unspecified superficial injury of right shoulder**

⑦**S40.912**   **Unspecified superficial injury of left shoulder**

⑦**S40.919**   **Unspecified superficial injury of unspecified shoulder**

S40.92   **Unspecified superficial injury of upper arm**

⑦**S40.921**   **Unspecified superficial injury of right upper arm**

⑦**S40.922**   **Unspecified superficial injury of left upper arm**

⑦**S40.929**   **Unspecified superficial injury of unspecified upper arm**

S41   **Open wound of shoulder and upper arm**

Code also any associated wound infection

Excludes1: traumatic amputation of shoulder and upper arm (S48.-)

Excludes2: open fracture of shoulder and upper arm (S42.- with 7th character B or C)

The appropriate 7th character is to be added to each code from category S41

A - initial encounter

D - subsequent encounter

S - sequela

S41.0   **Open wound of shoulder**

S41.00   **Unspecified open wound of shoulder**

⑦**S41.001**   **Unspecified open wound of right shoulder**

⑦**S41.002**   **Unspecified open wound of left shoulder**

⑦**S41.009**   **Unspecified open wound of unspecified shoulder**

S41.01   **Laceration without foreign body of shoulder**

⑦**S41.011**   **Laceration without foreign body of right shoulder**

⑦S41.012　Laceration without foreign body of left shoulder

⑦S41.019　Laceration without foreign body of unspecified shoulder

S41.02　Laceration with foreign body of shoulder

⑦S41.021　Laceration with foreign body of right shoulder

⑦S41.022　Laceration with foreign body of left shoulder

⑦S41.029　Laceration with foreign body of unspecified shoulder

S41.03　Puncture wound without foreign body of shoulder

⑦S41.031　Puncture wound without foreign body of right shoulder

⑦S41.032　Puncture wound without foreign body of left shoulder

⑦S41.039　Puncture wound without foreign body of unspecified shoulder

S41.04　Puncture wound with foreign body of shoulder

⑦S41.041　Puncture wound with foreign body of right shoulder

⑦S41.042　Puncture wound with foreign body of left shoulder

⑦S41.049　Puncture wound with foreign body of unspecified shoulder

S41.05　Open bite of shoulder

Bite of shoulder NOS

Excludes1: superficial bite of shoulder (S40.27)

⑦S41.051　Open bite of right shoulder

⑦S41.052　Open bite of left shoulder

⑦S41.059　Open bite of unspecified shoulder

S41.1　Open wound of upper arm

S41.10　Unspecified open wound of upper arm

⑦S41.101　Unspecified open wound of right upper arm

⑦S41.102　Unspecified open wound of left upper arm

⑦S41.109　Unspecified open wound of unspecified upper arm

S41.11　Laceration without foreign body of upper arm

⑦S41.111　Laceration without foreign body of right upper arm

⑦S41.112　Laceration without foreign body of left upper arm

⑦S41.119　Laceration without foreign body of unspecified upper arm

S41.12　Laceration with foreign body of upper arm

⑦S41.121　Laceration with foreign body of right upper arm

⑦S41.122　Laceration with foreign body of left upper arm

⑦S41.129　Laceration with foreign body of unspecified upper arm

S41.13　Puncture wound without foreign body of upper arm

⑦S41.131　Puncture wound without foreign body of right upper arm

⑦S41.132　Puncture wound without foreign body of left upper arm

⑦S41.139　Puncture wound without foreign body of unspecified upper arm

S41.14　Puncture wound with foreign body of upper arm

⑦S41.141　Puncture wound with foreign body of right upper arm

⑦S41.142　Puncture wound with foreign body of left upper arm

⑦S41.149　Puncture wound with foreign body of unspecified upper arm

S41.15　Open bite of upper arm

Bite of upper arm NOS

Excludes1: superficial bite of upper arm (S40.87)

⑦S41.151　Open bite of right upper arm

⑦S41.152　Open bite of left upper arm

⑦S41.159　Open bite of unspecified upper arm

S42　Fracture of shoulder and upper arm

Note: A fracture not indicated as displaced or nondisplaced should be coded to displaced

A fracture not indicated as open or closed should be coded to closed

Excludes1: traumatic amputation of shoulder and upper arm (S48.-)

The appropriate 7th character is to be added to all codes from category S42

A - initial encounter for closed fracture

B - initial encounter for open fracture

D - subsequent encounter for fracture with routine healing

G - subsequent encounter for fracture with delayed healing

K - subsequent encounter for fracture with nonunion

P - subsequent encounter for fracture with malunion

S - sequela

S42.0　Fracture of clavicle

S42.00　Fracture of unspecified part of clavicle

⑦S42.001　Fracture of unspecified part of right clavicle

⑦S42.002　Fracture of unspecified part of left clavicle

⑦S42.009　Fracture of unspecified part of unspecified clavicle

S42.01　Fracture of sternal end of clavicle

⑦S42.011　Anterior displaced fracture of sternal end of right clavicle

⑦S42.012　Anterior displaced fracture of sternal end of left clavicle

⑦S42.013　Anterior displaced fracture of sternal end of unspecified clavicle

Displaced fracture of sternal end of clavicle NOS

⑦S42.014　Posterior displaced fracture of sternal end of right clavicle

⑦S42.015　Posterior displaced fracture of sternal end of left clavicle

⑦S42.016　Posterior displaced fracture of sternal end of unspecified clavicle

⑦S42.017　Nondisplaced fracture of sternal end of right clavicle

⑦S42.018　Nondisplaced fracture of sternal end of left clavicle

⑦S42.019　Nondisplaced fracture of sternal end of unspecified clavicle

S42.02   Fracture of shaft of clavicle
　⑦S42.021   Displaced fracture of shaft of right clavicle
　⑦S42.022   Displaced fracture of shaft of left clavicle
　⑦S42.023   Displaced fracture of shaft of unspecified clavicle
　⑦S42.024   Nondisplaced fracture of shaft of right clavicle
　⑦S42.025   Nondisplaced fracture of shaft of left clavicle
　⑦S42.026   Nondisplaced fracture of shaft of unspecified clavicle

S42.03   Fracture of lateral end of clavicle
Fracture of acromial end of clavicle
　⑦S42.031   Displaced fracture of lateral end of right clavicle
　⑦S42.032   Displaced fracture of lateral end of left clavicle
　⑦S42.033   Displaced fracture of lateral end of unspecified clavicle
　⑦S42.034   Nondisplaced fracture of lateral end of right clavicle
　⑦S42.035   Nondisplaced fracture of lateral end of left clavicle
　⑦S42.036   Nondisplaced fracture of lateral end of unspecified clavicle

S42.1   Fracture of scapula
S42.10   Fracture of unspecified part of scapula
　⑦S42.101   Fracture of unspecified part of scapula, right shoulder
　⑦S42.102   Fracture of unspecified part of scapula, left shoulder
　⑦S42.109   Fracture of unspecified part of scapula, unspecified shoulder

S42.11   Fracture of body of scapula
　⑦S42.111   Displaced fracture of body of scapula, right shoulder
　⑦S42.112   Displaced fracture of body of scapula, left shoulder
　⑦S42.113   Displaced fracture of body of scapula, unspecified shoulder
　⑦S42.114   Nondisplaced fracture of body of scapula, right shoulder
　⑦S42.115   Nondisplaced fracture of body of scapula, left shoulder
　⑦S42.116   Nondisplaced fracture of body of scapula, unspecified shoulder

S42.12   Fracture of acromial process
　⑦S42.121   Displaced fracture of acromial process, right shoulder
　⑦S42.122   Displaced fracture of acromial process, left shoulder
　⑦S42.123   Displaced fracture of acromial process, unspecified shoulder
　⑦S42.124   Nondisplaced fracture of acromial process, right shoulder
　⑦S42.125   Nondisplaced fracture of acromial process, left shoulder
　⑦S42.126   Nondisplaced fracture of acromial process, unspecified shoulder

S42.13   Fracture of coracoid process
　⑦S42.131   Displaced fracture of coracoid process, right shoulder
　⑦S42.132   Displaced fracture of coracoid process, left shoulder
　⑦S42.133   Displaced fracture of coracoid process, unspecified shoulder
　⑦S42.134   Nondisplaced fracture of coracoid process, right shoulder
　⑦S42.135   Nondisplaced fracture of coracoid process, left shoulder
　⑦S42.136   Nondisplaced fracture of coracoid process, unspecified shoulder

S42.14   Fracture of glenoid cavity of scapula
　⑦S42.141   Displaced fracture of glenoid cavity of scapula, right shoulder
　⑦S42.142   Displaced fracture of glenoid cavity of scapula, left shoulder
　⑦S42.143   Displaced fracture of glenoid cavity of scapula, unspecified shoulder
　⑦S42.144   Nondisplaced fracture of glenoid cavity of scapula, right shoulder
　⑦S42.145   Nondisplaced fracture of glenoid cavity of scapula, left shoulder
　⑦S42.146   Nondisplaced fracture of glenoid cavity of scapula, unspecified shoulder

S42.15   Fracture of neck of scapula
　⑦S42.151   Displaced fracture of neck of scapula, right shoulder
　⑦S42.152   Displaced fracture of neck of scapula, left shoulder
　⑦S42.153   Displaced fracture of neck of scapula, unspecified shoulder
　⑦S42.154   Nondisplaced fracture of neck of scapula, right shoulder
　⑦S42.155   Nondisplaced fracture of neck of scapula, left shoulder
　⑦S42.156   Nondisplaced fracture of neck of scapula, unspecified shoulder

S42.19   Fracture of other part of scapula
　⑦S42.191   Fracture of other part of scapula, right shoulder
　⑦S42.192   Fracture of other part of scapula, left shoulder
　⑦S42.199   Fracture of other part of scapula, unspecified shoulder

S42.2   Fracture of upper end of humerus
Fracture of proximal end of humerus
Excludes2: fracture of shaft of humerus (S42.3-)
physeal fracture of upper end of humerus (S49.0-)

S42.20   Unspecified fracture of upper end of humerus
　⑦S42.201   Unspecified fracture of upper end of right humerus
　⑦S42.202   Unspecified fracture of upper end of left humerus

⑦ **S42.209** **Unspecified fracture of upper end of unspecified humerus**

S42.21 **Unspecified fracture of surgical neck of humerus**

Fracture of neck of humerus NOS

⑦ **S42.211** **Unspecified displaced fracture of surgical neck of right humerus**

⑦ **S42.212** **Unspecified displaced fracture of surgical neck of left humerus**

⑦ **S42.213** **Unspecified displaced fracture of surgical neck of unspecified humerus**

⑦ **S42.214** **Unspecified nondisplaced fracture of surgical neck of right humerus**

⑦ **S42.215** **Unspecified nondisplaced fracture of surgical neck of left humerus**

⑦ **S42.216** **Unspecified nondisplaced fracture of surgical neck of unspecified humerus**

S42.22 **2-part fracture of surgical neck of humerus**

⑦ **S42.221** **2-part displaced fracture of surgical neck of right humerus**

⑦ **S42.222** **2-part displaced fracture of surgical neck of left humerus**

⑦ **S42.223** **2-part displaced fracture of surgical neck of unspecified humerus**

⑦ **S42.224** **2-part nondisplaced fracture of surgical neck of right humerus**

⑦ **S42.225** **2-part nondisplaced fracture of surgical neck of left humerus**

⑦ **S42.226** **2-part nondisplaced fracture of surgical neck of unspecified humerus**

S42.23 **3-part fracture of surgical neck of humerus**

⑦ **S42.231** **3-part fracture of surgical neck of right humerus**

⑦ **S42.232** **3-part fracture of surgical neck of left humerus**

⑦ **S42.239** **3-part fracture of surgical neck of unspecified humerus**

S42.24 **4-part fracture of surgical neck of humerus**

⑦ **S42.241** **4-part fracture of surgical neck of right humerus**

⑦ **S42.242** **4-part fracture of surgical neck of left humerus**

⑦ **S42.249** **4-part fracture of surgical neck of unspecified humerus**

S42.25 **Fracture of greater tuberosity of humerus**

⑦ **S42.251** **Displaced fracture of greater tuberosity of right humerus**

⑦ **S42.252** **Displaced fracture of greater tuberosity of left humerus**

⑦ **S42.253** **Displaced fracture of greater tuberosity of unspecified humerus**

⑦ **S42.254** **Nondisplaced fracture of greater tuberosity of right humerus**

⑦ **S42.255** **Nondisplaced fracture of greater tuberosity of left humerus**

⑦ **S42.256** **Nondisplaced fracture of greater tuberosity of unspecified humerus**

S42.26 **Fracture of lesser tuberosity of humerus**

⑦ **S42.261** **Displaced fracture of lesser tuberosity of right humerus**

⑦ **S42.262** **Displaced fracture of lesser tuberosity of left humerus**

⑦ **S42.263** **Displaced fracture of lesser tuberosity of unspecified humerus**

⑦ **S42.264** **Nondisplaced fracture of lesser tuberosity of right humerus**

⑦ **S42.265** **Nondisplaced fracture of lesser tuberosity of left humerus**

⑦ **S42.266** **Nondisplaced fracture of lesser tuberosity of unspecified humerus**

S42.27 **Torus fracture of upper end of humerus**

The appropriate 7th character is to be added to all codes in subcategory S42.27

A - initial encounter for closed fracture

D - subsequent encounter for fracture with routine healing

G - subsequent encounter for fracture with delayed healing

K - subsequent encounter for fracture with nonunion

P - subsequent encounter for fracture with malunion S - sequela

⑦ **S42.271** **Torus fracture of upper end of right humerus**

⑦ **S42.272** **Torus fracture of upper end of left humerus**

⑦ **S42.279** **Torus fracture of upper end of unspecified humerus**

S42.29 **Other fracture of upper end of humerus**

Fracture of anatomical neck of humerus

Fracture of articular head of humerus

⑦ **S42.291** **Other displaced fracture of upper end of right humerus**

⑦ **S42.292** **Other displaced fracture of upper end of left humerus**

⑦ **S42.293** **Other displaced fracture of upper end of unspecified humerus**

⑦ **S42.294** **Other nondisplaced fracture of upper end of right humerus**

⑦ **S42.295** **Other nondisplaced fracture of upper end of left humerus**

⑦ **S42.296** **Other nondisplaced fracture of upper end of unspecified humerus**

S42.3 **Fracture of shaft of humerus**

Fracture of humerus NOS

Fracture of upper arm NOS

Excludes2: physeal fractures of upper end of humerus (S49.0-)

physeal fractures of lower end of humerus (S49.1-)

S42.30 **Unspecified fracture of shaft of humerus**

⑦ **S42.301** **Unspecified fracture of shaft of humerus, right arm**

⑦ **S42.302** **Unspecified fracture of shaft of humerus, left arm**

⑦ **S42.309** **Unspecified fracture of shaft of humerus, unspecified arm**

S42.31 **Greenstick fracture of shaft of humerus**

The appropriate 7th character is to be added to all codes in subcategory S42.31

A - initial encounter for closed fracture

D - subsequent encounter for fracture with routine healing

G - subsequent encounter for fracture with delayed healing

K - subsequent encounter for fracture with nonunion

P - subsequent encounter for fracture with malunion S - sequela

⑦**S42.311   Greenstick fracture of shaft of humerus, right arm**

⑦**S42.312   Greenstick fracture of shaft of humerus, left arm**

⑦**S42.319   Greenstick fracture of shaft of humerus, unspecified arm**

S42.32   Transverse fracture of shaft of humerus

⑦**S42.321   Displaced transverse fracture of shaft of humerus, right arm**

⑦**S42.322   Displaced transverse fracture of shaft of humerus, left arm**

⑦**S42.323   Displaced transverse fracture of shaft of humerus, unspecified arm**

⑦**S42.324   Nondisplaced transverse fracture of shaft of humerus, right arm**

⑦**S42.325   Nondisplaced transverse fracture of shaft of humerus, left arm**

⑦**S42.326   Nondisplaced transverse fracture of shaft of humerus, unspecified arm**

S42.33   Oblique fracture of shaft of humerus

⑦**S42.331   Displaced oblique fracture of shaft of humerus, right arm**

⑦**S42.332   Displaced oblique fracture of shaft of humerus, left arm**

⑦**S42.333   Displaced oblique fracture of shaft of humerus, unspecified arm**

⑦**S42.334   Nondisplaced oblique fracture of shaft of humerus, right arm**

⑦**S42.335   Nondisplaced oblique fracture of shaft of humerus, left arm**

⑦**S42.336   Nondisplaced oblique fracture of shaft of humerus, unspecified arm**

S42.34   ⑦Spiral fracture of shaft of humerus

⑦**S42.341   Displaced spiral fracture of shaft of humerus, right arm**

⑦**S42.342   Displaced spiral fracture of shaft of humerus, left arm**

⑦**S42.343   Displaced spiral fracture of shaft of humerus, unspecified arm**

⑦**S42.344   Nondisplaced spiral fracture of shaft of humerus, right arm**

⑦**S42.345   Nondisplaced spiral fracture of shaft of humerus, left arm**

⑦**S42.346   Nondisplaced spiral fracture of shaft of humerus, unspecified arm**

S42.35   Comminuted fracture of shaft of humerus

⑦**S42.351   Displaced comminuted fracture of shaft of humerus, right arm**

⑦**S42.352   Displaced comminuted fracture of shaft of humerus, left arm**

⑦**S42.353   Displaced comminuted fracture of shaft of humerus, unspecified arm**

⑦**S42.354   Nondisplaced comminuted fracture of shaft of humerus, right arm**

⑦**S42.355   Nondisplaced comminuted fracture of shaft of humerus, left arm**

⑦**S42.356   Nondisplaced comminuted fracture of shaft of humerus, unspecified arm**

S42.36   Segmental fracture of shaft of humerus

⑦**S42.361   Displaced segmental fracture of shaft of humerus, right arm**

⑦**S42.362   Displaced segmental fracture of shaft of humerus, left arm**

⑦**S42.363   Displaced segmental fracture of shaft of humerus, unspecified arm**

⑦**S42.364   Nondisplaced segmental fracture of shaft of humerus, right arm**

⑦**S42.365   Nondisplaced segmental fracture of shaft of humerus, left arm**

⑦**S42.366   Nondisplaced segmental fracture of shaft of humerus, unspecified arm**

S42.39   Other fracture of shaft of humerus

⑦**S42.391   Other fracture of shaft of right humerus**

⑦**S42.392   Other fracture of shaft of left humerus**

⑦**S42.399   Other fracture of shaft of unspecified humerus**

S42.4   Fracture of lower end of humerus

Fracture of distal end of humerus

Excludes2: fracture of shaft of humerus (S42.3-)

physeal fracture of lower end of humerus (S49.1-)

S42.40   Unspecified fracture of lower end of humerus

Fracture of elbow NOS

⑦**S42.401   Unspecified fracture of lower end of right humerus**

⑦**S42.402   Unspecified fracture of lower end of left humerus**

⑦**S42.409   Unspecified fracture of lower end of unspecified humerus**

S42.41   Simple supracondylar fracture without intercondylar fracture of humerus

⑦**S42.411   Displaced simple supracondylar fracture without intercondylar fracture of right humerus**

⑦**S42.412   Displaced simple supracondylar fracture without intercondylar fracture of left humerus**

⑦**S42.413   Displaced simple supracondylar fracture without intercondylar fracture of unspecified humerus**

⑦**S42.414   Nondisplaced simple supracondylar fracture without intercondylar fracture of right humerus**

⑦**S42.415   Nondisplaced simple supracondylar fracture without intercondylar fracture of left humerus**

⑦ **S42.416** Nondisplaced simple supracondylar fracture without intercondylar fracture of unspecified humerus

S42.42 Comminuted supracondylar fracture without intercondylar fracture of humerus

⑦ **S42.421** Displaced comminuted supracondylar fracture without intercondylar fracture of right humerus

⑦ **S42.422** Displaced comminuted supracondylar fracture without intercondylar fracture of left humerus

⑦ **S42.423** Displaced comminuted supracondylar fracture without intercondylar fracture of unspecified humerus

⑦ **S42.424** Nondisplaced comminuted supracondylar fracture without intercondylar fracture of right humerus

⑦ **S42.425** Nondisplaced comminuted supracondylar fracture without intercondylar fracture of left humerus

⑦ **S42.426** Nondisplaced comminuted supracondylar fracture without intercondylar fracture of unspecified humerus

S42.43 Fracture (avulsion) of lateral epicondyle of humerus

⑦ **S42.431** Displaced fracture (avulsion) of lateral epicondyle of right humerus

⑦ **S42.432** Displaced fracture (avulsion) of lateral epicondyle of left humerus

⑦ **S42.433** Displaced fracture (avulsion) of lateral epicondyle of unspecified humerus

⑦ **S42.434** Nondisplaced fracture (avulsion) of lateral epicondyle of right humerus

⑦ **S42.435** Nondisplaced fracture (avulsion) of lateral epicondyle of left humerus

⑦ **S42.436** Nondisplaced fracture (avulsion) of lateral epicondyle of unspecified humerus

S42.44 Fracture (avulsion) of medial epicondyle of humerus

⑦ **S42.441** Displaced fracture (avulsion) of medial epicondyle of right humerus

⑦ **S42.442** Displaced fracture (avulsion) of medial epicondyle of left humerus

⑦ **S42.443** Displaced fracture (avulsion) of medial epicondyle of unspecified humerus

⑦ **S42.444** Nondisplaced fracture (avulsion) of medial epicondyle of right humerus

⑦ **S42.445** Nondisplaced fracture (avulsion) of medial epicondyle of left humerus

⑦ **S42.446** Nondisplaced fracture (avulsion) of medial epicondyle of unspecified humerus

⑦ **S42.447** Incarcerated fracture (avulsion) of medial epicondyle of right humerus

⑦ **S42.448** Incarcerated fracture (avulsion) of medial epicondyle of left humerus

⑦ **S42.449** Incarcerated fracture (avulsion) of medial epicondyle of unspecified humerus

S42.45 Fracture of lateral condyle of humerus

Fracture of capitellum of humerus

⑦ **S42.451** Displaced fracture of lateral condyle of right humerus

⑦ **S42.452** Displaced fracture of lateral condyle of left humerus

⑦ **S42.453** Displaced fracture of lateral condyle of unspecified humerus

⑦ **S42.454** Nondisplaced fracture of lateral condyle of right humerus

⑦ **S42.455** Nondisplaced fracture of lateral condyle of left humerus

⑦ **S42.456** Nondisplaced fracture of lateral condyle of unspecified humerus

S42.46 Fracture of medial condyle of humerus

Trochlea fracture of humerus

⑦ **S42.461** Displaced fracture of medial condyle of right humerus

⑦ **S42.462** Displaced fracture of medial condyle of left humerus

⑦ **S42.463** Displaced fracture of medial condyle of unspecified humerus

⑦ **S42.464** Nondisplaced fracture of medial condyle of right humerus

⑦ **S42.465** Nondisplaced fracture of medial condyle of left humerus

⑦ **S42.466** Nondisplaced fracture of medial condyle of unspecified humerus

S42.47 Transcondylar fracture of humerus

⑦ **S42.471** Displaced transcondylar fracture of right humerus

⑦ **S42.472** Displaced transcondylar fracture of left humerus

⑦ **S42.473** Displaced transcondylar fracture of unspecified humerus

⑦ **S42.474** Nondisplaced transcondylar fracture of right humerus

⑦ **S42.475** Nondisplaced transcondylar fracture of left humerus

⑦ **S42.476** Nondisplaced transcondylar fracture of unspecified humerus

S42.48 Torus fracture of lower end of humerus

The appropriate 7th character is to be added to all codes in subcategory S42.48

A - initial encounter for closed fracture

D - subsequent encounter for fracture with routine healing

G - subsequent encounter for fracture with delayed healing

K - subsequent encounter for fracture with nonunion

P - subsequent encounter for fracture with malunion

S - sequela

● New code ▲ Revised code **Excludes1:** Not coded here **Excludes2:** Not included here ⊗ Placeholder required ⑦ 7ᵗʰ digit required

⑦S42.481   **Torus fracture of lower end of right humerus**

⑦S42.482   **Torus fracture of lower end of left humerus**

⑦S42.489   **Torus fracture of lower end of unspecified humerus**

S42.49   **Other fracture of lower end of humerus**

⑦S42.491   **Other displaced fracture of lower end of right humerus**

⑦S42.492   **Other displaced fracture of lower end of left humerus**

⑦S42.493   **Other displaced fracture of lower end of unspecified humerus**

⑦S42.494   **Other nondisplaced fracture of lower end of right humerus**

⑦S42.495   **Other nondisplaced fracture of lower end of left humerus**

⑦S42.496   **Other nondisplaced fracture of lower end of unspecified humerus**

S42.9   **Fracture of shoulder girdle, part unspecified**

Fracture of shoulder NOS

⊗⑦S42.90   **Fracture of unspecified shoulder girdle, part unspecified**

⊗⑦S42.91   **Fracture of right shoulder girdle, part unspecified**

⊗⑦S42.92   **Fracture of left shoulder girdle, part unspecified**

S43   **Dislocation and sprain of joints and ligaments of shoulder girdle**

Includes: avulsion of joint or ligament of shoulder girdle

laceration of cartilage, joint or ligament of shoulder girdle

sprain of cartilage, joint or ligament of shoulder girdle

traumatic hemarthrosis of joint or ligament of shoulder girdle

traumatic rupture of joint or ligament of shoulder girdle

traumatic subluxation of joint or ligament of shoulder girdle

traumatic tear of joint or ligament of shoulder girdle

Code also any associated open wound

Excludes2: strain of muscle, fascia and tendon of shoulder and upper arm (S46.-)

The appropriate 7th character is to be added to each code from category S43

A - initial encounter

D - subsequent encounter

S - sequela

S43.0   **Subluxation and dislocation of shoulder joint**

Dislocation of glenohumeral joint

Subluxation of glenohumeral joint

S43.00   **Unspecified subluxation and dislocation of shoulder joint**

Dislocation of humerus NOS

Subluxation of humerus NOS

⑦S43.001   **Unspecified subluxation of right shoulder joint**

⑦S43.002   **Unspecified subluxation of left shoulder joint**

⑦S43.003   **Unspecified subluxation of unspecified shoulder joint**

⑦S43.004   **Unspecified dislocation of right shoulder joint**

⑦S43.005   **Unspecified dislocation of left shoulder joint**

⑦S43.006   **Unspecified dislocation of unspecified shoulder joint**

S43.01   **Anterior subluxation and dislocation of humerus**

⑦S43.011   **Anterior subluxation of right humerus**

⑦S43.012   **Anterior subluxation of left humerus**

⑦S43.013   **Anterior subluxation of unspecified humerus**

⑦S43.014   **Anterior dislocation of right humerus**

⑦S43.015   **Anterior dislocation of left humerus**

⑦S43.016   **Anterior dislocation of unspecified humerus**

S43.02   **Posterior subluxation and dislocation of humerus**

⑦S43.021   **Posterior subluxation of right humerus**

⑦S43.022   **Posterior subluxation of left humerus**

⑦S43.023   **Posterior subluxation of unspecified humerus**

⑦S43.024   **Posterior dislocation of right humerus**

⑦S43.025   **Posterior dislocation of left humerus**

⑦S43.026   **Posterior dislocation of unspecified humerus**

S43.03   **Inferior subluxation and dislocation of humerus**

⑦S43.031   **Inferior subluxation of right humerus**

⑦S43.032   **Inferior subluxation of left humerus**

⑦S43.033   **Inferior subluxation of unspecified humerus**

⑦S43.034   **Inferior dislocation of right humerus**

⑦S43.035   **Inferior dislocation of left humerus**

⑦S43.036   **Inferior dislocation of unspecified humerus**

S43.08   **Other subluxation and dislocation of shoulder joint**

⑦S43.081   **Other subluxation of right shoulder joint**

⑦S43.082   **Other subluxation of left shoulder joint**

⑦S43.083   **Other subluxation of unspecified shoulder joint**

⑦S43.084   **Other dislocation of right shoulder joint**

⑦S43.085   **Other dislocation of left shoulder joint**

⑦S43.086   **Other dislocation of unspecified shoulder joint**

S43.1   **Subluxation and dislocation of acromioclavicular joint**

S43.10   **Unspecified dislocation of acromioclavicular joint**

   ⑦**S43.101**   **Unspecified dislocation of right acromioclavicular joint**

   ⑦**S43.102**   **Unspecified dislocation of left acromioclavicular joint**

   ⑦**S43.109**   **Unspecified dislocation of unspecified acromioclavicular joint**

S43.11   **Subluxation of acromioclavicular joint**

   ⑦**S43.111**   **Subluxation of right acromioclavicular joint**

   ⑦**S43.112**   **Subluxation of left acromioclavicular joint**

   ⑦**S43.119**   **Subluxation of unspecified acromioclavicular joint**

S43.12   **Dislocation of acromioclavicular joint, 100%-200% displacement**

   ⑦**S43.121**   **Dislocation of right acromioclavicular joint, 100%-200% displacement**

   ⑦**S43.122**   **Dislocation of left acromioclavicular joint, 100%-200% displacement**

   ⑦**S43.129**   **Dislocation of unspecified acromioclavicular joint, 100%-200% displacement**

S43.13   **Dislocation of acromioclavicular joint, greater than 200% displacement**

   ⑦**S43.131**   **Dislocation of right acromioclavicular joint, greater than 200% displacement**

   ⑦**S43.132**   **Dislocation of left acromioclavicular joint, greater than 200% displacement**

   ⑦**S43.139**   **Dislocation of unspecified acromioclavicular joint, greater than 200% displacement**

S43.14   **Inferior dislocation of acromioclavicular joint**

   ⑦**S43.141**   **Inferior dislocation of right acromioclavicular joint**

   ⑦**S43.142**   **Inferior dislocation of left acromioclavicular joint**

   ⑦**S43.149**   **Inferior dislocation of unspecified acromioclavicular joint**

S43.15   **Posterior dislocation of acromioclavicular joint**

   ⑦**S43.151**   **Posterior dislocation of right acromioclavicular joint**

   ⑦**S43.152**   **Posterior dislocation of left acromioclavicular joint**

   ⑦**S43.159**   **Posterior dislocation of unspecified acromioclavicular joint**

S43.2   **Subluxation and dislocation of sternoclavicular joint**

   S43.20   **Unspecified subluxation and dislocation of sternoclavicular joint**

     ⑦**S43.201**   **Unspecified subluxation of right sternoclavicular joint**

     ⑦**S43.202**   **Unspecified subluxation of left sternoclavicular joint**

     ⑦**S43.203**   **Unspecified subluxation of unspecified sternoclavicular joint**

     ⑦**S43.204**   **Unspecified dislocation of right sternoclavicular joint**

     ⑦**S43.205**   **Unspecified dislocation of left sternoclavicular joint**

     ⑦**S43.206**   **Unspecified dislocation of unspecified sternoclavicular joint**

   S43.21   **Anterior subluxation and dislocation of sternoclavicular joint**

     ⑦**S43.211**   **Anterior subluxation of right sternoclavicular joint**

     ⑦**S43.212**   **Anterior subluxation of left sternoclavicular joint**

     ⑦**S43.213**   **Anterior subluxation of unspecified sternoclavicular joint**

     ⑦**S43.214**   **Anterior dislocation of right sternoclavicular joint**

     ⑦**S43.215**   **Anterior dislocation of left sternoclavicular joint**

     ⑦**S43.216**   **Anterior dislocation of unspecified sternoclavicular joint**

   S43.22   **Posterior subluxation and dislocation of sternoclavicular joint**

     ⑦**S43.221**   **Posterior subluxation of right sternoclavicular joint**

     ⑦**S43.222**   **Posterior subluxation of left sternoclavicular joint**

     ⑦**S43.223**   **Posterior subluxation of unspecified sternoclavicular joint**

     ⑦**S43.224**   **Posterior dislocation of right sternoclavicular joint**

     ⑦**S43.225**   **Posterior dislocation of left sternoclavicular joint**

     ⑦**S43.226**   **Posterior dislocation of unspecified sternoclavicular joint**

S43.3   **Subluxation and dislocation of other and unspecified parts of shoulder girdle**

   S43.30   **Subluxation and dislocation of unspecified parts of shoulder girdle**

     Dislocation of shoulder girdle NOS

     Subluxation of shoulder girdle NOS

     ⑦**S43.301**   **Subluxation of unspecified parts of right shoulder girdle**

     ⑦**S43.302**   **Subluxation of unspecified parts of left shoulder girdle**

     ⑦**S43.303**   **Subluxation of unspecified parts of unspecified shoulder girdle**

     ⑦**S43.304**   **Dislocation of unspecified parts of right shoulder girdle**

     ⑦**S43.305**   **Dislocation of unspecified parts of left shoulder girdle**

     ⑦**S43.306**   **Dislocation of unspecified parts of unspecified shoulder girdle**

   S43.31   **Subluxation and dislocation of scapula**

     ⑦**S43.311**   **Subluxation of right scapula**

     ⑦**S43.312**   **Subluxation of left scapula**

     ⑦**S43.313**   **Subluxation of unspecified scapula**

     ⑦**S43.314**   **Dislocation of right scapula**

     ⑦**S43.315**   **Dislocation of left scapula**

     ⑦**S43.316**   **Dislocation of unspecified scapula**

   S43.39   **Subluxation and dislocation of other parts of shoulder girdle**

⑦**S43.391**   Subluxation of other parts of right shoulder girdle

⑦**S43.392**   Subluxation of other parts of left shoulder girdle

⑦**S43.393**   Subluxation of other parts of unspecified shoulder girdle

⑦**S43.394**   Dislocation of other parts of right shoulder girdle

⑦**S43.395**   Dislocation of other parts of left shoulder girdle

⑦**S43.396**   Dislocation of other parts of unspecified shoulder girdle

S43.4   **Sprain of shoulder joint**

S43.40   Unspecified sprain of shoulder joint

⑦**S43.401**   Unspecified sprain of right shoulder joint

⑦**S43.402**   Unspecified sprain of left shoulder joint

⑦**S43.409**   Unspecified sprain of unspecified shoulder joint

S43.41   Sprain of coracohumeral (ligament)

⑦**S43.411**   Sprain of right coracohumeral (ligament)

⑦**S43.412**   Sprain of left coracohumeral (ligament)

⑦**S43.419**   Sprain of unspecified coracohumeral (ligament)

S43.42   Sprain of rotator cuff capsule

Excludes1: rotator cuff syndrome (complete)(incomplete), not specified as traumatic (M75.1-)

Excludes2: injury of tendon of rotator cuff (S46.0-)

⑦**S43.421**   Sprain of right rotator cuff capsule

⑦**S43.422**   Sprain of left rotator cuff capsule

⑦**S43.429**   Sprain of unspecified rotator cuff capsule

S43.43   Superior glenoid labrum lesion

SLAP lesion

⑦**S43.431**   Superior glenoid labrum lesion of right shoulder

⑦**S43.432**   Superior glenoid labrum lesion of left shoulder

⑦**S43.439**   Superior glenoid labrum lesion of unspecified shoulder

S43.49   Other sprain of shoulder joint

⑦**S43.491**   Other sprain of right shoulder joint

⑦**S43.492**   Other sprain of left shoulder joint

⑦**S43.499**   Other sprain of unspecified shoulder joint

S43.5   **Sprain of acromioclavicular joint**

Sprain of acromioclavicular ligament

⊗⑦**S43.50**   Sprain of unspecified acromioclavicular joint

⊗⑦**S43.51**   Sprain of right acromioclavicular joint

⊗⑦**S43.52**   Sprain of left acromioclavicular joint

S43.6   **Sprain of sternoclavicular joint**

⊗⑦**S43.60**   Sprain of unspecified sternoclavicular joint

⊗⑦**S43.61**   Sprain of right sternoclavicular joint

⊗⑦**S43.62**   Sprain of left sternoclavicular joint

S43.8   **Sprain of other specified parts of shoulder girdle**

⊗⑦**S43.80**   Sprain of other specified parts of unspecified shoulder girdle

⊗⑦**S43.81**   Sprain of other specified parts of right shoulder girdle

⊗⑦**S43.82**   Sprain of other specified parts of left shoulder girdle

S43.9   **Sprain of unspecified parts of shoulder girdle**

⊗⑦**S43.90**   Sprain of unspecified parts of unspecified shoulder girdle

Sprain of shoulder girdle NOS

⊗⑦**S43.91**   Sprain of unspecified parts of right shoulder girdle

⊗⑦**S43.92**   Sprain of unspecified parts of left shoulder girdle

S44   **Injury of nerves at shoulder and upper arm level**

Code also any associated open wound (S41.-)

Excludes2: injury of brachial plexus (S14.3-)

The appropriate 7th character is to be added to each code from category S44

A - initial encounter

D - subsequent encounter

S - sequela

S44.0   **Injury of ulnar nerve at upper arm level**

Excludes1: ulnar nerve NOS (S54.0)

⊗⑦**S44.00**   Injury of ulnar nerve at upper arm level, unspecified arm

⊗⑦**S44.01**   Injury of ulnar nerve at upper arm level, right arm

⊗⑦**S44.02**   Injury of ulnar nerve at upper arm level, left arm

S44.1   **Injury of median nerve at upper arm level**

Excludes1: median nerve NOS (S54.1)

⊗⑦**S44.10**   Injury of median nerve at upper arm level, unspecified arm

⊗⑦**S44.11**   Injury of median nerve at upper arm level, right arm

⊗⑦**S44.12**   Injury of median nerve at upper arm level, left arm

S44.2   **Injury of radial nerve at upper arm level**

Excludes1: radial nerve NOS (S54.2)

⊗⑦**S44.20**   Injury of radial nerve at upper arm level, unspecified arm

⊗⑦**S44.21**   Injury of radial nerve at upper arm level, right arm

⊗⑦**S44.22**   Injury of radial nerve at upper arm level, left arm

S44.3   **Injury of axillary nerve**

⊗⑦**S44.30**   Injury of axillary nerve, unspecified arm

⊗⑦**S44.31**   Injury of axillary nerve, right arm

⊗⑦**S44.32**   Injury of axillary nerve, left arm

S44.4   **Injury of musculocutaneous nerve**

⊗⑦**S44.40**   Injury of musculocutaneous nerve, unspecified arm

⊗⑦**S44.41**   Injury of musculocutaneous nerve, right arm

⊗⑦**S44.42**   Injury of musculocutaneous nerve, left arm

S44.5   **Injury of cutaneous sensory nerve at shoulder and upper arm level**

⊗⑦S44.50 Injury of cutaneous sensory nerve at shoulder and upper arm level, unspecified arm

⊗⑦S44.51 Injury of cutaneous sensory nerve at shoulder and upper arm level, right arm

⊗⑦S44.52 Injury of cutaneous sensory nerve at shoulder and upper arm level, left arm

S44.8 Injury of other nerves at shoulder and upper arm level

  S44.8X Injury of other nerves at shoulder and upper arm level

    ⑦S44.8X1 Injury of other nerves at shoulder and upper arm level, right arm

    ⑦S44.8X2 Injury of other nerves at shoulder and upper arm level, left arm

    ⑦S44.8X9 Injury of other nerves at shoulder and upper arm level, unspecified arm

S44.9 Injury of unspecified nerve at shoulder and upper arm level

  ⊗⑦S44.90 Injury of unspecified nerve at shoulder and upper arm level, unspecified arm

  ⊗⑦S44.91 Injury of unspecified nerve at shoulder and upper arm level, right arm

  ⊗⑦S44.92 Injury of unspecified nerve at shoulder and upper arm level, left arm

S45 Injury of blood vessels at shoulder and upper arm level

Code also any associated open wound (S41.-)

Excludes2: injury of subclavian artery (S25.1)

  injury of subclavian vein (S25.3)

The appropriate 7th character is to be added to each code from category S45

A - initial encounter

D - subsequent encounter

S - sequela

S45.0 Injury of axillary artery

  S45.00 Unspecified injury of axillary artery

    ⑦S45.001 Unspecified injury of axillary artery, right side

    ⑦S45.002 Unspecified injury of axillary artery, left side

    ⑦S45.009 Unspecified injury of axillary artery, unspecified side

  S45.01 Laceration of axillary artery

    ⑦S45.011 Laceration of axillary artery, right side

    ⑦S45.012 Laceration of axillary artery, left side

    ⑦S45.019 Laceration of axillary artery, unspecified side

  S45.09 Other specified injury of axillary artery

    ⑦S45.091 Other specified injury of axillary artery, right side

    ⑦S45.092 Other specified injury of axillary artery, left side

    ⑦S45.099 Other specified injury of axillary artery, unspecified side

S45.1 Injury of brachial artery

  S45.10 Unspecified injury of brachial artery

    ⑦S45.101 Unspecified injury of brachial artery, right side

    ⑦S45.102 Unspecified injury of brachial artery, left side

    ⑦S45.109 Unspecified injury of brachial artery, unspecified side

  S45.11 Laceration of brachial artery

    ⑦S45.111 Laceration of brachial artery, right side

    ⑦S45.112 Laceration of brachial artery, left side

    ⑦S45.119 Laceration of brachial artery, unspecified side

  S45.19 Other specified injury of brachial artery

    ⑦S45.191 Other specified injury of brachial artery, right side

    ⑦S45.192 Other specified injury of brachial artery, left side

    ⑦S45.199 Other specified injury of brachial artery, unspecified side

S45.2 Injury of axillary or brachial vein

  S45.20 Unspecified injury of axillary or brachial vein

    ⑦S45.201 Unspecified injury of axillary or brachial vein, right side

    ⑦S45.202 Unspecified injury of axillary or brachial vein, left side

    ⑦S45.209 Unspecified injury of axillary or brachial vein, unspecified side

  S45.21 Laceration of axillary or brachial vein

    ⑦S45.211 Laceration of axillary or brachial vein, right side

    ⑦S45.212 Laceration of axillary or brachial vein, left side

    ⑦S45.219 Laceration of axillary or brachial vein, unspecified side

  S45.29 Other specified injury of axillary or brachial vein

    ⑦S45.291 Other specified injury of axillary or brachial vein, right side

    ⑦S45.292 Other specified injury of axillary or brachial vein, left side

    ⑦S45.299 Other specified injury of axillary or brachial vein, unspecified side

S45.3 Injury of superficial vein at shoulder and upper arm level

  S45.30 Unspecified injury of superficial vein at shoulder and upper arm level

    ⑦S45.301 Unspecified injury of superficial vein at shoulder and upper arm level, right arm

    ⑦S45.302 Unspecified injury of superficial vein at shoulder and upper arm level, left arm

    ⑦S45.309 Unspecified injury of superficial vein at shoulder and upper arm level, unspecified arm

  S45.31 Laceration of superficial vein at shoulder and upper arm level

    ⑦S45.311 Laceration of superficial vein at shoulder and upper arm level, right arm

⑦S45.312　　Laceration of superficial vein at shoulder and upper arm level, left arm

⑦S45.319　　Laceration of superficial vein at shoulder and upper arm level, unspecified arm

S45.39　　Other specified injury of superficial vein at shoulder and upper arm level

⑦S45.391　　Other specified injury of superficial vein at shoulder and upper arm level, right arm

⑦S45.392　　Other specified injury of superficial vein at shoulder and upper arm level, left arm

⑦S45.399　　Other specified injury of superficial vein at shoulder and upper arm level, unspecified arm

S45.8　　Injury of other specified blood vessels at shoulder and upper arm level

S45.80　　Unspecified injury of other specified blood vessels at shoulder and upper arm level

⑦S45.801　　Unspecified injury of other specified blood vessels at shoulder and upper arm level, right arm

⑦S45.802　　Unspecified injury of other specified blood vessels at shoulder and upper arm level, left arm

⑦S45.809　　Unspecified injury of other specified blood vessels at shoulder and upper arm level, unspecified arm

S45.81　　Laceration of other specified blood vessels at shoulder and upper arm level

⑦S45.811　　Laceration of other specified blood vessels at shoulder and upper arm level, right arm

⑦S45.812　　Laceration of other specified blood vessels at shoulder and upper arm level, left arm

⑦S45.819　　Laceration of other specified blood vessels at shoulder and upper arm level, unspecified arm

S45.89　　Other specified injury of other specified blood vessels at shoulder and upper arm level

⑦S45.891　　Other specified injury of other specified blood vessels at shoulder and upper arm level, right arm

⑦S45.892　　Other specified injury of other specified blood vessels at shoulder and upper arm level, left arm

⑦S45.899　　Other specified injury of other specified blood vessels at shoulder and upper arm level, unspecified arm

S45.9　　Injury of unspecified blood vessel at shoulder and upper arm level

S45.90　　Unspecified injury of unspecified blood vessel at shoulder and upper arm level

⑦S45.901　　Unspecified injury of unspecified blood vessel at shoulder and upper arm level, right arm

⑦S45.902　　Unspecified injury of unspecified blood vessel at shoulder and upper arm level, left arm

⑦S45.909　　Unspecified injury of unspecified blood vessel at shoulder and upper arm level, unspecified arm

S45.91　　Laceration of unspecified blood vessel at shoulder and upper arm level

⑦S45.911　　Laceration of unspecified blood vessel at shoulder and upper arm level, right arm

⑦S45.912　　Laceration of unspecified blood vessel at shoulder and upper arm level, left arm

⑦S45.919　　Laceration of unspecified blood vessel at shoulder and upper arm level, unspecified arm

S45.99　　Other specified injury of unspecified blood vessel at shoulder and upper arm level

⑦S45.991　　Other specified injury of unspecified blood vessel at shoulder and upper arm level, right arm

⑦S45.992　　Other specified injury of unspecified blood vessel at shoulder and upper arm level, left arm

⑦S45.999　　Other specified injury of unspecified blood vessel at shoulder and upper arm level, unspecified arm

S46　　Injury of muscle, fascia and tendon at shoulder and upper arm level

Code also any associated open wound (S41.-)

Excludes2: injury of muscle, fascia and tendon at elbow (S56.-)

sprain of joints and ligaments of shoulder girdle (S43.9)

The appropriate 7th character is to be added to each code from category S46

A - initial encounter

D - subsequent encounter

S - sequela

S46.0　　Injury of muscle(s) and tendon(s) of the rotator cuff of shoulder

S46.00　　Unspecified injury of muscle(s) and tendon(s) of the rotator cuff of shoulder

⑦S46.001　　Unspecified injury of muscle(s) and tendon(s) of the rotator cuff of right shoulder

⑦S46.002　　Unspecified injury of muscle(s) and tendon(s) of the rotator cuff of left shoulder

⑦S46.009　　Unspecified injury of muscle(s) and tendon(s) of the rotator cuff of unspecified shoulder

S46.01　　Strain of muscle(s) and tendon(s) of the rotator cuff of shoulder

⑦S46.011　　Strain of muscle(s) and tendon(s) of the rotator cuff of right shoulder

⑦S46.012　　Strain of muscle(s) and tendon(s) of the rotator cuff of left shoulder

⑦S46.019　　Strain of muscle(s) and tendon(s) of the rotator cuff of unspecified shoulder

S46.02　　Laceration of muscle(s) and tendon(s) of the rotator cuff of shoulder

⑦S46.021 Laceration of muscle(s) and tendon(s) of the rotator cuff of right shoulder

⑦S46.022 Laceration of muscle(s) and tendon(s) of the rotator cuff of left shoulder

⑦S46.029 Laceration of muscle(s) and tendon(s) of the rotator cuff of unspecified shoulder

S46.09 Other injury of muscle(s) and tendon(s) of the rotator cuff of shoulder

⑦S46.091 Other injury of muscle(s) and tendon(s) of the rotator cuff of right shoulder

⑦S46.092 Other injury of muscle(s) and tendon(s) of the rotator cuff of left shoulder

⑦S46.099 Other injury of muscle(s) and tendon(s) of the rotator cuff of unspecified shoulder

S46.1 Injury of muscle, fascia and tendon of long head of biceps

S46.10 Unspecified injury of muscle, fascia and tendon of long head of biceps

⑦S46.101 Unspecified injury of muscle, fascia and tendon of long head of biceps, right arm

⑦S46.102 Unspecified injury of muscle, fascia and tendon of long head of biceps, left arm

⑦S46.109 Unspecified injury of muscle, fascia and tendon of long head of biceps, unspecified arm

S46.11 Strain of muscle, fascia and tendon of long head of biceps

⑦S46.111 Strain of muscle, fascia and tendon of long head of biceps, right arm

⑦S46.112 Strain of muscle, fascia and tendon of long head of biceps, left arm

⑦S46.119 Strain of muscle, fascia and tendon of long head of biceps, unspecified arm

S46.12 Laceration of muscle, fascia and tendon of long head of biceps

⑦S46.121 Laceration of muscle, fascia and tendon of long head of biceps, right arm

⑦S46.122 Laceration of muscle, fascia and tendon of long head of biceps, left arm

⑦S46.129 Laceration of muscle, fascia and tendon of long head of biceps, unspecified arm

S46.19 Other injury of muscle, fascia and tendon of long head of biceps

⑦S46.191 Other injury of muscle, fascia and tendon of long head of biceps, right arm

⑦S46.192 Other injury of muscle, fascia and tendon of long head of biceps, left arm

⑦S46.199 Other injury of muscle, fascia and tendon of long head of biceps, unspecified arm

S46.2 Injury of muscle, fascia and tendon of other parts of biceps

S46.20 Unspecified injury of muscle, fascia and tendon of other parts of biceps

⑦S46.201 Unspecified injury of muscle, fascia and tendon of other parts of biceps, right arm

⑦S46.202 Unspecified injury of muscle, fascia and tendon of other parts of biceps, left arm

⑦S46.209 Unspecified injury of muscle, fascia and tendon of other parts of biceps, unspecified arm

S46.21 Strain of muscle, fascia and tendon of other parts of biceps

⑦S46.211 Strain of muscle, fascia and tendon of other parts of biceps, right arm

⑦S46.212 Strain of muscle, fascia and tendon of other parts of biceps, left arm

⑦S46.219 Strain of muscle, fascia and tendon of other parts of biceps, unspecified arm

S46.22 Laceration of muscle, fascia and tendon of other parts of biceps

⑦S46.221 Laceration of muscle, fascia and tendon of other parts of biceps, right arm

⑦S46.222 Laceration of muscle, fascia and tendon of other parts of biceps, left arm

⑦S46.229 Laceration of muscle, fascia and tendon of other parts of biceps, unspecified arm

S46.29 Other injury of muscle, fascia and tendon of other parts of biceps

⑦S46.291 Other injury of muscle, fascia and tendon of other parts of biceps, right arm

⑦S46.292 Other injury of muscle, fascia and tendon of other parts of biceps, left arm

⑦S46.299 Other injury of muscle, fascia and tendon of other parts of biceps, unspecified arm

S46.3 Injury of muscle, fascia and tendon of triceps

S46.30 Unspecified injury of muscle, fascia and tendon of triceps

⑦S46.301 Unspecified injury of muscle, fascia and tendon of triceps, right arm

⑦S46.302 Unspecified injury of muscle, fascia and tendon of triceps, left arm

⑦S46.309 Unspecified injury of muscle, fascia and tendon of triceps, unspecified arm

S46.31 Strain of muscle, fascia and tendon of triceps

⑦S46.311 Strain of muscle, fascia and tendon of triceps, right arm

⑦S46.312 Strain of muscle, fascia and tendon of triceps, left arm

⑦S46.319 Strain of muscle, fascia and tendon of triceps, unspecified arm

S46.32 Laceration of muscle, fascia and tendon of triceps

● New code ▲ Revised code **Excludes1:** Not coded here **Excludes2:** Not included here ⊗ Placeholder required ⑦7th digit required

⑦S46.321   Laceration of muscle, fascia and tendon of triceps, right arm

⑦S46.322   Laceration of muscle, fascia and tendon of triceps, left arm

⑦S46.329   Laceration of muscle, fascia and tendon of triceps, unspecified arm

S46.39   Other injury of muscle, fascia and tendon of triceps

⑦S46.391   Other injury of muscle, fascia and tendon of triceps, right arm

⑦S46.392   Other injury of muscle, fascia and tendon of triceps, left arm

⑦S46.399   Other injury of muscle, fascia and tendon of triceps, unspecified arm

S46.8   Injury of other muscles, fascia and tendons at shoulder and upper arm level

S46.80   Unspecified injury of other muscles, fascia and tendons at shoulder and upper arm level

⑦S46.801   Unspecified injury of other muscles, fascia and tendons at shoulder and upper arm level, right arm

⑦S46.802   Unspecified injury of other muscles, fascia and tendons at shoulder and upper arm level, left arm

⑦S46.809   Unspecified injury of other muscles, fascia and tendons at shoulder and upper arm level, unspecified arm

S46.81   Strain of other muscles, fascia and tendons at shoulder and upper arm level

⑦S46.811   Strain of other muscles, fascia and tendons at shoulder and upper arm level, right arm

⑦S46.812   Strain of other muscles, fascia and tendons at shoulder and upper arm level, left arm

⑦S46.819   Strain of other muscles, fascia and tendons at shoulder and upper arm level, unspecified arm

S46.82   Laceration of other muscles, fascia and tendons at shoulder and upper arm level

⑦S46.821   Laceration of other muscles, fascia and tendons at shoulder and upper arm level, right arm

⑦S46.822   Laceration of other muscles, fascia and tendons at shoulder and upper arm level, left arm

⑦S46.829   Laceration of other muscles, fascia and tendons at shoulder and upper arm level, unspecified arm

S46.89   Other injury of other muscles, fascia and tendons at shoulder and upper arm level

⑦S46.891   Other injury of other muscles, fascia and tendons at shoulder and upper arm level, right arm

⑦S46.892   Other injury of other muscles, fascia and tendons at shoulder and upper arm level, left arm

⑦S46.899   Other injury of other muscles, fascia and tendons at shoulder and upper arm level, unspecified arm

S46.9   Injury of unspecified muscle, fascia and tendon at shoulder and upper arm level

S46.90   Unspecified injury of unspecified muscle, fascia and tendon at shoulder and upper arm level

⑦S46.901   Unspecified injury of unspecified muscle, fascia and tendon at shoulder and upper arm level, right arm

⑦S46.902   Unspecified injury of unspecified muscle, fascia and tendon at shoulder and upper arm level, left arm

⑦S46.909   Unspecified injury of unspecified muscle, fascia and tendon at shoulder and upper arm level, unspecified arm

S46.91   Strain of unspecified muscle, fascia and tendon at shoulder and upper arm level

⑦S46.911   Strain of unspecified muscle, fascia and tendon at shoulder and upper arm level, right arm

⑦S46.912   Strain of unspecified muscle, fascia and tendon at shoulder and upper arm level, left arm

⑦S46.919   Strain of unspecified muscle, fascia and tendon at shoulder and upper arm level, unspecified arm

S46.92   Laceration of unspecified muscle, fascia and tendon at shoulder and upper arm level

⑦S46.921   Laceration of unspecified muscle, fascia and tendon at shoulder and upper arm level, right arm

⑦S46.922   Laceration of unspecified muscle, fascia and tendon at shoulder and upper arm level, left arm

⑦S46.929   Laceration of unspecified muscle, fascia and tendon at shoulder and upper arm level, unspecified arm

S46.99   Other injury of unspecified muscle, fascia and tendon at shoulder and upper arm level

⑦S46.991   Other injury of unspecified muscle, fascia and tendon at shoulder and upper arm level, right arm

⑦S46.992   Other injury of unspecified muscle, fascia and tendon at shoulder and upper arm level, left arm

⑦S46.999   Other injury of unspecified muscle, fascia and tendon at shoulder and upper arm level, unspecified arm

S47   Crushing injury of shoulder and upper arm

Use additional code for all associated injuries

Excludes2: crushing injury of elbow (S57.0-)

The appropriate 7th character is to be added to each code from category S47

A - initial encounter

D - subsequent encounter

S - sequela

⊗⑦S47.1   Crushing injury of right shoulder and upper arm

⊗⑦S47.2   Crushing injury of left shoulder and upper arm

⊗⑦S47.9   Crushing injury of shoulder and upper arm, unspecified arm

S48   Traumatic amputation of shoulder and upper arm

An amputation not identified as partial or complete should be coded to complete

Excludes1: traumatic amputation at elbow level (S58.0)

The appropriate 7th character is to be added to each code from category S48

A - initial encounter

D - subsequent encounter

S - sequela

S48.0   Traumatic amputation at shoulder joint

    S48.01   Complete traumatic amputation at shoulder joint

       ⑦ **S48.011   Complete traumatic amputation at right shoulder joint**

       ⑦ **S48.012   Complete traumatic amputation at left shoulder joint**

       ⑦ **S48.019   Complete traumatic amputation at unspecified shoulder joint**

    S48.02   Partial traumatic amputation at shoulder joint

       ⑦ **S48.021   Partial traumatic amputation at right shoulder joint**

       ⑦ **S48.022   Partial traumatic amputation at left shoulder joint**

       ⑦ **S48.029   Partial traumatic amputation at unspecified shoulder joint**

S48.1   Traumatic amputation at level between shoulder and elbow

    S48.11   Complete traumatic amputation at level between shoulder and elbow

       ⑦ **S48.111   Complete traumatic amputation at level between right shoulder and elbow**

       ⑦ **S48.112   Complete traumatic amputation at level between left shoulder and elbow**

       ⑦ **S48.119   Complete traumatic amputation at level between unspecified shoulder and elbow**

    S48.12   Partial traumatic amputation at level between shoulder and elbow

       ⑦ **S48.121   Partial traumatic amputation at level between right shoulder and elbow**

       ⑦ **S48.122   Partial traumatic amputation at level between left shoulder and elbow**

       ⑦ **S48.129   Partial traumatic amputation at level between unspecified shoulder and elbow**

S48.9   Traumatic amputation of shoulder and upper arm, level unspecified

    S48.91   Complete traumatic amputation of shoulder and upper arm, level unspecified

       ⑦ **S48.911   Complete traumatic amputation of right shoulder and upper arm, level unspecified**

       ⑦ **S48.912   Complete traumatic amputation of left shoulder and upper arm, level unspecified**

       ⑦ **S48.919   Complete traumatic amputation of unspecified shoulder and upper arm, level unspecified**

    S48.92   Partial traumatic amputation of shoulder and upper arm, level unspecified

       ⑦ **S48.921   Partial traumatic amputation of right shoulder and upper arm, level unspecified**

       ⑦ **S48.922   Partial traumatic amputation of left shoulder and upper arm, level unspecified**

       ⑦ **S48.929   Partial traumatic amputation of unspecified shoulder and upper arm, level unspecified**

S49   Other and unspecified injuries of shoulder and upper arm

The appropriate 7th character is to be added to each code from subcategories S49.0 and S49.1

A - initial encounter for closed fracture

D - subsequent encounter for fracture with routine healing

G - subsequent encounter for fracture with delayed healing

K - subsequent encounter for fracture with nonunion

P - subsequent encounter for fracture with malunion

S - sequela

S49.0   Physeal fracture of upper end of humerus

    S49.00   Unspecified physeal fracture of upper end of humerus

       ⑦ **S49.001   Unspecified physeal fracture of upper end of humerus, right arm**

       ⑦ **S49.002   Unspecified physeal fracture of upper end of humerus, left arm**

       ⑦ **S49.009   Unspecified physeal fracture of upper end of humerus, unspecified arm**

    S49.01   Salter-Harris Type I physeal fracture of upper end of humerus

       ⑦ **S49.011   Salter-Harris Type I physeal fracture of upper end of humerus, right arm**

       ⑦ **S49.012   Salter-Harris Type I physeal fracture of upper end of humerus, left arm**

       ⑦ **S49.019   Salter-Harris Type I physeal fracture of upper end of humerus, unspecified arm**

    S49.02   Salter-Harris Type II physeal fracture of upper end of humerus

       ⑦ **S49.021   Salter-Harris Type II physeal fracture of upper end of humerus, right arm**

       ⑦ **S49.022   Salter-Harris Type II physeal fracture of upper end of humerus, left arm**

       ⑦ **S49.029   Salter-Harris Type II physeal fracture of upper end of humerus, unspecified arm**

    S49.03   Salter-Harris Type III physeal fracture of upper end of humerus

       ▲⑦ **S49.031   Salter-Harris Type III physeal fracture of upper end of humerus, right arm**

       ▲⑦ **S49.032   Salter-Harris Type III physeal fracture of upper end of humerus, left arm**

▲⑦**S49.039**   **Salter-Harris Type III physeal fracture of upper end of humerus, unspecified arm**

S49.04   **Salter-Harris Type IV physeal fracture of upper end of humerus**

⑦**S49.041**   **Salter-Harris Type IV physeal fracture of upper end of humerus, right arm**

⑦**S49.042**   **Salter-Harris Type IV physeal fracture of upper end of humerus, left arm**

⑦**S49.049**   **Salter-Harris Type IV physeal fracture of upper end of humerus, unspecified arm**

S49.09   **Other physeal fracture of upper end of humerus**

⑦**S49.091**   **Other physeal fracture of upper end of humerus, right arm**

⑦**S49.092**   **Other physeal fracture of upper end of humerus, left arm**

⑦**S49.099**   **Other physeal fracture of upper end of humerus, unspecified arm**

S49.1   **Physeal fracture of lower end of humerus**

S49.10   **Unspecified physeal fracture of lower end of humerus**

⑦**S49.101**   **Unspecified physeal fracture of lower end of humerus, right arm**

⑦**S49.102**   **Unspecified physeal fracture of lower end of humerus, left arm**

⑦**S49.109**   **Unspecified physeal fracture of lower end of humerus, unspecified arm**

S49.11   **Salter-Harris Type I physeal fracture of lower end of humerus**

⑦**S49.111**   **Salter-Harris Type I physeal fracture of lower end of humerus, right arm**

⑦**S49.112**   **Salter-Harris Type I physeal fracture of lower end of humerus, left arm**

⑦**S49.119**   **Salter-Harris Type I physeal fracture of lower end of humerus, unspecified arm**

S49.12   **Salter-Harris Type II physeal fracture of lower end of humerus**

⑦**S49.121**   **Salter-Harris Type II physeal fracture of lower end of humerus, right arm**

⑦**S49.122**   **Salter-Harris Type II physeal fracture of lower end of humerus, left arm**

⑦**S49.129**   **Salter-Harris Type II physeal fracture of lower end of humerus, unspecified arm**

S49.13   **Salter-Harris Type III physeal fracture of lower end of humerus**

▲⑦**S49.131**   **Salter-Harris Type III physeal fracture of lower end of humerus, right arm**

▲⑦**S49.132**   **Salter-Harris Type III physeal fracture of lower end of humerus, left arm**

▲⑦**S49.139**   **Salter-Harris Type III physeal fracture of lower end of humerus, unspecified arm**

S49.14   **Salter-Harris Type IV physeal fracture of lower end of humerus**

⑦**S49.141**   **Salter-Harris Type IV physeal fracture of lower end of humerus, right arm**

⑦**S49.142**   **Salter-Harris Type IV physeal fracture of lower end of humerus, left arm**

⑦**S49.149**   **Salter-Harris Type IV physeal fracture of lower end of humerus, unspecified arm**

S49.19   **Other physeal fracture of lower end of humerus**

⑦**S49.191**   **Other physeal fracture of lower end of humerus, right arm**

⑦**S49.192**   **Other physeal fracture of lower end of humerus, left arm**

⑦**S49.199**   **Other physeal fracture of lower end of humerus, unspecified arm**

S49.8   **Other specified injuries of shoulder and upper arm**

The appropriate 7th character is to be added to each code in subcategory S49.8

A - initial encounter

D - subsequent encounter

S - sequela

⊗⑦**S49.80**   **Other specified injuries of shoulder and upper arm, unspecified arm**

⊗⑦**S49.81**   **Other specified injuries of right shoulder and upper arm**

⊗⑦**S49.82**   **Other specified injuries of left shoulder and upper arm**

S49.9   **Unspecified injury of shoulder and upper arm**

The appropriate 7th character is to be added to each code in subcategory S49.9

A - initial encounter

D - subsequent encounter

S - sequela

⊗⑦**S49.90**   **Unspecified injury of shoulder and upper arm, unspecified arm**

⊗⑦**S49.91**   **Unspecified injury of right shoulder and upper arm**

⊗⑦**S49.92**   **Unspecified injury of left shoulder and upper arm**

INJURIES TO THE ELBOW AND FOREARM (S50-S59)

Excludes2: burns and corrosions (T20-T32)

frostbite (T33-T34)

injuries of wrist and hand (S60-S69)

insect bite or sting, venomous (T63.4)

S50   **Superficial injury of elbow and forearm**

Excludes2: superficial injury of wrist and hand (S60.-)

The appropriate 7th character is to be added to each code from category S50

A - initial encounter

D - subsequent encounter

S - sequela

Add 4th-7th digits   Nonspecific code   Unspecified code   Manifestation code   **823**

S50.0   Contusion of elbow
 ⊗⑦**S50.00**   Contusion of unspecified elbow
 ⊗⑦**S50.01**   Contusion of right elbow
 ⊗⑦**S50.02**   Contusion of left elbow
S50.1   Contusion of forearm
 ⊗⑦**S50.10**   Contusion of unspecified forearm
 ⊗⑦**S50.11**   Contusion of right forearm
 ⊗⑦**S50.12**   Contusion of left forearm
S50.3   Other superficial injuries of elbow
 S50.31   Abrasion of elbow
  ⑦**S50.311**   Abrasion of right elbow
  ⑦**S50.312**   Abrasion of left elbow
  ⑦**S50.319**   Abrasion of unspecified elbow
 S50.32   Blister (nonthermal) of elbow
  ⑦**S50.321**   Blister (nonthermal) of right elbow
  ⑦**S50.322**   Blister (nonthermal) of left elbow
  ⑦**S50.329**   Blister (nonthermal) of unspecified elbow
 S50.34   External constriction of elbow
  ⑦**S50.341**   External constriction of right elbow
  ⑦**S50.342**   External constriction of left elbow
  ⑦**S50.349**   External constriction of unspecified elbow
 S50.35   Superficial foreign body of elbow
   Splinter in the elbow
  ⑦**S50.351**   Superficial foreign body of right elbow
  ⑦**S50.352**   Superficial foreign body of left elbow
  ⑦**S50.359**   Superficial foreign body of unspecified elbow
 S50.36   Insect bite (nonvenomous) of elbow
  ⑦**S50.361**   Insect bite (nonvenomous) of right elbow
  ⑦**S50.362**   Insect bite (nonvenomous) of left elbow
  ⑦**S50.369**   Insect bite (nonvenomous) of unspecified elbow
 S50.37   Other superficial bite of elbow
   Excludes1: open bite of elbow (S51.04)
  ⑦**S50.371**   Other superficial bite of right elbow
  ⑦**S50.372**   Other superficial bite of left elbow
  ⑦**S50.379**   Other superficial bite of unspecified elbow
S50.8   Other superficial injuries of forearm
 S50.81   Abrasion of forearm
  ⑦**S50.811**   Abrasion of right forearm
  ⑦**S50.812**   Abrasion of left forearm
  ⑦**S50.819**   Abrasion of unspecified forearm
 S50.82   Blister (nonthermal) of forearm
  ⑦**S50.821**   Blister (nonthermal) of right forearm
  ⑦**S50.822**   Blister (nonthermal) of left forearm
  ⑦**S50.829**   Blister (nonthermal) of unspecified forearm
 S50.84   External constriction of forearm

  ⑦**S50.841**   External constriction of right forearm
  ⑦**S50.842**   External constriction of left forearm
  ⑦**S50.849**   External constriction of unspecified forearm
 S50.85   Superficial foreign body of forearm
   Splinter in the forearm
  ⑦**S50.851**   Superficial foreign body of right forearm
  ⑦**S50.852**   Superficial foreign body of left forearm
  ⑦**S50.859**   Superficial foreign body of unspecified forearm
 S50.86   Insect bite (nonvenomous) of forearm
  ⑦**S50.861**   Insect bite (nonvenomous) of right forearm
  ⑦**S50.862**   Insect bite (nonvenomous) of left forearm
  ⑦**S50.869**   Insect bite (nonvenomous) of unspecified forearm
 S50.87   Other superficial bite of forearm
   Excludes1: open bite of forearm (S51.84)
  ⑦**S50.871**   Other superficial bite of right forearm
  ⑦**S50.872**   Other superficial bite of left forearm
  ⑦**S50.879**   Other superficial bite of unspecified forearm
S50.9   Unspecified superficial injury of elbow and forearm
 S50.90   Unspecified superficial injury of elbow
  ⑦**S50.901**   Unspecified superficial injury of right elbow
  ⑦**S50.902**   Unspecified superficial injury of left elbow
  ⑦**S50.909**   Unspecified superficial injury of unspecified elbow
 S50.91   Unspecified superficial injury of forearm
  ⑦**S50.911**   Unspecified superficial injury of right forearm
  ⑦**S50.912**   Unspecified superficial injury of left forearm
  ⑦**S50.919**   Unspecified superficial injury of unspecified forearm
S51   **Open wound of elbow and forearm**
   Code also any associated wound infection
   Excludes1: open fracture of elbow and forearm (S52.- with open fracture 7th character)
     traumatic amputation of elbow and forearm (S58.-)
   Excludes2: open wound of wrist and hand (S61.-)
   The appropriate 7th character is to be added to each code from category S51
   A - initial encounter
   D - subsequent encounter
   S - sequela
 S51.0   Open wound of elbow
  S51.00   Unspecified open wound of elbow
   ⑦**S51.001**   Unspecified open wound of right elbow

● New code   ▲ Revised code   **Excludes1:** Not coded here   **Excludes2:** Not included here   ⊗ Placeholder required   ⑦7th digit required

⑦S51.002   Unspecified open wound of left elbow

⑦S51.009   Unspecified open wound of unspecified elbow

Open wound of elbow NOS

S51.01   Laceration without foreign body of elbow

⑦S51.011   Laceration without foreign body of right elbow

⑦S51.012   Laceration without foreign body of left elbow

⑦S51.019   Laceration without foreign body of unspecified elbow

S51.02   Laceration with foreign body of elbow

⑦S51.021   Laceration with foreign body of right elbow

⑦S51.022   Laceration with foreign body of left elbow

⑦S51.029   Laceration with foreign body of unspecified elbow

S51.03   Puncture wound without foreign body of elbow

⑦S51.031   Puncture wound without foreign body of right elbow

⑦S51.032   Puncture wound without foreign body of left elbow

⑦S51.039   Puncture wound without foreign body of unspecified elbow

S51.04   Puncture wound with foreign body of elbow

⑦S51.041   Puncture wound with foreign body of right elbow

⑦S51.042   Puncture wound with foreign body of left elbow

⑦S51.049   Puncture wound with foreign body of unspecified elbow

S51.05   Open bite of elbow

Bite of elbow NOS

Excludes1: superficial bite of elbow (S50.36, S50.37)

⑦S51.051   Open bite, right elbow

⑦S51.052   Open bite, left elbow

⑦S51.059   Open bite, unspecified elbow

S51.8   Open wound of forearm

Excludes2: open wound of elbow (S51.0-)

S51.80   Unspecified open wound of forearm

⑦S51.801   Unspecified open wound of right forearm

⑦S51.802   Unspecified open wound of left forearm

⑦S51.809   Unspecified open wound of unspecified forearm

Open wound of forearm NOS

S51.81   Laceration without foreign body of forearm

⑦S51.811   Laceration without foreign body of right forearm

⑦S51.812   Laceration without foreign body of left forearm

⑦S51.819   Laceration without foreign body of unspecified forearm

S51.82   Laceration with foreign body of forearm

⑦S51.821   Laceration with foreign body of right forearm

⑦S51.822   Laceration with foreign body of left forearm

⑦S51.829   Laceration with foreign body of unspecified forearm

S51.83   Puncture wound without foreign body of forearm

⑦S51.831   Puncture wound without foreign body of right forearm

⑦S51.832   Puncture wound without foreign body of left forearm

⑦S51.839   Puncture wound without foreign body of unspecified forearm

S51.84   Puncture wound with foreign body of forearm

⑦S51.841   Puncture wound with foreign body of right forearm

⑦S51.842   Puncture wound with foreign body of left forearm

⑦S51.849   Puncture wound with foreign body of unspecified forearm

S51.85   Open bite of forearm

Bite of forearm NOS

Excludes1: superficial bite of forearm (S50.86, S50.87)

⑦S51.851   Open bite of right forearm

⑦S51.852   Open bite of left forearm

⑦S51.859   Open bite of unspecified forearm

S52   **Fracture of forearm**

Note: A fracture not indicated as displaced or nondisplaced should be coded to displaced

A fracture not indicated as open or closed should be coded to closed

The open fracture designations are based on the Gustilo open fracture classification

Excludes1: traumatic amputation of forearm (S58.-)

Excludes2: fracture at wrist and hand level (S62.-)

The appropriate 7th character is to be added to all codes from category S52

A - initial encounter for closed fracture

B - initial encounter for open fracture type I or II initial encounter for open fracture NOS

C - initial encounter for open fracture type IIIA, IIIB, or IIIC

D - subsequent encounter for closed fracture with routine healing

E - subsequent encounter for open fracture type I or II with routine healing

F - subsequent encounter for open fracture type IIIA, IIIB, or IIIC with routine healing

G - subsequent encounter for closed fracture with delayed healing

H - subsequent encounter for open fracture type I or II with delayed healing

J - subsequent encounter for open fracture type IIIA, IIIB, or IIIC with delayed healing

K - subsequent encounter for closed fracture with nonunion

M - subsequent encounter for open fracture type I or II with nonunion

N - subsequent encounter for open fracture type IIIA, IIIB, or IIIC with nonunion P - subsequent encounter for closed fracture with malunion

Q - subsequent encounter for open fracture type I or II with malunion

R - subsequent encounter for open fracture type IIIA, IIIB, or IIIC with malunion

S - sequela

S52.0   **Fracture of upper end of ulna**

Fracture of proximal end of ulna

Excludes2: fracture of elbow NOS (S42.40-)

fractures of shaft of ulna (S52.2-)

S52.00   **Unspecified fracture of upper end of ulna**

⑦**S52.001**   **Unspecified fracture of upper end of right ulna**

⑦**S52.002**   **Unspecified fracture of upper end of left ulna**

⑦**S52.009**   **Unspecified fracture of upper end of unspecified ulna**

S52.01   **Torus fracture of upper end of ulna**

The appropriate 7th character is to be added to all codes in subcategory S52.01

A - initial encounter for closed fracture

D - subsequent encounter for fracture with routine healing

G - subsequent encounter for fracture with delayed healing

K - subsequent encounter for fracture with nonunion

P - subsequent encounter for fracture with malunion S - sequela

⑦**S52.011**   **Torus fracture of upper end of right ulna**

⑦**S52.012**   **Torus fracture of upper end of left ulna**

⑦**S52.019**   **Torus fracture of upper end of unspecified ulna**

S52.02   **Fracture of olecranon process without intraarticular extension of ulna**

⑦**S52.021**   **Displaced fracture of olecranon process without intraarticular extension of right ulna**

⑦**S52.022**   **Displaced fracture of olecranon process without intraarticular extension of left ulna**

⑦**S52.023**   **Displaced fracture of olecranon process without intraarticular extension of unspecified ulna**

⑦**S52.024**   **Nondisplaced fracture of olecranon process without intraarticular extension of right ulna**

⑦**S52.025**   **Nondisplaced fracture of olecranon process without intraarticular extension of left ulna**

⑦**S52.026**   **Nondisplaced fracture of olecranon process without intraarticular extension of unspecified ulna**

S52.03   **Fracture of olecranon process with intraarticular extension of ulna**

⑦**S52.031**   **Displaced fracture of olecranon process with intraarticular extension of right ulna**

⑦**S52.032**   **Displaced fracture of olecranon process with intraarticular extension of left ulna**

⑦**S52.033**   **Displaced fracture of olecranon process with intraarticular extension of unspecified ulna**

⑦**S52.034**   **Nondisplaced fracture of olecranon process with intraarticular extension of right ulna**

⑦**S52.035**   **Nondisplaced fracture of olecranon process with intraarticular extension of left ulna**

⑦**S52.036**   **Nondisplaced fracture of olecranon process with intraarticular extension of unspecified ulna**

S52.04   **Fracture of coronoid process of ulna**

⑦**S52.041**   **Displaced fracture of coronoid process of right ulna**

⑦**S52.042**   **Displaced fracture of coronoid process of left ulna**

⑦**S52.043**   **Displaced fracture of coronoid process of unspecified ulna**

⑦**S52.044**   **Nondisplaced fracture of coronoid process of right ulna**

⑦**S52.045**   **Nondisplaced fracture of coronoid process of left ulna**

⑦**S52.046**   **Nondisplaced fracture of coronoid process of unspecified ulna**

S52.09   **Other fracture of upper end of ulna**

⑦**S52.091**   **Other fracture of upper end of right ulna**

⑦**S52.092**   **Other fracture of upper end of left ulna**

⑦**S52.099**   **Other fracture of upper end of unspecified ulna**

S52.1   **Fracture of upper end of radius**

Fracture of proximal end of radius

Excludes2: physeal fractures of upper end of radius (S59.2-)

fracture of shaft of radius (S52.3-)

S52.10   **Unspecified fracture of upper end of radius**

⑦**S52.101**   **Unspecified fracture of upper end of right radius**

⑦**S52.102**   **Unspecified fracture of upper end of left radius**

⑦**S52.109**   **Unspecified fracture of upper end of unspecified radius**

S52.11   **Torus fracture of upper end of radius**

The appropriate 7th character is to be added to all codes in subcategory S52.11

A - initial encounter for closed fracture

D - subsequent encounter for fracture with routine healing

G - subsequent encounter for fracture with delayed healing

K - subsequent encounter for fracture with nonunion

P - subsequent encounter for fracture with malunion S - sequela

⑦**S52.111** **Torus fracture of upper end of right radius**

● New code   ▲ Revised code   **Excludes1:** Not coded here   **Excludes2:** Not included here   ⊗ Placeholder required   ⑦7ᵗʰ digit required

⑦S52.112　Torus fracture of upper end of left radius

⑦S52.119　Torus fracture of upper end of unspecified radius

S52.12　Fracture of head of radius

⑦S52.121　Displaced fracture of head of right radius

⑦S52.122　Displaced fracture of head of left radius

⑦S52.123　Displaced fracture of head of unspecified radius

⑦S52.124　Nondisplaced fracture of head of right radius

⑦S52.125　Nondisplaced fracture of head of left radius

⑦S52.126　Nondisplaced fracture of head of unspecified radius

S52.13　Fracture of neck of radius

⑦S52.131　Displaced fracture of neck of right radius

⑦S52.132　Displaced fracture of neck of left radius

⑦S52.133　Displaced fracture of neck of unspecified radius

⑦S52.134　Nondisplaced fracture of neck of right radius

⑦S52.135　Nondisplaced fracture of neck of left radius

⑦S52.136　Nondisplaced fracture of neck of unspecified radius

S52.18　Other fracture of upper end of radius

⑦S52.181　Other fracture of upper end of right radius

⑦S52.182　Other fracture of upper end of left radius

⑦S52.189　Other fracture of upper end of unspecified radius

S52.2　Fracture of shaft of ulna

S52.20　Unspecified fracture of shaft of ulna

Fracture of ulna NOS

⑦S52.201　Unspecified fracture of shaft of right ulna

⑦S52.202　Unspecified fracture of shaft of left ulna

⑦S52.209　Unspecified fracture of shaft of unspecified ulna

S52.21　Greenstick fracture of shaft of ulna

The appropriate 7th character is to be added to all codes in subcategory S52.21

A - initial encounter for closed fracture

D - subsequent encounter for fracture with routine healing

G - subsequent encounter for fracture with delayed healing

K - subsequent encounter for fracture with nonunion

P - subsequent encounter for fracture with malunion

S - sequela

⑦S52.211　Greenstick fracture of shaft of right ulna

⑦S52.212　Greenstick fracture of shaft of left ulna

⑦S52.219　Greenstick fracture of shaft of unspecified ulna

S52.22　Transverse fracture of shaft of ulna

⑦S52.221　Displaced transverse fracture of shaft of right ulna

⑦S52.222　Displaced transverse fracture of shaft of left ulna

⑦S52.223　Displaced transverse fracture of shaft of unspecified ulna

⑦S52.224　Nondisplaced transverse fracture of shaft of right ulna

⑦S52.225　Nondisplaced transverse fracture of shaft of left ulna

⑦S52.226　Nondisplaced transverse fracture of shaft of unspecified ulna

S52.23　Oblique fracture of shaft of ulna

⑦S52.231　Displaced oblique fracture of shaft of right ulna

⑦S52.232　Displaced oblique fracture of shaft of left ulna

⑦S52.233　Displaced oblique fracture of shaft of unspecified ulna

⑦S52.234　Nondisplaced oblique fracture of shaft of right ulna

⑦S52.235　Nondisplaced oblique fracture of shaft of left ulna

⑦S52.236　Nondisplaced oblique fracture of shaft of unspecified ulna

S52.24　Spiral fracture of shaft of ulna

⑦S52.241　Displaced spiral fracture of shaft of ulna, right arm

⑦S52.242　Displaced spiral fracture of shaft of ulna, left arm

⑦S52.243　Displaced spiral fracture of shaft of ulna, unspecified arm

⑦S52.244　Nondisplaced spiral fracture of shaft of ulna, right arm

⑦S52.245　Nondisplaced spiral fracture of shaft of ulna, left arm

⑦S52.246　Nondisplaced spiral fracture of shaft of ulna, unspecified arm

S52.25　Comminuted fracture of shaft of ulna

⑦S52.251　Displaced comminuted fracture of shaft of ulna, right arm

⑦S52.252　Displaced comminuted fracture of shaft of ulna, left arm

⑦S52.253　Displaced comminuted fracture of shaft of ulna, unspecified arm

⑦S52.254　Nondisplaced comminuted fracture of shaft of ulna, right arm

⑦S52.255　Nondisplaced comminuted fracture of shaft of ulna, left arm

⑦S52.256　Nondisplaced comminuted fracture of shaft of ulna, unspecified arm

S52.26　Segmental fracture of shaft of ulna

⑦S52.261　Displaced segmental fracture of shaft of ulna, right arm

---

| | Add 4th-7th digits | | Nonspecific code | | Unspecified code | | Manifestation code | 827 |

⑦ **S52.262** **Displaced segmental fracture of shaft of ulna, left arm**

⑦ **S52.263** **Displaced segmental fracture of shaft of ulna, unspecified arm**

⑦ **S52.264** **Nondisplaced segmental fracture of shaft of ulna, right arm**

⑦ **S52.265** **Nondisplaced segmental fracture of shaft of ulna, left arm**

⑦ **S52.266** **Nondisplaced segmental fracture of shaft of ulna, unspecified arm**

S52.27 **Monteggia's fracture of ulna**

Fracture of upper shaft of ulna with dislocation of radial head

⑦ **S52.271** **Monteggia's fracture of right ulna**

⑦ **S52.272** **Monteggia's fracture of left ulna**

⑦ **S52.279** **Monteggia's fracture of unspecified ulna**

S52.28 **Bent bone of ulna**

⑦ **S52.281** **Bent bone of right ulna**

⑦ **S52.282** **Bent bone of left ulna**

⑦ **S52.283** **Bent bone of unspecified ulna**

S52.29 **Other fracture of shaft of ulna**

⑦ **S52.291** **Other fracture of shaft of right ulna**

⑦ **S52.292** **Other fracture of shaft of left ulna**

⑦ **S52.299** **Other fracture of shaft of unspecified ulna**

S52.3 **Fracture of shaft of radius**

S52.30 **Unspecified fracture of shaft of radius**

⑦ **S52.301** **Unspecified fracture of shaft of right radius**

⑦ **S52.302** **Unspecified fracture of shaft of left radius**

⑦ **S52.309** **Unspecified fracture of shaft of unspecified radius**

S52.31 **Greenstick fracture of shaft of radius**

The appropriate 7th character is to be added to all codes in subcategory S52.31

A - initial encounter for closed fracture

D - subsequent encounter for fracture with routine healing

G - subsequent encounter for fracture with delayed healing

K - subsequent encounter for fracture with nonunion

P - subsequent encounter for fracture with malunion S - sequela

⑦ **S52.311** **Greenstick fracture of shaft of radius, right arm**

⑦ **S52.312** **Greenstick fracture of shaft of radius, left arm**

⑦ **S52.319** **Greenstick fracture of shaft of radius, unspecified arm**

S52.32 **Transverse fracture of shaft of radius**

⑦ **S52.321** **Displaced transverse fracture of shaft of right radius**

⑦ **S52.322** **Displaced transverse fracture of shaft of left radius**

⑦ **S52.323** **Displaced transverse fracture of shaft of unspecified radius**

⑦ **S52.324** **Nondisplaced transverse fracture of shaft of right radius**

⑦ **S52.325** **Nondisplaced transverse fracture of shaft of left radius**

⑦ **S52.326** **Nondisplaced transverse fracture of shaft of unspecified radius**

S52.33 **Oblique fracture of shaft of radius**

⑦ **S52.331** **Displaced oblique fracture of shaft of right radius**

⑦ **S52.332** **Displaced oblique fracture of shaft of left radius**

⑦ **S52.333** **Displaced oblique fracture of shaft of unspecified radius**

⑦ **S52.334** **Nondisplaced oblique fracture of shaft of right radius**

⑦ **S52.335** **Nondisplaced oblique fracture of shaft of left radius**

⑦ **S52.336** **Nondisplaced oblique fracture of shaft of unspecified radius**

S52.34 **Spiral fracture of shaft of radius**

⑦ **S52.341** **Displaced spiral fracture of shaft of radius, right arm**

⑦ **S52.342** **Displaced spiral fracture of shaft of radius, left arm**

⑦ **S52.343** **Displaced spiral fracture of shaft of radius, unspecified arm**

⑦ **S52.344** **Nondisplaced spiral fracture of shaft of radius, right arm**

⑦ **S52.345** **Nondisplaced spiral fracture of shaft of radius, left arm**

⑦ **S52.346** **Nondisplaced spiral fracture of shaft of radius, unspecified arm**

S52.35 **Comminuted fracture of shaft of radius**

⑦ **S52.351** **Displaced comminuted fracture of shaft of radius, right arm**

⑦ **S52.352** **Displaced comminuted fracture of shaft of radius, left arm**

⑦ **S52.353** **Displaced comminuted fracture of shaft of radius, unspecified arm**

⑦ **S52.354** **Nondisplaced comminuted fracture of shaft of radius, right arm**

⑦ **S52.355** **Nondisplaced comminuted fracture of shaft of radius, left arm**

⑦ **S52.356** **Nondisplaced comminuted fracture of shaft of radius, unspecified arm**

S52.36 **Segmental fracture of shaft of radius**

⑦ **S52.361** **Displaced segmental fracture of shaft of radius, right arm**

⑦ **S52.362** **Displaced segmental fracture of shaft of radius, left arm**

⑦ **S52.363** **Displaced segmental fracture of shaft of radius, unspecified arm**

⑦ **S52.364** **Nondisplaced segmental fracture of shaft of radius, right arm**

⑦ **S52.365** **Nondisplaced segmental fracture of shaft of radius, left arm**

⑦ **S52.366** **Nondisplaced segmental fracture of shaft of radius, unspecified arm**

S52.37 **Galeazzi's fracture**

Fracture of lower shaft of radius with radioulnar joint dislocation

● New code   ▲ Revised code   **Excludes1:** Not coded here   **Excludes2:** Not included here   ⊗ Placeholder required   ⑦ 7th digit required

⑦S52.371   **Galeazzi's fracture of right radius**

⑦S52.372   **Galeazzi's fracture of left radius**

⑦S52.379   **Galeazzi's fracture of unspecified radius**

S52.38   **Bent bone of radius**

⑦S52.381   **Bent bone of right radius**

⑦S52.382   **Bent bone of left radius**

⑦S52.389   **Bent bone of unspecified radius**

S52.39   **Other fracture of shaft of radius**

⑦S52.391   **Other fracture of shaft of radius, right arm**

⑦S52.392   **Other fracture of shaft of radius, left arm**

⑦S52.399   **Other fracture of shaft of radius, unspecified arm**

S52.5   **Fracture of lower end of radius**

Fracture of distal end of radius

Excludes2: physeal fractures of lower end of radius (S59.2-)

S52.50   **Unspecified fracture of the lower end of radius**

⑦S52.501   **Unspecified fracture of the lower end of right radius**

⑦S52.502   **Unspecified fracture of the lower end of left radius**

⑦S52.509   **Unspecified fracture of the lower end of unspecified radius**

S52.51   **Fracture of radial styloid process**

⑦S52.511   **Displaced fracture of right radial styloid process**

⑦S52.512   **Displaced fracture of left radial styloid process**

⑦S52.513   **Displaced fracture of unspecified radial styloid process**

⑦S52.514   **Nondisplaced fracture of right radial styloid process**

⑦S52.515   **Nondisplaced fracture of left radial styloid process**

⑦S52.516   **Nondisplaced fracture of unspecified radial styloid process**

S52.52   **Torus fracture of lower end of radius**

The appropriate 7th character is to be added to all codes in subcategory S52.52

A - initial encounter for closed fracture

D - subsequent encounter for fracture with routine healing

G - subsequent encounter for fracture with delayed healing

K - subsequent encounter for fracture with nonunion

P - subsequent encounter for fracture with malunion

S - sequela

⑦S52.521   **Torus fracture of lower end of right radius**

⑦S52.522   **Torus fracture of lower end of left radius**

⑦S52.529   **Torus fracture of lower end of unspecified radius**

S52.53   **Colles' fracture**

⑦S52.531   **Colles' fracture of right radius**

⑦S52.532   **Colles' fracture of left radius**

⑦S52.539   **Colles' fracture of unspecified radius**

S52.54   **Smith's fracture**

⑦S52.541   **Smith's fracture of right radius**

⑦S52.542   **Smith's fracture of left radius**

⑦S52.549   **Smith's fracture of unspecified radius**

S52.55   **Other extraarticular fracture of lower end of radius**

⑦S52.551   **Other extraarticular fracture of lower end of right radius**

⑦S52.552   **Other extraarticular fracture of lower end of left radius**

⑦S52.559   **Other extraarticular fracture of lower end of unspecified radius**

S52.56   **Barton's fracture**

⑦S52.561   **Barton's fracture of right radius**

⑦S52.562   **Barton's fracture of left radius**

⑦S52.569   **Barton's fracture of unspecified radius**

S52.57   **Other intraarticular fracture of lower end of radius**

⑦S52.571   **Other intraarticular fracture of lower end of right radius**

⑦S52.572   **Other intraarticular fracture of lower end of left radius**

⑦S52.579   **Other intraarticular fracture of lower end of unspecified radius**

S52.59   **Other fractures of lower end of radius**

⑦S52.591   **Other fractures of lower end of right radius**

⑦S52.592   **Other fractures of lower end of left radius**

⑦S52.599   **Other fractures of lower end of unspecified radius**

S52.6   **Fracture of lower end of ulna**

S52.60   **Unspecified fracture of lower end of ulna**

⑦S52.601   **Unspecified fracture of lower end of right ulna**

⑦S52.602   **Unspecified fracture of lower end of left ulna**

⑦S52.609   **Unspecified fracture of lower end of unspecified ulna**

S52.61   **Fracture of ulna styloid process**

⑦S52.611   **Displaced fracture of right ulna styloid process**

⑦S52.612   **Displaced fracture of left ulna styloid process**

⑦S52.613   **Displaced fracture of unspecified ulna styloid process**

⑦S52.614   **Nondisplaced fracture of right ulna styloid process**

⑦S52.615   **Nondisplaced fracture of left ulna styloid process**

⑦S52.616   **Nondisplaced fracture of unspecified ulna styloid process**

S52.62   **Torus fracture of lower end of ulna**

The appropriate 7th character is to be added to all codes in subcategory S52.62

A - initial encounter for closed fracture

D - subsequent encounter for fracture with routine healing

G - subsequent encounter for fracture with delayed healing

K - subsequent encounter for fracture with nonunion

P - subsequent encounter for fracture with malunion

S - sequela

⑦ **S52.621** **Torus fracture of lower end of right ulna**

⑦ **S52.622** **Torus fracture of lower end of left ulna**

⑦ **S52.629** **Torus fracture of lower end of unspecified ulna**

S52.69 **Other fracture of lower end of ulna**

⑦ **S52.691** **Other fracture of lower end of right ulna**

⑦ **S52.692** **Other fracture of lower end of left ulna**

⑦ **S52.699** **Other fracture of lower end of unspecified ulna**

S52.9 **Unspecified fracture of forearm**

⊗⑦ **S52.90** **Unspecified fracture of unspecified forearm**

⊗⑦ **S52.91** **Unspecified fracture of right forearm**

⊗⑦ **S52.92** **Unspecified fracture of left forearm**

S53 **Dislocation and sprain of joints and ligaments of elbow**

Includes: avulsion of joint or ligament of elbow

laceration of cartilage, joint or ligament of elbow sprain of cartilage, joint or ligament of elbow

traumatic hemarthrosis of joint or ligament of elbow

traumatic rupture of joint or ligament of elbow

traumatic subluxation of joint or ligament of elbow

traumatic tear of joint or ligament of elbow

Code also any associated open wound

Excludes2: strain of muscle, fascia and tendon at forearm level (S56.-)

The appropriate 7th character is to be added to each code from category S53

A - initial encounter

D - subsequent encounter

S - sequela

S53.0 **Subluxation and dislocation of radial head**

Dislocation of radiohumeral joint

Subluxation of radiohumeral joint

Excludes1: Monteggia's fracture-dislocation (S52.27-)

S53.00 **Unspecified subluxation and dislocation of radial head**

⑦ **S53.001** **Unspecified subluxation of right radial head**

⑦ **S53.002** **Unspecified subluxation of left radial head**

⑦ **S53.003** **Unspecified subluxation of unspecified radial head**

⑦ **S53.004** **Unspecified dislocation of right radial head**

⑦ **S53.005** **Unspecified dislocation of left radial head**

⑦ **S53.006** **Unspecified dislocation of unspecified radial head**

S53.01 **Anterior subluxation and dislocation of radial head**

Anteriomedial subluxation and dislocation of radial head

⑦ **S53.011** **Anterior subluxation of right radial head**

⑦ **S53.012** **Anterior subluxation of left radial head**

⑦ **S53.013** **Anterior subluxation of unspecified radial head**

⑦ **S53.014** **Anterior dislocation of right radial head**

⑦ **S53.015** **Anterior dislocation of left radial head**

⑦ **S53.016** **Anterior dislocation of unspecified radial head**

S53.02 **Posterior subluxation and dislocation of radial head**

Posteriolateral subluxation and dislocation of radial head

⑦ **S53.021** **Posterior subluxation of right radial head**

⑦ **S53.022** **Posterior subluxation of left radial head**

⑦ **S53.023** **Posterior subluxation of unspecified radial head**

⑦ **S53.024** **Posterior dislocation of right radial head**

⑦ **S53.025** **Posterior dislocation of left radial head**

⑦ **S53.026** **Posterior dislocation of unspecified radial head**

S53.03 **Nursemaid's elbow**

⑦ **S53.031** **Nursemaid's elbow, right elbow**

⑦ **S53.032** **Nursemaid's elbow, left elbow**

⑦ **S53.033** **Nursemaid's elbow, unspecified elbow**

S53.09 **Other subluxation and dislocation of radial head**

⑦ **S53.091** **Other subluxation of right radial head**

⑦ **S53.092** **Other subluxation of left radial head**

⑦ **S53.093** **Other subluxation of unspecified radial head**

⑦ **S53.094** **Other dislocation of right radial head**

⑦ **S53.095** **Other dislocation of left radial head**

⑦ **S53.096** **Other dislocation of unspecified radial head**

S53.1 **Subluxation and dislocation of ulnohumeral joint**

Subluxation and dislocation of elbow NOS

Excludes1: dislocation of radial head alone (S53.0-)

● New code ▲ Revised code **Excludes1:** Not coded here **Excludes2:** Not included here ⊗ Placeholder required ⑦ 7th digit required

S53.10   Unspecified subluxation and dislocation of ulnohumeral joint

⑦S53.101   Unspecified subluxation of right ulnohumeral joint

⑦S53.102   Unspecified subluxation of left ulnohumeral joint

⑦S53.103   Unspecified subluxation of unspecified ulnohumeral joint

⑦S53.104   Unspecified dislocation of right ulnohumeral joint

⑦S53.105   Unspecified dislocation of left ulnohumeral joint

⑦S53.106   Unspecified dislocation of unspecified ulnohumeral joint

S53.11   Anterior subluxation and dislocation of ulnohumeral joint

⑦S53.111   Anterior subluxation of right ulnohumeral joint

⑦S53.112   Anterior subluxation of left ulnohumeral joint

⑦S53.113   Anterior subluxation of unspecified ulnohumeral joint

⑦S53.114   Anterior dislocation of right ulnohumeral joint

⑦S53.115   Anterior dislocation of left ulnohumeral joint

⑦S53.116   Anterior dislocation of unspecified ulnohumeral joint

S53.12   Posterior subluxation and dislocation of ulnohumeral joint

⑦S53.121   Posterior subluxation of right ulnohumeral joint

⑦S53.122   Posterior subluxation of left ulnohumeral joint

⑦S53.123   Posterior subluxation of unspecified ulnohumeral joint

⑦S53.124   Posterior dislocation of right ulnohumeral joint

⑦S53.125   Posterior dislocation of left ulnohumeral joint

⑦S53.126   Posterior dislocation of unspecified ulnohumeral joint

S53.13   Medial subluxation and dislocation of ulnohumeral joint

⑦S53.131   Medial subluxation of right ulnohumeral joint

⑦S53.132   Medial subluxation of left ulnohumeral joint

⑦S53.133   Medial subluxation of unspecified ulnohumeral joint

⑦S53.134   Medial dislocation of right ulnohumeral joint

⑦S53.135   Medial dislocation of left ulnohumeral joint

⑦S53.136   Medial dislocation of unspecified ulnohumeral joint

S53.14   Lateral subluxation and dislocation of ulnohumeral joint

⑦S53.141   Lateral subluxation of right ulnohumeral joint

⑦S53.142   Lateral subluxation of left ulnohumeral joint

⑦S53.143   Lateral subluxation of unspecified ulnohumeral joint

⑦S53.144   Lateral dislocation of right ulnohumeral joint

⑦S53.145   Lateral dislocation of left ulnohumeral joint

⑦S53.146   Lateral dislocation of unspecified ulnohumeral joint

S53.19   Other subluxation and dislocation of ulnohumeral joint

⑦S53.191   Other subluxation of right ulnohumeral joint

⑦S53.192   Other subluxation of left ulnohumeral joint

⑦S53.193   Other subluxation of unspecified ulnohumeral joint

⑦S53.194   Other dislocation of right ulnohumeral joint

⑦S53.195   Other dislocation of left ulnohumeral joint

⑦S53.196   Other dislocation of unspecified ulnohumeral joint

S53.2   Traumatic rupture of radial collateral ligament

Excludes1: sprain of radial collateral ligament NOS (S53.43-)

⊗⑦S53.20   Traumatic rupture of unspecified radial collateral ligament

⊗⑦S53.21   Traumatic rupture of right radial collateral ligament

⊗⑦S53.22   Traumatic rupture of left radial collateral ligament

S53.3   Traumatic rupture of ulnar collateral ligament

Excludes1: sprain of ulnar collateral ligament (S53.44-)

⊗⑦S53.30   Traumatic rupture of unspecified ulnar collateral ligament

⊗⑦S53.31   Traumatic rupture of right ulnar collateral ligament

⊗⑦S53.32   Traumatic rupture of left ulnar collateral ligament

S53.4   Sprain of elbow

Excludes2: traumatic rupture of radial collateral ligament (S53.2-)

traumatic rupture of ulnar collateral ligament (S53.3-)

S53.40   Unspecified sprain of elbow

⑦S53.401   Unspecified sprain of right elbow

⑦S53.402   Unspecified sprain of left elbow

⑦S53.409   Unspecified sprain of unspecified elbow

Sprain of elbow NOS

S53.41   Radiohumeral (joint) sprain

⑦S53.411   Radiohumeral (joint) sprain of right elbow

⑦S53.412   Radiohumeral (joint) sprain of left elbow

⑦S53.419   Radiohumeral (joint) sprain of unspecified elbow

S53.42   Ulnohumeral (joint) sprain

⑦S53.421   **Ulnohumeral (joint) sprain of right elbow**

⑦S53.422   **Ulnohumeral (joint) sprain of left elbow**

⑦S53.429   **Ulnohumeral (joint) sprain of unspecified elbow**

S53.43   **Radial collateral ligament sprain**

⑦S53.431   **Radial collateral ligament sprain of right elbow**

⑦S53.432   **Radial collateral ligament sprain of left elbow**

⑦S53.439   **Radial collateral ligament sprain of unspecified elbow**

S53.44   **Ulnar collateral ligament sprain**

⑦S53.441   **Ulnar collateral ligament sprain of right elbow**

⑦S53.442   **Ulnar collateral ligament sprain of left elbow**

⑦S53.449   **Ulnar collateral ligament sprain of unspecified elbow**

S53.49   **Other sprain of elbow**

⑦S53.491   **Other sprain of right elbow**

⑦S53.492   **Other sprain of left elbow**

⑦S53.499   **Other sprain of unspecified elbow**

S54   **Injury of nerves at forearm level**

Code also any associated open wound (S51.-)

Excludes2: injury of nerves at wrist and hand level (S64.-)

The appropriate 7th character is to be added to each code from category S54

A - initial encounter

D - subsequent encounter

S - sequela

S54.0   **Injury of ulnar nerve at forearm level**

Injury of ulnar nerve NOS

⊗⑦S54.00   **Injury of ulnar nerve at forearm level, unspecified arm**

⊗⑦S54.01   **Injury of ulnar nerve at forearm level, right arm**

⊗⑦S54.02   **Injury of ulnar nerve at forearm level, left arm**

S54.1   **Injury of median nerve at forearm level**

Injury of median nerve NOS

⊗⑦S54.10   **Injury of median nerve at forearm level, unspecified arm**

⊗⑦S54.11   **Injury of median nerve at forearm level, right arm**

⊗⑦S54.12   **Injury of median nerve at forearm level, left arm**

S54.2   **Injury of radial nerve at forearm level**

Injury of radial nerve NOS

⊗⑦S54.20   **Injury of radial nerve at forearm level, unspecified arm**

⊗⑦S54.21   **Injury of radial nerve at forearm level, right arm**

⊗⑦S54.22   **Injury of radial nerve at forearm level, left arm**

S54.3   **Injury of cutaneous sensory nerve at forearm level**

⊗⑦S54.30   **Injury of cutaneous sensory nerve at forearm level, unspecified arm**

⊗⑦S54.31   **Injury of cutaneous sensory nerve at forearm level, right arm**

⊗⑦S54.32   **Injury of cutaneous sensory nerve at forearm level, left arm**

S54.8   **Injury of other nerves at forearm level**

S54.8X   **Injury of other nerves at forearm level**

▲⑦S54.8X1   **Injury of other nerves at forearm level, right arm**

▲⑦S54.8X2   **Injury of other nerves at forearm level, left arm**

▲⑦S54.8X9   **Injury of other nerves at forearm level, unspecified arm**

S54.9   **Injury of unspecified nerve at forearm level**

⊗⑦S54.90   **Injury of unspecified nerve at forearm level, unspecified arm**

⊗⑦S54.91   **Injury of unspecified nerve at forearm level, right arm**

⊗⑦S54.92   **Injury of unspecified nerve at forearm level, left arm**

S55   **Injury of blood vessels at forearm level**

Code also any associated open wound (S51.-)

Excludes2: injury of blood vessels at wrist and hand level (S65.-)

injury of brachial vessels (S45.1-S45.2)

The appropriate 7th character is to be added to each code from category S55

A - initial encounter

D - subsequent encounter

S - sequela

S55.0   **Injury of ulnar artery at forearm level**

S55.00   **Unspecified injury of ulnar artery at forearm level**

⑦S55.001   **Unspecified injury of ulnar artery at forearm level, right arm**

⑦S55.002   **Unspecified injury of ulnar artery at forearm level, left arm**

⑦S55.009   **Unspecified injury of ulnar artery at forearm level, unspecified arm**

S55.01   **Laceration of ulnar artery at forearm level**

⑦S55.011   **Laceration of ulnar artery at forearm level, right arm**

⑦S55.012   **Laceration of ulnar artery at forearm level, left arm**

⑦S55.019   **Laceration of ulnar artery at forearm level, unspecified arm**

S55.09   **Other specified injury of ulnar artery at forearm level**

⑦S55.091   **Other specified injury of ulnar artery at forearm level, right arm**

⑦S55.092   **Other specified injury of ulnar artery at forearm level, left arm**

⑦S55.099   **Other specified injury of ulnar artery at forearm level, unspecified arm**

S55.1   **Injury of radial artery at forearm level**

S55.10   **Unspecified injury of radial artery at forearm level**

⑦S55.101   **Unspecified injury of radial artery at forearm level, right arm**

⑦S55.102   **Unspecified injury of radial artery at forearm level, left arm**

● New code   ▲ Revised code   **Excludes1:** Not coded here   **Excludes2:** Not included here   ⊗ Placeholder required   ⑦ 7th digit required

⑦S55.109   Unspecified injury of radial artery at forearm level, unspecified arm

S55.11   Laceration of radial artery at forearm level

⑦S55.111   Laceration of radial artery at forearm level, right arm

⑦S55.112   Laceration of radial artery at forearm level, left arm

⑦S55.119   Laceration of radial artery at forearm level, unspecified arm

S55.19   Other specified injury of radial artery at forearm level

⑦S55.191   Other specified injury of radial artery at forearm level, right arm

⑦S55.192   Other specified injury of radial artery at forearm level, left arm

⑦S55.199   Other specified injury of radial artery at forearm level, unspecified arm

S55.2   Injury of vein at forearm level

S55.20   Unspecified injury of vein at forearm level

⑦S55.201   Unspecified injury of vein at forearm level, right arm

⑦S55.202   Unspecified injury of vein at forearm level, left arm

⑦S55.209   Unspecified injury of vein at forearm level, unspecified arm

S55.21   Laceration of vein at forearm level

⑦S55.211   Laceration of vein at forearm level, right arm

⑦S55.212   Laceration of vein at forearm level, left arm

⑦S55.219   Laceration of vein at forearm level, unspecified arm

S55.29   Other specified injury of vein at forearm level

⑦S55.291   Other specified injury of vein at forearm level, right arm

⑦S55.292   Other specified injury of vein at forearm level, left arm

⑦S55.299   Other specified injury of vein at forearm level, unspecified arm

S55.8   Injury of other blood vessels at forearm level

S55.80   Unspecified injury of other blood vessels at forearm level

⑦S55.801   Unspecified injury of other blood vessels at forearm level, right arm

⑦S55.802   Unspecified injury of other blood vessels at forearm level, left arm

⑦S55.809   Unspecified injury of other blood vessels at forearm level, unspecified arm

S55.81   Laceration of other blood vessels at forearm level

⑦S55.811   Laceration of other blood vessels at forearm level, right arm

⑦S55.812   Laceration of other blood vessels at forearm level, left arm

⑦S55.819   Laceration of other blood vessels at forearm level, unspecified arm

S55.89   Other specified injury of other blood vessels at forearm level

⑦S55.891   Other specified injury of other blood vessels at forearm level, right arm

⑦S55.892   Other specified injury of other blood vessels at forearm level, left arm

⑦S55.899   Other specified injury of other blood vessels at forearm level, unspecified arm

S55.9   Injury of unspecified blood vessel at forearm level

S55.90   Unspecified injury of unspecified blood vessel at forearm level

⑦S55.901   Unspecified injury of unspecified blood vessel at forearm level, right arm

⑦S55.902   Unspecified injury of unspecified blood vessel at forearm level, left arm

⑦S55.909   Unspecified injury of unspecified blood vessel at forearm level, unspecified arm

S55.91   Laceration of unspecified blood vessel at forearm level

⑦S55.911   Laceration of unspecified blood vessel at forearm level, right arm

⑦S55.912   Laceration of unspecified blood vessel at forearm level, left arm

⑦S55.919   Laceration of unspecified blood vessel at forearm level, unspecified arm

S55.99   Other specified injury of unspecified blood vessel at forearm level

⑦S55.991   Other specified injury of unspecified blood vessel at forearm level, right arm

⑦S55.992   Other specified injury of unspecified blood vessel at forearm level, left arm

⑦S55.999   Other specified injury of unspecified blood vessel at forearm level, unspecified arm

S56   Injury of muscle, fascia and tendon at forearm level

Code also any associated open wound (S51.-)

Excludes2: injury of muscle, fascia and tendon at or below wrist (S66.-)

sprain of joints and ligaments of elbow (S53.4-)

The appropriate 7th character is to be added to each code from category S56

A - initial encounter

D - subsequent encounter

S - sequela

S56.0   Injury of flexor muscle, fascia and tendon of thumb at forearm level

S56.00   Unspecified injury of flexor muscle, fascia and tendon of thumb at forearm level

⑦S56.001   Unspecified injury of flexor muscle, fascia and tendon of right thumb at forearm level

⑦S56.002   Unspecified injury of flexor muscle, fascia and tendon of left thumb at forearm level

⑦ S56.009 Unspecified injury of flexor muscle, fascia and tendon of unspecified thumb at forearm level

S56.01 Strain of flexor muscle, fascia and tendon of thumb at forearm level

⑦ S56.011 Strain of flexor muscle, fascia and tendon of right thumb at forearm level

⑦ S56.012 Strain of flexor muscle, fascia and tendon of left thumb at forearm level

⑦ S56.019 Strain of flexor muscle, fascia and tendon of unspecified thumb at forearm level

S56.02 Laceration of flexor muscle, fascia and tendon of thumb at forearm level

⑦ S56.021 Laceration of flexor muscle, fascia and tendon of right thumb at forearm level

⑦ S56.022 Laceration of flexor muscle, fascia and tendon of left thumb at forearm level

⑦ S56.029 Laceration of flexor muscle, fascia and tendon of unspecified thumb at forearm level

S56.09 Other injury of flexor muscle, fascia and tendon of thumb at forearm level

⑦ S56.091 Other injury of flexor muscle, fascia and tendon of right thumb at forearm level

⑦ S56.092 Other injury of flexor muscle, fascia and tendon of left thumb at forearm level

⑦ S56.099 Other injury of flexor muscle, fascia and tendon of unspecified thumb at forearm level

S56.1 Injury of flexor muscle, fascia and tendon of other and unspecified finger at forearm level

S56.10 Unspecified injury of flexor muscle, fascia and tendon of other and unspecified finger at forearm level

⑦ S56.101 Unspecified injury of flexor muscle, fascia and tendon of right index finger at forearm level

⑦ S56.102 Unspecified injury of flexor muscle, fascia and tendon of left index finger at forearm level

⑦ S56.103 Unspecified injury of flexor muscle, fascia and tendon of right middle finger at forearm level

⑦ S56.104 Unspecified injury of flexor muscle, fascia and tendon of left middle finger at forearm level

⑦ S56.105 Unspecified injury of flexor muscle, fascia and tendon of right ring finger at forearm level

⑦ S56.106 Unspecified injury of flexor muscle, fascia and tendon of left ring finger at forearm level

⑦ S56.107 Unspecified injury of flexor muscle, fascia and tendon of right little finger at forearm level

⑦ S56.108 Unspecified injury of flexor muscle, fascia and tendon of left little finger at forearm level

⑦ S56.109 Unspecified injury of flexor muscle, fascia and tendon of unspecified finger at forearm level

S56.11 Strain of flexor muscle, fascia and tendon of other and unspecified finger at forearm level

⑦ S56.111 Strain of flexor muscle, fascia and tendon of right index finger at forearm level

⑦ S56.112 Strain of flexor muscle, fascia and tendon of left index finger at forearm level

⑦ S56.113 Strain of flexor muscle, fascia and tendon of right middle finger at forearm level

⑦ S56.114 Strain of flexor muscle, fascia and tendon of left middle finger at forearm level

⑦ S56.115 Strain of flexor muscle, fascia and tendon of right ring finger at forearm level

⑦ S56.116 Strain of flexor muscle, fascia and tendon of left ring finger at forearm level

⑦ S56.117 Strain of flexor muscle, fascia and tendon of right little finger at forearm level

⑦ S56.118 Strain of flexor muscle, fascia and tendon of left little finger at forearm level

⑦ S56.119 Strain of flexor muscle, fascia and tendon of finger of unspecified finger at forearm level

S56.12 Laceration of flexor muscle, fascia and tendon of other and unspecified finger at forearm level

⑦ S56.121 Laceration of flexor muscle, fascia and tendon of right index finger at forearm level

⑦ S56.122 Laceration of flexor muscle, fascia and tendon of left index finger at forearm level

⑦ S56.123 Laceration of flexor muscle, fascia and tendon of right middle finger at forearm level

⑦ S56.124 Laceration of flexor muscle, fascia and tendon of left middle finger at forearm level

⑦ S56.125 Laceration of flexor muscle, fascia and tendon of right ring finger at forearm level

⑦ S56.126 Laceration of flexor muscle, fascia and tendon of left ring finger at forearm level

⑦ S56.127 Laceration of flexor muscle, fascia and tendon of right little finger at forearm level

⑦ S56.128 Laceration of flexor muscle, fascia and tendon of left little finger at forearm level

● New code ▲ Revised code **Excludes1:** Not coded here **Excludes2:** Not included here ⊗ Placeholder required ⑦ 7ᵗʰ digit required

⑦S56.129　Laceration of flexor muscle, fascia and tendon of unspecified finger at forearm level

S56.19　Other injury of flexor muscle, fascia and tendon of other and unspecified finger at forearm level

⑦S56.191　Other injury of flexor muscle, fascia and tendon of right index finger at forearm level

⑦S56.192　Other injury of flexor muscle, fascia and tendon of left index finger at forearm level

⑦S56.193　Other injury of flexor muscle, fascia and tendon of right middle finger at forearm level

⑦S56.194　Other injury of flexor muscle, fascia and tendon of left middle finger at forearm level

⑦S56.195　Other injury of flexor muscle, fascia and tendon of right ring finger at forearm level

⑦S56.196　Other injury of flexor muscle, fascia and tendon of left ring finger at forearm level

⑦S56.197　Other injury of flexor muscle, fascia and tendon of right little finger at forearm level

⑦S56.198　Other injury of flexor muscle, fascia and tendon of left little finger at forearm level

⑦S56.199　Other injury of flexor muscle, fascia and tendon of unspecified finger at forearm level

S56.2　Injury of other flexor muscle, fascia and tendon at forearm level

S56.20　Unspecified injury of other flexor muscle, fascia and tendon at forearm level

⑦S56.201　Unspecified injury of other flexor muscle, fascia and tendon at forearm level, right arm

⑦S56.202　Unspecified injury of other flexor muscle, fascia and tendon at forearm level, left arm

⑦S56.209　Unspecified injury of other flexor muscle, fascia and tendon at forearm level, unspecified arm

S56.21　Strain of other flexor muscle, fascia and tendon at forearm level

⑦S56.211　Strain of other flexor muscle, fascia and tendon at forearm level, right arm

⑦S56.212　Strain of other flexor muscle, fascia and tendon at forearm level, left arm

⑦S56.219　Strain of other flexor muscle, fascia and tendon at forearm level, unspecified arm

S56.22　Laceration of other flexor muscle, fascia and tendon at forearm level

⑦S56.221　Laceration of other flexor muscle, fascia and tendon at forearm level, right arm

⑦S56.222　Laceration of other flexor muscle, fascia and tendon at forearm level, left arm

⑦S56.229　Laceration of other flexor muscle, fascia and tendon at forearm level, unspecified arm

S56.29　Other injury of other flexor muscle, fascia and tendon at forearm level

⑦S56.291　Other injury of other flexor muscle, fascia and tendon at forearm level, right arm

⑦S56.292　Other injury of other flexor muscle, fascia and tendon at forearm level, left arm

⑦S56.299　Other injury of other flexor muscle, fascia and tendon at forearm level, unspecified arm

S56.3　Injury of extensor or abductor muscles, fascia and tendons of thumb at forearm level

S56.30　Unspecified injury of extensor or abductor muscles, fascia and tendons of thumb at forearm level

⑦S56.301　Unspecified injury of extensor or abductor muscles, fascia and tendons of right thumb at forearm level

⑦S56.302　Unspecified injury of extensor or abductor muscles, fascia and tendons of left thumb at forearm level

⑦S56.309　Unspecified injury of extensor or abductor muscles, fascia and tendons of unspecified thumb at forearm level

S56.31　Strain of extensor or abductor muscles, fascia and tendons of thumb at forearm level

⑦S56.311　Strain of extensor or abductor muscles, fascia and tendons of right thumb at forearm level

⑦S56.312　Strain of extensor or abductor muscles, fascia and tendons of left thumb at forearm level

⑦S56.319　Strain of extensor or abductor muscles, fascia and tendons of unspecified thumb at forearm level

S56.32　Laceration of extensor or abductor muscles, fascia and tendons of thumb at forearm level

⑦S56.321　Laceration of extensor or abductor muscles, fascia and tendons of right thumb at forearm level

⑦S56.322　Laceration of extensor or abductor muscles, fascia and tendons of left thumb at forearm level

⑦S56.329　Laceration of extensor or abductor muscles, fascia and tendons of unspecified thumb at forearm level

S56.39　Other injury of extensor or abductor muscles, fascia and tendons of thumb at forearm level

⑦S56.391　Other injury of extensor or abductor muscles, fascia and tendons of right thumb at forearm level

⑦S56.392　Other injury of extensor or abductor muscles, fascia and

tendons of left thumb at forearm level

⑦ S56.399 **Other injury of extensor or abductor muscles, fascia and tendons of unspecified thumb at forearm level**

S56.4 **Injury of extensor muscle, fascia and tendon of other and unspecified finger at forearm level**

S56.40 **Unspecified injury of extensor muscle, fascia and tendon of other and unspecified finger at forearm level**

⑦ S56.401 **Unspecified injury of extensor muscle, fascia and tendon of right index finger at forearm level**

⑦ S56.402 **Unspecified injury of extensor muscle, fascia and tendon of left index finger at forearm level**

⑦ S56.403 **Unspecified injury of extensor muscle, fascia and tendon of right middle finger at forearm level**

⑦ S56.404 **Unspecified injury of extensor muscle, fascia and tendon of left middle finger at forearm level**

⑦ S56.405 **Unspecified injury of extensor muscle, fascia and tendon of right ring finger at forearm level**

⑦ S56.406 **Unspecified injury of extensor muscle, fascia and tendon of left ring finger at forearm level**

⑦ S56.407 **Unspecified injury of extensor muscle, fascia and tendon of right little finger at forearm level**

⑦ S56.408 **Unspecified injury of extensor muscle, fascia and tendon of left little finger at forearm level**

⑦ S56.409 **Unspecified injury of extensor muscle, fascia and tendon of unspecified finger at forearm level**

S56.41 **Strain of extensor muscle, fascia and tendon of other and unspecified finger at forearm level**

⑦ S56.411 **Strain of extensor muscle, fascia and tendon of right index finger at forearm level**

⑦ S56.412 **Strain of extensor muscle, fascia and tendon of left index finger at forearm level**

⑦ S56.413 **Strain of extensor muscle, fascia and tendon of right middle finger at forearm level**

⑦ S56.414 **Strain of extensor muscle, fascia and tendon of left middle finger at forearm level**

⑦ S56.415 **Strain of extensor muscle, fascia and tendon of right ring finger at forearm level**

⑦ S56.416 **Strain of extensor muscle, fascia and tendon of left ring finger at forearm level**

⑦ S56.417 **Strain of extensor muscle, fascia and tendon of right little finger at forearm level**

⑦ S56.418 **Strain of extensor muscle, fascia and tendon of left little finger at forearm level**

⑦ S56.419 **Strain of extensor muscle, fascia and tendon of finger, unspecified finger at forearm level**

S56.42 **Laceration of extensor muscle, fascia and tendon of other and unspecified finger at forearm level**

⑦ S56.421 **Laceration of extensor muscle, fascia and tendon of right index finger at forearm level**

⑦ S56.422 **Laceration of extensor muscle, fascia and tendon of left index finger at forearm level**

⑦ S56.423 **Laceration of extensor muscle, fascia and tendon of right middle finger at forearm level**

⑦ S56.424 **Laceration of extensor muscle, fascia and tendon of left middle finger at forearm level**

⑦ S56.425 **Laceration of extensor muscle, fascia and tendon of right ring finger at forearm level**

⑦ S56.426 **Laceration of extensor muscle, fascia and tendon of left ring finger at forearm level**

⑦ S56.427 **Laceration of extensor muscle, fascia and tendon of right little finger at forearm level**

⑦ S56.428 **Laceration of extensor muscle, fascia and tendon of left little finger at forearm level**

⑦ S56.429 **Laceration of extensor muscle, fascia and tendon of unspecified finger at forearm level**

S56.49 **Other injury of extensor muscle, fascia and tendon of other and unspecified finger at forearm level**

⑦ S56.491 **Other injury of extensor muscle, fascia and tendon of right index finger at forearm level**

⑦ S56.492 **Other injury of extensor muscle, fascia and tendon of left index finger at forearm level**

⑦ S56.493 **Other injury of extensor muscle, fascia and tendon of right middle finger at forearm level**

⑦ S56.494 **Other injury of extensor muscle, fascia and tendon of left middle finger at forearm level**

⑦ S56.495 **Other injury of extensor muscle, fascia and tendon of right ring finger at forearm level**

⑦ S56.496 **Other injury of extensor muscle, fascia and tendon of left ring finger at forearm level**

⑦ S56.497 **Other injury of extensor muscle, fascia and tendon of right little finger at forearm level**

⑦ S56.498 **Other injury of extensor muscle, fascia and tendon of left little finger at forearm level**

⑦ S56.499 **Other injury of extensor muscle, fascia and tendon of unspecified finger at forearm level**

● New code ▲ Revised code **Excludes1:** Not coded here **Excludes2:** Not included here ⊗ Placeholder required ⑦ 7th digit required

S56.5 Injury of other extensor muscle, fascia and tendon at forearm level

  S56.50 Unspecified injury of other extensor muscle, fascia and tendon at forearm level

    ⑦**S56.501** Unspecified injury of other extensor muscle, fascia and tendon at forearm level, right arm

    ⑦**S56.502** Unspecified injury of other extensor muscle, fascia and tendon at forearm level, left arm

    ⑦**S56.509** Unspecified injury of other extensor muscle, fascia and tendon at forearm level, unspecified arm

  S56.51 Strain of other extensor muscle, fascia and tendon at forearm level

    ⑦**S56.511** Strain of other extensor muscle, fascia and tendon at forearm level, right arm

    ⑦**S56.512** Strain of other extensor muscle, fascia and tendon at forearm level, left arm

    ⑦**S56.519** Strain of other extensor muscle, fascia and tendon at forearm level, unspecified arm

  S56.52 Laceration of other extensor muscle, fascia and tendon at forearm level

    ⑦**S56.521** Laceration of other extensor muscle, fascia and tendon at forearm level, right arm

    ⑦**S56.522** Laceration of other extensor muscle, fascia and tendon at forearm level, left arm

    ⑦**S56.529** Laceration of other extensor muscle, fascia and tendon at forearm level, unspecified arm

  S56.59 Other injury of other extensor muscle, fascia and tendon at forearm level

    ⑦**S56.591** Other injury of other extensor muscle, fascia and tendon at forearm level, right arm

    ⑦**S56.592** Other injury of other extensor muscle, fascia and tendon at forearm level, left arm

    ⑦**S56.599** Other injury of other extensor muscle, fascia and tendon at forearm level, unspecified arm

S56.8 Injury of other muscles, fascia and tendons at forearm level

  S56.80 Unspecified injury of other muscles, fascia and tendons at forearm level

    ⑦**S56.801** Unspecified injury of other muscles, fascia and tendons at forearm level, right arm

    ⑦**S56.802** Unspecified injury of other muscles, fascia and tendons at forearm level, left arm

    ⑦**S56.809** Unspecified injury of other muscles, fascia and tendons at forearm level, unspecified arm

  S56.81 Strain of other muscles, fascia and tendons at forearm level

    ⑦**S56.811** Strain of other muscles, fascia and tendons at forearm level, right arm

    ⑦**S56.812** Strain of other muscles, fascia and tendons at forearm level, left arm

    ⑦**S56.819** Strain of other muscles, fascia and tendons at forearm level, unspecified arm

  S56.82 Laceration of other muscles, fascia and tendons at forearm level

    ⑦**S56.821** Laceration of other muscles, fascia and tendons at forearm level, right arm

    ⑦**S56.822** Laceration of other muscles, fascia and tendons at forearm level, left arm

    ⑦**S56.829** Laceration of other muscles, fascia and tendons at forearm level, unspecified arm

  S56.89 Other injury of other muscles, fascia and tendons at forearm level

    ⑦**S56.891** Other injury of other muscles, fascia and tendons at forearm level, right arm

    ⑦**S56.892** Other injury of other muscles, fascia and tendons at forearm level, left arm

    ⑦**S56.899** Other injury of other muscles, fascia and tendons at forearm level, unspecified arm

S56.9 Injury of unspecified muscles, fascia and tendons at forearm level

  S56.90 Unspecified injury of unspecified muscles, fascia and tendons at forearm level

    ⑦**S56.901** Unspecified injury of unspecified muscles, fascia and tendons at forearm level, right arm

    ⑦**S56.902** Unspecified injury of unspecified muscles, fascia and tendons at forearm level, left arm

    ⑦**S56.909** Unspecified injury of unspecified muscles, fascia and tendons at forearm level, unspecified arm

  S56.91 Strain of unspecified muscles, fascia and tendons at forearm level

    ⑦**S56.911** Strain of unspecified muscles, fascia and tendons at forearm level, right arm

    ⑦**S56.912** Strain of unspecified muscles, fascia and tendons at forearm level, left arm

    ⑦**S56.919** Strain of unspecified muscles, fascia and tendons at forearm level, unspecified arm

  S56.92 Laceration of unspecified muscles, fascia and tendons at forearm level

    ⑦**S56.921** Laceration of unspecified muscles, fascia and tendons at forearm level, right arm

    ⑦**S56.922** Laceration of unspecified muscles, fascia and tendons at forearm level, left arm

    ⑦**S56.929** Laceration of unspecified muscles, fascia and tendons at forearm level, unspecified arm

  S56.99 Other injury of unspecified muscles, fascia and tendons at forearm level

⑦**S56.991** Other injury of unspecified muscles, fascia and tendons at forearm level, right arm

⑦**S56.992** Other injury of unspecified muscles, fascia and tendons at forearm level, left arm

⑦**S56.999** Other injury of unspecified muscles, fascia and tendons at forearm level, unspecified arm

S57 **Crushing injury of elbow and forearm**

Use additional code(s) for all associated injuries

Excludes2: crushing injury of wrist and hand (S67.-)

The appropriate 7th character is to be added to each code from category S57

A - initial encounter

D - subsequent encounter

S - sequela

S57.0 **Crushing injury of elbow**

⊗⑦**S57.00** Crushing injury of unspecified elbow

⊗⑦**S57.01** Crushing injury of right elbow

⊗⑦**S57.02** Crushing injury of left elbow

S57.8 **Crushing injury of forearm**

⊗⑦**S57.80** Crushing injury of unspecified forearm

⊗⑦**S57.81** Crushing injury of right forearm

⊗⑦**S57.82** Crushing injury of left forearm

S58 **Traumatic amputation of elbow and forearm**

An amputation not identified as partial or complete should be coded to complete

Excludes1: traumatic amputation of wrist and hand (S68.-)

The appropriate 7th character is to be added to each code from category S58

A - initial encounter

D - subsequent encounter

S - sequela

S58.0 **Traumatic amputation at elbow level**

S58.01 Complete traumatic amputation at elbow level

⑦**S58.011** Complete traumatic amputation at elbow level, right arm

⑦**S58.012** Complete traumatic amputation at elbow level, left arm

⑦**S58.019** Complete traumatic amputation at elbow level, unspecified arm

S58.02 Partial traumatic amputation at elbow level

⑦**S58.021** Partial traumatic amputation at elbow level, right arm

⑦**S58.022** Partial traumatic amputation at elbow level, left arm

⑦**S58.029** Partial traumatic amputation at elbow level, unspecified arm

S58.1 **Traumatic amputation at level between elbow and wrist**

S58.11 Complete traumatic amputation at level between elbow and wrist

⑦**S58.111** Complete traumatic amputation at level between elbow and wrist, right arm

⑦**S58.112** Complete traumatic amputation at level between elbow and wrist, left arm

⑦**S58.119** Complete traumatic amputation at level between elbow and wrist, unspecified arm

S58.12 Partial traumatic amputation at level between elbow and wrist

⑦**S58.121** Partial traumatic amputation at level between elbow and wrist, right arm

⑦**S58.122** Partial traumatic amputation at level between elbow and wrist, left arm

⑦**S58.129** Partial traumatic amputation at level between elbow and wrist, unspecified arm

S58.9 **Traumatic amputation of forearm, level unspecified**

Excludes1: traumatic amputation of wrist (S68.-)

S58.91 Complete traumatic amputation of forearm, level unspecified

⑦**S58.911** Complete traumatic amputation of right forearm, level unspecified

⑦**S58.912** Complete traumatic amputation of left forearm, level unspecified

⑦**S58.919** Complete traumatic amputation of unspecified forearm, level unspecified

S58.92 Partial traumatic amputation of forearm, level unspecified

⑦**S58.921** Partial traumatic amputation of right forearm, level unspecified

⑦**S58.922** Partial traumatic amputation of left forearm, level unspecified

⑦**S58.929** Partial traumatic amputation of unspecified forearm, level unspecified

S59 **Other and unspecified injuries of elbow and forearm**

Excludes2: Other and unspecified injuries of wrist and hand (S69.-)

The appropriate 7th character is to be added to each code from subcategories S59.0, S59.1, and S59.2

A - initial encounter for closed fracture

D - subsequent encounter for fracture with routine healing

G - subsequent encounter for fracture with delayed healing

K - subsequent encounter for fracture with nonunion

P - subsequent encounter for fracture with malunion

S - sequela

S59.0 **Physeal fracture of lower end of ulna**

S59.00 Unspecified physeal fracture of lower end of ulna

⑦**S59.001** Unspecified physeal fracture of lower end of ulna, right arm

⑦**S59.002** Unspecified physeal fracture of lower end of ulna, left arm

⑦**S59.009** Unspecified physeal fracture of lower end of ulna, unspecified arm

S59.01 Salter-Harris Type I physeal fracture of lower end of ulna

⑦**S59.011** Salter-Harris Type I physeal fracture of lower end of ulna, right arm

⑦S59.012   Salter-Harris Type I physeal fracture of lower end of ulna, left arm

⑦S59.019   Salter-Harris Type I physeal fracture of lower end of ulna, unspecified arm

S59.02   Salter-Harris Type II physeal fracture of lower end of ulna

⑦S59.021   Salter-Harris Type II physeal fracture of lower end of ulna, right arm

⑦S59.022   Salter-Harris Type II physeal fracture of lower end of ulna, left arm

⑦S59.029   Salter-Harris Type II physeal fracture of lower end of ulna, unspecified arm

S59.03   Salter-Harris Type III physeal fracture of lower end of ulna

⑦S59.031   Salter-Harris Type III physeal fracture of lower end of ulna, right arm

⑦S59.032   Salter-Harris Type III physeal fracture of lower end of ulna, left arm

⑦S59.039   Salter-Harris Type III physeal fracture of lower end of ulna, unspecified arm

S59.04   Salter-Harris Type IV physeal fracture of lower end of ulna

⑦S59.041   Salter-Harris Type IV physeal fracture of lower end of ulna, right arm

⑦S59.042   Salter-Harris Type IV physeal fracture of lower end of ulna, left arm

⑦S59.049   Salter-Harris Type IV physeal fracture of lower end of ulna, unspecified arm

S59.09   Other physeal fracture of lower end of ulna

⑦S59.091   Other physeal fracture of lower end of ulna, right arm

⑦S59.092   Other physeal fracture of lower end of ulna, left arm

⑦S59.099   Other physeal fracture of lower end of ulna, unspecified arm

S59.1   Physeal fracture of upper end of radius

S59.10   Unspecified physeal fracture of upper end of radius

⑦S59.101   Unspecified physeal fracture of upper end of radius, right arm

⑦S59.102   Unspecified physeal fracture of upper end of radius, left arm

⑦S59.109   Unspecified physeal fracture of upper end of radius, unspecified arm

S59.11   Salter-Harris Type I physeal fracture of upper end of radius

⑦S59.111   Salter-Harris Type I physeal fracture of upper end of radius, right arm

⑦S59.112   Salter-Harris Type I physeal fracture of upper end of radius, left arm

⑦S59.119   Salter-Harris Type I physeal fracture of upper end of radius, unspecified arm

S59.12   Salter-Harris Type II physeal fracture of upper end of radius

⑦S59.121   Salter-Harris Type II physeal fracture of upper end of radius, right arm

⑦S59.122   Salter-Harris Type II physeal fracture of upper end of radius, left arm

⑦S59.129   Salter-Harris Type II physeal fracture of upper end of radius, unspecified arm

S59.13   Salter-Harris Type III physeal fracture of upper end of radius

⑦S59.131   Salter-Harris Type III physeal fracture of upper end of radius, right arm

⑦S59.132   Salter-Harris Type III physeal fracture of upper end of radius, left arm

⑦S59.139   Salter-Harris Type III physeal fracture of upper end of radius, unspecified arm

S59.14   Salter-Harris Type IV physeal fracture of upper end of radius

⑦S59.141   Salter-Harris Type IV physeal fracture of upper end of radius, right arm

⑦S59.142   Salter-Harris Type IV physeal fracture of upper end of radius, left arm

⑦S59.149   Salter-Harris Type IV physeal fracture of upper end of radius, unspecified arm

S59.19   Other physeal fracture of upper end of radius

S59.191   Other physeal fracture of upper end of radius, right arm

⑦S59.192   Other physeal fracture of upper end of radius, left arm

⑦S59.199   Other physeal fracture of upper end of radius, unspecified arm

S59.2   Physeal fracture of lower end of radius

S59.20   Unspecified physeal fracture of lower end of radius

⑦S59.201   Unspecified physeal fracture of lower end of radius, right arm

⑦S59.202   Unspecified physeal fracture of lower end of radius, left arm

⑦S59.209   Unspecified physeal fracture of lower end of radius, unspecified arm

S59.21   Salter-Harris Type I physeal fracture of lower end of radius

⑦S59.211   Salter-Harris Type I physeal fracture of lower end of radius, right arm

⑦S59.212 **Salter-Harris Type I physeal fracture of lower end of radius, left arm**

⑦S59.219 **Salter-Harris Type I physeal fracture of lower end of radius, unspecified arm**

S59.22 **Salter-Harris Type II physeal fracture of lower end of radius**

⑦S59.221 **Salter-Harris Type II physeal fracture of lower end of radius, right arm**

⑦S59.222 **Salter-Harris Type II physeal fracture of lower end of radius, left arm**

⑦S59.229 **Salter-Harris Type II physeal fracture of lower end of radius, unspecified arm**

S59.23 **Salter-Harris Type III physeal fracture of lower end of radius**

⑦S59.231 **Salter-Harris Type III physeal fracture of lower end of radius, right arm**

⑦S59.232 **Salter-Harris Type III physeal fracture of lower end of radius, left arm**

⑦S59.239 **Salter-Harris Type III physeal fracture of lower end of radius, unspecified arm**

S59.24 **Salter-Harris Type IV physeal fracture of lower end of radius**

⑦S59.241 **Salter-Harris Type IV physeal fracture of lower end of radius, right arm**

⑦S59.242 **Salter-Harris Type IV physeal fracture of lower end of radius, left arm**

⑦S59.249 **Salter-Harris Type IV physeal fracture of lower end of radius, unspecified arm**

S59.29 **Other physeal fracture of lower end of radius**

⑦S59.291 **Other physeal fracture of lower end of radius, right arm**

⑦S59.292 **Other physeal fracture of lower end of radius, left arm**

⑦S59.299 **Other physeal fracture of lower end of radius, unspecified arm**

S59.8 **Other specified injuries of elbow and forearm**

The appropriate 7th character is to be added to each code in subcategory S59.8

A - initial encounter

D - subsequent encounter

S - sequela

S59.80 **Other specified injuries of elbow**

⑦S59.801 **Other specified injuries of right elbow**

⑦S59.802 **Other specified injuries of left elbow**

⑦S59.809 **Other specified injuries of unspecified elbow**

S59.81 **Other specified injuries of forearm**

⑦S59.811 **Other specified injuries right forearm**

⑦S59.812 **Other specified injuries left forearm**

⑦S59.819 **Other specified injuries unspecified forearm**

S59.9 **Unspecified injury of elbow and forearm**

The appropriate 7th character is to be added to each code in subcategory S59.9

A - initial encounter

D - subsequent encounter

S - sequela

S59.90 **Unspecified injury of elbow**

⑦S59.901 **Unspecified injury of right elbow**

⑦S59.902 **Unspecified injury of left elbow**

⑦S59.909 **Unspecified injury of unspecified elbow**

S59.91 **Unspecified injury of forearm**

⑦S59.911 **Unspecified injury of right forearm**

⑦S59.912 **Unspecified injury of left forearm**

⑦S59.919 **Unspecified injury of unspecified forearm**

INJURIES TO THE WRIST, HAND AND FINGERS (S60-S69)

Excludes2: burns and corrosions (T20-T32)

frostbite (T33-T34)

insect bite or sting, venomous (T63.4)

S60 Superficial injury of wrist, hand and fingers

The appropriate 7th character is to be added to each code from category S60

A - initial encounter

D - subsequent encounter

S - sequela

S60.0 **Contusion of finger without damage to nail**

Excludes1: contusion involving nail (matrix) (S60.1)

⊗⑦S60.00 **Contusion of unspecified finger without damage to nail**

Contusion of finger(s) NOS

S60.01 **Contusion of thumb without damage to nail**

⑦S60.011 **Contusion of right thumb without damage to nail**

⑦S60.012 **Contusion of left thumb without damage to nail**

⑦S60.019 **Contusion of unspecified thumb without damage to nail**

S60.02 **Contusion of index finger without damage to nail**

⑦S60.021 **Contusion of right index finger without damage to nail**

⑦S60.022 **Contusion of left index finger without damage to nail**

⑦S60.029 **Contusion of unspecified index finger without damage to nail**

S60.03 **Contusion of middle finger without damage to nail**

⑦S60.031 **Contusion of right middle finger without damage to nail**

⑦S60.032 **Contusion of left middle finger without damage to nail**

⑦S60.039 **Contusion of unspecified middle finger without damage to nail**

S60.04   Contusion of ring finger without damage to nail

   ⑦S60.041   Contusion of right ring finger without damage to nail

   ⑦S60.042   Contusion of left ring finger without damage to nail

   ⑦S60.049   Contusion of unspecified ring finger without damage to nail

S60.05   Contusion of little finger without damage to nail

   ⑦S60.051   Contusion of right little finger without damage to nail

   ⑦S60.052   Contusion of left little finger without damage to nail

   ⑦S60.059   Contusion of unspecified little finger without damage to nail

S60.1   **Contusion of finger with damage to nail**

  ⊗⑦S60.10   Contusion of unspecified finger with damage to nail

  S60.11   Contusion of thumb with damage to nail

   ⑦S60.111   Contusion of right thumb with damage to nail

   ⑦S60.112   Contusion of left thumb with damage to nail

   ⑦S60.119   Contusion of unspecified thumb with damage to nail

  S60.12   Contusion of index finger with damage to nail

   ⑦S60.121   Contusion of right index finger with damage to nail

   ⑦S60.122   Contusion of left index finger with damage to nail

   ⑦S60.129   Contusion of unspecified index finger with damage to nail

  S60.13   Contusion of middle finger with damage to nail

   ⑦S60.131   Contusion of right middle finger with damage to nail

   ⑦S60.132   Contusion of left middle finger with damage to nail

   ⑦S60.139   Contusion of unspecified middle finger with damage to nail

  S60.14   Contusion of ring finger with damage to nail

   ⑦S60.141   Contusion of right ring finger with damage to nail

   ⑦S60.142   Contusion of left ring finger with damage to nail

   ⑦S60.149   Contusion of unspecified ring finger with damage to nail

  S60.15   Contusion of little finger with damage to nail

   ⑦S60.151   Contusion of right little finger with damage to nail

   ⑦S60.152   Contusion of left little finger with damage to nail

   ⑦S60.159   Contusion of unspecified little finger with damage to nail

S60.2   **Contusion of wrist and hand**

  Excludes2: contusion of fingers (S60.0-, S60.1-)

  S60.21   Contusion of wrist

   ⑦S60.211   Contusion of right wrist

   ⑦S60.212   Contusion of left wrist

   ⑦S60.219   Contusion of unspecified wrist

  S60.22   Contusion of hand

   ⑦S60.221   Contusion of right hand

   ⑦S60.222   Contusion of left hand

   ⑦S60.229   Contusion of unspecified hand

S60.3   **Other superficial injuries of thumb**

  S60.31   Abrasion of thumb

   ⑦S60.311   Abrasion of right thumb

   ⑦S60.312   Abrasion of left thumb

   ⑦S60.319   Abrasion of unspecified thumb

  S60.32   Blister (nonthermal) of thumb

   ⑦S60.321   Blister (nonthermal) of right thumb

   ⑦S60.322   Blister (nonthermal) of left thumb

   ⑦S60.329   Blister (nonthermal) of unspecified thumb

  S60.34   External constriction of thumb

    Hair tourniquet syndrome of thumb

    Use additional cause code to identify the constricting item (W49.0-)

   ⑦S60.341   External constriction of right thumb

   ⑦S60.342   External constriction of left thumb

   ⑦S60.349   External constriction of unspecified thumb

  S60.35   Superficial foreign body of thumb

    Splinter in the thumb

   ⑦S60.351   Superficial foreign body of right thumb

   ⑦S60.352   Superficial foreign body of left thumb

   ⑦S60.359   Superficial foreign body of unspecified thumb

  S60.36   Insect bite (nonvenomous) of thumb

   ⑦S60.361   Insect bite (nonvenomous) of right thumb

   ⑦S60.362   Insect bite (nonvenomous) of left thumb

   ⑦S60.369   Insect bite (nonvenomous) of unspecified thumb

  S60.37   Other superficial bite of thumb

    Excludes1: open bite of thumb (S61.05-, S61.15-)

   ⑦S60.371   Other superficial bite of right thumb

   ⑦S60.372   Other superficial bite of left thumb

   ⑦S60.379   Other superficial bite of unspecified thumb

  S60.39   Other superficial injuries of thumb

   ⑦S60.391   Other superficial injuries of right thumb

   ⑦S60.392   Other superficial injuries of left thumb

   ⑦S60.399   Other superficial injuries of unspecified thumb

S60.4   **Other superficial injuries of other fingers**

  S60.41   Abrasion of fingers

   ⑦S60.410   Abrasion of right index finger

   ⑦S60.411   Abrasion of left index finger

   ▓ Add 4th-7th digits   ░ Nonspecific code   ░ Unspecified code   ▓ Manifestation code

⑦S60.412 **Abrasion of right middle finger**

⑦S60.413 **Abrasion of left middle finger**

⑦S60.414 **Abrasion of right ring finger**

⑦S60.415 **Abrasion of left ring finger**

⑦S60.416 **Abrasion of right little finger**

⑦S60.417 **Abrasion of left little finger**

⑦S60.418 **Abrasion of other finger**

Abrasion of specified finger with unspecified laterality

⑦S60.419 **Abrasion of unspecified finger**

S60.42 **Blister (nonthermal) of fingers**

⑦S60.420 **Blister (nonthermal) of right index finger**

⑦S60.421 **Blister (nonthermal) of left index finger**

⑦S60.422 **Blister (nonthermal) of right middle finger**

⑦S60.423 **Blister (nonthermal) of left middle finger**

⑦S60.424 **Blister (nonthermal) of right ring finger**

⑦S60.425 **Blister (nonthermal) of left ring finger**

⑦S60.426 **Blister (nonthermal) of right little finger**

⑦S60.427 **Blister (nonthermal) of left little finger**

⑦S60.428 **Blister (nonthermal) of other finger**

Blister (nonthermal) of specified finger with unspecified laterality

⑦S60.429 **Blister (nonthermal) of unspecified finger**

S60.44 **External constriction of fingers**

Hair tourniquet syndrome of finger

Use additional cause code to identify the constricting item (W49.0-)

⑦S60.440 **External constriction of right index finger**

⑦S60.441 **External constriction of left index finger**

⑦S60.442 **External constriction of right middle finger**

⑦S60.443 **External constriction of left middle finger**

⑦S60.444 **External constriction of right ring finger**

⑦S60.445 **External constriction of left ring finger**

⑦S60.446 **External constriction of right little finger**

⑦S60.447 **External constriction of left little finger**

⑦S60.448 **External constriction of other finger**

External constriction of specified finger with unspecified laterality

⑦S60.449 **External constriction of unspecified finger**

S60.45 **Superficial foreign body of fingers**

Splinter in the finger(s)

⑦S60.450 **Superficial foreign body of right index finger**

⑦S60.451 **Superficial foreign body of left index finger**

⑦S60.452 **Superficial foreign body of right middle finger**

⑦S60.453 **Superficial foreign body of left middle finger**

⑦S60.454 **Superficial foreign body of right ring finger**

⑦S60.455 **Superficial foreign body of left ring finger**

⑦S60.456 **Superficial foreign body of right little finger**

⑦S60.457 **Superficial foreign body of left little finger**

⑦S60.458 **Superficial foreign body of other finger**

Superficial foreign body of specified finger with unspecified laterality

⑦S60.459 **Superficial foreign body of unspecified finger**

S60.46 **Insect bite (nonvenomous) of fingers**

⑦S60.460 **Insect bite (nonvenomous) of right index finger**

⑦S60.461 **Insect bite (nonvenomous) of left index finger**

⑦S60.462 **Insect bite (nonvenomous) of right middle finger**

⑦S60.463 **Insect bite (nonvenomous) of left middle finger**

⑦S60.464 **Insect bite (nonvenomous) of right ring finger**

⑦S60.465 **Insect bite (nonvenomous) of left ring finger**

⑦S60.466 **Insect bite (nonvenomous) of right little finger**

⑦S60.467 **Insect bite (nonvenomous) of left little finger**

⑦S60.468 **Insect bite (nonvenomous) of other finger**

Insect bite (nonvenomous) of specified finger with unspecified laterality

⑦S60.469 **Insect bite (nonvenomous) of unspecified finger**

S60.47 **Other superficial bite of fingers**

Excludes1: open bite of fingers (S61.25-, S61.35-)

⑦S60.470 **Other superficial bite of right index finger**

⑦S60.471 **Other superficial bite of left index finger**

⑦S60.472 **Other superficial bite of right middle finger**

⑦S60.473 **Other superficial bite of left middle finger**

⑦S60.474 **Other superficial bite of right ring finger**

⑦S60.475 **Other superficial bite of left ring finger**

● New code ▲ Revised code **Excludes1:** Not coded here **Excludes2:** Not included here ⊗ Placeholder required ⑦7th digit required

⑦S60.476　Other superficial bite of right little finger

⑦S60.477　Other superficial bite of left little finger

⑦S60.478　Other superficial bite of other finger

　　　　　Other superficial bite of specified finger with unspecified laterality

⑦S60.479　Other superficial bite of unspecified finger

S60.5　Other superficial injuries of hand

　　Excludes2: superficial injuries of fingers (S60.3-, S60.4-)

　　S60.51　Abrasion of hand

　　　⑦S60.511　Abrasion of right hand

　　　⑦S60.512　Abrasion of left hand

　　　⑦S60.519　Abrasion of unspecified hand

　　S60.52　Blister (nonthermal) of hand

　　　⑦S60.521　Blister (nonthermal) of right hand

　　　⑦S60.522　Blister (nonthermal) of left hand

　　　⑦S60.529　Blister (nonthermal) of unspecified hand

　　S60.54　External constriction of hand

　　　⑦S60.541　External constriction of right hand

　　　⑦S60.542　External constriction of left hand

　　　⑦S60.549　External constriction of unspecified hand

　　S60.55　Superficial foreign body of hand

　　　　Splinter in the hand

　　　⑦S60.551　Superficial foreign body of right hand

　　　⑦S60.552　Superficial foreign body of left hand

　　　⑦S60.559　Superficial foreign body of unspecified hand

　　S60.56　Insect bite (nonvenomous) of hand

　　　⑦S60.561　Insect bite (nonvenomous) of right hand

　　　⑦S60.562　Insect bite (nonvenomous) of left hand

　　　⑦S60.569　Insect bite (nonvenomous) of unspecified hand

　　S60.57　Other superficial bite of hand

　　　　Excludes1: open bite of hand (S61.45-)

　　　⑦S60.571　Other superficial bite of hand of right hand

　　　⑦S60.572　Other superficial bite of hand of left hand

　　　⑦S60.579　Other superficial bite of hand of unspecified hand

S60.8　Other superficial injuries of wrist

　　S60.81　Abrasion of wrist

　　　⑦S60.811　Abrasion of right wrist

　　　⑦S60.812　Abrasion of left wrist

　　　⑦S60.819　Abrasion of unspecified wrist

　　S60.82　Blister (nonthermal) of wrist

　　　⑦S60.821　Blister (nonthermal) of right wrist

　　　⑦S60.822　Blister (nonthermal) of left wrist

　　　⑦S60.829　Blister (nonthermal) of unspecified wrist

S60.84　External constriction of wrist

　　⑦S60.841　External constriction of right wrist

　　⑦S60.842　External constriction of left wrist

　　⑦S60.849　External constriction of unspecified wrist

S60.85　Superficial foreign body of wrist

　　Splinter in the wrist

　　⑦S60.851　Superficial foreign body of right wrist

　　⑦S60.852　Superficial foreign body of left wrist

　　⑦S60.859　Superficial foreign body of unspecified wrist

S60.86　Insect bite (nonvenomous) of wrist

　　⑦S60.861　Insect bite (nonvenomous) of right wrist

　　⑦S60.862　Insect bite (nonvenomous) of left wrist

　　⑦S60.869　Insect bite (nonvenomous) of unspecified wrist

S60.87　Other superficial bite of wrist

　　Excludes1: open bite of wrist (S61.55)

　　⑦S60.871　Other superficial bite of right wrist

　　⑦S60.872　Other superficial bite of left wrist

　　⑦S60.879　Other superficial bite of unspecified wrist

S60.9　Unspecified superficial injury of wrist, hand and fingers

　　S60.91　Unspecified superficial injury of wrist

　　　⑦S60.911　Unspecified superficial injury of right wrist

　　　⑦S60.912　Unspecified superficial injury of left wrist

　　　⑦S60.919　Unspecified superficial injury of unspecified wrist

　　S60.92　Unspecified superficial injury of hand

　　　⑦S60.921　Unspecified superficial injury of right hand

　　　⑦S60.922　Unspecified superficial injury of left hand

　　　⑦S60.929　Unspecified superficial injury of unspecified hand

　　S60.93　Unspecified superficial injury of thumb

　　　⑦S60.931　Unspecified superficial injury of right thumb

　　　⑦S60.932　Unspecified superficial injury of left thumb

　　　⑦S60.939　Unspecified superficial injury of unspecified thumb

　　S60.94　Unspecified superficial injury of other fingers

　　　⑦S60.940　Unspecified superficial injury of right index finger

　　　⑦S60.941　Unspecified superficial injury of left index finger

　　　⑦S60.942　Unspecified superficial injury of right middle finger

　　　⑦S60.943　Unspecified superficial injury of left middle finger

　　　⑦S60.944　Unspecified superficial injury of right ring finger

⑦ S60.945 **Unspecified superficial injury of left ring finger**

⑦ S60.946 **Unspecified superficial injury of right little finger**

⑦ S60.947 **Unspecified superficial injury of left little finger**

⑦ S60.948 **Unspecified superficial injury of other finger**

Unspecified superficial injury of specified finger with unspecified laterality

⑦ S60.949 **Unspecified superficial injury of unspecified finger**

S61 **Open wound of wrist, hand and fingers**

Code also any associated wound infection

Excludes1: open fracture of wrist, hand and finger (S62.- with 7th character B)

traumatic amputation of wrist and hand (S68.-)

The appropriate 7th character is to be added to each code from category S61

A - initial encounter

D - subsequent encounter

S - sequela

S61.0 **Open wound of thumb without damage to nail**

Excludes1: open wound of thumb with damage to nail (S61.1-)

S61.00 **Unspecified open wound of thumb without damage to nail**

⑦ S61.001 **Unspecified open wound of right thumb without damage to nail**

⑦ S61.002 **Unspecified open wound of left thumb without damage to nail**

⑦ S61.009 **Unspecified open wound of unspecified thumb without damage to nail**

⑦ S61.01 **Laceration without foreign body of thumb without damage to nail**

⑦ S61.011 **Laceration without foreign body of right thumb without damage to nail**

⑦ S61.012 **Laceration without foreign body of left thumb without damage to nail**

⑦ S61.019 **Laceration without foreign body of unspecified thumb without damage to nail**

S61.02 **Laceration with foreign body of thumb without damage to nail**

⑦ S61.021 **Laceration with foreign body of right thumb without damage to nail**

⑦ S61.022 **Laceration with foreign body of left thumb without damage to nail**

⑦ S61.029 **Laceration with foreign body of unspecified thumb without damage to nail**

S61.03 **Puncture wound without foreign body of thumb without damage to nail**

⑦ S61.031 **Puncture wound without foreign body of right thumb without damage to nail**

⑦ S61.032 **Puncture wound without foreign body of left thumb without damage to nail**

⑦ S61.039 **Puncture wound without foreign body of unspecified thumb without damage to nail**

S61.04 **Puncture wound with foreign body of thumb without damage to nail**

⑦ S61.041 **Puncture wound with foreign body of right thumb without damage to nail**

⑦ S61.042 **Puncture wound with foreign body of left thumb without damage to nail**

⑦ S61.049 **Puncture wound with foreign body of unspecified thumb without damage to nail**

S61.05 **Open bite of thumb without damage to nail**

Bite of thumb NOS

Excludes1: superficial bite of thumb (S60.36-, S60.37-)

⑦ S61.051 **Open bite of right thumb without damage to nail**

⑦ S61.052 **Open bite of left thumb without damage to nail**

⑦ S61.059 **Open bite of unspecified thumb without damage to nail**

S61.1 **Open wound of thumb with damage to nail**

S61.10 **Unspecified open wound of thumb with damage to nail**

⑦ S61.101 **Unspecified open wound of right thumb with damage to nail**

⑦ S61.102 **Unspecified open wound of left thumb with damage to nail**

⑦ S61.109 **Unspecified open wound of unspecified thumb with damage to nail**

S61.11 **Laceration without foreign body of thumb with damage to nail**

⑦ S61.111 **Laceration without foreign body of right thumb with damage to nail**

⑦ S61.112 **Laceration without foreign body of left thumb with damage to nail**

⑦ S61.119 **Laceration without foreign body of unspecified thumb with damage to nail**

S61.12 **Laceration with foreign body of thumb with damage to nail**

⑦ S61.121 **Laceration with foreign body of right thumb with damage to nail**

⑦ S61.122 **Laceration with foreign body of left thumb with damage to nail**

⑦ S61.129 **Laceration with foreign body of unspecified thumb with damage to nail**

S61.13 **Puncture wound without foreign body of thumb with damage to nail**

⑦ S61.131 **Puncture wound without foreign body of right thumb with damage to nail**

⑦ S61.132 **Puncture wound without foreign body of left thumb with damage to nail**

⑦S61.139 **Puncture wound without foreign body of unspecified thumb with damage to nail**

S61.14 **Puncture wound with foreign body of thumb with damage to nail**

⑦S61.141 **Puncture wound with foreign body of right thumb with damage to nail**

⑦S61.142 **Puncture wound with foreign body of left thumb with damage to nail**

⑦S61.149 **Puncture wound with foreign body of unspecified thumb with damage to nail**

S61.15 **Open bite of thumb with damage to nail**

Bite of thumb with damage to nail NOS

Excludes1: superficial bite of thumb (S60.36-, S60.37-)

⑦S61.151 **Open bite of right thumb with damage to nail**

⑦S61.152 **Open bite of left thumb with damage to nail**

⑦S61.159 **Open bite of unspecified thumb with damage to nail**

S61.2 **Open wound of other finger without damage to nail**

Excludes1: open wound of finger involving nail (matrix) (S61.3-)

Excludes2: open wound of thumb without damage to nail (S61.0-)

S61.20 **Unspecified open wound of other finger without damage to nail**

⑦S61.200 **Unspecified open wound of right index finger without damage to nail**

⑦S61.201 **Unspecified open wound of left index finger without damage to nail**

⑦S61.202 **Unspecified open wound of right middle finger without damage to nail**

⑦S61.203 **Unspecified open wound of left middle finger without damage to nail**

⑦S61.204 **Unspecified open wound of right ring finger without damage to nail**

⑦S61.205 **Unspecified open wound of left ring finger without damage to nail**

⑦S61.206 **Unspecified open wound of right little finger without damage to nail**

⑦S61.207 **Unspecified open wound of left little finger without damage to nail**

⑦S61.208 **Unspecified open wound of other finger without damage to nail**

Unspecified open wound of specified finger with unspecified laterality without damage to nail

⑦S61.209 **Unspecified open wound of unspecified finger without damage to nail**

S61.21 **Laceration without foreign body of finger without damage to nail**

⑦S61.210 **Laceration without foreign body of right index finger without damage to nail**

⑦S61.211 **Laceration without foreign body of left index finger without damage to nail**

⑦S61.212 **Laceration without foreign body of right middle finger without damage to nail**

⑦S61.213 **Laceration without foreign body of left middle finger without damage to nail**

⑦S61.214 **Laceration without foreign body of right ring finger without damage to nail**

⑦S61.215 **Laceration without foreign body of left ring finger without damage to nail**

⑦S61.216 **Laceration without foreign body of right little finger without damage to nail**

⑦S61.217 **Laceration without foreign body of left little finger without damage to nail**

⑦S61.218 **Laceration without foreign body of other finger without damage to nail**

Laceration without foreign body of specified finger with unspecified laterality without damage to nail

⑦S61.219 **Laceration without foreign body of unspecified finger without damage to nail**

S61.22 **Laceration with foreign body of finger without damage to nail**

⑦S61.220 **Laceration with foreign body of right index finger without damage to nail**

⑦S61.221 **Laceration with foreign body of left index finger without damage to nail**

⑦S61.222 **Laceration with foreign body of right middle finger without damage to nail**

⑦S61.223 **Laceration with foreign body of left middle finger without damage to nail**

⑦S61.224 **Laceration with foreign body of right ring finger without damage to nail**

⑦S61.225 **Laceration with foreign body of left ring finger without damage to nail**

⑦S61.226 **Laceration with foreign body of right little finger without damage to nail**

⑦S61.227 **Laceration with foreign body of left little finger without damage to nail**

⑦S61.228 **Laceration with foreign body of other finger without damage to nail**

Laceration with foreign body of specified finger with unspecified laterality without damage to nail

⑦S61.229 **Laceration with foreign body of unspecified finger without damage to nail**

S61.23 **Puncture wound without foreign body of finger without damage to nail**

Add 4th-7th digits   Nonspecific code   Unspecified code   Manifestation code

⑦S61.230 **Puncture wound without foreign body of right index finger without damage to nail**

⑦S61.231 **Puncture wound without foreign body of left index finger without damage to nail**

⑦S61.232 **Puncture wound without foreign body of right middle finger without damage to nail**

⑦S61.233 **Puncture wound without foreign body of left middle finger without damage to nail**

⑦S61.234 **Puncture wound without foreign body of right ring finger without damage to nail**

⑦S61.235 **Puncture wound without foreign body of left ring finger without damage to nail**

⑦S61.236 **Puncture wound without foreign body of right little finger without damage to nail**

⑦S61.237 **Puncture wound without foreign body of left little finger without damage to nail**

⑦S61.238 **Puncture wound without foreign body of other finger without damage to nail**

Puncture wound without foreign body of specified finger with unspecified laterality without damage to nail

⑦S61.239 **Puncture wound without foreign body of unspecified finger without damage to nail**

S61.24 **Puncture wound with foreign body of finger without damage to nail**

⑦S61.240 **Puncture wound with foreign body of right index finger without damage to nail**

⑦S61.241 **Puncture wound with foreign body of left index finger without damage to nail**

⑦S61.242 **Puncture wound with foreign body of right middle finger without damage to nail**

⑦S61.243 **Puncture wound with foreign body of left middle finger without damage to nail**

⑦S61.244 **Puncture wound with foreign body of right ring finger without damage to nail**

⑦S61.245 **Puncture wound with foreign body of left ring finger without damage to nail**

⑦S61.246 **Puncture wound with foreign body of right little finger without damage to nail**

⑦S61.247 **Puncture wound with foreign body of left little finger without damage to nail**

⑦S61.248 **Puncture wound with foreign body of other finger without damage to nail**

Puncture wound with foreign body of specified finger with unspecified laterality without damage to nail

⑦S61.249 **Puncture wound with foreign body of unspecified finger without damage to nail**

S61.25 **Open bite of finger without damage to nail**

Bite of finger without damage to nail NOS

Excludes1: superficial bite of finger (S60.46-, S60.47-)

⑦S61.250 **Open bite of right index finger without damage to nail**

⑦S61.251 **Open bite of left index finger without damage to nail**

⑦S61.252 **Open bite of right middle finger without damage to nail**

⑦S61.253 **Open bite of left middle finger without damage to nail**

⑦S61.254 **Open bite of right ring finger without damage to nail**

⑦S61.255 **Open bite of left ring finger without damage to nail**

⑦S61.256 **Open bite of right little finger without damage to nail**

⑦S61.257 **Open bite of left little finger without damage to nail**

⑦S61.258 **Open bite of other finger without damage to nail**

Open bite of specified finger with unspecified laterality without damage to nail

⑦S61.259 **Open bite of unspecified finger without damage to nail**

S61.3 **Open wound of other finger with damage to nail**

S61.30 **Unspecified open wound of finger with damage to nail**

⑦S61.300 **Unspecified open wound of right index finger with damage to nail**

⑦S61.301 **Unspecified open wound of left index finger with damage to nail**

⑦S61.302 **Unspecified open wound of right middle finger with damage to nail**

⑦S61.303 **Unspecified open wound of left middle finger with damage to nail**

⑦S61.304 **Unspecified open wound of right ring finger with damage to nail**

⑦S61.305 **Unspecified open wound of left ring finger with damage to nail**

⑦S61.306 **Unspecified open wound of right little finger with damage to nail**

⑦S61.307 **Unspecified open wound of left little finger with damage to nail**

⑦S61.308 **Unspecified open wound of other finger with damage to nail**

Unspecified open wound of specified finger with unspecified laterality with damage to nail

⑦S61.309 **Unspecified open wound of unspecified finger with damage to nail**

S61.31 **Laceration without foreign body of finger with damage to nail**

● New code　▲ Revised code　Excludes1: Not coded here　Excludes2: Not included here　⊗ Placeholder required　⑦7th digit required

⑦S61.310 **Laceration without foreign body of right index finger with damage to nail**

⑦S61.311 **Laceration without foreign body of left index finger with damage to nail**

⑦S61.312 **Laceration without foreign body of right middle finger with damage to nail**

⑦S61.313 **Laceration without foreign body of left middle finger with damage to nail**

⑦S61.314 **Laceration without foreign body of right ring finger with damage to nail**

⑦S61.315 **Laceration without foreign body of left ring finger with damage to nail**

⑦S61.316 **Laceration without foreign body of right little finger with damage to nail**

⑦S61.317 **Laceration without foreign body of left little finger with damage to nail**

⑦S61.318 **Laceration without foreign body of other finger with damage to nail**

Laceration without foreign body of specified finger with unspecified laterality with damage to nail

⑦S61.319 **Laceration without foreign body of unspecified finger with damage to nail**

S61.32 **Laceration with foreign body of finger with damage to nail**

⑦S61.320 **Laceration with foreign body of right index finger with damage to nail**

⑦S61.321 **Laceration with foreign body of left index finger with damage to nail**

⑦S61.322 **Laceration with foreign body of right middle finger with damage to nail**

⑦S61.323 **Laceration with foreign body of left middle finger with damage to nail**

⑦S61.324 **Laceration with foreign body of right ring finger with damage to nail**

⑦S61.325 **Laceration with foreign body of left ring finger with damage to nail**

⑦S61.326 **Laceration with foreign body of right little finger with damage to nail**

⑦S61.327 **Laceration with foreign body of left little finger with damage to nail**

⑦S61.328 **Laceration with foreign body of other finger with damage to nail**

Laceration with foreign body of specified finger with unspecified laterality with damage to nail

⑦S61.329 **Laceration with foreign body of unspecified finger with damage to nail**

S61.33 **Puncture wound without foreign body of finger with damage to nail**

⑦S61.330 **Puncture wound without foreign body of right index finger with damage to nail**

⑦S61.331 **Puncture wound without foreign body of left index finger with damage to nail**

⑦S61.332 **Puncture wound without foreign body of right middle finger with damage to nail**

⑦S61.333 **Puncture wound without foreign body of left middle finger with damage to nail**

⑦S61.334 **Puncture wound without foreign body of right ring finger with damage to nail**

⑦S61.335 **Puncture wound without foreign body of left ring finger with damage to nail**

⑦S61.336 **Puncture wound without foreign body of right little finger with damage to nail**

⑦S61.337 **Puncture wound without foreign body of left little finger with damage to nail**

⑦S61.338 **Puncture wound without foreign body of other finger with damage to nail**

Puncture wound without foreign body of specified finger with unspecified laterality with damage to nail

⑦S61.339 **Puncture wound without foreign body of unspecified finger with damage to nail**

S61.34 **Puncture wound with foreign body of finger with damage to nail**

⑦S61.340 **Puncture wound with foreign body of right index finger with damage to nail**

⑦S61.341 **Puncture wound with foreign body of left index finger with damage to nail**

⑦S61.342 **Puncture wound with foreign body of right middle finger with damage to nail**

⑦S61.343 **Puncture wound with foreign body of left middle finger with damage to nail**

⑦S61.344 **Puncture wound with foreign body of right ring finger with damage to nail**

⑦S61.345 **Puncture wound with foreign body of left ring finger with damage to nail**

⑦S61.346 **Puncture wound with foreign body of right little finger with damage to nail**

⑦S61.347 **Puncture wound with foreign body of left little finger with damage to nail**

⑦S61.348 **Puncture wound with foreign body of other finger with damage to nail**

Puncture wound with foreign body of specified finger with unspecified laterality with damage to nail

⑦**S61.349** **Puncture wound with foreign body of unspecified finger with damage to nail**

S61.35 **Open bite of finger with damage to nail**

Bite of finger with damage to nail NOS

Excludes1: superficial bite of finger (S60.46-, S60.47-)

⑦**S61.350** **Open bite of right index finger with damage to nail**

⑦**S61.351** **Open bite of left index finger with damage to nail**

⑦**S61.352** **Open bite of right middle finger with damage to nail**

⑦**S61.353** **Open bite of left middle finger with damage to nail**

⑦**S61.354** **Open bite of right ring finger with damage to nail**

⑦**S61.355** **Open bite of left ring finger with damage to nail**

⑦**S61.356** **Open bite of right little finger with damage to nail**

⑦**S61.357** **Open bite of left little finger with damage to nail**

⑦**S61.358** **Open bite of other finger with damage to nail**

Open bite of specified finger with unspecified laterality with damage to nail

⑦**S61.359** **Open bite of unspecified finger with damage to nail**

S61.4 **Open wound of hand**

S61.40 **Unspecified open wound of hand**

⑦**S61.401** **Unspecified open wound of right hand**

⑦**S61.402** **Unspecified open wound of left hand**

⑦**S61.409** **Unspecified open wound of unspecified hand**

S61.41 **Laceration without foreign body of hand**

⑦**S61.411** **Laceration without foreign body of right hand**

⑦**S61.412** **Laceration without foreign body of left hand**

⑦**S61.419** **Laceration without foreign body of unspecified hand**

S61.42 **Laceration with foreign body of hand**

⑦**S61.421** **Laceration with foreign body of right hand**

⑦**S61.422** **Laceration with foreign body of left hand**

⑦**S61.429** **Laceration with foreign body of unspecified hand**

S61.43 **Puncture wound without foreign body of hand**

S61.431 **Puncture wound without foreign body of right hand**

⑦**S61.432** **Puncture wound without foreign body of left hand**

⑦**S61.439** **Puncture wound without foreign body of unspecified hand**

S61.44 **Puncture wound with foreign body of hand**

⑦**S61.441** **Puncture wound with foreign body of right hand**

⑦**S61.442** **Puncture wound with foreign body of left hand**

S61.449 **Puncture wound with foreign body of unspecified hand**

S61.45 **Open bite of hand**

Bite of hand NOS

Excludes1: superficial bite of hand (S60.56-, S60.57-)

⑦**S61.451** **Open bite of right hand**

⑦**S61.452** **Open bite of left hand**

⑦**S61.459** **Open bite of unspecified hand**

S61.5 **Open wound of wrist**

S61.50 **Unspecified open wound of wrist**

⑦**S61.501** **Unspecified open wound of right wrist**

⑦**S61.502** **Unspecified open wound of left wrist**

⑦**S61.509** **Unspecified open wound of unspecified wrist**

S61.51 **Laceration without foreign body of wrist**

⑦**S61.511** **Laceration without foreign body of right wrist**

⑦**S61.512** **Laceration without foreign body of left wrist**

⑦**S61.519** **Laceration without foreign body of unspecified wrist**

S61.52 **Laceration with foreign body of wrist**

⑦**S61.521** **Laceration with foreign body of right wrist**

⑦**S61.522** **Laceration with foreign body of left wrist**

⑦**S61.529** **Laceration with foreign body of unspecified wrist**

S61.53 **Puncture wound without foreign body of wrist**

⑦**S61.531** **Puncture wound without foreign body of right wrist**

⑦**S61.532** **Puncture wound without foreign body of left wrist**

⑦**S61.539** **Puncture wound without foreign body of unspecified wrist**

S61.54 **Puncture wound with foreign body of wrist**

⑦**S61.541** **Puncture wound with foreign body of right wrist**

⑦**S61.542** **Puncture wound with foreign body of left wrist**

⑦**S61.549** **Puncture wound with foreign body of unspecified wrist**

S61.55 **Open bite of wrist**

Bite of wrist NOS

Excludes1: superficial bite of wrist (S60.86-, S60.87-)

⑦**S61.551** **Open bite of right wrist**

⑦**S61.552** **Open bite of left wrist**

⑦**S61.559** **Open bite of unspecified wrist**

S62 **Fracture at wrist and hand level**

Note: A fracture not indicated as displaced or nondisplaced should be coded to displaced

● New code   ▲ Revised code   **Excludes1:** Not coded here   **Excludes2:** Not included here   ⊗ Placeholder required   ⑦7ᵗʰ digit required

A fracture not indicated as open or closed should be coded to closed

Excludes1: traumatic amputation of wrist and hand (S68.-)

Excludes2: fracture of distal parts of ulna and radius (S52.-)

The appropriate 7th character is to be added to each code from category S62

A - initial encounter for closed fracture

B - initial encounter for open fracture

D - subsequent encounter for fracture with routine healing

G - subsequent encounter for fracture with delayed healing

K - subsequent encounter for fracture with nonunion

P - subsequent encounter for fracture with malunion

S - sequela

S62.0   Fracture of navicular [scaphoid] bone of wrist

S62.00   Unspecified fracture of navicular [scaphoid] bone of wrist

⑦**S62.001   Unspecified fracture of navicular [scaphoid] bone of right wrist**

⑦**S62.002   Unspecified fracture of navicular [scaphoid] bone of left wrist**

⑦**S62.009   Unspecified fracture of navicular [scaphoid] bone of unspecified wrist**

S62.01   Fracture of distal pole of navicular [scaphoid] bone of wrist

Fracture of volar tuberosity of navicular [scaphoid] bone of wrist

⑦**S62.011   Displaced fracture of distal pole of navicular [scaphoid] bone of right wrist**

⑦**S62.012   Displaced fracture of distal pole of navicular [scaphoid] bone of left wrist**

⑦**S62.013   Displaced fracture of distal pole of navicular [scaphoid] bone of unspecified wrist**

⑦**S62.014   Nondisplaced fracture of distal pole of navicular [scaphoid] bone of right wrist**

⑦**S62.015   Nondisplaced fracture of distal pole of navicular [scaphoid] bone of left wrist**

⑦**S62.016   Nondisplaced fracture of distal pole of navicular [scaphoid] bone of unspecified wrist**

S62.02   Fracture of middle third of navicular [scaphoid] bone of wrist

⑦**S62.021   Displaced fracture of middle third of navicular [scaphoid] bone of right wrist**

⑦**S62.022   Displaced fracture of middle third of navicular [scaphoid] bone of left wrist**

⑦**S62.023   Displaced fracture of middle third of navicular [scaphoid] bone of unspecified wrist**

⑦**S62.024   Nondisplaced fracture of middle third of navicular [scaphoid] bone of right wrist**

⑦**S62.025   Nondisplaced fracture of middle third of navicular [scaphoid] bone of left wrist**

⑦**S62.026   Nondisplaced fracture of middle third of navicular [scaphoid] bone of unspecified wrist**

S62.03   Fracture of proximal third of navicular [scaphoid] bone of wrist

⑦**S62.031   Displaced fracture of proximal third of navicular [scaphoid] bone of right wrist**

⑦**S62.032   Displaced fracture of proximal third of navicular [scaphoid] bone of left wrist**

⑦**S62.033   Displaced fracture of proximal third of navicular [scaphoid] bone of unspecified wrist**

⑦**S62.034   Nondisplaced fracture of proximal third of navicular [scaphoid] bone of right wrist**

⑦**S62.035   Nondisplaced fracture of proximal third of navicular [scaphoid] bone of left wrist**

⑦**S62.036   Nondisplaced fracture of proximal third of navicular [scaphoid] bone of unspecified wrist**

S62.1   Fracture of other and unspecified carpal bone(s)

Excludes2: fracture of scaphoid of wrist (S62.0-)

S62.10   Fracture of unspecified carpal bone

Fracture of wrist NOS

⑦**S62.101   Fracture of unspecified carpal bone, right wrist**

⑦**S62.102   Fracture of unspecified carpal bone, left wrist**

⑦**S62.109   Fracture of unspecified carpal bone, unspecified wrist**

S62.11   Fracture of triquetrum [cuneiform] bone of wrist

⑦**S62.111   Displaced fracture of triquetrum [cuneiform] bone, right wrist**

⑦**S62.112   Displaced fracture of triquetrum [cuneiform] bone, left wrist**

⑦**S62.113   Displaced fracture of triquetrum [cuneiform] bone, unspecified wrist**

⑦**S62.114   Nondisplaced fracture of triquetrum [cuneiform] bone, right wrist**

⑦**S62.115   Nondisplaced fracture of triquetrum [cuneiform] bone, left wrist**

⑦**S62.116   Nondisplaced fracture of triquetrum [cuneiform] bone, unspecified wrist**

S62.12   Fracture of lunate [semilunar]

⑦**S62.121   Displaced fracture of lunate [semilunar], right wrist**

⑦**S62.122   Displaced fracture of lunate [semilunar], left wrist**

⑦**S62.123   Displaced fracture of lunate [semilunar], unspecified wrist**

⑦**S62.124   Nondisplaced fracture of lunate [semilunar], right wrist**

⑦**S62.125   Nondisplaced fracture of lunate [semilunar], left wrist**

⑦S62.126   Nondisplaced fracture of lunate [semilunar], unspecified wrist

S62.13   Fracture of capitate [os magnum] bone

⑦S62.131   Displaced fracture of capitate [os magnum] bone, right wrist

⑦S62.132   Displaced fracture of capitate [os magnum] bone, left wrist

⑦S62.133   Displaced fracture of capitate [os magnum] bone, unspecified wrist

⑦S62.134   Nondisplaced fracture of capitate [os magnum] bone, right wrist

⑦S62.135   Nondisplaced fracture of capitate [os magnum] bone, left wrist

⑦S62.136   Nondisplaced fracture of capitate [os magnum] bone, unspecified wrist

S62.14   Fracture of body of hamate [unciform] bone

    Fracture of hamate [unciform] bone NOS

⑦S62.141   Displaced fracture of body of hamate [unciform] bone, right wrist

⑦S62.142   Displaced fracture of body of hamate [unciform] bone, left wrist

⑦S62.143   Displaced fracture of body of hamate [unciform] bone, unspecified wrist

⑦S62.144   Nondisplaced fracture of body of hamate [unciform] bone, right wrist

⑦S62.145   Nondisplaced fracture of body of hamate [unciform] bone, left wrist

⑦S62.146   Nondisplaced fracture of body of hamate [unciform] bone, unspecified wrist

S62.15   Fracture of hook process of hamate [unciform] bone

    Fracture of unciform process of hamate [unciform] bone

⑦S62.151   Displaced fracture of hook process of hamate [unciform] bone, right wrist

⑦S62.152   Displaced fracture of hook process of hamate [unciform] bone, left wrist

⑦S62.153   Displaced fracture of hook process of hamate [unciform] bone, unspecified wrist

⑦S62.154   Nondisplaced fracture of hook process of hamate [unciform] bone, right wrist

⑦S62.155   Nondisplaced fracture of hook process of hamate [unciform] bone, left wrist

⑦S62.156   Nondisplaced fracture of hook process of hamate [unciform] bone, unspecified wrist

S62.16   Fracture of pisiform

⑦S62.161   Displaced fracture of pisiform, right wrist

⑦S62.162   Displaced fracture of pisiform, left wrist

⑦S62.163   Displaced fracture of pisiform, unspecified wrist

⑦S62.164   Nondisplaced fracture of pisiform, right wrist

⑦S62.165   Nondisplaced fracture of pisiform, left wrist

⑦S62.166   Nondisplaced fracture of pisiform, unspecified wrist

S62.17   Fracture of trapezium [larger multangular]

⑦S62.171   Displaced fracture of trapezium [larger multangular], right wrist

⑦S62.172   Displaced fracture of trapezium [larger multangular], left wrist

⑦S62.173   Displaced fracture of trapezium [larger multangular], unspecified wrist

⑦S62.174   Nondisplaced fracture of trapezium [larger multangular], right wrist

⑦S62.175   Nondisplaced fracture of trapezium [larger multangular], left wrist

⑦S62.176   Nondisplaced fracture of trapezium [larger multangular], unspecified wrist

S62.18   Fracture of trapezoid [smaller multangular]

⑦S62.181   Displaced fracture of trapezoid [smaller multangular], right wrist

⑦S62.182   Displaced fracture of trapezoid [smaller multangular], left wrist

⑦S62.183   Displaced fracture of trapezoid [smaller multangular], unspecified wrist

⑦S62.184   Nondisplaced fracture of trapezoid [smaller multangular], right wrist

⑦S62.185   Nondisplaced fracture of trapezoid [smaller multangular], left wrist

⑦S62.186   Nondisplaced fracture of trapezoid [smaller multangular], unspecified wrist

S62.2   Fracture of first metacarpal bone

S62.20   Unspecified fracture of first metacarpal bone

⑦S62.201   Unspecified fracture of first metacarpal bone, right hand

⑦S62.202   Unspecified fracture of first metacarpal bone, left hand

⑦S62.209   Unspecified fracture of first metacarpal bone, unspecified hand

S62.21   Bennett's fracture

⑦S62.211   Bennett's fracture, right hand

⑦S62.212   Bennett's fracture, left hand

⑦S62.213   Bennett's fracture, unspecified hand

S62.22   Rolando's fracture

⑦S62.221   Displaced Rolando's fracture, right hand

⑦S62.222   Displaced Rolando's fracture, left hand

⑦S62.223   Displaced Rolando's fracture, unspecified hand

⑦S62.224   Nondisplaced Rolando's fracture, right hand

⑦S62.225   Nondisplaced Rolando's fracture, left hand

⑦S62.226   Nondisplaced Rolando's fracture, unspecified hand

   ● New code   ▲ Revised code   **Excludes1:** Not coded here   **Excludes2:** Not included here   ⊗ Placeholder required   ⑦7th digit required

S62.23 Other fracture of base of first metacarpal bone

⑦ **S62.231** Other displaced fracture of base of first metacarpal bone, right hand

⑦ **S62.232** Other displaced fracture of base of first metacarpal bone, left hand

⑦ **S62.233** Other displaced fracture of base of first metacarpal bone, unspecified hand

⑦ **S62.234** Other nondisplaced fracture of base of first metacarpal bone, right hand

⑦ **S62.235** Other nondisplaced fracture of base of first metacarpal bone, left hand

⑦ **S62.236** Other nondisplaced fracture of base of first metacarpal bone, unspecified hand

S62.24 Fracture of shaft of first metacarpal bone

⑦ **S62.241** Displaced fracture of shaft of first metacarpal bone, right hand

⑦ **S62.242** Displaced fracture of shaft of first metacarpal bone, left hand

⑦ **S62.243** Displaced fracture of shaft of first metacarpal bone, unspecified hand

⑦ **S62.244** Nondisplaced fracture of shaft of first metacarpal bone, right hand

⑦ **S62.245** Nondisplaced fracture of shaft of first metacarpal bone, left hand

⑦ **S62.246** Nondisplaced fracture of shaft of first metacarpal bone, unspecified hand

S62.25 Fracture of neck of first metacarpal bone

⑦ **S62.251** Displaced fracture of neck of first metacarpal bone, right hand

⑦ **S62.252** Displaced fracture of neck of first metacarpal bone, left hand

⑦ **S62.253** Displaced fracture of neck of first metacarpal bone, unspecified hand

⑦ **S62.254** Nondisplaced fracture of neck of first metacarpal bone, right hand

⑦ **S62.255** Nondisplaced fracture of neck of first metacarpal bone, left hand

⑦ **S62.256** Nondisplaced fracture of neck of first metacarpal bone, unspecified hand

S62.29 Other fracture of first metacarpal bone

⑦ **S62.291** Other fracture of first metacarpal bone, right hand

⑦ **S62.292** Other fracture of first metacarpal bone, left hand

⑦ **S62.299** Other fracture of first metacarpal bone, unspecified hand

S62.3 Fracture of other and unspecified metacarpal bone

Excludes2: fracture of first metacarpal bone (S62.2-)

S62.30 Unspecified fracture of other metacarpal bone

⑦ **S62.300** Unspecified fracture of second metacarpal bone, right hand

⑦ **S62.301** Unspecified fracture of second metacarpal bone, left hand

⑦ **S62.302** Unspecified fracture of third metacarpal bone, right hand

⑦ **S62.303** Unspecified fracture of third metacarpal bone, left hand

⑦ **S62.304** Unspecified fracture of fourth metacarpal bone, right hand

⑦ **S62.305** Unspecified fracture of fourth metacarpal bone, left hand

⑦ **S62.306** Unspecified fracture of fifth metacarpal bone, right hand

⑦ **S62.307** Unspecified fracture of fifth metacarpal bone, left hand

⑦ **S62.308** Unspecified fracture of other metacarpal bone

Unspecified fracture of specified metacarpal bone with unspecified laterality

⑦ **S62.309** Unspecified fracture of unspecified metacarpal bone

S62.31 Displaced fracture of base of other metacarpal bone

⑦ **S62.310** Displaced fracture of base of second metacarpal bone, right hand

⑦ **S62.311** Displaced fracture of base of second metacarpal bone. left hand

⑦ **S62.312** Displaced fracture of base of third metacarpal bone, right hand

⑦ **S62.313** Displaced fracture of base of third metacarpal bone, left hand

⑦ **S62.314** Displaced fracture of base of fourth metacarpal bone, right hand

⑦ **S62.315** Displaced fracture of base of fourth metacarpal bone, left hand

⑦ **S62.316** Displaced fracture of base of fifth metacarpal bone, right hand

⑦ **S62.317** Displaced fracture of base of fifth metacarpal bone. left hand

⑦ **S62.318** Displaced fracture of base of other metacarpal bone

Displaced fracture of base of specified metacarpal bone with unspecified laterality

⑦ **S62.319** Displaced fracture of base of unspecified metacarpal bone

S62.32 Displaced fracture of shaft of other metacarpal bone

⑦ **S62.320** Displaced fracture of shaft of second metacarpal bone, right hand

⑦ **S62.321** Displaced fracture of shaft of second metacarpal bone, left hand

⑦ **S62.322** Displaced fracture of shaft of third metacarpal bone, right hand

⑦ **S62.323** Displaced fracture of shaft of third metacarpal bone, left hand

⑦ **S62.324** Displaced fracture of shaft of fourth metacarpal bone, right hand

⑦ **S62.325** Displaced fracture of shaft of fourth metacarpal bone, left hand

⑦ **S62.326** Displaced fracture of shaft of fifth metacarpal bone, right hand

⑦ **S62.327** Displaced fracture of shaft of fifth metacarpal bone, left hand

⑦ **S62.328** Displaced fracture of shaft of other metacarpal bone

Displaced fracture of shaft of specified metacarpal bone with unspecified laterality

⑦**S62.329** **Displaced fracture of shaft of unspecified metacarpal bone**

S62.33 **Displaced fracture of neck of other metacarpal bone**

⑦**S62.330** **Displaced fracture of neck of second metacarpal bone, right hand**

⑦**S62.331** **Displaced fracture of neck of second metacarpal bone, left hand**

⑦**S62.332** **Displaced fracture of neck of third metacarpal bone, right hand**

⑦**S62.333** **Displaced fracture of neck of third metacarpal bone, left hand**

⑦**S62.334** **Displaced fracture of neck of fourth metacarpal bone, right hand**

⑦**S62.335** **Displaced fracture of neck of fourth metacarpal bone, left hand**

⑦**S62.336** **Displaced fracture of neck of fifth metacarpal bone, right hand**

⑦**S62.337** **Displaced fracture of neck of fifth metacarpal bone, left hand**

⑦**S62.338** **Displaced fracture of neck of other metacarpal bone**

Displaced fracture of neck of specified metacarpal bone with unspecified laterality

⑦**S62.339** **Displaced fracture of neck of unspecified metacarpal bone**

S62.34 **Nondisplaced fracture of base of other metacarpal bone**

⑦**S62.340** **Nondisplaced fracture of base of second metacarpal bone, right hand**

⑦**S62.341** **Nondisplaced fracture of base of second metacarpal bone, left hand**

⑦**S62.342** **Nondisplaced fracture of base of third metacarpal bone, right hand**

⑦**S62.343** **Nondisplaced fracture of base of third metacarpal bone, left hand**

⑦**S62.344** **Nondisplaced fracture of base of fourth metacarpal bone, right hand**

⑦**S62.345** **Nondisplaced fracture of base of fourth metacarpal bone, left hand**

⑦**S62.346** **Nondisplaced fracture of base of fifth metacarpal bone, right hand**

⑦**S62.347** **Nondisplaced fracture of base of fifth metacarpal bone. left hand**

⑦**S62.348** **Nondisplaced fracture of base of other metacarpal bone**

Nondisplaced fracture of base of specified metacarpal bone with unspecified laterality

⑦**S62.349** **Nondisplaced fracture of base of unspecified metacarpal bone**

S62.35 **Nondisplaced fracture of shaft of other metacarpal bone**

⑦**S62.350** **Nondisplaced fracture of shaft of second metacarpal bone, right hand**

⑦**S62.351** **Nondisplaced fracture of shaft of second metacarpal bone, left hand**

⑦**S62.352** **Nondisplaced fracture of shaft of third metacarpal bone, right hand**

⑦**S62.353** **Nondisplaced fracture of shaft of third metacarpal bone, left hand**

⑦**S62.354** **Nondisplaced fracture of shaft of fourth metacarpal bone, right hand**

⑦**S62.355** **Nondisplaced fracture of shaft of fourth metacarpal bone, left hand**

⑦**S62.356** **Nondisplaced fracture of shaft of fifth metacarpal bone, right hand**

⑦**S62.357** **Nondisplaced fracture of shaft of fifth metacarpal bone, left hand**

⑦**S62.358** **Nondisplaced fracture of shaft of other metacarpal bone**

Nondisplaced fracture of shaft of specified metacarpal bone with unspecified laterality

⑦**S62.359** **Nondisplaced fracture of shaft of unspecified metacarpal bone**

S62.36 **Nondisplaced fracture of neck of other metacarpal bone**

⑦**S62.360** **Nondisplaced fracture of neck of second metacarpal bone, right hand**

⑦**S62.361** **Nondisplaced fracture of neck of second metacarpal bone, left hand**

⑦**S62.362** **Nondisplaced fracture of neck of third metacarpal bone, right hand**

⑦**S62.363** **Nondisplaced fracture of neck of third metacarpal bone, left hand**

⑦**S62.364** **Nondisplaced fracture of neck of fourth metacarpal bone, right hand**

⑦**S62.365** **Nondisplaced fracture of neck of fourth metacarpal bone, left hand**

⑦**S62.366** **Nondisplaced fracture of neck of fifth metacarpal bone, right hand**

⑦**S62.367** **Nondisplaced fracture of neck of fifth metacarpal bone, left hand**

⑦**S62.368** **Nondisplaced fracture of neck of other metacarpal bone**

Nondisplaced fracture of neck of specified metacarpal bone with unspecified laterality

⑦**S62.369** **Nondisplaced fracture of neck of unspecified metacarpal bone**

S62.39 **Other fracture of other metacarpal bone**

⑦**S62.390** **Other fracture of second metacarpal bone, right hand**

⑦**S62.391** **Other fracture of second metacarpal bone, left hand**

⑦**S62.392** **Other fracture of third metacarpal bone, right hand**

⑦**S62.393** **Other fracture of third metacarpal bone, left hand**

⑦**S62.394** **Other fracture of fourth metacarpal bone, right hand**

⑦**S62.395** **Other fracture of fourth metacarpal bone, left hand**

⑦**S62.396** **Other fracture of fifth metacarpal bone, right hand**

⑦**S62.397** **Other fracture of fifth metacarpal bone, left hand**

⑦S62.398 **Other fracture of other metacarpal bone**

Other fracture of specified metacarpal bone with unspecified laterality

⑦S62.399 **Other fracture of unspecified metacarpal bone**

S62.5 **Fracture of thumb**

S62.50 **Fracture of unspecified phalanx of thumb**

⑦S62.501 **Fracture of unspecified phalanx of right thumb**

⑦S62.502 **Fracture of unspecified phalanx of left thumb**

⑦S62.509 **Fracture of unspecified phalanx of unspecified thumb**

S62.51 **Fracture of proximal phalanx of thumb**

⑦S62.511 **Displaced fracture of proximal phalanx of right thumb**

⑦S62.512 **Displaced fracture of proximal phalanx of left thumb**

⑦S62.513 **Displaced fracture of proximal phalanx of unspecified thumb**

⑦S62.514 **Nondisplaced fracture of proximal phalanx of right thumb**

⑦S62.515 **Nondisplaced fracture of proximal phalanx of left thumb**

⑦S62.516 **Nondisplaced fracture of proximal phalanx of unspecified thumb**

S62.52 **Fracture of distal phalanx of thumb**

⑦S62.521 **Displaced fracture of distal phalanx of right thumb**

⑦S62.522 **Displaced fracture of distal phalanx of left thumb**

⑦S62.523 **Displaced fracture of distal phalanx of unspecified thumb**

⑦S62.524 **Nondisplaced fracture of distal phalanx of right thumb**

⑦S62.525 **Nondisplaced fracture of distal phalanx of left thumb**

⑦S62.526 **Nondisplaced fracture of distal phalanx of unspecified thumb**

S62.6 **Fracture of other and unspecified finger(s)**

Excludes2: fracture of thumb (S62.5-)

S62.60 **Fracture of unspecified phalanx of finger**

⑦S62.600 **Fracture of unspecified phalanx of right index finger**

⑦S62.601 **Fracture of unspecified phalanx of left index finger**

⑦S62.602 **Fracture of unspecified phalanx of right middle finger**

⑦S62.603 **Fracture of unspecified phalanx of left middle finger**

⑦S62.604 **Fracture of unspecified phalanx of right ring finger**

⑦S62.605 **Fracture of unspecified phalanx of left ring finger**

⑦S62.606 **Fracture of unspecified phalanx of right little finger**

⑦S62.607 **Fracture of unspecified phalanx of left little finger**

⑦S62.608 **Fracture of unspecified phalanx of other finger**

Fracture of unspecified phalanx of specified finger with unspecified laterality

⑦S62.609 **Fracture of unspecified phalanx of unspecified finger**

S62.61 **Displaced fracture of proximal phalanx of finger**

⑦S62.610 **Displaced fracture of proximal phalanx of right index finger**

⑦S62.611 **Displaced fracture of proximal phalanx of left index finger**

⑦S62.612 **Displaced fracture of proximal phalanx of right middle finger**

⑦S62.613 **Displaced fracture of proximal phalanx of left middle finger**

⑦S62.614 **Displaced fracture of proximal phalanx of right ring finger**

⑦S62.615 **Displaced fracture of proximal phalanx of left ring finger**

⑦S62.616 **Displaced fracture of proximal phalanx of right little finger**

⑦S62.617 **Displaced fracture of proximal phalanx of left little finger**

⑦S62.618 **Displaced fracture of proximal phalanx of other finger**

Displaced fracture of proximal phalanx of specified finger with unspecified laterality

⑦S62.619 **Displaced fracture of proximal phalanx of unspecified finger**

S62.62 **Displaced fracture of medial phalanx of finger**

⑦S62.620 **Displaced fracture of medial phalanx of right index finger**

⑦S62.621 **Displaced fracture of medial phalanx of left index finger**

⑦S62.622 **Displaced fracture of medial phalanx of right middle finger**

⑦S62.623 **Displaced fracture of medial phalanx of left middle finger**

⑦S62.624 **Displaced fracture of medial phalanx of right ring finger**

⑦S62.625 **Displaced fracture of medial phalanx of left ring finger**

⑦S62.626 **Displaced fracture of medial phalanx of right little finger**

⑦S62.627 **Displaced fracture of medial phalanx of left little finger**

⑦S62.628 **Displaced fracture of medial phalanx of other finger**

Displaced fracture of medial phalanx of specified finger with unspecified laterality

⑦S62.629 **Displaced fracture of medial phalanx of unspecified finger**

S62.63 **Displaced fracture of distal phalanx of finger**

⑦S62.630 **Displaced fracture of distal phalanx of right index finger**

⑦S62.631 **Displaced fracture of distal phalanx of left index finger**

⑦S62.632 **Displaced fracture of distal phalanx of right middle finger**

⑦S62.633 **Displaced fracture of distal phalanx of left middle finger**

⑦S62.634 **Displaced fracture of distal phalanx of right ring finger**

⑦S62.635 **Displaced fracture of distal phalanx of left ring finger**

⑦S62.636 **Displaced fracture of distal phalanx of right little finger**

⑦S62.637 **Displaced fracture of distal phalanx of left little finger**

⑦S62.638 **Displaced fracture of distal phalanx of other finger**

Displaced fracture of distal phalanx of specified finger with unspecified laterality

⑦S62.639 **Displaced fracture of distal phalanx of unspecified finger**

S62.64 **Nondisplaced fracture of proximal phalanx of finger**

⑦S62.640 **Nondisplaced fracture of proximal phalanx of right index finger**

⑦S62.641 **Nondisplaced fracture of proximal phalanx of left index finger**

⑦S62.642 **Nondisplaced fracture of proximal phalanx of right middle finger**

⑦S62.643 **Nondisplaced fracture of proximal phalanx of left middle finger**

⑦S62.644 **Nondisplaced fracture of proximal phalanx of right ring finger**

⑦S62.645 **Nondisplaced fracture of proximal phalanx of left ring finger**

⑦S62.646 **Nondisplaced fracture of proximal phalanx of right little finger**

⑦S62.647 **Nondisplaced fracture of proximal phalanx of left little finger**

⑦S62.648 **Nondisplaced fracture of proximal phalanx of other finger**

Nondisplaced fracture of proximal phalanx of specified finger with unspecified laterality

⑦S62.649 **Nondisplaced fracture of proximal phalanx of unspecified finger**

S62.65 **Nondisplaced fracture of medial phalanx of finger**

⑦S62.650 **Nondisplaced fracture of medial phalanx of right index finger**

⑦S62.651 **Nondisplaced fracture of medial phalanx of left index finger**

⑦S62.652 **Nondisplaced fracture of medial phalanx of right middle finger**

⑦S62.653 **Nondisplaced fracture of medial phalanx of left middle finger**

⑦S62.654 **Nondisplaced fracture of medial phalanx of right ring finger**

⑦S62.655 **Nondisplaced fracture of medial phalanx of left ring finger**

⑦S62.656 **Nondisplaced fracture of medial phalanx of right little finger**

⑦S62.657 **Nondisplaced fracture of medial phalanx of left little finger**

⑦S62.658 **Nondisplaced fracture of medial phalanx of other finger**

Nondisplaced fracture of medial phalanx of specified finger with unspecified laterality

⑦S62.659 **Nondisplaced fracture of medial phalanx of unspecified finger**

S62.66 **Nondisplaced fracture of distal phalanx of finger**

⑦S62.660 **Nondisplaced fracture of distal phalanx of right index finger**

⑦S62.661 **Nondisplaced fracture of distal phalanx of left index finger**

⑦S62.662 **Nondisplaced fracture of distal phalanx of right middle finger**

⑦S62.663 **Nondisplaced fracture of distal phalanx of left middle finger**

⑦S62.664 **Nondisplaced fracture of distal phalanx of right ring finger**

⑦S62.665 **Nondisplaced fracture of distal phalanx of left ring finger**

⑦S62.666 **Nondisplaced fracture of distal phalanx of right little finger**

⑦S62.667 **Nondisplaced fracture of distal phalanx of left little finger**

⑦S62.668 **Nondisplaced fracture of distal phalanx of other finger**

Nondisplaced fracture of distal phalanx of specified finger with unspecified laterality

⑦S62.669 **Nondisplaced fracture of distal phalanx of unspecified finger**

S62.9 **Unspecified fracture of wrist and hand**

⊗⑦S62.90 **Unspecified fracture of unspecified wrist and hand**

⊗⑦S62.91 **Unspecified fracture of right wrist and hand**

⊗⑦S62.92 **Unspecified fracture of left wrist and hand**

S63 **Dislocation and sprain of joints and ligaments at wrist and hand level**

Includes: avulsion of joint or ligament at wrist and hand level

laceration of cartilage, joint or ligament at wrist and hand level

sprain of cartilage, joint or ligament at wrist and hand level

traumatic hemarthrosis of joint or ligament at wrist and hand level

traumatic rupture of joint or ligament at wrist and hand level

traumatic subluxation of joint or ligament at wrist and hand level

traumatic tear of joint or ligament at wrist and hand level

Code also any associated open wound

Excludes2: strain of muscle, fascia and tendon of wrist and hand (S66.-)

The appropriate 7th character is to be added to each code from category S63

A - initial encounter

D - subsequent encounter

S - sequela

S63.0 **Subluxation and dislocation of wrist and hand joints**

S63.00 **Unspecified subluxation and dislocation of wrist and hand**

Dislocation of carpal bone NOS

Dislocation of distal end of radius NOS

Subluxation of carpal bone NOS

Subluxation of distal end of radius NOS

⑦**S63.001** **Unspecified subluxation of right wrist and hand**

⑦**S63.002** **Unspecified subluxation of left wrist and hand**

⑦**S63.003** **Unspecified subluxation of unspecified wrist and hand**

⑦**S63.004** **Unspecified dislocation of right wrist and hand**

⑦**S63.005** **Unspecified dislocation of left wrist and hand**

⑦**S63.006** **Unspecified dislocation of unspecified wrist and hand**

S63.01 **Subluxation and dislocation of distal radioulnar joint**

⑦**S63.011** **Subluxation of distal radioulnar joint of right wrist**

⑦**S63.012** **Subluxation of distal radioulnar joint of left wrist**

⑦**S63.013** **Subluxation of distal radioulnar joint of unspecified wrist**

⑦**S63.014** **Dislocation of distal radioulnar joint of right wrist**

⑦**S63.015** **Dislocation of distal radioulnar joint of left wrist**

⑦**S63.016** **Dislocation of distal radioulnar joint of unspecified wrist**

S63.02 **Subluxation and dislocation of radiocarpal joint**

⑦**S63.021** **Subluxation of radiocarpal joint of right wrist**

⑦**S63.022** **Subluxation of radiocarpal joint of left wrist**

⑦**S63.023** **Subluxation of radiocarpal joint of unspecified wrist**

⑦**S63.024** **Dislocation of radiocarpal joint of right wrist**

⑦**S63.025** **Dislocation of radiocarpal joint of left wrist**

⑦**S63.026** **Dislocation of radiocarpal joint of unspecified wrist**

S63.03 **Subluxation and dislocation of midcarpal joint**

⑦**S63.031** **Subluxation of midcarpal joint of right wrist**

⑦**S63.032** **Subluxation of midcarpal joint of left wrist**

⑦**S63.033** **Subluxation of midcarpal joint of unspecified wrist**

⑦**S63.034** **Dislocation of midcarpal joint of right wrist**

⑦**S63.035** **Dislocation of midcarpal joint of left wrist**

⑦**S63.036** **Dislocation of midcarpal joint of unspecified wrist**

S63.04 **Subluxation and dislocation of carpometacarpal joint of thumb**

Excludes2: interphalangeal subluxation and dislocation of thumb (S63.1-)

⑦**S63.041** **Subluxation of carpometacarpal joint of right thumb**

⑦**S63.042** **Subluxation of carpometacarpal joint of left thumb**

⑦**S63.043** **Subluxation of carpometacarpal joint of unspecified thumb**

⑦**S63.044** **Dislocation of carpometacarpal joint of right thumb**

⑦**S63.045** **Dislocation of carpometacarpal joint of left thumb**

⑦**S63.046** **Dislocation of carpometacarpal joint of unspecified thumb**

S63.05 **Subluxation and dislocation of other carpometacarpal joint**

Excludes2: subluxation and dislocation of carpometacarpal joint of thumb (S63.04-)

⑦**S63.051** **Subluxation of other carpometacarpal joint of right hand**

⑦**S63.052** **Subluxation of other carpometacarpal joint of left hand**

⑦**S63.053** **Subluxation of other carpometacarpal joint of unspecified hand**

⑦**S63.054** **Dislocation of other carpometacarpal joint of right hand**

⑦**S63.055** **Dislocation of other carpometacarpal joint of left hand**

⑦**S63.056** **Dislocation of other carpometacarpal joint of unspecified hand**

S63.06 **Subluxation and dislocation of metacarpal (bone), proximal end**

⑦**S63.061** **Subluxation of metacarpal (bone), proximal end of right hand**

⑦**S63.062** **Subluxation of metacarpal (bone), proximal end of left hand**

⑦**S63.063** **Subluxation of metacarpal (bone), proximal end of unspecified hand**

⑦**S63.064** **Dislocation of metacarpal (bone), proximal end of right hand**

⑦**S63.065** **Dislocation of metacarpal (bone), proximal end of left hand**

⑦**S63.066** **Dislocation of metacarpal (bone), proximal end of unspecified hand**

S63.07 **Subluxation and dislocation of distal end of ulna**

⑦**S63.071** **Subluxation of distal end of right ulna**

⑦**S63.072** **Subluxation of distal end of left ulna**

⑦**S63.073** **Subluxation of distal end of unspecified ulna**

⑦**S63.074** **Dislocation of distal end of right ulna**

⑦**S63.075** **Dislocation of distal end of left ulna**

⑦**S63.076** **Dislocation of distal end of unspecified ulna**

S63.09 **Other subluxation and dislocation of wrist and hand**

⑦S63.091   Other subluxation of right wrist and hand

⑦S63.092   Other subluxation of left wrist and hand

⑦S63.093   Other subluxation of unspecified wrist and hand

⑦S63.094   Other dislocation of right wrist and hand

⑦S63.095   Other dislocation of left wrist and hand

⑦S63.096   Other dislocation of unspecified wrist and hand

S63.1   **Subluxation and dislocation of thumb**

   S63.10   **Unspecified subluxation and dislocation of thumb**

     ⑦S63.101   Unspecified subluxation of right thumb

     ⑦S63.102   Unspecified subluxation of left thumb

     ⑦S63.103   Unspecified subluxation of unspecified thumb

     ⑦S63.104   Unspecified dislocation of right thumb

     ⑦S63.105   Unspecified dislocation of left thumb

     ⑦S63.106   Unspecified dislocation of unspecified thumb

   S63.11   **Subluxation and dislocation of metacarpophalangeal joint of thumb**

     ⑦S63.111   Subluxation of metacarpophalangeal joint of right thumb

     ⑦S63.112   Subluxation of metacarpophalangeal joint of left thumb

     ⑦S63.113   Subluxation of metacarpophalangeal joint of unspecified thumb

     ⑦S63.114   Dislocation of metacarpophalangeal joint of right thumb

     ⑦S63.115   Dislocation of metacarpophalangeal joint of left thumb

     ⑦S63.116   Dislocation of metacarpophalangeal joint of unspecified thumb

   S63.12   **Subluxation and dislocation of unspecified interphalangeal joint of thumb**

     ⑦S63.121   Subluxation of unspecified interphalangeal joint of right thumb

     ⑦S63.122   Subluxation of unspecified interphalangeal joint of left thumb

     ⑦S63.123   Subluxation of unspecified interphalangeal joint of unspecified thumb

     ⑦S63.124   Dislocation of unspecified interphalangeal joint of right thumb

     ⑦S63.125   Dislocation of unspecified interphalangeal joint of left thumb

     ⑦S63.126   Dislocation of unspecified interphalangeal joint of unspecified thumb

   S63.13   **Subluxation and dislocation of proximal interphalangeal joint of thumb**

⑦S63.131   Subluxation of proximal interphalangeal joint of right thumb

⑦S63.132   Subluxation of proximal interphalangeal joint of left thumb

⑦S63.133   Subluxation of proximal interphalangeal joint of unspecified thumb

⑦S63.134   Dislocation of proximal interphalangeal joint of right thumb

⑦S63.135   Dislocation of proximal interphalangeal joint of left thumb

⑦S63.136   Dislocation of proximal interphalangeal joint of unspecified thumb

   S63.14   **Subluxation and dislocation of distal interphalangeal joint of thumb**

     ⑦S63.141   Subluxation of distal interphalangeal joint of right thumb

     ⑦S63.142   Subluxation of distal interphalangeal joint of left thumb

     ⑦S63.143   Subluxation of distal interphalangeal joint of unspecified thumb

     ⑦S63.144   Dislocation of distal interphalangeal joint of right thumb

     ⑦S63.145   Dislocation of distal interphalangeal joint of left thumb

     ⑦S63.146   Dislocation of distal interphalangeal joint of unspecified thumb

S63.2   **Subluxation and dislocation of other finger(s)**

   Excludes2: subluxation and dislocation of thumb (S63.1-)

   S63.20   **Unspecified subluxation of other finger**

     ⑦S63.200   Unspecified subluxation of right index finger

     ⑦S63.201   Unspecified subluxation of left index finger

     ⑦S63.202   Unspecified subluxation of right middle finger

     ⑦S63.203   Unspecified subluxation of left middle finger

     ⑦S63.204   Unspecified subluxation of right ring finger

     ⑦S63.205   Unspecified subluxation of left ring finger

     ⑦S63.206   Unspecified subluxation of right little finger

     ⑦S63.207   Unspecified subluxation of left little finger

     ⑦S63.208   Unspecified subluxation of other finger

       Unspecified subluxation of specified finger with unspecified laterality

     ⑦S63.209   Unspecified subluxation of unspecified finger

   S63.21   **Subluxation of metacarpophalangeal joint of finger**

     ⑦S63.210   Subluxation of metacarpophalangeal joint of right index finger

     ⑦S63.211   Subluxation of metacarpophalangeal joint of left index finger

   ● New code   ▲ Revised code   **Excludes1:** Not coded here   **Excludes2:** Not included here   ⊗ Placeholder required   ⑦7th digit required

⑦S63.212 Subluxation of metacarpophalangeal joint of right middle finger

⑦S63.213 Subluxation of metacarpophalangeal joint of left middle finger

⑦S63.214 Subluxation of metacarpophalangeal joint of right ring finger

⑦S63.215 Subluxation of metacarpophalangeal joint of left ring finger

⑦S63.216 Subluxation of metacarpophalangeal joint of right little finger

⑦S63.217 Subluxation of metacarpophalangeal joint of left little finger

⑦S63.218 Subluxation of metacarpophalangeal joint of other finger

Subluxation of metacarpophalangeal joint of specified finger with unspecified laterality

⑦S63.219 Subluxation of metacarpophalangeal joint of unspecified finger

S63.22 Subluxation of unspecified interphalangeal joint of finger

⑦S63.220 Subluxation of unspecified interphalangeal joint of right index finger

⑦S63.221 Subluxation of unspecified interphalangeal joint of left index finger

⑦S63.222 Subluxation of unspecified interphalangeal joint of right middle finger

⑦S63.223 Subluxation of unspecified interphalangeal joint of left middle finger

⑦S63.224 Subluxation of unspecified interphalangeal joint of right ring finger

⑦S63.225 Subluxation of unspecified interphalangeal joint of left ring finger

⑦S63.226 Subluxation of unspecified interphalangeal joint of right little finger

⑦S63.227 Subluxation of unspecified interphalangeal joint of left little finger

⑦S63.228 Subluxation of unspecified interphalangeal joint of other finger

Subluxation of unspecified interphalangeal joint of specified finger with unspecified laterality

⑦S63.229 Subluxation of unspecified interphalangeal joint of unspecified finger

S63.23 Subluxation of proximal interphalangeal joint of finger

⑦S63.230 Subluxation of proximal interphalangeal joint of right index finger

⑦S63.231 Subluxation of proximal interphalangeal joint of left index finger

⑦S63.232 Subluxation of proximal interphalangeal joint of right middle finger

⑦S63.233 Subluxation of proximal interphalangeal joint of left middle finger

⑦S63.234 Subluxation of proximal interphalangeal joint of right ring finger

⑦S63.235 Subluxation of proximal interphalangeal joint of left ring finger

⑦S63.236 Subluxation of proximal interphalangeal joint of right little finger

⑦S63.237 Subluxation of proximal interphalangeal joint of left little finger

⑦S63.238 Subluxation of proximal interphalangeal joint of other finger

Subluxation of proximal interphalangeal joint of specified finger with unspecified laterality

⑦S63.239 Subluxation of proximal interphalangeal joint of unspecified finger

S63.24 Subluxation of distal interphalangeal joint of finger

⑦S63.240 Subluxation of distal interphalangeal joint of right index finger

⑦S63.241 Subluxation of distal interphalangeal joint of left index finger

⑦S63.242 Subluxation of distal interphalangeal joint of right middle finger

⑦S63.243 Subluxation of distal interphalangeal joint of left middle finger

⑦S63.244 Subluxation of distal interphalangeal joint of right ring finger

⑦S63.245 Subluxation of distal interphalangeal joint of left ring finger

⑦S63.246 Subluxation of distal interphalangeal joint of right little finger

⑦S63.247 Subluxation of distal interphalangeal joint of left little finger

⑦S63.248 Subluxation of distal interphalangeal joint of other finger

Subluxation of distal interphalangeal joint of specified finger with unspecified laterality

⑦S63.249   **Subluxation of distal interphalangeal joint of unspecified finger**

S63.25   **Unspecified dislocation of other finger**

  ⑦S63.250   **Unspecified dislocation of right index finger**

  ⑦S63.251   **Unspecified dislocation of left index finger**

  ⑦S63.252   **Unspecified dislocation of right middle finger**

  ⑦S63.253   **Unspecified dislocation of left middle finger**

  ⑦S63.254   **Unspecified dislocation of right ring finger**

  ⑦S63.255   **Unspecified dislocation of left ring finger**

  ⑦S63.256   **Unspecified dislocation of right little finger**

  ⑦S63.257   **Unspecified dislocation of left little finger**

  ⑦S63.258   **Unspecified dislocation of other finger**

    Unspecified dislocation of specified finger with unspecified laterality

  ⑦S63.259   **Unspecified dislocation of unspecified finger**

    Unspecified dislocation of specified finger with unspecified laterality

S63.26   **Dislocation of metacarpophalangeal joint of finger**

  ⑦S63.260   **Dislocation of metacarpophalangeal joint of right index finger**

  ⑦S63.261   **Dislocation of metacarpophalangeal joint of left index finger**

  ⑦S63.262   **Dislocation of metacarpophalangeal joint of right middle finger**

  ⑦S63.263   **Dislocation of metacarpophalangeal joint of left middle finger**

  ⑦S63.264   **Dislocation of metacarpophalangeal joint of right ring finger**

  ⑦S63.265   **Dislocation of metacarpophalangeal joint of left ring finger**

  ⑦S63.266   **Dislocation of metacarpophalangeal joint of right little finger**

  ⑦S63.267   **Dislocation of metacarpophalangeal joint of left little finger**

  ⑦S63.268   **Dislocation of metacarpophalangeal joint of other finger**

    Dislocation of metacarpophalangeal joint of specified finger with unspecified laterality

  ⑦S63.269   **Dislocation of metacarpophalangeal joint of unspecified finger**

S63.27   **Dislocation of unspecified interphalangeal joint of finger**

  ⑦S63.270   **Dislocation of unspecified interphalangeal joint of right index finger**

  ⑦S63.271   **Dislocation of unspecified interphalangeal joint of left index finger**

⑦S63.272   **Dislocation of unspecified interphalangeal joint of right middle finger**

⑦S63.273   **Dislocation of unspecified interphalangeal joint of left middle finger**

⑦S63.274   **Dislocation of unspecified interphalangeal joint of right ring finger**

⑦S63.275   **Dislocation of unspecified interphalangeal joint of left ring finger**

⑦S63.276   **Dislocation of unspecified interphalangeal joint of right little finger**

⑦S63.277   **Dislocation of unspecified interphalangeal joint of left little finger**

⑦S63.278   **Dislocation of unspecified interphalangeal joint of other finger**

  Dislocation of unspecified interphalangeal joint of specified finger with unspecified laterality

⑦S63.279   **Dislocation of unspecified interphalangeal joint of unspecified finger**

  Dislocation of unspecified interphalangeal joint of specified finger without specified laterality

S63.28   **Dislocation of proximal interphalangeal joint of finger**

  ⑦S63.280   **Dislocation of proximal interphalangeal joint of right index finger**

  ⑦S63.281   **Dislocation of proximal interphalangeal joint of left index finger**

  ⑦S63.282   **Dislocation of proximal interphalangeal joint of right middle finger**

  ⑦S63.283   **Dislocation of proximal interphalangeal joint of left middle finger**

  ⑦S63.284   **Dislocation of proximal interphalangeal joint of right ring finger**

  ⑦S63.285   **Dislocation of proximal interphalangeal joint of left ring finger**

  ⑦S63.286   **Dislocation of proximal interphalangeal joint of right little finger**

  ⑦S63.287   **Dislocation of proximal interphalangeal joint of left little finger**

  ⑦S63.288   **Dislocation of proximal interphalangeal joint of other finger**

    Dislocation of proximal interphalangeal joint of specified finger with unspecified laterality

  ⑦S63.289   **Dislocation of proximal interphalangeal joint of unspecified finger**

S63.29   Dislocation of distal interphalangeal joint of finger

⑦S63.290   Dislocation of distal interphalangeal joint of right index finger

⑦S63.291   Dislocation of distal interphalangeal joint of left index finger

⑦S63.292   Dislocation of distal interphalangeal joint of right middle finger

⑦S63.293   Dislocation of distal interphalangeal joint of left middle finger

⑦S63.294   Dislocation of distal interphalangeal joint of right ring finger

⑦S63.295   Dislocation of distal interphalangeal joint of left ring finger

⑦S63.296   Dislocation of distal interphalangeal joint of right little finger

⑦S63.297   Dislocation of distal interphalangeal joint of left little finger

⑦S63.298   Dislocation of distal interphalangeal joint of other finger

Dislocation of distal interphalangeal joint of specified finger with unspecified laterality

⑦S63.299   Dislocation of distal interphalangeal joint of unspecified finger

S63.3   Traumatic rupture of ligament of wrist

S63.30   Traumatic rupture of unspecified ligament of wrist

⑦S63.301   Traumatic rupture of unspecified ligament of right wrist

⑦S63.302   Traumatic rupture of unspecified ligament of left wrist

⑦S63.309   Traumatic rupture of unspecified ligament of unspecified wrist

S63.31   Traumatic rupture of collateral ligament of wrist

⑦S63.311   Traumatic rupture of collateral ligament of right wrist

⑦S63.312   Traumatic rupture of collateral ligament of left wrist

⑦S63.319   Traumatic rupture of collateral ligament of unspecified wrist

S63.32   Traumatic rupture of radiocarpal ligament

⑦S63.321   Traumatic rupture of right radiocarpal ligament

⑦S63.322   Traumatic rupture of left radiocarpal ligament

⑦S63.329   Traumatic rupture of unspecified radiocarpal ligament

S63.33   Traumatic rupture of ulnocarpal (palmar) ligament

⑦S63.331   Traumatic rupture of right ulnocarpal (palmar) ligament

⑦S63.332   Traumatic rupture of left ulnocarpal (palmar) ligament

⑦S63.339   Traumatic rupture of unspecified ulnocarpal (palmar) ligament

S63.39   Traumatic rupture of other ligament of wrist

⑦S63.391   Traumatic rupture of other ligament of right wrist

⑦S63.392   Traumatic rupture of other ligament of left wrist

⑦S63.399   Traumatic rupture of other ligament of unspecified wrist

S63.4   Traumatic rupture of ligament of finger at metacarpophalangeal and interphalangeal joint(s)

S63.40   Traumatic rupture of unspecified ligament of finger at metacarpophalangeal and interphalangeal joint

⑦S63.400   Traumatic rupture of unspecified ligament of right index finger at metacarpophalangeal and interphalangeal joint

⑦S63.401   Traumatic rupture of unspecified ligament of left index finger at metacarpophalangeal and interphalangeal joint

⑦S63.402   Traumatic rupture of unspecified ligament of right middle finger at metacarpophalangeal and interphalangeal joint

⑦S63.403   Traumatic rupture of unspecified ligament of left middle finger at metacarpophalangeal and interphalangeal joint

⑦S63.404   Traumatic rupture of unspecified ligament of right ring finger at metacarpophalangeal and interphalangeal joint

⑦S63.405   Traumatic rupture of unspecified ligament of left ring finger at metacarpophalangeal and interphalangeal joint

⑦S63.406   Traumatic rupture of unspecified ligament of right little finger at metacarpophalangeal and interphalangeal joint

⑦S63.407   Traumatic rupture of unspecified ligament of left little finger at metacarpophalangeal and interphalangeal joint

⑦S63.408   Traumatic rupture of unspecified ligament of other finger at metacarpophalangeal and interphalangeal joint

Traumatic rupture of unspecified ligament of specified finger with unspecified laterality at metacarpophalangeal and interphalangeal joint

⑦S63.409   Traumatic rupture of unspecified ligament of unspecified finger at metacarpophalangeal and interphalangeal joint

S63.41   Traumatic rupture of collateral ligament of finger at metacarpophalangeal and interphalangeal joint

⑦S63.410   Traumatic rupture of collateral ligament of right index finger at metacarpophalangeal and interphalangeal joint

⑦S63.411   Traumatic rupture of collateral ligament of left index finger at metacarpophalangeal and interphalangeal joint

⑦ S63.412 **Traumatic rupture of collateral ligament of right middle finger at metacarpophalangeal and interphalangeal joint**

⑦ S63.413 **Traumatic rupture of collateral ligament of left middle finger at metacarpophalangeal and interphalangeal joint**

⑦ S63.414 **Traumatic rupture of collateral ligament of right ring finger at metacarpophalangeal and interphalangeal joint**

⑦ S63.415 **Traumatic rupture of collateral ligament of left ring finger at metacarpophalangeal and interphalangeal joint**

⑦ S63.416 **Traumatic rupture of collateral ligament of right little finger at metacarpophalangeal and interphalangeal joint**

⑦ S63.417 **Traumatic rupture of collateral ligament of left little finger at metacarpophalangeal and interphalangeal joint**

⑦ S63.418 **Traumatic rupture of collateral ligament of other finger at metacarpophalangeal and interphalangeal joint**

Traumatic rupture of collateral ligament of specified finger with unspecified laterality at metacarpophalangeal and interphalangeal joint

⑦ S63.419 **Traumatic rupture of collateral ligament of unspecified finger at metacarpophalangeal and interphalangeal joint**

S63.42 **Traumatic rupture of palmar ligament of finger at metacarpophalangeal and interphalangeal joint**

⑦ S63.420 **Traumatic rupture of palmar ligament of right index finger at metacarpophalangeal and interphalangeal joint**

⑦ S63.421 **Traumatic rupture of palmar ligament of left index finger at metacarpophalangeal and interphalangeal joint**

⑦ S63.422 **Traumatic rupture of palmar ligament of right middle finger at metacarpophalangeal and interphalangeal joint**

⑦ S63.423 **Traumatic rupture of palmar ligament of left middle finger at metacarpophalangeal and interphalangeal joint**

⑦ S63.424 **Traumatic rupture of palmar ligament of right ring finger at metacarpophalangeal and interphalangeal joint**

⑦ S63.425 **Traumatic rupture of palmar ligament of left ring finger at metacarpophalangeal and interphalangeal joint**

⑦ S63.426 **Traumatic rupture of palmar ligament of right little finger at**

metacarpophalangeal and interphalangeal joint

⑦ S63.427 **Traumatic rupture of palmar ligament of left little finger at metacarpophalangeal and interphalangeal joint**

⑦ S63.428 **Traumatic rupture of palmar ligament of other finger at metacarpophalangeal and interphalangeal joint**

Traumatic rupture of palmar ligament of specified finger with unspecified laterality at metacarpophalangeal and interphalangeal joint

⑦ S63.429 **Traumatic rupture of palmar ligament of unspecified finger at metacarpophalangeal and interphalangeal joint**

S63.43 **Traumatic rupture of volar plate of finger at metacarpophalangeal and interphalangeal joint**

⑦ S63.430 **Traumatic rupture of volar plate of right index finger at metacarpophalangeal and interphalangeal joint**

⑦ S63.431 **Traumatic rupture of volar plate of left index finger at metacarpophalangeal and interphalangeal joint**

⑦ S63.432 **Traumatic rupture of volar plate of right middle finger at metacarpophalangeal and interphalangeal joint**

⑦ S63.433 **Traumatic rupture of volar plate of left middle finger at metacarpophalangeal and interphalangeal joint**

⑦ S63.434 **Traumatic rupture of volar plate of right ring finger at metacarpophalangeal and interphalangeal joint**

⑦ S63.435 **Traumatic rupture of volar plate of left ring finger at metacarpophalangeal and interphalangeal joint**

⑦ S63.436 **Traumatic rupture of volar plate of right little finger at metacarpophalangeal and interphalangeal joint**

⑦ S63.437 **Traumatic rupture of volar plate of left little finger at metacarpophalangeal and interphalangeal joint**

⑦ S63.438 **Traumatic rupture of volar plate of other finger at metacarpophalangeal and interphalangeal joint**

Traumatic rupture of volar plate of specified finger with unspecified laterality at metacarpophalangeal and interphalangeal joint

⑦ S63.439 **Traumatic rupture of volar plate of unspecified finger at metacarpophalangeal and interphalangeal joint**

● New code   ▲ Revised code   **Excludes1:** Not coded here   **Excludes2:** Not included here   ⊗ Placeholder required   ⑦ 7th digit required

S63.49   **Traumatic rupture of other ligament of finger at metacarpophalangeal and interphalangeal joint**

⑦S63.490   **Traumatic rupture of other ligament of right index finger at metacarpophalangeal and interphalangeal joint**

⑦S63.491   **Traumatic rupture of other ligament of left index finger at metacarpophalangeal and interphalangeal joint**

⑦S63.492   **Traumatic rupture of other ligament of right middle finger at metacarpophalangeal and interphalangeal joint**

⑦S63.493   **Traumatic rupture of other ligament of left middle finger at metacarpophalangeal and interphalangeal joint**

⑦S63.494   **Traumatic rupture of other ligament of right ring finger at metacarpophalangeal and interphalangeal joint**

⑦S63.495   **Traumatic rupture of other ligament of left ring finger at metacarpophalangeal and interphalangeal joint**

⑦S63.496   **Traumatic rupture of other ligament of right little finger at metacarpophalangeal and interphalangeal joint**

⑦S63.497   **Traumatic rupture of other ligament of left little finger at metacarpophalangeal and interphalangeal joint**

⑦S63.498   **Traumatic rupture of other ligament of other finger at metacarpophalangeal and interphalangeal joint**

Traumatic rupture of ligament of specified finger with unspecified laterality at metacarpophalangeal and interphalangeal joint

⑦S63.499   **Traumatic rupture of other ligament of unspecified finger at metacarpophalangeal and interphalangeal joint**

S63.5   **Other and unspecified sprain of wrist**

S63.50   **Unspecified sprain of wrist**

⑦S63.501   **Unspecified sprain of right wrist**

⑦S63.502   **Unspecified sprain of left wrist**

⑦S63.509   **Unspecified sprain of unspecified wrist**

S63.51   **Sprain of carpal (joint)**

⑦S63.511   **Sprain of carpal joint of right wrist**

⑦S63.512   **Sprain of carpal joint of left wrist**

⑦S63.519   **Sprain of carpal joint of unspecified wrist**

S63.52   **Sprain of radiocarpal joint**

Excludes1: traumatic rupture of radiocarpal ligament (S63.32-)

⑦S63.521   **Sprain of radiocarpal joint of right wrist**

⑦S63.522   **Sprain of radiocarpal joint of left wrist**

⑦S63.529   **Sprain of radiocarpal joint of unspecified wrist**

S63.59   **Other specified sprain of wrist**

⑦S63.591   **Other specified sprain of right wrist**

⑦S63.592   **Other specified sprain of left wrist**

⑦S63.599   **Other specified sprain of unspecified wrist**

S63.6   **Other and unspecified sprain of finger(s)**

Excludes1: traumatic rupture of ligament of finger at metacarpophalangeal and interphalangeal joint(s) (S63.4-)

S63.60   **Unspecified sprain of thumb**

⑦S63.601   **Unspecified sprain of right thumb**

⑦S63.602   **Unspecified sprain of left thumb**

⑦S63.609   **Unspecified sprain of unspecified thumb**

S63.61   **Unspecified sprain of other and unspecified finger(s)**

⑦S63.610   **Unspecified sprain of right index finger**

⑦S63.611   **Unspecified sprain of left index finger**

⑦S63.612   **Unspecified sprain of right middle finger**

⑦S63.613   **Unspecified sprain of left middle finger**

⑦S63.614   **Unspecified sprain of right ring finger**

⑦S63.615   **Unspecified sprain of left ring finger**

⑦S63.616   **Unspecified sprain of right little finger**

⑦S63.617   **Unspecified sprain of left little finger**

⑦S63.618   **Unspecified sprain of other finger**

Unspecified sprain of specified finger with unspecified laterality

⑦S63.619   **Unspecified sprain of unspecified finger**

S63.62   **Sprain of interphalangeal joint of thumb**

⑦S63.621   **Sprain of interphalangeal joint of right thumb**

⑦S63.622   **Sprain of interphalangeal joint of left thumb**

⑦S63.629   **Sprain of interphalangeal joint of unspecified thumb**

S63.63   **Sprain of interphalangeal joint of other and unspecified finger(s)**

⑦S63.630   **Sprain of interphalangeal joint of right index finger**

⑦S63.631   **Sprain of interphalangeal joint of left index finger**

⑦S63.632   **Sprain of interphalangeal joint of right middle finger**

⑦S63.633   **Sprain of interphalangeal joint of left middle finger**

⑦S63.634   **Sprain of interphalangeal joint of right ring finger**

⑦ S63.635　Sprain of interphalangeal joint of left ring finger

⑦ S63.636　Sprain of interphalangeal joint of right little finger

⑦ S63.637　Sprain of interphalangeal joint of left little finger

⑦ S63.638　Sprain of interphalangeal joint of other finger

⑦ S63.639　Sprain of interphalangeal joint of unspecified finger

S63.64　Sprain of metacarpophalangeal joint of thumb

⑦ S63.641　Sprain of metacarpophalangeal joint of right thumb

⑦ S63.642　Sprain of metacarpophalangeal joint of left thumb

S63.649　Sprain of metacarpophalangeal joint of unspecified thumb

S63.65　Sprain of metacarpophalangeal joint of other and unspecified finger(s)

⑦ S63.650　Sprain of metacarpophalangeal joint of right index finger

⑦ S63.651　Sprain of metacarpophalangeal joint of left index finger

⑦ S63.652　Sprain of metacarpophalangeal joint of right middle finger

⑦ S63.653　Sprain of metacarpophalangeal joint of left middle finger

⑦ S63.654　Sprain of metacarpophalangeal joint of right ring finger

⑦ S63.655　Sprain of metacarpophalangeal joint of left ring finger

⑦ S63.656　Sprain of metacarpophalangeal joint of right little finger

⑦ S63.657　Sprain of metacarpophalangeal joint of left little finger

⑦ S63.658　Sprain of metacarpophalangeal joint of other finger

Sprain of metacarpophalangeal joint of specified finger with unspecified laterality

⑦ S63.659　Sprain of metacarpophalangeal joint of unspecified finger

S63.68　Other sprain of thumb

⑦ S63.681　Other sprain of right thumb

⑦ S63.682　Other sprain of left thumb

⑦ S63.689　Other sprain of unspecified thumb

S63.69　Other sprain of other and unspecified finger(s)

⑦ S63.690　Other sprain of right index finger

⑦ S63.691　Other sprain of left index finger

⑦ S63.692　Other sprain of right middle finger

⑦ S63.693　Other sprain of left middle finger

⑦ S63.694　Other sprain of right ring finger

⑦ S63.695　Other sprain of left ring finger

⑦ S63.696　Other sprain of right little finger

⑦ S63.697　Other sprain of left little finger

⑦ S63.698　Other sprain of other finger

Other sprain of specified finger with unspecified laterality

⑦ S63.699　Other sprain of unspecified finger

S63.8　Sprain of other part of wrist and hand

S63.8X　Sprain of other part of wrist and hand

⑦ S63.8X1　Sprain of other part of right wrist and hand

⑦ S63.8X2　Sprain of other part of left wrist and hand

⑦ S63.8X9　Sprain of other part of unspecified wrist and hand

S63.9　Sprain of unspecified part of wrist and hand

⊗⑦ S63.90　Sprain of unspecified part of unspecified wrist and hand

⊗⑦ S63.91　Sprain of unspecified part of right wrist and hand

⊗⑦ S63.92　Sprain of unspecified part of left wrist and hand

S64　**Injury of nerves at wrist and hand level**

Code also any associated open wound (S61.-)

The appropriate 7th character is to be added to each code from category S64

A - initial encounter

D - subsequent encounter

S - sequela

S64.0　Injury of ulnar nerve at wrist and hand level

⊗⑦ S64.00　Injury of ulnar nerve at wrist and hand level of unspecified arm

⊗⑦ S64.01　Injury of ulnar nerve at wrist and hand level of right arm

⊗⑦ S64.02　Injury of ulnar nerve at wrist and hand level of left arm

S64.1　Injury of median nerve at wrist and hand level

⊗⑦ S64.10　Injury of median nerve at wrist and hand level of unspecified arm

⊗⑦ S64.11　Injury of median nerve at wrist and hand level of right arm

⊗⑦ S64.12　Injury of median nerve at wrist and hand level of left arm

S64.2　Injury of radial nerve at wrist and hand level

⊗⑦ S64.20　Injury of radial nerve at wrist and hand level of unspecified arm

⊗⑦ S64.21　Injury of radial nerve at wrist and hand level of right arm

⊗⑦ S64.22　Injury of radial nerve at wrist and hand level of left arm

S64.3　Injury of digital nerve of thumb

⊗⑦ S64.30　Injury of digital nerve of unspecified thumb

⊗⑦ S64.31　Injury of digital nerve of right thumb

⊗⑦ S64.32　Injury of digital nerve of left thumb

S64.4　Injury of digital nerve of other and unspecified finger

⊗⑦ S64.40　Injury of digital nerve of unspecified finger

S64.49　Injury of digital nerve of other finger

⑦ S64.490　Injury of digital nerve of right index finger

⑦ S64.491　Injury of digital nerve of left index finger

⑦ S64.492　Injury of digital nerve of right middle finger

⑦ S64.493　Injury of digital nerve of left middle finger

　● New code　▲ Revised code　**Excludes1:** Not coded here　**Excludes2:** Not included here　⊗ Placeholder required　⑦ 7th digit required

⑦S64.494   Injury of digital nerve of right ring finger

⑦S64.495   Injury of digital nerve of left ring finger

⑦S64.496   Injury of digital nerve of right little finger

⑦S64.497   Injury of digital nerve of left little finger

⑦S64.498   Injury of digital nerve of other finger

Injury of digital nerve of specified finger with unspecified laterality

S64.8   Injury of other nerves at wrist and hand level

  S64.8X   Injury of other nerves at wrist and hand level

    ⑦S64.8X1   Injury of other nerves at wrist and hand level of right arm

    ⑦S64.8X2   Injury of other nerves at wrist and hand level of left arm

    ⑦S64.8X9   Injury of other nerves at wrist and hand level of unspecified arm

S64.9   Injury of unspecified nerve at wrist and hand level

  ⊗⑦S64.90   Injury of unspecified nerve at wrist and hand level of unspecified arm

  ⊗⑦S64.91   Injury of unspecified nerve at wrist and hand level of right arm

  ⊗⑦S64.92   Injury of unspecified nerve at wrist and hand level of left arm

S65   Injury of blood vessels at wrist and hand level

Code also any associated open wound (S61.-)

The appropriate 7th character is to be added to each code from category S65

A - initial encounter

D - subsequent encounter

S - sequela

S65.0   Injury of ulnar artery at wrist and hand level

  S65.00   Unspecified injury of ulnar artery at wrist and hand level

    ⑦S65.001   Unspecified injury of ulnar artery at wrist and hand level of right arm

    ⑦S65.002   Unspecified injury of ulnar artery at wrist and hand level of left arm

    ⑦S65.009   Unspecified injury of ulnar artery at wrist and hand level of unspecified arm

  S65.01   Laceration of ulnar artery at wrist and hand level

    ⑦S65.011   Laceration of ulnar artery at wrist and hand level of right arm

    ⑦S65.012   Laceration of ulnar artery at wrist and hand level of left arm

    ⑦S65.019   Laceration of ulnar artery at wrist and hand level of unspecified arm

  S65.09   Other specified injury of ulnar artery at wrist and hand level

    ⑦S65.091   Other specified injury of ulnar artery at wrist and hand level of right arm

    ⑦S65.092   Other specified injury of ulnar artery at wrist and hand level of left arm

    ⑦S65.099   Other specified injury of ulnar artery at wrist and hand level of unspecified arm

S65.1   Injury of radial artery at wrist and hand level

  S65.10   Unspecified injury of radial artery at wrist and hand level

    ⑦S65.101   Unspecified injury of radial artery at wrist and hand level of right arm

    ⑦S65.102   Unspecified injury of radial artery at wrist and hand level of left arm

    ⑦S65.109   Unspecified injury of radial artery at wrist and hand level of unspecified arm

  S65.11   Laceration of radial artery at wrist and hand level

    ⑦S65.111   Laceration of radial artery at wrist and hand level of right arm

    ⑦S65.112   Laceration of radial artery at wrist and hand level of left arm

    ⑦S65.119   Laceration of radial artery at wrist and hand level of unspecified arm

  S65.19   Other specified injury of radial artery at wrist and hand level

    ⑦S65.191   Other specified injury of radial artery at wrist and hand level of right arm

    ⑦S65.192   Other specified injury of radial artery at wrist and hand level of left arm

    ⑦S65.199   Other specified injury of radial artery at wrist and hand level of unspecified arm

S65.2   Injury of superficial palmar arch

  S65.20   Unspecified injury of superficial palmar arch

    ⑦S65.201   Unspecified injury of superficial palmar arch of right hand

    ⑦S65.202   Unspecified injury of superficial palmar arch of left hand

    ⑦S65.209   Unspecified injury of superficial palmar arch of unspecified hand

  S65.21   Laceration of superficial palmar arch

    ⑦S65.211   Laceration of superficial palmar arch of right hand

    ⑦S65.212   Laceration of superficial palmar arch of left hand

    ⑦S65.219   Laceration of superficial palmar arch of unspecified hand

  S65.29   Other specified injury of superficial palmar arch

    ⑦S65.291   Other specified injury of superficial palmar arch of right hand

    ⑦S65.292   Other specified injury of superficial palmar arch of left hand

    ⑦S65.299   Other specified injury of superficial palmar arch of unspecified hand

S65.3   Injury of deep palmar arch

  S65.30   Unspecified injury of deep palmar arch

    ⑦S65.301   Unspecified injury of deep palmar arch of right hand

    ⑦S65.302   Unspecified injury of deep palmar arch of left hand

⑦ S65.309   **Unspecified injury of deep palmar arch of unspecified hand**

S65.31   **Laceration of deep palmar arch**

⑦ S65.311   **Laceration of deep palmar arch of right hand**

⑦ S65.312   **Laceration of deep palmar arch of left hand**

⑦ S65.319   **Laceration of deep palmar arch of unspecified hand**

S65.39   **Other specified injury of deep palmar arch**

⑦ S65.391   **Other specified injury of deep palmar arch of right hand**

⑦ S65.392   **Other specified injury of deep palmar arch of left hand**

⑦ S65.399   **Other specified injury of deep palmar arch of unspecified hand**

S65.4   **Injury of blood vessel of thumb**

S65.40   **Unspecified injury of blood vessel of thumb**

⑦ S65.401   **Unspecified injury of blood vessel of right thumb**

⑦ S65.402   **Unspecified injury of blood vessel of left thumb**

⑦ S65.409   **Unspecified injury of blood vessel of unspecified thumb**

S65.41   **Laceration of blood vessel of thumb**

⑦ S65.411   **Laceration of blood vessel of right thumb**

⑦ S65.412   **Laceration of blood vessel of left thumb**

⑦ S65.419   **Laceration of blood vessel of unspecified thumb**

S65.49   **Other specified injury of blood vessel of thumb**

⑦ S65.491   **Other specified injury of blood vessel of right thumb**

⑦ S65.492   **Other specified injury of blood vessel of left thumb**

⑦ S65.499   **Other specified injury of blood vessel of unspecified thumb**

S65.5   **Injury of blood vessel of other and unspecified finger**

S65.50   **Unspecified injury of blood vessel of other and unspecified finger**

⑦ S65.500   **Unspecified injury of blood vessel of right index finger**

⑦ S65.501   **Unspecified injury of blood vessel of left index finger**

⑦ S65.502   **Unspecified injury of blood vessel of right middle finger**

⑦ S65.503   **Unspecified injury of blood vessel of left middle finger**

⑦ S65.504   **Unspecified injury of blood vessel of right ring finger**

⑦ S65.505   **Unspecified injury of blood vessel of left ring finger**

⑦ S65.506   **Unspecified injury of blood vessel of right little finger**

⑦ S65.507   **Unspecified injury of blood vessel of left little finger**

⑦ S65.508   **Unspecified injury of blood vessel of other finger**

Unspecified injury of blood vessel of specified finger with unspecified laterality

⑦ S65.509   **Unspecified injury of blood vessel of unspecified finger**

S65.51   **Laceration of blood vessel of other and unspecified finger**

⑦ S65.510   **Laceration of blood vessel of right index finger**

⑦ S65.511   **Laceration of blood vessel of left index finger**

⑦ S65.512   **Laceration of blood vessel of right middle finger**

⑦ S65.513   **Laceration of blood vessel of left middle finger**

⑦ S65.514   **Laceration of blood vessel of right ring finger**

⑦ S65.515   **Laceration of blood vessel of left ring finger**

⑦ S65.516   **Laceration of blood vessel of right little finger**

⑦ S65.517   **Laceration of blood vessel of left little finger**

⑦ S65.518   **Laceration of blood vessel of other finger**

Laceration of blood vessel of specified finger with unspecified laterality

⑦ S65.519   **Laceration of blood vessel of unspecified finger**

S65.59   **Other specified injury of blood vessel of other and unspecified finger**

⑦ S65.590   **Other specified injury of blood vessel of right index finger**

⑦ S65.591   **Other specified injury of blood vessel of left index finger**

⑦ S65.592   **Other specified injury of blood vessel of right middle finger**

⑦ S65.593   **Other specified injury of blood vessel of left middle finger**

⑦ S65.594   **Other specified injury of blood vessel of right ring finger**

⑦ S65.595   **Other specified injury of blood vessel of left ring finger**

⑦ S65.596   **Other specified injury of blood vessel of right little finger**

⑦ S65.597   **Other specified injury of blood vessel of left little finger**

⑦ S65.598   **Other specified injury of blood vessel of other finger**

Other specified injury of blood vessel of specified finger with unspecified laterality

⑦ S65.599   **Other specified injury of blood vessel of unspecified finger**

S65.8   **Injury of other blood vessels at wrist and hand level**

S65.80   **Unspecified injury of other blood vessels at wrist and hand level**

⑦ S65.801   **Unspecified injury of other blood vessels at wrist and hand level of right arm**

⑦S65.802   Unspecified injury of other blood vessels at wrist and hand level of left arm

⑦S65.809   Unspecified injury of other blood vessels at wrist and hand level of unspecified arm

S65.81   Laceration of other blood vessels at wrist and hand level

⑦S65.811   Laceration of other blood vessels at wrist and hand level of right arm

⑦S65.812   Laceration of other blood vessels at wrist and hand level of left arm

⑦S65.819   Laceration of other blood vessels at wrist and hand level of unspecified arm

S65.89   Other specified injury of other blood vessels at wrist and hand level

⑦S65.891   Other specified injury of other blood vessels at wrist and hand level of right arm

⑦S65.892   Other specified injury of other blood vessels at wrist and hand level of left arm

⑦S65.899   Other specified injury of other blood vessels at wrist and hand level of unspecified arm

S65.9   Injury of unspecified blood vessel at wrist and hand level

S65.90   Unspecified injury of unspecified blood vessel at wrist and hand level

⑦S65.901   Unspecified injury of unspecified blood vessel at wrist and hand level of right arm

⑦S65.902   Unspecified injury of unspecified blood vessel at wrist and hand level of left arm

⑦S65.909   Unspecified injury of unspecified blood vessel at wrist and hand level of unspecified arm

S65.91   Laceration of unspecified blood vessel at wrist and hand level

⑦S65.911   Laceration of unspecified blood vessel at wrist and hand level of right arm

⑦S65.912   Laceration of unspecified blood vessel at wrist and hand level of left arm

⑦S65.919   Laceration of unspecified blood vessel at wrist and hand level of unspecified arm

S65.99   Other specified injury of unspecified blood vessel at wrist and hand level

⑦S65.991   Other specified injury of unspecified blood vessel at wrist and hand of right arm

⑦S65.992   Other specified injury of unspecified blood vessel at wrist and hand of left arm

⑦S65.999   Other specified injury of unspecified blood vessel at wrist and hand of unspecified arm

S66   Injury of muscle, fascia and tendon at wrist and hand level

Code also any associated open wound (S61.-)

Excludes2: sprain of joints and ligaments of wrist and hand (S63.-)

The appropriate 7th character is to be added to each code from category S66

A - initial encounter

D - subsequent encounter

S - sequela

S66.0   Injury of long flexor muscle, fascia and tendon of thumb at wrist and hand level

S66.00   Unspecified injury of long flexor muscle, fascia and tendon of thumb at wrist and hand level

⑦S66.001   Unspecified injury of long flexor muscle, fascia and tendon of right thumb at wrist and hand level

⑦S66.002   Unspecified injury of long flexor muscle, fascia and tendon of left thumb at wrist and hand level

⑦S66.009   Unspecified injury of long flexor muscle, fascia and tendon of unspecified thumb at wrist and hand level

S66.01   Strain of long flexor muscle, fascia and tendon of thumb at wrist and hand level

⑦S66.011   Strain of long flexor muscle, fascia and tendon of right thumb at wrist and hand level

⑦S66.012   Strain of long flexor muscle, fascia and tendon of left thumb at wrist and hand level

⑦S66.019   Strain of long flexor muscle, fascia and tendon of unspecified thumb at wrist and hand level

S66.02   Laceration of long flexor muscle, fascia and tendon of thumb at wrist and hand level

⑦S66.021   Laceration of long flexor muscle, fascia and tendon of right thumb at wrist and hand level

⑦S66.022   Laceration of long flexor muscle, fascia and tendon of left thumb at wrist and hand level

⑦S66.029   Laceration of long flexor muscle, fascia and tendon of unspecified thumb at wrist and hand level

S66.09   Other specified injury of long flexor muscle, fascia and tendon of thumb at wrist and hand level

⑦S66.091   Other specified injury of long flexor muscle, fascia and tendon of right thumb at wrist and hand level

⑦S66.092   Other specified injury of long flexor muscle, fascia and tendon of left thumb at wrist and hand level

⑦S66.099   Other specified injury of long flexor muscle, fascia and tendon of unspecified thumb at wrist and hand level

S66.1   Injury of flexor muscle, fascia and tendon of other and unspecified finger at wrist and hand level

Excludes2: Injury of long flexor muscle, fascia and tendon of thumb at wrist and hand level (S66.0-)

S66.10   Unspecified injury of flexor muscle, fascia and tendon of other and unspecified finger at wrist and hand level

⑦ **S66.100** Unspecified injury of flexor muscle, fascia and tendon of right index finger at wrist and hand level

⑦ **S66.101** Unspecified injury of flexor muscle, fascia and tendon of left index finger at wrist and hand level

⑦ **S66.102** Unspecified injury of flexor muscle, fascia and tendon of right middle finger at wrist and hand level

⑦ **S66.103** Unspecified injury of flexor muscle, fascia and tendon of left middle finger at wrist and hand level

⑦ **S66.104** Unspecified injury of flexor muscle, fascia and tendon of right ring finger at wrist and hand level

⑦ **S66.105** Unspecified injury of flexor muscle, fascia and tendon of left ring finger at wrist and hand level

⑦ **S66.106** Unspecified injury of flexor muscle, fascia and tendon of right little finger at wrist and hand level

⑦ **S66.107** Unspecified injury of flexor muscle, fascia and tendon of left little finger at wrist and hand level

⑦ **S66.108** Unspecified injury of flexor muscle, fascia and tendon of other finger at wrist and hand level

Unspecified injury of flexor muscle, fascia and tendon of specified finger with unspecified laterality at wrist and hand level

⑦ **S66.109** Unspecified injury of flexor muscle, fascia and tendon of unspecified finger at wrist and hand level

S66.11 Strain of flexor muscle, fascia and tendon of other and unspecified finger at wrist and hand level

⑦ **S66.110** Strain of flexor muscle, fascia and tendon of right index finger at wrist and hand level

⑦ **S66.111** Strain of flexor muscle, fascia and tendon of left index finger at wrist and hand level

⑦ **S66.112** Strain of flexor muscle, fascia and tendon of right middle finger at wrist and hand level

⑦ **S66.113** Strain of flexor muscle, fascia and tendon of left middle finger at wrist and hand level

⑦ **S66.114** Strain of flexor muscle, fascia and tendon of right ring finger at wrist and hand level

⑦ **S66.115** Strain of flexor muscle, fascia and tendon of left ring finger at wrist and hand level

⑦ **S66.116** Strain of flexor muscle, fascia and tendon of right little finger at wrist and hand level

⑦ **S66.117** Strain of flexor muscle, fascia and tendon of left little finger at wrist and hand level

⑦ **S66.118** Strain of flexor muscle, fascia and tendon of other finger at wrist and hand level

Strain of flexor muscle, fascia and tendon of specified finger with unspecified laterality at wrist and hand level

⑦ **S66.119** Strain of flexor muscle, fascia and tendon of unspecified finger at wrist and hand level

S66.12 Laceration of flexor muscle, fascia and tendon of other and unspecified finger at wrist and hand level

⑦ **S66.120** Laceration of flexor muscle, fascia and tendon of right index finger at wrist and hand level

⑦ **S66.121** Laceration of flexor muscle, fascia and tendon of left index finger at wrist and hand level

⑦ **S66.122** Laceration of flexor muscle, fascia and tendon of right middle finger at wrist and hand level

⑦ **S66.123** Laceration of flexor muscle, fascia and tendon of left middle finger at wrist and hand level

⑦ **S66.124** Laceration of flexor muscle, fascia and tendon of right ring finger at wrist and hand level

⑦ **S66.125** Laceration of flexor muscle, fascia and tendon of left ring finger at wrist and hand level

⑦ **S66.126** Laceration of flexor muscle, fascia and tendon of right little finger at wrist and hand level

⑦ **S66.127** Laceration of flexor muscle, fascia and tendon of left little finger at wrist and hand level

⑦ **S66.128** Laceration of flexor muscle, fascia and tendon of other finger at wrist and hand level

Laceration of flexor muscle, fascia and tendon of specified finger with unspecified laterality at wrist and hand level

⑦ **S66.129** Laceration of flexor muscle, fascia and tendon of unspecified finger at wrist and hand level

S66.19 Other injury of flexor muscle, fascia and tendon of other and unspecified finger at wrist and hand level

⑦ **S66.190** Other injury of flexor muscle, fascia and tendon of right index finger at wrist and hand level

⑦ **S66.191** Other injury of flexor muscle, fascia and tendon of left index finger at wrist and hand level

⑦ **S66.192** Other injury of flexor muscle, fascia and tendon of right middle finger at wrist and hand level

⑦ **S66.193** Other injury of flexor muscle, fascia and tendon of left middle finger at wrist and hand level

⑦ **S66.194** Other injury of flexor muscle, fascia and tendon of right ring finger at wrist and hand level

⑦ **S66.195** Other injury of flexor muscle, fascia and tendon of left ring finger at wrist and hand level

● New code   ▲ Revised code   **Excludes1:** Not coded here   **Excludes2:** Not included here   ⊗ Placeholder required   ⑦ 7th digit required

⑦**S66.196** Other injury of flexor muscle, fascia and tendon of right little finger at wrist and hand level

⑦**S66.197** Other injury of flexor muscle, fascia and tendon of left little finger at wrist and hand level

⑦**S66.198** Other injury of flexor muscle, fascia and tendon of other finger at wrist and hand level

Other injury of flexor muscle, fascia and tendon of specified finger with unspecified laterality at wrist and hand level

⑦**S66.199** Other injury of flexor muscle, fascia and tendon of unspecified finger at wrist and hand level

S66.2 **Injury of extensor muscle, fascia and tendon of thumb at wrist and hand level**

S66.20 **Unspecified injury of extensor muscle, fascia and tendon of thumb at wrist and hand level**

⑦**S66.201** Unspecified injury of extensor muscle, fascia and tendon of right thumb at wrist and hand level

⑦**S66.202** Unspecified injury of extensor muscle, fascia and tendon of left thumb at wrist and hand level

⑦**S66.209** Unspecified injury of extensor muscle, fascia and tendon of unspecified thumb at wrist and hand level

S66.21 **Strain of extensor muscle, fascia and tendon of thumb at wrist and hand level**

⑦**S66.211** Strain of extensor muscle, fascia and tendon of right thumb at wrist and hand level

⑦**S66.212** Strain of extensor muscle, fascia and tendon of left thumb at wrist and hand level

⑦**S66.219** Strain of extensor muscle, fascia and tendon of unspecified thumb at wrist and hand level

S66.22 **Laceration of extensor muscle, fascia and tendon of thumb at wrist and hand level**

⑦**S66.221** Laceration of extensor muscle, fascia and tendon of right thumb at wrist and hand level

⑦**S66.222** Laceration of extensor muscle, fascia and tendon of left thumb at wrist and hand level

⑦**S66.229** Laceration of extensor muscle, fascia and tendon of unspecified thumb at wrist and hand level

S66.29 **Other specified injury of extensor muscle, fascia and tendon of thumb at wrist and hand level**

⑦**S66.291** Other specified injury of extensor muscle, fascia and tendon of right thumb at wrist and hand level

⑦**S66.292** Other specified injury of extensor muscle, fascia and tendon of left thumb at wrist and hand level

⑦**S66.299** Other specified injury of extensor muscle, fascia and tendon of

unspecified thumb at wrist and hand level

S66.3 **Injury of extensor muscle, fascia and tendon of other and unspecified finger at wrist and hand level**

Excludes2: Injury of extensor muscle, fascia and tendon of thumb at wrist and hand level (S66.2-)

S66.30 **Unspecified injury of extensor muscle, fascia and tendon of other and unspecified finger at wrist and hand level**

⑦**S66.300** Unspecified injury of extensor muscle, fascia and tendon of right index finger at wrist and hand level

⑦**S66.301** Unspecified injury of extensor muscle, fascia and tendon of left index finger at wrist and hand level

⑦**S66.302** Unspecified injury of extensor muscle, fascia and tendon of right middle finger at wrist and hand level

⑦**S66.303** Unspecified injury of extensor muscle, fascia and tendon of left middle finger at wrist and hand level

⑦**S66.304** Unspecified injury of extensor muscle, fascia and tendon of right ring finger at wrist and hand level

⑦**S66.305** Unspecified injury of extensor muscle, fascia and tendon of left ring finger at wrist and hand level

⑦**S66.306** Unspecified injury of extensor muscle, fascia and tendon of right little finger at wrist and hand level

⑦**S66.307** Unspecified injury of extensor muscle, fascia and tendon of left little finger at wrist and hand level

⑦**S66.308** Unspecified injury of extensor muscle, fascia and tendon of other finger at wrist and hand level

Unspecified injury of extensor muscle, fascia and tendon of specified finger with unspecified laterality at wrist and hand level

⑦**S66.309** Unspecified injury of extensor muscle, fascia and tendon of unspecified finger at wrist and hand level

S66.31 **Strain of extensor muscle, fascia and tendon of other and unspecified finger at wrist and hand level**

⑦**S66.310** Strain of extensor muscle, fascia and tendon of right index finger at wrist and hand level

⑦**S66.311** Strain of extensor muscle, fascia and tendon of left index finger at wrist and hand level

⑦**S66.312** Strain of extensor muscle, fascia and tendon of right middle finger at wrist and hand level

⑦**S66.313** Strain of extensor muscle, fascia and tendon of left middle finger at wrist and hand level

⑦**S66.314** Strain of extensor muscle, fascia and tendon of right ring finger at wrist and hand level

⑦ S66.315 Strain of extensor muscle, fascia and tendon of left ring finger at wrist and hand level

⑦ S66.316 Strain of extensor muscle, fascia and tendon of right little finger at wrist and hand level

⑦ S66.317 Strain of extensor muscle, fascia and tendon of left little finger at wrist and hand level

⑦ S66.318 Strain of extensor muscle, fascia and tendon of other finger at wrist and hand level

Strain of extensor muscle, fascia and tendon of specified finger with unspecified laterality at wrist and hand level

⑦ S66.319 Strain of extensor muscle, fascia and tendon of unspecified finger at wrist and hand level

S66.32 Laceration of extensor muscle, fascia and tendon of other and unspecified finger at wrist and hand level

⑦ S66.320 Laceration of extensor muscle, fascia and tendon of right index finger at wrist and hand level

⑦ S66.321 Laceration of extensor muscle, fascia and tendon of left index finger at wrist and hand level

⑦ S66.322 Laceration of extensor muscle, fascia and tendon of right middle finger at wrist and hand level

⑦ S66.323 Laceration of extensor muscle, fascia and tendon of left middle finger at wrist and hand level

⑦ S66.324 Laceration of extensor muscle, fascia and tendon of right ring finger at wrist and hand level

⑦ S66.325 Laceration of extensor muscle, fascia and tendon of left ring finger at wrist and hand level

⑦ S66.326 Laceration of extensor muscle, fascia and tendon of right little finger at wrist and hand level

⑦ S66.327 Laceration of extensor muscle, fascia and tendon of left little finger at wrist and hand level

⑦ S66.328 Laceration of extensor muscle, fascia and tendon of other finger at wrist and hand level

Laceration of extensor muscle, fascia and tendon of specified finger with unspecified laterality at wrist and hand level

⑦ S66.329 Laceration of extensor muscle, fascia and tendon of unspecified finger at wrist and hand level

S66.39 Other injury of extensor muscle, fascia and tendon of other and unspecified finger at wrist and hand level

⑦ S66.390 Other injury of extensor muscle, fascia and tendon of right index finger at wrist and hand level

⑦ S66.391 Other injury of extensor muscle, fascia and tendon of left index finger at wrist and hand level

⑦ S66.392 Other injury of extensor muscle, fascia and tendon of right middle finger at wrist and hand level

⑦ S66.393 Other injury of extensor muscle, fascia and tendon of left middle finger at wrist and hand level

⑦ S66.394 Other injury of extensor muscle, fascia and tendon of right ring finger at wrist and hand level

⑦ S66.395 Other injury of extensor muscle, fascia and tendon of left ring finger at wrist and hand level

⑦ S66.396 Other injury of extensor muscle, fascia and tendon of right little finger at wrist and hand level

⑦ S66.397 Other injury of extensor muscle, fascia and tendon of left little finger at wrist and hand level

⑦ S66.398 Other injury of extensor muscle, fascia and tendon of other finger at wrist and hand level

Other injury of extensor muscle, fascia and tendon of specified finger with unspecified laterality at wrist and hand level

⑦ S66.399 Other injury of extensor muscle, fascia and tendon of unspecified finger at wrist and hand level

S66.4 Injury of intrinsic muscle, fascia and tendon of thumb at wrist and hand level

S66.40 Unspecified injury of intrinsic muscle, fascia and tendon of thumb at wrist and hand level

⑦ S66.401 Unspecified injury of intrinsic muscle, fascia and tendon of right thumb at wrist and hand level

⑦ S66.402 Unspecified injury of intrinsic muscle, fascia and tendon of left thumb at wrist and hand level

⑦ S66.409 Unspecified injury of intrinsic muscle, fascia and tendon of unspecified thumb at wrist and hand level

S66.41 Strain of intrinsic muscle, fascia and tendon of thumb at wrist and hand level

⑦ S66.411 Strain of intrinsic muscle, fascia and tendon of right thumb at wrist and hand level

⑦ S66.412 Strain of intrinsic muscle, fascia and tendon of left thumb at wrist and hand level

⑦ S66.419 Strain of intrinsic muscle, fascia and tendon of unspecified thumb at wrist and hand level

S66.42 Laceration of intrinsic muscle, fascia and tendon of thumb at wrist and hand level

⑦ S66.421 Laceration of intrinsic muscle, fascia and tendon of right thumb at wrist and hand level

⑦ S66.422 Laceration of intrinsic muscle, fascia and tendon of left thumb at wrist and hand level

⑦ S66.429 Laceration of intrinsic muscle, fascia and tendon of unspecified thumb at wrist and hand level

● New code   ▲ Revised code   **Excludes1:** Not coded here   **Excludes2:** Not included here   ⊗ Placeholder required   ⑦ 7ᵗʰ digit required

S66.49   Other specified injury of intrinsic muscle, fascia and tendon of thumb at wrist and hand level

⑦S66.491   Other specified injury of intrinsic muscle, fascia and tendon of right thumb at wrist and hand level

⑦S66.492   Other specified injury of intrinsic muscle, fascia and tendon of left thumb at wrist and hand level

⑦S66.499   Other specified injury of intrinsic muscle, fascia and tendon of unspecified thumb at wrist and hand level

S66.5   Injury of intrinsic muscle, fascia and tendon of other and unspecified finger at wrist and hand level

Excludes2: injury of intrinsic muscle, fascia and tendon of thumb at wrist and hand level (S66.4-)

S66.50   Unspecified injury of intrinsic muscle, fascia and tendon of other and unspecified finger at wrist and hand level

⑦S66.500   Unspecified injury of intrinsic muscle, fascia and tendon of right index finger at wrist and hand level

⑦S66.501   Unspecified injury of intrinsic muscle, fascia and tendon of left index finger at wrist and hand level

⑦S66.502   Unspecified injury of intrinsic muscle, fascia and tendon of right middle finger at wrist and hand level

⑦S66.503   Unspecified injury of intrinsic muscle, fascia and tendon of left middle finger at wrist and hand level

⑦S66.504   Unspecified injury of intrinsic muscle, fascia and tendon of right ring finger at wrist and hand level

⑦S66.505   Unspecified injury of intrinsic muscle, fascia and tendon of left ring finger at wrist and hand level

⑦S66.506   Unspecified injury of intrinsic muscle, fascia and tendon of right little finger at wrist and hand level

⑦S66.507   Unspecified injury of intrinsic muscle, fascia and tendon of left little finger at wrist and hand level

⑦S66.508   Unspecified injury of intrinsic muscle, fascia and tendon of other finger at wrist and hand level

Unspecified injury of intrinsic muscle, fascia and tendon of specified finger with unspecified laterality at wrist and hand level

⑦S66.509   Unspecified injury of intrinsic muscle, fascia and tendon of unspecified finger at wrist and hand level

S66.51   Strain of intrinsic muscle, fascia and tendon of other and unspecified finger at wrist and hand level

⑦S66.510   Strain of intrinsic muscle, fascia and tendon of right index finger at wrist and hand level

⑦S66.511   Strain of intrinsic muscle, fascia and tendon of left index finger at wrist and hand level

⑦S66.512   Strain of intrinsic muscle, fascia and tendon of right middle finger at wrist and hand level

⑦S66.513   Strain of intrinsic muscle, fascia and tendon of left middle finger at wrist and hand level

⑦S66.514   Strain of intrinsic muscle, fascia and tendon of right ring finger at wrist and hand level

⑦S66.515   Strain of intrinsic muscle, fascia and tendon of left ring finger at wrist and hand level

⑦S66.516   Strain of intrinsic muscle, fascia and tendon of right little finger at wrist and hand level

⑦S66.517   Strain of intrinsic muscle, fascia and tendon of left little finger at wrist and hand level

⑦S66.518   Strain of intrinsic muscle, fascia and tendon of other finger at wrist and hand level

Strain of intrinsic muscle, fascia and tendon of specified finger with unspecified laterality at wrist and hand level

⑦S66.519   Strain of intrinsic muscle, fascia and tendon of unspecified finger at wrist and hand level

S66.52   Laceration of intrinsic muscle, fascia and tendon of other and unspecified finger at wrist and hand level

⑦S66.520   Laceration of intrinsic muscle, fascia and tendon of right index finger at wrist and hand level

⑦S66.521   Laceration of intrinsic muscle, fascia and tendon of left index finger at wrist and hand level

⑦S66.522   Laceration of intrinsic muscle, fascia and tendon of right middle finger at wrist and hand level

⑦S66.523   Laceration of intrinsic muscle, fascia and tendon of left middle finger at wrist and hand level

⑦S66.524   Laceration of intrinsic muscle, fascia and tendon of right ring finger at wrist and hand level

⑦S66.525   Laceration of intrinsic muscle, fascia and tendon of left ring finger at wrist and hand level

⑦S66.526   Laceration of intrinsic muscle, fascia and tendon of right little finger at wrist and hand level

⑦S66.527   Laceration of intrinsic muscle, fascia and tendon of left little finger at wrist and hand level

⑦S66.528   Laceration of intrinsic muscle, fascia and tendon of other finger at wrist and hand level

Laceration of intrinsic muscle, fascia and tendon of specified finger with unspecified laterality at wrist and hand level

⑦ **S66.529** Laceration of intrinsic muscle, fascia and tendon of unspecified finger at wrist and hand level

S66.59 Other injury of intrinsic muscle, fascia and tendon of other and unspecified finger at wrist and hand level

⑦ **S66.590** Other injury of intrinsic muscle, fascia and tendon of right index finger at wrist and hand level

⑦ **S66.591** Other injury of intrinsic muscle, fascia and tendon of left index finger at wrist and hand level

⑦ **S66.592** Other injury of intrinsic muscle, fascia and tendon of right middle finger at wrist and hand level

⑦ **S66.593** Other injury of intrinsic muscle, fascia and tendon of left middle finger at wrist and hand level

⑦ **S66.594** Other injury of intrinsic muscle, fascia and tendon of right ring finger at wrist and hand level

⑦ **S66.595** Other injury of intrinsic muscle, fascia and tendon of left ring finger at wrist and hand level

⑦ **S66.596** Other injury of intrinsic muscle, fascia and tendon of right little finger at wrist and hand level

⑦ **S66.597** Other injury of intrinsic muscle, fascia and tendon of left little finger at wrist and hand level

⑦ **S66.598** Other injury of intrinsic muscle, fascia and tendon of other finger at wrist and hand level

Other injury of intrinsic muscle, fascia and tendon of specified finger with unspecified laterality at wrist and hand level

⑦ **S66.599** Other injury of intrinsic muscle, fascia and tendon of unspecified finger at wrist and hand level

S66.8 Injury of other specified muscles, fascia and tendons at wrist and hand level

S66.80 Unspecified injury of other specified muscles, fascia and tendons at wrist and hand level

⑦ **S66.801** Unspecified injury of other specified muscles, fascia and tendons at wrist and hand level, right hand

⑦ **S66.802** Unspecified injury of other specified muscles, fascia and tendons at wrist and hand level, left hand

⑦ **S66.809** Unspecified injury of other specified muscles, fascia and tendons at wrist and hand level, unspecified hand

S66.81 Strain of other specified muscles, fascia and tendons at wrist and hand level

⑦ **S66.811** Strain of other specified muscles, fascia and tendons at wrist and hand level, right hand

⑦ **S66.812** Strain of other specified muscles, fascia and tendons at wrist and hand level, left hand

⑦ **S66.819** Strain of other specified muscles, fascia and tendons at wrist and hand level, unspecified hand

S66.82 Laceration of other specified muscles, fascia and tendons at wrist and hand level

⑦ **S66.821** Laceration of other specified muscles, fascia and tendons at wrist and hand level, right hand

⑦ **S66.822** Laceration of other specified muscles, fascia and tendons at wrist and hand level, left hand

⑦ **S66.829** Laceration of other specified muscles, fascia and tendons at wrist and hand level, unspecified hand

S66.89 Other injury of other specified muscles, fascia and tendons at wrist and hand level

⑦ **S66.891** Other injury of other specified muscles, fascia and tendons at wrist and hand level, right hand

⑦ **S66.892** Other injury of other specified muscles, fascia and tendons at wrist and hand level, left hand

⑦ **S66.899** Other injury of other specified muscles, fascia and tendons at wrist and hand level, unspecified hand

S66.9 Injury of unspecified muscle, fascia and tendon at wrist and hand level

S66.90 Unspecified injury of unspecified muscle, fascia and tendon at wrist and hand level

⑦ **S66.901** Unspecified injury of unspecified muscle, fascia and tendon at wrist and hand level, right hand

⑦ **S66.902** Unspecified injury of unspecified muscle, fascia and tendon at wrist and hand level, left hand

⑦ **S66.909** Unspecified injury of unspecified muscle, fascia and tendon at wrist and hand level, unspecified hand

S66.91 Strain of unspecified muscle, fascia and tendon at wrist and hand level

⑦ **S66.911** Strain of unspecified muscle, fascia and tendon at wrist and hand level, right hand

⑦ **S66.912** Strain of unspecified muscle, fascia and tendon at wrist and hand level, left hand

⑦ **S66.919** Strain of unspecified muscle, fascia and tendon at wrist and hand level, unspecified hand

S66.92 Laceration of unspecified muscle, fascia and tendon at wrist and hand level

⑦ **S66.921** Laceration of unspecified muscle, fascia and tendon at wrist and hand level, right hand

⑦ **S66.922** Laceration of unspecified muscle, fascia and tendon at wrist and hand level, left hand

⑦ **S66.929** Laceration of unspecified muscle, fascia and tendon at wrist and hand level, unspecified hand

S66.99 Other injury of unspecified muscle, fascia and tendon at wrist and hand level

⑦ **S66.991** Other injury of unspecified muscle, fascia and tendon at wrist and hand level, right hand

● New code   ▲ Revised code   **Excludes1:** Not coded here   **Excludes2:** Not included here   ⊗ Placeholder required   ⑦ 7th digit required

⊘S66.992   **Other injury of unspecified muscle, fascia and tendon at wrist and hand level, left hand**

⊘S66.999   **Other injury of unspecified muscle, fascia and tendon at wrist and hand level, unspecified hand**

S67   **Crushing injury of wrist, hand and fingers**

<u>Use additional code</u> for all associated injuries, such as:

fracture of wrist and hand (S62.-) open wound of wrist and hand (S61.-)

The appropriate 7th character is to be added to each code from category S67

A - initial encounter

D - subsequent encounter

S - sequela

S67.0   **Crushing injury of thumb**

⊗⑦S67.00   **Crushing injury of unspecified thumb**

⊗⑦S67.01   **Crushing injury of right thumb**

⊗⑦S67.02   **Crushing injury of left thumb**

S67.1   **Crushing injury of other and unspecified finger(s)**

Excludes2: crushing injury of thumb (S67.0-)

⊗⑦S67.10   **Crushing injury of unspecified finger(s)**

S67.19   **Crushing injury of other finger(s)**

⑦S67.190   **Crushing injury of right index finger**

⑦S67.191   **Crushing injury of left index finger**

⑦S67.192   **Crushing injury of right middle finger**

⑦S67.193   **Crushing injury of left middle finger**

⑦S67.194   **Crushing injury of right ring finger**

⑦S67.195   **Crushing injury of left ring finger**

⑦S67.196   **Crushing injury of right little finger**

⑦S67.197   **Crushing injury of left little finger**

⑦S67.198   **Crushing injury of other finger**

Crushing injury of specified finger with unspecified laterality

S67.2   **Crushing injury of hand**

Excludes2: crushing injury of fingers (S67.1-)

crushing injury of thumb (S67.0-)

⊗⑦S67.20   **Crushing injury of unspecified hand**

⊗⑦S67.21   **Crushing injury of right hand**

⊗⑦S67.22   **Crushing injury of left hand**

S67.3   **Crushing injury of wrist**

⊗⑦S67.30   **Crushing injury of unspecified wrist**

⊗⑦S67.31   **Crushing injury of right wrist**

⊗⑦S67.32   **Crushing injury of left wrist**

S67.4   **Crushing injury of wrist and hand**

Excludes1: crushing injury of hand alone (S67.2-)

crushing injury of wrist alone (S67.3-)

Excludes2: crushing injury of fingers (S67.1-)

crushing injury of thumb (S67.0-)

⊗⑦S67.40   **Crushing injury of unspecified wrist and hand**

⊗⑦S67.41   **Crushing injury of right wrist and hand**

⊗⑦S67.42   **Crushing injury of left wrist and hand**

S67.9   **Crushing injury of unspecified part(s) of wrist, hand and fingers**

⊗⑦S67.90   **Crushing injury of unspecified part(s) of unspecified wrist, hand and fingers**

⊗⑦S67.91   **Crushing injury of unspecified part(s) of right wrist, hand and fingers**

⊗⑦S67.92   **Crushing injury of unspecified part(s) of left wrist, hand and fingers**

S68   **Traumatic amputation of wrist, hand and fingers**

An amputation not identified as partial or complete should be coded to complete

The appropriate 7th character is to be added to each code from category S68

A - initial encounter

D - subsequent encounter

S - sequela

S68.0   **Traumatic metacarpophalangeal amputation of thumb**

Traumatic amputation of thumb NOS

S68.01   **Complete traumatic metacarpophalangeal amputation of thumb**

⑦S68.011   **Complete traumatic metacarpophalangeal amputation of right thumb**

⑦S68.012   **Complete traumatic metacarpophalangeal amputation of left thumb**

⑦S68.019   **Complete traumatic metacarpophalangeal amputation of unspecified thumb**

S68.02   **Partial traumatic metacarpophalangeal amputation of thumb**

⑦S68.021   **Partial traumatic metacarpophalangeal amputation of right thumb**

⑦S68.022   **Partial traumatic metacarpophalangeal amputation of left thumb**

⑦S68.029   **Partial traumatic metacarpophalangeal amputation of unspecified thumb**

S68.1   **Traumatic metacarpophalangeal amputation of other and unspecified finger**

Traumatic amputation of finger NOS

Excludes2: traumatic metacarpophalangeal amputation of thumb (S68.0-)

S68.11   **Complete traumatic metacarpophalangeal amputation of other and unspecified finger**

⑦S68.110   **Complete traumatic metacarpophalangeal amputation of right index finger**

⑦S68.111   **Complete traumatic metacarpophalangeal amputation of left index finger**

⑦S68.112   **Complete traumatic metacarpophalangeal amputation of right middle finger**

⑦S68.113   **Complete traumatic metacarpophalangeal amputation of left middle finger**

⑦S68.114   **Complete traumatic metacarpophalangeal amputation of right ring finger**

⑦ S68.115   **Complete traumatic metacarpophalangeal amputation of left ring finger**

⑦ S68.116   **Complete traumatic metacarpophalangeal amputation of right little finger**

⑦ S68.117   **Complete traumatic metacarpophalangeal amputation of left little finger**

⑦ S68.118   **Complete traumatic metacarpophalangeal amputation of other finger**

Complete traumatic metacarpophalangeal amputation of specified finger with unspecified laterality

⑦ S68.119   **Complete traumatic metacarpophalangeal amputation of unspecified finger**

S68.12   **Partial traumatic metacarpophalangeal amputation of other and unspecified finger**

⑦ S68.120   **Partial traumatic metacarpophalangeal amputation of right index finger**

⑦ S68.121   **Partial traumatic metacarpophalangeal amputation of left index finger**

⑦ S68.122   **Partial traumatic metacarpophalangeal amputation of right middle finger**

⑦ S68.123   **Partial traumatic metacarpophalangeal amputation of left middle finger**

⑦ S68.124   **Partial traumatic metacarpophalangeal amputation of right ring finger**

⑦ S68.125   **Partial traumatic metacarpophalangeal amputation of left ring finger**

⑦ S68.126   **Partial traumatic metacarpophalangeal amputation of right little finger**

⑦ S68.127   **Partial traumatic metacarpophalangeal amputation of left little finger**

⑦ S68.128   **Partial traumatic metacarpophalangeal amputation of other finger**

Partial traumatic metacarpophalangeal amputation of specified finger with unspecified laterality

⑦ S68.129   **Partial traumatic metacarpophalangeal amputation of unspecified finger**

S68.4   **Traumatic amputation of hand at wrist level**

Traumatic amputation of hand NOS

Traumatic amputation of wrist

S68.41   **Complete traumatic amputation of hand at wrist level**

⑦ S68.411   **Complete traumatic amputation of right hand at wrist level**

⑦ S68.412   **Complete traumatic amputation of left hand at wrist level**

⑦ S68.419   **Complete traumatic amputation of unspecified hand at wrist level**

S68.42   **Partial traumatic amputation of hand at wrist level**

⑦ S68.421   **Partial traumatic amputation of right hand at wrist level**

⑦ S68.422   **Partial traumatic amputation of left hand at wrist level**

⑦ S68.429   **Partial traumatic amputation of unspecified hand at wrist level**

S68.5   **Traumatic transphalangeal amputation of thumb**

Traumatic interphalangeal joint amputation of thumb

S68.51   **Complete traumatic transphalangeal amputation of thumb**

⑦ S68.511   **Complete traumatic transphalangeal amputation of right thumb**

⑦ S68.512   **Complete traumatic transphalangeal amputation of left thumb**

⑦ S68.519   **Complete traumatic transphalangeal amputation of unspecified thumb**

S68.52   **Partial traumatic transphalangeal amputation of thumb**

⑦ S68.521   **Partial traumatic transphalangeal amputation of right thumb**

⑦ S68.522   **Partial traumatic transphalangeal amputation of left thumb**

⑦ S68.529   **Partial traumatic transphalangeal amputation of unspecified thumb**

S68.6   **Traumatic transphalangeal amputation of other and unspecified finger**

S68.61   **Complete traumatic transphalangeal amputation of other and unspecified finger(s)**

⑦ S68.610   **Complete traumatic transphalangeal amputation of right index finger**

⑦ S68.611   **Complete traumatic transphalangeal amputation of left index finger**

⑦ S68.612   **Complete traumatic transphalangeal amputation of right middle finger**

⑦ S68.613   **Complete traumatic transphalangeal amputation of left middle finger**

⑦ S68.614   **Complete traumatic transphalangeal amputation of right ring finger**

⑦ S68.615   **Complete traumatic transphalangeal amputation of left ring finger**

⑦ S68.616   **Complete traumatic transphalangeal amputation of right little finger**

⑦ S68.617   **Complete traumatic transphalangeal amputation of left little finger**

⑦ S68.618   **Complete traumatic transphalangeal amputation of other finger**

● New code   ▲ Revised code   **Excludes1:** Not coded here   **Excludes2:** Not included here   ⊗ Placeholder required   ⑦ 7th digit required

Complete traumatic transphalangeal amputation of specified finger with unspecified laterality

⑦S68.619 Complete traumatic transphalangeal amputation of unspecified finger

S68.62 Partial traumatic transphalangeal amputation of other and unspecified finger

⑦S68.620 Partial traumatic transphalangeal amputation of right index finger

⑦S68.621 Partial traumatic transphalangeal amputation of left index finger

⑦S68.622 Partial traumatic transphalangeal amputation of right middle finger

⑦S68.623 Partial traumatic transphalangeal amputation of left middle finger

⑦S68.624 Partial traumatic transphalangeal amputation of right ring finger

⑦S68.625 Partial traumatic transphalangeal amputation of left ring finger

⑦S68.626 Partial traumatic transphalangeal amputation of right little finger

⑦S68.627 Partial traumatic transphalangeal amputation of left little finger

⑦S68.628 Partial traumatic transphalangeal amputation of other finger

Partial traumatic transphalangeal amputation of specified finger with unspecified laterality

⑦S68.629 Partial traumatic transphalangeal amputation of unspecified finger

S68.7 Traumatic transmetacarpal amputation of hand

S68.71 Complete traumatic transmetacarpal amputation of hand

⑦S68.711 Complete traumatic transmetacarpal amputation of right hand

⑦S68.712 Complete traumatic transmetacarpal amputation of left hand

⑦S68.719 Complete traumatic transmetacarpal amputation of unspecified hand

S68.72 Partial traumatic transmetacarpal amputation of hand

⑦S68.721 Partial traumatic transmetacarpal amputation of right hand

⑦S68.722 Partial traumatic transmetacarpal amputation of left hand

⑦S68.729 Partial traumatic transmetacarpal amputation of unspecified hand

S69 Other and unspecified injuries of wrist, hand and finger(s)

The appropriate 7th character is to be added to each code from category S69

A - initial encounter

D - subsequent encounter

S - sequela

S69.8 Other specified injuries of wrist, hand and finger(s)

⊗⑦S69.80 Other specified injuries of unspecified wrist, hand and finger(s)

⊗⑦S69.81 Other specified injuries of right wrist, hand and finger(s)

⊗⑦S69.82 Other specified injuries of left wrist, hand and finger(s)

S69.9 Unspecified injury of wrist, hand and finger(s)

⊗⑦S69.90 Unspecified injury of unspecified wrist, hand and finger(s)

⊗⑦S69.91 Unspecified injury of right wrist, hand and finger(s)

⊗⑦S69.92 Unspecified injury of left wrist, hand and finger(s)

INJURIES TO THE HIP AND THIGH (S70-S79)

Excludes2: burns and corrosions (T20-T32)
frostbite (T33-T34) snake bite (T63.0-)
venomous insect bite or sting (T63.4-)

S70 Superficial injury of hip and thigh

The appropriate 7th character is to be added to each code from category S70

A - initial encounter

D - subsequent encounter

S - sequela

S70.0 Contusion of hip

⊗⑦S70.00 Contusion of unspecified hip

⊗⑦S70.01 Contusion of right hip

⊗⑦S70.02 Contusion of left hip

S70.1 Contusion of thigh

⊗⑦S70.10 Contusion of unspecified thigh

⊗⑦S70.11 Contusion of right thigh

⊗⑦S70.12 Contusion of left thigh

S70.2 Other superficial injuries of hip

S70.21 Abrasion of hip

⑦S70.211 Abrasion, right hip

⑦S70.212 Abrasion, left hip

⑦S70.219 Abrasion, unspecified hip

S70.22 Blister (nonthermal) of hip

⑦S70.221 Blister (nonthermal), right hip

⑦S70.222 Blister (nonthermal), left hip

⑦S70.229 Blister (nonthermal), unspecified hip

S70.24 External constriction of hip

⑦S70.241 External constriction, right hip

⑦S70.242 External constriction, left hip

⑦S70.249 External constriction, unspecified hip

S70.25 Superficial foreign body of hip

Splinter in the hip

⑦S70.251 Superficial foreign body, right hip

⑦S70.252 Superficial foreign body, left hip

⑦S70.259 Superficial foreign body, unspecified hip

S70.26 Insect bite (nonvenomous) of hip

⑦S70.261 Insect bite (nonvenomous), right hip

⑦S70.262 Insect bite (nonvenomous), left hip

⑦S70.269 Insect bite (nonvenomous), unspecified hip

S70.27　Other superficial bite of hip

　　Excludes1: open bite of hip (S71.05-)

　　⑦ S70.271　Other superficial bite of hip, right hip

　　⑦ S70.272　Other superficial bite of hip, left hip

　　⑦ S70.279　Other superficial bite of hip, unspecified hip

S70.3　Other superficial injuries of thigh

　S70.31　Abrasion of thigh

　　⑦ S70.311　Abrasion, right thigh

　　⑦ S70.312　Abrasion, left thigh

　　⑦ S70.319　Abrasion, unspecified thigh

　S70.32　Blister (nonthermal) of thigh

　　⑦ S70.321　Blister (nonthermal), right thigh

　　⑦ S70.322　Blister (nonthermal), left thigh

　　⑦ S70.329　Blister (nonthermal), unspecified thigh

　S70.34　External constriction of thigh

　　⑦ S70.341　External constriction, right thigh

　　⑦ S70.342　External constriction, left thigh

　　⑦ S70.349　External constriction, unspecified thigh

　S70.35　Superficial foreign body of thigh

　　Splinter in the thigh

　　⑦ S70.351　Superficial foreign body, right thigh

　　⑦ S70.352　Superficial foreign body, left thigh

　　⑦ S70.359　Superficial foreign body, unspecified thigh

　S70.36　Insect bite (nonvenomous) of thigh

　　⑦ S70.361　Insect bite (nonvenomous), right thigh

　　⑦ S70.362　Insect bite (nonvenomous), left thigh

　　⑦ S70.369　Insect bite (nonvenomous), unspecified thigh

　S70.37　Other superficial bite of thigh

　　Excludes1: open bite of thigh (S71.15)

　　⑦ S70.371　Other superficial bite of right thigh

　　⑦ S70.372　Other superficial bite of left thigh

　　⑦ S70.379　Other superficial bite of unspecified thigh

S70.9　Unspecified superficial injury of hip and thigh

　S70.91　Unspecified superficial injury of hip

　　⑦ S70.911　Unspecified superficial injury of right hip

　　⑦ S70.912　Unspecified superficial injury of left hip

　　⑦ S70.919　Unspecified superficial injury of unspecified hip

　S70.92　Unspecified superficial injury of thigh

　　⑦ S70.921　Unspecified superficial injury of right thigh

　　⑦ S70.922　Unspecified superficial injury of left thigh

　　⑦ S70.929　Unspecified superficial injury of unspecified thigh

S71　**Open wound of hip and thigh**

Code also any associated wound infection

Excludes1: open fracture of hip and thigh (S72.-)

　　traumatic amputation of hip and thigh (S78.-)

Excludes2: bite of venomous animal (T63.-)

　　open wound of ankle, foot and toes (S91.-)

　　open wound of knee and lower leg (S81.-)

The appropriate 7th character is to be added to each code from category S71

A - initial encounter

D - subsequent encounter

S - sequela

S71.0　Open wound of hip

　S71.00　Unspecified open wound of hip

　　⑦ S71.001　Unspecified open wound, right hip

　　⑦ S71.002　Unspecified open wound, left hip

　　⑦ S71.009　Unspecified open wound, unspecified hip

　S71.01　Laceration without foreign body of hip

　　⑦ S71.011　Laceration without foreign body, right hip

　　⑦ S71.012　Laceration without foreign body, left hip

　　⑦ S71.019　Laceration without foreign body, unspecified hip

　S71.02　Laceration with foreign body of hip

　　⑦ S71.021　Laceration with foreign body, right hip

　　⑦ S71.022　Laceration with foreign body, left hip

　　⑦ S71.029　Laceration with foreign body, unspecified hip

　S71.03　Puncture wound without foreign body of hip

　　⑦ S71.031　Puncture wound without foreign body, right hip

　　⑦ S71.032　Puncture wound without foreign body, left hip

　　⑦ S71.039　Puncture wound without foreign body, unspecified hip

　S71.04　Puncture wound with foreign body of hip

　　⑦ S71.041　Puncture wound with foreign body, right hip

　　⑦ S71.042　Puncture wound with foreign body, left hip

　　⑦ S71.049　Puncture wound with foreign body, unspecified hip

　S71.05　Open bite of hip

　　Bite of hip NOS

　　Excludes1: superficial bite of hip (S70.26, S70.27)

　　⑦ S71.051　Open bite, right hip

　　⑦ S71.052　Open bite, left hip

　　⑦ S71.059　Open bite, unspecified hip

S71.1　Open wound of thigh

　S71.10　Unspecified open wound of thigh

　　⑦ S71.101　Unspecified open wound, right thigh

　　⑦ S71.102　Unspecified open wound, left thigh

　● New code　▲ Revised code　Excludes1: Not coded here　Excludes2: Not included here　⊗ Placeholder required　⑦ 7th digit required

⑦**S71.109** **Unspecified open wound, unspecified thigh**

S71.11 **Laceration without foreign body of thigh**

⑦**S71.111** **Laceration without foreign body, right thigh**

⑦**S71.112** **Laceration without foreign body, left thigh**

⑦**S71.119** **Laceration without foreign body, unspecified thigh**

S71.12 **Laceration with foreign body of thigh**

⑦**S71.121** **Laceration with foreign body, right thigh**

⑦**S71.122** **Laceration with foreign body, left thigh**

⑦**S71.129** **Laceration with foreign body, unspecified thigh**

S71.13 **Puncture wound without foreign body of thigh**

⑦**S71.131** **Puncture wound without foreign body, right thigh**

⑦**S71.132** **Puncture wound without foreign body, left thigh**

⑦**S71.139** **Puncture wound without foreign body, unspecified thigh**

S71.14 **Puncture wound with foreign body of thigh**

⑦**S71.141** **Puncture wound with foreign body, right thigh**

⑦**S71.142** **Puncture wound with foreign body, left thigh**

⑦**S71.149** **Puncture wound with foreign body, unspecified thigh**

S71.15 **Open bite of thigh**

Bite of thigh NOS

Excludes1: superficial bite of thigh (S70.37-)

⑦**S71.151** **Open bite, right thigh**

⑦**S71.152** **Open bite, left thigh**

⑦**S71.159** **Open bite, unspecified thigh**

S72 **Fracture of femur**

Note: A fracture not indicated as displaced or nondisplaced should be coded to displaced

A fracture not indicated as open or closed should be coded to closed

The open fracture designations are based on the Gustilo open fracture classification

Excludes1: traumatic amputation of hip and thigh (S78.-)

Excludes2: fracture of lower leg and ankle (S82.-)

fracture of foot (S92.-)

periprosthetic fracture of prosthetic implant of hip (T84.040, T84.041)

The appropriate 7th character is to be added to all codes from category S72

A - initial encounter for closed fracture

B - initial encounter for open fracture type I or II initial encounter for open fracture NOS

C - initial encounter for open fracture type IIIA, IIIB, or IIIC

D - subsequent encounter for closed fracture with routine healing

E - subsequent encounter for open fracture type I or II with routine healing

F - subsequent encounter for open fracture type IIIA, IIIB, or IIIC with routine healing

G - subsequent encounter for closed fracture with delayed healing

H - subsequent encounter for open fracture type I or II with delayed healing

J - subsequent encounter for open fracture type IIIA, IIIB, or IIIC with delayed healing

K - subsequent encounter for closed fracture with nonunion

M - subsequent encounter for open fracture type I or II with nonunion

N - subsequent encounter for open fracture type IIIA, IIIB, or IIIC with nonunion

P - subsequent encounter for closed fracture with malunion

Q - subsequent encounter for open fracture type I or II with malunion

R - subsequent encounter for open fracture type IIIA, IIIB, or IIIC with malunion

S - sequela

S72.0 **Fracture of head and neck of femur**

Excludes2: physeal fracture of upper end of femur (S79.0-)

S72.00 **Fracture of unspecified part of neck of femur**

Fracture of hip NOS

Fracture of neck of femur NOS

⑦**S72.001** **Fracture of unspecified part of neck of right femur**

⑦**S72.002** **Fracture of unspecified part of neck of left femur**

⑦**S72.009** **Fracture of unspecified part of neck of unspecified femur**

S72.01 **Unspecified intracapsular fracture of femur**

Subcapital fracture of femur

⑦**S72.011** **Unspecified intracapsular fracture of right femur**

⑦**S72.012** **Unspecified intracapsular fracture of left femur**

⑦**S72.019** **Unspecified intracapsular fracture of unspecified femur**

S72.02 **Fracture of epiphysis (separation) (upper) of femur**

Transepiphyseal fracture of femur

Excludes1: capital femoral epiphyseal fracture (pediatric) of femur (S79.01-)

Salter-Harris Type I physeal fracture of upper end of femur (S79.01-)

⑦**S72.021** **Displaced fracture of epiphysis (separation) (upper) of right femur**

⑦**S72.022** **Displaced fracture of epiphysis (separation) (upper) of left femur**

⑦**S72.023** **Displaced fracture of epiphysis (separation) (upper) of unspecified femur**

⑦**S72.024** **Nondisplaced fracture of epiphysis (separation) (upper) of right femur**

⑦**S72.025** **Nondisplaced fracture of epiphysis (separation) (upper) of left femur**

⑦**S72.026** **Nondisplaced fracture of epiphysis (separation) (upper) of unspecified femur**

S72.03 **Midcervical fracture of femur**

Transcervical fracture of femur NOS

⑦**S72.031** **Displaced midcervical fracture of right femur**

⑦S72.032   **Displaced midcervical fracture of left femur**

⑦S72.033   **Displaced midcervical fracture of unspecified femur**

⑦S72.034   **Nondisplaced midcervical fracture of right femur**

⑦S72.035   **Nondisplaced midcervical fracture of left femur**

⑦S72.036   **Nondisplaced midcervical fracture of unspecified femur**

S72.04   **Fracture of base of neck of femur**

       Cervicotrochanteric fracture of femur

⑦S72.041   **Displaced fracture of base of neck of right femur**

⑦S72.042   **Displaced fracture of base of neck of left femur**

⑦S72.043   **Displaced fracture of base of neck of unspecified femur**

⑦S72.044   **Nondisplaced fracture of base of neck of right femur**

⑦S72.045   **Nondisplaced fracture of base of neck of left femur**

⑦S72.046   **Nondisplaced fracture of base of neck of unspecified femur**

S72.05   **Unspecified fracture of head of femur**

       Fracture of head of femur NOS

⑦S72.051   **Unspecified fracture of head of right femur**

⑦S72.052   **Unspecified fracture of head of left femur**

⑦S72.059   **Unspecified fracture of head of unspecified femur**

S72.06   **Articular fracture of head of femur**

⑦S72.061   **Displaced articular fracture of head of right femur**

⑦S72.062   **Displaced articular fracture of head of left femur**

⑦S72.063   **Displaced articular fracture of head of unspecified femur**

⑦S72.064   **Nondisplaced articular fracture of head of right femur**

⑦S72.065   **Nondisplaced articular fracture of head of left femur**

⑦S72.066   **Nondisplaced articular fracture of head of unspecified femur**

S72.09   **Other fracture of head and neck of femur**

⑦S72.091   **Other fracture of head and neck of right femur**

⑦S72.092   **Other fracture of head and neck of left femur**

⑦S72.099   **Other fracture of head and neck of unspecified femur**

S72.1   **Pertrochanteric fracture**

S72.10   **Unspecified trochanteric fracture of femur**

       Fracture of trochanter NOS

⑦S72.101   **Unspecified trochanteric fracture of right femur**

⑦S72.102   **Unspecified trochanteric fracture of left femur**

⑦S72.109   **Unspecified trochanteric fracture of unspecified femur**

S72.11   **Fracture of greater trochanter of femur**

⑦S72.111   **Displaced fracture of greater trochanter of right femur**

⑦S72.112   **Displaced fracture of greater trochanter of left femur**

⑦S72.113   **Displaced fracture of greater trochanter of unspecified femur**

⑦S72.114   **Nondisplaced fracture of greater trochanter of right femur**

⑦S72.115   **Nondisplaced fracture of greater trochanter of left femur**

⑦S72.116   **Nondisplaced fracture of greater trochanter of unspecified femur**

S72.12   **Fracture of lesser trochanter of femur**

⑦S72.121   **Displaced fracture of lesser trochanter of right femur**

⑦S72.122   **Displaced fracture of lesser trochanter of left femur**

⑦S72.123   **Displaced fracture of lesser trochanter of unspecified femur**

⑦S72.124   **Nondisplaced fracture of lesser trochanter of right femur**

⑦S72.125   **Nondisplaced fracture of lesser trochanter of left femur**

⑦S72.126   **Nondisplaced fracture of lesser trochanter of unspecified femur**

S72.13   **Apophyseal fracture of femur**

       Excludes1: chronic (nontraumatic) slipped upper femoral epiphysis (M93.0-)

⑦S72.131   **Displaced apophyseal fracture of right femur**

⑦S72.132   **Displaced apophyseal fracture of left femur**

⑦S72.133   **Displaced apophyseal fracture of unspecified femur**

⑦S72.134   **Nondisplaced apophyseal fracture of right femur**

⑦S72.135   **Nondisplaced apophyseal fracture of left femur**

⑦S72.136   **Nondisplaced apophyseal fracture of unspecified femur**

S72.14   **Intertrochanteric fracture of femur**

⑦S72.141   **Displaced intertrochanteric fracture of right femur**

⑦S72.142   **Displaced intertrochanteric fracture of left femur**

⑦S72.143   **Displaced intertrochanteric fracture of unspecified femur**

⑦S72.144   **Nondisplaced intertrochanteric fracture of right femur**

⑦S72.145   **Nondisplaced intertrochanteric fracture of left femur**

⑦S72.146   **Nondisplaced intertrochanteric fracture of unspecified femur**

S72.2   **Subtrochanteric fracture of femur**

⊗⑦S72.21   **Displaced subtrochanteric fracture of right femur**

⊗⑦S72.22   **Displaced subtrochanteric fracture of left femur**

⊗⑦S72.23 **Displaced subtrochanteric fracture of unspecified femur**

⊗⑦S72.24 **Nondisplaced subtrochanteric fracture of right femur**

⊗⑦S72.25 **Nondisplaced subtrochanteric fracture of left femur**

⊗⑦S72.26 **Nondisplaced subtrochanteric fracture of unspecified femur**

S72.3 **Fracture of shaft of femur**

S72.30 **Unspecified fracture of shaft of femur**

⑦S72.301 **Unspecified fracture of shaft of right femur**

⑦S72.302 **Unspecified fracture of shaft of left femur**

⑦S72.309 **Unspecified fracture of shaft of unspecified femur**

S72.32 **Transverse fracture of shaft of femur**

⑦S72.321 **Displaced transverse fracture of shaft of right femur**

⑦S72.322 **Displaced transverse fracture of shaft of left femur**

⑦S72.323 **Displaced transverse fracture of shaft of unspecified femur**

⑦S72.324 **Nondisplaced transverse fracture of shaft of right femur**

⑦S72.325 **Nondisplaced transverse fracture of shaft of left femur**

⑦S72.326 **Nondisplaced transverse fracture of shaft of unspecified femur**

S72.33 **Oblique fracture of shaft of femur**

⑦S72.331 **Displaced oblique fracture of shaft of right femur**

⑦S72.332 **Displaced oblique fracture of shaft of left femur**

⑦S72.333 **Displaced oblique fracture of shaft of unspecified femur**

⑦S72.334 **Nondisplaced oblique fracture of shaft of right femur**

⑦S72.335 **Nondisplaced oblique fracture of shaft of left femur**

⑦S72.336 **Nondisplaced oblique fracture of shaft of unspecified femur**

S72.34 **Spiral fracture of shaft of femur**

⑦S72.341 **Displaced spiral fracture of shaft of right femur**

⑦S72.342 **Displaced spiral fracture of shaft of left femur**

⑦S72.343 **Displaced spiral fracture of shaft of unspecified femur**

⑦S72.344 **Nondisplaced spiral fracture of shaft of right femur**

⑦S72.345 **Nondisplaced spiral fracture of shaft of left femur**

⑦S72.346 **Nondisplaced spiral fracture of shaft of unspecified femur**

S72.35 **Comminuted fracture of shaft of femur**

⑦S72.351 **Displaced comminuted fracture of shaft of right femur**

⑦S72.352 **Displaced comminuted fracture of shaft of left femur**

⑦S72.353 **Displaced comminuted fracture of shaft of unspecified femur**

⑦S72.354 **Nondisplaced comminuted fracture of shaft of right femur**

⑦S72.355 **Nondisplaced comminuted fracture of shaft of left femur**

⑦S72.356 **Nondisplaced comminuted fracture of shaft of unspecified femur**

S72.36 **Segmental fracture of shaft of femur**

⑦S72.361 **Displaced segmental fracture of shaft of right femur**

⑦S72.362 **Displaced segmental fracture of shaft of left femur**

⑦S72.363 **Displaced segmental fracture of shaft of unspecified femur**

⑦S72.364 **Nondisplaced segmental fracture of shaft of right femur**

⑦S72.365 **Nondisplaced segmental fracture of shaft of left femur**

⑦S72.366 **Nondisplaced segmental fracture of shaft of unspecified femur**

S72.39 **Other fracture of shaft of femur**

⑦S72.391 **Other fracture of shaft of right femur**

⑦S72.392 **Other fracture of shaft of left femur**

⑦S72.399 **Other fracture of shaft of unspecified femur**

S72.4 **Fracture of lower end of femur**

Fracture of distal end of femur

Excludes2: fracture of shaft of femur (S72.3-)

physeal fracture of lower end of femur (S79.1-)

S72.40 **Unspecified fracture of lower end of femur**

⑦S72.401 **Unspecified fracture of lower end of right femur**

⑦S72.402 **Unspecified fracture of lower end of left femur**

⑦S72.409 **Unspecified fracture of lower end of unspecified femur**

S72.41 **Unspecified condyle fracture of lower end of femur**

Condyle fracture of femur NOS

⑦S72.411 **Displaced unspecified condyle fracture of lower end of right femur**

⑦S72.412 **Displaced unspecified condyle fracture of lower end of left femur**

⑦S72.413 **Displaced unspecified condyle fracture of lower end of unspecified femur**

⑦S72.414 **Nondisplaced unspecified condyle fracture of lower end of right femur**

⑦S72.415 **Nondisplaced unspecified condyle fracture of lower end of left femur**

⑦S72.416 **Nondisplaced unspecified condyle fracture of lower end of unspecified femur**

S72.42 **Fracture of lateral condyle of femur**

⑦S72.421 **Displaced fracture of lateral condyle of right femur**

⑦S72.422 **Displaced fracture of lateral condyle of left femur**

⑦ **S72.423 Displaced fracture of lateral condyle of unspecified femur**

⑦ **S72.424 Nondisplaced fracture of lateral condyle of right femur**

⑦ **S72.425 Nondisplaced fracture of lateral condyle of left femur**

⑦ **S72.426 Nondisplaced fracture of lateral condyle of unspecified femur**

S72.43 Fracture of medial condyle of femur

⑦ **S72.431 Displaced fracture of medial condyle of right femur**

⑦ **S72.432 Displaced fracture of medial condyle of left femur**

⑦ **S72.433 Displaced fracture of medial condyle of unspecified femur**

⑦ **S72.434 Nondisplaced fracture of medial condyle of right femur**

⑦ **S72.435 Nondisplaced fracture of medial condyle of left femur**

⑦ **S72.436 Nondisplaced fracture of medial condyle of unspecified femur**

S72.44 Fracture of lower epiphysis (separation) of femur

Excludes1: Salter-Harris Type I physeal fracture of lower end of femur (S79.11-)

⑦ **S72.441 Displaced fracture of lower epiphysis (separation) of right femur**

⑦ **S72.442 Displaced fracture of lower epiphysis (separation) of left femur**

⑦ **S72.443 Displaced fracture of lower epiphysis (separation) of unspecified femur**

⑦ **S72.444 Nondisplaced fracture of lower epiphysis (separation) of right femur**

⑦ **S72.445 Nondisplaced fracture of lower epiphysis (separation) of left femur**

⑦ **S72.446 Nondisplaced fracture of lower epiphysis (separation) of unspecified femur**

S72.45 Supracondylar fracture without intracondylar extension of lower end of femur

Supracondylar fracture of lower end of femur NOS

Excludes1: supracondylar fracture with intracondylar extension of lower end of femur (S72.46-)

⑦ **S72.451 Displaced supracondylar fracture without intracondylar extension of lower end of right femur**

⑦ **S72.452 Displaced supracondylar fracture without intracondylar extension of lower end of left femur**

⑦ **S72.453 Displaced supracondylar fracture without intracondylar extension of lower end of unspecified femur**

⑦ **S72.454 Nondisplaced supracondylar fracture without intracondylar extension of lower end of right femur**

⑦ **S72.455 Nondisplaced supracondylar fracture without intracondylar extension of lower end of left femur**

⑦ **S72.456 Nondisplaced supracondylar fracture without intracondylar extension of lower end of unspecified femur**

S72.46 Supracondylar fracture with intracondylar extension of lower end of femur

Excludes1: supracondylar fracture without intracondylar extension of lower end of femur (S72.45-)

⑦ **S72.461 Displaced supracondylar fracture with intracondylar extension of lower end of right femur**

⑦ **S72.462 Displaced supracondylar fracture with intracondylar extension of lower end of left femur**

⑦ **S72.463 Displaced supracondylar fracture with intracondylar extension of lower end of unspecified femur**

⑦ **S72.464 Nondisplaced supracondylar fracture with intracondylar extension of lower end of right femur**

⑦ **S72.465 Nondisplaced supracondylar fracture with intracondylar extension of lower end of left femur**

⑦ **S72.466 Nondisplaced supracondylar fracture with intracondylar extension of lower end of unspecified femur**

S72.47 Torus fracture of lower end of femur

The appropriate 7th character is to be added to all codes in subcategory S72.47

A - initial encounter for closed fracture

D - subsequent encounter for fracture with routine healing

G - subsequent encounter for fracture with delayed healing

K - subsequent encounter for fracture with nonunion

P - subsequent encounter for fracture with malunion

S - sequela

⑦ **S72.471 Torus fracture of lower end of right femur**

⑦ **S72.472 Torus fracture of lower end of left femur**

⑦ **S72.479 Torus fracture of lower end of unspecified femur**

S72.49 Other fracture of lower end of femur

⑦ **S72.491 Other fracture of lower end of right femur**

⑦ **S72.492 Other fracture of lower end of left femur**

⑦ **S72.499 Other fracture of lower end of unspecified femur**

S72.8 Other fracture of femur

S72.8X Other fracture of femur

⑦ **S72.8X1 Other fracture of right femur**

⑦ **S72.8X2 Other fracture of left femur**

● New code ▲ Revised code **Excludes1:** Not coded here **Excludes2:** Not included here ⊗ Placeholder required ⑦ 7th digit required

⑦S72.8X9   **Other fracture of unspecified femur**

S72.9   **Unspecified fracture of femur**

Fracture of thigh NOS

Fracture of upper leg NOS

Excludes1: fracture of hip NOS (S72.00-, S72.01-)

⊗⑦S72.90   **Unspecified fracture of unspecified femur**

⊗⑦S72.91   **Unspecified fracture of right femur**

⊗⑦S72.92   **Unspecified fracture of left femur**

S73 **Dislocation and sprain of joint and ligaments of hip**

Includes: avulsion of joint or ligament of hip

laceration of cartilage, joint or ligament of hip sprain of cartilage, joint or ligament of hip

traumatic hemarthrosis of joint or ligament of hip

traumatic rupture of joint or ligament of hip

traumatic subluxation of joint or ligament of hip

traumatic tear of joint or ligament of hip

Code also any associated open wound

Excludes2: strain of muscle, fascia and tendon of hip and thigh (S76.-)

The appropriate 7th character is to be added to each code from category S73

A - initial encounter

D - subsequent encounter

S - sequela

S73.0   **Subluxation and dislocation of hip**

Excludes2: dislocation and subluxation of hip prosthesis (T84.020, T84.021)

S73.00   **Unspecified subluxation and dislocation of hip**

Dislocation of hip NOS Subluxation of hip NOS

⑦S73.001   **Unspecified subluxation of right hip**

⑦S73.002   **Unspecified subluxation of left hip**

⑦S73.003   **Unspecified subluxation of unspecified hip**

⑦S73.004   **Unspecified dislocation of right hip**

⑦S73.005   **Unspecified dislocation of left hip**

⑦S73.006   **Unspecified dislocation of unspecified hip**

S73.01   **Posterior subluxation and dislocation of hip**

⑦S73.011   **Posterior subluxation of right hip**

⑦S73.012   **Posterior subluxation of left hip**

⑦S73.013   **Posterior subluxation of unspecified hip**

⑦S73.014   **Posterior dislocation of right hip**

⑦S73.015   **Posterior dislocation of left hip**

⑦S73.016   **Posterior dislocation of unspecified hip**

S73.02   **Obturator subluxation and dislocation of hip**

⑦S73.021   **Obturator subluxation of right hip**

⑦S73.022   **Obturator subluxation of left hip**

⑦S73.023   **Obturator subluxation of unspecified hip**

⑦S73.024   **Obturator dislocation of right hip**

⑦S73.025   **Obturator dislocation of left hip**

⑦S73.026   **Obturator dislocation of unspecified hip**

S73.03   **Other anterior dislocation of hip**

⑦S73.031   **Other anterior subluxation of right hip**

⑦S73.032   **Other anterior subluxation of left hip**

⑦S73.033   **Other anterior subluxation of unspecified hip**

⑦S73.034   **Other anterior dislocation of right hip**

⑦S73.035   **Other anterior dislocation of left hip**

⑦S73.036   **Other anterior dislocation of unspecified hip**

S73.04   **Central dislocation of hip**

⑦S73.041   **Central subluxation of right hip**

⑦S73.042   **Central subluxation of left hip**

⑦S73.043   **Central subluxation of unspecified hip**

⑦S73.044   **Central dislocation of right hip**

⑦S73.045   **Central dislocation of left hip**

⑦S73.046   **Central dislocation of unspecified hip**

S73.1   **Sprain of hip**

S73.10   **Unspecified sprain of hip**

⑦S73.101   **Unspecified sprain of right hip**

⑦S73.102   **Unspecified sprain of left hip**

⑦S73.109   **Unspecified sprain of unspecified hip**

S73.11   **Iliofemoral ligament sprain of hip**

⑦S73.111   **Iliofemoral ligament sprain of right hip**

⑦S73.112   **Iliofemoral ligament sprain of left hip**

⑦S73.119   **Iliofemoral ligament sprain of unspecified hip**

S73.12   **Ischiocapsular (ligament) sprain of hip**

⑦S73.121   **Ischiocapsular ligament sprain of right hip**

⑦S73.122   **Ischiocapsular ligament sprain of left hip**

⑦S73.129   **Ischiocapsular ligament sprain of unspecified hip**

S73.19   **Other sprain of hip**

⑦S73.191   **Other sprain of right hip**

⑦S73.192   **Other sprain of left hip**

⑦S73.199   **Other sprain of unspecified hip**

S74 **Injury of nerves at hip and thigh level**

Code also any associated open wound (S71.-)

Excludes2: injury of nerves at ankle and foot level (S94.-)

injury of nerves at lower leg level (S84.-)

The appropriate 7th character is to be added to each code from category S74

A - initial encounter

D - subsequent encounter

S - sequela

S74.0   **Injury of sciatic nerve at hip and thigh level**

⊗⑦S74.00   **Injury of sciatic nerve at hip and thigh level, unspecified leg**

⊗⑦**S74.01** **Injury of sciatic nerve at hip and thigh level, right leg**

⊗⑦**S74.02** **Injury of sciatic nerve at hip and thigh level, left leg**

S74.1 **Injury of femoral nerve at hip and thigh level**

⊗⑦**S74.10** **Injury of femoral nerve at hip and thigh level, unspecified leg**

⊗⑦**S74.11** **Injury of femoral nerve at hip and thigh level, right leg**

⊗⑦**S74.12** **Injury of femoral nerve at hip and thigh level, left leg**

S74.2 **Injury of cutaneous sensory nerve at hip and thigh level**

⊗⑦**S74.20** **Injury of cutaneous sensory nerve at hip and thigh level, unspecified leg**

⊗⑦**S74.21** **Injury of cutaneous sensory nerve at hip and high level, right leg**

⊗⑦**S74.22** **Injury of cutaneous sensory nerve at hip and thigh level, left leg**

S74.8 **Injury of other nerves at hip and thigh level**

S74.8X **Injury of other nerves at hip and thigh level**

⑦**S74.8X1** **Injury of other nerves at hip and thigh level, right leg**

⑦**S74.8X2** **Injury of other nerves at hip and thigh level, left leg**

⑦**S74.8X9** **Injury of other nerves at hip and thigh level, unspecified leg**

S74.9 **Injury of unspecified nerve at hip and thigh level**

⊗⑦**S74.90** **Injury of unspecified nerve at hip and thigh level, unspecified leg**

⊗⑦**S74.91** **Injury of unspecified nerve at hip and thigh level, right leg**

⊗⑦**S74.92** **Injury of unspecified nerve at hip and thigh level, left leg**

S75 **Injury of blood vessels at hip and thigh level**

Code also any associated open wound (S71.-)

Excludes2: injury of blood vessels at lower leg level (S85.-)

injury of popliteal artery (S85.0)

The appropriate 7th character is to be added to each code from category S75

A - initial encounter

D - subsequent encounter

S - sequela

S75.0 **Injury of femoral artery**

S75.00 **Unspecified injury of femoral artery**

⑦**S75.001** **Unspecified injury of femoral artery, right leg**

⑦**S75.002** **Unspecified injury of femoral artery, left leg**

⑦**S75.009** **Unspecified injury of femoral artery, unspecified leg**

S75.01 **Minor laceration of femoral artery**

Incomplete transection of femoral artery

Laceration of femoral artery NOS

Superficial laceration of femoral artery

⑦**S75.011** **Minor laceration of femoral artery, right leg**

⑦**S75.012** **Minor laceration of femoral artery, left leg**

⑦**S75.019** **Minor laceration of femoral artery, unspecified leg**

S75.02 **Major laceration of femoral artery**

Complete transection of femoral artery

Traumatic rupture of femoral artery

⑦**S75.021** **Major laceration of femoral artery, right leg**

⑦**S75.022** **Major laceration of femoral artery, left leg**

⑦**S75.029** **Major laceration of femoral artery, unspecified leg**

S75.09 **Other specified injury of femoral artery**

⑦**S75.091** **Other specified injury of femoral artery, right leg**

⑦**S75.092** **Other specified injury of femoral artery, left leg**

⑦**S75.099** **Other specified injury of femoral artery, unspecified leg**

S75.1 **Injury of femoral vein at hip and thigh level**

S75.10 **Unspecified injury of femoral vein at hip and thigh level**

⑦**S75.101** **Unspecified injury of femoral vein at hip and thigh level, right leg**

⑦**S75.102** **Unspecified injury of femoral vein at hip and thigh level, left leg**

⑦**S75.109** **Unspecified injury of femoral vein at hip and thigh level, unspecified leg**

S75.11 **Minor laceration of femoral vein at hip and thigh level**

Incomplete transection of femoral vein at hip and thigh level

Laceration of femoral vein at hip and thigh level NOS

Superficial laceration of femoral vein at hip and thigh level

⑦**S75.111** **Minor laceration of femoral vein at hip and thigh level, right leg**

⑦**S75.112** **Minor laceration of femoral vein at hip and thigh level, left leg**

⑦**S75.119** **Minor laceration of femoral vein at hip and thigh level, unspecified leg**

S75.12 **Major laceration of femoral vein at hip and thigh level**

Complete transection of femoral vein at hip and thigh level

Traumatic rupture of femoral vein at hip and thigh level

⑦**S75.121** **Major laceration of femoral vein at hip and thigh level, right leg**

⑦**S75.122** **Major laceration of femoral vein at hip and thigh level, left leg**

⑦**S75.129** **Major laceration of femoral vein at hip and thigh level, unspecified leg**

S75.19 **Other specified injury of femoral vein at hip and thigh level**

⑦**S75.191** **Other specified injury of femoral vein at hip and thigh level, right leg**

⑦**S75.192** **Other specified injury of femoral vein at hip and thigh level, left leg**

● New code ▲ Revised code **Excludes1:** Not coded here **Excludes2:** Not included here ⊗ Placeholder required ⑦ 7th digit required

⑦**S75.199**   Other specified injury of femoral vein at hip and thigh level, unspecified leg

S75.2   **Injury of greater saphenous vein at hip and thigh level**

Excludes1: greater saphenous vein NOS (S85.3)

S75.20   Unspecified injury of greater saphenous vein at hip and thigh level

⑦**S75.201**   Unspecified injury of greater saphenous vein at hip and thigh level, right leg

⑦**S75.202**   Unspecified injury of greater saphenous vein at hip and thigh level, left leg

⑦**S75.209**   Unspecified injury of greater saphenous vein at hip and thigh level, unspecified leg

S75.21   Minor laceration of greater saphenous vein at hip and thigh level

Incomplete transection of greater saphenous vein at hip and thigh level

Laceration of greater saphenous vein at hip and thigh level NOS

Superficial laceration of greater saphenous vein at hip and thigh level

⑦**S75.211**   Minor laceration of greater saphenous vein at hip and thigh level, right leg

⑦**S75.212**   Minor laceration of greater saphenous vein at hip and thigh level, left leg

⑦**S75.219**   Minor laceration of greater saphenous vein at hip and thigh level, unspecified leg

S75.22   Major laceration of greater saphenous vein at hip and thigh level

Complete transection of greater saphenous vein at hip and thigh level

Traumatic rupture of greater saphenous vein at hip and thigh level

⑦**S75.221**   Major laceration of greater saphenous vein at hip and thigh level, right leg

⑦**S75.222**   Major laceration of greater saphenous vein at hip and thigh level, left leg

⑦**S75.229**   Major laceration of greater saphenous vein at hip and thigh level, unspecified leg

S75.29   Other specified injury of greater saphenous vein at hip and thigh level

⑦**S75.291**   Other specified injury of greater saphenous vein at hip and thigh level, right leg

⑦**S75.292**   Other specified injury of greater saphenous vein at hip and thigh level, left leg

⑦**S75.299**   Other specified injury of greater saphenous vein at hip and thigh level, unspecified leg

S75.8   **Injury of other blood vessels at hip and thigh level**

S75.80   Unspecified injury of other blood vessels at hip and thigh level

⑦**S75.801**   Unspecified injury of other blood vessels at hip and thigh level, right leg

⑦**S75.802**   Unspecified injury of other blood vessels at hip and thigh level, left leg

⑦**S75.809**   Unspecified injury of other blood vessels at hip and thigh level, unspecified leg

S75.81   Laceration of other blood vessels at hip and thigh level

⑦**S75.811**   Laceration of other blood vessels at hip and thigh level, right leg

⑦**S75.812**   Laceration of other blood vessels at hip and thigh level, left leg

⑦**S75.819**   Laceration of other blood vessels at hip and thigh level, unspecified leg

S75.89   Other specified injury of other blood vessels at hip and thigh level

⑦**S75.891**   Other specified injury of other blood vessels at hip and thigh level, right leg

⑦**S75.892**   Other specified injury of other blood vessels at hip and thigh level, left leg

⑦**S75.899**   Other specified injury of other blood vessels at hip and thigh level, unspecified leg

S75.9   **Injury of unspecified blood vessel at hip and thigh level**

S75.90   Unspecified injury of unspecified blood vessel at hip and thigh level

⑦**S75.901**   Unspecified injury of unspecified blood vessel at hip and thigh level, right leg

⑦**S75.902**   Unspecified injury of unspecified blood vessel at hip and thigh level, left leg

⑦**S75.909**   Unspecified injury of unspecified blood vessel at hip and thigh level, unspecified leg

S75.91   Laceration of unspecified blood vessel at hip and thigh level

⑦**S75.911**   Laceration of unspecified blood vessel at hip and thigh level, right leg

⑦**S75.912**   Laceration of unspecified blood vessel at hip and thigh level, left leg

⑦**S75.919**   Laceration of unspecified blood vessel at hip and thigh level, unspecified leg

S75.99   Other specified injury of unspecified blood vessel at hip and thigh level

⑦**S75.991**   Other specified injury of unspecified blood vessel at hip and thigh level, right leg

⑦**S75.992**   Other specified injury of unspecified blood vessel at hip and thigh level, left leg

⑦**S75.999**   Other specified injury of unspecified blood vessel at hip and thigh level, unspecified leg

S76   **Injury of muscle, fascia and tendon at hip and thigh level**

Code also any associated open wound (S71.-)

Excludes2: injury of muscle, fascia and tendon at lower leg level (S86)

sprain of joint and ligament of hip (S73.1)

The appropriate 7th character is to be added to each code from category S76

A - initial encounter

D - subsequent encounter

S - sequela

S76.0   Injury of muscle, fascia and tendon of hip

    S76.00   Unspecified injury of muscle, fascia and tendon of hip

       ⑦**S76.001   Unspecified injury of muscle, fascia and tendon of right hip**

       ⑦**S76.002   Unspecified injury of muscle, fascia and tendon of left hip**

       ⑦**S76.009   Unspecified injury of muscle, fascia and tendon of unspecified hip**

    S76.01   Strain of muscle, fascia and tendon of hip

       ⑦**S76.011   Strain of muscle, fascia and tendon of right hip**

       ⑦**S76.012   Strain of muscle, fascia and tendon of left hip**

       ⑦**S76.019   Strain of muscle, fascia and tendon of unspecified hip**

    S76.02   Laceration of muscle, fascia and tendon of hip

       ⑦**S76.021   Laceration of muscle, fascia and tendon of right hip**

       ⑦**S76.022   Laceration of muscle, fascia and tendon of left hip**

       ⑦**S76.029   Laceration of muscle, fascia and tendon of unspecified hip**

    S76.09   Other specified injury of muscle, fascia and tendon of hip

       ⑦**S76.091   Other specified injury of muscle, fascia and tendon of right hip**

       ⑦**S76.092   Other specified injury of muscle, fascia and tendon of left hip**

       ⑦**S76.099   Other specified injury of muscle, fascia and tendon of unspecified hip**

S76.1   Injury of quadriceps muscle, fascia and tendon

Injury of patellar ligament (tendon)

    S76.10   Unspecified injury of quadriceps muscle, fascia and tendon

       ⑦**S76.101   Unspecified injury of right quadriceps muscle, fascia and tendon**

       ⑦**S76.102   Unspecified injury of left quadriceps muscle, fascia and tendon**

       ⑦**S76.109   Unspecified injury of unspecified quadriceps muscle, fascia and tendon**

    S76.11   Strain of quadriceps muscle, fascia and tendon

       ⑦**S76.111   Strain of right quadriceps muscle, fascia and tendon**

       ⑦**S76.112   Strain of left quadriceps muscle, fascia and tendon**

       ⑦**S76.119   Strain of unspecified quadriceps muscle, fascia and tendon**

    S76.12   Laceration of quadriceps muscle, fascia and tendon

       ⑦**S76.121   Laceration of right quadriceps muscle, fascia and tendon**

       ⑦**S76.122   Laceration of left quadriceps muscle, fascia and tendon**

       ⑦**S76.129   Laceration of unspecified quadriceps muscle, fascia and tendon**

    S76.19   Other specified injury of quadriceps muscle, fascia and tendon

       ⑦**S76.191   Other specified injury of right quadriceps muscle, fascia and tendon**

       ⑦**S76.192   Other specified injury of left quadriceps muscle, fascia and tendon**

       ⑦**S76.199   Other specified injury of unspecified quadriceps muscle, fascia and tendon**

S76.2   Injury of adductor muscle, fascia and tendon of thigh

    S76.20   Unspecified injury of adductor muscle, fascia and tendon of thigh

       ⑦**S76.201   Unspecified injury of adductor muscle, fascia and tendon of right thigh**

       ⑦**S76.202   Unspecified injury of adductor muscle, fascia and tendon of left thigh**

       ⑦**S76.209   Unspecified injury of adductor muscle, fascia and tendon of unspecified thigh**

    S76.21   Strain of adductor muscle, fascia and tendon of thigh

       ⑦**S76.211   Strain of adductor muscle, fascia and tendon of right thigh**

       ⑦**S76.212   Strain of adductor muscle, fascia and tendon of left thigh**

       ⑦**S76.219   Strain of adductor muscle, fascia and tendon of unspecified thigh**

    S76.22   Laceration of adductor muscle, fascia and tendon of thigh

       ⑦**S76.221   Laceration of adductor muscle, fascia and tendon of right thigh**

       ⑦**S76.222   Laceration of adductor muscle, fascia and tendon of left thigh**

       ⑦**S76.229   Laceration of adductor muscle, fascia and tendon of unspecified thigh**

    S76.29   Other injury of adductor muscle, fascia and tendon of thigh

       ⑦**S76.291   Other injury of adductor muscle, fascia and tendon of right thigh**

       ⑦**S76.292   Other injury of adductor muscle, fascia and tendon of left thigh**

       ⑦**S76.299   Other injury of adductor muscle, fascia and tendon of unspecified thigh**

S76.3   Injury of muscle, fascia and tendon of the posterior muscle group at thigh level

    S76.30   Unspecified injury of muscle, fascia and tendon of the posterior muscle group at thigh level

⑦S76.301   Unspecified injury of muscle, fascia and tendon of the posterior muscle group at thigh level, right thigh

⑦S76.302   Unspecified injury of muscle, fascia and tendon of the posterior muscle group at thigh level, left thigh

⑦S76.309   Unspecified injury of muscle, fascia and tendon of the posterior muscle group at thigh level, unspecified thigh

S76.31   Strain of muscle, fascia and tendon of the posterior muscle group at thigh level

⑦S76.311   Strain of muscle, fascia and tendon of the posterior muscle group at thigh level, right thigh

⑦S76.312   Strain of muscle, fascia and tendon of the posterior muscle group at thigh level, left thigh

⑦S76.319   Strain of muscle, fascia and tendon of the posterior muscle group at thigh level, unspecified thigh

S76.32   Laceration of muscle, fascia and tendon of the posterior muscle group at thigh level

⑦S76.321   Laceration of muscle, fascia and tendon of the posterior muscle group at thigh level, right thigh

⑦S76.322   Laceration of muscle, fascia and tendon of the posterior muscle group at thigh level, left thigh

⑦S76.329   Laceration of muscle, fascia and tendon of the posterior muscle group at thigh level, unspecified thigh

S76.39   Other specified injury of muscle, fascia and tendon of the posterior muscle group at thigh level

⑦S76.391   Other specified injury of muscle, fascia and tendon of the posterior muscle group at thigh level, right thigh

⑦S76.392   Other specified injury of muscle, fascia and tendon of the posterior muscle group at thigh level, left thigh

⑦S76.399   Other specified injury of muscle, fascia and tendon of the posterior muscle group at thigh level, unspecified thigh

S76.8   Injury of other specified muscles, fascia and tendons at thigh level

S76.80   Unspecified injury of other specified muscles, fascia and tendons at thigh level

⑦S76.801   Unspecified injury of other specified muscles, fascia and tendons at thigh level, right thigh

⑦S76.802   Unspecified injury of other specified muscles, fascia and tendons at thigh level, left thigh

⑦S76.809   Unspecified injury of other specified muscles, fascia and tendons at thigh level, unspecified thigh

S76.81   Strain of other specified muscles, fascia and tendons at thigh level

⑦S76.811   Strain of other specified muscles, fascia and tendons at thigh level, right thigh

⑦S76.812   Strain of other specified muscles, fascia and tendons at thigh level, left thigh

⑦S76.819   Strain of other specified muscles, fascia and tendons at thigh level, unspecified thigh

S76.82   Laceration of other specified muscles, fascia and tendons at thigh level

⑦S76.821   Laceration of other specified muscles, fascia and tendons at thigh level, right thigh

⑦S76.822   Laceration of other specified muscles, fascia and tendons at thigh level, left thigh

⑦S76.829   Laceration of other specified muscles, fascia and tendons at thigh level, unspecified thigh

S76.89   Other injury of other specified muscles, fascia and tendons at thigh level

⑦S76.891   Other injury of other specified muscles, fascia and tendons at thigh level, right thigh

⑦S76.892   Other injury of other specified muscles, fascia and tendons at thigh level, left thigh

⑦S76.899   Other injury of other specified muscles, fascia and tendons at thigh level, unspecified thigh

S76.9   Injury of unspecified muscles, fascia and tendons at thigh level

S76.90   Unspecified injury of unspecified muscles, fascia and tendons at thigh level

⑦S76.901   Unspecified injury of unspecified muscles, fascia and tendons at thigh level, right thigh

⑦S76.902   Unspecified injury of unspecified muscles, fascia and tendons at thigh level, left thigh

⑦S76.909   Unspecified injury of unspecified muscles, fascia and tendons at thigh level, unspecified thigh

S76.91   Strain of unspecified muscles, fascia and tendons at thigh level

⑦S76.911   Strain of unspecified muscles, fascia and tendons at thigh level, right thigh

⑦S76.912   Strain of unspecified muscles, fascia and tendons at thigh level, left thigh

⑦S76.919   Strain of unspecified muscles, fascia and tendons at thigh level, unspecified thigh

S76.92   Laceration of unspecified muscles, fascia and tendons at thigh level

⑦S76.921   Laceration of unspecified muscles, fascia and tendons at thigh level, right thigh

⑦S76.922   Laceration of unspecified muscles, fascia and tendons at thigh level, left thigh

⑦S76.929 **Laceration of unspecified muscles, fascia and tendons at thigh level, unspecified thigh**

S76.99 **Other specified injury of unspecified muscles, fascia and tendons at thigh level**

⑦S76.991 **Other specified injury of unspecified muscles, fascia and tendons at thigh level, right thigh**

⑦S76.992 **Other specified injury of unspecified muscles, fascia and tendons at thigh level, left thigh**

⑦S76.999 **Other specified injury of unspecified muscles, fascia and tendons at thigh level, unspecified thigh**

S77 **Crushing injury of hip and thigh**

Use additional code(s) for all associated injuries

Excludes2: crushing injury of ankle and foot (S97.-)
crushing injury of lower leg (S87.-)

The appropriate 7th character is to be added to each code from category S77

A - initial encounter

D - subsequent encounter

S - sequela

S77.0 **Crushing injury of hip**

⊗⑦S77.00 **Crushing injury of unspecified hip**

⊗⑦S77.01 **Crushing injury of right hip**

⊗⑦S77.02 **Crushing injury of left hip**

S77.1 **Crushing injury of thigh**

⊗⑦S77.10 **Crushing injury of unspecified thigh**

⊗⑦S77.11 **Crushing injury of right thigh**

⊗⑦S77.12 **Crushing injury of left thigh**

S77.2 **Crushing injury of hip with thigh**

⊗⑦S77.20 **Crushing injury of unspecified hip with thigh**

⊗⑦S77.21 **Crushing injury of right hip with thigh**

⊗⑦S77.22 **Crushing injury of left hip with thigh**

S78 **Traumatic amputation of hip and thigh**

An amputation not identified as partial or complete should be coded to complete

Excludes1: traumatic amputation of knee (S88.0-)

The appropriate 7th character is to be added to each code from category S78

A - initial encounter

D - subsequent encounter

S - sequela

S78.0 **Traumatic amputation at hip joint**

S78.01 **Complete traumatic amputation at hip joint**

⑦S78.011 **Complete traumatic amputation at right hip joint**

⑦S78.012 **Complete traumatic amputation at left hip joint**

⑦S78.019 **Complete traumatic amputation at unspecified hip joint**

S78.02 **Partial traumatic amputation at hip joint**

⑦S78.021 **Partial traumatic amputation at right hip joint**

⑦S78.022 **Partial traumatic amputation at left hip joint**

⑦S78.029 **Partial traumatic amputation at unspecified hip joint**

S78.1 **Traumatic amputation at level between hip and knee**

Excludes1: traumatic amputation of knee (S88.0-)

S78.11 **Complete traumatic amputation at level between hip and knee**

⑦S78.111 **Complete traumatic amputation at level between right hip and knee**

⑦S78.112 **Complete traumatic amputation at level between left hip and knee**

⑦S78.119 **Complete traumatic amputation at level between unspecified hip and knee**

S78.12 **Partial traumatic amputation at level between hip and knee**

⑦S78.121 **Partial traumatic amputation at level between right hip and knee**

⑦S78.122 **Partial traumatic amputation at level between left hip and knee**

⑦S78.129 **Partial traumatic amputation at level between unspecified hip and knee**

S78.9 **Traumatic amputation of hip and thigh, level unspecified**

S78.91 **Complete traumatic amputation of hip and thigh, level unspecified**

⑦S78.911 **Complete traumatic amputation of right hip and thigh, level unspecified**

⑦S78.912 **Complete traumatic amputation of left hip and thigh, level unspecified**

⑦S78.919 **Complete traumatic amputation of unspecified hip and thigh, level unspecified**

S78.92 **Partial traumatic amputation of hip and thigh, level unspecified**

⑦S78.921 **Partial traumatic amputation of right hip and thigh, level unspecified**

⑦S78.922 **Partial traumatic amputation of left hip and thigh, level unspecified**

⑦S78.929 **Partial traumatic amputation of unspecified hip and thigh, level unspecified**

S79 **Other and unspecified injuries of hip and thigh**

Note: A fracture not indicated as open or closed should be coded to closed

The appropriate 7th character is to be added to each code from subcategories S79.0 and S79.1

A - initial encounter for closed fracture

D - subsequent encounter for fracture with routine healing

G - subsequent encounter for fracture with delayed healing

K - subsequent encounter for fracture with nonunion

P - subsequent encounter for fracture with malunion

S - sequela

S79.0 **Physeal fracture of upper end of femur**

Excludes1: apophyseal fracture of upper end of femur (S72.13-)

nontraumatic slipped upper femoral epiphysis (M93.0-)

● New code ▲ Revised code **Excludes1:** Not coded here **Excludes2:** Not included here ⊗ Placeholder required ⑦ 7th digit required

S79.00   Unspecified physeal fracture of upper end of femur

⑦ S79.001   Unspecified physeal fracture of upper end of right femur

⑦ S79.002   Unspecified physeal fracture of upper end of left femur

⑦ S79.009   Unspecified physeal fracture of upper end of unspecified femur

S79.01   Salter-Harris Type I physeal fracture of upper end of femur

Acute on chronic slipped capital femoral epiphysis (traumatic)

Acute slipped capital femoral epiphysis (traumatic)

Capital femoral epiphyseal fracture

Excludes1: chronic slipped upper femoral epiphysis (nontraumatic) (M93.02-)

⑦ S79.011   Salter-Harris Type I physeal fracture of upper end of right femur

⑦ S79.012   Salter-Harris Type I physeal fracture of upper end of left femur

⑦ S79.019   Salter-Harris Type I physeal fracture of upper end of unspecified femur

S79.09   Other physeal fracture of upper end of femur

⑦ S79.091   Other physeal fracture of upper end of right femur

⑦ S79.092   Other physeal fracture of upper end of left femur

⑦ S79.099   Other physeal fracture of upper end of unspecified femur

S79.1   Physeal fracture of lower end of femur

S79.10   Unspecified physeal fracture of lower end of femur

⑦ S79.101   Unspecified physeal fracture of lower end of right femur

⑦ S79.102   Unspecified physeal fracture of lower end of left femur

⑦ S79.109   Unspecified physeal fracture of lower end of unspecified femur

S79.11   Salter-Harris Type I physeal fracture of lower end of femur

⑦ S79.111   Salter-Harris Type I physeal fracture of lower end of right femur

⑦ S79.112   Salter-Harris Type I physeal fracture of lower end of left femur

⑦ S79.119   Salter-Harris Type I physeal fracture of lower end of unspecified femur

S79.12   Salter-Harris Type II physeal fracture of lower end of femur

⑦ S79.121   Salter-Harris Type II physeal fracture of lower end of right femur

⑦ S79.122   Salter-Harris Type II physeal fracture of lower end of left femur

⑦ S79.129   Salter-Harris Type II physeal fracture of lower end of unspecified femur

S79.13   Salter-Harris Type III physeal fracture of lower end of femur

⑦ S79.131   Salter-Harris Type III physeal fracture of lower end of right femur

⑦ S79.132   Salter-Harris Type III physeal fracture of lower end of left femur

⑦ S79.139   Salter-Harris Type III physeal fracture of lower end of unspecified femur

S79.14   Salter-Harris Type IV physeal fracture of lower end of femur

⑦ S79.141   Salter-Harris Type IV physeal fracture of lower end of right femur

⑦ S79.142   Salter-Harris Type IV physeal fracture of lower end of left femur

⑦ S79.149   Salter-Harris Type IV physeal fracture of lower end of unspecified femur

S79.19   Other physeal fracture of lower end of femur

⑦ S79.191   Other physeal fracture of lower end of right femur

⑦ S79.192   Other physeal fracture of lower end of left femur

⑦ S79.199   Other physeal fracture of lower end of unspecified femur

S79.8   Other specified injuries of hip and thigh

The appropriate 7th character is to be added to each code in subcategory S79.8

A - initial encounter

D - subsequent encounter

S - sequela

S79.81   Other specified injuries of hip

⑦ S79.811   Other specified injuries of right hip

⑦ S79.812   Other specified injuries of left hip

⑦ S79.819   Other specified injuries of unspecified hip

S79.82   Other specified injuries of thigh

⑦ S79.821   Other specified injuries of right thigh

⑦ S79.822   Other specified injuries of left thigh

⑦ S79.829   Other specified injuries of unspecified thigh

S79.9   Unspecified injury of hip and thigh

The appropriate 7th character is to be added to each code in subcategory S79.9

A - initial encounter

D - subsequent encounter

S - sequela

S79.91   Unspecified injury of hip

⑦ S79.911   Unspecified injury of right hip

⑦ S79.912   Unspecified injury of left hip

⑦ S79.919   Unspecified injury of unspecified hip

S79.92   Unspecified injury of thigh

⑦ S79.921   Unspecified injury of right thigh

⑦ S79.922   Unspecified injury of left thigh

⑦ S79.929   Unspecified injury of unspecified thigh

INJURIES TO THE KNEE AND LOWER LEG (S80-S89)

Excludes2: burns and corrosions (T20-T32)

frostbite (T33-T34)

injuries of ankle and foot, except fracture of ankle and malleolus (S90-S99)

insect bite or sting, venomous (T63.4)

S80 **Superficial injury of knee and lower leg**

Excludes2: superficial injury of ankle and foot (S90.-)

The appropriate 7th character is to be added to each code from category S80

A - initial encounter

D - subsequent encounter

S - sequela

S80.0 **Contusion of knee**

⊗⑦**S80.00** **Contusion of unspecified knee**

⊗⑦**S80.01** **Contusion of right knee**

⊗⑦**S80.02** **Contusion of left knee**

S80.1 **Contusion of lower leg**

⊗⑦**S80.10** **Contusion of unspecified lower leg**

⊗⑦**S80.11** **Contusion of right lower leg**

⊗⑦**S80.12** **Contusion of left lower leg**

S80.2 **Other superficial injuries of knee**

S80.21 **Abrasion of knee**

⑦**S80.211** **Abrasion, right knee**

⑦**S80.212** **Abrasion, left knee**

⑦**S80.219** **Abrasion, unspecified knee**

S80.22 **Blister (nonthermal) of knee**

⑦**S80.221** **Blister (nonthermal), right knee**

⑦**S80.222** **Blister (nonthermal), left knee**

⑦**S80.229** **Blister (nonthermal), unspecified knee**

S80.24 **External constriction of knee**

⑦**S80.241** **External constriction, right knee**

⑦**S80.242** **External constriction, left knee**

⑦**S80.249** **External constriction, unspecified knee**

S80.25 **Superficial foreign body of knee**

Splinter in the knee

⑦**S80.251** **Superficial foreign body, right knee**

⑦**S80.252** **Superficial foreign body, left knee**

⑦**S80.259** **Superficial foreign body, unspecified knee**

S80.26 **Insect bite (nonvenomous) of knee**

⑦**S80.261** **Insect bite (nonvenomous), right knee**

⑦**S80.262** **Insect bite (nonvenomous), left knee**

⑦**S80.269** **Insect bite (nonvenomous), unspecified knee**

S80.27 **Other superficial bite of knee**

Excludes1: open bite of knee (S81.05-)

⑦**S80.271** **Other superficial bite of right knee**

⑦**S80.272** **Other superficial bite of left knee**

⑦**S80.279** **Other superficial bite of unspecified knee**

S80.8 **Other superficial injuries of lower leg**

S80.81 **Abrasion of lower leg**

⑦**S80.811** **Abrasion, right lower leg**

⑦**S80.812** **Abrasion, left lower leg**

⑦**S80.819** **Abrasion, unspecified lower leg**

S80.82 **Blister (nonthermal) of lower leg**

⑦**S80.821** **Blister (nonthermal), right lower leg**

⑦**S80.822** **Blister (nonthermal), left lower leg**

⑦**S80.829** **Blister (nonthermal), unspecified lower leg**

S80.84 **External constriction of lower leg**

⑦**S80.841** **External constriction, right lower leg**

⑦**S80.842** **External constriction, left lower leg**

⑦**S80.849** **External constriction, unspecified lower leg**

S80.85 **Superficial foreign body of lower leg**

Splinter in the lower leg

⑦**S80.851** **Superficial foreign body, right lower leg**

⑦**S80.852** **Superficial foreign body, left lower leg**

⑦**S80.859** **Superficial foreign body, unspecified lower leg**

S80.86 **Insect bite (nonvenomous) of lower leg**

⑦**S80.861** **Insect bite (nonvenomous), right lower leg**

⑦**S80.862** **Insect bite (nonvenomous), left lower leg**

⑦**S80.869** **Insect bite (nonvenomous), unspecified lower leg**

S80.87 **Other superficial bite of lower leg**

Excludes1: open bite of lower leg (S81.85-)

⑦**S80.871** **Other superficial bite, right lower leg**

⑦**S80.872** **Other superficial bite, left lower leg**

⑦**S80.879** **Other superficial bite, unspecified lower leg**

S80.9 **Unspecified superficial injury of knee and lower leg**

S80.91 **Unspecified superficial injury of knee**

⑦**S80.911** **Unspecified superficial injury of right knee**

⑦**S80.912** **Unspecified superficial injury of left knee**

⑦**S80.919** **Unspecified superficial injury of unspecified knee**

S80.92 **Unspecified superficial injury of lower leg**

⑦**S80.921** **Unspecified superficial injury of right lower leg**

⑦**S80.922** **Unspecified superficial injury of left lower leg**

⑦**S80.929** **Unspecified superficial injury of unspecified lower leg**

S81 **Open wound of knee and lower leg**

Code also any associated wound infection

Excludes1: open fracture of knee and lower leg (S82.-)

traumatic amputation of lower leg (S88.-)

Excludes2: open wound of ankle and foot (S91.-)

The appropriate 7th character is to be added to each code from category S81

A - initial encounter

● New code ▲ Revised code **Excludes1:** Not coded here **Excludes2:** Not included here ⊗ Placeholder required ⑦7th digit required

D - subsequent encounter
S - sequela

S81.0 Open wound of knee

  S81.00 Unspecified open wound of knee

    ⑦**S81.001 Unspecified open wound, right knee**

    ⑦**S81.002 Unspecified open wound, left knee**

    ⑦**S81.009 Unspecified open wound, unspecified knee**

  S81.01 Laceration without foreign body of knee

    ⑦**S81.011 Laceration without foreign body, right knee**

    ⑦**S81.012 Laceration without foreign body, left knee**

    ⑦**S81.019 Laceration without foreign body, unspecified knee**

  S81.02 Laceration with foreign body of knee

    ⑦**S81.021 Laceration with foreign body, right knee**

    ⑦**S81.022 Laceration with foreign body, left knee**

    ⑦**S81.029 Laceration with foreign body, unspecified knee**

  S81.03 Puncture wound without foreign body of knee

    ⑦**S81.031 Puncture wound without foreign body, right knee**

    ⑦**S81.032 Puncture wound without foreign body, left knee**

    ⑦**S81.039 Puncture wound without foreign body, unspecified knee**

  S81.04 Puncture wound with foreign body of knee

    ⑦**S81.041 Puncture wound with foreign body, right knee**

    ⑦**S81.042 Puncture wound with foreign body, left knee**

    ⑦**S81.049 Puncture wound with foreign body, unspecified knee**

  S81.05 Open bite of knee

    Bite of knee NOS

    Excludes1: superficial bite of knee (S80.27-)

    ⑦**S81.051 Open bite, right knee**

    ⑦**S81.052 Open bite, left knee**

    ⑦**S81.059 Open bite, unspecified knee**

S81.8 Open wound of lower leg

  S81.80 Unspecified open wound of lower leg

    ⑦**S81.801 Unspecified open wound, right lower leg**

    ⑦**S81.802 Unspecified open wound, left lower leg**

    ⑦**S81.809 Unspecified open wound, unspecified lower leg**

  S81.81 Laceration without foreign body of lower leg

    ⑦**S81.811 Laceration without foreign body, right lower leg**

    ⑦**S81.812 Laceration without foreign body, left lower leg**

    ⑦**S81.819 Laceration without foreign body, unspecified lower leg**

  S81.82 Laceration with foreign body of lower leg

    ⑦**S81.821 Laceration with foreign body, right lower leg**

    ⑦**S81.822 Laceration with foreign body, left lower leg**

    ⑦**S81.829 Laceration with foreign body, unspecified lower leg**

  S81.83 Puncture wound without foreign body of lower leg

    ⑦**S81.831 Puncture wound without foreign body, right lower leg**

    ⑦**S81.832 Puncture wound without foreign body, left lower leg**

    ⑦**S81.839 Puncture wound without foreign body, unspecified lower leg**

  S81.84 Puncture wound with foreign body of lower leg

    ⑦**S81.841 Puncture wound with foreign body, right lower leg**

    ⑦**S81.842 Puncture wound with foreign body, left lower leg**

    ⑦**S81.849 Puncture wound with foreign body, unspecified lower leg**

  S81.85 Open bite of lower leg

    Bite of lower leg NOS

    Excludes1: superficial bite of lower leg (S80.86-S80.87-)

    ⑦**S81.851 Open bite, right lower leg**

    ⑦**S81.852 Open bite, left lower leg**

    ⑦**S81.859 Open bite, unspecified lower leg**

S82 Fracture of lower leg, including ankle

Note: A fracture not indicated as displaced or nondisplaced should be coded to displaced

A fracture not indicated as open or closed should be coded to closed

The open fracture designations are based on the Gustilo open fracture classification

Includes: fracture of malleolus

Excludes1: traumatic amputation of lower leg (S88.-)

Excludes2: fracture of foot, except ankle (S92.-)

periprosthetic fracture of prosthetic implant of knee (T84.042, T84.043)

The appropriate 7th character is to be added to all codes from category S82

A - initial encounter for closed fracture

B - initial encounter for open fracture type I or II initial encounter for open fracture NOS

C - initial encounter for open fracture type IIIA, IIIB, or IIIC

D - subsequent encounter for closed fracture with routine healing

E - subsequent encounter for open fracture type I or II with routine healing

F - subsequent encounter for open fracture type IIIA, IIIB, or IIIC with routine healing

G - subsequent encounter for closed fracture with delayed healing

H - subsequent encounter for open fracture type I or II with delayed healing

J - subsequent encounter for open fracture type IIIA, IIIB, or IIIC with delayed healing

K - subsequent encounter for closed fracture with nonunion

M - subsequent encounter for open fracture type I or II with nonunion

N - subsequent encounter for open fracture type IIIA, IIIB, or IIIC with nonunion

P - subsequent encounter for closed fracture with malunion

Q - subsequent encounter for open fracture type I or II with malunion

R - subsequent encounter for open fracture type IIIA, IIIB, or IIIC with malunion

S - sequela

S82.0   Fracture of patella
Knee cap

S82.00   Unspecified fracture of patella

⑦S82.001   **Unspecified fracture of right patella**

⑦S82.002   **Unspecified fracture of left patella**

⑦S82.009   **Unspecified fracture of unspecified patella**

S82.01   Osteochondral fracture of patella

⑦S82.011   **Displaced osteochondral fracture of right patella**

⑦S82.012   **Displaced osteochondral fracture of left patella**

⑦S82.013   **Displaced osteochondral fracture of unspecified patella**

⑦S82.014   **Nondisplaced osteochondral fracture of right patella**

⑦S82.015   **Nondisplaced osteochondral fracture of left patella**

⑦S82.016   **Nondisplaced osteochondral fracture of unspecified patella**

S82.02   Longitudinal fracture of patella

⑦S82.021   **Displaced longitudinal fracture of right patella**

⑦S82.022   **Displaced longitudinal fracture of left patella**

⑦S82.023   **Displaced longitudinal fracture of unspecified patella**

⑦S82.024   **Nondisplaced longitudinal fracture of right patella**

⑦S82.025   **Nondisplaced longitudinal fracture of left patella**

⑦S82.026   **Nondisplaced longitudinal fracture of unspecified patella**

S82.03   Transverse fracture of patella

⑦S82.031   **Displaced transverse fracture of right patella**

⑦S82.032   **Displaced transverse fracture of left patella**

⑦S82.033   **Displaced transverse fracture of unspecified patella**

⑦S82.034   **Nondisplaced transverse fracture of right patella**

⑦S82.035   **Nondisplaced transverse fracture of left patella**

⑦S82.036   **Nondisplaced transverse fracture of unspecified patella**

S82.04   Comminuted fracture of patella

⑦S82.041   **Displaced comminuted fracture of right patella**

⑦S82.042   **Displaced comminuted fracture of left patella**

⑦S82.043   **Displaced comminuted fracture of unspecified patella**

⑦S82.044   **Nondisplaced comminuted fracture of right patella**

⑦S82.045   **Nondisplaced comminuted fracture of left patella**

⑦S82.046   **Nondisplaced comminuted fracture of unspecified patella**

S82.09   Other fracture of patella

⑦S82.091   **Other fracture of right patella**

⑦S82.092   **Other fracture of left patella**

⑦S82.099   **Other fracture of unspecified patella**

S82.1   Fracture of upper end of tibia
Fracture of proximal end of tibia
Excludes2: fracture of shaft of tibia (S82.2-)
physeal fracture of upper end of tibia (S89.0-)

S82.10   Unspecified fracture of upper end of tibia

⑦S82.101   **Unspecified fracture of upper end of right tibia**

⑦S82.102   **Unspecified fracture of upper end of left tibia**

⑦S82.109   **Unspecified fracture of upper end of unspecified tibia**

S82.11   Fracture of tibial spine

⑦S82.111   **Displaced fracture of right tibial spine**

⑦S82.112   **Displaced fracture of left tibial spine**

⑦S82.113   **Displaced fracture of unspecified tibial spine**

⑦S82.114   **Nondisplaced fracture of right tibial spine**

⑦S82.115   **Nondisplaced fracture of left tibial spine**

⑦S82.116   **Nondisplaced fracture of unspecified tibial spine**

S82.12   Fracture of lateral condyle of tibia

⑦S82.121   **Displaced fracture of lateral condyle of right tibia**

⑦S82.122   **Displaced fracture of lateral condyle of left tibia**

⑦S82.123   **Displaced fracture of lateral condyle of unspecified tibia**

⑦S82.124   **Nondisplaced fracture of lateral condyle of right tibia**

⑦S82.125   **Nondisplaced fracture of lateral condyle of left tibia**

⑦S82.126   **Nondisplaced fracture of lateral condyle of unspecified tibia**

S82.13   Fracture of medial condyle of tibia

⑦S82.131   **Displaced fracture of medial condyle of right tibia**

⑦S82.132   **Displaced fracture of medial condyle of left tibia**

⑦S82.133   **Displaced fracture of medial condyle of unspecified tibia**

⑦S82.134   **Nondisplaced fracture of medial condyle of right tibia**

⑦S82.135 Nondisplaced fracture of medial condyle of left tibia

⑦S82.136 Nondisplaced fracture of medial condyle of unspecified tibia

S82.14 Bicondylar fracture of tibia

Fracture of tibial plateau NOS

⑦S82.141 Displaced bicondylar fracture of right tibia

⑦S82.142 Displaced bicondylar fracture of left tibia

⑦S82.143 Displaced bicondylar fracture of unspecified tibia

⑦S82.144 Nondisplaced bicondylar fracture of right tibia

⑦S82.145 Nondisplaced bicondylar fracture of left tibia

⑦S82.146 Nondisplaced bicondylar fracture of unspecified tibia

S82.15 Fracture of tibial tuberosity

⑦S82.151 Displaced fracture of right tibial tuberosity

⑦82.152 Displaced fracture of left tibial tuberosity

⑦S82.153 Displaced fracture of unspecified tibial tuberosity

⑦S82.154 Nondisplaced fracture of right tibial tuberosity

⑦S82.155 Nondisplaced fracture of left tibial tuberosity

⑦S82.156 Nondisplaced fracture of unspecified tibial tuberosity

S82.16 Torus fracture of upper end of tibia

The appropriate 7th character is to be added to all codes in subcategory S82.16

A - initial encounter for closed fracture

D - subsequent encounter for fracture with routine healing

G - subsequent encounter for fracture with delayed healing

K - subsequent encounter for fracture with nonunion

P - subsequent encounter for fracture with malunion

S - sequela

⑦S82.161 Torus fracture of upper end of right tibia

⑦S82.162 Torus fracture of upper end of left tibia

⑦S82.169 Torus fracture of upper end of unspecified tibia

S82.19 Other fracture of upper end of tibia

⑦S82.191 Other fracture of upper end of right tibia

⑦S82.192 Other fracture of upper end of left tibia

⑦S82.199 Other fracture of upper end of unspecified tibia

S82.2 Fracture of shaft of tibia

S82.20 Unspecified fracture of shaft of tibia

Fracture of tibia NOS

⑦S82.201 Unspecified fracture of shaft of right tibia

⑦S82.202 Unspecified fracture of shaft of left tibia

⑦S82.209 Unspecified fracture of shaft of unspecified tibia

S82.22 Transverse fracture of shaft of tibia

⑦S82.221 Displaced transverse fracture of shaft of right tibia

⑦S82.222 Displaced transverse fracture of shaft of left tibia

⑦S82.223 Displaced transverse fracture of shaft of unspecified tibia

⑦S82.224 Nondisplaced transverse fracture of shaft of right tibia

⑦S82.225 Nondisplaced transverse fracture of shaft of left tibia

⑦S82.226 Nondisplaced transverse fracture of shaft of unspecified tibia

S82.23 Oblique fracture of shaft of tibia

⑦S82.231 Displaced oblique fracture of shaft of right tibia

⑦S82.232 Displaced oblique fracture of shaft of left tibia

⑦S82.233 Displaced oblique fracture of shaft of unspecified tibia

⑦S82.234 Nondisplaced oblique fracture of shaft of right tibia

⑦S82.235 Nondisplaced oblique fracture of shaft of left tibia

⑦S82.236 Nondisplaced oblique fracture of shaft of unspecified tibia

S82.24 Spiral fracture of shaft of tibia

Toddler fracture

⑦S82.241 Displaced spiral fracture of shaft of right tibia

⑦S82.242 Displaced spiral fracture of shaft of left tibia

⑦S82.243 Displaced spiral fracture of shaft of unspecified tibia

⑦S82.244 Nondisplaced spiral fracture of shaft of right tibia

⑦S82.245 Nondisplaced spiral fracture of shaft of left tibia

⑦S82.246 Nondisplaced spiral fracture of shaft of unspecified tibia

S82.25 Comminuted fracture of shaft of tibia

⑦S82.251 Displaced comminuted fracture of shaft of right tibia

⑦S82.252 Displaced comminuted fracture of shaft of left tibia

⑦S82.253 Displaced comminuted fracture of shaft of unspecified tibia

⑦S82.254 Nondisplaced comminuted fracture of shaft of right tibia

⑦S82.255 Nondisplaced comminuted fracture of shaft of left tibia

⑦S82.256 Nondisplaced comminuted fracture of shaft of unspecified tibia

S82.26 Segmental fracture of shaft of tibia

⑦S82.261 Displaced segmental fracture of shaft of right tibia

⑦S82.262 Displaced segmental fracture of shaft of left tibia

⑦S82.263 Displaced segmental fracture of shaft of unspecified tibia

⑦S82.264 Nondisplaced segmental fracture of shaft of right tibia

⑦S82.265 Nondisplaced segmental fracture of shaft of left tibia

⑦S82.266 Nondisplaced segmental fracture of shaft of unspecified tibia

S82.29 Other fracture of shaft of tibia

⑦S82.291 Other fracture of shaft of right tibia

⑦S82.292 Other fracture of shaft of left tibia

⑦S82.299 Other fracture of shaft of unspecified tibia

S82.3 Fracture of lower end of tibia

Excludes1: bimalleolar fracture of lower leg (S82.84-)

fracture of medial malleolus alone (S82.5-)

Maisonneuve's fracture (S82.86-)

pilon fracture of distal tibia (S82.87-)

trimalleolar fractures of lower leg (S82.85-)

S82.30 Unspecified fracture of lower end of tibia

⑦S82.301 Unspecified fracture of lower end of right tibia

⑦S82.302 Unspecified fracture of lower end of left tibia

⑦S82.309 Unspecified fracture of lower end of unspecified tibia

S82.31 Torus fracture of lower end of tibia

The appropriate 7th character is to be added to all codes in subcategory S82.31

A - initial encounter for closed fracture

D - subsequent encounter for fracture with routine healing

G - subsequent encounter for fracture with delayed healing

K - subsequent encounter for fracture with nonunion

P - subsequent encounter for fracture with malunion

S - sequela

⑦S82.311 Torus fracture of lower end of right tibia

⑦S82.312 Torus fracture of lower end of left tibia

⑦S82.319 Torus fracture of lower end of unspecified tibia

S82.39 Other fracture of lower end of tibia

⑦S82.391 Other fracture of lower end of right tibia

⑦S82.392 Other fracture of lower end of left tibia

⑦S82.399 Other fracture of lower end of unspecified tibia

S82.4 Fracture of shaft of fibula

Excludes2: fracture of lateral malleolus alone (S82.6-)

S82.40 Unspecified fracture of shaft of fibula

⑦S82.401 Unspecified fracture of shaft of right fibula

⑦S82.402 Unspecified fracture of shaft of left fibula

⑦S82.409 Unspecified fracture of shaft of unspecified fibula

S82.42 Transverse fracture of shaft of fibula

⑦S82.421 Displaced transverse fracture of shaft of right fibula

⑦S82.422 Displaced transverse fracture of shaft of left fibula

⑦S82.423 Displaced transverse fracture of shaft of unspecified fibula

⑦S82.424 Nondisplaced transverse fracture of shaft of right fibula

⑦S82.425 Nondisplaced transverse fracture of shaft of left fibula

⑦S82.426 Nondisplaced transverse fracture of shaft of unspecified fibula

S82.43 Oblique fracture of shaft of fibula

⑦S82.431 Displaced oblique fracture of shaft of right fibula

⑦S82.432 Displaced oblique fracture of shaft of left fibula

⑦S82.433 Displaced oblique fracture of shaft of unspecified fibula

⑦S82.434 Nondisplaced oblique fracture of shaft of right fibula

⑦S82.435 Nondisplaced oblique fracture of shaft of left fibula

⑦S82.436 Nondisplaced oblique fracture of shaft of unspecified fibula

S82.44 Spiral fracture of shaft of fibula

⑦S82.441 Displaced spiral fracture of shaft of right fibula

⑦S82.442 Displaced spiral fracture of shaft of left fibula

⑦S82.443 Displaced spiral fracture of shaft of unspecified fibula

⑦S82.444 Nondisplaced spiral fracture of shaft of right fibula

⑦S82.445 Nondisplaced spiral fracture of shaft of left fibula

⑦S82.446 Nondisplaced spiral fracture of shaft of unspecified fibula

S82.45 Comminuted fracture of shaft of fibula

⑦S82.451 Displaced comminuted fracture of shaft of right fibula

⑦S82.452 Displaced comminuted fracture of shaft of left fibula

⑦S82.453 Displaced comminuted fracture of shaft of unspecified fibula

⑦S82.454 Nondisplaced comminuted fracture of shaft of right fibula

⑦S82.455 Nondisplaced comminuted fracture of shaft of left fibula

⑦S82.456 Nondisplaced comminuted fracture of shaft of unspecified fibula

S82.46 Segmental fracture of shaft of fibula

⑦S82.461 Displaced segmental fracture of shaft of right fibula

⑦S82.462 **Displaced segmental fracture of shaft of left fibula**

⑦S82.463 **Displaced segmental fracture of shaft of unspecified fibula**

⑦S82.464 **Nondisplaced segmental fracture of shaft of right fibula**

⑦S82.465 **Nondisplaced segmental fracture of shaft of left fibula**

⑦S82.466 **Nondisplaced segmental fracture of shaft of unspecified fibula**

S82.49 **Other fracture of shaft of fibula**

⑦S82.491 **Other fracture of shaft of right fibula**

⑦S82.492 **Other fracture of shaft of left fibula**

⑦S82.499 **Other fracture of shaft of unspecified fibula**

S82.5 **Fracture of medial malleolus**

Excludes1: pilon fracture of distal tibia (S82.87-)

Salter-Harris type III of lower end of tibia (S89.13-) Salter-Harris type IV of lower end of tibia (S89.14-)

⊗⑦S82.51 **Displaced fracture of medial malleolus of right tibia**

⊗⑦S82.52 **Displaced fracture of medial malleolus of left tibia**

⊗⑦S82.53 **Displaced fracture of medial malleolus of unspecified tibia**

⊗⑦S82.54 **Nondisplaced fracture of medial malleolus of right tibia**

⊗⑦S82.55 **Nondisplaced fracture of medial malleolus of left tibia**

⊗⑦S82.56 **Nondisplaced fracture of medial malleolus of unspecified tibia**

S82.6 **Fracture of lateral malleolus**

Excludes1: pilon fracture of distal tibia (S82.87-)

⊗⑦S82.61 **Displaced fracture of lateral malleolus of right fibula**

⊗⑦S82.62 **Displaced fracture of lateral malleolus of left fibula**

⊗⑦S82.63 **Displaced fracture of lateral malleolus of unspecified fibula**

⊗⑦S82.64 **Nondisplaced fracture of lateral malleolus of right fibula**

⊗⑦S82.65 **Nondisplaced fracture of lateral malleolus of left fibula**

⊗⑦S82.66 **Nondisplaced fracture of lateral malleolus of unspecified fibula**

S82.8 **Other fractures of lower leg**

S82.81 **Torus fracture of upper end of fibula**

The appropriate 7th character is to be added to all codes in subcategory S82.81

A - initial encounter for closed fracture

D - subsequent encounter for fracture with routine healing

G - subsequent encounter for fracture with delayed healing

K - subsequent encounter for fracture with nonunion

P - subsequent encounter for fracture with malunion

S - sequela

⑦S82.811 **Torus fracture of upper end of right fibula**

⑦S82.812 **Torus fracture of upper end of left fibula**

⑦S82.819 **Torus fracture of upper end of unspecified fibula**

S82.82 **Torus fracture of lower end of fibula**

The appropriate 7th character is to be added to all codes in subcategory S82.82

A - initial encounter for closed fracture

D - subsequent encounter for fracture with routine healing

G - subsequent encounter for fracture with delayed healing

K - subsequent encounter for fracture with nonunion

P - subsequent encounter for fracture with malunion

S - sequela

⑦S82.821 **Torus fracture of lower end of right fibula**

⑦S82.822 **Torus fracture of lower end of left fibula**

⑦S82.829 **Torus fracture of lower end of unspecified fibula**

S82.83 **Other fracture of upper and lower end of fibula**

⑦S82.831 **Other fracture of upper and lower end of right fibula**

⑦S82.832 **Other fracture of upper and lower end of left fibula**

⑦S82.839 **Other fracture of upper and lower end of unspecified fibula**

S82.84 **Bimalleolar fracture of lower leg**

⑦S82.841 **Displaced bimalleolar fracture of right lower leg**

⑦S82.842 **Displaced bimalleolar fracture of left lower leg**

⑦S82.843 **Displaced bimalleolar fracture of unspecified lower leg**

⑦S82.844 **Nondisplaced bimalleolar fracture of right lower leg**

⑦S82.845 **Nondisplaced bimalleolar fracture of left lower leg**

⑦S82.846 **Nondisplaced bimalleolar fracture of unspecified lower leg**

S82.85 **Trimalleolar fracture of lower leg**

⑦S82.851 **Displaced trimalleolar fracture of right lower leg**

⑦S82.852 **Displaced trimalleolar fracture of left lower leg**

⑦S82.853 **Displaced trimalleolar fracture of unspecified lower leg**

⑦S82.854 **Nondisplaced trimalleolar fracture of right lower leg**

⑦S82.855 **Nondisplaced trimalleolar fracture of left lower leg**

⑦S82.856 **Nondisplaced trimalleolar fracture of unspecified lower leg**

S82.86 **Maisonneuve's fracture**

⑦**S82.861** **Displaced Maisonneuve's fracture of right leg**

⑦**S82.862** **Displaced Maisonneuve's fracture of left leg**

⑦**S82.863** **Displaced Maisonneuve's fracture of unspecified leg**

⑦**S82.864** **Nondisplaced Maisonneuve's fracture of right leg**

⑦**S82.865** **Nondisplaced Maisonneuve's fracture of left leg**

⑦**S82.866** **Nondisplaced Maisonneuve's fracture of unspecified leg**

S82.87 **Pilon fracture of tibia**

⑦**S82.871** **Displaced pilon fracture of right tibia**

⑦**S82.872** **Displaced pilon fracture of left tibia**

⑦**S82.873** **Displaced pilon fracture of unspecified tibia**

⑦**S82.874** **Nondisplaced pilon fracture of right tibia**

⑦**S82.875** **Nondisplaced pilon fracture of left tibia**

⑦**S82.876** **Nondisplaced pilon fracture of unspecified tibia**

S82.89 **Other fractures of lower leg**

Fracture of ankle NOS

⑦**S82.891** **Other fracture of right lower leg**

⑦**S82.892** **Other fracture of left lower leg**

⑦**S82.899** **Other fracture of unspecified lower leg**

S82.9 **Unspecified fracture of lower leg**

⊗⑦**S82.90** **Unspecified fracture of unspecified lower leg**

⊗⑦**S82.91** **Unspecified fracture of right lower leg**

⊗⑦**S82.92** **Unspecified fracture of left lower leg**

S83 **Dislocation and sprain of joints and ligaments of knee**

Includes: avulsion of joint or ligament of knee

laceration of cartilage, joint or ligament of knee

sprain of cartilage, joint or ligament of knee

traumatic hemarthrosis of joint or ligament of knee

traumatic rupture of joint or ligament of knee

traumatic subluxation of joint or ligament of knee

traumatic tear of joint or ligament of knee

Code also any associated open wound

Excludes1: derangement of patella (M22.0-M22.3)

injury of patellar ligament (tendon) (S76.1-)

internal derangement of knee (M23.-)

old dislocation of knee (M24.36)

pathological dislocation of knee (M24.36)

recurrent dislocation of knee (M22.0)

Excludes2: strain of muscle, fascia and tendon of lower leg (S86.-)

The appropriate 7th character is to be added to each code from category S83

A - initial encounter

D - subsequent encounter

S - sequela

S83.0 **Subluxation and dislocation of patella**

S83.00 **Unspecified subluxation and dislocation of patella**

⑦**S83.001** **Unspecified subluxation of right patella**

⑦**S83.002** **Unspecified subluxation of left patella**

⑦**S83.003** **Unspecified subluxation of unspecified patella**

⑦**S83.004** **Unspecified dislocation of right patella**

⑦**S83.005** **Unspecified dislocation of left patella**

⑦**S83.006** **Unspecified dislocation of unspecified patella**

S83.01 **Lateral subluxation and dislocation of patella**

⑦**S83.011** **Lateral subluxation of right patella**

⑦**S83.012** **Lateral subluxation of left patella**

⑦**S83.013** **Lateral subluxation of unspecified patella**

⑦**S83.014** **Lateral dislocation of right patella**

⑦**S83.015** **Lateral dislocation of left patella**

⑦**S83.016** **Lateral dislocation of unspecified patella**

S83.09 **Other subluxation and dislocation of patella**

⑦**S83.091** **Other subluxation of right patella**

⑦**S83.092** **Other subluxation of left patella**

⑦**S83.093** **Other subluxation of unspecified patella**

⑦**S83.094** **Other dislocation of right patella**

⑦**S83.095** **Other dislocation of left patella**

⑦**S83.096** **Other dislocation of unspecified patella**

S83.1 **Subluxation and dislocation of knee**

Excludes2: instability of knee prosthesis (T84.022, T84.023)

S83.10 **Unspecified subluxation and dislocation of knee**

⑦**S83.101** **Unspecified subluxation of right knee**

⑦**S83.102** **Unspecified subluxation of left knee**

⑦**S83.103** **Unspecified subluxation of unspecified knee**

⑦**S83.104** **Unspecified dislocation of right knee**

⑦**S83.105** **Unspecified dislocation of left knee**

⑦**S83.106** **Unspecified dislocation of unspecified knee**

S83.11 **Anterior subluxation and dislocation of proximal end of tibia**

Posterior subluxation and dislocation of distal end of femur

⑦**S83.111** **Anterior subluxation of proximal end of tibia, right knee**

⑦**S83.112** **Anterior subluxation of proximal end of tibia, left knee**

⑦**S83.113** **Anterior subluxation of proximal end of tibia, unspecified knee**

⑦**S83.114** **Anterior dislocation of proximal end of tibia, right knee**

● New code ▲ Revised code **Excludes1:** Not coded here **Excludes2:** Not included here ⊗ Placeholder required ⑦7th digit required

⑦S83.115   **Anterior dislocation of proximal end of tibia, left knee**

⑦S83.116   **Anterior dislocation of proximal end of tibia, unspecified knee**

S83.12   **Posterior subluxation and dislocation of proximal end of tibia**

    Anterior dislocation of distal end of femur

⑦S83.121   **Posterior subluxation of proximal end of tibia, right knee**

⑦S83.122   **Posterior subluxation of proximal end of tibia, left knee**

⑦S83.123   **Posterior subluxation of proximal end of tibia, unspecified knee**

⑦S83.124   **Posterior dislocation of proximal end of tibia, right knee**

⑦S83.125   **Posterior dislocation of proximal end of tibia, left knee**

⑦S83.126   **Posterior dislocation of proximal end of tibia, unspecified knee**

S83.13   **Medial subluxation and dislocation of proximal end of tibia**

⑦S83.131   **Medial subluxation of proximal end of tibia, right knee**

⑦S83.132   **Medial subluxation of proximal end of tibia, left knee**

⑦S83.133   **Medial subluxation of proximal end of tibia, unspecified knee**

⑦S83.134   **Medial dislocation of proximal end of tibia, right knee**

⑦S83.135   **Medial dislocation of proximal end of tibia, left knee**

⑦S83.136   **Medial dislocation of proximal end of tibia, unspecified knee**

S83.14   **Lateral subluxation and dislocation of proximal end of tibia**

⑦S83.141   **Lateral subluxation of proximal end of tibia, right knee**

⑦S83.142   **Lateral subluxation of proximal end of tibia, left knee**

⑦S83.143   **Lateral subluxation of proximal end of tibia, unspecified knee**

⑦S83.144   **Lateral dislocation of proximal end of tibia, right knee**

⑦S83.145   **Lateral dislocation of proximal end of tibia, left knee**

⑦S83.146   **Lateral dislocation of proximal end of tibia, unspecified knee**

S83.19   **Other subluxation and dislocation of knee**

⑦S83.191   **Other subluxation of right knee**

⑦S83.192   **Other subluxation of left knee**

⑦S83.193   **Other subluxation of unspecified knee**

⑦S83.194   **Other dislocation of right knee**

⑦S83.195   **Other dislocation of left knee**

⑦S83.196   **Other dislocation of unspecified knee**

S83.2   **Tear of meniscus, current injury**

    Excludes1: old bucket-handle tear (M23.2)

S83.20   **Tear of unspecified meniscus, current injury**

    Tear of meniscus of knee NOS

⑦S83.200   **Bucket-handle tear of unspecified meniscus, current injury, right knee**

⑦S83.201   **Bucket-handle tear of unspecified meniscus, current injury, left knee**

⑦S83.202   **Bucket-handle tear of unspecified meniscus, current injury, unspecified knee**

⑦S83.203   **Other tear of unspecified meniscus, current injury, right knee**

⑦S83.204   **Other tear of unspecified meniscus, current injury, left knee**

⑦S83.205   **Other tear of unspecified meniscus, current injury, unspecified knee**

⑦S83.206   **Unspecified tear of unspecified meniscus, current injury, right knee**

⑦S83.207   **Unspecified tear of unspecified meniscus, current injury, left knee**

⑦S83.209   **Unspecified tear of unspecified meniscus, current injury, unspecified knee**

S83.21   **Bucket-handle tear of medial meniscus, current injury**

⑦S83.211   **Bucket-handle tear of medial meniscus, current injury, right knee**

⑦S83.212   **Bucket-handle tear of medial meniscus, current injury, left knee**

⑦S83.219   **Bucket-handle tear of medial meniscus, current injury, unspecified knee**

S83.22   **Peripheral tear of medial meniscus, current injury**

⑦S83.221   **Peripheral tear of medial meniscus, current injury, right knee**

⑦S83.222   **Peripheral tear of medial meniscus, current injury, left knee**

⑦S83.229   **Peripheral tear of medial meniscus, current injury, unspecified knee**

S83.23   **Complex tear of medial meniscus, current injury**

⑦S83.231   **Complex tear of medial meniscus, current injury, right knee**

⑦S83.232   **Complex tear of medial meniscus, current injury, left knee**

⑦S83.239   **Complex tear of medial meniscus, current injury, unspecified knee**

S83.24   **Other tear of medial meniscus, current injury**

⑦S83.241   **Other tear of medial meniscus, current injury, right knee**

⑦S83.242   **Other tear of medial meniscus, current injury, left knee**

⑦S83.249   **Other tear of medial meniscus, current injury, unspecified knee**

S83.25   **Bucket-handle tear of lateral meniscus, current injury**

⑦S83.251   **Bucket-handle tear of lateral meniscus, current injury, right knee**

⑦S83.252   **Bucket-handle tear of lateral meniscus, current injury, left knee**

⑦S83.259   **Bucket-handle tear of lateral meniscus, current injury, unspecified knee**

S83.26   **Peripheral tear of lateral meniscus, current injury**

⑦S83.261   Peripheral tear of lateral meniscus, current injury, right knee

⑦S83.262   Peripheral tear of lateral meniscus, current injury, left knee

⑦S83.269   Peripheral tear of lateral meniscus, current injury, unspecified knee

S83.27   **Complex tear of lateral meniscus, current injury**

⑦S83.271   Complex tear of lateral meniscus, current injury, right knee

⑦S83.272   Complex tear of lateral meniscus, current injury, left knee

⑦S83.279   Complex tear of lateral meniscus, current injury, unspecified knee

S83.28   **Other tear of lateral meniscus, current injury**

⑦S83.281   Other tear of lateral meniscus, current injury, right knee

⑦S83.282   Other tear of lateral meniscus, current injury, left knee

⑦S83.289   Other tear of lateral meniscus, current injury, unspecified knee

S83.3   **Tear of articular cartilage of knee, current**

⊗⑦S83.30   Tear of articular cartilage of unspecified knee, current

⊗⑦S83.31   Tear of articular cartilage of right knee, current

⊗⑦S83.32   Tear of articular cartilage of left knee, current

S83.4   **Sprain of collateral ligament of knee**

S83.40   **Sprain of unspecified collateral ligament of knee**

⑦S83.401   Sprain of unspecified collateral ligament of right knee

⑦S83.402   Sprain of unspecified collateral ligament of left knee

⑦S83.409   Sprain of unspecified collateral ligament of unspecified knee

S83.41   **Sprain of medial collateral ligament of knee**

Sprain of tibial collateral ligament

⑦S83.411   Sprain of medial collateral ligament of right knee

⑦S83.412   Sprain of medial collateral ligament of left knee

⑦S83.419   Sprain of medial collateral ligament of unspecified knee

S83.42   **Sprain of lateral collateral ligament of knee**

Sprain of fibular collateral ligament

⑦S83.421   Sprain of lateral collateral ligament of right knee

⑦S83.422   Sprain of lateral collateral ligament of left knee

⑦S83.429   Sprain of lateral collateral ligament of unspecified knee

S83.5   **Sprain of cruciate ligament of knee**

S83.50   **Sprain of unspecified cruciate ligament of knee**

⑦S83.501   Sprain of unspecified cruciate ligament of right knee

⑦S83.502   Sprain of unspecified cruciate ligament of left knee

⑦S83.509   Sprain of unspecified cruciate ligament of unspecified knee

S83.51   **Sprain of anterior cruciate ligament of knee**

⑦S83.511   Sprain of anterior cruciate ligament of right knee

⑦S83.512   Sprain of anterior cruciate ligament of left knee

⑦S83.519   Sprain of anterior cruciate ligament of unspecified knee

S83.52   **Sprain of posterior cruciate ligament of knee**

⑦S83.521   Sprain of posterior cruciate ligament of right knee

⑦S83.522   Sprain of posterior cruciate ligament of left knee

⑦S83.529   Sprain of posterior cruciate ligament of unspecified knee

S83.6   **Sprain of the superior tibiofibular joint and ligament**

⊗⑦S83.60   Sprain of the superior tibiofibular joint and ligament, unspecified knee

⊗⑦S83.61   Sprain of the superior tibiofibular joint and ligament, right knee

⊗⑦S83.62   Sprain of the superior tibiofibular joint and ligament, left knee

S83.8   **Sprain of other specified parts of knee**

S83.8X   **Sprain of other specified parts of knee**

⑦S83.8X1   Sprain of other specified parts of right knee

⑦S83.8X2   Sprain of other specified parts of left knee

⑦S83.8X9   Sprain of other specified parts of unspecified knee

S83.9   **Sprain of unspecified site of knee**

⊗⑦S83.90   Sprain of unspecified site of unspecified knee

⊗⑦S83.91   Sprain of unspecified site of right knee

⊗⑦S83.92   Sprain of unspecified site of left knee

S84   **Injury of nerves at lower leg level**

Code also any associated open wound (S81.-)

Excludes2: injury of nerves at ankle and foot level (S94.-)

The appropriate 7th character is to be added to each code from category S84

A - initial encounter

D - subsequent encounter

S - sequela

S84.0   **Injury of tibial nerve at lower leg level**

⊗⑦S84.00   Injury of tibial nerve at lower leg level, unspecified leg

⊗⑦S84.01   Injury of tibial nerve at lower leg level, right leg

⊗⑦S84.02   Injury of tibial nerve at lower leg level, left leg

S84.1   **Injury of peroneal nerve at lower leg level**

⊗⑦S84.10   Injury of peroneal nerve at lower leg level, unspecified leg

⊗⑦S84.11   Injury of peroneal nerve at lower leg level, right leg

⊗⑦S84.12   Injury of peroneal nerve at lower leg level, left leg

S84.2   **Injury of cutaneous sensory nerve at lower leg level**

⊗⑦**S84.20**   **Injury of cutaneous sensory nerve at lower leg level, unspecified leg**

⊗⑦**S84.21**   **Injury of cutaneous sensory nerve at lower leg level, right leg**

⊗⑦**S84.22**   **Injury of cutaneous sensory nerve at lower leg level, left leg**

S84.8   **Injury of other nerves at lower leg level**

   S84.80   **Injury of other nerves at lower leg level**

      ⑦**S84.801**   **Injury of other nerves at lower leg level, right leg**

      ⑦**S84.802**   **Injury of other nerves at lower leg level, left leg**

      ⑦**S84.809**   **Injury of other nerves at lower leg level, unspecified leg**

S84.9   **Injury of unspecified nerve at lower leg level**

   ⊗⑦**S84.90**   **Injury of unspecified nerve at lower leg level, unspecified leg**

   ⊗⑦**S84.91**   **Injury of unspecified nerve at lower leg level, right leg**

   ⊗⑦**S84.92**   **Injury of unspecified nerve at lower leg level, left leg**

S85   **Injury of blood vessels at lower leg level**

Code also any associated open wound (S81.-)

Excludes2: injury of blood vessels at ankle and foot level (S95.-)

The appropriate 7th character is to be added to each code from category S85

A - initial encounter

D - subsequent encounter

S - sequela

S85.0   **Injury of popliteal artery**

   S85.00   **Unspecified injury of popliteal artery**

      ⑦**S85.001**   **Unspecified injury of popliteal artery, right leg**

      ⑦**S85.002**   **Unspecified injury of popliteal artery, left leg**

      ⑦**S85.009**   **Unspecified injury of popliteal artery, unspecified leg**

   S85.01   **Laceration of popliteal artery**

      ⑦**S85.011**   **Laceration of popliteal artery, right leg**

      ⑦**S85.012**   **Laceration of popliteal artery, left leg**

      ⑦**S85.019**   **Laceration of popliteal artery, unspecified leg**

   S85.09   **Other specified injury of popliteal artery**

      ⑦**S85.091**   **Other specified injury of popliteal artery, right leg**

      ⑦**S85.092**   **Other specified injury of popliteal artery, left leg**

      ⑦**S85.099**   **Other specified injury of popliteal artery, unspecified leg**

S85.1   **Injury of tibial artery**

   S85.10   **Unspecified injury of unspecified tibial artery**

      Injury of tibial artery NOS

      ⑦**S85.101**   **Unspecified injury of unspecified tibial artery, right leg**

      ⑦**S85.102**   **Unspecified injury of unspecified tibial artery, left leg**

      ⑦**S85.109**   **Unspecified injury of unspecified tibial artery, unspecified leg**

   S85.11   **Laceration of unspecified tibial artery**

      ⑦**S85.111**   **Laceration of unspecified tibial artery, right leg**

      ⑦**S85.112**   **Laceration of unspecified tibial artery, left leg**

      ⑦**S85.119**   **Laceration of unspecified tibial artery, unspecified leg**

   S85.12   **Other specified injury of unspecified tibial artery**

      ⑦**S85.121**   **Other specified injury of unspecified tibial artery, right leg**

      ⑦**S85.122**   **Other specified injury of unspecified tibial artery, left leg**

      ⑦**S85.129**   **Other specified injury of unspecified tibial artery, unspecified leg**

   S85.13   **Unspecified injury of anterior tibial artery**

      ⑦**S85.131**   **Unspecified injury of anterior tibial artery, right leg**

      ⑦**S85.132**   **Unspecified injury of anterior tibial artery, left leg**

      ⑦**S85.139**   **Unspecified injury of anterior tibial artery, unspecified leg**

   S85.14   **Laceration of anterior tibial artery**

      ⑦**S85.141**   **Laceration of anterior tibial artery, right leg**

      ⑦**S85.142**   **Laceration of anterior tibial artery, left leg**

      ⑦**S85.149**   **Laceration of anterior tibial artery, unspecified leg**

   S85.15   **Other specified injury of anterior tibial artery**

      ⑦**S85.151**   **Other specified injury of anterior tibial artery, right leg**

      ⑦**S85.152**   **Other specified injury of anterior tibial artery, left leg**

      ⑦**S85.159**   **Other specified injury of anterior tibial artery, unspecified leg**

   S85.16   **Unspecified injury of posterior tibial artery**

      ⑦**S85.161**   **Unspecified injury of posterior tibial artery, right leg**

      ⑦**S85.162**   **Unspecified injury of posterior tibial artery, left leg**

      ⑦**S85.169**   **Unspecified injury of posterior tibial artery, unspecified leg**

   S85.17   **Laceration of posterior tibial artery**

      ⑦**S85.171**   **Laceration of posterior tibial artery, right leg**

      ⑦**S85.172**   **Laceration of posterior tibial artery, left leg**

      ⑦**S85.179**   **Laceration of posterior tibial artery, unspecified leg**

   S85.18   **Other specified injury of posterior tibial artery**

      ⑦**S85.181**   **Other specified injury of posterior tibial artery, right leg**

      ⑦**S85.182**   **Other specified injury of posterior tibial artery, left leg**

      ⑦**S85.189**   **Other specified injury of posterior tibial artery, unspecified leg**

S85.2 **Injury of peroneal artery**

  S85.20 **Unspecified injury of peroneal artery**

    ⑦S85.201 **Unspecified injury of peroneal artery, right leg**

    ⑦S85.202 **Unspecified injury of peroneal artery, left leg**

    ⑦S85.209 **Unspecified injury of peroneal artery, unspecified leg**

  S85.21 **Laceration of peroneal artery**

    ⑦S85.211 **Laceration of peroneal artery, right leg**

    ⑦S85.212 **Laceration of peroneal artery, left leg**

    ⑦S85.219 **Laceration of peroneal artery, unspecified leg**

  S85.29 **Other specified injury of peroneal artery**

    ⑦S85.291 **Other specified injury of peroneal artery, right leg**

    ⑦S85.292 **Other specified injury of peroneal artery, left leg**

    ⑦S85.299 **Other specified injury of peroneal artery, unspecified leg**

S85.3 **Injury of greater saphenous vein at lower leg level**

Injury of greater saphenous vein NOS

Injury of saphenous vein NOS

  S85.30 **Unspecified injury of greater saphenous vein at lower leg level**

    ⑦S85.301 **Unspecified injury of greater saphenous vein at lower leg level, right leg**

    ⑦S85.302 **Unspecified injury of greater saphenous vein at lower leg level, left leg**

    ⑦S85.309 **Unspecified injury of greater saphenous vein at lower leg level, unspecified leg**

  S85.31 **Laceration of greater saphenous vein at lower leg level**

    ⑦S85.311 **Laceration of greater saphenous vein at lower leg level, right leg**

    ⑦S85.312 **Laceration of greater saphenous vein at lower leg level, left leg**

    ⑦S85.319 **Laceration of greater saphenous vein at lower leg level, unspecified leg**

  S85.39 **Other specified injury of greater saphenous vein at lower leg level**

    ⑦S85.391 **Other specified injury of greater saphenous vein at lower leg level, right leg**

    ⑦S85.392 **Other specified injury of greater saphenous vein at lower leg level, left leg**

    ⑦S85.399 **Other specified injury of greater saphenous vein at lower leg level, unspecified leg**

S85.4 **Injury of lesser saphenous vein at lower leg level**

  S85.40 **Unspecified injury of lesser saphenous vein at lower leg level**

    ⑦S85.401 **Unspecified injury of lesser saphenous vein at lower leg level, right leg**

    ⑦S85.402 **Unspecified injury of lesser saphenous vein at lower leg level, left leg**

    ⑦S85.409 **Unspecified injury of lesser saphenous vein at lower leg level, unspecified leg**

  S85.41 **Laceration of lesser saphenous vein at lower leg level**

    ⑦S85.411 **Laceration of lesser saphenous vein at lower leg level, right leg**

    ⑦S85.412 **Laceration of lesser saphenous vein at lower leg level, left leg**

    ⑦S85.419 **Laceration of lesser saphenous vein at lower leg level, unspecified leg**

  S85.49 **Other specified injury of lesser saphenous vein at lower leg level**

    ⑦S85.491 **Other specified injury of lesser saphenous vein at lower leg level, right leg**

    ⑦S85.492 **Other specified injury of lesser saphenous vein at lower leg level, left leg**

    ⑦S85.499 **Other specified injury of lesser saphenous vein at lower leg level, unspecified leg**

S85.5 **Injury of popliteal vein**

  S85.50 **Unspecified injury of popliteal vein**

    ⑦S85.501 **Unspecified injury of popliteal vein, right leg**

    ⑦S85.502 **Unspecified injury of popliteal vein, left leg**

    ⑦S85.509 **Unspecified injury of popliteal vein, unspecified leg**

  S85.51 **Laceration of popliteal vein**

    ⑦S85.511 **Laceration of popliteal vein, right leg**

    ⑦S85.512 **Laceration of popliteal vein, left leg**

    ⑦S85.519 **Laceration of popliteal vein, unspecified leg**

  S85.59 **Other specified injury of popliteal vein**

    ⑦S85.591 **Other specified injury of popliteal vein, right leg**

    ⑦S85.592 **Other specified injury of popliteal vein, left leg**

    ⑦S85.599 **Other specified injury of popliteal vein, unspecified leg**

S85.8 **Injury of other blood vessels at lower leg level**

  S85.80 **Unspecified injury of other blood vessels at lower leg level**

    ⑦S85.801 **Unspecified injury of other blood vessels at lower leg level, right leg**

    ⑦S85.802 **Unspecified injury of other blood vessels at lower leg level, left leg**

    ⑦S85.809 **Unspecified injury of other blood vessels at lower leg level, unspecified leg**

  S85.81 **Laceration of other blood vessels at lower leg level**

● New code ▲ Revised code **Excludes1:** Not coded here **Excludes2:** Not included here ⊗ Placeholder required ⑦7th digit required

INJURY, POISONING AND CERTAIN OTHER CONSEQUENCES OF EXTERNAL CAUSES

⑦ **S85.811** Laceration of other blood vessels at lower leg level, right leg

⑦ **S85.812** Laceration of other blood vessels at lower leg level, left leg

⑦ **S85.819** Laceration of other blood vessels at lower leg level, unspecified leg

S85.89 Other specified injury of other blood vessels at lower leg level

⑦ **S85.891** Other specified injury of other blood vessels at lower leg level, right leg

⑦ **S85.892** Other specified injury of other blood vessels at lower leg level, left leg

⑦ **S85.899** Other specified injury of other blood vessels at lower leg level, unspecified leg

S85.9 Injury of unspecified blood vessel at lower leg level

S85.90 Unspecified injury of unspecified blood vessel at lower leg level

⑦ **S85.901** Unspecified injury of unspecified blood vessel at lower leg level, right leg

⑦ **S85.902** Unspecified injury of unspecified blood vessel at lower leg level, left leg

⑦ **S85.909** Unspecified injury of unspecified blood vessel at lower leg level, unspecified leg

S85.91 Laceration of unspecified blood vessel at lower leg level

⑦ **S85.911** Laceration of unspecified blood vessel at lower leg level, right leg

⑦ **S85.912** Laceration of unspecified blood vessel at lower leg level, left leg

⑦ **S85.919** Laceration of unspecified blood vessel at lower leg level, unspecified leg

S85.99 Other specified injury of unspecified blood vessel at lower leg level

⑦ **S85.991** Other specified injury of unspecified blood vessel at lower leg level, right leg

⑦ **S85.992** Other specified injury of unspecified blood vessel at lower leg level, left leg

⑦ **S85.999** Other specified injury of unspecified blood vessel at lower leg level, unspecified leg

S86 **Injury of muscle, fascia and tendon at lower leg level**

Code also any associated open wound (S81.-)

Excludes2: injury of muscle, fascia and tendon at ankle (S96.-)

injury of patellar ligament (tendon) (S76.1-)

sprain of joints and ligaments of knee (S83.-)

The appropriate 7th character is to be added to each code from category S86

A - initial encounter

D - subsequent encounter

S - sequela

S86.0 **Injury of Achilles tendon**

S86.00 Unspecified injury of Achilles tendon

⑦ **S86.001** Unspecified injury of right Achilles tendon

⑦ **S86.002** Unspecified injury of left Achilles tendon

⑦ **S86.009** Unspecified injury of unspecified Achilles tendon

S86.01 Strain of Achilles tendon

⑦ **S86.011** Strain of right Achilles tendon

⑦ **S86.012** Strain of left Achilles tendon

⑦ **S86.019** Strain of unspecified Achilles tendon

S86.02 Laceration of Achilles tendon

⑦ **S86.021** Laceration of right Achilles tendon

⑦ **S86.022** Laceration of left Achilles tendon

⑦ **S86.029** Laceration of unspecified Achilles tendon

S86.09 Other specified injury of Achilles tendon

⑦ **S86.091** Other specified injury of right Achilles tendon

⑦ **S86.092** Other specified injury of left Achilles tendon

⑦ **S86.099** Other specified injury of unspecified Achilles tendon

S86.1 Injury of other muscle(s) and tendon(s) of posterior muscle group at lower leg level

S86.10 Unspecified injury of other muscle(s) and tendon(s) of posterior muscle group at lower leg level

⑦ **S86.101** Unspecified injury of other muscle(s) and tendon(s) of posterior muscle group at lower leg level, right leg

⑦ **S86.102** Unspecified injury of other muscle(s) and tendon(s) of posterior muscle group at lower leg level, left leg

⑦ **S86.109** Unspecified injury of other muscle(s) and tendon(s) of posterior muscle group at lower leg level, unspecified leg

S86.11 Strain of other muscle(s) and tendon(s) of posterior muscle group at lower leg level

⑦ **S86.111** Strain of other muscle(s) and tendon(s) of posterior muscle group at lower leg level, right leg

⑦ **S86.112** Strain of other muscle(s) and tendon(s) of posterior muscle group at lower leg level, left leg

⑦ **S86.119** Strain of other muscle(s) and tendon(s) of posterior muscle group at lower leg level, unspecified leg

S86.12 Laceration of other muscle(s) and tendon(s) of posterior muscle group at lower leg level

⑦ **S86.121** Laceration of other muscle(s) and tendon(s) of posterior muscle group at lower leg level, right leg

⑦ **S86.122** Laceration of other muscle(s) and tendon(s) of posterior muscle group at lower leg level, left leg

⑦ **S86.129** Laceration of other muscle(s) and tendon(s) of posterior muscle group at lower leg level, unspecified leg

Add 4th-7th digits   Nonspecific code   Unspecified code   Manifestation code   897

S86.19 Other injury of other muscle(s) and tendon(s) of posterior muscle group at lower leg level

⑦ **S86.191** Other injury of other muscle(s) and tendon(s) of posterior muscle group at lower leg level, right leg

⑦ **S86.192** Other injury of other muscle(s) and tendon(s) of posterior muscle group at lower leg level, left leg

⑦ **S86.199** Other injury of other muscle(s) and tendon(s) of posterior muscle group at lower leg level, unspecified leg

S86.2 Injury of muscle(s) and tendon(s) of anterior muscle group at lower leg level

S86.20 Unspecified injury of muscle(s) and tendon(s) of anterior muscle group at lower leg level

⑦ **S86.201** Unspecified injury of muscle(s) and tendon(s) of anterior muscle group at lower leg level, right leg

⑦ **S86.202** Unspecified injury of muscle(s) and tendon(s) of anterior muscle group at lower leg level, left leg

⑦ **S86.209** Unspecified injury of muscle(s) and tendon(s) of anterior muscle group at lower leg level, unspecified leg

S86.21 Strain of muscle(s) and tendon(s) of anterior muscle group at lower leg level

⑦ **S86.211** Strain of muscle(s) and tendon(s) of anterior muscle group at lower leg level, right leg

⑦ **S86.212** Strain of muscle(s) and tendon(s) of anterior muscle group at lower leg level, left leg

⑦ **S86.219** Strain of muscle(s) and tendon(s) of anterior muscle group at lower leg level, unspecified leg

S86.22 Laceration of muscle(s) and tendon(s) of anterior muscle group at lower leg level

⑦ **S86.221** Laceration of muscle(s) and tendon(s) of anterior muscle group at lower leg level, right leg

⑦ **S86.222** Laceration of muscle(s) and tendon(s) of anterior muscle group at lower leg level, left leg

⑦ **S86.229** Laceration of muscle(s) and tendon(s) of anterior muscle group at lower leg level, unspecified leg

S86.29 Other injury of muscle(s) and tendon(s) of anterior muscle group at lower leg level

⑦ **S86.291** Other injury of muscle(s) and tendon(s) of anterior muscle group at lower leg level, right leg

⑦ **S86.292** Other injury of muscle(s) and tendon(s) of anterior muscle group at lower leg level, left leg

⑦ **S86.299** Other injury of muscle(s) and tendon(s) of anterior muscle group at lower leg level, unspecified leg

S86.3 Injury of muscle(s) and tendon(s) of peroneal muscle group at lower leg level

S86.30 Unspecified injury of muscle(s) and tendon(s) of peroneal muscle group at lower leg level

⑦ **S86.301** Unspecified injury of muscle(s) and tendon(s) of peroneal muscle group at lower leg level, right leg

⑦ **S86.302** Unspecified injury of muscle(s) and tendon(s) of peroneal muscle group at lower leg level, left leg

⑦ **S86.309** Unspecified injury of muscle(s) and tendon(s) of peroneal muscle group at lower leg level, unspecified leg

S86.31 Strain of muscle(s) and tendon(s) of peroneal muscle group at lower leg level

⑦ **S86.311** Strain of muscle(s) and tendon(s) of peroneal muscle group at lower leg level, right leg

⑦ **S86.312** Strain of muscle(s) and tendon(s) of peroneal muscle group at lower leg level, left leg

⑦ **S86.319** Strain of muscle(s) and tendon(s) of peroneal muscle group at lower leg level, unspecified leg

S86.32 Laceration of muscle(s) and tendon(s) of peroneal muscle group at lower leg level

⑦ **S86.321** Laceration of muscle(s) and tendon(s) of peroneal muscle group at lower leg level, right leg

⑦ **S86.322** Laceration of muscle(s) and tendon(s) of peroneal muscle group at lower leg level, left leg

⑦ **S86.329** Laceration of muscle(s) and tendon(s) of peroneal muscle group at lower leg level, unspecified leg

S86.39 Other injury of muscle(s) and tendon(s) of peroneal muscle group at lower leg level

⑦ **S86.391** Other injury of muscle(s) and tendon(s) of peroneal muscle group at lower leg level, right leg

⑦ **S86.392** Other injury of muscle(s) and tendon(s) of peroneal muscle group at lower leg level, left leg

⑦ **S86.399** Other injury of muscle(s) and tendon(s) of peroneal muscle group at lower leg level, unspecified leg

S86.8 Injury of other muscles and tendons at lower leg level

S86.80 Unspecified injury of other muscles and tendons at lower leg level

⑦ **S86.801** Unspecified injury of other muscle(s) and tendon(s) at lower leg level, right leg

⑦ **S86.802** Unspecified injury of other muscle(s) and tendon(s) at lower leg level, left leg

⑦ **S86.809** Unspecified injury of other muscle(s) and tendon(s) at lower leg level, unspecified leg

S86.81 Strain of other muscles and tendons at lower leg level

⑦ **S86.811** Strain of other muscle(s) and tendon(s) at lower leg level, right leg

⑦ **S86.812** Strain of other muscle(s) and tendon(s) at lower leg level, left leg

⑦ **S86.819** Strain of other muscle(s) and tendon(s) at lower leg level, unspecified leg

S86.82 Laceration of other muscles and tendons at lower leg level

● New code ▲ Revised code **Excludes1:** Not coded here **Excludes2:** Not included here ⊗ Placeholder required ⑦ 7th digit required

⑦ **S86.821** Laceration of other muscle(s) and tendon(s) at lower leg level, right leg

⑦ **S86.822** Laceration of other muscle(s) and tendon(s) at lower leg level, left leg

⑦ **S86.829** Laceration of other muscle(s) and tendon(s) at lower leg level, unspecified leg

S86.89 Other injury of other muscles and tendons at lower leg level

⑦ **S86.891** Other injury of other muscle(s) and tendon(s) at lower leg level, right leg

⑦ **S86.892** Other injury of other muscle(s) and tendon(s) at lower leg level, left leg

⑦ **S86.899** Other injury of other muscle(s) and tendon(s) at lower leg level, unspecified leg

S86.9 Injury of unspecified muscle and tendon at lower leg level

S86.90 Unspecified injury of unspecified muscle and tendon at lower leg level

⑦ **S86.901** Unspecified injury of unspecified muscle(s) and tendon(s) at lower leg level, right leg

⑦ **S86.902** Unspecified injury of unspecified muscle(s) and tendon(s) at lower leg level, left leg

⑦ **S86.909** Unspecified injury of unspecified muscle(s) and tendon(s) at lower leg level, unspecified leg

S86.91 Strain of unspecified muscle and tendon at lower leg level

⑦ **S86.911** Strain of unspecified muscle(s) and tendon(s) at lower leg level, right leg

⑦ **S86.912** Strain of unspecified muscle(s) and tendon(s) at lower leg level, left leg

⑦ **S86.919** Strain of unspecified muscle(s) and tendon(s) at lower leg level, unspecified leg

S86.92 Laceration of unspecified muscle and tendon at lower leg level

⑦ **S86.921** Laceration of unspecified muscle(s) and tendon(s) at lower leg level, right leg

⑦ **S86.922** Laceration of unspecified muscle(s) and tendon(s) at lower leg level, left leg

⑦ **S86.929** Laceration of unspecified muscle(s) and tendon(s) at lower leg level, unspecified leg

S86.99 Other injury of unspecified muscle and tendon at lower leg level

⑦ **S86.991** Other injury of unspecified muscle(s) and tendon(s) at lower leg level, right leg

⑦ **S86.992** Other injury of unspecified muscle(s) and tendon(s) at lower leg level, left leg

⑦ **S86.999** Other injury of unspecified muscle(s) and tendon(s) at lower leg level, unspecified leg

S87 **Crushing injury of lower leg**

Use additional code(s) for all associated injuries

Excludes2: crushing injury of ankle and foot (S97.-)

The appropriate 7th character is to be added to each code from category S87

A - initial encounter

D - subsequent encounter

S - sequela

S87.0 **Crushing injury of knee**

⊗⑦ **S87.00** Crushing injury of unspecified knee

⊗⑦ **S87.01** Crushing injury of right knee

⊗⑦ **S87.02** Crushing injury of left knee

S87.8 **Crushing injury of lower leg**

⊗⑦ **S87.80** Crushing injury of unspecified lower leg

⊗⑦ **S87.81** Crushing injury of right lower leg

⊗⑦ **S87.82** Crushing injury of left lower leg

S88 **Traumatic amputation of lower leg**

An amputation not identified as partial or complete should be coded to complete

Excludes1: traumatic amputation of ankle and foot (S98.-)

The appropriate 7th character is to be added to each code from category S88

A - initial encounter

D - subsequent encounter

S - sequela

S88.0 **Traumatic amputation at knee level**

S88.01 Complete traumatic amputation at knee level

⑦ **S88.011** Complete traumatic amputation at knee level, right lower leg

⑦ **S88.012** Complete traumatic amputation at knee level, left lower leg

⑦ **S88.019** Complete traumatic amputation at knee level, unspecified lower leg

S88.02 Partial traumatic amputation at knee level

⑦ **S88.021** Partial traumatic amputation at knee level, right lower leg

⑦ **S88.022** Partial traumatic amputation at knee level, left lower leg

⑦ **S88.029** Partial traumatic amputation at knee level, unspecified lower leg

S88.1 **Traumatic amputation at level between knee and ankle**

S88.11 Complete traumatic amputation at level between knee and ankle

⑦ **S88.111** Complete traumatic amputation at level between knee and ankle, right lower leg

⑦ **S88.112** Complete traumatic amputation at level between knee and ankle, left lower leg

⑦ **S88.119** Complete traumatic amputation at level between knee and ankle, unspecified lower leg

S88.12 Partial traumatic amputation at level between knee and ankle

⑦ **S88.121** Partial traumatic amputation at level between knee and ankle, right lower leg

⑦ **S88.122** Partial traumatic amputation at level between knee and ankle, left lower leg

⑦S88.129 **Partial traumatic amputation at level between knee and ankle, unspecified lower leg**

S88.9 **Traumatic amputation of lower leg, level unspecified**

S88.91 **Complete traumatic amputation of lower leg, level unspecified**

⑦S88.911 **Complete traumatic amputation of right lower leg, level unspecified**

⑦S88.912 **Complete traumatic amputation of left lower leg, level unspecified**

⑦S88.919 **Complete traumatic amputation of unspecified lower leg, level unspecified**

S88.92 **Partial traumatic amputation of lower leg, level unspecified**

⑦S88.921 **Partial traumatic amputation of right lower leg, level unspecified**

⑦S88.922 **Partial traumatic amputation of left lower leg, level unspecified**

⑦S88.929 **Partial traumatic amputation of unspecified lower leg, level unspecified**

S89 **Other and unspecified injuries of lower leg**

Note: A fracture not indicated as open or closed should be coded to closed

Excludes2: Other and unspecified injuries of ankle and foot (S99.-)

The appropriate 7th character is to be added to each code from subcategories S89.0, S89.1, S89.2, and S89.3

A - initial encounter for closed fracture

D - subsequent encounter for fracture with routine healing

G - subsequent encounter for fracture with delayed healing

K - subsequent encounter for fracture with nonunion

P - subsequent encounter for fracture with malunion

S - sequela

S89.0 **Physeal fracture of upper end of tibia**

S89.00 **Unspecified physeal fracture of upper end of tibia**

⑦S89.001 **Unspecified physeal fracture of upper end of right tibia**

⑦S89.002 **Unspecified physeal fracture of upper end of left tibia**

⑦S89.009 **Unspecified physeal fracture of upper end of unspecified tibia**

S89.01 **Salter-Harris Type I physeal fracture of upper end of tibia**

⑦S89.011 **Salter-Harris Type I physeal fracture of upper end of right tibia**

⑦S89.012 **Salter-Harris Type I physeal fracture of upper end of left tibia**

⑦S89.019 **Salter-Harris Type I physeal fracture of upper end of unspecified tibia**

S89.02 **Salter-Harris Type II physeal fracture of upper end of tibia**

⑦S89.021 **Salter-Harris Type II physeal fracture of upper end of right tibia**

⑦S89.022 **Salter-Harris Type II physeal fracture of upper end of left tibia**

⑦S89.029 **Salter-Harris Type II physeal fracture of upper end of unspecified tibia**

S89.03 **Salter-Harris Type III physeal fracture of upper end of tibia**

⑦S89.031 **Salter-Harris Type III physeal fracture of upper end of right tibia**

⑦S89.032 **Salter-Harris Type III physeal fracture of upper end of left tibia**

⑦S89.039 **Salter-Harris Type III physeal fracture of upper end of unspecified tibia**

S89.04 **Salter-Harris Type IV physeal fracture of upper end of tibia**

⑦S89.041 **Salter-Harris Type IV physeal fracture of upper end of right tibia**

⑦S89.042 **Salter-Harris Type IV physeal fracture of upper end of left tibia**

⑦S89.049 **Salter-Harris Type IV physeal fracture of upper end of unspecified tibia**

S89.09 **Other physeal fracture of upper end of tibia**

⑦S89.091 **Other physeal fracture of upper end of right tibia**

⑦S89.092 **Other physeal fracture of upper end of left tibia**

⑦S89.099 **Other physeal fracture of upper end of unspecified tibia**

S89.1 **Physeal fracture of lower end of tibia**

S89.10 **Unspecified physeal fracture of lower end of tibia**

⑦S89.101 **Unspecified physeal fracture of lower end of right tibia**

⑦S89.102 **Unspecified physeal fracture of lower end of left tibia**

⑦S89.109 **Unspecified physeal fracture of lower end of unspecified tibia**

S89.11 **Salter-Harris Type I physeal fracture of lower end of tibia**

⑦S89.111 **Salter-Harris Type I physeal fracture of lower end of right tibia**

⑦S89.112 **Salter-Harris Type I physeal fracture of lower end of left tibia**

⑦S89.119 **Salter-Harris Type I physeal fracture of lower end of unspecified tibia**

S89.12 **Salter-Harris Type II physeal fracture of lower end of tibia**

⑦S89.121 **Salter-Harris Type II physeal fracture of lower end of right tibia**

⑦S89.122 **Salter-Harris Type II physeal fracture of lower end of left tibia**

⑦S89.129 **Salter-Harris Type II physeal fracture of lower end of unspecified tibia**

S89.13 **Salter-Harris Type III physeal fracture of lower end of tibia**

Excludes1: fracture of medial malleolus (adult) (S82.5-)

⑦S89.131 **Salter-Harris Type III physeal fracture of lower end of right tibia**

⑦S89.132　Salter-Harris Type III physeal fracture of lower end of left tibia

⑦S89.139　Salter-Harris Type III physeal fracture of lower end of unspecified tibia

S89.14　Salter-Harris Type IV physeal fracture of lower end of tibia

Excludes1: fracture of medial malleolus (adult) (S82.5-)

⑦S89.141　Salter-Harris Type IV physeal fracture of lower end of right tibia

⑦S89.142　Salter-Harris Type IV physeal fracture of lower end of left tibia

⑦S89.149　Salter-Harris Type IV physeal fracture of lower end of unspecified tibia

S89.19　Other physeal fracture of lower end of tibia

⑦S89.191　Other physeal fracture of lower end of right tibia

⑦S89.192　Other physeal fracture of lower end of left tibia

⑦S89.199　Other physeal fracture of lower end of unspecified tibia

S89.2　Physeal fracture of upper end of fibula

S89.20　Unspecified physeal fracture of upper end of fibula

⑦S89.201　Unspecified physeal fracture of upper end of right fibula

⑦S89.202　Unspecified physeal fracture of upper end of left fibula

⑦S89.209　Unspecified physeal fracture of upper end of unspecified fibula

S89.21　Salter-Harris Type I physeal fracture of upper end of fibula

⑦S89.211　Salter-Harris Type I physeal fracture of upper end of right fibula

⑦S89.212　Salter-Harris Type I physeal fracture of upper end of left fibula

⑦S89.219　Salter-Harris Type I physeal fracture of upper end of unspecified fibula

S89.22　Salter-Harris Type II physeal fracture of upper end of fibula

⑦S89.221　Salter-Harris Type II physeal fracture of upper end of right fibula

⑦S89.222　Salter-Harris Type II physeal fracture of upper end of left fibula

⑦S89.229　Salter-Harris Type II physeal fracture of upper end of unspecified fibula

S89.29　Other physeal fracture of upper end of fibula

⑦S89.291　Other physeal fracture of upper end of right fibula

⑦S89.292　Other physeal fracture of upper end of left fibula

⑦S89.299　Other physeal fracture of upper end of unspecified fibula

S89.3　Physeal fracture of lower end of fibula

S89.30　Unspecified physeal fracture of lower end of fibula

⑦S89.301　Unspecified physeal fracture of lower end of right fibula

⑦S89.302　Unspecified physeal fracture of lower end of left fibula

⑦S89.309　Unspecified physeal fracture of lower end of unspecified fibula

S89.31　Salter-Harris Type I physeal fracture of lower end of fibula

⑦S89.311　Salter-Harris Type I physeal fracture of lower end of right fibula

⑦S89.312　Salter-Harris Type I physeal fracture of lower end of left fibula

⑦S89.319　Salter-Harris Type I physeal fracture of lower end of unspecified fibula

S89.32　Salter-Harris Type II physeal fracture of lower end of fibula

⑦S89.321　Salter-Harris Type II physeal fracture of lower end of right fibula

⑦S89.322　Salter-Harris Type II physeal fracture of lower end of left fibula

⑦S89.329　Salter-Harris Type II physeal fracture of lower end of unspecified fibula

S89.39　Other physeal fracture of lower end of fibula

⑦S89.391　Other physeal fracture of lower end of right fibula

⑦S89.392　Other physeal fracture of lower end of left fibula

⑦S89.399　Other physeal fracture of lower end of unspecified fibula

S89.8　Other specified injuries of lower leg

The appropriate 7th character is to be added to each code in subcategory S89.8

A - initial encounter

D - subsequent encounter

S - sequela

⊗⑦S89.80　Other specified injuries of unspecified lower leg

⊗⑦S89.81　Other specified injuries of right lower leg

⊗⑦S89.82　Other specified injuries of left lower leg

S89.9　Unspecified injury of lower leg

The appropriate 7th character is to be added to each code in subcategory S89.9

A - initial encounter

D - subsequent encounter

S - sequela

⊗⑦S89.90　Unspecified injury of unspecified lower leg

⊗⑦S89.91　Unspecified injury of right lower leg

⊗⑦S89.92　Unspecified injury of left lower leg

INJURIES TO THE ANKLE AND FOOT (S90-S99)

Excludes2: burns and corrosions (T20-T32)

fracture of ankle and malleolus (S82.-)

frostbite (T33-T34)

insect bite or sting, venomous (T63.4)

S90　Superficial injury of ankle, foot and toes

The appropriate 7th character is to be added to each code from category S90

Add 4th-7th digits　　　Nonspecific code　　　Unspecified code　　　Manifestation code

A - initial encounter

D - subsequent encounter

S - sequela

S90.0   Contusion of ankle

⊗⑦**S90.00   Contusion of unspecified ankle**

⊗⑦**S90.01   Contusion of right ankle**

⊗⑦**S90.02   Contusion of left ankle**

S90.1   Contusion of toe without damage to nail

S90.11   Contusion of great toe without damage to nail

⑦**S90.111   Contusion of right great toe without damage to nail**

⑦**S90.112   Contusion of left great toe without damage to nail**

⑦**S90.119   Contusion of unspecified great toe without damage to nail**

S90.12   Contusion of lesser toe without damage to nail

⑦**S90.121   Contusion of right lesser toe(s) without damage to nail**

⑦**S90.122   Contusion of left lesser toe(s) without damage to nail**

⑦**S90.129   Contusion of unspecified lesser toe(s) without damage to nail**

Contusion of toe NOS

S90.2   Contusion of toe with damage to nail

S90.21   Contusion of great toe with damage to nail

⑦**S90.211   Contusion of right great toe with damage to nail**

⑦**S90.212   Contusion of left great toe with damage to nail**

⑦**S90.219   Contusion of unspecified great toe with damage to nail**

S90.22   Contusion of lesser toe with damage to nail

⑦**S90.221   Contusion of right lesser toe(s) with damage to nail**

⑦**S90.222   Contusion of left lesser toe(s) with damage to nail**

⑦**S90.229   Contusion of unspecified lesser toe(s) with damage to nail**

S90.3   Contusion of foot

Excludes2: contusion of toes (S90.1-, S90.2-)

⊗⑦**S90.30   Contusion of unspecified foot**

Contusion of foot NOS

⊗⑦**S90.31   Contusion of right foot**

⊗⑦**S90.32   Contusion of left foot**

S90.4   Other superficial injuries of toe

S90.41   Abrasion of toe

⑦**S90.411   Abrasion, right great toe**

⑦**S90.412   Abrasion, left great toe**

⑦**S90.413   Abrasion, unspecified great toe**

⑦**S90.414   Abrasion, right lesser toe(s)**

⑦**S90.415   Abrasion, left lesser toe(s)**

⑦**S90.416   Abrasion, unspecified lesser toe(s)**

S90.42   Blister (nonthermal) of toe

⑦**S90.421   Blister (nonthermal), right great toe**

⑦**S90.422   Blister (nonthermal), left great toe**

⑦**S90.423   Blister (nonthermal), unspecified great toe**

⑦**S90.424   Blister (nonthermal), right lesser toe(s)**

⑦**S90.425   Blister (nonthermal), left lesser toe(s)**

⑦**S90.426   Blister (nonthermal), unspecified lesser toe(s)**

S90.44   External constriction of toe

Hair tourniquet syndrome of toe

⑦**S90.441   External constriction, right great toe**

⑦**S90.442   External constriction, left great toe**

⑦**S90.443   External constriction, unspecified great toe**

⑦**S90.444   External constriction, right lesser toe(s)**

⑦**S90.445   External constriction, left lesser toe(s)**

⑦**S90.446   External constriction, unspecified lesser toe(s)**

S90.45   Superficial foreign body of toe

Splinter in the toe

⑦**S90.451   Superficial foreign body, right great toe**

⑦**S90.452   Superficial foreign body, left great toe**

⑦**S90.453   Superficial foreign body, unspecified great toe**

⑦**S90.454   Superficial foreign body, right lesser toe(s)**

⑦**S90.455   Superficial foreign body, left lesser toe(s)**

⑦**S90.456   Superficial foreign body, unspecified lesser toe(s)**

S90.46   Insect bite (nonvenomous) of toe

⑦**S90.461   Insect bite (nonvenomous), right great toe**

⑦**S90.462   Insect bite (nonvenomous), left great toe**

⑦**S90.463   Insect bite (nonvenomous), unspecified great toe**

⑦**S90.464   Insect bite (nonvenomous), right lesser toe(s)**

⑦**S90.465   Insect bite (nonvenomous), left lesser toe(s)**

⑦**S90.466   Insect bite (nonvenomous), unspecified lesser toe(s)**

S90.47   Other superficial bite of toe

Excludes1: open bite of toe (S91.15-, S91.25-)

⑦**S90.471   Other superficial bite of right great toe**

⑦**S90.472   Other superficial bite of left great toe**

⑦**S90.473   Other superficial bite of unspecified great toe**

⑦**S90.474   Other superficial bite of right lesser toe(s)**

⑦**S90.475   Other superficial bite of left lesser toe(s)**

⑦**S90.476   Other superficial bite of unspecified lesser toe(s)**

S90.5 **Other superficial injuries of ankle**

S90.51 **Abrasion of ankle**

⑦ S90.511 **Abrasion, right ankle**

⑦ S90.512 **Abrasion, left ankle**

⑦ S90.519 **Abrasion, unspecified ankle**

S90.52 **Blister (nonthermal) of ankle**

⑦ S90.521 **Blister (nonthermal), right ankle**

⑦ S90.522 **Blister (nonthermal), left ankle**

⑦ S90.529 **Blister (nonthermal), unspecified ankle**

S90.54 **External constriction of ankle**

⑦ S90.541 **External constriction, right ankle**

⑦ S90.542 **External constriction, left ankle**

⑦ S90.549 **External constriction, unspecified ankle**

S90.55 **Superficial foreign body of ankle**

Splinter in the ankle

⑦ S90.551 **Superficial foreign body, right ankle**

⑦ S90.552 **Superficial foreign body, left ankle**

⑦ S90.559 **Superficial foreign body, unspecified ankle**

S90.56 **Insect bite (nonvenomous) of ankle**

⑦ S90.561 **Insect bite (nonvenomous), right ankle**

⑦ S90.562 **Insect bite (nonvenomous), left ankle**

⑦ S90.569 **Insect bite (nonvenomous), unspecified ankle**

S90.57 **Other superficial bite of ankle**

Excludes1: open bite of ankle (S91.05-)

⑦ S90.571 **Other superficial bite of ankle, right ankle**

⑦ S90.572 **Other superficial bite of ankle, left ankle**

⑦ S90.579 **Other superficial bite of ankle, unspecified ankle**

S90.8 **Other superficial injuries of foot**

S90.81 **Abrasion of foot**

⑦ S90.811 **Abrasion, right foot**

⑦ S90.812 **Abrasion, left foot**

⑦ S90.819 **Abrasion, unspecified foot**

S90.82 **Blister (nonthermal) of foot**

⑦ S90.821 **Blister (nonthermal), right foot**

⑦ S90.822 **Blister (nonthermal), left foot**

⑦ S90.829 **Blister (nonthermal), unspecified foot**

S90.84 **External constriction of foot**

⑦ S90.841 **External constriction, right foot**

⑦ S90.842 **External constriction, left foot**

⑦ S90.849 **External constriction, unspecified foot**

S90.85 **Superficial foreign body of foot**

Splinter in the foot

⑦ S90.851 **Superficial foreign body, right foot**

⑦ S90.852 **Superficial foreign body, left foot**

⑦ S90.859 **Superficial foreign body, unspecified foot**

S90.86 **Insect bite (nonvenomous) of foot**

⑦ S90.861 **Insect bite (nonvenomous), right foot**

⑦ S90.862 **Insect bite (nonvenomous), left foot**

⑦ S90.869 **Insect bite (nonvenomous), unspecified foot**

S90.87 **Other superficial bite of foot**

Excludes1: open bite of foot (S91.35-)

⑦ S90.871 **Other superficial bite of right foot**

⑦ S90.872 **Other superficial bite of left foot**

⑦ S90.879 **Other superficial bite of unspecified foot**

S90.9 **Unspecified superficial injury of ankle, foot and toe**

S90.91 **Unspecified superficial injury of ankle**

⑦ S90.911 **Unspecified superficial injury of right ankle**

⑦ S90.912 **Unspecified superficial injury of left ankle**

⑦ S90.919 **Unspecified superficial injury of unspecified ankle**

S90.92 **Unspecified superficial injury of foot**

⑦ S90.921 **Unspecified superficial injury of right foot**

⑦ S90.922 **Unspecified superficial injury of left foot**

⑦ S90.929 **Unspecified superficial injury of unspecified foot**

S90.93 **Unspecified superficial injury of toes**

⑦ S90.931 **Unspecified superficial injury of right great toe**

⑦ S90.932 **Unspecified superficial injury of left great toe**

⑦ S90.933 **Unspecified superficial injury of unspecified great toe**

⑦ S90.934 **Unspecified superficial injury of right lesser toe(s)**

⑦ S90.935 **Unspecified superficial injury of left lesser toe(s)**

⑦ S90.936 **Unspecified superficial injury of unspecified lesser toe(s)**

S91 **Open wound of ankle, foot and toes**

Code also any associated wound infection

Excludes1: open fracture of ankle, foot and toes (S92.-with 7th character B)

traumatic amputation of ankle and foot (S98.-)

The appropriate 7th character is to be added to each code from category S91

A - initial encounter

D - subsequent encounter

S - sequela

S91.0 **Open wound of ankle**

S91.00 **Unspecified open wound of ankle**

⑦ S91.001 **Unspecified open wound, right ankle**

⑦ S91.002 **Unspecified open wound, left ankle**

⑦ S91.009 **Unspecified open wound, unspecified ankle**

S91.01 Laceration without foreign body of ankle
   ⑦**S91.011** Laceration without foreign body, right ankle
   ⑦**S91.012** Laceration without foreign body, left ankle
   ⑦**S91.019** Laceration without foreign body, unspecified ankle

S91.02 Laceration with foreign body of ankle
   ⑦**S91.021** Laceration with foreign body, right ankle
   ⑦**S91.022** Laceration with foreign body, left ankle
   ⑦**S91.029** Laceration with foreign body, unspecified ankle

S91.03 Puncture wound without foreign body of ankle
   ⑦**S91.031** Puncture wound without foreign body, right ankle
   ⑦**S91.032** Puncture wound without foreign body, left ankle
   ⑦**S91.039** Puncture wound without foreign body, unspecified ankle

S91.04 Puncture wound with foreign body of ankle
   ⑦**S91.041** Puncture wound with foreign body, right ankle
   ⑦**S91.042** Puncture wound with foreign body, left ankle
   ⑦**S91.049** Puncture wound with foreign body, unspecified ankle

S91.05 Open bite of ankle
   Excludes1: superficial bite of ankle (S90.56-, S90.57-)
   ⑦**S91.051** Open bite, right ankle
   ⑦**S91.052** Open bite, left ankle
   ⑦**S91.059** Open bite, unspecified ankle

S91.1 Open wound of toe without damage to nail
  S91.10 Unspecified open wound of toe without damage to nail
   ⑦**S91.101** Unspecified open wound of right great toe without damage to nail
   ⑦**S91.102** Unspecified open wound of left great toe without damage to nail
   ⑦**S91.103** Unspecified open wound of unspecified great toe without damage to nail
   ⑦**S91.104** Unspecified open wound of right lesser toe(s) without damage to nail
   ⑦**S91.105** Unspecified open wound of left lesser toe(s) without damage to nail
   ⑦**S91.106** Unspecified open wound of unspecified lesser toe(s) without damage to nail
   ⑦**S91.109** Unspecified open wound of unspecified toe(s) without damage to nail

  S91.11 Laceration without foreign body of toe without damage to nail
   ⑦**S91.111** Laceration without foreign body of right great toe without damage to nail
   ⑦**S91.112** Laceration without foreign body of left great toe without damage to nail

   ⑦**S91.113** Laceration without foreign body of unspecified great toe without damage to nail
   ⑦**S91.114** Laceration without foreign body of right lesser toe(s) without damage to nail
   ⑦**S91.115** Laceration without foreign body of left lesser toe(s) without damage to nail
   ⑦**S91.116** Laceration without foreign body of unspecified lesser toe(s) without damage to nail
   ⑦**S91.119** Laceration without foreign body of unspecified toe without damage to nail

  S91.12 Laceration with foreign body of toe without damage to nail
   ⑦**S91.121** Laceration with foreign body of right great toe without damage to nail
   ⑦**S91.122** Laceration with foreign body of left great toe without damage to nail
   ⑦**S91.123** Laceration with foreign body of unspecified great toe without damage to nail
   ⑦**S91.124** Laceration with foreign body of right lesser toe(s) without damage to nail
   ⑦**S91.125** Laceration with foreign body of left lesser toe(s) without damage to nail
   ⑦**S91.126** Laceration with foreign body of unspecified lesser toe(s) without damage to nail
   ⑦**S91.129** Laceration with foreign body of unspecified toe(s) without damage to nail

  S91.13 Puncture wound without foreign body of toe without damage to nail
   ⑦**S91.131** Puncture wound without foreign body of right great toe without damage to nail
   ⑦**S91.132** Puncture wound without foreign body of left great toe without damage to nail
   ⑦**S91.133** Puncture wound without foreign body of unspecified great toe without damage to nail
   ⑦**S91.134** Puncture wound without foreign body of right lesser toe(s) without damage to nail
   ⑦**S91.135** Puncture wound without foreign body of left lesser toe(s) without damage to nail
   ⑦**S91.136** Puncture wound without foreign body of unspecified lesser toe(s) without damage to nail
   ⑦**S91.139** Puncture wound without foreign body of unspecified toe(s) without damage to nail

  S91.14 Puncture wound with foreign body of toe without damage to nail
   ⑦**S91.141** Puncture wound with foreign body of right great toe without damage to nail

⑦S91.142   Puncture wound with foreign body of left great toe without damage to nail

⑦S91.143   Puncture wound with foreign body of unspecified great toe without damage to nail

⑦S91.144   Puncture wound with foreign body of right lesser toe(s) without damage to nail

⑦S91.145   Puncture wound with foreign body of left lesser toe(s) without damage to nail

⑦S91.146   Puncture wound with foreign body of unspecified lesser toe(s) without damage to nail

⑦S91.149   Puncture wound with foreign body of unspecified toe(s) without damage to nail

S91.15   Open bite of toe without damage to nail

Bite of toe NOS

Excludes1: superficial bite of toe (S90.46-, S90.47-)

⑦S91.151   Open bite of right great toe without damage to nail

⑦S91.152   Open bite of left great toe without damage to nail

⑦S91.153   Open bite of unspecified great toe without damage to nail

⑦S91.154   Open bite of right lesser toe(s) without damage to nail

⑦S91.155   Open bite of left lesser toe(s) without damage to nail

⑦S91.156   Open bite of unspecified lesser toe(s) without damage to nail

⑦S91.159   Open bite of unspecified toe(s) without damage to nail

S91.2   **Open wound of toe with damage to nail**

S91.20   Unspecified open wound of toe with damage to nail

⑦S91.201   Unspecified open wound of right great toe with damage to nail

⑦S91.202   Unspecified open wound of left great toe with damage to nail

⑦S91.203   Unspecified open wound of unspecified great toe with damage to nail

⑦S91.204   Unspecified open wound of right lesser toe(s) with damage to nail

⑦S91.205   Unspecified open wound of left lesser toe(s) with damage to nail

⑦S91.206   Unspecified open wound of unspecified lesser toe(s) with damage to nail

⑦S91.209   Unspecified open wound of unspecified toe(s) with damage to nail

S91.21   Laceration without foreign body of toe with damage to nail

⑦S91.211   Laceration without foreign body of right great toe with damage to nail

⑦S91.212   Laceration without foreign body of left great toe with damage to nail

⑦S91.213   Laceration without foreign body of unspecified great toe with damage to nail

⑦S91.214   Laceration without foreign body of right lesser toe(s) with damage to nail

⑦S91.215   Laceration without foreign body of left lesser toe(s) with damage to nail

⑦S91.216   Laceration without foreign body of unspecified lesser toe(s) with damage to nail

⑦S91.219   Laceration without foreign body of unspecified toe(s) with damage to nail

S91.22   Laceration with foreign body of toe with damage to nail

⑦S91.221   Laceration with foreign body of right great toe with damage to nail

⑦S91.222   Laceration with foreign body of left great toe with damage to nail

⑦S91.223   Laceration with foreign body of unspecified great toe with damage to nail

⑦S91.224   Laceration with foreign body of right lesser toe(s) with damage to nail

⑦S91.225   Laceration with foreign body of left lesser toe(s) with damage to nail

⑦S91.226   Laceration with foreign body of unspecified lesser toe(s) with damage to nail

⑦S91.229   Laceration with foreign body of unspecified toe(s) with damage to nail

S91.23   Puncture wound without foreign body of toe with damage to nail

⑦S91.231   Puncture wound without foreign body of right great toe with damage to nail

⑦S91.232   Puncture wound without foreign body of left great toe with damage to nail

⑦S91.233   Puncture wound without foreign body of unspecified great toe with damage to nail

⑦S91.234   Puncture wound without foreign body of right lesser toe(s) with damage to nail

⑦S91.235   Puncture wound without foreign body of left lesser toe(s) with damage to nail

⑦S91.236   Puncture wound without foreign body of unspecified lesser toe(s) with damage to nail

⑦S91.239   Puncture wound without foreign body of unspecified toe(s) with damage to nail

S91.24   Puncture wound with foreign body of toe with damage to nail

⑦S91.241   Puncture wound with foreign body of right great toe with damage to nail

⑦S91.242   Puncture wound with foreign body of left great toe with damage to nail

⑦**S91.243** Puncture wound with foreign body of unspecified great toe with damage to nail

⑦**S91.244** Puncture wound with foreign body of right lesser toe(s) with damage to nail

⑦**S91.245** Puncture wound with foreign body of left lesser toe(s) with damage to nail

⑦**S91.246** Puncture wound with foreign body of unspecified lesser toe(s) with damage to nail

⑦**S91.249** Puncture wound with foreign body of unspecified toe(s) with damage to nail

S91.25 Open bite of toe with damage to nail

Bite of toe with damage to nail NOS

Excludes1: superficial bite of toe (S90.46-, S90.47-)

⑦**S91.251** Open bite of right great toe with damage to nail

⑦**S91.252** Open bite of left great toe with damage to nail

⑦**S91.253** Open bite of unspecified great toe with damage to nail

⑦**S91.254** Open bite of right lesser toe(s) with damage to nail

⑦**S91.255** Open bite of left lesser toe(s) with damage to nail

⑦**S91.256** Open bite of unspecified lesser toe(s) with damage to nail

⑦**S91.259** Open bite of unspecified toe(s) with damage to nail

S91.3 Open wound of foot

S91.30 Unspecified open wound of foot

⑦**S91.301** Unspecified open wound, right foot

⑦**S91.302** Unspecified open wound, left foot

⑦**S91.309** Unspecified open wound, unspecified foot

S91.31 Laceration without foreign body of foot

⑦**S91.311** Laceration without foreign body, right foot

⑦**S91.312** Laceration without foreign body, left foot

⑦**S91.319** Laceration without foreign body, unspecified foot

S91.32 Laceration with foreign body of foot

⑦**S91.321** Laceration with foreign body, right foot

⑦**S91.322** Laceration with foreign body, left foot

⑦**S91.329** Laceration with foreign body, unspecified foot

S91.33 Puncture wound without foreign body of foot

⑦**S91.331** Puncture wound without foreign body, right foot

⑦**S91.332** Puncture wound without foreign body, left foot

⑦**S91.339** Puncture wound without foreign body, unspecified foot

S91.34 Puncture wound with foreign body of foot

⑦**S91.341** Puncture wound with foreign body, right foot

⑦**S91.342** Puncture wound with foreign body, left foot

⑦**S91.349** Puncture wound with foreign body, unspecified foot

S91.35 Open bite of foot

Excludes1: superficial bite of foot (S90.86-, S90.87-)

⑦**S91.351** Open bite, right foot

⑦**S91.352** Open bite, left foot

⑦**S91.359** Open bite, unspecified foot

S92 Fracture of foot and toe, except ankle

Note: A fracture not indicated as displaced or nondisplaced should be coded to displaced

A fracture not indicated as open or closed should be coded to closed

Excludes1: traumatic amputation of ankle and foot (S98.-)

Excludes2: fracture of ankle (S82.-)

fracture of malleolus (S82.-)

The appropriate 7th character is to be added to each code from category S92

A - initial encounter for closed fracture

B - initial encounter for open fracture

D - subsequent encounter for fracture with routine healing

G - subsequent encounter for fracture with delayed healing

K - subsequent encounter for fracture with nonunion

P - subsequent encounter for fracture with malunion

S - sequela

S92.0 Fracture of calcaneus

Heel bone Os calcis

Excludes2: Physeal fracture of calcaneus (S99.0-)

S92.00 Unspecified fracture of calcaneus

⑦**S92.001** Unspecified fracture of right calcaneus

⑦**S92.002** Unspecified fracture of left calcaneus

⑦**S92.009** Unspecified fracture of unspecified calcaneus

S92.01 Fracture of body of calcaneus

⑦**S92.011** Displaced fracture of body of right calcaneus

⑦**S92.012** Displaced fracture of body of left calcaneus

⑦**S92.013** Displaced fracture of body of unspecified calcaneus

⑦**S92.014** Nondisplaced fracture of body of right calcaneus

⑦**S92.015** Nondisplaced fracture of body of left calcaneus

⑦**S92.016** Nondisplaced fracture of body of unspecified calcaneus

S92.02 Fracture of anterior process of calcaneus

⑦**S92.021** Displaced fracture of anterior process of right calcaneus

⑦**S92.022** Displaced fracture of anterior process of left calcaneus

⑦**S92.023** Displaced fracture of anterior process of unspecified calcaneus

⑦S92.024 Nondisplaced fracture of anterior process of right calcaneus

⑦S92.025 Nondisplaced fracture of anterior process of left calcaneus

⑦S92.026 Nondisplaced fracture of anterior process of unspecified calcaneus

S92.03 Avulsion fracture of tuberosity of calcaneus

⑦S92.031 Displaced avulsion fracture of tuberosity of right calcaneus

⑦S92.032 Displaced avulsion fracture of tuberosity of left calcaneus

⑦S92.033 Displaced avulsion fracture of tuberosity of unspecified calcaneus

⑦S92.034 Nondisplaced avulsion fracture of tuberosity of right calcaneus

⑦S92.035 Nondisplaced avulsion fracture of tuberosity of left calcaneus

⑦S92.036 Nondisplaced avulsion fracture of tuberosity of unspecified calcaneus

S92.04 Other fracture of tuberosity of calcaneus

⑦S92.041 Displaced other fracture of tuberosity of right calcaneus

⑦S92.042 Displaced other fracture of tuberosity of left calcaneus

⑦S92.043 Displaced other fracture of tuberosity of unspecified calcaneus

⑦S92.044 Nondisplaced other fracture of tuberosity of right calcaneus

⑦S92.045 Nondisplaced other fracture of tuberosity of left calcaneus

⑦S92.046 Nondisplaced other fracture of tuberosity of unspecified calcaneus

S92.05 Other extraarticular fracture of calcaneus

⑦S92.051 Displaced other extraarticular fracture of right calcaneus

⑦S92.052 Displaced other extraarticular fracture of left calcaneus

⑦S92.053 Displaced other extraarticular fracture of unspecified calcaneus

⑦S92.054 Nondisplaced other extraarticular fracture of right calcaneus

⑦S92.055 Nondisplaced other extraarticular fracture of left calcaneus

⑦S92.056 Nondisplaced other extraarticular fracture of unspecified calcaneus

S92.06 Intraarticular fracture of calcaneus

⑦S92.061 Displaced intraarticular fracture of right calcaneus

⑦S92.062 Displaced intraarticular fracture of left calcaneus

⑦S92.063 Displaced intraarticular fracture of unspecified calcaneus

⑦S92.064 Nondisplaced intraarticular fracture of right calcaneus

⑦S92.065 Nondisplaced intraarticular fracture of left calcaneus

⑦S92.066 Nondisplaced intraarticular fracture of unspecified calcaneus

S92.1 Fracture of talus
Astragalus

S92.10 Unspecified fracture of talus

⑦S92.101 Unspecified fracture of right talus

⑦S92.102 Unspecified fracture of left talus

⑦S92.109 Unspecified fracture of unspecified talus

S92.11 Fracture of neck of talus

⑦S92.111 Displaced fracture of neck of right talus

⑦S92.112 Displaced fracture of neck of left talus

⑦S92.113 Displaced fracture of neck of unspecified talus

⑦S92.114 Nondisplaced fracture of neck of right talus

⑦S92.115 Nondisplaced fracture of neck of left talus

⑦S92.116 Nondisplaced fracture of neck of unspecified talus

S92.12 Fracture of body of talus

⑦S92.121 Displaced fracture of body of right talus

⑦S92.122 Displaced fracture of body of left talus

⑦S92.123 Displaced fracture of body of unspecified talus

⑦S92.124 Nondisplaced fracture of body of right talus

⑦S92.125 Nondisplaced fracture of body of left talus

⑦S92.126 Nondisplaced fracture of body of unspecified talus

S92.13 Fracture of posterior process of talus

⑦S92.131 Displaced fracture of posterior process of right talus

⑦S92.132 Displaced fracture of posterior process of left talus

⑦S92.133 Displaced fracture of posterior process of unspecified talus

⑦S92.134 Nondisplaced fracture of posterior process of right talus

⑦S92.135 Nondisplaced fracture of posterior process of left talus

⑦S92.136 Nondisplaced fracture of posterior process of unspecified talus

S92.14 Dome fracture of talus

Excludes1: osteochondritis dissecans (M93.2)

⑦S92.141 Displaced dome fracture of right talus

⑦S92.142 Displaced dome fracture of left talus

⑦S92.143 Displaced dome fracture of unspecified talus

⑦S92.144 Nondisplaced dome fracture of right talus

⑦S92.145 Nondisplaced dome fracture of left talus

⑦S92.146 Nondisplaced dome fracture of unspecified talus

S92.15 Avulsion fracture (chip fracture) of talus

⑦S92.151 Displaced avulsion fracture (chip fracture) of right talus

⑦ S92.152   Displaced avulsion fracture (chip fracture) of left talus

⑦ S92.153   Displaced avulsion fracture (chip fracture) of unspecified talus

⑦ S92.154   Nondisplaced avulsion fracture (chip fracture) of right talus

⑦ S92.155   Nondisplaced avulsion fracture (chip fracture) of left talus

⑦ S92.156   Nondisplaced avulsion fracture (chip fracture) of unspecified talus

S92.19   Other fracture of talus

⑦ S92.191   Other fracture of right talus

⑦ S92.192   Other fracture of left talus

⑦ S92.199   Other fracture of unspecified talus

S92.2   Fracture of other and unspecified tarsal bone(s)

S92.20   Fracture of unspecified tarsal bone(s)

⑦ S92.201   Fracture of unspecified tarsal bone(s) of right foot

⑦ S92.202   Fracture of unspecified tarsal bone(s) of left foot

⑦ S92.209   Fracture of unspecified tarsal bone(s) of unspecified foot

S92.21   Fracture of cuboid bone

⑦ S92.211   Displaced fracture of cuboid bone of right foot

⑦ S92.212   Displaced fracture of cuboid bone of left foot

⑦ S92.213   Displaced fracture of cuboid bone of unspecified foot

⑦ S92.214   Nondisplaced fracture of cuboid bone of right foot

⑦ S92.215   Nondisplaced fracture of cuboid bone of left foot

⑦ S92.216   Nondisplaced fracture of cuboid bone of unspecified foot

S92.22   Fracture of lateral cuneiform

⑦ S92.221   Displaced fracture of lateral cuneiform of right foot

⑦ S92.222   Displaced fracture of lateral cuneiform of left foot

⑦ S92.223   Displaced fracture of lateral cuneiform of unspecified foot

⑦ S92.224   Nondisplaced fracture of lateral cuneiform of right foot

⑦ S92.225   Nondisplaced fracture of lateral cuneiform of left foot

⑦ S92.226   Nondisplaced fracture of lateral cuneiform of unspecified foot

S92.23   Fracture of intermediate cuneiform

⑦ S92.231   Displaced fracture of intermediate cuneiform of right foot

⑦ S92.232   Displaced fracture of intermediate cuneiform of left foot

⑦ S92.233   Displaced fracture of intermediate cuneiform of unspecified foot

⑦ S92.234   Nondisplaced fracture of intermediate cuneiform of right foot

⑦ S92.235   Nondisplaced fracture of intermediate cuneiform of left foot

⑦ S92.236   Nondisplaced fracture of intermediate cuneiform of unspecified foot

S92.24   Fracture of medial cuneiform

⑦ S92.241   Displaced fracture of medial cuneiform of right foot

⑦ S92.242   Displaced fracture of medial cuneiform of left foot

⑦ S92.243   Displaced fracture of medial cuneiform of unspecified foot

⑦ S92.244   Nondisplaced fracture of medial cuneiform of right foot

⑦ S92.245   Nondisplaced fracture of medial cuneiform of left foot

⑦ S92.246   Nondisplaced fracture of medial cuneiform of unspecified foot

S92.25   Fracture of navicular [scaphoid] of foot

⑦ S92.251   Displaced fracture of navicular [scaphoid] of right foot

⑦ S92.252   Displaced fracture of navicular [scaphoid] of left foot

⑦ S92.253   Displaced fracture of navicular [scaphoid] of unspecified foot

⑦ S92.254   Nondisplaced fracture of navicular [scaphoid] of right foot

⑦ S92.255   Nondisplaced fracture of navicular [scaphoid] of left foot

⑦ S92.256   Nondisplaced fracture of navicular [scaphoid] of unspecified foot

S92.3   Fracture of metatarsal bone(s)

Excludes2: Physeal fracture of metatarsal (S99.1-)

S92.30   Fracture of unspecified metatarsal bone(s)

⑦ S92.301   Fracture of unspecified metatarsal bone(s), right foot

⑦ S92.302   Fracture of unspecified metatarsal bone(s), left foot

⑦ S92.309   Fracture of unspecified metatarsal bone(s), unspecified foot

S92.31   Fracture of first metatarsal bone

⑦ S92.311   Displaced fracture of first metatarsal bone, right foot

⑦ S92.312   Displaced fracture of first metatarsal bone, left foot

⑦ S92.313   Displaced fracture of first metatarsal bone, unspecified foot

⑦ S92.314   Nondisplaced fracture of first metatarsal bone, right foot

⑦ S92.315   Nondisplaced fracture of first metatarsal bone, left foot

⑦ S92.316   Nondisplaced fracture of first metatarsal bone, unspecified foot

S92.32   Fracture of second metatarsal bone

⑦ S92.321   Displaced fracture of second metatarsal bone, right foot

⑦ S92.322   Displaced fracture of second metatarsal bone, left foot

⑦ S92.323   Displaced fracture of second metatarsal bone, unspecified foot

⑦ S92.324   Nondisplaced fracture of second metatarsal bone, right foot

⑦S92.325 Nondisplaced fracture of second metatarsal bone, left foot

⑦S92.326 Nondisplaced fracture of second metatarsal bone, unspecified foot

S92.33 Fracture of third metatarsal bone

⑦S92.331 Displaced fracture of third metatarsal bone, right foot

⑦S92.332 Displaced fracture of third metatarsal bone, left foot

⑦S92.333 Displaced fracture of third metatarsal bone, unspecified foot

⑦S92.334 Nondisplaced fracture of third metatarsal bone, right foot

⑦S92.335 Nondisplaced fracture of third metatarsal bone, left foot

⑦S92.336 Nondisplaced fracture of third metatarsal bone, unspecified foot

S92.34 Fracture of fourth metatarsal bone

⑦S92.341 Displaced fracture of fourth metatarsal bone, right foot

⑦S92.342 Displaced fracture of fourth metatarsal bone, left foot

⑦S92.343 Displaced fracture of fourth metatarsal bone, unspecified foot

⑦S92.344 Nondisplaced fracture of fourth metatarsal bone, right foot

⑦S92.345 Nondisplaced fracture of fourth metatarsal bone, left foot

⑦S92.346 Nondisplaced fracture of fourth metatarsal bone, unspecified foot

S92.35 Fracture of fifth metatarsal bone

⑦S92.351 Displaced fracture of fifth metatarsal bone, right foot

⑦S92.352 Displaced fracture of fifth metatarsal bone, left foot

⑦S92.353 Displaced fracture of fifth metatarsal bone, unspecified foot

⑦S92.354 Nondisplaced fracture of fifth metatarsal bone, right foot

⑦S92.355 Nondisplaced fracture of fifth metatarsal bone, left foot

⑦S92.356 Nondisplaced fracture of fifth metatarsal bone, unspecified foot

S92.4 Fracture of great toe

Excludes2: Physeal fracture of phalanx of toe (S99.2-)

S92.40 Unspecified fracture of great toe

⑦S92.401 Displaced unspecified fracture of right great toe

⑦S92.402 Displaced unspecified fracture of left great toe

⑦S92.403 Displaced unspecified fracture of unspecified great toe

⑦S92.404 Nondisplaced unspecified fracture of right great toe

⑦S92.405 Nondisplaced unspecified fracture of left great toe

⑦S92.406 Nondisplaced unspecified fracture of unspecified great toe

S92.41 Fracture of proximal phalanx of great toe

⑦S92.411 Displaced fracture of proximal phalanx of right great toe

⑦S92.412 Displaced fracture of proximal phalanx of left great toe

⑦S92.413 Displaced fracture of proximal phalanx of unspecified great toe

⑦S92.414 Nondisplaced fracture of proximal phalanx of right great toe

⑦S92.415 Nondisplaced fracture of proximal phalanx of left great toe

⑦S92.416 Nondisplaced fracture of proximal phalanx of unspecified great toe

S92.42 Fracture of distal phalanx of great toe

⑦S92.421 Displaced fracture of distal phalanx of right great toe

⑦S92.422 Displaced fracture of distal phalanx of left great toe

⑦S92.423 Displaced fracture of distal phalanx of unspecified great toe

⑦S92.424 Nondisplaced fracture of distal phalanx of right great toe

⑦S92.425 Nondisplaced fracture of distal phalanx of left great toe

⑦S92.426 Nondisplaced fracture of distal phalanx of unspecified great toe

S92.49 Other fracture of great toe

⑦S92.491 Other fracture of right great toe

⑦S92.492 Other fracture of left great toe

⑦S92.499 Other fracture of unspecified great toe

S92.5 Fracture of lesser toe(s)

Excludes2: Physeal fracture of phalanx of toe (S99.2-)

S92.50 Unspecified fracture of lesser toe(s)

⑦S92.501 Displaced unspecified fracture of right lesser toe(s)

⑦S92.502 Displaced unspecified fracture of left lesser toe(s)

⑦S92.503 Displaced unspecified fracture of unspecified lesser toe(s)

⑦S92.504 Nondisplaced unspecified fracture of right lesser toe(s)

⑦S92.505 Nondisplaced unspecified fracture of left lesser toe(s)

⑦S92.506 Nondisplaced unspecified fracture of unspecified lesser toe(s)

S92.51 Fracture of proximal phalanx of lesser toe(s)

⑦S92.511 Displaced fracture of proximal phalanx of right lesser toe(s)

⑦S92.512 Displaced fracture of proximal phalanx of left lesser toe(s)

⑦S92.513 Displaced fracture of proximal phalanx of unspecified lesser toe(s)

⑦S92.514 Nondisplaced fracture of proximal phalanx of right lesser toe(s)

⑦S92.515 Nondisplaced fracture of proximal phalanx of left lesser toe(s)

⑦S92.516 Nondisplaced fracture of proximal phalanx of unspecified lesser toe(s)

S92.52 Fracture of medial phalanx of lesser toe(s)

Add 4th-7th digits   Nonspecific code   Unspecified code   Manifestation code   909

⑦ **S92.521**   **Displaced fracture of medial phalanx of right lesser toe(s)**

⑦ **S92.522**   **Displaced fracture of medial phalanx of left lesser toe(s)**

⑦ **S92.523**   **Displaced fracture of medial phalanx of unspecified lesser toe(s)**

⑦ **S92.524**   **Nondisplaced fracture of medial phalanx of right lesser toe(s)**

⑦ **S92.525**   **Nondisplaced fracture of medial phalanx of left lesser toe(s)**

⑦ **S92.526**   **Nondisplaced fracture of medial phalanx of unspecified lesser toe(s)**

S92.53   **Fracture of distal phalanx of lesser toe(s)**

⑦ **S92.531**   **Displaced fracture of distal phalanx of right lesser toe(s)**

⑦ **S92.532**   **Displaced fracture of distal phalanx of left lesser toe(s)**

⑦ **S92.533**   **Displaced fracture of distal phalanx of unspecified lesser toe(s)**

⑦ **S92.534**   **Nondisplaced fracture of distal phalanx of right lesser toe(s)**

⑦ **S92.535**   **Nondisplaced fracture of distal phalanx of left lesser toe(s)**

⑦ **S92.536**   **Nondisplaced fracture of distal phalanx of unspecified lesser toe(s)**

S92.59   **Other fracture of lesser toe(s)**

⑦ **S92.591**   **Other fracture of right lesser toe(s)**

⑦ **S92.592**   **Other fracture of left lesser toe(s)**

⑦ **S92.599**   **Other fracture of unspecified lesser toe(s)**

S92.8   **Other fracture of foot, except ankle**

S92.81   **Other fracture of foot**

Sesamoid fracture of foot

● ⑦ **S92.811**   **Other fracture of right foot**

● ⑦ **S92.812**   **Other fracture of left foot**

● ⑦ **S92.819**   **Other fracture of unspecified foot**

S92.9   **Unspecified fracture of foot and toe**

S92.90   **Unspecified fracture of foot**

⑦ **S92.901**   **Unspecified fracture of right foot**

⑦ **S92.902**   **Unspecified fracture of left foot**

⑦ **S92.909**   **Unspecified fracture of unspecified foot**

S92.91   **Unspecified fracture of toe**

⑦ **S92.911**   **Unspecified fracture of right toe(s)**

⑦ **S92.912**   **Unspecified fracture of left toe(s)**

⑦ **S92.919**   **Unspecified fracture of unspecified toe(s)**

S93   **Dislocation and sprain of joints and ligaments at ankle, foot and toe level**

Includes: avulsion of joint or ligament of ankle, foot and toe

laceration of cartilage, joint or ligament of ankle, foot and toe

sprain of cartilage, joint or ligament of ankle, foot and toe

traumatic hemarthrosis of joint or ligament of ankle, foot and toe

traumatic rupture of joint or ligament of ankle, foot and toe

traumatic subluxation of joint or ligament of ankle, foot and toe

traumatic tear of joint or ligament of ankle, foot and toe

Code also any associated open wound

Excludes2: strain of muscle and tendon of ankle and foot (S96.-)

The appropriate 7th character is to be added to each code from category S93

A - initial encounter

D - subsequent encounter

S - sequela

S93.0   **Subluxation and dislocation of ankle joint**

Subluxation and dislocation of astragalus Subluxation and dislocation of fibula, lower end Subluxation and dislocation of talus Subluxation and dislocation of tibia, lower end

⊗⑦ **S93.01**   **Subluxation of right ankle joint**

⊗⑦ **S93.02**   **Subluxation of left ankle joint**

⊗⑦ **S93.03**   **Subluxation of unspecified ankle joint**

⊗⑦ **S93.04**   **Dislocation of right ankle joint**

⊗⑦ **S93.05**   **Dislocation of left ankle joint**

⊗⑦ **S93.06**   **Dislocation of unspecified ankle joint**

S93.1   **Subluxation and dislocation of toe**

S93.10   **Unspecified subluxation and dislocation of toe**

Dislocation of toe NOS Subluxation of toe NOS

⑦ **S93.101**   **Unspecified subluxation of right toe(s)**

⑦ **S93.102**   **Unspecified subluxation of left toe(s)**

⑦ **S93.103**   **Unspecified subluxation of unspecified toe(s)**

⑦ **S93.104**   **Unspecified dislocation of right toe(s)**

⑦ **S93.105**   **Unspecified dislocation of left toe(s)**

⑦ **S93.106**   **Unspecified dislocation of unspecified toe(s)**

S93.11   **Dislocation of interphalangeal joint**

⑦ **S93.111**   **Dislocation of interphalangeal joint of right great toe**

⑦ **S93.112**   **Dislocation of interphalangeal joint of left great toe**

⑦ **S93.113**   **Dislocation of interphalangeal joint of unspecified great toe**

⑦ **S93.114**   **Dislocation of interphalangeal joint of right lesser toe(s)**

⑦ **S93.115**   **Dislocation of interphalangeal joint of left lesser toe(s)**

⑦ **S93.116**   **Dislocation of interphalangeal joint of unspecified lesser toe(s)**

⑦ **S93.119**   **Dislocation of interphalangeal joint of unspecified toe(s)**

⑦ **S93.12 Dislocation of metatarsophalangeal joint**

⑦ **S93.121**   **Dislocation of metatarsophalangeal joint of right great toe**

⑦ **S93.122**   **Dislocation of metatarsophalangeal joint of left great toe**

⑦ **S93.123**   **Dislocation of metatarsophalangeal joint of unspecified great toe**

⑦ **S93.124**   **Dislocation of metatarsophalangeal joint of right lesser toe(s)**

⑦ **S93.125**   **Dislocation of metatarsophalangeal joint of left lesser toe(s)**

   ● New code   ▲ Revised code   **Excludes1:** Not coded here   **Excludes2:** Not included here   ⊗ Placeholder required   ⑦ 7th digit required

⑦S93.126 Dislocation of metatarsophalangeal joint of unspecified lesser toe(s)

⑦S93.129 Dislocation of metatarsophalangeal joint of unspecified toe(s)

S93.13 Subluxation of interphalangeal joint

⑦S93.131 Subluxation of interphalangeal joint of right great toe

⑦S93.132 Subluxation of interphalangeal joint of left great toe

⑦S93.133 Subluxation of interphalangeal joint of unspecified great toe

⑦S93.134 Subluxation of interphalangeal joint of right lesser toe(s)

⑦S93.135 Subluxation of interphalangeal joint of left lesser toe(s)

⑦S93.136 Subluxation of interphalangeal joint of unspecified lesser toe(s)

⑦S93.139 Subluxation of interphalangeal joint of unspecified toe(s)

S93.14 Subluxation of metatarsophalangeal joint

⑦S93.141 Subluxation of metatarsophalangeal joint of right great toe

⑦S93.142 Subluxation of metatarsophalangeal joint of left great toe

⑦S93.143 Subluxation of metatarsophalangeal joint of unspecified great toe

⑦S93.144 Subluxation of metatarsophalangeal joint of right lesser toe(s)

⑦S93.145 Subluxation of metatarsophalangeal joint of left lesser toe(s)

⑦S93.146 Subluxation of metatarsophalangeal joint of unspecified lesser toe(s)

⑦S93.149 Subluxation of metatarsophalangeal joint of unspecified toe(s)

S93.3 Subluxation and dislocation of foot

Excludes2: dislocation of toe (S93.1-)

S93.30 Unspecified subluxation and dislocation of foot

Dislocation of foot NOS

Subluxation of foot NOS

⑦S93.301 Unspecified subluxation of right foot

⑦S93.302 Unspecified subluxation of left foot

⑦S93.303 Unspecified subluxation of unspecified foot

⑦S93.304 Unspecified dislocation of right foot

⑦S93.305 Unspecified dislocation of left foot

⑦S93.306 Unspecified dislocation of unspecified foot

S93.31 Subluxation and dislocation of tarsal joint

⑦S93.311 Subluxation of tarsal joint of right foot

⑦S93.312 Subluxation of tarsal joint of left foot

⑦S93.313 Subluxation of tarsal joint of unspecified foot

⑦S93.314 Dislocation of tarsal joint of right foot

⑦S93.315 Dislocation of tarsal joint of left foot

⑦S93.316 Dislocation of tarsal joint of unspecified foot

S93.32 Subluxation and dislocation of tarsometatarsal joint

⑦S93.321 Subluxation of tarsometatarsal joint of right foot

⑦S93.322 Subluxation of tarsometatarsal joint of left foot

⑦S93.323 Subluxation of tarsometatarsal joint of unspecified foot

⑦S93.324 Dislocation of tarsometatarsal joint of right foot

⑦S93.325 Dislocation of tarsometatarsal joint of left foot

⑦S93.326 Dislocation of tarsometatarsal joint of unspecified foot

S93.33 Other subluxation and dislocation of foot

⑦S93.331 Other subluxation of right foot

⑦S93.332 Other subluxation of left foot

⑦S93.333 Other subluxation of unspecified foot

⑦S93.334 Other dislocation of right foot

⑦S93.335 Other dislocation of left foot

⑦S93.336 Other dislocation of unspecified foot

S93.4 Sprain of ankle

Excludes2: injury of Achilles tendon (S86.0-)

S93.40 Sprain of unspecified ligament of ankle

Sprain of ankle NOS

Sprained ankle NOS

⑦S93.401 Sprain of unspecified ligament of right ankle

⑦S93.402 Sprain of unspecified ligament of left ankle

⑦S93.409 Sprain of unspecified ligament of unspecified ankle

S93.41 Sprain of calcaneofibular ligament

⑦S93.411 Sprain of calcaneofibular ligament of right ankle

⑦S93.412 Sprain of calcaneofibular ligament of left ankle

⑦S93.419 Sprain of calcaneofibular ligament of unspecified ankle

S93.42 Sprain of deltoid ligament

⑦S93.421 Sprain of deltoid ligament of right ankle

⑦S93.422 Sprain of deltoid ligament of left ankle

⑦S93.429 Sprain of deltoid ligament of unspecified ankle

S93.43 Sprain of tibiofibular ligament

⑦S93.431 Sprain of tibiofibular ligament of right ankle

⑦S93.432 Sprain of tibiofibular ligament of left ankle

⑦S93.439 Sprain of tibiofibular ligament of unspecified ankle

S93.49 Sprain of other ligament of ankle

Sprain of internal collateral ligament

Sprain of talofibular ligament

⑦S93.491 Sprain of other ligament of right ankle

⑦S93.492   **Sprain of other ligament of left ankle**

⑦S93.499   **Sprain of other ligament of unspecified ankle**

S93.5   Sprain of toe

     S93.50   Unspecified sprain of toe

         ⑦S93.501   **Unspecified sprain of right great toe**

         ⑦S93.502   **Unspecified sprain of left great toe**

         ⑦S93.503   **Unspecified sprain of unspecified great toe**

         ⑦S93.504   **Unspecified sprain of right lesser toe(s)**

         ⑦S93.505   **Unspecified sprain of left lesser toe(s)**

         ⑦S93.506   **Unspecified sprain of unspecified lesser toe(s)**

         ⑦S93.509   **Unspecified sprain of unspecified toe(s)**

     S93.51   Sprain of interphalangeal joint of toe

         ⑦S93.511   **Sprain of interphalangeal joint of right great toe**

         ⑦S93.512   **Sprain of interphalangeal joint of left great toe**

         ⑦S93.513   **Sprain of interphalangeal joint of unspecified great toe**

         ⑦S93.514   **Sprain of interphalangeal joint of right lesser toe(s)**

         ⑦S93.515   **Sprain of interphalangeal joint of left lesser toe(s)**

         ⑦S93.516   **Sprain of interphalangeal joint of unspecified lesser toe(s)**

         ⑦S93.519   **Sprain of interphalangeal joint of unspecified toe(s)**

     S93.52   Sprain of metatarsophalangeal joint of toe

         ⑦S93.521   **Sprain of metatarsophalangeal joint of right great toe**

         ⑦S93.522   **Sprain of metatarsophalangeal joint of left great toe**

         ⑦S93.523   **Sprain of metatarsophalangeal joint of unspecified great toe**

         ⑦S93.524   **Sprain of metatarsophalangeal joint of right lesser toe(s)**

         ⑦S93.525   **Sprain of metatarsophalangeal joint of left lesser toe(s)**

         ⑦S93.526   **Sprain of metatarsophalangeal joint of unspecified lesser toe(s)**

         ⑦S93.529   **Sprain of metatarsophalangeal joint of unspecified toe(s)**

S93.6   Sprain of foot

     Excludes2: sprain of metatarsophalangeal joint of toe (S93.52-)

         sprain of toe (S93.5-)

     S93.60   Unspecified sprain of foot

         ⑦S93.601   **Unspecified sprain of right foot**

         ⑦S93.602   **Unspecified sprain of left foot**

         ⑦S93.609   **Unspecified sprain of unspecified foot**

     S93.61   Sprain of tarsal ligament of foot

         ⑦S93.611   **Sprain of tarsal ligament of right foot**

⑦S93.612   **Sprain of tarsal ligament of left foot**

⑦S93.619   **Sprain of tarsal ligament of unspecified foot**

     S93.62   Sprain of tarsometatarsal ligament of foot

         ⑦S93.621   **Sprain of tarsometatarsal ligament of right foot**

         ⑦S93.622   **Sprain of tarsometatarsal ligament of left foot**

         ⑦S93.629   **Sprain of tarsometatarsal ligament of unspecified foot**

     S93.69   Other sprain of foot

         ⑦S93.691   **Other sprain of right foot**

         ⑦S93.692   **Other sprain of left foot**

         ⑦S93.699   **Other sprain of unspecified foot**

S94   Injury of nerves at ankle and foot level

     <u>**Code also**</u> any associated open wound (S91.-)

     The appropriate 7th character is to be added to each code from category S94

     A - initial encounter

     D - subsequent encounter

     S - sequela

     S94.0   Injury of lateral plantar nerve

         ⊗S94.00   **Injury of lateral plantar nerve, unspecified leg**

         ⊗⑦S94.01   **Injury of lateral plantar nerve, right leg**

         ⊗⑦S94.02   **Injury of lateral plantar nerve, left leg**

     S94.1   Injury of medial plantar nerve

         ⊗⑦S94.10   **Injury of medial plantar nerve, unspecified leg**

         ⊗⑦S94.11   **Injury of medial plantar nerve, right leg**

         ⊗⑦S94.12   **Injury of medial plantar nerve, left leg**

     S94.2   Injury of deep peroneal nerve at ankle and foot level

         Injury of terminal, lateral branch of deep peroneal nerve

         ⊗⑦S94.20   **Injury of deep peroneal nerve at ankle and foot level, unspecified leg**

         ⊗⑦S94.21   **Injury of deep peroneal nerve at ankle and foot level, right leg**

         ⊗⑦S94.22   **Injury of deep peroneal nerve at ankle and foot level, left leg**

     S94.3   Injury of cutaneous sensory nerve at ankle and foot level

         ⊗⑦S94.30   **Injury of cutaneous sensory nerve at ankle and foot level, unspecified leg**

         ⊗⑦S94.31   **Injury of cutaneous sensory nerve at ankle and foot level, right leg**

         ⊗⑦S94.32   **Injury of cutaneous sensory nerve at ankle and foot level, left leg**

     S94.8   Injury of other nerves at ankle and foot level

     S94.8X   Injury of other nerves at ankle and foot level

         ⑦S94.8X1   **Injury of other nerves at ankle and foot level, right leg**

         ⑦S94.8X2   **Injury of other nerves at ankle and foot level, left leg**

         ⑦S94.8X9   **Injury of other nerves at ankle and foot level, unspecified leg**

     S94.9   Injury of unspecified nerve at ankle and foot level

         ⊗⑦S94.90   **Injury of unspecified nerve at ankle and foot level, unspecified leg**

         ⊗⑦S94.91   **Injury of unspecified nerve at ankle and foot level, right leg**

   ●   New code   ▲   Revised code   **Excludes1:** Not coded here   **Excludes2:** Not included here   ⊗ Placeholder required   ⑦7ᵗʰ digit required

⊗⑦**S94.92** **Injury of unspecified nerve at ankle and foot level, left leg**

S95 **Injury of blood vessels at ankle and foot level**

Code also any associated open wound (S91.-)

Excludes2: injury of posterior tibial artery and vein (S85.1-, S85.8-)

The appropriate 7th character is to be added to each code from category S95

A - initial encounter

D - subsequent encounter

S - sequela

S95.0 **Injury of dorsal artery of foot**

S95.00 **Unspecified injury of dorsal artery of foot**

⑦**S95.001** **Unspecified injury of dorsal artery of right foot**

⑦**S95.002** **Unspecified injury of dorsal artery of left foot**

⑦**S95.009** **Unspecified injury of dorsal artery of unspecified foot**

S95.01 **Laceration of dorsal artery of foot**

⑦**S95.011** **Laceration of dorsal artery of right foot**

⑦**S95.012** **Laceration of dorsal artery of left foot**

⑦**S95.019** **Laceration of dorsal artery of unspecified foot**

S95.09 **Other specified injury of dorsal artery of foot**

⑦**S95.091** **Other specified injury of dorsal artery of right foot**

⑦**S95.092** **Other specified injury of dorsal artery of left foot**

⑦**S95.099** **Other specified injury of dorsal artery of unspecified foot**

S95.1 **Injury of plantar artery of foot**

S95.10 **Unspecified injury of plantar artery of foot**

⑦**S95.101** **Unspecified injury of plantar artery of right foot**

⑦**S95.102** **Unspecified injury of plantar artery of left foot**

⑦**S95.109** **Unspecified injury of plantar artery of unspecified foot**

S95.11 **Laceration of plantar artery of foot**

⑦**S95.111** **Laceration of plantar artery of right foot**

⑦**S95.112** **Laceration of plantar artery of left foot**

⑦**S95.119** **Laceration of plantar artery of unspecified foot**

S95.19 **Other specified injury of plantar artery of foot**

⑦**S95.191** **Other specified injury of plantar artery of right foot**

⑦**S95.192** **Other specified injury of plantar artery of left foot**

⑦**S95.199** **Other specified injury of plantar artery of unspecified foot**

S95.2 **Injury of dorsal vein of foot**

S95.20 **Unspecified injury of dorsal vein of foot**

⑦**S95.201** **Unspecified injury of dorsal vein of right foot**

⑦**S95.202** **Unspecified injury of dorsal vein of left foot**

⑦**S95.209** **Unspecified injury of dorsal vein of unspecified foot**

S95.21 **Laceration of dorsal vein of foot**

⑦**S95.211** **Laceration of dorsal vein of right foot**

⑦**S95.212** **Laceration of dorsal vein of left foot**

⑦**S95.219** **Laceration of dorsal vein of unspecified foot**

S95.29 **Other specified injury of dorsal vein of foot**

⑦**S95.291** **Other specified injury of dorsal vein of right foot**

⑦**S95.292** **Other specified injury of dorsal vein of left foot**

⑦**S95.299** **Other specified injury of dorsal vein of unspecified foot**

S95.8 **Injury of other blood vessels at ankle and foot level**

S95.80 **Unspecified injury of other blood vessels at ankle and foot level**

⑦**S95.801** **Unspecified injury of other blood vessels at ankle and foot level, right leg**

⑦**S95.802** **Unspecified injury of other blood vessels at ankle and foot level, left leg**

⑦**S95.809** **Unspecified injury of other blood vessels at ankle and foot level, unspecified leg**

S95.81 **Laceration of other blood vessels at ankle and foot level**

⑦**S95.811** **Laceration of other blood vessels at ankle and foot level, right leg**

⑦**S95.812** **Laceration of other blood vessels at ankle and foot level, left leg**

⑦**S95.819** **Laceration of other blood vessels at ankle and foot level, unspecified leg**

S95.89 **Other specified injury of other blood vessels at ankle and foot level**

⑦**S95.891** **Other specified injury of other blood vessels at ankle and foot level, right leg**

⑦**S95.892** **Other specified injury of other blood vessels at ankle and foot level, left leg**

⑦**S95.899** **Other specified injury of other blood vessels at ankle and foot level, unspecified leg**

S95.9 **Injury of unspecified blood vessel at ankle and foot level**

S95.90 **Unspecified injury of unspecified blood vessel at ankle and foot level**

⑦**S95.901** **Unspecified injury of unspecified blood vessel at ankle and foot level, right leg**

⑦**S95.902** **Unspecified injury of unspecified blood vessel at ankle and foot level, left leg**

⑦**S95.909** **Unspecified injury of unspecified blood vessel at ankle and foot level, unspecified leg**

S95.91 **Laceration of unspecified blood vessel at ankle and foot level**

⑦ **S95.911** Laceration of unspecified blood vessel at ankle and foot level, right leg

⑦ **S95.912** Laceration of unspecified blood vessel at ankle and foot level, left leg

⑦ **S95.919** Laceration of unspecified blood vessel at ankle and foot level, unspecified leg

S95.99 Other specified injury of unspecified blood vessel at ankle and foot level

⑦ **S95.991** Other specified injury of unspecified blood vessel at ankle and foot level, right leg

⑦ **S95.992** Other specified injury of unspecified blood vessel at ankle and foot level, left leg

⑦ **S95.999** Other specified injury of unspecified blood vessel at ankle and foot level, unspecified leg

S96 **Injury of muscle and tendon at ankle and foot level**

Code also any associated open wound (S91.-)

Excludes2: injury of Achilles tendon (S86.0-)

sprain of joints and ligaments of ankle and foot (S93.-)

The appropriate 7th character is to be added to each code from category S96

A - initial encounter

D - subsequent encounter

S - sequela

S96.0 **Injury of muscle and tendon of long flexor muscle of toe at ankle and foot level**

S96.00 Unspecified injury of muscle and tendon of long flexor muscle of toe at ankle and foot level

⑦ **S96.001** Unspecified injury of muscle and tendon of long flexor muscle of toe at ankle and foot level, right foot

⑦ **S96.002** Unspecified injury of muscle and tendon of long flexor muscle of toe at ankle and foot level, left foot

⑦ **S96.009** Unspecified injury of muscle and tendon of long flexor muscle of toe at ankle and foot level, unspecified foot

S96.01 Strain of muscle and tendon of long flexor muscle of toe at ankle and foot level

⑦ **S96.011** Strain of muscle and tendon of long flexor muscle of toe at ankle and foot level, right foot

⑦ **S96.012** Strain of muscle and tendon of long flexor muscle of toe at ankle and foot level, left foot

⑦ **S96.019** Strain of muscle and tendon of long flexor muscle of toe at ankle and foot level, unspecified foot

S96.02 Laceration of muscle and tendon of long flexor muscle of toe at ankle and foot level

⑦ **S96.021** Laceration of muscle and tendon of long flexor muscle of toe at ankle and foot level, right foot

⑦ **S96.022** Laceration of muscle and tendon of long flexor muscle of toe at ankle and foot level, left foot

⑦ **S96.029** Laceration of muscle and tendon of long flexor muscle of toe at ankle and foot level, unspecified foot

S96.09 Other injury of muscle and tendon of long flexor muscle of toe at ankle and foot level

⑦ **S96.091** Other injury of muscle and tendon of long flexor muscle of toe at ankle and foot level, right foot

⑦ **S96.092** Other injury of muscle and tendon of long flexor muscle of toe at ankle and foot level, left foot

⑦ **S96.099** Other injury of muscle and tendon of long flexor muscle of toe at ankle and foot level, unspecified foot

S96.1 **Injury of muscle and tendon of long extensor muscle of toe at ankle and foot level**

S96.10 Unspecified injury of muscle and tendon of long extensor muscle of toe at ankle and foot level

⑦ **S96.101** Unspecified injury of muscle and tendon of long extensor muscle of toe at ankle and foot level, right foot

⑦ **S96.102** Unspecified injury of muscle and tendon of long extensor muscle of toe at ankle and foot level, left foot

⑦ **S96.109** Unspecified injury of muscle and tendon of long extensor muscle of toe at ankle and foot level, unspecified foot

S96.11 Strain of muscle and tendon of long extensor muscle of toe at ankle and foot level

⑦ **S96.111** Strain of muscle and tendon of long extensor muscle of toe at ankle and foot level, right foot

⑦ **S96.112** Strain of muscle and tendon of long extensor muscle of toe at ankle and foot level, left foot

⑦ **S96.119** Strain of muscle and tendon of long extensor muscle of toe at ankle and foot level, unspecified foot

S96.12 Laceration of muscle and tendon of long extensor muscle of toe at ankle and foot level

⑦ **S96.121** Laceration of muscle and tendon of long extensor muscle of toe at ankle and foot level, right foot

⑦ **S96.122** Laceration of muscle and tendon of long extensor muscle of toe at ankle and foot level, left foot

⑦ **S96.129** Laceration of muscle and tendon of long extensor muscle of toe at ankle and foot level, unspecified foot

S96.19 Other specified injury of muscle and tendon of long extensor muscle of toe at ankle and foot level

⑦ **S96.191** Other specified injury of muscle and tendon of long extensor muscle of toe at ankle and foot level, right foot

⑦ **S96.192** Other specified injury of muscle and tendon of long extensor muscle of toe at ankle and foot level, left foot

⑦ **S96.199** Other specified injury of muscle and tendon of long extensor muscle

of toe at ankle and foot level, unspecified foot

S96.2 **Injury of intrinsic muscle and tendon at ankle and foot level**

    S96.20 **Unspecified injury of intrinsic muscle and tendon at ankle and foot level**

      ⑦**S96.201** **Unspecified injury of intrinsic muscle and tendon at ankle and foot level, right foot**

      ⑦**S96.202** **Unspecified injury of intrinsic muscle and tendon at ankle and foot level, left foot**

      ⑦**S96.209** **Unspecified injury of intrinsic muscle and tendon at ankle and foot level, unspecified foot**

    S96.21 **Strain of intrinsic muscle and tendon at ankle and foot level**

      ⑦**S96.211** **Strain of intrinsic muscle and tendon at ankle and foot level, right foot**

      ⑦**S96.212** **Strain of intrinsic muscle and tendon at ankle and foot level, left foot**

      ⑦**S96.219** **Strain of intrinsic muscle and tendon at ankle and foot level, unspecified foot**

    S96.22 **Laceration of intrinsic muscle and tendon at ankle and foot level**

      ⑦**S96.221** **Laceration of intrinsic muscle and tendon at ankle and foot level, right foot**

      ⑦**S96.222** **Laceration of intrinsic muscle and tendon at ankle and foot level, left foot**

      ⑦**S96.229** **Laceration of intrinsic muscle and tendon at ankle and foot level, unspecified foot**

    S96.29 **Other specified injury of intrinsic muscle and tendon at ankle and foot level**

      ⑦**S96.291** **Other specified injury of intrinsic muscle and tendon at ankle and foot level, right foot**

      ⑦**S96.292** **Other specified injury of intrinsic muscle and tendon at ankle and foot level, left foot**

      ⑦**S96.299** **Other specified injury of intrinsic muscle and tendon at ankle and foot level, unspecified foot**

S96.8 **Injury of other specified muscles and tendons at ankle and foot level**

    S96.80 **Unspecified injury of other specified muscles and tendons at ankle and foot level**

      ⑦**S96.801** **Unspecified injury of other specified muscles and tendons at ankle and foot level, right foot**

      ⑦**S96.802** **Unspecified injury of other specified muscles and tendons at ankle and foot level, left foot**

      ⑦**S96.809** **Unspecified injury of other specified muscles and tendons at ankle and foot level, unspecified foot**

    S96.81 **Strain of other specified muscles and tendons at ankle and foot level**

      ⑦**S96.811** **Strain of other specified muscles and tendons at ankle and foot level, right foot**

      ⑦**S96.812** **Strain of other specified muscles and tendons at ankle and foot level, left foot**

      ⑦**S96.819** **Strain of other specified muscles and tendons at ankle and foot level, unspecified foot**

    S96.82 **Laceration of other specified muscles and tendons at ankle and foot level**

      ⑦**S96.821** **Laceration of other specified muscles and tendons at ankle and foot level, right foot**

      ⑦**S96.822** **Laceration of other specified muscles and tendons at ankle and foot level, left foot**

      ⑦**S96.829** **Laceration of other specified muscles and tendons at ankle and foot level, unspecified foot**

    S96.89 **Other specified injury of other specified muscles and tendons at ankle and foot level**

      ⑦**S96.891** **Other specified injury of other specified muscles and tendons at ankle and foot level, right foot**

      ⑦**S96.892** **Other specified injury of other specified muscles and tendons at ankle and foot level, left foot**

      ⑦**S96.899** **Other specified injury of other specified muscles and tendons at ankle and foot level, unspecified foot**

S96.9 **Injury of unspecified muscle and tendon at ankle and foot level**

    S96.90 **Unspecified injury of unspecified muscle and tendon at ankle and foot level**

      ⑦**S96.901** **Unspecified injury of unspecified muscle and tendon at ankle and foot level, right foot**

      ⑦**S96.902** **Unspecified injury of unspecified muscle and tendon at ankle and foot level, left foot**

      ⑦**S96.909** **Unspecified injury of unspecified muscle and tendon at ankle and foot level, unspecified foot**

    S96.91 **Strain of unspecified muscle and tendon at ankle and foot level**

      ⑦**S96.911** **Strain of unspecified muscle and tendon at ankle and foot level, right foot**

      ⑦**S96.912** **Strain of unspecified muscle and tendon at ankle and foot level, left foot**

      ⑦**S96.919** **Strain of unspecified muscle and tendon at ankle and foot level, unspecified foot**

    S96.92 **Laceration of unspecified muscle and tendon at ankle and foot level**

      ⑦**S96.921** **Laceration of unspecified muscle and tendon at ankle and foot level, right foot**

      ⑦**S96.922** **Laceration of unspecified muscle and tendon at ankle and foot level, left foot**

---

⑦ S96.929   Laceration of unspecified muscle and tendon at ankle and foot level, unspecified foot

   S96.99   Other specified injury of unspecified muscle and tendon at ankle and foot level

⑦ S96.991   Other specified injury of unspecified muscle and tendon at ankle and foot level, right foot

⑦ S96.992   Other specified injury of unspecified muscle and tendon at ankle and foot level, left foot

⑦ S96.999   Other specified injury of unspecified muscle and tendon at ankle and foot level, unspecified foot

S97   Crushing injury of ankle and foot

   <u>Use additional code</u>(s) for all associated injuries

   The appropriate 7th character is to be added to each code from category S97

   A - initial encounter

   D - subsequent encounter

   S - sequela

   S97.0   Crushing injury of ankle

⊗⑦ S97.00   Crushing injury of unspecified ankle

⊗⑦ S97.01   Crushing injury of right ankle

⊗⑦ S97.02   Crushing injury of left ankle

   S97.1   Crushing injury of toe

   S97.10   Crushing injury of unspecified toe(s)

⑦ S97.101   Crushing injury of unspecified right toe(s)

⑦ S97.102   Crushing injury of unspecified left toe(s)

⑦ S97.109   Crushing injury of unspecified toe(s)

     Crushing injury of toe NOS

   S97.11   Crushing injury of great toe

⑦ S97.111   Crushing injury of right great toe

⑦ S97.112   Crushing injury of left great toe

⑦ S97.119   Crushing injury of unspecified great toe

   S97.12   Crushing injury of lesser toe(s)

⑦ S97.121   Crushing injury of right lesser toe(s)

⑦ S97.122   Crushing injury of left lesser toe(s)

⑦ S97.129   Crushing injury of unspecified lesser toe(s)

   S97.8   Crushing injury of foot

⊗⑦ S97.80   Crushing injury of unspecified foot

     Crushing injury of foot NOS

⊗⑦ S97.81   Crushing injury of right foot

⊗⑦ S97.82   Crushing injury of left foot

S98   Traumatic amputation of ankle and foot

   An amputation not identified as partial or complete should be coded to complete

   The appropriate 7th character is to be added to each code from category ⑦ S98

   A - initial encounter

   D - subsequent encounter

   S - sequela

   S98.0   Traumatic amputation of foot at ankle level

   S98.01   Complete traumatic amputation of foot at ankle level

⑦ S98.011   Complete traumatic amputation of right foot at ankle level

⑦ S98.012   Complete traumatic amputation of left foot at ankle level

⑦ S98.019   Complete traumatic amputation of unspecified foot at ankle level

   S98.02   Partial traumatic amputation of foot at ankle level

⑦ S98.021   Partial traumatic amputation of right foot at ankle level

⑦ S98.022   Partial traumatic amputation of left foot at ankle level

⑦ S98.029   Partial traumatic amputation of unspecified foot at ankle level

   S98.1   Traumatic amputation of one toe

   S98.11   Complete traumatic amputation of great toe

⑦ S98.111   Complete traumatic amputation of right great toe

⑦ S98.112   Complete traumatic amputation of left great toe

⑦ S98.119   Complete traumatic amputation of unspecified great toe

   S98.12   Partial traumatic amputation of great toe

⑦ S98.121   Partial traumatic amputation of right great toe

⑦ S98.122   Partial traumatic amputation of left great toe

⑦ S98.129   Partial traumatic amputation of unspecified great toe

   S98.13   Complete traumatic amputation of one lesser toe

     Traumatic amputation of toe NOS

⑦ S98.131   Complete traumatic amputation of one right lesser toe

⑦ S98.132   Complete traumatic amputation of one left lesser toe

⑦ S98.139   Complete traumatic amputation of one unspecified lesser toe

   S98.14   Partial traumatic amputation of one lesser toe

⑦ S98.141   Partial traumatic amputation of one right lesser toe

⑦ S98.142   Partial traumatic amputation of one left lesser toe

⑦ S98.149   Partial traumatic amputation of one unspecified lesser toe

   S98.2   Traumatic amputation of two or more lesser toes

   S98.21   Complete traumatic amputation of two or more lesser toes

⑦ S98.211   Complete traumatic amputation of two or more right lesser toes

⑦ S98.212   Complete traumatic amputation of two or more left lesser toes

⑦ S98.219   Complete traumatic amputation of two or more unspecified lesser toes

   S98.22   Partial traumatic amputation of two or more lesser toes

   ● New code   ▲ Revised code   **Excludes1:** Not coded here   **Excludes2:** Not included here   ⊗ Placeholder required   ⑦ 7th digit required

⑦S98.221   **Partial traumatic amputation of two or more right lesser toes**

⑦S98.222   **Partial traumatic amputation of two or more left lesser toes**

⑦S98.229   **Partial traumatic amputation of two or more unspecified lesser toes**

S98.3   **Traumatic amputation of midfoot**

    S98.31   **Complete traumatic amputation of midfoot**

    ⑦S98.311   **Complete traumatic amputation of right midfoot**

    ⑦S98.312   **Complete traumatic amputation of left midfoot**

    ⑦S98.319   **Complete traumatic amputation of unspecified midfoot**

    S98.32   **Partial traumatic amputation of midfoot**

    ⑦S98.321   **Partial traumatic amputation of right midfoot**

    ⑦S98.322   **Partial traumatic amputation of left midfoot**

    ⑦S98.329   **Partial traumatic amputation of unspecified midfoot**

S98.9   **Traumatic amputation of foot, level unspecified**

    S98.91   **Complete traumatic amputation of foot, level unspecified**

    ⑦S98.911   **Complete traumatic amputation of right foot, level unspecified**

    ⑦S98.912   **Complete traumatic amputation of left foot, level unspecified**

    ⑦S98.919   **Complete traumatic amputation of unspecified foot, level unspecified**

    S98.92   **Partial traumatic amputation of foot, level unspecified**

    ⑦S98.921   **Partial traumatic amputation of right foot, level unspecified**

    ⑦S98.922   **Partial traumatic amputation of left foot, level unspecified**

    ⑦S98.929   **Partial traumatic amputation of unspecified foot, level unspecified**

S99   **Other and unspecified injuries of ankle and foot**

    S99.0   **Physeal fracture of calcaneus**

The appropriate 7th character is to be added to each code from subcategories S99.0

A - initial encounter for closed fracture

B - initial encounter for open fracture

D - subsequent encounter for fracture with routine healing

G - subsequent encounter for fracture with delayed healing

K - subsequent encounter for fracture with nonunion

P - subsequent encounter for fracture with malunion

S - sequela

    S99.00   **Unspecified physeal fracture of calcaneus**

    •⑦S99.001   **Unspecified physeal fracture of right calcaneus**

    •⑦S99.002   **Unspecified physeal fracture of left calcaneus**

    •⑦S99.009   **Unspecified physeal fracture of unspecified calcaneus**

    S99.01   **Salter-Harris Type I physeal fracture of calcaneus**

    •⑦S99.011   **Salter-Harris Type I physeal fracture of right calcaneus**

    •⑦S99.012   **Salter-Harris Type I physeal fracture of left calcaneus**

    •⑦S99.019   **Salter-Harris Type I physeal fracture of unspecified calcaneus**

    S99.02   **Salter-Harris Type II physeal fracture of calcaneus**

    •⑦S99.021   **Salter-Harris Type II physeal fracture of right calcaneus**

    •⑦S99.022   **Salter-Harris Type II physeal fracture of left calcaneus**

    •⑦S99.029   **Salter-Harris Type II physeal fracture of unspecified calcaneus**

    S99.03   **Salter-Harris Type III physeal fracture of calcaneus**

    •⑦S99.031   **Salter-Harris Type III physeal fracture of right calcaneus**

    •⑦S99.032   **Salter-Harris Type III physeal fracture of left calcaneus**

    •⑦S99.039   **Salter-Harris Type III physeal fracture of unspecified calcaneus**

    S99.04   **Salter-Harris Type IV physeal fracture of calcaneus**

    •⑦S99.041   **Salter-Harris Type IV physeal fracture of right calcaneus**

    •⑦S99.042   **Salter-Harris Type IV physeal fracture of left calcaneus**

    •⑦S99.049   **Salter-Harris Type IV physeal fracture of unspecified calcaneus**

    S99.09   **Other physeal fracture of calcaneus**

    •⑦S99.091   **Other physeal fracture of right calcaneus**

    •⑦S99.092   **Other physeal fracture of left calcaneus**

    •⑦S99.099   **Other physeal fracture of unspecified calcaneus**

    S99.1   **Physeal fracture of metatarsal**

The appropriate 7th character is to be added to each code from subcategories S99.1

A - initial encounter for closed fracture

B - initial encounter for open fracture

D - subsequent encounter for fracture with routine healing

G - subsequent encounter for fracture with delayed healing

K - subsequent encounter for fracture with nonunion

P - subsequent encounter for fracture with malunion

S - sequela

    S99.10   **Unspecified physeal fracture of metatarsal**

    •⑦S99.101   **Unspecified physeal fracture of right metatarsal**

    •⑦S99.102   **Unspecified physeal fracture of left metatarsal**

    •⑦S99.109   **Unspecified physeal fracture of unspecified metatarsal**

    S99.11   **Salter-Harris Type I physeal fracture of metatarsal**

    •⑦S99.111   **Salter-Harris Type I physeal fracture of right metatarsal**

    •⑦S99.112   **Salter-Harris Type I physeal fracture of left metatarsal**

- ⑦ **S99.119**   **Salter-Harris Type I physeal fracture of unspecified metatarsal**

S99.12   **Salter-Harris Type II physeal fracture of metatarsal**

- ⑦ **S99.121**   **Salter-Harris Type II physeal fracture of right metatarsal**
- ⑦ **S99.122**   **Salter-Harris Type II physeal fracture of left metatarsal**
- ⑦ **S99.129**   **Salter-Harris Type II physeal fracture of unspecified metatarsal**

S99.13   **Salter-Harris Type III physeal fracture of metatarsal**

- ⑦ **S99.131**   **Salter-Harris Type III physeal fracture of right metatarsal**
- ⑦ **S99.132**   **Salter-Harris Type III physeal fracture of left metatarsal**
- ⑦ **S99.139**   **Salter-Harris Type III physeal fracture of unspecified metatarsal**

S99.14   **Salter-Harris Type IV physeal fracture of metatarsal**

- ⑦ **S99.141**   **Salter-Harris Type IV physeal fracture of right metatarsal**
- ⑦ **S99.142**   **Salter-Harris Type IV physeal fracture of left metatarsal**
- ⑦ **S99.149**   **Salter-Harris Type IV physeal fracture of unspecified metatarsal**

S99.19   **Other physeal fracture of metatarsal**

- ⑦ **S99.191**   **Other physeal fracture of right metatarsal**
- ⑦ **S99.192**   **Other physeal fracture of left metatarsal**
- ⑦ **S99.199**   **Other physeal fracture of unspecified metatarsal**

S99.2   **Physeal fracture of phalanx of toe**

The appropriate 7th character is to be added to each code from subcategories S99.2

A - initial encounter for closed fracture

B - initial encounter for open fracture

D - subsequent encounter for fracture with routine healing

G - subsequent encounter for fracture with delayed healing

K - subsequent encounter for fracture with nonunion

P - subsequent encounter for fracture with malunion

S - sequela

S99.20   **Unspecified physeal fracture of phalanx of toe**

- ⑦ **S99.201**   **Unspecified physeal fracture of phalanx of right toe**
- ⑦ **S99.202**   **Unspecified physeal fracture of phalanx of left toe**
- ⑦ **S99.209**   **Unspecified physeal fracture of phalanx of unspecified toe**

S99.21   **Salter-Harris Type I physeal fracture of phalanx of toe**

- ⑦ **S99.211**   **Salter-Harris Type I physeal fracture of phalanx of right toe**
- ⑦ **S99.212**   **Salter-Harris Type I physeal fracture of phalanx of left toe**
- ⑦ **S99.219**   **Salter-Harris Type I physeal fracture of phalanx of unspecified toe**

S99.22   **Salter-Harris Type II physeal fracture of phalanx of toe**

- ⑦ **S99.221**   **Salter-Harris Type II physeal fracture of phalanx of right toe**
- ⑦ **S99.222**   **Salter-Harris Type II physeal fracture of phalanx of left toe**
- ⑦ **S99.229**   **Salter-Harris Type II physeal fracture of phalanx of unspecified toe**

S99.23   **Salter-Harris Type III physeal fracture of phalanx of toe**

- ⑦ **S99.231**   **Salter-Harris Type III physeal fracture of phalanx of right toe**
- ⑦ **S99.232**   **Salter-Harris Type III physeal fracture of phalanx of left toe**
- ⑦ **S99.239**   **Salter-Harris Type III physeal fracture of phalanx of unspecified toe**

S99.24   **Salter-Harris Type IV physeal fracture of phalanx of toe**

- ⑦ **S99.241**   **Salter-Harris Type IV physeal fracture of phalanx of right toe**
- ⑦ **S99.242**   **Salter-Harris Type IV physeal fracture of phalanx of left toe**
- ⑦ **S99.249**   **Salter-Harris Type IV physeal fracture of phalanx of unspecified toe**

S99.29   **Other physeal fracture of phalanx of toe**

- ⑦ **S99.291**   **Other physeal fracture of phalanx of right toe**
- ⑦ **S99.292**   **Other physeal fracture of phalanx of left toe**
- ⑦ **S99.299**   **Other physeal fracture of phalanx of unspecified toe**

S99.8   **Other specified injuries of ankle and foot**

The appropriate 7th character is to be added to each code from subcategory S99.8

A - initial encounter

D - subsequent encounter

S - sequela

S99.81   **Other specified injuries of ankle**

- ⑦ **S99.811**   **Other specified injuries of right ankle**
- ⑦ **S99.812**   **Other specified injuries of left ankle**
- ⑦ **S99.819**   **Other specified injuries of unspecified ankle**

S99.82   **Other specified injuries of foot**

- ⑦ **S99.821**   **Other specified injuries of right foot**
- ⑦ **S99.822**   **Other specified injuries of left foot**
- ⑦ **S99.829**   **Other specified injuries of unspecified foot**

S99.9   **Unspecified injury of ankle and foot**

The appropriate 7th character is to be added to each code from subcategory S99.9

A - initial encounter

D - subsequent encounter

S - sequela

S99.91   **Unspecified injury of ankle**

- ⑦ **S99.911**   **Unspecified injury of right ankle**

⑦S99.912   Unspecified injury of left ankle

⑦S99.919   Unspecified injury of unspecified ankle

S99.92   Unspecified injury of foot

⑦S99.921   Unspecified injury of right foot

⑦S99.922   Unspecified injury of left foot

⑦S99.929   Unspecified injury of unspecified foot

INJURY, POISONING AND CERTAIN OTHER CONSEQUENCES OF EXTERNAL CAUSES (T07-T88)

INJURIES INVOLVING MULTIPLE BODY REGIONS (T07)

Excludes1: burns and corrosions (T20-T32)

frostbite (T33-T34)

insect bite or sting, venomous (T63.4)

sunburn (L55.-)

T07   Unspecified multiple injuries

Excludes1: injury NOS (T14)

INJURY OF UNSPECIFIED BODY REGION (T14)

T14   Injury of unspecified body region

Excludes1: multiple unspecified injuries (T07)

T14.8   Other injury of unspecified body region

Abrasion NOS

Contusion NOS

Crush injury NOS

Fracture NOS

Skin injury NOS

Vascular injury NOS

T14.9   Unspecified injury

T14.90   Injury, unspecified

Injury NOS

T14.91   Suicide attempt

Attempted suicide NOS

EFFECTS OF FOREIGN BODY ENTERING THROUGH NATURAL ORIFICE (T15-T19)

Excludes2: foreign body accidentally left in operation wound (T81.5-)

foreign body in penetrating wound - See open wound by body region residual foreign body in soft tissue (M79.5)

splinter, without open wound - See superficial injury by body region

T15   Foreign body on external eye

Excludes2: foreign body in penetrating wound of orbit and eye ball (S05.4-, S05.5-)

open wound of eyelid and periocular area (S01.1-)

retained foreign body in eyelid (H02.8-)

retained (old) foreign body in penetrating wound of orbit and eye ball (H05.5-, H44.6-, H44.7-)

superficial foreign body of eyelid and periocular area (S00.25-)

The appropriate 7th character is to be added to each code from category T15

A - initial encounter

D - subsequent encounter

S - sequela

T15.0   Foreign body in cornea

⊗T15.00   Foreign body in cornea, unspecified eye

⊗T15.01   Foreign body in cornea, right eye

⊗T15.02   Foreign body in cornea, left eye

T15.1   Foreign body in conjunctival sac

⊗T15.10   Foreign body in conjunctival sac, unspecified eye

⊗T15.11   Foreign body in conjunctival sac, right eye

⊗T15.12   Foreign body in conjunctival sac, left eye

T15.8   Foreign body in other and multiple parts of external eye

Foreign body in lacrimal punctum

⊗T15.80   Foreign body in other and multiple parts of external eye, unspecified eye

⊗T15.81   Foreign body in other and multiple parts of external eye, right eye

⊗T15.82   Foreign body in other and multiple parts of external eye, left eye

T15.9   Foreign body on external eye, part unspecified

⊗T15.90   Foreign body on external eye, part unspecified, unspecified eye

⊗T15.91   Foreign body on external eye, part unspecified, right eye

⊗T15.92   Foreign body on external eye, part unspecified, left eye

T16   Foreign body in ear

Includes: foreign body in auditory canal

The appropriate 7th character is to be added to each code from category T16

A - initial encounter

D - subsequent encounter

S - sequela

⊗T16.1   Foreign body in right ear

⊗T16.2   Foreign body in left ear

⊗T16.9   Foreign body in ear, unspecified ear

T17   Foreign body in respiratory tract

The appropriate 7th character is to be added to each code from category T17

A - initial encounter

D - subsequent encounter

S - sequela

⊗T17.0   Foreign body in nasal sinus

⊗T17.1   Foreign body in nostril

Foreign body in nose NOS

T17.2   Foreign body in pharynx

Foreign body in nasopharynx

Foreign body in throat NOS

T17.20   Unspecified foreign body in pharynx

⑦T17.200   Unspecified foreign body in pharynx causing asphyxiation

⑦T17.208   Unspecified foreign body in pharynx causing other injury

T17.21   Gastric contents in pharynx

Aspiration of gastric contents into pharynx

Vomitus in pharynx

⑦T17.210   Gastric contents in pharynx causing asphyxiation

⑦T17.218   **Gastric contents in pharynx causing other injury**

T17.22   **Food in pharynx**

Bones in pharynx

Seeds in pharynx

⑦T17.220   **Food in pharynx causing asphyxiation**

⑦T17.228   **Food in pharynx causing other injury**

T17.29   **Other foreign object in pharynx**

⑦T17.290   **Other foreign object in pharynx causing asphyxiation**

⑦T17.298   **Other foreign object in pharynx causing other injury**

T17.3   **Foreign body in larynx**

T17.30   **Unspecified foreign body in larynx**

⑦T17.300   **Unspecified foreign body in larynx causing asphyxiation**

⑦T17.308   **Unspecified foreign body in larynx causing other injury**

T17.31   **Gastric contents in larynx**

Aspiration of gastric contents into larynx

Vomitus in larynx

⑦T17.310   **Gastric contents in larynx causing asphyxiation**

⑦T17.318   **Gastric contents in larynx causing other injury**

T17.32   **Food in larynx**

Bones in larynx

Seeds in larynx

⑦T17.320   **Food in larynx causing asphyxiation**

⑦T17.328   **Food in larynx causing other injury**

T17.39   **Other foreign object in larynx**

⑦T17.390   **Other foreign object in larynx causing asphyxiation**

⑦T17.398   **Other foreign object in larynx causing other injury**

T17.4   **Foreign body in trachea**

T17.40   **Unspecified foreign body in trachea**

⑦T17.400   **Unspecified foreign body in trachea causing asphyxiation**

⑦T17.408   **Unspecified foreign body in trachea causing other injury**

T17.41   **Gastric contents in trachea**

Aspiration of gastric contents into trachea

Vomitus in trachea

⑦T17.410   **Gastric contents in trachea causing asphyxiation**

⑦T17.418   **Gastric contents in trachea causing other injury**

T17.42   **Food in trachea**

Bones in trachea

Seeds in trachea

⑦T17.420   **Food in trachea causing asphyxiation**

⑦T17.428   **Food in trachea causing other injury**

T17.49   **Other foreign object in trachea**

⑦T17.490   **Other foreign object in trachea causing asphyxiation**

⑦T17.498   **Other foreign object in trachea causing other injury**

T17.5   **Foreign body in bronchus**

T17.50   **Unspecified foreign body in bronchus**

⑦T17.500   **Unspecified foreign body in bronchus causing asphyxiation**

⑦T17.508   **Unspecified foreign body in bronchus causing other injury**

T17.51   **Gastric contents in bronchus**

Aspiration of gastric contents into bronchus

Vomitus in bronchus

⑦T17.510   **Gastric contents in bronchus causing asphyxiation**

⑦T17.518   **Gastric contents in bronchus causing other injury**

T17.52   **Food in bronchus**

Bones in bronchus

Seeds in bronchus

⑦T17.520   **Food in bronchus causing asphyxiation**

⑦T17.528   **Food in bronchus causing other injury**

T17.59   **Other foreign object in bronchus**

⑦T17.590   **Other foreign object in bronchus causing asphyxiation**

⑦T17.598   **Other foreign object in bronchus causing other injury**

T17.8   **Foreign body in other parts of respiratory tract**

Foreign body in bronchioles

Foreign body in lung

T17.80   **Unspecified foreign body in other parts of respiratory tract**

⑦T17.800   **Unspecified foreign body in other parts of respiratory tract causing asphyxiation**

⑦T17.808   **Unspecified foreign body in other parts of respiratory tract causing other injury**

T17.81   **Gastric contents in other parts of respiratory tract**

Aspiration of gastric contents into other parts of respiratory tract

Vomitus in other parts of respiratory tract

⑦T17.810   **Gastric contents in other parts of respiratory tract causing asphyxiation**

⑦T17.818   **Gastric contents in other parts of respiratory tract causing other injury**

T17.82   **Food in other parts of respiratory tract**

Bones in other parts of respiratory tract

Seeds in other parts of respiratory tract

⑦T17.820   **Food in other parts of respiratory tract causing asphyxiation**

⑦T17.828   **Food in other parts of respiratory tract causing other injury**

T17.89   **Other foreign object in other parts of respiratory tract**

● New code   ▲ Revised code   **Excludes1:** Not coded here   **Excludes2:** Not included here   ⊗ Placeholder required   ⑦7th digit required

⑦**T17.890** **Other foreign object in other parts of respiratory tract causing asphyxiation**

⑦**T17.898** **Other foreign object in other parts of respiratory tract causing other injury**

T17.9 **Foreign body in respiratory tract, part unspecified**

T17.90 **Unspecified foreign body in respiratory tract, part unspecified**

⑦**T17.900** **Unspecified foreign body in respiratory tract, part unspecified causing asphyxiation**

⑦**T17.908** **Unspecified foreign body in respiratory tract, part unspecified causing other injury**

T17.91 **Gastric contents in respiratory tract, part unspecified**

Aspiration of gastric contents into respiratory tract, part unspecified

Vomitus in trachea respiratory tract, part unspecified

⑦**T17.910** **Gastric contents in respiratory tract, part unspecified causing asphyxiation**

⑦**T17.918** **Gastric contents in respiratory tract, part unspecified causing other injury**

T17.92 **Food in respiratory tract, part unspecified**

Bones in respiratory tract, part unspecified

Seeds in respiratory tract, part unspecified

⑦**T17.920** **Food in respiratory tract, part unspecified causing asphyxiation**

⑦**T17.928** **Food in respiratory tract, part unspecified causing other injury**

T17.99 **Other foreign object in respiratory tract, part unspecified**

⑦**T17.990** **Other foreign object in respiratory tract, part unspecified in causing asphyxiation**

⑦**T17.998** **Other foreign object in respiratory tract, part unspecified causing other injury**

T18 **Foreign body in alimentary tract**

Excludes2: foreign body in pharynx (T17.2-)

The appropriate 7th character is to be added to each code from category T18

A - initial encounter

D - subsequent encounter

S - sequela

⊗⑦**T18.0** **Foreign body in mouth**

T18.1 **Foreign body in esophagus**

Excludes2: foreign body in respiratory tract (T17.-)

T18.10 **Unspecified foreign body in esophagus**

⑦**T18.100** **Unspecified foreign body in esophagus causing compression of trachea**

Unspecified foreign body in esophagus causing obstruction of respiration

⑦**T18.108** **Unspecified foreign body in esophagus causing other injury**

T18.11 **Gastric contents in esophagus**

Vomitus in esophagus

⑦**T18.110** **Gastric contents in esophagus causing compression of trachea**

Gastric contents in esophagus causing obstruction of respiration

⑦**T18.118** **Gastric contents in esophagus causing other injury**

T18.12 **Food in esophagus**

Bones in esophagus

Seeds in esophagus

⑦**T18.120** **Food in esophagus causing compression of trachea**

Food in esophagus causing obstruction of respiration

⑦**T18.128** **Food in esophagus causing other injury**

T18.19 **Other foreign object in esophagus**

⑦**T18.190** **Other foreign object in esophagus causing compression of trachea**

Other foreign body in esophagus causing obstruction of respiration

⑦**T18.198** **Other foreign object in esophagus causing other injury**

⊗⑦**T18.2** **Foreign body in stomach**

⊗⑦**T18.3** **Foreign body in small intestine**

⊗⑦**T18.4** **Foreign body in colon**

⊗⑦**T18.5** **Foreign body in anus and rectum**

Foreign body in rectosigmoid (junction)

⊗⑦**T18.8** **Foreign body in other parts of alimentary tract**

⊗⑦**T18.9** **Foreign body of alimentary tract, part unspecified**

Foreign body in digestive system NOS

Swallowed foreign body NOS

T19 **Foreign body in genitourinary tract**

Excludes2: complications due to implanted mesh (T83.7-)

mechanical complications of contraceptive device (intrauterine) (vaginal) (T83.3-)

presence of contraceptive device (intrauterine) (vaginal) (Z97.5)

The appropriate 7th character is to be added to each code from category T19

A - initial encounter

D - subsequent encounter

S - sequela

⊗⑦**T19.0** **Foreign body in urethra**

⊗⑦**T19.1** **Foreign body in bladder**

⊗⑦**T19.2** **Foreign body in vulva and vagina**

⊗⑦**T19.3** **Foreign body in uterus**

⊗⑦**T19.4** **Foreign body in penis**

⊗⑦**T19.8** **Foreign body in other parts of genitourinary tract**

⊗⑦**T19.9** **Foreign body in genitourinary tract, part unspecified**

BURNS AND CORROSIONS (T20-T32)

Includes: burns (thermal) from electrical heating appliances

burns (thermal) from electricity

burns (thermal) from flame

burns (thermal) from friction

burns (thermal) from hot air and hot gases

burns (thermal) from hot objects

burns (thermal) from lightning

burns (thermal) from radiation

chemical burn [corrosion] (external) (internal) scalds

Excludes2: erythema [dermatitis] ab igne (L59.0)

radiation-related disorders of the skin and subcutaneous tissue (L55-L59)

sunburn (L55.-)

BURNS AND CORROSIONS OF EXTERNAL BODY SURFACE, SPECIFIED BY SITE (T20-T25)

Includes: burns and corrosions of first degree [erythema]

burns and corrosions of second degree [blisters][epidermal loss]

burns and corrosions of third degree [deep necrosis of underlying tissue] [full- thickness skin loss]

Use additional code from category T31 or T32 to identify extent of body surface involved

T20 **Burn and corrosion of head, face, and neck**

Excludes2: burn and corrosion of ear drum (T28.41, T28.91)

burn and corrosion of eye and adnexa (T26.-)

burn and corrosion of mouth and pharynx (T28.0)

The appropriate 7th character is to be added to each code from category T20

A - initial encounter

D - subsequent encounter

S - sequela

T20.0 **Burn of unspecified degree of head, face, and neck**

Use additional external cause code to identify the source, place and intent of the burn (X00-X19, X75-X77, X96-X98, Y92)

⊗⑦**T20.00** **Burn of unspecified degree of head, face, and neck, unspecified site**

T20.01 **Burn of unspecified degree of ear [any part, except ear drum]**

Excludes2: burn of ear drum (T28.41-)

⑦**T20.011** **Burn of unspecified degree of right ear [any part, except ear drum]**

⑦**T20.012** **Burn of unspecified degree of left ear [any part, except ear drum]**

⑦**T20.019** **Burn of unspecified degree of unspecified ear [any part, except ear drum]**

⊗⑦**T20.02** **Burn of unspecified degree of lip(s)**

⊗⑦**T20.03** **Burn of unspecified degree of chin**

⊗⑦**T20.04** **Burn of unspecified degree of nose (septum)**

⊗⑦**T20.05** **Burn of unspecified degree of scalp [any part]**

⊗⑦**T20.06** **Burn of unspecified degree of forehead and cheek**

⊗⑦**T20.07** **Burn of unspecified degree of neck**

⊗⑦**T20.09** **Burn of unspecified degree of multiple sites of head, face, and neck**

T20.1 **Burn of first degree of head, face, and neck**

Use additional external cause code to identify the source, place and intent of the burn (X00-X19, X75-X77, X96-X98, Y92)

⊗⑦**T20.10** **Burn of first degree of head, face, and neck, unspecified site**

T20.11 **Burn of first degree of ear [any part, except ear drum]**

Excludes2: burn of ear drum (T28.41-)

⑦**T20.111** **Burn of first degree of right ear [any part, except ear drum]**

⑦**T20.112** **Burn of first degree of left ear [any part, except ear drum]**

⑦**T20.119** **Burn of first degree of unspecified ear [any part, except ear drum]**

⊗⑦**T20.12** **Burn of first degree of lip(s)**

⊗⑦**T20.13** **Burn of first degree of chin**

⊗⑦**T20.14** **Burn of first degree of nose (septum)**

⊗⑦**T20.15** **Burn of first degree of scalp [any part]**

⊗⑦**T20.16** **Burn of first degree of forehead and cheek**

⊗⑦**T20.17** **Burn of first degree of neck**

⊗⑦**T20.19** **Burn of first degree of multiple sites of head, face, and neck**

T20.2 **Burn of second degree of head, face, and neck**

Use additional external cause code to identify the source, place and intent of the burn (X00-X19, X75-X77, X96-X98, Y92)

⊗⑦**T20.20** **Burn of second degree of head, face, and neck, unspecified site**

T20.21 **Burn of second degree of ear [any part, except ear drum]**

Excludes2: burn of ear drum (T28.41-)

⑦**T20.211** **Burn of second degree of right ear [any part, except ear drum]**

⑦**T20.212** **Burn of second degree of left ear [any part, except ear drum]**

⑦**T20.219** **Burn of second degree of unspecified ear [any part, except ear drum]**

⊗⑦**T20.22** **Burn of second degree of lip(s)**

⊗⑦**T20.23** **Burn of second degree of chin**

⊗⑦**T20.24** **Burn of second degree of nose (septum)**

⊗⑦**T20.25** **Burn of second degree of scalp [any part]**

⊗⑦**T20.26** **Burn of second degree of forehead and cheek**

⊗⑦**T20.27** **Burn of second degree of neck**

⊗⑦**T20.29** **Burn of second degree of multiple sites of head, face, and neck**

T20.3 **Burn of third degree of head, face, and neck**

Use additional external cause code to identify the source, place and intent of the burn (X00-X19, X75-X77, X96-X98, Y92)

⊗⑦**T20.30** **Burn of third degree of head, face, and neck, unspecified site**

T20.31 **Burn of third degree of ear [any part, except ear drum]**

Excludes2: burn of ear drum (T28.41-)

⑦**T20.311** **Burn of third degree of right ear [any part, except ear drum]**

⑦**T20.312** **Burn of third degree of left ear [any part, except ear drum]**

⑦**T20.319** **Burn of third degree of unspecified ear [any part, except ear drum]**

⊗⑦**T20.32** **Burn of third degree of lip(s)**

⊗⑦**T20.33** **Burn of third degree of chin**

⊗⑦**T20.34** **Burn of third degree of nose (septum)**

⊗⑦**T20.35**   **Burn of third degree of scalp [any part]**

⊗⑦**T20.36**   **Burn of third degree of forehead and cheek**

⊗⑦**T20.37**   **Burn of third degree of neck**

⊗⑦**T20.39**   **Burn of third degree of multiple sites of head, face, and neck**

T20.4   **Corrosion of unspecified degree of head, face, and neck**

Code first (T51-T65) to identify chemical and intent

Use additional external cause code to identify place (Y92)

⊗⑦**T20.40**   **Corrosion of unspecified degree of head, face, and neck, unspecified site**

T20.41   **Corrosion of unspecified degree of ear [any part, except ear drum]**

Excludes2: corrosion of ear drum (T28.91-)

⑦**T20.411**   **Corrosion of unspecified degree of right ear [any part, except ear drum]**

⑦**T20.412**   **Corrosion of unspecified degree of left ear [any part, except ear drum]**

⑦**T20.419**   **Corrosion of unspecified degree of unspecified ear [any part, except ear drum]**

⊗⑦**T20.42**   **Corrosion of unspecified degree of lip(s)**

⊗⑦**T20.43**   **Corrosion of unspecified degree of chin**

⊗⑦**T20.44**   **Corrosion of unspecified degree of nose (septum)**

⊗⑦**T20.45**   **Corrosion of unspecified degree of scalp [any part]**

⊗⑦**T20.46**   **Corrosion of unspecified degree of forehead and cheek**

⊗⑦**T20.47**   **Corrosion of unspecified degree of neck**

⊗⑦**T20.49**   **Corrosion of unspecified degree of multiple sites of head, face, and neck**

T20.5   **Corrosion of first degree of head, face, and neck**

Code first (T51-T65) to identify chemical and intent

Use additional external cause code to identify place (Y92)

⊗⑦**T20.50**   **Corrosion of first degree of head, face, and neck, unspecified site**

T20.51   **Corrosion of first degree of ear [any part, except ear drum]**

Excludes2: corrosion of ear drum (T28.91-)

⑦**T20.511**   **Corrosion of first degree of right ear [any part, except ear drum]**

⑦**T20.512**   **Corrosion of first degree of left ear [any part, except ear drum]**

⑦**T20.519**   **Corrosion of first degree of unspecified ear [any part, except ear drum]**

⊗⑦**T20.52**   **Corrosion of first degree of lip(s)**

⊗⑦**T20.53**   **Corrosion of first degree of chin**

⊗⑦**T20.54**   **Corrosion of first degree of nose (septum)**

⊗⑦**T20.55**   **Corrosion of first degree of scalp [any part]**

⊗⑦**T20.56**   **Corrosion of first degree of forehead and cheek**

⊗⑦**T20.57**   **Corrosion of first degree of neck**

⊗⑦**T20.59**   **Corrosion of first degree of multiple sites of head, face, and neck**

T20.6   **Corrosion of second degree of head, face, and neck**

Code first (T51-T65) to identify chemical and intent

Use additional external cause code to identify place (Y92)

⊗⑦**T20.60**   **Corrosion of second degree of head, face, and neck, unspecified site**

T20.61   **Corrosion of second degree of ear [any part, except ear drum]**

Excludes2: corrosion of ear drum (T28.91-)

⑦**T20.611**   **Corrosion of second degree of right ear [any part, except ear drum]**

⑦**T20.612**   **Corrosion of second degree of left ear [any part, except ear drum]**

⑦**T20.619**   **Corrosion of second degree of unspecified ear [any part, except ear drum]**

⊗⑦**T20.62**   **Corrosion of second degree of lip(s)**

⊗⑦**T20.63**   **Corrosion of second degree of chin**

⊗⑦**T20.64**   **Corrosion of second degree of nose (septum)**

⊗⑦**T20.65**   **Corrosion of second degree of scalp [any part]**

⊗⑦**T20.66**   **Corrosion of second degree of forehead and cheek**

⊗⑦**T20.67**   **Corrosion of second degree of neck**

⊗⑦**T20.69**   **Corrosion of second degree of multiple sites of head, face, and neck**

T20.7   **Corrosion of third degree of head, face, and neck**

Code first (T51-T65) to identify chemical and intent

Use additional external cause code to identify place (Y92)

⊗⑦**T20.70**   **Corrosion of third degree of head, face, and neck, unspecified site**

T20.71   **Corrosion of third degree of ear [any part, except ear drum]**

Excludes2: corrosion of ear drum (T28.91-)

⑦**T20.711**   **Corrosion of third degree of right ear [any part, except ear drum]**

⑦**T20.712**   **Corrosion of third degree of left ear [any part, except ear drum]**

⑦**T20.719**   **Corrosion of third degree of unspecified ear [any part, except ear drum]**

⊗⑦**T20.72**   **Corrosion of third degree of lip(s)**

⊗⑦**T20.73**   **Corrosion of third degree of chin**

⊗⑦**T20.74**   **Corrosion of third degree of nose (septum)**

⊗⑦**T20.75**   **Corrosion of third degree of scalp [any part]**

⊗⑦**T20.76**   **Corrosion of third degree of forehead and cheek**

⊗⑦**T20.77**   **Corrosion of third degree of neck**

⊗⑦**T20.79**   **Corrosion of third degree of multiple sites of head, face, and neck**

T21   **Burn and corrosion of trunk**

Includes: burns and corrosion of hip region

Excludes2: burns and corrosion of axilla (T22.- with fifth character 4)

burns and corrosion of scapular region (T22.- with fifth character 6)

burns and corrosion of shoulder (T22.- with fifth character 5)

The appropriate 7th character is to be added to each code from category T21

A - initial encounter

D - subsequent encounter

S - sequela

T21.0   **Burn of unspecified degree of trunk**

Add 4th-7th digits		Nonspecific code		Unspecified code		Manifestation code

Use additional external cause code to identify the source, place and intent of the burn (X00-X19, X75-X77, X96-X98, Y92)

⊗⑦**T21.00** **Burn of unspecified degree of trunk, unspecified site**

⊗⑦**T21.01** **Burn of unspecified degree of chest wall**

urn of of unspecified degree of breast

⊗⑦**T21.02** **Burn of unspecified degree of abdominal wall**

Burn of unspecified degree of flank

Burn of unspecified degree of groin

⊗⑦**T21.03** **Burn of unspecified degree of upper back**

urn of unspecified degree of interscapular region

⊗⑦**T21.04** **Burn of unspecified degree of lower back**

⊗⑦**T21.05** **Burn of unspecified degree of buttock**

urn of unspecified degree of anus

⊗⑦**T21.06** **Burn of unspecified degree of male genital region**

urn of unspecified degree of penis

urn of unspecified degree of scrotum

urn of unspecified degree of testis

⊗⑦**T21.07** **Burn of unspecified degree of female genital region**

urn of unspecified degree of labium (majus) (minus)

urn of unspecified degree of perineum

urn of unspecified degree of vulva

Excludes2: burn of vagina (T28.3)

⊗⑦**T21.09** **Burn of unspecified degree of other site of runk**

T21.1 **Burn of first degree of trunk**

Use additional external cause code to identify the source, place and intent of the burn (X00-X19, X75-X77, X96-X98, Y92)

⊗⑦**T21.10** **Burn of first degree of trunk, unspecified site**

⊗⑦**T21.11** **Burn of first degree of chest wall**

Burn of first degree of breast

⊗⑦**T21.12** **Burn of first degree of abdominal wall**

Burn of first degree of flank

Burn of first degree of groin

⊗⑦**T21.13** **Burn of first degree of upper back**

Burn of first degree of interscapular region

⊗⑦**T21.14** **Burn of first degree of lower back**

⊗⑦**T21.15** **Burn of first degree of buttock**

Burn of first degree of anus

⊗⑦**T21.16** **Burn of first degree of male genital region**

Burn of first degree of penis

Burn of f irst degree of scrotum

Burn of first degree of testis

⊗⑦**T21.17** **Burn of first degree of female genital region**

Burn of first degree of labium (majus) (minus)

Burn of first degree of perineum

Burn of first degree of vulva

Excludes2: burn of vagina (T28.3)

⊗⑦**T21.19** **Burn of first degree of other site of trunk**

T21.2 **Burn of second degree of trunk**

Use additional external cause code to identify the source, place and intent of the burn (X00-X19, X75-X77, X96-X98, Y92)

⊗⑦**T21.20** **Burn of second degree of trunk, unspecified site**

⊗⑦**T21.21** **Burn of second degree of chest wall**

Burn of second degree of breast

⊗⑦**T21.22** **Burn of second degree of abdominal wall**

Burn of second degree of flank

Burn of second degree of groin

T21.23 **Burn of second degree of upper back**

Burn of second degree of interscapular region

⊗⑦**T21.24** **Burn of second degree of lower back**

⊗⑦**T21.25** **Burn of second degree of buttock**

Burn of second degree of anus

⊗⑦**T21.26** **Burn of second degree of male genital region**

Burn of second degree of penis

Burn of second degree of scrotum

Burn of second degree of testis

⊗⑦**T21.27** **Burn of second degree of female genital region**

Burn of second degree of labium (majus) (minus)

Burn of second degree of perineum

Burn of second degree of vulva

Excludes2: burn of vagina (T28.3)

⊗⑦**T21.29** **Burn of second degree of other site of trunk**

T21.3 **Burn of third degree of trunk**

Use additional external cause code to identify the source, place and intent of the burn (X00-X19, X75-X77, X96-X98, Y92)

⊗⑦**T21.30** **Burn of third degree of trunk, unspecified site**

⊗⑦**T21.31** **Burn of third degree of chest wall**

Burn of third degree of breast

⊗⑦**T21.32** **Burn of third degree of abdominal wall**

Burn of third degree of flank

Burn of third degree of groin

⊗⑦**T21.33** **Burn of third degree of upper back**

Burn of third degree of interscapular region

⊗⑦**T21.34** **Burn of third degree of lower back**

⊗⑦**T21.35** **Burn of third degree of buttock**

Burn of third degree of anus

⊗⑦**T21.36** **Burn of third degree of male genital region**

Burn of third degree of penis

Burn of third degree of scrotum

Burn of third degree of testis

⊗⑦**T21.37** **Burn of third degree of female genital region**

Burn of third degree of labium (majus) (minus)

Burn of third degree of perineum

Burn of third degree of vulva

Excludes2: burn of vagina (T28.3)

⊗⑦**T21.39** **Burn of third degree of other site of trunk**

T21.4 **Corrosion of unspecified degree of trunk**

Code first (T51-T65) to identify chemical and intent

Use additional external cause code to identify place (Y92)

● New code ▲ Revised code **Excludes1:** Not coded here **Excludes2:** Not included here ⊗ Placeholder required ⑦ 7ᵗʰ digit required

⊗7 **T21.40** **Corrosion of unspecified degree of trunk, unspecified site**

⊗7 **T21.41** **Corrosion of unspecified degree of chest wall**

Corrosion of unspecified degree of breast

⊗7 **T21.42** **Corrosion of unspecified degree of abdominal wall**

Corrosion of unspecified degree of flank

Corrosion of unspecified degree of groin

⊗7 **T21.43** **Corrosion of unspecified degree of upper back**

Corrosion of unspecified degree of interscapular region

⊗7 **T21.44** **Corrosion of unspecified degree of lower back**

⊗7 **T21.45** **Corrosion of unspecified degree of buttock**

Corrosion of unspecified degree of anus

⊗7 **T21.46** **Corrosion of unspecified degree of male genital region**

Corrosion of unspecified degree of penis

Corrosion of unspecified degree of scrotum

Corrosion of unspecified degree of testis

⊗7 **T21.47** **Corrosion of unspecified degree of female genital region**

Corrosion of unspecified degree of labium (majus) (minus)

Corrosion of unspecified degree of perineum

Corrosion of unspecified degree of vulva

Excludes2: corrosion of vagina (T28.8)

⊗7 **T21.49** **Corrosion of unspecified degree of other site of trunk**

T21.5 **Corrosion of first degree of trunk**

Code first (T51-T65) to identify chemical and intent

Use additional external cause code to identify place (Y92)

⊗7 **T21.50** **Corrosion of first degree of trunk, unspecified site**

⊗7 **T21.51** **Corrosion of first degree of chest wall**

Corrosion of first degree of breast

⊗7 **T21.52** **Corrosion of first degree of abdominal wall**

Corrosion of first degree of flank

Corrosion of first degree of groin

⊗7 **T21.53** **Corrosion of first degree of upper back**

Corrosion of first degree of interscapular region

⊗7 **T21.54** **Corrosion of first degree of lower back**

⊗7 **T21.55** **Corrosion of first degree of buttock**

Corrosion of first degree of anus

⊗7 **T21.56** **Corrosion of first degree of male genital region**

Corrosion of first degree of penis

Corrosion of first degree of scrotum

Corrosion of first degree of testis

⊗7 **T21.57** **Corrosion of first degree of female genital region**

Corrosion of first degree of labium (majus) (minus)

Corrosion of first degree of perineum

Corrosion of first degree of vulva

Excludes2: corrosion of vagina (T28.8)

⊗7 **T21.59** **Corrosion of first degree of other site of trunk**

T21.6 **Corrosion of second degree of trunk**

Code first (T51-T65) to identify chemical and intent

Use additional external cause code to identify place (Y92)

⊗7 **T21.60** **Corrosion of second degree of trunk, unspecified site**

⊗7 **T21.61** **Corrosion of second degree of chest wall**

Corrosion of second degree of breast

⊗7 **T21.62** **Corrosion of second degree of abdominal wall**

Corrosion of second degree of flank

Corrosion of second degree of groin

⊗7 **T21.63** **Corrosion of second degree of upper back**

Corrosion of second degree of interscapular region

⊗7 **T21.64** **Corrosion of second degree of lower back**

⊗7 **T21.65** **Corrosion of second degree of buttock**

Corrosion of second degree of anus

⊗7 **T21.66** **Corrosion of second degree of male genital region**

Corrosion of second degree of penis

Corrosion of second degree of scrotum

Corrosion of second degree of testis

⊗7 **T21.67** **Corrosion of second degree of female genital region**

Corrosion of second degree of labium (majus) (minus)

Corrosion of second degree of perineum

Corrosion of second degree of vulva

Excludes2: corrosion of vagina (T28.8)

⊗7 **T21.69** **Corrosion of second degree of other site of trunk**

T21.7 **Corrosion of third degree of trunk**

Code first (T51-T65) to identify chemical and intent

Use additional external cause code to identify place (Y92)

⊗7 **T21.70** **Corrosion of third degree of trunk, unspecified site**

⊗7 **T21.71** **Corrosion of third degree of chest wall**

Corrosion of third degree of breast

⊗7 **T21.72** **Corrosion of third degree of abdominal wall**

Corrosion of third degree of flank

Corrosion of third degree of groin

⊗7 **T21.73** **Corrosion of third degree of upper back**

Corrosion of third degree of interscapular region

⊗7 **T21.74** **Corrosion of third degree of lower back**

⊗7 **T21.75** **Corrosion of third degree of buttock**

Corrosion of third degree of anus

⊗7 **T21.76** **Corrosion of third degree of male genital region**

Corrosion of third degree of penis

Corrosion of third degree of scrotum

Corrosion of third degree of testis

⊗7 **T21.77** **Corrosion of third degree of female genital region**

Corrosion of third degree of labium (majus) (minus)

Corrosion of third degree of perineum

Corrosion of third degree of vulva

Excludes2: corrosion of vagina (T28.8)

⊗⑦**T21.79**   Corrosion of third degree of other site of trunk

T22 **Burn and corrosion of shoulder and upper limb, except wrist and hand**

> Excludes2: burn and corrosion of interscapular region (T21.-)
>
> burn and corrosion of wrist and hand (T23.-)

The appropriate 7th character is to be added to each code from category T22

A - initial encounter

D - subsequent encounter

S - sequela

T22.0 **Burn of unspecified degree of shoulder and upper limb, except wrist and hand**

> **Use additional** external cause code to identify the source, place and intent of the burn (X00-X19, X75-X77, X96-X98, Y92)

⊗⑦**T22.00**   **Burn of unspecified degree of shoulder and upper limb, except wrist and hand, unspecified site**

T22.01   **Burn of unspecified degree of forearm**

⑦ **T22.011**   **Burn of unspecified degree of right forearm**

⑦ **T22.012**   **Burn of unspecified degree of left forearm**

⑦ **T22.019**   **Burn of unspecified degree of unspecified forearm**

T22.02   **Burn of unspecified degree of elbow**

⑦ **T22.021**   **Burn of unspecified degree of right elbow**

⑦ **T22.022**   **Burn of unspecified degree of left elbow**

⑦ **T22.029**   **Burn of unspecified degree of unspecified elbow**

T22.03   **Burn of unspecified degree of upper arm**

⑦ **T22.031**   **Burn of unspecified degree of right upper arm**

⑦ **T22.032**   **Burn of unspecified degree of left upper arm**

⑦ **T22.039**   **Burn of unspecified degree of unspecified upper arm**

T22.04   **Burn of unspecified degree of axilla**

⑦ **T22.041**   **Burn of unspecified degree of right axilla**

⑦ **T22.042**   **Burn of unspecified degree of left axilla**

⑦ **T22.049**   **Burn of unspecified degree of unspecified axilla**

T22.05   **Burn of unspecified degree of shoulder**

⑦ **T22.051**   **Burn of unspecified degree of right shoulder**

⑦ **T22.052**   **Burn of unspecified degree of left shoulder**

⑦ **T22.059**   **Burn of unspecified degree of unspecified shoulder**

T22.06   **Burn of unspecified degree of scapular region**

⑦ **T22.061**   **Burn of unspecified degree of right scapular region**

⑦ **T22.062**   **Burn of unspecified degree of left scapular region**

⑦ **T22.069**   **Burn of unspecified degree of unspecified scapular region**

T22.09   **Burn of unspecified degree of multiple sites of shoulder and upper limb, except wrist and hand**

⑦ **T22.091**   **Burn of unspecified degree of multiple sites of right shoulder and upper limb, except wrist and hand**

⑦ **T22.092**   **Burn of unspecified degree of multiple sites of left shoulder and upper limb, except wrist and hand**

⑦ **T22.099**   **Burn of unspecified degree of multiple sites of unspecified shoulder and upper limb, except wrist and hand**

T22.1 **Burn of first degree of shoulder and upper limb, except wrist and hand**

> **Use additional** external cause code to identify the source, place and intent of the burn (X00-X19, X75-X77, X96-X98, Y92)

⊗⑦**T22.10**   **Burn of first degree of shoulder and upper limb, except wrist and hand, unspecified site**

T22.11   **Burn of first degree of forearm**

⑦ **T22.111**   **Burn of first degree of right forearm**

⑦ **T22.112**   **Burn of first degree of left forearm**

⑦ **T22.119**   **Burn of first degree of unspecified forearm**

T22.12   **Burn of first degree of elbow**

⑦ **T22.121**   **Burn of first degree of right elbow**

⑦ **T22.122**   **Burn of first degree of left elbow**

⑦ **T22.129**   **Burn of first degree of unspecified elbow**

T22.13   **Burn of first degree of upper arm**

⑦ **T22.131**   **Burn of first degree of right upper arm**

⑦ **T22.132**   **Burn of first degree of left upper arm**

⑦ **T22.139**   **Burn of first degree of unspecified upper arm**

T22.14   **Burn of first degree of axilla**

⑦ **T22.141**   **Burn of first degree of right axilla**

⑦ **T22.142**   **Burn of first degree of left axilla**

⑦ **T22.149**   **Burn of first degree of unspecified axilla**

T22.15   **Burn of first degree of shoulder**

⑦ **T22.151**   **Burn of first degree of right shoulder**

⑦ **T22.152**   **Burn of first degree of left shoulder**

⑦ **T22.159**   **Burn of first degree of unspecified shoulder**

T22.16   **Burn of first degree of scapular region**

⑦ **T22.161**   **Burn of first degree of right scapular region**

⑦ **T22.162**   **Burn of first degree of left scapular region**

⑦ **T22.169**   **Burn of first degree of unspecified scapular region**

T22.19   **Burn of first degree of multiple sites of shoulder and upper limb, except wrist and hand**

● New code   ▲ Revised code   **Excludes1:** Not coded here   **Excludes2:** Not included here   ⊗ Placeholder required   ⑦ 7th digit required

⑦T22.191   Burn of first degree of multiple sites of right shoulder and upper limb, except wrist and hand

⑦T22.192   Burn of first degree of multiple sites of left shoulder and upper limb, except wrist and hand

⑦T22.199   Burn of first degree of multiple sites of unspecified shoulder and upper limb, except wrist and hand

T22.2   **Burn of second degree of shoulder and upper limb, except wrist and hand**

Use **additional** external cause code to identify the source, place and intent of the burn (X00-X19, X75-X77, X96-X98, Y92)

⊗⑦T22.20   **Burn of second degree of shoulder and upper limb, except wrist and hand, unspecified site**

T22.21   **Burn of second degree of forearm**

⑦T22.211   **Burn of second degree of right forearm**

⑦T22.212   **Burn of second degree of left forearm**

⑦T22.219   **Burn of second degree of unspecified forearm**

T22.22   **Burn of second degree of elbow**

⑦T22.221   **Burn of second degree of right elbow**

⑦T22.222   **Burn of second degree of left elbow**

⑦T22.229   **Burn of second degree of unspecified elbow**

T22.23   **Burn of second degree of upper arm**

⑦T22.231   **Burn of second degree of right upper arm**

⑦T22.232   **Burn of second degree of left upper arm**

⑦T22.239   **Burn of second degree of unspecified upper arm**

T22.24   **Burn of second degree of axilla**

⑦T22.241   **Burn of second degree of right axilla**

⑦T22.242   **Burn of second degree of left axilla**

⑦T22.249   **Burn of second degree of unspecified axilla**

T22.25   **Burn of second degree of shoulder**

⑦T22.251   **Burn of second degree of right shoulder**

⑦T22.252   **Burn of second degree of left shoulder**

⑦T22.259   **Burn of second degree of unspecified shoulder**

T22.26   **Burn of second degree of scapular region**

⑦T22.261   **Burn of second degree of right scapular region**

⑦T22.262   **Burn of second degree of left scapular region**

⑦T22.269   **Burn of second degree of unspecified scapular region**

T22.29   **Burn of second degree of multiple sites of shoulder and upper limb, except wrist and hand**

⑦T22.291   Burn of second degree of multiple sites of right shoulder and upper limb, except wrist and hand

⑦T22.292   Burn of second degree of multiple sites of left shoulder and upper limb, except wrist and hand

⑦T22.299   Burn of second degree of multiple sites of unspecified shoulder and upper limb, except wrist and hand

T22.3   **Burn of third degree of shoulder and upper limb, except wrist and hand**

Use **additional** external cause code to identify the source, place and intent of the burn (X00-X19, X75-X77, X96-X98, Y92)

⊗⑦T22.30   **Burn of third degree of shoulder and upper limb, except wrist and hand, unspecified site**

T22.31   **Burn of third degree of forearm**

⑦T22.311   **Burn of third degree of right forearm**

⑦T22.312   **Burn of third degree of left forearm**

⑦T22.319   **Burn of third degree of unspecified forearm**

T22.32   **Burn of third degree of elbow**

⑦T22.321   **Burn of third degree of right elbow**

⑦T22.322   **Burn of third degree of left elbow**

⑦T22.329   **Burn of third degree of unspecified elbow**

T22.33   **Burn of third degree of upper arm**

⑦T22.331   **Burn of third degree of right upper arm**

⑦T22.332   **Burn of third degree of left upper arm**

⑦T22.339   **Burn of third degree of unspecified upper arm**

T22.34   **Burn of third degree of axilla**

⑦T22.341   **Burn of third degree of right axilla**

⑦T22.342   **Burn of third degree of left axilla**

⑦T22.349   **Burn of third degree of unspecified axilla**

T22.35   **Burn of third degree of shoulder**

⑦T22.351   **Burn of third degree of right shoulder**

⑦T22.352   **Burn of third degree of left shoulder**

⑦T22.359   **Burn of third degree of unspecified shoulder**

T22.36   **Burn of third degree of scapular region**

⑦T22.361   **Burn of third degree of right scapular region**

⑦T22.362   **Burn of third degree of left scapular region**

⑦T22.369   **Burn of third degree of unspecified scapular region**

T22.39   **Burn of third degree of multiple sites of shoulder and upper limb, except wrist and hand**

⑦T22.391   Burn of third degree of multiple sites of right shoulder and upper limb, except wrist and hand

⑦T22.392   Burn of third degree of multiple sites of left shoulder and upper limb, except wrist and hand

⑦**T22.399** Burn of third degree of multiple sites of unspecified shoulder and upper limb, except wrist and hand

T22.4 **Corrosion of unspecified degree of shoulder and upper limb, except wrist and hand**

Code first (T51-T65) to identify chemical and intent

Use additional external cause code to identify place (Y92)

⊗⑦**T22.40** Corrosion of unspecified degree of shoulder and upper limb, except wrist and hand, unspecified site

T22.41 Corrosion of unspecified degree of forearm

⑦**T22.411** Corrosion of unspecified degree of right forearm

⑦**T22.412** Corrosion of unspecified degree of left forearm

⑦**T22.419** Corrosion of unspecified degree of unspecified forearm

T22.42 Corrosion of unspecified degree of elbow

⑦**T22.421** Corrosion of unspecified degree of right elbow

⑦**T22.422** Corrosion of unspecified degree of left elbow

⑦**T22.429** Corrosion of unspecified degree of unspecified elbow

T22.43 Corrosion of unspecified degree of upper arm

⑦**T22.431** Corrosion of unspecified degree of right upper arm

⑦**T22.432** Corrosion of unspecified degree of left upper arm

⑦**T22.439** Corrosion of unspecified degree of unspecified upper arm

T22.44 Corrosion of unspecified degree of axilla

⑦**T22.441** Corrosion of unspecified degree of right axilla

⑦**T22.442** Corrosion of unspecified degree of left axilla

⑦**T22.449** Corrosion of unspecified degree of unspecified axilla

T22.45 Corrosion of unspecified degree of shoulder

⑦**T22.451** Corrosion of unspecified degree of right shoulder

⑦**T22.452** Corrosion of unspecified degree of left shoulder

⑦**T22.459** Corrosion of unspecified degree of unspecified shoulder

T22.46 Corrosion of unspecified degree of scapular region

⑦**T22.461** Corrosion of unspecified degree of right scapular region

⑦**T22.462** Corrosion of unspecified degree of left scapular region

⑦**T22.469** Corrosion of unspecified degree of unspecified scapular region

T22.49 Corrosion of unspecified degree of multiple sites of shoulder and upper limb, except wrist and hand

⑦**T22.491** Corrosion of unspecified degree of multiple sites of right shoulder and upper limb, except wrist and hand

⑦**T22.492** Corrosion of unspecified degree of multiple sites of left shoulder and upper limb, except wrist and hand

⑦**T22.499** Corrosion of unspecified degree of multiple sites of unspecified shoulder and upper limb, except wrist and hand

T22.5 **Corrosion of first degree of shoulder and upper limb, except wrist and hand**

Code first (T51-T65) to identify chemical and intent

Use additional external cause code to identify place (Y92)

⊗⑦**T22.50** Corrosion of first degree of shoulder and upper limb, except wrist and hand unspecified site

T22.51 Corrosion of first degree of forearm

⑦**T22.511** Corrosion of first degree of right forearm

⑦**T22.512** Corrosion of first degree of left forearm

⑦**T22.519** Corrosion of first degree of unspecified forearm

T22.52 Corrosion of first degree of elbow

⑦**T22.521** Corrosion of first degree of right elbow

⑦**T22.522** Corrosion of first degree of left elbow

⑦**T22.529** Corrosion of first degree of unspecified elbow

T22.53 Corrosion of first degree of upper arm

⑦**T22.531** Corrosion of first degree of right upper arm

⑦**T22.532** Corrosion of first degree of left upper arm

⑦**T22.539** Corrosion of first degree of unspecified upper arm

T22.54 Corrosion of first degree of axilla

⑦**T22.541** Corrosion of first degree of right axilla

⑦**T22.542** Corrosion of first degree of left axilla

⑦**T22.549** Corrosion of first degree of unspecified axilla

T22.55 Corrosion of first degree of shoulder

⑦**T22.551** Corrosion of first degree of right shoulder

⑦**T22.552** Corrosion of first degree of left shoulder

⑦**T22.559** Corrosion of first degree of unspecified shoulder

T22.56 Corrosion of first degree of scapular region

⑦**T22.561** Corrosion of first degree of right scapular region

⑦**T22.562** Corrosion of first degree of left scapular region

⑦**T22.569** Corrosion of first degree of unspecified scapular region

T22.59 Corrosion of first degree of multiple sites of shoulder and upper limb, except wrist and hand

● New code ▲ Revised code **Excludes1:** Not coded here **Excludes2:** Not included here ⊗ Placeholder required ⑦ 7th digit required

⑦T22.591   Corrosion of first degree of multiple sites of right shoulder and upper limb, except wrist and hand

⑦T22.592   Corrosion of first degree of multiple sites of left shoulder and upper limb, except wrist and hand

⑦T22.599   Corrosion of first degree of multiple sites of unspecified shoulder and upper limb, except wrist and hand

T22.6   **Corrosion of second degree of shoulder and upper limb, except wrist and hand**

Code first (T51-T65) to identify chemical and intent

Use additional external cause code to identify place (Y92)

⊗⑦T22.60   Corrosion of second degree of shoulder and upper limb, except wrist and hand, unspecified site

T22.61   Corrosion of second degree of forearm

    ⑦T22.611   Corrosion of second degree of right forearm

    ⑦T22.612   Corrosion of second degree of left forearm

    ⑦T22.619   Corrosion of second degree of unspecified forearm

T22.62   Corrosion of second degree of elbow

    ⑦T22.621   Corrosion of second degree of right elbow

    ⑦T22.622   Corrosion of second degree of left elbow

    ⑦T22.629   Corrosion of second degree of unspecified elbow

T22.63   Corrosion of second degree of upper arm

    ⑦T22.631   Corrosion of second degree of right upper arm

    ⑦T22.632   Corrosion of second degree of left upper arm

    ⑦T22.639   Corrosion of second degree of unspecified upper arm

T22.64   Corrosion of second degree of axilla

    ⑦T22.641   Corrosion of second degree of right axilla

    ⑦T22.642   Corrosion of second degree of left axilla

    ⑦T22.649   Corrosion of second degree of unspecified axilla

T22.65   Corrosion of second degree of shoulder

    ⑦T22.651   Corrosion of second degree of right shoulder

    ⑦T22.652   Corrosion of second degree of left shoulder

    ⑦T22.659   Corrosion of second degree of unspecified shoulder

T22.66   Corrosion of second degree of scapular region

    ⑦T22.661   Corrosion of second degree of right scapular region

    ⑦T22.662   Corrosion of second degree of left scapular region

    ⑦T22.669   Corrosion of second degree of unspecified scapular region

T22.69   Corrosion of second degree of multiple sites of shoulder and upper limb, except wrist and hand

⑦T22.691   Corrosion of second degree of multiple sites of right shoulder and upper limb, except wrist and hand

⑦T22.692   Corrosion of second degree of multiple sites of left shoulder and upper limb, except wrist and hand

⑦T22.699   Corrosion of second degree of multiple sites of unspecified shoulder and upper limb, except wrist and hand

T22.7   **Corrosion of third degree of shoulder and upper limb, except wrist and hand**

Code first (T51-T65) to identify chemical and intent

Use additional external cause code to identify place (Y92)

⊗⑦T22.70   Corrosion of third degree of shoulder and upper limb, except wrist and hand, unspecified site

T22.71   Corrosion of third degree of forearm

    ⑦T22.711   Corrosion of third degree of right forearm

    ⑦T22.712   Corrosion of third degree of left forearm

    ⑦T22.719   Corrosion of third degree of unspecified forearm

T22.72   Corrosion of third degree of elbow

    ⑦T22.721   Corrosion of third degree of right elbow

    ⑦T22.722   Corrosion of third degree of left elbow

    ⑦T22.729   Corrosion of third degree of unspecified elbow

T22.73   Corrosion of third degree of upper arm

    ⑦T22.731   Corrosion of third degree of right upper arm

    ⑦T22.732   Corrosion of third degree of left upper arm

    ⑦T22.739   Corrosion of third degree of unspecified upper arm

T22.74   Corrosion of third degree of axilla

    ⑦T22.741   Corrosion of third degree of right axilla

    ⑦T22.742   Corrosion of third degree of left axilla

    ⑦T22.749   Corrosion of third degree of unspecified axilla

T22.75   Corrosion of third degree of shoulder

    ⑦T22.751   Corrosion of third degree of right shoulder

    ⑦T22.752   Corrosion of third degree of left shoulder

    ⑦T22.759   Corrosion of third degree of unspecified shoulder

T22.76   Corrosion of third degree of scapular region

    ⑦T22.761   Corrosion of third degree of right scapular region

    ⑦T22.762   Corrosion of third degree of left scapular region

    ⑦T22.769   Corrosion of third degree of unspecified scapular region

T22.79　**Corrosion of third degree of multiple sites of shoulder and upper limb, except wrist and hand**

⑦T22.791　**Corrosion of third degree of multiple sites of right shoulder and upper limb, except wrist and hand**

⑦T22.792　**Corrosion of third degree of multiple sites of left shoulder and upper limb, except wrist and hand**

⑦T22.799　**Corrosion of third degree of multiple sites of unspecified shoulder and upper limb, except wrist and hand**

T23　**Burn and corrosion of wrist and hand**

The appropriate 7th character is to be added to each code from category T23

A - initial encounter

D - subsequent encounter

S - sequela

T23.0　**Burn of unspecified degree of wrist and hand**

Use additional external cause code to identify the source, place and intent of the burn (X00-X19, X75-X77, X96-X98, Y92)

T23.00　**Burn of unspecified degree of hand, unspecified site**

⑦T23.001　**Burn of unspecified degree of right hand, unspecified site**

⑦T23.002　**Burn of unspecified degree of left hand, unspecified site**

⑦T23.009　**Burn of unspecified degree of unspecified hand, unspecified site**

T23.01　**Burn of unspecified degree of thumb (nail)**

⑦T23.011　**Burn of unspecified degree of right thumb (nail)**

⑦T23.012　**Burn of unspecified degree of left thumb (nail)**

⑦T23.019　**Burn of unspecified degree of unspecified thumb (nail)**

T23.02　**Burn of unspecified degree of single finger (nail) except thumb**

⑦T23.021　**Burn of unspecified degree of single right finger (nail) except thumb**

⑦T23.022　**Burn of unspecified degree of single left finger (nail) except thumb**

⑦T23.029　**Burn of unspecified degree of unspecified single finger (nail) except thumb**

T23.03　**Burn of unspecified degree of multiple fingers (nail), not including thumb**

⑦T23.031　**Burn of unspecified degree of multiple right fingers (nail), not including thumb**

⑦T23.032　**Burn of unspecified degree of multiple left fingers (nail), not including thumb**

⑦T23.039　**Burn of unspecified degree of unspecified multiple fingers (nail), not including thumb**

T23.04　**Burn of unspecified degree of multiple fingers (nail), including thumb**

⑦T23.041　**Burn of unspecified degree of multiple right fingers (nail), including thumb**

⑦T23.042　**Burn of unspecified degree of multiple left fingers (nail), including thumb**

⑦T23.049　**Burn of unspecified degree of unspecified multiple fingers (nail), including thumb**

T23.05　**Burn of unspecified degree of palm**

⑦T23.051　**Burn of unspecified degree of right palm**

⑦T23.052　**Burn of unspecified degree of left palm**

⑦T23.059　**Burn of unspecified degree of unspecified palm**

T23.06　**Burn of unspecified degree of back of hand**

⑦T23.061　**Burn of unspecified degree of back of right hand**

⑦T23.062　**Burn of unspecified degree of back of left hand**

⑦T23.069　**Burn of unspecified degree of back of unspecified hand**

T23.07　**Burn of unspecified degree of wrist**

⑦T23.071　**Burn of unspecified degree of right wrist**

⑦T23.072　**Burn of unspecified degree of left wrist**

⑦T23.079　**Burn of unspecified degree of unspecified wrist**

T23.09　**Burn of unspecified degree of multiple sites of wrist and hand**

⑦T23.091　**Burn of unspecified degree of multiple sites of right wrist and hand**

⑦T23.092　**Burn of unspecified degree of multiple sites of left wrist and hand**

⑦T23.099　**Burn of unspecified degree of multiple sites of unspecified wrist and hand**

T23.1　**Burn of first degree of wrist and hand**

Use additional external cause code to identify the source, place and intent of the burn (X00-X19, X75-X77, X96-X98, Y92)

T23.10　**Burn of first degree of hand, unspecified site**

⑦T23.101　**Burn of first degree of right hand, unspecified site**

⑦T23.102　**Burn of first degree of left hand, unspecified site**

⑦T23.109　**Burn of first degree of unspecified hand, unspecified site**

T23.11　**Burn of first degree of thumb (nail)**

⑦T23.111　**Burn of first degree of right thumb (nail)**

⑦T23.112　**Burn of first degree of left thumb (nail)**

⑦T23.119　**Burn of first degree of unspecified thumb (nail)**

T23.12　**Burn of first degree of single finger (nail) except thumb**

⑦T23.121   Burn of first degree of single right finger (nail) except thumb

⑦T23.122   Burn of first degree of single left finger (nail) except thumb

⑦T23.129   Burn of first degree of unspecified single finger (nail) except thumb

T23.13   Burn of first degree of multiple fingers (nail), not including thumb

⑦T23.131   Burn of first degree of multiple right fingers (nail), not including thumb

⑦T23.132   Burn of first degree of multiple left fingers (nail), not including thumb

⑦T23.139   Burn of first degree of unspecified multiple fingers (nail), not including thumb

T23.14   Burn of first degree of multiple fingers (nail), including thumb

⑦T23.141   Burn of first degree of multiple right fingers (nail), including thumb

⑦T23.142   Burn of first degree of multiple left fingers (nail), including thumb

⑦T23.149   Burn of first degree of unspecified multiple fingers (nail), including thumb

T23.15   Burn of first degree of palm

⑦T23.151   Burn of first degree of right palm

⑦T23.152   Burn of first degree of left palm

⑦T23.159   Burn of first degree of unspecified palm

T23.16   Burn of first degree of back of hand

⑦T23.161   Burn of first degree of back of right hand

⑦T23.162   Burn of first degree of back of left hand

⑦T23.169   Burn of first degree of back of unspecified hand

⑦T23.17   Burn of first degree of wrist

⑦T23.171   Burn of first degree of right wrist

⑦T23.172   Burn of first degree of left wrist

⑦T23.179   Burn of first degree of unspecified wrist

⑦T23.19   Burn of first degree of multiple sites of wrist and hand

⑦T23.191   Burn of first degree of multiple sites of right wrist and hand

⑦T23.192   Burn of first degree of multiple sites of left wrist and hand

⑦T23.199   Burn of first degree of multiple sites of unspecified wrist and hand

T23.2   Burn of second degree of wrist and hand

Use additional external cause code to identify the source, place and intent of the burn (X00-X19, X75-X77, X96-X98, Y92)

T23.20   Burn of second degree of hand, unspecified site

⑦T23.201   Burn of second degree of right hand, unspecified site

⑦T23.202   Burn of second degree of left hand, unspecified site

⑦T23.209   Burn of second degree of unspecified hand, unspecified site

T23.21   Burn of second degree of thumb (nail)

⑦T23.211   Burn of second degree of right thumb (nail)

⑦T23.212   Burn of second degree of left thumb (nail)

⑦T23.219   Burn of second degree of unspecified thumb (nail)

T23.22   Burn of second degree of single finger (nail) except thumb

⑦T23.221   Burn of second degree of single right finger (nail) except thumb

⑦T23.222   Burn of second degree of single left finger (nail) except thumb

⑦T23.229   Burn of second degree of unspecified single finger (nail) except thumb

T23.23   Burn of second degree of multiple fingers (nail), not including thumb

⑦T23.231   Burn of second degree of multiple right fingers (nail), not including thumb

⑦T23.232   Burn of second degree of multiple left fingers (nail), not including thumb

⑦T23.239   Burn of second degree of unspecified multiple fingers (nail), not including thumb

T23.24   Burn of second degree of multiple fingers (nail), including thumb

⑦T23.241   Burn of second degree of multiple right fingers (nail), including thumb

⑦T23.242   Burn of second degree of multiple left fingers (nail), including thumb

⑦T23.249   Burn of second degree of unspecified multiple fingers (nail), including thumb

T23.25   Burn of second degree of palm

⑦T23.251   Burn of second degree of right palm

⑦T23.252   Burn of second degree of left palm

⑦T23.259   Burn of second degree of unspecified palm

T23.26   Burn of second degree of back of hand

⑦T23.261   Burn of second degree of back of right hand

⑦T23.262   Burn of second degree of back of left hand

⑦T23.269   Burn of second degree of back of unspecified hand

T23.27   Burn of second degree of wrist

⑦T23.271   Burn of second degree of right wrist

⑦T23.272   Burn of second degree of left wrist

⑦T23.279   Burn of second degree of unspecified wrist

T23.29   Burn of second degree of multiple sites of wrist and hand

⑦T23.291   Burn of second degree of multiple sites of right wrist and hand

⑦T23.292   Burn of second degree of multiple sites of left wrist and hand

---

⑦T23.299   Burn of second degree of multiple sites of unspecified wrist and hand

T23.3   Burn of third degree of wrist and hand

Use additional external cause code to identify the source, place and intent of the burn (X00-X19, X75-X77, X96-X98, Y92)

T23.30   Burn of third degree of hand, unspecified site

⑦T23.301   Burn of third degree of right hand, unspecified site

⑦T23.302   Burn of third degree of left hand, unspecified site

⑦T23.309   Burn of third degree of unspecified hand, unspecified site

T23.31   Burn of third degree of thumb (nail)

⑦T23.311   Burn of third degree of right thumb (nail)

⑦T23.312   Burn of third degree of left thumb (nail)

⑦T23.319   Burn of third degree of unspecified thumb (nail)

T23.32   Burn of third degree of single finger (nail) except thumb

⑦T23.321   Burn of third degree of single right finger (nail) except thumb

⑦T23.322   Burn of third degree of single left finger (nail) except thumb

⑦T23.329   Burn of third degree of unspecified single finger (nail) except thumb

T23.33   Burn of third degree of multiple fingers (nail), not including thumb

⑦T23.331   Burn of third degree of multiple right fingers (nail), not including thumb

⑦T23.332   Burn of third degree of multiple left fingers (nail), not including thumb

⑦T23.339   Burn of third degree of unspecified multiple fingers (nail), not including thumb

T23.34   Burn of third degree of multiple fingers (nail), including thumb

⑦T23.341   Burn of third degree of multiple right fingers (nail), including thumb

⑦T23.342   Burn of third degree of multiple left fingers (nail), including thumb

⑦T23.349   Burn of third degree of unspecified multiple fingers (nail), including thumb

T23.35   Burn of third degree of palm

⑦T23.351   Burn of third degree of right palm

⑦T23.352   Burn of third degree of left palm

⑦T23.359   Burn of third degree of unspecified palm

T23.36   Burn of third degree of back of hand

⑦T23.361   Burn of third degree of back of right hand

⑦T23.362   Burn of third degree of back of left hand

⑦T23.369   Burn of third degree of back of unspecified hand

T23.37   Burn of third degree of wrist

⑦T23.371   Burn of third degree of right wrist

⑦T23.372   Burn of third degree of left wrist

⑦T23.379   Burn of third degree of unspecified wrist

T23.39   Burn of third degree of multiple sites of wrist and hand

⑦T23.391   Burn of third degree of multiple sites of right wrist and hand

⑦T23.392   Burn of third degree of multiple sites of left wrist and hand

⑦T23.399   Burn of third degree of multiple sites of unspecified wrist and hand

T23.4   Corrosion of unspecified degree of wrist and hand

Code first (T51-T65) to identify chemical and intent

Use additional external cause code to identify place (Y92)

T23.40   Corrosion of unspecified degree of hand, unspecified site

⑦T23.401   Corrosion of unspecified degree of right hand, unspecified site

⑦T23.402   Corrosion of unspecified degree of left hand, unspecified site

⑦T23.409   Corrosion of unspecified degree of unspecified hand, unspecified site

T23.41   Corrosion of unspecified degree of thumb (nail)

⑦T23.411   Corrosion of unspecified degree of right thumb (nail)

⑦T23.412   Corrosion of unspecified degree of left thumb (nail)

⑦T23.419   Corrosion of unspecified degree of unspecified thumb (nail)

T23.42   Corrosion of unspecified degree of single finger (nail) except thumb

⑦T23.421   Corrosion of unspecified degree of single right finger (nail) except thumb

⑦T23.422   Corrosion of unspecified degree of single left finger (nail) except thumb

⑦T23.429   Corrosion of unspecified degree of unspecified single finger (nail) except thumb

T23.43   Corrosion of unspecified degree of multiple fingers (nail), not including thumb

⑦T23.431   Corrosion of unspecified degree of multiple right fingers (nail), not including thumb

⑦T23.432   Corrosion of unspecified degree of multiple left fingers (nail), not including thumb

⑦T23.439   Corrosion of unspecified degree of unspecified multiple fingers (nail), not including thumb

T23.44   Corrosion of unspecified degree of multiple fingers (nail), including thumb

⑦T23.441   Corrosion of unspecified degree of multiple right fingers (nail), including thumb

⑦T23.442   Corrosion of unspecified degree of multiple left fingers (nail), including thumb

⑦T23.449   Corrosion of unspecified degree of unspecified multiple fingers (nail), including thumb

T23.45 Corrosion of unspecified degree of palm

⑦T23.451 Corrosion of unspecified degree of right palm

⑦T23.452 Corrosion of unspecified degree of left palm

⑦T23.459 Corrosion of unspecified degree of unspecified palm

T23.46 Corrosion of unspecified degree of back of hand

⑦T23.461 Corrosion of unspecified degree of back of right hand

⑦T23.462 Corrosion of unspecified degree of back of left hand

⑦T23.469 Corrosion of unspecified degree of back of unspecified hand

T23.47 Corrosion of unspecified degree of wrist

⑦T23.471 Corrosion of unspecified degree of right wrist

⑦T23.472 Corrosion of unspecified degree of left wrist

⑦T23.479 Corrosion of unspecified degree of unspecified wrist

T23.49 Corrosion of unspecified degree of multiple sites of wrist and hand

⑦T23.491 Corrosion of unspecified degree of multiple sites of right wrist and hand

⑦T23.492 Corrosion of unspecified degree of multiple sites of left wrist and hand

⑦T23.499 Corrosion of unspecified degree of multiple sites of unspecified wrist and hand

T23.5 Corrosion of first degree of wrist and hand

Code first (T51-T65) to identify chemical and intent

Use additional external cause code to identify place (Y92)

T23.50 Corrosion of first degree of hand, unspecified site

⑦T23.501 Corrosion of first degree of right hand, unspecified site

⑦T23.502 Corrosion of first degree of left hand, unspecified site

⑦T23.509 Corrosion of first degree of unspecified hand, unspecified site

T23.51 Corrosion of first degree of thumb (nail)

⑦T23.511 Corrosion of first degree of right thumb (nail)

⑦T23.512 Corrosion of first degree of left thumb (nail)

⑦T23.519 Corrosion of first degree of unspecified thumb (nail)

T23.52 Corrosion of first degree of single finger (nail) except thumb

⑦T23.521 Corrosion of first degree of single right finger (nail) except thumb

⑦T23.522 Corrosion of first degree of single left finger (nail) except thumb

⑦T23.529 Corrosion of first degree of unspecified single finger (nail) except thumb

T23.53 Corrosion of first degree of multiple fingers (nail), not including thumb

⑦T23.531 Corrosion of first degree of multiple right fingers (nail), not including thumb

⑦T23.532 Corrosion of first degree of multiple left fingers (nail), not including thumb

⑦T23.539 Corrosion of first degree of unspecified multiple fingers (nail), not including thumb

T23.54 Corrosion of first degree of multiple fingers (nail), including thumb

⑦T23.541 Corrosion of first degree of multiple right fingers (nail), including thumb

⑦T23.542 Corrosion of first degree of multiple left fingers (nail), including thumb

⑦T23.549 Corrosion of first degree of unspecified multiple fingers (nail), including thumb

T23.55 Corrosion of first degree of palm

⑦T23.551 Corrosion of first degree of right palm

⑦T23.552 Corrosion of first degree of left palm

⑦T23.559 Corrosion of first degree of unspecified palm

T23.56 Corrosion of first degree of back of hand

⑦T23.561 Corrosion of first degree of back of right hand

⑦T23.562 Corrosion of first degree of back of left hand

⑦T23.569 Corrosion of first degree of back of unspecified hand

T23.57 Corrosion of first degree of wrist

⑦T23.571 Corrosion of first degree of right wrist

⑦T23.572 Corrosion of first degree of left wrist

⑦T23.579 Corrosion of first degree of unspecified wrist

T23.59 Corrosion of first degree of multiple sites of wrist and hand

⑦T23.591 Corrosion of first degree of multiple sites of right wrist and hand

⑦T23.592 Corrosion of first degree of multiple sites of left wrist and hand

⑦T23.599 Corrosion of first degree of multiple sites of unspecified wrist and hand

T23.6 Corrosion of second degree of wrist and hand

Code first (T51-T65) to identify chemical and intent

Use additional external cause code to identify place (Y92)

T23.60 Corrosion of second degree of hand, unspecified site

⑦T23.601 Corrosion of second degree of right hand, unspecified site

⑦T23.602 Corrosion of second degree of left hand, unspecified site

⑦T23.609 Corrosion of second degree of unspecified hand, unspecified site

T23.61 Corrosion of second degree of thumb (nail)

⑦T23.611 Corrosion of second degree of right thumb (nail)

⑦T23.612   **Corrosion of second degree of left thumb (nail)**

⑦T23.619   **Corrosion of second degree of unspecified thumb (nail)**

T23.62   **Corrosion of second degree of single finger (nail) except thumb**

    ⑦T23.621   **Corrosion of second degree of single right finger (nail) except thumb**

    ⑦T23.622   **Corrosion of second degree of single left finger (nail) except thumb**

    ⑦T23.629   **Corrosion of second degree of unspecified single finger (nail) except thumb**

T23.63   **Corrosion of second degree of multiple fingers (nail), not including thumb**

    ⑦T23.631   **Corrosion of second degree of multiple right fingers (nail), not including thumb**

    ⑦T23.632   **Corrosion of second degree of multiple left fingers (nail), not including thumb**

    ⑦T23.639   **Corrosion of second degree of unspecified multiple fingers (nail), not including thumb**

T23.64   **Corrosion of second degree of multiple fingers (nail), including thumb**

    ⑦T23.641   **Corrosion of second degree of multiple right fingers (nail), including thumb**

    ⑦T23.642   **Corrosion of second degree of multiple left fingers (nail), including thumb**

    ⑦T23.649   **Corrosion of second degree of unspecified multiple fingers (nail), including thumb**

T23.65   **Corrosion of second degree of palm**

    ⑦T23.651   **Corrosion of second degree of right palm**

    ⑦T23.652   **Corrosion of second degree of left palm**

    ⑦T23.659   **Corrosion of second degree of unspecified palm**

T23.66   **Corrosion of second degree of back of hand**

    ⑦T23.661   **Corrosion of second degree back of right hand**

    ⑦T23.662   **Corrosion of second degree back of left hand**

    ⑦T23.669   **Corrosion of second degree back of unspecified hand**

T23.67   **Corrosion of second degree of wrist**

    ⑦T23.671   **Corrosion of second degree of right wrist**

    ⑦T23.672   **Corrosion of second degree of left wrist**

    ⑦T23.679   **Corrosion of second degree of unspecified wrist**

T23.69   **Corrosion of second degree of multiple sites of wrist and hand**

    ⑦T23.691   **Corrosion of second degree of multiple sites of right wrist and hand**

⑦T23.692   **Corrosion of second degree of multiple sites of left wrist and hand**

⑦T23.699   **Corrosion of second degree of multiple sites of unspecified wrist and hand**

T23.7   **Corrosion of third degree of wrist and hand**

    <u>Code first</u> (T51-T65) to identify chemical and intent

    Use additional external cause code to identify place (Y92)

T23.70   **Corrosion of third degree of hand, unspecified site**

    ⑦T23.701   **Corrosion of third degree of right hand, unspecified site**

    ⑦T23.702   **Corrosion of third degree of left hand, unspecified site**

    ⑦T23.709   **Corrosion of third degree of unspecified hand, unspecified site**

T23.71   **Corrosion of third degree of thumb (nail)**

    ⑦T23.711   **Corrosion of third degree of right thumb (nail)**

    ⑦T23.712   **Corrosion of third degree of left thumb (nail)**

    ⑦T23.719   **Corrosion of third degree of unspecified thumb (nail)**

T23.72   **Corrosion of third degree of single finger (nail) except thumb**

    ⑦T23.721   **Corrosion of third degree of single right finger (nail) except thumb**

    ⑦T23.722   **Corrosion of third degree of single left finger (nail) except thumb**

    ⑦T23.729   **Corrosion of third degree of unspecified single finger (nail) except thumb**

T23.73   **Corrosion of third degree of multiple fingers (nail), not including thumb**

    ⑦T23.731   **Corrosion of third degree of multiple right fingers (nail), not including thumb**

    ⑦T23.732   **Corrosion of third degree of multiple left fingers (nail), not including thumb**

    ⑦T23.739   **Corrosion of third degree of unspecified multiple fingers (nail), not including thumb**

T23.74   **Corrosion of third degree of multiple fingers (nail), including thumb**

    ⑦T23.741   **Corrosion of third degree of multiple right fingers (nail), including thumb**

    ⑦T23.742   **Corrosion of third degree of multiple left fingers (nail), including thumb**

    ⑦T23.749   **Corrosion of third degree of unspecified multiple fingers (nail), including thumb**

T23.75   **Corrosion of third degree of palm**

    ⑦T23.751   **Corrosion of third degree of right palm**

    ⑦T23.752   **Corrosion of third degree of left palm**

    ⑦T23.759   **Corrosion of third degree of unspecified palm**

T23.76   **Corrosion of third degree of back of hand**

   ● New code   ▲ Revised code   **Excludes1:** Not coded here   **Excludes2:** Not included here   ⊗ Placeholder required   ⑦ 7th digit required

⑦ **T23.761**   Corrosion of third degree of back of right hand

⑦ **T23.762**   Corrosion of third degree of back of left hand

⑦ **T23.769**   Corrosion of third degree back of unspecified hand

T23.77   Corrosion of third degree of wrist

⑦ **T23.771**   Corrosion of third degree of right wrist

⑦ **T23.772**   Corrosion of third degree of left wrist

⑦ **T23.779**   Corrosion of third degree of unspecified wrist

T23.79   Corrosion of third degree of multiple sites of wrist and hand

⑦ **T23.791**   Corrosion of third degree of multiple sites of right wrist and hand

⑦ **T23.792**   Corrosion of third degree of multiple sites of left wrist and hand

⑦ **T23.799**   Corrosion of third degree of multiple sites of unspecified wrist and hand

T24   **Burn and corrosion of lower limb, except ankle and foot**

Excludes2: burn and corrosion of ankle and foot (T25.-)

burn and corrosion of hip region (T21.-)

The appropriate 7th character is to be added to each code from category T24

A - initial encounter

D - subsequent encounter

S - sequela

T24.0   **Burn of unspecified degree of lower limb, except ankle and foot**

Use additional external cause code to identify the source, place and intent of the burn (X00-X19, X75-X77, X96-X98, Y92)

T24.00   Burn of unspecified degree of unspecified site of lower limb, except ankle and foot

⑦ **T24.001**   Burn of unspecified degree of unspecified site of right lower limb, except ankle and foot

⑦ **T24.002**   Burn of unspecified degree of unspecified site of left lower limb, except ankle and foot

⑦ **T24.009**   Burn of unspecified degree of unspecified site of unspecified lower limb, except ankle and foot

T24.01   Burn of unspecified degree of thigh

⑦ **T24.011**   Burn of unspecified degree of right thigh

⑦ **T24.012**   Burn of unspecified degree of left thigh

⑦ **T24.019**   Burn of unspecified degree of unspecified thigh

T24.02   Burn of unspecified degree of knee

⑦ **T24.021**   Burn of unspecified degree of right knee

⑦ **T24.022**   Burn of unspecified degree of left knee

⑦ **T24.029**   Burn of unspecified degree of unspecified knee

T24.03   Burn of unspecified degree of lower leg

⑦ **T24.031**   Burn of unspecified degree of right lower leg

⑦ **T24.032**   Burn of unspecified degree of left lower leg

⑦ **T24.039**   Burn of unspecified degree of unspecified lower leg

T24.09   Burn of unspecified degree of multiple sites of lower limb, except ankle and foot

⑦ **T24.091**   Burn of unspecified degree of multiple sites of right lower limb, except ankle and foot

⑦ **T24.092**   Burn of unspecified degree of multiple sites of left lower limb, except ankle and foot

⑦ **T24.099**   Burn of unspecified degree of multiple sites of unspecified lower limb, except ankle and foot

T24.1   **Burn of first degree of lower limb, except ankle and foot**

Use additional external cause code to identify the source, place and intent of the burn (X00-X19, X75-X77, X96-X98, Y92)

T24.10   Burn of first degree of unspecified site of lower limb, except ankle and foot

⑦ **T24.101**   Burn of first degree of unspecified site of right lower limb, except ankle and foot

⑦ **T24.102**   Burn of first degree of unspecified site of left lower limb, except ankle and foot

⑦ **T24.109**   Burn of first degree of unspecified site of unspecified lower limb, except ankle and foot

T24.11   Burn of first degree of thigh

⑦ **T24.111**   Burn of first degree of right thigh

⑦ **T24.112**   Burn of first degree of left thigh

⑦ **T24.119**   Burn of first degree of unspecified thigh

T24.12   Burn of first degree of knee

⑦ **T24.121**   Burn of first degree of right knee

⑦ **T24.122**   Burn of first degree of left knee

⑦ **T24.129**   Burn of first degree of unspecified knee

T24.13   Burn of first degree of lower leg

⑦ **T24.131**   Burn of first degree of right lower leg

⑦ **T24.132**   Burn of first degree of left lower leg

⑦ **T24.139**   Burn of first degree of unspecified lower leg

T24.19   Burn of first degree of multiple sites of lower limb, except ankle and foot

⑦ **T24.191**   Burn of first degree of multiple sites of right lower limb, except ankle and foot

⑦ **T24.192**   Burn of first degree of multiple sites of left lower limb, except ankle and foot

⑦ **T24.199**   Burn of first degree of multiple sites of unspecified lower limb, except ankle and foot

T24.2   Burn of second degree of lower limb, except ankle and foot

Use additional external cause code to identify the source, place and intent of the burn (X00-X19, X75-X77, X96-X98, Y92)

T24.20   Burn of second degree of unspecified site of lower limb, except ankle and foot

⑦**T24.201   Burn of second degree of unspecified site of right lower limb, except ankle and foot**

⑦**T24.202   Burn of second degree of unspecified site of left lower limb, except ankle and foot**

⑦**T24.209   Burn of second degree of unspecified site of unspecified lower limb, except ankle and foot**

T24.21   Burn of second degree of thigh

⑦**T24.211   Burn of second degree of right thigh**

⑦**T24.212   Burn of second degree of left thigh**

⑦**T24.219   Burn of second degree of unspecified thigh**

T24.22   Burn of second degree of knee

⑦**T24.221   Burn of second degree of right knee**

⑦**T24.222   Burn of second degree of left knee**

⑦**T24.229   Burn of second degree of unspecified knee**

T24.23   Burn of second degree of lower leg

⑦**T24.231   Burn of second degree of right lower leg**

⑦**T24.232   Burn of second degree of left lower leg**

⑦**T24.239   Burn of second degree of unspecified lower leg**

T24.29   Burn of second degree of multiple sites of lower limb, except ankle and foot

⑦**T24.291   Burn of second degree of multiple sites of right lower limb, except ankle and foot**

⑦**T24.292   Burn of second degree of multiple sites of left lower limb, except ankle and foot**

⑦**T24.299   Burn of second degree of multiple sites of unspecified lower limb, except ankle and foot**

T24.3   Burn of third degree of lower limb, except ankle and foot

Use additional external cause code to identify the source, place and intent of the burn (X00-X19, X75-X77, X96-X98, Y92)

T24.30   Burn of third degree of unspecified site of lower limb, except ankle and foot

⑦**T24.301   Burn of third degree of unspecified site of right lower limb, except ankle and foot**

⑦**T24.302   Burn of third degree of unspecified site of left lower limb, except ankle and foot**

⑦**T24.309   Burn of third degree of unspecified site of unspecified lower limb, except ankle and foot**

T24.31   Burn of third degree of thigh

⑦**T24.311   Burn of third degree of right thigh**

⑦**T24.312   Burn of third degree of left thigh**

⑦**T24.319   Burn of third degree of unspecified thigh**

T24.32   Burn of third degree of knee

⑦**T24.321   Burn of third degree of right knee**

⑦**T24.322   Burn of third degree of left knee**

⑦**T24.329   Burn of third degree of unspecified knee**

T24.33   Burn of third degree of lower leg

⑦**T24.331   Burn of third degree of right lower leg**

⑦**T24.332   Burn of third degree of left lower leg**

⑦**T24.339   Burn of third degree of unspecified lower leg**

T24.39   Burn of third degree of multiple sites of lower limb, except ankle and foot

⑦**T24.391   Burn of third degree of multiple sites of right lower limb, except ankle and foot**

⑦**T24.392   Burn of third degree of multiple sites of left lower limb, except ankle and foot**

⑦**T24.399   Burn of third degree of multiple sites of unspecified lower limb, except ankle and foot**

T24.4   Corrosion of unspecified degree of lower limb, except ankle and foot

Code first (T51-T65) to identify chemical and intent

Use additional external cause code to identify place (Y92)

T24.40   Corrosion of unspecified degree of unspecified site of lower limb, except ankle and foot

⑦**T24.401   Corrosion of unspecified degree of unspecified site of right lower limb, except ankle and foot**

⑦**T24.402   Corrosion of unspecified degree of unspecified site of left lower limb, except ankle and foot**

⑦**T24.409   Corrosion of unspecified degree of unspecified site of unspecified lower limb, except ankle and foot**

T24.41   Corrosion of unspecified degree of thigh

⑦**T24.411   Corrosion of unspecified degree of right thigh**

⑦**T24.412   Corrosion of unspecified degree of left thigh**

⑦**T24.419   Corrosion of unspecified degree of unspecified thigh**

T24.42   Corrosion of unspecified degree of knee

⑦**T24.421   Corrosion of unspecified degree of right knee**

⑦**T24.422   Corrosion of unspecified degree of left knee**

⑦**T24.429   Corrosion of unspecified degree of unspecified knee**

T24.43   Corrosion of unspecified degree of lower leg

⑦**T24.431   Corrosion of unspecified degree of right lower leg**

⑦**T24.432   Corrosion of unspecified degree of left lower leg**

⑦**T24.439** **Corrosion of unspecified degree of unspecified lower leg**

T24.49 **Corrosion of unspecified degree of multiple sites of lower limb, except ankle and foot**

⑦**T24.491** **Corrosion of unspecified degree of multiple sites of right lower limb, except ankle and foot**

⑦**T24.492** **Corrosion of unspecified degree of multiple sites of left lower limb, except ankle and foot**

⑦**T24.499** **Corrosion of unspecified degree of multiple sites of unspecified lower limb, except ankle and foot**

T24.5 **Corrosion of first degree of lower limb, except ankle and foot**

Code first (T51-T65) to identify chemical and intent

Use additional external cause code to identify place (Y92)

T24.50 **Corrosion of first degree of unspecified site of lower limb, except ankle and foot**

⑦**T24.501** **Corrosion of first degree of unspecified site of right lower limb, except ankle and foot**

⑦**T24.502** **Corrosion of first degree of unspecified site of left lower limb, except ankle and foot**

⑦**T24.509** **Corrosion of first degree of unspecified site of unspecified lower limb, except ankle and foot**

T24.51 **Corrosion of first degree of thigh**

⑦**T24.511** **Corrosion of first degree of right thigh**

⑦**T24.512** **Corrosion of first degree of left thigh**

⑦**T24.519** **Corrosion of first degree of unspecified thigh**

T24.52 **Corrosion of first degree of knee**

⑦**T24.521** **Corrosion of first degree of right knee**

⑦**T24.522** **Corrosion of first degree of left knee**

⑦**T24.529** **Corrosion of first degree of unspecified knee**

T24.53 **Corrosion of first degree of lower leg**

⑦**T24.531** **Corrosion of first degree of right lower leg**

⑦**T24.532** **Corrosion of first degree of left lower leg**

⑦**T24.539** **Corrosion of first degree of unspecified lower leg**

T24.59 **Corrosion of first degree of multiple sites of lower limb, except ankle and foot**

⑦**T24.591** **Corrosion of first degree of multiple sites of right lower limb, except ankle and foot**

⑦**T24.592** **Corrosion of first degree of multiple sites of left lower limb, except ankle and foot**

⑦**T24.599** **Corrosion of first degree of multiple sites of unspecified lower limb, except ankle and foot**

T24.6 **Corrosion of second degree of lower limb, except ankle and foot**

Code first (T51-T65) to identify chemical and intent

Use additional external cause code to identify place (Y92)

T24.60 **Corrosion of second degree of unspecified site of lower limb, except ankle and foot**

⑦**T24.601** **Corrosion of second degree of unspecified site of right lower limb, except ankle and foot**

⑦**T24.602** **Corrosion of second degree of unspecified site of left lower limb, except ankle and foot**

⑦**T24.609** **Corrosion of second degree of unspecified site of unspecified lower limb, except ankle and foot**

T24.61 **Corrosion of second degree of thigh**

⑦**T24.611** **Corrosion of second degree of right thigh**

⑦**T24.612** **Corrosion of second degree of left thigh**

⑦**T24.619** **Corrosion of second degree of unspecified thigh**

T24.62 **Corrosion of second degree of knee**

⑦**T24.621** **Corrosion of second degree of right knee**

⑦**T24.622** **Corrosion of second degree of left knee**

⑦**T24.629** **Corrosion of second degree of unspecified knee**

T24.63 **Corrosion of second degree of lower leg**

⑦**T24.631** **Corrosion of second degree of right lower leg**

⑦**T24.632** **Corrosion of second degree of left lower leg**

⑦**T24.639** **Corrosion of second degree of unspecified lower leg**

T24.69 **Corrosion of second degree of multiple sites of lower limb, except ankle and foot**

⑦**T24.691** **Corrosion of second degree of multiple sites of right lower limb, except ankle and foot**

⑦**T24.692** **Corrosion of second degree of multiple sites of left lower limb, except ankle and foot**

⑦**T24.699** **Corrosion of second degree of multiple sites of unspecified lower limb, except ankle and foot**

T24.7 **Corrosion of third degree of lower limb, except ankle and foot**

Code first (T51-T65) to identify chemical and intent

Use additional external cause code to identify place (Y92)

T24.70 **Corrosion of third degree of unspecified site of lower limb, except ankle and foot**

⑦**T24.701** **Corrosion of third degree of unspecified site of right lower limb, except ankle and foot**

⑦**T24.702** **Corrosion of third degree of unspecified site of left lower limb, except ankle and foot**

⑦**T24.709** **Corrosion of third degree of unspecified site of unspecified lower limb, except ankle and foot**

T24.71 **Corrosion of third degree of thigh**

⑦**T24.711** **Corrosion of third degree of right thigh**

---

⑦ **T24.712**   **Corrosion of third degree of left thigh**

⑦ **T24.719**   **Corrosion of third degree of unspecified thigh**

T24.72   **Corrosion of third degree of knee**

⑦ **T24.721**   **Corrosion of third degree of right knee**

⑦ **T24.722**   **Corrosion of third degree of left knee**

⑦ **T24.729**   **Corrosion of third degree of unspecified knee**

T24.73   **Corrosion of third degree of lower leg**

⑦ **T24.731**   **Corrosion of third degree of right lower leg**

⑦ **T24.732**   **Corrosion of third degree of left lower leg**

⑦ **T24.739**   **Corrosion of third degree of unspecified lower leg**

T24.79   **Corrosion of third degree of multiple sites of lower limb, except ankle and foot**

⑦ **T24.791**   **Corrosion of third degree of multiple sites of right lower limb, except ankle and foot**

⑦ **T24.792**   **Corrosion of third degree of multiple sites of left lower limb, except ankle and foot**

⑦ **T24.799**   **Corrosion of third degree of multiple sites of unspecified lower limb, except ankle and foot**

T25   **Burn and corrosion of ankle and foot**

The appropriate 7th character is to be added to each code from category T25

A - initial encounter

D - subsequent encounter

S - sequela

T25.0   **Burn of unspecified degree of ankle and foot**

Use additional external cause code to identify the source, place and intent of the burn (X00-X19, X75-X77, X96-X98, Y92)

T25.01   **Burn of unspecified degree of ankle**

⑦ **T25.011**   **Burn of unspecified degree of right ankle**

⑦ **T25.012**   **Burn of unspecified degree of left ankle**

⑦ **T25.019**   **Burn of unspecified degree of unspecified ankle**

T25.02   **Burn of unspecified degree of foot**

Excludes2: burn of unspecified degree of toe(s) (nail) (T25.03-)

⑦ **T25.021**   **Burn of unspecified degree of right foot**

⑦ **T25.022**   **Burn of unspecified degree of left foot**

⑦ **T25.029**   **Burn of unspecified degree of unspecified foot**

T25.03   **Burn of unspecified degree of toe(s) (nail)**

⑦ **T25.031**   **Burn of unspecified degree of right toe(s) (nail)**

⑦ **T25.032**   **Burn of unspecified degree of left toe(s) (nail)**

⑦ **T25.039**   **Burn of unspecified degree of unspecified toe(s) (nail)**

T25.09   **Burn of unspecified degree of multiple sites of ankle and foot**

⑦ **T25.091**   **Burn of unspecified degree of multiple sites of right ankle and foot**

⑦ **T25.092**   **Burn of unspecified degree of multiple sites of left ankle and foot**

⑦ **T25.099**   **Burn of unspecified degree of multiple sites of unspecified ankle and foot**

T25.1   **Burn of first degree of ankle and foot**

Use additional external cause code to identify the source, place and intent of the burn (X00-X19, X75-X77, X96-X98, Y92)

T25.11   **Burn of first degree of ankle**

⑦ **T25.111**   **Burn of first degree of right ankle**

⑦ **T25.112**   **Burn of first degree of left ankle**

⑦ **T25.119**   **Burn of first degree of unspecified ankle**

T25.12   **Burn of first degree of foot**

Excludes2: burn of first degree of toe(s) (nail) (T25.13-)

⑦ **T25.121**   **Burn of first degree of right foot**

⑦ **T25.122**   **Burn of first degree of left foot**

⑦ **T25.129**   **Burn of first degree of unspecified foot**

T25.13   **Burn of first degree of toe(s) (nail)**

⑦ **T25.131**   **Burn of first degree of right toe(s) (nail)**

⑦ **T25.132**   **Burn of first degree of left toe(s) (nail)**

⑦ **T25.139**   **Burn of first degree of unspecified toe(s) (nail)**

T25.19   **Burn of first degree of multiple sites of ankle and foot**

⑦ **T25.191**   **Burn of first degree of multiple sites of right ankle and foot**

⑦ **T25.192**   **Burn of first degree of multiple sites of left ankle and foot**

⑦ **T25.199**   **Burn of first degree of multiple sites of unspecified ankle and foot**

T25.2   **Burn of second degree of ankle and foot**

Use additional external cause code to identify the source, place and intent of the burn (X00-X19, X75-X77, X96-X98, Y92)

T25.21   **Burn of second degree of ankle**

⑦ **T25.211**   **Burn of second degree of right ankle**

⑦ **T25.212**   **Burn of second degree of left ankle**

⑦ **T25.219**   **Burn of second degree of unspecified ankle**

T25.22   **Burn of second degree of foot**

Excludes2: burn of second degree of toe(s) (nail) (T25.23-)

⑦ **T25.221**   **Burn of second degree of right foot**

⑦ **T25.222**   **Burn of second degree of left foot**

⑦**T25.229 Burn of second degree of unspecified foot**

T25.23 Burn of second degree of toe(s) (nail)

⑦**T25.231 Burn of second degree of right toe(s) (nail)**

⑦**T25.232 Burn of second degree of left toe(s) (nail)**

⑦**T25.239 Burn of second degree of unspecified toe(s) (nail)**

T25.29 Burn of second degree of multiple sites of ankle and foot

⑦**T25.291 Burn of second degree of multiple sites of right ankle and foot**

⑦**T25.292 Burn of second degree of multiple sites of left ankle and foot**

⑦**T25.299 Burn of second degree of multiple sites of unspecified ankle and foot**

T25.3 Burn of third degree of ankle and foot

Use additional external cause code to identify the source, place and intent of the burn (X00-X19, X75-X77, X96-X98, Y92)

T25.31 Burn of third degree of ankle

⑦**T25.311 Burn of third degree of right ankle**

⑦**T25.312 Burn of third degree of left ankle**

⑦**T25.319 Burn of third degree of unspecified ankle**

T25.32 Burn of third degree of foot

Excludes2: burn of third degree of toe(s) (nail) (T25.33-)

⑦**T25.321 Burn of third degree of right foot**

⑦**T25.322 Burn of third degree of left foot**

⑦**T25.329 Burn of third degree of unspecified foot**

T25.33 Burn of third degree of toe(s) (nail)

⑦**T25.331 Burn of third degree of right toe(s) (nail)**

⑦**T25.332 Burn of third degree of left toe(s) (nail)**

⑦**T25.339 Burn of third degree of unspecified toe(s) (nail)**

T25.39 Burn of third degree of multiple sites of ankle and foot

⑦**T25.391 Burn of third degree of multiple sites of right ankle and foot**

⑦**T25.392 Burn of third degree of multiple sites of left ankle and foot**

⑦**T25.399 Burn of third degree of multiple sites of unspecified ankle and foot**

T25.4 Corrosion of unspecified degree of ankle and foot

Code first (T51-T65) to identify chemical and intent

Use additional external cause code to identify place (Y92)

T25.41 Corrosion of unspecified degree of ankle

⑦**T25.411 Corrosion of unspecified degree of right ankle**

⑦**T25.412 Corrosion of unspecified degree of left ankle**

⑦**T25.419 Corrosion of unspecified degree of unspecified ankle**

T25.42 Corrosion of unspecified degree of foot

Excludes2: corrosion of unspecified degree of toe(s) (nail) (T25.43-)

⑦**T25.421 Corrosion of unspecified degree of right foot**

⑦**T25.422 Corrosion of unspecified degree of left foot**

⑦**T25.429 Corrosion of unspecified degree of unspecified foot**

T25.43 Corrosion of unspecified degree of toe(s) (nail)

⑦**T25.431 Corrosion of unspecified degree of right toe(s) (nail)**

⑦**T25.432 Corrosion of unspecified degree of left toe(s) (nail)**

⑦**T25.439 Corrosion of unspecified degree of unspecified toe(s) (nail)**

T25.49 Corrosion of unspecified degree of multiple sites of ankle and foot

⑦**T25.491 Corrosion of unspecified degree of multiple sites of right ankle and foot**

⑦**T25.492 Corrosion of unspecified degree of multiple sites of left ankle and foot**

⑦**T25.499 Corrosion of unspecified degree of multiple sites of unspecified ankle and foot**

T25.5 Corrosion of first degree of ankle and foot

Code first (T51-T65) to identify chemical and intent

Use additional external cause code to identify place (Y92)

T25.51 Corrosion of first degree of ankle

⑦**T25.511 Corrosion of first degree of right ankle**

⑦**T25.512 Corrosion of first degree of left ankle**

⑦**T25.519 Corrosion of first degree of unspecified ankle**

T25.52 Corrosion of first degree of foot

Excludes2: corrosion of first degree of toe(s) (nail) (T25.53-)

⑦**T25.521 Corrosion of first degree of right foot**

⑦**T25.522 Corrosion of first degree of left foot**

⑦**T25.529 Corrosion of first degree of unspecified foot**

T25.53 Corrosion of first degree of toe(s) (nail)

⑦**T25.531 Corrosion of first degree of right toe(s) (nail)**

⑦**T25.532 Corrosion of first degree of left toe(s) (nail)**

⑦**T25.539 Corrosion of first degree of unspecified toe(s) (nail)**

T25.59 Corrosion of first degree of multiple sites of ankle and foot

⑦**T25.591 Corrosion of first degree of multiple sites of right ankle and foot**

⑦**T25.592 Corrosion of first degree of multiple sites of left ankle and foot**

⑦**T25.599 Corrosion of first degree of multiple sites of unspecified ankle and foot**

T25.6 Corrosion of second degree of ankle and foot

Code first (T51-T65) to identify chemical and intent

Use additional external cause code to identify place (Y92)

T25.61   **Corrosion of second degree of ankle**

⑦T25.611   **Corrosion of second degree of right ankle**

⑦T25.612   **Corrosion of second degree of left ankle**

⑦T25.619   **Corrosion of second degree of unspecified ankle**

T25.62   **Corrosion of second degree of foot**

> **Excludes2:** corrosion of second degree of toe(s) (nail) (T25.63-)

⑦T25.621   **Corrosion of second degree of right foot**

⑦T25.622   **Corrosion of second degree of left foot**

⑦T25.629   **Corrosion of second degree of unspecified foot**

T25.63   **Corrosion of second degree of toe(s) (nail)**

⑦T25.631   **Corrosion of second degree of right toe(s) (nail)**

⑦T25.632   **Corrosion of second degree of left toe(s) (nail)**

⑦T25.639   **Corrosion of second degree of unspecified toe(s) (nail)**

⑦T25.69   **Corrosion of second degree of multiple sites of ankle and foot**

⑦T25.691   **Corrosion of second degree of right ankle and foot**

⑦T25.692   **Corrosion of second degree of left ankle and foot**

⑦T25.699   **Corrosion of second degree of unspecified ankle and foot**

T25.7   **Corrosion of third degree of ankle and foot**

> Code first (T51-T65) to identify chemical and intent
>
> Use additional external cause code to identify place (Y92)

T25.71   **Corrosion of third degree of ankle**

⑦T25.711   **Corrosion of third degree of right ankle**

⑦T25.712   **Corrosion of third degree of left ankle**

⑦T25.719   **Corrosion of third degree of unspecified ankle**

T25.72   **Corrosion of third degree of foot**

> **Excludes2:** corrosion of third degree of toe(s) (nail) (T25.73-)

⑦T25.721   **Corrosion of third degree of right foot**

⑦T25.722   **Corrosion of third degree of left foot**

⑦T25.729   **Corrosion of third degree of unspecified foot**

⑦T25.73   **Corrosion of third degree of toe(s) (nail)**

⑦T25.731   **Corrosion of third degree of right toe(s) (nail)**

⑦T25.732   **Corrosion of third degree of left toe(s) (nail)**

⑦T25.739   **Corrosion of third degree of unspecified toe(s) (nail)**

T25.79   **Corrosion of third degree of multiple sites of ankle and foot**

⑦T25.791   **Corrosion of third degree of multiple sites of right ankle and foot**

⑦T25.792   **Corrosion of third degree of multiple sites of left ankle and foot**

⑦T25.799   **Corrosion of third degree of multiple sites of unspecified ankle and foot**

BURNS AND CORROSIONS CONFINED TO EYE AND INTERNAL ORGANS (T26-T28)

T26   **Burn and corrosion confined to eye and adnexa**

> The appropriate 7th character is to be added to each code from category T26
>
> A - initial encounter
>
> D - subsequent encounter
>
> S - sequela

T26.0   **Burn of eyelid and periocular area**

> Use additional external cause code to identify the source, place and intent of the burn (X00-X19, X75-X77, X96-X98, Y92)

⊗⑦T26.00   **Burn of unspecified eyelid and periocular area**

⊗⑦T26.01   **Burn of right eyelid and periocular area**

⊗⑦T26.02   **Burn of left eyelid and periocular area**

T26.1   **Burn of cornea and conjunctival sac**

> Use additional external cause code to identify the source, place and intent of the burn (X00-X19, X75-X77, X96-X98, Y92)

⊗⑦T26.10   **Burn of cornea and conjunctival sac, unspecified eye**

⊗⑦T26.11   **Burn of cornea and conjunctival sac, right eye**

⊗⑦T26.12   **Burn of cornea and conjunctival sac, left eye**

T26.2   **Burn with resulting rupture and destruction of eyeball**

> Use additional external cause code to identify the source, place and intent of the burn (X00-X19, X75-X77, X96-X98, Y92)

⊗⑦T26.20   **Burn with resulting rupture and destruction of unspecified eyeball**

⊗⑦T26.21   **Burn with resulting rupture and destruction of right eyeball**

⊗⑦T26.22   **Burn with resulting rupture and destruction of left eyeball**

T26.3   **Burns of other specified parts of eye and adnexa**

> Use additional external cause code to identify the source, place and intent of the burn (X00-X19, X75-X77, X96-X98, Y92)

⊗⑦T26.30   **Burns of other specified parts of unspecified eye and adnexa**

⊗⑦T26.31   **Burns of other specified parts of right eye and adnexa**

⊗⑦T26.32   **Burns of other specified parts of left eye and adnexa**

T26.4   **Burn of eye and adnexa, part unspecified**

> Use additional external cause code to identify the source, place and intent of the burn (X00-X19, X75-X77, X96-X98, Y92)

⊗⑦T26.40   **Burn of unspecified eye and adnexa, part unspecified**

⊗⑦T26.41   **Burn of right eye and adnexa, part unspecified**

⊗⑦T26.42   **Burn of left eye and adnexa, part unspecified**

T26.5   **Corrosion of eyelid and periocular area**

● New code   ▲ Revised code   **Excludes1:** Not coded here   **Excludes2:** Not included here   ⊗ Placeholder required   ⑦7th digit required

Code first (T51-T65) to identify chemical and intent

Use additional external cause code to identify place (Y92)

⊗⑦**T26.50** **Corrosion of unspecified eyelid and periocular area**

⊗⑦**T26.51** **Corrosion of right eyelid and periocular area**

⊗⑦**T26.52** **Corrosion of left eyelid and periocular area**

T26.6 **Corrosion of cornea and conjunctival sac**

Code first (T51-T65) to identify chemical and intent

Use additional external cause code to identify place (Y92)

⊗⑦**T26.60** **Corrosion of cornea and conjunctival sac, unspecified eye**

⊗⑦**T26.61** **Corrosion of cornea and conjunctival sac, right eye**

⊗⑦**T26.62** **Corrosion of cornea and conjunctival sac, left eye**

T26.7 **Corrosion with resulting rupture and destruction of eyeball**

Code first (T51-T65) to identify chemical and intent

Use additional external cause code to identify place (Y92)

⊗⑦**T26.70** **Corrosion with resulting rupture and destruction of unspecified eyeball**

⊗⑦**T26.71** **Corrosion with resulting rupture and destruction of right eyeball**

⊗⑦**T26.72** **Corrosion with resulting rupture and destruction of left eyeball**

T26.8 **Corrosions of other specified parts of eye and adnexa**

Code first (T51-T65) to identify chemical and intent

Use additional external cause code to identify place (Y92)

⊗⑦**T26.80** **Corrosions of other specified parts of unspecified eye and adnexa**

⊗⑦**T26.81** **Corrosions of other specified parts of right eye and adnexa**

⊗⑦**T26.82** **Corrosions of other specified parts of left eye and adnexa**

⑦**T26.9** **Corrosion of eye and adnexa, part unspecified**

Code first (T51-T65) to identify chemical and intent

Use additional external cause code to identify place (Y92)

⊗⑦**T26.90** **Corrosion of unspecified eye and adnexa, part unspecified**

⊗⑦**T26.91** **Corrosion of right eye and adnexa, part unspecified**

⊗⑦**T26.92** **Corrosion of left eye and adnexa, part unspecified**

T27 **Burn and corrosion of respiratory tract**

Use additional external cause code to identify the source and intent of the burn (X00-X19, X75-X77, X96-X98)

Use additional external cause code to identify place (Y92)

The appropriate 7th character is to be added to each code from category T27

A - initial encounter

D - subsequent encounter

S - sequela

⊗⑦**T27.0** **Burn of larynx and trachea**

⊗⑦**T27.1** **Burn involving larynx and trachea with lung**

⊗⑦**T27.2** **Burn of other parts of respiratory tract**

Burn of thoracic cavity

⊗⑦**T27.3** **Burn of respiratory tract, part unspecified**

Code first (T51-T65) to identify chemical and intent for codes T27.4-T27.7

⊗⑦**T27.4** **Corrosion of larynx and trachea**

⊗⑦**T27.5** **Corrosion involving larynx and trachea with lung**

⊗⑦**T27.6** **Corrosion of other parts of respiratory tract**

⊗⑦**T27.7** **Corrosion of respiratory tract, part unspecified**

T28 **Burn and corrosion of other internal organs**

Use additional external cause code to identify the source and intent of the burn (X00-X19, X75-X77, X96-X98)

Use additional external cause code to identify place (Y92)

The appropriate 7th character is to be added to each code from category T28

A - initial encounter

D - subsequent encounter

S - sequela

⊗⑦**T28.0** **Burn of mouth and pharynx**

⊗⑦**T28.1** **Burn of esophagus**

⊗⑦**T28.2** **Burn of other parts of alimentary tract**

⊗⑦**T28.3** **Burn of internal genitourinary organs**

T28.4 **Burns of other and unspecified internal organs**

⊗⑦**T28.40** **Burn of unspecified internal organ**

T28.41 **Burn of ear drum**

⑦**T28.411** **Burn of right ear drum**

⑦**T28.412** **Burn of left ear drum**

⑦**T28.419** **Burn of unspecified ear drum**

⊗⑦**T28.49** **Burn of other internal organ**

Code first (T51-T65) to identify chemical and intent for T28.5-T28.9-

⊗⑦**T28.5** **Corrosion of mouth and pharynx**

⊗⑦**T28.6** **Corrosion of esophagus**

⊗⑦**T28.7** **Corrosion of other parts of alimentary tract**

⊗⑦**T28.8** **Corrosion of internal genitourinary organs**

T28.9 **Corrosions of other and unspecified internal organs**

⊗⑦**T28.90** **Corrosions of unspecified internal organs**

T28.91 **Corrosions of ear drum**

⑦**T28.911** **Corrosions of right ear drum**

⑦**T28.912** **Corrosions of left ear drum**

⑦**T28.919** **Corrosions of unspecified ear drum**

⊗⑦**T28.99** **Corrosions of other internal organs**

BURNS AND CORROSIONS OF MULTIPLE AND UNSPECIFIED BODY REGIONS (T30-T32)

T30 **Burn and corrosion, body region unspecified**

T30.0 **Burn of unspecified body region, unspecified degree**

This code is not for inpatient use. Code to specified site and degree of burns

Burn NOS

Multiple burns NOS

T30.4 **Corrosion of unspecified body region, unspecified degree**

This code is not for inpatient use. Code to specified site and degree of corrosion

Corrosion NOS

Multiple corrosion NOS

T31 **Burns classified according to extent of body surface involved**

Add 4th-7th digits   Nonspecific code   Unspecified code   Manifestation code

Note: This category is to be used as the primary code only when the site of the burn is unspecified. It should be used as a supplementary code with categories T20-T25 when the site is specified.

T31.0 **Burns involving less than 10% of body surface**

T31.1 **Burns involving 10-19% of body surface**

T31.10 **Burns involving 10-19% of body surface with 0% to 9% third degree burns**

Burns involving 10-19% of body surface NOS

T31.11 **Burns involving 10-19% of body surface with 10-19% third degree burns**

T31.2 **Burns involving 20-29% of body surface**

T31.20 **Burns involving 20-29% of body surface with 0% to 9% third degree burns**

Burns involving 20-29% of body surface NOS

T31.21 **Burns involving 20-29% of body surface with 10-19% third degree burns**

T31.22 **Burns involving 20-29% of body surface with 20-29% third degree burns**

T31.3 **Burns involving 30-39% of body surface**

T31.30 **Burns involving 30-39% of body surface with 0% to 9% third degree burns**

Burns involving 30-39% of body surface NOS

T31.31 **Burns involving 30-39% of body surface with 10-19% third degree burns**

T31.32 **Burns involving 30-39% of body surface with 20-29% third degree burns**

T31.33 **Burns involving 30-39% of body surface with 30-39% third degree burns**

T31.4 **Burns involving 40-49% of body surface**

T31.40 **Burns involving 40-49% of body surface with 0% to 9% third degree burns**

Burns involving 40-49% of body surface NOS

T31.41 **Burns involving 40-49% of body surface with 10-19% third degree burns**

T31.42 **Burns involving 40-49% of body surface with 20-29% third degree burns**

T31.43 **Burns involving 40-49% of body surface with 30-39% third degree burns**

T31.44 **Burns involving 40-49% of body surface with 40-49% third degree burns**

T31.5 **Burns involving 50-59% of body surface**

T31.50 **Burns involving 50-59% of body surface with 0% to 9% third degree burns**

Burns involving 50-59% of body surface NOS

T31.51 **Burns involving 50-59% of body surface with 10-19% third degree burns**

T31.52 **Burns involving 50-59% of body surface with 20-29% third degree burns**

T31.53 **Burns involving 50-59% of body surface with 30-39% third degree burns**

T31.54 **Burns involving 50-59% of body surface with 40-49% third degree burns**

T31.55 **Burns involving 50-59% of body surface with 50-59% third degree burns**

T31.6 **Burns involving 60-69% of body surface**

T31.60 **Burns involving 60-69% of body surface with 0% to 9% third degree burns**

Burns involving 60-69% of body surface NOS

T31.61 **Burns involving 60-69% of body surface with 10-19% third degree burns**

T31.62 **Burns involving 60-69% of body surface with 20-29% third degree burns**

T31.63 **Burns involving 60-69% of body surface with 30-39% third degree burns**

T31.64 **Burns involving 60-69% of body surface with 40-49% third degree burns**

T31.65 **Burns involving 60-69% of body surface with 50-59% third degree burns**

T31.66 **Burns involving 60-69% of body surface with 60-69% third degree burns**

T31.7 **Burns involving 70-79% of body surface**

T31.70 **Burns involving 70-79% of body surface with 0% to 9% third degree burns**

Burns involving 70-79% of body surface NOS

T31.71 **Burns involving 70-79% of body surface with 10-19% third degree burns**

T31.72 **Burns involving 70-79% of body surface with 20-29% third degree burns**

T31.73 **Burns involving 70-79% of body surface with 30-39% third degree burns**

T31.74 **Burns involving 70-79% of body surface with 40-49% third degree burns**

T31.75 **Burns involving 70-79% of body surface with 50-59% third degree burns**

T31.76 **Burns involving 70-79% of body surface with 60-69% third degree burns**

T31.77 **Burns involving 70-79% of body surface with 70-79% third degree burns**

T31.8 **Burns involving 80-89% of body surface**

T31.80 **Burns involving 80-89% of body surface with 0% to 9% third degree burns**

Burns involving 80-89% of body surface NOS

T31.81 **Burns involving 80-89% of body surface with 10-19% third degree burns**

T31.82 **Burns involving 80-89% of body surface with 20-29% third degree burns**

T31.83 **Burns involving 80-89% of body surface with 30-39% third degree burns**

T31.84 **Burns involving 80-89% of body surface with 40-49% third degree burns**

T31.85 **Burns involving 80-89% of body surface with 50-59% third degree burns**

T31.86 **Burns involving 80-89% of body surface with 60-69% third degree burns**

T31.87 **Burns involving 80-89% of body surface with 70-79% third degree burns**

T31.88 **Burns involving 80-89% of body surface with 80-89% third degree burns**

T31.9 **Burns involving 90% or more of body surface**

T31.90 **Burns involving 90% or more of body surface with 0% to 9% third degree burns**

Burns involving 90% or more of body surface NOS

T31.91 **Burns involving 90% or more of body surface with 10-19% third degree burns**

T31.92 **Burns involving 90% or more of body surface with 20-29% third degree burns**

T31.93 **Burns involving 90% or more of body surface with 30-39% third degree burns**

T31.94 **Burns involving 90% or more of body surface with 40-49% third degree burns**

T31.95   Burns involving 90% or more of body surface with 50-59% third degree burns

T31.96   Burns involving 90% or more of body surface with 60-69% third degree burns

T31.97   Burns involving 90% or more of body surface with 70-79% third degree burns

T31.98   Burns involving 90% or more of body surface with 80-89% third degree burns

T31.99   Burns involving 90% or more of body surface with 90% or more third degree burns

T32   **Corrosions classified according to extent of body surface involved**

Note: This category is to be used as the primary code only when the site of the corrosion is unspecified. It may be used as a supplementary code with categories T20-T25 when the site is specified.

T32.0   Corrosions involving less than 10% of body surface

T32.1   Corrosions involving 10-19% of body surface

    T32.10   Corrosions involving 10-19% of body surface with 0% to 9% third degree corrosion

        Corrosions involving 10-19% of body surface NOS

    T32.11   Corrosions involving 10-19% of body surface with 10-19% third degree corrosion

T32.2   Corrosions involving 20-29% of body surface

    T32.20   Corrosions involving 20-29% of body surface with 0% to 9% third degree corrosion

    T32.21   Corrosions involving 20-29% of body surface with 10-19% third degree corrosion

    T32.22   Corrosions involving 20-29% of body surface with 20-29% third degree corrosion

T32.3   Corrosions involving 30-39% of body surface

    T32.30   Corrosions involving 30-39% of body surface with 0% to 9% third degree corrosion

    T32.31   Corrosions involving 30-39% of body surface with 10-19% third degree corrosion

    T32.32   Corrosions involving 30-39% of body surface with 20-29% third degree corrosion

    T32.33   Corrosions involving 30-39% of body surface with 30-39% third degree corrosion

T32.4   Corrosions involving 40-49% of body surface

    T32.40   Corrosions involving 40-49% of body surface with 0% to 9% third degree corrosion

    T32.41   Corrosions involving 40-49% of body surface with 10-19% third degree corrosion

    T32.42   Corrosions involving 40-49% of body surface with 20-29% third degree corrosion

    T32.43   Corrosions involving 40-49% of body surface with 30-39% third degree corrosion

    T32.44   Corrosions involving 40-49% of body surface with 40-49% third degree corrosion

T32.5   Corrosions involving 50-59% of body surface

    T32.50   Corrosions involving 50-59% of body surface with 0% to 9% third degree corrosion

    T32.51   Corrosions involving 50-59% of body surface with 10-19% third degree corrosion

    T32.52   Corrosions involving 50-59% of body surface with 20-29% third degree corrosion

    T32.53   Corrosions involving 50-59% of body surface with 30-39% third degree corrosion

    T32.54   Corrosions involving 50-59% of body surface with 40-49% third degree corrosion

    T32.55   Corrosions involving 50-59% of body surface with 50-59% third degree corrosion

T32.6   Corrosions involving 60-69% of body surface

    T32.60   Corrosions involving 60-69% of body surface with 0% to 9% third degree corrosion

    T32.61   Corrosions involving 60-69% of body surface with 10-19% third degree corrosion

    T32.62   Corrosions involving 60-69% of body surface with 20-29% third degree corrosion

    T32.63   Corrosions involving 60-69% of body surface with 30-39% third degree corrosion

    T32.64   Corrosions involving 60-69% of body surface with 40-49% third degree corrosion

    T32.65   Corrosions involving 60-69% of body surface with 50-59% third degree corrosion

    T32.66   Corrosions involving 60-69% of body surface with 60-69% third degree corrosion

T32.7   Corrosions involving 70-79% of body surface

    T32.70   Corrosions involving 70-79% of body surface with 0% to 9% third degree corrosion

    T32.71   Corrosions involving 70-79% of body surface with 10-19% third degree corrosion

    T32.72   Corrosions involving 70-79% of body surface with 20-29% third degree corrosion

    T32.73   Corrosions involving 70-79% of body surface with 30-39% third degree corrosion

    T32.74   Corrosions involving 70-79% of body surface with 40-49% third degree corrosion

    T32.75   Corrosions involving 70-79% of body surface with 50-59% third degree corrosion

    T32.76   Corrosions involving 70-79% of body surface with 60-69% third degree corrosion

    T32.77   Corrosions involving 70-79% of body surface with 70-79% third degree corrosion

T32.8   Corrosions involving 80-89% of body surface

    T32.80   Corrosions involving 80-89% of body surface with 0% to 9% third degree corrosion

    T32.81   Corrosions involving 80-89% of body surface with 10-19% third degree corrosion

    T32.82   Corrosions involving 80-89% of body surface with 20-29% third degree corrosion

    T32.83   Corrosions involving 80-89% of body surface with 30-39% third degree corrosion

    T32.84   Corrosions involving 80-89% of body surface with 40-49% third degree corrosion

    T32.85   Corrosions involving 80-89% of body surface with 50-59% third degree corrosion

    T32.86   Corrosions involving 80-89% of body surface with 60-69% third degree corrosion

    T32.87   Corrosions involving 80-89% of body surface with 70-79% third degree corrosion

    T32.88   Corrosions involving 80-89% of body surface with 80-89% third degree corrosion

T32.9   Corrosions involving 90% or more of body surface

    T32.90   Corrosions involving 90% or more of body surface with 0% to 9% third degree corrosion

    T32.91   Corrosions involving 90% or more of body surface with 10-19% third degree corrosion

T32.92 Corrosions involving 90% or more of body surface with 20-29% third degree corrosion

T32.93 Corrosions involving 90% or more of body surface with 30-39% third degree corrosion

T32.94 Corrosions involving 90% or more of body surface with 40-49% third degree corrosion

T32.95 Corrosions involving 90% or more of body surface with 50-59% third degree corrosion

T32.96 Corrosions involving 90% or more of body surface with 60-69% third degree corrosion

T32.97 Corrosions involving 90% or more of body surface with 70-79% third degree corrosion

T32.98 Corrosions involving 90% or more of body surface with 80-89% third degree corrosion

T32.99 Corrosions involving 90% or more of body surface with 90% or more third degree corrosion

FROSTBITE (T33-T34)

Excludes2: hypothermia **and other** effects of reduced temperature (T68, T69.-)

T33 Superficial frostbite

Includes: frostbite with partial thickness skin loss

The appropriate 7th character is to be added to each code from category T33

A - initial encounter

D - subsequent encounter

S - sequela

T33.0 Superficial frostbite of head

    T33.01 Superficial frostbite of ear

      ⑦T33.011 Superficial frostbite of right ear

      ⑦T33.012 Superficial frostbite of left ear

      ⑦T33.019 Superficial frostbite of unspecified ear

⊗⑦T33.02 Superficial frostbite of nose

⊗⑦T33.09 Superficial frostbite of other part of head

⊗⑦T33.1 Superficial frostbite of neck

⊗⑦T33.2 Superficial frostbite of thorax

⊗⑦T33.3 Superficial frostbite of abdominal wall, lower back and pelvis

T33.4 Superficial frostbite of arm

    Excludes2: superficial frostbite of wrist and hand (T33.5-)

⊗⑦T33.40 Superficial frostbite of unspecified arm

⊗⑦T33.41 Superficial frostbite of right arm

⊗⑦T33.42 Superficial frostbite of left arm

T33.5 Superficial frostbite of wrist, hand, and fingers

    T33.51 Superficial frostbite of wrist

      ⑦T33.511 Superficial frostbite of right wrist

      ⑦T33.512 Superficial frostbite of left wrist

      ⑦T33.519 Superficial frostbite of unspecified wrist

    T33.52 Superficial frostbite of hand

    Excludes2: superficial frostbite of fingers (T33.53-)

      ⑦T33.521 Superficial frostbite of right hand

      ⑦T33.522 Superficial frostbite of left hand

      ⑦T33.529 Superficial frostbite of unspecified hand

    T33.53 Superficial frostbite of finger(s)

      ⑦T33.531 Superficial frostbite of right finger(s)

      ⑦T33.532 Superficial frostbite of left finger(s)

      ⑦T33.539 Superficial frostbite of unspecified finger(s)

T33.6 Superficial frostbite of hip and thigh

⊗⑦T33.60 Superficial frostbite of unspecified hip and thigh

⊗⑦T33.61 Superficial frostbite of right hip and thigh

⊗⑦T33.62 Superficial frostbite of left hip and thigh

T33.7 Superficial frostbite of knee and lower leg

    Excludes2: superficial frostbite of ankle and foot (T33.8-)

⊗⑦T33.70 Superficial frostbite of unspecified knee and lower leg

⊗⑦T33.71 Superficial frostbite of right knee and lower leg

⊗⑦T33.72 Superficial frostbite of left knee and lower leg

T33.8 Superficial frostbite of ankle, foot, and toe(s)

    T33.81 Superficial frostbite of ankle

      ⑦T33.811 Superficial frostbite of right ankle

      ⑦T33.812 Superficial frostbite of left ankle

      ⑦T33.819 Superficial frostbite of unspecified ankle

    T33.82 Superficial frostbite of foot

      ⑦T33.821 Superficial frostbite of right foot

      ⑦T33.822 Superficial frostbite of left foot

      ⑦T33.829 Superficial frostbite of unspecified foot

    T33.83 Superficial frostbite of toe(s)

      ⑦T33.831 Superficial frostbite of right toe(s)

      ⑦T33.832 Superficial frostbite of left toe(s)

      ⑦T33.839 Superficial frostbite of unspecified toe(s)

T33.9 Superficial frostbite of other and unspecified sites

⊗⑦T33.90 Superficial frostbite of unspecified sites

    Superficial frostbite NOS

⊗⑦T33.99 Superficial frostbite of other sites

    Superficial frostbite of leg NOS

    Superficial frostbite of trunk NOS

T34 Frostbite with tissue necrosis

The appropriate 7th character is to be added to each code from category T34

A - initial encounter

D - subsequent encounter

S - sequela

T34.0 Frostbite with tissue necrosis of head

    T34.01 Frostbite with tissue necrosis of ear

      ⑦T34.011 Frostbite with tissue necrosis of right ear

      ⑦T34.012 Frostbite with tissue necrosis of left ear

      ⑦T34.019 Frostbite with tissue necrosis of unspecified ear

⊗⑦T34.02 Frostbite with tissue necrosis of nose

⊗⑦T34.09 Frostbite with tissue necrosis of other part of head

⊗⑦**T34.1**   **Frostbite with tissue necrosis of neck**

⊗⑦**T34.2**   **Frostbite with tissue necrosis of thorax**

⊗⑦**T34.3**   **Frostbite with tissue necrosis of abdominal wall, lower back and pelvis**

T34.4   **Frostbite with tissue necrosis of arm**

> **Excludes2:** frostbite with tissue necrosis of wrist and hand (T34.5-)

⊗⑦**T34.40**   **Frostbite with tissue necrosis of unspecified arm**

⊗⑦**T34.41**   **Frostbite with tissue necrosis of right arm**

⊗⑦**T34.42**   **Frostbite with tissue necrosis of left arm**

T34.5   **Frostbite with tissue necrosis of wrist, hand, and finger(s)**

T34.51   **Frostbite with tissue necrosis of wrist**

⑦**T34.511**   **Frostbite with tissue necrosis of right wrist**

⑦**T34.512**   **Frostbite with tissue necrosis of left wrist**

⑦**T34.519**   **Frostbite with tissue necrosis of unspecified wrist**

T34.52   **Frostbite with tissue necrosis of hand**

> **Excludes2:** frostbite with tissue necrosis of finger(s) (T34.53-)

⑦**T34.521**   **Frostbite with tissue necrosis of right hand**

⑦**T34.522**   **Frostbite with tissue necrosis of left hand**

⑦**T34.529**   **Frostbite with tissue necrosis of unspecified hand**

T34.53   **Frostbite with tissue necrosis of finger(s)**

⑦**T34.531**   **Frostbite with tissue necrosis of right finger(s)**

⑦**T34.532**   **Frostbite with tissue necrosis of left finger(s)**

⑦**T34.539**   **Frostbite with tissue necrosis of unspecified finger(s)**

T34.6   **Frostbite with tissue necrosis of hip and thigh**

⊗⑦**T34.60**   **Frostbite with tissue necrosis of unspecified hip and thigh**

⊗⑦**T34.61**   **Frostbite with tissue necrosis of right hip and thigh**

⊗⑦**T34.62**   **Frostbite with tissue necrosis of left hip and thigh**

T34.7   **Frostbite with tissue necrosis of knee and lower leg**

> **Excludes2:** frostbite with tissue necrosis of ankle and foot (T34.8-)

⊗⑦**T34.70**   **Frostbite with tissue necrosis of unspecified knee and lower leg**

⊗⑦**T34.71**   **Frostbite with tissue necrosis of right knee and lower leg**

⊗⑦**T34.72**   **Frostbite with tissue necrosis of left knee and lower leg**

T34.8   **Frostbite with tissue necrosis of ankle, foot, and toe(s)**

T34.81   **Frostbite with tissue necrosis of ankle**

⑦**T34.811**   **Frostbite with tissue necrosis of right ankle**

⑦**T34.812**   **Frostbite with tissue necrosis of left ankle**

⑦**T34.819**   **Frostbite with tissue necrosis of unspecified ankle**

T34.82   **Frostbite with tissue necrosis of foot**

⑦**T34.821**   **Frostbite with tissue necrosis of right foot**

⑦**T34.822**   **Frostbite with tissue necrosis of left foot**

⑦**T34.829**   **Frostbite with tissue necrosis of unspecified foot**

T34.83   **Frostbite with tissue necrosis of toe(s)**

⑦**T34.831**   **Frostbite with tissue necrosis of right toe(s)**

⑦**T34.832**   **Frostbite with tissue necrosis of left toe(s)**

⑦**T34.839**   **Frostbite with tissue necrosis of unspecified toe(s)**

T34.9   **Frostbite with tissue necrosis of other and unspecified sites**

⊗⑦**T34.90**   **Frostbite with tissue necrosis of unspecified sites**

Frostbite with tissue necrosis NOS

⊗⑦**T34.99**   **Frostbite with tissue necrosis of other sites**

Frostbite with tissue necrosis of leg NOS

Frostbite with tissue necrosis of trunk NOS

POISONING BY, ADVERSE EFFECTS OF AND UNDERDOSING OF DRUGS, MEDICAMENTS AND BIOLOGICAL SUBSTANCES (T36-T50)

Includes: adverse effect of correct substance properly administered

poisoning by overdose of substance

poisoning by wrong substance given or taken in error underdosing by (inadvertently) (deliberately) taking less substance than prescribed or instructed

Code first, for adverse effects, the nature of the adverse effect, such as:

adverse effect NOS (T88.7)

aspirin gastritis (K29.-)

blood disorders (D56-D76)

contact dermatitis (L23-L25)

dermatitis due to substances taken internally (L27.-)

nephropathy (N14.0-N14.2)

Note: The drug giving rise to the adverse effect should be identified by use of codes from categories T36-T50 with fifth or sixth character 5.

Use additional code(s) to specify:

manifestations of poisoning

underdosing or failure in dosage during medical and surgical care (Y63.6, Y63.8-Y63.9)

underdosing of medication regimen (Z91.12-, Z91.13-)

Excludes1: toxic reaction to local anesthesia in pregnancy (O29.3-)

Excludes2: abuse and dependence of psychoactive substances (F10-F19)

abuse of non-dependence-producing substances (F55.-)

drug reaction and poisoning affecting newborn (P00-P96)

pathological drug intoxication (inebriation) (F10-F19)

T36   **Poisoning by, adverse effect of and underdosing of systemic antibiotics**

> **Excludes1:** antineoplastic antibiotics (T45.1-)
>
> locally applied antibiotic NEC (T49.0)
>
> topically used antibiotic for ear, nose and throat (T49.6)
>
> topically used antibiotic for eye (T49.5)

The appropriate 7th character is to be added to each code from category T36

A - initial encounter

D - subsequent encounter

S - sequela

T36.0   Poisoning by, adverse effect of and underdosing of penicillins

 T36.0X   Poisoning by, adverse effect of and underdosing of penicillins

  ⑦**T36.0X1   Poisoning by penicillins, accidental (unintentional)**

   Poisoning by penicillins NOS

  ⑦**T36.0X2   Poisoning by penicillins, intentional self-harm**

  ⑦**T36.0X3   Poisoning by penicillins, assault**

  ⑦**T36.0X4   Poisoning by penicillins, undetermined**

  ⑦**T36.0X5   Adverse effect of penicillins**

  ⑦**T36.0X6   Underdosing of penicillins**

T36.1   Poisoning by, adverse effect of and underdosing of cephalosporins and other beta-lactam antibiotics

 T36.1X   Poisoning by, adverse effect of and underdosing of cephalosporins and other beta-lactam antibiotics

  ⑦**T36.1X1   Poisoning by cephalosporins and other beta-lactam antibiotics, accidental (unintentional)**

   Poisoning by cephalosporins and other beta-lactam antibiotics NOS

  ⑦**T36.1X2   Poisoning by cephalosporins and other beta-lactam antibiotics, intentional self-harm**

  ⑦**T36.1X3   Poisoning by cephalosporins and other beta-lactam antibiotics, assault**

  ⑦**T36.1X4   Poisoning by cephalosporins and other beta-lactam antibiotics, undetermined**

  ⑦**T36.1X5   Adverse effect of cephalosporins and other beta-lactam antibiotics**

  ⑦**T36.1X6   Underdosing of cephalosporins and other beta-lactam antibiotics**

T36.2   Poisoning by, adverse effect of and underdosing of chloramphenicol group

 T36.2X   Poisoning by, adverse effect of and underdosing of chloramphenicol group

  ⑦**T36.2X1   Poisoning by chloramphenicol group, accidental (unintentional)**

   Poisoning by chloramphenicol group NOS

  ⑦**T36.2X2   Poisoning by chloramphenicol group, intentional self-harm**

  ⑦**T36.2X3   Poisoning by chloramphenicol group, assault**

  ⑦**T36.2X4   Poisoning by chloramphenicol group, undetermined**

  ⑦**T36.2X5   Adverse effect of chloramphenicol group**

  ⑦**T36.2X6   Underdosing of chloramphenicol group**

T36.3   Poisoning by, adverse effect of and underdosing of macrolides

 T36.3X   Poisoning by, adverse effect of and underdosing of macrolides

  ⑦**T36.3X1   Poisoning by macrolides, accidental (unintentional)**

   Poisoning by macrolides NOS

  ⑦**T36.3X2   Poisoning by macrolides, intentional self-harm**

  ⑦**T36.3X3   Poisoning by macrolides, assault**

  ⑦**T36.3X4   Poisoning by macrolides, undetermined**

  ⑦**T36.3X5   Adverse effect of macrolides**

  ⑦**T36.3X6   Underdosing of macrolides**

T36.4   Poisoning by, adverse effect of and underdosing of tetracyclines

 T36.4X   Poisoning by, adverse effect of and underdosing of tetracyclines

  ⑦**T36.4X1   Poisoning by tetracyclines, accidental (unintentional)**

   Poisoning by tetracyclines NOS

  ⑦**T36.4X2   Poisoning by tetracyclines, intentional self-harm**

  ⑦**T36.4X3   Poisoning by tetracyclines, assault**

  ⑦**T36.4X4   Poisoning by tetracyclines, undetermined**

  ⑦**T36.4X5   Adverse effect of tetracyclines**

  ⑦**T36.4X6   Underdosing of tetracyclines**

T36.5   Poisoning by, adverse effect of and underdosing of aminoglycosides

 Poisoning by, adverse effect of and underdosing of streptomycin

 T36.5X   Poisoning by, adverse effect of and underdosing of aminoglycosides

  ⑦**T36.5X1   Poisoning by aminoglycosides, accidental (unintentional)**

   Poisoning by aminoglycosides NOS

  ⑦**T36.5X2   Poisoning by aminoglycosides, intentional self-harm**

  ⑦**T36.5X3   Poisoning by aminoglycosides, assault**

  ⑦**T36.5X4   Poisoning by aminoglycosides, undetermined**

  ⑦**T36.5X5   Adverse effect of aminoglycosides**

  ⑦**T36.5X6   Underdosing of aminoglycosides**

T36.6   Poisoning by, adverse effect of and underdosing of rifampicins

 T36.6X   Poisoning by, adverse effect of and underdosing of rifampicins

  ⑦**T36.6X1   Poisoning by rifampicins, accidental (unintentional)**

   Poisoning by rifampicins NOS

  ⑦**T36.6X2   Poisoning by rifampicins, intentional self-harm**

  ⑦**T36.6X3   Poisoning by rifampicins, assault**

  ⑦**T36.6X4   Poisoning by rifampicins, undetermined**

  ⑦**T36.6X5   Adverse effect of rifampicins**

  ⑦**T36.6X6   Underdosing of rifampicins**

T36.7   Poisoning by, adverse effect of and underdosing of antifungal antibiotics, systemically used

● New code   ▲ Revised code   **Excludes1:** Not coded here   **Excludes2:** Not included here   ⊗ Placeholder required   ⑦7th digit required

T36.7X Poisoning by, adverse effect of and underdosing of antifungal antibiotics, systemically used

⑦T36.7X1 Poisoning by antifungal antibiotics, systemically used, accidental (unintentional)

Poisoning by antifungal antibiotics, systemically used NOS

⑦T36.7X2 Poisoning by antifungal antibiotics, systemically used, intentional self-harm

⑦T36.7X3 Poisoning by antifungal antibiotics, systemically used, assault

⑦T36.7X4 Poisoning by antifungal antibiotics, systemically used, undetermined

⑦T36.7X5 Adverse effect of antifungal antibiotics, systemically used

⑦T36.7X6 Underdosing of antifungal antibiotics, systemically used

T36.8 Poisoning by, adverse effect of and underdosing of other systemic antibiotics

T36.8X Poisoning by, adverse effect of and underdosing of other systemic antibiotics

⑦T36.8X1 Poisoning by other systemic antibiotics, accidental (unintentional)

Poisoning by other systemic antibiotics NOS

⑦T36.8X2 Poisoning by other systemic antibiotics, intentional self-harm

⑦T36.8X3 Poisoning by other systemic antibiotics, assault

⑦T36.8X4 Poisoning by other systemic antibiotics, undetermined

⑦T36.8X5 Adverse effect of other systemic antibiotics

⑦T36.8X6 Underdosing of other systemic antibiotics

T36.9 Poisoning by, adverse effect of and underdosing of unspecified systemic antibiotic

⊗⑦T36.91 Poisoning by unspecified systemic antibiotic, accidental (unintentional)

Poisoning by systemic antibiotic NOS

⊗⑦T36.92 Poisoning by unspecified systemic antibiotic, intentional self-harm

⊗⑦T36.93 Poisoning by unspecified systemic antibiotic, assault

⊗⑦T36.94 Poisoning by unspecified systemic antibiotic, undetermined

⊗⑦T36.95 Adverse effect of unspecified systemic antibiotic

⊗⑦T36.96 Underdosing of unspecified systemic antibiotic

T37 Poisoning by, adverse effect of and underdosing of other systemic anti- infectives and antiparasitics

Excludes1: anti-infectives topically used for ear, nose and throat (T49.6-)

anti-infectives topically used for eye (T49.5-)

locally applied anti-infectives NEC (T49.0-)

The appropriate 7th character is to be added to each code from category T37

A - initial encounter

D - subsequent encounter

S - sequela

T37.0 Poisoning by, adverse effect of and underdosing of sulfonamides

T37.0X Poisoning by, adverse effect of and underdosing of sulfonamides

⑦T37.0X1 Poisoning by sulfonamides, accidental (unintentional)

Poisoning by sulfonamides NOS

⑦T37.0X2 Poisoning by sulfonamides, intentional self-harm

⑦T37.0X3 Poisoning by sulfonamides, assault

⑦T37.0X4 Poisoning by sulfonamides, undetermined

⑦T37.0X5 Adverse effect of sulfonamides

⑦T37.0X6 Underdosing of sulfonamides

T37.1 Poisoning by, adverse effect of and underdosing of antimycobacterial drugs

Excludes1: rifampicins (T36.6-)

streptomycin (T36.5-)

T37.1X Poisoning by, adverse effect of and underdosing of antimycobacterial drugs

⑦T37.1X1 Poisoning by antimycobacterial drugs, accidental (unintentional)

Poisoning by antimycobacterial drugs NOS

⑦T37.1X2 Poisoning by antimycobacterial drugs, intentional self-harm

⑦T37.1X3 Poisoning by antimycobacterial drugs, assault

⑦T37.1X4 Poisoning by antimycobacterial drugs, undetermined

⑦T37.1X5 Adverse effect of antimycobacterial drugs

⑦T37.1X6 Underdosing of antimycobacterial drugs

T37.2 Poisoning by, adverse effect of and underdosing of antimalarials and drugs acting on other blood protozoa

Excludes1: hydroxyquinoline derivatives (T37.8-)

T37.2X Poisoning by, adverse effect of and underdosing of antimalarials and drugs acting on other blood protozoa

⑦T37.2X1 Poisoning by antimalarials and drugs acting on other blood protozoa, accidental (unintentional)

Poisoning by antimalarials and drugs acting on other blood protozoa NOS

⑦T37.2X2 Poisoning by antimalarials and drugs acting on other blood protozoa, intentional self-harm

⑦T37.2X3 Poisoning by antimalarials and drugs acting on other blood protozoa, assault

⑦T37.2X4 Poisoning by antimalarials and drugs acting on other blood protozoa, undetermined

⑦T37.2X5 Adverse effect of antimalarials and drugs acting on other blood protozoa

⑦**T37.2X6** Underdosing of antimalarials and drugs acting on other blood protozoa

T37.3 Poisoning by, adverse effect of and underdosing of other antiprotozoal drugs

   T37.3X Poisoning by, adverse effect of and underdosing of other antiprotozoal drugs

     ⑦**T37.3X1** Poisoning by other antiprotozoal drugs, accidental (unintentional)

        Poisoning by other antiprotozoal drugs NOS

     ⑦**T37.3X2** Poisoning by other antiprotozoal drugs, intentional self-harm

     ⑦**T37.3X3** Poisoning by other antiprotozoal drugs, assault

     ⑦**T37.3X4** Poisoning by other antiprotozoal drugs, undetermined

     ⑦**T37.3X5** Adverse effect of other antiprotozoal drugs

     ⑦**T37.3X6** Underdosing of other antiprotozoal drugs

T37.4 Poisoning by, adverse effect of and underdosing of anthelminthics

   T37.4X Poisoning by, adverse effect of and underdosing of anthelminthics

     ⑦**T37.4X1** Poisoning by anthelminthics, accidental (unintentional)

        Poisoning by anthelminthics NOS

     ⑦**T37.4X2** Poisoning by anthelminthics, intentional self-harm

     ⑦**T37.4X3** Poisoning by anthelminthics, assault

     ⑦**T37.4X4** Poisoning by anthelminthics, undetermined

     ⑦**T37.4X5** Adverse effect of anthelminthics

     ⑦**T37.4X6** Underdosing of anthelminthics

T37.5 Poisoning by, adverse effect of and underdosing of antiviral drugs

   Excludes1: amantadine (T42.8-)

      cytarabine (T45.1-)

   T37.5X Poisoning by, adverse effect of and underdosing of antiviral drugs

     ⑦**T37.5X1** Poisoning by antiviral drugs, accidental (unintentional)

        Poisoning by antiviral drugs NOS

     ⑦**T37.5X2** Poisoning by antiviral drugs, intentional self-harm

     ⑦**T37.5X3** Poisoning by antiviral drugs, assault

     ⑦**T37.5X4** Poisoning by antiviral drugs, undetermined

     ⑦**T37.5X5** Adverse effect of antiviral drugs

     ⑦**T37.5X6** Underdosing of antiviral drugs

T37.8 Poisoning by, adverse effect of and underdosing of other specified systemic anti-infectives and antiparasitics

   Poisoning by, adverse effect of and underdosing of hydroxyquinoline derivatives

   Excludes1: antimalarial drugs (T37.2-)

   T37.8X Poisoning by, adverse effect of and underdosing of other specified systemic anti-infectives and antiparasitics

⑦**T37.8X1** Poisoning by other specified systemic anti-infectives and antiparasitics, accidental (unintentional)

   Poisoning by other specified systemic anti-infectives and antiparasitics NOS

⑦**T37.8X2** Poisoning by other specified systemic anti-infectives and antiparasitics, intentional self-harm

⑦**T37.8X3** Poisoning by other specified systemic anti-infectives and antiparasitics, assault

⑦**T37.8X4** Poisoning by other specified systemic anti-infectives and antiparasitics, undetermined

⑦**T37.8X5** Adverse effect of other specified systemic anti-infectives and antiparasitics

⑦**T37.8X6** Underdosing of other specified systemic anti-infectives and antiparasitics

⑦**T37.9** Poisoning by, adverse effect of and underdosing of unspecified systemic anti-infective and antiparasitics

   ⊗⑦**T37.91** Poisoning by unspecified systemic anti-infective and antiparasitics, accidental (unintentional)

    Poisoning by, adverse effect of and underdosing of systemic anti-infective and antiparasitics NOS

   ⊗⑦**T37.92** Poisoning by unspecified systemic anti-infective and antiparasitics, intentional self-harm

   ⊗⑦**T37.93** Poisoning by unspecified systemic anti-infective and antiparasitics, assault

   ⊗⑦**T37.94** Poisoning by unspecified systemic anti-infective and antiparasitics, undetermined

   ⊗⑦**T37.95** Adverse effect of unspecified systemic anti-infective and antiparasitic

   ⊗⑦**T37.96** Underdosing of unspecified systemic anti-infectives and antiparasitics

T38 Poisoning by, adverse effect of and underdosing of hormones and their synthetic substitutes and antagonists, not elsewhere classified

   Excludes1: mineralocorticoids and their antagonists (T50.0-)

      oxytocic hormones (T48.0-)

      parathyroid hormones and derivatives (T50.9-)

The appropriate 7th character is to be added to each code from category T38

A - initial encounter

D - subsequent encounter

S - sequela

T38.0 Poisoning by, adverse effect of and underdosing of glucocorticoids and synthetic analogues

   Excludes1: glucocorticoids, topically used (T49.-)

   T38.0X Poisoning by, adverse effect of and underdosing of glucocorticoids and synthetic analogues

     ⑦**T38.0X1** Poisoning by glucocorticoids and synthetic analogues, accidental (unintentional)

        Poisoning by glucocorticoids and synthetic analogues NOS

⑦T38.0X2　Poisoning by glucocorticoids and synthetic analogues, intentional self-harm

⑦T38.0X3　Poisoning by glucocorticoids and synthetic analogues, assault

⑦T38.0X4　Poisoning by glucocorticoids and synthetic analogues, undetermined

⑦T38.0X5　Adverse effect of glucocorticoids and synthetic analogues

⑦T38.0X6　Underdosing of glucocorticoids and synthetic analogues

T38.1　Poisoning by, adverse effect of and underdosing of thyroid hormones and substitutes

　　T38.1X　Poisoning by, adverse effect of and underdosing of thyroid hormones and substitutes

　　　　⑦T38.1X1　Poisoning by thyroid hormones and substitutes, accidental (unintentional)

　　　　　　Poisoning by thyroid hormones and substitutes NOS

　　　　⑦T38.1X2　Poisoning by thyroid hormones and substitutes, intentional self-harm

　　　　⑦T38.1X3　Poisoning by thyroid hormones and substitutes, assault

　　　　⑦T38.1X4　Poisoning by thyroid hormones and substitutes, undetermined

　　　　⑦T38.1X5　Adverse effect of thyroid hormones and substitutes

　　　　⑦T38.1X6　Underdosing of thyroid hormones and substitutes

T38.2　Poisoning by, adverse effect of and underdosing of antithyroid drugs

　　T38.2X　Poisoning by, adverse effect of and underdosing of antithyroid drugs

　　　　⑦T38.2X1　Poisoning by antithyroid drugs, accidental (unintentional)

　　　　　　Poisoning by antithyroid drugs NOS

　　　　⑦T38.2X2　Poisoning by antithyroid drugs, intentional self-harm

　　　　⑦T38.2X3　Poisoning by antithyroid drugs, assault

　　　　⑦T38.2X4　Poisoning by antithyroid drugs, undetermined

　　　　⑦T38.2X5　Adverse effect of antithyroid drugs

　　　　⑦T38.2X6　Underdosing of antithyroid drugs

T38.3　Poisoning by, adverse effect of and underdosing of insulin and oral hypoglycemic [antidiabetic] drugs

　　T38.3X　Poisoning by, adverse effect of and underdosing of insulin and oral hypoglycemic [antidiabetic] drugs

　　　　⑦T38.3X1　Poisoning by insulin and oral hypoglycemic [antidiabetic] drugs, accidental (unintentional)

　　　　　　Poisoning by insulin and oral hypoglycemic [antidiabetic] drugs NOS

　　　　⑦T38.3X2　Poisoning by insulin and oral hypoglycemic [antidiabetic] drugs, intentional self-harm

⑦T38.3X3　Poisoning by insulin and oral hypoglycemic [antidiabetic] drugs, assault

⑦T38.3X4　Poisoning by insulin and oral hypoglycemic [antidiabetic] drugs, undetermined

⑦T38.3X5　Adverse effect of insulin and oral hypoglycemic [antidiabetic] drugs

⑦T38.3X6　Underdosing of insulin and oral hypoglycemic [antidiabetic] drugs

T38.4　Poisoning by, adverse effect of and underdosing of oral contraceptives

Poisoning by, adverse effect of and underdosing of multiple- and single-ingredient oral contraceptive preparations

　　T38.4X　Poisoning by, adverse effect of and underdosing of oral contraceptives

　　　　⑦T38.4X1　Poisoning by oral contraceptives, accidental (unintentional)

　　　　　　Poisoning by oral contraceptives NOS

　　　　⑦T38.4X2　Poisoning by oral contraceptives, intentional self-harm

　　　　⑦T38.4X3　Poisoning by oral contraceptives, assault

　　　　⑦T38.4X4　Poisoning by oral contraceptives, undetermined

　　　　⑦T38.4X5　Adverse effect of oral contraceptives

　　　　⑦T38.4X6　Underdosing of oral contraceptives

T38.5　Poisoning by, adverse effect of and underdosing of other estrogens and progestogens

Poisoning by, adverse effect of and underdosing of estrogens and progestogens mixtures and substitutes

　　T38.5X　Poisoning by, adverse effect of and underdosing of other estrogens and progestogens

　　　　⑦T38.5X1　Poisoning by other estrogens and progestogens, accidental (unintentional)

　　　　　　Poisoning by other estrogens and progestogens NOS

　　　　⑦T38.5X2　Poisoning by other estrogens and progestogens, intentional self-harm

　　　　⑦T38.5X3　Poisoning by other estrogens and progestogens, assault

　　　　⑦T38.5X4　Poisoning by other estrogens and progestogens, undetermined

　　　　⑦T38.5X5　Adverse effect of other estrogens and progestogens

　　　　⑦T38.5X6　Underdosing of other estrogens and progestogens

T38.6　Poisoning by, adverse effect of and underdosing of antigonadotrophins, antiestrogens, antiandrogens, not elsewhere classified

Poisoning by, adverse effect of and underdosing of tamoxifen

　　T38.6X　Poisoning by, adverse effect of and underdosing of antigonadotrophins, antiestrogens, antiandrogens, not elsewhere classified

　　　　⑦T38.6X1　Poisoning by antigonadotrophins, antiestrogens, antiandrogens, not

elsewhere classified, accidental (unintentional)

Poisoning by antigonadotrophins, antiestrogens, antiandrogens, not elsewhere classified NOS

⑦T38.6X2 **Poisoning by antigonadotrophins, antiestrogens, antiandrogens, not elsewhere classified, intentional self-harm**

⑦T38.6X3 **Poisoning by antigonadotrophins, antiestrogens, antiandrogens, not elsewhere classified, assault**

⑦T38.6X4 **Poisoning by antigonadotrophins, antiestrogens, antiandrogens, not elsewhere classified, undetermined**

⑦T38.6X5 **Adverse effect of antigonadotrophins, antiestrogens, antiandrogens, not elsewhere classified**

⑦T38.6X6 **Underdosing of antigonadotrophins, antiestrogens, antiandrogens, not elsewhere classified**

T38.7 **Poisoning by, adverse effect of and underdosing of androgens and anabolic congeners**

T38.7X **Poisoning by, adverse effect of and underdosing of androgens and anabolic congeners**

⑦T38.7X1 **Poisoning by androgens and anabolic congeners, accidental (unintentional)**

Poisoning by androgens and anabolic congeners NOS

⑦T38.7X2 **Poisoning by androgens and anabolic congeners, intentional self-harm**

⑦T38.7X3 **Poisoning by androgens and anabolic congeners, assault**

⑦T38.7X4 **Poisoning by androgens and anabolic congeners, undetermined**

⑦T38.7X5 **Adverse effect of androgens and anabolic congeners**

⑦T38.7X6 **Underdosing of androgens and anabolic congeners**

T38.8 **Poisoning by, adverse effect of and underdosing of other and unspecified hormones and synthetic substitutes**

⑦T38.80 **Poisoning by, adverse effect of and underdosing of unspecified hormones and synthetic substitutes**

⑦T38.801 **Poisoning by unspecified hormones and synthetic substitutes, accidental (unintentional)**

Poisoning by unspecified hormones and synthetic substitutes NOS

⑦T38.802 **Poisoning by unspecified hormones and synthetic substitutes, intentional self-harm**

⑦T38.803 **Poisoning by unspecified hormones and synthetic substitutes, assault**

⑦T38.804 **Poisoning by unspecified hormones and synthetic substitutes, undetermined**

⑦T38.805 **Adverse effect of unspecified hormones and synthetic substitutes**

⑦T38.806 **Underdosing of unspecified hormones and synthetic substitutes**

T38.81 **Poisoning by, adverse effect of and underdosing of anterior pituitary [adenohypophyseal] hormones**

⑦T38.811 **Poisoning by anterior pituitary [adenohypophyseal] hormones, accidental (unintentional)**

Poisoning by anterior pituitary [adenohypophyseal] hormones NOS

⑦T38.812 **Poisoning by anterior pituitary [adenohypophyseal] hormones, intentional self-harm**

⑦T38.813 **Poisoning by anterior pituitary [adenohypophyseal] hormones, assault**

⑦T38.814 **Poisoning by anterior pituitary [adenohypophyseal] hormones, undetermined**

⑦T38.815 **Adverse effect of anterior pituitary [adenohypophyseal] hormones**

⑦T38.816 **Underdosing of anterior pituitary [adenohypophyseal] hormones**

T38.89 **Poisoning by, adverse effect of and underdosing of other hormones and synthetic substitutes**

⑦T38.891 **Poisoning by other hormones and synthetic substitutes, accidental (unintentional)**

Poisoning by other hormones and synthetic substitutes NOS

⑦T38.892 **Poisoning by other hormones and synthetic substitutes, intentional self-harm**

⑦T38.893 **Poisoning by other hormones and synthetic substitutes, assault**

⑦T38.894 **Poisoning by other hormones and synthetic substitutes, undetermined**

⑦T38.895 **Adverse effect of other hormones and synthetic substitutes**

⑦T38.896 **Underdosing of other hormones and synthetic substitutes**

T38.9 **Poisoning by, adverse effect of and underdosing of other and unspecified hormone antagonists**

T38.90 **Poisoning by, adverse effect of and underdosing of unspecified hormone antagonists**

⑦T38.901 **Poisoning by unspecified hormone antagonists, accidental (unintentional)**

Poisoning by unspecified hormone antagonists NOS

⑦T38.902 **Poisoning by unspecified hormone antagonists, intentional self-harm**

⑦T38.903 **Poisoning by unspecified hormone antagonists, assault**

⑦T38.904 **Poisoning by unspecified hormone antagonists, undetermined**

⑦T38.905 **Adverse effect of unspecified hormone antagonists**

⑦T38.906 **Underdosing of unspecified hormone antagonists**

T38.99   Poisoning by, adverse effect of and underdosing of other hormone antagonists

⑦ T38.991   Poisoning by other hormone antagonists, accidental (unintentional)

Poisoning by other hormone antagonists NOS

⑦ T38.992   Poisoning by other hormone antagonists, intentional self-harm

⑦ T38.993   Poisoning by other hormone antagonists, assault

⑦ T38.994   Poisoning by other hormone antagonists, undetermined

⑦ T38.995   Adverse effect of other hormone antagonists

⑦ T38.996   Underdosing of other hormone antagonists

T39   Poisoning by, adverse effect of and underdosing of nonopioid analgesics, antipyretics and antirheumatics

The appropriate 7th character is to be added to each code from category T39

A - initial encounter

D - subsequent encounter

S - sequela

T39.0   Poisoning by, adverse effect of and underdosing of salicylates

T39.01   Poisoning by, adverse effect of and underdosing of aspirin

Poisoning by, adverse effect of and underdosing of acetylsalicylic acid

⑦ T39.011   Poisoning by aspirin, accidental (unintentional)

⑦ T39.012   Poisoning by aspirin, intentional self-harm

⑦ T39.013   Poisoning by aspirin, assault

⑦ T39.014   Poisoning by aspirin, undetermined

⑦ T39.015   Adverse effect of aspirin

⑦ T39.016   Underdosing of aspirin

T39.09   Poisoning by, adverse effect of and underdosing of other salicylates

⑦ T39.091   Poisoning by salicylates, accidental (unintentional)

Poisoning by salicylates NOS

⑦ T39.092   Poisoning by salicylates, intentional self-harm

⑦ T39.093   Poisoning by salicylates, assault

⑦ T39.094   Poisoning by salicylates, undetermined

⑦ T39.095   Adverse effect of salicylates

⑦ T39.096   Underdosing of salicylates

T39.1   Poisoning by, adverse effect of and underdosing of 4-Aminophenol derivatives

T39.1X   Poisoning by, adverse effect of and underdosing of 4-Aminophenol derivatives

⑦ T39.1X1   Poisoning by 4-Aminophenol derivatives, accidental (unintentional)

Poisoning by 4-Aminophenol derivatives NOS

⑦ T39.1X2   Poisoning by 4-Aminophenol derivatives, intentional self-harm

⑦ T39.1X3   Poisoning by 4-Aminophenol derivatives, assault

⑦ T39.1X4   Poisoning by 4-Aminophenol derivatives, undetermined

⑦ T39.1X5   Adverse effect of 4-Aminophenol derivatives

⑦ T39.1X6   Underdosing of 4-Aminophenol derivatives

T39.2   Poisoning by, adverse effect of and underdosing of pyrazolone derivatives

T39.2X   Poisoning by, adverse effect of and underdosing of pyrazolone derivatives

⑦ T39.2X1   Poisoning by pyrazolone derivatives, accidental (unintentional)

Poisoning by pyrazolone derivatives NOS

⑦ T39.2X2   Poisoning by pyrazolone derivatives, intentional self-harm

⑦ T39.2X3   Poisoning by pyrazolone derivatives, assault

⑦ T39.2X4   Poisoning by pyrazolone derivatives, undetermined

⑦ T39.2X5   Adverse effect of pyrazolone derivatives

⑦ T39.2X6   Underdosing of pyrazolone derivatives

T39.3   Poisoning by, adverse effect of and underdosing of other nonsteroidal anti-inflammatory drugs [NSAID]

T39.31   Poisoning by, adverse effect of and underdosing of propionic acid derivatives

Poisoning by, adverse effect of and underdosing of fenoprofen

Poisoning by, adverse effect of and underdosing of flurbiprofen

Poisoning by, adverse effect of and underdosing of ibuprofen

Poisoning by, adverse effect of and underdosing of ketoprofen

Poisoning by, adverse effect of and underdosing of naproxen

Poisoning by, adverse effect of and underdosing of oxaprozin

⑦ T39.311   Poisoning by propionic acid derivatives, accidental (unintentional)

⑦ T39.312   Poisoning by propionic acid derivatives, intentional self-harm

⑦ T39.313   Poisoning by propionic acid derivatives, assault

⑦ T39.314   Poisoning by propionic acid derivatives, undetermined

⑦ T39.315   Adverse effect of propionic acid derivatives

⑦ T39.316   Underdosing of propionic acid derivatives

T39.39   Poisoning by, adverse effect of and underdosing of other nonsteroidal anti-inflammatory drugs [NSAID]

⑦**T39.391** Poisoning by other nonsteroidal anti-inflammatory drugs [NSAID], accidental (unintentional)

Poisoning by other nonsteroidal anti-inflammatory drugs NOS

⑦**T39.392** Poisoning by other nonsteroidal anti-inflammatory drugs [NSAID], intentional self-harm

⑦**T39.393** Poisoning by other nonsteroidal anti-inflammatory drugs [NSAID], assault

⑦**T39.394** Poisoning by other nonsteroidal anti-inflammatory drugs [NSAID], undetermined

⑦**T39.395** Adverse effect of other nonsteroidal anti-inflammatory drugs [NSAID]

⑦**T39.396** Underdosing of other nonsteroidal anti-inflammatory drugs [NSAID]

T39.4 **Poisoning by, adverse effect of and underdosing of antirheumatics, not elsewhere classified**

Excludes1: poisoning by, adverse effect of and underdosing of glucocorticoids (T38.0-)

poisoning by, adverse effect of and underdosing of salicylates (T39.0-)

T39.4X **Poisoning by, adverse effect of and underdosing of antirheumatics, not elsewhere classified**

⑦**T39.4X1** Poisoning by antirheumatics, not elsewhere classified, accidental (unintentional)

Poisoning by antirheumatics, not elsewhere classified NOS

⑦**T39.4X2** Poisoning by antirheumatics, not elsewhere classified, intentional self-harm

⑦**T39.4X3** Poisoning by antirheumatics, not elsewhere classified, assault

⑦**T39.4X4** Poisoning by antirheumatics, not elsewhere classified, undetermined

⑦**T39.4X5** Adverse effect of antirheumatics, not elsewhere classified

⑦**T39.4X6** Underdosing of antirheumatics, not elsewhere classified

T39.8 **Poisoning by, adverse effect of and underdosing of other nonopioid analgesics and antipyretics, not elsewhere classified**

T39.8X **Poisoning by, adverse effect of and underdosing of other nonopioid analgesics and antipyretics, not elsewhere classified**

⑦**T39.8X1** Poisoning by other nonopioid analgesics and antipyretics, not elsewhere classified, accidental (unintentional)

Poisoning by other nonopioid analgesics and antipyretics, not elsewhere classified NOS

⑦**T39.8X2** Poisoning by other nonopioid analgesics and antipyretics, not elsewhere classified, intentional self-harm

⑦**T39.8X3** Poisoning by other nonopioid analgesics and antipyretics, not elsewhere classified, assault

⑦**T39.8X4** Poisoning by other nonopioid analgesics and antipyretics, not elsewhere classified, undetermined

⑦**T39.8X5** Adverse effect of other nonopioid analgesics and antipyretics, not elsewhere classified

⑦**T39.8X6** Underdosing of other nonopioid analgesics and antipyretics, not elsewhere classified

T39.9 **Poisoning by, adverse effect of and underdosing of unspecified nonopioid analgesic, antipyretic and antirheumatic**

⊗⑦**T39.91** Poisoning by unspecified nonopioid analgesic, antipyretic and antirheumatic, accidental (unintentional)

Poisoning by nonopioid analgesic, antipyretic and antirheumatic NOS

⊗⑦**T39.92** Poisoning by unspecified nonopioid analgesic, antipyretic and antirheumatic, intentional self-harm

⊗⑦**T39.93** Poisoning by unspecified nonopioid analgesic, antipyretic and antirheumatic, assault

⊗⑦**T39.94** Poisoning by unspecified nonopioid analgesic, antipyretic and antirheumatic, undetermined

⊗⑦**T39.95** Adverse effect of unspecified nonopioid analgesic, antipyretic and antirheumatic

⊗⑦**T39.96** Underdosing of unspecified nonopioid analgesic, antipyretic and antirheumatic

T40 **Poisoning by, adverse effect of and underdosing of narcotics and psychodysleptics [hallucinogens]**

Excludes2: drug dependence and related mental and behavioral disorders due to psychoactive substance use (F10.-F19.-)

The appropriate 7th character is to be added to each code from category T40

A - initial encounter

D - subsequent encounter

S - sequela

T40.0 **Poisoning by, adverse effect of and underdosing of opium**

T40.0X **Poisoning by, adverse effect of and underdosing of opium**

⑦**T40.0X1** Poisoning by opium, accidental (unintentional)

Poisoning by opium NOS

⑦**T40.0X2** Poisoning by opium, intentional self-harm

⑦**T40.0X3** Poisoning by opium, assault

⑦**T40.0X4** Poisoning by opium, undetermined

⑦**T40.0X5** Adverse effect of opium

⑦**T40.0X6** Underdosing of opium

T40.1 **Poisoning by and adverse effect of heroin**

T40.1X **Poisoning by and adverse effect of heroin**

⑦**T40.1X1** Poisoning by heroin, accidental (unintentional)

Poisoning by heroin NOS

⑦**T40.1X2** Poisoning by heroin, intentional self-harm

⑦**T40.1X3** Poisoning by heroin, assault

⑦**T40.1X4** Poisoning by heroin, undetermined

T40.2   **Poisoning by, adverse effect of and underdosing of other opioids**

  T40.2X   Poisoning by, adverse effect of and underdosing of other opioids

    ⑦T40.2X1   **Poisoning by other opioids, accidental (unintentional)**

      Poisoning by other opioids NOS

    ⑦T40.2X2   **Poisoning by other opioids, intentional self-harm**

    ⑦T40.2X3   **Poisoning by other opioids, assault**

    ⑦T40.2X4   **Poisoning by other opioids, undetermined**

    ⑦T40.2X5   **Adverse effect of other opioids**

    ⑦T40.2X6   **Underdosing of other opioids**

T40.3   **Poisoning by, adverse effect of and underdosing of methadone**

  T40.3X   Poisoning by, adverse effect of and underdosing of methadone

    ⑦T40.3X1   **Poisoning by methadone, accidental (unintentional)**

      Poisoning by methadone NOS

    ⑦T40.3X2   **Poisoning by methadone, intentional self-harm**

    ⑦T40.3X3   **Poisoning by methadone, assault**

    ⑦T40.3X4   **Poisoning by methadone, undetermined**

    ⑦T40.3X5   **Adverse effect of methadone**

    ⑦T40.3X6   **Underdosing of methadone**

T40.4   **Poisoning by, adverse effect of and underdosing of other synthetic narcotics**

  T40.4X   Poisoning by, adverse effect of and underdosing of other synthetic narcotics

    ⑦T40.4X1   **Poisoning by other synthetic narcotics, accidental (unintentional)**

      Poisoning by other synthetic narcotics NOS

    ⑦T40.4X2   **Poisoning by other synthetic narcotics, intentional self-harm**

    ⑦T40.4X3   **Poisoning by other synthetic narcotics, assault**

    ⑦T40.4X4   **Poisoning by other synthetic narcotics, undetermined**

    ⑦T40.4X5   **Adverse effect of other synthetic narcotics**

    ⑦T40.4X6   **Underdosing of other synthetic narcotics**

T40.5   **Poisoning by, adverse effect of and underdosing of cocaine**

  T40.5X   Poisoning by, adverse effect of and underdosing of cocaine

    ⑦T40.5X1   **Poisoning by cocaine, accidental (unintentional)**

      Poisoning by cocaine NOS

    ⑦T40.5X2   **Poisoning by cocaine, intentional self-harm**

    ⑦T40.5X3   **Poisoning by cocaine, assault**

    ⑦T40.5X4   **Poisoning by cocaine, undetermined**

    ⑦T40.5X5   **Adverse effect of cocaine**

    ⑦T40.5X6   **Underdosing of cocaine**

T40.6   **Poisoning by, adverse effect of and underdosing of other and unspecified narcotics**

  T40.60   Poisoning by, adverse effect of and underdosing of unspecified narcotics

    ⑦T40.601   **Poisoning by unspecified narcotics, accidental (unintentional)**

      Poisoning by narcotics NOS

    ⑦T40.602   **Poisoning by unspecified narcotics, intentional self-harm**

    ⑦T40.603   **Poisoning by unspecified narcotics, assault**

    ⑦T40.604   **Poisoning by unspecified narcotics, undetermined**

    ⑦T40.605   **Adverse effect of unspecified narcotics**

    ⑦T40.606   **Underdosing of unspecified narcotics**

  T40.69   Poisoning by, adverse effect of and underdosing of other narcotics

    ⑦T40.691   **Poisoning by other narcotics, accidental (unintentional)**

      Poisoning by other narcotics NOS

    ⑦T40.692   **Poisoning by other narcotics, intentional self-harm**

    ⑦T40.693   **Poisoning by other narcotics, assault**

    ⑦T40.694   **Poisoning by other narcotics, undetermined**

    ⑦T40.695   **Adverse effect of other narcotics**

    ⑦T40.696   **Underdosing of other narcotics**

T40.7   **Poisoning by, adverse effect of and underdosing of cannabis (derivatives)**

  T40.7X   Poisoning by, adverse effect of and underdosing of cannabis (derivatives)

    ⑦T40.7X1   **Poisoning by cannabis (derivatives), accidental (unintentional)**

      Poisoning by cannabis NOS

    ⑦T40.7X2   **Poisoning by cannabis (derivatives), intentional self-harm**

    ⑦T40.7X3   **Poisoning by cannabis (derivatives), assault**

    ⑦T40.7X4   **Poisoning by cannabis (derivatives), undetermined**

    ⑦T40.7X5   **Adverse effect of cannabis (derivatives)**

    ⑦T40.7X6   **Underdosing of cannabis (derivatives)**

T40.8   **Poisoning by and adverse effect of lysergide [LSD]**

  T40.8X   Poisoning by and adverse effect of lysergide [LSD]

    ⑦T40.8X1   **Poisoning by lysergide [LSD], accidental (unintentional)**

      Poisoning by lysergide [LSD]NOS

    ⑦T40.8X2   **Poisoning by lysergide [LSD], intentional self-harm**

    ⑦T40.8X3   **Poisoning by lysergide [LSD], assault**

    ⑦T40.8X4   **Poisoning by lysergide [LSD], undetermined**

T40.9 Poisoning by, adverse effect of and underdosing of other and unspecified psychodysleptics [hallucinogens]

  T40.90 Poisoning by, adverse effect of and underdosing of unspecified psychodysleptics [hallucinogens]

    ⑦T40.901 Poisoning by unspecified psychodysleptics [hallucinogens], accidental (unintentional)

    ⑦T40.902 Poisoning by unspecified psychodysleptics [hallucinogens], intentional self-harm

    ⑦T40.903 Poisoning by unspecified psychodysleptics [hallucinogens], assault

    ⑦T40.904 Poisoning by unspecified psychodysleptics [hallucinogens], undetermined

    ⑦T40.905 Adverse effect of unspecified psychodysleptics [hallucinogens]

    ⑦T40.906 Underdosing of unspecified psychodysleptics

  T40.99 Poisoning by, adverse effect of and underdosing of other psychodysleptics [hallucinogens]

    ⑦T40.991 Poisoning by other psychodysleptics [hallucinogens], accidental (unintentional)

    Poisoning by other psychodysleptics [hallucinogens] NOS

    ⑦T40.992 Poisoning by other psychodysleptics [hallucinogens], intentional self-harm

    ⑦T40.993 Poisoning by other psychodysleptics [hallucinogens], assault

    ⑦T40.994 Poisoning by other psychodysleptics [hallucinogens], undetermined

    ⑦T40.995 Adverse effect of other psychodysleptics [hallucinogens]

    ⑦T40.996 Underdosing of other psychodysleptics

T41 Poisoning by, adverse effect of and underdosing of anesthetics and therapeutic gases

Excludes1: benzodiazepines (T42.4-)

cocaine (T40.5-)

complications of anesthesia during pregnancy (O29.-)

complications of anesthesia during labor and delivery (O74.-)

complications of anesthesia during the puerperium (O89.-)

opioids (T40.0-T40.2-)

The appropriate 7th character is to be added to each code from category T41

A - initial encounter

D - subsequent encounter

S - sequela

T41.0 Poisoning by, adverse effect of and underdosing of inhaled anesthetics

Excludes1: oxygen (T41.5-)

  T41.0X Poisoning by, adverse effect of and underdosing of inhaled anesthetics

    ⑦T41.0X1 Poisoning by inhaled anesthetics, accidental (unintentional)

Poisoning by inhaled anesthetics NOS

    ⑦T41.0X2 Poisoning by inhaled anesthetics, intentional self-harm

    ⑦T41.0X3 Poisoning by inhaled anesthetics, assault

    ⑦T41.0X4 Poisoning by inhaled anesthetics, undetermined

    ⑦T41.0X5 Adverse effect of inhaled anesthetics

    ⑦T41.0X6 Underdosing of inhaled anesthetics

T41.1 Poisoning by, adverse effect of and underdosing of intravenous anesthetics

Poisoning by, adverse effect of and underdosing of thiobarbiturates

  T41.1X Poisoning by, adverse effect of and underdosing of intravenous anesthetics

    ⑦T41.1X1 Poisoning by intravenous anesthetics, accidental (unintentional)

Poisoning by intravenous anesthetics NOS

    ⑦T41.1X2 Poisoning by intravenous anesthetics, intentional self-harm

    ⑦T41.1X3 Poisoning by intravenous anesthetics, assault

    ⑦T41.1X4 Poisoning by intravenous anesthetics, undetermined

    ⑦T41.1X5 Adverse effect of intravenous anesthetics

    ⑦T41.1X6 Underdosing of intravenous anesthetics

T41.2 Poisoning by, adverse effect of and underdosing of other and unspecified general anesthetics

  T41.20 Poisoning by, adverse effect of and underdosing of unspecified general anesthetics

    ⑦T41.201 Poisoning by unspecified general anesthetics, accidental (unintentional)

Poisoning by general anesthetics NOS

    ⑦T41.202 Poisoning by unspecified general anesthetics, intentional self-harm

    ⑦T41.203 Poisoning by unspecified general anesthetics, assault

    ⑦T41.204 Poisoning by unspecified general anesthetics, undetermined

    ⑦T41.205 Adverse effect of unspecified general anesthetics

    ⑦T41.206 Underdosing of unspecified general anesthetics

  T41.29 Poisoning by, adverse effect of and underdosing of other general anesthetics

    ⑦T41.291 Poisoning by other general anesthetics, accidental (unintentional)

Poisoning by other general anesthetics NOS

    ⑦T41.292 Poisoning by other general anesthetics, intentional self-harm

    ⑦T41.293 Poisoning by other general anesthetics, assault

    ⑦T41.294 Poisoning by other general anesthetics, undetermined

⑦**T41.295**   **Adverse effect of other general anesthetics**

⑦**T41.296**   **Underdosing of other general anesthetics**

T41.3   **Poisoning by, adverse effect of and underdosing of local anesthetics**

Cocaine (topical)

Excludes2: poisoning by cocaine used as a central nervous system stimulant (T40.5X1-T40.5X4)

T41.3X   **Poisoning by, adverse effect of and underdosing of local anesthetics**

⑦**T41.3X1**   **Poisoning by local anesthetics, accidental (unintentional)**

Poisoning by local anesthetics NOS

⑦**T41.3X2**   **Poisoning by local anesthetics, intentional self-harm**

⑦**T41.3X3**   **Poisoning by local anesthetics, assault**

⑦**T41.3X4**   **Poisoning by local anesthetics, undetermined**

⑦**T41.3X5**   **Adverse effect of local anesthetics**

⑦**T41.3X6**   **Underdosing of local anesthetics**

T41.4   **Poisoning by, adverse effect of and underdosing of unspecified anesthetic**

⊗⑦**T41.41**   **Poisoning by unspecified anesthetic, accidental (unintentional)**

Poisoning by anesthetic NOS

⊗⑦**T41.42**   **Poisoning by unspecified anesthetic, intentional self-harm**

⊗⑦**T41.43**   **Poisoning by unspecified anesthetic, assault**

⊗⑦**T41.44**   **Poisoning by unspecified anesthetic, undetermined**

⊗⑦**T41.45**   **Adverse effect of unspecified anesthetic**

⊗⑦**T41.46**   **Underdosing of unspecified anesthetics**

T41.5   **Poisoning by, adverse effect of and underdosing of therapeutic gases**

T41.5X   **Poisoning by, adverse effect of and underdosing of therapeutic gases**

⑦**T41.5X1**   **Poisoning by therapeutic gases, accidental (unintentional)**

Poisoning by therapeutic gases NOS

⑦**T41.5X2**   **Poisoning by therapeutic gases, intentional self-harm**

⑦**T41.5X3**   **Poisoning by therapeutic gases, assault**

⑦**T41.5X4**   **Poisoning by therapeutic gases, undetermined**

⑦**T41.5X5**   **Adverse effect of therapeutic gases**

⑦**T41.5X6**   **Underdosing of therapeutic gases**

T42   **Poisoning by, adverse effect of and underdosing of antiepileptic, sedative- hypnotic and antiparkinsonism drugs**

Excludes2: drug dependence and related mental and behavioral disorders due to psychoactive substance use (F10.--F19.-)

The appropriate 7th character is to be added to each code from category T42

A - initial encounter

D - subsequent encounter

S - sequela

T42.0   **Poisoning by, adverse effect of and underdosing of hydantoin derivatives**

T42.0X   **Poisoning by, adverse effect of and underdosing of hydantoin derivatives**

⑦**T42.0X1**   **Poisoning by hydantoin derivatives, accidental (unintentional)**

Poisoning by hydantoin derivatives NOS

⑦**T42.0X2**   **Poisoning by hydantoin derivatives, intentional self-harm**

⑦**T42.0X3**   **Poisoning by hydantoin derivatives, assault**

⑦**T42.0X4**   **Poisoning by hydantoin derivatives, undetermined**

⑦**T42.0X5**   **Adverse effect of hydantoin derivatives**

⑦**T42.0X6**   **Underdosing of hydantoin derivatives**

T42.1   **Poisoning by, adverse effect of and underdosing of iminostilbenes**

Poisoning by, adverse effect of and underdosing of carbamazepine

T42.1X   **Poisoning by, adverse effect of and underdosing of iminostilbenes**

⑦**T42.1X1**   **Poisoning by iminostilbenes, accidental (unintentional)**

Poisoning by iminostilbenes NOS

⑦**T42.1X2**   **Poisoning by iminostilbenes, intentional self-harm**

⑦**T42.1X3**   **Poisoning by iminostilbenes, assault**

⑦**T42.1X4**   **Poisoning by iminostilbenes, undetermined**

⑦**T42.1X5**   **Adverse effect of iminostilbenes**

⑦**T42.1X6**   **Underdosing of iminostilbenes**

T42.2   **Poisoning by, adverse effect of and underdosing of succinimides and oxazolidinediones**

T42.2X   **Poisoning by, adverse effect of and underdosing of succinimides and oxazolidinediones**

⑦**T42.2X1**   **Poisoning by succinimides and oxazolidinediones, accidental (unintentional)**

Poisoning by succinimides and oxazolidinediones NOS

⑦**T42.2X2**   **Poisoning by succinimides and oxazolidinediones, intentional self-harm**

⑦**T42.2X3**   **Poisoning by succinimides and oxazolidinediones, assault**

⑦**T42.2X4**   **Poisoning by succinimides and oxazolidinediones, undetermined**

⑦**T42.2X5**   **Adverse effect of succinimides and oxazolidinediones**

⑦**T42.2X6**   **Underdosing of succinimides and oxazolidinediones**

T42.3   **Poisoning by, adverse effect of and underdosing of barbiturates**

Excludes1: poisoning by, adverse effect of and underdosing of thiobarbiturates (T41.1-)

T42.3X   **Poisoning by, adverse effect of and underdosing of barbiturates**

⑦ **T42.3X1** **Poisoning by barbiturates, accidental (unintentional)**

Poisoning by barbiturates NOS

⑦ **T42.3X2** **Poisoning by barbiturates, intentional self-harm**

⑦ **T42.3X3** **Poisoning by barbiturates, assault**

⑦ **T42.3X4** **Poisoning by barbiturates, undetermined**

⑦ **T42.3X5** **Adverse effect of barbiturates**

⑦ **T42.3X6** **Underdosing of barbiturates**

T42.4 **Poisoning by, adverse effect of and underdosing of benzodiazepines**

T42.4X **Poisoning by, adverse effect of and underdosing of benzodiazepines**

⑦ **T42.4X1** **Poisoning by benzodiazepines, accidental (unintentional)**

Poisoning by benzodiazepines NOS

⑦ **T42.4X2** **Poisoning by benzodiazepines, intentional self-harm**

⑦ **T42.4X3** **Poisoning by benzodiazepines, assault**

⑦ **T42.4X4** **Poisoning by benzodiazepines, undetermined**

⑦ **T42.4X5** **Adverse effect of benzodiazepines**

⑦ **T42.4X6** **Underdosing of benzodiazepines**

T42.5 **Poisoning by, adverse effect of and underdosing of mixed antiepileptics**

T42.5X **Poisoning by, adverse effect of and underdosing of antiepileptics**

⑦ **T42.5X1** **Poisoning by mixed antiepileptics, accidental (unintentional)**

Poisoning by mixed antiepileptics NOS

⑦ **T42.5X2** **Poisoning by mixed antiepileptics, intentional self-harm**

⑦ **T42.5X3** **Poisoning by mixed antiepileptics, assault**

⑦ **T42.5X4** **Poisoning by mixed antiepileptics, undetermined**

⑦ **T42.5X5** **Adverse effect of mixed antiepileptics**

⑦ **T42.5X6** **Underdosing of mixed antiepileptics**

T42.6 **Poisoning by, adverse effect of and underdosing of other antiepileptic and sedative-hypnotic drugs**

Poisoning by, adverse effect of and underdosing of methaqualone

Poisoning by, adverse effect of and underdosing of valproic acid

Excludes1: poisoning by, adverse effect of and underdosing of carbamazepine (T42.1-)

T42.6X **Poisoning by, adverse effect of and underdosing of other antiepileptic and sedative-hypnotic drugs**

⑦ **T42.6X1** **Poisoning by other antiepileptic and sedative-hypnotic drugs, accidental (unintentional)**

Poisoning by other antiepileptic and sedative-hypnotic drugs NOS

⑦ **T42.6X2** **Poisoning by other antiepileptic and sedative-hypnotic drugs, intentional self-harm**

⑦ **T42.6X3** **Poisoning by other antiepileptic and sedative-hypnotic drugs, assault**

⑦ **T42.6X4** **Poisoning by other antiepileptic and sedative-hypnotic drugs, undetermined**

⑦ **T42.6X5** **Adverse effect of other antiepileptic and sedative-hypnotic drugs**

⑦ **T42.6X6** **Underdosing of other antiepileptic and sedative-hypnotic drugs**

T42.7 **Poisoning by, adverse effect of and underdosing of unspecified antiepileptic and sedative-hypnotic drugs**

⊗⑦ **T42.71** **Poisoning by unspecified antiepileptic and sedative-hypnotic drugs, accidental (unintentional)**

Poisoning by antiepileptic and sedative-hypnotic drugs NOS

⊗⑦ **T42.72** **Poisoning by unspecified antiepileptic and sedative-hypnotic drugs, intentional self-harm**

⊗⑦ **T42.73** **Poisoning by unspecified antiepileptic and sedative-hypnotic drugs, assault**

⊗⑦ **T42.74** **Poisoning by unspecified antiepileptic and sedative-hypnotic drugs, undetermined**

⊗⑦ **T42.75** **Adverse effect of unspecified antiepileptic and sedative-hypnotic drugs**

⊗⑦ **T42.76** **Underdosing of unspecified antiepileptic and sedative-hypnotic drugs**

T42.8 **Poisoning by, adverse effect of and underdosing of antiparkinsonism drugs and other central muscle-tone depressants**

Poisoning by, adverse effect of and underdosing of amantadine

T42.8X **Poisoning by, adverse effect of and underdosing of antiparkinsonism drugs and other central muscle-tone depressants**

⑦ **T42.8X1** **Poisoning by antiparkinsonism drugs and other central muscle-tone depressants, accidental (unintentional)**

Poisoning by antiparkinsonism drugs and other central muscle-tone depressants NOS

⑦ **T42.8X2** **Poisoning by antiparkinsonism drugs and other central muscle-tone depressants, intentional self-harm**

⑦ **T42.8X3** **Poisoning by antiparkinsonism drugs and other central muscle-tone depressants, assault**

⑦ **T42.8X4** **Poisoning by antiparkinsonism drugs and other central muscle-tone depressants, undetermined**

⑦ **T42.8X5** **Adverse effect of antiparkinsonism drugs and other central muscle-tone depressants**

⑦ **T42.8X6** **Underdosing of antiparkinsonism drugs and other central muscle-tone depressants**

T43 **Poisoning by, adverse effect of and underdosing of psychotropic drugs, not elsewhere classified**

Excludes1: appetite depressants (T50.5-)

barbiturates (T42.3-)

benzodiazepines (T42.4-)

methaqualone (T42.6-)

psychodysleptics [hallucinogens] (T40.7-T40.9-)

Excludes2: drug dependence and related mental and behavioral disorders due to psychoactive substance use (F10.--F19.-)

The appropriate 7th character is to be added to each code from category T43

A - initial encounter

D - subsequent encounter

S - sequela

T43.0   **Poisoning by, adverse effect of and underdosing of tricyclic and tetracyclic antidepressants**

    T43.01   **Poisoning by, adverse effect of and underdosing of tricyclic antidepressants**

        ⑦T43.011   **Poisoning by tricyclic antidepressants, accidental (unintentional)**

            Poisoning by tricyclic antidepressants NOS

        ⑦T43.012   **Poisoning by tricyclic antidepressants, intentional self-harm**

        ⑦T43.013   **Poisoning by tricyclic antidepressants, assault**

        ⑦T43.014   **Poisoning by tricyclic antidepressants, undetermined**

        ⑦T43.015   **Adverse effect of tricyclic antidepressants**

        ⑦T43.016   **Underdosing of tricyclic antidepressants**

    T43.02   **Poisoning by, adverse effect of and underdosing of tetracyclic antidepressants**

        ⑦T43.021   **Poisoning by tetracyclic antidepressants, accidental (unintentional)**

            Poisoning by tetracyclic antidepressants NOS

        ⑦T43.022   **Poisoning by tetracyclic antidepressants, intentional self-harm**

        ⑦T43.023   **Poisoning by tetracyclic antidepressants, assault**

        ⑦T43.024   **Poisoning by tetracyclic antidepressants, undetermined**

        ⑦T43.025   **Adverse effect of tetracyclic antidepressants**

        ⑦T43.026   **Underdosing of tetracyclic antidepressants**

T43.1   **Poisoning by, adverse effect of and underdosing of monoamine-oxidase-inhibitor antidepressants**

    T43.1X   **Poisoning by, adverse effect of and underdosing of monoamine-oxidase-inhibitor antidepressants**

        ⑦T43.1X1   **Poisoning by monoamine-oxidase-inhibitor antidepressants, accidental (unintentional)**

            Poisoning by monoamine-oxidase-inhibitor antidepressants NOS

        ⑦T43.1X2   **Poisoning by monoamine-oxidase-inhibitor antidepressants, intentional self-harm**

        ⑦T43.1X3   **Poisoning by monoamine-oxidase-inhibitor antidepressants, assault**

        ⑦T43.1X4   **Poisoning by monoamine-oxidase-inhibitor antidepressants, undetermined**

        ⑦T43.1X5   **Adverse effect of monoamine-oxidase-inhibitor antidepressants**

        ⑦T43.1X6   **Underdosing of monoamine-oxidase-inhibitor antidepressants**

T43.2   **Poisoning by, adverse effect of and underdosing of other and unspecified antidepressants**

    T43.20   **Poisoning by, adverse effect of and underdosing of unspecified antidepressants**

        ⑦T43.201   **Poisoning by unspecified antidepressants, accidental (unintentional)**

            Poisoning by antidepressants NOS

        ⑦T43.202   **Poisoning by unspecified antidepressants, intentional self-harm**

        ⑦T43.203   **Poisoning by unspecified antidepressants, assault**

        ⑦T43.204   **Poisoning by unspecified antidepressants, undetermined**

        ⑦T43.205   **Adverse effect of unspecified antidepressants**

        ⑦T43.206   **Underdosing of unspecified antidepressants**

    T43.21   **Poisoning by, adverse effect of and underdosing of selective serotonin and norepinephrine reuptake inhibitors**

        Poisoning by, adverse effect of and underdosing of SSNRI antidepressants

        ⑦T43.211   **Poisoning by selective serotonin and norepinephrine reuptake inhibitors, accidental (unintentional)**

        ⑦T43.212   **Poisoning by selective serotonin and norepinephrine reuptake inhibitors, intentional self-harm**

        ⑦T43.213   **Poisoning by selective serotonin and norepinephrine reuptake inhibitors, assault**

        ⑦T43.214   **Poisoning by selective serotonin and norepinephrine reuptake inhibitors, undetermined**

        ⑦T43.215   **Adverse effect of selective serotonin and norepinephrine reuptake inhibitors**

        ⑦T43.216   **Underdosing of selective serotonin and norepinephrine reuptake inhibitors**

    T43.22   **Poisoning by, adverse effect of and underdosing of selective serotonin reuptake inhibitors**

        Poisoning by, adverse effect of and underdosing of SSRI antidepressants

        ⑦T43.221   **Poisoning by selective serotonin reuptake inhibitors, accidental (unintentional)**

        ⑦T43.222   **Poisoning by selective serotonin reuptake inhibitors, intentional self-harm**

        ⑦T43.223   **Poisoning by selective serotonin reuptake inhibitors, assault**

⑦ T43.224   **Poisoning by selective serotonin reuptake inhibitors, undetermined**

⑦ T43.225   **Adverse effect of selective serotonin reuptake inhibitors**

⑦ T43.226   **Underdosing of selective serotonin reuptake inhibitors**

    T43.29   **Poisoning by, adverse effect of and underdosing of other antidepressants**

⑦ T43.291   **Poisoning by other antidepressants, accidental (unintentional)**

         Poisoning by other antidepressants NOS

⑦ T43.292   **Poisoning by other antidepressants, intentional self-harm**

⑦ T43.293   **Poisoning by other antidepressants, assault**

⑦ T43.294   **Poisoning by other antidepressants, undetermined**

⑦ T43.295   **Adverse effect of other antidepressants**

⑦ T43.296   **Underdosing of other antidepressants**

T43.3   **Poisoning by, adverse effect of and underdosing of phenothiazine antipsychotics and neuroleptics**

    T43.3X   **Poisoning by, adverse effect of and underdosing of phenothiazine antipsychotics and neuroleptics**

⑦ T43.3X1   **Poisoning by phenothiazine antipsychotics and neuroleptics, accidental (unintentional)**

         Poisoning by phenothiazine antipsychotics and neuroleptics NOS

⑦ T43.3X2   **Poisoning by phenothiazine antipsychotics and neuroleptics, intentional self-harm**

⑦ T43.3X3   **Poisoning by phenothiazine antipsychotics and neuroleptics, assault**

⑦ T43.3X4   **Poisoning by phenothiazine antipsychotics and neuroleptics, undetermined**

⑦ T43.3X5   **Adverse effect of phenothiazine antipsychotics and neuroleptics**

⑦ T43.3X6   **Underdosing of phenothiazine antipsychotics and neuroleptics**

T43.4   **Poisoning by, adverse effect of and underdosing of butyrophenone and thiothixene neuroleptics**

    T43.4X   **Poisoning by, adverse effect of and underdosing of butyrophenone and thiothixene neuroleptics**

⑦ T43.4X1   **Poisoning by butyrophenone and thiothixene neuroleptics, accidental (unintentional)**

         Poisoning by butyrophenone and thiothixene neuroleptics NOS

⑦ T43.4X2   **Poisoning by butyrophenone and thiothixene neuroleptics, intentional self-harm**

⑦ T43.4X3   **Poisoning by butyrophenone and thiothixene neuroleptics, assault**

⑦ T43.4X4   **Poisoning by butyrophenone and thiothixene neuroleptics, undetermined**

⑦ T43.4X5   **Adverse effect of butyrophenone and thiothixene neuroleptics**

⑦ T43.4X6   **Underdosing of butyrophenone and thiothixene neuroleptics**

T43.5   **Poisoning by, adverse effect of and underdosing of other and unspecified antipsychotics and neuroleptics**

Excludes1: poisoning by, adverse effect of and underdosing of rauwolfia (T46.5-)

    T43.50   **Poisoning by, adverse effect of and underdosing of unspecified antipsychotics and neuroleptics**

⑦ T43.501   **Poisoning by unspecified antipsychotics and neuroleptics, accidental (unintentional)**

         Poisoning by antipsychotics and neuroleptics NOS

⑦ T43.502   **Poisoning by unspecified antipsychotics and neuroleptics, intentional self-harm**

⑦ T43.503   **Poisoning by unspecified antipsychotics and neuroleptics, assault**

⑦ T43.504   **Poisoning by unspecified antipsychotics and neuroleptics, undetermined**

⑦ T43.505   **Adverse effect of unspecified antipsychotics and neuroleptics**

⑦ T43.506   **Underdosing of unspecified antipsychotics and neuroleptics**

    T43.59   **Poisoning by, adverse effect of and underdosing of other antipsychotics and neuroleptics**

⑦ T43.591   **Poisoning by other antipsychotics and neuroleptics, accidental (unintentional)**

         Poisoning by other antipsychotics and neuroleptics NOS

⑦ T43.592   **Poisoning by other antipsychotics and neuroleptics, intentional self-harm**

⑦ T43.593   **Poisoning by other antipsychotics and neuroleptics, assault**

⑦ T43.594   **Poisoning by other antipsychotics and neuroleptics, undetermined**

⑦ T43.595   **Adverse effect of other antipsychotics and neuroleptics**

⑦ T43.596   **Underdosing of other antipsychotics and neuroleptics**

T43.6   **Poisoning by, adverse effect of and underdosing of psychostimulants**

Excludes1: poisoning by, adverse effect of and underdosing of cocaine (T40.5-)

    T43.60   **Poisoning by, adverse effect of and underdosing of unspecified psychostimulant**

⑦ T43.601   **Poisoning by unspecified psychostimulants, accidental (unintentional)**

         Poisoning by psychostimulants NOS

⑦ T43.602   **Poisoning by unspecified psychostimulants, intentional self-harm**

⑦ T43.603   **Poisoning by unspecified psychostimulants, assault**

  ● New code   ▲ Revised code   **Excludes1:** Not coded here   **Excludes2:** Not included here   ⊗ Placeholder required   ⑦ 7ᵗʰ digit required

⑦T43.604 Poisoning by unspecified psychostimulants, undetermined

⑦T43.605 Adverse effect of unspecified psychostimulants

⑦T43.606 Underdosing of unspecified psychostimulants

T43.61 Poisoning by, adverse effect of and underdosing of caffeine

⑦T43.611 Poisoning by caffeine, accidental (unintentional)

Poisoning by caffeine NOS

⑦T43.612 Poisoning by caffeine, intentional self-harm

⑦T43.613 Poisoning by caffeine, assault

⑦T43.614 Poisoning by caffeine, undetermined

⑦T43.615 Adverse effect of caffeine

⑦T43.616 Underdosing of caffeine

T43.62 Poisoning by, adverse effect of and underdosing of amphetamines

Poisoning by, adverse effect of and underdosing of methamphetamines

⑦T43.621 Poisoning by amphetamines, accidental (unintentional)

Poisoning by amphetamines NOS

⑦T43.622 Poisoning by amphetamines, intentional self-harm

⑦T43.623 Poisoning by amphetamines, assault

⑦T43.624 Poisoning by amphetamines, undetermined

⑦T43.625 Adverse effect of amphetamines

⑦T43.626 Underdosing of amphetamines

T43.63 Poisoning by, adverse effect of and underdosing of methylphenidate

⑦T43.631 Poisoning by methylphenidate, accidental (unintentional)

Poisoning by methylphenidate NOS

⑦T43.632 Poisoning by methylphenidate, intentional self-harm

⑦T43.633 Poisoning by methylphenidate, assault

⑦T43.634 Poisoning by methylphenidate, undetermined

⑦T43.635 Adverse effect of methylphenidate

⑦T43.636 Underdosing of methylphenidate

T43.69 Poisoning by, adverse effect of and underdosing of other psychostimulants

⑦T43.691 Poisoning by other psychostimulants, accidental (unintentional)

Poisoning by other psychostimulants NOS

⑦T43.692 Poisoning by other psychostimulants, intentional self-harm

⑦T43.693 Poisoning by other psychostimulants, assault

⑦T43.694 Poisoning by other psychostimulants, undetermined

⑦T43.695 Adverse effect of other psychostimulants

⑦T43.696 Underdosing of other psychostimulants

T43.8 Poisoning by, adverse effect of and underdosing of other psychotropic drugs

T43.8X Poisoning by, adverse effect of and underdosing of other psychotropic drugs

⑦T43.8X1 Poisoning by other psychotropic drugs, accidental (unintentional)

Poisoning by other psychotropic drugs NOS

⑦T43.8X2 Poisoning by other psychotropic drugs, intentional self-harm

⑦T43.8X3 Poisoning by other psychotropic drugs, assault

⑦T43.8X4 Poisoning by other psychotropic drugs, undetermined

⑦T43.8X5 Adverse effect of other psychotropic drugs

⑦T43.8X6 Underdosing of other psychotropic drugs

T43.9 Poisoning by, adverse effect of and underdosing of unspecified psychotropic drug

⊗⑦T43.91 Poisoning by unspecified psychotropic drug, accidental (unintentional)

Poisoning by psychotropic drug NOS

⊗⑦T43.92 Poisoning by unspecified psychotropic drug, intentional self-harm

⊗⑦T43.93 Poisoning by unspecified psychotropic drug, assault

⊗⑦T43.94 Poisoning by unspecified psychotropic drug, undetermined

⊗⑦T43.95 Adverse effect of unspecified psychotropic drug

⊗⑦T43.96 Underdosing of unspecified psychotropic drug

T44 Poisoning by, adverse effect of and underdosing of drugs primarily affecting the autonomic nervous system

The appropriate 7th character is to be added to each code from category T44

A - initial encounter

D - subsequent encounter

S - sequela

T44.0 Poisoning by, adverse effect of and underdosing of anticholinesterase agents

T44.0X Poisoning by, adverse effect of and underdosing of anticholinesterase agents

⑦T44.0X1 Poisoning by anticholinesterase agents, accidental (unintentional)

oisoning by anticholinesterase agents NOS

⑦T44.0X2 Poisoning by anticholinesterase agents, intentional self-harm

⑦T44.0X3 Poisoning by anticholinesterase agents, assault

⑦T44.0X4 Poisoning by anticholinesterase agents, undetermined

⑦T44.0X5 Adverse effect of anticholinesterase agents

⑦T44.0X6 Underdosing of anticholinesterase agents

T44.1 Poisoning by, adverse effect of and underdosing of other parasympathomimetics [cholinergics]

T44.1X Poisoning by, adverse effect of and underdosing of other parasympathomimetics [cholinergics]

⑦ T44.1X1 Poisoning by other parasympathomimetics [cholinergics], accidental (unintentional)

Poisoning by other parasympathomimetics [cholinergics] NOS

⑦ T44.1X2 Poisoning by other parasympathomimetics [cholinergics], intentional self-harm

⑦ T44.1X3 Poisoning by other parasympathomimetics [cholinergics], assault

⑦ T44.1X4 Poisoning by other parasympathomimetics [cholinergics], undetermined

⑦ T44.1X5 Adverse effect of other parasympathomimetics [cholinergics]

⑦ T44.1X6 Underdosing of other parasympathomimetics

T44.2 Poisoning by, adverse effect of and underdosing of ganglionic blocking drugs

T44.2X Poisoning by, adverse effect of and underdosing of ganglionic blocking drugs

⑦ T44.2X1 Poisoning by ganglionic blocking drugs, accidental (unintentional)

Poisoning by ganglionic blocking drugs NOS

⑦ T44.2X2 Poisoning by ganglionic blocking drugs, intentional self-harm

⑦ T44.2X3 Poisoning by ganglionic blocking drugs, assault

⑦ T44.2X4 Poisoning by ganglionic blocking drugs, undetermined

⑦ T44.2X5 Adverse effect of ganglionic blocking drugs

⑦ T44.2X6 Underdosing of ganglionic blocking drugs

T44.3 Poisoning by, adverse effect of and underdosing of other parasympatholytics [anticholinergics and antimuscarinics] and spasmolytics

Poisoning by, adverse effect of and underdosing of papaverine

T44.3X Poisoning by, adverse effect of and underdosing of other parasympatholytics [anticholinergics and antimuscarinics] and spasmolytics

⑦ T44.3X1 Poisoning by other parasympatholytics [anticholinergics and antimuscarinics] and spasmolytics, accidental (unintentional)

Poisoning by other parasympatholytics [anticholinergics and antimuscarinics] and spasmolytics NOS

⑦ T44.3X2 Poisoning by other parasympatholytics

[anticholinergics and antimuscarinics] and spasmolytics, intentional self-harm

⑦ T44.3X3 Poisoning by other parasympatholytics [anticholinergics and antimuscarinics] and spasmolytics, assault

⑦ T44.3X4 Poisoning by other parasympatholytics [anticholinergics and antimuscarinics] and spasmolytics, undetermined

⑦ T44.3X5 Adverse effect of other parasympatholytics [anticholinergics and antimuscarinics] and spasmolytics

⑦ T44.3X6 Underdosing of other parasympatholytics [anticholinergics and antimuscarinics] and spasmolytics

T44.4 Poisoning by, adverse effect of and underdosing of predominantly alpha-adrenoreceptor agonists

Poisoning by, adverse effect of and underdosing of metaraminol

T44.4X Poisoning by, adverse effect of and underdosing of predominantly alpha-adrenoreceptor agonists

⑦ T44.4X1 Poisoning by predominantly alpha-adrenoreceptor agonists, accidental (unintentional)

Poisoning by predominantly alpha-adrenoreceptor agonists NOS

⑦ T44.4X2 Poisoning by predominantly alpha-adrenoreceptor agonists, intentional self-harm

⑦ T44.4X3 Poisoning by predominantly alpha-adrenoreceptor agonists, assault

⑦ T44.4X4 Poisoning by predominantly alpha-adrenoreceptor agonists, undetermined

⑦ T44.4X5 Adverse effect of predominantly alpha-adrenoreceptor agonists

⑦ T44.4X6 Underdosing of predominantly alpha-adrenoreceptor agonists

T44.5 Poisoning by, adverse effect of and underdosing of predominantly beta-adrenoreceptor agonists

Excludes1: poisoning by, adverse effect of and underdosing of beta-adrenoreceptor agonists used in asthma therapy (T48.6-)

T44.5X Poisoning by, adverse effect of and underdosing of predominantly beta-adrenoreceptor agonists

⑦ T44.5X1 Poisoning by predominantly beta-adrenoreceptor agonists, accidental (unintentional)

Poisoning by predominantly beta-adrenoreceptor agonists NOS

⑦ T44.5X2 Poisoning by predominantly beta-adrenoreceptor agonists, intentional self-harm

⑦ T44.5X3 Poisoning by predominantly beta-adrenoreceptor agonists, assault

 ● New code　▲ Revised code　**Excludes1:** Not coded here　**Excludes2:** Not included here　⊗ Placeholder required　⑦ 7th digit required

⑦T44.5X4 **Poisoning by predominantly beta-adrenoreceptor agonists, undetermined**

⑦T44.5X5 **Adverse effect of predominantly beta-adrenoreceptor agonists**

⑦T44.5X6 **Underdosing of predominantly beta-adrenoreceptor agonists**

T44.6 **Poisoning by, adverse effect of and underdosing of alpha-adrenoreceptor antagonists**

Excludes1: poisoning by, adverse effect of and underdosing of ergot alkaloids (T48.0)

T44.6X **Poisoning by, adverse effect of and underdosing of alpha-adrenoreceptor antagonists**

⑦T44.6X1 **Poisoning by alpha-adrenoreceptor antagonists, accidental (unintentional)**

Poisoning by alpha-adrenoreceptor antagonists NOS

⑦T44.6X2 **Poisoning by alpha-adrenoreceptor antagonists, intentional self-harm**

⑦T44.6X3 **Poisoning by alpha-adrenoreceptor antagonists, assault**

⑦T44.6X4 **Poisoning by alpha-adrenoreceptor antagonists, undetermined**

⑦T44.6X5 **Adverse effect of alpha-adrenoreceptor antagonists**

⑦T44.6X6 **Underdosing of alpha-adrenoreceptor antagonists**

T44.7 **Poisoning by, adverse effect of and underdosing of beta-adrenoreceptor antagonists**

T44.7X **Poisoning by, adverse effect of and underdosing of beta-adrenoreceptor antagonists**

⑦T44.7X1 **Poisoning by beta-adrenoreceptor antagonists, accidental (unintentional)**

Poisoning by beta-adrenoreceptor antagonists NOS

⑦T44.7X2 **Poisoning by beta-adrenoreceptor antagonists, intentional self-harm**

⑦T44.7X3 **Poisoning by beta-adrenoreceptor antagonists, assault**

⑦T44.7X4 **Poisoning by beta-adrenoreceptor antagonists, undetermined**

⑦T44.7X5 **Adverse effect of beta-adrenoreceptor antagonists**

⑦T44.7X6 **Underdosing of beta-adrenoreceptor antagonists**

T44.8 **Poisoning by, adverse effect of and underdosing of centrally-acting and adrenergic-neuron- blocking agents**

Excludes1: poisoning by, adverse effect of and underdosing of clonidine (T46.5)

poisoning by, adverse effect of and underdosing of guanethidine (T46.5)

T44.8X **Poisoning by, adverse effect of and underdosing of centrally-acting and adrenergic- neuron-blocking agents**

⑦T44.8X1 **Poisoning by centrally-acting and adrenergic-neuron-blocking agents, accidental (unintentional)**

Poisoning by centrally-acting and adrenergic-neuron-blocking agents NOS

⑦T44.8X2 **Poisoning by centrally-acting and adrenergic-neuron-blocking agents, intentional self-harm**

⑦T44.8X3 **Poisoning by centrally-acting and adrenergic-neuron-blocking agents, assault**

⑦T44.8X4 **Poisoning by centrally-acting and adrenergic-neuron-blocking agents, undetermined**

⑦T44.8X5 **Adverse effect of centrally-acting and adrenergic-neuron-blocking agents**

⑦T44.8X6 **Underdosing of centrally-acting and adrenergic-neuron-blocking agents**

T44.9 **Poisoning by, adverse effect of and underdosing of other and unspecified drugs primarily affecting the autonomic nervous system**

Poisoning by, adverse effect of and underdosing of drug stimulating both alpha and beta-adrenoreceptors

T44.90 **Poisoning by, adverse effect of and underdosing of unspecified drugs primarily affecting the autonomic nervous system**

⑦T44.901 **Poisoning by unspecified drugs primarily affecting the autonomic nervous system, accidental (unintentional)**

Poisoning by unspecified drugs primarily affecting the autonomic nervous system NOS

⑦T44.902 **Poisoning by unspecified drugs primarily affecting the autonomic nervous system, intentional self-harm**

⑦T44.903 **Poisoning by unspecified drugs primarily affecting the autonomic nervous system, assault**

⑦T44.904 **Poisoning by unspecified drugs primarily affecting the autonomic nervous system, undetermined**

⑦T44.905 **Adverse effect of unspecified drugs primarily affecting the autonomic nervous system**

⑦T44.906 **Underdosing of unspecified drugs primarily affecting the autonomic nervous system**

T44.99 **Poisoning by, adverse effect of and underdosing of other drugs primarily affecting the autonomic nervous system**

⑦T44.991 **Poisoning by other drug primarily affecting the autonomic nervous system, accidental (unintentional)**

Poisoning by other drugs primarily affecting the autonomic nervous system NOS

⑦T44.992 **Poisoning by other drug primarily affecting the autonomic nervous system, intentional self-harm**

⑦T44.993 **Poisoning by other drug primarily affecting the autonomic nervous system, assault**

⑦**T44.994** **Poisoning by other drug primarily affecting the autonomic nervous system, undetermined**

⑦**T44.995** **Adverse effect of other drug primarily affecting the autonomic nervous system**

⑦**T44.996** **Underdosing of other drug primarily affecting the autonomic nervous system**

T45 **Poisoning by, adverse effect of and underdosing of primarily systemic and hematological agents, not elsewhere classified**

The appropriate 7th character is to be added to each code from category T45

A - initial encounter

D - subsequent encounter

S - sequela

T45.0 **Poisoning by, adverse effect of and underdosing of antiallergic and antiemetic drugs**

Excludes1: poisoning by, adverse effect of and underdosing of phenothiazine-based neuroleptics (T43.3)

T45.0X **Poisoning by, adverse effect of and underdosing of antiallergic and antiemetic drugs**

⑦**T45.0X1** **Poisoning by antiallergic and antiemetic drugs, accidental (unintentional)**

Poisoning by antiallergic and antiemetic drugs NOS

⑦**T45.0X2** **Poisoning by antiallergic and antiemetic drugs, intentional self-harm**

⑦**T45.0X3** **Poisoning by antiallergic and antiemetic drugs, assault**

⑦**T45.0X4** **Poisoning by antiallergic and antiemetic drugs, undetermined**

⑦**T45.0X5** **Adverse effect of antiallergic and antiemetic drugs**

⑦**T45.0X6** **Underdosing of antiallergic and antiemetic drugs**

T45.1 **Poisoning by, adverse effect of and underdosing of antineoplastic and immunosuppressive drugs**

Excludes1: poisoning by, adverse effect of and underdosing of tamoxifen (T38.6)

T45.1X **Poisoning by, adverse effect of and underdosing of antineoplastic and immunosuppressive drugs**

⑦**T45.1X1** **Poisoning by antineoplastic and immunosuppressive drugs, accidental (unintentional)**

Poisoning by antineoplastic and immunosuppressive drugs NOS

⑦**T45.1X2** **Poisoning by antineoplastic and immunosuppressive drugs, intentional self-harm**

⑦**T45.1X3** **Poisoning by antineoplastic and immunosuppressive drugs, assault**

⑦**T45.1X4** **Poisoning by antineoplastic and immunosuppressive drugs, undetermined**

⑦**T45.1X5** **Adverse effect of antineoplastic and immunosuppressive drugs**

⑦**T45.1X6** **Underdosing of antineoplastic and immunosuppressive drugs**

T45.2 **Poisoning by, adverse effect of and underdosing of vitamins**

Excludes2: poisoning by, adverse effect of and underdosing of nicotinic acid (derivatives) (T46.7)

poisoning by, adverse effect of and underdosing of iron (T45.4)

poisoning by, adverse effect of and underdosing of vitamin K (T45.7)

T45.2X **Poisoning by, adverse effect of and underdosing of vitamins**

⑦**T45.2X1** **Poisoning by vitamins, accidental (unintentional)**

Poisoning by vitamins NOS

⑦**T45.2X2** **Poisoning by vitamins, intentional self-harm**

⑦**T45.2X3** **Poisoning by vitamins, assault**

⑦**T45.2X4** **Poisoning by vitamins, undetermined**

⑦**T45.2X5** **Adverse effect of vitamins**

⑦**T45.2X6** **Underdosing of vitamins**

Excludes1: vitamin deficiencies (E50-E56)

T45.3 **Poisoning by, adverse effect of and underdosing of enzymes**

T45.3X **Poisoning by, adverse effect of and underdosing of enzymes**

⑦**T45.3X1** **Poisoning by enzymes, accidental (unintentional)**

Poisoning by enzymes NOS

⑦**T45.3X2** **Poisoning by enzymes, intentional self-harm**

⑦**T45.3X3** **Poisoning by enzymes, assault**

⑦**T45.3X4** **Poisoning by enzymes, undetermined**

⑦**T45.3X5** **Adverse effect of enzymes**

⑦**T45.3X6** **Underdosing of enzymes**

T45.4 **Poisoning by, adverse effect of and underdosing of iron and its compounds**

T45.4X **Poisoning by, adverse effect of and underdosing of iron and its compounds**

⑦**T45.4X1** **Poisoning by iron and its compounds, accidental (unintentional)**

Poisoning by iron and its compounds NOS

⑦**T45.4X2** **Poisoning by iron and its compounds, intentional self-harm**

⑦**T45.4X3** **Poisoning by iron and its compounds, assault**

⑦**T45.4X4** **Poisoning by iron and its compounds, undetermined**

⑦**T45.4X5** **Adverse effect of iron and its compounds**

⑦**T45.4X6** **Underdosing of iron and its compounds**

Excludes1: iron deficiency (E61.1)

T45.5 **Poisoning by, adverse effect of and underdosing of anticoagulants and antithrombotic drugs**

T45.51 **Poisoning by, adverse effect of and underdosing of anticoagulants**

⑦T45.511 **Poisoning by anticoagulants, accidental (unintentional)**

Poisoning by anticoagulants NOS

⑦T45.512 **Poisoning by anticoagulants, intentional self-harm**

⑦T45.513 **Poisoning by anticoagulants, assault**

⑦T45.514 **Poisoning by anticoagulants, undetermined**

⑦T45.515 **Adverse effect of anticoagulants**

⑦T45.516 **Underdosing of anticoagulants**

T45.52 **Poisoning by, adverse effect of and underdosing of antithrombotic drugs**

Poisoning by, adverse effect of and underdosing of antiplatelet drugs

Excludes2: poisoning by, adverse effect of and underdosing of aspirin (T39.01-)

poisoning by, adverse effect of and underdosing of acetylsalicylic acid (T39.01-)

⑦T45.521 **Poisoning by antithrombotic drugs, accidental (unintentional)**

Poisoning by antithrombotic drug NOS

⑦T45.522 **Poisoning by antithrombotic drugs, intentional self-harm**

⑦T45.523 **Poisoning by antithrombotic drugs, assault**

⑦T45.524 **Poisoning by antithrombotic drugs, undetermined**

⑦T45.525 **Adverse effect of antithrombotic drugs**

⑦T45.526 **Underdosing of antithrombotic drugs**

T45.6 **Poisoning by, adverse effect of and underdosing of fibrinolysis-affecting drugs**

T45.60 **Poisoning by, adverse effect of and underdosing of unspecified fibrinolysis-affecting drugs**

⑦T45.601 **Poisoning by unspecified fibrinolysis-affecting drugs, accidental (unintentional)**

Poisoning by fibrinolysis-affecting drug NOS

⑦T45.602 **Poisoning by unspecified fibrinolysis-affecting drugs, intentional self-harm**

⑦T45.603 **Poisoning by unspecified fibrinolysis-affecting drugs, assault**

⑦T45.604 **Poisoning by unspecified fibrinolysis-affecting drugs, undetermined**

⑦T45.605 **Adverse effect of unspecified fibrinolysis-affecting drugs**

⑦T45.606 **Underdosing of unspecified fibrinolysis-affecting drugs**

T45.61 **Poisoning by, adverse effect of and underdosing of thrombolytic drugs**

⑦T45.611 **Poisoning by thrombolytic drug, accidental (unintentional)**

Poisoning by thrombolytic drug NOS

⑦T45.612 **Poisoning by thrombolytic drug, intentional self-harm**

⑦T45.613 **Poisoning by thrombolytic drug, assault**

⑦T45.614 **Poisoning by thrombolytic drug, undetermined**

⑦T45.615 **Adverse effect of thrombolytic drugs**

⑦T45.616 **Underdosing of thrombolytic drugs**

T45.62 **Poisoning by, adverse effect of and underdosing of hemostatic drugs**

⑦T45.621 **Poisoning by hemostatic drug, accidental (unintentional)**

Poisoning by hemostatic drug NOS

⑦T45.622 **Poisoning by hemostatic drug, intentional self-harm**

⑦T45.623 **Poisoning by hemostatic drug, assault**

⑦T45.624 **Poisoning by hemostatic drug, undetermined**

⑦T45.625 **Adverse effect of hemostatic drug**

⑦T45.626 **Underdosing of hemostatic drugs**

T45.69 **Poisoning by, adverse effect of and underdosing of other fibrinolysis-affecting drugs**

⑦T45.691 **Poisoning by other fibrinolysis-affecting drugs, accidental (unintentional)**

Poisoning by other fibrinolysis-affecting drug NOS

⑦T45.692 **Poisoning by other fibrinolysis-affecting drugs, intentional self-harm**

⑦T45.693 **Poisoning by other fibrinolysis-affecting drugs, assault**

⑦T45.694 **Poisoning by other fibrinolysis-affecting drugs, undetermined**

⑦T45.695 **Adverse effect of other fibrinolysis-affecting drugs**

⑦T45.696 **Underdosing of other fibrinolysis-affecting drugs**

T45.7 **Poisoning by, adverse effect of and underdosing of anticoagulant antagonists, vitamin K and other coagulants**

T45.7X **Poisoning by, adverse effect of and underdosing of anticoagulant antagonists, vitamin K and other coagulants**

⑦T45.7X1 **Poisoning by anticoagulant antagonists, vitamin K and other coagulants, accidental (unintentional)**

Poisoning by anticoagulant antagonists, vitamin K and other coagulants NOS

⑦T45.7X2 **Poisoning by anticoagulant antagonists, vitamin K and other coagulants, intentional self-harm**

⑦T45.7X3 **Poisoning by anticoagulant antagonists, vitamin K and other coagulants, assault**

⑦ **T45.7X4** **Poisoning by anticoagulant antagonists, vitamin K and other coagulants, undetermined**

⑦ **T45.7X5** **Adverse effect of anticoagulant antagonists, vitamin K and other coagulants**

⑦ **T45.7X6** **Underdosing of anticoagulant antagonist, vitamin K and other coagulants**

Excludes1: vitamin K deficiency (E56.1)

T45.8 **Poisoning by, adverse effect of and underdosing of other primarily systemic and hematological agents**

Poisoning by, adverse effect of and underdosing of liver preparations **and other** antianemic agents

Poisoning by, adverse effect of and underdosing of natural blood and blood products

Poisoning by, adverse effect of and underdosing of plasma substitute

Excludes2: poisoning by, adverse effect of and underdosing of immunoglobulin (T50.Z1)

poisoning by, adverse effect of and underdosing of iron (T45.4) transfusion reactions (T80.-)

T45.8X **Poisoning by, adverse effect of and underdosing of other primarily systemic and hematological agents**

⑦ **T45.8X1** **Poisoning by other primarily systemic and hematological agents, accidental (unintentional)**

Poisoning by other primarily systemic and hematological agents NOS

⑦ **T45.8X2** **Poisoning by other primarily systemic and hematological agents, intentional self-harm**

⑦ **T45.8X3** **Poisoning by other primarily systemic and hematological agents, assault**

⑦ **T45.8X4** **Poisoning by other primarily systemic and hematological agents, undetermined**

⑦ **T45.8X5** **Adverse effect of other primarily systemic and hematological agents**

⑦ **T45.8X6** **Underdosing of other primarily systemic and hematological agents**

T45.9 **Poisoning by, adverse effect of and underdosing of unspecified primarily systemic and hematological agent**

T45.91 **Poisoning by unspecified primarily systemic and hematological agent, accidental (unintentional)**

Poisoning by primarily systemic and hematological agent NOS

T45.92 **Poisoning by unspecified primarily systemic and hematological agent, intentional self-harm**

T45.93 **Poisoning by unspecified primarily systemic and hematological agent, assault**

T45.94 **Poisoning by unspecified primarily systemic and hematological agent, undetermined**

T45.95 **Adverse effect of unspecified primarily systemic and hematological agent**

T45.96 **Underdosing of unspecified primarily systemic and hematological agent**

T46 **Poisoning by, adverse effect of and underdosing of agents primarily affecting the cardiovascular system**

Excludes1: poisoning by, adverse effect of and underdosing of metaraminol (T44.4)

The appropriate 7th character is to be added to each code from category T46

A - initial encounter

D - subsequent encounter

S - sequela

T46.0 **Poisoning by, adverse effect of and underdosing of cardiac-stimulant glycosides and drugs of similar action**

T46.0X **Poisoning by, adverse effect of and underdosing of cardiac-stimulant glycosides and drugs of similar action**

⑦ **T46.0X1** **Poisoning by cardiac-stimulant glycosides and drugs of similar action, accidental (unintentional)**

Poisoning by cardiac-stimulant glycosides and drugs of similar action NOS

⑦ **T46.0X2** **Poisoning by cardiac-stimulant glycosides and drugs of similar action, intentional self-harm**

⑦ **T46.0X3** **Poisoning by cardiac-stimulant glycosides and drugs of similar action, assault**

⑦ **T46.0X4** **Poisoning by cardiac-stimulant glycosides and drugs of similar action, undetermined**

⑦ **T46.0X5** **Adverse effect of cardiac-stimulant glycosides and drugs of similar action**

⑦ **T46.0X6** **Underdosing of cardiac-stimulant glycosides and drugs of similar action**

T46.1 **Poisoning by, adverse effect of and underdosing of calcium-channel blockers**

T46.1X **Poisoning by, adverse effect of and underdosing of calcium-channel blockers**

⑦ **T46.1X1** **Poisoning by calcium-channel blockers, accidental (unintentional)**

Poisoning by calcium-channel blockers NOS

⑦ **T46.1X2** **Poisoning by calcium-channel blockers, intentional self-harm**

⑦ **T46.1X3** **Poisoning by calcium-channel blockers, assault**

⑦ **T46.1X4** **Poisoning by calcium-channel blockers, undetermined**

⑦ **T46.1X5** **Adverse effect of calcium-channel blockers**

⑦ **T46.1X6** **Underdosing of calcium-channel blockers**

T46.2 **Poisoning by, adverse effect of and underdosing of other antidysrhythmic drugs, not elsewhere classified**

Excludes1: poisoning by, adverse effect of and underdosing of beta-adrenoreceptor antagonists (T44.7-)

T46.2X **Poisoning by, adverse effect of and underdosing of other antidysrhythmic drugs**

⑦ **T46.2X1** **Poisoning by other antidysrhythmic drugs, accidental (unintentional)**

Poisoning by other antidysrhythmic drugs NOS

● New code ▲ Revised code **Excludes1:** Not coded here **Excludes2:** Not included here ⊗ Placeholder required ⑦ 7th digit required

⑦**T46.2X2** **Poisoning by other antidysrhythmic drugs, intentional self-harm**

⑦**T46.2X3** **Poisoning by other antidysrhythmic drugs, assault**

⑦**T46.2X4** **Poisoning by other antidysrhythmic drugs, undetermined**

⑦**T46.2X5** **Adverse effect of other antidysrhythmic drugs**

⑦**T46.2X6** **Underdosing of other antidysrhythmic drugs**

T46.3 **Poisoning by, adverse effect of and underdosing of coronary vasodilators**

Poisoning by, adverse effect of and underdosing of dipyridamole

Excludes1: poisoning by, adverse effect of and underdosing of calcium-channel blockers (T46.1)

T46.3X **Poisoning by, adverse effect of and underdosing of coronary vasodilators**

⑦**T46.3X1** **Poisoning by coronary vasodilators, accidental (unintentional)**

Poisoning by coronary vasodilators NOS

⑦**T46.3X2** **Poisoning by coronary vasodilators, intentional self-harm**

⑦**T46.3X3** **Poisoning by coronary vasodilators, assault**

⑦**T46.3X4** **Poisoning by coronary vasodilators, undetermined**

⑦**T46.3X5** **Adverse effect of coronary vasodilators**

⑦**T46.3X6** **Underdosing of coronary vasodilators**

T46.4 **Poisoning by, adverse effect of and underdosing of angiotensin-converting-enzyme inhibitors**

T46.4X **Poisoning by, adverse effect of and underdosing of angiotensin-converting-enzyme inhibitors**

⑦**T46.4X1** **Poisoning by angiotensin-converting-enzyme inhibitors, accidental (unintentional)**

Poisoning by angiotensin-converting-enzyme inhibitors NOS

⑦**T46.4X2** **Poisoning by angiotensin-converting-enzyme inhibitors, intentional self-harm**

⑦**T46.4X3** **Poisoning by angiotensin-converting-enzyme inhibitors, assault**

⑦**T46.4X4** **Poisoning by angiotensin-converting-enzyme inhibitors, undetermined**

⑦**T46.4X5** **Adverse effect of angiotensin-converting-enzyme inhibitors**

⑦**T46.4X6** **Underdosing of angiotensin-converting-enzyme inhibitors**

T46.5 **Poisoning by, adverse effect of and underdosing of other antihypertensive drugs**

Excludes2: poisoning by, adverse effect of and underdosing of beta-adrenoreceptor antagonists (T44.7)

poisoning by, adverse effect of and underdosing of calcium-channel blockers (T46.1) \

poisoning by, adverse effect of and underdosing of diuretics (T50.0-T50.2)

T46.5X **Poisoning by, adverse effect of and underdosing of other antihypertensive drugs**

⑦**T46.5X1** **Poisoning by other antihypertensive drugs, accidental (unintentional)**

Poisoning by other antihypertensive drugs NOS

⑦**T46.5X2** **Poisoning by other antihypertensive drugs, intentional self-harm**

⑦**T46.5X3** **Poisoning by other antihypertensive drugs, assault**

⑦**T46.5X4** **Poisoning by other antihypertensive drugs, undetermined**

⑦**T46.5X5** **Adverse effect of other antihypertensive drugs**

⑦**T46.5X6** **Underdosing of other antihypertensive drugs**

T46.6 **Poisoning by, adverse effect of and underdosing of antihyperlipidemic and antiarteriosclerotic drugs**

T46.6X **Poisoning by, adverse effect of and underdosing of antihyperlipidemic and antiarteriosclerotic drugs**

⑦**T46.6X1** **Poisoning by antihyperlipidemic and antiarteriosclerotic drugs, accidental (unintentional)**

Poisoning by antihyperlipidemic and antiarteriosclerotic drugs NOS

⑦**T46.6X2** **Poisoning by antihyperlipidemic and antiarteriosclerotic drugs, intentional self-harm**

⑦**T46.6X3** **Poisoning by antihyperlipidemic and antiarteriosclerotic drugs, assault**

⑦**T46.6X4** **Poisoning by antihyperlipidemic and antiarteriosclerotic drugs, undetermined**

⑦**T46.6X5** **Adverse effect of antihyperlipidemic and antiarteriosclerotic drugs**

⑦**T46.6X6** **Underdosing of antihyperlipidemic and antiarteriosclerotic drugs**

T46.7 **Poisoning by, adverse effect of and underdosing of peripheral vasodilators**

Poisoning by, adverse effect of and underdosing of nicotinic acid (derivatives)

Excludes1: poisoning by, adverse effect of and underdosing of papaverine (T44.3)

T46.7X **Poisoning by, adverse effect of and underdosing of peripheral vasodilators**

⑦**T46.7X1** **Poisoning by peripheral vasodilators, accidental (unintentional)**

Poisoning by peripheral vasodilators NOS

⑦**T46.7X2** **Poisoning by peripheral vasodilators, intentional self-harm**

⑦**T46.7X3** **Poisoning by peripheral vasodilators, assault**

⑦**T46.7X4** **Poisoning by peripheral vasodilators, undetermined**

⑦**T46.7X5** **Adverse effect of peripheral vasodilators**

⑦ T46.7X6   Underdosing of peripheral vasodilators

T46.8   Poisoning by, adverse effect of and underdosing of antivaricose drugs, including sclerosing agents

T46.8X   Poisoning by, adverse effect of and underdosing of antivaricose drugs, including sclerosing agents

⑦ T46.8X1   Poisoning by antivaricose drugs, including sclerosing agents, accidental (unintentional)

Poisoning by antivaricose drugs, including sclerosing agents NOS

⑦ T46.8X2   Poisoning by antivaricose drugs, including sclerosing agents, intentional self-harm

⑦ T46.8X3   Poisoning by antivaricose drugs, including sclerosing agents, assault

⑦ T46.8X4   Poisoning by antivaricose drugs, including sclerosing agents, undetermined

⑦ T46.8X5   Adverse effect of antivaricose drugs, including sclerosing agents

⑦ T46.8X6   Underdosing of antivaricose drugs, including sclerosing agents

T46.9   Poisoning by, adverse effect of and underdosing of other and unspecified agents primarily affecting the cardiovascular system

T46.90   Poisoning by, adverse effect of and underdosing of unspecified agents primarily affecting the cardiovascular system

⑦ T46.901   Poisoning by unspecified agents primarily affecting the cardiovascular system, accidental (unintentional)

⑦ T46.902   Poisoning by unspecified agents primarily affecting the cardiovascular system, intentional self-harm

⑦ T46.903   Poisoning by unspecified agents primarily affecting the cardiovascular system, assault

⑦ T46.904   Poisoning by unspecified agents primarily affecting the cardiovascular system, undetermined

⑦ T46.905   Adverse effect of unspecified agents primarily affecting the cardiovascular system

⑦ T46.906   Underdosing of unspecified agents primarily affecting the cardiovascular system

T46.99   Poisoning by, adverse effect of and underdosing of other agents primarily affecting the cardiovascular system

⑦ T46.991   Poisoning by other agents primarily affecting the cardiovascular system, accidental (unintentional)

⑦ T46.992   Poisoning by other agents primarily affecting the cardiovascular system, intentional self-harm

⑦ T46.993   Poisoning by other agents primarily affecting the cardiovascular system, assault

⑦ T46.994   Poisoning by other agents primarily affecting the cardiovascular system, undetermined

⑦ T46.995   Adverse effect of other agents primarily affecting the cardiovascular system

⑦ T46.996   Underdosing of other agents primarily affecting the cardiovascular system

T47   Poisoning by, adverse effect of and underdosing of agents primarily affecting the gastrointestinal system

The appropriate 7th character is to be added to each code from category T47

A - initial encounter

D - subsequent encounter

S - sequela

T47.0   Poisoning by, adverse effect of and underdosing of histamine H2-receptor blockers

T47.0X   Poisoning by, adverse effect of and underdosing of histamine H2-receptor blockers

⑦ T47.0X1   Poisoning by histamine H2-receptor blockers, accidental (unintentional)

Poisoning by histamine H2-receptor blockers NOS

⑦ T47.0X2   Poisoning by histamine H2-receptor blockers, intentional self-harm

⑦ T47.0X3   Poisoning by histamine H2-receptor blockers, assault

⑦ T47.0X4   Poisoning by histamine H2-receptor blockers, undetermined

⑦ T47.0X5   Adverse effect of histamine H2-receptor blockers

⑦ T47.0X6   Underdosing of histamine H2-receptor blockers

T47.1   Poisoning by, adverse effect of and underdosing of other antacids and anti-gastric-secretion drugs

T47.1X   Poisoning by, adverse effect of and underdosing of other antacids and anti-gastric-secretion drugs

⑦ T47.1X1   Poisoning by other antacids and anti-gastric-secretion drugs, accidental (unintentional)

Poisoning by other antacids and anti-gastric-secretion drugs NOS

⑦ T47.1X2   Poisoning by other antacids and anti-gastric-secretion drugs, intentional self-harm

⑦ T47.1X3   Poisoning by other antacids and anti-gastric-secretion drugs, assault

⑦ T47.1X4   Poisoning by other antacids and anti-gastric-secretion drugs, undetermined

⑦ T47.1X5   Adverse effect of other antacids and anti-gastric-secretion drugs

⑦ T47.1X6   Underdosing of other antacids and anti-gastric-secretion drugs

T47.2   Poisoning by, adverse effect of and underdosing of stimulant laxatives

T47.2X   Poisoning by, adverse effect of and underdosing of stimulant laxatives

⑦T47.2X1 **Poisoning by stimulant laxatives, accidental (unintentional)**

Poisoning by stimulant laxatives NOS

⑦T47.2X2 **Poisoning by stimulant laxatives, intentional self-harm**

⑦T47.2X3 **Poisoning by stimulant laxatives, assault**

⑦T47.2X4 **Poisoning by stimulant laxatives, undetermined**

⑦T47.2X5 **Adverse effect of stimulant laxatives**

⑦T47.2X6 **Underdosing of stimulant laxatives**

T47.3 **Poisoning by, adverse effect of and underdosing of saline and osmotic laxatives**

  T47.3X **Poisoning by and adverse effect of saline and osmotic laxatives**

⑦T47.3X1 **Poisoning by saline and osmotic laxatives, accidental (unintentional)**

Poisoning by saline and osmotic laxatives NOS

⑦T47.3X2 **Poisoning by saline and osmotic laxatives, intentional self-harm**

⑦T47.3X3 **Poisoning by saline and osmotic laxatives, assault**

⑦T47.3X4 **Poisoning by saline and osmotic laxatives, undetermined**

⑦T47.3X5 **Adverse effect of saline and osmotic laxatives**

⑦T47.3X6 **Underdosing of saline and osmotic laxatives**

T47.4 **Poisoning by, adverse effect of and underdosing of other laxatives**

  T47.4X **Poisoning by, adverse effect of and underdosing of other laxatives**

⑦T47.4X1 **Poisoning by other laxatives, accidental (unintentional)**

Poisoning by other laxatives NOS

⑦T47.4X2 **Poisoning by other laxatives, intentional self-harm**

⑦T47.4X3 **Poisoning by other laxatives, assault**

⑦T47.4X4 **Poisoning by other laxatives, undetermined**

⑦T47.4X5 **Adverse effect of other laxatives**

⑦T47.4X6 **Underdosing of other laxatives**

T47.5 **Poisoning by, adverse effect of and underdosing of digestants**

  T47.5X **Poisoning by, adverse effect of and underdosing of digestants**

⑦T47.5X1 **Poisoning by digestants, accidental (unintentional)**

Poisoning by digestants NOS

⑦T47.5X2 **Poisoning by digestants, intentional self-harm**

⑦T47.5X3 **Poisoning by digestants, assault**

⑦T47.5X4 **Poisoning by digestants, undetermined**

⑦T47.5X5 **Adverse effect of digestants**

⑦T47.5X6 **Underdosing of digestants**

T47.6 **Poisoning by, adverse effect of and underdosing of antidiarrheal drugs**

Excludes2: poisoning by, adverse effect of and underdosing of systemic antibiotics **and other** anti-infectives (T36-T37)

  T47.6X **Poisoning by, adverse effect of and underdosing of antidiarrheal drugs**

⑦T47.6X1 **Poisoning by antidiarrheal drugs, accidental (unintentional)**

Poisoning by antidiarrheal drugs NOS

⑦T47.6X2 **Poisoning by antidiarrheal drugs, intentional self-harm**

⑦T47.6X3 **Poisoning by antidiarrheal drugs, assault**

⑦T47.6X4 **Poisoning by antidiarrheal drugs, undetermined**

⑦T47.6X5 **Adverse effect of antidiarrheal drugs**

⑦T47.6X6 **Underdosing of antidiarrheal drugs**

T47.7 **Poisoning by, adverse effect of and underdosing of emetics**

  T47.7X **Poisoning by, adverse effect of and underdosing of emetics**

⑦T47.7X1 **Poisoning by emetics, accidental (unintentional)**

Poisoning by emetics NOS

⑦T47.7X2 **Poisoning by emetics, intentional self-harm**

⑦T47.7X3 **Poisoning by emetics, assault**

⑦T47.7X4 **Poisoning by emetics, undetermined**

⑦T47.7X5 **Adverse effect of emetics**

⑦T47.7X6 **Underdosing of emetics**

T47.8 **Poisoning by, adverse effect of and underdosing of other agents primarily affecting gastrointestinal system**

  T47.8X **Poisoning by, adverse effect of and underdosing of other agents primarily affecting gastrointestinal system**

⑦T47.8X1 **Poisoning by other agents primarily affecting gastrointestinal system, accidental (unintentional)**

Poisoning by other agents primarily affected of any time gastrointestinal system NOS

⑦T47.8X2 **Poisoning by other agents primarily affecting gastrointestinal system, intentional self-harm**

⑦T47.8X3 **Poisoning by other agents primarily affecting gastrointestinal system, assault**

⑦T47.8X4 **Poisoning by other agents primarily affecting gastrointestinal system, undetermined**

⑦T47.8X5 **Adverse effect of other agents primarily affecting gastrointestinal system**

⑦T47.8X6 **Underdosing of other agents primarily affecting gastrointestinal system**

T47.9 **Poisoning by, adverse effect of and underdosing of unspecified agents primarily affecting the gastrointestinal system**

⊗⑦T47.91 **Poisoning by unspecified agents primarily affecting the gastrointestinal system, accidental (unintentional)**

Poisoning by agents primarily affecting the gastrointestinal system NOS

⊗⑦**T47.92** **Poisoning by unspecified agents primarily affecting the gastrointestinal system, intentional self-harm**

⊗⑦**T47.93** **Poisoning by unspecified agents primarily affecting the gastrointestinal system, assault**

⊗⑦**T47.94** **Poisoning by unspecified agents primarily affecting the gastrointestinal system, undetermined**

⊗⑦**T47.95** **Adverse effect of unspecified agents primarily affecting the gastrointestinal system**

⊗⑦**T47.96** **Underdosing of unspecified agents primarily affecting the gastrointestinal system**

T48 **Poisoning by, adverse effect of and underdosing of agents primarily acting on smooth and skeletal muscles and the respiratory system**

The appropriate 7th character is to be added to each code from category T48

A - initial encounter

D - subsequent encounter

S - sequela

T48.0 **Poisoning by, adverse effect of and underdosing of oxytocic drugs**

Excludes1: poisoning by, adverse effect of and underdosing of estrogens, progestogens and antagonists (T38.4-T38.6)

T48.0X **Poisoning by, adverse effect of and underdosing of oxytocic drugs**

⑦**T48.0X1** **Poisoning by oxytocic drugs, accidental (unintentional)**

Poisoning by oxytocic drugs NOS

⑦**T48.0X2** **Poisoning by oxytocic drugs, intentional self-harm**

⑦**T48.0X3** **Poisoning by oxytocic drugs, assault**

⑦**T48.0X4** **Poisoning by oxytocic drugs, undetermined**

⑦**T48.0X5** **Adverse effect of oxytocic drugs**

⑦**T48.0X6** **Underdosing of oxytocic drugs**

T48.1 **Poisoning by, adverse effect of and underdosing of skeletal muscle relaxants [neuromuscular blocking agents]**

T48.1X **Poisoning by, adverse effect of and underdosing of skeletal muscle relaxants [neuromuscular blocking agents]**

⑦**T48.1X1** **Poisoning by skeletal muscle relaxants [neuromuscular blocking agents], accidental (unintentional)**

Poisoning by skeletal muscle relaxants [neuromuscular blocking agents] NOS

⑦**T48.1X2** **Poisoning by skeletal muscle relaxants [neuromuscular blocking agents], intentional self-harm**

⑦**T48.1X3** **Poisoning by skeletal muscle relaxants [neuromuscular blocking agents], assault**

⑦**T48.1X4** **Poisoning by skeletal muscle relaxants [neuromuscular blocking agents], undetermined**

⑦**T48.1X5** **Adverse effect of skeletal muscle relaxants [neuromuscular blocking agents]**

⑦**T48.1X6** **Underdosing of skeletal muscle relaxants [neuromuscular blocking agents]**

T48.2 **Poisoning by, adverse effect of and underdosing of other and unspecified drugs acting on muscles**

T48.20 **Poisoning by, adverse effect of and underdosing of unspecified drugs acting on muscles**

⑦**T48.201** **Poisoning by unspecified drugs acting on muscles, accidental (unintentional)**

Poisoning by unspecified drugs acting on muscles NOS

⑦**T48.202** **Poisoning by unspecified drugs acting on muscles, intentional self-harm**

⑦**T48.203** **Poisoning by unspecified drugs acting on muscles, assault**

⑦**T48.204** **Poisoning by unspecified drugs acting on muscles, undetermined**

⑦**T48.205** **Adverse effect of unspecified drugs acting on muscles**

⑦**T48.206** **Underdosing of unspecified drugs acting on muscles**

T48.29 **Poisoning by, adverse effect of and underdosing of other drugs acting on muscles**

⑦**T48.291** **Poisoning by other drugs acting on muscles, accidental (unintentional)**

Poisoning by other drugs acting on muscles NOS

⑦**T48.292** **Poisoning by other drugs acting on muscles, intentional self-harm**

⑦**T48.293** **Poisoning by other drugs acting on muscles, assault**

⑦**T48.294** **Poisoning by other drugs acting on muscles, undetermined**

⑦**T48.295** **Adverse effect of other drugs acting on muscles**

⑦**T48.296** **Underdosing of other drugs acting on muscles**

T48.3 **Poisoning by, adverse effect of and underdosing of antitussives**

T48.3X **Poisoning by, adverse effect of and underdosing of antitussives**

⑦**T48.3X1** **Poisoning by antitussives, accidental (unintentional)**

Poisoning by antitussives NOS

⑦**T48.3X2** **Poisoning by antitussives, intentional self-harm**

⑦**T48.3X3** **Poisoning by antitussives, assault**

⑦**T48.3X4** **Poisoning by antitussives, undetermined**

⑦**T48.3X5** **Adverse effect of antitussives**

⑦**T48.3X6** **Underdosing of antitussives**

T48.4 **Poisoning by, adverse effect of and underdosing of expectorants**

T48.4X **Poisoning by, adverse effect of and underdosing of expectorants**

⑦**T48.4X1** **Poisoning by expectorants, accidental (unintentional)**

Poisoning by expectorants NOS

⑦T48.4X2   **Poisoning by expectorants, intentional self-harm**

⑦T48.4X3   **Poisoning by expectorants, assault**

⑦T48.4X4   **Poisoning by expectorants, undetermined**

⑦T48.4X5   **Adverse effect of expectorants**

⑦T48.4X6   **Underdosing of expectorants**

T48.5   **Poisoning by, adverse effect of and underdosing of other anti-common-cold drugs**

Poisoning by, adverse effect of and underdosing of decongestants

Excludes2: poisoning by, adverse effect of and underdosing of antipyretics, NEC (T39.9-)

poisoning by, adverse effect of and underdosing of non-steroidal antiinflammatory drugs (T39.3-)

poisoning by, adverse effect of and underdosing of salicylates (T39.0-)

T48.5X   **Poisoning by, adverse effect of and underdosing of other anti-common-cold drugs**

⑦T48.5X1   **Poisoning by other anti-common-cold drugs, accidental (unintentional)**

Poisoning by other anti-common-cold drugs NOS

⑦T48.5X2   **Poisoning by other anti-common-cold drugs, intentional self-harm**

⑦T48.5X3   **Poisoning by other anti-common-cold drugs, assault**

⑦T48.5X4   **Poisoning by other anti-common-cold drugs, undetermined**

⑦T48.5X5   **Adverse effect of other anti-common-cold drugs**

⑦T48.5X6   **Underdosing of other anti-common-cold drugs**

T48.6   **Poisoning by, adverse effect of and underdosing of antiasthmatics, not elsewhere classified**

Poisoning by, adverse effect of and underdosing of beta-adrenoreceptor agonists used in asthma therapy

Excludes1: poisoning by, adverse effect of and underdosing of beta-adrenoreceptor agonists not used in asthma therapy (T44.5)

poisoning by, adverse effect of and underdosing of anterior pituitary [adenohypophyseal] hormones (T38.8)

T48.6X   **Poisoning by, adverse effect of and underdosing of antiasthmatics**

⑦T48.6X1   **Poisoning by antiasthmatics, accidental (unintentional)**

Poisoning by antiasthmatics NOS

⑦T48.6X2   **Poisoning by antiasthmatics, intentional self-harm**

⑦T48.6X3   **Poisoning by antiasthmatics, assault**

⑦T48.6X4   **Poisoning by antiasthmatics, undetermined**

⑦T48.6X5   **Adverse effect of antiasthmatics**

⑦T48.6X6   **Underdosing of antiasthmatics**

T48.9   **Poisoning by, adverse effect of and underdosing of other and unspecified agents primarily acting on the respiratory system**

T48.90   **Poisoning by, adverse effect of and underdosing of unspecified agents primarily acting on the respiratory system**

⑦T48.901   **Poisoning by unspecified agents primarily acting on the respiratory system, accidental (unintentional)**

⑦T48.902   **Poisoning by unspecified agents primarily acting on the respiratory system, intentional self-harm**

⑦T48.903   **Poisoning by unspecified agents primarily acting on the respiratory system, assault**

⑦T48.904   **Poisoning by unspecified agents primarily acting on the respiratory system, undetermined**

⑦T48.905   **Adverse effect of unspecified agents primarily acting on the respiratory system**

⑦T48.906   **Underdosing of unspecified agents primarily acting on the respiratory system**

T48.99   **Poisoning by, adverse effect of and underdosing of other agents primarily acting on the respiratory system**

⑦T48.991   **Poisoning by other agents primarily acting on the respiratory system, accidental (unintentional)**

⑦T48.992   **Poisoning by other agents primarily acting on the respiratory system, intentional self-harm**

⑦T48.993   **Poisoning by other agents primarily acting on the respiratory system, assault**

⑦T48.994   **Poisoning by other agents primarily acting on the respiratory system, undetermined**

⑦T48.995   **Adverse effect of other agents primarily acting on the respiratory system**

⑦T48.996   **Underdosing of other agents primarily acting on the respiratory system**

T49   **Poisoning by, adverse effect of and underdosing of topical agents primarily affecting skin and mucous membrane and by ophthalmological, otorhinorlaryngological and dental drugs**

Includes: poisoning by, adverse effect of and underdosing of glucocorticoids, topically used

The appropriate 7th character is to be added to each code from category T49

A - initial encounter

D - subsequent encounter \

S - sequela

T49.0   **Poisoning by, adverse effect of and underdosing of local antifungal, anti-infective and anti-inflammatory drugs**

T49.0X   **Poisoning by, adverse effect of and underdosing of local antifungal, anti-infective and anti-inflammatory drugs**

⑦T49.0X1   **Poisoning by local antifungal, anti-infective and anti-inflammatory drugs, accidental (unintentional)**

Poisoning by local antifungal, anti-infective and anti-inflammatory drugs NOS

---

⑦T49.0X2 Poisoning by local antifungal, anti-infective and anti-inflammatory drugs, intentional self-harm

⑦T49.0X3 Poisoning by local antifungal, anti-infective and anti-inflammatory drugs, assault

⑦T49.0X4 Poisoning by local antifungal, anti-infective and anti-inflammatory drugs, undetermined

⑦T49.0X5 Adverse effect of local antifungal, anti-infective and anti-inflammatory drugs

⑦T49.0X6 Underdosing of local antifungal, anti-infective and anti-inflammatory drugs

T49.1 Poisoning by, adverse effect of and underdosing of antipruritics

 T49.1X Poisoning by, adverse effect of and underdosing of antipruritics

  ⑦T49.1X1 Poisoning by antipruritics, accidental (unintentional)

   Poisoning by antipruritics NOS

  ⑦T49.1X2 Poisoning by antipruritics, intentional self-harm

  ⑦T49.1X3 Poisoning by antipruritics, assault

  ⑦T49.1X4 Poisoning by antipruritics, undetermined

  ⑦T49.1X5 Adverse effect of antipruritics

  ⑦T49.1X6 Underdosing of antipruritics

T49.2 Poisoning by, adverse effect of and underdosing of local astringents and local detergents

 T49.2X Poisoning by, adverse effect of and underdosing of local astringents and local detergents

  ⑦T49.2X1 Poisoning by local astringents and local detergents, accidental (unintentional)

   Poisoning by local astringents and local detergents NOS

  ⑦T49.2X2 Poisoning by local astringents and local detergents, intentional self-harm

  ⑦T49.2X3 Poisoning by local astringents and local detergents, assault

  ⑦T49.2X4 Poisoning by local astringents and local detergents, undetermined

  ⑦T49.2X5 Adverse effect of local astringents and local detergents

  ⑦T49.2X6 Underdosing of local astringents and local detergents

T49.3 Poisoning by, adverse effect of and underdosing of emollients, demulcents and protectants

 T49.3X Poisoning by, adverse effect of and underdosing of emollients, demulcents and protectants

  ⑦T49.3X1 Poisoning by emollients, demulcents and protectants, accidental (unintentional)

   Poisoning by emollients, demulcents and protectants NOS

⑦T49.3X2 Poisoning by emollients, demulcents and protectants, intentional self-harm

⑦T49.3X3 Poisoning by emollients, demulcents and protectants, assault

⑦T49.3X4 Poisoning by emollients, demulcents and protectants, undetermined

⑦T49.3X5 Adverse effect of emollients, demulcents and protectants

⑦T49.3X6 Underdosing of emollients, demulcents and protectants

T49.4 Poisoning by, adverse effect of and underdosing of keratolytics, keratoplastics, and other hair treatment drugs and preparations

 T49.4X Poisoning by, adverse effect of and underdosing of keratolytics, keratoplastics, and other hair treatment drugs and preparations

  ⑦T49.4X1 Poisoning by keratolytics, keratoplastics, and other hair treatment drugs and preparations, accidental (unintentional)

   Poisoning by keratolytics, keratoplastics, **and other** hair treatment drugs and preparations NOS

  ⑦T49.4X2 Poisoning by keratolytics, keratoplastics, and other hair treatment drugs and preparations, intentional self-harm

  ⑦T49.4X3 Poisoning by keratolytics, keratoplastics, and other hair treatment drugs and preparations, assault

  ⑦T49.4X4 Poisoning by keratolytics, keratoplastics, and other hair treatment drugs and preparations, undetermined

  ⑦T49.4X5 Adverse effect of keratolytics, keratoplastics, and other hair treatment drugs and preparations

  ⑦T49.4X6 Underdosing of keratolytics, keratoplastics, and other hair treatment drugs and preparations

T49.5 Poisoning by, adverse effect of and underdosing of ophthalmological drugs and preparations

 T49.5X Poisoning by, adverse effect of and underdosing of ophthalmological drugs and preparations

  ⑦T49.5X1 Poisoning by ophthalmological drugs and preparations, accidental (unintentional)

   Poisoning by ophthalmological drugs and preparations NOS

  ⑦T49.5X2 Poisoning by ophthalmological drugs and preparations, intentional self-harm

  ⑦T49.5X3 Poisoning by ophthalmological drugs and preparations, assault

  ⑦T49.5X4 Poisoning by ophthalmological drugs and preparations, undetermined

  ⑦T49.5X5 Adverse effect of ophthalmological drugs and preparations

⑦T49.5X6 Underdosing of ophthalmological drugs and preparations

T49.6 Poisoning by, adverse effect of and underdosing of otorhinolaryngological drugs and preparations

T49.6X Poisoning by, adverse effect of and underdosing of otorhinolaryngological drugs and preparations

⑦T49.6X1 Poisoning by otorhinolaryngological drugs and preparations, accidental (unintentional)

Poisoning by otorhinolaryngological drugs and preparations NOS

⑦T49.6X2 Poisoning by otorhinolaryngological drugs and preparations, intentional self-harm

⑦T49.6X3 Poisoning by otorhinolaryngological drugs and preparations, assault

⑦T49.6X4 Poisoning by otorhinolaryngological drugs and preparations, undetermined

⑦T49.6X5 Adverse effect of otorhinolaryngological drugs and preparations

⑦T49.6X6 Underdosing of otorhinolaryngological drugs and preparations

T49.7 Poisoning by, adverse effect of and underdosing of dental drugs, topically applied

T49.7X Poisoning by, adverse effect of and underdosing of dental drugs, topically applied

⑦T49.7X1 Poisoning by dental drugs, topically applied, accidental (unintentional)

Poisoning by dental drugs, topically applied NOS

⑦T49.7X2 Poisoning by dental drugs, topically applied, intentional self-harm

⑦T49.7X3 Poisoning by dental drugs, topically applied, assault

⑦T49.7X4 Poisoning by dental drugs, topically applied, undetermined

⑦T49.7X5 Adverse effect of dental drugs, topically applied

⑦T49.7X6 Underdosing of dental drugs, topically applied

T49.8 Poisoning by, adverse effect of and underdosing of other topical agents

Poisoning by, adverse effect of and underdosing of spermicides

T49.8X Poisoning by, adverse effect of and underdosing of other topical agents

⑦T49.8X1 Poisoning by other topical agents, accidental (unintentional)

Poisoning by other topical agents NOS

⑦T49.8X2 Poisoning by other topical agents, intentional self-harm

⑦T49.8X3 Poisoning by other topical agents, assault

⑦T49.8X4 Poisoning by other topical agents, undetermined

⑦T49.8X5 Adverse effect of other topical agents

⑦T49.8X6 Underdosing of other topical agents

T49.9 Poisoning by, adverse effect of and underdosing of unspecified topical agent

⊗⑦T49.91 Poisoning by unspecified topical agent, accidental (unintentional)

⊗⑦T49.92 Poisoning by unspecified topical agent, intentional self-harm

⊗⑦T49.93 Poisoning by unspecified topical agent, assault

⊗⑦T49.94 Poisoning by unspecified topical agent, undetermined

⊗⑦T49.95 Adverse effect of unspecified topical agent

⊗⑦T49.96 Underdosing of unspecified topical agent

T50 Poisoning by, adverse effect of and underdosing of diuretics and other and unspecified drugs, medicaments and biological substances

The appropriate 7th character is to be added to each code from category T50

A - initial encounter

D - subsequent encounter

S - sequela

T50.0 Poisoning by, adverse effect of and underdosing of mineralocorticoids and their antagonists

T50.0X Poisoning by, adverse effect of and underdosing of mineralocorticoids and their antagonists

⑦T50.0X1 Poisoning by mineralocorticoids and their antagonists, accidental (unintentional)

Poisoning by mineralocorticoids and their antagonists NOS

⑦T50.0X2 Poisoning by mineralocorticoids and their antagonists, intentional self-harm

⑦T50.0X3 Poisoning by mineralocorticoids and their antagonists, assault

⑦T50.0X4 Poisoning by mineralocorticoids and their antagonists, undetermined

⑦T50.0X5 Adverse effect of mineralocorticoids and their antagonists

⑦T50.0X6 Underdosing of mineralocorticoids and their antagonists

T50.1 Poisoning by, adverse effect of and underdosing of loop [high-ceiling] diuretics

T50.1X Poisoning by, adverse effect of and underdosing of loop [high-ceiling] diuretics

⑦T50.1X1 Poisoning by loop [high-ceiling] diuretics, accidental (unintentional)

Poisoning by loop [high-ceiling] diuretics NOS

⑦T50.1X2 Poisoning by loop [high-ceiling] diuretics, intentional self-harm

⑦T50.1X3 Poisoning by loop [high-ceiling] diuretics, assault

⑦T50.1X4 Poisoning by loop [high-ceiling] diuretics, undetermined

⑦T50.1X5 Adverse effect of loop [high-ceiling] diuretics

⑦T50.1X6 Underdosing of loop [high-ceiling] diuretics

T50.2 **Poisoning by, adverse effect of and underdosing of carbonic-anhydrase inhibitors, benzothiadiazides and other diuretics**

Poisoning by, adverse effect of and underdosing of acetazolamide

T50.2X **Poisoning by, adverse effect of and underdosing of carbonic-anhydrase inhibitors, benzothiadiazides and other diuretics**

⑦ **T50.2X1** **Poisoning by carbonic-anhydrase inhibitors, benzothiadiazides and other diuretics, accidental (unintentional)**

Poisoning by carbonic-anhydrase inhibitors, benzothiadiazides and other diuretics NOS

⑦ **T50.2X2** **Poisoning by carbonic-anhydrase inhibitors, benzothiadiazides and other diuretics, intentional self-harm**

⑦ **T50.2X3** **Poisoning by carbonic-anhydrase inhibitors, benzothiadiazides and other diuretics, assault**

⑦ **T50.2X4** **Poisoning by carbonic-anhydrase inhibitors, benzothiadiazides and other diuretics, undetermined**

⑦ **T50.2X5** **Adverse effect of carbonic-anhydrase inhibitors, benzothiadiazides and other diuretics**

⑦ **T50.2X6** **Underdosing of carbonic-anhydrase inhibitors, benzothiadiazides and other diuretics**

T50.3 **Poisoning by, adverse effect of and underdosing of electrolytic, caloric and water-balance agents**

Poisoning by, adverse effect of and underdosing of oral rehydration salts

T50.3X **Poisoning by, adverse effect of and underdosing of electrolytic, caloric and water-balance agents**

⑦ **T50.3X1** **Poisoning by electrolytic, caloric and water-balance agents, accidental (unintentional)**

Poisoning by electrolytic, caloric and water-balance agents NOS

⑦ **T50.3X2** **Poisoning by electrolytic, caloric and water-balance agents, intentional self-harm**

⑦ **T50.3X3** **Poisoning by electrolytic, caloric and water-balance agents, assault**

⑦ **T50.3X4** **Poisoning by electrolytic, caloric and water-balance agents, undetermined**

⑦ **T50.3X5** **Adverse effect of electrolytic, caloric and water-balance agents**

⑦ **T50.3X6** **Underdosing of electrolytic, caloric and water-balance agents**

T50.4 **Poisoning by, adverse effect of and underdosing of drugs affecting uric acid metabolism**

T50.4X **Poisoning by, adverse effect of and underdosing of drugs affecting uric acid metabolism**

⑦ **T50.4X1** **Poisoning by drugs affecting uric acid metabolism, accidental (unintentional)**

Poisoning by drugs affecting uric acid metabolism NOS

⑦ **T50.4X2** **Poisoning by drugs affecting uric acid metabolism, intentional self-harm**

⑦ **T50.4X3** **Poisoning by drugs affecting uric acid metabolism, assault**

⑦ **T50.4X4** **Poisoning by drugs affecting uric acid metabolism, undetermined**

⑦ **T50.4X5** **Adverse effect of drugs affecting uric acid metabolism**

⑦ **T50.4X6** **Underdosing of drugs affecting uric acid metabolism**

T50.5 **Poisoning by, adverse effect of and underdosing of appetite depressants**

T50.5X **Poisoning by, adverse effect of and underdosing of appetite depressants**

⑦ **T50.5X1** **Poisoning by appetite depressants, accidental (unintentional)**

Poisoning by appetite depressants NOS

⑦ **T50.5X2** **Poisoning by appetite depressants, intentional self-harm**

⑦ **T50.5X3** **Poisoning by appetite depressants, assault**

⑦ **T50.5X4** **Poisoning by appetite depressants, undetermined**

⑦ **T50.5X5** **Adverse effect of appetite depressants**

⑦ **T50.5X6** **Underdosing of appetite depressants**

T50.6 **Poisoning by, adverse effect of and underdosing of antidotes and chelating agents**

Poisoning by, adverse effect of and underdosing of alcohol deterrents

T50.6X **Poisoning by, adverse effect of and underdosing of antidotes and chelating agents**

⑦ **T50.6X1** **Poisoning by antidotes and chelating agents, accidental (unintentional)**

Poisoning by antidotes and chelating agents NOS

⑦ **T50.6X2** **Poisoning by antidotes and chelating agents, intentional self-harm**

⑦ **T50.6X3** **Poisoning by antidotes and chelating agents, assault**

⑦ **T50.6X4** **Poisoning by antidotes and chelating agents, undetermined**

⑦ **T50.6X5** **Adverse effect of antidotes and chelating agents**

⑦ **T50.6X6** **Underdosing of antidotes and chelating agents**

T50.7 **Poisoning by, adverse effect of and underdosing of analeptics and opioid receptor antagonists**

T50.7X **Poisoning by, adverse effect of and underdosing of analeptics and opioid receptor antagonists**

⑦ **T50.7X1** **Poisoning by analeptics and opioid receptor antagonists, accidental (unintentional)**

● New code ▲ Revised code **Excludes1:** Not coded here **Excludes2:** Not included here ⊗ Placeholder required ⑦ 7th digit required

Poisoning by analeptics and opioid receptor antagonists NOS

⑦T50.7X2 **Poisoning by analeptics and opioid receptor antagonists, intentional self-harm**

⑦T50.7X3 **Poisoning by analeptics and opioid receptor antagonists, assault**

⑦T50.7X4 **Poisoning by analeptics and opioid receptor antagonists, undetermined**

⑦T50.7X5 **Adverse effect of analeptics and opioid receptor antagonists**

⑦T50.7X6 **Underdosing of analeptics and opioid receptor antagonists**

T50.8 **Poisoning by, adverse effect of and underdosing of diagnostic agents**

T50.8X **Poisoning by, adverse effect of and underdosing of diagnostic agents**

⑦T50.8X1 **Poisoning by diagnostic agents, accidental (unintentional)**

Poisoning by diagnostic agents NOS

⑦T50.8X2 **Poisoning by diagnostic agents, intentional self-harm**

⑦T50.8X3 **Poisoning by diagnostic agents, assault**

⑦T50.8X4 **Poisoning by diagnostic agents, undetermined**

⑦T50.8X5 **Adverse effect of diagnostic agents**

⑦T50.8X6 **Underdosing of diagnostic agents**

T50.A **Poisoning by, adverse effect of and underdosing of bacterial vaccines**

T50.A1 **Poisoning by, adverse effect of and underdosing of pertussis vaccine, including combinations with a pertussis component**

⑦T50.A11 **Poisoning by pertussis vaccine, including combinations with a pertussis component, accidental (unintentional)**

⑦T50.A12 **Poisoning by pertussis vaccine, including combinations with a pertussis component, intentional self-harm**

⑦T50.A13 **Poisoning by pertussis vaccine, including combinations with a pertussis component, assault**

⑦T50.A14 **Poisoning by pertussis vaccine, including combinations with a pertussis component, undetermined**

⑦T50.A15 **Adverse effect of pertussis vaccine, including combinations with a pertussis component**

⑦T50.A16 **Underdosing of pertussis vaccine, including combinations with a pertussis component**

T50.A2 **Poisoning by, adverse effect of and underdosing of mixed bacterial vaccines without a pertussis component**

⑦T50.A21 **Poisoning by mixed bacterial vaccines without a pertussis component, accidental (unintentional)**

⑦T50.A22 **Poisoning by mixed bacterial vaccines without a pertussis component, intentional self-harm**

⑦T50.A23 **Poisoning by mixed bacterial vaccines without a pertussis component, assault**

⑦T50.A24 **Poisoning by mixed bacterial vaccines without a pertussis component, undetermined**

⑦T50.A25 **Adverse effect of mixed bacterial vaccines without a pertussis component**

⑦T50.A26 **Underdosing of mixed bacterial vaccines without a pertussis component**

T50.A9 **Poisoning by, adverse effect of and underdosing of other bacterial vaccines**

⑦T50.A91 **Poisoning by other bacterial vaccines, accidental (unintentional)**

⑦T50.A92 **Poisoning by other bacterial vaccines, intentional self-harm**

⑦T50.A93 **Poisoning by other bacterial vaccines, assault**

⑦T50.A94 **Poisoning by other bacterial vaccines, undetermined**

⑦T50.A95 **Adverse effect of other bacterial vaccines**

⑦T50.A96 **Underdosing of other bacterial vaccines**

T50.B **Poisoning by, adverse effect of and underdosing of viral vaccines**

T50.B1 **Poisoning by, adverse effect of and underdosing of smallpox vaccines**

⑦T50.B11 **Poisoning by smallpox vaccines, accidental (unintentional)**

⑦T50.B12 **Poisoning by smallpox vaccines, intentional self-harm**

⑦T50.B13 **Poisoning by smallpox vaccines, assault**

⑦T50.B14 **Poisoning by smallpox vaccines, undetermined**

⑦T50.B15 **Adverse effect of smallpox vaccines**

⑦T50.B16 **Underdosing of smallpox vaccines**

T50.B9 **Poisoning by, adverse effect of and underdosing of other viral vaccines**

⑦T50.B91 **Poisoning by other viral vaccines, accidental (unintentional)**

⑦T50.B92 **Poisoning by other viral vaccines, intentional self-harm**

⑦T50.B93 **Poisoning by other viral vaccines, assault**

⑦T50.B94 **Poisoning by other viral vaccines, undetermined**

⑦T50.B95 **Adverse effect of other viral vaccines**

⑦T50.B96 **Underdosing of other viral vaccines**

T50.Z **Poisoning by, adverse effect of and underdosing of other vaccines and biological substances**

T50.Z1 **Poisoning by, adverse effect of and underdosing of immunoglobulin**

⑦T50.Z11 **Poisoning by immunoglobulin, accidental (unintentional)**

⑦T50.Z12 **Poisoning by immunoglobulin, intentional self-harm**

Add 4th-7th digits   Nonspecific code   Unspecified code   Manifestation code

⑦ **T50.Z13** **Poisoning by immunoglobulin, assault**

⑦ **T50.Z14** **Poisoning by immunoglobulin, undetermined**

⑦ **T50.Z15** **Adverse effect of immunoglobulin**

⑦ **T50.Z16** **Underdosing of immunoglobulin**

T50.Z9 **Poisoning by, adverse effect of and underdosing of other vaccines and biological substances**

⑦ **T50.Z91** **Poisoning by other vaccines and biological substances, accidental (unintentional)**

⑦ **T50.Z92** **Poisoning by other vaccines and biological substances, intentional self-harm**

⑦ **T50.Z93** **Poisoning by other vaccines and biological substances, assault**

⑦ **T50.Z94** **Poisoning by other vaccines and biological substances, undetermined**

⑦ **T50.Z95** **Adverse effect of other vaccines and biological substances**

⑦ **T50.Z96** **Underdosing of other vaccines and biological substances**

T50.9 **Poisoning by, adverse effect of and underdosing of other and unspecified drugs, medicaments and biological substances**

T50.90 **Poisoning by, adverse effect of and underdosing of unspecified drugs, medicaments and biological substances**

⑦ **T50.901** **Poisoning by unspecified drugs, medicaments and biological substances, accidental (unintentional)**

⑦ **T50.902** **Poisoning by unspecified drugs, medicaments and biological substances, intentional self-harm**

⑦ **T50.903** **Poisoning by unspecified drugs, medicaments and biological substances, assault**

⑦ **T50.904** **Poisoning by unspecified drugs, medicaments and biological substances, undetermined**

⑦ **T50.905** **Adverse effect of unspecified drugs, medicaments and biological substances**

⑦ **T50.906** **Underdosing of unspecified drugs, medicaments and biological substances**

T50.99 **Poisoning by, adverse effect of and underdosing of other drugs, medicaments and biological substances**

⑦ **T50.991** **Poisoning by other drugs, medicaments and biological substances, accidental (unintentional)**

⑦ **T50.992** **Poisoning by other drugs, medicaments and biological substances, intentional self-harm**

⑦ **T50.993** **Poisoning by other drugs, medicaments and biological substances, assault**

⑦ **T50.994** **Poisoning by other drugs, medicaments and biological substances, undetermined**

⑦ **T50.995** **Adverse effect of other drugs, medicaments and biological substances**

⑦ **T50.996** **Underdosing of other drugs, medicaments and biological substances**

TOXIC EFFECTS OF SUBSTANCES CHIEFLY NONMEDICINAL AS TO SOURCE (T51-T65)

Note: When no intent is indicated code to accidental. Undetermined intent is only for use when there is specific documentation in the record that the intent of the toxic effect cannot be determined.

<u>Use additional code</u>(s):

for all associated manifestations of toxic effect, such as: respiratory conditions due to external agents (J60-J70)

personal history of foreign body fully removed (Z87.821)

to identify any retained foreign body, if applicable (Z18.-)

Excludes1: contact with and (suspected) exposure to toxic substances (Z77.-)

T51 **Toxic effect of alcohol**

The appropriate 7th character is to be added to each code from category T51

A - initial encounter

D - subsequent encounter

S - sequela

T51.0 **Toxic effect of ethanol**

Toxic effect of ethyl alcohol

Excludes2: acute alcohol intoxication or 'hangover' effects (F10.129, F10.229, F10.929)

drunkenness (F10.129, F10.229, F10.929)

pathological alcohol intoxication (F10.129, F10.229, F10.929)

T51.0X **Toxic effect of ethanol**

⑦ **T51.0X1** **Toxic effect of ethanol, accidental (unintentional)**

Toxic effect of ethanol NOS

⑦ **T51.0X2** **Toxic effect of ethanol, intentional self-harm**

⑦ **T51.0X3** **Toxic effect of ethanol, assault**

⑦ **T51.0X4** **Toxic effect of ethanol, undetermined**

T51.1 **Toxic effect of methanol**

Toxic effect of methyl alcohol

T51.1X **Toxic effect of methanol**

⑦ **T51.1X1** **Toxic effect of methanol, accidental (unintentional)**

Toxic effect of methanol NOS

⑦ **T51.1X2** **Toxic effect of methanol, intentional self-harm**

⑦ **T51.1X3** **Toxic effect of methanol, assault**

⑦ **T51.1X4** **Toxic effect of methanol, undetermined**

T51.2 **Toxic effect of 2-Propanol**

Toxic effect of isopropyl alcohol

T51.2X **Toxic effect of 2-Propanol**

⑦ **T51.2X1** **Toxic effect of 2-Propanol, accidental (unintentional)**

Toxic effect of 2-Propanol NOS

⑦T51.2X2　Toxic effect of 2-Propanol, intentional self-harm

⑦T51.2X3　Toxic effect of 2-Propanol, assault

⑦T51.2X4　Toxic effect of 2-Propanol, undetermined

T51.3　Toxic effect of fusel oil

Toxic effect of amyl alcohol

Toxic effect of butyl [1-butanol] alcohol

Toxic effect of propyl [1-propanol] alcohol

T51.3X　Toxic effect of fusel oil

⑦T51.3X1　Toxic effect of fusel oil, accidental (unintentional)

Toxic effect of fusel oil NOS

⑦T51.3X2　Toxic effect of fusel oil, intentional self-harm

⑦T51.3X3　Toxic effect of fusel oil, assault

⑦T51.3X4　Toxic effect of fusel oil, undetermined

T51.8　Toxic effect of other alcohols

T51.8X　Toxic effect of other alcohols

⑦T51.8X1　Toxic effect of other alcohols, accidental (unintentional)

Toxic effect of other alcohols NOS

⑦T51.8X2　Toxic effect of other alcohols, intentional self-harm

⑦T51.8X3　Toxic effect of other alcohols, assault

⑦T51.8X4　Toxic effect of other alcohols, undetermined

T51.9　Toxic effect of unspecified alcohol

⊗⑦T51.91　Toxic effect of unspecified alcohol, accidental (unintentional)

⊗⑦T51.92　Toxic effect of unspecified alcohol, intentional self-harm

⊗⑦T51.93　Toxic effect of unspecified alcohol, assault

⊗⑦T51.94　Toxic effect of unspecified alcohol, undetermined

T52　Toxic effect of organic solvents

Excludes1: halogen derivatives of aliphatic and aromatic hydrocarbons (T53.-)

The appropriate 7th character is to be added to each code from category T52

A - initial encounter

D - subsequent encounter

S - sequela

⑦T52.0　Toxic effects of petroleum products

Toxic effects of gasoline [petrol]

Toxic effects of kerosene [paraffin oil]

Toxic effects of paraffin wax

Toxic effects of ether petroleum

Toxic effects of naphtha petroleum

Toxic effects of spirit petroleum

T52.0X　Toxic effects of petroleum products

⑦T52.0X1　Toxic effect of petroleum products, accidental (unintentional)

Toxic effects of petroleum products NOS

⑦T52.0X2　Toxic effect of petroleum products, intentional self-harm

⑦T52.0X3　Toxic effect of petroleum products, assault

⑦T52.0X4　Toxic effect of petroleum products, undetermined

T52.1　Toxic effects of benzene

Excludes1: homologues of benzene (T52.2)

nitroderivatives and aminoderivatives of benzene and its homologues (T65.3)

T52.1X　Toxic effects of benzene

⑦T52.1X1　Toxic effect of benzene, accidental (unintentional)

Toxic effects of benzene NOS

⑦T52.1X2　Toxic effect of benzene, intentional self-harm

⑦T52.1X3　Toxic effect of benzene, assault

⑦T52.1X4　Toxic effect of benzene, undetermined

T52.2　Toxic effects of homologues of benzene

Toxic effects of toluene [methylbenzene]

Toxic effects of xylene [dimethylbenzene]

T52.2X　Toxic effects of homologues of benzene

⑦T52.2X1　Toxic effect of homologues of benzene, accidental (unintentional)

Toxic effects of homologues of benzene NOS

⑦T52.2X2　Toxic effect of homologues of benzene, intentional self-harm

⑦T52.2X3　Toxic effect of homologues of benzene, assault

⑦T52.2X4　Toxic effect of homologues of benzene, undetermined

T52.3　Toxic effects of glycols

T52.3X　Toxic effects of glycols

⑦T52.3X1　Toxic effect of glycols, accidental (unintentional)

Toxic effects of glycols NOS

⑦T52.3X2　Toxic effect of glycols, intentional self-harm

⑦T52.3X3　Toxic effect of glycols, assault

⑦T52.3X4　Toxic effect of glycols, undetermined

T52.4　Toxic effects of ketones

T52.4X　Toxic effects of ketones

⑦T52.4X1　Toxic effect of ketones, accidental (unintentional)

Toxic effects of ketones NOS

⑦T52.4X2　Toxic effect of ketones, intentional self-harm

⑦T52.4X3　Toxic effect of ketones, assault

⑦T52.4X4　Toxic effect of ketones, undetermined

T52.8　Toxic effects of other organic solvents

T52.8X　Toxic effects of other organic solvents

⑦T52.8X1　Toxic effect of other organic solvents, accidental (unintentional)

Toxic effects of other organic solvents NOS

⑦ **T52.8X2** Toxic effect of other organic solvents, intentional self-harm

⑦ **T52.8X3** Toxic effect of other organic solvents, assault

⑦ **T52.8X4** Toxic effect of other organic solvents, undetermined

T52.9 **Toxic effects of unspecified organic solvent**

⊗⑦ **T52.91** Toxic effect of unspecified organic solvent, accidental (unintentional)

⊗⑦ **T52.92** Toxic effect of unspecified organic solvent, intentional self-harm

⊗⑦ **T52.93** Toxic effect of unspecified organic solvent, assault

⊗⑦ **T52.94** Toxic effect of unspecified organic solvent, undetermined

T53 **Toxic effect of halogen derivatives of aliphatic and aromatic hydrocarbons**

The appropriate 7th character is to be added to each code from category T53

A - initial encounter

D - subsequent encounter

S - sequela

T53.0 **Toxic effects of carbon tetrachloride**

Toxic effects of tetrachloromethane

T53.0X **Toxic effects of carbon tetrachloride**

⑦ **T53.0X1** Toxic effect of carbon tetrachloride, accidental (unintentional)

Toxic effects of carbon tetrachloride NOS

⑦ **T53.0X2** Toxic effect of carbon tetrachloride, intentional self-harm

⑦ **T53.0X3** Toxic effect of carbon tetrachloride, assault

⑦ **T53.0X4** Toxic effect of carbon tetrachloride, undetermined

T53.1 **Toxic effects of chloroform**

Toxic effects of trichloromethane

T53.1X **Toxic effects of chloroform**

⑦ **T53.1X1** Toxic effect of chloroform, accidental (unintentional)

Toxic effects of chloroform NOS

⑦ **T53.1X2** Toxic effect of chloroform, intentional self-harm

⑦ **T53.1X3** Toxic effect of chloroform, assault

⑦ **T53.1X4** Toxic effect of chloroform, undetermined

T53.2 **Toxic effects of trichloroethylene**

Toxic effects of trichloroethene

T53.2X **Toxic effects of trichloroethylene**

⑦ **T53.2X1** Toxic effect of trichloroethylene, accidental (unintentional)

Toxic effects of trichloroethylene NOS

⑦ **T53.2X2** Toxic effect of trichloroethylene, intentional self-harm

⑦ **T53.2X3** Toxic effect of trichloroethylene, assault

⑦ **T53.2X4** Toxic effect of trichloroethylene, undetermined

T53.3 **Toxic effects of tetrachloroethylene**

Toxic effects of perchloroethylene

Toxic effect of tetrachloroethene

T53.3X **Toxic effects of tetrachloroethylene**

⑦ **T53.3X1** Toxic effect of tetrachloroethylene, accidental (unintentional)

oxic effects of tetrachloroethylene NOS

⑦ **T53.3X2** Toxic effect of tetrachloroethylene, intentional self-harm

⑦ **T53.3X3** Toxic effect of tetrachloroethylene, assault

⑦ **T53.3X4** Toxic effect of tetrachloroethylene, undetermined

T53.4 **Toxic effects of dichloromethane**

Toxic effects of methylene chloride

T53.4X **Toxic effects of dichloromethane**

⑦ **T53.4X1** Toxic effect of dichloromethane, accidental (unintentional)

Toxic effects of dichloromethane NOS

⑦ **T53.4X2** Toxic effect of dichloromethane, intentional self-harm

⑦ **T53.4X3** Toxic effect of dichloromethane, assault

⑦ **T53.4X4** Toxic effect of dichloromethane, undetermined

T53.5 **Toxic effects of chlorofluorocarbons**

T53.5X **Toxic effects of chlorofluorocarbons**

⑦ **T53.5X1** Toxic effect of chlorofluorocarbons, accidental (unintentional)

Toxic effects of chlorofluorocarbons NOS

⑦ **T53.5X2** Toxic effect of chlorofluorocarbons, intentional self-harm

⑦ **T53.5X3** Toxic effect of chlorofluorocarbons, assault

⑦ **T53.5X4** Toxic effect of chlorofluorocarbons, undetermined

T53.6 **Toxic effects of other halogen derivatives of aliphatic hydrocarbons**

T53.6X **Toxic effects of other halogen derivatives of aliphatic hydrocarbons**

⑦ **T53.6X1** Toxic effect of other halogen derivatives of aliphatic hydrocarbons, accidental (unintentional)

Toxic effects of other halogen derivatives of aliphatic hydrocarbons NOS

⑦ **T53.6X2** Toxic effect of other halogen derivatives of aliphatic hydrocarbons, intentional self-harm

⑦ **T53.6X3** Toxic effect of other halogen derivatives of aliphatic hydrocarbons, assault

⑦ **T53.6X4** Toxic effect of other halogen derivatives of aliphatic hydrocarbons, undetermined

T53.7 **Toxic effects of other halogen derivatives of aromatic hydrocarbons**

● New code ▲ Revised code **Excludes1:** Not coded here **Excludes2:** Not included here ⊗ Placeholder required ⑦ 7th digit required

T53.7X **Toxic effects of other halogen derivatives of aromatic hydrocarbons**

⑦T53.7X1 **Toxic effect of other halogen derivatives of aromatic hydrocarbons, accidental (unintentional)**

Toxic effects **of other** halogen derivatives of aromatic hydrocarbons NOS

⑦T53.7X2 **Toxic effect of other halogen derivatives of aromatic hydrocarbons, intentional self-harm**

⑦T53.7X3 **Toxic effect of other halogen derivatives of aromatic hydrocarbons, assault**

⑦T53.7X4 **Toxic effect of other halogen derivatives of aromatic hydrocarbons, undetermined**

T53.9 **Toxic effects of unspecified halogen derivatives of aliphatic and aromatic hydrocarbons**

⊗⑦T53.91 **Toxic effect of unspecified halogen derivatives of aliphatic and aromatic hydrocarbons, accidental (unintentional)**

⊗⑦T53.92 **Toxic effect of unspecified halogen derivatives of aliphatic and aromatic hydrocarbons, intentional self-harm**

⊗⑦T53.93 **Toxic effect of unspecified halogen derivatives of aliphatic and aromatic hydrocarbons, assault**

⊗⑦T53.94 **Toxic effect of unspecified halogen derivatives of aliphatic and aromatic hydrocarbons, undetermined**

T54 **Toxic effect of corrosive substances**

The appropriate 7th character is to be added to each code from category T54

A - initial encounter

D - subsequent encounter

S - sequela

T54.0 **Toxic effects of phenol and phenol homologues**

T54.0X **Toxic effects of phenol and phenol homologues**

⑦T54.0X1 **Toxic effect of phenol and phenol homologues, accidental (unintentional)**

Toxic effects of phenol and phenol homologues NOS

⑦T54.0X2 **Toxic effect of phenol and phenol homologues, intentional self-harm**

⑦T54.0X3 **Toxic effect of phenol and phenol homologues, assault**

⑦T54.0X4 **Toxic effect of phenol and phenol homologues, undetermined**

T54.1 **Toxic effects of other corrosive organic compounds**

T54.1X **Toxic effects of other corrosive organic compounds**

⑦T54.1X1 **Toxic effect of other corrosive organic compounds, accidental (unintentional)**

Toxic effects **of other** corrosive organic compounds NOS

⑦T54.1X2 **Toxic effect of other corrosive organic compounds, intentional self-harm**

⑦T54.1X3 **Toxic effect of other corrosive organic compounds, assault**

⑦T54.1X4 **Toxic effect of other corrosive organic compounds, undetermined**

T54.2 **Toxic effects of corrosive acids and acid-like substances**

Toxic effects of hydrochloric acid

Toxic effects of sulfuric acid

T54.2X **Toxic effects of corrosive acids and acid-like substances**

⑦T54.2X1 **Toxic effect of corrosive acids and acid-like substances, accidental (unintentional)**

Toxic effects of corrosive acids and acid-like substances NOS

⑦T54.2X2 **Toxic effect of corrosive acids and acid-like substances, intentional self-harm**

⑦T54.2X3 **Toxic effect of corrosive acids and acid-like substances, assault**

⑦T54.2X4 **Toxic effect of corrosive acids and acid-like substances, undetermined**

T54.3 **Toxic effects of corrosive alkalis and alkali-like substances**

Toxic effects of potassium hydroxide

Toxic effects of sodium hydroxide

T54.3X **Toxic effects of corrosive alkalis and alkali-like substances**

⑦T54.3X1 **Toxic effect of corrosive alkalis and alkali-like substances, accidental (unintentional)**

Toxic effects of corrosive alkalis and alkali-like substances NOS

⑦T54.3X2 **Toxic effect of corrosive alkalis and alkali-like substances, intentional self-harm**

⑦T54.3X3 **Toxic effect of corrosive alkalis and alkali-like substances, assault**

⑦T54.3X4 **Toxic effect of corrosive alkalis and alkali-like substances, undetermined**

T54.9 **Toxic effects of unspecified corrosive substance**

⊗⑦T54.91 **Toxic effect of unspecified corrosive substance, accidental (unintentional)**

⊗⑦T54.92 **Toxic effect of unspecified corrosive substance, intentional self-harm**

⊗⑦T54.93 **Toxic effect of unspecified corrosive substance, assault**

⊗⑦T54.94 **Toxic effect of unspecified corrosive substance, undetermined**

T55 **Toxic effect of soaps and detergents**

The appropriate 7th character is to be added to each code from category T55

A - initial encounter

D - subsequent encounter

S - sequela

T55.0 **Toxic effect of soaps**

T55.0X **Toxic effect of soaps**

⑦T55.0X1 **Toxic effect of soaps, accidental (unintentional)**

Toxic effect of soaps NOS

⑦ **T55.0X2** **Toxic effect of soaps, intentional self-harm**

⑦ **T55.0X3** **Toxic effect of soaps, assault**

⑦ **T55.0X4** **Toxic effect of soaps, undetermined**

T55.1 **Toxic effect of detergents**

T55.1X **Toxic effect of detergents**

⑦ **T55.1X1** **Toxic effect of detergents, accidental (unintentional)**

Toxic effect of detergents NOS

⑦ **T55.1X2** **Toxic effect of detergents, intentional self-harm**

⑦ **T55.1X3** **Toxic effect of detergents, assault**

⑦ **T55.1X4** **Toxic effect of detergents, undetermined**

T56 **Toxic effect of metals**

Includes: toxic effects of fumes and vapors of metals

toxic effects of metals from all sources, except medicinal substances

Use additional code to identify any retained metal foreign body, if applicable (Z18.0-, T18.1-)

Excludes1: arsenic and its compounds (T57.0)

manganese and its compounds (T57.2)

The appropriate 7th character is to be added to each code from category T56

A - initial encounter

D - subsequent encounter

S - sequela

T56.0 **Toxic effects of lead and its compounds**

T56.0X **Toxic effects of lead and its compounds**

⑦ **T56.0X1** **Toxic effect of lead and its compounds, accidental (unintentional)**

Toxic effects of lead and its compounds NOS

⑦ **T56.0X2** **Toxic effect of lead and its compounds, intentional self-harm**

⑦ **T56.0X3** **Toxic effect of lead and its compounds, assault**

⑦ **T56.0X4** **Toxic effect of lead and its compounds, undetermined**

T56.1 **Toxic effects of mercury and its compounds**

⑦ **T56.1X** **Toxic effects of mercury and its compounds**

⑦ **T56.1X1** **Toxic effect of mercury and its compounds, accidental (unintentional)**

Toxic effects of mercury and its compounds NOS

⑦ **T56.1X2** **Toxic effect of mercury and its compounds, intentional self-harm**

⑦ **T56.1X3** **Toxic effect of mercury and its compounds, assault**

⑦ **T56.1X4** **Toxic effect of mercury and its compounds, undetermined**

T56.2 **Toxic effects of chromium and its compounds**

T56.2X **Toxic effects of chromium and its compounds**

⑦ **T56.2X1** **Toxic effect of chromium and its compounds, accidental (unintentional)**

Toxic effects of chromium and its compounds NOS

⑦ **T56.2X2** **Toxic effect of chromium and its compounds, intentional self-harm**

⑦ **T56.2X3** **Toxic effect of chromium and its compounds, assault**

⑦ **T56.2X4** **Toxic effect of chromium and its compounds, undetermined**

T56.3 **Toxic effects of cadmium and its compounds**

T56.3X **Toxic effects of cadmium and its compounds**

⑦ **T56.3X1** **Toxic effect of cadmium and its compounds, accidental (unintentional)**

Toxic effects of cadmium and its compounds NOS

⑦ **T56.3X2** **Toxic effect of cadmium and its compounds, intentional self-harm**

⑦ **T56.3X3** **Toxic effect of cadmium and its compounds, assault**

⑦ **T56.3X4** **Toxic effect of cadmium and its compounds, undetermined**

T56.4 **Toxic effects of copper and its compounds**

T56.4X **Toxic effects of copper and its compounds**

⑦ **T56.4X1** **Toxic effect of copper and its compounds, accidental (unintentional)**

Toxic effects of copper and its compounds NOS

⑦ **T56.4X2** **Toxic effect of copper and its compounds, intentional self-harm**

⑦ **T56.4X3** **Toxic effect of copper and its compounds, assault**

⑦ **T56.4X4** **Toxic effect of copper and its compounds, undetermined**

T56.5 **Toxic effects of zinc and its compounds**

T56.5X **Toxic effects of zinc and its compounds**

⑦ **T56.5X1** **Toxic effect of zinc and its compounds, accidental (unintentional)**

Toxic effects of zinc and its compounds NOS

⑦ **T56.5X2** **Toxic effect of zinc and its compounds, intentional self-harm**

⑦ **T56.5X3** **Toxic effect of zinc and its compounds, assault**

⑦ **T56.5X4** **Toxic effect of zinc and its compounds, undetermined**

T56.6 **Toxic effects of tin and its compounds**

T56.6X **Toxic effects of tin and its compounds**

⑦ **T56.6X1** **Toxic effect of tin and its compounds, accidental (unintentional)**

Toxic effects of tin and its compounds NOS

⑦ **T56.6X2** **Toxic effect of tin and its compounds, intentional self-harm**

⑦ **T56.6X3** **Toxic effect of tin and its compounds, assault**

⑦ **T56.6X4** **Toxic effect of tin and its compounds, undetermined**

T56.7 **Toxic effects of beryllium and its compounds**

● New code   ▲ Revised code   **Excludes1:** Not coded here   **Excludes2:** Not included here   ⊗ Placeholder required   ⑦ 7th digit required

T56.7X   Toxic effects of beryllium and its compounds

⑦ T56.7X1   Toxic effect of beryllium and its compounds, accidental (unintentional)

Toxic effects of beryllium and its compounds NOS

⑦ T56.7X2   Toxic effect of beryllium and its compounds, intentional self-harm

⑦ T56.7X3   Toxic effect of beryllium and its compounds, assault

⑦ T56.7X4   Toxic effect of beryllium and its compounds, undetermined

T56.8   Toxic effects of other metals

T56.81   Toxic effect of thallium

⑦ T56.811   Toxic effect of thallium, accidental (unintentional)

Toxic effect of thallium NOS

⑦ T56.812   Toxic effect of thallium, intentional self-harm

⑦ T56.813   Toxic effect of thallium, assault

⑦ T56.814   Toxic effect of thallium, undetermined

T56.89   Toxic effects of other metals

⑦ T56.891   Toxic effect of other metals, accidental (unintentional)

Toxic effects of other metals NOS

⑦ T56.892   Toxic effect of other metals, intentional self-harm

⑦ T56.893   Toxic effect of other metals, assault

⑦ T56.894   Toxic effect of other metals, undetermined

T56.9   Toxic effects of unspecified metal

⊗⑦ T56.91   Toxic effect of unspecified metal, accidental (unintentional)

⊗⑦ T56.92   Toxic effect of unspecified metal, intentional self-harm

⊗⑦ T56.93   Toxic effect of unspecified metal, assault

⊗⑦ T56.94   Toxic effect of unspecified metal, undetermined

T57   Toxic effect of other inorganic substances

The appropriate 7th character is to be added to each code from category T57

A - initial encounter

D - subsequent encounter

S - sequela

T57.0   Toxic effect of arsenic and its compounds

T57.0X   Toxic effect of arsenic and its compounds

⑦ T57.0X1   Toxic effect of arsenic and its compounds, accidental (unintentional)

Toxic effect of arsenic and its compounds NOS

⑦ T57.0X2   Toxic effect of arsenic and its compounds, intentional self-harm

⑦ T57.0X3   Toxic effect of arsenic and its compounds, assault

⑦ T57.0X4   Toxic effect of arsenic and its compounds, undetermined

T57.1   Toxic effect of phosphorus and its compounds

Excludes1: organophosphate insecticides (T60.0)

T57.1X   Toxic effect of phosphorus and its compounds

⑦ T57.1X1   Toxic effect of phosphorus and its compounds, accidental (unintentional)

Toxic effect of phosphorus and its compounds NOS

⑦ T57.1X2   Toxic effect of phosphorus and its compounds, intentional self-harm

⑦ T57.1X3   Toxic effect of phosphorus and its compounds, assault

⑦ T57.1X4   Toxic effect of phosphorus and its compounds, undetermined

T57.2   Toxic effect of manganese and its compounds

T57.2X   Toxic effect of manganese and its compounds

⑦ T57.2X1   Toxic effect of manganese and its compounds, accidental (unintentional)

Toxic effect of manganese and its compounds NOS

⑦ T57.2X2   Toxic effect of manganese and its compounds, intentional self-harm

⑦ T57.2X3   Toxic effect of manganese and its compounds, assault

⑦ T57.2X4   Toxic effect of manganese and its compounds, undetermined

T57.3   Toxic effect of hydrogen cyanide

T57.3X   Toxic effect of hydrogen cyanide

⑦ T57.3X1   Toxic effect of hydrogen cyanide, accidental (unintentional)

Toxic effect of hydrogen cyanide NOS

⑦ T57.3X2   Toxic effect of hydrogen cyanide, intentional self-harm

⑦ T57.3X3   Toxic effect of hydrogen cyanide, assault

⑦ T57.3X4   Toxic effect of hydrogen cyanide, undetermined

T57.8   Toxic effect of other specified inorganic substances

T57.8X   Toxic effect of other specified inorganic substances

⑦ T57.8X1   Toxic effect of other specified inorganic substances, accidental (unintentional)

Toxic effect of other specified inorganic substances NOS

⑦ T57.8X2   Toxic effect of other specified inorganic substances, intentional self-harm

⑦ T57.8X3   Toxic effect of other specified inorganic substances, assault

⑦ T57.8X4   Toxic effect of other specified inorganic substances, undetermined

T57.9   Toxic effect of unspecified inorganic substance

⊗⑦ T57.91   Toxic effect of unspecified inorganic substance, accidental (unintentional)

⊗⑦ T57.92   Toxic effect of unspecified inorganic substance, intentional self-harm

⊗⑦ T57.93   Toxic effect of unspecified inorganic substance, assault

⊗⑦T57.94 Toxic effect of unspecified inorganic
substance, undetermined

T58 **Toxic effect of carbon monoxide**

Includes: asphyxiation from carbon monoxide

toxic effect of carbon monoxide from all sources

The appropriate 7th character is to be added to each code from
category T58

A - initial encounter
D - subsequent encounter
S - sequela

T58.0 **Toxic effect of carbon monoxide from motor vehicle
exhaust**

Toxic effect of exhaust gas from gas engine

Toxic effect of exhaust gas from motor pump

⊗⑦T58.01 Toxic effect of carbon monoxide from motor
vehicle exhaust, accidental (unintentional)

⊗⑦T58.02 Toxic effect of carbon monoxide from motor
vehicle exhaust, intentional self-harm

⊗⑦T58.03 Toxic effect of carbon monoxide from motor
vehicle exhaust, assault

⊗⑦T58.04 Toxic effect of carbon monoxide from motor
vehicle exhaust, undetermined

T58.1 **Toxic effect of carbon monoxide from utility gas**

Toxic effect of acetylene

Toxic effect of gas NOS used for lighting, heating, cooking

Toxic effect of water gas

⊗⑦T58.11 Toxic effect of carbon monoxide from utility
gas, accidental (unintentional)

⊗⑦T58.12 Toxic effect of carbon monoxide from utility
gas, intentional self-harm

⊗⑦T58.13 Toxic effect of carbon monoxide from utility
gas, assault

⊗⑦T58.14 Toxic effect of carbon monoxide from utility
gas, undetermined

T58.2 **Toxic effect of carbon monoxide from incomplete
combustion of other domestic fuels**

Toxic effect of carbon monoxide from incomplete
combustion of coal, coke, kerosene, wood

T58.2X **Toxic effect of carbon monoxide from
incomplete combustion of other domestic fuels**

⑦T58.2X1 Toxic effect of carbon monoxide
from incomplete combustion of
other domestic fuels, accidental
(unintentional)

⑦T58.2X2 Toxic effect of carbon monoxide
from incomplete combustion of
other domestic fuels, intentional
self-harm

⑦T58.2X3 Toxic effect of carbon monoxide
from incomplete combustion of
other domestic fuels, assault

⑦T58.2X4 Toxic effect of carbon monoxide
from incomplete combustion of
other domestic fuels, undetermined

T58.8 **Toxic effect of carbon monoxide from other source**

Toxic effect of carbon monoxide from blast furnace gas

Toxic effect of carbon monoxide from fuels in industrial
use

Toxic effect of carbon monoxide from kiln vapor

T58.8X Toxic effect of carbon monoxide from other
source

⑦T58.8X1 Toxic effect of carbon monoxide
from other source, accidental
(unintentional)

⑦T58.8X2 Toxic effect of carbon monoxide
from other source, intentional self-
harm

⑦T58.8X3 Toxic effect of carbon monoxide
from other source, assault

⑦T58.8X4 Toxic effect of carbon monoxide
from other source, undetermined

T58.9 **Toxic effect of carbon monoxide from unspecified
source**

⊗⑦T58.91 Toxic effect of carbon monoxide from
unspecified source, accidental (unintentional)

⊗⑦T58.92 Toxic effect of carbon monoxide from
unspecified source, intentional self-harm

⊗⑦T58.93 Toxic effect of carbon monoxide from
unspecified source, assault

⊗⑦T58.94 Toxic effect of carbon monoxide from
unspecified source, undetermined

T59 **Toxic effect of other gases, fumes and vapors**

Includes: aerosol propellants

Excludes1: chlorofluorocarbons (T53.5)

The appropriate 7th character is to be added to each code from
category T59

A - initial encounter
D - subsequent encounter
S - sequela

T59.0 **Toxic effect of nitrogen oxides**

T59.0X Toxic effect of nitrogen oxides

⑦T59.0X1 Toxic effect of nitrogen oxides,
accidental (unintentional)

Toxic effect of nitrogen oxides NOS

⑦T59.0X2 Toxic effect of nitrogen oxides,
intentional self-harm

⑦T59.0X3 Toxic effect of nitrogen oxides,
assault

⑦T59.0X4 Toxic effect of nitrogen oxides,
undetermined

T59.1 **Toxic effect of sulfur dioxide**

T59.1X Toxic effect of sulfur dioxide

⑦T59.1X1 Toxic effect of sulfur dioxide,
accidental (unintentional)

Toxic effect of sulfur dioxide NOS

⑦T59.1X2 Toxic effect of sulfur dioxide,
intentional self-harm

⑦T59.1X3 Toxic effect of sulfur dioxide,
assault

⑦T59.1X4 Toxic effect of sulfur dioxide,
undetermined

T59.2 **Toxic effect of formaldehyde**

T59.2X Toxic effect of formaldehyde

⑦T59.2X1 Toxic effect of formaldehyde,
accidental (unintentional)

Toxic effect of formaldehyde NOS

⑦T59.2X2 Toxic effect of formaldehyde,
intentional self-harm

● New code ▲ Revised code **Excludes1:** Not coded here **Excludes2:** Not included here ⊗ Placeholder required ⑦7th digit required

⑦T59.2X3 **Toxic effect of formaldehyde, assault**

⑦T59.2X4 **Toxic effect of formaldehyde, undetermined**

T59.3 **Toxic effect of lacrimogenic gas**

Toxic effect of tear gas

T59.3X **Toxic effect of lacrimogenic gas**

⑦T59.3X1 **Toxic effect of lacrimogenic gas, accidental (unintentional)**

Toxic effect of lacrimogenic gas NOS

⑦T59.3X2 **Toxic effect of lacrimogenic gas, intentional self-harm**

⑦T59.3X3 **Toxic effect of lacrimogenic gas, assault**

⑦T59.3X4 **Toxic effect of lacrimogenic gas, undetermined**

T59.4 **Toxic effect of chlorine gas**

T59.4X **Toxic effect of chlorine gas**

⑦T59.4X1 **Toxic effect of chlorine gas, accidental (unintentional)**

Toxic effect of chlorine gas NOS

⑦T59.4X2 **Toxic effect of chlorine gas, intentional self-harm**

⑦T59.4X3 **Toxic effect of chlorine gas, assault**

⑦T59.4X4 **Toxic effect of chlorine gas, undetermined**

T59.5 **Toxic effect of fluorine gas and hydrogen fluoride**

T59.5X **Toxic effect of fluorine gas and hydrogen fluoride**

⑦T59.5X1 **Toxic effect of fluorine gas and hydrogen fluoride, accidental (unintentional)**

Toxic effect of fluorine gas and hydrogen fluoride NOS

⑦T59.5X2 **Toxic effect of fluorine gas and hydrogen fluoride, intentional self-harm**

⑦T59.5X3 **Toxic effect of fluorine gas and hydrogen fluoride, assault**

⑦T59.5X4 **Toxic effect of fluorine gas and hydrogen fluoride, undetermined**

T59.6 **Toxic effect of hydrogen sulfide**

T59.6X **Toxic effect of hydrogen sulfide**

⑦T59.6X1 **Toxic effect of hydrogen sulfide, accidental (unintentional)**

Toxic effect of hydrogen sulfide NOS

⑦T59.6X2 **Toxic effect of hydrogen sulfide, intentional self-harm**

⑦T59.6X3 **Toxic effect of hydrogen sulfide, assault**

⑦T59.6X4 **Toxic effect of hydrogen sulfide, undetermined**

T59.7 **Toxic effect of carbon dioxide**

T59.7X **Toxic effect of carbon dioxide**

⑦T59.7X1 **Toxic effect of carbon dioxide, accidental (unintentional)**

Toxic effect of carbon dioxide NOS

⑦T59.7X2 **Toxic effect of carbon dioxide, intentional self-harm**

⑦T59.7X3 **Toxic effect of carbon dioxide, assault**

⑦T59.7X4 **Toxic effect of carbon dioxide, undetermined**

T59.8 **Toxic effect of other specified gases, fumes and vapors**

T59.81 **Toxic effect of smoke**

Smoke inhalation

Excludes2: toxic effect of cigarette (tobacco) smoke (T65.22-)

⑦T59.811 **Toxic effect of smoke, accidental (unintentional)**

Toxic effect of smoke NOS

⑦T59.812 **Toxic effect of smoke, intentional self-harm**

⑦T59.813 **Toxic effect of smoke, assault**

⑦T59.814 **Toxic effect of smoke, undetermined**

T59.89 **Toxic effect of other specified gases, fumes and vapors**

⑦T59.891 **Toxic effect of other specified gases, fumes and vapors, accidental (unintentional)**

⑦T59.892 **Toxic effect of other specified gases, fumes and vapors, intentional self-harm**

⑦T59.893 **Toxic effect of other specified gases, fumes and vapors, assault**

⑦T59.894 **Toxic effect of other specified gases, fumes and vapors, undetermined**

T59.9 **Toxic effect of unspecified gases, fumes and vapors**

⊗⑦T59.91 **Toxic effect of unspecified gases, fumes and vapors, accidental (unintentional)**

⊗⑦T59.92 **Toxic effect of unspecified gases, fumes and vapors, intentional self-harm**

⊗⑦T59.93 **Toxic effect of unspecified gases, fumes and vapors, assault**

⊗⑦T59.94 **Toxic effect of unspecified gases, fumes and vapors, undetermined**

T60 **Toxic effect of pesticides**

Includes: toxic effect of wood preservatives

The appropriate 7th character is to be added to each code from category T60

A - initial encounter

D - subsequent encounter

S - sequela

T60.0 **Toxic effect of organophosphate and carbamate insecticides**

T60.0X **Toxic effect of organophosphate and carbamate insecticides**

⑦T60.0X1 **Toxic effect of organophosphate and carbamate insecticides, accidental (unintentional)**

Toxic effect of organophosphate and carbamate insecticides NOS

⑦T60.0X2 **Toxic effect of organophosphate and carbamate insecticides, intentional self-harm**

⑦T60.0X3 **Toxic effect of organophosphate and carbamate insecticides, assault**

⑦**T60.0X4** Toxic effect of organophosphate and carbamate insecticides, undetermined

T60.1 Toxic effect of halogenated insecticides
> **Excludes1:** chlorinated hydrocarbon (T53.-)

T60.1X Toxic effect of halogenated insecticides

⑦**T60.1X1** Toxic effect of halogenated insecticides, accidental (unintentional)
> Toxic effect of halogenated insecticides NOS

⑦**T60.1X2** Toxic effect of halogenated insecticides, intentional self-harm

⑦**T60.1X3** Toxic effect of halogenated insecticides, assault

⑦**T60.1X4** Toxic effect of halogenated insecticides, undetermined

T60.2 Toxic effect of other insecticides

T60.2X Toxic effect of other insecticides

⑦**T60.2X1** Toxic effect of other insecticides, accidental (unintentional)
> Toxic effect of other insecticides NOS

⑦**T60.2X2** Toxic effect of other insecticides, intentional self-harm

⑦**T60.2X3** Toxic effect of other insecticides, assault

⑦**T60.2X4** Toxic effect of other insecticides, undetermined

T60.3 Toxic effect of herbicides and fungicides

T60.3X Toxic effect of herbicides and fungicides

⑦**T60.3X1** Toxic effect of herbicides and fungicides, accidental (unintentional)
> Toxic effect of herbicides and fungicides NOS

⑦**T60.3X2** Toxic effect of herbicides and fungicides, intentional self-harm

⑦**T60.3X3** Toxic effect of herbicides and fungicides, assault

⑦**T60.3X4** Toxic effect of herbicides and fungicides, undetermined

T60.4 Toxic effect of rodenticides
> **Excludes1:** strychnine and its salts (T65.1)
> thallium (T56.81-)

T60.4X Toxic effect of rodenticides

⑦**T60.4X1** Toxic effect of rodenticides, accidental (unintentional)
> Toxic effect of rodenticides NOS

⑦**T60.4X2** Toxic effect of rodenticides, intentional self-harm

⑦**T60.4X3** Toxic effect of rodenticides, assault

⑦**T60.4X4** Toxic effect of rodenticides, undetermined

T60.8 Toxic effect of other pesticides

T60.8X Toxic effect of other pesticides

⑦**T60.8X1** Toxic effect of other pesticides, accidental (unintentional)
> Toxic effect of other pesticides NOS

⑦**T60.8X2** Toxic effect of other pesticides, intentional self-harm

⑦**T60.8X3** Toxic effect of other pesticides, assault

⑦**T60.8X4** Toxic effect of other pesticides, undetermined

T60.9 Toxic effect of unspecified pesticide

⊗⑦**T60.91** Toxic effect of unspecified pesticide, accidental (unintentional)

⊗⑦**T60.92** Toxic effect of unspecified pesticide, intentional self-harm

⊗⑦**T60.93** Toxic effect of unspecified pesticide, assault

⊗⑦**T60.94** Toxic effect of unspecified pesticide, undetermined

T61 Toxic effect of noxious substances eaten as seafood
> **Excludes1:** allergic reaction to food, such as:
> anaphylactic reaction or shock due to adverse food reaction (T78.0-)
> bacterial foodborne intoxications (A05.-)
> dermatitis (L23.6, L25.4, L27.2)
> food protein-induced enterocolitis syndrome (K52.21)
> food protein-induced enteropathy (K52.22)
> gastroenteritis (noninfective) (K52.29)
> toxic effect of aflatoxin **and other** mycotoxins (T64)
> toxic effect of cyanides (T65.0-)
> toxic effect of harmful algae bloom (T65.82-)
> toxic effect of hydrogen cyanide (T57.3-)
> toxic effect of mercury (T56.1-)
> toxic effect of red tide (T65.82-)

The appropriate 7th character is to be added to each code from category T61

A - initial encounter

D - subsequent encounter

S - sequela

T61.0 Ciguatera fish poisoning

⊗⑦**T61.01** Ciguatera fish poisoning, accidental (unintentional)

⊗⑦**T61.02** Ciguatera fish poisoning, intentional self-harm

⊗⑦**T61.03** Ciguatera fish poisoning, assault

⊗⑦**T61.04** Ciguatera fish poisoning, undetermined

T61.1 Scombroid fish poisoning
> Histamine-like syndrome

⊗⑦**T61.11** Scombroid fish poisoning, accidental (unintentional)

⊗⑦**T61.12** Scombroid fish poisoning, intentional self-harm

⊗⑦**T61.13** Scombroid fish poisoning, assault

⊗⑦**T61.14** Scombroid fish poisoning, undetermined

T61.7 Other fish and shellfish poisoning

T61.77 Other fish poisoning

⑦**T61.771** Other fish poisoning, accidental (unintentional)

⑦**T61.772** Other fish poisoning, intentional self-harm

⑦**T61.773** Other fish poisoning, assault

⑦**T61.774** Other fish poisoning, undetermined

T61.78 Other shellfish poisoning

⑦**T61.781** Other shellfish poisoning, accidental (unintentional)

● New code ▲ Revised code **Excludes1:** Not coded here **Excludes2:** Not included here ⊗ Placeholder required ⑦7th digit required

⑦ **T61.782** **Other shellfish poisoning, intentional self-harm**

⑦ **T61.783** **Other shellfish poisoning, assault**

⑦ **T61.784** **Other shellfish poisoning, undetermined**

T61.8 **Toxic effect of other seafood**

  T61.8X **Toxic effect of other seafood**

    ⑦ **T61.8X1** **Toxic effect of other seafood, accidental (unintentional)**

    ⑦ **T61.8X2** **Toxic effect of other seafood, intentional self-harm**

    ⑦ **T61.8X3** **Toxic effect of other seafood, assault**

    ⑦ **T61.8X4** **Toxic effect of other seafood, undetermined**

T61.9 **Toxic effect of unspecified seafood**

  ⊗⑦**T61.91** **Toxic effect of unspecified seafood, accidental (unintentional)**

  ⊗⑦**T61.92** **Toxic effect of unspecified seafood, intentional self-harm**

  ⊗⑦**T61.93** **Toxic effect of unspecified seafood, assault**

  ⊗⑦**T61.94** **Toxic effect of unspecified seafood, undetermined**

T62 **Toxic effect of other noxious substances eaten as food**

Excludes1: allergic reaction to food, such as:

anaphylactic shock (reaction) due to adverse food reaction (T78.0-)

acterial food borne intoxications (A05.-)

dermatitis (L23.6, L25.4, L27.2)

food protein-induced enterocolitis syndrome (K52.21)

food protein-induced enteropathy (K52.22)

gastroenteritis (noninfective) (K52.29)

toxic effect of aflatoxin **and other** mycotoxins (T64)

toxic effect of cyanides (T65.0-)

toxic effect of hydrogen cyanide (T57.3-)

toxic effect of mercury (T56.1-)

The appropriate 7th character is to be added to each code from category T62

A - initial encounter

D - subsequent encounter

S - sequela

T62.0 **Toxic effect of ingested mushrooms**

  T62.0X **Toxic effect of ingested mushrooms**

    ⑦ **T62.0X1** **Toxic effect of ingested mushrooms, accidental (unintentional)**

    Toxic effect of ingested mushrooms NOS

    ⑦ **T62.0X2** **Toxic effect of ingested mushrooms, intentional self-harm**

    ⑦ **T62.0X3** **Toxic effect of ingested mushrooms, assault**

    ⑦ **T62.0X4** **Toxic effect of ingested mushrooms, undetermined**

T62.1 **Toxic effect of ingested berries**

  T62.1X **Toxic effect of ingested berries**

    ⑦ **T62.1X1** **Toxic effect of ingested berries, accidental (unintentional)**

    Toxic effect of ingested berries NOS

⑦ **T62.1X2** **Toxic effect of ingested berries, intentional self-harm**

⑦ **T62.1X3** **Toxic effect of ingested berries, assault**

⑦ **T62.1X4** **Toxic effect of ingested berries, undetermined**

T62.2 **Toxic effect of other ingested (parts of) plant(s)**

  T62.2X **Toxic effect of other ingested (parts of) plant(s)**

    ⑦ **T62.2X1** **Toxic effect of other ingested (parts of) plant(s), accidental (unintentional)**

    Toxic effect of other ingested (parts of) plant(s) NOS

    ⑦ **T62.2X2** **Toxic effect of other ingested (parts of) plant(s), intentional self-harm**

    ⑦ **T62.2X3** **Toxic effect of other ingested (parts of) plant(s), assault**

    ⑦ **T62.2X4** **Toxic effect of other ingested (parts of) plant(s), undetermined**

T62.8 **Toxic effect of other specified noxious substances eaten as food**

  T62.8X **Toxic effect of other specified noxious substances eaten as food**

    ⑦ **T62.8X1** **Toxic effect of other specified noxious substances eaten as food, accidental (unintentional)**

    Toxic effect **of other** specified noxious substances eaten as food NOS

    ⑦ **T62.8X2** **Toxic effect of other specified noxious substances eaten as food, intentional self-harm**

    ⑦ **T62.8X3** **Toxic effect of other specified noxious substances eaten as food, assault**

    ⑦ **T62.8X4** **Toxic effect of other specified noxious substances eaten as food, undetermined**

T62.9 **Toxic effect of unspecified noxious substance eaten as food**

  ⊗⑦**T62.91** **Toxic effect of unspecified noxious substance eaten as food, accidental (unintentional)**

  Toxic effect of unspecified noxious substance eaten as food NOS

  ⊗⑦**T62.92** **Toxic effect of unspecified noxious substance eaten as food, intentional self-harm**

  ⊗⑦**T62.93** **Toxic effect of unspecified noxious substance eaten as food, assault**

  ⊗⑦**T62.94** **Toxic effect of unspecified noxious substance eaten as food, undetermined**

T63 **Toxic effect of contact with venomous animals and plants**

Includes: bite or touch of venomous animal

pricked or stuck by thorn or leaf

Excludes2: ingestion of toxic animal or plant (T61.-, T62.-)

The appropriate 7th character is to be added to each code from category T63

A - initial encounter

D - subsequent encounter

S - sequela

T63.0 **Toxic effect of snake venom**

  T63.00 **Toxic effect of unspecified snake venom**

⑦**T63.001** Toxic effect of unspecified snake venom, accidental (unintentional)

Toxic effect of unspecified snake venom NOS

⑦**T63.002** Toxic effect of unspecified snake venom, intentional self-harm

⑦**T63.003** Toxic effect of unspecified snake venom, assault

⑦**T63.004** Toxic effect of unspecified snake venom, undetermined

T63.01 Toxic effect of rattlesnake venom

⑦**T63.011** Toxic effect of rattlesnake venom, accidental (unintentional)

Toxic effect of rattlesnake venom NOS

⑦**T63.012** Toxic effect of rattlesnake venom, intentional self-harm

⑦**T63.013** Toxic effect of rattlesnake venom, assault

⑦**T63.014** Toxic effect of rattlesnake venom, undetermined

T63.02 Toxic effect of coral snake venom

⑦**T63.021** Toxic effect of coral snake venom, accidental (unintentional)

Toxic effect of coral snake venom NOS

⑦**T63.022** Toxic effect of coral snake venom, intentional self-harm

⑦**T63.023** Toxic effect of coral snake venom, assault

⑦**T63.024** Toxic effect of coral snake venom, undetermined

T63.03 Toxic effect of taipan venom

⑦**T63.031** Toxic effect of taipan venom, accidental (unintentional)

Toxic effect of taipan venom NOS

⑦**T63.032** Toxic effect of taipan venom, intentional self-harm

⑦**T63.033** Toxic effect of taipan venom, assault

⑦**T63.034** Toxic effect of taipan venom, undetermined

T63.04 Toxic effect of cobra venom

⑦**T63.041** Toxic effect of cobra venom, accidental (unintentional)

Toxic effect of cobra venom NOS

⑦**T63.042** Toxic effect of cobra venom, intentional self-harm

⑦**T63.043** Toxic effect of cobra venom, assault

⑦**T63.044** Toxic effect of cobra venom, undetermined

T63.06 Toxic effect of venom of other North and South American snake

⑦**T63.061** Toxic effect of venom of other North and South American snake, accidental (unintentional)

Toxic effect of venom of other North and South American snake NOS

⑦**T63.062** Toxic effect of venom of other North and South American snake, intentional self-harm

⑦**T63.063** Toxic effect of venom of other North and South American snake, assault

⑦**T63.064** Toxic effect of venom of other North and South American snake, undetermined

T63.07 Toxic effect of venom of other Australian snake

⑦**T63.071** Toxic effect of venom of other Australian snake, accidental (unintentional)

Toxic effect of venom of other Australian snake NOS

⑦**T63.072** Toxic effect of venom of other Australian snake, intentional self-harm

⑦**T63.073** Toxic effect of venom of other Australian snake, assault

⑦**T63.074** Toxic effect of venom of other Australian snake, undetermined

T63.08 Toxic effect of venom of other African and Asian snake

⑦**T63.081** Toxic effect of venom of other African and Asian snake, accidental (unintentional)

Toxic effect of venom of other African and Asian snake NOS

⑦**T63.082** Toxic effect of venom of other African and Asian snake, intentional self-harm

⑦**T63.083** Toxic effect of venom of other African and Asian snake, assault

⑦**T63.084** Toxic effect of venom of other African and Asian snake, undetermined

T63.09 Toxic effect of venom of other snake

⑦**T63.091** Toxic effect of venom of other snake, accidental (unintentional)

Toxic effect of venom of other snake NOS

⑦**T63.092** Toxic effect of venom of other snake, intentional self-harm

⑦**T63.093** Toxic effect of venom of other snake, assault

⑦**T63.094** Toxic effect of venom of other snake, undetermined

T63.1 Toxic effect of venom of other reptiles

T63.11 Toxic effect of venom of gila monster

⑦**T63.111** Toxic effect of venom of gila monster, accidental (unintentional)

Toxic effect of venom of gila monster NOS

⑦**T63.112** Toxic effect of venom of gila monster, intentional self-harm

⑦**T63.113** Toxic effect of venom of gila monster, assault

⑦**T63.114** Toxic effect of venom of gila monster, undetermined

T63.12 Toxic effect of venom of other venomous lizard

⑦**T63.121** Toxic effect of venom of other venomous lizard, accidental (unintentional)

Toxic effect of venom of other venomous lizard NOS

⑦ **T63.122** **Toxic effect of venom of other venomous lizard, intentional self-harm**

⑦ **T63.123** **Toxic effect of venom of other venomous lizard, assault**

⑦ **T63.124** **Toxic effect of venom of other venomous lizard, undetermined**

T63.19 **Toxic effect of venom of other reptiles**

⑦ **T63.191** **Toxic effect of venom of other reptiles, accidental (unintentional)**

Toxic effect of venom of other reptiles NOS

⑦ **T63.192** **Toxic effect of venom of other reptiles, intentional self-harm**

⑦ **T63.193** **Toxic effect of venom of other reptiles, assault**

⑦ **T63.194** **Toxic effect of venom of other reptiles, undetermined**

T63.2 **Toxic effect of venom of scorpion**

T63.2X **Toxic effect of venom of scorpion**

⑦ **T63.2X1** **Toxic effect of venom of scorpion, accidental (unintentional)**

Toxic effect of venom of scorpion NOS

⑦ **T63.2X2** **Toxic effect of venom of scorpion, intentional self-harm**

⑦ **T63.2X3** **Toxic effect of venom of scorpion, assault**

⑦ **T63.2X4** **Toxic effect of venom of scorpion, undetermined**

T63.3 **Toxic effect of venom of spider**

T63.30 **Toxic effect of unspecified spider venom**

⑦ **T63.301** **Toxic effect of unspecified spider venom, accidental (unintentional)**

⑦ **T63.302** **Toxic effect of unspecified spider venom, intentional self-harm**

⑦ **T63.303** **Toxic effect of unspecified spider venom, assault**

⑦ **T63.304** **Toxic effect of unspecified spider venom, undetermined**

T63.31 **Toxic effect of venom of black widow spider**

⑦ **T63.311** **Toxic effect of venom of black widow spider, accidental (unintentional)**

⑦ **T63.312** **Toxic effect of venom of black widow spider, intentional self-harm**

⑦ **T63.313** **Toxic effect of venom of black widow spider, assault**

⑦ **T63.314** **Toxic effect of venom of black widow spider, undetermined**

T63.32 **Toxic effect of venom of tarantula**

⑦ **T63.321** **Toxic effect of venom of tarantula, accidental (unintentional)**

⑦ **T63.322** **Toxic effect of venom of tarantula, intentional self-harm**

⑦ **T63.323** **Toxic effect of venom of tarantula, assault**

⑦ **T63.324** **Toxic effect of venom of tarantula, undetermined**

T63.33 **Toxic effect of venom of brown recluse spider**

⑦ **T63.331** **Toxic effect of venom of brown recluse spider, accidental (unintentional)**

⑦ **T63.332** **Toxic effect of venom of brown recluse spider, intentional self-harm**

⑦ **T63.333** **Toxic effect of venom of brown recluse spider, assault**

⑦ **T63.334** **Toxic effect of venom of brown recluse spider, undetermined**

T63.39 **Toxic effect of venom of other spider**

⑦ **T63.391** **Toxic effect of venom of other spider, accidental (unintentional)**

⑦ **T63.392** **Toxic effect of venom of other spider, intentional self-harm**

⑦ **T63.393** **Toxic effect of venom of other spider, assault**

⑦ **T63.394** **Toxic effect of venom of other spider, undetermined**

T63.4 **Toxic effect of venom of other arthropods**

T63.41 **Toxic effect of venom of centipedes and venomous millipedes**

⑦ **T63.411** **Toxic effect of venom of centipedes and venomous millipedes, accidental (unintentional)**

⑦ **T63.412** **Toxic effect of venom of centipedes and venomous millipedes, intentional self-harm**

⑦ **T63.413** **Toxic effect of venom of centipedes and venomous millipedes, assault**

⑦ **T63.414** **Toxic effect of venom of centipedes and venomous millipedes, undetermined**

T63.42 **Toxic effect of venom of ants**

⑦ **T63.421** **Toxic effect of venom of ants, accidental (unintentional)**

⑦ **T63.422** **Toxic effect of venom of ants, intentional self-harm**

⑦ **T63.423** **Toxic effect of venom of ants, assault**

⑦ **T63.424** **Toxic effect of venom of ants, undetermined**

T63.43 **Toxic effect of venom of caterpillars**

⑦ **T63.431** **Toxic effect of venom of caterpillars, accidental (unintentional)**

⑦ **T63.432** **Toxic effect of venom of caterpillars, intentional self-harm**

⑦ **T63.433** **Toxic effect of venom of caterpillars, assault**

⑦ **T63.434** **Toxic effect of venom of caterpillars, undetermined**

T63.44 **Toxic effect of venom of bees**

⑦ **T63.441** **Toxic effect of venom of bees, accidental (unintentional)**

⑦ **T63.442** **Toxic effect of venom of bees, intentional self-harm**

⑦ **T63.443** **Toxic effect of venom of bees, assault**

⑦ **T63.444** **Toxic effect of venom of bees, undetermined**

T63.45   **Toxic effect of venom of hornets**

⑦**T63.451**   **Toxic effect of venom of hornets, accidental (unintentional)**

⑦**T63.452**   **Toxic effect of venom of hornets, intentional self-harm**

⑦**T63.453**   **Toxic effect of venom of hornets, assault**

⑦**T63.454**   **Toxic effect of venom of hornets, undetermined**

T63.46   **Toxic effect of venom of wasps**

Toxic effect of yellow jacket

⑦**T63.461**   **Toxic effect of venom of wasps, accidental (unintentional)**

⑦**T63.462**   **Toxic effect of venom of wasps, intentional self-harm**

⑦**T63.463**   **Toxic effect of venom of wasps, assault**

⑦**T63.464**   **Toxic effect of venom of wasps, undetermined**

T63.48   **Toxic effect of venom of other arthropod**

⑦**T63.481**   **Toxic effect of venom of other arthropod, accidental (unintentional)**

⑦**T63.482**   **Toxic effect of venom of other arthropod, intentional self-harm**

⑦**T63.483**   **Toxic effect of venom of other arthropod, assault**

⑦**T63.484**   **Toxic effect of venom of other arthropod, undetermined**

T63.5   **Toxic effect of contact with venomous fish**

Excludes2: poisoning by ingestion of fish (T61.-)

T63.51   **Toxic effect of contact with stingray**

⑦**T63.511**   **Toxic effect of contact with stingray, accidental (unintentional)**

⑦**T63.512**   **Toxic effect of contact with stingray, intentional self-harm**

⑦**T63.513**   **Toxic effect of contact with stingray, assault**

⑦**T63.514**   **Toxic effect of contact with stingray, undetermined**

T63.59   **Toxic effect of contact with other venomous fish**

⑦**T63.591**   **Toxic effect of contact with other venomous fish, accidental (unintentional)**

⑦**T63.592**   **Toxic effect of contact with other venomous fish, intentional self-harm**

⑦**T63.593**   **Toxic effect of contact with other venomous fish, assault**

⑦**T63.594**   **Toxic effect of contact with other venomous fish, undetermined**

T63.6   **Toxic effect of contact with other venomous marine animals**

Excludes1: sea-snake venom (T63.09)

Excludes2: poisoning by ingestion of shellfish (T61.78-)

T63.61   **Toxic effect of contact with Portugese Man-o-war**

Toxic effect of contact with bluebottle

⑦**T63.611**   **Toxic effect of contact with Portugese Man-o-war, accidental (unintentional)**

⑦**T63.612**   **Toxic effect of contact with Portugese Man-o-war, intentional self-harm**

⑦**T63.613**   **Toxic effect of contact with Portugese Man-o-war, assault**

⑦**T63.614**   **Toxic effect of contact with Portugese Man-o-war, undetermined**

T63.62   **Toxic effect of contact with other jellyfish**

⑦**T63.621**   **Toxic effect of contact with other jellyfish, accidental (unintentional)**

⑦**T63.622**   **Toxic effect of contact with other jellyfish, intentional self-harm**

⑦**T63.623**   **Toxic effect of contact with other jellyfish, assault**

⑦**T63.624**   **Toxic effect of contact with other jellyfish, undetermined**

T63.63   **Toxic effect of contact with sea anemone**

⑦**T63.631**   **Toxic effect of contact with sea anemone, accidental (unintentional)**

⑦**T63.632**   **Toxic effect of contact with sea anemone, intentional self-harm**

⑦**T63.633**   **Toxic effect of contact with sea anemone, assault**

⑦**T63.634**   **Toxic effect of contact with sea anemone, undetermined**

T63.69   **Toxic effect of contact with other venomous marine animals**

⑦**T63.691**   **Toxic effect of contact with other venomous marine animals, accidental (unintentional)**

⑦**T63.692**   **Toxic effect of contact with other venomous marine animals, intentional self-harm**

⑦**T63.693**   **Toxic effect of contact with other venomous marine animals, assault**

⑦**T63.694**   **Toxic effect of contact with other venomous marine animals, undetermined**

T63.7   **Toxic effect of contact with venomous plant**

T63.71   **Toxic effect of contact with venomous marine plant**

⑦**T63.711**   **Toxic effect of contact with venomous marine plant, accidental (unintentional)**

⑦**T63.712**   **Toxic effect of contact with venomous marine plant, intentional self-harm**

⑦**T63.713**   **Toxic effect of contact with venomous marine plant, assault**

⑦**T63.714**   **Toxic effect of contact with venomous marine plant, undetermined**

T63.79   **Toxic effect of contact with other venomous plant**

⑦**T63.791**   **Toxic effect of contact with other venomous plant, accidental (unintentional)**

● New code   ▲ Revised code   Excludes1: Not coded here   Excludes2: Not included here   ⊗ Placeholder required   ⑦7th digit required

⑦ **T63.792** Toxic effect of contact with other venomous plant, intentional self-harm

⑦ **T63.793** Toxic effect of contact with other venomous plant, assault

⑦ **T63.794** Toxic effect of contact with other venomous plant, undetermined

T63.8 Toxic effect of contact with other venomous animals

   T63.81 Toxic effect of contact with venomous frog

      Excludes1: contact with nonvenomous frog (W62.0)

      ⑦ **T63.811** Toxic effect of contact with venomous frog, accidental (unintentional)

      ⑦ **T63.812** Toxic effect of contact with venomous frog, intentional self-harm

      ⑦ **T63.813** Toxic effect of contact with venomous frog, assault

      ⑦ **T63.814** Toxic effect of contact with venomous frog, undetermined

   T63.82 Toxic effect of contact with venomous toad

      Excludes1: contact with nonvenomous toad (W62.1)

      ⑦ **T63.821** Toxic effect of contact with venomous toad, accidental (unintentional)

      ⑦ **T63.822** Toxic effect of contact with venomous toad, intentional self-harm

      ⑦ **T63.823** Toxic effect of contact with venomous toad, assault

      ⑦ **T63.824** Toxic effect of contact with venomous toad, undetermined

   T63.83 Toxic effect of contact with other venomous amphibian

      Excludes1: contact with nonvenomous amphibian (W62.9)

      ⑦ **T63.831** Toxic effect of contact with other venomous amphibian, accidental (unintentional)

      ⑦ **T63.832** Toxic effect of contact with other venomous amphibian, intentional self-harm

      ⑦ **T63.833** Toxic effect of contact with other venomous amphibian, assault

      ⑦ **T63.834** Toxic effect of contact with other venomous amphibian, undetermined

   T63.89 Toxic effect of contact with other venomous animals

      ⑦ **T63.891** Toxic effect of contact with other venomous animals, accidental (unintentional)

      ⑦ **T63.892** Toxic effect of contact with other venomous animals, intentional self-harm

      ⑦ **T63.893** Toxic effect of contact with other venomous animals, assault

      ⑦ **T63.894** Toxic effect of contact with other venomous animals, undetermined

T63.9 Toxic effect of contact with unspecified venomous animal

   ⊗⑦ **T63.91** Toxic effect of contact with unspecified venomous animal, accidental (unintentional)

   ⊗⑦ **T63.92** Toxic effect of contact with unspecified venomous animal, intentional self-harm

   ⊗⑦ **T63.93** Toxic effect of contact with unspecified venomous animal, assault

   ⊗⑦ **T63.94** Toxic effect of contact with unspecified venomous animal, undetermined

T64 **Toxic effect of aflatoxin and other mycotoxin food contaminants**

The appropriate 7th character is to be added to each code from category T64

A - initial encounter

D - subsequent encounter

S - sequela

T64.0 Toxic effect of aflatoxin

   ⊗⑦ **T64.01** Toxic effect of aflatoxin, accidental (unintentional)

   ⊗⑦ **T64.02** Toxic effect of aflatoxin, intentional self-harm

   ⊗⑦ **T64.03** Toxic effect of aflatoxin, assault

   ⊗⑦ **T64.04** Toxic effect of aflatoxin, undetermined

T64.8 Toxic effect of other mycotoxin food contaminants

   ⊗⑦ **T64.81** Toxic effect of other mycotoxin food contaminants, accidental (unintentional)

   ⊗⑦ **T64.82** Toxic effect of other mycotoxin food contaminants, intentional self-harm

   ⊗⑦ **T64.83** Toxic effect of other mycotoxin food contaminants, assault

   ⊗⑦ **T64.84** Toxic effect of other mycotoxin food contaminants, undetermined

T65 **Toxic effect of other and unspecified substances**

The appropriate 7th character is to be added to each code from category T65

A - initial encounter

D - subsequent encounter

S - sequela

T65.0 Toxic effect of cyanides

   Excludes1: hydrogen cyanide (T57.3-)

   T65.0X Toxic effect of cyanides

      ⑦ **T65.0X1** Toxic effect of cyanides, accidental (unintentional)

          Toxic effect of cyanides NOS

      ⑦ **T65.0X2** Toxic effect of cyanides, intentional self-harm

      ⑦ **T65.0X3** Toxic effect of cyanides, assault

      ⑦ **T65.0X4** Toxic effect of cyanides, undetermined

   T65.1 Toxic effect of strychnine and its salts

      T65.1X Toxic effect of strychnine and its salts

      ⑦ **T65.1X1** Toxic effect of strychnine and its salts, accidental (unintentional)

         Toxic effect of strychnine and its salts NOS

      ⑦ **T65.1X2** Toxic effect of strychnine and its salts, intentional self-harm

      ⑦ **T65.1X3** Toxic effect of strychnine and its salts, assault

⑦ **T65.1X4** **Toxic effect of strychnine and its salts, undetermined**

T65.2 **Toxic effect of tobacco and nicotine**

Excludes2: nicotine dependence (F17.-)

T65.21 **Toxic effect of chewing tobacco**

⑦ **T65.211** **Toxic effect of chewing tobacco, accidental (unintentional)**

Toxic effect of chewing tobacco NOS

⑦ **T65.212** **Toxic effect of chewing tobacco, intentional self-harm**

⑦ **T65.213** **Toxic effect of chewing tobacco, assault**

⑦ **T65.214** **Toxic effect of chewing tobacco, undetermined**

T65.22 **Toxic effect of tobacco cigarettes**

Toxic effect of tobacco smoke

Use additional code for exposure to second hand tobacco smoke (Z57.31, Z77.22)

⑦ **T65.221** **Toxic effect of tobacco cigarettes, accidental (unintentional)**

Toxic effect of tobacco cigarettes NOS

⑦ **T65.222** **Toxic effect of tobacco cigarettes, intentional self-harm**

⑦ **T65.223** **Toxic effect of tobacco cigarettes, assault**

⑦ **T65.224** **Toxic effect of tobacco cigarettes, undetermined**

T65.29 **Toxic effect of other tobacco and nicotine**

⑦ **T65.291** **Toxic effect of other tobacco and nicotine, accidental (unintentional)**

Toxic effect of other tobacco and nicotine NOS

⑦ **T65.292** **Toxic effect of other tobacco and nicotine, intentional self-harm**

⑦ **T65.293** **Toxic effect of other tobacco and nicotine, assault**

⑦ **T65.294** **Toxic effect of other tobacco and nicotine, undetermined**

T65.3 **Toxic effect of nitroderivatives and aminoderivatives of benzene and its homologues**

Toxic effect of anilin [benzenamine]

Toxic effect of nitrobenzene

Toxic effect of trinitrotoluene

T65.3X **Toxic effect of nitroderivatives and aminoderivatives of benzene and its homologues**

⑦ **T65.3X1** **Toxic effect of nitroderivatives and aminoderivatives of benzene and its homologues, accidental (unintentional)**

Toxic effect of nitroderivatives and aminoderivatives of benzene and its homologues NOS

⑦ **T65.3X2** **Toxic effect of nitroderivatives and aminoderivatives of benzene and its homologues, intentional self-harm**

⑦ **T65.3X3** **Toxic effect of nitroderivatives and aminoderivatives of benzene and its homologues, assault**

⑦ **T65.3X4** **Toxic effect of nitroderivatives and aminoderivatives of benzene and its homologues, undetermined**

T65.4 **Toxic effect of carbon disulfide**

T65.4X **Toxic effect of carbon disulfide**

⑦ **T65.4X1** **Toxic effect of carbon disulfide, accidental (unintentional)**

Toxic effect of carbon disulfide NOS

⑦ **T65.4X2** **Toxic effect of carbon disulfide, intentional self-harm**

⑦ **T65.4X3** **Toxic effect of carbon disulfide, assault**

⑦ **T65.4X4** **Toxic effect of carbon disulfide, undetermined**

T65.5 **Toxic effect of nitroglycerin and other nitric acids and esters**

Toxic effect of 1,2,3-Propanetriol trinitrate

T65.5X **Toxic effect of nitroglycerin and other nitric acids and esters**

⑦ **T65.5X1** **Toxic effect of nitroglycerin and other nitric acids and esters, accidental (unintentional)**

Toxic effect of nitroglycerin and other nitric acids and esters NOS

⑦ **T65.5X2** **Toxic effect of nitroglycerin and other nitric acids and esters, intentional self-harm**

⑦ **T65.5X3** **Toxic effect of nitroglycerin and other nitric acids and esters, assault**

⑦ **T65.5X4** **Toxic effect of nitroglycerin and other nitric acids and esters, undetermined**

T65.6 **Toxic effect of paints and dyes, not elsewhere classified**

T65.6X **Toxic effect of paints and dyes, not elsewhere classified**

⑦ **T65.6X1** **Toxic effect of paints and dyes, not elsewhere classified, accidental (unintentional)**

Toxic effect of paints and dyes NOS

⑦ **T65.6X2** **Toxic effect of paints and dyes, not elsewhere classified, intentional self-harm**

⑦ **T65.6X3** **Toxic effect of paints and dyes, not elsewhere classified, assault**

⑦ **T65.6X4** **Toxic effect of paints and dyes, not elsewhere classified, undetermined**

T65.8 **Toxic effect of other specified substances**

T65.81 **Toxic effect of latex**

⑦ **T65.811** **Toxic effect of latex, accidental (unintentional)**

Toxic effect of latex NOS

⑦ **T65.812** **Toxic effect of latex, intentional self-harm**

⑦ **T65.813** **Toxic effect of latex, assault**

⑦ **T65.814** **Toxic effect of latex, undetermined**

T65.82 **Toxic effect of harmful algae and algae toxins**

Toxic effect of (harmful) algae bloom NOS

Toxic effect of blue-green algae bloom

Toxic effect of brown tide

Toxic effect of cyanobacteria bloom

● New code   ▲ Revised code   Excludes1: Not coded here   Excludes2: Not included here   ⊗ Placeholder required   ⑦ 7th digit required

Toxic effect of Florida red tide

Toxic effect of pfiesteria piscicida

Toxic effect of red tide

⑦**T65.821** **Toxic effect of harmful algae and algae toxins, accidental (unintentional)**

Toxic effect of harmful algae and algae toxins NOS

⑦**T65.822** **Toxic effect of harmful algae and algae toxins, intentional self-harm**

⑦**T65.823** **Toxic effect of harmful algae and algae toxins, assault**

⑦**T65.824** **Toxic effect of harmful algae and algae toxins, undetermined**

T65.83 **Toxic effect of fiberglass**

⑦**T65.831** **Toxic effect of fiberglass, accidental (unintentional)**

Toxic effect of fiberglass NOS

⑦**T65.832** **Toxic effect of fiberglass, intentional self-harm**

⑦**T65.833** **Toxic effect of fiberglass, assault**

⑦**T65.834** **Toxic effect of fiberglass, undetermined**

T65.89 **Toxic effect of other specified substances**

⑦**T65.891** **Toxic effect of other specified substances, accidental (unintentional)**

Toxic effect of other specified substances NOS

⑦**T65.892** **Toxic effect of other specified substances, intentional self-harm**

⑦**T65.893** **Toxic effect of other specified substances, assault**

⑦**T65.894** **Toxic effect of other specified substances, undetermined**

T65.9 **Toxic effect of unspecified substance**

⊗⑦**T65.91** **Toxic effect of unspecified substance, accidental (unintentional)**

Poisoning NOS

⊗⑦**T65.92** **Toxic effect of unspecified substance, intentional self-harm**

⊗⑦**T65.93** **Toxic effect of unspecified substance, assault**

⊗⑦**T65.94** **Toxic effect of unspecified substance, undetermined**

OTHER AND UNSPECIFIED EFFECTS OF EXTERNAL CAUSES (T66-T78)

⊗⑦**T66** **Radiation sickness, unspecified**

Excludes1: specified adverse effects of radiation, such as:

burns (T20-T31)

leukemia (C91-C95)

radiation gastroenteritis and colitis (K52.0)

radiation pneumonitis (J70.0)

radiation related disorders of the skin and subcutaneous tissue (L55-L59)

sunburn (L55.-)

The appropriate 7th character is to be added to code T66

A - initial encounter

D - subsequent encounter

S - sequela

T67 **Effects of heat and light**

Excludes1: erythema [dermatitis] ab igne (L59.0)

malignant hyperpyrexia due to anesthesia (T88.3)

radiation-related disorders of the skin and subcutaneous tissue (L55-L59)

Excludes2: burns (T20-T31)

sunburn (L55.-)

sweat disorder due to heat (L74-L75)

The appropriate 7th character is to be added to each code from category T67

A - initial encounter

D - subsequent encounter

S - sequela

⊗⑦**T67.0** **Heatstroke and sunstroke**

Heat apoplexy

Heat pyrexia

Siriasis

Thermoplegia

Use additional code(s) to identify any associated complications of heatstroke, such as:

coma and stupor (R40.-)

systemic inflammatory response syndrome (R65.1-)

⊗⑦**T67.1** **Heat syncope**

Heat collapse

⊗⑦**T67.2** **Heat cramp**

⊗⑦**T67.3** **Heat exhaustion, anhydrotic**

Heat prostration due to water depletion

Excludes1: heat exhaustion due to salt depletion (T67.4)

⊗⑦**T67.4** **Heat exhaustion due to salt depletion**

Heat prostration due to salt (and water) depletion

⊗⑦**T67.5** **Heat exhaustion, unspecified**

Heat prostration NOS

⊗⑦**T67.6** **Heat fatigue, transient**

⊗⑦**T67.7** **Heat edema**

⊗⑦**T67.8** **Other effects of heat and light**

⊗⑦**T67.9** **Effect of heat and light, unspecified**

⊗⑦**T68** **Hypothermia**

Accidental hypothermia

Hypothermia NOS

Use additional code to identify source of exposure:

Exposure to excessive cold of man-made origin (W93)

Exposure to excessive cold of natural origin (X31)

Excludes1: hypothermia following anesthesia (T88.51)

hypothermia not associated with low environmental temperature (R68.0)

hypothermia of newborn (P80.-)

Excludes2: frostbite (T33-T34)

The appropriate 7th character is to be added to code T68

A - initial encounter

D - subsequent encounter

S - sequela

T69 **Other effects of reduced temperature**

Use additional code to identify source of exposure:

Exposure to excessive cold of man-made origin (W93)

Exposure to excessive cold of natural origin (X31)

Excludes2: frostbite (T33-T34)

The appropriate 7th character is to be added to each code from category T69

A - initial encounter

D - subsequent encounter

S - sequela

T69.0 Immersion hand and foot

    T69.01 Immersion hand

      ⑦**T69.011 Immersion hand, right hand**

      ⑦**T69.012 Immersion hand, left hand**

      ⑦**T69.019 Immersion hand, unspecified hand**

    T69.02 Immersion foot

      Trench foot

      ⑦**T69.021 Immersion foot, right foot**

      ⑦**T69.022 Immersion foot, left foot**

      ⑦**T69.029 Immersion foot, unspecified foot**

⊗⑦**T69.1 Chilblains**

⊗⑦**T69.8 Other specified effects of reduced temperature**

⊗⑦**T69.9 Effect of reduced temperature, unspecified**

T70 Effects of air pressure and water pressure

The appropriate 7th character is to be added to each code from category T70

A - initial encounter

D - subsequent encounter

S - sequela

⊗⑦**T70.0 Otitic barotrauma**

    Aero-otitis media

    Effects of change in ambient atmospheric pressure or water pressure on ears

⊗⑦**T70.1 Sinus barotrauma**

    Aerosinusitis

    Effects of change in ambient atmospheric pressure on sinuses

T70.2 Other and unspecified effects of high altitude

    Excludes2: polycythemia due to high altitude (D75.1)

⊗⑦**T70.20 Unspecified effects of high altitude**

⊗⑦**T70.29 Other effects of high altitude**

    Alpine sickness

    Anoxia due to high altitude

    Barotrauma NOS

    Hypobaropathy

    Mountain sickness

⊗⑦**T70.3 Caisson disease [decompression sickness]**

    Compressed-air disease

    Diver's palsy or paralysis

⊗⑦**T70.4 Effects of high-pressure fluids**

    Hydraulic jet injection (industrial)

    Pneumatic jet injection (industrial)

    Traumatic jet injection (industrial)

⊗⑦**T70.8 Other effects of air pressure and water pressure**

⊗⑦**T70.9 Effect of air pressure and water pressure, unspecified**

T71 Asphyxiation

    Mechanical suffocation

    Traumatic suffocation

Excludes1: acute respiratory distress (syndrome) (J80)

anoxia due to high altitude (T70.2) asphyxia NOS (R09.01)

    asphyxia from carbon monoxide (T58.-)

    asphyxia from inhalation of food or foreign body (T17.-)

    asphyxia from other gases, fumes and vapors (T59.-)

    respiratory distress (syndrome) in newborn (P22.-)

The appropriate 7th character is to be added to each code from category T71

A - initial encounter

D - subsequent encounter

S - sequela

T71.1 Asphyxiation due to mechanical threat to breathing

    Suffocation due to mechanical threat to breathing

    T71.11 Asphyxiation due to smothering under pillow

      ⑦**T71.111 Asphyxiation due to smothering under pillow, accidental**

        Asphyxiation due to smothering under pillow NOS

      ⑦**T71.112 Asphyxiation due to smothering under pillow, intentional self-harm**

      ⑦**T71.113 Asphyxiation due to smothering under pillow, assault**

      ⑦**T71.114 Asphyxiation due to smothering under pillow, undetermined**

    T71.12 Asphyxiation due to plastic bag

      ⑦**T71.121 Asphyxiation due to plastic bag, accidental**

        Asphyxiation due to plastic bag NOS

      ⑦**T71.122 Asphyxiation due to plastic bag, intentional self-harm**

      ⑦**T71.123 Asphyxiation due to plastic bag, assault**

      ⑦**T71.124 Asphyxiation due to plastic bag, undetermined**

    T71.13 Asphyxiation due to being trapped in bed linens

      ⑦**T71.131 Asphyxiation due to being trapped in bed linens, accidental**

        Asphyxiation due to being trapped in bed linens NOS

      ⑦**T71.132 Asphyxiation due to being trapped in bed linens, intentional self-harm**

      ⑦**T71.133 Asphyxiation due to being trapped in bed linens, assault**

      ⑦**T71.134 Asphyxiation due to being trapped in bed linens, undetermined**

    T71.14 Asphyxiation due to smothering under another person's body (in bed)

      ⑦**T71.141 Asphyxiation due to smothering under another person's body (in bed), accidental**

        Asphyxiation due to smothering under another person's body (in bed) NOS

      ⑦**T71.143 Asphyxiation due to smothering under another person's body (in bed), assault**

      ⑦**T71.144 Asphyxiation due to smothering under another person's body (in bed), undetermined**

    T71.15 Asphyxiation due to smothering in furniture

● New code   ▲ Revised code   Excludes1: Not coded here   Excludes2: Not included here   ⊗ Placeholder required   ⑦ 7th digit required

⑦T71.151   **Asphyxiation due to smothering in furniture, accidental**

Asphyxiation due to smothering in furniture NOS

⑦T71.152   **Asphyxiation due to smothering in furniture, intentional self-harm**

⑦T71.153   **Asphyxiation due to smothering in furniture, assault**

⑦T71.154   **Asphyxiation due to smothering in furniture, undetermined**

T71.16   **Asphyxiation due to hanging**

Hanging by window shade cord

<u>Use additional code</u> for any associated injuries, such as:

crushing injury of neck (S17.-)

fracture of cervical vertebrae (S12.0-S12.2-)

open wound of neck (S11.-)

⑦T71.161   **Asphyxiation due to hanging, accidental**

Asphyxiation due to hanging NOS

Hanging NOS

⑦T71.162   **Asphyxiation due to hanging, intentional self-harm**

⑦T71.163   **Asphyxiation due to hanging, assault**

⑦T71.164   **Asphyxiation due to hanging, undetermined**

T71.19   **Asphyxiation due to mechanical threat to breathing due to other causes**

⑦T71.191   **Asphyxiation due to mechanical threat to breathing due to other causes, accidental**

Asphyxiation due **to other** causes NOS

⑦T71.192   **Asphyxiation due to mechanical threat to breathing due to other causes, intentional self-harm**

⑦T71.193   **Asphyxiation due to mechanical threat to breathing due to other causes, assault**

⑦T71.194   **Asphyxiation due to mechanical threat to breathing due to other causes, undetermined**

T71.2   **Asphyxiation due to systemic oxygen deficiency due to low oxygen content in ambient air**

Suffocation due to systemic oxygen deficiency due to low oxygen content in ambient air

⊗⑦T71.20   **Asphyxiation due to systemic oxygen deficiency due to low oxygen content in ambient air due to unspecified cause**

⊗⑦T71.21   **Asphyxiation due to cave-in or falling earth**

<u>Use additional code</u> for any associated cataclysm (X34-X38)

T71.22   **Asphyxiation due to being trapped in a car trunk**

⑦T71.221   **Asphyxiation due to being trapped in a car trunk, accidental**

⑦T71.222   **Asphyxiation due to being trapped in a car trunk, intentional self-harm**

⑦T71.223   **Asphyxiation due to being trapped in a car trunk, assault**

⑦T71.224   **Asphyxiation due to being trapped in a car trunk, undetermined**

T71.23   **Asphyxiation due to being trapped in a (discarded) refrigerator**

⑦T71.231   **Asphyxiation due to being trapped in a (discarded) refrigerator, accidental**

⑦T71.232   **Asphyxiation due to being trapped in a (discarded) refrigerator, intentional self-harm**

⑦T71.233   **Asphyxiation due to being trapped in a (discarded) refrigerator, assault**

⑦T71.234   **Asphyxiation due to being trapped in a (discarded) refrigerator, undetermined**

⊗⑦T71.29   **Asphyxiation due to being trapped in other low oxygen environment**

⊗⑦T71.9   **Asphyxiation due to unspecified cause**

Suffocation (by strangulation) due to unspecified cause

Suffocation NOS

Systemic oxygen deficiency due to low oxygen content in ambient air due to unspecified cause

Systemic oxygen deficiency due to mechanical threat to breathing due to unspecified cause

Traumatic asphyxia NOS

T73   Effects of other deprivation

The appropriate 7th character is to be added to each code from category T73

A - initial encounter

D - subsequent encounter

S - sequela

⊗⑦T73.0   **Starvation**

Deprivation of food

⊗⑦T73.1   **Deprivation of water**

⊗⑦T73.2   **Exhaustion due to exposure**

⊗⑦T73.3   **Exhaustion due to excessive exertion**

Exhaustion due to overexertion

⊗⑦T73.8   **Other effects of deprivation**

⊗⑦T73.9   **Effect of deprivation, unspecified**

T74   Adult and child abuse, neglect and other maltreatment, confirmed

<u>Use additional code</u>, if applicable, to identify any associated current injury

<u>Use additional</u> external cause code to identify perpetrator, if known (Y07.-)

Excludes1: abuse and maltreatment in pregnancy (O9A.3-, O9A.4-, O9A.5-)

adult and child maltreatment, suspected (T76.-)

The appropriate 7th character is to be added to each code from category T74

A - initial encounter

D - subsequent encounter

S - sequela

T74.0   **Neglect or abandonment, confirmed**

⊗⑦T74.01   **Adult neglect or abandonment, confirmed**

⊗⑦T74.02   **Child neglect or abandonment, confirmed**

T74.1   **Physical abuse, confirmed**

Excludes2: sexual abuse (T74.2-)

⊗⑦**T74.11**   **Adult physical abuse, confirmed**

⊗⑦**T74.12**   **Child physical abuse, confirmed**

       Excludes2: shaken infant syndrome (T74.4)

T74.2   **Sexual abuse, confirmed**

     Rape, confirmed

     Sexual assault, confirmed

⊗⑦**T74.21**   **Adult sexual abuse, confirmed**

⊗⑦**T74.22**   **Child sexual abuse, confirmed**

T74.3   **Psychological abuse, confirmed**

⊗⑦**T74.31**   **Adult psychological abuse, confirmed**

⊗⑦**T74.32**   **Child psychological abuse, confirmed**

T74.4   **Shaken infant syndrome**

T74.9   **Unspecified maltreatment, confirmed**

⊗⑦**T74.91**   **Unspecified adult maltreatment, confirmed**

⊗⑦**T74.92**   **Unspecified child maltreatment, confirmed**

T75   **Other and unspecified effects of other external causes**

Excludes1: adverse effects NEC (T78.-)

Excludes2: burns (electric) (T20-T31)

The appropriate 7th character is to be added to each code from category T75

A - initial encounter

D - subsequent encounter

S - sequela

T75.0   **Effects of lightning**

     Struck by lightning

⊗⑦**T75.00**   **Unspecified effects of lightning**

       Struck by lightning NOS

⊗⑦**T75.01**   **Shock due to being struck by lightning**

⊗⑦**T75.09**   **Other effects of lightning**

       Use additional code for other effects of lightning

⊗⑦**T75.1**   **Unspecified effects of drowning and nonfatal submersion**

     Immersion

       Excludes1: specified effects of drowning- code to effects

T75.2   **Effects of vibration**

⊗⑦**T75.20**   **Unspecified effects of vibration**

⊗⑦**T75.21**   **Pneumatic hammer syndrome**

⊗⑦**T75.22**   **Traumatic vasospastic syndrome**

⊗⑦**T75.23**   **Vertigo from infrasound**

       Excludes1: vertigo NOS (R42)

⊗⑦**T75.29**   **Other effects of vibration**

⊗⑦**T75.3**   **Motion sickness**

     Airsickness

     Seasickness

     Travel sickness

     Use additional external cause code to identify vehicle or type of motion (Y92.81-, Y93.5-)

⊗⑦**T75.4**   **Electrocution**

     Shock from electric current

     Shock from electroshock gun (taser)

T75.8   **Other specified effects of external causes**

⊗⑦**T75.81**   **Effects of abnormal gravitation [G] forces**

⊗⑦**T75.82**   **Effects of weightlessness**

⊗⑦**T75.89**   **Other specified effects of external causes**

T76   **Adult and child abuse, neglect and other maltreatment, suspected**

Use additional code, if applicable, to identify any associated current injury

Excludes1: adult and child maltreatment, confirmed (T74.-)

     suspected abuse and maltreatment in pregnancy (O9A.3-, O9A.4-, O9A.5-)

     suspected adult physical abuse, ruled out (Z04.71)

     suspected adult sexual abuse, ruled out (Z04.41)

     suspected child physical abuse, ruled out (Z04.72)

     suspected child sexual abuse, ruled out (Z04.42)

The appropriate 7th character is to be added to each code from category T76

A - initial encounter

D - subsequent encounter

S - sequela

T76.0   **Neglect or abandonment, suspected**

⊗⑦**T76.01**   **Adult neglect or abandonment, suspected**

⊗⑦**T76.02**   **Child neglect or abandonment, suspected**

T76.1   **Physical abuse, suspected**

⊗⑦**T76.11**   **Adult physical abuse, suspected**

⊗⑦**T76.12**   **Child physical abuse, suspected**

T76.2   **Sexual abuse, suspected**

     Rape, suspected

     Sexual abuse, suspected

       Excludes1: alleged abuse, ruled out (Z04.7)

⊗⑦**T76.21**   **Adult sexual abuse, suspected**

⊗⑦**T76.22**   **Child sexual abuse, suspected**

T76.3   **Psychological abuse, suspected**

⊗⑦**T76.31**   **Adult psychological abuse, suspected**

⊗⑦**T76.32**   **Child psychological abuse, suspected**

T76.9   **Unspecified maltreatment, suspected**

⊗⑦**T76.91**   **Unspecified adult maltreatment, suspected**

⊗⑦**T76.92**   **Unspecified child maltreatment, suspected**

T78   **Adverse effects, not elsewhere classified**

Excludes2: complications of surgical and medical care NEC (T80-T88)

The appropriate 7th character is to be added to each code from category T78

A - initial encounter

D - subsequent encounter

S - sequela

T78.0   **Anaphylactic reaction due to food**

     Anaphylactic reaction due to adverse food reaction

     Anaphylactic shock or reaction due to nonpoisonous foods

     Anaphylactoid reaction due to food

⊗⑦**T78.00**   **Anaphylactic reaction due to unspecified food**

⊗⑦**T78.01**   **Anaphylactic reaction due to peanuts**

⊗⑦**T78.02**   **Anaphylactic reaction due to shellfish (crustaceans)**

⊗⑦**T78.03**   **Anaphylactic reaction due to other fish**

⊗⑦**T78.04**   **Anaphylactic reaction due to fruits and vegetables**

⊗⑦**T78.05**   **Anaphylactic reaction due to tree nuts and seeds**

  ● New code   ▲ Revised code   Excludes1: Not coded here   Excludes2: Not included here   ⊗ Placeholder required   ⑦7th digit required

Excludes2: anaphylactic reaction due to peanuts (T78.01)

⊗⑦**T78.06** **Anaphylactic reaction due to food additives**

⊗⑦**T78.07** **Anaphylactic reaction due to milk and dairy products**

⊗⑦**T78.08** **Anaphylactic reaction due to eggs**

⊗⑦**T78.09** **Anaphylactic reaction due to other food products**

⊗⑦**T78.1** **Other adverse food reactions, not elsewhere classified**

Use additional code to identify the type of reaction, if applicable

Excludes1: anaphylactic reaction or shock due to adverse food reaction (T78.0-)

anaphylactic reaction due to food (T78.0-)

bacterial food borne intoxications (A05.-)

Excludes2: allergic and dietetic gastroenteritis and colitis (K52.29)

allergic rhinitis due to food (J30.5)

dermatitis due to food in contact with skin (L23.6, L24.6, L25.4)

dermatitis due to ingested food (L27.2)

food protein-induced enterocolitis syndrome (K52.21)

food protein-induced enteropathy (K52.22)

⊗⑦**T78.2** **Anaphylactic shock, unspecified**

Allergic shock

Anaphylactic reaction

Anaphylaxis

Excludes1: anaphylactic reaction or shock due to adverse effect of correct medicinal substance properly administered (T88.6)

anaphylactic reaction or shock due to adverse food reaction (T78.0-)

anaphylactic reaction or shock due to serum (T80.5-)

⊗⑦**T78.3** **Angioneurotic edema**

Allergic angioedema Giant urticaria Quincke's edema

Excludes1: serum urticaria (T80.6-)

urticaria (L50.-)

T78.4 **Other and unspecified allergy**

Excludes1: specified types of allergic reaction such as:

allergic diarrhea (K52.29)

allergic gastroenteritis and colitis (K52.29)

dermatitis (L23-L25, L27.-)

food protein-induced enterocolitis syndrome (K52.21)

food protein-induced enteropathy (K52.22)

hay fever (J30.1)

⊗⑦**T78.40** **Allergy, unspecified**

Allergic reaction NOS

Hypersensitivity NOS

⊗⑦**T78.41** **Arthus phenomenon**

Arthus reaction

⊗⑦**T78.49** **Other allergy**

⊗⑦**T78.8** **Other adverse effects, not elsewhere classified**

CERTAIN EARLY COMPLICATIONS OF TRAUMA (T79)

T79 **Certain early complications of trauma, not elsewhere classified**

Excludes2: acute respiratory distress syndrome (J80)

complications occurring during or following medical procedures (T80-T88)

complications of surgical and medical care NEC (T80-T88)

newborn respiratory distress syndrome (P22.0)

The appropriate 7th character is to be added to each code from category T79

A - initial encounter

D - subsequent encounter

S - sequela

⊗⑦**T79.0** **Air embolism (traumatic)**

Excludes1: air embolism complicating abortion or ectopic or molar pregnancy (O00-O07, O08.2)

air embolism complicating pregnancy, childbirth and the puerperium (O88.0)

air embolism following infusion, transfusion, and therapeutic injection (T80.0)

air embolism following procedure NEC (T81.7-)

⊗⑦**T79.1** **Fat embolism (traumatic)**

Excludes1: fat embolism complicating:

abortion or ectopic or molar pregnancy (O00-O07, O08.2)

pregnancy, childbirth and the puerperium (O88.8)

⊗⑦**T79.2** **Traumatic secondary and recurrent hemorrhage and seroma**

⊗⑦**T79.4** **Traumatic shock**

Shock (immediate) (delayed) following injury

Excludes1: anaphylactic shock due to adverse food reaction (T78.0-)

anaphylactic shock due to correct medicinal substance properly administered (T88.6)

anaphylactic shock due to serum (T80.5-)

anaphylactic shock NOS (T78.2)

anesthetic shock (T88.2)

electric shock (T75.4)

nontraumatic shock NEC (R57.-)

obstetric shock (O75.1)

postprocedural shock (T81.1-)

septic shock (R65.21)

shock complicating abortion or ectopic or molar pregnancy (O00-O07, O08.3)

shock due to lightning (T75.01)

shock NOS (R57.9)

⊗⑦**T79.5** **Traumatic anuria**

Crush syndrome

Renal failure following crushing

⊗⑦**T79.6** **Traumatic ischemia of muscle**

Traumatic rhabdomyolysis

Volkmann's ischemic contracture

Excludes2: anterior tibial syndrome (M76.8)

compartment syndrome (traumatic) (T79.A-)

nontraumatic ischemia of muscle (M62.2-)

⊗⑦**T79.7** **Traumatic subcutaneous emphysema**

Excludes1: emphysema NOS (J43)

emphysema (subcutaneous) resulting from a procedure (T81.82)

T79.A **Traumatic compartment syndrome**

Excludes1: fibromyalgia (M79.7)

nontraumatic compartment syndrome (M79.A-)

traumatic ischemic infarction of muscle (T79.6)

⊗⑦**T79.A0 Compartment syndrome, unspecified**

Compartment syndrome NOS

T79.A1 Traumatic compartment syndrome of upper extremity

Traumatic compartment syndrome of shoulder, arm, forearm, wrist, hand, and fingers

⑦**T79.A11 Traumatic compartment syndrome of right upper extremity**

⑦**T79.A12 Traumatic compartment syndrome of left upper extremity**

⑦**T79.A19 Traumatic compartment syndrome of unspecified upper extremity**

T79.A2 Traumatic compartment syndrome of lower extremity

Traumatic compartment syndrome of hip, buttock, thigh, leg, foot, and toes

⑦**T79.A21 Traumatic compartment syndrome of right lower extremity**

⑦**T79.A22 Traumatic compartment syndrome of left lower extremity**

⑦**T79.A29 Traumatic compartment syndrome of unspecified lower extremity**

⊗⑦**T79.A3 Traumatic compartment syndrome of abdomen**

⊗⑦**T79.A9 Traumatic compartment syndrome of other sites**

⊗⑦**T79.8 Other early complications of trauma**

⊗⑦**T79.9 Unspecified early complication of trauma**

COMPLICATIONS OF SURGICAL AND MEDICAL CARE, NOT ELSEWHERE CLASSIFIED (T80-T88)

Use additional code for adverse effect, if applicable, to identify drug (T36-T50 with fifth or sixth character 5)

Use additional code(s) to identify the specified condition resulting from the complication

Use additional code to identify devices involved and details of circumstances (Y62-Y82)

Excludes2: any encounters with medical care for postprocedural conditions in which no complications are present, such as:

artificial opening status (Z93.-) closure of external stoma (Z43.-)

fitting and adjustment of external prosthetic device (Z44.-)

burns and corrosions from local applications and irradiation (T20-T32)

complications of surgical procedures during pregnancy, childbirth and the puerperium (O00-O9A)

mechanical complication of respirator [ventilator] (J95.850)

poisoning and toxic effects of drugs and chemicals (T36-T65 with fifth or sixth character 1-4 or 6)

postprocedural fever (R50.82)

specified complications classified elsewhere, such as: cerebrospinal fluid leak from spinal puncture (G97.0)

colostomy malfunction (K94.0-)

disorders of fluid and electrolyte imbalance (E86-E87) f

unctional disturbances following cardiac surgery (I97.0-I97.1)

intraoperative and postprocedural complications of specified body systems (D78.-, E36.-, E89.-, G97.3-, G97.4, H59.3-, H59.-,

H95.2-, H95.3, I97.4-, I97.5, J95.6-, J95.7, K91.6-, L76.-, M96.-, N99.-)

ostomy complications (J95.0-, K94.-, N99.5-)

postgastric surgery syndromes (K91.1)

postlaminectomy syndrome NEC (M96.1)

postmastectomy lymphedema syndrome (I97.2)

postsurgical blind-loop syndrome (K91.2)

ventilator associated pneumonia (J95.851)

T80 Complications following infusion, transfusion and therapeutic injection

Includes: complications following perfusion

Excludes2: bone marrow transplant rejection (T86.01)

febrile nonhemolytic transfusion reaction (R50.84)

fluid overload due to transfusion (E87.71)

posttransfusion purpura (D69.51)

transfusion associated circulatory overload (TACO) (E87.71)

transfusion (red blood cell) associated hemochromatosis (E83.111)

transfusion related acute lung injury (TRALI) (J95.84)

The appropriate 7th character is to be added to each code from category T80

A - initial encounter

D - subsequent encounter

S - sequela

⊗⑦**T80.0 Air embolism following infusion, transfusion and therapeutic injection**

⊗⑦**T80.1 Vascular complications following infusion, transfusion and therapeutic injection**

Use additional code to identify the vascular complication

Excludes2: extravasation of vesicant agent (T80.81-)

infiltration of vesicant agent (T80.81-)

vascular complications specified as due to prosthetic devices, implants and grafts (T82.8-, T83.8-, T84.8-, T85.8-)

postprocedural vascular complications (T81.7-)

T80.2 Infections following infusion, transfusion and therapeutic injection

Use additional code to identify the specific infection, such as:

sepsis (A41.9)

Use additional code (R65.2-) to identify severe sepsis, if applicable

Excludes2: infections specified as due to prosthetic devices, implants and grafts (T82.6-T82.7, T83.5-T83.6, T84.5-T84.7, T85.7)

postprocedural infections (T81.4-)

T80.21 Infection due to central venous catheter

Infection due to pulmonary artery catheter (Swan-Ganz catheter)

⑦**T80.211 Bloodstream infection due to central venous catheter**

Catheter-related bloodstream infection (CRBSI) NOS

Central line-associated bloodstream infection (CLABSI)

Bloodstream infection due to Hickman catheter

Bloodstream infection due to peripherally inserted central catheter (PICC)

Bloodstream infection due to portacath (port-a-cath)

Bloodstream infection due to pulmonary artery catheter

Bloodstream infection due to triple lumen catheter

Bloodstream infection due to umbilical venous catheter

⑦T80.212 **Local infection due to central venous catheter**

Exit or insertion site infection

Local infection due to Hickman catheter

Local infection due to peripherally inserted central catheter (PICC)

Local infection due to portacath (port-a-cath)

Local infection due to pulmonary artery catheter

Local infection due to triple lumen catheter

Local infection due to umbilical venous catheter

Port or reservoir infection

Tunnel infection

⑦T80.218 **Other infection due to central venous catheter**

Other central line-associated infection

Other infection due to Hickman catheter

Other infection due to peripherally inserted central catheter (PICC)

Other infection due to portacath (port-a-cath)

Other infection due to pulmonary artery catheter

Other infection due to triple lumen catheter

Other infection due to umbilical venous catheter

⑦T80.219 **Unspecified infection due to central venous catheter**

Central line-associated infection NOS

Unspecified infection due to Hickman catheter

Unspecified infection due to peripherally inserted central catheter (PICC)

Unspecified infection due to portacath (port-a-cath)

Unspecified infection due to pulmonary artery catheter

Unspecified infection due to triple lumen catheter

Unspecified infection due to umbilical venous catheter

⊗⑦T80.22 **Acute infection following transfusion, infusion, or injection of blood and blood products**

⊗⑦T80.29 **Infection following other infusion, transfusion and therapeutic injection**

T80.3 **ABO incompatibility reaction due to transfusion of blood or blood products**

Excludes1: minor blood group antigens reactions (Duffy) (E) (K(ell)) (Kidd) (Lewis) (M) (N) (P) (S) (T80.A)

⊗⑦T80.30 **ABO incompatibility reaction due to transfusion of blood or blood products, unspecified**

ABO incompatibility blood transfusion NOS

Reaction to ABO incompatibility from transfusion NOS

T80.31 **ABO incompatibility with hemolytic transfusion reaction**

⑦T80.310 **ABO incompatibility with acute hemolytic transfusion reaction**

ABO incompatibility with hemolytic transfusion reaction less than 24 hours after transfusion

Acute hemolytic transfusion reaction (AHTR) due to ABO incompatibility

⑦T80.311 **ABO incompatibility with delayed hemolytic transfusion reaction**

ABO incompatibility with hemolytic transfusion reaction 24 hours or more after transfusion

Delayed hemolytic transfusion reaction (DHTR) due to ABO incompatibility

⑦T80.319 **ABO incompatibility with hemolytic transfusion reaction, unspecified**

ABO incompatibility with hemolytic transfusion reaction at unspecified time after transfusion

Hemolytic transfusion reaction (HTR) due to ABO incompatibility NOS

⑦T80.39 **Other ABO incompatibility reaction due to transfusion of blood or blood products**

Delayed serologic transfusion reaction (DSTR) from ABO incompatibility

Other ABO incompatible blood transfusion

Other reaction to ABO incompatible blood transfusion

T80.4 **Rh incompatibility reaction due to transfusion of blood or blood products**

Reaction due to incompatibility of Rh antigens (C) (c) (D) (E) (e)

⊗⑦T80.40 **Rh incompatibility reaction due to transfusion of blood or blood products, unspecified**

Reaction due to Rh factor in transfusion NOS

Rh incompatible blood transfusion NOS

T80.41 **Rh incompatibility with hemolytic transfusion reaction**

⑦T80.410 **Rh incompatibility with acute hemolytic transfusion reaction**

Acute hemolytic transfusion reaction (AHTR) due to Rh incompatibility

Rh incompatibility with hemolytic transfusion reaction less than 24 hours after transfusion

⑦T80.411 **Rh incompatibility with delayed hemolytic transfusion reaction**

Delayed hemolytic transfusion reaction (DHTR) due to Rh incompatibility

Rh incompatibility with hemolytic transfusion reaction 24 hours or more after transfusion

⑦ **T80.419** **Rh incompatibility with hemolytic transfusion reaction, unspecified**

Rh incompatibility with hemolytic transfusion reaction at unspecified time after transfusion

Hemolytic transfusion reaction (HTR) due to Rh incompatibility NOS

⊗⑦ **T80.49** **Other Rh incompatibility reaction due to transfusion of blood or blood products**

Delayed serologic transfusion reaction (DSTR) from Rh incompatibility

Other reaction to Rh incompatible blood transfusion

T80.A **Non-ABO incompatibility reaction due to transfusion of blood or blood products**

Reaction due to incompatibility of minor antigens (Duffy) (Kell) (Kidd) (Lewis) (M) (N) (P) (S)

⊗⑦ **T80.A0** **Non-ABO incompatibility reaction due to transfusion of blood or blood products, unspecified**

Non-ABO antigen incompatibility reaction from transfusion NOS

T80.A1 **Non-ABO incompatibility with hemolytic transfusion reaction**

⑦ **T80.A10** **Non-ABO incompatibility with acute hemolytic transfusion reaction**

Acute hemolytic transfusion reaction (AHTR) due to non-ABO incompatibility

Non-ABO incompatibility with hemolytic transfusion reaction less than 24 hours after transfusion

⑦ **T80.A11** **Non-ABO incompatibility with delayed hemolytic transfusion reaction**

Delayed hemolytic transfusion reaction (DHTR) due to non-ABO incompatibility

Non-ABO incompatibility with hemolytic transfusion reaction 24 or more hours after transfusion

⑦ **T80.A19** **Non-ABO incompatibility with hemolytic transfusion reaction, unspecified**

Hemolytic transfusion reaction (HTR) due to non-ABO incompatibility NOS

Non-ABO incompatibility with hemolytic transfusion reaction at unspecified time after transfusion

⊗⑦ **T80.A9** **Other non-ABO incompatibility reaction due to transfusion of blood or blood products**

Delayed serologic transfusion reaction (DSTR) from non-ABO incompatibility

Other reaction to non-ABO incompatible blood transfusion

T80.5 **Anaphylactic reaction due to serum**

Allergic shock due to serum

Anaphylactic shock due to serum

Anaphylactoid reaction due to serum

Anaphylaxis due to serum

Excludes1: ABO incompatibility reaction due to transfusion of blood or blood products (T80.3-)

allergic reaction or shock NOS (T78.2)

anaphylactic reaction or shock NOS (T78.2)

anaphylactic reaction or shock due to adverse effect of correct medicinal substance properly administered (T88.6) **Other** serum reaction (T80.6-)

⊗⑦ **T80.51** **Anaphylactic reaction due to administration of blood and blood products**

⊗⑦ **T80.52** **Anaphylactic reaction due to vaccination**

⊗⑦ **T80.59** **Anaphylactic reaction due to other serum**

T80.6 **Other serum reactions** intoxication by serum

Protein sickness

Serum rash

Serum sickness

Serum urticaria

Excludes2: serum hepatitis (B16-B19)

⊗⑦ **T80.61** **Other serum reaction due to administration of blood and blood products**

⊗⑦ **T80.62** **Other serum reaction due to vaccination**

⊗⑦ **T80.69** **Other serum reaction due to other serum**

T80.8 **Other complications following infusion, transfusion and therapeutic injection**

T80.81 **Extravasation of vesicant agent**

Infiltration of vesicant agent

⑦ **T80.810** **Extravasation of vesicant antineoplastic chemotherapy**

Infiltration of vesicant antineoplastic chemotherapy

⑦ **T80.818** **Extravasation of other vesicant agent**

Infiltration **of other** vesicant agent

⊗⑦ **T80.89** **Other complications following infusion, transfusion and therapeutic injection**

Delayed serologic transfusion reaction (DSTR), unspecified incompatibility

Use additional code to identify graft-versus-host reaction, if applicable, (D89.81-)

T80.9 **Unspecified complication following infusion, transfusion and therapeutic injection**

⊗⑦ **T80.90** **Unspecified complication following infusion and therapeutic injection**

T80.91 **Hemolytic transfusion reaction, unspecified incompatibility**

Excludes1: ABO incompatibility with hemolytic transfusion reaction (T80.31-)

Non-ABO incompatibility with hemolytic transfusion reaction (T80.A1-)

Rh incompatibility with hemolytic transfusion reaction (T80.41-)

⑦ **T80.910** **Acute hemolytic transfusion reaction, unspecified incompatibility**

● New code ▲ Revised code **Excludes1:** Not coded here **Excludes2:** Not included here ⊗ Placeholder required ⑦ 7th digit required

⑦ **T80.911**   **Delayed hemolytic transfusion reaction, unspecified incompatibility**

⑦ **T80.919**   **Hemolytic transfusion reaction, unspecified incompatibility, unspecified as acute or delayed**

Hemolytic transfusion reaction NOS

⊗⑦**T80.92**   **Unspecified transfusion reaction**

Transfusion reaction NOS

T81   **Complications of procedures, not elsewhere classified**

Use additional code for adverse effect, if applicable, to identify drug (T36-T50 with fifth or sixth character 5)

Excludes2: complications following immunization (T88.0-T88.1)

complications following infusion, transfusion and therapeutic injection (T80.-)

complications of transplanted organs and tissue (T86.-)

specified complications classified elsewhere, such as: complication of prosthetic devices, implants and grafts (T82-T85)

dermatitis due to drugs and medicaments (L23.3, L24.4, L25.1, L27.0-L27.1)

endosseous dental implant failure (M27.6-)

floppy iris syndrome (IFIS) (intraoperative) H21.81

intraoperative and postprocedural complications of specific body system (D78.-, E36.-, E89.-, G97.3-, G97.4, H59.3-, H59.-, H95.2-, H95.3, I97.4-, I97.5, J95, K91.-, L76.-, M96.-, N99.-)

ostomy complications (J95.0-, K94.-, N99.5-)

plateau iris syndrome (post-iridectomy) (postprocedural) H21.82

poisoning and toxic effects of drugs and chemicals (T36-T65 with fifth or sixth character 1-4 or 6)

The appropriate 7th character is to be added to each code from category T81

A - initial encounter

D - subsequent encounter

S - sequela

T81.1   **Postprocedural shock**

Shock during or resulting from a procedure, not elsewhere classified

Excludes1: anaphylactic shock NOS (T78.2)

anaphylactic shock due to correct substance properly administered (T88.6)

anaphylactic shock due to serum (T80.5-)

anesthetic shock (T88.2)

electric shock (T75.4)

obstetric shock (O75.1)

septic shock (R65.21)

shock following abortion or ectopic or molar pregnancy (O00-O07, O08.3)

traumatic shock (T79.4)

⊗⑦**T81.10**   **Postprocedural shock unspecified**

Collapse NOS during or resulting from a procedure, not elsewhere classified

Postprocedural failure of peripheral circulation

Postprocedural shock NOS

⊗⑦**T81.11**   **Postprocedural cardiogenic shock**

⊗⑦**T81.12**   **Postprocedural septic shock**

Postprocedural endotoxic shock resulting from a procedure, not elsewhere classified

Postprocedural gram-negative shock resulting from a procedure, not elsewhere classified

Code first underlying infection

Use additional code, to identify any associated acute organ dysfunction, if applicable

⊗⑦**T81.19**   **Other postprocedural shock**

Postprocedural hypovolemic shock

T81.3   **Disruption of wound, not elsewhere classified**

Disruption of any suture materials or other closure methods

Excludes1: breakdown (mechanical) of permanent sutures (T85.612)

displacement of permanent sutures (T85.622)

disruption of cesarean delivery wound (O90.0)

disruption of perineal obstetric wound (O90.1)

mechanical complication of permanent sutures NEC (T85.692)

⊗⑦**T81.30**   **Disruption of wound, unspecified**

Disruption of wound NOS

⊗⑦**T81.31**   **Disruption of external operation (surgical) wound, not elsewhere classified**

Dehiscence of operation wound NOS

Disruption of operation wound NOS

Disruption or dehiscence of closure of cornea

Disruption or dehiscence of closure of mucosa

Disruption or dehiscence of closure of skin and subcutaneous tissue

Full-thickness skin disruption or dehiscence

Superficial disruption or dehiscence of operation wound

Excludes1: dehiscence of amputation stump (T87.81)

⊗⑦**T81.32**   **Disruption of internal operation (surgical) wound, not elsewhere classified**

Deep disruption or dehiscence of operation wound NOS

Disruption or dehiscence of closure of internal organ or other internal tissue

Disruption or dehiscence of closure of muscle or muscle flap

Disruption or dehiscence of closure of ribs or rib cage

Disruption or dehiscence of closure of skull or craniotomy

Disruption or dehiscence of closure of sternum or sternotomy

Disruption or dehiscence of closure of tendon or ligament

Disruption or dehiscence of closure of superficial or muscular fascia

⊗⑦**T81.33**   **Disruption of traumatic injury wound repair**

Disruption or dehiscence of closure of traumatic laceration (external) (internal)

⊗⑦**T81.4**   **Infection following a procedure**

Intra-abdominal abscess following a procedure

Postprocedural infection, not elsewhere classified

Sepsis following a procedure

Stitch abscess following a procedure

Subphrenic abscess following a procedure

Wound abscess following a procedure

Use additional code to identify infection

Use additional code (R65.2-) to identify severe sepsis, if applicable

Excludes1: obstetric surgical wound infection (O86.0)

postprocedural fever NOS (R50.82)

postprocedural retroperitoneal abscess (K68.11)

Excludes2: bleb associated endophthalmitis (H59.4-)

infection due to infusion, transfusion and therapeutic injection (T80.2-)

infection due to prosthetic devices, implants and grafts (T82.6-T82.7, T83.5-T83.6, T84.5-T84.7, T85.7)

T81.5 Complications of foreign body accidentally left in body following procedure

T81.50 Unspecified complication of foreign body accidentally left in body following procedure

⑦**T81.500 Unspecified complication of foreign body accidentally left in body following surgical operation**

⑦**T81.501 Unspecified complication of foreign body accidentally left in body following infusion or transfusion**

⑦**T81.502 Unspecified complication of foreign body accidentally left in body following kidney dialysis**

⑦**T81.503 Unspecified complication of foreign body accidentally left in body following injection or immunization**

⑦**T81.504 Unspecified complication of foreign body accidentally left in body following endoscopic examination**

⑦**T81.505 Unspecified complication of foreign body accidentally left in body following heart catheterization**

⑦**T81.506 Unspecified complication of foreign body accidentally left in body following aspiration, puncture or other catheterization**

⑦**T81.507 Unspecified complication of foreign body accidentally left in body following removal of catheter or packing**

⑦**T81.508 Unspecified complication of foreign body accidentally left in body following other procedure**

⑦**T81.509 Unspecified complication of foreign body accidentally left in body following unspecified procedure**

T81.51 Adhesions due to foreign body accidentally left in body following procedure

⑦**T81.510 Adhesions due to foreign body accidentally left in body following surgical operation**

⑦**T81.511 Adhesions due to foreign body accidentally left in body following infusion or transfusion**

⑦**T81.512 Adhesions due to foreign body accidentally left in body following kidney dialysis**

⑦**T81.513 Adhesions due to foreign body accidentally left in body following injection or immunization**

⑦**T81.514 Adhesions due to foreign body accidentally left in body following endoscopic examination**

⑦**T81.515 Adhesions due to foreign body accidentally left in body following heart catheterization**

⑦**T81.516 Adhesions due to foreign body accidentally left in body following aspiration, puncture or other catheterization**

⑦**T81.517 Adhesions due to foreign body accidentally left in body following removal of catheter or packing**

⑦**T81.518 Adhesions due to foreign body accidentally left in body following other procedure**

⑦**T81.519 Adhesions due to foreign body accidentally left in body following unspecified procedure**

T81.52 Obstruction due to foreign body accidentally left in body following procedure

⑦**T81.520 Obstruction due to foreign body accidentally left in body following surgical operation**

⑦**T81.521 Obstruction due to foreign body accidentally left in body following infusion or transfusion**

⑦**T81.522 Obstruction due to foreign body accidentally left in body following kidney dialysis**

⑦**T81.523 Obstruction due to foreign body accidentally left in body following injection or immunization**

⑦**T81.524 Obstruction due to foreign body accidentally left in body following endoscopic examination**

⑦**T81.525 Obstruction due to foreign body accidentally left in body following heart catheterization**

⑦**T81.526 Obstruction due to foreign body accidentally left in body following aspiration, puncture or other catheterization**

⑦**T81.527 Obstruction due to foreign body accidentally left in body following removal of catheter or packing**

⑦**T81.528 Obstruction due to foreign body accidentally left in body following other procedure**

⑦**T81.529 Obstruction due to foreign body accidentally left in body following unspecified procedure**

T81.53 Perforation due to foreign body accidentally left in body following procedure

⑦**T81.530 Perforation due to foreign body accidentally left in body following surgical operation**

⑦**T81.531 Perforation due to foreign body accidentally left in body following infusion or transfusion**

⑦ **T81.532** **Perforation due to foreign body accidentally left in body following kidney dialysis**

⑦ **T81.533** **Perforation due to foreign body accidentally left in body following injection or immunization**

⑦ **T81.534** **Perforation due to foreign body accidentally left in body following endoscopic examination**

⑦ **T81.535** **Perforation due to foreign body accidentally left in body following heart catheterization**

⑦ **T81.536** **Perforation due to foreign body accidentally left in body following aspiration, puncture or other catheterization**

⑦ **T81.537** **Perforation due to foreign body accidentally left in body following removal of catheter or packing**

⑦ **T81.538** **Perforation due to foreign body accidentally left in body following other procedure**

⑦ **T81.539** **Perforation due to foreign body accidentally left in body following unspecified procedure**

T81.59 **Other complications of foreign body accidentally left in body following procedure**

Excludes2: obstruction or perforation due to prosthetic devices and implants intentionally left in body (T82.0-T82.5, T83.0-T83.4, T83.7, T84.0-T84.4, T85.0-T85.6)

⑦ **T81.590** **Other complications of foreign body accidentally left in body following surgical operation**

⑦ **T81.591** **Other complications of foreign body accidentally left in body following infusion or transfusion**

⑦ **T81.592** **Other complications of foreign body accidentally left in body following kidney dialysis**

⑦ **T81.593** **Other complications of foreign body accidentally left in body following injection or immunization**

⑦ **T81.594** **Other complications of foreign body accidentally left in body following endoscopic examination**

⑦ **T81.595** **Other complications of foreign body accidentally left in body following heart catheterization**

⑦ **T81.596** **Other complications of foreign body accidentally left in body following aspiration, puncture or other catheterization**

⑦ **T81.597** **Other complications of foreign body accidentally left in body following removal of catheter or packing**

⑦ **T81.598** **Other complications of foreign body accidentally left in body following other procedure**

⑦ **T81.599** **Other complications of foreign body accidentally left in body following unspecified procedure**

T81.6 **Acute reaction to foreign substance accidentally left during a procedure**

Excludes2: complications of foreign body accidentally left in body cavity or operation wound following procedure (T81.5-)

⊗⑦**T81.60** **Unspecified acute reaction to foreign substance accidentally left during a procedure**

⊗⑦**T81.61** **Aseptic peritonitis due to foreign substance accidentally left during a procedure**

Chemical peritonitis

⊗⑦**T81.69** **Other acute reaction to foreign substance accidentally left during a procedure**

T81.7 **Vascular complications following a procedure, not elsewhere classified**

Air embolism following procedure NEC

Phlebitis or thrombophlebitis resulting from a procedure

Excludes1: embolism complicating abortion or ectopic or molar pregnancy (O00-O07, O08.2)

embolism complicating pregnancy, childbirth and the puerperium (O88.-)

traumatic embolism (T79.0)

Excludes2: embolism due to prosthetic devices, implants and grafts (T82.8-, T83.81, T84.8-, T85.81-)

embolism following infusion, transfusion and therapeutic injection (T80.0)

T81.71 **Complication of artery following a procedure, not elsewhere classified**

⑦ **T81.710** **Complication of mesenteric artery following a procedure, not elsewhere classified**

⑦ **T81.711** **Complication of renal artery following a procedure, not elsewhere classified**

⑦ **T81.718** **Complication of other artery following a procedure, not elsewhere classified**

⑦ **T81.719** **Complication of unspecified artery following a procedure, not elsewhere classified**

⊗⑦**T81.72** **Complication of vein following a procedure, not elsewhere classified**

T81.8 **Other complications of procedures, not elsewhere classified**

Excludes2: hypothermia following anesthesia (T88.51)

malignant hyperpyrexia due to anesthesia (T88.3)

⊗⑦**T81.81** **Complication of inhalation therapy**

⊗⑦**T81.82** **Emphysema (subcutaneous) resulting from a procedure**

⊗⑦**T81.83** **Persistent postprocedural fistula**

⊗⑦**T81.89** **Other complications of procedures, not elsewhere classified**

Use additional code to specify complication, such as:

postprocedural delirium (F05)

⊗⑦**T81.9** **Unspecified complication of procedure**

T82 **Complications of cardiac and vascular prosthetic devices, implants and grafts**

Excludes2: failure and rejection of transplanted organs and tissue (T86.-)

The appropriate 7th character is to be added to each code from category T82

A - initial encounter

D - subsequent encounter

S - sequela

T82.0   Mechanical complication of heart valve prosthesis

Mechanical complication of artificial heart valve

Excludes1: mechanical complication of biological heart valve graft (T82.22-)

⊗⑦**T82.01   Breakdown (mechanical) of heart valve prosthesis**

⊗⑦**T82.02   Displacement of heart valve prosthesis**

Malposition of heart valve prosthesis

⊗⑦**T82.03   Leakage of heart valve prosthesis**

⊗⑦**T82.09   Other mechanical complication of heart valve prosthesis**

Obstruction (mechanical) of heart valve prosthesis

Perforation of heart valve prosthesis

Protrusion of heart valve prosthesis

T82.1   Mechanical complication of cardiac electronic device

T82.11   Breakdown (mechanical) of cardiac electronic device

⑦**T82.110   Breakdown (mechanical) of cardiac electrode**

⑦**T82.111   Breakdown (mechanical) of cardiac pulse generator (battery)**

⑦**T82.118   Breakdown (mechanical) of other cardiac electronic device**

⑦**T82.119   Breakdown (mechanical) of unspecified cardiac electronic device**

T82.12   Displacement of cardiac electronic device

Malposition of cardiac electronic device

⑦**T82.120   Displacement of cardiac electrode**

⑦**T82.121   Displacement of cardiac pulse generator (battery)**

⑦**T82.128   Displacement of other cardiac electronic device**

⑦**T82.129   Displacement of unspecified cardiac electronic device**

T82.19   Other mechanical complication of cardiac electronic device

Leakage of cardiac electronic device

Obstruction of cardiac electronic device

Perforation of cardiac electronic device

Protrusion of cardiac electronic device

⑦**T82.190   Other mechanical complication of cardiac electrode**

⑦**T82.191   Other mechanical complication of cardiac pulse generator (battery)**

⑦**T82.198   Other mechanical complication of other cardiac electronic device**

⑦**T82.199   Other mechanical complication of unspecified cardiac device**

T82.2   Mechanical complication of coronary artery bypass graft and biological heart valve graft

Excludes1: mechanical complication of artificial heart valve prosthesis (T82.0-)

T82.21   Mechanical complication of coronary artery bypass graft

⑦**T82.211   Breakdown (mechanical) of coronary artery bypass graft**

⑦**T82.212   Displacement of coronary artery bypass graft**

Malposition of coronary artery bypass graft

⑦**T82.213   Leakage of coronary artery bypass graft**

⑦**T82.218   Other mechanical complication of coronary artery bypass graft**

Obstruction, mechanical of coronary artery bypass graft

Perforation of coronary artery bypass graft

Protrusion of coronary artery bypass graft

T82.22   Mechanical complication of biological heart valve graft

⑦**T82.221   Breakdown (mechanical) of biological heart valve graft**

⑦**T82.222   Displacement of biological heart valve graft**

Malposition of biological heart valve graft

⑦**T82.223   Leakage of biological heart valve graft**

⑦**T82.228   Other mechanical complication of biological heart valve graft**

Obstruction of biological heart valve graft

Perforation of biological heart valve graft

Protrusion of biological heart valve graft

T82.3   Mechanical complication of other vascular grafts

T82.31   Breakdown (mechanical) of other vascular grafts

⑦**T82.310   Breakdown (mechanical) of aortic (bifurcation) graft (replacement)**

⑦**T82.311   Breakdown (mechanical) of carotid arterial graft (bypass)**

⑦**T82.312   Breakdown (mechanical) of femoral arterial graft (bypass)**

⑦**T82.318   Breakdown (mechanical) of other vascular grafts**

⑦**T82.319   Breakdown (mechanical) of unspecified vascular grafts**

T82.32   Displacement of other vascular grafts

Malposition of other vascular grafts

⑦**T82.320   Displacement of aortic (bifurcation) graft (replacement)**

⑦**T82.321   Displacement of carotid arterial graft (bypass)**

⑦**T82.322   Displacement of femoral arterial graft (bypass)**

⑦**T82.328   Displacement of other vascular grafts**

⑦**T82.329   Displacement of unspecified vascular grafts**

T82.33   Leakage of other vascular grafts

● New code   ▲ Revised code   **Excludes1:** Not coded here   **Excludes2:** Not included here   ⊗ Placeholder required   ⑦7th digit required

⑦T82.330　Leakage of aortic (bifurcation) graft (replacement)

⑦T82.331　Leakage of carotid arterial graft (bypass)

⑦T82.332　Leakage of femoral arterial graft (bypass)

⑦T82.338　Leakage of other vascular grafts

⑦T82.339　Leakage of unspecified vascular graft

T82.39　Other mechanical complication of other vascular grafts

Obstruction (mechanical) of other vascular grafts

Perforation of other vascular grafts

Protrusion of other vascular grafts

⑦T82.390　Other mechanical complication of aortic (bifurcation) graft (replacement)

⑦T82.391　Other mechanical complication of carotid arterial graft (bypass)

⑦T82.392　Other mechanical complication of femoral arterial graft (bypass)

⑦T82.398　Other mechanical complication of other vascular grafts

⑦T82.399　Other mechanical complication of unspecified vascular grafts

T82.4　Mechanical complication of vascular dialysis catheter

Mechanical complication of hemodialysis catheter

Excludes1: mechanical complication of intraperitoneal dialysis catheter (T85.62)

⊗⑦T82.41　Breakdown (mechanical) of vascular dialysis catheter

⊗⑦T82.42　Displacement of vascular dialysis catheter

Malposition of vascular dialysis catheter

⊗⑦T82.43　Leakage of vascular dialysis catheter

⊗⑦T82.49　Other complication of vascular dialysis catheter

Obstruction (mechanical) of vascular dialysis catheter

Perforation of vascular dialysis catheter

Protrusion of vascular dialysis catheter

T82.5　Mechanical complication of other cardiac and vascular devices and implants

Excludes2: mechanical complication of epidural and subdural infusion catheter (T85.61)

T82.51　Breakdown (mechanical) of other cardiac and vascular devices and implants

⑦T82.510　Breakdown (mechanical) of surgically created arteriovenous fistula

⑦T82.511　Breakdown (mechanical) of surgically created arteriovenous shunt

⑦T82.512　Breakdown (mechanical) of artificial heart

⑦T82.513　Breakdown (mechanical) of balloon (counterpulsation) device

⑦T82.514　Breakdown (mechanical) of infusion catheter

⑦T82.515　Breakdown (mechanical) of umbrella device

⑦T82.518　Breakdown (mechanical) of other cardiac and vascular devices and implants

⑦T82.519　Breakdown (mechanical) of unspecified cardiac and vascular devices and implants

T82.52　Displacement of other cardiac and vascular devices and implants

Malposition of other cardiac and vascular devices and implants

⑦T82.520　Displacement of surgically created arteriovenous fistula

⑦T82.521　Displacement of surgically created arteriovenous shunt

⑦T82.522　Displacement of artificial heart

⑦T82.523　Displacement of balloon (counterpulsation) device

⑦T82.524　Displacement of infusion catheter

⑦T82.525　Displacement of umbrella device

⑦T82.528　Displacement of other cardiac and vascular devices and implants

⑦T82.529　Displacement of unspecified cardiac and vascular devices and implants

T82.53　Leakage of other cardiac and vascular devices and implants

⑦T82.530　Leakage of surgically created arteriovenous fistula

⑦T82.531　Leakage of surgically created arteriovenous shunt

⑦T82.532　Leakage of artificial heart

⑦T82.533　Leakage of balloon (counterpulsation) device

⑦T82.534　Leakage of infusion catheter

⑦T82.535　Leakage of umbrella device

⑦T82.538　Leakage of other cardiac and vascular devices and implants

⑦T82.539　Leakage of unspecified cardiac and vascular devices and implants

T82.59　Other mechanical complication of other cardiac and vascular devices and implants

Obstruction (mechanical) of other cardiac and vascular devices and implants

Perforation of other cardiac and vascular devices and implants

Protrusion of other cardiac and vascular devices and implants

⑦T82.590　Other mechanical complication of surgically created arteriovenous fistula

⑦T82.591　Other mechanical complication of surgically created arteriovenous shunt

⑦T82.592　Other mechanical complication of artificial heart

⑦T82.593　Other mechanical complication of balloon (counterpulsation) device

⑦T82.594　Other mechanical complication of infusion catheter

⑦T82.595　Other mechanical complication of umbrella device

⑦ **T82.598** Other mechanical complication of other cardiac and vascular devices and implants

⑦ **T82.599** Other mechanical complication of unspecified cardiac and vascular devices and implants

⊗⑦**T82.6** Infection and inflammatory reaction due to cardiac valve prosthesis

<u>Use additional code</u> to identify infection

⊗⑦**T82.7** Infection and inflammatory reaction due to other cardiac and vascular devices, implants and grafts

<u>Use additional code</u> to identify infection

T82.8 Other specified complications of cardiac and vascular prosthetic devices, implants and grafts

T82.81 Embolism due to cardiac and vascular prosthetic devices, implants and grafts

▲⑦**T82.817** Embolism due to cardiac prosthetic devices, implants and grafts

▲⑦**T82.818** Embolism due to vascular prosthetic devices, implants and grafts

T82.82 Fibrosis due to cardiac and vascular prosthetic devices, implants and grafts

▲⑦**T82.827** Fibrosis due to cardiac prosthetic devices, implants and grafts

▲⑦**T82.828** Fibrosis due to vascular prosthetic devices, implants and grafts

T82.83 Hemorrhage due to cardiac and vascular prosthetic devices, implants and grafts

▲⑦**T82.837** Hemorrhage due to cardiac prosthetic devices, implants and grafts

▲⑦**T82.838** Hemorrhage due to vascular prosthetic devices, implants and grafts

T82.84 Pain due to cardiac and vascular prosthetic devices, implants and grafts

▲⑦**T82.847** Pain due to cardiac prosthetic devices, implants and grafts

▲⑦**T82.848** Pain due to vascular prosthetic devices, implants and grafts

T82.85 Stenosis due to cardiac and vascular prosthetic devices, implants and grafts

●⑦**T82.855** Stenosis of coronary artery stent

In-stent stenosis (restenosis) of coronary artery stent

Restenosis of coronary artery stent

●⑦**T82.856** Stenosis of peripheral vascular stent

In-stent stenosis (restenosis) of peripheral vascular stent

Restenosis of peripheral vascular stent

▲⑦**T82.857** Stenosis of other cardiac prosthetic devices, implants and grafts

▲⑦**T82.858** Stenosis of other vascular prosthetic devices, implants and grafts

T82.86 Thrombosis of cardiac and vascular prosthetic devices, implants and grafts

▲⑦**T82.867** Thrombosis due to cardiac prosthetic devices, implants and grafts

▲⑦**T82.868** Thrombosis due to vascular prosthetic devices, implants and grafts

T82.89 Other specified complication of cardiac and vascular prosthetic devices, implants and grafts

⑦**T82.897** Other specified complication of cardiac prosthetic devices, implants and grafts

⑦**T82.898** Other specified complication of vascular prosthetic devices, implants and grafts

⊗⑦**T82.9** Unspecified complication of cardiac and vascular prosthetic device, implant and graft

T83 Complications of genitourinary prosthetic devices, implants and grafts

Excludes2: failure and rejection of transplanted organs and tissue (T86.-)

The appropriate 7th character is to be added to each code from category T83

A - initial encounter

D - subsequent encounter

S - sequela

T83.0 Mechanical complication of urinary catheter

Excludes2: complications of stoma of urinary tract N99.5-)

T83.01 Breakdown (mechanical) of urinary catheter

⑦**T83.010** Breakdown (mechanical) of cystostomy catheter

●⑦**T83.011** Breakdown (mechanical) of indwelling urethral catheter

●⑦**T83.012** Breakdown (mechanical) of nephrostomy catheter

▲⑦**T83.018** Breakdown (mechanical) of other urinary catheter

Breakdown (mechanical) of Hopkins catheter

Breakdown (mechanical) of ileostomy catheter

Breakdown (mechanical) urostomy catheter

⑦**T83.02** Displacement of urinary catheter

Malposition of urinary catheter

⑦**T83.020** Displacement of cystostomy catheter

●⑦**T83.021** Displacement of indwelling urethral catheter

●⑦**T83.022** Displacement of nephrostomy catheter

▲⑦**T83.028** Displacement of other urinary catheter

Displacement of Hopkins catheter

Displacement of ileostomy catheter

Displacement of urostomy catheter

T83.03 Leakage of urinary catheter

⑦**T83.030** Leakage of cystostomy catheter

●⑦**T83.031** Leakage of indwelling urethral catheter

●⑦**T83.032** Leakage of nephrostomy catheter

▲⑦**T83.038** Leakage of other urinary catheter

Leakage of Hopkins catheter

Leakage of ileostomy catheter

Leakage of urostomy catheter

T83.09 **Other mechanical complication of urinary catheter**

Obstruction (mechanical) of urinary catheter

Perforation of urinary catheter

Protrusion of urinary catheter

⑦**T83.090** **Other mechanical complication of cystostomy catheter**

● ⑦**T83.091** **Other mechanical complication of indwelling urethral catheter**

● ⑦**T83.092** **Other mechanical complication of nephrostomy catheter**

▲ ⑦**T83.098** **Other mechanical complication of other urinary catheter**

Other mechanical complication of Hopkins catheter

Other mechanical complication of ileostomy catheter

Other mechanical complication of urostomy catheter

T83.1 **Mechanical complication of other urinary devices and implants**

T83.11 **Breakdown (mechanical) of other urinary devices and implants**

⑦**T83.110** **Breakdown (mechanical) of urinary electronic stimulator device**

Excludes2: Breakdown (mechanical) of electrode (lead) for sacral nerve neurostimulator (T85.111)

Breakdown (mechanical) of implanted electronic sacral neurostimulator, pulse generator or receiver (T85.113)

▲ ⑦**T83.111** **Breakdown (mechanical) of implanted urinary sphincter**

▲ ⑦**T83.112** **Breakdown (mechanical) of indwelling ureteral stent**

● ⑦**T83.113** **Breakdown (mechanical) of other urinary stents**

Breakdown (mechanical) of ileal conduit stent

Breakdown (mechanical) of nephroureteral stent

⑦**T83.118** **Breakdown (mechanical) of other urinary devices and implants**

T83.12 **Displacement of other urinary devices and implants**

Malposition of other urinary devices and implants

⑦**T83.120** **Displacement of urinary electronic stimulator device**

Excludes2: Displacement of electrode (lead) for sacral nerve neurostimulator (T85.121)

Displacement of implanted electronic sacral neurostimulator, pulse generator or receiver (T85.123)

▲ ⑦**T83.121** **Displacement of implanted urinary sphincter**

▲ ⑦**T83.122** **Displacement of indwelling ureteral stent**

● ⑦**T83.123** **Displacement of other urinary stents**

Displacement of ileal conduit stent

Displacement of nephroureteral stent

⑦**T83.128** **Displacement of other urinary devices and implants**

⑦**T83.19** **Other mechanical complication of other urinary devices and implants**

Leakage of other urinary devices and implants

Obstruction (mechanical) of other urinary devices and implants

Perforation of other urinary devices and implants

Protrusion of other urinary devices and implants

⑦**T83.190** **Other mechanical complication of urinary electronic stimulator device**

Excludes2: Other mechanical complication of electrode (lead) for sacral nerve neurostimulator (T85.191)

Other mechanical complication of implanted electronic sacral neurostimulator, pulse generator or receiver (T85.193)

▲ ⑦**T83.191** **Other mechanical complication of implanted urinary sphincter**

▲ ⑦**T83.192** **Other mechanical complication of indwelling ureteral stent**

● ⑦**T83.193** **Other mechanical complication of other urinary stent**

Other mechanical complication of ileal conduit stent

Other mechanical complication of nephroureteral stent

⑦**T83.198** **Other mechanical complication of other urinary devices and implants**

T83.2 **Mechanical complication of graft of urinary organ**

⊗⑦**T83.21** **Breakdown (mechanical) of graft of urinary organ**

⊗⑦**T83.22** **Displacement of graft of urinary organ**

Malposition of graft of urinary organ

⊗⑦**T83.23** **Leakage of graft of urinary organ**

● ⊗⑦**T83.24** **Erosion of graft of urinary organ**

● ⊗⑦**T83.25** **Exposure of graft of urinary organ**

⊗⑦**T83.29** **Other mechanical complication of graft of urinary organ**

Obstruction (mechanical) of graft of urinary organ

Perforation of graft of urinary organ

Protrusion of graft of urinary organ

T83.3 **Mechanical complication of intrauterine contraceptive device**

⊗⑦**T83.31** **Breakdown (mechanical) of intrauterine contraceptive device**

⊗⑦**T83.32** **Displacement of intrauterine contraceptive device**

Malposition of intrauterine contraceptive device

Missing string of intrauterine contraceptive device

⊗⑦ **T83.39**   **Other mechanical complication of intrauterine contraceptive device**

Leakage of intrauterine contraceptive device

Obstruction (mechanical) of intrauterine contraceptive device

Perforation of intrauterine contraceptive device

Protrusion of intrauterine contraceptive device

T83.4   **Mechanical complication of other prosthetic devices, implants and grafts of genital tract**

  T83.41   **Breakdown (mechanical) of other prosthetic devices, implants and grafts of genital tract**

    ▲⑦ **T83.410**   **Breakdown (mechanical) of implanted penile prosthesis**

Breakdown (mechanical) of penile prosthesis cylinder

Breakdown (mechanical) of penile prosthesis pump

Breakdown (mechanical) of penile prosthesis reservoir

    ▲⑦ **T83.411**   **Breakdown (mechanical) of implanted testicular prosthesis**

    ⑦ **T83.418**   **Breakdown (mechanical) of other prosthetic devices, implants and grafts of genital tract**

  T83.42   **Displacement of other prosthetic devices, implants and grafts of genital tract**

Malposition **of other** prosthetic devices, implants and grafts of genital tract

    ▲⑦ **T83.420**   **Displacement of implanted penile prosthesis**

Displacement of penile prosthesis cylinder

Displacement of penile prosthesis pump

Displacement of penile prosthesis reservoir

    ●⑦ **T83.421**   **Displacement of implanted testicular prosthesis**

    ⑦ **T83.428**   **Displacement of other prosthetic devices, implants and grafts of genital tract**

  T83.49   **Other mechanical complication of other prosthetic devices, implants and grafts of genital tract**

Leakage **of** other prosthetic devices, implants and grafts of genital tract

Obstruction, mechanical of other prosthetic devices, implants and grafts of genital tract

Perforation of other prosthetic devices, implants and grafts of genital tract

Protrusion **of other** prosthetic devices, implants and grafts of genital tract

    ▲⑦ **T83.490**   **Other mechanical complication of implanted penile prosthesis**

Other mechanical complication of penile prosthesis cylinder

Other mechanical complication of penile prosthesis pump

Other mechanical complication of penile prosthesis reservoir

    ●⑦ **T83.491**   **Other mechanical complication of implanted testicular prosthesis**

    ⑦ **T83.498**   **Other mechanical complication of other prosthetic devices, implants and grafts of genital tract**

T83.5   **Infection and inflammatory reaction due to prosthetic device, implant and graft in urinary system**

<u>Use additional code</u> to identify infection

  T83.51   **Infection and inflammatory reaction due to urinary catheter**

Excludes2: complications of stoma of urinary tract (N99.5-)

    ●⑦ **T83.510**   **Infection and inflammatory reaction due to cystostomy catheter**

    ●⑦ **T83.511**   **Infection and inflammatory reaction due to indwelling urethral catheter**

    ●⑦ **T83.512**   **Infection and inflammatory reaction due to nephrostomy catheter**

    ●⑦ **T83.518**   **Infection and inflammatory reaction due to other urinary catheter**

Infection and inflammatory reaction due to Hopkins catheter

Infection and inflammatory reaction due to ileostomy catheter

Infection and inflammatory reaction due to urostomy catheter

  T83.59   **Infection and inflammatory reaction due to prosthetic device, implant and graft in urinary system**

    ●⑦ **T83.590**   **Infection and inflammatory reaction due to implanted urinary neurostimulation device**

Excludes2: Infection and inflammatory reaction due to electrode lead of sacral nerve neurostimulator (T85.732)

Infection and inflammatory reaction due to pulse generator or receiver of sacral nerve neurostimulator (T85.734)

    ●⑦ **T83.591**   **Infection and inflammatory reaction due to implanted urinary sphincter**

    ●⑦ **T83.592**   **Infection and inflammatory reaction due to indwelling ureteral stent**

    ●⑦ **T83.593**   **Infection and inflammatory reaction due to other urinary stents**

Infection and inflammatory reaction due to ileal conduit stents

Infection and inflammatory reaction due to nephroureteral stent

    ●⑦ **T83.598**   **Infection and inflammatory reaction due to other prosthetic device, implant and graft in urinary system**

T83.6   **Infection and inflammatory reaction due to prosthetic device, implant and graft in genital tract**

<u>Use additional code</u> to identify infection

   ● New code   ▲ Revised code   **Excludes1:** Not coded here   **Excludes2:** Not included here   ⊗ Placeholder required   ⑦ 7th digit required

● ⊗⑦**T83.61** **Infection and inflammatory reaction due to implanted penile prosthesis**

Infection and inflammatory reaction due to penile prosthesis cylinder

Infection and inflammatory reaction due to penile prosthesis pump

Infection and inflammatory reaction due to penile prosthesis reservoir

● ⊗⑦**T83.62** **Infection and inflammatory reaction due to implanted testicular prosthesis**

● ⊗⑦**T83.69** **Infection and inflammatory reaction due to other prosthetic device, implant and graft in genital tract**

T83.7 **Complications due to implanted mesh and other prosthetic materials**

T83.71 **Erosion of implanted mesh and other prosthetic materials to surrounding organ or tissue**

▲ ⑦**T83.711** **Erosion of implanted vaginal mesh to surrounding organ or tissue**

Erosion of implanted vaginal mesh into pelvic floor muscles

● ⑦**T83.712** **Erosion of implanted urethral mesh to surrounding organ or tissue**

Erosion of implanted female urethral sling

Erosion of implanted male urethral sling

Erosion of implanted urethral mesh into pelvic floor muscles

● ⑦**T83.713** **Erosion of implanted urethral bulking agent to surrounding organ or tissue**

● ⑦**T83.714** **Erosion of implanted ureteral bulking agent to surrounding organ or tissue**

▲ ⑦**T83.718** **Erosion of other implanted mesh to organ or tissue**

● ⑦**T83.719** **Erosion of other prosthetic materials to surrounding organ or tissue**

T83.72 **Exposure of implanted mesh and other prosthetic materials into surrounding organ or tissue**

Extrusion of implanted mesh

▲ ⑦**T83.721** **Exposure of implanted vaginal mesh into vagina**

Exposure of implanted vaginal mesh through vaginal wall

● ⑦**T83.722** **Exposure of implanted urethral mesh into urethra**

Exposure of implanted female urethral sling

Exposure of implanted male urethral sling

Exposure of implanted urethral mesh through urethral wall

● ⑦**T83.723** **Exposure of implanted urethral bulking agent into urethra**

● ⑦**T83.724** **Exposure of implanted ureteral bulking agent into ureter**

▲ ⑦**T83.728** **Exposure of other implanted mesh into organ or tissue**

● ⑦**T83.729** **Exposure of other prosthetic materials into organ or tissue**

● ⊗⑦**T83.79** **Other specified complications due to other genitourinary prosthetic materials**

T83.8 **Other specified complications of genitourinary prosthetic devices, implants and grafts**

▲ ⊗⑦**T83.81** **Embolism due to genitourinary prosthetic devices, implants and grafts**

▲ ⊗⑦**T83.82** **Fibrosis due to genitourinary prosthetic devices, implants and grafts**

▲ ⊗⑦**T83.83** **Hemorrhage due to genitourinary prosthetic devices, implants and grafts**

▲ ⊗⑦**T83.84** **Pain due to genitourinary prosthetic devices, implants and grafts**

▲ ⊗⑦**T83.85** **Stenosis due to genitourinary prosthetic devices, implants and grafts**

▲ ⊗⑦**T83.86** **Thrombosis due to genitourinary prosthetic devices, implants and grafts**

⊗⑦**T83.89** **Other specified complication of genitourinary prosthetic devices, implants and grafts**

⑦**T83.9** **Unspecified complication of genitourinary prosthetic device, implant and graft**

T84 **Complications of internal orthopedic prosthetic devices, implants and grafts**

Excludes2: failure and rejection of transplanted organs and tissues (T86.-)

fracture of bone following insertion of orthopedic implant, joint prosthesis or bone plate (M96.6)

The appropriate 7th character is to be added to each code from category T84

A - initial encounter

D - subsequent encounter

S - sequela

T84.0 **Mechanical complication of internal joint prosthesis**

T84.01 **Broken internal joint prosthesis**

Breakage (fracture) of prosthetic joint

Broken prosthetic joint implant

Excludes1: periprosthetic joint implant fracture (T84.04)

⑦**T84.010** **Broken internal right hip prosthesis**

⑦**T84.011** **Broken internal left hip prosthesis**

⑦**T84.012** **Broken internal right knee prosthesis**

⑦**T84.013** **Broken internal left knee prosthesis**

⑦**T84.018** **Broken internal joint prosthesis, other site**

Use additional code to identify the joint (Z96.6-)

⑦**T84.019** **Broken internal joint prosthesis, unspecified site**

T84.02 **Dislocation of internal joint prosthesis**

Instability of internal joint prosthesis

Subluxation of internal joint prosthesis

⑦**T84.020** **Dislocation of internal right hip prosthesis**

⑦**T84.021** **Dislocation of internal left hip prosthesis**

⑦ **T84.022** **Instability of internal right knee prosthesis**

⑦ **T84.023** **Instability of internal left knee prosthesis**

⑦ **T84.028** **Dislocation of other internal joint prosthesis**

Use additional code to identify the joint (Z96.6-)

⑦ **T84.029** **Dislocation of unspecified internal joint prosthesis**

T84.03 **Mechanical loosening of internal prosthetic joint**

Aseptic loosening of prosthetic joint

⑦ **T84.030** **Mechanical loosening of internal right hip prosthetic joint**

⑦ **T84.031** **Mechanical loosening of internal left hip prosthetic joint**

⑦ **T84.032** **Mechanical loosening of internal right knee prosthetic joint**

⑦ **T84.033** **Mechanical loosening of internal left knee prosthetic joint**

⑦ **T84.038** **Mechanical loosening of other internal prosthetic joint**

Use additional code to identify the joint (Z96.6-)

⑦ **T84.039** **Mechanical loosening of unspecified internal prosthetic joint**

T84.05 **Periprosthetic osteolysis of internal prosthetic joint**

Use additional code to identify major osseous defect, if applicable (M89.7-)

⑦ **T84.050** **Periprosthetic osteolysis of internal prosthetic right hip joint**

⑦ **T84.051** **Periprosthetic osteolysis of internal prosthetic left hip joint**

⑦ **T84.052** **Periprosthetic osteolysis of internal prosthetic right knee joint**

⑦ **T84.053** **Periprosthetic osteolysis of internal prosthetic left knee joint**

⑦ **T84.058** **Periprosthetic osteolysis of other internal prosthetic joint**

Use additional code to identify the joint (Z96.6-)

⑦ **T84.059** **Periprosthetic osteolysis of unspecified internal prosthetic joint**

T84.06 **Wear of articular bearing surface of internal prosthetic joint**

⑦ **T84.060** **Wear of articular bearing surface of internal prosthetic right hip joint**

⑦ **T84.061** **Wear of articular bearing surface of internal prosthetic left hip joint**

⑦ **T84.062** **Wear of articular bearing surface of internal prosthetic right knee joint**

⑦ **T84.063** **Wear of articular bearing surface of internal prosthetic left knee joint**

⑦ **T84.068** **Wear of articular bearing surface of other internal prosthetic joint**

Use additional code to identify the joint (Z96.6-)

⑦ **T84.069** **Wear of articular bearing surface of unspecified internal prosthetic joint**

T84.09 **Other mechanical complication of internal joint prosthesis**

Prosthetic joint implant failure NOS

⑦ **T84.090** **Other mechanical complication of internal right hip prosthesis**

⑦ **T84.091** **Other mechanical complication of internal left hip prosthesis**

⑦ **T84.092** **Other mechanical complication of internal right knee prosthesis**

⑦ **T84.093** **Other mechanical complication of internal left knee prosthesis**

⑦ **T84.098** **Other mechanical complication of other internal joint prosthesis**

Use additional code to identify the joint (Z96.6-)

⑦ **T84.099** **Other mechanical complication of unspecified internal joint prosthesis**

T84.1 **Mechanical complication of internal fixation device of bones of limb**

Excludes2: mechanical complication of internal fixation device of bones of feet (T84.2-)

mechanical complication of internal fixation device of bones of fingers (T84.2-)

mechanical complication of internal fixation device of bones of hands (T84.2-)

mechanical complication of internal fixation device of bones of toes (T84.2-)

T84.11 **Breakdown (mechanical) of internal fixation device of bones of limb**

⑦ **T84.110** **Breakdown (mechanical) of internal fixation device of right humerus**

⑦ **T84.111** **Breakdown (mechanical) of internal fixation device of left humerus**

⑦ **T84.112** **Breakdown (mechanical) of internal fixation device of bone of right forearm**

⑦ **T84.113** **Breakdown (mechanical) of internal fixation device of bone of left forearm**

⑦ **T84.114** **Breakdown (mechanical) of internal fixation device of right femur**

⑦ **T84.115** **Breakdown (mechanical) of internal fixation device of left femur**

⑦ **T84.116** **Breakdown (mechanical) of internal fixation device of bone of right lower leg**

⑦ **T84.117** **Breakdown (mechanical) of internal fixation device of bone of left lower leg**

⑦ **T84.119** **Breakdown (mechanical) of internal fixation device of unspecified bone of limb**

T84.12 **Displacement of internal fixation device of bones of limb**

Malposition of internal fixation device of bones of limb

⑦ **T84.120** **Displacement of internal fixation device of right humerus**

⑦ **T84.121** **Displacement of internal fixation device of left humerus**

⑦ **T84.122** **Displacement of internal fixation device of bone of right forearm**

● New code   ▲ Revised code   **Excludes1:** Not coded here   **Excludes2:** Not included here   ⊗ Placeholder required   ⑦ 7th digit required

⑦T84.123   **Displacement of internal fixation device of bone of left forearm**

⑦T84.124   **Displacement of internal fixation device of right femur**

⑦T84.125   **Displacement of internal fixation device of left femur**

⑦T84.126   **Displacement of internal fixation device of bone of right lower leg**

⑦T84.127   **Displacement of internal fixation device of bone of left lower leg**

⑦T84.129   **Displacement of internal fixation device of unspecified bone of limb**

T84.19   **Other mechanical complication of internal fixation device of bones of limb**

Obstruction (mechanical) of internal fixation device of bones of limb

Perforation of internal fixation device of bones of limb

Protrusion of internal fixation device of bones of limb

⑦T84.190   **Other mechanical complication of internal fixation device of right humerus**

⑦T84.191   **Other mechanical complication of internal fixation device of left humerus**

⑦T84.192   **Other mechanical complication of internal fixation device of bone of right forearm**

⑦T84.193   **Other mechanical complication of internal fixation device of bone of left forearm**

⑦T84.194   **Other mechanical complication of internal fixation device of right femur**

⑦T84.195   **Other mechanical complication of internal fixation device of left femur**

⑦T84.196   **Other mechanical complication of internal fixation device of bone of right lower leg**

⑦T84.197   **Other mechanical complication of internal fixation device of bone of left lower leg**

⑦T84.199   **Other mechanical complication of internal fixation device of unspecified bone of limb**

T84.2   **Mechanical complication of internal fixation device of other bones**

T84.21   **Breakdown (mechanical) of internal fixation device of other bones**

⑦T84.210   **Breakdown (mechanical) of internal fixation device of bones of hand and fingers**

⑦T84.213   **Breakdown (mechanical) of internal fixation device of bones of foot and toes**

⑦T84.216   **Breakdown (mechanical) of internal fixation device of vertebrae**

⑦T84.218   **Breakdown (mechanical) of internal fixation device of other bones**

T84.22   **Displacement of internal fixation device of other bones**

Malposition of internal fixation device **of other** bones

⑦T84.220   **Displacement of internal fixation device of bones of hand and fingers**

⑦T84.223   **Displacement of internal fixation device of bones of foot and toes**

⑦T84.226   **Displacement of internal fixation device of vertebrae**

⑦T84.228   **Displacement of internal fixation device of other bones**

T84.29   **Other mechanical complication of internal fixation device of other bones**

Obstruction (mechanical) of internal fixation device **of other** bones

Perforation of internal fixation device **of other** bones

Protrusion of internal fixation device **of other** bones

⑦T84.290   **Other mechanical complication of internal fixation device of bones of hand and fingers**

⑦T84.293   **Other mechanical complication of internal fixation device of bones of foot and toes**

⑦T84.296   **Other mechanical complication of internal fixation device of vertebrae**

⑦T84.298   **Other mechanical complication of internal fixation device of other bones**

T84.3   **Mechanical complication of other bone devices, implants and grafts**

Excludes2: Other complications of bone graft (T86.83-)

T84.31   **Breakdown (mechanical) of other bone devices, implants and grafts**

⑦T84.310   **Breakdown (mechanical) of electronic bone stimulator**

⑦T84.318   **Breakdown (mechanical) of other bone devices, implants and grafts**

T84.32   **Displacement of other bone devices, implants and grafts**

Malposition **of other** bone devices, implants and grafts

⑦T84.320   **Displacement of electronic bone stimulator**

⑦T84.328   **Displacement of other bone devices, implants and grafts**

T84.39   **Other mechanical complication of other bone devices, implants and grafts**

Obstruction (mechanical) **of other** bone devices, implants and grafts

Perforation **of other** bone devices, implants and grafts

Protrusion **of other** bone devices, implants and grafts

⑦T84.390   **Other mechanical complication of electronic bone stimulator**

⑦T84.398   **Other mechanical complication of other bone devices, implants and grafts**

T84.4   **Mechanical complication of other internal orthopedic devices, implants and grafts**

T84.41 Breakdown (mechanical) of other internal orthopedic devices, implants and grafts

⑦ **T84.410** Breakdown (mechanical) of muscle and tendon graft

⑦ **T84.418** Breakdown (mechanical) of other internal orthopedic devices, implants and grafts

T84.42 Displacement of other internal orthopedic devices, implants and grafts

Malposition of other internal orthopedic devices, implants and grafts

⑦ **T84.420** Displacement of muscle and tendon graft

⑦ **T84.428** Displacement of other internal orthopedic devices, implants and grafts

T84.49 Other mechanical complication of other internal orthopedic devices, implants and grafts

Mechanical complication of other internal orthopedic devices, implants and grafts NOS

Obstruction (mechanical) of other internal orthopedic devices, implants and grafts

Perforation of other internal orthopedic devices, implants and grafts

Protrusion of other internal orthopedic devices, implants and grafts

⑦ **T84.490** Other mechanical complication of muscle and tendon graft

⑦ **T84.498** Other mechanical complication of other internal orthopedic devices, implants and grafts

T84.5 Infection and inflammatory reaction due to internal joint prosthesis

Use additional code to identify infection

⊗⑦ **T84.50** Infection and inflammatory reaction due to unspecified internal joint prosthesis

⊗⑦ **T84.51** Infection and inflammatory reaction due to internal right hip prosthesis

⊗⑦ **T84.52** Infection and inflammatory reaction due to internal left hip prosthesis

⊗⑦ **T84.53** Infection and inflammatory reaction due to internal right knee prosthesis

⊗⑦ **T84.54** Infection and inflammatory reaction due to internal left knee prosthesis

⊗⑦ **T84.59** Infection and inflammatory reaction due to other internal joint prosthesis

T84.6 Infection and inflammatory reaction due to internal fixation device

Use additional code to identify infection

⊗⑦ **T84.60** Infection and inflammatory reaction due to internal fixation device of unspecified site

T84.61 Infection and inflammatory reaction due to internal fixation device of arm

⑦ **T84.610** Infection and inflammatory reaction due to internal fixation device of right humerus

⑦ **T84.611** Infection and inflammatory reaction due to internal fixation device of left humerus

⑦ **T84.612** Infection and inflammatory reaction due to internal fixation device of right radius

⑦ **T84.613** Infection and inflammatory reaction due to internal fixation device of left radius

⑦ **T84.614** Infection and inflammatory reaction due to internal fixation device of right ulna

⑦ **T84.615** Infection and inflammatory reaction due to internal fixation device of left ulna

⑦ **T84.619** Infection and inflammatory reaction due to internal fixation device of unspecified bone of arm

T84.62 Infection and inflammatory reaction due to internal fixation device of leg

⑦ **T84.620** Infection and inflammatory reaction due to internal fixation device of right femur

⑦ **T84.621** Infection and inflammatory reaction due to internal fixation device of left femur

⑦ **T84.622** Infection and inflammatory reaction due to internal fixation device of right tibia

⑦ **T84.623** Infection and inflammatory reaction due to internal fixation device of left tibia

⑦ **T84.624** Infection and inflammatory reaction due to internal fixation device of right fibula

⑦ **T84.625** Infection and inflammatory reaction due to internal fixation device of left fibula

⑦ **T84.629** Infection and inflammatory reaction due to internal fixation device of unspecified bone of leg

⊗⑦ **T84.63** Infection and inflammatory reaction due to internal fixation device of spine

⊗⑦ **T84.69** Infection and inflammatory reaction due to internal fixation device of other site

⊗⑦ **T84.7** Infection and inflammatory reaction due to other internal orthopedic prosthetic devices, implants and grafts

Use additional code to identify infection

T84.8 Other specified complications of internal orthopedic prosthetic devices, implants and grafts

⊗⑦ **T84.81** Embolism due to internal orthopedic prosthetic devices, implants and grafts

⊗⑦ **T84.82** Fibrosis due to internal orthopedic prosthetic devices, implants and grafts

⊗⑦ **T84.83** Hemorrhage due to internal orthopedic prosthetic devices, implants and grafts

⊗⑦ **T84.84** Pain due to internal orthopedic prosthetic devices, implants and grafts

⊗⑦ **T84.85** Stenosis due to internal orthopedic prosthetic devices, implants and grafts

⊗⑦ **T84.86** Thrombosis due to internal orthopedic prosthetic devices, implants and grafts

⊗⑦ **T84.89** Other specified complication of internal orthopedic prosthetic devices, implants and grafts

● New code ▲ Revised code **Excludes1:** Not coded here **Excludes2:** Not included here ⊗ Placeholder required ⑦ 7th digit required

⊗⑦**T84.9**　**Unspecified complication of internal orthopedic prosthetic device, implant and graft**

T85　**Complications of other internal prosthetic devices, implants and grafts**

Excludes2: failure and rejection of transplanted organs and tissue (T86.-)

The appropriate 7th character is to be added to each code from category T85

A - initial encounter

D - subsequent encounter

S - sequela

T85.0　**Mechanical complication of ventricular intracranial (communicating) shunt**

⊗⑦**T85.01**　**Breakdown (mechanical) of ventricular intracranial (communicating) shunt**

⊗⑦**T85.02**　**Displacement of ventricular intracranial (communicating) shunt**

Malposition of ventricular intracranial (communicating) shunt

⊗⑦**T85.03**　**Leakage of ventricular intracranial (communicating) shunt**

⊗⑦**T85.09**　**Other mechanical complication of ventricular intracranial (communicating) shunt**

Obstruction (mechanical) of ventricular intracranial (communicating) shunt

Perforation of ventricular intracranial (communicating) shunt

Protrusion of ventricular intracranial (communicating) shunt

T85.1　**Mechanical complication of implanted electronic stimulator of nervous system**

T85.11　**Breakdown (mechanical) of implanted electronic stimulator of nervous system**

▲⑦**T85.110**　**Breakdown (mechanical) of implanted electronic neurostimulator of brain electrode (lead)**

▲⑦**T85.111**　**Breakdown (mechanical) of implanted electronic neurostimulator of peripheral nerve electrode (lead)**

Breakdown of electrode (lead) for cranial nerve neurostimulators

Breakdown of electrode (lead) for gastric neurostimulator

Breakdown of electrode (lead) for sacral nerve neurostimulator

Breakdown of electrode (lead) for vagal nerve neurostimulators

▲⑦**T85.112**　**Breakdown (mechanical) of implanted electronic neurostimulator of spinal cord electrode (lead)**

●⑦**T85.113**　**Breakdown (mechanical) of implanted electronic neurostimulator, generator**

Breakdown (mechanical) of implanted electronic neurostimuator generator, brain, peripheral, gastric, spinal

Breakdown (mechanical) of implanted electronic sacral neurostimulator, pulse generator or receiver

⑦**T85.118**　**Breakdown (mechanical) of other implanted electronic stimulator of nervous system**

T85.12　**Displacement of implanted electronic stimulator of nervous system**

Malposition of implanted electronic stimulator of nervous system

▲⑦**T85.120**　**Displacement of implanted electronic neurostimulator of brain electrode (lead)**

▲⑦**T85.121**　**Displacement of implanted electronic neurostimulator of peripheral nerve electrode (lead)**

Displacement of electrode (lead) for cranial nerve neurostimulators

Displacement of electrode (lead) for gastric neurostimulator

Displacement of electrode (lead) for sacral nerve neurostimulator

Displacement of electrode (lead) for vagal nerve neurostimulators

▲⑦**T85.122**　**Displacement of implanted electronic neurostimulator of spinal cord electrode (lead)**

●⑦**T85.123**　**Displacement of implanted electronic neurostimulator, generator**

Displacement of implanted electronic neurostimulator generator, brain, peripheral, gastric, spinal

Displacement of implanted electronic sacral neurostimulator, pulse generator or receiver

⑦**T85.128**　**Displacement of other implanted electronic stimulator of nervous system**

T85.19　**Other mechanical complication of implanted electronic stimulator of nervous system**

Leakage of implanted electronic stimulator of nervous system

Obstruction (mechanical) of implanted electronic stimulator of nervous system

Perforation of implanted electronic stimulator of nervous system

Protrusion of implanted electronic stimulator of nervous system

▲⑦**T85.190**　**Other mechanical complication of implanted electronic neurostimulator of brain electrode (lead)**

▲⑦**T85.191**　**Other mechanical complication of implanted electronic neurostimulator of peripheral nerve electrode (lead)**

Other mechanical complication of electrode (lead) for cranial nerve neurostimulators

Other mechanical complication of electrode (lead) for gastric neurostimulator

Other mechanical complication of electrode (lead) for sacral nerve neurostimulator

Other mechanical complication of electrode (lead) for vagal nerve neurostimulators

▲⑦ **T85.192** **Other mechanical complication of implanted electronic neurostimulator of spinal cord electrode (lead)**

●⑦ **T85.193** **Other mechanical complication of implanted electronic neurostimulator, generator**

Other mechanical complication of implanted electronic neurostimulator generator, brain, peripheral, gastric, spinal

Other mechanical complication of implanted electronic sacral neurostimulator, pulse generator or receiver

⑦ **T85.199** **Other mechanical complication of other implanted electronic stimulator of nervous system**

T85.2 **Mechanical complication of intraocular lens**

⊗⑦**T85.21** **Breakdown (mechanical) of intraocular lens**

⊗⑦**T85.22** **Displacement of intraocular lens**

Malposition of intraocular lens

⊗⑦**T85.29** **Other mechanical complication of intraocular lens**

Obstruction (mechanical) of intraocular lens

Perforation of intraocular lens

Protrusion of intraocular lens

T85.3 **Mechanical complication of other ocular prosthetic devices, implants and grafts**

Excludes2: Other complications of corneal graft (T86.84-)

T85.31 **Breakdown (mechanical) of other ocular prosthetic devices, implants and grafts**

⑦ **T85.310** **Breakdown (mechanical) of prosthetic orbit of right eye**

⑦ **T85.311** **Breakdown (mechanical) of prosthetic orbit of left eye**

⑦ **T85.318** **Breakdown (mechanical) of other ocular prosthetic devices, implants and grafts**

T85.32 **Displacement of other ocular prosthetic devices, implants and grafts**

Malposition **of other** ocular prosthetic devices, implants and grafts

⑦ **T85.320** **Displacement of prosthetic orbit of right eye**

⑦ **T85.321** **Displacement of prosthetic orbit of left eye**

⑦ **T85.328** **Displacement of other ocular prosthetic devices, implants and grafts**

T85.39 **Other mechanical complication of other ocular prosthetic devices, implants and grafts**

Obstruction (mechanical) of other ocular prosthetic devices, implants and grafts

Perforation of other ocular prosthetic devices, implants and grafts

Protrusion of other ocular prosthetic devices, implants and grafts

⑦ **T85.390** **Other mechanical complication of prosthetic orbit of right eye**

⑦ **T85.391** **Other mechanical complication of prosthetic orbit of left eye**

⑦ **T85.398** **Other mechanical complication of other ocular prosthetic devices, implants and grafts**

T85.4 **Mechanical complication of breast prosthesis and implant**

⊗⑦**T85.41** **Breakdown (mechanical) of breast prosthesis and implant**

⊗⑦**T85.42** **Displacement of breast prosthesis and implant**

Malposition of breast prosthesis and implant

⊗⑦**T85.43** **Leakage of breast prosthesis and implant**

⊗⑦**T85.44** **Capsular contracture of breast implant**

⊗⑦**T85.49** **Other mechanical complication of breast prosthesis and implant**

Obstruction (mechanical) of breast prosthesis and implant

Perforation of breast prosthesis and implant

Protrusion of breast prosthesis and implant

T85.5 **Mechanical complication of gastrointestinal prosthetic devices, implants and grafts**

T85.51 **Breakdown (mechanical) of gastrointestinal prosthetic devices, implants and grafts**

⑦ **T85.510** **Breakdown (mechanical) of bile duct prosthesis**

⑦ **T85.511** **Breakdown (mechanical) of esophageal anti-reflux device**

⑦ **T85.518** **Breakdown (mechanical) of other gastrointestinal prosthetic devices, implants and grafts**

T85.52 **Displacement of gastrointestinal prosthetic devices, implants and grafts**

Malposition of gastrointestinal prosthetic devices, implants and grafts

⑦ **T85.520** **Displacement of bile duct prosthesis**

⑦ **T85.521** **Displacement of esophageal anti-reflux device**

⑦ **T85.528** **Displacement of other gastrointestinal prosthetic devices, implants and grafts**

T85.59 **Other mechanical complication of gastrointestinal prosthetic devices, implants and**

Obstruction, mechanical of gastrointestinal prosthetic devices, implants and grafts

Perforation of gastrointestinal prosthetic devices, implants and grafts

Protrusion of gastrointestinal prosthetic devices, implants and grafts

⑦ **T85.590** **Other mechanical complication of bile duct prosthesis**

⑦ **T85.591** **Other mechanical complication of esophageal anti-reflux device**

⑦ **T85.598** **Other mechanical complication of other gastrointestinal prosthetic devices, implants and grafts**

T85.6 **Mechanical complication of other specified internal and external prosthetic devices, implants and grafts**

T85.61 **Breakdown (mechanical) of other specified internal prosthetic devices, implants and grafts**

▲ ⑦**T85.610** **Breakdown (mechanical) of cranial or spinal infusion catheter**

Breakdown (mechanical) of epidural infusion catheter

Breakdown (mechanical) of intrathecal infusion catheter

Breakdown (mechanical) of subarachnoid infusion catheter

Breakdown (mechanical) of subdural infusion catheter

⑦**T85.611** **Breakdown (mechanical) of intraperitoneal dialysis catheter**

Excludes1: mechanical complication of vascular dialysis catheter (T82.4-)

⑦**T85.612** **Breakdown (mechanical) of permanent sutures**

Excludes1: mechanical complication of permanent (wire) suture used in bone repair (T84.1-T84.2)

⑦**T85.613** **Breakdown (mechanical) of artificial skin graft and decellularized allodermis**

Failure of artificial skin graft and decellularized allodermis

Non-adherence of artificial skin graft and decellularized allodermis

Poor incorporation of artificial skin graft and decellularized allodermis

Shearing of artificial skin graft and decellularized allodermis

⑦**T85.614** **Breakdown (mechanical) of insulin pump**

• ⑦**T85.615** **Breakdown (mechanical) of other nervous system device, implant or graft**

Breakdown (mechanical) of intrathecal infusion pump

⑦**T85.618** **Breakdown (mechanical) of other specified internal prosthetic devices, implants and grafts**

T85.62 **Displacement of other specified internal prosthetic devices, implants and grafts**

Malposition **of other** specified internal prosthetic devices, implants and grafts

▲ ⑦**T85.620** **Displacement of cranial or spinal infusion catheter**

Displacement of epidural infusion catheter

Displacement of intrathecal infusion catheter

Displacement of subarachnoid infusion catheter

Displacement of subdural infusion catheter

⑦**T85.621** **Displacement of intraperitoneal dialysis catheter**

Excludes1: mechanical complication of vascular dialysis catheter (T82.4-)

⑦**T85.622** **Displacement of permanent sutures**

Excludes1: mechanical complication of permanent (wire) suture used in bone repair (T84.1-T84.2)

⑦**T85.623** **Displacement of artificial skin graft and decellularized allodermis**

Dislodgement of artificial skin graft and decellularized allodermis

Displacement of artificial skin graft and decellularized allodermis

⑦**T85.624** **Displacement of insulin pump**

• ⑦**T85.625** **Displacement of other nervous system device, implant or graft**

Displacement of intrathecal infusion pump

⑦**T85.628** **Displacement of other specified internal prosthetic devices, implants and grafts**

T85.63 **Leakage of other specified internal prosthetic devices, implants and grafts**

▲ ⑦**T85.630** **Leakage of cranial or spinal infusion catheter**

Leakage of epidural infusion catheter

Leakage of intrathecal infusion catheter infusion catheter

Leakage of subdural infusion catheter

Leakage of subarachnoid infusion catheter

⑦**T85.631** **Leakage of intraperitoneal dialysis catheter**

Excludes1: mechanical complication of vascular dialysis catheter (T82.4)

⑦**T85.633** **Leakage of insulin pump**

• ⑦**T85.635** **Leakage of other nervous system device, implant or graft**

Leakage of intrathecal infusion pump

⑦**T85.638** **Leakage of other specified internal prosthetic devices, implants and grafts**

T85.69 **Other mechanical complication of other specified internal prosthetic devices, implants and grafts**

Obstruction, mechanical of other specified internal prosthetic devices, implants and grafts

Perforation of other specified internal prosthetic devices, implants and grafts

Protrusion of other specified internal prosthetic devices, implants and grafts

▲ ⑦**T85.690** **Other mechanical complication of cranial or spinal infusion catheter**

Other mechanical complication of epidural infusion catheter **Other** mechanical complication of intrathecal infusion catheter **Other** mechanical complication of subarachnoid infusion catheter **Other** mechanical complication of subdural infusion catheter

⑦**T85.691** **Other mechanical complication of intraperitoneal dialysis catheter**

Excludes1: mechanical complication of vascular dialysis catheter (T82.4)

⑦ **T85.692** **Other mechanical complication of permanent sutures**

Excludes1: mechanical complication of permanent (wire) suture used in bone repair (T84.1-T84.2)

⑦ **T85.693** **Other mechanical complication of artificial skin graft and decellularized allodermis**

⑦ **T85.694** **Other mechanical complication of insulin pump**

●⑦ **T85.695** **Other mechanical complication of other nervous system device, implant or graft**

Other mechanical complication of intrathecal infusion pump

⑦ **T85.698** **Other mechanical complication of other specified internal prosthetic devices, implants and grafts**

Mechanical complication of nonabsorbable surgical material NOS

T85.7 **Infection and inflammatory reaction due to other internal prosthetic devices, implants and grafts**

Use additional code to identify infection

⊗⑦ **T85.71** **Infection and inflammatory reaction due to peritoneal dialysis catheter**

⊗⑦ **T85.72** **Infection and inflammatory reaction due to insulin pump**

T85.73 **Infection and inflammatory reaction due to nervous system devices, implants and graft**

●⑦ **T85.730** **Infection and inflammatory reaction due to ventricular intracranial (communicating) shunt**

●⑦ **T85.731** **Infection and inflammatory reaction due to implanted electronic neurostimulator of brain, electrode (lead)**

●⑦ **T85.732** **Infection and inflammatory reaction due to implanted electronic neurostimulator of peripheral nerve, electrode (lead)**

Infection and inflammatory reaction due to electrode (lead) for cranial nerve neurostimulators

Infection and inflammatory reaction due to electrode (lead) for gastric neurostimulator

Infection and inflammatory reaction due to electrode (lead) for sacral nerve neurostimulator

Infection and inflammatory reaction due to electrode (lead) for vagal nerve neurostimulators

●⑦ **T85.733** **Infection and inflammatory reaction due to implanted electronic neurostimulator of spinal cord, electrode (lead)**

●⑦ **T85.734** **Infection and inflammatory reaction due to implanted electronic neurostimulator, generator**

Generator pocket infection

●⑦ **T85.735** **Infection and inflammatory reaction due to cranial or spinal infusion catheter**

Infection and inflammatory reaction due to epidural catheter

Infection and inflammatory reaction due to intrathecal infusion catheter

Infection and inflammatory reaction due to subarachnoid catheter

Infection and inflammatory reaction due to subdural catheter

●⑦ **T85.738** **Infection and inflammatory reaction due to other nervous system device, implant or graft**

Infection and inflammatory reaction due to intrathecal infusion pump

⊗⑦ **T85.79** **Infection and inflammatory reaction due to other internal prosthetic devices, implants and grafts**

T85.8 **Other specified complications of internal prosthetic devices, implants and grafts, not elsewhere classified**

T85.81 **Embolism due to internal prosthetic devices, implants and grafts, not elsewhere classified**

●⑦ **T85.810** **Embolism due to nervous system prosthetic devices, implants and grafts**

●⑦ **T85.818** **Embolism due to other internal prosthetic devices, implants and grafts**

T85.82 **Fibrosis due to internal prosthetic devices, implants and grafts, not elsewhere classified**

●⑦ **T85.820** **Fibrosis due to nervous system prosthetic devices, implants and grafts**

●⑦ **T85.828** **Fibrosis due to other internal prosthetic devices, implants and grafts**

T85.83 **Hemorrhage due to internal prosthetic devices, implants and grafts, not elsewhere classified**

●⑦ **T85.830** **Hemorrhage due to nervous system prosthetic devices, implants and grafts**

●⑦ **T85.838** **Hemorrhage due to other internal prosthetic devices, implants and grafts**

T85.84 **Pain due to internal prosthetic devices, implants and grafts, not elsewhere classified**

●⑦ **T85.840** **Pain due to nervous system prosthetic devices, implants and grafts**

●⑦ **T85.848** **Pain due to other internal prosthetic devices, implants and grafts**

T85.85 **Stenosis due to internal prosthetic devices, implants and grafts, not elsewhere classified**

●⑦ **T85.850** **Stenosis due to nervous system prosthetic devices, implants and grafts**

●⑦ **T85.858** **Stenosis due to other internal prosthetic devices, implants and grafts**

T85.86 **Thrombosis due to internal prosthetic devices, implants and grafts, not elsewhere classified**

● ⑦T85.860　**Thrombosis due to nervous system prosthetic devices, implants and grafts**

● ⑦**T85.868**　**Thrombosis due to other internal prosthetic devices, implants and grafts**

T85.89　**Other specified complication of internal prosthetic devices, implants and grafts, not elsewhere classified**

Erosion or breakdown of subcutaneous device pocket

● ⑦**T85.890**　**Other specified complication of nervous system prosthetic devices, implants and grafts**

● ⑦**T85.898**　**Other specified complication of other internal prosthetic devices, implants and grafts**

⑦**T85.9**　**Unspecified complication of internal prosthetic device, implant and graft**

Complication of internal prosthetic device, implant and graft NOS

T86　**Complications of transplanted organs and tissue**

Use additional code to identify **Other** transplant complications, such as:

graft-versus-host disease (D89.81-)

malignancy associated with organ transplant (C80.2)

post-transplant lymphoproliferative disorders (PTLD) (D47.Z1)

T86.0　**Complications of bone marrow transplant**

T86.00　**Unspecified complication of bone marrow transplant**

T86.01　**Bone marrow transplant rejection**

T86.02　**Bone marrow transplant failure**

T86.03　**Bone marrow transplant infection**

T86.09　**Other complications of bone marrow transplant**

T86.1　**Complications of kidney transplant**

T86.10　**Unspecified complication of kidney transplant**

T86.11　**Kidney transplant rejection**

T86.12　**Kidney transplant failure**

T86.13　**Kidney transplant infection**

Use additional code to specify infection

T86.19　**Other complication of kidney transplant**

T86.2　**Complications of heart transplant**

Excludes1: complication of:

artificial heart device (T82.5) heart-lung transplant (T86.3)

T86.20　**Unspecified complication of heart transplant**

T86.21　**Heart transplant rejection**

T86.22　**Heart transplant failure**

T86.23　**Heart transplant infection**

Use additional code to specify infection

T86.29　**Other complications of heart transplant**

T86.290　**Cardiac allograft vasculopathy**

Excludes1: atherosclerosis of coronary arteries (I25.75-, I25.76-, I25.81-)

T86.298　**Other complications of heart transplant**

T86.3　**Complications of heart-lung transplant**

T86.30　**Unspecified complication of heart-lung transplant**

T86.31　**Heart-lung transplant rejection**

T86.32　**Heart-lung transplant failure**

T86.33　**Heart-lung transplant infection**

Use additional code to specify infection

T86.39　**Other complications of heart-lung transplant**

T86.4　**Complications of liver transplant**

T86.40　**Unspecified complication of liver transplant**

T86.41　**Liver transplant rejection**

T86.42　**Liver transplant failure**

T86.43　**Liver transplant infection**

Use additional code to identify infection, such as:

Cytomegalovirus (CMV) infection (B25.-)

T86.49　**Other complications of liver transplant**

T86.5　**Complications of stem cell transplant**

Complications from stem cells from peripheral blood

Complications from stem cells from umbilical cord

T86.8　**Complications of other transplanted organs and tissues**

T86.81　**Complications of lung transplant**

Excludes1: complication of heart-lung transplant (T86.3-)

T86.810　**Lung transplant rejection**

T86.811　**Lung transplant failure**

T86.812　**Lung transplant infection**

Use additional code to specify infection

T86.818　**Other complications of lung transplant**

T86.819　**Unspecified complication of lung transplant**

T86.82　**Complications of skin graft (allograft) (autograft)**

Excludes2: complication of artificial skin graft (T85.693)

T86.820　**Skin graft (allograft) rejection**

T86.821　**Skin graft (allograft) (autograft) failure**

T86.822　**Skin graft (allograft) (autograft) infection**

Use additional code to specify infection

T86.828　**Other complications of skin graft (allograft) (autograft)**

T86.829　**Unspecified complication of skin graft (allograft) (autograft)**

T86.83　**Complications of bone graft**

Excludes2: mechanical complications of bone graft (T84.3-)

T86.830　**Bone graft rejection**

T86.831　**Bone graft failure**

T86.832　**Bone graft infection**

Use additional code to specify infection

T86.838　**Other complications of bone graft**

T86.839　**Unspecified complication of bone graft**

T86.84 **Complications of corneal transplant**

Excludes2: mechanical complications of corneal graft (T85.3-)

T86.840 **Corneal transplant rejection**

T86.841 **Corneal transplant failure**

T86.842 **Corneal transplant infection**

Use additional code to specify infection

T86.848 **Other complications of corneal transplant**

T86.849 **Unspecified complication of corneal transplant**

T86.85 **Complication of intestine transplant**

T86.850 **Intestine transplant rejection**

T86.851 **Intestine transplant failure**

T86.852 **Intestine transplant infection**

Use additional code to specify infection

T86.858 **Other complications of intestine transplant**

T86.859 **Unspecified complication of intestine transplant**

T86.89 **Complications of other transplanted tissue**

Transplant failure or rejection of pancreas

T86.890 **Other transplanted tissue rejection**

T86.891 **Other transplanted tissue failure**

T86.892 **Other transplanted tissue infection**

Use additional code to specify infection

T86.898 **Other complications of other transplanted tissue**

T86.899 **Unspecified complication of other transplanted tissue**

T86.9 **Complication of unspecified transplanted organ and tissue**

T86.90 **Unspecified complication of unspecified transplanted organ and tissue**

T86.91 **Unspecified transplanted organ and tissue rejection**

T86.92 **Unspecified transplanted organ and tissue failure**

T86.93 **Unspecified transplanted organ and tissue infection**

Use additional code to specify infection

T86.99 **Other complications of unspecified transplanted organ and tissue**

T87 **Complications peculiar to reattachment and amputation**

T87.0 **Complications of reattached (part of) upper extremity**

T87.0X **Complications of reattached (part of) upper extremity**

T87.0X1 **Complications of reattached (part of) right upper extremity**

T87.0X2 **Complications of reattached (part of) left upper extremity**

T87.0X9 **Complications of reattached (part of) unspecified upper extremity**

T87.1 **Complications of reattached (part of) lower extremity**

T87.1X **Complications of reattached (part of) lower extremity**

T87.1X1 **Complications of reattached (part of) right lower extremity**

T87.1X2 **Complications of reattached (part of) left lower extremity**

T87.1X9 **Complications of reattached (part of) unspecified lower extremity**

T87.2 **Complications of other reattached body part**

T87.3 **Neuroma of amputation stump**

T87.30 **Neuroma of amputation stump, unspecified extremity**

T87.31 **Neuroma of amputation stump, right upper extremity**

T87.32 **Neuroma of amputation stump, left upper extremity**

T87.33 **Neuroma of amputation stump, right lower extremity**

T87.34 **Neuroma of amputation stump, left lower extremity**

T87.4 **Infection of amputation stump**

T87.40 **Infection of amputation stump, unspecified extremity**

T87.41 **Infection of amputation stump, right upper extremity**

T87.42 **Infection of amputation stump, left upper extremity**

T87.43 **Infection of amputation stump, right lower extremity**

T87.44 **Infection of amputation stump, left lower extremity**

T87.5 **Necrosis of amputation stump**

T87.50 **Necrosis of amputation stump, unspecified extremity**

T87.51 **Necrosis of amputation stump, right upper extremity**

T87.52 **Necrosis of amputation stump, left upper extremity**

T87.53 **Necrosis of amputation stump, right lower extremity**

T87.54 **Necrosis of amputation stump, left lower extremity**

T87.8 **Other complications of amputation stump**

T87.81 **Dehiscence of amputation stump**

T87.89 **Other complications of amputation stump**

Amputation stump contracture

Amputation stump contracture of next proximal joint

Amputation stump flexion

Amputation stump edema

Amputation stump hematoma

Excludes2: phantom limb syndrome (G54.6-G54.7)

T87.9 **Unspecified complications of amputation stump**

T88 **Other complications of surgical and medical care, not elsewhere classified**

Excludes2: complication following infusion, transfusion and therapeutic injection (T80.-)

complication following procedure NEC (T81.-)

complications of anesthesia in labor and delivery (O74.-)

complications of anesthesia in pregnancy (O29.-)

complications of anesthesia in puerperium (O89.-)

complications of devices, implants and grafts (T82-T85)

complications of obstetric surgery and procedure (O75.4)

dermatitis due to drugs and medicaments (L23.3, L24.4, L25.1, L27.0-L27.1)

poisoning and toxic effects of drugs and chemicals (T36-T65 with fifth or sixth character 1-4 or 6) specified complications classified elsewhere

The appropriate 7th character is to be added to each code from category T88

A - initial encounter

D - subsequent encounter

S - sequela

⊗⑦**T88.0** **Infection following immunization**

Sepsis following immunization

⊗⑦**T88.1** **Other complications following immunization, not elsewhere classified**

Generalized vaccinia

Rash following immunization

Excludes1: vaccinia not from vaccine (B08.011)

Excludes2: anaphylactic shock due to serum (T80.5-)

Other serum reactions (T80.6-)

postimmunization arthropathy (M02.2)

postimmunization encephalitis (G04.02)

postimmunization fever (R50.83)

⊗⑦**T88.2** **Shock due to anesthesia**

Use additional code for adverse effect, if applicable, to identify drug (T41.- with fifth or sixth character 5)

Excludes1: complications of anesthesia (in):

labor and delivery (O74.-)

pregnancy (O29.-)

puerperium (O89.-)

postprocedural shock NOS (T81.1-)

⊗⑦**T88.3** **Malignant hyperthermia due to anesthesia**

Use additional code for adverse effect, if applicable, to identify drug (T41.- with fifth or sixth character 5)

⊗⑦**T88.4** **Failed or difficult intubation**

T88.5 **Other complications of anesthesia**

Use additional code for adverse effect, if applicable, to identify drug (T41.- with fifth or sixth character 5)

⊗⑦**T88.51** **Hypothermia following anesthesia**

⊗⑦**T88.52** **Failed moderate sedation during procedure**

Failed conscious sedation during procedure

Excludes2: personal history of failed moderate sedation (Z92.83)

● ⊗⑦**T88.53** **Unintended awareness under general anesthesia during procedure**

Excludes2: personal history of unintended awareness under general anesthesia (Z92.84)

⊗⑦**T88.59** **Other complications of anesthesia**

⊗⑦**T88.6** **Anaphylactic reaction due to adverse effect of correct drug or medicament properly administered**

Anaphylactic shock due to adverse effect of correct drug or medicament properly administered

Anaphylactoid reaction NOS

Use additional code for adverse effect, if applicable, to identify drug (T36-T50 with fifth or sixth character 5)

Excludes1: anaphylactic reaction due to serum (T80.5-)

anaphylactic shock or reaction due to adverse food reaction (T78.0-)

⊗⑦**T88.7** **Unspecified adverse effect of drug or medicament**

Drug hypersensitivity NOS

Drug reaction NOS

Use additional code for adverse effect, if applicable, to identify drug (T36-T50 with fifth or sixth character 5)

Excludes1: specified adverse effects of drugs and medicaments (A00-R94 and T80-T88.6, T88.8)

⊗⑦**T88.8** **Other specified complications of surgical and medical care, not elsewhere classified**

Use additional code to identify the complication

⊗⑦**T88.9** **Complication of surgical and medical care, unspecified**

● New code ▲ Revised code **Excludes1:** Not coded here **Excludes2:** Not included here ⊗ Placeholder required ⑦ 7th digit required

Chapter 20: External Causes Of Morbidity (V00-Y99)

MULTIPLE CODING FOR A SINGLE CONDITION

In addition to the etiology/manifestation convention that requires two codes to fully describe a single condition that affects multiple body systems, there are other single conditions that also require more than one code. "Use additional code" notes are found in the Tabular List at codes that are not part of an etiology/manifestation pair where a secondary code is useful to fully describe a condition. The sequencing rule is the same as the etiology/manifestation pair, "use additional code" indicates that a secondary code should be added.

For example, for bacterial infections that are not included in chapter 1, a secondary code from category B95, Streptococcus, Staphylococcus, and Enterococcus, as the cause of diseases classified elsewhere, or B96, Other bacterial agents as the cause of diseases classified elsewhere, may be required to identify the bacterial organism causing the infection. A "use additional code" note will normally be found at the infectious disease code, indicating a need for the organism code to be added as a secondary code.

"Code first" notes are also under certain codes that are not specifically manifestation codes but may be due to an underlying cause. When there is a "code first" note and an underlying condition is present, the underlying condition should be sequenced first.

"Code, if applicable, any causal condition first", notes indicate that this code may be assigned as a principal diagnosis when the causal condition is unknown or not applicable. If a causal condition is known, then the code for that condition should be sequenced as the principal or first-listed diagnosis.

Multiple codes may be needed for sequela, complication codes and obstetric codes to more fully describe a condition. See the specific guidelines for these conditions for further instruction.

COMBINATION CODE

A combination code is a single code used to classify: Two diagnoses, or a diagnosis with an associated secondary process (manifestation) A diagnosis with an associated complication

Combination codes are identified by referring to subterm entries in the Alphabetic Index and by reading the inclusion and exclusion notes in the Tabular List.

Assign only the combination code when that code fully identifies the diagnostic conditions involved or when the Alphabetic Index so directs. Multiple coding should not be used when the classification provides a combination code that clearly identifies all of the elements documented in the diagnosis. When the combination code lacks necessary specificity in describing the manifestation or complication, an additional code should be used as a secondary code.

SEQUELA (LATE EFFECTS)

A sequela is the residual effect (condition produced) after the acute phase of an illness or injury has terminated. There is no time limit on when a sequela code can be used. The residual may be apparent early, such as in cerebral infarction, or it may occur months or years later, such as that due to a previous injury. Coding of sequela generally requires two codes sequenced in the following order: The condition or nature of the sequela is sequenced first.

The sequela code is sequenced second.

An exception to the above guidelines are those instances where the code for the sequela is followed by a manifestation code identified in the Tabular List and title, or the sequela code has been expanded (at the fourth, fifth or sixth character levels) to include the manifestation(s). The code for the acute phase of an illness or injury that led to the sequela is never used with a code for the late effect.

GENERAL

The external causes of morbidity codes should never be sequenced as the first-listed or principal diagnosis.

External cause codes are intended to provide data for injury research and evaluation of injury prevention strategies. These codes capture how the injury or health condition happened (cause), the intent (unintentional or accidental; or intentional, such as suicide or assault), the place where the event occurred the activity of the patient at the time of the event, and the person's status (e.g., civilian, military).

There is no national requirement for mandatory ICD-10-CM external cause code reporting. Unless a provider is subject to a state-based external cause code reporting mandate or these codes are required by a particular payer, reporting of ICD-10-CM codes in Chapter 20, External Causes of Morbidity, is not required. In the absence of a mandatory reporting requirement, providers are encouraged to voluntarily report external cause codes, as they provide valuable data for injury research and evaluation of injury prevention strategies.

The external causes of morbidity codes should never be sequenced as the first-listed or principal diagnosis.

External cause codes are intended to provide data for injury research and evaluation of injury prevention strategies. These codes capture how the injury or health condition happened (cause), the intent (unintentional or accidental; or intentional, such as suicide or assault), the place where the event occurred the activity of the patient at the time of the event, and the person's status (e.g., civilian, military).

There is no national requirement for mandatory ICD-10-CM external cause code reporting. Unless a provider is subject to a state-based external cause code reporting mandate or these codes are required by a particular payer, reporting of ICD-10-CM codes in Chapter 20, External Causes of Morbidity, is not required. In the absence of a mandatory reporting requirement, providers are encouraged to voluntarily report external cause codes, as they provide valuable data for injury research and evaluation of injury prevention strategies.

V00-Y99

| | Add 4th-7th digits | | Nonspecific code | | Unspecified code | | Manifestation code | 1017 |

GENERAL EXTERNAL CAUSE CODING GUIDELINES

1) **Used with any code in the range of A00.0-T88.9, Z00-Z99**

An external cause code may be used with any code in the range of A00.0-T88.9, Z00-Z99, classification that is a health condition due to an external cause. Though they are most applicable to injuries, they are also valid for use with such things as infections or diseases due to an external source, and other health conditions, such as a heart attack that occurs during strenuous physical activity.

2) **External cause code used for length of treatment**

Assign the external cause code, with the appropriate 7th character (initial encounter, subsequent encounter or sequela) for each encounter for which the injury or condition is being treated.

Most categories in chapter 20 have a 7th character requirement for each applicable code. Most categories in this chapter have three 7th character values: A, initial encounter, D, subsequent encounter and S, sequela. While the patient may be seen by a new or different provider over the course of treatment for an injury or condition, assignment of the 7th character for external cause should match the 7th character of the code assigned for the associated injury or condition for the encounter.

3) **Use the full range of external cause codes**

Use the full range of external cause codes to completely describe the cause, the intent, the place of occurrence, and if applicable, the activity of the patient at the time of the event, and the patient's status, for all injuries, and other health conditions due to an external cause.

4) **Assign as many external cause codes as necessary**

Assign as many external cause codes as necessary to fully explain each cause. If only one external code can be recorded, assign the code most related to the principal diagnosis.

5) **The selection of the appropriate external cause code**

The selection of the appropriate external cause code is guided by the Alphabetic Index of External Causes and by Inclusion and Exclusion notes in the Tabular List.

6) **External cause code can never be a principal diagnosis**

An external cause code can never be a principal (first-listed) diagnosis.

7) **Combination external cause codes**

Certain of the external cause codes are combination codes that identify sequential events that result in an injury, such as a fall which results in striking against an object. The injury may be due to either event or both. The combination external cause code used should correspond to the sequence of events regardless of which caused the most serious injury.

8) **No external cause code needed in certain circumstances**

No external cause code from Chapter 20 is needed if the external cause and intent are included in a code from another chapter (e.g. T36.0X1-Poisoning by penicillins, accidental (unintentional)).

PLACE OF OCCURRENCE GUIDELINE

Codes from category Y92, Place of occurrence of the external cause, are secondary codes for use after other external cause codes to identify the location of the patient at the time of injury or other condition.

Generally, a place of occurrence code is assigned only once, at the initial encounter for treatment. However, in the rare instance that a new injury occurs during hospitalization, an additional place of occurrence code may be assigned. No 7th characters are used for Y92.

Do not use place of occurrence code Y92.9 if the place is not stated or is not applicable.

ACTIVITY CODE

Assign a code from category Y93, Activity code, to describe the activity of the patient at the time the injury or other health condition occurred.

An activity code is used only once, at the initial encounter for treatment. Only one code from Y93 should be recorded on a medical record.

The activity codes are not applicable to poisonings, adverse effects, misadventures or sequela.

Do not assign Y93.9, Unspecified activity, if the activity is not stated.

A code from category Y93 is appropriate for use with external cause and intent codes if identifying the activity provides additional information about the event.

PLACE OF OCCURRENCE, ACTIVITY, AND STATUS CODES USED WITH OTHER EXTERNAL CAUSE CODE

When applicable, place of occurrence, activity, and external cause status codes are sequenced after the main external cause code(s). Regardless of the number of external cause codes assigned, generally there should be only one place of occurrence code, one activity code, and one external cause status code assigned to an encounter. However, in the rare instance that a new injury occurs during hospitalization, an additional place of occurrence code may be assigned.

IF THE REPORTING FORMAT LIMITS THE NUMBER OF EXTERNAL CAUSE CODES

If the reporting format limits the number of external cause codes that can be used in reporting clinical data, report the code for the cause/intent most related to the principal diagnosis. If the format permits capture of additional external cause codes, the cause/intent, including medical misadventures, of the additional events should be reported rather than the codes for place, activity, or external status.

MULTIPLE EXTERNAL CAUSE CODING GUIDELINES

More than one external cause code is required to fully describe the external cause of an illness or injury. The assignment of external cause codes should be sequenced in the following priority:

If two or more events cause separate injuries, an external cause code should be assigned for each cause. The first-listed external cause code will be selected in the following order:

External codes for child and adult abuse take priority over all other external cause codes.

See Section I.C.19., Child and Adult abuse guidelines.

External cause codes for terrorism events take priority over all other external cause codes except child and adult abuse.

External cause codes for cataclysmic events take priority over all other external cause codes except child and adult abuse and terrorism.

External cause codes for transport accidents take priority over all other external cause codes except cataclysmic events, child and adult abuse and terrorism.

Activity and external cause status codes are assigned following all causal (intent) external cause codes.

The first-listed external cause code should correspond to the cause of the most serious diagnosis due to an assault, accident, or self-harm, following the order of hierarchy listed above.

CHILD AND ADULT ABUSE GUIDELINE

Adult and child abuse, neglect and maltreatment are classified as assault. Any of the assault codes may be used to indicate the external cause of any injury resulting from the confirmed abuse.

For confirmed cases of abuse, neglect and maltreatment, when the perpetrator is known, a code from Y07, Perpetrator of maltreatment and neglect, should accompany any other assault codes.

See Section I.C.19. Adult and child abuse, neglect and other maltreatment

UNKNOWN OR UNDETERMINED INTENT GUIDELINE

If the intent (accident, self-harm, assault) of the cause of an injury or other condition is unknown or unspecified, code the intent as accidental intent. All transport accident categories assume accidental intent.

1) Use of undetermined intent

External cause codes for events of undetermined intent are only for use if the documentation in the record specifies that the intent cannot be determined.

SEQUELAE (LATE EFFECTS) OF EXTERNAL CAUSE GUIDELINES

1) Sequelae external cause codes

Sequela are reported using the external cause code with the 7th character "S" for sequela. These codes should be used with any report of a late effect or sequela resulting from a previous injury.

See Section I.B.10 Sequela (Late Effects)

2) Sequela external cause code with a related current injury

A sequela external cause code should never be used with a related current nature of injury code.

3) Use of sequela external cause codes for subsequent visits

Use a late effect external cause code for subsequent visits when a late effect of the initial injury is being treated. Do not use a late effect external cause code for subsequent visits for follow-up care (e.g., to assess healing, to receive rehabilitative therapy) of the injury when no late effect of the injury has been documented.

TERRORISM GUIDELINES

1) **Cause of injury identified by the Federal Government (FBI) as terrorism**

When the cause of an injury is identified by the Federal Government (FBI) as terrorism, the first-listed external cause code should be a code from category Y38, Terrorism. The definition of terrorism employed by the FBI is found at the inclusion note at the beginning of category Y38. Use additional code for place of occurrence (Y92.-). More than one Y38 code may be assigned if the injury is the result of more than one mechanism of terrorism.

2) **Cause of an injury is suspected to be the result of terrorism**

When the cause of an injury is suspected to be the result of terrorism a code from category Y38 should not be assigned. Suspected cases should be classified as assault.

3) **Code Y38.9, Terrorism, secondary effects**

Assign code Y38.9, Terrorism, secondary effects, for conditions occurring subsequent to the terrorist event. This code should not be assigned for conditions that are due to the initial terrorist act.

It is acceptable to assign code Y38.9 with another code from Y38 if there is an injury due to the initial terrorist event and an injury that is a subsequent result of the terrorist event.

EXTERNAL CAUSE STATUS

A code from category Y99, External cause status, should be assigned whenever any other external cause code is assigned for an encounter, including an Activity code, except for the events noted below. Assign a code from category Y99, External cause status, to indicate the work status of the person at the time the event occurred. The status code indicates whether the event occurred during military activity, whether a non-military person was at work, whether an individual including a student or volunteer was involved in a non-work activity at the time of the causal event.

A code from Y99, External cause status, should be assigned, when applicable, with other external cause codes, such as transport accidents and falls. The external cause status codes are not applicable to poisonings, adverse effects, misadventures or late effects.

Do not assign a code from category Y99 if no other external cause codes (cause, activity) are applicable for the encounter.

An external cause status code is used only once, at the initial encounter for treatment. Only one code from Y99 should be recorded on a medical record.

Do not assign code Y99.9, Unspecified external cause status, if the status is not stated.

Chapter 20
External Causes Of Morbidity (V00-Y99)

Note: This chapter permits the classification of environmental events and circumstances as the cause of injury, and other adverse effects. Where a code from this section is applicable, it is intended that it shall be used secondary to a code from another chapter of the Classification indicating the nature of the condition.

Most often, the condition will be classifiable to Chapter 19, Injury, poisoning and certain other consequences of external causes (S00-T88). Other conditions that may be stated to be due to external causes are classified in Chapters I to XVIII. For these conditions, codes from Chapter 20 should be used to provide additional information as to the cause of the condition.

This chapter contains the following blocks: V00-X58 Accidents

V00-V99	Transport accidents
V00-V09	Pedestrian injured in transport accident
V10-V19	Pedal cycle rider injured in transport accident
V20-V29	Motorcycle rider injured in transport accident
V30-V39	Occupant of three-wheeled motor vehicle injured in transport accident
V40-V49	Car occupant injured in transport accident
V50-V59	Occupant of pick-up truck or van injured in transport accident
V60-V69	Occupant of heavy transport vehicle injured in transport accident
V70-V79	Bus occupant injured in transport accident
V80-V89	Other land transport accidents
V90-V94	Water transport accidents
V95-V97	Air and space transport accidents
V98-V99	Other and unspecified transport accidents
W00-X58	Other external causes of accidental injury
W00-W19	Slipping, tripping, stumbling and falls
W20-W49	Exposure to inanimate mechanical forces
W50-W64	Exposure to animate mechanical forces
W65-W74	Accidental non-transport drowning and submersion
W85-W99	Exposure to electric current, radiation and extreme ambient air temperature and pressure
X00-X08	Exposure to smoke, fire and flames
X10-X19	Contact with heat and hot substances
X30-X39	Exposure to forces of nature
X50	Overexertion and strenuous or repetitive movements
X52-X58	Accidental exposure **to other** specified factors
X71-X83	Intentional self-harm
X92-Y09	Assault
Y21-Y33	Event of undetermined intent
Y35-Y38	Legal intervention, operations of war, military operations, and terrorism
Y62-Y84	Complications of medical and surgical care
Y62-Y69	Misadventures to patients during surgical and medical care
Y70-Y82	Medical devices associated with adverse incidents in diagnostic and therapeutic use
Y83-Y84	Surgical and other medical procedures as the cause of abnormal reaction of the patient, or of later complication, without mention of misadventure at the time of the procedure
Y90-Y99	Supplementary factors related to causes of morbidity classified elsewhere

ACCIDENTS (V00-X58)
TRANSPORT ACCIDENTS (V00-V99)

Note: This section is structured in 12 groups. Those relating to land transport accidents (V00-V89) reflect the victim's mode of transport and are subdivided to identify the victim's 'counterpart' or the type of event. The vehicle of which the injured person is an occupant is identified in the first two characters since it is seen as the most important factor to identify for prevention purposes. A transport accident is one in which the vehicle involved must be moving or running or in use for transport purposes at the time of the accident.

Use additional code to identify:

Airbag injury (W22.1)

Type of street or road (Y92.4-)

Use of cellular telephone and other electronic equipment at the time of the transport accident (Y93.C-)

Excludes1: agricultural vehicles in stationary use or maintenance (W31.-)

assault by crashing of motor vehicle (Y03.-)

automobile or motor cycle in stationary use or maintenance- code to type of accident crashing of motor vehicle, undetermined intent (Y32)

intentional self-harm by crashing of motor vehicle (X82)

Excludes2: transport accidents due to cataclysm (X34-X38)

Note: Definitions related to transport accidents:

a) A transport accident (V00-V99) is any accident involving a device designed primarily for, or used at the time primarily for, conveying persons or good from one place to another.

b) A public highway [trafficway] or street is the entire width between property lines (or other boundary lines) of land open to the public as a matter of right or custom for purposes of moving persons or property from one place to another. A roadway is that part of the public highway designed, improved and customarily used for vehicular traffic.

c) A traffic accident is any vehicle accident occurring on the public highway [i.e. originating on, terminating on, or involving a vehicle partially on the highway]. A vehicle accident is assumed to have occurred on the public highway unless another place is specified, except in the case of accidents involving only off-road motor vehicles, which are classified as nontraffic accidents unless the contrary is stated.

d) A nontraffic accident is any vehicle accident that occurs entirely in any place other than a public highway.

e) A pedestrian is any person involved in an accident who was not at the time of the accident riding in or on a motor vehicle, railway train, streetcar or animal-drawn or other vehicle, or on a pedal cycle or animal. This includes, a person changing a tire, working on a parked car, or a person on foot. It also includes the user of a pedestrian conveyance such as a babystroller, ice-skates, skis, sled, roller skates, a skateboard, nonmotorized or motorized wheelchair, motorized mobility scooter, or nonmotorized scooter.

f) A driver is an occupant of a transport vehicle who is operating or intending to operate it.

g) A passenger is any occupant of a transport vehicle other than the driver, except a person traveling on the outside of the vehicle.

h) A person on the outside of a vehicle is any person being transported by a vehicle but not occupying the space normally reserved for the driver or passengers, or the space intended for the transport of property. This includes a person travelling on the bodywork, bumper, fender, roof, running board or step of a vehicle, as well as, hanging on the outside of the vehicle.

i) A pedal cycle is any land transport vehicle operated solely by nonmotorized pedals including a bicycle or tricycle.

j) A pedal cyclist is any person riding a pedal cycle or in a sidecar or trailer attached to a pedal cycle.

k) A motorcycle is a two-wheeled motor vehicle with one or two riding saddles and sometimes with a third wheel for the support of a sidecar. The sidecar is considered part of the motorcycle. This includes a moped, motor scooter, or motorized bicycle.

l) A motorcycle rider is any person riding a motorcycle or in a sidecar or trailer attached to the motorcycle.

m) A three-wheeled motor vehicle is a motorized tricycle designed primarily for on-road use. This includes a motor-driven tricycle, a motorized rickshaw, or a three-wheeled motor car.

n) A car [automobile] is a four-wheeled motor vehicle designed primarily for carrying up to 7 persons. A trailer being towed by the car is considered part of the car. It does not include a van or minivan - see definition

o) A pick-up truck or van is a four or six-wheeled motor vehicle designed for carrying passengers as well as property or cargo weighing less than the local limit for classification as a heavy goods vehicle, and not requiring a special driver's license. This includes a minivan and a sport-utility vehicle (SUV).

p) A heavy transport vehicle is a motor vehicle designed primarily for carrying property, meeting local criteria for classification as a heavy goods vehicle in terms of weight and requiring a special driver's license.

q) A bus (coach) is a motor vehicle designed or adapted primarily for carrying more than 10 passengers, and requiring a special driver's license.

r) A railway train or railway vehicle is any device, with or without freight or passenger cars couple to it, designed for traffic on a railway track. This includes subterranean (subways) or elevated trains.

s) A streetcar, is a device designed and used primarily for transporting passengers within a municipality, running on rails, usually subject to normal traffic control signals, and operated principally on a right-of-way that forms part of the roadway. This includes a tram or trolley that runs on rails. A trailer being towed by a streetcar is considered part of the streetcar.

t) A special vehicle mainly used on industrial premises is a motor vehicle designed primarily for use within the buildings and premises of industrial or commercial establishments. This includes battery-powered airport passenger vehicles or baggage/mail trucks, forklifts, coal-cars in a coal mine, logging cars and trucks used in mines or quarries.

u) A special vehicle mainly used in agriculture is a motor vehicle designed specifically for use in farming and agriculture (horticulture), to work the land, tend and harvest crops and transport materials on the farm. This includes harvesters, farm machinery and tractor and trailers.

v) A special construction vehicle is a motor vehicle designed specifically for use on construction and demolition sites. This includes bulldozers, diggers, earth levellers, dump trucks. backhoes, front-end loaders, pavers, and mechanical shovels.

w) A special all-terrain vehicle is a motor vehicle of special design to enable it to negotiate over rough or soft terrain , snow or sand. Examples of special design are high construction, special wheels and tires, tracks, and support on a cushion of air. This includes snow mobiles, All-terrain vehicles (ATV), and dune buggies. It does not include passenger vehicle designated as Sport Utility Vehicles. (SUV)

x) A watercraft is any device designed for transporting passengers or goods on water. This includes motor or sail boats, ships, and hovercraft.

y) An aircraft is any device for transporting passengers or goods in the air. This includes hot-air balloons, gliders, helicopters and airplanes. (z) A military vehicle is any motorized vehicle operating on a public roadway owned by the military and being operated by a member of the military.

PEDESTRIAN INJURED IN TRANSPORT ACCIDENT (V00-V09)

Includes: person changing tire on transport vehicle

person examining engine of vehicle broken down in (on side of) road

Excludes1: fall due to non-transport collision with other person (W03)

pedestrian on foot falling (slipping) on ice and snow (W00.-)

struck or bumped by another person (W51)

V00   Pedestrian conveyance accident

Use additional place of occurrence and activity external cause codes, if known (Y92.-, Y93.-)

Excludes1: collision with another person without fall (W51)

fall due to person on foot colliding with another person on foot (W03)

fall from non-moving wheelchair, nonmotorized scooter and motorized mobility scooter without collision (W05.-)

pedestrian (conveyance) collision with other land transport vehicle (V01-V09)

pedestrian on foot falling (slipping) on ice and snow (W00.-)

The appropriate 7th character is to be added to each code from category V00

A - initial encounter

D - subsequent encounter

S - sequela

V00.0   Pedestrian on foot injured in collision with pedestrian conveyance

⊗⑦**V00.01   Pedestrian on foot injured in collision with roller-skater**

⊗⑦**V00.02   Pedestrian on foot injured in collision with skateboarder**

⊗⑦**V00.09   Pedestrian on foot injured in collision with other pedestrian conveyance**

V00.1   Rolling-type pedestrian conveyance accident

Excludes1: accident with babystroller (V00.82-)

accident with wheelchair (powered) (V00.81-)

accident with motorized mobility scooter (V00.83-)

V00.11   In-line roller-skate accident

⑦**V00.111   Fall from in-line roller-skates**

⑦**V00.112   In-line roller-skater colliding with stationary object**

⑦**V00.118   Other in-line roller-skate accident**

Excludes1: roller-skater collision with other land transport vehicle (V01-V09 with 5th character 1)

V00.12   Non-in- line roller-skate accident

⑦**V00.121   Fall from non-in-line roller-skates**

⑦**V00.122   Non-in-line roller-skater colliding with stationary object**

⑦**V00.128   Other non-in-line roller-skating accident**

Excludes1: roller-skater collision with other land transport vehicle (V01-V09 with 5th character 1)

V00.13   Skateboard accident

⑦**V00.131   Fall from skateboard**

⑦**V00.132   Skateboarder colliding with stationary object**

⑦**V00.138   Other skateboard accident**

Excludes1: skateboarder collision **with other** land transport vehicle (V01-V09 with 5th character 2)

V00.14   Scooter (nonmotorized) accident

    Excludes1: motorscooter accident (V20-V29)

⑦V00.141   **Fall from scooter (nonmotorized)**

⑦V00.142   **Scooter (nonmotorized) colliding with stationary object**

⑦V00.148   **Other scooter (nonmotorized) accident**

    Excludes1: scooter (nonmotorized) collision **with other** land transport vehicle (V01-V09 with fifth character 9)

V00.15   Heelies accident

    Rolling shoe Wheeled shoe Wheelies accident

⑦V00.151   **Fall from heelies**

⑦V00.152   **Heelies colliding with stationary object**

⑦V00.158   **Other heelies accident**

V00.18   Accident on other rolling-type pedestrian conveyance

⑦V00.181   **Fall from other rolling-type pedestrian conveyance**

⑦V00.182   **Pedestrian on other rolling-type pedestrian conveyance colliding with stationary object**

⑦V00.188   **Other accident on other rolling-type pedestrian conveyance**

V00.2   Gliding-type pedestrian conveyance accident

V00.21   Ice-skates accident

⑦V00.211   **Fall from ice-skates**

⑦V00.212   **Ice-skater colliding with stationary object**

⑦V00.218   **Other ice-skates accident**

    Excludes1: ice-skater collision **with other** land transport vehicle (V01-V09 with 5th digit 9)

V00.22   Sled accident

⑦V00.221   **Fall from sled**

⑦V00.222   **Sledder colliding with stationary object**

⑦V00.228   **Other sled accident**

    Excludes1: sled collision **with other** land transport vehicle (V01-V09 with 5th digit 9)

V00.28   Other gliding-type pedestrian conveyance accident

⑦V00.281   **Fall from other gliding-type pedestrian conveyance**

⑦V00.282   **Pedestrian on other gliding-type pedestrian conveyance colliding with stationary object**

⑦V00.288   **Other accident on other gliding-type pedestrian conveyance**

    Excludes1: gliding-type pedestrian conveyance collision **with other** land transport vehicle (V01-V09 with 5th digit 9)

V00.3   Flat-bottomed pedestrian conveyance accident

V00.31   Snowboard accident

⑦V00.311   **Fall from snowboard**

⑦V00.312   **Snowboarder colliding with stationary object**

⑦V00.318   **Other snowboard accident**

    Excludes1: snowboarder collision **with other** land transport vehicle (V01-V09 with 5th digit 9)

V00.32   Snow-ski accident

⑦V00.321   **Fall from snow-skis**

⑦V00.322   **Snow-skier colliding with stationary object**

⑦V00.328   **Other snow-ski accident**

    Excludes1: snow-skier collision **with other** land transport vehicle (V01-V09 with 5th digit 9)

V00.38   Other flat-bottomed pedestrian conveyance accident

⑦V00.381   **Fall from other flat-bottomed pedestrian conveyance**

⑦V00.382   **Pedestrian on other flat-bottomed pedestrian conveyance colliding with stationary object**

⑦V00.388   **Other accident on other flat-bottomed pedestrian conveyance**

V00.8   Accident on other pedestrian conveyance

V00.81   Accident with wheelchair (powered)

⑦V00.811   **Fall from moving wheelchair (powered)**

    Excludes1: fall from non-moving wheelchair (W05.0)

⑦V00.812   **Wheelchair (powered) colliding with stationary object**

⑦V00.818   **Other accident with wheelchair (powered)**

V00.82   Accident with babystroller

⑦V00.821   **Fall from babystroller**

⑦V00.822   **Babystroller colliding with stationary object**

⑦V00.828   **Other accident with babystroller**

V00.83   Accident with motorized mobility scooter

⑦V00.831   **Fall from motorized mobility scooter**

    Excludes1: fall from non-moving motorized mobility scooter (W05.2)

⑦V00.832   **Motorized mobility scooter colliding with stationary object**

⑦V00.838   **Other accident with motorized mobility scooter**

V00.89   Accident on other pedestrian conveyance

⑦V00.891   **Fall from other pedestrian conveyance**

⑦V00.892   **Pedestrian on other pedestrian conveyance colliding with stationary object**

⑦V00.898   **Other accident on other pedestrian conveyance**

    Excludes1: Other pedestrian (conveyance) collision **with other**

land transport vehicle (V01-V09 with 5th digit 9)

V01   Pedestrian injured in collision with pedal cycle

The appropriate 7th character is to be added to each code from category V01

A - initial encounter

D - subsequent encounter

S - sequela

V01.0   Pedestrian injured in collision with pedal cycle in nontraffic accident

⊗⑦**V01.00   Pedestrian on foot injured in collision with pedal cycle in nontraffic accident**

Pedestrian NOS injured in collision with pedal cycle in nontraffic accident

⊗⑦**V01.01   Pedestrian on roller-skates injured in collision with pedal cycle in nontraffic accident**

⊗⑦**V01.02   Pedestrian on skateboard injured in collision with pedal cycle in nontraffic accident**

⊗⑦**V01.09   Pedestrian with other conveyance injured in collision with pedal cycle in nontraffic accident**

Pedestrian with babystroller injured in collision with pedal cycle in nontraffic accident

Pedestrian on ice-skates injured in collision with pedal cycle in nontraffic accident

Pedestrian on nonmotorized scooter injured in collision with pedal cycle in nontraffic accident

Pedestrian on sled injured in collision with pedal cycle in nontraffic accident

Pedestrian on snowboard injured in collision with pedal cycle in nontraffic accident

Pedestrian on snow-skis injured in collision with pedal cycle in nontraffic accident

Pedestrian in wheelchair (powered) injured in collision with pedal cycle in nontraffic accident

Pedestrian in motorized mobility scooter injured in collision with pedal cycle in nontraffic accident

V01.1   Pedestrian injured in collision with pedal cycle in traffic accident

⊗⑦**V01.10   Pedestrian on foot injured in collision with pedal cycle in traffic accident**

Pedestrian NOS injured in collision with pedal cycle in traffic accident

⊗⑦**V01.11   Pedestrian on roller-skates injured in collision with pedal cycle in traffic accident**

⊗⑦**V01.12   Pedestrian on skateboard injured in collision with pedal cycle in traffic accident**

⊗⑦**V01.19   Pedestrian with other conveyance injured in collision with pedal cycle in traffic accident**

Pedestrian with babystroller injured in collision with pedal cycle in traffic accident

Pedestrian on ice-skates injured in collision with pedal cycle in traffic accident

Pedestrian on nonmotorized scooter injured in collision with pedal cycle in traffic accident

Pedestrian on sled injured in collision with pedal cycle in traffic accident

Pedestrian on snowboard injured in collision with pedal cycle in traffic accident

Pedestrian on snow-skis injured in collision with pedal cycle in traffic accident

Pedestrian in wheelchair (powered) injured in collision with pedal cycle in traffic accident

Pedestrian in motorized mobility scooter injured in collision with pedal cycle in traffic accident

V01.9   Pedestrian injured in collision with pedal cycle, unspecified whether traffic or nontraffic accident

⊗⑦**V01.90   Pedestrian on foot injured in collision with pedal cycle, unspecified whether traffic or nontraffic accident**

Pedestrian NOS injured in collision with pedal cycle, unspecified whether traffic or nontraffic accident

⊗⑦**V01.91   Pedestrian on roller-skates injured in collision with pedal cycle, unspecified whether traffic or nontraffic accident**

⊗⑦**V01.92   Pedestrian on skateboard injured in collision with pedal cycle, unspecified whether traffic or nontraffic accident**

⊗⑦**V01.99   Pedestrian with other conveyance injured in collision with pedal cycle, unspecified whether traffic or nontraffic accident**

Pedestrian with babystroller injured in collision with pedal cycle, unspecified whether traffic or nontraffic accident

Pedestrian on ice-skates injured in collision with pedal cycle unspecified, whether traffic or nontraffic accident

Pedestrian on nonmotorized scooter injured in collision with pedal cycle, unspecified whether traffic or nontraffic accident

Pedestrian on sled injured in collision with pedal cycle unspecified, whether traffic or nontraffic accident

Pedestrian on snowboard injured in collision with pedal cycle, unspecified whether traffic or nontraffic accident

Pedestrian on snow-skis injured in collision with pedal cycle, unspecified whether traffic or nontraffic accident

Pedestrian in wheelchair (powered) injured in collision with pedal cycle, unspecified whether traffic or nontraffic accident

Pedestrian in motorized mobility scooter injured in collision with pedal cycle, unspecified whether traffic or nontraffic accident

V02   Pedestrian injured in collision with two- or three-wheeled motor vehicle

The appropriate 7th character is to be added to each code from category V02

A - initial encounter

D - subsequent encounter

S - sequela

V02.0   Pedestrian injured in collision with two- or three-wheeled motor vehicle in nontraffic accident

⊗⑦**V02.00   Pedestrian on foot injured in collision with two- or three-wheeled motor vehicle in nontraffic accident**

Pedestrian NOS injured in collision with two- or three-wheeled motor vehicle in nontraffic accident

⊗⑦**V02.01   Pedestrian on roller-skates injured in collision with two- or three-wheeled motor vehicle in nontraffic accident**

⊗⑦**V02.02** **Pedestrian on skateboard injured in collision with two- or three-wheeled motor vehicle in nontraffic accident**

⊗⑦**V02.09** **Pedestrian with other conveyance injured in collision with two- or three-wheeled motor vehicle in nontraffic accident**

Pedestrian with babystroller injured in collision with two- or three-wheeled motor vehicle in nontraffic accident

Pedestrian on ice-skates injured in collision with two- or three-wheeled motor vehicle in nontraffic accident

Pedestrian on nonmotorized scooter injured in collision with two- or three-wheeled motor vehicle in nontraffic accident

Pedestrian on sled injured in collision with two- or three-wheeled motor vehicle in nontraffic accident

Pedestrian on snowboard injured in collision with two- or three-wheeled motor vehicle in nontraffic accident

Pedestrian on snow-skis injured in collision with two- or three-wheeled motor vehicle in nontraffic accident

Pedestrian in wheelchair (powered) injured in collision with two- or three-wheeled motor vehicle in nontraffic accident

Pedestrian in motorized mobility scooter injured in collision with two- or three-wheeled motor vehicle in nontraffic accident

V02.1 **Pedestrian injured in collision with two- or three-wheeled motor vehicle in traffic accident**

⊗⑦**V02.10** **Pedestrian on foot injured in collision with two- or three-wheeled motor vehicle in traffic accident**

Pedestrian NOS injured in collision with two- or three-wheeled motor vehicle in traffic accident

⊗⑦**V02.11** **Pedestrian on roller-skates injured in collision with two- or three-wheeled motor vehicle in traffic accident**

⊗⑦**V02.12** **Pedestrian on skateboard injured in collision with two- or three-wheeled motor vehicle in traffic accident**

⊗⑦**V02.19** **Pedestrian with other conveyance injured in collision with two- or three-wheeled motor vehicle in traffic accident**

Pedestrian with babystroller injured in collision with two- or three-wheeled motor vehicle in traffic accident

Pedestrian on ice-skates injured in collision with two- or three-wheeled motor vehicle in traffic accident

Pedestrian on nonmotorized scooter injured in collision with two- or three-wheeled motor vehicle in traffic accident

Pedestrian on sled injured in collision with two- or three-wheeled motor vehicle in traffic accident

Pedestrian on snowboard injured in collision with two- or three-wheeled motor vehicle in traffic accident

Pedestrian on snow-skis injured in collision with two- or three-wheeled motor vehicle in traffic accident

Pedestrian in wheelchair (powered) injured in collision with two- or three-wheeled motor vehicle in traffic accident

Pedestrian in motorized mobility scooter injured in collision with two- or three-wheeled motor vehicle in traffic accident

V02.9 **Pedestrian injured in collision with two- or three-wheeled motor vehicle, unspecified whether traffic or nontraffic accident**

⊗⑦**V02.90** **Pedestrian on foot injured in collision with two- or three-wheeled motor vehicle, unspecified whether traffic or nontraffic accident**

Pedestrian NOS injured in collision with two- or three-wheeled motor vehicle, unspecified whether traffic or nontraffic accident

⊗⑦**V02.91** **Pedestrian on roller-skates injured in collision with two- or three-wheeled motor vehicle, unspecified whether traffic or nontraffic accident**

⊗⑦**V02.92** **Pedestrian on skateboard injured in collision with two- or three-wheeled motor vehicle, unspecified whether traffic or nontraffic accident**

⊗⑦**V02.99** **Pedestrian with other conveyance injured in collision with two- or three-wheeled motor vehicle, unspecified whether traffic or nontraffic accident**

Pedestrian with babystroller injured in collision with two- or three-wheeled motor vehicle, unspecified whether traffic or nontraffic accident

Pedestrian on ice-skates injured in collision with two- or three-wheeled motor vehicle, unspecified whether traffic or nontraffic accident

Pedestrian on nonmotorized scooter injured in collision with two- or three-wheeled motor vehicle, unspecified whether traffic or nontraffic accident

Pedestrian on sled injured in collision with two- or three-wheeled motor vehicle, unspecified whether traffic or nontraffic accident

Pedestrian on snowboard injured in collision with two- or three-wheeled motor vehicle, unspecified whether traffic or nontraffic accident

Pedestrian on snow-skis injured in collision with two- or three-wheeled motor vehicle, unspecified whether traffic or nontraffic accident

Pedestrian in wheelchair (powered) injured in collision with two- or three-wheeled motor vehicle, unspecified whether traffic or nontraffic accident

Pedestrian in motorized mobility scooter injured in collision with two- or three-wheeled motor vehicle, unspecified whether traffic or nontraffic accident

V03 **Pedestrian injured in collision with car, pick-up truck or van**

The appropriate 7th character is to be added to each code from category V03

A - initial encounter

D - subsequent encounter

S - sequela

V03.0 **Pedestrian injured in collision with car, pick-up truck or van in nontraffic accident**

⊗⑦**V03.00** **Pedestrian on foot injured in collision with car, pick-up truck or van in nontraffic accident**

Pedestrian NOS injured in collision with car, pick-up truck or van in nontraffic accident

⊗⑦**V03.01** **Pedestrian on roller-skates injured in collision with car, pick-up truck or van in nontraffic accident**

⊗⑦**V03.02** **Pedestrian on skateboard injured in collision with car, pick-up truck or van in nontraffic accident**

⊗⑦**V03.09** **Pedestrian with other conveyance injured in collision with car, pick-up truck or van in nontraffic accident**

Pedestrian with babystroller injured in collision with car, pick-up truck or van in nontraffic accident

Pedestrian on ice-skates injured in collision with car, pick-up truck or van in nontraffic accident

Pedestrian on nonmotorized scooter injured in collision with car, pick-up truck or van in nontraffic accident

Pedestrian on sled injured in collision with car, pick-up truck or van in nontraffic accident

Pedestrian on snowboard injured in collision with car, pick-up truck or van in nontraffic accident

Pedestrian on snow-skis injured in collision with car, pick-up truck or van in nontraffic accident

Pedestrian in wheelchair (powered) injured in collision with car, pick-up truck or van in nontraffic accident

Pedestrian in motorized mobility scooter injured in collision with car, pick-up truck or van in nontraffic accident

V03.1 **Pedestrian injured in collision with car, pick-up truck or van in traffic accident**

⊗⑦**V03.10** **Pedestrian on foot injured in collision with car, pick-up truck or van in traffic accident**

Pedestrian NOS injured in collision with car, pick-up truck or van in traffic accident

⊗⑦**V03.11** **Pedestrian on roller-skates injured in collision with car, pick-up truck or van in traffic accident**

⊗⑦**V03.12** **Pedestrian on skateboard injured in collision with car, pick-up truck or van in traffic accident**

⊗⑦**V03.19** **Pedestrian with other conveyance injured in collision with car, pick-up truck or van in traffic accident**

Pedestrian with babystroller injured in collision with car, pick-up truck or van in traffic accident

Pedestrian on ice-skates injured in collision with car, pick-up truck or van in traffic accident

Pedestrian on nonmotorized scooter injured in collision with car, pick-up truck or van in traffic accident

Pedestrian on sled injured in collision with car, pick-up truck or van in traffic accident

Pedestrian on snowboard injured in collision with car, pick-up truck or van in traffic accident

Pedestrian on snow-skis injured in collision with car, pick-up truck or van in traffic accident

Pedestrian in wheelchair (powered) injured in collision with car, pick-up truck or van in traffic accident

Pedestrian in motorized mobility scooter injured in collision with car, pick-up truck or van in traffic accident

V03.9 **Pedestrian injured in collision with car, pick-up truck or van, unspecified whether traffic or nontraffic accident**

⊗⑦**V03.90** **Pedestrian on foot injured in collision with car, pick-up truck or van, unspecified whether traffic or nontraffic accident**

Pedestrian NOS injured in collision with car, pick-up truck or van, unspecified whether traffic or nontraffic accident

⊗⑦**V03.91** **Pedestrian on roller-skates injured in collision with car, pick-up truck or van, unspecified whether traffic or nontraffic accident**

⊗⑦**V03.92** **Pedestrian on skateboard injured in collision with car, pick-up truck or van, unspecified whether traffic or nontraffic accident**

⊗⑦**V03.99** **Pedestrian with other conveyance injured in collision with car, pick-up truck or van, unspecified whether traffic or nontraffic accident**

Pedestrian with babystroller injured in collision with car, pick-up truck or van, unspecified whether traffic or nontraffic accident

Pedestrian on ice-skates injured in collision with car, pick-up truck or van, unspecified whether traffic or nontraffic accident

Pedestrian on nonmotorized scooter injured in collision with car, pick-up truck or van, unspecified whether traffic or nontraffic accident

Pedestrian on sled injured in collision with car, pick-up truck or van in nontraffic accident

Pedestrian on snowboard injured in collision with car, pick-up truck or van, unspecified whether traffic or nontraffic accident

Pedestrian on snow-skis injured in collision with car, pick-up truck or van, unspecified whether traffic or nontraffic accident

Pedestrian in wheelchair (powered) injured in collision with car, pick-up truck or van, unspecified whether traffic or nontraffic accident

Pedestrian in motorized mobility scooter injured in collision with car, pick-up truck or van, unspecified whether traffic or nontraffic accident

V04 **Pedestrian injured in collision with heavy transport vehicle or bus**

Excludes1: pedestrian injured in collision with military vehicle (V09.01, V09.21)

The appropriate 7th character is to be added to each code from category V04

A - initial encounter

D - subsequent encounter

S - sequela

V04.0 **Pedestrian injured in collision with heavy transport vehicle or bus in nontraffic accident**

⊗⑦**V04.00** **Pedestrian on foot injured in collision with heavy transport vehicle or bus in nontraffic accident**

● New code ▲ Revised code **Excludes1:** Not coded here **Excludes2:** Not included here ⊗ Placeholder required ⑦ 7th digit required

Pedestrian NOS injured in collision with heavy transport vehicle or bus in nontraffic accident

⊗⑦**V04.01** **Pedestrian on roller-skates injured in collision with heavy transport vehicle or bus in nontraffic accident**

⊗⑦**V04.02** **Pedestrian on skateboard injured in collision with heavy transport vehicle or bus in nontraffic accident**

⊗⑦**V04.09** **Pedestrian with other conveyance injured in collision with heavy transport vehicle or bus in nontraffic accident**

Pedestrian with babystroller injured in collision with heavy transport vehicle or bus in nontraffic accident

Pedestrian on ice-skates injured in collision with heavy transport vehicle or bus in nontraffic accident

Pedestrian on nonmotorized scooter injured in collision with heavy transport vehicle or bus in nontraffic accident

Pedestrian on sled injured in collision with heavy transport vehicle or bus in nontraffic accident

Pedestrian on snowboard injured in collision with heavy transport vehicle or bus in nontraffic accident

Pedestrian on snow-skis injured in collision with heavy transport vehicle or bus in nontraffic accident

Pedestrian in wheelchair (powered) injured in collision with heavy transport vehicle or bus in nontraffic accident

Pedestrian in motorized mobility scooter injured in collision with heavy transport vehicle or bus in nontraffic accident

V04.1 **Pedestrian injured in collision with heavy transport vehicle or bus in traffic accident**

⊗⑦**V04.10** **Pedestrian on foot injured in collision with heavy transport vehicle or bus in traffic accident**

Pedestrian NOS injured in collision with heavy transport vehicle or bus in traffic accident

⊗⑦**V04.11** **Pedestrian on roller-skates injured in collision with heavy transport vehicle or bus in traffic accident**

⊗⑦**V04.12** **Pedestrian on skateboard injured in collision with heavy transport vehicle or bus in traffic accident**

⊗⑦**V04.19** **Pedestrian with other conveyance injured in collision with heavy transport vehicle or bus in traffic accident**

Pedestrian with babystroller injured in collision with heavy transport vehicle or bus in traffic accident

Pedestrian on ice-skates injured in collision with heavy transport vehicle or bus in traffic accident

Pedestrian on nonmotorized scooter injured in collision with heavy transport vehicle or bus in traffic accident

Pedestrian on sled injured in collision with heavy transport vehicle or bus in traffic accident

Pedestrian on snowboard injured in collision with heavy transport vehicle or bus in traffic accident

Pedestrian on snow-skis injured in collision with heavy transport vehicle or bus in traffic accident

Pedestrian in wheelchair (powered) injured in collision with heavy transport vehicle or bus in traffic accident

Pedestrian in motorized mobility scooter injured in collision with heavy transport vehicle or bus in traffic accident

V04.9 **Pedestrian injured in collision with heavy transport vehicle or bus, unspecified whether traffic or nontraffic accident**

⊗⑦**V04.90** **Pedestrian on foot injured in collision with heavy transport vehicle or bus, unspecified whether traffic or nontraffic accident**

Pedestrian NOS injured in collision with heavy transport vehicle or bus, unspecified whether traffic or nontraffic accident

⊗⑦**V04.91** **Pedestrian on roller-skates injured in collision with heavy transport vehicle or bus, unspecified whether traffic or nontraffic accident**

⊗⑦**V04.92** **Pedestrian on skateboard injured in collision with heavy transport vehicle or bus, unspecified whether traffic or nontraffic accident**

⊗⑦**V04.99** **Pedestrian with other conveyance injured in collision with heavy transport vehicle or bus, unspecified whether traffic or nontraffic accident**

Pedestrian with babystroller injured in collision with heavy transport vehicle or bus, unspecified whether traffic or nontraffic accident

Pedestrian on ice-skates injured in collision with heavy transport vehicle or bus, unspecified whether traffic or nontraffic accident

Pedestrian on nonmotorized scooter injured in collision with heavy transport vehicle or bus, unspecified whether traffic or nontraffic accident

Pedestrian on sled injured in collision with heavy transport vehicle or bus, unspecified whether traffic or nontraffic accident

Pedestrian on snowboard injured in collision with heavy transport vehicle or bus, unspecified whether traffic or nontraffic accident

Pedestrian on snow-skis injured in collision with heavy transport vehicle or bus, unspecified whether traffic or nontraffic accident

Pedestrian in wheelchair (powered) injured in collision with heavy transport vehicle or bus, unspecified whether traffic or nontraffic accident

Pedestrian in motorized mobility scooter injured in collision with heavy transport vehicle or bus, unspecified whether traffic or nontraffic accident

V05 **Pedestrian injured in collision with railway train or railway vehicle**

The appropriate 7th character is to be added to each code from category V05

A - initial encounter

D - subsequent encounter

S - sequela

V05.0 **Pedestrian injured in collision with railway train or railway vehicle in nontraffic accident**

⊗⑦**V05.00** **Pedestrian on foot injured in collision with railway train or railway vehicle in nontraffic accident**

Pedestrian NOS injured in collision with railway train or railway vehicle in nontraffic accident

⊗⑦**V05.01** **Pedestrian on roller-skates injured in collision with railway train or railway vehicle in nontraffic accident**

⊗⑦**V05.02** **Pedestrian on skateboard injured in collision with railway train or railway vehicle in nontraffic accident**

⊗⑦**V05.09** **Pedestrian with other conveyance injured in collision with railway train or railway vehicle in nontraffic accident**

Pedestrian with babystroller injured in collision with railway train or railway vehicle in nontraffic accident

Pedestrian on ice-skates injured in collision with railway train or railway vehicle in nontraffic accident

Pedestrian on nonmotorized scooter injured in collision with railway train or railway vehicle in nontraffic accident

Pedestrian on sled injured in collision with railway train or railway vehicle in nontraffic accident

Pedestrian on snowboard injured in collision with railway train or railway vehicle in nontraffic accident

Pedestrian on snow-skis injured in collision with railway train or railway vehicle in nontraffic accident

Pedestrian in wheelchair (powered) injured in collision with railway train or railway vehicle in nontraffic accident

Pedestrian in motorized mobility scooter injured in collision with railway train or railway vehicle in nontraffic accident

V05.1 **Pedestrian injured in collision with railway train or railway vehicle in traffic accident**

⊗⑦**V05.10** **Pedestrian on foot injured in collision with railway train or railway vehicle in traffic accident**

Pedestrian NOS injured in collision with railway train or railway vehicle in traffic accident

⊗⑦**V05.11** **Pedestrian on roller-skates injured in collision with railway train or railway vehicle in traffic accident**

⊗⑦**V05.12** **Pedestrian on skateboard injured in collision with railway train or railway vehicle in traffic accident**

⊗⑦**V05.19** **Pedestrian with other conveyance injured in collision with railway train or railway vehicle in traffic accident**

Pedestrian with babystroller injured in collision with railway train or railway vehicle in traffic accident

Pedestrian on ice-skates injured in collision with railway train or railway vehicle in traffic accident

Pedestrian on nonmotorized scooter injured in collision with railway train or railway vehicle in traffic accident

Pedestrian on sled injured in collision with railway train or railway vehicle in traffic accident

Pedestrian on snowboard injured in collision with railway train or railway vehicle in traffic accident

Pedestrian on snow-skis injured in collision with railway train or railway vehicle in traffic accident

Pedestrian in wheelchair (powered) injured in collision with railway train or railway vehicle in traffic accident

Pedestrian in motorized mobility scooter injured in collision with railway train or railway vehicle in traffic accident

V05.9 **Pedestrian injured in collision with railway train or railway vehicle, unspecified whether traffic or nontraffic accident**

⊗⑦**V05.90** **Pedestrian on foot injured in collision with railway train or railway vehicle, unspecified whether traffic or nontraffic accident**

Pedestrian NOS injured in collision with railway train or railway vehicle, unspecified whether traffic or nontraffic accident

⊗⑦**V05.91** **Pedestrian on roller-skates injured in collision with railway train or railway vehicle, unspecified whether traffic or nontraffic accident**

⊗⑦**V05.92** **Pedestrian on skateboard injured in collision with railway train or railway vehicle, unspecified whether traffic or nontraffic accident**

⊗⑦**V05.99** **Pedestrian with other conveyance injured in collision with railway train or railway vehicle, unspecified whether traffic or nontraffic accident**

Pedestrian with babystroller injured in collision with railway train or railway vehicle, unspecified whether traffic or nontraffic

Pedestrian on ice-skates injured in collision with railway train or railway vehicle, unspecified whether traffic or nontraffic

Pedestrian on nonmotorized scooter injured in collision with railway train or railway vehicle, unspecified whether traffic or nontraffic

Pedestrian on sled injured in collision with railway train or railway vehicle, unspecified whether traffic or nontraffic

Pedestrian on snowboard injured in collision with railway train or railway vehicle, unspecified whether traffic or nontraffic

Pedestrian on snow-skis injured in collision with railway train or railway vehicle, unspecified whether traffic or nontraffic

Pedestrian in wheelchair (powered) injured in collision with railway train or railway vehicle, unspecified whether traffic or nontraffic

Pedestrian in motorized mobility scooter injured in collision with railway train or railway vehicle, unspecified whether traffic or nontraffic

V06 **Pedestrian injured in collision with other nonmotor vehicle**

Includes: collision with animal-drawn vehicle, animal being ridden, nonpowered streetcar

Excludes1: pedestrian injured in collision with pedestrian conveyance (V00.0-)

The appropriate 7th character is to be added to each code from category V06

A - initial encounter

D - subsequent encounter

S - sequela

V06.0 **Pedestrian injured in collision with other nonmotor vehicle in nontraffic accident**

⊗⑦**V06.00** Pedestrian on foot injured in collision with other nonmotor vehicle in nontraffic accident

Pedestrian NOS injured in collision **with other** nonmotor vehicle in nontraffic accident

⊗⑦**V06.01** Pedestrian on roller-skates injured in collision with other nonmotor vehicle in nontraffic accident

⊗⑦**V06.02** Pedestrian on skateboard injured in collision with other nonmotor vehicle in nontraffic accident

⊗⑦**V06.09** Pedestrian with other conveyance injured in collision with other nonmotor vehicle in nontraffic accident

Pedestrian with babystroller injured in collision with other nonmotor vehicle in nontraffic accident

Pedestrian on ice-skates injured in collision with other nonmotor vehicle in nontraffic accident

Pedestrian on nonmotorized scooter injured in collision with other nonmotor vehicle in nontraffic accident

Pedestrian on sled injured in collision with other nonmotor vehicle in nontraffic accident

Pedestrian on snowboard injured in collision with other nonmotor vehicle in nontraffic accident

Pedestrian on snow-skis injured in collision with other nonmotor vehicle in nontraffic accident

Pedestrian in wheelchair (powered) injured in collision with other nonmotor vehicle in nontraffic accident

Pedestrian in motorized mobility scooter injured in collision with other nonmotor vehicle in nontraffic accident

V06.1 **Pedestrian injured in collision with other nonmotor vehicle in traffic accident**

⊗⑦**V06.10** Pedestrian on foot injured in collision with other nonmotor vehicle in traffic accident

Pedestrian NOS injured in collision with other nonmotor vehicle in traffic accident

⊗⑦**V06.11** Pedestrian on roller-skates injured in collision with other nonmotor vehicle in traffic accident

⊗⑦**V06.12** Pedestrian on skateboard injured in collision with other nonmotor vehicle in traffic accident

⊗⑦**V06.19** Pedestrian with other conveyance injured in collision with other nonmotor vehicle in traffic accident

Pedestrian with babystroller injured in collision **with other** nonmotor vehicle in nontraffic accident

Pedestrian on ice-skates injured in collision **with other** nonmotor vehicle in traffic accident

Pedestrian on nonmotorized scooter injured in collision **with other** nonmotor vehicle in traffic accident

Pedestrian on sled injured in collision **with other** nonmotor vehicle in traffic accident

Pedestrian on snowboard injured in collision **with other** nonmotor vehicle in traffic accident

Pedestrian on snow-skis injured in collision **with other** nonmotor vehicle in traffic accident

Pedestrian in wheelchair (powered) injured in collision **with other** nonmotor vehicle in traffic accident

Pedestrian in motorized mobility scooter injured in collision **with other** nonmotor vehicle in traffic accident

V06.9 **Pedestrian injured in collision with other nonmotor vehicle, unspecified whether traffic or nontraffic accident**

⊗⑦**V06.90** Pedestrian on foot injured in collision with other nonmotor vehicle, unspecified whether traffic or nontraffic accident

Pedestrian NOS injured in collision **with other** nonmotor vehicle, unspecified whether traffic or nontraffic accident

⊗⑦**V06.91** Pedestrian on roller-skates injured in collision with other nonmotor vehicle, unspecified whether traffic or nontraffic accident

⊗⑦**V06.92** Pedestrian on skateboard injured in collision with other nonmotor vehicle, unspecified whether traffic or nontraffic accident

⊗⑦**V06.99** Pedestrian with other conveyance injured in collision with other nonmotor vehicle, unspecified whether traffic or nontraffic accident

Pedestrian with babystroller injured in collision **with other** nonmotor vehicle, unspecified whether traffic or nontraffic accident

Pedestrian on ice-skates injured in collision **with other** nonmotor vehicle, unspecified whether traffic or nontraffic accident

Pedestrian on nonmotorized scooter injured in collision **with other** nonmotor vehicle, unspecified whether traffic or nontraffic accident

Pedestrian on sled injured in collision **with other** nonmotor vehicle, unspecified whether traffic or nontraffic accident

Pedestrian on snowboard injured in collision **with other** nonmotor vehicle, unspecified whether traffic or nontraffic accident

Pedestrian on snow-skis injured in collision **with other** nonmotor vehicle, unspecified whether traffic or nontraffic accident

Pedestrian in wheelchair (powered) injured in collision **with other** nonmotor vehicle, unspecified whether traffic or nontraffic accident

Pedestrian in motorized mobility scooter injured in collision **with other** nonmotor vehicle, unspecified whether traffic or nontraffic accident

V09 **Pedestrian injured in other and unspecified transport accidents**

The appropriate 7th character is to be added to each code from category V09

A - initial encounter

D - subsequent encounter

S - sequela

V09.0 **Pedestrian injured in nontraffic accident involving other and unspecified motor vehicles**

⊗⑦**V09.00** Pedestrian injured in nontraffic accident involving unspecified motor vehicles

⊗⑦**V09.01** Pedestrian injured in nontraffic accident involving military vehicle

⊗⑦**V09.09** Pedestrian injured in nontraffic accident involving other motor vehicles

Pedestrian injured in nontraffic accident by special vehicle

⊗⑦**V09.1**   **Pedestrian injured in unspecified nontraffic accident**

V09.2   **Pedestrian injured in traffic accident involving other and unspecified motor vehicles**

⊗⑦**V09.20**   **Pedestrian injured in traffic accident involving unspecified motor vehicles**

⊗⑦**V09.21**   **Pedestrian injured in traffic accident involving military vehicle**

⊗⑦**V09.29**   **Pedestrian injured in traffic accident involving other motor vehicles**

⊗⑦**V09.3**   **Pedestrian injured in unspecified traffic accident**

⊗⑦**V09.9**   **Pedestrian injured in unspecified transport accident**

PEDAL CYCLE RIDER INJURED IN TRANSPORT ACCIDENT (V10-V19)

Includes: any non-motorized vehicle, excluding an animal-drawn vehicle, or a sidecar or trailer attached to the pedal cycle

Excludes2: rupture of pedal cycle tire (W37.0)

V10   **Pedal cycle rider injured in collision with pedestrian or animal**

Excludes1: pedal cycle rider collision with animal-drawn vehicle or animal being ridden (V16.-)

The appropriate 7th character is to be added to each code from category V10

A - initial encounter

D - subsequent encounter

S - sequela

⊗⑦**V10.0**   **Pedal cycle driver injured in collision with pedestrian or animal in nontraffic accident**

⊗⑦**V10.1**   **Pedal cycle passenger injured in collision with pedestrian or animal in nontraffic accident**

⊗⑦**V10.2**   **Unspecified pedal cyclist injured in collision with pedestrian or animal in nontraffic accident**

⊗⑦**V10.3**   **Person boarding or alighting a pedal cycle injured in collision with pedestrian or animal**

⊗⑦**V10.4**   **Pedal cycle driver injured in collision with pedestrian or animal in traffic accident**

⊗⑦**V10.5**   **Pedal cycle passenger injured in collision with pedestrian or animal in traffic accident**

⊗⑦**V10.9**   **Unspecified pedal cyclist injured in collision with pedestrian or animal in traffic accident**

V11   **Pedal cycle rider injured in collision with other pedal cycle**

The appropriate 7th character is to be added to each code from category V11

A - initial encounter

D - subsequent encounter

S - sequela

⊗⑦**V11.0**   **Pedal cycle driver injured in collision with other pedal cycle in nontraffic accident**

⊗⑦**V11.1**   **Pedal cycle passenger injured in collision with other pedal cycle in nontraffic accident**

⊗⑦**V11.2**   **Unspecified pedal cyclist injured in collision with other pedal cycle in nontraffic accident**

⊗⑦**V11.3**   **Person boarding or alighting a pedal cycle injured in collision with other pedal cycle**

⊗⑦**V11.4**   **Pedal cycle driver injured in collision with other pedal cycle in traffic accident**

⊗⑦**V11.5**   **Pedal cycle passenger injured in collision with other pedal cycle in traffic accident**

⊗⑦**V11.9**   **Unspecified pedal cyclist injured in collision with other pedal cycle in traffic accident**

V12   **Pedal cycle rider injured in collision with two- or three-wheeled motor vehicle**

The appropriate 7th character is to be added to each code from category V12

A - initial encounter

D - subsequent encounter

S - sequela

⊗⑦**V12.0**   **Pedal cycle driver injured in collision with two- or three-wheeled motor vehicle in nontraffic accident**

⊗⑦**V12.1**   **Pedal cycle passenger injured in collision with two- or three-wheeled motor vehicle in nontraffic accident**

⊗⑦**V12.2**   **Unspecified pedal cyclist injured in collision with two- or three-wheeled motor vehicle in nontraffic accident**

⊗⑦**V12.3**   **Person boarding or alighting a pedal cycle injured in collision with two- or three-wheeled motor vehicle**

⊗⑦**V12.4**   **Pedal cycle driver injured in collision with two- or three-wheeled motor vehicle in traffic accident**

⊗⑦**V12.5**   **Pedal cycle passenger injured in collision with two- or three-wheeled motor vehicle in traffic accident**

⊗⑦**V12.9**   **Unspecified pedal cyclist injured in collision with two- or three-wheeled motor vehicle in traffic accident**

V13   **Pedal cycle rider injured in collision with car, pick-up truck or van**

The appropriate 7th character is to be added to each code from category V13

A - initial encounter

D - subsequent encounter

S - sequela

⊗⑦**V13.0**   **Pedal cycle driver injured in collision with car, pick-up truck or van in nontraffic accident**

⊗⑦**V13.1**   **Pedal cycle passenger injured in collision with car, pick-up truck or van in nontraffic accident**

⊗⑦**V13.2**   **Unspecified pedal cyclist injured in collision with car, pick-up truck or van in nontraffic accident**

⊗⑦**V13.3**   **Person boarding or alighting a pedal cycle injured in collision with car, pick-up truck or van**

⊗⑦**V13.4**   **Pedal cycle driver injured in collision with car, pick-up truck or van in traffic accident**

⊗⑦**V13.5**   **Pedal cycle passenger injured in collision with car, pick-up truck or van in traffic accident**

⊗⑦**V13.9**   **Unspecified pedal cyclist injured in collision with car, pick-up truck or van in traffic accident**

V14   **Pedal cycle rider injured in collision with heavy transport vehicle or bus**

Excludes1: pedal cycle rider injured in collision with military vehicle (V19.81)

The appropriate 7th character is to be added to each code from category V14

A - initial encounter

D - subsequent encounter

S - sequela

⊗⑦**V14.0**   **Pedal cycle driver injured in collision with heavy transport vehicle or bus in nontraffic accident**

⊗⑦**V14.1**   **Pedal cycle passenger injured in collision with heavy transport vehicle or bus in nontraffic accident**

⊗⑦**V14.2**   **Unspecified pedal cyclist injured in collision with heavy transport vehicle or bus in nontraffic accident**

⊗⑦V14.3   Person boarding or alighting a pedal cycle injured in collision with heavy transport vehicle or bus

⊗⑦V14.4   Pedal cycle driver injured in collision with heavy transport vehicle or bus in traffic accident

⊗⑦V14.5   Pedal cycle passenger injured in collision with heavy transport vehicle or bus in traffic accident

⊗⑦V14.9   Unspecified pedal cyclist injured in collision with heavy transport vehicle or bus in traffic accident

V15   Pedal cycle rider injured in collision with railway train or railway vehicle

The appropriate 7th character is to be added to each code from category V15

A - initial encounter

D - subsequent encounter

S - sequela

⊗⑦V15.0   Pedal cycle driver injured in collision with railway train or railway vehicle in nontraffic accident

⊗⑦V15.1   Pedal cycle passenger injured in collision with railway train or railway vehicle in nontraffic accident

⊗⑦V15.2   Unspecified pedal cyclist injured in collision with railway train or railway vehicle in nontraffic accident

⊗⑦V15.3   Person boarding or alighting a pedal cycle injured in collision with railway train or railway vehicle

⊗⑦V15.4   Pedal cycle driver injured in collision with railway train or railway vehicle in traffic accident

⊗⑦V15.5   Pedal cycle passenger injured in collision with railway train or railway vehicle in traffic accident

⊗⑦V15.9   Unspecified pedal cyclist injured in collision with railway train or railway vehicle in traffic accident

V16   Pedal cycle rider injured in collision with other nonmotor vehicle

Includes: collision with animal-drawn vehicle, animal being ridden, streetcar

The appropriate 7th character is to be added to each code from category V16

A - initial encounter

D - subsequent encounter

S - sequela

⊗⑦**V16.0**   Pedal cycle driver injured in collision with other nonmotor vehicle in nontraffic accident

⊗⑦**V16.1**   Pedal cycle passenger injured in collision with other nonmotor vehicle in nontraffic accident

⊗⑦**V16.2**   Unspecified pedal cyclist injured in collision with other nonmotor vehicle in nontraffic accident

⊗⑦**V16.3**   Person boarding or alighting a pedal cycle injured in collision with other nonmotor vehicle in nontraffic accident

⊗⑦**V16.4**   Pedal cycle driver injured in collision with other nonmotor vehicle in traffic accident

⊗⑦**V16.5**   Pedal cycle passenger injured in collision with other nonmotor vehicle in traffic accident

⊗⑦**V16.9**   Unspecified pedal cyclist injured in collision with other nonmotor vehicle in traffic accident

V17   Pedal cycle rider injured in collision with fixed or stationary object

The appropriate 7th character is to be added to each code from category V17

A - initial encounter

D - subsequent encounter

S - sequela

⊗⑦V17.0   Pedal cycle driver injured in collision with fixed or stationary object in nontraffic accident

⊗⑦V17.1   Pedal cycle passenger injured in collision with fixed or stationary object in nontraffic accident

⊗⑦V17.2   Unspecified pedal cyclist injured in collision with fixed or stationary object in nontraffic accident

⊗⑦V17.3   Person boarding or alighting a pedal cycle injured in collision with fixed or stationary object

⊗⑦V17.4   Pedal cycle driver injured in collision with fixed or stationary object in traffic accident

⊗⑦V17.5   Pedal cycle passenger injured in collision with fixed or stationary object in traffic accident

⊗⑦V17.9   Unspecified pedal cyclist injured in collision with fixed or stationary object in traffic accident

V18   Pedal cycle rider injured in noncollision transport accident

Includes: fall or thrown from pedal cycle (without antecedent collision)

overturning pedal cycle NOS overturning pedal cycle without collision

The appropriate 7th character is to be added to each code from category V18

A - initial encounter

D - subsequent encounter

S - sequela

⊗⑦**V18.0**   Pedal cycle driver injured in noncollision transport accident in nontraffic accident

⊗⑦**V18.1**   Pedal cycle passenger injured in noncollision transport accident in nontraffic accident

⊗⑦**V18.2**   Unspecified pedal cyclist injured in noncollision transport accident in nontraffic accident

⊗⑦**V18.3**   Person boarding or alighting a pedal cycle injured in noncollision transport accident

⊗⑦**V18.4**   Pedal cycle driver injured in noncollision transport accident in traffic accident

⊗⑦**V18.5**   Pedal cycle passenger injured in noncollision transport accident in traffic accident

⊗⑦**V18.9**   Unspecified pedal cyclist injured in noncollision transport accident in traffic accident

V19   Pedal cycle rider injured in other and unspecified transport accidents

The appropriate 7th character is to be added to each code from category V19

A - initial encounter

D - subsequent encounter

S - sequela

V19.0   Pedal cycle driver injured in collision with other and unspecified motor vehicles in nontraffic accident

⊗⑦V19.00   Pedal cycle driver injured in collision with unspecified motor vehicles in nontraffic accident

⊗⑦**V19.09**   Pedal cycle driver injured in collision with other motor vehicles in nontraffic accident

V19.1   Pedal cycle passenger injured in collision with other and unspecified motor vehicles in nontraffic accident

⊗⑦**V19.10**   Pedal cycle passenger injured in collision with unspecified motor vehicles in nontraffic accident

⊗⑦**V19.19**   Pedal cycle passenger injured in collision with other motor vehicles in nontraffic accident

V19.2   Unspecified pedal cyclist injured in collision with other and unspecified motor vehicles in nontraffic accident

⊗⑦**V19.20** Unspecified pedal cyclist injured in collision with unspecified motor vehicles in nontraffic accident

Pedal cycle collision NOS, nontraffic

⊗⑦**V19.29** Unspecified pedal cyclist injured in collision with other motor vehicles in nontraffic accident

⊗⑦**V19.3** Pedal cyclist (driver) (passenger) injured in unspecified nontraffic accident

Pedal cycle accident NOS, nontraffic

Pedal cyclist injured in nontraffic accident NOS

V19.4 Pedal cycle driver injured in collision with other and unspecified motor vehicles in traffic accident

⊗⑦**V19.40** Pedal cycle driver injured in collision with unspecified motor vehicles in traffic accident

⊗⑦**V19.49** Pedal cycle driver injured in collision with other motor vehicles in traffic accident

V19.5 Pedal cycle passenger injured in collision with other and unspecified motor vehicles in traffic accident

⊗⑦**V19.50** Pedal cycle passenger injured in collision with unspecified motor vehicles in traffic accident

⊗⑦**V19.59** Pedal cycle passenger injured in collision with other motor vehicles in traffic accident

V19.6 Unspecified pedal cyclist injured in collision with other and unspecified motor vehicles in traffic accident

⊗⑦**V19.60** Unspecified pedal cyclist injured in collision with unspecified motor vehicles in traffic accident

Pedal cycle collision NOS (traffic)

⊗⑦**V19.69** Unspecified pedal cyclist injured in collision with other motor vehicles in traffic accident

V19.8 Pedal cyclist (driver) (passenger) injured in other specified transport accidents

⊗⑦**V19.81** Pedal cyclist (driver) (passenger) injured in transport accident with military vehicle

⊗⑦**V19.88** Pedal cyclist (driver) (passenger) injured in other specified transport accidents

⊗⑦**V19.9** Pedal cyclist (driver) (passenger) injured in unspecified traffic accident

Pedal cycle accident NOS

MOTORCYCLE RIDER INJURED IN TRANSPORT ACCIDENT (V20-V29)

Includes: moped

motorcycle with sidecar motorized bicycle motor scooter

Excludes1: three-wheeled motor vehicle (V30-V39)

V20 Motorcycle rider injured in collision with pedestrian or animal

Excludes1: motorcycle rider collision with animal-drawn vehicle or animal being ridden (V26.-)

The appropriate 7th character is to be added to each code from category V20

A - initial encounter

D - subsequent encounter

S - sequela

⊗⑦**V20.0** Motorcycle driver injured in collision with pedestrian or animal in nontraffic accident

⊗⑦**V20.1** Motorcycle passenger injured in collision with pedestrian or animal in nontraffic accident

⊗⑦**V20.2** Unspecified motorcycle rider injured in collision with pedestrian or animal in nontraffic accident

⊗⑦**V20.3** Person boarding or alighting a motorcycle injured in collision with pedestrian or animal

⊗⑦**V20.4** Motorcycle driver injured in collision with pedestrian or animal in traffic accident

⊗⑦**V20.5** Motorcycle passenger injured in collision with pedestrian or animal in traffic accident

⊗⑦**V20.9** Unspecified motorcycle rider injured in collision with pedestrian or animal in traffic accident

V21 Motorcycle rider injured in collision with pedal cycle

The appropriate 7th character is to be added to each code from category V21

A - initial encounter

D - subsequent encounter

S - sequela

⊗⑦**V21.0** Motorcycle driver injured in collision with pedal cycle in nontraffic accident

⊗⑦**V21.1** Motorcycle passenger injured in collision with pedal cycle in nontraffic accident

⊗⑦**V21.2** Unspecified motorcycle rider injured in collision with pedal cycle in nontraffic accident

⊗⑦**V21.3** Person boarding or alighting a motorcycle injured in collision with pedal cycle

⊗⑦**V21.4** Motorcycle driver injured in collision with pedal cycle in traffic accident

⊗⑦**V21.5** Motorcycle passenger injured in collision with pedal cycle in traffic accident

⊗⑦**V21.9** Unspecified motorcycle rider injured in collision with pedal cycle in traffic accident

V22 Motorcycle rider injured in collision with two- or three-wheeled motor vehicle

The appropriate 7th character is to be added to each code from category V22

A - initial encounter

D - subsequent encounter

S - sequela

⊗⑦**V22.0** Motorcycle driver injured in collision with two- or three-wheeled motor vehicle in nontraffic accident

⊗⑦**V22.1** Motorcycle passenger injured in collision with two- or three-wheeled motor vehicle in nontraffic accident

⊗⑦**V22.2** Unspecified motorcycle rider injured in collision with two- or three-wheeled motor vehicle in nontraffic accident

⊗⑦**V22.3** Person boarding or alighting a motorcycle injured in collision with two- or three-wheeled motor vehicle

⊗⑦**V22.4** Motorcycle driver injured in collision with two- or three-wheeled motor vehicle in traffic accident

⊗⑦**V22.5** Motorcycle passenger injured in collision with two- or three-wheeled motor vehicle in traffic accident

⊗⑦**V22.9** Unspecified motorcycle rider injured in collision with two- or three-wheeled motor vehicle in traffic accident

V23 Motorcycle rider injured in collision with car, pick-up truck or van

The appropriate 7th character is to be added to each code from category V23

A - initial encounter

D - subsequent encounter

S - sequela

⊗⑦**V23.0** Motorcycle driver injured in collision with car, pick-up truck or van in nontraffic accident

⊗⑦**V23.1**   **Motorcycle passenger injured in collision with car, pick-up truck or van in nontraffic accident**

⊗⑦**V23.2**   **Unspecified motorcycle rider injured in collision with car, pick-up truck or van in nontraffic accident**

⊗⑦**V23.3**   **Person boarding or alighting a motorcycle injured in collision with car, pick-up truck or van**

⊗⑦**V23.4**   **Motorcycle driver injured in collision with car, pick-up truck or van in traffic accident**

⊗⑦**V23.5**   **Motorcycle passenger injured in collision with car, pick-up truck or van in traffic accident**

⊗⑦**V23.9**   **Unspecified motorcycle rider injured in collision with car, pick-up truck or van in traffic accident**

V24   **Motorcycle rider injured in collision with heavy transport vehicle or bus**

Excludes1: motorcycle rider injured in collision with military vehicle (V29.81)

The appropriate 7th character is to be added to each code from category V24

A - initial encounter

D - subsequent encounter

S - sequela

⊗⑦**V24.0**   **Motorcycle driver injured in collision with heavy transport vehicle or bus in nontraffic accident**

⊗⑦**V24.1**   **Motorcycle passenger injured in collision with heavy transport vehicle or bus in nontraffic accident**

⊗⑦**V24.2**   **Unspecified motorcycle rider injured in collision with heavy transport vehicle or bus in nontraffic accident**

⊗⑦**V24.3**   **Person boarding or alighting a motorcycle injured in collision with heavy transport vehicle or bus**

⊗⑦**V24.4**   **Motorcycle driver injured in collision with heavy transport vehicle or bus in traffic accident**

⊗⑦**V24.5**   **Motorcycle passenger injured in collision with heavy transport vehicle or bus in traffic accident**

⊗⑦**V24.9**   **Unspecified motorcycle rider injured in collision with heavy transport vehicle or bus in traffic accident**

V25   **Motorcycle rider injured in collision with railway train or railway vehicle**

The appropriate 7th character is to be added to each code from category V25

A - initial encounter

D - subsequent encounter

S - sequela

⊗⑦**V25.0**   **Motorcycle driver injured in collision with railway train or railway vehicle in nontraffic accident**

⊗⑦**V25.1**   **Motorcycle passenger injured in collision with railway train or railway vehicle in nontraffic accident**

⊗⑦**V25.2**   **Unspecified motorcycle rider injured in collision with railway train or railway vehicle in nontraffic accident**

⊗⑦**V25.3**   **Person boarding or alighting a motorcycle injured in collision with railway train or railway vehicle**

⊗⑦**V25.4**   **Motorcycle driver injured in collision with railway train or railway vehicle in traffic accident**

⊗⑦**V25.5**   **Motorcycle passenger injured in collision with railway train or railway vehicle in traffic accident**

⊗⑦**V25.9**   **Unspecified motorcycle rider injured in collision with railway train or railway vehicle in traffic accident**

V26   **Motorcycle rider injured in collision with other nonmotor vehicle**

Includes: collision with animal-drawn vehicle, animal being ridden, streetcar

The appropriate 7th character is to be added to each code from category V26

A - initial encounter

D - subsequent encounter

S - sequela

⊗⑦**V26.0**   **Motorcycle driver injured in collision with other nonmotor vehicle in nontraffic accident**

⊗⑦**V26.1**   **Motorcycle passenger injured in collision with other nonmotor vehicle in nontraffic accident**

⊗⑦**V26.2**   **Unspecified motorcycle rider injured in collision with other nonmotor vehicle in nontraffic accident**

⊗⑦**V26.3**   **Person boarding or alighting a motorcycle injured in collision with other nonmotor vehicle**

⊗⑦**V26.4**   **Motorcycle driver injured in collision with other nonmotor vehicle in traffic accident**

⊗⑦**V26.5**   **Motorcycle passenger injured in collision with other nonmotor vehicle in traffic accident**

⊗⑦**V26.9**   **Unspecified motorcycle rider injured in collision with other nonmotor vehicle in traffic accident**

V27   **Motorcycle rider injured in collision with fixed or stationary object**

The appropriate 7th character is to be added to each code from category V27

A - initial encounter

D - subsequent encounter

S - sequela

⊗⑦**V27.0**   **Motorcycle driver injured in collision with fixed or stationary object in nontraffic accident**

⊗⑦**V27.1**   **Motorcycle passenger injured in collision with fixed or stationary object in nontraffic accident**

⊗⑦**V27.2**   **Unspecified motorcycle rider injured in collision with fixed or stationary object in nontraffic accident**

⊗⑦**V27.3**   **Person boarding or alighting a motorcycle injured in collision with fixed or stationary object**

⊗⑦**V27.4**   **Motorcycle driver injured in collision with fixed or stationary object in traffic accident**

⊗⑦**V27.5**   **Motorcycle passenger injured in collision with fixed or stationary object in traffic accident**

⊗⑦**V27.9**   **Unspecified motorcycle rider injured in collision with fixed or stationary object in traffic accident**

V28   **Motorcycle rider injured in noncollision transport accident**

Includes: fall or thrown from motorcycle (without antecedent collision)

overturning motorcycle NOS overturning motorcycle without collision

The appropriate 7th character is to be added to each code from category V28

A - initial encounter

D - subsequent encounter

S - sequela

⊗⑦**V28.0**   **Motorcycle driver injured in noncollision transport accident in nontraffic accident**

⊗⑦**V28.1**   **Motorcycle passenger injured in noncollision transport accident in nontraffic accident**

⊗⑦**V28.2**   **Unspecified motorcycle rider injured in noncollision transport accident in nontraffic accident**

⊗⑦**V28.3**   **Person boarding or alighting a motorcycle injured in noncollision transport accident**

⊗⑦**V28.4**   **Motorcycle driver injured in noncollision transport accident in traffic accident**

⊗⑦**V28.5** Motorcycle passenger injured in noncollision transport accident in traffic accident

⊗⑦**V28.9** Unspecified motorcycle rider injured in noncollision transport accident in traffic accident

V29 Motorcycle rider injured in other and unspecified transport accidents

The appropriate 7th character is to be added to each code from category V29

A - initial encounter

D - subsequent encounter

S - sequela

V29.0 Motorcycle driver injured in collision with other and unspecified motor vehicles in nontraffic accident

⊗⑦**V29.00** Motorcycle driver injured in collision with unspecified motor vehicles in nontraffic accident

⊗⑦**V29.09** Motorcycle driver injured in collision with other motor vehicles in nontraffic accident

V29.1 Motorcycle passenger injured in collision with other and unspecified motor vehicles in nontraffic accident

⊗⑦**V29.10** Motorcycle passenger injured in collision with unspecified motor vehicles in nontraffic accident

⊗⑦**V29.19** Motorcycle passenger injured in collision with other motor vehicles in nontraffic accident

V29.2 Unspecified motorcycle rider injured in collision with other and unspecified motor vehicles in nontraffic accident

⊗⑦**V29.20** Unspecified motorcycle rider injured in collision with unspecified motor vehicles in nontraffic accident

Motorcycle collision NOS, nontraffic

⊗⑦**V29.29** Unspecified motorcycle rider injured in collision with other motor vehicles in nontraffic accident

⊗⑦**V29.3** Motorcycle rider (driver) (passenger) injured in unspecified nontraffic accident

Motorcycle accident NOS, nontraffic

Motorcycle rider injured in nontraffic accident NOS

V29.4 Motorcycle driver injured in collision with other and unspecified motor vehicles in traffic accident

⊗⑦**V29.40** Motorcycle driver injured in collision with unspecified motor vehicles in traffic accident

⊗⑦**V29.49** Motorcycle driver injured in collision with other motor vehicles in traffic accident

V29.5 Motorcycle passenger injured in collision with other and unspecified motor vehicles in traffic accident

⊗⑦**V29.50** Motorcycle passenger injured in collision with unspecified motor vehicles in traffic accident

⊗⑦**V29.59** Motorcycle passenger injured in collision with other motor vehicles in traffic accident

V29.6 Unspecified motorcycle rider injured in collision with other and unspecified motor vehicles in traffic accident

⊗⑦**V29.60** Unspecified motorcycle rider injured in collision with unspecified motor vehicles in traffic accident

Motorcycle collision NOS (traffic)

⊗⑦**V29.69** Unspecified motorcycle rider injured in collision with other motor vehicles in traffic accident

V29.8 Motorcycle rider (driver) (passenger) injured in other specified transport accidents

⊗⑦**V29.81** Motorcycle rider (driver) (passenger) injured in transport accident with military vehicle

⊗⑦**V29.88** Motorcycle rider (driver) (passenger) injured in other specified transport accidents

⊗⑦**V29.9** Motorcycle rider (driver) (passenger) injured in unspecified traffic accident

Motorcycle accident NOS

OCCUPANT OF THREE-WHEELED MOTOR VEHICLE INJURED IN TRANSPORT ACCIDENT (V30-V39)

Includes: motorized tricycle

motorized rickshaw three-wheeled motor car

Excludes1: all-terrain vehicles (V86.-)

motorcycle with sidecar (V20-V29)

vehicle designed primarily for off-road use (V86.-)

V30 Occupant of three-wheeled motor vehicle injured in collision with pedestrian or animal

Excludes1: three-wheeled motor vehicle collision with animal-drawn vehicle or animal being ridden (V36.-)

The appropriate 7th character is to be added to each code from category V30

A - initial encounter

D - subsequent encounter

S - sequela

⊗⑦**V30.0** Driver of three-wheeled motor vehicle injured in collision with pedestrian or animal in nontraffic accident

⊗⑦**V30.1** Passenger in three-wheeled motor vehicle injured in collision with pedestrian or animal in nontraffic accident

⊗⑦**V30.2** Person on outside of three-wheeled motor vehicle injured in collision with pedestrian or animal in nontraffic accident

⊗⑦**V30.3** Unspecified occupant of three-wheeled motor vehicle injured in collision with pedestrian or animal in nontraffic accident

⊗⑦**V30.4** Person boarding or alighting a three-wheeled motor vehicle injured in collision with pedestrian or animal

⊗⑦**V30.5** Driver of three-wheeled motor vehicle injured in collision with pedestrian or animal in traffic accident

⊗⑦**V30.6** Passenger in three-wheeled motor vehicle injured in collision with pedestrian or animal in traffic accident

⊗⑦**V30.7** Person on outside of three-wheeled motor vehicle injured in collision with pedestrian or animal in traffic accident

⊗⑦**V30.9** Unspecified occupant of three-wheeled motor vehicle injured in collision with pedestrian or animal in traffic accident

V31 Occupant of three-wheeled motor vehicle injured in collision with pedal cycle

The appropriate 7th character is to be added to each code from category V31

A - initial encounter

D - subsequent encounter

S - sequela

⊗⑦**V31.0** Driver of three-wheeled motor vehicle injured in collision with pedal cycle in nontraffic accident

⊗⑦V31.1 Passenger in three-wheeled motor vehicle injured in collision with pedal cycle in nontraffic accident

⊗⑦V31.2 Person on outside of three-wheeled motor vehicle injured in collision with pedal cycle in nontraffic accident

⊗⑦**V31.3** Unspecified occupant of three-wheeled motor vehicle injured in collision with pedal cycle in nontraffic accident

⊗⑦V31.4 Person boarding or alighting a three-wheeled motor vehicle injured in collision with pedal cycle

⊗⑦V31.5 Driver of three-wheeled motor vehicle injured in collision with pedal cycle in traffic accident

⊗⑦V31.6 Passenger in three-wheeled motor vehicle injured in collision with pedal cycle in traffic accident

⊗⑦V31.7 Person on outside of three-wheeled motor vehicle injured in collision with pedal cycle in traffic accident

⊗⑦**V31.9** Unspecified occupant of three-wheeled motor vehicle injured in collision with pedal cycle in traffic accident

V32 Occupant of three-wheeled motor vehicle injured in collision with two- or three-wheeled motor vehicle

The appropriate 7th character is to be added to each code from category V32

A - initial encounter

D - subsequent encounter

S - sequela

⊗⑦V32.0 Driver of three-wheeled motor vehicle injured in collision with two- or three-wheeled motor vehicle in nontraffic accident

⊗⑦V32.1 Passenger in three-wheeled motor vehicle injured in collision with two- or three-wheeled motor vehicle in nontraffic accident

⊗⑦V32.2 Person on outside of three-wheeled motor vehicle injured in collision with two- or three-wheeled motor vehicle in nontraffic accident

⊗⑦**V32.3** Unspecified occupant of three-wheeled motor vehicle injured in collision with two- or three-wheeled motor vehicle in nontraffic accident

⊗⑦V32.4 Person boarding or alighting a three-wheeled motor vehicle injured in collision with two- or three-wheeled motor vehicle

⊗⑦V32.5 Driver of three-wheeled motor vehicle injured in collision with two- or three-wheeled motor vehicle in traffic accident

⊗⑦V32.6 Passenger in three-wheeled motor vehicle injured in collision with two- or three-wheeled motor vehicle in traffic accident

⊗⑦V32.7 Person on outside of three-wheeled motor vehicle injured in collision with two- or three-wheeled motor vehicle in traffic accident

⊗⑦**V32.9** Unspecified occupant of three-wheeled motor vehicle injured in collision with two- or three-wheeled motor vehicle in traffic accident

V33 Occupant of three-wheeled motor vehicle injured in collision with car, pick-up truck or van

The appropriate 7th character is to be added to each code from category V33

A - initial encounter

D - subsequent encounter

S - sequela

⊗⑦**V33.0** Driver of three-wheeled motor vehicle injured in collision with car, pick-up truck or van in nontraffic accident

⊗⑦V33.1 Passenger in three-wheeled motor vehicle injured in collision with car, pick-up truck or van in nontraffic accident

⊗⑦V33.2 Person on outside of three-wheeled motor vehicle injured in collision with car, pick-up truck or van in nontraffic accident

⊗⑦**V33.3** Unspecified occupant of three-wheeled motor vehicle injured in collision with car, pick-up truck or van in nontraffic accident

⊗⑦V33.4 Person boarding or alighting a three-wheeled motor vehicle injured in collision with car, pick-up truck or van

⊗⑦V33.5 Driver of three-wheeled motor vehicle injured in collision with car, pick-up truck or van in traffic accident

⊗⑦V33.6 Passenger in three-wheeled motor vehicle injured in collision with car, pick-up truck or van in traffic accident

⊗⑦V33.7 Person on outside of three-wheeled motor vehicle injured in collision with car, pick-up truck or van in traffic accident

⊗⑦**V33.9** Unspecified occupant of three-wheeled motor vehicle injured in collision with car, pick-up truck or van in traffic accident

V34 Occupant of three-wheeled motor vehicle injured in collision with heavy transport vehicle or bus

Excludes1: occupant of three-wheeled motor vehicle injured in collision with military vehicle (V39.81)

The appropriate 7th character is to be added to each code from category V34

A - initial encounter

D - subsequent encounter

S - sequela

⊗⑦V34.0 Driver of three-wheeled motor vehicle injured in collision with heavy transport vehicle or bus in nontraffic accident

⊗⑦V34.1 Passenger in three-wheeled motor vehicle injured in collision with heavy transport vehicle or bus in nontraffic accident

⊗⑦V34.2 Person on outside of three-wheeled motor vehicle injured in collision with heavy transport vehicle or bus in nontraffic accident

⊗⑦**V34.3** Unspecified occupant of three-wheeled motor vehicle injured in collision with heavy transport vehicle or bus in nontraffic accident

⊗⑦V34.4 Person boarding or alighting a three-wheeled motor vehicle injured in collision with heavy transport vehicle or bus

⊗⑦V34.5 Driver of three-wheeled motor vehicle injured in collision with heavy transport vehicle or bus in traffic accident

⊗⑦V34.6 Passenger in three-wheeled motor vehicle injured in collision with heavy transport vehicle or bus in traffic accident

⊗⑦V34.7 Person on outside of three-wheeled motor vehicle injured in collision with heavy transport vehicle or bus in traffic accident

⊗⑦**V34.9** Unspecified occupant of three-wheeled motor vehicle injured in collision with heavy transport vehicle or bus in traffic accident

V35 Occupant of three-wheeled motor vehicle injured in collision with railway train or railway vehicle

The appropriate 7th character is to be added to each code from category V35

A - initial encounter

D - subsequent encounter

S - sequela

⊗⑦V35.0 **Driver of three-wheeled motor vehicle injured in collision with railway train or railway vehicle in nontraffic accident**

⊗⑦V35.1 **Passenger in three-wheeled motor vehicle injured in collision with railway train or railway vehicle in nontraffic accident**

⊗⑦V35.2 **Person on outside of three-wheeled motor vehicle injured in collision with railway train or railway vehicle in nontraffic accident**

⊗⑦V35.3 **Unspecified occupant of three-wheeled motor vehicle injured in collision with railway train or railway vehicle in nontraffic accident**

⊗⑦V35.4 **Person boarding or alighting a three-wheeled motor vehicle injured in collision with railway train or railway vehicle**

⊗⑦V35.5 **Driver of three-wheeled motor vehicle injured in collision with railway train or railway vehicle in traffic accident**

⊗⑦V35.6 **Passenger in three-wheeled motor vehicle injured in collision with railway train or railway vehicle in traffic accident**

⊗⑦V35.7 **Person on outside of three-wheeled motor vehicle injured in collision with railway train or railway vehicle in traffic accident**

⊗⑦V35.9 **Unspecified occupant of three-wheeled motor vehicle injured in collision with railway train or railway vehicle in traffic accident**

⊗⑦**V36** **Occupant of three-wheeled motor vehicle injured in collision with other nonmotor vehicle**

Includes: collision with animal-drawn vehicle, animal being ridden, streetcar

The appropriate 7th character is to be added to each code from category V36

A - initial encounter

D - subsequent encounter

S - sequela

⊗⑦V36.0 **Driver of three-wheeled motor vehicle injured in collision with other nonmotor vehicle in nontraffic accident**

⊗⑦V36.1 **Passenger in three-wheeled motor vehicle injured in collision with other nonmotor vehicle in nontraffic accident**

⊗⑦V36.2 **Person on outside of three-wheeled motor vehicle injured in collision with other nonmotor vehicle in nontraffic accident**

⊗⑦V36.3 **Unspecified occupant of three-wheeled motor vehicle injured in collision with other nonmotor vehicle in nontraffic accident**

⊗⑦V36.4 **Person boarding or alighting a three-wheeled motor vehicle injured in collision with other nonmotor vehicle**

⊗⑦V36.5 **Driver of three-wheeled motor vehicle injured in collision with other nonmotor vehicle in traffic accident**

⊗⑦V36.6 **Passenger in three-wheeled motor vehicle injured in collision with other nonmotor vehicle in traffic accident**

⊗⑦V36.7 **Person on outside of three-wheeled motor vehicle injured in collision with other nonmotor vehicle in traffic accident**

⊗⑦V36.9 **Unspecified occupant of three-wheeled motor vehicle injured in collision with other nonmotor vehicle in traffic accident**

V37 **Occupant of three-wheeled motor vehicle injured in collision with fixed or stationary object**

The appropriate 7th character is to be added to each code from category V37

A - initial encounter

D - subsequent encounter

S - sequela

⊗⑦V37.0 **Driver of three-wheeled motor vehicle injured in collision with fixed or stationary object in nontraffic accident**

⊗⑦V37.1 **Passenger in three-wheeled motor vehicle injured in collision with fixed or stationary object in nontraffic accident**

⊗⑦V37.2 **Person on outside of three-wheeled motor vehicle injured in collision with fixed or stationary object in nontraffic accident**

⊗⑦V37.3 **Unspecified occupant of three-wheeled motor vehicle injured in collision with fixed or stationary object in nontraffic accident**

⊗⑦V37.4 **Person boarding or alighting a three-wheeled motor vehicle injured in collision with fixed or stationary object**

⊗⑦V37.5 **Driver of three-wheeled motor vehicle injured in collision with fixed or stationary object in traffic accident**

⊗⑦V37.6 **Passenger in three-wheeled motor vehicle injured in collision with fixed or stationary object in traffic accident**

⊗⑦V37.7 **Person on outside of three-wheeled motor vehicle injured in collision with fixed or stationary object in traffic accident**

⊗⑦V37.9 **Unspecified occupant of three-wheeled motor vehicle injured in collision with fixed or stationary object in traffic accident**

V38 **Occupant of three-wheeled motor vehicle injured in noncollision transport accident**

Includes: fall or thrown from three-wheeled motor vehicle
overturning of three-wheeled motor vehicle NOS
overturning of three-wheeled motor vehicle without collision

The appropriate 7th character is to be added to each code from category V38

A - initial encounter

D - subsequent encounter

S - sequela

⊗⑦V38.0 **Driver of three-wheeled motor vehicle injured in noncollision transport accident in nontraffic accident**

⊗⑦V38.1 **Passenger in three-wheeled motor vehicle injured in noncollision transport accident in nontraffic accident**

⊗⑦V38.2 **Person on outside of three-wheeled motor vehicle injured in noncollision transport accident in nontraffic accident**

⊗⑦V38.3 **Unspecified occupant of three-wheeled motor vehicle injured in noncollision transport accident in nontraffic accident**

⊗⑦V38.4 **Person boarding or alighting a three-wheeled motor vehicle injured in noncollision transport accident**

⊗⑦V38.5 **Driver of three-wheeled motor vehicle injured in noncollision transport accident in traffic accident**

⊗⑦**V38.6** Passenger in three-wheeled motor vehicle injured in noncollision transport accident in traffic accident

⊗⑦**V38.7** Person on outside of three-wheeled motor vehicle injured in noncollision transport accident in traffic accident

⊗⑦**V38.9** Unspecified occupant of three-wheeled motor vehicle injured in noncollision transport accident in traffic accident

V39 **Occupant of three-wheeled motor vehicle injured in other and unspecified transport accidents**

The appropriate 7th character is to be added to each code from category V39

A - initial encounter

D - subsequent encounter

S - sequela

V39.0 Driver of three-wheeled motor vehicle injured in collision with other and unspecified motor vehicles in nontraffic accident

⊗⑦**V39.00** Driver of three-wheeled motor vehicle injured in collision with unspecified motor vehicles in nontraffic accident

⊗⑦**V39.09** Driver of three-wheeled motor vehicle injured in collision with other motor vehicles in nontraffic accident

V39.1 Passenger in three-wheeled motor vehicle injured in collision with other and unspecified motor vehicles in nontraffic accident

⊗⑦**V39.10** Passenger in three-wheeled motor vehicle injured in collision with unspecified motor vehicles in nontraffic accident

⊗⑦**V39.19** Passenger in three-wheeled motor vehicle injured in collision with other motor vehicles in nontraffic accident

V39.2 Unspecified occupant of three-wheeled motor vehicle injured in collision with other and unspecified motor vehicles in nontraffic accident

⊗⑦**V39.20** Unspecified occupant of three-wheeled motor vehicle injured in collision with unspecified motor vehicles in nontraffic accident

Collision NOS involving three-wheeled motor vehicle, nontraffic

⊗⑦**V39.29** Unspecified occupant of three-wheeled motor vehicle injured in collision with other motor vehicles in nontraffic accident

⊗⑦**V39.3** Occupant (driver) (passenger) of three-wheeled motor vehicle injured in unspecified nontraffic accident

Accident NOS involving three-wheeled motor vehicle, nontraffic

Occupant of three-wheeled motor vehicle injured in nontraffic accident NOS

V39.4 Driver of three-wheeled motor vehicle injured in collision with other and unspecified motor vehicles in traffic accident

⊗⑦**V39.40** Driver of three-wheeled motor vehicle injured in collision with unspecified motor vehicles in traffic accident

⊗⑦**V39.49** Driver of three-wheeled motor vehicle injured in collision with other motor vehicles in traffic accident

V39.5 Passenger in three-wheeled motor vehicle injured in collision with other and unspecified motor vehicles in traffic accident

⊗⑦**V39.50** Passenger in three-wheeled motor vehicle injured in collision with unspecified motor vehicles in traffic accident

⊗⑦**V39.59** Passenger in three-wheeled motor vehicle injured in collision with other motor vehicles in traffic accident

V39.6 Unspecified occupant of three-wheeled motor vehicle injured in collision with other and unspecified motor vehicles in traffic accident

⊗⑦**V39.60** Unspecified occupant of three-wheeled motor vehicle injured in collision with unspecified motor vehicles in traffic accident

Collision NOS involving three-wheeled motor vehicle (traffic)

⊗⑦**V39.69** Unspecified occupant of three-wheeled motor vehicle injured in collision with other motor vehicles in traffic accident

V39.8 Occupant (driver) (passenger) of three-wheeled motor vehicle injured in other specified transport accidents

⊗⑦**V39.81** Occupant (driver) (passenger) of three-wheeled motor vehicle injured in transport accident with military vehicle

⊗⑦**V39.89** Occupant (driver) (passenger) of three-wheeled motor vehicle injured in other specified transport accidents

⊗⑦**V39.9** Occupant (driver) (passenger) of three-wheeled motor vehicle injured in unspecified traffic accident

Accident NOS involving three-wheeled motor vehicle

CAR OCCUPANT INJURED IN TRANSPORT ACCIDENT (V40-V49)

Includes: a four-wheeled motor vehicle designed primarily for carrying passengers

automobile (pulling a trailer or camper)

Excludes1: bus (V50-V59)

minibus (V50-V59)

minivan (V50-V59)

motorcoach (V70-V79)

pick-up truck (V50-V59)

sport utility vehicle (SUV) (V50-V59)

V40 **Car occupant injured in collision with pedestrian or animal**

Excludes1: car collision with animal-drawn vehicle or animal being ridden (V46.-)

The appropriate 7th character is to be added to each code from category V40

A - initial encounter

D - subsequent encounter

S - sequela

⊗⑦**V40.0** Car driver injured in collision with pedestrian or animal in nontraffic accident

⊗⑦**V40.1** Car passenger injured in collision with pedestrian or animal in nontraffic accident

⊗⑦**V40.2** Person on outside of car injured in collision with pedestrian or animal in nontraffic accident

⊗⑦**V40.3** Unspecified car occupant injured in collision with pedestrian or animal in nontraffic accident

⊗⑦**V40.4** Person boarding or alighting a car injured in collision with pedestrian or animal

⊗⑦V40.5 Car driver injured in collision with pedestrian or animal in traffic accident

⊗⑦V40.6 Car passenger injured in collision with pedestrian or animal in traffic accident

⊗⑦V40.7 Person on outside of car injured in collision with pedestrian or animal in traffic accident

⊗⑦V40.9 Unspecified car occupant injured in collision with pedestrian or animal in traffic accident

V41 Car occupant injured in collision with pedal cycle

The appropriate 7th character is to be added to each code from category V41

A - initial encounter

D - subsequent encounter

S - sequela

⊗⑦V41.0 Car driver injured in collision with pedal cycle in nontraffic accident

⊗⑦V41.1 Car passenger injured in collision with pedal cycle in nontraffic accident

⊗⑦V41.2 Person on outside of car injured in collision with pedal cycle in nontraffic accident

⊗⑦V41.3 Unspecified car occupant injured in collision with pedal cycle in nontraffic accident

⊗⑦V41.4 Person boarding or alighting a car injured in collision with pedal cycle

⊗⑦V41.5 Car driver injured in collision with pedal cycle in traffic accident

⊗⑦V41.6 Car passenger injured in collision with pedal cycle in traffic accident

⊗⑦V41.7 Person on outside of car injured in collision with pedal cycle in traffic accident

⊗⑦V41.9 Unspecified car occupant injured in collision with pedal cycle in traffic accident

V42 Car occupant injured in collision with two- or three-wheeled motor vehicle

The appropriate 7th character is to be added to each code from category V42

A - initial encounter

D - subsequent encounter

S - sequela

⊗⑦V42.0 Car driver injured in collision with two- or three-wheeled motor vehicle in nontraffic accident

⊗⑦V42.1 Car passenger injured in collision with two- or three-wheeled motor vehicle in nontraffic accident

⊗⑦V42.2 Person on outside of car injured in collision with two- or three-wheeled motor vehicle in nontraffic accident

⊗⑦V42.3 Unspecified car occupant injured in collision with two- or three-wheeled motor vehicle in nontraffic accident

⊗⑦V42.4 Person boarding or alighting a car injured in collision with two- or three-wheeled motor vehicle

⊗⑦V42.5 Car driver injured in collision with two- or three-wheeled motor vehicle in traffic accident

⊗⑦V42.6 Car passenger injured in collision with two- or three-wheeled motor vehicle in traffic accident

⊗⑦V42.7 Person on outside of car injured in collision with two- or three-wheeled motor vehicle in traffic accident

⊗⑦V42.9 Unspecified car occupant injured in collision with two- or three-wheeled motor vehicle in traffic accident

V43 Car occupant injured in collision with car, pick-up truck or van

The appropriate 7th character is to be added to each code from category V43

A - initial encounter

D - subsequent encounter

S - sequela

V43.0 Car driver injured in collision with car, pick-up truck or van in nontraffic accident

⊗⑦V43.01 Car driver injured in collision with sport utility vehicle in nontraffic accident

⊗⑦V43.02 Car driver injured in collision with other type car in nontraffic accident

⊗⑦V43.03 Car driver injured in collision with pick-up truck in nontraffic accident

⊗⑦V43.04 Car driver injured in collision with van in nontraffic accident

V43.1 Car passenger injured in collision with car, pick-up truck or van in nontraffic accident

⊗⑦V43.11 Car passenger injured in collision with sport utility vehicle in nontraffic accident

⊗⑦V43.12 Car passenger injured in collision with other type car in nontraffic accident

⊗⑦V43.13 Car passenger injured in collision with pick-up in nontraffic accident

⊗⑦V43.14 Car passenger injured in collision with van in nontraffic accident

V43.2 Person on outside of car injured in collision with car, pick-up truck or van in nontraffic accident

⊗⑦V43.21 Person on outside of car injured in collision with sport utility vehicle in nontraffic accident

⊗⑦V43.22 Person on outside of car injured in collision with other type car in nontraffic accident

⊗⑦V43.23 Person on outside of car injured in collision with pick-up truck in nontraffic accident

⊗⑦V43.24 Person on outside of car injured in collision with van in nontraffic accident

V43.3 Unspecified car occupant injured in collision with car, pick-up truck or van in nontraffic accident

⊗⑦V43.31 Unspecified car occupant injured in collision with sport utility vehicle in nontraffic accident

⊗⑦V43.32 Unspecified car occupant injured in collision with other type car in nontraffic accident

⊗⑦V43.33 Unspecified car occupant injured in collision with pick-up truck in nontraffic accident

⊗⑦V43.34 Unspecified car occupant injured in collision with van in nontraffic accident

V43.4 Person boarding or alighting a car injured in collision with car, pick-up truck or van

⊗⑦V43.41 Person boarding or alighting a car injured in collision with sport utility vehicle

⊗⑦V43.42 Person boarding or alighting a car injured in collision with other type car

⊗⑦V43.43 Person boarding or alighting a car injured in collision with pick-up truck

⊗⑦V43.44 Person boarding or alighting a car injured in collision with van

V43.5 Car driver injured in collision with car, pick-up truck or van in traffic accident

⊗⑦V43.51 Car driver injured in collision with sport utility vehicle in traffic accident

⊗⑦V43.52 Car driver injured in collision with other type car in traffic accident

⊗⑦V43.53 Car driver injured in collision with pick-up truck in traffic accident

⊗⑦V43.54   Car driver injured in collision with van in traffic accident

V43.6   Car passenger injured in collision with car, pick-up truck or van in traffic accident

⊗⑦V43.61   Car passenger injured in collision with sport utility vehicle in traffic accident

⊗⑦V43.62   Car passenger injured in collision with other type car in traffic accident

⊗⑦V43.63   Car passenger injured in collision with pick-up truck in traffic accident

⊗⑦V43.64   Car passenger injured in collision with van in traffic accident

V43.7   Person on outside of car injured in collision with car, pick-up truck or van in traffic accident

⊗⑦V43.71   Person on outside of car injured in collision with sport utility vehicle in traffic accident

⊗⑦V43.72   Person on outside of car injured in collision with other type car in traffic accident

⊗⑦V43.73   Person on outside of car injured in collision with pick-up truck in traffic accident

⊗⑦V43.74   Person on outside of car injured in collision with van in traffic accident

V43.9   Unspecified car occupant injured in collision with car, pick-up truck or van in traffic accident

⊗⑦V43.91   Unspecified car occupant injured in collision with sport utility vehicle in traffic accident

⊗⑦V43.92   Unspecified car occupant injured in collision with other type car in traffic accident

⊗⑦V43.93   Unspecified car occupant injured in collision with pick-up truck in traffic accident

⊗⑦V43.94   Unspecified car occupant injured in collision with van in traffic accident

V44   Car occupant injured in collision with heavy transport vehicle or bus

Excludes1: car occupant injured in collision with military vehicle (V49.81)

The appropriate 7th character is to be added to each code from category V44

A - initial encounter

D - subsequent encounter

S - sequela

⊗⑦V44.0   Car driver injured in collision with heavy transport vehicle or bus in nontraffic accident

⊗⑦V44.1   Car passenger injured in collision with heavy transport vehicle or bus in nontraffic accident

⊗⑦V44.2   Person on outside of car injured in collision with heavy transport vehicle or bus in nontraffic accident

⊗⑦V44.3   Unspecified car occupant injured in collision with heavy transport vehicle or bus in nontraffic accident

⊗⑦V44.4   Person boarding or alighting a car injured in collision with heavy transport vehicle or bus

⊗⑦V44.5   Car driver injured in collision with heavy transport vehicle or bus in traffic accident

⊗⑦V44.6   Car passenger injured in collision with heavy transport vehicle or bus in traffic accident

⊗⑦V44.7   Person on outside of car injured in collision with heavy transport vehicle or bus in traffic accident

⊗⑦V44.9   Unspecified car occupant injured in collision with heavy transport vehicle or bus in traffic accident

V45   Car occupant injured in collision with railway train or railway vehicle

The appropriate 7th character is to be added to each code from category V45

A - initial encounter

D - subsequent encounter

S - sequela

⊗⑦V45.0   Car driver injured in collision with railway train or railway vehicle in nontraffic accident

⊗⑦V45.1   Car passenger injured in collision with railway train or railway vehicle in nontraffic accident

⊗⑦V45.2   Person on outside of car injured in collision with railway train or railway vehicle in nontraffic accident

⊗⑦V45.3   Unspecified car occupant injured in collision with railway train or railway vehicle in nontraffic accident

⊗⑦V45.4   Person boarding or alighting a car injured in collision with railway train or railway vehicle

⊗⑦V45.5   Car driver injured in collision with railway train or railway vehicle in traffic accident

⊗⑦V45.6   Car passenger injured in collision with railway train or railway vehicle in traffic accident

⊗⑦V45.7   Person on outside of car injured in collision with railway train or railway vehicle in traffic accident

⊗⑦V45.9   Unspecified car occupant injured in collision with railway train or railway vehicle in traffic accident

V46   Car occupant injured in collision with other nonmotor vehicle

Includes: collision with animal-drawn vehicle, animal being ridden, streetcar

The appropriate 7th character is to be added to each code from category V46

A - initial encounter

D - subsequent encounter

S - sequela

⊗⑦V46.0   Car driver injured in collision with other nonmotor vehicle in nontraffic accident

⊗⑦V46.1   Car passenger injured in collision with other nonmotor vehicle in nontraffic accident

⊗⑦V46.2   Person on outside of car injured in collision with other nonmotor vehicle in nontraffic accident

⊗⑦V46.3   Unspecified car occupant injured in collision with other nonmotor vehicle in nontraffic accident

⊗⑦V46.4   Person boarding or alighting a car injured in collision with other nonmotor vehicle

⊗⑦V46.5   Car driver injured in collision with other nonmotor vehicle in traffic accident

⊗⑦V46.6   Car passenger injured in collision with other nonmotor vehicle in traffic accident

⊗⑦V46.7   Person on outside of car injured in collision with other nonmotor vehicle in traffic accident

⊗⑦V46.9   Unspecified car occupant injured in collision with other nonmotor vehicle in traffic accident

V47   Car occupant injured in collision with fixed or stationary object

The appropriate 7th character is to be added to each code from category V47

A - initial encounter

D - subsequent encounter

S - sequela

• ⊗⑦V47.0   Car driver injured in collision with fixed or stationary object in nontraffic accident

• ⊗⑦V47.1   Car passenger injured in collision with fixed or stationary object in nontraffic accident

⊗⑦**V47.2** Person on outside of car injured in collision with fixed or stationary object in nontraffic accident

●⊗⑦**V47.3** Unspecified car occupant injured in collision with fixed or stationary object in nontraffic accident

⊗⑦**V47.4** Person boarding or alighting a car injured in collision with fixed or stationary object

●⊗⑦**V47.5** Car driver injured in collision with fixed or stationary object in traffic accident

●⊗⑦**V47.6** Car passenger injured in collision with fixed or stationary object in traffic accident

⊗⑦**V47.7** Person on outside of car injured in collision with fixed or stationary object in traffic accident

●⊗⑦**V47.9** Unspecified car occupant injured in collision with fixed or stationary object in traffic accident

V48 Car occupant injured in noncollision transport accident

Includes: overturning car NOS

overturning car without collision

The appropriate 7th character is to be added to each code from category ⊗⑦V48

A - initial encounter

D - subsequent encounter

S - sequela

⊗⑦**V48.0** Car driver injured in noncollision transport accident in nontraffic accident

⊗⑦**V48.1** Car passenger injured in noncollision transport accident in nontraffic accident

⊗⑦**V48.2** Person on outside of car injured in noncollision transport accident in nontraffic accident

⊗⑦**V48.3** Unspecified car occupant injured in noncollision transport accident in nontraffic accident

⊗⑦**V48.4** Person boarding or alighting a car injured in noncollision transport accident

⊗⑦**V48.5** Car driver injured in noncollision transport accident in traffic accident

⊗⑦**V48.6** Car passenger injured in noncollision transport accident in traffic accident

⊗⑦**V48.7** Person on outside of car injured in noncollision transport accident in traffic accident

⊗⑦**V48.9** Unspecified car occupant injured in noncollision transport accident in traffic accident

V49 Car occupant injured in other and unspecified transport accidents

The appropriate 7th character is to be added to each code from category V49

A - initial encounter

D - subsequent encounter

S - sequela

V49.0 Driver injured in collision with other and unspecified motor vehicles in nontraffic accident

⊗⑦**V49.00** Driver injured in collision with unspecified motor vehicles in nontraffic accident

⊗⑦**V49.09** Driver injured in collision with other motor vehicles in nontraffic accident

V49.1 Passenger injured in collision with other and unspecified motor vehicles in nontraffic accident

⊗⑦**V49.10** Passenger injured in collision with unspecified motor vehicles in nontraffic accident

⊗⑦**V49.19** Passenger injured in collision with other motor vehicles in nontraffic accident

V49.2 Unspecified car occupant injured in collision with other and unspecified motor vehicles in nontraffic accident

⊗⑦**V49.20** Unspecified car occupant injured in collision with unspecified motor vehicles in nontraffic accident

Car collision NOS, nontraffic

⊗⑦**V49.29** Unspecified car occupant injured in collision with other motor vehicles in nontraffic accident

⊗⑦**V49.3** Car occupant (driver) (passenger) injured in unspecified nontraffic accident

Car accident NOS, nontraffic

Car occupant injured in nontraffic accident NOS

V49.4 Driver injured in collision with other and unspecified motor vehicles in traffic accident

⊗⑦**V49.40** Driver injured in collision with unspecified motor vehicles in traffic accident

⊗⑦**V49.49** Driver injured in collision with other motor vehicles in traffic accident

V49.5 Passenger injured in collision with other and unspecified motor vehicles in traffic accident

⊗⑦**V49.50** Passenger injured in collision with unspecified motor vehicles in traffic accident

⊗⑦**V49.59** Passenger injured in collision with other motor vehicles in traffic accident

V49.6 Unspecified car occupant injured in collision with other and unspecified motor vehicles in traffic accident

⊗⑦**V49.60** Unspecified car occupant injured in collision with unspecified motor vehicles in traffic accident

Car collision NOS (traffic)

⊗⑦**V49.69** Unspecified car occupant injured in collision with other motor vehicles in traffic accident

V49.8 Car occupant (driver) (passenger) injured in other specified transport accidents

⊗⑦**V49.81** Car occupant (driver) (passenger) injured in transport accident with military vehicle

⊗⑦**V49.88** Car occupant (driver) (passenger) injured in other specified transport accidents

⊗⑦**V49.9** Car occupant (driver) (passenger) injured in unspecified traffic accident

Car accident NOS

OCCUPANT OF PICK-UP TRUCK OR VAN INJURED IN TRANSPORT ACCIDENT (V50-V59)

Includes: a four or six wheel motor vehicle designed primarily for carrying passengers and property but weighing less than the local limit for classification as a heavy goods vehicle

minibus

minivan

sport utility vehicle (SUV)

truck

van

Excludes1: heavy transport vehicle (V60-V69)

V50 Occupant of pick-up truck or van injured in collision with pedestrian or animal

Excludes1: pick-up truck or van collision with animal-drawn vehicle or animal being ridden (V56.-)

The appropriate 7th character is to be added to each code from category V50

A - initial encounter

D - subsequent encounter

S - sequela

⊗⑦**V50.0** Driver of pick-up truck or van injured in collision with pedestrian or animal in nontraffic accident

⊗⑦**V50.1** Passenger in pick-up truck or van injured in collision with pedestrian or animal in nontraffic accident

⊗⑦**V50.2** Person on outside of pick-up truck or van injured in collision with pedestrian or animal in nontraffic accident

⊗⑦**V50.3** Unspecified occupant of pick-up truck or van injured in collision with pedestrian or animal in nontraffic accident

⊗⑦**V50.4** Person boarding or alighting a pick-up truck or van injured in collision with pedestrian or animal

⊗⑦**V50.5** Driver of pick-up truck or van injured in collision with pedestrian or animal in traffic accident

⊗⑦**V50.6** Passenger in pick-up truck or van injured in collision with pedestrian or animal in traffic accident

⊗⑦**V50.7** Person on outside of pick-up truck or van injured in collision with pedestrian or animal in traffic accident

⊗⑦**V50.9** Unspecified occupant of pick-up truck or van injured in collision with pedestrian or animal in traffic accident

V51 Occupant of pick-up truck or van injured in collision with pedal cycle

The appropriate 7th character is to be added to each code from category V51

A - initial encounter

D - subsequent encounter

S - sequela

⊗⑦**V51.0** Driver of pick-up truck or van injured in collision with pedal cycle in nontraffic accident

⊗⑦**V51.1** Passenger in pick-up truck or van injured in collision with pedal cycle in nontraffic accident

⊗⑦**V51.2** Person on outside of pick-up truck or van injured in collision with pedal cycle in nontraffic accident

⊗⑦**V51.3** Unspecified occupant of pick-up truck or van injured in collision with pedal cycle in nontraffic accident

⊗⑦**V51.4** Person boarding or alighting a pick-up truck or van injured in collision with pedal cycle

⊗⑦**V51.5** Driver of pick-up truck or van injured in collision with pedal cycle in traffic accident

⊗⑦**V51.6** Passenger in pick-up truck or van injured in collision with pedal cycle in traffic accident

⊗⑦**V51.7** Person on outside of pick-up truck or van injured in collision with pedal cycle in traffic accident

⊗⑦**V51.9** Unspecified occupant of pick-up truck or van injured in collision with pedal cycle in traffic accident

V52 Occupant of pick-up truck or van injured in collision with two- or three-wheeled motor vehicle

The appropriate 7th character is to be added to each code from category V52

A - initial encounter

D - subsequent encounter

S - sequela

⊗⑦**V52.0** Driver of pick-up truck or van injured in collision with two- or three-wheeled motor vehicle in nontraffic accident

⊗⑦**V52.1** Passenger in pick-up truck or van injured in collision with two- or three-wheeled motor vehicle in nontraffic accident

⊗⑦**V52.2** Person on outside of pick-up truck or van injured in collision with two- or three-wheeled motor vehicle in nontraffic accident

⊗⑦**V52.3** Unspecified occupant of pick-up truck or van injured in collision with two- or three-wheeled motor vehicle in nontraffic accident

⊗⑦**V52.4** Person boarding or alighting a pick-up truck or van injured in collision with two- or three-wheeled motor vehicle

⊗⑦**V52.5** Driver of pick-up truck or van injured in collision with two- or three-wheeled motor vehicle in traffic accident

⊗⑦**V52.6** Passenger in pick-up truck or van injured in collision with two- or three-wheeled motor vehicle in traffic accident

⊗⑦**V52.7** Person on outside of pick-up truck or van injured in collision with two- or three-wheeled motor vehicle in traffic accident

⊗⑦**V52.9** Unspecified occupant of pick-up truck or van injured in collision with two- or three-wheeled motor vehicle in traffic accident

V53 Occupant of pick-up truck or van injured in collision with car, pick-up truck or van

The appropriate 7th character is to be added to each code from category V53

A - initial encounter

D - subsequent encounter

S - sequela

⊗⑦**V53.0** Driver of pick-up truck or van injured in collision with car, pick-up truck or van in nontraffic accident

⊗⑦**V53.1** Passenger in pick-up truck or van injured in collision with car, pick-up truck or van in nontraffic accident

⊗⑦**V53.2** Person on outside of pick-up truck or van injured in collision with car, pick-up truck or van in nontraffic accident

⊗⑦**V53.3** Unspecified occupant of pick-up truck or van injured in collision with car, pick-up truck or van in nontraffic accident

⊗⑦**V53.4** Person boarding or alighting a pick-up truck or van injured in collision with car, pick-up truck or van

⊗⑦**V53.5** Driver of pick-up truck or van injured in collision with car, pick-up truck or van in traffic accident

⊗⑦**V53.6** Passenger in pick-up truck or van injured in collision with car, pick-up truck or van in traffic accident

⊗⑦**V53.7** Person on outside of pick-up truck or van injured in collision with car, pick-up truck or van in traffic accident

⊗⑦**V53.9** Unspecified occupant of pick-up truck or van injured in collision with car, pick-up truck or van in traffic accident

V54 Occupant of pick-up truck or van injured in collision with heavy transport vehicle or bus

Excludes1: occupant of pick-up truck or van injured in collision with military vehicle (V59.81)

The appropriate 7th character is to be added to each code from category V54

A - initial encounter

D - subsequent encounter

S - sequela

⊗⑦**V54.0** Driver of pick-up truck or van injured in collision with heavy transport vehicle or bus in nontraffic accident

---

⊗⑦**V54.1** Passenger in pick-up truck or van injured in collision with heavy transport vehicle or bus in nontraffic accident

⊗⑦**V54.2** Person on outside of pick-up truck or van injured in collision with heavy transport vehicle or bus in nontraffic accident

⊗⑦**V54.3** Unspecified occupant of pick-up truck or van injured in collision with heavy transport vehicle or bus in nontraffic accident

⊗⑦**V54.4** Person boarding or alighting a pick-up truck or van injured in collision with heavy transport vehicle or bus

⊗⑦**V54.5** Driver of pick-up truck or van injured in collision with heavy transport vehicle or bus in traffic accident

⊗⑦**V54.6** Passenger in pick-up truck or van injured in collision with heavy transport vehicle or bus in traffic accident

⊗⑦**V54.7** Person on outside of pick-up truck or van injured in collision with heavy transport vehicle or bus in traffic accident

⊗⑦**V54.9** Unspecified occupant of pick-up truck or van injured in collision with heavy transport vehicle or bus in traffic accident

V55 Occupant of pick-up truck or van injured in collision with railway train or railway vehicle

The appropriate 7th character is to be added to each code from category V55

A - initial encounter

D - subsequent encounter

S - sequela

⊗⑦**V55.0** Driver of pick-up truck or van injured in collision with railway train or railway vehicle in nontraffic accident

⊗⑦**V55.1** Passenger in pick-up truck or van injured in collision with railway train or railway vehicle in nontraffic accident

⊗⑦**V55.2** Person on outside of pick-up truck or van injured in collision with railway train or railway vehicle in nontraffic accident

⊗⑦**V55.3** Unspecified occupant of pick-up truck or van injured in collision with railway train or railway vehicle in nontraffic accident

⊗⑦**V55.4** Person boarding or alighting a pick-up truck or van injured in collision with railway train or railway vehicle

⊗⑦**V55.5** Driver of pick-up truck or van injured in collision with railway train or railway vehicle in traffic accident

⊗⑦**V55.6** Passenger in pick-up truck or van injured in collision with railway train or railway vehicle in traffic accident

⊗⑦**V55.7** Person on outside of pick-up truck or van injured in collision with railway train or railway vehicle in traffic accident

⊗⑦**V55.9** Unspecified occupant of pick-up truck or van injured in collision with railway train or railway vehicle in traffic accident

V56 Occupant of pick-up truck or van injured in collision with other nonmotor vehicle

Includes: collision with animal-drawn vehicle, animal being ridden, streetcar

The appropriate 7th character is to be added to each code from category V56

A - initial encounter

D - subsequent encounter

S - sequela

⊗⑦**V56.0** Driver of pick-up truck or van injured in collision with other nonmotor vehicle in nontraffic accident

⊗⑦**V56.1** Passenger in pick-up truck or van injured in collision with other nonmotor vehicle in nontraffic accident

⊗⑦**V56.2** Person on outside of pick-up truck or van injured in collision with other nonmotor vehicle in nontraffic accident

⊗⑦**V56.3** Unspecified occupant of pick-up truck or van injured in collision with other nonmotor vehicle in nontraffic accident

⊗⑦**V56.4** Person boarding or alighting a pick-up truck or van injured in collision with other nonmotor vehicle

⊗⑦**V56.5** Driver of pick-up truck or van injured in collision with other nonmotor vehicle in traffic accident

⊗⑦**V56.6** Passenger in pick-up truck or van injured in collision with other nonmotor vehicle in traffic accident

⊗⑦**V56.7** Person on outside of pick-up truck or van injured in collision with other nonmotor vehicle in traffic accident

⊗⑦**V56.9** Unspecified occupant of pick-up truck or van injured in collision with other nonmotor vehicle in traffic accident

V57 Occupant of pick-up truck or van injured in collision with fixed or stationary object

The appropriate 7th character is to be added to each code from category V57

A - initial encounter

D - subsequent encounter

S - sequela

⊗⑦**V57.0** Driver of pick-up truck or van injured in collision with fixed or stationary object in nontraffic accident

⊗⑦**V57.1** Passenger in pick-up truck or van injured in collision with fixed or stationary object in nontraffic accident

⊗⑦**V57.2** Person on outside of pick-up truck or van injured in collision with fixed or stationary object in nontraffic accident

⊗⑦**V57.3** Unspecified occupant of pick-up truck or van injured in collision with fixed or stationary object in nontraffic accident

⊗⑦**V57.4** Person boarding or alighting a pick-up truck or van injured in collision with fixed or stationary object

⊗⑦**V57.5** Driver of pick-up truck or van injured in collision with fixed or stationary object in traffic accident

⊗⑦**V57.6** Passenger in pick-up truck or van injured in collision with fixed or stationary object in traffic accident

⊗⑦**V57.7** Person on outside of pick-up truck or van injured in collision with fixed or stationary object in traffic accident

⊗⑦**V57.9** Unspecified occupant of pick-up truck or van injured in collision with fixed or stationary object in traffic accident

V58 Occupant of pick-up truck or van injured in noncollision transport accident

Includes: overturning pick-up truck or van NOS

overturning pick-up truck or van without collision

The appropriate 7th character is to be added to each code from category V58

A - initial encounter

D - subsequent encounter

S - sequela

⊗⑦**V58.0** Driver of pick-up truck or van injured in noncollision transport accident in nontraffic accident

⊗⑦**V58.1** Passenger in pick-up truck or van injured in noncollision transport accident in nontraffic accident

⊗⑦V58.2 Person on outside of pick-up truck or van injured in noncollision transport accident in nontraffic accident

⊗⑦V58.3 Unspecified occupant of pick-up truck or van injured in noncollision transport accident in nontraffic accident

⊗⑦V58.4 Person boarding or alighting a pick-up truck or van injured in noncollision transport accident

⊗⑦V58.5 Driver of pick-up truck or van injured in noncollision transport accident in traffic accident

⊗⑦V58.6 Passenger in pick-up truck or van injured in noncollision transport accident in traffic accident

⊗⑦V58.7 Person on outside of pick-up truck or van injured in noncollision transport accident in traffic accident

⊗⑦V58.9 Unspecified occupant of pick-up truck or van injured in noncollision transport accident in traffic accident

V59 **Occupant of pick-up truck or van injured in other and unspecified transport accidents**

The appropriate 7th character is to be added to each code from category V59

A - initial encounter

D - subsequent encounter

S - sequela

V59.0 Driver of pick-up truck or van injured in collision with other and unspecified motor vehicles in nontraffic accident

⊗⑦V59.00 Driver of pick-up truck or van injured in collision with unspecified motor vehicles in nontraffic accident

⊗⑦V59.09 Driver of pick-up truck or van injured in collision with other motor vehicles in nontraffic accident

V59.1 Passenger in pick-up truck or van injured in collision with other and unspecified motor vehicles in nontraffic accident

⊗⑦V59.10 Passenger in pick-up truck or van injured in collision with unspecified motor vehicles in nontraffic accident

⊗⑦V59.19 Passenger in pick-up truck or van injured in collision with other motor vehicles in nontraffic accident

V59.2 Unspecified occupant of pick-up truck or van injured in collision with other and unspecified motor vehicles in nontraffic accident

⊗⑦V59.20 Unspecified occupant of pick-up truck or van injured in collision with unspecified motor vehicles in nontraffic accident

Collision NOS involving pick-up truck or van, nontraffic

⊗⑦V59.29 Unspecified occupant of pick-up truck or van injured in collision with other motor vehicles in nontraffic accident

⊗⑦V59.3 Occupant (driver) (passenger) of pick-up truck or van injured in unspecified nontraffic accident

Accident NOS involving pick-up truck or van, nontraffic

Occupant of pick-up truck or van injured in nontraffic accident NOS

V59.4 Driver of pick-up truck or van injured in collision with other and unspecified motor vehicles in traffic accident

⊗⑦V59.40 Driver of pick-up truck or van injured in collision with unspecified motor vehicles in traffic accident

⊗⑦V59.49 Driver of pick-up truck or van injured in collision with other motor vehicles in traffic accident

V59.5 Passenger in pick-up truck or van injured in collision with other and unspecified motor vehicles in traffic accident

⊗⑦V59.50 Passenger in pick-up truck or van injured in collision with unspecified motor vehicles in traffic accident

⊗⑦V59.59 Passenger in pick-up truck or van injured in collision with other motor vehicles in traffic accident

V59.6 Unspecified occupant of pick-up truck or van injured in collision with other and unspecified motor vehicles in traffic accident

⊗⑦V59.60 Unspecified occupant of pick-up truck or van injured in collision with unspecified motor vehicles in traffic accident

Collision NOS involving pick-up truck or van (traffic)

⊗⑦V59.69 Unspecified occupant of pick-up truck or van injured in collision with other motor vehicles in traffic accident

V59.8 Occupant (driver) (passenger) of pick-up truck or van injured in other specified transport accidents

⊗⑦V59.81 Occupant (driver) (passenger) of pick-up truck or van injured in transport accident with military vehicle

⊗⑦V59.88 Occupant (driver) (passenger) of pick-up truck or van injured in other specified transport accidents

⊗⑦V59.9 Occupant (driver) (passenger) of pick-up truck or van injured in unspecified traffic accident

Accident NOS involving pick-up truck or van

OCCUPANT OF HEAVY TRANSPORT VEHICLE INJURED IN TRANSPORT ACCIDENT (V60-V69)

Includes: 18 wheeler

armored car panel truck

Excludes1: bus

motorcoach

V60 **Occupant of heavy transport vehicle injured in collision with pedestrian or animal**

Excludes1: heavy transport vehicle collision with animal-drawn vehicle or animal being ridden (V66.-)

The appropriate 7th character is to be added to each code from category V60

A - initial encounter

D - subsequent encounter

S - sequela

⊗⑦V60.0 Driver of heavy transport vehicle injured in collision with pedestrian or animal in nontraffic accident

⊗⑦V60.1 Passenger in heavy transport vehicle injured in collision with pedestrian or animal in nontraffic accident

⊗⑦V60.2 Person on outside of heavy transport vehicle injured in collision with pedestrian or animal in nontraffic accident

⊗⑦V60.3 Unspecified occupant of heavy transport vehicle injured in collision with pedestrian or animal in nontraffic accident

⊗⑦V60.4 Person boarding or alighting a heavy transport vehicle injured in collision with pedestrian or animal

⊗⑦**V60.5** Driver of heavy transport vehicle injured in collision with pedestrian or animal in traffic accident

⊗⑦**V60.6** Passenger in heavy transport vehicle injured in collision with pedestrian or animal in traffic accident

⊗⑦**V60.7** Person on outside of heavy transport vehicle injured in collision with pedestrian or animal in traffic accident

⊗⑦**V60.9** Unspecified occupant of heavy transport vehicle injured in collision with pedestrian or animal in traffic accident

V61 Occupant of heavy transport vehicle injured in collision with pedal cycle

The appropriate 7th character is to be added to each code from category V61

A - initial encounter

D - subsequent encounter

S - sequela

⊗⑦**V61.0** Driver of heavy transport vehicle injured in collision with pedal cycle in nontraffic accident

⊗⑦**V61.1** Passenger in heavy transport vehicle injured in collision with pedal cycle in nontraffic accident

⊗⑦**V61.2** Person on outside of heavy transport vehicle injured in collision with pedal cycle in nontraffic accident

⊗⑦**V61.3** Unspecified occupant of heavy transport vehicle injured in collision with pedal cycle in nontraffic accident

⊗⑦**V61.4** Person boarding or alighting a heavy transport vehicle injured in collision with pedal cycle while boarding or alighting

⊗⑦**V61.5** Driver of heavy transport vehicle injured in collision with pedal cycle in traffic accident

⊗⑦**V61.6** Passenger in heavy transport vehicle injured in collision with pedal cycle in traffic accident

⊗⑦**V61.7** Person on outside of heavy transport vehicle injured in collision with pedal cycle in traffic accident

⊗⑦**V61.9** Unspecified occupant of heavy transport vehicle injured in collision with pedal cycle in traffic accident

V62 Occupant of heavy transport vehicle injured in collision with two- or three-wheeled motor vehicle

The appropriate 7th character is to be added to each code from category V62

A - initial encounter

D - subsequent encounter

S - sequela

⊗⑦**V62.0** Driver of heavy transport vehicle injured in collision with two- or three-wheeled motor vehicle in nontraffic accident

⊗⑦**V62.1** Passenger in heavy transport vehicle injured in collision with two- or three-wheeled motor vehicle in nontraffic accident

⊗⑦**V62.2** Person on outside of heavy transport vehicle injured in collision with two- or three-wheeled motor vehicle in nontraffic accident

⊗⑦**V62.3** Unspecified occupant of heavy transport vehicle injured in collision with two- or three-wheeled motor vehicle in nontraffic accident

⊗⑦**V62.4** Person boarding or alighting a heavy transport vehicle injured in collision with two- or three-way veh vehicle

⊗⑦**V62.5** Driver of heavy transport vehicle injured in collision with two- or three-wheeled motor vehicle in traffic accident

⊗⑦**V62.6** Passenger in heavy transport vehicle injured in collision with two- or three-wheeled motor vehicle in traffic accident

⊗⑦**V62.7** Person on outside of heavy transport vehicle injured in collision with two- or three-wheeled motor vehicle in traffic accident

⊗⑦**V62.9** Unspecified occupant of heavy transport vehicle injured in collision with two- or three-wheeled motor vehicle in traffic accident

V63 Occupant of heavy transport vehicle injured in collision with car, pick-up truck or van

The appropriate 7th character is to be added to each code from category V63

A - initial encounter

D - subsequent encounter

S - sequela

⊗⑦**V63.0** Driver of heavy transport vehicle injured in collision with car, pick-up truck or van in nontraffic accident

⊗⑦**V63.1** Passenger in heavy transport vehicle injured in collision with car, pick-up truck or van in nontraffic accident

⊗⑦**V63.2** Person on outside of heavy transport vehicle injured in collision with car, pick-up truck or van in nontraffic accident

⊗⑦**V63.3** Unspecified occupant of heavy transport vehicle injured in collision with car, pick-up truck or van in nontraffic accident

⊗⑦**V63.4** Person boarding or alighting a heavy transport vehicle injured in collision with car, pick-up truck or van

⊗⑦**V63.5** Driver of heavy transport vehicle injured in collision with car, pick-up truck or van in traffic accident

⊗⑦**V63.6** Passenger in heavy transport vehicle injured in collision with car, pick-up truck or van in traffic accident

⊗⑦**V63.7** Person on outside of heavy transport vehicle injured in collision with car, pick-up truck or van in traffic accident

⊗⑦**V63.9** Unspecified occupant of heavy transport vehicle injured in collision with car, pick-up truck or van in traffic accident

V64 Occupant of heavy transport vehicle injured in collision with heavy transport vehicle or bus

Excludes1: occupant of heavy transport vehicle injured in collision with military vehicle (V69.81)

The appropriate 7th character is to be added to each code from category V64

A - initial encounter

D - subsequent encounter

S - sequela

⊗⑦**V64.0** Driver of heavy transport vehicle injured in collision with heavy transport vehicle or bus in nontraffic accident

⊗⑦**V64.1** Passenger in heavy transport vehicle injured in collision with heavy transport vehicle or bus in nontraffic accident

⊗⑦**V64.2** Person on outside of heavy transport vehicle injured in collision with heavy transport vehicle or bus in nontraffic accident

⊗⑦**V64.3** Unspecified occupant of heavy transport vehicle injured in collision with heavy transport vehicle or bus in nontraffic accident

⊗⑦**V64.4** Person boarding or alighting a heavy transport vehicle injured in collision with heavy transport vehicle or bus while boarding or alighting

⊗⑦**V64.5** Driver of heavy transport vehicle injured in collision with heavy transport vehicle or bus in traffic accident

⊗⑦**V64.6** Passenger in heavy transport vehicle injured in collision with heavy transport vehicle or bus in traffic accident

⊗⑦**V64.7** Person on outside of heavy transport vehicle injured in collision with heavy transport vehicle or bus in traffic accident

⊗⑦**V64.9** Unspecified occupant of heavy transport vehicle injured in collision with heavy transport vehicle or bus in traffic accident

V65 Occupant of heavy transport vehicle injured in collision with railway train or railway vehicle

The appropriate 7th character is to be added to each code from category V65

A - initial encounter

D - subsequent encounter

S - sequela

⊗⑦**V65.0** Driver of heavy transport vehicle injured in collision with railway train or railway vehicle in nontraffic accident

⊗⑦**V65.1** Passenger in heavy transport vehicle injured in collision with railway train or railway vehicle in nontraffic accident

⊗⑦**V65.2** Person on outside of heavy transport vehicle injured in collision with railway train or railway vehicle in nontraffic accident

⊗⑦**V65.3** Unspecified occupant of heavy transport vehicle injured in collision with railway train or railway vehicle in nontraffic accident

⊗⑦**V65.4** Person boarding or alighting a heavy transport vehicle injured in collision with railway train or railway vehicle

⊗⑦**V65.5** Driver of heavy transport vehicle injured in collision with railway train or railway vehicle in traffic accident

⊗⑦**V65.6** Passenger in heavy transport vehicle injured in collision with railway train or railway vehicle in traffic accident

⊗⑦**V65.7** Person on outside of heavy transport vehicle injured in collision with railway train or railway vehicle in traffic accident

⊗⑦**V65.9** Unspecified occupant of heavy transport vehicle injured in collision with railway train or railway vehicle in traffic accident

V66 Occupant of heavy transport vehicle injured in collision with other nonmotor vehicle

Includes: collision with animal-drawn vehicle, animal being ridden, streetcar

The appropriate 7th character is to be added to each code from category V66

A - initial encounter

D - subsequent encounter

S - sequela

⊗⑦**V66.0** Driver of heavy transport vehicle injured in collision with other nonmotor vehicle in nontraffic accident

⊗⑦**V66.1** Passenger in heavy transport vehicle injured in collision with other nonmotor vehicle in nontraffic accident

⊗⑦**V66.2** Person on outside of heavy transport vehicle injured in collision with other nonmotor vehicle in nontraffic accident

⊗⑦**V66.3** Unspecified occupant of heavy transport vehicle injured in collision with other nonmotor vehicle in nontraffic accident

⊗⑦**V66.4** Person boarding or alighting a heavy transport vehicle injured in collision with other nonmotor vehicle

⊗⑦**V66.5** Driver of heavy transport vehicle injured in collision with other nonmotor vehicle in traffic accident

⊗⑦**V66.6** Passenger in heavy transport vehicle injured in collision with other nonmotor vehicle in traffic accident

⊗⑦**V66.7** Person on outside of heavy transport vehicle injured in collision with other nonmotor vehicle in traffic accident

⊗⑦**V66.9** Unspecified occupant of heavy transport vehicle injured in collision with other nonmotor vehicle in traffic accident

V67 Occupant of heavy transport vehicle injured in collision with fixed or stationary object

The appropriate 7th character is to be added to each code from category V67

A - initial encounter

D - subsequent encounter

S - sequela

⊗⑦**V67.0** Driver of heavy transport vehicle injured in collision with fixed or stationary object in nontraffic accident

⊗⑦**V67.1** Passenger in heavy transport vehicle injured in collision with fixed or stationary object in nontraffic accident

⊗⑦**V67.2** Person on outside of heavy transport vehicle injured in collision with fixed or stationary object in nontraffic accident

⊗⑦**V67.3** Unspecified occupant of heavy transport vehicle injured in collision with fixed or stationary object in nontraffic accident

⊗⑦**V67.4** Person boarding or alighting a heavy transport vehicle injured in collision with fixed or stationary object vehicle injured in collision with other motor vehicles in nontraffic accident

V69.2 Unspecified occupant of heavy transport vehicle injured in collision with other and unspecified motor vehicles in nontraffic accident

⊗⑦**V69.20** Unspecified occupant of heavy transport vehicle injured in collision with unspecified motor vehicles in nontraffic accident

Collision NOS involving heavy transport vehicle, nontraffic

⊗⑦**V69.29** Unspecified occupant of heavy transport vehicle injured in collision with other motor vehicles in nontraffic accident

⊗⑦**V69.3** Occupant (driver) (passenger) of heavy transport vehicle injured in unspecified nontraffic accident

Accident NOS involving heavy transport vehicle, nontraffic

Occupant of heavy transport vehicle injured in nontraffic accident NOS

V69.4 Driver of heavy transport vehicle injured in collision with other and unspecified motor vehicles in traffic accident

⊗⑦**V69.40** Driver of heavy transport vehicle injured in collision with unspecified motor vehicles in traffic accident

⊗⑦**V69.49** Driver of heavy transport vehicle injured in collision with other motor vehicles in traffic accident

V69.5 Passenger in heavy transport vehicle injured in collision with other and unspecified motor vehicles in traffic accident

⊗⑦**V69.50** Passenger in heavy transport vehicle injured in collision with unspecified motor vehicles in traffic accident

⊗⑦**V69.59** Passenger in heavy transport vehicle injured in collision with other motor vehicles in traffic accident

TABULAR LIST

V69.6 Unspecified occupant of heavy transport vehicle injured in collision with other and unspecified motor vehicles in traffic accident

⊗⑦**V69.60** Unspecified occupant of heavy transport vehicle injured in collision with unspecified motor vehicles in traffic accident

Collision NOS involving heavy transport vehicle (traffic)

⊗⑦**V69.69** Unspecified occupant of heavy transport vehicle injured in collision with other motor vehicles in traffic accident

V69.8 Occupant (driver) (passenger) of heavy transport vehicle injured in other specified transport accidents

⊗⑦**V69.81** Occupant (driver) (passenger) of heavy transport vehicle injured in transport accidents with military vehicle

⊗⑦**V69.88** Occupant (driver) (passenger) of heavy transport vehicle injured in other specified transport accidents

⊗⑦**V69.9** Occupant (driver) (passenger) of heavy transport vehicle injured in unspecified traffic accident

Accident NOS involving heavy transport vehicle

BUS OCCUPANT INJURED IN TRANSPORT ACCIDENT (V70-V79)

Includes: motorcoach

Excludes1: minibus (V50-V59)

V70 Bus occupant injured in collision with pedestrian or animal

The appropriate 7th character is to be added to each code from category V70

A - initial encounter

D - subsequent encounter

S - sequela

Excludes1: bus collision with animal-drawn vehicle or animal being ridden (V76.-)

⊗⑦**V70.0** Driver of bus injured in collision with pedestrian or animal in nontraffic accident

⊗⑦**V70.1** Passenger on bus injured in collision with pedestrian or animal in nontraffic accident

⊗⑦**V70.2** Person on outside of bus injured in collision with pedestrian or animal in nontraffic accident

⊗⑦**V70.3** Unspecified occupant of bus injured in collision with pedestrian or animal in nontraffic accident

⊗⑦**V70.4** Person boarding or alighting from bus injured in collision with pedestrian or animal

⊗⑦**V70.5** Driver of bus injured in collision with pedestrian or animal in traffic accident

⊗⑦**V70.6** Passenger on bus injured in collision with pedestrian or animal in traffic accident

⊗⑦**V70.7** Person on outside of bus injured in collision with pedestrian or animal in traffic accident

⊗⑦**V70.9** Unspecified occupant of bus injured in collision with pedestrian or animal in traffic accident

V71 Bus occupant injured in collision with pedal cycle

The appropriate 7th character is to be added to each code from category V71

A - initial encounter

D - subsequent encounter

S - sequela

⊗⑦**V71.0** Driver of bus injured in collision with pedal cycle in nontraffic accident

⊗⑦**V71.1** Passenger on bus injured in collision with pedal cycle in nontraffic accident

⊗⑦**V71.2** Person on outside of bus injured in collision with pedal cycle in nontraffic accident

⊗⑦**V71.3** Unspecified occupant of bus injured in collision with pedal cycle in nontraffic accident

⊗⑦**V71.4** Person boarding or alighting from bus injured in collision with pedal cycle

⊗⑦**V71.5** Driver of bus injured in collision with pedal cycle in traffic accident

⊗⑦**V71.6** Passenger on bus injured in collision with pedal cycle in traffic accident

⊗⑦**V71.7** Person on outside of bus injured in collision with pedal cycle in traffic accident

⊗⑦**V71.9** Unspecified occupant of bus injured in collision with pedal cycle in traffic accident

V72 Bus occupant injured in collision with two- or three-wheeled motor vehicle

The appropriate 7th character is to be added to each code from category V72

A - initial encounter

D - subsequent encounter

S - sequela

⊗⑦**V72.0** Driver of bus injured in collision with two- or three-wheeled motor vehicle in nontraffic accident

⊗⑦**V72.1** Passenger on bus injured in collision with two- or three-wheeled motor vehicle in nontraffic accident

⊗⑦**V72.2** Person on outside of bus injured in collision with two- or three-wheeled motor vehicle in nontraffic accident

⊗⑦**V72.3** Unspecified occupant of bus injured in collision with two- or three-wheeled motor vehicle in nontraffic accident

⊗⑦**V72.4** Person boarding or alighting from bus injured in collision with two- or three-wheeled motor vehicle

⊗⑦**V72.5** Driver of bus injured in collision with two- or three-wheeled motor vehicle in traffic accident

⊗⑦**V72.6** Passenger on bus injured in collision with two- or three-wheeled motor vehicle in traffic accident

⊗⑦**V72.7** Person on outside of bus injured in collision with two- or three-wheeled motor vehicle in traffic accident

⊗⑦**V72.9** Unspecified occupant of bus injured in collision with two- or three-wheeled motor vehicle in traffic accident

V73 Bus occupant injured in collision with car, pick-up truck or van

The appropriate 7th character is to be added to each code from category V73

A - initial encounter

D - subsequent encounter

S - sequela

⊗⑦**V73.0** Driver of bus injured in collision with car, pick-up truck or van in nontraffic accident

⊗⑦**V73.1** Passenger on bus injured in collision with car, pick-up truck or van in nontraffic accident

⊗⑦**V73.2** Person on outside of bus injured in collision with car, pick-up truck or van in nontraffic accident

⊗⑦**V73.3** Unspecified occupant of bus injured in collision with car, pick-up truck or van in nontraffic accident

⊗⑦**V73.4** Person boarding or alighting from bus injured in collision with car, pick-up truck or van

⊗⑦**V73.5** Driver of bus injured in collision with car, pick-up truck or van in traffic accident

⊗⑦**V73.6** Passenger on bus injured in collision with car, pick-up truck or van in traffic accident

⊗⑦**V73.7** Person on outside of bus injured in collision with car, pick-up truck or van in traffic accident

⊗⑦**V73.9** Unspecified occupant of bus injured in collision with car, pick-up truck or van in traffic accident

V74 Bus occupant injured in collision with heavy transport vehicle or bus

Excludes1: bus occupant injured in collision with military vehicle (V79.81)

The appropriate 7th character is to be added to each code from category V74

A - initial encounter

D - subsequent encounter

S - sequela

⊗⑦**V74.0** Driver of bus injured in collision with heavy transport vehicle or bus in nontraffic accident

⊗⑦**V74.1** Passenger on bus injured in collision with heavy transport vehicle or bus in nontraffic accident

⊗⑦**V74.2** Person on outside of bus injured in collision with heavy transport vehicle or bus in nontraffic accident

⊗⑦**V74.3** Unspecified occupant of bus injured in collision with heavy transport vehicle or bus in nontraffic accident

⊗⑦**V74.4** Person boarding or alighting from bus injured in collision with heavy transport vehicle or bus

⊗⑦**V74.5** Driver of bus injured in collision with heavy transport vehicle or bus in traffic accident

⊗⑦**V74.6** Passenger on bus injured in collision with heavy transport vehicle or bus in traffic accident

⊗⑦**V74.7** Person on outside of bus injured in collision with heavy transport vehicle or bus in traffic accident

⊗⑦**V74.9** Unspecified occupant of bus injured in collision with heavy transport vehicle or bus in traffic accident

V75 Bus occupant injured in collision with railway train or railway vehicle

The appropriate 7th character is to be added to each code from category V75

A - initial encounter

D - subsequent encounter

S - sequela

⊗⑦**V75.0** Driver of bus injured in collision with railway train or railway vehicle in nontraffic accident

⊗⑦**V75.1** Passenger on bus injured in collision with railway train or railway vehicle in nontraffic accident

⊗⑦**V75.2** Person on outside of bus injured in collision with railway train or railway vehicle in nontraffic accident

⊗⑦**V75.3** Unspecified occupant of bus injured in collision with railway train or railway vehicle in nontraffic accident

⊗⑦**V75.4** Person boarding or alighting from bus injured in collision with railway train or railway vehicle

⊗⑦**V75.5** Driver of bus injured in collision with railway train or railway vehicle in traffic accident

⊗⑦**V75.6** Passenger on bus injured in collision with railway train or railway vehicle in traffic accident

⊗⑦**V75.7** Person on outside of bus injured in collision with railway train or railway vehicle in traffic accident

⊗⑦**V75.9** Unspecified occupant of bus injured in collision with railway train or railway vehicle in traffic accident

V76 Bus occupant injured in collision with other nonmotor vehicle

Includes: collision with animal-drawn vehicle, animal being ridden, streetcar

The appropriate 7th character is to be added to each code from category V76

A - initial encounter

D - subsequent encounter

S - sequela

⊗⑦**V76.0** Driver of bus injured in collision with other nonmotor vehicle in nontraffic accident

⊗⑦**V76.1** Passenger on bus injured in collision with other nonmotor vehicle in nontraffic accident

⊗⑦**V76.2** Person on outside of bus injured in collision with other nonmotor vehicle in nontraffic accident

⊗⑦**V76.3** Unspecified occupant of bus injured in collision with other nonmotor vehicle in nontraffic accident

⊗⑦**V76.4** Person boarding or alighting from bus injured in collision with other nonmotor vehicle

⊗⑦**V76.5** Driver of bus injured in collision with other nonmotor vehicle in traffic accident

⊗⑦**V76.6** Passenger on bus injured in collision with other nonmotor vehicle in traffic accident

⊗⑦**V76.7** Person on outside of bus injured in collision with other nonmotor vehicle in traffic accident

⊗⑦**V76.9** Unspecified occupant of bus injured in collision with other nonmotor vehicle in traffic accident

V77 Bus occupant injured in collision with fixed or stationary object

The appropriate 7th character is to be added to each code from category V77

A - initial encounter

D - subsequent encounter

S - sequela

⊗⑦**V77.0** Driver of bus injured in collision with fixed or stationary object in nontraffic accident

⊗⑦**V77.1** Passenger on bus injured in collision with fixed or stationary object in nontraffic accident

⊗⑦**V77.2** Person on outside of bus injured in collision with fixed or stationary object in nontraffic accident

⊗⑦**V77.3** Unspecified occupant of bus injured in collision with fixed or stationary object in nontraffic accident

⊗⑦**V77.4** Person boarding or alighting from bus injured in collision with fixed or stationary object

⊗⑦**V77.5** Driver of bus injured in collision with fixed or stationary object in traffic accident

⊗⑦**V77.6** Passenger on bus injured in collision with fixed or stationary object in traffic accident

⊗⑦**V77.7** Person on outside of bus injured in collision with fixed or stationary object in traffic accident

⊗⑦**V77.9** Unspecified occupant of bus injured in collision with fixed or stationary object in traffic accident

V78 Bus occupant injured in noncollision transport accident

Includes: overturning bus NOS

overturning bus without collision

The appropriate 7th character is to be added to each code from category V78

A - initial encounter

D - subsequent encounter

S - sequela

⊗⑦**V78.0** Driver of bus injured in noncollision transport accident in nontraffic accident

⊗⑦**V78.1** Passenger on bus injured in noncollision transport accident in nontraffic accident

⊗⑦**V78.2** Person on outside of bus injured in noncollision transport accident in nontraffic accident

⊗⑦**V78.3** Unspecified occupant of bus injured in noncollision transport accident in nontraffic accident

⊗⑦**V78.4** Person boarding or alighting from bus injured in noncollision transport accident

⊗⑦**V78.5** Driver of bus injured in noncollision transport accident in traffic accident

⊗⑦**V78.6** Passenger on bus injured in noncollision transport accident in traffic accident

⊗⑦**V78.7** Person on outside of bus injured in noncollision transport accident in traffic accident

⊗⑦**V78.9** Unspecified occupant of bus injured in noncollision transport accident in traffic accident

V79 Bus occupant injured in other and unspecified transport accidents

The appropriate 7th character is to be added to each code from category V79

A - initial encounter

D - subsequent encounter

S - sequela

V79.0 Driver of bus injured in collision with other and unspecified motor vehicles in nontraffic accident

⊗⑦**V79.00** Driver of bus injured in collision with unspecified motor vehicles in nontraffic accident

⊗⑦**V79.09** Driver of bus injured in collision with other motor vehicles in nontraffic accident

V79.1 Passenger on bus injured in collision with other and unspecified motor vehicles in nontraffic accident

⊗⑦**V79.10** Passenger on bus injured in collision with unspecified motor vehicles in nontraffic accident

⊗⑦**V79.19** Passenger on bus injured in collision with other motor vehicles in nontraffic accident

V79.2 Unspecified bus occupant injured in collision with other and unspecified motor vehicles in nontraffic accident

⊗⑦**V79.20** Unspecified bus occupant injured in collision with unspecified motor vehicles in nontraffic accident

Bus collision NOS, nontraffic

⊗⑦**V79.29** Unspecified bus occupant injured in collision with other motor vehicles in nontraffic accident

V79.3 Bus occupant (driver) (passenger) injured in unspecified nontraffic accident

Bus accident NOS, nontraffic

Bus occupant injured in nontraffic accident NOS

V79.4 Driver of bus injured in collision with other and unspecified motor vehicles in traffic accident

⊗⑦**V79.40** Driver of bus injured in collision with unspecified motor vehicles in traffic accident

⊗⑦**V79.49** Driver of bus injured in collision with other motor vehicles in traffic accident

V79.5 Passenger on bus injured in collision with other and unspecified motor vehicles in traffic accident

⊗⑦**V79.50** Passenger on bus injured in collision with unspecified motor vehicles in traffic accident

⊗⑦**V79.59** Passenger on bus injured in collision with other motor vehicles in traffic accident

V79.6 Unspecified bus occupant injured in collision with other and unspecified motor vehicles in traffic accident

⊗⑦**V79.60** Unspecified bus occupant injured in collision with unspecified motor vehicles in traffic accident

Bus collision NOS (traffic)

⊗⑦**V79.69** Unspecified bus occupant injured in collision with other motor vehicles in traffic accident

V79.8 Bus occupant (driver) (passenger) injured in other specified transport accidents

⊗⑦**V79.81** Bus occupant (driver) (passenger) injured in transport accidents with military vehicle

⊗⑦**V79.88** Bus occupant (driver) (passenger) injured in other specified transport accidents

⊗⑦**V79.9** Bus occupant (driver) (passenger) injured in unspecified traffic accident

Bus accident NOS

OTHER LAND TRANSPORT ACCIDENTS (V80-V89)

V80 Animal-rider or occupant of animal-drawn vehicle injured in transport accident

The appropriate 7th character is to be added to each code from category V80

A - initial encounter

D - subsequent encounter

S - sequela

V80.0 Animal-rider or occupant of animal drawn vehicle injured by fall from or being thrown from animal or animal-drawn vehicle in noncollision accident

V80.01 Animal-rider injured by fall from or being thrown from animal in noncollision accident

⑦**V80.010** Animal-rider injured by fall from or being thrown from horse in noncollision accident

⑦**V80.018** Animal-rider injured by fall from or being thrown from other animal in noncollision accident

⊗⑦**V80.02** Occupant of animal-drawn vehicle injured by fall from or being thrown from animal-drawn vehicle in noncollision accident

Overturning animal-drawn vehicle NOS

Overturning animal-drawn vehicle without collision

V80.1 Animal-rider or occupant of animal-drawn vehicle injured in collision with pedestrian or animal

Excludes1: animal-rider or animal-drawn vehicle collision with animal-drawn vehicle or animal being ridden (V80.7)

⊗⑦**V80.11** Animal-rider injured in collision with pedestrian or animal

⊗⑦**V80.12** Occupant of animal-drawn vehicle injured in collision with pedestrian or animal

V80.2 Animal-rider or occupant of animal-drawn vehicle injured in collision with pedal cycle

⊗⑦**V80.21** Animal-rider injured in collision with pedal cycle

● New code ▲ Revised code **Excludes1:** Not coded here **Excludes2:** Not included here ⊗ Placeholder required ⑦7th digit required

⊗⑦V80.22 Occupant of animal-drawn vehicle injured in collision with pedal cycle

V80.3 Animal-rider or occupant of animal-drawn vehicle injured in collision with two- or three-wheeled motor vehicle

⊗⑦V80.31 Animal-rider injured in collision with two- or three-wheeled motor vehicle

⊗⑦V80.32 Occupant of animal-drawn vehicle injured in collision with two- or three-wheeled motor vehicle

V80.4 Animal-rider or occupant of animal-drawn vehicle injured in collision with car, pick-up truck, van, heavy transport vehicle or bus

Excludes1: animal-rider injured in collision with military vehicle (V80.910)

occupant of animal-drawn vehicle injured in collision with military vehicle (V80.920)

⊗⑦V80.41 Animal-rider injured in collision with car, pick-up truck, van, heavy transport vehicle or bus

⊗⑦V80.42 Occupant of animal-drawn vehicle injured in collision with car, pick-up truck, van, heavy transport vehicle or bus

V80.5 Animal-rider or occupant of animal-drawn vehicle injured in collision with other specified motor vehicle

⊗⑦V80.51 Animal-rider injured in collision with other specified motor vehicle

⊗⑦V80.52 Occupant of animal-drawn vehicle injured in collision with other specified motor vehicle

V80.6 Animal-rider or occupant of animal-drawn vehicle injured in collision with railway train or railway vehicle

⊗⑦V80.61 Animal-rider injured in collision with railway train or railway vehicle

⊗⑦V80.62 Occupant of animal-drawn vehicle injured in collision with railway train or railway vehicle

V80.7 Animal-rider or occupant of animal-drawn vehicle injured in collision with other nonmotor vehicles

V80.71 Animal-rider or occupant of animal-drawn vehicle injured in collision with animal being ridden

⑦V80.710 Animal-rider injured in collision with other animal being ridden

⑦V80.711 Occupant of animal-drawn vehicle injured in collision with animal being ridden

V80.72 Animal-rider or occupant of animal-drawn vehicle injured in collision with other animal-drawn vehicle

⑦V80.720 Animal-rider injured in collision with animal-drawn vehicle

⑦V80.721 Occupant of animal-drawn vehicle injured in collision with other animal-drawn vehicle

V80.73 Animal-rider or occupant of animal-drawn vehicle injured in collision with streetcar

⑦V80.730 Animal-rider injured in collision with streetcar

⑦V80.731 Occupant of animal-drawn vehicle injured in collision with streetcar

V80.79 Animal-rider or occupant of animal-drawn vehicle injured in collision with other nonmotor vehicles

⑦V80.790 Animal-rider injured in collision with other nonmotor vehicles

⑦V80.791 Occupant of animal-drawn vehicle injured in collision with other nonmotor vehicles

V80.8 Animal-rider or occupant of animal-drawn vehicle injured in collision with fixed or stationary object

⊗⑦V80.81 Animal-rider injured in collision with fixed or stationary object

⊗⑦V80.82 Occupant of animal-drawn vehicle injured in collision with fixed or stationary object

V80.9 Animal-rider or occupant of animal-drawn vehicle injured in other and unspecified transport accidents

V80.91 Animal-rider injured in other and unspecified transport accidents

⑦V80.910 Animal-rider injured in transport accident with military vehicle

⑦V80.918 Animal-rider injured in other transport accident

⑦V80.919 Animal-rider injured in unspecified transport accident

Animal rider accident NOS

V80.92 Occupant of animal-drawn vehicle injured in other and unspecified transport accidents

⑦V80.920 Occupant of animal-drawn vehicle injured in transport accident with military vehicle

⑦V80.928 Occupant of animal-drawn vehicle injured in other transport accident

⑦V80.929 Occupant of animal-drawn vehicle injured in unspecified transport accident

Animal-drawn vehicle accident NOS

V81 Occupant of railway train or railway vehicle injured in transport accident

Includes: derailment of railway train or railway vehicle

person on outside of train

Excludes1: streetcar (V82.-)

The appropriate 7th character is to be added to each code from category V81

A - initial encounter

D - subsequent encounter

S - sequela

⊗⑦V81.0 Occupant of railway train or railway vehicle injured in collision with motor vehicle in nontraffic accident

Excludes1: Occupant of railway train or railway vehicle injured due to collision with military vehicle (V81.83)

⊗⑦V81.1 Occupant of railway train or railway vehicle injured in collision with motor vehicle in traffic accident

Excludes1: Occupant of railway train or railway vehicle injured due to collision with military vehicle (V81.83)

⊗⑦V81.2 Occupant of railway train or railway vehicle injured in collision with or hit by rolling stock

⊗⑦V81.3 Occupant of railway train or railway vehicle injured in collision with other object

Railway collision NOS

⊗⑦V81.4 Person injured while boarding or alighting from railway train or railway vehicle

⊗⑦V81.5 Occupant of railway train or railway vehicle injured by fall in railway train or railway vehicle

⊗⑦**V81.6** **Occupant of railway train or railway vehicle injured by fall from railway train or railway vehicle**

⊗⑦**V81.7** **Occupant of railway train or railway vehicle injured in derailment without antecedent collision**

V81.8 **Occupant of railway train or railway vehicle injured in other specified railway accidents**

  ⊗⑦**V81.81** **Occupant of railway train or railway vehicle injured due to explosion or fire on train**

  ⊗⑦**V81.82** **Occupant of railway train or railway vehicle injured due to object falling onto train**

    Occupant of railway train or railway vehicle injured due to falling earth onto train

    Occupant of railway train or railway vehicle injured due to falling rocks onto train

    Occupant of railway train or railway vehicle injured due to falling snow onto train

    Occupant of railway train or railway vehicle injured due to falling trees onto train

  ⊗⑦**V81.83** **Occupant of railway train or railway vehicle injured due to collision with military vehicle**

  ⊗⑦**V81.89** **Occupant of railway train or railway vehicle injured due to other specified railway accident**

⊗⑦**V81.9** **Occupant of railway train or railway vehicle injured in unspecified railway accident**

  Railway accident NOS

V82 **Occupant of powered streetcar injured in transport accident**

Includes: interurban electric car

person on outside of streetcar tram (car)

trolley (car)

Excludes1: bus (V70-V79)

  motorcoach (V70-V79)

  nonpowered streetcar (V76.-) train (V81.-)

The appropriate 7th character is to be added to each code from category V82

A - initial encounter

D - subsequent encounter

S - sequela

⊗⑦**V82.0** **Occupant of streetcar injured in collision with motor vehicle in nontraffic accident**

⊗⑦**V82.1** **Occupant of streetcar injured in collision with motor vehicle in traffic accident**

⊗⑦**V82.2** **Occupant of streetcar injured in collision with or hit by rolling stock**

⊗⑦**V82.3** **Occupant of streetcar injured in collision with other object**

  Excludes1: collision with animal-drawn vehicle or animal being ridden (V82.8)

⊗⑦**V82.4** **Person injured while boarding or alighting from streetcar**

⊗⑦**V82.5** **Occupant of streetcar injured by fall in streetcar**

  Excludes1: fall in streetcar:

    while boarding or alighting (V82.4)

    with antecedent collision (V82.0-V82.3)

⊗⑦**V82.6** **Occupant of streetcar injured by fall from streetcar**

  Excludes1: fall from streetcar:

    while boarding or alighting (V82.4)

    with antecedent collision (V82.0-V82.3)

⊗⑦**V82.7** **Occupant of streetcar injured in derailment without antecedent collision**

  Excludes1: occupant of streetcar injured in derailment with antecedent collision (V82.0-V82.3)

⊗⑦**V82.8** **Occupant of streetcar injured in other specified transport accidents**

  Streetcar collision with military vehicle

  Streetcar collision with train or nonmotor vehicles

⊗⑦**V82.9** **Occupant of streetcar injured in unspecified traffic accident**

  Streetcar accident NOS

V83 **Occupant of special vehicle mainly used on industrial premises injured in transport accident**

Includes: battery-powered airport passenger vehicle

  battery-powered truck (baggage) (mail)

  coal-car in mine

  forklift (truck)

  logging car

  self-propelled industrial truck

  station baggage truck (powered)

  tram, truck, or tub (powered) in mine or quarry

Excludes1: special construction vehicles (V85.-)

  special industrial vehicle in stationary use or maintenance (W31.-)

The appropriate 7th character is to be added to each code from category V83

A - initial encounter

D - subsequent encounter

S - sequela

⊗⑦**V83.0** **Driver of special industrial vehicle injured in traffic accident**

⊗⑦**V83.1** **Passenger of special industrial vehicle injured in traffic accident**

⊗⑦**V83.2** **Person on outside of special industrial vehicle injured in traffic accident**

⊗⑦**V83.3** **Unspecified occupant of special industrial vehicle injured in traffic accident**

⊗⑦**V83.4** **Person injured while boarding or alighting from special industrial vehicle**

⊗⑦**V83.5** **Driver of special industrial vehicle injured in nontraffic accident**

⊗⑦**V83.6** **Passenger of special industrial vehicle injured in nontraffic accident**

⊗⑦**V83.7** **Person on outside of special industrial vehicle injured in nontraffic accident**

⊗⑦**V83.9** **Unspecified occupant of special industrial vehicle injured in nontraffic accident**

  Special-industrial-vehicle accident NOS

V84 **Occupant of special vehicle mainly used in agriculture injured in transport accident**

Includes: self-propelled farm machinery

tractor (and trailer)

Excludes1: animal-powered farm machinery accident (W30.8-)

  contact with combine harvester (W30.0)

  special agricultural vehicle in stationary use or maintenance (W30.-)

The appropriate 7th character is to be added to each code from category V84

A - initial encounter

D - subsequent encounter

 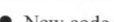

S - sequela

⊗⑦**V84.0** **Driver of special agricultural vehicle injured in traffic accident**

⊗⑦**V84.1** **Passenger of special agricultural vehicle injured in traffic accident**

⊗⑦**V84.2** **Person on outside of special agricultural vehicle injured in traffic accident**

⊗⑦**V84.3** **Unspecified occupant of special agricultural vehicle injured in traffic accident**

⊗⑦**V84.4** **Person injured while boarding or alighting from special agricultural vehicle**

⊗⑦**V84.5** **Driver of special agricultural vehicle injured in nontraffic accident**

⊗⑦**V84.6** **Passenger of special agricultural vehicle injured in nontraffic accident**

⊗⑦**V84.7** **Person on outside of special agricultural vehicle injured in nontraffic accident**

⊗⑦**V84.9** **Unspecified occupant of special agricultural vehicle injured in nontraffic accident**

Special-agricultural vehicle accident NOS

V85 **Occupant of special construction vehicle injured in transport accident**

Includes: bulldozer

digger dump truck

earth-leveller mechanical shovel road-roller

Excludes1: special industrial vehicle (V83.-)

special construction vehicle in stationary use or maintenance (W31.-)

The appropriate 7th character is to be added to each code from category V85

A - initial encounter

D - subsequent encounter

S - sequela

⊗⑦**V85.0** **Driver of special construction vehicle injured in traffic accident**

⊗⑦**V85.1** **Passenger of special construction vehicle injured in traffic accident**

⊗⑦**V85.2** **Person on outside of special construction vehicle injured in traffic accident**

⊗⑦**V85.3** **Unspecified occupant of special construction vehicle injured in traffic accident**

⊗⑦**V85.4** **Person injured while boarding or alighting from special construction vehicle**

⊗⑦**V85.5** **Driver of special construction vehicle injured in nontraffic accident**

⊗⑦**V85.6** **Passenger of special construction vehicle injured in nontraffic accident**

⊗⑦**V85.7** **Person on outside of special construction vehicle injured in nontraffic accident**

⊗⑦**V85.9** **Unspecified occupant of special construction vehicle injured in nontraffic accident**

Special-construction-vehicle accident NOS

V86 **Occupant of special all-terrain or other off-road motor vehicle, injured in transport accident**

Excludes1: special all-terrain vehicle in stationary use or maintenance (W31.-)

sport-utility vehicle (V50-V59)

three-wheeled motor vehicle designed for on-road use (V30-V39)

The appropriate 7th character is to be added to each code from category V86

A - initial encounter

D - subsequent encounter

S - sequela

V86.0 **Driver of special all-terrain or other off-road motor vehicle injured in traffic accident**

⊗⑦**V86.01** **Driver of ambulance or fire engine injured in traffic accident**

⊗⑦**V86.02** **Driver of snowmobile injured in traffic accident**

⊗⑦**V86.03** **Driver of dune buggy injured in traffic accident**

⊗⑦**V86.04** **Driver of military vehicle injured in traffic accident**

⊗⑦**V86.09** **Driver of other special all-terrain or other off-road motor vehicle injured in traffic accident**

Driver of dirt bike injured in traffic accident

Driver of go cart injured in traffic accident

Driver of golf cart injured in traffic accident

V86.1 **Passenger of special all-terrain or other off-road motor vehicle injured in traffic accident**

⊗⑦**V86.11** **Passenger of ambulance or fire engine injured in traffic accident**

⊗⑦**V86.12** **Passenger of snowmobile injured in traffic accident**

⊗⑦**V86.13** **Passenger of dune buggy injured in traffic accident**

⊗⑦**V86.14** **Passenger of military vehicle injured in traffic accident**

⊗⑦**V86.19** **Passenger of other special all-terrain or other off-road motor vehicle injured in traffic accident**

Passenger of dirt bike injured in traffic accident

Passenger of go cart injured in traffic accident

Passenger of golf cart injured in traffic accident

V86.2 **Person on outside of special all-terrain or other off-road motor vehicle injured in traffic accident**

⊗⑦**V86.21** **Person on outside of ambulance or fire engine injured in traffic accident**

⊗⑦**V86.22** **Person on outside of snowmobile injured in traffic accident**

⊗⑦**V86.23** **Person on outside of dune buggy injured in traffic accident**

⊗⑦**V86.24** **Person on outside of military vehicle injured in traffic accident**

⊗⑦**V86.29** **Person on outside of other special all-terrain or other off-road motor vehicle injured in traffic accident**

Person on outside of dirt bike injured in traffic accident

Person on outside of go cart in traffic accident

Person on outside of golf cart injured in traffic accident

V86.3 **Unspecified occupant of special all-terrain or other off-road motor vehicle injured in traffic accident**

⊗⑦**V86.31** **Unspecified occupant of ambulance or fire engine injured in traffic accident**

⊗⑦**V86.32** **Unspecified occupant of snowmobile injured in traffic accident**

⊗⑦**V86.33** **Unspecified occupant of dune buggy injured in traffic accident**

⊗⑦**V86.34** **Unspecified occupant of military vehicle injured in traffic accident**

⊗⑦**V86.39** **Unspecified occupant of other special all-terrain or other off-road motor vehicle injured in traffic accident**

Unspecified occupant of dirt bike injured in traffic accident

Unspecified occupant of go cart injured in traffic accident

Unspecified occupant of golf cart injured in traffic accident

V86.4 **Person injured while boarding or alighting from special all-terrain or other off-road motor vehicle**

⊗⑦**V86.41** **Person injured while boarding or alighting from ambulance or fire engine**

⊗⑦**V86.42** **Person injured while boarding or alighting from snowmobile**

⊗⑦**V86.43** **Person injured while boarding or alighting from dune buggy**

⊗⑦**V86.44** **Person injured while boarding or alighting from military vehicle**

⊗⑦**V86.49** **Person injured while boarding or alighting from other special all-terrain or other off-road motor vehicle**

Person injured while boarding or alighting from dirt bike

Person injured while boarding or alighting from go cart

Person injured while boarding or alighting from golf cart

V86.5 **Driver of special all-terrain or other off-road motor vehicle injured in nontraffic accident**

⊗⑦**V86.51** **Driver of ambulance or fire engine injured in nontraffic accident**

⊗⑦**V86.52** **Driver of snowmobile injured in nontraffic accident**

⊗⑦**V86.53** **Driver of dune buggy injured in nontraffic accident**

⊗⑦**V86.54** **Driver of military vehicle injured in nontraffic accident**

⊗⑦**V86.59** **Driver of other special all-terrain or other off-road motor vehicle injured in nontraffic accident**

Driver of dirt bike injured in nontraffic accident

Driver of go cart injured in nontraffic accident

Driver of golf cart injured in nontraffic accident

V86.6 **Passenger of special all-terrain or other off-road motor vehicle injured in nontraffic accident**

⊗⑦**V86.61** **Passenger of ambulance or fire engine injured in nontraffic accident**

⊗⑦**V86.62** **Passenger of snowmobile injured in nontraffic accident**

⊗⑦**V86.63** **Passenger of dune buggy injured in nontraffic accident**

⊗⑦**V86.64** **Passenger of military vehicle injured in nontraffic accident**

⊗⑦**V86.69** **Passenger of other special all-terrain or other off-road motor vehicle injured in nontraffic accident**

Passenger of dirt bike injured in nontraffic accident

Passenger of go cart injured in nontraffic accident

Passenger of golf cart injured in nontraffic accident

V86.7 **Person on outside of special all-terrain or other off-road motor vehicle injured in nontraffic accident**

⊗⑦**V86.71** **Person on outside of ambulance or fire engine injured in nontraffic accident**

⊗⑦**V86.72** **Person on outside of snowmobile injured in nontraffic accident**

⊗⑦**V86.73** **Person on outside of dune buggy injured in nontraffic accident**

⊗⑦**V86.74** **Person on outside of military vehicle injured in nontraffic accident**

⊗⑦**V86.79** **Person on outside of other special all-terrain or other off-road motor vehicles injured in nontraffic accident**

Person on outside of dirt bike injured in nontraffic accident

Person on outside of go cart injured in nontraffic accident

Person on outside of golf cart injured in nontraffic accident

V86.9 **Unspecified occupant of special all-terrain or other off-road motor vehicle injured in nontraffic accident**

⊗⑦**V86.91** **Unspecified occupant of ambulance or fire engine injured in nontraffic accident**

⊗⑦**V86.92** **Unspecified occupant of snowmobile injured in nontraffic accident**

⊗⑦**V86.93** **Unspecified occupant of dune buggy injured in nontraffic accident**

⊗⑦**V86.94** **Unspecified occupant of military vehicle injured in nontraffic accident**

⊗⑦**V86.99** **Unspecified occupant of other special all-terrain or other off-road motor vehicle injured in nontraffic accident**

All-terrain motor-vehicle accident NOS

Off-road motor-vehicle accident NOS

Other motor-vehicle accident NOS

Unspecified occupant of dirt bike injured in nontraffic accident

Unspecified occupant of go cart injured in nontraffic accident

Unspecified occupant of golf cart injured in nontraffic accident

V87 **Traffic accident of specified type but victim's mode of transport unknown**

Excludes1: collision involving:

pedal cycle (V10-V19) pedestrian (V01-V09)

The appropriate 7th character is to be added to each code from category V87

A - initial encounter

D - subsequent encounter

S - sequela

⊗⑦**V87.0** **Person injured in collision between car and two- or three-wheeled powered vehicle (traffic)**

⊗⑦**V87.1** **Person injured in collision between other motor vehicle and two- or three-wheeled motor vehicle (traffic)**

⊗⑦**V87.2** **Person injured in collision between car and pick-up truck or van (traffic)**

⊗⑦**V87.3** **Person injured in collision between car and bus (traffic)**

⊗⑦**V87.4** **Person injured in collision between car and heavy transport vehicle (traffic)**

⊗⑦**V87.5** **Person injured in collision between heavy transport vehicle and bus (traffic)**

⊗⑦**V87.6** **Person injured in collision between railway train or railway vehicle and car (traffic)**

⊗⑦**V87.7** **Person injured in collision between other specified motor vehicles (traffic)**

⊗⑦**V87.8** **Person injured in other specified noncollision transport accidents involving motor vehicle (traffic)**

⊗⑦**V87.9** **Person injured in other specified (collision)(noncollision) transport accidents involving nonmotor vehicle (traffic)**

V88 **Nontraffic accident of specified type but victim's mode of transport unknown**

Excludes1: collision involving:

pedal cycle (V10-V19) pedestrian (V01-V09)

The appropriate 7th character is to be added to each code from category V88

A - initial encounter

D - subsequent encounter

S - sequela

V88.0 **Person injured in collision between car and two- or three-wheeled motor vehicle, nontraffic**

⊗⑦**V88.1** **Person injured in collision between other motor vehicle and two- or three-wheeled motor vehicle, nontraffic**

⊗⑦**V88.2** **Person injured in collision between car and pick-up truck or van, nontraffic**

⊗⑦**V88.3** **Person injured in collision between car and bus, nontraffic**

⊗⑦**V88.4** **Person injured in collision between car and heavy transport vehicle, nontraffic**

⊗⑦**V88.5** **Person injured in collision between heavy transport vehicle and bus, nontraffic**

⊗⑦**V88.6** **Person injured in collision between railway train or railway vehicle and car, nontraffic**

⊗⑦**V88.7** **Person injured in collision between other specified motor vehicle, nontraffic**

⊗⑦**V88.8** **Person injured in other specified noncollision transport accidents involving motor vehicle, nontraffic**

⊗⑦**V88.9** **Person injured in other specified (collision)(noncollision) transport accidents involving nonmotor vehicle, nontraffic**

V89 **Motor- or nonmotor-vehicle accident, type of vehicle unspecified**

The appropriate 7th character is to be added to each code from category V89

A - initial encounter

D - subsequent encounter

S - sequela

⊗⑦**V89.0** **Person injured in unspecified motor-vehicle accident, nontraffic**

Motor-vehicle accident NOS, nontraffic

⊗⑦**V89.1** **Person injured in unspecified nonmotor-vehicle accident, nontraffic**

Nonmotor-vehicle accident NOS (nontraffic)

⊗⑦**V89.2** **Person injured in unspecified motor-vehicle accident, traffic**

Motor-vehicle accident [MVA] NOS

Road (traffic) accident [RTA] NOS

⊗⑦**V89.3** **Person injured in unspecified nonmotor-vehicle accident, traffic**

Nonmotor-vehicle traffic accident NOS

⊗⑦**V89.9** **Person injured in unspecified vehicle accident**

Collision NOS

WATER TRANSPORT ACCIDENTS (V90-V94)

V90 **Drowning and submersion due to accident to watercraft**

Excludes1: civilian water transport accident involving military watercraft (V94.81-)

fall into water not from watercraft (W16.-)

military watercraft accident in military or war operations (Y36.0-, Y37.0-)

water-transport-related drowning or submersion without accident to watercraft (V92.-)

The appropriate 7th character is to be added to each code from category V90

A - initial encounter

D - subsequent encounter

S - sequela

V90.0 **Drowning and submersion due to watercraft overturning**

⊗⑦**V90.00** **Drowning and submersion due to merchant ship overturning**

⊗⑦**V90.01** **Drowning and submersion due to passenger ship overturning**

Drowning and submersion due to Ferry-boat overturning

Drowning and submersion due to Liner overturning

⊗⑦**V90.02** **Drowning and submersion due to fishing boat overturning**

⊗⑦**V90.03** **Drowning and submersion due to other powered watercraft overturning**

Drowning and submersion due to Hovercraft (on open water) overturning

Drowning and submersion due to Jet ski overturning

⊗⑦**V90.04** **Drowning and submersion due to sailboat overturning**

⊗⑦**V90.05** **Drowning and submersion due to canoe or kayak overturning**

⊗⑦**V90.06** **Drowning and submersion due to (nonpowered) inflatable craft overturning**

⊗⑦**V90.08** **Drowning and submersion due to other unpowered watercraft overturning**

Drowning and submersion due to windsurfer overturning

⊗⑦**V90.09** **Drowning and submersion due to unspecified watercraft overturning**

Drowning and submersion due to boat NOS overturning

Drowning and submersion due to ship NOS overturning

Drowning and submersion due to watercraft NOS overturning

V90.1 Drowning and submersion due to watercraft sinking

⊗⑦**V90.10   Drowning and submersion due to merchant ship sinking**

⊗⑦**V90.11   Drowning and submersion due to passenger ship sinking**

Drowning and submersion due to Ferry-boat sinking

Drowning and submersion due to Liner sinking

⊗⑦**V90.12   Drowning and submersion due to fishing boat sinking**

⊗⑦**V90.13   Drowning and submersion due to other powered watercraft sinking**

Drowning and submersion due to Hovercraft (on open water) sinking

Drowning and submersion due to Jet ski sinking

⊗⑦**V90.14   Drowning and submersion due to sailboat sinking**

⊗⑦**V90.15   Drowning and submersion due to canoe or kayak sinking**

⊗⑦**V90.16   Drowning and submersion due to (nonpowered) inflatable craft sinking**

⊗⑦**V90.18   Drowning and submersion due to other unpowered watercraft sinking**

⊗⑦**V90.19   Drowning and submersion due to unspecified watercraft sinking**

Drowning and submersion due to boat NOS sinking

Drowning and submersion due to ship NOS sinking

Drowning and submersion due to watercraft NOS sinking

V90.2 Drowning and submersion due to falling or jumping from burning watercraft

⊗⑦**V90.20   Drowning and submersion due to falling or jumping from burning merchant ship**

⊗⑦**V90.21   Drowning and submersion due to falling or jumping from burning passenger ship**

Drowning and submersion due to falling or jumping from burning Ferry-boat

Drowning and submersion due to falling or jumping from burning Liner

⊗⑦**V90.22   Drowning and submersion due to falling or jumping from burning fishing boat**

⊗⑦**V90.23   Drowning and submersion due to falling or jumping from other burning powered watercraft**

Drowning and submersion due to falling and jumping from burning Hovercraft (on open water)

Drowning and submersion due to falling and jumping from burning Jet ski

⊗⑦**V90.24   Drowning and submersion due to falling or jumping from burning sailboat**

⊗⑦**V90.25   Drowning and submersion due to falling or jumping from burning canoe or kayak**

⊗⑦**V90.26   Drowning and submersion due to falling or jumping from burning (nonpowered) inflatable craft**

⊗⑦**V90.27   Drowning and submersion due to falling or jumping from burning water-skis**

⊗⑦**V90.28   Drowning and submersion due to falling or jumping from other burning unpowered watercraft**

Drowning and submersion due to falling and jumping from burning surf-board

Drowning and submersion due to falling and jumping from burning windsurfer

⊗⑦**V90.29   Drowning and submersion due to falling or jumping from unspecified burning watercraft**

Drowning and submersion due to falling or jumping from burning boat NOS

Drowning and submersion due to falling or jumping from burning ship NOS

Drowning and submersion due to falling or jumping from burning watercraft NOS

V90.3 Drowning and submersion due to falling or jumping from crushed watercraft

⊗⑦**V90.30   Drowning and submersion due to falling or jumping from crushed merchant ship**

⊗⑦**V90.31   Drowning and submersion due to falling or jumping from crushed passenger ship**

Drowning and submersion due to falling and jumping from crushed Ferry boat

Drowning and submersion due to falling and jumping from crushed Liner

⊗⑦**V90.32   Drowning and submersion due to falling or jumping from crushed fishing boat**

⊗⑦**V90.33   Drowning and submersion due to falling or jumping from other crushed powered watercraft**

Drowning and submersion due to falling and jumping from crushed Hovercraft

Drowning and submersion due to falling and jumping from crushed Jet ski

⊗⑦**V90.34   Drowning and submersion due to falling or jumping from crushed sailboat**

⊗⑦**V90.35   Drowning and submersion due to falling or jumping from crushed canoe or kayak**

⊗⑦**V90.36   Drowning and submersion due to falling or jumping from crushed (nonpowered) inflatable craft**

⊗⑦**V90.37   Drowning and submersion due to falling or jumping from crushed water-skis**

⊗⑦**V90.38   Drowning and submersion due to falling or jumping from other crushed unpowered watercraft**

Drowning and submersion due to falling and jumping from crushed surf-board

Drowning and submersion due to falling and jumping from crushed windsurfer

⊗⑦**V90.39   Drowning and submersion due to falling or jumping from crushed unspecified watercraft**

Drowning and submersion due to falling and jumping from crushed boat NOS

Drowning and submersion due to falling and jumping from crushed ship NOS

Drowning and submersion due to falling and jumping from crushed watercraft NOS

V90.8 Drowning and submersion due to other accident to watercraft

⊗⑦**V90.80   Drowning and submersion due to other accident to merchant ship**

⊗⑦**V90.81** **Drowning and submersion due to other accident to passenger ship**

Drowning and submersion due to other accident to Ferry-boat

Drowning and submersion due to other accident to Liner

⊗⑦**V90.82** **Drowning and submersion due to other accident to fishing boat**

⊗⑦**V90.83** **Drowning and submersion due to other accident to other powered watercraft**

Drowning and submersion due to other accident to Hovercraft (on open water)

Drowning and submersion due to other accident to Jet ski

⊗⑦**V90.84** **Drowning and submersion due to other accident to sailboat**

⊗⑦**V90.85** **Drowning and submersion due to other accident to canoe or kayak**

⊗⑦**V90.86** **Drowning and submersion due to other accident to (nonpowered) inflatable craft**

⊗⑦**V90.87** **Drowning and submersion due to other accident to water-skis**

⊗⑦**V90.88** **Drowning and submersion due to other accident to other unpowered watercraft**

Drowning and submersion due to other accident to surf-board

Drowning and submersion due to other accident to windsurfer

⊗⑦**V90.89** **Drowning and submersion due to other accident to unspecified watercraft**

Drowning and submersion due to other accident to boat NOS

Drowning and submersion due to other accident to ship NOS

Drowning and submersion due to other accident to watercraft NOS

V91 **Other injury due to accident to watercraft**

Includes: any injury except drowning and submersion as a result of an accident to watercraft

Excludes1: civilian water transport accident involving military watercraft (V94.81-)

military watercraft accident in military or war operations (Y36, Y37.-)

Excludes2: drowning and submersion due to accident to watercraft (V90.-)

The appropriate 7th character is to be added to each code from category V91

A - initial encounter
D - subsequent encounter
S - sequela

V91.0 **Burn due to watercraft on fire**

Excludes1: burn from localized fire or explosion on board ship without accident to watercraft (V93.-)

⊗⑦**V91.00** **Burn due to merchant ship on fire**

⊗⑦**V91.01** **Burn due to passenger ship on fire**

Burn due to Ferry-boat on fire

Burn due to Liner on fire

⊗⑦**V91.02** **Burn due to fishing boat on fire**

⊗⑦**V91.03** **Burn due to other powered watercraft on fire**

Burn due to Hovercraft (on open water) on fire

Burn due to Jet ski on fire

⊗⑦**V91.04** **Burn due to sailboat on fire**

⊗⑦**V91.05** **Burn due to canoe or kayak on fire**

⊗⑦**V91.06** **Burn due to (nonpowered) inflatable craft on fire**

⊗⑦**V91.07** **Burn due to water-skis on fire**

⊗⑦**V91.08** **Burn due to other unpowered watercraft on fire**

⊗⑦**V91.09** **Burn due to unspecified watercraft on fire**

Burn due to boat NOS on fire

Burn due to ship NOS on fire

Burn due to watercraft NOS on fire

V91.1 **Crushed between watercraft and other watercraft or other object due to collision**

Crushed by lifeboat after abandoning ship in a collision

Note: select the specified type of watercraft that the victim was on at the time of the collision

⊗⑦**V91.10** **Crushed between merchant ship and other watercraft or other object due to collision**

⊗⑦**V91.11** **Crushed between passenger ship and other watercraft or other object due to collision**

Crushed between Ferry-boat and other watercraft or other object due to collision

Crushed between Liner and other watercraft or other object due to collision

⊗⑦**V91.12** **Crushed between fishing boat and other watercraft or other object due to collision**

⊗⑦**V91.13** **Crushed between other powered watercraft and other watercraft or other object due to collision**

Crushed between Hovercraft (on open water) and other watercraft or other object due to collision

Crushed between Jet ski and other watercraft or other object due to collision

⊗⑦**V91.14** **Crushed between sailboat and other watercraft or other object due to collision**

⊗⑦**V91.15** **Crushed between canoe or kayak and other watercraft or other object due to collision**

⊗⑦**V91.16** **Crushed between (nonpowered) inflatable craft and other watercraft or other object due to collision**

⊗⑦**V91.18** **Crushed between other unpowered watercraft and other watercraft or other object due to collision**

Crushed between surfboard and other watercraft or other object due to collision

Crushed between windsurfer and other watercraft or other object due to collision

⊗⑦**V91.19** **Crushed between unspecified watercraft and other watercraft or other object due to collision**

Crushed between boat NOS and other watercraft or other object due to collision

Crushed between ship NOS and other watercraft or other object due to collision

Crushed between watercraft NOS and other watercraft or other object due to collision

V91.2 **Fall due to collision between watercraft and other watercraft or other object**

Fall while remaining on watercraft after collision

Note: select the specified type of watercraft that the victim was on at the time of the collision

Excludes1: crushed between watercraft and other watercraft and other object due to collision (V91.1-)

drowning and submersion due to falling from crushed watercraft (V90.3-)

⊗⑦**V91.20 Fall due to collision between merchant ship and other watercraft or other object**

⊗⑦**V91.21 Fall due to collision between passenger ship and other watercraft or other object**

Fall due to collision between Ferry-boat and other watercraft or other object

Fall due to collision between Liner and other watercraft or other object

⊗⑦**V91.22 Fall due to collision between fishing boat and other watercraft or other object**

⊗⑦**V91.23 Fall due to collision between other powered watercraft and other watercraft or other object**

Fall due to collision between Hovercraft (on open water) and other watercraft or other object

Fall due to collision between Jet ski and other watercraft or other object

⊗⑦**V91.24 Fall due to collision between sailboat and other watercraft or other object**

⊗⑦**V91.25 Fall due to collision between canoe or kayak and other watercraft or other object**

⊗⑦**V91.26 Fall due to collision between (nonpowered) inflatable craft and other watercraft or other object**

⊗⑦**V91.29 Fall due to collision between unspecified watercraft and other watercraft or other object**

Fall due to collision between boat NOS and other watercraft or other object

Fall due to collision between ship NOS and other watercraft or other object

Fall due to collision between watercraft NOS and other watercraft or other object

V91.3 Hit or struck by falling object due to accident to watercraft

Hit or struck by falling object (part of damaged watercraft or other object) after falling or jumping from damaged watercraft

Excludes2: drowning or submersion due to fall or jumping from damaged watercraft (V90.2-, V90.3-)

⊗⑦**V91.30 Hit or struck by falling object due to accident to merchant ship**

⊗⑦**V91.31 Hit or struck by falling object due to accident to passenger ship**

Hit or struck by falling object due to accident to Ferry-boat

Hit or struck by falling object due to accident to Liner

⊗⑦**V91.32 Hit or struck by falling object due to accident to fishing boat**

⊗⑦**V91.33 Hit or struck by falling object due to accident to other powered watercraft**

Hit or struck by falling object due to accident to Hovercraft (on open water)

Hit or struck by falling object due to accident to Jet ski

⊗⑦**V91.34 Hit or struck by falling object due to accident to sailboat**

⊗⑦**V91.35 Hit or struck by falling object due to accident to canoe or kayak**

⊗⑦**V91.36 Hit or struck by falling object due to accident to (nonpowered) inflatable craft**

⊗⑦**V91.37 Hit or struck by falling object due to accident to water-skis**

Hit by water-skis after jumping off of waterskis

⊗⑦**V91.38 Hit or struck by falling object due to accident to other unpowered watercraft**

Hit or struck by surf-board after falling off damaged surf-board

Hit or struck by object after falling off damaged windsurfer

⊗⑦**V91.39 Hit or struck by falling object due to accident to unspecified watercraft**

Hit or struck by falling object due to accident to boat NOS

Hit or struck by falling object due to accident to ship NOS

Hit or struck by falling object due to accident to watercraft NOS

V91.8 Other injury due to other accident to watercraft

⊗⑦**V91.80 Other injury due to other accident to merchant ship**

⊗⑦**V91.81 Other injury due to other accident to passenger ship**

Other injury due to other accident to Ferry-boat
Other injury due to other accident to Liner

⊗⑦**V91.82 Other injury due to other accident to fishing boat**

⊗⑦**V91.83 Other injury due to other accident to other powered watercraft**

Other injury due to other accident to Hovercraft (on open water)

Other injury due to other accident to Jet ski

⊗⑦**V91.84 Other injury due to other accident to sailboat**

⊗⑦**V91.85 Other injury due to other accident to canoe or kayak**

⊗⑦**V91.86 Other injury due to other accident to (nonpowered) inflatable craft**

⊗⑦**V91.87 Other injury due to other accident to water-skis**

⊗⑦**V91.88 Other injury due to other accident to other unpowered watercraft**

Other injury due to other accident to surf-board
Other injury due to other accident to windsurfer

⊗⑦**V91.89 Other injury due to other accident to unspecified watercraft**

Other injury due to other accident to boat NOS
Other injury due to other accident to ship NOS
Other injury due to other accident to watercraft NOS

V92 Drowning and submersion due to accident on board watercraft, without accident to watercraft

Excludes1: civilian water transport accident involving military watercraft (V94.81-)

drowning or submersion due to accident to watercraft (V90-V91)

● New code   ▲ Revised code   **Excludes1:** Not coded here   **Excludes2:** Not included here   ⊗ Placeholder required   ⑦7th digit required

drowning or submersion of diver who voluntarily jumps from boat not involved in an accident (W16.711, W16.721)

fall into water without watercraft (W16.-)

military watercraft accident in military or war operations (Y36, Y37)

The appropriate 7th character is to be added to each code from category V92

A - initial encounter

D - subsequent encounter

S - sequela

V92.0   Drowning and submersion due to fall off watercraft

Drowning and submersion due to fall from gangplank of watercraft

Drowning and submersion due to fall overboard watercraft

Excludes2: hitting head on object or bottom of body of water due to fall from watercraft (V94.0-)

⊗⑦**V92.00   Drowning and submersion due to fall off merchant ship**

⊗⑦**V92.01   Drowning and submersion due to fall off passenger ship**

Drowning and submersion due to fall off Ferryboat

Drowning and submersion due to fall off Liner

⊗⑦**V92.02   Drowning and submersion due to fall off fishing boat**

⊗⑦**V92.03   Drowning and submersion due to fall off other powered watercraft**

Drowning and submersion due to fall off Hovercraft (on open water)

Drowning and submersion due to fall off Jet ski

⊗⑦**V92.04   Drowning and submersion due to fall off sailboat**

⊗⑦**V92.05   Drowning and submersion due to fall off canoe or kayak**

⊗⑦**V92.06   Drowning and submersion due to fall off (nonpowered) inflatable craft**

⊗⑦**V92.07   Drowning and submersion due to fall off water-skis**

Excludes1: drowning and submersion due to falling off burning water-skis (V90.27)

drowning and submersion due to falling off crushed water-skis (V90.37)

hit by boat while water-skiing NOS (V94.X)

⊗⑦**V92.08   Drowning and submersion due to fall off other unpowered watercraft**

Drowning and submersion due to fall off surfboard

Drowning and submersion due to fall off windsurfer

Excludes1: drowning and submersion due to fall off burning unpowered watercraft (V90.28)

drowning and submersion due to fall off crushed unpowered watercraft (V90.38)

drowning and submersion due to fall off damaged unpowered watercraft (V90.88)

rowning and submersion due to rider of nonpowered watercraft being hit by other watercraft (V94.-)

Other injury due to rider of nonpowered watercraft being hit by other watercraft (V94.-)

⊗⑦**V92.09   Drowning and submersion due to fall off unspecified watercraft**

Drowning and submersion due to fall off boat NOS

Drowning and submersion due to fall off ship

Drowning and submersion due to fall off watercraft NOS

V92.1   Drowning and submersion due to being thrown overboard by motion of watercraft

Excludes1: drowning and submersion due to fall off surfboard (V92.08)

drowning and submersion due to fall off water-skis (V92.07)

drowning and submersion due to fall off windsurfer (V92.08)

⊗⑦**V92.10   Drowning and submersion due to being thrown overboard by motion of merchant ship**

⊗⑦**V92.11   Drowning and submersion due to being thrown overboard by motion of passenger ship**

Drowning and submersion due to being thrown overboard by motion of Ferry-boat

Drowning and submersion due to being thrown overboard by motion of Liner

⊗⑦**V92.12   Drowning and submersion due to being thrown overboard by motion of fishing boat**

⊗⑦**V92.13   Drowning and submersion due to being thrown overboard by motion of other powered watercraft**

Drowning and submersion due to being thrown overboard by motion of Hovercraft

⊗⑦**V92.14   Drowning and submersion due to being thrown overboard by motion of sailboat**

⊗⑦**V92.15   Drowning and submersion due to being thrown overboard by motion of canoe or kayak**

⊗⑦**V92.16   Drowning and submersion due to being thrown overboard by motion of (nonpowered) inflatable craft**

⊗⑦**V92.19   Drowning and submersion due to being thrown overboard by motion of unspecified watercraft**

Drowning and submersion due to being thrown overboard by motion of boat NOS

Drowning and submersion due to being thrown overboard by motion of ship NOS

Drowning and submersion due to being thrown overboard by motion of watercraft NOS

V92.2   Drowning and submersion due to being washed overboard from watercraft

Code first any associated cataclysm (X37.0-)

⊗⑦**V92.20   Drowning and submersion due to being washed overboard from merchant ship**

⊗⑦**V92.21   Drowning and submersion due to being washed overboard from passenger ship**

Drowning and submersion due to being washed overboard from Ferry-boat

Drowning and submersion due to being washed overboard from Liner

⊗⑦**V92.22** **Drowning and submersion due to being washed overboard from fishing boat**

⊗⑦**V92.23** **Drowning and submersion due to being washed overboard from other powered watercraft**

Drowning and submersion due to being washed overboard from Hovercraft (on open water)

Drowning and submersion due to being washed overboard from Jet ski

⊗⑦**V92.24** **Drowning and submersion due to being washed overboard from sailboat**

⊗⑦**V92.25** **Drowning and submersion due to being washed overboard from canoe or kayak**

⊗⑦**V92.26** **Drowning and submersion due to being washed overboard from (nonpowered) inflatable craft**

⊗⑦**V92.27** **Drowning and submersion due to being washed overboard from water-skis**

Excludes1: drowning and submersion due to fall off water-skis (V92.07)

⊗⑦**V92.28** **Drowning and submersion due to being washed overboard from other unpowered watercraft**

Drowning and submersion due to being washed overboard from surf-board

Drowning and submersion due to being washed overboard from windsurfer

⊗⑦**V92.29** **Drowning and submersion due to being washed overboard from unspecified watercraft**

Drowning and submersion due to being washed overboard from boat NOS

Drowning and submersion due to being washed overboard from ship NOS

Drowning and submersion due to being washed overboard from watercraft NOS

V93 **Other injury due to accident on board watercraft, without accident to watercraft**

Excludes1: civilian water transport accident involving military watercraft (V94.81-)

Other injury due to accident to watercraft (V91.-)

military watercraft accident in military or war operations (Y36, Y37.-)

Excludes2: drowning and submersion due to accident on board watercraft, without accident to watercraft (V92.-)

The appropriate 7th character is to be added to each code from category V93

A - initial encounter

D - subsequent encounter

S - sequela

V93.0 **Burn due to localized fire on board watercraft**

Excludes1: burn due to watercraft on fire (V91.0-)

⊗⑦**V93.00** **Burn due to localized fire on board merchant vessel**

⊗⑦**V93.01** **Burn due to localized fire on board passenger vessel**

Burn due to localized fire on board Ferry-boat

Burn due to localized fire on board Liner

⊗⑦**V93.02** **Burn due to localized fire on board fishing boat**

⊗⑦**V93.03** **Burn due to localized fire on board other powered watercraft**

Burn due to localized fire on board Hovercraft

Burn due to localized fire on board Jet ski

⊗⑦**V93.04** **Burn due to localized fire on board sailboat**

⊗⑦**V93.09** **Burn due to localized fire on board unspecified watercraft**

Burn due to localized fire on board boat NOS

Burn due to localized fire on board ship NOS

Burn due to localized fire on board watercraft NOS

V93.1 **Other burn on board watercraft**

Burn due to source **Other** than fire on board watercraft

Excludes1: burn due to watercraft on fire (V91.0-)

⊗⑦**V93.10** **Other burn on board merchant vessel**

⊗⑦**V93.11** **Other burn on board passenger vessel**

Other burn on board Ferry-boat

Other burn on board Liner

⊗⑦**V93.12** **Other burn on board fishing boat**

⊗⑦**V93.13** **Other burn on board other powered watercraft**

Other burn on board Hovercraft

Other burn on board Jet ski

⊗⑦**V93.14** **Other burn on board sailboat**

⊗⑦**V93.19** **Other burn on board unspecified watercraft**

Other burn on board boat NOS

Other burn on board ship NOS

Other burn on board watercraft NOS

V93.2 **Heat exposure on board watercraft**

Excludes1: exposure to man-made heat not aboard watercraft (W92)

exposure to natural heat while on board watercraft (X30)

exposure to sunlight while on board watercraft (X32)

Excludes2: burn due to fire on board watercraft (V93.0-)

⊗⑦**V93.20** **Heat exposure on board merchant ship**

⊗⑦**V93.21** **Heat exposure on board passenger ship**

Heat exposure on board Ferry-boat

Heat exposure on board Liner

⊗⑦**V93.22** **Heat exposure on board fishing boat**

⊗⑦**V93.23** **Heat exposure on board other powered watercraft**

Heat exposure on board hovercraft

⊗⑦**V93.24** **Heat exposure on board sailboat**

⊗⑦**V93.29** **Heat exposure on board unspecified watercraft**

Heat exposure on board boat NOS

Heat exposure on board ship NOS

Heat exposure on board watercraft NOS

V93.3 **Fall on board watercraft**

Excludes1: fall due to collision of watercraft (V91.2-)

⊗⑦**V93.30** **Fall on board merchant ship**

⊗⑦**V93.31** **Fall on board passenger ship**

Fall on board Ferry-boat Fall on board Liner

⊗⑦**V93.32** **Fall on board fishing boat**

⊗⑦**V93.33** **Fall on board other powered watercraft**

Fall on board Hovercraft (on open water)

Fall on board Jet ski

⊗⑦**V93.34** **Fall on board sailboat**

⊗⑦**V93.35** **Fall on board canoe or kayak**

⊗⑦**V93.36** **Fall on board (nonpowered) inflatable craft**

⊗⑦**V93.38** **Fall on board other unpowered watercraft**

⊗⑦**V93.39** **Fall on board unspecified watercraft**

Fall on board boat NOS Fall on board ship NOS

Fall on board watercraft NOS

V93.4 **Struck by falling object on board watercraft**

Hit by falling object on board watercraft

Excludes1: struck by falling object due to accident to watercraft (V91.3)

⊗⑦**V93.40** **Struck by falling object on merchant ship**

⊗⑦**V93.41** **Struck by falling object on passenger ship**

Struck by falling object on Ferry-boat

Struck by falling object on Liner

⊗⑦**V93.42** **Struck by falling object on fishing boat**

⊗⑦**V93.43** **Struck by falling object on other powered watercraft**

Struck by falling object on Hovercraft

⊗⑦**V93.44** **Struck by falling object on sailboat**

⊗⑦**V93.48** **Struck by falling object on other unpowered watercraft**

⊗⑦**V93.49** **Struck by falling object on unspecified watercraft**

V93.5 **Explosion on board watercraft**

Boiler explosion on steamship

Excludes2: fire on board watercraft (V93.0-)

⊗⑦**V93.50** **Explosion on board merchant ship**

⊗⑦**V93.51** **Explosion on board passenger ship**

Explosion on board Ferry-boat

Explosion on board Liner

⊗⑦**V93.52** **Explosion on board fishing boat**

⊗⑦**V93.53** **Explosion on board other powered watercraft**

Explosion on board Hovercraft

Explosion on board Jet ski

⊗⑦**V93.54** **Explosion on board sailboat**

⊗⑦**V93.59** **Explosion on board unspecified watercraft**

Explosion on board boat NOS

Explosion on board ship NOS

Explosion on board watercraft NOS

V93.6 **Machinery accident on board watercraft**

Excludes1: machinery explosion on board watercraft (V93.4-)

machinery fire on board watercraft (V93.0-)

⊗⑦**V93.60** **Machinery accident on board merchant ship**

⊗⑦**V93.61** **Machinery accident on board passenger ship**

Machinery accident on board Ferry-boat

Machinery accident on board Liner

⊗⑦**V93.62** **Machinery accident on board fishing boat**

⊗⑦**V93.63** **Machinery accident on board other powered watercraft**

Machinery accident on board Hovercraft

⊗⑦**V93.64** **Machinery accident on board sailboat**

⊗⑦**V93.69** **Machinery accident on board unspecified watercraft**

Machinery accident on board boat NOS

Machinery accident on board ship NOS

Machinery accident on board watercraft NOS

V93.8 **Other injury due to other accident on board watercraft**

Accidental poisoning by gases or fumes on watercraft

⊗⑦**V93.80** **Other injury due to other accident on board merchant ship**

⊗⑦**V93.81** **Other injury due to other accident on board passenger ship**

Other injury due to other accident on board Ferry-boat

Other injury due to other accident on board Liner

⊗⑦**V93.82** **Other injury due to other accident on board fishing boat**

⊗⑦**V93.83** **Other injury due to other accident on board other powered watercraft**

Other injury due to other accident on board Hovercraft

Other injury due to other accident on board Jet ski

⊗⑦**V93.84** **Other injury due to other accident on board sailboat**

⊗⑦**V93.85** **Other injury due to other accident on board canoe or kayak**

⊗⑦**V93.86** **Other injury due to other accident on board (nonpowered) inflatable craft**

⊗⑦**V93.87** **Other injury due to other accident on board water-skis**

Hit or struck by object while waterskiing

⊗⑦**V93.88** **Other injury due to other accident on board other unpowered watercraft**

Hit or struck by object while surfing

Hit or struck by object while on board windsurfer

⊗⑦**V93.89** **Other injury due to other accident on board unspecified watercraft**

Other injury due to other accident on board boat NOS

Other injury due to other accident on board ship NOS

Other injury due to other accident on board watercraft NOS

V94 **Other and unspecified water transport accidents**

Excludes1: military watercraft accidents in military or war operations (Y36, Y37)

The appropriate 7th character is to be added to each code from category V94

A - initial encounter

D - subsequent encounter

S - sequela

⊗⑦**V94.0** **Hitting object or bottom of body of water due to fall from watercraft**

Excludes2: drowning and submersion due to fall from watercraft (V92.0-)

⊗⑦**V94.1**　**Bather struck by watercraft**

　　Swimmer hit by watercraft

⊗⑦**V94.11**　**Bather struck by powered watercraft**

⊗⑦**V94.12**　**Bather struck by nonpowered watercraft**

V94.2　**Rider of nonpowered watercraft struck by other watercraft**

⊗⑦**V94.21**　**Rider of nonpowered watercraft struck by other nonpowered watercraft**

　　Canoer hit by other nonpowered watercraft

　　Surfer hit by other nonpowered watercraft

　　Windsurfer hit by other nonpowered watercraft

⊗⑦**V94.22**　**Rider of nonpowered watercraft struck by powered watercraft**

　　Canoer hit by motorboat

　　Surfer hit by motorboat

　　Windsurfer hit by motorboat

V94.3　**Injury to rider of (inflatable) watercraft being pulled behind other watercraft**

⊗⑦**V94.31**　**Injury to rider of (inflatable) recreational watercraft being pulled behind other watercraft**

　　Injury to rider of inner-tube pulled behind motor boat

⊗⑦**V94.32**　**Injury to rider of non-recreational watercraft being pulled behind other watercraft**

　　Injury to occupant of dingy being pulled behind boat or ship

　　Injury to occupant of life-raft being pulled behind boat or ship

⊗⑦**V94.4**　**Injury to barefoot water-skier**

　　Injury to person being pulled behind boat or ship

V94.8　**Other water transport accident**

V94.81　**Water transport accident involving military watercraft**

⑦**V94.810**　**Civilian watercraft involved in water transport accident with military watercraft**

　　Passenger on civilian watercraft injured due to accident with military watercraft

⑦**V94.811**　**Civilian in water injured by military watercraft**

⑦**V94.818**　**Other water transport accident involving military watercraft**

⊗⑦**V94.89**　**Other water transport accident**

⊗⑦**V94.9**　**Unspecified water transport accident**

　　Water transport accident NOS

AIR AND SPACE TRANSPORT ACCIDENTS (V95-V97)

Excludes1: military aircraft accidents in military or war operations (Y36, Y37)

V95　**Accident to powered aircraft causing injury to occupant**

　　The appropriate 7th character is to be added to each code from category V95

　　A - initial encounter

　　D - subsequent encounter

　　S - sequela

V95.0　**Helicopter accident injuring occupant**

⊗⑦**V95.00**　**Unspecified helicopter accident injuring occupant**

⊗⑦**V95.01**　**Helicopter crash injuring occupant**

⊗⑦**V95.02**　**Forced landing of helicopter injuring occupant**

⊗⑦**V95.03**　**Helicopter collision injuring occupant**

　　Helicopter collision with any object, fixed, movable or moving

⊗⑦**V95.04**　**Helicopter fire injuring occupant**

⊗⑦**V95.05**　**Helicopter explosion injuring occupant**

⊗⑦**V95.09**　**Other helicopter accident injuring occupant**

V95.1　**Ultralight, microlight or powered-glider accident injuring occupant**

⊗⑦**V95.10**　**Unspecified ultralight, microlight or powered-glider accident injuring occupant**

⊗⑦**V95.11**　**Ultralight, microlight or powered-glider crash injuring occupant**

⊗⑦**V95.12**　**Forced landing of ultralight, microlight or powered-glider injuring occupant**

⊗⑦**V95.13**　**Ultralight, microlight or powered-glider collision injuring occupant**

　　Ultralight, microlight or powered-glider collision with any object, fixed, movable or moving

⊗⑦**V95.14**　**Ultralight, microlight or powered-glider fire injuring occupant**

⊗⑦**V95.15**　**Ultralight, microlight or powered-glider explosion injuring occupant**

⊗⑦**V95.19**　**Other ultralight, microlight or powered-glider accident injuring occupant**

V95.2　**Other private fixed-wing aircraft accident injuring occupant**

⊗⑦**V95.20**　**Unspecified accident to other private fixed-wing aircraft, injuring occupant**

⊗⑦**V95.21**　**Other private fixed-wing aircraft crash injuring occupant**

⊗⑦**V95.22**　**Forced landing of other private fixed-wing aircraft injuring occupant**

⊗⑦**V95.23**　**Other private fixed-wing aircraft collision injuring occupant**

　　Other private fixed-wing aircraft collision with any object, fixed, movable or moving

⊗⑦**V95.24**　**Other private fixed-wing aircraft fire injuring occupant**

⊗⑦**V95.25**　**Other private fixed-wing aircraft explosion injuring occupant**

⊗⑦**V95.29**　**Other accident to other private fixed-wing aircraft injuring occupant**

V95.3　**Commercial fixed-wing aircraft accident injuring occupant**

⊗⑦**V95.30**　**Unspecified accident to commercial fixed-wing aircraft injuring occupant**

⊗⑦**V95.31**　**Commercial fixed-wing aircraft crash injuring occupant**

⊗⑦**V95.32**　**Forced landing of commercial fixed-wing aircraft injuring occupant**

⊗⑦**V95.33**　**Commercial fixed-wing aircraft collision injuring occupant**

　　Commercial fixed-wing aircraft collision with any object, fixed, movable or moving

⊗⑦**V95.34**　**Commercial fixed-wing aircraft fire injuring occupant**

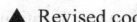

⊗⑦**V95.35 Commercial fixed-wing aircraft explosion injuring occupant**

⊗⑦**V95.39 Other accident to commercial fixed-wing aircraft injuring occupant**

V95.4 Spacecraft accident injuring occupant

⊗⑦**V95.40 Unspecified spacecraft accident injuring occupant**

⊗⑦**V95.41 Spacecraft crash injuring occupant**

⊗⑦**V95.42 Forced landing of spacecraft injuring occupant**

⊗⑦**V95.43 Spacecraft collision injuring occupant**

Spacecraft collision with any object, fixed, moveable or moving

⊗⑦**V95.44 Spacecraft fire injuring occupant**

⊗⑦**V95.45 Spacecraft explosion injuring occupant**

⊗⑦**V95.49 Other spacecraft accident injuring occupant**

⊗**V95.8 Other powered aircraft accidents injuring occupant**

⊗⑦**V95.9 Unspecified aircraft accident injuring occupant**

Aircraft accident NOS

Air transport accident NOS

V96 Accident to nonpowered aircraft causing injury to occupant

The appropriate 7th character is to be added to each code from category V96

A - initial encounter

D - subsequent encounter

S - sequela

V96.0 Balloon accident injuring occupant

⊗⑦**V96.00 Unspecified balloon accident injuring occupant**

⊗⑦**V96.01 Balloon crash injuring occupant**

⊗⑦**V96.02 Forced landing of balloon injuring occupant**

⊗⑦**V96.03 Balloon collision injuring occupant**

Balloon collision with any object, fixed, moveable or moving

⊗⑦**V96.04 Balloon fire injuring occupant**

⊗⑦**V96.05 Balloon explosion injuring occupant**

⊗⑦**V96.09 Other balloon accident injuring occupant**

V96.1 Hang-glider accident injuring occupant

⊗⑦**V96.10 Unspecified hang-glider accident injuring occupant**

⊗⑦**V96.11 Hang-glider crash injuring occupant**

⊗⑦**V96.12 Forced landing of hang-glider injuring occupant**

⊗⑦**V96.13 Hang-glider collision injuring occupant**

Hang-glider collision with any object, fixed, moveable or moving

⊗⑦**V96.14 Hang-glider fire injuring occupant**

⊗⑦**V96.15 Hang-glider explosion injuring occupant**

⊗⑦**V96.19 Other hang-glider accident injuring occupant**

V96.2 Glider (nonpowered) accident injuring occupant

⊗⑦**V96.20 Unspecified glider (nonpowered) accident injuring occupant**

⊗⑦**V96.21 Glider (nonpowered) crash injuring occupant**

⊗⑦**V96.22 Forced landing of glider (nonpowered) injuring occupant**

⊗⑦**V96.23 Glider (nonpowered) collision injuring occupant**

Glider (nonpowered) collision with any object, fixed, moveable or moving

⊗⑦**V96.24 Glider (nonpowered) fire injuring occupant**

⊗⑦**V96.25 Glider (nonpowered) explosion injuring occupant**

⊗⑦**V96.29 Other glider (nonpowered) accident injuring occupant**

⊗⑦**V96.8 Other nonpowered-aircraft accidents injuring occupant**

Kite carrying a person accident injuring occupant

⊗⑦**V96.9 Unspecified nonpowered-aircraft accident injuring occupant**

Nonpowered-aircraft accident NOS

V97 Other specified air transport accidents

The appropriate 7th character is to be added to each code from category V97

A - initial encounter

D - subsequent encounter

S - sequela

⊗⑦**V97.0 Occupant of aircraft injured in other specified air transport accidents**

Fall in, on or from aircraft in air transport accident

Excludes1: accident while boarding or alighting aircraft (V97.1)

⊗⑦**V97.1 Person injured while boarding or alighting from aircraft**

V97.2 Parachutist accident

⊗⑦**V97.21 Parachutist entangled in object**

Parachutist landing in tree

⊗⑦**V97.22 Parachutist injured on landing**

⊗⑦**V97.29 Other parachutist accident**

V97.3 Person on ground injured in air transport accident

⊗⑦**V97.31 Hit by object falling from aircraft**

Hit by crashing aircraft

Injured by aircraft hitting house

Injured by aircraft hitting car

⊗⑦**V97.32 Injured by rotating propeller**

⊗⑦**V97.33 Sucked into jet engine**

⊗⑦**V97.39 Other injury to person on ground due to air transport accident**

⊗⑦**V97.8 Other air transport accidents, not elsewhere classified**

Excludes1: aircraft accident NOS (V95.9)

exposure to changes in air pressure during ascent or descent (W94.-)

V97.81 Air transport accident involving military aircraft

⑦**V97.810 Civilian aircraft involved in air transport accident with military aircraft**

Passenger in civilian aircraft injured due to accident with military aircraft

⑦**V97.811 Civilian injured by military aircraft**

⑦**V97.818 Other air transport accident involving military aircraft**

⊗⑦**V97.89 Other air transport accidents, not elsewhere classified**

Injury from machinery on aircraft

OTHER AND UNSPECIFIED TRANSPORT ACCIDENTS

Add 4th-7th digits   Nonspecific code   Unspecified code   Manifestation code   1061

(V98-V99)

Excludes1: vehicle accident, type of vehicle unspecified (V89.-)

V98   Other specified transport accidents

The appropriate 7th character is to be added to each code from category V98

A - initial encounter

D - subsequent encounter

S - sequela

⊗⑦**V98.0   Accident to, on or involving cable-car, not on rails**

Caught or dragged by cable-car, not on rails

Fall or jump from cable-car, not on rails

Object thrown from or in cable-car, not on rails

⊗⑦**V98.1   Accident to, on or involving land-yacht**

⊗⑦**V98.2   Accident to, on or involving ice yacht**

⊗⑦**V98.3   Accident to, on or involving ski lift**

Accident to, on or involving ski chair-lift

Accident to, on or involving ski-lift with gondola

⊗⑦**V98.8   Other specified transport accidents**

⊗⑦**V99   Unspecified transport accident**

The appropriate 7th character is to be added to code V99

A - initial encounter

D - subsequent encounter

S - sequela

OTHER EXTERNAL CAUSES OF ACCIDENTAL INJURY (W00-X58)

SLIPPING, TRIPPING, STUMBLING AND FALLS (W00-W19)

Excludes1: assault involving a fall (Y01-Y02)

fall from animal (V80.-)

fall (in) (from) machinery (in operation) (W28-W31)

fall (in) (from) transport vehicle (V01-V99)

intentional self-harm involving a fall (X80-X81)

Excludes2: at risk for fall (history of fall) Z91.81

fall (in) (from) burning building (X00.-)

fall into fire (X00-X04, X08-X09)

W00   Fall due to ice and snow

Includes: pedestrian on foot falling (slipping) on ice and snow

Excludes1: fall on (from) ice and snow involving pedestrian conveyance (V00.-)

fall from stairs and steps not due to ice and snow (W10.-)

The appropriate 7th character is to be added to each code from category W00

A - initial encounter

D - subsequent encounter

S - sequela

⊗⑦**W00.0   Fall on same level due to ice and snow**

⊗⑦**W00.1   Fall from stairs and steps due to ice and snow**

⊗⑦**W00.2   Other fall from one level to another due to ice and snow**

⊗⑦**W00.9   Unspecified fall due to ice and snow**

W01   Fall on same level from slipping, tripping and stumbling

Includes: fall on moving sidewalk

Excludes1: fall due to bumping (striking) against object (W18.0-)

fall in shower or bathtub (W18.2-)

fall on same level NOS (W18.30)

fall on same level from slipping, tripping and stumbling due to ice or snow (W00.0)

fall off or from toilet (W18.1-)

slipping, tripping and stumbling NOS (W18.40)

slipping, tripping and stumbling without falling (W18.4-)

The appropriate 7th character is to be added to each code from category W01

A - initial encounter

D - subsequent encounter

S - sequela

⊗⑦**W01.0   Fall on same level from slipping, tripping and stumbling without subsequent striking against object**

Falling over animal

W01.1   Fall on same level from slipping, tripping and stumbling with subsequent striking against object

⊗⑦**W01.10   Fall on same level from slipping, tripping and stumbling with subsequent striking against unspecified object**

W01.11   Fall on same level from slipping, tripping and stumbling with subsequent striking against sharp object

⑦**W01.110   Fall on same level from slipping, tripping and stumbling with subsequent striking against sharp glass**

⑦**W01.111   Fall on same level from slipping, tripping and stumbling with subsequent striking against power tool or machine**

⑦**W01.118   Fall on same level from slipping, tripping and stumbling with subsequent striking against other sharp object**

⑦**W01.119   Fall on same level from slipping, tripping and stumbling with subsequent striking against unspecified sharp object**

W01.19   Fall on same level from slipping, tripping and stumbling with subsequent striking against other object

⑦**W01.190   Fall on same level from slipping, tripping and stumbling with subsequent striking against furniture**

⑦**W01.198   Fall on same level from slipping, tripping and stumbling with subsequent striking against other object**

⊗⑦**W03   Other fall on same level due to collision with another person**

Fall due to non-transport collision **with other** person

Excludes1: collision with another person without fall (W51)

crushed or pushed by a crowd or human stampede (W52)

fall involving pedestrian conveyance (V00-V09)

fall due to ice or snow (W00)

fall on same level NOS (W18.30)

The appropriate 7th character is to be added to code W03

A - initial encounter

D - subsequent encounter

S - sequela

⊗⑦**W04   Fall while being carried or supported by other persons**

Accidentally dropped while being carried

The appropriate 7th character is to be added to code W04

A - initial encounter

D - subsequent encounter

S - sequela

W05 **Fall from non-moving wheelchair, nonmotorized scooter and motorized mobility scooter**

Excludes1: fall from moving wheelchair (powered) (V00.811)

fall from moving motorized mobility scooter (V00.831)

fall from nonmotorized scooter (V00.141)

The appropriate 7th character is to be added to each code from category W05

A - initial encounter

D - subsequent encounter

S - sequela

⊗⑦**W05.0** **Fall from non-moving wheelchair**

⊗⑦**W05.1** **Fall from non-moving nonmotorized scooter**

⊗⑦**W05.2** **Fall from non-moving motorized mobility scooter**

⊗⑦**W06** **Fall from bed**

The appropriate 7th character is to be added to code W06

A - initial encounter

D - subsequent encounter

S - sequela

⊗⑦**W07** **Fall from chair**

The appropriate 7th character is to be added to code W07

A - initial encounter

D - subsequent encounter

S - sequela

⊗⑦**W08** **Fall from other furniture**

The appropriate 7th character is to be added to code W08

A - initial encounter

D - subsequent encounter

S - sequela

W09 **Fall on and from playground equipment**

Excludes1: fall involving recreational machinery (W31)

The appropriate 7th character is to be added to each code from category W09

A - initial encounter

D - subsequent encounter

S - sequela

⊗⑦**W09.0** **Fall on or from playground slide**

⊗⑦**W09.1** **Fall from playground swing**

⊗⑦**W09.2** **Fall on or from jungle gym**

⊗⑦**W09.8** **Fall on or from other playground equipment**

W10 **Fall on and from stairs and steps**

Excludes1: Fall from stairs and steps due to ice and snow (W00.1)

The appropriate 7th character is to be added to each code from category W10

A - initial encounter

D - subsequent encounter

S - sequela

⊗⑦**W10.0** **Fall (on)(from) escalator**

⊗⑦**W10.1** **Fall (on)(from) sidewalk curb**

⊗⑦**W10.2** **Fall (on)(from) incline**

Fall (on) (from) ramp

⊗⑦**W10.8** **Fall (on) (from) other stairs and steps**

⊗⑦**W10.9** **Fall (on) (from) unspecified stairs and steps**

⊗⑦**W11** **Fall on and from ladder**

The appropriate 7th character is to be added to code W11

A - initial encounter

D - subsequent encounter

S - sequela

⊗⑦**W12** **Fall on and from scaffolding**

The appropriate 7th character is to be added to code W12

A - initial encounter

D - subsequent encounter

S - sequela

W13 **Fall from, out of or through building or structure**

The appropriate 7th character is to be added to each code from category W13

A - initial encounter

D - subsequent encounter

S - sequela

⊗⑦**W13.0** **Fall from, out of or through balcony**

Fall from, out of or through railing

⊗⑦**W13.1** **Fall from, out of or through bridge**

⊗⑦**W13.2** **Fall from, out of or through roof**

⊗⑦**W13.3** **Fall through floor**

⊗⑦**W13.4** **Fall from, out of or through window**

Excludes2: fall with subsequent striking against sharp glass (W01.110)

⊗⑦**W13.8** **Fall from, out of or through other building or structure**

Fall from, out of or through viaduct

Fall from, out of or through wall

Fall from, out of or through flag-pole

⊗⑦**W13.9** **Fall from, out of or through building, not otherwise specified**

Excludes1: collapse of a building or structure (W20.-)

fall or jump from burning building or structure (X00.-)

⊗⑦**W14** **Fall from tree**

The appropriate 7th character is to be added to code W14

A - initial encounter

D - subsequent encounter

S - sequela

⊗⑦**W15** **Fall from cliff**

The appropriate 7th character is to be added to code W15

A - initial encounter

D - subsequent encounter

S - sequela

W16 **Fall, jump or diving into water**

Excludes1: accidental non-watercraft drowning and submersion not involving fall (W65-W74)

effects of air pressure from diving (W94.-)

fall into water from watercraft (V90-V94)

hitting an object or against bottom when falling from watercraft (V94.0)

Excludes2: striking or hitting diving board (W21.4)

The appropriate 7th character is to be added to each code from category W16

A - initial encounter

D - subsequent encounter

S - sequela

W16.0 Fall into swimming pool

Fall into swimming pool NOS

Excludes1: fall into empty swimming pool (W17.3)

W16.01 Fall into swimming pool striking water surface

⑦**W16.011   Fall into swimming pool striking water surface causing drowning and submersion**

Excludes1: drowning and submersion while in swimming pool without fall (W67)

⑦**W16.012   Fall into swimming pool striking water surface causing other injury**

W16.02 Fall into swimming pool striking bottom

⑦**W16.021   Fall into swimming pool striking bottom causing drowning and submersion**

Excludes1: drowning and submersion while in swimming pool without fall (W67)

⑦**W16.022   Fall into swimming pool striking bottom causing other injury**

W16.03 Fall into swimming pool striking wall

⑦**W16.031   Fall into swimming pool striking wall causing drowning and submersion**

Excludes1: drowning and submersion while in swimming pool without fall (W67)

⑦**W16.032   Fall into swimming pool striking wall causing other injury**

W16.1 Fall into natural body of water

Fall into lake

Fall into open sea Fall into river

Fall into stream

W16.11 Fall into natural body of water striking water surface

⑦**W16.111   Fall into natural body of water striking water surface causing drowning and submersion**

Excludes1: drowning and submersion while in natural body of water without fall (W69)

⑦**W16.112   Fall into natural body of water striking water surface causing other injury**

W16.12 Fall into natural body of water striking bottom

⑦**W16.121   Fall into natural body of water striking bottom causing drowning and submersion**

Excludes1: drowning and submersion while in natural body of water without fall (W69)

⑦**W16.122   Fall into natural body of water striking bottom causing other injury**

W16.13 Fall into natural body of water striking side

⊗⑦**W16.131 Fall into natural body of water striking side causing drowning and submersion**

Excludes1: drowning and submersion while in natural body of water without fall (W69)

⑦**W16.132   Fall into natural body of water striking side causing other injury**

W16.2 Fall in (into) filled bathtub or bucket of water

W16.21 Fall in (into) filled bathtub

Excludes1: fall into empty bathtub (W18.2)

⑦**W16.211   Fall in (into) filled bathtub causing drowning and submersion**

Excludes1: drowning and submersion while in filled bathtub without fall (W65)

⑦**W16.212   Fall in (into) filled bathtub causing other injury**

W16.22 Fall in (into) bucket of water

⑦**W16.221   Fall in (into) bucket of water causing drowning and submersion**

⑦**W16.222   Fall in (into) bucket of water causing other injury**

W16.3 Fall into other water

Fall into fountain Fall into reservoir

W16.31 Fall into other water striking water surface

⑦**W16.311   Fall into other water striking water surface causing drowning and submersion**

Excludes1: drowning and submersion while in other water without fall (W73)

⑦**W16.312   Fall into other water striking water surface causing other injury**

W16.32 Fall into other water striking bottom

⑦**W16.321   Fall into other water striking bottom causing drowning and submersion**

Excludes1: drowning and submersion while in other water without fall (W73)

⑦**W16.322   Fall into other water striking bottom causing other injury**

W16.33 Fall into other water striking wall

⑦**W16.331   Fall into other water striking wall causing drowning and submersion**

Excludes1: drowning and submersion while in other water without fall (W73)

⑦**W16.332   Fall into other water striking wall causing other injury**

W16.4 Fall into unspecified water

⊗⑦**W16.41 Fall into unspecified water causing drowning and submersion**

⊗⑦**W16.42 Fall into unspecified water causing other injury**

W16.5 Jumping or diving into swimming pool

⊗⑦**W16.51 Jumping or diving into swimming pool striking water surface**

⑦**W16.511   Jumping or diving into swimming pool striking water surface causing drowning and submersion**

Excludes1: drowning and submersion while in swimming pool without jumping or diving (W67)

⑦**W16.512** Jumping or diving into swimming pool striking water surface causing other injury

W16.52 Jumping or diving into swimming pool striking bottom

⑦**W16.521** Jumping or diving into swimming pool striking bottom causing drowning and submersion

Excludes1: drowning and submersion while in swimming pool without jumping or diving (W67)

⑦**W16.522** Jumping or diving into swimming pool striking bottom causing other injury

W16.53 Jumping or diving into swimming pool striking wall

⑦**W16.531** Jumping or diving into swimming pool striking wall causing drowning and submersion

Excludes1: drowning and submersion while in swimming pool without jumping or diving (W67)

⑦**W16.532** Jumping or diving into swimming pool striking wall causing other injury

W16.6 Jumping or diving into natural body of water

Jumping or diving into lake

Jumping or diving into open sea

Jumping or diving into river

Jumping or diving into stream

W16.61 Jumping or diving into natural body of water striking water surface

⑦**W16.611** Jumping or diving into natural body of water striking water surface causing drowning and submersion

Excludes1: drowning and submersion while in natural body of water without jumping or diving (W69)

⑦**W16.612** Jumping or diving into natural body of water striking water surface causing other injury

W16.62 Jumping or diving into natural body of water striking bottom

⑦**W16.621** Jumping or diving into natural body of water striking bottom causing drowning and submersion

Excludes1: drowning and submersion while in natural body of water without jumping or diving (W69)

⑦**W16.622** Jumping or diving into natural body of water striking bottom causing other injury

W16.7 Jumping or diving from boat

Excludes1: Fall from boat into water -see watercraft accident (V90-V94)

W16.71 Jumping or diving from boat striking water surface

⑦**W16.711** Jumping or diving from boat striking water surface causing drowning and submersion

⑦**W16.712** Jumping or diving from boat striking water surface causing other injury

W16.72 Jumping or diving from boat striking bottom

⑦**W16.721** Jumping or diving from boat striking bottom causing drowning and submersion

⑦**W16.722** Jumping or diving from boat striking bottom causing other injury

W16.8 Jumping or diving into other water

Jumping or diving into fountain

Jumping or diving into reservoir

W16.81 Jumping or diving into other water striking water surface

⑦**W16.811** Jumping or diving into other water striking water surface causing drowning and submersion

Excludes1: drowning and submersion while **in other** water without jumping or diving (W73)

⑦**W16.812** Jumping or diving into other water striking water surface causing other injury

W16.82 Jumping or diving into other water striking bottom

⑦**W16.821** Jumping or diving into other water striking bottom causing drowning and submersion

Excludes1: drowning and submersion while **in other** water without jumping or diving (W73)

⑦**W16.822** Jumping or diving into other water striking bottom causing other injury

W16.83 Jumping or diving into other water striking wall

⑦**W16.831** Jumping or diving into other water striking wall causing drowning and submersion

Excludes1: drowning and submersion while **in other** water without jumping or diving (W73)

⑦**W16.832** Jumping or diving into other water striking wall causing other injury

W16.9 Jumping or diving into unspecified water

⊗⑦**W16.91** Jumping or diving into unspecified water causing drowning and submersion

⊗⑦**W16.92** Jumping or diving into unspecified water causing other injury

W17 Other fall from one level to another

The appropriate 7th character is to be added to each code from category W17

A - initial encounter

D - subsequent encounter

S - sequela

⊗⑦**W17.0** Fall into well

⊗⑦**W17.1** Fall into storm drain or manhole

⊗⑦**W17.2** Fall into hole

Fall into pit

⊗⑦**W17.3** Fall into empty swimming pool

⊗⑦**W18.43** **Slipping, tripping and stumbling without falling due to stepping from one level to another**

⊗⑦**W18.49** **Other slipping, tripping and stumbling without falling**

⊗⑦**W19** **Unspecified fall**

Accidental fall NOS

The appropriate 7th character is to be added to code W19

A - initial encounter

D - subsequent encounter

S - sequela

EXPOSURE TO INANIMATE MECHANICAL FORCES (W20-W49)

Excludes1: assault (X92-Y09)

contact or collision with animals or persons (W50-W64)

exposure to inanimate mechanical forces involving military or war operations (Y36.-, Y37.-)

intentional self-harm (X71-X83)

W20 **Struck by thrown, projected or falling object**

Code first any associated:

cataclysm (X34-X39)

lightning strike (T75.00)

Excludes1: falling object in machinery accident (W24, W28-W31)

falling object in transport accident (V01-V99)

object set in motion by explosion (W35-W40)

object set in motion by firearm (W32-W34)

struck by thrown sports equipment (W21.-)

The appropriate 7th character is to be added to each code from categoryW20

A - initial encounter

D - subsequent encounter

S - sequela

⊗⑦**W20.0** **Struck by falling object in cave-in**

Excludes2: asphyxiation due to cave-in (T71.21)

⊗⑦**W20.1** **Struck by object due to collapse of building**

Excludes1: struck by object due to collapse of burning building (X00.2, X02.2)

⊗⑦**W20.8** **Other cause of strike by thrown, projected or falling object**

Excludes1: struck by thrown sports equipment (W21.-)

W21 **Striking against or struck by sports equipment**

Excludes1: assault with sports equipment (Y08.0-)

striking against or struck by sports equipment with subsequent fall (W18.01)

The appropriate 7th character is to be added to each code from category W21

A - initial encounter

D - subsequent encounter

S - sequela

W21.0 **Struck by hit or thrown ball**

⊗⑦**W21.00** **Struck by hit or thrown ball, unspecified type**

⊗⑦**W21.01** **Struck by football**

⊗⑦**W21.02** **Struck by soccer ball**

⊗⑦**W21.03** **Struck by baseball**

⊗⑦**W21.04** **Struck by golf ball**

Excludes1: fall into filled swimming pool (W16.0-)

⊗⑦**W17.4** **Fall from dock**

W17.8 **Other fall from one level to another**

⊗⑦**W17.81** **Fall down embankment (hill)**

⊗⑦**W17.82** **Fall from (out of) grocery cart**

Fall due to grocery cart tipping over

⊗⑦**W17.89** **Other fall from one level to another**

Fall from cherry picker Fall from lifting device

Fall from mobile elevated work platform [MEWP]

Fall from sky lift

W18 **Other slipping, tripping and stumbling and falls**

The appropriate 7th character is to be added to each code from category W18

A - initial encounter

D - subsequent encounter

S - sequela

W18.0 **Fall due to bumping against object**

Striking against object with subsequent fall

Excludes1: fall on same level due to slipping, tripping, or stumbling with subsequent striking against object (W01.1-)

⊗⑦**W18.00** **Striking against unspecified object with subsequent fall**

⊗⑦**W18.01** **Striking against sports equipment with subsequent fall**

⊗⑦**W18.02** **Striking against glass with subsequent fall**

⊗⑦**W18.09** **Striking against other object with subsequent fall**

W18.1 **Fall from or off toilet**

⊗⑦**W18.11** **Fall from or off toilet without subsequent striking against object**

Fall from (off) toilet NOS

⊗⑦**W18.12** **Fall from or off toilet with subsequent striking against object**

⊗⑦**W18.2** **Fall in (into) shower or empty bathtub**

Excludes1: fall in full bathtub causing drowning or submersion (W16.21-)

W18.3 **Other and unspecified fall on same level**

⊗⑦**W18.30** **Fall on same level, unspecified**

⊗⑦**W18.31** **Fall on same level due to stepping on an object**

Fall on same level due to stepping on an animal

Excludes1: slipping, tripping and stumbling without fall due to stepping on animal (W18.41)

⊗⑦**W18.39** **Other fall on same level**

W18.4 **Slipping, tripping and stumbling without falling**

Excludes1: collision with another person without fall (W51)

⊗⑦**W18.40** **Slipping, tripping and stumbling without falling, unspecified**

⊗⑦**W18.41** **Slipping, tripping and stumbling without falling due to stepping on object**

Slipping, tripping and stumbling without falling due to stepping on animal

Excludes1: slipping, tripping and stumbling with fall due to stepping on animal (W18.31)

⊗⑦**W18.42** **Slipping, tripping and stumbling without falling due to stepping into hole or opening**

⊗⑦**W21.05** **Struck by basketball**

⊗⑦**W21.06** **Struck by volleyball**

⊗⑦**W21.07** **Struck by softball**

⊗⑦**W21.09** **Struck by other hit or thrown ball**

W21.1 **Struck by bat, racquet or club**

⊗⑦**W21.11** **Struck by baseball bat**

⊗⑦**W21.12** **Struck by tennis racquet**

⊗⑦**W21.13** **Struck by golf club**

⊗⑦**W21.19** **Struck by other bat, racquet or club**

W21.2 **Struck by hockey stick or puck**

W21.21 **Struck by hockey stick**

⑦**W21.210** **Struck by ice hockey stick**

⑦**W21.211** **Struck by field hockey stick**

W21.22 **Struck by hockey puck**

⑦**W21.220** **Struck by ice hockey puck**

⑦**W21.221** **Struck by field hockey puck**

W21.3 **Struck by sports foot wear**

⊗⑦**W21.31** **Struck by shoe cleats**

Stepped on by shoe cleats

⊗⑦**W21.32** **Struck by skate blades**

Skated over by skate blades

⊗⑦**W21.39** **Struck by other sports foot wear**

⊗⑦**W21.4** **Striking against diving board**

<u>Use additional code</u> for subsequent falling into water, if applicable (W16.-)

W21.8 **Striking against or struck by other sports equipment**

⊗⑦**W21.81** **Striking against or struck by football helmet**

⊗⑦**W21.89** **Striking against or struck by other sports equipment**

⊗⑦**W21.9** **Striking against or struck by unspecified sports equipment**

W22 **Striking against or struck by other objects**

Excludes1: striking against or struck by object with subsequent fall (W18.09)

The appropriate 7th character is to be added to each code from category W22

A - initial encounter

D - subsequent encounter

S - sequela

W22.0 **Striking against stationary object**

Excludes1: striking against stationary sports equipment (W21.8)

⊗⑦**W22.01** **Walked into wall**

⊗⑦**W22.02** **Walked into lamppost**

⊗⑦**W22.03** **Walked into furniture**

W22.04 **Striking against wall of swimming pool**

⑦**W22.041** **Striking against wall of swimming pool causing drowning and submersion**

Excludes1: drowning and submersion while swimming without striking against wall (W67)

⑦**W22.042** **Striking against wall of swimming pool causing other injury**

⊗⑦**W22.09** **Striking against other stationary object**

W22.1 **Striking against or struck by automobile airbag**

⊗⑦**W22.10** **Striking against or struck by unspecified automobile airbag**

⊗⑦**W22.11** **Striking against or struck by driver side automobile airbag**

⊗⑦**W22.12** **Striking against or struck by front passenger side automobile airbag**

⊗⑦**W22.19** **Striking against or struck by other automobile airbag**

⊗⑦**W22.8** **Striking against or struck by other objects**

Striking against or struck by object NOS

Excludes1: struck by thrown, projected or falling object (W20.-)

W23 **Caught, crushed, jammed or pinched in or between objects**

Excludes1: injury caused by cutting or piercing instruments (W25-W27)

injury caused by firearms malfunction (W32.1, W33.1-, W34.1-)

injury caused by lifting and transmission devices (W24.-)

injury caused by machinery (W28-W31)

injury caused by nonpowered hand tools (W27.-)

injury caused by transport vehicle being used as a means of transportation (V01-V99)

injury caused by struck by thrown, projected or falling object (W20.-)

The appropriate 7th character is to be added to each code from category W23

A - initial encounter

D - subsequent encounter

S - sequela

⊗⑦**W23.0** **Caught, crushed, jammed, or pinched between moving objects**

⊗⑦**W23.1** **Caught, crushed, jammed, or pinched between stationary objects**

W24 **Contact with lifting and transmission devices, not elsewhere classified**

Excludes1: transport accidents (V01-V99)

The appropriate 7th character is to be added to each code from category W24

A - initial encounter

D - subsequent encounter

S - sequela

⊗⑦**W24.0** **Contact with lifting devices, not elsewhere classified**

Contact with chain hoist

Contact with drive belt

Contact with pulley (block)

⊗⑦**W24.1** **Contact with transmission devices, not elsewhere classified**

Contact with transmission belt or cable

⊗⑦**W25** **Contact with sharp glass**

<u>Code first</u> any associated:

injury due to flying glass from explosion or firearm discharge (W32-W40)

transport accident (V00-V99)

Excludes1: fall on same level due to slipping, tripping and stumbling with subsequent striking against sharp glass (W01.10)

striking against sharp glass with subsequent fall (W18.02)

Excludes2: glass embedded in skin (W45)

The appropriate 7th character is to be added to code W25

A - initial encounter

D - subsequent encounter

S - sequela

W26   **Contact with other sharp objects**

Excludes2: sharp object(s) embedded in skin (W45)

The appropriate 7th character is to be added to each code from category W26

A - initial encounter

D - subsequent encounter

S - sequela

⊗⑦**W26.0**   **Contact with knife**

Excludes1: contact with electric knife (W29.1)

⊗⑦**W26.1**   **Contact with sword or dagger**

●⊗⑦**W26.2**   **Contact with edge of stiff paper**

Paper cut

●⊗⑦**W26.8**   **Contact with other sharp object(s), not elsewhere classified**

Contact with tin can lid

●⊗⑦**W26.9**   **Contact with unspecified sharp object(s)**

W27   **Contact with nonpowered hand tool**

The appropriate 7th character is to be added to each code from category W27

A - initial encounter

D - subsequent encounter

S - sequela

⊗⑦**W27.0**   **Contact with workbench tool**

Contact with auger

Contact with axe

Contact with chisel

Contact with handsaw

Contact with screwdriver

⊗⑦**W27.1**   **Contact with garden tool**

Contact with hoe

Contact with nonpowered lawn mower

Contact with pitchfork

Contact with rake

⊗⑦**W27.2**   **Contact with scissors**

⊗⑦**W27.3**   **Contact with needle (sewing)**

Excludes1: contact with hypodermic needle (W46.-)

⊗⑦**W27.4**   **Contact with kitchen utensil**

Contact with fork

Contact with ice-pick

Contact with can-opener NOS

⊗⑦**W27.5**   **Contact with paper-cutter**

⊗⑦**W27.8**   **Contact with other nonpowered hand tool**

Contact with nonpowered sewing machine

Contact with shovel

⊗⑦**W28**   **Contact with powered lawn mower**

Powered lawn mower (commercial) (residential)

Excludes1: contact with nonpowered lawn mower (W27.1)

Excludes2: exposure to electric current (W86.-)

The appropriate 7th character is to be added to code W28

A - initial encounter

D - subsequent encounter

S - sequela

W29   **Contact with other powered hand tools and household machinery**

Excludes1: contact with commercial machinery (W31.82)

contact with hot household appliance (X15)

contact with nonpowered hand tool (W27.-)

exposure to electric current (W86)

The appropriate 7th character is to be added to each code from category W29

A - initial encounter

D - subsequent encounter

S - sequela

⊗⑦**W29.0**   **Contact with powered kitchen appliance**

Contact with blender

Contact with can-opener

Contact with garbage disposal

Contact with mixer

⊗⑦**W29.1**   **Contact with electric knife**

⊗⑦**W29.2**   **Contact with other powered household machinery**

Contact with electric fan

Contact with powered dryer (clothes) (powered) (spin)

Contact with washing-machine

Contact with sewing machine

⊗⑦**W29.3**   **Contact with powered garden and outdoor hand tools and machinery**

Contact with chainsaw

Contact with edger

Contact with garden cultivator (tiller)

Contact with hedge trimmer

Contact with other powered garden tool

Excludes1: contact with powered lawn mower (W28)

⊗⑦**W29.4**   **Contact with nail gun**

⊗⑦**W29.8**   **Contact with other powered powered hand tools and household machinery**

Contact with do-it-yourself tool NOS

W30   **Contact with agricultural machinery**

Includes: animal-powered farm machine

Excludes1: agricultural transport vehicle accident (V01-V99)

explosion of grain store (W40.8)

exposure to electric current (W86.-)

The appropriate 7th character is to be added to each code from category W30

A - initial encounter

D - subsequent encounter

S - sequela

⊗⑦**W30.0**   **Contact with combine harvester**

Contact with reaper

Contact with thresher

⊗⑦**W30.1**   **Contact with power take-off devices (PTO)**

⊗⑦**W30.2**   **Contact with hay derrick**

⊗⑦**W30.3**   **Contact with grain storage elevator** **Excludes1:** explosion of grain store (W40.8)

W30.8   **Contact with other specified agricultural machinery**

⊗⑦**W30.81 Contact with agricultural transport vehicle in stationary use**

Contact with agricultural transport vehicle under repair, not on public roadway

Excludes1: agricultural transport vehicle accident (V01-V99)

⊗⑦**W30.89 Contact with other specified agricultural machinery**

⊗⑦**W30.9 Contact with unspecified agricultural machinery**

Contact with farm machinery NOS

W31 Contact with other and unspecified machinery

Excludes1: contact with agricultural machinery (W30.-)

contact with machinery in transport under own power or being towed by a vehicle (V01-V99) exposure to electric current (W86)

The appropriate 7th character is to be added to each code from category W31

A - initial encounter

D - subsequent encounter

S - sequela

⊗⑦**W31.0 Contact with mining and earth-drilling machinery**

Contact with bore or drill (land) (seabed)

Contact with shaft hoist

Contact with shaft lift

Contact with undercutter

⊗⑦**W31.1 Contact with metalworking machines**

Contact with abrasive wheel

Contact with forging machine

Contact with lathe

Contact with mechanical shears

Contact with metal drilling machine

Contact with milling machine

Contact with power press

Contact with rolling-mill

Contact with metal sawing machine

⊗⑦**W31.2 Contact with powered woodworking and forming machines**

Contact with band saw

Contact with bench saw

Contact with circular saw

Contact with molding machine

Contact with overhead plane

Contact with powered saw

Contact with radial saw

Contact with sander

Excludes1: nonpowered woodworking tools (W27.0)

⊗⑦**W31.3 Contact with prime movers**

Contact with gas turbine

Contact with internal combustion engine

Contact with steam engine

Contact with water driven turbine

W31.8 Contact with other specified machinery

⊗⑦**W31.81 Contact with recreational machinery**

Contact with roller coaster

⊗⑦**W31.82 Contact with other commercial machinery**

Contact with commercial electric fan

Contact with commercial kitchen appliances

Contact with commercial powered dryer (clothes) (powered) (spin)

Contact with commercial washing-machine

Contact with commercial sewing machine

Excludes1: contact with household machinery (W29.-)

contact with powered lawn mower (W28)

⊗⑦**W31.83 Contact with special construction vehicle in stationary use**

Contact with special construction vehicle under repair, not on public roadway

Excludes1: special construction vehicle accident (V01-V99)

⊗⑦**W31.89 Contact with other specified machinery**

⊗⑦**W31.9 Contact with unspecified machinery**

Contact with machinery NOS

W32 Accidental handgun discharge and malfunction

Includes: accidental discharge and malfunction of gun for single hand use

accidental discharge and malfunction of pistol accidental discharge and malfunction of revolver

Handgun discharge and malfunction NOS

Excludes1: accidental airgun discharge and malfunction (W34.010, W34.110)

accidental BB gun discharge and malfunction (W34.010, W34.110)

accidental pellet gun discharge and malfunction (W34.010, W34.110)

accidental shotgun discharge and malfunction (W33.01, W33.11)

assault by handgun discharge (X93)

handgun discharge involving legal intervention (Y35.0-)

handgun discharge involving military or war operations (Y36.4-)

intentional self-harm by handgun discharge (X72)

Very pistol discharge and malfunction (W34.09, W34.19)

The appropriate 7th character is to be added to each code from category W32

A - initial encounter

D - subsequent encounter

S - sequela

⊗⑦**W32.0 Accidental handgun discharge**

⊗⑦**W32.1 Accidental handgun malfunction**

Injury due to explosion of handgun (parts)

Injury due to malfunction of mechanism or component of handgun

Injury due to recoil of handgun

Powder burn from handgun

W33 Accidental rifle, shotgun and larger firearm discharge and malfunction

Includes: rifle, shotgun and larger firearm discharge and malfunction NOS

Excludes1: accidental airgun discharge and malfunction (W34.010, W34.110)

accidental BB gun discharge and malfunction (W34.010, W34.110)

accidental handgun discharge and malfunction (W32.-)

accidental pellet gun discharge and malfunction (W34.010, W34.110)

assault by rifle, shotgun and larger firearm discharge (X94)

firearm discharge involving legal intervention (Y35.0-)

firearm discharge involving military or war operations (Y36.4-)

intentional self-harm by rifle, shotgun and larger firearm discharge (X73)

The appropriate 7th character is to be added to each code from category W33

A - initial encounter

D - subsequent encounter

S - sequela

W33.0 Accidental rifle, shotgun and larger firearm discharge

⊗⑦**W33.00 Accidental discharge of unspecified larger firearm**

Discharge of unspecified larger firearm NOS

⊗⑦**W33.01 Accidental discharge of shotgun**

Discharge of shotgun NOS

⊗⑦**W33.02 Accidental discharge of hunting rifle**

Discharge of hunting rifle NOS

⊗⑦**W33.03 Accidental discharge of machine gun**

Discharge of machine gun NOS

⊗⑦**W33.09 Accidental discharge of other larger firearm**

Discharge **of other** larger firearm NOS

W33.1 Accidental rifle, shotgun and larger firearm malfunction

Injury due to explosion of rifle, shotgun and larger firearm (parts)

Injury due to malfunction of mechanism or component of rifle, shotgun and larger firearm

Injury due to piercing, cutting, crushing or pinching due to (by) slide trigger mechanism, scope or other gun part

Injury due to recoil of rifle, shotgun and larger firearm

Powder burn from rifle, shotgun and larger firearm

⊗⑦**W33.10 Accidental malfunction of unspecified larger firearm**

Malfunction of unspecified larger firearm NOS

⊗⑦**W33.11 Accidental malfunction of shotgun**

Malfunction of shotgun NOS

⊗⑦**W33.12 Accidental malfunction of hunting rifle**

Malfunction of hunting rifle NOS

⊗⑦**W33.13 Accidental malfunction of machine gun**

Malfunction of machine gun NOS

⊗⑦**W33.19 Accidental malfunction of other larger firearm**

Malfunction **of other** larger firearm NOS

W34 Accidental discharge and malfunction from other and unspecified firearms and guns

The appropriate 7th character is to be added to each code from category W34

A - initial encounter

D - subsequent encounter

S - sequela

W34.0 Accidental discharge from other and unspecified firearms and guns

⊗⑦**W34.00 Accidental discharge from unspecified firearms or gun**

Discharge from firearm NOS

Gunshot wound NOS

Shot NOS

W34.01 Accidental discharge of gas, air or spring-operated guns

⑦**W34.010 Accidental discharge of airgun**

Accidental discharge of BB gun

Accidental discharge of pellet gun

⑦**W34.011 Accidental discharge of paintball gun**

Accidental injury due to paintball discharge

⑦**W34.018 Accidental discharge of other gas, air or spring-operated gun**

⊗⑦**W34.09 Accidental discharge from other specified firearms**

Accidental discharge from Very pistol [flare]

W34.1 Accidental malfunction from other and unspecified firearms and guns

⊗⑦**W34.10 Accidental malfunction from unspecified firearms or gun**

Firearm malfunction NOS

W34.11 Accidental malfunction of gas, air or spring-operated guns

⑦**W34.110 Accidental malfunction of airgun**

Accidental malfunction of BB gun

Accidental malfunction of pellet gun

⑦**W34.111 Accidental malfunction of paintball gun**

Accidental injury due to paintball gun malfunction

⑦**W34.118 Accidental malfunction of other gas, air or spring-operated gun**

⊗⑦**W34.19 Accidental malfunction from other specified firearms**

Accidental malfunction from Very pistol [flare]

⊗⑦**W35 Explosion and rupture of boiler**

Excludes1: explosion and rupture of boiler on watercraft (V93.4)

The appropriate 7th character is to be added to code W35

A - initial encounter

D - subsequent encounter

S - sequela

W36 Explosion and rupture of gas cylinder

The appropriate 7th character is to be added to each code from category W36

A - initial encounter

D - subsequent encounter

S - sequela

⊗⑦**W36.1 Explosion and rupture of aerosol can**

⊗⑦**W36.2 Explosion and rupture of air tank**

⊗⑦**W36.3 Explosion and rupture of pressurized-gas tank**

⊗⑦**W36.8 Explosion and rupture of other gas cylinder**

⊗⑦**W36.9 Explosion and rupture of unspecified gas cylinder**

W37 Explosion and rupture of pressurized tire, pipe or hose

The appropriate 7th character is to be added to each code from category W37

A - initial encounter

D - subsequent encounter

S - sequela

⊗⑦**W37.0** **Explosion of bicycle tire**

⊗⑦**W37.8** **Explosion and rupture of other pressurized tire, pipe or hose**

⊗⑦**W38** **Explosion and rupture of other specified pressurized devices**

The appropriate 7th character is to be added to code W38

A - initial encounter

D - subsequent encounter

S - sequela

⊗⑦**W39** **Discharge of firework**

The appropriate 7th character is to be added to code W39

A - initial encounter

D - subsequent encounter

S - sequela

W40 **Explosion of other materials**

Excludes1: assault by explosive material (X96)

explosion involving legal intervention (Y35.1-)

explosion involving military or war operations (Y36.0-, Y36.2-)

intentional self-harm by explosive material (X75)

The appropriate 7th character is to be added to each code from category W40

A - initial encounter

D - subsequent encounter

S - sequela

⊗⑦**W40.0** **Explosion of blasting material**

Explosion of blasting cap

Explosion of detonator

Explosion of dynamite

Explosion of explosive (any) used in blasting operations

⊗⑦**W40.1** **Explosion of explosive gases**

Explosion of acetylene

Explosion of butane

Explosion of coal gas

Explosion in mine NOS

Explosion of explosive gas

Explosion of fire damp

Explosion of gasoline fumes

Explosion of methane

Explosion of propane

⊗⑦**W40.8** **Explosion of other specified explosive materials**

Explosion in dump NOS

Explosion in factory NOS

Explosion in grain store

Explosion in munitions

Excludes1: explosion involving legal intervention (Y35.1-)

explosion involving military or war operations (Y36.0-, Y36.2-)

⊗⑦**W40.9** **Explosion of unspecified explosive materials**

Explosion NOS

W42 **Exposure to noise**

The appropriate 7th character is to be added to each code from category W42

A - initial encounter

D - subsequent encounter

S - sequela

⊗⑦**W42.0** **Exposure to supersonic waves**

⊗⑦**W42.9** **Exposure to other noise**

Exposure to sound waves NOS

W45 **Foreign body or object entering through skin**

Includes: foreign body or object embedded in skin

nail embedded in skin

Excludes2: contact with hand tools (nonpowered) (powered) (W27-W29)

contact with other sharp object(s) (W26.-)

contact with sharp glass (W25.-)

struck by objects (W20-W22)

The appropriate 7th character is to be added to each code from category W45

A - initial encounter

D - subsequent encounter

S - sequela

⊗⑦**W45.0** **Nail entering through skin**

⊗⑦**W45.8** **Other foreign body or object entering through skin**

Splinter in skin NOS

W46 **Contact with hypodermic needle**

The appropriate 7th character is to be added to each code from category W46

A - initial encounter

D - subsequent encounter

S - sequela

⊗⑦**W46.0** **Contact with hypodermic needle**

Hypodermic needle stick NOS

⊗⑦**W46.1** **Contact with contaminated hypodermic needle**

W49 **Exposure to other inanimate mechanical forces**

Includes: exposure to abnormal gravitational [G] forces

exposure to inanimate mechanical forces NEC

Excludes1: exposure to inanimate mechanical forces involving military or war operations (Y36.-, Y37.-)

The appropriate 7th character is to be added to each code from category W49

A - initial encounter

D - subsequent encounter

S - sequela

W49.0 **Item causing external constriction**

⊗⑦**W49.01** **Hair causing external constriction**

⊗⑦**W49.02** **String or thread causing external constriction**

⊗⑦**W49.03** **Rubber band causing external constriction**

⊗⑦**W49.04** **Ring or other jewelry causing external constriction**

⊗⑦**W49.09** **Other specified item causing external constriction**

⊗⑦**W49.9** **Exposure to other inanimate mechanical forces**

EXPOSURE TO ANIMATE MECHANICAL FORCES (W50-W64)

Excludes1: Toxic effect of contact with venomous animals and plants (T63.-)

W50 **Accidental hit, strike, kick, twist, bite or scratch by another person**

Includes: hit, strike, kick, twist, bite, or scratch by another person NOS

Excludes1: assault by bodily force (Y04)

struck by objects (W20-22)

The appropriate 7th character is to be added to each code from category W50

A - initial encounter

D - subsequent encounter

S - sequela

- ⊗⑦**W50.0 Accidental hit or strike by another person**

  Hit or strike by another person NOS

- ⊗⑦**W50.1 Accidental kick by another person**

  Kick by another person NOS

⊗⑦**W50.2 Accidental twist by another person**

  Twist by another person NOS

- ⊗⑦**W50.3 Accidental bite by another person**

  Human bite

  Bite by another person NOS

⊗⑦**W50.4 Accidental scratch by another person**

  Scratch by another person NOS

⊗⑦**W51 Accidental striking against or bumped into by another person**

  Excludes1: assault by striking against or bumping into by another person (Y04.2)

  fall due to collision with another person (W03)

The appropriate 7th character is to be added to code W51

A - initial encounter

D - subsequent encounter

S - sequela

⊗⑦**W52 Crushed, pushed or stepped on by crowd or human stampede**

  Crushed, pushed or stepped on by crowd or human stampede with or without fall

The appropriate 7th character is to be added to code W52

A - initial encounter

D - subsequent encounter

S - sequela

W53 Contact with rodent

  Includes: contact with saliva, feces or urine of rodent

The appropriate 7th character is to be added to each code from category W53

A - initial encounter

D - subsequent encounter

S - sequela

W53.0 Contact with mouse

  ⊗⑦**W53.01 Bitten by mouse**

  ⊗⑦**W53.09 Other contact with mouse**

W53.1 Contact with rat

  ⊗⑦**W53.11 Bitten by rat**

  ⊗⑦**W53.19 Other contact with rat**

W53.2 Contact with squirrel

  ⊗⑦**W53.21 Bitten by squirrel**

  ⊗⑦**W53.29 Other contact with squirrel**

W53.8 Contact with other rodent

  ⊗⑦**W53.81 Bitten by other rodent**

  ⊗⑦**W53.89 Other contact with other rodent**

W54 Contact with dog

  Includes: contact with saliva, feces or urine of dog

The appropriate 7th character is to be added to each code from category W54

A - initial encounter

D - subsequent encounter

S - sequela

⊗⑦**W54.0 Bitten by dog**

⊗⑦**W54.1 Struck by dog**

  Knocked over by dog

⊗⑦**W54.8 Other contact with dog**

W55 Contact with other mammals

  Includes: contact with saliva, feces or urine of mammal

  Excludes1: animal being ridden- see transport accidents

  bitten or struck by dog (W54)

  bitten or struck by rodent (W53.-)

  contact with marine mammals (W56.-)

The appropriate 7th character is to be added to each code from category W55

A - initial encounter

D - subsequent encounter

S - sequela

W55.0 Contact with cat

  ⊗⑦**W55.01 Bitten by cat**

  ⊗⑦**W55.03 Scratched by cat**

  ⊗⑦**W55.09 Other contact with cat**

W55.1 Contact with horse

  ⊗⑦**W55.11 Bitten by horse**

  ⊗⑦**W55.12 Struck by horse**

  ⊗⑦**W55.19 Other contact with horse**

W55.2 Contact with cow

  Contact with bull

  ⊗⑦**W55.21 Bitten by cow**

  ⊗⑦**W55.22 Struck by cow**

  Gored by bull

  ⊗⑦**W55.29 Other contact with cow**

W55.3 Contact with other hoof stock

  Contact with goats

  Contact with sheep

  ⊗⑦**W55.31 Bitten by other hoof stock**

  ⊗⑦**W55.32 Struck by other hoof stock**

  Gored by goat

  Gored by ram

  ⊗⑦**W55.39 Other contact with other hoof stock**

W55.4 Contact with pig

  ⊗⑦**W55.41 Bitten by pig**

  ⊗⑦**W55.42 Struck by pig**

  ⊗⑦**W55.49 Other contact with pig**

W55.5 Contact with raccoon

  ⊗⑦**W55.51 Bitten by raccoon**

  ⊗⑦**W55.52 Struck by raccoon**

  ⊗⑦**W55.59 Other contact with raccoon**

W55.8 Contact with other mammals

  ⊗⑦**W55.81 Bitten by other mammals**

  ⊗⑦**W55.82 Struck by other mammals**

  ⊗⑦**W55.89 Other contact with other mammals**

W56 Contact with nonvenomous marine animal

  Excludes1: contact with venomous marine animal (T63.-)

The appropriate 7th character is to be added to each code from category W56

A - initial encounter

D - subsequent encounter

S - sequela

W56.0 Contact with dolphin

⊗⑦**W56.01 Bitten by dolphin**

⊗⑦**W56.02 Struck by dolphin**

⊗⑦**W56.09 Other contact with dolphin**

W56.1 Contact with sea lion

⊗⑦**W56.11 Bitten by sea lion**

⊗⑦**W56.12 Struck by sea lion**

⊗⑦**W56.19 Other contact with sea lion**

W56.2 Contact with orca

Contact with killer whale

⊗⑦**W56.21 Bitten by orca**

⊗⑦**W56.22 Struck by orca**

⊗⑦**W56.29 Other contact with orca**

W56.3 Contact with other marine mammals

⊗⑦**W56.31 Bitten by other marine mammals**

⊗⑦**W56.32 Struck by other marine mammals**

⊗⑦**W56.39 Other contact with other marine mammals**

W56.4 Contact with shark

⊗⑦**W56.41 Bitten by shark**

⊗⑦**W56.42 Struck by shark**

⊗⑦**W56.49 Other contact with shark**

W56.5 Contact with other fish

⊗⑦**W56.51 Bitten by other fish**

⊗⑦**W56.52 Struck by other fish**

⊗⑦**W56.59 Other contact with other fish**

W56.8 Contact with other nonvenomous marine animals

⊗⑦**W56.81 Bitten by other nonvenomous marine animals**

⊗⑦**W56.82 Struck by other nonvenomous marine animals**

⊗⑦**W56.89 Other contact with other nonvenomous marine animals**

⊗⑦**W57 Bitten or stung by nonvenomous insect and other nonvenomous arthropods**

Excludes1: contact with venomous insects and arthropods (T63.2-, T63.3-, T63.4-)

The appropriate 7th character is to be added to code W57

A - initial encounter

D - subsequent encounter

S - sequela

W58 Contact with crocodile or alligator

The appropriate 7th character is to be added to each code from category W58

A - initial encounter

D - subsequent encounter

S - sequela

W58.0 Contact with alligator

⊗⑦**W58.01 Bitten by alligator**

⊗⑦**W58.02 Struck by alligator**

⊗⑦**W58.03 Crushed by alligator**

⊗⑦**W58.09 Other contact with alligator**

W58.1 Contact with crocodile

⊗⑦**W58.11 Bitten by crocodile**

⊗⑦**W58.12 Struck by crocodile**

⊗⑦**W58.13 Crushed by crocodile**

⊗⑦**W58.19 Other contact with crocodile**

W59 Contact with other nonvenomous reptiles

Excludes1: contact with venomous reptile (T63.0-, T63.1-)

The appropriate 7th character is to be added to each code from category W59

A - initial encounter

D - subsequent encounter

S - sequela

W59.0 Contact with nonvenomous lizards

⊗⑦**W59.01 Bitten by nonvenomous lizards**

⊗⑦**W59.02 Struck by nonvenomous lizards**

⊗⑦**W59.09 Other contact with nonvenomous lizards**

Exposure to nonvenomous lizards

W59.1 Contact with nonvenomous snakes

⊗⑦**W59.11 Bitten by nonvenomous snake**

⊗⑦**W59.12 Struck by nonvenomous snake**

⊗⑦**W59.13 Crushed by nonvenomous snake**

⊗⑦**W59.19 Other contact with nonvenomous snake**

W59.2 Contact with turtles

Excludes1: contact with tortoises (W59.8-)

⊗⑦**W59.21 Bitten by turtle**

⊗⑦**W59.22 Struck by turtle**

⊗⑦**W59.29 Other contact with turtle**

Exposure to turtles

W59.8 Contact with other nonvenomous reptiles

⊗⑦**W59.81 Bitten by other nonvenomous reptiles**

⊗⑦**W59.82 Struck by other nonvenomous reptiles**

⊗⑦**W59.83 Crushed by other nonvenomous reptiles**

⊗⑦**W59.89 Other contact with other nonvenomous reptiles**

⊗⑦**W60 Contact with nonvenomous plant thorns and spines and sharp leaves**

Excludes1: Contact with venomous plants (T63.7-)

The appropriate 7th character is to be added to code W60

A - initial encounter

D - subsequent encounter

S - sequela

W61 Contact with birds (domestic) (wild)

Includes: contact with excreta of birds

The appropriate 7th character is to be added to each code from category W61

A - initial encounter

D - subsequent encounter

S - sequela

W61.0 Contact with parrot

⊗⑦**W61.01 Bitten by parrot**

⊗⑦**W61.02 Struck by parrot**

⊗⑦**W61.09 Other contact with parrot**

Exposure to parrots

W61.1 Contact with macaw

⊗⑦**W61.11 Bitten by macaw**

⊗⑦**W61.12 Struck by macaw**

⊗⑦**W61.19**　**Other contact with macaw**
　　　　　　Exposure to macaws

W61.2　**Contact with other psittacines**
　⊗⑦**W61.21**　**Bitten by other psittacines**
　⊗⑦**W61.22**　**Struck by other psittacines**
　⊗⑦**W61.29**　**Other contact with other psittacines**
　　　　　　Exposure to other psittacines

W61.3　**Contact with chicken**
　⊗⑦**W61.32**　**Struck by chicken**
　⊗⑦**W61.33**　**Pecked by chicken**
　⊗⑦**W61.39**　**Other contact with chicken**
　　　　　　Exposure to chickens

W61.4　**Contact with turkey**
　⊗⑦**W61.42**　**Struck by turkey**
　⊗⑦**W61.43**　**Pecked by turkey**
　⊗⑦**W61.49**　**Other contact with turkey**

W61.5　**Contact with goose**
　⊗⑦**W61.51**　**Bitten by goose**
　⊗⑦**W61.52**　**Struck by goose**
　⊗⑦**W61.59**　**Other contact with goose**

W61.6　**Contact with duck**
　⊗⑦**W61.61**　**Bitten by duck**
　⊗⑦**W61.62**　**Struck by duck**
　⊗⑦**W61.69**　**Other contact with duck**

W61.9　**Contact with other birds**
　⊗⑦**W61.91**　**Bitten by other birds**
　⊗⑦**W61.92**　**Struck by other birds**
　⊗⑦**W61.99**　**Other contact with other birds**
　　　　　　Contact with bird NOS

W62　**Contact with nonvenomous amphibians**
　Excludes1: contact with venomous amphibians (T63.81-R63.83)
　The appropriate 7th character is to be added to each code from category W62
　A - initial encounter
　D - subsequent encounter
　S - sequela

　⊗⑦**W62.0**　**Contact with nonvenomous frogs**
　⊗⑦**W62.1**　**Contact with nonvenomous toads**
　⊗⑦**W62.9**　**Contact with other nonvenomous amphibians**

⊗⑦**W64**　**Exposure to other animate mechanical forces**
　Includes: exposure to nonvenomous animal NOS
　Excludes1: contact with venomous animal (T63.-)
　The appropriate 7th character is to be added to code ⊗⑦W64
　A - initial encounter
　D - subsequent encounter
　S - sequela

ACCIDENTAL NON-TRANSPORT DROWNING AND SUBMERSION (W65-W74)
Excludes1: accidental drowning and submersion due to fall into water (W16.-)
　accidental drowning and submersion due to water transport accident (V90.-, V92.-)
Excludes2: accidental drowning and submersion due to cataclysm (X34-X39)

⊗⑦**W65**　**Accidental drowning and submersion while in bath-tub**
　Excludes1: accidental drowning and submersion due to fall in (into) bathtub (W16.211)
　The appropriate 7th character is to be added to code W65
　A - initial encounter
　D - subsequent encounter
　S - sequela

⊗⑦**W67**　**Accidental drowning and submersion while in swimming-pool**
　Excludes1: accidental drowning and submersion due to fall into swimming pool (W16.011, W16.021, W16.031)
　　accidental drowning and submersion due to striking into wall of swimming pool (W22.041)
　The appropriate 7th character is to be added to code W67
　A - initial encounter
　D - subsequent encounter
　S - sequela

⊗⑦**W69**　**Accidental drowning and submersion while in natural water**
　Accidental drowning and submersion while in lake
　Accidental drowning and submersion while in open sea
　Accidental drowning and submersion while in river
　Accidental drowning and submersion while in stream
　Excludes1: accidental drowning and submersion due to fall into natural body of water (W16.111, W16.121, W16.131)
　The appropriate 7th character is to be added to code W69
　A - initial encounter
　D - subsequent encounter
　S - sequela

⊗⑦**W73**　**Other specified cause of accidental non-transport drowning and submersion**
　Accidental drowning and submersion while in quenching tank
　Accidental drowning and submersion while in reservoir
　Excludes1: accidental drowning and submersion due to fall into other water (W16.311, W16.321, W16.331)
　The appropriate 7th character is to be added to code W73
　A - initial encounter
　D - subsequent encounter
　S - sequela

⊗⑦**W74**　**Unspecified cause of accidental drowning and submersion**
　Drowning NOS
　The appropriate 7th character is to be added to code W74
　A - initial encounter
　D - subsequent encounter
　S - sequela

EXPOSURE TO ELECTRIC CURRENT, RADIATION AND EXTREME AMBIENT AIR TEMPERATURE AND PRESSURE (W85-W99)
Excludes1: exposure to:
　failure in dosage of radiation or temperature during surgical and medical care (Y63.2-Y63.5)
　lightning (T75.0-)
　natural cold (X31)
　natural heat (X30)
　natural radiation NOS (X39)
　radiological procedure and radiotherapy (Y84.2)
　sunlight (X32)

⊗⑦**W85 Exposure to electric transmission lines**

Broken power line

The appropriate 7th character is to be added to code W85

A - initial encounter

D - subsequent encounter

S - sequela

W86 Exposure to other specified electric current

The appropriate 7th character is to be added to each code from category W86

A - initial encounter

D - subsequent encounter

S - sequela

⊗⑦**W86.0 Exposure to domestic wiring and appliances**

⊗⑦**W86.1 Exposure to industrial wiring, appliances and electrical machinery**

Exposure to conductors

Exposure to control apparatus

Exposure to electrical equipment and machinery

Exposure to transformers

⊗⑦**W86.8 Exposure to other electric current**

Exposure to wiring and appliances in or on farm (not farmhouse)

Exposure to wiring and appliances outdoors

Exposure to wiring and appliances in or on public building

Exposure to wiring and appliances in or on residential institutions

Exposure to wiring and appliances in or on schools

W88 Exposure to ionizing radiation

Excludes1: exposure to sunlight (X32)

The appropriate 7th character is to be added to each code from category W88

A - initial encounter

D - subsequent encounter

S - sequela

⊗⑦**W88.0 Exposure to X-rays**

⊗⑦**W88.1 Exposure to radioactive isotopes**

⊗⑦**W88.8 Exposure to other ionizing radiation**

W89 Exposure to man-made visible and ultraviolet light

Includes: exposure to welding light (arc)

Excludes1: exposure to sunlight (X32)

The appropriate 7th character is to be added to each code from category W89

A - initial encounter

D - subsequent encounter

S - sequela

⊗⑦**W89.0 Exposure to welding light (arc)**

⊗⑦**W89.1 Exposure to tanning bed**

⊗⑦**W89.8 Exposure to other man-made visible and ultraviolet light**

⊗⑦**W89.9 Exposure to unspecified man-made visible and ultraviolet light**

W90 Exposure to other nonionizing radiation

Excludes1: exposure to sunlight (X32)

The appropriate 7th character is to be added to each code from category W90

A - initial encounter

D - subsequent encounter

S - sequela

⊗⑦**W90.0 Exposure to radiofrequency**

⊗⑦**W90.1 Exposure to infrared radiation**

⊗⑦**W90.2 Exposure to laser radiation**

⊗⑦**W90.8 Exposure to other nonionizing radiation**

⊗⑦**W92 Exposure to excessive heat of man-made origin**

The appropriate 7th character is to be added to code W92

A - initial encounter

D - subsequent encounter

S - sequela

W93 Exposure to excessive cold of man-made origin

The appropriate 7th character is to be added to each code from category W93

A - initial encounter

D - subsequent encounter

S - sequela

W93.0 Contact with or inhalation of dry ice

⊗⑦**W93.01 Contact with dry ice**

⊗⑦**W93.02 Inhalation of dry ice**

W93.1 Contact with or inhalation of liquid air

⊗⑦**W93.11 Contact with liquid air**

Contact with liquid hydrogen

Contact with liquid nitrogen

⊗⑦**W93.12 Inhalation of liquid air**

Inhalation of liquid hydrogen

Inhalation of liquid nitrogen

⊗⑦**W93.2 Prolonged exposure in deep freeze unit or refrigerator**

⊗⑦**W93.8 Exposure to other excessive cold of man-made origin**

⊗⑦**W94 Exposure to high and low air pressure and changes in air pressure**

The appropriate 7th character is to be added to each code from category W94

A - initial encounter

D - subsequent encounter

S - sequela

⊗⑦**W94.0 Exposure to prolonged high air pressure**

W94.1 Exposure to prolonged low air pressure

⊗⑦**W94.11 Exposure to residence or prolonged visit at high altitude**

⊗⑦**W94.12 Exposure to other prolonged low air pressure**

W94.2 Exposure to rapid changes in air pressure during ascent

⊗⑦**W94.21 Exposure to reduction in atmospheric pressure while surfacing from deep-water diving**

⊗⑦**W94.22 Exposure to reduction in atmospheric pressure while surfacing from underground**

⊗⑦**W94.23 Exposure to sudden change in air pressure in aircraft during ascent**

⊗⑦**W94.29 Exposure to other rapid changes in air pressure during ascent**

W94.3 Exposure to rapid changes in air pressure during descent

⊗⑦**W94.31 Exposure to sudden change in air pressure in aircraft during descent**

⊗⑦**W94.32** **Exposure to high air pressure from rapid descent in water**

⊗⑦**W94.39** **Exposure to other rapid changes in air pressure during descent**

⊗⑦**W99** **Exposure to other man-made environmental factors**

The appropriate 7th character is to be added to code W99

A - initial encounter

D - subsequent encounter

S - sequela

EXPOSURE TO SMOKE, FIRE AND FLAMES (X00-X08)

Excludes1: arson (X97)

Excludes2: explosions (W35-W40)

lightning (T75.0-)

transport accident (V01-V99)

X00 **Exposure to uncontrolled fire in building or structure**

Includes: conflagration in building or structure

Code first any associated cataclysm

Excludes2: Exposure to ignition or melting of nightwear (X05)

Exposure to ignition or melting **of other** clothing and apparel (X06.-)

Exposure **to other** specified smoke, fire and flames (X08.-)

The appropriate 7th character is to be added to each code from category X00

A - initial encounter

D - subsequent encounter

S - sequela

⊗⑦**X00.0** **Exposure to flames in uncontrolled fire in building or structure**

⊗⑦**X00.1** **Exposure to smoke in uncontrolled fire in building or structure**

⊗⑦**X00.2** **Injury due to collapse of burning building or structure in uncontrolled fire**

Excludes1: injury due to collapse of building not on fire (W20.1)

⊗⑦**X00.3** **Fall from burning building or structure in uncontrolled fire**

⊗⑦**X00.4** **Hit by object from burning building or structure in uncontrolled fire**

⊗⑦**X00.5** **Jump from burning building or structure in uncontrolled fire**

⊗⑦**X00.8** **Other exposure to uncontrolled fire in building or structure**

X01 **Exposure to uncontrolled fire, not in building or structure**

Includes: exposure to forest fire

The appropriate 7th character is to be added to each code from category X01

A - initial encounter

D - subsequent encounter

S - sequela

⊗⑦**X01.0** **Exposure to flames in uncontrolled fire, not in building or structure**

⊗⑦**X01.1** **Exposure to smoke in uncontrolled fire, not in building or structure**

⊗⑦**X01.3** **Fall due to uncontrolled fire, not in building or structure**

⊗⑦**X01.4** **Hit by object due to uncontrolled fire, not in building or structure**

⊗⑦**X01.8** **Other exposure to uncontrolled fire, not in building or structure**

X02 **Exposure to controlled fire in building or structure**

Includes: exposure to fire in fireplace

exposure to fire in stove

The appropriate 7th character is to be added to each code from category X02

A - initial encounter

D - subsequent encounter

S - sequela

⊗⑦**X02.0** **Exposure to flames in controlled fire in building or structure**

⊗⑦**X02.1** **Exposure to smoke in controlled fire in building or structure**

⊗⑦**X02.2** **Injury due to collapse of burning building or structure in controlled fire**

Excludes1: injury due to collapse of building not on fire (W20.1)

⊗⑦**X02.3** **Fall from burning building or structure in controlled fire**

⊗⑦**X02.4** **Hit by object from burning building or structure in controlled fire**

⊗⑦**X02.5** **Jump from burning building or structure in controlled fire**

⊗⑦**X02.8** **Other exposure to controlled fire in building or structure**

X03 **Exposure to controlled fire, not in building or structure**

Includes: exposure to bon fire

exposure to camp-fire

exposure to trash fire

The appropriate 7th character is to be added to each code from category X03

A - initial encounter

D - subsequent encounter

S - sequela

⊗⑦**X03.0** **Exposure to flames in controlled fire, not in building or structure**

⊗⑦**X03.1** **Exposure to smoke in controlled fire, not in building or structure**

⊗⑦**X03.3** **Fall due to controlled fire, not in building or structure**

⊗⑦**X03.4** **Hit by object due to controlled fire, not in building or structure**

⊗⑦**X03.8** **Other exposure to controlled fire, not in building or structure**

X04 **Exposure to ignition of highly flammable material**

Exposure to ignition of gasoline

Exposure to ignition of kerosene

Exposure to ignition of petrol

Excludes2: exposure to ignition or melting of nightwear (X05)

exposure to ignition or melting **of other** clothing and apparel (X06)

The appropriate 7th character is to be added to code X04

A - initial encounter

D - subsequent encounter

S - sequela

⊗⑦**X05** **Exposure to ignition or melting of nightwear**

● New code ▲ Revised code **Excludes1:** Not coded here **Excludes2:** Not included here ⊗ Placeholder required ⑦ 7th digit required

Excludes2: exposure to uncontrolled fire in building or structure (X00.-)

exposure to uncontrolled fire, not in building or structure (X01.-)

exposure to controlled fire in building or structure (X02.-)

exposure to controlled fire, not in building or structure (X03.-)

exposure to ignition of highly flammable materials (X04.-)

The appropriate 7th character is to be added to code X05

A - initial encounter

D - subsequent encounter

S - sequela

X06 **Exposure to ignition or melting of other clothing and apparel**

Excludes2: exposure to uncontrolled fire in building or structure (X00.-)

exposure to uncontrolled fire, not in building or structure (X01.-)
exposure to controlled fire in building or structure (X02.-) exposure to controlled fire, not in building or structure (X03.-) exposure to ignition of highly flammable materials (X04.-)

The appropriate 7th character is to be added to each code from category X06

A - initial encounter

D - subsequent encounter

S - sequela

⊗⑦**X06.0** **Exposure to ignition of plastic jewelry**

⊗⑦**X06.1** **Exposure to melting of plastic jewelry**

⊗⑦**X06.2** **Exposure to ignition of other clothing and apparel**

⊗⑦**X06.3** **Exposure to melting of other clothing and apparel**

X08 **Exposure to other specified smoke, fire and flames**

The appropriate 7th character is to be added to each code from category X08

A - initial encounter

D - subsequent encounter

S - sequela

X08.0 **Exposure to bed fire**

Exposure to mattress fire

⊗⑦**X08.00** **Exposure to bed fire due to unspecified burning material**

⊗⑦**X08.01** **Exposure to bed fire due to burning cigarette**

⊗⑦**X08.09** **Exposure to bed fire due to other burning material**

X08.1 **Exposure to sofa fire**

⊗⑦**X08.10** **Exposure to sofa fire due to unspecified burning material**

⊗⑦**X08.11** **Exposure to sofa fire due to burning cigarette**

⊗⑦**X08.19** **Exposure to sofa fire due to other burning material**

X08.2 **Exposure to other furniture fire**

⊗⑦**X08.20** **Exposure to other furniture fire due to unspecified burning material**

⊗⑦**X08.21** **Exposure to other furniture fire due to burning cigarette**

⊗⑦**X08.29** **Exposure to other furniture fire due to other burning material**

⊗⑦**X08.8** **Exposure to other specified smoke, fire and flames**

CONTACT WITH HEAT AND HOT SUBSTANCES (X10-X19)

Excludes1: exposure to excessive natural heat (X30)

exposure to fire and flames (X00-X09)

X10 **Contact with hot drinks, food, fats and cooking oils**

The appropriate 7th character is to be added to each code from category X10

A - initial encounter

D - subsequent encounter

S - sequela

⊗⑦**X10.0** **Contact with hot drinks**

⊗⑦**X10.1** **Contact with hot food**

⊗⑦**X10.2** **Contact with fats and cooking oils**

X11 **Contact with hot tap-water**

Includes: contact with boiling tap-water

contact with boiling water NOS

Excludes1: contact with water heated on stove (X12)

The appropriate 7th character is to be added to each code from category X11

A - initial encounter

D - subsequent encounter

S - sequela

⊗⑦**X11.0** **Contact with hot water in bath or tub**

Excludes1: contact with running hot water in bath or tub (X11.1)

⊗⑦**X11.1** **Contact with running hot water**

Contact with hot water running out of hose

Contact with hot water running out of tap

⊗⑦**X11.8** **Contact with other hot tap-water**

Contact with hot water in bucket

Contact with hot tap-water NOS

X12 **Contact with other hot fluids**

Contact with water heated on stove

Excludes1: hot (liquid) metals (X18)

The appropriate 7th character is to be added to code X12

A - initial encounter

D - subsequent encounter

S - sequela

X13 **Contact with steam and other hot vapors**

The appropriate 7th character is to be added to each code from category X13

A - initial encounter

D - subsequent encounter

S - sequela

⊗⑦**X13.0** **Inhalation of steam and other hot vapors**

⊗⑦**X13.1** **Other contact with steam and other hot vapors**

X14 **Contact with hot air and other hot gases**

The appropriate 7th character is to be added to each code from category X14

A - initial encounter

D - subsequent encounter

S - sequela

⊗⑦**X14.0** **Inhalation of hot air and gases**

⊗⑦**X14.1** **Other contact with hot air and other hot gases**

X15 **Contact with hot household appliances**

Excludes1: contact with heating appliances (X16)

contact with powered household appliances (W29.-)

exposure to controlled fire in building or structure due to household appliance (X02.8) exposure to household appliances electrical current (W86.0)

Add 4th-7th digits   Nonspecific code   Unspecified code   Manifestation code

The appropriate 7th character is to be added to each code from category X15

A - initial encounter

D - subsequent encounter

S - sequela

⊗⑦**X15.0** **Contact with hot stove (kitchen)**

⊗⑦**X15.1** **Contact with hot toaster**

⊗⑦**X15.2** **Contact with hotplate**

⊗⑦**X15.3** **Contact with hot saucepan or skillet**

⊗⑦**X15.8** **Contact with other hot household appliances**

Contact with cooker

Contact with kettle

Contact with light bulbs

⊗⑦**X16** **Contact with hot heating appliances, radiators and pipes**

Excludes1: contact with powered appliances (W29.-)

exposure to controlled fire in building or structure due to appliance (X02.8)

exposure to industrial appliances electrical current (W86.1)

The appropriate 7th character is to be added to code X16

A - initial encounter

D - subsequent encounter

S - sequela

⊗⑦**X17** **Contact with hot engines, machinery and tools**

Excludes1: contact with hot heating appliances, radiators and pipes (X16)

contact with hot household appliances (X15)

The appropriate 7th character is to be added to code X17

A - initial encounter

D - subsequent encounter

S - sequela

⊗⑦**X18** **Contact with other hot metals**

Contact with liquid metal

The appropriate 7th character is to be added to code X18

A - initial encounter

D - subsequent encounter

S - sequela

⊗⑦**X19** **Contact with other heat and hot substances**

Excludes1: objects that are not normally hot, e.g., an object made hot by a house fire (X00-X09)

The appropriate 7th character is to be added to code X19

A - initial encounter

D - subsequent encounter

S - sequela

EXPOSURE TO FORCES OF NATURE (X30-X39)

⊗⑦**X30** **Exposure to excessive natural heat**

Exposure to excessive heat as the cause of sunstroke

Exposure to heat NOS

Excludes1: excessive heat of man-made origin (W92)

exposure to man-made radiation (W89)

exposure to sunlight (X32)

exposure to tanning bed (W89)

The appropriate 7th character is to be added to code X30

A - initial encounter

D - subsequent encounter

S - sequela

⊗⑦**X31** **Exposure to excessive natural cold**

Excessive cold as the cause of chilblains NOS

Excessive cold as the cause of immersion foot or hand

Exposure to cold NOS

Exposure to weather conditions

Excludes1: cold of man-made origin (W93.-)

contact with or inhalation of dry ice (W93.-)

contact with or inhalation of liquefied gas (W93.-)

The appropriate 7th character is to be added to code X31

A - initial encounter

D - subsequent encounter

S - sequela

⊗⑦**X32** **Exposure to sunlight**

Excludes1: man-made radiation (tanning bed) (W89)

The appropriate 7th character is to be added to code X32

A - initial encounter

D - subsequent encounter

S - sequela

⊗⑦**X34** **Earthquake**

Excludes2: tidal wave (tsunami) due to earthquake (X37.41)

The appropriate 7th character is to be added to code X34

A - initial encounter

D - subsequent encounter

S - sequela

⊗⑦**X35** **Volcanic eruption**

Excludes2: tidal wave (tsunami) due to volcanic eruption (X37.41)

The appropriate 7th character is to be added to code X35

A - initial encounter

D - subsequent encounter

S - sequela

X36 **Avalanche, landslide and other earth movements**

Includes: victim of mudslide of cataclysmic nature

Excludes1: earthquake (X34)

Excludes2: transport accident involving collision with avalanche or landslide not in motion (V01-V99)

The appropriate 7th character is to be added to each code from category X36

A - initial encounter

D - subsequent encounter

S - sequela

⊗⑦**X36.0** **Collapse of dam or man-made structure causing earth movement**

⊗⑦**X36.1** **Avalanche, landslide, or mudslide**

X37 **Cataclysmic storm**

The appropriate 7th character is to be added to each code from category X37

A - initial encounter

D - subsequent encounter

S - sequela

⊗⑦**X37.0** **Hurricane**

Storm surge

Typhoon

⊗⑦**X37.1** **Tornado**

Cyclone

Twister

⊗⑦**X37.2** **Blizzard (snow)(ice)**

⊗⑦**X37.3** **Dust storm**

X37.4 **Tidalwave**

⊗⑦**X37.41** **Tidal wave due to earthquake or volcanic eruption**

Tidal wave NOS

Tsunami

⊗⑦**X37.42** **Tidal wave due to storm**

⊗⑦**X37.43** **Tidal wave due to landslide**

⊗⑦**X37.8** **Other cataclysmic storms**

Cloudburst

Torrential rain

Excludes2: flood (X38)

⊗⑦**X37.9** **Unspecified cataclysmic storm**

Storm NOS

Excludes1: collapse of dam or man-made structure causing earth movement (X39.0)

⊗⑦**X38** **Flood**

Flood arising from remote storm

Flood of cataclysmic nature arising from melting snow

Flood resulting directly from storm

Excludes1: collapse of dam or man-made structure causing earth movement (X39.0)

tidal wave NOS (X37.41)

tidal wave caused by storm (X37.2)

The appropriate 7th character is to be added to code X38

A - initial encounter

D - subsequent encounter

S - sequela

X39 **Exposure to other forces of nature**

The appropriate 7th character is to be added to each code from category X39

A - initial encounter

D - subsequent encounter

S - sequela

⊗⑦**X39.0** **Exposure to natural radiation**

Excludes1: contact with and (suspected) exposure to radon and other naturally occuring radiation (Z77.123)

exposure to man-made radiation (W88-W90)

exposure to sunlight (X32)

⊗⑦**X39.01** **Exposure to radon**

⊗⑦**X39.08** **Exposure to other natural radiation**

⊗⑦**X39.8** **Other exposure to forces of nature**

OVEREXERTION AND STRENUOUS OR REPETITIVE MOVEMENTS (X50)

X50 **Overexertion and strenuous or repetitive movements**

The appropriate 7th character is to be added to each code from category X50

A - initial encounter

D - subsequent encounter

S - sequela

•⊗⑦**X50.0** **Overexertion from strenuous movement or load**

Lifting heavy objects

Lifting weights

•⊗⑦**X50.1** **Overexertion from prolonged static or awkward postures**

Prolonged bending

Prolonged kneeling

Prolonged reaching

Prolonged sitting

Prolonged standing

Prolonged twisting

Static bending

Static kneeling

Static reaching

Static sitting

Static standing

Static twisting

•⊗⑦**X50.3** **Overexertion from repetitive movements**

Use of hand as hammer

Excludes2: Overuse from prolonged static or awkward postures (X50.1)

•⊗⑦**X50.9** **Other and unspecified overexertion or strenuous movements or postures**

Contact pressure

Contact stress

ACCIDENTAL EXPOSURE TO OTHER SPECIFIED FACTORS (X52-X58)

⊗⑦**X52** **Prolonged stay in weightless environment**

Weightlessness in spacecraft (simulator)

The appropriate 7th character is to be added to code X52

A - initial encounter

D - subsequent encounter

S - sequela

⊗⑦**X58** **Exposure to other specified factors**

Accident NOS

Exposure NOS

The appropriate 7th character is to be added to code X58

A - initial encounter

D - subsequent encounter

S - sequela

INTENTIONAL SELF-HARM (X71-X83)

Purposely self-inflicted injury Suicide (attempted)

X71 **Intentional self-harm by drowning and submersion**

The appropriate 7th character is to be added to each code from category X71

A - initial encounter

D - subsequent encounter

S - sequela

⊗⑦**X71.0** **Intentional self-harm by drowning and submersion while in bathtub**

⊗⑦**X71.1** **Intentional self-harm by drowning and submersion while in swimming pool**

⊗⑦**X71.2** **Intentional self-harm by drowning and submersion after jump into swimming pool**

⊗⑦**X71.3** **Intentional self-harm by drowning and submersion in natural water**

Add 4th-7th digits	Nonspecific code	Unspecified code	Manifestation code

⊗⑦**X71.8** **Other intentional self-harm by drowning and submersion**

⊗⑦**X71.9** **Intentional self-harm by drowning and submersion, unspecified**

⊗⑦**X72** **Intentional self-harm by handgun discharge**

Intentional self-harm by gun for single hand use

Intentional self-harm by pistol

Intentional self-harm by revolver

Excludes1: Very pistol (X74.8)

The appropriate 7th character is to be added to code X72

A - initial encounter

D - subsequent encounter

S - sequela

X73 **Intentional self-harm by rifle, shotgun and larger firearm discharge**

Excludes1: airgun (X74.01)

The appropriate 7th character is to be added to each code from category X73

A - initial encounter

D - subsequent encounter

S - sequela

⊗⑦**X73.0** **Intentional self-harm by shotgun discharge**

⊗⑦**X73.1** **Intentional self-harm by hunting rifle discharge**

⊗⑦**X73.2** **Intentional self-harm by machine gun discharge**

⊗⑦**X73.8** **Intentional self-harm by other larger firearm discharge**

⊗⑦**X73.9** **Intentional self-harm by unspecified larger firearm discharge**

X74 **Intentional self-harm by other and unspecified firearm and gun discharge**

The appropriate 7th character is to be added to each code from category X74

A - initial encounter

D - subsequent encounter

S - sequela

X74.0 **Intentional self-harm by gas, air or spring-operated guns**

⊗⑦**X74.01** **Intentional self-harm by airgun**

Intentional self-harm by BB gun discharge

Intentional self-harm by pellet gun discharge

⊗⑦**X74.02** **Intentional self-harm by paintball gun**

⊗⑦**X74.09** **Intentional self-harm by other gas, air or spring-operated gun**

⊗⑦**X74.8** **Intentional self-harm by other firearm discharge**

Intentional self-harm by Very pistol [flare] discharge

⊗⑦**X74.9** **Intentional self-harm by unspecified firearm discharge**

⊗⑦**X75** **Intentional self-harm by explosive material**

The appropriate 7th character is to be added to code X75

A - initial encounter

D - subsequent encounter

S - sequela

⊗⑦**X76** **Intentional self-harm by smoke, fire and flames**

The appropriate 7th character is to be added to code X76

A - initial encounter

D - subsequent encounter

S - sequela

X77 **Intentional self-harm by steam, hot vapors and hot objects**

The appropriate 7th character is to be added to each code from category X77

A - initial encounter

D - subsequent encounter

S - sequela

⊗⑦**X77.0** **Intentional self-harm by steam or hot vapors**

⊗⑦**X77.1** **Intentional self-harm by hot tap water**

⊗⑦**X77.2** **Intentional self-harm by other hot fluids**

⊗⑦**X77.3** **Intentional self-harm by hot household appliances**

⊗⑦**X77.8** **Intentional self-harm by other hot objects**

⊗⑦**X77.9** **Intentional self-harm by unspecified hot objects**

X78 **Intentional self-harm by sharp object**

The appropriate 7th character is to be added to each code from category X78

A - initial encounter

D - subsequent encounter

S - sequela

⊗⑦**X78.0** **Intentional self-harm by sharp glass**

⊗⑦**X78.1** **Intentional self-harm by knife**

⊗⑦**X78.2** **Intentional self-harm by sword or dagger**

⊗⑦**X78.8** **Intentional self-harm by other sharp object**

⊗⑦**X78.9** **Intentional self-harm by unspecified sharp object**

⊗⑦**X79** **Intentional self-harm by blunt object**

The appropriate 7th character is to be added to code X79

A - initial encounter

D - subsequent encounter

S - sequela

⊗⑦**X80** **Intentional self-harm by jumping from a high place**

Intentional fall from one level to another

The appropriate 7th character is to be added to code X80

A - initial encounter

D - subsequent encounter

S - sequela

X81 **Intentional self-harm by jumping or lying in front of moving object**

The appropriate 7th character is to be added to each code from category X81

A - initial encounter

D - subsequent encounter

S - sequela

⊗⑦**X81.0** **Intentional self-harm by jumping or lying in front of motor vehicle**

⊗⑦**X81.1** **Intentional self-harm by jumping or lying in front of (subway) train**

⊗⑦**X81.8** **Intentional self-harm by jumping or lying in front of other moving object**

X82 **Intentional self-harm by crashing of motor vehicle**

The appropriate 7th character is to be added to each code from category X82

A - initial encounter

D - subsequent encounter

S - sequela

⊗⑦**X82.0** **Intentional collision of motor vehicle with other motor vehicle**

⊗⑦**X82.1** **Intentional collision of motor vehicle with train**

⊗⑦**X82.2** **Intentional collision of motor vehicle with tree**

⊗⑦**X82.8** **Other intentional self-harm by crashing of motor vehicle**

X83 **Intentional self-harm by other specified means**

Excludes1: intentional self-harm by poisoning or contact with toxic substance- See Table of Drugs and Chemicals

The appropriate 7th character is to be added to each code from category X83

A - initial encounter

D - subsequent encounter

S - sequela

⊗⑦**X83.0** **Intentional self-harm by crashing of aircraft**

⊗⑦**X83.1** **Intentional self-harm by electrocution**

⊗⑦**X83.2** **Intentional self-harm by exposure to extremes of cold**

⊗⑦**X83.8** **Intentional self-harm by other specified means**

ASSAULT (X92-Y09)

Includes: homicide

injuries inflicted by another person with intent to injure or kill, by any means

Excludes1: injuries due to legal intervention (Y35.-)

injuries due to operations of war (Y36.-)

injuries due to terrorism (Y38.-)

X92 **Assault by drowning and submersion**

The appropriate 7th character is to be added to each code from category X92

A - initial encounter

D - subsequent encounter

S - sequela

⊗⑦**X92.0** **Assault by drowning and submersion while in bathtub**

⊗⑦**X92.1** **Assault by drowning and submersion while in swimming pool**

⊗⑦**X92.2** **Assault by drowning and submersion after push into swimming pool**

⊗⑦**X92.3** **Assault by drowning and submersion in natural water**

⊗⑦**X92.8** **Other assault by drowning and submersion**

⊗⑦**X92.9** **Assault by drowning and submersion, unspecified**

⊗⑦**X93** **Assault by handgun discharge**

Assault by discharge of gun for single hand use

Assault by discharge of pistol

Assault by discharge of revolver

Excludes1: Very pistol (X95.8)

The appropriate 7th character is to be added to code X93

A - initial encounter

D - subsequent encounter

S - sequela

X94 **Assault by rifle, shotgun and larger firearm discharge**

Excludes1: airgun (X95.01)

The appropriate 7th character is to be added to each code from category X94

A - initial encounter

D - subsequent encounter

S - sequela

⊗⑦**X94.0** **Assault by shotgun**

⊗⑦**X94.1** **Assault by hunting rifle**

⊗⑦**X94.2** **Assault by machine gun**

⊗⑦**X94.8** **Assault by other larger firearm discharge**

⊗⑦**X94.9** **Assault by unspecified larger firearm discharge**

X95 **Assault by other and unspecified firearm and gun discharge**

The appropriate 7th character is to be added to each code from category X95

A - initial encounter

D - subsequent encounter

S - sequela

X95.0 **Assault by gas, air or spring-operated guns**

⊗⑦**X95.01** **Assault by airgun discharge**

Assault by BB gun discharge

Assault by pellet gun discharge

⊗⑦**X95.02** **Assault by paintball gun discharge**

⊗⑦**X95.09** **Assault by other gas, air or spring-operated gun**

⊗⑦**X95.8** **Assault by other firearm discharge**

Assault by very pistol [flare] discharge

⊗⑦**X95.9** **Assault by unspecified firearm discharge**

X96 **Assault by explosive material**

Excludes1: incendiary device (X97)

terrorism involving explosive material (Y38.2-)

The appropriate 7th character is to be added to each code from category X96

A - initial encounter

D - subsequent encounter

S - sequela

⊗⑦**X96.0** **Assault by antipersonnel bomb**

Excludes1: antipersonnel bomb use in military or war (Y36.2-)

⊗⑦**X96.1** **Assault by gasoline bomb**

⊗⑦**X96.2** **Assault by letter bomb**

⊗⑦**X96.3** **Assault by fertilizer bomb**

⊗⑦**X96.4** **Assault by pipe bomb**

⊗⑦**X96.8** **Assault by other specified explosive**

⊗⑦**X96.9** **Assault by unspecified explosive**

⊗⑦**X97** **Assault by smoke, fire and flames**

Assault by arson

Assault by cigarettes

Assault by incendiary device

The appropriate 7th character is to be added to code X97

A - initial encounter

D - subsequent encounter

S - sequela

X98 **Assault by steam, hot vapors and hot objects**

The appropriate 7th character is to be added to each code from category X98

A - initial encounter

D - subsequent encounter

S - sequela

⊗⑦**X98.0** **Assault by steam or hot vapors**

⊗⑦**X98.1** **Assault by hot tap water**

⊗⑦**X98.2** **Assault by hot fluids**

⊗⑦**X98.3** **Assault by hot household appliances**

⊗⑦**X98.8** **Assault by other hot objects**

⊗⑦**X98.9** **Assault by unspecified hot objects**

X99 **Assault by sharp object**

Excludes1: assault by strike by sports equipment (Y08.0-)

The appropriate 7th character is to be added to each code from category X99

A - initial encounter

D - subsequent encounter

S - sequela

⊗⑦**X99.0 Assault by sharp glass**

⊗⑦**X99.1 Assault by knife**

⊗⑦**X99.2 Assault by sword or dagger**

⊗⑦**X99.8 Assault by other sharp object**

⊗⑦**X99.9 Assault by unspecified sharp object**

Assault by stabbing NOS

⊗⑦**Y00 Assault by blunt object**

Excludes1: assault by strike by sports equipment (Y08.0-)

The appropriate 7th character is to be added to code Y00

A - initial encounter

D - subsequent encounter

S - sequela

⊗⑦**Y01 Assault by pushing from high place**

The appropriate 7th character is to be added to code Y01

A - initial encounter

D - subsequent encounter

S - sequela

Y02 Assault by pushing or placing victim in front of moving object

The appropriate 7th character is to be added to each code from category Y02

A - initial encounter

D - subsequent encounter

S - sequela

⊗⑦**Y02.0 Assault by pushing or placing victim in front of motor vehicle**

⊗⑦**Y02.1 Assault by pushing or placing victim in front of (subway) train**

⊗⑦**Y02.8 Assault by pushing or placing victim in front of other moving object**

Y03 Assault by crashing of motor vehicle

The appropriate 7th character is to be added to each code from category Y03

A - initial encounter

D - subsequent encounter

S - sequela

⊗⑦**Y03.0 Assault by being hit or run over by motor vehicle**

⊗⑦**Y03.8 Other assault by crashing of motor vehicle**

Y04 Assault by bodily force

Excludes1: assault by:

submersion (X92.-)

use of weapon (X93-X95, X99, Y00)

The appropriate 7th character is to be added to each code from category Y04

A - initial encounter

D - subsequent encounter

S - sequela

⊗⑦**Y04.0 Assault by unarmed brawl or fight**

⊗⑦**Y04.1 Assault by human bite**

⊗⑦**Y04.2 Assault by strike against or bumped into by another person**

⊗⑦**Y04.8 Assault by other bodily force**

Assault by bodily force NOS

Y07 Perpetrator of assault, maltreatment and neglect

Note: Codes from this category are for use only in cases of confirmed abuse (T74.-)

Selection of the correct perpetrator code is based on the relationship between the perpetrator and the victim

Includes: perpetrator of abandonment

perpetrator of emotional neglect perpetrator of mental cruelty

perpetrator of physical abuse perpetrator of physical neglect

perpetrator of sexual abuse perpetrator of torture

Y07.0 Spouse or partner, perpetrator of maltreatment and neglect

Spouse or partner, perpetrator of maltreatment and neglect against spouse or partner

Y07.01 Husband, perpetrator of maltreatment and neglect

Y07.02 Wife, perpetrator of maltreatment and neglect

Y07.03 Male partner, perpetrator of maltreatment and neglect

Y07.04 Female partner, perpetrator of maltreatment and neglect

Y07.1 Parent (adoptive) (biological), perpetrator of maltreatment and neglect

Y07.11 Biological father, perpetrator of maltreatment and neglect

Y07.12 Biological mother, perpetrator of maltreatment and neglect

Y07.13 Adoptive father, perpetrator of maltreatment and neglect

Y07.14 Adoptive mother, perpetrator of maltreatment and neglect

Y07.4 Other family member, perpetrator of maltreatment and neglect

Y07.41 Sibling, perpetrator of maltreatment and neglect

Excludes1: stepsibling, perpetrator of maltreatment and neglect (Y07.435, Y07.436)

Y07.410 Brother, perpetrator of maltreatment and neglect

Y07.411 Sister, perpetrator of maltreatment and neglect

Y07.42 Foster parent, perpetrator of maltreatment and neglect

Y07.420 Foster father, perpetrator of maltreatment and neglect

Y07.421 Foster mother, perpetrator of maltreatment and neglect

Y07.43 Stepparent or stepsibling, perpetrator of maltreatment and neglect

Y07.430 Stepfather, perpetrator of maltreatment and neglect

Y07.432 Male friend of parent (co-residing in household), perpetrator of maltreatment and neglect

Y07.433 Stepmother, perpetrator of maltreatment and neglect

Y07.434 Female friend of parent (co-residing in household), perpetrator of maltreatment and neglect

Y07.435 Stepbrother, perpetrator or maltreatment and neglect

Y07.436 Stepsister, perpetrator of maltreatment and neglect

Y07.49 Other family member, perpetrator of maltreatment and neglect

Y07.490 Male cousin, perpetrator of maltreatment and neglect

Y07.491 Female cousin, perpetrator of maltreatment and neglect

Y07.499 Other family member, perpetrator of maltreatment and neglect

Y07.5 Non-family member, perpetrator of maltreatment and neglect

Y07.50 Unspecified non-family member, perpetrator of maltreatment and neglect

Y07.51 Daycare provider, perpetrator of maltreatment and neglect

Y07.510 At-home childcare provider, perpetrator of maltreatment and neglect

Y07.511 Daycare center childcare provider, perpetrator of maltreatment and neglect

Y07.512 At-home adultcare provider, perpetrator of maltreatment and neglect

Y07.513 Adultcare center provider, perpetrator of maltreatment and neglect

Y07.519 Unspecified daycare provider, perpetrator of maltreatment and neglect

Y07.52 Healthcare provider, perpetrator of maltreatment and neglect

Y07.521 Mental health provider, perpetrator of maltreatment and neglect

Y07.528 Other therapist or healthcare provider, perpetrator of maltreatment and neglect

Nurse perpetrator of maltreatment and neglect

Occupational therapist perpetrator of maltreatment and neglect

Physical therapist perpetrator of maltreatment and neglect

Speech therapist perpetrator of maltreatment and neglect

Y07.529 Unspecified healthcare provider, perpetrator of maltreatment and neglect

Y07.53 Teacher or instructor, perpetrator of maltreatment and neglect

Coach, perpetrator of maltreatment and neglect

Y07.59 Other non-family member, perpetrator of maltreatment and neglect

Y07.9 Unspecified perpetrator of maltreatment and neglect

Y08 Assault by other specified means

The appropriate 7th character is to be added to each code from category Y08

A - initial encounter

D - subsequent encounter

S - sequela

Y08.0 Assault by strike by sport equipment

⊗⑦**Y08.01** Assault by strike by hockey stick

⊗⑦**Y08.02** Assault by strike by baseball bat

⊗⑦**Y08.09** Assault by strike by other specified type of sport equipment

Y08.8 Assault by other specified means

⊗⑦**Y08.81** Assault by crashing of aircraft

⊗⑦**Y08.89** Assault by other specified means

Y09 Assault by unspecified means

Assassination (attempted) NOS

Homicide (attempted) NOS

Manslaughter (attempted) NOS

Murder (attempted) NOS

EVENT OF UNDETERMINED INTENT (Y21-Y33)

Undetermined intent is only for use when there is specific documentation in the record that the intent of the injury cannot be determined. If no such documentation is present, code to accidental (unintentional)

Y21 Drowning and submersion, undetermined intent

The appropriate 7th character is to be added to each code from category Y21

A - initial encounter

D - subsequent encounter

S - sequela

⊗⑦**Y21.0** Drowning and submersion while in bathtub, undetermined intent

⊗⑦**Y21.1** Drowning and submersion after fall into bathtub, undetermined intent

⊗⑦**Y21.2** Drowning and submersion while in swimming pool, undetermined intent

⊗⑦**Y21.3** Drowning and submersion after fall into swimming pool, undetermined intent

⊗⑦**Y21.4** Drowning and submersion in natural water, undetermined intent

⊗⑦**Y21.8** Other drowning and submersion, undetermined intent

⊗⑦**Y21.9** Unspecified drowning and submersion, undetermined intent

⊗⑦**Y22** Handgun discharge, undetermined intent

Discharge of gun for single hand use, undetermined intent

Discharge of pistol, undetermined intent

Discharge of revolver, undetermined intent

Excludes2: very pistol (Y24.8)

The appropriate 7th character is to be added to code Y22

A - initial encounter

D - subsequent encounter

S - sequela

Y23 Rifle, shotgun and larger firearm discharge, undetermined intent

Excludes2: airgun (Y24.0)

The appropriate 7th character is to be added to each code from category Y23

A - initial encounter

Add 4th-7th digits   Nonspecific code   Unspecified code   Manifestation code

D - subsequent encounter

S - sequela

⊗⑦**Y23.0**   **Shotgun discharge, undetermined intent**

⊗⑦**Y23.1**   **Hunting rifle discharge, undetermined intent**

⊗⑦**Y23.2**   **Military firearm discharge, undetermined intent**

⊗⑦**Y23.3**   **Machine gun discharge, undetermined intent**

⊗⑦**Y23.8**   **Other larger firearm discharge, undetermined intent**

⊗⑦**Y23.9**   **Unspecified larger firearm discharge, undetermined intent**

Y24   **Other and unspecified firearm discharge, undetermined intent**

The appropriate 7th character is to be added to each code from category Y24

A - initial encounter

D - subsequent encounter

S - sequela

⊗⑦**Y24.0**   **Airgun discharge, undetermined intent**

BB gun discharge, undetermined intent

Pellet gun discharge, undetermined intent

⊗⑦**Y24.8**   **Other firearm discharge, undetermined intent**

Paintball gun discharge, undetermined intent

Very pistol [flare] discharge, undetermined intent

⊗⑦**Y24.9**   **Unspecified firearm discharge, undetermined intent**

⊗⑦**Y25**   **Contact with explosive material, undetermined intent**

The appropriate 7th character is to be added to code Y25

A - initial encounter

D - subsequent encounter

S - sequela

⊗⑦**Y26**   **Exposure to smoke, fire and flames, undetermined intent**

The appropriate 7th character is to be added to code Y26

A - initial encounter

D - subsequent encounter

S - sequela

Y27   **Contact with steam, hot vapors and hot objects, undetermined intent**

The appropriate 7th character is to be added to each code from category Y27

A - initial encounter

D - subsequent encounter

S - sequela

⊗⑦**Y27.0**   **Contact with steam and hot vapors, undetermined intent**

⊗⑦**Y27.1**   **Contact with hot tap water, undetermined intent**

⊗⑦**Y27.2**   **Contact with hot fluids, undetermined intent**

⊗⑦**Y27.3**   **Contact with hot household appliance, undetermined intent**

⊗⑦**Y27.8**   **Contact with other hot objects, undetermined intent**

⊗⑦**Y27.9**   **Contact with unspecified hot objects, undetermined intent**

Y28   **Contact with sharp object, undetermined intent**

The appropriate 7th character is to be added to each code from category Y28

A - initial encounter

D - subsequent encounter

S - sequela

⊗⑦**Y28.0**   **Contact with sharp glass, undetermined intent**

⊗⑦**Y28.1**   **Contact with knife, undetermined intent**

⊗⑦**Y28.2**   **Contact with sword or dagger, undetermined intent**

⊗⑦**Y28.8**   **Contact with other sharp object, undetermined intent**

⊗⑦**Y28.9**   **Contact with unspecified sharp object, undetermined intent**

⊗⑦**Y29**   **Contact with blunt object, undetermined intent**

The appropriate 7th character is to be added to code Y29

A - initial encounter

D - subsequent encounter

S - sequela

⊗⑦**Y30**   **Falling, jumping or pushed from a high place, undetermined intent**

Victim falling from one level to another, undetermined intent

The appropriate 7th character is to be added to code Y30

A - initial encounter

D - subsequent encounter

S - sequela

⊗⑦**Y31**   **Falling, lying or running before or into moving object, undetermined intent**

The appropriate 7th character is to be added to code Y31

A - initial encounter

D - subsequent encounter

S - sequela

⊗⑦**Y32**   **Crashing of motor vehicle, undetermined intent**

The appropriate 7th character is to be added to code Y32

A - initial encounter

D - subsequent encounter

S - sequela

⊗⑦**Y33**   **Other specified events, undetermined intent**

The appropriate 7th character is to be added to code Y33

A - initial encounter

D - subsequent encounter

S - sequela

LEGAL INTERVENTION, OPERATIONS OF WAR, MILITARY OPERATIONS, AND TERRORISM (Y35-Y38)

Y35   **Legal intervention**

Includes: any injury sustained as a result of an encounter with any law enforcement official, serving in any capacity at the time of the encounter, whether on-duty or off-duty.

Includes: injury to law enforcement official, suspect and bystander

The appropriate 7th character is to be added to each code from category Y35

A - initial encounter

D - subsequent encounter

S - sequela

Y35.0   **Legal intervention involving firearm discharge**

Y35.00   **Legal intervention involving unspecified firearm discharge**

Legal intervention involving gunshot wound

Legal intervention involving shot NOS

⑦**Y35.001**   **Legal intervention involving unspecified firearm discharge, law enforcement official injured**

⑦**Y35.002**   **Legal intervention involving unspecified firearm discharge, bystander injured**

● New code   ▲ Revised code   **Excludes1:** Not coded here   **Excludes2:** Not included here   ⊗ Placeholder required   ⑦ 7th digit required

⑦Y35.003 **Legal intervention involving unspecified firearm discharge, suspect injured**

Y35.01 **Legal intervention involving injury by machine gun**

⑦Y35.011 **Legal intervention involving injury by machine gun, law enforcement official injured**

⑦Y35.012 **Legal intervention involving injury by machine gun, bystander injured**

⑦Y35.013 **Legal intervention involving injury by machine gun, suspect injured**

Y35.02 **Legal intervention involving injury by handgun**

⑦Y35.021 **Legal intervention involving injury by handgun, law enforcement official injured**

⑦Y35.022 **Legal intervention involving injury by handgun, bystander injured**

⑦Y35.023 **Legal intervention involving injury by handgun, suspect injured**

Y35.03 **Legal intervention involving injury by rifle pellet**

⑦Y35.031 **Legal intervention involving injury by rifle pellet, law enforcement official injured**

⑦Y35.032 **Legal intervention involving injury by rifle pellet, bystander injured**

⑦Y35.033 **Legal intervention involving injury by rifle pellet, suspect injured**

Y35.04 **Legal intervention involving injury by rubber bullet**

⑦Y35.041 **Legal intervention involving injury by rubber bullet, law enforcement official injured**

⑦Y35.042 **Legal intervention involving injury by rubber bullet, bystander injured**

⑦Y35.043 **Legal intervention involving injury by rubber bullet, suspect injured**

Y35.09 **Legal intervention involving other firearm discharge**

⑦Y35.091 **Legal intervention involving other firearm discharge, law enforcement official injured**

⑦Y35.092 **Legal intervention involving other firearm discharge, bystander injured**

⑦Y35.093 **Legal intervention involving other firearm discharge, suspect injured**

Y35.1 **Legal intervention involving explosives**

Y35.10 **Legal intervention involving unspecified explosives**

⑦Y35.101 **Legal intervention involving unspecified explosives, law enforcement official injured**

⑦Y35.102 **Legal intervention involving unspecified explosives, bystander injured**

⑦Y35.103 **Legal intervention involving unspecified explosives, suspect injured**

Y35.11 **Legal intervention involving injury by dynamite**

⑦Y35.111 **Legal intervention involving injury by dynamite, law enforcement official injured**

⑦Y35.112 **Legal intervention involving injury by dynamite, bystander injured**

⑦Y35.113 **Legal intervention involving injury by dynamite, suspect injured**

Y35.12 **Legal intervention involving injury by explosive shell**

⑦Y35.121 **Legal intervention involving injury by explosive shell, law enforcement official injured**

⑦Y35.122 **Legal intervention involving injury by explosive shell, bystander injured**

⑦Y35.123 **Legal intervention involving injury by explosive shell, suspect injured**

Y35.19 **Legal intervention involving other explosives**

Legal intervention involving injury by grenade
Legal intervention involving injury by mortar bomb

⑦Y35.191 **Legal intervention involving other explosives, law enforcement official injured**

⑦Y35.192 **Legal intervention involving other explosives, bystander injured**

⑦Y35.193 **Legal intervention involving other explosives, suspect injured**

Y35.2 **Legal intervention involving gas**

Legal intervention involving asphyxiation by gas
Legal intervention involving poisoning by gas

Y35.20 **Legal intervention involving unspecified gas**

⑦Y35.201 **Legal intervention involving unspecified gas, law enforcement official injured**

⑦Y35.202 **Legal intervention involving unspecified gas, bystander injured**

⑦Y35.203 **Legal intervention involving unspecified gas, suspect injured**

Y35.21 **Legal intervention involving injury by tear gas**

⑦Y35.211 **Legal intervention involving injury by tear gas, law enforcement official injured**

⑦Y35.212 **Legal intervention involving injury by tear gas, bystander injured**

⑦Y35.213 **Legal intervention involving injury by tear gas, suspect injured**

Y35.29 **Legal intervention involving other gas**

⑦Y35.291 **Legal intervention involving other gas, law enforcement official injured**

⑦Y35.292 **Legal intervention involving other gas, bystander injured**

⑦Y35.293 **Legal intervention involving other gas, suspect injured**

Y35.3 **Legal intervention involving blunt objects**

Legal intervention involving being hit or struck by blunt object

Y35.30 **Legal intervention involving unspecified blunt objects**

---

⑦**Y35.301** Legal intervention involving unspecified blunt objects, law enforcement official injured

⑦**Y35.302** Legal intervention involving unspecified blunt objects, bystander injured

⑦**Y35.303** Legal intervention involving unspecified blunt objects, suspect injured

Y35.31 Legal intervention involving baton

⑦**Y35.311** Legal intervention involving baton, law enforcement official injured

⑦**Y35.312** Legal intervention involving baton, bystander injured

⑦**Y35.313** Legal intervention involving baton, suspect injured

Y35.39 Legal intervention involving other blunt objects

⑦**Y35.391** Legal intervention involving other blunt objects, law enforcement official injured

⑦**Y35.392** Legal intervention involving other blunt objects, bystander injured

⑦**Y35.393** Legal intervention involving other blunt objects, suspect injured

Y35.4 Legal intervention involving sharp objects

Legal intervention involving being cut by sharp objects

Legal intervention involving being stabbed by sharp objects

Y35.40 Legal intervention involving unspecified sharp objects

⑦**Y35.401** Legal intervention involving unspecified sharp objects, law enforcement official injured

⑦**Y35.402** Legal intervention involving unspecified sharp objects, bystander injured

⑦**Y35.403** Legal intervention involving unspecified sharp objects, suspect injured

Y35.41 Legal intervention involving bayonet

⑦**Y35.411** Legal intervention involving bayonet, law enforcement official injured

⑦**Y35.412** Legal intervention involving bayonet, bystander injured

⑦**Y35.413** Legal intervention involving bayonet, suspect injured

Y35.49 Legal intervention involving other sharp objects

⑦**Y35.491** Legal intervention involving other sharp objects, law enforcement official injured

⑦**Y35.492** Legal intervention involving other sharp objects, bystander injured

⑦**Y35.493** Legal intervention involving other sharp objects, suspect injured

Y35.8 Legal intervention involving other specified means

Y35.81 Legal intervention involving manhandling

⑦**Y35.811** Legal intervention involving manhandling, law enforcement official injured

⑦**Y35.812** Legal intervention involving manhandling, bystander injured

⑦**Y35.813** Legal intervention involving manhandling, suspect injured

Y35.89 Legal intervention involving other specified means

⑦**Y35.891** Legal intervention involving other specified means, law enforcement official injured

⑦**Y35.892** Legal intervention involving other specified means, bystander injured

⑦**Y35.893** Legal intervention involving other specified means, suspect injured

Y35.9 Legal intervention, means unspecified

⊗⑦**Y35.91** Legal intervention, means unspecified, law enforcement official injured

⊗⑦**Y35.92** Legal intervention, means unspecified, bystander injured

⊗⑦**Y35.93** Legal intervention, means unspecified, suspect injured

Y36 **Operations of war**

Includes: injuries to military personnel and civilians caused by war, civil insurrection, and peacekeeping missions

Excludes1: injury to military personnel occurring during peacetime military operations (Y37.-)

military vehicles involved in transport accidents with non-military vehicle during peacetime (V09.01, V09.21, V19.81, V29.81, V39.81, V49.81, V59.81, V69.81, V79.81)

The appropriate 7th character is to be added to each code from category Y36

A - initial encounter

D - subsequent encounter

S - sequela

Y36.0 War operations involving explosion of marine weapons

Y36.00 War operations involving explosion of unspecified marine weapon

War operations involving underwater blast NOS

⑦**Y36.000** War operations involving explosion of unspecified marine weapon, military personnel

⑦**Y36.001** War operations involving explosion of unspecified marine weapon, civilian

Y36.01 War operations involving explosion of depth-charge

⑦**Y36.010** War operations involving explosion of depth-charge, military personnel

⑦**Y36.011** War operations involving explosion of depth-charge, civilian

Y36.02 War operations involving explosion of marine mine

War operations involving explosion of marine mine, at sea or in harbor

⑦**Y36.020** War operations involving explosion of marine mine, military personnel

⑦**Y36.021** War operations involving explosion of marine mine, civilian

Y36.03 War operations involving explosion of sea-based artillery shell

⑦**Y36.030** War operations involving explosion of sea-based artillery shell, military personnel

⑦**Y36.031** War operations involving explosion of sea-based artillery shell, civilian

Y36.04 War operations involving explosion of torpedo

⑦**Y36.040** War operations involving explosion of torpedo, military personnel

⑦**Y36.041** War operations involving explosion of torpedo, civilian

Y36.05 War operations involving accidental detonation of onboard marine weapons

⑦**Y36.050** War operations involving accidental detonation of onboard marine weapons, military personnel

⑦**Y36.051** War operations involving accidental detonation of onboard marine weapons, civilian

Y36.09 War operations involving explosion of other marine weapons

⑦**Y36.090** War operations involving explosion of other marine weapons, military personnel

⑦**Y36.091** War operations involving explosion of other marine weapons, civilian

Y36.1 War operations involving destruction of aircraft

Y36.10 War operations involving unspecified destruction of aircraft

⑦**Y36.100** War operations involving unspecified destruction of aircraft, military personnel

⑦**Y36.101** War operations involving unspecified destruction of aircraft, civilian

Y36.11 War operations involving destruction of aircraft due to enemy fire or explosives

War operations involving destruction of aircraft due to air to air missile

War operations involving destruction of aircraft due to explosive placed on aircraft

War operations involving destruction of aircraft due to rocket propelled grenade [RPG]

War operations involving destruction of aircraft due to small arms fire

War operations involving destruction of aircraft due to surface to air missile

⑦**Y36.110** War operations involving destruction of aircraft due to enemy fire or explosives, military personnel

⑦**Y36.111** War operations involving destruction of aircraft due to enemy fire or explosives, civilian

Y36.12 War operations involving destruction of aircraft due to collision with other aircraft

⑦**Y36.120** War operations involving destruction of aircraft due to collision with other aircraft, military personnel

⑦**Y36.121** War operations involving destruction of aircraft due to collision with other aircraft, civilian

Y36.13 War operations involving destruction of aircraft due to onboard fire

⑦**Y36.130** War operations involving destruction of aircraft due to onboard fire, military personnel

⑦**Y36.131** War operations involving destruction of aircraft due to onboard fire, civilian

Y36.14 War operations involving destruction of aircraft due to accidental detonation of onboard munitions and explosives

⑦**Y36.140** War operations involving destruction of aircraft due to accidental detonation of onboard munitions and explosives, military personnel

⑦**Y36.141** War operations involving destruction of aircraft due to accidental detonation of onboard munitions and explosives, civilian

Y36.19 War operations involving other destruction of aircraft

⑦**Y36.190** War operations involving other destruction of aircraft, military personnel

⑦**Y36.191** War operations involving other destruction of aircraft, civilian

Y36.2 War operations involving other explosions and fragments

Excludes1: war operations involving explosion of aircraft (Y36.1-)

war operations involving explosion of marine weapons (Y36.0-)

war operations involving explosion of nuclear weapons (Y36.5-)

war operations involving explosion occurring after cessation of hostilities (Y36.8-)

Y36.20 War operations involving unspecified explosion and fragments

War operations involving air blast NOS

War operations involving blast NOS

War operations involving blast fragments NOS

War operations involving blast wave NOS

War operations involving blast wind NOS

War operations involving explosion NOS

War operations involving explosion of bomb NOS

⑦**Y36.200** War operations involving unspecified explosion and fragments, military personnel

⑦**Y36.201** War operations involving unspecified explosion and fragments, civilian

Y36.21 War operations involving explosion of aerial bomb

⑦**Y36.210** War operations involving explosion of aerial bomb, military personnel

⑦**Y36.211** War operations involving explosion of aerial bomb, civilian

Y36.22 War operations involving explosion of guided missile

⑦Y36.220   **War operations involving explosion of guided missile, military personnel**

⑦Y36.221   **War operations involving explosion of guided missile, civilian**

Y36.23   **War operations involving explosion of improvised explosive device [IED]**

War operations involving explosion of person-borne improvised explosive device [IED]

War operations involving explosion of vehicle-borne improvised explosive device [IED]

War operations involving explosion of roadside improvised explosive device [IED]

⑦Y36.230   **War operations involving explosion of improvised explosive device [IED], military personnel**

⑦Y36.231   **War operations involving explosion of improvised explosive device [IED], civilian**

Y36.24   **War operations involving explosion due to accidental detonation and discharge of own munitions or munitions launch device**

⑦Y36.240   **War operations involving explosion due to accidental detonation and discharge of own munitions or munitions launch device, military personnel**

⑦Y36.241   **War operations involving explosion due to accidental detonation and discharge of own munitions or munitions launch device, civilian**

Y36.25   **War operations involving fragments from munitions**

⑦Y36.250   **War operations involving fragments from munitions, military personnel**

⑦Y36.251   **War operations involving fragments from munitions, civilian**

Y36.26   **War operations involving fragments of improvised explosive device [IED]**

War operations involving fragments of person-borne improvised explosive device [IED]

War operations involving fragments of vehicle-borne improvised explosive device [IED]

War operations involving fragments of roadside improvised explosive device [IED]

⑦Y36.260   **War operations involving fragments of improvised explosive device [IED], military personnel**

⑦Y36.261   **War operations involving fragments of improvised explosive device [IED], civilian**

Y36.27   **War operations involving fragments from weapons**

⑦Y36.270   **War operations involving fragments from weapons, military personnel**

⑦Y36.271   **War operations involving fragments from weapons, civilian**

Y36.29   **War operations involving other explosions and fragments**

War operations involving explosion of grenade
War operations involving explosions of land mine War operations involving shrapnel NOS

⑦Y36.290   **War operations involving other explosions and fragments, military personnel**

⑦Y36.291   **War operations involving other explosions and fragments, civilian**

Y36.3   **War operations involving fires, conflagrations and hot substances**

War operations involving smoke, fumes, and heat from fires, conflagrations and hot substances

Excludes1: war operations involving fires and conflagrations aboard military aircraft (Y36.1-)

war operations involving fires and conflagrations aboard military watercraft (Y36.0-)

war operations involving fires and conflagrations caused indirectly by conventional weapons (Y36.2-)

war operations involving fires and thermal effects of nuclear weapons (Y36.53-)

Y36.30   **War operations involving unspecified fire, conflagration and hot substance**

⑦Y36.300   **War operations involving unspecified fire, conflagration and hot substance, military personnel**

⑦Y36.301   **War operations involving unspecified fire, conflagration and hot substance, civilian**

Y36.31   **War operations involving gasoline bomb**

War operations involving incendiary bomb

War operations involving petrol bomb

⑦Y36.310   **War operations involving gasoline bomb, military personnel**

⑦Y36.311   **War operations involving gasoline bomb, civilian**

Y36.32   **War operations involving incendiary bullet**

⑦Y36.320   **War operations involving incendiary bullet, military personnel**

⑦Y36.321   **War operations involving incendiary bullet, civilian**

Y36.33   **War operations involving flamethrower**

⑦Y36.330   **War operations involving flamethrower, military personnel**

⑦Y36.331   **War operations involving flamethrower, civilian**

Y36.39   **War operations involving other fires, conflagrations and hot substances**

⑦Y36.390   **War operations involving other fires, conflagrations and hot substances, military personnel**

⑦Y36.391   **War operations involving other fires, conflagrations and hot substances, civilian**

Y36.4   **War operations involving firearm discharge and other forms of conventional warfare**

Y36.41   **War operations involving rubber bullets**

⑦Y36.410   **War operations involving rubber bullets, military personnel**

⑦Y36.411   **War operations involving rubber bullets, civilian**

Y36.42   **War operations involving firearms pellets**

● New code   ▲ Revised code   **Excludes1:** Not coded here   **Excludes2:** Not included here   ⊗ Placeholder required   ⑦7th digit required

⑦Y36.420   **War operations involving firearms pellets, military personnel**

⑦Y36.421   **War operations involving firearms pellets, civilian**

Y36.43   **War operations involving other firearms discharge**

War operations involving bullets NOS

> **Excludes1:** war operations involving munitions fragments (Y36.25-)
>
> war operations involving incendiary bullets (Y36.32-)

⑦Y36.430   **War operations involving other firearms discharge, military personnel**

⑦Y36.431   **War operations involving other firearms discharge, civilian**

Y36.44   **War operations involving unarmed hand to hand combat**

> **Excludes1:** war operations involving combat using blunt or piercing object (Y36.45-)
>
> war operations involving intentional restriction of air and airway (Y36.46-)
>
> war operations involving unintentional restriction of air and airway (Y36.47-)

⑦Y36.440   **War operations involving unarmed hand to hand combat, military personnel**

⑦Y36.441   **War operations involving unarmed hand to hand combat, civilian**

Y36.45   **War operations involving combat using blunt or piercing object**

⑦Y36.450   **War operations involving combat using blunt or piercing object, military personnel**

⑦Y36.451   **War operations involving combat using blunt or piercing object, civilian**

Y36.46   **War operations involving intentional restriction of air and airway**

⑦Y36.460   **War operations involving intentional restriction of air and airway, military personnel**

⑦Y36.461   **War operations involving intentional restriction of air and airway, civilian**

Y36.47   **War operations involving unintentional restriction of air and airway**

⑦Y36.470   **War operations involving unintentional restriction of air and airway, military personnel**

⑦Y36.471   **War operations involving unintentional restriction of air and airway, civilian**

Y36.49   **War operations involving other forms of conventional warfare**

⑦Y36.490   **War operations involving other forms of conventional warfare, military personnel**

⑦Y36.491   **War operations involving other forms of conventional warfare, civilian**

Y36.5   **War operations involving nuclear weapons**

War operations involving dirty bomb NOS

Y36.50   **War operations involving unspecified effect of nuclear weapon**

⑦Y36.500   **War operations involving unspecified effect of nuclear weapon, military personnel**

⑦Y36.501   **War operations involving unspecified effect of nuclear weapon, civilian**

Y36.51   **War operations involving direct blast effect of nuclear weapon**

War operations involving blast pressure of nuclear weapon

⑦Y36.510   **War operations involving direct blast effect of nuclear weapon, military personnel**

⑦Y36.511   **War operations involving direct blast effect of nuclear weapon, civilian**

Y36.52   **War operations involving indirect blast effect of nuclear weapon**

War operations involving being thrown by blast of nuclear weapon

War operations involving being struck or crushed by blast debris of nuclear weapon

⑦Y36.520   **War operations involving indirect blast effect of nuclear weapon, military personnel**

⑦Y36.521   **War operations involving indirect blast effect of nuclear weapon, civilian**

Y36.53   **War operations involving thermal radiation effect of nuclear weapon**

War operations involving direct heat from nuclear weapon

War operation involving fireball effects from nuclear weapon

⑦Y36.530   **War operations involving thermal radiation effect of nuclear weapon, military personnel**

⑦Y36.531   **War operations involving thermal radiation effect of nuclear weapon, civilian**

Y36.54   **War operation involving nuclear radiation effects of nuclear weapon**

War operation involving acute radiation exposure from nuclear weapon

War operation involving exposure to immediate ionizing radiation from nuclear weapon

War operation involving fallout exposure from nuclear weapon

War operation involving secondary effects of nuclear weapon

⑦Y36.540   **War operation involving nuclear radiation effects of nuclear weapon, military personnel**

⑦Y36.541   **War operation involving nuclear radiation effects of nuclear weapon, civilian**

Y36.59   **War operation involving other effects of nuclear weapons**

---

⑦**Y36.590** War operation involving other effects of nuclear weapons, military personnel

⑦**Y36.591** War operation involving other effects of nuclear weapons, civilian

Y36.6 War operations involving biological weapons

Y36.6X War operations involving biological weapons

⑦**Y36.6X0** War operations involving biological weapons, military personnel

⑦**Y36.6X1** War operations involving biological weapons, civilian

Y36.7 War operations involving chemical weapons and other forms of unconventional warfare

Excludes1: war operations involving incendiary devices (Y36.3-, Y36.5-)

Y36.7X War operations involving chemical weapons and other forms of unconventional warfare

⑦**Y36.7X0** War operations involving chemical weapons and other forms of unconventional warfare, military personnel

⑦**Y36.7X1** War operations involving chemical weapons and other forms of unconventional warfare, civilian

Y36.8 War operations occurring after cessation of hostilities

War operations classifiable to categories Y36.0-Y36.8 but occurring after cessation of hostilities

Y36.81 Explosion of mine placed during war operations but exploding after cessation of hostilities

⑦**Y36.810** Explosion of mine placed during war operations but exploding after cessation of hostilities, military personnel

⑦**Y36.811** Explosion of mine placed during war operations but exploding after cessation of hostilities, civilian

Y36.82 Explosion of bomb placed during war operations but exploding after cessation of hostilities

⑦**Y36.820** Explosion of bomb placed during war operations but exploding after cessation of hostilities, military personnel

⑦**Y36.821** Explosion of bomb placed during war operations but exploding after cessation of hostilities, civilian

Y36.88 Other war operations occurring after cessation of hostilities

⑦**Y36.880** Other war operations occurring after cessation of hostilities, military personnel

⑦**Y36.881** Other war operations occurring after cessation of hostilities, civilian

Y36.89 Unspecified war operations occurring after cessation of hostilities

⑦**Y36.890** Unspecified war operations occurring after cessation of hostilities, military personnel

⑦**Y36.891** Unspecified war operations occurring after cessation of hostilities, civilian

Y36.9 Other and unspecified war operations

⊗⑦**Y36.90** War operations, unspecified

⊗⑦**Y36.91** War operations involving unspecified weapon of mass destruction [WMD]

⊗⑦**Y36.92** War operations involving friendly fire

Y37 **Military operations**

Includes: injuries to military personnel and civilians occurring during peacetime on military property and during routine military exercises and operations

Excludes1: military aircraft involved in aircraft accident with civilian aircraft (V97.81-)

military vehicles involved in transport accident with civilian vehicle (V09.01, V09.21, V19.81, V29.81, V39.81, V49.81, V59.81, V69.81, V79.81)

military watercraft involved in water transport accident with civilian watercraft (V94.81-) war operations (Y36.-)

The appropriate 7th character is to be added to each code from category Y37

A - initial encounter

D - subsequent encounter

S - sequela

Y37.0 Military operations involving explosion of marine weapons

Y37.00 Military operations involving explosion of unspecified marine weapon

Military operations involving underwater blast NOS

⑦**Y37.000** Military operations involving explosion of unspecified marine weapon, military personnel

⑦**Y37.001** Military operations involving explosion of unspecified marine weapon, civilian

Y37.01 Military operations involving explosion of depth-charge

⑦**Y37.010** Military operations involving explosion of depth-charge, military personnel

⑦**Y37.011** Military operations involving explosion of depth-charge, civilian

Y37.02 Military operations involving explosion of marine mine

Military operations involving explosion of marine mine, at sea or in harbor

⑦**Y37.020** Military operations involving explosion of marine mine, military personnel

⑦**Y37.021** Military operations involving explosion of marine mine, civilian

Y37.03 Military operations involving explosion of sea-based artillery shell

⑦**Y37.030** Military operations involving explosion of sea-based artillery shell, military personnel

⑦**Y37.031** Military operations involving explosion of sea-based artillery shell, civilian

Y37.04 Military operations involving explosion of torpedo

⑦**Y37.040** Military operations involving explosion of torpedo, military personnel

● New code ▲ Revised code **Excludes1:** Not coded here **Excludes2:** Not included here ⊗ Placeholder required ⑦7th digit required

⑦**Y37.041** **Military operations involving explosion of torpedo, civilian**

Y37.05 **Military operations involving accidental detonation of onboard marine weapons**

⑦**Y37.050** **Military operations involving accidental detonation of onboard marine weapons, military personnel**

⑦**Y37.051** **Military operations involving accidental detonation of onboard marine weapons, civilian**

Y37.09 **Military operations involving explosion of other marine weapons**

⑦**Y37.090** **Military operations involving explosion of other marine weapons, military personnel**

⑦**Y37.091** **Military operations involving explosion of other marine weapons, civilian**

Y37.1 **Military operations involving destruction of aircraft**

Y37.10 **Military operations involving unspecified destruction of aircraft**

⑦**Y37.100** **Military operations involving unspecified destruction of aircraft, military personnel**

⑦**Y37.101** **Military operations involving unspecified destruction of aircraft, civilian**

Y37.11 **Military operations involving destruction of aircraft due to enemy fire or explosives**

Military operations involving destruction of aircraft due to air to air missile

Military operations involving destruction of aircraft due to explosive placed on aircraft

Military operations involving destruction of aircraft due to rocket propelled grenade [RPG]

Military operations involving destruction of aircraft due to small arms fire

Military operations involving destruction of aircraft due to surface to air missile

⑦**Y37.110** **Military operations involving destruction of aircraft due to enemy fire or explosives, military personnel**

⑦**Y37.111** **Military operations involving destruction of aircraft due to enemy fire or explosives, civilian**

Y37.12 **Military operations involving destruction of aircraft due to collision with other aircraft**

⑦**Y37.120** **Military operations involving destruction of aircraft due to collision with other aircraft, military personnel**

⑦**Y37.121** **Military operations involving destruction of aircraft due to collision with other aircraft, civilian**

Y37.13 **Military operations involving destruction of aircraft due to onboard fire**

⑦**Y37.130** **Military operations involving destruction of aircraft due to onboard fire, military personnel**

⑦**Y37.131** **Military operations involving destruction of aircraft due to onboard fire, civilian**

Y37.14 **Military operations involving destruction of aircraft due to accidental detonation of onboard munitions and explosives**

⑦**Y37.140** **Military operations involving destruction of aircraft due to accidental detonation of onboard munitions and explosives, military personnel**

⑦**Y37.141** **Military operations involving destruction of aircraft due to accidental detonation of onboard munitions and explosives, civilian**

Y37.19 **Military operations involving other destruction of aircraft**

⑦**Y37.190** **Military operations involving other destruction of aircraft, military personnel**

⑦**Y37.191** **Military operations involving other destruction of aircraft, civilian**

Y37.2 **Military operations involving other explosions and fragments**

Excludes1: military operations involving explosion of aircraft (Y37.1-)

military operations involving explosion of marine weapons (Y37.0-)

military operations involving explosion of nuclear weapons (Y37.5-)

Y37.20 **Military operations involving unspecified explosion and fragments**

Military operations involving air blast NOS

Military operations involving blast NOS

Military operations involving blast fragments NOS

Military operations involving blast wave NOS

Military operations involving blast wind NOS

Military operations involving explosion NOS

Military operations involving explosion of bomb NOS

⑦**Y37.200** **Military operations involving unspecified explosion and fragments, military personnel**

⑦**Y37.201** **Military operations involving unspecified explosion and fragments, civilian**

Y37.21 **Military operations involving explosion of aerial bomb**

⑦**Y37.210** **Military operations involving explosion of aerial bomb, military personnel**

⑦**Y37.211** **Military operations involving explosion of aerial bomb, civilian**

Y37.22 **Military operations involving explosion of guided missile**

⑦**Y37.220** **Military operations involving explosion of guided missile, military personnel**

⑦**Y37.221** **Military operations involving explosion of guided missile, civilian**

Y37.23 **Military operations involving explosion of improvised explosive device [IED]**

Military operations involving explosion of person-borne improvised explosive device [IED]

Military operations involving explosion of vehicle-borne improvised explosive device [IED]

Military operations involving explosion of roadside improvised explosive device [IED]

⑦**Y37.230** **Military operations involving explosion of improvised explosive device [IED], military personnel**

⑦**Y37.231** **Military operations involving explosion of improvised explosive device [IED], civilian**

Y37.24 **Military operations involving explosion due to accidental detonation and discharge of own munitions or munitions launch device**

⑦**Y37.240** **Military operations involving explosion due to accidental detonation and discharge of own munitions or munitions launch device, military personnel**

⑦**Y37.241** **Military operations involving explosion due to accidental detonation and discharge of own munitions or munitions launch device, civilian**

Y37.25 **Military operations involving fragments from munitions**

⑦**Y37.250** **Military operations involving fragments from munitions, military personnel**

⑦**Y37.251** **Military operations involving fragments from munitions, civilian**

Y37.26 **Military operations involving fragments of improvised explosive device [IED]**

Military operations involving fragments of person-borne improvised explosive device [IED]

Military operations involving fragments of vehicle-borne improvised explosive device [IED]

Military operations involving fragments of roadside improvised explosive device [IED]

⑦**Y37.260** **Military operations involving fragments of improvised explosive device [IED], military personnel**

⑦**Y37.261** **Military operations involving fragments of improvised explosive device [IED], civilian**

Y37.27 **Military operations involving fragments from weapons**

⑦**Y37.270** **Military operations involving fragments from weapons, military personnel**

⑦**Y37.271** **Military operations involving fragments from weapons, civilian**

Y37.29 **Military operations involving other explosions and fragments**

Military operations involving explosion of grenade

Military operations involving explosions of land mine

Military operations involving shrapnel NOS

⑦**Y37.290** **Military operations involving other explosions and fragments, military personnel**

⑦**Y37.291** **Military operations involving other explosions and fragments, civilian**

Y37.3 **Military operations involving fires, conflagrations and hot substances**

Military operations involving smoke, fumes, and heat from fires, conflagrations and hot substances

Excludes1: military operations involving fires and conflagrations aboard military aircraft (Y37.1-)

military operations involving fires and conflagrations aboard military watercraft (Y37.0-)

military operations involving fires and conflagrations caused indirectly by conventional weapons (Y37.2-)

military operations involving fires and thermal effects of nuclear weapons (Y36.53-)

Y37.30 **Military operations involving unspecified fire, conflagration and hot substance**

⑦**Y37.300** **Military operations involving unspecified fire, conflagration and hot substance, military personnel**

⑦**Y37.301** **Military operations involving unspecified fire, conflagration and hot substance, civilian**

Y37.31 **Military operations involving gasoline bomb**

Military operations involving incendiary bomb

Military operations involving petrol bomb

⑦**Y37.310** **Military operations involving gasoline bomb, military personnel**

⑦**Y37.311** **Military operations involving gasoline bomb, civilian**

Y37.32 **Military operations involving incendiary bullet**

⑦**Y37.320** **Military operations involving incendiary bullet, military personnel**

⑦**Y37.321** **Military operations involving incendiary bullet, civilian**

Y37.33 **Military operations involving flamethrower**

⑦**Y37.330** **Military operations involving flamethrower, military personnel**

⑦**Y37.331** **Military operations involving flamethrower, civilian**

Y37.39 **Military operations involving other fires, conflagrations and hot substances**

⑦**Y37.390** **Military operations involving other fires, conflagrations and hot substances, military personnel**

⑦**Y37.391** **Military operations involving other fires, conflagrations and hot substances, civilian**

Y37.4 **Military operations involving firearm discharge and other forms of conventional warfare**

Y37.41 **Military operations involving rubber bullets**

⑦**Y37.410** **Military operations involving rubber bullets, military personnel**

⑦**Y37.411** **Military operations involving rubber bullets, civilian**

Y37.42 **Military operations involving firearms pellets**

⑦**Y37.420** **Military operations involving firearms pellets, military personnel**

⑦**Y37.421** **Military operations involving firearms pellets, civilian**

Y37.43 **Military operations involving other firearms discharge**

Military operations involving bullets NOS

Excludes1: military operations involving munitions fragments (Y37.25-)

military operations involving incendiary bullets (Y37.32-)

⑦**Y37.430** **Military operations involving other firearms discharge, military personnel**

⑦**Y37.431** **Military operations involving other firearms discharge, civilian**

Y37.44 **Military operations involving unarmed hand to hand combat**

Excludes1: military operations involving combat using blunt or piercing object (Y37.45-)

military operations involving intentional restriction of air and airway (Y37.46-)

military operations involving unintentional restriction of air and airway (Y37.47-)

⑦**Y37.440** **Military operations involving unarmed hand to hand combat, military personnel**

⑦**Y37.441** **Military operations involving unarmed hand to hand combat, civilian**

Y37.45 **Military operations involving combat using blunt or piercing object**

⑦**Y37.450** **Military operations involving combat using blunt or piercing object, military personnel**

⑦**Y37.451** **Military operations involving combat using blunt or piercing object, civilian**

Y37.46 **Military operations involving intentional restriction of air and airway**

⑦**Y37.460** **Military operations involving intentional restriction of air and airway, military personnel**

⑦**Y37.461** **Military operations involving intentional restriction of air and airway, civilian**

Y37.47 **Military operations involving unintentional restriction of air and airway**

⑦**Y37.470** **Military operations involving unintentional restriction of air and airway, military personnel**

⑦**Y37.471** **Military operations involving unintentional restriction of air and airway, civilian**

Y37.49 **Military operations involving other forms of conventional warfare**

⑦**Y37.490** **Military operations involving other forms of conventional warfare, military personnel**

⑦**Y37.491** **Military operations involving other forms of conventional warfare, civilian**

Y37.5 **Military operations involving nuclear weapons**

Military operation involving dirty bomb NOS

Y37.50 **Military operations involving unspecified effect of nuclear weapon**

⑦**Y37.500** **Military operations involving unspecified effect of nuclear weapon, military personnel**

⑦**Y37.501** **Military operations involving unspecified effect of nuclear weapon, civilian**

Y37.51 **Military operations involving direct blast effect of nuclear weapon**

Military operations involving blast pressure of nuclear weapon

⑦**Y37.510** **Military operations involving direct blast effect of nuclear weapon, military personnel**

⑦**Y37.511** **Military operations involving direct blast effect of nuclear weapon, civilian**

Y37.52 **Military operations involving indirect blast effect of nuclear weapon**

Military operations involving being thrown by blast of nuclear weapon

Military operations involving being struck or crushed by blast debris of nuclear weapon

⑦**Y37.520** **Military operations involving indirect blast effect of nuclear weapon, military personnel**

⑦**Y37.521** **Military operations involving indirect blast effect of nuclear weapon, civilian**

Y37.53 **Military operations involving thermal radiation effect of nuclear weapon**

Military operations involving direct heat from nuclear weapon

Military operation involving fireball effects from nuclear weapon

⑦**Y37.530** **Military operations involving thermal radiation effect of nuclear weapon, military personnel**

⑦**Y37.531** **Military operations involving thermal radiation effect of nuclear weapon, civilian**

Y37.54 **Military operation involving nuclear radiation effects of nuclear weapon**

Military operation involving acute radiation exposure from nuclear weapon

Military operation involving exposure to immediate ionizing radiation from nuclear weapon

Military operation involving fallout exposure from nuclear weapon

Military operation involving secondary effects of nuclear weapons

⑦**Y37.540** **Military operation involving nuclear radiation effects of nuclear weapon, military personnel**

⑦**Y37.541** **Military operation involving nuclear radiation effects of nuclear weapon, civilian**

Y37.59 **Military operation involving other effects of nuclear weapons**

---

⑦**Y37.590**   **Military operation involving other effects of nuclear weapons, military personnel**

⑦**Y37.591**   **Military operation involving other effects of nuclear weapons, civilian**

Y37.6   Military operations involving biological weapons

Y37.6X   Military operations involving biological weapons

⑦**Y37.6X0**   **Military operations involving biological weapons, military personnel**

⑦**Y37.6X1**   **Military operations involving biological weapons, civilian**

Y37.7   Military operations involving chemical weapons and other forms of unconventional warfare

Excludes1: military operations involving incendiary devices (Y36.3-, Y36.5-)

Y37.7X   Military operations involving chemical weapons and other forms of unconventional warfare

⑦**Y37.7X0**   **Military operations involving chemical weapons and other forms of unconventional warfare, military personnel**

⑦**Y37.7X1**   **Military operations involving chemical weapons and other forms of unconventional warfare, civilian**

Y37.9   Other and unspecified military operations

⊗⑦**Y37.90**   **Military operations, unspecified**

⊗⑦**Y37.91**   **Military operations involving unspecified weapon of mass destruction [WMD]**

⊗⑦**Y37.92**   **Military operations involving friendly fire**

Y38   Terrorism

These codes are for use to identify injuries resulting from the unlawful use of force or violence against persons or property to intimidate or coerce a Government, the civilian population, or any segment thereof, in furtherance of political or social objective

Use additional code for place of occurrence (Y92.-)

The appropriate 7th character is to be added to each code from category Y38

A - initial encounter

D - subsequent encounter

S - sequela

Y38.0   Terrorism involving explosion of marine weapons

Terrorism involving depth-charge

Terrorism involving marine mine

Terrorism involving mine NOS, at sea or in harbor

Terrorism involving sea-based artillery shell

Terrorism involving torpedo

Terrorism involving underwater blast

Y38.0X   Terrorism involving explosion of marine weapons

⑦**Y38.0X1**   **Terrorism involving explosion of marine weapons, public safety official injured**

⑦**Y38.0X2**   **Terrorism involving explosion of marine weapons, civilian injured**

⑦**Y38.0X3**   **Terrorism involving explosion of marine weapons, terrorist injured**

Y38.1   Terrorism involving destruction of aircraft

Terrorism involving aircraft burned

Terrorism involving aircraft exploded

Terrorism involving aircraft being shot down

Terrorism involving aircraft used as a weapon

Y38.1X   Terrorism involving destruction of aircraft

⑦**Y38.1X1**   **Terrorism involving destruction of aircraft, public safety official injured**

⑦**Y38.1X2**   **Terrorism involving destruction of aircraft, civilian injured**

⑦**Y38.1X3**   **Terrorism involving destruction of aircraft, terrorist injured**

Y38.2   Terrorism involving other explosions and fragments

Terrorism involving antipersonnel (fragments) bomb

Terrorism involving blast NOS

Terrorism involving explosion NOS

Terrorism involving explosion of breech block

Terrorism involving explosion of cannon block

Terrorism involving explosion (fragments) of artillery shell

Terrorism involving explosion (fragments) of bomb

Terrorism involving explosion (fragments) of grenade

Terrorism involving explosion (fragments) of guided missile

Terrorism involving explosion (fragments) of land mine

Terrorism involving explosion of mortar bomb

Terrorism involving explosion of munitions

Terrorism involving explosion (fragments) of rocket

Terrorism involving explosion (fragments) of shell

Terrorism involving shrapnel

Terrorism involving mine NOS, on land

Excludes1: terrorism involving explosion of nuclear weapon (Y38.5)

terrorism involving suicide bomber (Y38.81)

Y38.2X   Terrorism involving other explosions and fragments

⑦**Y38.2X1**   **Terrorism involving other explosions and fragments, public safety official injured**

⑦**Y38.2X2**   **Terrorism involving other explosions and fragments, civilian injured**

⑦**Y38.2X3**   **Terrorism involving other explosions and fragments, terrorist injured**

Y38.3   Terrorism involving fires, conflagration and hot substances

Terrorism involving conflagration NOS

Terrorism involving fire NOS

Terrorism involving petrol bomb

Excludes1: terrorism involving fire or heat of nuclear weapon (Y38.5)

Y38.3X   Terrorism involving fires, conflagration and hot substances

⑦**Y38.3X1**   **Terrorism involving fires, conflagration and hot substances, public safety official injured**

⑦**Y38.3X2**   **Terrorism involving fires, conflagration and hot substances, civilian injured**

● New code   ▲ Revised code   **Excludes1:** Not coded here   **Excludes2:** Not included here   ⊗ Placeholder required   ⑦7th digit required

⑦**Y38.3X3** **Terrorism involving fires, conflagration and hot substances, terrorist injured**

Y38.4 **Terrorism involving firearms**

Terrorism involving carbine bullet

Terrorism involving machine gun bullet

Terrorism involving pellets (shotgun)

Terrorism involving pistol bullet

Terrorism involving rifle bullet

Terrorism involving rubber (rifle) bullet

Y38.4X **Terrorism involving firearms**

⑦**Y38.4X1** **Terrorism involving firearms, public safety official injured**

⑦**Y38.4X2** **Terrorism involving firearms, civilian injured**

⑦**Y38.4X3** **Terrorism involving firearms, terrorist injured**

Y38.5 **Terrorism involving nuclear weapons**

Terrorism involving blast effects of nuclear weapon

Terrorism involving exposure to ionizing radiation from nuclear weapon

Terrorism involving fireball effect of nuclear weapon

Terrorism involving heat from nuclear weapon

Y38.5X **Terrorism involving nuclear weapons**

⑦**Y38.5X1** **Terrorism involving nuclear weapons, public safety official injured**

⑦**Y38.5X2** **Terrorism involving nuclear weapons, civilian injured**

⑦**Y38.5X3** **Terrorism involving nuclear weapons, terrorist injured**

Y38.6 **Terrorism involving biological weapons**

Terrorism involving anthrax

Terrorism involving cholera

Terrorism involving smallpox

Y38.6X **Terrorism involving biological weapons**

⑦**Y38.6X1** **Terrorism involving biological weapons, public safety official injured**

⑦**Y38.6X2** **Terrorism involving biological weapons, civilian injured**

⑦**Y38.6X3** **Terrorism involving biological weapons, terrorist injured**

Y38.7 **Terrorism involving chemical weapons**

Terrorism involving gases, fumes, chemicals

Terrorism involving hydrogen cyanide

Terrorism involving phosgene

Terrorism involving sarin

Y38.7X **Terrorism involving chemical weapons**

⑦**Y38.7X1** **Terrorism involving chemical weapons, public safety official injured**

⑦**Y38.7X2** **Terrorism involving chemical weapons, civilian injured**

⑦**Y38.7X3** **Terrorism involving chemical weapons, terrorist injured**

Y38.8 **Terrorism involving other and unspecified means**

⊗⑦**Y38.80** **Terrorism involving unspecified means**

Terrorism NOS

Y38.81 **Terrorism involving suicide bomber**

⑦**Y38.811** **Terrorism involving suicide bomber, public safety official injured**

⑦**Y38.812** **Terrorism involving suicide bomber, civilian injured**

Y38.89 **Terrorism involving other means**

Terrorism involving drowning and submersion

Terrorism involving lasers

Terrorism involving piercing or stabbing instruments

⑦**Y38.891** **Terrorism involving other means, public safety official injured**

⑦**Y38.892** **Terrorism involving other means, civilian injured**

⑦**Y38.893** **Terrorism involving other means, terrorist injured**

Y38.9 **Terrorism, secondary effects**

Note: This code is for use to identify conditions occurring subsequent to a terrorist attack not those that are due to the initial terrorist attack

Y38.9X **Terrorism, secondary effects**

⑦**Y38.9X1** **Terrorism, secondary effects, public safety official injured**

⑦**Y38.9X2** **Terrorism, secondary effects, civilian injured**

COMPLICATIONS OF MEDICAL AND SURGICAL CARE (Y62-Y84)

Includes: complications of medical devices

surgical and medical procedures as the cause of abnormal reaction of the patient, or of later complication, without mention of misadventure at the time of the procedure

MISADVENTURES TO PATIENTS DURING SURGICAL AND MEDICAL CARE (Y62-Y69)

Excludes1: surgical and medical procedures as the cause of abnormal reaction of the patient, without mention of misadventure at the time of the procedure (Y83-Y84)

Excludes2: breakdown or malfunctioning of medical device (during procedure) (after implantation) (ongoing use) (Y70-Y82)

Y62 **Failure of sterile precautions during surgical and medical care**

Y62.0 **Failure of sterile precautions during surgical operation**

Y62.1 **Failure of sterile precautions during infusion or transfusion**

Y62.2 **Failure of sterile precautions during kidney dialysis and other perfusion**

Y62.3 **Failure of sterile precautions during injection or immunization**

Y62.4 **Failure of sterile precautions during endoscopic examination**

Y62.5 **Failure of sterile precautions during heart catheterization**

Y62.6 **Failure of sterile precautions during aspiration, puncture and other catheterization**

Y62.8 **Failure of sterile precautions during other surgical and medical care**

Y62.9 **Failure of sterile precautions during unspecified surgical and medical care**

Y63 Failure in dosage during surgical and medical care

Excludes2: accidental overdose of drug or wrong drug given in error (T36-T50)

Y63.0 Excessive amount of blood or other fluid given during transfusion or infusion

Y63.1 Incorrect dilution of fluid used during infusion

Y63.2 Overdose of radiation given during therapy

Y63.3 Inadvertent exposure of patient to radiation during medical care

Y63.4 Failure in dosage in electroshock or insulin-shock therapy

Y63.5 Inappropriate temperature in local application and packing

Y63.6 Underdosing and nonadministration of necessary drug, medicament or biological substance

Y63.8 Failure in dosage during other surgical and medical care

Y63.9 Failure in dosage during unspecified surgical and medical care

Y64 Contaminated medical or biological substances

Y64.0 Contaminated medical or biological substance, transfused or infused

Y64.1 Contaminated medical or biological substance, injected or used for immunization

Y64.8 Contaminated medical or biological substance administered by other means

Y64.9 Contaminated medical or biological substance administered by unspecified means

Administered contaminated medical or biological substance NOS

Y65 Other misadventures during surgical and medical care

Y65.0 Mismatched blood in transfusion

Y65.1 Wrong fluid used in infusion

Y65.2 Failure in suture or ligature during surgical operation

Y65.3 Endotracheal tube wrongly placed during anesthetic procedure

Y65.4 Failure to introduce or to remove other tube or instrument

Y65.5 Performance of wrong procedure (operation)

Y65.51 Performance of wrong procedure (operation) on correct patient

Wrong device implanted into correct surgical site

Excludes1: performance of correct procedure (operation) on wrong side or body part (Y65.53)

Y65.52 Performance of procedure (operation) on patient not scheduled for surgery

Performance of procedure (operation) intended for another patient

Performance of procedure (operation) on wrong patient

Y65.53 Performance of correct procedure (operation) on wrong side or body part

Performance of correct procedure (operation) on wrong side

Performance of correct procedure (operation) on wrong site

Y65.8 Other specified misadventures during surgical and medical care

Y66 Nonadministration of surgical and medical care

Premature cessation of surgical and medical care

Excludes1: DNR status (Z66)

palliative care (Z51.5)

Y69 Unspecified misadventure during surgical and medical care

MEDICAL DEVICES ASSOCIATED WITH ADVERSE INCIDENTS IN DIAGNOSTIC AND THERAPEUTIC USE (Y70-Y82)

Includes: breakdown or malfunction of medical devices (during use) (after implantation) (ongoing use)

Excludes2: breakdown or malfunctioning of medical device (after implantation) (during procedure) (ongoing use) (Y70-Y82)

later complications following use of medical devices without breakdown or malfunctioning of device (Y83-Y84)

misadventure to patients during surgical and medical care, classifiable to (Y62-Y69)

surgical and other medical procedures as the cause of abnormal reaction of the patient, or of later complication, without mention of misadventure at the time of the procedure (Y83-Y84)

Y70 Anesthesiology devices associated with adverse incidents

Y70.0 Diagnostic and monitoring anesthesiology devices associated with adverse incidents

Y70.1 Therapeutic (nonsurgical) and rehabilitative anesthesiology devices associated with adverse incidents

Y70.2 Prosthetic and other implants, materials and accessory anesthesiology devices associated with adverse incidents

Y70.3 Surgical instruments, materials and anesthesiology devices (including sutures) associated with adverse incidents

Y70.8 Miscellaneous anesthesiology devices associated with adverse incidents, not elsewhere classified

Y71 Cardiovascular devices associated with adverse incidents

Y71.0 Diagnostic and monitoring cardiovascular devices associated with adverse incidents

Y71.1 Therapeutic (nonsurgical) and rehabilitative cardiovascular devices associated with adverse incidents

Y71.2 Prosthetic and other implants, materials and accessory cardiovascular devices associated with adverse incidents

Y71.3 Surgical instruments, materials and cardiovascular devices (including sutures) associated with adverse incidents

Y71.8 Miscellaneous cardiovascular devices associated with adverse incidents, not elsewhere classified

Y72 Otorhinolaryngological devices associated with adverse incidents

Y72.0 Diagnostic and monitoring otorhinolaryngological devices associated with adverse incidents

Y72.1 Therapeutic (nonsurgical) and rehabilitative otorhinolaryngological devices associated with adverse incidents

Y72.2 Prosthetic and other implants, materials and accessory otorhinolaryngological devices associated with adverse incidents

Y72.3 Surgical instruments, materials and otorhinolaryngological devices (including sutures) associated with adverse incidents

Y72.8 Miscellaneous otorhinolaryngological devices associated with adverse incidents, not elsewhere classified

Y73 Gastroenterology and urology devices associated with adverse incidents

● New code ▲ Revised code Excludes1: Not coded here Excludes2: Not included here ⊗ Placeholder required ⑦7th digit required

Y73.0   Diagnostic and monitoring gastroenterology and urology devices associated with adverse incidents

Y73.1   Therapeutic (nonsurgical) and rehabilitative gastroenterology and urology devices associated with adverse incidents

Y73.2   Prosthetic and other implants, materials and accessory gastroenterology and urology devices associated with adverse incidents

Y73.3   Surgical instruments, materials and gastroenterology and urology devices (including sutures) associated with adverse incidents

Y73.8   Miscellaneous gastroenterology and urology devices associated with adverse incidents, not elsewhere classified

Y74   General hospital and personal-use devices associated with adverse incidents

Y74.0   Diagnostic and monitoring general hospital and personal-use devices associated with adverse incidents

Y74.1   Therapeutic (nonsurgical) and rehabilitative general hospital and personal-use devices associated with adverse incidents

Y74.2   Prosthetic and other implants, materials and accessory general hospital and personal-use devices associated with adverse incidents

Y74.3   Surgical instruments, materials and general hospital and personal-use devices (including sutures) associated with adverse incidents

Y74.8   Miscellaneous general hospital and personal-use devices associated with adverse incidents, not elsewhere classified

Y75   Neurological devices associated with adverse incidents

Y75.0   Diagnostic and monitoring neurological devices associated with adverse incidents

Y75.1   Therapeutic (nonsurgical) and rehabilitative neurological devices associated with adverse incidents

Y75.2   Prosthetic and other implants, materials and neurological devices associated with adverse incidents

Y75.3   Surgical instruments, materials and neurological devices (including sutures) associated with adverse incidents

Y75.8   Miscellaneous neurological devices associated with adverse incidents, not elsewhere classified

Y76   Obstetric and gynecological devices associated with adverse incidents

Y76.0   Diagnostic and monitoring obstetric and gynecological devices associated with adverse incidents

Y76.1   Therapeutic (nonsurgical) and rehabilitative obstetric and gynecological devices associated with adverse incidents

Y76.2   Prosthetic and other implants, materials and accessory obstetric and gynecological devices associated with adverse incidents

Y76.3   Surgical instruments, materials and obstetric and gynecological devices (including sutures) associated with adverse incidents

Y76.8   Miscellaneous obstetric and gynecological devices associated with adverse incidents, not elsewhere classified

Y77   Ophthalmic devices associated with adverse incidents

Y77.0   Diagnostic and monitoring ophthalmic devices associated with adverse incidents

Y77.1   Therapeutic (nonsurgical) and rehabilitative ophthalmic devices associated with adverse incidents

Y77.2   Prosthetic and other implants, materials and accessory ophthalmic devices associated with adverse incidents

Y77.3   Surgical instruments, materials and ophthalmic devices (including sutures) associated with adverse incidents

Y77.8   Miscellaneous ophthalmic devices associated with adverse incidents, not elsewhere classified

Y78   Radiological devices associated with adverse incidents

Y78.0   Diagnostic and monitoring radiological devices associated with adverse incidents

Y78.1   Therapeutic (nonsurgical) and rehabilitative radiological devices associated with adverse incidents

Y78.2   Prosthetic and other implants, materials and accessory radiological devices associated with adverse incidents

Y78.3   Surgical instruments, materials and radiological devices (including sutures) associated with adverse incidents

Y78.8   Miscellaneous radiological devices associated with adverse incidents, not elsewhere classified

Y79   Orthopedic devices associated with adverse incidents

Y79.0   Diagnostic and monitoring orthopedic devices associated with adverse incidents

Y79.1   Therapeutic (nonsurgical) and rehabilitative orthopedic devices associated with adverse incidents

Y79.2   Prosthetic and other implants, materials and accessory orthopedic devices associated with adverse incidents

Y79.3   Surgical instruments, materials and orthopedic devices (including sutures) associated with adverse incidents

Y79.8   Miscellaneous orthopedic devices associated with adverse incidents, not elsewhere classified

Y80   Physical medicine devices associated with adverse incidents

Y80.0   Diagnostic and monitoring physical medicine devices associated with adverse incidents

Y80.1   Therapeutic (nonsurgical) and rehabilitative physical medicine devices associated with adverse incidents

Y80.2   Prosthetic and other implants, materials and accessory physical medicine devices associated with adverse incidents

Y80.3   Surgical instruments, materials and physical medicine devices (including sutures) associated with adverse incidents

Y80.8   Miscellaneous physical medicine devices associated with adverse incidents, not elsewhere classified

Y81   General- and plastic-surgery devices associated with adverse incidents

Y81.0   Diagnostic and monitoring general- and plastic-surgery devices associated with adverse incidents

Y81.1   Therapeutic (nonsurgical) and rehabilitative general- and plastic-surgery devices associated with adverse incidents

Y81.2   Prosthetic and other implants, materials and accessory general- and plastic-surgery devices associated with adverse incidents

Y81.3   Surgical instruments, materials and general- and plastic-surgery devices (including sutures) associated with adverse incidents

Y81.8   Miscellaneous general- and plastic-surgery devices associated with adverse incidents, not elsewhere classified

Y82   Other and unspecified medical devices associated with adverse incidents

Y82.8   Other medical devices associated with adverse incidents

Y82.9   Unspecified medical devices associated with adverse incidents

---

Add 4th-7th digits   Nonspecific code   Unspecified code   Manifestation code

SURGICAL AND OTHER MEDICAL PROCEDURES AS THE CAUSE OF ABNORMAL REACTION OF THE PATIENT, OR OF LATER COMPLICATION, WITHOUT MENTION OF MISADVENTURE AT THE TIME OF THE PROCEDURE (Y83-Y84)

Excludes1: misadventures to patients during surgical and medical care, classifiable to (Y62-Y69)

Excludes2: breakdown or malfunctioning of medical device (after implantation) (during procedure) (ongoing use) (Y70-Y82)

Y83 Surgical operation and other surgical procedures as the cause of abnormal reaction of the patient, or of later complication, without mention of misadventure at the time of the procedure

Y83.0 Surgical operation with transplant of whole organ as the cause of abnormal reaction of the patient, or of later complication, without mention of misadventure at the time of the procedure

Y83.1 Surgical operation with implant of artificial internal device as the cause of abnormal reaction of the patient, or of later complication, without mention of misadventure at the time of the procedure

Y83.2 Surgical operation with anastomosis, bypass or graft as the cause of abnormal reaction of the patient, or of later complication, without mention of misadventure at the time of the procedure

Y83.3 Surgical operation with formation of external stoma as the cause of abnormal reaction of the patient, or of later complication, without mention of misadventure at the time of the procedure

Y83.4 Other reconstructive surgery as the cause of abnormal reaction of the patient, or of later complication, without mention of misadventure at the time of the procedure

Y83.5 Amputation of limb(s) as the cause of abnormal reaction of the patient, or of later complication, without mention of misadventure at the time of the procedure

Y83.6 Removal of other organ (partial) (total) as the cause of abnormal reaction of the patient, or of later complication, without mention of misadventure at the time of the procedure

Y83.8 Other surgical procedures as the cause of abnormal reaction of the patient, or of later complication, without mention of misadventure at the time of the procedure

Y83.9 Surgical procedure, unspecified as the cause of abnormal reaction of the patient, or of later complication, without mention of misadventure at the time of the procedure

Y84 Other medical procedures as the cause of abnormal reaction of the patient, or of later complication, without mention of misadventure at the time of the procedure

Y84.0 Cardiac catheterization as the cause of abnormal reaction of the patient, or of later complication, without mention of misadventure at the time of the procedure

Y84.1 Kidney dialysis as the cause of abnormal reaction of the patient, or of later complication, without mention of misadventure at the time of the procedure

Y84.2 Radiological procedure and radiotherapy as the cause of abnormal reaction of the patient, or of later complication, without mention of misadventure at the time of the procedure

Y84.3 Shock therapy as the cause of abnormal reaction of the patient, or of later complication, without mention of misadventure at the time of the procedure

Y84.4 Aspiration of fluid as the cause of abnormal reaction of the patient, or of later complication, without mention of misadventure at the time of the procedure

Y84.5 Insertion of gastric or duodenal sound as the cause of abnormal reaction of the patient, or of later complication, without mention of misadventure at the time of the procedure

Y84.6 Urinary catheterization as the cause of abnormal reaction of the patient, or of later complication, without mention of misadventure at the time of the procedure

Y84.7 Blood-sampling as the cause of abnormal reaction of the patient, or of later complication, without mention of misadventure at the time of the procedure

Y84.8 Other medical procedures as the cause of abnormal reaction of the patient, or of later complication, without mention of misadventure at the time of the procedure

Y84.9 Medical procedure, unspecified as the cause of abnormal reaction of the patient, or of later complication, without mention of misadventure at the time of the procedure

SUPPLEMENTARY FACTORS RELATED TO CAUSES OF MORBIDITY CLASSIFIED ELSEWHERE (Y90-Y99)

Note: These categories may be used to provide supplementary information concerning causes of morbidity. They are not to be used for single-condition coding.

Y90 Evidence of alcohol involvement determined by blood alcohol level

Code first any associated alcohol related disorders (F10)

Y90.0 Blood alcohol level of less than 20 mg/100 ml

Y90.1 Blood alcohol level of 20-39 mg/100 ml

Y90.2 Blood alcohol level of 40-59 mg/100 ml

Y90.3 Blood alcohol level of 60-79 mg/100 ml

Y90.4 Blood alcohol level of 80-99 mg/100 ml

Y90.5 Blood alcohol level of 100-119 mg/100 ml

Y90.6 Blood alcohol level of 120-199 mg/100 ml

Y90.7 Blood alcohol level of 200-239 mg/100 ml

Y90.8 Blood alcohol level of 240 mg/100 ml or more

Y90.9 Presence of alcohol in blood, level not specified

Y92 Place of occurrence of the external cause

The following category is for use, when relevant, to identify the place of occurrence of the external cause. Use in conjunction with an activity code.

Place of occurrence should be recorded only at the initial encounter for treatment

Y92.0 Non-institutional (private) residence as the place of occurrence of the external cause

Excludes1: abandoned or derelict house (Y92.89)

home under construction but not yet occupied (Y92.6-)

institutional place of residence (Y92.1-)

Y92.00 Unspecified non-institutional (private) residence as the place of occurrence of the external cause

Y92.000 Kitchen of unspecified non-institutional (private) residence as the place of occurrence of the external cause

Y92.001 Dining room of unspecified non-institutional (private) residence as the place of occurrence of the external cause

Y92.002 Bathroom of unspecified non-institutional (private) residence

single-family (private) house as the place of occurrence of the external cause

Y92.003 Bedroom of unspecified non-institutional (private) residence as the place of occurrence of the external cause

Y92.007 Garden or yard of unspecified non-institutional (private) residence as the place of occurrence of the external cause

Y92.008 Other place in unspecified non-institutional (private) residence as the place of occurrence of the external cause

Y92.009 Unspecified place in unspecified non-institutional (private) residence as the place of occurrence of the external cause

Home (NOS) as the place of occurrence of the external cause

Y92.01 Single-family non-institutional (private) house as the place of occurrence of the external cause

Farmhouse as the place of occurrence of the external cause

Excludes1: barn (Y92.71)

chicken coop or hen house (Y92.72)

farm field (Y92.73)

orchard (Y92.74)

single family mobile home or trailer (Y92.02-)

slaughter house (Y92.86)

Y92.010 Kitchen of single-family (private) house as the place of occurrence of the external cause

Y92.011 Dining room of single-family (private) house as the place of occurrence of the external cause

Y92.012 Bathroom of single-family (private) house as the place of occurrence of the external cause

Y92.013 Bedroom of single-family (private) house as the place of occurrence of the external cause

Y92.014 Private driveway to single-family (private) house as the place of occurrence of the external cause

Y92.015 Private garage of single-family (private) house as the place of occurrence of the external cause

Y92.016 Swimming-pool in single-family (private) house or garden as the place of occurrence of the external cause

Y92.017 Garden or yard in single-family (private) house as the place of occurrence of the external cause

Y92.018 Other place in single-family (private) house as the place of occurrence of the external cause

Y92.019 Unspecified place in single-family (private) house as the place of occurrence of the external cause

Y92.02 Mobile home as the place of occurrence of the external cause

Y92.020 Kitchen in mobile home as the place of occurrence of the external cause

Y92.021 Dining room in mobile home as the place of occurrence of the external cause

Y92.022 Bathroom in mobile home as the place of occurrence of the external cause

Y92.023 Bedroom in mobile home as the place of occurrence of the external cause

Y92.024 Driveway of mobile home as the place of occurrence of the external cause

Y92.025 Garage of mobile home as the place of occurrence of the external cause

Y92.026 Swimming-pool of mobile home as the place of occurrence of the external cause

Y92.027 Garden or yard of mobile home as the place of occurrence of the external cause

Y92.028 Other place in mobile home as the place of occurrence of the external cause

Y92.029 Unspecified place in mobile home as the place of occurrence of the external cause

Y92.03 Apartment as the place of occurrence of the external cause

Condominium as the place of occurrence of the external cause

Co-op apartment as the place of occurrence of the external cause

Y92.030 Kitchen in apartment as the place of occurrence of the external cause

Y92.031 Bathroom in apartment as the place of occurrence of the external cause

Y92.032 Bedroom in apartment as the place of occurrence of the external cause

Y92.038 Other place in apartment as the place of occurrence of the external cause

Y92.039 Unspecified place in apartment as the place of occurrence of the external cause

Y92.04 Boarding-house as the place of occurrence of the external cause

Y92.040 Kitchen in boarding-house as the place of occurrence of the external cause

Y92.041 Bathroom in boarding-house as the place of occurrence of the external cause

Y92.042 Bedroom in boarding-house as the place of occurrence of the external cause

Y92.043 Driveway of boarding-house as the place of occurrence of the external cause

Y92.044 Garage of boarding-house as the place of occurrence of the external cause

Y92.045 Swimming-pool of boarding-house as the place of occurrence of the external cause

Y92.046 Garden or yard of boarding-house as the place of occurrence of the external cause

Y92.048 Other place in boarding-house as the place of occurrence of the external cause

Y92.049 Unspecified place in boarding-house as the place of occurrence of the external cause

Y92.09 Other non-institutional residence as the place of occurrence of the external cause

Y92.090 Kitchen in other non-institutional residence as the place of occurrence of the external cause

Y92.091 Bathroom in other non-institutional residence as the place of occurrence of the external cause

Y92.092 Bedroom in other non-institutional residence as the place of occurrence of the external cause

Y92.093 Driveway of other non-institutional residence as the place of occurrence of the external cause

Y92.094 Garage of other non-institutional residence as the place of occurrence of the external cause

Y92.095 Swimming-pool of other non-institutional residence as the place of occurrence of the external cause

Y92.096 Garden or yard of other non-institutional residence as the place of occurrence of the external cause

Y92.098 Other place in other non-institutional residence as the place of occurrence of the external cause

Y92.099 Unspecified place in other non-institutional residence as the place of occurrence of the external cause

Y92.1 Institutional (nonprivate) residence as the place of occurrence of the external cause

Y92.10 Unspecified residential institution as the place of occurrence of the external cause

Y92.11 Children's home and orphanage as the place of occurrence of the external cause

Y92.110 Kitchen in children's home and orphanage as the place of occurrence of the external cause

Y92.111 Bathroom in children's home and orphanage as the place of occurrence of the external cause

Y92.112 Bedroom in children's home and orphanage as the place of occurrence of the external cause

Y92.113 Driveway of children's home and orphanage as the place of occurrence of the external cause

Y92.114 Garage of children's home and orphanage as the place of occurrence of the external cause

Y92.115 Swimming-pool of children's home and orphanage as the place of occurrence of the external cause

Y92.116 Garden or yard of children's home and orphanage as the place of occurrence of the external cause

Y92.118 Other place in children's home and orphanage as the place of occurrence of the external cause

Y92.119 Unspecified place in children's home and orphanage as the place of occurrence of the external cause

Y92.12 Nursing home as the place of occurrence of the external cause

Home for the sick as the place of occurrence of the external cause

Hospice as the place of occurrence of the external cause

Y92.120 Kitchen in nursing home as the place of occurrence of the external cause

Y92.121 Bathroom in nursing home as the place of occurrence of the external cause

Y92.122 Bedroom in nursing home as the place of occurrence of the external cause

Y92.123 Driveway of nursing home as the place of occurrence of the external cause

Y92.124 Garage of nursing home as the place of occurrence of the external cause

Y92.125 Swimming-pool of nursing home as the place of occurrence of the external cause

Y92.126 Garden or yard of nursing home as the place of occurrence of the external cause

Y92.128 Other place in nursing home as the place of occurrence of the external cause

Y92.129 Unspecified place in nursing home as the place of occurrence of the external cause

Y92.13 Military base as the place of occurrence of the external cause

Excludes1: military training grounds (Y92.83)

Y92.130 Kitchen on military base as the place of occurrence of the external cause

Y92.131 Mess hall on military base as the place of occurrence of the external cause

Y92.133 Barracks on military base as the place of occurrence of the external cause

Y92.135 Garage on military base as the place of occurrence of the external cause

Y92.136   Swimming-pool on military base as the place of occurrence of the external cause

Y92.137   Garden or yard on military base as the place of occurrence of the external cause

Y92.138   Other place on military base as the place of occurrence of the external cause

Y92.139   Unspecified place military base as the place of occurrence of the external cause

Y92.14   Prison as the place of occurrence of the external cause

Y92.140   Kitchen in prison as the place of occurrence of the external cause

Y92.141   Dining room in prison as the place of occurrence of the external cause

Y92.142   Bathroom in prison as the place of occurrence of the external cause

Y92.143   Cell of prison as the place of occurrence of the external cause

Y92.146   Swimming-pool of prison as the place of occurrence of the external cause

Y92.147   Courtyard of prison as the place of occurrence of the external cause

Y92.148   Other place in prison as the place of occurrence of the external cause

Y92.149   Unspecified place in prison as the place of occurrence of the external cause

Y92.15   Reform school as the place of occurrence of the external cause

Y92.150   Kitchen in reform school as the place of occurrence of the external cause

Y92.151   Dining room in reform school as the place of occurrence of the external cause

Y92.152   Bathroom in reform school as the place of occurrence of the external cause

Y92.153   Bedroom in reform school as the place of occurrence of the external cause

Y92.154   Driveway of reform school as the place of occurrence of the external cause

Y92.155   Garage of reform school as the place of occurrence of the external cause

Y92.156   Swimming-pool of reform school as the place of occurrence of the external cause

Y92.157   Garden or yard of reform school as the place of occurrence of the external cause

Y92.158   Other place in reform school as the place of occurrence of the external cause

Y92.159   Unspecified place in reform school as the place of occurrence of the external cause

Y92.16   School dormitory as the place of occurrence of the external cause

Excludes1: reform school as the place of occurrence of the external cause (Y92.15-)

school buildings and grounds as the place of occurrence of the external cause (Y92.2-)

school sports and athletic areas as the place of occurrence of the external cause (Y92.3-)

Y92.160   Kitchen in school dormitory as the place of occurrence of the external cause

Y92.161   Dining room in school dormitory as the place of occurrence of the external cause

Y92.162   Bathroom in school dormitory as the place of occurrence of the external cause

Y92.163   Bedroom in school dormitory as the place of occurrence of the external cause

Y92.168   Other place in school dormitory as the place of occurrence of the external cause

Y92.169   Unspecified place in school dormitory as the place of occurrence of the external cause

Y92.19   Other specified residential institution as the place of occurrence of the external cause

Y92.190   Kitchen in other specified residential institution as the place of occurrence of the external cause

Y92.191   Dining room in other specified residential institution as the place of occurrence of the external cause

Y92.192   Bathroom in other specified residential institution as the place of occurrence of the external cause

Y92.193   Bedroom in other specified residential institution as the place of occurrence of the external cause

Y92.194   Driveway of other specified residential institution as the place of occurrence of the external cause

Y92.195   Garage of other specified residential institution as the place of occurrence of the external cause

Y92.196   Pool of other specified residential institution as the place of occurrence of the external cause

Y92.197   Garden or yard of other specified residential institution as the place of occurrence of the external cause

Y92.198   Other place in other specified residential institution as the place of occurrence of the external cause

Y92.199   Unspecified place in other specified residential institution as the place of occurrence of the external cause

Y92.2   School, other institution and public administrative area as the place of occurrence of the external cause

Building and adjacent grounds used by the general public or by a particular group of the public

Excludes1: building under construction as the place of occurrence of the external cause (Y92.6)

residential institution as the place of occurrence of the external cause (Y92.1)

school dormitory as the place of occurrence of the external cause (Y92.16-)

sports and athletics area of schools as the place of occurrence of the external cause (Y92.3-)

Y92.21   School (private) (public) (state) as the place of occurrence of the external cause

Y92.210   Daycare center as the place of occurrence of the external cause

Y92.211   Elementary school as the place of occurrence of the external cause

Kindergarten as the place of occurrence of the external cause

Y92.212   Middle school as the place of occurrence of the external cause

Y92.213   High school as the place of occurrence of the external cause

Y92.214   College as the place of occurrence of the external cause

University as the place of occurrence of the external cause

Y92.215   Trade school as the place of occurrence of the external cause

Y92.218   Other school as the place of occurrence of the external cause

Y92.219   Unspecified school as the place of occurrence of the external cause

Y92.22   Religious institution as the place of occurrence of the external cause

Church as the place of occurrence of the external cause

Mosque as the place of occurrence of the external cause

Synagogue as the place of occurrence of the external cause

Y92.23   Hospital as the place of occurrence of the external cause

Excludes1: ambulatory (outpatient) health services establishments (Y92.53-)

home for the sick as the place of occurrence of the external cause (Y92.12-)

hospice as the place of occurrence of the external cause (Y92.12-)

nursing home as the place of occurrence of the external cause (Y92.12-)

Y92.230   Patient room in hospital as the place of occurrence of the external cause

Y92.231   Patient bathroom in hospital as the place of occurrence of the external cause

Y92.232   Corridor of hospital as the place of occurrence of the external cause

Y92.233   Cafeteria of hospital as the place of occurrence of the external cause

Y92.234   Operating room of hospital as the place of occurrence of the external cause

Y92.238   Other place in hospital as the place of occurrence of the external cause

Y92.239   Unspecified place in hospital as the place of occurrence of the external cause

Y92.24   Public administrative building as the place of occurrence of the external cause

Y92.240   Courthouse as the place of occurrence of the external cause

Y92.241   Library as the place of occurrence of the external cause

Y92.242   Post office as the place of occurrence of the external cause

Y92.243   City hall as the place of occurrence of the external cause

Y92.248   Other public administrative building as the place of occurrence of the external cause

Y92.25   Cultural building as the place of occurrence of the external cause

Y92.250   Art Gallery as the place of occurrence of the external cause

Y92.251   Museum as the place of occurrence of the external cause

Y92.252   Music hall as the place of occurrence of the external cause

Y92.253   Opera house as the place of occurrence of the external cause

Y92.254   Theater (live) as the place of occurrence of the external cause

Y92.258   Other cultural public building as the place of occurrence of the external cause

Y92.26   Movie house or cinema as the place of occurrence of the external cause

Y92.29   Other specified public building as the place of occurrence of the external cause

Assembly hall as the place of occurrence of the external cause

Clubhouse as the place of occurrence of the external cause

Y92.3   Sports and athletics area as the place of occurrence of the external cause

Y92.31   Athletic court as the place of occurrence of the external cause

Excludes1: tennis court in private home or garden (Y92.09)

Y92.310   Basketball court as the place of occurrence of the external cause

Y92.311   Squash court as the place of occurrence of the external cause

Y92.312   Tennis court as the place of occurrence of the external cause

Y92.318   Other athletic court as the place of occurrence of the external cause

Y92.32   Athletic field as the place of occurrence of the external cause

Y92.320   Baseball field as the place of occurrence of the external cause

Y92.321 Football field as the place of occurrence of the external cause

Y92.322 Soccer field as the place of occurrence of the external cause

Y92.328 Other athletic field as the place of occurrence of the external cause

Cricket field as the place of occurrence of the external cause

Hockey field as the place of occurrence of the external cause

Y92.33 Skating rink as the place of occurrence of the external cause

Y92.330 Ice skating rink (indoor) (outdoor) as the place of occurrence of the external cause

Y92.331 Roller skating rink as the place of occurrence of the external cause

Y92.34 Swimming pool (public) as the place of occurrence of the external cause

Excludes1: swimming pool in private home or garden (Y92.016)

Y92.39 Other specified sports and athletic area as the place of occurrence of the external cause

Golf-course as the place of occurrence of the external cause

Gymnasium as the place of occurrence of the external cause

Riding-school as the place of occurrence of the external cause

Stadium as the place of occurrence of the external cause

Y92.4 Street, highway and other paved roadways as the place of occurrence of the external cause

Excludes1: private driveway of residence (Y92.014, Y92.024, Y92.043, Y92.093, Y92.113, Y92.123, Y92.154, Y92.194)

Y92.41 Street and highway as the place of occurrence of the external cause

Y92.410 Unspecified street and highway as the place of occurrence of the external cause

Road NOS as the place of occurrence of the external cause

Y92.411 Interstate highway as the place of occurrence of the external cause

Freeway as the place of occurrence of the external cause

Motorway as the place of occurrence of the external cause

Y92.412 Parkway as the place of occurrence of the external cause

Y92.413 State road as the place of occurrence of the external cause

Y92.414 Local residential or business street as the place of occurrence of the external cause

Y92.415 Exit ramp or entrance ramp of street or highway as the place of occurrence of the external cause

Y92.48 Other paved roadways as the place of occurrence of the external cause

Y92.480 Sidewalk as the place of occurrence of the external cause

Y92.481 Parking lot as the place of occurrence of the external cause

Y92.482 Bike path as the place of occurrence of the external cause

Y92.488 Other paved roadways as the place of occurrence of the external cause

Y92.5 Trade and service area as the place of occurrence of the external cause

Excludes1: garage in private home (Y92.015)

schools and other public administration buildings (Y92.2-)

Y92.51 Private commercial establishments as the place of occurrence of the external cause

Y92.510 Bank as the place of occurrence of the external cause

Y92.511 Restaurant or café as the place of occurrence of the external cause

Y92.512 Supermarket, store or market as the place of occurrence of the external cause

Y92.513 Shop (commercial) as the place of occurrence of the external cause

Y92.52 Service areas as the place of occurrence of the external cause

Y92.520 Airport as the place of occurrence of the external cause

Y92.521 Bus station as the place of occurrence of the external cause

Y92.522 Railway station as the place of occurrence of the external cause

Y92.523 Highway rest stop as the place of occurrence of the external cause

Y92.524 Gas station as the place of occurrence of the external cause

Petroleum station as the place of occurrence of the external cause

Service station as the place of occurrence of the external cause

Y92.53 Ambulatory health services establishments as the place of occurrence of the external cause

Y92.530 Ambulatory surgery center as the place of occurrence of the external cause

Outpatient surgery center, including that connected with a hospital as the place of occurrence of the external cause

Same day surgery center, including that connected with a hospital as the place of occurrence of the external cause

Y92.531 Health care provider office as the place of occurrence of the external cause

Physician office as the place of occurrence of the external cause

Y92.532 Urgent care center as the place of occurrence of the external cause

Y92.538 Other ambulatory health services establishments as the place of occurrence of the external cause

Y92.59 Other trade areas as the place of occurrence of the external cause

Office building as the place of occurrence of the external cause

Casino as the place of occurrence of the external cause

Garage (commercial) as the place of occurrence of the external cause

Hotel as the place of occurrence of the external cause

Radio or television station as the place of occurrence of the external cause

Shopping mall as the place of occurrence of the external cause

Warehouse as the place of occurrence of the external cause

Y92.6 Industrial and construction area as the place of occurrence of the external cause

Y92.61 Building [any] under construction as the place of occurrence of the external cause

Y92.62 Dock or shipyard as the place of occurrence of the external cause

Dockyard as the place of occurrence of the external cause

Dry dock as the place of occurrence of the external cause

Shipyard as the place of occurrence of the external cause

Y92.63 Factory as the place of occurrence of the external cause

Factory building as the place of occurrence of the external cause

Factory premises as the place of occurrence of the external cause

Industrial yard as the place of occurrence of the external cause

Y92.64 Mine or pit as the place of occurrence of the external cause

Mine as the place of occurrence of the external cause

Y92.65 Oil rig as the place of occurrence of the external cause

Pit (coal) (gravel) (sand) as the place of occurrence of the external cause

Y92.69 Other specified industrial and construction area as the place of occurrence of the external cause

Gasworks as the place of occurrence of the external cause

Power-station (coal) (nuclear) (oil) as the place of occurrence of the external cause

Tunnel under construction as the place of occurrence of the external cause

Workshop as the place of occurrence of the external cause

Y92.7 Farm as the place of occurrence of the external cause

Ranch as the place of occurrence of the external cause

Excludes1: farmhouse and home premises of farm (Y92.01-)

Y92.71 Barn as the place of occurrence of the external cause

Y92.72 Chicken coop as the place of occurrence of the external cause

Hen house as the place of occurrence of the external cause

Y92.73 Farm field as the place of occurrence of the external cause

Y92.74 Orchard as the place of occurrence of the external cause

Y92.79 Other farm location as the place of occurrence of the external cause

Y92.8 Other places as the place of occurrence of the external cause

Y92.81 Transport vehicle as the place of occurrence of the external cause

Excludes1: transport accidents (V00-V99)

Y92.810 Car as the place of occurrence of the external cause

Y92.811 Bus as the place of occurrence of the external cause

Y92.812 Truck as the place of occurrence of the external cause

Y92.813 Airplane as the place of occurrence of the external cause

Y92.814 Boat as the place of occurrence of the external cause

Y92.815 Train as the place of occurrence of the external cause

Y92.816 Subway car as the place of occurrence of the external cause

Y92.818 Other transport vehicle as the place of occurrence of the external cause

Y92.82 Wilderness area

Y92.820 Desert as the place of occurrence of the external cause

Y92.821 Forest as the place of occurrence of the external cause

Y92.828 Other wilderness area as the place of occurrence of the external cause

Swamp as the place of occurrence of the external cause

Mountain as the place of occurrence of the external cause

Marsh as the place of occurrence of the external cause

Prairie as the place of occurrence of the external cause

Y92.83 Recreation area as the place of occurrence of the external cause

Y92.830 Public park as the place of occurrence of the external cause

Y92.831 Amusement park as the place of occurrence of the external cause

Y92.832 Beach as the place of occurrence of the external cause

Seashore as the place of occurrence of the external cause

 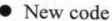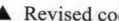

Y92.833	**Campsite as the place of occurrence of the external cause**
Y92.834	**Zoological garden (Zoo) as the place of occurrence of the external cause**
Y92.838	**Other recreation area as the place of occurrence of the external cause**
Y92.84	**Military training ground as the place of occurrence of the external cause**
Y92.85	**Railroad track as the place of occurrence of the external cause**
Y92.86	**Slaughter house as the place of occurrence of the external cause**
Y92.89	**Other specified places as the place of occurrence of the external cause**

Derelict house as the place of occurrence of the external cause

Y92.9 Unspecified place or not applicable

Y93 Activity codes

Note: Category Y93 is provided for use to indicate the activity of the person seeking healthcare for an injury or health condition, such as a heart attack while shoveling snow, which resulted from, or was contributed to, by the activity. These codes are appropriate for use for both acute injuries, such as those from chapter 19, and conditions that are due to the long-term, cumulative effects of an activity, such as those from chapter 13. They are also appropriate for use with external cause codes for cause and intent if identifying the activity provides additional information on the event. These codes should be used in conjunction with codes for external cause status (Y99) and place of occurrence (Y92).

This section contains the following broad activity categories: Y93.0

Activities involving walking and running Y93.1

Activities involving water and water craft Y93.2

Activities involving ice and snow Y93.3

Activities involving climbing, rappelling, and jumping off Y93.4

Activities involving dancing and other rhythmic movement Y93.5

Activities involving other sports and athletics played individually Y93.6

Activities involving other sports and athletics played as a team or group Y93.7

Activities involving other specified sports and athletics Y93.A

Activities involving other cardiorespiratory exercise Y93.B

Activities involving other muscle strengthening exercises Y93.C

Activities involving computer technology and electronic devices Y93.D

Activities involving arts and handcrafts Y93.E

Activities involving personal hygiene and interior property and clothing maintenance Y93.F

Activities involving caregiving Y93.G

Activities involving food preparation, cooking and grilling Y93.H

Activities involving exterior property and land maintenance, building and construction Y93.I

Activities involving roller coasters and other types of external motion Y93.J

Activities involving playing musical instrument Y93.K

Activities involving animal care Y93.8

Activities, other specified Y93.9

Activity, unspecified

Y93.0 Activities involving walking and running

Excludes1: activity, walking an animal (Y93.K1)

activity, walking or running on a treadmill (Y93.A1)

Y93.01 Activity, walking, marching and hiking

Activity, walking, marching and hiking on level or elevated terrain

Excludes1: activity, mountain climbing (Y93.31)

Y93.02 Activity, running

Y93.1 Activities involving water and water craft

Excludes1: activities involving ice (Y93.2-)

Y93.11 Activity, swimming

Y93.12 Activity, springboard and platform diving

Y93.13 Activity, water polo

Y93.14 Activity, water aerobics and water exercise

Y93.15 Activity, underwater diving and snorkeling

Activity, SCUBA diving

Y93.16 Activity, rowing, canoeing, kayaking, rafting and tubing

Activity, canoeing, kayaking, rafting and tubing in calm and turbulent water

Y93.17 Activity, water skiing and wake boarding

Y93.18 Activity, surfing, windsurfing and boogie boarding

Activity, water sliding

Y93.19 Activity, other involving water and watercraft

Activity involving water NOS

Activity, parasailing

Activity, water survival training and testing

Y93.2 Activities involving ice and snow

Excludes1: activity, shoveling ice and snow (Y93.H1)

Y93.21 Activity, ice skating

Activity, figure skating (singles) (pairs)

Activity, ice dancing

Excludes1: activity, ice hockey (Y93.22)

Y93.22 Activity, ice hockey

Y93.23 Activity, snow (alpine) (downhill) skiing, snow boarding, sledding, tobogganing and snow tubing

Excludes1: activity, cross country skiing (Y93.24)

Y93.24 Activity, cross country skiing

Activity, nordic skiing

Y93.29 Activity, other involving ice and snow

Activity involving ice and snow NOS

Y93.3 Activities involving climbing, rappelling and jumping off

Excludes1: activity, hiking on level or elevated terrain (Y93.01)

activity, jumping rope (Y93.56)

activity, trampoline jumping (Y93.44)

Y93.31 Activity, mountain climbing, rock climbing and wall climbing

Y93.32 Activity, rappelling

Y93.33 Activity, BASE jumping

Activity, Building, Antenna, Span, Earth jumping

Y93.34 Activity, bungee jumping

Y93.35 Activity, hang gliding

Y93.39 Activity, other involving climbing, rappelling and jumping off

Y93.4 Activities involving dancing and other rhythmic movement

Excludes1: activity, martial arts (Y93.75)

Y93.41 Activity, dancing

Y93.42 Activity, yoga

Y93.43 Activity, gymnastics

Activity, rhythmic gymnastics

Excludes1: activity, trampolining (Y93.44)

Y93.44 Activity, trampolining

Y93.45 Activity, cheerleading

Y93.49 Activity, other involving dancing and other rhythmic movements

Y93.5 Activities involving other sports and athletics played individually

Excludes1: activity, dancing (Y93.41)

activity, gymnastic (Y93.43)

activity, trampolining (Y93.44)

activity, yoga (Y93.42)

Y93.51 Activity, roller skating (inline) and skateboarding

Y93.52 Activity, horseback riding

Y93.53 Activity, golf

Y93.54 Activity, bowling

Y93.55 Activity, bike riding

Y93.56 Activity, jumping rope

Y93.57 Activity, non-running track and field events

Excludes1: activity, running (any form) (Y93.02)

Y93.59 Activity, other involving other sports and athletics played individually

Excludes1: activities involving climbing, rappelling, and jumping (Y93.3-)

activities involving ice and snow (Y93.2-)

activities involving walking and running (Y93.0-)

activities involving water and watercraft (Y93.1-)

Y93.6 Activities involving other sports and athletics played as a team or group

Excludes1: activity, ice hockey (Y93.22)

activity, water polo (Y93.13)

Y93.61 Activity, american tackle football

Activity, football NOS

Y93.62 Activity, american flag or touch football

Y93.63 Activity, rugby

Y93.64 Activity, baseball

Activity, softball

Y93.65 Activity, lacrosse and field hockey

Y93.66 Activity, soccer

Y93.67 Activity, basketball

Y93.68 Activity, volleyball (beach) (court)

Y93.6A Activity, physical games generally associated with school recess, summer camp and children

Activity, capture the flag

Activity, dodge ball

Activity, four square

Activity, kickball

Y93.69 Activity, other involving other sports and athletics played as a team or group

Activity, cricket

Y93.7 Activities involving other specified sports and athletics

Y93.71 Activity, boxing

Y93.72 Activity, wrestling

Y93.73 Activity, racquet and hand sports

Activity, handball

Activity, racquetball

Activity, squash

Activity, tennis

Y93.74 Activity, frisbee

Activity, ultimate frisbee

Y93.75 Activity, martial arts

Activity, combatives

Y93.79 Activity, other specified sports and athletics

Excludes1: sports and athletics activities specified in categories Y93.0-Y93.6

Y93.A Activities involving other cardiorespiratory exercise

Activities involving physical training

Y93.A1 Activity, exercise machines primarily for cardiorespiratory conditioning

Activity, elliptical and stepper machines

Activity, stationary bike

Activity, treadmill

Y93.A2 Activity, calisthenics

Activity, jumping jacks

Activity, warm up and cool down

Y93.A3 Activity, aerobic and step exercise

Y93.A4 Activity, circuit training

Y93.A5 Activity, obstacle course

Activity, challenge course

Activity, confidence course

Y93.A6 Activity, grass drills

Activity, guerilla drills

Y93.A9 Activity, other involving cardiorespiratory exercise

Excludes1: activities involving cardiorespiratory exercise specified in categories Y93.0-Y93.7

Y93.B Activities involving other muscle strengthening exercises

Y93.B1 Activity, exercise machines primarily for muscle strengthening

Y93.B2 Activity, push-ups, pull-ups, sit-ups

Y93.B3 Activity, free weights

Activity, barbells

Activity, dumbbells

Y93.B4 Activity, pilates

Y93.B9 Activity, other involving muscle strengthening exercises

Excludes1: activities involving muscle strengthening specified in categories Y93.0-Y93.A

Y93.C Activities involving computer technology and electronic devices

Excludes1: activity, electronic musical keyboard or instruments (Y93.J-)

Y93.C1 Activity, computer keyboarding

Activity, electronic game playing using keyboard or other stationary device

Y93.C2 Activity, hand held interactive electronic device

Activity, cellular telephone and communication device

Activity, electronic game playing using interactive device

Excludes1: activity, electronic game playing using keyboard or other stationary device (Y93.C1)

Y93.C9 Activity, other involving computer technology and electronic devices

Y93.D Activities involving arts and handcrafts

Excludes1: activities involving playing musical instrument (Y93.J-)

Y93.D1 Activity, knitting and crocheting

Y93.D2 Activity, sewing

Y93.D3 Activity, furniture building and finishing

Activity, furniture repair

Y93.D9 Activity, other involving arts and handcrafts

Y93.E Activities involving personal hygiene and interior property and clothing maintenance

Excludes1: activities involving cooking and grilling (Y93.G-)

activities involving exterior property and land maintenance, building and construction (Y93.H-)

activities involving caregiving (Y93.F-)

activity, dishwashing (Y93.G1)

activity, food preparation (Y93.G1)

activity, gardening (Y93.H2)

Y93.E1 Activity, personal bathing and showering

Y93.E2 Activity, laundry

Y93.E3 Activity, vacuuming

Y93.E4 Activity, ironing

Y93.E5 Activity, floor mopping and cleaning

Y93.E6 Activity, residential relocation

Activity, packing up and unpacking involved in moving to a new residence

Y93.E8 Activity, other personal hygiene

Y93.E9 Activity, other interior property and clothing maintenance

Y93.F Activities involving caregiving

Activity involving the provider of caregiving

Y93.F1 Activity, caregiving, bathing

Y93.F2 Activity, caregiving, lifting

Y93.F9 Activity, other caregiving

Y93.G Activities involving food preparation, cooking and grilling

Y93.G1 Activity, food preparation and clean up

Activity, dishwashing

Y93.G2 Activity, grilling and smoking food

Y93.G3 Activity, cooking and baking

Activity, use of stove, oven and microwave oven

Y93.G9 Activity, other involving cooking and grilling

Y93.H Activities involving exterior property and land maintenance, building and construction

Y93.H1 Activity, digging, shoveling and raking

Activity, dirt digging

Activity, raking leaves

Activity, snow shoveling

Y93.H2 Activity, gardening and landscaping

Activity, pruning, trimming shrubs, weeding

Y93.H3 Activity, building and construction

Y93.H9 Activity, other involving exterior property and land maintenance, building and construction

Y93.I Activities involving roller coasters and other types of external motion

Y93.I1 Activity, roller coaster riding

Y93.I9 Activity, other involving external motion

Y93.J Activities involving playing musical instrument

Activity involving playing electric musical instrument

Y93.J1 Activity, piano playing

Activity, musical keyboard (electronic) playing

Y93.J2 Activity, drum and other percussion instrument playing

Y93.J3 Activity, string instrument playing

Y93.J4 Activity, winds and brass instrument playing

Y93.K Activities involving animal care

Excludes1: activity, horseback riding (Y93.52)

Y93.K1 Activity, walking an animal

Y93.K2 Activity, milking an animal

Y93.K3 Activity, grooming and shearing an animal

Y93.K9 Activity, other involving animal care

Y93.8 Activities, other specified

Y93.81 Activity, refereeing a sports activity

Y93.82 Activity, spectator at an event

Y93.83 Activity, rough housing and horseplay

Y93.84 Activity, sleeping

●**Y93.85 Activity, choking game**

Activity, blackout game

Activity, fainting game

Activity, pass out game

Y93.89 Activity, other specified

Y93.9 Activity, unspecified

Y95 Nosocomial condition

Y99 External cause status

Note: A single code from category Y99 should be used in conjunction with the external cause code(s) assigned to a record to indicate the status of the person at the time the event occurred.

Y99.0 Civilian activity done for income or pay

Civilian activity done for financial or other compensation

Excludes1: military activity (Y99.1)

volunteer activity (Y99.2)

Y99.1 Military activity

Excludes1: activity of off duty military personnel (Y99.8)

Y99.2 Volunteer activity

Excludes1: activity of child or other family member assisting in compensated work **of other** family member (Y99.8)

Y99.8 Other external cause status

Add 4th-7th digits   Nonspecific code   Unspecified code   Manifestation code   1107

Activity NEC

Activity of child or other family member assisting in compensated work **of other** family member

Hobby not done for income

Leisure activity

Off-duty activity of military personnel

Recreation or sport not for income or while a student

Student activity

Excludes1: civilian activity done for income or compensation (Y99.0)

military activity (Y99.1)

Y99.9 **Unspecified external cause status**

Chapter 21; Factors Influencing Health Status And Contact With Health Services (Z00-Z99)

DEFINITIONS

This chapter includes definitions of selected key words, terms and phrases and coding alerts for adding points to the clinical domain, and references to coding late effects where appropriate. An example from this chapter is as follows:

Z14   Genetic carrier
    Definition: A genetic carrier (or just carrier), is a person who has inherited a genetic trait or mutation but does not display that trait or show symptoms of the disease. Carriers are, however, able to pass the gene onto their offspring, who may then express the gene.

MULTIPLE CODING FOR A SINGLE CONDITION

In addition to the etiology/manifestation convention that requires two codes to fully describe a single condition that affects multiple body systems, there are other single conditions that also require more than one code. "Use additional code" notes are found in the Tabular List at codes that are not part of an etiology/manifestation pair where a secondary code is useful to fully describe a condition. The sequencing rule is the same as the etiology/manifestation pair, "use additional code" indicates that a secondary code should be added.

For example, for bacterial infections that are not included in chapter 1, a secondary code from category B95, Streptococcus, Staphylococcus, and Enterococcus, as the cause of diseases classified elsewhere, or B96, Other bacterial agents as the cause of diseases classified elsewhere, may be required to identify the bacterial organism causing the infection. A "use additional code" note will normally be found at the infectious disease code, indicating a need for the organism code to be added as a secondary code.

"Code first" notes are also under certain codes that are not specifically manifestation codes but may be due to an underlying cause. When there is a "code first" note and an underlying condition is present, the underlying condition should be sequenced first.

"Code, if applicable, any causal condition first", notes indicate that this code may be assigned as a principal diagnosis when the causal condition is unknown or not applicable. If a causal condition is known, then the code for that condition should be sequenced as the principal or first-listed diagnosis.

Multiple codes may be needed for sequela, complication codes and obstetric codes to more fully describe a condition. See the specific guidelines for these conditions for further instruction.

COMBINATION CODE

A combination code is a single code used to classify: Two diagnoses, or a diagnosis with an associated secondary process (manifestation) A diagnosis with an associated complication

Combination codes are identified by referring to subterm entries in the Alphabetic Index and by reading the inclusion and exclusion notes in the Tabular List.

Assign only the combination code when that code fully identifies the diagnostic conditions involved or when the Alphabetic Index so directs. Multiple coding should not be used when the classification provides a combination code that clearly identifies all of the elements documented in the diagnosis. When the combination code lacks necessary specificity in describing the manifestation or complication, an additional code should be used as a secondary code.

SEQUELA (LATE EFFECTS)

A sequela is the residual effect (condition produced) after the acute phase of an illness or injury has terminated. There is no time limit on when a sequela code can be used. The residual may be apparent early, such as in cerebral infarction, or it may occur months or years later, such as that due to a previous injury. Coding of sequela generally requires two codes sequenced in the following order: The condition or nature of the sequela is sequenced first.

The sequela code is sequenced second.

An exception to the above guidelines are those instances where the code for the sequela is followed by a manifestation code identified in the Tabular List and title, or the sequela code has been expanded (at the fourth, fifth or sixth character levels) to include the manifestation(s). The code for the acute phase of an illness or injury that led to the sequela is never used with a code for the late effect.

Note: The chapter specific guidelines provide additional information about the use of Z codes for specified encounters.

USE OF Z CODES IN ANY HEALTHCARE SETTING

Z codes are for use in any healthcare setting. Z codes may be used as either a first-listed (principal diagnosis code in the inpatient setting) or secondary code, depending on the circumstances of the encounter. Certain Z codes may only be used as first-listed or principal diagnosis.

Z CODES INDICATE A REASON FOR AN ENCOUNTER

Z codes are not procedure codes. A corresponding procedure code must accompany a Z code to describe any procedure performed.

CATEGORIES OF Z CODES

1) Contact/Exposure

Category Z20 indicates contact with, and suspected exposure to, communicable diseases. These codes are for patients who do not show any sign or symptom of a disease but are suspected to have been exposed to it by close personal contact with an infected individual or are in an area where a disease is epidemic.

Category Z77, Other contact with and (suspected) exposures hazardous to health, indicates contact with and suspected exposures hazardous to health.

Contact/exposure codes may be used as a first-listed code to explain an encounter for testing, or, more commonly, as a secondary code to identify a potential risk.

2) Inoculations and vaccinations

Code Z23 is for encounters for inoculations and vaccinations. It indicates that a patient is being seen to receive a prophylactic inoculation against a disease. Procedure codes are required to identify the actual administration of the injection and the type(s) of immunizations given. Code Z23 may be used as a secondary code if the inoculation is given as a routine part of preventive health care, such as a well-baby visit.

3) Status

Status codes indicate that a patient is either a carrier of a disease or has the sequelae or residual of a past disease or condition. This includes such things as the presence of prosthetic or mechanical devices resulting from past treatment. A status code is informative, because the status may affect the course of treatment and its outcome. A status code is distinct from a history code. The history code indicates that the patient no longer has the condition.

A status code should not be used with a diagnosis code from one of the body system chapters, if the diagnosis code includes the information provided by the status code. For example, code Z94.1, Heart transplant status, should not be used with a code from subcategory T86.2, Complications of heart transplant. The status code does not provide additional information. The complication code indicates that the patient is a heart transplant patient.

For encounters for weaning from a mechanical ventilator, assign a code from subcategory J96.1, Chronic respiratory failure, followed by code Z99.11, Dependence on respirator [ventilator] status.

The status Z codes/categories are:

Z14   Genetic carrier

Genetic carrier status indicates that a person carries a gene, associated with a particular disease, which may be passed to offspring who may develop that disease. The person does not have the disease and is not at risk of developing the disease.

Z15   Genetic susceptibility to disease

Genetic susceptibility indicates that a person has a gene that increases the risk of that person developing the disease.

Codes from category Z15 should not be used as principal or first-listed codes. If the patient has the condition to which he/she is susceptible, and that condition is the reason for the encounter, the code for the current condition should be sequenced first. If the patient is being seen for follow-up after completed treatment for this condition, and the condition no longer exists, a follow-up code should be sequenced first, followed by the appropriate personal history and genetic susceptibility codes. If the purpose of the encounter is genetic counseling associated with procreative management, code Z31.5, Encounter for genetic counseling, should be assigned as the first-listed code, followed by a code from category Z15. Additional codes should be assigned for any applicable family or personal history.

Z16   Resistance to antimicrobial drugs

This code indicates that a patient has a condition that is resistant to antimicrobial drug treatment. Sequence the infection code first.

Z17   Estrogen receptor status

Z18   Retained foreign body fragments

Z19   Hormone sensitivity malignancy status

Z21   Asymptomatic HIV infection status

This code indicates that a patient has tested positive for HIV but has manifested no signs or symptoms of the disease.

Z22   Carrier of infectious disease

Carrier status indicates that a person harbors the specific organisms of a disease without manifest symptoms and is capable of transmitting the infection.

Z28.3   Underimmunization status

Z33.1   Pregnant state, incidental

This code is a secondary code only for use when the pregnancy is in no way complicating the reason for visit. Otherwise, a code from the obstetric chapter is required.

Z66   Do not resuscitate

This code may be used when it is documented by the provider that a patient is on do not resuscitate status at any time during the stay.

Z67   Blood type

Z68   Body mass index (BMI)

As with all other secondary diagnosis codes, the BMI codes should only be assigned when they meet the definition of a reportable diagnosis (see Section III, Reporting Additional Diagnoses).

Z74.01   Bed confinement status

Z76.82   Awaiting organ transplant status

Z78   Other specified health status

Code Z78.1, Physical restraint status, may be used when it is documented by the provider that a patient has been put in restraints during the current encounter. Please note that this code should not be reported when it is documented by the provider that a patient is temporarily restrained during a procedure.

Z79   Long-term (current) drug therapy

Codes from this category indicate a patient's continuous use of a prescribed drug (including such things as aspirin therapy) for the long-term treatment of a condition or for prophylactic use. It is not for use for patients who have addictions to drugs. This subcategory is not for use of medications for detoxification or maintenance programs to prevent withdrawal symptoms in patients with drug dependence (e.g., methadone maintenance for opiate dependence). Assign the appropriate code for the drug dependence instead.

Assign a code from Z79 if the patient is receiving a medication for an extended period as a prophylactic measure (such as for the prevention of deep vein thrombosis) or as treatment of a chronic condition (such as arthritis) or a disease requiring a lengthy course of treatment (such as cancer). Do not assign a code from category Z79 for medication being administered for a brief period of time to treat an acute illness or injury (such as a course of antibiotics to treat acute bronchitis).

Z88   Allergy status to drugs, medicaments and biological substances

Except: Z88.9, Allergy status to unspecified drugs, medicaments and biological substances status

Z89   Acquired absence of limb

Z90   Acquired absence of organs, not elsewhere classified

Z91.0-   Allergy status, other than to drugs and biological substances

Z92.82   Status post administration of tPA (rtPA) in a different facility within the last 24 hours prior to admission to a current facility

Assign code Z92.82, Status post administration of tPA (rtPA) in a different facility within the last 24 hours prior to admission to current facility, as a secondary diagnosis when a patient is received by transfer into a facility and documentation indicates they were administered tissue plasminogen activator (tPA) within the last 24 hours prior to admission to the current facility.

This guideline applies even if the patient is still receiving the tPA at the time they are received into the current facility.

The appropriate code for the condition for which the tPA was administered (such as cerebrovascular disease or myocardial infarction) should be assigned first.

Code Z92.82 is only applicable to the receiving facility record and not to the transferring facility record.

Z93   Artificial opening status

Z94   Transplanted organ and tissue status

Z95   Presence of cardiac and vascular implants and grafts

Z96   Presence of other functional implants

Z97   Presence of other devices

Z98   Other postprocedural states

> Assign code Z98.85, Transplanted organ removal status, to indicate that a transplanted organ has been previously removed. This code should not be assigned for the encounter in which the transplanted organ is removed. The complication necessitating removal of the transplant organ should be assigned for that encounter.
>
> *See section I.C19. for information on the coding of organ transplant complications.*

Z99   Dependence on enabling machines and devices, not elsewhere classified

Note: Categories Z89-Z90 and Z93-Z99 are for use only if there are no complications or malfunctions of the organ or tissue replaced, the amputation site or the equipment on which the patient is dependent.

4) History (of)

There are two types of history Z codes, personal and family. Personal history codes explain a patient's past medical condition that no longer exists and is not receiving any treatment, but that has the potential for recurrence, and therefore may require continued monitoring.

Family history codes are for use when a patient has a family member(s) who has had a particular disease that causes the patient to be at higher risk of also contracting the disease.

Personal history codes may be used in conjunction with follow-up codes and family history codes may be used in conjunction with screening codes to explain the need for a test or procedure. History codes are also acceptable on any medical record regardless of the reason for visit. A history of an illness, even if no longer present, is important information that may alter the type of treatment ordered.

The history Z code categories are:

Z80   Family history of primary malignant neoplasm

Z81   Family history of mental and behavioral disorders

Z82   Family history of certain disabilities and chronic diseases (leading to disablement)

Z83   Family history of other specific disorders

Z84   Family history of other conditions

Z85   Personal history of malignant neoplasm

Z86   Personal history of certain other diseases

Z87   Personal history of other diseases and conditions

Z91.4-   Personal history of psychological trauma, not elsewhere classified

Z91.5   Personal history of self-harm

Z91.8-   Other specified personal risk factors, not elsewhere classified Exception:

Z91.83, Wandering in diseases classified elsewhere

Z92   Personal history of medical treatment

> Except: Z92.0, Personal history of contraception Except: Z92.82, Status post administration of tPA (rtPA) in a different facility within the last 24 hours prior to admission to a current facility

5) Screening

Screening is the testing for disease or disease precursors in seemingly well individuals so that early detection and treatment can be provided for those who test positive for the disease (e.g., screening mammogram).

The testing of a person to rule out or confirm a suspected diagnosis because the patient has some sign or symptom is a diagnostic examination, not a screening. In these cases, the sign or symptom is used to explain the reason for the test.

A screening code may be a first-listed code if the reason for the visit is specifically the screening exam. It may also be used as an additional code if the screening is done during an office visit for other health problems. A screening code is not necessary if the screening is inherent to a routine examination, such as a pap smear done during a routine pelvic examination.

Should a condition be discovered during the screening then the code for the condition may be assigned as an additional diagnosis.

The Z code indicates that a screening exam is planned. A procedure code is required to confirm that the screening was performed.

The screening Z codes/categories:

Z11   Encounter for screening for infectious and parasitic diseases

Z12   Encounter for screening for malignant neoplasms

Z13   Encounter for screening for other diseases and disorders

       Except: Z13.9, Encounter for screening, unspecified

Z36   Encounter for antenatal screening for mother

6)   Observation

There are three observation Z code categories. They are for use in very limited circumstances when a person is being observed for a suspected condition that is ruled out. The observation codes are not for use if an injury or illness or any signs or symptoms related to the suspected condition are present. In such cases the diagnosis/symptom code is used with the corresponding external cause code.

The observation codes are to be used as principal diagnosis only. The only exception to this is when the principal diagnosis is required to be a code from category Z38, Liveborn infants according to place of birth and type of delivery. Then a code from category Z05, Encounter for observation and evaluation of newborn for suspected diseases and conditions ruled out, is sequenced after the Z38 code. Additional codes may be used in addition to the observation code, but only if they are unrelated to the suspected condition being observed.

Codes from subcategory Z03.7, Encounter for suspected maternal and fetal conditions ruled out, may either be used as a first-listed or as an additional code assignment depending on the case. They are for use in very limited circumstances on a maternal record when an encounter is for a suspected maternal or fetal condition that is ruled out during that encounter (for example, a maternal or fetal condition may be suspected due to an abnormal test result). These codes should not be used when the condition is confirmed. In those cases, the confirmed condition should be coded. In addition, these codes are not for use if an illness or any signs or symptoms related to the suspected condition or problem are present. In such cases the diagnosis/symptom code is used.

Additional codes may be used in addition to the code from subcategory Z03.7, but only if they are unrelated to the suspected condition being evaluated.

Codes from subcategory Z03.7 may not be used for encounters for antenatal screening of mother. *See Section I.C.21. Screening.*

For encounters for suspected fetal condition that are inconclusive following testing and evaluation, assign the appropriate code from category O35, O36, O40 or O41.

The observation Z code categories:

Z03   Encounter for medical observation for suspected diseases and conditions ruled out

Z04   Encounter for examination and observation for other reasons

       Except: Z04.9, Encounter for examination and observation for unspecified reason

Z05   Encounter for observation and evaluation of newborn for suspected diseases and conditions ruled out

7)   Aftercare

Aftercare visit codes cover situations when the initial treatment of a disease has been performed and the patient requires continued care during the healing or recovery phase, or for the long-term consequences of the disease. The aftercare Z code should not be used if treatment is directed at a current, acute disease. The diagnosis code is to be used in these cases. Exceptions to this rule are codes Z51.0, Encounter for antineoplastic radiation therapy, and codes from subcategory Z51.1, Encounter for antineoplastic chemotherapy and immunotherapy. These codes are to be first-listed, followed by the diagnosis code when a patient's encounter is solely to receive radiation therapy, chemotherapy, or immunotherapy for the treatment of a neoplasm. If the reason for the encounter is more than one type of antineoplastic therapy, code Z51.0 and a code from subcategory Z51.1 may be assigned together, in which case one of these codes would be reported as a secondary diagnosis.

The aftercare Z codes should also not be used for aftercare for injuries. For aftercare of an injury, assign the acute injury code with the appropriate 7th character (for subsequent encounter).

The aftercare codes are generally first-listed to explain the specific reason for the encounter. An aftercare code may be used as an additional code when some type of aftercare is provided in addition to the reason for admission and no diagnosis code is applicable. An example of this would be the closure of a colostomy during an encounter for treatment of another condition.

Aftercare codes should be used in conjunction with other aftercare codes or diagnosis codes to provide better detail on the specifics of an aftercare encounter visit, unless otherwise directed by the classification. Should a patient receive multiple types of antineoplastic therapy during the same encounter, code Z51.0, Encounter for antineoplastic radiation therapy, and codes from subcategory Z51.1, Encounter for antineoplastic chemotherapy and immunotherapy, may be used together on a record. The sequencing of multiple aftercare codes depends on the circumstances of the encounter.

Certain aftercare Z code categories need a secondary diagnosis code to describe the resolving condition or sequelae. For others, the condition is included in the code title.

Additional Z code aftercare category terms include fitting and adjustment, and attention to artificial openings.

Status Z codes may be used with aftercare Z codes to indicate the nature of the aftercare. For example code Z95.1, Presence of aortocoronary bypass graft, may be used with code Z48.812, Encounter for surgical aftercare following surgery on the circulatory system, to indicate the surgery for which the aftercare is being performed. A status code should not be used when the aftercare code indicates the type of status, such as using Z43.0, Encounter for attention to tracheostomy, with Z93.0, Tracheostomy status.

The aftercare Z category/codes:

Z42   Encounter for plastic and reconstructive surgery following medical procedure or healed injury

Z43   Encounter for attention to artificial openings Z44 Encounter for fitting and adjustment of external prosthetic device

Z45   Encounter for adjustment and management of implanted device

Z46   Encounter for fitting and adjustment of other devices

Z47   Orthopedic aftercare

Z48   Encounter for other postprocedural aftercare

Z49   Encounter for care involving renal dialysis

Z51   Encounter for other aftercare and medical care

8) Follow-up

The follow-up codes are used to explain continuing surveillance following completed treatment of a disease, condition, or injury. They imply that the condition has been fully treated and no longer exists. They should not be confused with aftercare codes, or injury codes with a 7th character for subsequent encounter, that explain ongoing care of a healing condition or its sequelae. Follow-up codes may be used in conjunction with history codes to provide the full picture of the healed condition and its treatment. The follow-up code is sequenced first, followed by the history code.

A follow-up code may be used to explain multiple visits. Should a condition be found to have recurred on the follow-up visit, then the diagnosis code for the condition should be assigned in place of the follow-up code.

The follow-up Z code categories:

Z08   Encounter for follow-up examination after completed treatment for malignant neoplasm

Z09   Encounter for follow-up examination after completed treatment for conditions other than malignant neoplasm

Z39   Encounter for maternal postpartum care and examination

9) Donor

Codes in category Z52, Donors of organs and tissues, are used for living individuals who are donating blood or other body tissue. These codes are only for individuals donating for others, not for self-donations. They are not used to identify cadaveric donations.

10) Counseling

Counseling Z codes are used when a patient or family member receives assistance in the aftermath of an illness or injury, or when support is required in coping with family or social problems. They are not used in conjunction with a diagnosis code when the counseling component of care is considered integral to standard treatment.

The counseling Z codes/categories:

Z30.0- Encounter for general counseling and advice on contraception

Z31.5   Encounter for genetic counseling

Z31.6-	Encounter for general counseling and advice on procreation
Z32.2	Encounter for childbirth instruction
Z32.3	Encounter for childcare instruction
Z69	Encounter for mental health services for victim and perpetrator of abuse
Z70	Counseling related to sexual attitude, behavior and orientation
Z71	Persons encountering health services for other counseling and medical advice, not elsewhere classified
Z76.81	Expectant mother prebirth pediatrician visit

11) Encounters for Obstetrical and Reproductive Services

See Section I.C.15. Pregnancy, Childbirth, and the Puerperium, for further instruction on the use of these codes.

Z codes for pregnancy are for use in those circumstances when none of the problems or complications included in the codes from the Obstetrics chapter exist (a routine prenatal visit or postpartum care). Codes in category Z34, Encounter for supervision of normal pregnancy, are always first-listed and are not to be used with any other code from the OB chapter.

Codes in category Z3A, Weeks of gestation, may be assigned to provide additional information about the pregnancy. Category Z3A codes should not be assigned for pregnancies with abortive outcomes (categories O00-O08), elective termination of pregnancy (code Z33.32), nor for postpartum conditions, as category Z3A is not applicable to these conditions. The date of the admission should be used to determine weeks of gestation for inpatient admissions that encompass more than one gestational week.

The outcome of delivery, category Z37, should be included on all maternal delivery records. It is always a secondary code. Codes in category Z37 should not be used on the newborn record.

Z codes for family planning (contraceptive) or procreative management and counseling should be included on an obstetric record either during the pregnancy or the postpartum stage, if applicable.

Z codes/categories for obstetrical and reproductive services:

Z30	Encounter for contraceptive management
Z31	Encounter for procreative management
Z32.2	Encounter for childbirth instruction
Z32.3	Encounter for childcare instruction
Z33	Pregnant state
Z34	Encounter for supervision of normal pregnancy
Z36	Encounter for antenatal screening of mother
Z3A	Weeks of gestation
Z37	Outcome of delivery
Z39	Encounter for maternal postpartum care and examination
Z76.81	Expectant mother prebirth pediatrician visit

12) Newborns and Infants

See Section I.C.16. Newborn (Perinatal) Guidelines, for further instruction on the use of these codes.

Newborn Z codes/categories:

Z76.1	Encounter for health supervision and care of foundling
Z00.1-	Encounter for routine child health examination
Z38	Liveborn infants according to place of birth and type of delivery

13) Routine and administrative examinations

The Z codes allow for the description of encounters for routine examinations, such as, a general check-up, or, examinations for administrative purposes, such as, a pre-employment physical. The codes are not to be used if the examination is for diagnosis of a suspected condition or for treatment purposes. In such cases the diagnosis code is used. During a routine exam, should a diagnosis or condition be discovered, it should be coded as an additional code. Pre-existing and chronic conditions and history codes may also be included as additional codes as long as the examination is for administrative purposes and not focused on any particular condition.

Some of the codes for routine health examinations distinguish between "with" and "without" abnormal findings. Code assignment depends on the information that is known at the time the encounter is being coded. For example, if no abnormal findings were found during the examination, but the encounter is being coded before test results are back, it is acceptable to assign the code for "without abnormal findings." When assigning a code for "with abnormal findings," additional code(s) should be assigned to identify the specific abnormal finding(s).

Pre-operative examination and pre-procedural laboratory examination Z codes are for use only in those situations when a patient is being cleared for a procedure or surgery and no treatment is given.

The Z codes/categories for routine and administrative examinations:

Z00   Encounter for general examination without complaint, suspected or reported diagnosis

Z01   Encounter for other special examination without complaint, suspected or reported diagnosis

Z02   Encounter for administrative examination

     Except: Z02.9, Encounter for administrative examinations, unspecified

Z32.0- Encounter for pregnancy test

14) Miscellaneous Z codes

The miscellaneous Z codes capture a number of other health care encounters that do not fall into one of the other categories. Certain of these codes identify the reason for the encounter; others are for use as additional codes that provide useful information on circumstances that may affect a patient's care and treatment.

Prophylactic Organ Removal

For encounters specifically for prophylactic removal of an organ (such as prophylactic removal of breasts due to a genetic susceptibility to cancer or a family history of cancer), the principal or first-listed code should be a code from category Z40, Encounter for prophylactic surgery, followed by the appropriate codes to identify the associated risk factor (such as genetic susceptibility or family history).

If the patient has a malignancy of one site and is having prophylactic removal at another site to prevent either a new primary malignancy or metastatic disease, a code for the malignancy should also be assigned in addition to a code from subcategory Z40.0, Encounter for prophylactic surgery for risk factors related to malignant neoplasms. A Z40.0 code should not be assigned if the patient is having organ removal for treatment of a malignancy, such as the removal of the testes for the treatment of prostate cancer.

Miscellaneous Z codes/categories:

Z28   Immunization not carried out

     Except: Z28.3, Underimmunization status

Z29   Encounter for other prophylactic measures

Z40   Encounter for prophylactic surgery

Z41   Encounter for procedures for purposes other than remedying health state

     Except: Z41.9, Encounter for procedure for purposes other than remedying health state, unspecified

Z53   Persons encountering health services for specific procedures and treatment, not carried out

Z55   Problems related to education and literacy

Z56   Problems related to employment and unemployment

Z57   Occupational exposure to risk factors

Z58   Problems related to physical environment

Z59   Problems related to housing and economic circumstances

Z60   Problems related to social environment

Z62   Problems related to upbringing

Z63   Other problems related to primary support group, including family circumstances

Z64   Problems related to certain psychosocial circumstances

Z65   Problems related to other psychosocial circumstances

Z72   Problems related to lifestyle

Note: These codes should be assigned only when the documentation specifies that the patient has an associated problem

Z73   Problems related to life management difficulty

Z74   Problems related to care provider dependency

Except: Z74.01, Bed confinement status

Z75   Problems related to medical facilities and other health care

Z76.0   Encounter for issue of repeat prescription

Z76.3   Healthy person accompanying sick person

Z76.4   Other boarder to healthcare facility

Z76.5   Malingerer [conscious simulation]

Z91.1-   Patient's noncompliance with medical treatment and regimen

Z91.83   Wandering in diseases classified elsewhere

Z91.89   Other specified personal risk factors, not elsewhere classified

15) Nonspecific Z codes

Certain Z codes are so non-specific, or potentially redundant with other codes in the classification, that there can be little justification for their use in the inpatient setting. Their use in the outpatient setting should be limited to those instances when there is no further documentation to permit more precise coding. Otherwise, any sign or symptom or any other reason for visit that is captured in another code should be used.

Nonspecific Z codes/categories:

Z02.9   Encounter for administrative examinations, unspecified

Z04.9   Encounter for examination and observation for unspecified reason

Z13.9   Encounter for screening, unspecified

Z41.9   Encounter for procedure for purposes other than remedying health state, unspecified

Z52.9   Donor of unspecified organ or tissue

Z86.59   Personal history of other mental and behavioral disorders

Z88.9   Allergy status to unspecified drugs, medicaments and biological substances status

Z92.0   Personal history of contraception

16) Z Codes That May Only be Principal/First-Listed Diagnosis

The following Z codes/categories may only be reported as the principal/first-listed diagnosis, except when there are multiple encounters on the same day and the medical records for the encounters are combined:

Z00   Encounter for general examination without complaint, suspected or reported diagnosis

Except: Z00.6

Z01   Encounter for other special examination without complaint, suspected or reported diagnosis

Z02   Encounter for administrative examination

Z03   Encounter for medical observation for suspected diseases and conditions ruled out

Z04   Encounter for examination and observation for other reasons

Z33.2 Encounter for elective termination of pregnancy

Z31.81 Encounter for male factor infertility in female patient

Z31.83 Encounter for assisted reproductive fertility procedure cycle

Z31.84 Encounter for fertility preservation procedure

Z34   Encounter for supervision of normal pregnancy

Z39   Encounter for maternal postpartum care and examination

Z38   Liveborn infants according to place of birth and type of delivery

Z42   Encounter for plastic and reconstructive surgery following medical procedure or healed injury

Z51.0 Encounter for antineoplastic radiation therapy

Z51.1- Encounter for antineoplastic chemotherapy and immunotherapy

Z52   Donors of organs and tissues

      Except: Z52.9, Donor of unspecified organ or tissue

Z76.1 Encounter for health supervision and care of foundling

Z76.2 Encounter for health supervision and care of other healthy infant and child

Z99.12 Encounter for respirator [ventilator] dependence during power failure

● New code ▲ Revised code **Excludes1:** Not coded here **Excludes2:** Not included here ⊗ Placeholder required ⑦ 7th digit required

Chapter 21

Factors Influencing Health Status And Contact With Health Services (Z00-Z99)

Note: Z codes represent reasons for encounters. A corresponding procedure code must accompany a Z code if a procedure is performed. Categories Z00-Z99 are provided for occasions when circumstances other than a disease, injury or external cause classifiable to categories A00-Y89 are recorded as 'diagnoses' or 'problems'. This can arise in two main ways: (a) When a person who may or may not be sick encounters the health services for some specific purpose, such as to receive limited care or service for a current condition, to donate an organ or tissue, to receive prophylactic vaccination (immunization), or to discuss a problem which is in itself not a disease or injury. (b) When some circumstance or problem is present which influences the person's health status but is not in itself a current illness or injury.

This chapter contains the following blocks:

Z00-Z13	Persons encountering health services for examinations
Z14-Z15	Genetic carrier and genetic susceptibility to disease
Z16	Resistance to antimicrobial drugs
Z17	Estrogen receptor status
Z18	Retained foreign body fragments
Z19	Hormone sensitivity malignancy status
Z20-Z29	Persons with potential health hazards related to communicable diseases
Z30-Z39	Persons encountering health services in circumstances related to reproduction
Z40-Z53	Encounters for other specific health care
Z55-Z65	Persons with potential health hazards related to socioeconomic and psychosocial circumstances
Z66	Do not resuscitate status
Z67	Blood type
Z68	Body mass index (BMI)
Z69-Z76	Persons encountering health services **in other** circumstances
Z77-Z99	Persons with potential health hazards related to family and personal history and certain conditions influencing health status

PERSONS ENCOUNTERING HEALTH SERVICES FOR EXAMINATIONS (Z00-Z13)

Note: Nonspecific abnormal findings disclosed at the time of these examinations are classified to categories R70-R94.

Excludes1: examinations related to pregnancy and reproduction (Z30-Z36, Z39.-)

Z00 **Encounter for general examination without complaint, suspected or reported diagnosis**

Excludes1: encounter for examination for administrative purposes (Z02.-)

Excludes2: encounter for pre-procedural examinations (Z01.81-)
special screening examinations (Z11-Z13)

Z00.0 **Encounter for general adult medical examination**

Encounter for adult periodic examination (annual) (physical) and any associated laboratory and radiologic examinations

Excludes1: encounter for examination of sign or symptom-code to sign or symptom

general health check-up of infant or child (Z00.12-)

Z00.00 **Encounter for general adult medical examination without abnormal findings**

Encounter for adult health check-up NOS

Z00.01 **Encounter for general adult medical examination with abnormal findings**

Use additional code to identify abnormal findings

Z00.1 **Encounter for newborn, infant and child health examinations**

Z00.11 **Newborn health examination**

Health check for child under 29 days old

Use additional code to identify any abnormal findings

Excludes1: health check for child over 28 days old (Z00.12-)

Z00.110 **Health examination for newborn under 8 days old**

Health check for newborn under 8 days old

Z00.111 **Health examination for newborn 8 to 28 days old**

Health check for newborn 8 to 28 days old Newborn weight check

Z00.12 **Encounter for routine child health examination**

Encounter for development testing of infant or child

Health check (routine) for child over 28 days old

Excludes1: health check for child under 29 days old (Z00.11-)

health supervision of foundling or other healthy infant or child (Z76.1-Z76.2)

newborn health examination (Z00.11-)

Z00.121 **Encounter for routine child health examination with abnormal findings**

Use additional code to identify abnormal findings

Z00.129 **Encounter for routine child health examination without abnormal findings**

Encounter for routine child health examination NOS

Z00.2 **Encounter for examination for period of rapid growth in childhood**

Z00.3 **Encounter for examination for adolescent development state**

Encounter for puberty development state

Z00.5 **Encounter for examination of potential donor of organ and tissue**

Z00.6 **Encounter for examination for normal comparison and control in clinical research program**

Examination of participant or control in clinical research program

Z00.7 **Encounter for examination for period of delayed growth in childhood**

Z00.70 **Encounter for examination for period of delayed growth in childhood without abnormal findings**

Z00.71 **Encounter for examination for period of delayed growth in childhood with abnormal findings**

Use additional code to identify abnormal findings

Z00.8 **Encounter for other general examination**

Encounter for health examination in population surveys

Z01 **Encounter for other special examination without complaint, suspected or reported diagnosis**

Includes: routine examination of specific system

Note: Codes from category Z01 represent the reason for the encounter. A separate procedure code is required to identify any examinations or procedures performed

Excludes1: encounter for examination for administrative purposes (Z02.-)

encounter for examination for suspected conditions, proven not to exist (Z03.-)

encounter for laboratory and radiologic examinations as a component of general medical examinations (Z00.0-)

encounter for laboratory, radiologic and imaging examinations for sign(s) and symptom(s) - code to the sign(s) or symptom(s)

Excludes2: screening examinations (Z11-Z13)

Z01.0 **Encounter for examination of eyes and vision**

Excludes1: examination for driving license (Z02.4)

Z01.00 **Encounter for examination of eyes and vision without abnormal findings**

Encounter for examination of eyes and vision NOS

Z01.01 **Encounter for examination of eyes and vision with abnormal findings**

Use additional code to identify abnormal findings

Z01.1 **Encounter for examination of ears and hearing**

Z01.10 **Encounter for examination of ears and hearing without abnormal findings**

Encounter for examination of ears and hearing NOS

Z01.11 **Encounter for examination of ears and hearing with abnormal findings**

Z01.110 **Encounter for hearing examination following failed hearing screening**

Z01.118 **Encounter for examination of ears and hearing with other abnormal findings**

Use additional code to identify abnormal findings

Z01.12 **Encounter for hearing conservation and treatment**

Z01.2 **Encounter for dental examination and cleaning**

Z01.20 **Encounter for dental examination and cleaning without abnormal findings**

Encounter for dental examination and cleaning NOS

Z01.21 **Encounter for dental examination and cleaning with abnormal findings**

Use additional code to identify abnormal findings

Z01.3 **Encounter for examination of blood pressure**

Z01.30 **Encounter for examination of blood pressure without abnormal findings**

Encounter for examination of blood pressure NOS

Z01.31 **Encounter for examination of blood pressure with abnormal findings**

Use additional code to identify abnormal findings

Z01.4 **Encounter for gynecological examination**

Excludes2: pregnancy examination or test (Z32.0-)

routine examination for contraceptive maintenance (Z30.4-)

Z01.41 **Encounter for routine gynecological examination**

Encounter for general gynecological examination with or without cervical smear

Encounter for gynecological examination (general) (routine) NOS

Encounter for pelvic examination (annual) (periodic)

Use additional code:

for screening for human papillomavirus, if applicable, (Z11.51)

for screening vaginal pap smear, if applicable (Z12.72)

to identify acquired absence of uterus, if applicable (Z90.71-)

Excludes1: gynecologic examination status-post hysterectomy for malignant condition (Z08)

screening cervical pap smear not a part of a routine gynecological examination (Z12.4)

Z01.411 **Encounter for gynecological examination (general) (routine) with abnormal findings**

Use additional code to identify abnormal findings

Z01.419 **Encounter for gynecological examination (general) (routine) without abnormal findings**

Z01.42 **Encounter for cervical smear to confirm findings of recent normal smear following initial abnormal smear**

Z01.8 **Encounter for other specified special examinations**

Z01.81 **Encounter for preprocedural examinations**

Encounter for preoperative examinations

Encounter for radiological and imaging examinations as part of preprocedural examination

Z01.810 **Encounter for preprocedural cardiovascular examination**

Z01.811 **Encounter for preprocedural respiratory examination**

Z01.812 **Encounter for preprocedural laboratory examination**

Blood and urine tests prior to treatment or procedure

Z01.818 **Encounter for other preprocedural examination**

Encounter for preprocedural examination NOS

Encounter for examinations prior to antineoplastic chemotherapy

Z01.82 Encounter for allergy testing

Excludes1: encounter for antibody response examination (Z01.84)

Z01.83 Encounter for blood typing

Encounter for Rh typing

Z01.84 Encounter for antibody response examination

Encounter for immunity status testing

Excludes1: encounter for allergy testing (Z01.82)

Z01.89 Encounter for other specified special examinations

Z02 Encounter for administrative examination

Z02.0 Encounter for examination for admission to educational institution

Encounter for examination for admission to preschool (education)

Encounter for examination for re-admission to school following illness or medical treatment

Z02.1 Encounter for pre-employment examination

Z02.2 Encounter for examination for admission to residential institution

Excludes1: examination for admission to prison (Z02.89)

Z02.3 Encounter for examination for recruitment to armed forces

Z02.4 Encounter for examination for driving license

Z02.5 Encounter for examination for participation in sport

Excludes1: blood-alcohol and blood-drug test (Z02.83)

Z02.6 Encounter for examination for insurance purposes

Z02.7 Encounter for issue of medical certificate

Excludes1: encounter for general medical examination (Z00-Z01, Z02.0-Z02.6, Z02.8-Z02.9,)

Z02.71 Encounter for disability determination

Encounter for issue of medical certificate of incapacity

Encounter for issue of medical certificate of invalidity

Z02.79 Encounter for issue of other medical certificate

Z02.8 Encounter for other administrative examinations

Z02.81 Encounter for paternity testing

Z02.82 Encounter for adoption services

Z02.83 Encounter for blood-alcohol and blood-drug test

Use additional code for findings of alcohol or drugs in blood (R78.-)

Z02.89 Encounter for other administrative examinations

Encounter for examination for admission to prison

Encounter for examination for admission to summer camp

Encounter for immigration examination

Encounter for naturalization examination

Encounter for premarital examination

Excludes1: health supervision of foundling or other healthy infant or child (Z76.1-Z76.2)

Z02.9 Encounter for administrative examinations, unspecified

Z03 Encounter for medical observation for suspected diseases and conditions ruled out

This category is to be used when a person without a diagnosis is suspected of having an abnormal condition, without signs or symptoms, which requires study, but after examination and observation, is ruled out. This category is also for use for administrative and legal observation status.

Excludes1: contact with and (suspected) exposures hazardous to health (Z77.-)

newborn observation for suspected condition, ruled out (P00-P04) person with feared complaint in whom no diagnosis is made (Z71.1) signs or symptoms under study- code to signs or symptoms

Z03.6 Encounter for observation for suspected toxic effect from ingested substance ruled out

Encounter for observation for suspected adverse effect from drug

Encounter for observation for suspected poisoning

Z03.7 Encounter for suspected maternal and fetal conditions ruled out

Encounter for suspected maternal and fetal conditions not found

Excludes1: known or suspected fetal anomalies affecting management of mother, not ruled out (O26.-, O35.-, O36.-, O40.-, O41.-)

Z03.71 Encounter for suspected problem with amniotic cavity and membrane ruled out

Encounter for suspected oligohydramnios ruled out

Encounter for suspected polyhydramnios ruled out

Z03.72 Encounter for suspected placental problem ruled out

Z03.73 Encounter for suspected fetal anomaly ruled out

Z03.74 Encounter for suspected problem with fetal growth ruled out

Z03.75 Encounter for suspected cervical shortening ruled out

Z03.79 Encounter for other suspected maternal and fetal conditions ruled out

Z03.8 Encounter for observation for other suspected diseases and conditions ruled out

Z03.81 Encounter for observation for suspected exposure to biological agents ruled out

Z03.810 Encounter for observation for suspected exposure to anthrax ruled out

Z03.818 Encounter for observation for suspected exposure to other biological agents ruled out

Z03.89 Encounter for observation for other suspected diseases and conditions ruled out

Z04 Encounter for examination and observation for other reasons

Includes: encounter for examination for medicolegal reasons

This category is to be used when a person without a diagnosis is suspected of having an abnormal condition, without signs or symptoms, which requires study, but after examination and observation, is ruled-out. This category is also for use for administrative and legal observation status.

Z04.1 Encounter for examination and observation following transport accident

Excludes1: encounter for examination and observation following work accident (Z04.2)

Z04.2 **Encounter for examination and observation following work accident**

Z04.3 **Encounter for examination and observation following other accident**

Z04.4 **Encounter for examination and observation following alleged rape**

Encounter for examination and observation of victim following alleged rape

Encounter for examination and observation of victim following alleged sexual abuse

Z04.41 **Encounter for examination and observation following alleged adult rape**

Suspected adult rape, ruled out

Suspected adult sexual abuse, ruled out

Z04.42 **Encounter for examination and observation following alleged child rape**

Suspected child rape, ruled out

Suspected child sexual abuse, ruled out

Z04.6 **Encounter for general psychiatric examination, requested by authority**

Z04.7 **Encounter for examination and observation following alleged physical abuse**

Z04.71 **Encounter for examination and observation following alleged adult physical abuse**

Suspected adult physical abuse, ruled out

Excludes1: confirmed case of adult physical abuse (T74.-)

encounter for examination and observation following alleged adult sexual abuse (Z04.41)

suspected case of adult physical abuse, not ruled out (T76.-)

Z04.72 **Encounter for examination and observation following alleged child physical abuse**

Suspected child physical abuse, ruled out

Excludes1: confirmed case of child physical abuse (T74.-)

encounter for examination and observation following alleged child sexual abuse (Z04.42)

suspected case of child physical abuse, not ruled out (T76.-)

Z04.8 **Encounter for examination and observation for other specified reasons**

Encounter for examination and observation for request for expert evidence

Z04.9 **Encounter for examination and observation for unspecified reason**

Encounter for observation NOS

Z05 **Encounter for observation and evaluation of newborn for suspected diseases and conditions ruled out**

This category is to be used for newborns, within the neonatal period (the first 28 days of life), who are suspected of having an abnormal condition unrelated to exposure from the mother or the birth process, but without signs or symptoms, and which, after examination and observation, is ruled out.

Excludes2: newborn observation for suspected condition, related to exposure from the mother or birth process (P00-P04)

● **Z05.0** **Observation and evaluation of newborn for suspected cardiac condition ruled out**

● **Z05.1** **Observation and evaluation of newborn for suspected infectious condition ruled out**

● **Z05.2** **Observation and evaluation of newborn for suspected neurological condition ruled out**

● **Z05.3** **Observation and evaluation of newborn for suspected respiratory condition ruled out**

Z05.4 **Observation and evaluation of newborn for suspected genetic, metabolic or immunologic condition ruled out**

● **Z05.41** **Observation and evaluation of newborn for suspected genetic condition ruled out**

● **Z05.42** **Observation and evaluation of newborn for suspected metabolic condition ruled out**

● **Z05.43** **Observation and evaluation of newborn for suspected immunologic condition ruled out**

● **Z05.5** **Observation and evaluation of newborn for suspected gastrointestinal condition ruled out**

● **Z05.6** **Observation and evaluation of newborn for suspected genitourinary condition ruled out**

Z05.7 **Observation and evaluation of newborn for suspected skin, subcutaneous, musculoskeletal and connective tissue condition ruled out**

● **Z05.71** **Observation and evaluation of newborn for suspected skin and subcutaneous tissue condition ruled out**

● **Z05.72** **Observation and evaluation of newborn for suspected musculoskeletal condition ruled out**

● **Z05.73** **Observation and evaluation of newborn for suspected connective tissue condition ruled out**

● **Z05.8** **Observation and evaluation of newborn for other specified suspected condition ruled out**

● **Z05.9** **Observation and evaluation of newborn for unspecified suspected condition ruled out**

Z08 **Encounter for follow-up examination after completed treatment for malignant neoplasm**

Medical surveillance following completed treatment

Use additional code to identify any acquired absence of organs (Z90.-)

Use additional code to identify the personal history of malignant neoplasm (Z85.-)

Excludes1: aftercare following medical care (Z43-Z49, Z51)

Z09 **Encounter for follow-up examination after completed treatment for conditions other than malignant neoplasm**

Medical surveillance following completed treatment

Use additional code to identify any applicable history of disease code (Z86.-. Z87.-)

Excludes1: aftercare following medical care (Z43-Z49, Z51)

surveillance of contraception (Z30.4-)

surveillance of prosthetic and other medical devices (Z44-Z46)

Z11 **Encounter for screening for infectious and parasitic diseases**

Screening is the testing for disease or disease precursors in asymptomatic individuals so that early detection and

treatment can be provided for those who test positive for the disease.

Excludes1: encounter for diagnostic examination-code to sign or symptom

Z11.0 **Encounter for screening for intestinal infectious diseases**

Z11.1 **Encounter for screening for respiratory tuberculosis**

Z11.2 **Encounter for screening for other bacterial diseases**

Z11.3 **Encounter for screening for infections with a predominantly sexual mode of transmission**

Excludes2: encounter for screening for human immunodeficiency virus [HIV] (Z11.4)

encounter for screening for human papillomavirus (Z11.51)

Z11.4 **Encounter for screening for human immunodeficiency virus [HIV]**

Z11.5 **Encounter for screening for other viral diseases**

Excludes2: encounter for screening for viral intestinal disease (Z11.0)

Z11.51 **Encounter for screening for human papillomavirus (HPV)**

Z11.59 **Encounter for screening for other viral diseases**

Z11.6 **Encounter for screening for other protozoal diseases and helminthiases**

Excludes2: encounter for screening for protozoal intestinal disease (Z11.0)

Z11.8 **Encounter for screening for other infectious and parasitic diseases**

Encounter for screening for chlamydia

Encounter for screening for rickettsial

Encounter for screening for spirochetal

Encounter for screening for mycoses

Z11.9 **Encounter for screening for infectious and parasitic diseases, unspecified**

Z12 **Encounter for screening for malignant neoplasms**

Screening is the testing for disease or disease precursors in asymptomatic individuals so that early detection and

treatment can be provided for those who test positive for the disease.

Use additional code to identify any family history of malignant neoplasm (Z80.-)

Excludes1: encounter for diagnostic examination-code to sign or symptom

Z12.0 **Encounter for screening for malignant neoplasm of stomach**

Z12.1 **Encounter for screening for malignant neoplasm of intestinal tract**

Z12.10 **Encounter for screening for malignant neoplasm of intestinal tract, unspecified**

Z12.11 **Encounter for screening for malignant neoplasm of colon**

Encounter for screening colonoscopy NOS

Z12.12 **Encounter for screening for malignant neoplasm of rectum**

Z12.13 **Encounter for screening for malignant neoplasm of small intestine**

Z12.2 **Encounter for screening for malignant neoplasm of respiratory organs**

Z12.3 **Encounter for screening for malignant neoplasm of breast**

Z12.31 **Encounter for screening mammogram for malignant neoplasm of breast**

Excludes1: inconclusive mammogram (R92.2)

Z12.39 **Encounter for other screening for malignant neoplasm of breast**

Z12.4 **Encounter for screening for malignant neoplasm of cervix**

Encounter for screening pap smear for malignant neoplasm of cervix

Excludes1: when screening is part of general gynecological examination (Z01.4-)

Excludes2: encounter for screening for human papillomavirus (Z11.51)

Z12.5 **Encounter for screening for malignant neoplasm of prostate**

Z12.6 **Encounter for screening for malignant neoplasm of bladder**

Z12.7 **Encounter for screening for malignant neoplasm of other genitourinary organs**

Z12.71 **Encounter for screening for malignant neoplasm of testis**

Z12.72 **Encounter for screening for malignant neoplasm of vagina**

Vaginal pap smear status-post hysterectomy for non-malignant condition

Use additional code to identify acquired absence of uterus (Z90.71-)

Excludes1: vaginal pap smear status-post hysterectomy for malignant conditions (Z08)

Z12.73 **Encounter for screening for malignant neoplasm of ovary**

Z12.79 **Encounter for screening for malignant neoplasm of other genitourinary organs**

Z12.8 **Encounter for screening for malignant neoplasm of other sites**

Z12.81 **Encounter for screening for malignant neoplasm of oral cavity**

Z12.82 **Encounter for screening for malignant neoplasm of nervous system**

Z12.83 **Encounter for screening for malignant neoplasm of skin**

Z12.89 **Encounter for screening for malignant neoplasm of other sites**

Z12.9 **Encounter for screening for malignant neoplasm, site unspecified**

Z13 **Encounter for screening for other diseases and disorders**

Screening is the testing for disease or disease precursors in asymptomatic individuals so that early detection and treatment can be provided for those who test positive for the disease.

Excludes1: encounter for diagnostic examination-code to sign or symptom

Z13.0 **Encounter for screening for diseases of the blood and blood-forming organs and certain disorders involving the immune mechanism**

Z13.1 **Encounter for screening for diabetes mellitus**

Z13.2 **Encounter for screening for nutritional, metabolic and other endocrine disorders**

Z13.21 **Encounter for screening for nutritional disorder**

Z13.22 **Encounter for screening for metabolic disorder**

Z13.220 **Encounter for screening for lipoid disorders**

Encounter for screening for cholesterol level

Encounter for screening for hypercholesterolemia

Encounter for screening for hyperlipidemia

Z13.228   Encounter for screening for other metabolic disorders

Z13.29   Encounter for screening for other suspected endocrine disorder

Excludes1: encounter for screening for diabetes mellitus (Z13.1)

Z13.4   Encounter for screening for certain developmental disorders in childhood

Encounter for screening for developmental handicaps in early childhood

Excludes1: routine development testing of infant or child (Z00.1-)

Z13.5   Encounter for screening for eye and ear disorders

Excludes2: encounter for general hearing examination (Z01.1-)

encounter for general vision examination (Z01.0-)

Z13.6   Encounter for screening for cardiovascular disorders

Z13.7   Encounter for screening for genetic and chromosomal anomalies

Excludes1: genetic testing for procreative management (Z31.4-)

Z13.71   Encounter for nonprocreative screening for genetic disease carrier status

Z13.79   Encounter for other screening for genetic and chromosomal anomalies

Z13.8   Encounter for screening for other specified diseases and disorders

Excludes2: screening for malignant neoplasms (Z12.-)

Z13.81   Encounter for screening for digestive system disorders

Z13.810   Encounter for screening for upper gastrointestinal disorder

Z13.811   Encounter for screening for lower gastrointestinal disorder

Excludes1: encounter for screening for intestinal infectious disease (Z11.0)

Z13.818   Encounter for screening for other digestive system disorders

Z13.82   Encounter for screening for musculoskeletal disorder

Z13.820   Encounter for screening for osteoporosis

Z13.828   Encounter for screening for other musculoskeletal disorder

Z13.83   Encounter for screening for respiratory disorder NEC

Excludes1: encounter for screening for respiratory tuberculosis (Z11.1)

Z13.84   Encounter for screening for dental disorders

Z13.85   Encounter for screening for nervous system disorders

Z13.850   Encounter for screening for traumatic brain injury

Z13.858   Encounter for screening for other nervous system disorders

Z13.88   Encounter for screening for disorder due to exposure to contaminants

Excludes1: those exposed to contaminants without suspected disorders (Z57.-, Z77.-)

Z13.89   Encounter for screening for other disorder

Encounter for screening for genitourinary disorders

Z13.9   Encounter for screening, unspecified

GENETIC CARRIER AND GENETIC SUSCEPTIBILITY TO DISEASE (Z14-Z15)

Z14   Genetic carrier

Definition: A genetic carrier is a person who has inherited a genetic trait or mutation but does not display that trait or show symptoms of the disease. Genetic carriers are, however, able to pass the gene onto their offspring, who may then express the gene.

Z14.0   Hemophilia A carrier

Z14.01   Asymptomatic hemophilia A carrier

Z14.02   Symptomatic hemophilia A carrier

Z14.1   Cystic fibrosis carrier

Z14.8   Genetic carrier of other disease

Z15   Genetic susceptibility to disease

Includes: confirmed abnormal gene

Use additional code, if applicable, for any associated family history of the disease (Z80-Z84)

Excludes1: chromosomal anomalies (Q90-Q99)

Z15.0   Genetic susceptibility to malignant neoplasm

Code first, if applicable, any current malignant neoplasm (C00-C75, C81-C96)

Use additional code, if applicable, for any personal history of malignant neoplasm (Z85.-)

Z15.01   Genetic susceptibility to malignant neoplasm of breast

Z15.02   Genetic susceptibility to malignant neoplasm of ovary

Z15.03   Genetic susceptibility to malignant neoplasm of prostate

Z15.04   Genetic susceptibility to malignant neoplasm of endometrium

Z15.09   Genetic susceptibility to other malignant neoplasm

Z15.8   Genetic susceptibility to other disease

Z15.81   Genetic susceptibility to multiple endocrine neoplasia [MEN]

Excludes1: multiple endocrine neoplasia [MEN] syndromes (E31.2-)

Z15.89   Genetic susceptibility to other disease

RESISTANCE TO ANTIMICROBIAL DRUGS (Z16)

Definition: An antimicrobial is an agent that kills microorganisms or inhibits their growth. Antimicrobial drugs can be grouped according to the microorganisms they act primarily against.

Z16   Resistance to antimicrobial drugs

Note: The codes in this category are provided for use as additional codes to identify the resistance and non-responsiveness of a condition to antimicrobial drugs.

Code first the infection

Excludes1: Methicillin resistant Staphylococcus aureus infection (A49.02)

Methicillin resistant Staphylococcus aureus infection in diseases classified elsewhere (B95.62)

Methicillin resistant Staphylococcus aureus pneumonia (J15.212)

Sepsis due to Methicillin resistant Staphylococcus aureus (A41.02)

Z16.1 Resistance to beta lactam antibiotics

Z16.10 Resistance to unspecified beta lactam antibiotics

Z16.11 Resistance to penicillins

Resistance to amoxicillin

Resistance to ampicillin

Z16.12 Extended spectrum beta lactamase (ESBL) resistance

Z16.19 Resistance to other specified beta lactam antibiotics

Resistance to cephalosporins

Z16.2 Resistance to other antibiotics

Z16.20 Resistance to unspecified antibiotic

Resistance to antibiotics NOS

Z16.21 Resistance to vancomycin

Z16.22 Resistance to vancomycin related antibiotics

Z16.23 Resistance to quinolones and fluoroquinolones

Z16.24 Resistance to multiple antibiotics

Z16.29 Resistance to other single specified antibiotic

Resistance to aminoglycosides

Resistance to macrolides

Resistance to sulfonamides

Resistance to tetracyclines

Z16.3 Resistance to other antimicrobial drugs

Excludes1: resistance to antibiotics (Z16.1-, Z16.2-)

Z16.30 Resistance to unspecified antimicrobial drugs

Drug resistance NOS

Z16.31 Resistance to antiparasitic drug(s)

Resistance to quinine and related compounds

Z16.32 Resistance to antifungal drug(s)

Z16.33 Resistance to antiviral drug(s)

Z16.34 Resistance to antimycobacterial drug(s)

Resistance to tuberculostatics

Z16.341 Resistance to single antimycobacterial drug

Resistance to antimycobacterial drug NOS

Z16.342 Resistance to multiple antimycobacterial drugs

Z16.35 Resistance to multiple antimicrobial drugs

Excludes1: Resistance to multiple antibiotics only (Z16.24)

Z16.39 Resistance to other specified antimicrobial drug

ESTROGEN RECEPTOR STATUS (Z17)

Z17 Estrogen receptor status

Code first malignant neoplasm of breast (C50.-)

Z17.0 Estrogen receptor positive status [ER+]

Z17.1 Estrogen receptor negative status [ER-]

RETAINED FOREIGN BODY FRAGMENTS (Z18)

Z18 Retained foreign body fragments

Includes: embedded fragment (status)

embedded splinter (status) retained foreign body status

Excludes1: artificial joint prosthesis status (Z96.6-)

foreign body accidentally left during a procedure (T81.5-)

foreign body entering through orifice (T15-T19)

in situ cardiac device (Z95.-)

organ or tissue replaced by means other than transplant (Z96.-, Z97.-)

organ or tissue replaced by transplant (Z94.-)

personal history of retained foreign body fully removed Z87.821

superficial foreign body (non-embedded splinter) - code to superficial foreign body, by site

Z18.0 Retained radioactive fragments

Z18.01 Retained depleted uranium fragments

Z18.09 Other retained radioactive fragments

Other retained depleted isotope fragments

Retained nontherapeutic radioactive fragments

Z18.1 Retained metal fragments

Excludes1: retained radioactive metal fragments (Z18.01-Z18.09)

Z18.10 Retained metal fragments, unspecified

Retained metal fragment NOS

Z18.11 Retained magnetic metal fragments

Z18.12 Retained nonmagnetic metal fragments

Z18.2 Retained plastic fragments

Acrylics fragments

Diethylhexylphthalates fragments

Isocyanate fragments

Z18.3 Retained organic fragments

Z18.31 Retained animal quills or spines

Z18.32 Retained tooth

Z18.33 Retained wood fragments

Z18.39 Other retained organic fragments

Z18.8 Other specified retained foreign body

Z18.81 Retained glass fragments

Z18.83 Retained stone or crystalline fragments

Retained concrete or cement fragments

Z18.89 Other specified retained foreign body fragments

Z18.9 Retained foreign body fragments, unspecified material

HORMONE SENSITIVITY MALIGNANCY STATUS (Z19)

Z19 Hormone sensitivity malignancy status

Code first malignant neoplasm - see Table of Neoplasms, by site, malignant

●**Z19.1 Hormone sensitive malignancy status**

●**Z19.2 Hormone resistant malignancy status**

Castrate resistant prostate malignancy status

PERSONS WITH POTENTIAL HEALTH HAZARDS RELATED TO COMMUNICABLE DISEASES (Z20-Z29)

Z20 Contact with and (suspected) exposure to communicable diseases

Excludes1: carrier of infectious disease (Z22.-)

diagnosed current infectious or parasitic disease -see Alphabetic Index

Excludes2: personal history of infectious and parasitic diseases (Z86.1-)

Z20.0 **Contact with and (suspected) exposure to intestinal infectious diseases**

    Z20.01 **Contact with and (suspected) exposure to intestinal infectious diseases due to Escherichia coli (E. coli)**

    Z20.09 **Contact with and (suspected) exposure to other intestinal infectious diseases**

Z20.1 **Contact with and (suspected) exposure to tuberculosis**

Z20.2 **Contact with and (suspected) exposure to infections with a predominantly sexual mode of transmission**

Z20.3 **Contact with and (suspected) exposure to rabies**

Z20.4 **Contact with and (suspected) exposure to rubella**

Z20.5 **Contact with and (suspected) exposure to viral hepatitis**

Z20.6 **Contact with and (suspected) exposure to human immunodeficiency virus [HIV]**

    Excludes1: asymptomatic human immunodeficiency virus [HIV]

    HIV infection status (Z21)

Z20.7 **Contact with and (suspected) exposure to pediculosis, acariasis and other infestations**

Z20.8 **Contact with and (suspected) exposure to other communicable diseases**

    Z20.81 **Contact with and (suspected) exposure to other bacterial communicable diseases**

        Z20.810 **Contact with and (suspected) exposure to anthrax**

        Z20.811 **Contact with and (suspected) exposure to meningococcus**

        Z20.818 **Contact with and (suspected) exposure to other bacterial communicable diseases**

    Z20.82 **Contact with and (suspected) exposure to other viral communicable diseases**

        Z20.820 **Contact with and (suspected) exposure to varicella**

        Z20.828 **Contact with and (suspected) exposure to other viral communicable diseases**

    Z20.89 **Contact with and (suspected) exposure to other communicable diseases**

Z20.9 **Contact with and (suspected) exposure to unspecified communicable disease**

Z21 **Asymptomatic human immunodeficiency virus [HIV] infection status**

HIV positive NOS

Code first Human immunodeficiency virus [HIV] disease complicating pregnancy, childbirth and the puerperium, if applicable (O98.7-)

Excludes1: acquired immunodeficiency syndrome (B20)

    contact with human immunodeficiency virus [HIV] (Z20.6)

    exposure to human immunodeficiency virus [HIV] (Z20.6)

    human immunodeficiency virus [HIV] disease (B20)

    inconclusive laboratory evidence of human immunodeficiency virus [HIV] (R75)

Z22 **Carrier of infectious disease**

Includes: colonization status

    suspected carrier

Excludes2: carrier of viral hepatitis (B18.-)

Z22.0 **Carrier of typhoid**

Z22.1 **Carrier of other intestinal infectious diseases**

Z22.2 **Carrier of diphtheria**

Z22.3 **Carrier of other specified bacterial diseases**

    Z22.31 **Carrier of bacterial disease due to meningococci**

    Z22.32 **Carrier of bacterial disease due to staphylococci**

        Z22.321 **Carrier or suspected carrier of Methicillin susceptible Staphylococcus aureus**

        MSSA colonization

        Z22.322 **Carrier or suspected carrier of Methicillin resistant Staphylococcus aureus**

        MRSA colonization

    Z22.33 **Carrier of bacterial disease due to streptococci**

        Z22.330 **Carrier of Group B streptococcus**

        Excludes1: Carrier of streptococcus group B (GBS) complicating pregnancy, childbirth and the puerperium (O99.82-)

        Z22.338 **Carrier of other streptococcus**

    Z22.39 **Carrier of other specified bacterial diseases**

Z22.4 **Carrier of infections with a predominantly sexual mode of transmission**

Z22.6 **Carrier of human T-lymphotropic virus type-1 [HTLV-1] infection**

Z22.8 **Carrier of other infectious diseases**

Z22.9 **Carrier of infectious disease, unspecified**

Z23 **Encounter for immunization**

Code first any routine childhood examination

Note: procedure codes are required to identify the types of immunizations given

Z28 **Immunization not carried out and underimmunization status**

Includes: vaccination not carried out

Z28.0 **Immunization not carried out because of contraindication**

    Z28.01 **Immunization not carried out because of acute illness of patient**

    Z28.02 **Immunization not carried out because of chronic illness or condition of patient**

    Z28.03 **Immunization not carried out because of immune compromised state of patient**

    Z28.04 **Immunization not carried out because of patient allergy to vaccine or component**

    Z28.09 **Immunization not carried out because of other contraindication**

Z28.1 **Immunization not carried out because of patient decision for reasons of belief or group pressure**

    Immunization not carried out because of religious belief

Z28.2 **Immunization not carried out because of patient decision for other and unspecified reason**

    Z28.20 **Immunization not carried out because of patient decision for unspecified reason**

Z28.21 Immunization not carried out because of patient refusal

Z28.29 Immunization not carried out because of patient decision for other reason

Z28.3 Underimmunization status

Delinquent immunization status Lapsed immunization schedule status

Z28.8 Immunization not carried out for other reason

Z28.81 Immunization not carried out due to patient having had the disease

Z28.82 Immunization not carried out because of caregiver refusal

Immunization not carried out because of guardian refusal

Immunization not carried out because of parent refusal

Excludes1: immunization not carried out because of caregiver refusal because of religious belief (Z28.1)

Z28.89 Immunization not carried out for other reason

Z28.9 Immunization not carried out for unspecified reason

Z29 Encounter for other prophylactic measures

Excludes 1: desensitization to allergens (Z51.6)
prophylactic surgery (Z40.-)

Z29.1 Encounter for prophylactic immunotherapy

Encounter for administration of immunoglobulin

●**Z29.11** Encounter for prophylactic immunotherapy for respiratory syncytial virus (RSV)

●**Z29.12** Encounter for prophylactic antivenin

●**Z29.13** Encounter for prophylactic Rho(D) immune globulin

●**Z29.14** Encounter for prophylactic rabies immune globin

●**Z29.3** Encounter for prophylactic fluoride administration

●**Z29.8** Encounter for other specified prophylactic measures

●**Z29.9** Encounter for prophylactic measures, unspecified

PERSONS ENCOUNTERING HEALTH SERVICES IN CIRCUMSTANCES RELATED TO REPRODUCTION (Z30-Z39)

Z30 Encounter for contraceptive management

Z30.0 Encounter for general counseling and advice on contraception

Z30.01 Encounter for initial prescription of contraceptives

Excludes1: encounter for surveillance of contraceptives (Z30.4-)

Z30.011 Encounter for initial prescription of contraceptive pills

Z30.012 Encounter for prescription of emergency contraception

Encounter for postcoital contraception

Z30.013 Encounter for initial prescription of injectable contraceptive

Z30.014 Encounter for initial prescription of intrauterine contraceptive device

Excludes1: encounter for insertion of intrauterine contraceptive device (Z30.430, Z30.432)

●**Z30.015** Encounter for initial prescription of vaginal ring hormonal contraceptive

●**Z30.016** Encounter for initial prescription of transdermal patch hormonal contraceptive device

●**Z30.017** Encounter for initial prescription of implantable subdermal contraceptive

Z30.018 Encounter for initial prescription of other contraceptives

Encounter for initial prescription of barrier contraception

Encounter for initial prescription of diaphragm

Z30.019 Encounter for initial prescription of contraceptives, unspecified

Z30.02 Counseling and instruction in natural family planning to avoid pregnancy

Z30.09 Encounter for other general counseling and advice on contraception

Encounter for family planning advice NOS

Z30.2 Encounter for sterilization

Z30.4 Encounter for surveillance of contraceptives

Z30.40 Encounter for surveillance of contraceptives, unspecified

Z30.41 Encounter for surveillance of contraceptive pills

Encounter for repeat prescription for contraceptive pill

Z30.42 Encounter for surveillance of injectable contraceptive

Z30.43 Encounter for surveillance of intrauterine contraceptive device

Z30.430 Encounter for insertion of intrauterine contraceptive device

Z30.431 Encounter for routine checking of intrauterine contraceptive device

Z30.432 Encounter for removal of intrauterine contraceptive device

Z30.433 Encounter for removal and reinsertion of intrauterine contraceptive device

Encounter for replacement of intrauterine contraceptive device

●**Z30.44** Encounter for surveillance of vaginal ring hormonal contraceptive device

●**Z30.45** Encounter for surveillance of transdermal patch hormonal contraceptive device

●**Z30.46** Encounter for surveillance of implantable subdermal contraceptive

Encounter for checking, reinsertion or removal of implantable subdermal contraceptive

Z30.49 Encounter for surveillance of other contraceptives

Encounter for surveillance of barrier contraception

Encounter for surveillance of diaphragm

Z30.8 Encounter for other contraceptive management

Encounter for postvasectomy sperm count

Encounter for routine examination for contraceptive maintenance

Excludes1: sperm count following sterilization reversal (Z31.42)

sperm count for fertility testing (Z31.41)

Z30.9 **Encounter for contraceptive management, unspecified**

Z31 **Encounter for procreative management**

Excludes1: complications associated with artificial fertilization (N98.-)

female infertility (N97.-)

male infertility (N46.-)

Z31.0 **Encounter for reversal of previous sterilization**

Z31.4 **Encounter for procreative investigation and testing**

Excludes1: postvasectomy sperm count (Z30.8)

Z31.41 **Encounter for fertility testing**

Encounter for fallopian tube patency testing

Encounter for sperm count for fertility testing

Z31.42 **Aftercare following sterilization reversal**

Sperm count following sterilization reversal

Z31.43 **Encounter for genetic testing of female for procreative management**

Use additional code for recurrent pregnancy loss, if applicable (N96, O26.2-)

Excludes1: nonprocreative genetic testing (Z13.7-)

Z31.430 **Encounter of female for testing for genetic disease carrier status for procreative management**

Z31.438 **Encounter for other genetic testing of female for procreative management**

Z31.44 **Encounter for genetic testing of male for procreative management**

Excludes1: nonprocreative genetic testing (Z13.7-)

Z31.440 **Encounter of male for testing for genetic disease carrier status for procreative management**

Z31.441 **Encounter for testing of male partner of patient with recurrent pregnancy loss**

Z31.448 **Encounter for other genetic testing of male for procreative management**

Z31.49 **Encounter for other procreative investigation and testing**

Z31.5 **Encounter for genetic counseling**

Z31.6 **Encounter for general counseling and advice on procreation**

Z31.61 **Procreative counseling and advice using natural family planning**

Z31.62 **Encounter for fertility preservation counseling**

Encounter for fertility preservation counseling prior to cancer therapy

Encounter for fertility preservation counseling prior to surgical removal of gonads

Z31.69 **Encounter for other general counseling and advice on procreation**

●**Z31.7** **Encounter for procreative management and counseling for gestational carrier**

Excludes1: pregnant state, gestational carrier (Z33.3)

Z31.8 **Encounter for other procreative management**

Z31.81 **Encounter for male factor infertility in female patient**

Z31.82 **Encounter for Rh incompatibility status**

Z31.83 **Encounter for assisted reproductive fertility procedure cycle**

Patient undergoing in vitro fertilization cycle

Use additional code to identify the type of infertility

Excludes1: pre-cycle diagnosis and testing - code to reason for encounter

Z31.84 **Encounter for fertility preservation procedure**

Encounter for fertility preservation procedure prior to cancer therapy

Encounter for fertility preservation procedure prior to surgical removal of gonads

Z31.89 **Encounter for other procreative management**

Z31.9 **Encounter for procreative management, unspecified**

Z32 **Encounter for pregnancy test and childbirth and childcare instruction**

Z32.0 **Encounter for pregnancy test**

Z32.00 **Encounter for pregnancy test, result unknown**

Encounter for pregnancy test NOS

Z32.01 **Encounter for pregnancy test, result positive**

Z32.02 **Encounter for pregnancy test, result negative**

Z32.2 **Encounter for childbirth instruction**

Z32.3 **Encounter for childcare instruction**

Encounter for prenatal or postpartum childcare instruction

Z33 **Pregnant state**

Z33.1 **Pregnant state, incidental**

Pregnant state NOS

Excludes1: complications of pregnancy (O00-O9A)

pregnant state, gestational carrier (Z33.3)

Z33.2 **Encounter for elective termination of pregnancy**

Excludes1: early fetal death with retention of dead fetus (O02.1)

late fetal death (O36.4) spontaneous abortion (O03)

●**Z33.3** **Pregnant state, gestational carrier**

Excludes1: encounter for procreative management and counseling for gestational carrier (Z31.7)

Z34 **Encounter for supervision of normal pregnancy**

Excludes1: any complication of pregnancy (O00-O9A)

encounter for pregnancy test (Z32.0-)

encounter for supervision of high risk pregnancy (O09.-)

Z34.0 **Encounter for supervision of normal first pregnancy**

Z34.00 **Encounter for supervision of normal first pregnancy, unspecified trimester**

Z34.01 **Encounter for supervision of normal first pregnancy, first trimester**

Z34.02 **Encounter for supervision of normal first pregnancy, second trimester**

Z34.03 **Encounter for supervision of normal first pregnancy, third trimester**

Z34.8 **Encounter for supervision of other normal pregnancy**

Z34.80   Encounter for supervision of other normal pregnancy, unspecified trimester

Z34.81   Encounter for supervision of other normal pregnancy, first trimester

Z34.82   Encounter for supervision of other normal pregnancy, second trimester

Z34.83   Encounter for supervision of other normal pregnancy, third trimester

Z34.9   Encounter for supervision of normal pregnancy, unspecified

Z34.90   Encounter for supervision of normal pregnancy, unspecified, unspecified trimester

Z34.91   Encounter for supervision of normal pregnancy, unspecified, first trimester

Z34.92   Encounter for supervision of normal pregnancy, unspecified, second trimester

Z34.93   Encounter for supervision of normal pregnancy, unspecified, third trimester

Z36   Encounter for antenatal screening of mother

Excludes1: abnormal findings on antenatal screening of mother (O28.-)

diagnostic examination- code to sign or symptom

encounter for suspected maternal and fetal conditions ruled out (Z03.7-)

suspected fetal condition affecting management of pregnancy - code to condition in Chapter 15

Excludes2: genetic counseling and testing (Z31.43-, Z31.5)

routine prenatal care (Z34)

Z3A   Weeks of gestation

Note: Codes from category Z3A are for use, only on the maternal record, to indicate the weeks of gestation of the pregnancy, if known.

Code first complications of pregnancy, childbirth and the puerperium (O00-O9A)

Z3A.0   Weeks of gestation of pregnancy, unspecified or less than 10 weeks

Z3A.00   Weeks of gestation of pregnancy not specified

Z3A.01   Less than 8 weeks gestation of pregnancy

Z3A.08   8 weeks gestation of pregnancy

Z3A.09   9 weeks gestation of pregnancy

Z3A.1   Weeks of gestation of pregnancy, weeks 10-19

Z3A.10   10 weeks gestation of pregnancy

Z3A.11   11 weeks gestation of pregnancy

Z3A.12   12 weeks gestation of pregnancy

Z3A.13   13 weeks gestation of pregnancy

Z3A.14   14 weeks gestation of pregnancy

Z3A.15   15 weeks gestation of pregnancy

Z3A.16   16 weeks gestation of pregnancy

Z3A.17   17 weeks gestation of pregnancy

Z3A.18   18 weeks gestation of pregnancy

Z3A.19   19 weeks gestation of pregnancy

Z3A.2   Weeks of gestation of pregnancy, weeks 20-29

Z3A.20   20 weeks gestation of pregnancy

Z3A.21   21 weeks gestation of pregnancy

Z3A.22   22 weeks gestation of pregnancy

Z3A.23   23 weeks gestation of pregnancy

Z3A.24   24 weeks gestation of pregnancy

Z3A.25   25 weeks gestation of pregnancy

Z3A.26   26 weeks gestation of pregnancy

Z3A.27   27 weeks gestation of pregnancy

Z3A.28   28 weeks gestation of pregnancy

Z3A.29   29 weeks gestation of pregnancy

Z3A.3   Weeks of gestation of pregnancy, weeks 30-39

Z3A.30   30 weeks gestation of pregnancy

Z3A.31   31 weeks gestation of pregnancy

Z3A.32   32 weeks gestation of pregnancy

Z3A.33   33 weeks gestation of pregnancy

Z3A.34   34 weeks gestation of pregnancy

Z3A.35   35 weeks gestation of pregnancy

Z3A.36   36 weeks gestation of pregnancy

Z3A.37   37 weeks gestation of pregnancy

Z3A.38   38 weeks gestation of pregnancy

Z3A.39   39 weeks gestation of pregnancy

Z3A.4   Weeks of gestation of pregnancy, weeks 40 or greater

Z3A.40   40 weeks gestation of pregnancy

Z3A.41   41 weeks gestation of pregnancy

Z3A.42   42 weeks gestation of pregnancy

Z3A.49   Greater than 42 weeks gestation of pregnancy

Z37   Outcome of delivery

This category is intended for use as an additional code to identify the outcome of delivery on the mother's record. It is not for use on the newborn record.

Excludes1: stillbirth (P95)

Z37.0   Single live birth

Z37.1   Single stillbirth

Z37.2   Twins, both liveborn

Z37.3   Twins, one liveborn and one stillborn

Z37.4   Twins, both stillborn

Z37.5   Other multiple births, all liveborn

Z37.50   Multiple births, unspecified, all liveborn

Z37.51   Triplets, all liveborn

Z37.52   Quadruplets, all liveborn

Z37.53   Quintuplets, all liveborn

Z37.54   Sextuplets, all liveborn

Z37.59   Other multiple births, all liveborn

Z37.6   Other multiple births, some liveborn

Z37.60   Multiple births, unspecified, some liveborn

Z37.61   Triplets, some liveborn

Z37.62   Quadruplets, some liveborn

Z37.63   Quintuplets, some liveborn

Z37.64   Sextuplets, some liveborn

Z37.69   Other multiple births, some liveborn

Z37.7   Other multiple births, all stillborn

Z37.9   Outcome of delivery, unspecified

Multiple birth NOS

Single birth NOS

Z38   Liveborn infants according to place of birth and type of delivery

This category is for use as the principal code on the initial record of a newborn baby. It is to be used for the initial birth record only. It is not to be used on the mother's record.

Z38.0   Single liveborn infant, born in hospital

Single liveborn infant, born in birthing center or other health care facility

Z38.00   Single liveborn infant, delivered vaginally

Z38.01   Single liveborn infant, delivered by cesarean

Z38.1   Single liveborn infant, born outside hospital

Z38.2   Single liveborn infant, unspecified as to place of birth

Single liveborn infant NOS

Z38.3   Twin liveborn infant, born in hospital

Z38.30   Twin liveborn infant, delivered vaginally

Z38.31   Twin liveborn infant, delivered by cesarean

Z38.4   Twin liveborn infant, born outside hospital

Z38.5   Twin liveborn infant, unspecified as to place of birth

Z38.6   Other multiple liveborn infant, born in hospital

Z38.61   Triplet liveborn infant, delivered vaginally

Z38.62   Triplet liveborn infant, delivered by cesarean

Z38.63   Quadruplet liveborn infant, delivered vaginally

Z38.64   Quadruplet liveborn infant, delivered by cesarean

Z38.65   Quintuplet liveborn infant, delivered vaginally

Z38.66   Quintuplet liveborn infant, delivered by cesarean

Z38.68   Other multiple liveborn infant, delivered vaginally

Z38.69   Other multiple liveborn infant, delivered by cesarean

Z38.7   Other multiple liveborn infant, born outside hospital

Z38.8   Other multiple liveborn infant, unspecified as to place of birth

Z39   Encounter for maternal postpartum care and examination

Z39.0   Encounter for care and examination of mother immediately after delivery

Care and observation in uncomplicated cases when the delivery occurs outside a healthcare facility

Excludes1: care for postpartum complication- see Alphabetic index

Z39.1   Encounter for care and examination of lactating mother

Encounter for supervision of lactation

Excludes1: disorders of lactation (O92.-)

Z39.2   Encounter for routine postpartum follow-up

ENCOUNTERS FOR OTHER SPECIFIC HEALTH CARE (Z40-Z53)

Categories Z40-Z53 are intended for use to indicate a reason for care. They may be used for patients who have already been treated for a disease or injury, but who are receiving aftercare or prophylactic care, or care to consolidate the treatment, or to deal with a residual state

Excludes2: follow-up examination for medical surveillance after treatment (Z08-Z09)

Z40   Encounter for prophylactic surgery

Excludes1: organ donations (Z52.-)

therapeutic organ removal-code to condition

Z40.0   Encounter for prophylactic surgery for risk factors related to malignant neoplasms

Admission for prophylactic organ removal

Use additional code to identify risk factor

Z40.00   Encounter for prophylactic removal of unspecified organ

Z40.01   Encounter for prophylactic removal of breast

Z40.02   Encounter for prophylactic removal of ovary

Z40.09   Encounter for prophylactic removal of other organ

Z40.8   Encounter for other prophylactic surgery

Z40.9   Encounter for prophylactic surgery, unspecified

Z41   Encounter for procedures for purposes other than remedying health state

Z41.1   Encounter for cosmetic surgery

Encounter for cosmetic breast implant

Encounter for cosmetic procedure

Excludes1: encounter for plastic and reconstructive surgery following medical procedure or healed injury (Z42.-)

encounter for post-mastectomy breast implantation (Z42.1)

Z41.2   Encounter for routine and ritual male circumcision

Z41.3   Encounter for ear piercing

Z41.8   Encounter for other procedures for purposes other than remedying health state

Z41.9   Encounter for procedure for purposes other than remedying health state, unspecified

Z42   Encounter for plastic and reconstructive surgery following medical procedure or healed injury

Excludes1: encounter for cosmetic plastic surgery (Z41.1)

encounter for plastic surgery for treatment of current injury - code to relevent injury

Z42.1   Encounter for breast reconstruction following mastectomy

Excludes1: deformity and disproportion of reconstructed breast (N65.1-)

Z42.8   Encounter for other plastic and reconstructive surgery following medical procedure or healed injury

Z43   Encounter for attention to artificial openings

Includes: closure of artificial openings

passage of sounds or bougies through artificial openings

reforming artificial openings

removal of catheter from artificial openings toilet or cleansing of artificial openings

Excludes1: artificial opening status only, without need for care (Z93.-)

complications of external stoma (J95.0-, K94.-, N99.5-)

Excludes2: fitting and adjustment of prosthetic **and other** devices (Z44-Z46)

Z43.0   Encounter for attention to tracheostomy

Z43.1   Encounter for attention to gastrostomy

Z43.2   Encounter for attention to ileostomy

Z43.3   Encounter for attention to colostomy

Z43.4   Encounter for attention to other artificial openings of digestive tract

Z43.5   Encounter for attention to cystostomy

Z43.6   Encounter for attention to other artificial openings of urinary tract

Encounter for attention to nephrostomy

Encounter for attention to ureterostomy

Encounter for attention to urethrostomy

Z43.7   Encounter for attention to artificial vagina

Z43.8 Encounter for attention to other artificial openings

Z43.9 Encounter for attention to unspecified artificial opening

Z44 Encounter for fitting and adjustment of external prosthetic device

Includes: removal or replacement of external prosthetic device

Excludes1: malfunction or other complications of device - see Alphabetical Index

presence of prosthetic device (Z97.-)

Z44.0 Encounter for fitting and adjustment of artificial arm

Z44.00 Encounter for fitting and adjustment of unspecified artificial arm

Z44.001 Encounter for fitting and adjustment of unspecified right artificial arm

Z44.002 Encounter for fitting and adjustment of unspecified left artificial arm

Z44.009 Encounter for fitting and adjustment of unspecified artificial arm, unspecified arm

Z44.01 Encounter for fitting and adjustment of complete artificial arm

Z44.011 Encounter for fitting and adjustment of complete right artificial arm

Z44.012 Encounter for fitting and adjustment of complete left artificial arm

Z44.019 Encounter for fitting and adjustment of complete artificial arm, unspecified arm

Z44.02 Encounter for fitting and adjustment of partial artificial arm

Z44.021 Encounter for fitting and adjustment of partial artificial right arm

Z44.022 Encounter for fitting and adjustment of partial artificial left arm

Z44.029 Encounter for fitting and adjustment of partial artificial arm, unspecified arm

Z44.1 Encounter for fitting and adjustment of artificial leg

Z44.10 Encounter for fitting and adjustment of unspecified artificial leg

Z44.101 Encounter for fitting and adjustment of unspecified right artificial leg

Z44.102 Encounter for fitting and adjustment of unspecified left artificial leg

Z44.109 Encounter for fitting and adjustment of unspecified artificial leg, unspecified leg

Z44.11 Encounter for fitting and adjustment of complete artificial leg

Z44.111 Encounter for fitting and adjustment of complete right artificial leg

Z44.112 Encounter for fitting and adjustment of complete left artificial leg

Z44.119 Encounter for fitting and adjustment of complete artificial leg, unspecified leg

Z44.12 Encounter for fitting and adjustment of partial artificial leg

Z44.121 Encounter for fitting and adjustment of partial artificial right leg

Z44.122 Encounter for fitting and adjustment of partial artificial left leg

Z44.129 Encounter for fitting and adjustment of partial artificial leg, unspecified leg

Z44.2 Encounter for fitting and adjustment of artificial eye

Excludes1: mechanical complication of ocular prosthesis (T85.3)

Z44.20 Encounter for fitting and adjustment of artificial eye, unspecified

Z44.21 Encounter for fitting and adjustment of artificial right eye

Z44.22 Encounter for fitting and adjustment of artificial left eye

Z44.3 Encounter for fitting and adjustment of external breast prosthesis

Excludes1: complications of breast implant (T85.4-)

encounter for adjustment or removal of breast implant (Z45.81-)

encounter for initial breast implant insertion for cosmetic breast augmentation (Z41.1)

encounter for breast reconstruction following mastectomy (Z42.1)

Z44.30 Encounter for fitting and adjustment of external breast prosthesis, unspecified breast

Z44.31 Encounter for fitting and adjustment of external right breast prosthesis

Z44.32 Encounter for fitting and adjustment of external left breast prosthesis

Z44.8 Encounter for fitting and adjustment of other external prosthetic devices

Z44.9 Encounter for fitting and adjustment of unspecified external prosthetic device

Z45 Encounter for adjustment and management of implanted device

Includes: removal or replacement of implanted device

Excludes1: malfunction or other complications of device - see Alphabetical Index

presence of prosthetic and other devices (Z95-Z97)

Excludes2: encounter for fitting and adjustment of non-implanted device (Z46.-)

Z45.0 Encounter for adjustment and management of cardiac device

Z45.01 Encounter for adjustment and management of cardiac pacemaker

Encounter for adjustment and management of cardiac resynchronization therapy pacemaker (CRT-P)

Excludes1: encounter for adjustment and management of automatic implantable cardiac defibrillator with synchronous cardiac pacemaker (Z45.02)

Z45.010 **Encounter for checking and testing of cardiac pacemaker pulse generator [battery]**
Encounter for replacing cardiac pacemaker pulse generator [battery]

Z45.018 **Encounter for adjustment and management of other part of cardiac pacemaker**

Z45.02 **Encounter for adjustment and management of automatic implantable cardiac defibrillator**
Encounter for adjustment and management of automatic implantable cardiac defibrillator with synchronous cardiac pacemaker
Encounter for adjustment and management of cardiac resynchronization therapy defibrillator (CRT-D)

Z45.09 **Encounter for adjustment and management of other cardiac device**

Z45.1 **Encounter for adjustment and management of infusion pump**

Z45.2 **Encounter for adjustment and management of vascular access device**
Encounter for adjustment and management of vascular catheters
Excludes1: encounter for adjustment and management of renal dialysis catheter (Z49.01)

Z45.3 **Encounter for adjustment and management of implanted devices of the special senses**

Z45.31 **Encounter for adjustment and management of implanted visual substitution device**

Z45.32 **Encounter for adjustment and management of implanted hearing device**
Excludes1: Encounter for fitting and adjustment of hearing aide (Z46.1)

Z45.320 **Encounter for adjustment and management of bone conduction device**

Z45.321 **Encounter for adjustment and management of cochlear device**

Z45.328 **Encounter for adjustment and management of other implanted hearing device**

Z45.4 **Encounter for adjustment and management of implanted nervous system device**

Z45.41 **Encounter for adjustment and management of cerebrospinal fluid drainage device**
Encounter for adjustment and management of cerebral ventricular (communicating) shunt

Z45.42 **Encounter for adjustment and management of neuropacemaker (brain) (peripheral nerve) (spinal cord)**

Z45.49 **Encounter for adjustment and management of other implanted nervous system device**

Z45.8 **Encounter for adjustment and management of other implanted devices**

Z45.81 **Encounter for adjustment or removal of breast implant**
Encounter for elective implant exchange (different material) (different size)
Encounter removal of tissue expander without synchronous insertion of permanent implant
Excludes1: complications of breast implant (T85.4-)

encounter for initial breast implant insertion for cosmetic breast augmentation (Z41.1)
encounter for breast reconstruction following mastectomy (Z42.1)

Z45.811 **Encounter for adjustment or removal of right breast implant**

Z45.812 **Encounter for adjustment or removal of left breast implant**

Z45.819 **Encounter for adjustment or removal of unspecified breast implant**

Z45.82 **Encounter for adjustment or removal of myringotomy device (stent) (tube)**

Z45.89 **Encounter for adjustment and management of other implanted devices**

Z45.9 **Encounter for adjustment and management of unspecified implanted device**

Z46 **Encounter for fitting and adjustment of other devices**
Includes: removal or replacement of other device
Excludes1: malfunction or other complications of device - see Alphabetical Index
Excludes2: encounter for fitting and management of implanted devices (Z45.-)
issue of repeat prescription only (Z76.0)
presence of prosthetic and other devices (Z95-Z97)

Z46.0 **Encounter for fitting and adjustment of spectacles and contact lenses**

Z46.1 **Encounter for fitting and adjustment of hearing aid**
Excludes1: encounter for adjustment and management of implanted hearing device (Z45.32-)

Z46.2 **Encounter for fitting and adjustment of other devices related to nervous system and special senses**
Excludes2: encounter for adjustment and management of implanted nervous system device (Z45.4-)
encounter for adjustment and management of implanted visual substitution device (Z45.31)

Z46.3 **Encounter for fitting and adjustment of dental prosthetic device**
Encounter for fitting and adjustment of dentures

Z46.4 **Encounter for fitting and adjustment of orthodontic device**

Z46.5 **Encounter for fitting and adjustment of other gastrointestinal appliance and device**
Excludes1: encounter for attention to artificial openings of digestive tract (Z43.1-Z43.4)

Z46.51 **Encounter for fitting and adjustment of gastric lap band**

Z46.59 **Encounter for fitting and adjustment of other gastrointestinal appliance and device**

Z46.6 **Encounter for fitting and adjustment of urinary device**
Excludes2: attention to artificial openings of urinary tract (Z43.5, Z43.6)

Z46.8 **Encounter for fitting and adjustment of other specified devices**

Z46.81 **Encounter for fitting and adjustment of insulin pump**
Encounter for insulin pump instruction and training
Encounter for insulin pump titration

Z46.82 Encounter for fitting and adjustment of non-vascular catheter

Z46.89 Encounter for fitting and adjustment of other specified devices

Encounter for fitting and adjustment of wheelchair

Z46.9 Encounter for fitting and adjustment of unspecified device

Z47 Orthopedic aftercare

Excludes1: aftercare for healing fracture-code to fracture with 7th character D

Z47.1 Aftercare following joint replacement surgery

Use additional code to identify the joint (Z96.6-)

Z47.2 Encounter for removal of internal fixation device

Excludes1: encounter for adjustment of internal fixation device for fracture treatment- code to fracture with appropriate 7th character

encounter for removal of external fixation device- code to fracture with 7th character D infection or inflammatory reaction to internal fixation device (T84.6-)

mechanical complication of internal fixation device (T84.1-)

Z47.3 Aftercare following explantation of joint prosthesis

Aftercare following explantation of joint prosthesis, staged procedure

Encounter for joint prosthesis insertion following prior explantation of joint prosthesis

Z47.31 Aftercare following explantation of shoulder joint prosthesis

Excludes1: acquired absence of shoulder joint following prior explantation of shoulder joint prosthesis (Z89.23-)

shoulder joint prosthesis explantation status (Z89.23-)

Z47.32 Aftercare following explantation of hip joint prosthesis

Excludes1: acquired absence of hip joint following prior explantation of hip joint prosthesis (Z89.62-)

hip joint prosthesis explantation status (Z89.62-)

Z47.33 Aftercare following explantation of knee joint prosthesis

Excludes1: acquired absence of knee joint following prior explantation of knee prosthesis (Z89.52-

knee joint prosthesis explantation status (Z89.52-)

Z47.8 Encounter for other orthopedic aftercare

Z47.81 Encounter for orthopedic aftercare following surgical amputation

Use additional code to identify the limb amputated (Z89.-)

Z47.82 Encounter for orthopedic aftercare following scoliosis surgery

Z47.89 Encounter for other orthopedic aftercare

Z48 Encounter for other postprocedural aftercare

Excludes1: encounter for follow-up examination after completed treatment (Z08-Z09)

Excludes2: encounter for attention to artificial openings (Z43.-)

encounter for fitting and adjustment of prosthetic **and other** devices (Z44-Z46)

Z48.0 Encounter for attention to dressings, sutures and drains

Excludes1: encounter for planned postprocedural wound closure (Z48.1)

Z48.00 Encounter for change or removal of nonsurgical wound dressing

Encounter for change or removal of wound dressing NOS

Z48.01 Encounter for change or removal of surgical wound dressing

Z48.02 Encounter for removal of sutures

Encounter for removal of staples

Z48.03 Encounter for change or removal of drains

Z48.1 Encounter for planned postprocedural wound closure

Excludes1: encounter for attention to dressings and sutures (Z48.0-)

Z48.2 Encounter for aftercare following organ transplant

Z48.21 Encounter for aftercare following heart transplant

Z48.22 Encounter for aftercare following kidney transplant

Z48.23 Encounter for aftercare following liver transplant

Z48.24 Encounter for aftercare following lung transplant

Z48.28 Encounter for aftercare following multiple organ transplant

Z48.280 Encounter for aftercare following heart-lung transplant

Z48.288 Encounter for aftercare following multiple organ transplant

Z48.29 Encounter for aftercare following other organ transplant

Z48.290 Encounter for aftercare following bone marrow transplant

Z48.298 Encounter for aftercare following other organ transplant

Z48.3 Aftercare following surgery for neoplasm

Use additional code to identify the neoplasm

Z48.8 Encounter for other specified postprocedural aftercare

Z48.81 Encounter for surgical aftercare following surgery on specified body systems

These codes identify the body system requiring aftercare. They are for use in conjunction with other aftercare codes to fully explain the aftercare encounter. The condition treated should also be coded if still present.

Excludes1: aftercare for injury- code the injury with 7th character D

aftercare following surgery for neoplasm (Z48.3)

Excludes2: aftercare following organ transplant (Z48.2-)

orthopedic aftercare (Z47.-)

Z48.810 Encounter for surgical aftercare following surgery on the sense organs

Z48.811 Encounter for surgical aftercare following surgery on the nervous system

Excludes2: encounter for surgical aftercare following surgery on the sense organs (Z48.810)

Z48.812 **Encounter for surgical aftercare following surgery on the circulatory system**

Z48.813 **Encounter for surgical aftercare following surgery on the respiratory system**

Z48.814 **Encounter for surgical aftercare following surgery on the teeth or oral cavity**

Z48.815 **Encounter for surgical aftercare following surgery on the digestive system**

Z48.816 **Encounter for surgical aftercare following surgery on the genitourinary system**

Excludes1: encounter for aftercare following sterilization reversal (Z31.42)

Z48.817 **Encounter for surgical aftercare following surgery on the skin and subcutaneous tissue**

Z48.89 **Encounter for other specified surgical aftercare**

Z49 **Encounter for care involving renal dialysis**

Code also associated end stage renal disease (N18.6)

Z49.0 **Preparatory care for renal dialysis**

Encounter for dialysis instruction and training

Z49.01 **Encounter for fitting and adjustment of extracorporeal dialysis catheter**

Removal or replacement of renal dialysis catheter

Toilet or cleansing of renal dialysis catheter

Z49.02 **Encounter for fitting and adjustment of peritoneal dialysis catheter**

Z49.3 **Encounter for adequacy testing for dialysis**

Z49.31 **Encounter for adequacy testing for hemodialysis**

Z49.32 **Encounter for adequacy testing for peritoneal dialysis**

Encounter for peritoneal equilibration test

Z51 **Encounter for other aftercare and medical care**

Code also condition requiring care

Excludes1: follow-up examination after treatment (Z08-Z09)

Z51.0 **Encounter for antineoplastic radiation therapy**

Z51.1 **Encounter for antineoplastic chemotherapy and immunotherapy**

Excludes2: encounter for chemotherapy and immunotherapy for nonneoplastic condition - code to condition

Z51.11 **Encounter for antineoplastic chemotherapy**

Z51.12 **Encounter for antineoplastic immunotherapy**

Z51.5 **Encounter for palliative care**

●Z51.6 **Encounter for desensitization to allergens**

Z51.8 **Encounter for other specified aftercare**

Excludes1: holiday relief care (Z75.5)

Z51.81 **Encounter for therapeutic drug level monitoring**

Code also any long-term (current) drug therapy (Z79.-)

Excludes1: encounter for blood-drug test for administrative or medicolegal reasons (Z02.83)

Z51.89 **Encounter for other specified aftercare**

Z52 **Donors of organs and tissues**

Includes: autologous and other living donors

Excludes1: cadaveric donor - omit code examination of potential donor (Z00.5)

Z52.0 **Blood donor**

Z52.00 **Unspecified blood donor**

Z52.000 **Unspecified donor, whole blood**

Z52.001 **Unspecified donor, stem cells**

Z52.008 **Unspecified donor, other blood**

Z52.01 **Autologous blood donor**

Z52.010 **Autologous donor, whole blood**

Z52.011 **Autologous donor, stem cells**

Z52.018 **Autologous donor, other blood**

Z52.09 **Other blood donor** Volunteer donor

Z52.090 **Other blood donor, whole blood**

Z52.091 **Other blood donor, stem cells**

Z52.098 **Other blood donor, other blood**

Z52.1 **Skin donor**

Z52.10 **Skin donor, unspecified**

Z52.11 **Skin donor, autologous**

Z52.19 **Skin donor, other**

Z52.2 **Bone donor**

Z52.20 **Bone donor, unspecified**

Z52.21 **Bone donor, autologous**

Z52.29 **Bone donor, other**

Z52.3 **Bone marrow donor**

Z52.4 **Kidney donor**

Z52.5 **Cornea donor**

Z52.6 **Liver donor**

Z52.8 **Donor of other specified organs or tissues**

Z52.81 **Egg (Oocyte) donor**

Z52.810 **Egg (Oocyte) donor under age 35, anonymous recipient**

Egg donor under age 35 NOS

Z52.811 **Egg (Oocyte) donor under age 35, designated recipient**

Z52.812 **Egg (Oocyte) donor age 35 and over, anonymous recipient**

Egg donor age 35 and over NOS

Z52.813 **Egg (Oocyte) donor age 35 and over, designated recipient**

Z52.819 **Egg (Oocyte) donor, unspecified**

Z52.89 **Donor of other specified organs or tissues**

Z52.9 **Donor of unspecified organ or tissue**

Donor NOS

Z53 **Persons encountering health services for specific procedures and treatment, not carried out**

Z53.0 **Procedure and treatment not carried out because of contraindication**

Z53.01 **Procedure and treatment not carried out due to patient smoking**

Z53.09 **Procedure and treatment not carried out because of other contraindication**

Z53.1 Procedure and treatment not carried out because of patient's decision for reasons of belief and group pressure

Z53.2 Procedure and treatment not carried out because of patient's decision for other and unspecified reasons

Z53.20 Procedure and treatment not carried out because of patient's decision for unspecified reasons

Z53.21 Procedure and treatment not carried out due to patient leaving prior to being seen by health care provider

Z53.29 Procedure and treatment not carried out because of patient's decision for other reasons

Z53.3 Procedure converted to open procedure

●**Z53.31** Laparoscopic surgical procedure converted to open procedure

●**Z53.32** Thoracoscopic surgical procedure converted to open procedure

●**Z53.33** Arthroscopic surgical procedure converted to open procedure

●**Z53.39** Other specified procedure converted to open procedure

Z53.8 Procedure and treatment not carried out for other reasons

Z53.9 Procedure and treatment not carried out, unspecified reason

PERSONS WITH POTENTIAL HEALTH HAZARDS RELATED TO SOCIOECONOMIC AND PSYCHOSOCIAL CIRCUMSTANCES (Z55-Z65)

Z55 Problems related to education and literacy

Excludes1: disorders of psychological development (F80-F89)

Z55.0 Illiteracy and low-level literacy

Z55.1 Schooling unavailable and unattainable

Z55.2 Failed school examinations

Z55.3 Underachievement in school

Z55.4 Educational maladjustment and discord with teachers and classmates

Z55.8 Other problems related to education and literacy

Problems related to inadequate teaching

Z55.9 Problems related to education and literacy, unspecified

Academic problems NOS

Z56 Problems related to employment and unemployment

Excludes2: occupational exposure to risk factors (Z57.-)

problems related to housing and economic circumstances (Z59.-)

Z56.0 Unemployment, unspecified

Z56.1 Change of job

Z56.2 Threat of job loss

Z56.3 Stressful work schedule

Z56.4 Discord with boss and workmates

Z56.5 Uncongenial work environment

Difficult conditions at work

Z56.6 Other physical and mental strain related to work

Z56.8 Other problems related to employment

Z56.81 Sexual harassment on the job

Z56.82 Military deployment status

Individual (civilian or military) currently deployed in theater or in support of military war, peacekeeping and humanitarian operations

Z56.89 Other problems related to employment

Z56.9 Unspecified problems related to employment

Occupational problems NOS

Z57 Occupational exposure to risk factors

Z57.0 Occupational exposure to noise

Z57.1 Occupational exposure to radiation

Z57.2 Occupational exposure to dust

Z57.3 Occupational exposure to other air contaminants

Z57.31 Occupational exposure to environmental tobacco smoke

Excludes2: exposure to environmental tobacco smoke (Z77.22)

Z57.39 Occupational exposure to other air contaminants

Z57.4 Occupational exposure to toxic agents in agriculture

Occupational exposure to solids, liquids, gases or vapors in agriculture

Z57.5 Occupational exposure to toxic agents in other industries

Occupational exposure to solids, liquids, gases or vapors in other industries

Z57.6 Occupational exposure to extreme temperature

Z57.7 Occupational exposure to vibration

Z57.8 Occupational exposure to other risk factors

Z57.9 Occupational exposure to unspecified risk factor

Z59 Problems related to housing and economic circumstances

Excludes2: problems related to upbringing (Z62.-)

Z59.0 Homelessness

Z59.1 Inadequate housing

Lack of heating

Restriction of space

Technical defects in home preventing adequate care

Unsatisfactory surroundings

Excludes1: problems related to the natural and physical environment (Z77.1-)

Z59.2 Discord with neighbors, lodgers and landlord

Z59.3 Problems related to living in residential institution

Boarding-school resident

Excludes1: institutional upbringing (Z62.2)

Z59.4 Lack of adequate food and safe drinking water

Inadequate drinking water supply

Excludes1: effects of hunger (T73.0)

inappropriate diet or eating habits (Z72.4)

malnutrition (E40-E46)

Z59.5 Extreme poverty

Z59.6 Low income

Z59.7 Insufficient social insurance and welfare support

Z59.8 Other problems related to housing and economic circumstances

Foreclosure on loan

Isolated dwelling

Problems with creditors

Z59.9 Problem related to housing and economic circumstances, unspecified

---

Add 4th-7th digits   Nonspecific code   Unspecified code   Manifestation code

Z60 Problems related to social environment

Z60.0 **Problems of adjustment to life-cycle transitions**
Empty nest syndrome
Phase of life problem
Problem with adjustment to retirement [pension]

Z60.2 **Problems related to living alone**

Z60.3 **Acculturation difficulty**
Problem with migration
Problem with social transplantation

Z60.4 **Social exclusion and rejection**
Exclusion and rejection on the basis of personal characteristics, such as unusual physical appearance, illness or behavior.
Excludes1: target of adverse discrimination such as for racial or religious reasons (Z60.5)

Z60.5 **Target of (perceived) adverse discrimination and persecution**
Excludes1: social exclusion and rejection (Z60.4)

Z60.8 **Other problems related to social environment**

Z60.9 **Problem related to social environment, unspecified**

Z62 Problems related to upbringing
Includes: current and past negative life events in childhood
current and past problems of a child related to upbringing
Excludes2: maltreatment syndrome (T74.-)
problems related to housing and economic circumstances (Z59.-)

Z62.0 **Inadequate parental supervision and control**

Z62.1 **Parental overprotection**

Z62.2 **Upbringing away from parents**
Excludes1: problems with boarding school (Z59.3)

Z62.21 **Child in welfare custody**
Child in care of non-parental family member
Child in foster care
Excludes2: problem for parent due to child in welfare custody (Z63.5)

Z62.22 **Institutional upbringing**
Child living in orphanage or group home

Z62.29 **Other upbringing away from parents**

Z62.3 **Hostility towards and scapegoating of child**

Z62.6 **Inappropriate (excessive) parental pressure**

Z62.8 **Other specified problems related to upbringing**

Z62.81 **Personal history of abuse in childhood**

Z62.810 **Personal history of physical and sexual abuse in childhood**
Excludes1: current child physical abuse (T74.12, T76.12)
current child sexual abuse (T74.22, T76.22)

Z62.811 **Personal history of psychological abuse in childhood**
Excludes1: current child psychological abuse (T74.32, T76.32)

Z62.812 **Personal history of neglect in childhood**
Excludes1: current child neglect (T74.02, T76.02)

Z62.819 **Personal history of unspecified abuse in childhood**
Excludes1: current child abuse NOS (T74.92, T76.92)

Z62.82 **Parent-child conflict**

Z62.820 **Parent-biological child conflict**
Parent-child problem NOS

Z62.821 **Parent-adopted child conflict**

Z62.822 **Parent-foster child conflict**

Z62.89 **Other specified problems related to upbringing**

Z62.890 **Parent-child estrangement NEC**

Z62.891 **Sibling rivalry**

Z62.898 **Other specified problems related to upbringing**

Z62.9 **Problem related to upbringing, unspecified**

Z63 Other problems related to primary support group, including family circumstances
Excludes2: maltreatment syndrome (T74.-, T76)
parent-child problems (Z62.-)
problems related to negative life events in childhood (Z62.-)
problems related to upbringing (Z62.-)

Z63.0 **Problems in relationship with spouse or partner**
Excludes1: counseling for spousal or partner abuse problems (Z69.1)
counseling related to sexual attitude, behavior, and orientation (Z70.-)

Z63.1 **Problems in relationship with in-laws**

Z63.3 **Absence of family member**
Excludes1: absence of family member due to disappearance and death (Z63.4)
absence of family member due to separation and divorce (Z63.5)

Z63.31 **Absence of family member due to military deployment**
Individual or family affected by other family member being on military deployment
Excludes1: family disruption due to return of family member from military deployment (Z63.71)

Z63.32 **Other absence of family member**

Z63.4 **Disappearance and death of family member**
Assumed death of family member
Bereavement

Z63.5 **Disruption of family by separation and divorce**
Marital estrangement

Z63.6 **Dependent relative needing care at home**

Z63.7 **Other stressful life events affecting family and household**

Z63.71 **Stress on family due to return of family member from military deployment**
Individual or family affected by family member having returned from military deployment (current or past conflict)

Z63.72 **Alcoholism and drug addiction in family**

Z63.79 **Other stressful life events affecting family and household**

Anxiety (normal) about sick person in family

Health problems within family

Ill or disturbed family member

Isolated family

Z63.8 Other specified problems related to primary support group

Family discord NOS Family estrangement NOS

High expressed emotional level within family

Inadequate family support NOS

Inadequate or distorted communication within family

Z63.9 Problem related to primary support group, unspecified

Relationship disorder NOS

Z64 Problems related to certain psychosocial circumstances

Z64.0 Problems related to unwanted pregnancy

Z64.1 Problems related to multiparity

Z64.4 Discord with counselors

Discord with probation officer

Discord with social worker

Z65 Problems related to other psychosocial circumstances

Z65.0 Conviction in civil and criminal proceedings without imprisonment

Z65.1 Imprisonment and other incarceration

Z65.2 Problems related to release from prison

Z65.3 Problems related to other legal circumstances

Arrest

Child custody or support proceedings Litigation

Prosecution

Z65.4 Victim of crime and terrorism

Victim of torture

Z65.5 Exposure to disaster, war and other hostilities

Excludes1: target of perceived discrimination or persecution (Z60.5)

Z65.8 Other specified problems related to psychosocial circumstances

Z65.9 Problem related to unspecified psychosocial circumstances

DO NOT RESUSCITATE STATUS (Z66)

Z66 Do not resuscitate

DNR status

BLOOD TYPE (Z67)

Z67 Blood type

Z67.1 Type A blood

Z67.10 Type A blood, Rh positive

Z67.11 Type A blood, Rh negative

Z67.2 Type B blood

Z67.20 Type B blood, Rh positive

Z67.21 Type B blood, Rh negative

Z67.3 Type AB blood

Z67.30 Type AB blood, Rh positive

Z67.31 Type AB blood, Rh negative

Z67.4 Type O blood

Z67.40 Type O blood, Rh positive

Z67.41 Type O blood, Rh negative

Z67.9 Unspecified blood type

Z67.90 Unspecified blood type, Rh positive

Z67.91 Unspecified blood type, Rh negative

BODY MASS INDEX [BMI] (Z68)

Definition: Body Mass Index is a measure of body fat that is the ratio of the weight of the body in kilograms to the square of its height in meters.

Z68 Body mass index [BMI]

Kilograms per meters squared

Note: BMI adult codes are for use for persons 21 years of age or older

BMI pediatric codes are for use for persons 2-20 years of age. These percentiles are based on the growth charts published by the Centers for Disease Control and Prevention (CDC)

Z68.1 Body mass index (BMI) 19 or less, adult

Z68.2 Body mass index (BMI) 20-29, adult

Z68.20 Body mass index (BMI) 20.0-20.9, adult

Z68.21 Body mass index (BMI) 21.0-21.9, adult

Z68.22 Body mass index (BMI) 22.0-22.9, adult

Z68.23 Body mass index (BMI) 23.0-23.9, adult

Z68.24 Body mass index (BMI) 24.0-24.9, adult

Z68.25 Body mass index (BMI) 25.0-25.9, adult

Z68.26 Body mass index (BMI) 26.0-26.9, adult

Z68.27 Body mass index (BMI) 27.0-27.9, adult

Z68.28 Body mass index (BMI) 28.0-28.9, adult

Z68.29 Body mass index (BMI) 29.0-29.9, adult

Z68.3 Body mass index (BMI) 30-39, adult

Z68.30 Body mass index (BMI) 30.0-30.9, adult

Z68.31 Body mass index (BMI) 31.0-31.9, adult

Z68.32 Body mass index (BMI) 32.0-32.9, adult

Z68.33 Body mass index (BMI) 33.0-33.9, adult

Z68.34 Body mass index (BMI) 34.0-34.9, adult

Z68.35 Body mass index (BMI) 35.0-35.9, adult

Z68.36 Body mass index (BMI) 36.0-36.9, adult

Z68.37 Body mass index (BMI) 37.0-37.9, adult

Z68.38 Body mass index (BMI) 38.0-38.9, adult

Z68.39 Body mass index (BMI) 39.0-39.9, adult

Z68.4 Body mass index (BMI) 40 or greater, adult

Z68.41 Body mass index (BMI) 40.0-44.9, adult

Z68.42 Body mass index (BMI) 45.0-49.9, adult

Z68.43 Body mass index (BMI) 50-59.9, adult

Z68.44 Body mass index (BMI) 60.0-69.9, adult

Z68.45 Body mass index (BMI) 70 or greater, adult

Z68.5 Body mass index (BMI) pediatric

Z68.51 Body mass index (BMI) pediatric, less than 5th percentile for age

Z68.52 Body mass index (BMI) pediatric, 5th percentile to less than 85th percentile for age

Z68.53 Body mass index (BMI) pediatric, 85th percentile to less than 95th percentile for age

Z68.54 Body mass index (BMI) pediatric, greater than or equal to 95th percentile for age

PERSONS ENCOUNTERING HEALTH SERVICES IN OTHER CIRCUMSTANCES (Z69-Z76)

Z69 **Encounter for mental health services for victim and perpetrator of abuse**

Includes: counseling for victims and perpetrators of abuse

Z69.0 **Encounter for mental health services for child abuse problems**

Z69.01 **Encounter for mental health services for parental child abuse**

Z69.010 **Encounter for mental health services for victim of parental child abuse**

Z69.011 **Encounter for mental health services for perpetrator of parental child abuse**

Excludes1: encounter for mental health services for non-parental child abuse (Z69.02-)

Z69.02 **Encounter for mental health services for non-parental child abuse**

Z69.020 **Encounter for mental health services for victim of non-parental child abuse**

Z69.021 **Encounter for mental health services for perpetrator of non-parental child abuse**

Z69.1 **Encounter for mental health services for spousal or partner abuse problems**

Z69.11 **Encounter for mental health services for victim of spousal or partner abuse**

Z69.12 **Encounter for mental health services for perpetrator of spousal or partner abuse**

Z69.8 **Encounter for mental health services for victim or perpetrator of other abuse**

Z69.81 **Encounter for mental health services for victim of other abuse**

Encounter for rape victim counseling

Z69.82 **Encounter for mental health services for perpetrator of other abuse**

Z70 **Counseling related to sexual attitude, behavior and orientation**

Includes: encounter for mental health services for sexual attitude, behavior and orientation

Excludes2: contraceptive or procreative counseling (Z30-Z31)

Z70.0 **Counseling related to sexual attitude**

Z70.1 **Counseling related to patient's sexual behavior and orientation**

Patient concerned regarding impotence

Patient concerned regarding non-responsiveness

Patient concerned regarding promiscuity

Patient concerned regarding sexual orientation

Z70.2 **Counseling related to sexual behavior and orientation of third party**

Advice sought regarding sexual behavior and orientation of child

Advice sought regarding sexual behavior and orientation of partner

Advice sought regarding sexual behavior and orientation of spouse

Z70.3 **Counseling related to combined concerns regarding sexual attitude, behavior and orientation**

Z70.8 **Other sex counseling**

Encounter for sex education

Z70.9 **Sex counseling, unspecified**

Z71 **Persons encountering health services for other counseling and medical advice, not elsewhere classified**

Excludes2: contraceptive or procreation counseling (Z30-Z31)

sex counseling (Z70.-)

Z71.0 **Person encountering health services to consult on behalf of another person**

Person encountering health services to seek advice or treatment for non-attending third party

Excludes2: anxiety (normal) about sick person in family (Z63.7)

expectant (adoptive) parent(s) pre-birth pediatrician visit (Z76.81)

Z71.1 **Person with feared health complaint in whom no diagnosis is made**

Person encountering health services with feared condition which was not demonstrated

Person encountering health services in which problem was normal state

'Worried well'

Excludes1: medical observation for suspected diseases and conditions proven not to exist (Z03.-)

Z71.2 **Person consulting for explanation of examination or test findings**

Z71.3 **Dietary counseling and surveillance**

Use additional code for any associated underlying medical condition

Use additional code to identify body mass index (BMI), if known (Z68.-)

Z71.4 **Alcohol abuse counseling and surveillance**

Use additional code for alcohol abuse or dependence (F10.-)

Z71.41 **Alcohol abuse counseling and surveillance of alcoholic**

Z71.42 **Counseling for family member of alcoholic**

Counseling for significant **Other**, partner, or friend of alcoholic

Z71.5 **Drug abuse counseling and surveillance**

Use additional code for drug abuse or dependence (F11-F16, F18-F19)

Z71.51 **Drug abuse counseling and surveillance of drug abuser**

Z71.52 **Counseling for family member of drug abuser**

Counseling for significant **Other**, partner, or friend of drug abuser

Z71.6 **Tobacco abuse counseling**

Use additional code for nicotine dependence (F17.-)

Z71.7 **Human immunodeficiency virus [HIV] counseling**

Z71.8 **Other specified counseling**

Excludes2: counseling for contraception (Z30.0-)

counseling for genetics (Z31.5)

counseling for procreative management (Z31.6-)

Z71.81 **Spiritual or religious counseling**

Z71.89 **Other specified counseling**

Z71.9 **Counseling, unspecified**

Encounter for medical advice NOS

Z72 **Problems related to lifestyle**

Excludes2: problems related to life-management difficulty (Z73.-)

problems related to socioeconomic and psychosocial circumstances (Z55-Z65)

Z72.0 **Tobacco use**

Tobacco use NOS

Excludes1: history of tobacco dependence (Z87.891)

nicotine dependence (F17.2-)

tobacco dependence (F17.2-)

tobacco use during pregnancy (O99.33-)

Z72.3 **Lack of physical exercise**

Z72.4 **Inappropriate diet and eating habits**

Excludes1: behavioral eating disorders of infancy or childhood (F98.2.-F98.3)

eating disorders (F50.-)

lack of adequate food (Z59.4)

malnutrition and other nutritional deficiencies (E40-E64)

Z72.5 **High risk sexual behavior**

Promiscuity

Excludes1: paraphilias (F65)

Z72.51 **High risk heterosexual behavior**

Z72.52 **High risk homosexual behavior**

Z72.53 **High risk bisexual behavior**

Z72.6 **Gambling and betting**

Excludes1: compulsive or pathological gambling (F63.0)

Z72.8 **Other problems related to lifestyle**

Z72.81 **Antisocial behavior**

Excludes1: conduct disorders (F91.-)

Z72.810 **Child and adolescent antisocial behavior** Antisocial behavior (child) (adolescent) without manifest psychiatric disorder

Delinquency NOS

Group delinquency

Offenses in the context of gang membership

Stealing in company with others

Truancy from school

Z72.811 **Adult antisocial behavior** Adult antisocial behavior without manifest psychiatric disorder

Z72.82 **Problems related to sleep**

Z72.820 **Sleep deprivation**

Lack of adequate sleep

Excludes1: insomnia (G47.0-)

Z72.821 **Inadequate sleep hygiene**

Bad sleep habits

Irregular sleep habits

Unhealthy sleep wake schedule

Excludes1: insomnia (F51.0-, G47.0-)

Z72.89 **Other problems related to lifestyle**

Self-damaging behavior

Z72.9 **Problem related to lifestyle, unspecified**

Z73 **Problems related to life management difficulty**

Excludes2: problems related to socioeconomic and psychosocial circumstances (Z55-Z65)

Z73.0 **Burn-out**

Z73.1 **Type A behavior pattern**

Z73.2 **Lack of relaxation and leisure**

Z73.3 **Stress, not elsewhere classified**

Physical and mental strain NOS

Excludes1: stress related to employment or unemployment (Z56.-)

Z73.4 **Inadequate social skills, not elsewhere classified**

Z73.5 **Social role conflict, not elsewhere classified**

Z73.6 **Limitation of activities due to disability**

Excludes1: care-provider dependency (Z74.-)

Z73.8 **Other problems related to life management difficulty**

Z73.81 **Behavioral insomnia of childhood**

Z73.810 **Behavioral insomnia of childhood, sleep-onset association type**

Z73.811 **Behavioral insomnia of childhood, limit setting type**

Z73.812 **Behavioral insomnia of childhood, combined type**

Z73.819 **Behavioral insomnia of childhood, unspecified type**

Z73.82 **Dual sensory impairment**

Z73.89 **Other problems related to life management difficulty**

Z73.9 **Problem related to life management difficulty, unspecified**

Z74 **Problems related to care provider dependency**

Excludes2: dependence on enabling machines or devices NEC (Z99.-)

Z74.0 **Reduced mobility**

Z74.01 **Bed confinement status**

Bedridden

Z74.09 **Other reduced mobility**

Chairridden

Reduced mobility NOS

Excludes2: wheelchair dependence (Z99.3)

Z74.1 **Need for assistance with personal care**

Z74.2 **Need for assistance at home and no other household member able to render care**

Z74.3 **Need for continuous supervision**

Z74.8 **Other problems related to care provider dependency**

Z74.9 **Problem related to care provider dependency, unspecified**

Z75 **Problems related to medical facilities and other health care**

Z75.0 **Medical services not available in home**

Excludes1: no Other household member able to render care (Z74.2)

Z75.1 **Person awaiting admission to adequate facility elsewhere**

Z75.2 **Other waiting period for investigation and treatment**

Z75.3 **Unavailability and inaccessibility of health-care facilities**

Excludes1: bed unavailable (Z75.1)

Z75.4 **Unavailability and inaccessibility of other helping agencies**

Z75.5 **Holiday relief care**

Z75.8 **Other problems related to medical facilities and other health care**

Z75.9 **Unspecified problem related to medical facilities and other health care**

Z76 **Persons encountering health services in other circumstances**

Z76.0 **Encounter for issue of repeat prescription**

Encounter for issue of repeat prescription for appliance

Encounter for issue of repeat prescription for medicaments

Encounter for issue of repeat prescription for spectacles

Excludes2: issue of medical certificate (Z02.7)

repeat prescription for contraceptive (Z30.4-)

Z76.1 **Encounter for health supervision and care of foundling**

Z76.2 **Encounter for health supervision and care of other healthy infant and child**

Encounter for medical or nursing care or supervision of healthy infant under circumstances such as adverse socioeconomic conditions at home

Encounter for medical or nursing care or supervision of healthy infant under circumstances such as awaiting foster or adoptive placement

Encounter for medical or nursing care or supervision of healthy infant under circumstances such as maternal illness

Encounter for medical or nursing care or supervision of healthy infant under circumstances such as number of children at home preventing or interfering with normal care

Z76.3 **Healthy person accompanying sick person**

Z76.4 **Other boarder to healthcare facility**

Excludes1: homelessness (Z59.0)

Z76.5 **Malingerer [conscious simulation]**

Person feigning illness (with obvious motivation)

Excludes1: factitious disorder (F68.1-)

peregrinating patient (F68.1-)

Z76.8 **Persons encountering health services in other specified circumstances**

Z76.81 **Expectant parent(s) prebirth pediatrician visit**

Pre-adoption pediatrician visit for adoptive parent(s)

Z76.82 **Awaiting organ transplant status**

Patient waiting for organ availability

Z76.89 **Persons encountering health services in other specified circumstances**

Persons encountering health services NOS

PERSONS WITH POTENTIAL HEALTH HAZARDS RELATED TO FAMILY AND PERSONAL HISTORY AND CERTAIN CONDITIONS INFLUENCING HEALTH STATUS (Z77-Z99)

Code also any follow-up examination (Z08-Z09)

Z77 **Other contact with and (suspected) exposures hazardous to health**

Includes: contact with and (suspected) exposures to potential hazards to health

Excludes2: contact with and (suspected) exposure to communicable diseases (Z20.-)

exposure to (parental) (environmental) tobacco smoke in the perinatal period (P96.81)

newborn affected by noxious substances transmitted via placenta or breast milk (P04.-)

occupational exposure to risk factors (Z57.-)

retained foreign body (Z18.-)

retained foreign body fully removed (Z87.821)

toxic effects of substances chiefly nonmedicinal as to source (T51-T65)

Z77.0 **Contact with and (suspected) exposure to hazardous, chiefly nonmedicinal, chemicals**

Z77.01 **Contact with and (suspected) exposure to hazardous metals**

Z77.010 **Contact with and (suspected) exposure to arsenic**

Z77.011 **Contact with and (suspected) exposure to lead**

Z77.012 **Contact with and (suspected) exposure to uranium**

Excludes1: retained depleted uranium fragments (Z18.01)

Z77.018 **Contact with and (suspected) exposure to other hazardous metals**

Contact with and (suspected) exposure to chromium compounds

Contact with and (suspected) exposure to nickel dust

Z77.02 **Contact with and (suspected) exposure to hazardous aromatic compounds**

Z77.020 **Contact with and (suspected) exposure to aromatic amines**

Z77.021 **Contact with and (suspected) exposure to benzene**

Z77.028 **Contact with and (suspected) exposure to other hazardous aromatic compounds**

Aromatic dyes NOS

Polycyclic aromatic hydrocarbons

Z77.09 **Contact with and (suspected) exposure to other hazardous, chiefly nonmedicinal, chemicals**

Z77.090 **Contact with and (suspected) exposure to asbestos**

Z77.098 **Contact with and (suspected) exposure to other hazardous, chiefly nonmedicinal, chemicals** Dyes NOS

Z77.1 **Contact with and (suspected) exposure to environmental pollution and hazards in the physical environment**

Z77.11 **Contact with and (suspected) exposure to environmental pollution**

Z77.110 **Contact with and (suspected) exposure to air pollution**

Z77.111 **Contact with and (suspected) exposure to water pollution**

Z77.112 **Contact with and (suspected) exposure to soil pollution**

Z77.118 **Contact with and (suspected) exposure to other environmental pollution**

Z77.12 **Contact with and (suspected) exposure to hazards in the physical environment**

Z77.120 **Contact with and (suspected) exposure to mold (toxic)**

Z77.121 **Contact with and (suspected) exposure to harmful algae and algae toxins**

Contact with and (suspected) exposure to (harmful) algae bloom NOS

Contact with and (suspected) exposure to blue-green algae bloom

Contact with and (suspected) exposure to brown tide

Contact with and (suspected) exposure to cyanobacteria bloom

Contact with and (suspected) exposure to Florida red tide

Contact with and (suspected) exposure to pfiesteria piscicida

Contact with and (suspected) exposure to red tide

Z77.122 Contact with and (suspected) exposure to noise

Z77.123 Contact with and (suspected) exposure to radon and other naturally occuring radiation

Excludes2: radiation exposure as the cause of a confirmed condition (W88-W90, X39.0-)

radiation sickness NOS (T66)

Z77.128 Contact with and (suspected) exposure to other hazards in the physical environment

Z77.2 Contact with and (suspected) exposure to other hazardous substances

Z77.21 Contact with and (suspected) exposure to potentially hazardous body fluids

Z77.22 Contact with and (suspected) exposure to environmental tobacco smoke (acute) (chronic)

Exposure to second hand tobacco smoke (acute) (chronic)

Passive smoking (acute) (chronic)

Excludes1: nicotine dependence (F17.-)

tobacco use (Z72.0)

Excludes2: occupational exposure to environmental tobacco smoke (Z57.31)

Z77.29 Contact with and (suspected) exposure to other hazardous substances

Z77.9 Other contact with and (suspected) exposures hazardous to health

Z78 Other specified health status

Excludes2: asymptomatic human immunodeficiency virus [HIV] infection status (Z21)

postprocedural status (Z93-Z99)

sex reassignment status (Z87.890)

Z78.0 Asymptomatic menopausal state

Menopausal state NOS

Postmenopausal status NOS

Excludes2: symptomatic menopausal state (N95.1)

Z78.1 Physical restraint status

Excludes1: physical restraint due to a procedure - omit code

Z78.9 Other specified health status

Z79 Long term (current) drug therapy

Includes: long term (current) drug use for prophylactic purposes

Code also any therapeutic drug level monitoring (Z51.81)

Excludes2: drug abuse and dependence (F11-F19)

drug use complicating pregnancy, childbirth, and the puerperium (O99.32-)

long term (current) use of oral antidiabetic drugs (Z79.84)

long term (current) use of oral hypoglycemic drugs (Z79.84)

Z79.0 Long term (current) use of anticoagulants and antithrombotics/antiplatelets

Excludes2: long term (current) use of aspirin (Z79.82)

Z79.01 Long term (current) use of anticoagulants

Z79.02 Long term (current) use of antithrombotics/antiplatelets

Z79.1 Long term (current) use of non-steroidal anti-inflammatories (NSAID)

Excludes2: long term (current) use of aspirin (Z79.82)

Z79.2 Long term (current) use of antibiotics

Z79.3 Long term (current) use of hormonal contraceptives

Long term (current) use of birth control pill or patch

Z79.4 Long term (current) use of insulin

Z79.5 Long term (current) use of steroids

Z79.51 Long term (current) use of inhaled steroids

Z79.52 Long term (current) use of systemic steroids

Z79.8 Other long term (current) drug therapy

Z79.81 Long term (current) use of agents affecting estrogen receptors and estrogen levels

Code first, if applicable:

malignant neoplasm of breast (C50.-)

malignant neoplasm of prostate (C61)

Use additional code, if applicable, to identify:

estrogen receptor positive status (Z17.0)

family history of breast cancer (Z80.3)

genetic susceptibility to malignant neoplasm (cancer) (Z15.0-)

personal history of breast cancer (Z85.3)

personal history of prostate cancer (Z85.46)

postmenopausal status (Z78.0)

Excludes1: hormone replacement therapy (postmenopausal) (Z79.890)

Z79.810 Long term (current) use of selective estrogen receptor modulators (SERMs)

Long term (current) use of raloxifene (Evista)

Long term (current) use of tamoxifen (Nolvadex)

Long term (current) use of toremifene (Fareston)

Z79.811 Long term (current) use of aromatase inhibitors

Long term (current) use of anastrozole (Arimidex)

Long term (current) use of exemestane (Aromasin)

Long term (current) use of letrozole (Femara)

Z79.818 Long term (current) use of other agents affecting estrogen receptors and estrogen levels

Long term (current) use of estrogen receptor downregulators

Long term (current) use of fulvestrant (Faslodex)

Long term (current) use of gonadotropin-releasing hormone (GnRH) agonist

Long term (current) use of goserelin acetate (Zoladex)

Long term (current) use of leuprolide acetate (leuprorelin) (Lupron)

Long term (current) use of megestrol acetate (Megace)

Z79.82 **Long term (current) use of aspirin**

Z79.83 **Long term (current) use of bisphosphonates**

•**Z79.84** **Long term (current) use of oral hypoglycemic drugs**

Long term (current) use of oral antidiabetic drugs

Excludes2: long term (current) use of insulin (Z79.4)

Z79.89 **Other long term (current) drug therapy**

Z79.890 **Hormone replacement therapy (postmenopausal)**

Z79.891 **Long term (current) use of opiate analgesic**

Long term (current) use of methadone for pain management

Excludes1: methadone use NOS (F11.9-)

use of methodone for treatment of heroin addiction (F11.2-)

Z79.899 **Other long term (current) drug therapy**

Z80 **Family history of primary malignant neoplasm**

Z80.0 **Family history of malignant neoplasm of digestive organs**

Conditions classifiable to C15-C26

Z80.1 **Family history of malignant neoplasm of trachea, bronchus and lung**

Conditions classifiable to C33-C34

Z80.2 **Family history of malignant neoplasm of other respiratory and intrathoracic organs**

Conditions classifiable to C30-C32, C37-C39

Z80.3 **Family history of malignant neoplasm of breast**

Conditions classifiable to C50.-

Z80.4 **Family history of malignant neoplasm of genital organs**

Conditions classifiable to C51-C63

Z80.41 **Family history of malignant neoplasm of ovary**

Z80.42 **Family history of malignant neoplasm of prostate**

Z80.43 **Family history of malignant neoplasm of testis**

Z80.49 **Family history of malignant neoplasm of other genital organs**

Z80.5 **Family history of malignant neoplasm of urinary tract**

Conditions classifiable to C64-C68

Z80.51 **Family history of malignant neoplasm of kidney**

Z80.52 **Family history of malignant neoplasm of bladder**

Z80.59 **Family history of malignant neoplasm of other urinary tract organ**

Z80.6 **Family history of leukemia**

Conditions classifiable to C91-C95

Z80.7 **Family history of other malignant neoplasms of lymphoid, hematopoietic and related tissues**

Conditions classifiable to C81-C90, C96.-

Z80.8 **Family history of malignant neoplasm of other organs or systems**

Conditions classifiable to C00-C14, C40-C49, C69-C79

Z80.9 **Family history of malignant neoplasm, unspecified**

Conditions classifiable to C80.1

Z81 **Family history of mental and behavioral disorders**

Z81.0 **Family history of intellectual disabilities**

Conditions classifiable to F70-F79

Z81.1 **Family history of alcohol abuse and dependence**

Conditions classifiable to F10.-

Z81.2 **Family history of tobacco abuse and dependence**

Conditions classifiable to F17.-

Z81.3 **Family history of other psychoactive substance abuse and dependence**

Conditions classifiable to F11-F16, F18-F19

Z81.4 **Family history of other substance abuse and dependence**

Conditions classifiable to F55

Z81.8 **Family history of other mental and behavioral disorders**

Conditions classifiable elsewhere in F01-F99

Z82 **Family history of certain disabilities and chronic diseases (leading to disablement)**

Z82.0 **Family history of epilepsy and other diseases of the nervous system**

Conditions classifiable to G00-G99

Z82.1 **Family history of blindness and visual loss**

Conditions classifiable to H54.-

Z82.2 **Family history of deafness and hearing loss**

Conditions classifiable to H90-H91

Z82.3 **Family history of stroke**

Conditions classifiable to I60-I64

Z82.4 **Family history of ischemic heart disease and other diseases of the circulatory system**

Conditions classifiable to I00-I52, I65-I99

Z82.41 **Family history of sudden cardiac death**

Z82.49 **Family history of ischemic heart disease and other diseases of the circulatory system**

Z82.5 **Family history of asthma and other chronic lower respiratory diseases**

Conditions classifiable to J40-J47

Excludes2: family history of other diseases of the respiratory system (Z83.6)

Z82.6 **Family history of arthritis and other diseases of the musculoskeletal system and connective tissue**

Conditions classifiable to M00-M99

Z82.61 **Family history of arthritis**

Z82.62 **Family history of osteoporosis**

Z82.69 **Family history of other diseases of the musculoskeletal system and connective tissue**

Z82.7 **Family history of congenital malformations, deformations and chromosomal abnormalities**

Conditions classifiable to Q00-Q99

Z82.71   **Family history of polycystic kidney**

Z82.79   **Family history of other congenital malformations, deformations and chromosomal abnormalities**

Z82.8   **Family history of other disabilities and chronic diseases leading to disablement, not elsewhere classified**

Z83   **Family history of other specific disorders**

     Excludes2: contact with and (suspected) exposure to communicable disease in the family (Z20.-)

Z83.0   **Family history of human immunodeficiency virus [HIV] disease**

Conditions classifiable to B20

Z83.1   **Family history of other infectious and parasitic diseases**

Conditions classifiable to A00-B19, B25-B94, B99

Z83.2   **Family history of diseases of the blood and blood-forming organs and certain disorders involving the immune mechanism**

Conditions classifiable to D50-D89

Z83.3   **Family history of diabetes mellitus**

Conditions classifiable to E08-E13

Z83.4   **Family history of other endocrine, nutritional and metabolic diseases**

Conditions classifiable to E00-E07, E15-E88

Z83.41   **Family history of multiple endocrine neoplasia [MEN] syndrome**

●**Z83.42**   **Family history of familial hypercholesterolemia**

Z83.49   **Family history of other endocrine, nutritional and metabolic diseases**

Z83.5   **Family history of eye and ear disorders**

Z83.51   **Family history of eye disorders**

Conditions classifiable to H00-H53, H55-H59

     Excludes2: family history of blindness and visual loss (Z82.1)

Z83.511   **Family history of glaucoma**

Z83.518   **Family history of other specified eye disorder**

Z83.52   **Family history of ear disorders**

Conditions classifiable to H60-H83, H92-H95

     Excludes2: family history of deafness and hearing loss (Z82.2)

Z83.6   **Family history of other diseases of the respiratory system**

Conditions classifiable to J00-J39, J60-J99

     Excludes2: family history of asthma **and other** chronic lower respiratory diseases (Z82.5)

Z83.7   **Family history of diseases of the digestive system**

Conditions classifiable to K00-K93

Z83.71   **Family history of colonic polyps**

     Excludes1: family history of malignant neoplasm of digestive organs (Z80.0)

Z83.79   **Family history of other diseases of the digestive system**

Z84   **Family history of other conditions**

Z84.0   **Family history of diseases of the skin and subcutaneous tissue**

Conditions classifiable to L00-L99

Z84.1   **Family history of disorders of kidney and ureter**

Conditions classifiable to N00-N29

Z84.2   **Family history of other diseases of the genitourinary system**

Conditions classifiable to N30-N99

Z84.3   **Family history of consanguinity**

Z84.8   **Family history of other specified conditions**

Z84.81   **Family history of carrier of genetic disease**

●**Z84.82**   **Family history of sudden infant death syndrome**

Family history of SIDS

Z84.89   **Family history of other specified conditions**

Z85   **Personal history of malignant neoplasm**

<u>**Code first**</u> any follow-up examination after treatment of malignant neoplasm (Z08)

<u>**Use additional code**</u> to identify:

alcohol use and dependence (F10.-)

exposure to environmental tobacco smoke (Z77.22)

history of tobacco dependence (Z87.891)

occupational exposure to environmental tobacco smoke (Z57.31)

tobacco dependence (F17.-)

tobacco use (Z72.0)

Excludes2: personal history of benign neoplasm (Z86.01-)

     personal history of carcinoma-in-situ (Z86.00-)

Z85.0   **Personal history of malignant neoplasm of digestive organs**

Z85.00   **Personal history of malignant neoplasm of unspecified digestive organ**

Z85.01   **Personal history of malignant neoplasm of esophagus**

Conditions classifiable to C15

Z85.02   **Personal history of malignant neoplasm of stomach**

Z85.020   **Personal history of malignant carcinoid tumor of stomach**

Conditions classifiable to C7A.092

Z85.028   **Personal history of other malignant neoplasm of stomach**

Conditions classifiable to C16

Z85.03   **Personal history of malignant neoplasm of large intestine**

Z85.030   **Personal history of malignant carcinoid tumor of large intestine**

Conditions classifiable to C7A.022-C7A.025, C7A.029

Z85.038   **Personal history of other malignant neoplasm of large intestine**

Conditions classifiable to C18

Z85.04   **Personal history of malignant neoplasm of rectum, rectosigmoid junction, and anus**

Z85.040   **Personal history of malignant carcinoid tumor of rectum**

Conditions classifiable to C7A.026

Z85.048   **Personal history of other malignant neoplasm of rectum, rectosigmoid junction, and anus**

Conditions classifiable to C19-C21

Z85.05 **Personal history of malignant neoplasm of liver**

Conditions classifiable to C22

Z85.06 **Personal history of malignant neoplasm of small intestine**

Z85.060 **Personal history of malignant carcinoid tumor of small intestine**

Conditions classifiable to C7A.01-

Z85.068 **Personal history of other malignant neoplasm of small intestine**

Conditions classifiable to C17

Z85.07 **Personal history of malignant neoplasm of pancreas**

Conditions classifiable to C25

Z85.09 **Personal history of malignant neoplasm of other digestive organs**

Z85.1 **Personal history of malignant neoplasm of trachea, bronchus and lung**

Z85.11 **Personal history of malignant neoplasm of bronchus and lung**

Z85.110 **Personal history of malignant carcinoid tumor of bronchus and lung**

Conditions classifiable to C7A.090

Z85.118 **Personal history of other malignant neoplasm of bronchus and lung**

Conditions classifiable to C34

Z85.12 **Personal history of malignant neoplasm of trachea**

Conditions classifiable to C33

Z85.2 **Personal history of malignant neoplasm of other respiratory and intrathoracic organs**

Z85.20 **Personal history of malignant neoplasm of unspecified respiratory organ**

Z85.21 **Personal history of malignant neoplasm of larynx**

Conditions classifiable to C32

Z85.22 **Personal history of malignant neoplasm of nasal cavities, middle ear, and accessory sinuses**

Conditions classifiable to C30-C31

Z85.23 **Personal history of malignant neoplasm of thymus**

Z85.230 **Personal history of malignant carcinoid tumor of thymus**

Conditions classifiable to C7A.091

Z85.238 **Personal history of other malignant neoplasm of thymus**

Conditions classifiable to C37

Z85.29 **Personal history of malignant neoplasm of other respiratory and intrathoracic organs**

Z85.3 **Personal history of malignant neoplasm of breast**

Conditions classifiable to C50.-

Z85.4 **Personal history of malignant neoplasm of genital organs**

Conditions classifiable to C51-C63

Z85.40 **Personal history of malignant neoplasm of unspecified female genital organ**

Z85.41 **Personal history of malignant neoplasm of cervix uteri**

Z85.42 **Personal history of malignant neoplasm of other parts of uterus**

Z85.43 **Personal history of malignant neoplasm of ovary**

Z85.44 **Personal history of malignant neoplasm of other female genital organs**

Z85.45 **Personal history of malignant neoplasm of unspecified male genital organ**

Z85.46 **Personal history of malignant neoplasm of prostate**

Z85.47 **Personal history of malignant neoplasm of testis**

Z85.48 **Personal history of malignant neoplasm of epididymis**

Z85.49 **Personal history of malignant neoplasm of other male genital organs**

Z85.5 **Personal history of malignant neoplasm of urinary tract**

Conditions classifiable to C64-C68

Z85.50 **Personal history of malignant neoplasm of unspecified urinary tract organ**

Z85.51 **Personal history of malignant neoplasm of bladder**

Z85.52 **Personal history of malignant neoplasm of kidney**

Excludes1: personal history of malignant neoplasm of renal pelvis (Z85.53)

Z85.520 **Personal history of malignant carcinoid tumor of kidney**

Conditions classifiable to C7A.093

Z85.528 **Personal history of other malignant neoplasm of kidney**

Conditions classifiable to C64

Z85.53 **Personal history of malignant neoplasm of renal pelvis**

Z85.54 **Personal history of malignant neoplasm of ureter**

Z85.59 **Personal history of malignant neoplasm of other urinary tract organ**

Z85.6 **Personal history of leukemia**

Conditions classifiable to C91-C95

Excludes1: leukemia in remission C91.0-C95.9 with 5th character 1

Z85.7 **Personal history of other malignant neoplasms of lymphoid, hematopoietic and related tissues**

Z85.71 **Personal history of Hodgkin lymphoma**

Conditions classifiable to C81

Z85.72 **Personal history of non-Hodgkin lymphomas**

Conditions classifiable to C82-C85

Z85.79 **Personal history of other malignant neoplasms of lymphoid, hematopoietic and related tissues**

Conditions classifiable to C88-C90, C96

Excludes1: multiple myeloma in remission (C90.01)

plasma cell leukemia in remission (C90.11)

plasmacytoma in remission (C90.21)

Z85.8 **Personal history of malignant neoplasms of other organs and systems**

Conditions classifiable to C00-C14, C40-C49, C69-C75, C7A.098, C76-C79

Z85.81 **Personal history of malignant neoplasm of lip, oral cavity, and pharynx**

    Z85.810 **Personal history of malignant neoplasm of tongue**

    Z85.818 **Personal history of malignant neoplasm of other sites of lip, oral cavity, and pharynx**

    Z85.819 **Personal history of malignant neoplasm of unspecified site of lip, oral cavity, and pharynx**

Z85.82 **Personal history of malignant neoplasm of skin**

    Z85.820 **Personal history of malignant melanoma of skin**

      Conditions classifiable to C43

    Z85.821 **Personal history of Merkel cell carcinoma**

      Conditions classifiable to C4A

    Z85.828 **Personal history of other malignant neoplasm of skin**

      Conditions classifiable to C44

Z85.83 **Personal history of malignant neoplasm of bone and soft tissue**

    Z85.830 **Personal history of malignant neoplasm of bone**

    Z85.831 **Personal history of malignant neoplasm of soft tissue**

    Excludes2: personal history of malignant neoplasm of skin (Z85.82-)

Z85.84 **Personal history of malignant neoplasm of eye and nervous tissue**

    Z85.840 **Personal history of malignant neoplasm of eye**

    Z85.841 **Personal history of malignant neoplasm of brain**

    Z85.848 **Personal history of malignant neoplasm of other parts of nervous tissue**

Z85.85 **Personal history of malignant neoplasm of endocrine glands**

    Z85.850 **Personal history of malignant neoplasm of thyroid**

    Z85.858 **Personal history of malignant neoplasm of other endocrine glands**

Z85.89 **Personal history of malignant neoplasm of other organs and systems**

Z85.9 **Personal history of malignant neoplasm, unspecified**

Conditions classifiable to C7A.00, C80.1

Z86 **Personal history of certain other diseases**

Code first any follow-up examination after treatment (Z09)

Z86.0 **Personal history of in-situ and benign neoplasms and neoplasms of uncertain behavior**

    Excludes2: personal history of malignant neoplasms (Z85.-)

Z86.00 **Personal history of in-situ neoplasm**

Conditions classifiable to D00-D09

    Z86.000 **Personal history of in-situ neoplasm of breast**

    Z86.001 **Personal history of in-situ neoplasm of cervix uteri**

Personal history of cervical intraepithelial neoplasia III [CIN III]

    Z86.008 **Personal history of in-situ neoplasm of other site**

Personal history of vaginal intraepithelial neoplasia III [VAIN III]

Personal history of vulvar intraepithelial neoplasia III [VIN III]

Z86.01 **Personal history of benign neoplasm**

    Z86.010 **Personal history of colonic polyps**

    Z86.011 **Personal history of benign neoplasm of the brain**

    Z86.012 **Personal history of benign carcinoid tumor**

    Z86.018 **Personal history of other benign neoplasm**

Z86.03 **Personal history of neoplasm of uncertain behavior**

Z86.1 **Personal history of infectious and parasitic diseases**

Conditions classifiable to A00-B89, B99

    Excludes1: personal history of infectious diseases specific to a body system

sequelae of infectious and parasitic diseases (B90-B94)

Z86.11 **Personal history of tuberculosis**

Z86.12 **Personal history of poliomyelitis**

Z86.13 **Personal history of malaria**

Z86.14 **Personal history of Methicillin resistant Staphylococcus aureus infection**

Personal history of MRSA infection

Z86.19 **Personal history of other infectious and parasitic diseases**

Z86.2 **Personal history of diseases of the blood and blood-forming organs and certain disorders involving the immune mechanism**

Conditions classifiable to D50-D89

Z86.3 **Personal history of endocrine, nutritional and metabolic diseases**

Conditions classifiable to E00-E88

Z86.31 **Personal history of diabetic foot ulcer**

    Excludes2: current diabetic foot ulcer (E08.621, E09.621, E10.621, E11.621, E13.621)

Z86.32 **Personal history of gestational diabetes**

Personal history of conditions classifiable to O24.4-

    Excludes1: gestational diabetes mellitus in current pregnancy (O24.4-)

Z86.39 **Personal history of other endocrine, nutritional and metabolic disease**

Z86.5 **Personal history of mental and behavioral disorders**

Conditions classifiable to F40-F59

Z86.51 **Personal history of combat and operational stress reaction**

Z86.59 **Personal history of other mental and behavioral disorders**

Z86.6 **Personal history of diseases of the nervous system and sense organs**

Conditions classifiable to G00-G99, H00-H95

�∎ Add 4th-7th digits	Nonspecific code	Unspecified code	Manifestation code

Z86.61   Personal history of infections of the central nervous system

Personal history of encephalitis

Personal history of meningitis

Z86.69   Personal history of other diseases of the nervous system and sense organs

Z86.7   Personal history of diseases of the circulatory system

Conditions classifiable to I00-I99

Excludes2: old myocardial infarction (I25.2)

personal history of anaphylactic shock (Z87.892)

postmyocardial infarction syndrome (I24.1)

Z86.71   Personal history of venous thrombosis and embolism

Z86.711   Personal history of pulmonary embolism

Z86.718   Personal history of other venous thrombosis and embolism

Z86.72   Personal history of thrombophlebitis

Z86.73   Personal history of transient ischemic attack (TIA), and cerebral infarction without residual deficits

Personal history of prolonged reversible ischemic neurological deficit (PRIND)

Personal history of stroke NOS without residual deficits

Excludes1: personal history of traumatic brain injury (Z87.820)

sequelae of cerebrovascular disease (I69.-)

Z86.74   Personal history of sudden cardiac arrest

Personal history of sudden cardiac death successfully resuscitated

Z86.79   Personal history of other diseases of the circulatory system

Z87   Personal history of other diseases and conditions

Code first any follow-up examination after treatment (Z09)

Z87.0   Personal history of diseases of the respiratory system

Conditions classifiable to J00-J99

Z87.01   Personal history of pneumonia (recurrent)

Z87.09   Personal history of other diseases of the respiratory system

Z87.1   Personal history of diseases of the digestive system

Conditions classifiable to K00-K93

Z87.11   Personal history of peptic ulcer disease

Z87.19   Personal history of other diseases of the digestive system

Z87.2   Personal history of diseases of the skin and subcutaneous tissue

Conditions classifiable to L00-L99

Excludes2: personal history of diabetic foot ulcer (Z86.31)

Z87.3   Personal history of diseases of the musculoskeletal system and connective tissue

Conditions classifiable to M00-M99

Excludes2: personal history of (healed) traumatic fracture (Z87.81)

Z87.31   Personal history of (healed) nontraumatic fracture

Z87.310   Personal history of (healed) osteoporosis fracture

Personal history of (healed) fragility fracture

Personal history of (healed) collapsed vertebra due to osteoporosis

Z87.311   Personal history of (healed) other pathological fracture

Personal history of (healed) collapsed vertebra NOS

Excludes2: personal history of osteoporosis fracture (Z87.310)

Z87.312   Personal history of (healed) stress fracture

Personal history of (healed) fatigue fracture

Z87.39   Personal history of other diseases of the musculoskeletal system and connective tissue

Z87.4   Personal history of diseases of genitourinary system

Conditions classifiable to N00-N99

Z87.41   Personal history of dysplasia of the female genital tract

Excludes1: personal history of intraepithelial neoplasia III of female genital tract (Z87.001, Z87.008)

personal history of malignant neoplasm of female genital tract (Z85.40-Z85.44)

Z87.410   Personal history of cervical dysplasia

Z87.411   Personal history of vaginal dysplasia

Z87.412   Personal history of vulvar dysplasia

Z87.42   Personal history of other diseases of the female genital tract

Z87.43   Personal history of diseases of male genital organs

Z87.430   Personal history of prostatic dysplasia

Excludes1: personal history of malignant neoplasm of prostate (Z85.46)

Z87.438   Personal history of other diseases of male genital organs

Z87.44   Personal history of diseases of urinary system

Excludes1: personal history of malignant neoplasm of cervix uteri (Z85.41)

Z87.440   Personal history of urinary (tract) infections

Z87.441   Personal history of nephrotic syndrome

Z87.442   Personal history of urinary calculi

Personal history of kidney stones

Z87.448   Personal history of other diseases of urinary system

Z87.5   Personal history of complications of pregnancy, childbirth and the puerperium

Conditions classifiable to O00-O9A

Excludes2: recurrent pregnancy loss (N96)

Z87.51   Personal history of pre-term labor Excludes1: current pregnancy with history of pre-term labor (O09.21-)

Z87.59   Personal history of other complications of pregnancy, childbirth and the puerperium

Personal history of trophoblastic disease

Z87.7 Personal history of (corrected) congenital malformations

Conditions classifiable to Q00-Q89 that have been repaired or corrected

Excludes1: congenital malformations that have been partially corrected or repair but which still require medical treatment - code to condition

Excludes2: Other postprocedural states (Z98.-)

personal history of medical treatment (Z92.-)

presence of cardiac and vascular implants and grafts (Z95.-) presence of other devices (Z97.-)

presence of other functional implants (Z96.-) transplanted organ and tissue status (Z94.-)

Z87.71 Personal history of (corrected) congenital malformations of genitourinary system

Z87.710 Personal history of (corrected) hypospadias

Z87.718 Personal history of other specified (corrected) congenital malformations of genitourinary system

Z87.72 Personal history of (corrected) congenital malformations of nervous system and sense organs

Z87.720 Personal history of (corrected) congenital malformations of eye

Z87.721 Personal history of (corrected) congenital malformations of ear

Z87.728 Personal history of other specified (corrected) congenital malformations of nervous system and sense organs

Z87.73 Personal history of (corrected) congenital malformations of digestive system

Z87.730 Personal history of (corrected) cleft lip and palate

Z87.738 Personal history of other specified (corrected) congenital malformations of digestive system

Z87.74 Personal history of (corrected) congenital malformations of heart and circulatory system

Z87.75 Personal history of (corrected) congenital malformations of respiratory system

Z87.76 Personal history of (corrected) congenital malformations of integument, limbs and musculoskeletal system

Z87.79 Personal history of other (corrected) congenital malformations

Z87.790 Personal history of (corrected) congenital malformations of face and neck

Z87.798 Personal history of other (corrected) congenital malformations

Z87.8 Personal history of other specified conditions

Excludes2: personal history of self harm (Z91.5)

Z87.81 Personal history of (healed) traumatic fracture

Excludes2: personal history of (healed) nontraumatic fracture (Z87.31-)

Z87.82 Personal history of other (healed) physical injury and trauma

Conditions classifiable to S00-T88, except traumatic fractures

Z87.820 Personal history of traumatic brain injury

Excludes1: personal history of transient ischemic attack (TIA), and cerebral infarction without residual deficits (Z86.73)

Z87.821 Personal history of retained foreign body fully removed

Z87.828 Personal history of other (healed) physical injury and trauma

Z87.89 Personal history of other specified conditions

Z87.890 Personal history of sex reassignment

Z87.891 Personal history of nicotine dependence

Excludes1: current nicotine dependence (F17.2-)

Z87.892 Personal history of anaphylaxis

Code also allergy status such as:

allergy status to drugs, medicaments and biological substances (Z88.-)

allergy status, **other** than to drugs and biological substances (Z91.0-)

Z87.898 Personal history of other specified conditions

Z88 Allergy status to drugs, medicaments and biological substances

Excludes2: Allergy status, **other** than to drugs and biological substances (Z91.0-)

Z88.0 Allergy status to penicillin

Z88.1 Allergy status to other antibiotic agents status

Z88.2 Allergy status to sulfonamides status

Z88.3 Allergy status to other anti-infective agents status

Z88.4 Allergy status to anesthetic agent status

Z88.5 Allergy status to narcotic agent status

Z88.6 Allergy status to analgesic agent status

Z88.7 Allergy status to serum and vaccine status

Z88.8 Allergy status to other drugs, medicaments and biological substances status

Z88.9 Allergy status to unspecified drugs, medicaments and biological substances status

Z89 Acquired absence of limb

Includes: amputation status

postprocedural loss of limb post-traumatic loss of limb

Excludes1: acquired deformities of limbs (M20-M21)

congenital absence of limbs (Q71-Q73)

Z89.0 Acquired absence of thumb and other finger(s)

Z89.01 Acquired absence of thumb

Z89.011 Acquired absence of right thumb

Z89.012 Acquired absence of left thumb

Z89.019 Acquired absence of unspecified thumb

Z89.02 Acquired absence of other finger(s)

Excludes2: acquired absence of thumb (Z89.01-)

Z89.021 Acquired absence of right finger(s)

Z89.022 Acquired absence of left finger(s)

Z89.029 Acquired absence of unspecified finger(s)

Z89.1   **Acquired absence of hand and wrist**

     Z89.11   **Acquired absence of hand**

         Z89.111   **Acquired absence of right hand**

         Z89.112   **Acquired absence of left hand**

         Z89.119   **Acquired absence of unspecified hand**

     Z89.12   **Acquired absence of wrist**

         Disarticulation at wrist

         Z89.121   **Acquired absence of right wrist**

         Z89.122   **Acquired absence of left wrist**

         Z89.129   **Acquired absence of unspecified wrist**

Z89.2   **Acquired absence of upper limb above wrist**

     Z89.20   **Acquired absence of upper limb, unspecified level**

         Z89.201   **Acquired absence of right upper limb, unspecified level**

         Z89.202   **Acquired absence of left upper limb, unspecified level**

         Z89.209   **Acquired absence of unspecified upper limb, unspecified level**

         Acquired absence of arm NOS

     Z89.21   **Acquired absence of upper limb below elbow**

         Z89.211   **Acquired absence of right upper limb below elbow**

         Z89.212   **Acquired absence of left upper limb below elbow**

         Z89.219   **Acquired absence of unspecified upper limb below elbow**

     Z89.22   **Acquired absence of upper limb above elbow**

         Disarticulation at elbow

         Z89.221   **Acquired absence of right upper limb above elbow**

         Z89.222   **Acquired absence of left upper limb above elbow**

         Z89.229   **Acquired absence of unspecified upper limb above elbow**

     Z89.23   **Acquired absence of shoulder**

         Acquired absence of shoulder joint following explanation of shoulder joint prosthesis, with or without presence of antibiotic-impregnated cement spacer

         Z89.231   **Acquired absence of right shoulder**

         Z89.232   **Acquired absence of left shoulder**

         Z89.239   **Acquired absence of unspecified shoulder**

Z89.4   **Acquired absence of toe(s), foot, and ankle**

     Z89.41   **Acquired absence of great toe**

         Z89.411   **Acquired absence of right great toe**

         Z89.412   **Acquired absence of left great toe**

         Z89.419   **Acquired absence of unspecified great toe**

     Z89.42   **Acquired absence of other toe(s)**

         Excludes2: acquired absence of great toe (Z89.41-)

         Z89.421   **Acquired absence of other right toe(s)**

         Z89.422   **Acquired absence of other left toe(s)**

         Z89.429   **Acquired absence of other toe(s), unspecified side**

     Z89.43   **Acquired absence of foot**

         Z89.431   **Acquired absence of right foot**

         Z89.432   **Acquired absence of left foot**

         Z89.439   **Acquired absence of unspecified foot**

     Z89.44   **Acquired absence of ankle**

         Disarticulation of ankle

         Z89.441   **Acquired absence of right ankle**

         Z89.442   **Acquired absence of left ankle**

         Z89.449   **Acquired absence of unspecified ankle**

Z89.5   **Acquired absence of leg below knee**

     Z89.51   **Acquired absence of leg below knee**

         Z89.511   **Acquired absence of right leg below knee**

         Z89.512   **Acquired absence of left leg below knee**

         Z89.519   **Acquired absence of unspecified leg below knee**

     Z89.52   **Acquired absence of knee**

         Acquired absence of knee joint following explanation of knee joint prosthesis, with or without presence of antibiotic-impregnated cement spacer

         Z89.521   **Acquired absence of right knee**

         Z89.522   **Acquired absence of left knee**

         Z89.529   **Acquired absence of unspecified knee**

Z89.6   **Acquired absence of leg above knee**

     Z89.61   **Acquired absence of leg above knee**

         Acquired absence of leg NOS

         Disarticulation at knee

         Z89.611   **Acquired absence of right leg above knee**

         Z89.612   **Acquired absence of left leg above knee**

         Z89.619   **Acquired absence of unspecified leg above knee**

     Z89.62   **Acquired absence of hip**

         Acquired absence of hip joint following explanation of hip joint prosthesis, with or without presence of antibiotic-impregnated cement spacer

         Disarticulation at hip

         Z89.621   **Acquired absence of right hip joint**

         Z89.622   **Acquired absence of left hip joint**

         Z89.629   **Acquired absence of unspecified hip joint**

Z89.9   **Acquired absence of limb, unspecified**

Z90   **Acquired absence of organs, not elsewhere classified**

     Includes: postprocedural or post-traumatic loss of body part NEC

     Excludes1: congenital absence - see Alphabetical Index

     Excludes2: postprocedural absence of endocrine glands (E89.-)

     Z90.0   **Acquired absence of part of head and neck**

         Z90.01   **Acquired absence of eye**

         Z90.02   **Acquired absence of larynx**

Z90.09 **Acquired absence of other part of head and neck**

Acquired absence of nose

Excludes2: teeth (K08.1)

Z90.1 **Acquired absence of breast and nipple**

Z90.10 **Acquired absence of unspecified breast and nipple**

Z90.11 **Acquired absence of right breast and nipple**

Z90.12 **Acquired absence of left breast and nipple**

Z90.13 **Acquired absence of bilateral breasts and nipples**

Z90.2 **Acquired absence of lung [part of]**

Z90.3 **Acquired absence of stomach [part of]**

Z90.4 **Acquired absence of other specified parts of digestive tract**

Z90.41 **Acquired absence of pancreas**

Code also exocrine pancreatic insufficiency (K86.81)

Use additional code to identify any associated:

insulin use (Z79.4)

diabetes mellitus, postpancreatectomy (E13.-)

Z90.410 **Acquired total absence of pancreas**

Acquired absence of pancreas NOS

Z90.411 **Acquired partial absence of pancreas**

Z90.49 **Acquired absence of other specified parts of digestive tract**

Z90.5 **Acquired absence of kidney**

Z90.6 **Acquired absence of other parts of urinary tract**

Acquired absence of bladder

Z90.7 **Acquired absence of genital organ(s)**

Excludes1: personal history of sex reassignment (Z87.890)

Excludes2: female genital mutilation status (N90.81-)

Z90.71 **Acquired absence of cervix and uterus**

Z90.710 **Acquired absence of both cervix and uterus**

Acquired absence of uterus NOS

Status post total hysterectomy

Z90.711 **Acquired absence of uterus with remaining cervical stump**

Status post partial hysterectomy with remaining cervical stump

Z90.712 **Acquired absence of cervix with remaining uterus**

Z90.72 **Acquired absence of ovaries**

Z90.721 **Acquired absence of ovaries, unilateral**

Z90.722 **Acquired absence of ovaries, bilateral**

Z90.79 **Acquired absence of other genital organ(s)**

Z90.8 **Acquired absence of other organs**

Z90.81 **Acquired absence of spleen**

Z90.89 **Acquired absence of other organs**

Z91 **Personal risk factors, not elsewhere classified**

Excludes2: contact with and (suspected) exposures hazardous to health (Z77.-)

exposure to pollution **and other** problems related to physical environment (Z77.1-)

personal history of physical injury and trauma (Z87.81, Z87.82-)

occupational exposure to risk factors (Z57.-)

Z91.0 **Allergy status, other than to drugs and biological substances**

Excludes2: Allergy status to drugs, medicaments, and biological substances (Z88.-)

Z91.01 **Food allergy status**

Excludes2: food additives allergy status (Z91.02)

Z91.010 **Allergy to peanuts**

Z91.011 **Allergy to milk products**

Excludes1: lactose intolerance (E73.-)

Z91.012 **Allergy to eggs**

Z91.013 **Allergy to seafood**

Allergy to shellfish

Allergy to octopus or squid ink

Z91.018 **Allergy to other foods**

Allergy to nuts other than peanuts

Z91.02 **Food additives allergy status**

Z91.03 **Insect allergy status**

Z91.030 **Bee allergy status**

Z91.038 **Other insect allergy status**

Z91.04 **Nonmedicinal substance allergy status**

Z91.040 **Latex allergy status**

Latex sensitivity status

Z91.041 **Radiographic dye allergy status**

Allergy status to contrast media used for diagnostic X-ray procedure

Z91.048 **Other nonmedicinal substance allergy status**

Z91.09 **Other allergy status, other than to drugs and biological substances**

Z91.1 **Patient's noncompliance with medical treatment and regimen**

Z91.11 **Patient's noncompliance with dietary regimen**

Z91.12 **Patient's intentional underdosing of medication regimen**

Code first underdosing of medication (T36-T50) with fifth or sixth character 6

Excludes1: adverse effect of prescribed drug taken as directed- code to adverse effect poisoning (overdose) -code to poisoning

Z91.120 **Patient's intentional underdosing of medication regimen due to financial hardship**

Z91.128 **Patient's intentional underdosing of medication regimen for other reason**

Z91.13 **Patient's unintentional underdosing of medication regimen**

Code first underdosing of medication (T36-T50) with fifth or sixth character 6

Excludes1: adverse effect of prescribed drug taken as directed- code to adverse effect poisoning (overdose) -code to poisoning

Z91.130 **Patient's unintentional underdosing of medication regimen due to age-related debility**

Z91.138 Patient's unintentional underdosing of medication regimen for other reason

Z91.14 Patient's other noncompliance with medication regimen

Patient's underdosing of medication NOS

Z91.15 Patient's noncompliance with renal dialysis

Z91.19 Patient's noncompliance with other medical treatment and regimen

Z91.4 Personal history of psychological trauma, not elsewhere classified

Z91.41 Personal history of adult abuse

Excludes2: personal history of abuse in childhood (Z62.81-)

Z91.410 Personal history of adult physical and sexual abuse

Excludes1: current adult physical abuse (T74.11, T76.11)

current adult sexual abuse (T74.21, T76.11)

Z91.411 Personal history of adult psychological abuse

Z91.412 Personal history of adult neglect

Excludes1: current adult neglect (T74.01, T76.01)

Z91.419 Personal history of unspecified adult abuse

Z91.49 Other personal history of psychological trauma, not elsewhere classified

Z91.5 Personal history of self-harm

Personal history of parasuicide

Personal history of self-poisoning

Personal history of suicide attempt

Z91.8 Other specified personal risk factors, not elsewhere classified

Z91.81 History of falling

At risk for falling

Z91.82 Personal history of military deployment

Individual (civilian or military) with past history of military war, peacekeeping and humanitarian deployment (current or past conflict)

Returned from military deployment

Z91.83 Wandering in diseases classified elsewhere

Code first underlying disorder such as:

Alzheimer's disease (G30.-)

autism or pervasive developmental disorder (F84.-)

intellectual disabilities (F70-F79)

unspecified dementia with behavioral disturbance (F03.9-)

Z91.89 Other specified personal risk factors, not elsewhere classified

Z92 Personal history of medical treatment

Excludes2: postprocedural states (Z98.-)

Z92.0 Personal history of contraception

Excludes1: counseling or management of current contraceptive practices (Z30.-)

long term (current) use of contraception (Z79.3)

presence of (intrauterine) contraceptive device (Z97.5)

Z92.2 Personal history of drug therapy

Excludes2: long term (current) drug therapy (Z79.-)

Z92.21 Personal history of antineoplastic chemotherapy

Z92.22 Personal history of monoclonal drug therapy

Z92.23 Personal history of estrogen therapy

Z92.24 Personal history of steroid therapy

Z92.240 Personal history of inhaled steroid therapy

Z92.241 Personal history of systemic steroid therapy

Personal history of steroid therapy NOS

Z92.25 Personal history of immunosupression therapy

Excludes2: personal history of steroid therapy (Z92.24)

Z92.29 Personal history of other drug therapy

Z92.3 Personal history of irradiation

Personal history of exposure to therapeutic radiation

Excludes1: exposure to radiation in the physical environment (Z77.12)

occupational exposure to radiation (Z57.1)

Z92.8 Personal history of other medical treatment

Z92.81 Personal history of extracorporeal membrane oxygenation (ECMO)

Z92.82 Status post administration of tPA (rtPA) in a different facility within the last 24 hours prior to admission to current facility

Code first condition requiring tPA administration, such as:

acute cerebral infarction (I63.-)

acute myocardial infarction (I21.-, I22.-)

Z92.83 Personal history of failed moderate sedation

Personal history of failed conscious sedation

Excludes2: failed moderate sedation during procedure (T88.52)

•**Z92.84** Personal history of unintended awareness under general anesthesia

Excludes2: unintended awareness under general anesthesia during procedure (T88.53)

Z92.89 Personal history of other medical treatment

Z93 Artificial opening status

Excludes1: artificial openings requiring attention or management (Z43.-)

complications of external stoma (J95.0-, K94.-, N99.5-)

Z93.0 Tracheostomy status

Z93.1 Gastrostomy status

Z93.2 Ileostomy status

Z93.3 Colostomy status

Z93.4 Other artificial openings of gastrointestinal tract status

Z93.5 Cystostomy status

Z93.50 Unspecified cystostomy status

Z93.51 Cutaneous-vesicostomy status

Z93.52 Appendico-vesicostomy status

Z93.59 Other cystostomy status

Z93.6 Other artificial openings of urinary tract status

Nephrostomy status

Ureterostomy status

Urethrostomy status

Z93.8   **Other artificial opening status**

Z93.9   **Artificial opening status, unspecified**

Z94   **Transplanted organ and tissue status**

Includes: organ or tissue replaced by heterogenous or homogenous transplant

Excludes1: complications of transplanted organ or tissue - see Alphabetical Index

Excludes2: presence of vascular grafts (Z95.-)

Z94.0   **Kidney transplant status**

Z94.1   **Heart transplant status**

Excludes1: artificial heart status (Z95.812)

heart-valve replacement status (Z95.2-Z95.4)

Z94.2   **Lung transplant status**

Z94.3   **Heart and lungs transplant status**

Z94.4   **Liver transplant status**

Z94.5   **Skin transplant status**

Autogenous skin transplant status

Z94.6   **Bone transplant status**

Z94.7   **Corneal transplant status**

Z94.8   **Other transplanted organ and tissue status**

Z94.81   **Bone marrow transplant status**

Z94.82   **Intestine transplant status**

Z94.83   **Pancreas transplant status**

Z94.84   **Stem cells transplant status**

Z94.89   **Other transplanted organ and tissue status**

Z94.9   **Transplanted organ and tissue status, unspecified**

Z95   **Presence of cardiac and vascular implants and grafts**

Excludes1: complications of cardiac and vascular devices, implants and grafts (T82.-)

Z95.0   **Presence of cardiac pacemaker**

Presence of cardiac resynchronization therapy (CRT-P) pacemaker

Excludes1: adjustment or management of cardiac device (Z45.0-)

adjustment or management of cardiac pacemaker (Z45.0)

presence of automatic (implantable) cardiac defibrillator with synchronous cardiac pacemaker (Z95.810)

Z95.1   **Presence of aortocoronary bypass graft**

Presence of coronary artery bypass graft

Z95.2   **Presence of prosthetic heart valve**

Presence of heart valve NOS

Z95.3   **Presence of xenogenic heart valve**

Z95.4   **Presence of other heart-valve replacement**

Z95.5   **Presence of coronary angioplasty implant and graft**

Excludes1: coronary angioplasty status without implant and graft (Z98.61)

Z95.8   **Presence of other cardiac and vascular implants and grafts**

Z95.81   **Presence of other cardiac implants and grafts**

Z95.810   **Presence of automatic (implantable) cardiac defibrillator**

Presence of automatic (implantable) cardiac defibrillator with synchronous cardiac pacemaker

Presence of cardiac resynchronization therapy defibrillator (CRT-D)

Presence of cardioverter-defibrillator (ICD)

Z95.811   **Presence of heart assist device**

Z95.812   **Presence of fully implantable artificial heart**

Z95.818   **Presence of other cardiac implants and grafts**

Z95.82   **Presence of other vascular implants and grafts**

Z95.820   **Peripheral vascular angioplasty status with implants and grafts**

Excludes1: peripheral vascular angioplasty without implant and graft (Z98.62)

Z95.828   **Presence of other vascular implants and grafts**

Presence of intravascular prosthesis NEC

Z95.9   **Presence of cardiac and vascular implant and graft, unspecified**

Z96   **Presence of other functional implants**

Excludes2: complications of internal prosthetic devices, implants and grafts (T82-T85)

fitting and adjustment of prosthetic and other devices (Z44-Z46)

Z96.0   **Presence of urogenital implants**

Z96.1   **Presence of intraocular lens**

Presence of pseudophakia

Z96.2   **Presence of otological and audiological implants**

Z96.20   **Presence of otological and audiological implant, unspecified**

Z96.21   **Cochlear implant status**

Z96.22   **Myringotomy tube(s) status**

Z96.29   **Presence of other otological and audiological implants**

Presence of bone-conduction hearing device

Presence of eustachian tube stent

Stapes replacement

Z96.3   **Presence of artificial larynx**

Z96.4   **Presence of endocrine implants**

Z96.41   **Presence of insulin pump (external) (internal)**

Z96.49   **Presence of other endocrine implants**

Z96.5   **Presence of tooth-root and mandibular implants**

Z96.6   **Presence of orthopedic joint implants**

Z96.60   **Presence of unspecified orthopedic joint implant**

Z96.61   **Presence of artificial shoulder joint**

Z96.611   **Presence of right artificial shoulder joint**

Z96.612   **Presence of left artificial shoulder joint**

Z96.619   **Presence of unspecified artificial shoulder joint**

Z96.62   **Presence of artificial elbow joint**

Z96.621   **Presence of right artificial elbow joint**

Z96.622   **Presence of left artificial elbow joint**

Z96.629   **Presence of unspecified artificial elbow joint**

Z96.63   **Presence of artificial wrist joint**

Z96.631   Presence of right artificial wrist joint

Z96.632   Presence of left artificial wrist joint

Z96.639   Presence of unspecified artificial wrist joint

Z96.64   Presence of artificial hip joint

Hip-joint replacement (partial) (total)

Z96.641   Presence of right artificial hip joint

Z96.642   Presence of left artificial hip joint

Z96.643   Presence of artificial hip joint, bilateral

Z96.649   Presence of unspecified artificial hip joint

Z96.65   Presence of artificial knee joint

Z96.651   Presence of right artificial knee joint

Z96.652   Presence of left artificial knee joint

Z96.653   Presence of artificial knee joint, bilateral

Z96.659   Presence of unspecified artificial knee joint

Z96.66   Presence of artificial ankle joint

Z96.661   Presence of right artificial ankle joint

Z96.662   Presence of left artificial ankle joint

Z96.669   Presence of unspecified artificial ankle joint

Z96.69   Presence of other orthopedic joint implants

Z96.691   Finger-joint replacement of right hand

Z96.692   Finger-joint replacement of left hand

Z96.693   Finger-joint replacement, bilateral

Z96.698   Presence of other orthopedic joint implants

Z96.7   Presence of other bone and tendon implants

Presence of skull plate

Z96.8   Presence of other specified functional implants

Z96.81   Presence of artificial skin

Z96.89   Presence of other specified functional implants

Z96.9   Presence of functional implant, unspecified

Z97   **Presence of other devices**

Excludes1: complications of internal prosthetic devices, implants and grafts (T82-T85)

fitting and adjustment of prosthetic **and other** devices (Z44-Z46)

Excludes2: presence of cerebrospinal fluid drainage device (Z98.2)

Z97.0   Presence of artificial eye

Z97.1   Presence of artificial limb (complete) (partial)

Z97.10   Presence of artificial limb (complete) (partial), unspecified

Z97.11   Presence of artificial right arm (complete) (partial)

Z97.12   Presence of artificial left arm (complete) (partial)

Z97.13   Presence of artificial right leg (complete) (partial)

Z97.14   Presence of artificial left leg (complete) (partial)

Z97.15   Presence of artificial arms, bilateral (complete) (partial)

Z97.16   Presence of artificial legs, bilateral (complete) (partial)

Z97.2   Presence of dental prosthetic device (complete) (partial)

Presence of dentures (complete) (partial)

Z97.3   Presence of spectacles and contact lenses

Z97.4   Presence of external hearing-aid

Z97.5   Presence of (intrauterine) contraceptive device

Excludes1: checking, reinsertion or removal of implantable subdermal contraceptive (Z30.46)

checking, reinsertion or removal of intrauterine contraceptive device (Z30.43-)

Z97.8   Presence of other specified devices

Z98   **Other postprocedural states**

Excludes2: aftercare (Z43-Z49, Z51)

follow-up medical care (Z08-Z09)

postprocedural complication - see Alphabetical Index

Z98.0   Intestinal bypass and anastomosis status

Excludes2: bariatric surgery status (Z98.84)

gastric bypass status (Z98.84)

obesity surgery status (Z98.84)

Z98.1   Arthrodesis status

Z98.2   Presence of cerebrospinal fluid drainage device

Presence of CSF shunt

Z98.3   Post therapeutic collapse of lung status

Code first underlying disease

Z98.4   Cataract extraction status

Use additional code to identify intraocular lens implant status (Z96.1)

Excludes1: aphakia (H27.0)

Z98.41   Cataract extraction status, right eye

Z98.42   Cataract extraction status, left eye

Z98.49   Cataract extraction status, unspecified eye

Z98.5   Sterilization status

Excludes1: female infertility (N97.-)

male infertility (N46.-)

Z98.51   Tubal ligation status

Z98.52   Vasectomy status

Z98.6   Angioplasty status

Z98.61   Coronary angioplasty status

Excludes1: coronary angioplasty status with implant and graft (Z95.5)

Z98.62   Peripheral vascular angioplasty status

Excludes1: peripheral vascular angioplasty status with implant and graft (Z95.820)

Z98.8   Other specified postprocedural states

Z98.81   Dental procedure status

Z98.810   Dental sealant status

Z98.811   Dental restoration status

Dental crown status

Dental fillings status

Z98.818   Other dental procedure status

Z98.82   Breast implant status

Excludes1: breast implant removal status (Z98.86)

Z98.83 **Filtering (vitreous) bleb after glaucoma surgery status**

Excludes1: Inflammation (infection) of postprocedural bleb (H59.4-)

Z98.84 **Bariatric surgery status**

Gastric banding status

Gastric bypass status for obesity

Obesity surgery status

Excludes1: bariatric surgery status complicating pregnancy, childbirth, or the puerperium (O99.84)

Excludes2: intestinal bypass and anastomosis status (Z98.0)

Z98.85 **Transplanted organ removal status**

Transplanted organ previously removed due to complication, failure, rejection or infection

Excludes1: encounter for removal of transplanted organ -code to complication of transplanted organ (T86.-)

Z98.86 **Personal history of breast implant removal**

Z98.87 **Personal history of in utero procedure**

Z98.870 **Personal history of in utero procedure during pregnancy**

Excludes2: complications from in utero procedure for current pregnancy (O35.7)

supervision of current pregnancy with history of in utero procedure during previous pregnancy (O09.82-)

Z98.871 **Personal history of in utero procedure while a fetus**

Z98.89 **Other specified postprocedural states**

• **Z98.890** **Other specified postprocedural states**

Personal history of surgery, not elsewhere classified

• **Z98.891** **History of uterine scar from previous surgery**

Excludes1: Maternal care due to uterine scar from previous surgery (O34.2-)

Z99 **Dependence on enabling machines and devices, not elsewhere classified**

Excludes1: cardiac pacemaker status (Z95.0)

Z99.0 **Dependence on aspirator**

Z99.1 **Dependence on respirator** Dependence on ventilator

Z99.11 **Dependence on respirator [ventilator] status**

Z99.12 **Encounter for respirator [ventilator] dependence during power failure**

Excludes1: mechanical complication of respirator [ventilator] (J95.850)

Z99.2 **Dependence on renal dialysis**

Hemodialysis status

Peritoneal dialysis status

Presence of arteriovenous shunt for dialysis

Renal dialysis status NOS

Excludes1: encounter for fitting and adjustment of dialysis catheter (Z49.0-)

Excludes2: noncompliance with renal dialysis (Z91.15)

Z99.3 **Dependence on wheelchair**

Wheelchair confinement status

Code first cause of dependence, such as:

muscular dystrophy (G71.0) obesity (E66.-)

Z99.8 **Dependence on other enabling machines and devices**

Z99.81 **Dependence on supplemental oxygen**

Dependence on long-term oxygen

Z99.89 **Dependence on other enabling machines and devices**

Dependence on machine or device NOS

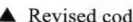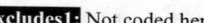

Alphabetic Index To Diseases And Injuries

The Alphabetic Index is an alphabetical list of ICD-10-CM terms and their corresponding code that helps determine which section to refer to in the Tabular List. The Alphabetic Index has two parts; the Index to Diseases and Injuries; and the Index to External Causes of Injury. The Alphabetic Index is folled by the Table of Neoplasms and the Table of Drugs and Chemicals. The ICD-10-CM Official Guidelines for Coding and Reporting include important references to the proper use of the Alphabetic Index which are listed below.

LOCATING A CODE IN THE ICD-10-CM

To select a code in the classification that corresponds to a diagnosis or reason for visit documented in a medical record, first locate the term in the Alphabetic Index, and then verify the code in the Tabular List. Read and be guided by instructional notations that appear in both the Alphabetic Index and the Tabular List.

It is essential to use both the Alphabetic Index and Tabular List when locating and assigning a code. The Alphabetic Index does not always provide the full code. Selection of the full code, including laterality and any applicable 7th character can only be done in the Tabular List. A dash (-) at the end of an Alphabetic Index entry indicates that additional characters are required. Even if a dash is not included at the Alphabetic Index entry, it is necessary to refer to the Tabular List to verify that no 7th character is required.

ALPHABETIC INDEX ABBREVIATIONS

NEC "Not elsewhere classifiable"

This abbreviation in the Alphabetic Index represents "other specified." When a specific code is not available for a condition, the Alphabetic Index directs the coder to the "other specified" code in the Tabular List.

NOS "Not otherwise specified"

This abbreviation is the equivalent of unspecified.

PUNCTUATION

[ ]   Brackets are used in the Alphabetic Index to identify manifestation codes.

( )   Parentheses are used in the Alphabetic Index to enclose supplementary words that may be present or absent in the statement of a disease or procedure without affecting the code number to which it is assigned. The terms within the parentheses are referred to as nonessential modifiers. The nonessential modifiers in the Alphabetic Index to Diseases apply to subterms following a main term except when a nonessential modifier and a subentry are mutually exclusive, the subentry takes precedence.

OTHER CODES

Codes titled "other" or "other specified" are for use when the information in the medical record provides detail for which a specific code does not exist. Alphabetic Index entries with NEC in the line designate "other" codes in the Tabular List. These Alphabetic Index entries represent specific disease entities for which no specific code exists so the term is included within an "other" code.

ETIOLOGY/MANIFESTATION CONVENTION

Certain conditions have both an underlying etiology and multiple body system manifestations due to the underlying etiology. For such conditions, the ICD-10-CM has a coding convention that requires the underlying condition be sequenced first, if applicable, followed by the manifestation.

In addition to the notes in the Tabular List, these conditions also have a specific Alphabetic Index entry structure. In the Alphabetic Index both conditions are listed together with the etiology code first followed by the manifestation codes in brackets. The code in brackets is always to be sequenced second.

WITH

The word "with" should be interpreted to mean "associated with" or "due to" when it appears in a code title, the Alphabetic Index, or an instructional note in the Tabular List. The classification presumes a causal relationship between the two conditions linked by these terms in the Alphabetic Index or Tabular List.

SEE AND SEE ALSO

The "see" instruction following a main term in the Alphabetic Index indicates that another term should be referenced. It is necessary to go to the main term referenced with the "see" note to locate the correct code.

A "see also" instruction following a main term in the Alphabetic Index instructs that there is another main term that may also be referenced that may provide additional Alphabetic Index entries that may be useful. It is not necessary to follow the "see also" note when the original main term provides the necessary code.

DEFAULT CODES

A code listed next to a main term in the ICD-10-CM Alphabetic Index is referred to as a default code. The default code represents that condition that is most commonly associated with the main term, or is the unspecified code for the condition. If a condition is documented in a medical record without any additional information, such as acute or chronic, the default code should be assigned.

ACUTE AND CHRONIC CONDITIONS

If the same condition is described as both acute (subacute) and chronic, and separate subentries exist in the Alphabetic Index at the same indentation level, code both and sequence the acute (subacute) code first.

COMBINATION CODE

A combination code is a single code used to classify:

- Two diagnoses, or
- A diagnosis with an associated secondary process (manifestation)
- A diagnosis with an associated complication

Combination codes are identified by referring to subterm entries in the Alphabetic Index and by reading the inclusion and exclusion notes in the Tabular List.

Assign only the combination code when that code fully identifies the diagnostic conditions involved or when the Alphabetic Index so directs.

SYNDROMES

Follow the Alphabetic Index guidance when coding syndromes. In the absence of Alphabetic Index guidance, assign codes for the documented manifestations of the syndrome.

NEOPLASMS

The Table of Neoplasms provides the proper code based on histology of the neoplasm and site. The neoplasm table following the Alphabetic Index should be referenced first. However, if the histological term is documented, that term should be referenced first, rather than going immediately to the Neoplasm Table, in order to determine which column in the Neoplasm Table is appropriate. For example, if the documentation indicates "adenoma," refer to the term in the Alphabetic Index to review the entries under this term and the instructional note to "see also neoplasm, by site, benign." The table provides the proper code based on the type of neoplasm and the site. It is important to select the proper column in the table that corresponds to the type of neoplasm. The Tabular List should then be referenced to verify that the correct code has been selected from the table and that a more specific site code does not exist.

A

Aarskog's syndrome Q87.1
Abandonment -see Maltreatment
Abasia (astasia) (hysterical) F44.4
Abderhalden-Kaufmann-Lignac syndrome
  (cystinosis) E72.04
Abdomen, abdominal -see also condition
  acute R10.0
  angina K55.1
  muscle deficiency syndrome Q79.4
Abdominalgia -see Pain, abdominal
Abduction contracture, hip or other joint -
  see Contraction, joint
Aberrant (congenital) -see also Malposition,
  congenital
  adrenal gland Q89.1
  artery (peripheral) Q27.8
    basilar NEC Q28.1
    cerebral Q28.3
    coronary Q24.5
    digestive system Q27.8
    eye Q15.8
    lower limb Q27.8
    precerebral Q28.1
    pulmonary Q25.79
    renal Q27.2
    retina Q14.1
    specified site NEC Q27.8
    subclavian Q27.8
    upper limb Q27.8
    vertebral Q28.1
  breast Q83.8
  endocrine gland NEC Q89.2
  hepatic duct Q44.5
  pancreas Q45.3
  parathyroid gland Q89.2
  pituitary gland Q89.2
  sebaceous glands, mucous membrane, mouth,
    congenital Q38.6
  spleen Q89.09
  subclavian artery Q27.8
  thymus (gland) Q89.2
  thyroid gland Q89.2
  vein (peripheral) NEC Q27.8
    cerebral Q28.3
    digestive system Q27.8
    lower limb Q27.8
    precerebral Q28.1
    specified site NEC Q27.8
    upper limb Q27.8
Aberration
  distantal -see Disturbance, visual
  mental F99
Abetalipoproteinemia E78.6
Abiotrophy R68.89
Ablatio, ablation
  retinae -see Detachment, retina
Ablepharia, ablepharon Q10.3
Abnormal, abnormality, abnormalities -see
  also Anomaly
  acid-base balance (mixed) E87.4
  albumin R77.0
  alphafetoprotein R77.2
  alveolar ridge K08.9
  anatomical relationship Q89.9
  apertures, congenital, diaphragm Q79.1
  auditory perception H93.29
    diplacusis -see Diplacusis
    hyperacusis -see Hyperacusis
    recruitment -see Recruitment, auditory

Abnormal, abnormality, abnormalities --
  continued
    threshold shift -see Shift, auditory threshold
  autosomes Q99.9
    fragile site Q95.5
  basal metabolic rate R94.8
  biosynthesis, testicular androgen E29.1
  bleeding time R79.1
  blood-gas level R79.81
  blood level (of)
    cobalt R79.0
    copper R79.0
    iron R79.0
    lithium R78.89
    magnesium R79.0
    mineral NEC R79.0
    zinc R79.0
  blood pressure
    elevated R03.0
    low reading (nonspecific) R03.1
  blood sugar R73.09
  bowel sounds R19.15
    absent R19.11
    hyperactive R19.12
  brain scan R94.02
  breathing R06.9
  caloric test R94.138
  cerebrospinal fluid R83.9
    cytology R83.6
    drug level R83.2
    enzyme level R83.0
    hormones R83.1
    immunology R83.4
    microbiology R83.5
    nonmedicinal level R83.3
    specified type NEC R83.8
  chemistry, blood R79.9
    C-reactive protein R79.82
    drugs -see Findings, abnormal, in blood
    gas level R79.81
    minerals R79.0
    pancytopenia D61.818
    PTT R79.1
    specified NEC R79.89
    toxins -see Findings, abnormal, in blood
  chest sounds (friction) (rales) R09.89
  chromosome, chromosomal Q99.9
    with more than three X chromosomes,
    female Q97.1
    analysis result R89.8
      bronchial washings R84.8
      cerebrospinal fluid R83.8
      cervix uteri NEC R87.89
      nasal secretions R84.8
      nipple discharge R89.8
      peritoneal fluid R85.89
      pleural fluid R84.8
      prostatic secretions R86.8
      saliva R85.89
      seminal fluid R86.8
      sputum R84.8
      synovial fluid R89.8
      throat scrapings R84.8
      vagina R87.89
      vulva R87.89
      wound secretions R89.8
    dicentric replacement Q93.2
    ring replacement Q93.2
    sex Q99.8
      female phenotype Q97.9
        specified NEC Q97.8

Abnormal, abnormality, abnormalities --
  continued
    male phenotype Q98.9
      specified NEC Q98.8
      structural male Q98.6
    specified NEC Q99.8
  clinical findings NEC R68.89
  coagulation D68.9
    newborn, transient P61.6
    profile R79.1
    time R79.1
  communication -see Fistula
  conjunctiva, vascular H11.41
  coronary artery Q24.5
  cortisol-binding globulin E27.8
  course, eustachian tube Q17.8
  creatinine clearance R94.4
  cytology
    anus R85.619
      atypical squamous cells cannot exclude
        high grade squamous intraepithelial lesion
        (ASC-H) R85.611
      atypical squamous cells of undetermined
        significance (ASC-US) R85.610
      cytologic evidence of malignancy R85.614
      high grade squamous intraepithelial lesion
        (HGSIL) R85.613
      human papillomavirus (HPV) DNA test
        high risk positive R85.81
        low risk positive R85.82
      inadequate smear R85.615
      low grade squamous intraepithelial lesion
        (LGSIL) R85.612
      satisfactory anal smear but lacking
        transformation zone R85.616
      specified NEC R85.618
      unsatisfactory smear R85.615
    female genital organs -see Abnormal,
      Papanicolaou (smear)
  dark adaptation curve H53.61
  dentofacial NEC -see Anomaly, dentofacial
  development, developmental Q89.9
    central nervous system Q07.9
  diagnostic imaging
    abdomen, abdominal region NEC R93.5
    biliary tract R93.2
    bladder R93.41
    breast R92.8
    central nervous system NEC R90.89
    cerebrovascular NEC R90.89
    coronary circulation R93.1
    digestive tract NEC R93.3
    gastrointestinal (tract) R93.3
    genitourinary organs R93.8
    head R93.0
    heart R93.1
    intrathoracic organ NEC R93.8
    kidney R93.42
    limbs R93.6
    liver R93.2
    lung (field) R91.8
    musculoskeletal system NEC R93.7
    renal pelvis R93.41
    retroperitoneum R93.5
    site specified NEC R93.8
    skin and subcutaneous tissue R93.8
    skull R93.0
    urinary organs specified NEC R93.49
    ureter R93.41
  direction, teeth, fully erupted M26.30
  ear ossicles, acquired NEC H74.39

Abnormal, abnormality, abnormalities --
continued
  ankylosis -*see* Ankylosis, ear ossicles
  discontinuity -*see* Discontinuity, ossicles, ear
  partial loss -*see* Loss, ossicles, ear (partial)
  Ebstein Q22.5
  echocardiogram R93.1
  echoencephalogram R90.81
  echogram -*see* Abnormal, diagnostic imaging
  electrocardiogram [ECG] [EKG] R94.31
  electroencephalogram [EEG] R94.01
  electrolyte -*see* Imbalance, electrolyte
  electromyogram [EMG] R94.131
  electro-oculogram [EOG] R94.110
  electrophysiological intracardiac studies R94.39
  electroretinogram [ERG] R94.111
  erythrocytes
    congenital, with perinatal jaundice D58.9
  feces (color) (contents) (mucus) R19.5
  finding -*see* Findings, abnormal, without diagnosis
  fluid
    amniotic -*see* Abnormal, specimen, specified
    cerebrospinal -*see* Abnormal, cerebrospinal fluid
    peritoneal -*see* Abnormal, specimen, digestive organs
    pleural -*see* Abnormal, specimen, respiratory organs
    synovial -*see* Abnormal, specimen, specified
    thorax (bronchial washings) (pleural fluid) -*see* Abnormal, specimen, respiratory organs
    vaginal -*see* Abnormal, specimen, female genital organs
  form
    teeth K00.2
    uterus -*see* Anomaly, uterus
  function studies
    auditory R94.120
    bladder R94.8
    brain R94.09
    cardiovascular R94.30
    ear R94.128
    endocrine NEC R94.7
    eye NEC R94.118
    kidney R94.4
    liver R94.5
    nervous system
      central NEC R94.09
      peripheral NEC R94.138
    pancreas R94.8
    placenta R94.8
    pulmonary R94.2
    special senses NEC R94.128
    spleen R94.8
    thyroid R94.6
    vestibular R94.121
  gait -*see* Gait
    hysterical F44.4
  gastrin secretion E16.4
  globulin R77.1
    cortisol-binding E27.8
    thyroid-binding E07.89
  glomerular, minor -*see also* N00 N07 with fourth character .0 N05.0
  glucagon secretion E16.3
  glucose tolerance (test) (non-fasting) R73.09

Abnormal, abnormality, abnormalities --
continued
  gravitational (G) forces or states (effect of) T75.81
  hair (color) (shaft) L67.9
    specified NEC L67.8
  hard tissue formation in pulp (dental) K04.3
  head movement R25.0
  heart
    rate R00.9
      specified NEC R00.8
    shadow R93.1
    sounds NEC R01.2
  hemoglobin (disease) -*see also* Disease, hemoglobin D58.2
    trait -*see* Trait, hemoglobin, abnormal
  histology NEC R89.7
  immunological findings R89.4
    in serum R76.9
      specified NEC R76.8
  increase in appetite R63.2
  involuntary movement -*see* Abnormal, movement, involuntary
  jaw closure M26.51
  karyotype R89.8
  kidney function test R94.4
  knee jerk R29.2
  leukocyte (cell) (differential) NEC D72.9
  liver
    loss of
      height R29.890
      weight R63.4
  mammogram NEC R92.8
    calcification (calculus) R92.1
    microcalcification R92.0
  Mantoux test R76.11
  movement (disorder) -*see also* Disorder, movement
    head R25.0
    involuntary R25.9
      fasciculation R25.3
      of head R25.0
      spasm R25.2
      specified type NEC R25.8
      tremor R25.1
  myoglobin (Aberdeen) (Annapolis) R89.7
  neonatal screening P09
  oculomotor study R94.113
  palmar creases Q82.8
  Papanicolaou (smear)
    anus R85.619
      atypical squamous cells cannot exclude high grade squamous intraepithelial lesion (ASC-H) R85.611
      atypical squamous cells of undetermined significance (ASC-US) R85.610
      cytologic evidence of malignancy R85.614
      high grade squamous intraepithelial lesion (HGSIL) R85.613
      human papillomavirus (HPV) DNA test
        high risk positive R85.81
        low risk positive R85.82
      inadequate smear R85.615
      low grade squamous intraepithelial lesion (LGSIL) R85.612
      satisfactory anal smear but lacking transformation zone R85.616
      specified NEC R85.618
      unsatisfactory smear R85.615
    bronchial washings R84.6
    cerebrospinal fluid R83.6

Abnormal, abnormality, abnormalities --
continued
  cervix R87.619
    atypical squamous cells cannot exclude high grade squamous intraepithelial lesion (ASC-H) R87.611
    atypical squamous cells of undetermined significance (ASC-US) R87.610
    cytologic evidence of malignancy R87.614
    high grade squamous intraepithelial lesion (HGSIL) R87.613
    inadequate smear R87.615
    low grade squamous intraepithelial lesion (LGSIL) R87.612
    non-atypical endometrial cells R87.618
    satisfactory cervical smear but lacking transformation zone R87.616
    specified NEC R87.618
    thin preparation R87.619
    unsatisfactory smear R87.615
  nasal secretions R84.6
  nipple discharge R89.6
  peritoneal fluid R85.69
  pleural fluid R84.6
  prostatic secretions R86.6
  saliva R85.69
  seminal fluid R86.6
  sites NEC R89.6
  sputum R84.6
  synovial fluid R89.6
  throat scrapings R84.6
  vagina R87.629
    atypical squamous cells cannot exclude high grade squamous intraepithelial lesion (ASC-H) R87.621
    atypical squamous cells of undetermined significance (ASC-US) R87.620
    cytologic evidence of malignancy R87.624
    high grade squamous intraepithelial lesion (HGSIL) R87.623
    inadequate smear R87.625
    low grade squamous intraepithelial lesion (LGSIL) R87.622
    specified NEC R87.628
    thin preparation R87.629
    unsatisfactory smear R87.625
  vulva R87.69
  wound secretions R89.6
  partial thromboplastin time (PTT) R79.1
  pelvis (bony) -*see* Deformity, pelvis
  percussion, chest (tympany) R09.89
  periods (grossly) -*see* Menstruation
  phonocardiogram R94.39
  plantar reflex R29.2
  plasma
    protein R77.9
      specified NEC R77.8
    viscosity R70.1
  pleural (folds) Q34.0
  posture R29.3
  product of conception O02.9
    specified type NEC O02.89
  prothrombin time (PT) R79.1
  pulmonary
    artery, congenital Q25.79
    function, newborn P28.89
    test results R94.2
  pulsations in neck R00.2
  pupillary H21.56
    function (reaction) (reflex) -*see* Anomaly, pupil, function

Abnormal, abnormality, abnormalities --
continued
radiological examination -*see* Abnormal, diagnostic imaging
red blood cell(s) (morphology) (volume) R71.8
reflex -*see* Reflex
renal function test R94.4
response to nerve stimulation R94.130
retinal correspondence H53.31
retinal function study R94.111
rhythm, heart -*see also* Arrhythmia
saliva -*see* Abnormal, specimen, digestive organs
scan
  kidney R94.4
  liver R93.2
  thyroid R94.6
secretion
  gastrin E16.4
  glucagon E16.3
semen, seminal fluid -*see* Abnormal, specimen, male genital organs
serum level (of)
  acid phosphatase R74.8
  alkaline phosphatase R74.8
  amylase R74.8
  enzymes R74.9
    specified NEC R74.8
  lipase R74.8
  triacylglycerol lipase R74.8
shape
  gravid uterus -*see* Anomaly, uterus
sinus venosus Q21.1
size, tooth, teeth K00.2
spacing, tooth, teeth, fully erupted M26.30
specimen
  digestive organs (peritoneal fluid) (saliva) R85.9
    cytology R85.69
    drug level R85.2
    enzyme level R85.0
    histology R85.7
    hormones R85.1
    immunology R85.4
    microbiology R85.5
    nonmedicinal level R85.3
    specified type NEC R85.89
  female genital organs (secretions) (smears) R87.9
    cytology R87.69
      cervix R87.619
        human papillomavirus (HPV) DNA test
          high risk positive R87.810
          low risk positive R87.820
        inadequate (unsatisfactory) smear R87.615
        non-atypical endometrial cells R87.618
        specified NEC R87.618
      vagina R87.629
        human papillomavirus (HPV) DNA test
          high risk positive R87.811
          low risk positive R87.821
        inadequate (unsatisfactory) smear R87.625
      vulva R87.69
    drug level R87.2
    enzyme level R87.0
    histological R87.7
    hormones R87.1
    immunology R87.4

Abnormal, abnormality, abnormalities --
continued
    microbiology R87.5
    nonmedicinal level R87.3
    specified type NEC R87.89
  male genital organs (prostatic secretions) (semen) R86.9
    cytology R86.6
    drug level R86.2
    enzyme level R86.0
    histological R86.7
    hormones R86.1
    immunology R86.4
    microbiology R86.5
    nonmedicinal level R86.3
    specified type NEC R86.8
  nipple discharge -*see* Abnormal, specimen, specified
  respiratory organs (bronchial washings) (nasal secretions) (pleural fluid) (sputum) R84.9
    cytology R84.6
    drug level R84.2
    enzyme level R84.0
    histology R84.7
    hormones R84.1
    immunology R84.4
    microbiology R84.5
    nonmedicinal level R84.3
    specified type NEC R84.8
  specified organ, system and tissue NOS R89.9
    cytology R89.6
    drug level R89.2
    enzyme level R89.0
    histology R89.7
    hormones R89.1
    immunology R89.4
    microbiology R89.5
    nonmedicinal level R89.3
    specified type NEC R89.8
  synovial fluid -*see* Abnormal, specimen, specified
  thorax (bronchial washings) (pleural fluids) -*see* Abnormal, specimen, respiratory organs
  vagina (secretion) (smear) R87.629
  vulva (secretion) (smear) R87.69
  wound secretion -*see* Abnormal, specimen, specified
spermatozoa -*see* Abnormal, specimen, male genital organs
sputum (amount) (color) (odor) R09.3
stool (color) (contents) (mucus) R19.5
  bloody K92.1
  guaiac positive R19.5
synchondrosis Q78.8
thermography -*see also* Abnormal, diagnostic imaging R93.8
thyroid-binding globulin E07.89
tooth, teeth (form) (size) K00.2
toxicology (findings) R78.9
transport protein E88.09
tumor marker NEC R97.8
ultrasound results -*see* Abnormal, diagnostic imaging
umbilical cord complicating delivery O69.9
urination NEC R39.198
urine (constituents) R82.90
  bile R82.2
  cytological examination R82.8

Abnormal, abnormality, abnormalities --
continued
  drugs R82.5
  fat R82.0
  glucose R81
  heavy metals R82.6
  hemoglobin R82.3
  histological examination R82.8
  ketones R82.4
  microbiological examination (culture) R82.79
  myoglobin R82.1
  positive culture R82.79
  protein -*see* Proteinuria
  specified substance NEC R82.99
    chromoabnormality NEC R82.91
  substances nonmedical R82.6
uterine hemorrhage -*see* Hemorrhage, uterus
vectorcardiogram R94.39
visually evoked potential (VEP) R94.112
white blood cells D72.9
  specified NEC D72.89
X ray examination -*see* Abnormal, diagnostic imaging
Abnormity (any organ or part) -*see* Anomaly
Abocclusion M26.29
  hemolytic disease (newborn) P55.1
  incompatibility reaction ABO -*see* Complication(s), transfusion, incompatibility reaction, ABO
Abolition, language R48.8
Aborter, habitual or recurrent -*see* Loss (of), pregnancy, recurrent
Abortion (complete) (spontaneous) O03.9
with
  retained products of conception -*see* Abortion, incomplete
attempted (elective) (failed) O07.4
  complicated by O07.30
    afibrinogenemia O07.1
    cardiac arrest O07.36
    chemical damage of pelvic organ(s) O07.34
    circulatory collapse O07.31
    cystitis O07.38
    defibrination syndrome O07.1
    electrolyte imbalance O07.33
    embolism (air) (amniotic fluid) (blood clot) (fat) (pulmonary) (septic) (soap) O07.2
    endometritis O07.0
    genital tract and pelvic infection O07.0
    hemolysis O07.1
    hemorrhage (delayed) (excessive) O07.1
    infection
      genital tract or pelvic O07.0
      urinary tract O07.38
    intravascular coagulation O07.1
    laceration of pelvic organ(s) O07.34
    metabolic disorder O07.33
    oliguria O07.32
    oophoritis O07.0
    parametritis O07.0
    pelvic peritonitis O07.0
    perforation of pelvic organ(s) O07.34
    renal failure or shutdown O07.32
    salpingitis or salpingo-oophoritis O07.0
    sepsis O07.37
    shock O07.31
    specified condition NEC O07.39
    tubular necrosis (renal) O07.32
    uremia O07.32
    urinary tract infection O07.38

Abortion (complete) (spontaneous) -- *continued*
    venous complication NEC O07.35
      embolism (air) (amniotic fluid) (blood clot) (fat) (pulmonary) (septic) (soap) O07.2
  complicated (by) (following) O03.80
    afibrinogenemia O03.6
    cardiac arrest O03.86
    chemical damage of pelvic organ(s) O03.84
    circulatory collapse O03.81
    cystitis O03.88
    defibrination syndrome O03.6
    electrolyte imbalance O03.83
    embolism (air) (amniotic fluid) (blood clot) (fat) (pulmonary) (septic) (soap) O03.7
    endometritis O03.5
    genital tract and pelvic infection O03.5
    hemolysis O03.6
    hemorrhage (delayed) (excessive) O03.6
    infection
      genital tract or pelvic O03.5
      urinary tract O03.88
    intravascular coagulation O03.6
    laceration of pelvic organ(s) O03.84
    metabolic disorder O03.83
    oliguria O03.82
    oophoritis O03.5
    parametritis O03.5
    pelvic peritonitis O03.5
    perforation of pelvic organ(s) O03.84
    renal failure or shutdown O03.82
    salpingitis or salpingo-oophoritis O03.5
    sepsis O03.87
    shock O03.81
    specified condition NEC O03.89
    tubular necrosis (renal) O03.82
    uremia O03.82
    urinary tract infection O03.88
    venous complication NEC O03.85
      embolism (air) (amniotic fluid) (blood clot) (fat) (pulmonary) (septic) (soap) O03.7
  failed -*see* Abortion, attempted
  habitual or recurrent N96
    with current abortion -*see* categories O03 O06
    without current pregnancy N96
    care in current pregnancy O26.2
  incomplete (spontaneous) O03.4
    complicated (by) (following) O03.30
      afibrinogenemia O03.1
      cardiac arrest O03.36
      chemical damage of pelvic organ(s) O03.34
      circulatory collapse O03.31
      cystitis O03.38
      defibrination syndrome O03.1
      electrolyte imbalance O03.33
      embolism (air) (amniotic fluid) (blood clot) (fat) (pulmonary) (septic) (soap) O03.2
      endometritis O03.0
      genital tract and pelvic infection O03.0
      hemolysis O03.1
      hemorrhage (delayed) (excessive) O03.1
      infection
        genital tract or pelvic O03.0
        urinary tract O03.38
      intravascular coagulation O03.1
      laceration of pelvic organ(s) O03.34
      metabolic disorder O03.33
      oliguria O03.32
      oophoritis O03.0

Abortion (complete) (spontaneous) -- *continued*
    parametritis O03.0
    pelvic peritonitis O03.0
    perforation of pelvic organ(s) O03.34
    renal failure or shutdown O03.32
    salpingitis or salpingo-oophoritis O03.0
    sepsis O03.37
    shock O03.31
    specified condition NEC O03.39
    tubular necrosis (renal) O03.32
    uremia O03.32
    urinary infection O03.38
    venous complication NEC O03.35
      embolism (air) (amniotic fluid) (blood clot) (fat) (pulmonary) (septic) (soap) O03.2
  induced (encounter for) Z33.2
    complicated by O04.80
      afibrinogenemia O04.6
      cardiac arrest O04.86
      chemical damage of pelvic organ(s) O04.84
      circulatory collapse O04.81
      cystitis O04.88
      defibrination syndrome O04.6
      electrolyte imbalance O04.83
      embolism (air) (amniotic fluid) (blood clot) (fat) (pulmonary) (septic) (soap) O04.7
      endometritis O04.5
      genital tract and pelvic infection O04.5
      hemolysis O04.6
      hemorrhage (delayed) (excessive) O04.6
      infection
        genital tract or pelvic O04.5
        urinary tract O04.88
      intravascular coagulation O04.6
      laceration of pelvic organ(s) O04.84
      metabolic disorder O04.83
      oliguria O04.82
      oophoritis O04.5
      parametritis O04.5
      pelvic peritonitis O04.5
      perforation of pelvic organ(s) O04.84
      renal failure or shutdown O04.82
      salpingitis or salpingo-oophoritis O04.5
      sepsis O04.87
      shock O04.81
      specified condition NEC O04.89
      tubular necrosis (renal) O04.82
      uremia O04.82
      urinary tract infection O04.88
      venous complication NEC O04.85
        embolism (air) (amniotic fluid) (blood clot) (fat) (pulmonary) (septic) (soap) O04.7
  missed O02.1
  spontaneous -*see* Abortion (complete) (spontaneous)
    threatened O20.0
  threatened (spontaneous) O20.0
  tubal O00.10
    with intrauterine pregnancy O00.11
Abortus fever A23.1
Aboulomania F60.7
Abrami's disease D59.8
Abramov-Fiedler myocarditis (acute isolated myocarditis) I40.1
Abrasion T14.8
  abdomen, abdominal (wall) S30.811
  alveolar process S00.512
  ankle S90.51
  antecubital space -*see* Abrasion, elbow

Abrasion -*continued*
  anus S30.817
  arm (upper) S40.81
  auditory canal -*see* Abrasion, ear
  auricle -*see* Abrasion, ear
  axilla -*see* Abrasion, arm
  back, lower S30.810
  breast S20.11
  brow S00.81
  buttock S30.810
  calf -*see* Abrasion, leg
  canthus -*see* Abrasion, eyelid
  cheek S00.81
    internal S00.512
  chest wall -*see* Abrasion, thorax
  chin S00.81
  clitoris S30.814
  cornea S05.0
  costal region -*see* Abrasion, thorax
  dental K03.1
  digit(s)
    foot -*see* Abrasion, toe
    hand -*see* Abrasion, finger
  ear S00.41
  elbow S50.31
  epididymis S30.813
  epigastric region S30.811
  epiglottis S10.11
  esophagus (thoracic) S27.818
    cervical S10.11
  eyebrow -*see* Abrasion, eyelid
  eyelid S00.21
  face S00.81
  finger(s) S60.41
    index S60.41
    little S60.41
    middle S60.41
    ring S60.41
  flank S30.811
  foot (except toe(s) alone) S90.81
    toe -*see* Abrasion, toe
  forearm S50.81
    elbow only -*see* Abrasion, elbow
  forehead S00.81
  genital organs, external
    female S30.816
    male S30.815
  groin S30.811
  gum S00.512
  hand S60.51
  head S00.91
    ear -*see* Abrasion, ear
    eyelid -*see* Abrasion, eyelid
    lip S00.511
    nose S00.31
    oral cavity S00.512
    scalp S00.01
    specified site NEC S00.81
  heel -*see* Abrasion, foot
  hip S70.21
  inguinal region S30.811
  interscapular region S20.419
  jaw S00.81
  knee S80.21
  labium (majus) (minus) S30.814
  larynx S10.11
  leg (lower) S80.81
    knee -*see* Abrasion, knee
    upper -*see* Abrasion, thigh
  lip S00.511
  lower back S30.810

Abrasion --*continued*

lumbar region S30.810
malar region S00.81
mammary -*see* Abrasion, breast
mastoid region S00.81
mouth S00.512
nail
  finger -*see* Abrasion, finger
  toe -*see* Abrasion, toe
nape S10.81
nasal S00.31
neck S10.91
  specified site NEC S10.81
  throat S10.11
nose S00.31
occipital region S00.01
oral cavity S00.512
orbital region -*see* Abrasion, eyelid
palate S00.512
palm -*see* Abrasion, hand
parietal region S00.01
pelvis S30.810
penis S30.812
perineum
  female S30.814
  male S30.810
periocular area -*see* Abrasion, eyelid
phalanges
  finger -*see* Abrasion, finger
  toe -*see* Abrasion, toe
pharynx S10.11
pinna -*see* Abrasion, ear
popliteal space -*see* Abrasion, knee
prepuce S30.812
pubic region S30.810
pudendum
  female S30.816
  male S30.815
sacral region S30.810
scalp S00.01
scapular region -*see* Abrasion, shoulder
scrotum S30.813
shin -*see* Abrasion, leg
shoulder S40.21
skin NEC T14.8
sternal region S20.319
submaxillary region S00.81
submental region S00.81
subungual
  finger(s) -*see* Abrasion, finger
  toe(s) -*see* Abrasion, toe
supraclavicular fossa S10.81
supraorbital S00.81
temple S00.81
temporal region S00.81
testis S30.813
thigh S70.31
thorax, thoracic (wall) S20.91
  back S20.41
  front S20.31
throat S10.11
thumb S60.31   toe(s) (lesser) S90.416
  great S90.41
tongue S00.512
tooth, teeth (dentifrice) (habitual) (hard
  tissues) (occupational) (ritual) (traditional)
  K03.1
trachea S10.11
tunica vaginalis S30.813
tympanum, tympanic membrane -*see*
  Abrasion, ear

Abrasion --*continued*

uvula S00.512
vagina S30.814
vocal cords S10.11
vulva S30.814
wrist S60.81
Abrism -*see* Poisoning, food, noxious, plant
Abruptio placentae O45.9
with
  afibrinogenemia O45.01
  coagulation defect O45.00
    specified NEC O45.09
  disseminated intravascular coagulation
    O45.02
  hypofibrinogenemia O45.01
  specified NEC O45.8
Abruption, placenta -*see* Abruptio placentae
Abscess (connective tissue) (embolic)
  (fistulous) (infective) (metastatic) (multiple)
  (pernicious) (pyogenic) (septic) L02.91
with
  diverticular disease (intestine) K57.80
    with bleeding K57.81
    large intestine K57.20
    with
      bleeding K57.21
      small intestine K57.40
        with bleeding K57.41
    small intestine K57.00
    with
      bleeding K57.01
      large intestine K57.40
        with bleeding K57.41
  lymphangitis
code by site under Abscess
abdomen, abdominal
  cavity K65.1
  wall L02.211
abdominopelvic K65.1
accessory sinus -*see* Sinusitis
adrenal (capsule) (gland) E27.8
alveolar K04.7
  with sinus K04.6
amebic A06.4
  brain (and liver or lung abscess) A06.6
  genitourinary tract A06.82
  liver (without mention of brain or lung
    abscess) A06.4
  lung (and liver) (without mention of brain
    abscess) A06.5
  specified site NEC A06.89
  spleen A06.89
anaerobic A48.0
ankle -*see* Abscess, lower limb
anorectal K61.2
antecubital space -*see* Abscess, upper limb
antrum (chronic) (Highmore) -*see* Sinusitis,
  maxillary
anus K61.0
apical (tooth) K04.7
  with sinus (alveolar) K04.6
appendix K35.3
areola (acute) (chronic) (nonpuerperal) N61.1
  puerperal, postpartum or gestational -*see*
  Infection, nipple
arm (any part) -*see* Abscess, upper limb
artery (wall) I77.89
atheromatous I77.2
auricle, ear -*see* Abscess, ear, external
axilla (region) L02.41
  lymph gland or node L04.2

Abscess --*continued*

back (any part, except buttock) L02.212
Bartholin's gland N75.1
  with
    abortion -*see* Abortion, by type
      complicated by, sepsis
    ectopic or molar pregnancy O08.0
    following ectopic or molar pregnancy O08.0
Bezold's -*see* Mastoiditis, acute
bilharziasis B65.1
bladder (wall) -*see* Cystitis, specified type
  NEC
bone (subperiosteal) -*see also* Osteomyelitis,
  specified type NEC
  accessory sinus (chronic) -*see* Sinusitis
  chronic or old -*see* Osteomyelitis, chronic
  jaw (lower) (upper) M27.2
  mastoid -*see* Mastoiditis, acute,
    subperiosteal
  petrous -*see* Petrositis
  spinal (tuberculous) A18.01
    nontuberculous -*see* Osteomyelitis,
    vertebra
bowel K63.0
brain (any part) (cystic) (otogenic) G06.0
  amebic (with abscess of any other site)
  A06.6
  gonococcal A54.82
  pheomycotic (chromomycotic) B43.1
  tuberculous A17.81
breast (acute) (chronic) (nonpuerperal) N61.1
  newborn P39.0
  puerperal, postpartum, gestational -*see*
    Mastitis, obstetric, purulent
broad ligament N73.2
  acute N73.0
  chronic N73.1
Brodie's (localized) (chronic) M86.8X
bronchi J98.09
buccal cavity K12.2
bulbourethral gland N34.0
bursa M71.00
  ankle M71.07
  elbow M71.02
  foot M71.07
  hand M71.04
  hip M71.05
  knee M71.06
  multiple sites M71.09
  pharyngeal J39.1
  shoulder M71.01
  specified site NEC M71.08
  wrist M71.03
buttock L02.31
canthus -*see* Blepharoconjunctivitis
cartilage -*see* Disorder, cartilage, specified
  type NEC
cecum K35.3
cerebellum, cerebellar G06.0
  sequelae G09
cerebral (embolic) G06.0
  sequelae G09
cervical (meaning neck) L02.11
  lymph gland or node L04.0
cervix (stump) (uteri) -*see* Cervicitis
cheek (external) L02.01
  inner K12.2
chest J86.9
  with fistula J86.0
  wall L02.213
chin L02.01

Abscess --*continued*
  choroid -*see* Inflammation, chorioretinal
  circumtonsillar J36
  cold (lung) (tuberculous) -*see also*
    Tuberculosis, abscess, lung
      articular -*see* Tuberculosis, joint
  colon (wall) K63.0
  colostomy K94.02
  conjunctiva -*see* Conjunctivitis, acute
  cornea H16.31
  corpus
    cavernosum N48.21
    luteum -*see* Oophoritis
  Cowper's gland N34.0
  cranium G06.0
  cul-de-sac (Douglas') (posterior) -*see*
    Peritonitis, pelvic, female
  cutaneous -*see* Abscess, by site
  dental K04.7
    with sinus (alveolar) K04.6
  dentoalveolar K04.7
    with sinus K04.6
  diaphragm, diaphragmatic K65.1
  Douglas' cul-de-sac or pouch -*see* Peritonitis,
    pelvic, female
  Dubois A50.59
  ear (middle) -*see also* Otitis, media,
    suppurative
      acute -*see* Otitis, media, suppurative, acute
      external H60.0
  entamebic -*see* Abscess, amebic
  enterostomy K94.12
  epididymis N45.4
  epidural G06.2
    brain G06.0
    spinal cord G06.1
  epiglottis J38.7
  epiploon, epiploic K65.1
  erysipelatous -*see* Erysipelas
  esophagus K20.8
  ethmoid (bone) (chronic) (sinus) J32.2
  external auditory canal -*see* Abscess, ear,
    external
  extradural G06.2
    brain G06.0
      sequelae G09
    spinal cord G06.1
  extraperitoneal K68.19
  eye -*see* Endophthalmitis, purulent
  eyelid H00.03
  face (any part, except ear, eye and nose)
    L02.01
  fallopian tube -*see* Salpingitis
  fascia M72.8
  fauces J39.1
  fecal K63.0
  femoral (region) -*see* Abscess, lower limb
  filaria, filarial -*see* Infestation, filarial
  finger (any) -*see also* Abscess, hand
    nail -*see* Cellulitis, finger
  foot L02.61
  forehead L02.01
  frontal sinus (chronic) J32.1
  gallbladder K81.0
  genital organ or tract
    female (external) N76.4
    male N49.9
      multiple sites N49.8
      specified NEC N49.8
  gestational mammary O91.11
  gestational subareolar O91.11

Abscess --*continued*
  gingival -*see* Peridontitis, aggressive,
    localized
  gland, glandular (lymph) (acute) -*see*
    Lymphadenitis, acute
  gluteal (region) L02.31
  gonorrheal -*see* Gonococcus
  groin L02.214
  gum -*see* Peridontitis, aggressive, localized
  hand L02.51
  head NEC L02.811
    face (any part, except ear, eye and nose)
      L02.01
  heart -*see* Carditis
  heel -*see* Abscess, foot
  helminthic -*see* Infestation, helminth
  hepatic (cholangitic) (hematogenic)
    (lymphogenic) (pylephlebitic) K75.0
    amebic A06.4
  hip (region) -*see* Abscess, lower limb
  ileocecal K35.3
  ileostomy (bud) K94.12
  iliac (region) L02.214
    fossa K35.3
  infraclavicular (fossa) -*see* Abscess, upper
    limb
  inguinal (region) L02.214
    lymph gland or node L04.1
  intestine, intestinal NEC K63.0
    rectal K61.1
  intra-abdominal -*see also* Abscess,
    peritoneum K65.1
    postprocedural T81.43
      retroperitoneal K68.11
  intracranial G06.0
  intramammary -*see* Abscess, breast
  intra-muscular, postprocedural T81.42
  intraorbital -*see* Abscess, orbit
  intraperitoneal K65.1
  intrasphincteric (anus) K61.4
  intraspinal G06.1
  intratonsillar J36
  ischiorectal (fossa) K61.3
  jaw (bone) (lower) (upper) M27.2
  joint -*see* Arthritis, pyogenic or pyemic
    spine (tuberculous) A18.01
      nontuberculous -*see* Spondylopathy,
      infective
  kidney N15.1
    with calculus N20.0
      with hydronephrosis N13.6
    puerperal (postpartum) O86.21
  knee -*see also* Abscess, lower limb
    joint M00.9
  labium (majus) (minus) N76.4
  lacrimal
    caruncle -*see* Inflammation, lacrimal,
      passages, acute
    gland -*see* Dacryoadenitis
    passages (duct) (sac) -*see* Inflammation,
      lacrimal, passages, acute
  lacunar N34.0
  larynx J38.7
  lateral (alveolar) K04.7
    with sinus K04.6
  leg (any part) -*see* Abscess, lower limb
  lens H27.8
  lingual K14.0
    tonsil J36
  lip K13.0
  Littre's gland N34.0

Abscess --*continued*
  liver (cholangitic) (hematogenic)
    (lymphogenic) (pylephlebitic) (pyogenic)
    K75.0
    amebic (due to Entamoeba histolytica)
      (dysenteric) (tropical) A06.4
      with
        brain abscess (and liver or lung abscess)
          A06.6
        lung abscess A06.5
  loin (region) L02.211
  lower limb L02.41
  lumbar (tuberculous) A18.01
    nontuberculous L02.212
  lung (miliary) (putrid) J85.2
    with pneumonia J85.1
      due to specified organism (see Pneumonia,
        in (due to))
    amebic (with liver abscess) A06.5
      with
        brain abscess A06.6
        pneumonia A06.5
  lymph, lymphatic, gland or node (acute) -*see*
    also Lymphadenitis, acute
  mesentery I88.0
  malar M27.2
  mammary gland -*see* Abscess, breast
  marginal, anus K61.0
  mastoid -*see* Mastoiditis, acute
  maxilla, maxillary M27.2
    molar (tooth) K04.7
      with sinus K04.6
    premolar K04.7
    sinus (chronic) J32.0
  mediastinum J85.3
  meibomian gland -*see* Hordeolum
  meninges G06.2
  mesentery, mesenteric K65.1
  mesosalpinx -*see* Salpingitis
  mons pubis L02.215
  mouth (floor) K12.2
  muscle -*see* Myositis, infective
  myocardium I40.0
  nabothian (follicle) -*see* Cervicitis
  nasal J32.9
  nasopharyngeal J39.1
  navel L02.216
    newborn P38.9
      with mild hemorrhage P38.1
      without hemorrhage P38.9
  neck (region) L02.11
    lymph gland or node L04.0
  nephritic -*see* Abscess, kidney   nipple N61.1
    associated with
      lactation -*see* Pregnancy, complicated by
      pregnancy -*see* Pregnancy, complicated by
  nose (external) (fossa) (septum) J34.0
    sinus (chronic) -*see* Sinusitis
  omentum K65.1
  operative wound T81.40
  orbit, orbital -*see* Cellulitis, orbit
  otogenic G06.0
  ovary, ovarian (corpus luteum) -*see*
    Oophoritis
  oviduct -*see* Oophoritis
  palate (soft) K12.2
    hard M27.2
  palmar (space) -*see* Abscess, hand
  pancreas (duct) -*see* Pancreatitis, acute
  parafrenal N48.21

Abscess --continued
  parametric, parametrium N73.2
    acute N73.0
    chronic N73.1
  paranephric N15.1
  parapancreatic -see Pancreatitis, acute
  parapharyngeal J39.0
  pararectal K61.1
  parasinus -see Sinusitis
  parauterine -see also Disease, pelvis,
    inflammatory N73.2
  paravaginal -see Vaginitis
  parietal region (scalp) L02.811
  parodontal -see Peridontitis, aggressive,
    localized
  parotid (duct) (gland) K11.3
    region K12.2
Abscess --continued
  pectoral (region) L02.213
  pelvis, pelvic
    female -see Disease, pelvis, inflammatory
    male, peritoneal K65.1
  penis N48.21
    gonococcal (accessory gland) (periurethral)
    A54.1
  perianal K61.0
  periapical K04.7
    with sinus (alveolar) K04.6
  periappendicular K35.3
  pericardial I30.1
  pericecal K35.3
  pericemental -see Peridontitis, aggressive,
    localized
  pericholecystic -see Cholecystitis, acute
  pericoronal -see Peridontitis, aggressive,
    localized
  peridental -see Peridontitis, aggressive,
    localized
  perimetric -see also Disease, pelvis,
    inflammatory N73.2
  perinephric, perinephritic -see Abscess,
    kidney
  perineum, perineal (superficial) L02.215
    urethra N34.0
  periodontal (parietal) -see Peridontitis,
    aggressive, localized
    apical K04.7
  periosteum, periosteal -see also
    Osteomyelitis, specified type NEC
    with osteomyelitis -see also Osteomyelitis,
    specified type NEC
      acute -see Osteomyelitis, acute
      chronic -see Osteomyelitis, chronic
  peripharyngeal J39.0
  peripleuritic J86.9
    with fistula J86.0
  periprostatic N41.2
  perirectal K61.1
  perirenal (tissue) -see Abscess, kidney
  perisinuous (nose) -see Sinusitis
  peritoneum, peritoneal (perforated) (ruptured)
    K65.1
    with appendicitis K35.3
    pelvic
      female -see Peritonitis, pelvic, female
      male K65.1
    postoperative T81.43
    puerperal, postpartum, childbirth O85
    tuberculous A18.31
  peritonsillar J36
  perityphlic K35.3

Abscess --continued
  periureteral N28.89
  periurethral N34.0
    gonococcal (accessory gland) (periurethral)
    A54.1
  periuterine -see also Disease, pelvis,
    inflammatory N73.2
  perivesical -see Cystitis, specified type NEC
  petrous bone -see Petrositis
  phagedenic NOS L02.91
    chancroid A57
  pharynx, pharyngeal (lateral) J39.1
  pilonidal L05.01
  pituitary (gland) E23.6
  pleura J86.9
    with fistula J86.0
  popliteal -see Abscess, lower limb
  postcecal K35.3
  postlaryngeal J38.7
  postnasal J34.0
  postoperative (any site) T81.40
    retroperitoneal K68.11
  postpharyngeal J39.0
  posttonsillar J36
  post-typhoid A01.09
  pouch of Douglas -see Peritonitis, pelvic,
    female
  premammary -see Abscess, breast
  prepatellar -see Abscess, lower limb
  prostate N41.2
    gonococcal (acute) (chronic) A54.22
  psoas muscle K68.12
  puerperal
  code by site under Puerperal, abscess
  pulmonary -see Abscess, lung
  pulp, pulpal (dental) K04.01
    irreversible K04.02
    reversible K04.01
  rectovaginal septum K63.0
  rectovesical -see Cystitis, specified type NEC
  rectum K61.1
  renal -see Abscess, kidney
  retina -see Inflammation, chorioretinal
  retrobulbar -see Abscess, orbit
  retrocecal K65.1
  retrolaryngeal J38.7
  retromammary -see Abscess, breast
  retroperitoneal NEC K68.19
    postprocedural K68.11
  retropharyngeal J39.0
  retrouterine -see Peritonitis, pelvic, female
  retrovesical -see Cystitis, specified type NEC
  root, tooth K04.7
    with sinus (alveolar) K04.6
  round ligament -see also Disease, pelvis,
    inflammatory N73.2
  rupture (spontaneous) NOS L02.91
  sacrum (tuberculous) A18.01
    nontuberculous M46.28
  salivary (duct) (gland) K11.3
  scalp (any part) L02.811
  scapular -see Osteomyelitis, specified type
    NEC
  sclera -see Scleritis
  scrofulous (tuberculous) A18.2
  scrotum N49.2
  seminal vesicle N49.0
  septal, dental K04.7
    with sinus (alveolar) K04.6
  serous -see Periostitis
  shoulder (region) -see Abscess, upper limb

Abscess --continued
  sigmoid K63.0
  sinus (accessory) (chronic) (nasal) -see also
    Sinusitis
    intracranial venous (any) G06.0
  Skene's duct or gland N34.0
  skin -see Abscess, by site
  specified site NEC L02.818
  spermatic cord N49.1
  sphenoidal (sinus) (chronic) J32.3
  spinal cord (any part) (staphylococcal) G06.1
    tuberculous A17.81
  spine (column) (tuberculous) A18.01
    epidural G06.1
    nontuberculous -see Osteomyelitis, vertebra
  spleen D73.3
    amebic A06.89
  stitch T81.48
  subarachnoid G06.2
    brain G06.0
    spinal cord G06.1
  subareolar -see Abscess, breast
  subcecal K35.3
  subcutaneous -see also Abscess, by site
    pheomycotic (chromomycotic) B43.2
    postprocedural T81.41
  subdiaphragmatic K65.1
  subdural G06.2
    brain G06.0
      sequelae G09
    spinal cord G06.1
  subgaleal L02.811
  subhepatic K65.1
  sublingual K12.2
    gland K11.3
  submammary -see Abscess, breast
  submandibular (region) (space) (triangle)
    K12.2
    gland K11.3
  submaxillary (region) L02.01
    gland K11.3
  submental L02.01
    gland K11.3
  subperiosteal -see Osteomyelitis, specified
    type NEC
  subphrenic K65.1
    postoperative T81.43
  suburethral N34.0
  sudoriparous L75.8
  supraclavicular (fossa) -see Abscess, upper
    limb
  suprapelvic, acute N73.0
  suprarenal (capsule) (gland) E27.8
  sweat gland L74.8
  tear duct -see Inflammation, lacrimal,
    passages, acute
  temple L02.01
  temporal region L02.01
  temporosphenoidal G06.0
  tendon (sheath) M65.00
    ankle M65.07
    foot M65.07
    forearm M65.03
    hand M65.04
    lower leg M65.06
    pelvic region M65.05
    shoulder region M65.01
    specified site NEC M65.08
    thigh M65.05
    upper arm M65.02
  testis N45.4

Abscess --continued
  thigh -see Abscess, lower limb
  thorax J86.9
    with fistula J86.0
  throat J39.1
  thumb -see also Abscess, hand
    nail -see Cellulitis, finger
  thymus (gland) E32.1
  thyroid (gland) E06.0
  toe (any) -see also Abscess, foot
    nail -see Cellulitis, toe
  tongue (staphylococcal) K14.0
  tonsil(s) (lingual) J36
  tonsillopharyngeal J36
  tooth, teeth (root) K04.7
    with sinus (alveolar) K04.6
    supporting structures NEC -see Peridontitis,
      aggressive, localized
  trachea J39.8
  trunk L02.219
    abdominal wall L02.211
    back L02.212
    chest wall L02.213
    groin L02.214
    perineum L02.215
    umbilicus L02.216
  tubal -see Salpingitis
  tuberculous -see Tuberculosis, abscess
  tubo-ovarian -see Salpingo-oophoritis
  tunica vaginalis N49.1
  umbilicus L02.216
  upper
    limb L02.41
    respiratory J39.8
  urethral (gland) N34.0
  urinary N34.0
  uterus, uterine (wall) -see also Endometritis
    ligament -see also Disease, pelvis,
      inflammatory N73.2
    neck -see Cervicitis
  uvula K12.2
  vagina (wall) -see Vaginitis
  vaginorectal -see Vaginitis
  vas deferens N49.1
  vermiform appendix K35.3
  vertebra (column) (tuberculous) A18.01
    nontuberculous -see Osteomyelitis, vertebra
  vesical -see Cystitis, specified type NEC
  vesico-uterine pouch -see Peritonitis, pelvic,
    female
  vitreous (humor) -see Endophthalmitis,
    purulent
  vocal cord J38.3
  von Bezold's -see Mastoiditis, acute
  vulva N76.4
  vulvovaginal gland N75.1
  web space -see Abscess, hand
  wound T81.40
  wrist -see Abscess, upper limb
**Absence (of) (organ or part) (complete or
partial)**
  adrenal (gland) (congenital) Q89.1
    acquired E89.6
  albumin in blood E88.09
  alimentary tract (congenital) Q45.8
    upper Q40.8
  alveolar process (acquired) -see Anomaly,
    alveolar
  ankle (acquired) Z89.44
  anus (congenital) Q42.3
    with fistula Q42.2

**Absence (of) (organ or part) (complete or
partial)** --continued
  aorta (congenital) Q25.41
  appendix, congenital Q42.8
  arm (acquired) Z89.20
    above elbow Z89.22
      congenital (with hand present) -see
        Agenesis, arm, with hand present
        and hand -see Agenesis, forearm, and
          hand
    below elbow Z89.21
      congenital (with hand present) -see
        Agenesis, arm, with hand present
        and hand -see Agenesis, forearm, and
          hand
    congenital -see Defect, reduction, upper
      limb
    shoulder (following explanation of shoulder
      joint prosthesis) (joint) (with or without
      presence of antibiotic-impregnated cement
      spacer) Z89.23
      congenital (with hand present) -see
        Agenesis, arm, with hand present
  artery (congenital) (peripheral) Q27.8
    brain Q28.3
    coronary Q24.5
    pulmonary Q25.79
    specified NEC Q27.8
    umbilical Q27.0
  atrial septum (congenital) Q21.1
  auditory canal (congenital) (external) Q16.1
  auricle (ear), congenital Q16.0
  bile, biliary duct, congenital Q44.5
  bladder (acquired) Z90.6
    congenital Q64.5
  bowel sounds R19.11
  brain Q00.0
    part of Q04.3
  breast(s) (and nipple(s)) (acquired) Z90.1
    congenital Q83.8
  broad ligament Q50.6
  bronchus (congenital) Q32.4
  canaliculus lacrimalis, congenital Q10.4
  cerebellum (vermis) Q04.3
  cervix (acquired) (with uterus) Z90.710
    with remaining uterus Z90.712
    congenital Q51.5
  chin, congenital Q18.8
  cilia (congenital) Q10.3
    acquired -see Madarosis
  clitoris (congenital) Q52.6
  coccyx, congenital Q76.49
  cold sense R20.8
  congenital
    lumen -see Atresia
    organ or site NEC -see Agenesis
    septum -see Imperfect, closure
  corpus callosum Q04.0
  cricoid cartilage, congenital Q31.8
  diaphragm (with hernia), congenital Q79.1
  digestive organ(s) or tract, congenital Q45.8
    acquired NEC Z90.49
    upper Q40.8
  ductus arteriosus Q28.8
  duodenum (acquired) Z90.49
    congenital Q41.0
  ear, congenital Q16.9
    acquired H93.8
    auricle Q16.0
    external Q16.0
    inner Q16.5

**Absence (of) (organ or part) (complete or
partial)** --continued
  lobe, lobule Q17.8
    middle, except ossicles Q16.4
      ossicles Q16.3
    ossicles Q16.3
  ejaculatory duct (congenital) Q55.4
  endocrine gland (congenital) NEC Q89.2
    acquired E89.89
  epididymis (congenital) Q55.4
    acquired Z90.79
  epiglottis, congenital Q31.8
  esophagus (congenital) Q39.8
    acquired (partial) Z90.49
  eustachian tube (congenital) Q16.2
  extremity (acquired) Z89.9
    congenital Q73.0
    knee (following explanation of knee joint
      prosthesis) (joint) (with or without
      presence of antibiotic-impregnated cement
      spacer) Z89.52
    lower (above knee) Z89.619
      below knee Z89.51
    upper -see Absence, arm
  eye (acquired) Z90.01
    congenital Q11.1
    muscle (congenital) Q10.3
  eyeball (acquired) Z90.01
  eyelid (fold) (congenital) Q10.3
    acquired Z90.01
  face, specified part NEC Q18.8
  fallopian tube(s) (acquired) Z90.79
    congenital Q50.6
  family member (causing problem in home)
    NEC -see also Disruption, family Z63.32
  femur, congenital -see Defect, reduction,
    lower limb, longitudinal, femur
  fibrinogen (congenital) D68.2
    acquired D65
  finger(s) (acquired) Z89.02
    congenital -see Agenesis, hand
  foot (acquired) Z89.43
    congenital -see Agenesis, foot
  forearm (acquired) -see Absence, arm, below
    elbow
  gallbladder (acquired) Z90.49
    congenital Q44.0
  gamma globulin in blood D80.1
    hereditary D80.0
  genital organs
    acquired (female) (male) Z90.79
    female, congenital Q52.8
      external Q52.71
      internal NEC Q52.8
    male, congenital Q55.8
  genitourinary organs, congenital NEC
    female Q52.8
    male Q55.8
  globe (acquired) Z90.01
    congenital Q11.1
  glottis, congenital Q31.8
  hand and wrist (acquired) Z89.11
    congenital -see Agenesis, hand
  head, part (acquired) NEC Z90.09
  heat sense R20.8
  hip (following explanation of hip joint
    prosthesis) (joint) (with or without presence
    of antibiotic-impregnated cement spacer)
    Z89.62
  hymen (congenital) Q52.4
  ileum (acquired) Z90.49

Absence (of) (organ or part) (complete or partial) --*continued*
  congenital Q41.2
  immunoglobulin, isolated NEC D80.3
    IgA D80.2
    IgG D80.3
    IgM D80.4
  incus (acquired) -*see* Loss, ossicles, ear
    congenital Q16.3
  inner ear, congenital Q16.5
  intestine (acquired) (small) Z90.49
    congenital Q41.9
      specified NEC Q41.8
    large Z90.49
      congenital Q42.9
        specified NEC Q42.8
  iris, congenital Q13.1
  jejunum (acquired) Z90.49
    congenital Q41.1
  joint
    acquired
      hip (following explantation of hip joint prosthesis) (with or without presence of antibiotic-impregnated cement spacer) Z89.62
      knee (following explantation of knee joint prosthesis) (with or without presence of antibiotic-impregnated cement spacer) Z89.52
      shoulder (following explantation of shoulder joint prosthesis) (with or without presence of antibiotic-impregnated cement spacer) Z89.23
    congenital NEC Q74.8
  kidney(s) (acquired) Z90.5
    congenital Q60.2
      bilateral Q60.1
      unilateral Q60.0
  knee (following explantation of knee joint prosthesis) (joint) (with or without presence of antibiotic-impregnated cement spacer) Z89.52
  labyrinth, membranous Q16.5
  larynx (congenital) Q31.8
    acquired Z90.02
  leg (acquired) (above knee) Z89.61
    below knee (acquired) Z89.51
    congenital -*see* Defect, reduction, lower limb
  lens (acquired) -*see also* Aphakia
    congenital Q12.3
    post cataract extraction Z98.4
  limb (acquired) -*see* Absence, extremity
  lip Q38.6
  liver (congenital) Q44.7
  lung (fissure) (lobe) (bilateral) (unilateral) (congenital) Q33.3
    acquired (any part) Z90.2
  menstruation -*see* Amenorrhea
  muscle (congenital) (pectoral) Q79.8
    ocular Q10.3
  neck, part Q18.8
  neutrophil -*see* Agranulocytosis
  nipple(s) (with breast(s)) (acquired) Z90.1
    congenital Q83.2
  nose (congenital) Q30.1
    acquired Z90.09
  organ
    of Corti, congenital Q16.5
    or site, congenital NEC Q89.8
      acquired NEC Z90.89

Absence (of) (organ or part) (complete or partial) --*continued*
  osseous meatus (ear) Q16.4
  ovary (acquired)
    bilateral Z90.722
    congenital
      bilateral Q50.02
      unilateral Q50.01
    unilateral Z90.721
  oviduct (acquired)
    bilateral Z90.722
    congenital Q50.6
    unilateral Z90.721
  pancreas (congenital) Q45.0
    acquired Z90.410
      complete Z90.410
      partial Z90.411
      total Z90.410
  parathyroid gland (acquired) E89.2
    congenital Q89.2
  patella, congenital Q74.1
  penis (congenital) Q55.5
    acquired Z90.79
  pericardium (congenital) Q24.8
  pituitary gland (congenital) Q89.2
    acquired E89.3
  prostate (acquired) Z90.79
    congenital Q55.4
  pulmonary valve Q22.0
  punctum lacrimale (congenital) Q10.4
  radius, congenital -*see* Defect, reduction, upper limb, longitudinal, radius
  rectum (congenital) Q42.1
    with fistula Q42.0
    acquired Z90.49
  respiratory organ NOS Q34.9
  rib (acquired) Z90.89
    congenital Q76.6
  sacrum, congenital Q76.49
  salivary gland(s), congenital Q38.4
  scrotum, congenital Q55.29
  seminal vesicles (congenital) Q55.4
    acquired Z90.79
  septum
    atrial (congenital) Q21.1
    between aorta and pulmonary artery Q21.4
    ventricular (congenital) Q20.4
  sex chromosome
    female phenotype Q97.8
    male phenotype Q98.8
  skull bone (congenital) Q75.8
    with
      anencephaly Q00.0
      encephalocele -*see* Encephalocele
      hydrocephalus Q03.9
        with spina bifida -*see* Spina bifida, by site, with hydrocephalus
      microcephaly Q02
  spermatic cord, congenital Q55.4
  spine, congenital Q76.49
  spleen (congenital) Q89.01
    acquired Z90.81
  sternum, congenital Q76.7
  stomach (acquired) (partial) Z90.3
    congenital Q40.2
  superior vena cava, congenital Q26.8
  teeth, tooth (congenital) K00.0
    acquired (complete) K08.109
      class I K08.101
      class II K08.102
      class III K08.103

Absence (of) (organ or part) (complete or partial) --*continued*
      class IV K08.104
      due to
        caries K08.139
          class I K08.131
          class II K08.132
          class III K08.133
          class IV K08.134
        periodontal disease K08.129
          class I K08.121
          class II K08.122
          class III K08.123
          class IV K08.124
        specified NEC K08.199
          class I K08.191
          class II K08.192
          class III K08.193
          class IV K08.194
        trauma K08.119
          class I K08.111
          class II K08.112
          class III K08.113
          class IV K08.114
    partial K08.409
      class I K08.401
      class II K08.402
      class III K08.403
      class IV K08.404
      due to
        caries K08.439
          class I K08.431
          class II K08.432
          class III K08.433
          class IV K08.434
        periodontal disease K08.429
          class I K08.421
          class II K08.422
          class III K08.423
          class IV K08.424
        specified NEC K08.499
          class I K08.491
          class II K08.492
          class III K08.493
          class IV K08.494
        trauma K08.419
          class I K08.411
          class II K08.412
          class III K08.413
          class IV K08.414
  tendon (congenital) Q79.8
  testis (congenital) Q55.0
    acquired Z90.79
  thumb (acquired) Z89.01
    congenital -*see* Agenesis, hand
  thymus gland Q89.2
  thyroid (gland) (acquired) E89.0
    cartilage, congenital Q31.8
    congenital E03.1
  toe(s) (acquired) Z89.42
    with foot -*see* Absence, foot and ankle
    congenital -*see* Agenesis, foot
    great Z89.41
  tongue, congenital Q38.3
  trachea (cartilage), congenital Q32.1
  transverse aortic arch, congenital Q25.49
  tricuspid valve Q22.4
  umbilical artery, congenital Q27.0
  upper arm and forearm with hand present, congenital -*see* Agenesis, arm, with hand present

Absence (of) (organ or part) (complete or partial) --*continued*
  ureter (congenital) Q62.4
    acquired Z90.6
  urethra, congenital Q64.5
  uterus (acquired) Z90.710
    with cervix Z90.710
    with remaining cervical stump Z90.711
    congenital Q51.0
  uvula, congenital Q38.5
  vagina, congenital Q52.0
  vas deferens (congenital) Q55.4
    acquired Z90.79
  vein (peripheral) congenital NEC Q27.8
    cerebral Q28.3
    digestive system Q27.8
    great Q26.8
    lower limb Q27.8
    portal Q26.5
    precerebral Q28.1
    specified site NEC Q27.8
    upper limb Q27.8
  vena cava (inferior) (superior), congenital Q26.8
  ventricular septum Q20.4
  vertebra, congenital Q76.49
  vulva, congenital Q52.71
  wrist (acquired) Z89.12
Absorbent system disease I87.8
Absorption
  carbohydrate, disturbance K90.49
  chemical -*see* Table of Drugs and Chemicals
    through placenta (newborn) P04.9
      environmental substance P04.6
      nutritional substance P04.5
      obstetric anesthetic or analgesic drug P04.0
  drug NEC -*see* Table of Drugs and Chemicals
    addictive
      through placenta (newborn) P04.49
        cocaine P04.41
      medicinal
        through placenta (newborn) P04.1
    through placenta (newborn) P04.1
      obstetric anesthetic or analgesic drug P04.0
  fat, disturbance K90.49
    pancreatic K90.3
  noxious substance -*see* Table of Drugs and Chemicals
  protein, disturbance K90.49
  starch, disturbance K90.49
  toxic substance -*see* Table of Drugs and Chemicals
  uremic -*see* Uremia
Abstinence symptoms, syndrome
  alcohol F10.239
    with delirium F10.231
  cocaine F14.23
  neonatal P96.1
  nicotine -*see* Dependence, drug, nicotine, with, withdrawal
  opioid F11.93
    with dependence F11.23
Abstinence symptoms, syndrome --*continued*- psychoactive NEC F19.939
  with
    delirium F19.931
    dependence F19.239
      with
        delirium F19.231
        perceptual disturbance F19.232
      uncomplicated F19.230

Abstinence symptoms, syndrome --*continued*
    perceptual disturbance F19.932
    uncomplicated F19.930
  sedative F13.939
    with
      delirium F13.931
      dependence F13.239
        with
          delirium F13.231
          perceptual disturbance F13.232
        uncomplicated F13.230
      perceptual disturbance F13.932
    uncomplicated F13.930
  stimulant NEC F15.93
    with dependence F15.23
Abulia R68.89
Abulomania F60.7
Abuse
  adult -*see* Maltreatment, adult
    as reason for
      couple seeking advice (including offender) Z63.0
  alcohol (non-dependent) F10.10
    with
      anxiety disorder F10.180
      intoxication F10.129
        with delirium F10.121
        uncomplicated F10.120
      mood disorder F10.14
      other specified disorder F10.188
      psychosis F10.159
        delusions F10.150
        hallucinations F10.151
      sexual dysfunction F10.181
      sleep disorder F10.182
      unspecified disorder F10.19
    counseling and surveillance Z71.41
  amphetamine (or related substance) -*see* Abuse, drug, stimulant NEC
  analgesics (non-prescribed) (over the counter) F55.8
  antacids F55.0
  antidepressants -*see* Abuse, drug, psychoactive NEC
  anxiolytic -*see* Abuse, drug, sedative
  barbiturates -*see* Abuse, drug, sedative
  caffeine -*see* Abuse, drug, stimulant NEC
  cannabis, cannabinoids -*see* Abuse, drug, cannabis
  child -*see* Maltreatment, child
  cocaine -*see* Abuse, drug, cocaine
  drug NEC (non-dependent) F19.10
    with sleep disorder F19.182
    amphetamine type -*see* Abuse, drug, stimulant NEC
    analgesics (non-prescribed) (over the counter) F55.8
    antacids F55.0
    antidepressants -*see* Abuse, drug, psychoactive NEC
    anxiolytics -*see* Abuse, drug, sedative
    barbiturates -*see* Abuse, drug, sedative
    caffeine -*see* Abuse, drug, stimulant NEC
    cannabis F12.10
      with
        anxiety disorder F12.180
        intoxication F12.129
          with
            delirium F12.121
            perceptual disturbance F12.122

Abuse --*continued*
      uncomplicated F12.120
      other specified disorder F12.188
      psychosis F12.159
        delusions F12.150
        hallucinations F12.151
      unspecified disorder F12.19
    cocaine F14.10
      with
        anxiety disorder F14.180
        intoxication F14.129
          with
            delirium F14.121
            perceptual disturbance F14.122
          uncomplicated F14.120
        mood disorder F14.14
        other specified disorder F14.188
        psychosis F14.159
          delusions F14.150
          hallucinations F14.151
        sexual dysfunction F14.181
        sleep disorder F14.182
        unspecified disorder F14.19
      counseling and surveillance Z71.51
    hallucinogen F16.10
      with
        anxiety disorder F16.180
        flashbacks F16.183
        intoxication F16.129
          with
            delirium F16.121
            perceptual disturbance F16.122
          uncomplicated F16.120
        mood disorder F16.14
        other specified disorder F16.188
        perception disorder, persisting F16.183
        psychosis F16.159
          delusions F16.150
          hallucinations F16.151
        unspecified disorder F16.19
    hashish -*see* Abuse, drug, cannabis
    herbal or folk remedies F55.1
    hormones F55.3
    hypnotics -*see* Abuse, drug, sedative
    inhalant F18.10
      with
        anxiety disorder F18.180
        dementia, persisting F18.17
        intoxication F18.129
          with delirium F18.121
          uncomplicated F18.120
        mood disorder F18.14
        other specified disorder F18.188
        psychosis F18.159
          delusions F18.150
          hallucinations F18.151
        unspecified disorder F18.19
    laxatives F55.2
    LSD -*see* Abuse, drug, hallucinogen
    marihuana -*see* Abuse, drug, cannabis
    morphine type (opioids) -*see* Abuse, drug, opioid
    opioid F11.10
      with
        intoxication F11.129
          with
            delirium F11.121
            perceptual disturbance F11.122
          uncomplicated F11.120
        mood disorder F11.14
        other specified disorder F11.188

Abuse --*continued*
- psychosis F11.159
  - delusions F11.150
  - hallucinations F11.151
- sexual dysfunction F11.181
- sleep disorder F11.182
- unspecified disorder F11.19
- PCP (phencyclidine) (or related substance) - *see* Abuse, drug, hallucinogen
- psychoactive NEC F19.10
  - with
    - amnestic disorder F19.16
    - anxiety disorder F19.180
    - dementia F19.17
    - intoxication F19.129
      - with
        - delirium F19.121
        - perceptual disturbance F19.122
      - uncomplicated F19.120
    - mood disorder F19.14
    - other specified disorder F19.188
    - psychosis F19.159
      - delusions F19.150
      - hallucinations F19.151
    - sexual dysfunction F19.181
    - sleep disorder F19.182
    - unspecified disorder F19.19
- sedative, hypnotic or anxiolytic F13.10
  - with
    - anxiety disorder F13.180
    - intoxication F13.129
      - with delirium F13.121
      - uncomplicated F13.120
    - mood disorder F13.14
    - other specified disorder F13.188
    - psychosis F13.159
      - delusions F13.150
      - hallucinations F13.151
    - sexual dysfunction F13.181
    - sleep disorder F13.182
    - unspecified disorder F13.19
- solvent *-see* Abuse, drug, inhalant
- steroids F55.3
- stimulant NEC F15.10
  - with
    - anxiety disorder F15.180
    - intoxication F15.129
      - with
        - delirium F15.121
        - perceptual disturbance F15.122
      - uncomplicated F15.120
    - mood disorder F15.14
    - other specified disorder F15.188
    - psychosis F15.159
      - delusions F15.150
      - hallucinations F15.151
    - sexual dysfunction F15.181
    - sleep disorder F15.182
    - unspecified disorder F15.19
- tranquilizers *-see* Abuse, drug, sedative
- vitamins F55.4
- hallucinogens *-see* Abuse, drug, hallucinogen
- hashish *-see* Abuse, drug, cannabis
- herbal or folk remedies F55.1
- hormones F55.3
- hypnotic *-see* Abuse, drug, sedative
- inhalant *-see* Abuse, drug, inhalant
- laxatives F55.2
- LSD *-see* Abuse, drug, hallucinogen
- marihuana *-see* Abuse, drug, cannabis

Abuse --*continued*
- morphine type (opioids) *-see* Abuse, drug, opioid
- non-psychoactive substance NEC F55.8
  - antacids F55.0
  - folk remedies F55.1
  - herbal remedies F55.1
  - hormones F55.3
  - laxatives F55.2
  - steroids F55.3
  - vitamins F55.4
- opioids *-see* Abuse, drug, opioid
- PCP (phencyclidine) (or related substance) - *see* Abuse, drug, hallucinogen
- physical (adult) (child) *-see* Maltreatment
- psychoactive substance *-see* Abuse, drug, psychoactive NEC
- psychological (adult) (child) *-see* Maltreatment
- sedative *-see* Abuse, drug, sedative
- sexual *-see* Maltreatment
- solvent *-see* Abuse, drug, inhalant
- steroids F55.3
- vitamins F55.4

Acalculia R48.8
- developmental F81.2

Acanthamebiasis (with) B60.10
- conjunctiva B60.12
- keratoconjunctivitis B60.13
- meningoencephalitis B60.11
- other specified B60.19

Acanthocephaliasis B83.8

Acanthocheilonemiasis B74.4

Acanthocytosis E78.6

Acantholysis L11.9

Acanthosis (acquired) (nigricans) L83
- benign Q82.8
- congenital Q82.8
- seborrheic L82.1
  - inflamed L82.0
- tongue K14.3

Acapnia E87.3

Acarbia E87.2

Acardia, acardius Q89.8

Acardiacus amorphus Q89.8

Acardiotrophia I51.4

Acariasis B88.0
- scabies B86

Acarodermatitis (urticarioides) B88.0

Acarophobia F40.218

Acatalasemia, acatalasia E80.3

Acathisia (drug induced) G25.71

Accelerated atrioventricular conduction I45.6

Accentuation of personality traits (type A) Z73.1

Accessory (congenital)
- adrenal gland Q89.1
- anus Q43.4
- appendix Q43.4
- atrioventricular conduction I45.6
- auditory ossicles Q16.3
- auricle (ear) Q17.0
- biliary duct or passage Q44.5
- bladder Q64.79
- blood vessels NEC Q27.9
  - coronary Q24.5
- bone NEC Q79.8
- breast tissue, axilla Q83.1
- carpal bones Q74.0
- cecum Q43.4

- chromosome(s) NEC (nonsex) Q92.9
  - with complex rearrangements NEC Q92.5
    - seen only at prometaphase Q92.8
  - partial Q92.9
  - sex
    - female phenotype Q97.8
    - 13 *-see* Trisomy, 13
    - 18 *-see* Trisomy, 18
    - 21 *-see* Trisomy, 21
- coronary artery Q24.5
- cusp(s), heart valve NEC Q24.8
  - pulmonary Q22.3
- cystic duct Q44.5
- digit(s) Q69.9
- ear (auricle) (lobe) Q17.0
- endocrine gland NEC Q89.2
- eye muscle Q10.3
- eyelid Q10.3
- face bone(s) Q75.8
- fallopian tube (fimbria) (ostium) Q50.6
- finger(s) Q69.0
- foreskin N47.8
- frontonasal process Q75.8
- gallbladder Q44.1
- genital organ(s)
  - female Q52.8
    - external Q52.79
    - internal NEC Q52.8
  - male Q55.8
- genitourinary organs NEC Q89.8
  - female Q52.8
  - male Q55.8
- hallux Q69.2
- heart Q24.8
  - valve NEC Q24.8
    - pulmonary Q22.3
- hepatic ducts Q44.5
- hymen Q52.4
- intestine (large) (small) Q43.4
- kidney Q63.0
- lacrimal canal Q10.6
- leaflet, heart valve NEC Q24.8
- ligament, broad Q50.6
- liver Q44.7
  - duct Q44.5
- lobule (ear) Q17.0
- lung (lobe) Q33.1
- muscle Q79.8
- navicular of carpus Q74.0
- nervous system, part NEC Q07.8
- nipple Q83.3
- nose Q30.8
- organ or site not listed *-see* Anomaly, by site
- ovary Q50.31
- oviduct Q50.6
- pancreas Q45.3
- parathyroid gland Q89.2
- parotid gland (and duct) Q38.4
- pituitary gland Q89.2
- preauricular appendage Q17.0
- prepuce N47.8
- renal arteries (multiple) Q27.2
- rib Q76.6
  - cervical Q76.5
- roots (teeth) K00.2
- salivary gland Q38.4
- sesamoid bones Q74.8
  - foot Q74.2
  - hand Q74.0
- skin tags Q82.8

Accessory (congenital) --*continued*
spleen Q89.09
sternum Q76.7
submaxillary gland Q38.4
tarsal bones Q74.2
teeth, tooth K00.1
tendon Q79.8
thumb Q69.1
thymus gland Q89.2
thyroid gland Q89.2
toes Q69.2
tongue Q38.3
tooth, teeth K00.1
tragus Q17.0
ureter Q62.5
urethra Q64.79
urinary organ or tract NEC Q64.8
uterus Q51.2
vagina Q52.10
valve, heart NEC Q24.8
pulmonary Q22.3
vertebra Q76.49
vocal cords Q31.8
vulva Q52.79
Accident
birth -*see* Birth, injury
cardiac -*see* Infarct, myocardium
cerebral I63.9
cerebrovascular (embolic) (ischemic)
(thrombotic) I63.9
aborted I63.9
hemorrhagic -*see* Hemorrhage, intracranial,
intracerebral
old (without sequelae) Z86.73
with sequelae (of) -*see* Sequelae,
infarction, cerebral
coronary -*see* Infarct, myocardium
craniovascular I63.9
vascular, brain I63.9
Accidental -*see* condition
Accommodation (disorder) -*see also*
condition
hysterical paralysis of F44.89
insufficiency of H52.4
paresis -*see* Paresis, of accommodation
spasm -*see* Spasm, of accommodation
Accouchement -*see* Delivery
Accreta placenta O43.21
Accretio cordis (nonrheumatic) I31.0
Accretions, tooth, teeth K03.6
Acculturation difficulty Z60.3
Accumulation secretion, prostate N42.89
Acephalia, acephalism, acephalus, acephaly
Q00.0
Acephalobrachia monster Q89.8
Acephalochirus monster Q89.8
Acephalogaster Q89.8
Acephalostomus monster Q89.8
Acephalothorax Q89.8
Acerophobia F40.298
Acetonemia R79.89
in Type 1 diabetes E10.10
with coma E10.11
Acetonuria R82.4
Achalasia (cardia) (esophagus) K22.0
congenital Q39.5
pylorus Q40.0
sphincteral NEC K59.8
Ache(s) -*see* Pain
Acheilia Q38.6
Achillobursitis -*see* Tendinitis, Achilles

Achillodynia -*see* Tendinitis, Achilles
Achlorhydria, achlorhydric (neurogenic)
K31.83
anemia D50.8
diarrhea K31.83
psychogenic F45.8
secondary to vagotomy K91.1
Achluophobia F40.228
Acholia K82.8
Acholuric jaundice (familial)
(splenomegalic) -*see also* Spherocytosis
acquired D59.8
Achondrogenesis Q77.0
Achondroplasia (osteosclerosis congenita)
Q77.4
Achroma, cutis L80
Achromat (ism), achromatopsia (acquired)
(congenital) H53.51
Achromia, congenital -*see* Albinism
Achromia parasitica B36.0
Achylia gastrica K31.89
psychogenic F45.8
Acid
burn -*see* Corrosion
deficiency
amide nicotinic E52
ascorbic E54
folic E53.8
nicotinic E52
pantothenic E53.8
intoxication E87.2
peptic disease K30
phosphatase deficiency E83.39
stomach K30
psychogenic F45.8
Acidemia E87.2
argininosuccinic E72.22
isovaleric E71.110
metabolic (newborn) P19.9
first noted before onset of labor P19.0
first noted during labor P19.1
noted at birth P19.2
methylmalonic E71.120
pipecolic E72.3
propionic E71.121
Acidity, gastric (high) K30
psychogenic F45.8
Acidocytopenia -*see* Agranulocytosis
Acidocytosis D72.1
Acidopenia -*see* Agranulocytosis
Acidosis (lactic) (respiratory) E87.2
in Type 1 diabetes E10.10
with coma E10.11
kidney, tubular N25.89
lactic E87.2
metabolic NEC E87.2
with respiratory acidosis E87.4
late, of newborn P74.0
mixed metabolic and respiratory, newborn
P84
newborn P84
renal (hyperchloremic) (tubular) N25.89
respiratory E87.2
complicated by
metabolic
acidosis E87.4
alkalosis E87.4
Aciduria
argininosuccinic E72.22
glutaric (type I) E72.3
type II E71.313

Aciduria- *continued*
type III E71.5
orotic (congenital) (hereditary) (pyrimidine
deficiency) E79.8
anemia D53.0
Acladiosis (skin) B36.0
Aclasis, diaphyseal Q78.6
Acleistocardia Q21.1
Aclusion -*see* Anomaly, dentofacial,
malocclusion
Acne L70.9
artificialis L70.8
atrophica L70.2
cachecticorum (Hebra) L70.8
conglobata L70.1
cystic L70.0
decalvans L66.2
excoriée (des jeunes filles) L70.5
frontalis L70.2
indurata L70.0
infantile L70.4
keloid L73.0
lupoid L70.2
necrotic, necrotica (miliaris) L70.2
neonatal L70.4
nodular L70.0
occupational L70.8
picker's L70.5
pustular L70.0
rodens L70.2
rosacea L71.9
specified NEC L70.8
tropica L70.3
varioliformis L70.2
vulgaris L70.0
Acnitis (primary) A18.4
Acosta's disease T70.29
Acoustic -*see* condition
Acousticophobia F40.298
Acquired -*see also* condition
immunodeficiency syndrome (AIDS) B20
Acrania Q00.0
Acroangiodermatitis I78.9
Acroasphyxia, chronic I73.89
Acrobystitis N47.7
Acrocephalopolysyndactyly Q87.0
Acrocephalosyndactyly Q87.0
Acrocephaly Q75.0
Acrochondrohyperplasia -*see* Syndrome,
Marfan's
Acrocyanosis I73.8
newborn P28.2
meaning transient blue hands and feet
omit code
Acrodermatitis L30.8
atrophicans (chronica) L90.4
continua (Hallopeau) L40.2
enteropathica (hereditary) E83.2
Hallopeau's L40.2
infantile papular L44.4
perstans L40.2
pustulosa continua L40.2
recalcitrant pustular L40.2
Acrodynia -*see* Poisoning, mercury
Acromegaly, acromegalia E22.0
Acromelalgia I73.81
Acromicria, acromicria Q79.8
Acronyx L60.0
Acropachy, thyroid -*see* Thyrotoxicosis
Acroparesthesia (simple) (vasomotor) I73.89
Acropathy, thyroid -*see* Thyrotoxicosis

Acrophobia F40.241
Acroposthitis N47.7
Acroscleriasis, acroscleroderma,
  acrosclerosis -see Sclerosis, systemic
Acrosphacelus I96
Acrospiroma, eccrine -see Neoplasm, skin,
  benign
Acrostealgia -see Osteochondropathy
Acrotrophodynia -see Immersion
ACTH ectopic syndrome E24.3
Actinic -see condition
Actinobacillosis, actinobacillus A28.8
  mallei A24.0
  muris A25.1
Actinomyces israelii (infection) -see
  Actinomycosis
Actinomycetoma (foot) B47.1
Actinomycosis, actinomycotic A42.9
  with pneumonia A42.0
  abdominal A42.1
  cervicofacial A42.2
  cutaneous A42.89
  gastrointestinal A42.1
  pulmonary A42.0
  sepsis A42.7
  specified site NEC A42.89
Actinoneuritis G62.82
Action, heart
  disorder I49.9
  irregular I49.9
    psychogenic F45.8
Activated protein C resistance D68.51
Activation
  mast cell (disorder) (syndrome) D89.40
    idiopathic D89.42
    monoclonal D89.41
    secondary D89.43
    specified type NEC D89.49
Active -see condition
Acute -see also condition
  abdomen R10.0
  gallbladder -see Cholecystitis, acute
Acyanotic heart disease (congenital) Q24.9
Acystia Q64.5
Adair-Dighton syndrome (brittle bones and
  blue sclera, deafness) Q78.0
Adamantinoblastoma -see Ameloblastoma
Adamantinoma -see also Cyst, calcifying
  odontogenic
  long bones C40.90
    lower limb C40.2
    upper limb C40.0
  malignant C41.1
    jaw (bone) (lower) C41.1
      upper C41.0
  tibial C40.2
Adamantoblastoma -see Ameloblastoma
Adams-Stokes (Morgagni) disease or
  syndrome I45.9
Adaption reaction -see Disorder, adjustment
Addiction -see also Dependence F19.20
  alcohol, alcoholic (ethyl) (methyl) (wood)
    (without remission) F10.20
    with remission F10.21
  drug -see Dependence, drug
  ethyl alcohol (without remission) F10.20
    with remission F10.21
  heroin -see Dependence, drug, opioid
  methyl alcohol (without remission) F10.20
    with remission F10.21
  methylated spirit (without remission) F10.20

Addiction - continued
  with remission F10.21
  morphine (like substances) -see Dependence,
    drug, opioid
  nicotine -see Dependence, drug, nicotine
  opium and opioids -see Dependence, drug,
    opioid
  tobacco -see Dependence, drug, nicotine
Addisonian crisis E27.2
Addison's
  anemia (pernicious) D51.0
  disease (bronze) or syndrome E27.1
    tuberculous A18.7
  keloid L94.0
Addison-Biermer anemia (pernicious) D51.0
Addison-Schilder complex E71.528
Additional -see also Accessory
  chromosome(s) Q99.8
  sex -see Abnormal, chromosome, sex
  21
  -see Trisomy, 21
Adduction contracture, hip or other joint -
  see Contraction, joint
Adenitis -see also Lymphadenitis
  acute, unspecified site L04.9
  axillary I88.9
    acute L04.2
    chronic or subacute I88.1
  Bartholin's gland N75.8
  bulbourethral gland -see Urethritis
  cervical I88.9
    acute L04.0
    chronic or subacute I88.1
  chancroid (Hemophilus ducreyi) A57
  chronic, unspecified site I88.1
  Cowper's gland -see Urethritis
  due to Pasteurella multocida (p. septica)
    A28.0
  epidemic, acute B27.09
  gangrenous L04.9
  gonorrheal NEC A54.89
  groin I88.9
    acute L04.1
    chronic or subacute I88.1
  infectious (acute) (epidemic) B27.09
  inguinal I88.9
    acute L04.1
    chronic or subacute I88.1
  lymph gland or node, except mesenteric I88.9
    acute -see Lymphadenitis, acute
    chronic or subacute I88.1
  mesenteric (acute) (chronic) (nonspecific)
    (subacute) I88.0
  parotid gland (suppurative) -see Sialoadenitis
  salivary gland (any) (suppurative) -see
    Sialoadenitis
  scrofulous (tuberculous) A18.2
  Skene's duct or gland -see Urethritis
  strumous, tuberculous A18.2
  subacute, unspecified site I88.1
  sublingual gland (suppurative) -see
    Sialoadenitis
  submandibular gland (suppurative) -see
    Sialoadenitis
  submaxillary gland (suppurative) -see
    Sialoadenitis
  tuberculous -see Tuberculosis, lymph gland
  urethral gland -see Urethritis
  Wharton's duct (suppurative) -see
    Sialoadenitis

Adenoacanthoma -see Neoplasm, malignant,
  by site
Adenoameloblastoma -see Cyst, calcifying
  odontogenic
Adenocarcinoid (tumor) -see Neoplasm,
  malignant, by site
Adenocarcinoma -see also Neoplasm,
  malignant, by site
  acidophil
    specified site -see Neoplasm, malignant, by
      site
    unspecified site C75.1
  adrenal cortical C74.0
  alveolar -see Neoplasm, lung, malignant
  apocrine
    breast -see Neoplasm, breast, malignant
    in situ
      breast D05.8
      specified site NEC -see Neoplasm, skin, in
        situ
      unspecified site D04.9
    specified site NEC -see Neoplasm, skin,
      malignant
    unspecified site C44.99
  basal cell
    specified site -see Neoplasm, skin,
      malignant
    unspecified site C08.9
  basophil
    specified site -see Neoplasm, malignant, by
      site
    unspecified site C75.1
  bile duct type C22.1
    liver C22.1
    specified site NEC -see Neoplasm,
      malignant, by site
    unspecified site C22.1
  bronchiolar -see Neoplasm, lung, malignant
  bronchioloalveolar -see Neoplasm, lung,
    malignant
  ceruminous C44.29
  cervix, in situ -see also Carcinoma, cervix
    uteri, in situ D06.9
  chromophobe
    specified site -see Neoplasm, malignant, by
      site
    unspecified site C75.1
  diffuse type
    specified site -see Neoplasm, malignant, by
      site
    unspecified site C16.9
  duct
    infiltrating
      with Paget's disease -see Neoplasm, breast,
        malignant
      specified site -see Neoplasm, malignant, by
        site
      unspecified site (female) C50.91
        male C50.92
    specified site -see Neoplasm, malignant,
      by site
    unspecified site
      female C56.9
      male C61
  eosinophil
    specified site -see Neoplasm, malignant, by
      site
    unspecified site C75.1
  follicular
    with papillary C73
    moderately differentiated C73

Adenocarcinoma - *continued*
  specified site *-see* Neoplasm, malignant, by
    site
  trabecular C73
  unspecified site C73
  well differentiated C73
  Hürthle cell C73
  in
    adenomatous
      polyposis coli C18.9
  infiltrating duct
    with Paget's disease *-see* Neoplasm, breast,
      malignant
    specified site *-see* Neoplasm, by site,
      malignant
    unspecified site (female) C50.91
      male C50.92
  inflammatory
    specified site *-see* Neoplasm, by site,
      malignant
    unspecified site (female) C50.91
      male C50.92
  intestinal type
    specified site *-see* Neoplasm, by site,
      malignant
    unspecified site C16.9
  intracystic papillary
  intraductal
    breast D05.1
    noninfiltrating
      breast D05.1
      papillary
        with invasion
          specified site *-see* Neoplasm, by site,
            malignant
          unspecified site (female) C50.91
            male C50.92
        breast D05.1
        specified site NEC *-see* Neoplasm, in
          situ, by site
        unspecified site D05.1
    specified site NEC *-see* Neoplasm, in situ,
      by site
    unspecified site D05.1
  papillary
    with invasion
      specified site *-see* Neoplasm, malignant,
        by site
      unspecified site (female) C50.91
        male C50.92
    breast D05.1
    specified site *-see* Neoplasm, in situ, by
      site
    unspecified site D05.1
  specified site NEC *-see* Neoplasm, in situ,
    by site
  unspecified site D05.1
  islet cell
    with exocrine, mixed
      specified site *-see* Neoplasm, malignant, by
        site
      unspecified site C25.9
    pancreas C25.4
    specified site NEC *-see* Neoplasm,
      malignant, by site
    unspecified site C25.4
  lobular
    in situ
      breast D05.0
      specified site NEC *-see* Neoplasm, in situ,
        by site

Adenocarcinoma - *continued*
  unspecified site D05.0
  specified site *-see* Neoplasm, malignant, by
    site
  unspecified site (female) C50.91
    male C50.92
  mucoid *-see also* Neoplasm, malignant, by
    site
  cell
    specified site *-see* Neoplasm, malignant, by
      site
    unspecified site C75.1
  nonencapsulated sclerosing C73
  papillary
    with follicular C73
    follicular variant C73
    intraductal (noninfiltrating)
      with invasion
        specified site *-see* Neoplasm, malignant,
          by site
        unspecified site (female) C50.91
          male C50.92
      breast D05.1
      specified site NEC *-see* Neoplasm, in situ,
        by site
      unspecified site D05.1
    serous
      specified site *-see* Neoplasm, malignant, by
        site
      unspecified site C56.9
  papillocystic
    specified site *-see* Neoplasm, malignant, by
      site
    unspecified site C56.9
  pseudomucinous
    specified site *-see* Neoplasm, malignant, by
      site
    unspecified site C56.9
  renal cell C64
  sebaceous *-see* Neoplasm, skin, malignant
  serous *-see also* Neoplasm, malignant, by site
    papillary
      specified site *-see* Neoplasm, malignant, by
        site
      unspecified site C56.9
  sweat gland *-see* Neoplasm, skin, malignant
  water-clear cell C75.0
Adenocarcinoma-in-situ *-see also* Neoplasm,
  in situ, by site
  breast D05.9
Adenofibroma
  clear cell *-see* Neoplasm, benign, by site
  endometrioid D27.9
    borderline malignancy D39.10
    malignant C56
  mucinous
    specified site *-see* Neoplasm, benign, by site
    unspecified site D27.9
  papillary
    specified site *-see* Neoplasm, benign, by site
    unspecified site D27.9
  prostate *-see* Enlargement, enlarged, prostate
  serous
    specified site *-see* Neoplasm, benign, by site
    unspecified site D27.9
  specified site *-see* Neoplasm, benign, by site
  unspecified site D27.9
Adenofibrosis
  breast *-see* Fibroadenosis, breast
  endometrioid N80.0

Adenoiditis (chronic) J35.02
  with tonsillitis J35.03
  acute J03.90
    recurrent J03.91
    specified organism NEC J03.80
      recurrent J03.81
    staphylococcal J03.80
      recurrent J03.81
    streptococcal J03.00
      recurrent J03.01
Adenoids *-see* condition
Adenolipoma *-see* Neoplasm, benign, by site
Adenolipomatosis, Launois-Bensaude E88.89
Adenolymphoma
  specified site *-see* Neoplasm, benign, by site
  unspecified site D11.9
Adenoma *-see also* Neoplasm, benign, by site
  acidophil
    specified site *-see* Neoplasm, benign, by site
    unspecified site D35.2
  acidophil-basophil, mixed
    specified site *-see* Neoplasm, benign, by site
    unspecified site D35.2
  adrenal (cortical) D35.00
    clear cell D35.00
    compact cell D35.00
    glomerulosa cell D35.00
    heavily pigmented variant D35.00
    mixed cell D35.00
  alpha-cell
    pancreas D13.7
    specified site NEC *-see* Neoplasm, benign,
      by site
    unspecified site D13.7
  alveolar D14.30
  apocrine
    breast D24
    specified site NEC *-see* Neoplasm, skin,
      benign, by site
    unspecified site D23.9
  basal cell D11.9
  basophil
    specified site *-see* Neoplasm, benign, by site
    unspecified site D35.2
  basophil-acidophil, mixed
    specified site *-see* Neoplasm, benign, by site
    unspecified site D35.2
  beta-cell
    pancreas D13.7
    specified site NEC *-see* Neoplasm, benign,
      by site
    unspecified site D13.7
  bile duct D13.4
    common D13.5
    extrahepatic D13.5
    intrahepatic D13.4
    specified site NEC *-see* Neoplasm, benign,
      by site
    unspecified site D13.4
  black D35.00
  bronchial D38.1
    cylindroid type *-see* Neoplasm, lung,
  malignant
  ceruminous D23.2
  chief cell D35.1
  chromophobe
    specified site *-see* Neoplasm, benign, by site
    unspecified site D35.2
  colloid
    specified site *-see* Neoplasm, benign, by site
    unspecified site D34

Adenoma - *continued*
 duct
  eccrine, papillary -*see* Neoplasm, skin, benign
  endocrine, multiple
   single specified site -*see* Neoplasm,
    uncertain behavior, by site
   two or more specified sites D44
   unspecified site D44.9
  endometrioid -*see also* Neoplasm, benign
   borderline malignancy -*see* Neoplasm,
    uncertain behavior, by site
  eosinophil
   specified site -*see* Neoplasm, benign, by site
   unspecified site D35.2
  fetal
   specified site -*see* Neoplasm, benign, by site
   unspecified site D34
  follicular
   specified site -*see* Neoplasm, benign, by site
   unspecified site D34
  hepatocellular D13.4
  Hürthle cell D34
  islet cell
   pancreas D13.7
   specified site NEC -*see* Neoplasm, benign,
    by site
   unspecified site D13.7
  liver cell D13.4
  macrofollicular
   specified site -*see* Neoplasm, benign, by site
   unspecified site D34
  malignant, malignum -*see* Neoplasm,
   malignant, by site
  microcystic
   pancreas D13.6
   specified site NEC -*see* Neoplasm, benign,
    by site
   unspecified site D13.6
  microfollicular
   specified site -*see* Neoplasm, benign, by site
   unspecified site D34
  mucoid cell
   specified site -*see* Neoplasm, benign, by site
   unspecified site D35.2
  multiple endocrine
   single specified site -*see* Neoplasm,
    uncertain behavior, by site
   two or more specified sites D44
   unspecified site D44.9
  nipple D24
  papillary -*see also* Neoplasm, benign, by site
   eccrine -*see* Neoplasm, skin, benign, by site
  Pick's tubular
   specified site -*see* Neoplasm, benign, by site
   unspecified site
    female D27.9
    male D29.20
  pleomorphic
   carcinoma in -*see* Neoplasm, salivary gland,
    malignant
    specified site -*see* Neoplasm, malignant, by
     site
    unspecified site C08.9
  polypoid -*see also* Neoplasm, benign
   adenocarcinoma in -*see* Neoplasm,
    malignant, by site
   adenocarcinoma in situ -*see* Neoplasm, in
    situ, by site
  prostate -*see* Neoplasm, benign, prostate
  rete cell D29.20
  sebaceous -*see* Neoplasm, skin, benign

Adenoma - *continued*
 Sertoli cell
  specified site -*see* Neoplasm, benign, by site
  unspecified site
   female D27.9
   male D29.20
 skin appendage -*see* Neoplasm, skin, benign
 sudoriferous gland -*see* Neoplasm, skin,
  benign
 sweat gland -*see* Neoplasm, skin, benign
 testicular
  specified site -*see* Neoplasm, benign, by site
  unspecified site
   female D27.9
   male D29.20
 tubular -*see also* Neoplasm, benign, by site
  adenocarcinoma in -*see* Neoplasm,
   malignant, by site
  adenocarcinoma in situ -*see* Neoplasm, in
   situ, by site
  Pick's
   specified site -*see* Neoplasm, benign, by
    site
   unspecified site
    female D27.9
    male D29.20
 tubulovillous -*see also* Neoplasm, benign, by
  site
  adenocarcinoma in -*see* Neoplasm,
   malignant, by site
  adenocarcinoma in situ -*see* Neoplasm, in
   situ, by site
 villous -*see* Neoplasm, uncertain behavior, by
  site
  adenocarcinoma in -*see* Neoplasm,
   malignant, by site
  adenocarcinoma in situ -*see* Neoplasm, in
   situ, by site
 water-clear cell D35.1
Adenomatosis
 endocrine (multiple) E31.20
  single specified site -*see* Neoplasm,
   uncertain behavior, by site
 erosive of nipple D24
 pluriendocrine -*see* Adenomatosis, endocrine
 pulmonary D38.1
  malignant -*see* Neoplasm, lung, malignant
 specified site -*see* Neoplasm, benign, by site
 unspecified site D12.6
Adenomatous
 goiter (nontoxic) E04.9
  with hyperthyroidism -*see* Hyperthyroidism,
   with, goiter, nodular
  toxic -*see* Hyperthyroidism, with, goiter,
   nodular
Adenomyoma -*see also* Neoplasm, benign, by
 site
 prostate -*see* Enlarged, prostate
Adenomyometritis N80.0
Adenomyosis N80.0
Adenopathy (lymph gland) R59.9
 generalized R59.1
 inguinal R59.0
 localized R59.0
 mediastinal R59.0
 mesentery R59.0
 syphilitic (secondary) A51.49
 tracheobronchial R59.0
  tuberculous A15.4
   primary (progressive) A15.7

Adenopathy (lymph gland) --*continued*
 tuberculous -*see also* Tuberculosis, lymph
  gland
   tracheobronchial A15.4
    primary (progressive) A15.7
Adenosalpingitis -*see* Salpingitis
Adenosarcoma -*see* Neoplasm, malignant, by
 site
Adenosclerosis I88.8
Adenosis (sclerosing) breast -*see*
 Fibroadenosis, breast
**Adenovirus, as cause of disease classified
 elsewhere** B97.0
Adentia (complete) (partial) -*see* Absence,
 teeth
Adherent -*see also* Adhesions
 labia (minora) N90.89
 pericardium (nonrheumatic) I31.0
  rheumatic I09.2
 placenta (with hemorrhage) O72.0
  without hemorrhage O73.0
 prepuce, newborn N47.0
 scar (skin) L90.5
 tendon in scar L90.5
Adhesions, adhesive (postinfective) K66.0
 with intestinal obstruction K56.5
 abdominal (wall) -*see* Adhesions, peritoneum
 appendix K38.8
 bile duct (common) (hepatic) K83.8
 bladder (sphincter) N32.89
 bowel -*see* Adhesions, peritoneum
 cardiac I31.0
  rheumatic I09.2
 cecum -*see* Adhesions, peritoneum
 cervicovaginal N88.1
  congenital Q52.8
  postpartal O90.89
   old N88.1
 cervix N88.1
 ciliary body NEC -*see* Adhesions, iris
 clitoris N90.89
 colon -*see* Adhesions, peritoneum
 common duct K83.8
 congenital -*see also* Anomaly, by site
  fingers -*see* Syndactylism, complex, fingers
  omental, anomalous Q43.3
  peritoneal Q43.3
  tongue (to gum or roof of mouth) Q38.3
 conjunctiva (acquired) H11.21
  congenital Q15.8
 cystic duct K82.8
 diaphragm -*see* Adhesions, peritoneum
 due to foreign body -*see* Foreign body
 duodenum -*see* Adhesions, peritoneum
 ear
  middle H74.1
 epididymis N50.89
 epidural -*see* Adhesions, meninges
 epiglottis J38.7
 eyelid H02.59
 female pelvis N73.6
 gallbladder K82.8
 globe H44.89
 heart I31.0
  rheumatic I09.2
 ileocecal (coil) -*see* Adhesions, peritoneum
 ileum -*see* Adhesions, peritoneum
 intestine -*see also* Adhesions, peritoneum
  with obstruction K56.5
 intra-abdominal -*see* Adhesions, peritoneum
 iris H21.50

Adhesions, adhesive (postinfective) --
continued
    anterior H21.51
    goniosynechiae H21.52
    posterior H21.54
    to corneal graft T85.898
  joint -see Ankylosis
    knee M23.8X
    temporomandibular M26.61
  labium (majus) (minus), congenital Q52.5
  liver -see Adhesions, peritoneum
  lung J98.4
  mediastinum J98.59
  meninges (cerebral) (spinal) G96.12
    congenital Q07.8
    tuberculous (cerebral) (spinal) A17.0
  mesenteric -see Adhesions, peritoneum
  nasal (septum) (to turbinates) J34.89
  ocular muscle -see Strabismus, mechanical
  omentum -see Adhesions, peritoneum
  ovary N73.6
    congenital (to cecum, kidney or omentum)
      Q50.39
  paraovarian N73.6
  pelvic (peritoneal)
    female N73.6
      postprocedural N99.4
    male -see Adhesions, peritoneum
    postpartal (old) N73.6
    tuberculous A18.17
  penis to scrotum (congenital) Q55.8
  periappendiceal -see also Adhesions,
    peritoneum
  pericardium (nonrheumatic) I31.0
    focal I31.8
    rheumatic I09.2
    tuberculous A18.84
  pericholecystic K82.8
  perigastric -see Adhesions, peritoneum
  periovarian N73.6
  periprostatic N42.89
  perirectal -see Adhesions, peritoneum
  perirenal N28.89
  peritoneum, peritoneal (postinfective)
    (postprocedural) K66.0
    with obstruction (intestinal) K56.5
    congenital Q43.3
    pelvic, female N73.6
      postprocedural N99.4
    postpartal, pelvic N73.6
    to uterus N73.6
  peritubal N73.6
  periureteral N28.89
  periuterine N73.6
  perivesical N32.89
  perivesicular (seminal vesicle) N50.89
  pleura, pleuritic J94.8
    tuberculous NEC A15.6
  pleuropericardial J94.8
  postoperative (gastrointestinal tract) K66.0
    with obstruction K91.3
    due to foreign body accidentally left in
      wound -see Foreign body, accidentally left
      during a procedure
    pelvic peritoneal N99.4
    urethra -see Stricture, urethra,
      postprocedural
    vagina N99.2
  postpartal, old (vulva or perineum) N90.89
  preputial, prepuce N47.5
  pulmonary J98.4

Adhesions, adhesive (postinfective) --
continued
  pylorus -see Adhesions, peritoneum
  sciatic nerve -see Lesion, nerve, sciatic
  seminal vesicle N50.89
  shoulder (joint) -see Capsulitis, adhesive
  sigmoid flexure -see Adhesions, peritoneum
  spermatic cord (acquired) N50.89
    congenital Q55.4
  spinal canal G96.12
  stomach -see Adhesions, peritoneum
  subscapular -see Capsulitis, adhesive
  temporomandibular M26.61
  tendinitis -see also Tenosynovitis, specified
    type NEC
    shoulder -see Capsulitis, adhesive
  testis N44.8
  tongue, congenital (to gum or roof of mouth)
    Q38.3
    acquired K14.8
  trachea J39.8
  tubo-ovarian N73.6
  tunica vaginalis N44.8
  uterus N73.6
    internal N85.6
    to abdominal wall N73.6
  vagina (chronic) N89.5
    postoperative N99.2
  vitreomacular H43.82
  vitreous H43.89
  vulva N90.89
Adiaspiromycosis B48.8
Adie (Holmes) pupil or syndrome -see
  Anomaly, pupil, function, tonic pupil
Adiponecrosis neonatorum P83.8
Adiposis -see also Obesity   cerebralis E23.6
  dolorosa E88.2
Adiposity -see also Obesity
  heart -see Degeneration, myocardial
  localized E65
Adiposogenital dystrophy E23.6
Adjustment
  disorder -see Disorder, adjustment
  implanted device -see Encounter (for),
    adjustment (of)
  prosthesis, external -see Fitting
  reaction -see Disorder, adjustment
**Administration of tPA (rtPA) in a different
facility within the last 24 hours prior to
admission to current facility** Z92.82
Admission (for) -see also Encounter (for)
  adjustment (of)
    artificial
      arm Z44.00
        complete Z44.01
        partial Z44.02
      eye Z44.2
      leg Z44.10
        complete Z44.11
        partial Z44.12
    brain neuropacemaker Z46.2
      implanted Z45.42
    breast
      implant Z45.81
      prosthesis (external) Z44.3
    colostomy belt Z46.89
    contact lenses Z46.0
    cystostomy device Z46.6
    dental prosthesis Z46.3
    device NEC
      abdominal Z46.89

Admission (for) --continued
    implanted Z45.89
    cardiac Z45.09
      defibrillator (with synchronous cardiac
        pacemaker) Z45.02
      pacemaker (cardiac resynchronization
        therapy (CRT-P)) Z45.018
        pulse generator Z45.010
      resynchronization therapy defibrillator
        (CRT-D) Z45.02
    hearing device Z45.328
      bone conduction Z45.320
      cochlear Z45.321
    infusion pump Z45.1
    nervous system Z45.49
      CSF drainage Z45.41
      hearing device -see Admission,
        adjustment, device, implanted, hearing
        device
      neuropacemaker Z45.42
      visual substitution Z45.31
    specified NEC Z45.89
    vascular access Z45.2
    visual substitution Z45.31
  nervous system Z46.2
    implanted -see Admission, adjustment,
      device, implanted, nervous system
  orthodontic Z46.4
  prosthetic Z44.9
    arm -see Admission, adjustment,
      artificial, arm
    breast Z44.3
    dental Z46.3
    eye Z44.2
    leg -see Admission, adjustment, artificial,
      leg
    specified type NEC Z44.8
  substitution
    auditory Z46.2
      implanted -see Admission, adjustment,
        device, implanted, hearing device
    nervous system Z46.2
      implanted -see Admission, adjustment,
        device, implanted, nervous system
    visual Z46.2
      implanted Z45.31
  urinary Z46.6
  hearing aid Z46.1
    implanted -see Admission, adjustment,
      device, implanted, hearing device
  ileostomy device Z46.89
  intestinal appliance or device NEC Z46.89
  neuropacemaker (brain) (peripheral nerve)
    (spinal cord) Z46.2
    implanted Z45.42
  orthodontic device Z46.4
  orthopedic (brace) (cast) (device) (shoes)
    Z46.89
  pacemaker (cardiac resynchronization
  therapy (CRT-P))
    cardiac Z45.018
      pulse generator Z45.010
    nervous system Z46.2
      implanted Z45.42
  portacath (port-a-cath) Z45.2
  prosthesis Z44.9
    arm -see Admission, adjustment, artificial,
      arm
    breast Z44.3
    dental Z46.3
    eye Z44.2

Admission (for) --*continued*
    leg -*see* Admission, adjustment, artificial, leg
        specified NEC Z44.8
        spectacles Z46.0
    aftercare -*see also* Aftercare Z51.89
      postpartum
        immediately after delivery Z39.0
        routine follow-up Z39.2
      radiation therapy (antineoplastic) Z51.0
    attention to artificial opening (of) Z43.9
      artificial vagina Z43.7
      colostomy Z43.3
      cystostomy Z43.5
      enterostomy Z43.4
      gastrostomy Z43.1
      ileostomy Z43.2
      jejunostomy Z43.4
      nephrostomy Z43.6
      specified site NEC Z43.8
        intestinal tract Z43.4
        urinary tract Z43.6
      tracheostomy Z43.0
      ureterostomy Z43.6
      urethrostomy Z43.6
    breast augmentation or reduction Z41.1
    breast reconstruction following mastectomy Z42.1
    change of
      dressing (nonsurgical) Z48.00
      neuropacemaker device (brain) (peripheral nerve) (spinal cord) Z46.2
        implanted Z45.42
      surgical dressing Z48.01
    circumcision, ritual or routine (in absence of diagnosis) Z41.2
    clinical research investigation (control) (normal comparison) (participant) Z00.6
    contraceptive management Z30.9
    cosmetic surgery NEC Z41.1
    counseling -*see also* Counseling
      dietary Z71.3
      gestational carrier Z31.7
      HIV Z71.7
      human immunodeficiency virus Z71.7
      nonattending third party Z71.0
      procreative management NEC Z31.69
    delivery, full-term, uncomplicated O80
      cesarean, without indication O82
    desensitization to allergens Z51.6
    dietary surveillance and counseling Z71.3
    ear piercing Z41.3
    examination at health care facility (adult) -*see also* Examination Z00.00
      with abnormal findings Z00.01
      clinical research investigation (control) (normal comparison) (participant) Z00.6
      dental Z01.20
        with abnormal findings Z01.21
      donor (potential) Z00.5
      ear Z01.10
        with abnormal findings NEC Z01.118
      eye Z01.00
        with abnormal findings Z01.01
      general, specified reason NEC Z00.8
      hearing Z01.10
        with abnormal findings NEC Z01.118
      postpartum checkup Z39.2
      psychiatric (general) Z00.8
        requested by authority Z04.6
      vision Z01.00

Admission (for) --*continued*
      with abnormal findings Z01.01
    fitting (of)
      artificial
        arm -*see* Admission, adjustment, artificial, arm
        eye Z44.2
        leg -*see* Admission, adjustment, artificial, leg
      brain neuropacemaker Z46.2
        implanted Z45.42
      breast prosthesis (external) Z44.3
      colostomy belt Z46.89
      contact lenses Z46.0
      cystostomy device Z46.6
      dental prosthesis Z46.3
      dentures Z46.3
      device NEC
        abdominal Z46.89
        nervous system Z46.2
          implanted -*see* Admission, adjustment, device, implanted, nervous system
        orthodontic Z46.4
        prosthetic Z44.9
          breast Z44.3
          dental Z46.3
          eye Z44.2
        substitution
          auditory Z46.2
            implanted -*see* Admission, adjustment, device, implanted, hearing device
          nervous system Z46.2
            implanted -*see* Admission, adjustment, device, implanted, nervous system
          visual Z46.2
            implanted Z45.31
      hearing aid Z46.1
      ileostomy device Z46.89
      intestinal appliance or device NEC Z46.89
      neuropacemaker (brain) (peripheral nerve) (spinal cord) Z46.2
        implanted Z45.42
      orthodontic device Z46.4
      orthopedic device (brace) (cast) (shoes) Z46.89
      prosthesis Z44.9
        arm -*see* Admission, adjustment, artificial, arm
        breast Z44.3
        dental Z46.3
        eye Z44.2
        leg -*see* Admission, adjustment, artificial, leg
        specified type NEC Z44.8
        spectacles Z46.0
    follow-up examination Z09
    intrauterine device management Z30.431
      initial prescription Z30.014
    mental health evaluation Z00.8
      requested by authority Z04.6
    observation -*see* Observation
    Papanicolaou smear, cervix Z12.4
      for suspected malignant neoplasm Z12.4
    plastic and reconstructive surgery following medical procedure or healed injury NEC Z42.8
    plastic surgery, cosmetic NEC Z41.1
    postpartum observation
      immediately after delivery Z39.0
      routine follow-up Z39.2
    poststerilization (for restoration) Z31.0

Admission (for) --*continued*
    aftercare Z31.42
    procreative management Z31.9
    prophylactic (measure) -*see also* Encounter, prophylactic measures
      organ removal Z40.00
        breast Z40.01
        ovary Z40.02
        specified organ NEC Z40.09
        testes Z40.09
      vaccination Z23
    psychiatric examination (general) Z00.8
      requested by authority Z04.6
    radiation therapy (antineoplastic) Z51.0
    reconstructive surgery following medical procedure or healed injury NEC Z42.8
    removal of
      cystostomy catheter Z43.5
      drains Z48.03
      dressing (nonsurgical) Z48.00
      implantable subdermal contraceptive Z30.46
      intrauterine contraceptive device Z30.432
      neuropacemaker (brain) (peripheral nerve) (spinal cord) Z46.2
        implanted Z45.42
      staples Z48.02
      surgical dressing Z48.01
      sutures Z48.02
      ureteral stent Z46.6
    respirator [ventilator] use during power failure Z99.12
    restoration of organ continuity (poststerilization) Z31.0
      aftercare Z31.42
    sensitivity test -*see also* Test, skin
      allergy NEC Z01.82
      Mantoux Z11.1
    tuboplasty following previous sterilization Z31.0
      aftercare Z31.42
    vasoplasty following previous sterilization Z31.0
      aftercare Z31.42
    vision examination Z01.00
      with abnormal findings Z01.01
    waiting period for admission to other facility Z75.1

Adnexitis (suppurative) -*see* Salpingo-oophoritis
Adolescent X linked adrenoleukodystrophy E71.521
Adrenal (gland) -*see* condition
Adrenalism, tuberculous A18.7
Adrenalitis, adrenitis E27.8
    autoimmune E27.1
    meningococcal, hemorrhagic A39.1
Adrenarche, premature E27.0
Adrenocortical syndrome -*see* Cushing's, syndrome
Adrenogenital syndrome E25.9
    acquired E25.8
    congenital E25.0
    salt loss E25.0
Adrenogenitalism, congenital E25.0
Adrenoleukodystrophy E71.529
    neonatal E71.511
    X linked E71.529
      Addison only phenotype E71.528
      Addison-Schilder E71.528
      adolescent E71.521
      adrenomyeloneuropathy E71.522

Adrenoleukodystrophy *--continued*
  childhood cerebral E71.520
  other specified E71.528
Adrenomyeloneuropathy E71.522
Adventitious bursa *-see* Bursopathy, specified
  type NEC
Adverse effect *-see* Table of Drugs and
  Chemicals, categories T36 T50, with 6th
  character 5
Advice *-see* Counseling
Adynamia (episodica) (hereditary) (periodic)
  G72.3
Aeration lung imperfect, newborn *-see*
  Atelectasis
Aerobullosis T70.3
Aerocele *-see* Embolism, air
Aerodermectasia
  subcutaneous (traumatic) T79.7
Aerodontalgia T70.29
Aeroembolism T70.3
Aerogenes capsulatus infection A48.0
Aero-otitis media T70.0
Aerophagy, aerophagia (psychogenic) F45.8
Aerophobia F40.228
Aerosinusitis T70.1
Aerotitis T70.0
Affection *-see* Disease
Afibrinogenemia *-see also* Defect, coagulation
  D68.8
  acquired D65
  congenital D68.2
  following ectopic or molar pregnancy O08.1
  in abortion *-see* Abortion, by type,
    complicated by, afibrinogenemia
  puerperal O72.3
African
  sleeping sickness B56.9
  tick fever A68.1
  trypanosomiasis B56.9
    Gambian B56.0
    Rhodesian B56.1
Aftercare *-see also* Care Z51.89
  following surgery (for) (on)
    amputation Z47.81
    attention to
      drains Z48.03
      dressings (nonsurgical) Z48.00
        surgical Z48.01
      sutures Z48.02
    circulatory system Z48.812
    delayed (planned) wound closure Z48.1
    digestive system Z48.815
    explantation of joint prosthesis (staged
      procedure)
      hip Z47.32
      knee Z47.33
      shoulder Z47.31
    genitourinary system Z48.816
    joint replacement Z47.1
    neoplasm Z48.3
    nervous system Z48.811
    oral cavity Z48.814
    organ transplant
      bone marrow Z48.290
      heart Z48.21
      heart-lung Z48.280
      kidney Z48.22
      liver Z48.23
      lung Z48.24
      multiple organs NEC Z48.288
      specified NEC Z48.298

Aftercare *--continued*
  orthopedic NEC Z47.89
  planned wound closure Z48.1
  removal of internal fixation device Z47.2
  respiratory system Z48.813
  scoliosis Z47.82
  sense organs Z48.810
  skin and subcutaneous tissue Z48.817
  specified body system
    circulatory Z48.812
    digestive Z48.815
    genitourinary Z48.816
    nervous Z48.811
    oral cavity Z48.814
    respiratory Z48.813
    sense organs Z48.810
    skin and subcutaneous tissue Z48.817
    teeth Z48.814
  specified NEC Z48.89
  spinal Z48.89
  teeth Z48.814
  fracture
  code to fracture with seventh character D
  involving
    removal of
      drains Z48.03
      dressings (nonsurgical) Z48.00
      staples Z48.02
      surgical dressings Z48.01
      sutures Z48.02
  neuropacemaker (brain) (peripheral nerve)
  (spinal cord) Z46.2
    implanted Z45.42
  orthopedic NEC Z47.89
  postprocedural *-see* Aftercare, following
  surgery
After-cataract *-see* Cataract, secondary
Agalactia (primary) O92.3
  elective, secondary or therapeutic O92.5
Agammaglobulinemia (acquired
(secondary)) (nonfamilial) D80.1
  with
    immunoglobulin-bearing B-lymphocytes
      D80.1
    lymphopenia D81.9
  autosomal recessive (Swiss type) D80.0
  Bruton's X linked D80.0
  common variable (CVA gamma) D80.1
  congenital sex linked D80.0
  hereditary D80.0
  lymphopenic D81.9
  Swiss type (autosomal recessive) D80.0
  X linked (with growth hormone deficiency)
    (Bruton) D80.0
Aganglionosis (bowel) (colon) Q43.1
Age (old) *-see* Senility
Agenesis
  adrenal (gland) Q89.1
  alimentary tract (complete) (partial) NEC
    Q45.8
    upper Q40.8
  anus, anal (canal) Q42.3
    with fistula Q42.2
  aorta Q25.41
  appendix Q42.8
  arm (complete) Q71.0
    with hand present Q71.1
  artery (peripheral) Q27.9
    brain Q28.3
    coronary Q24.5
    pulmonary Q25.79

Agenesis - *continued*
    specified NEC Q27.8
    umbilical Q27.0
  auditory (canal) (external) Q16.1
  auricle (ear) Q16.0
  bile duct or passage Q44.5
  bladder Q64.5
  bone Q79.9
  brain Q00.0
    part of Q04.3
  breast (with nipple present) Q83.8
    with absent nipple Q83.0
  bronchus Q32.4
  canaliculus lacrimalis Q10.4
  carpus *-see* Agenesis, hand
  cartilage Q79.9
  cecum Q42.8
  cerebellum Q04.3
  cervix Q51.5
  chin Q18.8
  cilia Q10.3
  circulatory system, part NOS Q28.9
  clavicle Q74.0
  clitoris Q52.6
  coccyx Q76.49
  colon Q42.9
    specified NEC Q42.8
  corpus callosum Q04.0
  cricoid cartilage Q31.8
  diaphragm (with hernia) Q79.1
  digestive organ(s) or tract (complete) (partial)
    NEC Q45.8
    upper Q40.8
  ductus arteriosus Q28.8
  duodenum Q41.0
  ear Q16.9
    auricle Q16.0
    lobe Q17.8
  ejaculatory duct Q55.4
  endocrine (gland) NEC Q89.2
  epiglottis Q31.8
  esophagus Q39.8
  eustachian tube Q16.2
  eye Q11.1
    adnexa Q15.8
  eyelid (fold) Q10.3
  face
    bones NEC Q75.8
    specified part NEC Q18.8
  fallopian tube Q50.6
  femur *-see* Defect, reduction, lower limb,
    longitudinal, femur
  fibula *-see* Defect, reduction, lower limb,
    longitudinal, fibula
  finger (complete) (partial) *-see* Agenesis,
    hand
  foot (and toes) (complete) (partial) Q72.3
  forearm (with hand present) *-see* Agenesis,
  arm, with hand present
    and hand Q71.2
  gallbladder Q44.0
  gastric Q40.2
  genitalia, genital (organ(s))
    female Q52.8
      external Q52.71
      internal NEC Q52.8
    male Q55.8
  glottis Q31.8
  hair Q84.0
  hand (and fingers) (complete) (partial) Q71.3
  heart Q24.8

Agenesis - *continued*
  valve NEC Q24.8
    pulmonary Q22.0
  hepatic Q44.7
  humerus -*see* Defect, reduction, upper limb
  hymen Q52.4
  ileum Q41.2
  incus Q16.3
  intestine (small) Q41.9
    large Q42.9
      specified NEC Q42.8
  iris (dilator fibers) Q13.1
  jaw M26.09
  jejunum Q41.1
  kidney(s) (partial) Q60.2
    bilateral Q60.1
    unilateral Q60.0
  labium (majus) (minus) Q52.71
  labyrinth, membranous Q16.5
  lacrimal apparatus Q10.4
  larynx Q31.8
  leg (complete) Q72.0
    with foot present Q72.1
    lower leg (with foot present) -*see* Agenesis, leg, with foot present
      and foot Q72.2
  lens Q12.3
  limb (complete) Q73.0
    lower -*see* Agenesis, leg
    upper -*see* Agenesis, arm
  lip Q38.0
  liver Q44.7
  lung (fissure) (lobe) (bilateral) (unilateral) Q33.3
  mandible, maxilla M26.09
  metacarpus -*see* Agenesis, hand
  metatarsus -*see* Agenesis, foot
  muscle Q79.8
    eyelid Q10.3
    ocular Q15.8
  musculoskeletal system NEC Q79.8
  nail(s) Q84.3
  neck, part Q18.8
  nerve Q07.8
  nervous system, part NEC Q07.8
  nipple Q83.2
  nose Q30.1
  nuclear Q07.8
  organ
    of Corti Q16.5
    or site not listed -*see* Anomaly, by site
  osseous meatus (ear) Q16.1
  ovary
    bilateral Q50.02
    unilateral Q50.01
  oviduct Q50.6
  pancreas Q45.0
  parathyroid (gland) Q89.2
  parotid gland(s) Q38.4
  patella Q74.1
  pelvic girdle (complete) (partial) Q74.2
  penis Q55.5
  pericardium Q24.8
  pituitary (gland) Q89.2
  prostate Q55.4
  punctum lacrimale Q10.4
  radioulnar -*see* Defect, reduction, upper limb
  radius -*see* Defect, reduction, upper limb, longitudinal, radius
  rectum Q42.1
    with fistula Q42.0

Agenesis - *continued*
  renal Q60.2
    bilateral Q60.1
    unilateral Q60.0
  respiratory organ NEC Q34.8
  rib Q76.6
  roof of orbit Q75.8
  round ligament Q52.8
  sacrum Q76.49
  salivary gland Q38.4
  scapula Q74.0
  scrotum Q55.29
  seminal vesicles Q55.4
  septum
    atrial Q21.1
    between aorta and pulmonary artery Q21.4
    ventricular Q20.4
  shoulder girdle (complete) (partial) Q74.0
  skull (bone) Q75.8
    with
      anencephaly Q00.0
      encephalocele -*see* Encephalocele
      hydrocephalus Q03.9
        with spina bifida -*see* Spina bifida, by site, with hydrocephalus
      microcephaly Q02
  spermatic cord Q55.4
  spinal cord Q06.0
  spine Q76.49
  spleen Q89.01
  sternum Q76.7
  stomach Q40.2
  submaxillary gland(s) (congenital) Q38.4
  tarsus -*see* Agenesis, foot
  tendon Q79.8
  testicle Q55.0
  thymus (gland) Q89.2
  thyroid (gland) E03.1
    cartilage Q31.8
  tibia -*see* Defect, reduction, lower limb, longitudinal, tibia
  tibiofibular -*see* Defect, reduction, lower limb, specified type NEC
  toe (and foot) (complete) (partial) -*see* Agenesis, foot
  tongue Q38.3
  trachea (cartilage) Q32.1
  ulna -*see* Defect, reduction, upper limb, longitudinal, ulna
  upper limb -*see* Agenesis, arm
  ureter Q62.4
  urethra Q64.5
  urinary tract NEC Q64.8
  uterus Q51.0
  uvula Q38.5
  vagina Q52.0
  vas deferens Q55.4
  vein(s) (peripheral) Q27.9
    brain Q28.3
    great NEC Q26.8
    portal Q26.5
  vena cava (inferior) (superior) Q26.8
  vermis of cerebellum Q04.3
  vertebra Q76.49
  vulva Q52.71
Ageusia R43.2
Agitated -*see* condition **Agitation** R45.1
Aglossia (congenital) Q38.3
Aglossia-adactylia syndrome Q87.0
Aglycogenosis E74.00

Agnosia (body image) (other senses) (tactile) R48.1
  developmental F88
  verbal R48.1
    auditory R48.1
      developmental F80.2
    developmental F80.2
  visual (object) R48.3
Agoraphobia F40.00
  with panic disorder F40.01
  without panic disorder F40.02
Agrammatism R48.8
Agranulocytopenia -*see* Agranulocytosis
Agranulocytosis (chronic) (cyclical) (genetic) (infantile) (periodic) (pernicious) -*see also* Neutropenia D70.9
  congenital D70.0
  cytoreductive cancer chemotherapy sequela D70.1
  drug-induced D70.2
    due to cytoreductive cancer chemotherapy D70.1
  due to infection D70.3
  secondary D70.4
    drug-induced D70.2
    due to cytoreductive cancer chemotherapy D70.1
Agraphia (absolute) R48.8
  with alexia R48.0
  developmental F81.81
Ague (dumb) -*see* Malaria
Agyria Q04.3
Ahumada-del Castillo syndrome E23.0
Aichmophobia F40.298
AIDS (related complex) B20
Ailment heart -*see* Disease, heart
Ailurophobia F40.218
Ainhum (disease) L94.6
AIN -*see* Neoplasia, intraepithelial, anal
AIPHI (acute idiopathic pulmonary hemorrhage in infants (over 28 days old)) R04.81
Air
  anterior mediastinum J98.2
  compressed, disease T70.3
  conditioner lung or pneumonitis J67.7
  embolism (artery) (cerebral) (any site) T79.0
    with ectopic or molar pregnancy O08.2
    due to implanted device NEC -*see* Complications, by site and type, specified NEC
    following
      abortion -*see* Abortion by type, complicated by, embolism
      ectopic or molar pregnancy O08.2
    infusion, therapeutic injection or transfusion T80.0
    in pregnancy, childbirth or puerperium -*see* Embolism, obstetric
    traumatic T79.0
  hunger, psychogenic F45.8
  rarefied, effects of -*see* Effect, adverse, high altitude
  sickness T75.3
Airplane sickness T75.3
Akathisia (drug-induced) (treatment-induced) G25.71
  neuroleptic induced (acute) G25.71
Akinesia R29.898
Akinetic mutism R41.89
Akureyri's disease G93.3

Alactasia, congenital E73.0
Alagille's syndrome Q44.7
Alastrim B03
Albers-Schönberg syndrome Q78.2
Albert's syndrome -*see* Tendinitis, Achilles
Albinism, albino E70.30
  with hematologic abnormality E70.339
    Chédiak-Higashi syndrome E70.330
    Hermansky Pudlak syndrome E70.331
    other specified E70.338
  I E70.320
  II E70.321
  ocular E70.319
    autosomal recessive E70.311
    other specified E70.318
    X linked E70.310
  oculocutaneous E70.329
    other specified E70.328
    tyrosinase (ty) negative E70.320
    tyrosinase (ty) positive E70.321
  other specified E70.39
Albinismus E70.30
Albright (McCune)(Sternberg) syndrome
  Q78.1
Albuminous -*see* condition
Albuminuria, albuminuric (acute) (chronic)
  (subacute) -*see also* Proteinuria R80.9
  complicating pregnancy -*see* Proteinuria,
  gestational
    with
      gestational hypertension -*see* Pre-
        eclampsia
      pre-existing hypertension -*see*
        Hypertension, complicating pregnancy,
        pre-existing, with, pre-eclampsia
  gestational -*see* Proteinuria, gestational
    with
      gestational hypertension -*see* Pre-
        eclampsia
      pre-existing hypertension -*see*
        Hypertension, complicating pregnancy,
        pre-existing, with, pre-eclampsia
  orthostatic R80.2
  postural R80.2
  pre-eclamptic -*see* Pre-eclampsia
  scarlatinal A38.8
Albuminurophobia F40.298
Alcaptonuria E70.29
Alcohol, alcoholic, alcohol-induced
  addiction (without remission) F10.20
    with remission F10.21
  amnestic disorder, persisting F10.96
    with dependence F10.26
  anxiety disorder F10.980
  bipolar and related disorder F10.94
  depressive disorder F10.94
  major neurocognitive disorder, amnestic-
    confabulatory type F10.96
  major neurocognitive disorder, nonamnestic-
    confabulatory type F10.97
  mild neurocognitive disorder F10.988
  psychotic disorder F10.959
  sexual dysfunction F10.981
  sleep disorder F10.982
  brain syndrome, chronic F10.97
    with dependence F10.27
  cardiopathy I42.6
  counseling and surveillance Z71.41
    family member Z71.42
  delirium (acute) (tremens) (withdrawal)
    F10.231

Alcohol, alcoholic, alcohol-induced
--*continued*
  with intoxication F10.921
  in
    abuse F10.121
    dependence F10.221
  dementia F10.97
    with dependence F10.27
  deterioration F10.97
    with dependence F10.27
  hallucinosis (acute) F10.951
  in
    abuse F10.151
    dependence F10.251
  insanity F10.959
  intoxication (acute) (without dependence)
    F10.129
    with
      delirium F10.121
      dependence F10.229
        with delirium F10.221
        uncomplicated F10.220
      uncomplicated F10.120
  jealousy F10.988
  Korsakoff's, Korsakov's, Korsakow's F10.26
  liver K70.9
    acute -*see* Disease, liver, alcoholic, hepatitis
  mania (acute) (chronic) F10.959
  paranoia, paranoid (type) psychosis F10.950
  pellagra E52
  poisoning, accidental (acute) NEC -*see* Table
    of Drugs and Chemicals, alcohol, poisoning
  psychosis -*see* Psychosis, alcoholic
  withdrawal (without convulsions) F10.239
    with delirium F10.231
Alcoholism (chronic) (without remission)
  F10.20
  with
    psychosis -*see* Psychosis, alcoholic
    remission F10.21
  Korsakov's F10.96
    with dependence F10.26
Alder (Reilly) anomaly or syndrome
  (leukocyte granulation) D72.0
Aldosteronism E26.9
  familial (type I) E26.02
  glucocorticoid-remediable E26.02
  primary (due to (bilateral) adrenal
    hyperplasia) E26.09
  primary NEC E26.09
  secondary E26.1
  specified NEC E26.89
Aldosteronoma D44.10
Aldrich (Wiskott) syndrome (eczema-
  thrombocytopenia) D82.0
Alektorophobia F40.218
Aleppo boil B55.1
Aleukemic -*see* condition
Aleukia
  congenital D70.0
  hemorrhagica D61.9
    congenital D61.09
  splenica D73.1
Alexia R48.0
  developmental F81.0
  secondary to organic lesion R48.0
Algoneurodystrophy M89.00
  ankle M89.07
  foot M89.07
  forearm M89.03
  hand M89.04

Algoneurodystrophy --*continued*
  lower leg M89.06
  multiple sites M89.0
  shoulder M89.01
  specified site NEC M89.08
  thigh M89.05
  upper arm M89.02
Algophobia F40.298
Alienation, mental -*see* Psychosis
Alkalemia E87.3
Alkalosis E87.3
  metabolic E87.3
    with respiratory acidosis E87.4
  respiratory E87.3
Alkaptonuria E70.29
Allen-Masters syndrome N83.8
Allergy, allergic (reaction) (to) T78.40
  air-borne substance NEC (rhinitis) J30.89
  alveolitis (extrinsic) J67.9
    due to
      Aspergillus clavatus J67.4
      Cryptostroma corticale J67.6
      organisms (fungal, thermophilic
        actinomycete) growing in ventilation (air
        conditioning) systems J67.7
    specified type NEC J67.8
  anaphylactic reaction or shock T78.2
  angioneurotic edema T78.3
  animal (dander) (epidermal) (hair) (rhinitis)
    J30.81
  bee sting (anaphylactic shock) -*see* Toxicity,
    venom, arthropod, bee
  biological -*see* Allergy, drug
  colitis -*see also* Colitis, allergic K52.29
  dander (animal) (rhinitis) J30.81
  dandruff (rhinitis) J30.81
  dental restorative material (existing) K08.55
  dermatitis -*see* Dermatitis, contact, allergic
  diathesis -*see* History, allergy
  drug, medicament & biological (any)
    (external) (internal) T78.40
    correct substance properly administered -*see*
      Table of Drugs and Chemicals, by drug,
      adverse effect
    wrong substance given or taken NEC (by
      accident) -*see* Table of Drugs and
      Chemicals, by drug, poisoning
  due to pollen J30.1
  dust (house) (stock) (rhinitis) J30.89
    with asthma -*see* Asthma, allergic extrinsic
  eczema -*see* Dermatitis, contact, allergic
  epidermal (animal) (rhinitis) J30.81
  feathers (rhinitis) J30.89
  food (any) (ingested) NEC T78.1
    anaphylactic shock -*see* Shock,
      anaphylactic, due to food
    dermatitis -*see* Dermatitis, due to, food
    dietary counseling and surveillance Z71.3
    in contact with skin L23.6
    rhinitis J30.5
    status (without reaction) Z91.018
      eggs Z91.012
      milk products Z91.011
      peanuts Z91.010
      seafood Z91.013
      specified NEC Z91.018
  gastrointestinal -*see also* specific type of
    allergic reaction
    meaning colitis -*see also* Colitis, allergic
  K52.29

Allergy, allergic (reaction) (to) --*continued*
  meaning gastroenteritis -*see also*
    Gastroenteritis, allergic K52.29
  meaning other adverse food reaction not
    elsewhere classified T78.1
  grain J30.1
  grass (hay fever) (pollen) J30.1
    asthma -*see* Asthma, allergic extrinsic
  hair (animal) (rhinitis) J30.81
  history (of) -*see* History, allergy
  horse serum -*see* Allergy, serum
  inhalant (rhinitis) J30.89
    pollen J30.1
  kapok (rhinitis) J30.89
  medicine -*see* Allergy, drug
  milk protein -*see also* Allergy, food Z91.011
    anaphylactic reaction T78.07
    dermatitis L27.2
    enterocolitis syndrome K52.21
    enteropathy K52.22
    gastroenteritis K52.29
    gastroesophageal reflux -*see also* Reaction,
    adverse, food K21.9
      with esophagitis K21.0
    proctocolitis K52.82
  nasal, seasonal due to pollen J30.1
  pneumonia J82
  pollen (any) (hay fever) J30.1
    asthma -*see* Asthma, allergic extrinsic
  primrose J30.1
  primula J30.1
  proctocolitis K52.82
  purpura D69.0
  ragweed (hay fever) (pollen) J30.1
    asthma -*see* Asthma, allergic extrinsic
  rose (pollen) J30.1
  seasonal NEC J30.2
  Senecio jacobae (pollen) J30.1
  serum -*see also* Reaction, serum T80.69
    anaphylactic shock T80.59
  shock (anaphylactic) T78.2
    due to
      administration of blood and blood products
        T80.51
      adverse effect of correct medicinal
        substance properly administered T88.6
      immunization T80.52
      serum NEC T80.59
      vaccination T80.52
  specific NEC T78.49
  tree (any) (hay fever) (pollen) J30.1
    asthma -*see* Asthma, allergic extrinsic
  upper respiratory J30.9
  urticaria L50.0
  vaccine -*see* Allergy, serum
  wheat -*see* Allergy, food
Allescheriasis B48.2
Alligator skin disease Q80.9
Allocheiria, allochiria R20.8
Almeida's disease -*see*
  Paracoccidioidomycosis
Alopecia (hereditaria) (seborrheica) L65.9
  androgenic L64.9
    drug-induced L64.0
    specified NEC L64.8
  areata L63.9
    ophiasis L63.2
    specified NEC L63.8
    totalis L63.0
    universalis L63.1
  cicatricial L66.9

Allergy, allergic (reaction) (to) --*continued*
  specified NEC L66.8
  circumscripta L63.9
  congenital, congenitalis Q84.0
  due to cytotoxic drugs NEC L65.8
  mucinosa L65.2
  postinfective NEC L65.8
  postpartum L65.0
  premature L64.8
  specific (syphilitic) A51.32
  specified NEC L65.8
  syphilitic (secondary) A51.32
  totalis (capitis) L63.0
  universalis (entire body) L63.1
  X ray L58.1
Alpers' disease G31.81
Alpine sickness T70.29
Alport syndrome Q87.81
ALTE (apparent life threatening event) in
  newborn and infant R68.13
Alteration (of), Altered
  awareness
    transient R40.4
    unintended under general anesthesia, during
      procedure T88.53
  mental status R41.82
  pattern of family relationships affecting child
    Z62.898
  sensation
    following
      cerebrovascular disease I69.998
        cerebral infarction I69.398
        intracerebral hemorrhage I69.198
        nontraumatic intracranial hemorrhage
          NEC I69.298
        specified disease NEC I69.898
        subarachnoid hemorrhage I69.098
Alternating -*see* condition
Altitude, high (effects) -*see* Effect, adverse,
  high altitude
Aluminosis (of lung) J63.0
Alveolitis
  allergic (extrinsic) -*see* Pneumonitis,
    hypersensitivity due to
      Aspergillus clavatus J67.4
      Cryptostroma corticale J67.6
  fibrosing (cryptogenic) (idiopathic) J84.112
  jaw M27.3
  sicca dolorosa M27.3
Alveolus, alveolar -*see* condition
Alymphocytosis D72.810
  thymic (with immunodeficiency) D82.1
Alymphoplasia, thymic D82.1
Alzheimer's disease or sclerosis -*see* Disease,
  Alzheimer's
Amastia (with nipple present) Q83.8
  with absent nipple Q83.0
Amathophobia F40.228
Amaurosis (acquired) (congenital) -*see also*
  Blindness
  fugax G45.3
  hysterical F44.6
  Leber's congenital H35.50
  uremic -*see* Uremia
Amaurotic idiocy (infantile) (juvenile) (late)
  E75.4
Amaxophobia F40.248
Ambiguous genitalia Q56.4
Amblyopia (congenital) (ex anopsia) (partial)
  (suppression) H53.00
  anisometropic -*see* Amblyopia, refractive

Amblyopia - *continued*
  deprivation H53.01
  hysterical F44.6
  nocturnal -*see also* Blindness, night
    vitamin A deficiency E50.5
  refractive H53.02
  strabismic H53.03
  suspect H53.04
  tobacco H53.8
  toxic NEC H53.8
  uremic -*see* Uremia
Ameba, amebic (histolytica) -*see also*
  Amebiasis
  abscess (liver) A06.4
Amebiasis A06.9
  with abscess -*see* Abscess, amebic
  acute A06.0
  chronic (intestine) A06.1
    with abscess -*see* Abscess, amebic
  cutaneous A06.7
  cutis A06.7
  cystitis A06.81
  genitourinary tract NEC A06.82
  hepatic -*see* Abscess, liver, amebic
  intestine A06.0
  nondysenteric colitis A06.2
  skin A06.7
  specified site NEC A06.89
Ameboma (of intestine) A06.3
Amelia Q73.0
  lower limb -*see* Agenesis, leg
  upper limb -*see* Agenesis, arm
Ameloblastoma -*see also* Cyst, calcifying
  odontogenic
  long bones C40.9
    lower limb C40.2
    upper limb C40.0
  malignant C41.1
    jaw (bone) (lower) C41.1
      upper C41.0
  tibial C40.2
Amelogenesis imperfecta K00.5
  nonhereditaria (segmentalis) K00.4
Amenorrhea N91.2
  hyperhormonal E28.8
  primary N91.0
  secondary N91.1
Amentia -*see* Disability, intellectual
  Meynert's (nonalcoholic) F04
American
  leishmaniasis B55.2
  mountain tick fever A93.2
Ametropia -*see* Disorder, refraction
AMH (asymptomatic microscopic
  hematuria) R31.21
Amianthosis J61
Amimia R48.8
Amino-acid disorder E72.9
  anemia D53.0
Aminoacidopathy E72.9
Aminoaciduria E72.9
Amnes (t)ic syndrome (post-traumatic) F04
  induced by
    alcohol F10.96
      with dependence F10.26
    psychoactive NEC F19.96
      with
        abuse F19.16
        dependence F19.26
    sedative F13.96
      with dependence F13.26

Amnesia R41.3
  anterograde R41.1
  auditory R48.8
  dissociative F44.0
    with dissociative fugue F44.1
  hysterical F44.0
  postictal in epilepsy -*see* Epilepsy
  psychogenic F44.0
  retrograde R41.2
  transient global G45.4
Amnion, amniotic -*see* condition
Amnionitis -*see* Pregnancy, complicated by
Amok F68.8
Amoral traits F60.89
Amphetamine (or other stimulant) induced
  anxiety disorder F15.980
  bipolar and related disorder F15.94
  delirium F15.921
  depressive disorder F15.94
  obsessive-compulsive and related disorder
    F15.988
  psychotic disorder F15.959
  sexual dysfunction F15.981
  sleep disorder F15.982
  stimulant withdrawal F15.23
Ampulla
  lower esophagus K22.8
  phrenic K22.8
Amputation -*see also* Absence, by site,
    acquired
  neuroma (postoperative) (traumatic) -*see*
    Complications, amputation stump, neuroma
  stump (surgical)
    abnormal, painful, or with complication
      (late) -*see* Complications, amputation
      stump
    healed or old NOS Z89.9
  traumatic (complete) (partial)
    arm (upper) (complete) S48.91
      at
        elbow S58.01
          partial S58.02
        shoulder joint (complete) S48.01
          partial S48.02
      between
        elbow and wrist (complete) S58.11
          partial S58.12
        shoulder and elbow (complete) S48.11
          partial S48.12
      partial S48.92
    breast (complete) S28.21
      partial S28.22
    clitoris (complete) S38.211
      partial S38.212
    ear (complete) S08.11
      partial S08.12
    finger (complete) (metacarpophalangeal)
      S68.11
      index S68.11
      little S68.11
      middle S68.11
      partial S68.12
        index S68.12
        little S68.12
        middle S68.12
        ring S68.12
      ring S68.11
      thumb -*see* Amputation, traumatic, thumb
      transphalangeal (complete) S68.61
        index S68.61
        little S68.61
        middle S68.61

Amputation --*continued*
    partial S68.62
      index S68.62
      little S68.62
      middle S68.62
      ring S68.62
    ring S68.61
  foot (complete) S98.91
    at ankle level S98.01
      partial S98.02
    midfoot S98.31
      partial S98.32
    partial S98.92
  forearm (complete) S58.91
    at elbow level (complete) S58.01
      partial S58.02
    between elbow and wrist (complete)
      S58.11
      partial S58.12
    partial S58.92
  genital organ(s) (external)
    female (complete) S38.211
      partial S38.212
    male
      penis (complete) S38.221
        partial S38.222
      scrotum (complete) S38.231
        partial S38.232
      testes (complete) S38.231
        partial S38.232
  hand (complete) (wrist level) S68.41
    finger(s) alone -*see* Amputation, traumatic,
      finger
    partial S68.42
    thumb alone -*see* Amputation, traumatic,
      thumb
    transmetacarpal (complete) S68.71
      partial S68.72
  head
    ear -*see* Amputation, traumatic, ear
    nose (partial) S08.812
      complete S08.811
    part S08.89
      scalp S08.0
  hip (and thigh) (complete) S78.91
    at hip joint (complete) S78.01
      partial S78.02
    between hip and knee (complete) S78.11
      partial S78.12
    partial S78.92
  labium (majus) (minus) (complete) S38.21
    partial S38.21
  leg (lower) S88.91
    at knee level S88.01
      partial S88.02
    between knee and ankle S88.11
      partial S88.12
    partial S88.92
  nose (partial) S08.812
    complete S08.811
  penis (complete) S38.221
    partial S38.222
  scrotum (complete) S38.231
    partial S38.232
  shoulder -*see* Amputation, traumatic, arm
    at shoulder joint -*see* Amputation,
      traumatic, arm, at shoulder joint
  testes (complete) S38.231
    partial S38.232
  thigh -*see* Amputation, traumatic, hip
  thorax, part of S28.1

Amputation --*continued*
    breast -*see* Amputation, traumatic, breast
    thumb (complete) (metacarpophalangeal)
      S68.01
      partial S68.02
      transphalangeal (complete) S68.51
        partial S68.52
    toe (lesser) S98.13
      great S98.11
        partial S98.12
      more than one S98.21
        partial S98.22
      partial S98.14
    vulva (complete) S38.211
      partial S38.212
Amputee (bilateral) (old) Z89.9
Amsterdam dwarfism Q87.1
Amusia R48.8
  developmental F80.89
Amyelencephalus, amyelencephaly Q00.0
Amyelia Q06.0
Amygdalitis -*see* Tonsillitis
Amygdalolith J35.8
Amyloid heart (disease) E85.4 [*I43*]
Amyloidosis (generalized) (primary) E85.9
  with lung involvement E85.4 [*J99*]
  familial E85.2
  genetic E85.2
  heart E85.4 [*I43*]
  hemodialysis-associated E85.3
  liver E85.4 [*K77*]
  localized E85.4
  neuropathic heredofamilial E85.1
  non-neuropathic heredofamilial E85.0
  organ limited E85.4
  Portuguese E85.1
  pulmonary E85.4 [*J99*]
  secondary systemic E85.3
  skin (lichen) (macular) E85.4 [*L99*]
  specified NEC E85.8
  subglottic E85.4 [*J99*]
Amylopectinosis (brancher enzyme
    deficiency) E74.03
Amylophagia -*see* Pica
Amyoplasia congenita Q79.8
Amyotonia M62.89
  congenita G70.2
Amyotrophia, amyotrophy, amyotrophic
    G71.8
  congenita Q79.8
  diabetic -*see* Diabetes, amyotrophy
  lateral sclerosis G12.21
  neuralgic G54.5
  spinal progressive G12.21
Anacidity, gastric K31.83
  psychogenic F45.8
Anaerosis of newborn P28.89
Analbuminemia E88.09
Analgesia -*see* Anesthesia
Analphalipoproteinemia E78.6
Anaphylactic
  purpura D69.0
  shock or reaction -*see* Shock, anaphylactic
Anaphylactoid shock or reaction -*see* Shock,
    anaphylactic
Anaphylactoid syndrome of pregnancy
    O88.01
Anaphylaxis -*see* Shock, anaphylactic
Anaplasia cervix -*see also* Dysplasia, cervix
    N87.9
Anaplasmosis, human A77.49

Anarthria R47.1
Anasarca R60.1
  cardiac -see Failure, heart, congestive
  lung J18.2
  newborn P83.2
  nutritional E43
  pulmonary J18.2
  renal N04.9
Anastomosis
  aneurysmal -see Aneurysm
  arteriovenous ruptured brain I60.8
  intestinal K63.89
    complicated NEC K91.89
      involving urinary tract N99.89
  retinal and choroidal vessels (congenital)
    Q14.8
Anatomical narrow angle H40.03
Ancylostoma, ancylostomiasis (braziliense) (caninum) (ceylanicum) (duodenale) B76.0
  Necator americanus B76.1
Andersen's disease (glycogen storage) E74.09
Anderson-Fabry disease E75.21
Andes disease T70.29
Andrews' disease (bacterid) L08.89
Androblastoma
  benign
    specified site -see Neoplasm, benign, by site
    unspecified site
      female D27.9
      male D29.20
  malignant
    specified site -see Neoplasm, malignant, by site
    unspecified site
      female C56.9
      male C62.90
  specified site -see Neoplasm, uncertain behavior, by site
  tubular
    with lipid storage
      specified site -see Neoplasm, benign, by site
      unspecified site
        female D27.9
        male D29.20
    specified site -see Neoplasm, benign, by site
    unspecified site
      female D27.9
      male D29.20
  unspecified site
    female D39.10
    male D40.10
Androgen insensitivity syndrome -see also Syndrome, androgen insensitivity E34.50
Androgen resistance syndrome -see also Syndrome, androgen insensitivity E34.50
Android pelvis Q74.2
  with disproportion (fetopelvic) O33.3
    causing obstructed labor O65.3
Androphobia F40.290
Anectasis, pulmonary (newborn) -see Atelectasis
Anemia (essential) (general) (hemoglobin deficiency) (infantile) (primary) (profound) D64.9
  with (due to) (in)
    disorder of
      anaerobic glycolysis D55.2
      pentose phosphate pathway D55.1
    koilonychia D50.9
  achlorhydric D50.8

Anemia - continued
  achrestic D53.1
  Addison (Biermer) (pernicious) D51.0
  agranulocytic -see Agranulocytosis
  amino-acid-deficiency D53.0
  aplastic D61.9
    congenital D61.09
    drug-induced D61.1
    due to
      drugs D61.1
      external agents NEC D61.2
      infection D61.2
      radiation D61.2
    idiopathic D61.3
    red cell (pure) D60.9
      chronic D60.0
      congenital D61.01
      specified type NEC D60.8
      transient D60.1
    specified type NEC D61.89
    toxic D61.2
  aregenerative
    congenital D61.09
  asiderotic D50.9
  atypical (primary) D64.9
  Baghdad spring D55.0
  Balantidium coli A07.0
  Biermer's (pernicious) D51.0
  blood loss (chronic) D50.0
    acute D62
  bothriocephalus B70.0 [D63.8]
  brickmaker's B76.9 [D63.8]
  cerebral I67.89
  childhood D58.9
  chlorotic D50.8
  chronic
    blood loss D50.0
    hemolytic D58.9
      idiopathic D59.9
    simple D53.9
  chronica congenita aregenerativa D61.09
  combined system disease NEC D51.0 [G32.0]
    due to dietary vitamin B12 deficiency D51.3 [G32.0]
  complicating pregnancy, childbirth or puerperium -see Pregnancy, complicated by (management affected by), anemia
  congenital P61.4
    aplastic D61.09
    due to isoimmunization NOS P55.9
    dyserythropoietic, dyshematopoietic D64.4
    following fetal blood loss P61.3
    Heinz body D58.2
    hereditary hemolytic NOS D58.9
    pernicious D51.0
    spherocytic D58.0
  Cooley's (erythroblastic) D56.1
  cytogenic D51.0
  deficiency D53.9
    2, 3 diphosphoglycerate mutase D55.2
    2, 3 PG D55.2
    6 phosphogluconate dehydrogenase D55.1
    6 PGD D55.1
    amino-acid D53.0
    combined B12 and folate D53.1
    enzyme D55.9
      drug-induced (hemolytic) D59.2
      glucose-6 phosphate dehydrogenase (G6PD) D55.0
      glycolytic D55.2
      nucleotide metabolism D55.3

Anemia - continued
  related to hexose monophosphate (HMP) shunt pathway NEC D55.1
    specified type NEC D55.8
  erythrocytic glutathione D55.1
  folate D52.9
    dietary D52.0
    drug-induced D52.1
  folic acid D52.9
    dietary D52.0
    drug-induced D52.1
  G SH D55.1
  GGS-R D55.1
  glucose-6 phosphate dehydrogenase D55.0
  glutathione reductase D55.1
  glyceraldehyde phosphate dehydrogenase D55.2
  G6PD D55.0
  hexokinase D55.2
  iron D50.9
    secondary to blood loss (chronic) D50.0
  nutritional D53.9
    with
      poor iron absorption D50.8
      specified deficiency NEC D53.8
  phosphofructo-aldolase D55.2
  phosphoglycerate kinase D55.2
  PK D55.2
  protein D53.0
  pyruvate kinase D55.2
  transcobalamin II D51.2
  triose-phosphate isomerase D55.2
  vitamin B12 NOS D51.9
    dietary D51.3
    due to
      intrinsic factor deficiency D51.0
      selective vitamin B12 malabsorption with proteinuria D51.1
    pernicious D51.0
    specified type NEC D51.8
  Diamond-Blackfan (congenital hypoplastic) D61.01
  dibothriocephalus B70.0 [D63.8]
  dimorphic D53.1
  diphasic D53.1
  Diphyllobothrium (Dibothriocephalus) B70.0 [D63.8]
  due to (in) (with)
    antineoplastic chemotherapy D64.81
    blood loss (chronic) D50.0
      acute D62
    chemotherapy, antineoplastic D64.81
    chronic disease classified elsewhere NEC D63.8
    chronic kidney disease D63.1
    deficiency
      amino-acid D53.0
      copper D53.8
      folate (folic acid) D52.9
        dietary D52.0
        drug-induced D52.1
      molybdenum D53.8
      protein D53.0
      zinc D53.8
    dietary vitamin B12 deficiency D51.3
    disorder of
      glutathione metabolism D55.1
      nucleotide metabolism D55.3
    drug -see Anemia, by type -see also Table of Drugs and Chemicals

Anemia - *continued*
  end stage renal disease D63.1
  enzyme disorder D55.9
  fetal blood loss P61.3
  fish tapeworm (D. Latum) infestation B70.0
    [D63.8]
  hemorrhage (chronic) D50.0
    acute D62
  impaired absorption D50.9
  loss of blood (chronic) D50.0
    acute D62
  myxedema E03.9 [D63.8]
  Necator americanus B76.1 [D63.8]
  prematurity P61.2
  selective vitamin B12 malabsorption with
    proteinuria D51.1
  transcobalamin II deficiency D51.2
  Dyke-Young type (secondary) (symptomatic)
    D59.1
  dyserythropoietic (congenital) D64.4
  dyshematopoietic (congenital) D64.4
  Egyptian B76.9 [D63.8]
  elliptocytosis -*see* Elliptocytosis
  enzyme-deficiency, drug-induced D59.2
  epidemic -*see also* Ancylostomiasis B76.9
    [D63.8]
  erythroblastic
    familial D56.1
    newborn -*see also* Disease, hemolytic P55.9
    of childhood D56.1
  erythrocytic glutathione deficiency D55.1
  erythropoietin-resistant anemia (EPO resistant
    anemia) D63.1
  Faber's (achlorhydric anemia) D50.9
  factitious (self-induced blood letting) D50.0
  familial erythroblastic D56.1
  Fanconi's (congenital pancytopenia) D61.09
  favism D55.0
  fish tapeworm (D. latum) infestation B70.0
    [D63.8]
  folate (folic acid) deficiency D52.9
  glucose-6 phosphate dehydrogenase (G6PD)
    deficiency D55.0
  glutathione-reductase deficiency D55.1
  goat's milk D52.0
  granulocytic -*see* Agranulocytosis
  Heinz body, congenital D58.2
  hemolytic D58.9
    acquired D59.9
      with hemoglobinuria NEC D59.6
      autoimmune NEC D59.1
      infectious D59.4
      specified type NEC D59.8
      toxic D59.4
    acute D59.9
      due to enzyme deficiency specified type
        NEC D55.8
      Lederer's D59.1
    autoimmune D59.1
      drug-induced D59.0
    chronic D58.9
      idiopathic D59.9
    cold type (secondary) (symptomatic) D59.1
    congenital (spherocytic) -*see* Spherocytosis
    due to
      cardiac conditions D59.4
      drugs (nonautoimmune) D59.2
        autoimmune D59.0
      enzyme disorder D55.9
        drug-induced D59.2

Anemia - *continued*
    presence of shunt or other internal
      prosthetic device D59.4
    familial D58.9
    hereditary D58.9
      due to enzyme disorder D55.9
        specified type NEC D55.8
      specified type NEC D58.8
    idiopathic (chronic) D59.9
    mechanical D59.4
    microangiopathic D59.4
    nonautoimmune D59.4
      drug-induced D59.2
    nonspherocytic
      congenital or hereditary NEC D55.8
        glucose-6 phosphate dehydrogenase
          deficiency D55.0
        pyruvate kinase deficiency D55.2
        type
          I D55.1
          II D55.2
      type
        I D55.1
        II D55.2
    secondary D59.4
      autoimmune D59.1
    specified (hereditary) type NEC D58.8
    Stransky Regala type -*see also*
      Hemoglobinopathy D58.8
    symptomatic D59.4
      autoimmune D59.1
    toxic D59.4
    warm type (secondary) (symptomatic) D59.1
  hemorrhagic (chronic) D50.0
    acute D62
  Herrick's D57.1
  hexokinase deficiency D55.2
  hookworm B76.9 [D63.8]
  hypochromic (idiopathic) (microcytic)
  (normoblastic) D50.9
    due to blood loss (chronic) D50.0
      acute D62
    familial sex linked D64.0
    pyridoxine-responsive D64.3
    sideroblastic, sex linked D64.0
  hypoplasia, red blood cells D61.9
    congenital or familial D61.01
  hypoplastic (idiopathic) D61.9
    congenital or familial (of childhood) D61.01
  hypoproliferative (refractive) D61.9
  idiopathic D64.9
    aplastic D61.3
    hemolytic, chronic D59.9
  in (due to) (with)
    chronic kidney disease D63.1
    end stage renal disease D63.1
    failure, kidney (renal) D63.1
    neoplastic disease -*see also* Neoplasm D63.0
  intertropical -*see also* Ancylostomiasis D63.8
  iron deficiency D50.9
    secondary to blood loss (chronic) D50.0
      acute D62
    specified type NEC D50.8
  Joseph-Diamond-Blackfan (congenital
    hypoplastic) D61.01
  Lederer's (hemolytic) D59.1
  leukoerythroblastic D61.82
  macrocytic D53.9
    nutritional D52.0
    tropical D52.8
  malarial -*see also* Malaria B54 [D63.8]

Anemia - *continued*
  malignant (progressive) D51.0
  malnutrition D53.9
  marsh -*see also* Malaria B54 [D63.8]
  Mediterranean (with other hemoglobinopathy)
    D56.9
  megaloblastic D53.1
    combined B12 and folate deficiency D53.1
    hereditary D51.1
    nutritional D52.0
    orotic aciduria D53.0
    refractory D53.1
    specified type NEC D53.1
  megalocytic D53.1
  microcytic (hypochromic) D50.9
    due to blood loss (chronic) D50.0
      acute D62
    familial D56.8
  microdrepanocytosis D57.40
  microelliptopoikilocytic (Rietti-Grippe-
    Micheli) D56.9
  miner's B76.9 [D63.8]
  myelodysplastic D46.9
  myelofibrosis D75.81
  myelogenous D64.89
  myelopathic D64.89
  myelophthisic D61.82
  myeloproliferative D47.Z9
  newborn P61.4
    due to
      ABO (antibodies, isoimmunization,
        maternal/fetal incompatibility) P55.1
      Rh (antibodies, isoimmunization,
        maternal/fetal incompatibility) P55.0
    following fetal blood loss P61.3
    posthemorrhagic (fetal) P61.3
  nonspherocytic hemolytic -*see* Anemia,
    hemolytic, nonspherocytic
  normocytic (infectional) D64.9
    due to blood loss (chronic) D50.0
      acute D62
    myelophthisic D61.82
  nutritional (deficiency) D53.9
    with
      poor iron absorption D50.8
      specified deficiency NEC D53.8
    megaloblastic D52.0
  of prematurity P61.2
  orotaciduric (congenital) (hereditary) D53.0
  osteosclerotic D64.89
  ovalocytosis (hereditary) -*see* Elliptocytosis
  paludal -*see also* Malaria B54 [D63.8]
  pernicious (congenital) (malignant)
    (progressive) D51.0
  pleochromic D64.89
    of sprue D52.8
  posthemorrhagic (chronic) D50.0
    acute D62
    newborn P61.3
  postoperative (postprocedural)
    due to (acute) blood loss D62
      chronic blood loss D50.0
    specified NEC D64.9
  postpartum O90.81
  pressure D64.89
  progressive D64.9
    malignant D51.0
    pernicious D51.0
  protein-deficiency D53.0
  pseudoleukemica infantum D64.89
  pure red cell D60.9

Anemia - *continued*
  congenital D61.01
pyridoxine-responsive D64.3
pyruvate kinase deficiency D55.2
refractory D46.4
  with
    excess of blasts D46.20
      1 (RAEB 1) D46.21
      2 (RAEB 2) D46.22
      in transformation (RAEB T) *-see*
        Leukemia, acute myeloblastic
    hemochromatosis D46.1
    sideroblasts (ring) (RARS) D46.1
    megaloblastic D53.1
    sideroblastic D46.1
    sideropenic D50.9
    without ring sideroblasts, so stated D46.0
    without sideroblasts without excess of blasts
      D46.0
  Rietti-Grippe-Micheli D56.9
  scorbutic D53.2
  secondary to
    blood loss (chronic) D50.0
      acute D62
    hemorrhage (chronic) D50.0
      acute D62
  semiplastic D61.89
  sickle-cell *-see* Disease, sickle-cell
  sideroblastic D64.3
    hereditary D64.0
    hypochromic, sex linked D64.0
    pyridoxine-responsive NEC D64.3
    refractory D46.1
    secondary (due to)
      disease D64.1
      drugs and toxins D64.2
    specified type NEC D64.3
  sideropenic (refractory) D50.9
    due to blood loss (chronic) D50.0
      acute D62
  simple chronic D53.9
  specified type NEC D64.89
  spherocytic (hereditary) *-see* Spherocytosis
  splenic D64.89
  splenomegalic D64.89
  stomatocytosis D58.8
  syphilitic (acquired) (late) A52.79 [*D63.8*]
  target cell D64.89
  thalassemia D56.9
  thrombocytopenic *-see* Thrombocytopenia
  toxic D61.2
  tropical B76.9 [*D63.8*]
    macrocytic D52.8
  tuberculous A18.89 [*D63.8*]
  vegan D51.3
  vitamin
    B6 responsive D64.3
    B12 deficiency (dietary) pernicious D51.0
  von Jaksch's D64.89
  Witts' (achlorhydric anemia) D50.8
Anemophobia F40.228
Anencephalus, anencephaly Q00.0
Anergasia *-see* Psychosis, organic
Anesthesia, anesthetic R20.0
  complication or reaction NEC *-see also*
    Complications, anesthesia T88.59
    due to
      correct substance properly administered -
        see Table of Drugs and Chemicals, by drug,
        adverse effect

Anesthesia, anesthetic *--continued*
      overdose or wrong substance given *-see*
        Table of Drugs and Chemicals, by drug,
        poisoning
    unintended awareness under general
      anesthesia during procedure T88.53
      personal history of Z92.84
  cornea H18.81
  dissociative F44.6
  functional (hysterical) F44.6
  hyperesthetic, thalamic G89.0
  hysterical F44.6
  local skin lesion R20.0
  sexual (psychogenic) F52.1
  shock (due to) T88.2
  skin R20.0
  testicular N50.9
Anetoderma (maculosum) (of) L90.8
  Jadassohn-Pellizzari L90.2
  Schweniger-Buzzi L90.1
Aneurin deficiency E51.9
Aneurysm (anastomotic) (artery) (cirsoid)
  (diffuse) (false) (fusiform) (multiple)
  (saccular) I72.9
  abdominal (aorta) I71.4
    ruptured I71.3
    syphilitic A52.01
  aorta, aortic (nonsyphilitic) I71.9
    abdominal I71.4
      ruptured I71.3
    arch I71.2
      ruptured I71.1
    arteriosclerotic I71.9
      ruptured I71.8
    ascending I71.2
      ruptured I71.1
    congenital Q25.43
    descending I71.9
      abdominal I71.4
        ruptured I71.3
      ruptured I71.8
      thoracic I71.2
        ruptured I71.1
    root Q25.43
    ruptured I71.8
    sinus, congenital Q25.43
    syphilitic A52.01
    thoracic I71.2
      ruptured I71.1
    thoracoabdominal I71.6
      ruptured I71.5
    thorax, thoracic (arch) I71.2
      ruptured I71.1
    transverse I71.2
      ruptured I71.1
    valve (heart) *-see also* Endocarditis, aortic
      I35.8
  arteriosclerotic I72.9
    cerebral I67.1
      ruptured *-see* Hemorrhage, intracranial,
        subarachnoid
  arteriovenous (congenital) *-see also*
    Malformation, arteriovenous
    acquired I77.0
      brain I67.1
      coronary I25.41
      pulmonary I28.0
    brain Q28.2
      ruptured I60.8
    peripheral *-see* Malformation, arteriovenous,
      peripheral

Aneurysm - *continued*
  precerebral vessels Q28.0
  specified site NEC *-see also* Malformation,
    arteriovenous
    acquired I77.0
  basal *-see* Aneurysm, brain
  basilar (trunk) I72.5
  berry (congenital) (nonruptured) I67.1
    ruptured I60.7
  brain I67.1
    arteriosclerotic I67.1
      ruptured *-see* Hemorrhage, intracranial,
        subarachnoid
    arteriovenous (congenital) (nonruptured)
      Q28.2
      acquired I67.1
        ruptured I60.8
      ruptured I60.8
    berry (congenital) (nonruptured) I67.1
      ruptured *-see also* Hemorrhage,
        intracranial, subarachnoid I60.7
    congenital Q28.3
      ruptured I60.7
    meninges I67.1
      ruptured I60.8
    miliary (congenital) (nonruptured) I67.1
      ruptured *-see also* Hemorrhage,
        intracranial, subarachnoid I60.7
    mycotic I33.0
      ruptured *-see* Hemorrhage, intracranial,
        subarachnoid
    syphilitic (hemorrhage) A52.05
  cardiac (false) *-see also* Aneurysm, heart
    I25.3
  carotid artery (common) (external) I72.0
    internal (intracranial) I67.1
      extracranial portion I72.0
    ruptured into brain I60.0
    syphilitic A52.09
      intracranial A52.05
  cavernous sinus I67.1
    arteriovenous (congenital) (nonruptured)
      Q28.3
      ruptured I60.8
  celiac I72.8
  central nervous system, syphilitic A52.05
  cerebral *-see* Aneurysm, brain
  chest *-see* Aneurysm, thorax - circle of Willis
    I67.1
    congenital Q28.3
      ruptured I60.6
    ruptured I60.6
  common iliac artery I72.3
  congenital (peripheral) Q27.8
    aorta (root) (sinus) Q25.43
    brain Q28.3
      ruptured I60.7
    coronary Q24.5
    digestive system Q27.8
    lower limb Q27.8
    pulmonary Q25.79
    retina Q14.1
    specified site NEC Q27.8
    upper limb Q27.8
  conjunctiva *-see* Abnormality, conjunctiva,
    vascular
  conus arteriosus *-see* Aneurysm, heart
  coronary (arteriosclerotic) (artery) I25.41
    arteriovenous, congenital Q24.5
    congenital Q24.5
    ruptured *-see* Infarct, myocardium

Aneurysm - *continued*
syphilitic A52.06
vein I25.89
cylindroid (aorta) I71.9
ruptured I71.8
syphilitic A52.01
ductus arteriosus Q25.0
endocardial, infective (any valve) I33.0
femoral (artery) (ruptured) I72.4
gastroduodenal I72.8
gastroepiploic I72.8
heart (wall) (chronic or with a stated duration
of over 4 weeks) I25.3
valve -*see* Endocarditis
hepatic I72.8
iliac (common) (artery) (ruptured) I72.3
infective I72.9
endocardial (any valve) I33.0
innominate (nonsyphilitic) I72.8
syphilitic A52.09
interauricular septum -*see* Aneurysm, heart
interventricular septum -*see* Aneurysm, heart
intrathoracic (nonsyphilitic) I71.2
ruptured I71.1
syphilitic A52.01
lower limb I72.4
lung (pulmonary artery) I28.1
mediastinal (nonsyphilitic) I72.8
syphilitic A52.09
miliary (congenital) I67.1
ruptured -*see* Hemorrhage, intracerebral,
subarachnoid, intracranial
mitral (heart) (valve) I34.8
mural -*see* Aneurysm, heart
mycotic I72.9
endocardial (any valve) I33.0
ruptured, brain -*see* Hemorrhage,
intracerebral, subarachnoid
myocardium -*see* Aneurysm, heart
neck I72.0
pancreaticoduodenal I72.8
patent ductus arteriosus Q25.0
peripheral NEC I72.8
congenital Q27.8
digestive system Q27.8
lower limb Q27.8
specified site NEC Q27.8
upper limb Q27.8
popliteal (artery) (ruptured) I72.4
precerebral
congenital (nonruptured) Q28.1
specified site, NEC I72.5
pulmonary I28.1
arteriovenous Q25.72
acquired I28.0
syphilitic A52.09
valve (heart) -*see* Endocarditis, pulmonary
racemose (peripheral) I72.9
congenital -*see* Aneurysm, congenital
radial I72.1
Rasmussen NEC A15.0
renal (artery) I72.2
retina -*see also* Disorder, retina,
microaneurysms
congenital Q14.1
diabetic -*see* Diabetes, microaneurysms,
retinal
sinus of Valsalva Q25.49
specified NEC I72.8
spinal (cord) I72.8

Aneurysm - *continued*
syphilitic (hemorrhage) A52.09
splenic I72.8
subclavian (artery) (ruptured) I72.8
syphilitic A52.09
superior mesenteric I72.8
syphilitic (aorta) A52.01
central nervous system A52.05
congenital (late) A50.54 [*I79.0*]
spine, spinal A52.09
thoracoabdominal (aorta) I71.6
ruptured I71.5
syphilitic A52.01
thorax, thoracic (aorta) (arch) (nonsyphilitic)
I71.2
ruptured I71.1
syphilitic A52.01
traumatic (complication) (early), specified site
-*see* Injury, blood vessel
tricuspid (heart) (valve) I07.8
ulnar I72.1
upper limb (ruptured) I72.1
valve, valvular -*see* Endocarditis
venous -*see also* Varix I86.8
congenital Q27.8
digestive system Q27.8
lower limb Q27.8
specified site NEC Q27.8
upper limb Q27.8
ventricle -*see* Aneurysm, heart
vertebral artery I72.6
visceral NEC I72.8
Angelman syndrome Q93.5
Anger R45.4
Angiectasis, angiectopia I99.8
Angiitis I77.6
allergic granulomatous M30.1
hypersensitivity M31.0
necrotizing M31.9
specified NEC M31.8
nervous system, granulomatous I67.7
Angina (attack) (cardiac) (chest) (heart)
(pectoris) (syndrome) (vasomotor) I20.9
with
atherosclerotic heart disease -*see*
Arteriosclerosis, coronary (artery),
documented spasm I20.1
abdominal K55.1
accelerated -*see* Angina, unstable
agranulocytic -*see* Agranulocytosis
angiospastic -*see* Angina, with documented
spasm
aphthous B08.5
crescendo -*see* Angina, unstable
croupous J05.0
cruris I73.9
de novo effort -*see* Angina, unstable
diphtheritic, membranous A36.0
equivalent I20.8
exudative, chronic J37.0
following acute myocardial infarction I23.7
gangrenous diphtheritic A36.0
intestinal K55.1
Ludovici K12.2
Ludwig's K12.2
malignant diphtheritic A36.0
membranous J05.0
diphtheritic A36.0
Vincent's A69.1
mesenteric K55.1
monocytic -*see* Mononucleosis, infectious

Angina - *continued*
of effort -*see* Angina, specified NEC
phlegmonous J36
diphtheritic A36.0
post-infarctional I23.7
pre-infarctional -*see* Angina, unstable
Prinzmetal -*see* Angina, with documented
spasm
progressive -*see* Angina, unstable
pseudomembranous A69.1
pultaceous, diphtheritic A36.0
spasm-induced -*see* Angina, with documented
spasm
specified NEC I20.8
stable I20.8
stenocardia -*see* Angina, specified NEC
stridulous, diphtheritic A36.2
tonsil J36
trachealis J05.0
unstable I20.0
variant -*see* Angina, with documented spasm
Vincent's A69.1
worsening effort -*see* Angina, unstable
Angioblastoma -*see* Neoplasm, connective
tissue, uncertain behavior
Angiocholecystitis -*see* Cholecystitis, acute
Angiocholitis -*see also* Cholecystitis, acute
K83.0
Angiodysgenesis spinalis G95.19
Angiodysplasia (cecum) (colon) K55.20
with bleeding K55.21
duodenum (and stomach) K31.819
with bleeding K31.811
stomach (and duodenum) K31.819
with bleeding K31.811
Angioedema (allergic) (any site) (with
urticaria) T78.3
hereditary D84.1
Angioendothelioma -*see* Neoplasm, uncertain
behavior, by site
benign D18.00
intra-abdominal D18.03
intracranial D18.02
skin D18.01
specified site NEC D18.09
bone -*see* Neoplasm, bone, malignant
Ewing's -*see* Neoplasm, bone, malignant
Angioendotheliomatosis C85.8
Angiofibroma -*see also* Neoplasm, benign, by
site
juvenile
specified site -*see* Neoplasm, benign, by site
unspecified site D10.6
Angiohemophilia (A) (B) D68.0
Angioid streaks (choroid) (macula) (retina)
H35.33
Angiokeratoma -*see* Neoplasm, skin, benign
corporis diffusum E75.21
Angioleiomyoma -*see* Neoplasm, connective
tissue, benign
Angiolipoma -*see also* Lipoma
infiltrating -*see* Lipoma
Angioma -*see also* Hemangioma, by site
capillary I78.1
hemorrhagicum hereditaria I78.0
intra-abdominal D18.03
intracranial D18.02
malignant -*see* Neoplasm, connective tissue,
malignant
plexiform D18.00
intra-abdominal D18.03

Angioma – *continued*
  intracranial D18.02
  skin D18.01
  specified site NEC D18.09
  senile I78.1
  serpiginosum L81.7
  skin D18.01
  specified site NEC D18.09
  spider I78.1
  stellate I78.1
  venous Q28.3
Angiomatosis Q82.8
  bacillary A79.89
  encephalotrigeminal Q85.8
  hemorrhagic familial I78.0
  hereditary familial I78.0
  liver K76.4
Angiomyolipoma -*see* Lipoma
Angiomyoliposarcoma -*see* Neoplasm,
  connective tissue, malignant
Angiomyoma -*see* Neoplasm, connective
  tissue, benign
Angiomyosarcoma -*see* Neoplasm, connective
  tissue, malignant
Angiomyxoma -*see* Neoplasm, connective
  tissue, uncertain behavior
Angioneurosis F45.8
Angioneurotic edema (allergic) (any site)
  (with urticaria) T78.3
  hereditary D84.1
Angiopathia, angiopathy I99.9
  cerebral I67.9
    amyloid E85.4 [*I68.0*]
  diabetic (peripheral) -*see* Diabetes,
    angiopathy
  peripheral I73.9
    diabetic -*see* Diabetes, angiopathy
    specified type NEC I73.89
  retinae syphilitica A52.05
  retinalis (juvenilis)
    diabetic -*see* Diabetes, retinopathy
    proliferative -*see* Retinopathy, proliferative
Angiosarcoma -*see also* Neoplasm, connective
  tissue, malignant
  liver C22.3
Angiosclerosis -*see* Arteriosclerosis
Angiospasm (peripheral) (traumatic) (vessel)
  I73.9
  brachial plexus G54.0
  cerebral G45.9
  cervical plexus G54.2
  nerve
    arm -*see* Mononeuropathy, upper limb
      axillary G54.0
      median -*see* Lesion, nerve, median
      ulnar -*see* Lesion, nerve, ulnar
    axillary G54.0
    leg -*see* Mononeuropathy, lower limb
    median -*see* Lesion, nerve, median
    plantar -*see* Lesion, nerve, plantar
    ulnar -*see* Lesion, nerve, ulnar
Angiospastic disease or edema I73.9
Angiostrongyliasis
  due to
    Parastrongylus
      cantonensis B83.2
      costaricensis B81.3
  intestinal B81.3
Anguillulosis -*see* Strongyloidiasis
Angulation
  cecum -*see* Obstruction, intestine

Angulation - *continued*
  coccyx (acquired) -*see also* subcategory
  M43.8
    congenital NEC Q76.49
  femur (acquired) -*see also* Deformity, limb,
  specified type NEC, thigh
    congenital Q74.2
  intestine (large) (small) -*see* Obstruction,
    intestine
  sacrum (acquired) -*see also* subcategory
  M43.8
    congenital NEC Q76.49
  sigmoid (flexure) -*see* Obstruction, intestine
  spine -*see* Dorsopathy, deforming, specified
    NEC
  tibia (acquired) -*see also* Deformity, limb,
  specified type NEC, lower leg
    congenital Q74.2
  ureter N13.5
    with infection N13.6
  wrist (acquired) -*see also* Deformity, limb,
  specified type NEC, forearm
    congenital Q74.0
Angulus infectiosus (lips) K13.0
Anhedonia R45.84
  sexual F52.0
Anhidrosis L74.4
Anhydration E86.0
Anhydremia E86.0
Anidrosis L74.4
Aniridia (congenital) Q13.1
Anisakiasis (infection) (infestation) B81.0
Anisakis larvae infestation B81.0
Aniseikonia H52.32
Anisocoria (pupil) H57.02
  congenital Q13.2
Anisocytosis R71.8
Anisometropia (congenital) H52.31
Ankle -*see* condition
Ankyloblepharon (eyelid) (acquired) -*see*
  also Blepharophimosis
  filiforme (adnatum) (congenital) Q10.3
  total Q10.3
Ankyloglossia Q38.1
Ankylosis (fibrous) (osseous) (joint) M24.60
  ankle M24.67
  arthrodesis status Z98.1
  cricoarytenoid (cartilage) (joint) (larynx)
    J38.7
  dental K03.5
  ear ossicles H74.31
  elbow M24.62
  foot M24.67
  hand M24.64
  hip M24.65
  incostapedial joint (infectional) -*see*
    Ankylosis, ear ossicles
  jaw (temporomandibular) M26.61
  knee M24.66
  lumbosacral (joint) M43.27
  postoperative (status) Z98.1
  produced by surgical fusion, status Z98.1
  sacro-iliac (joint) M43.28
  shoulder M24.61
  spine (joint) -*see also* Fusion, spine
    spondylitic -*see* Spondylitis, ankylosing
  surgical Z98.1
  temporomandibular M26.61
  tooth, teeth (hard tissues) K03.5
  wrist M24.63

Ankylostoma -*see* Ancylostoma
Ankylostomiasis -*see* Ancylostomiasis
Ankylurethria -*see* Stricture, urethra
Annular -*see also* condition
  detachment, cervix N88.8
  organ or site, congenital NEC -*see* Distortion
  pancreas (congenital) Q45.1
Anodontia (complete) (partial) (vera) K00.0
  acquired K08.10
Anomaly, anomalous (congenital)
  (unspecified type) Q89.9
  abdominal wall NEC Q79.59
  acoustic nerve Q07.8
  adrenal (gland) Q89.1
  Alder (Reilly) (leukocyte granulation) D72.0
  alimentary tract Q45.9
    upper Q40.9
  alveolar M26.70
    hyperplasia M26.79
      mandibular M26.72
      maxillary M26.71
    hypoplasia M26.79
      mandibular M26.74
      maxillary M26.73
    ridge (process) M26.79
    specified NEC M26.79
  ankle (joint) Q74.2
  anus Q43.9
  aorta (arch) NEC Q25.40
    coarctation (preductal) (postductal) Q25.1
  aortic cusp or valve Q23.9
  appendix Q43.8
  apple peel syndrome Q41.1
  aqueduct of Sylvius Q03.0
    with spina bifida -*see* Spina bifida, with
  hydrocephalus
  arm Q74.0
  arteriovenous NEC
    coronary Q24.5
    gastrointestinal Q27.33
      acquired -*see* Angiodysplasia
  artery (peripheral) Q27.9
    basilar NEC Q28.1
    cerebral Q28.3
    coronary Q24.5
    digestive system Q27.8
    eye Q15.8
    great Q25.9
      specified NEC Q25.8
    lower limb Q27.8
    peripheral Q27.9
      specified NEC Q27.8
    pulmonary NEC Q25.79
    renal Q27.2
    retina Q14.1
    specified site NEC Q27.8
    subclavian Q27.8
      origin Q25.48
    umbilical Q27.0
    upper limb Q27.8
    vertebral NEC Q28.1
  aryteno-epiglottic folds Q31.8
  atrial
    bands or folds Q20.8
    septa Q21.1
  atrioventricular
    excitation I45.6
    septum Q21.0
  auditory canal Q17.8
  auricle
    ear Q17.8

Anomaly, anomalous - *continued*
causing impairment of hearing Q16.9
heart Q20.8
Axenfeld's Q15.0
back Q89.9
band
atrial Q20.8
heart Q24.8
ventricular Q24.8
Bartholin's duct Q38.4
biliary duct or passage Q44.5
bladder Q64.70
absence Q64.5
diverticulum Q64.6
exstrophy Q64.10
cloacal Q64.12
extroversion Q64.19
specified type NEC Q64.19
supravesical fissure Q64.11
neck obstruction Q64.31
specified type NEC Q64.79
bone Q79.9
arm Q74.0
face Q75.9
leg Q74.2
pelvic girdle Q74.2
shoulder girdle Q74.0
skull Q75.9
with
anencephaly Q00.0
encephalocele -*see* Encephalocele
hydrocephalus Q03.9
with spina bifida -*see* Spina bifida, by
site, with hydrocephalus
microcephaly Q02
brain (multiple) Q04.9
vessel Q28.3
breast Q83.9
broad ligament Q50.6
bronchus Q32.4
bulbus cordis Q21.9
bursa Q79.9
canal of Nuck Q52.4
canthus Q10.3
capillary Q27.9
cardiac Q24.9
chambers Q20.9
specified NEC Q20.8
septal closure Q21.9
specified NEC Q21.8
valve NEC Q24.8
pulmonary Q22.3
cardiovascular system Q28.8
carpus Q74.0
caruncle, lacrimal Q10.6
cascade stomach Q40.2
cauda equina Q06.3
cecum Q43.9
cerebral Q04.9
vessels Q28.3
cervix Q51.9
Chédiak-Higashi (Steinbrinck) (congenital
gigantism of peroxidase granules) E70.330
cheek Q18.9
chest wall Q67.8
bones Q76.9
chin Q18.9
chordae tendineae Q24.8
choroid Q14.3
plexus Q07.8
chromosomes, chromosomal Q99.9

Anomaly, anomalous - *continued*
D (1) -*see* condition, chromosome 13
E (3) -*see* condition, chromosome 18
G -*see* condition, chromosome 21
sex
female phenotype Q97.8
gonadal dysgenesis (pure) Q99.1
Klinefelter's Q98.4
male phenotype Q98.9
Turner's Q96.9
specified NEC Q99.8
cilia Q10.3
circulatory system Q28.9
clavicle Q74.0
clitoris Q52.6
coccyx Q76.49
colon Q43.9
common duct Q44.5
communication
coronary artery Q24.5
left ventricle with right atrium Q21.0
concha (ear) Q17.3
connection
portal vein Q26.5
pulmonary venous Q26.4
partial Q26.3
total Q26.2
renal artery with kidney Q27.2
cornea (shape) Q13.4
coronary artery or vein Q24.5
cranium -*see* Anomaly, skull
cricoid cartilage Q31.8
cystic duct Q44.5
dental
alveolar -*see* Anomaly, alveolar
arch relationship M26.20
specified NEC M26.29
dentofacial M26.9
alveolar -*see* Anomaly, alveolar
dental arch relationship M26.20
specified NEC M26.29
functional M26.50
specified NEC M26.59
jaw-cranial base relationship M26.10
asymmetry M26.12
maxillary M26.11
specified type NEC M26.19
jaw size M26.00
macrogenia M26.05
mandibular
hyperplasia M26.03
hypoplasia M26.04
maxillary
hyperplasia M26.01
hypoplasia M26.02
microgenia M26.06
specified type NEC M26.09
malocclusion M26.4
dental arch relationship NEC M26.29
jaw-cranial base relationship -*see*
Anomaly, dentofacial, jaw-cranial base
relationship
jaw size -*see* Anomaly, dentofacial, jaw
size
specified type NEC M26.89
temporomandibular joint M26.60
adhesions M26.61
ankylosis M26.61
arthralgia M26.62
articular disc M26.63
specified type NEC M26.69

Anomaly, anomalous - *continued*
tooth position, fully erupted M26.30
specified NEC M26.39
dermatoglyphic Q82.8
diaphragm (apertures) NEC Q79.1
digestive organ(s) or tract Q45.9
lower Q43.9
upper Q40.9
distance, interarch (excessive) (inadequate)
M26.25
distribution, coronary artery Q24.5
ductus
arteriosus Q25.0
botalli Q25.0
duodenum Q43.9
dura (brain) Q04.9
spinal cord Q06.9
ear (external) Q17.9
causing impairment of hearing Q16.9
inner Q16.5
middle (causing impairment of hearing)
Q16.4
ossicles Q16.3
Ebstein's (heart) (tricuspid valve) Q22.5
ectodermal Q82.9
Eisenmenger's (ventricular septal defect)
Q21.8
ejaculatory duct Q55.4
elbow Q74.0
endocrine gland NEC Q89.2
epididymis Q55.4
epiglottis Q31.8
esophagus Q39.9
eustachian tube Q17.8
eye Q15.9
anterior segment Q13.9
specified NEC Q13.89
posterior segment Q14.9
specified NEC Q14.8
ptosis (eyelid) Q10.0
specified NEC Q15.8
eyebrow Q18.8
eyelid Q10.3
ptosis Q10.0
face Q18.9
bone(s) Q75.9
fallopian tube Q50.6
fascia Q79.9
femur NEC Q74.2
fibula NEC Q74.2
finger Q74.0
fixation, intestine Q43.3
flexion (joint) NOS Q74.9
hip or thigh Q65.89
foot NEC Q74.2
varus (congenital) Q66.3
foramen
Botalli Q21.1
ovale Q21.1
forearm Q74.0
forehead Q75.8
form, teeth K00.2
fovea centralis Q14.1
frontal bone -*see* Anomaly, skull
gallbladder (position) (shape) (size) Q44.1
Gartner's duct Q52.4
gastrointestinal tract Q45.9
genitalia, genital organ(s) or system
female Q52.9
external Q52.70
internal NOS Q52.9

Anomaly, anomalous - *continued*
  male Q55.9
    hydrocele P83.5
    specified NEC Q55.8
  genitourinary NEC
    female Q52.9
    male Q55.9
  Gerbode Q21.0
  glottis Q31.8
  granulation or granulocyte, genetic
  (constitutional) (leukocyte) D72.0
  gum Q38.6
  gyri Q07.9
  hair Q84.2
  hand Q74.0
  hard tissue formation in pulp K04.3
  head -*see* Anomaly, skull
  heart Q24.9
    auricle Q20.8
    bands or folds Q24.8
    fibroelastosis cordis I42.4
    obstructive NEC Q22.6
    patent ductus arteriosus (Botalli) Q25.0
    septum Q21.9
      auricular Q21.1
      interatrial Q21.1
      interventricular Q21.0
        with pulmonary stenosis or atresia,
  dextroposition of aorta and hypertrophy of
  right ventricle Q21.3
      specified NEC Q21.8
      ventricular Q21.0
        with pulmonary stenosis or atresia,
  dextroposition of aorta and hypertrophy of
  right ventricle Q21.3
    tetralogy of Fallot Q21.3
    valve NEC Q24.8
      aortic
        bicuspid valve Q23.1
        insufficiency Q23.1
        stenosis Q23.0
          subaortic Q24.4
      mitral
        insufficiency Q23.3
        stenosis Q23.2
      pulmonary Q22.3
        atresia Q22.0
        insufficiency Q22.2
        stenosis Q22.1
          infundibular Q24.3
          subvalvular Q24.3
      tricuspid
        atresia Q22.4
        stenosis Q22.4
    ventricle Q20.8
  heel NEC Q74.2
  Hegglin's D72.0
  hemianencephaly Q00.0
  hemicephaly Q00.0
  hemicrania Q00.0
  hepatic duct Q44.5
  hip NEC Q74.2
  hourglass stomach Q40.2
  humerus Q74.0
  hydatid of Morgagni
    female Q50.5
    male (epididymal) Q55.4
      testicular Q55.29
  hymen Q52.4
  hypersegmentation of neutrophils, hereditary
  D72.0

Anomaly, anomalous - *continued*
  hypophyseal Q89.2
  ileocecal (coil) (valve) Q43.9
  ileum Q43.9
  ilium NEC Q74.2
  integument Q84.9
    specified NEC Q84.8
  interarch distance (excessive) (inadequate)
  M26.25
  intervertebral cartilage or disc Q76.49
  intestine (large) (small) Q43.9
    with anomalous adhesions, fixation or
    malrotation Q43.3
  iris Q13.2
  ischium NEC Q74.2
  jaw -*see* Anomaly, dentofacial
    alveolar -*see* Anomaly, alveolar
  jaw-cranial base relationship -*see* Anomaly,
  dentofacial, jaw-cranial base relationship
  jejunum Q43.8
  joint Q74.9
    specified NEC Q74.8
  Jordan's D72.0
  kidney(s) (calyx) (pelvis) Q63.9
    artery Q27.2
    specified NEC Q63.8
  Klippel-Feil (brevicollis) Q76.1
  knee Q74.1
  labium (majus) (minus) Q52.70
  labyrinth, membranous Q16.5
  lacrimal apparatus or duct Q10.6
  larynx, laryngeal (muscle) Q31.9
    web (bed) Q31.0
  lens Q12.9
  leukocytes, genetic D72.0
    granulation (constitutional) D72.0
  lid (fold) Q10.3
  ligament Q79.9
    broad Q50.6
    round Q52.8
  limb Q74.9
    lower NEC Q74.2
      reduction deformity -*see* Defect, reduction,
  lower limb
    upper Q74.0
  lip Q38.0
  liver Q44.7
    duct Q44.5
  lower limb NEC Q74.2
  lumbosacral (joint) (region) Q76.49
    kyphosis -*see* Kyphosis, congenital
    lordosis -*see* Lordosis, congenital
  lung (fissure) (lobe) Q33.9
  mandible -*see* Anomaly, dentofacial
  maxilla -*see* Anomaly, dentofacial
  May (Hegglin) D72.0
  meatus urinarius NEC Q64.79
  meningeal bands or folds Q07.9
    constriction of Q07.8
    spinal Q06.9
  meninges Q07.9
    cerebral Q04.8
    spinal Q06.9
  meningocele Q05.9
  mesentery Q45.9
  metacarpus Q74.0
  metatarsus NEC Q74.2
  middle ear Q16.4
    ossicles Q16.3
  mitral (leaflets) (valve) Q23.9
    insufficiency Q23.3

Anomaly, anomalous - *continued*
    specified NEC Q23.8
    stenosis Q23.2
  mouth Q38.6
  Müllerian -*see also* Anomaly, by site
    uterus NEC Q51.818
  multiple NEC Q89.7
  muscle Q79.9
    eyelid Q10.3
  musculoskeletal system, except limbs Q79.9
  myocardium Q24.8
  nail Q84.6
  narrowness, eyelid Q10.3
  nasal sinus (wall) Q30.8
  neck (any part) Q18.9
  nerve Q07.9
    acoustic Q07.8
    optic Q07.8
  nervous system (central) Q07.9
  nipple Q83.9
  nose, nasal (bones) (cartilage) (septum)
  (sinus) Q30.9
    specified NEC Q30.8
  ocular muscle Q15.8
  omphalomesenteric duct Q43.0
  opening, pulmonary veins Q26.4
  optic
    disc Q14.2
    nerve Q07.8
  opticociliary vessels Q13.2
  orbit (eye) Q10.7
  organ Q89.9
    of Corti Q16.5
  origin
    artery
      innominate Q25.8
      pulmonary Q25.79
      renal Q27.2
      subclavian Q25.48
  osseous meatus (ear) Q16.1
  ovary Q50.39
  oviduct Q50.6
  palate (hard) (soft) NEC Q38.5
  pancreas or pancreatic duct Q45.3
  papillary muscles Q24.8
  parathyroid gland Q89.2
  paraurethral ducts Q64.79
  parotid (gland) Q38.4
  patella Q74.1
  Pelger-Huët (hereditary hyposegmentation)
  D72.0
  pelvic girdle NEC Q74.2
  pelvis (bony) NEC Q74.2
    rachitic E64.3
  penis (glans) Q55.69
  pericardium Q24.8
  peripheral vascular system Q27.9
  Peter's Q13.4
  pharynx Q38.8
  pigmentation L81.9
    congenital Q82.8
  pituitary (gland) Q89.2
  pleural (folds) Q34.0
  portal vein Q26.5
    connection Q26.5
  position, tooth, teeth, fully erupted M26.30
    specified NEC M26.39
  precerebral vessel Q28.1
  prepuce Q55.69
  prostate Q55.4
  pulmonary Q33.9

Anomaly, anomalous - *continued*

artery NEC Q25.79
valve Q22.3
atresia Q22.0
insufficiency Q22.2
specified type NEC Q22.3
stenosis Q22.1
infundibular Q24.3
subvalvular Q24.3
venous connection Q26.4
partial Q26.3
total Q26.2
pupil Q13.2
function H57.00
anisocoria H57.02
Argyll Robertson pupil H57.01
miosis H57.03
mydriasis H57.04
specified type NEC H57.09
tonic pupil H57.05
pylorus Q40.3
radius Q74.0
rectum Q43.9
reduction (extremity) (limb)
femur (longitudinal) -*see* Defect, reduction, lower limb, longitudinal, femur
fibula (longitudinal) -*see* Defect, reduction, lower limb, longitudinal, fibula
lower limb -*see* Defect, reduction, lower limb
radius (longitudinal) -*see* Defect, reduction, upper limb, longitudinal, radius
tibia (longitudinal) -*see* Defect, reduction, lower limb, longitudinal, tibia
ulna (longitudinal) -*see* Defect, reduction, upper limb, longitudinal, ulna
upper limb -*see* Defect, reduction, upper limb
refraction -*see* Disorder, refraction
renal Q63.9
artery Q27.2
pelvis Q63.9
specified NEC Q63.8
respiratory system Q34.9
specified NEC Q34.8
retina Q14.1
rib Q76.6
cervical Q76.5
Rieger's Q13.81
rotation -*see* Malrotation
hip or thigh Q65.89
round ligament Q52.8
sacroiliac (joint) NEC Q74.2
sacrum NEC Q76.49
kyphosis -*see* Kyphosis, congenital
lordosis -*see* Lordosis, congenital
saddle nose, syphilitic A50.57
salivary duct or gland Q38.4
scapula Q74.0
scrotum -*see* Malformation, testis and scrotum
sebaceous gland Q82.9
seminal vesicles Q55.4
sense organs NEC Q07.8
sex chromosomes NEC -*see also* Anomaly, chromosomes
female phenotype Q97.8
male phenotype Q98.9
shoulder (girdle) (joint) Q74.0
sigmoid (flexure) Q43.9
simian crease Q82.8
sinus of Valsalva Q25.49

Anomaly, anomalous - *continued*

skeleton generalized Q78.9
skin (appendage) Q82.9
skull Q75.9
with
anencephaly Q00.0
encephalocele -*see* Encephalocele
hydrocephalus Q03.9
with spina bifida -*see* Spina bifida, by site, with hydrocephalus
microcephaly Q02
specified organ or site NEC Q89.8
spermatic cord Q55.4
spine, spinal NEC Q76.49
column NEC Q76.49
kyphosis -*see* Kyphosis, congenital
lordosis -*see* Lordosis, congenital
cord Q06.9
nerve root Q07.8
spleen Q89.09
agenesis Q89.01
stenonian duct Q38.4
sternum NEC Q76.7
stomach Q40.3
submaxillary gland Q38.4
tarsus NEC Q74.2
tendon Q79.9
testis -*see* Malformation, testis and scrotum
thigh NEC Q74.2
thorax (wall) Q67.8
bony Q76.9
throat Q38.8
thumb Q74.0
thymus gland Q89.2
thyroid (gland) Q89.2
cartilage Q31.8
tibia NEC Q74.2
saber A50.56
toe Q74.2
tongue Q38.3
tooth, teeth K00.9
eruption K00.6
position, fully erupted M26.30
spacing, fully erupted M26.30
trachea (cartilage) Q32.1
tragus Q17.9
tricuspid (leaflet) (valve) Q22.9
atresia or stenosis Q22.4
Ebstein's Q22.5
Uhl's (hypoplasia of myocardium, right ventricle) Q24.8
ulna Q74.0
umbilical artery Q27.0
union
cricoid cartilage and thyroid cartilage Q31.8
thyroid cartilage and hyoid bone Q31.8
trachea with larynx Q31.8
upper limb Q74.0
urachus Q64.4
ureter Q62.8
obstructive NEC Q62.39
cecoureterocele Q62.32
orthotopic ureterocele Q62.31
urethra Q64.70
absence Q64.5
double Q64.74
fistula to rectum Q64.73
obstructive Q64.39
stricture Q64.32
prolapse Q64.71
specified type NEC Q64.79

Anomaly, anomalous - *continued*

urinary tract Q64.9
uterus Q51.9
with only one functioning horn Q51.4
uvula Q38.5
vagina Q52.4
valleculae Q31.8
valve (heart) NEC Q24.8
coronary sinus Q24.5
inferior vena cava Q24.8
pulmonary Q22.3
sinus coronario Q24.5
venae cavae inferioris Q24.8
vas deferens Q55.4
vascular Q27.9
brain Q28.3
ring Q25.45
vein(s) (peripheral) Q27.9
brain Q28.3
cerebral Q28.3
coronary Q24.5
developmental Q28.3
great Q26.9
specified NEC Q26.8
vena cava (inferior) (superior) Q26.9
venous -*see* Anomaly, vein(s)
venous return Q26.8
ventricular
bands or folds Q24.8
septa Q21.0
vertebra Q76.49
kyphosis -*see* Kyphosis, congenital
lordosis -*see* Lordosis, congenital
vesicourethral orifice Q64.79
vessel(s) Q27.9
optic papilla Q14.2
precerebral Q28.1
vitelline duct Q43.0
vitreous body or humor Q14.0
vulva Q52.70
wrist (joint) Q74.0
Anomia R48.8
Anonychia (congenital) Q84.3
acquired L60.8
Anophthalmos, anophthalmus (congenital) (globe) Q11.1
acquired Z90.01
Anopia, anopsia H53.46
quadrant H53.46
Anorchia, anorchism, anorchidism Q55.0
Anorexia R63.0
hysterical F44.89
nervosa F50.00
atypical F50.9
binge-eating type F50.2
with purging F50.02
restricting type F50.01
Anorgasmy, psychogenic (female) F52.31
male F52.32
Anosmia R43.0
hysterical F44.6
postinfectional J39.8
Anosognosia R41.89
Anosteoplasia Q78.9
Anovulatory cycle N97.0
Anoxemia R09.02
newborn P84
Anoxia (pathological) R09.02
altitude T70.29
cerebral G93.1
complicating

Anoxia - *continued*
  anesthesia (general) (local) or other
sedation T88.59
    in labor and delivery O74.3
    in pregnancy O29.21
    postpartum, puerperal O89.2
  delivery (cesarean) (instrumental) O75.4
  during a procedure G97.81
  newborn P84
  resulting from a procedure G97.82
  due to
    drowning T75.1
    high altitude T70.29
  heart -*see* Insufficiency, coronary
  intrauterine P84
  myocardial -*see* Insufficiency, coronary
  newborn P84
  spinal cord G95.11
  systemic (by suffocation) (low content in
  atmosphere) -*see* Asphyxia, traumatic
Anteflexion -*see* Anteversion
Antenatal
  care (normal pregnancy) Z34.90
  screening (encounter for) of mother Z36
Antepartum -*see* condition
Anterior -*see* condition
Antero-occlusion M26.220
Anteversion
  cervix -*see* Anteversion, uterus
  femur (neck), congenital Q65.89
  uterus, uterine (cervix) (postinfectional)
  (postpartal, old) N85.4
    congenital Q51.818
    in pregnancy or childbirth -*see* Pregnancy,
  complicated by
Anthophobia F40.228
Anthracosilicosis J60
Anthracosis (lung) (occupational) J60
  lingua K14.3
Anthrax A22.9
  with pneumonia A22.1
  cerebral A22.8
  colitis A22.2
  cutaneous A22.0
  gastrointestinal A22.2
  inhalation A22.1
  intestinal A22.2
  meningitis A22.8
  pulmonary A22.1
  respiratory A22.1
  sepsis A22.7
  specified manifestation NEC A22.8
Anthropoid pelvis Q74.2
  with disproportion (fetopelvic) O33.0
Anthropophobia F40.10
  generalized F40.11
Antibodies, maternal (blood group) -*see*
  Isoimmunization, affecting management of
  pregnancy anti-D -*see* Isoimmunization,
  affecting management of pregnancy, Rh
  newborn P55.0
Antibody
  anticardiolipin R76.0
    with
      hemorrhagic disorder D68.312
      hypercoagulable state D68.61
  antiphosphatidylglycerol R76.0
    with
      hemorrhagic disorder D68.312
      hypercoagulable state D68.61
  antiphosphatidylinositol R76.0

Antibody --*continued*
  with
      hemorrhagic disorder D68.312
      hypercoagulable state D68.61
  antiphosphatidylserine R76.0
    with
      hemorrhagic disorder D68.312
      hypercoagulable state D68.61
  antiphospholipid R76.0
    with
      hemorrhagic disorder D68.312
      hypercoagulable state D68.61
Anticardiolipin syndrome D68.61
Anticoagulant, circulating (intrinsic) -*see*
  also - Disorder, hemorrhagic D68.318
  drug-induced (extrinsic) -*see also* - Disorder,
  hemorrhagic D68.32
  iatrogenic D68.32
Antidiuretic hormone syndrome E22.2
Antimonial cholera -*see* Poisoning, antimony
Antiphospholipid
  antibody
    with hemorrhagic disorder D68.312
    syndrome D68.61
Antisocial personality F60.2
Antithrombinemia -*see* Circulating
  anticoagulants
Antithromboplastinemia D68.318
Antithromboplastinogenemia D68.318
Antitoxin complication or reaction -*see*
  Complications, vaccination
Antlophobia F40.228
Antritis J32.0
  maxilla J32.0
    acute J01.00
      recurrent J01.01
  stomach K29.60
    with bleeding K29.61
Antrum, antral -*see* condition
Anuria R34
  calculous (impacted) (recurrent) -*see also*
  Calculus, urinary N20.9
  following
    abortion -*see* Abortion by type complicated
      by, renal failure
    ectopic or molar pregnancy O08.4
  newborn P96.0
  postprocedural N99.0
  postrenal N13.8
  traumatic (following crushing) T79.5
Anus, anal -*see* condition
Anusitis K62.89
Anxiety F41.9
  depression F41.8
  episodic paroxysmal F41.0
  generalized F41.1
  hysteria F41.8
  neurosis F41.1
  panic type F41.0
  reaction F41.1
  separation, abnormal (of childhood) F93.0
  specified NEC F41.8
  state F41.1
Aorta, aortic -*see* condition
Aortectasia -*see* Ectasia, aorta
  with aneurysm -*see* Aneurysm, aorta
Aortitis (nonsyphilitic) (calcific) I77.6
  arteriosclerotic I70.0
  Doehle-Heller A52.02
  luetic A52.02
  rheumatic -*see* Endocarditis, acute, rheumatic

Aortitis - *continued*
  specific (syphilitic) A52.02
  syphilitic A52.02
    congenital A50.54 [*I79.1*]
Apathetic thyroid storm -*see* Thyrotoxicosis
Apathy R45.3
Apeirophobia F40.228
Apepsia K30
  psychogenic F45.8
Aperistalsis, esophagus K22.0
Apertognathia M26.29
Apert's syndrome Q87.0
Aphagia R13.0
  psychogenic F50.9
Aphakia (acquired) (postoperative) H27.0
  congenital Q12.3
**Aphasia (amnestic) (global) (nominal)
  (semantic) (syntactic)** R47.01
  acquired, with epilepsy (Landau-Kleffner
    syndrome) -*see* Epilepsy, specified NEC
  auditory (developmental) F80.2
  developmental (receptive type) F80.2
    expressive type F80.1
    Wernicke's F80.2
  following
    cerebrovascular disease I69.920
      cerebral infarction I69.320
      intracerebral hemorrhage I69.120
      nontraumatic intracranial hemorrhage NEC
        I69.220
      specified disease NEC I69.820
      subarachnoid hemorrhage I69.020
  primary progressive G31.01 [*F02.80*]
    with behavioral disturbance G31.01
      [*F02.81*]
  progressive isolated G31.01 [*F02.80*]
    with behavioral disturbance G31.01
      [*F02.81*]
  sensory F80.2
  syphilis, tertiary A52.19
  Wernicke's (developmental) F80.2
Aphonia (organic) R49.1
  hysterical F44.4
  psychogenic F44.4
Aphthae, aphthous -*see also* condition
  Bednar's K12.0
  cachectic K14.0
  epizootic B08.8
  fever B08.8
  oral (recurrent) K12.0
  stomatitis (major) (minor) K12.0
  thrush B37.0
  ulcer (oral) (recurrent) K12.0
    genital organ(s) NEC
      female N76.6
      male N50.89
    larynx J38.7
Apical -*see* condition
Apiphobia F40.218
Aplasia -*see also* Agenesis
  abdominal muscle syndrome Q79.4
  alveolar process (acquired) -*see* Anomaly,
  alveolar
    congenital Q38.6
  aorta (congenital) Q25.41
  axialis extracorticalis (congenita) E75.29
  bone marrow (myeloid) D61.9
    congenital D61.01
  brain Q00.0
    part of Q04.3
  bronchus Q32.4

Aplasia - *continued*
  cementum K00.4
  cerebellum Q04.3
  cervix (congenital) Q51.5
  congenital pure red cell D61.01
  corpus callosum Q04.0
  cutis congenita Q84.8
  erythrocyte congenital D61.01
  extracortical axial E75.29
  eye Q11.1
  fovea centralis (congenital) Q14.1
  gallbladder, congenital Q44.0
  iris Q13.1
  labyrinth, membranous Q16.5
  limb (congenital) Q73.8
    lower -*see* Defect, reduction, lower limb
    upper -*see* Agenesis, arm
  lung, congenital (bilateral) (unilateral) Q33.3
  pancreas Q45.0
  parathyroid-thymic D82.1
  Pelizaeus-Merzbacher E75.29
  penis Q55.5
  prostate Q55.4
  red cell (with thymoma) D60.9
    acquired D60.9
      due to drugs D60.9
    adult D60.9
    chronic D60.0
    congenital D61.01
    constitutional D61.01
    due to drugs D60.9
    hereditary D61.01
    of infants D61.01
    primary D61.01
    pure D61.01
      due to drugs D60.9
    specified type NEC D60.8
    transient D60.1
  round ligament Q52.8
  skin Q84.8
  spermatic cord Q55.4
  spleen Q89.01
  testicle Q55.0
  thymic, with immunodeficiency D82.1
  thyroid (congenital) (with myxedema) E03.1
  uterus Q51.0
  ventral horn cell Q06.1
Apnea, apneic (of) (spells) R06.81
  newborn NEC P28.4
    obstructive P28.4
    sleep (central) (obstructive) (primary) P28.3
  prematurity P28.4
  sleep G47.30
    central (primary) G47.31
      in conditions classified elsewhere G47.37
    obstructive (adult) (pediatric) G47.33
    primary central G47.31
    specified NEC G47.39
Apneumatosis, newborn P28.0
Apocrine metaplasia (breast) -*see* Dysplasia,
  mammary, specified type NEC
Apophysitis (bone) -*see also*
  Osteochondropathy
  calcaneus M92.8
  juvenile M92.9
Apoplectiform convulsions (cerebral
  ischemia) I67.82
Apoplexia, apoplexy, apoplectic
  adrenal A39.1
  heart (auricle) (ventricle) -*see* Infarct,
  myocardium

Apoplexia, apoplexy, apoplectic --*continued*
  heat T67.0
  hemorrhagic (stroke) -*see* Hemorrhage,
  intracranial
  meninges, hemorrhagic -*see* Hemorrhage,
  intracranial, subarachnoid
  uremic N18.9 [*I68.8*]
Appearance
  bizarre R46.1
  specified NEC R46.89
  very low level of personal hygiene R46.0
Appendage
  epididymal (organ of Morgagni) Q55.4
  intestine (epiploic) Q43.8
  preauricular Q17.0
  testicular (organ of Morgagni) Q55.29
Appendicitis (pneumococcal) (retrocecal)
  K37
  with
    perforation or rupture K35.2
    peritoneal abscess K35.3
    peritonitis NEC K35.3
      generalized (with perforation or rupture)
      K35.2
      localized (with perforation or rupture)
      K35.3
  acute (catarrhal) (fulminating) (gangrenous)
    (obstructive) (retrocecal) (suppurative)
    K35.80
    with
      peritoneal abscess K35.3
      peritonitis NEC K35.3
        generalized (with perforation or rupture)
        K35.2
        localized (with perforation or rupture)
        K35.3
      specified NEC K35.89
  amebic A06.89
  chronic (recurrent) K36
  exacerbation -*see* Appendicitis, acute
  gangrenous -*see* Appendicitis, acute
  healed (obliterative) K36
  interval K36
  neurogenic K36
  obstructive K36
  recurrent K36
  relapsing K36
  subacute (adhesive) K36
  subsiding K36
  suppurative -*see* Appendicitis, acute
  tuberculous A18.32
Appendicopathia oxyurica B80
Appendix, appendicular -*see also* condition
  epididymis Q55.4
  Morgagni
    female Q50.5
    male (epididymal) Q55.4
      testicular Q55.29
  testis Q55.29
Appetite
  depraved -*see* Pica
  excessive R63.2
  lack or loss -*see also* Anorexia R63.0
    nonorganic origin F50.89
    psychogenic F50.89
  perverted (hysterical) -*see* Pica
Apple peel syndrome Q41.1
Apprehension state F41.1
Apprehensiveness, abnormal F41.9
Approximal wear K03.0

Apraxia (classic) (ideational) (ideokinetic)
  (ideomotor) (motor) (verbal) R48.2
  following
    cerebrovascular disease I69.990
      cerebral infarction I69.390
      intracerebral hemorrhage I69.190
      nontraumatic intracranial hemorrhage NEC
      I69.290
      specified disease NEC I69.890
      subarachnoid hemorrhage I69.090
  oculomotor, congenital H51.8
Aptyalism K11.7
Apudoma -*see* Neoplasm, uncertain behavior,
  by site
Aqueous misdirection H40.83
Arabicum elephantiasis -*see* Infestation,
  filarial
Arachnitis -*see* Meningitis
Arachnodactyly -*see* Syndrome, Marfan's
Arachnoiditis (acute) (adhesive) (basal)
  (brain) (cerebrospinal) -*see* Meningitis
Arachnophobia F40.210
Arboencephalitis, Australian A83.4
Arborization block (heart) I45.5
ARC (AIDS-related complex) B20
Arches -*see* condition
Arcuate uterus Q51.810
Arcuatus uterus Q51.810
Arcus (cornea) senilis -*see* Degeneration,
  cornea, senile
Arc-welder's lung J63.4
Areflexia R29.2
Areola -*see* condition
Argentaffinoma -*see also* Neoplasm, uncertain
  behavior, by site
  malignant -*see* Neoplasm, malignant, by site
  syndrome E34.0
Argininemia E72.21
Arginosuccinic aciduria E72.22
Argyll Robertson phenomenon, pupil or
  syndrome (syphilitic) A52.19
  atypical H57.09
  nonsyphilitic H57.09
Argyria, argyriasis
  conjunctival H11.13
  from drug or medicament -*see* Table of Drugs
  and Chemicals, by substance
Argyrosis, conjunctival H11.13
Arhinencephaly Q04.1
Ariboflavinosis E53.0
Arm -*see* condition
Arnold-Chiari disease, obstruction or
  syndrome (type II) Q07.00
  with
    hydrocephalus Q07.02
      with spina bifida Q07.03
    spina bifida Q07.01
      with hydrocephalus Q07.03
  type III -*see* Encephalocele
  type IV Q04.8
Aromatic amino-acid metabolism disorder
  E70.9
  specified NEC E70.8
Arousals, confusional G47.51
Arrest, arrested
  cardiac I46.9
    complicating
      abortion -*see* Abortion, by type,
  complicated by, cardiac arrest

Arrest, arrested --*continued*
  anesthesia (general) (local) or other
  sedation -*see* Table of Drugs and Chemicals,
  by drug,
    in labor and delivery O74.2
    in pregnancy O29.11
    postpartum, puerperal O89.1
    delivery (cesarean) (instrumental) O75.4
  due to
    cardiac condition I46.2
    specified condition NEC I46.8
  intraoperative I97.71
  newborn P29.81
  postprocedural I97.12
    obstetric procedure O75.4
  cardiorespiratory -*see* Arrest, cardiac
  circulatory -*see* Arrest, cardiac
  deep transverse O64.0
  development or growth
    bone -*see* Disorder, bone, development or
  growth
    child R62.50
    tracheal rings Q32.1
  epiphyseal
    complete
      femur M89.15
      humerus M89.12
      tibia M89.16
      ulna M89.13
      forearm M89.13
        specified NEC M89.13
        ulna -*see* Arrest, epiphyseal, by type, ulna
      lower leg M89.16
        specified NEC M89.168
        tibia -*see* Arrest, epiphyseal, by type, tibia
    partial
      femur M89.15
      humerus M89.12
      tibia M89.16
      ulna M89.13
      specified NEC M89.18
  granulopoiesis -*see* Agranulocytosis
  growth plate -*see* Arrest, epiphyseal
  heart -*see* Arrest, cardiac
  legal, anxiety concerning Z65.3
  physeal -*see* Arrest, epiphyseal
  respiratory R09.2
    newborn P28.81
  sinus I45.5
  spermatogenesis (complete) -*see*
  Azoospermia
    incomplete -*see* Oligospermia
  transverse (deep) O64.0
Arrhenoblastoma
  benign
    specified site -*see* Neoplasm, benign, by site
    unspecified site
      female D27.9
      male D29.20
  malignant
    specified site -*see* Neoplasm, malignant, by
  site
    unspecified site
      female C56.9
      male C62.90
  specified site -*see* Neoplasm, uncertain
  behavior, by site
  unspecified site
    female D39.10
    male D40.10

Arrhythmia (auricle) (cardiac)
(juvenile)(nodal) (reflex) (sinus)
(supraventricular)(transitory)(ventricle) I49.9
  block I45.9
  extrasystolic I49.49
  newborn
    bradycardia P29.12
    occurring before birth P03.819
      before onset of labor P03.810
      during labor P03.811
    tachycardia P29.11
  psychogenic F45.8
  specified NEC I49.8
  vagal R55
  ventricular re-entry I47.0
**Arrillaga-Ayerza syndrome (pulmonary
sclerosis with pulmonary hypertension)**
I27.0
Arsenical pigmentation L81.8
  from drug or medicament -*see* Table of Drugs
  and Chemicals
Arsenism -*see* Poisoning, arsenic
Arterial -*see* condition
Arteriofibrosis -*see* Arteriosclerosis
Arteriolar sclerosis -*see* Arteriosclerosis
Arteriolith -*see* Arteriosclerosis
Arteriolitis I77.6
  necrotizing, kidney I77.5
  renal -*see* Hypertension, kidney
Arteriolosclerosis -*see* Arteriosclerosis
Arterionephrosclerosis -*see* Hypertension,
kidney
Arteriopathy I77.9
Arteriosclerosis, arteriosclerotic (diffuse)
(obliterans) (of) (senile) (with calcification)
I70.90
  aorta I70.0
  arteries of extremities -*see* Arteriosclerosis,
    extremities
  brain I67.2
  bypass graft
    coronary -*see* Arteriosclerosis, coronary,
    bypass graft
    extremities -*see* Arteriosclerosis,
    extremities, bypass graft
  cardiac -*see* Disease, heart, ischemic,
    atherosclerotic
  cardiopathy -*see* Disease, heart, ischemic,
    atherosclerotic
  cardiorenal -*see* Hypertension, cardiorenal
  cardiovascular -*see* Disease, heart, ischemic,
    atherosclerotic
  carotid -*see also* Occlusion, artery, carotid
    I65.2
  central nervous system I67.2
  cerebral I67.2
  cerebrovascular I67.2
  coronary (artery) I25.10
    due to
      calcified coronary lesion (severely) I25.84
      lipid rich plaque I25.83
    bypass graft I25.810
      with
        angina pectoris I25.709
          with documented spasm I25.701
          specified type NEC I25.708
          unstable I25.700
        ischemic chest pain I25.709
      autologous artery I25.810
        with
          angina pectoris I25.729

Arteriosclerosis, arteriosclerotic --*continued*
          with documented spasm I25.721
          specified type I25.728
          unstable I25.720
        ischemic chest pain I25.729
      autologous vein I25.810
        with
          angina pectoris I25.719
            with documented spasm I25.711
            specified type I25.718
            unstable I25.710
          ischemic chest pain I25.719
      nonautologous biological I25.810
        with
          angina pectoris I25.739
            with documented spasm I25.731
            specified type I25.738
            unstable I25.730
          ischemic chest pain I25.739
      specified type NEC I25.810
        with
          angina pectoris I25.799
            with documented spasm I25.791
            specified type I25.798
            unstable I25.790
          ischemic chest pain I25.799
    native vessel
      with
        angina pectoris I25.119
          with documented spasm I25.111
          specified type NEC I25.118
          unstable I25.110
        ischemic chest pain I25.119
    transplanted heart I25.811
      bypass graft I25.812
        with
          angina pectoris I25.769
            with documented spasm I25.761
            specified type I25.768
            unstable I25.760
          ischemic chest pain I25.769
      native coronary artery I25.811
        with
          angina pectoris I25.759
            with documented spasm I25.751
            specified type I25.758
            unstable I25.750
          ischemic chest pain I25.759
  extremities (native arteries) I70.209
    bypass graft I70.309
      autologous vein graft I70.409
      leg I70.409
        with
          gangrene (and intermittent
          claudication, rest pain and ulcer)
          I70.469
          intermittent claudication I70.419
          rest pain (and intermittent
          claudication) I70.429
      bilateral I70.403
        with
          gangrene (and intermittent
          claudication, rest pain and ulcer)
          I70.463
          intermittent claudication I70.413
          rest pain (and intermittent
          claudication) I70.423
          specified type NEC I70.493
      left I70.402
        with

Arteriosclerosis, arteriosclerotic --*continued*
    gangrene (and intermittent
      claudication, rest pain and ulcer)
      I70.462
    intermittent claudication I70.412
    rest pain (and intermittent
      claudication) I70.422
    ulceration (and intermittent
      claudication and rest pain) I70.449
      ankle I70.443
      calf I70.442
      foot site NEC I70.445
      heel I70.444
      lower leg NEC I70.448
      midfoot I70.444
      thigh I70.441
    specified type NEC I70.492
   right I70.401
    with
      gangrene (and intermittent
        claudication, rest pain and ulcer)
        I70.461
      intermittent claudication I70.411
      rest pain (and intermittent
        claudication) I70.421
      ulceration (and intermittent
        claudication and rest pain) I70.439
        ankle I70.433
        calf I70.432
        foot site NEC I70.435
        heel I70.434
        lower leg NEC I70.438
        midfoot I70.434
        thigh I70.431
      specified type NEC I70.491
    specified type NEC I70.499
   specified NEC I70.408
    with
      gangrene (and intermittent
        claudication, rest pain and ulcer)
        I70.468
      intermittent claudication I70.418
      rest pain (and intermittent
        claudication) I70.428
      ulceration (and intermittent
        claudication and rest pain) I70.45
      specified type NEC I70.498
   leg I70.309
    with
      gangrene (and intermittent claudication,
      rest pain and ulcer) I70.369
      intermittent claudication I70.319
      rest pain (and intermittent claudication)
        I70.329
   bilateral I70.303
    with
      gangrene (and intermittent
        claudication, rest pain and ulcer)
        I70.363
      intermittent claudication I70.313
      rest pain (and intermittent
        claudication) I70.323
      specified type NEC I70.393
   left I70.302
    with
      gangrene (and intermittent
        claudication, rest pain and ulcer)
        I70.362
      intermittent claudication I70.312

Arteriosclerosis, arteriosclerotic --*continued*
    rest pain (and intermittent
      claudication) I70.322
    ulceration (and intermittent
    claudication and rest pain) I70.349
      ankle I70.343
      calf I70.342
      foot site NEC I70.345
      heel I70.344
      lower leg NEC I70.348
      midfoot I70.344
      thigh I70.341
    specified type NEC I70.392
   right I70.301
    with
      gangrene (and intermittent
        claudication, rest pain and ulcer)
        I70.361
      intermittent claudication I70.311
      rest pain (and intermittent
        claudication) I70.321
      ulceration (and intermittent
        claudication and rest pain) I70.339
        ankle I70.333
        calf I70.332
        foot site NEC I70.335
        heel I70.334
        lower leg NEC I70.338
        midfoot I70.334
        thigh I70.331
      specified type NEC I70.391
    specified type NEC I70.399
   nonautologous biological graft I70.509
    leg I70.509
      with
        gangrene (and intermittent
          claudication, rest pain and ulcer)
          I70.569
        intermittent claudication I70.519
        rest pain (and intermittent
          claudication) I70.529
    bilateral I70.503
      with
        gangrene (and intermittent
          claudication, rest pain and ulcer)
          I70.563
        intermittent claudication I70.513
        rest pain (and intermittent
          claudication) I70.523
        specified type NEC I70.593
    left I70.502
      with
        gangrene (and intermittent
          claudication, rest pain and ulcer)
          I70.562
        intermittent claudication I70.512
        rest pain (and intermittent
          claudication) I70.522
        ulceration (and intermittent
        claudication and rest pain) I70.549
        ankle I70.543
        calf I70.542
        foot site NEC I70.545
        heel I70.544
        lower leg NEC I70.548
        midfoot I70.544
        thigh I70.541
      specified type NEC I70.592
    right I70.501
      with

Arteriosclerosis, arteriosclerotic --*continued*
    gangrene (and intermittent
      claudication, rest pain and ulcer)
      I70.561
    intermittent claudication I70.511
    rest pain (and intermittent
      claudication) I70.521
    ulceration (and intermittent
    claudication and rest pain) I70.539
      ankle I70.533
      calf I70.532
      foot site NEC I70.535
      heel I70.534
      lower leg NEC I70.538
      midfoot I70.534
      thigh I70.531
    specified type NEC I70.591
   specified type NEC I70.599
  specified NEC I70.508
    with
      gangrene (and intermittent
        claudication, rest pain and ulcer)
        I70.568
      intermittent claudication I70.518
      rest pain (and intermittent
        claudication) I70.528
      ulceration (and intermittent
        claudication and rest pain) I70.55
      specified type NEC I70.598
  nonbiological graft I70.609
   leg I70.609
    with
      gangrene (and intermittent
        claudication, rest pain and ulcer)
        I70.669
      intermittent claudication I70.619
      rest pain (and intermittent
        claudication) I70.629
   bilateral I70.603
    with
      gangrene (and intermittent
        claudication, rest pain and ulcer)
        I70.663
      intermittent claudication I70.613
      rest pain (and intermittent
        claudication) I70.623
      specified type NEC I70.693
   left I70.602
    with
      gangrene (and intermittent
        claudication, rest pain and ulcer)
        I70.662
      intermittent claudication I70.612
      rest pain (and intermittent
        claudication) I70.622
      ulceration (and intermittent
      claudication and rest pain) I70.649
        ankle I70.643
        calf I70.642
        foot site NEC I70.645
        heel I70.644
        lower leg NEC I70.648
        midfoot I70.644
        thigh I70.641
      specified type NEC I70.692
   right I70.601
    with
      gangrene (and intermittent
        claudication, rest pain and ulcer)
        I70.661
      intermittent claudication I70.611

Arteriosclerosis, arteriosclerotic --*continued*
    rest pain (and intermittent claudication) I70.621
    ulceration (and intermittent claudication and rest pain) I70.639
      ankle I70.633
      calf I70.632
      foot site NEC I70.635
      heel I70.634
      lower leg NEC I70.638
      midfoot I70.634
      thigh I70.631
    specified type NEC I70.691
    specified type NEC I70.699
  specified NEC I70.608
    with
      gangrene (and intermittent claudication, rest pain and ulcer) I70.668
      intermittent claudication I70.618
      rest pain (and intermittent claudication) I70.628
      ulceration (and intermittent claudication and rest pain) I70.65
    specified type NEC I70.698
  specified graft NEC I70.709
  leg I70.709
    with
      gangrene (and intermittent claudication, rest pain and ulcer) I70.769
      intermittent claudication I70.719
      rest pain (and intermittent claudication) I70.729
    bilateral I70.703
      with
        gangrene (and intermittent claudication, rest pain and ulcer) I70.763
        intermittent claudication I70.713
        rest pain (and intermittent claudication) I70.723
      specified type NEC I70.793
    left I70.702
      with
        gangrene (and intermittent claudication, rest pain and ulcer) I70.762
        intermittent claudication I70.712
        rest pain (and intermittent claudication) I70.722
        ulceration (and intermittent claudication and rest pain) I70.749
          ankle I70.743
          calf I70.742
          foot site NEC I70.745
          heel I70.744
          lower leg NEC I70.748
          midfoot I70.744
          thigh I70.741
      specified type NEC I70.792
    right I70.701
      with
        gangrene (and intermittent claudication, rest pain and ulcer) I70.761
        intermittent claudication I70.711
        rest pain (and intermittent claudication) I70.721
        ulceration (and intermittent claudication and rest pain) I70.739

Arteriosclerosis, arteriosclerotic --*continued*
          ankle I70.733
          calf I70.732
          foot site NEC I70.735
          heel I70.734
          lower leg NEC I70.738
          midfoot I70.734
          thigh I70.731
      specified type NEC I70.791
    specified type NEC I70.799
  specified NEC I70.708
    with
      gangrene (and intermittent claudication, rest pain and ulcer) I70.768
      intermittent claudication I70.718
      rest pain (and intermittent claudication) I70.728
      ulceration (and intermittent claudication and rest pain) I70.75
    specified type NEC I70.798
  specified NEC I70.308
    with
      gangrene (and intermittent claudication, rest pain and ulcer) I70.368
      intermittent claudication I70.318
      rest pain (and intermittent claudication) I70.328
      ulceration (and intermittent claudication and rest pain) I70.35
    specified type NEC I70.398
  leg I70.209
    with
      gangrene (and intermittent claudication, rest pain and ulcer) I70.269
      intermittent claudication I70.219
      rest pain (and intermittent claudication) I70.229
    bilateral I70.203
      with
        gangrene (and intermittent claudication, rest pain and ulcer) I70.263
        intermittent claudication I70.213
        rest pain (and intermittent claudication) I70.223
      specified type NEC I70.293
    left I70.202
      with
        gangrene (and intermittent claudication, rest pain and ulcer) I70.262
        intermittent claudication I70.212
        rest pain (and intermittent claudication) I70.222
        ulceration (and intermittent claudication and rest pain) I70.249
          ankle I70.243
          calf I70.242
          foot site NEC I70.245
          heel I70.244
          lower leg NEC I70.248
          midfoot I70.244
          thigh I70.241
      specified type NEC I70.292
    right I70.201
      with
        gangrene (and intermittent claudication, rest pain and ulcer) I70.261
        intermittent claudication I70.211
        rest pain (and intermittent claudication) I70.221

Arteriosclerosis, arteriosclerotic --*continued*
  ulceration (and intermittent claudication and rest pain) I70.239
    ankle I70.233
    calf I70.232
    foot site NEC I70.235
    heel I70.234
    lower leg NEC I70.238
    midfoot I70.234
    thigh I70.231
  specified type NEC I70.291
  specified type NEC I70.299
  specified site NEC I70.208
    with
      gangrene (and intermittent claudication, rest pain and ulcer) I70.268
      intermittent claudication I70.218
      rest pain (and intermittent claudication) I70.228
      ulceration (and intermittent claudication and rest pain) I70.25
    specified type NEC I70.298
  generalized I70.91
  heart (disease) -*see* Arteriosclerosis, coronary (artery),   kidney -*see* Hypertension, kidney
  medial -*see* Arteriosclerosis, extremities
  mesenteric (artery) K55.1
  Mönckeberg's -*see* Arteriosclerosis, extremities
  myocarditis I51.4
  peripheral (of extremities) -*see* Arteriosclerosis, extremities
  pulmonary (idiopathic) I27.0
  renal (arterioles) -*see also* Hypertension, kidney
    artery I70.1
  retina (vascular) I70.8 [*H35.0*]
  specified artery NEC I70.8
  spinal (cord) G95.19
  vertebral (artery) I67.2
Arteriospasm I73.9
Arteriovenous -*see* condition
Arteritis I77.6
  allergic M31.0
  aorta (nonsyphilitic) I77.6
    syphilitic A52.02
  aortic arch M31.4
  brachiocephalic M31.4
  brain I67.7
    syphilitic A52.04
  cerebral I67.7
    in
      diseases classified elsewhere I68.2
      systemic lupus erythematosus M32.19
    listerial A32.89
    syphilitic A52.04
    tuberculous A18.89
  coronary (artery) I25.89
    rheumatic I01.8
      chronic I09.89
    syphilitic A52.06
  cranial (left) (right), giant cell M31.6
  deformans -*see* Arteriosclerosis
  giant cell NEC M31.6
    with polymyalgia rheumatica M31.5
  necrosing or necrotizing M31.9
    specified NEC M31.8
  nodosa M30.0
  obliterans -*see* Arteriosclerosis
  pulmonary I28.8
  rheumatic -*see* Fever, rheumatic

Arteritis - *continued*
senile *-see* Arteriosclerosis
suppurative I77.2
syphilitic (general) A52.09
  brain A52.04
  coronary A52.06
  spinal A52.09
temporal, giant cell M31.6
young female aortic arch syndrome M31.4
Artery, arterial *-see also* condition
abscess I77.89
single umbilical Q27.0
Arthralgia (allergic) *-see also* Pain, joint
in caisson disease T70.3
temporomandibular M26.62
Arthritis, arthritic (acute) (chronic)
(nonpyogenic) (subacute) M19.90
allergic *-see* Arthritis, specified form NEC
ankylosing (crippling) (spine) *-see also*
Spondylitis, ankylosing
  sites other than spine *-see* Arthritis, specified
  form NEC
atrophic *-see* Osteoarthritis
  spine *-see* Spondylitis, ankylosing
back *-see* Spondylopathy, inflammatory
blennorrhagic (gonococcal) A54.42
Charcot's *-see* Arthropathy, neuropathic
  diabetic *-see* Diabetes, arthropathy,
  neuropathic
syringomyelic G95.0
chylous (filarial) *-see also* category M01
B74.9
climacteric (any site) NEC *-see* Arthritis,
  specified form NEC
crystal (induced) *-see* Arthritis, in, crystals
deformans *-see* Osteoarthritis
degenerative *-see* Osteoarthritis
due to or associated with
  acromegaly E22.0
  brucellosis *-see* Brucellosis
  caisson disease T70.3
  diabetes *-see* Diabetes, arthropathy
  dracontiasis *-see also* category M01 B72
  enteritis NEC
    regional *-see* Enteritis, regional
  erysipelas *-see also* category M01 A46
  erythema
    epidemic A25.1
    nodosum L52
  filariasis NOS B74.9
  glanders A24.0
  helminthiasis *-see also* category M01 B83.9
  hemophilia D66 *[M36.2]*
  Henoch- (Schönlein) purpura D69.0 *[M36.4]*
  human parvovirus *-see also* category M01
  B97.6
  infectious disease NEC *-see* category M01
  leprosy (see also category M01) *-see also*
  Leprosy A30.9
  Lyme disease A69.23
  mycobacteria *-see also* category M01 A31.8
  parasitic disease NEC *-see also* category
  M01 B89
  paratyphoid fever (see also category M01) -
  see also Fever, paratyphoid A01.4
  rat bite fever *-see also* category M01 A25.1
  regional enteritis *-see* Enteritis, regional
  respiratory disorder NOS J98.9
  serum sickness *-see also* Reaction, serum
  T80.69
  syringomyelia G95.0

Arthritis, arthritic *--continued*
typhoid fever A01.04
epidemic erythema A25.1
febrile *-see* Fever, rheumatic
gonococcal A54.42
gouty (acute) *-see* Gout
in (due to)
  acromegaly *-see also* subcategory M14.8
  E22.0
  amyloidosis *-see also* subcategory M14.8
  E85.4
  bacterial disease *-see also* subcategory M01
  A49.9
  Behçet's syndrome M35.2
  caisson disease *-see also* subcategory
  M14.8 T70.3
  coliform bacilli (Escherichia coli) *-see*
  Arthritis, in, pyogenic organism NEC
  crystals M11.9
    dicalcium phosphate *-see* Arthritis, in,
crystals, specified type NEC
    hydroxyapatite M11.0
    pyrophosphate *-see* Arthritis, in, crystals,
specified type NEC
    specified type NEC M11.80
      ankle M11.87
      elbow M11.82
      foot joint M11.87
      hand joint M11.84
      hip M11.85
      knee M11.86
      multiple sites M11.8
      shoulder M11.81
      vertebrae M11.88
      wrist M11.83
  dermatoarthritis, lipoid E78.81
  dracontiasis (dracunculiasis) *-see also*
  category M01 B72
  endocrine disorder NEC *-see also*
  subcategory M14.8 E34.9
  enteritis, infectious NEC *-see also* category
  M01 A09
    specified organism NEC *-see also* category
    M01 A08.8
  erythema
    multiforme *-see also* subcategory M14.8
    L51.9
    nodosum *-see also* subcategory M14.8
    L52
  gout *-see* Gout
  helminthiasis NEC *-see also* category M01
  B83.9
  hemochromatosis *-see also* subcategory
  M14.8 E83.118
  hemoglobinopathy NEC D58.2 *[M36.3]*
  hemophilia NEC D66 *[M36.2]*
  Hemophilus influenzae M00.8 *[B96.3]*
  Henoch (Schönlein) purpura D69.0 *[M36.4]*
  hyperparathyroidism NEC *-see also*
  subcategory M14.8 E21.3
  hypersensitivity reaction NEC T78.49
  [M36.4]
  hypogammaglobulinemia *-see also*
  subcategory M14.8 D80.1
  hypothyroidism NEC *-see also* subcategory
  M14.8 E03.9
  infection *-see* Arthritis, pyogenic or pyemic
    spine *-see* Spondylopathy, infective
  infectious disease NEC *-see* category M01
  leprosy *-see also* category M01 A30.9
  leukemia NEC C95.9 *[M36.1]*

Arthritis, arthritic *--continued*
lipoid dermatoarthritis E78.81
Lyme disease A69.23
Mediterranean fever, familial *-see also*
subcategory M14.8 M04.1
Meningococcus A39.83
metabolic disorder NEC *-see also*
subcategory M14.8 E88.9
multiple myelomatosis C90.0 *[M36.1]*
mumps B26.85
mycosis NEC *-see also* category M01 B49
myelomatosis (multiple) C90.0 *[M36.1]*
neurological disorder NEC G98.0
ochronosis *-see also* subcategory M14.8
E70.29
O'nyong-nyong *-see also* category M01
A92.1
parasitic disease NEC *-see also* category
M01 B89
paratyphoid fever *-see also* category M01
A01.4
Pseudomonas *-see* Arthritis, pyogenic,
bacterial NEC
psoriasis L40.50
pyogenic organism NEC *-see* Arthritis,
pyogenic, bacterial NEC
Reiter's disease *-see* Reiter's disease
respiratory disorder NEC *-see also*
subcategory M14.8 J98.9
reticulosis, malignant *-see also* subcategory
M14.8 C86.0
rubella B06.82
Salmonella (arizonae) (cholerae-suis)
(enteritidis) (typhimurium) A02.23
sarcoidosis D86.86
specified bacteria NEC *-see* Arthritis,
pyogenic, bacterial NEC
sporotrichosis B42.82
syringomyelia G95.0
thalassemia NEC D56.9 *[M36.3]*
tuberculosis *-see* Tuberculosis, arthritis
typhoid fever A01.04
urethritis, Reiter's *-see* Reiter's disease
viral disease NEC *-see also* category M01
B34.9
infectious or infective *-see also* Arthritis,
pyogenic or pyemic
spine *-see* Spondylopathy, infective
juvenile M08.90
  with systemic onset *-see* Still's disease
  ankle M08.97
  elbow M08.92
  foot joint M08.97
  hand joint M08.94
  hip M08.95
  knee M08.96
  multiple site M08.99
  pauciarticular M08.40
    ankle M08.47
    elbow M08.42
    foot joint M08.47
    hand joint M08.44
    hip M08.45
    knee M08.46
    shoulder M08.41
    vertebrae M08.48
    wrist M08.43
  psoriatic L40.54
  rheumatoid *-see* Arthritis, rheumatoid,
  juvenile
  shoulder M08.91

Arthritis, arthritic --*continued*
  vertebra M08.98
  specified type NEC M08.80
    ankle M08.87
    elbow M08.82
    foot joint M08.87
    hand joint M08.84
    hip M08.85
    knee M08.86
    multiple site M08.89
    shoulder M08.81
    specified joint NEC M08.88
    vertebrae M08.88
    wrist M08.83
  wrist M08.93
  meaning osteoarthritis -*see* Osteoarthritis
  meningococcal A39.83
  menopausal (any site) NEC -*see* Arthritis,
    specified form NEC
  mutilans (psoriatic) L40.52
  mycotic NEC -*see also* category M01 B49
  neuropathic (Charcot) -*see* Arthropathy,
    neuropathic
    diabetic -*see* Diabetes, arthropathy,
      neuropathic
    nonsyphilitic NEC G98.0
    syringomyelic G95.0
  ochronotic -*see also* subcategory M14.8
    E70.29
  palindromic (any site) -*see* Rheumatism,
    palindromic
  pneumococcal M00.10
    ankle M00.17
    elbow M00.12
    foot joint -*see* Arthritis, pneumococcal,
      ankle
    hand joint M00.14
    hip M00.15
    knee M00.16
    multiple site M00.19
    shoulder M00.11
    vertebra M00.18
    wrist M00.13
  postdysenteric -*see* Arthropathy,
    postdysenteric
  postmeningococcal A39.84
  postrheumatic, chronic -*see* Arthropathy,
    postrheumatic, chronic
  primary progressive -*see also* Arthritis,
    specified form NEC
    spine -*see* Spondylitis, ankylosing
  psoriatic L40.50
  purulent (any site except spine) -*see* Arthritis,
    pyogenic or pyemic
    spine -*see* Spondylopathy, infective
  pyogenic or pyemic (any site except spine)
    M00.9
    bacterial NEC M00.80
      ankle M00.87
      elbow M00.82
      foot joint -*see* Arthritis, pyogenic, bacterial
        NEC, ankle
      hand joint M00.84
      hip M00.85
      knee M00.86
      multiple site M00.89
      shoulder M00.81
      vertebra M00.88
      wrist M00.83
    pneumococcal -*see* Arthritis, pneumococcal
    spine -*see* Spondylopathy, infective

Arthritis, arthritic --*continued*
  staphylococcal -*see* Arthritis, staphylococcal
  streptococcal -*see* Arthritis, streptococcal
    NEC
    pneumococcal -*see* Arthritis,
      pneumococcal
  reactive -*see* Reiter's disease
  rheumatic -*see also* Arthritis, rheumatoid
    acute or subacute -*see* Fever, rheumatic
  rheumatoid M06.9
    with
      carditis -*see* Rheumatoid, carditis
      endocarditis -*see* Rheumatoid, carditis
      heart involvement NEC -*see* Rheumatoid,
        carditis
      lung involvement -*see* Rheumatoid, lung
      myocarditis -*see* Rheumatoid, carditis
      myopathy -*see* Rheumatoid, myopathy
      pericarditis -*see* Rheumatoid, carditis
      polyneuropathy -*see* Rheumatoid,
        polyneuropathy
      rheumatoid factor -*see* Arthritis,
        rheumatoid, seropositive
      splenoadenomegaly and leukopenia -*see*
        Felty's syndrome
      vasculitis -*see* Rheumatoid, vasculitis
      visceral involvement NEC -*see*
        Rheumatoid, arthritis, with involvement
        of organs NEC
    juvenile (with or without rheumatoid factor)
      M08.00
      ankle M08.07
      elbow M08.02
      foot joint M08.07
      hand joint M08.04
      hip M08.05
      knee M08.06
      multiple site M08.09
      shoulder M08.01
      vertebra M08.08
      wrist M08.03
    seronegative M06.00
      ankle M06.07
      elbow M06.02
      foot joint M06.07
      hand joint M06.04
      hip M06.05
      knee M06.06
      multiple site M06.09
      shoulder M06.01
      vertebra M06.08
      wrist M06.03
    seropositive M05.9
      specified NEC M05.80
        ankle M05.87
        elbow M05.82
        foot joint M05.87
        hand joint M05.84
        hip M05.85
        knee M05.86
        multiple sites M05.89
        shoulder M05.81
        vertebra -*see* Spondylitis, ankylosing
        wrist M05.83
      without organ involvement M05.70
        ankle M05.77
        elbow M05.72
        foot joint M05.77
        hand joint M05.74
        hip M05.75
        knee M05.76

Arthritis, arthritic --*continued*
      multiple sites M05.79
      shoulder M05.71
      vertebra -*see* Spondylitis, ankylosing
      wrist M05.73
    specified type NEC M06.80
      ankle M06.87
      elbow M06.82
      foot joint M06.87
      hand joint M06.84
      hip M06.85
      knee M06.86
      multiple site M06.89
      shoulder M06.81
      vertebra M06.88
      wrist M06.83
    spine -*see* Spondylitis, ankylosing
  rubella B06.82
  scorbutic -*see also* subcategory M14.8 E54
  senile or senescent -*see* Osteoarthritis
  septic (any site except spine) -*see* Arthritis,
    pyogenic or pyemic
    spine -*see* Spondylopathy, infective
  serum (nontherapeutic) (therapeutic) -*see*
    Arthropathy, postimmunization
  specified form NEC M13.80
    ankle M13.87
    elbow M13.82
    foot joint M13.87
    hand joint M13.84
    hip M13.85
    knee M13.86
    multiple site M13.89
    shoulder M13.81
    specified joint NEC M13.88
    wrist M13.83
  spine -*see also* Spondylopathy, inflammatory
    infectious or infective NEC -*see*
      Spondylopathy, infective
    Marie-Strümpell -*see* Spondylitis,
      ankylosing
    pyogenic -*see* Spondylopathy, infective
    rheumatoid -*see* Spondylitis, ankylosing
    traumatic (old) -*see* Spondylopathy,
      traumatic
    tuberculous A18.01
  staphylococcal M00.00
    ankle M00.07
    elbow M00.02
    foot joint -*see* Arthritis, staphylococcal,
  ankle
    hand joint M00.04
    hip M00.05
    knee M00.06
    multiple site M00.09
    shoulder M00.01
    vertebra M00.08
    wrist M00.03
  streptococcal NEC M00.20
    ankle M00.27
    elbow M00.22
    foot joint -*see* Arthritis, streptococcal, ankle
    hand joint M00.24
    hip M00.25
    knee M00.26
    multiple site M00.29
    shoulder M00.21
    vertebra M00.28
    wrist M00.23
  suppurative -*see* Arthritis, pyogenic or pyemic
  syphilitic (late) A52.16

Arthritis, arthritic --*continued*
   congenital A50.55 [*M12.80*]
   syphilitica deformans (Charcot) A52.16
   temporomandibular M26.69
   toxic of menopause (any site) -*see* Arthritis, specified form NEC
   transient -*see* Arthropathy, specified form NEC
   traumatic (chronic) -*see* Arthropathy, traumatic
   tuberculous A18.02
      spine A18.01
   uratic -*see* Gout
   urethritica (Reiter's) -*see* Reiter's disease
   vertebral -*see* Spondylopathy, inflammatory
   villous (any site) -*see* Arthropathy, specified form NEC
Arthrocele -*see* Effusion, joint
Arthrodesis status Z98.1
Arthrodynia -*see also* Pain, joint
Arthrodysplasia Q74.9
Arthrofibrosis, joint -*see* Ankylosis
Arthrogryposis (congenital) Q68.8
   multiplex congenita Q74.3
Arthrokatadysis M24.7
Arthropathy -*see also* Arthritis M12.9
   Charcot's -*see* Arthropathy, neuropathic
      diabetic -*see* Diabetes, arthropathy, neuropathic
      syringomyelic G95.0
   cricoarytenoid J38.7
   crystal (induced) -*see* Arthritis, in, crystals
   diabetic NEC -*see* Diabetes, arthropathy
   distal interphalangeal, psoriatic L40.51
   enteropathic M07.60
      ankle M07.67
      elbow M07.62
      foot joint M07.67
      hand joint M07.64
      hip M07.65
      knee M07.66
      multiple site M07.69
      shoulder M07.61
      vertebra M07.68
      wrist M07.63
   following intestinal bypass M02.00
      ankle M02.07
      elbow M02.02
      foot joint M02.07
      hand joint M02.04
      hip M02.05
      knee M02.06
      multiple site M02.09
      shoulder M02.01
      vertebra M02.08
      wrist M02.03
   gouty -*see also* Gout
      in (due to)
         Lesch-Nyhan syndrome E79.1 [*M14.8*]
         sickle-cell disorders D57 [*M14.8*]
   hemophilic NEC D66 [*M36.2*]
      in (due to)
         hyperparathyroidism NEC E21.3 [*M14.8*]
         metabolic disease NOS E88.9 [*M14.8*]
   in (due to)
      acromegaly E22.0 [*M14.8*]
      amyloidosis E85.4 [*M14.8*]
      blood disorder NOS D75.9 [*M36.3*]
      diabetes -*see* Diabetes, arthropathy
      endocrine disease NOS E34.9 [*M14.8*]
      erythema

Arthropathy --*continued*
      multiforme L51.9 [*M14.8*]
         nodosum L52 [*M14.8*]
      hemochromatosis E83.118 [*M14.8*]
      hemoglobinopathy NEC D58.2 [*M36.3*]
      hemophilia NEC D66 [*M36.2*]
      Henoch-Schönlein purpura D69.0 [*M36.4*]
      hyperthyroidism E05.90 [*M14.8*]
      hypothyroidism E03.9 [*M14.8*]
      infective endocarditis I33.0 [*M12.80*]
      leukemia NEC C95.9 [*M36.1*]
      malignant histiocytosis C96.A [*M36.1*]
      metabolic disease NOS E88.9 [*M14.8*]
      multiple myeloma C90.0 [*M36.1*]
      neoplastic disease NOS (see also Neoplasm) D49.9 [*M36.1*]
      nutritional deficiency -*see also* subcategory M14.8 E63.9
      psoriasis NOS L40.50
      sarcoidosis D86.86
      syphilis (late) A52.77
         congenital A50.55 [*M12.80*]
      thyrotoxicosis -*see also* subcategory M14.8 E05.90
      ulcerative colitis K51.90 [*M07.60*]
      viral hepatitis (postinfectious) NEC B19.9 [*M12.80*]
      Whipple's disease -*see also* subcategory M14.8 K90.81
   Jaccoud -*see* Arthropathy, postrheumatic, chronic
   juvenile -*see* Arthritis, juvenile
      psoriatic L40.54
   mutilans (psoriatic) L40.52
   neuropathic (Charcot) M14.60
      ankle M14.67
      diabetic -*see* Diabetes, arthropathy, neuropathic
      elbow M14.62
      foot joint M14.67
      hand joint M14.64
      hip M14.65
      knee M14.66
      multiple site M14.69
      nonsyphilitic NEC G98.0
      shoulder M14.61
      syringomyelic G95.0
      vertebra M14.68
      wrist M14.63
   osteopulmonary -*see* Osteoarthropathy, hypertrophic, specified NEC
   postdysenteric M02.10
      ankle M02.17
      elbow M02.12
      foot joint M02.17
      hand joint M02.14
      hip M02.15
      knee M02.16
      multiple site M02.19
      shoulder M02.11
      vertebra M02.18
      wrist M02.13
   postimmunization M02.20
      ankle M02.27
      elbow M02.22
      foot joint M02.27
      hand joint M02.24
      hip M02.25
      knee M02.26
      multiple site M02.29
      shoulder M02.21

Arthropathy --*continued*
   vertebra M02.28
   wrist M02.23
   postinfectious NEC B99 [*M12.80*]
      in (due to)
         enteritis due to Yersinia enterocolitica A04.6 [*M12.80*]
         syphilis A52.77
         viral hepatitis NEC B19.9 [*M12.80*]
   postrheumatic, chronic (Jaccoud) M12.00
      ankle M12.07
      elbow M12.02
      foot joint M12.07
      hand joint M12.04
      hip M12.05
      knee M12.06
      multiple site M12.09
      shoulder M12.01
      specified joint NEC M12.08
      vertebrae M12.08
      wrist M12.03
   psoriatic NEC L40.59
      interphalangeal, distal L40.51
   reactive M02.9
      in (due to)
         infective endocarditis I33.0 [*M02.9*]
      specified type NEC M02.80
         ankle M02.87
         elbow M02.82
         foot joint M02.87
         hand joint M02.84
         hip M02.85
         knee M02.86
         multiple site M02.89
         shoulder M02.81
         vertebra M02.88
         wrist M02.83
   specified form NEC M12.80
      ankle M12.87
      elbow M12.82
      foot joint M12.87
      hand joint M12.84
      hip M12.85
      knee M12.86
      multiple site M12.89
      shoulder M12.81
      specified joint NEC M12.88
      vertebrae M12.88
      wrist M12.83
   syringomyelic G95.0
   tabes dorsalis A52.16
   tabetic A52.16
   transient -*see* Arthropathy, specified form NEC
   traumatic M12.50
      ankle M12.57
      elbow M12.52
      foot joint M12.57
      hand joint M12.54
      hip M12.55
      knee M12.56
      multiple site M12.59
      shoulder M12.51
      specified joint NEC M12.58
      vertebrae M12.58
      wrist M12.53
Arthropyosis -*see* Arthritis, pyogenic or pyemic
Arthrosis (deformans) (degenerative) (localized) -*see also* Osteoarthritis M19.90
   spine -*see* Spondylosis

Arthus' phenomenon or reaction T78.41
  due to
    drug -*see* Table of Drugs and Chemicals, by
    drug
Articular -*see* condition
Articulation, reverse (teeth) M26.24
Artificial
  insemination complication -*see*
  Complications, artificial, fertilization
  opening status (functioning) (without
  complication) Z93.9
    anus (colostomy) Z93.3
    colostomy Z93.3
    cystostomy Z93.50
      appendico-vesicostomy Z93.52
      cutaneous Z93.51
      specified NEC Z93.59
    enterostomy Z93.4
    gastrostomy Z93.1
    ileostomy Z93.2
    intestinal tract NEC Z93.4
    jejunostomy Z93.4
    nephrostomy Z93.6
    specified site NEC Z93.8
    tracheostomy Z93.0
    ureterostomy Z93.6
    urethrostomy Z93.6
    urinary tract NEC Z93.6
    vagina Z93.8
  vagina status Z93.8
Arytenoid -*see* condition
Asbestosis (occupational) J61
**ASC-H (atypical squamous cells cannot
  exclude high grade squamous
  intraepithelial lesion on cytologic smear)**
    anus R85.611
    cervix R87.611
    vagina R87.621
**ASC-US (atypical squamous cells of
  undetermined significance on cytologic
  smear)**
    anus R85.610
    cervix R87.610
    vagina R87.620
Ascariasis B77.9
  with
    complications NEC B77.89
    intestinal complications B77.0
    pneumonia, pneumonitis B77.81
Ascaridosis, ascaridiasis -*see* Ascariasis
**Ascaris (infection) (infestation)
  (lumbricoides)** -*see* Ascariasis
Ascending -*see* condition
Aschoff's bodies -*see* Myocarditis, rheumatic
Ascites (abdominal) R18.8
  cardiac I50.9
  chylous (nonfilarial) I89.8
    filarial -*see* Infestation, filarial
  due to
    cirrhosis, alcoholic K70.31
    hepatitis
      alcoholic K70.11
      chronic active K71.51
    S. japonicum B65.2
  heart I50.9
  malignant R18.0
  pseudochylous R18.8
  syphilitic A52.74
  tuberculous A18.31
Aseptic -*see* condition
Asherman's syndrome N85.6

Asialia K11.7
Asiatic cholera -*see* Cholera
Asimultagnosia (simultanagnosia) R48.3
Askin's tumor -*see* Neoplasm, connective
  tissue, malignant
Asocial personality F60.2
Asomatognosia R41.4
Aspartylglucosaminuria E77.1
Asperger's disease or syndrome F84.5
Aspergilloma -*see* Aspergillosis
Aspergillosis (with pneumonia) B44.9
  bronchopulmonary, allergic B44.81
  disseminated B44.7
  generalized B44.7
  pulmonary NEC B44.1
    allergic B44.81
    invasive B44.0
  specified NEC B44.89
  tonsillar B44.2
**Aspergillus (flavus) (fumigatus) (infection)
  (terreus)** -*see* Aspergillosis
Aspermatogenesis -*see* Azoospermia
Aspermia (testis) -*see* Azoospermia
Asphyxia, asphyxiation (by) R09.01
  antenatal P84
  birth P84
  bunny bag -*see* Asphyxia, due to, mechanical
    threat to breathing, trapped in bed clothes
  crushing S28.0
  drowning T75.1
  gas, fumes, or vapor -*see* Table of Drugs and
    Chemicals
  inhalation -*see* Inhalation
  intrauterine P84
  local I73.00
    with gangrene I73.01
  mucus -*see also* Foreign body, respiratory
    tract, causing asphyxia
  newborn P84
  pathological R09.01
  postnatal P84
    mechanical -*see* Asphyxia, due to,
      mechanical threat to breathing
  prenatal P84
  reticularis R23.1
  strangulation -*see* Asphyxia, due to,
    mechanical threat to breathing
  submersion T75.1
  traumatic T71.9
    due to
      crushed chest S28.0
      foreign body (in) -*see* Foreign body,
    respiratory tract, causing asphyxia
      low oxygen content of ambient air T71.20
        due to
          being trapped in
            low oxygen environment T71.29
            in car trunk T71.221
              circumstances undetermined
                T71.224
              done with intent to harm by
                another person T71.223
                self T71.222
            in refrigerator T71.231
              circumstances undetermined
                T71.234
              done with intent to harm by
                another person T71.233
                self T71.232
          cave-in T71.21

Asphyxia, asphyxiation --*continued*
  mechanical threat to breathing (accidental)
    T71.191
    circumstances undetermined T71.194
    done with intent to harm by
      another person T71.193
      self T71.192
    hanging T71.161
      circumstances undetermined T71.164
      done with intent to harm by
        another person T71.163
        self T71.162
    plastic bag T71.121
      circumstances undetermined T71.124
      done with intent to harm by
        another person T71.123
        self T71.122
    smothering
      in furniture T71.151
        circumstances undetermined T71.154
        done with intent to harm by
          another person T71.153
          self T71.152
      under
        another person's body T71.141
          circumstances undetermined T71.144
          done with intent to harm T71.143
        pillow T71.111
          circumstances undetermined T71.114
          done with intent to harm by
            another person T71.113
            self T71.112
      trapped in bed clothes T71.131
        circumstances undetermined T71.134
        done with intent to harm by
          another person T71.133
          self T71.132
  vomiting, vomitus -*see* Foreign body,
    respiratory tract, causing asphyxia
Aspiration
  amniotic (clear) fluid (newborn) P24.10
    with
      pneumonia (pneumonitis) P24.11
      respiratory symptoms P24.11
  blood
    newborn (without respiratory symptoms)
      P24.20
      with
        pneumonia (pneumonitis) P24.21
        respiratory symptoms P24.21
    specified age NEC -*see* Foreign body,
  respiratory tract
  bronchitis J69.0
  food or foreign body (with asphyxiation) -*see*
    Asphyxia, food - liquor (amnii) (newborn)
  P24.10
    with
      pneumonia (pneumonitis) P24.11
      respiratory symptoms P24.11
  meconium (newborn) (without respiratory
  symptoms) P24.00
    with
      pneumonitis (pneumonitis) P24.01
      respiratory symptoms P24.01
  milk (newborn) (without respiratory
  symptoms) P24.30
    with
      pneumonia (pneumonitis) P24.31
      respiratory symptoms P24.31
  specified age NEC -*see* Foreign body,
  respiratory tract

Aspiration - *continued*
mucus *-see also* Foreign body, by site,
causing asphyxia
newborn P24.10
with
pneumonia (pneumonitis) P24.11
respiratory symptoms P24.11
neonatal P24.9
specific NEC (without respiratory
symptoms) P24.80
with
pneumonia (pneumonitis) P24.81
respiratory symptoms P24.81
newborn P24.9
specific NEC (without respiratory
symptoms) P24.80
with
pneumonia (pneumonitis) P24.81
respiratory symptoms P24.81
pneumonia J69.0
pneumonitis J69.0
syndrome of newborn *-see* Aspiration, by
substance, with pneumonia
vernix caseosa (newborn) P24.80
with
pneumonia (pneumonitis) P24.81
respiratory symptoms P24.81
vomitus *-see also* Foreign body, respiratory
tract
newborn (without respiratory symptoms)
P24.30
with
pneumonia (pneumonitis) P24.31
respiratory symptoms P24.31
Asplenia (congenital) Q89.01
postsurgical Z90.81
Assam fever B55.0
Assault, sexual *-see* Maltreatment
Assmann's focus NEC A15.0
Astasia (abasia) (hysterical) F44.4
Asteatosis cutis L85.3
Astereognosia, astereognosis R48.1
Asterixis R27.8
in liver disease K71.3
Asteroid hyalitis *-see* Deposit, crystalline
Asthenia, asthenic R53.1
cardiac *-see also* Failure, heart I50.9
psychogenic F45.8
cardiovascular *-see also* Failure, heart I50.9
psychogenic F45.8
heart *-see also* Failure, heart I50.9
psychogenic F45.8
hysterical F44.4
myocardial *-see also* Failure, heart I50.9
psychogenic F45.8
nervous F48.8
neurocirculatory F45.8
neurotic F48.8
psychogenic F48.8
psychoneurotic F48.8
psychophysiologic F48.8
reaction (psychophysiologic) F48.8
senile R54
Asthenopia *-see also* Discomfort, visual
hysterical F44.6
psychogenic F44.6
Asthenospermia *-see* Abnormal, specimen,
male genital organs
Asthma, asthmatic (bronchial) (catarrh)
(spasmodic) J45.909
with

Asthma, asthmatic *--continued*
chronic obstructive bronchitis J44.9
with
acute lower respiratory infection J44.0
exacerbation (acute) J44.1
chronic obstructive pulmonary disease J44.9
with
acute lower respiratory infection J44.0
exacerbation (acute) J44.1
exacerbation (acute) J45.901
hay fever *-see* Asthma, allergic extrinsic
rhinitis, allergic *-see* Asthma, allergic
extrinsic
status asthmaticus J45.902
allergic extrinsic J45.909
with
exacerbation (acute) J45.901
status asthmaticus J45.902
atopic *-see* Asthma, allergic extrinsic
cardiac *-see* Failure, ventricular, left
cardiobronchial I50.1
childhood J45.909
with
exacerbation (acute) J45.901
status asthmaticus J45.902
chronic obstructive J44.9
with
acute lower respiratory infection J44.0
exacerbation (acute) J44.1
collier's J60
cough variant J45.991
detergent J69.8
due to
detergent J69.8
inhalation of fumes J68.3
eosinophilic J82
extrinsic, allergic *-see* Asthma, allergic
extrinsic
grinder's J62.8
hay *-see* Asthma, allergic extrinsic
heart I50.1
idiosyncratic *-see* Asthma, nonallergic
intermittent (mild) J45.20
with
exacerbation (acute) J45.21
status asthmaticus J45.22
intrinsic, nonallergic *-see* Asthma, nonallergic
Kopp's E32.8
late-onset J45.909
with
exacerbation (acute) J45.901
status asthmaticus J45.902
mild intermittent J45.20
with
exacerbation (acute) J45.21
status asthmaticus J45.22
mild persistent J45.30
with
exacerbation (acute) J45.31
status asthmaticus J45.32
Millar's (laryngismus stridulus) J38.5
miner's J60
mixed J45.909
with
exacerbation (acute) J45.901
status asthmaticus J45.902
moderate persistent J45.40
with
exacerbation (acute) J45.41
status asthmaticus J45.42
nervous *-see* Asthma, nonallergic

Asthma, asthmatic *--continued*
nonallergic (intrinsic) J45.909
with
exacerbation (acute) J45.901
status asthmaticus J45.902
persistent
mild J45.30
with
exacerbation (acute) J45.31
status asthmaticus J45.32
moderate J45.40
with
exacerbation (acute) J45.41
status asthmaticus J45.42
severe J45.50
with
exacerbation (acute) J45.51
status asthmaticus J45.52
platinum J45.998
pneumoconiotic NEC J64
potter's J62.8
predominantly allergic J45.909
psychogenic F54
pulmonary eosinophilic J82
red cedar J67.8
Rostan's I50.1
sandblaster's J62.8
sequoiosis J67.8
severe persistent J45.50
with
exacerbation (acute) J45.51
status asthmaticus J45.52
specified NEC J45.998
stonemason's J62.8
thymic E32.8
tuberculous *-see* Tuberculosis, pulmonary
Wichmann's (laryngismus stridulus) J38.5
wood J67.8
Astigmatism (compound) (congenital)
H52.20
irregular H52.21
regular H52.22
Astraphobia F40.220
Astroblastoma
specified site *-see* Neoplasm, malignant, by
site
unspecified site C71.9
Astrocytoma (cystic)
anaplastic
specified site *-see* Neoplasm, malignant, by
site
unspecified site C71.9
fibrillary
specified site *-see* Neoplasm, malignant, by
site
unspecified site C71.9
fibrous
specified site *-see* Neoplasm, malignant, by
site
unspecified site C71.9
gemistocytic
specified site *-see* Neoplasm, malignant, by
site
unspecified site C71.9
juvenile
specified site *-see* Neoplasm, malignant, by
site
unspecified site C71.9
pilocytic
specified site *-see* Neoplasm, malignant, by
site

Astrocytoma (cystic) --*continued*
  unspecified site C71.9
  piloid
    specified site -*see* Neoplasm, malignant, by site
    unspecified site C71.9
  protoplasmic
    specified site -*see* Neoplasm, malignant, site
    unspecified site C71.9
  specified site NEC -*see* Neoplasm, malignant, by site
  subependymal D43.2
    giant cell
      specified site -*see* Neoplasm, uncertain behavior, by site
      unspecified site D43.2
    specified site -*see* Neoplasm, uncertain behavior, by site
    unspecified site D43.2
  unspecified site C71.9
Astroglioma
  specified site -*see* Neoplasm, malignant, by site
  unspecified site C71.9
Asymbolia R48.8
Asymmetry -*see also* Distortion
  between native and reconstructed breast N65.1
  face Q67.0
  jaw (lower) -*see* Anomaly, dentofacial, jaw-cranial base relationship, asymmetry
Asynergia, asynergy R27.8
  ventricular I51.89
Asystole (heart) -*see* Arrest, cardiac
At risk
  for falling Z91.81
Ataxia, ataxy, ataxic R27.0
  acute R27.8
  brain (hereditary) G11.9
  cerebellar (hereditary) G11.9
    with defective DNA repair G11.3
    alcoholic G31.2
    early onset G11.1
    in
      alcoholism G31.2
      myxedema E03.9 [*G13.2*]
      neoplastic disease -*see also* Neoplasm D49.9 [*G32.81*]
      specified disease NEC G32.81
    late-onset (Marie's) G11.2
  cerebral (hereditary) G11.9
  congenital nonprogressive G11.0
  family, familial -*see* Ataxia, hereditary
  following
    cerebrovascular disease I69.993
      cerebral infarction I69.393
      intracerebral hemorrhage I69.193
      nontraumatic intracranial hemorrhage NEC I69.293
      specified disease NEC I69.893
      subarachnoid hemorrhage I69.093
  Friedreich's (heredofamilial) (cerebellar) (spinal) G11.1
  gait R26.0
    hysterical F44.4
  general R27.8
  gluten M35.9 [*G32.81*]
    with celiac disease K90.0 [*G32.81*]
  hereditary G11.9
    with neuropathy G60.2

Ataxia, ataxy, ataxic --*continued*
  cerebellar -*see* Ataxia, cerebellar
  spastic G11.4
    specified NEC G11.8
    spinal (Friedreich's) G11.1
  heredofamilial -*see* Ataxia, hereditary
  Hunt's G11.1
  hysterical F44.4
  locomotor (progressive) (syphilitic) (partial) (spastic) A52.11
    diabetic -*see* Diabetes, ataxia
  Marie's (cerebellar) (heredofamilial) (late-onset) G11.2
  nonorganic origin F44.4
  nonprogressive, congenital G11.0
  psychogenic F44.4
  Roussy Lévy G60.0
  Sanger-Brown's (hereditary) G11.2
  spastic hereditary G11.4
  spinal
    hereditary (Friedreich's) G11.1
    progressive (syphilitic) A52.11
  spinocerebellar, X linked recessive G11.1
  telangiectasia (Louis-Bar) G11.3
Ataxia-telangiectasia (Louis-Bar) G11.3
Atelectasis (massive) (partial) (pressure) (pulmonary) J98.11
  newborn P28.10
    due to resorption P28.11
    partial P28.19
    primary P28.0
    secondary P28.19
  primary (newborn) P28.0
  tuberculous -*see* Tuberculosis, pulmonary
Atelocardia Q24.9
Atelomyelia Q06.1
Atheroembolism
  of
    extremities
      lower I75.02
      upper I75.01
    kidney I75.81
    specified NEC I75.89
Atheroma, atheromatous -*see also*
  Arteriosclerosis I70.90
  aorta, aortic I70.0
    valve -*see also* Endocarditis, aortic I35.8
  aorto-iliac I70.0
  artery -*see* Arteriosclerosis
  basilar (artery) I67.2
  carotid (artery) (common) (internal) I67.2
  cerebral (arteries) I67.2
  coronary (artery) I25.10
    with angina pectoris -*see* Arteriosclerosis, coronary (artery),
    degeneration -*see* Arteriosclerosis
  heart, cardiac -*see* Disease, heart, ischemic, atherosclerotic
  mitral (valve) I34.8
  myocardium, myocardial -*see* Disease, heart, ischemic, atherosclerotic
  pulmonary valve (heart) -*see also*
    Endocarditis, pulmonary I37.8
  tricuspid (heart) (valve) I36.8
  valve, valvular -*see* Endocarditis
  vertebral (artery) I67.2
Atheromatosis -*see* Arteriosclerosis
Atherosclerosis -*see also* Arteriosclerosis
  coronary
    artery I25.10

Atherosclerosis - *continued*
  with angina pectoris -*see* Arteriosclerosis, coronary (artery),
    due to
      calcified coronary lesion (severely) I25.84
      lipid rich plaque I25.83
  transplanted heart I25.811
    bypass graft I25.812
      with angina pectoris -*see* Arteriosclerosis, coronary (artery),
    native coronary artery I25.811
      with angina pectoris -*see* Arteriosclerosis, coronary (artery),
Athetosis (acquired) R25.8
  bilateral (congenital) G80.3
  congenital (bilateral) (double) G80.3
  double (congenital) G80.3
  unilateral R25.8
Athlete's
  foot B35.3
  heart I51.7
Athrepsia E41
Athyrea (acquired) -*see also* Hypothyroidism
  congenital E03.1
Atonia, atony, atonic
  bladder (sphincter) (neurogenic) N31.2
  capillary I78.8
  cecum K59.8
    psychogenic F45.8
  colon -*see* Atony, intestine
  congenital P94.2
  esophagus K22.8
  intestine K59.8
    psychogenic F45.8
  stomach K31.89
    neurotic or psychogenic F45.8
  uterus (during labor) O62.2
    with hemorrhage (postpartum) O72.1
    postpartum (with hemorrhage) O72.1
      without hemorrhage O75.89
Atopy -*see* History, allergy
Atransferrinemia, congenital E88.09
Atresia, atretic
  alimentary organ or tract NEC Q45.8
    upper Q40.8
  ani, anus, anal (canal) Q42.3
    with fistula Q42.2
  aorta (ring) Q25.29
  aortic (orifice) (valve) Q23.0
    arch Q25.21
    congenital with hypoplasia of ascending aorta and defective development of left ventricle (with mitral stenosis) Q23.4
    in hypoplastic left heart syndrome Q23.4
  aqueduct of Sylvius Q03.0
    with spina bifida -*see* Spina bifida, with hydrocephalus
  artery NEC Q27.8
    cerebral Q28.3
    coronary Q24.5
    digestive system Q27.8
    eye Q15.8
    lower limb Q27.8
    pulmonary Q25.5
    specified site NEC Q27.8
    umbilical Q27.0
    upper limb Q27.8
  auditory canal (external) Q16.1
  bile duct (common) (congenital) (hepatic) Q44.2

Atresia, atretic --*continued*
  acquired -*see* Obstruction, bile duct
  bladder (neck) Q64.39
    obstruction Q64.31
  bronchus Q32.4
  cecum Q42.8
  cervix (acquired) N88.2
    congenital Q51.828
    in pregnancy or childbirth -*see* Anomaly,
    cervix, in pregnancy or childbirth
      causing obstructed labor O65.5
  choana Q30.0
  colon Q42.9
    specified NEC Q42.8
  common duct Q44.2
  cricoid cartilage Q31.8
  cystic duct Q44.2
    acquired K82.8
      with obstruction K82.0
  digestive organs NEC Q45.8
  duodenum Q41.0
  ear canal Q16.1
  ejaculatory duct Q55.4
  epiglottis Q31.8
  esophagus Q39.0
    with tracheoesophageal fistula Q39.1
  eustachian tube Q17.8
  fallopian tube (congenital) Q50.6
    acquired N97.1
  follicular cyst N83.0
  foramen of
    Luschka Q03.1
      with spina bifida -*see* Spina bifida, with
      hydrocephalus
    Magendie Q03.1
      with spina bifida -*see* Spina bifida, with
    hydrocephalus
  gallbladder Q44.1
  genital organ
    external
      female Q52.79
      male Q55.8
    internal
      female Q52.8
      male Q55.8
  glottis Q31.8
  gullet Q39.0
    with tracheoesophageal fistula Q39.1
  heart valve NEC Q24.8
    pulmonary Q22.0
    tricuspid Q22.4
  hymen Q52.3
    acquired (postinfective) N89.6
  ileum Q41.2
  intestine (small) Q41.9
    large Q42.9
      specified NEC Q42.8
  iris, filtration angle Q15.0
  jejunum Q41.1
  lacrimal apparatus Q10.4
  larynx Q31.8
  meatus urinarius Q64.33
  mitral valve Q23.2
    in hypoplastic left heart syndrome Q23.4
  nares (anterior) (posterior) Q30.0
  nasopharynx Q34.8
  nose, nostril Q30.0
    acquired J34.89
  organ or site NEC Q89.8
  osseous meatus (ear) Q16.1
  oviduct (congenital) Q50.6

Atresia, atretic --*continued*
  acquired N97.1
  parotid duct Q38.4
    acquired K11.8
  pulmonary (artery) Q25.5
    valve Q22.0
  pulmonic Q22.0
  pupil Q13.2
  rectum Q42.1
    with fistula Q42.0
  salivary duct Q38.4
    acquired K11.8
  sublingual duct Q38.4
    acquired K11.8
  submandibular duct Q38.4
    acquired K11.8
  submaxillary duct Q38.4
    acquired K11.8
  thyroid cartilage Q31.8
  trachea Q32.1
  tricuspid valve Q22.4
  ureter Q62.10
    pelvic junction Q62.11
    vesical orifice Q62.12
  ureteropelvic junction Q62.11
  ureterovesical orifice Q62.12
  urethra (valvular) Q64.39
    stricture Q64.32
  urinary tract NEC Q64.8
  uterus Q51.818
    acquired N85.8
  vagina (congenital) Q52.4
    acquired (postinfectional) (senile) N89.5
  vas deferens Q55.3
  vascular NEC Q27.8
    cerebral Q28.3
    digestive system Q27.8
    lower limb Q27.8
    specified site NEC Q27.8
    upper limb Q27.8
  vein NEC Q27.8
    digestive system Q27.8
    great Q26.8
    lower limb Q27.8
    portal Q26.5
    pulmonary Q26.3
    specified site NEC Q27.8
    upper limb Q27.8
  vena cava (inferior) (superior) Q26.8
  vesicourethral orifice Q64.31
  vulva Q52.79
    acquired N90.5
Atrichia, atrichosis -*see* Alopecia
Atrophia -*see also* Atrophy
  cutis senilis L90.8
    due to radiation L57.8
  gyrata of choroid and retina H31.23
  senilis R54
    dermatological L90.8
      due to radiation (nonionizing) (solar) L57.8
  unguium L60.3
    congenita Q84.6
Atrophie blanche (en plaque) (de Milian)
L95.0
Atrophoderma, atrophodermia (of) L90.9
  diffusum (idiopathic) L90.4
  maculatum L90.8
    et striatum L90.8
      due to syphilis A52.79
    syphilitic A51.39
  neuriticum L90.8

Atrophoderma, atrophodermia (of) --
continued
  Pasini and Pierini L90.3
  pigmentosum Q82.1
  reticulatum symmetricum faciei L66.4
  senile L90.8
    due to radiation (nonionizing) (solar) L57.8
  vermiculata (cheeks) L66.4
Atrophy, atrophic (of)
  adrenal (capsule) (gland) E27.49
    primary (autoimmune) E27.1
  alveolar process or ridge (edentulous) K08.20
  anal sphincter (disuse) N81.84
  appendix K38.8
  arteriosclerotic -*see* Arteriosclerosis
  bile duct (common) (hepatic) K83.8
  bladder N32.89
    neurogenic N31.8
  blanche (en plaque) (of Milian) L95.0
  bone (senile) NEC -*see also* Disorder, bone,
  specified type NEC
    due to
      tabes dorsalis (neurogenic) A52.11
  brain (cortex) (progressive) G31.9
    frontotemporal circumscribed G31.01
      [F02.80]
      with behavioral disturbance G31.01
      [F02.81]
    senile NEC G31.1
  breast N64.2
    obstetric -*see* Disorder, breast, specified type
  NEC
  buccal cavity K13.79
  cardiac -*see* Degeneration, myocardial
  cartilage (infectional) (joint) -*see* Disorder,
  cartilage, specified NEC
  cerebellar -*see* Atrophy, brain
  cerebral -*see* Atrophy, brain
  cervix (mucosa) (senile) (uteri) N88.8
    menopausal N95.8
  Charcot-Marie-Tooth G60.0
  choroid (central) (macular) (myopic) (retina)
  H31.10
    diffuse secondary H31.12
    gyrate H31.23
    senile H31.11
  ciliary body -*see* Atrophy, iris
  conjunctiva (senile) H11.89
  corpus cavernosum N48.89
  cortical -*see* Atrophy, brain
  cystic duct K82.8
  Déjérine-Thomas G23.8
  disuse NEC -*see* Atrophy, muscle
  Duchenne-Aran G12.21
  ear H93.8
  edentulous alveolar ridge K08.20
  endometrium (senile) N85.8
    cervix N88.8
  enteric K63.89
  epididymis N50.89
  eyeball -*see* Disorder, globe, degenerated
  condition, atrophy
  eyelid (senile) -*see* Disorder, eyelid,
  degenerative
  facial (skin) L90.9
  fallopian tube (senile) N83.32
    with ovary N83.33
  fascioscapulohumeral (Landouzy Déjérine)
  G71.0
  fatty, thymus (gland) E32.8
  gallbladder K82.8

Atrophy, atrophic (of) --*continued*
- gastric K29.40
  - with bleeding K29.41
- gastrointestinal K63.89
- glandular I89.8
- globe H44.52
- gum -*see also* Recession, gingival K06.0
- hair L67.8
- heart (brown) -*see* Degeneration, myocardial
- hemifacial Q67.4
  - Romberg G51.8
- infantile E41
  - paralysis, acute -*see* Poliomyelitis, paralytic
- intestine K63.89
- iris (essential) (progressive) H21.26
  - specified NEC H21.29
- kidney (senile) (terminal) -*see also* Sclerosis, renal N26.1
  - congenital or infantile Q60.5
    - bilateral Q60.4
    - unilateral Q60.3
  - hydronephrotic -*see* Hydronephrosis
- lacrimal gland (primary) H04.14
  - secondary H04.15
- Landouzy Déjérine G71.0
- laryngitis, infective J37.0
- larynx J38.7
- Leber's optic (hereditary) H47.22
- lip K13.0
- liver (yellow) K72.90
  - with coma K72.91
  - acute, subacute K72.00
    - with coma K72.01
  - chronic K72.10
    - with coma K72.11
- lung (senile) J98.4
- macular (dermatological) L90.8
  - syphilitic, skin A51.39
    - striated A52.79
- mandible (edentulous) K08.20
  - minimal K08.21
  - moderate K08.22
  - severe K08.23
- maxilla K08.20
  - minimal K08.24
  - moderate K08.25
  - severe K08.26
- muscle, muscular (diffuse) (general) (idiopathic) (primary) M62.50
  - ankle M62.57
  - Duchenne-Aran G12.21
  - foot M62.57
  - forearm M62.53
  - hand M62.54
  - infantile spinal G12.0
  - lower leg M62.56
  - multiple sites M62.59
  - myelopathic -*see* Atrophy, muscle, spinal
  - myotonic G71.11
  - neuritic G58.9
  - neuropathic (peroneal) (progressive) G60.0
  - pelvic (disuse) N81.84
  - peroneal G60.0
  - progressive (bulbar) G12.21
    - adult G12.1
    - infantile (spinal) G12.0
    - spinal G12.9
      - adult G12.1
      - infantile G12.0
  - pseudohypertrophic G71.0
  - shoulder region M62.51

Atrophy, atrophic (of) --*continued*
- specified site NEC M62.58
- spinal G12.9
  - adult form G12.1
  - Aran-Duchenne G12.21
  - childhood form, type II G12.1
  - distal G12.1
  - hereditary NEC G12.1
  - infantile, type I (Werdnig-Hoffmann) G12.0
  - juvenile form, type III (Kugelberg-Welander) G12.1
  - progressive G12.21
  - scapuloperoneal form G12.1
  - specified NEC G12.8
  - syphilitic A52.78
  - thigh M62.55
  - upper arm M62.52
- myocardium -*see* Degeneration, myocardial
- myometrium (senile) N85.8
  - cervix N88.8
- myopathic NEC -*see* Atrophy, muscle
- myotonia G71.11
- nail L60.3
- nasopharynx J31.1
- nerve -*see also* Disorder, nerve
  - abducens -*see* Strabismus, paralytic, sixth nerve
  - accessory G52.8
  - acoustic or auditory -*see* subcategory H93.3
  - cranial G52.9
    - eighth (auditory) -*see* subcategory H93.3
    - eleventh (accessory) G52.8
    - fifth (trigeminal) G50.8
    - first (olfactory) G52.0
    - fourth (trochlear) -*see* Strabismus, paralytic, fourth nerve
    - second (optic) H47.20
    - sixth (abducens) -*see* Strabismus, paralytic, sixth nerve
    - tenth (pneumogastric) (vagus) G52.2
    - third (oculomotor) -*see* Strabismus, paralytic, third nerve
    - twelfth (hypoglossal) G52.3
  - hypoglossal G52.3
  - oculomotor -*see* Strabismus, paralytic, third nerve
  - olfactory G52.0
  - optic (papillomacular bundle)
    - syphilitic (late) A52.15
      - congenital A50.44
  - pneumogastric G52.2
  - trigeminal G50.8
  - trochlear -*see* Strabismus, paralytic, fourth nerve
  - vagus (pneumogastric) G52.2
- neurogenic, bone, tabetic A52.11
- nutritional E41
- old age R54
- olivopontocerebellar G23.8
- optic (nerve) H47.20
  - glaucomatous H47.23
  - hereditary H47.22
  - primary H47.21
  - specified type NEC H47.29
  - syphilitic (late) A52.15
    - congenital A50.44
- orbit H05.31
- ovary (senile) N83.31
  - with fallopian tube N83.33

Atrophy, atrophic (of) --*continued*
- oviduct (senile) -*see* Atrophy, fallopian tube -
  - palsy, diffuse (progressive) G12.22
- pancreas (duct) (senile) K86.89
- parotid gland K11.0
- pelvic muscle N81.84
- penis N48.89
- pharynx J39.2
- pluriglandular E31.8
  - autoimmune E31.0
- polyarthritis M15.9
- prostate N42.89
- pseudohypertrophic (muscle) G71.0
- renal -*see also* Sclerosis, renal N26.1
- retina, retinal (postinfectional) H35.89
- rhinitis J31.0
- salivary gland K11.0
- scar L90.5
- sclerosis, lobar (of brain) G31.09   [*F02.80*]
  - with behavioral disturbance G31.09 [*F02.81*]
- scrotum N50.89
- seminal vesicle N50.89
- senile R54
  - due to radiation (nonionizing) (solar) L57.8
- skin (patches) (spots) L90.9
  - degenerative (senile) L90.8
  - due to radiation (nonionizing) (solar) L57.8
  - senile L90.8
- spermatic cord N50.89
- spinal (acute) (cord) G95.89
  - muscular -*see* Atrophy, muscle, spinal
  - paralysis G12.20
    - acute -*see* Poliomyelitis, paralytic
    - meaning progressive muscular atrophy G12.21
- spine (column) -*see* Spondylopathy, specified NEC
- spleen (senile) D73.0
- stomach K29.40
  - with bleeding K29.41
- striate (skin) L90.6
  - syphilitic A52.79
- subcutaneous L90.9
- sublingual gland K11.0
- submandibular gland K11.0
- submaxillary gland K11.0
- Sudeck's -*see* Algoneurodystrophy
- suprarenal (capsule) (gland) E27.49
  - primary E27.1
- systemic affecting central nervous system in
  - myxedema E03.9 [*G13.2*]
  - neoplastic disease -*see also* Neoplasm D49.9 [*G13.1*]
  - specified disease NEC G13.8
- tarso-orbital fascia, congenital Q10.3
- testis N50.0
- thenar, partial -*see* Syndrome, carpal tunnel
- thymus (fatty) E32.8
- thyroid (gland) (acquired) E03.4
  - with cretinism E03.1
  - congenital (with myxedema) E03.1
- tongue (senile) K14.8
  - papillae K14.4
- trachea J39.8
- tunica vaginalis N50.89
- turbinate J34.89
- tympanic membrane (nonflaccid) H73.82
  - flaccid H73.81
- upper respiratory tract J39.8

Atrophy, atrophic (of) --*continued*
  uterus, uterine (senile) N85.8
    cervix N88.8
      due to radiation (intended effect) N85.8
        adverse effect or misadventure N99.89
  vagina (senile) N95.2
  vas deferens N50.89
  vascular I99.8
  vertebra (senile) -*see* Spondylopathy,
    specified NEC
  vulva (senile) N90.5
  Werdnig-Hoffmann G12.0
  yellow -*see* Failure, hepatic
Attack, attacks
  with alteration of consciousness (with
    automatisms) -*see* Epilepsy, localization-
    related, symptomatic, with complex
  partial seizures
    Adams-Stokes I45.9
    akinetic -*see* Epilepsy, generalized, specified
      NEC
    angina -*see* Angina
    atonic -*see* Epilepsy, generalized, specified
      NEC
    benign shuddering G25.83
    cataleptic -*see* Catalepsy
    coronary -*see* Infarct, myocardium
    cyanotic, newborn P28.2
    drop NEC R55
    epileptic -*see* Epilepsy
    heart -*see* infarct, myocardium
    hysterical F44.9
    jacksonian -*see* Epilepsy, localization-related,
      symptomatic, with simple partial seizures
    myocardium, myocardial -*see* Infarct,
      myocardium
    myoclonic -*see* Epilepsy, generalized,
      specified NEC
    panic F41.0
    psychomotor -*see* Epilepsy, localization-
      related, symptomatic, with complex partial
      seizures
    salaam -*see* Epilepsy, spasms
    schizophreniform, brief F23
    shuddering, benign G25.83
    Stokes-Adams I45.9
    syncope R55
    transient ischemic (TIA) G45.9
      specified NEC G45.8
    unconsciousness R55
      hysterical F44.89
    vasomotor R55
    vasovagal (paroxysmal) (idiopathic) R55
    without alteration of consciousness -*see*
      Epilepsy, localization-related, symptomatic,
      with simple partial seizures
Attention (to)
  artificial
    opening (of) Z43.9
      digestive tract NEC Z43.4
        colon Z43.3
        ilium Z43.2
        stomach Z43.1
      specified NEC Z43.8
      trachea Z43.0
      urinary tract NEC Z43.6
        cystostomy Z43.5
        nephrostomy Z43.6
        ureterostomy Z43.6
        urethrostomy Z43.6
      vagina Z43.7

Attention (to) --*continued*
  colostomy Z43.3
  cystostomy Z43.5
  deficit disorder or syndrome F98.8
    with hyperactivity -*see* Disorder, attention-
      deficit hyperactivity gastrostomy Z43.1
  ileostomy Z43.2
  jejunostomy Z43.4
  nephrostomy Z43.6
  surgical dressings Z48.01
  sutures Z48.02
  tracheostomy Z43.0
  ureterostomy Z43.6
  urethrostomy Z43.6
Attrition
  gum -*see also* Recession, gingival K06.0
  tooth, teeth (excessive) (hard tissues) K03.0
Atypical, atypism -*see also* condition
  cells (on cytological smear) (endocervical)
    (endometrial) (glandular)
      cervix R87.619
      vagina R87.629
  cervical N87.9
  endometrium N85.9
    hyperplasia N85.00
  parenting situation Z62.9
Auditory -*see* condition
Aujeszky's disease B33.8
Aurantiasis, cutis E67.1
Auricle, auricular -*see also* condition
  cervical Q18.2
Auriculotemporal syndrome G50.8
Austin Flint murmur (aortic insufficiency)
  I35.1
Australian
  Q fever A78
  X disease A83.4
Autism, autistic (childhood) (infantile) F84.0
  atypical F84.9
  spectrum disorder F84.0
Autodigestion R68.89
Autoerythrocyte sensitization (syndrome)
  D69.2
Autographism L50.3
Autoimmune
  disease (systemic) M35.9
  inhibitors to clotting factors D68.311
  lymphoproliferative syndrome [ALPS]
    D89.82
  thyroiditis E06.3
Autointoxication R68.89
Automatism G93.89
  with temporal sclerosis G93.81
  epileptic -*see* Epilepsy, localization-related,
    symptomatic, with complex partial seizures
  paroxysmal, idiopathic -*see* Epilepsy,
    localization-related, symptomatic, with
    complex partial seizures
Autonomic, autonomous
  bladder (neurogenic) N31.2
  hysteria seizure F44.5
Autosensitivity, erythrocyte D69.2
Autosensitization, cutaneous L30.2
Autosome -*see* condition by chromosome
  involved
Autotopagnosia R48.1
Autotoxemia R68.89
Autumn -*see* condition
Avellis' syndrome G46.8

Aversion
  oral R63.3
    newborn P92.
    nonorganic origin F98.2
  sexual F52.1
Aviator's
  disease or sickness -*see* Effect, adverse, high
    altitude
  ear T70.0
Avitaminosis (multiple) -*see also* Deficiency,
  vitamin E56.9
  B E53.9
    with
      beriberi E51.11
      pellagra E52
  B2 E53.0
  B6 E53.1
  B12 E53.8
  D E55.9
    with rickets E55.0
  G E53.0
  K E56.1
  nicotinic acid E52
AVNRT (atrioventricular nodal re-entrant
  tachycardia) I47.1
AVRT (atrioventricular nodal re-entrant
  tachycardia) I47.1
Avulsion (traumatic)
  blood vessel -*see* Injury, blood vessel
  bone -*see* Fracture, by site
  cartilage -*see also* Dislocation, by site
    symphyseal (inner), complicating delivery
      O71.6
  external site other than limb -*see* Wound,
    open, by site
  eye S05.7
  head (intracranial)
    external site NEC S08.89
    scalp S08.0
  internal organ or site -*see* Injury, by site
  joint -*see also* Dislocation, by site
    capsule -*see* Sprain, by site
  kidney S37.06
  ligament -*see* Sprain, by site
  limb -*see also* Amputation, traumatic, by site
    skin and subcutaneous tissue -*see* Wound,
      open, by site
  muscle -*see* Injury, muscle
  nerve (root) -*see* Injury, nerve
  scalp S08.0
  skin and subcutaneous tissue -*see* Wound,
    open, by site
  spleen S36.032
  symphyseal cartilage (inner), complicating
    delivery O71.6
  tendon -*see* Injury, muscle
  tooth S03.2
Awareness of heart beat R00.2
Axenfeld's
  anomaly or syndrome Q15.0
  degeneration (calcareous) Q13.4
Axilla, axillary -*see also* condition
  breast Q83.1
Axonotmesis -*see* Injury, nerve
Ayerza's disease or syndrome (pulmonary
  artery sclerosis with pulmonary
  hypertension) I27.0
Azoospermia (organic) N46.01
  due to
    drug therapy N46.021
    efferent duct obstruction N46.023

Azoospermia (organic) --continued
  infection N46.022
  radiation N46.024
  specified cause NEC N46.029
  systemic disease N46.025
Azotemia R79.89
  meaning uremia N19
Aztec ear Q17.3
Azygos
  continuation inferior vena cava Q26.8
  lobe (lung) Q33.1

B

Baastrup's disease -see Kissing spine
Babesiosis B60.0
Babington's disease (familial hemorrhagic telangiectasia) I78.0
Babinski's syndrome A52.79
Baby
  crying constantly R68.11
  floppy (syndrome) P94.2
Bacillary -see condition
Bacilluria R82.71
Bacillus -see also Infection, bacillus
  abortus infection A23.1
  anthracis infection A22.9
  coli infection -see also Escherichia coli B96.20
  Flexner's A03.1
  mallei infection A24.0
  Shiga's A03.0
  suipestifer infection -see Infection, salmonella
Back -see condition
Backache (postural) M54.9
  sacroiliac M53.3
  specified NEC M54.89
Backflow -see Reflux
Backward reading (dyslexia) F81.0
Bacteremia R78.81
  with sepsis -see Sepsis
Bactericholia -see Cholecystitis, acute
Bacterid, bacteride (pustular) L40.3
Bacterium, bacteria, bacterial
  agent NEC, as cause of disease classified elsewhere B96.89
  in blood -see Bacteremia
  in urine -see Bacteriuria
Bacteriuria, bacteruria R82.71
  asymptomatic R82.71
Bacteroides
  fragilis, as cause of disease classified elsewhere B96.6
Bad
  heart -see Disease, heart
  trip
    due to drug abuse -see Abuse, drug, hallucinogen
    due to drug dependence -see Dependence, drug, hallucinogen
Baelz's disease (cheilitis glandularis apostematosa) K13.0
Baerensprung's disease (eczema marginatum) B35.6
Bagasse disease or pneumonitis J67.1
Bagassosis J67.1
Baker's cyst -see Cyst, Baker's
Bakwin-Krida syndrome (metaphyseal dysplasia) Q78.5
Balancing side interference M26.56

Balanitis (circinata) (erosiva) (gangrenosa) (phagedenic) (vulgaris) N48.1
  amebic A06.82
  candidal B37.42
  due to Haemophilus ducreyi A57
  gonococcal (acute) (chronic) A54.09
  xerotica obliterans N48.0
Balanoposthitis N47.6
  gonococcal (acute) (chronic) A54.09
  ulcerative (specific) A63.8
Balanorrhagia -see Balanitis
Balantidiasis, balantidiosis A07.0
Bald tongue K14.4
Baldness -see also Alopecia
  male-pattern -see Alopecia, androgenic
Balkan grippe A78
Balloon disease -see Effect, adverse, high altitude
Balo's disease (concentric sclerosis) G37.5
Bamberger-Marie disease -see Osteoarthropathy, hypertrophic, specified type NEC
Bancroft's filariasis B74.0
Band(s)
  adhesive -see Adhesions, peritoneum
  anomalous or congenital -see also Anomaly, by site
    heart (atrial) (ventricular) Q24.8
    intestine Q43.3
    omentum Q43.3
  cervix N88.1
  constricting, congenital Q79.8
  gallbladder (congenital) Q44.1
  intestinal (adhesive) -see Adhesions, peritoneum
  obstructive
    intestine K56.5
    peritoneum K56.5
  periappendiceal, congenital Q43.3
  peritoneal (adhesive) -see Adhesions, peritoneum
  uterus N73.6
    internal N85.6
  vagina N89.5
Bandemia D72.825
Bandl's ring (contraction), complicating delivery O62.4
Bangkok hemorrhagic fever A91
Bang's disease (brucella abortus) A23.1
Bankruptcy, anxiety concerning Z59.8
Bannister's disease T78.3
  hereditary D84.1
Banti's disease or syndrome (with cirrhosis) (with portal hypertension) K76.6
Bar, median, prostate -see Enlargement, enlarged, prostate
Barcoo disease or rot -see Ulcer, skin
Barlow's disease E54
Barodontalgia T70.29
Baron Münchausen syndrome -see Disorder, factitious
Barosinusitis T70.1
Barotitis T70.0
Barotrauma T70.29
  odontalgia T70.29
  otitic T70.0
  sinus T70.1
Barraquer (Simons) disease or syndrome (progressive lipodystrophy) E88.1
Barré Guillain disease or syndrome G61.0

Barré Liéou syndrome (posterior cervical sympathetic) M53.0
Barrel chest M95.4
Barrett's
  disease -see Barrett's, esophagus
  esophagus K22.70
    with dysplasia K22.719
      high grade K22.711
      low grade K22.710
    without dysplasia K22.70
  syndrome -see Barrett's, esophagus
  ulcer K22.10
    with bleeding K22.11
    without bleeding K22.10
Bársony (Polgár) (Teschendorf) syndrome (corkscrew esophagus) K22.4
Bartholinitis (suppurating) N75.8
  gonococcal (acute) (chronic) (with abscess) A54.1
Barth syndrome E78.71
Bartonellosis A44.9
  cutaneous A44.1
  mucocutaneous A44.1
  specified NEC A44.8
  systemic A44.0
Barton's fracture S52.56
Bartter's syndrome E26.81
Basal -see condition
Basan's (hidrotic) ectodermal dysplasia Q82.4
Baseball finger -see Dislocation, finger
Basedow's disease (exophthalmic goiter) -see Hyperthyroidism, with, goiter
Basic -see condition
Basilar -see condition
Bason's (hidrotic) ectodermal dysplasia Q82.4
Basopenia -see Agranulocytosis
Basophilia D72.824
Basophilism (cortico-adrenal) (Cushing's) (pituitary) E24.0
Bassen-Kornzweig disease or syndrome E78.6
Bat ear Q17.5
Bateman's
  disease B08.1
  purpura (senile) D69.2
Bathing cramp T75.1
Bathophobia F40.248
Batten (Mayou) disease E75.4
  retina E75.4 [H36]
Batten-Steinert syndrome G71.11
Battered -see Maltreatment
Battey Mycobacterium infection A31.0
Battle exhaustion F43.0
Battledore placenta O43.19
Baumgarten-Cruveilhier cirrhosis, disease or syndrome K74.69
Bauxite fibrosis (of lung) J63.1
Bayle's disease (general paresis) A52.17
Bazin's disease (primary) (tuberculous) A18.4
Beach ear -see Swimmer's, ear
Beaded hair (congenital) Q84.1
Béal conjunctivitis or syndrome B30.2
Beard's disease (neurasthenia) F48.8
Beat(s)
  atrial, premature I49.1
  ectopic I49.49
  elbow -see Bursitis, elbow
  escaped, heart I49.49

Beat(s) – continued
hand -*see* Bursitis, hand
knee -*see* Bursitis, knee - premature I49.40
  atrial I49.1
  auricular I49.1
  supraventricular I49.1
Beau's
disease or syndrome -*see* Degeneration, myocardial
lines (transverse furrows on fingernails) L60.4
Bechterev's syndrome -*see* Spondylitis, ankylosing
Beck's syndrome (anterior spinal artery occlusion) I65.8
Becker's
cardiomyopathy I42.8
disease
  idiopathic mural endomyocardial disease I42.3
  myotonia congenita, recessive form G71.12
dystrophy G71.0
pigmented hairy nevus D22.5
Beckwith-Wiedemann syndrome Q87.3
Bed confinement status Z74.01
Bed sore -*see* Ulcer, pressure, by site
Bedbug bite(s) -*see* Bite(s), by site, superficial, insect
Bedclothes, asphyxiation or suffocation by - *see* Asphyxia, traumatic, due to, mechanical, trapped
Bednar's
aphthae K12.0
tumor -*see* Neoplasm, malignant, by site
Bedridden Z74.01
Bedsore -*see* Ulcer, pressure, by site
Bedwetting -*see* Enuresis
Bee sting (with allergic or anaphylactic shock) -*see* Toxicity, venom, arthropod, bee
Beer drinker's heart (disease) I42.6
Begbie's disease (exophthalmic goiter) -*see* Hyperthyroidism, with, goiter
Behavior
antisocial
  adult Z72.811
  child or adolescent Z72.810
disorder, disturbance -*see* Disorder, conduct
disruptive -*see* Disorder, conduct
drug seeking Z76.5
inexplicable R46.2
marked evasiveness R46.5
obsessive-compulsive R46.81
overactivity R46.3
poor responsiveness R46.4
self-damaging (life-style) Z72.89
sleep-incompatible Z72.821
slowness R46.4
specified NEC R46.89
strange (and inexplicable) R46.2
suspiciousness R46.5
type A pattern Z73.1
undue concern or preoccupation with stressful events R46.6
verbosity and circumstantial detail obscuring reason for contact R46.7
Behçet's disease or syndrome M35.2
Behr's disease -*see* Degeneration, macula
Beigel's disease or morbus (white piedra) B36.2
Bejel A65
Bekhterev's syndrome -*see* Spondylitis, ankylosing

Belching -*see* Eructation
Bell's
mania F30.8
palsy, paralysis G51.0
  infant or newborn P11.3
spasm G51.3
Bence Jones albuminuria or proteinuria NEC R80.3
Bends T70.3
Benedikt's paralysis or syndrome G46.3
Benign -*see also* condition
prostatic hyperplasia -*see* Hyperplasia, prostate
Bennett's fracture (displaced) S62.21
Benson's disease -*see* Deposit, crystalline
Bent
back (hysterical) F44.4
nose M95.0
  congenital Q67.4
Bereavement (uncomplicated) Z63.4
Bergeron's disease (hysterical chorea) F44.4
Berger's disease -*see* Nephropathy, IgA
Beriberi (dry) E51.11
heart (disease) E51.12
polyneuropathy E51.11
wet E51.12
  involving circulatory system E51.11
Berlin's disease or edema (traumatic) S05.8X
Berlock (berloque) dermatitis L56.2
Bernard-Horner syndrome G90.2
Bernard-Soulier disease or thrombopathia D69.1
Bernhardt (Roth) disease -*see* Mononeuropathy, lower limb, meralgia paresthetica
Bernheim's syndrome -*see* Failure, heart, congestive
Bertielliasis B71.8
Berylliosis (lung) J63.2
Besnier-Boeck (Schaumann) disease -*see* Sarcoidosis
Besnier's
lupus pernio D86.3
prurigo L20.0
Bestiality F65.89
Best's disease H35.50
Beta-mercaptolactate-cysteine disulfiduria E72.09
Betalipoproteinemia, broad or floating E78.2
Betting and gambling Z72.6
pathological (compulsive) F63.0
Bezoar T18.9
intestine T18.3
stomach T18.2
Bezold's abscess -*see* Mastoiditis, acute
Bianchi's syndrome R48.8
Bicornate or bicornis uterus Q51.3
in pregnancy or childbirth O34.0
  causing obstructed labor O65.5
Bicuspid aortic valve Q23.1
Biedl-Bardet syndrome Q87.89
Bielschowsky (Jansky) disease E75.4
Biermer's (pernicious) anemia or disease D51.0
Biett's disease L93.0
Bifid (congenital)
apex, heart Q24.8
clitoris Q52.6
kidney Q63.8
nose Q30.2

Bifid (congenital) --*continued*
patella Q74.1
scrotum Q55.29
toe NEC Q74.2
tongue Q38.3
ureter Q62.8
uterus Q51.3
uvula Q35.7
Biforis uterus (suprasimplex) Q51.3
Bifurcation (congenital)
gallbladder Q44.1
kidney pelvis Q63.8
renal pelvis Q63.8
rib Q76.6
tongue, congenital Q38.3
trachea Q32.1
ureter Q62.8
urethra Q64.74
vertebra Q76.49
Big spleen syndrome D73.1
Bigeminal pulse R00.8
Bilateral -*see* condition
Bile
duct -*see* condition
pigments in urine R82.2
Bilharziasis -*see also* Schistosomiasis
chyluria B65.0
cutaneous B65.3
galacturia B65.0
hematochyluria B65.0
intestinal B65.1
lipemia B65.9
lipuria B65.0
oriental B65.2
piarhemia B65.9
pulmonary NOS B65.9 [*J99*]
  pneumonia B65.9 [*J17*]
tropical hematuria B65.0
vesical B65.0
Biliary -*see* condition
Bilirubin metabolism disorder E80.7
specified NEC E80.6
Bilirubinemia, familial nonhemolytic E80.4
Bilirubinuria R82.2
Biliuria R82.2
Bilocular stomach K31.2
Biparta, bipartite
carpal scaphoid Q74.0
patella Q74.1
vagina Q52.10
Bird
face Q75.8
fancier's disease or lung J67.2
Birt-Hogg-Dube syndrome Q87.89
Birth
complications in mother -*see* Delivery, complicated
compression during NOS P15.9
defect -*see* Anomaly
immature (less than 37
completed weeks) -*see* Preterm, newborn
  extremely (less than 28 completed weeks) - *see* Immaturity, extreme
inattention, at or after -*see* Maltreatment, child, neglect
injury NOS P15.9
  basal ganglia P11.1
  brachial plexus NEC P14.3
  brain (compression) (pressure) P11.2
  central nervous system NOS P11.9

Birth --continued
  cerebellum P11.1
  cerebral hemorrhage P10.1
  external genitalia P15.5
  eye P15.3
  face P15.4
  fracture
    bone P13.9
      specified NEC P13.8
    clavicle P13.4
    femur P13.2
    humerus P13.3
    long bone, except femur P13.3
    radius and ulna P13.3
    skull P13.0
    spine P11.5
    tibia and fibula P13.3
  intracranial P11.2
    laceration or hemorrhage P10.9
      specified NEC P10.8
  intraventricular hemorrhage P10.2
  laceration
    brain P10.1
    by scalpel P15.8
    peripheral nerve P14.9
  liver P15.0
  meninges
    brain P11.1
    spinal cord P11.5
  nerve
    brachial plexus P14.3
    cranial NEC (except facial) P11.4
    facial P11.3
    peripheral P14.9
    phrenic (paralysis) P14.2
  paralysis
    facial nerve P11.3
    spinal P11.5
  penis P15.5
  rupture
    spinal cord P11.5
  scalp P12.9
  scalpel wound P15.8
  scrotum P15.5
  skull NEC P13.1
    fracture P13.0
  specified type NEC P15.8
  spinal cord P11.5
  spine P11.5
  spleen P15.1
  sternomastoid (hematoma) P15.2
  subarachnoid hemorrhage P10.3
  subcutaneous fat necrosis P15.6
  subdural hemorrhage P10.0
  tentorial tear P10.4
  testes P15.5
  vulva P15.5
lack of care, at or after -see Maltreatment,
  child, neglect
neglect, at or after -see Maltreatment, child,
  neglect
palsy or paralysis, newborn, NOS (birth
  injury) P14.9
premature (infant) -see Preterm, newborn
shock, newborn P96.89
trauma -see Birth, injury   weight
  low (2499 grams or less) -see Low,
    birthweight
      extremely (999 grams or less) -see Low,
        birthweight, extreme
  4000 grams to 4499 grams P08.1

Birth – continued --continued
  4500 grams or more P08.0
Birthmark Q82.5
Bisalbuminemia E88.09
Biskra's button B55.1
Bite(s) (animal) (human)
  abdomen, abdominal
    wall S31.159
      with penetration into peritoneal cavity
        S31.659
      epigastric region S31.152
        with penetration into peritoneal cavity
          S31.652
      left
        lower quadrant S31.154
          with penetration into peritoneal cavity
            S31.654
        upper quadrant S31.151
          with penetration into peritoneal cavity
            S31.651
      periumbilic region S31.155
        with penetration into peritoneal cavity
          S31.655
      right
        lower quadrant S31.153
          with penetration into peritoneal cavity
            S31.653
        upper quadrant S31.150
          with penetration into peritoneal cavity
            S31.650
      superficial NEC S30.871
        insect S30.861
  alveolar (process) -see Bite, oral cavity
  amphibian (venomous) -see Venom, bite,
    amphibian
  animal -see also Bite, by site
    venomous -see Venom
  ankle S91.05
    superficial NEC S90.57
      insect S90.56
  antecubital space -see Bite, elbow
  anus S31.835
    superficial NEC S30.877
      insect S30.867
  arm (upper) S41.15
    lower -see Bite, forearm
    superficial NEC S40.87
      insect S40.86
  arthropod NEC -see Venom, bite, arthropod
  auditory canal (external) (meatus) -see Bite,
    ear
  auricle, ear -see Bite, ear
  axilla -see Bite, arm
  back -see also Bite, thorax, back
    lower S31.050
      with penetration into retroperitoneal space
        S31.051
      superficial NEC S30.870
        insect S30.860
  bedbug -see Bite(s), by site, superficial, insect
  breast S21.05
    superficial NEC S20.17
      insect S20.16
  brow -see Bite, head, specified site NEC
  buttock S31.805
    left S31.825
    right S31.815
    superficial NEC S30.870
      insect S30.860
  calf -see Bite, leg
  canaliculus lacrimalis -see Bite, eyelid

Bite(s) (animal) (human) --continued
  canthus, eye -see Bite, eyelid
  centipede -see Toxicity, venom, arthropod,
    centipede
  cheek (external) S01.45
    superficial NEC S00.87
      insect S00.86
    internal -see Bite, oral cavity   chest wall -
      see Bite, thorax
  chigger B88.0
  chin -see Bite, head, specified site NEC
  clitoris -see Bite, vulva
  costal region -see Bite, thorax - digit(s)
    hand -see Bite, finger
    toe -see Bite, toe
  ear (canal) (external) S01.35
    superficial NEC S00.47
      insect S00.46
  elbow S51.05
    superficial NEC S50.37
      insect S50.36
  epididymis -see Bite, testis
  epigastric region -see Bite, abdomen
  epiglottis -see Bite, neck, specified site NEC
  esophagus, cervical S11.25
    superficial NEC S10.17
      insect S10.16
  eyebrow -see Bite, eyelid
  eyelid S01.15
    superficial NEC S00.27
      insect S00.26
  face NEC -see Bite, head, specified site NEC
  finger(s) S61.259
    with
      damage to nail S61.359
    index S61.258
      with
        damage to nail S61.358
      left S61.251
        with
          damage to nail S61.351
      right S61.250
        with
          damage to nail S61.350
      superficial NEC S60.478
        insect S60.46
    little S61.25
      with
        damage to nail S61.35
      superficial NEC S60.47
        insect S60.46
    middle S61.25
      with
        damage to nail S61.35
      superficial NEC S60.47
        insect S60.46
    ring S61.25
      with
        damage to nail S61.35
      superficial NEC S60.47
        insect S60.46
    superficial NEC S60.479
      insect S60.469
    thumb -see Bite, thumb
  flank -see Bite, abdomen, wall
  flea -see Bite, by site, superficial, insect
  foot (except toe(s) alone) S91.35
    superficial NEC S90.87
      insect S90.86
    toe -see Bite, toe - forearm S51.85
      elbow only -see Bite, elbow

Bite(s) (animal) (human) --*continued*
  superficial NEC S50.87
    insect S50.86
  forehead -*see* Bite, head, specified site NEC
  genital organs, external
    female S31.552
      superficial NEC S30.876
        insect S30.866
      vagina and vulva -*see* Bite, vulva
    male S31.551
      penis -*see* Bite, penis
      scrotum -*see* Bite, scrotum
      superficial NEC S30.875
        insect S30.865
      testes -*see* Bite, testis
  groin -*see* Bite, abdomen, wall
  gum -*see* Bite, oral cavity
  hand S61.45
    finger -*see* Bite, finger
    superficial NEC S60.57
      insect S60.56
    thumb -*see* Bite, thumb
  head S01.95
    cheek -*see* Bite, cheek
    ear -*see* Bite, ear
    eyelid -*see* Bite, eyelid
    lip -*see* Bite, lip
    nose -*see* Bite, nose
    oral cavity -*see* Bite, oral cavity
    scalp -*see* Bite, scalp
    specified site NEC S01.85
      superficial NEC S00.87
        insect S00.86
    superficial NEC S00.97
      insect S00.96
    temporomandibular area -*see* Bite, cheek
  heel -*see* Bite, foot
  hip S71.05
    superficial NEC S70.27
      insect S70.26
  hymen S31.45
  hypochondrium -*see* Bite, abdomen, wall
  hypogastric region -*see* Bite, abdomen, wall
  inguinal region -*see* Bite, abdomen, wall
  insect -*see* Bite, by site, superficial, insect
  instep -*see* Bite, foot
  interscapular region -*see* Bite, thorax, back
  jaw -*see* Bite, head, specified site NEC
  knee S81.05
    superficial NEC S80.27
      insect S80.26
  labium (majus) (minus) -*see* Bite, vulva
  lacrimal duct -*see* Bite, eyelid
  larynx S11.015
    superficial NEC S10.17
      insect S10.16
  leg (lower) S81.85
    ankle -*see* Bite, ankle
    foot -*see* Bite, foot
    knee -*see* Bite, knee
    superficial NEC S80.87
      insect S80.86
    toe -*see* Bite, toe
    upper -*see* Bite, thigh
  lip S01.551
    superficial NEC S00.571
      insect S00.561
  lizard (venomous) -*see* Venom, bite, reptile
  loin -*see* Bite, abdomen, wall
  lower back -*see* Bite, back, lower
  lumbar region -*see* Bite, back, lower

Bite(s) (animal) (human) --*continued*
  malar region -*see* Bite, head, specified site
    NEC
  mammary -*see* Bite, breast
  marine animals (venomous) -*see* Toxicity,
    venom, marine animal
  mastoid region -*see* Bite, head, specified site
    NEC
  mouth -*see* Bite, oral cavity nail
    finger -*see* Bite, finger
    toe -*see* Bite, toe
  nape -*see* Bite, neck, specified site NEC
  nasal (septum) (sinus) -*see* Bite, nose
  nasopharynx -*see* Bite, head, specified site
    NEC
  neck S11.95
    involving
      cervical esophagus -*see* Bite, esophagus,
      cervical
      larynx -*see* Bite, larynx
      pharynx -*see* Bite, pharynx
      thyroid gland S11.15
      trachea -*see* Bite, trachea
    specified site NEC S11.85
      superficial NEC S10.87
        insect S10.86
    superficial NEC S10.97
      insect S10.96
    throat S11.85
      superficial NEC S10.17
        insect S10.16
  nose (septum) (sinus) S01.25
    superficial NEC S00.37
      insect S00.36
  occipital region -*see* Bite, scalp
  oral cavity S01.552
    superficial NEC S00.572
      insect S00.562
  orbital region -*see* Bite, eyelid
  palate -*see* Bite, oral cavity
  palm -*see* Bite, hand
  parietal region -*see* Bite, scalp
  pelvis S31.050
    with penetration into retroperitoneal space
    S31.051
    superficial NEC S30.870
      insect S30.860
  penis S31.25
    superficial NEC S30.872
      insect S30.862
  perineum
    female -*see* Bite, vulva
    male -*see* Bite, pelvis
  periocular area (with or without lacrimal
    passages) -*see* Bite, eyelid
  phalanges
    finger -*see* Bite, finger
    toe -*see* Bite, toe
  pharynx S11.25
    superficial NEC S10.17
      insect S10.16
  pinna -*see* Bite, ear
  poisonous -*see* Venom
  popliteal space -*see* Bite, knee - prepuce -*see*
    Bite, penis
  pubic region -*see* Bite, abdomen, wall
  rectovaginal septum -*see* Bite, vulva
  red bug B88.0
  reptile NEC -*see also* Venom, bite, reptile
    nonvenomous -*see* Bite, by site
    snake -*see* Venom, bite, snake

Bite(s) (animal) (human) --*continued*
  sacral region -*see* Bite, back, lower
  sacroiliac region -*see* Bite, back, lower
  salivary gland -*see* Bite, oral cavity
  scalp S01.05
    superficial NEC S00.07
      insect S00.06
  scapular region -*see* Bite, shoulder
  scrotum S31.35
    superficial NEC S30.873
      insect S30.863
  sea-snake (venomous) -*see* Toxicity, venom,
    snake, sea snake - shin -*see* Bite, leg
  shoulder S41.05
    superficial NEC S40.27
      insect S40.26
  snake -*see also* Venom, bite, snake
    nonvenomous -*see* Bite, by site
  spermatic cord -*see* Bite, testis
  spider (venomous) -*see* Toxicity, venom,
    spider
    nonvenomous -*see* Bite, by site, superficial,
    insect
  sternal region -*see* Bite, thorax, front
  submaxillary region -*see* Bite, head, specified
    site NEC
  submental region -*see* Bite, head, specified
    site NEC
  subungual
    finger(s) -*see* Bite, finger
    toe -*see* Bite, toe
  superficial -*see* Bite, by site, superficial
  supraclavicular fossa S11.85
  supraorbital -*see* Bite, head, specified site
    NEC
  temple, temporal region -*see* Bite, head,
    specified site NEC
  temporomandibular area -*see* Bite, cheek
  testis S31.35
    superficial NEC S30.873
      insect S30.863
  thigh S71.15
    superficial NEC S70.37
      insect S70.36
  thorax, thoracic (wall) S21.95
    back S21.25
      with penetration into thoracic cavity
      S21.45
    breast -*see* Bite, breast
    front S21.15
      with penetration into thoracic cavity
      S21.35
    superficial NEC S20.97
      back S20.47
      front S20.37
      insect S20.96
        back S20.46
        front S20.36
  throat -*see* Bite, neck, throat
  thumb S61.05
    with
      damage to nail S61.15
    superficial NEC S60.37
      insect S60.36
  thyroid S11.15
    superficial NEC S10.87
      insect S10.86
  toe(s) S91.15
    with
      damage to nail S91.25
    great S91.15

Bite(s) (animal) (human) --*continued*
  with
    damage to nail S91.25
  lesser S91.15
    with
      damage to nail S91.25
  superficial NEC S90.47
    great S90.47
    insect S90.46
      great S90.46
  tongue S01.552
  trachea S11.025
    superficial NEC S10.17
    insect S10.16
  tunica vaginalis -*see* Bite, testis
  tympanum, tympanic membrane -*see* Bite, ear
  umbilical region S31.155
  uvula -*see* Bite, oral cavity   vagina -*see* Bite, vulva
  venomous -*see* Venom
  vocal cords S11.035
    superficial NEC S10.17
    insect S10.16
  vulva S31.45
    superficial NEC S30.874
    insect S30.864
  wrist S61.55
    superficial NEC S60.87
    insect S60.86
Biting, cheek or lip K13.1
Biventricular failure (heart) I50.9
Björck (Thorson) syndrome (malignant carcinoid) E34.0
Black
  death A20.9
  eye S00.1
  hairy tongue K14.3
  heel (foot) S90.3
  lung (disease) J60
  palm (hand) S60.22
Blackfan-Diamond anemia or syndrome (congenital hypoplastic anemia) D61.01
Blackhead L70.0
Blackout R55
Bladder -*see* condition
Blast (air) (hydraulic) (immersion) (underwater)
  blindness S05.8X
  injury
    abdomen or thorax -*see* Injury, by site
    ear (acoustic nerve trauma) -*see* Injury, nerve, acoustic, specified type NEC
    syndrome NEC T70.8
Blastoma -*see* Neoplasm, malignant, by site
  pulmonary -*see* Neoplasm, lung, malignant
Blastomycosis, blastomycotic B40.9
  Brazilian -*see* Paracoccidioidomycosis
  cutaneous B40.3
  disseminated B40.7
  European -*see* Cryptococcosis
  generalized B40.7
  keloidal B48.0
  North American B40.9
  primary pulmonary B40.0
  pulmonary B40.2
    acute B40.0
    chronic B40.1
  skin B40.3
  South American -*see* Paracoccidioidomycosis
  specified NEC B40.89

Bleb(s) R23.8
  emphysematous (lung) (solitary) J43.9
  endophthalmitis H59.43
  filtering (vitreous), after glaucoma surgery Z98.83
  inflamed (infected), postprocedural H59.40
    stage 1H59.41
    stage 2H59.42
    stage 3H59.43
  lung (ruptured) J43.9
    congenital -*see* Atelectasis
    newborn P25.8
  subpleural (emphysematous) J43.9
Blebitis, postprocedural H59.40
  stage 1 H59.41
  stage 2 H59.42
  stage 3 H59.43
Bleeder (familial) (hereditary) -*see* Hemophilia
Bleeding -*see also* Hemorrhage
  anal K62.5
  anovulatory N97.0
  atonic, following delivery O72.1
  capillary I78.8
    puerperal O72.2
  contact (postcoital) N93.0
  due to uterine subinvolution N85.3
  ear -*see* Otorrhagia
  excessive, associated with menopausal onset N92.4
  familial -*see* Defect, coagulation
  following intercourse N93.0
  gastrointestinal K92.2
  hemorrhoids -*see* Hemorrhoids
  intermenstrual (regular) N92.3
    irregular N92.1
  intraoperative -*see* Complication, intraoperative, hemorrhage
  irregular N92.6
  menopausal N92.4
  newborn, intraventricular -*see* Newborn, affected by, hemorrhage, intraventricular
  nipple N64.59
  nose R04.0
  ovulation N92.3
  postclimacteric N95.0
  postcoital N93.0
  postmenopausal N95.0
  postoperative -*see* Complication, postprocedural, hemorrhage
  preclimacteric N92.4
  pre-pubertal vaginal N93.1
  puberty (excessive, with onset of menstrual periods) N92.2
  rectum, rectal K62.5
    newborn P54.2
  tendencies -*see* Defect, coagulation
  throat R04.1
  tooth socket (post-extraction) K91.840
  umbilical stump P51.9
  uterus, uterine NEC N93.9
    climacteric N92.4
    dysfunctional of functional N93.8
    menopausal N92.4
    preclimacteric or premenopausal N92.4
    unrelated to menstrual cycle N93.9
  vagina, vaginal (abnormal) N93.9
    dysfunctional or functional N93.8
    newborn P54.6
    pre-pubertal N93.1
  vicarious N94.89

Blennorrhagia, blennorrhagic -*see* Gonorrhea
Blennorrhea (acute) (chronic) -*see also* Gonorrhea
  inclusion (neonatal) (newborn) P39.1
  lower genitourinary tract (gonococcal) A54.00
  neonatorum (gonococcal ophthalmia) A54.31
Blepharelosis -*see* Entropion
Blepharitis (angularis) (ciliaris) (eyelid) (marginal) (nonulcerative) H01.009
  herpes zoster B02.39
  left H01.006
    lower H01.005
    upper H01.004
  right H01.003
    lower H01.002
    upper H01.001
  squamous H01.029
    left H01.026
      lower H01.025
      upper H01.024
    right H01.023
      lower H01.022
      upper H01.021
  ulcerative H01.019
    left H01.016
      lower H01.015
      upper H01.014
    right H01.013
      lower H01.012
      upper H01.011
Blepharochalasis H02.30
  congenital Q10.0
  left H02.36
    lower H02.35
    upper H02.34
  right H02.33
    lower H02.32
    upper H02.31
Blepharoclonus H02.59
Blepharoconjunctivitis H10.50
  angular H10.52
  contact H10.53
  ligneous H10.51
Blepharophimosis (eyelid) H02.529
  congenital Q10.3
  left H02.526
    lower H02.525
    upper H02.524
  right H02.523
    lower H02.522
    upper H02.521
Blepharoptosis H02.40
  congenital Q10.0
  mechanical H02.41
  myogenic H02.42
  neurogenic H02.43
  paralytic H02.43
Blepharopyorrhea, gonococcal A54.39
Blepharospasm G24.5
  drug induced G24.01
Blighted ovum O02.0
Blind -*see also* Blindness
  bronchus (congenital) Q32.4
  loop syndrome K90.2
    congenital Q43.8
  sac, fallopian tube (congenital) Q50.6
  spot, enlarged -*see* Defect, visual field, localized, scotoma, blind spot area
  tract or tube, congenital NEC -*see* Atresia, by site

Blindness (acquired) (congenital) (both eyes)
H54.0
  blast S05.8X
  color -see Deficiency, color vision
  concussion S05.8X
  cortical H47.619
    left brain H47.612
    right brain H47.611
  day H53.11
  due to injury (current episode) S05.9
    sequelae - code to injury with seventh
      character S
  eclipse (total) -see Retinopathy, solar
  emotional (hysterical) F44.6
  face H53.16
  hysterical F44.6
  legal (both eyes) (USA definition) H54.8
  mind R48.8
  night H53.60
    abnormal dark adaptation curve H53.61
    acquired H53.62
    congenital H53.63
    specified type NEC H53.69
    vitamin A deficiency E50.5
  one eye (other eye normal) H54.40
    left (normal vision on right) H54.42
      low vision on right H54.12
    low vision, other eye H54.10
    right (normal vision on left) H54.41
      low vision on left H54.11
  psychic R48.8
  river B73.01
  snow -see Photokeratitis
  sun, solar -see Retinopathy, solar
  transient -see Disturbance, vision, subjective,
    loss, transient
  traumatic (current episode) S05.9
  word (developmental) F81.0
    acquired R48.0
    secondary to organic lesion R48.0
Blister (nonthermal)
  abdominal wall S30.821
  alveolar process S00.522
  ankle S90.52
  antecubital space -see Blister, elbow
  anus S30.827
  arm (upper) S40.82
  auditory canal -see Blister, ear
  auricle -see Blister, ear
  axilla -see Blister, arm
  back, lower S30.820
  beetle dermatitis L24.89
  breast S20.12
  brow S00.82
  calf -see Blister, leg
  canthus -see Blister, eyelid
  cheek S00.82
    internal S00.522
  chest wall -see Blister, thorax - chin S00.82
  costal region -see Blister, thorax - digit(s)
    foot -see Blister, toe
    hand -see Blister, finger
  due to burn -see Burn, by site, second degree -
    ear S00.42
  elbow S50.32
  epiglottis S10.12
  esophagus, cervical S10.12
  eyebrow -see Blister, eyelid
  eyelid S00.22
  face S00.82
  fever B00.1

Blister (nonthermal) --continued
  finger(s) S60.429
    index S60.42
    little S60.42
    middle S60.42
    ring S60.42
  foot (except toe(s) alone) S90.82
    toe -see Blister, toe
  forearm S50.82
    elbow only -see Blister, elbow
  forehead S00.82
  fracture
  omit code
  genital organ
    female S30.826
    male S30.825
  gum S00.522
  hand S60.52
  head S00.92
    ear -see Blister, ear
    eyelid -see Blister, eyelid
    lip S00.521
    nose S00.32
    oral cavity S00.522
    scalp S00.02
    specified site NEC S00.82
  heel -see Blister, foot
  hip S70.22
  interscapular region S20.429
  jaw S00.82
  knee S80.22
  larynx S10.12
  leg (lower) S80.82
    knee -see Blister, knee
    upper -see Blister, thigh
  lip S00.521
  malar region S00.82
  mammary -see Blister, breast
  mastoid region S00.82
  mouth S00.522
  multiple, skin, nontraumatic R23.8
  nail
    finger -see Blister, finger
    toe -see Blister, toe
  nasal S00.32
  neck S10.92
    specified site NEC S10.82
    throat S10.12
  nose S00.32
  occipital region S00.02
  oral cavity S00.522
  orbital region -see Blister, eyelid
  palate S00.522
  palm -see Blister, hand
  parietal region S00.02
  pelvis S30.820
  penis S30.822
  periocular area -see Blister, eyelid
  phalanges
    finger -see Blister, finger
    toe -see Blister, toe
  pharynx S10.12
  pinna -see Blister, ear
  popliteal space -see Blister, knee - scalp
    S00.02
  scapular region -see Blister, shoulder
  scrotum S30.823
  shin -see Blister, leg
  shoulder S40.22
  sternal region S20.329
  submaxillary region S00.82

Blister (nonthermal) --continued
  submental region S00.82
  subungual
    finger(s) -see Blister, finger
    toe(s) -see Blister, toe
  supraclavicular fossa S10.82
  supraorbital S00.82
  temple S00.82
  temporal region S00.82
  testis S30.823
  thermal -see Burn, second degree, by site
  thigh S70.32
  thorax, thoracic (wall) S20.92
    back S20.42
    front S20.32
  throat S10.12
  thumb S60.32
  toe(s) S90.42
    great S90.42
  tongue S00.522
  trachea S10.12
  tympanum, tympanic membrane -see Blister,
    ear
  upper arm -see Blister, arm (upper)
  uvula S00.522
  vagina S30.824
  vocal cords S10.12
  vulva S30.824
  wrist S60.82
Bloating R14.0
Bloch-Sulzberger disease or syndrome Q82.3
Block, blocked
  alveolocapillary J84.10
  arborization (heart) I45.5
  arrhythmic I45.9
  atrioventricular (incomplete) (partial) I44.30
    with atrioventricular dissociation I44.2
    complete I44.2
      congenital Q24.6
    congenital Q24.6
    first degree I44.0
    second degree (types I and II) I44.1
    specified NEC I44.39
    third degree I44.2
    types I and II I44.1
  auriculoventricular -see Block,
    atrioventricular
  bifascicular (cardiac) I45.2
  bundle-branch (complete) (false) (incomplete)
    I45.4
    bilateral I45.2
    left I44.7
      with right bundle branch block I45.2
      hemiblock I44.60
        anterior I44.4
        posterior I44.5
      incomplete I44.7
        with right bundle branch block I45.2
    right I45.10
      with
        left bundle branch block I45.2
        left fascicular block I45.2
        specified NEC I45.19
    Wilson's type I45.19
  cardiac I45.9
  conduction I45.9
    complete I44.2
  fascicular (left) I44.60
    anterior I44.4
    posterior I44.5
    right I45.0

Block, blocked --continued
  specified NEC I44.69
  foramen Magendie (acquired) G91.1
  congenital Q03.1
    with spina bifida -see Spina bifida, by site,
  with hydrocephalus
  heart I45.9
    bundle branch I45.4
      bilateral I45.2
    complete (atrioventricular) I44.2
    congenital Q24.6
    first degree (atrioventricular) I44.0
    second degree (atrioventricular) I44.1
    specified type NEC I45.5
    third degree (atrioventricular) I44.2
  hepatic vein I82.0
  intraventricular (nonspecific) I45.4
    bundle branch
      bilateral I45.2
  kidney N28.9
    postcystoscopic or postprocedural N99.0
  Mobitz (types I and II) I44.1
  myocardial -see Block, heart
  nodal I45.5
  organ or site, congenital NEC -see Atresia, by
  site
  portal (vein) I81
  second degree (types I and II) I44.1
  sinoatrial I45.5
  sinoauricular I45.5
  third degree I44.2
  trifascicular I45.3
  tubal N97.1
  vein NOS I82.90
  Wenckebach (types I and II) I44.1
Blockage -see Obstruction
Blocq's disease F44.4
Blood
  constituents, abnormal R78.9
  disease D75.9
  donor -see Donor, blood - dyscrasia D75.9
    with
      abortion -see Abortion, by type,
  complicated by, hemorrhage
    ectopic pregnancy O08.1
    molar pregnancy O08.1
    following ectopic or molar pregnancy O08.1
    newborn P61.9
    puerperal, postpartum O72.3
  flukes NEC -see Schistosomiasis
  in
    feces K92.1
      occult R19.5
    urine -see Hematuria
  mole O02.0
  occult in feces R19.5
  pressure
    decreased, due to shock following injury
    T79.4
    examination only Z01.30
    fluctuating I99.8
    high -see Hypertension
      borderline R03.0
      incidental reading, without diagnosis of
      hypertension R03.0
    low -see also Hypotension
      incidental reading, without diagnosis of
      hypotension R03.1
  spitting -see Hemoptysis
  staining cornea -see Pigmentation, cornea,
  stromal

Blood – continued
  transfusion
    reaction or complication -see Complications,
    transfusion
    type
      A (Rh positive) Z67.10
        Rh negative Z67.11
      AB (Rh positive) Z67.30
        Rh negative Z67.31
      B (Rh positive) Z67.20
        Rh negative Z67.21
      O (Rh positive) Z67.40
        Rh negative Z67.41
      Rh (positive) Z67.90
        negative Z67.91
  vessel rupture -see Hemorrhage
  vomiting -see Hematemesis
Blood-forming organs, disease D75.9
Bloodgood's disease -see Mastopathy, cystic
Bloom (Machacek)(Torre) syndrome Q82.8
Blount's disease or osteochondrosis -see
  Osteochondrosis, juvenile, tibia
Blue
  baby Q24.9
  diaper syndrome E72.09
  dome cyst (breast) -see Cyst, breast
  dot cataract Q12.0
  nevus D22.9
  sclera Q13.5
    with fragility of bone and deafness Q78.0
  toe syndrome I75.02
Blueness -see Cyanosis
Blues, postpartal O90.6
  baby O90.6
Blurring, visual H53.8
Blushing (abnormal) (excessive) R23.2
BMI -see Body, mass index
Boarder, hospital NEC Z76.4
  accompanying sick person Z76.3
  healthy infant or child Z76.2
    foundling Z76.1
Bockhart's impetigo L01.02
**Bodechtel-Guttman disease (subacute
  sclerosing panencephalitis)** A81.1
**Boder-Sedgwick syndrome (ataxia-
  telangiectasia)** G11.3
Body, bodies
  Aschoff's -see Myocarditis, rheumatic
  asteroid, vitreous -see Deposit, crystalline
  cytoid (retina) -see Occlusion, artery, retina
  drusen (degenerative) (macula) (retinal) -see
  also Degeneration, macula, drusen
    optic disc -see Drusen, optic disc
  foreign -see Foreign body
  loose
    joint, except knee -see Loose, body, joint
    knee M23.4
    sheath, tendon -see Disorder, tendon,
    specified type NEC
  mass index (BMI)
    adult
      19 or less Z68.1
      20.0 20.9 Z68.20
      21.0 21.9 Z68.21
      22.0 22.9 Z68.22
      23.0 23.9 Z68.23
      24.0 24.9 Z68.24
      25.0 25.9 Z68.25
      26.0 26.9 Z68.26
      27.0 27.9 Z68.27
      28.0 28.9 Z68.28

Body, bodies - continued
      29.0 29.9 Z68.29
      30.0 30.9 Z68.30
      31.0 31.9 Z68.31
      32.0 32.9 Z68.32
      33.0 33.9 Z68.33
      34.0 34.9 Z68.34
      35.0 35.9 Z68.35
      36.0 36.9 Z68.36
      37.0 37.9 Z68.37
      38.0 38.9 Z68.38
      39.0 39.9 Z68.39
      40.0 44.9 Z68.41
      45.0 49.9 Z68.42
      50.0 59.9 Z68.43
      60.0 69.9 Z68.44
      70 and over Z68.45
    pediatric
      5th percentile to less than 85th percentile
      for age Z68.52
      85th percentile to less than 95th percentile
      for age Z68.53
      greater than or equal to ninety fifth
      percentile for age Z68.54
      less than fifth percentile for age Z68.51
  Mooser's A75.2
  rice -see also Loose, body, joint
    knee M23.4
  rocking F98.4
Boeck's
  disease or sarcoid -see Sarcoidosis
  lupoid (miliary) D86.3
**Boerhaave's syndrome (spontaneous
  esophageal rupture)** K22.3
Boggy
  cervix N88.8
  uterus N85.8
Boil -see also Furuncle, by site
  Aleppo B55.1
  Baghdad B55.1
  Delhi B55.1
  lacrimal
    gland -see Dacryoadenitis
    passages (duct) (sac) -see Inflammation,
  lacrimal, passages, acute
  Natal B55.1
  orbit, orbital -see Abscess, orbit
  tropical B55.1
Bold hives -see Urticaria
Bombé, iris -see Membrane, pupillary
Bone -see condition
Bonnevie-Ullrich syndrome -see also Turner's
  syndrome Q87.1
Bonnier's syndrome -see subcategory H81.8
Bonvale dam fever T73.3
Bony block of joint -see Ankylosis
**BOOP (bronchiolitis obliterans organized
  pneumonia)** J84.89
Borderline
  diabetes mellitus R73.03
  hypertension R03.0
  osteopenia M85.8
  pelvis, with obstruction during labor O65.1
  personality F60.3
Borna disease A83.9
Bornholm disease B33.0
Boston exanthem A88.0
Botalli, ductus (patent) (persistent) Q25.0
Bothriocephalus latus infestation B70.0

Botulism (foodborne intoxication) A05.1
  infant A48.51
  non-foodborne A48.52
  wound A48.52
Bouba -*see* Yaws
Bouchard's nodes (with arthropathy) M15.2
Bouffée délirante F23
Bouillaud's disease or syndrome (rheumatic heart disease) I01.9
Bourneville's disease Q85.1
Boutonniere deformity (finger) -*see* Deformity, finger, boutonniere
Bouveret (Hoffmann) syndrome (paroxysmal tachycardia) I47.9
Bovine heart -*see* Hypertrophy, cardiac
Bowel -*see* condition
Bowen's
  dermatosis (precancerous) -*see* Neoplasm, skin, in situ
  disease -*see* Neoplasm, skin, in situ
  epithelioma -*see* Neoplasm, skin, in situ
  type
    epidermoid carcinoma-in-situ -*see* Neoplasm, skin, in situ
    intraepidermal squamous cell carcinoma - *see* Neoplasm, skin, in situ
Bowing
  femur -*see also* Deformity, limb, specified type NEC, thigh
    congenital Q68.3
  fibula -*see also* Deformity, limb, specified type NEC, lower leg
    congenital Q68.4
  forearm -*see* Deformity, limb, specified type NEC, forearm
  leg(s), long bones, congenital Q68.5
  radius -*see* Deformity, limb, specified type NEC, forearm
  tibia -*see also* Deformity, limb, specified type NEC, lower leg
    congenital Q68.4
Bowleg(s) (acquired) M21.16
  congenital Q68.5
  rachitic E64.3
Boyd's dysentery A03.2
Brachial -*see* condition
Brachycardia R00.1
Brachycephaly Q75.0
Bradley's disease A08.19
Bradyarrhythmia, cardiac I49.8
Bradycardia (sinoatrial) (sinus) (vagal) R00.1
  neonatal P29.12
  reflex G90.09
  tachycardia syndrome I49.5
Bradykinesia R25.8
Bradypnea R06.89
Bradytachycardia I49.5
Brailsford's disease or osteochondrosis -*see* Osteochondrosis, juvenile, radius
Brain -*see also* condition
  death G93.82
  syndrome -*see* Syndrome, brain
Branched-chain amino-acid disorder E71.2
Branchial -*see* condition
  cartilage, congenital Q18.2
Branchiogenic remnant (in neck) Q18.0
Brandt's syndrome (acrodermatitis enteropathica) E83.2
Brash (water) R12

Bravais-jacksonian epilepsy -*see* Epilepsy, localization-related, symptomatic, with simple partial seizures
Braxton Hicks contractions -*see* False, labor
Brazilian leishmaniasis B55.2
BRBPR K62.5
Break, retina (without detachment) H33.30
  with retinal detachment -*see* Detachment, retina
  horseshoe tear H33.31
  multiple H33.33
  round hole H33.32
Breakdown
  device, graft or implant -*see also* Complications, by site and type, mechanical T85.618
    arterial graft NEC -*see* Complication, cardiovascular device, mechanical, vascular
    breast (implant) T85.41
    catheter NEC T85.618
      cystostomy T83.010
      Hopkins T83.018
      ileostomy T83.018
      dialysis (renal) T82.41
        intraperitoneal T85.611
      infusion NEC T82.514
        cranial T85.610
        epidural T85.610
        intrathecal T85.610
        spinal T85.610
        subarachnoid T85.610
        subdural T85.610
      nephrostomy T83.012
      urethral indwelling T83.011
      urinary NEC T83.018
      urostomy T83.018
    electronic (electrode) (pulse generator) (stimulator)
      bone T84.310
      cardiac T82.119
        electrode T82.110
        pulse generator T82.111
        specified type NEC T82.118
      nervous system -*see* Complication, prosthetic device, mechanical, electronic nervous system stimulator
      urinary -*see* Complication, genitourinary, device, urinary, mechanical
    fixation, internal (orthopedic) NEC -*see* Complication, fixation device, mechanical
    gastrointestinal -*see* Complications, prosthetic device, mechanical, gastrointestinal device
    genital NEC T83.418
      intrauterine contraceptive device T83.31
      penile prosthesis (cylinder) (implanted) (pump) (reservoir) T83.410
      testicular prosthesis T83.411
    heart NEC -*see* Complication, cardiovascular device, mechanical
    intrathecal infusion pump T85.615
    joint prosthesis -*see* Complications..., joint prosthesis, internal, mechanical, by site
    nervous system, specified device NEC T85.615
    ocular NEC -*see* Complications, prosthetic device, mechanical, ocular device
    orthopedic NEC -*see* Complication, orthopedic, device, mechanical
    specified NEC T85.618
    subcutaneous device pocket

Breakdown - *continued*
    nervous system prosthetic device, implant, or graft T85.890
    other internal prosthetic device, implant, or graft T85.898
    sutures, permanent T85.612
      used in bone repair -*see* Complications, fixation device, internal (orthopedic), mechanical
    urinary NEC T83.118
      graft T83.21
      sphincter, implanted T83.111
      stent (ileal conduit) (nephroureteral) T83.113
      ureteral indwelling T83.112
    vascular NEC -*see* Complication, cardiovascular device, mechanical
    ventricular intracranial shunt T85.01
  nervous F48.8
  perineum O90.1
  respirator J95.850
    specified NEC J95.859
  ventilator J95.850
    specified NEC J95.859
Breast -*see also* condition
  buds E30.1
    in newborn P96.89
  dense R92.2
  nodule N63
Breath
  foul R19.6
  holder, child R06.89
  holding spell R06.89
  shortness R06.02
Breathing
  labored -*see* Hyperventilation
  mouth R06.5
    causing malocclusion M26.5
  periodic R06.3
    high altitude G47.32
Breathlessness R06.81
Breda's disease -*see* Yaws
Breech presentation (mother) O32.1
  causing obstructed labor O64.1
  footling O32.8
    causing obstructed labor O64.8
  incomplete O32.8
    causing obstructed labor O64.8
Breisky's disease N90.4
Brennemann's syndrome I88.0
Brenner
  tumor (benign) D27.9
    borderline malignancy D39.1
    malignant C56
    proliferating D39.1
Bretonneau's disease or angina A36.0
Breus' mole O02.0
Brevicollis Q76.49
Brickmakers' anemia B76.9 [*D63.8*]
Bridge, myocardial Q24.5
Bright red blood per rectum (BRBPR) K62.5
Bright's disease -*see also* Nephritis
  arteriosclerotic -*see* Hypertension, kidney
Brill (Zinsser) disease (recrudescent typhus) A75.1
  flea-borne A75.2
  louse-borne A75.1
Brill-Symmers' disease C82.90
Brion-Kayser disease -*see* Fever, parathyroid
Briquet's disorder or syndrome F45.0

Brissaud's
  infantilism or dwarfism E23.0
  motor-verbal tic F95.2
Brittle
  bones disease Q78.0
  nails L60.3
    congenital Q84.6
Broad -see also condition
  beta disease E78.2
  ligament laceration syndrome N83.8
Broad- or floating-betalipoproteinemia
  E78.2
Brock's syndrome (atelectasis due to enlarged lymph nodes) J98.19
Brocq-Duhring disease (dermatitis herpetiformis) L13.0
Brodie's abscess or disease M86.8X
Broken
  arches -see also Deformity, limb, flat foot
  arm (meaning upper limb) -see Fracture, arm
  back -see Fracture, vertebra
  bone -see Fracture
  implant or internal device -see Complications, by site and type, mechanical
  leg (meaning lower limb) -see Fracture, leg
  nose S02.2
  tooth, teeth -see Fracture, tooth
Bromhidrosis, bromidrosis L75.0
Bromidism, bromism G92
  due to
    correct substance properly administered -see Table of Drugs and Chemicals, by drug, adverse effect
    overdose or wrong substance given or taken -see Table of Drugs and Chemicals, by drug, poisoning
  chronic (dependence) F13.20
Bromidrosiphobia F40.298
Bronchi, bronchial -see condition
Bronchiectasis (cylindrical) (diffuse) (fusiform) (localized) (saccular) J47.9
  with
    acute
      bronchitis J47.0
      lower respiratory infection J47.0
    exacerbation (acute) J47.1
  congenital Q33.4
  tuberculous NEC -see Tuberculosis, pulmonary
Bronchiolectasis -see Bronchiectasis
Bronchiolitis (acute) (infective) (subacute) J21.9
  with
    bronchospasm or obstruction J21.9
    influenza, flu or grippe -see Influenza, with, respiratory manifestations NEC
  chemical (chronic) J68.4
    acute J68.0
  chronic (fibrosing) (obliterative) J44.9
  due to
    external agent -see Bronchitis, acute, due to
    human metapneumovirus J21.1
    respiratory syncytial virus J21.0
    specified organism NEC J21.8
  fibrosa obliterans J44.9
  influenzal -see Influenza, with, respiratory manifestations NEC
  obliterans J42
    with organizing pneumonia (BOOP) J84.89
  obliterative (chronic) (subacute) J44.9
    due to fumes or vapors J68.4

Bronchiolitis --continued
  due to chemicals, gases, fumes or vapors (inhalation) J68.4
  respiratory, interstitial lung disease J84.115
Bronchitis (diffuse) (fibrinous) (hypostatic) (infective) (membranous) J40
  with
    influenza, flu or grippe -see Influenza, with, respiratory manifestations NEC
    obstruction (airway) (lung) J44.9
    tracheitis (15 years of age and above) J40
      acute or subacute J20.9
      chronic J42
    under 15 years of age J20.9
  acute or subacute (with bronchospasm or obstruction) J20.9
    with
      bronchiectasis J47.0
      chronic obstructive pulmonary disease J44.0
    chemical (due to gases, fumes or vapors) J68.0
    due to
      fumes or vapors J68.0
      Haemophilus influenzae J20.1
      Mycoplasma pneumoniae J20.0
      radiation J70.0
      specified organism NEC J20.8
      Streptococcus J20.2
      virus
        coxsackie J20.3
        echovirus J20.7
        parainfluenzae J20.4
        respiratory syncytial J20.5
        rhinovirus J20.6
      viral NEC J20.8
  allergic (acute) J45.909
    with
      exacerbation (acute) J45.901
      status asthmaticus J45.902
  arachidic T17.528
  aspiration (due to fumes or vapors) J68.0
  asthmatic J45.9
    chronic J44.9
      with
        acute lower respiratory infection J44.0
        exacerbation (acute) J44.1
  capillary -see Pneumonia, broncho
  caseous (tuberculous) A15.5
  Castellani's A69.8
  catarrhal (15 years of age and above) J40
    acute -see Bronchitis, acute
    chronic J41.0
    under 15
  years of age J20.9
    chemical (acute) (subacute) J68.0
      chronic J68.4
      due to fumes or vapors J68.0
        chronic J68.4
  chronic J42
    with
      airways obstruction J44.9
      tracheitis (chronic) J42
    asthmatic (obstructive) J44.9
    catarrhal J41.0
    chemical (due to fumes or vapors) J68.4
    due to
      chemicals, gases, fumes or vapors (inhalation) J68.4
      radiation J70.1
      tobacco smoking J41.0

Bronchitis --continued
  emphysematous J44.9
  mucopurulent J41.1
  non-obstructive J41.0
  obliterans J44.9
  obstructive J44.9
  purulent J41.1
  simple J41.0
  croupous -see Bronchitis, acute
  due to gases, fumes or vapors (chemical) J68.0
  emphysematous (obstructive) J44.9
  exudative -see Bronchitis, acute
  fetid J41.1
  grippal -see Influenza, with, respiratory manifestations NEC
  in those under 15 years age -see Bronchitis, acute
    chronic -see Bronchitis, chronic
  influenzal -see Influenza, with, respiratory manifestations NEC
  mixed simple and mucopurulent J41.8
  moulder's J62.8
  mucopurulent (chronic) (recurrent) J41.1
    acute or subacute J20.9
    simple (mixed) J41.8
  obliterans (chronic) J44.9
  obstructive (chronic) (diffuse) J44.9
  pituitous J41.1
  pneumococcal, acute or subacute J20.2
  pseudomembranous, acute or subacute -see Bronchitis, acute
  purulent (chronic) (recurrent) J41.1
    acute or subacute -see Bronchitis, acute
  putrid J41.1
  senile (chronic) J42
  simple and mucopurulent (mixed) J41.8
  smokers' J41.0
  spirochetal NEC A69.8
  subacute -see Bronchitis, acute
  suppurative (chronic) J41.1
    acute or subacute -see Bronchitis, acute
  tuberculous A15.5
  under 15 years of age -see Bronchitis, acute
    chronic -see Bronchitis, chronic
  viral NEC, acute or subacute -see also Bronchitis, acute J20.8
Bronchoalveolitis J18.0
Bronchoaspergillosis B44.1
Bronchocele meaning goiter E04.0
Broncholithiasis J98.09
  tuberculous NEC A15.5
Bronchomalacia J98.09
  congenital Q32.2
Bronchomycosis NOS B49 [J99]
  candidal B37.1
Bronchopleuropneumonia -see Pneumonia, broncho
Bronchopneumonia -see Pneumonia, broncho
Bronchopneumonitis -see Pneumonia, broncho
Bronchopulmonary -see condition
Bronchopulmonitis -see Pneumonia, broncho
Bronchorrhagia (see Hemoptysis)
Bronchorrhea J98.09
  acute J20.9
  chronic (infective) (purulent) J42
Bronchospasm (acute) J98.01
  with
    bronchiolitis, acute J21.9

Bronchospasm - *continued*
bronchitis, acute (conditions in J20) -*see*
Bronchitis, acute
due to external agent -*see* condition,
respiratory, acute, due to
exercise induced J45.990
Bronchospirochetosis A69.8
Castellani A69.8
Bronchostenosis J98.09
Bronchus -*see* condition
Brontophobia F40.220
Bronze baby syndrome P83.8
Brooke's tumor -*see* Neoplasm, skin, benign
Brown enamel of teeth (hereditary) K00.5
Brown's sheath syndrome H50.61
**Brown-Séquard disease, paralysis or
syndrome** G83.81
Bruce sepsis A23.0
Brucellosis (infection) A23.9
abortus A23.1
canis A23.3
dermatitis A23.9
melitensis A23.0
mixed A23.8
sepsis A23.9
melitensis A23.0
specified NEC A23.8
suis A23.2
Bruck-de Lange disease Q87.1
Bruck's disease -*see* Deformity, limb
Brugsch's syndrome Q82.8
Bruise (skin surface intact) -*see also*
Contusion
with
open wound -*see* Wound, open
internal organ -*see* Injury, by site
newborn P54.5
scalp, due to birth injury, newborn P12.3
umbilical cord O69.5
Bruit (arterial) R09.89
cardiac R01.1
Brush burn -*see* Abrasion, by site
Bruton's X linked agammaglobulinemia
D80.0
Bruxism
psychogenic F45.8
sleep related G47.63
Bubbly lung syndrome P27.0
Bubo I88.8
blennorrhagic (gonococcal) A54.89
chancroidal A57
climatic A55
due to Haemophilus ducreyi A57
gonococcal A54.89
indolent (nonspecific) I88.8
inguinal (nonspecific) I88.8
chancroidal A57
climatic A55
due to H. ducreyi A57
infective I88.8
scrofulous (tuberculous) A18.2
soft chancre A57
suppurating -*see* Lymphadenitis, acute
syphilitic (primary) A51.0
congenital A50.07
tropical A55
virulent (chancroidal) A57
Bubonic plague A20.0
Bubonocele -*see* Hernia, inguinal
Buccal -*see* condition

Buchanan's disease or osteochondrosis
M91.0
Buchem's syndrome (hyperostosis corticalis)
M85.2
**Bucket-handle fracture or tear (semilunar
cartilage)** -*see* Tear, meniscus
**Budd-Chiari syndrome (hepatic vein
thrombosis)** I82.0
Budgerigar fancier's disease or lung J67.2
Buds
breast E30.1
in newborn P96.89
**Buerger's disease (thromboangiitis
obliterans)** I73.1
Bulbar -*see* condition
Bulbus cordis (left ventricle) (persistent)
Q21.8
Bulimia (nervosa) F50.2
atypical F50.9
normal weight F50.9
Bulky
stools R19.5
uterus N85.2
Bulla (e) R23.8
lung (emphysematous) (solitary) J43.9
newborn P25.8
Bullet wound -*see also* Wound, open
fracture
code as Fracture, by site
internal organ -*see* Injury, by site
Bundle
branch block (complete) (false) (incomplete) -
see Block, bundle-branch
of His -*see* condition
Bunion M21.61
tailor's M21.62
Bunionette M21.62
Buphthalmia, buphthalmos (congenital)
Q15.0
Burdwan fever B55.0
Bürger-Grütz disease or syndrome E78.3
Buried
penis (congenital) Q55.64
acquired N48.83
roots K08.3
Burke's syndrome K86.89
Burkitt
cell leukemia C91.0
lymphoma (malignant) C83.7
small noncleaved, diffuse C83.7
spleen C83.77
undifferentiated C83.7
tumor C83.7
type
acute lymphoblastic leukemia C91.0
undifferentiated C83.7
Burn (electricity) (flame) (hot gas, liquid or
hot object) (radiation) (steam) (thermal) T30.0
abdomen, abdominal (muscle) (wall) T21.02
first degree T21.12
second degree T21.22
third degree T21.32
above elbow T22.039
first degree T22.139
left T22.032
first degree T22.132
second degree T22.232
third degree T22.332
right T22.031
first degree T22.131
second degree T22.231

Burn - *continued*
third degree T22.331
second degree T22.239
third degree T22.339
acid (caustic) (external) (internal) -*see*
Corrosion, by site
alimentary tract NEC T28.2
esophagus T28.1
mouth T28.0
pharynx T28.0
alkaline (caustic) (external) (internal) -*see*
Corrosion, by site
ankle T25.019
first degree T25.119
left T25.012
first degree T25.112
second degree T25.212
third degree T25.312
multiple with foot -*see* Burn, lower, limb,
multiple, ankle and foot
right T25.011
first degree T25.111
second degree T25.211
third degree T25.311
second degree T25.219
third degree T25.319
anus -*see* Burn, buttock
arm (lower) (upper) -*see* Burn, upper, limb
axilla T22.049
first degree T22.149
left T22.042
first degree T22.142
second degree T22.242
third degree T22.342
right T22.041
first degree T22.141
second degree T22.241
third degree T22.341
second degree T22.249
third degree T22.349
back (lower) T21.04
first degree T21.14
second degree T21.24
third degree T21.34
upper T21.03
first degree T21.13
second degree T21.23
third degree T21.33
blisters
code as Burn, second degree, by site
breast(s) -*see* Burn, chest wall
buttock(s) T21.05
first degree T21.15
second degree T21.25
third degree T21.35
calf T24.039
first degree T24.139
left T24.032
first degree T24.132
second degree T24.232
third degree T24.332
right T24.031
first degree T24.131
second degree T24.231
third degree T24.331
second degree T24.239
third degree T24.339
canthus (eye) -*see* Burn, eyelid
caustic acid or alkaline -*see* Corrosion, by site
cervix T28.3
cheek T20.06

Burn - *continued*

first degree T20.16
second degree T20.26
third degree T20.36
chemical (acids) (alkalines) (caustics)
(external) (internal) *-see* Corrosion, by site
chest wall T21.01
first degree T21.11
second degree T21.21
third degree T21.31
chin T20.03
first degree T20.13
second degree T20.23
third degree T20.33
colon T28.2
conjunctiva (and cornea) *-see* Burn, cornea
cornea (and conjunctiva) T26.1
chemical *-see* Corrosion, cornea
corrosion (external) (internal) *-see* Corrosion,
by site
deep necrosis of underlying tissue - code as
Burn, third degree, by site
dorsum of hand T23.069
first degree T23.169
left T23.062
first degree T23.162
second degree T23.262
third degree T23.362
right T23.061
first degree T23.161
second degree T23.261
third degree T23.361
second degree T23.269
third degree T23.369
due to ingested chemical agent *-see*
Corrosion, by site
ear (auricle) (external) (canal) T20.01
first degree T20.11
second degree T20.21
third degree T20.31
elbow T22.029
first degree T22.129
left T22.022
first degree T22.122
second degree T22.222
third degree T22.322
right T22.021
first degree T22.121
second degree T22.221
third degree T22.321
second degree T22.229
third degree T22.329
epidermal loss
code as Burn, second degree, by site
erythema, erythematous
code as Burn, first degree, by site
esophagus T28.1
extent (percentage of body surface)
less than 10 percent T31.0
10 19 percent T31.10
with 0 9 percent third degree burns T31.10
with 10 19 percent third degree burns
T31.11
20 29 percent T31.20
with 0 9 percent third degree burns T31.20
with 10 19 percent third degree burns
T31.21
with 20 29 percent third degree burns
T31.22
30 39 percent T31.30
with 0 9 percent third degree burns T31.30

Burn - *continued*

with 10 19 percent third degree burns
T31.31
with 20 29 percent third degree burns
T31.32
with 30 39 percent third degree burns
T31.33
40 49 percent T31.40
with 0 9 percent third degree burns T31.40
with 10 19 percent third degree burns
T31.41
with 20 29 percent third degree burns
T31.42
with 30 39 percent third degree burns
T31.43
with 40 49 percent third degree burns
T31.44
50 59 percent T31.50
with 0 9 percent third degree burns T31.50
with 10 19 percent third degree burns
T31.51
with 20 29 percent third degree burns
T31.52
with 30 39 percent third degree burns
T31.53
with 40 49 percent third degree burns
T31.54
with 50 59 percent third degree burns
T31.55
60 69 percent T31.60
with 0 9 percent third degree burns T31.60
with 10 19 percent third degree burns
T31.61
with 20 29 percent third degree burns
T31.62
with 30 39 percent third degree burns
T31.63
with 40 49 percent third degree burns
T31.64
with 50 59 percent third degree burns
T31.65
with 60 69 percent third degree burns
T31.66
70 79 percent T31.70
with 0 9 percent third degree burns T31.70
with 10 19 percent third degree burns
T31.71
with 20 29 percent third degree burns
T31.72
with 30 39 percent third degree burns
T31.73
with 40 49 percent third degree burns
T31.74
with 50 59 percent third degree burns
T31.75
with 60 69 percent third degree burns
T31.76
with 70 79 percent third degree burns
T31.77
80 89 percent T31.80
with 0 9 percent third degree burns T31.80
with 10 19 percent third degree burns
T31.81
with 20 29 percent third degree burns
T31.82
with 30 39 percent third degree burns
T31.83
with 40 49 percent third degree burns
T31.84
with 50 59 percent third degree burns
T31.85

Burn - *continued*

with 60 69 percent third degree burns
T31.86
with 70 79 percent third degree burns
T31.87
with 80 89 percent third degree burns
T31.88
90 percent or more T31.90
with 0 9 percent third degree burns T31.90
with 10 19 percent third degree burns
T31.91
with 20 29 percent third degree burns
T31.92
with 30 39 percent third degree burns
T31.93
with 40 49 percent third degree burns
T31.94
with 50 59 percent third degree burns
T31.95
with 60 69 percent third degree burns
T31.96
with 70 79 percent third degree burns
T31.97
with 80 89 percent third degree burns
T31.98
with 90 percent or more third degree burns
T31.99
extremity *-see* Burn, limb
eye(s) and adnexa T26.4
with resulting rupture and destruction of
eyeball T26.2
conjunctival sac *-see* Burn, cornea
cornea *-see* Burn, cornea
lid *-see* Burn, eyelid
periocular area *-see* Burn, eyelid
specified site NEC T26.3
eyeball *-see* Burn, eye - eyelid(s) T26.0
chemical *-see* Corrosion, eyelid
face *-see* Burn, head
finger T23.029
first degree T23.129
left T23.022
first degree T23.122
second degree T23.222
third degree T23.322
multiple sites (without thumb) T23.039
with thumb T23.049
first degree T23.149
left T23.042
first degree T23.142
second degree T23.242
third degree T23.342
right T23.041
first degree T23.141
second degree T23.241
third degree T23.341
second degree T23.249
third degree T23.349
first degree T23.139
left T23.032
first degree T23.132
second degree T23.232
third degree T23.332
right T23.031
first degree T23.131
second degree T23.231
third degree T23.331
second degree T23.239
third degree T23.339
right T23.021
first degree T23.121

Burn - *continued*

second degree T23.221
third degree T23.321
second degree T23.229
third degree T23.329
flank -*see* Burn, abdominal wall
foot T25.029
first degree T25.129
left T25.022
first degree T25.122
second degree T25.222
third degree T25.322
multiple with ankle -*see* Burn, lower, limb, multiple, ankle and foot
right T25.021
first degree T25.121
second degree T25.221
third degree T25.321
second degree T25.229
third degree T25.329
forearm T22.019
first degree T22.119
left T22.012
first degree T22.112
second degree T22.212
third degree T22.312
right T22.011
first degree T22.111
second degree T22.211
third degree T22.311
second degree T22.219
third degree T22.319
forehead T20.06
first degree T20.16
second degree T20.26
third degree T20.36
fourth degree - code as Burn, third degree, by site
friction -*see* Burn, by site
from swallowing caustic or corrosive substance NEC -*see* Corrosion, by site
full thickness skin loss
code as Burn, third degree, by site
gastrointestinal tract NEC T28.2
from swallowing caustic or corrosive substance T28.7
genital organs
external
female T21.07
first degree T21.17
second degree T21.27
third degree T21.37
male T21.06
first degree T21.16
second degree T21.26
third degree T21.36
internal T28.3
from caustic or corrosive substance T28.8
groin -*see* Burn, abdominal wall
hand(s) T23.009
back -*see* Burn, dorsum of hand
finger -*see* Burn, finger
first degree T23.109
left T23.002
first degree T23.102
second degree T23.202
third degree T23.302
multiple sites with wrist T23.099
first degree T23.199
left T23.092
first degree T23.192

Burn - *continued*

second degree T23.292
third degree T23.392
right T23.091
first degree T23.191
second degree T23.291
third degree T23.391
second degree T23.299
third degree T23.399
palm -*see* Burn, palm
right T23.001
first degree T23.101
second degree T23.201
third degree T23.301
second degree T23.209
third degree T23.309
thumb -*see* Burn, thumb
head (and face) (and neck) T20.00
cheek -*see* Burn, cheek
chin -*see* Burn, chin
ear -*see* Burn, ear
eye(s) only -*see* Burn, eye
first degree T20.10
forehead -*see* Burn, forehead
lip -*see* Burn, lip
multiple sites T20.09
first degree T20.19
second degree T20.29
third degree T20.39
neck -*see* Burn, neck
nose -*see* Burn, nose
scalp -*see* Burn, scalp
second degree T20.20
third degree T20.30
hip(s) -*see* Burn, thigh
inhalation -*see* Burn, respiratory tract
caustic or corrosive substance (fumes) -*see* Corrosion, respiratory tract
internal organ(s) T28.40
alimentary tract T28.2
esophagus T28.1
eardrum T28.41
esophagus T28.1
from caustic or corrosive substance (swallowing) NEC -*see* Corrosion, by site
genitourinary T28.3
mouth T28.0
pharynx T28.0
respiratory tract -*see* Burn, respiratory tract
specified organ NEC T28.49
interscapular region -*see* Burn, back, upper
intestine (large) (small) T28.2
knee T24.029
first degree T24.129
left T24.022
first degree T24.122
second degree T24.222
third degree T24.322
right T24.021
first degree T24.121
second degree T24.221
third degree T24.321
second degree T24.229
third degree T24.329
labium (majus) (minus) -*see* Burn, genital organs, external, female
lacrimal apparatus, duct, gland or sac -*see* Burn, eye, specified site NEC
larynx T27.0
with lung T27.1
leg(s) (lower) (upper) -*see* Burn, lower, limb

Burn - *continued*

lightning -*see* Burn, by site
limb(s)
lower (except ankle or foot alone) -*see* Burn, lower, limb
upper -*see* Burn, upper limb
lip(s) T20.02
first degree T20.12
second degree T20.22
third degree T20.32
lower
back -*see* Burn, back
limb T24.009
ankle -*see* Burn, ankle
calf -*see* Burn, calf
first degree T24.109
foot -*see* Burn, foot
hip -*see* Burn, thigh
knee -*see* Burn, knee
left T24.002
first degree T24.102
second degree T24.202
third degree T24.302
multiple sites, except ankle and foot T24.099
ankle and foot T25.099
first degree T25.199
left T25.092
first degree T25.192
second degree T25.292
third degree T25.392
right T25.091
first degree T25.191
second degree T25.291
third degree T25.391
second degree T25.299
third degree T25.399
first degree T24.199
left T24.092
first degree T24.192
second degree T24.292
third degree T24.392
right T24.091
first degree T24.191
second degree T24.291
third degree T24.391
second degree T24.299
third degree T24.399
right T24.001
first degree T24.101
second degree T24.201
third degree T24.301
second degree T24.209
thigh -*see* Burn, thigh
third degree T24.309
toe -*see* Burn, toe
lung (with larynx and trachea) T27.1
mouth T28.0
neck T20.07
first degree T20.17
second degree T20.27
third degree T20.37
nose (septum) T20.04
first degree T20.14
second degree T20.24
third degree T20.34
ocular adnexa -*see* Burn, eye - orbit region -*see* Burn, eyelid
palm T23.059
first degree T23.159
left T23.052

Burn - *continued*
    first degree T23.152
    second degree T23.252
    third degree T23.352
  right T23.051
    first degree T23.151
    second degree T23.251
    third degree T23.351
  second degree T23.259
  third degree T23.359
  partial thickness
  code as Burn, unspecified degree, by site
  pelvis *-see* Burn, trunk
  penis *-see* Burn, genital organs, external, male
  perineum
    female *-see* Burn, genital organs, external, female
    male *-see* Burn, genital organs, external, male
  periocular area *-see* Burn, eyelid
  pharynx T28.0
  rectum T28.2
  respiratory tract T27.3
    larynx *-see* Burn, larynx
    specified part NEC T27.2
    trachea *-see* Burn, trachea
  sac, lacrimal *-see* Burn, eye, specified site NEC
  scalp T20.05
    first degree T20.15
    second degree T20.25
    third degree T20.35
  scapular region T22.069
    first degree T22.169
    left T22.062
      first degree T22.162
      second degree T22.262
      third degree T22.362
    right T22.061
      first degree T22.161
      second degree T22.261
      third degree T22.361
    second degree T22.269
    third degree T22.369
  sclera *-see* Burn, eye, specified site NEC
  scrotum *-see* Burn, genital organs, external, male
  shoulder T22.059
    first degree T22.159
    left T22.052
      first degree T22.152
      second degree T22.252
      third degree T22.352
    right T22.051
      first degree T22.151
      second degree T22.251
      third degree T22.351
    second degree T22.259
    third degree T22.359
  stomach T28.2
  temple *-see* Burn, head
  testis *-see* Burn, genital organs, external, male
  thigh T24.019
    first degree T24.119
    left T24.012
      first degree T24.112
      second degree T24.212
      third degree T24.312
    right T24.011
      first degree T24.111
      second degree T24.211

Burn - *continued*
    third degree T24.311
    second degree T24.219
    third degree T24.319
  thorax (external) *-see* Burn, trunk
  throat (meaning pharynx) T28.0
  thumb(s) T23.019
    first degree T23.119
    left T23.012
      first degree T23.112
      second degree T23.212
      third degree T23.312
    multiple sites with fingers T23.049
      first degree T23.149
      left T23.042
        first degree T23.142
        second degree T23.242
        third degree T23.342
      right T23.041
        first degree T23.141
        second degree T23.241
        third degree T23.341
      second degree T23.249
      third degree T23.349
    right T23.011
      first degree T23.111
      second degree T23.211
      third degree T23.311
    second degree T23.219
    third degree T23.319
  toe T25.039
    first degree T25.139
    left T25.032
      first degree T25.132
      second degree T25.232
      third degree T25.332
    right T25.031
      first degree T25.131
      second degree T25.231
      third degree T25.331
    second degree T25.239
    third degree T25.339
  tongue T28.0
  tonsil(s) T28.0
  trachea T27.0
    with lung T27.1
  trunk T21.00
    abdominal wall *-see* Burn, abdominal wall
    anus *-see* Burn, buttock
    axilla *-see* Burn, upper limb
    back *-see* Burn, back
    breast *-see* Burn, chest wall
    buttock *-see* Burn, buttock
    chest wall *-see* Burn, chest wall
    first degree T21.10
    flank *-see* Burn, abdominal wall
    genital
      female *-see* Burn, genital organs, external, female
      male *-see* Burn, genital organs, external, male
    groin *-see* Burn, abdominal wall
    interscapular region *-see* Burn, back, upper
    labia *-see* Burn, genital organs, external, female
    lower back *-see* Burn, back
    penis *-see* Burn, genital organs, external, male
    perineum
      female *-see* Burn, genital organs, external, female

Burn - *continued*
    male *-see* Burn, genital organs, external, male
  scapula region *-see* Burn, scapular region
  scrotum *-see* Burn, genital organs, external, male
  second degree T21.20
  specified site NEC T21.09
    first degree T21.19
    second degree T21.29
    third degree T21.39
  testes *-see* Burn, genital organs, external, male
  third degree T21.30
  upper back *-see* Burn, back, upper
  vulva *-see* Burn, genital organs, external, female
  unspecified site with extent of body surface involved specified
    less than 10 percent T31.0
    10 19 percent (0 9 percent third degree) T31.10
      with 10 19 percent third degree T31.11
    20 29 percent (0 9 percent third degree) T31.20
      with
        10 19 percent third degree T31.21
        20 29 percent third degree T31.22
    30 39 percent (0 9 percent third degree) T31.30
      with
        10 19 percent third degree T31.31
        20 29 percent third degree T31.32
        30 39 percent third degree T31.33
    40 49 percent (0 9 percent third degree) T31.40
      with
        10 19 percent third degree T31.41
        20 29 percent third degree T31.42
        30 39 percent third degree T31.43
        40 49 percent third degree T31.44
    50 59 percent (0 9 percent third degree) T31.50
      with
        10 19 percent third degree T31.51
        20 29 percent third degree T31.52
        30 39 percent third degree T31.53
        40 49 percent third degree T31.54
        50 59 percent third degree T31.55
    60 69 percent (0 9 percent third degree) T31.60
      with
        10 19 percent third degree T31.61
        20 29 percent third degree T31.62
        30 39 percent third degree T31.63
        40 49 percent third degree T31.64
        50 59 percent third degree T31.65
        60 69 percent third degree T31.66
    70 79 percent (0 9 percent third degree) T31.70
      with
        10 19 percent third degree T31.71
        20 29 percent third degree T31.72
        30 39 percent third degree T31.73
        40 49 percent third degree T31.74
        50 59 percent third degree T31.75
        60 69 percent third degree T31.76
        70 79 percent third degree T31.77
    80 89 percent (0 9 percent third degree) T31.80
      with

Burn - *continued*

    10 19 percent third degree T31.81
    20 29 percent third degree T31.82
    30 39 percent third degree T31.83
    40 49 percent third degree T31.84
    50 59 percent third degree T31.85
    60 69 percent third degree T31.86
    70 79 percent third degree T31.87
    80 89 percent third degree T31.88
  90 percent or more (0 9 percent third degree) T31.90
    with
      10 19 percent third degree T31.91
      20 29 percent third degree T31.92
      30 39 percent third degree T31.93
      40 49 percent third degree T31.94
      50 59 percent third degree T31.95
      60 69 percent third degree T31.96
      70 79 percent third degree T31.97
      80 89 percent third degree T31.98
      90 99 percent third degree T31.99
upper limb T22.00
  above elbow *-see* Burn, above elbow
  axilla *-see* Burn, axilla
  elbow *-see* Burn, elbow
  first degree T22.10
  forearm *-see* Burn, forearm
  hand *-see* Burn, hand
  interscapular region *-see* Burn, back, upper
  multiple sites T22.099
    first degree T22.199
    left T22.092
      first degree T22.192
      second degree T22.292
      third degree T22.392
    right T22.091
      first degree T22.191
      second degree T22.291
      third degree T22.391
    second degree T22.299
    third degree T22.399
  scapular region *-see* Burn, scapular region
  second degree T22.20
  shoulder *-see* Burn, shoulder
  third degree T22.30
  wrist *-see* Burn, wrist
uterus T28.3
vagina T28.3
vulva *-see* Burn, genital organs, external, female
wrist T23.079
  first degree T23.179
  left T23.072
    first degree T23.172
    second degree T23.272
    third degree T23.372
  multiple sites with hand T23.099
    first degree T23.199
    left T23.092
      first degree T23.192
      second degree T23.292
      third degree T23.392
    right T23.091
      first degree T23.191
      second degree T23.291
      third degree T23.391
    second degree T23.299
    third degree T23.399
  right T23.071
    first degree T23.171
    second degree T23.271

Burn - *continued*

  third degree T23.371
  second degree T23.279
  third degree T23.379
Burnett's syndrome E83.52
Burning
  feet syndrome E53.9
  sensation R20.8
  tongue K14.6
Burn-out (state) Z73.0
Burns' disease or osteochondrosis *-see* Osteochondrosis, juvenile, ulna
Bursa *-see* condition
Bursitis M71.9
  Achilles *-see* Tendinitis, Achilles
  adhesive *-see* Bursitis, specified NEC
  ankle *-see* Enthesopathy, lower limb, ankle, specified type NEC
  calcaneal *-see* Enthesopathy, foot, specified type NEC
  collateral ligament, tibial *-see* Bursitis, tibial collateral
  due to use, overuse, pressure *-see also* Disorder, soft tissue, due to use, specified type NEC
    specified NEC *-see* Disorder, soft tissue, due to use, specified NEC
  Duplay's M75.0
  elbow NEC M70.3
    olecranon M70.2
  finger *-see* Disorder, soft tissue, due to use, specified type NEC, hand
  foot *-see* Enthesopathy, foot, specified type NEC
  gonococcal A54.49
  gouty *-see* Gout
  hand M70.1
  hip NEC M70.7
    trochanteric M70.6
  infective NEC M71.10
    abscess *-see* Abscess, bursa
    ankle M71.17
    elbow M71.12
    foot M71.17
    hand M71.14
    hip M71.15
    knee M71.16
    multiple sites M71.19
    shoulder M71.11
    specified site NEC M71.18
    wrist M71.13
  ischial *-see* Bursitis, hip
  knee NEC M70.5
    prepatellar M70.4
  occupational NEC *-see also* Disorder, soft tissue, due to, use
  olecranon *-see* Bursitis, elbow, olecranon
  pharyngeal J39.1
  popliteal *-see* Bursitis, knee - prepatellar M70.4
  radiohumeral M77.8
  rheumatoid M06.20
    ankle M06.27
    elbow M06.22
    foot joint M06.27
    hand joint M06.24
    hip M06.25
    knee M06.26
    multiple site M06.29
    shoulder M06.21
    vertebra M06.28

Bursitis *--continued*

  wrist M06.23
  scapulohumeral *-see* Bursitis, shoulder
  semimembranous muscle (knee) *-see* Bursitis, knee
  shoulder M75.5
    adhesive *-see* Capsulitis, adhesive
  specified NEC M71.50
    ankle M71.57
    due to use, overuse or pressure *-see* Disorder, soft tissue, due to, use
    elbow M71.52
    foot M71.57
    hand M71.54
    hip M71.55
    knee M71.56
    shoulder *-see* Bursitis, shoulder
    specified site NEC M71.58
    tibial collateral M76.4
    wrist M71.53
  subacromial *-see* Bursitis, shoulder
  subcoracoid *-see* Bursitis, shoulder
  subdeltoid *-see* Bursitis, shoulder
  syphilitic A52.78
  Thornwaldt, Tornwaldt J39.2
  tibial collateral M76.4
  toe *-see* Enthesopathy, foot, specified type NEC
  trochanteric (area) *-see* Bursitis, hip, trochanteric
  wrist *-see* Bursitis, hand
Bursopathy M71.9
  specified type NEC M71.80
    ankle M71.87
    elbow M71.82
    foot M71.87
    hand M71.84
    hip M71.85
    knee M71.86
    multiple sites M71.89
    shoulder M71.81
    specified site NEC M71.88
    wrist M71.83
Burst stitches or sutures (complication of surgery) T81.31
  external operation wound T81.31
  internal operation wound T81.32
Buruli ulcer A31.1
Bury's disease L95.1
Buschke's
  disease B45.3
  scleredema *-see* Sclerosis, systemic
Busse-Buschke disease B45.3
Buttock *-see* condition
Button
  Biskra B55.1
  Delhi B55.1
  oriental B55.1
Buttonhole deformity (finger) *-see* Deformity, finger, boutonniere
Bwamba fever A92.8
Byssinosis J66.0
Bywaters' syndrome T79.5

C

Cachexia R64
  cancerous R64
  cardiac *-see* Disease, heart
  dehydration E86.0
  due to malnutrition R64

Cachexia - *continued*
exophthalmic -*see* Hyperthyroidism
heart -*see* Disease, heart
hypophyseal E23.0
hypopituitary E23.0
lead -*see* Poisoning, lead
malignant R64
marsh -*see* Malaria
nervous F48.8
old age R54
paludal -*see* Malaria
pituitary E23.0
renal N28.9
saturnine -*see* Poisoning, lead
senile R54
Simmonds' E23.0
splenica D73.0
strumipriva E03.4
tuberculous NEC -*see* Tuberculosis
Café, au lait spots L81.3
Caffeine-induced
anxiety disorder F15.980
sleep disorder F15.982
Caffey's syndrome Q78.8
Caisson disease T70.3
Cake kidney Q63.1
Caked breast (puerperal, postpartum)
O92.79
Calabar swelling B74.3
Calcaneal spur -*see* Spur, bone, calcaneal
Calcaneo-apophysitis M92.8
Calcareous -*see* condition
Calcicosis J62.8
Calciferol (vitamin D) deficiency E55.9
with rickets E55.0
Calcification
adrenal (capsule) (gland) E27.49
tuberculous E35 [*B90.8*]
aorta I70.0
artery (annular) -*see* Arteriosclerosis
auricle (ear) -*see* Disorder, pinna, specified
type NEC
basal ganglia G23.8
bladder N32.89
due to Schistosoma hematobium B65.0
brain (cortex) -*see* Calcification, cerebral
bronchus J98.09
bursa M71.40
ankle M71.47
elbow M71.42
foot M71.47
hand M71.44
hip M71.45
knee M71.46
multiple sites M71.49
shoulder M75.3
specified site NEC M71.48
wrist M71.43
cardiac -*see* Degeneration, myocardial
cerebral (cortex) G93.89
artery I67.2
cervix (uteri) N88.8
choroid plexus G93.89
conjunctiva -*see* Concretion, conjunctiva
corpora cavernosa (penis) N48.89
cortex (brain) -*see* Calcification, cerebral
dental pulp (nodular) K04.2
dentinal papilla K00.4
fallopian tube N83.8
falx cerebri G96.19
gallbladder K82.8

Calcification - *continued*
general E83.59
heart -*see also* Degeneration, myocardial
valve -*see* Endocarditis
idiopathic infantile arterial (IIAC) Q28.8
intervertebral cartilage or disc (postinfective)
-*see* Disorder, disc, specified NEC
intracranial -*see* Calcification, cerebral
joint -*see* Disorder, joint, specified type NEC
kidney N28.89
tuberculous N29 [*B90.1*]
larynx (senile) J38.7
lens -*see* Cataract, specified NEC
lung (active) (postinfectional) J98.4
tuberculous B90.9
lymph gland or node (postinfectional) I89.8
tuberculous -*see also* Tuberculosis, lymph
gland B90.8
mammographic R92.1
massive (paraplegic) -*see* Myositis, ossificans,
in, quadriplegia
medial -*see* Arteriosclerosis, extremities
meninges (cerebral) (spinal) G96.19
metastatic E83.59
Mönckeberg's -*see* Arteriosclerosis,
extremities
muscle M61.9
due to burns -*see* Myositis, ossificans, in,
burns
paralytic -*see* Myositis, ossificans, in,
quadriplegia
specified type NEC M61.40
ankle M61.47
foot M61.47
forearm M61.43
hand M61.44
lower leg M61.46
multiple sites M61.49
pelvic region M61.45
shoulder region M61.41
specified site NEC M61.48
thigh M61.45
upper arm M61.42
myocardium, myocardial -*see* Degeneration,
myocardial
ovary N83.8
pancreas K86.89
penis N48.89
periarticular -*see* Disorder, joint, specified
type NEC
pericardium -*see also* Pericarditis I31.1
pineal gland E34.8
pleura J94.8
postinfectional J94.8
tuberculous NEC B90.9
pulpal (dental) (nodular) K04.2
sclera H15.89
spleen D73.89
subcutaneous L94.2
suprarenal (capsule) (gland) E27.49
tendon (sheath) -*see also* Tenosynovitis,
specified type NEC
with bursitis, synovitis or tenosynovitis -*see*
Tendinitis, calcific
trachea J39.8
ureter N28.89
uterus N85.8
vitreous -*see* Deposit, crystalline
Calcified -*see* Calcification

Calcinosis (interstitial) (tumoral) (universalis)
E83.59
with Raynaud's phenomenon, esophageal
dysfunction, sclerodactyly, telangiectasia
(CREST syndrome) M34.1
circumscripta (skin) L94.2
cutis L94.2
Calciphylaxis -*see also* Calcification, by site
E83.59
Calcium
deposits -*see* Calcification, by site
metabolism disorder E83.50
salts or soaps in vitreous -*see* Deposit,
crystalline
Calciuria R82.99
Calculi -*see* Calculus
Calculosis, intrahepatic -*see* Calculus, bile
duct
Calculus, calculi, calculous
ampulla of Vater -*see* Calculus, bile duct
anuria (impacted) (recurrent) -*see also*
Calculus, urinary N20.9
appendix K38.1
bile duct (common) (hepatic) K80.50
with
calculus of gallbladder -*see* Calculus,
gallbladder and bile duct
cholangitis K80.30
with
cholecystitis -*see* Calculus, bile duct,
with cholecystitis
obstruction K80.31
acute K80.32
with
chronic cholangitis K80.36
with obstruction K80.37
obstruction K80.33
chronic K80.34
with
acute cholangitis K80.36
with obstruction K80.37
obstruction K80.35
cholecystitis (with cholangitis) K80.40
with obstruction K80.41
acute K80.42
with
chronic cholecystitis K80.46
with obstruction K80.47
obstruction K80.43
chronic K80.44
with
acute cholecystitis K80.46
with obstruction K80.47
obstruction K80.45
obstruction K80.51
biliary -*see also* Calculus, gallbladder
specified NEC K80.80
with obstruction K80.81
bilirubin, multiple -*see* Calculus, gallbladder
bladder (encysted) (impacted) (urinary)
(diverticulum) N21.0
bronchus J98.09
calyx (kidney) (renal) -*see* Calculus, kidney
cholesterol (pure) (solitary) -*see* Calculus,
gallbladder
common duct (bile) -*see* Calculus, bile duct
conjunctiva -*see* Concretion, conjunctiva
cystic N21.0
duct -*see* Calculus, gallbladder
dental (subgingival) (supragingival) K03.6
diverticulum

Calculus, calculi, calculous - *continued*
  bladder N21.0
  kidney N20.0
  epididymis N50.89
  gallbladder K80.20
    with
      bile duct calculus -*see* Calculus,
  gallbladder and bile duct
      cholecystitis K80.10
        with obstruction K80.11
        acute K80.00
          with
            chronic cholecystitis K80.12
              with obstruction K80.13
              obstruction K80.01
          chronic K80.10
            with
              acute cholecystitis K80.12
                with obstruction K80.13
                obstruction K80.11
          specified NEC K80.18
            with obstruction K80.19
        obstruction K80.21
  gallbladder and bile duct K80.70
    with
      cholecystitis K80.60
        with obstruction K80.61
        acute K80.62
          with
            chronic cholecystitis K80.66
              with obstruction K80.67
              obstruction K80.63
          chronic K80.64
            with
              acute cholecystitis K80.66
                with obstruction K80.67
                obstruction K80.65
        obstruction K80.71
  hepatic (duct) -*see* Calculus, bile duct
  hepatobiliary K80.80
    with obstruction K80.81
  ileal conduit N21.8
  intestinal (impaction) (obstruction) K56.49
  kidney (impacted) (multiple) (pelvis)
    (recurrent) (staghorn) N20.0
    with calculus, ureter N20.2
    congenital Q63.8
  lacrimal passages -*see* Dacryolith
  liver (impacted) -*see* Calculus, bile duct
  lung J98.4
  mammographic R92.1
  nephritic (impacted) (recurrent) -*see* Calculus,
    kidney nose J34.89
  pancreas (duct) K86.89
  parotid duct or gland K11.5
  pelvis, encysted -*see* Calculus, kidney
    prostate N42.0
  pulmonary J98.4
  pyelitis (impacted) (recurrent) N20.0
    with hydronephrosis N13.2
  pyelonephritis (impacted) (recurrent) -*see*
    category N20
    with hydronephrosis N13.2
  renal (impacted) (recurrent) -*see* Calculus,
    kidney salivary (duct) (gland) K11.5
  seminal vesicle N50.89
  staghorn -*see* Calculus, kidney Stensen's
    duct K11.5
  stomach K31.89
  sublingual duct or gland K11.5
    congenital Q38.4

Calculus, calculi, calculous - *continued*
  submandibular duct, gland or region K11.5
  submaxillary duct, gland or region K11.5
  suburethral N21.8
  tonsil J35.8
  tooth, teeth (subgingival) (supragingival)
    K03.6
  tunica vaginalis N50.89
  ureter (impacted) (recurrent) N20.1
    with calculus, kidney N20.2
      with hydronephrosis N13.2
        with infection N13.6
  urethra (impacted) N21.1
  urinary (duct) (impacted) (passage) (tract)
    N20.9
    with hydronephrosis N13.2
      with infection N13.6
    in (due to)
    lower N21.9
      specified NEC N21.8
  vagina N89.8
  vesical (impacted) N21.0
  Wharton's duct K11.5
  xanthine E79.8 [*N22*]
Calicectasis N28.89
Caliectasis N28.89
California
  disease B38.9
  encephalitis A83.5
Caligo cornea -*see* Opacity, cornea, central
Callositas, callosity (infected) L84
Callus (infected) L84
  bone -*see* Osteophyte
    excessive, following fracture
  code as Sequelae of fracture
**CALME (childhood asymmetric labium
  majus enlargement)** N90.61
Calorie deficiency or malnutrition -*see also*
  Malnutrition E46
Calvé Perthes disease -*see* Legg-Calvé
  Perthes disease
Calvé's disease -*see* Osteochondrosis, juvenile,
  spine
Calvities -*see* Alopecia, androgenic
Cameroon fever -*see* Malaria
Camptocormia (hysterical) F44.4
Camurati-Engelmann syndrome Q78.3
Canal -*see also* condition
  atrioventricular common Q21.2
Canaliculitis (lacrimal) (acute) (subacute)
  H04.33
  Actinomyces A42.89
  chronic H04.42 **Canavan's disease** E75.29
Canceled procedure (surgical) Z53.9
  because of
    contraindication Z53.09
      smoking Z53.01
    left against medical advice (AMA) Z53.21
    patient's decision Z53.20
      for reasons of belief or group pressure
        Z53.1
      specified reason NEC Z53.29
    specified reason NEC Z53.8
Cancer -*see also* Neoplasm, by site, malignant
  bile duct type liver C22.1
  blood -*see* Leukemia
  breast -*see also* Neoplasm, breast, malignant
    C50.91
  hepatocellular C22.0
  lung -*see also* Neoplasm, lung, malignant
    C34.90

Cancer - *continued*
  ovarian -*see also* Neoplasm ovary, malignant
    C56.9
  unspecified site (primary) C80.1
Cancer (o) phobia F45.29
Cancerous -*see* Neoplasm, malignant, by site
Cancrum oris A69.0
Candidiasis, candidal B37.9
  balanitis B37.42
  bronchitis B37.1
  cheilitis B37.83
  congenital P37.5
  cystitis B37.41
  disseminated B37.7
  endocarditis B37.6
  enteritis B37.82
  esophagitis B37.81
  intertrigo B37.2
  lung B37.1
  meningitis B37.5
  mouth B37.0
  nails B37.2
  neonatal P37.5
  onychia B37.2
  oral B37.0
  osteomyelitis B37.89
  otitis externa B37.84
  paronychia B37.2
  perionyxis B37.2
  pneumonia B37.1
  proctitis B37.82
  pulmonary B37.1
  pyelonephritis B37.49
  sepsis B37.7
  skin B37.2
  specified site NEC B37.89
  stomatitis B37.0
  systemic B37.7
  urethritis B37.41
  urogenital site NEC B37.49
  vagina B37.3
  vulva B37.3
  vulvovaginitis B37.3
Candidid L30.2
Candidosis -*see* Candidiasis
Candiru infection or infestation B88.8
Canities (premature) L67.1
  congenital Q84.2
Canker (mouth) (sore) K12.0
  rash A38.9
Cannabinosis J66.2
Cannabis induced
  anxiety disorder F12.980
  psychotic disorder F12.959
  sleep disorder F12.988
Canton fever A75.9
Cantrell's syndrome Q87.89
Capillariasis (intestinal) B81.1
  hepatic B83.8
Capillary -*see* condition
Caplan's syndrome -*see* Rheumatoid, lung
Capsule -*see* condition
Capsulitis (joint) -*see also* Enthesopathy
  adhesive (shoulder) M75.0
  hepatic K65.8
  labyrinthine -*see* Otosclerosis, specified NEC
  thyroid E06.9
Caput
  crepitus Q75.8
  medusae I86.8
  succedaneum P12.81

Car sickness T75.3
Carapata (disease) A68.0
Carate *-see* Pinta
Carbon lung J60
Carbuncle L02.93
  abdominal wall L02.231
  anus K61.0
  auditory canal, external *-see* Abscess, ear,
    external
  auricle ear *-see* Abscess, ear, external
  axilla L02.43
  back (any part) L02.232
  breast N61.1
  buttock L02.33
  cheek (external) L02.03
  chest wall L02.233
  chin L02.03
  corpus cavernosum N48.21
  ear (any part) (external) (middle) *-see*
    Abscess, ear, external
  external auditory canal *-see* Abscess, ear,
    external
  eyelid *-see* Abscess, eyelid
  face NEC L02.03
  femoral (region) *-see* Carbuncle, lower limb
  finger *-see* Carbuncle, hand
  flank L02.231
  foot L02.63
  forehead L02.03
  genital *-see* Abscess, genital
  gluteal (region) L02.33
  groin L02.234
  hand L02.53
  head NEC L02.831
  heel *-see* Carbuncle, foot
  hip *-see* Carbuncle, lower limb
  kidney *-see* Abscess, kidney
  knee *-see* Carbuncle, lower limb
  labium (majus) (minus) N76.4
  lacrimal
    gland *-see* Dacryoadenitis
    passages (duct) (sac) *-see* Inflammation,
      lacrimal, passages, acute
  leg *-see* Carbuncle, lower limb
  lower limb L02.43
  malignant A22.0
  navel L02.236
  neck L02.13
  nose (external) (septum) J34.0
  orbit, orbital *-see* Abscess, orbit
  palmar (space) *-see* Carbuncle, hand
  partes posteriores L02.33
  pectoral region L02.233
  penis N48.21
  perineum L02.235
  pinna *-see* Abscess, ear, external
  popliteal *-see* Carbuncle, lower limb
  scalp L02.831
  seminal vesicle N49.0
  shoulder *-see* Carbuncle, upper limb
  specified site NEC L02.838
  temple (region) L02.03
  thumb *-see* Carbuncle, hand
  toe *-see* Carbuncle, foot
  trunk L02.239
    abdominal wall L02.231
    back L02.232
    chest wall L02.233
    groin L02.234
    perineum L02.235
    umbilicus L02.236

Carbuncle *--continued*
  umbilicus L02.236
  upper limb L02.43
  urethra N34.0
  vulva N76.4
Carbunculus *-see* Carbuncle
Carcinoid (tumor) *-see* Tumor, carcinoid
Carcinoidosis E34.0
Carcinoma (malignant) *-see also* Neoplasm,
 by site, malignant
  acidophil
    specified site *-see* Neoplasm, malignant, by
      site
    unspecified site C75.1
  acidophil-basophil, mixed
    specified site *-see* Neoplasm, malignant, by
      site
    unspecified site C75.1
  adnexal (skin) *-see* Neoplasm, skin, malignant
  adrenal cortical C74.0
  alveolar *-see* Neoplasm, lung, malignant
    cell *-see* Neoplasm, lung, malignant
  ameloblastic C41.1
    upper jaw (bone) C41.0
  apocrine
    breast *-see* Neoplasm, breast, malignant
    specified site NEC *-see* Neoplasm, skin,
      malignant
    unspecified site C44.99
  basal cell (pigmented) (see also Neoplasm,
    skin, malignant) C44.91
    fibro-epithelial *-see* Neoplasm, skin,
      malignant
    morphea *-see* Neoplasm, skin, malignant
    multicentric *-see* Neoplasm, skin, malignant
  basaloid
  basal-squamous cell, mixed *-see* Neoplasm,
    skin, malignant
  basophil
    specified site *-see* Neoplasm, malignant, by
    site
    unspecified site C75.1
  basophil-acidophil, mixed
    specified site *-see* Neoplasm, malignant, by
      site
    unspecified site C75.1
  basosquamous *-see* Neoplasm, skin,
  malignant
  bile duct
    with hepatocellular, mixed C22.0
    liver C22.1
    specified site NEC *-see* Neoplasm,
      malignant, by site
    unspecified site C22.1
  branchial or branchiogenic C10.4
  bronchial or bronchogenic *-see* Neoplasm,
    lung, malignant
  bronchiolar *-see* Neoplasm, lung, malignant
  bronchioloalveolar *-see* Neoplasm, lung,
  malignant
  C cell
    specified site *-see* Neoplasm, malignant, by
      site
    unspecified site C73
  ceruminous C44.29
  cervix uteri
    in situ D06.9
      endocervix D06.0
      exocervix D06.1
      specified site NEC D06.7
  chorionic

Carcinoma *--continued*
    specified site *-see* Neoplasm, malignant, by
      site
    unspecified site
      female C58
      male C62.90
  chromophobe
    specified site *-see* Neoplasm, malignant, by
      site
    unspecified site C75.1
  cloacogenic
    specified site *-see* Neoplasm, malignant, by
      site
    unspecified site C21.2
  diffuse type
    specified site *-see* Neoplasm, malignant, by
      site
    unspecified site C16.9
  duct (cell)
    with Paget's disease *-see* Neoplasm, breast,
      malignant
    infiltrating
      with lobular carcinoma (in situ)
        specified site *-see* Neoplasm, malignant,
          by site
        unspecified site (female) C50.91
          male C50.92
      specified site *-see* Neoplasm, malignant, by
      site
        unspecified site (female) C50.91
          male C50.92
  ductal
    with lobular
      specified site *-see* Neoplasm, malignant, by
        site
      unspecified site (female) C50.91
        male C50.92
  ductular, infiltrating
    specified site *-see* Neoplasm, malignant, by
      site
    unspecified site (female) C50.91
      male C50.92
  embryonal
    liver C22.7
  endometrioid
    specified site *-see* Neoplasm, malignant, by
      site
    unspecified site
      female C56.9
      male C61
  eosinophil
    specified site *-see* Neoplasm, malignant, by
      site
    unspecified site C75.1
  epidermoid *-see also* Neoplasm, skin
  malignant
    in situ, Bowen's type *-see* Neoplasm, skin, in
      situ
    fibroepithelial, basal cell *-see* Neoplasm, skin,
      malignant
  follicular
    with papillary (mixed) C73
    moderately differentiated C73
    pure follicle C73
    specified site *-see* Neoplasm, malignant, by
      site
    trabecular C73
    unspecified site C73
    well differentiated C73
  generalized, with unspecified primary site
    C80.0

Carcinoma *--continued*
   glycogen-rich *-see* Neoplasm, breast,
      malignant
   granulosa cell C56
   hepatic cell C22.0
   hepatocellular C22.0
      with bile duct, mixed C22.0
      fibrolamellar C22.0
   hepatocholangiolitic C22.0
   Hürthle cell C73
   in
      adenomatous
         polyposis coli C18.9
      pleomorphic adenoma *-see* Neoplasm,
         salivary glands, malignant
      situ *-see* Carcinoma-in-situ
   infiltrating
      duct
         with lobular
            specified site *-see* Neoplasm, malignant,
               by site
            unspecified site (female) C50.91
               male C50.92
         with Paget's disease *-see* Neoplasm,
            breast, malignant
         specified site *-see* Neoplasm, malignant
         unspecified site (female) C50.91
            male C50.92
      ductular
         specified site *-see* Neoplasm, malignant
         unspecified site (female) C50.91
            male C50.92
      lobular
         specified site *-see* Neoplasm, malignant
         unspecified site (female) C50.91
            male C50.92
   inflammatory
      specified site *-see* Neoplasm, malignant
      unspecified site (female) C50.91
         male C50.92
   intestinal type
      specified site *-see* Neoplasm, malignant, by
         site
      unspecified site C16.9
   intracystic
      noninfiltrating *-see* Neoplasm, in situ, by
         site
   intraductal (noninfiltrating)
      with Paget's disease *-see* Neoplasm, breast,
      malignant
      breast D05.1
      papillary
         with invasion
            specified site *-see* Neoplasm, malignant,
               by site
            unspecified site (female) C50.91
               male C50.92
         breast D05.1
         specified site NEC *-see* Neoplasm, in situ,
            by site
         unspecified site (female) D05.1
      specified site NEC *-see* Neoplasm, in situ,
         by site
      unspecified site (female) D05.1
   intraepidermal *-see* Neoplasm, in situ
      squamous cell, Bowen's type *-see* Neoplasm,
         skin, in situ
   intraepithelial *-see* Neoplasm, in situ, by site
      squamous cell *-see* Neoplasm, in situ, by site
   intraosseous C41.1
      upper jaw (bone) C41.0

Carcinoma *--continued*
   islet cell
      with exocrine, mixed
         specified site *-see* Neoplasm, malignant, by
            site
         unspecified site C25.9
      pancreas C25.4
      specified site NEC *-see* Neoplasm,
         malignant, by site
      unspecified site C25.4
   juvenile, breast *-see* Neoplasm, breast,
   malignant
   large cell
      small cell
         specified site *-see* Neoplasm, malignant, by
            site
         unspecified site C34.90
   Leydig cell (testis)
      specified site *-see* Neoplasm, malignant, by
      site
      unspecified site
         female C56.9
         male C62.90
   lipid-rich (female) C50.91
      male C50.92
   liver cell C22.0
   liver NEC C22.7
   lobular (infiltrating)
      with intraductal
         specified site *-see* Neoplasm, malignant, by
            site
         unspecified site (female) C50.91
            male C50.92
      noninfiltrating
         breast D05.0
         specified site NEC *-see* Neoplasm, in situ,
            by site
         unspecified site D05.0
      specified site *-see* Neoplasm, malignant, by
         site
      unspecified site (female) C50.91
         male C50.92
   medullary
      with
         amyloid stroma
            specified site *-see* Neoplasm, malignant,
               by site
            unspecified site C73
         lymphoid stroma
            specified site *-see* Neoplasm, malignant,
               by site
            unspecified site (female) C50.91
               male C50.92
   Merkel cell C4A.9
      anal margin C4A.51
      anal skin C4A.51
      canthus C4A.1
      ear and external auricular canal C4A.2
      external auricular canal C4A.2
      eyelid, including canthus C4A.1
      face C4A.30
         specified NEC C4A.39
      hip C4A.7
      lip C4A.0
      lower limb, including hip C4A.7
      neck C4A.4
      nodal presentation C7B.1
      nose C4A.31
      overlapping sites C4A.8
      perianal skin C4A.51
      scalp C4A.4

Carcinoma *--continued*
      secondary C7B.1
      shoulder C4A.6
      skin of breast C4A.52
      trunk NEC C4A.59
      upper limb, including shoulder C4A.6
      visceral metastatic C7B.1
   metastatic *-see* Neoplasm, secondary, by site
   metatypical *-see* Neoplasm, skin, malignant
   morphea, basal cell *-see* Neoplasm, skin,
      malignant
   mucoid
      cell
         specified site *-see* Neoplasm, malignant, by
            site
         unspecified site C75.1
   neuroendocrine *-see also* Tumor,
   neuroendocrine
      high grade, any site C7A.1
      poorly differentiated, any site C7A.1
   nonencapsulated sclerosing C73
   noninfiltrating
      intracystic *-see* Neoplasm, in situ, by site
      intraductal
         breast D05.1
         papillary
            breast D05.1
            specified site NEC *-see* Neoplasm, in
               situ, by site
            unspecified site D05.1
         specified site *-see* Neoplasm, in situ, by
            site
         unspecified site D05.1
      lobular
         breast D05.0
         specified site NEC *-see* Neoplasm, in situ,
            by site
         unspecified site (female) D05.0
   oat cell
      specified site *-see* Neoplasm, malignant, by
         site
      unspecified site C34.90
   odontogenic C41.1
      upper jaw (bone) C41.0
   papillary
      with follicular (mixed) C73
      follicular variant C73
      intraductal (noninfiltrating)
         with invasion
            specified site *-see* Neoplasm, malignant,
               by site
            unspecified site (female) C50.91
               male C50.92
         breast D05.1
         specified site NEC *-see* Neoplasm, in situ,
            by site
         unspecified site D05.1
      serous
         specified site *-see* Neoplasm, malignant, by
            site
      surface
         specified site *-see* Neoplasm, malignant,
            by site
         unspecified site C56.9
      unspecified site C56.9
   papillocystic
      specified site *-see* Neoplasm, malignant, by
         site
      unspecified site C56.9
   parafollicular cell

Carcinoma --*continued*
  specified site -*see* Neoplasm, malignant, by
    site
  unspecified site C73
  pilomatrix -*see* Neoplasm, skin, malignant
  pseudomucinous
    specified site -*see* Neoplasm, malignant, by
      site
    unspecified site C56.9
  renal cell C64
  Schmincke -*see* Neoplasm, nasopharynx,
    malignant
  Schneiderian
    specified site -*see* Neoplasm, malignant, by
      site
    unspecified site C30.0
  sebaceous -*see* Neoplasm, skin, malignant
  secondary -*see also* Neoplasm, secondary, by
    site
    Merkel cell C7B.1
  secretory, breast -*see* Neoplasm, breast,
    malignant
  serous
    papillary
      specified site -*see* Neoplasm, malignant, by
        site
      unspecified site C56.9
    surface, papillary
      specified site -*see* Neoplasm, malignant, by
        site
      unspecified site C56.9
  Sertoli cell
    specified site -*see* Neoplasm, malignant, by
      site
    unspecified site C62.90
      female C56.9
      male C62.90
  skin appendage -*see* Neoplasm, skin,
    malignant
  small cell
    fusiform cell
      specified site -*see* Neoplasm, malignant, by
        site
      unspecified site C34.90
    intermediate cell
      specified site -*see* Neoplasm, malignant, by
        site
      unspecified site C34.90
    large cell
      specified site -*see* Neoplasm, malignant, by
        site
      unspecified site C34.90
  solid
    with amyloid stroma
      specified site -*see* Neoplasm, malignant, by
        site
      unspecified site C73
    microinvasive
      specified site -*see* Neoplasm, malignant, by
        site
      unspecified site C53.9
  sweat gland -*see* Neoplasm, skin, malignant
  theca cell C56.
  thymic C37
  unspecified site (primary) C80.1
  water-clear cell C75.0
Carcinoma-in-situ -*see also* Neoplasm, in situ,
  by site
  breast NOS D05.9
    specified type NEC D05.8

Carcinoma-in-situ --*continued*
  epidermoid -*see also* Neoplasm, in situ, by
    site
    with questionable stromal invasion
      cervix D06.9
      specified site NEC -*see* Neoplasm, in situ,
        by site
      unspecified site D06.9
    Bowen's type -*see* Neoplasm, skin, in situ
  intraductal
    breast D05.1
    specified site NEC -*see* Neoplasm, in situ,
      by site
    unspecified site D05.1
  lobular
    with
      infiltrating duct
        breast (female) C50.91
          male C50.92
        specified site NEC -*see* Neoplasm,
          malignant
        unspecified site (female) C50.91
          male C50.92
      intraductal
        breast D05.8
        specified site NEC -*see* Neoplasm, in
          situ, by site
        unspecified site (female) D05.8
    breast D05.0
    specified site NEC -*see* Neoplasm, in situ,
      by site
    unspecified site D05.0
  squamous cell -*see also* Neoplasm, in situ, by
    site
    with questionable stromal invasion
      cervix D06.9
      specified site NEC -*see* Neoplasm, in situ,
        by site
      unspecified site D06.9
Carcinomaphobia F45.29
Carcinomatosis C80.0
  peritonei C78.6
  unspecified site (primary) (secondary) C80.0
Carcinosarcoma -*see* Neoplasm, malignant,
  by site
  embryonal -*see* Neoplasm, malignant, by site
Cardia, cardial -*see* condition
Cardiac -*see also* condition
  death, sudden -*see* Arrest, cardiac
  pacemaker
    in situ Z95.0
    management or adjustment Z45.018
  tamponade I31.4
Cardialgia -*see* Pain, precordial
Cardiectasis -*see* Hypertrophy, cardiac
Cardiochalasia K21.9
Cardiomalacia I51.5
Cardiomegalia glycogenica diffusa E74.02
  [I43]
Cardiomegaly -*see also* Hypertrophy, cardiac
  congenital Q24.8
  glycogen E74.02 *[I43]*
  idiopathic I51.7
Cardiomyoliposis I51.5
Cardiomyopathy (familial) (idiopathic) I42.9
  alcoholic I42.6
  amyloid E85.4 *[I43]*
  arteriosclerotic -*see* Disease, heart, ischemic,
    atherosclerotic
  beriberi E51.12
  cobalt-beer I42.6

Cardiomyopathy --*continued*
  congenital I42.4
  congestive I42.0
  constrictive NOS I42.5
  dilated I42.0
  due to
    alcohol I42.6
    beriberi E51.12
    cardiac glycogenosis E74.02 *[I43]*
    drugs I42.7
    external agents NEC I42.7
    Friedreich's ataxia G11.1
    myotonia atrophica G71.11 *[I43]*
    progressive muscular dystrophy G71.0
  glycogen storage E74.02 *[I43]*
  hypertensive -*see* Hypertension, heart
  hypertrophic (nonobstructive) I42.2
    obstructive I42.1
      congenital Q24.8
  in
    Chagas' disease (chronic) B57.2
      acute B57.0
    sarcoidosis D86.85
  ischemic I25.5
  metabolic E88.9 *[I43]*
    thyrotoxic E05.90 *[I43]*
      with thyroid storm E05.91 *[I43]*
  newborn I42.8
    congenital I42.4
  nutritional E63.9 *[I43]*
    beriberi E51.12
  obscure of Africa I42.8
  peripartum O90.3
  postpartum O90.3
  restrictive NEC I42.5
  rheumatic I09.0
  secondary I42.9
  stress induced I51.81
  takotsubo I51.81
  thyrotoxic E05.90 *[I43]*
    with thyroid storm E05.91 *[I43]*
  toxic NEC I42.7
  tuberculous A18.84
  viral B33.24
Cardionephritis -*see* Hypertension,
  cardiorenal
Cardionephropathy -*see* Hypertension,
  cardiorenal
Cardionephrosis -*see* Hypertension,
  cardiorenal
Cardiopathia nigra I27.0
Cardiopathy -*see also* Disease, heart I51.9
  idiopathic I42.9
  mucopolysaccharidosis E76.3 *[I52]*
Cardiopericarditis -*see* Pericarditis
Cardiophobia F45.29
Cardiorenal -*see* condition
Cardiorrhexis -*see* Infarct, myocardium
Cardiosclerosis -*see* Disease, heart, ischemic,
  atherosclerotic
Cardiosis -*see* Disease, heart
Cardiospasm (esophagus) (reflex) (stomach)
  K22.0
  congenital Q39.5
    with megaesophagus Q39.5
Cardiostenosis -*see* Disease, heart
Cardiosymphysis I31.0
Cardiovascular -*see* condition
Carditis (acute) (bacterial) (chronic)
  (subacute) I51.89
  meningococcal A39.50

Carditis - *continued*
rheumatic -*see* Disease, heart, rheumatic
rheumatoid -*see* Rheumatoid, carditis
viral B33.20
Care (of) (for) (following)
child (routine) Z76.2
family member (handicapped) (sick)
creating problem for family Z63.6
provided away from home for holiday relief
Z75.5
unavailable, due to
absence (person rendering care) (sufferer)
Z74.2
inability (any reason) of person rendering
care Z74.2
foundling Z76.1
holiday relief Z75.5
improper -*see* Maltreatment
lack of (at or after birth) (infant) -*see*
Maltreatment, child, neglect
lactating mother Z39.1
palliative Z51.5
postpartum
immediately after delivery Z39.0
routine follow-up Z39.2
respite Z75.5
unavailable, due to
absence of person rendering care Z74.2
inability (any reason) of person rendering
care Z74.2
well-baby Z76.2
Caries
bone NEC A18.03
dental (dentino enamel junction) (early
childhood) (of dentine) (pre-eruptive)
(recurrent) (to the pulp) K02.9
arrested (coronal) (root) K02.3
chewing surface
limited to enamel K02.51
penetrating into dentin K02.52
penetrating into pulp K02.53
coronal surface
chewing surface
limited to enamel K02.51
penetrating into dentin K02.52
penetrating into pulp K02.53
pit and fissure surface
limited to enamel K02.51
penetrating into dentin K02.52
penetrating into pulp K02.53
smooth surface
limited to enamel K02.61
penetrating into dentin K02.62
penetrating into pulp K02.63
pit and fissure surface
limited to enamel K02.51
penetrating into dentin K02.52
penetrating into pulp K02.53
primary, cervical origin K02.52
root K02.7
smooth surface
limited to enamel K02.61
penetrating into dentin K02.62
penetrating into pulp K02.63
external meatus -*see* Disorder, ear, external,
specified type NEC
hip (tuberculous) A18.02
initial (tooth)
chewing surface K02.51
pit and fissure surface K02.51
smooth surface K02.61

Caries - *continued*
knee (tuberculous) A18.02
labyrinth -*see* subcategory H83.8
limb NEC (tuberculous) A18.03
mastoid process (chronic) -*see* Mastoiditis,
chronic
tuberculous A18.03
middle ear -*see* subcategory H74.8
nose (tuberculous) A18.03
orbit (tuberculous) A18.03
ossicles, ear -*see* Abnormal, ear ossicles
petrous bone -*see* Petrositis
root (dental) (tooth) K02.7
sacrum (tuberculous) A18.01
spine, spinal (column) (tuberculous) A18.01
syphilitic A52.77
congenital (early) A50.02 [*M90.80*]
tooth, teeth -*see* Caries, dental
tuberculous A18.03
vertebra (column) (tuberculous) A18.01
Carious teeth -*see* Caries, dental
Carneous mole O02.0
Carnitine insufficiency E71.40
Carotid body or sinus syndrome G90.01
Carotidynia G90.01
Carotinemia (dietary) E67.1
Carotinosis (cutis) (skin) E67.1
Carpal tunnel syndrome -*see* Syndrome,
carpal tunnel
Carpenter's syndrome Q87.0
Carpopedal spasm -*see* Tetany
Carr-Barr-Plunkett syndrome Q97.1
Carrier (suspected) of
amebiasis Z22.1
bacterial disease NEC Z22.39
diphtheria Z22.2
intestinal infectious NEC Z22.1
typhoid Z22.0
meningococcal Z22.31
sexually transmitted Z22.4
specified NEC Z22.39
staphylococcal (Methicillin susceptible)
Z22.321
Methicillin resistant Z22.322
streptococcal Z22.338
group B Z22.330
complicating pregnancy or delivery
O99.82
typhoid Z22.0
cholera Z22.1
diphtheria Z22.2
gastrointestinal pathogens NEC Z22.1
genetic Z14.8
cystic fibrosis Z14.1
hemophilia A (asymptomatic) Z14.01
symptomatic Z14.02
gestational, pregnant Z33.1
gonorrhea Z22.4
HAA (hepatitis Australian-antigen) B18.8
HB (c)(s) AG B18.1
hepatitis (viral) B18.9
Australia-antigen (HAA) B18.8
B surface antigen (HBsAg) B18.1
with acute delta- (super) infection B17.0
C B18.2
specified NEC B18.8
human T-cell lymphotropic virus type-1
(HTLV-1) infection Z22.6
infectious organism Z22.9
specified NEC Z22.8
meningococci Z22.31

Carrier (suspected) of --*continued*
Salmonella typhosa Z22.0
serum hepatitis -*see* Carrier, hepatitis
staphylococci (Methicillin susceptible)
Z22.321
Methicillin resistant Z22.322
streptococci Z22.338
group B Z22.330
complicating pregnancy or delivery
O99.82
syphilis Z22.4
typhoid Z22.0
venereal disease NEC Z22.4
Carrion's disease A44.0
Carter's relapsing fever (Asiatic) A68.1
Cartilage -*see* condition
Caruncle (inflamed)
conjunctiva (acute) -*see* Conjunctivitis, acute
labium (majus) (minus) N90.89
lacrimal -*see* Inflammation, lacrimal, passages
myrtiform N89.8
urethral (benign) N36.2
Cascade stomach K31.2
Caseation lymphatic gland (tuberculous)
A18.2
**Cassidy (Scholte) syndrome (malignant
carcinoid)** E34.0
Castellani's disease A69.8
Castration, traumatic, male S38.231
Casts in urine R82.99
Cat
cry syndrome Q93.4
ear Q17.3
eye syndrome Q92.8
Catabolism, senile R54
Catalepsy (hysterical) F44.2
schizophrenic F20.2
Cataplexy (idiopathic) -*see* Narcolepsy
Cataract (cortical) (immature) (incipient)
H26.9
with
neovascularization -*see* Cataract,
complicated
age-related -*see* Cataract, senile
anterior
and posterior axial embryonal Q12.0
pyramidal Q12.0
associated with
galactosemia E74.21 [*H28*]
myotonic disorders G71.19 [*H28*]
blue Q12.0
central Q12.0
cerulean Q12.0
complicated H26.20
with
neovascularization H26.21
ocular disorder H26.22
glaucomatous flecks H26.23
congenital Q12.0
coralliform Q12.0
coronary Q12.0
crystalline Q12.0
diabetic -*see* Diabetes, cataract
drug-induced H26.3
due to
ocular disorder -*see* Cataract, complicated
radiation H26.8
electric H26.8
extraction status Z98.4
glass-blower's H26.8
heat ray H26.8

Cataract - *continued*
  heterochromic -*see* Cataract, complicated
  hypermature -*see* Cataract, senile, morgagnian
  type - in (due to)
    chronic iridocyclitis -*see* Cataract,
      complicated
    diabetes -*see* Diabetes, cataract
    endocrine disease E34.9 [*H28*]
    eye disease -*see* Cataract, complicated
    hypoparathyroidism E20.9 [*H28*]
    malnutrition-dehydration E46 [*H28*]
    metabolic disease E88.9 [*H28*]
    myotonic disorders G71.19 [*H28*]
    nutritional disease E63.9 [*H28*]
  infantile -*see* Cataract, presenile
  irradiational -*see* Cataract, specified NEC
  juvenile -*see* Cataract, presenile
  malnutrition-dehydration E46 [*H28*]
  morgagnian -*see* Cataract, senile, morgagnian
    type - myotonic G71.19 [*H28*]
  myxedema E03.9 [*H28*]
  nuclear
    embryonal Q12.0
    sclerosis -*see* Cataract, senile, nuclear
  presenile H26.00
    combined forms H26.06
    cortical H26.01
    lamellar -*see* Cataract, presenile, cortical
    nuclear H26.03
    specified NEC H26.09
    subcapsular polar (anterior) H26.04
      posterior H26.05
    zonular -*see* Cataract, presenile, cortical
  secondary H26.40
    Soemmering's ring H26.41
    specified NEC H26.49
    to eye disease -*see* Cataract, complicated -
      senile H25.9
  brunescens -*see* Cataract, senile, nuclear
  combined forms H25.81
  coronary -*see* Cataract, senile, incipient
  cortical H25.01
  hypermature -*see* Cataract, senile,
    morgagnian type
  incipient (mature) (total) H25.09
    cortical -*see* Cataract, senile, cortical
    subcapsular -*see* Cataract, senile,
      subcapsular
  morgagnian type (hypermature) H25.2
  nuclear (sclerosis) H25.1
  polar subcapsular (anterior) (posterior) -*see*
    Cataract, senile, incipient
  punctate -*see* Cataract, senile, incipient
  specified NEC H25.89
  subcapsular polar (anterior) H25.03
    posterior H25.04
  snowflake -*see* Diabetes, cataract
  specified NEC H26.8
  toxic -*see* Cataract, drug-induced - traumatic
    H26.10
    localized H26.11
    partially resolved H26.12
    total H26.13
  zonular (perinuclear) Q12.0
Cataracta -*see also* Cataract
  brunescens -*see* Cataract, senile, nuclear
  centralis pulverulenta Q12.0
  cerulea Q12.0
  complicata -*see* Cataract, complicated
  congenita Q12.0
  coralliformis Q12.0

Cataracta - *continued*
  coronaria Q12.0
  diabetic -*see* Diabetes, cataract
  membranacea
    accreta -*see* Cataract, secondary
    congenita Q12.0
  nigra -*see* Cataract, senile, nuclear
  sunflower -*see* Cataract, complicated
Catarrh, catarrhal (acute) (febrile)
  (infectious) (inflammation) -*see also*
    condition J00
  bronchial -*see* Bronchitis
  chest -*see* Bronchitis
  chronic J31.0
  due to congenital syphilis A50.03
  enteric -*see* Enteritis
  eustachian H68.009
  fauces -*see* Pharyngitis
  gastrointestinal -*see* Enteritis
  gingivitis K05.00
    nonplaque induced K05.01
    plaque induced K05.00
  hay -*see* Fever, hay
  intestinal -*see* Enteritis
  larynx, chronic J37.0
  liver B15.9
    with hepatic coma B15.0
  lung -*see* Bronchitis
  middle ear, chronic -*see* Otitis, media,
    nonsuppurative, chronic, serous
  mouth K12.1
  nasal (chronic) -*see* Rhinitis
  nasobronchial J31.1
  nasopharyngeal (chronic) J31.1
    acute J00
  pulmonary -*see* Bronchitis
  spring (eye) (vernal) -*see* Conjunctivitis,
    acute, atopic
  summer (hay) -*see* Fever, hay
  throat J31.2
  tubotympanal -*see also* Otitis, media,
    nonsuppurative
    chronic -*see* Otitis, media, nonsuppurative,
      chronic, serous
Catatonia (schizophrenic) F20.2
Catatonic
  disorder due to known physiologic condition
    F06.1
  schizophrenia F20.2
  stupor R40.1
Cat-scratch -*see also* Abrasion
  disease or fever A28.1
Cauda equina -*see* condition
Cauliflower ear M95.1
Causalgia (upper limb) G56.4
  lower limb G57.7
Cause
  external, general effects T75.89
Caustic burn -*see* Corrosion, by site
Cavare's disease (familial periodic paralysis)
  G72.3
Cave-in, injury
  crushing (severe) -*see* Crush
  suffocation -*see* Asphyxia, traumatic, due to
    low oxygen, due to cave-in
Cavernitis (penis) N48.29
Cavernositis N48.29
Cavernous -*see* condition
Cavitation of lung -*see also* Tuberculosis,
  pulmonary
  nontuberculous J98.4

Cavities, dental -*see* Caries, dental
Cavity
  lung -*see* Cavitation of lung
  optic papilla Q14.2
  pulmonary -*see* Cavitation of lung
Cavovarus foot, congenital Q66.1
Cavus foot (congenital) Q66.7
  acquired -*see* Deformity, limb, foot, specified
    NEC
Cazenave's disease L10.2
Cecitis K52.9
  with perforation, peritonitis, or rupture K65.8
Cecum -*see* condition
Celiac
  artery compression syndrome I77.4
  disease (with steatorrhea) K90.0
  infantilism K90.0
Cell(s), cellular -*see also* condition
  in urine R82.99
Cellulitis (diffuse) (phlegmonous) (septic)
  (suppurative) L03.90
  abdominal wall L03.311
  anaerobic A48.0
  ankle -*see* Cellulitis, lower limb
  anus K61.0
  arm -*see* Cellulitis, upper limb
  auricle (ear) -*see* Cellulitis, ear
  axilla L03.11
  back (any part) L03.312
  breast (acute) (nonpuerperal) (subacute)
    N61.0
    nipple N61.0
  broad ligament
    acute N73.0
  buttock L03.317
  cervical (meaning neck) L03.221
  cervix (uteri) -*see* Cervicitis
  cheek (external) L03.211
    internal K12.2
  chest wall L03.313
  chronic L03.90
  clostridial A48.0
  corpus cavernosum N48.22
  digit
    finger -*see* Cellulitis, finger
    toe -*see* Cellulitis, toe
  Douglas' cul-de-sac or pouch
    acute N73.0
  drainage site (following operation) T81.48
  ear (external) H60.1
  eosinophilic (granulomatous) L98.3
  erysipelatous -*see* Erysipelas
  external auditory canal -*see* Cellulitis, ear
  eyelid -*see* Abscess, eyelid
  face NEC L03.211
  finger (intrathecal) (periosteal)
    (subcutaneous) (subcuticular) L03.01
  foot -*see* Cellulitis, lower limb
  gangrenous -*see* Gangrene
  genital organ NEC
    female (external) N76.4
    male N49.9
      multiple sites N49.8
      specified NEC N49.8
  gluteal (region) L03.317
  gonococcal A54.89
  groin L03.314
  hand -*see* Cellulitis, upper limb
  head NEC L03.811
    face (any part, except ear, eye and nose)
      L03.211

Cellulitis - *continued*
 heel -*see* Cellulitis, lower limb
 hip -*see* Cellulitis, lower limb
 jaw (region) L03.211
 knee -*see* Cellulitis, lower limb
 labium (majus) (minus) -*see* Vulvitis
 lacrimal passages -*see* Inflammation, lacrimal,
  passages
 larynx J38.7
 leg -*see* Cellulitis, lower limb
 lip K13.0
 lower limb L03.11
  toe -*see* Cellulitis, toe - mouth (floor) K12.2
 multiple sites, so stated L03.90
 nasopharynx J39.1
 navel L03.316
  newborn P38.9
   with mild hemorrhage P38.1
   without hemorrhage P38.9
 neck (region) L03.221
 nipple (acute) (nonpuerperal) (subacute)
  N61.0
 nose (septum) (external) J34.0
 orbit, orbital H05.01
 palate (soft) K12.2
 pectoral (region) L03.313
 pelvis, pelvic (chronic)
  female -*see also* Disease, pelvis,
  inflammatory N73.2
   acute N73.0
  following ectopic or molar pregnancy O08.0
  male K65.0
 penis N48.22
 perineal, perineum L03.315
 periorbital L03.213
 perirectal K61.1
 peritonsillar J36
 periurethral N34.0
 periuterine -*see also* Disease, pelvis,
  inflammatory N73.2
   acute N73.0
 pharynx J39.1
 preseptal L03.213
 rectum K61.1
 retroperitoneal K68.9
 round ligament
  acute N73.0
 scalp (any part) L03.811
 scrotum N49.2
 seminal vesicle N49.0
 shoulder -*see* Cellulitis, upper limb
 specified site NEC L03.818
 submandibular (region) (space) (triangle)
  K12.2
  gland K11.3
 submaxillary (region) K12.2
  gland K11.3
 thigh -*see* Cellulitis, lower limb
 thumb (intrathecal) (periosteal)
  (subcutaneous) (subcuticular) -*see* Cellulitis,
  finger
 toe (intrathecal) (periosteal) (subcutaneous)
  (subcuticular) L03.03
 tonsil J36
 trunk L03.319
  abdominal wall L03.311
  back (any part) L03.312
  buttock L03.317
  chest wall L03.313
  groin L03.314
  perineal, perineum L03.315

Cellulitis - *continued*
  umbilicus L03.316
  tuberculous (primary) A18.4
  umbilicus L03.316
 upper limb L03.11
  axilla -*see* Cellulitis, axilla
  finger -*see* Cellulitis, finger
  thumb -*see* Cellulitis, finger
 vaccinal T88.0
 vocal cord J38.3
 vulva -*see* Vulvitis
 wrist -*see* Cellulitis, upper limb
Cementoblastoma, benign -*see* Cyst,
 calcifying odontogenic
Cementoma -*see* Cyst, calcifying odontogenic
Cementoperiostitis -*see* Periodontitis
Cementosis K03.4
Central auditory processing disorder H93.25
Central pain syndrome G89.0
Cephalematocele, cephal (o) hematocele
 newborn P52.8
  birth injury P10.8
 traumatic -*see* Hematoma, brain
**Cephalematoma, cephalhematoma
(calcified)**
 newborn (birth injury) P12.0
 traumatic -*see* Hematoma, brain
Cephalgia, cephalalgia -*see also* Headache -
 histamine G44.009
  intractable G44.001
  not intractable G44.009
 trigeminal autonomic (TAC) NEC G44.099
  intractable G44.091
  not intractable G44.099
Cephalic -*see* condition
Cephalitis -*see* Encephalitis
Cephalocele -*see* Encephalocele
Cephalomenia N94.89
Cephalopelvic -*see* condition
**Cerclage (with cervical incompetence) in
 pregnancy -***see* Incompetence, cervix, in
 pregnancy
Cerebellitis -*see* Encephalitis
Cerebellum, cerebellar -*see* condition
Cerebral -*see* condition
Cerebritis -*see* Encephalitis
Cerebro-hepato-renal syndrome Q87.89
Cerebromalacia -*see* Softening, brain
 sequelae of cerebrovascular disease I69.398
Cerebroside lipidosis E75.22
Cerebrospasticity (congenital) G80.1
Cerebrospinal -*see* condition
Cerebrum -*see* condition
Ceroid-lipofuscinosis, neuronal E75.4
Cerumen (accumulation) (impacted) H61.2
Cervical -*see also* condition
 auricle Q18.2
 dysplasia in pregnancy -*see* Abnormal, cervix,
 in pregnancy or childbirth
 erosion in pregnancy -*see* Abnormal, cervix,
 in pregnancy or childbirth
 fibrosis in pregnancy -*see* Abnormal, cervix,
 in pregnancy or childbirth
 fusion syndrome Q76.1
 rib Q76.5
 shortening (complicating pregnancy) O26.87
Cervicalgia M54.2
Cervicitis (acute) (chronic) (nonvenereal)
 (senile (atrophic)) (subacute) (with ulceration)
 N72
 with

Cervicitis - *continued-* abortion -*see*
 Abortion, by type complicated by genital tract
 and pelvic infection
  ectopic pregnancy O08.0
  molar pregnancy O08.0
 chlamydial A56.09
 gonococcal A54.03
 herpesviral A60.03
 puerperal (postpartum) O86.11
 syphilitic A52.76
 trichomonal A59.09
 tuberculous A18.16
Cervicocolpitis (emphysematosa) (see also
 Cervicitis) N72
Cervix -*see* condition
**Cesarean delivery, previous, affecting
 management of pregnancy** O34.219
 classical (vertical) scar O34.212
 low transverse scar O34.211
Céstan (Chenais) paralysis or syndrome
 G46.3
Céstan-Raymond syndrome I65.8
Cestode infestation B71.9
 specified type NEC B71.8
Cestodiasis B71.9
Chabert's disease A22.9
Chacaleh E53.8
Chafing L30.4
Chagas' (Mazza) disease (chronic) B57.2
 with
  cardiovascular involvement NEC B57.2
  digestive system involvement B57.30
   megacolon B57.32
   megaesophagus B57.31
   other specified B57.39
  megacolon B57.32
  megaesophagus B57.31
  myocarditis B57.2
  nervous system involvement B57.40
   meningitis B57.41
   meningoencephalitis B57.42
   other specified B57.49
  specified organ involvement NEC B57.5
 acute (with) B57.1
  cardiovascular NEC B57.0
  myocarditis B57.0
Chagres fever B50.9
Chair ridden Z74.09
Chalasia (cardiac sphincter) K21.9
Chalazion H00.19
 left H00.16
  lower H00.15
  upper H00.14
 right H00.13
  lower H00.12
  upper H00.11
Chalcosis -*see also* Disorder, globe,
 degenerative, chalcosis
 cornea -*see* Deposit, cornea
 crystalline lens -*see* Cataract, complicated -
 retina H35.89
Chalicosis (pulmonum) J62.8
Chancre (any genital site) (hard) (hunterian)
 (mixed) (primary) (seronegative)
 (seropositive) (syphilitic) A51.0
 congenital A50.07
 conjunctiva NEC A51.2
 Ducrey's A57
 extragenital A51.2
 eyelid A51.2
 lip A51.2

Chancre --*continued*
nipple A51.2
Nisbet's A57
of
carate A67.0
pinta A67.0
yaws A66.0
palate, soft A51.2
phagedenic A57
simple A57
soft A57
bubo A57
palate A51.2
urethra A51.0
yaws A66.0
Chancroid (anus) (genital) (penis) (perineum) (rectum) (urethra) (vulva) A57
Chandler's disease (osteochondritis dissecans, hip) -*see* Osteochondritis, dissecans, hip
Change(s) (in) (of) -*see also* Removal
arteriosclerotic -*see* Arteriosclerosis
bone -*see also* Disorder, bone
diabetic -*see* Diabetes, bone change
bowel habit R19.4
cardiorenal (vascular) -*see* Hypertension, cardiorenal
cardiovascular -*see* Disease, cardiovascular
circulatory I99.9
cognitive (mild) (organic) R41.89
color, tooth, teeth
during formation K00.8
posteruptive K03.7
contraceptive device Z30.433
corneal membrane H18.30
Bowman's membrane fold or rupture H18.31
Descemet's membrane
fold H18.32
rupture H18.33
coronary -*see* Disease, heart, ischemic
degenerative, spine or vertebra -*see* Spondylosis
dental pulp, regressive K04.2
dressing (nonsurgical) Z48.00
surgical Z48.01
heart -*see* Disease, heart
hip joint -*see* Derangement, joint, hip
hyperplastic larynx J38.7
hypertrophic
nasal sinus J34.89
turbinate, nasal J34.3
upper respiratory tract J39.8
indwelling catheter Z46.6
inflammatory -*see also* Inflammation
sacroiliac M46.1
job, anxiety concerning Z56.1
joint -*see* Derangement, joint
life -*see* Menopause
mental status R41.82
minimal (glomerular) -*see also* N00 N07 with fourth character .0 N05.0
myocardium, myocardial -*see* Degeneration, myocardial
of life -*see* Menopause - pacemaker Z45.018
pulse generator Z45.010
personality (enduring) F68.8
due to (secondary to)
general medical condition F07.0
secondary (nonspecific) F60.89
regressive, dental pulp K04.2
renal -*see* Disease, renal

Change(s) (in) (of) retina H35.9 --*continued*
myopic H44.2
sacroiliac joint M53.3
senile -*see also* condition R54
sensory R20.8
skin R23.9
acute, due to ultraviolet radiation L56.9
specified NEC L56.8
chronic, due to nonionizing radiation L57.9
specified NEC L57.8
cyanosis R23.0
flushing R23.2
pallor R23.1
petechiae R23.3
specified change NEC R23.8
swelling -*see* Mass, localized
texture R23.4
trophic
arm -*see* Mononeuropathy, upper limb
leg -*see* Mononeuropathy, lower limb
vascular I99.9
vasomotor I73.9
voice R49.9
psychogenic F44.4
specified NEC R49.8
Changing sleep-work schedule, affecting sleep G47.26
Changuinola fever A93.1
Chapping skin T69.8
Charcot-Marie-Tooth disease, paralysis or syndrome G60.0
Charcot's
arthropathy -*see* Arthropathy, neuropathic
cirrhosis K74.3
disease (tabetic arthropathy) A52.16
joint (disease) (tabetic) A52.16
diabetic -*see* Diabetes, with, arthropathy
syringomyelic G95.0
syndrome (intermittent claudication) I73.9
CHARGE association Q89.8
Charley horse (quadriceps) M62.831
traumatic (quadriceps) S76.11
Charlouis' disease -*see* Yaws
Cheadle's disease E54
Checking (of)
cardiac pacemaker (battery) (electrode(s)) Z45.018
pulse generator Z45.010
implantable subdermal contraceptive Z30.46
intrauterine contraceptive device Z30.431
Check-up -*see* Examination
Chédiak-Higashi (Steinbrinck) syndrome (congenital gigantism of peroxidase granules) E70.330
Cheek -*see* condition
Cheese itch B88.0
Cheese-washer's lung J67.8
Cheese-worker's lung J67.8
Cheilitis (acute) (angular) (catarrhal) (chronic) (exfoliative) (gangrenous) (glandular) (infectional) (suppurative) (ulcerative) (vesicular) K13.0
actinic (due to sun) L56.8
other than from sun L59.8
candidal B37.83
Cheilodynia K13.0
Cheiloschisis -*see* Cleft, lip
Cheilosis (angular) K13.0
with pellagra E52
due to
vitamin B2 (riboflavin) deficiency E53.0

Cheiromegaly M79.89
Cheiropompholyx L30.1
Cheloid -*see* Keloid
Chemical burn -*see* Corrosion, by site
Chemodectoma -*see* Paraganglioma, nonchromaffin
Chemosis, conjunctiva -*see* Edema, conjunctiva
Chemotherapy (session) (for)
cancer Z51.11
neoplasm Z51.11
Cherubism M27.8
Chest -*see* condition
Cheyne-Stokes breathing (respiration) R06.3
Chiari's
disease or syndrome (hepatic vein thrombosis) I82.0
malformation
type I G93.5
type II -*see* Spina bifida
net Q24.8
Chicago disease B40.9
Chickenpox -*see* Varicella
Chiclero ulcer or sore B55.1
Chigger (infestation) B88.0
Chignon (disease) B36.8
newborn (from vacuum extraction) (birth injury) P12.1
Chilaiditi's syndrome (subphrenic displacement, colon) Q43.3
Chilblain(s) (lupus) T69.1
Child
custody dispute Z65.3
Childbirth -*see* Delivery
Childhood
cerebral X linked adrenoleukodystrophy E71.520
period of rapid growth Z00.2
Chill(s) R68.83
with fever R50.9
congestive in malarial regions B54
without fever R68.83
Chilomastigiasis A07.8
Chimera 46,XX/46,XY Q99.0
Chin -*see* condition
Chinese dysentery A03.9
Chionophobia F40.228
Chitral fever A93.1
Chlamydia, chlamydial A74.9
cervicitis A56.09
conjunctivitis A74.0
cystitis A56.01
endometritis A56.11
epididymitis A56.19
female
pelvic inflammatory disease A56.11
pelviperitonitis A56.11
orchitis A56.19
peritonitis A74.81
pharyngitis A56.4
proctitis A56.3
psittaci (infection) A70
salpingitis A56.11
sexually transmitted infection NEC A56.8
specified NEC A74.89
urethritis A56.01
vulvovaginitis A56.02
Chlamydiosis -*see* Chlamydia
Chloasma (skin) (idiopathic) (symptomatic) L81.1
eyelid H02.719

Chloasma - *continued*
hyperthyroid E05.90 [*H02.719*]
with thyroid storm E05.91 [*H02.719*]
left H02.716
lower H02.715
upper H02.714
right H02.713
lower H02.712
upper H02.711
Chloroma C92.3
Chlorosis D50.9
Egyptian B76.9 [*D63.8*]
miner's B76.9 [*D63.8*]
Chlorotic anemia D50.8
Chocolate cyst (ovary) N80.1
Choked
disc or disk -*see* Papilledema
on food, phlegm, or vomitus NOS -*see*
Foreign body, by site
while vomiting NOS -*see* Foreign body, by
site
Chokes (resulting from bends) T70.3
Choking sensation R09.89
Cholangiectasis K83.8
Cholangiocarcinoma
with hepatocellular carcinoma, combined
C22.0
liver C22.1
specified site NEC -*see* Neoplasm, malignant,
by site
unspecified site C22.1
Cholangiohepatitis K83.8
due to fluke infestation B66.1
Cholangiohepatoma C22.0
Cholangiolitis (acute) (chronic) (extrahepatic)
(gangrenous) (intrahepatic) K83.0
paratyphoidal -*see* Fever, paratyphoid
typhoidal A01.09
Cholangioma D13.4
malignant -*see* Cholangiocarcinoma
Cholangitis (ascending) (primary) (recurrent)
(sclerosing) (secondary) (stenosing)
(suppurative) K83.0
with calculus, bile duct -*see* Calculus, bile
duct, with cholangitis
chronic nonsuppurative destructive K74.3
Cholecystectasia K82.8
Cholecystitis K81.9
with
calculus, stones in
bile duct (common) (hepatic) -*see*
Calculus, bile duct, with cholecystitis
cystic duct -*see* Calculus, gallbladder, with
cholecystitis
gallbladder -*see* Calculus, gallbladder, with
cholecystitis
choledocholithiasis -*see* Calculus, bile duct,
with cholecystitis
cholelithiasis -*see* Calculus, gallbladder,
with cholecystitis
acute (emphysematous) (gangrenous)
(suppurative) K81.0
with
calculus, stones in
cystic duct -*see* Calculus, gallbladder,
with cholecystitis, acute
gallbladder -*see* Calculus, gallbladder,
with cholecystitis, acute
choledocholithiasis -*see* Calculus, bile
duct, with cholecystitis, acute

Cholecystitis --*continued*
cholelithiasis -*see* Calculus, gallbladder,
with cholecystitis, acute
chronic cholecystitis K81.2
with gallbladder calculus K80.12
with obstruction K80.13
chronic K81.1
with acute cholecystitis K81.2
with gallbladder calculus K80.12
with obstruction K80.13
emphysematous (acute) -*see* Cholecystitis,
acute
gangrenous -*see* Cholecystitis, acute
paratyphoidal, current A01.4
suppurative -*see* Cholecystitis, acute
typhoidal A01.09
Cholecystolithiasis -*see* Calculus, gallbladder
Choledochitis (suppurative) K83.0
Choledocholith -*see* Calculus, bile duct
**Choledocholithiasis (common duct) (hepatic
duct)** -*see* Calculus, bile duct
cystic -*see* Calculus, gallbladder
typhoidal A01.09
Cholelithiasis (cystic duct) (gallbladder)
(impacted) (multiple) -*see* Calculus,
gallbladder
bile duct (common) (hepatic) -*see* Calculus,
bile duct
hepatic duct -*see* Calculus, bile duct
specified NEC K80.80
with obstruction K80.81
Cholemia -*see also* Jaundice
familial (simple) (congenital) E80.4
Gilbert's E80.4
Choleperitoneum, choleperitonitis K65.3
Cholera (Asiatic) (epidemic) (malignant)
A00.9
antimonial -*see* Poisoning, antimony
classical A00.0
due to Vibrio cholerae 01 A00.9
biovar cholerae A00.0
biovar eltor A00.1
el tor A00.1
el tor A00.1
Cholerine -*see* Cholera
Cholestasis NEC K83.1
with hepatocyte injury K71.0
due to total parenteral nutrition (TPN) K76.89
pure K71.0
Cholesteatoma (ear) (middle) (with reaction)
H71.9
attic H71.0
external ear (canal) H60.4
mastoid H71.2
postmastoidectomy cavity (recurrent) -*see*
Complications, postmastoidectomy,
recurrent cholesteatoma
recurrent (postmastoidectomy) -*see*
Complications, postmastoidectomy,
recurrent cholesteatoma
tympanum H71.1
Cholesteatosis, diffuse H71.3
Cholesteremia E78.00
Cholesterin in vitreous -*see* Deposit,
crystalline
Cholesterol
deposit
retina H35.89
vitreous -*see* Deposit, crystalline
elevated (high) E78.00
with elevated (high) triglycerides E78.2

Cholesterol - *continued*
screening for Z13.220
imbibition of gallbladder K82.4
Cholesterolemia (essential) (pure) E78.00
familial E78.01
hereditary E78.01
Cholesterolosis, cholesterosis (gallbladder)
K82.4
cerebrotendinous E75.5
Cholocolic fistula K82.3
Choluria R82.2
Chondritis M94.8X9
auricle H61.03
costal (Tietze's) M94.0
external ear H61.03
patella, posttraumatic -*see* Chondromalacia,
patella
pinna H61.03
purulent M94.8X
tuberculous NEC A18.02
intervertebral A18.01
Chondroblastoma -*see also* Neoplasm, bone,
benign
malignant -*see* Neoplasm, bone, malignant
Chondrocalcinosis M11.20
ankle M11.27
elbow M11.22
familial M11.10
ankle M11.17
elbow M11.12
foot joint M11.17
hand joint M11.14
hip M11.15
knee M11.16
multiple site M11.19
shoulder M11.11
vertebrae M11.18
wrist M11.13
foot joint M11.27
hand joint M11.24
hip M11.25
knee M11.26
multiple site M11.29
shoulder M11.21
vertebrae M11.28
specified type NEC M11.20
ankle M11.27
elbow M11.22
foot joint M11.27
hand joint M11.24
hip M11.25
knee M11.26
multiple site M11.29
shoulder M11.21
vertebrae M11.28
wrist M11.23
wrist M11.23
**Chondrodermatitis nodularis helicis or
anthelicis** -*see* Perichondritis, ear
Chondrodysplasia Q78.9
with hemangioma Q78.4
calcificans congenita Q77.3
fetalis Q77.4
metaphyseal (Jansen's) (McKusick's)
(Schmid's) Q78.8
punctata Q77.3
Chondrodystrophy, chondrodystrophia
(familial) (fetalis) (hypoplastic) Q78.9
calcificans congenita Q77.3
myotonic (congenital) G71.13
punctata Q77.3

Chondroectodermal dysplasia Q77.6
Chondrogenesis imperfecta Q77.4
Chondrolysis M94.35
Chondroma -see also Neoplasm, cartilage,
    benign
    juxtacortical -see Neoplasm, bone, benign
    periosteal -see Neoplasm, bone, benign
Chondromalacia (systemic) M94.20
    acromioclavicular joint M94.21
    ankle M94.27
    elbow M94.22
    foot joint M94.27
    glenohumeral joint M94.21
    hand joint M94.24
    hip M94.25
    knee M94.26
        patella M22.4
    multiple sites M94.29
    patella M22.4
    rib M94.28
    sacroiliac joint M94.259
    shoulder M94.21
    sternoclavicular joint M94.21
    vertebral joint M94.28
    wrist M94.23
Chondromatosis -see also Neoplasm,
    cartilage, uncertain behavior
    internal Q78.4
Chondromyxosarcoma -see Neoplasm,
    cartilage, malignant
**Chondro-osteodysplasia (Morquio-
    Brailsford type)** E76.219
Chondro-osteodystrophy E76.29
Chondro-osteoma -see Neoplasm, bone,
    benign
Chondropathia tuberosa M94.0
Chondrosarcoma -see Neoplasm, cartilage,
    malignant
    juxtacortical -see Neoplasm, bone, malignant
    mesenchymal -see Neoplasm, connective
        tissue, malignant
    myxoid -see Neoplasm, cartilage, malignant
Chordee (nonvenereal) N48.89
    congenital Q54.4
    gonococcal A54.09
Chorditis (fibrinous) (nodosa) (tuberosa) J38.2
Chordoma -see Neoplasm, vertebral (column),
    malignant
**Chorea (chronic) (gravis) (posthemiplegic)
    (senile) (spasmodic)** G25.5
    with
        heart involvement I02.0
            active or acute (conditions in I01) I02.0
                rheumatic I02.9
                    with valvular disorder I02.0
            rheumatic heart disease (chronic)
    (inactive)(quiescent)   code to rheumatic heart
    condition involved - drug-induced G25.4
        habit F95.8
        hereditary G10
        Huntington's G10
        hysterical F44.4
        minor I02.9
            with heart involvement I02.0
        progressive G25.5
            hereditary G10
        rheumatic (chronic) I02.9
            with heart involvement I02.0
        Sydenham's I02.9
            with heart involvement -see Chorea, with
                rheumatic heart disease
            nonrheumatic G25.5

Choreoathetosis (paroxysmal) G25.5
Chorioadenoma (destruens) D39.2
Chorioamnionitis O41.12
Chorioangioma D26.7
Choriocarcinoma -see Neoplasm, malignant,
    by site
    combined with
        embryonal carcinoma -see Neoplasm,
            malignant, by site
        other germ cell elements -see Neoplasm,
            malignant, by site
        teratoma -see Neoplasm, malignant, by site
    specified site -see Neoplasm, malignant, by
    site
    unspecified site
        female C58
        male C62.90
**Chorioencephalitis (acute) (lymphocytic)
    (serous)** A87.2
Chorioepithelioma -see Choriocarcinoma
**Choriomeningitis (acute) (lymphocytic)
    (serous)** A87.2
Chorionepithelioma -see Choriocarcinoma
Chorioretinitis -see also Inflammation,
    chorioretinal
    disseminated -see also Inflammation,
        chorioretinal, disseminated
        in neurosyphilis A52.19
    Egyptian B76.9 [D63.8]
    focal -see also Inflammation, chorioretinal,
        focal
    histoplasmic B39.9 [H32]
    in (due to)
        histoplasmosis B39.9 [H32]
        syphilis (secondary) A51.43
            late A52.71
        toxoplasmosis (acquired) B58.01
            congenital (active) P37.1 [H32]
        tuberculosis A18.53
    juxtapapillary, juxtapapillaris -see
        Inflammation, chorioretinal, focal,
        juxtapapillary
    leprous A30.9 [H32]
    miner's B76.9 [D63.8]
    progressive myopia (degeneration) H44.2
    syphilitic (secondary) A51.43
        congenital (early) A50.01 [H32]
            late A50.32
        late A52.71
    tuberculous A18.53
Chorioretinopathy, central serous H35.71
Choroid -see condition
Choroideremia H31.21
Choroiditis -see Chorioretinitis
Choroidopathy -see Disorder, choroid
Choroidoretinitis -see Chorioretinitis
Choroidoretinopathy, central serous -see
    Chorioretinopathy, central serous
Christian-Weber disease M35.6
Christmas disease D67
Chromaffinoma -see also Neoplasm, benign,
    by site
    malignant -see Neoplasm, malignant, by site
Chromatopsia -see Deficiency, color vision
Chromhidrosis, chromidrosis L75.1
Chromoblastomycosis -see Chromomycosis
Chromoconversion R82.91
Chromomycosis B43.9
    brain abscess B43.1
    cerebral B43.1
    cutaneous B43.0

Chromomycosis - continued
    skin B43.0
    specified NEC B43.8
    subcutaneous abscess or cyst B43.2
Chromophytosis B36.0
Chromosome -see condition by chromosome
    involved
    D (1) -see condition, chromosome 13
    E (3) -see condition, chromosome 18
    G -see condition, chromosome 21
Chromotrichomycosis B36.8
Chronic -see condition
    fracture -see Fracture, pathological
Churg-Strauss syndrome M30.1
Chyle cyst, mesentery I89.8
Chylocele (nonfilarial) I89.8
    filarial -see also Infestation, filarial B74.9
        [N51]
    tunica vaginalis N50.89
        filarial -see also Infestation, filarial B74.9
        [N51]
**Chylomicronemia (fasting) (with
    hyperprebetalipoproteinemia)** E78.3
Chylopericardium I31.3
    acute I30.9
Chylothorax (nonfilarial) I89.8
    filarial -see also Infestation, filarial B74.9
    [J91.8]
Chylous -see condition
Chyluria (nonfilarial) R82.0
    due to
        bilharziasis B65.0
        Brugia (malayi) B74.1
            timori B74.2
        schistosomiasis (bilharziasis) B65.0
        Wuchereria (bancrofti) B74.0
    filarial -see Infestation, filarial
Cicatricial (deformity) -see Cicatrix
**Cicatrix (adherent) (contracted) (painful)
    (vicious)** -see also Scar L90.5
    adenoid (and tonsil) J35.8
    alveolar process M26.79
    anus K62.89
    auricle -see Disorder, pinna, specified type
        NEC
    bile duct (common) (hepatic) K83.8
    bladder N32.89
    bone -see Disorder, bone, specified type NEC
    brain G93.89
    cervix (postoperative) (postpartal) N88.1
    common duct K83.8
    cornea H17.9
        tuberculous A18.59
    duodenum (bulb), obstructive K31.5
    esophagus K22.2
    eyelid -see Disorder, eyelid function
    hypopharynx J39.2
    lacrimal passages -see Obstruction, lacrimal
    larynx J38.7
    lung J98.4
    middle ear -see subcategory H74.8
    mouth K13.79
    muscle M62.89
        with contracture -see Contraction, muscle
        NEC
    nasopharynx J39.2
    palate (soft) K13.79
    penis N48.89
    pharynx J39.2
    prostate N42.89
    rectum K62.89

Cicatrix - *continued*
retina -*see* Scar, chorioretinal
semilunar cartilage -*see* Derangement, meniscus
seminal vesicle N50.89
skin L90.5
infected L08.89
postinfective L90.5
tuberculous B90.8
specified site NEC L90.5
throat J39.2
tongue K14.8
tonsil (and adenoid) J35.8
trachea J39.8
tuberculous NEC B90.9
urethra N36.8
uterus N85.8
vagina N89.8
postoperative N99.2
vocal cord J38.3
wrist, constricting (annular) L90.5
CIDP (chronic inflammatory demyelinating polyneuropathy) G61.81
CIN -*see* Neoplasia, intraepithelial, cervix
CINCA (chronic infantile neurological, cutaneous and articular syndrome) M04.2
Cinchonism -*see* Deafness, ototoxic
correct substance properly administered -*see* Table of Drugs and Chemicals, by drug, adverse effect
overdose or wrong substance given or taken -*see* Table of Drugs and Chemicals, by drug, poisoning
Circle of Willis -*see* condition
Circular -*see* condition
Circulating anticoagulants -*see also* -Disorder, hemorrhagic D68.318
due to drugs -*see also* - Disorder, hemorrhagic D68.32
following childbirth O72.3
Circulation
collateral, any site I99.8
defective (lower extremity) I99.8
congenital Q28.9
embryonic Q28.9
failure (peripheral) R57.9
newborn P29.89
fetal, persistent P29.3
heart, incomplete Q28.9
Circulatory system -*see* condition
Circulus senilis (cornea) -*see* Degeneration, cornea, senile
Circumcision (in absence of medical indication) (ritual) (routine) Z41.2
Circumscribed -*see* condition
Circumvallate placenta O43.11
Cirrhosis, cirrhotic (hepatic) (liver) K74.60
alcoholic K70.30
with ascites K70.31
atrophic -*see* Cirrhosis, liver
Baumgarten-Cruveilhier K74.69
biliary (cholangiolitic) (cholangitic) (hypertrophic) (obstructive) (pericholangiolitic) K74.5
due to
Clonorchiasis B66.1
flukes B66.3
primary K74.3
secondary K74.4
cardiac (of liver) K76.1
Charcot's K74.3

Cirrhosis, cirrhotic --*continued*
cholangiolitic, cholangitic, cholestatic (primary) K74.3
congestive K76.1
Cruveilhier-Baumgarten K74.69
cryptogenic (liver) K74.69
due to
hepatolenticular degeneration E83.01
Wilson's disease E83.01
xanthomatosis E78.2
fatty K76.0
alcoholic K70.0
Hanot's (hypertrophic) K74.3
hepatic -*see* Cirrhosis, liver
hypertrophic K74.3
Indian childhood K74.69
kidney -*see* Sclerosis, renal
Laennec's K70.30
with ascites K70.31
alcoholic K70.30
with ascites K70.31
nonalcoholic K74.69
liver K74.60
alcoholic K70.30
with ascites K70.31
fatty K70.0
congenital P78.81
syphilitic A52.74
lung (chronic) J84.10
macronodular K74.69
alcoholic K70.30
with ascites K70.31
micronodular K74.69
alcoholic K70.30
with ascites K70.31
mixed type K74.69
monolobular K74.3
nephritis -*see* Sclerosis, renal
nutritional K74.69
alcoholic K70.30
with ascites K70.31
obstructive -*see* Cirrhosis, biliary
ovarian N83.8
pancreas (duct) K86.89
pigmentary E83.110
portal K74.69
alcoholic K70.30
with ascites K70.31
postnecrotic K74.69
alcoholic K70.30
with ascites K70.31
pulmonary J84.10
renal -*see* Sclerosis, renal
spleen D73.2
stasis K76.1
Todd's K74.3
unilobar K74.3
xanthomatous (biliary) K74.5
due to xanthomatosis (familial) (metabolic) (primary) E78.2
Cistern, subarachnoid R93.0
Citrullinemia E72.23
Citrullinuria E72.23
Civatte's disease or poikiloderma L57.3
Clam digger's itch B65.3
Clammy skin R23.1
Clap -*see* Gonorrhea
Clarke-Hadfield syndrome (pancreatic infantilism) K86.89
Clark's paralysis G80.9
Clastothrix L67.8

Claude Bernard-Horner syndrome G90.2
traumatic -*see* Injury, nerve, cervical sympathetic
Claude's disease or syndrome G46.3
Claudication (intermittent) I73.9
cerebral (artery) G45.9
spinal cord (arteriosclerotic) G95.19
syphilitic A52.09
venous (axillary) I87.8
Claudication venosa intermittens I87.8
Claustrophobia F40.240
Clavus (infected) L84
Clawfoot (congenital) Q66.89
acquired -*see* Deformity, limb, clawfoot
Clawhand (acquired) -*see also* Deformity, limb, clawhand
congenital Q68.1
Claw toe (congenital) Q66.89
acquired -*see* Deformity, toe, specified NEC
Clay eating -*see* Pica
Cleansing of artificial opening -*see* Attention to, artificial, opening
Cleft (congenital) -*see also* Imperfect, closure
alveolar process M26.79
branchial (cyst) (persistent) Q18.2
cricoid cartilage, posterior Q31.8
foot Q72.7
hand Q71.6
lip (unilateral) Q36.9
with cleft palate Q37.9
hard Q37.1
with soft Q37.5
soft Q37.3
with hard Q37.5
bilateral Q36.0
with cleft palate Q37.8
hard Q37.0
with soft Q37.4
soft Q37.2
with hard Q37.4
median Q36.1
nose Q30.2
palate Q35.9
with cleft lip (unilateral) Q37.9
bilateral Q37.8
hard Q35.1
with
cleft lip (unilateral) Q37.1
bilateral Q37.0
soft Q35.5
with cleft lip (unilateral) Q37.5
bilateral Q37.4
medial Q35.5
soft Q35.3
with
cleft lip (unilateral) Q37.3
bilateral Q37.2
hard Q35.5
with cleft lip (unilateral) Q37.5
bilateral Q37.4
penis Q55.69
scrotum Q55.29
thyroid cartilage Q31.8
uvula Q35.7
Cleidocranial dysostosis Q74.0
Cleptomania F63.2
Clicking hip (newborn) R29.4
Climacteric (female) -*see also* Menopause
arthritis (any site) NEC -*see* Arthritis, specified form NEC
depression (single episode) F32.89

Climacteric (female) --*continued*
  recurrent episode F33.8
  melancholia (single episode) F32.89
    recurrent episode F33.8
  male (symptoms) (syndrome) NEC N50.89
  paranoid state F22
  polyarthritis NEC -*see* Arthritis, specified
    form NEC
  symptoms (female) N95.1
Clinical research investigation (clinical trial)
  (control subject) (normal comparison)
  (participant) Z00.6
Clitoris -*see* condition
Cloaca (persistent) Q43.7
Clonorchiasis, Clonorchis infection (liver)
  B66.1
Clonus R25.8
Closed bite M26.29
Clostridium (C.) perfringens, as cause of
  disease classified elsewhere B96.7
Closure
  congenital, nose Q30.0
  cranial sutures, premature Q75.0
  defective or imperfect NEC -*see* Imperfect,
    closure
  fistula, delayed -*see* Fistula
  foramen ovale, imperfect Q21.1
  hymen N89.6
  interauricular septum, defective Q21.1
  interventricular septum, defective Q21.0
  lacrimal duct -*see also* Stenosis, lacrimal, duct
    congenital Q10.5
  nose (congenital) Q30.0
    acquired M95.0
  of artificial opening -*see* Attention to,
    artificial, opening
  primary angle, without glaucoma damage
    H40.06
  vagina N89.5
  valve -*see* Endocarditis
  vulva N90.5
Clot (blood) -*see also* Embolism
  artery (obstruction) (occlusion) -*see*
    Embolism
  bladder N32.89
  brain (intradural or extradural) -*see*
    Occlusion, artery, cerebral
  circulation I74.9
  heart -*see also* Infarct, myocardium
    not resulting in infarction I51.3
  vein -*see* Thrombosis
Clouded state R40.1
  epileptic -*see* Epilepsy, specified NEC
  paroxysmal -*see* Epilepsy, specified NEC
Cloudy antrum, antra J32.0
Clouston's (hidrotic) ectodermal dysplasia
  Q82.4
Clubbed nail pachydermoperiostosis M89.40
  [*L62*]
Clubbing of finger(s) (nails) R68.3
Club finger R68.3
  congenital Q68.1
Clubfoot (congenital) Q66.89
  acquired -*see* Deformity, limb, clubfoot
  equinovarus Q66.0
  paralytic -*see* Deformity, limb, clubfoot
Clubhand (congenital) (radial) Q71.4
  acquired -*see* Deformity, limb, clubhand
Club nail R68.3
  congenital Q84.6
Clump, kidney Q63.1

Clumsiness, clumsy child syndrome F82
Cluttering F80.81
Clutton's joints A50.51 [*M12.80*]
Coagulation, intravascular (diffuse)
  (disseminated) -*see also* Defibrination
  syndrome
  complicating abortion -*see* Abortion, by type,
    complicated by, intravascular coagulation
  following ectopic or molar pregnancy O08.1
Coagulopathy -*see also* Defect, coagulation
  consumption D65
  intravascular D65
  newborn P60
Coalition
  calcaneo-scaphoid Q66.89
  tarsal Q66.89
Coalminer's
  elbow -*see* Bursitis, elbow, olecranon
  lung or pneumoconiosis J60
Coalworker's lung or pneumoconiosis J60
Coarctation
  aorta (preductal) (postductal) Q25.1
  pulmonary artery Q25.71
Coated tongue K14.3
Coats' disease (exudative retinopathy) -*see*
  Retinopathy, exudative
Cocaine-induced
  anxiety disorder F14.980
  bipolar and related disorder F14.94
  depressive disorder F14.94
  obsessive-compulsive and related disorder
    F14.988
  psychotic disorder F14.959
  sleep disorder F14.982
  sexual dysfunction F14.981
Cocainism -*see* Disorder, cocaine use
Coccidioidomycosis B38.9
  cutaneous B38.3
  disseminated B38.7
  generalized B38.7
  meninges B38.4
  prostate B38.81
  pulmonary B38.2
    acute B38.0
    chronic B38.1
  skin B38.3
  specified NEC B38.89
Coccidioidosis -*see* Coccidioidomycosis
Coccidiosis (intestinal) A07.3
Coccydynia, coccygodynia M53.3
Coccyx -*see* condition
Cochin-China diarrhea K90.1
Cockayne's syndrome Q87.1
Cocked up toe -*see* Deformity, toe, specified
  NEC
Cock's peculiar tumor L72.3
Codman's tumor -*see* Neoplasm, bone, benign
Coenurosis B71.8
Coffee-worker's lung J67.8
Cogan's syndrome H16.32
  oculomotor apraxia H51.8
Coitus, painful (female) N94.10
  male N53.12
  psychogenic F52.6
Cold J00
  with influenza, flu, or grippe -*see* Influenza,
    with, respiratory manifestations NEC
  agglutinin disease or hemoglobinuria
    (chronic) D59.1
  bronchial -*see* Bronchitis
  chest -*see* Bronchitis

Cold --*continued*
  common (head) J00
  effects of T69.9
    specified effect NEC T69.8
  excessive, effects of T69.9
    specified effect NEC T69.8
  exhaustion from T69.8
  exposure to T69.9
    specified effect NEC T69.8
  head J00
  injury syndrome (newborn) P80.0
  on lung -*see* Bronchitis
  rose J30.1
  sensitivity, auto-immune D59.1
  virus J00
Cold sore B00.1
Colibacillosis A49.8
  as the cause of other disease -*see also*
    Escherichia coli B96.20
  generalized A41.50
Colic (bilious) (infantile) (intestinal)
  (recurrent) (spasmodi**c**) R10.83
  abdomen R10.83
    psychogenic F45.8
  appendix, appendicular K38.8
  bile duct -*see* Calculus, bile duct
  biliary -*see* Calculus, bile duct
  common duct -*see* Calculus, bile duct
  cystic duct -*see* Calculus, gallbladder
  Devonshire NEC -*see* Poisoning, lead
  gallbladder -*see* Calculus, gallbladder
  gallstone -*see* Calculus, gallbladder
    gallbladder or cystic duct -*see* Calculus,
      gallbladder
  hepatic (duct) -*see* Calculus, bile duct
  hysterical F45.8
  kidney N23
  lead NEC -*see* Poisoning, lead
  mucous K58.9
    with diarrhea K58.0
    psychogenic F54
  nephritic N23
  painter's NEC -*see* Poisoning, lead
  pancreas K86.89
  psychogenic F45.8
  renal N23
  saturnine NEC -*see* Poisoning, lead
  ureter N23
  urethral N36.8
    due to calculus N21.1
  uterus NEC N94.89
    menstrual -*see* Dysmenorrhea
  worm NOS B83.9
Colicystitis -*see* Cystitis
Colitis (acute) (catarrhal) (chronic)
  (noninfective) (hemorrhagic) -*see also*
  Enteritis K52.9
  allergic K52.29
    with
      food protein-induced enterocolitis
        syndrome K52.21
      proctocolitis K52.82
  amebic (acute) -*see also* Amebiasis A06.0
    nondysenteric A06.2
  anthrax A22.2
  bacillary -*see* Infection, Shigella
  balantidial A07.0
  Clostridium difficile A04.7
  coccidial A07.3
  collagenous K52.831
  cystica superficialis K52.89

Colitis - *continued*
  dietary counseling and surveillance (for) Z71.3
  dietetic -*see also* Colitis, allergic K52.29
  drug-induced K52.1
  due to radiation K52.0
  eosinophilic K52.82
  food hypersensitivity -*see also* Colitis, allergic K52.29
  giardial A07.1
  granulomatous -*see* Enteritis, regional, large intestine
  indeterminate, so stated K52.3
  infectious -*see* Enteritis, infectious
  ischemic K55.9
    acute (subacute) -*see also* Ischemia, intestine, acute K55.039
    chronic K55.1
    due to mesenteric artery insufficiency K55.1
    fulminant (acute) -*see also* Ischemia, intestine, acute K55.039
  left sided K51.50
    with
      abscess K51.514
      complication K51.519
        specified NEC K51.518
      fistula K51.513
      obstruction K51.512
      rectal bleeding K51.511
  lymphocytic K52.832
  membranous
    psychogenic F54
  microscopic K52.839
    specified NEC K52.838
  mucous -*see* Syndrome, irritable, bowel
    psychogenic F54
  noninfective K52.9
    specified NEC K52.89
  polyposa -*see* Polyp, colon, inflammatory
  protozoal A07.9
  pseudomembranous A04.7
  pseudomucinous -*see* Syndrome, irritable, bowel
  regional -*see* Enteritis, regional, large intestine
  segmental -*see* Enteritis, regional, large intestine
  septic -*see* Enteritis, infectious
  spastic K58.9
    with diarrhea K58.0
    psychogenic F54
  staphylococcal A04.8
    foodborne A05.0
  subacute ischemic -*see also* Ischemia, intestine, acute K55.039
  thromboulcerative -*see also* Ischemia, intestine, acute K55.039
  toxic NEC K52.1
    due to Clostridium difficile A04.7
  transmural -*see* Enteritis, regional, large intestine
  trichomonal A07.8
  tuberculous (ulcerative) A18.32
  ulcerative (chronic) K51.90
    with
      complication K51.919
        abscess K51.914
        fistula K51.913
        obstruction K51.912
        rectal bleeding K51.911
        specified complication NEC K51.918

Colitis - *continued*
    enterocolitis -*see* Enterocolitis, ulcerative
    ileocolitis -*see* Ileocolitis, ulcerative
    mucosal proctocolitis -*see* Proctocolitis, mucosal
    proctitis -*see* Proctitis, ulcerative
    pseudopolyposis -*see* Polyp, colon, inflammatory
    psychogenic F54
    rectosigmoiditis -*see* Rectosigmoiditis, ulcerative
    specified type NEC K51.80
      with
        complication K51.819
          abscess K51.814
          fistula K51.813
          obstruction K51.812
          rectal bleeding K51.811
          specified complication NEC K51.818
Collagenosis, collagen disease (nonvascular) (vascular) M35.9
  cardiovascular I42.8
  reactive perforating L87.1
  specified NEC M35.8
Collapse R55
  adrenal E27.2
  cardiorespiratory R57.0
  cardiovascular R57.0
    newborn P29.89
  circulatory (peripheral) R57.9
    during or after labor and delivery O75.1
    following ectopic or molar pregnancy O08.3
    newborn P29.89
  during or
    after labor and delivery O75.1
    resulting from a procedure, not elsewhere classified T81.10
  external ear canal -*see* Stenosis, external ear canal
  general R55
  heart -*see* Disease, heart
  heat T67.1
  hysterical F44.89
  labyrinth, membranous (congenital) Q16.5
  lung (massive) -*see also* Atelectasis J98.19
    pressure due to anesthesia (general) (local) or other sedation T88.2
      during labor and delivery O74.1
      in pregnancy O29.02
      postpartum, puerperal O89.09
  myocardial -*see* Disease, heart
  nervous F48.8
  neurocirculatory F45.8
  nose M95.0
  postoperative T81.10
  pulmonary -*see also* Atelectasis J98.19
    newborn -*see* Atelectasis
  trachea J39.8
  tracheobronchial J98.09
  valvular -*see* Endocarditis
  vascular (peripheral) R57.9
    during or after labor and delivery O75.1
    following ectopic or molar pregnancy O08.3
    newborn P29.89
  vertebra M48.50
    cervical region M48.52
    cervicothoracic region M48.53
    in (due to)
      metastasis -*see* Collapse, vertebra, in, specified disease NEC

Collapse --*continued*
    osteoporosis -*see also* Osteoporosis M80.88
      cervical region M80.88
      cervicothoracic region M80.88
      lumbar region M80.88
      lumbosacral region M80.88
      multiple sites M80.88
      occipito-atlanto-axial region M80.88
      sacrococcygeal region M80.88
      thoracic region M80.88
      thoracolumbar region M80.88
    specified disease NEC M48.50
      cervical region M48.52
      cervicothoracic region M48.53
      lumbar region M48.56
      lumbosacral region M48.57
      occipito-atlanto-axial region M48.51
      sacrococcygeal region M48.58
      thoracic region M48.54
      thoracolumbar region M48.55
    lumbar region M48.56
    lumbosacral region M48.57
    occipito-atlanto-axial region M48.51
    sacrococcygeal region M48.58
    thoracic region M48.54
    thoracolumbar region M48.55
Collateral -*see also* condition
  circulation (venous) I87.8
  dilation, veins I87.8
Colles' fracture S52.53
Collet (Sicard) syndrome G52.7
Collier's asthma or lung J60
Collodion baby Q80.2
Colloid nodule (of thyroid) (cystic) E04.1
Coloboma (iris) Q13.0
  eyelid Q10.3
  fundus Q14.8
  lens Q12.2
  optic disc (congenital) Q14.2
    acquired H47.31
Coloenteritis -*see* Enteritis
Colon -*see* condition
Colonization
  MRSA (Methicillin resistant Staphylococcus aureus) Z22.322
  MSSA (Methicillin susceptible Staphylococcus aureus) Z22.321
  status -*see* Carrier (suspected) of
Coloptosis K63.4
Color blindness -*see* Deficiency, color vision
Colostomy
  attention to Z43.3
  fitting or adjustment Z46.89
  malfunctioning K94.03
  status Z93.3
Colpitis (acute) -*see* Vaginitis
Colpocele N81.5
Colpocystitis -*see* Vaginitis
Colpospasm N94.2
Column, spinal, vertebral -*see* condition
Coma R40.20
  with
    motor response (none) R40.231
      abnormal R40.233
      extension R40.232
      flexion withdrawal R40.234
      localizes pain R40.235
      obeys commands R40.236
    opening of eyes (never) R40.211
      in response to

Coma - *continued*
    pain R40.212
    sound R40.213
    spontaneous R40.214
    verbal response (none) R40.221
      confused conversation R40.224
      inappropriate words R40.223
      incomprehensible words R40.222
      oriented R40.225
  eclamptic -*see* Eclampsia
  epileptic -*see* Epilepsy
  Glasgow, scale score -*see* Glasgow coma scale
  hepatic -*see* Failure, hepatic, by type, with coma
  hyperglycemic (diabetic) -*see* Diabetes, by type, with hyperosmolarity, with coma
  hyperosmolar (diabetic) -*see* Diabetes, by type, with hyperosmolarity, with coma
  hypoglycemic (diabetic) -*see* Diabetes, by type, with hypoglycemia, with coma nondiabetic E15
  in diabetes -*see* Diabetes, coma
  insulin-induced -*see* Coma, hypoglycemic
  myxedematous E03.5
  newborn P91.5
  persistent vegetative state R40.3
  specified NEC, without documented Glasgow coma scale score, or with partial Glasgow coma scale score reported R40.244
Comatose -*see* Coma
Combat fatigue F43.0
Combined -*see* condition
Comedo, comedones (giant) L70.0
Comedocarcinoma -*see also* Neoplasm, breast, malignant
  noninfiltrating
    breast D05.8
    specified site -*see* Neoplasm, in situ, by site unspecified site D05.8
Comedomastitis -*see* Ectasia, mammary duct
Comminuted fracture code as Fracture, closed Common
  arterial trunk Q20.0
  atrioventricular canal Q21.2
  atrium Q21.1
  cold (head) J00
  truncus (arteriosus) Q20.0
  variable immunodeficiency -*see* Immunodeficiency, common variable
  ventricle Q20.4
Commotio, commotion (current)
  brain -*see* Injury, intracranial, concussion
  cerebri -*see* Injury, intracranial, concussion
  retinae S05.8X
  spinal cord -*see* Injury, spinal cord, by region
  spinalis -*see* Injury, spinal cord, by region
Communication
  between
    base of aorta and pulmonary artery Q21.4
    left ventricle and right atrium Q20.5
    pericardial sac and pleural sac Q34.8
    pulmonary artery and pulmonary vein, congenital Q25.72
  congenital between uterus and digestive or urinary tract Q51.7
Compartment syndrome (deep) (posterior) (traumatic) T79.A0
  abdomen T79.A3
  lower extremity (hip, buttock, thigh, leg, foot, toes) T79.A2

Compartment syndrome --*continued*
  nontraumatic
    abdomen M79.A3
    lower extremity (hip, buttock, thigh, leg, foot, toes) M79.A2
    specified site NEC M79.A9
    upper extremity (shoulder, arm, forearm, wrist, hand, fingers) M79.A1
  specified site NEC T79.A9
  upper extremity (shoulder, arm, forearm, wrist, hand, fingers) T79.A1
Compensation
  failure -*see* Disease, heart
  neurosis, psychoneurosis -*see* Disorder, factitious
Complaint -*see also* Disease
  bowel, functional K59.9
    psychogenic F45.8
  intestine, functional K59.9
    psychogenic F45.8
  kidney -*see* Disease, renal
  miners' J60
Complete -*see* condition
Complex
  Addison-Schilder E71.528
  cardiorenal -*see* Hypertension, cardiorenal
  Costen's M26.69
  disseminated mycobacterium avium-intracellulare (DMAC) A31.2
  Eisenmenger's (ventricular septal defect) I27.89
  hypersexual F52.8
  jumped process, spine -*see* Dislocation, vertebra
  primary, tuberculous A15.7
  Schilder-Addison E71.528
  subluxation (vertebral) M99.19
    abdomen M99.19
    acromioclavicular M99.17
    cervical region M99.11
    cervicothoracic M99.11
    costochondral M99.18
    costovertebral M99.18
    head region M99.10
    hip M99.15
    lower extremity M99.16
    lumbar region M99.13
    lumbosacral M99.13
    occipitocervical M99.10
    pelvic region M99.15
    pubic M99.15
    rib cage M99.18
    sacral region M99.14
    sacrococcygeal M99.14
    sacroiliac M99.14
    specified NEC M99.19
    sternochondral M99.18
    sternoclavicular M99.17
    thoracic region M99.12
    thoracolumbar M99.12
    upper extremity M99.17
  Taussig-Bing (transposition, aorta and overriding pulmonary artery) Q20.1
Complication(s) (from) (of)
  accidental puncture or laceration during a procedure (of) -*see* Complications, intraoperative (intraprocedural), puncture or laceration
  amputation stump (surgical) (late) NEC T87.9
    dehiscence T87.81
    infection or inflammation T87.40

Complication(s) (from) (of) --*continued*
    lower limb T87.4
    upper limb T87.4
    necrosis T87.50
      lower limb T87.5
      upper limb T87.5
    neuroma T87.30
      lower limb T87.3
      upper limb T87.3
    specified type NEC T87.89
  anastomosis (and bypass) -*see also* Complications, prosthetic device or implant
    intestinal (internal) NEC K91.89
      involving urinary tract N99.89
    urinary tract (involving intestinal tract) N99.89
    vascular -*see* Complications, cardiovascular device or implant
  anesthesia, anesthetic -*see also* Anesthesia, complication T88.59
    brain, postpartum, puerperal O89.2
    cardiac
      in
        labor and delivery O74.2
        pregnancy O29.19
      postpartum, puerperal O89.1
    central nervous system
      in
        labor and delivery O74.3
        pregnancy O29.29
      postpartum, puerperal O89.2
    difficult or failed intubation T88.4
      in pregnancy O29.6
    failed sedation (conscious) (moderate) during procedure T88.52
    general, unintended awareness during procedure T88.53
    hyperthermia, malignant T88.3
    hypothermia T88.51
    intubation failure T88.4
    malignant hyperthermia T88.3
    pulmonary
      in
        labor and delivery O74.1
        pregnancy NEC O29.09
      postpartum, puerperal O89.09
    shock T88.2
    spinal and epidural
      in
        labor and delivery NEC O74.6
          headache O74.5
        pregnancy NEC O29.5X
      postpartum, puerperal NEC O89.5
        headache O89.4
    unintended awareness under general anesthesia during procedure T88.53
  anti-reflux device -*see* Complications, esophageal anti-reflux device
  aortic (bifurcation) graft -*see* Complications, graft, vascular
  aortocoronary (bypass) graft -*see* Complications, coronary artery (bypass) graft
  aortofemoral (bypass) graft -*see* Complications, extremity artery (bypass) graft
  arteriovenous
    fistula, surgically created T82.9
      embolism T82.818
      fibrosis T82.828
      hemorrhage T82.838
      infection or inflammation T82.7
      mechanical

Complication(s) (from) (of) --*continued*
    breakdown T82.510
    displacement T82.520
    leakage T82.530
    malposition T82.520
    obstruction T82.590
    perforation T82.590
    protrusion T82.590
   pain T82.848
   specified type NEC T82.898
   stenosis T82.858
   thrombosis T82.868
  shunt, surgically created T82.9
   embolism T82.818
   fibrosis T82.828
   hemorrhage T82.838
   infection or inflammation T82.7
   mechanical
    breakdown T82.511
    displacement T82.521
    leakage T82.531
    malposition T82.521
    obstruction T82.591
    perforation T82.591
    protrusion T82.591
   pain T82.848
   specified type NEC T82.898
   stenosis T82.858
   thrombosis T82.868
  arthroplasty -*see* Complications, joint
  prosthesis
  artificial
   fertilization or insemination N98.9
    attempted introduction (of)
     embryo in embryo transfer N98.3
     ovum following in vitro fertilization
     N98.2
    hyperstimulation of ovaries N98.1
    infection N98.0
    specified NEC N98.8
  heart T82.9
   embolism T82.817
   fibrosis T82.827
   hemorrhage T82.837
   infection or inflammation T82.7
   mechanical
    breakdown T82.512
    displacement T82.522
    leakage T82.532
    malposition T82.522
    obstruction T82.592
    perforation T82.592
    protrusion T82.592
   pain T82.847
   specified type NEC T82.897
   stenosis T82.857
   thrombosis T82.867
  opening
   cecostomy -*see* Complications, colostomy
   colostomy -*see* Complications, colostomy
   cystostomy -*see* Complications,
    cystostomy
   enterostomy -*see* Complications,
    enterostomy
   gastrostomy -*see* Complications,
    gastrostomy
   ileostomy -*see* Complications, enterostomy
   jejunostomy -*see* Complications,
    enterostomy
   nephrostomy -*see* Complications, stoma,
   urinary tract

Complication(s) (from) (of) --*continued*
   tracheostomy -*see* Complications,
    tracheostomy
   ureterostomy -*see* Complications, stoma,
    urinary tract
   urethrostomy -*see* Complications, stoma,
    urinary tract
  balloon implant or device
   gastrointestinal T85.9
    embolism T85.818
    fibrosis T85.828
    hemorrhage T85.838
    infection and inflammation T85.79
    pain T85.848
    specified type NEC T85.898
    stenosis T85.858
    thrombosis T85.868
   vascular (counterpulsation) T82.9
    embolism T82.818
    fibrosis T82.828
    hemorrhage T82.838
    infection or inflammation T82.7
    mechanical
     breakdown T82.513
     displacement T82.523
     leakage T82.533
     malposition T82.523
     obstruction T82.593
     perforation T82.593
     protrusion T82.593
    pain T82.848
    specified type NEC T82.898
    stenosis T82.858
    thrombosis T82.868
  bariatric procedure
   gastric band procedure K95.09
    infection K95.01
   specified procedure NEC K95.89
    infection K95.81
  bile duct implant (prosthetic) T85.9
   embolism T85.818
   fibrosis T85.828
   hemorrhage T85.838
   infection and inflammation T85.79
   mechanical
    breakdown T85.510
    displacement T85.520
    malfunction T85.510
    malposition T85.520
    obstruction T85.590
    perforation T85.590
    protrusion T85.590
    specified NEC T85.590
   pain T85.848
   specified type NEC T85.898
   stenosis T85.858
   thrombosis T85.868
  bladder device (auxiliary) -*see* Complications,
  genitourinary, device or implant, urinary
  system
  bleeding (postoperative) -*see* Complication,
  postoperative, hemorrhage
   intraoperative -*see* Complication,
   intraoperative, hemorrhage
  blood vessel graft -*see* Complications, graft,
  vascular
  bone
   device NEC T84.9
    embolism T84.81
    fibrosis T84.82
    hemorrhage T84.83

Complication(s) (from) (of) --*continued*
    infection or inflammation T84.7
    mechanical
     breakdown T84.318
     displacement T84.328
     malposition T84.328
     obstruction T84.398
     perforation T84.398
     protrusion T84.398
    pain T84.84
    specified type NEC T84.89
    stenosis T84.85
    thrombosis T84.86
   graft -*see* Complications, graft, bone
   growth stimulator (electrode) -*see*
    Complications, electronic stimulator
    device, bone
   marrow transplant -*see* Complications,
    transplant, bone, marrow
  brain neurostimulator (electrode) -*see*
   Complications, electronic stimulator device,
   brain
  breast implant (prosthetic) T85.9
   capsular contracture T85.44
   embolism T85.818
   fibrosis T85.828
   hemorrhage T85.838
   infection and inflammation T85.79
   mechanical
    breakdown T85.41
    displacement T85.42
    leakage T85.43
    malposition T85.42
    obstruction T85.49
    perforation T85.49
    protrusion T85.49
    specified NEC T85.49
   pain T85.848
   specified type NEC T85.898
   stenosis T85.858
   thrombosis T85.868
  bypass -*see also* Complications, prosthetic
  device or implant
   aortocoronary -*see* Complications, coronary
    artery (bypass) graft
   arterial -*see also* Complications, graft,
    vascular
    extremity -*see* Complications, extremity
    artery (bypass) graft
   cardiac -*see also* Disease, heart
   device, implant or graft T82.9
    embolism T82.817
    fibrosis T82.827
    hemorrhage T82.837
    infection or inflammation T82.7
    valve prosthesis T82.6
    mechanical
     breakdown T82.519
      specified device NEC T82.518
     displacement T82.529
      specified device NEC T82.528
     leakage T82.539
      specified device NEC T82.538
     malposition T82.529
      specified device NEC T82.528
     obstruction T82.599
      specified device NEC T82.598
     perforation T82.599
      specified device NEC T82.598
     protrusion T82.599
      specified device NEC T82.598

Complication(s) (from) (of) *--continued*
  pain T82.847
  specified type NEC T82.897
  stenosis T82.857
  thrombosis T82.867
cardiovascular device, graft or implant T82.9
  aortic graft *-see* Complications, graft,
    vascular
  arteriovenous
    fistula, artificial *-see* Complication,
      arteriovenous, fistula, surgically created
    shunt *-see* Complication, arteriovenous,
      shunt, surgically created
  artificial heart *-see* Complication, artificial,
    heart
  balloon (counterpulsation) device *-see*
    Complication, balloon implant, vascular
  carotid artery graft *-see* Complications,
    graft, vascular
  coronary bypass graft *-see* Complication,
    coronary artery (bypass) graft
  dialysis catheter (vascular) *-see*
    Complication, catheter, dialysis
  electronic T82.9
    electrode T82.9
      embolism T82.817
      fibrosis T82.827
      hemorrhage T82.837
      infection T82.7
      mechanical
        breakdown T82.110
        displacement T82.120
        leakage T82.190
        obstruction T82.190
        perforation T82.190
        protrusion T82.190
        specified type NEC T82.190
      pain T82.847
      specified NEC T82.897
      stenosis T82.857
      thrombosis T82.867
    embolism T82.817
    fibrosis T82.827
    hemorrhage T82.837
    infection T82.7
    mechanical
      breakdown T82.119
      displacement T82.129
      leakage T82.199
      obstruction T82.199
      perforation T82.199
      protrusion T82.199
      specified type NEC T82.199
    pain T82.847
    pulse generator T82.9
      embolism T82.817
      fibrosis T82.827
      hemorrhage T82.837
      infection T82.7
      mechanical
        breakdown T82.111
        displacement T82.121
        leakage T82.191
        obstruction T82.191
        perforation T82.191
        protrusion T82.191
        specified type NEC T82.191
      pain T82.847
      specified NEC T82.897
      stenosis T82.857
      thrombosis T82.867

Complication(s) (from) (of) *--continued*
  specified condition NEC T82.897
  specified device NEC T82.9
    embolism T82.817
    fibrosis T82.827
    hemorrhage T82.837
    infection T82.7
    mechanical
      breakdown T82.118
      displacement T82.128
      leakage T82.198
      obstruction T82.198
      perforation T82.198
      protrusion T82.198
      specified type NEC T82.198
    pain T82.847
    specified NEC T82.897
    stenosis T82.857
    thrombosis T82.867
  stenosis T82.857
  thrombosis T82.867
extremity artery graft *-see* Complication,
    extremity artery (bypass) graft
femoral artery graft *-see* Complication,
    extremity artery (bypass) graft
heart-lung transplant *-see* Complication,
    transplant, heart, with lung
heart
    transplant *-see* Complication, transplant,
      heart
    valve *-see* Complication, prosthetic device,
      heart valve
    graft *-see* Complication, heart, valve,
      graft
  infection or inflammation T82.7
  umbrella device *-see* Complication, umbrella
    device, vascular
  vascular graft (or anastomosis) *-see*
    Complication, graft, vascular
carotid artery (bypass) graft *-see*
  Complications, graft, vascular
catheter (device) NEC *-see also*
Complications, prosthetic device or implant
  cranial infusion
    infection and inflammation T85.735
    mechanical
      breakdown T85.610
      displacement T85.620
      leakage T85.630
      malfunction T85.690
      malposition T85.620
      obstruction T85.690
      perforation T85.690
      protrusion T85.690
      specified NEC T85.690
  cystostomy T83.9
    embolism T83.81
    fibrosis T83.82
    hemorrhage T83.83
    infection and inflammation T83.510
    mechanical
      breakdown T83.010
      displacement T83.020
      leakage T83.030
      malposition T83.020
      obstruction T83.090
      perforation T83.090
      protrusion T83.090
      specified NEC T83.090
    pain T83.84
    specified type NEC T83.89

Complication(s) (from) (of) *--continued*
  stenosis T83.85
  thrombosis T83.86
dialysis (vascular) T82.9
  embolism T82.818
  fibrosis T82.828
  hemorrhage T82.838
  infection and inflammation T82.7
  intraperitoneal *-see* Complications,
    catheter, intraperitoneal
  mechanical
    breakdown T82.41
    displacement T82.42
    leakage T82.43
    malposition T82.42
    obstruction T82.49
    perforation T82.49
    protrusion T82.49
  pain T82.848
  specified type NEC T82.898
  stenosis T82.858
  thrombosis T82.868
epidural infusion T85.9
  embolism T85.810
  fibrosis T85.820
  hemorrhage T85.830
  infection and inflammation T85.735
  mechanical
    breakdown T85.610
    displacement T85.620
    leakage T85.630
    malfunction T85.610
    malposition T85.620
    obstruction T85.690
    perforation T85.690
    protrusion T85.690
    specified NEC T85.690
  pain T85.840
  specified type NEC T85.890
  stenosis T85.850
  thrombosis T85.860
intraperitoneal dialysis T85.9
  embolism T85.818
  fibrosis T85.828
  hemorrhage T85.838
  infection and inflammation T85.71
  mechanical
    breakdown T85.611
    displacement T85.621
    leakage T85.631
    malfunction T85.611
    malposition T85.621
    obstruction T85.691
    perforation T85.691
    protrusion T85.691
    specified NEC T85.691
  pain T85.848
  specified type NEC T85.898
  stenosis T85.858
  thrombosis T85.868
intrathecal infusion
  infection and inflammation T85.735
  mechanical
    breakdown T85.610
    displacement T85.620
    leakage T85.630
    malfunction T85.690
    malposition T85.620
    obstruction T85.690
    perforation T85.690
    protrusion T85.690

Complication(s) (from) (of) --*continued*
  specified NEC T85.690
  intravenous infusion T82.9
    embolism T82.818
    fibrosis T82.828
    hemorrhage T82.838
    infection or inflammation T82.7
    mechanical
      breakdown T82.514
      displacement T82.524
      leakage T82.534
      malposition T82.524
      obstruction T82.594
      perforation T82.594
      protrusion T82.594
    pain T82.848
    specified type NEC T82.898
    stenosis T82.858
    thrombosis T82.868
  spinal infusion
    infection and inflammation T85.735
    mechanical
      breakdown T85.610
      displacement T85.620
      leakage T85.630
      malfunction T85.690
      malposition T85.620
      obstruction T85.690
      perforation T85.690
      protrusion T85.690
      specified NEC T85.690
  subarachnoid infusion
    infection and inflammation T85.735
    mechanical
      breakdown T85.610
      displacement T85.620
      leakage T85.630
      malfunction T85.690
      malposition T85.620
      obstruction T85.690
      perforation T85.690
      protrusion T85.690
      specified NEC T85.690
  subdural infusion T85.9
    embolism T85.810
    fibrosis T85.820
    hemorrhage T85.830
    infection and inflammation T85.735
    mechanical
      breakdown T85.610
      displacement T85.620
      leakage T85.630
      malfunction T85.610
      malposition T85.620
      obstruction T85.690
      perforation T85.690
      protrusion T85.690
      specified NEC T85.690
    pain T85.840
    specified type NEC T85.890
    stenosis T85.850
    thrombosis T85.860
  urethral T83.9
    displacement T83.028
    embolism T83.81
    fibrosis T83.82
    hemorrhage T83.83
    indwelling
      breakdown T83.011
      displacement T83.021
      infection and inflammation T83.511

Complication(s) (from) (of) --*continued*
      leakage T83.031
      specified complication NEC T83.091
    infection and inflammation T83.511
    leakage T83.038
    malposition T83.028
    mechanical
      breakdown T83.011
    obstruction (mechanical) T83.091
    pain T83.84
    perforation T83.091
    protrusion T83.091
    specified type NEC T83.091
    stenosis T83.85
    thrombosis T83.86
  urinary NEC
    breakdown T83.018
    displacement T83.028
    infection and inflammation T83.518
    leakage T83.038
    specified complication NEC T83.098
  cecostomy (stoma) -*see* Complications,
  colostomy
  cesarean delivery wound NEC O90.89
    disruption O90.0
    hematoma O90.2
    infection (following delivery) O86.0
  chemotherapy (antineoplastic) NEC T88.7
  chin implant (prosthetic) -*see* Complication,
  prosthetic device or implant, specified NEC
  circulatory system I99.8
    intraoperative I97.88
    postprocedural I97.89
      following cardiac surgery I97.19
        postcardiotomy syndrome I97.0
      hypertension I97.3
      lymphedema after mastectomy I97.2
      postcardiotomy syndrome I97.0
      specified NEC I97.89
  colostomy (stoma) K94.00
    hemorrhage K94.01
    infection K94.02
    malfunction K94.03
    mechanical K94.03
    specified complication NEC K94.09
  contraceptive device, intrauterine -*see*
  Complications, intrauterine, contraceptive
  device
  cord (umbilical) -*see* Complications,
  umbilical cord
  corneal graft -*see* Complications, graft, cornea
  coronary artery (bypass) graft T82.9
    atherosclerosis -*see* Arteriosclerosis,
    coronary (artery),   embolism T82.818
    fibrosis T82.828
    hemorrhage T82.838
    infection and inflammation T82.7
    mechanical
      breakdown T82.211
      displacement T82.212
      leakage T82.213
      malposition T82.212
      obstruction T82.218
      perforation T82.218
      protrusion T82.218
      specified NEC T82.218
    pain T82.848
    specified type NEC T82.898
    stenosis T82.858
    thrombosis T82.868

Complication(s) (from) (of) --*continued*
  counterpulsation device (balloon), intra-
    aortic -*see* Complications, balloon implant,
    vascular
  cystostomy (stoma) N99.518
    catheter -*see* Complications, catheter,
    cystostomy
    hemorrhage N99.510
    infection N99.511
    malfunction N99.512
    specified type NEC N99.518
  delivery -*see also* Complications, obstetric
  O75.9
    procedure (instrumental) (manual) (surgical)
    O75.4
    specified NEC O75.89
  dialysis (peritoneal) (renal) -*see also*
  Complications, infusion
    catheter (vascular) -*see* Complication,
    catheter, dialysis
      peritoneal, intraperitoneal -*see*
      Complications, catheter, intraperitoneal
  dorsal column (spinal) neurostimulator -*see*
  Complications, electronic stimulator device,
  spinal cord
  drug NEC T88.7
  ear procedure -*see also* Disorder, ear
    intraoperative H95.88
      hematoma -*see* Complications,
      intraoperative, hemorrhage (hematoma)
      (of), ear
      hemorrhage -*see* Complications,
      intraoperative, hemorrhage (hematoma)
      (of), ear
      laceration -*see* Complications,
      intraoperative, puncture or laceration...,
      ear
      specified NEC H95.88
    postoperative H95.89
      external ear canal stenosis H95.81
      hematoma -*see* Complications,
      postprocedural, hematoma (of), ear
      hemorrhage -*see* Complications,
      postprocedural, hemorrhage (of), ear
      postmastoidectomy -*see* Complications,
      postmastoidectomy
      seroma -*see* Complications,
      postprocedural, seroma (of), mastoid
      process
      specified NEC H95.89
  ectopic pregnancy O08.9
    damage to pelvic organs O08.6
    embolism O08.2
    genital infection O08.0
    hemorrhage (delayed) (excessive) O08.1
    metabolic disorder O08.5
    renal failure O08.4
    shock O08.3
    specified type NEC O08.0
    venous complication NEC O08.7
  electronic stimulator device
    bladder (urinary) -*see* Complications,
  electronic stimulator device, urinary
    bone T84.9
      breakdown T84.310
      displacement T84.320
      embolism T84.81
      fibrosis T84.82
      hemorrhage T84.83
      infection or inflammation T84.7
      malfunction T84.310
      malposition T84.320

Complication(s) (from) (of) *--continued*
  mechanical NEC T84.390
  obstruction T84.390
  pain T84.84
  perforation T84.390
  protrusion T84.390
  specified type NEC T84.89
  stenosis T84.85
  thrombosis T84.86
  brain T85.9
   embolism T85.810
   fibrosis T85.820
   hemorrhage T85.830
   infection and inflammation T85.731
   mechanical
    breakdown T85.110
    displacement T85.120
    leakage T85.190
    malposition T85.120
    obstruction T85.190
    perforation T85.190
    protrusion T85.190
    specified NEC T85.190
   pain T85.840
   specified type NEC T85.890
   stenosis T85.850
   thrombosis T85.860
  cardiac (defibrillator) (pacemaker) *-see*
  Complications, cardiovascular device or
  implant, electronic
  generator (brain) (gastric) (peripheral)
  (sacral) (spinal)
   breakdown T85.113
   displacement T85.123
   leakage T85.193
   malposition T85.123
   obstruction T85.193
   perforation T85.193
   protrusion T85.193
   specified type NEC T85.193
  muscle T84.9
   breakdown T84.418
   displacement T84.428
   embolism T84.81
   fibrosis T84.82
   hemorrhage T84.83
   infection or inflammation T84.7
   mechanical NEC T84.498
   pain T84.84
   specified type NEC T84.89
   stenosis T84.85
   thrombosis T84.86
  nervous system T85.9
   brain *-see* Complications, electronic
    stimulator device, brain
   cranial nerve *-see* Complications,
    electronic stimulator device, peripheral
    nerve
   embolism T85.810
   fibrosis T85.820
   gastric nerve *-see* Complications,
    electronic stimulator device, peripheral
    nerve
   hemorrhage T85.830
   infection and inflammation T85.738
   mechanical
    breakdown T85.118
    displacement T85.128
    leakage T85.199
    malposition T85.128
    obstruction T85.199
    perforation T85.199
    protrusion T85.199

Complication(s) (from) (of) *--continued*
    specified NEC T85.199
   pain T85.840
   peripheral nerve *-see* Complications,
    electronic stimulator device, peripheral
    nerve
   sacral nerve *-see* Complications, electronic
    stimulator device, peripheral nerve
   specified type NEC T85.890
   spinal cord *-see* Complications, electronic
    stimulator device, spinal cord
   stenosis T85.850
   thrombosis T85.860
   vagal nerve *-see* Complications, electronic
    stimulator device, peripheral nerve
   peripheral nerve T85.9
   embolism T85.810
   fibrosis T85.820
   hemorrhage T85.830
   infection and inflammation T85.732
   mechanical
    breakdown T85.111
    displacement T85.121
    leakage T85.191
    malposition T85.121
    obstruction T85.191
    perforation T85.191
    protrusion T85.191
    specified NEC T85.191
   pain T85.840
   specified type NEC T85.890
   stenosis T85.850
   thrombosis T85.860
  spinal cord T85.9
   embolism T85.810
   fibrosis T85.820
   hemorrhage T85.830
   infection and inflammation T85.733
   mechanical
    breakdown T85.112
    displacement T85.122
    leakage T85.192
    malposition T85.122
    obstruction T85.192
    perforation T85.192
    protrusion T85.192
    specified NEC T85.192
   pain T85.840
   specified type NEC T85.890
   stenosis T85.850
   thrombosis T85.860
  urinary T83.9
   embolism T83.81
   fibrosis T83.82
   hemorrhage T83.83
   infection and inflammation T83.598
   mechanical
    breakdown T83.110
    displacement T83.120
    malposition T83.120
    perforation T83.190
    protrusion T83.190
    specified NEC T83.190
   pain T83.84
   specified type NEC T83.89
   stenosis T83.85
   thrombosis T83.86
  electroshock therapy T88.9
   specified NEC T88.8
  endocrine E34.9

Complication(s) (from) (of) *--continued*
  postprocedural
   adrenal hypofunction E89.6
   hypoinsulinemia E89.1
   hypoparathyroidism E89.2
   hypopituitarism E89.3
   hypothyroidism E89.0
   ovarian failure E89.40
    asymptomatic E89.40
    symptomatic E89.41
   specified NEC E89.89
   testicular hypofunction E89.5
  endodontic treatment NEC M27.59
  enterostomy (stoma) K94.10
   hemorrhage K94.11
   infection K94.12
   malfunction K94.13
   mechanical K94.13
   specified complication NEC K94.19
  episiotomy, disruption O90.1
  esophageal anti-reflux device T85.9
   embolism T85.818
   fibrosis T85.828
   hemorrhage T85.838
   infection and inflammation T85.79
   mechanical
    breakdown T85.511
    displacement T85.521
    malfunction T85.511
    malposition T85.521
    obstruction T85.591
    perforation T85.591
    protrusion T85.591
    specified NEC T85.591
   pain T85.848
   specified type NEC T85.898
   stenosis T85.858
   thrombosis T85.868
  esophagostomy K94.30
   hemorrhage K94.31
   infection K94.32
   malfunction K94.33
   mechanical K94.33
   specified complication NEC K94.39
  extracorporeal circulation T80.90
  extremity artery (bypass) graft T82.9
   arteriosclerosis *-see* Arteriosclerosis,
    extremities, bypass graft
   embolism T82.818
   fibrosis T82.828
   hemorrhage T82.838
   infection and inflammation T82.7
   mechanical
    breakdown T82.318
     femoral artery T82.312
    displacement T82.328
     femoral artery T82.322
    leakage T82.338
     femoral artery T82.332
    malposition T82.328
     femoral artery T82.322
    obstruction T82.398
     femoral artery T82.392
    perforation T82.398
     femoral artery T82.392
    protrusion T82.398
     femoral artery T82.392
   pain T82.848
   specified type NEC T82.898
   stenosis T82.858
   thrombosis T82.868

Complication(s) (from) (of) --*continued*
eye H57.9
corneal graft -*see* Complications, graft, cornea
implant (prosthetic) T85.9
embolism T85.818
fibrosis T85.828
hemorrhage T85.838
infection and inflammation T85.79
mechanical
breakdown T85.318
displacement T85.328
leakage T85.398
malposition T85.328
obstruction T85.398
perforation T85.398
protrusion T85.398
specified NEC T85.398
pain T85.848
specified type NEC T85.898
stenosis T85.858
thrombosis T85.868
intraocular lens -*see* Complications, intraocular lens
orbital prosthesis -*see* Complications, orbital prosthesis
female genital N94.9
device, implant or graft NEC -*see* Complications, genitourinary, device or implant, genital tract
femoral artery (bypass) graft -*see* Complication, extremity artery (bypass) graft
fixation device, internal (orthopedic) T84.9
infection and inflammation T84.60
arm T84.61
humerus T84.61
radius T84.61
ulna T84.61
leg T84.629
femur T84.62
fibula T84.62
tibia T84.62
specified site NEC T84.69
spine T84.63
mechanical
breakdown
limb T84.119
carpal T84.210
femur T84.11
fibula T84.11
humerus T84.11
metacarpal T84.210
metatarsal T84.213
phalanx
foot T84.213
hand T84.210
radius T84.11
tarsal T84.213
tibia T84.11
ulna T84.11
specified bone NEC T84.218
spine T84.216
displacement
limb T84.129
carpal T84.220
femur T84.12
fibula T84.12
humerus T84.12
metacarpal T84.220
metatarsal T84.223
phalanx

Complication(s) (from) (of) --*continued*
foot T84.223
hand T84.220
radius T84.12
tarsal T84.223
tibia T84.12
ulna T84.12
specified bone NEC T84.228
spine T84.226
malposition -*see* Complications, fixation device, internal, mechanical, displacement
obstruction -*see* Complications, fixation device, internal, mechanical, specified type NEC
perforation -*see* Complications, fixation device, internal, mechanical, specified type NEC
protrusion -*see* Complications, fixation device, internal, mechanical, specified type NEC
specified type NEC
limb T84.199
carpal T84.290
femur T84.19
fibula T84.19
humerus T84.19
metacarpal T84.290
metatarsal T84.293
phalanx
foot T84.293
hand T84.290
radius T84.19
tarsal T84.293
tibia T84.19
ulna T84.19
specified bone NEC T84.298
vertebra T84.296
specified type NEC T84.89
embolism T84.81
fibrosis T84.82
hemorrhage T84.83
pain T84.84
specified complication NEC T84.89
stenosis T84.85
thrombosis T84.86
following
acute myocardial infarction NEC I23.8
aneurysm (false) (of cardiac wall) (of heart wall) (ruptured) I23.3
angina I23.7
atrial
septal defect I23.1
thrombosis I23.6
cardiac wall rupture I23.3
chordae tendinae rupture I23.4
defect
septal
atrial (heart) I23.1
ventricular (heart) I23.2
hemopericardium I23.0
papillary muscle rupture I23.5
rupture
cardiac wall I23.3
with hemopericardium I23.0
chordae tendineae I23.4
papillary muscle I23.5
specified NEC I23.8
thrombosis
atrium I23.6
auricular appendage I23.6
ventricle (heart) I23.6

Complication(s) (from) (of) --*continued*
ventricular
septal defect I23.2
thrombosis I23.6
ectopic or molar pregnancy O08.9
cardiac arrest O08.81
sepsis O08.82
specified type NEC O08.89
urinary tract infection O08.83
termination of pregnancy -*see* Abortion
gastrointestinal K92.9
bile duct prosthesis -*see* Complications, bile duct implant
esophageal anti-reflux device -*see* Complications, esophageal anti-reflux device
postoperative
colostomy -*see* Complications, colostomy
dumping syndrome K91.1
enterostomy -*see* Complications, enterostomy
gastrostomy -*see* Complications, gastrostomy
malabsorption NEC K91.2
obstruction K91.3
postcholecystectomy syndrome K91.5
specified NEC K91.89
vomiting after GI surgery K91.0
prosthetic device or implant
bile duct prosthesis -*see* Complications, bile duct implant
esophageal anti-reflux device -*see* Complications, esophageal anti-reflux device
specified type NEC
embolism T85.818
fibrosis T85.828
hemorrhage T85.838
mechanical
breakdown T85.518
displacement T85.528
malfunction T85.518
malposition T85.528
obstruction T85.598
perforation T85.598
protrusion T85.598
specified NEC T85.598
pain T85.848
specified complication NEC T85.898
stenosis T85.858
thrombosis T85.868
gastrostomy (stoma) K94.20
hemorrhage K94.21
infection K94.22
malfunction K94.23
mechanical K94.23
specified complication NEC K94.29
genitourinary
device or implant T83.9
genital tract T83.9
infection or inflammation T83.69
intrauterine contraceptive device -*see* Complications, intrauterine, contraceptive device
mechanical -*see* Complications, by device, mechanical
mesh -*see* Complications, mesh
penile prosthesis -*see* Complications, prosthetic device, penile
specified type NEC T83.89
embolism T83.81

Complication(s) (from) (of) --*continued*
    fibrosis T83.82
    hemorrhage T83.83
    pain T83.84
    specified complication NEC T83.89
    stenosis T83.85
    thrombosis T83.86
    vaginal mesh -*see* Complications, mesh
  urinary system T83.9
    cystostomy catheter -*see* Complication, catheter, cystostomy
    electronic stimulator -*see* Complications, electronic stimulator device, urinary
    indwelling urethral catheter -*see* Complications, catheter, urethral, indwelling
    infection or inflammation T83.598
      indwelling urethral catheter T83.511
    kidney transplant -*see* Complication, transplant, kidney
    organ graft -*see* Complication, graft, urinary organ
    specified type NEC T83.89
      embolism T83.81
      fibrosis T83.82
      hemorrhage T83.83
      mechanical T83.198
        breakdown T83.118
        displacement T83.128
        malfunction T83.118
        malposition T83.128
        obstruction T83.198
        perforation T83.198
        protrusion T83.198
        specified NEC T83.198
      sphincter, implanted T83.191
      stent (ileal conduit) (nephroureteral) T83.193
        ureteral indwelling T83.192
      pain T83.84
      specified complication NEC T83.89
      stenosis T83.85
      thrombosis T83.86
    sphincter implant -*see* Complications, implant, urinary sphincter
  postprocedural
    pelvic peritoneal adhesions N99.4
    renal failure N99.0
    specified NEC N99.89
    stoma -*see* Complications, stoma, urinary tract
    urethral stricture -*see* Stricture, urethra, postprocedural
    vaginal
      adhesions N99.2
      vault prolapse N99.3
 graft (bypass) (patch) -*see also* Complications, prosthetic device or implant
  aorta -*see* Complications, graft, vascular
  arterial -*see* Complication, graft, vascular
  bone T86.839
    failure T86.831
    infection T86.832
    mechanical T84.318
      breakdown T84.318
      displacement T84.328
      protrusion T84.398
      specified type NEC T84.398
    rejection T86.830
    specified type NEC T86.838

Complication(s) (from) (of) --*continued*
  carotid artery -*see* Complications, graft, vascular
  cornea T86.849
    failure T86.841
    infection T86.842
    mechanical T85.398
      breakdown T85.318
      displacement T85.328
      protrusion T85.398
      specified type NEC T85.398
    rejection T86.840
    retroprosthetic membrane T85.398
    specified type NEC T86.848
  femoral artery (bypass) -*see* Complication, extremity artery (bypass) graft
  genital organ or tract -*see* Complications, genitourinary, device or implant, genital tract
  muscle T84.9
    breakdown T84.410
    displacement T84.420
    embolism T84.81
    fibrosis T84.82
    hemorrhage T84.83
    infection and inflammation T84.7
    mechanical NEC T84.490
    pain T84.84
    specified type NEC T84.89
    stenosis T84.85
    thrombosis T84.86
  nerve -*see* Complication, prosthetic device or implant, specified NEC
  skin -*see* Complications, prosthetic device or implant, skin graft
  tendon T84.9
    breakdown T84.410
    displacement T84.420
    embolism T84.81
    fibrosis T84.82
    hemorrhage T84.83
    infection and inflammation T84.7
    mechanical NEC T84.490
    pain T84.84
    specified type NEC T84.89
    stenosis T84.85
    thrombosis T84.86
  urinary organ T83.9
    embolism T83.81
    fibrosis T83.82
    hemorrhage T83.83
    infection and inflammation T83.598
      indwelling urethral catheter T83.511
    mechanical
      breakdown T83.21
      displacement T83.22
      erosion T83.24
      exposure T83.25
      leakage T83.23
      malposition T83.22
      obstruction T83.29
      perforation T83.29
      protrusion T83.29
      specified NEC T83.29
    pain T83.84
    specified type NEC T83.89
    stenosis T83.85
    thrombosis T83.86
  vascular T82.9
    embolism T82.818

Complication(s) (from) (of) --*continued*
  femoral artery -*see* Complication, extremity artery (bypass) graft
    fibrosis T82.828
    hemorrhage T82.838
    mechanical
      breakdown T82.319
        aorta (bifurcation) T82.310
        carotid artery T82.311
        specified vessel NEC T82.318
      displacement T82.329
        aorta (bifurcation) T82.320
        carotid artery T82.321
        specified vessel NEC T82.328
      leakage T82.339
        aorta (bifurcation) T82.330
        carotid artery T82.331
        specified vessel NEC T82.338
      malposition T82.329
        aorta (bifurcation) T82.320
        carotid artery T82.321
        specified vessel NEC T82.328
      obstruction T82.399
        aorta (bifurcation) T82.390
        carotid artery T82.391
        specified vessel NEC T82.398
      perforation T82.399
        aorta (bifurcation) T82.390
        carotid artery T82.391
        specified vessel NEC T82.398
      protrusion T82.399
        aorta (bifurcation) T82.390
        carotid artery T82.391
        specified vessel NEC T82.398
    pain T82.848
    specified complication NEC T82.898
    stenosis T82.858
    thrombosis T82.868
 heart I51.9
  assist device
    infection and inflammation T82.7
  following acute myocardial infarction -*see* Complications, following, acute myocardial infarction
  postoperative -*see* Complications, circulatory system
  transplant -*see* Complication, transplant, heart
    and lung(s) -*see* Complications, transplant, heart, with lung
  valve
    graft (biological) T82.9
      embolism T82.817
      fibrosis T82.827
      hemorrhage T82.837
      infection and inflammation T82.7
      mechanical T82.228
        breakdown T82.221
        displacement T82.222
        leakage T82.223
        malposition T82.222
        obstruction T82.228
        perforation T82.228
        protrusion T82.228
      pain T82.847
      specified type NEC T82.897
      stenosis T82.857
      thrombosis T82.867
    prosthesis T82.9
      embolism T82.817
      fibrosis T82.827

Complication(s) (from) (of) --*continued*
    hemorrhage T82.837
    infection or inflammation T82.6
    mechanical T82.09
      breakdown T82.01
      displacement T82.02
      leakage T82.03
      malposition T82.02
      obstruction T82.09
      perforation T82.09
      protrusion T82.09
    pain T82.847
    specified type NEC T82.897
      mechanical T82.09
    stenosis T82.857
    thrombosis T82.867
  hematoma
    intraoperative -*see* Complication,
      intraoperative, hemorrhage
    postprocedural -*see* Complication,
      postprocedural, hematoma
  hemodialysis -*see* Complications, dialysis
  hemorrhage
    intraoperative -*see* Complication,
      intraoperative, hemorrhage
    postprocedural -*see* Complication,
      postprocedural, hemorrhage
  ileostomy (stoma) -*see* Complications,
    enterostomy
  immunization (procedure) -*see*
    Complications, vaccination
  implant -*see also* Complications, by site and
  type
    urinary sphincter T83.9
      embolism T83.81
      fibrosis T83.82
      hemorrhage T83.83
      infection and inflammation T83.591
      mechanical
        breakdown T83.111
        displacement T83.121
        leakage T83.191
        malposition T83.121
        obstruction T83.191
        perforation T83.191
        protrusion T83.191
        specified NEC T83.191
      pain T83.84
      specified type NEC T83.89
      stenosis T83.85
      thrombosis T83.86
  infusion (procedure) T80.90
    air embolism T80.0
    blood -*see* Complications, transfusion
    catheter -*see* Complications, catheter
    infection T80.29
    pump -*see* Complications, cardiovascular,
      device or implant
    sepsis T80.29
    serum reaction -*see also* Reaction, serum
    T80.69
      anaphylactic shock -*see also* Shock,
      anaphylactic T80.59
    specified type NEC T80.89
  inhalation therapy NEC T81.81
  injection (procedure) T80.90
    drug reaction -*see* Reaction, drug
    infection T80.29
    sepsis T80.29
    serum (prophylactic) (therapeutic) -*see*
    Complications, vaccination

Complication(s) (from) (of) --*continued*
    specified type NEC T80.89
    vaccine (any) -*see* Complications,
      vaccination
  inoculation (any) -*see* Complications,
  vaccination
  insulin pump
    infection and inflammation T85.72
    mechanical
      breakdown T85.614
      displacement T85.624
      leakage T85.633
      malposition T85.624
      obstruction T85.694
      perforation T85.694
      protrusion T85.694
      specified NEC T85.694
  intestinal pouch NEC K91.858
  intraocular lens (prosthetic) T85.9
    embolism T85.818
    fibrosis T85.828
    hemorrhage T85.838
    infection and inflammation T85.79
    mechanical
      breakdown T85.21
      displacement T85.22
      malposition T85.22
      obstruction T85.29
      perforation T85.29
      protrusion T85.29
      specified NEC T85.29
    pain T85.848
    specified type NEC T85.898
    stenosis T85.858
    thrombosis T85.868
  intraoperative (intraprocedural)
    cardiac arrest
      during cardiac surgery I97.710
      during other surgery I97.711
    cardiac functional disturbance NEC
      during cardiac surgery I97.790
      during other surgery I97.791
    hemorrhage (hematoma) (of)
      circulatory system organ or structure
        during cardiac bypass I97.411
        during cardiac catheterization I97.410
        during other circulatory system procedure
        I97.418
        during other procedure I97.42
      digestive system organ
        during procedure on digestive system
        K91.61
        during procedure on other organ K91.62
      ear
        during procedure on ear and mastoid
        process H95.21
        during procedure on other organ H95.22
      endocrine system organ or structure
        during procedure on endocrine system
        organ or structure E36.01
        during procedure on other organ E36.02
      eye and adnexa
        during ophthalmic procedure H59.11
        during other procedure H59.12
      genitourinary organ or structure
        during procedure on genitourinary organ
        or structure N99.61
        during procedure on other organ N99.62
      mastoid process
        during procedure on ear and mastoid
        process H95.21

Complication(s) (from) (of) --*continued*
        during procedure on other organ H95.22
      musculoskeletal structure
        during musculoskeletal surgery M96.810
        during non-orthopedic surgery M96.811
        during orthopedic surgery M96.810
      nervous system
        during a nervous system procedure
        G97.31
        during other procedure G97.32
      respiratory system
        during other procedure J95.62
        during procedure on respiratory system
        organ or structure J95.61
      skin and subcutaneous tissue
        during a dermatologic procedure L76.01
        during a procedure on other organ L76.02
      spleen
        during a procedure on other organ D78.02
        during a procedure on the spleen D78.01
    puncture or laceration (accidental)
    (unintentional) (of)
      brain
        during a nervous system procedure
        G97.48
        during other procedure G97.49
      circulatory system organ or structure
        during circulatory system procedure
        I97.51
        during other procedure I97.52
      digestive system
        during procedure on digestive system
        K91.71
        during procedure on other organ K91.72
      ear
        during procedure on ear and mastoid
        process H95.31
        during procedure on other organ H95.32
      endocrine system organ or structure
        during procedure on endocrine system
        organ or structure E36.11
        during procedure on other organ E36.12
      eye and adnexa
        during ophthalmic procedure H59.21
        during other procedure H59.22
      genitourinary organ or structure
        during procedure on genitourinary organ
        or structure N99.71
        during procedure on other organ N99.72
      mastoid process
        during procedure on ear and mastoid
        process H95.31
        during procedure on other organ H95.32
      musculoskeletal structure
        during musculoskeletal surgery M96.820
        during non-orthopedic surgery M96.821
        during orthopedic surgery M96.820
      nervous system
        during a nervous system procedure
        G97.48
        during other procedure G97.49
      respiratory system
        during other procedure J95.72
        during procedure on respiratory system
        organ or structure J95.71
      skin and subcutaneous tissue
        during a dermatologic procedure L76.11
        during a procedure on other organ L76.12
      spleen
        during a procedure on other organ D78.12
        during a procedure on the spleen D78.11

Complication(s) (from) (of) --*continued*
  specified NEC
    circulatory system I97.88
    digestive system K91.81
    ear H95.88
    endocrine system E36.8
    eye and adnexa H59.88
    genitourinary system N99.81
    mastoid process H95.88
    musculoskeletal structure M96.89
    nervous system G97.81
    respiratory system J95.88
    skin and subcutaneous tissue L76.81
    spleen D78.81
  intraperitoneal catheter (dialysis) (infusion) -
see Complications, catheter, intraperitoneal
  intrathecal infusion pump
    infection and inflammation T85.738
    mechanical
      breakdown T85.615
      displacement T85.625
      leakage T85.635
      malfunction T85.695
      malposition T85.625
      obstruction T85.695
      perforation T85.695
      protrusion T85.695
      specified NEC T85.695
  intrauterine
    contraceptive device
      embolism T83.81
      fibrosis T83.82
      hemorrhage T83.83
      infection and inflammation T83.69
      mechanical
        breakdown T83.31
        displacement T83.32
        malposition T83.32
        obstruction T83.39
        perforation T83.39
        protrusion T83.39
        specified NEC T83.39
      pain T83.84
      specified type NEC T83.89
      stenosis T83.85
      thrombosis T83.86
    procedure (fetal), to newborn P96.5
  jejunostomy (stoma) -*see* Complications,
enterostomy
  joint prosthesis, internal T84.9
    breakage (fracture) T84.01
    dislocation T84.02
    fracture T84.01
    infection or inflammation T84.50
      hip T84.5
      knee T84.5
      specified joint NEC T84.59
    instability T84.02
    malposition -*see* Complications, joint
prosthesis, mechanical, displacement
    mechanical
      breakage, broken T84.01
      dislocation T84.02
      fracture T84.01
      instability T84.02
      leakage -*see* Complications, joint
prosthesis, mechanical, specified NEC
      loosening T84.039
        hip T84.03
        knee T84.03
        specified joint NEC T84.038

Complication(s) (from) (of) --*continued*
    obstruction -*see* Complications, joint
prosthesis, mechanical, specified NEC
    perforation -*see* Complications, joint
prosthesis, mechanical, specified NEC
      osteolysis T84.059
        hip T84.05
        knee T84.05
        other specified joint T84.058
    protrusion -*see* Complications, joint
prosthesis, mechanical, specified NEC
      specified complication NEC T84.099
        hip T84.09
        knee T84.09
        other specified joint T84.098
      subluxation T84.02
      wear of articular bearing surface T84.069
        hip T84.06
        knee T84.06
        other specified joint T84.068
    specified joint NEC T84.89
      embolism T84.81
      fibrosis T84.82
      hemorrhage T84.83
      pain T84.84
      specified complication NEC T84.89
      stenosis T84.85
      thrombosis T84.86
    subluxation T84.02
  kidney transplant -*see* Complications,
transplant, kidney   labor O75.9
    specified NEC O75.89
  liver transplant (immune or nonimmune) -*see*
Complications, transplant, liver
  lumbar puncture G97.1
    cerebrospinal fluid leak G97.0
    headache or reaction G97.1
  lung transplant -*see* Complications, transplant,
lung
    and heart -*see* Complications, transplant,
lung, with heart
  male genital N50.9
    device, implant or graft -*see* Complications,
genitourinary, device or implant, genital
tract
    postprocedural or postoperative -*see*
Complications, genitourinary,
postprocedural
    specified NEC N99.89
  mastoid (process) procedure
    intraoperative H95.88
      hematoma -*see* Complications,
intraoperative, hemorrhage (hematoma)
(of), mastoid process
      hemorrhage -*see* Complications,
intraoperative, hemorrhage (hematoma)
(of), mastoid process
      laceration -*see* Complications,
intraoperative, puncture or laceration...,
mastoid process
      specified NEC H95.88
    postmastoidectomy -*see* Complications,
postmastoidectomy
    postoperative H95.89
      external ear canal stenosis H95.81
      hematoma -*see* Complications...,
postprocedural, hematoma (of), mastoid
process
      hemorrhage -*see* Complications...,
postprocedural, hemorrhage (of), mastoid
process

Complication(s) (from) (of) --*continued*
      postmastoidectomy -*see* Complications,
postmastoidectomy
      seroma -*see* Complications,
postprocedural, seroma (of), mastoid
process
      specified NEC H95.89
    mastoidectomy cavity -*see* Complications,
postmastoidectomy
  mechanical -*see* Complications, by site and
type, mechanical
  medical procedures -*see also* Complication(s),
intraoperative T88.9
  metabolic E88.9
    postoperative E89.89
      specified NEC E89.89
  molar pregnancy NOS O08.9
    damage to pelvic organs O08.6
    embolism O08.2
    genital infection O08.0
    hemorrhage (delayed) (excessive) O08.1
    metabolic disorder O08.5
    renal failure O08.4
    shock O08.3
    specified type NEC O08.0
    venous complication NEC O08.7
  musculoskeletal system -*see also*
Complication, intraoperative
(intraprocedural), by site
    device, implant or graft NEC -*see*
Complications, orthopedic, device or
implant
    internal fixation (nail) (plate) (rod) -*see*
Complications, fixation device, internal
    joint prosthesis -*see* Complications, joint
prosthesis
    postoperative (postprocedural) M96.89
      with osteoporosis -*see* Osteoporosis
      fracture following insertion of device -*see*
Fracture, following insertion of
orthopedic implant, joint prosthesis or
bone plate
      joint instability after prosthesis removal
M96.89
      lordosis M96.4
      postlaminectomy syndrome NEC M96.1
        kyphosis M96.3
      pseudarthrosis M96.0
      specified complication NEC M96.89
    post radiation M96.89
      kyphosis M96.2
      scoliosis M96.5
      specified complication NEC M96.89
  nephrostomy (stoma) -*see* Complications,
stoma, urinary tract, external NEC
  nervous system G98.8
    central G96.9
    device, implant or graft -*see also*
Complication, prosthetic device or implant,
specified NEC
      electronic stimulator (electrode(s)) -*see*
Complications, electronic stimulator device
      specified NEC
        infection and inflammation T85.738
        mechanical T85.695
          breakdown T85.615
          displacement T85.625
          leakage T85.635
          malfunction T85.695
          malposition T85.625
          obstruction T85.695
          perforation T85.695

Complication(s) (from) (of) --*continued*
    protrusion T85.695
      specified NEC T85.695
    ventricular shunt -*see* Complications,
      ventricular shunt
  electronic stimulator (electrode(s)) -*see*
    Complications, electronic stimulator device
  postprocedural G97.82
    intracranial hypotension G97.2
    specified NEC G97.82
    spinal fluid leak G97.0
  newborn, due to intrauterine (fetal) procedure
    P96.5
  nonabsorbable (permanent) sutures -*see*
    Complication, sutures, permanent
  obstetric O75.9
    procedure (instrumental) (manual) (surgical)
    specified NEC O75.4
    specified NEC O75.89
    surgical wound NEC O90.89
      hematoma O90.2
      infection O86.0
  ocular lens implant -*see* Complications,
    intraocular lens
  ophthalmologic
    postprocedural bleb -*see* Blebitis
  orbital prosthesis T85.9
    embolism T85.818
    fibrosis T85.828
    hemorrhage T85.838
    infection and inflammation T85.79
    mechanical
      breakdown T85.31
      displacement T85.32
      malposition T85.32
      obstruction T85.39
      perforation T85.39
      protrusion T85.39
      specified NEC T85.39
    pain T85.848
    specified type NEC T85.898
    stenosis T85.858
    thrombosis T85.868
  organ or tissue transplant (partial) (total) -*see*
    Complications, transplant
  orthopedic -*see also* Disorder, soft tissue
    device or implant T84.9
      bone
        device or implant -*see* Complication,
        bone, device NEC
        graft -*see* Complication, graft, bone
      breakdown T84.418
      displacement T84.428
      electronic bone stimulator -*see*
        Complications, electronic stimulator
        device, bone
      embolism T84.81
      fibrosis T84.82
      fixation device -*see* Complication, fixation
        device, internal
      hemorrhage T84.83
      infection or inflammation T84.7
      joint prosthesis -*see* Complication, joint
        prosthesis, internal
      malfunction T84.418
      malposition T84.428
      mechanical NEC T84.498
      muscle graft -*see* Complications, graft,
        muscle
      obstruction T84.498
      pain T84.84

Complication(s) (from) (of) --*continued*
    perforation T84.498
    protrusion T84.498
    specified complication NEC T84.89
    stenosis T84.85
    tendon graft -*see* Complications, graft,
      tendon
    thrombosis T84.86
    fracture (following insertion of device) -*see*
      Fracture, following insertion of orthopedic
      implant, joint prosthesis or bone plate
    postprocedural M96.89
      fracture -*see* Fracture, following insertion
        of orthopedic implant, joint prosthesis or
        bone plate
      postlaminectomy syndrome NEC M96.1
        kyphosis M96.3
        lordosis M96.4
      postradiation
        kyphosis M96.2
        scoliosis M96.5
      pseudarthrosis post-fusion M96.0
      specified type NEC M96.89
  pacemaker (cardiac) -*see* Complications,
    cardiovascular device or implant, electronic
  pancreas transplant -*see* Complications,
    transplant, pancreas
  penile prosthesis (implant) -*see*
    Complications, prosthetic device, penile
  perfusion NEC T80.90
  perineal repair (obstetrical) NEC O90.89
    disruption O90.1
    hematoma O90.2
    infection (following delivery) O86.0
  phototherapy T88.9
    specified NEC T88.8
  postmastoidectomy NEC H95.19
    cyst, mucosal H95.13
    granulation H95.12
    inflammation, chronic H95.11
    recurrent cholesteatoma H95.0
  postoperative -*see* Complications,
    postprocedural
    circulatory -*see* Complications, circulatory
      system
    ear -*see* Complications, ear
    endocrine -*see* Complications, endocrine
    eye -*see* Complications, eye
    lumbar puncture G97.1
      cerebrospinal fluid leak G97.0
    nervous system (central) (peripheral) -*see*
      Complications, nervous system
    respiratory system -*see* Complications,
      respiratory system
  postprocedural -*see also* Complications,
  surgical procedure
    cardiac arrest
      following cardiac surgery I97.120
      following other surgery I97.121
    cardiac functional disturbance NEC
      following cardiac surgery I97.190
      following other surgery I97.191
    cardiac insufficiency
      following cardiac surgery I97.110
      following other surgery I97.111
    chorioretinal scars following retinal surgery
      H59.81
    following cataract surgery
      cataract (lens) fragments H59.02
      cystoid macular edema H59.03
      specified NEC H59.09

Complication(s) (from) (of) --*continued*
  vitreous (touch) syndrome H59.01
  heart failure
    following cardiac surgery I97.130
    following other surgery I97.131
  hematoma (of)
    circulatory system organ or structure
      following cardiac bypass I97.631
      following cardiac catheterization I97.630
      following other circulatory system
        procedure I97.638
      following other procedure I97.621
    digestive system
      following procedure on digestive system
        K91.870
      following procedure on other organ
        K91.871
    ear
      following other procedure H95.52
      following procedure on ear and mastoid
        process H95.51
    endocrine system
      following endocrine system procedure
        E89.820
      following other procedure E89.821
    eye and adnexa
      following ophthalmic procedure H59.33
      following other procedure H59.34
    genitourinary organ or structure
      following procedure on genitourinary
        organ or structure N99.840
      following procedure on other organ
        N99.841
    mastoid process
      following other procedure H95.52
      following procedure on ear and mastoid
        process H95.51
    musculoskeletal structure
      following musculoskeletal surgery
        M96.840
      following non-orthopedic surgery
        M96.841
      following orthopedic surgery M96.840
    nervous system
      following nervous system procedure
        G97.61
      following other procedure G97.62
    respiratory system
      following other procedure J95.861
      following procedure on respiratory
      system organ or structure J95.860
    skin and subcutaneous tissue
      following dermatologic procedure L76.31
      following procedure on other organ
        L76.32
    spleen
      following procedure on other organ
        D78.32
      following procedure on the spleen
        D78.31
  hemorrhage (of)
    circulatory system organ or structure
      following cardiac bypass I97.611
      following cardiac catheterization I97.610
      following other circulatory system
      procedure I97.618
      following other procedure I97.620
    digestive system
      following procedure on digestive system
        K91.840

Complication(s) (from) (of) --*continued*

following procedure on other organ
K91.841
ear
following other procedure H95.42
following procedure on ear and mastoid
process H95.41
endocrine system
following endocrine system procedure
E89.810
following other procedure E89.811
eye and adnexa
following ophthalmic procedure H59.31
following other procedure H59.32
genitourinary organ or structure
following procedure on genitourinary
organ or structure N99.820
following procedure on other organ
N99.821
mastoid process
following other procedure H95.42
following procedure on ear and mastoid
process H95.41
musculoskeletal structure
following musculoskeletal surgery
M96.830
following non-orthopedic surgery
M96.831
following orthopedic surgery M96.830
nervous system
following nervous system procedure
G97.51
following other procedure G97.52
respiratory system
following other procedure J95.831
following procedure on respiratory
system organ or structure J95.830
skin and subcutaneous tissue
following dermatologic procedure L76.21
following a procedure on other organ
L76.22
spleen
following procedure on other organ
D78.22
following procedure on the spleen
D78.21
seroma (of)
circulatory system organ or structure
following cardiac bypass I97.641
following cardiac catheterization I97.640
following other circulatory system
procedure I97.648
following other procedure I97.622
digestive system
following procedure on digestive system
K91.872
following procedure on other organ
K91.873
ear
following other procedure H95.54
following procedure on ear and mastoid
process H95.53
endocrine system
following endocrine system procedure
E89.822
following other procedure E89.823
eye and adnexa
following ophthalmic procedure H59.35
following other procedure H59.36
genitourinary organ or structure

Complication(s) (from) (of) --*continued*

following procedure on genitourinary
organ or structure N99.842
following procedure on other organ
N99.843
mastoid process
following other procedure H95.54
following procedure on ear and mastoid
process H95.53
musculoskeletal structure
following musculoskeletal surgery
M96.842
following non-orthopedic surgery
M96.843
following orthopedic surgery M96.842
nervous system
following nervous system procedure
G97.63
following other procedure G97.64
respiratory system
following other procedure J95.863
following procedure on respiratory
system organ or structure J95.862
skin and subcutaneous tissue
following dermatologic procedure L76.33
following procedure on other organ
L76.34
spleen
following procedure on other organ
D78.34
following procedure on the spleen
D78.33
specified NEC
circulatory system I97.89
digestive K91.89
ear H95.89
endocrine E89.89
eye and adnexa H59.89
genitourinary N99.89
mastoid process H95.89
metabolic E89.89
musculoskeletal structure M96.89
nervous system G97.82
respiratory system J95.89
skin and subcutaneous tissue L76.82
spleen D78.89
pregnancy NEC -*see* Pregnancy, complicated
by
prosthetic device or implant T85.9
bile duct -*see* Complications, bile duct
implant
breast -*see* Complications, breast implant
bulking agent
ureteral
erosion T83.714
exposure T83.724
urethral
erosion T83.713
exposure T83.723
cardiac and vascular NEC -*see*
Complications, cardiovascular device or
implant
corneal transplant -*see* Complications, graft,
cornea
electronic nervous system stimulator -*see*
Complications, electronic stimulator device
epidural infusion catheter -*see*
Complications, catheter, epidural
esophageal anti-reflux device -*see*
Complications, esophageal anti-reflux
device

Complication(s) (from) (of) --*continued*

genital organ or tract -*see* Complications,
genitourinary, device or implant, genital
tract
specified NEC T83.79
heart valve -*see* Complications, heart, valve,
prosthesis
infection or inflammation T85.79
intestine transplant T86.892
liver transplant T86.43
lung transplant T86.812
pancreas transplant T86.892
skin graft T86.822
intraocular lens -*see* Complications,
intraocular lens
intraperitoneal (dialysis) catheter -*see*
Complications, catheter, intraperitoneal
joint -*see* Complications, joint prosthesis,
internal
mechanical NEC T85.698
dialysis catheter (vascular) -*see also*
Complication, catheter, dialysis,
mechanical
peritoneal -*see* Complication, catheter,
intraperitoneal, mechanical
gastrointestinal device T85.598
ocular device T85.398
subdural (infusion) catheter T85.690
suture, permanent T85.692
that for bone repair -*see* Complications,
fixation device, internal (orthopedic),
mechanical
ventricular shunt
breakdown T85.01
displacement T85.02
leakage T85.03
malposition T85.02
obstruction T85.09
perforation T85.09
protrusion T85.09
specified NEC T85.09
mesh
erosion (to surrounding organ or tissue)
T83.717
urethral (into pelvic floor muscles)
T83.712
vaginal (into pelvic floor muscles)
T83.711
exposure (into surrounding organ or tissue)
T83.727
urethral (through urethral wall) T83.722
vaginal (into vagina) (through vaginal
wall) T83.721
orbital -*see* Complications, orbital prosthesis
penile T83.9
embolism T83.81
fibrosis T83.82
hemorrhage T83.83
infection and inflammation T83.61
mechanical
breakdown T83.410
displacement T83.420
leakage T83.490
malposition T83.420
obstruction T83.490
perforation T83.490
protrusion T83.490
specified NEC T83.490
pain T83.84
specified type NEC T83.89
stenosis T83.85

Complication(s) (from) (of) --*continued*
  thrombosis T83.86
  prosthetic materials NEC
    erosion (to surrounding organ or tissue)
      T83.718
    exposure (into surrounding organ or tissue)
      T83.728
  skin graft T86.829
    artificial skin or decellularized allodermis
      embolism T85.818
      fibrosis T85.828
      hemorrhage T85.838
      infection and inflammation T85.79
      mechanical
        breakdown T85.613
        displacement T85.623
        malfunction T85.613
        malposition T85.623
        obstruction T85.693
        perforation T85.693
        protrusion T85.693
        specified NEC T85.693
      pain T85.848
      specified type NEC T85.898
      stenosis T85.858
      thrombosis T85.868
    failure T86.821
    infection T86.822
    rejection T86.820
    specified NEC T86.828
  sling
    urethral (female) (male)
      erosion T83.712
      exposure T83.722
  specified NEC T85.9
    embolism T85.818
    fibrosis T85.828
    hemorrhage T85.838
    infection and inflammation T85.79
    mechanical
      breakdown T85.618
      displacement T85.628
      leakage T85.638
      malfunction T85.618
      malposition T85.628
      obstruction T85.698
      perforation T85.698
      protrusion T85.698
      specified NEC T85.698
    pain T85.848
    specified type NEC T85.898
    stenosis T85.858
    thrombosis T85.868
  subdural infusion catheter -*see*
    Complications, catheter, subdural
  sutures -*see* Complications, sutures
  urinary organ or tract NEC -*see*
    Complications, genitourinary, device or
    implant, urinary system
  vascular -*see* Complications, cardiovascular
    device or implant
  ventricular shunt -*see* Complications,
    ventricular shunt (device)
  puerperium -*see* Puerperal
  puncture, spinal G97.1
    cerebrospinal fluid leak G97.0
    headache or reaction G97.1
  pyelogram N99.89
  radiation
    kyphosis M96.2
    scoliosis M96.5

Complication(s) (from) (of) --*continued*
  reattached
    extremity (infection) (rejection)
      lower T87.1X
      upper T87.0X
    specified body part NEC T87.2
  reconstructed breast
    asymmetry between native and
      reconstructed breast N65.1
    deformity N65.0
    disproportion between native and
      reconstructed breast N65.1
    excess tissue N65.0
    misshapen N65.0
  reimplant NEC -*see also* Complications,
  prosthetic device or implant
    limb (infection) (rejection) -*see*
      Complications, reattached, extremity
    organ (partial) (total) -*see* Complications,
      transplant
    prosthetic device NEC -*see* Complications,
      prosthetic device
  renal N28.9
    allograft -*see* Complications, transplant,
      kidney
    dialysis -*see* Complications, dialysis
  respirator
    mechanical J95.850
      specified NEC J95.859
  respiratory system J98.9
    device, implant or graft -*see* Complication,
      prosthetic device or implant, specified
      NEC
    lung transplant -*see* Complications,
      prosthetic device or implant, lung
      transplant
    postoperative J95.89
      air leak J95.812
      Mendelson's syndrome (chemical
        pneumonitis) J95.4
      pneumothorax J95.811
      pulmonary insufficiency (acute) (after
        nonthoracic surgery) J95.2
        chronic J95.3
        following thoracic surgery J95.1
      respiratory failure (acute) J95.821
        acute and chronic J95.822
      specified NEC J95.89
      subglottic stenosis J95.5
      tracheostomy complication -*see*
        Complications, tracheostomy
    therapy T81.89
  sedation during labor and delivery O74.9
    cardiac O74.2
    central nervous system O74.3
    pulmonary NEC O74.1
  shunt -*see also* Complications, prosthetic
  device or implant
    arteriovenous -*see* Complications,
      arteriovenous, shunt
    ventricular (communicating) -*see*
      Complications, ventricular shunt
  skin
    graft T86.829
      failure T86.821
      infection T86.822
      rejection T86.820
      specified type NEC T86.828
  spinal
    anesthesia -*see* Complications, anesthesia,
      spinal
    catheter (epidural) (subdural) -*see*
      Complications, catheter

Complication(s) (from) (of) --*continued*
  puncture or tap G97.1
    cerebrospinal fluid leak G97.0
    headache or reaction G97.1
  stent
    bile duct -*see* Complications, bile duct
    prosthesis
    ureteral indwelling
      breakdown T83.112
      displacement T83.122
      leakage T83.192
      malposition T83.122
      obstruction T83.192
      perforation T83.192
      protrusion T83.192
      specified NEC T83.192
    urinary NEC (ileal conduit) (nephroureteral)
      T83.193
      embolism T83.81
      fibrosis T83.82
      hemorrhage T83.83
      infection and inflammation T83.593
      mechanical
        breakdown T83.113
        displacement T83.123
        leakage T83.193
        malposition T83.123
        obstruction T83.193
        perforation T83.193
        protrusion T83.193
        specified NEC T83.193
      pain T83.84
      specified type NEC T83.89
      stenosis T83.85
      thrombosis T83.86
    vascular
      end stent stenosis -*see* Restenosis, stent
      in stent stenosis -*see* Restenosis, stent
  stoma
    digestive tract
      colostomy -*see* Complications, colostomy
      enterostomy -*see* Complications,
        enterostomy
      esophagostomy -*see* Complications,
        esophagostomy
      gastrostomy -*see* Complications,
        gastrostomy
    urinary tract N99.528
      continent N99.538
        hemorrhage N99.530
        herniation N99.533
        infection N99.531
        malfunction N99.532
        specified type NEC N99.538
        stenosis N99.534
      cystostomy -*see* Complications,
        cystostomy
      external NOS N99.528
      hemorrhage N99.520
      herniation N99.523
      incontinent N99.528
        hemorrhage N99.520
        herniation N99.523
        infection N99.521
        malfunction N99.522
        specified type NEC N99.528
        stenosis N99.524
      infection N99.521
      malfunction N99.522
      specified type NEC N99.528
      stenosis N99.524

Complication(s) (from) (of) --*continued*
stomach banding -*see* Complication(s),
  bariatric procedure
stomach stapling -*see* Complication(s),
  bariatric procedure
surgical material, nonabsorbable -*see*
  Complication, suture, permanent
surgical procedure (on) T81.9
  amputation stump (late) -*see* Complications,
    amputation stump
  cardiac -*see* Complications, circulatory
    system
  cholesteatoma, recurrent -*see* Complications,
    postmastoidectomy, recurrent
    cholesteatoma
  circulatory (early) -*see* Complications,
    circulatory system
  digestive system -*see* Complications,
    gastrointestinal
  dumping syndrome (postgastrectomy) K91.1
  ear -*see* Complications, ear
  elephantiasis or lymphedema I97.89
    postmastectomy I97.2
  emphysema (surgical) T81.82
  endocrine -*see* Complications, endocrine
  eye -*see* Complications, eye
  fistula (persistent postoperative) T81.83
  foreign body inadvertently left in wound
    (sponge) (suture) (swab) -*see* Foreign
    body, accidentally left during a procedure
  gastrointestinal -*see* Complications,
    gastrointestinal
  genitourinary NEC N99.89
  hematoma
    intraoperative -*see* Complication,
      intraoperative, hemorrhage
    postprocedural -*see* Complication,
      postprocedural, hematoma
  hemorrhage
    intraoperative -*see* Complication,
      intraoperative, hemorrhage
    postprocedural -*see* Complication,
      postprocedural, hemorrhage
  hepatic failure K91.82
  hyperglycemia (postpancreatectomy) E89.1
  hypoinsulinemia (postpancreatectomy)
    E89.1
  hypoparathyroidism
    (postparathyroidectomy) E89.2
  hypopituitarism (posthypophysectomy)
    E89.3
  hypothyroidism (post-thyroidectomy) E89.0
  intestinal obstruction K91.3
  intracranial hypotension following
    ventricular shunting (ventriculostomy)
    G97.2
  lymphedema I97.89
    postmastectomy I97.2
  malabsorption (postsurgical) NEC K91.2
    osteoporosis -*see* Osteoporosis,
      postsurgical malabsorption
  mastoidectomy cavity NEC -*see*
    Complications, postmastoidectomy
  metabolic E89.89
    specified NEC E89.89
  musculoskeletal -*see* Complications,
    musculoskeletal system
  nervous system (central) (peripheral) -*see*
    Complications, nervous system
  ovarian failure E89.40
    asymptomatic E89.40
    symptomatic E89.41

Complication(s) (from) (of) --*continued*
  peripheral vascular -*see* Complications,
    surgical procedure, vascular
  postcardiotomy syndrome I97.0
  postcholecystectomy syndrome K91.5
  postcommissurotomy syndrome I97.0
  postgastrectomy dumping syndrome K91.1
  postlaminectomy syndrome NEC M96.1
    kyphosis M96.3
  postmastectomy lymphedema syndrome
    I97.2
  postmastoidectomy cholesteatoma -*see*
    Complications, postmastoidectomy,
    recurrent cholesteatoma
  postvagotomy syndrome K91.1
  postvalvulotomy syndrome I97.0
  pulmonary insufficiency (acute) J95.2
    chronic J95.3
    following thoracic surgery J95.1
  reattached body part -*see* Complications,
    reattached
  respiratory -*see* Complications, respiratory
    system
  shock (hypovolemic) T81.19
  spleen (postoperative) D78.89
    intraoperative D78.81
  stitch abscess T81.48
  subglottic stenosis (postsurgical) J95.5
  testicular hypofunction E89.5
  transplant -*see* Complications, organ or
    tissue transplant
  urinary NEC N99.89
  vaginal vault prolapse (posthysterectomy)
    N99.3
  vascular (peripheral)
    artery T81.719
      mesenteric T81.710
      renal T81.711
      specified NEC T81.718
    vein T81.72
  wound infection T81.40
suture, permanent (wire) NEC T85.9
  with repair of bone -*see* Complications,
    fixation device, internal
  embolism T85.818
  fibrosis T85.828
  hemorrhage T85.838
  infection and inflammation T85.79
  mechanical
    breakdown T85.612
    displacement T85.622
    malfunction T85.612
    malposition T85.622
    obstruction T85.692
    perforation T85.692
    protrusion T85.692
    specified NEC T85.692
  pain T85.848
  specified type NEC T85.898
  stenosis T85.858
  thrombosis T85.868
tracheostomy J95.00
  granuloma J95.09
  hemorrhage J95.01
  infection J95.02
  malfunction J95.03
  mechanical J95.03
  obstruction J95.03
  specified type NEC J95.09
  tracheo-esophageal fistula J95.04

Complication(s) (from) (of) --*continued*
transfusion (blood) (lymphocytes) (plasma)
  T80.92
  air embolism T80.0
  circulatory overload E87.71
  febrile nonhemolytic transfusion reaction
    R50.84
  hemolysis T80.89
  hemochromatosis E83.111
  hemolytic reaction (antigen unspecified)
    T80.919
  incompatibility reaction (antigen
  unspecified) T80.919
    ABO T80.30
      delayed serologic (DSTR) T80.39
      hemolytic transfusion reaction (HTR)
        (unspecified time after transfusion)
        T80.319
        acute (AHTR) (less than 24 hours after
          transfusion) T80.310
        delayed (DHTR) (24 hours or more after
          transfusion) T80.311
      specified NEC T80.39
    acute (antigen unspecified) T80.910
    delayed (antigen unspecified) T80.911
    delayed serologic (DSTR) T80.89
    Non-ABO (minor antigens (Duffy) (Kell)
      (Kidd) (Lewis) (M) (N) (P) (S)) T80.A0
      delayed serologic (DSTR) T80.A9
      hemolytic transfusion reaction (HTR)
        (unspecified time after transfusion)
        T80.A19
        acute (AHTR) (less than 24 hours after
          transfusion) T80.A10
        delayed (DHTR) (24 hours or more after
          transfusion) T80.A11
      specified NEC T80.A9
    Rh (antigens (C) (c) (D) (E) (e)) (factor)
      T80.40
      delayed serologic (DSTR) T80.49
      hemolytic transfusion reaction (HTR)
        (unspecified time after transfusion)
        T80.419
        acute (AHTR) (less than 24 hours after
          transfusion) T80.410
        delayed (DHTR) (24 hours or more after
          transfusion) T80.411
      specified NEC T80.49
  infection T80.29
    acute T80.22
  reaction NEC T80.89
  sepsis T80.29
  shock T80.89
transplant T86.90
  bone T86.839
    failure T86.831
    infection T86.832
    rejection T86.830
    specified type NEC T86.838
  bone marrow T86.00
    failure T86.02
    infection T86.03
    rejection T86.01
    specified type NEC T86.09
  cornea T86.849
    failure T86.841
    infection T86.842
    rejection T86.840
    specified type NEC T86.848
  failure T86.92
  heart T86.20

Complication(s) (from) (of) --*continued*
with lung T86.30
cardiac allograft vasculopathy T86.290
failure T86.32
infection T86.33
rejection T86.31
specified type NEC T86.39
failure T86.22
infection T86.23
rejection T86.21
specified type NEC T86.298
infection T86.93
intestine T86.859
failure T86.851
infection T86.852
rejection T86.850
specified type NEC T86.858
kidney T86.10
failure T86.12
infection T86.13
rejection T86.11
specified type NEC T86.19
liver T86.40
failure T86.42
infection T86.43
rejection T86.41
specified type NEC T86.49
lung T86.819
with heart T86.30
failure T86.32
infection T86.33
rejection T86.31
specified type NEC T86.39
failure T86.811
infection T86.812
rejection T86.810
specified type NEC T86.818
malignant neoplasm C80.2
pancreas T86.899
failure T86.891
infection T86.892
rejection T86.890
specified type NEC T86.898
peripheral blood stem cells T86.5
post-transplant lymphoproliferative disorder (PTLD) D47.Z1
rejection T86.91
skin T86.829
failure T86.821
infection T86.822
rejection T86.820
specified type NEC T86.828
specified
tissue T86.899
failure T86.891
infection T86.892
rejection T86.890
specified type NEC T86.898
type NEC T86.99
stem cell (from peripheral blood) (from umbilical cord) T86.5
umbilical cord stem cells T86.5
trauma (early) T79.9
specified NEC T79.8
ultrasound therapy NEC T88.9
umbilical cord NEC
complicating delivery O69.9
specified NEC O69.89
umbrella device, vascular T82.9
embolism T82.818
fibrosis T82.828

Complication(s) (from) (of) --*continued*
hemorrhage T82.838
infection or inflammation T82.7
mechanical
breakdown T82.515
displacement T82.525
leakage T82.535
malposition T82.525
obstruction T82.595
perforation T82.595
protrusion T82.595
pain T82.848
specified type NEC T82.898
stenosis T82.858
thrombosis T82.868
urethral catheter -*see* Complications, catheter, urethral, indwelling
vaccination T88.1
anaphylaxis NEC T80.52
arthropathy -*see* Arthropathy, postimmunization
cellulitis T88.0
encephalitis or encephalomyelitis G04.02
infection (general) (local) NEC T88.0
meningitis G03.8
myelitis G04.02
protein sickness T80.62
rash T88.1
reaction (allergic) T88.1
serum T80.62
sepsis T88.0
serum intoxication, sickness, rash, or other serum reaction NEC T80.62
anaphylactic shock T80.52
shock (allergic) (anaphylactic) T80.52
vaccinia (generalized) (localized) T88.1
vas deferens device or implant -*see* Complications, genitourinary, device or implant, genital tract
vascular I99.9
device or implant T82.9
embolism T82.818
fibrosis T82.828
hemorrhage T82.838
infection or inflammation T82.7
mechanical
breakdown T82.519
specified device NEC T82.518
displacement T82.529
specified device NEC T82.528
leakage T82.539
specified device NEC T82.538
malposition T82.529
specified device NEC T82.528
obstruction T82.599
specified device NEC T82.598
perforation T82.599
specified device NEC T82.598
protrusion T82.599
specified device NEC T82.598
pain T82.848
specified type NEC T82.898
stenosis T82.858
thrombosis T82.868
dialysis catheter -*see* Complication, catheter, dialysis
following infusion, therapeutic injection or transfusion T80.1
graft T82.9
embolism T82.818
fibrosis T82.828

Complication(s) (from) (of) --*continued*
hemorrhage T82.838
mechanical
breakdown T82.319
aorta (bifurcation) T82.310
carotid artery T82.311
specified vessel NEC T82.318
displacement T82.329
aorta (bifurcation) T82.320
carotid artery T82.321
specified vessel NEC T82.328
leakage T82.339
aorta (bifurcation) T82.330
carotid artery T82.331
specified vessel NEC T82.338
malposition T82.329
aorta (bifurcation) T82.320
carotid artery T82.321
specified vessel NEC T82.328
obstruction T82.399
aorta (bifurcation) T82.390
carotid artery T82.391
specified vessel NEC T82.398
perforation T82.399
aorta (bifurcation) T82.390
carotid artery T82.391
specified vessel NEC T82.398
protrusion T82.399
aorta (bifurcation) T82.390
carotid artery T82.391
specified vessel NEC T82.398
pain T82.848
specified complication NEC T82.898
stenosis T82.858
thrombosis T82.868
postoperative -*see* Complications, postoperative, circulatory
vena cava device (filter) (sieve) (umbrella) -*see* Complications, umbrella device, vascular
ventilation therapy NEC T81.81
ventilator
mechanical J95.850
specified NEC J95.859
ventricular (communicating) shunt (device) T85.9
embolism T85.810
fibrosis T85.820
hemorrhage T85.830
infection and inflammation T85.730
mechanical
breakdown T85.01
displacement T85.02
leakage T85.03
malposition T85.02
obstruction T85.09
perforation T85.09
protrusion T85.09
specified NEC T85.09
pain T85.840
specified type NEC T85.890
stenosis T85.850
thrombosis T85.860
wire suture, permanent (implanted) -*see* Complications, suture, permanent
Compressed air disease T70.3
Compression
with injury   code by Nature of injury   artery I77.1
celiac, syndrome I77.4
brachial plexus G54.0
brain (stem) G93.5

Compression - *continued*

due to

contusion (diffuse) -*see* Injury, intracranial, diffuse

focal -*see* Injury, intracranial, focal

injury NEC -*see* Injury, intracranial, diffuse

traumatic -*see* Injury, intracranial, diffuse

bronchus J98.09

cauda equina G83.4

celiac (artery) (axis) I77.4

cerebral -*see* Compression, brain

cervical plexus G54.2

cord

spinal -*see* Compression, spinal

umbilical -*see* Compression, umbilical cord

cranial nerve G52.9

eighth -*see* subcategory H93.3

eleventh G52.8

fifth G50.8

first G52.0

fourth -*see* Strabismus, paralytic, fourth nerve

ninth G52.1

second -*see* Disorder, nerve, optic

seventh G52.8

sixth -*see* Strabismus, paralytic, sixth nerve

tenth G52.2

third -*see* Strabismus, paralytic, third nerve

twelfth G52.3

diver's squeeze T70.3

during birth (newborn) P15.9

esophagus K22.2

eustachian tube -*see* Obstruction, eustachian tube, cartilaginous

facies Q67.1

fracture

nontraumatic NOS -*see* Collapse, vertebra

pathological -*see* Fracture, pathological

traumatic -*see* Fracture, traumatic

heart -*see* Disease, heart

intestine -*see* Obstruction, intestine

laryngeal nerve, recurrent G52.2

with paralysis of vocal cords and larynx J38.00

bilateral J38.02

unilateral J38.01

lumbosacral plexus G54.1

lung J98.4

lymphatic vessel I89.0

medulla -*see* Compression, brain

nerve -*see also* Disorder, nerve G58.9

arm NEC -*see* Mononeuropathy, upper limb

axillary G54.0

cranial -*see* Compression, cranial nerve

leg NEC -*see* Mononeuropathy, lower limb

median (in carpal tunnel) -*see* Syndrome, carpal tunnel

optic -*see* Disorder, nerve, optic

plantar -*see* Lesion, nerve, plantar

posterior tibial (in tarsal tunnel) -*see* Syndrome, tarsal tunnel

root or plexus NOS (in) G54.9

intervertebral disc disorder NEC -*see* Disorder, disc, with, radiculopathy

with myelopathy -*see* Disorder, disc, with, myelopathy

neoplastic disease -*see also* Neoplasm D49.9 [*G55*]

spondylosis -*see* Spondylosis, with radiculopathy

Compression - *continued*

sciatic (acute) -*see* Lesion, nerve, sciatic

sympathetic G90.8

traumatic -*see* Injury, nerve

ulnar -*see* Lesion, nerve, ulnar

upper extremity NEC -*see* Mononeuropathy, upper limb

spinal (cord) G95.20

by displacement of intervertebral disc NEC -*see also* Disorder, disc, with, myelopathy

nerve root NOS G54.9

due to displacement of intervertebral disc NEC -*see* Disorder, disc, with, radiculopathy

with myelopathy -*see* Disorder, disc, with, myelopathy

specified NEC G95.29

spondylogenic (cervical) (lumbar, lumbosacral) (thoracic) -*see* Spondylosis, with myelopathy NEC

anterior -*see* Syndrome, anterior, spinal artery, compression

traumatic -*see* Injury, spinal cord, by region

subcostal nerve (syndrome) -*see* Mononeuropathy, upper limb, specified NEC

sympathetic nerve NEC G90.8

syndrome T79.5

trachea J39.8

ulnar nerve (by scar tissue) -*see* Lesion, nerve, ulnar

umbilical cord

complicating delivery O69.2

cord around neck O69.1

prolapse O69.0

specified NEC O69.2

ureter N13.5

vein I87.1

vena cava (inferior) (superior) I87.1

Compulsion, compulsive

gambling F63.0

neurosis F42.8

personality F60.5

states F42.8

swearing F42.8

in Gilles de la Tourette's syndrome F95.2

tics and spasms F95.9

Concato's disease (pericardial polyserositis) A19.9

nontubercular I31.1

pleural -*see* Pleurisy, with effusion

Concavity chest wall M95.4

Concealed penis Q55.69

Concern (normal) about sick person in family Z63.6

Concrescence (teeth) K00.2

Concretio cordis I31.1

rheumatic I09.2

Concretion -*see also* Calculus

appendicular K38.1

canaliculus -*see* Dacryolith

clitoris N90.89

conjunctiva H11.12

eyelid -*see* Disorder, eyelid, specified type NEC

lacrimal passages -*see* Dacryolith

prepuce (male) N47.8

salivary gland (any) K11.5

seminal vesicle N50.89

tonsil J35.8

Concussion (brain) (cerebral) (current) S06.0X9

with

Concussion --*continued*

loss of consciousness of 30 minutes or less S06.0X1

loss of consciousness of unspecified durationS06.0X9

blast (air) (hydraulic) (immersion) (underwater)

abdomen or thorax -*see* Injury, blast, by site

ear with acoustic nerve injury -*see* Injury, nerve, acoustic, specified type NEC

cauda equina S34.3

conus medullaris S34.02

ocular S05.8X

spinal (cord)

cervical S14.0

lumbar S34.01

sacral S34.02

thoracic S24.0

syndrome F07.81

without loss of consciousness S06.0X0

Condition -*see* Disease

Conditions arising in the perinatal period -*see* Newborn, affected by

Conduct disorder -*see* Disorder, conduct

Condyloma A63.0

acuminatum A63.0

gonorrheal A54.09

latum A51.31

syphilitic A51.31

congenital A50.07

venereal, syphilitic A51.31

Conflagration -*see also* Burn

asphyxia (by inhalation of gases, fumes or vapors) -*see also* Table of Drugs and Chemicals T59.9

Conflict (with) -*see also* Discord

family Z73.9

marital Z63.0

involving divorce or estrangement Z63.5

parent-child Z62.820

parent-adopted child Z62.821

parent-biological child Z62.820

parent-foster child Z62.822

social role NEC Z73.5

Confluent -*see* condition

Confusion, confused R41.0

epileptic F05

mental state (psychogenic) F44.89

psychogenic F44.89

reactive (from emotional stress, psychological trauma) F44.89

Confusional arousals G47.51

Congelation T69.9

Congenital -*see also* condition

aortic septum Q25.49

intrinsic factor deficiency D51.0

malformation -*see* Anomaly

Congestion, congestive

bladder N32.89

bowel K63.89

brain G93.89

breast N64.59

bronchial J98.09

catarrhal J31.0

chest R09.89

chill, malarial -*see* Malaria

circulatory NEC I99.8

duodenum K31.89

eye -*see* Hyperemia, conjunctiva

facial, due to birth injury P15.4

general R68.89

glottis J37.0

Congestion, congestive
 heart -see Failure, heart, congestive
 hepatic K76.1
 hypostatic (lung) -see Edema, lung
 intestine K63.89
 kidney N28.89
 labyrinth -see subcategory H83.8
 larynx J37.0
 liver K76.1
 lung R09.89
  active or acute -see Pneumonia
 malaria, malarial -see Malaria
 nasal R09.81
 nose R09.81
 orbit, orbital -see also Exophthalmos
  inflammatory (chronic) -see Inflammation, orbit
 ovary N83.8
 pancreas K86.89
 pelvic, female N94.89
 pleural J94.8
 prostate (active) N42.1
 pulmonary -see Congestion, lung
 renal N28.89
 retina H35.81
 seminal vesicle N50.1
 spinal cord G95.19
 spleen (chronic) D73.2
 stomach K31.89
 trachea -see Tracheitis
 urethra N36.8
 uterus N85.8
  with subinvolution N85.3
 venous (passive) I87.8
 viscera R68.89
Congestive -see Congestion
Conical
 cervix (hypertrophic elongation) N88.4
 cornea -see Keratoconus
 teeth K00.2
Conjoined twins Q89.4
Conjugal maladjustment Z63.0
 involving divorce or estrangement Z63.5
Conjunctiva -see condition
Conjunctivitis (staphylococcal) (streptococcal)
 NOS H10.9
 Acanthamoeba B60.12
 acute H10.3
  atopic H10.1
  mucopurulent H10.02
   follicular H10.01
  chemical -see also Corrosion, cornea
  H10.21
  pseudomembranous H10.22
  serous except viral H10.23
   viral -see Conjunctivitis, viral
  toxic H10.21
 adenoviral (acute) (follicular) B30.1
 allergic (acute) -see Conjunctivitis, acute, atopic
  chronic H10.45
   vernal H10.44
 anaphylactic -see Conjunctivitis, acute, atopic
 Apollo B30.3
 atopic (acute) -see Conjunctivitis, acute, atopic
 Béal's B30.2
 blennorrhagic (gonococcal) (neonatorum) A54.31
 chemical (acute) -see also Corrosion, cornea
 H10.21

Conjunctivitis --continued
 chlamydial A74.0 --continued
  due to trachoma A71.1
  neonatal P39.1
 chronic (nodosa) (petrificans) (phlyctenular) H10.40
  allergic H10.45
   vernal H10.44
  follicular H10.43
  giant papillary H10.41
  simple H10.42
  vernal H10.44
 coxsackievirus 24 B30.3
 diphtheritic A36.86
 due to
  dust -see Conjunctivitis, acute, atopic
  filariasis B74.9
  mucocutaneous leishmaniasis B55.2
 enterovirus type 70 (hemorrhagic) B30.3
 epidemic (viral) B30.9
  hemorrhagic B30.3
 gonococcal (neonatorum) A54.31
 granular (trachomatous) A71.1
  sequelae (late effect) B94.0
 hemorrhagic (acute) (epidemic) B30.3
 herpes zoster B02.31
 in (due to)
  Acanthamoeba B60.12
  adenovirus (acute) (follicular) B30.1
  Chlamydia A74.0
  coxsackievirus 24 B30.3
  diphtheria A36.86
  enterovirus type 70 (hemorrhagic) B30.3
  filariasis B74.9
  gonococci A54.31
  herpes (simplex) virus B00.53
   zoster B02.31
  infectious disease NEC B99
  meningococci A39.89
  mucocutaneous leishmaniasis B55.2
  rosacea L71.9
  syphilis (late) A52.71
  zoster B02.31
 inclusion A74.0
 infantile P39.1
  gonococcal A54.31
 Koch-Weeks' -see Conjunctivitis, acute, mucopurulent
 light -see Conjunctivitis, acute, atopic
 ligneous -see Blepharoconjunctivitis, ligneous
 meningococcal A39.89
 mucopurulent -see Conjunctivitis, acute, mucopurulent
 neonatal P39.1
  gonococcal A54.31
 Newcastle B30.8
 of Béal B30.2
 parasitic
  filariasis B74.9
  mucocutaneous leishmaniasis B55.2
 Parinaud's H10.89
 petrificans H10.89
 rosacea L71.9
 specified NEC H10.89
 swimming-pool B30.1
 trachomatous A71.1
  acute A71.0
  sequelae (late effect) B94.0
 traumatic NEC H10.89
 tuberculous A18.59
 tularemic A21.1

Conjunctivitis --continued
 tularensis A21.1
 viral B30.9
  due to
   adenovirus B30.1
   enterovirus B30.3
  specified NEC B30.8
Conjunctivochalasis H11.82
Connective tissue -see condition
Conn's syndrome E26.01
Conradi (Hunermann) disease Q77.3
Consanguinity Z84.3
 counseling Z71.89
Conscious simulation (of illness) Z76.5
Consecutive -see condition
Consolidation lung (base) -see Pneumonia, lobar
Constipation (atonic) (neurogenic) (simple) (spastic) K59.00
 chronic K59.09
  idiopathic K59.04
 drug-induced K59.03
 functional K59.04
 outlet dysfunction K59.02
 psychogenic F45.8
 slow transit K59.01
 specified NEC K59.09
Constitutional -see also condition
 substandard F60.7
Constitutionally substandard F60.7
Constriction -see also Stricture
 auditory canal -see Stenosis, external ear canal
 bronchial J98.09
 duodenum K31.5
 esophagus K22.2
 external
  abdomen, abdominal (wall) S30.841
  alveolar process S00.542
  ankle S90.54
  antecubital space -see Constriction, external, forearm
  arm (upper) S40.84
  auricle -see Constriction, external, ear
  axilla -see Constriction, external, arm
  back, lower S30.840
  breast S20.14
  brow S00.84
  buttock S30.840
  calf -see Constriction, external, leg
  canthus -see Constriction, external, eyelid
  cheek S00.84
   internal S00.542
  chest wall -see Constriction, external, thorax
  chin S00.84
  clitoris S30.844
  costal region -see Constriction, external, thorax
  digit(s)
   foot -see Constriction, external, toe
   hand -see Constriction, external, finger
  ear S00.44
  elbow S50.34
  epididymis S30.843
  epigastric region S30.841
  esophagus, cervical S10.14
  eyebrow -see Constriction, external, eyelid
  eyelid S00.24
  face S00.84
  finger(s) S60.44
   index S60.44

Constriction - *continued*

little S60.44
middle S60.44
ring S60.44
flank S30.841
foot (except toe(s) alone) S90.84
toe -*see* Constriction, external, toe
forearm S50.84
elbow only -*see* Constriction, external,
elbow
forehead S00.84
genital organs, external
female S30.846
male S30.845
groin S30.841
gum S00.542
hand S60.54
head S00.94
ear -*see* Constriction, external, ear
eyelid -*see* Constriction, external, eyelid
lip S00.541
nose S00.34
oral cavity S00.542
scalp S00.04
specified site NEC S00.84
heel -*see* Constriction, external, foot
hip S70.24
inguinal region S30.841
interscapular region S20.449
jaw S00.84
knee S80.24
labium (majus) (minus) S30.844
larynx S10.14
leg (lower) S80.84
knee -*see* Constriction, external, knee
upper -*see* Constriction, external, thigh
lip S00.541
lower back S30.840
lumbar region S30.840
malar region S00.84
mammary -*see* Constriction, external, breast
mastoid region S00.84
mouth S00.542
nail
finger -*see* Constriction, external, finger
toe -*see* Constriction, external, toe
nasal S00.34
neck S10.94
specified site NEC S10.84
throat S10.14
nose S00.34
occipital region S00.04
oral cavity S00.542
orbital region -*see* Constriction, external,
eyelid
palate S00.542
palm -*see* Constriction, external, hand
parietal region S00.04
pelvis S30.840
penis S30.842
perineum
female S30.844
male S30.840
periocular area -*see* Constriction, external,
eyelid
phalanges
finger -*see* Constriction, external, finger
toe -*see* Constriction, external, toe
pharynx S10.14
pinna -*see* Constriction, external, ear

Constriction - *continued*

popliteal space -*see* Constriction, external,
knee
prepuce S30.842
pubic region S30.840
pudendum
female S30.846
male S30.845
sacral region S30.840
scalp S00.04
scapular region -*see* Constriction, external,
shoulder
scrotum S30.843
shin -*see* Constriction, external, leg
shoulder S40.24
sternal region S20.349
submaxillary region S00.84
submental region S00.84
subungual
finger(s) -*see* Constriction, external, finger
toe(s) -*see* Constriction, external, toe
supraclavicular fossa S10.84
supraorbital S00.84
temple S00.84
temporal region S00.84
testis S30.843
thigh S70.34
thorax, thoracic (wall) S20.94
back S20.44
front S20.34
throat S10.14
thumb S60.34
toe(s) (lesser) S90.44
great S90.44
tongue S00.542
trachea S10.14
tunica vaginalis S30.843
uvula S00.542
vagina S30.844
vulva S30.844
wrist S60.84
gallbladder -*see* Obstruction, gallbladder
intestine -*see* Obstruction, intestine
larynx J38.6
congenital Q31.8
specified NEC Q31.8
subglottic Q31.1
organ or site, congenital NEC -*see* Atresia, by
site
prepuce (acquired) (congenital) N47.1
pylorus (adult hypertrophic) K31.1
congenital or infantile Q40.0
newborn Q40.0
ring dystocia (uterus) O62.4
spastic -*see also* Spasm
ureter N13.5
ureter N13.5
with infection N13.6
urethra -*see* Stricture, urethra
visual field (peripheral) (functional) -*see*
Defect, visual field
Constrictive -*see* condition
Consultation
medical -*see* Counseling, medical
religious Z71.81
specified reason NEC Z71.89
spiritual Z71.81
without complaint or sickness Z71.9
feared complaint unfounded Z71.1
specified reason NEC Z71.89
Consumption -*see* Tuberculosis

Contact (with) -*see also* Exposure (to)
acariasis Z20.7
AIDS virus Z20.6
air pollution Z77.110
algae and algae toxins Z77.121
algae bloom Z77.121
anthrax Z20.810
aromatic amines Z77.020
aromatic (hazardous) compounds NEC
Z77.028
aromatic dyes NOS Z77.028
arsenic Z77.010
asbestos Z77.090
bacterial disease NEC Z20.818
benzene Z77.021
blue-green algae bloom Z77.121
body fluids (potentially hazardous) Z77.21
brown tide Z77.121
chemicals (chiefly nonmedicinal) (hazardous)
NEC Z77.098
cholera Z20.09
chromium compounds Z77.018
communicable disease Z20.9
bacterial NEC Z20.818
specified NEC Z20.89
viral NEC Z20.828
cyanobacteria bloom Z77.121
dyes Z77.098
Escherichia coli (E. coli) Z20.01
fiberglass -*see* Table of Drugs and Chemicals,
fiberglass
German measles Z20.4
gonorrhea Z20.2
hazardous metals NEC Z77.018
hazardous substances NEC Z77.29
hazards in the physical environment NEC
Z77.128
hazards to health NEC Z77.9
HIV Z20.6
HTLV-III/LAV Z20.6
human immunodeficiency virus (HIV) Z20.6
infection Z20.9
specified NEC Z20.89
infestation (parasitic) NEC Z20.7
intestinal infectious disease NEC Z20.09
Escherichia coli (E. coli) Z20.01
lead Z77.011
meningococcus Z20.811
mold (toxic) Z77.120
nickel dust Z77.018
noise Z77.122
parasitic disease Z20.7
pediculosis Z20.7
pfiesteria piscicida Z77.121
poliomyelitis Z20.89
pollution
air Z77.110
environmental NEC Z77.118
soil Z77.112
water Z77.111
polycyclic aromatic hydrocarbons Z77.028
rabies Z20.3
radiation, naturally occurring NEC Z77.123
radon Z77.123
red tide (Florida) Z77.121
rubella Z20.4
sexually transmitted disease Z20.2
smallpox (laboratory) Z20.89
syphilis Z20.2
tuberculosis Z20.1
uranium Z77.012

Contact (with) --*continued*
  varicella Z20.820
  venereal disease Z20.2
  viral disease NEC Z20.828
  viral hepatitis Z20.5
  water pollution Z77.111
Contamination, food -*see* Intoxication,
  foodborne
Contraception, contraceptive
  advice Z30.09
  counseling Z30.09
  device (intrauterine) (in situ) Z97.5
    causing menorrhagia T83.83
    checking Z30.431
    complications -*see* Complications,
  intrauterine, contraceptive device
    in place Z97.5
    initial prescription Z30.014
    reinsertion Z30.433
    removal Z30.432
    replacement Z30.433
  emergency (postcoital) Z30.012
  initial prescription Z30.019
    barrier Z30.018
    diaphragm Z30.018
    injectable Z30.013
    intrauterine device Z30.014
    pills Z30.011
    postcoital (emergency) Z30.012
    specified type NEC Z30.018
    subdermal implantable Z30.017
    transdermal patch hormonal Z30.016
    vaginal ring hormonal Z30.015
  maintenance Z30.40
    barrier Z30.49
    diaphragm Z30.49
    examination Z30.8
    injectable Z30.42
    intrauterine device Z30.431
    pills Z30.41
    specified type NEC Z30.49
    subdermal implantable Z30.46
    transdermal patch hormonal Z30.45
    vaginal ring hormonal Z30.44
  management Z30.9
    specified NEC Z30.8
  postcoital (emergency) Z30.012
  prescription Z30.019
    repeat Z30.40
  sterilization Z30.2
  surveillance (drug) -*see* Contraception,
  maintenance
Contraction(s), contracture, contracted
  Achilles tendon -*see also* Short, tendon,
  Achilles
    congenital Q66.89
  amputation stump (surgical) (flexion) (late)
  (next proximal joint) T87.89
  anus K59.8
  bile duct (common) (hepatic) K83.8
  bladder N32.89
    neck or sphincter N32.0
  bowel, cecum, colon or intestine, any part -*see*
  Obstruction, intestine
  Braxton Hicks -*see* False, labor
  breast implant, capsular T85.44
  bronchial J98.09
  burn (old) -*see* Cicatrix
  cervix -*see* Stricture, cervix
  cicatricial -*see* Cicatrix
  conjunctiva, trachomatous, active A71.1

Contraction(s), contracture, contracted
--*continued*
    sequelae (late effect) B94.0
  Dupuytren's M72.0
  eyelid -*see* Disorder, eyelid function
  fascia (lata) (postural) M72.8
    Dupuytren's M72.0
    palmar M72.0
    plantar M72.2
  finger NEC -*see also* Deformity, finger
    congenital Q68.1
    joint -*see* Contraction, joint, hand
  flaccid -*see* Contraction, paralytic
  gallbladder K82.0
  heart valve -*see* Endocarditis
  hip -*see* Contraction, joint, hip
  hourglass
    bladder N32.89
      congenital Q64.79
    gallbladder K82.0
      congenital Q44.1
    stomach K31.89
      congenital Q40.2
      psychogenic F45.8
    uterus (complicating delivery) O62.4
  hysterical F44.4
  internal os -*see* Stricture, cervix
  joint (abduction) (acquired) (adduction)
  (flexion) (rotation) M24.50
    ankle M24.57
    congenital NEC Q68.8
      hip Q65.89
    elbow M24.52
    foot joint M24.57
    hand joint M24.54
    hip M24.55
      congenital Q65.89
    hysterical F44.4
    knee M24.56
    shoulder M24.51
    wrist M24.53
  kidney (granular) (secondary) N26.9
    congenital Q63.8
    hydronephritic -*see* Hydronephrosis
  Page N26.2
    pyelonephritic -*see* Pyelitis, chronic
    tuberculous A18.11
  ligament -*see also* Disorder, ligament
    congenital Q79.8
  muscle (postinfective) (postural) NEC
  M62.40
    with contracture of joint -*see* Contraction,
  joint
    ankle M62.47
    congenital Q79.8
      sternocleidomastoid Q68.0
    extraocular -*see* Strabismus
    eye (extrinsic) -*see* Strabismus
    foot M62.47
    forearm M62.43
    hand M62.44
    hysterical F44.4
    ischemic (Volkmann's) T79.6
    lower leg M62.46
    multiple sites M62.49
    pelvic region M62.45
    posttraumatic -*see* Strabismus, paralytic
    psychogenic F45.8
      conversion reaction F44.4
    shoulder region M62.41
    specified site NEC M62.48

Contraction(s), contracture, contracted
--*continued*
    thigh M62.45
    upper arm M62.42
  neck -*see* Torticollis
  ocular muscle -*see* Strabismus
  organ or site, congenital NEC -*see* Atresia, by
  site
  outlet (pelvis) -*see* Contraction, pelvis
  palmar fascia M72.0
  paralytic
    joint -*see* Contraction, joint
    muscle -*see also* Contraction, muscle NEC
      ocular -*see* Strabismus, paralytic
  pelvis (acquired) (general) M95.5
    with disproportion (fetopelvic) O33.1
      causing obstructed labor O65.1
    inlet O33.2
    mid-cavity O33.3
    outlet O33.3
  plantar fascia M72.2
  premature
    atrium I49.1
    auriculoventricular I49.49
    heart I49.49
    junctional I49.2
    supraventricular I49.1
    ventricular I49.3
  prostate N42.89
  pylorus NEC -*see also* Pylorospasm
    psychogenic F45.8
  rectum, rectal (sphincter) K59.8
  ring (Bandl's) (complicating delivery) O62.4
  scar -*see* Cicatrix
  spine -*see* Dorsopathy, deforming
  sternocleidomastoid (muscle), congenital
  Q68.0
  stomach K31.89
    hourglass K31.89
      congenital Q40.2
      psychogenic F45.8
    psychogenic F45.8
  tendon (sheath) M62.40
    with contracture of joint -*see* Contraction,
  joint
    Achilles -*see* Short, tendon, Achilles
    ankle M62.47
      Achilles -*see* Short, tendon, Achilles
    foot M62.47
    forearm M62.43
    hand M62.44
    lower leg M62.46
    multiple sites M62.49
    neck M62.48
    pelvic region M62.45
    shoulder region M62.41
    specified site NEC M62.48
    thigh M62.45
    thorax M62.48
    trunk M62.48
    upper arm M62.42
  toe -*see* Deformity, toe, specified NEC
  ureterovesical orifice (postinfectional) N13.5
    with infection N13.6
  urethra -*see also* Stricture, urethra
    orifice N32.0
  uterus N85.8
    abnormal NEC O62.9
    clonic (complicating delivery) O62.4
    dyscoordinate (complicating delivery) O62.4
    hourglass (complicating delivery) O62.4

Contraction(s), contracture, contracted
--*continued*
  hypertonic O62.4
  hypotonic NEC O62.2
  inadequate
    primary O62.0
    secondary O62.1
  incoordinate (complicating delivery) O62.4
  poor O62.2
  tetanic (complicating delivery) O62.4
  vagina (outlet) N89.5
  vesical N32.89
    neck or urethral orifice N32.0
  visual field -*see* Defect, visual field,
  generalized
  Volkmann's (ischemic) T79.6
Contusion (skin surface intact) T14.8
  abdomen, abdominal (muscle) (wall) S30.1
  adnexa, eye NEC S05.8X
  adrenal gland S37.812
  alveolar process S00.532
  ankle S90.0
  antecubital space -*see* Contusion, forearm
  anus S30.3
  arm (upper) S40.02
    lower (with elbow) -*see* Contusion, forearm
  auditory canal -*see* Contusion, ear
  auricle -*see* Contusion, ear
  axilla -*see* Contusion, arm, upper
  back -*see also* Contusion, thorax, back
    lower S30.0
  bile duct S36.13
  bladder S37.22
  bone NEC T14.8
  brain (diffuse) -*see* Injury, intracranial,
  diffuse
    focal -*see* Injury, intracranial, focal
  brainstem S06.38
  breast S20.0
  broad ligament S37.892
  brow S00.83
  buttock S30.0
  canthus, eye S00.1
  cauda equina S34.3
  cerebellar, traumatic S06.37
  cerebral S06.33
    left side S06.32
    right side S06.31
  cheek S00.83
    internal S00.532
  chest (wall) -*see* Contusion, thorax - chin
  S00.83
  clitoris S30.23
  colon -*see* Injury, intestine, large, contusion
  common bile duct S36.13
  conjunctiva S05.1
    with foreign body (in conjunctival sac) -*see*
    Foreign body, conjunctival sac
  conus medullaris (spine) S34.139
  cornea -*see* Contusion, eyeball
    with foreign body -*see* Foreign body, cornea
  corpus cavernosum S30.21
  cortex (brain) (cerebral) -*see* Injury,
  intracranial, diffuse
    focal -*see* Injury, intracranial, focal
  costal region -*see* Contusion, thorax - cystic
  duct S36.13
  diaphragm S27.802
  duodenum S36.420
  ear S00.43
  elbow S50.0

Contusion --*continued*
  with forearm -*see* Contusion, forearm
  epididymis S30.22
  epigastric region S30.1
  epiglottis S10.0
  esophagus (thoracic) S27.812
    cervical S10.0
  eyeball S05.1
  eyebrow S00.1
  eyelid (and periocular area) S00.1
  face NEC S00.83
  fallopian tube S37.529
    bilateral S37.522
    unilateral S37.521
  femoral triangle S30.1
  finger(s) S60.00
    with damage to nail (matrix) S60.10
    index S60.02
      with damage to nail S60.12
    little S60.05
      with damage to nail S60.15
    middle S60.03
      with damage to nail S60.13
    ring S60.04
      with damage to nail S60.14
    thumb -*see* Contusion, thumb
  flank S30.1
  foot (except toe(s) alone) S90.3
    toe -*see* Contusion, toe
  forearm S50.1
    elbow only -*see* Contusion, elbow
  forehead S00.83
  gallbladder S36.122
  genital organs, external
    female S30.202
    male S30.201
  globe (eye) -*see* Contusion, eyeball
  groin S30.1
  gum S00.532
  hand S60.22
    finger(s) -*see* Contusion, finger
    wrist -*see* Contusion, wrist
  head S00.93
    ear -*see* Contusion, ear
    eyelid -*see* Contusion, eyelid
    lip S00.531
    nose S00.33
    oral cavity S00.532
    scalp S00.03
    specified part NEC S00.83
  heart -*see also* Injury, heart S26.91
  heel -*see* Contusion, foot
  hepatic duct S36.13
  hip S70.0
  ileum S36.428
  iliac region S30.1
  inguinal region S30.1
  interscapular region S20.229
  intra-abdominal organ S36.92
    colon -*see* Injury, intestine, large, contusion
    liver S36.112
    pancreas -*see* Contusion, pancreas
    rectum S36.62
    small intestine -*see* Injury, intestine, small,
    contusion
    specified organ NEC S36.892
    spleen -*see* Contusion, spleen
    stomach S36.32
  iris (eye) -*see* Contusion, eyeball
  jaw S00.83
  jejunum S36.428

Contusion --*continued*
  kidney S37.01
    major (greater than 2 cm) S37.02
    minor (less than 2 cm) S37.01
  knee S80.0
  labium (majus) (minus) S30.23
  lacrimal apparatus, gland or sac S05.8X
  larynx S10.0
  leg (lower) S80.1
    knee -*see* Contusion, knee - lens -*see*
    Contusion, eyeball
  lip S00.531
  liver S36.112
  lower back S30.0
  lumbar region S30.0
  lung S27.329
    bilateral S27.322
    unilateral S27.321
  malar region S00.83
  mastoid region S00.83
  membrane, brain -*see* Injury, intracranial,
  diffuse
    focal -*see* Injury, intracranial, focal
  mesentery S36.892
  mesosalpinx S37.892
  mouth S00.532
  muscle -*see* Contusion, by site
  nail
    finger -*see* Contusion, finger, with damage
    to nail
    toe -*see* Contusion, toe, with damage to nail
  nasal S00.33
  neck S10.93
    specified site NEC S10.83
    throat S10.0
  nerve -*see* Injury, nerve
  newborn P54.5
  nose S00.33
  occipital
    lobe (brain) -*see* Injury, intracranial, diffuse
    focal -*see* Injury, intracranial, focal
    region (scalp) S00.03
  orbit (region) (tissues) S05.1
  ovary S37.429
    bilateral S37.422
    unilateral S37.421
  palate S00.532
  pancreas S36.229
    body S36.221
    head S36.220
    tail S36.222
  parietal
    lobe (brain) -*see* Injury, intracranial, diffuse
    focal -*see* Injury, intracranial, focal
    region (scalp) S00.03
  pelvic organ S37.92
    adrenal gland S37.812
    bladder S37.22
    fallopian tube -*see* Contusion, fallopian tube
    kidney -*see* Contusion, kidney
    ovary -*see* Contusion, ovary
    prostate S37.822
    specified organ NEC S37.892
    ureter S37.12
    urethra S37.32
    uterus S37.62
  pelvis S30.0
  penis S30.21
  perineum
    female S30.23
    male S30.0

Contusion --*continued*
periocular area S00.1
peritoneum S36.81
periurethral tissue -*see* Contusion, urethra
pharynx S10.0
pinna -*see* Contusion, ear
popliteal space -*see* Contusion, knee -
prepuce S30.21
prostate S37.822
pubic region S30.1
pudendum
  female S30.202
  male S30.201
quadriceps femoris -*see* Contusion, thigh
rectum S36.62
retroperitoneum S36.892
round ligament S37.892
sacral region S30.0
scalp S00.03
  due to birth injury P12.3
scapular region -*see* Contusion, shoulder
sclera -*see* Contusion, eyeball
scrotum S30.22
seminal vesicle S37.892
shoulder S40.01
skin NEC T14.8
small intestine -*see* Injury, intestine, small, contusion
spermatic cord S30.22
spinal cord -*see* Injury, spinal cord, by region
  cauda equina S34.3
  conus medullaris S34.139
spleen S36.029
  major S36.021
  minor S36.020
sternal region S20.219
stomach S36.32
subconjunctival S05.1
subcutaneous NEC T14.8
submaxillary region S00.83
submental region S00.83
subperiosteal NEC T14.8
subungual
  finger -*see* Contusion, finger, with damage to nail
  toe -*see* Contusion, toe, with damage to nail
supraclavicular fossa S10.83
supraorbital S00.83
suprarenal gland S37.812
temple (region) S00.83
temporal
  lobe (brain) -*see* Injury, intracranial, diffuse
  focal -*see* Injury, intracranial, focal
  region S00.83
testis S30.22
thigh S70.1
thorax (wall) S20.20
  back S20.22
  front S20.21
throat S10.0
thumb S60.01
  with damage to nail S60.11
toe(s) (lesser) S90.12
  with damage to nail S90.22
  great S90.11
    with damage to nail S90.21
    specified type NEC S90.221
tongue S00.532
trachea (cervical) S10.0
  thoracic S27.52
tunica vaginalis S30.22

Contusion --*continued*
tympanum, tympanic membrane -*see* Contusion, ear
ureter S37.12
urethra S37.32
urinary organ NEC S37.892
uterus S37.62
uvula S00.532
vagina S30.23
vas deferens S37.892
vesical S37.22
vocal cord(s) S10.0
vulva S30.23
wrist S60.21
Conus (congenital) (any type) Q14.8
cornea -*see* Keratoconus
medullaris syndrome G95.81
Conversion hysteria, neurosis or reaction F44.9
Converter, tuberculosis (test reaction) R76.11
Conviction (legal), anxiety concerning Z65.0
with imprisonment Z65.1
Convulsions (idiopathic) -*see also* Seizure(s) R56.9
apoplectiform (cerebral ischemia) I67.82
dissociative F44.5
epileptic -*see* Epilepsy
epileptiform, epileptoid -*see* Seizure, epileptiform
ether (anesthetic) -*see* Table of Drugs and Chemicals, by drug
febrile R56.00
  with status epilepticus G40.901
  complex R56.01
    with status epilepticus G40.901
  simple R56.00
hysterical F44.5
infantile P90
  epilepsy -*see* Epilepsy
jacksonian -*see* Epilepsy, localization-related, symptomatic, with simple partial seizures
myoclonic G25.3
newborn P90
obstetrical (nephritic) (uremic) -*see* Eclampsia
paretic A52.17
post traumatic R56.1
psychomotor -*see* Epilepsy, localization-related, symptomatic, with complex partial seizures
recurrent R56.9
reflex R25.8
scarlatinal A38.8
tetanus, tetanic -*see* Tetanus
thymic E32.8
Convulsive -*see also* Convulsions
Cooley's anemia D56.1
Coolie itch B76.9
Cooper's
disease -*see* Mastopathy, cystic
hernia -*see* Hernia, abdomen, specified site NEC
Copra itch B88.0
Coprophagy F50.89
Coprophobia F40.298
Coproporphyria, hereditary E80.29
Cor
biloculare Q20.8
bovis, bovinum -*see* Hypertrophy, cardiac
pulmonale (chronic) I27.81
  acute I26.09

Cor - *continued*
triatriatum, triatrium Q24.2
triloculare Q20.8
  biatrium Q20.4
  biventriculare Q21.1
Corbus' disease (gangrenous balanitis) N48.1
Cord -*see also* condition
around neck (tightly) (with compression)
  complicating delivery O69.1
bladder G95.89
  tabetic A52.19
Cordis ectopia Q24.8
Corditis (spermatic) N49.1
Corectopia Q13.2
Cori's disease (glycogen storage) E74.03
Cork handler's disease or lung J67.3
Corkscrew esophagus K22.4
Cork worker's disease or lung J67.3
Corn (infected) L84
Cornea -*see also* condition
donor Z52.5
plana Q13.4
Cornelia de Lange syndrome Q87.1
Cornu cutaneum L85.8
Cornual gestation or pregnancy O00.80
with intrauterine pregnancy O00.81
Coronary (artery) -*see* condition
Coronavirus, as cause of disease classified elsewhere B97.29
SARS-associated B97.21
Corpora -*see also* condition
amylacea, prostate N42.89
cavernosa -*see* condition
Corpulence -*see* Obesity
Corpus -*see* condition
Corrected transposition Q20.5
Corrosion (injury) (acid) (caustic) (chemical) (lime) (external) (internal) T30.4
abdomen, abdominal (muscle) (wall) T21.42
  first degree T21.52
  second degree T21.62
  third degree T21.72
above elbow T22.439
  first degree T22.539
  left T22.432
    first degree T22.532
    second degree T22.632
    third degree T22.732
  right T22.431
    first degree T22.531
    second degree T22.631
    third degree T22.731
  second degree T22.639
  third degree T22.739
alimentary tract NEC T28.7
ankle T25.419
  first degree T25.519
  left T25.412
    first degree T25.512
    second degree T25.612
    third degree T25.712
  multiple with foot -*see* Corrosion, lower, limb, multiple, ankle and foot
  right T25.411
    first degree T25.511
    second degree T25.611
    third degree T25.711
  second degree T25.619
  third degree T25.719
anus -*see* Corrosion, buttock

Corrosion - *continued*
arm(s) (meaning upper limb(s)) -*see*
Corrosion, upper limb
axilla T22.449
first degree T22.549
left T22.442
first degree T22.542
second degree T22.642
third degree T22.742
right T22.441
first degree T22.541
second degree T22.641
third degree T22.741
second degree T22.649
third degree T22.749
back (lower) T21.44
first degree T21.54
second degree T21.64
third degree T21.74
upper T21.43
first degree T21.53
second degree T21.63
third degree T21.73
blisters
code as Corrosion, second degree, by site
breast(s) -*see* Corrosion, chest wall
buttock(s) T21.45
first degree T21.55
second degree T21.65
third degree T21.75
calf T24.439
first degree T24.539
left T24.432
first degree T24.532
second degree T24.632
third degree T24.732
right T24.431
first degree T24.531
second degree T24.631
third degree T24.731
second degree T24.639
third degree T24.739
canthus (eye) -*see* Corrosion, eyelid
cervix T28.8
cheek T20.46
first degree T20.56
second degree T20.66
third degree T20.76
chest wall T21.41
first degree T21.51
second degree T21.61
third degree T21.71
chin T20.43
first degree T20.53
second degree T20.63
third degree T20.73
colon T28.7
conjunctiva (and cornea) -*see* Corrosion,
cornea
cornea (and conjunctiva) T26.6
deep necrosis of underlying tissue - code as
Corrosion, third degree, by site
dorsum of hand T23.469
first degree T23.569
left T23.462
first degree T23.562
second degree T23.662
third degree T23.762
right T23.461
first degree T23.561
second degree T23.661

Corrosion - *continued*
third degree T23.761
second degree T23.669
third degree T23.769
ear (auricle) (external) (canal) T20.41
drum T28.91
first degree T20.51
second degree T20.61
third degree T20.71
elbow T22.429
first degree T22.529
left T22.422
first degree T22.522
second degree T22.622
third degree T22.722
right T22.421
first degree T22.521
second degree T22.621
third degree T22.721
second degree T22.629
third degree T22.729
entire body -*see* Corrosion, multiple body
regions
epidermal loss
code as Corrosion, second degree, by site
epiglottis T27.4
erythema, erythematous
code as Corrosion, first degree, by site
esophagus T28.6
extent (percentage of body surface)
less than 10 percent T32.0
10 19 percent (0 9 percent third degree)
T32.10
with 10 19 percent third degree T32.11
20 29 percent (0 9 percent third degree)
T32.20
with
10 19 percent third degree T32.21
20 29 percent third degree T32.22
30 39 percent (0 9 percent third degree)
T32.30
with
10 19 percent third degree T32.31
20 29 percent third degree T32.32
30 39 percent third degree T32.33
40 49 percent (0 9 percent third degree)
T32.40
with
10 19 percent third degree T32.41
20 29 percent third degree T32.42
30 39 percent third degree T32.43
40 49 percent third degree T32.44
50 59 percent (0 9 percent third degree)
T32.50
with
10 19 percent third degree T32.51
20 29 percent third degree T32.52
30 39 percent third degree T32.53
40 49 percent third degree T32.54
50 59 percent third degree T32.55
60 69 percent (0 9 percent third degree)
T32.60
with
10 19 percent third degree T32.61
20 29 percent third degree T32.62
30 39 percent third degree T32.63
40 49 percent third degree T32.64
50 59 percent third degree T32.65
60 69 percent third degree T32.66
70 79 percent (0 9 percent third degree)
T32.70

Corrosion - *continued*
with
10 19 percent third degree T32.71
20 29 percent third degree T32.72
30 39 percent third degree T32.73
40 49 percent third degree T32.74
50 59 percent third degree T32.75
60 69 percent third degree T32.76
70 79 percent third degree T32.77
80 89 percent (0 9 percent third degree)
T32.80
with
10 19 percent third degree T32.81
20 29 percent third degree T32.82
30 39 percent third degree T32.83
40 49 percent third degree T32.84
50 59 percent third degree T32.85
60 69 percent third degree T32.86
70 79 percent third degree T32.87
80 89 percent third degree T32.88
90 percent or more (0 9 percent third
degree) T32.90
with
10 19 percent third degree T32.91
20 29 percent third degree T32.92
30 39 percent third degree T32.93
40 49 percent third degree T32.94
50 59 percent third degree T32.95
60 69 percent third degree T32.96
70 79 percent third degree T32.97
80 89 percent third degree T32.98
90 99 percent third degree T32.99
extremity -*see* Corrosion, limb
eye(s) and adnexa T26.9
with resulting rupture and destruction of
eyeball T26.7
conjunctival sac -*see* Corrosion, cornea
cornea -*see* Corrosion, cornea
lid -*see* Corrosion, eyelid
periocular area -*see* Corrosion eyelid
specified site NEC T26.8
eyeball -*see* Corrosion, eye - eyelid(s) T26.5
face -*see* Corrosion, head - finger T23.429
first degree T23.529
left T23.422
first degree T23.522
second degree T23.622
third degree T23.722
multiple sites (without thumb) T23.439
with thumb T23.449
first degree T23.549
left T23.442
first degree T23.542
second degree T23.642
third degree T23.742
right T23.441
first degree T23.541
second degree T23.641
third degree T23.741
second degree T23.649
third degree T23.749
first degree T23.539
left T23.432
first degree T23.532
second degree T23.632
third degree T23.732
right T23.431
first degree T23.531
second degree T23.631
third degree T23.731
second degree T23.639

Corrosion - *continued*
  third degree T23.739
  right T23.421
    first degree T23.521
    second degree T23.621
    third degree T23.721
    second degree T23.629
    third degree T23.729
  flank -*see* Corrosion, abdomen
  foot T25.429
    first degree T25.529
    left T25.422
      first degree T25.522
      second degree T25.622
      third degree T25.722
    multiple with ankle -*see* Corrosion, lower,
  limb, multiple, ankle and foot
    right T25.421
      first degree T25.521
      second degree T25.621
      third degree T25.721
    second degree T25.629
    third degree T25.729
  forearm T22.419
    first degree T22.519
    left T22.412
      first degree T22.512
      second degree T22.612
      third degree T22.712
    right T22.411
      first degree T22.511
      second degree T22.611
      third degree T22.711
    second degree T22.619
    third degree T22.719
  forehead T20.46
    first degree T20.56
    second degree T20.66
    third degree T20.76
  fourth degree - code as Corrosion, third
  degree, by site
  full thickness skin loss
  code as Corrosion, third degree, by site
  gastrointestinal tract NEC T28.7
  genital organs
    external
      female T21.47
        first degree T21.57
        second degree T21.67
        third degree T21.77
      male T21.46
        first degree T21.56
        second degree T21.66
        third degree T21.76
    internal T28.8
  groin -*see* Corrosion, abdominal wall
  hand(s) T23.409
    back -*see* Corrosion, dorsum of hand
    finger -*see* Corrosion, finger
    first degree T23.509
    left T23.402
      first degree T23.502
      second degree T23.602
      third degree T23.702
    multiple sites with wrist T23.499
      first degree T23.599
      left T23.492
        first degree T23.592
        second degree T23.692
        third degree T23.792
      right T23.491

Corrosion - *continued*
    first degree T23.591
    second degree T23.691
    third degree T23.791
    second degree T23.699
    third degree T23.799
  palm -*see* Corrosion, palm
  right T23.401
    first degree T23.501
    second degree T23.601
    third degree T23.701
  second degree T23.609
  third degree T23.709
  thumb -*see* Corrosion, thumb
  head (and face) (and neck) T20.40
    cheek -*see* Corrosion, cheek
    chin -*see* Corrosion, chin
    ear -*see* Corrosion, ear
    eye(s) only -*see* Corrosion, eye
    first degree T20.50
    forehead -*see* Corrosion, forehead
    lip -*see* Corrosion, lip
    multiple sites T20.49
      first degree T20.59
      second degree T20.69
      third degree T20.79
    neck -*see* Corrosion, neck
    nose -*see* Corrosion, nose
    scalp -*see* Corrosion, scalp
    second degree T20.60
    third degree T20.70
  hip(s) -*see* Corrosion, lower, limb
  inhalation -*see* Corrosion, respiratory tract
  internal organ(s) -*see also* Corrosion, by site
  T28.90
    alimentary tract T28.7
      esophagus T28.6
    esophagus T28.6
    genitourinary T28.8
    mouth T28.5
    pharynx T28.5
    specified organ NEC T28.99
  interscapular region -*see* Corrosion, back,
  upper
  intestine (large) (small) T28.7
  knee T24.429
    first degree T24.529
    left T24.422
      first degree T24.522
      second degree T24.622
      third degree T24.722
    right T24.421
      first degree T24.521
      second degree T24.621
      third degree T24.721
    second degree T24.629
    third degree T24.729
  labium (majus) (minus) -*see* Corrosion,
  genital organs, external, female
  lacrimal apparatus, duct, gland or sac -*see*
  Corrosion, eye, specified site NEC
  larynx T27.4
    with lung T27.5
  leg(s) (meaning lower limb(s)) -*see*
  Corrosion, lower limb
  limb(s)
    lower -*see* Corrosion, lower, limb
    upper -*see* Corrosion, upper limb
  lip(s) T20.42
    first degree T20.52
    second degree T20.62

Corrosion - *continued*
    third degree T20.72
  lower
    back -*see* Corrosion, back
    limb T24.409
      ankle -*see* Corrosion, ankle
      calf -*see* Corrosion, calf
      first degree T24.509
      foot -*see* Corrosion, foot
      knee -*see* Corrosion, knee
      left T24.402
        first degree T24.502
        second degree T24.602
        third degree T24.702
      multiple sites, except ankle and foot
      T24.499
        ankle and foot T25.499
          first degree T25.599
          left T25.492
            first degree T25.592
            second degree T25.692
            third degree T25.792
          right T25.491
            first degree T25.591
            second degree T25.691
            third degree T25.791
          second degree T25.699
          third degree T25.799
        first degree T24.599
        left T24.492
          first degree T24.592
          second degree T24.692
          third degree T24.792
        right T24.491
          first degree T24.591
          second degree T24.691
          third degree T24.791
        second degree T24.699
        third degree T24.699
      right T24.401
        first degree T24.501
        second degree T24.601
        third degree T24.701
      second degree T24.609
      hip -*see* Corrosion, thigh
      thigh -*see* Corrosion, thigh
      third degree T24.709
  lung (with larynx and trachea) T27.5
  mouth T28.5
  neck T20.47
    first degree T20.57
    second degree T20.67
    third degree T20.77
  nose (septum) T20.44
    first degree T20.54
    second degree T20.64
    third degree T20.74
  ocular adnexa -*see* Corrosion, eye - orbit
  region -*see* Corrosion, eyelid
  palm T23.459
    first degree T23.559
    left T23.452
      first degree T23.552
      second degree T23.652
      third degree T23.752
    right T23.451
      first degree T23.551
      second degree T23.651
      third degree T23.751
    second degree T23.659
    third degree T23.759

Corrosion - *continued*

20 29 percent third degree T32.82
30 39 percent third degree T32.83
40 49 percent third degree T32.84
50 59 percent third degree T32.85
60 69 percent third degree T32.86
70 79 percent third degree T32.87
80 89 percent third degree T32.88
90 percent or more (0 9 percent third degree) T32.90
  with
    10 19 percent third degree T32.91
    20 29 percent third degree T32.92
    30 39 percent third degree T32.93
    40 49 percent third degree T32.94
    50 59 percent third degree T32.95
    60 69 percent third degree T32.96
    70 79 percent third degree T32.97
    80 89 percent third degree T32.98
    90 99 percent third degree T32.99
upper limb (axilla) (scapular region) T22.40
above elbow -*see* Corrosion, above elbow
axilla -*see* Corrosion, axilla
elbow -*see* Corrosion, elbow
first degree T22.50
forearm -*see* Corrosion, forearm
hand -*see* Corrosion, hand
interscapular region -*see* Corrosion, back, upper
multiple sites T22.499
  first degree T22.599
  left T22.492
    first degree T22.592
    second degree T22.692
    third degree T22.792
  right T22.491
    first degree T22.591
    second degree T22.691
    third degree T22.791
  second degree T22.699
  third degree T22.799
scapular region -*see* Corrosion, scapular region
second degree T22.60
shoulder -*see* Corrosion, shoulder
third degree T22.70
wrist -*see* Corrosion, hand
uterus T28.8
vagina T28.8
vulva -*see* Corrosion, genital organs, external, female
wrist T23.479
first degree T23.579
left T23.472
  first degree T23.572
  second degree T23.672
  third degree T23.772
multiple sites with hand T23.499
  first degree T23.599
  left T23.492
    first degree T23.592
    second degree T23.692
    third degree T23.792
  right T23.491
    first degree T23.591
    second degree T23.691
    third degree T23.791
  second degree T23.699
  third degree T23.799
right T23.471
  first degree T23.571

Corrosion - *continued*

second degree T23.671
  third degree T23.771
second degree T23.679
  third degree T23.779
Corrosive burn -*see* Corrosion
Corsican fever -*see* Malaria
Cortical -*see* condition
Cortico-adrenal -*see* condition
Coryza (acute) J00
with grippe or influenza -*see* Influenza, with, respiratory manifestations NEC
syphilitic
  congenital (chronic) A50.05
Costen's syndrome or complex M26.69
Costiveness -*see* Constipation
Costochondritis M94.0
Cotard's syndrome F22
Cot death R99
Cotia virus B08.8
Cotton wool spots (retinal) H35.81
Cotugno's disease -*see* Sciatica
Cough (affected) (chronic) (epidemic) (nervous) R05
with hemorrhage -*see* Hemoptysis
bronchial R05
  with grippe or influenza -*see* Influenza, with, respiratory manifestations NEC
functional F45.8
hysterical F45.8
laryngeal, spasmodic R05
psychogenic F45.8
smokers' J41.0
tea taster's B49
Counseling (for) Z71.9
abuse NEC
  perpetrator Z69.82
  victim Z69.81
alcohol abuser Z71.41
  family Z71.42
child abuse
  nonparental
    perpetrator Z69.021
    victim Z69.020
  parental
    perpetrator Z69.011
    victim Z69.010
consanguinity Z71.89
contraceptive Z30.09
dietary Z71.3
drug abuser Z71.51
  family member Z71.52
family Z71.89
fertility preservation (prior to cancer therapy) (prior to removal of gonads) Z31.62
for non-attending third party Z71.0
  related to sexual behavior or orientation Z70.2
genetic NEC Z31.5
gestational carrier Z31.7
health (advice) (education) (instruction) -*see* Counseling, medical
human immunodeficiency virus (HIV) Z71.7
impotence Z70.1
insulin pump use Z46.81
medical (for) Z71.9
  boarding school resident Z59.3
  consanguinity Z71.89
  feared complaint and no disease found Z71.1
  human immunodeficiency virus (HIV) Z71.7
  institutional resident Z59.3

Counseling --*continued*

on behalf of another Z71.0
  related to sexual behavior or orientation Z70.2
person living alone Z60.2
specified reason NEC Z71.89
natural family planning
  procreative Z31.61
  to avoid pregnancy Z30.02
perpetrator (of)
  abuse NEC Z69.82
  child abuse
    non-parental Z69.021
    parental Z69.011
  rape NEC Z69.82
  spousal abuse Z69.12
procreative NEC Z31.69
  fertility preservation (prior to cancer therapy) (prior to removal of gonads) Z31.62
  using natural family planning Z31.61
promiscuity Z70.1
rape victim Z69.81
religious Z71.81
sex, sexual (related to) Z70.9
  attitude(s) Z70.0
  behavior or orientation Z70.1
  combined concerns Z70.3
  non-responsiveness Z70.1
  on behalf of third party Z70.2
  specified reason NEC Z70.8
specified reason NEC Z71.89
spiritual Z71.81
spousal abuse (perpetrator) Z69.12
  victim Z69.11
substance abuse Z71.89
  alcohol Z71.41
  drug Z71.51
  tobacco Z71.6
tobacco use Z71.6
use (of)
  insulin pump Z46.81
victim (of)
  abuse Z69.81
  child abuse
    by parent Z69.010
    non-parental Z69.020
  rape NEC Z69.81
Coupled rhythm R00.8
Couvelaire syndrome or uterus (complicating delivery) O45.8X
Cowperitis -*see* Urethritis
Cowper's gland -*see* condition
Cowpox B08.010
due to vaccination T88.1
Coxa
magna M91.4
plana M91.2
valga (acquired) -*see also* Deformity, limb, specified type NEC, thigh
  congenital Q65.81
  sequelae (late effect) of rickets E64.3
vara (acquired) -*see also* Deformity, limb, specified type NEC, thigh
  congenital Q65.82
  sequelae (late effect) of rickets E64.3
Coxalgia, coxalgic (nontuberculous) -*see also* Pain, joint, hip
tuberculous A18.02
Coxitis -*see* Monoarthritis, hip
Coxsackie (virus) (infection) B34.1

Coxsackie (virus) (infection) --*continued*
   as cause of disease classified elsewhere
      B97.11
   carditis B33.20
   central nervous system NEC A88.8
   endocarditis B33.21
   enteritis A08.39
   meningitis (aseptic) A87.0
   myocarditis B33.22
   pericarditis B33.23
   pharyngitis B08.5
   pleurodynia B33.0
   specific disease NEC B33.8
Crabs, meaning pubic lice B85.3
Crack baby P04.41
Cracked nipple N64.0
   associated with
      lactation O92.13
      pregnancy O92.11
      puerperium O92.12
Cracked tooth K03.81
Cradle cap L21.0
Craft neurosis F48.8
Cramp(s) R25.2
   abdominal -*see* Pain, abdominal
   bathing T75.1
   colic R10.83
      psychogenic F45.8
   due to immersion T75.1
   fireman T67.2
   heat T67.2
   immersion T75.1
   intestinal -*see* Pain, abdominal
      psychogenic F45.8
   leg, sleep related G47.62
   limb (lower) (upper) NEC R25.2
      sleep related G47.62
   linotypist's F48.8
      organic G25.89
   muscle (limb) (general) R25.2
      due to immersion T75.1
      psychogenic F45.8
   occupational (hand) F48.8
      organic G25.89
   salt-depletion E87.1
   sleep related, leg G47.62
   stoker's T67.2
   swimmer's T75.1
   telegrapher's F48.8
      organic G25.89
   typist's F48.8
      organic G25.89
   uterus N94.89
      menstrual -*see* Dysmenorrhea
   writer's F48.8
      organic G25.89
Cranial -*see* condition
Craniocleidodysostosis Q74.0
Craniofenestria (skull) Q75.8
Craniolacunia (skull) Q75.8
Craniopagus Q89.4
Craniopathy, metabolic M85.2
Craniopharyngeal -*see* condition
Craniopharyngioma D44.4
Craniorachischisis (totalis) Q00.1
Cranioschisis Q75.8
Craniostenosis Q75.0
Craniosynostosis Q75.0
Craniotabes (cause unknown) M83.8
   neonatal P96.3
   rachitic E64.3
   syphilitic A50.56

Cranium -*see* condition
Craw-craw -*see* Onchocerciasis
Creaking joint -*see* Derangement, joint,
   specified type NEC
Creeping
   eruption B76.9
   palsy or paralysis G12.22
Crenated tongue K14.8
Creotoxism A05.9
Crepitus
   caput Q75.8
   joint -*see* Derangement, joint, specified type
   NEC
Crescent or conus choroid, congenital Q14.3
CREST syndrome M34.1
Cretin, cretinism (congenital) (endemic)
   (nongoitrous) (sporadic) E00.9
   pelvis
      with disproportion (fetopelvic) O33.0
         causing obstructed labor O65.0
   type
      hypothyroid E00.1
      mixed E00.2
      myxedematous E00.1
      neurological E00.0
Creutzfeldt-Jakob disease or syndrome
   (with dementia) A81.00
   familial A81.09
   iatrogenic A81.09
   specified NEC A81.09
   sporadic A81.09
   variant (vCJD) A81.01
Crib death R99
Cribriform hymen Q52.3
Cri-du-chat syndrome Q93.4
Crigler-Najjar disease or syndrome E80.5
Crime, victim of Z65.4
Criminalism F60.2
Crisis
   abdomen R10.0
   acute reaction F43.0
   addisonian E27.2
   adrenal (cortical) E27.2
   celiac K90.0
   Dietl's N13.8
   emotional -*see also* Disorder, adjustment
      acute reaction to stress F43.0
      specific to childhood and adolescence F93.8
   glaucomatocyclitic -*see* Glaucoma,
   secondary, inflammation
   heart -*see* Failure, heart
   nitritoid I95.2
      correct substance properly administered -*see*
      Table of Drugs and Chemicals, by drug,
      adverse effect
      overdose or wrong substance given or taken
      -*see* Table of Drugs and Chemicals, by drug,
      poisoning
   oculogyric H51.8
      psychogenic F45.8
   Pel's (tabetic) A52.11
   psychosexual identity F64.2
   renal N28.0
   sickle-cell D57.00
      with
         acute chest syndrome D57.01
         splenic sequestration D57.02
   state (acute reaction) F43.0
   tabetic A52.11
   thyroid -*see* Thyrotoxicosis with thyroid
   storm

Crisis - *continued*
   thyrotoxic -*see* Thyrotoxicosis with thyroid
   storm
Crocq's disease (acrocyanosis) I73.89
Crohn's disease -*see* Enteritis, regional
Crooked septum, nasal J34.2
Cross syndrome E70.328
Crossbite (anterior) (posterior) M26.24
Cross-eye -*see* Strabismus, convergent
   concomitant
Croup, croupous (catarrhal) (infectious)
   (inflammatory) (non diphtheritic) J05.0
   bronchial J20.9
   diphtheritic A36.2
   false J38.5
   spasmodic J38.5
      diphtheritic A36.2
   stridulous J38.5
      diphtheritic A36.2
Crouzon's disease Q75.1
Crowding, tooth, teeth, fully erupted M26.31
CRST syndrome M34.1
Cruchet's disease A85.8
Cruelty in children -*see also* Disorder,
   conduct
Crural ulcer -*see* Ulcer, lower limb
Crush, crushed, crushing T14.8
   abdomen S38.1
   ankle S97.0
   arm (upper) (and shoulder) S47.   axilla -*see*
   Crush, arm
   back, lower S38.1
   buttock S38.1
   cheek S07.0
   chest S28.0
   cranium S07.1
   ear S07.0
   elbow S57.0
   extremity
      lower
         ankle -*see* Crush, ankle
         below knee -*see* Crush, leg
         foot -*see* Crush, foot
         hip -*see* Crush, hip
         knee -*see* Crush, knee
         thigh -*see* Crush, thigh
         toe -*see* Crush, toe
      upper
         below elbow S67.9
         elbow -*see* Crush, elbow
         finger -*see* Crush, finger
         forearm -*see* Crush, forearm
         hand -*see* Crush, hand
         thumb -*see* Crush, thumb
         upper arm -*see* Crush, arm
         wrist -*see* Crush, wrist
   face S07.0
   finger(s) S67.1
      with hand (and wrist) -*see* Crush, hand,
      specified site NEC
      index S67.19
      little S67.19
      middle S67.19
      ring S67.19
      thumb -*see* Crush, thumb
   foot S97.8
      toe -*see* Crush, toe - forearm S57.8
   genitalia, external
      female S38.002
         vagina S38.03
         vulva S38.03

Crush, crushed, crushing --*continued*
  male S38.001
    penis S38.01
    scrotum S38.02
    testis S38.02
  hand (except fingers alone) S67.2
    with wrist S67.4
  head S07.9
    specified NEC S07.8
  heel -*see* Crush, foot
  hip S77.0
    with thigh S77.2
  internal organ (abdomen, chest, or pelvis)
    NEC T14.8
  knee S87.0
  labium (majus) (minus) S38.03
  larynx S17.0
  leg (lower) S87.8
    knee -*see* Crush, knee - lip S07.0
  lower
    back S38.1
    leg -*see* Crush, leg
  neck S17.9
  nerve -*see* Injury, nerve
  nose S07.0
  pelvis S38.1
  penis S38.01
  scalp S07.8
  scapular region -*see* Crush, arm
  scrotum S38.02
  severe, unspecified site T14.8
  shoulder (and upper arm) -*see* Crush, arm
  skull S07.1
  syndrome (complication of trauma) T79.5
  testis S38.02
  thigh S77.1
    with hip S77.2
  throat S17.8
  thumb S67.0
    with hand (and wrist) -*see* Crush, hand,
    specified site NEC
  toe(s) S97.10
    great S97.11
    lesser S97.12
  trachea S17.0
  vagina S38.03
  vulva S38.03
  wrist S67.3
    with hand S67.4
Crusta lactea L21.0
Crusts R23.4
Crutch paralysis -*see* Injury, brachial plexus
Cruveilhier-Baumgarten cirrhosis, disease
or syndrome K74.69
Cruveilhier's atrophy or disease G12.8
Crying (constant) (continuous) (excessive)
  child, adolescent, or adult R45.83
  infant (baby) (newborn) R68.11
Cryofibrinogenemia D89.2
Cryoglobulinemia (essential) (idiopathic)
(mixed) (primary) (purpura) (secondary)
(vasculitis) D89.1
  with lung involvement D89.1 [*J99*]
Cryptitis (anal) (rectal) K62.89
Cryptococcosis, cryptococcus (infection)
(neoformans) B45.9
  bone B45.3
  cerebral B45.1
  cutaneous B45.2
  disseminated B45.7
  generalized B45.7

Cryptococcosis, cryptococcus --*continued*
  meningitis B45.1
  meningocerebralis B45.1
  osseous B45.3
  pulmonary B45.0
  skin B45.2
  specified NEC B45.8
Cryptopapillitis (anus) K62.89
Cryptophthalmos Q11.2
  syndrome Q87.0
Cryptorchid, cryptorchism, cryptorchidism
  Q53.9
  bilateral Q53.20
    abdominal Q53.21
    perineal Q53.22
  unilateral Q53.10
    abdominal Q53.11
    perineal Q53.12
Cryptosporidiosis A07.2
  hepatobiliary B88.8
  respiratory B88.8
Cryptostromosis J67.6
Crystalluria R82.99
Cubitus
  congenital Q68.8
  valgus (acquired) M21.0
    congenital Q68.8
    sequelae (late effect) of rickets E64.3
  varus (acquired) M21.1
    congenital Q68.8
    sequelae (late effect) of rickets E64.3
Cultural deprivation or shock Z60.3
Curling esophagus K22.4
Curling's ulcer -*see* Ulcer, peptic, acute
Curschmann (Batten) (Steinert) disease or
syndrome G71.11
Curse, Ondine's -*see* Apnea, sleep
Curvature
  organ or site, congenital NEC -*see* Distortion
  penis (lateral) Q55.61
  Pott's (spinal) A18.01
  radius, idiopathic, progressive (congenital)
  Q74.0
  spine (acquired) (angular) (idiopathic)
  (incorrect) (postural) -*see* Dorsopathy,
  deforming
    congenital Q67.5
    due to or associated with
      Charcot-Marie-Tooth disease -*see also*
      subcategory M49.8 G60.0
      osteitis
        deformans M88.88
        fibrosa cystica -*see also* subcategory
        M49.8 E21.0
      tuberculosis (Pott's curvature) A18.01
    sequelae (late effect) of rickets E64.3
    tuberculous A18.01
Cushingoid due to steroid therapy E24.2
  correct substance properly administered -*see*
  Table of Drugs and Chemicals, by drug,
  adverse effect
  overdose or wrong substance given or taken -
  see Table of Drugs and Chemicals, by drug,
  poisoning
Cushing's
  syndrome or disease E24.9
    drug-induced E24.2
    iatrogenic E24.2
    pituitary dependent E24.0
    specified NEC E24.8
  ulcer -*see* Ulcer, peptic, acute

Cusp, Carabelli omit code
Cut (external) -*see also* Laceration
  muscle -*see* Injury, muscle
Cutaneous -*see also* condition
  hemorrhage R23.3
  larva migrans B76.9
Cutis -*see also* condition
  hyperelastica Q82.8
    acquired L57.4
  laxa (hyperelastica) -*see* Dermatolysis
  marmorata R23.8
  osteosis L94.2
  pendula -*see* Dermatolysis
  rhomboidalis nuchae L57.2
  verticis gyrata Q82.8
    acquired L91.8
Cyanosis R23.0
  due to
    patent foramen botalli Q21.1
    persistent foramen ovale Q21.1
  enterogenous D74.8
  paroxysmal digital -*see* Raynaud's disease
    with gangrene I73.01
  retina, retinal H35.89
Cyanotic heart disease I24.9
  congenital Q24.9
Cycle
  anovulatory N97.0
  menstrual, irregular N92.6
Cyclencephaly Q04.9
Cyclical vomiting -*see also* Vomiting, cyclical
  G43.A0
  psychogenic F50.89
Cyclitis -*see also* Iridocyclitis H20.9
  chronic -*see* Iridocyclitis, chronic
  Fuchs' heterochromic H20.81
  granulomatous -*see* Iridocyclitis, chronic
  lens-induced -*see* Iridocyclitis, lens-induced
  posterior H30.2
Cycloid personality F34.0
Cyclophoria H50.54
Cyclopia, cyclops Q87.0
Cyclopism Q87.0
Cyclosporiasis A07.4
Cyclothymia F34.0
Cyclothymic personality F34.0
Cyclotropia H50.41
Cylindroma -*see also* Neoplasm, malignant,
  by site
  eccrine dermal -*see* Neoplasm, skin, benign
  skin -*see* Neoplasm, skin, benign
Cylindruria R82.99
Cynanche
  diphtheritic A36.2
  tonsillaris J36
Cynophobia F40.218
Cynorexia R63.2
Cyphosis -*see* Kyphosis
Cyprus fever -*see* Brucellosis
Cyst (colloid) (mucous) (simple) (retention)
  adenoid (infected) J35.8
  adrenal gland E27.8
    congenital Q89.1
  air, lung J98.4
  allantoic Q64.4
  alveolar process (jaw bone) M27.40
  amnion, amniotic O41.8X
  aneurysmal M27.49
  anterior
    chamber (eye) -*see* Cyst, iris
    nasopalatine K09.1

Cyst - *continued*
antrum J34.1
anus K62.89
apical (tooth) (periodontal) K04.8
appendix K38.8
arachnoid, brain (acquired) G93.0
  congenital Q04.6
arytenoid J38.7
Baker's M71.2
  ruptured M66.0
  tuberculous A18.02
Bartholin's gland N75.0
bile duct (common) (hepatic) K83.5
bladder (multiple) (trigone) N32.89
blue dome (breast) -*see* Cyst, breast
bone (local) NEC M85.60
  aneurysmal M85.50
    ankle M85.57
    foot M85.57
    forearm M85.53
    hand M85.54
    jaw M27.49
    lower leg M85.56
    multiple site M85.59
    neck M85.58
    rib M85.58
    shoulder M85.51
    skull M85.58
    specified site NEC M85.58
    thigh M85.55
    toe M85.57
    upper arm M85.52
    vertebra M85.58
  solitary M85.40
    ankle M85.47
    fibula M85.46
    foot M85.47
    hand M85.44
    humerus M85.42
    jaw M27.49
    neck M85.48
    pelvis M85.45
    radius M85.43
    rib M85.48
    shoulder M85.41
    skull M85.48
    specified site NEC M85.48
    tibia M85.46
    toe M85.47
    ulna M85.43
    vertebra M85.48
  specified type NEC M85.60
    ankle M85.67
    foot M85.67
    forearm M85.63
    hand M85.64
    jaw M27.40
      developmental (nonodontogenic) K09.1
        odontogenic K09.0
      latent M27.0
    lower leg M85.66
    multiple site M85.69
    neck M85.68
    rib M85.68
    shoulder M85.61
    skull M85.68
    specified site NEC M85.68
    thigh M85.65
    toe M85.67
    upper arm M85.62
    vertebra M85.68

Cyst - *continued*
brain (acquired) G93.0
  congenital Q04.6
  hydatid B67.99 [*G94]*
  third ventricle (colloid), congenital Q04.6
branchial (cleft) Q18.0
branchiogenic Q18.0
breast (benign) (blue dome) (pedunculated)
(solitary) N60.0
  involution -*see* Dysplasia, mammary,
specified type NEC
  sebaceous -*see* Dysplasia, mammary,
specified type NEC
broad ligament (benign) N83.8
bronchogenic (mediastinal) (sequestration)
J98.4
  congenital Q33.0
buccal K09.8
bulbourethral gland N36.8
bursa, bursal NEC M71.30
  with rupture -*see* Rupture, synovium
  ankle M71.37
  elbow M71.32
  foot M71.37
  hand M71.34
  hip M71.35
  multiple sites M71.39
  pharyngeal J39.2
  popliteal space -*see* Cyst, Baker's
  shoulder M71.31
  specified site NEC M71.38
  wrist M71.33
calcifying odontogenic D16.5
  upper jaw (bone) (maxilla) D16.4
canal of Nuck (female) N94.89
  congenital Q52.4
canthus -*see* Cyst, conjunctiva
carcinomatous -*see* Neoplasm, malignant, by
site
cauda equina G95.89
cavum septi pellucidi -*see* Cyst, brain
celomic (pericardium) Q24.8
cerebellopontine (angle) -*see* Cyst, brain
cerebellum -*see* Cyst, brain
cerebral -*see* Cyst, brain
cervical lateral Q18.0
cervix NEC N88.8
  embryonic Q51.6
  nabothian N88.8
chiasmal optic NEC -*see* Disorder, optic,
chiasm
chocolate (ovary) N80.1
choledochus, congenital Q44.4
chorion O41.8X
choroid plexus G93.0
ciliary body -*see* Cyst, iris
clitoris N90.7
colon K63.89
common (bile) duct K83.5
congenital NEC Q89.8
  adrenal gland Q89.1
  epiglottis Q31.8
  esophagus Q39.8
  fallopian tube Q50.4
  kidney Q61.00
    more than one (multiple) Q61.02
      specified as polycystic Q61.3
        adult type Q61.2
        infantile type NEC Q61.19
          collecting duct dilation Q61.11
    solitary Q61.01

Cyst - *continued*
larynx Q31.8
liver Q44.6
lung Q33.0
mediastinum Q34.1
ovary Q50.1
oviduct Q50.4
periurethral (tissue) Q64.79
prepuce Q55.69
salivary gland (any) Q38.4
sublingual Q38.6
submaxillary gland Q38.6
thymus (gland) Q89.2
tongue Q38.3
ureterovesical orifice Q62.8
vulva Q52.79
conjunctiva H11.44
cornea H18.89
corpora quadrigemina G93.0
corpus
  albicans N83.29
  luteum (hemorrhagic) (ruptured) N83.1
Cowper's gland (benign) (infected) N36.8
cranial meninges G93.0
craniobuccal pouch E23.6
craniopharyngeal pouch E23.6
cystic duct K82.8
Cysticercus -*see* Cysticercosis
Dandy Walker Q03.1
  with spina bifida -*see* Spina bifida
dental (root) K04.8
  developmental K09.0
  eruption K09.0
  primordial K09.0
dentigerous (mandible) (maxilla) K09.0
dermoid -*see* Neoplasm, benign, by site
  with malignant transformation C56.
  implantation
    external area or site (skin) NEC L72.0
    iris -*see* Cyst, iris, implantation
    vagina N89.8
    vulva N90.7
  mouth K09.8
  oral soft tissue K09.8
  sacrococcygeal -*see* Cyst, pilonidal
developmental K09.1
  odontogenic K09.0
  oral region (nonodontogenic) K09.1
  ovary, ovarian Q50.1
dura (cerebral) G93.0
  spinal G96.19
ear (external) Q18.1
echinococcal -*see* Echinococcus
embryonic
  cervix uteri Q51.6
  fallopian tube Q50.4
  vagina Q51.6
endometrium, endometrial (uterus) N85.8
  ectopic -*see* Endometriosis
enterogenous Q43.8
epidermal, epidermoid (inclusion) (see also
Cyst, skin) L72.0
  mouth K09.8
  oral soft tissue K09.8
epididymis N50.3
epiglottis J38.7
epiphysis cerebri E34.8
epithelial (inclusion) L72.0
epoophoron Q50.5
eruption K09.0
esophagus K22.8

Cyst - *continued*
ethmoid sinus J34.1
external female genital organs NEC N90.7
eye NEC H57.8
  congenital Q15.8
eyelid (sebaceous) H02.829
  infected -*see* Hordeolum
  left H02.826
    lower H02.825
    upper H02.824
  right H02.823
    lower H02.822
    upper H02.821
fallopian tube N83.8
  congenital Q50.4
fimbrial (twisted) Q50.4
fissural (oral region) K09.1
follicle (graafian) (hemorrhagic) N83.0
  nabothian N88.8
follicular (atretic) (hemorrhagic) (ovarian) N83.0
  dentigerous K09.0
  odontogenic K09.0
  skin L72.9
    specified NEC L72.8
frontal sinus J34.1
gallbladder K82.8
ganglion -*see* Ganglion
Gartner's duct Q52.4
gingiva K09.0
gland of Moll -*see* Cyst, eyelid
globulomaxillary K09.1
graafian follicle (hemorrhagic) N83.0
granulosal lutein (hemorrhagic) N83.1
hemangiomatous D18.00
  intra-abdominal D18.03
  intracranial D18.02
  skin D18.01
  specified site NEC D18.09
hemorrhagic M27.49
hydatid -*see also* Echinococcus B67.90
  brain B67.99 *[G94]*
  liver -*see also* Cyst, liver, hydatid B67.8
  lung NEC B67.99 *[J99]*
  Morgagni
    female Q50.5
    male (epididymal) Q55.4
      testicular Q55.29
  specified site NEC B67.99
hymen N89.8
  embryonic Q52.4
hypopharynx J39.2
hypophysis, hypophyseal (duct) (recurrent) E23.6
  cerebri E23.6
implantation (dermoid)
  external area or site (skin) NEC L72.0
  iris -*see* Cyst, iris, implantation
  vagina N89.8
  vulva N90.7
incisive canal K09.1
inclusion (epidermal) (epithelial) (epidermoid) (squamous) L72.0
  not of skin
    code under Cyst, by site
intestine (large) (small) K63.89
intracranial -*see* Cyst, brain
intraligamentous -*see also* Disorder, ligament
  knee -*see* Derangement, knee
intrasellar E23.6
iris H21.309

Cyst - *continued*
exudative H21.31
  idiopathic H21.30
  implantation H21.32
  parasitic H21.33
  pars plana (primary) H21.34
    exudative H21.35
jaw (bone) M27.40
  aneurysmal M27.49
  hemorrhagic M27.49
  traumatic M27.49
  developmental (odontogenic) K09.0
  fissural K09.1
joint NEC -*see* Disorder, joint, specified type NEC
kidney (acquired) N28.1
  calyceal -*see* Hydronephrosis
  congenital Q61.00
    more than one (multiple) Q61.02
      specified as polycystic Q61.3
        adult type (autosomal dominant) Q61.2
        infantile type (autosomal recessive) NEC Q61.19
          collecting duct dilation Q61.11
  pyelogenic -*see* Hydronephrosis
  simple N28.1
  solitary (single) Q61.01
    acquired N28.1
labium (majus) (minus) N90.7
  sebaceous N90.7
lacrimal -*see also* Disorder, lacrimal system, specified NEC
  gland H04.13
  passages or sac -*see* Disorder, lacrimal system, specified NEC
larynx J38.7
lateral periodontal K09.0
lens H27.8
  congenital Q12.8
lip (gland) K13.0
liver (idiopathic) (simple) K76.89
  congenital Q44.6
  hydatid B67.8
    granulosus B67.0
    multilocularis B67.5
lung J98.4
  congenital Q33.0
  giant bullous J43.9
lutein N83.1
lymphangiomatous D18.1
lymphoepithelial, oral soft tissue K09.8
macula -*see* Degeneration, macula, hole
malignant -*see* Neoplasm, malignant, by site
mammary gland -*see* Cyst, breast
mandible M27.40
  dentigerous K09.0
  radicular K04.8
maxilla M27.40
  dentigerous K09.0
  radicular K04.8
medial, face and neck Q18.8
median
  anterior maxillary K09.1
  palatal K09.1
mediastinum, congenital Q34.1
meibomian (gland) -*see* Chalazion
  infected -*see* Hordeolum
membrane, brain G93.0
meninges (cerebral) G93.0
  spinal G96.19

Cyst - *continued*
meniscus, knee -*see* Derangement, knee, meniscus, cystic
mesentery, mesenteric K66.8
  chyle I89.8
mesonephric duct
  female Q50.5
  male Q55.4
milk N64.89
Morgagni (hydatid)
  female Q50.5
  male (epididymal) Q55.4
    testicular Q55.29
mouth K09.8
Müllerian duct Q50.4
  appendix testis Q55.29
  cervix Q51.6
  fallopian tube Q50.4
  female Q50.4
  male Q55.29
  prostatic utricle Q55.4
  vagina (embryonal) Q52.4
multilocular (ovary) D39.10
  benign -*see* Neoplasm, benign, by site
myometrium N85.8
nabothian (follicle) (ruptured) N88.8
nasoalveolar K09.1
nasolabial K09.1
nasopalatine (anterior) (duct) K09.1
nasopharynx J39.2
neoplastic -*see* Neoplasm, uncertain behavior, by site
  benign -*see* Neoplasm, benign, by site
nervous system NEC G96.8
neuroenteric (congenital) Q06.8
nipple -*see* Cyst, breast
nose (turbinates) J34.1
  sinus J34.1
odontogenic, developmental K09.0
omentum (lesser) K66.8
  congenital Q45.8
ora serrata -*see* Cyst, retina, ora serrata
oral
  region K09.9
    developmental (nonodontogenic) K09.1
    specified NEC K09.8
  soft tissue K09.9
    specified NEC K09.8
orbit H05.81
ovary, ovarian (twisted) N83.20
  adherent N83.20
  chocolate N80.1
  corpus
    albicans N83.29
    luteum (hemorrhagic) N83.1
  dermoid D27.9
  developmental Q50.1
  due to failure of involution NEC N83.20
  endometrial N80.1
  follicular (graafian) (hemorrhagic) N83.0
  hemorrhagic N83.20
  in pregnancy or childbirth O34.8
    with obstructed labor O65.5
  multilocular D39.10
  pseudomucinous D27.9
  retention N83.29
  serous N83.20
  specified NEC N83.29
  theca lutein (hemorrhagic) N83.1
  tuberculous A18.18
oviduct N83.8

Cyst - *continued*
palate (median) (fissural) K09.1
palatine papilla (jaw) K09.1
pancreas, pancreatic (hemorrhagic) (true)
K86.2
  congenital Q45.2
  false K86.3
paralabral
  hip M24.85
  shoulder S43.43
paramesonephric duct Q50.4
  female Q50.4
  male Q55.29
paranephric N28.1
paraphysis, cerebri, congenital Q04.6
parasitic B89
parathyroid (gland) E21.4
paratubal N83.8
paraurethral duct N36.8
paroophoron Q50.5
parotid gland K11.6
parovarian Q50.5
pelvis, female N94.89
  in pregnancy or childbirth O34.8
    causing obstructed labor O65.5
penis (sebaceous) N48.89
periapical K04.8
pericardial (congenital) Q24.8
  acquired (secondary) I31.8
pericoronal K09.0
periodontal K04.8
  lateral K09.0
peripelvic (lymphatic) N28.1
peritoneum K66.8
  chylous I89.8
periventricular, acquired, newborn P91.1
pharynx (wall) J39.2
pilar L72.11
pilonidal (infected) (rectum) L05.91
  with abscess L05.01
  malignant C44.59
pituitary (duct) (gland) E23.6
placenta O43.19
pleura J94.8
popliteal -*see* Cyst, Baker's
porencephalic Q04.6
  acquired G93.0
postanal (infected) -*see* Cyst, pilonidal
postmastoidectomy cavity (mucosal) -*see*
Complications, postmastoidectomy, cyst
preauricular Q18.1
prepuce N47.4
  congenital Q55.69
primordial (jaw) K09.0
prostate N42.83
pseudomucinous (ovary) D27.9
pupillary, miotic H21.27
radicular (residual) K04.8
radiculodental K04.8
ranular K11.8
Rathke's pouch E23.6
rectum (epithelium) (mucous) K62.89
renal -*see* Cyst, kidney
residual (radicular) K04.8
retention (ovary) N83.29
  salivary gland K11.6
retina H33.19
  ora serrata H33.11
  parasitic H33.12
retroperitoneal K68.9
sacrococcygeal (dermoid) -*see* Cyst, pilonidal

Cyst - *continued*
salivary gland or duct (mucous extravasation
or retention) K11.6
Sampson's N80.1
sclera H15.89
scrotum L72.9
  sebaceous L72.3
sebaceous (duct) (gland) L72.3
  breast -*see* Dysplasia, mammary, specified
type NEC
  eyelid -*see* Cyst, eyelid
  genital organ NEC
    female N94.89
    male N50.89
  scrotum L72.3
semilunar cartilage (knee) (multiple) -*see*
Derangement, knee, meniscus, cystic
seminal vesicle N50.89
serous (ovary) N83.20
sinus (accessory) (nasal) J34.1
Skene's gland N36.8
skin L72.9
  breast -*see* Dysplasia, mammary, specified
type NEC
  epidermal, epidermoid L72.0
  epithelial L72.0
  eyelid -*see* Cyst, eyelid
  genital organ NEC
    female N90.7
    male N50.89
  inclusion L72.0
  scrotum L72.9
  sebaceous L72.3
  sweat gland or duct L74.8
solitary
  bone -*see* Cyst, bone, solitary
  jaw M27.40
  kidney N28.1
spermatic cord N50.89
sphenoid sinus J34.1
spinal meninges G96.19
spleen NEC D73.4
  congenital Q89.09
  hydatid -*see also* Echinococcus B67.99
[D77]
Stafne's M27.0
subarachnoid intrasellar R93.0
subcutaneous, pheomycotic (chromomycotic)
B43.2
subdural (cerebral) G93.0
  spinal cord G96.19
sublingual gland K11.6
submandibular gland K11.6
submaxillary gland K11.6
suburethral N36.8
suprarenal gland E27.8
suprasellar -*see* Cyst, brain
sweat gland or duct L74.8
synovial -*see also* Cyst, bursa
  ruptured -*see* Rupture, synovium
tarsal -*see* Chalazion
tendon (sheath) -*see* Disorder, tendon,
specified type NEC
testis N44.2
  tunica albuginea N44.1
theca lutein (ovary) N83.1
Thornwaldt's J39.2
thymus (gland) E32.8
thyroglossal duct (infected) (persistent) Q89.2
thyrolingual duct (infected) (persistent) Q89.2
thyroid (gland) E04.1

Cyst - *continued*
tongue K14.8
tonsil J35.8
tooth -*see* Cyst, dental
Tornwaldt's J39.2
trichilemmal (proliferating) L72.12
trichodermal L72.12
tubal (fallopian) N83.8
  inflammatory -*see* Salpingitis, chronic
tubo-ovarian N83.8
  inflammatory N70.13
tunica
  albuginea testis N44.1
  vaginalis N50.89
turbinate (nose) J34.1
Tyson's gland N48.89
urachus, congenital Q64.4
ureter N28.89
ureterovesical orifice N28.89
urethra, urethral (gland) N36.8
uterine ligament N83.8
uterus (body) (corpus) (recurrent) N85.8
  embryonic Q51.818
  cervix Q51.6
vagina, vaginal (implantation) (inclusion)
(squamous cell) (wall) N89.8
  embryonic Q52.4
vallecula, vallecular (epiglottis) J38.7
vesical (orifice) N32.89
vitreous body H43.89
vulva (implantation) (inclusion) N90.7
  congenital Q52.79
  sebaceous gland N90.7
vulvovaginal gland N90.7
wolffian
  female Q50.5
  male Q55.4
Cystadenocarcinoma -*see* Neoplasm,
malignant, by site
bile duct C22.1
endometrioid -*see* Neoplasm, malignant, by
site
  specified site -*see* Neoplasm, malignant, by
site
  unspecified site
    female C56.9
    male C61
mucinous
  papillary
    specified site -*see* Neoplasm, malignant, by
site
    unspecified site C56.9
  specified site -*see* Neoplasm, malignant, by
site
  unspecified site C56.9
papillary
  mucinous
    specified site -*see* Neoplasm, malignant, by
site
    unspecified site C56.9
  pseudomucinous
    specified site -*see* Neoplasm, malignant, by
site
    unspecified site C56.9
  serous
    specified site -*see* Neoplasm, malignant, by
site
    unspecified site C56.9
  specified site -*see* Neoplasm, malignant, by
site
  unspecified site C56.9

Cystadenocarcinoma - *continued*
  pseudomucinous
    papillary
      specified site -*see* Neoplasm, malignant, by site
      unspecified site C56.9
    specified site -*see* Neoplasm, malignant, by site
    unspecified site C56.9
  serous
    papillary
      specified site -*see* Neoplasm, malignant, by site
      unspecified site C56.9
    specified site -*see* Neoplasm, malignant, by site
    unspecified site C56.9

Cystadenofibroma
  clear cell -*see* Neoplasm, benign, by site
  endometrioid D27.9
    borderline malignancy D39.1
    malignant C56.
  mucinous
    specified site -*see* Neoplasm, benign, by site
    unspecified site D27.9
  serous
    specified site -*see* Neoplasm, benign, by site
    unspecified site D27.9
  specified site -*see* Neoplasm, benign, by site
  unspecified site D27.9

Cystadenoma -*see also* Neoplasm, benign, by site
  bile duct D13.4
  endometrioid -*see* Neoplasm, benign, by site
    borderline malignancy -*see* Neoplasm, uncertain behavior, by site
  malignant -*see* Neoplasm, malignant, by site
  mucinous
    borderline malignancy
      ovary C56.
      specified site NEC -*see* Neoplasm, uncertain behavior, by site
      unspecified site C56.9
    papillary
      borderline malignancy
        ovary C56.
        specified site NEC -*see* Neoplasm, uncertain behavior, by site
        unspecified site C56.9
      specified site -*see* Neoplasm, benign, by site
      unspecified site D27.9
    specified site -*see* Neoplasm, benign, by site
    unspecified site D27.9
  papillary
    borderline malignancy
      ovary C56.
      specified site NEC -*see* Neoplasm, uncertain behavior, by site
      unspecified site C56.9
    lymphomatosum
      specified site -*see* Neoplasm, benign, by site
      unspecified site D11.9
    mucinous
      borderline malignancy
        ovary C56.
        specified site NEC -*see* Neoplasm, uncertain behavior, by site
        unspecified site C56.9

Cystadenoma - *continued*
      specified site -*see* Neoplasm, benign, by site
      unspecified site D27.9
    pseudomucinous
      borderline malignancy
        ovary C56.
        specified site NEC -*see* Neoplasm, uncertain behavior, by site
        unspecified site C56.9
      specified site -*see* Neoplasm, benign, by site
      unspecified site D27.9
    serous
      borderline malignancy
        ovary C56.
        specified site NEC -*see* Neoplasm, uncertain behavior, by site
        unspecified site C56.9
      specified site -*see* Neoplasm, benign, by site
      unspecified site D27.9
  specified site -*see* Neoplasm, benign, by site
  unspecified site D27.9
  pseudomucinous
    borderline malignancy
      ovary C56.
      specified site NEC -*see* Neoplasm, uncertain behavior, by site
      unspecified site C56.9
    papillary
      borderline malignancy
        ovary C56.
        specified site NEC -*see* Neoplasm, uncertain behavior, by site
        unspecified site C56.9
      specified site -*see* Neoplasm, benign, by site
      unspecified site D27.9
    specified site -*see* Neoplasm, benign, by site
    unspecified site D27.9
  serous
    borderline malignancy
      ovary C56.
      specified site NEC -*see* Neoplasm, uncertain behavior, by site
      unspecified site C56.9
    papillary
      borderline malignancy
        ovary C56.
        specified site NEC -*see* Neoplasm, uncertain behavior, by site
        unspecified site C56.9
      specified site -*see* Neoplasm, benign, by site
      unspecified site D27.9
    specified site -*see* Neoplasm, benign, by site
    unspecified site D27.9

Cystathionine synthase deficiency E72.11
Cystathioninemia E72.19
Cystathioninuria E72.19
Cystic -*see also* condition
  breast (chronic) -*see* Mastopathy, cystic
  corpora lutea (hemorrhagic) N83.1
  duct -*see* condition
  eyeball (congenital) Q11.0
  fibrosis -*see* Fibrosis, cystic
  kidney (congenital) Q61.9
    adult type Q61.2
    infantile type NEC Q61.19
      collecting duct dilatation Q61.11

Cystic --*continued*
  medullary Q61.5
  liver, congenital Q44.6
  lung disease J98.4
    congenital Q33.0
  mastitis, chronic -*see* Mastopathy, cystic
  medullary, kidney Q61.5
  meniscus -*see* Derangement, knee, meniscus, cystic
  ovary N83.20
Cysticercosis, cysticerciasis B69.9
  with
    epileptiform fits B69.0
    myositis B69.81
  brain B69.0
  central nervous system B69.0
  cerebral B69.0
  ocular B69.1
  specified NEC B69.89
Cysticercus cellulose infestation -*see* Cysticercosis
Cystinosis (malignant) E72.04
Cystinuria E72.01
Cystitis (exudative) (hemorrhagic) (septic) (suppurative) N30.90
  with
    fibrosis -*see* Cystitis, chronic, interstitial
    hematuria N30.91
    leukoplakia -*see* Cystitis, chronic, interstitial
    malakoplakia -*see* Cystitis, chronic, interstitial
    metaplasia -*see* Cystitis, chronic, interstitial
    prostatitis N41.3
  acute N30.00
    with hematuria N30.01
    of trigone N30.30
      with hematuria N30.31
  allergic -*see* Cystitis, specified type NEC
  amebic A06.81
  bilharzial B65.9 [*N33*]
  blennorrhagic (gonococcal) A54.01
  bullous -*see* Cystitis, specified type NEC
  calculous N21.0
  chlamydial A56.01
  chronic N30.20
    with hematuria N30.21
    interstitial N30.10
      with hematuria N30.11
    of trigone N30.30
      with hematuria N30.31
    specified NEC N30.20
      with hematuria N30.21
  cystic (a) -*see* Cystitis, specified type NEC
  diphtheritic A36.85
  echinococcal
    granulosus B67.39
    multilocularis B67.69
  emphysematous -*see* Cystitis, specified type NEC
  encysted -*see* Cystitis, specified type NEC
  eosinophilic -*see* Cystitis, specified type NEC
  follicular -*see* Cystitis, of trigone
  gangrenous -*see* Cystitis, specified type NEC
  glandularis -*see* Cystitis, specified type NEC
  gonococcal A54.01
  incrusted -*see* Cystitis, specified type NEC
  interstitial (chronic) -*see* Cystitis, chronic, interstitial
  irradiation N30.40
    with hematuria N30.41
  irritation -*see* Cystitis, specified type NEC

Cystitis - *continued*
  malignant *-see* Cystitis, specified type NEC
  of trigone N30.30
    with hematuria N30.31
  panmural *-see* Cystitis, chronic, interstitial
  polyposa *-see* Cystitis, specified type NEC
  prostatic N41.3
  puerperal (postpartum) O86.22
  radiation *-see* Cystitis, irradiation
  specified type NEC N30.80
    with hematuria N30.81
  subacute *-see* Cystitis, chronic
  submucous *-see* Cystitis, chronic, interstitial
  syphilitic (late) A52.76
  trichomonal A59.03
  tuberculous A18.12
  ulcerative *-see* Cystitis, chronic, interstitial
Cystocele (urethrocele)
  female N81.10
    with prolapse of uterus *-see* Prolapse, uterus
    lateral N81.12
    midline N81.11
    paravaginal N81.12
  in pregnancy or childbirth O34.8
    causing obstructed labor O65.5
  male N32.89
Cystolithiasis N21.0
Cystoma *-see also* Neoplasm, benign, by site
  endometrial, ovary N80.1
  mucinous
    specified site *-see* Neoplasm, benign, by site
    unspecified site D27.9
  serous
    specified site *-see* Neoplasm, benign, by site
    unspecified site D27.9
  simple (ovary) N83.29
Cystoplegia N31.2
Cystoptosis N32.89
Cystopyelitis *-see* Pyelonephritis
Cystorrhagia N32.89
Cystosarcoma phyllodes D48.6
  benign D24
  malignant *-see* Neoplasm, breast, malignant
Cystostomy
  attention to Z43.5
  complication *-see* Complications, cystostomy
  status Z93.50
    appendico-vesicostomy Z93.52
    cutaneous Z93.51
    specified NEC Z93.59
Cystourethritis *-see* Urethritis
Cystourethrocele *-see also* Cystocele
  female N81.10
    with uterine prolapse *-see* Prolapse, uterus
    lateral N81.12
    midline N81.11
    paravaginal N81.12
  male N32.89
Cytomegalic inclusion disease congenital
  P35.1
Cytomegalovirus infection B25.9
Cytomycosis (reticuloendothelial) B39.4
Cytopenia D75.9
  refractory
    with multilineage dysplasia D46.A
      and ring sideroblasts (RCMD RS) D46.B
**Czerny's disease (periodic hydrarthrosis of
the knee)** *-see* Effusion, joint, knee

D

**Daae (Finsen) disease (epidemic
pleurodynia)** B33.0
Da Costa's syndrome F45.8
Dabney's grip B33.0
Dacryoadenitis, dacryadenitis H04.00
  acute H04.01
  chronic H04.02
Dacryocystitis H04.30
  acute H04.32
  chronic H04.41
  neonatal P39.1
  phlegmonous H04.31
  syphilitic A52.71
    congenital (early) A50.01
  trachomatous, active A71.1
    sequelae (late effect) B94.0
Dacryocystoblennorrhea *-see* Inflammation,
  lacrimal, passages, chronic
Dacryocystocele *-see* Disorder, lacrimal
  system, changes
Dacryolith, dacryolithiasis H04.51
Dacryoma *-see* Disorder, lacrimal system,
  changes
Dacryopericystitis *-see* Dacryocystitis
Dacryops H04.11
Dacryostenosis *-see also* Stenosis, lacrimal
  congenital Q10.5
Dactylitis
  bone *-see* Osteomyelitis
  sickle-cell D57.00
    Hb C D57.219
    Hb SS D57.00
    specified NEC D57.819
  skin L08.9
  syphilitic A52.77
  tuberculous A18.03
Dactylolysis spontanea (ainhum) L94.6
Dactylosymphysis Q70.9
  fingers *-see* Syndactylism, complex, fingers
  toes *-see* Syndactylism, complex, toes
Damage
  arteriosclerotic *-see* Arteriosclerosis
  brain (nontraumatic) G93.9
    anoxic, hypoxic G93.1
      resulting from a procedure G97.82
    child NEC G80.9
    due to birth injury P11.2
  cardiorenal (vascular) *-see* Hypertension,
  cardiorenal
  cerebral NEC *-see* Damage, brain
  coccyx, complicating delivery O71.6
  coronary *-see* Disease, heart, ischemic
  eye, birth injury P15.3
  liver (nontraumatic) K76.9
    alcoholic K70.9
    due to drugs *-see* Disease, liver, toxic
    toxic *-see* Disease, liver, toxic
  medication T88.7
  pelvic
    joint or ligament, during delivery O71.6
    organ NEC
      during delivery O71.5
      following ectopic or molar pregnancy
      O08.6
  renal *-see* Disease, renal
  subendocardium, subendocardial *-see*
  Degeneration, myocardial
  vascular I99.9

**Dana-Putnam syndrome (subacute
combined sclerosis with pernicious anemia)**
  -see Degeneration, combined
**Danbolt (Cross) syndrome (acrodermatitis
enteropathica)** E83.2
Dandruff L21.0
Dandy Walker syndrome Q03.1
  with spina bifida *-see* Spina bifida
Danlos' syndrome Q79.6
Darier (White) disease (congenital) Q82.8
  meaning erythema annulare centrifugum
  L53.1
Darier-Roussy sarcoid D86.3
Darling's disease or histoplasmosis B39.4
Darwin's tubercle Q17.8
Dawson's (inclusion body) encephalitis A81.1
De Beurmanni (Gougerot) disease B42.1
De la Tourette's syndrome F95.2
De Lange's syndrome Q87.1
De Morgan's spots (senile angiomas) I78.1
De Quervain's
  disease (tendon sheath) M65.4
  syndrome E34.51
  thyroiditis (subacute granulomatous
  thyroiditis) E06.1
De Toni-Fanconi (Debré) syndrome E72.09
  with cystinosis E72.04
Dead
  fetus, retained (mother) O36.4
    early pregnancy O02.1
  labyrinth *-see* subcategory H83.2
  ovum, retained O02.0
Deaf nonspeaking NEC H91.3
Deafmutism (acquired) (congenital) NEC
  H91.3
  hysterical F44.6
  syphilitic, congenital *-see also* subcategory
  H94.8 A50.09
**Deafness (acquired) (complete) (hereditary)
(partial)** H91.9
  with blue sclera and fragility of bone Q78.0
  auditory fatigue *-see* Deafness, specified type
  NEC
  aviation T70.0
    nerve injury *-see* Injury, nerve, acoustic,
  specified type NEC
  boilermaker's *-see* subcategory H83.3
  central *-see* Deafness, sensorineural
  conductive H90.2
    and sensorineural
      mixed H90.8
        bilateral H90.6
      bilateral H90.0
      unilateral H90.1
        with restricted hearing on the contralateral
  side H90.A- congenital H90.5
      with blue sclera and fragility of bone Q78.0
  due to toxic agents *-see* Deafness, ototoxic
  emotional (hysterical) F44.6
  functional (hysterical) F44.6
  high frequency H91.9
  hysterical F44.6
  low frequency H91.9
  mental R48.8
  mixed conductive and sensorineural H90.8
    bilateral H90.6
    unilateral H90.7
  nerve *-see* Deafness, sensorineural
  neural *-see* Deafness, sensorineural
  noise-induced *-see also* subcategory H83.3

Deafness - *continued*
  nerve injury *-see* Injury, nerve, acoustic,
  specified type NEC
  nonspeaking H91.3
  ototoxic *-see* subcategory H91.0
  perceptive *-see* Deafness, sensorineural
  psychogenic (hysterical) F44.6
  sensorineural H90.5
    and conductive
      mixed H90.8
        bilateral H90.6
      bilateral H90.3
      unilateral H90.4
        with restricted hearing on the contralateral
        side H90.A- sensory *-see* Deafness,
        sensorineural
  specified type NEC *-see* subcategory H91.8
  sudden (idiopathic) H91.2
  syphilitic A52.15
  transient ischemic H93.01
  traumatic *-see* Injury, nerve, acoustic,
  specified type NEC
  word (developmental) H93.25
Death (cause unknown) (of) (unexplained)
(unspecified cause) R99
  brain G93.82
  cardiac (sudden) (with successful
  resuscitation)
  code to underlying disease
    family history of Z82.41
    personal history of Z86.74
  family member (assumed) Z63.4
Debility (chronic) (general) (nervous) R53.81
  congenital or neonatal NOS P96.9
  nervous R53.81
  old age R54
  senile R54
Debove's disease (splenomegaly) R16.1
Decalcification
  bone *-see* Osteoporosis
  teeth K03.89
Decapsulation, kidney N28.89
Decay
  dental *-see* Caries, dental
  senile R54
  tooth, teeth *-see* Caries, dental **Deciduitis**
  (acute)
  following ectopic or molar pregnancy O08.0
Decline (general) *-see* Debility
  cognitive, age-associated R41.81
Decompensation
  cardiac (acute) (chronic) *-see* Disease, heart
  cardiovascular *-see* Disease, cardiovascular
  heart *-see* Disease, heart
  hepatic *-see* Failure, hepatic
  myocardial (acute) (chronic) *-see* Disease,
  heart
  respiratory J98.8
Decompression sickness T70.3
Decrease (d)
  absolute neutrophile count *-see* Neutropenia
  blood
    platelets *-see* Thrombocytopenia
    pressure R03.1
      due to shock following
        injury T79.4
        operation T81.19
  estrogen E28.39
    postablative E89.40
      asymptomatic E89.40
      symptomatic E89.41

Decrease (d) *--continued*
  fragility of erythrocytes D58.8
  function
    lipase (pancreatic) K90.3
    ovary in hypopituitarism E23.0
    parenchyma of pancreas K86.89
    pituitary (gland) (anterior) (lobe) E23.0
      posterior (lobe) E23.0
  functional activity R68.89
  glucose R73.09
  hematocrit R71.0
  hemoglobin R71.0
  leukocytes D72.819
    specified NEC D72.818
  libido R68.82
  lymphocytes D72.810
  platelets D69.6
  respiration, due to shock following injury
  T79.4
  sexual desire R68.82
  tear secretion NEC *-see* Syndrome, dry eye -
  tolerance
    fat K90.49
    glucose R73.09
    pancreatic K90.3
    salt and water E87.8
  vision NEC H54.7
  white blood cell count D72.819
    specified NEC D72.818
Decubitus (ulcer) *-see* Ulcer, pressure, by site
  cervix N86
Deepening acetabulum *-see* Derangement,
joint, specified type NEC, hip
Defect, defective Q89.9
  3 beta-hydroxysteroid dehydrogenase E25.0
  11 hydroxylase E25.0
  21 hydroxylase E25.0
  abdominal wall, congenital Q79.59
  antibody immunodeficiency D80.9
  aorticopulmonary septum Q21.4
  atrial septal (ostium secundum type) Q21.1
    following acute myocardial infarction
    (current complication) I23.1
    ostium primum type Q21.2
  atrioventricular
    canal Q21.2
    septum Q21.2
  auricular septal Q21.1
  bilirubin excretion NEC E80.6
  biosynthesis, androgen (testicular) E29.1
  bulbar septum Q21.0
  catalase E80.3
  cell membrane receptor complex (CR3) D71
  circulation I99.9
    congenital Q28.9
    newborn Q28.9
  coagulation (factor) *-see also* Deficiency,
  factor D68.9
    with
      ectopic pregnancy O08.1
      molar pregnancy O08.1
    acquired D68.4
    antepartum with hemorrhage *-see*
    Hemorrhage, antepartum, with coagulation
    defect
    due to
      liver disease D68.4
      vitamin K deficiency D68.4
    hereditary NEC D68.2
    intrapartum O67.0
    newborn, transient P61.6

Defect, defective *--continued*
  postpartum O72.3
    specified type NEC D68.8
  complement system D84.1
  conduction (heart) I45.9
    bone *-see* Deafness, conductive
  congenital, organ or site not listed *-see*
  Anomaly, by site
  coronary sinus Q21.1
  cushion, endocardial Q21.2
  degradation, glycoprotein E77.1
  dental bridge, crown, fillings *-see* Defect,
  dental restoration
  dental restoration K08.50
    specified NEC K08.59
  dentin (hereditary) K00.5
  Descemet's membrane, congenital Q13.89
  developmental *-see also* Anomaly
    cauda equina Q06.3
  diaphragm
    with elevation, eventration or hernia *-see*
    Hernia, diaphragm
    congenital Q79.1
      with hernia Q79.0
      gross (with hernia) Q79.0
  ectodermal, congenital Q82.9
  Eisenmenger's Q21.8
  enzyme
    catalase E80.3
    peroxidase E80.3
  esophagus, congenital Q39.9
  extensor retinaculum M62.89
  fibrin polymerization D68.2
  filling
    bladder R93.41
    kidney R93.42
    renal pelvis R93.41
    stomach R93.3
    ureter R93.41
    urinary organs, specified NEC R93.49
  Gerbode Q21.0
  glycoprotein degradation E77.1
  Hageman (factor) D68.2
  hearing *-see* Deafness
  high grade F70
  interatrial septal Q21.1
  interauricular septal Q21.1
  interventricular septal Q21.0
    with dextroposition of aorta, pulmonary
    stenosis and hypertrophy of right ventricle
    Q21.3
    in tetralogy of Fallot Q21.3
  learning (specific) *-see* Disorder, learning
  lymphocyte function antigen-1 (LFA-1)
  D84.0
  lysosomal enzyme, post-translational
  modification E77.0
  major osseous M89.70
    ankle M89.77
    carpus M89.74
    clavicle M89.71
    femur M89.75
    fibula M89.76
    fingers M89.74
    foot M89.77
    forearm M89.73
    hand M89.74
    humerus M89.72
    lower leg M89.76
    metacarpus M89.74
    metatarsus M89.77

Defect, defective --*continued*
  multiple sites M89.79
  pelvic region M89.75
  pelvis M89.75
  radius M89.73
  scapula M89.71
  shoulder region M89.71
  specified NEC M89.78
  tarsus M89.77
  thigh M89.75
  tibia M89.76
  toes M89.77
  ulna M89.73
  mental -*see* Disability, intellectual
  modification, lysosomal enzymes, post-
    translational E77.0
  obstructive, congenital
    renal pelvis Q62.39
    ureter Q62.39
      atresia -*see* Atresia, ureter
      cecoureterocele Q62.32
      megaureter Q62.2
      orthotopic ureterocele Q62.31
  osseous, major M89.70
    ankle M89.77
    carpus M89.74
    clavicle M89.71
    femur M89.75
    fibula M89.76
    fingers M89.74
    foot M89.77
    forearm M89.73
    hand M89.74
    humerus M89.72
    lower leg M89.76
    metacarpus M89.74
    metatarsus M89.77
    multiple sites M89.9
    pelvic region M89.75
    pelvis M89.75
    radius M89.73
    scapula M89.71
    shoulder region M89.71
    specified NEC M89.78
    tarsus M89.77
    thigh M89.75
    tibia M89.76
    toes M89.77
    ulna M89.73
  osteochondral NEC -*see also* Deformity
    M95.8
  ostium
    primum Q21.2
    secundum Q21.1
  peroxidase E80.3
  placental blood supply -*see* Insufficiency,
    placental
  platelets, qualitative D69.1
    constitutional D68.0
  postural NEC, spine -*see* Dorsopathy,
    deforming
  reduction
    limb Q73.8
      lower Q72.9
        absence -*see* Agenesis, leg
          foot -*see* Agenesis, foot
        longitudinal
          femur Q72.4
          fibula Q72.6
          tibia Q72.5
      specified type NEC Q72.89

Defect, defective --*continued*
  split foot Q72.7
  specified type NEC Q73.8
  upper Q71.9
    absence -*see* Agenesis, arm
      forearm -*see* Agenesis, forearm
      hand -*see* Agenesis, hand
    lobster-claw hand Q71.6
    longitudinal
      radius Q71.4
      ulna Q71.5
    specified type NEC Q71.89
  renal pelvis Q63.8
    obstructive Q62.39
  respiratory system, congenital Q34.9
  restoration, dental K08.50
    specified NEC K08.59
  retinal nerve bundle fibers H35.89
  septal (heart) NOS Q21.9
    acquired (atrial) (auricular) (ventricular)
    (old) I51.0
    atrial Q21.1
      concurrent with acute myocardial
        infarction -*see* Infarct, myocardium
      following acute myocardial infarction
        (current complication) I23.1
      ventricular -*see also* Defect, ventricular
    septal Q21.0
  sinus venosus Q21.1
  speech R47.9
    developmental F80.9
    specified NEC R47.89
  Taussig-Bing (aortic transposition and
    overriding pulmonary artery) Q20.1
  teeth, wedge K03.1
  vascular (local) I99.9
    congenital Q27.9
  ventricular septal Q21.0
    concurrent with acute myocardial infarction
    -*see* Infarct, myocardium
      following acute myocardial infarction
        (current complication) I23.2
      in tetralogy of Fallot Q21.3
  vision NEC H54.7
  visual field H53.40
    bilateral
      heteronymous H53.47
      homonymous H53.46
    generalized contraction H53.48
    localized
      arcuate H53.43
      scotoma (central area) H53.41
        blind spot area H53.42
      sector H53.43
    specified type NEC H53.45
  voice R49.9
    specified NEC R49.8
  wedge, tooth, teeth (abrasion) K03.1
Deferentitis N49.1
  gonorrheal (acute) (chronic) A54.23
Defibrination (syndrome) D65
  antepartum -*see* Hemorrhage, antepartum,
    with coagulation defect, disseminated
    intravascular coagulation
  following ectopic or molar pregnancy O08.1
  intrapartum O67.0
  newborn P60
  postpartum O72.3
Deficiency, deficient
  3 beta hydroxysteroid dehydrogenase E25.0

Deficiency, deficient - *continued*
  5 alpha reductase (with male
    pseudohermaphroditism) E29.1
  11 hydroxylase E25.0
  21 hydroxylase E25.0
  abdominal muscle syndrome Q79.4
  accelerator globulin (Ac G) (blood) D68.2
  AC globulin (congenital) (hereditary) D68.2
    acquired D68.4
  acid phosphatase E83.39
  activating factor (blood) D68.2
  adenosine deaminase (ADA) D81.3
  aldolase (hereditary) E74.19
  alpha-1 antitrypsin E88.01
  amino-acids E72.9
  anemia -*see* Anemia
  aneurin E51.9
  antibody with
    hyperimmunoglobulinemia D80.6
    near-normal immunoglobins D80.6
  antidiuretic hormone E23.2
  anti-hemophilic
    factor (A) D66
      B D67
      C D68.1
    globulin (AHG) NEC D66
  antithrombin (antithrombin III) D68.59
  ascorbic acid E54
  attention (disorder) (syndrome) F98.8
    with hyperactivity -*see* Disorder, attention-
  deficit hyperactivity   autoprothrombin
    I D68.2
    II D67
    C D68.2
  beta-glucuronidase E76.29
  biotin E53.8
  biotin-dependent carboxylase D81.819
  biotinidase D81.810
  brancher enzyme (amylopectinosis) E74.03
  calciferol E55.9
    with
      adult osteomalacia M83.8
      rickets -*see* Rickets
  calcium (dietary) E58
  calorie, severe E43
    with marasmus E41
      and kwashiorkor E42
  cardiac -*see* Insufficiency, myocardial
  carnitine E71.40
    due to
      hemodialysis E71.43
      inborn errors of metabolism E71.42
      Valproic acid therapy E71.43
    iatrogenic E71.43
    muscle palmitoyltransferase E71.314
    primary E71.41
    secondary E71.448
  carotene E50.9
  central nervous system G96.8
  ceruloplasmin (Wilson) E83.01
  choline E53.8
  Christmas factor D67
  chromium E61.4
  clotting (blood) -*see also* Deficiency,
    coagulation factor D68.9
  clotting factor NEC (hereditary) -*see also*
    Deficiency, factor D68.2
  coagulation NOS D68.9
    with
      ectopic pregnancy O08.1
      molar pregnancy O08.1

Deficiency, deficient - *continued*
  acquired (any) D68.4
  antepartum hemorrhage -*see* Hemorrhage,
  antepartum, with coagulation defect
  clotting factor NEC -*see also* Deficiency,
  factor D68.2
  due to
    hyperprothrombinemia D68.4
    liver disease D68.4
    vitamin K deficiency D68.4
  newborn, transient P61.6
  postpartum O72.3
  specified NEC D68.8
cognitive F09
color vision H53.50
  achromatopsia H53.51
  acquired H53.52
  deuteranomaly H53.53
  protanomaly H53.54
  specified type NEC H53.59
  tritanomaly H53.55
combined glucocorticoid and
  mineralocorticoid E27.49
contact factor D68.2
copper (nutritional) E61.0
corticoadrenal E27.40
  primary E27.1
craniofacial axis Q75.0
cyanocobalamin E53.8
C1 esterase inhibitor (C1 INH) D84.1
debrancher enzyme (limit dextrinosis) E74.03
dehydrogenase
  long chain/very long chain acyl CoA
    E71.310
  medium chain acyl CoA E71.311
  short chain acyl CoA E71.312
diet E63.9
dihydropyrimidine dehydrogenase (DPD)
  E88.89
disaccharidase E73.9
edema -*see* Malnutrition, severe
endocrine E34.9
energy supply -*see* Malnutrition
enzymes, circulating NEC E88.09
ergosterol E55.9
  with
    adult osteomalacia M83.8
    rickets -*see* Rickets
essential fatty acid (EFA) E63.0
factor -*see also* Deficiency, coagulation
  Hageman D68.2
  I (congenital) (hereditary) D68.2
  II (congenital) (hereditary) D68.2
  IX (congenital) (functional) (hereditary)
    (with functional defect) D67
  multiple (congenital) D68.8
    acquired D68.4
  V (congenital) (hereditary) D68.2
  VII (congenital) (hereditary) D68.2
  VIII (congenital) (functional) (hereditary)
    (with functional defect) D66
    with vascular defect D68.0
  X (congenital) (hereditary) D68.2
  XI (congenital) (hereditary) D68.1
  XII (congenital) (hereditary) D68.2
  XIII (congenital) (hereditary) D68.2
femoral, proximal focal (congenital) -*see*
  Defect, reduction, lower limb, longitudinal,
  femur
fibrin-stabilizing factor (congenital)
  (hereditary) D68.2

Deficiency, deficient - *continued*
  acquired D68.4
  fibrinase D68.2
  fibrinogen (congenital) (hereditary) D68.2
    acquired D65
  folate E53.8
  folic acid E53.8
  foreskin N47.3
  fructokinase E74.11
  fructose 1,6 diphosphatase E74.19
  fructose-1 phosphate aldolase E74.19
  galactokinase E74.29
  galactose-1 phosphate uridyl transferase
    E74.29
  gammaglobulin in blood D80.1
    hereditary D80.0
  glass factor D68.2
  glucocorticoid E27.49
    mineralocorticoid E27.49
  glucose-6 phosphatase E74.01
  glucose-6 phosphate dehydrogenase anemia
    D55.0
  glucuronyl transferase E80.5
  glycogen synthetase E74.09
  gonadotropin (isolated) E23.0
  growth hormone (idiopathic) (isolated) E23.0
  Hageman factor D68.2
  hemoglobin D64.9
  hepatophosphorylase E74.09
  homogentisate 1,2 dioxygenase E70.29
  hormone
    anterior pituitary (partial) NEC E23.0
      growth E23.0
    growth (isolated) E23.0
    pituitary E23.0
    testicular E29.1
  hypoxanthine- (guanine)
    phosphoribosyltransferase (HG- PRT) (total
    H-PRT) E79.1
  immunity D84.9
    cell-mediated D84.8
      with thrombocytopenia and eczema D82.0
    combined D81.9
    humoral D80.9
    IgA (secretory) D80.2
    IgG D80.3
    IgM D80.4
  immuno -*see* Immunodeficiency
  immunoglobulin, selective
    A (IgA) D80.2
    G (IgG) (subclasses) D80.3
    M (IgM) D80.4
  inositol (B complex) E53.8
  intrinsic
    factor (congenital) D51.0
    sphincter N36.42
      with urethral hypermobility N36.43
  iodine E61.8
    congenital syndrome -*see* Syndrome, iodine-
    deficiency, congenital
  iron E61.1
    anemia D50.9
  kalium E87.6
  kappa-light chain D80.8
  labile factor (congenital) (hereditary) D68.2
    acquired D68.4
  lacrimal fluid (acquired) -*see also* Syndrome,
  dry eye
    congenital Q10.6
    congenital E73.0
    secondary E73.1

Deficiency, deficient - *continued*
  lactase
    Laki-Lorand factor D68.2
  lecithin cholesterol acyltransferase E78.6
  lipocaic K86.89
  lipoprotein (familial) (high density) E78.6
  liver phosphorylase E74.09
  lysosomal alpha-1, 4 glucosidase E74.02
  magnesium E61.2
  major histocompatibility complex
    class I D81.6
    class II D81.7
  manganese E61.3
  menadione (vitamin K) E56.1
    newborn P53
  mental (familial) (hereditary) -*see* Disability,
    intellectual
  methylenetetrahydrofolate reductase
    (MTHFR) E72.12
  mevalonate kinase M04.1
  mineral NEC E61.8
  mineralocorticoid E27.49
    with glucocorticoid E27.49
  molybdenum (nutritional) E61.5
  moral F60.2
  multiple nutrient elements E61.7
  muscle
    carnitine (palmitoyltransferase) E71.314
    phosphofructokinase E74.09
  myoadenylate deaminase E79.2
  myocardial -*see* Insufficiency, myocardial
  myophosphorylase E74.04
  NADH diaphorase or reductase (congenital)
    D74.0
  NADH-methemoglobin reductase (congenital)
    D74.0
  natrium E87.1
  niacin (amide) (tryptophan) E52
  nicotinamide E52
  nicotinic acid E52
  number of teeth -*see* Anodontia
  nutrient element E61.9
    multiple E61.7
    specified NEC E61.8
  nutrition, nutritional E63.9
    sequelae -*see* Sequelae, nutritional
    deficiency
    specified NEC E63.8
  of interleukin 1
  receptor antagonist [DIRA] M04.8
  ornithine transcarbamylase E72.4
  ovarian E28.39
  oxygen -*see* Anoxia
  pantothenic acid E53.8
  parathyroid (gland) E20.9
  perineum (female) N81.89
  phenylalanine hydroxylase E70.1
  phosphoenolpyruvate carboxykinase E74.4
  phosphofructokinase E74.19
  phosphomannomutase E74.8
  phosphomannose isomerase E74.8
  phosphomannosyl mutase E74.8
  phosphorylase kinase, liver E74.09
  pituitary hormone (isolated) E23.0
  plasma thromboplastin
    antecedent (PTA) D68.1
    component (PTC) D67
  platelet NEC D69.1
    constitutional D68.0
  polyglandular E31.8
    autoimmune E31.0

Deficiency, deficient - *continued*
  potassium (K) E87.6
  prepuce N47.3
  proaccelerin (congenital) (hereditary) D68.2
    acquired D68.4
  proconvertin factor (congenital) (hereditary)
      D68.2
    acquired D68.4
  protein *-see also* Malnutrition E46
    anemia D53.0
    C D68.59
    S D68.59
  prothrombin (congenital) (hereditary) D68.2
    acquired D68.4
  Prower factor D68.2
  pseudocholinesterase E88.09
  PTA (plasma thromboplastin antecedent)
      D68.1
  PTC (plasma thromboplastin component) D67
  purine nucleoside phosphorylase (PNP) D81.5
  pyracin (alpha) (beta) E53.1
  pyridoxal E53.1
  pyridoxamine E53.1
  pyridoxine (derivatives) E53.1
  pyruvate
    carboxylase E74.4
    dehydrogenase E74.4
  riboflavin (vitamin B2) E53.0
  salt E87.1
  secretion
    ovary E28.39
    salivary gland (any) K11.7
    urine R34
  selenium (dietary) E59
  serum antitrypsin, familial E88.01
  short stature homeobox gene (SHOX)
    with
      dyschondrosteosis Q78.8
      short stature (idiopathic) E34.3
      Turner's syndrome Q96.9
  sodium (Na) E87.1
  SPCA (factor VII) D68.2
  sphincter, intrinsic N36.42
    with urethral hypermobility N36.43
  stable factor (congenital) (hereditary) D68.2
    acquired D68.4
  Stuart-Prower (factor X) D68.2
  sucrase E74.39
  sulfatase E75.29
  sulfite oxidase E72.19
  thiamin, thiaminic (chloride) E51.9
    beriberi (dry) E51.11
      wet E51.12
  thrombokinase D68.2
    newborn P53
  thyroid (gland) *-see* Hypothyroidism
  tocopherol E56.0
  tooth bud K00.0
  transcobalamine II (anemia) D51.2
  vanadium E61.6
  vascular I99.9
  vasopressin E23.2
  vertical ridge K06.8
  viosterol *-see* Deficiency, calciferol
  vitamin (multiple) NOS E56.9
    A E50.9
      with
        Bitot's spot (corneal) E50.1
        follicular keratosis E50.8
        keratomalacia E50.4
        manifestations NEC E50.8

      night blindness E50.5
      scar of cornea, xerophthalmic E50.6
      xeroderma E50.8
      xerophthalmia E50.7
      xerosis
        conjunctival E50.0
          and Bitot's spot E50.1
        cornea E50.2
          and ulceration E50.3
      sequelae E64.1
    B (complex) NOS E53.9
      with
        beriberi (dry) E51.11
          wet E51.12
        pellagra E52
    B1 NOS E51.9
      beriberi (dry) E51.11
        with circulatory system manifestations
            E51.11
        wet E51.12
    B12 E53.8
    B2 (riboflavin) E53.0
    B6 E53.1
    C E54
      sequelae E64.2
    D E55.9
      with
        adult osteomalacia M83.8
        rickets *-see* Rickets
        25 hydroxylase E83.32
    E E56.0
    folic acid E53.8
    G E53.0
    group B E53.9
      specified NEC E53.8
    H (biotin) E53.8
    K E56.1
      of newborn P53
    nicotinic E52
    P E56.8
    PP (pellagra-preventing) E52
    specified NEC E56.8
    thiamin E51.9
      beriberi *-see* Beriberi
  zinc, dietary E60
Deficit *-see also* Deficiency
  attention and concentration R41.840
    following
      cerebral infarction I69.310
      cerebrovascular disease I69.910
        specified disease NEC I69.810
      nontraumatic
        intracerebral hemorrhage I69.110
        specified intracranial hemorrhage NEC
            I69.210
        subarachnoid hemorrhage I69.010
  disorder *-see* Attention, deficit
  cognitive
    communication R41.841
    emotional
      following
        cerebral infarction I69.315
        cerebrovascular disease I69.915
          specified disease NEC I69.815
        nontraumatic
          intracerebral hemorrhage I69.115
          specified intracranial hemorrhage NEC
              I69.215
      cerebral infarction I69.319
      cerebrovascular disease I69.919
        subarachnoid hemorrhage I69.015

Deficit *--continued*
  following
    specified disease NEC I69.819
    nontraumatic
      intracerebral hemorrhage I69.119
      specified intracranial hemorrhage NEC
          I69.219
      subarachnoid hemorrhage I69.019
  social
    following
      cerebral infarction I69.315
      cerebrovascular disease I69.915
        specified disease NEC I69.815
      nontraumatic
        intracerebral hemorrhage I69.115
        specified intracranial hemorrhage NEC
            I69.215
        subarachnoid hemorrhage I69.015
  cognitive NEC R41.89
    following
      cerebral infarction I69.318
      cerebrovascular disease I69.918
        specified disease NEC I69.818
      nontraumatic
        intracerebral hemorrhage I69.118
        specified intracranial hemorrhage NEC
            I69.218
        subarachnoid hemorrhage I69.018
  concentration R41.840
  executive function R41.844
    following
      cerebral infarction I69.314
      cerebrovascular disease I69.914
        specified disease NEC I69.814
      nontraumatic
        intracerebral hemorrhage I69.114
        specified intracranial hemorrhage NEC
            I69.214
        subarachnoid hemorrhage I69.014
  frontal lobe R41.844
    following
      cerebral infarction I69.314
      cerebrovascular disease I69.914
        specified disease NEC I69.814
      nontraumatic
        intracerebral hemorrhage I69.114
        specified intracranial hemorrhage NEC
            I69.214
        subarachnoid hemorrhage I69.014
  memory
    following
      cerebral infarction I69.311
      cerebrovascular disease I69.911
        specified disease NEC I69.811
      nontraumatic
        intracerebral hemorrhage I69.111
        specified intracranial hemorrhage NEC
            I69.211
        subarachnoid hemorrhage I69.011
  neurologic NEC R29.818
    ischemic
      reversible (RIND) I63.9
        prolonged (PRIND) I63.9
  oxygen R09.02
  prolonged reversible ischemic neurologic
      (PRIND) I63.9
  psychomotor R41.843
    following
      cerebral infarction I69.313
      cerebrovascular disease I69.913
        specified disease NEC I69.813

Deficit --*continued*
  nontraumatic
    intracerebral hemorrhage I69.113
    specified intracranial hemorrhage NEC
      I69.213
    subarachnoid hemorrhage I69.013
  visuospatial R41.842
  following
    cerebral infarction I69.312
    cerebrovascular disease I69.912
      specified disease NEC I69.812
    nontraumatic
      intracerebral hemorrhage I69.112
      specified intracranial hemorrhage NEC
        I69.212
      subarachnoid hemorrhage I69.012

Deflection
  radius -*see* Deformity, limb, specified type
    NEC, forearm
  septum (acquired) (nasal) (nose) J34.2
  spine -*see* Curvature, spine
  turbinate (nose) J34.2

Defluvium
  capillorum -*see* Alopecia
  ciliorum -*see* Madarosis
  unguium L60.8

Deformity Q89.9
  abdomen, congenital Q89.9
  abdominal wall
    acquired M95.8
    congenital Q79.59
  acquired (unspecified site) M95.9
  adrenal gland Q89.1
  alimentary tract, congenital Q45.9
    upper Q40.9
  ankle (joint) (acquired) -*see also* Deformity,
    limb, lower leg
    abduction -*see* Contraction, joint, ankle
    congenital Q68.8
    contraction -*see* Contraction, joint, ankle
    specified type NEC -*see* Deformity, limb,
      foot, specified NEC
  anus (acquired) K62.89
    congenital Q43.9
  aorta (arch) (congenital) Q25.40
    acquired I77.89
  aortic
    arch, acquired I77.89
    cusp or valve (congenital) Q23.8
      acquired -*see also* Endocarditis, aortic
        I35.8
  arm (acquired) (upper) -*see also* Deformity,
    limb, upper arm
    congenital Q68.8
    forearm -*see* Deformity, limb, forearm
  artery (congenital) (peripheral) NOS Q27.9
    acquired I77.89
    coronary (acquired) I25.9
      congenital Q24.5
    umbilical Q27.0
  atrial septal Q21.1
  auditory canal (external) (congenital) -*see
    also* Malformation, ear, external
    acquired -*see* Disorder, ear, external,
      specified type NEC
  auricle
    ear (congenital) -*see also* Malformation, ear,
      external
      acquired -*see* Disorder, pinna, deformity
  bile duct (common) (congenital) (hepatic)
    Q44.5

Deformity --*continued*
  back -*see* Dorsopathy, deforming
    acquired K83.8
  biliary duct or passage (congenital) Q44.5
    acquired K83.8
  bladder (neck) (trigone) (sphincter) (acquired)
    N32.89
    congenital Q64.79
  bone (acquired) NOS M95.9
    congenital Q79.9
    turbinate M95.0
  brain (congenital) Q04.9
    acquired G93.89
    reduction Q04.3
  breast (acquired) N64.89
    congenital Q83.9
    reconstructed N65.0
  bronchus (congenital) Q32.4
    acquired NEC J98.09
  bursa, congenital Q79.9
  canaliculi (lacrimalis) (acquired) -*see also*
    Disorder, lacrimal system, changes
    congenital Q10.6
  canthus, acquired -*see* Disorder, eyelid,
    specified type NEC
  capillary (acquired) I78.8
  cardiovascular system, congenital Q28.9
  caruncle, lacrimal (acquired) -*see also*
    Disorder, lacrimal system, changes
    congenital Q10.6
  cascade, stomach K31.2
  cecum (congenital) Q43.9
    acquired K63.89
  cerebral, acquired G93.89
    congenital Q04.9
  cervix (uterus) (acquired) NEC N88.8
    congenital Q51.9
  cheek (acquired) M95.2
    congenital Q18.9
  chest (acquired) (wall) M95.4
    congenital Q67.8
    sequelae (late effect) of rickets E64.3
  chin (acquired) M95.2
    congenital Q18.9
  choroid (congenital) Q14.3
    acquired H31.8
    plexus Q07.8
      acquired G96.19
  cicatricial -*see* Cicatrix
  cilia, acquired -*see* Disorder, eyelid, specified
    type NEC
  clavicle (acquired) M95.8
    congenital Q68.8
  clitoris (congenital) Q52.6
    acquired N90.89
  clubfoot -*see* Clubfoot
  coccyx (acquired) -*see* subcategory M43.8
  colon (congenital) Q43.9
    acquired K63.89
  concha (ear), congenital -*see also*
    Malformation, ear, external
    acquired -*see* Disorder, pinna, deformity
  cornea (acquired) H18.70
    congenital Q13.4
    descemetocele -*see* Descemetocele
    ectasia -*see* Ectasia, cornea
    specified NEC H18.79
    staphyloma -*see* Staphyloma, cornea
  coronary artery (acquired) I25.9
  cranium (acquired) -*see* Deformity, skull
  cricoid cartilage (congenital) Q31.8

Deformity --*continued*
  congenital Q24.5
    acquired J38.7
  cystic duct (congenital) Q44.5
    acquired K82.8
  Dandy Walker Q03.1
    with spina bifida -*see* Spina bifida
  diaphragm (congenital) Q79.1
    acquired J98.6
  digestive organ NOS Q45.9
  ductus arteriosus Q25.0
  duodenal bulb K31.89
  duodenum (congenital) Q43.9
    acquired K31.89
  dura -*see* Deformity, meninges
  ear (acquired) -*see also* Disorder, pinna,
    deformity
    congenital (external) Q17.9
    internal Q16.5
    middle Q16.4
      ossicles Q16.3
    ossicles Q16.3
  ectodermal (congenital) NEC Q84.9
  ejaculatory duct (congenital) Q55.4
    acquired N50.89
  elbow (joint) (acquired) -*see also* Deformity,
    limb, upper arm
    congenital Q68.8
    contraction -*see* Contraction, joint, elbow
  endocrine gland NEC Q89.2
  epididymis (congenital) Q55.4
    acquired N50.89
  epiglottis (congenital) Q31.8
    acquired J38.7
  esophagus (congenital) Q39.9
    acquired K22.8
  eustachian tube (congenital) NEC Q17.8
  eye, congenital Q15.9
  eyebrow (congenital) Q18.8
  eyelid (acquired) -*see also* Disorder, eyelid,
    specified type NEC
    congenital Q10.3
  face (acquired) M95.2
    congenital Q18.9
  fallopian tube, acquired N83.8
  femur (acquired) -*see* Deformity, limb,
    specified type NEC, thigh
  fetal
    with fetopelvic disproportion O33.7
    causing obstructed labor O66.3
  finger (acquired) M20.00
    boutonniere M20.02
    congenital Q68.1
    flexion contracture -*see* Contraction, joint,
      hand
    mallet finger M20.01
    specified NEC M20.09
    swan-neck M20.03
  flexion (joint) (acquired) -*see also* Deformity,
    limb, flexion M21.20
    congenital NOS Q74.9
    hip Q65.89
  foot (acquired) -*see also* Deformity, limb,
    lower leg
    cavovarus (congenital) Q66.1
    congenital NOS Q66.9
    specified type NEC Q66.89
    specified type NEC -*see* Deformity, limb,
      foot, specified NEC
    varus (congenital) NEC Q66.3

Deformity --continued
　acquired -see Deformity, varus, ankle
　forearm (acquired) -see also Deformity, limb,
　forearm
　　congenital Q68.8
　forehead (acquired) M95.2
　　congenital Q75.8
　frontal bone (acquired) M95.2
　　congenital Q75.8
　gallbladder (congenital) Q44.1
　　acquired K82.8
　gastrointestinal tract (congenital) NOS Q45.9
　　acquired K63.89
　genitalia, genital organ(s) or system NEC
　　female (congenital) Q52.9
　　　acquired N94.89
　　　external Q52.70
　　male (congenital) Q55.9
　　　acquired N50.89
　globe (eye) (congenital) Q15.8
　　acquired H44.89
　gum, acquired NEC K06.8
　hand (acquired) -see Deformity, limb, hand
　　congenital Q68.1
　head (acquired) M95.2
　　congenital Q75.8
　heart (congenital) Q24.9
　　septum Q21.9
　　　auricular Q21.1
　　　ventricular Q21.0
　　valve (congenital) NEC Q24.8
　　　acquired -see Endocarditis
　heel (acquired) -see Deformity, foot
　hepatic duct (congenital) Q44.5
　　acquired K83.8
　hip (joint) (acquired) -see also Deformity,
　limb, thigh
　　congenital Q65.9
　　due to (previous) juvenile osteochondrosis -
　　　see Coxa, plana
　　flexion -see Contraction, joint, hip
　hourglass -see Contraction, hourglass
　humerus (acquired) M21.82
　　congenital Q74.0
　hypophyseal (congenital) Q89.2
　ileocecal (coil) (valve) (acquired) K63.89
　　congenital Q43.9
　ileum (congenital) Q43.9
　　acquired K63.89
　ilium (acquired) M95.5
　　congenital Q74.2
　integument (congenital) Q84.9
　intervertebral cartilage or disc (acquired) -see
　　Disorder, disc, specified NEC
　intestine (large) (small) (congenital) NOS
　Q43.9
　　acquired K63.89
　intrinsic minus or plus (hand) -see Deformity,
　limb, specified type NEC, forearm
　iris (acquired) H21.89
　　congenital Q13.2
　ischium (acquired) M95.5
　　congenital Q74.2
　jaw (acquired) (congenital) M26.9
　joint (acquired) NEC M21.90
　　congenital Q68.8
　　elbow M21.92
　　hand M21.94
　　shoulder M21.92
　　wrist M21.93
　　hip M21.95

Deformity --continued
　knee M21.96
　kidney(s) (calyx) (pelvis) (congenital) Q63.9
　　acquired N28.89
　　artery (congenital) Q27.2
　　　acquired I77.89
　Klippel-Feil (brevicollis) Q76.1
　knee (acquired) NEC -see also Deformity,
　limb, lower leg
　　congenital Q68.2
　labium (majus) (minus) (congenital) Q52.79
　　acquired N90.89
　lacrimal passages or duct (congenital) NEC
　Q10.6
　　acquired -see Disorder, lacrimal system,
　changes
　larynx (muscle) (congenital) Q31.8
　　acquired J38.7
　　web (glottic) Q31.0
　leg (upper) (acquired) NEC -see also
　Deformity, limb, thigh
　　congenital Q68.8
　　lower leg -see Deformity, limb, lower leg
　lens (acquired) H27.8
　　congenital Q12.9
　lid (fold) (acquired) -see also Disorder,
　eyelid, specified type NEC
　　congenital Q10.3
　ligament (acquired) -see Disorder, ligament
　　congenital Q79.9
　limb (acquired) M21.90
　　clawfoot M21.53
　　clawhand M21.51
　　clubfoot M21.54
　　clubhand M21.52
　　congenital, except reduction deformity
　Q74.9
　　flat foot M21.4
　　flexion M21.20
　　　ankle M21.27
　　　elbow M21.22
　　　finger M21.24
　　　hip M21.25
　　　knee M21.26
　　　shoulder M21.21
　　　toe M21.27
　　　wrist M21.23
　　foot
　　　claw -see Deformity, limb, clawfoot
　　　club -see Deformity, limb, clubfoot
　　　drop M21.37
　　　flat -see Deformity, limb, flat foot
　　　specified NEC M21.6X
　　forearm M21.93
　　hand M21.94
　　lower leg M21.96
　　specified type NEC M21.80
　　　forearm M21.83
　　　lower leg M21.86
　　　thigh M21.85
　　　upper arm M21.82
　　thigh M21.95
　　unequal length M21.70
　　　short site is
　　　　femur M21.75
　　　　fibula M21.76
　　　　humerus M21.72
　　　　radius M21.73
　　upper arm M21.92
　　valgus -see Deformity, valgus
　　varus -see Deformity, varus

Deformity --continued
　　tibia M21.76
　　ulna M21.73
　　wrist drop M21.33
　lip (acquired) NEC K13.0
　　congenital Q38.0
　liver (congenital) Q44.7
　　acquired K76.89
　lumbosacral (congenital) (joint) (region)
　Q76.49
　　acquired -see subcategory M43.8
　　kyphosis -see Kyphosis, congenital
　　lordosis -see Lordosis, congenital
　lung (congenital) Q33.9
　　acquired J98.4
　lymphatic system, congenital Q89.9
　Madelung's (radius) Q74.0
　mandible (acquired) (congenital) M26.9
　maxilla (acquired) (congenital) M26.9
　meninges or membrane (congenital) Q07.9
　　cerebral Q04.8
　　　acquired G96.19
　　spinal cord (congenital) G96.19
　　　acquired G96.19
　metacarpus (acquired) -see Deformity, limb,
　forearm
　　congenital Q74.0
　metatarsus (acquired) -see Deformity, foot
　　congenital Q66.9
　middle ear (congenital) Q16.4
　　ossicles Q16.3
　mitral (leaflets) (valve) I05.8
　　parachute Q23.2
　　stenosis, congenital Q23.2
　mouth (acquired) K13.79
　　congenital Q38.6
　multiple, congenital NEC Q89.7
　muscle (acquired) M62.89
　　congenital Q79.9
　　sternocleidomastoid Q68.0
　musculoskeletal system (acquired) M95.9
　　congenital Q79.9
　　specified NEC M95.8
　nail (acquired) L60.8
　　congenital Q84.6
　nasal -see Deformity, nose - neck (acquired)
　M95.3
　　congenital Q18.9
　　sternocleidomastoid Q68.0
　nervous system (congenital) Q07.9
　nipple (congenital) Q83.9
　　acquired N64.89
　nose (acquired) (cartilage) M95.0
　　bone (turbinate) M95.0
　　congenital Q30.9
　　　bent or squashed Q67.4
　　saddle M95.0
　　　syphilitic A50.57
　　septum (acquired) J34.2
　　　congenital Q30.8
　　sinus (wall) (congenital) Q30.8
　　　acquired M95.0
　　syphilitic (congenital) A50.57
　　　late A52.73
　ocular muscle (congenital) Q10.3
　　acquired -see Strabismus, mechanical
　opticociliary vessels (congenital) Q13.2
　orbit (eye) (acquired) H05.30
　　atrophy -see Atrophy, orbit
　　congenital Q10.7
　　due to

Deformity *--continued*
    bone disease NEC H05.32
      trauma or surgery H05.33
    enlargement -*see* Enlargement, orbit
    exostosis -*see* Exostosis, orbit
    organ of Corti (congenital) Q16.5
    ovary (congenital) Q50.39
      acquired N83.8
    oviduct, acquired N83.8
    palate (congenital) Q38.5
      acquired M27.8
      cleft (congenital) -*see* Cleft, palate
    pancreas (congenital) Q45.3
      acquired K86.89
    parathyroid (gland) Q89.2
    parotid (gland) (congenital) Q38.4
      acquired K11.8
    patella (acquired) -*see* Disorder, patella, specified NEC
    pelvis, pelvic (acquired) (bony) M95.5
      with disproportion (fetopelvic) O33.0
        causing obstructed labor O65.0
      congenital Q74.2
      rachitic sequelae (late effect) E64.3
    penis (glans) (congenital) Q55.69
      acquired N48.89
    pericardium (congenital) Q24.8
      acquired -*see* Pericarditis
    pharynx (congenital) Q38.8
      acquired J39.2
    pinna, acquired -*see also* Disorder, pinna, deformity
      congenital Q17.9
    pituitary (congenital) Q89.2
    posture -*see* Dorsopathy, deforming
    prepuce (congenital) Q55.69
      acquired N47.8
    prostate (congenital) Q55.4
      acquired N42.89
    pupil (congenital) Q13.2
      acquired -*see* Abnormality, pupillary
    pylorus (congenital) Q40.3
      acquired K31.89
    rachitic (acquired), old or healed E64.3
    radius (acquired) -*see also* Deformity, limb, forearm
      congenital Q68.8
    rectum (congenital) Q43.9
      acquired K62.89
    reduction (extremity) (limb), congenital -*see also* condition and site Q73.8
      brain Q04.3
      lower -*see* Defect, reduction, lower limb
      upper -*see* Defect, reduction, upper limb
    renal -*see* Deformity, kidney
    respiratory system (congenital) Q34.9
    rib (acquired) M95.4
      congenital Q76.6
        cervical Q76.5
    rotation (joint) (acquired) -*see* Deformity, limb, specified site NEC
      congenital Q74.9
      hip -*see* Deformity, limb, specified type NEC, thigh
        congenital Q65.89
    sacroiliac joint (congenital) Q74.2
      acquired -*see* subcategory M43.8
    sacrum (acquired) -*see* subcategory M43.8
      nose M95.0
        syphilitic A50.57
    saddle

Deformity *--continued*
    back -*see* Lordosis
    salivary gland or duct (congenital) Q38.4
      acquired K11.8
    scapula (acquired) M95.8
      congenital Q68.8
    scrotum (congenital) -*see also* Malformation, testis and scrotum
      acquired N50.89
    seminal vesicles (congenital) Q55.4
      acquired N50.89
    septum, nasal (acquired) J34.2
    shoulder (joint) (acquired) -*see* Deformity, limb, upper arm
      congenital Q74.0
      contraction -*see* Contraction, joint, shoulder
    sigmoid (flexure) (congenital) Q43.9
      acquired K63.89
    skin (congenital) Q82.9
    skull (acquired) M95.2
      congenital Q75.8
        with
          anencephaly Q00.0
          encephalocele -*see* Encephalocele
          hydrocephalus Q03.9
            with spina bifida -*see* Spina bifida, by site, with hydrocephalus
          microcephaly Q02
    soft parts, organs or tissues (of pelvis)
      in pregnancy or childbirth NEC O34.8
        causing obstructed labor O65.5
    spermatic cord (congenital) Q55.4
      acquired N50.89
      torsion -*see* Torsion, spermatic cord
    spinal -*see* Dorsopathy, deforming
      column (acquired) -*see* Dorsopathy, deforming
        congenital Q67.5
      cord (congenital) Q06.9
        acquired G95.89
      nerve root (congenital) Q07.9
    spine (acquired) -*see also* Dorsopathy, deforming
      congenital Q67.5
      rachitic E64.3
      specified NEC -*see* Dorsopathy, deforming, specified NEC
    spleen
      acquired D73.89
      congenital Q89.09
    Sprengel's (congenital) Q74.0
    sternocleidomastoid (muscle), congenital Q68.0
    sternum (acquired) M95.4
      congenital NEC Q76.7
    stomach (congenital) Q40.3
      acquired K31.89
    submandibular gland (congenital) Q38.4
    submaxillary gland (congenital) Q38.4
      acquired K11.8
    talipes -*see* Talipes
    testis (congenital) -*see also* Malformation, testis and scrotum
      acquired N44.8
      torsion -*see* Torsion, testis
    thigh (acquired) -*see also* Deformity, limb, thigh
      congenital NEC Q68.8
      sequelae of rickets E64.3
    thumb (acquired) -*see also* Deformity, finger
      congenital NEC Q68.1

Deformity *--continued*
    thorax (acquired) (wall) M95.4
      congenital Q67.8
    thymus (tissue) (congenital) Q89.2
    thyroid (gland) (congenital) Q89.2
      cartilage Q31.8
        acquired J38.7
    tibia (acquired) -*see also* Deformity, limb, specified type NEC, lower leg
      congenital NEC Q68.8
      saber (syphilitic) A50.56
    toe (acquired) M20.6
      congenital Q66.9
      hallux rigidus M20.2
      hallux valgus M20.1
      hallux varus M20.3
      hammer toe M20.4
      specified NEC M20.5X
    tongue (congenital) Q38.3
      acquired K14.8
    tooth, teeth K00.2
    trachea (rings) (congenital) Q32.1
      acquired J39.8
    transverse aortic arch (congenital) Q25.49
    tricuspid (leaflets) (valve) I07.8
      atresia or stenosis Q22.4
      Ebstein's Q22.5
    trunk (acquired) M95.8
      congenital Q89.9
    ulna (acquired) -*see also* Deformity, limb, forearm
      congenital NEC Q68.8
    urachus, congenital Q64.4
    ureter (opening) (congenital) Q62.8
      acquired N28.89
    urethra (congenital) Q64.79
      acquired N36.8
    urinary tract (congenital) Q64.9
      urachus Q64.4
    uterus (congenital) Q51.9
      acquired N85.8
    uvula (congenital) Q38.5
    vagina (acquired) N89.8
      congenital Q52.4
    valgus NEC M21.00
      ankle M21.07
      elbow M21.02
      hip M21.05
      knee M21.06
    valve, valvular (congenital) (heart) Q24.8
      acquired -*see* Endocarditis
    varus NEC M21.10
      ankle M21.17
      elbow M21.12
      hip M21.15
      knee M21.16
      tibia -*see* Osteochondrosis, juvenile, tibia
    vas deferens (congenital) Q55.4
      acquired N50.89
    vein (congenital) Q27.9
      great Q26.9
    vertebra -*see* Dorsopathy, deforming
    vertical talus (congenital) Q66.80
      left foot Q66.82
      right foot Q66.81
    vesicourethral orifice (acquired) N32.89
      congenital NEC Q64.79
    vessels of optic papilla (congenital) Q14.2
    visual field (contraction) -*see* Defect, visual field
    vitreous body, acquired H43.89

Deformity --*continued*
  vulva (congenital) Q52.79
    acquired N90.89
  wrist (joint) (acquired) -*see also* Deformity, limb, forearm
    congenital Q68.8
    contraction -*see* Contraction, joint, wrist

Degeneration, degenerative
  adrenal (capsule) (fatty) (gland) (hyaline) (infectional) E27.8
  amyloid -*see also* Amyloidosis E85.9
  anterior cornua, spinal cord G12.29
  anterior labral S43.49
  aorta, aortic I70.0
    fatty I77.89
  aortic valve (heart) -*see* Endocarditis, aortic
  arteriovascular -*see* Arteriosclerosis
  artery, arterial (atheromatous) (calcareous) - *see also* Arteriosclerosis
    cerebral, amyloid E85.4 [*I68.0*]
    medial -*see* Arteriosclerosis, extremities
  articular cartilage NEC -*see* Derangement, joint, articular cartilage, by site
  atheromatous -*see* Arteriosclerosis
  basal nuclei or ganglia G23.9
    specified NEC G23.8
  bone NEC -*see* Disorder, bone, specified type NEC
  brachial plexus G54.0
  brain (cortical) (progressive) G31.9
    alcoholic G31.2
    arteriosclerotic I67.2
    childhood G31.9
      specified NEC G31.89
    cystic G31.89
      congenital Q04.6
    in
      alcoholism G31.2
      beriberi E51.2
      cerebrovascular disease I67.9
      congenital hydrocephalus Q03.9
        with spina bifida -*see also* Spina bifida
      Fabry Anderson disease E75.21
      Gaucher's disease E75.22
      Hunter's syndrome E76.1
      lipidosis
        cerebral E75.4
        generalized E75.6
      mucopolysaccharidosis -*see* Mucopolysaccharidosis
      myxedema E03.9 [*G32.89*]
      neoplastic disease -*see also* Neoplasm D49.6 [*G32.89*]
      Niemann-Pick disease E75.249 [*G32.89*]
      sphingolipidosis E75.3 [*G32.89*]
      vitamin B12 deficiency E53.8 [*G32.89*]
    senile NEC G31.1
  breast N64.89
  Bruch's membrane -*see* Degeneration, choroid
  capillaries (fatty) I78.8
    amyloid E85.8 [*I79.8*]
  cardiac -*see also* Degeneration, myocardial
    valve, valvular -*see* Endocarditis
  cardiorenal -*see* Hypertension, cardiorenal
  cardiovascular -*see also* Disease, cardiovascular
    renal -*see* Hypertension, cardiorenal
  cerebellar NOS G31.9
  cerebral -*see* Degeneration, brain
  cerebrovascular I67.9
    due to hypertension I67.4

Degeneration, degenerative --*continued*
    alcoholic G31.2
    primary (hereditary) (sporadic) G11.9
  cervical plexus G54.2
  cervix N88.8
    due to radiation (intended effect) N88.8
      adverse effect or misadventure N99.89
  chamber angle H21.21
  changes, spine or vertebra -*see* Spondylosis
  chorioretinal -*see also* Degeneration, choroid
    hereditary H31.20
  choroid (colloid) (drusen) H31.10
    atrophy -*see* Atrophy, choroidal
    hereditary -*see* Dystrophy, choroidal, hereditary
  ciliary body H21.22
  cochlear -*see* subcategory H83.8
  combined (spinal cord) (subacute) E53.8 [*G32.0*]
    with anemia (pernicious) D51.0 [*G32.0*]
      due to dietary vitamin B12 deficiency D51.3 [*G32.0*]
    in (due to)
      vitamin B12 deficiency E53.8 [*G32.0*]
        anemia D51.9 [*G32.0*]
  conjunctiva H11.10
    concretions -*see* Concretion, conjunctiva
    deposits -*see* Deposit, conjunctiva
    pigmentations -*see* Pigmentation, conjunctiva
    pinguecula -*see* Pinguecula
    xerosis -*see* Xerosis, conjunctiva
  cornea H18.40
    calcereous H18.43
      band keratopathy H18.42
    familial, hereditary -*see* Dystrophy, cornea
    hyaline (of old scars) H18.49
    keratomalacia -*see* Keratomalacia
    nodular H18.45
    peripheral H18.46
    senile H18.41
    specified type NEC H18.49
  cortical (cerebellar) (parenchymatous) G31.89
    alcoholic G31.2
    diffuse, due to arteriopathy I67.2
  corticobasal G31.85
  cutis L98.8
    amyloid E85.4 [*L99*]
  dental pulp K04.2
  disc disease -*see* Degeneration, intervertebral disc NEC
  dorsolateral (spinal cord) -*see* Degeneration, combined
  extrapyramidal G25.9
  eye, macular -*see also* Degeneration, macula
    congenital or hereditary -*see* Dystrophy, retina
  facet joints -*see* Spondylosis
  fatty
    liver NEC K76.0
      alcoholic K70.0
  grey matter (brain) (Alpers') G31.81
  heart -*see also* Degeneration, myocardial
    amyloid E85.4 [*I43*]
    atheromatous -*see* Disease, heart, ischemic, atherosclerotic
    ischemic -*see* Disease, heart, ischemic
  hepatolenticular (Wilson's) E83.01
    localized -*see* Degeneration, by site
  infrapatellar fat pad M79.4
  intervertebral disc NOS

Degeneration, degenerative --*continued*
  hepatorenal K76.7
  hyaline (diffuse) (generalized)
    with
      myelopathy -*see* Disorder, disc, with, myelopathy
      radiculitis or radiculopathy -*see* Disorder, disc, with, radiculopathy
    cervical, cervicothoracic -*see* Disorder, disc, cervical, degeneration
      with
        myelopathy -*see* Disorder, disc, cervical, with myelopathy
        neuritis, radiculitis or radiculopathy -*see* Disorder, disc, cervical, with neuritis
    lumbar region M51.36
      with
        myelopathy M51.06
        neuritis, radiculitis, radiculopathy or sciatica M51.16
    lumbosacral region M51.37
      with
        neuritis, radiculitis, radiculopathy or sciatica M51.17
    sacrococcygeal region M53.3
    thoracic region M51.34
      with
        myelopathy M51.04
        neuritis, radiculitis, radiculopathy M51.14
    thoracolumbar region M51.35
      with
        myelopathy M51.05
        neuritis, radiculitis, radiculopathy M51.15
  intestine, amyloid E85.4
  iris (pigmentary) H21.23
  ischemic -*see* Ischemia
  joint disease -*see* Osteoarthritis
  kidney N28.89
    amyloid E85.4 [*N29*]
    cystic, congenital Q61.9
    fatty N28.89
    polycystic Q61.3
      adult type (autosomal dominant) Q61.2
      infantile type (autosomal recessive) NEC Q61.19
        collecting duct dilatation Q61.11
  Kuhnt-Junius -*see also* Degeneration, macula H35.32
  lens -*see* Cataract
  lenticular (familial) (progressive) (Wilson's) (with cirrhosis of liver) E83.01
  liver (diffuse) NEC K76.89
    amyloid E85.4 [*K77*]
    cystic K76.89
      congenital Q44.6
    fatty NEC K76.0
      alcoholic K70.0
    hypertrophic K76.89
    parenchymatous, acute or subacute K72.00
      with coma K72.01
    pigmentary K76.89
    toxic (acute) K71.9
  lung J98.4
  lymph gland I89.8
    hyaline I89.8
  macula, macular (acquired) (age-related) (senile) H35.30
    angioid streaks H35.33
    atrophic age-related H35.31

Degeneration, degenerative --*continued*
  congenital or hereditary -*see* Dystrophy, retina
    cystoid H35.35
    drusen H35.36
    dry age-related H35.31
    exudative H35.32
    hole H35.34
    nonexudative H35.31
    puckering H35.37
    toxic H35.38
    wet age-related H35.32
  membranous labyrinth, congenital (causing impairment of hearing) Q16.5
  meniscus -*see* Derangement, meniscus
  mitral -*see* Insufficiency, mitral
  Mönckeberg's -*see* Arteriosclerosis, extremities
  motor centers, senile G31.1
  multi-system G90.3
  mural -*see* Degeneration, myocardial
  muscle (fatty) (fibrous) (hyaline) (progressive) M62.89
    heart -*see* Degeneration, myocardial
  myelin, central nervous system G37.9
  myocardial, myocardium (fatty) (hyaline) (senile) I51.5
    with rheumatic fever (conditions in I00) I09.0
      active, acute or subacute I01.2
        with chorea I02.0
      inactive or quiescent (with chorea) I09.0
    hypertensive -*see* Hypertension, heart
    rheumatic -*see* Degeneration, myocardial, with rheumatic fever
    syphilitic A52.06
  nasal sinus (mucosa) J32.9
    frontal J32.1
    maxillary J32.0
  nerve -*see* Disorder, nerve
  nervous system G31.9
    alcoholic G31.2
    amyloid E85.4 [*G99.8*]
    autonomic G90.9
    fatty G31.89
    specified NEC G31.89
  nipple N64.89
  olivopontocerebellar (hereditary) (familial) G23.8
  osseous labyrinth -*see* subcategory H83.8
  ovary N83.8
    cystic N83.20
    microcystic N83.20
  pallidal pigmentary (progressive) G23.0
  pancreas K86.89
    tuberculous A18.83
  penis N48.89
  pigmentary (diffuse) (general)
    localized -*see* Degeneration, by site
    pallidal (progressive) G23.0
  pineal gland E34.8
  pituitary (gland) E23.6
  popliteal fat pad M79.4
  posterolateral (spinal cord) -*see* Degeneration, combined
  pulmonary valve (heart) I37.8
  pulp (tooth) K04.2
  pupillary margin H21.24
  renal -*see* Degeneration, kidney   retina H35.9
    hereditary (cerebroretinal) (congenital)

Degeneration, degenerative --*continued*
  (juvenile) (macula) (peripheral) (pigmentary) -*see* Dystrophy, retina
    Kuhnt-Junius -*see also* Degeneration, macula H35.32
    macula (cystic) (exudative) (hole) (nonexudative) (pseudohole) (senile) (toxic) -*see* Degeneration, macula
    peripheral H35.40
      lattice H35.41
      microcystoid H35.42
      paving stone H35.43
      secondary
        pigmentary H35.45
        vitreoretinal H35.46
      senile reticular H35.44
    pigmentary (primary) -*see also* Dystrophy, retina
      secondary -*see* Degeneration, retina, peripheral, secondary
    posterior pole -*see* Degeneration, macula
  saccule, congenital (causing impairment of hearing) Q16.5
  senile R54
    brain G31.1
    cardiac, heart or myocardium -*see* Degeneration, myocardial
    motor centers G31.1
    vascular -*see* Arteriosclerosis
  sinus (cystic) -*see also* Sinusitis
    polypoid J33.1
  skin L98.8
    amyloid E85.4 [*L99*]
    colloid L98.8
  spinal (cord) G31.89
    amyloid E85.4 [*G32.89*]
    combined (subacute) -*see* Degeneration, combined
    dorsolateral -*see* Degeneration, combined
    familial NEC G31.89
    fatty G31.89
    funicular -*see* Degeneration, combined
    posterolateral -*see* Degeneration, combined
    subacute combined -*see* Degeneration, combined
    tuberculous A17.81
  spleen D73.0
    amyloid E85.4 [*D77*]
  stomach K31.89
  striatonigral G23.2
  suprarenal (capsule) (gland) E27.8
  synovial membrane (pulpy) -*see* Disorder, synovium, specified type NEC
  tapetoretinal -*see* Dystrophy, retina
  thymus (gland) E32.8
    fatty E32.8
  thyroid (gland) E07.89
  tricuspid (heart) (valve) I07.9
  tuberculous NEC -*see* Tuberculosis
  turbinate J34.89
  uterus (cystic) N85.8
  vascular (senile) -*see* Arteriosclerosis
    hypertensive -*see* Hypertension
  vitreoretinal, secondary -*see* Degeneration, retina, peripheral, secondary, vitreoretinal
  vitreous (body) H43.81
  Wallerian -*see* Disorder, nerve
  Wilson's hepatolenticular E83.01
Deglutition
  paralysis R13.0
    hysterical F44.4
  pneumonia J69.0

Degos' disease I77.89
Dehiscence (of)
  amputation stump T87.81
  cesarean wound O90.0
  closure of
    cornea T81.31
    craniotomy T81.32
    fascia (muscular) (superficial) T81.32
    internal organ or tissue T81.32
    laceration (external) (internal) T81.33
    ligament T81.32
    mucosa T81.31
    muscle or muscle flap T81.32
    ribs or rib cage T81.32
    skin and subcutaneous tissue (full-thickness) (superficial) T81.31
    skull T81.32
    sternum (sternotomy) T81.32
    tendon T81.32
    traumatic laceration (external) (internal) T81.33
  episiotomy O90.1
  operation wound NEC T81.31
    external operation wound (superficial) T81.31
    internal operation wound (deep) T81.32
  perineal wound (postpartum) O90.1
  traumatic injury wound repair T81.33
  wound T81.30
    traumatic repair T81.33
Dehydration E86.0
  newborn P74.1
Déjérine-Roussy syndrome G89.0
Déjérine-Sottas disease or neuropathy (hypertrophic) G60.0
Déjérine-Thomas atrophy G23.8
Delay, delayed
  any plane in pelvis
    complicating delivery O66.9
  birth or delivery NOS O63.9
  closure, ductus arteriosus (Botalli) P29.3
  coagulation -*see* Defect, coagulation
  conduction (cardiac) (ventricular) I45.9
  delivery, second twin, triplet, etc O63.2
  development R62.50
    global F88
    intellectual (specific) F81.9
    language F80.9
      due to hearing loss F80.4
    learning F81.9
    pervasive F84.9
    physiological R62.50
      specified stage NEC R62.0
    reading F81.0
    sexual E30.0
    speech F80.9
      due to hearing loss F80.4
    spelling F81.81
  ejaculation F52.32
  gastric emptying K30
  menarche E30.0
  menstruation (cause unknown) N91.0
  milestone R62.0
  passage of meconium (newborn) P76.0
  primary respiration P28.9
  puberty (constitutional) E30.0
  separation of umbilical cord P96.82   sexual maturation, female E30.0
  sleep phase syndrome G47.21
  union, fracture -*see* Fracture, by site
  vaccination Z28.9

Deletion(s)
autosome Q93.9
  identified by fluorescence in situ
    hybridization (FISH) Q93.89
  identified by in situ hybridization (ISH)
    Q93.89
chromosome
  with complex rearrangements NEC Q93.7
  part of NEC Q93.5
  seen only at prometaphase Q93.89
  short arm
    4 Q93.3
    5p Q93.4
    22q11.2 Q93.81
  specified NEC Q93.89
long arm chromosome 18 or 21 Q93.89
  with complex rearrangements NEC Q93.7
microdeletions NEC Q93.88
Delhi boil or button B55.1
Delinquency (juvenile) (neurotic) F91.8
group Z72.810
Delinquent immunization status Z28.3
**Delirium, delirious (acute or subacute) (not
alcohol- or drug-induced) (with dementia)**
R41.0
alcoholic (acute) (tremens) (withdrawal)
  F10.921
  with intoxication F10.921
    in
      abuse F10.121
      dependence F10.221
due to (secondary to)
  alcohol
    intoxication F10.921
      in
        abuse F10.121
        dependence F10.221
    withdrawal F10.231
  amphetamine intoxication F15.921
    in
      abuse F15.121
      dependence F15.221
  anxiolytic
    intoxication F13.921
      in
        abuse F13.121
        dependence F13.221
    withdrawal F13.231
  cannabis intoxication (acute) F12.921
    in
      abuse F12.121
      dependence F12.221
  cocaine intoxication (acute) F14.921
    in
      abuse F14.121
      dependence F14.221
  general medical condition F05
  hallucinogen intoxication F16.921
    in
      abuse F16.121
      dependence F16.221
  hypnotic
    intoxication F13.921
      in
        abuse F13.121
        dependence F13.221
    withdrawal F13.231
  inhalant intoxication (acute) F18.921
    in
      abuse F18.121
      dependence F18.221

Delirium, delirious --*continued*
multiple etiologies F05
opioid intoxication (acute) F11.921
  in
    abuse F11.121
    dependence F11.221
other (or unknown) substance F19.921
phencyclidine intoxication (acute) F16.921
  in
    abuse F16.121
    dependence F16.221
psychoactive substance NEC intoxication
  (acute) F19.921
  in
    abuse F19.121
    dependence F19.221
sedative
  intoxication F13.921
    in
      abuse F13.121
      dependence F13.221
  withdrawal F13.231
unknown etiology F05
exhaustion F43.0
hysterical F44.89
postprocedural (postoperative) F05
puerperal F05
thyroid -*see* Thyrotoxicosis with thyroid
storm
traumatic -*see* Injury, intracranial
tremens (alcohol-induced) F10.231
  sedative-induced F13.231
Delivery (childbirth) (labor)
arrested active phase O62.1
cesarean (for)
  abnormal
    pelvis (bony) (deformity) (major) NEC
      with disproportion (fetopelvic) O33.0
        with obstructed labor O65.0
      presentation or position O32.9
  abruptio placentae -*see also* Abruptio
    placentae O45.9
  acromion presentation O32.2
  atony, uterus O62.2
  breech presentation O32.1
    incomplete O32.8
  brow presentation O32.3
  cephalopelvic disproportion O33.9
  cerclage O34.3
  chin presentation O32.3
  cicatrix of cervix O34.4
  contracted pelvis (general)
    inlet O33.2
    outlet O33.3
  cord presentation or prolapse O69.0
  cystocele O34.8
  deformity (acquired) (congenital)
    pelvic organs or tissues NEC O34.8
    pelvis (bony) NEC O33.0
  disproportion NOS O33.9
  eclampsia -*see* Eclampsia
  face presentation O32.3
  failed
    forceps O66.5
    induction of labor O61.9
      instrumental O61.1
      mechanical O61.1
      medical O61.0
      specified NEC O61.8
      surgical O61.1
    trial of labor NOS O66.40

Delivery (childbirth) (labor) --*continued*
following previous cesarean delivery
  O66.41
vacuum extraction O66.5
ventouse O66.5
fetal-maternal hemorrhage O43.01
hemorrhage (intrapartum) O67.9
  with coagulation defect O67.0
  specified cause NEC O67.8
high head at term O32.4
hydrocephalic fetus O33.6
incarceration of uterus O34.51
incoordinate uterine action O62.4
increased size, fetus O33.5
inertia, uterus O62.2
  primary O62.0
  secondary O62.1
lateroversion, uterus O34.59
mal lie O32.9
malposition
  fetus O32.9
  pelvic organs or tissues NEC O34.8
  uterus NEC O34.59
malpresentation NOS O32.9
oblique presentation O32.2
occurring after 37 completed weeks of
  gestation but before 39 completed weeks
  gestation due to (spontaneous) onset of labor
  O75.82
oversize fetus O33.5
pelvic tumor NEC O34.8
placenta previa O44.0
  complete O44.0
    with hemorrhage O44.1
placental insufficiency O36.51
planned, occurring after 37 completed weeks
  of gestation but before 39 completed weeks
  gestation due to (spontaneous) onset of labor
  O75.82
polyp, cervix O34.4
  causing obstructed labor O65.5
poor dilatation, cervix O62.0
pre-eclampsia O14.94
  mild O14.04
  moderate O14.04
  severe O14.14
    with hemolysis, elevated liver enzymes
      and low platelet count (HELLP) O14.24
previous
  cesarean delivery O34.219
    classical (vertical) scar O34.212
    low transverse scar O34.211
  surgery (to)
    cervix O34.4
    gynecological NEC O34.8
    rectum O34.7
    uterus O34.29
    vagina O34.6
prolapse
  arm or hand O32.2
  uterus O34.52
prolonged labor NOS O63.9
rectocele O34.8
retroversion
  uterus O34.53
rigid- cervix O34.4
    pelvic floor O34.8
    perineum O34.7
    vagina O34.6
    vulva O34.7

Delivery (childbirth) (labor) --*continued*
- sacculation, pregnant uterus O34.59
- scar(s)
  - cervix O34.4
  - cesarean delivery O34.219
    - classical (vertical) O34.212
    - low transverse O34.211
  - transmural uterine O34.29
  - uterus O34.29
- Shirodkar suture in situ O34.3
- shoulder presentation O32.2
- stenosis or stricture, cervix O34.4
- streptococcus group B (GBS) carrier state O99.824
- transmural uterine scar O34.29
- transverse presentation or lie O32.2
- tumor, pelvic organs or tissues NEC O34.8
  - cervix O34.4
- umbilical cord presentation or prolapse O69.0
- without indication O82
- completely normal case O80
- complicated O75.9
  - by
    - abnormal, abnormality (of)
      - forces of labor O62.9
        - specified type NEC O62.8
      - glucose O99.814
      - uterine contractions NOS O62.9
    - abruptio placentae -*see also* Abruptio placentae O45.9
    - abuse
      - physical O9A.32
      - psychological O9A.52
      - sexual O9A.42
    - adherent placenta O72.0
      - without hemorrhage O73.0
    - alcohol use O99.314
    - anemia (pre-existing) O99.02
    - anesthetic death O74.8
    - annular detachment of cervix O71.3
    - atony, uterus O62.2
    - attempted vacuum extraction and forceps O66.5
    - Bandl's ring O62.4
    - bariatric surgery status O99.844
    - biliary tract disorder O26.62
    - bleeding -*see* Delivery, complicated by, hemorrhage
    - blood disorder NEC O99.12
    - cervical dystocia (hypotonic) O62.2
      - primary O62.0
      - secondary O62.1
    - circulatory system disorder O99.42
    - compression of cord (umbilical) NEC O69.2
    - condition NEC O99.89
    - contraction, contracted ring O62.4
    - cord (umbilical)
      - around neck
        - with compression O69.1
        - without compression O69.81
      - bruising O69.5
      - complication O69.9
        - specified NEC O69.89
      - compression NEC O69.2
      - entanglement O69.2
        - without compression O69.82
      - hematoma O69.5
      - presentation O69.0
      - prolapse O69.0

Delivery (childbirth) (labor) --*continued*
- short O69.3
- thrombosis (vessels) O69.5
- vascular lesion O69.5
- Couvelaire uterus O45.8X
- damage to (injury to) NEC
  - perineum O71.82
  - periurethral tissue O71.82
  - vulva O71.82
- delay following rupture of membranes (spontaneous) -*see* Pregnancy, complicated by, premature rupture of membranes
- depressed fetal heart tones O76
- diabetes O24.92
  - gestational O24.429
    - diet controlled O24.420
    - insulin controlled O24.424
    - oral drug controlled (antidiabetic) (hypoglycemic) O24.425
  - pre-existing O24.32
    - specified NEC O24.82
    - type 1 O24.02
    - type 2 O24.12
- diastasis recti (abdominis) O71.89
- dilatation
  - bladder O66.8
  - cervix incomplete, poor or slow O62.0
- disease NEC O99.89
- disruptio uteri -*see* Delivery, complicated by, rupture, uterus
- drug use O99.324
- dysfunction, uterus NOS O62.9
  - hypertonic O62.4
  - hypotonic O62.2
    - primary O62.0
    - secondary O62.1
  - incoordinate O62.4
- eclampsia O15.1
- embolism (pulmonary) -*see* Embolism, obstetric
- endocrine, nutritional or metabolic disease NEC O99.284
- failed
  - attempted vaginal birth after previous cesarean delivery O66.41
  - induction of labor O61.9
    - instrumental O61.1
    - mechanical O61.1
    - medical O61.0
    - specified NEC O61.8
    - surgical O61.1
  - trial of labor O66.40
- female genital mutilation O65.5
- fetal
  - abnormal acid-base balance O68
  - acidemia O68
  - acidosis O68
  - alkalosis O68
  - death, early O02.1
  - deformity O66.3
  - heart rate or rhythm (abnormal) (non-reassuring) O76
  - hypoxia O77.8
  - stress O77.9
    - due to drug administration O77.1
    - electrocardiographic evidence of O77.8
    - specified NEC O77.8
    - ultrasound evidence of O77.8
- fever during labor O75.2
- gastric banding status O99.844

Delivery (childbirth) (labor) --*continued*
- gastric bypass status O99.844
- gastrointestinal disease NEC O99.62
- gestational
  - diabetes O24.429
    - diet controlled O24.420
    - insulin (and diet) controlled O24.424
    - oral drug controlled (antidiabetic) (hypoglycemic) O24.425
  - edema O12.04
    - with proteinuria O12.24
  - proteinuria O12.14
  - gonorrhea O98.22
  - hematoma O71.7
    - ischial spine O71.7
    - pelvic O71.7
    - vagina O71.7
    - vulva or perineum O71.7
- hemorrhage (uterine) O67.9
  - associated with
    - afibrinogenemia O67.0
    - coagulation defect O67.0
    - hyperfibrinolysis O67.0
    - hypofibrinogenemia O67.0
  - due to
    - low implantation of placenta O44.5
    - low lying placenta O44.5
    - placenta previa O44.1
      - marginal O44.3
      - partial O44.3
    - premature separation of placenta (normally implanted) -*see also* Abruptio placentae O45.9
    - retained placenta O72.0
    - uterine leiomyoma O67.8
  - placenta NEC O67.8
  - postpartum NEC (atonic) (immediate) O72.1
    - with retained or trapped placenta O72.0
    - delayed O72.2
    - secondary O72.2
    - third stage O72.0
- hourglass contraction, uterus O62.4
- hypertension, hypertensive (pre-existing) -*see* Hypertension, complicated by, childbirth (labor)
- hypotension O26.5
- incomplete dilatation (cervix) O62.0
- incoordinate uterus contractions O62.4
- inertia, uterus O62.2
  - during latent phase of labor O62.0
  - primary O62.0
  - secondary O62.1
- infection (maternal) O98.92
  - carrier state NEC O99.834
  - gonorrhea O98.22
  - human immunodeficiency virus (HIV) O98.72
  - sexually transmitted NEC O98.32
  - specified NEC O98.82
  - syphilis O98.12
  - tuberculosis O98.02
  - viral hepatitis O98.42
  - viral NEC O98.52
- injury (to mother) -*see also* Delivery, complicated, by, damage to O71.9
  - nonobstetric O9A.22
  - caused by abuse -*see* Delivery, complicated by, abuse
- intrauterine fetal death, early O02.1
- inversion, uterus O71.2

Delivery (childbirth) (labor) --*continued*
  laceration (perineal) O70.9
    anus (sphincter) O70.4
      with third degree laceration -*see also*
      Delivery, complicated, by, laceration,
      perineum, third degree O70.20
        with mucosa O70.3
      without third degree laceration O70.4
    bladder (urinary) O71.5
    bowel O71.5
    cervix (uteri) O71.3
    fourchette O70.0
    hymen O70.0
    labia O70.0
    pelvic
      floor O70.1
      organ NEC O71.5
    perineum, perineal O70.9
      first degree O70.0
      fourth degree O70.3
      muscles O70.1
      second degree O70.1
      skin O70.0
      slight O70.0
      third degree O70.20
        with
          both external anal sphincter (EAS)
          and internal anal sphincter (IAS) torn
          (IIIc) O70.23
          less than 50% of external anal
          sphincter (EAS) thickness torn (IIIa)
          O70.21
          more than 50% external anal
          sphincter (EAS) thickness torn (IIIb)
          O70.22
        IIIa O70.21
        IIIb O70.22
        IIIc O70.23
    peritoneum (pelvic) O71.5
    rectovaginal (septum) (without perineal
    laceration) O71.4
      with perineum -*see also* Delivery,
      complicated, by, laceration, perineum,
      third degree O70.20
        with anal or rectal mucosa O70.3
    specified NEC O71.89
    sphincter ani -*see* Delivery, complicated,
    by, laceration, anus (sphincter)
    urethra O71.5
    uterus O71.81
      before labor O71.81
    vagina, vaginal (deep) (high) (without
    perineal laceration) O71.4
      with perineum O70.0
        muscles, with perineum O70.1
    vulva O70.0
  liver disorder O26.62
  malignancy O9A.12
  malnutrition O25.2
  malposition, malpresentation
    placenta O44.0
      with hemorrhage O44.1
    uterus or cervix O65.5
    without obstruction -*see also* Delivery,
    complicated by, obstruction O32.9
      breech O32.1
      compound O32.6
      face (brow) (chin) O32.3
      footling O32.8
      high head O32.4
      oblique O32.2

Delivery (childbirth) (labor) --*continued*
    specified NEC O32.8
    transverse O32.2
    unstable lie O32.0
  meconium in amniotic fluid O77.0
  mental disorder NEC O99.344
  metrorrhexis -*see* Delivery, complicated
  by, rupture, uterus
  nervous system disorder O99.354
  obesity (pre-existing) O99.214
  obesity surgery status O99.844
  obstetric trauma O71.9
    specified NEC O71.89
  obstructed labor
    due to
      breech (complete) (frank) presentation
      O64.1
        incomplete O64.8
      brow presentation O64.3
      buttock presentation O64.1
      chin presentation O64.2
      compound presentation O64.5
      contracted pelvis O65.1
      deep transverse arrest O64.0
      deformed pelvis O65.0
      dystocia (fetal) O66.9
        due to
          conjoined twins O66.3
          fetal
            abnormality NEC O66.3
            ascites O66.3
            hydrops O66.3
            meningomyelocele O66.3
            sacral teratoma O66.3
            tumor O66.3
          hydrocephalic fetus O66.3
        shoulder O66.0
      face presentation O64.2
      fetopelvic disproportion O65.4
      footling presentation O64.8
      impacted shoulders O66.0
      incomplete rotation of fetal head O64.0
      large fetus O66.2
      locked twins O66.1
      malposition O64.9
        specified NEC O64.8
      malpresentation O64.9
        specified NEC O64.8
      multiple fetuses NEC O66.6
      pelvic
        abnormality (maternal) O65.9
          organ O65.5
          specified NEC O65.8
        contraction
          inlet O65.2
          mid-cavity O65.3
          outlet O65.3
      persistent (position)
        occipitoiliac O64.0
        occipitoposterior O64.0
        occipitosacral O64.0
        occipitotransverse O64.0
      prolapsed arm O64.4
      shoulder presentation O64.4
    specified NEC O66.8
  pathological retraction ring, uterus O62.4
  penetration, pregnant uterus by instrument
  O71.1
  perforation -*see* Delivery, complicated by,
  laceration
  placenta, placental

Delivery (childbirth) (labor) --*continued*
  ablatio -*see also* Abruptio placentae
    O45.9
  abnormality O43.9
    specified NEC O43.89
  abruptio -*see also* Abruptio placentae
    O45.9
  accreta O43.21
  adherent (with hemorrhage) O72.0
    without hemorrhage O73.0
  detachment (premature) -*see also*
    Abruptio placentae O45.9
  disorder O43.9
    specified NEC O43.89
  hemorrhage NEC O67.8
  increta O43.22
  low (implantation) (lying) O44.4
    with hemorrhage O44.5
  malformation O43.10
  malposition O44.0
    without hemorrhage O44.1
  percreta O43.23
  previa (central) (complete) (lateral) (total)
    O44.0
    with hemorrhage O44.1
    marginal O44.2
      with hemorrhage O44.3
    partial O44.2
      with hemorrhage O44.3
  retained (with hemorrhage) O72.0
    without hemorrhage O73.0
  separation (premature) O45.9
    specified NEC O45.8X
  vicious insertion O44.1
  precipitate labor O62.3
  premature rupture, membranes -*see also*
  Pregnancy, complicated by, premature
  rupture of membranes O42.90
  prolapse
    arm or hand O32.2
    cord (umbilical) O69.0
    foot or leg O32.8
    uterus O34.52
  prolonged labor O63.9
    first stage O63.0
    second stage O63.1
  protozoal disease (maternal) O98.62
  respiratory disease NEC O99.52
  retained membranes or portions of placenta
  O72.2
    without hemorrhage O73.1
  retarded birth O63.9
  retention of secundines (with hemorrhage)
  O72.0
    without hemorrhage O73.0
    partial O72.2
      without hemorrhage O73.1
  rupture
    bladder (urinary) O71.5
    cervix O71.3
    pelvic organ NEC O71.5
    urethra O71.5
    uterus (during or after labor) O71.1
      before labor O71.0
  separation, pubic bone (symphysis pubis)
    O71.6   shock O75.1
  shoulder presentation O64.4
  skin disorder NEC O99.72
  spasm, cervix O62.4
  stenosis or stricture, cervix O65.5

Delivery (childbirth) (labor) --*continued*
　streptococcus group B (GBS) carrier state
　　O99.824
　subluxation of symphysis (pubis) O26.72
　syphilis (maternal) O98.12
　tear -*see* Delivery, complicated by,
　　laceration
　tetanic uterus O62.4
　trauma (obstetrical) -*see also* Delivery,
　　complicated, by, damage to O71.9
　　non-obstetric O9A.22
　　periurethral O71.82
　　specified NEC O71.89
　tuberculosis (maternal) O98.02
　tumor, pelvic organs or tissues NEC O65.5
　umbilical cord around neck
　　with compression O69.1
　　without compression O69.81
　uterine inertia O62.2
　　during latent phase of labor O62.0
　　primary O62.0
　　secondary O62.1
　vasa previa O69.4
　velamentous insertion of cord O43.12
　specified complication NEC O75.89
delayed NOS O63.9
　following rupture of membranes
　　artificial O75.5
　second twin, triplet, etc. O63.2
forceps, low following failed vacuum
　extraction O66.5
missed (at or near term) O36.4
normal O80
obstructed -*see* Delivery, complicated by,
　obstruction
precipitate O62.3
preterm -*see also* Pregnancy, complicated by,
　preterm labor O60.10
spontaneous O80
term pregnancy NOS O80
uncomplicated O80
vaginal, following previous cesarean delivery
　O34.219
　classical (vertical) scar O34.212
　low transverse scar O34.211
Delusions (paranoid) -*see* Disorder, delusional
Dementia (degenerative (primary)) (old age)
(persisting) F03.90
　with
　　aggressive behavior F03.91
　　behavioral disturbance F03.91
　　combative behavior F03.91
　　Lewy bodies G31.83 [*F02.80*]
　　　with behavioral disturbance G31.83
　　　[*F02.81*]
　　Parkinsonism G31.83 [*F02.80*]
　　　with behavioral disturbance G31.83
　　　[*F02.81*]
　　Parkinson's disease G20 [*F02.80*]
　　　with behavioral disturbance G20 [*F02.81*]
　　violent behavior F03.91
　alcoholic F10.97
　　with dependence F10.27
　Alzheimer's type -*see* Disease, Alzheimer's
　arteriosclerotic -*see* Dementia, vascular
　atypical, Alzheimer's type -*see* Disease,
　　Alzheimer's, specified NEC
　congenital -*see* Disability, intellectual
　frontal (lobe) G31.09 [*F02.80*]
　　with behavioral disturbance G31.09
　　[*F02.81*]

Dementia --*continued*
　frontotemporal G31.09 [*F02.80*]
　　with behavioral disturbance G31.09
　　[*F02.81*]
　　specified NEC G31.09 [*F02.80*]
　　　with behavioral disturbance G31.09
　　　[*F02.81*]
　in (due to)
　　alcohol F10.97
　　　with dependence F10.27
　　Alzheimer's disease -*see* Disease,
　　　Alzheimer's
　　arteriosclerotic brain disease -*see* Dementia,
　　　vascular
　　cerebral lipidoses E75. [*F02.80*]
　　　with behavioral disturbance E75. [*F02.81*]
　　Creutzfeldt-Jakob disease -*see also*
　　　Creutzfeldt-Jakob disease or syndrome (with
　　　dementia) A81.00
　　epilepsy G40. [*F02.80*]
　　　with behavioral disturbance G40.
　　　[*F02.81*]
　　hepatolenticular degeneration E83.01
　　　[*F02.80*]
　　　with behavioral disturbance E83.01
　　　[*F02.81*]
　　human immunodeficiency virus (HIV)
　　disease B20 [*F02.80*]
　　　with behavioral disturbance B20 [*F02.81*]
　　Huntington's disease or chorea G10
　　hypercalcemia E83.52 [*F02.80*]
　　　with behavioral disturbance E83.52
　　　[*F02.81*]
　　hypothyroidism, acquired E03.9 [*F02.80*]
　　　with behavioral disturbance E03.9
　　　[*F02.81*]
　　　due to iodine deficiency E01.8 [*F02.80*]
　　　　with behavioral disturbance E01.8
　　　　[*F02.81*]
　　inhalants F18.97
　　　with dependence F18.27
　　multiple
　　　etiologies F03
　　　sclerosis G35 [*F02.80*]
　　　　with behavioral disturbance G35
　　　　[*F02.81*]
　　neurosyphilis A52.17 [*F02.80*]
　　　with behavioral disturbance A52.17
　　　[*F02.81*]
　　juvenile A50.49 [*F02.80*]
　　　with behavioral disturbance A50.49
　　　[*F02.81*]
　　niacin deficiency E52 [*F02.80*]
　　　with behavioral disturbance E52 [*F02.81*]
　　paralysis agitans G20 [*F02.80*]
　　　with behavioral disturbance G20 [*F02.81*]
　　Parkinson's disease G20 [*F02.80*]
　　pellagra E52 [*F02.80*]
　　　with behavioral disturbance E52 [*F02.81*]
　　Pick's G31.01 [*F02.80*]
　　　with behavioral disturbance G31.01
　　　[*F02.81*]
　　polyarteritis nodosa M30.0 [*F02.80*]
　　　with behavioral disturbance M30.0
　　　[*F02.81*]
　　psychoactive drug F19.97
　　　with dependence F19.27
　　inhalants F18.97
　　　with dependence F18.27
　　sedatives, hypnotics or anxiolytics F13.97
　　　with dependence F13.27

Dementia --*continued*
　　sedatives, hypnotics or anxiolytics F13.97
　　　with dependence F13.27
　　systemic lupus erythematosus M32.
　　　[*F02.80*]
　　　with behavioral disturbance M32.
　　　[*F02.81*]
　　trypanosomiasis
　　　African B56.9 [*F02.80*]
　　　　with behavioral disturbance B56.9
　　　　[*F02.81*]
　　unknown etiology F03
　　vitamin B12
　deficiency E53.8 [*F02.80*]
　　with behavioral disturbance E53.8
　　[*F02.81*]
　　volatile solvents F18.97
　　　with dependence F18.27
　　with behavioral disturbance G31.83
　　[*F02.81*]
　infantile, infantilis F84.3
　Lewy body G31.83 [*F02.80*]
　　with behavioral disturbance G31.83
　　[*F02.81*]
　multi-infarct -*see* Dementia, vascular
　paralytica, paralytic (syphilitic) A52.17
　　[*F02.80*]
　　with behavioral disturbance A52.17
　　[*F02.81*]
　　juvenilis A50.45
　paretic A52.17
　praecox -*see* Schizophrenia
　presenile F03
　　Alzheimer's type -*see* Disease, Alzheimer's,
　　　early onset
　primary degenerative F03
　progressive, syphilitic A52.17
　senile F03
　　with acute confusional state F05
　　Alzheimer's type -*see* Disease, Alzheimer's,
　　　late onset
　　depressed or paranoid type F03
　vascular (acute onset) (mixed) (multi-infarct)
　　(subcortical) F01.50
　　with behavioral disturbance F01.51
Demineralization, bone -*see* Osteoporosis
Demodex folliculorum (infestation) B88.0
Demophobia F40.248
Demoralization R45.3
Demyelination, demyelinization
　central nervous system G37.9
　　specified NEC G37.8
　corpus callosum (central) G37.1
　disseminated, acute G36.9
　　specified NEC G36.8
　global G35
　in optic neuritis G36.0
Dengue (classical) (fever) A90
　hemorrhagic A91
　sandfly A93.1
Dennie-Marfan syphilitic syndrome A50.45
Dens evaginatus, in dente or invaginatus
　K00.2
Dense breasts R92.2
Density
　increased, bone (disseminated) (generalized)
　　(spotted) -*see* Disorder, bone, density and
　　structure, specified type NEC
　lung (nodular) J98.4

Dental -*see also* condition
  examination Z01.20
    with abnormal findings Z01.21
  restoration
    aesthetically inadequate or displeasing
      K08.56
    defective K08.50
      specified NEC K08.59
    failure of marginal integrity K08.51
    failure of periodontal anatomical integrity
      K08.54
Dentia praecox K00.6
Denticles (pulp) K04.2
Dentigerous cyst K09.0
Dentin
  irregular (in pulp) K04.3
  opalescent K00.5
  secondary (in pulp) K04.3
  sensitive K03.89
Dentinogenesis imperfecta K00.5
Dentinoma -*see* Cyst, calcifying odontogenic
Dentition (syndrome) K00.7
  delayed K00.6
  difficult K00.7
  precocious K00.6
  premature K00.6
  retarded K00.6
Dependence (on) (syndrome) F19.20
  with remission F19.21
  alcohol (ethyl) (methyl) (without remission)
    F10.20
    with
      amnestic disorder, persisting F10.26
      anxiety disorder F10.280
      dementia, persisting F10.27
      intoxication F10.229
        with delirium F10.221
        uncomplicated F10.220
      mood disorder F10.24
      psychotic disorder F10.259
        with
          delusions F10.250
          hallucinations F10.251
      remission F10.21
      sexual dysfunction F10.281
      sleep disorder F10.282
      specified disorder NEC F10.288
      withdrawal F10.239
        with
          delirium F10.231
          perceptual disturbance F10.232
        uncomplicated F10.230
    counseling and surveillance Z71.41
  amobarbital -*see* Dependence, drug, sedative
  amphetamine(s) (type) -*see* Dependence,
    drug, stimulant NEC
  amytal (sodium) -*see* Dependence, drug,
    sedative
  analgesic NEC F55.8
  anesthetic (agent) (gas) (general) (local) NEC
    -*see* Dependence, drug, psychoactive NEC
  anxiolytic NEC -*see* Dependence, drug,
    sedative
  barbital(s) -*see* Dependence, drug, sedative
  barbiturate(s) (compounds) (drugs classifiable
    to T42) -*see* Dependence, drug, sedative
  benzedrine -*see* Dependence, drug, stimulant
    NEC
  bhang -*see* Dependence, drug, cannabis
  bromide(s) NEC -*see* Dependence, drug,
    sedative

Dependence (on) (syndrome) --*continued*
  caffeine -*see* Dependence, drug, stimulant
    NEC
  cannabis (sativa) (indica) (resin) (derivatives)
    (type) -*see* Dependence, drug, cannabis
  chloral (betaine) (hydrate) -*see* Dependence,
    drug, sedative
  chlordiazepoxide -*see* Dependence, drug,
    sedative
  coca (leaf) (derivatives) -*see* Dependence,
    drug, cocaine
  cocaine -*see* Dependence, drug, cocaine
  codeine -*see* Dependence, drug, opioid
  combinations of drugs F19.20
  dagga -*see* Dependence, drug, cannabis
  demerol -*see* Dependence, drug, opioid
  dexamphetamine -*see* Dependence, drug,
    stimulant NEC
  dexedrine -*see* Dependence, drug, stimulant
    NEC
  dextromethorphan -*see* Dependence, drug,
    opioid
  dextromoramide -*see* Dependence, drug,
    opioid
  dextro-nor-pseudo-ephedrine -*see*
    Dependence, drug, stimulant NEC
  dextrorphan -*see* Dependence, drug, opioid
  diazepam -*see* Dependence, drug, sedative
  dilaudid -*see* Dependence, drug, opioid
  D-lysergic acid diethylamide -*see*
    Dependence, drug, hallucinogen
  drug NEC F19.20
    with sleep disorder F19.282
    cannabis F12.20
      with
        anxiety disorder F12.280
        intoxication F12.229
          with
            delirium F12.221
            perceptual disturbance F12.222
          uncomplicated F12.220
        other specified disorder F12.288
        psychosis F12.259
          delusions F12.250
          hallucinations F12.251
        unspecified disorder F12.29
      in remission F12.21
    cocaine F14.20
      with
        anxiety disorder F14.280
        intoxication F14.229
          with
            delirium F14.221
            perceptual disturbance F14.222
          uncomplicated F14.220
        mood disorder F14.24
        other specified disorder F14.288
        psychosis F14.259
          delusions F14.250
          hallucinations F14.251
        sexual dysfunction F14.281
        sleep disorder F14.282
        unspecified disorder F14.29
        withdrawal F14.23
      in remission F14.21
      withdrawal symptoms in newborn P96.1
    counseling and surveillance Z71.51
    hallucinogen F16.20
      with
        anxiety disorder F16.280
        flashbacks F16.283

Dependence (on) (syndrome) --*continued*
      intoxication F16.229
        with delirium F16.221
        uncomplicated F16.220
      mood disorder F16.24
      other specified disorder F16.288
      perception disorder, persisting F16.283
      psychosis F16.259
        delusions F16.250
        hallucinations F16.251
      unspecified disorder F16.29
    in remission F16.21
  in remission F19.21
  inhalant F18.20
    with
      anxiety disorder F18.280
      dementia, persisting F18.27
      intoxication F18.229
        with delirium F18.221
        uncomplicated F18.220
      mood disorder F18.24
      other specified disorder F18.288
      psychosis F18.259
        delusions F18.250
        hallucinations F18.251
      unspecified disorder F18.29
    in remission F18.21
  nicotine F17.200
    with disorder F17.209
      remission F17.201
      specified disorder NEC F17.208
      withdrawal F17.203
    chewing tobacco F17.220
      with disorder F17.229
        remission F17.221
        specified disorder NEC F17.228
        withdrawal F17.223
    cigarettes F17.210
      with disorder F17.219
        remission F17.211
        specified disorder NEC F17.218
        withdrawal F17.213
    specified product NEC F17.290
      with disorder F17.299
        remission F17.291
        specified disorder NEC F17.298
        withdrawal F17.293
  opioid F11.20
    with
      intoxication F11.229
        with
          delirium F11.221
          perceptual disturbance F11.222
        uncomplicated F11.220
      mood disorder F11.24
      other specified disorder F11.288
      psychosis F11.259
        delusions F11.250
        hallucinations F11.251
      sexual dysfunction F11.281
      sleep disorder F11.282
      unspecified disorder F11.29
      withdrawal F11.23
    in remission F11.21
  psychoactive NEC F19.20
    with
      amnestic disorder F19.26
      anxiety disorder F19.280
      dementia F19.27
      intoxication F19.229
        with

Dependence (on) (syndrome) --*continued*
 delirium F19.221
  perceptual disturbance F19.222
  uncomplicated F19.220
 mood disorder F19.24
 other specified disorder F19.288
 psychosis F19.259
  delusions F19.250
  hallucinations F19.251
 sexual dysfunction F19.281
 sleep disorder F19.282
 unspecified disorder F19.29
 withdrawal F19.239
  with
   delirium F19.231
   perceptual disturbance F19.232
   uncomplicated F19.230
sedative, hypnotic or anxiolytic F13.20
 with
  amnestic disorder F13.26
  anxiety disorder F13.280
  dementia, persisting F13.27
  intoxication F13.229
   with delirium F13.221
   uncomplicated F13.220
  mood disorder F13.24
  other specified disorder F13.288
  psychosis F13.259
   delusions F13.250
   hallucinations F13.251
  sexual dysfunction F13.281
  sleep disorder F13.282
  unspecified disorder F13.29
  withdrawal F13.239
   with
    delirium F13.231
    perceptual disturbance F13.232
    uncomplicated F13.230
 in remission F13.21
stimulant NEC F15.20
 with
  anxiety disorder F15.280
  intoxication F15.229
   with
    delirium F15.221
    perceptual disturbance F15.222
   uncomplicated F15.220
  mood disorder F15.24
  other specified disorder F15.288
  psychosis F15.259
   delusions F15.250
   hallucinations F15.251
  sexual dysfunction F15.281
  sleep disorder F15.282
  unspecified disorder F15.29
  withdrawal F15.23
 in remission F15.21
ethyl
 alcohol (without remission) F10.20
  with remission F10.21
 bromide -*see* Dependence, drug, sedative
 carbamate F19.20
 chloride F19.20
 morphine -*see* Dependence, drug, opioid
ganja -*see* Dependence, drug, cannabis
glue (airplane) (sniffing) -*see* Dependence,
 drug, inhalant
glutethimide -*see* Dependence, drug, sedative
hallucinogenics -*see* Dependence, drug,
 hallucinogen
hashish -*see* Dependence, drug, cannabis

Dependence (on) (syndrome) --*continued*
hemp -*see* Dependence, drug, cannabis
heroin (salt) (any) -*see* Dependence, drug,
 opioid
hypnotic NEC -*see* Dependence, drug,
 sedative
Indian hemp -*see* Dependence, drug, cannabis
inhalants -*see* Dependence, drug, inhalant
khat -*see* Dependence, drug, stimulant NEC
laudanum -*see* Dependence, drug, opioid
LSD (25) (derivatives) -*see* Dependence,
 drug, hallucinogen
luminal -*see* Dependence, drug, sedative
lysergic acid -*see* Dependence, drug,
 hallucinogen
maconha -*see* Dependence, drug, cannabis
marihuana -*see* Dependence, drug, cannabis
meprobamate -*see* Dependence, drug, sedative
mescaline -*see* Dependence, drug,
 hallucinogen
methadone -*see* Dependence, drug, opioid
methamphetamine(s) -*see* Dependence, drug,
 stimulant NEC
methaqualone -*see* Dependence, drug,
 sedative
methyl
 alcohol (without remission) F10.20
  with remission F10.21
 bromide -*see* Dependence, drug, sedative
 morphine -*see* Dependence, drug, opioid
 phenidate -*see* Dependence, drug, stimulant
  NEC
 sulfonal -*see* Dependence, drug, sedative
morphine (sulfate) (sulfite) (type) -*see*
 Dependence, drug, opioid
narcotic (drug) NEC -*see* Dependence, drug,
 opioid
nembutal -*see* Dependence, drug, sedative
neraval -*see* Dependence, drug, sedative
neravan -*see* Dependence, drug, sedative
neurobarb -*see* Dependence, drug, sedative
nicotine -*see* Dependence, drug, nicotine
nitrous oxide F19.20
nonbarbiturate sedatives and tranquilizers
 with similar effect -*see* Dependence, drug,
 sedative
on
 artificial heart (fully implantable)
  (mechanical) Z95.812
 aspirator Z99.0
 care provider (because of) Z74.9
  impaired mobility Z74.09
  need for
   assistance with personal care Z74.1
   continuous supervision Z74.3
  no other household member able to render
   care Z74.2
  specified reason NEC Z74.8
 machine Z99.89
  enabling NEC Z99.89
  specified type NEC Z99.89
 renal dialysis (hemodialysis) (peritoneal)
  Z99.2
 respirator Z99.11
 ventilator Z99.11
 wheelchair Z99.3
opiate -*see* Dependence, drug, opioid
opioids -*see* Dependence, drug, opioid
opium (alkaloids) (derivatives) (tincture) -*see*
 Dependence, drug, opioid
oxygen (long-term) (supplemental) Z99.81

Dependence (on) (syndrome) --*continued*
paraldehyde -*see* Dependence, drug, sedative
paregoric -*see* Dependence, drug, opioid
PCP (phencyclidine) (or related substance) -
 see Dependence, drug, hallucinogen
pentobarbital -*see* Dependence, drug, sedative
pentobarbitone (sodium) -*see* Dependence,
 drug, sedative
pentothal -*see* Dependence, drug, sedative
peyote -*see* Dependence, drug, hallucinogen
phencyclidine (PCP) (or related substance) -
 see Dependence, drug, hallucinogen
phenmetrazine -*see* Dependence, drug,
 stimulant NEC
phenobarbital -*see* Dependence, drug,
 sedative
polysubstance F19.20
psilocybin, psilocin, psilocin, psilocyline -*see*
 Dependence, drug, hallucinogen
psychostimulant NEC -*see* Dependence, drug,
 stimulant NEC
secobarbital -*see* Dependence, drug, sedative
seconal -*see* Dependence, drug, sedative
sedative NEC -*see* Dependence, drug,
 sedative
specified drug NEC -*see* Dependence, drug
stimulant NEC -*see* Dependence, drug,
 stimulant NEC
substance NEC -*see* Dependence, drug
supplemental oxygen Z99.81
tobacco -*see* Dependence, drug, nicotine
 counseling and surveillance Z71.6
tranquilizer NEC -*see* Dependence, drug,
 sedative
vitamin B6 E53.1
volatile solvents -*see* Dependence, drug,
 inhalant
Dependency
care-provider Z74.9
passive F60.7
reactions (persistent) F60.7
Depersonalization (in neurotic state)
(neurotic) (syndrome) F48.1
Depletion
extracellular fluid E86.9
plasma E86.1
potassium E87.6
 nephropathy N25.89
salt or sodium E87.1
 causing heat exhaustion or prostration T67.4
 nephropathy N28.9
volume NOS E86.9
Deployment (current) (military) status
Z56.82
in theater or in support of military war,
 peacekeeping and humanitarian operations
 Z56.82
personal history of Z91.82
 military war, peacekeeping and
  humanitarian deployment (current or past
  conflict) Z91.82
 returned from Z91.82
Depolarization, premature I49.40
atrial I49.1
junctional I49.2
specified NEC I49.49
ventricular I49.3
Deposit
bone in Boeck's sarcoid D86.89
calcareous, calcium -*see* Calcification
cholesterol
 retina H35.89

Deposit - *continued*
  vitreous (body) (humor) -*see* Deposit, crystalline
  conjunctiva H11.11
  cornea H18.00
    argentous H18.02
    due to metabolic disorder H18.03
    Kayser-Fleischer ring H18.04
    pigmentation -*see* Pigmentation, cornea
  crystalline, vitreous (body) (humor) H43.2
  hemosiderin in old scars of cornea -*see* Pigmentation, cornea, stromal
  metallic in lens -*see* Cataract, specified NEC
  skin R23.8
  tooth, teeth (betel) (black) (green) (materia alba) (orange) (tobacco) K03.6
  urate, kidney -*see* Calculus, kidney
Depraved appetite -*see* Pica
Depressed
  HDL cholesterol E78.6
Depression (acute) (mental) F32.9
  agitated (single episode) F32.2
  anaclitic -*see* Disorder, adjustment
  anxiety F41.8
    persistent F34.1
  arches -*see also* Deformity, limb, flat foot
  atypical (single episode) F32.89
    recurrent episode F33.8
  basal metabolic rate R94.8
  bone marrow D75.89
  central nervous system R09.2
  cerebral R29.818
    newborn P91.4
  cerebrovascular I67.9
  chest wall M95.4
  climacteric (single episode) F32.89
    recurrent episode F33.8
  endogenous (without psychotic symptoms) F33.2
    with psychotic symptoms F33.3
  functional activity R68.89
  hysterical F44.89
  involutional (single episode) F32.89
    recurrent episode F33.8
  major F32.9
    with psychotic symptoms F32.3
    recurrent -*see* Disorder, depressive, recurrent
  manic-depressive -*see* Disorder, depressive, recurrent
  masked (single episode) F32.89
  medullary G93.89
  menopausal (single episode) F32.89
    recurrent episode F33.8
  metatarsus -*see* Depression, arches
  monopolar F33.9
  nervous F34.1
  neurotic F34.1
  nose M95.0
  postnatal F53
  postpartum F53
  post-psychotic of schizophrenia F32.89
  post-schizophrenic F32.89
  psychogenic (reactive) (single episode) F32.9
  psychoneurotic F34.1
  psychotic (single episode) F32.3
    recurrent F33.3
  reactive (psychogenic) (single episode) F32.9
    psychotic (single episode) F32.3
  recurrent -*see* Disorder, depressive, recurrent
  respiratory center G93.89

Depression - *continued*
  seasonal -*see* Disorder, depressive, recurrent
  senile F03
  severe, single episode F32.2
  situational F43.21
  skull Q67.4
  specified NEC (single episode) F32.89
  sternum M95.4
  visual field -*see* Defect, visual field
  vital (recurrent) (without psychotic symptoms) F33.2
    with psychotic symptoms F33.3
    single episode F32.2
Deprivation
  cultural Z60.3
  effects NOS T73.9
    specified NEC T73.8
  emotional NEC Z65.8
    affecting infant or child -*see* Maltreatment, child, psychological
  food T73.0
  protein -*see* Malnutrition
  sleep Z72.820
  social Z60.4
    affecting infant or child -*see* Maltreatment, child, psychological
  specified NEC T73.8
  vitamins -*see* Deficiency, vitamin
  water T73.1
Derangement
  ankle (internal) -*see* Derangement, joint, ankle
  cartilage (articular) NEC -*see* Derangement, joint, articular cartilage, by site
    recurrent -*see* Dislocation, recurrent
  cruciate ligament, anterior, current injury -*see* Sprain, knee, cruciate, anterior
  elbow (internal) -*see* Derangement, joint, elbow
  hip (joint) (internal) (old) -*see* Derangement, joint, hip
  joint (internal) M24.9
    ankylosis -*see* Ankylosis
    articular cartilage M24.10
      ankle M24.17
      elbow M24.12
      foot M24.17
      hand M24.14
      hip M24.15
      knee NEC M23.9
      loose body -*see* Loose, body
      shoulder M24.11
      wrist M24.13
    contracture -*see* Contraction, joint
    current injury -*see also* Dislocation
      knee, meniscus or cartilage -*see* Tear, meniscus
    dislocation
      pathological -*see* Dislocation, pathological
      recurrent -*see* Dislocation, recurrent
    knee -*see* Derangement, knee
    ligament -*see* Disorder, ligament
    loose body -*see* Loose, body
    recurrent -*see* Dislocation, recurrent
    specified type NEC M24.80
      ankle M24.87
      elbow M24.82
      foot joint M24.87
      hand joint M24.84
      hip M24.85
      shoulder M24.81

Derangement - *continued*
  wrist M24.83
  temporomandibular M26.69
  knee (recurrent) M23.9
    ligament disruption, spontaneous M23.60
      anterior cruciate M23.61
      capsular M23.67
      instability, chronic M23.5
      lateral collateral M23.64
      medial collateral M23.63
      posterior cruciate M23.62
    loose body M23.4
    meniscus M23.30
      cystic M23.00
        lateral M23.002
          anterior horn M23.04
          posterior horn M23.05
          specified NEC M23.06
        medial M23.005
          anterior horn M23.01
          posterior horn M23.02
          specified NEC M23.03
      degenerate -*see* Derangement, knee, meniscus, specified NEC
      detached -*see* Derangement, knee, meniscus, specified NEC
      due to old tear or injury M23.20
        lateral M23.20
          anterior horn M23.24
          posterior horn M23.25
          specified NEC M23.26
        medial M23.20
          anterior horn M23.21
          posterior horn M23.22
          specified NEC M23.23
      retained -*see* Derangement, knee, meniscus, specified NEC
      specified NEC M23.30
        lateral M23.30
          anterior horn M23.34
          posterior horn M23.35
          specified NEC M23.36
        medial M23.30
          anterior horn M23.31
          posterior horn M23.32
          specified NEC M23.33
      old M23.8X
    specified NEC -*see* subcategory M23.8
  low back NEC -*see* Dorsopathy, specified NEC
  meniscus -*see* Derangement, knee, meniscus
  mental -*see* Psychosis
  patella, specified NEC -*see* Disorder, patella, derangement NEC
  semilunar cartilage (knee) -*see* Derangement, knee, meniscus, specified NEC
  shoulder (internal) -*see* Derangement, joint, shoulder
Dercum's disease E88.2
Derealization (neurotic) F48.1
Dermal -*see* condition **Dermaphytid -***see* Dermatophytosis
Dermatitis (eczematous) L30.9
  ab igne L59.0
  acarine B88.0
  actinic (due to sun) L57.8
    other than from sun L59.8 allergic -*see* Dermatitis, contact, allergic
  ambustionis, due to burn or scald -*see* Burn
  amebic A06.7
  ammonia L22

Dermatitis - *continued*
  arsenical (ingested) L27.8
  artefacta L98.1
    psychogenic F54
  atopic L20.9
    psychogenic F54
    specified NEC L20.89
  autoimmune progesterone L30.8
  berlock, berloque L56.2
  blastomycotic B40.3
  blister beetle L24.89
  bullous, bullosa L13.9
    mucosynechial, atrophic L12.1
    seasonal L30.8
    specified NEC L13.8
  calorica L59.0
    due to burn or scald -*see* Burn
  caterpillar L24.89
  cercarial B65.3
  combustionis L59.0
    due to burn or scald -*see* Burn
  congelationis T69.1
  contact (occupational) L25.9
    allergic L23.9
      due to
        adhesives L23.1
        cement L23.5
        chemical products NEC L23.5
        chromium L23.0
        cosmetics L23.2
        dander (cat) (dog) L23.81
        drugs in contact with skin L23.3
        dyes L23.4
        food in contact with skin L23.6
        hair (cat) (dog) L23.81
        insecticide L23.5
        metals L23.0
        nickel L23.0
        plants, non-food L23.7
        plastic L23.5
        rubber L23.5
        specified agent NEC L23.89
    due to
      cement L25.3
      chemical products NEC L25.3
      cosmetics L25.0
      dander (cat) (dog) L23.81
      drugs in contact with skin L25.1
      dyes L25.2
      food in contact with skin L25.4
      hair (cat) (dog) L23.81
      plants, non-food L25.5
      specified agent NEC L25.8
    irritant L24.9
      due to
        cement L24.5
        chemical products NEC L24.5
        cosmetics L24.3
        detergents L24.0
        drugs in contact with skin L24.4
        food in contact with skin L24.6
        oils and greases L24.1
        plants, non-food L24.7
        solvents L24.2
        specified agent NEC L24.89
  contusiformis L52
Dermatitis - *continued*
  diabetic -*see* E08 E13 with .620
  diaper L22
  diphtheritica A36.3
  dry skin L85.3

Dermatitis - *continued*
  due to
    acetone (contact) (irritant) L24.2
    acids (contact) (irritant) L24.5
    adhesive(s) (allergic) (contact) (plaster)
      L23.1
        irritant L24.5
    alcohol (irritant) (skin contact) (substances
      in category T51) L24.2
        taken internally L27.8
    alkalis (contact) (irritant) L24.5
    arsenic (ingested) L27.8
    carbon disulfide (contact) (irritant) L24.2
    caustics (contact) (irritant) L24.5
    cement (contact) L25.3
    cereal (ingested) L27.2
    chemical(s) NEC L25.3
        taken internally L27.8
    chlorocompounds L24.2
    chromium (contact) (irritant) L24.81
    coffee (ingested) L27.2
    cold weather L30.8
    cosmetics (contact) L25.0
        allergic L23.2
        irritant L24.3
    cyclohexanes L24.2
    dander (cat) (dog) L23.81
    Demodex species B88.0
    Dermanyssus gallinae B88.0
    detergents (contact) (irritant) L24.0
    dichromate L24.81
    drugs and medicaments (generalized)
      (internal use) L27.0
        external -*see* Dermatitis, due to, drugs, in
          contact with skin
        in contact with skin L25.1
          allergic L23.3
          irritant L24.4
        localized skin eruption L27.1
        specified substance -*see* Table of Drugs
          and Chemicals
    dyes (contact) L25.2
        allergic L23.4
        irritant L24.89
    epidermophytosis -*see* Dermatophytosis
    esters L24.2
    external irritant NEC L24.9
    fish (ingested) L27.2
    flour (ingested) L27.2
    food (ingested) L27.2
        in contact with skin L25.4
    fruit (ingested) L27.2
    furs (allergic) (contact) L23.81
    glues -*see* Dermatitis, due to, adhesives
    glycols L24.2
    greases NEC (contact) (irritant) L24.1
    hair (cat) (dog) L23.81
    hot
        objects and materials -*see* Burn
        weather or places L59.0
    hydrocarbons L24.2
    infrared rays L59.8
    ingestion, ingested substance L27.9
        chemical NEC L27.8
        drugs and medicaments -*see* Dermatitis,
          due to, drugs
        food L27.2
        specified NEC L27.8
    insecticide in contact with skin L24.5
    internal agent L27.9

Dermatitis - *continued*
    drugs and medicaments (generalized) -*see*
      Dermatitis, due to, drugs
      food L27.2
    irradiation -*see* Dermatitis, due to,
      radioactive substance
    ketones L24.2
    lacquer tree (allergic) (contact) L23.7
    light (sun) NEC L57.8
      acute L56.8
      other L59.8
    Liponyssoides sanguineus B88.0
    low temperature L30.8
    meat (ingested) L27.2
    metals, metal salts (contact) (irritant) L24.81
    milk (ingested) L27.2
    nickel (contact) (irritant) L24.81
    nylon (contact) (irritant) L24.5
    oils NEC (contact) (irritant) L24.1
    paint solvent (contact) (irritant) L24.2
    petroleum products (contact) (irritant)
      (substances in T52.0) L24.2
    plants NEC (contact) L25.5
      allergic L23.7
      irritant L24.7
    plasters (adhesive) (any) (allergic) (contact)
      L23.1
        irritant L24.5
    plastic (contact) L25.3
    preservatives (contact) -*see* Dermatitis, due
      to, chemical, in contact with skin
    primrose (allergic) (contact) L23.7
    primula (allergic) (contact) L23.7
    radiation L59.8
      nonionizing (chronic exposure) L57.8
      sun NEC L57.8
        acute L56.8
    radioactive substance L58.9
      acute L58.0
      chronic L58.1
    radium L58.9
      acute L58.0
      chronic L58.1
    ragweed (allergic) (contact) L23.7
    Rhus (allergic) (contact) (diversiloba)
      (radicans) (toxicodendron) (venenata)
      (verniciflua) L23.7
    rubber (contact) L24.5
    Senecio jacobaea (allergic) (contact) L23.7
    solvents (contact) (irritant) (substances in
      categories T52) L24.2
    specified agent NEC (contact) L25.8
      allergic L23.89
      irritant L24.89
    sunshine NEC L57.8
      acute L56.8
    tetrachlorethylene (contact) (irritant) L24.2
    toluene (contact) (irritant) L24.2
    turpentine (contact) L24.2
    ultraviolet rays (sun NEC) (chronic
      exposure) L57.8
      acute L56.8
    vaccine or vaccination L27.0
      specified substance -*see* Table of Drugs
        and Chemicals
    varicose veins -*see* Varix, leg, with,
  inflammation- X rays L58.9
      acute L58.0
      chronic L58.1
  dyshidrotic L30.1

Dermatitis - *continued*
dysmenorrheica N94.6
escharotica -*see* Burn
exfoliative, exfoliativa (generalized) L26
   neonatorum L00
eyelid -*see also* Dermatosis, eyelid
   allergic H01.119
      left H01.116
         lower H01.115
         upper H01.114
      right H01.113
         lower H01.112
         upper H01.111
   contact -*see* Dermatitis, eyelid, allergic
   due to
      Demodex species B88.0
      herpes (zoster) B02.39
         simplex B00.59
   eczematous H01.139
      left H01.136
         lower H01.135
         upper H01.134
      right H01.133
         lower H01.132
         upper H01.131
facta, factitia, factitial L98.1
   psychogenic F54
flexural NEC L20.82
friction L30.4
fungus B36.9
   specified type NEC B36.8
gangrenosa, gangrenous infantum L08.0
harvest mite B88.0
heat L59.0
herpesviral, vesicular (ear) (lip) B00.1
herpetiformis (bullous) (erythematous)
   (pustular) (vesicular) L13.0
      juvenile L12.2
      senile L12.0
hiemalis L30.8
hypostatic, hypostatica -*see* Varix, leg, with,
   inflammation
infectious eczematoid L30.3
infective L30.3
irritant -*see* Dermatitis, contact, irritant
Jacquet's (diaper dermatitis) L22
Leptus B88.0
lichenified NEC L28.0
medicamentosa (generalized) (internal use) -
   see Dermatitis, due to drugs
mite B88.0
multiformis L13.0
   juvenile L12.2
napkin L22
neurotica L13.0
nummular L30.0
papillaris capillitii L73.0
pellagrous E52
perioral L71.0
photocontact L56.2
polymorpha dolorosa L13.0
pruriginosa L13.0
pruritic NEC L30.8
psychogenic F54
purulent L08.0
pustular
   contagious B08.02
   subcorneal L13.1
pyococcal L08.0
pyogenica L08.0
repens L40.2

Dermatitis - *continued*
Ritter's (exfoliativa) L00
Schamberg's L81.7
schistosome B65.3
seasonal bullous L30.8
seborrheic L21.9
   infantile L21.1
   specified NEC L21.8
sensitization NOS L23.9
septic L08.0
solare L57.8
specified NEC L30.8
stasis I87.2
   with
      varicose ulcer -*see* Varix, leg, with ulcer,
         with inflammation
      varicose veins -*see* Varix, leg, with,
         inflammation
   due to postthrombotic syndrome -*see*
      Syndrome, postthrombotic
suppurative L08.0
traumatic NEC L30.4
trophoneurotica L13.0
ultraviolet (sun) (chronic exposure) L57.8
   acute L56.8
varicose -*see* Varix, leg, with, inflammation
vegetans L10.1
verrucosa B43.0
vesicular, herpesviral B00.1
Dermatoarthritis, lipoid E78.81
Dermatochalasis, eyelid H02.839
   left H02.836
      lower H02.835
      upper H02.834
   right H02.833
      lower H02.832
      upper H02.831
Dermatofibroma (lenticulare) -*see* Neoplasm,
skin, benign
   protuberans -*see* Neoplasm, skin, uncertain
   behavior
Dermatofibrosarcoma (pigmented)
   (protuberans) -*see* Neoplasm, skin,
   malignant
Dermatographia L50.3
Dermatolysis (exfoliativa) (congenital) Q82.8
   acquired L57.4
   eyelids -*see* Blepharochalasis
   palpebrarum -*see* Blepharochalasis
   senile L57.4
Dermatomegaly NEC Q82.8
Dermatomucosomyositis M33.10
   with
      myopathy M33.12
      respiratory involvement M33.11
      specified organ involvement NEC M33.19
Dermatomycosis B36.9
   furfuracea B36.0
   specified type NEC B36.8
Dermatomyositis (acute) (chronic) -*see also*
   Dermatopolymyositis
   in (due to) neoplastic disease -*see also*
      Neoplasm D49.9 [*M36.0*]
Dermatoneuritis of children -*see* Poisoning,
mercury
Dermatophilosis A48.8

Dermatophytid L30.2
Dermatophytide -*see* Dermatophytosis
Dermatophytosis (epidermophyton)
   (infection) (Microsporum) (tinea)
   (Trichophyton) B35.9
   beard B35.0
   body B35.4
   capitis B35.0
   corporis B35.4
   deep-seated B35.8
   disseminated B35.8
   foot B35.3
   granulomatous B35.8
   groin B35.6
   hand B35.2
   nail B35.1
   perianal (area) B35.6
   scalp B35.0
   specified NEC B35.8
Dermatopolymyositis M33.90
   with
      myopathy M33.92
      respiratory involvement M33.91
      specified organ involvement NEC M33.99
   in neoplastic disease -*see also* Neoplasm
      D49.9 [*M36.0*]
   juvenile M33.00
      with
         myopathy M33.02
         respiratory involvement M33.01
         specified organ involvement NEC M33.09
   specified NEC M33.10
      myopathy M33.12
      respiratory involvement M33.11
      specified organ involvement NEC M33.19
Dermatopolyneuritis -*see* Poisoning, mercury
Dermatorrhexis Q79.6
   acquired L57.4
Dermatosclerosis -*see also* Scleroderma
   localized L94.0
Dermatosis L98.9
   Andrews' L08.89
   Bowen's -*see* Neoplasm, skin, in situ
   bullous L13.9
      specified NEC L13.8
   exfoliativa L26
   eyelid (noninfectious)
      dermatitis -*see* Dermatitis, eyelid
      discoid lupus erythematosus -*see* Lupus,
         erythematosus, eyelid
      xeroderma -*see* Xeroderma, acquired, eyelid
   factitial L98.1
   febrile neutrophilic L98.2
   gonococcal A54.89
   herpetiformis L13.0
      juvenile L12.2
   linear IgA L13.8
   menstrual NEC L98.8
   neutrophilic, febrile L98.2
   occupational -*see* Dermatitis, contact
   papulosa nigra L82.1
   pigmentary L81.9
      progressive L81.7
         Schamberg's L81.7
   psychogenic F54
   purpuric, pigmented L81.7
   pustular, subcorneal L13.1
   transient acantholytic L11.1
Dermographia, dermographism L50.3
Dermoid (cyst) -*see also* Neoplasm, benign, by
site
   with malignant transformation C56
   due to radiation (nonionizing) L57.8

Dermopathy
infiltrative with thyrotoxicosis -*see*
Thyrotoxicosis
nephrogenic fibrosing L90.8
Dermophytosis -*see* Dermatophytosis
Descemetocele H18.73
Descemet's membrane -*see* condition
Descending -*see* condition
Descensus uteri -*see* Prolapse, uterus
Desert
rheumatism B38.0
sore -*see* Ulcer, skin
Desertion (newborn) -*see* Maltreatment
Desmoid (extra-abdominal) (tumor) -*see*
Neoplasm, connective tissue, uncertain
behavior
abdominal D48.1
Despondency F32.9
Desquamation, skin R23.4
Destruction, destructive -*see also* Damage
articular facet -*see also* Derangement, joint,
specified type NEC
knee M23.8X
vertebra -*see* Spondylosis
bone -*see also* Disorder, bone, specified type
NEC
syphilitic A52.77
joint -*see also* Derangement, joint, specified
type NEC
sacroiliac M53.3
rectal sphincter K62.89
septum (nasal) J34.89
tuberculous NEC -*see* Tuberculosis
tympanum, tympanic membrane
(nontraumatic) -*see* Disorder, tympanic
membrane, specified NEC
vertebral disc -*see* Degeneration,
intervertebral disc
Destructiveness -*see also* Disorder, conduct
adjustment reaction -*see* Disorder, adjustment
Desultory labor O62.2
Detachment
cartilage -*see* Sprain
cervix, annular N88.8
complicating delivery O71.3
choroid (old) (postinfectional) (simple)
(spontaneous) H31.40
hemorrhagic H31.41
serous H31.42
ligament -*see* Sprain
meniscus (knee) -*see also* Derangement, knee,
meniscus, specified NEC
current injury -*see* Tear, meniscus
due to old tear or injury -*see* Derangement,
knee, meniscus, due to old tear
retina (without retinal break) (serous) H33.2
with retinal:
break H33.00
giant H33.03
multiple H33.02
single H33.01
dialysis H33.04
pigment epithelium -*see* Degeneration,
retina, separation of layers, pigment
epithelium detachment
rhegmatogenous -*see* Detachment, retina,
with retinal, break
specified NEC H33.8
total H33.05
traction H33.4
vitreous (body) H43.81

Detergent asthma J69.8
Deterioration
epileptic F06.8
general physical R53.81
heart, cardiac -*see* Degeneration, myocardial
mental -*see* Psychosis
myocardial, myocardium -*see* Degeneration,
myocardial
senile (simple) R54
Deuteranomaly (anomalous trichromat)
H53.53
Deuteranopia (complete) (incomplete)
H53.53
Development
abnormal, bone Q79.9
arrested R62.50
bone -*see* Arrest, development or growth,
bone
child R62.50
due to malnutrition E45
defective, congenital -*see also* Anomaly, by
site
cauda equina Q06.3
left ventricle Q24.8
in hypoplastic left heart syndrome Q23.4
valve Q24.8
pulmonary Q22.3
delayed -*see also* Delay, development R62.50
arithmetical skills F81.2
language (skills) (expressive) F80.1
learning skill F81.9
mixed skills F88
motor coordination F82
reading F81.0
specified learning skill NEC F81.89
speech F80.9
spelling F81.81
written expression F81.81
imperfect, congenital -*see also* Anomaly, by
site
heart Q24.9
lungs Q33.6
incomplete
bronchial tree Q32.4
organ or site not listed -*see* Hypoplasia, by
site
respiratory system Q34.9
sexual, precocious NEC E30.1
tardy, mental -*see also* Disability, intellectual
F79
Developmental -*see* condition
testing, infant or child -*see* Examination, child
Devergie's disease (pityriasis rubra pilaris)
L44.0
Deviation (in)
conjugate palsy (eye) (spastic) H51.0
esophagus (acquired) K22.8
eye, skew H51.8
midline (jaw) (teeth) (dental arch) M26.29
specified site NEC -*see* Malposition
nasal septum J34.2
congenital Q67.4
opening and closing of the mandible M26.53
organ or site, congenital NEC -*see*
Malposition, congenital
septum (nasal) (acquired) J34.2
congenital Q67.4
sexual F65.9
bestiality F65.89
erotomania F52.8
exhibitionism F65.2

Deviation (in) --*continued*
fetishism, fetishistic F65.0
transvestism F65.1
frotteurism F65.81
masochism F65.51
multiple F65.89
necrophilia F65.89
nymphomania F52.8
pederosis F65.4
pedophilia F65.4
sadism, sadomasochism F65.52
satyriasis F52.8
specified type NEC F65.89
transvestism F64.1
voyeurism F65.3
teeth, midline M26.29
trachea J39.8
ureter, congenital Q62.61
Device
cerebral ventricle (communicating) in situ
Z98.2
contraceptive -*see* Contraceptive, device
drainage, cerebrospinal fluid, in situ Z98.2
Devic's disease G36.0
Devil's
grip B33.0
pinches (purpura simplex) D69.2
Devitalized tooth K04.99
Devonshire colic -*see* Poisoning, lead
Dextraposition, aorta Q20.3
in tetralogy of Fallot Q21.3
**Dextrinosis, limit (debrancher enzyme
deficiency)** E74.03
Dextrocardia (true) Q24.0
with
complete transposition of viscera Q89.3
situs inversus Q89.3
Dextrotransposition, aorta Q20.3
d-glycericacidemia E72.59
Dhat syndrome F48.8
Dhobi itch B35.6
Di George's syndrome D82.1
Di Guglielmo's disease C94.0
Diabetes, diabetic (mellitus) (sugar) E11.9
with
amyotrophy E11.44
arthropathy NEC E11.618
autonomic (poly) neuropathy E11.43
cataract E11.36
Charcot's joints E11.610
chronic kidney disease E11.22
circulatory complication NEC E11.59
complication E11.8
specified NEC E11.69
dermatitis E11.620
foot ulcer E11.621
gangrene E11.52
gastroparalysis E11.43
gastroparesis E11.43
glomerulonephrosis, intracapillary E11.21
glomerulosclerosis, intercapillary E11.21
hyperglycemia E11.65
hyperosmolarity E11.00
with coma E11.01
hypoglycemia E11.649
with coma E11.641
kidney complications NEC E11.29
Kimmelstiel-Wilson disease E11.21
loss of protective sensation (LOPS) -*see*
Diabetes, by type, with neuropathy
mononeuropathy E11.41

Diabetes, diabetic *--continued*
  myasthenia E11.44
  necrobiosis lipoidica E11.620
  nephropathy E11.21
  neuralgia E11.42
  neurologic complication NEC E11.49
  neuropathic arthropathy E11.610
  neuropathy E11.40
  ophthalmic complication NEC E11.39
  oral complication NEC E11.638
  osteomyelitis E11.69
  periodontal disease E11.630
  peripheral angiopathy E11.51
    with gangrene E11.52
  polyneuropathy E11.42
  renal complication NEC E11.29
  renal tubular degeneration E11.29
  retinopathy E11.319
    with macular edema E11.311
      resolved following treatment E11.37
    nonproliferative E11.329
      with macular edema E11.321
      mild E11.329
        with macular edema E11.321
      moderate E11.339
        with macular edema E11.331
      severe E11.349
        with macular edema E11.341
    proliferative E11.359
      with
        combined traction retinal detachment
          and rhegmatogenous retinal
          detachment E11.354
        macular edema E11.351
        stable proliferative diabetic retinopathy
          E11.355
        traction retinal detachment involving the
          macula E11.352
        traction retinal detachment not
          involving the macula E11.353
  skin complication NEC E11.628
  skin ulcer NEC E11.622
  brittle *-see* Diabetes, type 1
  bronzed E83.110
  complicating pregnancy *-see* Pregnancy,
    complicated by, diabetes
  dietary counseling and surveillance Z71.3
  due to
    autoimmune process *-see* Diabetes, type 1
    immune mediated pancreatic islet beta-cell
      destruction *-see* Diabetes, type 1
  due to drug or chemical E09.9
    with
      amyotrophy E09.44
      arthropathy NEC E09.618
      autonomic (poly) neuropathy E09.43
      cataract E09.36
      Charcot's joints E09.610
      chronic kidney disease E09.22
      circulatory complication NEC E09.59
      complication E09.8
        specified NEC E09.69
      dermatitis E09.620
      foot ulcer E09.621
      gangrene E09.52
      gastroparalysis E09.43
      gastroparesis E09.43
      glomerulonephrosis, intracapillary E09.21
      glomerulosclerosis, intercapillary E09.21
      hyperglycemia E09.65
      hyperosmolarity E09.00

Diabetes, diabetic *--continued*
      with coma E09.01
    hypoglycemia E09.649
      with coma E09.641
    ketoacidosis E09.10
      with coma E09.11
    kidney complications NEC E09.29
    Kimmelstiel-Wilson disease E09.21
    mononeuropathy E09.41
    myasthenia E09.44
    necrobiosis lipoidica E09.620
    nephropathy E09.21
    neuralgia E09.42
    neurologic complication NEC E09.49
    neuropathic arthropathy E09.610
    neuropathy E09.40
    ophthalmic complication NEC E09.39
    oral complication NEC E09.638
    periodontal disease E09.630
    peripheral angiopathy E09.51
      with gangrene E09.52
    polyneuropathy E09.42
    renal complication NEC E09.29
    renal tubular degeneration E09.29
    retinopathy E09.319
      with macular edema E09.311
      resolved following treatment E09.37
      nonproliferative E09.329
        with macular edema E09.321
        mild E09.329
          with macular edema E09.321
        moderate E09.339
          with macular edema E09.331
        severe E09.349
          with macular edema E09.341
      proliferative E09.359
        with
          combined traction retinal detachment
          and rhegmatogenous retinal
          detachment E09.354
          macular edema E09.351
          stable proliferative diabetic
          retinopathy E09.355
          traction retinal detachment involving
          the macula E09.352
          traction retinal detachment not
          involving the macula E09.353
    skin complication NEC E09.628
    skin ulcer NEC E09.622
  due to underlying condition E08.9
    with
      amyotrophy E08.44
      arthropathy NEC E08.618
      autonomic (poly) neuropathy E08.43
      cataract E08.36
      Charcot's joints E08.610
      chronic kidney disease E08.22
      circulatory complication NEC E08.59
      complication E08.8
        specified NEC E08.69
      dermatitis E08.620
      foot ulcer E08.621
      gangrene E08.52
      gastroparalysis E08.43
      gastroparesis E08.43
      glomerulonephrosis, intracapillary E08.21
      glomerulosclerosis, intercapillary E08.21
      hyperglycemia E08.65
      hyperosmolarity E08.00
        with coma E08.01
      hypoglycemia E08.649

Diabetes, diabetic *--continued*
      with coma E08.641
    ketoacidosis E08.10
      with coma E08.11
    kidney complications NEC E08.29
    Kimmelstiel-Wilson disease E08.21
    mononeuropathy E08.41
    myasthenia E08.44
    necrobiosis lipoidica E08.620
    nephropathy E08.21
    neuralgia E08.42
    neurologic complication NEC E08.49
    neuropathic arthropathy E08.610
    neuropathy E08.40
    ophthalmic complication NEC E08.39
    oral complication NEC E08.638
    periodontal disease E08.630
    peripheral angiopathy E08.51
      with gangrene E08.52
    polyneuropathy E08.42
    renal complication NEC E08.29
    renal tubular degeneration E08.29
    retinopathy E08.319
      with macular edema E08.311
      resolved following treatment E08.37
      nonproliferative E08.329
        with macular edema E08.321
        mild E08.329
          with macular edema E08.321
        moderate E08.339
          with macular edema E08.331
        severe E08.349
          with macular edema E08.341
      proliferative E08.359
        with
          combined traction retinal detachment
          and rhegmatogenous retinal
          detachment E08.354
          macular edema E08.351
          stable proliferative diabetic
          retinopathy E08.355
          traction retinal detachment involving
          the macula E08.352
          traction retinal detachment not
          involving the macula E08.353
    skin complication NEC E08.628
    skin ulcer NEC E08.622
  gestational (in pregnancy) O24.419
    affecting newborn P70.0
    diet controlled O24.410
    in childbirth O24.429
      diet controlled O24.420
      insulin (and diet) controlled O24.424
      oral drug controlled (antidiabetic)
        (hypoglycemic) O24.425
    insulin (and diet) controlled O24.414
    oral drug controlled (antidiabetic)
      (hypoglycemic) O24.415
    puerperal O24.439
      diet controlled O24.430
      insulin (and diet) controlled O24.434
      oral drug controlled (antidiabetic)
        (hypoglycemic) O24.435
  hepatogenous E13.9
  idiopathic *-see* Diabetes, type 1
  inadequately controlled - code to Diabetes, by
    type, with hyperglycemia
  insipidus E23.2
    nephrogenic N25.1
    pituitary E23.2
    vasopressin resistant N25.1

Diabetes, diabetic --continued
insulin dependent - code to type of diabetes
juvenile-onset -see Diabetes, type 1
ketosis-prone -see Diabetes, type 1
latent R73.03
neonatal (transient) P70.2
non-insulin dependent
code to type of diabetes
out of control
code to Diabetes, by type, with hyperglycemia
phosphate E83.39
poorly controlled - code to Diabetes, by type,
with hyperglycemia
postpancreatectomy -see Diabetes, specified
type NEC
postprocedural -see Diabetes, specified type
NEC
secondary diabetes mellitus NEC -see
Diabetes, specified type NEC
specified type NEC E13.9
with
amyotrophy E13.44
arthropathy NEC E13.618
autonomic (poly) neuropathy E13.43
cataract E13.36
Charcot's joints E13.610
chronic kidney disease E13.22
circulatory complication NEC E13.59
complication E13.8
specified NEC E13.69
dermatitis E13.620
foot ulcer E13.621
gangrene E13.52
gastroparalysis E13.43
gastroparesis E13.43
glomerulonephrosis, intracapillary E13.21
glomerulosclerosis, intercapillary E13.21
hyperglycemia E13.65
hyperosmolarity E13.00
with coma E13.01
hypoglycemia E13.649
with coma E13.641
ketoacidosis E13.10
with coma E13.11
kidney complications NEC E13.29
Kimmelstiel-Wilson disease E13.21
mononeuropathy E13.41
myasthenia E13.44
necrobiosis lipoidica E13.620
nephropathy E13.21
neuralgia E13.42
neurologic complication NEC E13.49
neuropathic arthropathy E13.610
neuropathy E13.40
ophthalmic complication NEC E13.39
oral complication NEC E13.638
periodontal disease E13.630
peripheral angiopathy E13.51
with gangrene E13.52
polyneuropathy E13.42
renal complication NEC E13.29
renal tubular degeneration E13.29
retinopathy E13.319
with macular edema E13.311
resolved following treatment E13.37
nonproliferative E13.329
with macular edema E13.321
mild E13.329
with macular edema E13.321
moderate E13.339
with macular edema E13.331

severe E13.349
with macular edema E13.341
proliferative E13.359
with
combined traction retinal detachment
and rhegmatogenous retinal
detachment E13.354
macular edema E13.351
stable proliferative diabetic
retinopathy E13.355
traction retinal detachment involving
the macula E13.352
traction retinal detachment not
involving the macula E13.353
skin complication NEC E13.628
skin ulcer NEC E13.622
steroid-induced -see Diabetes, due to, drug or
chemical
type 1 E10.9
with
amyotrophy E10.44
arthropathy NEC E10.618
autonomic (poly) neuropathy E10.43
cataract E10.36
Charcot's joints E10.610
chronic kidney disease E10.22
circulatory complication NEC E10.59
complication E10.8
specified NEC E10.69
dermatitis E10.620
foot ulcer E10.621
gangrene E10.52
gastroparalysis E10.43
gastroparesis E10.43
glomerulonephrosis, intracapillary E10.21
glomerulosclerosis, intercapillary E10.21
hyperglycemia E10.65
hypoglycemia E10.649
with coma E10.641
ketoacidosis E10.10
with coma E10.11
kidney complications NEC E10.29
Kimmelstiel-Wilson disease E10.21
mononeuropathy E10.41
myasthenia E10.44
necrobiosis lipoidica E10.620
nephropathy E10.21
neuralgia E10.42
neurologic complication NEC E10.49
neuropathic arthropathy E10.610
neuropathy E10.40
ophthalmic complication NEC E10.39
oral complication NEC E10.638
periodontal disease E10.630
peripheral angiopathy E10.51
with gangrene E10.52
polyneuropathy E10.42
renal complication NEC E10.29
renal tubular degeneration E10.29
retinopathy E10.319
with macular edema E10.311
resolved following treatment E10.37
nonproliferative E10.329
with macular edema E10.321
mild E10.329
with macular edema E10.321
moderate E10.339
with macular edema E10.331
severe E10.349
with macular edema E10.341

proliferative E10.359
with
combined traction retinal detachment
and rhegmatogenous retinal
detachment E10.354
macular edema E10.351
stable proliferative diabetic
retinopathy E10.355
traction retinal detachment involving
the macula E10.352
traction retinal detachment not
involving the macula E10.353
skin complication NEC E10.628
skin ulcer NEC E10.622
type 2 E11.9
with
amyotrophy E11.44
arthropathy NEC E11.618
autonomic (poly) neuropathy E11.43
cataract E11.36
Charcot's joints E11.610
chronic kidney disease E11.22
circulatory complication NEC E11.59
complication E11.8
specified NEC E11.69
dermatitis E11.620
foot ulcer E11.621
gangrene E11.52
gastroparalysis E11.43
gastroparesis E11.43
glomerulonephrosis, intracapillary E11.21
glomerulosclerosis, intercapillary E11.21
hyperglycemia E11.65
hyperosmolarity E11.00
with coma E11.01
hypoglycemia E11.649
with coma E11.641
kidney complications NEC E11.29
Kimmelstiel-Wilson disease E11.21
mononeuropathy E11.41
myasthenia E11.44
necrobiosis lipoidica E11.620
nephropathy E11.21
neuralgia E11.42
neurologic complication NEC E11.49
neuropathic arthropathy E11.610
neuropathy E11.40
ophthalmic complication NEC E11.39
oral complication NEC E11.638
periodontal disease E11.630
peripheral angiopathy E11.51
with gangrene E11.52
polyneuropathy E11.42
renal complication NEC E11.29
renal tubular degeneration E11.29
retinopathy E11.319
with macular edema E11.311
resolved following treatment E11.37
nonproliferative E11.329
with macular edema E11.321
mild E11.329
with macular edema E11.321
moderate E11.339
with macular edema E11.331
severe E11.349
with macular edema E11.341
proliferative E11.359
with

Diabetes, diabetic --continued
    combined traction retinal detachment
      and rhegmatogenous retinal
      detachment E11.354
    macular edema E11.351
    stable proliferative diabetic
      retinopathy E11.355
    traction retinal detachment involving
      the macula E11.352
    traction retinal detachment not
      involving the macula E11.353
  skin complication NEC E11.628
  skin ulcer NEC E11.622
 uncontrolled
  meaning
    hyperglycemia -*see* Diabetes, by type,
      with, hyperglycemia
    hypoglycemia -*see* Diabetes, by type, with,
      hypoglycemia
Diacyclothrombopathia D69.1
Diagnosis deferred R69
Dialysis (intermittent) (treatment)
 noncompliance (with) Z91.15
 renal (hemodialysis) (peritoneal), status Z99.2
 retina, retinal -*see* Detachment, retina, with
  retinal, dialysis
Diamond-Blackfan anemia (congenital
  hypoplastic) D61.01
Diamond-Gardener syndrome
  (autoerythrocyte sensitization) D69.2
Diaper rash L22
Diaphoresis (excessive) R61
Diaphragm -*see* condition
Diaphragmalgia R07.1
Diaphragmatitis, diaphragmitis J98.6
Diaphysial aclasis Q78.6
Diaphysitis -*see* Osteomyelitis, specified type
NEC
Diarrhea, diarrheal (disease) (infantile)
  (inflammatory) R19.7
 achlorhydric K31.83
 allergic K52.29
  due to
    colitis -*see* Colitis, allergic
    enteritis -*see* Enteritis, allergic
 amebic -*see also* Amebiasis A06.0
  with abscess -*see* Abscess, amebic
  acute A06.0
  chronic A06.1
  nondysenteric A06.2
 bacillary -*see* Dysentery, bacillary
 balantidial A07.0
 cachectic NEC K52.89
 Chilomastix A07.8
 choleriformis A00.1
 chronic (noninfectious) K52.9
 coccidial A07.3
 Cochin-China K90.1
  strongyloidiasis B78.0
 Dientamoeba A07.8
 dietetic -*see also* Diarrhea, allergic K52.29
 drug-induced K52.1
 due to
  bacteria A04.9
    specified NEC A04.8
  Campylobacter A04.5
  Capillaria philippinensis B81.1
  Clostridium difficile A04.7
  Clostridium perfringens (C) (F) A04.8
  Cryptosporidium A07.2
  drugs K52.1

Diarrhea, diarrheal --continued
  Escherichia coli A04.4
    enteroaggregative A04.4
    enterohemorrhagic A04.3
    enteroinvasive A04.2
    enteropathogenic A04.0
    enterotoxigenic A04.1
    specified NEC A04.4
  food hypersensitivity -*see also* Diarrhea,
    allergic K52.29
  Necator americanus B76.1
  S. japonicum B65.2
  specified organism NEC A08.8
    bacterial A04.8
    viral A08.39
  Staphylococcus A04.8
  Trichuris trichiura B79
  virus -*see* Enteritis, viral
  Yersinia enterocolitica A04.6
 dysenteric A09
 endemic A09
 epidemic A09
 flagellate A07.9
 Flexner's (ulcerative) A03.1
 functional K59.1
  following gastrointestinal surgery K91.89
  psychogenic F45.8
 Giardia lamblia A07.1
 giardial A07.1
 hill K90.1
 infectious A09
 malarial -*see* Malaria
 mite B88.0
 mycotic NEC B49
 neonatal (noninfectious) P78.3
 nervous F45.8
 neurogenic K59.1
 noninfectious K52.9
 postgastrectomy K91.1
 postvagotomy K91.1
 protozoal A07.9
  specified NEC A07.8
 psychogenic F45.8
 specified
  bacterium NEC A04.8
  virus NEC A08.39
 strongyloidiasis B78.0
 toxic K52.1
 trichomonal A07.8
 tropical K90.1
 tuberculous A18.32
 viral -*see* Enteritis, viral
Diastasis
 cranial bones M84.88
  congenital NEC Q75.8
 joint (traumatic) -*see* Dislocation
 muscle M62.00
  ankle M62.07
  congenital Q79.8
  foot M62.07
  forearm M62.03
  hand M62.04
  lower leg M62.06
  pelvic region M62.05
  shoulder region M62.01
  specified site NEC M62.08
  thigh M62.05
  upper arm M62.02
 recti (abdomen)
  complicating delivery O71.89
  congenital Q79.59

Diastema, tooth, teeth, fully erupted M26.32
Diastematomyelia Q06.2
Diataxia, cerebral G80.4
Diathesis
 allergic -*see* History, allergy bleeding
  (familial) D69.9
 cystine (familial) E72.00
 gouty -*see* Gout
 hemorrhagic (familial) D69.9
  newborn NEC P53
 spasmophilic R29.0
Diaz's disease or osteochondrosis (juvenile)
  (talus) -*see* Osteochondrosis, juvenile, tarsus
Dibothriocephalus, dibothriocephaliasis
  (latus) (infection) (infestation) B70.0
 larval B70.1
Dicephalus, dicephaly Q89.4
Dichotomy, teeth K00.2
Dichromat, dichromatopsia (congenital) -*see*
  Deficiency, color vision
Dichuchwa A65
Dicroceliasis B66.2
Didelphia, didelphys -*see* Double uterus
Didymitis N45.1
 with orchitis N45.3
Dietary
 inadequacy or deficiency E63.9
 surveillance and counseling Z71.3
Dietl's crisis N13.8
Dieulafoy lesion (hemorrhagic)
 duodenum K31.82
 esophagus K22.8
 intestine (colon) K63.81
 stomach K31.82
Difficult, difficulty (in)
 acculturation Z60.3
 feeding R63.3
  newborn P92.9
    breast P92.5
    specified NEC P92.8
  nonorganic (infant or child) F98.29
 intubation, in anesthesia T88.4
 mechanical, gastroduodenal stoma K91.89
  causing obstruction K91.3
 micturition
  need to immediately re-void R39.191
  position dependent R39.192
  specified NEC R39.198
 reading (developmental) F81.0
  secondary to emotional disorders F93.9
 spelling (specific) F81.81
  with reading disorder F81.89
  due to inadequate teaching Z55.8
 swallowing -*see* Dysphagia
 walking R26.2
 work
  conditions NEC Z56.5
  schedule Z56.3
Diffuse -*see* condition
Digeorge's syndrome (thymic hypoplasia)
  D82.1
Digestive -*see* condition
Dihydropyrimidine dehydrogenase disease
  (DPD) E88.89
Diktyoma -*see* Neoplasm, malignant, by site
Dilaceration, tooth K00.4
Dilatation
 anus K59.8
  venule -*see* Hemorrhoids
 aorta (focal) (general) -*see* Ectasia, aorta
  with aneurysm -*see* Aneurysm, aorta

Dilatation - *continued*
  congenital Q25.44
  artery *-see* Aneurysm
  bladder (sphincter) N32.89
    congenital Q64.79
  blood vessel I99.8
  bronchial J47.9
    with
      exacerbation (acute) J47.1
      lower respiratory infection J47.0
  calyx (due to obstruction) *-see*
  Hydronephrosis
  capillaries I78.8
  cardiac (acute) (chronic) *-see also*
  Hypertrophy, cardiac
    congenital Q24.8
      valve NEC Q24.8
        pulmonary Q22.3
    valve *-see* Endocarditis
  cavum septi pellucidi Q06.8
  cervix (uteri) *-see also* Incompetency, cervix
    incomplete, poor, slow complicating
    delivery O62.0
  colon K59.39
    congenital Q43.1
    psychogenic F45.8
    toxic K59.31
  common duct (acquired) K83.8
    congenital Q44.5
  cystic duct (acquired) K82.8
    congenital Q44.5
  duct, mammary *-see* Ectasia, mammary duct
  duodenum K59.8
  esophagus K22.8
    congenital Q39.5
    due to achalasia K22.0
  eustachian tube, congenital Q17.8
  gallbladder K82.8
  gastric *-see* Dilatation, stomach
  heart (acute) (chronic) *-see also* Hypertrophy,
  cardiac
    congenital Q24.8
    valve *-see* Endocarditis
  ileum K59.8
    psychogenic F45.8
  jejunum K59.8
    psychogenic F45.8
  kidney (calyx) (collecting structures) (cystic)
    (parenchyma) (pelvis) (idiopathic) N28.89
  lacrimal passages or duct *-see* Disorder,
  lacrimal system, changes
  lymphatic vessel I89.0
  mammary duct *-see* Ectasia, mammary duct
  Meckel's diverticulum (congenital) Q43.0
    malignant *-see* Table of Neoplasms, small
    intestine, malignant
  myocardium (acute) (chronic) *-see*
  Hypertrophy, cardiac
  organ or site, congenital NEC *-see* Distortion
  pancreatic duct K86.89
  pericardium *-see* Pericarditis
  pharynx J39.2
  prostate N42.89
  pulmonary
    artery (idiopathic) I28.8
    valve, congenital Q22.3
  pupil H57.04
  rectum K59.39
  saccule, congenital Q16.5
  salivary gland (duct) K11.8
  sphincter ani K62.89

Dilatation - *continued*
  stomach K31.89
    acute K31.0
    psychogenic F45.8
  submaxillary duct K11.8
  trachea, congenital Q32.1
  ureter (idiopathic) N28.82
    congenital Q62.2
    due to obstruction N13.4
  urethra (acquired) N36.8
  vasomotor I73.9
  vein I86.8
  ventricular, ventricle (acute) (chronic) *-see*
  also Hypertrophy, cardiac
    cerebral, congenital Q04.8
  venule NEC I86.8
  vesical orifice N32.89
Dilated, dilation *-see* Dilatation
Diminished, diminution
  hearing (acuity) *-see* Deafness
  sense or sensation (cold) (heat) (tactile)
    (vibratory) R20.8
  vision NEC H54.7
  vital capacity R94.2
Diminuta taenia B71.0
Dimitri-Sturge-Weber disease Q85.8
Dimple
  congenital sacral Q82.6
  parasacral Q82.6
  pilonidal or postanal *-see* Cyst, pilonidal
Dioctophyma renalis (infection) (infestation)
  B83.8
Dipetalonemiasis B74.4
Diphallus Q55.69
Diphtheria, diphtheritic (gangrenous)
  (hemorrhagic) A36.9
  carrier (suspected) Z22.2
  cutaneous A36.3
  faucial A36.0
  infection of wound A36.3
  laryngeal A36.2
  myocarditis A36.81
  nasal, anterior A36.89
  nasopharyngeal A36.1
  neurological complication A36.89
  pharyngeal A36.0
  specified site NEC A36.89
  tonsillar A36.0
Diphyllobothriasis (intestine) B70.0
  larval B70.1
Diplacusis H93.22
Diplegia (upper limbs) G83.0
  congenital (cerebral) G80.8
  facial G51.0
  lower limbs G82.20
  spastic G80.1
Diplococcus, diplococcal *-see* condition
Diplopia H53.2
Dipsomania F10.20
  with
    psychosis *-see* Psychosis, alcoholic
    remission F10.21
Dipylidiasis B71.1
DIRA (deficiency of interleukin 1
receptor antagonist) M04.8
Direction, teeth, abnormal, fully erupted
  M26.30
Dirofilariasis B74.8
Dirt-eating child F98.3
Disability, disabilities
  heart *-see* Disease, heart

Disability, disabilities - *continued*
  intellectual F79
    with
      autistic features F84.9
    mild (I.Q.50 69) F70
    moderate (I.Q.35 49) F71
    profound (I.Q. under 20) F73
    severe (I.Q.20 34) F72
    specified level NEC F78
  knowledge acquisition F81.9
  learning F81.9
  limiting activities Z73.6
  spelling, specific F81.81
Disappearance of family member Z63.4
Disarticulation *-see* Amputation
  meaning traumatic amputation *-see*
  Amputation, traumatic
Discharge (from)
  abnormal finding in *-see* Abnormal, specimen
  breast (female) (male) N64.52
  diencephalic autonomic idiopathic *-see*
  Epilepsy, specified NEC
  ear *-see also* Otorrhea
    blood *-see* Otorrhagia
  excessive urine R35.8
  nipple N64.52
  penile R36.9
  postnasal R09.82
  prison, anxiety concerning Z65.2
  urethral R36.9
    without blood R36.0
    hematospermia R36.1
  vaginal N89.8
Discitis, diskitis M46.40
  cervical region M46.42
  cervicothoracic region M46.43
  lumbar region M46.46
  lumbosacral region M46.47
  multiple sites M46.49
  occipito-atlanto-axial region M46.41
  pyogenic *-see* Infection, intervertebral disc,
  pyogenic
  sacrococcygeal region M46.48
  thoracic region M46.44
  thoracolumbar region M46.45
Discoid
  meniscus (congenital) Q68.6
  semilunar cartilage (congenital) *-see*
  Derangement, knee, meniscus, specified NEC
Discoloration
  nails L60.8
  teeth (posteruptive) K03.7
    during formation K00.8
Discomfort
  chest R07.89
  visual H53.14
Discontinuity, ossicles, ear H74.2
Discord (with)
  boss Z56.4
  classmates Z55.4
  counselor Z64.4
  employer Z56.4
  family Z63.8
  fellow employees Z56.4
  in-laws Z63.1
  landlord Z59.2
  lodgers Z59.2
  neighbors Z59.2
  probation officer Z64.4
  social worker Z64.4
  teachers Z55.4
  workmates Z56.4

Discordant connection
atrioventricular (congenital) Q20.5
ventriculoarterial Q20.3
Discrepancy
centric occlusion maximum intercuspation
M26.55
leg length (acquired) -*see* Deformity, limb,
unequal length
  congenital -*see* Defect, reduction, lower
  limb
uterine size date O26.84
Discrimination
ethnic Z60.5
political Z60.5
racial Z60.5
religious Z60.5
sex Z60.5
Disease, diseased -*see also* Syndrome -
absorbent system I87.8
acid-peptic K30
Acosta's T70.29
Adams-Stokes (Morgagni) (syncope with
heart block) I45.9
Addison's anemia (pernicious) D51.0
adenoids (and tonsils) J35.9
adrenal (capsule) (cortex) (gland) (medullary)
E27.9
  hyperfunction E27.0
  specified NEC E27.8
ainhum L94.6
airway
  obstructive, chronic J44.9
    due to
      cotton dust J66.0
      specific organic dusts NEC J66.8
  reactive -*see* Asthma
akamushi (scrub typhus) A75.3
Albers-Schönberg (marble bones) Q78.2
Albert's -*see* Tendinitis, Achilles
alimentary canal K63.9
alligator-skin Q80.9
  acquired L85.0
alpha heavy chain C88.3
alpine T70.29
altitude T70.20
alveolar ridge
  edentulous K06.9
    specified NEC K06.8
alveoli, teeth K08.9
Alzheimer's G30.9 *[F02.80]*
  with behavioral disturbance G30.9 *[F02.81]*
  early onset G30.0 *[F02.80]*
    with behavioral disturbance G30.0
    [F02.81]
  late onset G30.1 *[F02.80]*
    with behavioral disturbance G30.1
    [F02.81]
  specified NEC G30.8 *[F02.80]*
    with behavioral disturbance G30.8
    [F02.81]
amyloid -*see* Amyloidosis
Andersen's (glycogenosis IV) E74.09
Andes T70.29
Andrews' (bacterid) L08.89
angiospastic I73.9
  cerebral G45.9
  vein I87.8
anterior
  chamber H21.9
  horn cell G12.29

Disease, diseased -*continued*
antiglomerular basement membrane (anti-
GBM) antibody M31.0
  tubulo-interstitial nephritis N12
antral -*see* Sinusitis, maxillary
anus K62.9
  specified NEC K62.89
aorta (nonsyphilitic) I77.9
  syphilitic NEC A52.02
aortic (heart) (valve) I35.9
  rheumatic I06.9
Apollo B30.3
aponeuroses -*see* Enthesopathy
appendix K38.9
  specified NEC K38.8
aqueous (chamber) H21.9
Arnold-Chiari -*see* Arnold-Chiari disease -
arterial I77.9
  occlusive -*see* Occlusion, by site
    due to stricture or stenosis I77.1
arteriocardiorenal -*see* Hypertension,
cardiorenal
arteriolar (generalized) (obliterative) I77.9
arteriorenal -*see* Hypertension, kidney
arteriosclerotic -*see also* Arteriosclerosis
  cardiovascular -*see* Disease, heart, ischemic,
    atherosclerotic
  coronary (artery) -*see* Disease, heart,
    ischemic, atherosclerotic
  heart -*see* Disease, heart, ischemic,
    atherosclerotic
artery I77.9
  cerebral I67.9
  coronary I25.10
    with angina pectoris -*see* Arteriosclerosis,
coronary (artery),
arthropod-borne NOS (viral) A94
  specified type NEC A93.8
atticoantral, chronic H66.20
  left H66.22
    with right H66.23
  right H66.21
    with left H66.23
auditory canal -*see* Disorder, ear, external
auricle, ear NEC -*see* Disorder, pinna
Australian X A83.4
autoimmune (systemic) NOS M35.9
  hemolytic (cold type) (warm type) D59.1
    drug-induced D59.0
  thyroid E06.3
aviator's -*see* Effect, adverse, high altitude
Ayerza's (pulmonary artery sclerosis with
pulmonary hypertension) I27.0
Babington's (familial hemorrhagic
telangiectasia) I78.0
bacterial A49.9
  specified NEC A48.8
  zoonotic A28.9
    specified type NEC A28.8
Baelz's (cheilitis glandularis apostematosa)
K13.0
bagasse J67.1
balloon -*see* Effect, adverse, high altitude
Bang's (brucella abortus) A23.1
Bannister's T78.3
barometer makers' -*see* Poisoning, mercury
Barraquer (Simons') (progressive
lipodystrophy) E88.1
Barrett's -*see* Barrett's, esophagus
Bartholin's gland N75.9
basal ganglia G25.9

Disease, diseased -*continued*
degenerative G23.9
  specified NEC G23.8
  specified NEC G25.89
Basedow's (exophthalmic goiter) -*see*
Hyperthyroidism, with, goiter (diffuse)
Bateman's B08.1
Batten-Steinert G71.11
Battey A31.0
Beard's (neurasthenia) F48.8
Becker
  idiopathic mural endomyocardial I42.3
  myotonia congenita G71.12
Begbie's (exophthalmic goiter) -*see*
Hyperthyroidism, with, goiter (diffuse)
behavioral, organic F07.9
Beigel's (white piedra) B36.2
Benson's -*see* Deposit, crystalline
Bernard-Soulier (thrombopathy) D69.1
Bernhardt (Roth) -*see* Mononeuropathy,
lower limb, meralgia paresthetica
Biermer's (pernicious anemia) D51.0
bile duct (common) (hepatic) K83.9
  with calculus, stones -*see* Calculus, bile duct
  specified NEC K83.8
biliary (tract) K83.9
  specified NEC K83.8
Billroth's -*see* Spina bifida
bird fancier's J67.2
black lung J60
bladder N32.9
  in (due to)
    schistosomiasis (bilharziasis) B65.0 *[N33]*
  specified NEC N32.89
bleeder's D66
blood D75.9
  forming organs D75.9
  vessel I99.9
Bloodgood's -*see* Mastopathy, cystic
Bodechtel-Guttmann (subacute sclerosing
panencephalitis) A81.1
bone -*see also* Disorder, bone
  aluminum M83.4
  fibrocystic NEC
  jaw M27.49
bone-marrow D75.9
Borna A83.9
Bornholm (epidemic pleurodynia) B33.0
Bouchard's (myopathic dilatation of the
stomach) K31.0
Bouillaud's (rheumatic heart disease) I01.9
Bourneville (Brissaud) (tuberous sclerosis)
Q85.1
Bouveret (Hoffmann) (paroxysmal
tachycardia) I47.9
bowel K63.9
  functional K59.9
    psychogenic F45.8
brain G93.9
  arterial, artery I67.9
    arteriosclerotic I67.2
  congenital Q04.9
  degenerative -*see* Degeneration, brain
  inflammatory -*see* Encephalitis
  organic G93.9
    arteriosclerotic I67.2
  parasitic NEC B71.9 *[G94]*
  senile NEC G31.1
  specified NEC G93.89
breast -*see also* Disorder, breast N64.9
  cystic (chronic) -*see* Mastopathy, cystic

Disease, diseased --*continued*
  fibrocystic -*see* Mastopathy, cystic
  Paget's
    female, unspecified side C50.91
    male, unspecified side C50.92
    specified NEC N64.89
  Breda's -*see* Yaws
  Bretonneau's (diphtheritic malignant angina)
    A36.0
  Bright's -*see* Nephritis
    arteriosclerotic -*see* Hypertension, kidney
  Brill's (recrudescent typhus) A75.1
  Brill-Zinsser (recrudescent typhus) A75.1
  Brion-Kayser -*see* Fever, paratyphoid
  broad
    beta E78.2
    ligament (noninflammatory) N83.9
      inflammatory -*see* Disease, pelvis,
  inflammatory
      specified NEC N83.8
  Brocq-Duhring (dermatitis herpetiformis)
    L13.0
  Brocq's
    meaning
      dermatitis herpetiformis L13.0
      prurigo L28.2
  bronchopulmonary J98.4
  bronchus NEC J98.09
  bronze Addison's E27.1
    tuberculous A18.7
  budgerigar fancier's J67.2
  bullous L13.9
    chronic of childhood L12.2
    specified NEC L13.8
  Buerger's (thromboangiitis obliterans) I73.1
  Bürger-Grütz (essential familial
    hyperlipemia) E78.3
  bursa -*see* Bursopathy
  caisson T70.3
  California -*see* Coccidioidomycosis
  capillaries I78.9
    specified NEC I78.8
  Carapata A68.0
  cardiac -*see* Disease, heart
  cardiopulmonary, chronic I27.9
  cardiorenal (hepatic) (hypertensive) (vascular)
    -*see* Hypertension, cardiorenal
  cardiovascular (atherosclerotic) I25.10
    with angina pectoris -*see* Arteriosclerosis,
      coronary (artery),   congenital Q28.9
    newborn P29.9
      specified NEC P29.89
    hypertensive -*see* Hypertension, heart
    renal (hypertensive) -*see* Hypertension,
      cardiorenal
    syphilitic (asymptomatic) A52.00
  cartilage -*see* Disorder, cartilage
  Castellani's A69.8
  Castleman (unicentric) (multicentric) D47.Z2
    HHV-8 associated -*see also* Herpesvirus,
      human, 8 D47.Z2
  cat-scratch A28.1
  Cavare's (familial periodic paralysis) G72.3
  cecum K63.9
  celiac (adult) (infantile) (with steatorrhea)
    K90.0
  cellular tissue L98.9
  central core G71.2
  cerebellar, cerebellum -*see* Disease, brain
  cerebral -*see also* Disease, brain
    degenerative -*see* Degeneration, brain

Disease, diseased --*continued*
  cerebrospinal G96.9
  cerebrovascular I67.9
    acute I67.89
      embolic I63.4
      thrombotic I63.3
    arteriosclerotic I67.2
    specified NEC I67.89
  cervix (uteri) (noninflammatory) N88.9
    inflammatory -*see* Cervicitis
    specified NEC N88.8
  Chabert's A22.9
  Chandler's (osteochondritis dissecans, hip) -
    see Osteochondritis, dissecans, hip
  Charlouis -*see* Yaws
  Chédiak-Steinbrinck (Higashi) (congenital
    gigantism of peroxidase granules) E70.330
  chest J98.9
  Chiari's (hepatic vein thrombosis) I82.0
  Chicago B40.9
  Chignon B36.8
  chigo, chigoe B88.1
  childhood granulomatous D71
  Chinese liver fluke B66.1
  chlamydial A74.9
    specified NEC A74.89
  cholecystic K82.9
  choroid H31.9
    specified NEC H31.8
  Christmas D67
  chronic bullous of childhood L12.2
  chylomicron retention E78.3
  ciliary body H21.9
    specified NEC H21.89
  circulatory (system) NEC I99.8
    newborn P29.9
    syphilitic A52.00
      congenital A50.54
  coagulation factor deficiency (congenital) -*see*
    Defect, coagulation
  coccidioidal -*see* Coccidioidomycosis
  cold
    agglutinin or hemoglobinuria D59.1
      paroxysmal D59.6
    hemagglutinin (chronic) D59.1
  collagen NOS (nonvascular) (vascular) M35.9
    specified NEC M35.8
  colon K63.9
    functional K59.9
      congenital Q43.2
    ischemic -*see also* Ischemia, intestine, acute
      K55.039
  colonic inflammatory bowel, unclassified
    (IBDU) K52.3
  combined system -*see* Degeneration,
    combined
  compressed air T70.3
  Concato's (pericardial polyserositis) A19.9
    nontubercular I31.1
    pleural -*see* Pleurisy, with effusion
  conjunctiva H11.9
    chlamydial A74.0
    specified NEC H11.89
    viral B30.9
      specified NEC B30.8
  connective tissue, systemic (diffuse) M35.9
    in (due to)
      hypogammaglobulinemia D80.1 [*M36.8*]
      ochronosis E70.29 [*M36.8*]
    specified NEC M35.8
  Conor and Bruch's (boutonneuse fever) A77.1

Disease, diseased --*continued*
  Cooper's -*see* Mastopathy, cystic
  Cori's (glycogenosis III) E74.03
  cork handler's or cork worker's J67.3
  cornea H18.9
    specified NEC H18.89
  coronary (artery) -*see* Disease, heart,
    ischemic, atherosclerotic
    congenital Q24.5
    ostial, syphilitic (aortic) (mitral)
      (pulmonary) A52.03
  corpus cavernosum N48.9
    specified NEC N48.89
  Cotugno's -*see* Sciatica
  coxsackie (virus) NEC B34.1
  cranial nerve NOS G52.9
  Creutzfeldt-Jakob -*see* Creutzfeldt-Jakob
    disease or syndrome - Crocq's
    (acrocyanosis) I73.89
  Crohn's -*see* Enteritis, regional
  Curschmann G71.11
  cystic
    breast (chronic) -*see* Mastopathy, cystic
    kidney, congenital Q61.9
    liver, congenital Q44.6
    lung J98.4
      congenital Q33.0
  cytomegalic inclusion (generalized) B25.9
    with pneumonia B25.0
    congenital P35.1
  cytomegaloviral B25.9
    specified NEC B25.8
  Czerny's (periodic hydrarthrosis of the knee) -
    see Effusion, joint, knee - Daae (Finsen)
    (epidemic pleurodynia) B33.0
  Darling's -*see* Histoplasmosis capsulati
  Debove's (splenomegaly) R16.1
  deer fly -*see* Tularemia
  Degos' I77.89
  demyelinating, demyelinizating (nervous
  system) G37.9
    multiple sclerosis G35
    specified NEC G37.8
  dense deposit -*see also* N00 N07 with fourth
  character .6 N05.6
  deposition, hydroxyapatite -*see* Disease,
    hydroxyapatite deposition
  de Quervain's (tendon sheath) M65.4
    thyroid (subacute granulomatous thyroiditis)
    E06.1
  Devergie's (pityriasis rubra pilaris) L44.0
  Devic's G36.0
  diaphorase deficiency D74.0
  diaphragm J98.6
  diarrheal, infectious NEC A09
  digestive system K92.9
    specified NEC K92.89
  disc, degenerative -*see* Degeneration,
    intervertebral disc
  discogenic -*see also* Displacement,
  intervertebral disc NEC
    with myelopathy -*see* Disorder, disc, with,
  myelopathy
  diverticular -*see* Diverticula
  Dubois (thymus) A50.59 [*E35*]
  Duchenne-Griesinger G71.0
  Duchenne's
    muscular dystrophy G71.0
    pseudohypertrophy, muscles G71.0
  ductless glands E34.9
  Duhring's (dermatitis herpetiformis) L13.0

Disease, diseased *--continued*

duodenum K31.9
  specified NEC K31.89
Dupré's (meningism) R29.1
Dupuytren's (muscle contracture) M72.0
Durand-Nicholas-Favre (climatic bubo) A55
Duroziez's (congenital mitral stenosis) Q23.2
ear -*see* Disorder, ear
Eberth's -*see* Fever, typhoid
Ebola (virus) A98.4
Ebstein's heart Q22.5
Echinococcus -*see* Echinococcus
echovirus NEC B34.1
Eddowes' (brittle bones and blue sclera)
  Q78.0
edentulous (alveolar) ridge K06.9
  specified NEC K06.8
Edsall's T67.2
Eichstedt's (pityriasis versicolor) B36.0
Ellis-van Creveld (chondroectodermal
  dysplasia) Q77.6
end stage renal (ESRD) N18.6
  due to hypertension I12.0
endocrine glands or system NEC E34.9
endomyocardial (eosinophilic) I42.3
English (rickets) E55.0
enteroviral, enterovirus NEC B34.1
  central nervous system NEC A88.8
epidemic B99.9
  specified NEC B99.8
epididymis N50.9
Erb (Landouzy) G71.0
Erdheim-Chester (ECD) E88.89
esophagus K22.9
  functional K22.4
  psychogenic F45.8
  specified NEC K22.8
Eulenburg's (congenital paramyotonia)
  G71.19
eustachian tube -*see* Disorder, eustachian tube
  - external
  auditory canal -*see* Disorder, ear, external
  ear -*see* Disorder, ear, external
extrapyramidal G25.9
  specified NEC G25.89
eye H57.9
  anterior chamber H21.9
  inflammatory NEC H57.8
  muscle (external) -*see* Strabismus
  specified NEC H57.8
  syphilitic -*see* Oculopathy, syphilitic
eyeball H44.9
  specified NEC H44.89
eyelid -*see* Disorder, eyelid
  specified NEC -*see* Disorder, eyelid,
  specified type NEC
eyeworm of Africa B74.3
facial nerve (seventh) G51.9
  newborn (birth injury) P11.3
Fahr (of brain) G23.8
Fahr Volhard (of kidney) I12.
fallopian tube (noninflammatory) N83.9
  inflammatory -*see* Salpingo-oophoritis
  specified NEC N83.8
familial periodic paralysis G72.3
Fanconi's (congenital pancytopenia) D61.09
fascia NEC -*see also* Disorder, muscle
  inflammatory -*see* Myositis
  specified NEC M62.89
Fauchard's (periodontitis) -*see* Periodontitis
Favre-Durand-Nicolas (climatic bubo) A55

Disease, diseased *--continued*

Fede's K14.0
Feer's -*see* Poisoning, mercury
female pelvic inflammatory -*see also* Disease,
  pelvis, inflammatory N73.9
  syphilitic (secondary) A51.42
  tuberculous A18.17
Fernels' (aortic aneurysm) I71.9
fibrocaseous of lung -*see* Tuberculosis,
  pulmonary
fibrocystic -*see* Fibrocystic disease
Fiedler's (leptospiral jaundice) A27.0
fifth B08.3
file-cutter's -*see* Poisoning, lead - fish-skin
  Q80.9
  acquired L85.0
Flajani (Basedow) (exophthalmic goiter) -*see*
  Hyperthyroidism, with, goiter (diffuse)
flax dresser's J66.1
fluke -*see* Infestation, fluke - foot and mouth
  B08.8
foot process N04.9
Forbes' (glycogenosis III) E74.03
Fordyce-Fox (apocrine miliaria) L75.2
Fordyce's (ectopic sebaceous glands) (mouth)
  Q38.6
Forestier's (rhizomelic pseudopolyarthritis)
  M35.3
  meaning ankylosing hyperostosis -*see*
  Hyperostosis, ankylosing
Fothergill's
  neuralgia -*see* Neuralgia, trigeminal
  scarlatina anginosa A38.9
Fournier (gangrene) N49.3
  female N76.89
fourth B08.8
Fox (Fordyce) (apocrine miliaria) L75.2
Francis' -*see* Tularemia
Franklin C88.2
Frei's (climatic bubo) A55
Friedreich's
  combined systemic or ataxia G11.1
  myoclonia G25.3
frontal sinus -*see* Sinusitis, frontal
fungus NEC B49
Gaisböck's (polycythemia hypertonica) D75.1
gallbladder K82.9
  calculus -*see* Calculus, gallbladder
  cholecystitis -*see* Cholecystitis
  cholesterolosis K82.4
  fistula -*see* Fistula, gallbladder
  hydrops K82.1
  obstruction -*see* Obstruction, gallbladder
  perforation K82.2
  specified NEC K82.8
gamma heavy chain C88.2
Gamna's (siderotic splenomegaly) D73.2
Gamstorp's (adynamia episodica hereditaria)
  G72.3
Gandy Nanta (siderotic splenomegaly) D73.2
ganister J62.8
gastric -*see* Disease, stomach
gastroesophageal reflux (GERD) K21.9
  with esophagitis K21.0
gastrointestinal (tract) K92.9
  amyloid E85.4
  functional K59.9
  psychogenic F45.8
  specified NEC K92.89
Gee (Herter) (Heubner) (Thaysen)
  (nontropical sprue) K90.0

Disease, diseased *--continued*

genital organs
  female N94.9
  male N50.9
Gerhardt's (erythromelalgia) I73.81
Gibert's (pityriasis rosea) L42
Gierke's (glycogenosis I) E74.01
Gilles de la Tourette's (motor-verbal tic)
  F95.2
gingiva K06.9
  plaque induced K05.00
  specified NEC K06.8
gland (lymph) I89.9
Glanzmann's (hereditary hemorrhagic
  thrombasthenia) D69.1
glass-blower's (cataract) -*see* Cataract,
  specified NEC
  salivary gland hypertrophy K11.1
Glisson's -*see* Rickets
globe H44.9
  specified NEC H44.89
glomerular -*see also* Glomerulonephritis
  with edema -*see* Nephrosis
  acute -*see* Nephritis, acute
  chronic -*see* Nephritis, chronic
  minimal change N05.0
  rapidly progressive N01.9
glycogen storage E74.00
  Andersen's E74.09
  Cori's E74.03
  Forbes' E74.03
  generalized E74.00
  glucose-6 phosphatase deficiency E74.01
  heart E74.02 [143]
  hepatorenal E74.09
  Hers' E74.09
  liver and kidney E74.09
  McArdle's E74.04
  muscle phosphofructokinase E74.09
  myocardium E74.02 [143]
  Pompe's E74.02
  Tauri's E74.09
  type 0 E74.09
  type I E74.01
  type II E74.02
  type III E74.03
  type IV E74.09
  type V E74.04
  type VI-XI E74.09
  Von Gierke's E74.01
Goldstein's (familial hemorrhagic
  telangiectasia) I78.0
gonococcal NOS A54.9
graft-versus-host (GVH) D89.813
  acute D89.810
  acute on chronic D89.812
  chronic D89.811
grain handler's J67.8
granulomatous (childhood) (chronic) D71
Graves' (exophthalmic goiter) -*see*
  Hyperthyroidism, with, goiter (diffuse)
Griesinger's -*see* Ancylostomiasis
Grisel's M43.6
Gruby's (tinea tonsurans) B35.0
Guillain-Barré G61.0
Guinon's (motor-verbal tic) F95.2
gum K06.9
gynecological N94.9
H (Hartnup's) E72.02
Haff -*see* Poisoning, mercury

Disease, diseased --*continued*
Hageman (congenital factor XII deficiency)
D68.2
hair (color) (shaft) L67.9
follicles L73.9
specified NEC L73.8
Hamman's (spontaneous mediastinal
emphysema) J98.2
hand, foot and mouth B08.4
Hansen's -*see* Leprosy
Hantavirus, with pulmonary manifestations
B33.4
with renal manifestations A98.5
Harada's H30.81
Hartnup (pellagra-cerebellar ataxia-renal
aminoaciduria) E72.02
Hart's (pellagra-cerebellar ataxia-renal
aminoaciduria) E72.02
Hashimoto's (struma lymphomatosa) E06.3
Hb -*see* Disease, hemoglobin
heart (organic) I51.9
with
pulmonary edema (acute) -*see also* Failure,
ventricular, left I50.1
rheumatic fever (conditions in I00)
active I01.9
with chorea I02.0
specified NEC I01.8
inactive or quiescent (with chorea) I09.9
specified NEC I09.89
amyloid E85.4 [*I43*]
aortic (valve) I35.9
arteriosclerotic or sclerotic (senile) -*see*
Disease, heart, ischemic, atherosclerotic
artery, arterial -*see* Disease, heart, ischemic,
atherosclerotic
beer drinkers' I42.6
beriberi (wet) E51.12
black I27.0
congenital Q24.9
cyanotic Q24.9
specified NEC Q24.8
coronary -*see* Disease, heart, ischemic
cryptogenic I51.9
fibroid -*see* Myocarditis
functional I51.89
psychogenic F45.8
glycogen storage E74.02 [*I43*]
gonococcal A54.83
hypertensive -*see* Hypertension, heart
hyperthyroid -*see also* Hyperthyroidism
E05.90 [*I43*]
with thyroid storm E05.91 [*I43*]
ischemic (chronic or with a stated duration
of over 4 weeks) I25.9
atherosclerotic (of) I25.10
with angina pectoris -*see* Arteriosclerosis,
coronary (artery)
coronary artery bypass graft -*see*
Arteriosclerosis, coronary (artery),
cardiomyopathy I25.5
diagnosed on ECG or other special
investigation, but currently presenting no
symptoms I25.6
silent I25.6
specified form NEC I25.89
kyphoscoliotic I27.1
meningococcal A39.50
endocarditis A39.51
myocarditis A39.52
pericarditis A39.53

Disease, diseased --*continued*
mitral I05.9
specified NEC I05.8
muscular -*see* Degeneration, myocardial
psychogenic (functional) F45.8
pulmonary (chronic) I27.9
in schistosomiasis B65.9 [*152*]
specified NEC I27.89
rheumatic (chronic) (inactive) (old)
(quiescent) (with chorea) I09.9
active or acute I01.9
with chorea (acute) (rheumatic)
(Sydenham's) I02.0
specified NEC I09.89
senile -*see* Myocarditis
syphilitic A52.06
aortic A52.03
aneurysm A52.01
congenital A50.54 [*152*]
thyrotoxic -*see also* Thyrotoxicosis E05.90
[*143*]
with thyroid storm E05.91 [*143*]
valve, valvular (obstructive) (regurgitant) -
see also Endocarditis
congenital NEC Q24.8
pulmonary Q22.3
vascular -*see* Disease, cardiovascular
heavy chain NEC C88.2
alpha C88.3
gamma C88.2
mu C88.2
Hebra's
pityriasis
maculata et circinata L42
rubra pilaris L44.0
prurigo L28.2
hematopoietic organs D75.9
hemoglobin or Hb
abnormal (mixed) NEC D58.2
with thalassemia D56.9
AS genotype D57.3
Bart's D56.0
C (Hb-C) D58.2
with other abnormal hemoglobin NEC
D58.2
elliptocytosis D58.1
Hb-S D57.2
sickle-cell D57.2
thalassemia D56.8
Constant Spring D58.2
D (Hb-D) D58.2
E (Hb-E) D58.2
E-beta thalassemia D56.5
elliptocytosis D58.1
H (Hb-H) (thalassemia) D56.0
with other abnormal hemoglobin NEC
D56.9
Constant Spring D56.0
I thalassemia D56.9
M D74.0
S or SS D57.1
SC D57.2
SD D57.8
SE D57.8
spherocytosis D58.0
unstable, hemolytic D58.2
hemolytic (newborn) P55.9
autoimmune (cold type) (warm type) D59.1
drug-induced D59.0
due to or with
incompatibility

Disease, diseased --*continued*
ABO (blood group) P55.1
blood (group) (Duffy) (K(ell)) (Kidd)
(Lewis) (M) (S) NEC P55.8
Rh (blood group) (factor) P55.0
Rh negative mother P55.0
specified type NEC P55.8
unstable hemoglobin D58.2
hemorrhagic D69.9
newborn P53
Henoch (Schönlein) (purpura nervosa) D69.0
hepatic -*see* Disease, liver
hepatobiliary K83.9
toxic K71.9
hepatolenticular E83.01
heredodegenerative NEC
spinal cord G95.89
herpesviral, disseminated B00.7
Hers' (glycogenosis VI) E74.09
Herter (Gee) (Heubner) (nontropical sprue)
K90.0
Heubner-Herter (nontropical sprue) K90.0
high fetal gene or hemoglobin thalassemia
D56.9
Hildebrand's -*see* Typhus
hip (joint) M25.9
congenital Q65.89
suppurative M00.9
tuberculous A18.02
His (Werner) (trench fever) A79.0
Hodgson's I71.2
ruptured I71.1
Holla -*see* Spherocytosis
hookworm B76.9
specified NEC B76.8
host-versus-graft D89.813
acute D89.810
acute on chronic D89.812
chronic D89.811
human immunodeficiency virus (HIV) B20
Huntington's G10
Hutchinson's (cheiropompholyx) -*see*
Hutchinson's disease - hyaline (diffuse)
(generalized)
membrane (lung) (newborn) P22.0
adult J80
hydatid -*see* Echinococcus
hydroxyapatite deposition M11.00
ankle M11.07
elbow M11.02
foot joint M11.07
hand joint M11.04
hip M11.05
knee M11.06
multiple site M11.09
shoulder M11.01
vertebra M11.08
wrist M11.03
hyperkinetic -*see* Hyperkinesia
hypertensive -*see* Hypertension
hypophysis E23.7
Iceland G93.3
I-cell E77.0
immune D89.9
immunoproliferative (malignant) C88.9
small intestinal C88.3
specified NEC C88.8
inclusion B25.9
salivary gland B25.9
infectious, infective B99.9
congenital P37.9

Disease, diseased --*continued*
  specified NEC P37.8
  viral P35.9
    specified type NEC P35.8
  specified NEC B99.8
  inflammatory
    penis N48.29
      abscess N48.21
      cellulitis N48.22
    prepuce N47.7
      balanoposthitis N47.6
    tubo-ovarian -*see* Salpingo-oophoritis
  intervertebral disc -*see also* Disorder, disc
    with myelopathy -*see* Disorder, disc, with, myelopathy
    cervical, cervicothoracic -*see* Disorder, disc, cervical
      with
        myelopathy -*see* Disorder, disc, cervical, with myelopathy
        neuritis, radiculitis or radiculopathy -*see* Disorder, disc, cervical, with neuritis
        specified NEC -*see* Disorder, disc, cervical, specified type NEC
    lumbar (with)
      myelopathy M51.06
      neuritis, radiculitis, radiculopathy or sciatica M51.16
      specified NEC M51.86
    lumbosacral (with)
      neuritis, radiculitis, radiculopathy or sciatica M51.17
      specified NEC M51.87
    specified NEC -*see* Disorder, disc, specified NEC
    thoracic (with)
      myelopathy M51.04
      neuritis, radiculitis or radiculopathy M51.14
      specified NEC M51.84
    thoracolumbar (with)
      myelopathy M51.05
      neuritis, radiculitis or radiculopathy M51.15
      specified NEC M51.85
  intestine K63.9
    functional K59.9
      psychogenic F45.8
      specified NEC K59.8
    organic K63.9
    protozoal A07.9
    specified NEC K63.89
  iris H21.9
    specified NEC H21.89
  iron metabolism or storage E83.10
  island (scrub typhus) A75.3
  itai-itai -*see* Poisoning, cadmium
  Jakob-Creutzfeldt -*see* Creutzfeldt-Jakob
  disease or syndrome - jaw M27.9
    fibrocystic M27.49
    specified NEC M27.8
  jigger B88.1
  joint -*see also* Disorder, joint
    Charcot's -*see* Arthropathy, neuropathic (Charcot)
    degenerative -*see* Osteoarthritis
      multiple M15.9
      spine -*see* Spondylosis
    hypertrophic -*see* Osteoarthritis
    sacroiliac M53.3

Disease, diseased --*continued*
    specified NEC -*see* Disorder, joint, specified type NEC
    spine NEC -*see* Dorsopathy
    suppurative -*see* Arthritis, pyogenic or pyemic
  Jourdain's (acute gingivitis) K05.00
    nonplaque induced K05.01
    plaque induced K05.00
  Kaschin-Beck (endemic polyarthritis) M12.10
    ankle M12.17
    elbow M12.12
    foot joint M12.17
    hand joint M12.14
    hip M12.15
    knee M12.16
    multiple site M12.19
    shoulder M12.11
    vertebra M12.18
    wrist M12.13
  Katayama B65.2
  Kedani (scrub typhus) A75.3
  Keshan E59
  kidney (functional) (pelvis) N28.9
    chronic N18.9
      hypertensive -*see* Hypertension, kidney
      stage 1N18.1
      stage 2(mild) N18.2
      stage 3(moderate) N18.3
      stage 4(severe) N18.4
      stage 5N18.5
    complicating pregnancy -*see* Pregnancy, complicated by, renal disease
    cystic (congenital) Q61.9
    diabetic -*see* E08 E13 with .22
    fibrocystic (congenital) Q61.8
    hypertensive -*see* Hypertension, kidney
    in (due to)
      schistosomiasis (bilharziasis) B65.9 [*N29*]
    multicystic Q61.4
    polycystic Q61.3
      adult type Q61.2
      childhood type NEC Q61.19
        collecting duct dilatation Q61.11
  Kimmelstiel (Wilson) (intercapillary polycystic (congenital) glomerulosclerosis) -*see* E08 E13 with .21
  Kimura D21.9
    specified site (see Neoplasm, connective tissue benign)
  Kinnier Wilson's (hepatolenticular degeneration) E83.01
  kissing -*see* Mononucleosis, infectious
  Klebs' -*see also* Glomerulonephritis N05.
  Klippel-Feil (brevicollis) Q76.1
  Köhler-Pellegrini-Stieda (calcification, knee joint) -*see* Bursitis, tibial collateral
  Kok Q89.8
  Koenig's (osteochondritis dissecans) -*see* Osteochondritis, dissecans
  Korsakoff's (nonalcoholic) F04
    alcoholic F10.96
      with dependence F10.26
  Kostmann's (infantile genetic agranulocytosis) D70.0
  kuru A81.81
  Kyasanur Forest A98.2
  labyrinth, ear -*see* Disorder, ear, inner
  lacrimal system -*see* Disorder, lacrimal system
  Lafora's -*see* Epilepsy, generalized, idiopathic

Disease, diseased --*continued*
  Lancereaux Mathieu (leptospiral jaundice) A27.0
  Landry's G61.0
  Larrey Weil (leptospiral jaundice) A27.0
  larynx J38.7
  legionnaires' A48.1
    nonpneumonic A48.2
  Lenegre's I44.2
  lens H27.9
    specified NEC H27.8
  Lev's (acquired complete heart block) I44.2
  Lewy body (dementia) G31.83 [*F02.80]*
    with behavioral disturbance G31.83 [*F02.81]*
  Lichtheim's (subacute combined sclerosis with pernicious anemia) D51.0
  Lightwood's (renal tubular acidosis) N25.89
  Lignac's (cystinosis) E72.04
  lip K13.0
  lipid-storage E75.6
    specified NEC E75.5
  Lipschütz's N76.6
  liver (chronic) (organic) K76.9
    alcoholic (chronic) K70.9
      acute -*see* Disease, liver, alcoholic, hepatitis
      cirrhosis K70.30
        with ascites K70.31
      failure K70.40
        with coma K70.41
      fatty liver K70.0
      fibrosis K70.2
      hepatitis K70.10
        with ascites K70.11
      sclerosis K70.2
    cystic, congenital Q44.6
    drug-induced (idiosyncratic) (toxic) (predictable) (unpredictable) -*see* Disease, liver, toxic
    end stage K72.90
      due to hepatitis -*see* Hepatitis
    fatty, nonalcoholic (NAFLD) K76.0
      alcoholic K70.0
    fibrocystic (congenital) Q44.6
    fluke
      Chinese B66.1
      oriental B66.1
      sheep B66.3
    glycogen storage E74.09 [*K77*]
    in (due to)
      schistosomiasis (bilharziasis) B65.9 [*K77*]
    inflammatory K75.9
      alcoholic K70.1
      specified NEC K75.89
    polycystic (congenital) Q44.6
    toxic K71.9
      with
        cholestasis K71.0
        cirrhosis (liver) K71.7
        fibrosis (liver) K71.7
        focal nodular hyperplasia K71.8
        hepatic granuloma K71.8
        hepatic necrosis K71.10
          with coma K71.11
        hepatitis NEC K71.6
          acute K71.2
          chronic
            active K71.50
              with ascites K71.51
            lobular K71.4

Disease, diseased --*continued*
  persistent K71.3
    lupoid K71.50
      with ascites K71.51
    peliosis hepatis K71.8
    veno-occlusive disease (VOD) of liver K71.8
  veno-occlusive K76.5
  Lobo's (keloid blastomycosis) B48.0
  Lobstein's (brittle bones and blue sclera) Q78.0
  Ludwig's (submaxillary cellulitis) K12.2
  lumbosacral region M53.87
  lung J98.4
    black J60
    congenital Q33.9
    cystic J98.4
      congenital Q33.0
    fibroid (chronic) -*see* Fibrosis, lung
    fluke B66.4
      oriental B66.4
    in
      amyloidosis E85.4 [*J99*]
      sarcoidosis D86.0
      Sjögren's syndrome M35.02
      systemic
        lupus erythematosus M32.13
        sclerosis M34.81
    interstitial J84.9
      of childhood, specified NEC J84.848
      respiratory bronchiolitis J84.115
      specified NEC J84.89
    obstructive (chronic) J44.9
      with
        acute
          bronchitis J44.0
          exacerbation NEC J44.1
          lower respiratory infection J44.0
        alveolitis, allergic J67.9
        asthma J44.9
        bronchiectasis J47.9
          with
            exacerbation (acute) J47.1
            lower respiratory infection J47.0
        bronchitis J44.9
          with
            exacerbation (acute) J44.1
            lower respiratory infection J44.0
        emphysema J44.9
        hypersensitivity pneumonitis J67.9
      decompensated J44.1
        with
          exacerbation (acute) J44.1
    polycystic J98.4
      congenital Q33.0
    rheumatoid (diffuse) (interstitial) -*see*
Rheumatoid, lung
  Lutembacher's (atrial septal defect with mitral stenosis) Q21.1
  Lyme A69.20
  lymphatic (gland) (system) (channel) (vessel) I89.9
  lymphoproliferative D47.9
    specified NEC D47.Z9
    T-gamma D47.Z9
    X linked D82.3
  Magitot's M27.2
  malarial -*see* Malaria
  malignant -*see also* Neoplasm, malignant, by site
  Manson's B65.1

Disease, diseased --*continued*
  maple bark J67.6
  maple-syrup-urine E71.0
  Marburg (virus) A98.3
  Marion's (bladder neck obstruction) N32.0
  Marsh's (exophthalmic goiter) -*see*
Hyperthyroidism, with, goiter (diffuse)
  mastoid (process) -*see* Disorder, ear, middle
  Mathieu's (leptospiral jaundice) A27.0
  Maxcy's A75.2
  McArdle (Schmid-Pearson) (glycogenosis V) E74.04
  mediastinum J98.59
  medullary center (idiopathic) (respiratory) G93.89
  Meige's (chronic hereditary edema) Q82.0
  meningococcal -*see* Infection, meningococcal
  mental F99
    organic F09
  mesenchymal M35.9
  mesenteric embolic -*see also* Ischemia, intestine, acute K55.039
  metabolic, metabolism E88.9
    bilirubin E80.7
  metal-polisher's J62.8
  metastatic -*see also* Neoplasm, secondary, by site C79.9
  microvascular
  code to condition
  microvillus
    atrophy Q43.8
    inclusion (MVD) Q43.8
  middle ear -*see* Disorder, ear, middle
  Mikulicz' (dryness of mouth, absent or decreased lacrimation) K11.8
  Milroy's (chronic hereditary edema) Q82.0
  Minamata -*see* Poisoning, mercury minicore G71.2
  Minor's G95.19
  Minot's (hemorrhagic disease, newborn) P53
  Minot-von Willebrand-Jürgens (angiohemophilia) D68.0
  Mitchell's (erythromelalgia) I73.81
  mitral (valve) I05.9
    nonrheumatic I34.9
  mixed connective tissue M35.1
  moldy hay J67.0
  Monge's T70.29
  Morgagni-Adams-Stokes (syncope with heart block) I45.9
  Morgagni's (syndrome) (hyperostosis frontalis interna) M85.2
  Morton's (with metatarsalgia) -*see* Lesion, nerve, plantar
  Morvan's G60.8
  motor neuron (bulbar) (familial) (mixed type) (spinal) G12.20
    amyotrophic lateral sclerosis G12.21
    progressive bulbar palsy G12.22
    specified NEC G12.29
  moyamoya I67.5
  mu heavy chain disease C88.2
  multicore G71.2
  muscle -*see also* Disorder, muscle
    inflammatory -*see* Myositis
    ocular (external) -*see* Strabismus
  musculoskeletal system, soft tissue -*see also* Disorder, soft tissue
    specified NEC -*see* Disorder, soft tissue, specified type NEC
  mushroom workers' J67.5

Disease, diseased --*continued*
  mycotic B49
  myelodysplastic, not classified C94.6
  myeloproliferative, not classified C94.6
    chronic D47.1
  myocardium, myocardial -*see also*
Degeneration, myocardial I51.5
    primary (idiopathic) I42.9
  myoneural G70.9
  Naegeli's D69.1
  nails L60.9
    specified NEC L60.8
  Nairobi (sheep virus) A93.8
  nasal J34.9
  nemaline body G71.2
  nerve -*see* Disorder, nerve
  nervous system G98.8
    autonomic G90.9
    central G96.9
      specified NEC G96.8
    congenital Q07.9
    parasympathetic G90.9
    specified NEC G98.8
    sympathetic G90.9
    vegetative G90.9
  neuromuscular system G70.9
  Newcastle B30.8
  Nicolas (Durand) Favre (climatic bubo) A55
  nipple N64.9
    Paget's C50.01
      female C50.01
      male C50.02
  Nishimoto (Takeuchi) I67.5
  nonarthropod-borne NOS (viral) B34.9
    enterovirus NEC B34.1
  nonautoimmune hemolytic D59.4
    drug-induced D59.2
  Nonne-Milroy Meige (chronic hereditary edema) Q82.0
  nose J34.9
  nucleus pulposus -*see* Disorder, disc
  nutritional E63.9
  oast-house-urine E72.19
  ocular
    herpesviral B00.50
    zoster B02.30
  obliterative vascular I77.1
  Ohara's -*see* Tularemia
  Opitz's (congestive splenomegaly) D73.2
  Oppenheim-Urbach (necrobiosis lipoidica diabeticorum) -*see* E08 E13 with .620
  optic nerve NEC -*see* Disorder, nerve, optic
  orbit -*see* Disorder, orbit
  Oriental liver fluke B66.1
  Oriental lung fluke B66.4
  Ormond's N13.5
  Oropouche virus A93.0
  Osler-Rendu (familial hemorrhagic telangiectasia) I78.0
  osteofibrocystic E21.0
  Otto's M24.7
  outer ear -*see* Disorder, ear, external
  ovary (noninflammatory) N83.9
    cystic N83.20
    inflammatory -*see* Salpingo-oophoritis
    polycystic E28.2
    specified NEC N83.8
  Owren's (congenital) -*see* Defect, coagulation
  pancreas K86.9
    cystic K86.2
    fibrocystic E84.9

Disease, diseased *--continued*
 specified NEC K86.89
 panvalvular I08.9
  specified NEC I08.8
 parametrium (noninflammatory) N83.9
 parasitic B89
  cerebral NEC B71.9 [*G94*]
  intestinal NOS B82.9
  mouth B37.0
  skin NOS B88.9
  specified type *-see* Infestation
  tongue B37.0
 parathyroid (gland) E21.5
  specified NEC E21.4
 Parkinson's G20
 parodontal K05.6
 Parrot's (syphilitic osteochondritis) A50.02
 Parry's (exophthalmic goiter) *-see*
  Hyperthyroidism, with, goiter (diffuse)
 Parson's (exophthalmic goiter) *-see*
  Hyperthyroidism, with, goiter (diffuse)
 Paxton's (white piedra) B36.2
 pearl-worker's *-see* Osteomyelitis, specified
  type NEC
 Pellegrini-Stieda (calcification, knee joint) -
  see Bursitis, tibial collateral
 pelvis, pelvic
  female NOS N94.9
   specified NEC N94.89
  gonococcal (acute) (chronic) A54.24
  inflammatory (female) N73.9
   acute N73.0
   chlamydial A56.11
   chronic N73.1
   specified NEC N73.8
   syphilitic (secondary) A51.42
    late A52.76
   tuberculous A18.17
  organ, female N94.9
  peritoneum, female NEC N94.89
 penis N48.9
  inflammatory N48.29
   abscess N48.21
   cellulitis N48.22
   specified NEC N48.89
 periapical tissues NOS K04.90
 periodontal K05.6
  specified NEC K05.5
 periosteum *-see* Disorder, bone, specified type
  NEC
 peripheral
  arterial I73.9
  autonomic nervous system G90.9
  nerves *-see* Polyneuropathy
  vascular NOS I73.9
 peritoneum K66.9
  pelvic, female NEC N94.89
  specified NEC K66.8
 persistent mucosal (middle ear) H66.20
  left H66.22
   with right H66.23
  right H66.21
   with left H66.23
 Petit's *-see* Hernia, abdomen, specified site
  NEC
 pharynx J39.2
  specified NEC J39.2
 Phocas' *-see* Mastopathy, cystic
 photochromogenic (acid-fast bacilli)
  (pulmonary) A31.0
  nonpulmonary A31.9

Disease, diseased *--continued*
 Pick's G31.01 [*F02.80*]
  with behavioral disturbance G31.01
  [*F02.81*]
  brain G31.01 [F*02.80*]
   with behavioral disturbance G31.01
   [*F02.81*]
  of pericardium (pericardial pseudocirrhosis)
  of liver) I31.1
 pigeon fancier's J67.2
 pineal gland E34.8
 pink *-see* Poisoning, mercury Pinkus' (lichen
  nitidus) L44.1
 pinworm B80
 Piry virus A93.8
 pituitary (gland) E23.7
 pituitary snuff-taker's J67.8
 pleura (cavity) J94.9
  specified NEC J94.8
 pneumatic drill (hammer) T75.21
 Pollitzer's (hidradenitis suppurativa) L73.2
 polycystic
  kidney or renal Q61.3
   adult type Q61.2
   childhood type NEC Q61.19
    collecting duct dilatation Q61.11
  liver or hepatic Q44.6
  lung or pulmonary J98.4
   congenital Q33.0
  ovary, ovaries E28.2
  spleen Q89.09
 polyethylene T84.05
 Pompe's (glycogenosis II) E74.02
 Posadas-Wernicke B38.9
 Potain's (pulmonary edema) *-see* Edema, lung
 prepuce N47.8
  inflammatory N47.7
   balanoposthitis N47.6
 Pringle's (tuberous sclerosis) Q85.1
 prion, central nervous system A81.9
  specified NEC A81.89
 prostate N42.9
  specified NEC N42.89
 protozoal B64
  acanthamebiasis *-see* Acanthamebiasis
  African trypanosomiasis *-see* African
  trypanosomiasis
  babesiosis B60.0
  Chagas disease *-see* Chagas disease
  intestine, intestinal A07.9
  leishmaniasis *-see* Leishmaniasis
  malaria *-see* Malaria
  naegleriasis B60.2
  pneumocystosis B59
  specified organism NEC B60.8
  toxoplasmosis *-see* Toxoplasmosis
 pseudo-Hurler's E77.0
 psychiatric F99
 psychotic *-see* Psychosis
 Puente's (simple glandular cheilitis) K13.0
 puerperal *-see also* Puerperal O90.89
 pulmonary *-see also* Disease, lung
  artery I28.9
  chronic obstructive J44.9
   with
    acute bronchitis J44.0
    exacerbation (acute) J44.1
    lower respiratory infection (acute) J44.0
   decompensated J44.1
    with
     exacerbation (acute) J44.1

Disease, diseased *--continued*
  heart I27.9
   specified NEC I27.89
  hypertensive (vascular) I27.0
  valve I37.9
   rheumatic I09.89
 pulp (dental) NOS K04.90
 pulseless M31.4
 Putnam's (subacute combined sclerosis with
  pernicious anemia) D51.0
 Pyle (Cohn) (metaphyseal dysplasia) Q78.5
 ragpicker's or ragsorter's A22.1
 Raynaud's *-see* Raynaud's disease - reactive
  airway *-see* Asthma
 Reclus' (cystic) *-see* Mastopathy, cystic
 rectum K62.9
  specified NEC K62.89
 Refsum's (heredopathia atactica
  polyneuritiformis) G60.1
 renal (functional) (pelvis) *-see also* Disease,
  kidney N28.9
  with
   edema *-see* Nephrosis
   glomerular lesion *-see* Glomerulonephritis
    with edema *-see* Nephrosis
   interstitial nephritis N12
  acute N28.9
  chronic *-see also* Disease, kidney, chronic
  N18.9
  cystic, congenital Q61.9
  diabetic *-see* E08 E13 with .22
  end-stage (failure) N18.6
   due to hypertension I12.0
  fibrocystic (congenital) Q61.8
  hypertensive *-see* Hypertension, kidney
  lupus M32.14
  phosphate-losing (tubular) N25.0
  polycystic (congenital) Q61.3
   adult type Q61.2
   childhood type NEC Q61.19
    collecting duct dilatation Q61.11
  rapidly progressive N01.9
  subacute N01.9
 Rendu-Osler-Weber (familial hemorrhagic
  telangiectasia) I78.0
 renovascular (arteriosclerotic) *-see*
  Hypertension, kidney
 respiratory (tract) J98.9
  acute or subacute NOS J06.9
   due to
    chemicals, gases, fumes or vapors
    (inhalation) J68.3
    external agent J70.9
     specified NEC J70.8
    radiation J70.0
    smoke inhalation J70.5
   noninfectious J39.8
  chronic NOS J98.9
   due to
    chemicals, gases, fumes or vapors J68.4
    external agent J70.9
     specified NEC J70.8
    radiation J70.1
  newborn P27.9
   specified NEC P27.8
  due to
   chemicals, gases, fumes or vapors J68.9
    acute or subacute NEC J68.3
    chronic J68.4
   external agent J70.9
    specified NEC J70.8

Disease, diseased --*continued*
  newborn P28.9
    specified type NEC P28.89
  upper J39.9
    acute or subacute J06.9
    noninfectious NEC J39.8
    specified NEC J39.8
    streptococcal J06.9
  retina, retinal H35.9
    Batten's or Batten-Mayou E75.4 [*H36*]
    specified NEC H35.89
  rheumatoid -*see* Arthritis, rheumatoid
  rickettsial NOS A79.9
    specified type NEC A79.89
  Riga (Fede) (cachectic aphthae) K14.0
  Riggs' (compound periodontitis) -*see*
    Periodontitis
  Ritter's L00
  Rivalta's (cervicofacial actinomycosis) A42.2
  Robles' (onchocerciasis) B73.01
  Roger's (congenital interventricular septal
    defect) Q21.0
  Rosenthal's (factor XI deficiency) D68.1
  Rossbach's (hyperchlorhydria) K30
  Ross River B33.1
  Rotes Quérol -*see* Hyperostosis, ankylosing
  Roth (Bernhardt) -*see* Mononeuropathy,
    lower limb, meralgia paresthetica
  Runeberg's (progressive pernicious anemia)
    D51.0
  sacroiliac NEC M53.3
  salivary gland or duct K11.9
    inclusion B25.9
    specified NEC K11.8
    virus B25.9
  sandworm B76.9
  Schimmelbusch's -*see* Mastopathy, cystic
  Schmorl's -*see* Schmorl's disease or nodes
  Schönlein (Henoch) (purpura rheumatica)
    D69.0
  Schottmüller's -*see* Fever, paratyphoid
  Schultz's (agranulocytosis) -*see*
    Agranulocytosis
  Schwalbe-Ziehen-Oppenheim G24.1
  Schwartz Jampel G71.13
  sclera H15.9
    specified NEC H15.89
  scrofulous (tuberculous) A18.2
  scrotum N50.9
  sebaceous glands L73.9
  semilunar cartilage, cystic -*see also*
    Derangement, knee, meniscus, cystic
  seminal vesicle N50.9
  serum NEC -*see also* Reaction, serum T80.69
  sexually transmitted A64
    anogenital
      herpesviral infection -*see* Herpes,
    anogenital
      warts A63.0
    chancroid A57
    chlamydial infection -*see* Chlamydia
    gonorrhea -*see* Gonorrhea
    granuloma inguinale A58
    specified organism NEC A63.8
    syphilis -*see* Syphilis
    trichomoniasis -*see* Trichomoniasis
  Sézary C84.1
  shimamushi (scrub typhus) A75.3
  shipyard B30.0
  sickle-cell D57.1
    with crisis (vasoocclusive pain) D57.00

Disease, diseased --*continued*
  with
    acute chest syndrome D57.01
    splenic sequestration D57.02
  elliptocytosis D57.8
  Hb-C D57.20
    with crisis (vasoocclusive pain) D57.219
      with
        acute chest syndrome D57.211
        splenic sequestration D57.212
    without crisis D57.20
  Hb-SD D57.80
    with crisis D57.819
      with
        acute chest syndrome D57.811
        splenic sequestration D57.812
  Hb-SE D57.80
    with crisis D57.819
      with
        acute chest syndrome D57.811
        splenic sequestration D57.812
  specified NEC D57.80
    with crisis D57.819
      with
        acute chest syndrome D57.811
        splenic sequestration D57.812
  spherocytosis D57.80
    with crisis D57.819
      with
        acute chest syndrome D57.811
        splenic sequestration D57.812
  thalassemia D57.40
    with crisis (vasoocclusive pain) D57.419
      with
        acute chest syndrome D57.411
        splenic sequestration D57.412
    without crisis D57.40
  silo-filler's J68.8
    bronchitis J68.0
    pneumonitis J68.0
    pulmonary edema J68.1
  simian B B00.4
  Simons' (progressive lipodystrophy) E88.1
  sin nombre virus B33.4
  sinus -*see* Sinusitis
  Sirkari's B55.0
  sixth B08.20
    due to human herpesvirus 6 B08.21
    due to human herpesvirus 7 B08.22
  skin L98.9
    due to metabolic disorder NEC E88.9 [*L99*]
    specified NEC L98.8
  slim (HIV) B20
  small vessel I73.9
  Sneddon-Wilkinson (subcorneal pustular
    dermatosis) L13.1
  South African creeping B88.0
  spinal (cord) G95.9
    congenital Q06.9
    specified NEC G95.89
  spine -*see also* Spondylopathy
    joint -*see* Dorsopathy
    tuberculous A18.01
  spinocerebellar (hereditary) G11.9
    specified NEC G11.8
  spleen D73.9
    amyloid E85.4 [*D77*]
    organic D73.9
    polycystic Q89.09
    postinfectional D73.89

Disease, diseased --*continued*
  sponge-diver's -*see* Toxicity, venom, marine
    animal, sea anemone
  Startle Q89.8
  Steinert's G71.11
  Sticker's (erythema infectiosum) B08.3
  Stieda's (calcification, knee joint) -*see*
    Bursitis, tibial collateral
  Stokes' (exophthalmic goiter) -*see*
    Hyperthyroidism, with, goiter (diffuse)
  Stokes-Adams (syncope with heart block)
    I45.9
  stomach K31.9
    functional, psychogenic F45.8
    specified NEC K31.89
  stonemason's J62.8
  storage
    glycogen -*see* Disease, glycogen storage
    mucopolysaccharide -*see*
      Mucopolysaccharidosis
  striatopallidal system NEC G25.89
  Stuart-Prower (congenital factor X
    deficiency) D68.2
  Stuart's (congenital factor X deficiency)
    D68.2
  subcutaneous tissue -*see* Disease, skin
  supporting structures of teeth K08.9
    specified NEC K08.89
  suprarenal (capsule) (gland) E27.9
    hyperfunction E27.0
    specified NEC E27.8
  sweat glands L74.9
    specified NEC L74.8
  Sweeley Klionsky E75.21
  Swift (Feer) -*see* Poisoning, mercury
  swimming-pool granuloma A31.1
  Sylvest's (epidemic pleurodynia) B33.0
  sympathetic nervous system G90.9
  synovium -*see* Disorder, synovium
  syphilitic -*see* Syphilis
  systemic tissue mast cell C96.2
  tanapox (virus) B08.71
  Tangier E78.6
  Tarral-Besnier (pityriasis rubra pilaris) L44.0
  Tauri's E74.09
  tear duct -*see* Disorder, lacrimal system
  tendon, tendinous -*see also* Disorder, tendon
    nodular -*see* Trigger finger
  terminal vessel I73.9
  testis N50.9
  thalassemia Hb-S -*see* Disease, sickle-cell,
    thalassemia
  Thaysen-Gee (nontropical sprue) K90.0
  Thomsen G71.12
  throat J39.2
    septic J02.0
  thromboembolic -*see* Embolism
  thymus (gland) E32.9
    specified NEC E32.8
  thyroid (gland) E07.9
    heart -*see also* Hyperthyroidism E05.90
    [*I43*]
      with thyroid storm E05.91 [*I43*]
    specified NEC E07.89
  Tietze's M94.0
  tongue K14.9
    specified NEC K14.8
  tonsils, tonsillar (and adenoids) J35.9
  tooth, teeth K08.9
    hard tissues K03.9
      specified NEC K03.89

Disease, diseased --*continued*
pulp NEC K04.99
specified NEC K08.89
Tourette's F95.2
trachea NEC J39.8
tricuspid I07.9
nonrheumatic I36.9
triglyceride-storage E75.5
trophoblastic -*see* Mole, hydatidiform
tsutsugamushi A75.3
tube (fallopian) (noninflammatory) N83.9
inflammatory -*see* Salpingitis
specified NEC N83.8
tuberculous NEC -*see* Tuberculosis
tubo-ovarian (noninflammatory) N83.9
inflammatory -*see* Salpingo-oophoritis
specified NEC N83.8
tubotympanic, chronic -*see* Otitis, media,
suppurative, chronic, tubotympanic
tubulo-interstitial N15.9
specified NEC N15.8
tympanum -*see* Disorder, tympanic membrane
Uhl's Q24.8
Underwood's (sclerema neonatorum) P83.0
Unverricht (Lundborg) -*see* Epilepsy,
generalized, idiopathic
Urbach-Oppenheim (necrobiosis lipoidica
diabeticorum) -*see* E08 E13 with .620
ureter N28.9
in (due to)
schistosomiasis (bilharziasis) B65.0 [*N29*]
urethra N36.9
specified NEC N36.8
urinary (tract) N39.9
bladder N32.9
specified NEC N32.89
specified NEC N39.8
uterus (noninflammatory) N85.9
infective -*see* Endometritis
inflammatory -*see* Endometritis
specified NEC N85.8
uveal tract (anterior) H21.9
posterior H31.9
vagabond's B85.1
vagina, vaginal (noninflammatory) N89.9
inflammatory NEC N76.89
specified NEC N89.8
valve, valvular I38
multiple I08.9
specified NEC I08.8
van Creveld-von Gierke (glycogenosis I)
E74.01
vas deferens N50.9
vascular I99.9
arteriosclerotic -*see* Arteriosclerosis
ciliary body NEC -*see* Disorder, iris,
vascular
hypertensive -*see* Hypertension
iris NEC -*see* Disorder, iris, vascular
obliterative I77.1
peripheral I73.9
occlusive I99.8
peripheral (occlusive) I73.9
in diabetes mellitus -*see* E08 E13 with .51
vasomotor I73.9
vasospastic I73.9
vein I87.9
venereal -*see also* Disease, sexually
transmitted A64
chlamydial NEC A56.8
anus A56.3

Disease, diseased --*continued*
genitourinary NOS A56.2
pharynx A56.4
rectum A56.3
fifth A55
sixth A55
specified nature or type NEC A63.8
vertebra, vertebral -*see also* Spondylopathy
disc -*see* Disorder, disc
vibration -*see* Vibration, adverse effects
viral, virus -*see also* Disease, by type of virus
B34.9
arbovirus NOS A94
arthropod-borne NOS A94
congenital P35.9
specified NEC P35.8
Hanta (with renal manifestations) (Dobrava)
(Puumala) (Seoul) A98.5
with pulmonary manifestations (Andes)
(Bayou) (Bermejo) (Black Creek Canal)
(Choclo) (Juquitiba) (Laguna
negra)(Lechiguanas) (New York) (Oran)
(Sin nombre) B33.4
Hantaan (Korean hemorrhagic fever) A98.5
human immunodeficiency (HIV) B20
Kunjin A83.4
nonarthropod-borne NOS B34.9
Powassan A84.8
Rocio (encephalitis) A83.6
Sin nombre (Hantavirus) (cardio) pulmonary
syndrome) B33.4
Tahyna B33.8
vesicular stomatitis A93.8
vitreous H43.9
specified NEC H43.89
vocal cord J38.3
Volkmann's, acquired T79.6
von Eulenburg's (congenital paramyotonia)
G71.19
von Gierke's (glycogenosis I) E74.01
von Graefe's -*see* Strabismus, paralytic,
ophthalmoplegia, progressive
von Willebrand (Jürgens) (angiohemophilia)
D68.0
Vrolik's (osteogenesis imperfecta) Q78.0
vulva (noninflammatory) N90.9
inflammatory NEC N76.89
specified NEC N90.89
Wallgren's (obstruction of splenic vein with
collateral circulation) I87.8
Wassilieff's (leptospiral jaundice) A27.0
wasting NEC R64
due to malnutrition E41
Waterhouse-Friderichsen A39.1
Wegner's (syphilitic osteochondritis) A50.02
Weil's (leptospiral jaundice of lung) A27.0
Weir Mitchell's (erythromelalgia) I73.81
Werdnig-Hoffmann G12.0
Wermer's E31.21
Werner-His (trench fever) A79.0
Werner-Schultz (neutropenic splenomegaly)
D73.81
Wernicke-Posadas B38.9
whipworm B79
white blood cells D72.9
specified NEC D72.89
white matter R90.82
white-spot, meaning lichen sclerosus et
atrophicus L90.0
penis N48.0
vulva N90.4

Disease, diseased --*continued*
Wilkie's K55.1
Wilkinson-Sneddon (subcorneal pustular
dermatosis) L13.1
Willis' -*see* Diabetes
Wilson's (hepatolenticular degeneration)
E83.01
woolsorter's A22.1
yaba monkey tumor B08.72
yaba pox (virus) B08.72
Zika virus A92.5
zoonotic, bacterial A28.9
specified type NEC A28.8
Disfigurement (due to scar) L90.5
Disgerminoma -*see* Dysgerminoma
**DISH (diffuse idiopathic skeletal
hyperostosis)** -*see* Hyperostosis, ankylosing
Disinsertion, retina -*see* Detachment, retina
Dislocatable hip, congenital Q65.6
Dislocation (articular)
with fracture -*see* Fracture
acromioclavicular (joint) S43.10
with displacement
100% 200% S43.12
more than 200% S43.13
inferior S43.14
posterior S43.15
ankle S93.0
astragalus -*see* Dislocation, ankle
atlantoaxial S13.121
atlantooccipital S13.111
atloido-occipital S13.111
breast bone S23.29
capsule, joint
code by site under Dislocation
carpal (bone) -*see* Dislocation, wrist
carpometacarpal (joint) NEC S63.05
thumb S63.04
cartilage (joint)
code by site under Dislocation
cervical spine (vertebra) -*see* Dislocation,
vertebra, cervical
chronic -*see* Dislocation, recurrent
clavicle -*see* Dislocation, acromioclavicular
joint
coccyx S33.2
congenital NEC Q68.8
coracoid -*see* Dislocation, shoulder
costal cartilage S23.29
costochondral S23.29
cricoarytenoid articulation S13.29
cricothyroid articulation S13.29
dorsal vertebra -*see* Dislocation, vertebra,
thoracic
ear ossicle -*see* Discontinuity, ossicles, ear
elbow S53.10
congenital Q68.8
pathological -*see* Dislocation, pathological
NEC, elbow
radial head alone -*see* Dislocation, radial
head
recurrent -*see* Dislocation, recurrent, elbow
traumatic S53.10
anterior S53.11
lateral S53.14
medial S53.13
posterior S53.12
specified type NEC S53.19
eye, nontraumatic -*see* Luxation, globe
eyeball, nontraumatic -*see* Luxation, globe -
femur

Dislocation (articular) --*continued*
  distal end -*see* Dislocation, knee
  proximal end -*see* Dislocation, hip
fibula
  distal end -*see* Dislocation, ankle
  proximal end -*see* Dislocation, knee - finger
    S63.25
  index S63.25
  interphalangeal S63.27
    distal S63.29
      index S63.29
      little S63.29
      middle S63.29
      ring S63.29
    index S63.27
    little S63.27
    middle S63.27
    proximal S63.28
      index S63.28
      little S63.28
      middle S63.28
      ring S63.28
    ring S63.27
  little S63.25
  metacarpophalangeal S63.26
    index S63.26
    little S63.26
    middle S63.26
    ring S63.26
  middle S63.25
  recurrent -*see* Dislocation, recurrent, finger
  ring S63.25
  thumb -*see* Dislocation, thumb
foot S93.30
  recurrent -*see* Dislocation, recurrent, foot
  specified site NEC S93.33
  tarsal joint S93.31
  tarsometatarsal joint S93.32
  toe -*see* Dislocation, toe
fracture -*see* Fracture
glenohumeral (joint) -*see* Dislocation,
    shoulder
glenoid -*see* Dislocation, shoulder
habitual -*see* Dislocation, recurrent
hip S73.00
  anterior S73.03
    obturator S73.02
  central S73.04
  congenital (total) Q65.2
    bilateral Q65.1
    partial Q65.5
      bilateral Q65.4
      unilateral Q65.3
    unilateral Q65.0
  developmental M24.85
  pathological -*see* Dislocation, pathological
    NEC, hip
  posterior S73.01
  recurrent -*see* Dislocation, recurrent, hip
humerus, proximal end -*see* Dislocation,
    shoulder
incomplete -*see* Subluxation, by site
incus -*see* Discontinuity, ossicles, ear
infracoracoid -*see* Dislocation, shoulder
innominate (pubic junction) (sacral junction)
    S33.39
  acetabulum -*see* Dislocation, hip
interphalangeal (joint(s))
  finger S63.279
    distal S63.29
      index S63.29

Dislocation (articular) --*continued*
    little S63.29
    middle S63.29
    ring S63.29
  index S63.27
  little S63.27
  middle S63.27
  proximal S63.28
    index S63.28
    little S63.28
    middle S63.28
    ring S63.28
  ring S63.27
  foot or toe -*see* Dislocation, toe
  thumb S63.12
    distal joint S63.14
    proximal joint S63.13
jaw (cartilage) (meniscus) S03.0
joint prosthesis -*see* Complications, joint
  prosthesis, mechanical, displacement, by site
knee S83.106
  cap -*see* Dislocation, patella
  congenital Q68.2
  old M23.8X
  patella -*see* Dislocation, patella
  pathological -*see* Dislocation, pathological
    NEC, knee
  proximal tibia
    anteriorly S83.11
    laterally S83.14
    medially S83.13
    posteriorly S83.12
  recurrent -*see also* Derangement, knee,
    specified NEC
  specified type NEC S83.19
lacrimal gland H04.16
lens (complete) H27.10
  anterior H27.12
  congenital Q12.1
  ocular implant -*see* Complications,
    intraocular lens
  partial H27.11
  posterior H27.13
  traumatic S05.8X
ligament
  code by site under Dislocation
lumbar (vertebra) -*see* Dislocation, vertebra,
  lumbar
lumbosacral (vertebra) -*see also* Dislocation,
  vertebra, lumbar
  congenital Q76.49
mandible S03.0
meniscus (knee) -*see* Tear, meniscus
  other sites
  code by site under Dislocation
metacarpal (bone)
  distal end -*see* Dislocation, finger
  proximal end S63.06
metacarpophalangeal (joint)
  finger S63.26
    index S63.26
    little S63.26
    middle S63.26
    ring S63.26
  thumb S63.11
metatarsal (bone) -*see* Dislocation, foot
metatarsophalangeal (joint(s)) -*see*
  Dislocation, toe - midcarpal (joint) S63.03
midtarsal (joint) -*see* Dislocation, foot
neck S13.20
  specified site NEC S13.29

Dislocation (articular) --*continued*
  vertebra -*see* Dislocation, vertebra, cervical
nose (septal cartilage) S03.1
occipitoatloid S13.111
old -*see* Derangement, joint, specified type
    NEC
ossicles, ear -*see* Discontinuity, ossicles, ear
partial -*see* Subluxation, by site
patella S83.006
  congenital Q74.1
  lateral S83.01
  recurrent (nontraumatic) M22.0
    incomplete M22.1
  specified type NEC S83.09
pathological NEC M24.30
  ankle M24.37
  elbow M24.32
  foot joint M24.37
  hand joint M24.34
  hip M24.35
  knee M24.36
  lumbosacral joint -*see* subcategory M53.2
  pelvic region -*see* Dislocation, pathological,
    hip
  sacroiliac -*see* subcategory M53.2
  shoulder M24.31
  wrist M24.33
pelvis NEC S33.30
  specified NEC S33.39
phalanx
  finger or hand -*see* Dislocation, finger
  foot or toe -*see* Dislocation, toe
prosthesis, internal -*see* Complications,
  prosthetic device, by site, mechanical
radial head S53.006
  anterior S53.01
  posterior S53.02
  specified type NEC S53.09
radiocarpal (joint) S63.02
radiohumeral (joint) -*see* Dislocation, radial
head - radioulnar (joint)
  distal S63.01
  proximal -*see* Dislocation, elbow
radius
  distal end -*see* Dislocation, wrist
  proximal end -*see* Dislocation, radial head -
recurrent M24.40
  ankle M24.47
  elbow M24.42
  finger M24.44
  foot joint M24.47
  hand joint M24.44
  hip M24.45
  knee M24.46
    patella -*see* Dislocation, patella, recurrent
  patella -*see* Dislocation, patella, recurrent
  sacroiliac -*see* subcategory M53.2
  shoulder M24.41
  toe M24.47
  vertebra -*see also* subcategory M43.5
    atlantoaxial M43.4
      with myelopathy M43.3
  wrist M24.43
rib (cartilage) S23.29
sacrococcygeal S33.2
sacroiliac (joint) (ligament) S33.2
  congenital Q74.2
  recurrent -*see* subcategory M53.2
sacrum S33.2
scaphoid (bone) (hand) (wrist) -*see*
Dislocation, wrist

Dislocation (articular) --*continued*

foot -*see* Dislocation, foot
scapula -*see* Dislocation, shoulder, girdle, scapula
semilunar cartilage, knee -*see* Tear, meniscus
septal cartilage (nose) S03.1
septum (nasal) (old) J34.2
sesamoid bone
code by site under Dislocation
shoulder (blade) (ligament) (joint) (traumatic) S43.006
  acromioclavicular -*see* Dislocation, acromioclavicular
  chronic -*see* Dislocation, recurrent, shoulder
  congenital Q68.8
  girdle S43.30
    scapula S43.31
    specified site NEC S43.39
  humerus S43.00
    anterior S43.01
    inferior S43.03
    posterior S43.02
  pathological -*see* Dislocation, pathological NEC, shoulder
  recurrent -*see* Dislocation, recurrent, shoulder
  specified type NEC S43.08
spine
  cervical -*see* Dislocation, vertebra, cervical
  congenital Q76.49
  due to birth trauma P11.5
  lumbar -*see* Dislocation, vertebra, lumbar
  thoracic -*see* Dislocation, vertebra, thoracic
spontaneous -*see* Dislocation, pathological
sternoclavicular (joint) S43.206
  anterior S43.21
  posterior S43.22
sternum S23.29
subglenoid -*see* Dislocation, shoulder
symphysis pubis S33.4
talus -*see* Dislocation, ankle
tarsal (bone(s)) (joint(s)) -*see* Dislocation, foot
tarsometatarsal (joint(s)) -*see* Dislocation, foot
temporomandibular (joint) S03.0
thigh, proximal end -*see* Dislocation, hip
thorax S23.20
  specified site NEC S23.29
  vertebra -*see* Dislocation, vertebra
thumb S63.10
  interphalangeal joint -*see* Dislocation, interphalangeal (joint), thumb
  metacarpophalangeal joint -*see* Dislocation, metacarpophalangeal (joint), thumb
thyroid cartilage S13.29
tibia
  distal end -*see* Dislocation, ankle
  proximal end -*see* Dislocation, knee - tibiofibular (joint)
  distal -*see* Dislocation, ankle
  superior -*see* Dislocation, knee - toe(s) S93.106
  great S93.10
    interphalangeal joint S93.11
    metatarsophalangeal joint S93.12
  interphalangeal joint S93.119
  lesser S93.106
    interphalangeal joint S93.11
    metatarsophalangeal joint S93.12
  metatarsophalangeal joint S93.12

Dislocation (articular) --*continued*

tooth S03.2
trachea S23.29
ulna
  distal end S63.07
  proximal end -*see* Dislocation, elbow
ulnohumeral (joint) -*see* Dislocation, elbow
vertebra (articular process) (body) (traumatic)
  cervical S13.101
    atlantoaxial joint S13.121
    atlantooccipital joint S13.111
    atloido-occipital joint S13.111
    joint between
      C0 and C1 S13.111
      C1 and C2 S13.121
      C2 and C3 S13.131
      C3 and C4 S13.141
      C4 and C5 S13.151
      C5and C6 S13.161
      C6and C7 S13.171
      C7and T1 S13.181
    occipitoatloid joint S13.111
  congenital Q76.49
  lumbar S33.101
    joint between
      L1 and L2 S33.111
      L2 and L3 S33.121
      L3 and L4 S33.131
      L4 and L5 S33.141
  nontraumatic -*see* Displacement, intervertebral disc
  partial -*see* Subluxation, by site
  recurrent NEC -*see* subcategory M43.5
  thoracic S23.101
    joint between
      T1 and T2 S23.111
      T2 and T3 S23.121
      T3 and T4 S23.123
      T4 and T5 S23.131
      T5 and T6 S23.133
      T6 and T7 S23.141
      T7 and T8 S23.143
      T8 and T9 S23.151
      T9 and T10 S23.153
      T10 and T11 S23.161
      T11 and T12 S23.163
      T12 and L1 S23.171
wrist (carpal bone) S63.006
  carpometacarpal joint -*see* Dislocation, carpometacarpal (joint)
  distal radioulnar joint -*see* Dislocation, radioulnar (joint), distal
  metacarpal bone, proximal -*see* Dislocation, metacarpal (bone), proximal end
  midcarpal -*see* Dislocation, midcarpal (joint)
  radiocarpal joint -*see* Dislocation, radiocarpal (joint)
  recurrent -*see* Dislocation, recurrent, wrist
  specified site NEC S63.09
  ulna -*see* Dislocation, ulna, distal end
xiphoid cartilage S23.29

Disorder (of) -*see also* Disease - acantholytic L11.9
  specified NEC L11.8
acute
  psychotic -*see* Psychosis, acute
  stress F43.0
adjustment (grief) F43.20
  with
    anxiety F43.22
      with depressed mood F43.23

Disorder (of) *continued*

conduct disturbance F43.24
  with emotional disturbance F43.25
  depressed mood F43.21
    with anxiety F43.23
  other specified symptom F43.29
adrenal (capsule) (gland) (medullary) E27.9
  specified NEC E27.8
adrenogenital E25.9
  drug-induced E25.8
  iatrogenic E25.8
  idiopathic E25.8
adult personality (and behavior) F69
  specified NEC F68.8
affective (mood) -*see* Disorder, mood
aggressive, unsocialized F91.1
alcohol-related F10.99
  with
    amnestic disorder, persisting F10.96
    anxiety disorder F10.980
    dementia, persisting F10.97
    intoxication F10.929
      with delirium F10.921
      uncomplicated F10.920
    mood disorder F10.94
    other specified F10.988
    psychotic disorder F10.959
      with
        delusions F10.950
        hallucinations F10.951
    sexual dysfunction F10.981
    sleep disorder F10.982
alcohol use
  mild F10.10
    with
      alcohol-induced
        anxiety disorder F10.180
        bipolar and related disorder F10.14
        depressive disorder F10.14
        psychotic disorder F10.159
        sexual dysfunction F10.181
        sleep disorder F10.182
      alcohol intoxication F10.129
        delirium F10.121
  moderate or severe F10.20
    with
      alcohol-induced
        anxiety disorder F10.280
        bipolar and related disorder F10.24
        depressive disorder F10.24
        major neurocognitive disorder, amnestic-confabulatory type F10.26
        major neurocognitive disorder, nonamnestic-confabulatory type F10.27
        mild neurocognitive disorder F10.288
        psychotic disorder F10.259
        sexual dysfunction F10.281
        sleep disorder F10.282
      alcohol intoxication F10.229
        delirium F10.221
allergic -*see* Allergy
alveolar NEC J84.09
amino-acid
  cystathioninuria E72.19
  cystinosis E72.04
  cystinuria E72.01
  glycinuria E72.09
  homocystinuria E72.11
  metabolism -*see* Disturbance, metabolism, amino-acid
    specified NEC E72.8

Disorder (of) *continued*
  neonatal, transitory P74.8
  renal transport NEC E72.09
  transport NEC E72.09
amnesic, amnestic
  alcohol-induced F10.96
    with dependence F10.26
  due to (secondary to) general medical
    condition F04
  psychoactive NEC-induced F19.96
    with
      abuse F19.16
      dependence F19.26
  sedative, hypnotic or anxiolytic-induced
    F13.96
    with dependence F13.26
amphetamine-type substance use
  mild F15.10
  moderate F15.20
  severe F15.20
amphetamine (or other stimulant) use
  mild
    with
      amphetamine (or other stimulant)
      induced
        anxiety disorder F15.180
        bipolar and related disorder F15.14
        depressive disorder F15.14
        obsessive-compulsive and related
          disorder F15.188
        psychotic disorder F15.159
        sexual dysfunction F15.181
      amphetamine, cocaine, or other stimulant
      intoxication
        with perceptual disturbances F15.122
        without perceptual disturbances F15.129
      intoxication delirium F15.121
  moderate or severe
    with
      amphetamine (or other stimulant)
      induced
        anxiety disorder F15.280
        obsessive-compulsive and related
          disorder F15.288
        sexual dysfunction F15.281
        bipolar and related disorder F15.24
        depressive disorder F15.24
        psychotic disorder F15.259
      amphetamine, cocaine, or other stimulant
      intoxication
        with perceptual disturbances F15.222
        without perceptual disturbances F15.229
      intoxication delirium F15.221
anaerobic glycolysis with anemia D55.2
anxiety F41.9
  due to (secondary to)
    alcohol F10.980
    amphetamine F15.980
    in
      abuse F15.180
      dependence F15.280
    anxiolytic F13.980
    in
      abuse F13.180
      dependence F13.280
    caffeine F15.980
    in
      abuse F15.180
      dependence F15.280
    cannabis F12.980
    in

Disorder (of) *continued*
    abuse F12.180
    dependence F12.280
  cocaine F14.980
  in
    abuse F14.180
    dependence F14.180
  general medical condition F06.4
  hallucinogen F16.980
  in
    abuse F16.180
    dependence F16.280
  hypnotic F13.980
  in
    abuse F13.180
    dependence F13.280
  inhalant F18.980
  in
    abuse F18.180
    dependence F18.280
  phencyclidine F16.980
  in
    abuse F16.180
    dependence F16.280
  psychoactive substance NEC F19.980
  in
    abuse F19.180
    dependence F19.280
  sedative F13.980
  in
    abuse F13.180
    dependence F13.280
  volatile solvents F18.980
  in
    abuse F18.180
    dependence F18.280
  generalized F41.1
  illness F45.21
  mixed
    with depression (mild) F41.8
    specified NEC F41.3
  organic F06.4
  phobic F40.9
    of childhood F40.8
  specified NEC F41.8
aortic valve -*see* Endocarditis, aortic
aromatic amino-acid metabolism E70.9
  specified NEC E70.8
arteriole NEC I77.89
artery NEC I77.89
articulation -*see* Disorder, joint
attachment (childhood)
  disinhibited F94.2
  reactive F94.1
attention-deficit hyperactivity (adolescent)
(adult) (child) F90.9
  combined type F90.2
  hyperactive type F90.1
  inattentive type F90.0
  specified type NEC F90.8
attention-deficit without hyperactivity
  (adolescent) (adult) (child) F98.8
auditory processing (central) H93.25
autistic F84.0
autism spectrum F84.0
autonomic nervous system G90.9
  specified NEC G90.8
avoidant
  child or adolescent F40.10
  restrictive food intake F50.89
balance

Disorder (of) *continued*
  acid-base E87.8
    mixed E87.4
  electrolyte E87.8
  fluid NEC E87.8
behavioral (disruptive) -*see* Disorder, conduct
beta-amino-acid metabolism E72.8
bile acid and cholesterol metabolism E78.70
  Barth syndrome E78.71
  other specified E78.79
  Smith-Lemli-Opitz syndrome E78.72
bilirubin excretion E80.6
binge eating F50.81
binocular
  movement H51.9
    convergence
      excess H51.12
      insufficiency H51.11
    internuclear ophthalmoplegia -*see*
      Ophthalmoplegia, internuclear
    palsy of conjugate gaze H51.0
    specified type NEC H51.8
  vision NEC -*see* Disorder, vision, binocular
bipolar (I) F31.9
  current episode
    depressed F31.9
      with psychotic features F31.5
      without psychotic features F31.30
        mild F31.31
        moderate F31.32
        severe (without psychotic features)
          F31.4
          with psychotic features F31.5
    hypomanic F31.0
    manic F31.9
      with psychotic features F31.2
      without psychotic features F31.10
        mild F31.11
        moderate F31.12
        severe (without psychotic features)
          F31.13
          with psychotic features F31.2
    mixed F31.60
      mild F31.61
      moderate F31.62
      severe (without psychotic features)
        F31.63
        with psychotic features F31.64
    severe depression (without psychotic
      features) F31.4
      with psychotic features F31.5
  in remission (currently) F31.70
  in full remission
    most recent episode
      depressed F31.76
      hypomanic F31.72
      manic F31.74
      mixed F31.78
  in partial remission
    most recent episode
      depressed F31.75
      hypomanic F31.71
      manic F31.73
      mixed F31.77
  specified NEC F31.89
  II F31.81
  organic F06.30
  single manic episode F30.9
    mild F30.11
    moderate F30.12

Disorder (of) *continued*
  severe (without psychotic symptoms)
    F30.13
    with psychotic symptoms F30.2
  bladder N32.9
    functional NEC N31.9
    in schistosomiasis B65.0 [*N33*]
    specified NEC N32.89
  bleeding D68.9
  blood D75.9
    in congenital early syphilis A50.09 [*D77*]
  body dysmorphic F45.22
  bone M89.9
    continuity M84.9
      specified type NEC M84.80
        ankle M84.87
        fibula M84.86
        foot M84.87
        hand M84.84
        humerus M84.82
        neck M84.88
        pelvis M84.859
        radius M84.83
        rib M84.88
        shoulder M84.81
        skull M84.88
        thigh M84.85
        tibia M84.86
        ulna M84.83
        vertebra M84.88
    density and structure M85.9
    cyst -*see also* Cyst, bone, specified type
      NEC
      aneurysmal -*see* Cyst, bone, aneurysmal
      solitary -*see* Cyst, bone, solitary
    diffuse idiopathic skeletal hyperostosis -*see*
      Hyperostosis, ankylosing
    fibrous dysplasia (monostotic) -*see*
      Dysplasia, fibrous, bone
    fluorosis -*see* Fluorosis, skeletal
    hyperostosis of skull M85.2
    osteitis condensans -*see* Osteitis,
      condensans
    specified type NEC M85.8
      ankle M85.87
      foot M85.87
      forearm M85.83
      hand M85.84
      lower leg M85.86
      multiple sites M85.89
      neck M85.88
      rib M85.88
      shoulder M85.81
      skull M85.88
      thigh M85.85
      upper arm M85.82
      vertebra M85.88
    development and growth NEC M89.20
      carpus M89.24
      clavicle M89.21
      femur M89.25
      fibula M89.26
      finger M89.24
      humerus M89.22
      ilium M89.259
      ischium M89.259
      metacarpus M89.24
      metatarsus M89.27
      multiple sites M89.29
      neck M89.28
      radius M89.23

Disorder (of) *continued*
  rib M89.28
  scapula M89.21
  skull M89.28
  tarsus M89.27
  tibia M89.26
  toe M89.27
  ulna M89.23
  vertebra M89.28
    specified type NEC M89.8X   brachial
  plexus G54.0
  branched-chain amino-acid metabolism E71.2
    specified NEC E71.19
  breast N64.9
    agalactia -*see* Agalactia
    associated with
      lactation O92.70
        specified NEC O92.79
      pregnancy O92.20
        specified NEC O92.29
      puerperium O92.20
        specified NEC O92.29
    cracked nipple -*see* Cracked nipple
    galactorrhea -*see* Galactorrhea
    hypogalactia O92.4
    lactation disorder NEC O92.79
    mastitis -*see* Mastitis
    nipple infection -*see* Infection, nipple
    retracted nipple -*see* Retraction, nipple
    specified type NEC N64.89
  Briquet's F45.0
  bullous, in diseases classified elsewhere L14
  caffeine use
    mild
      with
        caffeine-induced
          anxiety disorder F15.180
          sleep disorder F15.182
    moderate or severe
      with
        caffeine-induced
          anxiety disorder F15.280
          sleep disorder F15.282
  cannabis use
    mild F12.10
      with
        cannabis-induced
          anxiety disorder F12.180
          psychotic disorder F12.159
          sleep disorder F12.188
        cannabis intoxication delirium F12.121
          with perceptual disturbances F12.122
          without perceptual disturbances F12.129
    moderate or severe F12.20
      with
        cannabis-induced
          anxiety disorder F12.280
          psychotic disorder F12.259
          sleep disorder F12.288
        cannabis intoxication
          with perceptual disturbances F12.222
          without perceptual disturbances F12.229
          delirium F12.221
  carbohydrate
    absorption, intestinal NEC E74.39
    metabolism (congenital) E74.9
      specified NEC E74.8
  cardiac, functional I51.89
  carnitine metabolism E71.40
  cartilage M94.9

Disorder (of) *continued*
  articular NEC -*see* Derangement, joint,
    articular cartilage
    chondrocalcinosis -*see* Chondrocalcinosis
  specified type NEC M94.8X
    articular -*see* Derangement, joint, articular
      cartilage
    multiple sites M94.8X0
  catatonia (due to known physiological
    condition) (with another mental disorder)
    F06.1
  catatonic
    due to (secondary to) known physiological
      condition F06.1
    organic F06.1
  central auditory processing H93.25
  cervical
    region NEC M53.82
    root (nerve) NEC G54.2
  character NOS F60.9
  childhood disintegrative NEC F84.3
  cholesterol and bile acid metabolism E78.70
    Barth syndrome E78.71
    other specified E78.79
    Smith-Lemli-Opitz syndrome E78.72
  choroid H31.9
    atrophy -*see* Atrophy, choroid
    degeneration -*see* Degeneration, choroid
    detachment -*see* Detachment, choroid
    dystrophy -*see* Dystrophy, choroid
    hemorrhage -*see* Hemorrhage, choroid
    rupture -*see* Rupture, choroid
    scar -*see* Scar, chorioretinal
    solar retinopathy -*see* Retinopathy, solar
    specified type NEC H31.8
  ciliary body -*see* Disorder, iris
    degeneration -*see* Degeneration, ciliary body
  coagulation (factor) -*see also* Defect,
  coagulation D68.9
    newborn, transient P61.6
  cocaine use
    mild F14.10
      with
        amphetamine, cocaine, or other stimulant
          intoxication
          with perceptual disturbances F14.122
          without perceptual disturbances F14.129
        cocaine-induced
          anxiety disorder F14.180
          bipolar and related disorder F14.14
          depressive disorder F14.14
          obsessive-compulsive and related
            disorder F14.188
          psychotic disorder F14.159
          sexual dysfunction F14.181
          sleep disorder F14.182
        cocaine intoxication delirium F14.121
    moderate or severe F14.20
      with
        amphetamine, cocaine, or other stimulant
          intoxication
          with perceptual disturbances F14.222
          without perceptual disturbances F14.229
        cocaine-induced
          anxiety disorder F14.280
          bipolar and related disorder F14.24
          depressive disorder F14.24
          obsessive-compulsive and related
            disorder F14.288
          psychotic disorder F14.259
          sexual dysfunction F14.281

Disorder (of) *continued*
- sleep disorder F14.282
- cocaine intoxication delirium F14.221
- coccyx NEC M53.3
- cognitive F09
  - due to (secondary to) general medical condition F09
  - persisting R41.89
    - due to
      - alcohol F10.97
        - with dependence F10.27
      - anxiolytics F13.97
        - with dependence F13.27
      - hypnotics F13.97
        - with dependence F13.27
      - sedatives F13.97
        - with dependence F13.27
      - specified substance NEC F19.97
        - with
          - abuse F19.17
          - dependence F19.27
- communication F80.9
  - social pragmatic F80.82
- conduct (childhood) F91.9
  - adjustment reaction -*see* Disorder, adjustment
  - adolescent onset type F91.2
  - childhood onset type F91.1
  - compulsive F63.9
  - confined to family context F91.0
  - depressive F91.8
  - group type F91.2
  - hyperkinetic -*see* Disorder, attention-deficit hyperactivity
  - oppositional defiance F91.3
  - socialized F91.2
  - solitary aggressive type F91.1
  - specified NEC F91.8
  - unsocialized (aggressive) F91.1
- conduction, heart I45.9
- congenital glycosylation (CDG) E74.8
- conjunctiva H11.9
  - infection -*see* Conjunctivitis
- connective tissue, localized L94.9
  - specified NEC L94.8
- conversion (functional neurological symptom disorder)
  - with
    - abnormal movement F44.4
    - anesthesia or sensory loss F44.6
    - attacks or seizures F44.5
    - mixed symptoms F44.7
    - special sensory symptoms F44.6
    - speech symptoms F44.4
    - swallowing symptoms F44.4
    - weakness or paralysis F44.4
- convulsive (secondary) -*see* Convulsions
- cornea H18.9
  - deformity -*see* Deformity, cornea
  - degeneration -*see* Degeneration, cornea
  - deposits -*see* Deposit, cornea
  - due to contact lens H18.82
    - specified as edema -*see* Edema, cornea
  - edema -*see* Edema, cornea
  - keratitis -*see* Keratitis
  - keratoconjunctivitis -*see* Keratoconjunctivitis
  - membrane change -*see* Change, corneal membrane
  - neovascularization -*see* Neovascularization, cornea

Disorder (of) *continued*
- scar -*see* Opacity, cornea
- specified type NEC H18.89
- ulcer -*see* Ulcer, cornea
- corpus cavernosum N48.9
- cranial nerve -*see* Disorder, nerve, cranial
- cyclothymic F34.0
- defiant oppositional F91.3
- delusional (persistent) (systematized) F22
  - induced F24
- depersonalization F48.1
- depressive F32.9
  - major F32.9
    - with psychotic symptoms F32.3
    - in remission (full) F32.5
      - partial F32.4
    - recurrent F33.9
    - single episode F32.9
      - mild F32.0
      - moderate F32.1
      - severe (without psychotic symptoms) F32.2
        - with psychotic symptoms F32.3
  - organic F06.31
  - persistent F34.1
  - recurrent F33.9
    - current episode
      - mild F33.0
      - moderate F33.1
      - severe (without psychotic symptoms) F33.2
        - with psychotic symptoms F33.3
    - in remission F33.40
      - full F33.42
      - partial F33.41
    - specified NEC F33.8
  - single episode -*see* Episode, depressive
  - specified NEC F32.89
- developmental F89
  - arithmetical skills F81.2
  - coordination (motor) F82
  - expressive writing F81.81
  - language F80.9
    - expressive F80.1
    - mixed receptive and expressive F80.2
    - receptive type F80.2
    - specified NEC F80.89
  - learning F81.9
    - arithmetical F81.2
    - reading F81.0
  - mixed F88
  - motor coordination or function F82
  - pervasive F84.9
    - specified NEC F84.8
  - phonological F80.0
  - reading F81.0
  - scholastic skills -*see also* Disorder, learning
    - mixed F81.89
  - specified NEC F88
  - speech F80.9
    - articulation F80.0
    - specified NEC F80.89
  - written expression F81.81
- diaphragm J98.6
- digestive (system) K92.9
  - newborn P78.9
    - specified NEC P78.89
  - postprocedural -*see* Complication, gastrointestinal
- psychogenic F45.8
- disc (intervertebral) M51.9

Disorder (of) *continued*
- with
  - myelopathy
    - cervical region M50.00
    - cervicothoracic region M50.03
    - high cervical region M50.01
    - lumbar region M51.06
    - mid-cervical region M50.020
    - sacrococcygeal region M53.3
    - thoracic region M51.04
    - thoracolumbar region M51.05
  - radiculopathy
    - cervical region M50.10
    - cervicothoracic region M50.13
    - high cervical region M50.11
    - lumbar region M51.16
    - lumbosacral region M51.17
    - mid-cervical region M50.120
    - sacrococcygeal region M53.3
    - thoracic region M51.14
    - thoracolumbar region M51.15
- cervical M50.90
  - with
    - myelopathy M50.00
      - C2 C3 M50.01
      - C3 C4 M50.01
      - C4 C5 M50.021
      - C5 C6 M50.022
      - C6 C7 M50.023
      - C7 T1 M50.03
      - cervicothoracic region M50.03
      - high cervical region M50.01
      - mid-cervical region M50.020
    - neuritis, radiculitis or radiculopathy M50.10
      - C2 C3 M50.11
      - C3 C4 M50.11
      - C4 C5 M50.121
      - C5 C6 M50.122
      - C6 C7 M50.123
      - C7 T1 M50.13
      - cervicothoracic region M50.13
      - high cervical region M50.11
      - mid-cervical region M50.120
  - C2 C3 M50.91
  - C3 C4 M50.91
  - C4 C5 M50.921
  - C5 C6 M50.922
  - C6 C7 M50.923
  - C7 T1 M50.93
  - cervicothoracic region M50.93
  - degeneration M50.30
    - C2 C3 M50.31
    - C3 C4 M50.31
    - C4 C5 M50.321
    - C5 C6 M50.322
    - C6 C7 M50.323
    - C7 T1 M50.33
    - cervicothoracic region M50.33
    - high cervical region M50.31
    - mid-cervical region M50.320
  - displacement M50.20
    - C2 C3 M50.21
    - C3 C4 M50.21
    - C4 C5 M50.221
    - C5 C6 M50.222
    - C6 C7 M50.223
    - C7 T1 M50.23
    - cervicothoracic region M50.23
    - high cervical region M50.21
    - mid-cervical region M50.220

Disorder (of) *continued*

    high cervical region M50.91
    mid-cervical region M50.920
    specified type NEC M50.80
        C2 C3 M50.81
        C3 C4 M50.81
        C4 C5 M50.821
        C5 C6 M50.822
        C6 C7 M50.823
        C7 T1 M50.83
        cervicothoracic region M50.83
        high cervical region M50.81
        mid-cervical region M50.820
    specified NEC
        lumbar region M51.86
        lumbosacral region M51.87
        sacrococcygeal region M53.3
        thoracic region M51.84
        thoracolumbar region M51.85
  disinhibited attachment (childhood) F94.2
  disintegrative, childhood NEC F84.3
  disruptive F91.9
    mood dysregulation F34.81
    specified NEC F91.8
  disruptive behavior F91.9
  dissocial personality F60.2
  dissociative F44.9
    affecting
      motor function F44.4
        and sensation F44.7
      sensation F44.6
        and motor function F44.7
    brief reactive F43.0
    due to (secondary to) general medical
  condition F06.8
    mixed F44.7
    organic F06.8
    other specified NEC F44.89
  double heterozygous sickling -*see* Disease,
  sickle-cell
  dream anxiety F51.5
  drug induced hemorrhagic D68.32
  drug related F19.99
    abuse -*see* Abuse, drug
    dependence -*see* Dependence, drug
  dysmorphic body F45.22
  dysthymic F34.1
  ear H93.9
    bleeding -*see* Otorrhagia
    deafness -*see* Deafness
    degenerative H93.09
    discharge -*see* Otorrhea
    external H61.9
      auditory canal stenosis -*see* Stenosis,
    external ear canal
      exostosis -*see* Exostosis, external ear canal
      impacted cerumen -*see* Impaction,
    cerumen
      otitis -*see* Otitis, externa
      perichondritis -*see* Perichondritis, ear
      pinna -*see* Disorder, pinna
      specified type NEC H61.89
        in diseases classified elsewhere H62.8X
    inner H83.9
      vestibular dysfunction -*see* Disorder,
    vestibular function
    middle H74.9
      adhesive H74.1
      ossicle -*see* Abnormal, ear ossicles
      polyp -*see* Polyp, ear (middle)

Disorder (of) *continued*

    specified NEC, in diseases classified
    elsewhere H75.8
    postprocedural -*see* Complications, ear,
  procedure
    specified NEC, in diseases classified
    elsewhere H94.8
  eating (adult) (psychogenic) F50.9
    anorexia -*see* Anorexia
    binge F50.81
    bulimia F50.2
    child F98.29
      pica F98.3
      rumination disorder F98.21
    pica F50.89
      childhood F98.3
  electrolyte (balance) NEC E87.8
    with
      abortion -*see* Abortion by type complicated
      by specified condition NEC
      ectopic pregnancy O08.5
      molar pregnancy O08.5
    acidosis (metabolic) (respiratory) E87.2
    alkalosis (metabolic) (respiratory) E87.3
  elimination, transepidermal L87.9
    specified NEC L87.8
  emotional (persistent) F34.9
    of childhood F93.9
      specified NEC F93.8
  endocrine E34.9
    postprocedural E89.89
      specified NEC E89.89
  erectile (male) (organic) -*see also*
  Dysfunction, sexual, male, erectile N52.9
    nonorganic F52.21
  erythematous -*see* Erythema
  esophagus K22.9
    functional K22.4
    psychogenic F45.8
  eustachian tube H69.9
    infection -*see* Salpingitis, eustachian
    obstruction -*see* Obstruction, eustachian tube
    patulous -*see* Patulous, eustachian tube
    specified NEC H69.8
  extrapyramidal G25.9
    in diseases classified elsewhere - see
  category G26
    specified type NEC G25.89
  eye H57.9
    postprocedural -*see* Complication,
  postprocedural, eye - eyelid H02.9
    cyst -*see* Cyst, eyelid
    degenerative H02.70
      chloasma -*see* Chloasma, eyelid
      madarosis -*see* Madarosis
      specified type NEC H02.79
      vitiligo -*see* Vitiligo, eyelid
      xanthelasma -*see* Xanthelasma
    dermatochalasis -*see* Dermatochalasis
    edema -*see* Edema, eyelid
    elephantiasis -*see* Elephantiasis, eyelid
    foreign body, retained -*see* Foreign body,
  retained, eyelid
    function H02.59
      abnormal innervation syndrome -*see*
    Syndrome, abnormal innervation
      blepharochalasis -*see* Blepharochalasis
      blepharoclonus -*see* Blepharoclonus
      blepharophimosis -*see* Blepharophimosis
      blepharoptosis -*see* Blepharoptosis
      lagophthalmos -*see* Lagophthalmos

Disorder (of) *continued*

    lid retraction -*see* Retraction, lid
    hypertrichosis -*see* Hypertrichosis, eyelid
    specified type NEC H02.89
    vascular H02.879
      left H02.876
        lower H02.875
        upper H02.874
      right H02.873
        lower H02.872
        upper H02.871
  factitious F68.10
    with predominantly
      psychological symptoms F68.11
        with physical symptoms F68.13
      physical symptoms F68.12
        with psychological symptoms F68.13
  factor, coagulation -*see* Defect, coagulation
  fatty acid
    metabolism E71.30
      specified NEC E71.39
    oxidation
      LCAD E71.310
      MCAD E71.311
      SCAD E71.312
      specified deficiency NEC E71.318
  feeding (infant or child) -*see also* Disorder,
  eating R63.3
  feigned (with obvious motivation) Z76.5
    without obvious motivation -*see* Disorder,
  factitious
  female
    hypoactive sexual desire F52.0
    orgasmic F52.31
    sexual arousal F52.22
  fibroblastic M72.9
    specified NEC M72.8
  fluency
    adult onset F98.5
    childhood onset F80.81
    following
      cerebral infarction I69.323
      cerebrovascular disease I69.923
        specified disease NEC I69.823
      intracerebral hemorrhage I69.123
      nontraumatic intracranial hemorrhage NEC
  I69.223
      subarachnoid hemorrhage I69.023
    in conditions classified elsewhere R47.82
  fluid balance E87.8
  follicular (skin) L73.9
    specified NEC L73.8
  fructose metabolism E74.10
    essential fructosuria E74.11
    fructokinase deficiency E74.11
    fructose-1, 6 diphosphatase deficiency
  E74.19
    hereditary fructose intolerance E74.12
    other specified E74.19
  functional polymorphonuclear neutrophils
  D71
  gallbladder, biliary tract and pancreas in
  diseases classified elsewhere K87
  gamma-glutamyl cycle E72.8
  gastric (functional) K31.9
    motility K30
    psychogenic F45.8
    secretion K30
  gastrointestinal (functional) NOS K92.9
    newborn P78.9
    psychogenic F45.8

Disorder (of) *continued*
gender-identity or -role F64.9
childhood F64.2
effect on relationship F66
of adolescence or adulthood F64.0
nontranssexual F64.8
specified NEC F64.8
uncertainty F66
genito-pelvic pain penetration F52.6
genitourinary system
female N94.9
male N50.9
psychogenic F45.8
globe H44.9
degenerated condition H44.50
absolute glaucoma H44.51
atrophy H44.52
leucocoria H44.53
degenerative H44.30
chalcosis H44.31
myopia H44.2
siderosis H44.32
specified type NEC H44.39
endophthalmitis *-see* Endophthalmitis
foreign body, retained *-see* Foreign body, intraocular, old, retained
hemophthalmos *-see* Hemophthalmos
hypotony H44.40
due to
ocular fistula H44.42
specified disorder NEC H44.43
flat anterior chamber H44.41
primary H44.44
luxation *-see* Luxation, globe
specified type NEC H44.89
glomerular (in) N05.9
amyloidosis E85.4 *[N08]*
cryoglobulinemia D89.1 *[N08]*
disseminated intravascular coagulation D65 *[N08]*
Fabry's disease E75.21 *[N08]*
familial lecithin cholesterol acyltransferase deficiency E78.6 *[N08]*
Goodpasture's syndrome M31.0
hemolytic-uremic syndrome D59.3
Henoch (Schönlein) purpura D69.0 *[N08]*
malariae malaria B52.0
microscopic polyangiitis M31.7 *[N08]*
multiple myeloma C90.0 *[N08]*
mumps B26.83
schistosomiasis B65.9 *[N08]*
sepsis NEC A41. *[N08]*
streptococcal A40. *[N08]*
sickle-cell disorders D57. *[N08]*
strongyloidiasis B78.9 *[N08]*
subacute bacterial endocarditis I33.0 *[N08]*
syphilis A52.75
systemic lupus erythematosus M32.14
thrombotic thrombocytopenic purpura M31.1 *[N08]*
Waldenström macroglobulinemia C88.0 *[N08]*
Wegener's granulomatosis M31.31
gluconeogenesis E74.4
glucosaminoglycan metabolism *-see* Disorder, metabolism, glucosaminoglycan
glycine metabolism E72.50
d-glycericacidemia E72.59
hyperhydroxyprolinemia E72.59
hyperoxaluria E72.53
hyperprolinemia E72.59

Disorder (of) *continued*
non-ketotic hyperglycinemia E72.51
oxalosis E72.53
oxaluria E72.53
sarcosinemia E72.59
trimethylaminuria E72.52
glycoprotein metabolism E77.9
specified NEC E77.8
habit (and impulse) F63.9
involving sexual behavior NEC F65.9
specified NEC F63.89
hallucinogen use
mild F16.10
with
hallucinogen-induced
anxiety disorder F16.180
bipolar and related disorder F16.14
depressive disorder F16.14
psychotic disorder F16.159
hallucinogen intoxication delirium F16.121
other hallucinogen intoxication F16.129
moderate or severe F16.20
with
hallucinogen-induced
anxiety disorder F16.280
bipolar and related disorder F16.24
depressive disorder F16.24
psychotic disorder F16.259
hallucinogen intoxication delirium F16.221
other hallucinogen intoxication F16.229
heart action I49.9
hematological D75.9
newborn (transient) P61.9
specified NEC P61.8
hematopoietic organs D75.9
hemorrhagic NEC D69.9
drug-induced D68.32
due to
extrinsic circulating anticoagulants D68.32
increase in
anti-IIa D68.32
anti-Xa D68.32
intrinsic
circulating anticoagulants D68.318
increase in
antithrombin D68.318
anti-VIIIa D68.318
anti-IXa D68.318
anti-XIa D68.318
following childbirth O72.3
hemostasis *-see* Defect, coagulation
histidine metabolism E70.40
histidinemia E70.41
other specified E70.49
hoarding F42.3
hyperkinetic *-see* Disorder, attention-deficit hyperactivity hyperleucine-isoleucinemia E71.19
hypervalinemia E71.19
hypoactive sexual desire F52.0
hypochondriacal F45.20
body dysmorphic F45.22
neurosis F45.21
other specified F45.29
identity
dissociative F44.81
of childhood F93.8
illness anxiety F45.21
immune mechanism (immunity) D89.9

Disorder (of) *continued*
specified type NEC D89.89
impaired renal tubular function N25.9
specified NEC N25.89
impulse (control) F63.9
inflammatory
pelvic, in diseases classified elsewhere - see category N74
penis N48.29
abscess N48.21
cellulitis N48.22
inhalant use
mild F18.10
with
inhalant-induced
anxiety disorder F18.180
depressive disorder F18.14
major neurocognitive disorder F18.17
mild neurocognitive disorder F18.188
psychotic disorder F18.159
inhalant intoxication F18.129
inhalant intoxication delirium F18.121
moderate or severe F18.20
with
inhalant-induced
anxiety disorder F18.280
depressive disorder F18.24
major neurocognitive disorder F18.27
mild neurocognitive disorder F18.288
psychotic disorder F18.259
inhalant intoxication F18.229
inhalant intoxication delirium F18.221
integument, newborn P83.9
specified NEC P83.8
intermittent explosive F63.81
internal secretion pancreas *-see* Increased, secretion, pancreas, endocrine
intestine, intestinal
carbohydrate absorption NEC E74.39
postoperative K91.2
functional NEC K59.9
postoperative K91.89
psychogenic F45.8
vascular K55.9
chronic K55.1
specified NEC K55.8
intraoperative (intraprocedural) *-see* Complications, intraoperative
involuntary emotional expression (IEED) F48.2
iris H21.9
adhesions *-see* Adhesions, iris
atrophy *-see* Atrophy, iris
chamber angle recession *-see* Recession, chamber angle
cyst *-see* Cyst, iris
degeneration *-see* Degeneration, iris
in diseases classified elsewhere H22
iridodialysis *-see* Iridodialysis
iridoschisis *-see* Iridoschisis
miotic pupillary cyst *-see* Cyst, pupillary
pupillary
abnormality *-see* Abnormality, pupillary
membrane *-see* Membrane, pupillary
specified type NEC H21.89
vascular NEC H21.1X
iron metabolism E83.10
specified NEC E83.19
isovaleric acidemia E71.110
jaw, developmental M27.0

Disorder (of) *continued*
  temporomandibular -*see also* Anomaly, dentofacial, temporomandibular joint M26.60
  joint M25.9
    derangement -*see* Derangement, joint
    effusion -*see* Effusion, joint
    fistula -*see* Fistula, joint
    hemarthrosis -*see* Hemarthrosis
    instability -*see* Instability, joint
    osteophyte -*see* Osteophyte
    pain -*see* Pain, joint
    psychogenic F45.8
    specified type NEC M25.80
      ankle M25.87
      elbow M25.82
      foot joint M25.87
      hand joint M25.84
      hip M25.85
      knee M25.86
      shoulder M25.81
      wrist M25.83
    stiffness -*see* Stiffness, joint
  ketone metabolism E71.32
  kidney N28.9
    functional (tubular) N25.9
    in
      schistosomiasis B65.9 [*N29*]
    tubular function N25.9
    specified NEC N25.89
  lacrimal system H04.9
    changes H04.69
    fistula -*see* Fistula, lacrimal
    gland H04.19
      atrophy -*see* Atrophy, lacrimal gland
      cyst -*see* Cyst, lacrimal, gland
      dacryops -*see* Dacryops
      dislocation -*see* Dislocation, lacrimal gland
      dry eye syndrome -*see* Syndrome, dry eye
      infection -*see* Dacryoadenitis
    granuloma -*see* Granuloma, lacrimal
    inflammation -*see* Inflammation, lacrimal
    obstruction -*see* Obstruction, lacrimal
    specified NEC H04.89
  lactation NEC O92.79
  language (developmental) F80.9
    expressive F80.1
    mixed receptive and expressive F80.2
    receptive F80.2
  late luteal phase dysphoric N94.89
  learning (specific) F81.9
    acalculia R48.8
    alexia R48.0
    mathematics F81.2
    reading F81.0
    specified NEC F81.89
    spelling F81.81
    written expression F81.81
  lens H27.9
    aphakia -*see* Aphakia
    cataract -*see* Cataract
    dislocation -*see* Dislocation, lens
    specified type NEC H27.8
  ligament M24.20
    ankle M24.27
    attachment, spine -*see* Enthesopathy, spinal
    elbow M24.22
    foot joint M24.27
    hand joint M24.24
    hip M24.25
    knee -*see* Derangement, knee, specified NEC

Disorder (of) *continued*
    shoulder M24.21
    vertebra M24.28
    wrist M24.23
  ligamentous attachments -*see also* Enthesopathy
    spine -*see* Enthesopathy, spinal
  lipid
    metabolism, congenital E78.9
    storage E75.6
      specified NEC E75.5
  lipoprotein
    deficiency (familial) E78.6
    metabolism E78.9
      specified NEC E78.89
  liver K76.9
    malarial B54 [*K77*]
  low back -*see also* Dorsopathy, specified NEC
  lumbosacral
    plexus G54.1
    root (nerve) NEC G54.4
  lung, interstitial, drug-induced J70.4
    acute J70.2
    chronic J70.3
  lymphoproliferative, post-transplant (PTLD) D47.Z1
  lysine and hydroxylysine metabolism E72.3
  major neurocognitive -*see* Dementia, in (due to)
  male
    erectile (organic) -*see also* Dysfunction, sexual, male, erectile N52.9
      nonorganic F52.21
    hypoactive sexual desire F52.0
    orgasmic F52.32
  manic F30.9
    organic F06.33
  mast cell activation -*see* Activation, mast cell
  mastoid -*see also* Disorder, ear, middle
    postprocedural -*see* Complications, ear, procedure
  meniscus -*see* Derangement, knee, meniscus
  menopausal N95.9
    specified NEC N95.8
  menstrual N92.6
    psychogenic F45.8
    specified NEC N92.5
  mental (or behavioral) (nonpsychotic) F99
    due to (secondary to)
      amphetamine
        due to drug abuse -*see* Abuse, drug, stimulant
        due to drug dependence -*see* Dependence, drug, stimulant
      brain disease, damage and dysfunction F09
      caffeine use
        due to drug abuse -*see* Abuse, drug, stimulant
        due to drug dependence -*see* Dependence, drug, stimulant
      cannabis use
        due to drug abuse -*see* Abuse, drug, cannabis
        due to drug dependence -*see* Dependence, drug, cannabis
      general medical condition F09
      sedative or hypnotic use
        due to drug abuse -*see* Abuse, drug, sedative

Disorder (of) *continued*
        due to drug dependence -*see* Dependence, drug, sedative
      tobacco (nicotine) use -*see* Dependence, drug, nicotine
    following organic brain damage F07.9
      frontal lobe syndrome F07.0
      personality change F07.0
      postconcussional syndrome F07.81
      specified NEC F07.89
    infancy, childhood or adolescence F98.9
    neurotic -*see* Neurosis
    organic or symptomatic F09
    presenile, psychotic F03
    problem NEC
    psychoneurotic -*see* Neurosis
    psychotic -*see* Psychosis
    puerperal F53
    senile, psychotic NEC F03
  metabolic, amino acid, transitory, newborn P74.8
  metabolism NOS E88.9
    amino-acid E72.9
      aromatic E70.9
        albinism -*see* Albinism
        histidine E70.40
          histidinemia E70.41
          other specified E70.49
        hyperphenylalaninemia E70.1
          classical phenylketonuria E70.0
        other specified E70.8
        tryptophan E70.5
        tyrosine E70.20
          hypertyrosinemia E70.21
          other specified E70.29
      branched chain E71.2
        3 methylglutaconic aciduria E71.111
        hyperleucine-isoleucinemia E71.19
        hypervalinemia E71.19
        isovaleric acidemia E71.110
        maple syrup urine disease E71.0
        methylmalonic acidemia E71.120
        organic aciduria NEC E71.118
        other specified E71.19
        propionate NEC E71.128
        propionic acidemia E71.121
      glycine E72.50
        d-glycericacidemia E72.59
        hyperhydroxyprolinemia E72.59
        hyperoxaluria E72.53
        hyperprolinemia E72.59
        non-ketotic hyperglycinemia E72.51
        other specified E72.59
        sarcosinemia E72.59
        trimethylaminuria E72.52
      hydroxylysine E72.3
      lysine E72.3
      ornithine E72.4
      other specified E72.8
        beta-amino acid E72.8
        gamma-glutamyl cycle E72.8
        straight-chain E72.8
      sulfur-bearing E72.10
        homocystinuria E72.11
        methylenetetrahydrofolate reductase deficiency E72.12
        other specified E72.19
    bile acid and cholesterol metabolism E78.70
    bilirubin E80.7
      specified NEC E80.6
    calcium E83.50

Disorder (of) *continued*

   hypercalcemia E83.52
   hypocalcemia E83.51
   other specified E83.59
  carbohydrate E74.9
   specified NEC E74.8
  cholesterol and bile acid metabolism E78.70
  congenital E88.9
  copper E83.00
   Wilson's disease E83.01
   specified type NEC E83.09
  cystinuria E72.01
  fructose E74.10
  galactose E74.20
  glucosaminoglycan E76.9
   mucopolysaccharidosis -*see*
    Mucopolysaccharidosis
   specified NEC E76.8
  glutamine E72.8
  glycine E72.50
  glycogen storage (hepatorenal) E74.09
  glycoprotein E77.9
   specified NEC E77.8
  glycosaminoglycan E76.9
   specified NEC E76.8
  in labor and delivery O75.89
  iron E83.10
  isoleucine E71.19
  leucine E71.19
  lipoid E78.9
  lipoprotein E78.9
   specified NEC E78.89
  magnesium E83.40
   hypermagnesemia E83.41
   hypomagnesemia E83.42
   other specified E83.49
  mineral E83.9
   specified NEC E83.89
  mitochondrial E88.40
   MELAS syndrome E88.41
   MERRF syndrome (myoclonic epilepsy
    associated with ragged-red fibers) E88.42
   other specified E88.49
  ornithine E72.4
  phosphatases E83.30
  phosphorus E83.30
   acid phosphatase deficiency E83.39
   hypophosphatasia E83.39
   hypophosphatemia E83.39
    familial E83.31
   other specified E83.39
   pseudovitamin D deficiency E83.32
  plasma protein NEC E88.09
  porphyrin -*see* Porphyria
  postprocedural E89.89
   specified NEC E89.89
  purine E79.9
   specified NEC E79.8
  pyrimidine E79.9
   specified NEC E79.8
  pyruvate E74.4
  serine E72.8
  sodium E87.8
  specified NEC E88.89
  threonine E72.8
  valine E71.19
  zinc E83.2
 methylmalonic acidemia E71.120
 micturition NEC -*see also* Difficulty,
 micturition R39.198
  feeling of incomplete emptying R39.14

Disorder (of) *continued*

  hesitancy R39.11
  poor stream R39.12
  psychogenic F45.8
  split stream R39.13
  straining R39.16
  urgency R39.15
 mild neurocognitive G31.84
 mitochondrial metabolism E88.40
 mitral (valve) -*see* Endocarditis, mitral
 mixed
  anxiety and depressive F41.8
  of scholastic skills (developmental) F81.89
  receptive expressive language F80.2
 mood F39
 bipolar -*see* Disorder, bipolar
 depressive -*see* Disorder, depressive
 due to (secondary to)
  alcohol F10.94
  amphetamine F15.94
   in
    abuse F15.14
    dependence F15.24
  anxiolytic F13.94
   in
    abuse F13.14
    dependence F13.24
  cocaine F14.94
   in
    abuse F14.14
    dependence F14.24
  general medical condition F06.30
  hallucinogen F16.94
   in
    abuse F16.14
    dependence F16.24
  hypnotic F13.94
   in
    abuse F13.14
    dependence F13.24
  inhalant F18.94
   in
    abuse F18.14
    dependence F18.24
  opioid F11.94
   in
    abuse F11.14
    dependence F11.24
  phencyclidine (PCP) F16.94
   in
    abuse F16.14
    dependence F16.24
  physiological condition F06.30
   with
    depressive features F06.31
    major depressive-like episode F06.32
    manic features F06.33
    mixed features F06.34
  psychoactive substance NEC F19.94
   in
    abuse F19.14
    dependence F19.24
  sedative F13.94
   in
    abuse F13.14
    dependence F13.24
  volatile solvents F18.94
   in
    abuse F18.14
    dependence F18.24
 manic episode F30.9

Disorder (of) *continued*

  with psychotic symptoms F30.2
  in remission (full) F30.4
   partial F30.3
  specified type NEC F30.8
  without psychotic symptoms F30.10
   mild F30.11
   moderate F30.12
   severe F30.13
  organic F06.30
   right hemisphere F07.89
  persistent F34.9
   cyclothymia F34.0
   dysthymia F34.1
   specified type NEC F34.89
  recurrent F39
  right hemisphere organic F07.89
 movement G25.9
  drug-induced G25.70
   akathisia G25.71
   specified NEC G25.79
  hysterical F44.4
  in diseases classified elsewhere - see
 category G26
  periodic limb G47.61
   sleep related G47.61
  specified NEC G25.89
  sleep related NEC G47.69
  stereotyped F98.4
  treatment-induced G25.9
 multiple personality F44.81
 muscle M62.9
  attachment, spine -*see* Enthesopathy, spinal
  in trichinellosis -*see* Trichinellosis, with
   muscle disorder
  psychogenic F45.8
  specified type NEC M62.89
  tone, newborn P94.9
   specified NEC P94.8
 muscular
  attachments -*see also* Enthesopathy
   spine -*see* Enthesopathy, spinal
  urethra N36.44
 musculoskeletal system, soft tissue -*see*
 Disorder, soft tissue
  postprocedural M96.89
  psychogenic F45.8
 myoneural G70.9
  due to lead G70.1
  specified NEC G70.89
  toxic G70.1
 myotonic NEC G71.19
 nail, in diseases classified elsewhere L62
 neck region NEC -*see* Dorsopathy, specified
 NEC
 neonatal onset multisystemic inflammatory
 (NOMID) M04.2
 nerve G58.9
  abducent NEC -*see* Strabismus, paralytic,
 sixth nerve
  accessory G52.8
  acoustic -*see* subcategory H93.3
  auditory -*see* subcategory H93.3
  auriculotemporal G50.8
  axillary G54.0
  cerebral -*see* Disorder, nerve, cranial
  cranial G52.9
   eighth -*see* subcategory H93.3
   eleventh G52.8
   fifth G50.9
   first G52.0

Disorder (of) *continued*
- fourth NEC -*see* Strabismus, paralytic, fourth nerve
- multiple G52.7
- ninth G52.1
- second NEC -*see* Disorder, nerve, optic
- seventh NEC G51.8
- sixth NEC -*see* Strabismus, paralytic, sixth nerve
- specified NEC G52.8
- tenth G52.2
- third NEC -*see* Strabismus, paralytic, third nerve
- twelfth G52.3
- entrapment -*see* Neuropathy, entrapment
- facial G51.9
  - specified NEC G51.8
- femoral -*see* Lesion, nerve, femoral
- glossopharyngeal NEC G52.1
- hypoglossal G52.3
- intercostal G58.0
- lateral
  - cutaneous of thigh -*see* Mononeuropathy, lower limb, meralgia paresthetica
  - popliteal -*see* Lesion, nerve, popliteal
- lower limb -*see* Mononeuropathy, lower limb
- medial popliteal -*see* Lesion, nerve, popliteal, medial
- median NEC -*see* Lesion, nerve, median
- multiple G58.7
- oculomotor NEC -*see* Strabismus, paralytic, third nerve
- olfactory G52.0
- optic NEC H47.09
  - hemorrhage into sheath -*see* Hemorrhage, optic nerve
  - ischemic H47.01
- peroneal -*see* Lesion, nerve, popliteal
- phrenic G58.8
- plantar -*see* Lesion, nerve, plantar
- pneumogastric G52.2
- posterior tibial -*see* Syndrome, tarsal tunnel
- radial -*see* Lesion, nerve, radial
- recurrent laryngeal G52.2
- root G54.9
  - cervical G54.2
  - lumbosacral G54.1
  - specified NEC G54.8
  - thoracic G54.3
- sciatic NEC -*see* Lesion, nerve, sciatic
- specified NEC G58.8
  - lower limb -*see* Mononeuropathy, lower limb, specified NEC
  - upper limb -*see* Mononeuropathy, upper limb, specified NEC
- sympathetic G90.9
- tibial -*see* Lesion, nerve, popliteal, medial
- trigeminal G50.9
  - specified NEC G50.8
- trochlear NEC -*see* Strabismus, paralytic, fourth nerve
- ulnar -*see* Lesion, nerve, ulnar
- upper limb -*see* Mononeuropathy, upper limb
- vagus G52.2
- nervous system G98.8
  - autonomic (peripheral) G90.9
    - specified NEC G90.8
  - central G96.9
    - specified NEC G96.8

Disorder (of) *continued*
- parasympathetic G90.9
  - specified NEC G98.8
- sympathetic G90.9
- vegetative G90.9
- neurocognitive
  - major
    - with
      - aggressive behavior F01.51
      - combative behavior F01.51
      - violent behavior F01.51
    - due to vascular disease, with behavioral disturbance F01.51
    - in (due to) (other diseases classified elsewhere) -*see also* Dementia, in (due to) F02.80
      - with
        - aggressive behavior F02.81
        - combative behavior F02.81
        - violent behavior F02.81
      - without behavioral disturbance F01.50
  - mild G31.84
- neurodevelopmental F89
  - specified NEC F88
- neurohypophysis NEC E23.3
- neurological NEC R29.818
- neuromuscular G70.9
  - hereditary NEC G71.9
  - specified NEC G70.89
  - toxic G70.1
- neurotic F48.9
  - specified NEC F48.8
- neutrophil, polymorphonuclear D71
- nicotine use -*see* Dependence, drug, nicotine
- nightmare F51.5
- nose J34.9
  - specified NEC J34.89
- obsessive-compulsive F42.9
- odontogenesis NOS K00.9
- opioid use
  - with
    - opioid-induced psychotic disorder F11.959
      - with
        - delusions F11.950
        - hallucinations F11.951
  - due to drug abuse -*see* Abuse, drug, opioid
  - due to drug dependence -*see* Dependence, drug, opioid
  - mild F11.10
    - with
      - opioid-induced
        - anxiety disorder F11.188
        - depressive disorder F11.14
        - sexual dysfunction F11.181
      - opioid intoxication
        - with perceptual disturbances F11.122
        - delirium F11.121
        - without perceptual disturbances F11.129
  - moderate or severe F11.20
    - with
      - opioid-induced
        - anxiety disorder F11.288
        - anxiety disorder F11.988
        - depressive disorder F11.24
        - depressive disorder F11.94
        - sexual dysfunction F11.281
        - sexual dysfunction F11.981
      - opioid intoxication
        - with perceptual disturbances F11.222
        - delirium F11.221
        - without perceptual disturbances F11.229

Disorder (of) *continued*
- oppositional defiant F91.3
- optic
  - chiasm H47.49
    - due to
      - inflammatory disorder H47.41
      - neoplasm H47.42
      - vascular disorder H47.43
  - disc H47.39
    - coloboma -*see* Coloboma, optic disc
    - drusen -*see* Drusen, optic disc
    - pseudopapilledema -*see* Pseudopapilledema
  - radiations -*see* Disorder, visual, pathway
  - tracts -*see* Disorder, visual, pathway orbit H05.9
  - cyst -*see* Cyst, orbit
  - deformity -*see* Deformity, orbit
  - edema -*see* Edema, orbit
  - enophthalmos -*see* Enophthalmos
  - exophthalmos -*see* Exophthalmos
  - hemorrhage -*see* Hemorrhage, orbit
  - inflammation -*see* Inflammation, orbit
  - myopathy -*see* Myopathy, extraocular muscles
  - retained foreign body -*see* Foreign body, orbit, old
  - specified type NEC H05.89
- organic
  - anxiety F06.4
  - catatonic F06.1
  - delusional F06.2
  - dissociative F06.8
  - emotionally labile (asthenic) F06.8
  - mood (affective) F06.30
  - schizophrenia-like F06.2
- orgasmic (female) F52.31
  - male F52.32
- ornithine metabolism E72.4
- overanxious F41.1
  - of childhood F93.8
- pain
  - with related psychological factors F45.42
  - exclusively related to psychological factors F45.41
  - genito-pelvic penetration disorder F52.6
- pancreatic internal secretion E16.9
  - specified NEC E16.8
- panic F41.0
  - with agoraphobia F40.01
- papulosquamous L44.9
  - in diseases classified elsewhere L45
  - specified NEC L44.8
- paranoid F22
  - induced F24
  - shared F24
- parathyroid (gland) E21.5
  - specified NEC E21.4
- parietoalveolar NEC J84.09
- paroxysmal, mixed R56.9
- patella M22.9
  - chondromalacia -*see* Chondromalacia, patella
  - derangement NEC M22.3X
  - recurrent
    - dislocation -*see* Dislocation, patella, recurrent
    - subluxation -*see* Dislocation, patella, recurrent, incomplete
  - specified NEC M22.8X
- patellofemoral M22.2X

Disorder (of) *continued*

pentose phosphate pathway with anemia D55.1

perception, due to hallucinogens F16.983

in
abuse F16.183
dependence F16.283

peripheral nervous system NEC G64

peroxisomal E71.50
biogenesis
neonatal adrenoleukodystrophy E71.511
specified disorder NEC E71.518
Zellweger syndrome E71.510
rhizomelic chondrodysplasia punctata E71.540
specified form NEC E71.548
group 1 E71.518
group 2 E71.53
group 3 E71.542
X linked adrenoleukodystrophy E71.529
adolescent E71.521
adrenomyeloneuropathy E71.522
childhood E71.520
specified form NEC E71.528
Zellweger-like syndrome E71.541

persistent
(somatoform) pain F45.41
affective (mood) F34.9

personality -*see also* Personality F60.9
affective F34.0
aggressive F60.3
amoral F60.2
anankastic F60.5
antisocial F60.2
anxious F60.6
asocial F60.2
asthenic F60.7
avoidant F60.6
borderline F60.3
change (secondary) due to general medical condition F07.0
compulsive F60.5
cyclothymic F34.0
dependent (passive) F60.7
depressive F34.1
dissocial F60.2
emotional instability F60.3
expansive paranoid F60.0
explosive F60.3
following organic brain damage F07.9
histrionic F60.4
hyperthymic F34.0
hypothymic F34.1
hysterical F60.4
immature F60.89
inadequate F60.7
labile F60.3
mixed (nonspecific) F60.89
moral deficiency F60.2
narcissistic F60.81
negativistic F60.89
obsessional F60.5
obsessive (compulsive) F60.5
organic F07.9
overconscientious F60.5
paranoid F60.0
passive (dependent) F60.7
passive-aggressive F60.89
pathological NEC F60.9
pseudosocial F60.2
psychopathic F60.2

Disorder (of) *continued*

schizoid F60.1
schizotypal F21
self-defeating F60.7
specified NEC F60.89
type A F60.5
unstable (emotional) F60.3

pervasive, developmental F84.9

phencyclidine use
mild F16.10
with
phencyclidine-induced
anxiety disorder F16.180
bipolar and related disorder F16.14
depressive disorder F16.14
psychotic disorder F16.159
phencyclidine intoxication F16.129
phencyclidine intoxication delirium F16.121
moderate or severe F16.20
with
phencyclidine-induced
anxiety disorder F16.280
bipolar and related disorder F16.24
depressive disorder F16.24
psychotic disorder F16.259
phencyclidine intoxication F16.229
phencyclidine intoxication delirium F16.221

phobic anxiety, childhood F40.8

phosphate-losing tubular N25.0

pigmentation L81.9
choroid, congenital Q14.3
diminished melanin formation L81.6
iron L81.8
specified NEC L81.8

pinna (noninfective) H61.10
deformity, acquired H61.11
hematoma H61.12
perichondritis -*see* Perichondritis, ear
specified type NEC H61.19

pituitary gland E23.7
iatrogenic (postprocedural) E89.3
specified NEC E23.6

platelets D69.1

plexus G54.9
specified NEC G54.8

polymorphonuclear neutrophils D71

porphyrin metabolism -*see* Porphyria

postconcussional F07.81

posthallucinogen perception F16.983
in
abuse F16.183
dependence F16.283

postmenopausal N95.9
specified NEC N95.8

postprocedural (postoperative) -*see* Complications, postprocedural

post-transplant lymphoproliferative D47.Z1

post-traumatic stress (PTSD) F43.10
acute F43.11
chronic F43.12

premenstrual dysphoric (PMDD) F32.81

prepuce N47.8

propionic acidemia E71.121

prostate N42.9
specified NEC N42.89

psychogenic NOS -*see also* condition F45.9
anxiety F41.8
appetite F50.9
asthenic F48.8

Disorder (of) *continued*

cardiovascular (system) F45.8
compulsive F42.8
cutaneous F54
depressive F32.9
digestive (system) F45.8
dysmenorrheic F45.8
dyspneic F45.8
endocrine (system) F54
eye NEC F45.8
feeding -*see* Disorder, eating
functional NEC F45.8
gastric F45.8
gastrointestinal (system) F45.8
genitourinary (system) F45.8
heart (function) (rhythm) F45.8
hyperventilatory F45.8
hypochondriacal -*see* Disorder, hypochondriacal
intestinal F45.8
joint F45.8
learning F81.9
limb F45.8
lymphatic (system) F45.8
menstrual F45.8
micturition F45.8
monoplegic NEC F44.4
motor F44.4
muscle F45.8
musculoskeletal F45.8
neurocirculatory F45.8
obsessive F42.8
occupational F48.8
organ or part of body NEC F45.8
paralytic NEC F44.4
phobic F40.9
physical NEC F45.8
rectal F45.8
respiratory (system) F45.8
rheumatic F45.8
sexual (function) F52.9
skin (allergic) (eczematous) F54
sleep F51.9
specified part of body NEC F45.8
stomach F45.8

psychological F99
associated with
disease classified elsewhere F54
sexual
development F66
relationship F66
uncertainty about gender identity F64.9

psychomotor NEC F44.4
hysterical F44.4

psychoneurotic -*see also* Neurosis
mixed NEC F48.8

psychophysiologic -*see* Disorder, somatoform

psychosexual F65.9
development F66
identity of childhood F64.2

psychosomatic NOS -*see* Disorder, somatoform
multiple F45.0
undifferentiated F45.1

psychotic -*see* Psychosis
transient (acute) F23

puberty E30.9
specified NEC E30.8

pulmonary (valve) -*see* Endocarditis, pulmonary

purine metabolism E79.9

Disorder (of) *continued*
pyrimidine metabolism E79.9
pyruvate metabolism E74.4
reactive attachment (childhood) F94.1
reading R48.0
  developmental (specific) F81.0
receptive language F80.2
receptor, hormonal, peripheral -*see also*
  Syndrome, androgen insensitivity E34.50
recurrent brief depressive F33.8
reflex R29.2
refraction H52.7
  aniseikonia H52.32
  anisometropia H52.31
  astigmatism -*see* Astigmatism
  hypermetropia -*see* Hypermetropia
  myopia -*see* Myopia
  presbyopia H52.4
  specified NEC H52.6
relationship F68.8
  due to sexual orientation F66
REM sleep behavior G47.52
renal function, impaired (tubular) N25.9
resonance R49.9
  specified NEC R49.8
respiratory function, impaired -*see also*
Failure, respiration
  postprocedural -*see* Complication,
  postoperative, respiratory system
  psychogenic F45.8
retina H35.9
  angioid streaks H35.33
  changes in vascular appearance H35.01
  degeneration -*see* Degeneration, retina
  dystrophy (hereditary) -*see* Dystrophy,
  retina
  edema H35.81
  hemorrhage -*see* Hemorrhage, retina
  ischemia H35.82
  macular degeneration -*see* Degeneration,
  macula
  microaneurysms H35.04
  microvascular abnormality NEC H35.09
  neovascularization -*see* Neovascularization,
  retina
  retinopathy -*see* Retinopathy
  separation of layers H35.70
    central serous chorioretinopathy H35.71
    pigment epithelium detachment (serous)
  H35.72
      hemorrhagic H35.73
  specified type NEC H35.89
  telangiectasis -*see* Telangiectasis, retina
  vasculitis -*see* Vasculitis, retina
retroperitoneal K68.9
right hemisphere organic affective F07.89
rumination (infant or child) F98.21
sacrum, sacrococcygeal NEC M53.3
schizoaffective F25.9
  bipolar type F25.0
  depressive type F25.1
  manic type F25.0
  mixed type F25.0
  specified NEC F25.8
schizoid of childhood F84.5
schizophreniform F20.81
  brief F23
schizotypal (personality) F21
secretion, thyrocalcitonin E07.0
sedative, hypnotic, or anxiolytic use
  mild F13.10

Disorder (of) *continued*
  with
    sedative, hypnotic, or anxiolytic-induced
      anxiety disorder F13.180
      bipolar and related disorder F13.14
      depressive disorder F13.14
      psychotic disorder F13.159
      sexual dysfunction F13.181
    sedative, hypnotic, or anxiolytic
      intoxication F13.129
    sedative, hypnotic, or anxiolytic
      intoxication delirium F13.121
  moderate or severe F13.20
    with
      sedative, hypnotic, or anxiolytic-induced
        anxiety disorder F13.280
        bipolar and related disorder F13.24
        depressive disorder F13.24
        major neurocognitive disorder F13.27
        mild neurocognitive disorder F13.288
        psychotic disorder F13.259
        sexual dysfunction F13.281
      sedative, hypnotic, or anxiolytic
        intoxication F13.229
      sedative, hypnotic, or anxiolytic
        intoxication delirium F13.221
seizure -*see also* Epilepsy G40.909
  intractable G40.919
    with status epilepticus G40.911
semantic pragmatic F80.89
  with autism F84.0
sense of smell R43.1
  psychogenic F45.8
separation anxiety, of childhood F93.0
sexual
  arousal, female F52.22
  aversion F52.1
  function, psychogenic F52.9
  maturation F66
  nonorganic F52.9
  preference -*see also* Deviation, sexual F65.9
    fetishistic transvestism F65.1
  relationship F66
shyness, of childhood and adolescence F40.10
sibling rivalry F93.8
sickle-cell (sickling) (homozygous) -*see*
Disease, sickle-cell
  heterozygous D57.3
  specified type NEC D57.8
  trait D57.3
sinus (nasal) J34.9
  specified NEC J34.89
skin L98.9
  atrophic L90.9
    specified NEC L90.8
  granulomatous L92.9
    specified NEC L92.8
  hypertrophic L91.9
    specified NEC L91.8
  infiltrative NEC L98.6
  newborn P83.9
    specified NEC P83.8
  picking F42.4
  psychogenic (allergic) (eczematous) F54
sleep G47.9
  breathing-related -*see* Apnea, sleep
  circadian rhythm G47.20
    advance sleep phase type G47.22
    delayed sleep phase type G47.21
    due to
      alcohol

Disorder (of) *continued*
        abuse F10.182
        dependence F10.282
        use F10.982
      amphetamines
        abuse F15.182
        dependence F15.282
        use F15.982
      caffeine
        abuse F15.182
        dependence F15.282
        use F15.982
      cocaine
        abuse F14.182
        dependence F14.282
        use F14.982
      drug NEC
        abuse F19.182
        dependence F19.282
        use F19.982
      opioid
        abuse F11.182
        dependence F11.282
        use F11.982
      psychoactive substance NEC
        abuse F19.182
        dependence F19.282
        use F19.982
      sedative, hypnotic, or anxiolytic
        abuse F13.182
        dependence F13.282
        use F13.982
      stimulant NEC
        abuse F15.182
        dependence F15.282
        use F15.982
    free running type G47.24
    in conditions classified elsewhere G47.27
    irregular sleep wake type G47.23
    jet lag type G47.25
    shift work type G47.26
    specified NEC G47.29
  due to
    alcohol
      abuse F10.182
      dependence F10.282
      use F10.982
    amphetamine
      abuse F15.182
      dependence F15.282
      use F15.982
    anxiolytic
      abuse F13.182
      dependence F13.282
      use F13.982
    caffeine
      abuse F15.182
      dependence F15.282
      use F15.982
    cocaine
      abuse F14.182
      dependence F14.282
      use F14.982
    drug NEC
      abuse F19.182
      dependence F19.282
      use F19.982
    hypnotic
      abuse F13.182
      dependence F13.282
      use F13.982

Disorder (of) *continued*
  opioid
    abuse F11.182
    dependence F11.282
    use F11.982
  psychoactive substance NEC
    abuse F19.182
    dependence F19.282
    use F19.982
  sedative
    abuse F13.182
    dependence F13.282
    use F13.982
  stimulant NEC
    abuse F15.182
    dependence F15.282
    use F15.982
  emotional F51.9
  excessive somnolence -*see* Hypersomnia
  hypersomnia type -*see* Hypersomnia
  initiating or maintaining -*see* Insomnia
  nightmares F51.5
  nonorganic F51.9
    specified NEC F51.8
  parasomnia type G47.50
  specified NEC G47.8
  terrors F51.4
  walking F51.3
sleep-wake pattern or schedule -*see* Disorder,
sleep, circadian rhythm
social
  anxiety of childhood F40.10
  functioning in childhood F94.9
    specified NEC F94.8
  pragmatic F80.82
soft tissue M79.9
  ankle M79.9
  due to use, overuse and pressure M70.90
    ankle M70.97
    bursitis -*see* Bursitis
    foot M70.97
    forearm M70.93
    hand M70.94
    lower leg M70.96
    multiple sites M70.99
    pelvic region M70.95
    shoulder region M70.91
    specified site NEC M70.98
    specified type NEC M70.80
      ankle M70.87
      foot M70.87
      forearm M70.83
      hand M70.84
      lower leg M70.86
      multiple sites M70.89
      pelvic region M70.85
      shoulder region M70.81
      specified site NEC M70.88
      thigh M70.85
      upper arm M70.82
    thigh M70.95
    upper arm M70.92
  foot M79.9
  forearm M79.9
  hand M79.9
  lower leg M79.9
  multiple sites M79.9
  occupational -*see* Disorder, soft tissue, due
  to use, overuse and pressure
  pelvic region M79.9
  shoulder region M79.9

Disorder (of) *continued*
    specified type NEC M79.89
    thigh M79.9
    upper arm M79.9
  somatic symptom F45.1
  somatization F45.0
  somatoform F45.9
    pain (persistent) F45.41
    somatization (multiple) (long-lasting) F45.0
    specified NEC F45.8
    undifferentiated F45.1
  somnolence, excessive -*see* Hypersomnia
  specific
    arithmetical F81.2
    developmental, of motor F82
    reading F81.0
    speech and language F80.9
    spelling F81.81
    written expression F81.81
  speech R47.9
    articulation (functional) (specific) F80.0
    developmental F80.9
    specified NEC R47.89
  speech-sound F80.0
  spelling (specific) F81.81
  spine -*see also* Dorsopathy
    ligamentous or muscular attachments,
    peripheral -*see* Enthesopathy, spinal
    specified NEC -*see* Dorsopathy, specified
    NEC
  stereotyped, habit or movement F98.4
  stimulant use (other) (unspecified)
    mild F15.10
    moderate or severe F15.20
  stomach (functional) -*see* Disorder, gastric
  stress F43.9
    acute F43.0
    post-traumatic F43.10
      acute F43.11
      chronic F43.12
  substance use (other) (unknown)
    mild F19.10
      with substance-induced
        anxiety disorder F19.180
        bipolar and related disorder F19.14
        depressive disorder F19.14
        major neurocognitive disorder F19.17
        mild neurocognitive disorder F19.188
        obsessive-compulsive and related
        disorder F19.188
        sexual dysfunction F19.181
      substance intoxication F19.129
      substance intoxication delirium F19.121
    moderate or severe F19.20
      with substance-induced
        anxiety disorder F19.280
        bipolar and related disorder F19.24
        depressive disorder F19.24
        major neurocognitive disorder F19.27
        mild neurocognitive disorder F19.288
        obsessive-compulsive and related
        disorder F19.288
        sexual dysfunction F19.281
      substance intoxication F19.229
      substance intoxication delirium F19.221
  sulfur-bearing amino-acid metabolism E72.10
  sweat gland (eccrine) L74.9
    apocrine L75.9
      specified NEC L75.8
    specified NEC L74.8
  synovium M67.90

Disorder (of) *continued*
  acromioclavicular M67.91
  ankle M67.97
  elbow M67.92
  foot M67.97
  forearm M67.93
  hand M67.94
  hip M67.95
  knee M67.96
  multiple sites M67.99
  rupture -*see* Rupture, synovium
  shoulder M67.91
  specified type NEC M67.80
    acromioclavicular M67.81
    ankle M67.87
    elbow M67.82
    foot M67.87
    hand M67.84
    hip M67.85
    knee M67.86
    multiple sites M67.89
    wrist M67.83
  synovitis -*see* Synovitis
  upper arm M67.92
  wrist M67.93
temperature regulation, newborn P81.9
  specified NEC P81.8
temporomandibular joint M26.60
tendon M67.90
  acromioclavicular M67.91
  ankle M67.97
  contracture -*see* Contracture, tendon
  elbow M67.92
  foot M67.97
  forearm M67.93
  hand M67.94
  hip M67.95
  knee M67.96
  multiple sites M67.99
  rupture -*see* Rupture, tendon
  shoulder M67.91
  specified type NEC M67.80
    acromioclavicular M67.81
    ankle M67.87
    elbow M67.82
    foot M67.87
    hand M67.84
    hip M67.85
    knee M67.86
    multiple sites M67.89
    trunk M67.88
    wrist M67.83
  synovitis -*see* Synovitis
  tendinitis -*see* Tendinitis
  tenosynovitis -*see* Tenosynovitis
  trunk M67.98
  upper arm M67.92
  wrist M67.93
thoracic root (nerve) NEC G54.3
thyrocalcitonin hypersecretion E07.0
thyroid (gland) E07.9
  function NEC, neonatal, transitory P72.2
  iodine-deficiency related E01.8
  specified NEC E07.89
tic -*see* Tic
tobacco use
  mild Z72.0
  moderate F17.200
  severe F17.200
tooth K08.9
  development K00.9

Disorder (of) *continued*
　　specified NEC K00.8
　　eruption K00.6
　Tourette's F95.2
　trance and possession F44.89
　trauma and stressor-related F43.9
　　other specified F43.8
　tricuspid (valve) -*see* Endocarditis, tricuspid
　tryptophan metabolism E70.5
　tubular, phosphate-losing N25.0
　tubulo-interstitial (in)
　　brucellosis A23.9 *[N16]*
　　cystinosis E72.04
　　diphtheria A36.84
　　glycogen storage disease E74.00 *[N16]*
　　leukemia NEC C95.9 *[N16]*
　　lymphoma NEC C85.9 *[N16]*
　　mixed cryoglobulinemia D89.1 *[N16]*
　　multiple myeloma C90.0 *[N16]*
　　Salmonella infection A02.25
　　sarcoidosis D86.84
　　sepsis A41.9 *[N16]*
　　　streptococcal A40.9 *[N16]*
　　systemic lupus erythematosus M32.15
　　toxoplasmosis B58.83
　　transplant rejection T86.91 *[N16]*
　　Wilson's disease E83.01 *[N16]*
　tubulo-renal function, impaired N25.9
　　specified NEC N25.89
　tympanic membrane H73.9
　　atrophy -*see* Atrophy, tympanic membrane
　　infection -*see* Myringitis
　　perforation -*see* Perforation, tympanum
　　specified NEC H73.89
　unsocialized aggressive F91.1
　urea cycle metabolism E72.20
　　argininemia E72.21
　　arginosuccinic aciduria E72.22
　　citrullinemia E72.23
　　ornithine transcarbamylase deficiency E72.4
　　other specified E72.29
　ureter (in) N28.9
　　schistosomiasis B65.0 *[N29]*
　　tuberculosis A18.11
　urethra N36.9
　　specified NEC N36.8
　urinary system N39.9
　　specified NEC N39.8
　valve, heart
　　aortic -*see* Endocarditis, aortic
　　mitral -*see* Endocarditis, mitral
　　pulmonary -*see* Endocarditis, pulmonary
　　rheumatic
　　　aortic -*see* Endocarditis, aortic, rheumatic
　　　mitral -*see* Endocarditis, mitral
　　　pulmonary -*see* Endocarditis, pulmonary,
　　rheumatic
　　　tricuspid -*see* Endocarditis, tricuspid
　　tricuspid -*see* Endocarditis, tricuspid
　vestibular function H81.9
　　specified NEC -*see* subcategory H81.8
　　　in diseases classified elsewhere H82.
　　vertigo -*see* Vertigo
　vision, binocular H53.30
　　abnormal retinal correspondence H53.31
　　diplopia H53.2
　　fusion with defective stereopsis H53.32
　　simultaneous perception H53.33
　　suppression H53.34
　visual
　　cortex

Disorder (of) *continued*
　blindness H47.619
　　left brain H47.612
　　right brain H47.611
　　due to
　　　inflammatory disorder H47.629
　　　　left brain H47.622
　　　　right brain H47.621
　　　neoplasm H47.639
　　　　left brain H47.632
　　　　right brain H47.631
　　　vascular disorder H47.649
　　　　left brain H47.642
　　　　right brain H47.641
　　pathway H47.9
　　　due to
　　　　inflammatory disorder H47.51
　　　　neoplasm H47.52
　　　　vascular disorder H47.53
　　　optic chiasm -*see* Disorder, optic, chiasm
　vitreous body H43.9
　　crystalline deposits -*see* Deposit, crystalline
　　degeneration -*see* Degeneration, vitreous
　　hemorrhage -*see* Hemorrhage, vitreous
　　opacities -*see* Opacity, vitreous
　　prolapse -*see* Prolapse, vitreous
　　specified type NEC H43.89
　voice R49.9
　　specified type NEC R49.8
　volatile solvent use
　　due to drug abuse -*see* Abuse, drug, inhalant
　　due to drug dependence -*see* Dependence,
　　drug, inhalant
　white blood cells D72.9
　　specified NEC D72.89
　withdrawing, child or adolescent F40.10
Disorientation R41.0
Displacement, displaced
　acquired traumatic of bone, cartilage, joint,
　tendon NEC -*see* Dislocation
　adrenal gland (congenital) Q89.1
　appendix, retrocecal (congenital) Q43.8
　auricle (congenital) Q17.4
　bladder (acquired) N32.89
　　congenital Q64.19
　brachial plexus (congenital) Q07.8
　brain stem, caudal (congenital) Q04.8
　canaliculus (lacrimalis), congenital Q10.6
　cardia through esophageal hiatus (congenital)
　Q40.1
　cerebellum, caudal (congenital) Q04.8
　cervix -*see* Malposition, uterus
　colon (congenital) Q43.3
　device, implant or graft -*see also*
　Complications, by site and type, mechanical
　T85.628
　　arterial graft NEC -*see* Complication,
　cardiovascular device, mechanical, vascular
　　breast (implant) T85.42
　　catheter NEC T85.628
　　　dialysis (renal) T82.42
　　　　intraperitoneal T85.621
　　　infusion NEC T82.524
　　　　spinal (epidural) (subdural) T85.620
　　　urinary
　　　　cystostomy T83.020
　　　　Hopkins T83.028
　　　　ileostomy T83.028
　　　　indwelling T83.021
　　　　nephrostomy T83.022
　　　　specified NEC T83.028

Displacement, displaced --*continued*
　　urostomy T83.028
　electronic (electrode) (pulse generator)
　　(stimulator) -*see* Complication, electronic
　　stimulator
　fixation, internal (orthopedic) NEC -*see*
　　Complication, fixation device, mechanical
　gastrointestinal -*see* Complications,
　　prosthetic device, mechanical,
　　gastrointestinal device
　genital NEC T83.428
　　intrauterine contraceptive device (string)
　　T83.32
　　penile prosthesis (cylinder) (implanted)
　　(pump) (reservoir) T83.420
　　testicular prosthesis T83.421
　heart NEC -*see* Complication,
　　cardiovascular device, mechanical
　joint prosthesis -*see* Complications, joint
　　prosthesis, mechanical
　ocular -*see* Complications, prosthetic device,
　　mechanical, ocular device
　orthopedic NEC -*see* Complication,
　　orthopedic, device or graft, mechanical
　specified NEC T85.628
　urinary NEC T83.128
　　graft T83.22
　　sphincter, implanted T83.121
　　stent (ileal conduit) (nephroureteral)
　　T83.123
　　　ureteral indwelling T83.122
　vascular NEC -*see* Complication,
　　cardiovascular device, mechanical
　ventricular intracranial shunt T85.02
　electronic stimulator
　bone T84.320
　cardiac -*see* Complications, cardiac device,
　　electronic
　nervous system -*see* Complication,
　　prosthetic device, mechanical, electronic
　　nervous system stimulator
　urinary -*see* Complications, electronic
　　stimulator, urinary
　esophageal mucosa into cardia of stomach,
　　congenital Q39.8
　esophagus (acquired) K22.8
　　congenital Q39.8
　eyeball (acquired) (lateral) (old) -*see*
　Displacement, globe
　　congenital Q15.8
　　current -*see* Avulsion, eye
　fallopian tube (acquired) N83.4
　　congenital Q50.6
　　opening (congenital) Q50.6
　gallbladder (congenital) Q44.1
　gastric mucosa (congenital) Q40.2
　globe (acquired) (old) (lateral) H05.21
　　current -*see* Avulsion, eye
　heart (congenital) Q24.8
　　acquired I51.89
　hymen (upward) (congenital) Q52.4
　intervertebral disc NEC
　　with myelopathy -*see* Disorder, disc, with,
　　myelopathy
　　cervical, cervicothoracic (with) M50.20
　　　myelopathy -*see* Disorder, disc, cervical,
　　　with myelopathy
　　　neuritis, radiculitis or radiculopathy -*see*
　　　Disorder, disc, cervical, with neuritis
　　due to trauma -*see* Dislocation, vertebra
　　lumbar region M51.26

Displacement, displaced
with
myelopathy M51.06
neuritis, radiculitis, radiculopathy or
sciatica M51.16
lumbosacral region M51.27
with
neuritis, radiculitis, radiculopathy or
sciatica M51.17
sacrococcygeal region M53.3
thoracic region M51.24
with
myelopathy M51.04
neuritis, radiculitis, radiculopathy
M51.14
thoracolumbar region M51.25
with
myelopathy M51.05
neuritis, radiculitis, radiculopathy
M51.15
intrauterine device (string) T83.32
kidney (acquired) N28.83
congenital Q63.2
lachrymal, lacrimal apparatus or duct
(congenital) Q10.6
lens, congenital Q12.1
macula (congenital) Q14.1
Meckel's diverticulum Q43.0
malignant -see Table of Neoplasms, small
intestine, malignant
nail (congenital) Q84.6
acquired L60.8
opening of Wharton's duct in mouth Q38.4
organ or site, congenital NEC -see
Malposition, congenital
ovary (acquired) N83.4
congenital Q50.39
free in peritoneal cavity (congenital) Q50.39
into hernial sac N83.4
oviduct (acquired) N83.4
congenital Q50.6
parathyroid (gland) E21.4
parotid gland (congenital) Q38.4
punctum lacrimale (congenital) Q10.6
sacro-iliac (joint) (congenital) Q74.2
current injury S33.2
old -see subcategory M53.2
salivary gland (any) (congenital) Q38.4
spleen (congenital) Q89.09
stomach, congenital Q40.2
sublingual duct Q38.4
tongue (downward) (congenital) Q38.3
tooth, teeth, fully erupted M26.30
horizontal M26.33
vertical M26.34
trachea (congenital) Q32.1
ureter or ureteric opening or orifice
(congenital) Q62.62
uterine opening of oviducts or fallopian tubes
Q50.6
uterus, uterine -see Malposition, uterus
ventricular septum Q21.0
with rudimentary ventricle Q20.4
Disproportion
between native and reconstructed breast
N65.1
fiber-type G71.2
Disruptio uteri -see Rupture, uterus
Disruption (of)
ciliary body NEC H21.89
closure of

Disruption (of) --continued
cornea T81.31
craniotomy T81.32
fascia (muscular) (superficial) T81.32
internal organ or tissue T81.32
laceration (external) (internal) T81.33
ligament T81.32
mucosa T81.31
muscle or muscle flap T81.32
ribs or rib cage T81.32
skin and subcutaneous tissue (full-thickness)
(superficial) T81.31
skull T81.32
sternum (sternotomy) T81.32
tendon T81.32
traumatic laceration (external) (internal)
T81.33
family Z63.8
due to
absence of family member due to military
deployment Z63.31
absence of family member NEC Z63.32
alcoholism and drug addiction in family
Z63.72
bereavement Z63.4
death (assumed) or disappearance of
family member Z63.4
divorce or separation Z63.5
drug addiction in family Z63.72
return of family member from military
deployment (current or past conflict)
Z63.71
stressful life events NEC Z63.79
iris NEC H21.89
ligament(s) -see also Sprain
knee
current injury -see Dislocation, knee
old (chronic) -see Derangement, knee,
ligament, instability, chronic
spontaneous NEC -see Derangement, knee,
disruption ligament
ossicular chain -see Discontinuity, ossicles,
ear
pelvic ring (stable) S32.810
unstable S32.811
wound T81.30
episiotomy O90.1
operation T81.31
cesarean O90.0
external operation wound (superficial)
T81.31
internal operation wound (deep) T81.32
perineal (obstetric) O90.1
traumatic injury repair T81.33
traumatic injury wound repair T81.33
Dissatisfaction with
employment Z56.9
school environment Z55.4
Dissecting -see condition
Dissection
aorta I71.00
abdominal I71.02
thoracic I71.01
thoracoabdominal I71.03
artery I77.70
basilar (trunk) I77.75
carotid I77.71
cerebral (nonruptured) I67.0
ruptured -see Hemorrhage, intracranial,
subarachnoid
coronary I25.42

Dissection - continued
extremity
lower I77.77
upper I77.76
iliac I77.72
precerebral
congenital (nonruptured) Q28.1
specified site NEC I77.75
renal I77.73
specified NEC I77.79
vertebral I77.74
traumatic -see Wound, open, by site
vascular I99.8
wound -see Wound, open
Disseminated -see condition
Dissociation
auriculoventricular or atrioventricular (AV)
(any degree) (isorhythmic) I45.89
with heart block I44.2
interference I45.89
Dissociative reaction, state F44.9
Dissolution, vertebra -see Osteoporosis
Distension, distention
abdomen R14.0
bladder N32.89
cecum K63.89
colon K63.89
gallbladder K82.8
intestine K63.89
kidney N28.89
liver K76.89
seminal vesicle N50.89
stomach K31.89
acute K31.0
psychogenic F45.8
ureter -see Dilatation, ureter
uterus N85.8
Distoma hepaticum infestation B66.3
Distomiasis B66.9
bile passages B66.3
hemic B65.9
hepatic B66.3
due to Clonorchis sinensis B66.1
intestinal B66.5
liver B66.3
due to Clonorchis sinensis B66.1
lung B66.4
pulmonary B66.4
Distomolar (fourth molar) K00.1
Disto-occlusion (Division I) (Division II)
M26.212
Distortion(s) (congenital)
adrenal (gland) Q89.1
arm NEC Q68.8
bile duct or passage Q44.5
bladder Q64.79
brain Q04.9
cervix (uteri) Q51.9
chest (wall) Q67.8
bones Q76.8
clavicle Q74.0
clitoris Q52.6
coccyx Q76.49
common duct Q44.5
coronary Q24.5
cystic duct Q44.5
ear (auricle) (external) Q17.3
inner Q16.5
middle Q16.4
ossicles Q16.3
endocrine NEC Q89.2
eustachian tube Q17.8

Distortion(s) (congenital)

eye (adnexa) Q15.8
face bone(s) NEC Q75.8
fallopian tube Q50.6
femur NEC Q68.8
fibula NEC Q68.8
finger(s) Q68.1
foot Q66.9
genitalia, genital organ(s)
  female Q52.8
    external Q52.79
    internal NEC Q52.8
gyri Q04.8
hand bone(s) Q68.1
heart (auricle) (ventricle) Q24.8
  valve (cusp) Q24.8
hepatic duct Q44.5
humerus NEC Q68.8
hymen Q52.4
intrafamilial communications Z63.8
jaw NEC M26.89
labium (majus) (minus) Q52.79
leg NEC Q68.8
lens Q12.8
liver Q44.7
lumbar spine Q76.49
  with disproportion O33.8
    causing obstructed labor O65.0
lumbosacral (joint) (region) Q76.49
  kyphosis -see Kyphosis, congenital
  lordosis -see Lordosis, congenital
nerve Q07.8
nose Q30.8
organ
  of Corti Q16.5
  or site not listed -see Anomaly, by site
ossicles, ear Q16.3
oviduct Q50.6
pancreas Q45.3
parathyroid (gland) Q89.2
pituitary (gland) Q89.2
radius NEC Q68.8
sacroiliac joint Q74.2
sacrum Q76.49
scapula Q74.0
shoulder girdle Q74.0
skull bone(s) NEC Q75.8
  with
    anencephalus Q00.0
    encephalocele -see Encephalocele
    hydrocephalus Q03.9
      with spina bifida -see Spina bifida, with
        hydrocephalus
    microcephaly Q02
spinal cord Q06.8
spine Q76.49
  kyphosis -see Kyphosis, congenital
  lordosis -see Lordosis, congenital
spleen Q89.09
sternum NEC Q76.7
thorax (wall) Q67.8
  bony Q76.8
thymus (gland) Q89.2
thyroid (gland) Q89.2
tibia NEC Q68.8
toe(s) Q66.9
tongue Q38.3
trachea (cartilage) Q32.1
ulna NEC Q68.8
ureter Q62.8
urethra Q64.79

Distortion(s) (congenital) --continued

causing obstruction Q64.39
uterus Q51.9
vagina Q52.4
vertebra Q76.49
  kyphosis -see Kyphosis, congenital
  lordosis -see Lordosis, congenital
visual -see also Disturbance, vision
  shape and size H53.15
vulva Q52.79
wrist (bones) (joint) Q68.8

Distress

abdomen -see Pain, abdominal
acute respiratory R06.00
  syndrome (adult) (child) J80
epigastric R10.13
fetal P84
  complicating pregnancy -see Stress, fetal
gastrointestinal (functional) K30
  psychogenic F45.8
intestinal (functional) NOS K59.9
  psychogenic F45.8
maternal, during labor and delivery O75.0
respiratory (adult) (child) R06.00
  newborn P22.9
    specified NEC P22.8
  orthopnea R06.01
  psychogenic F45.8
  shortness of breath R06.02
  specified type NEC R06.09

Distribution vessel, atypical Q27.9

coronary artery Q24.5
precerebral Q28.1

Distichiasis L68.8

Disturbance(s) -see also Disease - absorption K90.9

calcium E58
carbohydrate K90.49
fat K90.49
  pancreatic K90.3
protein K90.49
starch K90.49
vitamin -see Deficiency, vitamin
acid-base equilibrium E87.8
  mixed E87.4
activity and attention (with hyperkinesis) -see
  Disorder, attention-deficit hyperactivity
amino acid transport E72.00
assimilation, food K90.9
auditory nerve, except deafness -see
  subcategory H93.3
behavior -see Disorder, conduct
blood clotting (mechanism) -see also Defect,
  coagulation D68.9
cerebral
  nerve -see Disorder, nerve, cranial
  status, newborn P91.9
    specified NEC P91.8
circulatory I99.9
conduct -see also Disorder, conduct F91.9
  adjustment reaction -see Disorder,
    adjustment
  compulsive F63.9
  disruptive F91.9
  hyperkinetic -see Disorder, attention-deficit
    hyperactivity
  socialized F91.2
  specified NEC F91.8
  unsocialized F91.1
coordination R27.8
cranial nerve -see Disorder, nerve, cranial

Disturbance(s) --continued

deep sensibility -see Disturbance, sensation
digestive K30
  psychogenic F45.8
electrolyte -see also Imbalance, electrolyte
  newborn, transitory P74.4
    hyperammonemia P74.6
    potassium balance P74.3
    sodium balance P74.2
    specified type NEC P74.4
emotions specific to childhood and
adolescence F93.9
  with
    anxiety and fearfulness NEC F93.8
    elective mutism F94.0
    oppositional disorder F91.3
    sensitivity (withdrawal) F40.10
    shyness F40.10
    social withdrawal F40.10
  involving relationship problems F93.8
  mixed F93.8
  specified NEC F93.8
endocrine (gland) E34.9
  neonatal, transitory P72.9
    specified NEC P72.8
equilibrium R42
fructose metabolism E74.10
gait -see Gait
  hysterical F44.4
  psychogenic F44.4
gastrointestinal (functional) K30
  psychogenic F45.8
habit, child F98.9
hearing, except deafness and tinnitus -see
  Abnormal, auditory perception
heart, functional (conditions in I44 I50)
  due to presence of (cardiac) prosthesis
    I97.19
  postoperative I97.89
    cardiac surgery I97.19
hormones E34.9
innervation uterus (parasympathetic)
  (sympathetic) N85.8
keratinization NEC
  gingiva K05.10
    nonplaque induced K05.11
    plaque induced K05.10
  lip K13.0
  oral (mucosa) (soft tissue) K13.29
  tongue K13.29
learning (specific) -see Disorder, learning
memory -see Amnesia
  mild, following organic brain damage F06.8
mental F99
  associated with diseases classified elsewhere
    F54
metabolism E88.9
  with
    abortion -see Abortion, by type with other
      specified complication
    ectopic pregnancy O08.5
    molar pregnancy O08.5
  amino-acid E72.9
    aromatic E70.9
    branched-chain E71.2
    straight-chain E72.8
    sulfur-bearing E72.10
  ammonia E72.20
  arginine E72.21
  arginosuccinic acid E72.22
  carbohydrate E74.9

Disturbance(s) *--continued*
cholesterol E78.9
citrulline E72.23
cystathionine E72.19
general E88.9
glutamine E72.8
histidine E70.40
homocystine E72.19
hydroxylysine E72.3
in labor or delivery O75.89
iron E83.10
lipoid E78.9
lysine E72.3
methionine E72.19
neonatal, transitory P74.9
calcium and magnesium P71.9
specified type NEC P71.8
carbohydrate metabolism P70.9
specified type NEC P70.8
specified NEC P74.8
ornithine E72.4
phosphate E83.39
sodium NEC E87.8
threonine E72.8
tryptophan E70.5
tyrosine E70.20
urea cycle E72.20
motor R29.2
nervous, functional R45.0
neuromuscular mechanism (eye), due to
syphilis A52.15
nutritional E63.9
nail L60.3
ocular motion H51.9
psychogenic F45.8
oculogyric H51.8
psychogenic F45.8
oculomotor H51.9
psychogenic F45.8
olfactory nerve R43.1
optic nerve NEC *-see* Disorder, nerve, optic
oral epithelium, including tongue NEC
K13.29
perceptual due to
alcohol withdrawal F10.232
amphetamine intoxication F15.922
in
abuse F15.122
dependence F15.222
anxiolytic withdrawal F13.232
cannabis intoxication (acute) F12.922
in
abuse F12.122
dependence F12.222
cocaine intoxication (acute) F14.922
in
abuse F14.122
dependence F14.222
hypnotic withdrawal F13.232
opioid intoxication (acute) F11.922
in
abuse F11.122
dependence F11.222
phencyclidine intoxication (acute) F16.122
sedative withdrawal F13.232
personality (pattern) (trait) *-see also* Disorder,
personality F60.9
following organic brain damage F07.9
polyglandular E31.9
specified NEC E31.8
potassium balance, newborn P74.3

Disturbance(s) *--continued*
psychogenic F45.9
psychomotor F44.4
psychophysical visual H53.16
pupillary *-see* Anomaly, pupil, function
reflex R29.2
rhythm, heart I49.9
salivary secretion K11.7
sensation (cold) (heat) (localization) (tactile
discrimination) (texture) (vibratory) NEC
R20.9
hysterical F44.6
skin R20.9
anesthesia R20.0
hyperesthesia R20.3
hypoesthesia R20.1
paresthesia R20.2
specified type NEC R20.8
smell R43.9
and taste (mixed) R43.8
anosmia R43.0
parosmia R43.1
specified NEC R43.8
taste R43.9
and smell (mixed) R43.8
parageusia R43.2
specified NEC R43.8
sensory *-see* Disturbance, sensation
situational (transient) *-see also* Disorder,
adjustment
acute F43.0
sleep G47.9
nonorganic origin F51.9
smell *-see* Disturbance, sensation, smell
sociopathic F60.2
sodium balance, newborn P74.2
speech R47.9
developmental F80.9
specified NEC R47.89
stomach (functional) K31.9
sympathetic (nerve) G90.9
taste *-see* Disturbance, sensation, taste
temperature
regulation, newborn P81.9
specified NEC P81.8
sense R20.8
hysterical F44.6
tooth
eruption K00.6
formation K00.4
structure, hereditary NEC K00.5
touch *-see* Disturbance, sensation
vascular I99.9
arteriosclerotic *-see* Arteriosclerosis
vasomotor I73.9
vasospastic I73.9
vision, visual H53.9
following
cerebral infarction I69.398
cerebrovascular disease I69.998
specified NEC I69.898
intracerebral hemorrhage I69.198
nontraumatic intracranial hemorrhage NEC
I69.298
specified disease NEC I69.898
subarachnoid hemorrhage I69.098
psychophysical H53.16
specified NEC H53.8
subjective H53.10
day blindness H53.11
discomfort H53.14

Disturbance(s) *--continued*
distortions of shape and size H53.15
loss
sudden H53.13
transient H53.12
specified type NEC H53.19
voice R49.9
psychogenic F44.4
specified NEC R49.8
Diuresis R35.8
Diver's palsy, paralysis or squeeze T70.3
Diverticulitis (acute) K57.92
bladder *-see* Cystitis
ileum *-see* Diverticulitis, intestine, small
intestine K57.92
with
abscess, perforation or peritonitis K57.80
with bleeding K57.81
bleeding K57.93
congenital Q43.8
large K57.32
with
abscess, perforation or peritonitis K57.20
with bleeding K57.21
bleeding K57.33
small intestine K57.52
with
abscess, perforation or peritonitis
K57.40
with bleeding K57.41
bleeding K57.53
small K57.12
with
abscess, perforation or peritonitis K57.00
with bleeding K57.01
bleeding K57.13
large intestine K57.52
with
abscess, perforation or peritonitis
K57.40
with bleeding K57.41
bleeding K57.53
Diverticulosis K57.90
with bleeding K57.91
large intestine K57.30
with
bleeding K57.31
small intestine K57.50
with bleeding K57.51
small intestine K57.10
with
bleeding K57.11
large intestine K57.50
with bleeding K57.51
Diverticulum, diverticula (multiple) K57.90
appendix (noninflammatory) K38.2
bladder (sphincter) N32.3
congenital Q64.6
bronchus (congenital) Q32.4
acquired J98.09
calyx, calyceal (kidney) N28.89
cardia (stomach) K31.4
cecum *-see* Diverticulosis, intestine, large
congenital Q43.8
colon *-see* Diverticulosis, intestine, large
congenital Q43.8
duodenum *-see* Diverticulosis, intestine, small
congenital Q43.8
epiphrenic (esophagus) K22.5
esophagus (congenital) Q39.6

Diverticulum, diverticula - *continued*
  acquired (epiphrenic) (pulsion) (traction)
    K22.5
  eustachian tube -*see* Disorder, eustachian
    tube, specified NEC
  fallopian tube N83.8
  gastric K31.4
  heart (congenital) Q24.8
  ileum -*see* Diverticulosis, intestine, small
  jejunum -*see* Diverticulosis, intestine, small
  kidney (pelvis) (calyces) N28.89
    with calculus -*see* Calculus, kidney
  Meckel's (displaced) (hypertrophic) Q43.0
    malignant -*see* Table of Neoplasms, small
      intestine, malignant
  midthoracic K22.5
  organ or site, congenital NEC -*see* Distortion
  pericardium (congenital) (cyst) Q24.8
    acquired I31.8
  pharyngoesophageal (congenital) Q39.6
    acquired K22.5
  pharynx (congenital) Q38.7
  rectosigmoid -*see* Diverticulosis, intestine,
    large
    congenital Q43.8
  rectum -*see* Diverticulosis, intestine, large
  Rokitansky's K22.5
  seminal vesicle N50.89
  sigmoid -*see* Diverticulosis, intestine, large
    congenital Q43.8
  stomach (acquired) K31.4
    congenital Q40.2
  trachea (acquired) J39.8
  ureter (acquired) N28.89
    congenital Q62.8
  ureterovesical orifice N28.89
  urethra (acquired) N36.1
    congenital Q64.79
  ventricle, left (congenital) Q24.8
  vesical N32.3
    congenital Q64.6
  Zenker's (esophagus) K22.5
Division
  cervix uteri (acquired) N88.8
  glans penis Q55.69
  labia minora (congenital) Q52.79
  ligament (partial or complete) (current) -*see*
    also Sprain
    with open wound -*see* Wound, open
  muscle (partial or complete) (current) -*see*
    also Injury, muscle
    with open wound -*see* Wound, open
  nerve (traumatic) -*see* Injury, nerve
  spinal cord -*see* Injury, spinal cord, by region
  vein I87.8
Divorce, causing family disruption Z63.5
Dix Hallpike neurolabyrinthitis -*see*
  Neuronitis, vestibular
Dizziness R42
  hysterical F44.89
  psychogenic F45.8
**DMAC (disseminated mycobacterium
  avium- intracellulare complex)** A31.2
DNR (do not resuscitate) Z66
**Doan-Wiseman syndrome (primary splenic
  neutropenia) -***see* Agranulocytosis
Doehle-Heller aortitis A52.02
Dog bite -*see* Bite
Dohle body panmyelopathic syndrome D72.0
Dolichocephaly Q67.2
Dolichocolon Q43.8

Dolichostenomelia -*see* Syndrome, Marfan's
Donohue's syndrome E34.8
Donor (organ or tissue) Z52.9
  blood (whole) Z52.000
    autologous Z52.010
    specified component (lymphocytes)
      (platelets) NEC Z52.008
      autologous Z52.018
        specified donor NEC Z52.098
    specified donor NEC Z52.090
    stem cells Z52.001
      autologous Z52.011
      specified donor NEC Z52.091
  bone Z52.20
    autologous Z52.21
    marrow Z52.3
    specified type NEC Z52.29
  cornea Z52.5
  egg (Oocyte) Z52.819
    age 35 and over Z52.812
      anonymous recipient Z52.812
      designated recipient Z52.813
    under age 35 Z52.810
      anonymous recipient Z52.810
      designated recipient Z52.811
  kidney Z52.4
  liver Z52.6
  lung Z52.89
  lymphocyte -*see* Donor, blood, specified
    components NEC
  Oocyte -*see* Donor, egg
  platelets Z52.008
  potential, examination of Z00.5
  semen Z52.89
  skin Z52.10
    autologous Z52.11
    specified type NEC Z52.19
  specified organ or tissue NEC Z52.89
  sperm Z52.89
Donovanosis A58
Dorsalgia M54.9
  psychogenic F45.41
  specified NEC M54.89
Dorsopathy M53.9
  deforming M43.9
    specified NEC -*see* subcategory M43.8
  specified NEC M53.80
    cervical region M53.82
    cervicothoracic region M53.83
    lumbar region M53.86
    lumbosacral region M53.87
    occipito-atlanto-axial region M53.81
    sacrococcygeal region M53.88
    thoracic region M53.84
    thoracolumbar region M53.85
Double
  albumin E88.09
  aortic arch Q25.45
  auditory canal Q17.8
  auricle (heart) Q20.8
  bladder Q64.79
  cervix Q51.820
    with doubling of uterus (and vagina) Q51.10
      with obstruction Q51.11
  inlet ventricle Q20.4
  kidney with double pelvis (renal) Q63.0
  meatus urinarius Q64.75
  monster Q89.4
  outlet
    left ventricle Q20.2
    right ventricle Q20.1

Double --*continued*
  pelvis (renal) with double ureter Q62.5
  tongue Q38.3
  ureter (one or both sides) Q62.5
    with double pelvis (renal) Q62.5
  urethra Q64.74
  urinary meatus Q64.75
  uterus Q51.2
    with
      doubling of cervix (and vagina) Q51.10
        with obstruction Q51.11
      in pregnancy or childbirth O34.59
        causing obstructed labor O65.5
  vagina Q52.10
    with doubling of uterus (and cervix) Q51.10
      with obstruction Q51.11
  vision H53.2
  vulva Q52.79
Douglas' pouch, cul-de-sac -*see* condition
Down syndrome Q90.9
  meiotic nondisjunction Q90.0
  mitotic nondisjunction Q90.1
  mosaicism Q90.1
  translocation Q90.2
**DPD (dihydropyrimidine dehydrogenase
  deficiency)** E88.89
Dracontiasis B72
Dracunculiasis, dracunculosis B72
Dream state, hysterical F44.89
Dreschlera (hawaiiensis) (infection) B43.8
Drepanocytic anemia -*see* Disease, sickle-cell
Dresbach's syndrome (elliptocytosis) D58.1
Dressler's syndrome I24.1
Drift, ulnar -*see* Deformity, limb, specified
  type NEC, forearm
Drinking (alcohol)
  excessive, to excess NEC (without
    dependence) F10.10
    habitual (continual) (without remission)
      F10.20
        with remission F10.21
Drip, postnasal (chronic) R09.82
  due to
    allergic rhinitis -*see* Rhinitis, allergic
    common cold J00
    gastroesophageal reflux -*see* Reflux,
      gastroesophageal
    nasopharyngitis -*see* Nasopharyngitis
    other know condition
      code to condition
    sinusitis -*see* Sinusitis
Droop
  facial R29.810
    cerebrovascular disease I69.992
      cerebral infarction I69.392
      intracerebral hemorrhage I69.192
      nontraumatic intracranial hemorrhage NEC
        I69.292
      specified disease NEC I69.892
      subarachnoid hemorrhage I69.092
Drop (in)
  attack NEC R55
  finger -*see* Deformity, finger
  foot -*see* Deformity, limb, foot, drop
  hematocrit (precipitous) R71.0
  hemoglobin R71.0
  toe -*see* Deformity, toe, specified NEC
  wrist -*see* Deformity, limb, wrist drop
Dropped heart beats I45.9

Dropsy, dropsical -*see also* Hydrops
   abdomen R18.8
   brain -*see* Hydrocephalus
   cardiac, heart -*see* Failure, heart, congestive
   gangrenous -*see* Gangrene
   heart -*see* Failure, heart, congestive
   kidney -*see* Nephrosis
   lung -*see* Edema, lung
   newborn due to isoimmunization P56.0
   pericardium -*see* Pericarditis
Drowned, drowning (near) T75.1
Drowsiness R40.0
Drug
   abuse counseling and surveillance Z71.51
   addiction -*see* Dependence
   dependence -*see* Dependence
   habit -*see* Dependence
   harmful use -*see* Abuse, drug
   induced fever R50.2
   overdose -*see* Table of Drugs and Chemicals,
      by drug, poisoning
   poisoning -*see* Table of Drugs and Chemicals,
      by drug, poisoning
   resistant organism infection -*see also*
      Resistant, organism, to, drug Z16.30
   therapy
      long term (current) (prophylactic) -*see*
         Therapy, drug long-term (current)
         (prophylactic)
      short term
   omit code
   wrong substance given or taken in error -*see*
      Table of Drugs and Chemicals, by drug,
      poisoning
Drunkenness (without dependence) F10.129
   acute in alcoholism F10.229
   chronic (without remission) F10.20
      with remission F10.21
   pathological (without dependence) F10.129
      with dependence F10.229
   sleep F51.9
Drusen
   macula (degenerative) (retina) -*see*
      Degeneration, macula, drusen
   optic disc H47.32
Dry, dryness -*see also* condition
   larynx J38.7
   mouth R68.2
      due to dehydration E86.0
   nose J34.89
   socket (teeth) M27.3
   throat J39.2
DSAP L56.5
Duane's syndrome H50.81
Dubin-Johnson disease or syndrome E80.6
Dubois' disease (thymus gland) A50.59 [*E35*]
Dubowitz' syndrome Q87.1
Duchenne-Aran muscular atrophy G12.21
Duchenne-Griesinger disease G71.0
Duchenne's
   disease or syndrome
      motor neuron disease G12.22
      muscular dystrophy G71.0
   locomotor ataxia (syphilitic) A52.11
   paralysis
      birth injury P14.0
      due to or associated with
         motor neuron disease G12.22
         muscular dystrophy G71.0
Ducrey's chancre A57
Duct, ductus -*see* condition

Duhring's disease (dermatitis herpetiformis)
   L13.0
Dullness, cardiac (decreased) (increased)
   R01.2
Dumb ague -*see* Malaria
Dumbness -*see* Aphasia
Dumdum fever B55.0
Dumping syndrome (postgastrectomy) K91.1
Duodenitis (nonspecific) (peptic) K29.80
   with bleeding K29.81
Duodenocholangitis -*see* Cholangitis
Duodenum, duodenal -*see* condition
Duplay's bursitis or periarthritis -*see*
   Tendinitis, calcific, shoulder
Duplication, duplex -*see also* Accessory
   alimentary tract Q45.8
   anus Q43.4
   appendix (and cecum) Q43.4
   biliary duct (any) Q44.5
   bladder Q64.79
   cecum (and appendix) Q43.4
   cervix Q51.820
   chromosome NEC
      with complex rearrangements NEC Q92.5
      seen only at prometaphase Q92.8
   cystic duct Q44.5
   digestive organs Q45.8
   esophagus Q39.8
   frontonasal process Q75.8
   intestine (large) (small) Q43.4
   kidney Q63.0
   liver Q44.7
   pancreas Q45.3
   penis Q55.69
   respiratory organs NEC Q34.8
   salivary duct Q38.4
   spinal cord (incomplete) Q06.2
   stomach Q40.2
Dupré's disease (meningism) R29.1
Dupuytren's contraction or disease M72.0
Durand-Nicolas-Favre disease A55
Durotomy (inadvertent) (incidental) G97.41
Duroziez's disease (congenital mitral
   stenosis) Q23.2
Dutton's relapsing fever (West African)
   A68.1
Dwarfism E34.3
   achondroplastic Q77.4
   congenital E34.3
   constitutional E34.3
   hypochondroplastic Q77.4
   hypophyseal E23.0
   infantile E34.3
   Laron-type E34.3
   Lorain (Levi) type E23.0
   metatropic Q77.8
   nephrotic-glycosuric (with hypophosphatemic
   rickets) E72.09
   nutritional E45
   pancreatic K86.89
   pituitary E23.0
   renal N25.0
   thanatophoric Q77.1
Dyke-Young anemia (secondary)
   (symptomatic) D59.1
Dysacusis -*see* Abnormal, auditory perception
Dysadrenocortism E27.9
   hyperfunction E27.0
Dysarthria R47.1
   following
      cerebral infarction I69.322

Dysarthria --*continued*
   cerebrovascular disease I69.922
      specified disease NEC I69.822
   intracerebral hemorrhage I69.122
   nontraumatic intracranial hemorrhage NEC
      I69.222
   subarachnoid hemorrhage I69.022
Dysautonomia (familial) G90.1
Dysbarism T70.3
Dysbasia R26.2
   angiosclerotica intermittens I73.9
   hysterical F44.4
   lordotica (progressiva) G24.1
   nonorganic origin F44.4
   psychogenic F44.4
Dysbetalipoproteinemia (familial) E78.2
Dyscalculia R48.8
   developmental F81.2
Dyschezia K59.00
Dyschondroplasia (with hemangiomata)
   Q78.4
Dyschromia (skin) L81.9
Dyscollagenosis M35.9
Dyscranio-pygo-phalangy Q87.0
Dyscrasia
   blood (with) D75.9
      antepartum hemorrhage -*see* Hemorrhage,
         antepartum, with coagulation defect
      newborn P61.9
         specified type NEC P61.8
      intrapartum hemorrhage O67.0
      puerperal, postpartum O72.3
   polyglandular, plurigalndular E31.9
Dysendocrinism E34.9
Dysentery, dysenteric (catarrhal) (diarrhea)
   (epidemic) (hemorrhagic) (infectious)
   (sporadic) (tropical) A09
   abscess, liver A06.4
   amebic -*see also* Amebiasis A06.0
      with abscess -*see* Abscess, amebic
      acute A06.0
      chronic A06.1
   arthritis -*see also* category M01 A09
      bacillary -*see also* category M01 A03.9
   bacillary A03.9
      arthritis -*see also* category M01 A03.9
      Boyd A03.2
      Flexner A03.1
      Schmitz (Stutzer) A03.0
      Shiga (Kruse) A03.0
      Shigella A03.9
         boydii A03.2
         dysenteriae A03.0
         flexneri A03.1
         group A A03.0
         group B A03.1
         group C A03.2
         group D A03.3
         sonnei A03.3
         specified type NEC A03.8
      Sonne A03.3
      specified type NEC A03.8
   balantidial A07.0
   Balantidium coli A07.0
   Boyd's A03.2
   candidal B37.82
   Chilomastix A07.8
   Chinese A03.9
   coccidial A07.3
   Dientamoeba (fragilis) A07.8
   Embadomonas A07.8

Dysentery, dysenteric --*continued*
  Entamoeba, entamebic -*see* Dysentery,
  amebic
  Flexner-Boyd A03.2
  Flexner's A03.1
  Giardia lamblia A07.1
  Hiss-Russell A03.1
  Lamblia A07.1
  leishmanial B55.0
  malarial -*see* Malaria
  metazoal B82.0
  monilial B37.82
  protozoal A07.9
  Salmonella A02.0
  schistosomal B65.1
  Schmitz (Stutzer) A03.0
  Shiga (Kruse) A03.0
  Shigella NOS -*see* Dysentery, bacillary
  Sonne A03.3
  strongyloidiasis B78.0
  trichomonal A07.8
  viral -*see also* Enteritis, viral A08.4
Dysequilibrium R42
Dysesthesia R20.8
  hysterical F44.6
Dysfibrinogenemia (congenital) D68.2
Dysfunction
  adrenal E27.9
    hyperfunction E27.0
  autonomic
    due to alcohol G31.2
    somatoform F45.8
  bladder N31.9
    neurogenic NOS -*see* Dysfunction, bladder,
    neuromuscular
    neuromuscular NOS N31.9
      atonic (motor) (sensory) N31.2
      autonomous N31.2
      flaccid N31.2
      nonreflex N31.2
      reflex N31.1
      specified NEC N31.8
      uninhibited N31.0
  bleeding, uterus N93.8
  cerebral G93.89
  colon K59.9
    psychogenic F45.8
  colostomy K94.03
  cystic duct K82.8
  cystostomy (stoma) -*see* Complications,
    cystostomy
  ejaculatory N53.19
    anejaculatory orgasm N53.13
    painful N53.12
    premature F52.4
    retarded N53.11
  endocrine NOS E34.9
  endometrium N85.8
  enterostomy K94.13
  erectile -*see* Dysfunction, sexual, male,
    erectile
  gallbladder K82.8
  gastrostomy (stoma) K94.23
  gland, glandular NOS E34.9
  heart I51.89
  hemoglobin D75.89
  hepatic K76.89
  hypophysis E23.7
  hypothalamic NEC E23.3
  ileostomy (stoma) K94.13
  jejunostomy (stoma) K94.13

Dysfunction - *continued*
  kidney -*see* Disease, renal
  labyrinthine - see subcategory H83.2
  left ventricular, following sudden emotional
    stress I51.81
  liver K76.89
  male -*see* Dysfunction, sexual, male
  orgasmic (female) F52.31
    male F52.32
  ovary E28.9
    specified NEC E28.8
  papillary muscle I51.89
  parathyroid E21.4
  physiological NEC R68.89
    psychogenic F59
  pineal gland E34.8
  pituitary (gland) E23.3
  platelets D69.1
  polyglandular E31.9
    specified NEC E31.8
  psychophysiologic F59
  psychosexual F52.9
    with
      dyspareunia F52.6
      premature ejaculation F52.4
      vaginismus F52.5
  pylorus K31.9
  rectum K59.9
    psychogenic F45.8
  reflex (sympathetic) -*see* Syndrome, pain,
    complex regional I
  segmental -*see* Dysfunction, somatic
  senile R54
  sexual (due to) R37
    alcohol F10.981
    amphetamine F15.981
      in
        abuse F15.181
        dependence F15.281
    anxiolytic F13.981
      in
        abuse F13.181
        dependence F13.281
    cocaine F14.981
      in
        abuse F14.181
        dependence F14.281
    excessive sexual drive F52.8
    failure of genital response (male) F52.21
      female F52.22
    female N94.9
      aversion F52.1
      dyspareunia N94.10
        psychogenic F52.6
      frigidity F52.22
      nymphomania F52.8
      orgasmic F52.31
      psychogenic F52.9
        aversion F52.1
        dyspareunia F52.6
        frigidity F52.22
        nymphomania F52.8
        orgasmic F52.31
        vaginismus F52.5
      vaginismus N94.2
        psychogenic F52.5
    hypnotic F13.981
      in
        abuse F13.181
        dependence F13.281
    inhibited orgasm (female) F52.31

Dysfunction - *continued*
  male F52.32
  lack
    of sexual enjoyment F52.1
    or loss of sexual desire F52.0
  male N53.9
    anejaculatory orgasm N53.13
    ejaculatory N53.19
      painful N53.12
      premature F52.4
      retarded N53.11
    erectile N52.9
      drug induced N52.2
      due to
        disease classified elsewhere N52.1
        drug N52.2
      postoperative (postprocedural) N52.39
        following
          cryotherapy N52.37
          interstitial seed therapy N52.36
          prostate ablative therapy N52.37
          prostatectomy N52.34
            radical N52.31
          radiation therapy N52.35
          radical cystectomy N52.32
          ultrasound ablative therapy N52.37
          urethral surgery N52.33
      psychogenic F52.21
      specified cause NEC N52.8
      vasculogenic
        arterial insufficiency N52.01
          with corporo-venous occlusive N52.03
        corporo-venous occlusive N52.02
          with arterial insufficiency N52.03
    impotence -*see* Dysfunction, sexual, male,
      erectile
    psychogenic F52.9
      aversion F52.1
      erectile F52.21
      orgasmic F52.32
      premature ejaculation F52.4
      satyriasis F52.8
      specified type NEC F52.8
    specified type NEC N53.8
  nonorganic F52.9
    specified NEC F52.8
  opioid F11.981
    in
      abuse F11.181
      dependence F11.281
  orgasmic dysfunction (female) F52.31
    male F52.32
  premature ejaculation F52.4
  psychoactive substances NEC F19.981
    in
      abuse F19.181
      dependence F19.281
  psychogenic F52.9
  sedative F13.981
    in
      abuse F13.181
      dependence F13.281
  sexual aversion F52.1
  vaginismus (nonorganic) (psychogenic)
    F52.5
  sinoatrial node I49.5
  somatic M99.09
    abdomen M99.09
    acromioclavicular M99.07
    cervical region M99.01
    cervicothoracic M99.01

Dysfunction - *continued*
  costochondral M99.08
  costovertebral M99.08
  head region M99.00
  hip M99.05
  lower extremity M99.06
  lumbar region M99.03
  lumbosacral M99.03
  occipitocervical M99.00
  pelvic region M99.05
  pubic M99.05
  rib cage M99.08
  sacral region M99.04
  sacrococcygeal M99.04
  sacroiliac M99.04
  specified NEC M99.09
  sternochondral M99.08
  sternoclavicular M99.07
  thoracic region M99.02
  thoracolumbar M99.02
  upper extremity M99.07
  somatoform autonomic F45.8
  stomach K31.89
    psychogenic F45.8
  suprarenal E27.9
    hyperfunction E27.0
  symbolic R48.9
    specified type NEC R48.8
  temporomandibular (joint) M26.69
    joint-pain syndrome M26.62
  testicular (endocrine) E29.9
    specified NEC E29.8
  thymus E32.9
  thyroid E07.9
  ureterostomy (stoma) -*see* Complications, stoma, urinary tract
  uterus, complicating delivery O62.9
    hypertonic O62.4
    hypotonic O62.2
      primary O62.0
      secondary O62.1
  ventricular I51.9
    with congestive heart failure I50.9   left, reversible, following sudden emotional stress I51.81
Dysgenesis
  gonadal (due to chromosomal anomaly) Q96.9
    pure Q99.1
  renal Q60.5
    bilateral Q60.4
    unilateral Q60.3
  reticular D72.0
  tidal platelet D69.3
Dysgerminoma
  specified site -*see* Neoplasm, malignant, by site
  unspecified site
    female C56.9
    male C62.90
Dysgeusia R43.2
Dysgraphia R27.8
Dyshidrosis, dysidrosis L30.1
Dyskaryotic cervical smear R87.619
Dyskeratosis L85.8
  cervix -*see* Dysplasia, cervix
  congenital Q82.8
  uterus NEC N85.8
Dyskinesia G24.9
  biliary (cystic duct or gallbladder) K82.8
  drug induced

Dyskinesia - *continued*
  orofacial G24.01
  esophagus K22.4
  hysterical F44.4
  intestinal K59.8
  nonorganic origin F44.4
  orofacial (idiopathic) G24.4
    drug induced G24.01
  psychogenic F44.4
  subacute, drug induced G24.01
  tardive G24.01
    neuroleptic induced G24.01
  trachea J39.8
  tracheobronchial J98.09
Dyslalia (developmental) F80.0
Dyslexia R48.0
  developmental F81.0
Dyslipidemia E78.5
  depressed HDL cholesterol E78.6
  elevated fasting triglycerides E78.1
Dysmaturity -*see also* Light for dates
  pulmonary (newborn) (Wilson-Mikity) P27.0
Dysmenorrhea (essential) (exfoliative) N94.6
  congestive (syndrome) N94.6
  primary N94.4
  psychogenic F45.8
  secondary N94.5
Dysmetabolic syndrome X E88.81
Dysmetria R27.8
Dysmorphism (due to)
  alcohol Q86.0
  exogenous cause NEC Q86.8
  hydantoin Q86.1
  warfarin Q86.2
Dysmorphophobia (nondelusional) F45.22
  delusional F22
Dysnomia R47.01
Dysorexia R63.0
  psychogenic F50.89
Dysostosis
  cleidocranial, cleidocranialis Q74.0
  craniofacial Q75.1
  Fairbank's (idiopathic familial generalized osteophytosis) Q78.9
  mandibulofacial (incomplete) Q75.4
  multiplex E76.01
  oculomandibular Q75.5
Dyspareunia (female) N94.10
  deep N94.12
  male N53.12
  nonorganic F52.6
  psychogenic F52.6
  secondary N94.19
  specified NEC N94.19
  superficial (introital) N94.11
Dyspepsia R10.13
  atonic K30
  functional (allergic) (congenital) (gastrointestinal) (occupational) (reflex) K30
  intestinal K59.8
  nervous F45.8
  neurotic F45.8
  psychogenic F45.8
Dysphagia R13.10
  cervical R13.19
  following
    cerebral infarction I69.391
    cerebrovascular disease I69.991
      specified NEC I69.891
    intracerebral hemorrhage I69.191

Dysphagia --*continued*
    nontraumatic intracranial hemorrhage NEC I69.291
    specified disease NEC I69.891
    subarachnoid hemorrhage I69.091
  functional (hysterical) F45.8
  hysterical F45.8
  nervous (hysterical) F45.8
  neurogenic R13.19
  oral phase R13.11
  oropharyngeal phase R13.12
  pharyngeal phase R13.13
  pharyngoesophageal phase R13.14
  psychogenic F45.8
  sideropenic D50.1
  spastica K22.4
  specified NEC R13.19
Dysphagocytosis, congenital D71
Dysphasia R47.02
  developmental
    expressive type F80.1
    receptive type F80.2
  following
    cerebrovascular disease I69.921
      cerebral infarction I69.321
      intracerebral hemorrhage I69.121
      nontraumatic intracranial hemorrhage NEC I69.221
      specified disease NEC I69.821
      subarachnoid hemorrhage I69.021
Dysphonia R49.0
  functional F44.4
  hysterical F44.4
  psychogenic F44.4
  spastica J38.3
Dysphoria
  gender
    in
      adolescence and adulthood F64.0
      children F64.2
    postpartal O90.6
Dyspituitarism E23.3
Dysplasia -*see also* Anomaly
  acetabular, congenital Q65.89
  alveolar capillary, with vein misalignment J84.843
  anus (histologically confirmed) (mild) (moderate) K62.82
    severe D01.3
  arrhythmogenic right ventricular I42.8
  arterial, fibromuscular I77.3
  asphyxiating thoracic (congenital) Q77.2
  brain Q07.9
  bronchopulmonary, perinatal P27.1
  cervix (uteri) N87.9
    mild N87.0
    moderate N87.1
    severe D06.9
  chondroectodermal Q77.6
  colon D12.6
  craniometaphyseal Q78.8
  dentinal K00.5
  diaphyseal, progressive Q78.3
  dystrophic Q77.5
  ectodermal (anhidrotic) (congenital) (hereditary) Q82.4
    hydrotic Q82.8
  epithelial, uterine cervix -*see* Dysplasia, cervix
  eye (congenital) Q11.2
  fibrous

Dysplasia - *continued*
bone NEC (monostotic) M85.00
ankle M85.07
foot M85.07
forearm M85.03
hand M85.04
lower leg M85.06
multiple site M85.09
neck M85.08
rib M85.08
shoulder M85.01
skull M85.08
specified site NEC M85.08
thigh M85.05
toe M85.07
upper arm M85.02
vertebra M85.08
diaphyseal, progressive Q78.3
jaw M27.8
polyostotic Q78.1
florid osseous -*see also* Cyst, calcifying
odontogenic
high grade, focal D12.6
hip, congenital Q65.89
joint, congenital Q74.8
kidney Q61.4
multicystic Q61.4
leg Q74.2
lung, congenital (not associated with short
gestation) Q33.6
mammary (gland) (benign) N60.9
cyst (solitary) -*see* Cyst, breast
cystic -*see* Mastopathy, cystic
duct ectasia -*see* Ectasia, mammary duct
fibroadenosis -*see* Fibroadenosis, breast
fibrosclerosis -*see* Fibrosclerosis, breast
specified type NEC N60.8
metaphyseal Q78.5
muscle Q79.8
oculodentodigital Q87.0
periapical (cemental) (cemento-osseous) -*see*
Cyst, calcifying odontogenic
periosteum -*see* Disorder, bone, specified type
NEC
polyostotic fibrous Q78.1
prostate -*see also* Neoplasia, intraepithelial,
prostate N42.30
severe D07.5
specified NEC N42.39
renal Q61.4
multicystic Q61.4
retinal, congenital Q14.1
right ventricular, arrhythmogenic I42.8
septo-optic Q04.4
skin L98.8
spinal cord Q06.1
spondyloepiphyseal Q77.7
thymic, with immunodeficiency D82.1
vagina N89.3
mild N89.0
moderate N89.1
severe NEC D07.2
vulva N90.3
mild N90.0
moderate N90.1
severe NEC D07.1
Dyspnea (nocturnal) (paroxysmal) R06.00
asthmatic (bronchial) J45.909
with
exacerbation (acute) J45.901
bronchitis J45.909

Dyspnea --*continued*
with
exacerbation (acute) J45.901
status asthmaticus J45.902
chronic J44.9
status asthmaticus J45.902
cardiac -*see* Failure, ventricular, left
cardiac -*see* Failure, ventricular, left
functional F45.8
hyperventilation R06.4
hysterical F45.8
newborn P28.89
orthopnea R06.01
psychogenic F45.8
shortness of breath R06.02
specified type NEC R06.09
Dyspraxia R27.8
developmental (syndrome) F82
Dysproteinemia E88.09
Dysreflexia, autonomic G90.4
Dysrhythmia
cardiac I49.9
newborn
bradycardia P29.12
occurring before birth P03.819
before onset of labor P03.810
during labor P03.811
tachycardia P29.11
postoperative I97.89
cerebral or cortical -*see* Epilepsy
Dyssomnia -*see* Disorder, sleep
Dyssynergia
biliary K83.8
bladder sphincter N36.44
cerebellaris myoclonica (Hunt's ataxia) G11.1
Dysthymia F34.1
Dysthyroidism E07.9
Dystocia O66.9
affecting newborn P03.1
cervical (hypotonic) O62.2
affecting newborn P03.6
primary O62.0
secondary O62.1
contraction ring O62.4
fetal O66.9
abnormality NEC O66.3
conjoined twins O66.3
oversize O66.2
maternal O66.9
positional O64.9
shoulder (girdle) O66.0
causing obstructed labor O66.0
uterine NEC O62.4
Dystonia G24.9
deformans progressiva G24.1
drug induced NEC G24.09
acute G24.02
specified NEC G24.09
familial G24.1
idiopathic G24.1
familial G24.1
nonfamilial G24.2
orofacial G24.4
lenticularis G24.8
musculorum deformans G24.1
neuroleptic induced (acute) G24.02
orofacial (idiopathic) G24.4
oromandibular G24.4
due to drug G24.01
specified NEC G24.8
torsion (familial) (idiopathic) G24.1

Dystonia - *continued*
acquired G24.8
genetic G24.1
symptomatic (nonfamilial) G24.2
Dystonic movements R25.8
Dystrophy, dystrophia
adiposogenital E23.6
Becker's type G71.0
cervical sympathetic G90.2
choroid (hereditary) H31.20
central areolar H31.22
choroideremia H31.21
gyrate atrophy H31.23
specified type NEC H31.29
cornea (hereditary) H18.50
endothelial H18.51
epithelial H18.52
granular H18.53
lattice H18.54
macular H18.55
specified type NEC H18.59
Duchenne's type G71.0
due to malnutrition E45
Erb's G71.0
Fuchs' H18.51
Gower's muscular G71.0
hair L67.8
infantile neuraxonal G31.89
Landouzy Déjérine G71.0
Leyden-Möbius G71.0
muscular G71.0
benign (Becker type) G71.0
congenital (hereditary) (progressive) (with
specific morphological abnormalities of
the muscle fiber) G71.0
myotonic G71.11
distal G71.0
Duchenne type G71.0
Emery Dreifuss G71.0
Erb type G71.0
facioscapulohumeral G71.0
Gower's G71.0
hereditary (progressive) G71.0
Landouzy Déjérine type G71.0
limb-girdle G71.0
myotonic G71.11
progressive (hereditary) G71.0
Charcot-Marie (Tooth) type G60.0
pseudohypertrophic (infantile) G71.0
severe (Duchenne type) G71.0
myocardium, myocardial -*see* Degeneration,
myocardial
myotonic, myotonica G71.11
nail L60.3
congenital Q84.6
nutritional E45
ocular G71.0
oculocerebrorenal E72.03
oculopharyngeal G71.0
ovarian N83.8
polyglandular E31.8
reflex (neuromuscular) (sympathetic) -*see*
Syndrome, pain, complex regional I
retinal (hereditary) H35.50
in
lipid storage disorders E75.6 [*H36*]
systemic lipidoses E75.6 [*H36*]
involving
pigment epithelium H35.54
sensory area H35.53
pigmentary H35.52

Dystrophy, dystrophia - *continued*
  vitreoretinal H35.51
  Salzmann's nodular -*see* Degeneration,
    cornea, nodular
  scapuloperoneal G71.0
  skin NEC L98.8
  sympathetic (reflex) -*see* Syndrome, pain,
    complex regional I
     cervical G90.2
  tapetoretinal H35.54
  thoracic, asphyxiating Q77.2
  unguium L60.3
    congenital Q84.6
  vitreoretinal H35.51
  vulva N90.4
  yellow (liver) -*see* Failure, hepatic
Dysuria R30.0
  psychogenic F45.8

E

Eales' disease H35.06
Ear -*see also* condition
  piercing Z41.3
  tropical NEC B36.9 [*H62.40*]
    in
     aspergillosis B44.89
     candidiasis B37.84
     moniliasis B37.84
  wax (impacted) H61.20
    left H61.22
     with right H61.23
    right H61.21
     with left H61.23
Earache -*see* subcategory H92.0
Early satiety R68.81
Eaton-Lambert syndrome -*see* Syndrome,
  Lambert-Eaton
Eberth's disease (typhoid fever) A01.00
Ebola virus disease A98.4
Ebstein's anomaly or syndrome (heart)
  Q22.5
Eccentro-osteochondrodysplasia E76.29
Ecchondroma -*see* Neoplasm, bone, benign
Ecchondrosis D48.0
Ecchymosis R58
  conjunctiva -*see* Hemorrhage, conjunctiva
  eye (traumatic) -*see* Contusion, eyeball
  eyelid (traumatic) -*see* Contusion, eyelid
  newborn P54.5
  spontaneous R23.3
  traumatic -*see* Contusion
Echinococciasis -*see* Echinococcus
Echinococcosis -*see* Echinococcus
Echinococcus (infection) B67.90
  granulosus B67.4
    bone B67.2
    liver B67.0
    lung B67.1
    multiple sites B67.32
    specified site NEC B67.39
    thyroid B67.31
  liver NOS B67.8
    granulosus B67.0
    multilocularis B67.5
  lung NEC B67.99
    granulosus B67.1
    multilocularis B67.69
  multilocularis B67.7
    liver B67.5
    multiple sites B67.61

Echinococcus (infection) --*continued*
    specified site NEC B67.69
  specified site NEC B67.99
    granulosus B67.39
    multilocularis B67.69
  thyroid NEC B67.99
    granulosus B67.31
    multilocularis B67.69 [*E35*]
Echinorhynchiasis B83.8
Echinostomiasis B66.8
Echolalia R48.8
Echovirus, as cause of disease classified
  elsewhere B97.12
Eclampsia, eclamptic (coma) (convulsions)
  (delirium) (with hypertension) NEC O15.9
  complicating
    labor and delivery O15.1
    postpartum O15.2
    pregnancy O15.0
    puerperium O15.2
Economic circumstances affecting care Z59.9
Economo's disease A85.8
Ectasia, ectasis
  annuloaortic I35.8
  aorta I77.819
    with aneurysm -*see* Aneurysm, aorta
    abdominal I77.811
    thoracic I77.810
    thoracoabdominal I77.812
  breast -*see* Ectasia, mammary duct
  capillary I78.8
  cornea H18.71
  gastric antral vascular (GAVE) K31.819
    with hemorrhage K31.811
    without hemorrhage K31.819
  mammary duct N60.4
  salivary gland (duct) K11.8
  sclera -*see* Sclerectasia
Ecthyma L08.0
  contagiosum B08.02
  gangrenosum L08.0
  infectiosum B08.02
Ectocardia Q24.8
Ectodermal dysplasia (anhidrotic) Q82.4
Ectodermosis erosiva pluriorificialis L51.1
Ectopic, ectopia (congenital)
  abdominal viscera Q45.8
    due to defect in anterior abdominal wall
     Q79.59
  ACTH syndrome E24.3
  adrenal gland Q89.1
  anus Q43.5
  atrial beats I49.1
  beats I49.49
    atrial I49.1
    ventricular I49.3
  bladder Q64.10
  bone and cartilage in lung Q33.5
  brain Q04.8
  breast tissue Q83.8
  cardiac Q24.8
  cerebral Q04.8
  cordis Q24.8
  endometrium -*see* Endometriosis
  gastric mucosa Q40.2
  gestation -*see* Pregnancy, by site
  heart Q24.8
  hormone secretion NEC E34.2
  kidney (crossed) (pelvis) Q63.2
  lens, lentis Q12.1
  mole -*see* Pregnancy, by site

Ectopic, ectopia - *continued*
  organ or site NEC -*see* Malposition,
    congenital
  pancreas Q45.3
  pregnancy -*see* Pregnancy, ectopic
  pupil -*see* Abnormality, pupillary
  renal Q63.2
  sebaceous glands of mouth Q38.6
  spleen Q89.09
  testis Q53.00
    bilateral Q53.02
    unilateral Q53.01
  thyroid Q89.2
  tissue in lung Q33.5
  ureter Q62.63
  ventricular beats I49.3
  vesicae Q64.10
Ectromelia Q73.8
  lower limb -*see* Defect, reduction, limb,
    lower, specified type NEC
  upper limb -*see* Defect, reduction, limb,
    upper, specified type NEC
Ectropion H02.109
  cervix N86
    with cervicitis N72
  congenital Q10.1
  eyelid (paralytic) H02.109
    cicatricial H02.119
     left H02.116
      lower H02.115
      upper H02.114
     right H02.113
      lower H02.112
      upper H02.111
    congenital Q10.1
    left H02.106
     lower H02.105
     upper H02.104
    mechanical H02.129
     left H02.126
      lower H02.125
      upper H02.124
     right H02.123
      lower H02.122
      upper H02.121
    right H02.103
     lower H02.102
     upper H02.101
    senile H02.139
     left H02.136
      lower H02.135
      upper H02.134
     right H02.133
      lower H02.132
      upper H02.131
    spastic H02.149
     left H02.146
      lower H02.145
      upper H02.144
     right H02.143
      lower H02.142
      upper H02.141
  iris H21.89
  lip (acquired) K13.0
    congenital Q38.0
  urethra N36.8
  uvea H21.89
Eczema (acute) (chronic) (erythematous)
  (fissum) (rubrum) (squamous) -*see also*
  Dermatitis L30.9
  contact -*see* Dermatitis, contact

Eczema - *continued*
dyshidrotic L30.1
external ear -*see* Otitis, externa, acute, eczematoid
flexural L20.82
herpeticum B00.0
hypertrophicum L28.0
hypostatic -*see* Varix, leg, with, inflammation
impetiginous L01.1
infantile (due to any substance) L20.83
  intertriginous L21.1
  seborrheic L21.1
intertriginous NEC L30.4
  infantile L21.1
intrinsic (allergic) L20.84
lichenified NEC L28.0
marginatum (hebrae) B35.6
pustular L30.3
stasis I87.2
  with varicose veins -*see* Varix, leg, with, inflammation
vaccination, vaccinatum T88.1
varicose -*see* Varix, leg, with, inflammation
Eczematid L30.2
Eddowes (Spurway) syndrome Q78.0
Edema, edematous (infectious) (pitting) (toxic) R60.9
with nephritis -*see* Nephrosis
allergic T78.3
amputation stump (surgical) (sequelae (late effect)) T87.89
angioneurotic (allergic) (any site) (with urticaria) T78.3
  hereditary D84.1
angiospastic I73.9
Berlin's (traumatic) S05.8X
brain (cytotoxic) (vasogenic) G93.6
  due to birth injury P11.0
  newborn (anoxia or hypoxia) P52.4
    birth injury P11.0
  traumatic -*see* Injury, intracranial, cerebral edema
cardiac -*see* Failure, heart, congestive
cardiovascular -*see* Failure, heart, congestive
cerebral -*see* Edema, brain
cerebrospinal -*see* Edema, brain
cervix (uteri) (acute) N88.8
  puerperal, postpartum O90.89
chronic hereditary Q82.0
circumscribed, acute T78.3
  hereditary D84.1
conjunctiva H11.42
cornea H18.2
  idiopathic H18.22
  secondary H18.23
    due to contact lens H18.21
due to
  lymphatic obstruction I89.0
  salt retention E87.0
epiglottis -*see* Edema, glottis
essential, acute T78.3
  hereditary D84.1
extremities, lower -*see* Edema, legs
eyelid NEC H02.849
  left H02.846
    lower H02.845
    upper H02.844
  right H02.843
    lower H02.842
    upper H02.841
familial, hereditary Q82.0

Edema, edematous --*continued*
famine -*see* Malnutrition, severe
generalized R60.1
glottis, glottic, glottidis (obstructive) (passive) J38.4
  allergic T78.3
    hereditary D84.1
heart -*see* Failure, heart, congestive
heat T67.7
hereditary Q82.0
inanition -*see* Malnutrition, severe
intracranial G93.6
iris H21.89
joint -*see* Effusion, joint
larynx -*see* Edema, glottis
legs R60.0
  due to venous obstruction I87.1
  hereditary Q82.0
localized R60.0
  due to venous obstruction I87.1
lower limbs -*see* Edema, legs
lung J81.1
  with heart condition or failure -*see* Failure, ventricular, left
  acute J81.0
  chemical (acute) J68.1
    chronic J68.1
  chronic J81.1
    due to
      chemicals, gases, fumes or vapors (inhalation) J68.1
      external agent J70.9
        specified NEC J70.8
      radiation J70.1
  due to
    chemicals, fumes or vapors (inhalation) J68.1
    external agent J70.9
      specified NEC J70.8
    high altitude T70.29
    near drowning T75.1
    radiation J70.0
  meaning failure, left ventricle I50.1
lymphatic I89.0
  due to mastectomy I97.2
macula H35.81
  cystoid, following cataract surgery -*see* Complications, postprocedural, following cataract surgery
  diabetic -*see* Diabetes, by type, with, retinopathy, with macular edema
malignant -*see* Gangrene, gas
Milroy's Q82.0
nasopharynx J39.2
newborn P83.30
  hydrops fetalis -*see* Hydrops, fetalis
  specified NEC P83.39
nutritional -*see also* Malnutrition, severe
  with dyspigmentation, skin and hair E40
optic disc or nerve -*see* Papilledema
orbit H05.22
pancreas K86.89
papilla, optic -*see* Papilledema
penis N48.89
periodic T78.3
  hereditary D84.1
pharynx J39.2
pulmonary -*see* Edema, lung
Quincke's T78.3
  hereditary D84.1
renal -*see* Nephrosis

Edema, edematous --*continued*
retina H35.81
  diabetic -*see* Diabetes, by type, with, retinopathy, with macular edema
salt E87.0
scrotum N50.89
seminal vesicle N50.89
spermatic cord N50.89
spinal (cord) (vascular) (nontraumatic) G95.19
starvation -*see* Malnutrition, severe
stasis -*see* Hypertension, venous, (chronic)
subglottic -*see* Edema, glottis
supraglottic -*see* Edema, glottis
testis N44.8
tunica vaginalis N50.89
vas deferens N50.89
vulva (acute) N90.89
Edentulism -*see* Absence, teeth, acquired
Edsall's disease T67.2
Educational handicap Z55.9
specified NEC Z55.8
Edward's syndrome -*see* Trisomy, 18
Effect, adverse
abnormal gravitational (G) forces or states T75.81
abuse -*see* Maltreatment
air pressure T70.9
  specified NEC T70.8
altitude (high) -*see* Effect, adverse, high altitude
anesthesia -*see also* Anesthesia T88.59
  in labor and delivery O74.9
  local, toxic
    in labor and delivery O74.4
    in pregnancy NEC O29.3
    postpartum, puerperal O89.3
  postpartum, puerperal O89.9
  specified NEC T88.59
    in labor and delivery O74.8
    postpartum, puerperal O89.8
  spinal and epidural T88.59
    headache T88.59
      in labor and delivery O74.5
      postpartum, puerperal O89.4
    specified NEC
      in labor and delivery O74.6
      postpartum, puerperal O89.5
antitoxin -*see* Complications, vaccination
atmospheric pressure T70.9
  due to explosion T70.8
  high T70.3
  low -*see* Effect, adverse, high altitude
  specified effect NEC T70.8
biological, correct substance properly administered -*see* Effect, adverse, drug
blood (derivatives) (serum) (transfusion) -*see* Complications, transfusion
chemical substance -*see* Table of Drugs and Chemicals
cold (temperature) (weather) T69.9
  chilblains T69.1
  frostbite -*see* Frostbite
  specified effect NEC T69.8
drugs and medicaments T88.7
  specified drug -*see* Table of Drugs and Chemicals, by drug, adverse effect
  specified effect
code to condition
electric current, electricity (shock) T75.4
  burn -*see* Burn

Effect, adverse --*continued*
  exertion (excessive) T73.3
  exposure -*see* Exposure
  external cause NEC T75.89
  foodstuffs T78.1
    allergic reaction -*see* Allergy, food
      causing anaphylaxis -*see* Shock,
      anaphylactic, due to food
    noxious -*see* Poisoning, food, noxious
  gases, fumes, or vapors T59.9
    specified agent -*see* Table of Drugs and
    Chemicals
  glue (airplane) sniffing
    due to drug abuse -*see* Abuse, drug, inhalant
    due to drug dependence -*see* Dependence,
    drug, inhalant
  heat -*see* Heat
  high altitude NEC T70.29
    anoxia T70.29
    on
      ears T70.0
      sinuses T70.1
    polycythemia D75.1
  high pressure fluids T70.4
  hot weather -*see* Heat
  hunger T73.0
  immersion, foot -*see* Immersion
  immunization -*see* Complications, vaccination
  immunological agents -*see* Complications,
    vaccination
  infrared (radiation) (rays) NOS T66
    dermatitis or eczema L59.8
  infusion -*see* Complications, infusion
  lack of care of infants -*see* Maltreatment,
    child
  lightning -*see* Lightning
  medical care T88.9
    specified NEC T88.8
  medicinal substance, correct, properly
    administered -*see* Effect, adverse, drug
  motion T75.3
  noise, on inner ear -*see* subcategory H83.3
  overheated places -*see* Heat
  psychosocial, of work environment Z56.5
  radiation (diagnostic) (infrared) (natural
  source) (therapeutic) (ultraviolet) (X ray)
  NOS T66
    dermatitis or eczema -*see* Dermatitis, due to,
      radiation
    fibrosis of lung J70.1
    pneumonitis J70.0
    pulmonary manifestations
      acute J70.0
      chronic J70.1
    skin L59.9
  radioactive substance NOS
    dermatitis or eczema -*see* Radiodermatitis
  reduced temperature T69.9
    immersion foot or hand -*see* Immersion
    specified effect NEC T69.8
  serum NEC -*see also* Reaction, serum T80.69
  specified NEC T78.8
    external cause NEC T75.89
  strangulation -*see* Asphyxia, traumatic
  submersion T75.1
  thirst T73.1
  toxic -*see* Toxicity
  transfusion -*see* Complications, transfusion
  ultraviolet (radiation) (rays) NOS T66
    burn -*see* Burn

Effect, adverse --*continued*
    dermatitis or eczema -*see* Dermatitis, due to,
    ultraviolet rays
      acute L56.8
  vaccine (any) -*see* Complications, vaccination
  vibration -*see* Vibration, adverse effects
  water pressure NEC T70.9
    specified NEC T70.8
  weightlessness T75.82
  whole blood -*see* Complications, transfusion
  work environment Z56.5
Effect(s) (of) (from) -*see* Effect, adverse NEC
Effects, late -*see* Sequelae
Effluvium
  anagen L65.1
  telogen L65.0
Effort syndrome (psychogenic) F45.8
Effusion
  amniotic fluid -*see* Pregnancy, complicated
  by, premature rupture of membranes
  brain (serous) G93.6
  bronchial -*see* Bronchitis
  cerebral G93.6
  cerebrospinal -*see also* Meningitis
    vessel G93.6
  chest -*see* Effusion, pleura
  chylous, chyliform (pleura) J94.0
  intracranial G93.6
  joint M25.40
    ankle M25.47
    elbow M25.42
    foot joint M25.47
    hand joint M25.44
    hip M25.45
    knee M25.46
    shoulder M25.41
    specified joint NEC M25.48
    wrist M25.43
  malignant pleural J91.0
  meninges -*see* Meningitis
  pericardium, pericardial (noninflammatory)
  I31.3
    acute -*see* Pericarditis, acute
  peritoneal (chronic) R18.8
  pleura, pleurisy, pleuritic, pleuropericardial
  J90
    chylous, chyliform J94.0
    due to systemic lupus erythematosus
    M32.13
    influenzal -*see* Influenza, with, respiratory
  manifestations NEC
    malignant J91.0
    newborn P28.89
    tuberculous NEC A15.6
      primary (progressive) A15.7
  spinal -*see* Meningitis
  thorax, thoracic -*see* Effusion, pleura
Egg shell nails L60.3
  congenital Q84.6
Egyptian splenomegaly B65.1
Ehrlichiosis A77.40
  due to
    E. chafeensis A77.41
    E. sennetsu A79.81
    specified organism NEC A77.49
Ehlers-Danlos syndrome Q79.6
Eichstedt's disease B36.0
Eisenmenger's
  complex or syndrome I27.89
  defect Q21.8
Ejaculation
  delayed F52.32

Ejaculation - *continued*
  painful N53.12
  premature F52.4
  retarded N53.11
  retrograde N53.14
  semen, painful N53.12
    psychogenic F52.6
Ekbom's syndrome (restless legs) G25.81
**Ekman's syndrome (brittle bones and blue
sclera)** Q78.0
Elastic skin Q82.8
  acquired L57.4
Elastofibroma -*see* Neoplasm, connective
tissue, benign
Elastoma (juvenile) Q82.8
  Miescher's L87.2
Elastomyofibrosis I42.4
Elastosis
  actinic, solar L57.8
  atrophicans (senile) L57.4
  perforans serpiginosa L87.2
  senilis L57.4
Elbow -*see* condition
**Electric current, electricity, effects
(concussion) (fatal) (nonfatal) (shock)** T75.4
  burn -*see* Burn
Electric feet syndrome E53.8
Electrocution T75.4
  from electroshock gun (taser) T75.4
Electrolyte imbalance E87.8
  with
    abortion -*see* Abortion by type, complicated
      by, electrolyte imbalance
    ectopic pregnancy O08.5
    molar pregnancy O08.5
Elephantiasis (nonfilarial) I89.0
  arabicum -*see* Infestation, filarial
  bancroftian B74.0
  congenital (any site) (hereditary) Q82.0
  due to
    Brugia (malayi) B74.1
      timori B74.2
    mastectomy I97.2
    Wuchereria (bancrofti) B74.0
  eyelid H02.859
    left H02.856
      lower H02.855
      upper H02.854
    right H02.853
      lower H02.852
      upper H02.851
  filarial, filariensis -*see* Infestation, filarial
  glandular I89.0
  graecorum A30.9
  lymphangiectatic I89.0
  lymphatic vessel I89.0
    due to mastectomy I97.2
  scrotum (nonfilarial) I89.0
  streptococcal I89.0
  surgical I97.89
    postmastectomy I97.2
  telangiectodes I89.0
  vulva (nonfilarial) N90.89
Elevated, elevation
  antibody titer R76.0
  basal metabolic rate R94.8
  blood pressure -*see also* Hypertension
    reading (incidental) (isolated) (nonspecific),
    no diagnosis of hypertension R03.0
  blood sugar R73.9
  body temperature (of unknown origin) R50.9

Elevated, elevation - *continued*
  C-reactive protein (CRP) R79.82
  cancer antigen 125 [CA 125] R97.1
  carcinoembryonic antigen [CEA] R97.0
  cholesterol E78.00
    with high triglycerides E78.2
  conjugate, eye H51.0
  diaphragm, congenital Q79.1
  erythrocyte sedimentation rate R70.0
  fasting glucose R73.01
  fasting triglycerides E78.1
  finding on laboratory examination -*see*
    Findings, abnormal, inconclusive, without
    diagnosis, by type of exam
  GFR (glomerular filtration rate) -*see* Findings,
    abnormal, inconclusive, without diagnosis,
    by type of exam
  glucose tolerance (oral) R73.02
  immunoglobulin level R76.8
  indoleacetic acid R82.5
  lactic acid dehydrogenase (LDH) level R74.0
  leukocytes D72.829
  lipoprotein a level E78.8
  liver function
    study R94.5
    test R79.89
      alkaline phosphatase R74.8
      aminotransferase R74.0
      bilirubin R17
      hepatic enzyme R74.8
      lactate dehydrogenase R74.0
  lymphocytes D72.820
  prostate specific antigen [PSA] R97.20
  Rh titer -*see* Complication(s), transfusion,
    incompatibility reaction, Rh (factor)
  scapula, congenital Q74.0
  sedimentation rate R70.0
  SGOT R74.0
  SGPT R74.0
  transaminase level R74.0
  triglycerides E78.1
    with high cholesterol E78.2
  tumor associated antigens [TAA] NEC R97.8
  tumor specific antigens [TSA] NEC R97.8
  urine level of
    catecholamine R82.5
    indoleacetic acid R82.5
    17 ketosteroids R82.5
    steroids R82.5
    vanillylmandelic acid (VMA) R82.5
  venous pressure I87.8
  white blood cell count D72.829
    specified NEC D72.828
Elliptocytosis (congenital) (hereditary) D58.1
  Hb C (disease) D58.1
  hemoglobin disease D58.1
  sickle-cell (disease) D57.8
    trait D57.3
Ellison-Zollinger syndrome E16.4
Ellis-van Creveld syndrome
  (chondroectodermal dysplasia) Q77.6
Elongated, elongation (congenital) -*see also*
  Distortion
  bone Q79.9
  cervix (uteri) Q51.828
    acquired N88.4
    hypertrophic N88.4
  colon Q43.8
  common bile duct Q44.5
  cystic duct Q44.5
  frenulum, penis Q55.69

Elongated, elongation - *continued*
  labia minora (acquired) N90.69
  ligamentum patellae Q74.1
  petiolus (epiglottidis) Q31.8
  tooth, teeth K00.2
  uvula Q38.6
Eltor cholera A00.1
Emaciation (due to malnutrition) E41
Embadomoniasis A07.8
Embedded tooth, teeth K01.0
  root only K08.3
Embolic -*see* condition
Embolism (multiple) (paradoxical) I74.9
  air (any site) (traumatic) T79.0
    following
      abortion -*see* Abortion by type complicated
        by embolism
      ectopic pregnancy O08.2
      infusion, therapeutic injection or
        transfusion T80.0
      molar pregnancy O08.2
      procedure NEC
        artery T81.719
          mesenteric T81.710
          renal T81.711
          specified NEC T81.718
        vein T81.72
    in pregnancy, childbirth or puerperium -*see*
      Embolism, obstetric
  amniotic fluid (pulmonary) -*see also*
    Embolism, obstetric
    following
      abortion -*see* Abortion by type complicated
        by embolism
      ectopic pregnancy O08.2
      molar pregnancy O08.2
  aorta, aortic I74.10
    abdominal I74.09
      saddle I74.01
    bifurcation I74.09
    saddle I74.01
    thoracic I74.11
  artery I74.9
    auditory, internal I65.8
    basilar -*see* Occlusion, artery, basilar
    carotid (common) (internal) -*see* Occlusion,
      artery, carotid
    cerebellar (anterior inferior) (posterior
      inferior) (superior) I66.3
    cerebral -*see* Occlusion, artery, cerebral
    choroidal (anterior) I66.8
    communicating posterior I66.8
    coronary -*see also* Infarct, myocardium
      not resulting in infarction I24.0
    extremity I74.4
      lower I74.3
      upper I74.2
    hypophyseal I66.8
    iliac I74.5
    limb I74.4
      lower I74.3
      upper I74.2
    mesenteric (with gangrene) -*see also*
      Ischemia, intestine, acute K55.059
    ophthalmic -*see* Occlusion, artery, retina
    peripheral I74.4
    pontine I66.8
    precerebral -*see* Occlusion, artery,
      precerebral
    pulmonary -*see* Embolism, pulmonary
    renal N28.0

Embolism --*continued*
  retinal -*see* Occlusion, artery, retina
  septic I76
  specified NEC I74.8
  vertebral -*see* Occlusion, artery, vertebral
  basilar (artery) I65.1
  blood clot
    following
      abortion -*see* Abortion by type complicated
        by embolism
      ectopic or molar pregnancy O08.2
    in pregnancy, childbirth or puerperium -*see*
      Embolism, obstetric
  brain -*see also* Occlusion, artery, cerebral
    following
      abortion -*see* Abortion by type complicated
        by embolism
      ectopic or molar pregnancy O08.2
    puerperal, postpartum, childbirth -*see*
      Embolism, obstetric
  capillary I78.8
  cardiac -*see also* Infarct, myocardium
    not resulting in infarction I51.3
  carotid (artery) (common) (internal) -*see*
    Occlusion, artery, carotid
  cavernous sinus (venous) -*see* Embolism,
    intracranial venous sinus
  cerebral -*see* Occlusion, artery, cerebral
  cholesterol -*see* Atheroembolism
  coronary (artery or vein) (systemic) -*see*
    Occlusion, coronary
  due to device, implant or graft -*see also*
  Complications, by site and type, specified
  NEC
    arterial graft NEC T82.818
    breast (implant) T85.818
    catheter NEC T85.818
      dialysis (renal) T82.818
        intraperitoneal T85.818
      infusion NEC T82.818
        spinal (epidural) (subdural) T85.810
      urinary (indwelling) T83.81
    electronic (electrode) (pulse generator)
      (stimulator)
        bone T84.81
        cardiac T82.817
        nervous system (brain) (peripheral nerve)
          (spinal) T85.810
        urinary T83.81
    fixation, internal (orthopedic) NEC T84.81
    gastrointestinal (bile duct) (esophagus)
      T85.818
    genital NEC T83.81
    heart (graft) (valve) T82.817
    joint prosthesis T84.81
    ocular (corneal graft) (orbital implant)
      T85.818
    orthopedic (bone graft) NEC T86.838
    specified NEC T85.818
    urinary (graft) NEC T83.81
    vascular NEC T82.818
    ventricular intracranial shunt T85.810
  extremities
    lower -*see* Embolism, vein, lower extremity
      arterial I74.3
    upper I74.2
  eye H34.9
  fat (cerebral) (pulmonary) (systemic) T79.1
    following
      abortion -*see* Abortion by type complicated
        by embolism

Embolism --*continued*
- ectopic or molar pregnancy O08.2
- complicating delivery -*see* Embolism, obstetric
- following
  - abortion -*see* Abortion by type complicated by embolism
  - ectopic or molar pregnancy O08.2
  - infusion, therapeutic injection or transfusion air T80.0
- heart (fatty) -*see also* Infarct, myocardium
  - not resulting in infarction I51.3
- hepatic (vein) I82.0
- in pregnancy, childbirth or puerperium -*see* Embolism, obstetric
- intestine (artery) (vein) (with gangrene) -*see also* Ischemia, intestine, acute K55.039
- intracranial -*see also* Occlusion, artery, cerebral
  - venous sinus (any) G08
    - nonpyogenic I67.6
- intraspinal venous sinuses or veins G08
  - nonpyogenic G95.19
- kidney (artery) N28.0
- lateral sinus (venous) -*see* Embolism, intracranial, venous sinus
- leg -*see* Embolism, vein, lower extremity
  - arterial I74.3
- longitudinal sinus (venous) -*see* Embolism, intracranial, venous sinus
- lung (massive) -*see* Embolism, pulmonary
- meninges I66.8
- mesenteric (artery) (vein) (with gangrene) -*see also* Ischemia, intestine, acute K55.059
- obstetric (in) (pulmonary)
  - childbirth O88.22
    - air O88.02
    - amniotic fluid O88.12
    - blood clot O88.22
    - fat O88.82
    - pyemic O88.32
    - septic O88.32
    - specified type NEC O88.82
  - pregnancy O88.21
    - air O88.01
    - amniotic fluid O88.11
    - blood clot O88.21
    - fat O88.81
    - pyemic O88.31
    - septic O88.31
    - specified type NEC O88.81
  - puerperal O88.23
    - air O88.03
    - amniotic fluid O88.13
    - blood clot O88.23
    - fat O88.83
    - pyemic O88.33
    - septic O88.33
    - specified type NEC O88.83
- ophthalmic -*see* Occlusion, artery, retina
- penis N48.81
- peripheral artery NOS I74.4
- pituitary E23.6
- popliteal (artery) I74.3
- portal (vein) I81
- postoperative, postprocedural
  - artery T81.719
    - mesenteric T81.710
    - renal T81.711
    - specified NEC T81.718
  - vein T81.72

Embolism --*continued*
- precerebral artery -*see* Occlusion, artery, precerebral
- puerperal -*see* Embolism, obstetric
- pulmonary (acute) (artery) (vein) I26.99
  - with acute cor pulmonale I26.09
  - chronic I27.82
  - following
    - abortion -*see* Abortion by type complicated by embolism
    - ectopic or molar pregnancy O08.2
  - healed or old Z86.711
  - in pregnancy, childbirth or puerperium -*see* Embolism, obstetric
  - personal history of Z86.711
  - saddle I26.92
    - with acute cor pulmonale I26.02
  - septic I26.90
    - with acute cor pulmonale I26.01
- pyemic (multiple) I76
  - following
    - abortion -*see* Abortion by type complicated by embolism
    - ectopic or molar pregnancy O08.2
  - Hemophilus influenzae A41.3
  - pneumococcal A40.3
    - with pneumonia J13
  - puerperal, postpartum, childbirth (any organism) -*see* Embolism, obstetric
  - specified organism NEC A41.89
  - staphylococcal A41.2
  - streptococcal A40.9
- renal (artery) N28.0
  - vein I82.3
- retina, retinal -*see* Occlusion, artery, retina
- saddle
  - abdominal aorta I74.01
  - pulmonary artery I26.92
    - with acute cor pulmonale I26.02
- septic (arterial) I76
  - complicating abortion -*see* Abortion, by type, complicated by, embolism
- sinus -*see* Embolism, intracranial, venous sinus
- soap complicating abortion -*see* Abortion, by type, complicated by, embolism
- spinal cord G95.19
  - pyogenic origin G06.1
- spleen, splenic (artery) I74.8
- upper extremity I74.2
- vein (acute) I82.90
  - antecubital I82.61
    - chronic I82.71
  - axillary I82.A1
    - chronic I82.A2
  - basilic I82.61
    - chronic I82.71
  - brachial I82.62
    - chronic I82.72
  - brachiocephalic (innominate) I82.290
    - chronic I82.291
  - cephalic I82.61
    - chronic I82.71
  - chronic I82.91
  - deep (DVT) I82.40
    - calf I82.4Z
      - chronic I82.5Z
    - lower leg I82.4Z
      - chronic I82.5Z
    - thigh I82.4Y
      - chronic I82.5Y

Embolism --*continued*
- upper leg I82.4Y
  - chronic I82.5Y
- femoral I82.41
  - chronic I82.51
- iliac (iliofemoral) I82.42
  - chronic I82.52
- innominate I82.290
  - chronic I82.291
- internal jugular I82.C1
  - chronic I82.C2
- lower extremity
  - deep I82.40
    - chronic I82.50
  - specified NEC I82.49
    - chronic NEC I82.59
  - distal
    - deep I82.4Z
  - proximal
    - deep I82.4Y
      - chronic I82.5Y
  - superficial I82.81
- popliteal I82.43
  - chronic I82.53
- radial I82.62
  - chronic I82.72
- renal I82.3
- saphenous (greater) (lesser) I82.81
- specified NEC I82.890
  - chronic NEC I82.891
- subclavian I82.B1
  - chronic I82.B2
- thoracic NEC I82.290
  - chronic I82.291
- tibial I82.44
  - chronic I82.54
- ulnar I82.62
  - chronic I82.72
- upper extremity I82.60
  - chronic I82.70
  - deep I82.62
    - chronic I82.72
  - superficial I82.61
    - chronic I82.71
- vena cava
  - inferior (acute) I82.220
    - chronic I82.221
  - superior (acute) I82.210
    - chronic I82.211
- venous sinus G08
- vessels of brain -*see* Occlusion, artery, cerebral

Embolus -*see* Embolism

Embryoma -*see also* Neoplasm, uncertain behavior, by site
- benign -*see* Neoplasm, benign, by site
- kidney C64.
- liver C22.0
- malignant -*see also* Neoplasm, malignant, by site
  - kidney C64.
  - liver C22.0
  - testis C62.9
    - descended (scrotal) C62.1
    - undescended C62.0
- testis C62.9
  - descended (scrotal) C62.1
  - undescended C62.0

Embryonic
- circulation Q28.9
- heart Q28.9
- vas deferens Q55.4

Embryopathia NOS Q89.9
Embryotoxon Q13.4
Emesis -*see* Vomiting
Emotional lability R45.86
Emotionality, pathological F60.3
Emotogenic disease -*see* Disorder,
  psychogenic
Emphysema (atrophic) (bullous) (chronic)
  (interlobular) (lung) (obstructive)
  (pulmonary) (senile) (vesicular) J43.9
  cellular tissue (traumatic) T79.7
    surgical T81.82
  centrilobular J43.2
  compensatory J98.3
  congenital (interstitial) P25.0
  conjunctiva H11.89
  connective tissue (traumatic) T79.7
    surgical T81.82
  due to chemicals, gases, fumes or vapors
    J68.4
  eyelid(s) -*see* Disorder, eyelid, specified type
    NEC
    surgical T81.82
    traumatic T79.7
  interstitial J98.2
    congenital P25.0
    perinatal period P25.0
  laminated tissue T79.7
    surgical T81.82
  mediastinal J98.2
    newborn P25.2
  orbit, orbital -*see* Disorder, orbit, specified
    type NEC
  panacinar J43.1
  panlobular J43.1
  specified NEC J43.8
  subcutaneous (traumatic) T79.7
    nontraumatic J98.2
    postprocedural T81.82
    surgical T81.82
  surgical T81.82
  thymus (gland) (congenital) E32.8
  traumatic (subcutaneous) T79.7
  unilateral J43.0
Empty nest syndrome Z60.0
Empyema (acute) (chest) (double) (pleura)
  (supradiaphragmatic) (thorax) J86.9
  with fistula J86.0
  accessory sinus (chronic) -*see* Sinusitis
  antrum (chronic) -*see* Sinusitis, maxillary
  brain (any part) -*see* Abscess, brain
  ethmoidal (chronic) (sinus) -*see* Sinusitis,
    ethmoidal
  extradural -*see* Abscess, extradural
  frontal (chronic) (sinus) -*see* Sinusitis, frontal
  gallbladder K81.0
  mastoid (process) (acute) -*see* Mastoiditis,
    acute
  maxilla, maxillary M27.2
    sinus (chronic) -*see* Sinusitis, maxillary
  nasal sinus (chronic) -*see* Sinusitis
  sinus (accessory) (chronic) (nasal) -*see*
    Sinusitis
  sphenoidal (sinus) (chronic) -*see* Sinusitis,
    sphenoidal
  subarachnoid -*see* Abscess, extradural
  subdural -*see* Abscess, subdural
  tuberculous A15.6
  ureter -*see* Ureteritis
  ventricular -*see* Abscess, brain
En coup de sabre lesion L94.1

Enamel pearls K00.2
Enameloma K00.2
Enanthema, viral B09
Encephalitis (chronic) (hemorrhagic)
  (idiopathic) (nonepidemic) (spurious)
  (subacute) G04.90
  acute -*see also* Encephalitis, viral A86
    disseminated G04.00
      infectious G04.01
      noninfectious G04.81
      postimmunization (postvaccination)
        G04.02
      postinfectious G04.01
    inclusion body A85.8
    necrotizing hemorrhagic G04.30
      postimmunization G04.32
      postinfectious G04.31
      specified NEC G04.39
  arboviral, arbovirus NEC A85.2
  arthropod-borne NEC (viral) A85.2
  Australian A83.4
  California (virus) A83.5
  Central European (tick-borne) A84.1
  Czechoslovakian A84.1
  Dawson's (inclusion body) A81.1
  diffuse sclerosing A81.1
  disseminated, acute G04.00
  due to
    cat scratch disease A28.1
    human immunodeficiency virus (HIV)
      disease B20 [*G05.3*]
    malaria -*see* Malaria
    rickettsiosis -*see* Rickettsiosis
    smallpox inoculation G04.02
    typhus -*see* Typhus
  Eastern equine A83.2
  endemic (viral) A86
  epidemic NEC (viral) A86
  equine (acute) (infectious) (viral) A83.9
    Eastern A83.2
    Venezuelan A92.2
    Western A83.1
  Far Eastern (tick-borne) A84.0
  following vaccination or other immunization
    procedure G04.02
  herpes zoster B02.0
  herpesviral B00.4
    due to herpesvirus 6 B10.01
    due to herpesvirus 7 B10.09
    specified NEC B10.09
  Ilhéus (virus) A83.8
  inclusion body A81.1
  in (due to)
    actinomycosis A42.82
    adenovirus A85.1
    African trypanosomiasis B56.9 [*G05.3*]
    Chagas' disease (chronic) B57.42
    cytomegalovirus B25.8
    enterovirus A85.0
    herpes (simplex) virus B00.4
      due to herpesvirus 6 B10.01
      due to herpesvirus 7 B10.09
      specified NEC B10.09
    infectious disease NEC B99 [*G05.3*]
    influenza -*see* Influenza, with,
      encephalopathy
    listeriosis A32.12
    measles B05.0
    mumps B26.2
    naegleriasis B60.2
    parasitic disease NEC B89 [*G05.3*]

Encephalitis --*continued*
  poliovirus A80.9 [*G05.3*]
  rubella B06.01
  syphilis
    congenital A50.42
    late A52.14
  systemic lupus erythematosus M32.19
  toxoplasmosis (acquired) B58.2
    congenital P37.1
  tuberculosis A17.82
  zoster B02.0
  infectious (acute) (virus) NEC A86
  Japanese (B type) A83.0
  La Crosse A83.5
  lead -*see* Poisoning, lead
  lethargica (acute) (infectious) A85.8
  louping ill A84.8
  lupus erythematosus, systemic M32.19
  lymphatica A87.2
  Mengo A85.8
  meningococcal A39.81
  Murray Valley A83.4
  otitic NEC H66.40 [*G05.3*]
  parasitic NOS B71.9
  periaxial G37.0
  periaxialis (concentrica) (diffuse) G37.5
  post chickenpox B01.11
  postexanthematous NEC B09
  postimmunization G04.02
  postinfectious NEC G04.01
  postmeasles B05.0
  postvaccinal G04.02
  post varicella B01.11
  postviral NEC A86
  Powassan A84.8
  Rasmussen G04.81
  Rio Bravo A85.8
  Russian
    autumnal A83.0
    spring-summer (taiga) A84.0
  saturnine -*see* Poisoning, lead - specified
    NEC G04.81
  St. Louis A83.3
  subacute sclerosing A81.1
  summer A83.0
  suppurative G04.81
  tick-borne A84.9
  Torula, torular (cryptococcal) B45.1
  toxic NEC G92
  trichinosis B75 [*G05.3*]
  type
    B A83.0
    C A83.3
  van Bogaert's A81.1
  Venezuelan equine A92.2
  Vienna A85.8
  viral, virus A86
    arthropod-borne NEC A85.2
    mosquito-borne A83.9
      Australian X disease A83.4
      California virus A83.5
      Eastern equine A83.2
      Japanese (B type) A83.0
      Murray Valley A83.4
      specified NEC A83.8
      St. Louis A83.3
      type B A83.0
      type C A83.3
      Western equine A83.1
    tick-borne A84.9
      biundulant A84.1

Encephalitis --*continued*
  central European A84.1
  Czechoslovakian A84.1
  diphasic meningoencephalitis A84.1
  Far Eastern A84.0
  Russian spring-summer (taiga) A84.0
  specified NEC A84.8
  specified type NEC A85.8
  Western equine A83.1
Encephalocele Q01.9
  frontal Q01.0
  nasofrontal Q01.1
  occipital Q01.2
  specified NEC Q01.8
Encephalocystocele -*see* Encephalocele
Encephaloduroarteriomyosynangiosis (EDAMS) I67.5
Encephalomalacia (brain) (cerebellar) (cerebral) -*see* Softening, brain
Encephalomeningitis -*see* Meningoencephalitis
Encephalomeningocele -*see* Encephalocele
Encephalomeningomyelitis -*see* Meningoencephalitis
Encephalomyelitis -*see also* Encephalitis G04.90
  acute disseminated G04.00
    infectious G04.01
    noninfectious G04.81
    postimmunization G04.02
    postinfectious G04.01
  acute necrotizing hemorrhagic G04.30
    postimmunization G04.32
    postinfectious G04.31
    specified NEC G04.39
  benign myalgic G93.3
  equine A83.9
    Eastern A83.2
    Venezuelan A92.2
    Western A83.1
  in diseases classified elsewhere G05.3
  myalgic, benign G93.3
  post chickenpox B01.11
  postinfectious NEC G04.01
  postmeasles B05.0
  postvaccinal G04.02
  post varicella B01.11
  rubella B06.01
  specified NEC G04.81
  Venezuelan equine A92.2
Encephalomyelocele -*see* Encephalocele
Encephalomyelomeningitis -*see* Meningoencephalitis
Encephalomyelopathy G96.9
Encephalomyeloradiculitis (acute) G61.0
Encephalomyeloradiculoneuritis (acute) (Guillain-Barré) G61.0
Encephalomyeloradiculopathy G96.9
Encephalopathia hyperbilirubinemic, newborn P57.9
  due to isoimmunization (conditions in P55) P57.0
Encephalopathy (acute) G93.40
  acute necrotizing hemorrhagic G04.30
    postimmunization G04.32
    postinfectious G04.31
    specified NEC G04.39
  alcoholic G31.2
  anoxic -*see* Damage, brain, anoxic
  arteriosclerotic I67.2
  centrolobar progressive (Schilder) G37.0

Encephalopathy (acute) --*continued*
  congenital Q07.9
  degenerative, in specified disease NEC G32.89
  demyelinating callosal G37.1
  due to
    drugs - -*see also* Table of Drugs and Chemicals G92
  hepatic -*see* Failure, hepatic
  hyperbilirubinemic, newborn P57.9
    due to isoimmunization (conditions in P55) P57.0
  hypertensive I67.4
  hypoglycemic E16.2
  hypoxic -*see* Damage, brain, anoxic
  hypoxic ischemic P91.60
    mild P91.61
    moderate P91.62
    severe P91.63
  in (due to) (with)
    birth injury P11.1
    hyperinsulinism E16.1 *[G94]*
    influenza -*see* Influenza, with, encephalopathy
    lack of vitamin -*see also* Deficiency, vitamin E56.9 *[G32.89]*
    neoplastic disease (see also Neoplasm) D49.9 *[G13.1]*
    serum -*see also* Reaction, serum T80.69
    syphilis A52.17
    trauma (postconcussional) F07.81
      current injury -*see* Injury, intracranial
    vaccination G04.02
  lead -*see* Poisoning, lead - metabolic G93.41
    drug induced G92
    toxic G92
  myoclonic, early, symptomatic -*see* Epilepsy, generalized, specified NEC
  necrotizing, subacute (Leigh) G31.82
  pellagrous E52 *[G32.89]*
  portosystemic -*see* Failure, hepatic
  postcontusional F07.81
    current injury -*see* Injury, intracranial, diffuse - posthypoglycemic (coma) E16.1 *[G94]*
  postradiation G93.89
  saturnine -*see* Poisoning, lead - septic G93.41
  specified NEC G93.49
  spongiform, subacute (viral) A81.09
  toxic G92
    metabolic G92
  traumatic (postconcussional) F07.81
    current injury -*see* Injury, intracranial
  vitamin B deficiency NEC E53.9 *[G32.89]*
    vitamin B1 E51.2
  Wernicke's E51.2
Encephalorrhagia -*see* Hemorrhage, intracranial, intracerebral
Encephalosis, posttraumatic F07.81
Enchondroma -*see also* Neoplasm, bone, benign
Enchondromatosis (cartilaginous) (multiple) Q78.4
Encopresis R15.9
  functional F98.1
  nonorganic origin F98.1
  psychogenic F98.1
Encounter (with health service) (for) Z76.89
  adjustment and management (of)
    breast implant Z45.81
    implanted device NEC Z45.89

Encounter (with health service) (for) -- *continued*
    myringotomy device (stent) (tube) Z45.82
  administrative purpose only Z02.9
    examination for
      adoption Z02.82
      armed forces Z02.3
      disability determination Z02.71
      driving license Z02.4
      employment Z02.1
      insurance Z02.6
      medical certificate NEC Z02.79
      paternity testing Z02.81
      residential institution admission Z02.2
      school admission Z02.0
      sports Z02.5
      specified reason NEC Z02.89
  aftercare -*see* Aftercare
  antenatal screening Z36
  assisted reproductive fertility procedure cycle Z31.83
  blood typing Z01.83
    Rh typing Z01.83
  breast augmentation or reduction Z41.1
  breast implant exchange (different material) (different size) Z45.81
  breast reconstruction following mastectomy Z42.1
  check-up -*see* Examination
  chemotherapy for neoplasm Z51.11
  colonoscopy, screening Z12.11
  counseling -*see* Counseling
  delivery, full-term, uncomplicated O80
    cesarean, without indication O82
  desensitization to allergens Z51.6
  ear piercing Z41.3
  examination -*see* Examination
  expectant parent(s) (adoptive) pre-birth pediatrician visit Z76.81
  fertility preservation procedure (prior to cancer therapy) (prior to removal of gonads) Z31.84
  fitting (of) -*see* Fitting (and adjustment) (of)
  genetic
    counseling Z31.5
    testing -*see* Test, genetic
  hearing conservation and treatment Z01.12
  immunotherapy for neoplasm Z51.12
  in vitro fertilization cycle Z31.83
  instruction (in)
    childbirth Z32.2
    child care (postpartal) (prenatal) Z32.3
    natural family planning
      procreative Z31.61
      to avoid pregnancy Z30.02
  insulin pump titration Z46.81
  joint prosthesis insertion following prior explantation of joint prosthesis (staged procedure)
    hip Z47.32
    knee Z47.33
    shoulder Z47.31
  laboratory (as part of a general medical examination) Z00.00
    with abnormal findings Z00.01
  mental health services (for)
    abuse NEC
      perpetrator Z69.82
      victim Z69.81
    child abuse
      nonparental

Encounter (with health service) (for)
--continued
  perpetrator Z69.021
  victim Z69.020
 parental
  perpetrator Z69.011
  victim Z69.010
 spousal or partner abuse
  perpetrator Z69.12
  victim Z69.11
observation (for) (ruled out)
 exposure to (suspected)
  anthrax Z03.810
  biological agent NEC Z03.818
pediatrician visit, by expectant parent(s) (adoptive) Z76.81
plastic and reconstructive surgery following medical procedure or healed injury NEC Z42.8
pregnancy
 supervision of -see Pregnancy, supervision of
 test Z32.00
  result negative Z32.02
  result positive Z32.01
procreative management and counseling for gestational carrier Z31.7
prophylactic measures Z29.9
 antivenin Z29.12
 fluoride administration Z29.3
 immunotherapy for respiratory syncytial virus (RSV) Z29.11
 rabies immune globin Z29.14
 Rho (D) immune globulin Z29.13
 specified NEC Z29.8
radiation therapy (antineoplastic) Z51.0
radiological (as part of a general medical examination) Z00.00
 with abnormal findings Z00.01
reconstructive surgery following medical procedure or healed injury NEC Z42.8
removal (of) -see also Removal
 artificial
  arm Z44.00
   complete Z44.01
   partial Z44.02
  eye Z44.2
  leg Z44.10
   complete Z44.11
   partial Z44.12
 breast implant Z45.81
 tissue expander (without synchronous insertion of permanent implant) Z45.81
 device Z46.9
  specified NEC Z46.89
 external
  fixation device
   code to fracture with seventh character D
 prosthesis, prosthetic device Z44.9
  breast Z44.3
  specified NEC Z44.8
 implanted device NEC Z45.89
 insulin pump Z46.81
 internal fixation device Z47.2
 myringotomy device (stent) (tube) Z45.82
 nervous system device NEC Z46.2
  brain neuropacemaker Z46.2
  visual substitution device Z46.2
   implanted Z45.31
 non-vascular catheter Z46.82
 orthodontic device Z46.4

Encounter (with health service) (for)
--continued
 stent
  ureteral Z46.6
 urinary device Z46.6
repeat cervical smear to confirm findings of recent normal smear following initial abnormal smear Z01.42
respirator [ventilator] use during power failure Z99.12
Rh typing Z01.83
screening -see Screening
specified NEC Z76.89
sterilization Z30.2
suspected condition, ruled out
 amniotic cavity and membrane Z03.71
 cervical shortening Z03.75
 fetal anomaly Z03.73
 fetal growth Z03.74
 maternal and fetal conditions NEC Z03.79
 oligohydramnios Z03.71
 placental problem Z03.72
 polyhydramnios Z03.71
suspected exposure (to), ruled out
 anthrax Z03.810
 biological agents NEC Z03.818
termination of pregnancy, elective Z33.2
testing -see Test
therapeutic drug level monitoring Z51.81
titration, insulin pump Z46.81
to determine fetal viability of pregnancy O36.80
training
 insulin pump Z46.81
X ray of chest (as part of a general medical examination) Z00.00
 with abnormal findings Z00.01
Encystment -see Cyst
Endarteritis (bacterial, subacute) (infective) I77.6
brain I67.7
cerebral or cerebrospinal I67.7
deformans -see Arteriosclerosis
embolic -see Embolism
obliterans -see also Arteriosclerosis
 pulmonary I28.8
pulmonary I28.8
retina -see Vasculitis, retina
senile -see Arteriosclerosis
syphilitic A52.09
 brain or cerebral A52.04
 congenital A50.54 [I79.8]
tuberculous A18.89
Endemic -see condition
Endocarditis (chronic) (marantic) (nonbacterial) (thrombotic) (valvular) I38
with rheumatic fever (conditions in I00)
 active -see Endocarditis, acute, rheumatic
 inactive or quiescent (with chorea) I09.1
acute or subacute I33.9
 infective I33.0
 rheumatic (aortic) (mitral) (pulmonary) (tricuspid) I01.1
  with chorea (acute) (rheumatic) (Sydenham's) I02.0
aortic (heart) (nonrheumatic) (valve) I35.8
 with
  mitral disease I08.0
   with tricuspid (valve) disease I08.3
   active or acute I01.1

Endocarditis - continued
 with chorea (acute) (rheumatic) (Sydenham's) I02.0
 rheumatic fever (conditions in I00)
  active -see Endocarditis, acute, rheumatic
  inactive or quiescent (with chorea) I06.9
 tricuspid (valve) disease I08.2
  with mitral (valve) disease I08.3
acute or subacute I33.9
arteriosclerotic I35.8
rheumatic I06.9
 with mitral disease I08.0
  with tricuspid (valve) disease I08.3
  active or acute I01.1
   with chorea (acute) (rheumatic) (Sydenham's) I02.0
 active or acute I01.1
  with chorea (acute) (rheumatic) (Sydenham's) I02.0
 specified NEC I06.8
specified cause NEC I35.8
syphilitic A52.03
arteriosclerotic I38
atypical verrucous (Libman-Sacks) M32.11
bacterial (acute) (any valve) (subacute) I33.0
candidal B37.6
congenital Q24.8
constrictive I33.0
Coxiella burnetii A78 [I39]
Coxsackie B33.21
due to
 prosthetic cardiac valve T82.6
 Q fever A78 [I39]
 Serratia marcescens I33.0
 typhoid (fever) A01.02
gonococcal A54.83
infectious or infective (acute) (any valve) (subacute) I33.0
lenta (acute) (any valve) (subacute) I33.0
Libman-Sacks M32.11
listerial A32.82
Löffler's I42.3
malignant (acute) (any valve) (subacute) I33.0
meningococcal A39.51
mitral (chronic) (double) (fibroid) (heart) (inactive) (valve) (with chorea) I05.9
 with
  aortic (valve) disease I08.0
   with tricuspid (valve) disease I08.3
   active or acute I01.1
    with chorea (acute) (rheumatic) (Sydenham's) I02.0
  rheumatic fever (conditions in I00)
   active -see Endocarditis, acute, rheumatic
   inactive or quiescent (with chorea) I05.9
  tricuspid (valve) disease I08.1
   with aortic (valve) disease I08.3
 active or acute I01.1
  with chorea (acute) (rheumatic) (Sydenham's) I02.0
 bacterial I33.0
arteriosclerotic I34.8
nonrheumatic I34.8
 acute or subacute I33.9
specified NEC I05.8
monilial B37.6
multiple valves I08.9
 specified disorders I08.8
mycotic (acute) (any valve) (subacute) I33.0
pneumococcal (acute) (any valve) (subacute) I33.0

Endocarditis - *continued*
pulmonary (chronic) (heart) (valve) I37.8
  with rheumatic fever (conditions in I00)
    active -*see* Endocarditis, acute, rheumatic
    inactive or quiescent (with chorea) I09.89
      with aortic, mitral or tricuspid disease
        I08.8
  acute or subacute I33.9
    rheumatic I01.1
      with chorea (acute) (rheumatic)
        (Sydenham's) I02.0
  arteriosclerotic I37.8
  congenital Q22.2
  rheumatic (chronic) (inactive) (with chorea)
    I09.89
    active or acute I01.1
      with chorea (acute) (rheumatic)
        (Sydenham's) I02.0
  syphilitic A52.03
  purulent (acute) (any valve) (subacute) I33.0
  Q fever A78 [139]
  rheumatic (chronic) (inactive) (with chorea)
    I09.1
    active or acute (aortic) (mitral) (pulmonary)
      (tricuspid) I01.1
      with chorea (acute) (rheumatic)
        (Sydenham's) I02.0
  rheumatoid -*see* Rheumatoid, carditis
  septic (acute) (any valve) (subacute) I33.0
  streptococcal (acute) (any valve) (subacute)
    I33.0
  subacute -*see* Endocarditis, acute
  suppurative (acute) (any valve) (subacute)
    I33.0
  syphilitic A52.03
  toxic I33.9
  tricuspid (chronic) (heart) (inactive)
    (rheumatic) (valve) (with chorea) I07.9
    with
      aortic (valve) disease I08.2
        mitral (valve) disease I08.3
      mitral (valve) disease I08.1
        aortic (valve) disease I08.3
      rheumatic fever (conditions in I00)
        active -*see* Endocarditis, acute, rheumatic
        inactive or quiescent (with chorea) I07.8
    active or acute I01.1
      with chorea (acute) (rheumatic)
        (Sydenham's) I02.0
  arteriosclerotic I36.8
  nonrheumatic I36.8
    acute or subacute I33.9
  specified cause, except rheumatic I36.8
  tuberculous -*see* Tuberculosis, endocarditis
  typhoid A01.02
  ulcerative (acute) (any valve) (subacute) I33.0
  vegetative (acute) (any valve) (subacute)
    I33.0
  verrucous (atypical) (nonbacterial)
    (nonrheumatic) M32.11
Endocardium, endocardial -*see also*
  condition
  cushion defect Q21.2
Endocervicitis -*see also* Cervicitis
  due to intrauterine (contraceptive) device
    T83.69
  hyperplastic N72
Endocrine -*see* condition
Endocrinopathy, pluriglandular E31.9
Endodontic
  overfill M27.52
  underfill M27.53

Endodontitis K04.01
  irreversible K04.02
  reversible K04.01
Endomastoiditis -*see* Mastoiditis
Endometrioma N80.9
Endometriosis N80.9
  appendix N80.5
  bladder N80.8
  bowel N80.5
  broad ligament N80.3
  cervix N80.0
  colon N80.5
  cul-de-sac (Douglas') N80.3
  exocervix N80.0
  fallopian tube N80.2
  female genital organ NEC N80.8
  gallbladder N80.8
  in scar of skin N80.6
  internal N80.0
  intestine N80.5
  lung N80.8
  myometrium N80.0
  ovary N80.1
  parametrium N80.3
  pelvic peritoneum N80.3
  peritoneal (pelvic) N80.3
  rectovaginal septum N80.4
  rectum N80.5
  round ligament N80.3
  skin (scar) N80.6
  specified site NEC N80.8
  stromal D39.0
  umbilicus N80.8
  uterus (internal) N80.0
  vagina N80.4
  vulva N80.8
Endometritis (decidual) (nonspecific)
(purulent) (senile) (atrophic) (suppurative)
N71.9
  with ectopic pregnancy O08.0
  acute N71.0
  blenorrhagic (gonococcal) (acute) (chronic)
    A54.24
  cervix, cervical (with erosion or ectropion) -
    see also Cervicitis
    hyperplastic N72
  chlamydial A56.11
  chronic N71.1
  following
    abortion -*see* Abortion by type complicated
  by genital infection
    ectopic or molar pregnancy O08.0
  gonococcal, gonorrheal (acute) (chronic)
    A54.24
  hyperplastic -*see also* Hyperplasia,
  endometrial N85.00
    cervix N72
  puerperal, postpartum, childbirth O86.12
  subacute N71.0
  tuberculous A18.17
Endometrium -*see* condition
Endomyocardiopathy, South African I42.3
Endomyocarditis -*see* Endocarditis
Endomyofibrosis I42.3
Endomyometritis -*see* Endometritis
Endopericarditis -*see* Endocarditis
Endoperineuritis -*see* Disorder, nerve
Endophlebitis -*see* Phlebitis
Endophthalmia -*see* Endophthalmitis,
  purulent

Endophthalmitis (acute) (infective)
(metastatic) (subacute) H44.009
  bleb associated H59.4 -*see also* Bleb,
    inflamed (infected), postprocedural
  gonorrheal A54.39
  in (due to)
    cysticercosis B69.1
    onchocerciasis B73.01
    toxocariasis B83.0
  panuveitis -*see* Panuveitis
  parasitic H44.12
  purulent H44.00
    panophthalmitis -*see* Panophthalmitis
    vitreous abscess H44.02
  specified NEC H44.19
  sympathetic -*see* Uveitis, sympathetic
Endosalpingoma D28.2
Endosalpingiosis N94.89
Endosteitis -*see* Osteomyelitis
Endothelioma, bone -*see* Neoplasm, bone,
  malignant
Endotheliosis (hemorrhagic infectional)
  D69.8
Endotoxemia - code to condition
Endotrachelitis -*see* Cervicitis
Engelmann (Camurati) syndrome Q78.3
English disease -*see* Rickets
Engman's disease L30.3
Engorgement
  breast N64.59
    newborn P83.4
    puerperal, postpartum O92.79
  lung (passive) -*see* Edema, lung
  pulmonary (passive) -*see* Edema, lung
  stomach K31.89
  venous, retina -*see* Occlusion, retina, vein,
    engorgement
Enlargement, enlarged -*see also* Hypertrophy
  adenoids J35.2
    with tonsils J35.3
  alveolar ridge K08.89
    congenital -*see* Anomaly, alveolar
  apertures of diaphragm (congenital) Q79.1
  gingival K06.1
  heart, cardiac -*see* Hypertrophy, cardiac
  labium majus, childhood asymmetric
    (CALME) N90.61
  lacrimal gland, chronic H04.03
  liver -*see* Hypertrophy, liver
  lymph gland or node R59.9
    generalized R59.1
    localized R59.0
  orbit H05.34
  organ or site, congenital NEC -*see* Anomaly,
    by site
  parathyroid (gland) E21.0
  pituitary fossa R93.0
  prostate N40.0
    with lower urinary tract symptoms (LUTS)
      N40.1
    without lower urinary tract symptoms
      (LUTS) N40.0
  sella turcica R93.0
  spleen -*see* Splenomegaly
  thymus (gland) (congenital) E32.0
  thyroid (gland) -*see* Goiter
  tongue K14.8
  tonsils J35.1
    with adenoids J35.3
  uterus N85.2

Enophthalmos H05.40
  due to
    orbital tissue atrophy H05.41
    trauma or surgery H05.42
Enostosis M27.8
Entamebic, entamebiasis -*see* Amebiasis
Entanglement
  umbilical cord(s) O69.2
    with compression O69.2
      without compression O69.82
    around neck (with compression) O69.1
      without compression O69.81
    of twins in monoamniotic sac O69.2
Enteralgia -*see* Pain, abdominal
Enteric -*see* condition
Enteritis (acute) (diarrheal) (hemorrhagic)
(noninfective) K52.9
  adenovirus A08.2
  aertrycke infection A02.0
  allergic K52.29
    with
      eosinophilic gastritis or gastroenteritis
      K52.81
      food protein-induced enterocolitis
      syndrome K52.21
      food protein-induced enteropathy K52.22
  amebic (acute) A06.0
    with abscess -*see* Abscess, amebic
    chronic A06.1
      with abscess -*see* Abscess, amebic
      nondysenteric A06.2
    nondysenteric A06.2
  astrovirus A08.32
  bacillary NOS A03.9
  bacterial A04.9
    specified NEC A04.8
  calicivirus A08.31
  candidal B37.82
  Chilomastix A07.8
  choleriformis A00.1
  chronic (noninfectious) K52.9
    ulcerative -*see* Colitis, ulcerative
  cicatrizing (chronic) -*see* Enteritis, regional,
  small intestine
  Clostridium
    botulinum (food poisoning) A05.1
    difficile A04.7
  coccidial A07.3
  coxsackie virus A08.39
  dietetic -*see also* Enteritis, allergic K52.29
  drug-induced K52.1
  due to
    astrovirus A08.32
    calicivirus A08.31
    coxsackie virus A08.39
    drugs K52.1
    echovirus A08.39
    enterovirus NEC A08.39
    food hypersensitivity -*see also* Enteritis,
    allergic K52.29
    infectious organism (bacterial) (viral) -*see*
    Enteritis, infectious
    torovirus A08.39
    Yersinia enterocolitica A04.6
  echovirus A08.39
  eltor A00.1
  enterovirus NEC A08.39
  eosinophilic K52.81
  epidemic (infectious) A09
  fulminant -*see also* Ischemia, intestine, acute
  K55.019

Endodontic --*continued*
  gangrenous -*see* Enteritis, infectious
  giardial A07.1
  infectious NOS A09
    due to
      adenovirus A08.2
      Aerobacter aerogenes A04.8
      Arizona (bacillus) A02.0
      bacteria NOS A04.9
        specified NEC A04.8
      Campylobacter A04.5
      Clostridium difficile A04.7
      Clostridium perfringens A04.8
      Enterobacter aerogenes A04.8
      enterovirus A08.39
      Escherichia coli A04.4
        enteroaggregative A04.4
        enterohemorrhagic A04.3
        enteroinvasive A04.2
        enteropathogenic A04.0
        enterotoxigenic A04.1
        specified NEC A04.4
      specified
        bacteria NEC A04.8
        virus NEC A08.39
      Staphylococcus A04.8
      virus NEC A08.4
        specified type NEC A08.39
      Yersinia enterocolitica A04.6
      specified organism NEC A08.8
  influenzal -*see* Influenza, with, digestive
  manifestations
  ischemic K55.9
    acute -*see also* Ischemia, intestine, acute
    K55.019
    chronic K55.1
  microsporidial A07.8
  mucomembranous, myxomembranous -*see*
  Syndrome, irritable bowel
  mucous -*see* Syndrome, irritable bowel
  necroticans A05.2
  necrotizing of newborn -*see* Enterocolitis,
  necrotizing, in newborn
  neurogenic -*see* Syndrome, irritable bowel
  newborn necrotizing -*see* Enterocolitis,
  necrotizing, in newborn
  noninfectious K52.9
  norovirus A08.11
  parasitic NEC B82.9
  paratyphoid (fever) -*see* Fever, paratyphoid
  protozoal A07.9
    specified NEC A07.8
  radiation K52.0
  regional (of) K50.90
    with
      complication K50.919
        abscess K50.914
        fistula K50.913
        intestinal obstruction K50.912
        rectal bleeding K50.911
        specified complication NEC K50.918
    colon -*see* Enteritis, regional, large intestine
    duodenum -*see* Enteritis, regional, small
    intestine
    ileum -*see* Enteritis, regional, small intestine
    jejunum -*see* Enteritis, regional, small
    intestine
    large bowel -*see* Enteritis, regional, large
    intestine
    large intestine (colon) (rectum) K50.10
      with

Endodontic --*continued*
      complication K50.119
        abscess K50.114
        fistula K50.113
        intestinal obstruction K50.112
        rectal bleeding K50.111
        small intestine (duodenum) (ileum)
        (jejunum) involvement K50.80
          with
            complication K50.819
              abscess K50.814
              fistula K50.813
              intestinal obstruction K50.812
              rectal bleeding K50.811
              specified complication NEC
              K50.818
        specified complication NEC K50.118
    rectum -*see* Enteritis, regional, large
    intestine
    small intestine (duodenum) (ileum)
    (jejunum) K50.00
      with
        complication K50.019
          abscess K50.014
          fistula K50.013
          intestinal obstruction K50.012
        large intestine (colon) (rectum)
        involvement K50.80
          with
            complication K50.819
              abscess K50.814
              fistula K50.813
              intestinal obstruction K50.812
              rectal bleeding K50.811
              specified complication NEC
              K50.818
        rectal bleeding K50.011
        specified complication NEC K50.018
  Rotaviral A08.0
  Salmonella, salmonellosis (arizonae)
  (cholerae-suis) (enteritidis) (typhimurium)
  A02.0
  segmental -*see* Enteritis, regional
  septic A09
  Shigella -*see* Infection, Shigella
  small round structured NEC A08.19
  spasmodic, spastic -*see* Syndrome, irritable
  bowel
  staphylococcal A04.8
    due to food A05.0
  torovirus A08.39
  toxic NEC K52.1
    due to Clostridium difficile A04.7
  trichomonal A07.8
  tuberculous A18.32
  typhosa A01.00
  ulcerative (chronic) -*see* Colitis, ulcerative
  viral A08.4
    adenovirus A08.2
    enterovirus A08.39
    Rotavirus A08.0
    small round structured NEC A08.19
    specified NEC A08.39
    virus specified NEC A08.39
Enterobiasis B80
Enterobius vermicularis (infection)
(infestation) B80
Enterocele -*see also* Hernia, abdomen
  pelvic, pelvis (acquired) (congenital) N81.5
  vagina, vaginal (acquired) (congenital) NEC
  N81.5

Enterocolitis -*see also* Enteritis K52.9
  due to Clostridium difficile A04.7
  fulminant ischemic -*see also* Ischemia,
    intestine, acute K55.059
  granulomatous -*see* Enteritis, regional
  hemorrhagic (acute) -*see also* Ischemia,
    intestine, acute K55.059
    chronic K55.1
  infectious NEC A09
  ischemic K55.9
  necrotizing K55.30
    with
      perforation K55.33
      pneumatosis K55.32
        and perforation K55.33
    due to Clostridium difficile A04.7
    in non-newborn K55.30
      stage 1 (without pneumatosis, without
        perforation) K55.31
      stage 2 (with pneumatosis, without
        perforation) K55.32
      stage 3 (with pneumatosis, with
        perforation) K55.33
    in newborn P77.9
      stage 1 (without pneumatosis, without
        perforation) P77.1
      stage 2 (with pneumatosis, without
        perforation) P77.2
      stage 3 (with pneumatosis, with
        perforation) P77.3
    without pneumatosis or perforation K55.31
  noninfectious K52.9
  newborn -*see* Enterocolitis, necrotizing, in
    newborn
  pseudomembranous (newborn) A04.7
  radiation K52.0
  newborn -*see* Enterocolitis, necrotizing, in
    newborn
  ulcerative (chronic) -*see* Pancolitis, ulcerative
    (chronic)
Enterogastritis -*see* Enteritis
Enteropathy K63.9
  food protein-induced enterocolitis K52.22
  gluten-sensitive K90.0
    non-celiac K90.41
  hemorrhagic, terminal -*see also* Ischemia,
    intestine, acute K55.059
  protein-losing K90.49
Enteroperitonitis -*see* Peritonitis
Enteroptosis K63.4
Enterorrhagia K92.2
Enterospasm -*see also* Syndrome, irritable,
  bowel
  psychogenic F45.8
Enterostenosis -*see also* Obstruction, intestine
  K56.69
Enterostomy
  complication -*see* Complication, enterostomy
  status Z93.4
**Enterovirus, as cause of disease classified
  elsewhere** B97.10
  coxsackievirus B97.11
  echovirus B97.12
  other specified B97.19
Enthesopathy (peripheral) M77.9
  Achilles tendinitis -*see* Tendinitis, Achilles
  ankle and tarsus M77.9
    specified type NEC -*see* Enthesopathy, foot,
      specified type NEC
  anterior tibial syndrome M76.81
  calcaneal spur -*see* Spur, bone, calcaneal

Enthesopathy --*continued*
  elbow region M77.8
    lateral epicondylitis -*see* Epicondylitis,
      lateral
    medial epicondylitis -*see* Epicondylitis,
      medial
  foot NEC M77.9
    metatarsalgia -*see* Metatarsalgia
    specified type NEC M77.5
  forearm M77.9
  gluteal tendinitis -*see* Tendinitis, gluteal
  hand M77.9
  hip -*see* Enthesopathy, lower limb, specified
    type NEC
  iliac crest spur -*see* Spur, bone, iliac crest
  iliotibial band syndrome -*see* Syndrome,
    iliotibial band
  knee -*see* Enthesopathy, lower limb, lower
    leg, specified type NEC
  lateral epicondylitis -*see* Epicondylitis, lateral
  lower limb (excluding foot) M76.9
    Achilles tendinitis -*see* Tendinitis, Achilles
    anterior tibial syndrome M76.81
    gluteal tendinitis -*see* Tendinitis, gluteal
    iliac crest spur -*see* Spur, bone, iliac crest
    iliotibial band syndrome -*see* Syndrome,
      iliotibial band
    patellar tendinitis -*see* Tendinitis, patellar
    pelvic region -*see* Enthesopathy, lower limb,
      specified type NEC
    peroneal tendinitis -*see* Tendinitis, peroneal
    posterior tibial syndrome M76.82
    psoas tendinitis -*see* Tendinitis, psoas
    shoulder M77.9
    specified type NEC M76.89
    tibial collateral bursitis -*see* Bursitis, tibial
      collateral
  medial epicondylitis -*see* Epicondylitis,
    medial
  metatarsalgia -*see* Metatarsalgia
  multiple sites M77.9
  patellar tendinitis -*see* Tendinitis, patellar
  pelvis M77.9
  periarthritis of wrist -*see* Periarthritis, wrist
  peroneal tendinitis -*see* Tendinitis, peroneal
  posterior tibial syndrome M76.82
  psoas tendinitis -*see* Tendinitis, psoas
  shoulder region -*see* Lesion, shoulder
  specified site NEC M77.9
  specified type NEC M77.8
  spinal M46.00
    cervical region M46.02
    cervicothoracic region M46.03
    lumbar region M46.06
    lumbosacral region M46.07
    multiple sites M46.09
    occipito-atlanto-axial region M46.01
    sacrococcygeal region M46.08
    thoracic region M46.04
    thoracolumbar region M46.05
  tibial collateral bursitis -*see* Bursitis, tibial
    collateral
  upper arm M77.9
  wrist and carpus NEC M77.8
    calcaneal spur -*see* Spur, bone, calcaneal
    periarthritis of wrist -*see* Periarthritis, wrist
Entomophobia F40.218
Entomophthoromycosis B46.8
Entrance, air into vein -*see* Embolism, air
Entrapment, nerve -*see* Neuropathy,
  entrapment

Entropion (eyelid) (paralytic) H02.009
  cicatricial H02.019
    left H02.016
      lower H02.015
      upper H02.014
    right H02.013
      lower H02.012
      upper H02.011
  congenital Q10.2
    left H02.006
      lower H02.005
      upper H02.004
  mechanical H02.029
    left H02.026
      lower H02.025
      upper H02.024
    right H02.023
      lower H02.022
      upper H02.021
  senile H02.039
    left H02.036
      lower H02.035
      upper H02.034
    right H02.033
      lower H02.032
      upper H02.031
  spastic H02.049
    left H02.046
      lower H02.045
      upper H02.044
    right H02.043
      lower H02.042
      upper H02.041
Enucleated eye (traumatic, current) S05.7
Enuresis R32
  functional F98.0
  habit disturbance F98.0
  nocturnal N39.44
    psychogenic F98.0
  nonorganic origin F98.0
  psychogenic F98.0
Eosinopenia -*see* Agranulocytosis
**Eosinophilia (allergic) (hereditary)
  (idiopathic) (secondary)** D72.1
  with
    angiolymphoid hyperplasia (ALHE) D18.01
  infiltrative J82
  Löffler's J82
  peritoneal -*see* Peritonitis, eosinophilic
  pulmonary NEC J82
  tropical (pulmonary) J82
Eosinophilia-myalgia syndrome M35.8
**Ependymitis (acute) (cerebral) (chronic)
  (granular)** -*see* Encephalomyelitis
Ependymoblastoma
  specified site -*see* Neoplasm, malignant, by
    site
  unspecified site C71.9
Ependymoma (epithelial) (malignant)
  anaplastic
    specified site -*see* Neoplasm, malignant, by
      site
    unspecified site C71.9
  benign
    specified site -*see* Neoplasm, benign, by site
    unspecified site D33.2
  myxopapillary D43.2

Ependymoma - *continued*
  specified site *-see* Neoplasm, uncertain
    behavior, by site
  unspecified site D43.2
  papillary D43.2
    specified site *-see* Neoplasm, uncertain
      behavior, by site
    unspecified site D43.2
  specified site *-see* Neoplasm, malignant, by
    site
  unspecified site C71.9
Ependymopathy G93.89
Ephelis, ephelides L81.2
Epiblepharon (congenital) Q10.3
Epicanthus, epicanthic fold (eyelid)
  (congenital) Q10.3
Epicondylitis (elbow)
  lateral M77.1
  medial M77.0
Epicystitis *-see* Cystitis
Epidemic *-see* condition
Epidermidalization, cervix *-see* Dysplasia,
  cervix
Epidermis, epidermal *-see* condition
Epidermodysplasia verruciformis B07.8
Epidermolysis
  bullosa (congenital) Q81.9
    acquired L12.30
      drug-induced L12.31
      specified cause NEC L12.35
    dystrophica Q81.2
    letalis Q81.1
    simplex Q81.0
    specified NEC Q81.8
  necroticans combustiformis L51.2
    due to drug *-see* Table of Drugs and
      Chemicals, by drug
Epidermophytid *-see* Dermatophytosis
Epidermophytosis (infected) *-see*
  Dermatophytosis
Epididymis *-see* condition
Epididymitis (acute) (nonvenereal)
  (recurrent) (residual) N45.1
  with orchitis N45.3
  blennorrhagic (gonococcal) A54.23
  caseous (tuberculous) A18.15
  chlamydial A56.19
  filarial *-see also* Infestation, filarial B74.9
    [N51]
  gonococcal A54.23
  syphilitic A52.76
  tuberculous A18.15
Epididymo-orchitis *-see also* Epididymitis
  N45.3
Epidural *-see* condition
Epigastrium, epigastric *-see* condition
Epigastrocele *-see* Hernia, ventral
Epiglottis *-see* condition
Epiglottitis, epiglottiditis (acute) J05.10
  with obstruction J05.11
  chronic J37.0
Epignathus Q89.4
Epilepsia partialis continua *-see also*
  Kozhevnikov's epilepsy G40.1
Epilepsy, epileptic, epilepsia (attack)
  (cerebral) (convulsion) (fit) (seizure)
  G40.909
  Note: the following terms are to be considered
  equivalent to intractable: pharmacoresistent
  (pharmacologically resistant), treatment

Epilepsy, epileptic, epilepsia - *continued*
  resistant, refractory (medically) and poorly
  controlled
  with
    complex partial seizures *-see* Epilepsy,
      localization-related, symptomatic, with
      complex partial seizures
    grand mal seizures on awakening *-see*
      Epilepsy, generalized, specified NEC
    myoclonic absences *-see* Epilepsy,
      generalized, specified NEC
    myoclonic-astatic seizures *-see* Epilepsy,
      generalized, specified NEC
    simple partial seizures *-see* Epilepsy,
      localization-related, symptomatic, with
      simple partial seizures
  akinetic *-see* Epilepsy, generalized, specified
    NEC
  benign childhood with centrotemporal EEG
    spikes *-see* Epilepsy, localization-related,
    idiopathic
  benign myoclonic in infancy G40.80
  Bravais-jacksonian *-see* Epilepsy,
    localization-related, symptomatic, with
    simple partial seizures
  childhood
    with occipital EEG paroxysms *-see*
      Epilepsy, localization-related, idiopathic
    absence G40.A09
      intractable G40.A19
        with status epilepticus G40.A11
        without status epilepticus G40.A19
      not intractable G40.A09
        with status epilepticus G40.A01
        without status epilepticus G40.A09
  climacteric *-see* Epilepsy, specified NEC
  cysticercosis B69.0
  deterioration (mental) F06.8
  due to syphilis A52.19
  focal *-see* Epilepsy, localization-related,
    symptomatic, with simple partial seizures
  generalized
    idiopathic G40.309
      intractable G40.319
        with status epilepticus G40.311
        without status epilepticus G40.319
      not intractable G40.309
        with status epilepticus G40.301
        without status epilepticus G40.309
    specified NEC G40.409
      intractable G40.419
        with status epilepticus G40.411
        without status epilepticus G40.419
      not intractable G40.409
        with status epilepticus G40.401
        without status epilepticus G40.409
  impulsive petit mal *-see* Epilepsy, juvenile
    myoclonic
  intractable G40.919
    with status epilepticus G40.911
    without status epilepticus G40.919
  juvenile absence G40.A09
    intractable G40.A19
      with status epilepticus G40.A11
      without status epilepticus G40.A19
    not intractable G40.A09
      with status epilepticus G40.A01
      without status epilepticus G40.A09
  juvenile myoclonic G40.B09
    intractable G40.B19
      with status epilepticus G40.B11

Epilepsy, epileptic, epilepsia - *continued*
    without status epilepticus G40.B19
  not intractable G40.B09
    with status epilepticus G40.B01
    without status epilepticus G40.B09
  localization-related (focal) (partial)
    idiopathic G40.009
      with seizures of localized onset G40.009
        intractable G40.019
          with status epilepticus G40.011
          without status epilepticus G40.019
        not intractable G40.009
          with status epilepticus G40.001
          without status epilepticus G40.009
    symptomatic
      with complex partial seizures G40.209
        intractable G40.219
          with status epilepticus G40.211
          without status epilepticus G40.219
        not intractable G40.209
          with status epilepticus G40.201
          without status epilepticus G40.209
      with simple partial seizures G40.109
        intractable G40.119
          with status epilepticus G40.111
          without status epilepticus G40.119
        not intractable G40.109
          with status epilepticus G40.101
          without status epilepticus G40.109
  myoclonus, myoclonic *-see* Epilepsy,
    generalized, specified NEC
    progressive *-see* Epilepsy, generalized,
      idiopathic
  not intractable G40.909
    with status epilepticus G40.901
    without status epilepticus G40.909
  on awakening *-see* Epilepsy, generalized,
    specified NEC
  parasitic NOS B71.9 [G94]
  partialis continua *-see also* Kozhevnikov's
    epilepsy G40.1
  peripheral *-see* Epilepsy, specified NEC
  procursiva *-see* Epilepsy, localization-related,
    symptomatic, with simple partial seizures
  progressive (familial) myoclonic *-see*
    Epilepsy, generalized, idiopathic
  reflex *-see* Epilepsy, specified NEC
  related to
    alcohol G40.509
      not intractable G40.509
        with status epilepticus G40.501
        without status epilepticus G40.509
    drugs G40.509
      not intractable G40.509
        with status epilepticus G40.501
        without status epilepticus G40.509
    external causes G40.509
      not intractable G40.509
        with status epilepticus G40.501
        without status epilepticus G40.509
    hormonal changes G40.509
      not intractable G40.509
        with status epilepticus G40.501
        without status epilepticus G40.509
    sleep deprivation G40.509
      not intractable G40.509
        with status epilepticus G40.501
        without status epilepticus G40.509
    stress G40.509
      not intractable G40.509
        with status epilepticus G40.501

Epilepsy, epileptic, epilepsia - *continued*
  without status epilepticus G40.509
  somatomotor *-see* Epilepsy, localization-
    related, symptomatic, with simple partial
    seizures
  somatosensory *-see* Epilepsy, localization-
    related, symptomatic, with simple partial
    seizures
  spasms G40.822
    intractable G40.824
      with status epilepticus G40.823
      without status epilepticus G40.824
    not intractable G40.822
      with status epilepticus G40.821
      without status epilepticus G40.822
    specified NEC G40.802
      intractable G40.804
        with status epilepticus G40.803
        without status epilepticus G40.804
      not intractable G40.802
        with status epilepticus G40.801
        without status epilepticus G40.802
  syndromes
    generalized
      idiopathic G40.309
        intractable G40.319
          with status epilepticus G40.311
          without status epilepticus G40.319
        not intractable G40.309
          with status epilepticus G40.301
          without status epilepticus G40.309
      specified NEC G40.409
        intractable G40.419
          with status epilepticus G40.411
          without status epilepticus G40.419
        not intractable G40.409
          with status epilepticus G40.401
          without status epilepticus G40.409
    localization-related (focal) (partial)
      idiopathic G40.009
        with seizures of localized onset G40.009
          intractable G40.019
            with status epilepticus G40.011
            without status epilepticus G40.019
          not intractable G40.009
            with status epilepticus G40.001
            without status epilepticus G40.009
      symptomatic
        with complex partial seizures G40.209
          intractable G40.219
            with status epilepticus G40.211
            without status epilepticus G40.219
          not intractable G40.209
            with status epilepticus G40.201
            without status epilepticus G40.209
        with simple partial seizures G40.109
          intractable G40.119
            with status epilepticus G40.111
            without status epilepticus G40.119
          not intractable G40.109
            with status epilepticus G40.101
            without status epilepticus G40.109
    specified NEC G40.802
      intractable G40.804
        with status epilepticus G40.803
        without status epilepticus G40.804
      not intractable G40.802
        with status epilepticus G40.801
        without status epilepticus G40.802
  tonic (clonic) *-see* Epilepsy, generalized,
    specified NEC

Epilepsy, epileptic, epilepsia - *continued*
  twilight F05
  uncinate (gyrus) *-see* Epilepsy, localization-
    related, symptomatic, with complex partial
    seizures
  Unverricht (Lundborg) (familial myoclonic) -
    see Epilepsy, generalized, idiopathic
  visceral *-see* Epilepsy, specified NEC
  visual *-see* Epilepsy, specified NEC
Epiloia Q85.1
Epimenorrhea N92.0
Epipharyngitis *-see* Nasopharyngitis
Epiphora H04.20
  due to
    excess lacrimation H04.21
    insufficient drainage H04.22
Epiphyseal arrest *-see* Arrest, epiphyseal
Epiphyseolysis, epiphysiolysis *-see*
  Osteochondropathy
Epiphysitis *-see also* Osteochondropathy
  juvenile M92.9
  syphilitic (congenital) A50.02
Epiplocele *-see* Hernia, abdomen
Epiploitis *-see* Peritonitis
Epiplosarcomphalocele *-see* Hernia,
  umbilicus
Episcleritis (suppurative) H15.10
  in (due to)
    syphilis A52.71
    tuberculosis A18.51
  nodular H15.12
  periodica fugax H15.11
    angioneurotic *-see* Edema, angioneurotic
  syphilitic (late) A52.71
  tuberculous A18.51
Episode
  affective, mixed F39
  depersonalization (in neurotic state) F48.1
  depressive F32.9
    major F32.9
      mild F32.0
      moderate F32.1
      severe (without psychotic symptoms)
      F32.2
        with psychotic symptoms F32.3
    recurrent F33.9
      brief F33.8
    specified NEC F32.89
  hypomanic F30.8
  manic F30.9
    with
      psychotic symptoms F30.2
      remission (full) F30.4
        partial F30.3
    other specified F30.8
    recurrent F31.89
    without psychotic symptoms F30.10
      mild F30.11
      moderate F30.12
      severe (without psychotic symptoms)
      F30.13
        with psychotic symptoms F30.2
  psychotic F23
    organic F06.8
  schizophrenic (acute) NEC, brief F23
Epispadias (female) (male) Q64.0
Episplenitis D73.89
Epistaxis (multiple) R04.0
  hereditary I78.0
  vicarious menstruation N94.89

Epithelioma (malignant) *-see also* Neoplasm,
  malignant, by site
  adenoides cysticum *-see* Neoplasm, skin,
    benign
  basal cell *-see* Neoplasm, skin, malignant
  benign *-see* Neoplasm, benign, by site
  Bowen's *-see* Neoplasm, skin, in situ
  calcifying, of Malherbe *-see* Neoplasm, skin,
    benign
  external site *-see* Neoplasm, skin, malignant
  intraepidermal, Jadassohn *-see* Neoplasm,
    skin, benign
  squamous cell *-see* Neoplasm, malignant, by
    site
Epitheliomatosis pigmented Q82.1
Epitheliopathy, multifocal placoid pigment
  H30.14
Epithelium, epithelial *-see* condition
Epituberculosis (with atelectasis) (allergic)
  A15.7
Eponychia Q84.6
Epstein's
  nephrosis or syndrome *-see* Nephrosis
  pearl K09.8
Epulis (gingiva) (fibrous) (giant cell) K06.8
Equinia A24.0
Equinovarus (congenital) (talipes) Q66.0
  acquired *-see* Deformity, limb, clubfoot
Equivalent
  convulsive (abdominal) *-see* Epilepsy,
    specified NEC
  epileptic (psychic) *-see* Epilepsy, localization-
    related, symptomatic, with complex partial
    seizures
Erb (Duchenne) paralysis (birth injury)
  (newborn) P14.0
Erb-Goldflam disease or syndrome G70.00
  with exacerbation (acute) G70.01
  in crisis G70.01
Erb's
  disease G71.0
  palsy, paralysis (brachial) (birth) (newborn)
    P14.0
    spinal (spastic) syphilitic A52.17
  pseudohypertrophic muscular dystrophy
    G71.0
Erdheim's syndrome (acromegalic
  macrospondylitis) E22.0
Erection, painful (persistent) *-see* Priapism
Ergosterol deficiency (vitamin D) E55.9
  with
    adult osteomalacia M83.8
    rickets *-see* Rickets
Ergotism *-see also* Poisoning, food, noxious,
  plant
  from ergot used as drug (migraine therapy) -
    see Table of Drugs and Chemicals
Erosio interdigitalis blastomycetica B37.2
Erosion
  artery I77.2
    without rupture I77.89
  bone *-see* Disorder, bone, density and
    structure, specified NEC
  bronchus J98.09
  cartilage (joint) *-see* Disorder, cartilage,
    specified type NEC
  cervix (uteri) (acquired) (chronic) (congenital)
    N86
    with cervicitis N72
  cornea (nontraumatic) *-see* Ulcer, cornea
    recurrent H18.83

Erosion
traumatic -*see* Abrasion, cornea
dental (idiopathic) (occupational) (due to diet, drugs or vomiting) K03.2
duodenum, postpyloric -*see* Ulcer, duodenum
esophagus K22.10
    with bleeding K22.11
gastric -*see* Ulcer, stomach
gastrojejunal -*see* Ulcer, gastrojejunal
implanted mesh -*see* Complications, mesh
intestine K63.3
lymphatic vessel I89.8
pylorus, pyloric (ulcer) -*see* Ulcer, stomach
spine, aneurysmal A52.09
stomach -*see* Ulcer, stomach
subcutaneous device pocket
    nervous system prosthetic device, implant, or graft T85.890
    other internal prosthetic device, implant, or graft T85.898
teeth (idiopathic) (occupational) (due to diet, drugs or vomiting) K03.2
urethra N36.8
uterus N85.8
Erotomania F52.8
Error
metabolism, inborn - se Disorder, metabolism
refractive -*see* Disorder, refraction
Eructation R14.2
nervous or psychogenic F45.8
Eruption
creeping B76.9
drug (generalized) (taken internally) L27.0
    fixed L27.1
    in contact with skin -*see* Dermatitis, due to drugs
        localized L27.1
Hutchinson, summer L56.4
Kaposi's varicelliform B00.0
napkin L22
polymorphous light (sun) L56.4
recalcitrant pustular L13.8
ringed R23.8
skin (nonspecific) R21
    creeping (meaning hookworm) B76.9
    due to inoculation/vaccination (generalized) -*see also* Dermatitis, due to, vaccine L27.0
        localized L27.1
    erysipeloid A26.0
    feigned L98.1
    Kaposi's varicelliform B00.0
    lichenoid L28.0
    meaning dermatitis -*see* Dermatitis
    toxic NEC L53.0
tooth, teeth, abnormal (incomplete) (late) (premature) (sequence) K00.6
vesicular R23.8
Erysipelas (gangrenous) (infantile) (newborn) (phlegmonous) (suppurative) A46
external ear A46 [*H62.40*]
puerperal, postpartum O86.89
Erysipeloid A26.9
cutaneous (Rosenbach's) A26.0
disseminated A26.8
sepsis A26.7
specified NEC A26.8
Erythema, erythematous (infectional) (inflammation) L53.9
ab igne L59.0

Erythema, erythematous - *continued*
annulare (centrifugum) (rheumaticum) L53.1
arthriticum epidemicum A25.1
brucellum -*see* Brucellosis
chronic figurate NEC L53.3
chronicum migrans (Borrelia burgdorferi) A69.20
diaper L22
due to
    chemical NEC L53.0
        in contact with skin L24.5
    drug (internal use) -*see* Dermatitis, due to, drugs
elevatum diutinum L95.1
endemic E52
epidemic, arthritic A25.1
figuratum perstans L53.3
gluteal L22
heat
    code by site under Burn, first degree - ichthyosiforme congenitum bullous Q80.3
in diseases classified elsewhere L54
induratum (nontuberculous) L52
    tuberculous A18.4
infectiosum B08.3
intertrigo L30.4
iris L51.9
marginatum L53.2
    in (due to) acute rheumatic fever I00
medicamentosum -*see* Dermatitis, due to, drugs
migrans A26.0
    chronicum A69.20
    tongue K14.1
multiforme (major) (minor) L51.9
    bullous, bullosum L51.1
    conjunctiva L51.1
    nonbullous L51.0
    pemphigoides L12.0
    specified NEC L51.8
napkin L22
neonatorum P83.8
    toxic P83.1
nodosum L52
    tuberculous A18.4
palmar L53.8
pernio T69.1
rash, newborn P83.8
scarlatiniform (recurrent) (exfoliative) L53.8
solare L55.0
specified NEC L53.8
toxic, toxicum NEC L53.0
    newborn P83.1
tuberculous (primary) A18.4
Erythematous, erythematosus -*see* condition
Erythermalgia (primary) I73.81
Erythralgia I73.81
Erythrasma L08.1
Erythredema (polyneuropathy) -*see* Poisoning, mercury
Erythremia (acute) C94.0
chronic D45
secondary D75.1
Erythroblastopenia -*see also* Aplasia, red cell D60.9
congenital D61.01

Erythroblastophthisis D61.09
Erythroblastosis (fetalis) (newborn) P55.9
due to
    ABO (antibodies) (incompatibility) (isoimmunization) P55.1
    Rh (antibodies) (incompatibility) (isoimmunization) P55.0
Erythrocyanosis (crurum) I73.89
Erythrocythemia -*see* Erythremia
Erythrocytosis (megalosplenic) (secondary) D75.1
familial D75.0
oval, hereditary -*see* Elliptocytosis
secondary D75.1
stress D75.1
Erythroderma (secondary) -*see also* Erythema L53.9
bullous ichthyosiform, congenital Q80.3
desquamativum L21.1
ichthyosiform, congenital (bullous) Q80.3
neonatorum P83.8
psoriaticum L40.8
Erythrodysesthesia, palmar plantar (PPE) L27.1
Erythrogenesis imperfecta D61.09
Erythroleukemia C94.0
Erythromelalgia I73.81
Erythrophagocytosis D75.89
Erythrophobia F40.298
Erythroplakia, oral epithelium, and tongue K13.29
Erythroplasia (Queyrat) D07.4
specified site -*see* Neoplasm, skin, in situ
unspecified site D07.4
Escherichia coli (E. coli), as cause of disease classified elsewhere B96.20
non-O157 Shiga toxin-producing (with known O group) B96.22
non-Shiga toxin-producing B96.29
O157 with confirmation of Shiga toxin when H antigen is unknown, or is not H7 B96.21
O157:H- (nonmotile) with confirmation of Shiga toxin B96.21
O157:H7 with or without confirmation of Shiga toxin-production B96.21
Shiga toxin-producing (with unspecified O group) (STEC) B96.23
    O157 B96.21
    O157:H7 with or without confirmation of Shiga toxin-production B96.21
    specified NEC B96.22
specified NEC B96.29
Esophagismus K22.4
Esophagitis (acute) (alkaline) (chemical) (chronic) (infectional) (necrotic) (peptic) (postoperative) K20.9
candidal B37.81
due to gastrointestinal reflux disease K21.0
eosinophilic K20.0
reflux K21.0
specified NEC K20.8
tuberculous A18.83
ulcerative K22.10
    with bleeding K22.11
Esophagocele K22.5
Esophagomalacia K22.8
Esophagospasm K22.4
Esophagostenosis K22.2
Esophagostomiasis B81.8
Esophagotracheal -*see* condition
Esophagus -*see* condition

Esophoria H50.51
  convergence, excess H51.12
  divergence, insufficiency H51.8
Esotropia -*see* Strabismus, convergent
  concomitant
Espundia B55.2
Essential -*see* condition
Esthesioneuroblastoma C30.0
Esthesioneurocytoma C30.0
Esthesioneuroepithelioma C30.0
Esthiomene A55
Estivo-autumnal malaria (fever) B50.9
Estrangement (marital) Z63.5
  parent-child NEC Z62.890
Estriasis -*see* Myiasis
Ethanolism -*see* Alcoholism
Etherism -*see* Dependence, drug, inhalant
Ethmoid, ethmoidal -*see* condition
Ethmoiditis (chronic) (nonpurulent)
  (purulent) -*see also* Sinusitis, ethmoidal
  influenzal -*see* Influenza, with, respiratory
  manifestations NEC
  Woakes' J33.1
Ethylism -*see* Alcoholism
Eulenburg's disease (congenital
  paramyotonia) G71.19
Eumycetoma B47.0
Eunuchoidism E29.1
  hypogonadotropic E23.0
European blastomycosis -*see* Cryptococcosis
Eustachian -*see* condition
Evaluation (for) (of)
  development state
    adolescent Z00.3
    period of
      delayed growth in childhood Z00.70
        with abnormal findings Z00.71
      rapid growth in childhood Z00.2
      puberty Z00.3
  growth and developmental state (period of
    rapid growth) Z00.2
    delayed growth Z00.70
      with abnormal findings Z00.71
  mental health (status) Z00.8
    requested by authority Z04.6
  period of
    delayed growth in childhood Z00.70
      with abnormal findings Z00.71
    rapid growth in childhood Z00.2
  suspected condition -*see* Observation
Evans syndrome D69.41
Event, apparent life threatening in newborn
  and infant (ALTE) R68.13
Eventration -*see also* Hernia, ventral
  colon into chest -*see* Hernia, diaphragm
  diaphragm (congenital) Q79.1
Eversion
  bladder N32.89
  cervix (uteri) N86
    with cervicitis N72
  foot NEC -*see also* Deformity, valgus, ankle
    congenital Q66.6
  punctum lacrimale (postinfectional) (senile)
    H04.52
  ureter (meatus) N28.89
  urethra (meatus) N36.8
  uterus N81.4

Evidence
  cytologic
    of malignancy on anal smear R85.614
    of malignancy on cervical smear R87.614
    of malignancy on vaginal smear R87.624
Evisceration
  birth injury P15.8
  traumatic NEC
    eye -*see* Enucleated eye
Evulsion -*see* Avulsion
Ewing's sarcoma or tumor
  -*see* Neoplasm, bone, malignant
Examination (for) (following) (general) (of)
  (routine) Z00.00
  with abnormal findings Z00.01
  abuse, physical (alleged), ruled out
    adult Z04.71
    child Z04.72
  adolescent (development state) Z00.3
  alleged rape or sexual assault (victim), ruled
    out
    adult Z04.41
    child Z04.42
  allergy Z01.82
  annual (adult) (periodic) (physical) Z00.00
    with abnormal findings Z00.01
    gynecological Z01.419
      with abnormal findings Z01.411
  antibody response Z01.84
  blood -*see* Examination, laboratory   blood
  pressure Z01.30
    with abnormal findings Z01.31
  cancer staging -*see* Neoplasm, malignant, by
  site
  cervical Papanicolaou smear Z12.4
    as part of routine gynecological examination
    Z01.419
      with abnormal findings Z01.411
  child (over 28 days old) Z00.129
    with abnormal findings Z00.121
    under 28 days old -*see* Newborn,
  examination
  clinical research control or normal
  comparison (control) (participant) Z00.6
  contraceptive (drug) maintenance (routine)
  Z30.8
    device (intrauterine) Z30.431
  dental Z01.20
    with abnormal findings Z01.21
  developmental -*see* Examination, child -
    donor (potential) Z00.5
  ear Z01.10
    with abnormal findings NEC Z01.118
  eye Z01.00
    with abnormal findings Z01.01
  following
    accident NEC Z04.3
      transport Z04.1
      work Z04.2
    assault, alleged, ruled out
      adult Z04.71
      child Z04.72
    motor vehicle accident Z04.1
    treatment (for) Z09
      combined NEC Z09
        fracture Z09
        malignant neoplasm Z08
      malignant neoplasm Z08
      mental disorder Z09
      specified condition NEC Z09
  follow-up (routine) (following) Z09

Examination - *continued*
  chemotherapy NEC Z09
    malignant neoplasm Z08
  fracture Z09
  malignant neoplasm Z08
  postpartum Z39.2
  psychotherapy Z09
  radiotherapy NEC Z09
    malignant neoplasm Z08
  surgery NEC Z09
    malignant neoplasm Z08
  gynecological Z01.419
    with abnormal findings Z01.411
    for contraceptive maintenance Z30.8
  health -*see* Examination, medical
  hearing Z01.10
    with abnormal findings NEC Z01.118
    following failed hearing screening Z01.110
  immunity status testing Z01.84
  laboratory (as part of a general medical
  examination) Z00.00
    with abnormal findings Z00.01
    preprocedural Z01.812
  lactating mother Z39.1
  medical (adult) (for) (of) Z00.00
    with abnormal findings Z00.01
    administrative purpose only Z02.9
      specified NEC Z02.89
    admission to
      armed forces Z02.3
      old age home Z02.2
      prison Z02.89
      residential institution Z02.2
      school Z02.0
        following illness or medical treatment
        Z02.0
      summer camp Z02.89
    adoption Z02.82
    blood alcohol or drug level Z02.83
    camp (summer) Z02.89
    clinical research, normal subject (control)
      (participant) Z00.6
    control subject in clinical research (normal
  comparison) (participant) Z00.6
    donor (potential) Z00.5
    driving license Z02.4
    general (adult) Z00.00
      with abnormal findings Z00.01
    immigration Z02.89
    insurance purposes Z02.6
    marriage Z02.89
    medicolegal reasons NEC Z04.8
    naturalization Z02.89
    participation in sport Z02.5
    paternity testing Z02.81
    population survey Z00.8
    pre-employment Z02.1
    pre-operative -*see* Examination, pre-
  procedural
    pre-procedural
      cardiovascular Z01.810
      respiratory Z01.811
      specified NEC Z01.818
    preschool children
      for admission to school Z02.0
    prisoners
      for entrance into prison Z02.89
    recruitment for armed forces Z02.3
    specified NEC Z00.8
    sport competition Z02.5
  medicolegal reason NEC Z04.8

Examination - *continued*
newborn -*see* Newborn, examination
pelvic (annual) (periodic) Z01.419
  with abnormal findings Z01.411
period of rapid growth in childhood Z00.2
periodic (adult) (annual) (routine) Z00.00
  with abnormal findings Z00.01
physical (adult) -*see also* Examination,
medical Z00.00
  sports Z02.5
postpartum
  immediately after delivery Z39.0
  routine follow-up Z39.2
prenatal (normal pregnancy) -*see also*
Pregnancy, normal Z34.9
pre-chemotherapy (antineoplastic) Z01.818
pre-procedural (pre-operative)
  cardiovascular Z01.810
  laboratory Z01.812
  respiratory Z01.811
  specified NEC Z01.818
prior to chemotherapy (antineoplastic)
  Z01.818
psychiatric NEC Z00.8
  follow-up not needing further care Z09
  requested by authority Z04.6
radiological (as part of a general medical
examination) Z00.00
  with abnormal findings Z00.01
repeat cervical smear to confirm findings of
recent normal smear following initial
abnormal smear Z01.42
skin (hypersensitivity) Z01.82
special -*see also* Examination, by type Z01.89
  specified type NEC Z01.89
  specified type or reason NEC Z04.8
teeth Z01.20
  with abnormal findings Z01.21
urine -*see* Examination, laboratory   vision
Z01.00
  with abnormal findings Z01.01

Exanthem, exanthema -*see also* Rash
with enteroviral vesicular stomatitis B08.4
Boston A88.0
epidemic with meningitis A88.0 [*G02*]
subitum B08.20
  due to human herpesvirus 6 B08.21
  due to human herpesvirus 7 B08.22
viral, virus B09
  specified type NEC B08.8

Excess, excessive, excessively   alcohol level
in blood R78.0
androgen (ovarian) E28.1
attrition, tooth, teeth K03.0
carotene, carotin (dietary) E67.1
cold, effects of T69.9
  specified effect NEC T69.8
convergence H51.12
crying
  in child, adolescent, or adult R45.83
  in infant R68.11
development, breast N62
divergence H51.8
drinking (alcohol) NEC (without dependence)
F10.10
  habitual (continual) (without remission)
  F10.20
eating R63.2
estrogen E28.0
fat -*see also* Obesity
  in heart -*see* Degeneration, myocardial

Excess, excessive, excessively --*continued*
localized E65
foreskin N47.8
gas R14.0
glucagon E16.3
heat -*see* Heat
intermaxillary vertical dimension of fully
  erupted teeth M26.37
interocclusal distance of fully erupted teeth
  M26.37
kalium E87.5
large
  colon K59.39
    congenital Q43.8
  infant P08.0
  organ or site, congenital NEC -*see* Anomaly,
  by site
long
  organ or site, congenital NEC -*see* Anomaly,
  by site
menstruation (with regular cycle) N92.0
  with irregular cycle N92.1
napping Z72.821
natrium E87.0
number of teeth K00.1
nutrient (dietary) NEC R63.2
potassium (K) E87.5
salivation K11.7
secretion -*see also* Hypersecretion
  milk O92.6
  sputum R09.3
  sweat R61
sexual drive F52.8
short
  organ or site, congenital NEC -*see* Anomaly,
  by site
  umbilical cord in labor or delivery O69.3
skin L98.7
  and subcutaneous tissue L98.7
  eyelid (acquired) -*see* Blepharochalasis
    congenital Q10.3
sodium (Na) E87.0
spacing of fully erupted teeth M26.32
sputum R09.3
sweating R61
thirst R63.1
  due to deprivation of water T73.1
tuberosity of jaw M26.07
vitamin
  A (dietary) E67.0
    administered as drug (prolonged intake) -
    see Table of Drugs and Chemicals,
    vitamins, adverse effect
    overdose or wrong substance given or
    taken -*see* Table of Drugs and Chemicals,
    vitamins, poisoning
  D (dietary) E67.3
    administered as drug (prolonged intake) -
    see Table of Drugs and Chemicals,
    vitamins, adverse effect
    overdose or wrong substance given or
    taken -*see* Table of Drugs and Chemicals,
    vitamins, poisoning
weight
  gain R63.5
  loss R63.4

**Excitability, abnormal, under minor stress
(personality disorder)** F60.3
Excitation
anomalous atrioventricular I45.6
psychogenic F30.8
reactive (from emotional stress, psychological
trauma) F30.8
Excitement
hypomanic F30.8
manic F30.9
mental, reactive (from emotional stress,
psychological trauma) F30.8
state, reactive (from emotional stress,
psychological trauma) F30.8
Excoriation (traumatic) -*see also* Abrasion
neurotic L98.1
skin picking disorder F42.4
Exfoliation
due to erythematous conditions according to
extent of body surface involved L49.0
  10 19 percent of body surface L49.1
  20 29 percent of body surface L49.2
  30 39 percent of body surface L49.3
  40 49 percent of body surface L49.4
  50 59 percent of body surface L49.5
  60 69 percent of body surface L49.6
  70 79 percent of body surface L49.7
  80 89 percent of body surface L49.8
  90 99 percent of body surface L49.9
  less than 10 percent of body surface L49.0
teeth, due to systemic causes K08.0
Exfoliative -*see* condition
Exhaustion, exhaustive (physical NEC)
R53.83
battle F43.0
cardiac -*see* Failure, heart
delirium F43.0
due to
  cold T69.8
  excessive exertion T73.3
  exposure T73.2
  neurasthenia F48.8
heart -*see* Failure, heart
heat -*see also* Heat, exhaustion T67.5
  due to
    salt depletion T67.4
    water depletion T67.3
maternal, complicating delivery O75.81
mental F48.8
myocardium, myocardial -*see* Failure, heart
nervous F48.8
old age R54
psychogenic F48.8
psychosis F43.0
senile R54
vital NEC Z73.0
Exhibitionism F65.2
Exocervicitis -*see* Cervicitis
Exomphalos Q79.2
meaning hernia -*see* Hernia, umbilicus
Exophoria H50.52
convergence, insufficiency H51.11
divergence, excess H51.8
Exophthalmos H05.2
congenital Q15.8
constant NEC H05.24
displacement, globe -*see* Displacement, globe
due to thyrotoxicosis (hyperthyroidism) -*see*
  Hyperthyroidism, with, goiter (diffuse)
dysthyroid -*see* Hyperthyroidism, with, goiter
(diffuse)

Exophthalmos - *continued*
goiter -*see* Hyperthyroidism, with, goiter (diffuse)
intermittent NEC H05.25
malignant -*see* Hyperthyroidism, with, goiter (diffuse)
orbital
edema -*see* Edema, orbit
hemorrhage -*see* Hemorrhage, orbit
pulsating NEC H05.26
thyrotoxic, thyrotropic -*see* Hyperthyroidism, with, goiter (diffuse)
Exostosis -*see also* Disorder, bone
cartilaginous -*see* Neoplasm, bone, benign
congenital (multiple) Q78.6
external ear canal H61.81
gonococcal A54.49
jaw (bone) M27.8
multiple, congenital Q78.6
orbit H05.35
osteocartilaginous -*see* Neoplasm, bone, benign
syphilitic A52.77
Exotropia -*see* Strabismus, divergent concomitant
Explanation of
investigation finding Z71.2
medication Z71.89
Exposure (to) -*see also* Contact, with T75.89
acariasis Z20.7
AIDS virus Z20.6
air pollution Z77.110
algae and algae toxins Z77.121
algae bloom Z77.121
anthrax Z20.810
aromatic amines Z77.020
aromatic (hazardous) compounds NEC Z77.028
aromatic dyes NOS Z77.028
arsenic Z77.010
asbestos Z77.090
bacterial disease NEC Z20.818
benzene Z77.021
blue-green algae bloom Z77.121
body fluids (potentially hazardous) Z77.21
brown tide Z77.121
chemicals (chiefly nonmedicinal) (hazardous) NEC Z77.098
cholera Z20.09
chromium compounds Z77.018
cold, effects of T69.9
specified effect NEC T69.8
communicable disease Z20.9
bacterial NEC Z20.818
specified NEC Z20.89
viral NEC Z20.828
cyanobacteria bloom Z77.121
disaster Z65.5
discrimination Z60.5
dyes Z77.098
effects of T73.9
environmental tobacco smoke (acute) (chronic) Z77.22
Escherichia coli (E. coli) Z20.01
exhaustion due to T73.2
fiberglass -*see* Table of Drugs and Chemicals, fiberglass
German measles Z20.4
gonorrhea Z20.2
hazardous metals NEC Z77.018
hazardous substances NEC Z77.29

Exposure (to) --*continued*
hazards in the physical environment NEC Z77.128
hazards to health NEC Z77.9
human immunodeficiency virus (HIV) Z20.6
human T-lymphotropic virus type-1 (HTLV-1) Z20.89
implanted
mesh -*see* Complications, mesh
prosthetic materials NEC -*see* Complications, prosthetic materials NEC
infestation (parasitic) NEC Z20.7
intestinal infectious disease NEC Z20.09
Escherichia coli (E. coli) Z20.01
lead Z77.011
meningococcus Z20.811
mold (toxic) Z77.120
nickel dust Z77.018
noise Z77.122
occupational
air contaminants NEC Z57.39
dust Z57.2
environmental tobacco smoke Z57.31
extreme temperature Z57.6
noise Z57.0
radiation Z57.1
risk factors Z57.9
specified NEC Z57.8
toxic agents (gases) (liquids) (solids) (vapors) in agriculture Z57.4
toxic agents (gases) (liquids) (solids) (vapors) in industry NEC Z57.5
vibration Z57.7
parasitic disease NEC Z20.7
pediculosis Z20.7
persecution Z60.5
pfiesteria piscicida Z77.121
poliomyelitis Z20.89
polycyclic aromatic hydrocarbons Z77.028
pollution
air Z77.110
environmental NEC Z77.118
soil Z77.112
water Z77.111
prenatal (drugs) (toxic chemicals) -*see* Newborn, affected by, noxious substances transmitted via placenta or breast milk
rabies Z20.3
radiation, naturally occurring NEC Z77.123
radon Z77.123
red tide (Florida) Z77.121
rubella Z20.4
second hand tobacco smoke (acute) (chronic) Z77.22
in the perinatal period P96.81
sexually transmitted disease Z20.2
smallpox (laboratory) Z20.89
syphilis Z20.2
terrorism Z65.4
torture Z65.4
tuberculosis Z20.1
uranium Z77.012
varicella Z20.820
venereal disease Z20.2
viral disease NEC Z20.828
war Z65.5
water pollution Z77.111
Exsanguination -*see* Hemorrhage
Exstrophy
abdominal contents Q45.8
bladder Q64.10

Exstrophy --*continued*
cloacal Q64.12
specified type NEC Q64.19
supravesical fissure Q64.11
Extensive -*see* condition
Extra -*see also* Accessory
marker chromosomes (normal individual) Q92.61
in abnormal individual Q92.62
rib Q76.6
cervical Q76.5
Extrasystoles (supraventricular) I49.49
atrial I49.1
auricular I49.1
junctional I49.2
ventricular I49.3
Extrauterine gestation or pregnancy -*see* Pregnancy, by site
Extravasation
blood R58
chyle into mesentery I89.8
pelvicalyceal N13.8
pyelosinus N13.8
urine (from ureter) R39.0
vesicant agent
antineoplastic chemotherapy T80.810
other agent NEC T80.818
Extremity -*see* condition, limb
Extrophy -*see* Exstrophy
Extroversion
bladder Q64.19
uterus N81.4
complicating delivery O71.2
postpartal (old) N81.4
Extruded tooth (teeth) M26.34
Extrusion
breast implant (prosthetic) T85.42
eye implant (globe) (ball) T85.328
intervertebral disc -*see* Displacement, intervertebral disc
ocular lens implant (prosthetic) -*see* Complications, intraocular lens
vitreous -*see* Prolapse, vitreous
Exudate
pleural -*see* Effusion, pleura
retina H35.89
Exudative -*see* condition
Eye, eyeball, eyelid -*see* condition
Eyestrain -*see* Disturbance, vision, subjective
Eyeworm disease of Africa B74.3

F

Faber's syndrome (achlorhydric anemia) D50.9
Fabry (Anderson) disease E75.21
Faciocephalalgia, autonomic -*see also* Neuropathy, peripheral, autonomic G90.09
Factor(s)
psychic, associated with diseases classified elsewhere F54
psychological
affecting physical conditions F54
or behavioral
affecting general medical condition F54
associated with disorders or diseases classified elsewhere F54
Fahr disease (of brain) G23.8
Fahr Volhard disease (of kidney) I12.

Failure, failed
abortion -*see* Abortion, attempted
aortic (valve) I35.8
  rheumatic I06.8
attempted abortion -*see* Abortion, attempted
biventricular I50.9
bone marrow -*see* Anemia, aplastic
cardiac -*see* Failure, heart
cardiorenal (chronic) I50.9
  hypertensive I13.2
cardiorespiratory -*see also* Failure, heart
  R09.2
cardiovascular (chronic) -*see* Failure, heart
cerebrovascular I67.9
cervical dilatation in labor O62.0
circulation, circulatory (peripheral) R57.9
  newborn P29.89
compensation -*see* Disease, heart
compliance with medical treatment or
  regimen -*see* Noncompliance
congestive -*see* Failure, heart, congestive
dental implant (endosseous) M27.69
  due to
    failure of dental prosthesis M27.63
    lack of attached gingiva M27.62
    occlusal trauma (poor prosthetic design)
      M27.62
    parafunctional habits M27.62
    periodontal infection (peri-implantitis)
      M27.62
    poor oral hygiene M27.62
  osseointegration M27.61
    due to
      complications of systemic disease
        M27.61
      poor bone quality M27.61
    iatrogenic M27.61
  post-osseointegration
    biological M27.62
    due to complications of systemic disease
      M27.62
    iatrogenic M27.62
    mechanical M27.63
  pre-integration M27.61
  pre-osseointegration M27.61
  specified NEC M27.69
descent of head (at term) of pregnancy
  (mother) O32.4
endosseous dental implant -*see* Failure, dental
  implant
engagement of head (term of pregnancy)
  (mother) O32.4
erection (penile) -*see also* Dysfunction,
  sexual, male, erectile N52.9
    nonorganic F52.21
examination(s), anxiety concerning Z55.2
expansion terminal respiratory units
  (newborn) (primary) P28.0
forceps NOS (with subsequent cesarean
  delivery) O66.5
gain weight (child over 28 days old) R62.51
  adult R62.7
  newborn P92.6
genital response (male) F52.21
  female F52.22
heart (acute) (senile) (sudden) I50.9
  with
    acute pulmonary edema -*see* Failure,
      ventricular, left
    decompensation -*see* Failure, heart,
      congestive

Failure, failed --*continued*
  dilatation -*see* Disease, heart
  arteriosclerotic I70.90
  biventricular I50.9
  combined left-right sided I50.9
  compensated I50.9
  complicating
    anesthesia (general) (local) or other
      sedation
      in labor and delivery O74.2
      in pregnancy O29.12
      postpartum, puerperal O89.1
    delivery (cesarean) (instrumental) O75.4
  congestive (compensated) (decompensated)
    I50.9
    with rheumatic fever (conditions in I00)
      active I01.8
      inactive or quiescent (with chorea) I09.81
    newborn P29.0
    rheumatic (chronic) (inactive) (with
      chorea) I09.81
      active or acute I01.8
        with chorea I02.0
  decompensated I50.9
  degenerative -*see* Degeneration, myocardial
  diastolic (congestive) I50.30
    acute (congestive) I50.31
      and (on) chronic (congestive) I50.33
    chronic (congestive) I50.32
      and (on) acute (congestive) I50.33
    combined with systolic (congestive) I50.40
      acute (congestive) I50.41
        and (on) chronic (congestive) I50.43
      chronic (congestive) I50.42
        and (on) acute (congestive) I50.43
  due to presence of cardiac prosthesis I97.13
  following cardiac surgery I97.13
  high output NOS I50.9
  hypertensive -*see* Hypertension, heart
  left (ventricular) -*see* Failure, ventricular,
    left
  low output (syndrome) NOS I50.9
  newborn P29.0
  organic -*see* Disease, heart
  peripartum O90.3
  postprocedural I97.13
  rheumatic (chronic) (inactive) I09.9
  right (ventricular) (secondary to left heart
    failure) -*see* Failure, heart, congestive
  systolic (congestive) I50.20
    acute (congestive) I50.21
      and (on) chronic (congestive) I50.23
    chronic (congestive) I50.22
      and (on) acute (congestive) I50.23
    combined with diastolic (congestive)
      I50.40
      acute (congestive) I50.41
        and (on) chronic (congestive) I50.43
      chronic (congestive) I50.42
        and (on) acute (congestive) I50.43
  thyrotoxic -*see also* Thyrotoxicosis E05.90
    [143]
    with thyroid storm E05.91 [143]
  valvular -*see* Endocarditis
hepatic K72.90
  with coma K72.91
  acute or subacute K72.00
    with coma K72.01
    due to drugs K71.10
      with coma K71.11

Failure, failed --*continued*
  alcoholic (acute) (chronic) (subacute)
    K70.40
    with coma K70.41
  chronic K72.10
    with coma K72.11
    due to drugs (acute) (subacute) (chronic)
      K71.10
      with coma K71.11
    due to drugs (acute) (subacute) (chronic)
      K71.10
      with coma K71.11
  postprocedural K91.82
hepatorenal K76.7
induction (of labor) O61.9
  abortion -*see* Abortion, attempted
  by
    oxytocic drugs O61.0
    prostaglandins O61.0
  instrumental O61.1
  mechanical O61.1
  medical O61.0
  specified NEC O61.8
  surgical O61.1
intubation during anesthesia T88.4
  in pregnancy O29.6
  labor and delivery O74.7
  postpartum, puerperal O89.6
involution, thymus (gland) E32.0
kidney -*see also* Disease, kidney, chronic N19
  acute -*see also* Failure, renal, acute N17.9
  diabetic -*see* E08 E13 with .22
lactation (complete) O92.3
  partial O92.4
Leydig's cell, adult E29.1
liver -*see* Failure, hepatic
menstruation at puberty N91.0
mitral I05.8
myocardial, myocardium -*see also* Failure,
  heart I50.9
  chronic -*see also* Failure, heart, congestive
    I50.9
  congestive -*see also* Failure, heart,
    congestive I50.9
orgasm (female) (psychogenic) F52.31
  male F52.32
ovarian (primary) E28.39
  iatrogenic E89.40
    asymptomatic E89.40
    symptomatic E89.41
  postprocedural (postablative)
    (postirradiation) (postsurgical) E89.40
    asymptomatic E89.40
    symptomatic E89.41
ovulation causing infertility N97.0
polyglandular, autoimmune E31.0
prosthetic joint implant -*see* Complications,
  joint prosthesis, mechanical, breakdown, by
  site
renal N19
  with
    tubular necrosis (acute) N17.0
  acute N17.9
    with
      cortical necrosis N17.1
      medullary necrosis N17.2
      tubular necrosis N17.0
    specified NEC N17.8
  chronic N18.9
    hypertensive -*see* Hypertension, kidney
  congenital P96.0

Failure, failed --*continued*
  end stage (chronic) N18.6
    due to hypertension I12.0
  following
    abortion -*see* Abortion by type complicated
      by specified condition NEC
    crushing T79.5
    ectopic or molar pregnancy O08.4
    labor and delivery (acute) O90.4
  hypertensive -*see* Hypertension, kidney
  postprocedural N99.0
  respiration, respiratory J96.90
    with
      hypercapnia J96.92
      hypoxia J96.91
    acute J96.00
      with
        hypercapnia J96.02
        hypoxia J96.01
    center G93.89
    acute and (on) chronic J96.20
      with
        hypercapnia J96.22
        hypoxia J96.21
    chronic J96.10
      with
        hypercapnia J96.12
        hypoxia J96.11
    newborn P28.5
    postprocedural (acute) J95.821
      acute and chronic J95.822
  rotation
    cecum Q43.3
    colon Q43.3
    intestine Q43.3
    kidney Q63.2
  sedation (conscious) (moderate) during
  procedure T88.52
    history of Z92.83
  segmentation -*see also* Fusion
    fingers -*see* Syndactylism, complex, fingers
    vertebra Q76.49
      with scoliosis Q76.3
  seminiferous tubule, adult E29.1
  senile (general) R54
  sexual arousal (male) F52.21
    female F52.22
  testicular endocrine function E29.1
  to thrive (child over 28 days old) R62.51
    adult R62.7
    newborn P92.6
  transplant T86.92
    bone T86.831
      marrow T86.02
    cornea T86.841
    heart T86.22
      with lung(s) T86.32
    intestine T86.851
    kidney T86.12
    liver T86.42
    lung(s) T86.811
      with heart T86.32
    pancreas T86.891
    skin (allograft) (autograft) T86.821
    specified organ or tissue NEC T86.891
    stem cell (peripheral blood) (umbilical cord)
      T86.5
  trial of labor (with subsequent cesarean
  delivery) O66.40
    following previous cesarean delivery O66.41
  tubal ligation N99.89

Failure, failed --*continued*
  urinary -*see* Disease, kidney, chronic
  vacuum extraction NOS (with subsequent
    cesarean delivery) O66.5
  vasectomy N99.89
  ventouse NOS (with subsequent cesarean
    delivery) O66.5
  ventricular -*see also* Failure, heart I50.9
    left I50.1
      with rheumatic fever (conditions in I00)
        active I01.8
          with chorea I02.0
        inactive or quiescent (with chorea) I09.81
      rheumatic (chronic) (inactive) (with
        chorea) I09.81
        active or acute I01.8
          with chorea I02.0
    right -*see also* Failure, heart, congestive
      I50.9
  vital centers, newborn P91.8
Fainting (fit) R55
Fallen arches -*see* Deformity, limb, flat foot
Falling, falls (repeated) R29.6
  any organ or part -*see* Prolapse
Fallopian
  insufflation Z31.41
  tube -*see* condition
Fallot's
  pentalogy Q21.8
  tetrad or tetralogy Q21.3
  triad or trilogy Q22.3
False -*see also* condition
  croup J38.5
  joint -*see* Nonunion, fracture
  labor (pains) O47.9
    at or after 37 completed weeks of gestation
      O47.1
    before 37 completed weeks of gestation
      O47.0
  passage, urethra (prostatic) N36.5
  pregnancy F45.8
Family, familial -*see also* condition
  disruption Z63.8
    involving divorce or separation Z63.5
  Li-Fraumeni (syndrome) Z15.01
  planning advice Z30.09
  problem Z63.9
    specified NEC Z63.8
  retinoblastoma C69.2
Famine (effects of) T73.0
  edema -*see* Malnutrition, severe
Fanconi (de Toni)(Debré) syndrome E72.09
  with cystinosis E72.04
Fanconi's anemia (congenital pancytopenia)
  D61.09
Farber's disease or syndrome E75.29
Farcy A24.0
Farmer's
  lung J67.0
  skin L57.8
Farsightedness -*see* Hypermetropia
Fascia -*see* condition
Fasciculation R25.3
Fasciitis M72.9
  diffuse (eosinophilic) M35.4
  infective M72.8
    necrotizing M72.6
  necrotizing M72.6
  nodular M72.4
  perirenal (with ureteral obstruction) N13.5
    with infection N13.6

Fasciitis - *continued*
  plantar M72.2
  specified NEC M72.8
  traumatic (old) M72.8
    current
    code by site under Sprain
Fascioliasis B66.3
Fasciolopsis, fasciolopsiasis (intestinal) B66.5
Fascioscapulohumeral myopathy G71.0
Fast pulse R00.0
Fat
  embolism -*see* Embolism, fat
  excessive -*see also* Obesity
    in heart -*see* Degeneration, myocardial
  in stool R19.5
  localized (pad) E65
    heart -*see* Degeneration, myocardial
    knee M79.4
    retropatellar M79.4
  necrosis
    breast N64.1
    mesentery K65.4
    omentum K65.4
  pad E65
    knee M79.4
Fatigue R53.83
  auditory deafness -*see* Deafness
  chronic R53.82
  combat F43.0
  general R53.83
    psychogenic F48.8
  heat (transient) T67.6
  muscle M62.89
  myocardium -*see* Failure, heart
  neoplasm-related R53.0
  nervous, neurosis F48.8
  operational F48.8
  psychogenic (general) F48.8
  senile R54
  voice R49.8
Fatness -*see* Obesity
Fatty -*see also* condition
  apron E65
  degeneration -*see* Degeneration, fatty
  heart (enlarged) -*see* Degeneration,
    myocardial
  liver NEC K76.0
    alcoholic K70.0
    nonalcoholic K76.0
  necrosis -*see* Degeneration, fatty
Fauces -*see* condition
Fauchard's disease (periodontitis) -*see*
  Periodontitis
Faucitis J02.9
Favism (anemia) D55.0
Favus -*see* Dermatophytosis
Fazio-Londe disease or syndrome G12.1
Fear complex or reaction F40.9
Fear of -*see* Phobia
Feared complaint unfounded Z71.1
Febris, febrile -*see also* Fever
  flava -*see also* Fever, yellow A95.9
  melitensis A23.0
  pestis -*see* Plague
  recurrens -*see* Fever, relapsing
  rubra A38.9
Fecal
  incontinence R15.9
  smearing R15.1
  soiling R15.1
  urgency R15.2

Fecalith (impaction) K56.41
  appendix K38.1
  congenital P76.8
Fede's disease K14.0
Feeble rapid pulse due to shock following injury T79.4
Feeble-minded F70
Feeding
  difficulties R63.3
  problem R63.3
    newborn P92.9
      specified NEC P92.8
    nonorganic (adult) -see Disorder, eating
Feeling (of)
  foreign body in throat R09.89
Feer's disease -see Poisoning, mercury
Feet -see condition
Feigned illness Z76.5
Feil-Klippel syndrome (brevicollis) Q76.1
Feinmesser's (hidrotic) ectodermal dysplasia Q82.4
Felinophobia F40.218
Felon -see also Cellulitis, digit
  with lymphangitis -see Lymphangitis, acute, digit
Felty's syndrome M05.00
  ankle M05.07
  elbow M05.02
  foot joint M05.07
  hand joint M05.04
  hip M05.05
  knee M05.06
  multiple site M05.09
  shoulder M05.01
  vertebra -see Spondylitis, ankylosing
  wrist M05.03
Female genital cutting status -see Female genital mutilation status (FGM)
Female genital mutilation status (FGM) N90.810
  specified NEC N90.818
  type I (clitorectomy status) N90.811
  type II (clitorectomy with excision of labia minora status) N90.812
  type III (infibulation status) N90.813
  type IV N90.818
Femur, femoral -see condition
Fenestration, fenestrated -see also Imperfect, closure
  aortico-pulmonary Q21.4
  cusps, heart valve NEC Q24.8
    pulmonary Q22.3
  pulmonic cusps Q22.3
Fernell's disease (aortic aneurysm) I71.9
Fertile eunuch syndrome E23.0
Fetid
  breath R19.6
  sweat L75.0
Fetishism F65.0
  transvestic F65.1
Fetus, fetal -see also condition
  alcohol syndrome (dysmorphic) Q86.0
  compressus O31.0
  hydantoin syndrome Q86.1
  lung tissue P28.0
  papyraceous O31.0
Fever (inanition) (of unknown origin) (persistent) (with chills) (with rigor) R50.9
  abortus A23.1
  Aden (dengue) A90
  African tick-borne A68.1

Fever --continued
  American
    mountain (tick) A93.2
    spotted A77.0
  aphthous B08.8
  arbovirus, arboviral A94
    hemorrhagic A94
    specified NEC A93.8
  Argentinian hemorrhagic A96.0
  Assam B55.0
  Australian Q A78
  Bangkok hemorrhagic A91
  Barmah forest A92.8
  Bartonella A44.0
  bilious, hemoglobinuric B50.8
  blackwater B50.8
  blister B00.1
  Bolivian hemorrhagic A96.1
  Bonvale dam T73.3
  boutonneuse A77.1
  brain -see Encephalitis
  Brazilian purpuric A48.4
  breakbone A90
  Bullis A77.0
  Bunyamwera A92.8
  Burdwan B55.0
  Bwamba A92.8
  Cameroon -see Malaria
  Canton A75.9
  catarrhal (acute) J00
    chronic J31.0
  cat-scratch A28.1
  Central Asian hemorrhagic A98.0
  cerebral -see Encephalitis
  cerebrospinal meningococcal A39.0
  Chagres B50.9
  Chandipura A92.8
  Changuinola A93.1
  Charcot's (biliary) (hepatic) (intermittent) see Calculus, bile duct
  Chikungunya (viral) (hemorrhagic) A92.0
  Chitral A93.1
  Colombo -see Fever, paratyphoid
  Colorado tick (virus) A93.2
  congestive (remittent) -see Malaria
  Congo virus A98.0
  continued malarial B50.9
  Corsican -see Malaria
  Crimean-Congo hemorrhagic A98.0
  Cyprus -see Brucellosis
  dandy A90
  deer fly -see Tularemia
  dengue (virus) A90
    hemorrhagic A91
    sandfly A93.1
  desert B38.0
  drug induced R50.2
  due to
    conditions classified elsewhere R50.81
    heat T67.0
  enteric A01.00
  enteroviral exanthematous (Boston exanthem) A88.0
  ephemeral (of unknown origin) R50.9
  epidemic hemorrhagic A98.5
  erysipelatous -see Erysipelas
  estivo-autumnal (malarial) B50.9
  famine A75.0
  five day A79.0
  following delivery O86.4
  Fort Bragg A27.89

Fever --continued
  gastroenteric A01.00
  gastromalarial -see Malaria
  Gibraltar -see Brucellosis
  glandular -see Mononucleosis, infectious
  Guama (viral) A92.8
  Haverhill A25.1
  hay (allergic) J30.1
    with asthma (bronchial) J45.909
    with
      exacerbation (acute) J45.901
      status asthmaticus J45.902
    due to
      allergen other than pollen J30.89
      pollen, any plant or tree J30.1
  heat (effects) T67.0
  hematuric, bilious B50.8
  hemoglobinuric (malarial) (bilious) B50.8
  hemorrhagic (arthropod-borne) NOS A94
    with renal syndrome A98.5
    arenaviral A96.9
      specified NEC A96.8
    Argentinian A96.0
    Bangkok A91
    Bolivian A96.1
    Central Asian A98.0
    Chikungunya A92.0
    Crimean-Congo A98.0
    dengue (virus) A91
    epidemic A98.5
    Junin (virus) A96.0
    Korean A98.5
    Kyasanur forest A98.2
    Machupo (virus) A96.1
    mite-borne A93.8
    mosquito-borne A92.8
    Omsk A98.1
    Philippine A91
    Russian A98.5
    Singapore A91
    Southeast Asia A91
    Thailand A91
    tick-borne NEC A93.8
    viral A99
      specified NEC A98.8
  hepatic -see Cholecystitis
  herpetic -see Herpes
  icterohemorrhagic A27.0
  Indiana A93.8
  infective B99.9
    specified NEC B99.8
  intermittent (bilious) -see also Malaria
    of unknown origin R50.9
    pernicious B50.9
  iodide R50.2
  Japanese river A75.3
  jungle -see also Malaria
    yellow A95.0
  Junin (virus) hemorrhagic A96.0
  Katayama B65.2
  kedani A75.3
  Kenya (tick) A77.1
  Kew Garden A79.1
  Korean hemorrhagic A98.5
  Lassa A96.2
  Lone Star A77.0
  Machupo (virus) hemorrhagic A96.1
  malaria, malarial -see Malaria
  Malta A23.9
  Marseilles A77.1
  marsh -see Malaria

Fever --*continued*
Mayaro (viral) A92.8
Mediterranean -*see also* Brucellosis A23.9
  familial M04.1
  tick A77.1
meningeal -*see* Meningitis
Meuse A79.0
Mexican A75.2
mianeh A68.1
miasmatic -*see* Malaria
mosquito-borne (viral) A92.9
  hemorrhagic A92.8
mountain -*see also* Brucellosis
  meaning Rocky Mountain spotted fever
    A77.0
  tick (American) (Colorado) (viral) A93.2
Mucambo (viral) A92.8
mud A27.9
Neapolitan -*see* Brucellosis
neutropenic D70.9
newborn P81.9
  environmental P81.0
Nine-Mile A78
non-exanthematous tick A93.2
North Asian tick-borne A77.2
Omsk hemorrhagic A98.1
O'nyong-nyong (viral) A92.1
Oropouche (viral) A93.0
Oroya A44.0
paludal -*see* Malaria
Panama (malarial) B50.9
Pappataci A93.1
paratyphoid A01.4
  A A01.1
  B A01.2
  C A01.3
parrot A70
periodic (Mediterranean) M04.1
persistent (of unknown origin) R50.9
petechial A39.0
pharyngoconjunctival B30.2
Philippine hemorrhagic A91
phlebotomus A93.1
Piry (virus) A93.8
Pixuna (viral) A92.8
Plasmodium ovale B53.0
polioviral (nonparalytic) A80.4
Pontiac A48.2
postimmunization R50.83
postoperative R50.82
  due to infection T81.40
posttransfusion R50.84
postvaccination R50.83
presenting with conditions classified
  elsewhere R50.81
pretibial A27.89
puerperal O86.4
Q A78
quadrilateral A78
quartan (malaria) B52.9
Queensland (coastal) (tick) A77.3
quintan A79.0
rabbit -*see* Tularemia
rat-bite A25.9
  due to
    Spirillum A25.0
    Streptobacillus moniliformis A25.1
recurrent -*see* Fever, relapsing
relapsing (Borrelia) A68.9
  Carter's (Asiatic) A68.1
  Dutton's (West African) A68.1

Fever --*continued*
Koch's A68.9
louse-borne A68.0
Novy's
  louse-borne A68.0
  tick-borne A68.1
Obermeyer's (European) A68.0
tick-borne A68.1
remittent (bilious) (congestive) (gastric) -*see*
  Malaria
rheumatic (active) (acute) (chronic)
(subacute) I00
  with central nervous system involvement
    I02.9
  active with heart involvement -*see* category
    I01
  inactive or quiescent with
    cardiac hypertrophy I09.89
    carditis I09.9
    endocarditis I09.1
      aortic (valve) I06.9
        with mitral (valve) disease I08.0
      mitral (valve) I05.9
        with aortic (valve) disease I08.0
      pulmonary (valve) I09.89
      tricuspid (valve) I07.8
    heart disease NEC I09.89
    heart failure (congestive) (conditions in
      I50.9) I09.81
    left ventricular failure (conditions in I50.1)
      I09.81
    myocarditis, myocardial degeneration
      (conditions in I51.4) I09.0
    pancarditis I09.9
    pericarditis I09.2
Rift Valley (viral) A92.4
Rocky Mountain spotted A77.0
rose J30.1
Ross River B33.1
Russian hemorrhagic A98.5
San Joaquin (Valley) B38.0
sandfly A93.1
Sao Paulo A77.0
scarlet A38.9
seven day (leptospirosis) (autumnal)
  (Japanese) A27.89
  dengue A90
shin-bone A79.0
Singapore hemorrhagic A91
solar A90
Songo A98.5
sore B00.1
South African tick-bite A68.1
Southeast Asia hemorrhagic A91
spinal -*see* Meningitis
spirillary A25.0
splenic -*see* Anthrax - spotted A77.9
  American A77.0
  Brazilian A77.0
  cerebrospinal meningitis A39.0
  Colombian A77.0
  due to Rickettsia
    australis A77.3
    conorii A77.1
    rickettsii A77.0
    sibirica A77.2
    specified type NEC A77.8
  Ehrlichiosis A77.40
    due to
      E. chafeensis A77.41
      specified organism NEC A77.49

Fever --*continued*
Rocky Mountain A77.0
steroid R50.2
streptobacillary A25.1
subtertian B50.9
Sumatran mite A75.3
sun A90
swamp A27.9
swine A02.8
sylvatic, yellow A95.0
Tahyna B33.8
tertian -*see* Malaria, tertian
Thailand hemorrhagic A91
thermic T67.0
three-day A93.1
tick
  American mountain A93.2
  Colorado A93.2
  Kemerovo A93.8
  Mediterranean A77.1
  mountain A93.2
  nonexanthematous A93.2
  Quaranfil A93.8
tick-bite NEC A93.8
tick-borne (hemorrhagic) NEC A93.8
trench A79.0
tsutsugamushi A75.3
typhogastric A01.00
typhoid (abortive) (hemorrhagic)
  (intermittent) (malignant) A01.00
  complicated by
    arthritis A01.04
    heart involvement A01.02
    meningitis A01.01
    osteomyelitis A01.05
    pneumonia A01.03
    specified NEC A01.09
typhomalarial -*see* Malaria
typhus -*see* Typhus (fever)
undulant -*see* Brucellosis
unknown origin R50.9
uveoparotid D86.89
valley B38.0
Venezuelan equine A92.2
vesicular stomatitis A93.8
viral hemorrhagic -*see* Fever, hemorrhagic, by
type of virus
Volhynian A79.0
Wesselsbron (viral) A92.8
West
  African B50.8
  Nile (viral) A92.30
    with
      complications NEC A92.39
      cranial nerve disorders A92.32
      encephalitis A92.31
      encephalomyelitis A92.31
      neurologic manifestation NEC A92.32
      optic neuritis A92.32
      polyradiculitis A92.32
Whitmore's -*see* Melioidosis
Wolhynian A79.0
worm B83.9
yellow A95.9
  jungle A95.0
  sylvatic A95.0
  urban A95.1
Zika virus A92.5
Fibrillation
atrial or auricular (established) I48.91
  chronic I48.2

Fibrillation - *continued*
  paroxysmal I48.0
  permanent I48.2
  persistent I48.1
  cardiac I49.8
  heart I49.8
  muscular M62.89
  ventricular I49.01
Fibrin
  ball or bodies, pleural (sac) J94.1
  chamber, anterior (eye) (gelatinous exudate) -
  see Iridocyclitis, acute
Fibrinogenolysis *-see* Fibrinolysis
Fibrinogenopenia D68.8
  acquired D65
  congenital D68.2
Fibrinolysis (hemorrhagic) (acquired) D65
  antepartum hemorrhage *-see* Hemorrhage,
  antepartum, with coagulation defect
  following
    abortion *-see* Abortion by type complicated
  by hemorrhage
    ectopic or molar pregnancy O08.1
  intrapartum O67.0
  newborn, transient P60
  postpartum O72.3
Fibrinopenia (hereditary) D68.2
  acquired D68.4
Fibrinopurulent *-see* condition
Fibrinous *-see* condition
Fibroadenoma
  cellular intracanalicular D24
  giant D24
  intracanalicular
    cellular D24
    giant D24
    specified site *-see* Neoplasm, benign, by site
    unspecified site D24
  juvenile D24
  pericanalicular
    specified site *-see* Neoplasm, benign, by site
    unspecified site D24
  phyllodes D24
  prostate D29.1
  specified site NEC *-see* Neoplasm, benign, by
  site
  unspecified site D24
Fibroadenosis, breast (chronic) (cystic)
  (diffuse) (periodic) (segmental) N60.2
Fibroangioma *-see also* Neoplasm, benign, by
  site
  juvenile
    specified site *-see* Neoplasm, benign, by site
    unspecified site D10.6
Fibrochondrosarcoma *-see* Neoplasm,
  cartilage, malignant
Fibrocystic
  disease *-see also* Fibrosis, cystic
    breast *-see* Mastopathy, cystic
    jaw M27.49
    kidney (congenital) Q61.8
    liver Q44.6
    pancreas E84.9
    kidney (congenital) Q61.8
Fibrodysplasia ossificans progressiva - *-see*
  Myositis, ossificans, progressiva
Fibroelastosis (cordis) (endocardial)
  (endomyocardial) I42.4
Fibroid (tumor) *-see also* Neoplasm,
  connective tissue, benign
  disease, lung (chronic) *-see* Fibrosis, lung

Fibroid *--continued*
  heart (disease) *-see* Myocarditis
  in pregnancy or childbirth O34.1
    causing obstructed labor O65.5
  induration, lung (chronic) *-see* Fibrosis, lung
  lung *-see* Fibrosis, lung
  pneumonia (chronic) *-see* Fibrosis, lung
  uterus D25.9
Fibrolipoma *-see* Lipoma
Fibroliposarcoma *-see* Neoplasm, connective
  tissue, malignant
Fibroma *-see also* Neoplasm, connective
  tissue, benign
  ameloblastic *-see* Cyst, calcifying
  odontogenic
  bone (nonossifying) *-see* Disorder, bone,
  specified type NEC
    ossifying *-see* Neoplasm, bone, benign
  cementifying *-see* Neoplasm, bone, benign
  chondromyxoid *-see* Neoplasm, bone, benign
  desmoplastic *-see* Neoplasm, connective
  tissue, uncertain behavior
  durum *-see* Neoplasm, connective tissue,
  benign
  fascial *-see* Neoplasm, connective tissue,
  benign
  invasive *-see* Neoplasm, connective tissue,
  uncertain behavior
  molle *-see* Lipoma
  myxoid *-see* Neoplasm, connective tissue,
  benign
  nasopharynx, nasopharyngeal (juvenile)
  D10.6
  nonosteogenic (nonossifying) *-see* Dysplasia,
  fibrous
  odontogenic (central) *-see* Cyst, calcifying
  odontogenic
  ossifying *-see* Neoplasm, bone, benign
  periosteal *-see* Neoplasm, bone, benign
  soft *-see* Lipoma
Fibromatosis M72.9
  abdominal *-see* Neoplasm, connective tissue,
  uncertain behavior
  aggressive *-see* Neoplasm, connective tissue,
  uncertain behavior
  congenital generalized *-see* Neoplasm,
  connective tissue, uncertain behavior
  Dupuytren's M72.0
  gingival K06.1
  palmar (fascial) M72.0
  plantar (fascial) M72.2
  pseudosarcomatous (proliferative)
  (subcutaneous) M72.4
  retroperitoneal D48.3
  specified NEC M72.8
Fibromyalgia M79.7
Fibromyoma *-see also* Neoplasm, connective
  tissue, benign
  uterus (corpus) *-see also* Leiomyoma, uterus
    in pregnancy or childbirth *-see* Fibroid, in
  pregnancy or childbirth
    causing obstructed labor O65.5
Fibromyositis M79.7
Fibromyxolipoma D17.9
Fibromyxoma *-see* Neoplasm, connective
  tissue, benign
Fibromyxosarcoma *-see* Neoplasm,
  connective tissue, malignant
Fibro-odontoma, ameloblastic *-see* Cyst,
  calcifying odontogenic
Fibro-osteoma *-see* Neoplasm, bone, benign

Fibroplasia, retrolental H35.17
Fibropurulent *-see* condition
Fibrosarcoma *-see also* Neoplasm, connective
  tissue, malignant
  ameloblastic C41.1
    upper jaw (bone) C41.0
  congenital *-see* Neoplasm, connective tissue,
  malignant
  fascial *-see* Neoplasm, connective tissue,
  malignant
  infantile *-see* Neoplasm, connective tissue,
  malignant
  odontogenic C41.1
    upper jaw (bone) C41.0
  periosteal *-see* Neoplasm, bone, malignant
Fibrosclerosis
  breast N60.3
  multifocal M35.5
  penis (corpora cavernosa) N48.6
Fibrosis, fibrotic
  adrenal (gland) E27.8
  amnion O41.8X
  anal papillae K62.89
  arteriocapillary *-see* Arteriosclerosis
  bladder N32.89
    interstitial *-see* Cystitis, chronic, interstitial
    localized submucosal *-see* Cystitis, chronic,
  interstitial
    panmural *-see* Cystitis, chronic, interstitial
  breast *-see* Fibrosclerosis, breast
  capillary *-see also* Arteriosclerosis I70.90
    lung (chronic) *-see* Fibrosis, lung
  cardiac *-see* Myocarditis
  cervix N88.8
  chorion O41.8X
  corpus cavernosum (sclerosing) N48.6
  cystic (of pancreas) E84.9
    with
      distal intestinal obstruction syndrome
      E84.19
      fecal impaction E84.19
      intestinal manifestations NEC E84.19
      pulmonary manifestations E84.0
      specified manifestations NEC E84.8
  due to device, implant or graft *-see also*
  Complications, by site and type, specified
  NEC T85.828
    arterial graft NEC T82.828
    breast (implant) T85.828
    catheter NEC T85.828
      dialysis (renal) T82.828
        intraperitoneal T85.828
      infusion NEC T82.828
        spinal (epidural) (subdural) T85.820
      urinary (indwelling) T83.82
    electronic (electrode) (pulse generator)
    (stimulator)
      bone T84.82
      cardiac T82.827
      nervous system (brain) (peripheral nerve)
      (spinal) T85.820
      urinary T83.82
    fixation, internal (orthopedic) NEC T84.82
    gastrointestinal (bile duct) (esophagus)
    T85.828
    genital NEC T83.82
    heart NEC T82.827
    joint prosthesis T84.82
    ocular (corneal graft) (orbital implant) NEC
    T85.828
    orthopedic NEC T84.82

Fibrosis, fibrotic --continued

specified NEC T85.828
   urinary NEC T83.82
   vascular NEC T82.828
   ventricular intracranial shunt T85.820
ejaculatory duct N50.89
endocardium -see Endocarditis
endomyocardial (tropical) I42.3
epididymis N50.89
eye muscle -see Strabismus, mechanical
heart -see Myocarditis
hepatic -see Fibrosis, liver
hepatolienal (portal hypertension) K76.6
hepatosplenic (portal hypertension) K76.6
infrapatellar fat pad M79.4
intrascrotal N50.89
kidney N26.9
liver K74.0
   with sclerosis K74.2
   alcoholic K70.2
lung (atrophic) (chronic) (confluent)
(massive) (perialveolar) (peribronchial)
J84.10
   with
      anthracosilicosis J60
      anthracosis J60
      asbestosis J61
      bagassosis J67.1
      bauxite J63.1
      berylliosis J63.2
      byssinosis J66.0
      calcicosis J62.8
      chalicosis J62.8
      dust reticulation J64
      farmer's lung J67.0
      ganister disease J62.8
      graphite J63.3
      pneumoconiosis NOS J64
      siderosis J63.4
      silicosis J62.8
   capillary J84.10
   congenital P27.8
   diffuse (idiopathic) J84.10
      chemicals, gases, fumes or vapors
         (inhalation) J68.4
      interstitial J84.10
         acute J84.114
      talc J62.0
   following radiation J70.1
   idiopathic J84.112
   postinflammatory J84.10
   silicotic J62.8
   tuberculous -see Tuberculosis, pulmonary
lymphatic gland I89.8
median bar -see Hyperplasia, prostate
mediastinum (idiopathic) J98.59
meninges G96.19
myocardium, myocardial -see Myocarditis
ovary N83.8
oviduct N83.8
pancreas K86.89
penis NEC N48.6
pericardium I31.0
perineum, in pregnancy or childbirth O34.7
   causing obstructed labor O65.5
pleura J94.1
popliteal fat pad M79.4
prostate (chronic) -see Hyperplasia, prostate
pulmonary -see also Fibrosis, lung J84.10
   congenital P27.8
   idiopathic J84.112

Fibrosis, fibrotic --continued

rectal sphincter K62.89
retroperitoneal, idiopathic (with ureteral
obstruction) N13.5
   with infection N13.6
sclerosing mesenteric (idiopathic) K65.4
scrotum N50.89
seminal vesicle N50.89
senile R54
skin L90.5
spermatic cord N50.89
spleen D73.89
   in schistosomiasis (bilharziasis) B65.9
   [D77]
subepidermal nodular -see Neoplasm, skin,
benign
submucous (oral) (tongue) K13.5
testis N44.8
   chronic, due to syphilis A52.76
thymus (gland) E32.8
tongue, submucous K13.5
tunica vaginalis N50.89
uterus (non-neoplastic) N85.8
vagina N89.8
valve, heart -see Endocarditis
vas deferens N50.89
vein I87.8

Fibrositis (periarticular) M79.7

nodular, chronic (Jaccoud's) (rheumatoid) -see
Arthropathy, postrheumatic, chronic

Fibrothorax J94.1

Fibrotic -see Fibrosis

Fibrous -see condition

Fibroxanthoma -see also Neoplasm,

connective tissue, benign
atypical -see Neoplasm, connective tissue,
uncertain behavior
malignant -see Neoplasm, connective tissue,
malignant

Fibroxanthosarcoma -see Neoplasm,

connective tissue, malignant

Fiedler's

disease (icterohemorrhagic leptospirosis)
A27.0
myocarditis (acute) I40.1

Fifth disease B08.3

venereal A55

Filaria, filarial, filariasis -see Infestation,

filarial

Filatov's disease -see Mononucleosis,

infectious

File-cutter's disease -see Poisoning, lead

Filling defect

biliary tract R93.2
bladder R93.41
duodenum R93.3
gallbladder R93.2
gastrointestinal tract R93.3
intestine R93.3
kidney R93.42
stomach R93.3
ureter R93.41
urinary organs, specified NEC R93.49

Fimbrial cyst Q50.4

Financial problem affecting care NOS Z59.9

bankruptcy Z59.8
foreclosure on loan Z59.8

Findings, abnormal, inconclusive, without

diagnosis -see also Abnormal
17 ketosteroids, elevated R82.5
acetonuria R82.4

Findings - continued

alcohol in blood R78.0
anisocytosis R71.8
antenatal screening of mother O28.9
   biochemical O28.1
   chromosomal O28.5
   cytological O28.2
   genetic O28.5
   hematological O28.0
   radiological O28.4
   specified NEC O28.8
   ultrasonic O28.3
antibody titer, elevated R76.0
anticardiolipin antibody R76.0
antiphosphatidylglycerol antibody R76.0
antiphosphatidylinositol antibody R76.0
antiphosphatidylserine antibody R76.0
antiphospholipid antibody R76.0
bacteriuria R82.71
bicarbonate E87.8
bile in urine R82.2
blood sugar R73.09
   high R73.9
   low (transient) E16.2
body fluid or substance, specified NEC R88.8
casts, urine R82.99
catecholamines R82.5
cells, urine R82.99
chloride E87.8
cholesterol E78.9
   high E78.00
      with high triglycerides E78.2
chyluria R82.0
cloudy
   dialysis effluent R88.0
   urine R82.90
creatinine clearance R94.4
crystals, urine R82.99
culture
   blood R78.81
   positive -see Positive, culture
echocardiogram R93.1
electrolyte level, urinary R82.99
function study NEC R94.8
   bladder R94.8
   endocrine NEC R94.7
      thyroid R94.6
   kidney R94.4
   liver R94.5
   pancreas R94.8
   placenta R94.8
   pulmonary R94.2
   spleen R94.8
gallbladder, nonvisualization R93.2
glucose (tolerance test) (non-fasting) R73.09
glycosuria R81
heart
   shadow R93.1
   sounds R01.2
hematinuria R82.3
hematocrit drop (precipitous) R71.0
hemoglobinuria R82.3
human papillomavirus (HPV) DNA test
positive
   cervix
      high risk R87.810
      low risk R87.820
   vagina
      high risk R87.811
      low risk R87.821

Findings - *continued*
in blood (of substance not normally found in blood) R78.9
addictive drug NEC R78.4
alcohol (excessive level) R78.0
cocaine R78.2
hallucinogen R78.3
heavy metals (abnormal level) R78.79
lead R78.71
lithium (abnormal level) R78.89
opiate drug R78.1
psychotropic drug R78.5
specified substance NEC R78.89
steroid agent R78.6
indoleacetic acid, elevated R82.5
ketonuria R82.4
lactic acid dehydrogenase (LDH) R74.0
liver function test R79.89
mammogram NEC R92.8
calcification (calculus) R92.1
inconclusive result (due to dense breasts) R92.2
microcalcification R92.0
mediastinal shift R93.8
melanin, urine R82.99
myoglobinuria R82.1
neonatal screening P09
nonvisualization of gallbladder R93.2
odor of urine NOS R82.90
Papanicolaou cervix R87.619
non-atypical endometrial cells R87.618
pneumoencephalogram R93.0
poikilocytosis R71.8
potassium (deficiency) E87.6
excess E87.5
PPD R76.11
radiologic (X ray) R93.8
abdomen R93.5
biliary tract R93.2
breast R92.8
gastrointestinal tract R93.3
genitourinary organs R93.8
head R93.0
inconclusive due to excess body fat of patient R93.9
intrathoracic organs NEC R93.1
placenta R93.8
retroperitoneum R93.5
skin R93.8
skull R93.0
subcutaneous tissue R93.8
red blood cell (count) (morphology) (sickling) (volume) R71.8
scan NEC R94.8
bladder R94.8
bone R94.8
kidney R94.4
liver R93.2
lung R94.2
pancreas R94.8
placental R94.8
spleen R94.8
thyroid R94.6
sedimentation rate, elevated R70.0
SGOT R74.0
SGPT R74.0
sodium (deficiency) E87.1
excess E87.0
specified body fluid NEC R88.8
stress test R94.39

Findings - *continued*
thyroid (function) (metabolic rate) (scan) (uptake) R94.6
transaminase (level) R74.0
triglycerides E78.9
high E78.1
with high cholesterol E78.2
tuberculin skin test (without active tuberculosis) R76.11
urine R82.90
acetone R82.4
bacteria R82.71
bile R82.2
casts or cells R82.99
chyle R82.0
culture positive R82.79
glucose R81
hemoglobin R82.3
ketone R82.4
sugar R81
vanillylmandelic acid (VMA), elevated R82.5
vectorcardiogram (VCG) R94.39
ventriculogram R93.0
white blood cell (count) (differential) (morphology) D72.9
xerography R92.8
Finger -*see* condition
Fire, Saint Anthony's -*see* Erysipelas
Fire-setting
pathological (compulsive) F63.1
Fish hook stomach K31.89
Fishmeal-worker's lung J67.8
Fissure, fissured
anus, anal K60.2
acute K60.0
chronic K60.1
congenital Q43.8
ear, lobule, congenital Q17.8
epiglottis (congenital) Q31.8
larynx J38.7
congenital Q31.8
lip K13.0
congenital -*see* Cleft, lip
nipple N64.0
associated with
lactation O92.13
pregnancy O92.11
puerperium O92.12
nose Q30.2
palate (congenital) -*see* Cleft, palate
skin R23.4
spine (congenital) -*see also* Spina bifida
with hydrocephalus -*see* Spina bifida, by site, with hydrocephalus
tongue (acquired) K14.5
congenital Q38.3
Fistula (cutaneous) L98.8
abdomen (wall) K63.2
bladder N32.2
intestine NEC K63.2
ureter N28.89
uterus N82.5
abdominorectal K63.2
abdominosigmoidal K63.2
abdominothoracic J86.0
abdominouterine N82.5
congenital Q51.7
abdominovesical N32.2
accessory sinuses -*see* Sinusitis
actinomycotic -*see* Actinomycosis
alveolar antrum -*see* Sinusitis, maxillary

Fistula (cutaneous) --*continued*
alveolar process K04.6
anorectal K60.5
antrobuccal -*see* Sinusitis, maxillary
antrum -*see* Sinusitis, maxillary
anus, anal (recurrent) (infectional) K60.3
congenital Q43.6
with absence, atresia and stenosis Q42.2
tuberculous A18.32
aorta-duodenal I77.2
appendix, appendicular K38.3
arteriovenous (acquired) (nonruptured) I77.0
brain I67.1
congenital Q28.2
ruptured I60.8
ruptured I60.8
cerebral -*see* Fistula, arteriovenous, brain
congenital (peripheral) -*see also* Malformation, arteriovenous
brain Q28.2
ruptured I60.8
coronary Q24.5
pulmonary Q25.72
coronary I25.41
congenital Q24.5
pulmonary I28.0
congenital Q25.72
surgically created (for dialysis) Z99.2
complication -*see* Complication, arteriovenous, fistula, surgically created
traumatic -*see* Injury, blood vessel
artery I77.2
aural (mastoid) -*see* Mastoiditis, chronic
auricle -*see also* Disorder, pinna, specified type NEC
congenital Q18.1
Bartholin's gland N82.8
bile duct (common) (hepatic) K83.3
with calculus, stones -*see* Calculus, bile duct
biliary (tract) -*see* Fistula, bile duct
bladder (sphincter) NEC -*see also* Fistula, vesico- N32.2
into seminal vesicle N32.2
bone -*see also* Disorder, bone, specified type NEC
with osteomyelitis, chronic -*see* Osteomyelitis, chronic, with draining sinus
brain G93.89
arteriovenous (acquired) I67.1
congenital Q28.2
branchial (cleft) Q18.0
branchiogenous Q18.0
breast N61.0
puerperal, postpartum or gestational, due to mastitis (purulent) -*see* Mastitis, obstetric, purulent
bronchial J86.0
bronchocutaneous, bronchomediastinal, bronchopleural, bronchopleuromediastinal (infective) J86.0
tuberculous NEC A15.5
bronchoesophageal J86.0
congenital Q39.2
with atresia of esophagus Q39.1
bronchovisceral J86.0
buccal cavity (infective) K12.2
cecosigmoidal K63.2
cecum K63.2
cerebrospinal (fluid) G96.0
cervical, lateral Q18.1
cervicoaural Q18.1

Fistula (cutaneous) --*continued*
- cervicosigmoidal N82.4
- cervicovesical N82.1
- cervix N82.8
- chest (wall) J86.0
- cholecystenteric -*see* Fistula, gallbladder
- cholecystocolic -*see* Fistula, gallbladder
- cholecystocolonic -*see* Fistula, gallbladder
- cholecystoduodenal -*see* Fistula, gallbladder
- cholecystogastric -*see* Fistula, gallbladder
- cholecystointestinal -*see* Fistula, gallbladder
- choledochoduodenal -*see* Fistula, bile duct
- cholocolic K82.3
- coccyx -*see* Sinus, pilonidal
- colon K63.2
- colostomy K94.09
- common duct -*see* Fistula, bile duct
- congenital, site not listed -*see* Anomaly, by site
- coronary, arteriovenous I25.41
  - congenital Q24.5
- costal region J86.0
- cul-de-sac, Douglas' N82.8
- cystic duct -*see also* Fistula, gallbladder
  - congenital Q44.5
- dental K04.6
- diaphragm J86.0
- duodenum K31.6
- ear (external) (canal) -*see* Disorder, ear, external, specified type NEC
- enterocolic K63.2
- enterocutaneous K63.2
- enterouterine N82.4
  - congenital Q51.7
- enterovaginal N82.4
  - congenital Q52.2
  - large intestine N82.3
  - small intestine N82.2
- enterovesical N32.1
- epididymis N50.89
  - tuberculous A18.15
- esophagobronchial J86.0
  - congenital Q39.2
    - with atresia of esophagus Q39.1
- esophagocutaneous K22.8
- esophagopleural-cutaneous J86.0
- esophagotracheal J86.0
  - congenital Q39.2
    - with atresia of esophagus Q39.1
- esophagus K22.8
  - congenital Q39.2
    - with atresia of esophagus Q39.1
- ethmoid -*see* Sinusitis, ethmoidal
- eyeball (cornea) (sclera) -*see* Disorder, globe, hypotony   eyelid H01.8
- fallopian tube, external N82.5
- fecal K63.2
  - congenital Q43.6
- from periapical abscess K04.6
- frontal sinus -*see* Sinusitis, frontal
- gallbladder K82.3
  - with calculus, cholelithiasis, stones -*see* Calculus, gallbladder
- gastric K31.6
- gastrocolic K31.6
  - congenital Q40.2
  - tuberculous A18.32
- gastroenterocolic K31.6
- gastroesophageal K31.6
- gastrojejunal K31.6
- gastrojejunocolic K31.6

Fistula (cutaneous) --*continued*
- genital tract (female) N82.9
  - specified NEC N82.8
  - to intestine NEC N82.4
  - to skin N82.5
- hepatic artery portal vein, congenital Q26.6
- hepatopleural J86.0
- hepatopulmonary J86.0
- ileorectal or ileosigmoidal K63.2
- ileovaginal N82.2
- ileovesical N32.1
- ileum K63.2
- in ano K60.3
  - tuberculous A18.32
- inner ear (labyrinth) -*see* subcategory H83.1
- intestine NEC K63.2
- intestinocolic (abdominal) K63.2
- intestinoureteral N28.89
- intestinouterine N82.4
- intestinovaginal N82.4
  - large intestine N82.3
  - small intestine N82.2
- intestinovesical N32.1
- ischiorectal (fossa) K61.3
- jejunum K63.2
- joint M25.10
  - ankle M25.17
  - elbow M25.12
  - foot joint M25.17
  - hand joint M25.14
  - hip M25.15
  - knee M25.16
  - shoulder M25.11
  - specified joint NEC M25.18
  - tuberculous -*see* Tuberculosis, joint
  - vertebrae M25.18
  - wrist M25.13
- kidney N28.89
- labium (majus) (minus) N82.8
- labyrinth -*see* subcategory H83.1
- lacrimal (gland) (sac) H04.61
- lacrimonasal duct -*see* Fistula, lacrimal
- laryngotracheal, congenital Q34.8
- larynx J38.7
- lip K13.0
  - congenital Q38.0
- lumbar, tuberculous A18.01
- lung J86.0
- lymphatic I89.8
- mammary (gland) N61.0
- mastoid (process) (region) -*see* Mastoiditis, chronic
- maxillary J32.0
- medial, face and neck Q18.8
- mediastinal J86.0
- mediastinobronchial J86.0
- mediastinocutaneous J86.0
- middle ear -*see* subcategory H74.8
- mouth K12.2
- nasal J34.89
  - sinus -*see* Sinusitis
- nasopharynx J39.2
- nipple N64.0
- nose J34.89
- oral (cutaneous) K12.2
  - maxillary J32.0
  - nasal (with cleft palate) -*see* Cleft, palate
- orbit, orbital -*see* Disorder, orbit, specified type NEC
- oroantral J32.0
- oviduct, external N82.5

Fistula (cutaneous) --*continued*
- palate (hard) M27.8
- pancreatic K86.89
- pancreaticoduodenal K86.89
- parotid (gland) K11.4
  - region K12.2
- penis N48.89
- perianal K60.3
- pericardium (pleura) (sac) -*see* Pericarditis
- pericecal K63.2
- perineorectal K60.4
- perineosigmoidal K63.2
- perineum, perineal (with urethral involvement) NEC N36.0
  - tuberculous A18.13
  - ureter N28.89
- perirectal K60.4
  - tuberculous A18.32
- peritoneum K65.9
- pharyngoesophageal J39.2
- pharynx J39.2
  - branchial cleft (congenital) Q18.0
- pilonidal (infected) (rectum) -*see* Sinus, pilonidal
- pleura, pleural, pleurocutaneous, pleuroperitoneal J86.0
  - tuberculous NEC A15.6
- pleuropericardial I31.8
- portal vein-hepatic artery, congenital Q26.6
- postauricular H70.81
- postoperative, persistent T81.83
  - specified site -*see* Fistula, by site
- preauricular (congenital) Q18.1
- prostate N42.89
- pulmonary J86.0
  - arteriovenous I28.0
    - congenital Q25.72
  - tuberculous -*see* Tuberculosis, pulmonary
- pulmonoperitoneal J86.0
- rectolabial N82.4
- rectosigmoid (intercommunicating) K63.2
- rectoureteral N28.89
- rectourethral N36.0
  - congenital Q64.73
- rectouterine N82.4
  - congenital Q51.7
- rectovaginal N82.3
  - congenital Q52.2
  - tuberculous A18.18
- rectovesical N32.1
  - congenital Q64.79
- rectovesicovaginal N82.3
- rectovulval N82.4
  - congenital Q52.79
- rectum (to skin) K60.4
  - congenital Q43.6
    - with absence, atresia and stenosis Q42.0
  - tuberculous A18.32
- renal N28.89
- retroauricular -*see* Fistula, postauricular
- salivary duct or gland (any) K11.4
  - congenital Q38.4
- scrotum (urinary) N50.89
  - tuberculous A18.15
- semicircular canals -*see* subcategory H83.1
- sigmoid K63.2
  - to bladder N32.1
- sinus -*see* Sinusitis
- skin L98.8
  - to genital tract (female) N82.5
- splenocolic D73.89

Fistula (cutaneous) --*continued*
  stercoral K63.2
  stomach K31.6
  sublingual gland K11.4
  submandibular gland K11.4
  submaxillary (gland) K11.4
    region K12.2
  thoracic J86.0
    duct I89.8
  thoracoabdominal J86.0
  thoracogastric J86.0
  thoracointestinal J86.0
  thorax J86.0
  thyroglossal duct Q89.2
  thyroid E07.89
  trachea, congenital (external) (internal) Q32.1
  tracheoesophageal J86.0
    congenital Q39.2
      with atresia of esophagus Q39.1
    following tracheostomy J95.04
  traumatic arteriovenous -*see* Injury, blood
    vessel, by site
  tuberculous
  code by site under Tuberculosis
  typhoid A01.09
  umbilicourinary Q64.8
  urachus, congenital Q64.4
  ureter (persistent) N28.89
  ureteroabdominal N28.89
  ureterorectal N28.89
  ureterosigmoido-abdominal N28.89
  ureterovaginal N82.1
  ureterovesical N32.2
  urethra N36.0
    congenital Q64.79
    tuberculous A18.13
  urethroperineal N36.0
  urethroperineovesical N32.2
  urethrorectal N36.0
    congenital Q64.73
  urethroscrotal N50.89
  urethrovaginal N82.1
  urethrovesical N32.2
  urinary (tract) (persistent) (recurrent) N36.0
  uteroabdominal N82.5
    congenital Q51.7
  uteroenteric, uterointestinal N82.4
    congenital Q51.7
  uterorectal N82.4
    congenital Q51.7
  uteroureteric N82.1
  uterourethral Q51.7
  uterovaginal N82.8
  uterovesical N82.1
    congenital Q51.7
  uterus N82.8
  vagina (postpartal) (wall) N82.8
  vaginocutaneous (postpartal) N82.5
  vaginointestinal NEC N82.4
    large intestine N82.3
    small intestine N82.2
  vaginoperineal N82.5
  vasocutaneous, congenital Q55.7
  vesical NEC N32.2
  vesicoabdominal N32.2
  vesicocervicovaginal N82.1
  vesicocolic N32.1
  vesicocutaneous N32.2
  vesicoenteric N32.1
  vesicointestinal N32.1
  vesicometrorectal N82.4

Fistula (cutaneous) --*continued*
  vesicoperineal N32.2
  vesicorectal N32.1
    congenital Q64.79
  vesicosigmoidal N32.1
  vesicosigmoidovaginal N82.3
  vesicoureteral N32.2
  vesicoureterovaginal N82.1
  vesicourethral N32.2
  vesicourethrorectal N32.1
  vesicouterine N82.1
    congenital Q51.7
  vesicovaginal N82.0
  vulvorectal N82.4
    congenital Q52.79
Fit R56.9
  epileptic -*see* Epilepsy
  fainting R55
  hysterical F44.5
  newborn P90
Fitting (and adjustment) (of)
  artificial
    arm -*see* Admission, adjustment, artificial,
    arm
    breast Z44.3
    eye Z44.2
    leg -*see* Admission, adjustment, artificial,
    leg
  automatic implantable cardiac defibrillator
    (with synchronous cardiac pacemaker)
    Z45.02
  brain neuropacemaker Z46.2
    implanted Z45.42
  cardiac defibrillator -*see* Fitting (and
    adjustment) (of), automatic implantable
    cardiac defibrillator
  catheter, non-vascular Z46.82
  colostomy belt Z46.89
  contact lenses Z46.0
  CRT-D (resynchronization therapy
    defibrillator) Z45.02
  CRT-P (cardiac resynchronization therapy
    pacemaker) Z45.018
    pulse generator Z45.010
  cystostomy device Z46.6
  defibrillator, cardiac -*see* Fitting (and
    adjustment) (of), automatic implantable
    cardiac defibrillator
  dentures Z46.3
  device NOS Z46.9
    abdominal Z46.89
    gastrointestinal NEC Z46.59
    implanted NEC Z45.89
    nervous system Z46.2
      implanted -*see* Admission, adjustment,
      device, implanted, nervous system
    orthodontic Z46.4
    orthoptic Z46.0
    orthotic Z46.89
    prosthetic (external) Z44.9
      breast Z44.3
      dental Z46.3
      eye Z44.2
      specified NEC Z44.8
    specified NEC Z46.89
    substitution
      auditory Z46.2
        implanted -*see* Admission, adjustment,
        device, implanted, hearing device
      nervous system Z46.2

Fitting (and adjustment) (of)
--*continued*
    implanted -*see* Admission, adjustment,
  device, implanted, nervous system
    visual Z46.2
      implanted Z45.31
    urinary Z46.6
  gastric lap band Z46.51
  gastrointestinal appliance NEC Z46.59
  glasses (reading) Z46.0
  hearing aid Z46.1
  ileostomy device Z46.89
  insulin pump Z46.81
  intestinal appliance NEC Z46.89
  myringotomy device (stent) (tube) Z45.82
  neuropacemaker Z46.2
    implanted Z45.42
  non-vascular catheter Z46.82
  orthodontic device Z46.4
  orthopedic device (brace) (cast) (corset)
    (shoes) Z46.89
  pacemaker (cardiac) (cardiac
    resynchronization therapy (CRT-P))
    Z45.018
    nervous system (brain) (peripheral nerve)
    (spinal cord) Z46.2
      implanted Z45.42
    pulse generator Z45.010
  portacath (port-a-cath) Z45.2
  prosthesis (external) Z44.9
    arm -*see* Admission, adjustment, artificial,
    arm
    breast Z44.3
    dental Z46.3
    eye Z44.2
    leg -*see* Admission, adjustment, artificial,
    leg
    specified NEC Z44.8
  spectacles Z46.0
  wheelchair Z46.89
Fitzhugh-Curtis syndrome
  due to
    Chlamydia trachomatis A74.81
    Neisseria gonorrhorea (gonococcal
  peritonitis) A54.85
**Fitz's syndrome (acute hemorrhagic
pancreatitis)** -*see also* Pancreatitis, acute
K85.80
Fixation
  joint -*see* Ankylosis
  larynx J38.7
  stapes -*see* Ankylosis, ear ossicles
    deafness -*see* Deafness, conductive
  uterus (acquired) -*see* Malposition, uterus
  vocal cord J38.3
Flabby ridge K06.8
Flaccid -*see also* condition
  palate, congenital Q38.5
Flail
  chest S22.5
    newborn (birth injury) P13.8
  joint (paralytic) M25.20
    ankle M25.27
    elbow M25.22
    foot joint M25.27
    hand joint M25.24
    hip M25.25
    knee M25.26
    shoulder M25.21
    specified joint NEC M25.28
    wrist M25.23

Flajani's disease -see Hyperthyroidism, with, goiter (diffuse)
Flap, liver K71.3
Flashbacks (residual to hallucinogen use) F16.283
Flat
  chamber (eye) -see Disorder, globe, hypotony, flat anterior chamber
  chest, congenital Q67.8
  foot (acquired) (fixed type) (painful) (postural) -see also Deformity, limb, flat foot
    congenital (rigid) (spastic (everted)) Q66.5
    rachitic sequelae (late effect) E64.3
  organ or site, congenital NEC -see Anomaly, by site
  pelvis M95.5
    with disproportion (fetopelvic) O33.0
      causing obstructed labor O65.0
    congenital Q74.2
Flatau-Schilder disease G37.0
Flatback syndrome M40.30
  lumbar region M40.36
  lumbosacral region M40.37
  thoracolumbar region M40.35
Flattening
  head, femur M89.8X5
  hip -see Coxa, plana
  lip (congenital) Q18.8
  nose (congenital) Q67.4
    acquired M95.0
Flatulence R14.3
  psychogenic F45.8
Flatus R14.3
  vaginalis N89.8
Flax dresser's disease J66.1
Flea bite -see Injury, bite, by site, superficial, insect
Flecks, glaucomatous (subcapsular) -see Cataract, complicated
Fleischer (Kayser) ring (cornea) H18.04
Fleshy mole O02.0
Flexibilitas cerea -see Catalepsy
Flexion
  amputation stump (surgical) T87.89
  cervix -see Malposition, uterus
  contracture, joint -see Contraction, joint
  deformity, joint -see also Deformity, limb, flexion M21.20
    hip, congenital Q65.89
  uterus -see also Malposition, uterus
    lateral -see Lateroversion, uterus
Flexner-Boyd dysentery A03.2
Flexner's dysentery A03.1
Flexure -see Flexion
Flint murmur (aortic insufficiency) I35.1
Floater, vitreous -see Opacity, vitreous
Floating
  cartilage (joint) -see also Loose, body, joint
  knee -see Derangement, knee, loose body
  gallbladder, congenital Q44.1
  kidney N28.89
    congenital Q63.8
  spleen D73.89
Flooding N92.0
Floor -see condition
Floppy
  baby syndrome (nonspecific) P94.2
  iris syndrome (intraoperative) (IFIS) H21.81
  nonrheumatic mitral valve syndrome I34.1

Flu -see also Influenza
  avian -see also Influenza, due to, identified novel influenza A virus J09.X2
  bird -see also Influenza, due to, identified novel influenza A virus J09.X2
  intestinal NEC A08.4
  swine (viruses that normally cause infections in pigs) -see also Influenza, due to, identified novel influenza A virus J09.X2
Fluctuating blood pressure I99.8
Fluid
  abdomen R18.8
  chest J94.8
  heart -see Failure, heart, congestive
  joint -see Effusion, joint
  loss (acute) E86.9
  lung -see Edema, lung
  overload E87.70
    specified NEC E87.79
  peritoneal cavity R18.8
  pleural cavity J94.8
  retention R60.9
Flukes NEC -see also Infestation, fluke -
  blood NEC -see Schistosomiasis
  liver B66.3
Fluor (vaginalis) N89.8
  trichomonal or due to Trichomonas (vaginalis) A59.00
Fluorosis
  dental K00.3
  skeletal M85.10
    ankle M85.17
    foot M85.17
    forearm M85.13
    hand M85.14
    lower leg M85.16
    multiple site M85.19
    neck M85.18
    rib M85.18
    shoulder M85.11
    skull M85.18
    specified site NEC M85.18
    thigh M85.15
    toe M85.17
    upper arm M85.12
    vertebra M85.18
Flush syndrome E34.0
Flushing R23.2
  menopausal N95.1
Flutter
  atrial or auricular I48.92
    atypical I48.4
    type I I48.3
    type II I48.4
    typical I48.3
  heart I49.8
  atrial or auricular I48.92
    atypical I48.4
    type I I48.3
    type II I48.4
    typical I48.3
  ventricular I49.02
  ventricular I49.02
FNHTR (febrile nonhemolytic transfusion reaction) R50.84
Fochier's abscess - code by site under Abscess
Focus, Assmann's -see Tuberculosis, pulmonary
Fogo selvagem L10.3
Foix Alajouanine syndrome G95.19

Fold, folds (anomalous) -see also Anomaly, by site
  Descemet's membrane -see Change, corneal membrane, Descemet's, fold
  epicanthic Q10.3
  heart Q24.8
Folie à deux F24
Follicle
  cervix (nabothian) (ruptured) N88.8
  graafian, ruptured, with hemorrhage N83.0
  nabothian N88.8
Follicular -see condition
Folliculitis (superficial) L73.9
  abscedens et suffodiens L66.3
  cyst N83.0
  decalvans L66.2
  deep -see Furuncle, by site
  gonococcal (acute) (chronic) A54.01
  keloid, keloidalis L73.0
  pustular L01.02
  ulerythematosa reticulata L66.4
Folliculome lipidique
  specified site -see Neoplasm, benign, by site
  unspecified site
    female D27.9
    male D29.20
Følling's disease E70.0
Follow-up -see Examination, follow-up
Fong's syndrome (hereditary osteo-onychodysplasia) Q87.2
Food
  allergy L27.2
  asphyxia (from aspiration or inhalation) -see Foreign body, by site
  choked on -see Foreign body, by site
  deprivation T73.0
    specified kind of food NEC E63.8
  intoxication -see Poisoning, food
  lack of T73.0
  poisoning -see Poisoning, food
  rejection NEC -see Disorder, eating
  strangulation or suffocation -see Foreign body, by site
  toxemia -see Poisoning, food
Foot -see condition
Foramen ovale (nonclosure) (patent) (persistent) Q21.1
Forbes' glycogen storage disease E74.03
Fordyce-Fox disease L75.2
Fordyce's disease (mouth) Q38.6
Forearm -see condition
Foreign body
  with
    laceration -see Laceration, by site, with foreign body
    puncture wound -see Puncture, by site, with foreign body
  accidentally left following a procedure T81.509
    aspiration T81.506
      resulting in
        adhesions T81.516
        obstruction T81.526
        perforation T81.536
        specified complication NEC T81.596
    cardiac catheterization T81.505
      resulting in
        acute reaction T81.60
          aseptic peritonitis T81.61
          specified NEC T81.69
        adhesions T81.515

Foreign body *--continued*
- obstruction T81.525
  - perforation T81.535
  - specified complication NEC T81.595
- causing
  - acute reaction T81.60
    - aseptic peritonitis T81.61
    - specified complication NEC T81.69
  - adhesions T81.519
  - aseptic peritonitis T81.61
  - obstruction T81.529
  - perforation T81.539
  - specified complication NEC T81.599
- endoscopy T81.504
  - resulting in
    - adhesions T81.514
    - obstruction T81.524
    - perforation T81.534
    - specified complication NEC T81.594
- immunization T81.503
  - resulting in
    - adhesions T81.513
    - obstruction T81.523
    - perforation T81.533
    - specified complication NEC T81.593
- infusion T81.501
  - resulting in
    - adhesions T81.511
    - obstruction T81.521
    - perforation T81.531
    - specified complication NEC T81.591
- injection T81.503
  - resulting in
    - adhesions T81.513
    - obstruction T81.523
    - perforation T81.533
    - specified complication NEC T81.593
- kidney dialysis T81.502
  - resulting in
    - adhesions T81.512
    - obstruction T81.522
    - perforation T81.532
    - specified complication NEC T81.592
- packing removal T81.507
  - resulting in
    - acute reaction T81.60
      - aseptic peritonitis T81.61
      - specified NEC T81.69
    - adhesions T81.517
    - obstruction T81.527
    - perforation T81.537
    - specified complication NEC T81.597
- puncture T81.506
  - resulting in
    - adhesions T81.516
    - obstruction T81.526
    - perforation T81.536
    - specified complication NEC T81.596
- specified procedure NEC T81.508
  - resulting in
    - acute reaction T81.60
      - aseptic peritonitis T81.61
      - specified NEC T81.69
    - adhesions T81.518
    - obstruction T81.528
    - perforation T81.538
    - specified complication NEC T81.598
- surgical operation T81.500
  - resulting in
    - acute reaction T81.60
      - aseptic peritonitis T81.61

Foreign body *--continued*
- specified NEC T81.69
  - adhesions T81.510
  - obstruction T81.520
  - perforation T81.530
  - specified complication NEC T81.590
- transfusion T81.501
  - resulting in
    - adhesions T81.511
    - obstruction T81.521
    - perforation T81.531
    - specified complication NEC T81.591
- alimentary tract T18.9
  - anus T18.5
  - colon T18.4
  - esophagus *-see* Foreign body, esophagus
  - mouth T18.0
  - multiple sites T18.8
  - rectosigmoid (junction) T18.5
  - rectum T18.5
  - small intestine T18.3
  - specified site NEC T18.8
  - stomach T18.2
- anterior chamber (eye) S05.5
- auditory canal *-see* Foreign body, entering through orifice, ear
- bronchus T17.508
  - causing
    - asphyxiation T17.500
      - food (bone) (seed) T17.520
      - gastric contents (vomitus) T17.510
      - specified type NEC T17.590
    - injury NEC T17.508
      - food (bone) (seed) T17.528
      - gastric contents (vomitus) T17.518
      - specified type NEC T17.598
- canthus *-see* Foreign body, conjunctival sac -
  - ciliary body (eye) S05.5
- conjunctival sac T15.1
- cornea T15.0
- entering through orifice
  - accessory sinus T17.0
  - alimentary canal T18.9
    - multiple parts T18.8
    - specified part NEC T18.8
  - alveolar process T18.0
  - antrum (Highmore's) T17.0
  - anus T18.5
  - appendix T18.4
  - auditory canal *-see* Foreign body, entering through orifice, ear
  - auricle *-see* Foreign body, entering through orifice, ear
  - bladder T19.1
  - bronchioles *-see* Foreign body, respiratory tract, specified site NEC
  - bronchus (main) *-see* Foreign body, bronchus
  - buccal cavity T18.0
  - canthus (inner) *-see* Foreign body, conjunctival sac
  - cecum T18.4
  - cervix (canal) (uteri) T19.3
  - colon T18.4
  - conjunctival sac *-see* Foreign body, conjunctival sac
  - cornea *-see* Foreign body, cornea
  - digestive organ or tract NOS T18.9
    - multiple parts T18.8
    - specified part NEC T18.8
  - duodenum T18.3

Foreign body *--continued*
- ear (external) T16.
- esophagus *-see* Foreign body, esophagus
- eye (external) NOS T15.9
  - conjunctival sac *-see* Foreign body, conjunctival sac
  - cornea *-see* Foreign body, cornea
  - specified part NEC T15.8
- eyeball *-see also* Foreign body, entering through orifice, eye, specified part NEC
  - with penetrating wound *-see* Puncture, eyeball
- eyelid *-see also* Foreign body, conjunctival sac
  - with
    - laceration *-see* Laceration, eyelid, with foreign body
    - puncture *-see* Puncture, eyelid, with foreign body
    - superficial injury *-see* Foreign body, superficial, eyelid
- gastrointestinal tract T18.9
  - multiple parts T18.8
  - specified part NEC T18.8
- genitourinary tract T19.9
  - multiple parts T19.8
  - specified part NEC T19.8
- globe *-see* Foreign body, entering through orifice, eyeball
- gum T18.0
- Highmore's antrum T17.0
- hypopharynx *-see* Foreign body, pharynx
- ileum T18.3
- intestine (small) T18.3
  - large T18.4
- lacrimal apparatus (punctum) *-see* Foreign body, entering through orifice, eye, specified part NEC
- large intestine T18.4
- larynx *-see* Foreign body, larynx
- lung *-see* Foreign body, respiratory tract, specified site NEC
- maxillary sinus T17.0
- mouth T18.0
- nasal sinus T17.0
- nasopharynx *-see* Foreign body, pharynx
- nose (passage) T17.1
- nostril T17.1
- oral cavity T18.0
- palate T18.0
- penis T19.4
- pharynx *-see* Foreign body, pharynx
- piriform sinus *-see* Foreign body, pharynx
- rectosigmoid (junction) T18.5
- rectum T18.5
- respiratory tract *-see* Foreign body, respiratory tract
- sinus (accessory) (frontal) (maxillary) (nasal) T17.0
  - piriform *-see* Foreign body, pharynx
- small intestine T18.3
- stomach T18.2
- suffocation by *-see* Foreign body, by site
- tear ducts or glands *-see* Foreign body, entering through orifice, eye, specified part NEC
- throat *-see* Foreign body, pharynx
- tongue T18.0
- tonsil, tonsillar (fossa) *-see* Foreign body, pharynx
- trachea *-see* Foreign body, trachea

Foreign body --*continued*
  ureter T19.8
  urethra T19.0
  uterus (any part) T19.3
  vagina T19.2
  vulva T19.2
  esophagus T18.108
    causing
      injury NEC T18.108
        food (bone) (seed) T18.128
        gastric contents (vomitus) T18.118
        specified type NEC T18.198
      tracheal compression T18.100
        food (bone) (seed) T18.120
        gastric contents (vomitus) T18.110
        specified type NEC T18.190
  felling of, in throat R09.89
  fragment -*see* Retained, foreign body
    fragments (type of)
  genitourinary tract T19.9
    bladder T19.1
    multiple parts T19.8
    penis T19.4
    specified site NEC T19.8
    urethra T19.0
    uterus T19.3
      IUD Z97.5
    vagina T19.2
      contraceptive device Z97.5
    vulva T19.2
  granuloma (old) (soft tissue) -*see also*
    Granuloma, foreign body
    skin L92.3
  in
    laceration -*see* Laceration, by site, with
    foreign body
    puncture wound -*see* Puncture, by site, with
    foreign body
    soft tissue (residual) M79.5
  inadvertently left in operation wound -*see*
    Foreign body, accidentally left during a
    procedure
  ingestion, ingested NOS T18.9
  inhalation or inspiration -*see* Foreign body, by
    site
  internal organ, not entering through a natural
    orifice
    code as specific injury with foreign body
  intraocular S05.5
    old, retained (nonmagnetic) H44.70
      anterior chamber H44.71
      ciliary body H44.72
      iris H44.72
      lens H44.73
      magnetic H44.60
        anterior chamber H44.61
        ciliary body H44.62
        iris H44.62
        lens H44.63
        posterior wall H44.64
        specified site NEC H44.69
        vitreous body H44.65
      posterior wall H44.74
      specified site NEC H44.79
      vitreous body H44.75
  iris -*see* Foreign body, intraocular
  lacrimal punctum -*see* Foreign body, entering
    through orifice, eye, specified part NEC
  larynx T17.308
    causing
      asphyxiation T17.300

Foreign body --*continued*
      food (bone) (seed) T17.320
      gastric contents (vomitus) T17.310
      specified type NEC T17.390
    injury NEC T17.308
      food (bone) (seed) T17.328
      gastric contents (vomitus) T17.318
      specified type NEC T17.398
  lens -*see* Foreign body, intraocular
  ocular muscle S05.4
    old, retained -*see* Foreign body, orbit, old -
  old or residual
    soft tissue (residual) M79.5
  operation wound, left accidentally -*see*
  Foreign body, accidentally left during a
  procedure
  orbit S05.4
    old, retained H05.5
  pharynx T17.208
    causing
      asphyxiation T17.200
        food (bone) (seed) T17.220
        gastric contents (vomitus) T17.210
        specified type NEC T17.290
      injury NEC T17.208
        food (bone) (seed) T17.228
        gastric contents (vomitus) T17.218
        specified type NEC T17.298
  respiratory tract T17.908
    bronchioles -*see* Foreign body, respiratory
  tract, specified site NEC
    bronchus -*see* Foreign body, bronchus
    causing
      asphyxiation T17.900
        food (bone) (seed) T17.920
        gastric contents (vomitus) T17.910
        specified type NEC T17.990
      injury NEC T17.908
        food (bone) (seed) T17.928
        gastric contents (vomitus) T17.918
        specified type NEC T17.998
    larynx -*see* Foreign body, larynx
    lung -*see* Foreign body, respiratory tract,
  specified site NEC
    multiple parts -*see* Foreign body, respiratory
  tract, specified site NEC
    nasal sinus T17.0
    nasopharynx -*see* Foreign body, pharynx
    nose T17.1
    nostril T17.1
    pharynx -*see* Foreign body, pharynx
    specified site NEC T17.808
      causing
        asphyxiation T17.800
          food (bone) (seed) T17.820
          gastric contents (vomitus) T17.810
          specified type NEC T17.890
        injury NEC T17.808
          food (bone) (seed) T17.828
          gastric contents (vomitus) T17.818
          specified type NEC T17.898
    throat -*see* Foreign body, pharynx
    trachea -*see* Foreign body, trachea
  retained (old) (nonmagnetic) (in)
    anterior chamber (eye) -*see* Foreign body,
  intraocular, old, retained, anterior chamber
      magnetic -*see* Foreign body, intraocular,
  old, retained, magnetic, anterior chamber
    ciliary body -*see* Foreign body, intraocular,
  old, retained, ciliary body

Foreign body --*continued*
    magnetic -*see* Foreign body, intraocular,
    old, retained, magnetic, ciliary body
  eyelid H02.819
    left H02.816
      lower H02.815
      upper H02.814
    right H02.813
      lower H02.812
      upper H02.811
  fragments -*see* Retained, foreign body
    fragments (type of)
  globe -*see* Foreign body, intraocular, old,
    retained
    magnetic -*see* Foreign body, intraocular,
    old, retained, magnetic
  intraocular -*see* Foreign body, intraocular,
    old, retained
    magnetic -*see* Foreign body, intraocular,
    old, retained, magnetic
  iris -*see* Foreign body, intraocular, old,
    retained, iris
    magnetic -*see* Foreign body, intraocular,
    old, retained, magnetic, iris
  lens -*see* Foreign body, intraocular, old,
    retained, lens
    magnetic -*see* Foreign body, intraocular,
    old, retained, magnetic, lens
  muscle -*see* Foreign body, retained, soft
    tissue
  orbit -*see* Foreign body, orbit, old
  posterior wall of globe -*see* Foreign body,
    intraocular, old, retained, posterior wall
    magnetic -*see* Foreign body, intraocular,
    old, retained, magnetic, posterior wall
  retrobulbar -*see* Foreign body, orbit, old,
    retrobulbar
  soft tissue M79.5
  vitreous -*see* Foreign body, intraocular, old,
    retained, vitreous body
    magnetic -*see* Foreign body, intraocular,
    old, retained, magnetic, vitreous body
  retina S05.5
  superficial, without open wound
    abdomen, abdominal (wall) S30.851
    alveolar process S00.552
    ankle S90.55
    antecubital space -*see* Foreign body,
    superficial, forearm
    anus S30.857
    arm (upper) S40.85
    auditory canal -*see* Foreign body,
    superficial, ear
    auricle -*see* Foreign body, superficial, ear
    axilla -*see* Foreign body, superficial, arm
    back, lower S30.850
    breast S20.15
    brow S00.85
    buttock S30.850
    calf -*see* Foreign body, superficial, leg
    canthus -*see* Foreign body, superficial,
    eyelid
    cheek S00.85
      internal S00.552
    chest wall -*see* Foreign body, superficial,
    thorax
    chin S00.85
    clitoris S30.854
    costal region -*see* Foreign body, superficial,
    thorax
    digit(s)

Foreign body --*continued*
    hand -*see* Foreign body, superficial, finger
    foot -*see* Foreign body, superficial, toe
    ear S00.45
    elbow S50.35
    epididymis S30.853
    epigastric region S30.851
    epiglottis S10.15
    esophagus, cervical S10.15
    eyebrow -*see* Foreign body, superficial, eyelid
    eyelid S00.25
    face S00.85
    finger(s) S60.459
      index S60.45
      little S60.45
      middle S60.45
      ring S60.45
    flank S30.851
    foot (except toe(s) alone) S90.85
      toe -*see* Foreign body, superficial, toe
    forearm S50.85
      elbow only -*see* Foreign body, superficial, elbow
    forehead S00.85
    genital organs, external
      female S30.856
      male S30.855
    groin S30.851
    gum S00.552
    hand S60.55
    head S00.95
      ear -*see* Foreign body, superficial, ear
      eyelid -*see* Foreign body, superficial, eyelid
      lip S00.551
      nose S00.35
      oral cavity S00.552
      scalp S00.05
      specified site NEC S00.85
    heel -*see* Foreign body, superficial, foot
    hip S70.25
    inguinal region S30.851
    interscapular region S20.459
    jaw S00.85
    knee S80.25
    labium (majus) (minus) S30.854
    larynx S10.15
    leg (lower) S80.85
      knee -*see* Foreign body, superficial, knee
      upper -*see* Foreign body, superficial, thigh
    lip S00.551
    lower back S30.850
    lumbar region S30.850
    malar region S00.85
    mammary -*see* Foreign body, superficial, breast
    mastoid region S00.85
    mouth S00.552
    nail
      finger -*see* Foreign body, superficial, finger
      toe -*see* Foreign body, superficial, toe
    nape S10.85
    nasal S00.35
    neck S10.95
      specified site NEC S10.85
      throat S10.15
    nose S00.35
    occipital region S00.05
    oral cavity S00.552

Foreign body --*continued*
    orbital region -*see* Foreign body, superficial, eyelid
    palate S00.552
    palm -*see* Foreign body, superficial, hand
    parietal region S00.05
    pelvis S30.850
    penis S30.852
    perineum
      female S30.854
      male S30.850
    periocular area -*see* Foreign body, superficial, eyelid
    phalanges
      finger -*see* Foreign body, superficial, finger
      toe -*see* Foreign body, superficial, toe
    pharynx S10.15
    pinna -*see* Foreign body, superficial, ear
    popliteal space -*see* Foreign body, superficial, knee
    prepuce S30.852
    pubic region S30.850
    pudendum
      female S30.856
      male S30.855
    sacral region S30.850
    scalp S00.05
    scapular region -*see* Foreign body, superficial, shoulder
    scrotum S30.853
    shin -*see* Foreign body, superficial, leg
    shoulder S40.25
    sternal region S20.359
    submaxillary region S00.85
    submental region S00.85
    subungual
      finger(s) -*see* Foreign body, superficial, finger
      toe(s) -*see* Foreign body, superficial, toe
    supraclavicular fossa S10.85
    supraorbital S00.85
    temple S00.85
    temporal region S00.85
    testis S30.853
    thigh S70.35
    thorax, thoracic (wall) S20.95
      back S20.45
      front S20.35
    throat S10.15
    thumb S60.35
    toe(s) (lesser) S90.456
      great S90.45
    tongue S00.552
    trachea S10.15
    tunica vaginalis S30.853
    tympanum, tympanic membrane -*see* Foreign body, superficial, ear
    uvula S00.552
    vagina S30.854
    vocal cords S10.15
    vulva S30.854
    wrist S60.85
    swallowed T18.9
    trachea T17.408
      causing
        asphyxiation T17.400
        food (bone) (seed) T17.420
        gastric contents (vomitus) T17.410
        specified type NEC T17.490
        injury NEC T17.408

Foreign body --*continued*
      food (bone) (seed) T17.428
      gastric contents (vomitus) T17.418
      specified type NEC T17.498
    type of fragment -*see* Retained, foreign body fragments (type of)
    vitreous (humor) S05.5
Forestier's disease (rhizomelic pseudopolyarthritis) M35.3
    meaning ankylosing hyperostosis -*see* Hyperostosis, ankylosing
Formation
    hyalin in cornea -*see* Degeneration, cornea
    sequestrum in bone (due to infection) -*see* Osteomyelitis, chronic
    valve
      colon, congenital Q43.8
      ureter (congenital) Q62.39
Formication R20.2
Fort Bragg fever A27.89
Fossa -*see also* condition
    pyriform -*see* condition
Foster-Kennedy syndrome H47.14
Fothergill's
    disease (trigeminal neuralgia) -*see also* Neuralgia, trigeminal
    scarlatina anginosa A38.9
Foul breath R19.6
Foundling Z76.1
Fournier disease or gangrene N49.3
    female N76.89
Fourth
    cranial nerve -*see* condition
    molar K00.1
Foville's (peduncular) disease or syndrome G46.3
Fox (Fordyce) disease (apocrine miliaria) L75.2
Fracture, burst -*see* Fracture, traumatic, by site
Fracture, chronic -*see* Fracture, pathological
Fracture, insufficiency -*see* Fracture, pathologic, by site
Fracture, nontraumatic, NEC
    atypical
      femur M84.750
        complete
          oblique M84.759
            left side M84.758
            right side M84.757
          transverse M84.756
            left side M84.755
            right side M84.754
        incomplete M84.753
          left side M84.752
          right side M84.751
Fracture, pathological (pathologic) -*see also* Fracture, traumatic M84.40
    ankle M84.47
    carpus M84.44
    clavicle M84.41
    compression (not due to trauma) -*see also* Collapse, vertebra M48.50
    dental implant M27.63
    dental restorative material K08.539
      with loss of material K08.531
      without loss of material K08.530
    due to
      neoplastic disease NEC -*see also* Neoplasm M84.50
        ankle M84.57

Fracture, pathological - *continued*
carpus M84.54
clavicle M84.51
femur M84.55
fibula M84.56
finger M84.54
hip M84.559
humerus M84.52
ilium M84.550
ischium M84.550
metacarpus M84.54
metatarsus M84.57
neck M84.58
pelvis M84.550
radius M84.53
rib M84.58
scapula M84.51
skull M84.58
specified site NEC M84.58
tarsus M84.57
tibia M84.56
toe M84.57
ulna M84.53
vertebra M84.58
osteoporosis M80.00
disuse -*see* Osteoporosis, specified type
NEC, with pathological fracture
drug-induced -*see* Osteoporosis, drug
induced, with pathological fracture
idiopathic -*see* Osteoporosis, specified type
NEC, with pathological fracture
postmenopausal -*see* Osteoporosis,
postmenopausal, with pathological
fracture
postoophorectomy -*see* Osteoporosis,
postoophorectomy, with pathological
fracture
postsurgical malabsorption -*see*
Osteoporosis, specified type NEC, with
pathological fracture
specified cause NEC -*see* Osteoporosis,
specified type NEC, with pathological
fracture
specified disease NEC M84.60
ankle M84.67
carpus M84.64
clavicle M84.61
femur M84.65
fibula M84.66
finger M84.64
hip M84.65
humerus M84.62
ilium M84.650
ischium M84.650
metacarpus M84.64
metatarsus M84.67
neck M84.68
radius M84.63
rib M84.68
scapula M84.61
skull M84.68
tarsus M84.67
tibia M84.66
toe M84.67
ulna M84.63
vertebra M84.68
femur M84.45
fibula M84.46
finger M84.44
hip M84.459
humerus M84.42

Fracture, pathological - *continued*
ilium M84.454
ischium M84.454
joint prosthesis -*see* Complications, joint
prosthesis, mechanical, breakdown, by site
periprosthetic -*see* Fracture, pathological,
periprosthetic
metacarpus M84.44
metatarsus M84.47
neck M84.48
pelvis M84.454
periprosthetic M97.9
ankle M97.2
elbow M97.4
finger M97.8
hip M97.0
knee M97.1
other specified joint M97.8
shoulder M97.3
spinal joint M97.8
toe joint M97.8
wrist joint M97.8
radius M84.43
restorative material (dental) K08.539
with loss of material K08.531
without loss of material K08.530
rib M84.48
scapula M84.41
skull M84.48
tarsus M84.47
tibia M84.46
toe M84.47
ulna M84.43
vertebra M84.48
Fracture, traumatic (abduction) (adduction)
(separation) -*see also* Fracture, pathological
T14.8
acetabulum S32.40
column
anterior (displaced) (iliopubic) S32.43
nondisplaced S32.436
posterior (displaced) (ilioischial) S32.443
nondisplaced S32.44
dome (displaced) S32.48
nondisplaced S32.48
specified NEC S32.49
transverse (displaced) S32.45
with associated posterior wall fracture
(displaced) S32.46
nondisplaced S32.46
nondisplaced S32.45
wall
anterior (displaced) S32.41
nondisplaced S32.41
medial (displaced) S32.47
nondisplaced S32.47
posterior (displaced) S32.42
with associated transverse fracture
(displaced) S32.46
nondisplaced S32.46
nondisplaced S32.42
acromion -*see* Fracture, scapula, acromial
process
ankle S82.899
bimalleolar (displaced) S82.84
nondisplaced S82.84
lateral malleolus only (displaced) S82.6
nondisplaced S82.6
medial malleolus (displaced) S82.5
associated with Maisonneuve's fracture -
see Fracture, Maisonneuve's

Fracture, pathological - *continued*
nondisplaced S82.5
talus -*see* Fracture, tarsal, talus
trimalleolar (displaced) S82.85
nondisplaced S82.85
arm (upper) -*see also* Fracture, humerus, shaft
humerus -*see* Fracture, humerus
radius -*see* Fracture, radius
ulna -*see* Fracture, ulna
astragalus -*see* Fracture, tarsal, talus
atlas -*see* Fracture, neck, cervical vertebra,
first
axis -*see* Fracture, neck, cervical vertebra,
second
back -*see* Fracture, vertebra
Barton's -*see* Barton's fracture
base of skull -*see* Fracture, skull, base
basicervical (basal) (femoral) S72.0
Bennett's -*see* Bennett's fracture
bimalleolar -*see* Fracture, ankle, bimalleolar
blow-out S02.3
bone NEC T14.8
birth injury P13.9
following insertion of orthopedic implant,
joint prosthesis or bone plate -*see* Fracture,
following insertion of orthopedic implant,
joint prosthesis or bone plate
in (due to) neoplastic disease NEC -*see*
Fracture, pathological, due to, neoplastic
disease
pathological (cause unknown) -*see* Fracture,
pathological
breast bone -*see* Fracture, sternum
bucket handle (semilunar cartilage) -*see* Tear,
meniscus
burst -*see* Fracture, traumatic, by site
calcaneus -*see* Fracture, tarsal, calcaneus
carpal bone(s) S62.10
capitate (displaced) S62.13
nondisplaced S62.13
cuneiform -*see* Fracture, carpal bone,
triquetrum
hamate (body) (displaced) S62.143
hook process (displaced) S62.15
nondisplaced S62.15
nondisplaced S62.14
larger multangular -*see* Fracture, carpal
bones, trapezium
lunate (displaced) S62.12
nondisplaced S62.12
navicular S62.00
distal pole (displaced) S62.01
nondisplaced S62.01
middle third (displaced) S62.02
nondisplaced S62.02
proximal third (displaced) S62.03
nondisplaced S62.03
volar tuberosity -*see* Fracture, carpal
bones, navicular, distal pole
os magnum -*see* Fracture, carpal bones,
capitate
pisiform (displaced) S62.16
nondisplaced S62.16
semilunar -*see* Fracture, carpal bones, lunate
smaller multangular -*see* Fracture, carpal
bones, trapezoid
trapezium (displaced) S62.17
nondisplaced S62.17
trapezoid (displaced) S62.18
nondisplaced S62.18
triquetrum (displaced) S62.11

Fracture, pathological - *continued*

nondisplaced S62.11

unciform -*see* Fracture, carpal bones, hamate

cervical -*see* Fracture, vertebra, cervical

clavicle S42.00

  acromial end (displaced) S42.03

    nondisplaced S42.03

  birth injury P13.4

  lateral end -*see* Fracture, clavicle, acromial end

  shaft (displaced) S42.02

    nondisplaced S42.02

  sternal end (anterior) (displaced) S42.01

    nondisplaced S42.01

    posterior S42.01

coccyx S32.2

collapsed -*see* Collapse, vertebra

collar bone -*see* Fracture, clavicle

Colles' -*see* Colles' fracture

coronoid process -*see* Fracture, ulna, upper end, coronoid process

corpus cavernosum penis S39.840

costochondral cartilage S23.41

costochondral, costosternal junction -*see* Fracture, rib

cranium -*see* Fracture, skull

cricoid cartilage S12.8

cuboid (ankle) -*see* Fracture, tarsal, cuboid

cuneiform

  foot -*see* Fracture, tarsal, cuneiform

  wrist -*see* Fracture, carpal, triquetrum

delayed union -*see* Delay, union, fracture

dental restorative material K08.539

  with loss of material K08.531

  without loss of material K08.530

due to

  birth injury -*see* Birth, injury, fracture

  osteoporosis -*see* Osteoporosis, with fracture

Dupuytren's -*see* Fracture, ankle, lateral malleolus

elbow S42.40

ethmoid (bone) (sinus) -*see* Fracture, skull, base

face bone S02.92

fatigue -*see also* Fracture, stress

  vertebra M48.40

    cervical region M48.42

    cervicothoracic region M48.43

    lumbar region M48.46

    lumbosacral region M48.47

    occipito-atlanto-axial region M48.41

    sacrococcygeal region M48.48

    thoracic region M48.44

    thoracolumbar region M48.45

femur, femoral S72.9

  basicervical (basal) S72.0

  birth injury P13.2

  capital epiphyseal S79.01

  condyles, epicondyles -*see* Fracture, femur, lower end

  distal end -*see* Fracture, femur, lower end

  epiphysis

    head -*see* Fracture, femur, upper end, epiphysis

    lower -*see* Fracture, femur, lower end, epiphysis

    upper -*see* Fracture, femur, upper end, epiphysis

  following insertion of implant, prosthesis or plate M96.66

  head -*see* Fracture, femur, upper end, head

Fracture, pathological - *continued*

intertrochanteric -*see* Fracture, femur, trochanteric

intratrochanteric -*see* Fracture, femur, trochanteric

lower end S72.40

  condyle (displaced) S72.41

    lateral (displaced) S72.42

      nondisplaced S72.42

    medial (displaced) S72.43

      nondisplaced S72.43

    nondisplaced S72.41

  epiphysis (displaced) S72.44

    nondisplaced S72.44

  physeal S79.10

    Salter-Harris

      Type I S79.11

      Type II S79.12

      Type III S79.13

      Type IV S79.14

    specified NEC S79.19

  specified NEC S72.49

  supracondylar (displaced) S72.45

    with intracondylar extension (displaced) S72.46

      nondisplaced S72.46

    nondisplaced S72.45

  torus S72.47

neck -*see* Fracture, femur, upper end, neck

pertrochanteric -*see* Fracture, femur, trochanteric

shaft (lower third) (middle third) (upper third) S72.30

  comminuted (displaced) S72.35

    nondisplaced S72.35

  oblique (displaced) S72.33

    nondisplaced S72.33

  segmental (displaced) S72.36

    nondisplaced S72.36

  specified NEC S72.39

  spiral (displaced) S72.34

    nondisplaced S72.34

  transverse (displaced) S72.32

    nondisplaced S72.32

specified site NEC -*see* subcategory S72.8

subcapital (displaced) S72.01

subtrochanteric (region) (section) (displaced) S72.2

  nondisplaced S72.2

transcervical -*see* Fracture, femur, upper end, neck

transtrochanteric -*see* Fracture, femur, trochanteric

trochanteric S72.10

  apophyseal (displaced) S72.13

    nondisplaced S72.13

  greater trochanter (displaced) S72.11

    nondisplaced S72.11

  intertrochanteric (displaced) S72.14

    nondisplaced S72.14

  lesser trochanter (displaced) S72.12

    nondisplaced S72.12

upper end S72.00

  apophyseal (displaced) S72.13

    nondisplaced S72.13

  cervicotrochanteric -*see* Fracture, femur, upper end, neck, base

  epiphysis (displaced) S72.02

    nondisplaced S72.02

  head S72.05

    articular (displaced) S72.06

Fracture, pathological - *continued*

    nondisplaced S72.06

    specified NEC S72.09

  intertrochanteric (displaced) S72.14

    nondisplaced S72.14

  intracapsular S72.01

  midcervical (displaced) S72.03

    nondisplaced S72.03

  neck S72.00

    base (displaced) S72.04

      nondisplaced S72.04

    specified NEC S72.09

  pertrochanteric -*see* Fracture, femur, upper end, trochanteric

  physeal S79.00

    Salter-Harris type I S79.01

    specified NEC S79.09

  subcapital (displaced) S72.01

  subtrochanteric (displaced) S72.2

    nondisplaced S72.2

  transcervical -*see* Fracture, femur, upper end, midcervical

  trochanteric S72.10

    greater (displaced) S72.11

      nondisplaced S72.11

    lesser (displaced) S72.12

      nondisplaced S72.12

fibula (shaft) (styloid) S82.40

  comminuted (displaced) S82.45

    nondisplaced S82.45

  following insertion of implant, prosthesis or plate M96.67

  involving ankle or malleolus -*see* Fracture, fibula, lateral malleolus

  lateral malleolus (displaced) S82.6

    nondisplaced S82.6

  lower end

    physeal S89.30

      Salter-Harris

        Type I S89.31

        Type II S89.32

        specified NEC S89.39

    specified NEC S82.83

    torus S82.82

  oblique (displaced) S82.43

    nondisplaced S82.43

  segmental (displaced) S82.46

    nondisplaced S82.46

  specified NEC S82.49

  spiral (displaced) S82.44

    nondisplaced S82.44

  transverse (displaced) S82.42

    nondisplaced S82.42

  upper end

    physeal S89.20

      Salter-Harris

        Type I S89.21

        Type II S89.22

      specified NEC S89.29

    specified NEC S82.83

    torus S82.81

finger (except thumb) S62.60

  distal phalanx (displaced) S62.63

    nondisplaced S62.66

  index S62.60

    distal phalanx (displaced) S62.63

      nondisplaced S62.66

    medial phalanx (displaced) S62.62

      nondisplaced S62.65

    proximal phalanx (displaced) S62.61

      nondisplaced S62.64

Fracture, pathological - *continued*
  little S62.60
    distal phalanx (displaced) S62.63
      nondisplaced S62.66
    medial phalanx (displaced) S62.62
      nondisplaced S62.65
    proximal phalanx (displaced) S62.61
      nondisplaced S62.64
  medial phalanx (displaced) S62.62
    nondisplaced S62.65
  middle S62.60
    distal phalanx (displaced) S62.63
      nondisplaced S62.66
    medial phalanx (displaced) S62.62
      nondisplaced S62.65
    proximal phalanx (displaced) S62.61
      nondisplaced S62.64
  proximal phalanx (displaced) S62.61
    nondisplaced S62.64
  ring S62.60
    distal phalanx (displaced) S62.63
      nondisplaced S62.66
    medial phalanx (displaced) S62.62
      nondisplaced S62.65
    proximal phalanx (displaced) S62.61
      nondisplaced S62.64
  thumb -*see* Fracture, thumb
  following insertion (intraoperative)
  (postoperative) of orthopedic implant, joint
  prosthesis or bone plate M96.69
    femur M96.66
    fibula M96.67
    humerus M96.62
    pelvis M96.65
    radius M96.63
    specified bone NEC M96.69
    tibia M96.67
    ulna M96.63
  foot S92.90
    astragalus -*see* Fracture, tarsal, talus
    calcaneus -*see* Fracture, tarsal, calcaneus
    cuboid -*see* Fracture, tarsal, cuboid
    cuneiform -*see* Fracture, tarsal, cuneiform
    metatarsal -*see* Fracture, metatarsal
    navicular -*see* Fracture, tarsal, navicular
    sesamoid S92.81
    specified NEC S92.81
    talus -*see* Fracture, tarsal, talus
    tarsal -*see* Fracture, tarsal
    toe -*see* Fracture, toe
  forearm S52.9
    radius -*see* Fracture, radius
    ulna -*see* Fracture, ulna
  fossa (anterior) (middle) (posterior) S02.19
  frontal (bone) (skull) S02.0
    sinus S02.19
  glenoid (cavity) (scapula) -*see* Fracture,
    scapula, glenoid cavity   greenstick -*see*
    Fracture, by site
  hallux -*see* Fracture, toe, great
  hand S62.9
    carpal -*see* Fracture, carpal bone
    finger (except thumb) -*see* Fracture, finger
    metacarpal -*see* Fracture, metacarpal
    navicular (scaphoid) (hand) -*see* Fracture,
      carpal bone, navicular
    thumb -*see* Fracture, thumb
  healed or old
    with complications
  code by Nature of the complication
  heel bone -*see* Fracture, tarsal, calcaneus

Fracture, pathological - *continued*
  Hill-Sachs S42.29
  hip -*see* Fracture, femur, neck
  humerus S42.30
    anatomical neck -*see* Fracture, humerus,
      upper end
    articular process -*see* Fracture, humerus,
      lower end
    capitellum -*see* Fracture, humerus, lower
      end, condyle, lateral
    distal end -*see* Fracture, humerus, lower end
    epiphysis
      lower -*see* Fracture, humerus, lower end,
        physeal
      upper -*see* Fracture, humerus, upper end,
        physeal
    external condyle -*see* Fracture, humerus,
      lower end, condyle, lateral
    following insertion of implant, prosthesis or
      plate M96.62
    great tuberosity -*see* Fracture, humerus,
      upper end, greater tuberosity
    intercondylar -*see* Fracture, humerus, lower
      end
    internal epicondyle -*see* Fracture, humerus,
      lower end, epicondyle, medial
    lesser tuberosity -*see* Fracture, humerus,
      upper end, lesser tuberosity
    lower end S42.40
      condyle
        lateral (displaced) S42.45
          nondisplaced S42.45
        medial (displaced) S42.46
          nondisplaced S42.46
      epicondyle
        lateral (displaced) S42.43
          nondisplaced S42.43
        medial (displaced) S42.44
          incarcerated S42.44
          nondisplaced S42.44
      physeal S49.10
        Salter-Harris
          Type I S49.11
          Type II S49.12
          Type III S49.13
          Type IV S49.14
        specified NEC S49.19
      specified NEC (displaced) S42.49
        nondisplaced S42.49
      supracondylar (simple) (displaced) S42.41
        with intercondylar fracture -*see* Fracture,
          humerus, lower end
        comminuted (displaced) S42.42
          nondisplaced S42.42
        nondisplaced S42.41
      torus S42.48
      transcondylar (displaced) S42.47
        nondisplaced S42.47
    proximal end -*see* Fracture, humerus, upper
      end
    shaft S42.30
      comminuted (displaced) S42.35
        nondisplaced S42.35
      greenstick S42.31
      oblique (displaced) S42.33
        nondisplaced S42.33
      segmental (displaced) S42.36
        nondisplaced S42.36
      specified NEC S42.39
      spiral (displaced) S42.34
        nondisplaced S42.34

Fracture, pathological - *continued*
    transverse (displaced) S42.32
      nondisplaced S42.32
    supracondylar -*see* Fracture, humerus, lower
      end
    surgical neck -*see* Fracture, humerus, upper
      end, surgical neck
    trochlea -*see* Fracture, humerus, lower end,
      condyle, medial
    tuberosity -*see* Fracture, humerus, upper end
    upper end S42.20
      anatomical neck -*see* Fracture, humerus,
        upper end, specified NEC
      articular head -*see* Fracture, humerus,
        upper end, specified NEC
      epiphysis -*see* Fracture, humerus, upper
        end, physeal
      greater tuberosity (displaced) S42.25
        nondisplaced S42.25
      lesser tuberosity (displaced) S42.26
        nondisplaced S42.26
      physeal S49.00
        Salter-Harris
          Type I S49.01
          Type II S49.02
          Type III S49.03
          Type IV S49.04
        specified NEC S49.09
      specified NEC (displaced) S42.29
        nondisplaced S42.29
      surgical neck (displaced) S42.21
        four-part S42.24
        nondisplaced S42.21
        three-part S42.23
        two-part (displaced) S42.22
          nondisplaced S42.22
      torus S42.27
    transepiphyseal -*see* Fracture, humerus,
    upper end, physeal
  hyoid bone S12.8
  ilium S32.30
    with disruption of pelvic ring -*see*
      Disruption, pelvic ring
    avulsion (displaced) S32.31
      nondisplaced S32.31
    specified NEC S32.39
  impaction, impacted - code as Fracture, by
  site
  innominate bone -*see* Fracture, ilium
  instep -*see* Fracture, foot
  ischium S32.60
    with disruption of pelvic ring -*see*
      Disruption, pelvic ring
    avulsion (displaced) S32.61
      nondisplaced S32.61
    specified NEC S32.69
  jaw (bone) (lower) -*see* Fracture, mandible
    upper -*see* Fracture, maxilla
  joint prosthesis -*see* Complications, joint
  prosthesis, mechanical, breakdown, by site
    periprosthetic -*see* Fracture, traumatic,
    periprosthetic
  knee cap -*see* Fracture, patella
  larynx S12.8
  late effects -*see* Sequelae, fracture
  leg (lower) S82.9
    ankle -*see* Fracture, ankle
    femur -*see* Fracture, femur
    fibula -*see* Fracture, fibula
    malleolus -*see* Fracture, ankle
    patella -*see* Fracture, patella

Fracture, pathological - *continued*
    specified site NEC S82.89
    tibia *-see* Fracture, tibia
  lumbar spine *-see* Fracture, vertebra, lumbar
  lumbosacral spine S32.9
  Maisonneuve's (displaced) S82.86
    nondisplaced S82.86
  malar bone *-see also* Fracture, maxilla
    S02.400
    left side S02.40B
    right side S02.40A
  malleolus *-see* Fracture, ankle
  malunion *-see* Fracture, by site
  mandible (lower jaw (bone)) S02.609
    alveolus S02.67
    angle (of jaw) S02.65
    body, unspecified S02.600
      left side S02.602
      right side S02.601
    condylar process S02.61
    coronoid process S02.63
    ramus, unspecified S02.64
    specified site NEC S02.69
    subcondylar process S02.62
    symphysis S02.66
  manubrium (sterni) S22.21
    dissociation from sternum S22.23
  march *-see* Fracture, traumatic, stress, by site
  maxilla, maxillary (bone) (sinus) (superior)
  (upper jaw) S02.401
    alveolus S02.42
    inferior *-see* Fracture, mandible
    LeFort I S02.411
    LeFort II S02.412
    LeFort III S02.413
    left side S02.40D
    right side S02.40C - metacarpal S62.309
    base (displaced) S62.319
      nondisplaced S62.349
    fifth S62.30
      base (displaced) S62.31
        nondisplaced S62.34
      neck (displaced) S62.33
        nondisplaced S62.36
      shaft (displaced) S62.32
        nondisplaced S62.35
      specified NEC S62.398
    first S62.20
      base NEC (displaced) S62.23
        nondisplaced S62.23
      Bennett's *-see* Bennett's fracture
      neck (displaced) S62.25
        nondisplaced S62.25
      shaft (displaced) S62.24
        nondisplaced S62.24
      specified NEC S62.29
    fourth S62.30
      base (displaced) S62.31
        nondisplaced S62.34
      neck (displaced) S62.33
        nondisplaced S62.36
      shaft (displaced) S62.32
        nondisplaced S62.35
      specified NEC S62.39
    neck (displaced) S62.33
      nondisplaced S62.36
    Rolando's *-see* Rolando's fracture
    second S62.30
      base (displaced) S62.31
        nondisplaced S62.34
      neck (displaced) S62.33

Fracture, pathological - *continued*
      nondisplaced S62.36
      shaft (displaced) S62.32
        nondisplaced S62.35
      specified NEC S62.39
    shaft (displaced) S62.32
      nondisplaced S62.35
    third S62.30
      base (displaced) S62.31
        nondisplaced S62.34
      neck (displaced) S62.33
        nondisplaced S62.36
      shaft (displaced) S62.32
        nondisplaced S62.35
      specified NEC S62.39
    specified NEC S62.399
  metastatic *-see* Fracture, pathological, due to,
  neoplastic disease *-see also* Neoplasm
  metatarsal bone S92.30
    fifth (displaced) S92.35
      nondisplaced S92.35
    first (displaced) S92.31
      nondisplaced S92.31
    fourth (displaced) S92.34
      nondisplaced S92.34
    physeal S99.10
      Salter-Harris
        Type I S99.11
        Type II S99.12
        Type III S99.13
        Type IV S99.14
      specified NEC S99.19
    second (displaced) S92.32
      nondisplaced S92.32
    third (displaced) S92.33
      nondisplaced S92.33
  Monteggia's *-see* Monteggia's fracture
  multiple
    hand (and wrist) NEC *-see* Fracture, by site
    ribs *-see* Fracture, rib, multiple
  nasal (bone(s)) S02.2
  navicular (scaphoid) (foot) *-see also* Fracture,
    tarsal, navicular
    hand *-see* Fracture, carpal, navicular
  neck S12.9
    cervical vertebra S12.9
      fifth (displaced) S12.400
        nondisplaced S12.401
        specified type NEC (displaced) S12.490
          nondisplaced S12.491
      first (displaced) S12.000
        burst (stable) S12.01
          unstable S12.02
        lateral mass (displaced) S12.040
          nondisplaced S12.041
        nondisplaced S12.001
        posterior arch (displaced) S12.030
          nondisplaced S12.031
        specified type NEC (displaced) S12.090
          nondisplaced S12.091
      fourth (displaced) S12.300
        nondisplaced S12.301
        specified type NEC (displaced) S12.390
          nondisplaced S12.391
      second (displaced) S12.100
        nondisplaced S12.101
        dens (anterior) (displaced) (type II)
        S12.110
          nondisplaced S12.112
          posterior S12.111
        specified type NEC (displaced) S12.120

Fracture, pathological - *continued*
        nondisplaced S12.121
      specified type NEC (displaced) S12.190
        nondisplaced S12.191
      seventh (displaced) S12.600
        nondisplaced S12.601
        specified type NEC (displaced) S12.690
          nondisplaced S12.691
      sixth (displaced) S12.500
        nondisplaced S12.501
        specified type NEC (displaced) S12.590
          nondisplaced S12.591
      third (displaced) S12.200
        nondisplaced S12.201
        specified type NEC (displaced) S12.290
          nondisplaced S12.291
    hyoid bone S12.8
    larynx S12.8
    specified site NEC S12.8
    thyroid cartilage S12.8
    trachea S12.8
  neoplastic NEC *-see* Fracture, pathological,
    due to, neoplastic disease
  neural arch *-see* Fracture, vertebra
  newborn *-see* Birth, injury, fracture
  nontraumatic *-see* Fracture, pathological
  nonunion *-see* Nonunion, fracture
  nose, nasal (bone) (septum) S02.2
  occiput *-see* Fracture, skull, base, occiput
  odontoid process *-see* Fracture, neck, cervical
    vertebra, second
  olecranon (process) (ulna) *-see* Fracture, ulna,
    upper end, olecranon process
  orbit, orbital (bone) (region) S02.8
    floor (blow-out) S02.3
    roof S02.19
  os
    calcis *-see* Fracture, tarsal, calcaneus
    magnum *-see* Fracture, carpal, capitate
    pubis *-see* Fracture, pubis
  palate S02.8
  parietal bone (skull) S02.0
  patella S82.00
    comminuted (displaced) S82.04
      nondisplaced S82.04
    longitudinal (displaced) S82.02
      nondisplaced S82.02
    osteochondral (displaced) S82.01
      nondisplaced S82.01
    specified NEC S82.09
    transverse (displaced) S82.03
      nondisplaced S82.03
  pedicle (of vertebral arch) *-see* Fracture,
    vertebra
  pelvis, pelvic (bone) S32.9
    acetabulum *-see* Fracture, acetabulum
    circle *-see* Disruption, pelvic ring
    following insertion of implant, prosthesis or
      plate M96.65
    ilium *-see* Fracture, ilium
    ischium *-see* Fracture, ischium
    multiple
      with disruption of pelvic ring (circle) *-see*
        Disruption, pelvic ring
      without disruption of pelvic ring (circle)
        S32.82
    pubis *-see* Fracture, pubis
    specified site NEC S32.89
    sacrum *-see* Fracture, sacrum
  periprosthetic, around internal prosthetic joint
    M97.9

Fracture, pathological - *continued*
  ankle M97.2
  elbow M97.4
  finger M97.8
  hip M97.0
  knee M97.1
  shoulder M97.3
  specified joint NEC M97.8
  spine M97.8
  toe M97.8
  wrist M97.8
  phalanx
    foot -*see* Fracture, toe
    hand -*see* Fracture, finger
  pisiform -*see* Fracture, carpal, pisiform
  pond -*see* Fracture, skull
  prosthetic device, internal -*see* Complications, prosthetic device, by site, mechanical
  pubis S32.50
    with disruption of pelvic ring -*see* Disruption, pelvic ring
    specified site NEC S32.59
    superior rim S32.51
  radius S52.9
    distal end -*see* Fracture, radius, lower end
    following insertion of implant, prosthesis or plate M96.63
    head -*see* Fracture, radius, upper end, head
    lower end S52.50
      Barton's -*see* Barton's fracture
      Colles' -*see* Colles' fracture
      extraarticular NEC S52.55
      intraarticular NEC S52.57
      physeal S59.20
        Salter-Harris
          Type I S59.21
          Type II S59.22
          Type III S59.23
          Type IV S59.24
        specified NEC S59.29
      Smith's -*see* Smith's fracture
      specified NEC S52.59
      styloid process (displaced) S52.51
        nondisplaced S52.51
      torus S52.52
    neck -*see* Fracture, radius, upper end
    proximal end -*see* Fracture, radius, upper end
    shaft S52.30
      bent bone S52.38
      comminuted (displaced) S52.35
        nondisplaced S52.35
      Galeazzi's -*see* Galeazzi's fracture
      greenstick S52.31
      oblique (displaced) S52.33
        nondisplaced S52.33
      segmental (displaced) S52.36
        nondisplaced S52.36
      specified NEC S52.39
      spiral (displaced) S52.34
        nondisplaced S52.34
      transverse (displaced) S52.32
        nondisplaced S52.32
    upper end S52.10
      head (displaced) S52.12
        nondisplaced S52.12
      neck (displaced) S52.13
        nondisplaced S52.13
      specified NEC S52.18
      physeal S59.10
        Salter-Harris

Fracture, pathological - *continued*
      Type I S59.11
      Type II S59.12
      Type III S59.13
      Type IV S59.14
     specified NEC S59.19
    torus S52.11
  ramus
    inferior or superior, pubis -*see* Fracture, pubis
    mandible -*see* Fracture, mandible
  restorative material (dental) K08.539
    with loss of material K08.531
    without loss of material K08.530
  rib S22.3
    with flail chest -*see* Flail, chest
    multiple S22.4
      with flail chest -*see* Flail, chest
  root, tooth -*see* Fracture, tooth
  sacrum S32.10
    specified NEC S32.19
    Type
      1 S32.14
      2 S32.15
      3 S32.16
      4 S32.17
    Zone
      I S32.119
        displaced (minimally) S32.111
          severely S32.112
        nondisplaced S32.110
      II S32.129
        displaced (minimally) S32.121
          severely S32.122
        nondisplaced S32.120
      III S32.139
        displaced (minimally) S32.131
          severely S32.132
        nondisplaced S32.130
  scaphoid (hand) -*see also* Fracture, carpal, navicular
    foot -*see* Fracture, tarsal, navicular
  scapula S42.10
    acromial process (displaced) S42.12
      nondisplaced S42.12
    body (displaced) S42.11
      nondisplaced S42.11
    coracoid process (displaced) S42.13
      nondisplaced S42.13
    glenoid cavity (displaced) S42.14
      nondisplaced S42.14
    neck (displaced) S42.15
      nondisplaced S42.15
    specified NEC S42.19
  semilunar bone, wrist -*see* Fracture, carpal, lunate
  sequelae -*see* Sequelae, fracture
  sesamoid bone
    foot S92.81
    hand -*see* Fracture, carpal
    other -*see* Fracture, traumatic, by site
  shepherd's -*see* Fracture, tarsal, talus
  shoulder (girdle) S42.9
    blade -*see* Fracture, scapula
  sinus (ethmoid) (frontal) S02.19
  skull S02.91
    base S02.10
      occiput S02.119
        condyle S02.113
          type I S02.110
            left side S02.11B

Fracture, pathological - *continued*
            right side S02.11A
          type II S02.111
            left side S02.11D
            right side S02.11C
          type III S02.112
            left side S02.11F
            right side S02.11E
          specified NEC S02.118
            left side S02.11H
            right side S02.11G
      specified NEC S02.19
    birth injury P13.0
    frontal bone S02.0
    parietal bone S02.0
    specified site NEC S02.8
    temporal bone S02.19
    vault S02.0
  Smith's -*see* Smith's fracture
  sphenoid (bone) (sinus) S02.19
  spine -*see* Fracture, vertebra
  spinous process -*see* Fracture, vertebra
  spontaneous (cause unknown) -*see* Fracture, pathological
  stave (of thumb) -*see* Fracture, metacarpal, first
  sternum S22.20
    with flail chest -*see* Flail, chest
    body S22.22
    manubrium S22.21
    xiphoid (process) S22.24
  stress M84.30
    ankle M84.37
    carpus M84.34
    clavicle M84.31
    femoral neck M84.359
    femur M84.35
    fibula M84.36
    finger M84.34
    hip M84.359
    humerus M84.32
    ilium M84.350
    ischium M84.350
    metacarpus M84.34
    metatarsus M84.37
    neck -*see* Fracture, fatigue, vertebra
    pelvis M84.350
    radius M84.33
    rib M84.38
    scapula M84.31
    skull M84.38
    tarsus M84.37
    tibia M84.36
    toe M84.37
    ulna M84.33
    vertebra -*see* Fracture, fatigue, vertebra
  supracondylar, elbow -*see* Fracture, humerus, lower end, supracondylar
  symphysis pubis -*see* Fracture, pubis
  talus (ankle bone) -*see* Fracture, tarsal, talus
  tarsal bone(s) S92.20
    astragalus -*see* Fracture, tarsal, talus
    calcaneus S92.00
      anterior process (displaced) S92.02
        nondisplaced S92.02
      body (displaced) S92.01
        nondisplaced S92.01
      extraarticular NEC (displaced) S92.05
        nondisplaced S92.05
      intraarticular (displaced) S92.06
        nondisplaced S92.06

Fracture, pathological - *continued*
  physeal S99.00
    Salter-Harris
      Type I S99.01
      Type II S99.02
      Type III S99.03
      Type IV S99.04
      specified NEC S99.09
    tuberosity (displaced) S92.04
      avulsion (displaced) S92.03
        nondisplaced S92.03
      nondisplaced S92.04
    cuboid (displaced) S92.21
      nondisplaced S92.21
    cuneiform
      intermediate (displaced) S92.23
        nondisplaced S92.23
      lateral (displaced) S92.22
        nondisplaced S92.22
      medial (displaced) S92.24
        nondisplaced S92.24
    navicular (displaced) S92.25
      nondisplaced S92.25
    scaphoid *-see* Fracture, tarsal, navicular
    talus S92.10
      avulsion (displaced) S92.15
        nondisplaced S92.15
      body (displaced) S92.12
        nondisplaced S92.12
      dome (displaced) S92.14
        nondisplaced S92.14
      head (displaced) S92.12
        nondisplaced S92.12
      lateral process (displaced) S92.14
        nondisplaced S92.14
      neck (displaced) S92.11
        nondisplaced S92.11
      posterior process (displaced) S92.13
        nondisplaced S92.13
      specified NEC S92.19
    temporal bone (styloid) S02.19
    thorax (bony) S22.9
      with flail chest *-see* Flail, chest
      rib S22.3
        multiple S22.4
          with flail chest *-see* Flail, chest
      sternum S22.20
        body S22.22
        manubrium S22.21
        xiphoid process S22.24
      vertebra (displaced) S22.009
        burst (stable) S22.001
          unstable S22.002
        eighth S22.069
          burst (stable) S22.061
            unstable S22.062
          specified type NEC S22.068
          wedge compression S22.060
        eleventh S22.089
          burst (stable) S22.081
            unstable S22.082
          specified type NEC S22.088
          wedge compression S22.080
        fifth S22.059
          burst (stable) S22.051
            unstable S22.052
          specified type NEC S22.058
          wedge compression S22.050
        first S22.019
          burst (stable) S22.011
            unstable S22.012

Fracture, pathological - *continued*
        specified type NEC S22.018
        wedge compression S22.010
      fourth S22.049
        burst (stable) S22.041
          unstable S22.042
        specified type NEC S22.048
        wedge compression S22.040
      ninth S22.079
        burst (stable) S22.071
          unstable S22.072
        specified type NEC S22.078
        wedge compression S22.070
      nondisplaced S22.001
      second S22.029
        burst (stable) S22.021
          unstable S22.022
        specified type NEC S22.028
        wedge compression S22.020
      seventh S22.069
        burst (stable) S22.061
          unstable S22.062
        specified type NEC S22.068
        wedge compression S22.060
      sixth S22.059
        burst (stable) S22.051
          unstable S22.052
        specified type NEC S22.058
        wedge compression S22.050
      specified type NEC S22.008
      tenth S22.079
        burst (stable) S22.071
          unstable S22.072
        specified type NEC S22.078
        wedge compression S22.070
      third S22.039
        burst (stable) S22.031
          unstable S22.032
        specified type NEC S22.038
        wedge compression S22.030
      twelfth S22.089
        burst (stable) S22.081
          unstable S22.082
        specified type NEC S22.088
        wedge compression S22.080
      wedge compression S22.000
    thumb S62.50
      distal phalanx (displaced) S62.52
        nondisplaced S62.52
      proximal phalanx (displaced) S62.51
        nondisplaced S62.51
    thyroid cartilage S12.8
    tibia (shaft) S82.20
      comminuted (displaced) S82.25
        nondisplaced S82.25
      condyles *-see* Fracture, tibia, upper end
      distal end *-see* Fracture, tibia, lower end
      epiphysis
        lower *-see* Fracture, tibia, lower end
        upper *-see* Fracture, tibia, upper end
      following insertion of implant, prosthesis or
      plate M96.67
      head (involving knee joint) *-see* Fracture,
      tibia, upper end
      intercondyloid eminence *-see* Fracture, tibia,
      upper end
      involving ankle or malleolus *-see* Fracture,
      ankle, medial malleolus
      lower end S82.30
        physeal S89.10
          Salter-Harris

Fracture, pathological - *continued*
      Type I S89.11
      Type II S89.12
      Type III S89.13
      Type IV S89.14
      specified NEC S89.19
    pilon (displaced) S82.87
      nondisplaced S82.87
    specified NEC S82.39
    torus S82.31
    malleolus *-see* Fracture, ankle, medial
    malleolus
    oblique (displaced) S82.23
      nondisplaced S82.23
    pilon *-see* Fracture, tibia, lower end, pilon
    proximal end *-see* Fracture, tibia, upper end
    segmental (displaced) S82.26
      nondisplaced S82.26
    specified NEC S82.29
    spine *-see* Fracture, upper end, spine
    spiral (displaced) S82.24
      nondisplaced S82.24
    transverse (displaced) S82.22
      nondisplaced S82.22
    tuberosity *-see* Fracture, tibia, upper end,
    tuberosity
    upper end S82.10
      bicondylar (displaced) S82.14
        nondisplaced S82.14
      lateral condyle (displaced) S82.12
        nondisplaced S82.12
      medial condyle (displaced) S82.13
        nondisplaced S82.13
      physeal S89.00
        Salter-Harris
          Type I S89.01
          Type II S89.02
          Type III S89.03
          Type IV S89.04
          specified NEC S89.09
      plateau *-see* Fracture, tibia, upper end,
      bicondylar
      spine (displaced) S82.11
        nondisplaced S82.11
      torus S82.16
      specified NEC S82.19
      tuberosity (displaced) S82.15
        nondisplaced S82.15
    toe S92.91
      great (displaced) S92.40
        distal phalanx (displaced) S92.42
          nondisplaced S92.42
        nondisplaced S92.40
        proximal phalanx (displaced) S92.41
          nondisplaced S92.41
        specified NEC S92.49
      lesser (displaced) S92.50
        distal phalanx (displaced) S92.53
          nondisplaced S92.53
        medial phalanx (displaced) S92.52
          nondisplaced S92.52
        nondisplaced S92.50
        proximal phalanx (displaced) S92.51
          nondisplaced S92.51
        specified NEC S92.59
      physeal
        phalanx S99.20
          Salter-Harris
            Type I S99.21
            Type II S99.22
            Type III S99.23

Fracture, pathological - *continued*
  Type IV S99.24
    specified NEC S99.29
 tooth (root) S02.5
 trachea (cartilage) S12.8
 transverse process -*see* Fracture, vertebra
 trapezium or trapezoid bone -*see* Fracture, carpal
 trimalleolar -*see* Fracture, ankle, trimalleolar
 triquetrum (cuneiform of carpus) -*see* Fracture, carpal, triquetrum
 trochanter -*see* Fracture, femur, trochanteric
 tuberosity (external) -*see* Fracture, traumatic, by site
 ulna (shaft) S52.20
  bent bone S52.28
  coronoid process -*see* Fracture, ulna, upper end, coronoid process
  distal end -*see* Fracture, ulna, lower end
  following insertion of implant, prosthesis or plate M96.63
  head S52.00
  lower end S52.60
    physeal S59.00
    Salter-Harris
      Type I S59.01
      Type II S59.02
      Type III S59.03
      Type IV S59.04
      specified NEC S59.09
    specified NEC S52.69
    styloid process (displaced) S52.61
      nondisplaced S52.61
    torus S52.62
  proximal end -*see* Fracture, ulna, upper end
  shaft S52.20
    comminuted (displaced) S52.25
      nondisplaced S52.25
    greenstick S52.21
    Monteggia's -*see* Monteggia's fracture
    oblique (displaced) S52.23
      nondisplaced S52.23
    segmental (displaced) S52.26
      nondisplaced S52.26
    specified NEC S52.29
    spiral (displaced) S52.24
      nondisplaced S52.24
    transverse (displaced) S52.22
      nondisplaced S52.22
  upper end S52.00
    coronoid process (displaced) S52.04
      nondisplaced S52.04
    olecranon process (displaced) S52.02
      with intraarticular extension S52.03
      nondisplaced S52.02
        with intraarticular extension S52.03
    specified NEC S52.09
    torus S52.01
 unciform -*see* Fracture, carpal, hamate
 vault of skull S02.0
 vertebra, vertebral (arch) (body) (column) (neural arch) (pedicle) (spinous process) (transverse process)
  atlas -*see* Fracture, neck, cervical vertebra, first
  axis -*see* Fracture, neck, cervical vertebra, second
  cervical (teardrop) S12.9
    axis -*see* Fracture, neck, cervical vertebra, second

Fracture, pathological - *continued*
  first (atlas) -*see* Fracture, neck, cervical vertebra, first
  second (axis) -*see* Fracture, neck, cervical vertebra, second
 chronic M84.48
 coccyx S32.2
 dorsal -*see* Fracture, thorax, vertebra
 lumbar S32.009
  burst (stable) S32.001
    unstable S32.002
  fifth S32.059
    burst (stable) S32.051
      unstable S32.052
    specified type NEC S32.058
    wedge compression S32.050
  first S32.019
    burst (stable) S32.011
      unstable S32.012
    specified type NEC S32.018
    wedge compression S32.010
  fourth S32.049
    burst (stable) S32.041
      unstable S32.042
    specified type NEC S32.048
    wedge compression S32.040
  second S32.029
    burst (stable) S32.021
      unstable S32.022
    specified type NEC S32.028
    wedge compression S32.020
  specified type NEC S32.008
  third S32.039
    burst (stable) S32.031
      unstable S32.032
    specified type NEC S32.038
    wedge compression S32.030
  wedge compression S32.000
 metastatic -*see* Collapse, vertebra, in,
 specified disease NEC -*see also* Neoplasm
 newborn (birth injury) P11.5
 sacrum S32.10
  specified NEC S32.19
  Type
    1 S32.14
    2 S32.15
    3 S32.16
    4 S32.17
  Zone
    I S32.119
      displaced (minimally) S32.111
        severely S32.112
      nondisplaced S32.110
    II S32.129
      displaced (minimally) S32.121
        severely S32.122
      nondisplaced S32.120
    III S32.139
      displaced (minimally) S32.131
        severely S32.132
      nondisplaced S32.130
 thoracic -*see* Fracture, thorax, vertebra
 vertex S02.0
 vomer (bone) S02.2
 wrist S62.10
  carpal -*see* Fracture, carpal bone
  navicular (scaphoid) (hand) -*see* Fracture, carpal, navicular
 xiphisternum, xiphoid (process) S22.24
 zygoma S02.402
  left side S02.40F
  right side S02.40E

Fragile, fragility
 autosomal site Q95.5
 bone, congenital (with blue sclera) Q78.0
 capillary (hereditary) D69.8
 hair L67.8
 nails L60.3
 non-sex chromosome site Q95.5
 X chromosome Q99.2
Fragilitas
 crinium L67.8
 ossium (with blue sclerae) (hereditary) Q78.0
 unguium L60.3
  congenital Q84.6
Fragments, cataract (lens), following cataract surgery H59.02
 retained foreign body -*see* Retained, foreign body fragments (type of)
Frailty (frail) R54
 mental R41.81
Frambesia, frambesial (tropica) -*see also* Yaws
 initial lesion or ulcer A66.0
 primary A66.0
Frambeside
 gummatous A66.4
 of early yaws A66.2
Frambesioma A66.1
Franceschetti-Klein (Wildervanck) disease or syndrome Q75.4
Francis' disease -*see* Tularemia
Franklin disease C88.2
Frank's essential thrombocytopenia D69.3
Fraser's syndrome Q87.0
Freckle(s) L81.2
 malignant melanoma in -*see* Melanoma
 melanotic (Hutchinson's) -*see* Melanoma, in situ
 retinal D49.81
Frederickson's hyperlipoproteinemia, type
 I and V E78.3
 IIA E78.00
 IIB and III E78.2
 IV E78.1
Freeman Sheldon syndrome Q87.0
Freezing -*see also* Effect, adverse, cold T69.9
Freiberg's disease (infraction of metatarsal head or osteochondrosis) -*see* Osteochondrosis, juvenile, metatarsus
Frei's disease A55
Fremitus, friction, cardiac R01.2
Frenum, frenulum
 external os Q51.828
 tongue (shortening) (congenital) Q38.1
Frequency micturition (nocturnal) R35.0
 psychogenic F45.8
Frey's syndrome
 auriculotemporal G50.8
 hyperhidrosis L74.52
Friction
 burn -*see* Burn, by site
 fremitus, cardiac R01.2
 precordial R01.2
 sounds, chest R09.89
Friderichsen-Waterhouse syndrome or disease A39.1
Friedländer's B (bacillus) NEC -*see also* condition A49.8
Friedreich's
 ataxia G11.1
 combined systemic disease G11.1
 facial hemihypertrophy Q67.4
 sclerosis (cerebellum) (spinal cord) G11.1

Frigidity F52.22
Fröhlich's syndrome E23.6
Frontal -see also condition
lobe syndrome F07.0
Frostbite (superficial) T33.90
with
partial thickness skin loss -see Frostbite
(superficial), by site
tissue necrosis T34.90
abdominal wall T33.3
with tissue necrosis T34.3
ankle T33.81
with tissue necrosis T34.81
arm T33.4
with tissue necrosis T34.4
finger(s) -see Frostbite, finger
hand -see Frostbite, hand
wrist -see Frostbite, wrist
ear T33.01
with tissue necrosis T34.01
face T33.09
with tissue necrosis T34.09
finger T33.53
with tissue necrosis T34.53
foot T33.82
with tissue necrosis T34.82
hand T33.52
with tissue necrosis T34.52
head T33.09
with tissue necrosis T34.09
ear -see Frostbite, ear
nose -see Frostbite, nose - hip (and thigh)
T33.6
with tissue necrosis T34.6
knee T33.7
with tissue necrosis T34.7
leg T33.9
with tissue necrosis T34.9
ankle -see Frostbite, ankle
foot -see Frostbite, foot
knee -see Frostbite, knee
lower T33.7
with tissue necrosis T34.7
thigh -see Frostbite, hip
toe -see Frostbite, toe
limb
lower T33.99
with tissue necrosis T34.99
upper -see Frostbite, arm
neck T33.1
with tissue necrosis T34.1
nose T33.02
with tissue necrosis T34.02
pelvis T33.3
with tissue necrosis T34.3
specified site NEC T33.99
with tissue necrosis T34.99
thigh -see Frostbite, hip
thorax T33.2
with tissue necrosis T34.2
toes T33.83
with tissue necrosis T34.83
trunk T33.99
with tissue necrosis T34.99
wrist T33.51
with tissue necrosis T34.51
Frotteurism F65.81
Frozen -see also Effect, adverse, cold T69.9
pelvis (female) N94.89
male K66.8
shoulder -see Capsulitis, adhesive

Fructokinase deficiency E74.11
Fructose 1,6
diphosphatase deficiency E74.19
Fructosemia (benign) (essential) E74.12
Fructosuria (benign) (essential) E74.11
Fuchs'
black spot (myopic) H44.2
dystrophy (corneal endothelium) H18.51
heterochromic cyclitis -see Cyclitis, Fuchs'
heterochromic
Fucosidosis E77.1
Fugue R68.89
dissociative F44.1
hysterical (dissociative) F44.1
postictal in epilepsy -see Epilepsy
reaction to exceptional stress (transient) F43.0
Fulminant, fulminating -see condition
Functional -see also condition
bleeding (uterus) N93.8
Functioning, intellectual, borderline R41.83
Fundus -see condition
Fungemia NOS B49
Fungus, fungous
cerebral G93.89
disease NOS B49
infection -see Infection, fungus
Funiculitis (acute) (chronic) (endemic) N49.1
gonococcal (acute) (chronic) A54.23
tuberculous A18.15
Funnel
breast (acquired) M95.4
congenital Q67.6
sequelae (late effect) of rickets E64.3
chest (acquired) M95.4
congenital Q67.6
sequelae (late effect) of rickets E64.3
pelvis (acquired) M95.5
with disproportion (fetopelvic) O33.3
causing obstructed labor O65.3
congenital Q74.2
FUO (fever of unknown origin) R50.9
Furfur L21.0
microsporon B36.0
Furrier's lung J67.8
Furrowed K14.5
nail(s) (transverse) L60.4
congenital Q84.6
tongue K14.5
congenital Q38.3
Furuncle L02.92
abdominal wall L02.221
ankle -see Furuncle, lower limb
anus K61.0
antecubital space -see Furuncle, upper limb
arm -see Furuncle, upper limb
auditory canal, external -see Abscess, ear,
external
auricle (ear) -see Abscess, ear, external
axilla (region) L02.42
back (any part) L02.222
breast N61.1
buttock L02.32
cheek (external) L02.02
chest wall L02.223
chin L02.02
corpus cavernosum N48.21
ear, external -see Abscess, ear, external
external auditory canal -see Abscess, ear,
external
eyelid -see Abscess, eyelid
face L02.02

Furuncle --continued
femoral (region) -see Furuncle, lower limb
finger -see Furuncle, hand
flank L02.221
foot L02.62
forehead L02.02
gluteal (region) L02.32
groin L02.224
hand L02.52
head L02.821
face L02.02
hip -see Furuncle, lower limb
kidney -see Abscess, kidney
knee -see Furuncle, lower limb
labium (majus) (minus) N76.4
lacrimal
gland -see Dacryoadenitis
passages (duct) (sac) -see Inflammation,
lacrimal, passages, acute
leg (any part) -see Furuncle, lower limb
lower limb L02.42
malignant A22.0
mouth K12.2
navel L02.226
neck L02.12
nose J34.0
orbit, orbital -see Abscess, orbit
palmar (space) -see Furuncle, hand
partes posteriores L02.32
pectoral region L02.223
penis N48.21
perineum L02.225
pinna -see Abscess, ear, external
popliteal -see Furuncle, lower limb
prepatellar -see Furuncle, lower limb
scalp L02.821
seminal vesicle N49.0
shoulder -see Furuncle, upper limb
specified site NEC L02.828
submandibular K12.2
temple (region) L02.02
thumb -see Furuncle, hand
toe -see Furuncle, foot
trunk L02.229
abdominal wall L02.221
back L02.222
chest wall L02.223
groin L02.224
perineum L02.225
umbilicus L02.226
umbilicus L02.226
upper limb L02.42
vulva N76.4
Furunculosis -see Furuncle
Fused -see Fusion, fused
Fusion, fused (congenital)
astragaloscaphoid Q74.2
atria Q21.1
auditory canal Q16.1
auricles, heart Q21.1
binocular with defective stereopsis H53.32
bone Q79.8
cervical spine M43.22
choanal Q30.0
commissure, mitral valve Q23.2
cusps, heart valve NEC Q24.8
mitral Q23.2
pulmonary Q22.1
tricuspid Q22.4
ear ossicles Q16.3
fingers Q70.0

Fusion, fused --*continued*
  hymen Q52.3
  joint (acquired) -*see also* Ankylosis
    congenital Q74.8
  kidneys (incomplete) Q63.1
  labium (majus) (minus) Q52.5
  larynx and trachea Q34.8
  limb, congenital Q74.8
    lower Q74.2
    upper Q74.0
  lobes, lung Q33.8
  lumbosacral (acquired) M43.27
    arthrodesis status Z98.1
    congenital Q76.49
    postprocedural status Z98.1
  nares, nose, nasal, nostril(s) Q30.0
  organ or site not listed -*see* Anomaly, by site
  ossicles Q79.9
    auditory Q16.3
  pulmonic cusps Q22.1
  ribs Q76.6
  sacroiliac (joint) (acquired) M43.28
    arthrodesis status Z98.1
    congenital Q74.2
    postprocedural status Z98.1
  spine (acquired) NEC M43.20
    arthrodesis status Z98.1
    cervical region M43.22
    cervicothoracic region M43.23
    congenital Q76.49
    lumbar M43.26
    lumbosacral region M43.27
    occipito-atlanto-axial region M43.21
    postoperative status Z98.1
    sacrococcygeal region M43.28
    thoracic region M43.24
    thoracolumbar region M43.25
  sublingual duct with submaxillary duct at
    opening in mouth Q38.4
  testes Q55.1
  toes Q70.2
  tooth, teeth K00.2
  trachea and esophagus Q39.8
  twins Q89.4
  vagina Q52.4
  ventricles, heart Q21.0
  vertebra (arch) -*see* Fusion, spine
  vulva Q52.5
Fusospirillosis (mouth) (tongue) (tonsil)
  A69.1
Fussy baby R68.12

G

Gain in weight (abnormal) (excessive) -*see
  also* Weight, gain
**Gaisböck's disease (polycythemia
  hypertonica)** D75.1
Gait abnormality R26.9
  ataxic R26.0
  falling R29.6
  hysterical (ataxic) (staggering) F44.4
  paralytic R26.1
  spastic R26.1
  specified type NEC R26.89
  staggering R26.0
  unsteadiness R26.81
  walking difficulty NEC R26.2
Galactocele (breast) N64.89
  puerperal, postpartum O92.79
Galactokinase deficiency E74.29

Galactophoritis N61.0
  gestational, puerperal, postpartum O91.2
Galactorrhea O92.6
  not associated with childbirth N64.3
Galactosemia (classic) (congenital) E74.21
Galactosuria E74.29
Galacturia R82.0
  schistosomiasis (bilharziasis) B65.0
Galeazzi's fracture S52.37
Galen's vein -*see* condition
Galeophobia F40.218
Gall duct -*see* condition
Gallbladder -*see also* condition
  acute K81.0
Gallop rhythm R00.8
**Gallstone (colic) (cystic duct) (gallbladder)
  (impacted) (multiple)** -*see also* Calculus,
  gallbladder
  with
    cholecystitis -*see* Calculus, gallbladder, with
    cholecystitis
  bile duct (common) (hepatic) -*see* Calculus,
    bile duct
  causing intestinal obstruction K56.3
  specified NEC K80.80
    with obstruction K80.81
Gambling Z72.6
  pathological (compulsive) F63.0
**Gammopathy (of undetermined significance
  [MGUS])** D47.2
  associated with lymphoplasmacytic dyscrasia
    D47.2
  monoclonal D47.2
  polyclonal D89.0
Gamna's disease (siderotic splenomegaly)
  D73.1
Gamophobia F40.298
Gampsodactylia (congenital) Q66.7
**Gamstorp's disease (adynamia episodica
  hereditaria)** G72.3
**Gandy Nanta disease (siderotic
  splenomegaly)** D73.1
Gang
  membership offenses Z72.810
Gangliocytoma D36.10
Ganglioglioma -*see* Neoplasm, uncertain
  behavior, by site
**Ganglion (compound) (diffuse) (joint)
  (tendon (sheath))** M67.40
  ankle M67.47
  foot M67.47
  forearm M67.43
  hand M67.44
  lower leg M67.46
  multiple sites M67.49
  of yaws (early) (late) A66.6
  pelvic region M67.45
  periosteal -*see* Periostitis
  shoulder region M67.41
  specified site NEC M67.48
  thigh region M67.45
  tuberculous A18.09
  upper arm M67.42
  wrist M67.43
Ganglioneuroblastoma -*see* Neoplasm, nerve,
  malignant
Ganglioneuroma D36.10
  malignant -*see* Neoplasm, nerve, malignant
Ganglioneuromatosis D36.10
Ganglionitis
  fifth nerve -*see* Neuralgia, trigeminal

Ganglionitis --*continued*
  gasserian (postherpetic) (postzoster) B02.21
  geniculate G51.1
    newborn (birth injury) P11.3
    postherpetic, postzoster B02.21
  herpes zoster B02.21
  postherpetic geniculate B02.21
Gangliosidosis E75.10
  GM1E75.19
  GM2E75.00
    other specified E75.09
    Sandhoff disease E75.01
    Tay Sachs disease E75.02
  GM3E75.19
  mucolipidosis IV E75.11
Gangosa A66.5
**Gangrene, gangrenous (connective tissue)
  (dropsical) (dry) (moist) (skin) (ulcer)** -*see
  also* Necrosis I96
  with diabetes (mellitus) -*see* Diabetes,
    gangrene
  abdomen (wall) I96
  alveolar M27.3
  appendix K35.80
    with
      perforation or rupture K35.2
      peritoneal abscess K35.3
      peritonitis NEC K35.3
        generalized (with perforation or rupture)
          K35.2
        localized (with perforation or rupture)
          K35.3
  arteriosclerotic (general) (senile) -*see*
    Arteriosclerosis, extremities, with, gangrene
  auricle I96
  Bacillus welchii A48.0
  bladder (infectious) -*see* Cystitis, specified
    type NEC
  bowel, cecum, or colon -*see* Gangrene,
    intestine
  Clostridium perfringens or welchii A48.0
  cornea H18.89
  corpora cavernosa N48.29
    noninfective N48.89
  cutaneous, spreading I96
  decubital -*see* Ulcer, pressure, by site
  diabetic (any site) -*see* Diabetes, gangrene
  epidemic -*see* Poisoning, food, noxious, plant
  epididymis (infectional) N45.1
  erysipelas -*see* Erysipelas
  emphysematous -*see* Gangrene, gas
  extremity (lower) (upper) I96
  Fournier N49.3
    female N76.89
  fusospirochetal A69.0
  gallbladder -*see* Cholecystitis, acute
  gas (bacillus) A48.0
    following
      abortion -*see* Abortion by type complicated
        by infection
      ectopic or molar pregnancy O08.0
  glossitis K14.0
  hernia -*see* Hernia, by site, with gangrene
  intestine, intestinal (hemorrhagic) (massive) -
    see also Infarct, intestine K55.069
    with
      mesenteric embolism -*see also* Infarct,
        intestine K55.069
      obstruction -*see* Obstruction, intestine
  laryngitis J04.0
  limb (lower) (upper) I96

Gangrene, gangrenous - *continued*
  lung J85.0
    spirochetal A69.8
  lymphangitis I89.1
  Meleney's (synergistic) -*see* Ulcer, skin
  mesentery -*see also* Infarct, intestine K55.069
    with
      embolism -*see also* Infarct, intestine
        K55.069
      intestinal obstruction -*see* Obstruction,
        intestine
  mouth A69.0
  ovary -*see* Oophoritis
  pancreas -*see* Pancreatitis, acute
  penis N48.29
    noninfective N48.89
  perineum I96
  pharynx -*see also* Pharyngitis
    Vincent's A69.1
  presenile I73.1
  progressive synergistic -*see* Ulcer, skin
  pulmonary J85.0
  pulpal (dental) K04.1
  quinsy J36
  Raynaud's (symmetric gangrene) I73.01
  retropharyngeal J39.2
  scrotum N49.3
    noninfective N50.89
  senile (atherosclerotic) -*see* Arteriosclerosis,
    extremities, with, gangrene
  spermatic cord N49.1
    noninfective N50.89
  spine I96
  spirochetal NEC A69.8
  spreading cutaneous I96
  stomatitis A69.0
  symmetrical I73.01
  testis (infectional) N45.2
    noninfective N44.8
  throat -*see also* Pharyngitis
    diphtheritic A36.0
    Vincent's A69.1
  thyroid (gland) E07.89
  tooth (pulp) K04.1
  tuberculous NEC -*see* Tuberculosis
  tunica vaginalis N49.1
    noninfective N50.89
  umbilicus I96
  uterus -*see* Endometritis
  uvulitis K12.2
  vas deferens N49.1
    noninfective N50.89
  vulva N76.89
Ganister disease J62.8
Ganser's syndrome (hysterical) F44.89
**Gardner-Diamond syndrome
  (autoerythrocyte sensitization)** D69.2
Gargoylism E76.01
**Garré's disease, osteitis (sclerosing),
  osteomyelitis** -*see* Osteomyelitis, specified
  type NEC
Garrod's pad, knuckle M72.1
Gartner's duct
  cyst Q52.4
  persistent Q50.6
Gas R14.3
  asphyxiation, inhalation, poisoning,
    suffocation NEC -*see* Table of Drugs and
    Chemicals
  excessive R14.0
  gangrene A48.0

Gas - *continued*
  following
    abortion -*see* Abortion by type complicated
  by infection
    ectopic or molar pregnancy O08.0
  on stomach R14.0
  pains R14.1
Gastralgia -*see also* Pain, abdominal
Gastrectasis K31.0
  psychogenic F45.8
Gastric -*see* condition
Gastrinoma
  malignant
    pancreas C25.4
    specified site NEC -*see* Neoplasm,
  malignant, by site
    unspecified site C25.4
  specified site -*see* Neoplasm, uncertain
  behavior
  unspecified site D37.9
Gastritis (simple) K29.70
  with bleeding K29.71
  acute (erosive) K29.00
    with bleeding K29.01
  alcoholic K29.20
    with bleeding K29.21
  allergic K29.60
    with bleeding K29.61
  atrophic (chronic) K29.40
    with bleeding K29.41
  chronic (antral) (fundal) K29.50
    with bleeding K29.51
    atrophic K29.40
      with bleeding K29.41
    superficial K29.30
      with bleeding K29.31
  dietary counseling and surveillance Z71.3
  due to diet deficiency E63.9
  eosinophilic K52.81
  giant hypertrophic K29.60
    with bleeding K29.61
  granulomatous K29.60
    with bleeding K29.61
  hypertrophic (mucosa) K29.60
    with bleeding K29.61
  nervous F54
  spastic K29.60
    with bleeding K29.61
  specified NEC K29.60
    with bleeding K29.61
  superficial chronic K29.30
    with bleeding K29.31
  tuberculous A18.83
  viral NEC A08.4
Gastrocarcinoma -*see* Neoplasm, malignant,
  stomach
Gastrocolic -*see* condition
Gastrodisciasis, gastrodiscoidiasis B66.8
Gastroduodenitis K29.90
  with bleeding K29.91
  virus, viral A08.4
    specified type NEC A08.39
Gastrodynia -*see* Pain, abdominal
**Gastroenteritis (acute) (chronic)
  (noninfectious)** -*see also* Enteritis K52.9
  allergic K52.29
    with
      eosinophilic gastritis or gastroenteritis
        K52.81
      food protein-induced enterocolitis
        syndrome K52.21

Gastroenteritis --*continued*
    food protein-induced enteropathy K52.22
  dietetic -*see also* Gastroenteritis, allergic
    K52.29
  drug-induced K52.1
  due to
    Cryptosporidium A07.2
    drugs K52.1
    food poisoning -*see* Intoxication, foodborne
    radiation K52.0
  eosinophilic K52.81
  epidemic (infectious) A09
  food hypersensitivity -*see also*
    Gastroenteritis, allergic K52.29
  infectious -*see* Enteritis, infectious
  influenzal -*see* Influenza, with gastroenteritis
  noninfectious K52.9
    specified NEC K52.89
  Rotaviral A08.0
  Salmonella A02.0
  toxic K52.1
  viral NEC A08.4
    acute infectious A08.39
      type Norwalk A08.11
    infantile (acute) A08.39
    Norwalk agent A08.11
    Rotaviral A08.0
    severe of infants A08.39
    specified type NEC A08.39
Gastroenteropathy -*see also* Gastroenteritis
  K52.9
  acute, due to Norwalk agent A08.11
  acute, due to Norovirus A08.11
  infectious A09
Gastroenteroptosis K63.4
**Gastroesophageal laceration- hemorrhage
  syndrome** K22.6
Gastrointestinal -*see* condition
Gastrojejunal -*see* condition
Gastrojejunitis -*see also* Enteritis K52.9
Gastrojejunocolic -*see* condition
Gastroliths K31.89
Gastromalacia K31.89
Gastroparalysis K31.84
  diabetic -*see* Diabetes, gastroparalysis
Gastroparesis K31.84
  diabetic -*see* Diabetes, by type, with
    gastroparesis
Gastropathy K31.9
  congestive portal K31.89
  erythematous K29.70
  exudative K90.89
  portal hypertensive K31.89
Gastroptosis K31.89
Gastrorrhagia K92.2
  psychogenic F45.8
Gastroschisis (congenital) Q79.3
Gastrospasm (neurogenic) (reflex) K31.89
  neurotic F45.8
  psychogenic F45.8
Gastrostaxis -*see* Gastritis, with bleeding
Gastrostenosis K31.89
Gastrostomy
  attention to Z43.1
  status Z93.1
**Gastrosuccorrhea (continuous)
  (intermittent)** K31.89
  neurotic F45.8
  psychogenic F45.8
Gatophobia F40.218

GHI

Gaucher's disease or splenomegaly (adult) (infantile) E75.22
Gee (Herter)(Thaysen) disease (nontropical sprue) K90.0
Gélineau's syndrome G47.419
with cataplexy G47.411
Gemination, tooth, teeth K00.2
Gemistocytoma
specified site -*see* Neoplasm, malignant, by site
unspecified site C71.9
General, generalized -*see* condition
Genetic
carrier (status)
cystic fibrosis Z14.1
hemophilia A (asymptomatic) Z14.01
symptomatic Z14.02
specified NEC Z14.8
susceptibility to disease NEC Z15.89
malignant neoplasm Z15.09
breast Z15.01
endometrium Z15.04
ovary Z15.02
prostate Z15.03
specified NEC Z15.09
multiple endocrine neoplasia Z15.81
Genital -*see* condition
Genito-anorectal syndrome A55
Genitourinary system -*see* condition
Genu
congenital Q74.1
extrorsum (acquired) -*see also* Deformity, varus, knee
congenital Q74.1
sequelae (late effect) of rickets E64.3
introrsum (acquired) -*see also* Deformity, valgus, knee
congenital Q74.1
sequelae (late effect) of rickets E64.3
rachitic (old) E64.3
recurvatum (acquired) -*see also* Deformity, limb, specified type NEC, lower leg
congenital Q68.2
sequelae (late effect) of rickets E64.3
valgum (acquired) (knock-knee) M21.06
congenital Q74.1
sequelae (late effect) of rickets E64.3
varum (acquired) (bowleg) M21.16
congenital Q74.1
sequelae (late effect) of rickets E64.3
Geographic tongue K14.1
Geophagia -*see* Pica **Geotrichosis** B48.3
stomatitis B48.3
Gephyrophobia F40.242
Gerbode defect Q21.0
GERD (gastroesophageal reflux disease) K21.9
Gerhardt's
disease (erythromelalgia) I73.81
syndrome (vocal cord paralysis) J38.00
bilateral J38.02
unilateral J38.01
German measles -*see also* Rubella
exposure to Z20.4
Germinoblastoma (diffuse) C85.9
follicular C82.9
Germinoma -*see* Neoplasm, malignant, by site
Gerontoxon -*see* Degeneration, cornea, senile
Gerstmann-Sträussler-Scheinker syndrome (GSS) A81.82

Gerstmann's syndrome R48.8
developmental F81.2
Gestation (period) -*see also* Pregnancy
ectopic -*see* Pregnancy, by site
multiple O30.9
greater than quadruplets -*see* Pregnancy, multiple (gestation), specified NEC
specified NEC -*see* Pregnancy, multiple (gestation), specified NEC
Gestational
mammary abscess O91.11
purulent mastitis O91.11
subareolar abscess O91.11
Ghon tubercle, primary infection A15.7
Ghost
teeth K00.4
vessels (cornea) H16.41 **Ghoul hand** A66.3
Gianotti-Crosti disease L44.4
Giant
cell
epulis K06.8
peripheral granuloma K06.8
esophagus, congenital Q39.5
kidney, congenital Q63.3
urticaria T78.3
hereditary D84.1
Giardiasis A07.1
Gibert's disease or pityriasis L42
Giddiness R42
hysterical F44.89
psychogenic F45.8
Gierke's disease (glycogenosis I) E74.01
Gigantism (cerebral) (hypophyseal) (pituitary) E22.0
constitutional E34.4
Gilbert's disease or syndrome E80.4
Gilchrist's disease B40.9
Gilford-Hutchinson disease E34.8
Gilles de la Tourette's disease or syndrome (motor-verbal tic) F95.2
Gingivitis K05.10
acute (catarrhal) K05.00
necrotizing A69.1
nonplaque induced K05.01
plaque induced K05.00
chronic (desquamative) (hyperplastic) (simple marginal) (pregnancy associated) (ulcerative) K05.10
nonplaque induced K05.11
plaque induced K05.10
expulsiva -*see* Periodontitis
necrotizing ulcerative (acute) A69.1
pellagrous E52
acute necrotizing A69.1
Vincent's A69.1
Gingivoglossitis K14.0
Gingivopericementitis -*see* Periodontitis
Gingivosis -*see* Gingivitis, chronic
Gingivostomatitis K05.10
herpesviral B00.2
necrotizing ulcerative (acute) A69.1
Gland, glandular -*see* condition
Glanders A24.0
Glanzmann (Naegeli) disease or thrombasthenia D69.1
Glasgow coma scale
total score
3 8 R40.243
9 12 R40.242
13 15 R40.241

Glass-blower's disease (cataract) -*see* Cataract, specified NEC
Glaucoma H40.9
with
increased episcleral venous pressure H40.81
pseudoexfoliation of lens -*see* Glaucoma, open angle, primary, capsular
absolute H44.51
angle-closure (primary) H40.20
acute (attack) (crisis) H40.21
chronic H40.22
intermittent H40.23
residual stage H40.24
borderline H40.00
capsular (with pseudoexfoliation of lens) -*see* Glaucoma, open angle, primary, capsular
childhood Q15.0
closed angle -*see* Glaucoma, angle-closure
congenital Q15.0
corticosteroid-induced -*see* Glaucoma, secondary, drugs
hypersecretion H40.82
in (due to)
amyloidosis E85.4 [*H42*]
aniridia Q13.1 [*H42*]
concussion of globe -*see* Glaucoma, secondary, trauma
dislocation of lens -*see* Glaucoma, secondary
disorder of lens NEC -*see* Glaucoma, secondary
drugs -*see* Glaucoma, secondary, drugs
endocrine disease NOS E34.9 [*H42*]
eye
inflammation -*see* Glaucoma, secondary, inflammation
trauma -*see* Glaucoma, secondary, trauma
hypermature cataract -*see* Glaucoma, secondary
iridocyclitis -*see* Glaucoma, secondary, inflammation
lens disorder -*see* Glaucoma, secondary, Lowe's syndrome E72.03 [*H42*]
metabolic disease NOS E88.9 [*H42*]
ocular disorders NEC -*see* Glaucoma, secondary
onchocerciasis B73.02
pupillary block -*see* Glaucoma, secondary
retinal vein occlusion -*see* Glaucoma, secondary
Rieger's anomaly Q13.81 [*H42*]
rubeosis of iris -*see* Glaucoma, secondary
tumor of globe -*see* Glaucoma, secondary
infantile Q15.0
low tension -*see* Glaucoma, open angle, primary, low-tension
malignant H40.83
narrow angle -*see* Glaucoma, angle-closure
newborn Q15.0
noncongestive (chronic) -*see* Glaucoma, open angle
nonobstructive -*see* Glaucoma, open angle
obstructive -*see also* Glaucoma, angle-closure
due to lens changes -*see* Glaucoma, secondary
open angle H40.10
primary H40.11
capsular (with pseudoexfoliation of lens) H40.14
low-tension H40.12

Glaucoma- *continued*
   pigmentary H40.13
    residual stage H40.15
  phacolytic *-see* Glaucoma, secondary
  pigmentary *-see* Glaucoma, open angle,
   primary, pigmentary
  postinfectious *-see* Glaucoma, secondary,
  inflammation
  secondary (to) H40.5
   drugs H40.6
   inflammation H40.4
   trauma H40.3
  simple (chronic) H40.11
  simplex H40.11
  specified type NEC H40.89
  suspect H40.00
  syphilitic A52.71
  traumatic *-see also* Glaucoma, secondary,
  trauma
   newborn (birth injury) P15.3
  tuberculous A18.59
Glaucomatous flecks (subcapsular) *-see*
Cataract, complicated
Glazed tongue K14.4
Gleet (gonococcal) A54.01
Glénard's disease K63.4
Glioblastoma (multiforme)
  with sarcomatous component
   specified site *-see* Neoplasm, malignant, by
  site
   unspecified site C71.9
  giant cell
   specified site *-see* Neoplasm, malignant, by
  site
   unspecified site C71.9
  specified site *-see* Neoplasm, malignant, by
  site
  unspecified site C71.9
Glioma (malignant)
  astrocytic
   specified site *-see* Neoplasm, malignant, by
   site
   unspecified site C71.9
  mixed
   specified site *-see* Neoplasm, malignant, by
   site
   unspecified site C71.9
  nose Q30.8
  specified site NEC *-see* Neoplasm, malignant,
  by site
  subependymal D43.2
   specified site *-see* Neoplasm, uncertain
   behavior, by site
   unspecified site D43.2
  unspecified site C71.9
Gliomatosis cerebri C71.0
Glioneuroma *-see* Neoplasm, uncertain
behavior, by site
Gliosarcoma
  specified site *-see* Neoplasm, malignant, by
  site
  unspecified site C71.9
Gliosis (cerebral) G93.89
  spinal G95.89
Glisson's disease *-see* Rickets
Globinuria R82.3
Globus (hystericus) F45.8
Glomangioma D18.00
  intra-abdominal D18.03
  intracranial D18.02
  skin D18.01
  specified site NEC D18.09

Glomangiomyoma D18.00
  intra-abdominal D18.03
  intracranial D18.02
  skin D18.01
  specified site NEC D18.09
Glomangiosarcoma *-see* Neoplasm,
connective tissue, malignant
Glomerular
  disease in syphilis A52.75
  nephritis *-see* Glomerulonephritis
Glomerulitis *-see* Glomerulonephritis
Glomerulonephritis *-see also* Nephritis N05.9
  with
   edema *-see* Nephrosis
   minimal change N05.0
   minor glomerular abnormality N05.0
  acute N00.9
  chronic N03.9
  crescentic (diffuse) NEC *-see also* N00 N07
  with fourth character .7 N05.7
  dense deposit *-see also* N00 N07 with fourth
  character .6 N05.6
  diffuse
   crescentic *-see also* N00 N07 with fourth
  character .7 N05.7
   endocapillary proliferative *-see also* N00
  N07 with fourth character .4 N05.4
   membranous *-see also* N00 N07 with fourth
  character .2 N05.2
   mesangial proliferative *-see also* N00 N07
  with fourth character .3 N05.3
   mesangiocapillary *-see also* N00 N07 with
  fourth character .5 N05.5
   sclerosing N05.8
  endocapillary proliferative (diffuse) NEC *-see*
  also N00 N07 with fourth character .4 N05.4
  extracapillary NEC *-see also* N00 N07 with
  fourth character .7 N05.7
  focal (and segmental) *-see also* N00 N07 with
  fourth character .1 N05.1
  hypocomplementemic *-see*
  Glomerulonephritis, membranoproliferative
  IgA *-see* Nephropathy, IgA
  immune complex (circulating) NEC N05.8
  in (due to)
   amyloidosis E85.4 *[N08]*
   bilharziasis B65.9 *[N08]*
   cryoglobulinemia D89.1 *[N08]*
   defibrination syndrome D65 *[N08]*
   diabetes mellitus *-see* Diabetes,
  glomerulosclerosis
   disseminated intravascular coagulation D65
  [N08]
   Fabry (Anderson) disease E75.21 *[N08]*
   Goodpasture's syndrome M31.0
   hemolytic-uremic syndrome D59.3
   Henoch (Schönlein) purpura D69.0 *[N08]*
   lecithin cholesterol acyltransferase
  deficiency E78.6 *[N08]*
   microscopic polyangiitis M31.7 *[N08]*
   multiple myeloma C90.0 *[N08]*
   Plasmodium malariae B52.0
   schistosomiasis B65.9 *[N08]*
   sepsis A41.9 *[N08]*
    streptococcal A40 *[N08]*
   sickle-cell disorders D57. *[N08]*
   strongyloidiasis B78.9 *[N08]*
   subacute bacterial endocarditis I33.0 *[N08]*
   syphilis (late) congenital A50.59 *[N08]*
   systemic lupus erythematosus M32.14

Glomerulonephritis - *continued*
   thrombotic thrombocytopenic purpura
   M31.1 *[N08]*
   typhoid fever A01.09
   Waldenström macroglobulinemia C88.0
   [N08]
   Wegener's granulomatosis M31.31
  latent or quiescent N03.9
  lobular, lobulonodular *-see*
  Glomerulonephritis, membranoproliferative
  membranoproliferative (diffuse)(type 1 or 3) -
  see also N00 N07 with fourth character .5
  N05.5
   dense deposit (type 2) NEC *-see also* N00
   N07 with fourth character .6 N05.6
  membranous (diffuse) NEC *-see also* N00
  N07 with fourth character .2 N05.2
  mesangial
   IgA/IgG *-see* Nephropathy, IgA
   proliferative (diffuse) NEC *-see also* N00
   N07 with fourth character .3 N05.3
  mesangiocapillary (diffuse) NEC *-see also*
  N00 N07 with fourth character .5 N05.5
  necrotic, necrotizing NEC *-see also* N00 N07
  with fourth character .8 N05.8
  nodular *-see* Glomerulonephritis,
  membranoproliferative
  poststreptococcal NEC N05.9
   acute N00.9
   chronic N03.9
   rapidly progressive N01.9
  proliferative NEC *-see also* N00 N07 with
   fourth character .8 N05.8
   diffuse (lupus) M32.14
  rapidly progressive N01.9
  sclerosing, diffuse N05.8
  specified pathology NEC *-see also* N00 N07
   with fourth character .8 N05.8
  subacute N01.9
Glomerulopathy *-see* Glomerulonephritis
Glomerulosclerosis *-see also* Sclerosis, renal
  intercapillary (nodular) (with diabetes) *-see*
  Diabetes, glomerulosclerosis
  intracapillary *-see* Diabetes,
  glomerulosclerosis
Glossagra K14.6
Glossalgia K14.6
Glossitis (chronic superficial) (gangrenous)
(Moeller's) K14.0
  areata exfoliativa K14.1
  atrophic K14.4
  benign migratory K14.1
  cortical superficial, sclerotic K14.0
  Hunter's D51.0
  interstitial, sclerous K14.0
  median rhomboid K14.2
  pellagrous E52
  superficial, chronic K14.0
Glossocele K14.8
Glossodynia K14.6
  exfoliativa K14.4
Glossoncus K14.8
Glossopathy K14.9
Glossophytia K14.3
Glossoplegia K14.8
Glossoptosis K14.8
Glossopyrosis K14.6
Glossotrichia K14.3
Glossy skin L90.8
Glottis *-see* condition
Glottitis *-see also* Laryngitis J04.0

Glucagonoma
  pancreas
    benign D13.7
    malignant C25.4
    uncertain behavior D37.8
  specified site NEC
    benign -see Neoplasm, benign, by site
    malignant -see Neoplasm, malignant, by site
    uncertain behavior -see Neoplasm, uncertain
    behavior, by site
  unspecified site
    benign D13.7
    malignant C25.4
    uncertain behavior D37.8
Glucoglycinuria E72.51
Glucose-galactose malabsorption E74.39
Glue
  ear -see Otitis, media, nonsuppurative,
  chronic, mucoid
  sniffing (airplane) -see Abuse, drug, inhalant
    dependence -see Dependence, drug, inhalant
Glutaric aciduria E72.3
Glycinemia E72.51
Glycinuria (renal) (with ketosis) E72.09
Glycogen
  infiltration -see Disease, glycogen storage
  storage disease -see Disease, glycogen storage
Glycogenosis (diffuse) (generalized) -see also
  Disease, glycogen storage
  cardiac E74.02 [143]
  diabetic, secondary -see Diabetes,
  glycogenosis, secondary
  pulmonary interstitial J84.842
Glycopenia E16.2
Glycosuria R81
  renal E74.8
Gnathostoma spinigerum (infection)
  (infestation), gnathostomiasis (wandering
  swelling) B83.1
Goiter (plunging) (substernal) E04.9
  with
    hyperthyroidism (recurrent) -see
    Hyperthyroidism, with, goiter
    thyrotoxicosis -see Hyperthyroidism, with,
    goiter
  adenomatous -see Goiter, nodular
  cancerous C73
  congenital (nontoxic) E03.0
    diffuse E03.0
    parenchymatous E03.0
    transitory, with normal functioning P72.0
  cystic E04.2
    due to iodine-deficiency E01.1
  due to
    enzyme defect in synthesis of thyroid
  hormone E07.1
    iodine-deficiency (endemic) E01.2
  dyshormonogenetic (familial) E07.1
  endemic (iodine-deficiency) E01.2
    diffuse E01.0
    multinodular E01.1
  exophthalmic -see Hyperthyroidism, with,
  goiter
  iodine-deficiency (endemic) E01.2
    diffuse E01.0
    multinodular E01.1
    nodular E01.1
  lingual Q89.2
  lymphadenoid E06.3
  malignant C73
  multinodular (cystic) (nontoxic) E04.2

Goiter --continued
  toxic or with hyperthyroidism E05.20
    with thyroid storm E05.21
  neonatal NEC P72.0
  nodular (nontoxic) (due to) E04.9
    with
      hyperthyroidism E05.20
        with thyroid storm E05.21
      thyrotoxicosis E05.20
        with thyroid storm E05.21
    endemic E01.1
    iodine-deficiency E01.1
    sporadic E04.9
    toxic E05.20
      with thyroid storm E05.21
  nontoxic E04.9
    diffuse (colloid) E04.0
    multinodular E04.2
    simple E04.0
    specified NEC E04.8
    uninodular E04.1
  simple E04.0
  toxic -see Hyperthyroidism, with, goiter
  uninodular (nontoxic) E04.1
    toxic or with hyperthyroidism E05.10
      with thyroid storm E05.11
Goiter-deafness syndrome E07.1
Goldberg syndrome Q89.8
Goldberg-Maxwell syndrome E34.51
Goldblatt's hypertension or kidney I70.1
Goldenhar (Gorlin) syndrome Q87.0
Goldflam-Erb disease or syndrome G70.00
  with exacerbation (acute) G70.01
  in crisis G70.01
Goldscheider's disease Q81.8
Goldstein's disease (familial hemorrhagic
  telangiectasia) I78.0
Golfer's elbow -see Epicondylitis, medial
Gonadoblastoma
  specified site -see Neoplasm, uncertain
  behavior, by site
  unspecified site
    female D39.10
    male D40.10
Gonecystitis -see Vesiculitis
Gongylonemiasis B83.8
Goniosynechiae -see Adhesions, iris,
  goniosynechiae
Gonococcemia A54.86
Gonococcus, gonococcal (disease) (infection)
  -see also condition A54.9
  anus A54.6
  bursa, bursitis A54.49
  conjunctiva, conjunctivitis (neonatorum)
  A54.31
  endocardium A54.83
  eye A54.30
    conjunctivitis A54.31
    iridocyclitis A54.32
    keratitis A54.33
    newborn A54.31
    other specified A54.39
  fallopian tubes (acute) (chronic) A54.24
  genitourinary (organ) (system) (tract) (acute)
    lower A54.00
      with abscess (accessory gland)
  (periurethral) A54.1
    upper -see also condition A54.29
  heart A54.83
  iridocyclitis A54.32
  joint A54.42

Gonococcus, gonococcal - *continued*
  lymphatic (gland) (node) A54.89
  meninges, meningitis A54.81
  musculoskeletal A54.40
    arthritis A54.42
    osteomyelitis A54.43
    other specified A54.49
    spondylopathy A54.41
  pelviperitonitis A54.24
  pelvis (acute) (chronic) A54.24
  pharynx A54.5
  proctitis A54.6
  pyosalpinx (acute) (chronic) A54.24
  rectum A54.6
  skin A54.89
  specified site NEC A54.89
  tendon sheath A54.49
  throat A54.5
  urethra (acute) (chronic) A54.01
    with abscess (accessory gland) (periurethral)
    A54.1
  vulva (acute) (chronic) A54.02
Gonocytoma
  specified site -see Neoplasm, uncertain
  behavior, by site
  unspecified site
    female D39.10
    male D40.10
Gonorrhea (acute) (chronic) A54.9
  Bartholin's gland (acute) (chronic) (purulent)
  A54.02
    with abscess (accessory gland) (periurethral)
    A54.1
  bladder A54.01
  cervix A54.03
  conjunctiva, conjunctivitis (neonatorum)
  A54.31
  contact Z20.2
  Cowper's gland (with abscess) A54.1
  exposure to Z20.2
  fallopian tube (acute) (chronic) A54.24
  kidney (acute) (chronic) A54.21
  lower genitourinary tract A54.00
    with abscess (accessory gland) (periurethral)
    A54.1
  ovary (acute) (chronic) A54.24
  pelvis (acute) (chronic) A54.24
    female pelvic inflammatory disease A54.24
  penis A54.09
  prostate (acute) (chronic) A54.22
  seminal vesicle (acute) (chronic) A54.23
  specified site not listed -see also Gonococcus
  A54.89
  spermatic cord (acute) (chronic) A54.23
  urethra A54.01
    with abscess (accessory gland) (periurethral)
    A54.1
  vagina A54.02
  vas deferens (acute) (chronic) A54.23
  vulva A54.02
Goodall's disease A08.19
Goodpasture's syndrome M31.0
Gopalan's syndrome (burning feet) E53.0
Gorlin-Chaudry Moss syndrome Q87.0
Gottron's papules L94.4
Gougerot's syndrome (trisymptomatic)
  L81.7
Gougerot-Blum syndrome (pigmented
  purpuric lichenoid dermatitis) L81.7
Gougerot-Carteaud disease or syndrome
  (confluent reticulate papillomatosis) L83

Gouley's syndrome (constrictive pericarditis) I31.1
Goundou A66.6
Gout, gouty (acute) (attack) (flare) -see also
  Gout, chronic M10.9
  drug-induced M10.20
    ankle M10.27
    elbow M10.22
    foot joint M10.27
    hand joint M10.24
    hip M10.25
    knee M10.26
    multiple site M10.29
    shoulder M10.21
    vertebrae M10.28
    wrist M10.23
  idiopathic M10.00
    ankle M10.07
    elbow M10.02
    foot joint M10.07
    hand joint M10.04
    hip M10.05
    knee M10.06
    multiple site M10.09
    shoulder M10.01
    vertebrae M10.08
    wrist M10.03
  in (due to) renal impairment M10.30
    ankle M10.37
    elbow M10.32
    foot joint M10.37
    hand joint M10.34
    hip M10.35
    knee M10.36
    multiple site M10.39
    shoulder M10.31
    vertebrae M10.38
    wrist M10.33
  lead-induced M10.10
    ankle M10.17
    elbow M10.12
    foot joint M10.17
    hand joint M10.14
    hip M10.15
    knee M10.16
    multiple site M10.19
    shoulder M10.11
    vertebrae M10.18
    wrist M10.13
  primary -see Gout, idiopathic
  saturnine -see Gout, lead-induced - secondary NEC M10.40
    ankle M10.47
    elbow M10.42
    foot joint M10.47
    hand joint M10.44
    hip M10.45
    knee M10.46
    multiple site M10.49
    shoulder M10.41
    vertebrae M10.48
    wrist M10.43
  syphilitic -see also subcategory M14.8 A52.77
  tophi -see Gout, chronic
Gout, chronic -see also Gout, gouty M1A.9
  drug-induced M1A.20
    ankle M1A.27
    elbow M1A.22
    foot joint M1A.27
    hand joint M1A.24

Gout, chronic --continued
    hip M1A.25
    knee M1A.26
    multiple site M1A.29
    shoulder M1A.21
    vertebrae M1A.28
    wrist M1A.23
  idiopathic M1A.00
    ankle M1A.07
    elbow M1A.02
    foot joint M1A.07
    hand joint M1A.04
    hip M1A.05
    knee M1A.06
    multiple site M1A.09
    shoulder M1A.01
    vertebrae M1A.08
    wrist M1A.03
  in (due to) renal impairment M1A.30
    ankle M1A.37
    elbow M1A.32
    foot joint M1A.37
    hand joint M1A.34
    hip M1A.35
    knee M1A.36
    multiple site M1A.39
    shoulder M1A.31
    vertebrae M1A.38
    wrist M1A.33
  lead-induced M1A.10
    ankle M1A.17
    elbow M1A.12
    foot joint M1A.17
    hand joint M1A.14
    hip M1A.15
    knee M1A.16
    multiple site M1A.19
    shoulder M1A.11
    vertebrae M1A.18
    wrist M1A.13
  primary -see Gout, chronic, idiopathic
  saturnine -see Gout, chronic, lead-induced -
  secondary NEC M1A.40
    ankle M1A.47
    elbow M1A.42
    foot joint M1A.47
    hand joint M1A.44
    hip M1A.45
    knee M1A.46
    multiple site M1A.49
    shoulder M1A.41
    vertebrae M1A.48
    wrist M1A.43
  syphilitic -see also subcategory M14.8 A52.77
  tophi M1A.9
Gower's
  muscular dystrophy G71.0
  syndrome (vasovagal attack) R55
Gradenigo's syndrome -see Otitis, media, suppurative, acute
Graefe's disease -see Strabismus, paralytic, ophthalmoplegia, progressive
Graft-versus-host disease D89.813
  acute D89.810
  acute on chronic D89.812
  chronic D89.811
Grainhandler's disease or lung J67.8
Grain mite (itch) B88.0
Grand mal -see Epilepsy, generalized, specified NEC

Grand multipara status only (not pregnant) Z64.1
  pregnant -see Pregnancy, complicated by, grand multiparity
Granite worker's lung J62.8
Granular -see also condition
  inflammation, pharynx J31.2
  kidney (contracting) -see Sclerosis, renal
  liver K74.69
Granulation tissue (abnormal) (excessive) L92.9
  postmastoidectomy cavity -see Complications, postmastoidectomy, granulation
Granulocytopenia (primary) (malignant) -see Agranulocytosis
Granuloma L92.9
  abdomen K66.8
    from residual foreign body L92.3
    pyogenicum L98.0
  actinic L57.5
  annulare (perforating) L92.0
  apical K04.5
  aural -see Otitis, externa, specified NEC
  beryllium (skin) L92.3
  bone
    eosinophilic C96.6
    from residual foreign body -see Osteomyelitis, specified type NEC
    lung C96.6
  brain (any site) G06.0
    schistosomiasis B65.9 [G07]
  canaliculus lacrimalis -see Granuloma, lacrimal
  candidal (cutaneous) B37.2
  cerebral (any site) G06.0
  coccidioidal (primary) (progressive) B38.7
    lung B38.1
    meninges B38.4
  colon K63.89
  conjunctiva H11.22
  dental K04.5
  ear, middle -see Cholesteatoma
  eosinophilic C96.6
    bone C96.6
    lung C96.6
    oral mucosa K13.4
    skin L92.2
  eyelid H01.8
  facial (e) L92.2
  foreign body (in soft tissue) NEC M60.20
    ankle M60.27
    foot M60.27
    forearm M60.23
    hand M60.24
    in operation wound -see Foreign body, accidentally left during a procedure
    lower leg M60.26
    pelvic region M60.25
    shoulder region M60.21
    skin L92.3
    specified site NEC M60.28
    subcutaneous tissue L92.3
    thigh M60.25
    upper arm M60.22
  gangraenescens M31.2
  genito-inguinale A58
  giant cell (central) (reparative) (jaw) M27.1
    gingiva (peripheral) K06.8
  gland (lymph) I88.8
  hepatic NEC K75.3

Granuloma - *continued*
in (due to)
berylliosis J63.2 [*K77*]
sarcoidosis D86.89
Hodgkin C81.9
ileum K63.89
infectious B99.9
specified NEC B99.8
inguinale (Donovan) (venereal) A58
intestine NEC K63.89
intracranial (any site) G06.0
intraspinal (any part) G06.1
iridocyclitis -*see* Iridocyclitis, chronic
jaw (bone) (central) M27.1
reparative giant cell M27.1
kidney -*see also* Infection, kidney N15.8
lacrimal H04.81
larynx J38.7
lethal midline (faciale(e)) M31.2
liver NEC -*see* Granuloma, hepatic
lung (infectious) -*see also* Fibrosis, lung
coccidioidal B38.1
eosinophilic C96.6
Majocchi's B35.8
malignant (facial(e)) M31.2
mandible (central) M27.1
midline (lethal) M31.2
monilial (cutaneous) B37.2
nasal sinus -*see* Sinusitis
operation wound T81.89
foreign body -*see* Foreign body, accidentally
left during a procedure
stitch T81.89
talc -*see* Foreign body, accidentally left
during a procedure
oral mucosa K13.4
orbit, orbital H05.11
paracoccidioidal B41.8
penis, venereal A58
periapical K04.5
peritoneum K66.8
due to ova of helminths NOS -*see also*
Helminthiasis B83.9 [*K67*]
postmastoidectomy cavity -*see*
Complications, postmastoidectomy, recurrent
cholesteatoma
prostate N42.89
pudendi (ulcerating) A58
pulp, internal (tooth) K03.3
pyogenic, pyogenicum (of) (skin) L98.0
gingiva K06.8
maxillary alveolar ridge K04.5
oral mucosa K13.4
rectum K62.89
reticulohistiocytic D76.3
rubrum nasi L74.8
Schistosoma -*see* Schistosomiasis
septic (skin) L98.0
silica (skin) L92.3
sinus (accessory) (infective) (nasal) -*see*
Sinusitis
skin L92.9
from residual foreign body L92.3
pyogenicum L98.0
spine
syphilitic (epidural) A52.19
tuberculous A18.01
stitch (postoperative) T81.89
suppurative (skin) L98.0
swimming pool A31.1
talc -*see also* Granuloma, foreign body

Granuloma - *continued*
in operation wound -*see* Foreign body,
accidentally left during a procedure
telangiectaticum (skin) L98.0
tracheostomy J95.09
trichophyticum B35.8
tropicum A66.4
umbilicus L92.9
urethra N36.8
uveitis -*see* Iridocyclitis, chronic
vagina A58
venereum A58
vocal cord J38.3
Granulomatosis L92.9
lymphoid C83.8
miliary (listerial) A32.89
necrotizing, respiratory M31.30
progressive septic D71
specified NEC L92.8
Wegener's M31.30
with renal involvement M31.31
Granulomatous tissue (abnormal) (excessive)
L92.9
Granulosis rubra nasi L74.8
Graphite fibrosis (of lung) J63.3
Graphospasm F48.8
organic G25.89
Grating scapula M89.8X1
Gravel (urinary) -*see* Calculus, urinary
Graves' disease -*see* Hyperthyroidism, with,
goiter
Gravis -*see* condition
Grawitz tumor C64.
Gray syndrome (newborn) P93.0
Grayness, hair (premature) L67.1
congenital Q84.2
Green sickness D50.8
Greenfield's disease
meaning
concentric sclerosis (encephalitis periaxialis
concentrica) G37.5
metachromatic leukodystrophy E75.25
Greenstick fracture
code as Fracture, by site **Grey syndrome**
(newborn) P93.0
Grief F43.21
prolonged F43.29
reaction -*see also* Disorder, adjustment
F43.20
Griesinger's disease B76.9
Grinder's lung or pneumoconiosis J62.8
Grinding, teeth
psychogenic F45.8
sleep related G47.63
Grip
Dabney's B33.0
devil's B33.0
Grippe, grippal -*see also* Influenza
Balkan A78
summer, of Italy A93.1
Grisel's disease M43.6
Groin -*see* condition
Grooved tongue K14.5
Ground itch B76.9
Grover's disease or syndrome L11.1
Growing pains, children R29.898
Growth (fungoid) (neoplastic) (new) -*see also*
Neoplasm
adenoid (vegetative) J35.8
benign -*see* Neoplasm, benign, by site
malignant -*see* Neoplasm, malignant, by site
rapid, childhood Z00.2
secondary -*see* Neoplasm, secondary, by site

Gruby's disease B35.0
Gubler-Millard paralysis or syndrome G46.3
Guerin-Stern syndrome Q74.3
Guidance, insufficient anterior (occlusal)
M26.54
Guillain-Barré disease or syndrome G61.0
sequelae G65.0
Guinea worms (infection) (infestation) B72
Guinon's disease (motor-verbal tic) F95.2
Gull's disease E03.4
Gum -*see* condition
Gumboil K04.7
with sinus K04.6
Gumma (syphilitic) A52.79
artery A52.09
cerebral A52.04
bone A52.77
of yaws (late) A66.6
brain A52.19
cauda equina A52.19
central nervous system A52.3
ciliary body A52.71
congenital A50.59
eyelid A52.71
heart A52.06
intracranial A52.19
iris A52.71
kidney A52.75
larynx A52.73
leptomeninges A52.19
liver A52.74
meninges A52.19
myocardium A52.06
nasopharynx A52.73
neurosyphilitic A52.3
nose A52.73
orbit A52.71
palate (soft) A52.79
penis A52.76
pericardium A52.06
pharynx A52.73
pituitary A52.79
scrofulous (tuberculous) A18.4
skin A52.79
specified site NEC A52.79
spinal cord A52.19
tongue A52.79
tonsil A52.73
trachea A52.73
tuberculous A18.4
ulcerative due to yaws A66.4
ureter A52.75
yaws A66.4
bone A66.6
Gunn's syndrome Q07.8
Gunshot wound -*see also* Wound, open
fracture
code as Fracture, by site
internal organs -*see* Injury, by site
Gynandrism Q56.0
Gynandroblastoma
specified site -*see* Neoplasm, uncertain
behavior, by site
unspecified site
female D39.10
male D40.10
Gynecological examination (periodic)
(routine) Z01.419
with abnormal findings Z01.411
Gynecomastia N62
Gynephobia F40.291
Gyrate scalp Q82.8

H

H (Hartnup's) disease E72.02
Haas' disease or osteochondrosis (juvenile)
  (head of humerus) -see Osteochondrosis,
  juvenile, humerus
Habit, habituation
  bad sleep Z72.821
  chorea F95.8
  disturbance, child F98.9
  drug -see Dependence, drug
  irregular sleep Z72.821
  laxative F55.2
  spasm -see Tic
  tic -see Tic
Haemophilus (H.) influenzae, as cause of
  disease classified elsewhere B96.3
Haff disease -see Poisoning, mercury
Hageman's factor defect, deficiency or
  disease D68.2
Haglund's disease or osteochondrosis
  (juvenile) (os tibiale externum) -see
  Osteochondrosis, juvenile, tarsus
Hailey Hailey disease Q82.8
Hair -see also condition
  plucking F63.3
    in stereotyped movement disorder F98.4
  tourniquet syndrome -see also Constriction,
    external, by site
      finger S60.44
      penis S30.842
      thumb S60.34
      toe S90.44
Hairball in stomach T18.2
Hair-pulling, pathological (compulsive)
  F63.3
Hairy black tongue K14.3
Half vertebra Q76.49
Halitosis R19.6
Hallerman-Streiff syndrome Q87.0
Hallervorden-Spatz disease G23.0
Hallopeau's acrodermatitis or disease L40.2
Hallucination R44.3
  auditory R44.0
  gustatory R44.2
  olfactory R44.2
  specified NEC R44.2
  tactile R44.2
  visual R44.1
Hallucinosis (chronic) F28
  alcoholic (acute) F10.951
    in
      abuse F10.151
      dependence F10.251
  drug-induced F19.951
    cannabis F12.951
    cocaine F14.951
    hallucinogen F16.151
      in
        abuse F19.151
          cannabis F12.151
          cocaine F14.151
          hallucinogen F16.151
          inhalant F18.151
          opioid F11.151
          sedative, anxiolytic or hypnotic F13.151
          stimulant NEC F15.151
        dependence F19.251
          cannabis F12.251
          hallucinogen F16.251
          inhalant F18.251

Hallucinosis - continued
    cocaine F14.251
    opioid F11.251
    sedative, anxiolytic or hypnotic F13.251
    stimulant NEC F15.251
  inhalant F18.951
  opioid F11.951
  sedative, anxiolytic or hypnotic F13.951
  stimulant NEC F15.951
  organic F06.0
Hallux
  deformity (acquired) NEC M20.5X   limitus
    M20.5X
  malleus (acquired) NEC M20.3
  rigidus (acquired) M20.2
    congenital Q74.2
    sequelae (late effect) of rickets E64.3
  valgus (acquired) M20.1
    congenital Q66.6
  varus (acquired) M20.3
    congenital Q66.3
Halo, visual H53.19
Hamartoma, hamartoblastoma Q85.9
  epithelial (gingival), odontogenic, central or
    peripheral -see Cyst, calcifying odontogenic
Hamartoses Q85.9
Hamman-Rich syndrome J84.114
Hammer toe (acquired) NEC -see also
  Deformity, toe, hammer toe
  congenital Q66.89
  sequelae (late effect) of rickets E64.3
Hand -see condition
Hand-foot syndrome L27.1
Handicap, handicapped
  educational Z55.9
    specified NEC Z55.8
Hand-Schüller-Christian disease or
  syndrome C96.5
Hanging (asphyxia) (strangulation)
  (suffocation) -see Asphyxia, traumatic, due to
  mechanical threat
Hangnail -see also Cellulitis, digit
  with lymphangitis -see Lymphangitis, acute,
  digit
Hangover (alcohol) F10.129
Hanhart's syndrome Q87.0
Hanot-Chauffard (Troisier) syndrome
  E83.19
Hanot's cirrhosis or disease K74.3
Hansen's disease -see Leprosy
Hantaan virus disease (Korean hemorrhagic
  fever) A98.5
Hantavirus disease (with renal
  manifestations) (Dobrava) (Puumala)
  (Seoul) A98.5
  with pulmonary manifestations (Andes)
  (Bayou) (Bermejo) (Black Creek Canal)
  (Choclo) (Juquitiba) (Laguna negra)
  (Lechiguanas) (New York) (Oran) (Sin
  nombre) B33.4
Happy puppet syndrome Q93.5
Harada's disease or syndrome H30.81
Hardening
  artery -see Arteriosclerosis
  brain G93.89
Harelip (complete) (incomplete) -see Cleft,
  lip
Harlequin (newborn) Q80.4
Harley's disease D59.6
Harmful use (of)
  alcohol F10.10

anxiolytics -see Abuse, drug, sedative
cannabinoids -see Abuse, drug, cannabis
cocaine -see Abuse, drug, cocaine
drug -see Abuse, drug
hallucinogens -see Abuse, drug, hallucinogen
hypnotics -see Abuse, drug, sedative
opioids -see Abuse, drug, opioid
PCP (phencyclidine) -see Abuse, drug,
  hallucinogen
sedatives -see Abuse, drug, sedative
stimulants NEC -see Abuse, drug, stimulant
Harris' lines -see Arrest, epiphyseal
Hartnup's disease E72.02
Harvester's lung J67.0
Harvesting ovum for in vitro fertilization
  Z31.83
Hashimoto's disease or thyroiditis E06.3
Hashitoxicosis (transient) E06.3
Hassal-Henle bodies or warts (cornea)
  H18.49
Haut mal -see Epilepsy, generalized, specified
  NEC
Haverhill fever A25.1
Hay fever -see also Fever, hay J30.1
Hayem-Widal syndrome D59.8
Haygarth's nodes M15.8
Haymaker's lung J67.0
Hb (abnormal)
  Bart's disease D56.0
  disease -see Disease, hemoglobin
  trait -see Trait
Head -see condition
Headache R51
  allergic NEC G44.89
  associated with sexual activity G44.82
  chronic daily R51
  cluster G44.009
    chronic G44.029
      intractable G44.021
      not intractable G44.029
    episodic G44.019
      intractable G44.011
      not intractable G44.019
    intractable G44.001
    not intractable G44.009
  cough (primary) G44.83
  daily chronic R51
  drug-induced NEC G44.40
    intractable G44.41
    not intractable G44.40
  exertional (primary) G44.84
  histamine G44.009
    intractable G44.001
    not intractable G44.009
  hypnic G44.81
  lumbar puncture G97.1
  medication overuse G44.40
    intractable G44.41
    not intractable G44.40
  menstrual -see Migraine, menstrual
  migraine (type) -see also Migraine G43.909
  nasal septum R51
  neuralgiform, short lasting unilateral, with
    conjunctival injection and tearing (SUNCT)
    G44.059
      intractable G44.051
      not intractable G44.059
  new daily persistent (NDPH) G44.52
  orgasmic G44.82

Headache --*continued*
  periodic syndromes in adults and children G43.C0
    with refractory migraine G43.C1
    intractable G43.C1
    not intractable G43.C0
    without refractory migraine G43.C0
  postspinal puncture G97.1
  post-traumatic G44.309
    acute G44.319
      intractable G44.311
      not intractable G44.319
    chronic G44.329
      intractable G44.321
      not intractable G44.329
    intractable G44.301
    not intractable G44.309
  pre-menstrual -*see* Migraine, menstrual
  preorgasmic G44.82
  primary
    cough G44.83
    exertional G44.84
    stabbing G44.85
    thunderclap G44.53
  rebound G44.40
    intractable G44.41
    not intractable G44.40
  short lasting unilateral neuralgiform, with conjunctival injection and tearing (SUNCT) G44.059
    intractable G44.051
    not intractable G44.059
  specified syndrome NEC G44.89
  spinal and epidural anesthesia induced T88.59
    in labor and delivery O74.5
    in pregnancy O29.4
    postpartum, puerperal O89.4
  spinal fluid loss (from puncture) G97.1
  stabbing (primary) G44.85
  tension (type) G44.209
    chronic G44.229
      intractable G44.221
      not intractable G44.229
    episodic G44.219
      intractable G44.211
      not intractable G44.219
    intractable G44.201
    not intractable G44.209
  thunderclap (primary) G44.53
  vascular NEC G44.1

Healthy
  infant
    accompanying sick mother Z76.3
    receiving care Z76.2
  person accompanying sick person Z76.3
Hearing examination Z01.10
  with abnormal findings NEC Z01.118
  following failed hearing screening Z01.110
  for hearing conservation and treatment Z01.12
Heart -*see* condition
Heart beat
  abnormality R00.9
    specified NEC R00.8
  awareness R00.2
  rapid R00.0
  slow R00.1
Heartburn R12
  psychogenic F45.8
Heat (effects) T67.9
  apoplexy T67.0

Heat (effects) --*continued*
  burn -*see also* Burn L55.9
  collapse T67.1
  cramps T67.2
  dermatitis or eczema L59.0
  edema T67.7
  erythem*a* - code by site under Burn, first degree
  excessive T67.9
    specified effect NEC T67.8
  exhaustion T67.5
    anhydrotic T67.3
    due to
      salt (and water) depletion T67.4
      water depletion T67.3
        with salt depletion T67.4
  fatigue (transient) T67.6
  fever T67.0
  hyperpyrexia T67.0
  prickly L74.0
  prostration -*see* Heat, exhaustion
  pyrexia T67.0
  rash L74.0
  specified effect NEC T67.8
  stroke T67.0
  sunburn -*see* Sunburn
  syncope T67.1
Heavy for-dates NEC (infant) (4000g to 4499g) P08.1
  exceptionally (4500g or more) P08.0
Hebephrenia, hebephrenic (schizophrenia) F20.1
Heberden's disease or nodes (with arthropathy) M15.1
Hebra's
  pityriasis L26
  prurigo L28.2
Heel -*see* condition Heerfordt's disease D86.89
Hegglin's anomaly or syndrome D72.0
Heilmeyer-Schoner disease D45
Heine-Medin disease A80.9
Heinz body anemia, congenital D58.2
Heliophobia F40.228
Heller's disease or syndrome F84.3
HELLP syndrome (hemolysis, elevated liver enzymes and low platelet count) O14.2
  complicating
    childbirth O14.24
    puerperium O14.25
Helminthiasis -*see also* Infestation, helminth
  Ancylostoma B76.0
  intestinal B82.0
    mixed types (types classifiable to more than one of the titles B65.0 B81.3 and B81.8) B81.4
    specified type NEC B81.8
  mixed types (intestinal) (types classifiable to more than one of the titles B65.0 B81.3 and B81.8) B81.4
  Necator (americanus) B76.1
  specified type NEC B83.8
Heloma L84
Hemangioblastoma -*see* Neoplasm, connective tissue, uncertain behavior
  malignant -*see* Neoplasm, connective tissue, malignant
Hemangioendothelioma -*see also* Neoplasm, uncertain behavior, by site
  benign D18.00
    intra-abdominal D18.03

Hemangioendothelioma --*continued*
    intracranial D18.02
    skin D18.01
    specified site NEC D18.09
  bone (diffuse) -*see* Neoplasm, bone, malignant
  epithelioid -*see also* Neoplasm, uncertain behavior, by site
    malignant -*see* Neoplasm, malignant, by site
  malignant -*see* Neoplasm, connective tissue, malignant
Hemangiofibroma -*see* Neoplasm, benign, by site
Hemangiolipoma -*see* Lipoma
Hemangioma D18.00
  arteriovenous D18.00
    intra-abdominal D18.03
    intracranial D18.02
    skin D18.01
    specified site NEC D18.09
  capillary D18.00
    intra-abdominal D18.03
    intracranial D18.02
    skin D18.01
    specified site NEC D18.09
  cavernous D18.00
    intra-abdominal D18.03
    intracranial D18.02
    skin D18.01
    specified site NEC D18.09
  epithelioid D18.00
    intra-abdominal D18.03
    intracranial D18.02
    skin D18.01
    specified site NEC D18.09
  histiocytoid D18.00
    intra-abdominal D18.03
    intracranial D18.02
    skin D18.01
    specified site NEC D18.09
  infantile D18.00
    intra-abdominal D18.03
    intracranial D18.02
    skin D18.01
    specified site NEC D18.09
  intra-abdominal D18.03
  intracranial D18.02
  intramuscular D18.00
    intra-abdominal D18.03
    intracranial D18.02
    skin D18.01
    specified site NEC D18.09
  intrathoracic structures D18.09
  juvenile D18.00
  malignant -*see* Neoplasm, connective tissue, malignant
  plexiform D18.00
    intra-abdominal D18.03
    intracranial D18.02
    skin D18.01
    specified site NEC D18.09
  racemose D18.00
    intra-abdominal D18.03
    intracranial D18.02
    skin D18.01
    specified site NEC D18.09
  sclerosing -*see* Neoplasm, skin, benign
  simplex D18.00
    intra-abdominal D18.03
    intracranial D18.02
    skin D18.01

Hemangioma - *continued*
  specified site NEC D18.09
  skin D18.01
  specified site NEC D18.09
  venous D18.00
    intra-abdominal D18.03
    intracranial D18.02
    skin D18.01
    specified site NEC D18.09
  verrucous keratotic D18.00
    intra-abdominal D18.03
    intracranial D18.02
    skin D18.01
    specified site NEC D18.09
Hemangiomatosis (systemic) I78.8
  involving single site -*see* Hemangioma
Hemangiopericytoma -*see also* Neoplasm,
  connective tissue, uncertain behavior
  benign -*see* Neoplasm, connective tissue,
  benign
  malignant -*see* Neoplasm, connective tissue,
  malignant
Hemangiosarcoma -*see* Neoplasm, connective
  tissue, malignant
Hemarthrosis (nontraumatic) M25.00
  ankle M25.07
  elbow M25.02
  foot joint M25.07
  hand joint M25.04
  hip M25.05
  in hemophilic arthropathy -*see* Arthropathy,
  hemophilic
  knee M25.06
  shoulder M25.01
  specified joint NEC M25.08
  traumatic -*see* Sprain, by site
  vertebrae M25.08
  wrist M25.03
Hematemesis K92.0
  with ulcer
  code by site under Ulcer, with hemorrhage
  K27.4
  newborn, neonatal P54.0
    due to swallowed maternal blood P78.2
Hematidrosis L74.8
Hematinuria -*see also* Hemoglobinuria
  malarial B50.8
Hematobilia K83.8
Hematocele
  female NEC N94.89
    with ectopic pregnancy O00.90
      with intrauterine pregnancy O00.91
    ovary N83.8
  male N50.1
Hematochezia -*see also* Melena K92.1
Hematochyluria -*see also* Infestation, filarial
  schistosomiasis (bilharziasis) B65.0
**Hematocolpos (with hematometra or
  hematosalpinx)** N89.7
Hematocornea -*see* Pigmentation, cornea,
  stromal
Hematogenous -*see* condition
Hematoma (traumatic) (skin surface intact) -
  see also Contusion
  with
    injury of internal organs -*see* Injury, by site
    open wound -*see* Wound, open
  amputation stump (surgical) (late) T87.89
  aorta, dissecting I71.00
    abdominal I71.02
    thoracic I71.01

Hematoma - *continued*
  thoracoabdominal I71.03
  aortic intramural -*see* Dissection, aorta
  arterial (complicating trauma) -*see* Injury,
  blood vessel, by site
  auricle -*see* Contusion, ear
    nontraumatic -*see* Disorder, pinna,
  hematoma
  birth injury NEC P15.8
  brain (traumatic)
    with
      cerebral laceration or contusion (diffuse) -
      see Injury, intracranial, diffuse
        focal -*see* Injury, intracranial, focal
      cerebellar, traumatic S06.37
    newborn NEC P52.4
      birth injury P10.1
    intracerebral, traumatic -*see* Injury,
  intracranial, intracerebral hemorrhage
    nontraumatic -*see* Hemorrhage, intracranial
    subarachnoid, arachnoid, traumatic -*see*
  Injury, intracranial, subarachnoid hemorrhage
    subdural, traumatic -*see* Injury, intracranial,
  subdural hemorrhage
  breast (nontraumatic) N64.89
  broad ligament (nontraumatic) N83.7
    traumatic S37.892
  cerebellar, traumatic S06.37
  cerebral -*see* Hematoma, brain
  cerebrum S06.36
    left S06.35
    right S06.34
  cesarean delivery wound O90.2
  complicating delivery (perineal) (pelvic)
  (vagina) (vulva) O71.7
  corpus cavernosum (nontraumatic) N48.89
  epididymis (nontraumatic) N50.1
  epidural (traumatic) -*see* Injury, intracranial,
  epidural hemorrhage
    spinal -*see* Injury, spinal cord, by region
  episiotomy O90.2
  face, birth injury P15.4
  genital organ NEC (nontraumatic)
    female (nonobstetric) N94.89
      traumatic S30.202
    male N50.1
      traumatic S30.201
  internal organs -*see* Injury, by site
  intracerebral, traumatic -*see* Injury,
  intracranial, intracerebral hemorrhage
  intraoperative -*see* Complications,
  intraoperative, hemorrhage
  labia (nontraumatic) (nonobstetric) N90.89
  liver (subcapsular) (nontraumatic) K76.89
    birth injury P15.0
  mediastinum -*see* Injury, intrathoracic
  mesosalpinx (nontraumatic) N83.7
    traumatic S37.898
  muscle
  code by site under Contusion
  nontraumatic
    muscle M79.81
    soft tissue M79.81
  obstetrical surgical wound O90.2
  orbit, orbital (nontraumatic) -*see also*
  Hemorrhage, orbit
    traumatic -*see* Contusion, orbit
  pelvis (female) (nontraumatic) (nonobstetric)
  N94.89
    obstetric O71.7
    traumatic -*see* Injury, by site

Hematoma - *continued*
  penis (nontraumatic) N48.89
    birth injury P15.5
  perianal (nontraumatic) K64.5
  perineal S30.23
    complicating delivery O71.7
  perirenal -*see* Injury, kidney
  pinna -*see* Contusion, ear
    nontraumatic -*see* Disorder, pinna,
  hematoma
  placenta O43.89
  postoperative (postprocedural) -*see*
  Complication, postprocedural, hematoma
  retroperitoneal (nontraumatic) K66.1
    traumatic S36.892
  scrotum, superficial S30.22
    birth injury P15.5
  seminal vesicle (nontraumatic) N50.1
    traumatic S37.892
  spermatic cord (traumatic) S37.892
    nontraumatic N50.1
  spinal (cord) (meninges) -*see also* Injury,
  spinal cord, by region
    newborn (birth injury) P11.5
  spleen D73.5
    intraoperative -*see* Complications,
    intraoperative, hemorrhage, spleen
    postprocedural (postoperative) -*see*
    Complications, postprocedural,
    hemorrhage, spleen
  sternocleidomastoid, birth injury P15.2
  sternomastoid, birth injury P15.2
  subarachnoid (traumatic) -*see* Injury,
  intracranial, subarachnoid hemorrhage
    newborn (nontraumatic) P52.5
      due to birth injury P10.3
    nontraumatic -*see* Hemorrhage, intracranial,
  subarachnoid
  subdural (traumatic) -*see* Injury, intracranial,
  subdural hemorrhage
    newborn (localized) P52.8
      birth injury P10.0
    nontraumatic -*see* Hemorrhage, intracranial,
  subdural
  superficial, newborn P54.5
  testis (nontraumatic) N50.1
    birth injury P15.5
  tunica vaginalis (nontraumatic) N50.1
  umbilical cord, complicating delivery O69.5
  uterine ligament (broad) (nontraumatic)
  N83.7
    traumatic S37.892
  vagina (ruptured) (nontraumatic) N89.8
    complicating delivery O71.7
  vas deferens (nontraumatic) N50.1
    traumatic S37.892
  vitreous -*see* Hemorrhage, vitreous
  vulva (nontraumatic) (nonobstetric) N90.89
    complicating delivery O71.7
    newborn (birth injury) P15.5
Hematometra N85.7
  with hematocolpos N89.7
Hematomyelia (central) G95.19
  newborn (birth injury) P11.5
  traumatic T14.8
Hematomyelitis G04.90
Hematoperitoneum -*see* Hemoperitoneum
Hematophobia F40.230
Hematopneumothorax (see Hemothorax)
Hematopoiesis, cyclic D70.4
Hematoporphyria -*see* Porphyria

Hematorachis, hematorrhachis G95.19
  newborn (birth injury) P11.5
Hematosalpinx N83.6
  with
    hematocolpos N89.7
    hematometra N85.7
      with hematocolpos N89.7
  infectional -*see* Salpingitis
Hematospermia R36.1
Hematothorax (see Hemothorax)
Hematuria R31.9
  due to sulphonamide, sulfonamide -*see* Table
    of Drugs and Chemicals, by drug
  benign (familial) (of childhood) -*see also*
    Hematuria, idiopathic
    essential microscopic R31.1
  endemic -*see also* Schistosomiasis B65.0
  gross R31.0
  idiopathic N02.9
    with glomerular lesion
      crescentic (diffuse) glomerulonephritis
        N02.7
      dense deposit disease N02.6
      endocapillary proliferative
        glomerulonephritis N02.4
      focal and segmental hyalinosis or sclerosis
        N02.1
      membranoproliferative (diffuse) N02.5
      membranous (diffuse) N02.2
      mesangial proliferative (diffuse) N02.3
      mesangiocapillary (diffuse) N02.5
      minor abnormality N02.0
      proliferative NEC N02.8
      specified pathology NEC N02.8
  intermittent -*see* Hematuria, idiopathic
  malarial B50.8
  microscopic NEC (with symptoms) R31.29
    asymptomatic R31.21
    benign essential R31.1
  paroxysmal -*see also* Hematuria, idiopathic
    nocturnal D59.5
  persistent -*see* Hematuria, idiopathic
  recurrent -*see* Hematuria, idiopathic
  tropical -*see also* Schistosomiasis B65.0
  tuberculous A18.13
Hemeralopia (day blindness) H53.11
  vitamin A deficiency E50.5
Hemi-akinesia R41.4
Hemianalgesia R20.0
Hemianencephaly Q00.0
Hemianesthesia R20.0
Hemianopia, hemianopsia (heteronymous)
  H53.47
  homonymous H53.46
  syphilitic A52.71
Hemiathetosis R25.8
Hemiatrophy R68.89
  cerebellar G31.9
  face, facial, progressive (Romberg) G51.8
  tongue K14.8
Hemiballism (us) G25.5
Hemicardia Q24.8
Hemicephalus, hemicephaly Q00.0
Hemichorea G25.5
Hemicolitis, left -*see* Colitis, left sided
Hemicrania
  congenital malformation Q00.0
  continua G44.51
  meaning migraine -*see also* Migraine
    G43.909
  paroxysmal G44.039

Hemicrania - *continued*
  chronic G44.049
    intractable G44.041
    not intractable G44.049
  episodic G44.039
    intractable G44.031
    not intractable G44.039
  intractable G44.031
  not intractable G44.039
Hemidystrophy -*see* Hemiatrophy
Hemiectromelia Q73.8
Hemihypalgesia R20.8
Hemihypesthesia R20.1
Hemi-inattention R41.4
Hemimelia Q73.8
  lower limb -*see* Defect, reduction, lower limb,
    specified type NEC
  upper limb -*see* Defect, reduction, upper limb,
    specified type NEC
Hemiparalysis -*see* Hemiplegia
Hemiparesis -*see* Hemiplegia
Hemiparesthesia R20.2
Hemiparkinsonism G20
Hemiplegia G81.9
  alternans facialis G83.89
  ascending NEC G81.90
    spinal G95.89
  congenital (cerebral) G80.8
    spastic G80.2
  embolic (current episode) I63.4
  flaccid G81.0
  following
    cerebrovascular disease I69.959
      cerebral infarction I69.35
      intracerebral hemorrhage I69.15
      nontraumatic intracranial hemorrhage NEC
        I69.25
      specified disease NEC I69.85
      stroke NOS I69.35
      subarachnoid hemorrhage I69.05
  hysterical F44.4
  newborn NEC P91.8
    birth injury P11.9
  spastic G81.1
    congenital G80.2
  thrombotic (current episode) I63.3
Hemisection, spinal cord -*see* Injury, spinal
  cord, by region
Hemispasm (facial) R25.2
Hemisporosis B48.8
Hemitremor R25.1
Hemivertebra Q76.49
  failure of segmentation with scoliosis Q76.3
  fusion with scoliosis Q76.3
Hemochromatosis E83.119
  with refractory anemia D46.1
  due to repeated red blood cell transfusion
    E83.111
  hereditary (primary) E83.110
  primary E83.110
  specified NEC E83.118
Hemoglobin -*see also* condition
  abnormal (disease) -*see* Disease, hemoglobin
  AS genotype D57.3
  Constant Spring D58.2
  E-beta thalassemia D56.5
  fetal, hereditary persistence (HPFH) D56.4
  H Constant Spring D56.0
  low NOS D64.9
  S (Hb S), heterozygous D57.3

Hemoglobinemia D59.9
  due to blood transfusion T80.89
  paroxysmal D59.6
    nocturnal D59.5
Hemoglobinopathy (mixed) D58.2
  with thalassemia D56.8
  sickle-cell D57.1
    with thalassemia D57.40
      with crisis (vasoocclusive pain) D57.419
        with
          acute chest syndrome D57.411
          splenic sequestration D57.412
      without crisis D57.40
Hemoglobinuria R82.3
  with anemia, hemolytic, acquired (chronic)
    NEC D59.6
  cold (agglutinin) (paroxysmal) (with
    Raynaud's syndrome) D59.6
  due to exertion or hemolysis NEC D59.6
  intermittent D59.6
  malarial B50.8
  march D59.6
  nocturnal (paroxysmal) D59.5
  paroxysmal (cold) D59.6
    nocturnal D59.5
Hemolymphangioma D18.1
Hemolysis
  intravascular
    with
      abortion -*see* Abortion, by type,
        complicated by, hemorrhage
      ectopic or molar pregnancy O08.1
      hemorrhage
        antepartum -*see* Hemorrhage, antepartum,
          with coagulation defect
        intrapartum -*see also* Hemorrhage,
          complicating, delivery O67.0
        postpartum O72.3
  neonatal (excessive) P58.9
    specified NEC P58.8
Hemolytic -*see* condition
Hemopericardium I31.2
  following acute myocardial infarction (current
    complication) I23.0
  newborn P54.8
  traumatic -*see* Injury, heart, with
    hemopericardium
Hemoperitoneum K66.1
  infectional K65.9
  traumatic S36.899
    with open wound -*see* Wound, open, with
      penetration into peritoneal cavity
Hemophilia (classical) (familial) (hereditary)
  D66
  A D66
  B D67
  C D68.1
  acquired D68.311
  autoimmune D68.311
  calcipriva -*see also* Defect, coagulation D68.4
  nonfamilial -*see also* Defect, coagulation
    D68.4
  secondary D68.311
  vascular D68.0
Hemophthalmos H44.81
Hemopneumothorax -*see also* Hemothorax -
  traumatic S27.2
Hemoptysis R04.2
  newborn P26.9
  tuberculous -*see* Tuberculosis, pulmonary

Hemorrhage, hemorrhagic (concealed) R58
abdomen R58
accidental antepartum -*see* Hemorrhage, antepartum
acute idiopathic pulmonary, in infants R04.81
adenoid J35.8
adrenal (capsule) (gland) E27.49
  medulla E27.8
  newborn P54.4
after delivery -*see* Hemorrhage, postpartum
alveolar
  lung, newborn P26.8
  process K08.89
alveolus K08.89
amputation stump (surgical) T87.89
anemia (chronic) D50.0
  acute D62
antepartum (with) O46.90
  with coagulation defect O46.00
    afibrinogenemia O46.01
    disseminated intravascular coagulation O46.02
    hypofibrinogenemia O46.01
    specified defect NEC O46.09
  before 20
weeks gestation O20.9
    specified type NEC O20.8
    threatened abortion O20.0
  due to
    abruptio placenta -*see also* Abruptio
placentae O45.9
    leiomyoma, uterus -*see* Hemorrhage,
antepartum, specified cause NEC
      placenta previa O44.1
    specified cause NEC -*see* subcategory
O46.8X
anus (sphincter) K62.5
apoplexy (stroke) -*see* Hemorrhage,
intracranial, intracerebral
arachnoid -*see* Hemorrhage, intracranial,
subarachnoid
artery R58
  brain -*see* Hemorrhage, intracranial,
intracerebral
basilar (ganglion) I61.0
bladder N32.89
bowel K92.2
  newborn P54.3
brain (miliary) (nontraumatic) -*see*
Hemorrhage, intracranial, intracerebral
  due to
    birth injury P10.1
    syphilis A52.05
  epidural or extradural (traumatic) -*see*
Injury, intracranial, epidural hemorrhage
  newborn P52.4
    birth injury P10.1
  subarachnoid -*see* Hemorrhage, intracranial,
subarachnoid
  subdural -*see* Hemorrhage, intracranial,
subdural
brainstem (nontraumatic) I61.3
  traumatic S06.38
breast N64.59
bronchial tube -*see* Hemorrhage, lung
bronchopulmonary -*see* Hemorrhage, lung
bronchus -*see* Hemorrhage, lung
bulbar I61.5
capillary I78.8
  primary D69.8
cecum K92.2

Hemorrhage, hemorrhagic --*continued*
cerebellar, cerebellum (nontraumatic) I61.4
  newborn P52.6
  traumatic S06.37
cerebral, cerebrum -*see also* Hemorrhage,
intracranial, intracerebral
  newborn (anoxic) P52.4
    birth injury P10.1
  lobe I61.1
cerebromeningeal I61.8
cerebrospinal -*see* Hemorrhage, intracranial,
intracerebral
cervix (uteri) (stump) NEC N88.8
chamber, anterior (eye) -*see* Hyphema
childbirth -*see* Hemorrhage, complicating,
delivery   choroid H31.30
  expulsive H31.31
ciliary body -*see* Hyphema
cochlea -*see* subcategory H83.8
colon K92.2
complicating
  abortion -*see* Abortion, by type, complicated
by, hemorrhage
  delivery O67.9
    associated with coagulation defect
(afibrinogenemia) (DIC)
(hyperfibrinolysis) O67.0
    specified cause NEC O67.8
  surgical procedure -*see* Hemorrhage,
intraoperative
conjunctiva H11.3
  newborn P54.8
cord, newborn (stump) P51.9
corpus luteum (ruptured) cyst N83.1
cortical (brain) I61.1
cranial -*see* Hemorrhage, intracranial
cutaneous R23.3
  due to autosensitivity, erythrocyte D69.2
  newborn P54.5
delayed
  following ectopic or molar pregnancy O08.1
  postpartum O72.2
diathesis (familial) D69.9
disease D69.9
  newborn P53
  specified type NEC D69.8
due to or associated with
  afibrinogenemia or other coagulation defect
(conditions in categories D65 D69)
    antepartum -*see* Hemorrhage, antepartum,
with coagulation defect
    intrapartum O67.0
  dental implant M27.61
  device, implant or graft -*see also*
Complications, by site and type, specified
NEC T85.838
    arterial graft NEC T82.838
    breast T85.838
    catheter NEC T85.838
      dialysis (renal) T82.838
        intraperitoneal T85.838
      infusion NEC T82.838
        spinal (epidural) (subdural) T85.830
      urinary (indwelling) T83.83
    electronic (electrode) (pulse generator)
(stimulator)
      bone T84.83
      cardiac T82.837
      nervous system (brain) (peripheral nerve)
(spinal) T85.830
      urinary T83.83

Hemorrhage, hemorrhagic --*continued*
    fixation, internal (orthopedic) NEC T84.83
    gastrointestinal (bile duct) (esophagus)
T85.838
    genital NEC T83.83
    heart NEC T82.837
    joint prosthesis T84.83
    ocular (corneal graft) (orbital implant)
NEC T85.838
    orthopedic NEC T84.83
      bone graft T86.838
    specified NEC T85.838
    urinary NEC T83.83
    vascular NEC T82.838
    ventricular intracranial shunt T85.830
duodenum, duodenal K92.2
  ulcer -*see* Ulcer, duodenum, with
hemorrhage
dura mater -*see* Hemorrhage, intracranial,
subdural
endotracheal -*see* Hemorrhage, lung
epicranial subaponeurotic (massive), birth
injury P12.2
epidural (traumatic) -*see also* Injury,
intracranial, epidural hemorrhage
  nontraumatic I62.1
esophagus K22.8
  varix I85.01
    secondary I85.11
excessive, following ectopic gestation
(subsequent episode) O08.1
extradural (traumatic) -*see* Injury, intracranial,
epidural hemorrhage
  birth injury P10.8
  newborn (anoxic) (nontraumatic) P52.8
  nontraumatic I62.1
eye NEC H57.8
  fundus -*see* Hemorrhage, retina
  lid -*see* Disorder, eyelid, specified type NEC
fallopian tube N83.6
fibrinogenolysis -*see* Fibrinolysis
fibrinolytic (acquired) -*see* Fibrinolysis
from
  ear (nontraumatic) -*see* Otorrhagia
  tracheostomy stoma J95.01
fundus, eye -*see* Hemorrhage, retina
funis -*see* Hemorrhage, umbilicus, cord
gastric -*see* Hemorrhage, stomach
gastroenteric K92.2
  newborn P54.3
gastrointestinal (tract) K92.2
  newborn P54.3
genital organ, male N50.1
genitourinary (tract) NOS R31.9
gingiva K06.8
globe (eye) -*see* Hemophthalmos
graafian follicle cyst (ruptured) N83.0
gum K06.8
heart I51.89
hypopharyngeal (throat) R04.1
intermenstrual (regular) N92.3
  irregular N92.1
internal (organs) NEC R58
  capsule I61.0
  ear -*see* subcategory H83.8
  newborn P54.8
intestine K92.2
  newborn P54.3
intra-abdominal R58
intra-alveolar (lung), newborn P26.8

Hemorrhage, hemorrhagic --*continued*
  intracerebral (nontraumatic) -*see* Hemorrhage,
    intracranial, intracerebral
  intracranial (nontraumatic) I62.9
    birth injury P10.9
    epidural, nontraumatic I62.1
    extradural, nontraumatic I62.1
    newborn P52.9
      specified NEC P52.8
    intracerebral (nontraumatic) (in) I61.9
      brain stem I61.3
      cerebellum I61.4
      newborn P52.4
        birth injury P10.1
      hemisphere I61.2
        cortical (superficial) I61.1
        subcortical (deep) I61.0
      intraoperative
        during a nervous system procedure
          G97.31
        during other procedure G97.32
      intraventricular I61.5
      multiple localized I61.6
      postprocedural
        following a nervous system procedure
          G97.51
        following other procedure G97.52
      specified NEC I61.8
      superficial I61.1
      traumatic (diffuse) -*see* Injury, intracranial,
        diffuse
        focal -*see* Injury, intracranial, focal
    subarachnoid (nontraumatic) (from) I60.9
      newborn P52.5
        birth injury P10.3
      intracranial (cerebral) artery I60.7
        anterior communicating I60.2
        basilar I60.4
        carotid siphon and bifurcation I60.0
        communicating I60.7
          anterior I60.2
          posterior I60.3
        middle cerebral I60.1
        posterior communicating I60.3
        specified artery NEC I60.6
        vertebral I60.5
      specified NEC I60.8
      traumatic S06.6X
    subdural (nontraumatic) I62.00
      acute I62.01
      birth injury P10.0
      chronic I62.03
      newborn (anoxic) (hypoxic) P52.8
        birth injury P10.0
      spinal G95.19
      subacute I62.02
      traumatic -*see* Injury, intracranial, subdural
    hemorrhage
    traumatic -*see* Injury, intracranial, focal
  brain injury
  intramedullary NEC G95.19
  intraocular -*see* Hemophthalmos
  intraoperative, intraprocedural -*see*
    Complication, hemorrhage (hematoma),
    intraoperative (intraprocedural), by site
  intrapartum -*see* Hemorrhage, complicating,
    delivery
  intrapelvic
    female N94.89
    male K66.1
  intraperitoneal K66.1

Hemorrhage, hemorrhagic --*continued*
  intrapontine I61.3
  intraprocedural -*see* Complication,
    hemorrhage (hematoma), intraoperative
    (intraprocedural), by site
  intrauterine N85.7
    complicating delivery -*see also* Hemorrhage,
      complicating, delivery O67.9
    postpartum -*see* Hemorrhage, postpartum
  intraventricular I61.5
    newborn (nontraumatic) -*see also* Newborn,
      affected by, hemorrhage P52.3
      due to birth injury P10.2
      grade
        1 P52.0
        2 P52.1
        3 P52.21
        4 P52.22
  intravesical N32.89
  iris (postinfectional) (postinflammatory)
    (toxic) -*see* Hyphema
  joint (nontraumatic) -*see* Hemarthrosis
  kidney N28.89
  knee (joint) (nontraumatic) -*see* Hemarthrosis,
    knee
  labyrinth -*see* subcategory H83.8
  lenticular striate artery I61.0
  ligature, vessel -*see* Hemorrhage,
    postoperative
  liver K76.89
  lung R04.89
    newborn P26.9
      massive P26.1
      specified NEC P26.8
    tuberculous -*see* Tuberculosis, pulmonary
  massive umbilical, newborn P51.0
  mediastinum -*see* Hemorrhage, lung
  medulla I61.3
  membrane (brain) I60.8
    spinal cord -*see* Hemorrhage, spinal cord
  meninges, meningeal (brain) (middle) I60.8
    spinal cord -*see* Hemorrhage, spinal cord
  mesentery K66.1
  metritis -*see* Endometritis
  mouth K13.79
  mucous membrane NEC R58
    newborn P54.8
  muscle M62.89
  nail (subungual) L60.8
  nasal turbinate R04.0
    newborn P54.8
  navel, newborn P51.9
  newborn P54.9
    specified NEC P54.8
  nipple N64.59
  nose R04.0
    newborn P54.8
  omentum K66.1
  optic nerve (sheath) H47.02
  orbit, orbital H05.23
  ovary NEC N83.8
  oviduct N83.6
  pancreas K86.89
  parathyroid (gland) (spontaneous) E21.4
  parturition -*see* Hemorrhage, complicating,
    delivery penis N48.89
  pericardium, pericarditis I31.2
  peritoneum, peritoneal K66.1
  peritonsillar tissue J35.8
    due to infection J36
  petechial R23.3

Hemorrhage, hemorrhagic --*continued*
  due to autosensitivity, erythrocyte D69.2
  pituitary (gland) E23.6
  pleura -*see* Hemorrhage, lung
  polioencephalitis, superior E51.2
  polymyositis -*see* Polymyositis
  pons, pontine I61.3
  posterior fossa (nontraumatic) I61.8
    newborn P52.6
  postmenopausal N95.0
  postnasal R04.0
  postoperative -*see* Complications,
    postprocedural, hemorrhage, by site
  postpartum NEC (following delivery of
    placenta) O72.1
    delayed or secondary O72.2
    retained placenta O72.0
    third stage O72.0
  pregnancy -*see* Hemorrhage, antepartum
  preretinal -*see* Hemorrhage, retina
  prostate N42.1
  puerperal -*see* Hemorrhage, postpartum
    delayed or secondary O72.2
  pulmonary R04.89
    newborn P26.9
      massive P26.1
      specified NEC P26.8
    tuberculous -*see* Tuberculosis, pulmonary
  purpura (primary) D69.3
  rectum (sphincter) K62.5
    newborn P54.2
  recurring, following initial hemorrhage at
    time of injury T79.2
  renal N28.89
  respiratory passage or tract R04.9
    specified NEC R04.89
  retina, retinal (vessels) H35.6
    diabetic -*see* Diabetes, retinal, hemorrhage
  retroperitoneal R58
  scalp R58
  scrotum N50.1
  secondary (nontraumatic) R58
    following initial hemorrhage at time of
      injury T79.2
  seminal vesicle N50.1
  skin R23.3
    newborn P54.5
  slipped umbilical ligature P51.8
  spermatic cord N50.1
  spinal (cord) G95.19
    newborn (birth injury) P11.5
  spleen D73.5
    intraoperative -*see* Complications,
      intraoperative, hemorrhage, spleen
    postprocedural -*see* Complications,
      postprocedural, hemorrhage, spleen
  stomach K92.2
    newborn P54.3
    ulcer -*see* Ulcer, stomach, with hemorrhage
  subarachnoid (nontraumatic) -*see*
    Hemorrhage, intracranial, subarachnoid
  subconjunctival -*see also* Hemorrhage,
    conjunctiva
    birth injury P15.3
  subcortical (brain) I61.0
  subcutaneous R23.3
  subdiaphragmatic R58
  subdural (acute) (nontraumatic) -*see*
    Hemorrhage, intracranial, subdural
  subependymal
    newborn P52.0

Hemorrhage, hemorrhagic --*continued*
  with intraventricular extension P52.1
    and intracerebral extension P52.22
  subgaleal P12.2
  subhyaloid -*see* Hemorrhage, retina
  subperiosteal -*see* Disorder, bone, specified
    type NEC
  subretinal -*see* Hemorrhage, retina
  subtentorial -*see* Hemorrhage, intracranial,
    subdural
  subungual L60.8
  suprarenal (capsule) (gland) E27.49
    newborn P54.4
  tentorium (traumatic) NEC -*see* Hemorrhage,
    brain
    newborn (birth injury) P10.4
  testis N50.1
  third stage (postpartum) O72.0
  thorax -*see* Hemorrhage, lung
  throat R04.1
  thymus (gland) E32.8
  thyroid (cyst) (gland) E07.89
  tongue K14.8
  tonsil J35.8
  trachea -*see* Hemorrhage, lung
  tracheobronchial R04.89
    newborn P26.0
  traumatic
  code to specific injury
    cerebellar -*see* Hemorrhage, brain
    intracranial -*see* Hemorrhage, brain
    recurring or secondary (following initial
      hemorrhage at time of injury) T79.2
  tuberculous NEC -*see also* Tuberculosis,
    pulmonary A15.0
  tunica vaginalis N50.1
  ulcer
  code by site under Ulcer, with hemorrhage
    K27.4
  umbilicus, umbilical
    cord
      after birth, newborn P51.9
      complicating delivery O69.5
      newborn P51.9
        massive P51.0
        slipped ligature P51.8
      stump P51.9
  urethra (idiopathic) N36.8
  uterus, uterine (abnormal) N93.9
    climacteric N92.4
    complicating delivery -*see* Hemorrhage,
    complicating, delivery
    dysfunctional or functional N93.8
    intermenstrual (regular) N92.3
      irregular N92.1
    postmenopausal N95.0
    postpartum -*see* Hemorrhage, postpartum
    preclimacteric or premenopausal N92.4
    prepubertal N93.8
    pubertal N92.2
  vagina (abnormal) N93.9
    newborn P54.6
  vas deferens N50.1
  vasa previa O69.4
  ventricular I61.5
  vesical N32.89
  viscera NEC R58
    newborn P54.8
  vitreous (humor) (intraocular) H43.1
  vulva N90.89

Hemorrhoids (bleeding) (without mention of degree) K64.9
  1st degree (grade/stage I) (without prolapse
    outside of anal canal) K64.0
  2nd degree (grade/stage II) (that prolapse with
    straining but retract spontaneously) K64.1
  3rd degree (grade/stage III) (that prolapse
    with straining and require manual
    replacement back inside anal canal) K64.2
  4th degree (grade/stage IV) (with prolapsed
    tissue that cannot be manually replaced)
    K64.3
  complicating
    pregnancy O22.4
    puerperium O87.2
  external K64.4
    with
      thrombosis K64.5
  internal (without mention of degree) K64.8
  prolapsed K64.8
  skin tags
    anus K64.4
    residual K64.4
  specified NEC K64.8
  strangulated -*see also* Hemorrhoids, by degree
    K64.8
  thrombosed -*see also* Hemorrhoids, by degree
    K64.5
  ulcerated -*see also* Hemorrhoids, by degree
    K64.8
Hemosalpinx N83.6
  with
    hematocolpos N89.7
    hematometra N85.7
      with hematocolpos N89.7
Hemosiderosis (dietary) E83.19
  pulmonary, idiopathic E83.1 *[J84.03]*
  transfusion T80.89
Hemothorax (bacterial) (nontuberculous)
J94.2
  newborn P54.8
  traumatic S27.1
    with pneumothorax S27.2
  tuberculous NEC A15.6
**Henoch (Schönlein) disease or syndrome
(purpura)** D69.0
Henpue, henpuye A66.6
Hepar lobatum (syphilitic) A52.74
Hepatalgia K76.89
Hepatitis K75.9
  acute B17.9
    with coma K72.01
    with hepatic failure -*see* Failure, hepatic
    alcoholic -*see* Hepatitis, alcoholic
    infectious B17.9
    non-viral K72.0
    viral B17.9
  alcoholic (acute) (chronic) K70.10
    with ascites K70.11
  amebic -*see* Abscess, liver, amebic
  anicteric, (viral) -*see* Hepatitis, viral
  antigen-associated (HAA) -*see* Hepatitis, B
  Australia-antigen (positive) -*see* Hepatitis, B
  autoimmune K75.4
  B B19.10
    with hepatic coma B19.11
    acute B16.9
      with
        delta-agent (coinfection) (without hepatic
        coma) B16.1
          with hepatic coma B16.0

Hepatitis - *continued*
  hepatic coma (without delta-agent
    coinfection) B16.2
  chronic B18.1
    with delta-agent B18.0
  bacterial NEC K75.89
  C (viral) B19.20
    with hepatic coma B19.21
    acute B17.10
      with hepatic coma B17.11
    chronic B18.2
  catarrhal (acute) B15.9
    with hepatic coma B15.0
  cholangiolitic K75.89
  cholestatic K75.89
  chronic K73.9
    active NEC K73.2
    lobular NEC K73.1
    persistent NEC K73.0
    specified NEC K73.8
  cytomegaloviral B25.1
  due to ethanol (acute) (chronic) -*see* Hepatitis,
    alcoholic
  epidemic B15.9
    with hepatic coma B15.0
  fulminant NEC (viral) -*see* Hepatitis, viral
  neonatal giant cell P59.29
  granulomatous NEC K75.3
  herpesviral B00.81
  history of
    B Z86.19
    C Z86.19
  homologous serum -*see* Hepatitis, viral, type
    B
  in (due to)
    mumps B26.81
    toxoplasmosis (acquired) B58.1
      congenital (active) P37.1 *[K77]*
  infectious, infective B15.9
    acute (subacute) B17.9
    chronic B18.9
  inoculation -*see* Hepatitis, viral, type B
  interstitial (chronic) K74.69
  lupoid NEC K75.4
  malignant NEC (with hepatic failure) K72.90
    with coma K72.91
  neonatal (idiopathic) (toxic) P59.29
  newborn P59.29
  postimmunization -*see* Hepatitis, viral, type B
  post-transfusion -*see* Hepatitis, viral, type B
  reactive, nonspecific K75.2
  serum -*see* Hepatitis, viral, type B
  specified type NEC
    with hepatic failure -*see* Failure, hepatic
  syphilitic (late) A52.74
    congenital (early) A50.08 *[K77]*
      late A50.59 *[K77]*
    secondary A51.45
  toxic -*see also* Disease, liver, toxic K71.6
  tuberculous A18.83
  viral, virus B19.9
    with hepatic coma B19.0
    acute B17.9
    chronic B18.9
      specified NEC B18.8
    type
      B B18.1
        with delta-agent B18.0
      C B18.2
    congenital P35.3
    coxsackie B33.8 *[K77]*

Hepatitis - *continued*
  cytomegalic inclusion B25.1
  in remission, any type - code to Hepatitis, chronic, by type
  non-A, non-B B17.8
  specified type NEC (with or without coma) B17.8
  type
    A B15.9
      with hepatic coma B15.0
    B B19.10
      with hepatic coma B19.11
      acute B16.9
        with
          delta-agent (coinfection) (without hepatic coma) B16.1
            with hepatic coma B16.0
          hepatic coma (without delta-agent coinfection) B16.2
      chronic B18.1
        with delta-agent B18.0
    C B19.20
      with hepatic coma B19.21
      acute B17.10
        with hepatic coma B17.11
      chronic B18.2
    E B17.2
    non-A, non-B B17.8
Hepatization lung (acute) -*see* Pneumonia, lobar
Hepatoblastoma C22.2
Hepatocarcinoma C22.0
Hepatocholangiocarcinoma C22.0
Hepatocholangioma, benign D13.4
Hepatocholangitis K75.89
Hepatolenticular degeneration E83.01
Hepatoma (malignant) C22.0
  benign D13.4
  embryonal C22.0
Hepatomegaly -*see also* Hypertrophy, liver
  with splenomegaly R16.2
  congenital Q44.7
  in mononucleosis
    gammaherpesviral B27.09
    infectious specified NEC B27.89
Hepatoptosis K76.89
Hepatorenal syndrome following labor and delivery O90.4
Hepatosis K76.89
Hepatosplenomegaly R16.2
  hyperlipemic (Bürger-Grütz type) E78.3
    [K77]
Hereditary -*see* condition
Heredodegeneration, macular -*see* Dystrophy, retina
Heredopathia atactica polyneuritiformis G60.1
Heredosyphilis -*see* Syphilis, congenital
Herlitz' syndrome Q81.1
Hermansky Pudlak syndrome E70.331
Hermaphrodite, hermaphroditism (true) Q56.0
  46,XX with streak gonads Q99.1
  46,XX/46,XY Q99.0
  46,XY with streak gonads Q99.1
  chimera 46,XX/46,XY Q99.0
Hernia, hernial (acquired) (recurrent) K46.9
  with
    gangrene -*see* Hernia, by site, with, gangrene

Hernia, hernial - *continued*
    incarceration -*see* Hernia, by site, with, obstruction
      irreducible -*see* Hernia, by site, with, obstruction
      obstruction -*see* Hernia, by site, with, obstruction
      strangulation -*see* Hernia, by site, with, obstruction
  abdomen, abdominal K46.9
    with
      gangrene (and obstruction) K46.1
      obstruction K46.0
    femoral -*see* Hernia, femoral
    incisional -*see* Hernia, incisional
    inguinal -*see* Hernia, inguinal
    specified site NEC K45.8
      with
        gangrene (and obstruction) K45.1
        obstruction K45.0
    umbilical -*see* Hernia, umbilical
    wall -*see* Hernia, ventral
  appendix -*see* Hernia, abdomen
  bladder (mucosa) (sphincter)
    congenital (female) (male) Q79.51
    female -*see* Cystocele
    male N32.89
  brain, congenital -*see* Encephalocele
  cartilage, vertebra -*see* Displacement, intervertebral disc - cerebral, congenital -*see also* Encephalocele
    endaural Q01.8
  ciliary body (traumatic) S05.2
  colon -*see* Hernia, abdomen
  Cooper's -*see* Hernia, abdomen, specified site NEC
  crural -*see* Hernia, femoral
  diaphragm, diaphragmatic K44.9
    with
      gangrene (and obstruction) K44.1
      obstruction K44.0
    congenital Q79.0
  direct (inguinal) -*see* Hernia, inguinal
  diverticulum, intestine -*see* Hernia, abdomen
  double (inguinal) -*see* Hernia, inguinal, bilateral
  due to adhesions (with obstruction) K56.5
  epigastric -*see also* Hernia, ventral K43.9
  esophageal hiatus -*see* Hernia, hiatal
  external (inguinal) -*see* Hernia, inguinal
  fallopian tube N83.4
  fascia M62.89
  femoral K41.90
    with
      gangrene (and obstruction) K41.40
        not specified as recurrent K41.40
        recurrent K41.41
      obstruction K41.30
        not specified as recurrent K41.30
        recurrent K41.31
    bilateral K41.20
      with
        gangrene (and obstruction) K41.10
          not specified as recurrent K41.10
          recurrent K41.11
        obstruction K41.00
          not specified as recurrent K41.00
          recurrent K41.01
      not specified as recurrent K41.20
      recurrent K41.21
    unilateral K41.90

Hernia, hernial - *continued*
    with
      gangrene (and obstruction) K41.40
        not specified as recurrent K41.40
        recurrent K41.41
      obstruction K41.30
        not specified as recurrent K41.30
        recurrent K41.31
    not specified as recurrent K41.90
    recurrent K41.91
    not specified as recurrent K41.90
    recurrent K41.91
  foramen magnum G93.5
    congenital Q01.8
  funicular (umbilical) -*see also* Hernia, umbilicus
    spermatic (cord) -*see* Hernia, inguinal
  gastrointestinal tract -*see* Hernia, abdomen
  Hesselbach's -*see* Hernia, femoral, specified site NEC
  hiatal (esophageal) (sliding) K44.9
    with
      gangrene (and obstruction) K44.1
      obstruction K44.0
    congenital Q40.1
  hypogastric -*see* Hernia, ventral
  incarcerated -*see also* Hernia, by site, with obstruction
    with gangrene -*see* Hernia, by site, with gangrene
  incisional K43.2
    with
      gangrene (and obstruction) K43.1
      obstruction K43.0
  indirect (inguinal) -*see* Hernia, inguinal
  inguinal (direct) (external) (funicular) (indirect) (internal) (oblique) (scrotal) (sliding) K40.90
    with
      gangrene (and obstruction) K40.40
        not specified as recurrent K40.40
        recurrent K40.41
      obstruction K40.30
        not specified as recurrent K40.30
        recurrent K40.31
    not specified as recurrent K40.90
    recurrent K40.91
    bilateral K40.20
      with
        gangrene (and obstruction) K40.10
          not specified as recurrent K40.10
          recurrent K40.11
        obstruction K40.00
          not specified as recurrent K40.00
          recurrent K40.01
      not specified as recurrent K40.20
      recurrent K40.21
    unilateral K40.90
      with
        gangrene (and obstruction) K40.40
          not specified as recurrent K40.40
          recurrent K40.41
        obstruction K40.30
          not specified as recurrent K40.30
          recurrent K40.31
      not specified as recurrent K40.90
      recurrent K40.91
  internal -*see also* Hernia, abdomen
  inguinal -*see* Hernia, inguinal
  interstitial -*see* Hernia, abdomen

Hernia, hernial - *continued*
intervertebral cartilage or disc -*see*
  Displacement, intervertebral disc - intestine,
  intestinal -*see* Hernia, by site
intra-abdominal -*see* Hernia, abdomen
iris (traumatic) S05.2
irreducible -*see also* Hernia, by site, with
  obstruction
    with gangrene -*see* Hernia, by site, with
    gangrene
ischiatic -*see* Hernia, abdomen, specified site
  NEC
ischiorectal -*see* Hernia, abdomen, specified
  site NEC
lens (traumatic) S05.2
linea (alba) (semilunaris) -*see* Hernia, ventral
Littre's -*see* Hernia, abdomen
lumbar -*see* Hernia, abdomen, specified site
  NEC
lung (subcutaneous) J98.4
mediastinum J98.59
mesenteric (internal) -*see* Hernia, abdomen
midline -*see* Hernia, ventral
muscle (sheath) M62.89
nucleus pulposus -*see* Displacement,
  intervertebral disc - oblique (inguinal) -*see*
  Hernia, inguinal
obstructive -*see also* Hernia, by site, with
  obstruction
    with gangrene -*see* Hernia, by site, with
    gangrene
obturator -*see* Hernia, abdomen, specified site
  NEC
omental -*see* Hernia, abdomen
ovary N83.4
oviduct N83.4
paraesophageal -*see also* Hernia, diaphragm
  congenital Q40.1
parastomal K43.5
  with
    gangrene (and obstruction) K43.4
    obstruction K43.3
paraumbilical -*see* Hernia, umbilicus
perineal -*see* Hernia, abdomen, specified site
  NEC
Petit's -*see* Hernia, abdomen, specified site
  NEC
postoperative -*see* Hernia, incisional
pregnant uterus -*see* Abnormal, uterus in
  pregnancy or childbirth
prevesical N32.89
properitoneal -*see* Hernia, abdomen, specified
  site NEC
pudendal -*see* Hernia, abdomen, specified site
  NEC
rectovaginal N81.6
retroperitoneal -*see* Hernia, abdomen,
  specified site NEC
Richter's -*see* Hernia, abdomen, with
  obstruction
Rieux's, Riex's -*see* Hernia, abdomen,
  specified site NEC
sac condition (adhesion) (dropsy)
  (inflammation) (laceration) (suppuration)
code by site under Hernia
sciatic -*see* Hernia, abdomen, specified site
  NEC
scrotum, scrotal -*see* Hernia, inguinal
sliding (inguinal) -*see also* Hernia, inguinal
  hiatus -*see* Hernia, hiatal
spigelian -*see* Hernia, ventral

Hernia, hernial - *continued*
spinal -*see* Spina bifida
strangulated -*see also* Hernia, by site, with
  obstruction
    with gangrene -*see* Hernia, by site, with
    gangrene
subxiphoid -*see* Hernia, ventral
supra-umbilicus -*see* Hernia, ventral
tendon -*see* Disorder, tendon, specified type
  NEC
Treitz's (fossa) -*see* Hernia, abdomen,
  specified site NEC
tunica vaginalis Q55.29
umbilicus, umbilical K42.9
  with
    gangrene (and obstruction) K42.1
    obstruction K42.0
ureter N28.89
urethra, congenital Q64.79
urinary meatus, congenital Q64.79
uterus N81.4
  pregnant -*see* Abnormal, uterus in
  pregnancy or childbirth
vaginal (anterior) (wall) -*see* Cystocele
Velpeau's -*see* Hernia, femoral
ventral K43.9
  with
    gangrene (and obstruction) K43.7
    obstruction K43.6
  recurrent -*see* Hernia, incisional
  incisional K43.2
    with
      gangrene (and obstruction) K43.1
      obstruction K43.0
  specified NEC K43.9
    with
      gangrene (and obstruction) K43.7
      obstruction K43.6
vesical
  congenital (female) (male) Q79.51
  female -*see* Cystocele
  male N32.89
vitreous (into wound) S05.2
  into anterior chamber -*see* Prolapse, vitreous
Herniation -*see also* Hernia
brain (stem) G93.5
cerebral G93.5
mediastinum J98.59
nucleus pulposus -*see* Displacement,
intervertebral disc
Herpangina B08.5
Herpes, herpesvirus, herpetic B00.9
anogenital A60.9
  perianal skin A60.1
  rectum A60.1
  urogenital tract A60.00
    cervix A60.03
    male genital organ NEC A60.02
    penis A60.01
    specified site NEC A60.09
    vagina A60.04
    vulva A60.04
blepharitis (zoster) B02.39
  simplex B00.59
circinatus B35.4
  bullosus L12.0
conjunctivitis (simplex) B00.53
  zoster B02.31
cornea B02.33
encephalitis B00.4
  due to herpesvirus 6 B10.01

Herpes, herpesvirus, herpetic --*continued*
due to herpesvirus 7 B10.09
  specified NEC B10.09
eye (zoster) B02.30
  simplex B00.50
eyelid (zoster) B02.39
  simplex B00.59
facialis B00.1
febrilis B00.1
geniculate ganglionitis B02.21
genital, genitalis A60.00
  female A60.09
  male A60.02
gestational, gestationis O26.4
gingivostomatitis B00.2
human B00.9
  1 -*see* Herpes, simplex
  2 -*see* Herpes, simplex
  3 -*see* Varicella
  4 -*see* Mononucleosis, Epstein-Barr (virus)
  5 -*see* Disease, cytomegalic inclusion
    (generalized)
  6
    encephalitis B10.01
    specified NEC B10.81
  7
    encephalitis B10.09
    specified NEC B10.82
  8 B10.89
infection NEC B10.89
  Kaposi's sarcoma associated B10.89
iridocyclitis (simplex) B00.51
  zoster B02.32
iris (vesicular erythema multiforme) L51.9
iritis (simplex) B00.51
  Kaposi's sarcoma associated B10.89
keratitis (simplex) (dendritic) (disciform)
  (interstitial) B00.52
  zoster (interstitial) B02.33
keratoconjunctivitis (simplex) B00.52
  zoster B02.33
labialis B00.1
lip B00.1
meningitis (simplex) B00.3
  zoster B02.1
ophthalmicus (zoster) NEC B02.30
  simplex B00.50
penis A60.01
perianal skin A60.1
pharyngitis, pharyngotonsillitis B00.2
rectum A60.1
scrotum A60.02
sepsis B00.7
simplex B00.9
  complicated NEC B00.89
  congenital P35.2
  conjunctivitis B00.53
  external ear B00.1
  eyelid B00.59
  hepatitis B00.81
  keratitis (interstitial) B00.52
  myelitis B00.82
  specified complication NEC B00.89
  visceral B00.89
stomatitis B00.2
tonsurans B35.0
visceral B00.89
vulva A60.04
whitlow B00.89
zoster -*see also* condition B02.9
  auricularis B02.21

Herpes, herpesvirus, herpetic *--continued*
  complicated NEC B02.8
  conjunctivitis B02.31
  disseminated B02.7
  encephalitis B02.0
  eye (lid) B02.39
  geniculate ganglionitis B02.21
  keratitis (interstitial) B02.33
  meningitis B02.1
  myelitis B02.24
  neuritis, neuralgia B02.29
  ophthalmicus NEC B02.30
  oticus B02.21
  polyneuropathy B02.23
  specified complication NEC B02.8
  trigeminal neuralgia B02.22
Herpesvirus (human) *-see* Herpes
Herpetophobia F40.218
Herrick's anemia *-see* Disease, sickle-cell
Hers' disease E74.09
Herter-Gee syndrome K90.0
Herxheimer's reaction R68.89
Hesitancy
  of micturition R39.11
  urinary R39.11
Hesselbach's hernia *-see* Hernia, femoral, specified site NEC
Heterochromia (congenital) Q13.2
  cataract *-see* Cataract, complicated
  cyclitis (Fuchs) *-see* Cyclitis, Fuchs' heterochromic
  hair L67.1
  iritis *-see* Cyclitis, Fuchs' heterochromic
  retained metallic foreign body (nonmagnetic) *-see* Foreign body, intraocular, old, retained
    magnetic *-see* Foreign body, intraocular, old, retained, magnetic
  uveitis *-see* Cyclitis, Fuchs' heterochromic
Heterophoria *-see* Strabismus, heterophoria
Heterophyes, heterophyiasis (small intestine) B66.8
Heterotopia, heterotopic *-see also* Malposition, congenital
  cerebralis Q04.8
Heterotropia *-see* Strabismus
Heubner-Herter disease K90.0
Hexadactylism Q69.9
HGSIL (cytology finding) (high grade squamous intraepithelial lesion on cytologic smear) (Pap smear finding)
  anus R85.613
  cervix R87.613
    biopsy (histology) finding *-see* Neoplasia, intraepithelial, cervix, grade II or grade III
  vagina R87.623
    biopsy (histology) finding *-see* Neoplasia, intraepithelial, vagina, grade II or grade III
Hibernoma *-see* Lipoma
Hiccup, hiccough R06.6
  epidemic B33.0
  psychogenic F45.8
Hidden penis (congenital) Q55.64
  acquired N48.83
Hidradenitis (axillaris) (suppurative) L73.2
Hidradenoma (nodular) *-see also* Neoplasm, skin, benign
  clear cell *-see* Neoplasm, skin, benign
  papillary *-see* Neoplasm, skin, benign
Hidrocystoma *-see* Neoplasm, skin, benign

High
  altitude effects T70.20
    anoxia T70.29
    on
      ears T70.0
      sinuses T70.1
    polycythemia D75.1
  arch
    foot Q66.7
    palate, congenital Q38.5
  arterial tension *-see* Hypertension
  basal metabolic rate R94.8
  blood pressure *-see also* Hypertension
    borderline R03.0
    reading (incidental) (isolated) (nonspecific), without diagnosis of hypertension R03.0
  cholesterol E78.00
    with high triglycerides E78.2
  diaphragm (congenital) Q79.1
  expressed emotional level within family Z63.8
  head at term O32.4
  palate, congenital Q38.5
  risk
    infant NEC Z76.2
    sexual behavior (heterosexual) Z72.51
      bisexual Z72.53
      homosexual Z72.52
  temperature (of unknown origin) R50.9
  thoracic rib Q76.6
  triglycerides E78.1
    with high cholesterol E78.2
Hildebrand's disease A75.0
Hilum *-see* condition
Hip *-see* condition
Hippel's disease Q85.8
Hippophobia F40.218
Hippus H57.09
Hirschsprung's disease or megacolon Q43.1
Hirsutism, hirsuties L68.0
Hirudiniasis
  external B88.3
  internal B83.4
Hiss-Russell dysentery A03.1
Histidinemia, histidinuria E70.41
Histiocytoma *-see also* Neoplasm, skin, benign
  fibrous *-see also* Neoplasm, skin, benign
    atypical *-see* Neoplasm, connective tissue, uncertain behavior
    malignant *-see* Neoplasm, connective tissue, malignant
Histiocytosis D76.3
  acute differentiated progressive C96.0
  Langerhans' cell NEC C96.6
    multifocal X
      multisystemic (disseminated) C96.0
      unisystemic C96.5
    pulmonary, adult (adult PLCH) J84.82
    unifocal (X) C96.6
  lipid, lipoid D76.3
    essential E75.29
  malignant C96.A
  mononuclear phagocytes NEC D76.1
    Langerhans' cells C96.6
  non-Langerhans cell D76.3
  polyostotic sclerosing D76.3
  sinus, with massive lymphadenopathy D76.3
  syndrome NEC D76.3
  X NEC C96.6
    acute (progressive) C96.0
    chronic C96.6

Histiocytosis - *continued*
  multifocal C96.5
  multisystemic C96.0
  unifocal C96.6
Histoplasmosis B39.9
  with pneumonia NEC B39.2
  African B39.5
  American *-see* Histoplasmosis, capsulati
  capsulati B39.4
    disseminated B39.3
    generalized B39.3
    pulmonary B39.2
      acute B39.0
      chronic B39.1
  Darling's B39.4
  duboisii B39.5
  lung NEC B39.2
History
  family (of) *-see also* History, personal (of)
    alcohol abuse Z81.1
    allergy NEC Z84.89
    anemia Z83.2
    arthritis Z82.61
    asthma Z82.5
    blindness Z82.1
    cardiac death (sudden) Z82.41
    carrier of genetic disease Z84.81
    chromosomal anomaly Z82.79
    chronic
      disabling disease NEC Z82.8
      lower respiratory disease Z82.5
    colonic polyps Z83.71
    congenital malformations and deformations Z82.79
      polycystic kidney Z82.71
    consanguinity Z84.3
    deafness Z82.2
    diabetes mellitus Z83.3
    disability NEC Z82.8
    disease or disorder (of)
      allergic NEC Z84.89
      behavioral NEC Z81.8
      blood and blood-forming organs Z83.2
      cardiovascular NEC Z82.49
      chronic disabling NEC Z82.8
      digestive Z83.79
      ear NEC Z83.52
      endocrine NEC Z83.49
      eye NEC Z83.518
        glaucoma Z83.511
      familial hypercholesterolemia Z83.42
      genitourinary NEC Z84.2
      glaucoma Z83.511
      hematological Z83.2
      immune mechanism Z83.2
      infectious NEC Z83.1
      ischemic heart Z82.49
      kidney Z84.1
      mental NEC Z81.8
      metabolic Z83.49
      musculoskeletal NEC Z82.69
      neurological NEC Z82.0
      nutritional Z83.49
      parasitic NEC Z83.1
      psychiatric NEC Z81.8
      respiratory NEC Z83.6
      skin and subcutaneous tissue NEC Z84.0
      specified NEC Z84.89
    drug abuse NEC Z81.3
    epilepsy Z82.0
    familial hypercholesterolemia Z83.42

History --*continued*

genetic disease carrier Z84.81
glaucoma Z83.511
hearing loss Z82.2
human immunodeficiency virus (HIV)
  infection Z83.0
Huntington's chorea Z82.0
intellectual disability Z81.0
leukemia Z80.6
malignant neoplasm (of) NOS Z80.9
  bladder Z80.52
  breast Z80.3
  bronchus Z80.1
  digestive organ Z80.0
  gastrointestinal tract Z80.0
  genital organ Z80.49
    ovary Z80.41
    prostate Z80.42
    specified organ NEC Z80.49
    testis Z80.43
  hematopoietic NEC Z80.7
  intrathoracic organ NEC Z80.2
  kidney Z80.51
  lung Z80.1
  lymphatic NEC Z80.7
  ovary Z80.41
  prostate Z80.42
  respiratory organ NEC Z80.2
  specified site NEC Z80.8
  testis Z80.43
  trachea Z80.1
  urinary organ or tract Z80.59
    bladder Z80.52
    kidney Z80.51
mental
  disorder NEC Z81.8
multiple endocrine neoplasia (MEN)
syndrome Z83.41
osteoporosis Z82.62
polycystic kidney Z82.71
polyps (colon) Z83.71
psychiatric disorder Z81.8
psychoactive substance abuse NEC Z81.3
respiratory condition NEC Z83.6
  asthma and other lower respiratory
  conditions Z82.5
self-harmful behavior Z81.8
SIDS (sudden infant death syndrome)
  Z84.82
skin condition Z84.0
specified condition NEC Z84.89
stroke (cerebrovascular) Z82.3
substance abuse NEC Z81.4
  alcohol Z81.1
  drug NEC Z81.3
  psychoactive NEC Z81.3
  tobacco Z81.2
sudden
  cardiac death Z82.41
  infant death syndrome (SIDS) Z84.82
tobacco abuse Z81.2
violence, violent behavior Z81.8
visual loss Z82.1
personal (of) -*see also* History, family (of)
abuse
  childhood Z62.819
    physical Z62.810
    psychological Z62.811
    sexual Z62.810
  adult Z91.419
    physical and sexual Z91.410

History --*continued*

    psychological Z91.411
alcohol dependence F10.21
allergy (to) Z88.9
  analgesic agent NEC Z88.6
  anesthetic Z88.4
  antibiotic agent NEC Z88.1
  anti-infective agent NEC Z88.3
  contrast media Z91.041
  drugs, medicaments and biological
  substances Z88.9
    specified NEC Z88.8
  food Z91.018
    additives Z91.02
    eggs Z91.012
    milk products Z91.011
    peanuts Z91.010
    seafood Z91.013
    specified food NEC Z91.018
  insect Z91.038
    bee Z91.030
  latex Z91.040
  medicinal agents Z88.9
    specified NEC Z88.8
  narcotic agent NEC Z88.5
  nonmedicinal agents Z91.048
  penicillin Z88.0
  serum Z88.7
  specified NEC Z91.09
  sulfonamides Z88.2
  vaccine Z88.7
anaphylactic shock Z87.892
anaphylaxis Z87.892
behavioral disorders Z86.59
benign carcinoid tumor Z86.012
benign neoplasm Z86.018
  carcinoid Z86.012
  brain Z86.011
  colonic polyps Z86.010
brain injury (traumatic) Z87.820
breast implant removal Z98.86
calculi, renal Z87.442
cancer -*see* History, personal (of), malignant
neoplasm (of)
cardiac arrest (death), successfully
resuscitated Z86.74
  cerebral infarction without residual deficit
  Z86.73
  cervical dysplasia Z87.410
  chemotherapy for neoplastic condition
  Z92.21
  childhood abuse -*see* History, personal (of),
  abuse
  cleft lip (corrected) Z87.730
  cleft palate (corrected) Z87.730
  collapsed vertebra (healed) Z87.311
    due to osteoporosis Z87.310
  combat and operational stress reaction
  Z86.51
  congenital malformation (corrected)
  Z87.798
    circulatory system (corrected) Z87.74
    digestive system (corrected) NEC Z87.738
    ear (corrected) Z87.720
    eye (corrected) Z87.721
    face and neck (corrected) Z87.790
    genitourinary system (corrected) NEC
    Z87.718
    heart (corrected) Z87.74
    integument (corrected) Z87.76
    limb(s) (corrected) Z87.76

History --*continued*

    musculoskeletal system (corrected) Z87.76
    neck (corrected) Z87.790
    nervous system (corrected) NEC Z87.728
    respiratory system (corrected) Z87.75
    sense organs (corrected) NEC Z87.728
    specified NEC Z87.798
contraception Z92.0
deployment (military) Z91.82
diabetic foot ulcer Z86.31
disease or disorder (of) Z87.898
  blood and blood-forming organs Z86.2
  circulatory system Z86.79
    specified condition NEC Z86.79
  connective tissue NEC Z87.39
  digestive system Z87.19
    colonic polyp Z86.010
    peptic ulcer disease Z87.11
    specified condition NEC Z87.19
  ear Z86.69
  endocrine Z86.39
    diabetic foot ulcer Z86.31
    gestational diabetes Z86.32
    specified type NEC Z86.39
  eye Z86.69
  genital (track) system NEC
    female Z87.42
    male Z87.438
  hematological Z86.2
  Hodgkin Z85.71
  immune mechanism Z86.2
  infectious Z86.19
    malaria Z86.13
    Methicillin resistant Staphylococcus
      aureus (MRSA) Z86.14
    poliomyelitis Z86.12
    specified NEC Z86.19
    tuberculosis Z86.11
  mental NEC Z86.59
  metabolic Z86.39
    diabetic foot ulcer Z86.31
    gestational diabetes Z86.32
    specified type NEC Z86.39
  musculoskeletal NEC Z87.39
  nervous system Z86.69
  nutritional Z86.39
  parasitic Z86.19
  respiratory system NEC Z87.09
  sense organs Z86.69
  skin Z87.2
  specified site or type NEC Z87.898
  subcutaneous tissue Z87.2
  trophoblastic Z87.59
  urinary system NEC Z87.448
drug dependence -*see* Dependence, drug, by
type, in remission
drug therapy
  antineoplastic chemotherapy Z92.21
  estrogen Z92.23
  immunosuppression Z92.25
  inhaled steroids Z92.240
  monoclonal drug Z92.22
  specified NEC Z92.29
  steroid Z92.241
  systemic steroids Z92.241
dysplasia
  cervical (mild) (moderate) Z87.410
    severe (grade III) Z86.001
  prostatic Z87.430
  vaginal (mild) (moderate) Z87.411
    severe (grade III) Z86.008

History --continued
 vulvar (mild) (moderate) Z87.412
  severe (grade III) Z86.008
 embolism (venous) Z86.718
  pulmonary Z86.711
 encephalitis Z86.61
 estrogen therapy Z92.23
 extracorporeal membrane oxygenation (ECMO) Z92.81
 failed moderate sedation Z92.83
 failed conscious sedation Z92.83
 fall, falling Z91.81
 fracture (healed)
  fatigue Z87.312
  fragility Z87.310
  osteoporosis Z87.310
  pathological NEC Z87.311
  stress Z87.312
  traumatic Z87.81
 gestational diabetes Z86.32
 hepatitis
  B Z86.19
  C Z86.19
 Hodgkin disease Z85.71
 hyperthermia, malignant Z88.4
 hypospadias (corrected) Z87.710
 hysterectomy Z90.710
 immunosuppression therapy Z92.25
 in situ neoplasm
  breast Z86.000
  cervix uteri Z86.001
  specified NEC Z86.008
 infection NEC Z86.19
  central nervous system Z86.61
  Methicillin resistant Staphylococcus aureus (MRSA) Z86.14
  urinary (recurrent) (tract) Z87.440
 injury NEC Z87.828
 in utero procedure during pregnancy Z98.870
 in utero procedure while a fetus Z98.871
 irradiation Z92.3
 kidney stones Z87.442
 leukemia Z85.6
 lymphoma (non-Hodgkin) Z85.72
 malignant melanoma (skin) Z85.820
 malignant neoplasm (of) Z85.9
  accessory sinuses Z85.22
  anus NEC Z85.048
   carcinoid Z85.040
  bladder Z85.51
  bone Z85.830
  brain Z85.841
  breast Z85.3
  bronchus NEC Z85.118
   carcinoid Z85.110
  carcinoid -see History, personal (of), malignant neoplasm, by site, carcinoid
  cervix Z85.41
  colon NEC Z85.038
   carcinoid Z85.030
  digestive organ Z85.00
   specified NEC Z85.09
  endocrine gland NEC Z85.858
  epididymis Z85.48
  esophagus Z85.01
  eye Z85.840
  gastrointestinal tract -see History, malignant neoplasm, digestive organ
  genital organ
   female Z85.40

History --continued
   specified NEC Z85.44
   male Z85.45
    specified NEC Z85.49
  hematopoietic NEC Z85.79
  intrathoracic organ Z85.20
  kidney NEC Z85.528
   carcinoid Z85.520
  large intestine NEC Z85.038
   carcinoid Z85.030
  larynx Z85.21
  liver Z85.05
  lung NEC Z85.118
   carcinoid Z85.110
  mediastinum Z85.29
  Merkel cell Z85.821
  middle ear Z85.22
  nasal cavities Z85.22
  nervous system NEC Z85.848
  oral cavity Z85.819
   specified site NEC Z85.818
  ovary Z85.43
  pancreas Z85.07
  pharynx Z85.819
   specified site NEC Z85.818
  pelvis Z85.53
  pleura Z85.29
  prostate Z85.46
  rectosigmoid junction NEC Z85.048
   carcinoid Z85.040
  rectum NEC Z85.048
   carcinoid Z85.040
  respiratory organ Z85.20
  sinuses, accessory Z85.22
  skin NEC Z85.828
   melanoma Z85.820
   Merkel cell Z85.821
  small intestine NEC Z85.068
   carcinoid Z85.060
  soft tissue Z85.831
  specified site NEC Z85.89
  stomach NEC Z85.028
   carcinoid Z85.020
  testis Z85.47
  thymus NEC Z85.238
   carcinoid Z85.230
  thyroid Z85.850
  tongue Z85.810
  trachea Z85.12
  ureter Z85.54
  urinary organ or tract Z85.50
   specified NEC Z85.59
  uterus Z85.42
 maltreatment Z91.89
 medical treatment NEC Z92.89
 melanoma (malignant) (skin) Z85.820
 meningitis Z86.61
 mental disorder Z86.59
 Merkel cell carcinoma (skin) Z85.821
 Methicillin resistant Staphylococcus aureus (MRSA) Z86.14
 military deployment Z91.82
 military war, peacekeeping and humanitarian deployment (current or past conflict) Z91.82
 myocardial infarction (old) I25.2
 neglect (in)
  adult Z91.412
  childhood Z62.812
 neoplasm
  benign Z86.018

History --continued
  brain Z86.011
  colon polyp Z86.010
  in situ
   breast Z86.000
   cervix uteri Z86.001
   specified NEC Z86.008
  malignant -see History of, malignant neoplasm
  uncertain behavior Z86.03
 nephrotic syndrome Z87.441
 nicotine dependence Z87.891
 noncompliance with medical treatment or regimen -see Noncompliance
 nutritional deficiency Z86.39
 obstetric complications Z87.59
  childbirth Z87.59
  pregnancy Z87.59
  pre-term labor Z87.51
  puerperium Z87.59
 osteoporosis fractures Z87.31
 parasuicide (attempt) Z91.5
 physical trauma NEC Z87.828
  self-harm or suicide attempt Z91.5
 poisoning NEC Z91.89
  self-harm or suicide attempt Z91.5
 poor personal hygiene Z91.89
 pneumonia (recurrent) Z87.01
 preterm labor Z87.51
 prolonged reversible ischemic neurologic deficit (PRIND) Z86.73
 procedure during pregnancy Z98.870
 procedure while a fetus Z98.871
 prostatic dysplasia Z87.430
 psychological
  abuse
   adult Z91.411
   child Z62.811
  trauma, specified NEC Z91.49
 radiation therapy Z92.3
 removal
  implant
   breast Z98.86
 renal calculi Z87.442
 respiratory condition NEC Z87.09
 retained foreign body fully removed Z87.821
 risk factors NEC Z91.89
 self-harm Z91.5
 self-poisoning attempt Z91.5
 sex reassignment Z87.890
 sleep-wake cycle problem Z72.821
 specified NEC Z87.898
 steroid therapy (systemic) Z92.241
  inhaled Z92.240
 stroke without residual deficits Z86.73
 substance abuse NEC F10 F19 with fifth character 1
 sudden cardiac arrest Z86.74
 sudden cardiac death successfully resuscitated Z86.74
 suicide attempt Z91.5
 surgery NEC Z98.890
  with uterine scar Z98.891
  sex reassignment Z87.890
  transplant -see Transplant
 thrombophlebitis Z86.72
 thrombosis (venous) Z86.718
  pulmonary Z86.711
 tobacco dependence Z87.891

History *--continued*
> transient ischemic attack (TIA) without
residual deficits Z86.73
> trauma (physical) NEC Z87.828
>> psychological NEC Z91.49
>> self-harm Z91.5
> traumatic brain injury Z87.820
> unhealthy sleep-wake cycle Z72.821
> unintended awareness under general
anesthesia Z92.84
> urinary calculi Z87.442
> urinary (recurrent) (tract) infection(s)
Z87.440
> uterine scar from previous surgery Z98.891
> vaginal dysplasia Z87.411
> venous thrombosis or embolism Z86.718
>> pulmonary Z86.711
> vulvar dysplasia Z87.412
His-Werner disease A79.0
HIV *-see also* Human, immunodeficiency virus
B20
> laboratory evidence (nonconclusive) R75
> positive, seropositive Z21
> nonconclusive test (in infants) R75
Hives (bold) *-see* Urticaria
Hoarseness R49.0
Hobo Z59.0
Hodgkin disease *-see* Lymphoma, Hodgkin
Hodgson's disease I71.2
> ruptured I71.1
Hoffa-Kastert disease E88.89
Hoffa's disease E88.89
Hoffmann-Bouveret syndrome I47.9
Hoffmann's syndrome E03.9 *[G73.7]*
Hole (round)
> macula H35.34
> retina (without detachment) *-see* Break,
retina, round hole
>> with detachment *-see* Detachment, retina,
with retinal, break
Holiday relief care Z75.5
Hollenhorst's plaque *-see* Occlusion, artery,
retina
Hollow foot (congenital) Q66.7
> acquired *-see* Deformity, limb, foot, specified
NEC
Holoprosencephaly Q04.2
Holt-Oram syndrome Q87.2
Homelessness Z59.0
Homesickness *-see* Disorder, adjustment
Homocystinemia, homocystinuria E72.11
Homogentisate 1,2 dioxygenase deficiency
E70.29
Homologous serum hepatitis (prophylactic)
(therapeutic) *-see* Hepatitis, viral, type B
Honeycomb lung J98.4
> congenital Q33.0
Hooded
> clitoris Q52.6
> penis Q55.69
Hookworm (anemia) (disease) (infection)
(infestation) B76.9
> specified NEC B76.8
Hordeolum (eyelid) (externum) (recurrent)
H00.019
> internum H00.029
>> left H00.026
>>> lower H00.025
>>> upper H00.024
>> right H00.023
>>> lower H00.022

Hordeolum - *continued*
>> upper H00.021
> left H00.016
>> lower H00.015
>> upper H00.014
> right H00.013
>> lower H00.012
>> upper H00.011
Horn
> cutaneous L85.8
> nail L60.2
>> congenital Q84.6
Horner (Claude Bernard) syndrome G90.2
> traumatic *-see* Injury, nerve, cervical
sympathetic
Horseshoe kidney (congenital) Q63.1
Horton's headache or neuralgia G44.099
> intractable G44.091
> not intractable G44.099
Hospital hopper syndrome *-see* Disorder,
factitious
Hospitalism in children *-see* Disorder,
adjustment
Hostility R45.5
> towards child Z62.3
Hot flashes
> menopausal N95.1
Hourglass (contracture) *-see also*
Contraction, hourglass
> stomach K31.89
>> congenital Q40.2
>> stricture K31.2
Household, housing circumstance affecting
care Z59.9
> specified NEC Z59.8
Housemaid's knee *-see* Bursitis, prepatellar
Hudson (Stähli) line (cornea) *-see*
Pigmentation, cornea, anterior
Human
> bite (open wound) *-see also* Bite
>> intact skin surface *-see* Bite, superficial
> herpesvirus *-see* Herpes
> immunodeficiency virus (HIV) disease
(infection) B20
>> asymptomatic status Z21
>> contact Z20.6
>> counseling Z71.7
>> dementia B20 *[F02.80]*
>>> with behavioral disturbance B20 *[F02.81]*
>> exposure to Z20.6
>> laboratory evidence R75
>> type-2 (HIV 2) as cause of disease classified
elsewhere B97.35
> papillomavirus (HPV)
>> DNA test positive
>>> high risk
>>>> cervix R87.810
>>>> vagina R87.811
>>> low risk
>>>> cervix R87.820
>>>> vagina R87.821
>> screening for Z11.51
> T-cell lymphotropic virus
>> type-1 (HTLV-I) infection B33.3
>>> as cause of disease classified elsewhere
B97.33
>>> carrier Z22.6
>> type-2 (HTLV-II) as cause of disease
classified elsewhere B97.34
Humidifier lung or pneumonitis J67.7

Humiliation (experience) in childhood
Z62.898
Humpback (acquired) *-see* Kyphosis
Hunchback (acquired) *-see* Kyphosis
Hunger T73.0
> air, psychogenic F45.8
Hungry bone syndrome E83.81
Hunner's ulcer *-see* Cystitis, chronic,
interstitial
Hunter's
> glossitis D51.0
> syndrome E76.1
Huntington's disease or chorea G10
> with dementia G10 *[F02.80]*
>> with behavioral disturbance G10 *[F02.81]*
Hunt's
> disease or syndrome (herpetic geniculate
ganglionitis) B02.21
>> dyssynergia cerebellaris myoclonica G11.1
> neuralgia B02.21
Hurler (Scheie) disease or syndrome E76.02
Hurst's disease G36.1
Hürthle cell
> adenocarcinoma C73
> adenoma D34
> carcinoma C73
> tumor D34
Hutchinson-Boeck disease or syndrome *-see*
Sarcoidosis
Hutchinson-Gilford disease or syndrome
E34.8
Hutchinson's
> disease, meaning
>> angioma serpiginosum L81.7
>> pompholyx (cheiropompholyx) L30.1
>> prurigo estivalis L56.4
>> summer eruption or summer prurigo L56.4
> melanotic freckle *-see* Melanoma, in situ
>> malignant melanoma in *-see* Melanoma
> teeth or incisors (congenital syphilis) A50.52
> triad (congenital syphilis) A50.53
Hyalin plaque, sclera, senile H15.89
Hyaline membrane (disease) (lung)
(pulmonary) (newborn) P22.0
Hyalinosis
> cutis (et mucosae) E78.89
> focal and segmental (glomerular) *-see also*
N00 N07 with fourth character .1N05.1
Hyalitis, hyalosis, asteroid *-see also* Deposit,
crystalline
> syphilitic (late) A52.71
Hydatid
> cyst or tumor *-see* Echinococcus
> mole *-see* Hydatidiform mole
> Morgagni
>> female Q50.5
>> male (epididymal) Q55.4
>>> testicular Q55.29
Hydatidiform mole (benign) (complicating
pregnancy) (delivered) (undelivered) O01.9
> classical O01.0
> complete O01.0
> incomplete O01.1
> invasive D39.2
> malignant D39.2
> partial O01.1
Hydatidosis *-see* Echinococcus
Hydradenitis (axillaris) (suppurative) L73.2
Hydradenoma *-see* Hidradenoma
Hydramnios O40.

Hydrancephaly, hydranencephaly Q04.3
  with spina bifida -*see* Spina bifida, with
  hydrocephalus
Hydrargyrism NEC -*see* Poisoning, mercury
Hydrarthrosis -*see also* Effusion, joint
  gonococcal A54.42
  intermittent M12.40
    ankle M12.47
    elbow M12.42
    foot joint M12.47
    hand joint M12.44
    hip M12.45
    knee M12.46
    multiple site M12.49
    shoulder M12.41
    specified joint NEC M12.48
    wrist M12.43
  of yaws (early) (late) -*see also* subcategory
  M14.8 A66.6
  syphilitic (late) A52.77
    congenital A50.55 [*M12.80*]
Hydremia D64.89
Hydrencephalocele (congenital) -*see*
  Encephalocele
Hydrencephalomeningocele (congenital) -*see*
  Encephalocele
Hydroa R23.8
  aestivale L56.4
  vacciniforme L56.4
Hydroadenitis (axillaris) (suppurative) L73.2
Hydrocalycosis -*see* Hydronephrosis
**Hydrocele (spermatic cord) (testis) (tunica
  vaginalis)** N43.3
  canal of Nuck N94.89
  communicating N43.2
    congenital P83.5
  congenital P83.5
  encysted N43.0
  female NEC N94.89
  infected N43.1
  newborn P83.5
  round ligament N94.89
  specified NEC N43.2
  spinalis -*see* Spina bifida
  vulva N90.89
**Hydrocephalus (acquired) (external)
  (internal) (malignant) (recurrent)** G91.9
  aqueduct Sylvius stricture Q03.0
  causing disproportion O33.6
    with obstructed labor O66.3
  communicating G91.0
  congenital (external) (internal) Q03.9
    with spina bifida Q05.4
      cervical Q05.0
      dorsal Q05.1
      lumbar Q05.2
      lumbosacral Q05.2
      sacral Q05.3
      thoracic Q05.1
      thoracolumbar Q05.1
    specified NEC Q03.8
  due to toxoplasmosis (congenital) P37.1
  foramen Magendie block (acquired) G91.1
    congenital -*see also* Hydrocephalus,
    congenital Q03.1
  in (due to)
    infectious disease NEC B89 [*G91.4*]
    neoplastic disease NEC (see also Neoplasm)
    G91.4
    parasitic disease B89 [*G91.4*]
  newborn Q03.9

Hydrocephalus - *continued*
  with spina bifida -*see* Spina bifida, with
  hydrocephalus
  noncommunicating G91.1
  normal pressure G91.2
    secondary G91.0
  obstructive G91.1
  otitic G93.2
  post-traumatic NEC G91.3
  secondary G91.4
    post-traumatic G91.3
  specified NEC G91.8
  syphilitic, congenital A50.49
Hydrocolpos (congenital) N89.8
Hydrocystoma -*see* Neoplasm, skin, benign
Hydroencephalocele (congenital) -*see*
  Encephalocele
Hydroencephalomeningocele (congenital) -
  see Encephalocele
Hydrohematopneumothorax -*see*
  Hemothorax
Hydromeningitis -*see* Meningitis
Hydromeningocele (spinal) -*see also* Spina
  bifida
  cranial -*see* Encephalocele
Hydrometra N85.8
Hydrometrocolpos N89.8
Hydromicrocephaly Q02
Hydromphalus (since birth) Q45.8
Hydromyelia Q06.4
Hydromyelocele -*see* Spina bifida
**Hydronephrosis (atrophic) (early)
  (functionless) (intermittent) (primary)
  (secondary) NEC** N13.30
  with
    infection N13.6
    obstruction (by) (of)
      renal calculus N13.2
        with infection N13.6
      ureteral NEC N13.1
        with infection N13.6
        calculus N13.2
          with infection N13.6
      ureteropelvic junction (congenital) Q62.0
        acquired N13.0
          with infection N13.6
      ureteral stricture NEC N13.1
        with infection N13.6
  congenital Q62.0
  due to acquired occlusion of ureteropelvic
  junction N13.0
  specified type NEC N13.39
  tuberculous A18.11
Hydropericarditis -*see* Pericarditis
Hydropericardium -*see* Pericarditis
Hydroperitoneum R18.8
Hydrophobia -*see* Rabies
Hydrophthalmos Q15.0
Hydropneumohemothorax -*see* Hemothorax
Hydropneumopericarditis -*see* Pericarditis
Hydropneumopericardium -*see* Pericarditis
Hydropneumothorax J94.8
  traumatic -*see* Injury, intrathoracic, lung
  tuberculous NEC A15.6
Hydrops R60.9
  abdominis R18.8
  articulorum intermittens -*see* Hydrarthrosis,
  intermittent
  cardiac -*see* Failure, heart, congestive
  causing obstructed labor (mother) O66.3
  endolymphatic H81.0

Hydrops - *continued*
  fetal -*see* Pregnancy, complicated by,
  hydrops, fetalis
  fetalis P83.2
    due to
      ABO isoimmunization P56.0
      alpha thalassemia D56.0
      hemolytic disease P56.90
        specified NEC P56.99
      isoimmunization (ABO) (Rh) P56.0
      other specified nonhemolytic disease NEC
      P83.2
      Rh incompatibility P56.0
  during pregnancy -*see* Pregnancy,
  complicated by, hydrops, fetalis
  gallbladder K82.1
  joint -*see* Effusion, joint
  labyrinth H81.0
  newborn (idiopathic) P83.2
    due to
      ABO isoimmunization P56.0
      alpha thalassemia D56.0
      hemolytic disease P56.90
        specified NEC P56.99
      isoimmunization (ABO) (Rh) P56.0
      Rh incompatibility P56.0
  nutritional -*see* Malnutrition, severe
  pericardium -*see* Pericarditis
  pleura -*see* Hydrothorax
  spermatic cord -*see* Hydrocele
Hydropyonephrosis N13.6
Hydrorachis Q06.4
Hydrorrhea (nasal) J34.89
  pregnancy -*see* Rupture, membranes,
  premature
Hydrosadenitis (axillaris) (suppurative)
  L73.2
Hydrosalpinx (fallopian tube) (follicularis)
  N70.11
Hydrothorax (double) (pleura) J94.8
  chylous (nonfilarial) I89.8
    filarial -*see also* Infestation, filarial B74.9
    [*J91.8*]
  traumatic -*see* Injury, intrathoracic
  tuberculous NEC (non primary) A15.6
Hydroureter -*see also* Hydronephrosis N13.4
  with infection N13.6
  congenital Q62.39
Hydroureteronephrosis -*see* Hydronephrosis
Hydrourethra N36.8
Hydroxykynureninuria E70.8
Hydroxylysinemia E72.3
Hydroxyprolinemia E72.59
Hygiene, sleep
  abuse Z72.821
  inadequate Z72.821
  poor Z72.821
Hygroma (congenital) (cystic) D18.1
  praepatellare, prepatellar -*see* Bursitis,
  prepatellar
Hymen -*see* condition
**Hymenolepis, hymenolepiasis (diminuta)
  (infection) (infestation) (nana)** B71.0
Hypalgesia R20.8
Hyperacidity (gastric) K31.89
  psychogenic F45.8
Hyperactive, hyperactivity F90.9
  basal cell, uterine cervix -*see* Dysplasia,
  cervix
  bowel sounds R19.12
  cervix epithelial (basal) -*see* Dysplasia, cervix

Hyperactive, hyperactivity --*continued*
  child F90.9
    attention deficit -*see* Disorder, attention-deficit hyperactivity   detrusor muscle N32.81
  gastrointestinal K31.89
    psychogenic F45.8
  nasal mucous membrane J34.3
  stomach K31.89
  thyroid (gland) -*see* Hyperthyroidism
Hyperacusis H93.23
Hyperadrenalism E27.5
Hyperadrenocorticism E24.9
  congenital E25.0
  iatrogenic E24.2
    correct substance properly administered -*see* Table of Drugs and Chemicals, by drug, adverse effect
    overdose or wrong substance given or taken -*see* Table of Drugs and Chemicals, by drug, poisoning
  not associated with Cushing's syndrome E27.0
  pituitary dependent E24.0
Hyperaldosteronism E26.9
  familial (type I) E26.02
  glucocorticoid-remediable E26.02
  primary (due to (bilateral) adrenal hyperplasia) E26.09
  primary NEC E26.09
  secondary E26.1
  specified NEC E26.89
Hyperalgesia R20.8
Hyperalimentation R63.2
  carotene, carotin E67.1
  specified NEC E67.8
  vitamin
    A E67.0
    D E67.3
Hyperaminoaciduria - arginine E72.21
  cystine E72.01
  lysine E72.3
  ornithine E72.4
Hyperammonemia (congenital) E72.20
Hyperazotemia -*see* Uremia
Hyperbetalipoproteinemia (familial) E78.00
  with prebetalipoproteinemia E78.2
Hyperbilirubinemia
  constitutional E80.6
  familial conjugated E80.6
  neonatal (transient) -*see* Jaundice, newborn
Hypercalcemia, hypocalciuric, familial E83.52
Hypercalciuria, idiopathic E83.52
Hypercapnia R06.89
  newborn P84
Hypercarotenemia, hypercarotenemia (dietary) E67.1
Hypercementosis K03.4
Hyperchloremia E87.8
Hyperchlorhydria K31.89
  neurotic F45.8
  psychogenic F45.8
Hypercholesterinemia -*see* Hypercholesterolemia
Hypercholesterolemia (essential) (primary) (pure) E78.00
  with hyperglyceridemia, endogenous E78.2
  dietary counseling and surveillance Z71.3
  familial E78.01
  hereditary E78.01
Hyperchylia gastrica, psychogenic F45.8

Hyperchylomicronemia (familial) (primary) E78.3
  with hyperbetalipoproteinemia E78.3
Hypercoagulable (state) D68.59
  activated protein C resistance D68.51
  antithrombin (III) deficiency D68.59
  factor V Leiden mutation D68.51
  primary NEC D68.59
  protein C deficiency D68.59
  protein S deficiency D68.59
  prothrombin gene mutation D68.52
  secondary D68.69
  specified NEC D68.69
Hypercoagulation (state) D68.59
Hypercorticalism, pituitary dependent E24.0
Hypercorticosolism -*see* Cushing's, syndrome
Hypercorticosteronism E24.2
  correct substance properly administered -*see* Table of Drugs and Chemicals, by drug, adverse effect
  overdose or wrong substance given or taken -*see* Table of Drugs and Chemicals, by drug, poisoning
Hypercortisonism E24.2
  correct substance properly administered -*see* Table of Drugs and Chemicals, by drug, adverse effect
  overdose or wrong substance given or taken -*see* Table of Drugs and Chemicals, by drug, poisoning **H**
hyperekplexia Q89.8
Hyperelectrolytemia E87.8
Hyperemesis R11.10
  with nausea R11.2
  gravidarum (mild) O21.0
    with
      carbohydrate depletion O21.1
      dehydration O21.1
      electrolyte imbalance O21.1
      metabolic disturbance O21.1
      severe (with metabolic disturbance) O21.1
  projectile R11.12
  psychogenic F45.8
Hyperemia (acute) (passive) R68.89
  anal mucosa K62.89
  bladder N32.89
  cerebral I67.89
  conjunctiva H11.43
  ear internal, acute - see subcategory H83.0
  enteric K59.8
  eye -*see* Hyperemia, conjunctiva
  eyelid (active) (passive) -*see* Disorder, eyelid, specified type NEC
  intestine K59.8
  iris -*see* Disorder, iris, vascular
  kidney N28.89
  labyrinth -*see* subcategory H83.0
  liver (active) K76.89
  lung (passive) -*see* Edema, lung
  pulmonary (passive) -*see* Edema, lung
  renal N28.89
  retina H35.89
  stomach K31.89
Hyperesthesia (body surface) R20.3
  larynx (reflex) J38.7
    hysterical F44.89
  pharynx (reflex) J39.2
    hysterical F44.89
Hyperestrogenism (drug-induced) (iatrogenic) E28.0
Hyperexplexia Q89.8

Hyperfibrinolysis -*see* Fibrinolysis
Hyperfructosemia E74.19
Hyperfunction
  adrenal cortex, not associated with Cushing's syndrome E27.0
    medulla E27.5
      adrenomedullary E27.5
    virilism E25.9
      congenital E25.0
  ovarian E28.8
  pancreas K86.89
  parathyroid (gland) E21.3
  pituitary (gland) (anterior) E22.9
    specified NEC E22.8
  polyglandular E31.1
  testicular E29.0
Hypergammaglobulinemia D89.2
  polyclonal D89.0
  Waldenström D89.0
Hypergastrinemia E16.4
Hyperglobulinemia R77.1
Hyperglycemia, hyperglycemic (transient) R73.9
  coma -*see* Diabetes, by type, with coma
  postpancreatectomy E89.1
Hyperglyceridemia (endogenous) (essential) (familial) (hereditary) (pure) E78.1
  mixed E78.3
Hyperglycinemia (non-ketotic) E72.51
Hypergonadism
  ovarian E28.8
  testicular (primary) (infantile) E29.0
Hyperheparinemia D68.32
Hyperhidrosis, hyperidrosis R61
  focal
    primary L74.519
      axilla L74.510
      face L74.511
      palms L74.512
      soles L74.513
    secondary L74.52
  generalized R61
  localized
    primary L74.519
      axilla L74.510
      face L74.511
      palms L74.512
      soles L74.513
    secondary L74.52
  psychogenic F45.8
  secondary R61
    focal L74.52
Hyperhistidinemia E70.41
Hyperhomocysteinemia E72.11
Hyperhydroxyprolinemia E72.59
Hyperinsulinism (functional) E16.1
  with
    coma (hypoglycemic) E15
    encephalopathy E16.1 [*G94*]
  ectopic E16.1
  therapeutic misadventure (from administration of insulin) -*see* subcategory T38.3
Hyperkalemia E87.5
Hyperkeratosis -*see also* Keratosis L85.9
  cervix N88.0
  due to yaws (early) (late) (palmar or plantar) A66.3
  follicularis Q82.8
    penetrans (in cutem) L87.0
  palmoplantaris climacterica L85.1

Hyperkeratosis - *continued*
 pinta A67.1
 senile (with pruritus) L57.0
 universalis congenita Q80.8
 vocal cord J38.3
 vulva N90.4
Hyperkinesia, hyperkinetic (disease)
 (reaction) (syndrome) (childhood)
 (adolescence) -*see also* Disorder, attention-
 deficit hyperactivity
 heart I51.89
Hyperleucine-isoleucinemia E71.19
Hyperlipemia, hyperlipidemia E78.5
 combined E78.2
 familial E78.4
 group
 A E78.00
 B E78.1
 C E78.2
 D E78.3
 mixed E78.2
 specified NEC E78.4
Hyperlipidosis E75.6
 hereditary NEC E75.5
Hyperlipoproteinemia E78.5
 Fredrickson's type
 I E78.3
 IIa E78.00
 IIb E78.2
 III E78.2
 IV E78.1
 V E78.3
 low-density lipoprotein-type (LDL) E78.00
 very low-density lipoprotein-type (VLDL)
 E78.1
Hyperlucent lung, unilateral J43.0
Hyperlysinemia E72.3
Hypermagnesemia E83.41
 neonatal P71.8
Hypermenorrhea N92.0
Hypermethioninemia E72.19
Hypermetropia (congenital) H52.0
Hypermobility, hypermotility
 cecum -*see* Syndrome, irritable bowel
 coccyx -*see* subcategory M53.2
 colon -*see* Syndrome, irritable bowel
 psychogenic F45.8
 ileum K58.9
 intestine -*see also* Syndrome, irritable bowel
 K58.9
 psychogenic F45.8
 meniscus (knee) -*see* Derangement, knee,
 meniscus
 scapula -*see* Instability, joint, shoulder
 stomach K31.89
 psychogenic F45.8
 syndrome M35.7
 urethra N36.41
 with intrinsic sphincter deficiency N36.43
Hypernasality R49.21
Hypernatremia E87.0
Hypernephroma C64. **Hyperopia** -*see*
 Hypermetropia
Hyperorexia nervosa F50.2
Hyperornithinemia E72.4
Hyperosmia R43.1
Hyperosmolality E87.0
Hyperostosis (monomelic) -*see also* Disorder,
 bone, density and structure, specified NEC
 ankylosing (spine) M48.10
 cervical region M48.12

Hyperostosis - *continued*
 cervicothoracic region M48.13
 lumbar region M48.16
 lumbosacral region M48.17
 multiple sites M48.19
 occipito-atlanto-axial region M48.11
 sacrococcygeal region M48.18
 thoracic region M48.14
 thoracolumbar region M48.15
 cortical (skull) M85.2
 infantile M89.8X
 frontal, internal of skull M85.2
 interna frontalis M85.2
 skeletal, diffuse idiopathic -*see* Hyperostosis,
 ankylosing
 skull M85.2
 congenital Q75.8
 vertebral, ankylosing -*see* Hyperostosis,
 ankylosing
Hyperovarism E28.8
Hyperoxaluria (primary) E72.53
Hyperparathyroidism E21.3
 primary E21.0
 secondary (renal) N25.81
 non-renal E21.1
 specified NEC E21.2
 tertiary E21.2
Hyperpathia R20.8
Hyperperistalsis R19.2
 psychogenic F45.8
Hyperpermeability, capillary I78.8
Hyperphagia R63.2
Hyperphenylalaninemia NEC E70.1
Hyperphoria (alternating) H50.53
Hyperphosphatemia E83.39
Hyperpiesis, hyperpiesia -*see* Hypertension
Hyperpigmentation -*see also* Pigmentation
 melanin NEC L81.4
 postinflammatory L81.0
Hyperpinealism E34.8
Hyperpituitarism E22.9
Hyperplasia, hyperplastic
 adenoids J35.2
 adrenal (capsule) (cortex) (gland) E27.8
 with
 sexual precocity (male) E25.9
 congenital E25.0
 virilism, adrenal E25.9
 congenital E25.0
 virilization (female) E25.9
 congenital E25.0
 congenital E25.0
 salt-losing E25.0
 adrenomedullary E27.5
 angiolymphoid, eosinophilia (ALHE) D18.01
 appendix (lymphoid) K38.0
 artery, fibromuscular I77.3
 bone -*see also* Hypertrophy, bone
 marrow D75.89
 breast -*see also* Hypertrophy, breast
 ductal (atypical) N60.9
 C-cell, thyroid E07.0
 cementation (tooth) (teeth) K03.4
 cervical gland R59.0
 cervix (uteri) (basal cell) (endometrium)
 (polypoid) -*see also* Dysplasia, cervix
 congenital Q51.828
 clitoris, congenital Q52.6
 denture K06.2
 endocervicitis N72

Hyperplasia, hyperplastic --*continued*
 endometrium, endometrial (adenomatous)
 (benign) (cystic) (glandular) (glandular-
 cystic) (polypoid) N85.00
 with atypia N85.02
 cervix -*see* Dysplasia, cervix
 complex (without atypia) N85.01
 simple (without atypia) N85.01
 epithelial L85.9
 focal, oral, including tongue K13.29
 nipple N62
 skin L85.9
 tongue K13.29
 vaginal wall N89.3
 erythroid D75.89
 fibromuscular of artery (carotid) (renal) I77.3
 genital
 female NEC N94.89
 male N50.89
 gingiva K06.1
 glandularis cystica uteri (interstitialis) -*see
 also* Hyperplasia, endometrial N85.00
 gum K06.1
 hymen, congenital Q52.4
 irritative, edentulous (alveolar) K06.2
 jaw M26.09
 alveolar M26.79
 lower M26.03
 alveolar M26.72
 upper M26.01
 alveolar M26.71
 kidney (congenital) Q63.3
 labia N90.69
 epithelial N90.3
 liver (congenital) Q44.7
 nodular, focal K76.89
 lymph gland or node R59.9
 mandible, mandibular M26.03
 alveolar M26.72
 unilateral condylar M27.8
 maxilla, maxillary M26.01
 alveolar M26.71
 myometrium, myometrial N85.2
 neuroendocrine cell, of infancy J84.841
 nose
 lymphoid J34.89
 polypoid J33.9
 oral mucosa (irritative) K13.6
 organ or site, congenital NEC -*see* Anomaly,
 by site
 ovary N83.8
 palate, papillary (irritative) K13.6
 pancreatic islet cells E16.9
 alpha E16.8
 with excess
 gastrin E16.4
 glucagon E16.3
 beta E16.1
 parathyroid (gland) E21.0
 pharynx (lymphoid) J39.2
 prostate (adenofibromatous) (nodular) N40.0
 with lower urinary tract symptoms (LUTS)
 N40.1
 without lower urinary tract symptoms
 (LUTS) N40.0
 renal artery I77.89
 reticulo-endothelial (cell) D75.89
 salivary gland (any) K11.1
 Schimmelbusch's -*see* Mastopathy, cystic
 suprarenal capsule (gland) E27.8
 thymus (gland) (persistent) E32.0

Hyperplasia, hyperplastic --*continued*
  thyroid (gland) -*see* Goiter
  tonsils (faucial) (infective) (lingual)
  (lymphoid) J35.1
    with adenoids J35.3
  unilateral condylar M27.8
  uterus, uterine N85.2
    endometrium (glandular) -*see also*
    Hyperplasia, endometrial N85.00
  vulva N90.69
    epithelial N90.3
Hyperpnea -*see* Hyperventilation
Hyperpotassemia E87.5
Hyperprebetalipoproteinemia (familial)
  E78.1
Hyperprolactinemia E22.1
Hyperprolinemia (type I) (type II) E72.59
Hyperproteinemia E88.09
Hyperprothrombinemia, causing
  coagulation factor deficiency D68.4
Hyperpyrexia R50.9
  heat (effects) T67.0
  malignant, due to anesthetic T88.3
  rheumatic -*see* Fever, rheumatic
  unknown origin R50.9
Hyper-reflexia R29.2
Hypersalivation K11.7
Hypersecretion
  ACTH (not associated with Cushing's
  syndrome) E27.0
    pituitary E24.0
  adrenaline E27.5
  adrenomedullary E27.5
  androgen (testicular) E29.0
    ovarian (drug-induced) (iatrogenic) E28.1
  calcitonin E07.0
  catecholamine E27.5
  corticoadrenal E24.9
  cortisol E24.9
  epinephrine E27.5
  estrogen E28.0
  gastric K31.89
    psychogenic F45.8
  gastrin E16.4
  glucagon E16.3
  hormone(s)
    ACTH (not associated with Cushing's
    syndrome) E27.0
      pituitary E24.0
    antidiuretic E22.2
    growth E22.0
    intestinal NEC E34.1
    ovarian androgen E28.1
    pituitary E22.9
    testicular E29.0
    thyroid stimulating E05.80
      with thyroid storm E05.81
  insulin -*see* Hyperinsulinism
  lacrimal glands -*see* Epiphora
  medulloadrenal E27.5
  milk O92.6
  ovarian androgens E28.1
  salivary gland (any) K11.7
  thyrocalcitonin E07.0
  upper respiratory J39.8
Hypersegmentation, leukocytic, hereditary
  D72.0
Hypersensitive, hypersensitiveness,
  hypersensitivity -*see also* Allergy carotid
  sinus G90.01
  colon -*see* Irritable, colon

Hypersensitive --*continued*
  drug T88.7
  gastrointestinal K52.29
    immediate K52.29
    psychogenic F45.8
  labyrinth -*see* subcategory H83.2
  pain R20.8
  pneumonitis -*see* Pneumonitis, allergic
  reaction T78.40
    upper respiratory tract NEC J39.3
Hypersomnia (organic) G47.10
  due to
    alcohol
      abuse F10.182
      dependence F10.282
      use F10.982
    amphetamines
      abuse F15.182
      dependence F15.282
      use F15.982
    caffeine
      abuse F15.182
      dependence F15.282
      use F15.982
    cocaine
      abuse F14.182
      dependence F14.282
      use F14.982
    drug NEC
      abuse F19.182
      dependence F19.282
      use F19.982
    medical condition G47.14
    mental disorder F51.13
    opioid
      abuse F11.182
      dependence F11.282
      use F11.982
    psychoactive substance NEC
      abuse F19.182
      dependence F19.282
      use F19.982
    sedative, hypnotic, or anxiolytic
      abuse F13.182
      dependence F13.282
      use F13.982
    stimulant NEC
      abuse F15.182
      dependence F15.282
      use F15.982
  idiopathic G47.11
    with long sleep time G47.11
    without long sleep time G47.12
  menstrual related G47.13
  nonorganic origin F51.11
    specified NEC F51.19
  not due to a substance or known physiological
  condition F51.11
    specified NEC F51.19
  primary F51.11
  recurrent G47.13
  specified NEC G47.19
Hypersplenia, hypersplenism D73.1
Hyperstimulation, ovaries (associated with
  induced ovulation) N98.1
Hypersusceptibility -*see* Allergy
Hypertelorism (ocular) (orbital) Q75.2
Hypertension, hypertensive (accelerated)
  (benign) (essential) (idiopathic) (malignant)
  (systemic) I10
  with

Hypertension, hypertensive --*continued*
  heart involvement (conditions in I51.4 I51.9
    due to hypertension) -*see* Hypertension,
    heart
  kidney involvement -*see* Hypertension,
    kidney
  benign, intracranial G93.2
  borderline R03.0
  cardiorenal (disease) I13.10
    with heart failure I13.0
      with stage 1 through stage 4 chronic
        kidney disease I13.0
      with stage 5 or end stage renal disease
        I13.2
    without heart failure I13.10
      with stage 1 through stage 4 chronic
        kidney disease I13.10
      with stage 5 or end stage renal disease
        I13.11
  cardiovascular
    disease (arteriosclerotic) (sclerotic) -*see*
    Hypertension, heart
    renal (disease) -*see* Hypertension,
    cardiorenal
  chronic venous -*see* Hypertension, venous
  (chronic)
  complicating
    childbirth (labor) O16.4
      pre-existing O10.92
        with
          heart disease O10.12
            with renal disease O10.32
          pre-eclampsia O11.4
          renal disease O10.22
            with heart disease O10.32
      essential O10.02
      secondary O10.42
    pregnancy O16.
      with edema -*see also* Pre-eclampsia O14.9
      gestational (pregnancy induced) (without
      proteinuria) O13.
      with proteinuria O14.9
        mild pre-eclampsia O14.0
        moderate pre-eclampsia O14.0
        severe pre-eclampsia O14.1
          with hemolysis, elevated liver
          enzymes and low platelet count
          (HELLP) O14.2
      pre-existing O10.91
        with
          heart disease O10.11
            with renal disease O10.31
          pre-eclampsi*a* -*see* category O11
          renal disease O10.21
            with heart disease O10.31
        essential O10.01
        secondary O10.41
      transient O13.
    puerperium, pre-existing O16.5
      pre-existing
        with
          heart disease O10.13
            with renal disease O10.33
          pre-eclampsia O11.5
          renal disease O10.23
            with heart disease O10.33
        essential O10.03
      pregnancy induced O13.9
      secondary O10.43
  crisis I16.9
  due to

Hypertension, hypertensive --*continued*
  endocrine disorders I15.2
    pheochromocytoma I15.2
  renal disorders NEC I15.1
    arterial I15.0
  renovascular disorders I15.0
  specified disease NEC I15.8
  emergency I16.2
  encephalopathy I67.4
  gestational (without significant proteinuria)
    (pregnancy induced) (transient) O13.
    with significant proteinuria -*see* Pre-
    eclampsia
    complicating
      delivery O13.4
      puerperium O13.5
  Goldblatt's I70.1
  heart (disease) (conditions in I51.4 I51.9 due
  to hypertension) I11.9
    with
      heart failure (congestive) I11.0
      kidney disease (chronic) -*see*
      Hypertension, cardiorenal
  intracranial (benign) G93.2
  kidney I12.9
    with
      heart disease -*see* Hypertension,
        cardiorenal
      stage 5 chronic kidney disease (CKD) or
        end stage renal disease (ESRD) I12.0
      stage 1 through stage 4 chronic kidney
        disease I12.9
  lesser circulation I27.0
  maternal O16.
  newborn P29.2
    pulmonary (persistent) P29.3
  ocular H40.05
  pancreatic duct
  code to underlying condition
    with chronic pancreatitis K86.1
  portal (due to chronic liver disease)
    (idiopathic) K76.6
    gastropathy K31.89
    in (due to) schistosomiasis (bilharziasis)
      B65.9 [*K77*]
  postoperative I97.3
  psychogenic F45.8
  pulmonary (artery) (secondary) NEC I27.2
    with
      cor pulmonale (chronic) I27.2
        acute I26.09
      right heart ventricular strain/failure I27.2
        acute I26.09
    of newborn (persistent) P29.3
    primary (idiopathic) I27.0
  renal -*see* Hypertension, kidney
  renovascular I15.0
  secondary NEC I15.9
    due to
      endocrine disorders I15.2
        pheochromocytoma I15.2
      renal disorders NEC I15.1
        arterial I15.0
      renovascular disorders I15.0
    specified NEC I15.8
  transient, of pregnancy O13.   urgency I16.0
  venous (chronic)
    due to
      deep vein thrombosis -*see* Syndrome,
  postthrombotic
    idiopathic I87.309

Hypertension, hypertensive --*continued*
  with
    inflammation I87.32
      with ulcer I87.33
    specified complication NEC I87.39
    ulcer I87.31
      with inflammation I87.33
    asymptomatic I87.30
Hypertensive urgency -*see* Hypertension
Hyperthecosis ovary E28.8
Hyperthermia (of unknown origin) -*see also*
  Hyperpyrexia
  malignant, due to anesthesia T88.3
  newborn P81.9
    environmental P81.0
Hyperthyroid (recurrent) -*see*
  Hyperthyroidism
Hyperthyroidism (latent) (pre-adult)
  (recurrent) E05.90
  with
    goiter (diffuse) E05.00
      with thyroid storm E05.01
    nodular (multinodular) E05.20
      with thyroid storm E05.21
      uninodular E05.10
        with thyroid storm E05.11
    storm E05.91
  due to ectopic thyroid tissue E05.30
    with thyroid storm E05.31
  neonatal, transitory P72.1
  specified NEC E05.80
    with thyroid storm E05.81
Hypertony, hypertonia, hypertonicity
  bladder N31.8
  congenital P94.1
  stomach K31.89
    psychogenic F45.8
  uterus, uterine (contractions) (complicating
  delivery) O62.4
Hypertrichosis L68.9
  congenital Q84.2
  eyelid H02.869
    left H02.866
      lower H02.865
      upper H02.864
    right H02.863
      lower H02.862
      upper H02.861
  lanuginosa Q84.2
    acquired L68.1
  localized L68.2
  specified NEC L68.8
Hypertriglyceridemia, essential E78.1
Hypertrophy, hypertrophic
  adenofibromatous, prostate -*see* Enlargement,
    enlarged, prostate
  adenoids (infective) J35.2
    with tonsils J35.3
  adrenal cortex E27.8
  alveolar process or ridge -*see* Anomaly,
    alveolar
  anal papillae K62.89
  artery I77.89
    congenital NEC Q27.8
      digestive system Q27.8
      lower limb Q27.8
      specified site NEC Q27.8
      upper limb Q27.8
  auricular -*see* Hypertrophy, cardiac -
  Bartholin's gland N75.8
  bile duct (common) (hepatic) K83.8

Hypertrophy, hypertrophic --*continued*
  bladder (sphincter) (trigone) N32.89
  bone M89.30
    carpus M89.34
    clavicle M89.31
    femur M89.35
    fibula M89.36
    finger M89.34
    humerus M89.32
    ilium M89.359
    ischium M89.359
    metacarpus M89.34
    metatarsus M89.37
    multiple sites M89.39
    neck M89.38
    radius M89.33
    rib M89.38
    scapula M89.31
    skull M89.38
    tarsus M89.37
    tibia M89.36
    toe M89.37
    ulna M89.33
    vertebra M89.38
  brain G93.89
  breast N62
    cystic -*see* Mastopathy, cystic
    newborn P83.4
    pubertal, massive N62
    puerperal, postpartum -*see* Disorder, breast,
  specified type NEC
    senile (parenchymatous) N62
  cardiac (chronic) (idiopathic) I51.7
    with rheumatic fever (conditions in I00)
      active I01.8
      inactive or quiescent (with chorea) I09.89
    congenital NEC Q24.8
    fatty -*see* Degeneration, myocardial
    hypertensive -*see* Hypertension, heart
    rheumatic (with chorea) I09.89
      active or acute I01.8
        with chorea I02.0
    valve -*see* Endocarditis
  cartilage -*see* Disorder, cartilage, specified
  type NEC
  cecum -*see* Megacolon
  cervix (uteri) N88.8
    congenital Q51.828
    elongation N88.4
  clitoris (cirrhotic) N90.89
    congenital Q52.6
  colon -*see also* Megacolon
    congenital Q43.2
  conjunctiva, lymphoid H11.89
  corpora cavernosa N48.89
  cystic duct K82.8
  duodenum K31.89
  endometrium (glandular) -*see also*
  Hyperplasia, endometrial N85.00
    cervix N88.8
  epididymis N50.89
  esophageal hiatus (congenital) Q79.1
    with hernia -*see* Hernia, hiatal
  eyelid -*see* Disorder, eyelid, specified type
  NEC
  fat pad E65
    knee (infrapatellar) (popliteal) (prepatellar)
  (retropatellar) M79.4
  foot (congenital) Q74.2
  frenulum, frenum (tongue) K14.8
    lip K13.0

Hypertrophy, hypertrophic --*continued*

gallbladder K82.8

gastric mucosa K29.60
  with bleeding K29.61

gland, glandular R59.9
  generalized R59.1
  localized R59.0

gum (mucous membrane) K06.1

heart (idiopathic) -*see also* Hypertrophy, cardiac
  valve -*see also* Endocarditis I38

hemifacial Q67.4

hepatic -*see* Hypertrophy, liver

hiatus (esophageal) Q79.1

hilus gland R59.0

hymen, congenital Q52.4

ileum K63.89

intestine NEC K63.89

jejunum K63.89

kidney (compensatory) N28.81
  congenital Q63.3

labium (majus) (minus) N90.60

ligament -*see* Disorder, ligament

lingual tonsil (infective) J35.1
  with adenoids J35.3

lip K13.0
  congenital Q18.6

liver R16.0
  acute K76.89
  congenital Q44.7
  cirrhotic -*see* Cirrhosis, liver
  fatty -*see* Fatty, liver

lymph, lymphatic gland R59.9
  generalized R59.1
  localized R59.0
  tuberculous -*see* Tuberculosis, lymph gland

mammary gland -*see* Hypertrophy, breast

Meckel's diverticulum (congenital) Q43.0
  malignant -*see* Table of Neoplasms, small intestine, malignant

median bar -*see* Hyperplasia, prostate

meibomian gland -*see* Chalazion

meniscus, knee, congenital Q74.1

metatarsal head -*see* Hypertrophy, bone, metatarsus

metatarsus -*see* Hypertrophy, bone, metatarsus

mucous membrane
  alveolar ridge K06.2
  gum K06.1
  nose (turbinate) J34.3

muscle M62.89

muscular coat, artery I77.89

myocardium -*see also* Hypertrophy, cardiac
  idiopathic I42.2

myometrium N85.2

nail L60.2
  congenital Q84.5

nasal J34.89
  alae J34.89
  bone J34.89
  cartilage J34.89
  mucous membrane (septum) J34.3
  sinus J34.89
  turbinate J34.3

nasopharynx, lymphoid (infectional) (tissue) (wall) J35.2

nipple N62

organ or site, congenital NEC -*see* Anomaly, by site

ovary N83.8

Hypertrophy, hypertrophic --*continued*

palate (hard) M27.8
  soft K13.79

pancreas, congenital Q45.3

parathyroid (gland) E21.0

parotid gland K11.1

penis N48.89

pharyngeal tonsil J35.2

pharynx J39.2
  lymphoid (infectional) (tissue) (wall) J35.2

pituitary (anterior) (fossa) (gland) E23.6

prepuce (congenital) N47.8
  female N90.89

prostate -*see* Enlargement, enlarged, prostate
  congenital Q55.4

pseudomuscular G71.0

pylorus (adult) (muscle) (sphincter) K31.1
  congenital or infantile Q40.0

rectal, rectum (sphincter) K62.89

rhinitis (turbinate) J31.0

salivary gland (any) K11.1
  congenital Q38.4

scaphoid (tarsal) -*see* Hypertrophy, bone, tarsus

scar L91.0

scrotum N50.89

seminal vesicle N50.89

sigmoid -*see* Megacolon

skin L91.9
  specified NEC L91.8

spermatic cord N50.89

spleen -*see* Splenomegaly

spondylitis -*see* Spondylosis

stomach K31.89

sublingual gland K11.1

submandibular gland K11.1

suprarenal cortex (gland) E27.8

synovial NEC M67.20
  acromioclavicular M67.21
  ankle M67.27
  elbow M67.22
  foot M67.27
  hand M67.24
  hip M67.25
  knee M67.26
  multiple sites M67.29
  specified site NEC M67.28
  wrist M67.23

tendon -*see* Disorder, tendon, specified type NEC

testis N44.8
  congenital Q55.29

thymic, thymus (gland) (congenital) E32.0

thyroid (gland) -*see* Goiter

toe (congenital) Q74.2
  acquired -*see also* Deformity, toe, specified NEC

tongue K14.8
  congenital Q38.2
  papillae (foliate) K14.3

tonsils (faucial) (infective) (lingual) (lymphoid) J35.1
  with adenoids J35.3

tunica vaginalis N50.89

ureter N28.89

urethra N36.8

uterus N85.2
  neck (with elongation) N88.4
  puerperal O90.89

uvula K13.79

vagina N89.8

Hypertrophy, hypertrophic --*continued*

vas deferens N50.89

vein I87.8

ventricle, ventricular (heart) -*see also* Hypertrophy, cardiac
  congenital Q24.8
  in tetralogy of Fallot Q21.3

verumontanum N36.8

vocal cord J38.3

vulva N90.60
  stasis (nonfilarial) N90.69

Hypertropia H50.2

Hypertyrosinemia E70.21

Hyperuricemia (asymptomatic) E79.0

Hypervalinemia E71.19

Hyperventilation (tetany) R06.4
  hysterical F45.8
  psychogenic F45.8
  syndrome F45.8

Hypervitaminosis (dietary) NEC E67.8
  A E67.0
    administered as drug (prolonged intake) -*see* Table of Drugs and Chemicals, vitamins, adverse effect
    overdose or wrong substance given or taken -*see* Table of Drugs and Chemicals, vitamins, poisoning
  B6 E67.2
  D E67.3
    administered as drug (prolonged intake) -*see* Table of Drugs and Chemicals, vitamins, adverse effect
    overdose or wrong substance given or taken -*see* Table of Drugs and Chemicals, vitamins, poisoning
  K E67.8
    administered as drug (prolonged intake) -*see* Table of Drugs and Chemicals, vitamins, adverse effect
    overdose or wrong substance given or taken -*see* Table of Drugs and Chemicals, vitamins, poisoning

Hypervolemia E87.70
  specified NEC E87.79

Hypesthesia R20.1
  cornea -*see* Anesthesia, cornea

Hyphema H21.0
  traumatic S05.1

Hypoacidity, gastric K31.89
  psychogenic F45.8

Hypoadrenalism, hypoadrenia E27.40
  primary E27.1
  tuberculous A18.7

Hypoadrenocorticism E27.40
  pituitary E23.0
  primary E27.1

Hypoalbuminemia E88.09

Hypoaldosteronism E27.40

Hypoalphalipoproteinemia E78.6

Hypobarism T70.29

Hypobaropathy T70.29

Hypobetalipoproteinemia (familial) E78.6

Hypocalcemia E83.51
  dietary E58
  neonatal P71.1
    due to cow's milk P71.0
  phosphate-loading (newborn) P71.1

Hypochloremia E87.8

Hypochlorhydria K31.89
  neurotic F45.8
  psychogenic F45.8

Hypochondria, hypochondriac, hypochondriasis (reaction) F45.21
  sleep F51.03
Hypochondrogenesis Q77.0
Hypochondroplasia Q77.4
Hypochromasia, blood cells D50.8
Hypodontia -see Anodontia
Hypoeosinophilia D72.89
Hypoesthesia R20.1
Hypofibrinogenemia D68.8
  acquired D65
  congenital (hereditary) D68.2
Hypofunction
  adrenocortical E27.40
    drug-induced E27.3
    postprocedural E89.6
    primary E27.1
  adrenomedullary, postprocedural E89.6
  cerebral R29.818
  corticoadrenal NEC E27.40
  intestinal K59.8
  labyrinth -see subcategory H83.2
  ovary E28.39
  pituitary (gland) (anterior) E23.0
  testicular E29.1
    postprocedural (postsurgical) (postirradiation) (iatrogenic) E89.5
Hypogalactia O92.4
Hypogammaglobulinemia -see also
  Agammaglobulinemia D80.1
  hereditary D80.0
  nonfamilial D80.1
  transient, of infancy D80.7
Hypogenitalism (congenital) -see
  Hypogonadism
Hypoglossia Q38.3
Hypoglycemia (spontaneous) E16.2
  coma E15
    diabetic -see Diabetes, coma
  diabetic -see Diabetes, hypoglycemia
  dietary counseling and surveillance Z71.3
  drug-induced E16.0
    with coma (nondiabetic) E15
  due to insulin E16.0
    with coma (nondiabetic) E15
    therapeutic misadventure - see subcategory T38.3
  functional, nonhyperinsulinemic E16.1
  iatrogenic E16.0
    with coma (nondiabetic) E15
  in infant of diabetic mother P70.1
    gestational diabetes P70.0
  infantile E16.1
  leucine-induced E71.19
  neonatal (transitory) P70.4
    iatrogenic P70.3
  reactive (not drug-induced) E16.1
  transitory neonatal P70.4
Hypogonadism
  female E28.39
  hypogonadotropic E23.0
  male E29.1
  ovarian (primary) E28.39
  pituitary E23.0
  testicular (primary) E29.1
Hypohidrosis, hypoidrosis L74.4
Hypoinsulinemia, postprocedural E89.1
Hypokalemia E87.6
Hypoleukocytosis -see Agranulocytosis
Hypolipoproteinemia (alpha) (beta) E78.6

Hypomagnesemia E83.42
  neonatal P71.2
Hypomania, hypomanic reaction F30.8
Hypomenorrhea -see Oligomenorrhea
Hypometabolism R63.8
Hypomotility
  gastrointestinal (tract) K31.89
    psychogenic F45.8
  intestine K59.8
    psychogenic F45.8
  stomach K31.89
    psychogenic F45.8
Hyponasality R49.22
Hyponatremia E87.1
Hypo-osmolality E87.1
Hypo-ovarianism, hypo-ovarism E28.39
Hypoparathyroidism E20.9
  familial E20.8
  idiopathic E20.0
  neonatal, transitory P71.4
  postprocedural E89.2
  specified NEC E20.8
Hypoperfusion (in)
  newborn P96.89
Hypopharyngitis -see Laryngopharyngitis
Hypophoria H50.53
Hypophosphatemia, hypophosphatasia (acquired) (congenital) (renal) E83.39
  familial E83.31
Hypophyseal, hypophysis -see also condition
  dwarfism E23.0
  gigantism E22.0
Hypopiesis -see Hypotension
Hypopinealism E34.8
Hypopituitarism (juvenile) E23.0
  drug-induced E23.1
  due to
    hypophysectomy E89.3
    radiotherapy E89.3
  iatrogenic NEC E23.1
  postirradiation E89.3
  postpartum O99.285
  postprocedural E89.3
Hypoplasia, hypoplastic
  adrenal (gland), congenital Q89.1
  alimentary tract, congenital Q45.8
    upper Q40.8
  anus, anal (canal) Q42.3
    with fistula Q42.2
  aorta, aortic Q25.42
    ascending, in hypoplastic left heart syndrome Q23.4
    valve Q23.1
      in hypoplastic left heart syndrome Q23.4
  areola, congenital Q83.8
  arm (congenital) -see Defect, reduction, upper limb
  artery (peripheral) Q27.8
    brain (congenital) Q28.3
    coronary Q24.5
    digestive system Q27.8
    lower limb Q27.8
    pulmonary Q25.79
      functional, unilateral J43.0
    retinal (congenital) Q14.1
    specified site NEC Q27.8
    umbilical Q27.0
    upper limb Q27.8
  auditory canal Q17.8
    causing impairment of hearing Q16.9
  biliary duct or passage Q44.5

Hypoplasia, hypoplastic --continued
  bone NOS Q79.9
    face Q75.8
    marrow D61.9
      megakaryocytic D69.49
    skull -see Hypoplasia, skull
  brain Q02
    gyri Q04.3
    part of Q04.3
  breast (areola) N64.82
  bronchus Q32.4
  cardiac Q24.8
  carpus -see Defect, reduction, upper limb, specified type NEC
  cartilage hair Q78.8
  cecum Q42.8
  cementum K00.4
  cephalic Q02
  cerebellum Q04.3
  cervix (uteri), congenital Q51.821
  clavicle (congenital) Q74.0
  coccyx Q76.49
  colon Q42.9
    specified NEC Q42.8
  corpus callosum Q04.0
  cricoid cartilage Q31.2
  digestive organ(s) or tract NEC Q45.8
    upper (congenital) Q40.8
  ear (auricle) (lobe) Q17.2
    middle Q16.4
  enamel of teeth (neonatal) (postnatal) (prenatal) K00.4
  endocrine (gland) NEC Q89.2
  endometrium N85.8
  epididymis (congenital) Q55.4
  epiglottis Q31.2
  erythroid, congenital D61.01
  esophagus (congenital) Q39.8
  eustachian tube Q17.8
  eye Q11.2
  eyelid (congenital) Q10.3
  face Q18.8
    bone(s) Q75.8
  femur (congenital) -see Defect, reduction, lower limb, specified type NEC
  fibula (congenital) -see Defect, reduction, lower limb, specified type NEC
  finger (congenital) -see Defect, reduction, upper limb, specified type NEC
  focal dermal Q82.8
  foot -see Defect, reduction, lower limb, specified type NEC
  gallbladder Q44.0
  genitalia, genital organ(s)
    female, congenital Q52.8
      external Q52.79
      internal NEC Q52.8
    in adiposogenital dystrophy E23.6
  glottis Q31.2
  hair Q84.2
  hand (congenital) -see Defect, reduction, upper limb, specified type NEC
  heart Q24.8
  humerus (congenital) -see Defect, reduction, upper limb, specified type NEC
  intestine (small) Q41.9
    large Q42.9
      specified NEC Q42.8
  jaw M26.09
    alveolar M26.79
      lower M26.04

Hypoplasia, hypoplastic --*continued*
  alveolar M26.74
    upper M26.02
    alveolar M26.73
  kidney(s) Q60.5
    bilateral Q60.4
    unilateral Q60.3
  labium (majus) (minus), congenital Q52.79
  larynx Q31.2
  left heart syndrome Q23.4
  leg (congenital) -*see* Defect, reduction, lower limb
  limb Q73.8
    lower (congenital) -*see* Defect, reduction, lower limb
    upper (congenital) -*see* Defect, reduction, upper limb
  liver Q44.7
  lung (lobe) (not associated with short gestation) Q33.6
    associated with immaturity, low birth weight, prematurity, or short gestation P28.0
  mammary (areola), congenital Q83.8
  mandible, mandibular M26.04
    alveolar M26.74
    unilateral condylar M27.8
  maxillary M26.02
    alveolar M26.73
  medullary D61.9
  megakaryocytic D69.49
  metacarpus -*see* Defect, reduction, upper limb, specified type NEC
  metatarsus -*see* Defect, reduction, lower limb, specified type NEC
  muscle Q79.8
  nail(s) Q84.6
  nose, nasal Q30.1
  optic nerve H47.03
  osseous meatus (ear) Q17.8
  ovary, congenital Q50.39
  pancreas Q45.0
  parathyroid (gland) Q89.2
  parotid gland Q38.4
  patella Q74.1
  pelvis, pelvic girdle Q74.2
  penis (congenital) Q55.62
  peripheral vascular system Q27.8
    digestive system Q27.8
    lower limb Q27.8
    specified site NEC Q27.8
    upper limb Q27.8
  pituitary (gland) (congenital) Q89.2
  pulmonary (not associated with short gestation) Q33.6
    artery, functional J43.0
    associated with short gestation P28.0
  radioulnar -*see* Defect, reduction, upper limb, specified type NEC
  radius -*see* Defect, reduction, upper limb
  rectum Q42.1
    with fistula Q42.0
  respiratory system NEC Q34.8
  rib Q76.6
  right heart syndrome Q22.6
  sacrum Q76.49
  scapula Q74.0
  scrotum Q55.1
  shoulder girdle Q74.0
  skin Q82.8
  skull (bone) Q75.8
    with

Hypoplasia, hypoplastic --*continued*
  anencephaly Q00.0
  encephalocele -*see* Encephalocele
  hydrocephalus Q03.9
    with spina bifida -*see* Spina bifida, by site, with hydrocephalus
  microcephaly Q02
  spinal (cord) (ventral horn cell) Q06.1
  spine Q76.49
  sternum Q76.7
  tarsus -*see* Defect, reduction, lower limb, specified type NEC
  testis Q55.1
  thymic, with immunodeficiency D82.1
  thymus (gland) Q89.2
    with immunodeficiency D82.1
  thyroid (gland) E03.1
    cartilage Q31.2
  tibiofibular (congenital) -*see* Defect, reduction, lower limb, specified type NEC
  toe -*see* Defect, reduction, lower limb, specified type NEC
  tongue Q38.3
  Turner's K00.4
  ulna (congenital) -*see* Defect, reduction, upper limb
  umbilical artery Q27.0
  unilateral condylar M27.8
  ureter Q62.8
  uterus, congenital Q51.811
  vagina Q52.4
  vascular NEC peripheral Q27.8
    brain Q28.3
    digestive system Q27.8
    lower limb Q27.8
    specified site NEC Q27.8
    upper limb Q27.8
  vein(s) (peripheral) Q27.8
    brain Q28.3
    digestive system Q27.8
    great Q26.8
    lower limb Q27.8
    specified site NEC Q27.8
    upper limb Q27.8
  vena cava (inferior) (superior) Q26.8
  vertebra Q76.49
  vulva, congenital Q52.79
  zonule (ciliary) Q12.8
Hypopotassemia E87.6
Hypoproconvertinemia, congenital (hereditary) D68.2
Hypoproteinemia E77.8
Hypoprothrombinemia (congenital) (hereditary) (idiopathic) D68.2
  acquired D68.4
  newborn, transient P61.6
Hypoptyalism K11.7
Hypopyon (eye) (anterior chamber) -*see* Iridocyclitis, acute, hypopyon
Hypopyrexia R68.0
Hyporeflexia R29.2
Hyposecretion
  ACTH E23.0
  antidiuretic hormone E23.2
  ovary E28.39
  salivary gland (any) K11.7
  vasopressin E23.2
Hyposegmentation, leukocytic, hereditary D72.0
Hyposiderinemia D50.9

Hypospadias Q54.9
  balanic Q54.0
  coronal Q54.0
  glandular Q54.0
  penile Q54.1
  penoscrotal Q54.2
  perineal Q54.3
  specified NEC Q54.8
Hypospermatogenesis -*see* Oligospermia
Hyposplenism D73.0
Hypostasis pulmonary, passive -*see* Edema, lung
Hypostatic -*see* condition
Hyposthenuria N28.89
Hypotension (arterial) (constitutional) I95.9
  chronic I95.89
  due to (of) hemodialysis I95.3
  drug-induced I95.2
  iatrogenic I95.89
  idiopathic (permanent) I95.0
  intracranial, following ventricular shunting (ventriculostomy) G97.2
  intra-dialytic I95.3
  maternal, syndrome (following labor and delivery) O26.5
  neurogenic, orthostatic G90.3
  orthostatic (chronic) I95.1
    due to drugs I95.2
    neurogenic G90.3
  postoperative I95.81
  postural I95.1
  specified NEC I95.89
Hypothermia (accidental) T68
  due to anesthesia, anesthetic T88.51
  low environmental temperature T68
  neonatal P80.9
    environmental (mild) NEC P80.8
    mild P80.8
    severe (chronic) (cold injury syndrome) P80.0
    specified NEC P80.8
  not associated with low environmental temperature R68.0
Hypothyroidism (acquired) E03.9
  congenital (without goiter) E03.1
    with goiter (diffuse) E03.0
  due to
    exogenous substance NEC E03.2
    iodine-deficiency, acquired E01.8
      subclinical E02
    irradiation therapy E89.0
    medicament NEC E03.2
    P-aminosalicylic acid (PAS) E03.2
    phenylbutazone E03.2
    resorcinol E03.2
    sulfonamide E03.2
    surgery E89.0
    thiourea group drugs E03.2
  iatrogenic NEC E03.2
  iodine-deficiency (acquired) E01.8
    congenital -*see* Syndrome, iodine-deficiency, congenital
    subclinical E02
  neonatal, transitory P72.2
  postinfectious E03.3
  postirradiation E89.0
  postprocedural E89.0
  postsurgical E89.0
  specified NEC E03.8
  subclinical, iodine-deficiency related E02

Hypotonia, hypotonicity, hypotony
bladder N31.2
congenital (benign) P94.2
eye -see Disorder, globe, hypotony
Hypotrichosis -see Alopecia
Hypotropia H50.2
Hypoventilation R06.89
congenital central alveolar G47.35
sleep related
idiopathic nonobstructive alveolar G47.34
in conditions classified elsewhere G47.36
Hypovitaminosis -see Deficiency, vitamin
Hypovolemia E86.1
surgical shock T81.19
traumatic (shock) T79.4
Hypoxemia R09.02
newborn P84
sleep related, in conditions classified
elsewhere G47.36
Hypoxia -see also Anoxia R09.02
cerebral, during a procedure NEC G97.81
postprocedural NEC G97.82
intrauterine P84
myocardial -see Insufficiency, coronary
newborn P84
sleep-related G47.34
Hypsarhythmia -see Epilepsy, generalized,
specified NEC
Hysteralgia, pregnant uterus O26.89
Hysteria, hysterical (conversion)
(dissociative state) F44.9
anxiety F41.8
convulsions F44.5
psychosis, acute F44.9
Hysteroepilepsy F44.5

I

IBDU (colonic inflammatory bowel disease
unclassified) K52.3
Ichthyoparasitism due to Vandellia cirrhosa
B88.8
Ichthyosis (congenital) Q80.9
acquired L85.0
fetalis Q80.4
hystrix Q80.8
lamellar Q80.2
lingual K13.29
palmaris and plantaris Q82.8
simplex Q80.0
vera Q80.8
vulgaris Q80.0
X linked Q80.1
Ichthyotoxism -see Poisoning, fish
bacterial -see Intoxication, foodborne
Icteroanemia, hemolytic (acquired) D59.9
congenital -see Spherocytosis
Icterus -see also Jaundice
conjunctiva R17
newborn P59.9
gravis, newborn P55.0
hematogenous (acquired) D59.9
hemolytic (acquired) D59.9
congenital -see Spherocytosis
hemorrhagic (acute) (leptospiral) (spirochetal)
A27.0
newborn P53
infectious B15.9
with hepatic coma B15.0
leptospiral A27.0
spirochetal A27.0
neonatorum -see Jaundice, newborn
spirochetal A27.0

Ictus solaris, solis T67.0
Ideation
homicidal R45.850
suicidal R45.851
Identity disorder (child) F64.9
gender role F64.2
psychosexual F64.2
Id reaction (due to bacteria) L30.2
Idioglossia F80.0
Idiopathic -see condition
Idiot, idiocy (congenital) F73
amaurotic (Bielschowsky(Jansky)) (family)
(infantile (late)) (juvenile (late)) (Vogt-
Spielmeyer) E75.4
microcephalic Q02
IgE asthma J45.909
IIAC (idiopathic infantile arterial
calcification) Q28.8
Ileitis (chronic) (noninfectious) -see also
Enteritis K52.9
backwash -see Pancolitis, ulcerative (chronic)
infectious A09
regional (ulcerative) -see Enteritis, regional,
small intestine
segmental -see Enteritis, regional
terminal (ulcerative) -see Enteritis, regional,
small intestine
Ileocolitis -see also Enteritis K52.9
regional -see Enteritis, regional
infectious A09
Ileostomy
attention to Z43.2
malfunctioning K94.13
status Z93.2
with complication -see Complications,
enterostomy
Ileotyphus -see Typhoid
Ileum -see condition
Ileus (bowel) (colon) (inhibitory) (intestine)
K56.7
adynamic K56.0
due to gallstone (in intestine) K56.3
duodenal (chronic) K31.5
gallstone K56.3
mechanical NEC K56.69
meconium P76.0
in cystic fibrosis E84.11
meaning meconium plug (without cystic
fibrosis) P76.0
myxedema K59.8
neurogenic K56.0
Hirschsprung's disease or megacolon Q43.1
newborn
due to meconium P76.0
in cystic fibrosis E84.11
meaning meconium plug (without cystic
fibrosis) P76.0
transitory P76.1
obstructive K56.69
paralytic K56.0
Iliac -see condition
Iliotibial band syndrome M76.3
Illiteracy Z55.0
Illness -see also Disease R69
manic-depressive -see Disorder, bipolar
Imbalance R26.89
autonomic G90.8
constituents of food intake E63.1
electrolyte E87.8
with

Imbalance --continued
abortion -see Abortion by type,
complicated by, electrolyte imbalance
molar pregnancy O08.5
due to hyperemesis gravidarum O21.1
following ectopic or molar pregnancy O08.5
neonatal, transitory NEC P74.4
potassium P74.3
sodium P74.2
endocrine E34.9
eye muscle NOS H50.9
hormone E34.9
hysterical F44.4
labyrinth -see subcategory H83.2
posture R29.3
protein-energy -see Malnutrition
sympathetic G90.8
Imbecile, imbecility (I.Q.35 49) F71
Imbedding, intrauterine device T83.39
Imbibition, cholesterol (gallbladder) K82.4
Imbrication, teeth,, fully erupted M26.30
Imerslund (Gräsbeck) syndrome D51.1
Immature -see also Immaturity
birth (less than 37
completed weeks) -see Preterm, newborn
extremely (less than 28
completed weeks) -see Immaturity, extreme -
personality F60.89
Immaturity (less than 37
completed weeks) -see also Preterm, newborn
extreme of newborn (less than 28
completed weeks of gestation) (less than 196
completed days of gestation)
(unspecified weeks of gestation) P07.20
gestational age
23 completed weeks (23 weeks, 0 days
through 23 weeks, 6 days) P07.22
24 completed weeks (24 weeks, 0 days
through 24 weeks, 6 days) P07.23
25 completed weeks (25 weeks, 0 days
through 25 weeks, 6 days) P07.24
26 completed weeks (26 weeks, 0 days
through 26 weeks, 6 days) P07.25
27 completed weeks (27 weeks, 0 days
through 27 weeks, 6 days) P07.26
less than 23 completed weeks P07.21
fetus or infant light-for-dates -see Light-for-
dates
lung, newborn P28.0
organ or site NEC -see Hypoplasia
pulmonary, newborn P28.0
reaction F60.89
sexual (female) (male), after puberty E30.0
Immersion T75.1
hand T69.01
foot T69.02
Immobile, immobility
complete, due to severe physical disability or
frailty R53.2
intestine K59.8
syndrome (paraplegic) M62.3
Immune reconstitution (inflammatory)
syndrome [IRIS] D89.3
Immunization -see also Vaccination
ABO -see Incompatibility, ABO
in newborn P55.1
complication -see Complications, vaccination
encounter for Z23
not done (not carried out) Z28.9
because (of)
acute illness of patient Z28.01

Immunization - *continued*
   allergy to vaccine (or component) Z28.04
   caregiver refusal Z28.82
   chronic illness of patient Z28.02
   contraindication NEC Z28.09
   group pressure Z28.1
   guardian refusal Z28.82
   immune compromised state of patient
      Z28.03
   parent refusal Z28.82
   patient's belief Z28.1
   patient had disease being vaccinated
      against Z28.81
   patient refusal Z28.21
   religious beliefs of patient Z28.1
   specified reason NEC Z28.89
      of patient Z28.29
   unspecified patient reason Z28.20
Rh factor
   affecting management of pregnancy NEC
      O36.09
      anti-D antibody O36.01
   from transfusion -*see* Complication(s),
   transfusion, incompatibility reaction, Rh
   (factor)
Immunocytoma C83.0
Immunodeficiency D84.9
with
   adenosine-deaminase deficiency D81.3
   antibody defects D80.9
      specified type NEC D80.8
   hyperimmunoglobulinemia D80.6
   increased immunoglobulin M (IgM) D80.5
   major defect D82.9
      specified type NEC D82.8
   partial albinism D82.8
   short-limbed stature D82.2
   thrombocytopenia and eczema D82.0
antibody with
   hyperimmunoglobulinemia D80.6
   near-normal immunoglobulins D80.6
autosomal recessive, Swiss type D80.0
combined D81.9
   biotin-dependent carboxylase D81.819
      biotinidase D81.810
      holocarboxylase synthetase D81.818
      specified type NEC D81.818
   severe (SCID) D81.9
      with
         low or normal B-cell numbers D81.2
         low T- and B-cell numbers D81.1
         reticular dysgenesis D81.0
   specified type NEC D81.89
common variable D83.9
   with
      abnormalities of B-cell numbers and
         function D83.0
      autoantibodies to B- or T-cells D83.2
      immunoregulatory T-cell disorders D83.1
   specified type NEC D83.8
following hereditary defective response to
   Epstein-Barr virus (EBV) D82.3
selective, immunoglobulin
   A (IgA) D80.2
   G (IgG) (subclasses) D80.3
   M (IgM) D80.4
severe combined (SCID) D81.9
specified type NEC D84.8
X linked, with increased IgM D80.5
Immunotherapy (encounter for)
   antineoplastic Z51.12

Impaction, impacted
   bowel, colon, rectum -*see also* Impaction,
      fecal K56.49
      by gallstone K56.3
   calculus -*see* Calculus
   cerumen (ear) (external) H61.2
   cuspid -*see* Impaction, tooth
   dental (same or adjacent tooth) K01.1
   fecal, feces K56.41
   fracture -*see* Fracture, by site
   gallbladder -*see* Calculus, gallbladder
   gallstone(s) -*see* Calculus, gallbladder
      bile duct (common) (hepatic) -*see* Calculus,
         bile duct
      cystic duct -*see* Calculus, gallbladder
      in intestine, with obstruction (any part)
         K56.3
   intestine (calculous) NEC -*see also*
      Impaction, fecal K56.49
      gallstone, with ileus K56.3
   intrauterine device (IUD) T83.39
   molar -*see* Impaction, tooth
   shoulder, causing obstructed labor O66.0
   tooth, teeth K01.1
   turbinate J34.89
Impaired, impairment (function)
   auditory discrimination -*see* Abnormal,
      auditory perception
   cognitive, mild, so stated G31.84
   dual sensory Z73.82
   fasting glucose R73.01
   glucose tolerance (oral) R73.02
   hearing -*see* Deafness
   heart -*see* Disease, heart
   kidney N28.9
      disorder resulting from N25.9
         specified NEC N25.89
   liver K72.90
      with coma K72.91
   mastication K08.89
   mild cognitive, so stated G31.84
   mobility
      ear ossicles -*see* Ankylosis, ear ossicles
      requiring care provider Z74.09
   myocardium, myocardial -*see* Insufficiency,
      myocardial
   rectal sphincter R19.8
   renal (acute) (chronic) N28.9
      disorder resulting from N25.9
         specified NEC N25.89
   vision NEC H54.7
      both eyes H54.3
Impediment, speech R47.9
   psychogenic (childhood) F98.8
   slurring R47.81
   specified NEC R47.89
Impending
   coronary syndrome I20.0
   delirium tremens F10.239
   myocardial infarction I20.0
Imperception auditory (acquired) -*see also*
   Deafness
   congenital H93.25
Imperfect
   aeration, lung (newborn) NEC -*see*
      Atelectasis
   closure (congenital)
      alimentary tract NEC Q45.8
         lower Q43.8
         upper Q40.8
      atrioventricular ostium Q21.2

Imperfect - *continued*
   atrium (secundum) Q21.1
   branchial cleft or sinus Q18.0
   choroid Q14.3
   cricoid cartilage Q31.8
   cusps, heart valve NEC Q24.8
      pulmonary Q22.3
   ductus
      arteriosus Q25.0
      Botalli Q25.0
   ear drum (causing impairment of hearing)
      Q16.4
   esophagus with communication to bronchus
      or trachea Q39.1
   eyelid Q10.3
   foramen
      botalli Q21.1
      ovale Q21.1
   genitalia, genital organ(s) or system
      female Q52.8
         external Q52.79
         internal NEC Q52.8
      male Q55.8
   glottis Q31.8
   interatrial ostium or septum Q21.1
   interauricular ostium or septum Q21.1
   interventricular ostium or septum Q21.0
   larynx Q31.8
   lip -*see* Cleft, lip
   nasal septum Q30.3
   nose Q30.2
   omphalomesenteric duct Q43.0
   optic nerve entry Q14.2
   organ or site not listed -*see* Anomaly, by site
   ostium
      interatrial Q21.1
      interauricular Q21.1
      interventricular Q21.0
   palate -*see* Cleft, palate
   preauricular sinus Q18.1
   retina Q14.1
   roof of orbit Q75.8
   sclera Q13.5
   septum
      aorticopulmonary Q21.4
      atrial (secundum) Q21.1
      between aorta and pulmonary artery Q21.4
      heart Q21.9
      interatrial (secundum) Q21.1
      interauricular (secundum) Q21.1
      interventricular Q21.0
         in tetralogy of Fallot Q21.3
      nasal Q30.3
      ventricular Q21.0
         with pulmonary stenosis or atresia,
            dextroposition of aorta, and hypertrophy
            of right ventricle Q21.3
         in tetralogy of Fallot Q21.3
   skull Q75.0
      with
         anencephaly Q00.0
         encephalocele -*see* Encephalocele
         hydrocephalus Q03.9
            with spina bifida -*see* Spina bifida, by
               site, with hydrocephalus
         microcephaly Q02
   spine (with meningocele) -*see* Spina bifida
   trachea Q32.1
   tympanic membrane (causing impairment of
      hearing) Q16.4
   uterus Q51.818

Imperfect - *continued*
  vitelline duct Q43.0
  erection -*see* Dysfunction, sexual, male,
    erectile
  fusion -*see* Imperfect, closure
  inflation, lung (newborn) -*see* Atelectasis
  posture R29.3
  rotation, intestine Q43.3
  septum, ventricular Q21.0
Imperfectly descended testis -*see* Cryptorchid
Imperforate (congenital) -*see also* Atresia
  anus Q42.3
    with fistula Q42.2
  cervix (uteri) Q51.828
  esophagus Q39.0
    with tracheoesophageal fistula Q39.1
  hymen Q52.3
  jejunum Q41.1
  pharynx Q38.8
  rectum Q42.1
    with fistula Q42.0
  urethra Q64.39
  vagina Q52.4
Impervious (congenital) -*see also* Atresia
  anus Q42.3
    with fistula Q42.2
  bile duct Q44.2
  esophagus Q39.0
    with tracheoesophageal fistula Q39.1
  intestine (small) Q41.9
    large Q42.9
      specified NEC Q42.8
  rectum Q42.1
    with fistula Q42.0
  ureter -*see* Atresia, ureter
  urethra Q64.39
Impetiginization of dermatoses L01.1
Impetigo (any organism) (any site)
  (circinate) (contagiosa) (simplex) (vulgaris)
  L01.00
  Bockhart's L01.02
  bullous, bullosa L01.03
  external ear L01.00 [*H62.40*]
  follicularis L01.02
  furfuracea L30.5
  herpetiformis L40.1
    nonobstetrical L40.1
  neonatorum L01.03
  nonbullous L01.01
  specified type NEC L01.09
  ulcerative L01.09
Impingement (on teeth)
  soft tissue
    anterior M26.81
    posterior M26.82
Implant, endometrial N80.9
Implantation
  anomalous -*see* Anomaly, by site
    ureter Q62.63
  cyst
    external area or site (skin) NEC L72.0
    iris -*see* Cyst, iris, implantation
    vagina N89.8
    vulva N90.7
  dermoid (cyst) -*see* Implantation, cyst
Impotence (sexual) N52.9
  counseling Z70.1
  organic origin -*see also* Dysfunction, sexual,
    male, erectile N52.9
  psychogenic F52.21
Impression, basilar Q75.8

Imprisonment, anxiety concerning Z65.1
Improper care (child) (newborn) -*see*
  Maltreatment
Improperly tied umbilical cord (causing
  hemorrhage) P51.8
Impulsiveness (impulsive) R45.87
Inability to swallow -*see* Aphagia
Inaccessible, inaccessibility
  health care NEC Z75.3
    due to
      waiting period Z75.2
        for admission to facility elsewhere Z75.1
    other helping agencies Z75.4
Inactive -*see* condition
Inadequate, inadequacy
  aesthetics of dental restoration K08.56
  biologic, constitutional, functional, or social
    F60.7
  development
    child R62.50
    genitalia
      after puberty NEC E30.0
      congenital
        female Q52.8
          external Q52.79
          internal Q52.8
        male Q55.8
    lungs Q33.6
      associated with short gestation P28.0
    organ or site not listed -*see* Anomaly, by site
  diet (causing nutritional deficiency) E63.9
  eating habits Z72.4
  environment, household Z59.1
  family support Z63.8
  food (supply) NEC Z59.4
    hunger effects T73.0
  functional F60.7
  household care, due to
    family member
      handicapped or ill Z74.2
      on vacation Z75.5
      temporarily away from home Z74.2
    technical defects in home Z59.1
    temporary absence from home of person
    rendering care Z74.2
  housing (heating) (space) Z59.1
  income (financial) Z59.6
  intrafamilial communication Z63.8
  material resources Z59.9
  mental -*see* Disability, intellectual
  parental supervision or control of child Z62.0
  personality F60.7
  pulmonary
    function R06.89
      newborn P28.5
    ventilation, newborn P28.5
  sample of cytologic smear
    anus R85.615
    cervix R87.615
    vagina R87.625
  social F60.7
    insurance Z59.7
    skills NEC Z73.4
  supervision of child by parent Z62.0
  teaching affecting education Z55.8
  welfare support Z59.7
Inanition R64
  with edema -*see* Malnutrition, severe
  due to
    deprivation of food T73.0
    malnutrition -*see* Malnutrition
  fever R50.9

Inappropriate
  change in quantitative human chorionic
    gonadotropin (hCG) in early pregnancy
    O02.81
  diet or eating habits Z72.4
  level of quantitative human chorionic
    gonadotropin (hCG) for gestational age in
    early pregnancy O02.81
  secretion
    antidiuretic hormone (ADH) (excessive)
    E22.2
    deficiency E23.2
    pituitary (posterior) E22.2
Inattention at or after birth -*see* Neglect
Incarceration, incarcerated
  enterocele K46.0
    gangrenous K46.1
  epiplocele K46.0
    gangrenous K46.1
  exomphalos K42.0
    gangrenous K42.1
  hernia -*see also* Hernia, by site, with
    obstruction
    with gangrene -*see* Hernia, by site, with
    gangrene
  iris, in wound -*see* Injury, eye, laceration,
    with prolapse
  lens, in wound -*see* Injury, eye, laceration,
    with prolapse
  omphalocele K42.0
  prison, anxiety concerning Z65.1
  rupture -*see* Hernia, by site
  sarcoepiplocele K46.0
    gangrenous K46.1
  sarcoepiplomphalocele K42.0
    with gangrene K42.1
  uterus N85.8
    gravid O34.51
      causing obstructed labor O65.5
Incised wound
  external -*see* Laceration
  internal organs -*see* Injury, by site
Incision, incisional
  hernia K43.2
    with
      gangrene (and obstruction) K43.1
      obstruction K43.0
  surgical, complication -*see* Complications,
    surgical procedure
  traumatic
    external -*see* Laceration
    internal organs -*see* Injury, by site
Inclusion
  azurophilic leukocytic D72.0
  blennorrhea (neonatal) (newborn) P39.1
  gallbladder in liver (congenital) Q44.1
Incompatibility
  ABO
    affecting management of pregnancy O36.11
      anti-A sensitization O36.11
      anti-B sensitization O36.19
      specified NEC O36.19
    infusion or transfusion reaction -*see*
    Complication(s), transfusion, incompatibility
    reaction, ABO
    newborn P55.1
  blood (group) (Duffy) (K(ell)) (Kidd) (Lewis)
    (M) (S) NEC
    affecting management of pregnancy O36.11
      anti-A sensitization O36.11
      anti-B sensitization O36.19

Incompatibility --*continued*
   infusion or transfusion reaction T80.89
      newborn P55.8
   divorce or estrangement Z63.5
   Rh (blood group) (factor) Z31.82
      affecting management of pregnancy NEC
         O36.09
         anti-D antibody O36.01
      infusion or transfusion reaction -*see*
         Complication(s), transfusion,
         incompatibility reaction, Rh (factor)
      newborn P55.0
   rhesus -*see* Incompatibility, Rh
Incompetency, incompetent, incompetence
   annular
      aortic (valve) -*see* Insufficiency, aortic
      mitral (valve) I34.0
      pulmonary valve (heart) I37.1
   aortic (valve) -*see* Insufficiency, aortic
   cardiac valve -*see* Endocarditis
   cervix, cervical (os) N88.3
      in pregnancy O34.3
   chronotropic I45.89
      with
         autonomic dysfunction G90.8
         ischemic heart disease I25.89
         left ventricular dysfunction I51.89
         sinus node dysfunction I49.8
   esophagogastric (junction) (sphincter) K22.0
   mitral (valve) -*see* Insufficiency, mitral
   pelvic fundus N81.89
   pubocervical tissue N81.82
   pulmonary valve (heart) I37.1
      congenital Q22.3
   rectovaginal tissue N81.83
   tricuspid (annular) (valve) -*see* Insufficiency,
      tricuspid
   valvular -*see* Endocarditis
      congenital Q24.8
   vein, venous (saphenous) (varicose) -*see*
      Varix, leg
Incomplete -*see also* condition
   bladder, emptying R33.9
   defecation R15.0
   expansion lungs (newborn) NEC -*see*
      Atelectasis
   rotation, intestine Q43.3
Inconclusive
   diagnostic imaging due to excess body fat of
      patient R93.9
   findings on diagnostic imaging of breast NEC
      R92.8
   mammogram (due to dense breasts) R92.2
Incontinence R32
   anal sphincter R15.9
   coital N39.491
   feces R15.9
      nonorganic origin F98.1
   insensible (urinary) N39.42
   overflow N39.490
   postural (urinary) N39.492
   psychogenic F45.8
   rectal R15.9
   reflex N39.498
   stress (female) (male) N39.3
      and urge N39.46
   urethral sphincter R32
   urge N39.41
      and stress (female) (male) N39.46
   urine (urinary) R32
      continuous N39.45

Incontinence --*continued*
   due to cognitive impairment, or severe
      physical disability or immobility R39.81
   functional R39.81
   insensible N39.42
   mixed (stress and urge) N39.46
   nocturnal N39.44
   nonorganic origin F98.0
   overflow N39.490
   post dribbling N39.43
   postural N39.492
   reflex N39.498
   specified NEC N39.498
   stress (female) (male) N39.3
      and urge N39.46
   total N39.498
   unaware N39.42
   urge N39.41
      and stress (female) (male) N39.46
Incontinentia pigmenti Q82.3
Incoordinate, incoordination
   esophageal-pharyngeal (newborn) -*see*
   Dysphagia
   muscular R27.8
   uterus (action) (contractions) (complicating
   delivery) O62.4
Increase, increased
   abnormal, in development R63.8
   androgens (ovarian) E28.1
   anticoagulants (antithrombin) (anti-VIIIa)
      (anti-IXa) (anti-Xa) (anti-XIa) -*see*
      Circulating anticoagulants
   cold sense R20.8
   estrogen E28.0
   function
      adrenal
         cortex -*see* Cushing's, syndrome
         medulla E27.5
      pituitary (gland) (anterior) (lobe) E22.9
         posterior E22.2
   heat sense R20.8
   intracranial pressure (benign) G93.2
   permeability, capillaries I78.8
   pressure, intracranial G93.2
   secretion
      gastrin E16.4
      glucagon E16.3
      pancreas, endocrine E16.9
         growth hormone-releasing hormone E16.8
         pancreatic polypeptide E16.8
         somatostatin E16.8
         vasoactive-intestinal polypeptide E16.8
   sphericity, lens Q12.4
   splenic activity D73.1
   venous pressure I87.8
      portal K76.6
Increta placenta O43.22
Incrustation, cornea, foreign body
   (lead)(zinc) -*see* Foreign body, cornea
Incyclophoria H50.54
Incyclotropia -*see* Cyclotropia **Indeterminate**
   sex Q56.4
India rubber skin Q82.8
Indigestion (acid) (bilious) (functional) K30
   catarrhal K31.89
   due to decomposed food NOS A05.9
   nervous F45.8
   psychogenic F45.8
Indirect -*see* condition
Induration penis plastica N48.6

Induration, indurated
   brain G93.89
   breast (fibrous) N64.51
      puerperal, postpartum O92.29
   broad ligament N83.8
   chancre
      anus A51.1
      congenital A50.07
      extragenital NEC A51.2
   corpora cavernosa (penis) (plastic) N48.6
   liver (chronic) K76.89
   lung (black) (chronic) (fibroid) -*see also*
      Fibrosis, lung J84.10
      essential brown J84.03
   penile (plastic) N48.6
   phlebitic -*see* Phlebitis
   skin R23.4
Inebriety (without dependence) -*see* Alcohol,
   intoxication
Inefficiency, kidney N28.9
Inelasticity, skin R23.4
Inequality, leg (length) (acquired) -*see also*
   Deformity, limb, unequal length
   congenital -*see* Defect, reduction, lower limb
   lower leg -*see* Deformity, limb, unequal
      length
Inertia
   bladder (neurogenic) N31.2
   stomach K31.89
      psychogenic F45.8
   uterus, uterine during labor O62.2
      during latent phase of labor O62.0
      primary O62.0
      secondary O62.1
   vesical (neurogenic) N31.2
Infancy, infantile, infantilism -*see also*
   condition
   celiac K90.0
   genitalia, genitals (after puberty) E30.0
   Herter's (nontropical sprue) K90.0
   intestinal K90.0
   Lorain E23.0
   pancreatic K86.89
   pelvis M95.5
      with disproportion (fetopelvic) O33.1
         causing obstructed labor O65.1
   pituitary E23.0
   renal N25.0
   uterus -*see* Infantile, genitalia
Infant(s) -*see also* Infancy
   excessive crying R68.11
   irritable child R68.12
   lack of care -*see* Neglect
   liveborn (singleton) Z38.2
      born in hospital Z38.00
         by cesarean Z38.01
      born outside hospital Z38.1
      multiple NEC Z38.8
         born in hospital Z38.68
            by cesarean Z38.69
         born outside hospital Z38.7
      quadruplet Z38.8
         born in hospital Z38.63
            by cesarean Z38.64
         born outside hospital Z38.7
      quintuplet Z38.8
         born in hospital Z38.65
            by cesarean Z38.66
         born outside hospital Z38.7
      triplet Z38.8
         born in hospital Z38.61

Infant(s) --*continued*
 by cesarean Z38.62
 born outside hospital Z38.7
 twin Z38.5
 born in hospital Z38.30
  by cesarean Z38.31
 born outside hospital Z38.4
 of diabetic mother (syndrome of) P70.1
 gestational diabetes P70.0
Infantile -*see also* condition
 genitalia, genitals E30.0
 os, uterine E30.0
 penis E30.0
 testis E29.1
 uterus E30.0
Infantilism -*see* Infancy
Infarct, infarction
 adrenal (capsule) (gland) E27.49
 appendices epiploicae -*see also* Infarct,
  intestine K55.069
 bowel -*see also* Infarct, intestine K55.069
 brain (stem) -*see* Infarct, cerebral
 breast N64.89
 brewer's (kidney) N28.0
 cardiac -*see* Infarct, myocardium
 cerebellar -*see* Infarct, cerebral
 cerebral -*see also* Occlusion, artery cerebral
 or precerebral, with infarction I63.9
  aborted I63.9
  cortical I63.9
  due to
   cerebral venous thrombosis, nonpyogenic
    I63.6
   embolism
    cerebral arteries I63.4
    precerebral arteries I63.1
   occlusion NEC
    cerebral arteries I63.5
    precerebral arteries I63.2
   stenosis NEC
    cerebral arteries I63.5
    precerebral arteries I63.2
   thrombosis
    cerebral artery I63.3
    precerebral artery I63.0
  intraoperative
   during cardiac surgery I97.810
   during other surgery I97.811
  postprocedural
   following cardiac surgery I97.820
   following other surgery I97.821
  specified NEC I63.8
 colon (acute) (agnogenic) (embolic)
  (hemorrhagic) (nonocclusive)
  (nonthrombotic) (occlusive) (segmental)
  (thrombotic)(with gangrene) -*see also*
  Infarct, intestine K55.049
 coronary artery -*see* Infarct, myocardium
 embolic -*see* Embolism
 fallopian tube N83.8
 gallbladder K82.8
 heart -*see* Infarct, myocardium
 hepatic K76.3
 hypophysis (anterior lobe) E23.6
 impending (myocardium) I20.0
 intestine (acute) (agnogenic) (embolic)
  (hemorrhagic) (nonocclusive)
  (nonthrombotic) (occlusive) (thrombotic)
  (with
 gangrene) K55.069
  diffuse K55.062

Infarct, infarction - *continued*
 focal K55.061
 large K55.049
  diffuse K55.042
  focal K55.041
 small K55.029
  diffuse K55.022
  focal K55.021
 kidney N28.0
 liver K76.3
 lung (embolic) (thrombotic) -*see* Embolism,
  pulmonary
 lymph node I89.8
 mesentery, mesenteric (embolic) (thrombotic)
  (with gangrene) -*see also* Infarct, intestine
  K55.069
 muscle (ischemic) M62.20
  ankle M62.27
  foot M62.27
  forearm M62.23
  hand M62.24
  lower leg M62.26
  pelvic region M62.25
  shoulder region M62.21
  specified site NEC M62.28
  thigh M62.25
  upper arm M62.22
 myocardium, myocardial (acute) (with stated
 duration of 4weeks or less) I21.3
 diagnosed on ECG, but presenting no
  symptoms I25.2
 healed or old I25.2
 intraoperative
  during cardiac surgery I97.790
  during other surgery I97.791
 non-Q wave I21.4
 non-ST elevation (NSTEMI) I21.4
  subsequent I22.2
 nontransmural I21.4
 past (diagnosed on ECG or other
  investigation, but currently presenting no
  symptoms) I25.2
 postprocedural
  following cardiac surgery I97.190
  following other surgery I97.191
 Q wave (see also, Infarct, myocardium, by
  site) I21.3
 ST elevation (STEMI) I21.3
  anterior (anteroapical) (anterolateral)
   (anteroseptal) (Q wave) (wall) I21.09
   subsequent I22.0
  inferior (diaphragmatic) (inferolateral)
   (inferoposterior) (wall) NEC I21.19
   subsequent I22.1
  inferoposterior transmural (Q wave) I21.11
  involving
   coronary artery of anterior wall NEC
    I21.09
   coronary artery of inferior wall NEC
    I21.19
   diagonal coronary artery I21.02
   left anterior descending coronary artery
    I21.02
   left circumflex coronary artery I21.21
   left main coronary artery I21.01
   oblique marginal coronary artery I21.21
   right coronary artery I21.11
  lateral (apical-lateral) (basal-lateral) (high)
   I21.29
   subsequent I22.8

Infarct, infarction - *continued*
 posterior (posterobasal) (posterolateral)
  (posteroseptal) (true) I21.29
  subsequent I22.8
 septal I21.29
  subsequent I22.8
 specified NEC I21.29
  subsequent I22.8
 subsequent I22.9
 subsequent (recurrent) (reinfarction) I22.9
  anterior (anteroapical) (anterolateral)
   (anteroseptal) (wall) I22.0
  diaphragmatic (wall) I22.1
  inferior (diaphragmatic) (inferolateral)
   (inferoposterior) (wall) I22.1
  lateral (apical-lateral) (basal-lateral) (high)
   I22.8
  non-ST elevation (NSTEMI) I22.2
  posterior (posterobasal) (posterolateral)
   (posteroseptal) (true) I22.8
  septal I22.8
  specified NEC I22.8
  ST elevation I22.9
   anterior (anteroapical) (anterolateral)
    (anteroseptal) (wall) I22.0
   inferior (diaphragmatic) (inferolateral)
    (inferoposterior) (wall) I22.1
   specified NEC I22.8
  subendocardial I22.2
  transmural I22.9
   anterior (anteroapical) (anterolateral)
    (anteroseptal) (wall) I22.0
   diaphragmatic (wall) I22.1
   inferior (diaphragmatic) (inferolateral)
    (inferoposterior) (wall) I22.1
   lateral (apical-lateral) (basal-lateral)
    (high) I22.8
   posterior (posterobasal) (posterolateral)
    (posteroseptal) (true) I22.8
   specified NEC I22.8
 syphilitic A52.06
 transmural I21.3
  anterior (anteroapical) (anterolateral)
   (anteroseptal) (Q wave) (wall) NEC
   I21.09
  inferior (diaphragmatic) (inferolateral)
   (inferoposterior) (Q wave) (wall) NEC
   I21.19
  inferoposterior (Q wave) I21.11
  lateral (apical-lateral) (basal-lateral) (high)
   NEC I21.29
  posterior (posterobasal) (posterolateral)
   (posteroseptal) (true) NEC I21.29
  septal NEC I21.29
  specified NEC I21.29
 nontransmural I21.4
 omentum -*see also* Infarct, intestine K55.069
 ovary N83.8
 pancreas K86.89
 papillary muscle -*see* Infarct, myocardium
 parathyroid gland E21.4
 pituitary (gland) E23.6
 placenta O43.81
 prostate N42.89
 pulmonary (artery) (vein) (hemorrhagic) -*see*
  Embolism, pulmonary
 renal (embolic) (thrombotic) N28.0
 retina, retinal (artery) -*see* Occlusion, artery,
  retina
 spinal (cord) (acute) (embolic) (nonembolic)
  G95.11

Infarct, infarction - *continued*
spleen D73.5
  embolic or thrombotic I74.8
subendocardial (acute) (nontransmural) I21.4
suprarenal (capsule) (gland) E27.49
testis N50.1
thrombotic -*see also* Thrombosis
  artery, arterial -*see* Embolism
thyroid (gland) E07.89
ventricle (heart) -*see* Infarct, myocardium
Infecting -*see* condition
Infection, infected, infective (opportunistic)
B99.9
with
  drug resistant organism -*see* Resistance (to),
    drug -*see also* specific organism
  lymphangitis -*see* Lymphangitis
  organ dysfunction (acute) R65.20
    with septic shock R65.21
abscess (skin)
code by site under Abscess
Absidia -*see* Mucormycosis
Acanthamoeba -*see* Acanthamebiasis
Acanthocheilonema (perstans) (streptocerca)
  B74.4
accessory sinus (chronic) -*see* Sinusitis
achorion -*see* Dermatophytosis
Acremonium falciforme B47.0
acromioclavicular M00.9
Actinobacillus (actinomycetem-comitans)
  A28.8
  mallei A24.0
  muris A25.1
Actinomadura B47.1
Actinomyces (israelii) -*see also*
  Actinomycosis A42.9
Actinomycetales -*see* Actinomycosis
actinomycotic NOS -*see* Actinomycosis
adenoid (and tonsil) J03.90
  chronic J35.02
adenovirus NEC
  as cause of disease classified elsewhere
    B97.0
  unspecified nature or site B34.0
aerogenes capsulatus A48.0
aertrycke -*see* Infection, salmonella
alimentary canal NOS -*see* Enteritis,
  infectious
Allescheria boydii B48.2
Alternaria B48.8
alveolus, alveolar (process) K04.7
Ameba, amebic (histolytica) -*see* Amebiasis
amniotic fluid, sac or cavity O41.10
  chorioamnionitis O41.12
  placentitis O41.14
amputation stump (surgical) -*see*
  Complication, amputation stump, infection
Ancylostoma (duodenalis) B76.0
Anisakiasis, Anisakis larvae B81.0
anthrax -*see* Anthrax
antrum (chronic) -*see* Sinusitis, maxillary
anus, anal (papillae) (sphincter) K62.89
arbovirus (arbor virus) A94
  specified type NEC A93.8
artificial insemination N98.0
Ascaris lumbricoides -*see* Ascariasis
Ascomycetes B47.0
Aspergillus (flavus) (fumigatus) (terreus) -*see*
  Aspergillosis
atypical

Infection, infected, infective continued
acid-fast (bacilli) -*see* Mycobacterium,
  atypical
  mycobacteria -*see* Mycobacterium, atypical
  virus A81.9
    specified type NEC A81.89
auditory meatus (external) -*see* Otitis, externa,
  infective
auricle (ear) -*see* Otitis, externa, infective
axillary gland (lymph) L04.2
Bacillus A49.9
  abortus A23.1
  anthracis -*see* Anthrax
  Ducrey's (any location) A57
  Flexner's A03.1
  Friedländer's NEC A49.8
  gas (gangrene) A48.0
  mallei A24.0
  melitensis A23.0
  paratyphoid, paratyphosus A01.4
    A A01.1
    B A01.2
    C A01.3
  Shiga (Kruse) A03.0
  suipestifer -*see* Infection, salmonella
  swimming pool A31.1
  typhosa A01.00
  welchii -*see* Gangrene, gas
bacterial NOS A49.9
  as cause of disease classified elsewhere
    B96.89
    Clostridium perfringens [C. perfringens]
      B96.7
    Bacteroides fragilis [B. fragilis] B96.6
    Enterobacter sakazakii B96.89
    Enterococcus B95.2
    Escherichia coli [E. coli]
  -*see also* Escherichia coli B96.20
    Helicobacter pylori [H. pylori] B96.81
    Hemophilus influenzae [H. influenzae]
      B96.3
    Klebsiella pneumoniae [K. pneumoniae]
      B96.1
    Mycoplasma pneumoniae [M.
      pneumoniae] B96.0
    Proteus (mirabilis) (morganii) B96.4
    Pseudomonas (aeruginosa) (mallei)
      (pseudomallei) B96.5
    Staphylococcus B95.8
      aureus (methicillin susceptible) (MSSA)
      B95.61
        methicillin resistant (MRSA) B95.62
      specified NEC B95.7
    Streptococcus B95.5
      group A B95.0
      group B B95.1
      pneumoniae B95.3
      specified NEC B95.4
    Vibrio vulnificus B96.82
    specified NEC A48.8
Bacterium
  paratyphosum A01.4
    A A01.1
    B A01.2
    C A01.3
  typhosum A01.00
Bacteroides NEC A49.8
  fragilis, as cause of disease classified
    elsewhere B96.6
Balantidium coli A07.0
Bartholin's gland N75.8

Infection, infected, infective continued
Basidiobolus B46.8
bile duct (common) (hepatic) -*see* Cholangitis
bladder -*see* Cystitis
Blastomyces, blastomycotic -*see also*
Blastomycosis
  brasiliensis -*see* Paracoccidioidomycosis
  dermatitidis -*see* Blastomycosis
  European -*see* Cryptococcosis
  Loboi B48.0
  North American B40.9
  South American -*see*
    Paracoccidioidomycosis
bleb, postprocedure -*see* Blebitis
bone -*see* Osteomyelitis
Bordetella -*see* Whooping cough
Borrelia bergdorfi A69.20
brain -*see also* Encephalitis G04.90
  membranes -*see* Meningitis
  septic G06.0
  meninges -*see* Meningitis, bacterial
branchial cyst Q18.0
breast -*see* Mastitis
bronchus -*see* Bronchitis
Brucella A23.9
  abortus A23.1
  canis A23.3
  melitensis A23.0
  mixed A23.8
  specified NEC A23.8
  suis A23.2
Brugia (malayi) B74.1
  timori B74.2
bursa -*see* Bursitis, infective
buttocks (skin) L08.9
Campylobacter, intestinal A04.5
  as cause of disease classified elsewhere
    B96.81
Candida (albicans) (tropicalis) -*see*
Candidiasis
candiru B88.8
Capillaria (intestinal) B81.1
  hepatica B83.8
  philippinensis B81.1
cartilage -*see* Disorder, cartilage, specified
  type NEC
catheter-related bloodstream (CRBSI)
  T80.211
cat liver fluke B66.0
cellulitis
code by site under Cellulitis
central line-associated T80.219
  bloodstream (CLABSI) T80.211
  specified NEC T80.218
Cephalosporium falciforme B47.0
cerebrospinal -*see* Meningitis
cervical gland (lymph) L04.0
cervix -*see* Cervicitis
cesarean delivery wound (puerperal) O86.0
cestodes -*see* Infestation, cestodes
chest J22
Chilomastix (intestinal) A07.8
Chlamydia, chlamydial A74.9
  anus A56.3
  genitourinary tract A56.2
    lower A56.00
    specified NEC A56.19
  lymphogranuloma A55
  pharynx A56.4
  psittaci A70
  rectum A56.3

Infection, infected, infective *continued*
  sexually transmitted NEC A56.8
  cholera -*see* Cholera
  Cladosporium
    bantianum (brain abscess) B43.1
    carrionii B43.0
    castellanii B36.1
    trichoides (brain abscess) B43.1
    werneckii B36.1
  Clonorchis (sinensis) (liver) B66.1
  Clostridium NEC
    bifermentans A48.0
    botulinum (food poisoning) A05.1
      infant A48.51
      wound A48.52
    difficile
      as cause of disease classified elsewhere B96.89
      foodborne (disease) A04.7
      gas gangrene A48.0
      necrotizing enterocolitis A04.7
      sepsis A41.4
    gas-forming NEC A48.0
    histolyticum A48.0
    novyi, causing gas gangrene A48.0
    oedematiens A48.0
    perfringens
      as cause of disease classified elsewhere B96.7
      due to food A05.2
      foodborne (disease) A05.2
      gas gangrene A48.0
      sepsis A41.4
    septicum, causing gas gangrene A48.0
    sordellii, causing gas gangrene A48.0
    welchii
      as cause of disease classified elsewhere B96.7
      foodborne (disease) A05.2
      gas gangrene A48.0
      necrotizing enteritis A05.2
      sepsis A41.4
  Coccidioides (immitis) -*see* Coccidioidomycosis
  colon -*see* Enteritis, infectious
  colostomy K94.02
  common duct -*see* Cholangitis
  congenital P39.9
    Candida (albicans) P37.5
    cytomegalovirus P35.1
    hepatitis, viral P35.3
    herpes simplex P35.2
    infectious or parasitic disease P37.9
      specified NEC P37.8
    listeriosis (disseminated) P37.2
    malaria NEC P37.4
      falciparum P37.3
    Plasmodium falciparum P37.3
    poliomyelitis P35.8
    rubella P35.0
    skin P39.4
    toxoplasmosis (acute) (subacute) (chronic) P37.1
    tuberculosis P37.0
    urinary (tract) P39.3
    vaccinia P35.8
    virus P35.9
      specified type NEC P35.8
  Conidiobolus B46.8
  coronavirus NEC B34.2

Infection, infected, infective *continued*
  as cause of disease classified elsewhere B97.29
    severe acute respiratory syndrome (SARS associated) B97.21
  corpus luteum -*see* Salpingo-oophoritis
  Corynebacterium diphtheriae -*see* Diphtheria
  cotia virus B08.8
  Coxiella burnetii A78
  coxsackie -*see* Coxsackie
  Cryptococcus neoformans -*see* Cryptococcosis
  Cryptosporidium A07.2
  Cunninghamella -*see* Mucormycosis
  cyst -*see* Cyst
  cystic duct -*see also* Cholecystitis K81.9
  Cysticercus cellulosae -*see* Cysticercosis
  cytomegalovirus, cytomegaloviral B25.9
    congenital P35.1
    maternal, maternal care for (suspected) damage to fetus O35.3
    mononucleosis B27.10
      with
        complication NEC B27.19
        meningitis B27.12
        polyneuropathy B27.11
  delta-agent (acute), in hepatitis B carrier B17.0
  dental (pulpal origin) K04.7
  Deuteromycetes B47.0
  Dicrocoelium dendriticum B66.2
  Dipetalonema (perstans) (streptocerca) B74.4
  diphtherial -*see* Diphtheria
  Diphyllobothrium (adult) (latum) (pacificum) B70.0
    larval B70.1
  Diplogonoporus (grandis) B71.8
  Dipylidium caninum B67.4
  Dirofilaria B74.8
  Dracunculus medinensis B72
  Drechslera (hawaiiensis) B43.8
  Ducrey Haemophilus (any location) A57
  due to or resulting from
    artificial insemination N98.0
    central venous catheter T80.219
      bloodstream T80.211
      exit or insertion site T80.212
      localized T80.212
      port or reservoir T80.212
      specified NEC T80.218
      tunnel T80.212
    device, implant or graft -*see also*
  Complications, by site and type, infection or inflammation T85.79
      arterial graft NEC T82.7
      breast (implant) T85.79
      catheter NEC T85.79
        dialysis (renal) T82.7
          intraperitoneal T85.71
        infusion NEC T82.7
          cranial T85.735
          intrathecal T85.735
          spinal (epidural) (subdural) T85.735
          subarachnoid T85.735
        urinary T83.518
          cystostomy T83.510
          Hopkins T83.518
          ileostomy T83.518
          nephrostomy T83.512
          specified NEC T83.518
          urethral indwelling T83.511

Infection, infected, infective *continued*
      urostomy T83.518
    electronic (electrode) (pulse generator) (stimulator)
      bone T84.7
      cardiac T82.7
      nervous system T85.738
        brain T85.731
        cranial nerve T85.732
        gastric nerve T85.732
        generator pocket T85.734
        neurostimulator generator T85.734
        peripheral nerve T85.732
        sacral nerve T85.732
        spinal cord T85.733
        vagal nerve T85.732
      urinary T83.590
    fixation, internal (orthopedic) NEC -*see* Complication, fixation device, infection
    gastrointestinal (bile duct) (esophagus) T85.79
      neurostimulator electrode (lead) T85.732
    genital NEC T83.69
    heart NEC T82.7
      valve (prosthesis) T82.6
      graft T82.7
    joint prosthesis -*see* Complication, joint prosthesis, infection
    ocular (corneal graft) (orbital implant) NEC T85.79
    orthopedic NEC T84.7
    penile (cylinder) (pump) (reservoir) T83.61
    specified NEC T85.79
    testicular T83.62
    urinary NEC T83.598
      ileal conduit stent T83.593
      implanted neurostimulation T83.590
      implanted sphincter T83.591
      indwelling ureteral stent T83.592
      nephroureteral stent T83.593
      specified stent NEC T83.593
    vascular NEC T82.7
    ventricular intracranial (communicating) shunt T85.730
    Hickman catheter T80.219
      bloodstream T80.211
      localized T80.212
      specified NEC T80.218
    immunization or vaccination T88.0
    infusion, injection or transfusion NEC T80.29
      acute T80.22
    injury NEC
  code by site under Wound, open
    peripherally inserted central catheter (PICC) T80.219
      bloodstream T80.211
      localized T80.212
      specified NEC T80.218
    portacath (port-a-cath) T80.219
      bloodstream T80.211
      localized T80.212
      specified NEC T80.218
    pulmonary artery catheter -*see* Infection, due to or resulting from, central venous catheter
    surgery T81.40
    Swan Ganz catheter -*see* Infection, due to or resulting from, central venous catheter
    triple lumen catheter T80.219
      bloodstream T80.211

Infection, infected, infective *continued*
    localized T80.212
    specified NEC T80.218
    umbilical venous catheter T80.219
      bloodstream T80.211
      localized T80.212
      specified NEC T80.218
  during labor NEC O75.3
  ear (middle) -*see also* Otitis media
    external -*see* Otitis, externa, infective
    inner -*see* subcategory H83.0
  Eberthella typhosa A01.00
  Echinococcus -*see* Echinococcus
  echovirus
    as cause of disease classified elsewhere
      B97.12
    unspecified nature or site B34.1
  endocardium I33.0
  endocervix -*see* Cervicitis
  Entamoeba -*see* Amebiasis
  enteric -*see* Enteritis, infectious
  Enterobacter sakazakii B96.89
  Enterobius vermicularis B80
  enterostomy K94.12
  enterovirus B34.1
    as cause of disease classified elsewhere
      B97.10
      coxsackievirus B97.11
      echovirus B97.12
      specified NEC B97.19
  Entomophthora B46.8
  Epidermophyton -*see* Dermatophytosis
  epididymis -*see* Epididymitis
  episiotomy (puerperal) O86.0
  Erysipelothrix (insidiosa) (rhusiopathiae) -*see*
    Erysipeloid
  erythema infectiosum B08.3
  Escherichia (E.) coli NEC A49.8
    as cause of disease classified elsewhere -*see*
      also Escherichia coli B96.20
    congenital P39.8
      sepsis P36.4
    generalized A41.51
    intestinal -*see* Enteritis, infectious, due to,
      Escherichia coli
  ethmoidal (chronic) (sinus) -*see* Sinusitis,
    ethmoidal
  eustachian tube (ear) -*see* Salpingitis,
    eustachian
  external auditory canal (meatus) NEC -*see*
    Otitis, externa, infective
  eye (purulent) -*see* Endophthalmitis, purulent
  eyelid -*see* Inflammation, eyelid
  fallopian tube -*see* Salpingo-oophoritis
  Fasciola (gigantica) (hepatica) (indica) B66.3
  Fasciolopsis (buski) B66.5
  filarial -*see* Infestation, filarial
  finger (skin) L08.9
    nail L03.01
      fungus B35.1
  fish tapeworm B70.0
    larval B70.1
  flagellate, intestinal A07.9
  fluke -*see* Infestation, fluke
  focal
    teeth (pulpal origin) K04.7
    tonsils J35.01
  Fonsecaea (compactum) (pedrosoi) B43.0
  food -*see* Intoxication, foodborne
  foot (skin) L08.9
    dermatophytic fungus B35.3

Infection, infected, infective *continued*
  Francisella tularensis -*see* Tularemia
  frontal (sinus) (chronic) -*see* Sinusitis, frontal
  fungus NOS B49
    beard B35.0
    dermatophytic -*see* Dermatophytosis
    foot B35.3
    groin B35.6
    hand B35.2
    nail B35.1
    pathogenic to compromised host only B48.8
    perianal (area) B35.6
    scalp B35.0
    skin B36.9
      foot B35.3
      hand B35.2
      toenails B35.1
  Fusarium B48.8
  gallbladder -*see* Cholecystitis
  gas bacillus -*see* Gangrene, gas
  gastrointestinal -*see* Enteritis, infectious
  generalized NEC -*see* Sepsis
  generator pocket, implanted electronic
    neurostimulator T85.734
  genital organ or tract
    female -*see* Disease, pelvis, inflammatory
    male N49.9
      multiple sites N49.8
      specified NEC N49.8
  Ghon tubercle, primary A15.7
  Giardia lamblia A07.1
  gingiva (chronic) K05.10
    acute K05.00
      nonplaque induced K05.01
      plaque induced K05.00
    nonplaque induced K05.11
    plaque induced K05.10
  glanders A24.0
  glenosporosis B48.0
  Gnathostoma (spinigerum) B83.1
  Gongylonema B83.8
  gonococcal -*see* Gonococcus
  gram-negative bacilli NOS A49.9
  guinea worm B72
  gum (chronic) K05.10
    acute K05.00
      nonplaque induced K05.01
      plaque induced K05.00
    nonplaque induced K05.11
    plaque induced K05.10
  Haemophilus -*see* Infection, Hemophilus
  heart -*see* Carditis
  Helicobacter pylori A04.8
    as cause of disease classified elsewhere
      B96.81
  helminths B83.9
    intestinal B82.0
      mixed (types classifiable to more than one
        of the titles B65.0 B81.3 and B81.8)
        B81.4
      specified type NEC B81.8
    specified type NEC B83.8
  Hemophilus
    aegyptius, systemic A48.4
    Ducrey (any location) A57
    influenzae NEC A49.2
      as cause of disease classified elsewhere
        B96.3
      generalized A41.3
  herpes (simplex) -*see also* Herpes
    congenital P35.2

Infection, infected, infective *continued*
    disseminated B00.7
    zoster B02.9
  herpesvirus, herpesviral -*see* Herpes
  hip (joint) NEC M00.9
    due to internal joint prosthesis
      left T84.52
      right T84.51
    skin NEC L08.9
  Heterophyes (heterophyes) B66.8
  Histoplasma -*see* Histoplasmosis
    American B39.4
    capsulatum B39.4
  hookworm B76.9
  Hymenolepis B71.0
  hypopharynx -*see* Pharyngitis
  human
    papilloma virus A63.0
    T-cell lymphotropic virus type-1(HTLV-1)
      B33.3
  hydrocele N43.0
  Hymenolepis B71.0
  hypopharynx -*see* Pharyngitis
  inguinal (lymph) glands L04.1
    due to soft chancre A57
  intervertebral disc, pyogenic M46.30
    cervical region M46.32
    cervicothoracic region M46.33
    lumbar region M46.36
    lumbosacral region M46.37
    multiple sites M46.39
    occipito-atlanto-axial region M46.31
    sacrococcygeal region M46.38
    thoracic region M46.34
    thoracolumbar region M46.35
  intestine, intestinal -*see* Enteritis, infectious
    specified NEC A08.8
  intra-amniotic affecting newborn NEC P39.2
  Isospora belli or hominis A07.3
  Japanese B encephalitis A83.0
  jaw (bone) (lower) (upper) M27.2
  joint NEC M00.9
    due to internal joint prosthesis T84.50
  kidney (cortex) (hematogenous) N15.9
    with calculus N20.0
      with hydronephrosis N13.6
    following ectopic gestation O08.83
    pelvis and ureter (cystic) N28.85
    puerperal (postpartum) O86.21
    specified NEC N15.8
  Klebsiella (K.) pneumoniae NEC A49.8
    as cause of disease classified elsewhere
      B96.1
  knee (joint) NEC M00.9
    joint M00.9
    due to internal joint prosthesis
      left T84.54
      right T84.53
    skin L08.9
  Koch's -*see* Tuberculosis
  labia (majora) (minora) (acute) -*see* Vulvitis
  lacrimal
    gland -*see* Dacryoadenitis
    passages (duct) (sac) -*see* Inflammation,
    lacrimal, passages
  lancet fluke B66.2
  larynx NEC J38.7
  leg (skin) NOS L08.9
  Legionella pneumophila A48.1
    nonpneumonic A48.2
  Leishmania -*see also* Leishmaniasis
    aethiopica B55.1
    braziliensis B55.2

Infection, infected, infective continued
- chagasi B55.0
- donovani B55.0
- infantum B55.0
- major B55.1
- mexicana B55.1
- tropica B55.1
- lentivirus, as cause of disease classified elsewhere B97.31
- Leptosphaeria senagalensis B47.0
- Leptospira interrogans A27.9
  - autumnalis A27.89
  - canicola A27.89
  - hebdomadis A27.89
  - icterohaemorrhagiae A27.0
  - pomona A27.89
  - specified type NEC A27.89
- leptospirochetal NEC -see Leptospirosis
- Listeria monocytogenes -see also Listeriosis
  - congenital P37.2
- Loa loa B74.3
  - with conjunctival infestation B74.3
  - eyelid B74.3
- Loboa loboi B48.0
- local, skin (staphylococcal) (streptococcal) L08.9
  - abscess
  - code by site under Abscess
  - cellulitis
  - code by site under Cellulitis
  - specified NEC L08.89
  - ulcer -see Ulcer, skin
- Loefflerella mallei A24.0
- lung -see also Pneumonia J18.9
  - atypical Mycobacterium A31.0
  - spirochetal A69.8
  - tuberculous -see Tuberculosis, pulmonary
  - virus -see Pneumonia, viral
- lymph gland -see also Lymphadenitis, acute
  - mesenteric I88.0
- lymphoid tissue, base of tongue or posterior pharynx, NEC (chronic) J35.03
- Madurella (grisea) (mycetomii) B47.0
- major
  - following ectopic or molar pregnancy O08.0
  - puerperal, postpartum, childbirth O85
- Malassezia furfur B36.0
- Malleomyces
  - mallei A24.0
  - pseudomallei (whitmori) -see Melioidosis
- mammary gland N61.0
- Mansonella (ozzardi) (perstans) (streptocerca) B74.4
- mastoid -see Mastoiditis
- maxilla, maxillary M27.2
- sinus (chronic) -see Sinusitis, maxillary
- mediastinum J98.51
- Medina (worm) B72
- meibomian cyst or gland -see Hordeolum
- meninges -see Meningitis, bacterial
- meningococcal -see also condition A39.9
  - adrenals A39.1
  - brain A39.81
  - cerebrospinal A39.0
  - conjunctiva A39.89
  - endocardium A39.51
  - heart A39.50
    - endocardium A39.51
    - myocardium A39.52
    - pericardium A39.53
  - joint A39.83

Infection, infected, infective continued
- meninges A39.0
- meningococcemia A39.4
  - acute A39.2
  - chronic A39.3
- myocardium A39.52
- pericardium A39.53
- retrobulbar neuritis A39.82
- specified site NEC A39.89
- mesenteric lymph nodes or glands NEC I88.0
- Metagonimus B66.8
- metatarsophalangeal M00.9
- methicillin
  - resistant Staphylococcus aureus (MRSA) A49.02
  - susceptible Staphylococcus aureus (MSSA) A49.01
- Microsporum, microsporic -see Dermatophytosis
- mixed flora (bacterial) NEC A49.8
- Monilia -see Candidiasis
- Monosporium apiospermum B48.2
- mouth, parasitic B37.0
- Mucor -see Mucormycosis
- muscle NEC -see Myositis, infective
- mycelium NOS B49
- mycetoma B47.9
  - actinomycotic NEC B47.1
  - mycotic NEC B47.0
- Mycobacterium, mycobacterial -see Mycobacterium
- Mycoplasma NEC A49.3
  - pneumoniae, as cause of disease classified elsewhere B96.0
- mycotic NOS B49
  - pathogenic to compromised host only B48.8
  - skin NOS B36.9
- myocardium NEC I40.0
- nail (chronic)
  - with lymphangitis -see Lymphangitis, acute, digit
  - finger L03.01
    - fungus B35.1
  - ingrowing L60.0
  - toe L03.03
    - fungus B35.1
- nasal sinus (chronic) -see Sinusitis
- nasopharynx -see Nasopharyngitis
- navel L08.82
- Necator americanus B76.1
- Neisseria -see Gonococcus
- Neotestudina rosatii B47.0
- newborn P39.9
  - intra-amniotic NEC P39.2
  - skin P39.4
  - specified type NEC P39.8
- nipple N61.0
  - associated with
    - lactation O91.03
    - pregnancy O91.01
    - puerperium O91.02
- Nocardia -see Nocardiosis
- obstetrical surgical wound (puerperal) O86.0
- Oesophagostomum (apiostomum) B81.8
- Oestrus ovis -see Myiasis
- Oidium albicans B37.9
- Onchocerca (volvulus) -see Onchocerciasis
- oncovirus, as cause of disease classified elsewhere B97.32
- operation wound T81.40
- Opisthorchis (felineus) (viverrini) B66.0

Infection, infected, infective continued
- orbit, orbital -see Inflammation, orbit
- orthopoxvirus NEC B08.09
- ovary -see Salpingo-oophoritis
- Oxyuris vermicularis B80
- pancreas (acute) -see Pancreatitis, acute
  - abscess -see Pancreatitis, acute
  - specified NEC -see also Pancreatitis, acute K85.80
- papillomavirus, as cause of disease classified elsewhere B97.7
- papovavirus NEC B34.4
- Paracoccidioides brasiliensis -see Paracoccidioidomycosis
- Paragonimus (westermani) B66.4
- parainfluenza virus B34.8
- parameningococcus NOS A39.9
- parapoxvirus B08.60
  - specified NEC B08.69
- parasitic B89
- Parastrongylus
  - cantonensis B83.2
  - costaricensis B81.3
- paratyphoid A01.4
  - Type A A01.1
  - Type B A01.2
  - Type C A01.3
- paraurethral ducts N34.2
- parotid gland -see Sialoadenitis
- parvovirus NEC B34.3
  - as cause of disease classified elsewhere B97.6
- Pasteurella NEC A28.0
  - multocida A28.0
  - pestis -see Plague
  - pseudotuberculosis A28.0
  - septica (cat bite) (dog bite) A28.0
  - tularensis -see Tularemia
- pelvic, female -see Disease, pelvis, inflammatory Penicillium (marneffei) B48.4
- penis (glans) (retention) NEC N48.29
- periapical K04.5
- peridental, periodontal K05.20
  - generalized -see Peridontitis, aggressive, generalized
  - localized -see Peridontitis, aggressive, localized
- perinatal period P39.9
  - specified type NEC P39.8
- perineal repair (puerperal) O86.0
- periorbital -see Inflammation, orbit
- perirectal K62.89
- perirenal -see Infection, kidney peritoneal -see Peritonitis
- periureteral N28.89
- Petriellidium boydii B48.2
- pharynx -see also Pharyngitis
  - coxsackievirus B08.5
  - posterior, lymphoid (chronic) J35.03
- Phialophora
  - gougerotii (subcutaneous abscess or cyst) B43.2
  - jeanselmei (subcutaneous abscess or cyst) B43.2
  - verrucosa (skin) B43.0
- Piedraia hortae B36.3
- pinta A67.9
  - intermediate A67.1
  - late A67.2
  - mixed A67.3

Infection, infected, infective *continued*
  primary A67.0
  pinworm B80
  pityrosporum furfur B36.0
  pleuro-pneumonia-like organism (PPLO)
    NEC A49.3
    as cause of disease classified elsewhere
      B96.0
  pneumococcus, pneumococcal NEC A49.1
    as cause of disease classified elsewhere
      B95.3
    generalized (purulent) A40.3
      with pneumonia J13
  Pneumocystis carinii (pneumonia) B59
  Pneumocystis jiroveci (pneumonia) B59
  port or reservoir T80.212
  postoperative T81.40
  postoperative wound T81.40
  postprocedural T81.40
    deep incisional surgical site T81.42
    organ and space surgical site T81.43
    sepsis T81.49
    specified surgical site NEC T81.48
    superficial incisional surgical site T81.41
  postvaccinal T88.0
  prepuce NEC N47.7
    with penile inflammation N47.6
  prion -*see* Disease, prion, central nervous
    system
  prostate (capsule) -*see* Prostatitis
  Proteus (mirabilis) (morganii) (vulgaris) NEC
    A49.8
    as cause of disease classified elsewhere
      B96.4
  protozoal NEC B64
    intestinal A07.9
      specified NEC A07.8
    specified NEC B60.8
  Pseudoallescheria boydii B48.2
  Pseudomonas NEC A49.8
    as cause of disease classified elsewhere
      B96.5
    mallei A24.0
    pneumonia J15.1
    pseudomallei -*see* Melioidosis
  puerperal O86.4
    genitourinary tract NEC O86.89
    major or generalized O85
    minor O86.4
    specified NEC O86.89
  pulmonary -*see* Infection, lung
  purulent -*see* Abscess
  Pyrenochaeta romeroi B47.0
  Q fever A78
  rectum (sphincter) K62.89
  renal -*see also* Infection, kidney
    pelvis and ureter (cystic) N28.85
  reovirus, as cause of disease classified
    elsewhere B97.5
  respiratory (tract) NEC J98.8
    acute J22
    chronic J98.8
    influenzal (upper) (acute) -*see* Influenza,
      with, respiratory manifestations NEC
    lower (acute) J22
      chronic -*see* Bronchitis, chronic
    rhinovirus J00
    syncytial virus, as cause of disease classified
      elsewhere B97.4
    upper (acute) NOS J06.9
      chronic J39.8

Infection, infected, infective *continued*
    streptococcal J06.9
    viral NOS J06.9
  resulting from
    presence of internal prosthesis, implant,
      graft -*see* Complications, by site and type,
      infection
  retortamoniasis A07.8
  retroperitoneal NEC K68.9
  retrovirus B33.3
    as cause of disease classified elsewhere
      B97.30
      human
        immunodeficiency, type 2 (HIV 2)
          B97.35
        T-cell lymphotropic
          type I (HTLV-I) B97.33
          type II (HTLV-II) B97.34
      lentivirus B97.31
      oncovirus B97.32
      specified NEC B97.39
  Rhinosporidium (seeberi) B48.1
  rhinovirus
    as cause of disease classified elsewhere
      B97.89
    unspecified nature or site B34.8
  Rhizopus -*see* Mucormycosis
  rickettsial NOS A79.9
  roundworm (large) NEC B82.0
    Ascariasis -*see also* Ascariasis B77.9
  rubella -*see* Rubella
  Saccharomyces -*see* Candidiasis
  salivary duct or gland (any) -*see* Sialoadenitis
  Salmonella (aertrycke) (arizonae)
    (callinarum) (cholerae-suis) (enteritidis)
    (suipestifer) (typhimurium) A02.9
    with
      (gastro) enteritis A02.0
      sepsis A02.1
      specified manifestation NEC A02.8
    due to food (poisoning) A02.9
    hirschfeldii A01.3
    localized A02.20
      arthritis A02.23
      meningitis A02.21
      osteomyelitis A02.24
      pneumonia A02.22
      pyelonephritis A02.25
      specified NEC A02.29
    paratyphi A01.4
      A A01.1
      B A01.2
      C A01.3
    schottmuelleri A01.2
    typhi, typhosa -*see* Typhoid
  Sarcocystis A07.8
  scabies B86
  Schistosoma -*see* Infestation, Schistosoma
  scrotum (acute) NEC N49.2
  seminal vesicle -*see* Vesiculitis
  septic
    localized, skin -*see* Abscess
  sheep liver fluke B66.3
  Shigella A03.9
    boydii A03.2
    dysenteriae A03.0
    flexneri A03.1
    group
      A A03.0
      B A03.1
      C A03.2

Infection, infected, infective *continued*
    D A03.3
    Schmitz (Stutzer) A03.0
    schmitzii A03.0
    shigae A03.0
    sonnei A03.3
    specified NEC A03.8
  shoulder (joint) NEC M00.9
    due to internal joint prosthesis T84.59
    skin NEC L08.9
  sinus (accessory) (chronic) (nasal) -*see also*
    Sinusitis
    pilonidal -*see* Sinus, pilonidal
    skin NEC L08.89
  Skene's duct or gland -*see* Urethritis
  skin (local) (staphylococcal) (streptococcal)
    L08.9
    abscess
      code by site under Abscess
    cellulitis
      code by site under Cellulitis
    due to fungus B36.9
      specified type NEC B36.8
    mycotic B36.9
      specified type NEC B36.8
    newborn P39.4
    ulcer -*see* Ulcer, skin
  slow virus A81.9
    specified NEC A81.89
  Sparganum (mansoni) (proliferum) (baxteri)
    B70.1
  specific -*see also* Syphilis
    to perinatal period -*see* Infection, congenital
  specified NEC B99.8
  spermatic cord NEC N49.1
  sphenoidal (sinus) -*see* Sinusitis, sphenoidal
  spinal cord NOS -*see also* Myelitis G04.91
    abscess G06.1
    meninges -*see* Meningitis
    streptococcal G04.89
  Spirillum A25.0
  spirochetal NOS A69.9
    lung A69.8
    specified NEC A69.8
  Spirometra larvae B70.1
  spleen D73.89
  Sporotrichum, Sporothrix (schenckii) -*see*
    Sporotrichosis
  staphylococcal, unspecified site
    aureus (methicillin susceptible) (MSSA)
      A49.01
      methicillin resistant (MRSA) A49.02
    as cause of disease classified elsewhere
      B95.8
      aureus (methicillin susceptible) (MSSA)
        B95.61
        methicillin resistant (MRSA) B95.62
        specified NEC B95.7
    food poisoning A05.0
    generalized (purulent) A41.2
    pneumonia -*see* Pneumonia, staphylococcal
  Stellantchasmus falcatus B66.8
  streptobacillus moniliformis A25.1
  streptococcal NEC A49.1
    as cause of disease classified elsewhere
      B95.5
    B genitourinary complicating
      childbirth O98.82
      pregnancy O98.81
      puerperium O98.83
    congenital

Infection, infected, infective continued

  sepsis P36.10
    group B P36.0
    specified NEC P36.19
  generalized (purulent) A40.9
  Streptomyces B47.1
  Strongyloides (stercoralis) -see
    Strongyloidiasis
  stump (amputation) (surgical) -see
    Complication, amputation stump, infection
  subcutaneous tissue, local L08.9
  suipestifer -see Infection, salmonella
  swimming pool bacillus A31.1
  Taenia -see Infestation, Taenia
  Taeniarhynchus saginatus B68.1
  tapeworm -see Infestation, tapeworm
  tendon (sheath) -see Tenosynovitis, infective
    NEC
  Ternidens diminutus B81.8
  testis -see Orchitis
  threadworm B80
  throat -see Pharyngitis
  thyroglossal duct K14.8
  toe (skin) L08.9
    cellulitis L03.03
      fungus B35.1
    nail L03.03
      fungus B35.1
  tongue NEC K14.0
    parasitic B37.0
  tonsil (and adenoid) (faucial) (lingual)
    (pharyngeal) -see Tonsillitis
  tooth, teeth K04.7
    periapical K04.7
    peridental, periodontal K05.20
      generalized -see Peridontitis, aggressive,
      generalized
      localized -see Peridontitis, aggressive,
      localized
    pulp K04.01
    irreversible K04.02
    reversible K04.01
    socket M27.3
  TORCH -see Infection, congenital
    without active infection P00.2
  Torula histolytica -see Cryptococcosis
  Toxocara (canis) (cati) (felis) B83.0
  Toxoplasma gondii -see Toxoplasma
  trachea, chronic J42
  trematode NEC -see Infestation, fluke
  trench fever A79.0
  Treponema pallidum -see Syphilis
  Trichinella (spiralis) B75
  Trichomonas A59.9
    cervix A59.09
    intestine A07.8
    prostate A59.02
    specified site NEC A59.8
    urethra A59.03
    urogenitalis A59.00
    vagina A59.01
    vulva A59.01
  Trichophyton, trichophytic -see
    Dermatophytosis
  Trichosporon (beigelii) cutaneum B36.2
  Trichostrongylus B81.2
  Trichuris (trichiura) B79
  Trombicula (irritans) B88.0
  Trypanosoma
    brucei
      gambiense B56.0

Infection, infected, infective continued

    rhodesiense B56.1
    cruzi -see Chagas' disease
  tubal -see Salpingo-oophoritis
  tuberculous NEC -see Tuberculosis
  tubo-ovarian -see Salpingo-oophoritis
  tunnel T80.212
  tunica vaginalis N49.1
  tympanic membrane NEC -see Myringitis
  typhoid (abortive) (ambulant) (bacillus) -see
    Typhoid
  typhus A75.9
    flea-borne A75.2
    mite-borne A75.3
    recrudescent A75.1
    tick-borne A77.9
      African A77.1
      North Asian A77.2
  umbilicus L08.82
  ureter N28.86
  urethra -see Urethritis
  urinary (tract) N39.0
    bladder -see Cystitis
    complicating
      pregnancy O23.4
        specified type NEC O23.3
    kidney -see Infection, kidney
    newborn P39.3
    puerperal (postpartum) O86.20
    tuberculous A18.13
    urethra -see Urethritis
  uterus, uterine -see Endometritis
  vaccination T88.0
  vaccinia not from vaccination B08.011
  vagina (acute) -see Vaginitis
  varicella B01.9
  varicose veins -see Varix
  vas deferens NEC N49.1
  vesical -see Cystitis
  Vibrio
    cholerae A00.0
      El Tor A00.1
    parahaemolyticus (food poisoning) A05.3
    vulnificus
      as cause of disease classified elsewhere
      B96.82
      foodborne intoxication A05.5
  Vincent's (gum) (mouth) (tonsil) A69.1
  virus, viral NOS B34.9
    adenovirus
      as cause of disease classified elsewhere
      B97.0
      unspecified nature or site B34.0
    arborvirus, arbovirus arthropod-borne A94
    as cause of disease classified elsewhere
    B97.89
      adenovirus B97.0
      coronavirus B97.29
        SARS-associated B97.21
      coxsackievirus B97.11
      echovirus B97.12
      enterovirus B97.10
        coxsackievirus B97.11
        echovirus B97.12
        specified NEC B97.19
    human
      immunodeficiency, type 2 (HIV 2)
      B97.35
      T-cell lymphotropic,
        type I (HTLV-I) B97.33
        type II (HTLV-II) B97.34

Infection, infected, infective continued

    metapneumovirus B97.81
    papillomavirus B97.7
    parvovirus B97.6
    reovirus B97.5
    respiratory syncytial B97.4
    retrovirus B97.30
      human
        immunodeficiency, type 2 (HIV 2)
        B97.35
        T-cell lymphotropic,
          type I (HTLV-I) B97.33
          type II (HTLV-II) B97.34
      lentivirus B97.31
      oncovirus B97.32
      specified NEC B97.39
    specified NEC B97.89
    central nervous system A89
      atypical A81.9
        specified NEC A81.89
      enterovirus NEC A88.8
        meningitis A87.0
      slow virus A81.9
        specified NEC A81.89
      specified NEC A88.8
    chest J98.8
    cotia B08.8
    coxsackie -see also Infection, coxsackie
    B34.1
      as cause of disease classified elsewhere
      B97.11
    ECHO
      as cause of disease classified elsewhere
      B97.12
      unspecified nature or site B34.1
    encephalitis, tick-borne A84.9
    enterovirus, as cause of disease classified
    elsewhere B97.10
      coxsackievirus B97.11
      echovirus B97.12
      specified NEC B97.19
    exanthem NOS B09
    human papilloma as cause of disease
    classified elsewhere B97.7
    human metapneumovirus as cause of disease
    classified elsewhere B97.81
    intestine -see Enteritis, viral
    respiratory syncytial
      as cause of disease classified elsewhere
      B97.4
      bronchopneumonia J12.1
      common cold syndrome J00
      nasopharyngitis (acute) J00
    rhinovirus
      as cause of disease classified elsewhere
      B97.89
      unspecified nature or site B34.8
    slow A81.9
      specified NEC A81.89
    specified type NEC B33.8
      as cause of disease classified elsewhere
      B97.89
      unspecified nature or site B34.8
    unspecified nature or site B34.9
    West Nile -see Virus, West Nile
  vulva (acute) -see Vulvitis
  West Nile -see Virus, West Nile
  whipworm B79
  worms B83.9
    specified type NEC B83.8
  Wuchereria (bancrofti) B74.0

Infection, infected, infective continued
  malayi B74.1
  yatapoxvirus B08.70
    specified NEC B08.79
  yeast -see also Candidiasis B37.9
  yellow fever -see Fever, yellow
  Yersinia
    enterocolitica (intestinal) A04.6
    pestis -see Plague
    pseudotuberculosis A28.2
  Zeis' gland -see Hordeolum
  Zika virus A92.5
  zoonotic bacterial NOS A28.9
  Zofia senagalensis B47.0
Infective, infectious -see condition
Infertility
  female N97.9
    age-related N97.8
    associated with
      anovulation N97.0
      cervical (mucus) disease or anomaly N88.3
      congenital anomaly
        cervix N88.3
        fallopian tube N97.1
        uterus N97.2
        vagina N97.8
      dysmucorrhea N88.3
      fallopian tube disease or anomaly N97.1
      pituitary hypothalamic origin E23.0
      specified origin NEC N97.8
      Stein-Leventhal syndrome E28.2
      uterine disease or anomaly N97.2
      vaginal disease or anomaly N97.8
    due to
      cervical anomaly N88.3
      fallopian tube anomaly N97.1
      ovarian failure E28.39
      Stein-Leventhal syndrome E28.2
      uterine anomaly N97.2
      vaginal anomaly N97.8
    nonimplantation N97.2
    origin
      cervical N88.3
      tubal (block) (occlusion) (stenosis) N97.1
      uterine N97.2
      vaginal N97.8
  male N46.9
    azoospermia N46.01
      extratesticular cause N46.029
        drug therapy N46.021
        efferent duct obstruction N46.023
        infection N46.022
        radiation N46.024
        specified cause NEC N46.029
        systemic disease N46.025
    oligospermia N46.11
      extratesticular cause N46.129
        drug therapy N46.121
        efferent duct obstruction N46.123
        infection N46.122
        radiation N46.124
        specified cause NEC N46.129
        systemic disease N46.125
    specified type NEC N46.8
Infestation B88.9
  Acanthocheilonema (perstans) (streptocerca) B74.4
  Acariasis B88.0
    demodex folliculorum B88.0
    sarcoptes scabiei B86
    trombiculae B88.0

Infestation - continued
  Agamofilaria streptocerca B74.4
  Ancylostoma, ankylostoma (braziliense) (caninum) (ceylanicum) (duodenale) B76.0
    americanum B76.1
    new world B76.1
  Anisakis larvae, anisakiasis B81.0
  arthropod NEC B88.2
  Ascaris lumbricoides -see Ascariasis
  Balantidium coli A07.0
  beef tapeworm B68.1
  Bothriocephalus (latus) B70.0
    larval B70.1
  broad tapeworm B70.0
    larval B70.1
  Brugia (malayi) B74.1
    timori B74.2
  candiru B88.8
  Capillaria
    hepatica B83.8
    philippinensis B81.1
  cat liver fluke B66.0
  cestodes B71.9
    diphyllobothrium -see Infestation, diphyllobothrium
    dipylidiasis B71.1
    hymenolepiasis B71.0
    specified type NEC B71.8
  chigger B88.0
  chigo, chigoe B88.1
  Clonorchis (sinensis) (liver) B66.1
  coccidial A07.3
  crab-lice B85.3
  Cysticercus cellulosae -see Cysticercosis
  Demodex (folliculorum) B88.0
  Dermanyssus gallinae B88.0
  Dermatobia (hominis) -see Myiasis
  Dibothriocephalus (latus) B70.0
    larval B70.1
  Dicrocoelium dendriticum B66.2
  Diphyllobothrium (adult) (latum) (intestinal) (pacificum) B70.0
    larval B70.1
  Diplogonoporus (grandis) B71.8
  Dipylidium caninum B67.4
  Distoma hepaticum B66.3
  dog tapeworm B67.4
  Dracunculus medinensis B72
  dragon worm B72
  dwarf tapeworm B71.0
  Echinococcus -see Echinococcus
  Echinostomum ilocanum B66.8
  Entamoeba (histolytica) -see Infection, Ameba
  Enterobius vermicularis B80
  eyelid
    in (due to)
      leishmaniasis B55.1
      loiasis B74.3
      onchocerciasis B73.09
      phthiriasis B85.3
      parasitic NOS B89
  eyeworm B74.3
  Fasciola (gigantica) (hepatica) (indica) B66.3
  Fasciolopsis (buski) (intestine) B66.5
  filarial B74.9
    bancroftian B74.0
    conjunctiva B74.9
    due to
      Acanthocheilonema (perstans) (streptocerca) B74.4

Infestation - continued
  Brugia (malayi) B74.1
    timori B74.2
  Dracunculus medinensis B72
  guinea worm B72
  loa loa B74.3
  Mansonella (ozzardi) (perstans) (streptocerca) B74.4
  Onchocerca volvulus B73.00
    eye B73.00
    eyelid B73.09
  Wuchereria (bancrofti) B74.0
  Malayan B74.1
  ozzardi B74.4
  specified type NEC B74.8
  fish tapeworm B70.0
    larval B70.1
  fluke B66.9
    blood NOS -see Schistosomiasis
    cat liver B66.0
    intestinal B66.5
    liver (sheep) B66.3
      cat B66.0
      Chinese B66.1
      due to clonorchiasis B66.1
      oriental B66.1
    lancet B66.2
    lung (oriental) B66.4
    sheep liver B66.3
    specified type NEC B66.8
  fly larvae -see Myiasis
  Gasterophilus (intestinalis) -see Myiasis
  Gastrodiscoides hominis B66.8
  Giardia lamblia A07.1
  Gnathostoma (spinigerum) B83.1
  Gongylonema B83.8
  guinea worm B72
  helminth B83.9
    angiostrongyliasis B83.2
      intestinal B81.3
    gnathostomiasis B83.1
    hirudiniasis, internal B83.4
    intestinal B82.0
      angiostrongyliasis B81.3
      anisakiasis B81.0
      ascariasis -see Ascariasis
      capillariasis B81.1
      cysticercosis -see Cysticercosis
      diphyllobothriasis -see Infestation, diphyllobothriasis
      dracunculiasis B72
      echinococcus -see Echinococcosis
      enterobiasis B80
      filariasis
      -see Infestation, filarial
      fluke -see Infestation, fluke
      hookworm -see Infestation, hookworm
      mixed (types classifiable to more than one of the titles B65.0 B81.3 and B81.8) B81.4
      onchocerciasis -see Onchocerciasis
      schistosomiasis -see Infestation, schistosoma
      specified
        cestode NEC -see Infestation, cestode type NEC B81.8
      strongyloidiasis -see Strongyloidiasis
      taenia -see Infestation, taenia
      trichinellosis B75
      trichostrongyliasis B81.2
      trichuriasis B79

Infestation - *continued*
specified type NEC B83.8
syngamiasis B83.3
visceral larva migrans B83.0
Heterophyes (heterophyes) B66.8
hookworm B76.9
ancylostomiasis B76.0
necatoriasis B76.1
specified type NEC B76.8
Hymenolepis (diminuta) (nana) B71.0
intestinal NEC B82.9
leeches (aquatic) (land) -*see* Hirudiniasis
Leishmania -*see* Leishmaniasis
lice, louse -*see* Infestation, Pediculus
Linguatula B88.8
Liponyssoides sanguineus B88.0
Loa loa B74.3
conjunctival B74.3
eyelid B74.3
louse -*see* Infestation, Pediculus
maggots -*see* Myiasis
Mansonella (ozzardi) (perstans) (streptocerca)
B74.4
Medina (worm) B72
Metagonimus (yokogawai) B66.8
microfilaria streptocerca -*see* Onchocerciasis
eye B73.00
eyelid B73.09
mites B88.9
scabic B86
Monilia (albicans) -*see* Candidiasis
mouth B37.0
Necator americanus B76.1
nematode NEC (intestinal) B82.0
Ancylostoma B76.0
conjunctiva NEC B83.9
Enterobius vermicularis B80
Gnathostoma spinigerum B83.1
physaloptera B80
specified NEC B81.8
trichostrongylus B81.2
trichuris (trichuria) B79
Oesophagostomum (apiostomum) B81.8
Oestrus ovis -*see also* Myiasis B87.9
Onchocerca (volvulus) -*see* Onchocerciasis
Opisthorchis (felineus) (viverrini) B66.0
orbit, parasitic NOS B89
Oxyuris vermicularis B80
Paragonimus (westermani) B66.4
parasite, parasitic B89
eyelid B89
intestinal NOS B82.9
mouth B37.0
skin B88.9
tongue B37.0
Parastrongylus
cantonensis B83.2
costaricensis B81.3
Pediculus B85.2
body B85.1
capitis (humanus) (any site) B85.0
corporis (humanus) (any site) B85.1
head B85.0
mixed (classifiable to more than one of the
titles B85.0 B85.3) B85.4
pubis (any site) B85.3
Pentastoma B88.8
Phthirus (pubis) (any site) B85.3
with any infestation classifiable to B85.0
B85.2 B85.4
pinworm B80

Infestation - *continued*
pork tapeworm (adult) B68.0
protozoal NEC B64
intestinal A07.9
specified NEC A07.8
specified NEC B60.8
pubic, louse B85.3
rat tapeworm B71.0
red bug B88.0
roundworm (large) NEC B82.0
Ascariasis -*see also* Ascariasis B77.9
sandflea B88.1
Sarcoptes scabiei B86
scabies B86
Schistosoma B65.9
bovis B65.8
cercariae B65.3
haematobium B65.0
intercalatum B65.8
japonicum B65.2
mansoni B65.1
mattheei B65.8
mekongi B65.8
specified type NEC B65.8
spindale B65.8
screw worms -*see* Myiasis
skin NOS B88.9
Sparganum (mansoni) (proliferum) (baxteri)
B70.1
larval B70.1
specified type NEC B88.8
Spirometra larvae B70.1
Stellantchasmus falcatus B66.8
Strongyloides stercoralis -*see* Strongyloidiasis
Taenia B68.9
diminuta B71.0
echinococcus -*see* Echinococcus
mediocanellata B68.1
nana B71.0
saginata B68.1
solium (intestinal form) B68.0
larval form -*see* Cysticercosis
Taeniarhynchus saginatus B68.1
tapeworm B71.9
beef B68.1
broad B70.0
larval B70.1
dog B67.4
dwarf B71.0
fish B70.0
larval B70.1
pork B68.0
rat B71.0
Ternidens diminutus B81.8
Tetranychus molestissimus B88.0
threadworm B80
tongue B37.0
Toxocara (canis) (cati) (felis) B83.0
trematode(s) NEC -*see* Infestation, fluke
Trichinella (spiralis) B75
Trichocephalus B79
Trichomonas -*see* Trichomoniasis
Trichostrongylus B81.2
Trichuris (trichiura) B79
Trombicula (irritans) B88.0
Tunga penetrans B88.1
Uncinaria americana B76.1
Vandellia cirrhosa B88.8
whipworm B79
worms B83.9
intestinal B82.0
Wuchereria (bancrofti) B74.0

Infiltrate, infiltration
amyloid (generalized) (localized) -*see*
Amyloidosis
calcareous NEC R89.7
localized -*see* Degeneration, by site
calcium salt R89.7
cardiac
fatty -*see* Degeneration, myocardial
glycogenic E74.02 [*143*]
corneal -*see* Edema, cornea
eyelid -*see* Inflammation, eyelid
glycogen, glycogenic -*see* Disease, glycogen
storage
heart, cardiac
fatty -*see* Degeneration, myocardial
glycogenic E74.02 [*143*]
inflammatory in vitreous H43.89
kidney N28.89
leukemic -*see* Leukemia
liver K76.89
fatty -*see* Fatty, liver NEC
glycogen -*see also* Disease, glycogen
storage E74.03 [*K77*]
lung R91.8
eosinophilic J82
lymphatic -*see also* Leukemia, lymphatic
C91.9
gland I88.9
muscle, fatty M62.89
myocardium, myocardial
fatty -*see* Degeneration, myocardial
glycogenic E74.02 [*143*]
on chest x ray R91.8
pulmonary R91.8
with eosinophilia J82
skin (lymphocytic) L98.6
thymus (gland) (fatty) E32.8
urine R39.0
vesicant agent
antineoplastic chemotherapy T80.810
other agent NEC T80.818
vitreous body H43.89
Infirmity R68.89
senile R54
**Inflammation, inflamed, inflammatory (with
exudation)**
abducent (nerve) -*see* Strabismus, paralytic,
sixth nerve
accessory sinus (chronic) -*see* Sinusitis
adrenal (gland) E27.8
alveoli, teeth M27.3
scorbutic E54
anal canal, anus K62.89
antrum (chronic) -*see* Sinusitis, maxillary
appendix -*see* Appendicitis
arachnoid -*see* Meningitis
areola N61.0
puerperal, postpartum or gestational -*see*
Infection, nipple
areolar tissue NOS L08.9
artery -*see* Arteritis
auditory meatus (external) -*see* Otitis, externa
Bartholin's gland N75.8
bile duct (common) (hepatic) or passage -*see*
Cholangitis
bladder -*see* Cystitis
bone -*see* Osteomyelitis
brain -*see also* Encephalitis
membrane -*see* Meningitis
breast N61.0

Inflammation, inflamed, inflammatory --
continued
  puerperal, postpartum, gestational -*see*
    Mastitis, obstetric
  broad ligament -*see* Disease, pelvis,
    inflammatory
  bronchi -*see* Bronchitis
  catarrhal J00
  cecum -*see* Appendicitis
  cerebral -*see also* Encephalitis
    membrane -*see* Meningitis
  cerebrospinal
    meningococcal A39.0
  cervix (uteri) -*see* Cervicitis
  chest J98.8
  chorioretinal H30.9
    cyclitis -*see* Cyclitis
    disseminated H30.10
      generalized H30.13
      peripheral H30.12
      posterior pole H30.11
    epitheliopathy -*see* Epitheliopathy
    focal H30.00
      juxtapapillary H30.01
      macular H30.04
      paramacular -*see* Inflammation,
        chorioretinal, focal, macular
      peripheral H30.03
      posterior pole H30.02
    specified type NEC H30.89
  choroid -*see* Inflammation, chorioretinal
  chronic, postmastoidectomy cavity -*see*
    Complications, postmastoidectomy,
    inflammation
  colon -*see* Enteritis
  connective tissue (diffuse) NEC -*see*
    Disorder, soft tissue, specified type NEC
  cornea -*see* Keratitis
  corpora cavernosa N48.29
  cranial nerve -*see* Disorder, nerve, cranial
  Douglas' cul-de-sac or pouch (chronic) N73.0
  due to device, implant or graft -*see also*
    Complications, by site and type, infection or
    inflammation
    arterial graft T82.7
    breast (implant) T85.79
    catheter T85.79
      dialysis (renal) T82.7
        intraperitoneal T85.71
      infusion T82.7
        cranial T85.735
        intrathecal T85.735
        spinal (epidural) (subdural) T85.735
        subarachnoid T85.735
      urinary T83.518
        cystostomy T83.510
        Hopkins T83.518
        ileostomy T83.518
        nephrostomy T83.512
        specified NEC T83.518
        urethral indwelling T83.511
        urostomy T83.518
    electronic (electrode) (pulse generator)
    (stimulator)
      bone T84.7
      cardiac T82.7
      nervous system T85.738
        brain T85.731
        cranial nerve T85.732
        gastric nerve T85.732
        neurostimulator generator T85.734

Inflammation, inflamed, inflammatory --
continued
        peripheral nerve T85.732
        sacral nerve T85.732
        spinal cord T85.733
        vagal nerve T85.732
      urinary T83.590
    fixation, internal (orthopedic) NEC -*see*
      Complication, fixation device, infection
    gastrointestinal (bile duct) (esophagus)
      T85.79
      neurostimulator electrode (lead) T85.732
    genital NEC T83.69
    heart NEC T82.7
      valve (prosthesis) T82.6
        graft T82.7
    joint prosthesis -*see* Complication, joint
      prosthesis, infection
    ocular (corneal graft) (orbital implant) NEC
      T85.79
    orthopedic NEC T84.7
    penile (cylinder) (pump) (reservoir) T83.61
    specified NEC T85.79
    testicular T83.62
    urinary NEC T83.598
      ileal conduit stent T83.593
      implanted neurostimulation T83.590
      implanted sphincter T83.591
      indwelling ureteral stent T83.592
      nephroureteral stent T83.593
      specified stent NEC T83.593
    vascular NEC T82.7
    ventricular intracranial (communicating)
    shunt T85.730
  duodenum K29.80
    with bleeding K29.81
  dura mater -*see* Meningitis
  ear (middle) -*see also* Otitis, media
    external -*see* Otitis, externa
    inner -*see* subcategory H83.0
  epididymis -*see* Epididymitis
  esophagus K20.9
  ethmoidal (sinus) (chronic) -*see* Sinusitis,
    ethmoidal
  eustachian tube (catarrhal) -*see* Salpingitis,
    eustachian
  eyelid H01.9
    abscess -*see* Abscess, eyelid
    blepharitis -*see* Blepharitis
    chalazion -*see* Chalazion
    dermatosis (noninfectious) -*see* Dermatosis,
      eyelid
    hordeolum -*see* Hordeolum
    specified NEC H01.8
  fallopian tube -*see* Salpingo-oophoritis
  fascia -*see* Myositis
  follicular, pharynx J31.2
  frontal (sinus) (chronic) -*see* Sinusitis, frontal
  gallbladder -*see* Cholecystitis
  gastric -*see* Gastritis
  gastrointestinal -*see* Enteritis
  genital organ (internal) (diffuse)
    female -*see* Disease, pelvis, inflammatory
    male N49.9
      multiple sites N49.8
      specified NEC N49.8
  gland (lymph) -*see* Lymphadenitis
  glottis -*see* Laryngitis
  granular, pharynx J31.2
  gum K05.10
    nonplaque induced K05.11

Inflammation, inflamed, inflammatory --
continued
  plaque induced K05.10
  heart -*see* Carditis
  hepatic duct -*see* Cholangitis
  ileoanal (internal) pouch K91.850
  ileum -*see also* Enteritis
    regional or terminal -*see* Enteritis, regional
  intestine (any part) -*see* Enteritis
  intestinal pouch K91.850
  jaw (acute) (bone) (chronic) (lower)
    (suppurative) (upper) M27.2
  joint NEC -*see* Arthritis
    sacroiliac M46.1
  kidney -*see* Nephritis
  knee (joint) M13.169
    tuberculous A18.02
  labium (majus) (minus) -*see* Vulvitis
  lacrimal
    gland -*see* Dacryoadenitis
    passages (duct) (sac) -*see also*
      Dacryocystitis
      canaliculitis -*see* Canaliculitis, lacrimal
  larynx -*see* Laryngitis
  leg NOS L08.9
  lip K13.0
  liver (capsule) -*see also* Hepatitis
    chronic K73.9
    suppurative K75.0
  lung (acute) -*see also* Pneumonia
    chronic J98.4
  lymph gland or node -*see* Lymphadenitis
  lymphatic vessel -*see* Lymphangitis
  maxilla, maxillary M27.2
    sinus (chronic) -*see* Sinusitis, maxillary
  membranes of brain or spinal cord -*see*
    Meningitis
  meninges -*see* Meningitis
  mouth K12.1
  muscle -*see* Myositis
  myocardium -*see* Myocarditis
  nasal sinus (chronic) -*see* Sinusitis
  nasopharynx -*see* Nasopharyngitis
  navel L08.82
  nerve NEC -*see* Neuralgia
  nipple N61.0
    puerperal, postpartum or gestational -*see*
      Infection, nipple
  nose -*see* Rhinitis
  oculomotor (nerve) -*see* Strabismus, paralytic,
    third nerve
  optic nerve -*see* Neuritis, optic
  orbit (chronic) H05.10
    acute H05.00
      abscess -*see* Abscess, orbit
      cellulitis -*see* Cellulitis, orbit
      osteomyelitis -*see* Osteomyelitis, orbit
      periostitis -*see* Periostitis, orbital
      tenonitis -*see* Tenonitis, eye
    granuloma -*see* Granuloma, orbit
    myositis -*see* Myositis, orbital
  ovary -*see* Salpingo-oophoritis
  oviduct -*see* Salpingo-oophoritis
  pancreas (acute) -*see* Pancreatitis
  parametrium N73.0
  parotid region L08.9
  pelvis, female -*see* Disease, pelvis,
    inflammatory penis (corpora cavernosa)
    N48.29
  perianal K62.89
  pericardium -*see* Pericarditis

Inflammation, inflamed, inflammatory --
continued
perineum (female) (male) L08.9
perirectal K62.89
peritoneum -*see* Peritonitis
periuterine -*see* Disease, pelvis, inflammatory
perivesical -*see* Cystitis
petrous bone (acute) (chronic) -*see* Petrositis
pharynx (acute) -*see* Pharyngitis
pia mater -*see* Meningitis
pleura -*see* Pleurisy
polyp, colon -*see also* Polyp, colon,
   inflammatory K51.40
prostate -*see also* Prostatitis
   specified type NEC N41.8
rectosigmoid -*see* Rectosigmoiditis
rectum -*see also* Proctitis K62.89
respiratory, upper -*see also* Infection,
   respiratory, upper J06.9
   acute, due to radiation J70.0
   chronic, due to external agent -*see* condition,
      respiratory, chronic, due to
   due to
      chemicals, gases, fumes or vapors
         (inhalation) J68.2
      radiation J70.1
retina -*see* Chorioretinitis
retrocecal -*see* Appendicitis
retroperitoneal -*see* Peritonitis
salivary duct or gland (any) (suppurative) -*see*
   Sialoadenitis
scorbutic, alveoli, teeth E54
scrotum N49.2
seminal vesicle -*see* Vesiculitis
sigmoid -*see* Enteritis
sinus -*see* Sinusitis
Skene's duct or gland -*see* Urethritis
skin L08.9
spermatic cord N49.1
sphenoidal (sinus) -*see* Sinusitis, sphenoidal
spinal
   cord -*see* Encephalitis
   membrane -*see* Meningitis
   nerve -*see* Disorder, nerve
spine -*see* Spondylopathy, inflammatory
spleen (capsule) D73.89
stomach -*see* Gastritis
subcutaneous tissue L08.9
suprarenal (gland) E27.8
synovial -*see* Tenosynovitis
tendon (sheath) NEC -*see* Tenosynovitis
testis -*see* Orchitis
throat (acute) -*see* Pharyngitis
thymus (gland) E32.8
thyroid (gland) -*see* Thyroiditis
tongue K14.0
tonsil -*see* Tonsillitis
trachea -*see* Tracheitis
trochlear (nerve) -*see* Strabismus, paralytic,
   fourth nerve
tubal -*see* Salpingo-oophoritis
tuberculous NEC -*see* Tuberculosis
tubo-ovarian -*see* Salpingo-oophoritis
tunica vaginalis N49.1
tympanic membrane -*see* Tympanitis
umbilicus, umbilical L08.82
uterine ligament -*see* Disease, pelvis,
   inflammatory   uterus (catarrhal) -*see*
   Endometritis
uveal tract (anterior) NOS -*see also*
Iridocyclitis

Inflammation, inflamed, inflammatory --
continued
posterior -*see* Chorioretinitis
vagina -*see* Vaginitis
vas deferens N49.1
vein -*see also* Phlebitis
   intracranial or intraspinal (septic) G08
   thrombotic I80.9
      leg -*see* Phlebitis, leg
      lower extremity -*see* Phlebitis, leg
vocal cord J38.3
vulva -*see* Vulvitis
Wharton's duct (suppurative) -*see*
Sialoadenitis
Inflation, lung, imperfect (newborn) -*see*
Atelectasis
**Influenza (bronchial) (epidemic)
(respiratory (upper)) (unidentified
influenza virus)** J11.1
with
   digestive manifestations J11.2
   encephalopathy J11.81
   enteritis J11.2
   gastroenteritis J11.2
   gastrointestinal manifestations J11.2
   laryngitis J11.1
   myocarditis J11.82
   otitis media J11.83
   pharyngitis J11.1
   pneumonia J11.00
      specified type J11.08
   respiratory manifestations NEC J11.1
   specified manifestation NEC J11.89
A/H5N1
-*see also* Influenza, due to, identified novel
   influenza A virus J09.X2
avian -*see also* Influenza, due to, identified
   novel influenza A virus J09.X2
bird -*see also* Influenza, due to, identified
   novel influenza A virus J09.X2
novel (2009) H1N1
influenza -*see also* Influenza, due to, identified
   influenza virus NEC J10.1
novel influenza A/H1N1
-*see also* Influenza, due to, identified influenza
   virus NEC J10.1
due to
   avian -*see also* Influenza, due to, identified
      novel influenza A virus J09.X2
   identified influenza virus NEC J10.1
      with
         digestive manifestations J10.2
         encephalopathy J10.81
         enteritis J10.2
         gastroenteritis J10.2
         gastrointestinal manifestations J10.2
         laryngitis J10.1
         myocarditis J10.82
         otitis media J10.83
         pharyngitis J10.1
         pneumonia (unspecified type) J10.00
            with same identified influenza virus
               J10.01
            specified type NEC J10.08
         respiratory manifestations NEC J10.1
         specified manifestation NEC J10.89
   identified novel influenza A virus J09.X2
      with
         digestive manifestations J09.X3
         encephalopathy J09.X9
         enteritis J09.X3

Influenza - *continued*
   gastroenteritis J09.X3
   gastrointestinal manifestations J09.X3
   laryngitis J09.X2
   myocarditis J09.X9
   otitis media J09.X9
   pharyngitis J09.X2
   pneumonia J09.X1
   respiratory manifestations NEC J09.X2
   specified manifestation NEC J09.X9
   upper respiratory symptoms J09.X2
of other animal origin, not bird or swine -*see
   also* Influenza, due to, identified novel
   influenza A virus J09.X2
swine (viruses that normally cause infections
   in pigs) -*see also* Influenza, due to,
   identified novel influenza A virus J09.X2
Influenza-like disease -*see* Influenza
Influenzal -*see* Influenza
Infraction, Freiberg's (metatarsal head) -*see*
Osteochondrosis, juvenile, metatarsus
Infraeruption of tooth (teeth) M26.34
**Infusion complication, misadventure, or
reaction** -*see* Complications, infusion
Ingestion
chemical -*see* Table of Drugs and Chemicals,
   by substance, poisoning
drug or medicament
   correct substance properly administered -*see*
      Table of Drugs and Chemicals, by drug,
      adverse effect
   overdose or wrong substance given or taken
      -*see* Table of Drugs and Chemicals, by drug,
      poisoning
foreign body -*see* Foreign body, alimentary
   tract
tularemia A21.3
Ingrowing
hair (beard) L73.1
nail (finger) (toe) L60.0
Inguinal -*see also* condition
testicle Q53.9
   bilateral Q53.21
   unilateral Q53.11
Inhalant-induced
anxiety disorder F18.980
depressive disorder F18.94
major neurocognitive disorder F18.97
mild neurocognitive disorder F18.988
psychotic disorder F18.959
Inhalation
anthrax A22.1
flame T27.3
food or foreign body -*see* Foreign body, by
   site
gases, fumes, or vapors NEC T59.9
   specified agent -*see* Table of Drugs and
      Chemicals, by substance
liquid or vomitus -*see* Asphyxia
meconium (newborn) P24.00
   with
      pneumonia (pneumonitis) P24.01
      with respiratory symptoms P24.01
mucus -*see* Asphyxia, mucus
oil or gasoline (causing suffocation) -*see*
   Foreign body, by site
smoke J70.5
due to chemicals, gases, fumes and vapors
   J68.9
steam -*see* Toxicity, vapors

Inhalation ---*continued*
　stomach contents or secretions -*see* Foreign
　　body, by site
　　due to anesthesia (general) (local) or other
　　　sedation T88.59
　　　　in labor and delivery O74.0
　　　　in pregnancy O29.01
　　　　postpartum, puerperal O89.01
Inhibition, orgasm
　female F52.31
　male F52.32
**Inhibitor, systemic lupus erythematosus
　(presence of)** D68.62
Iniencephalus, iniencephaly Q00.2
**Injection, traumatic jet (air) (industrial)
　(water) (paint or dye)** T70.4
Injury -*see also* specified injury type T14.90
　abdomen, abdominal S39.91
　　blood vessel -*see* Injury, blood vessel,
　　　abdomen
　　cavity -*see* Injury, intra-abdominal
　　contusion S30.1
　　internal -*see* Injury, intra-abdominal
　　intra-abdominal organ -*see* Injury, intra-
　　　abdominal
　　nerve -*see* Injury, nerve, abdomen
　　open -*see* Wound, open, abdomen
　　specified NEC S39.81
　　superficial -*see* Injury, superficial, abdomen
　Achilles tendon S86.00
　　laceration S86.02
　　specified type NEC S86.09
　　strain S86.01
　acoustic, resulting in deafness -*see* Injury,
　　nerve, acoustic
　adrenal (gland) S37.819
　　contusion S37.812
　　laceration S37.813
　　specified type NEC S37.818
　alveolar (process) S09.93
　ankle S99.91
　　contusion -*see* Contusion, ankle
　　dislocation -*see* Dislocation, ankle
　　fracture -*see* Fracture, ankle
　　nerve -*see* Injury, nerve, ankle
　　open -*see* Wound, open, ankle
　　specified type NEC S99.81
　　sprain -*see* Sprain, ankle
　　superficial -*see* Injury, superficial, ankle
　anterior chamber, eye -*see* Injury, eye,
　　specified site NEC
　anus -*see* Injury, abdomen
　aorta (thoracic) S25.00
　　abdominal S35.00
　　　laceration (minor) (superficial) S35.01
　　　　major S35.02
　　　specified type NEC S35.09
　　laceration (minor) (superficial) S25.01
　　　major S25.02
　　specified type NEC S25.09
　arm (upper) S49.9
　　blood vessel -*see* Injury, blood vessel, arm
　　contusion -*see* Contusion, arm, upper
　　fracture -*see* Fracture, humerus
　　lower -*see* Injury, forearm
　　muscle -*see* Injury, muscle, shoulder
　　nerve -*see* Injury, nerve, arm
　　open -*see* Wound, open, arm
　　specified type NEC S49.8
　　superficial -*see* Injury, superficial, arm

Injury --*continued*
　artery (complicating trauma) -*see also* Injury,
　　blood vessel, by site
　　cerebral or meningeal -*see* Injury,
　　　intracranial
　auditory canal (external) (meatus) S09.91
　auricle, auris, ear S09.91
　axilla -*see* Injury, shoulder
　back -*see* Injury, back, lower
　bile duct S36.13
　birth -*see also* Birth, injury P15.9
　bladder (sphincter) S37.20
　　at delivery O71.5
　　contusion S37.22
　　laceration S37.23
　　obstetrical trauma O71.5
　　specified type NEC S37.29
　blast (air) (hydraulic) (immersion)
　　(underwater) NEC T14.8
　　acoustic nerve trauma -*see* Injury, nerve,
　　　acoustic
　　bladder -*see* Injury, bladder
　　brain -*see* Concussion
　　colon -*see* Injury, intestine, large, blast
　　　injury
　　ear (primary) S09.31
　　　secondary S09.39
　　generalized T70.8
　　lung -*see* Injury, intrathoracic, lung, blast
　　　injury
　　multiple body organs T70.8
　　peritoneum S36.81
　　rectum S36.61
　　retroperitoneum S36.898
　　small intestine S36.419
　　　duodenum S36.410
　　　specified site NEC S36.418
　　specified
　　　intra-abdominal organ NEC S36.898
　　　pelvic organ NEC S37.899
　blood vessel NEC T14.8
　　abdomen S35.9
　　　aorta -*see* Injury, aorta, abdominal
　　　celiac artery -*see* Injury, blood vessel,
　　　　celiac artery
　　　iliac vessel -*see* Injury, blood vessel, iliac
　　　laceration S35.91
　　　mesenteric vessel -*see* Injury, mesenteric
　　　portal vein -*see* Injury, blood vessel, portal
　　　　vein
　　　renal vessel -*see* Injury, blood vessel, renal
　　　specified vessel NEC S35.8X
　　　splenic vessel -*see* Injury, blood vessel,
　　　　splenic
　　　vena cava -*see* Injury, vena cava, inferior
　　ankle -*see* Injury, blood vessel, foot
　　aorta (abdominal) (thoracic) -*see* Injury,
　　　aorta
　　arm (upper) NEC S45.90
　　　forearm -*see* Injury, blood vessel, forearm
　　　laceration S45.91
　　　specified
　　　　site NEC S45.80
　　　　　laceration S45.81
　　　　　specified type NEC S45.89
　　　　type NEC S45.99
　　　superficial vein S45.30
　　　　laceration S45.31
　　　　specified type NEC S45.39
　　axillary
　　　artery S45.00

Injury --*continued*
　　　laceration S45.01
　　　specified type NEC S45.09
　　vein S45.20
　　　laceration S45.21
　　　specified type NEC S45.29
　　azygos vein -*see* Injury, blood vessel,
　　　thoracic, specified site NEC
　　brachial
　　　artery S45.10
　　　　laceration S45.11
　　　　specified type NEC S45.19
　　　vein S45.20
　　　　laceration S45.219
　　　　specified type NEC S45.29
　　carotid artery (common) (external) (internal,
　　　extracranial) S15.00
　　　internal, intracranial S06.8
　　　laceration (minor) (superficial) S15.01
　　　　major S15.02
　　　specified type NEC S15.09
　　celiac artery S35.219
　　　branch S35.299
　　　　laceration (minor) (superficial) S35.291
　　　　　major S35.292
　　　　specified NEC S35.298
　　　laceration (minor) (superficial) S35.211
　　　　major S35.212
　　　specified type NEC S35.218
　　cerebral -*see* Injury, intracranial
　　deep plantar -*see* Injury, blood vessel,
　　　plantar artery
　　digital (hand) -*see* Injury, blood vessel,
　　　finger
　　dorsal
　　　artery (foot) S95.00
　　　　laceration S95.01
　　　　specified type NEC S95.09
　　　vein (foot) S95.20
　　　　laceration S95.21
　　　　specified type NEC S95.29
　　due to accidental laceration during
　　　procedure -*see* Laceration, accidental
　　　complicating surgery
　　extremity -*see* Injury, blood vessel, limb
　　femoral
　　　artery (common) (superficial) S75.00
　　　　laceration (minor) (superficial) S75.01
　　　　　major S75.02
　　　　specified type NEC S75.09
　　　vein (hip level) (thigh level) S75.10
　　　　laceration (minor) (superficial) S75.11
　　　　　major S75.12
　　　　specified type NEC S75.19
　　finger S65.50
　　　index S65.50
　　　　laceration S65.51
　　　　specified type NEC S65.59
　　　laceration S65.51
　　　little S65.50
　　　　laceration S65.51
　　　　specified type NEC S65.59
　　　middle S65.50
　　　　laceration S65.51
　　　　specified type NEC S65.59
　　　specified type NEC S65.59
　　　thumb -*see* Injury, blood vessel, thumb
　　foot S95.90
　　　dorsal
　　　　artery -*see* Injury, blood vessel, dorsal,
　　　　　artery

Injury --*continued*

vein -*see* Injury, blood vessel, dorsal, vein
laceration S95.91
plantar artery -*see* Injury, blood vessel, plantar artery
specified
site NEC S95.80
laceration S95.81
specified type NEC S95.89
specified type NEC S95.99
forearm S55.90
laceration S55.91
radial artery -*see* Injury, blood vessel, radial artery
specified
site NEC S55.80
laceration S55.81
specified type NEC S55.89
type NEC S55.99
ulnar artery -*see* Injury, blood vessel, ulnar artery
vein S55.20
laceration S55.21
specified type NEC S55.29
gastric
artery -*see* Injury, mesenteric, artery, branch
vein -*see* Injury, blood vessel, abdomen
gastroduodenal artery -*see* Injury, mesenteric, artery, branch
greater saphenous vein (lower leg level) S85.30
hip (and thigh) level S75.20
laceration (minor) (superficial) S75.21
major S75.22
specified type NEC S75.29
laceration S85.31
specified type NEC S85.39
hand (level) S65.90
finger -*see* Injury, blood vessel, finger
laceration S65.91
palmar arch -*see* Injury, blood vessel, palmar arch
radial artery -*see* Injury, blood vessel, radial artery, hand
specified
site NEC S65.80
laceration S65.81
specified type NEC S65.89
type NEC S65.99
thumb -*see* Injury, blood vessel, thumb
ulnar artery -*see* Injury, blood vessel, ulnar artery, hand
head S09.0
intracranial -*see* Injury, intracranial
multiple S09.0
hepatic
artery -*see* Injury, mesenteric, artery
vein -*see* Injury, vena cava, inferior
hip S75.90
femoral artery -*see* Injury, blood vessel, femoral, artery
femoral vein -*see* Injury, blood vessel, femoral, vein
greater saphenous vein -*see* Injury, blood vessel, greater saphenous, hip level
laceration S75.91
specified
site NEC S75.80
laceration S75.81

specified type NEC S75.89
type NEC S75.99
hypogastric (artery) (vein) -*see* Injury, blood vessel, iliac
iliac S35.5
artery S35.51
specified vessel NEC S35.5
uterine vessel -*see* Injury, blood vessel, uterine
vein S35.51
innominate -*see* Injury, blood vessel, thoracic, innominate
intercostal (artery) (vein) -*see* Injury, blood vessel, thoracic, intercostal
jugular vein (external) S15.20
internal S15.30
laceration (minor) (superficial) S15.31
major S15.32
specified type NEC S15.39
laceration (minor) (superficial) S15.21
major S15.22
specified type NEC S15.29
leg (level) (lower) S85.90
greater saphenous -*see* Injury, blood vessel, greater saphenous
laceration S85.91
lesser saphenous -*see* Injury, blood vessel, lesser saphenous
peroneal artery -*see* Injury, blood vessel, peroneal artery
popliteal
artery -*see* Injury, blood vessel, popliteal, artery
vein -*see* Injury, blood vessel, popliteal, vein
specified
site NEC S85.80
laceration S85.81
specified type NEC S85.89
type NEC S85.99
thigh -*see* Injury, blood vessel, hip
tibial artery -*see* Injury, blood vessel, tibial artery
lesser saphenous vein (lower leg level) S85.40
laceration S85.41
specified type NEC S85.49
limb
lower -*see* Injury, blood vessel, leg
upper -*see* Injury, blood vessel, arm
lower back -*see* Injury, blood vessel, abdomen
specified NEC -*see* Injury, blood vessel, abdomen, specified, site NEC
mammary (artery) (vein) -*see* Injury, blood vessel, thoracic, specified site NEC
mesenteric (inferior) (superior)
artery -*see* Injury, mesenteric, artery
vein -*see* Injury, mesenteric, vein
neck S15.9
specified site NEC S15.8
ovarian (artery) (vein) -*see* subcategory S35.8
palmar arch (superficial) S65.20
deep S65.30
laceration S65.31
specified type NEC S65.39
laceration S65.21
specified type NEC S65.29
pelvis -*see* Injury, blood vessel, abdomen

specified NEC -*see* Injury, blood vessel, abdomen, specified, site NEC
peroneal artery S85.20
laceration S85.21
specified type NEC S85.29
plantar artery (deep) (foot) S95.10
laceration S95.11
specified type NEC S95.19
popliteal
artery S85.00
laceration S85.01
specified type NEC S85.09
vein S85.50
laceration S85.51
specified type NEC S85.59
portal vein S35.319
laceration S35.311
specified type NEC S35.318
precerebral -*see* Injury, blood vessel, neck
pulmonary (artery) (vein) -*see* Injury, blood vessel, thoracic, pulmonary
radial artery (forearm level) S55.10
hand and wrist (level) S65.10
laceration S65.11
specified type NEC S65.19
laceration S55.11
specified type NEC S55.19
renal
artery S35.40
laceration S35.41
specified NEC S35.49
vein S35.40
laceration S35.41
specified NEC S35.49
saphenous vein (greater) (lower leg level) -*see* Injury, blood vessel, greater saphenous
hip and thigh level -*see* Injury, blood vessel, greater saphenous, hip level
lesser -*see* Injury, blood vessel, lesser saphenous
shoulder
specified NEC -*see* Injury, blood vessel, arm, specified site NEC
superficial vein -*see* Injury, blood vessel, arm, superficial vein
specified NEC T14.8
splenic
artery -*see* Injury, blood vessel, celiac artery, branch
vein S35.329
laceration S35.321
specified NEC S35.328
subclavian -*see* Injury, blood vessel, thoracic, innominate
thigh -*see* Injury, blood vessel, hip
thoracic S25.90
aorta S25.00
laceration (minor) (superficial) S25.01
major S25.02
specified type NEC S25.09
azygos vein -*see* Injury, blood vessel, thoracic, specified, site NEC
innominate
artery S25.10
laceration (minor) (superficial) S25.11
major S25.12
specified type NEC S25.19
vein S25.30
laceration (minor) (superficial) S25.31
major S25.32

Injury --*continued*

    specified type NEC S25.39
  intercostal S25.50
    laceration S25.51
    specified type NEC S25.59
  laceration S25.91
  mammary vessel -*see* Injury, blood vessel,
thoracic, specified, site NEC
  pulmonary S25.40
    laceration (minor) (superficial) S25.41
      major S25.42
    specified type NEC S25.49
  specified
    site NEC S25.80
      laceration S25.81
      specified type NEC S25.89
    type NEC S25.99
  subclavian -*see* Injury, blood vessel,
thoracic, innominate
  vena cava (superior) S25.20
    laceration (minor) (superficial) S25.21
      major S25.22
    specified type NEC S25.29
  thumb S65.40
    laceration S65.41
    specified type NEC S65.49
  tibial artery S85.10
    anterior S85.13
      laceration S85.14
      specified injury NEC S85.15
    laceration S85.11
    posterior S85.16
      laceration S85.17
      specified injury NEC S85.18
    specified injury NEC S85.12
  ulnar artery (forearm level) S55.00
    hand and wrist (level) S65.00
      laceration S65.01
      specified type NEC S65.09
    laceration S55.01
    specified type NEC S55.09
  upper arm (level) -*see* Injury, blood vessel,
arm
    superficial vein -*see* Injury, blood vessel,
arm, superficial vein
  uterine S35.5
    artery S35.53
    vein S35.53
  vena cava -*see* Injury, vena cava
  vertebral artery S15.10
    laceration (minor) (superficial) S15.11
      major S15.12
    specified type NEC S15.19
  wrist (level) -*see* Injury, blood vessel, hand
brachial plexus S14.3
  newborn P14.3
brain (traumatic) S06.9
  diffuse (axonal) S06.2X
  focal S06.30
brainstem S06.38
breast NOS S29.9
broad ligament -*see* Injury, pelvic organ,
specified site NEC
bronchus, bronchi -*see* Injury, intrathoracic,
bronchus
brow S09.90
buttock S39.92
canthus, eye S05.90
cardiac plexus -*see* Injury, nerve, thorax,
sympathetic
cauda equina S34.3

Injury --*continued*

cavernous sinus -*see* Injury, intracranial
cecum -*see* Injury, colon
celiac ganglion or plexus -*see* Injury, nerve,
lumbosacral, sympathetic
cerebellum -*see* Injury, intracranial
cerebral -*see* Injury, intracranial
cervix (uteri) -*see* Injury, uterus
cheek (wall) S09.93
chest -*see* Injury, thorax
childbirth (newborn) -*see also* Birth, injury
  maternal NEC O71.9
chin S09.93
choroid (eye) -*see* Injury, eye, specified site
NEC
clitoris S39.94
coccyx -*see also* Injury, back, lower
  complicating delivery O71.6
colon -*see* Injury, intestine, large
common bile duct -*see* Injury, liver
conjunctiva (superficial) -*see* Injury, eye,
conjunctiva
conus medullaris -*see* Injury, spinal, sacral
cord
  spermatic (pelvic region) S37.898
    scrotal region S39.848
  spinal -*see* Injury, spinal cord, by region
cornea -*see* Injury, eye, specified site NEC
  abrasion -*see* Injury, eye, cornea, abrasion
cortex (cerebral) -*see also* Injury, intracranial
  visual -*see* Injury, nerve, optic
costal region NEC S29.9
costochondral NEC S29.9
cranial
  cavity -*see* Injury, intracranial
  nerve -*see* Injury, nerve, cranial
crushing -*see* Crush
cutaneous sensory nerve
cystic duct -*see* Injury, liver
deep tissue -*see* Contusion, by site
  meaning pressure ulcer -*see* Ulcer, pressure,
unstageable, by site
delivery (newborn) P15.9
  maternal NEC O71.9
Descemet's membrane -*see* Injury, eyeball,
penetrating
diaphragm -*see* Injury, intrathoracic,
diaphragm
duodenum -*see* Injury, intestine, small,
duodenum
ear (auricle) (external) (canal) S09.91
  abrasion -*see* Abrasion, ear
  bite -*see* Bite, ear
  blister -*see* Blister, ear
  bruise -*see* Contusion, ear
  contusion -*see* Contusion, ear
  external constriction -*see* Constriction,
external, ear
  hematoma -*see* Hematoma, ear
  inner -*see* Injury, ear, middle
  laceration -*see* Laceration, ear
  middle S09.30
    blast -*see* Injury, blast, ear
    specified NEC S09.39
  puncture -*see* Puncture, ear
  superficial -*see* Injury, superficial, ear
  eighth cranial nerve (acoustic or auditory) -
see Injury, nerve, acoustic
elbow S59.90
  contusion -*see* Contusion, elbow
  dislocation -*see* Dislocation, elbow

Injury --*continued*

  fracture -*see* Fracture, ulna, upper end
  open -*see* Wound, open, elbow
  specified NEC S59.80
  sprain -*see* Sprain, elbow
  superficial -*see* Injury, superficial, elbow
eleventh cranial nerve (accessory) -*see* Injury,
nerve, accessory   epididymis S39.94
epigastric region S39.91
epiglottis NEC S19.89
esophageal plexus -*see* Injury, nerve, thorax,
sympathetic
esophagus (thoracic part) -*see also* Injury,
intrathoracic, esophagus
  cervical NEC S19.85
eustachian tube S09.30
eye S05.9
  avulsion S05.7
  ball -*see* Injury, eyeball
  conjunctiva S05.0
  cornea
    abrasion S05.0
    laceration S05.3
      with prolapse S05.2
  lacrimal apparatus S05.8X
  orbit penetration S05.4
  specified site NEC S05.8X   eyeball
S05.8X
  contusion S05.1
  penetrating S05.6
    with
      foreign body S05.5
      prolapse or loss of intraocular tissue
S05.2
      without prolapse or loss of intraocular
tissue S05.3
  specified type NEC S05.8
eyebrow S09.93
eyelid S09.93
  abrasion -*see* Abrasion, eyelid
  contusion -*see* Contusion, eyelid
  open -*see* Wound, open, eyelid
face S09.93
fallopian tube S37.509
  bilateral S37.502
    blast injury S37.512
    contusion S37.522
    laceration S37.532
    specified type NEC S37.592
  blast injury (primary) S37.519
    bilateral S37.512
    secondary -*see* Injury, fallopian tube,
specified type NEC
    unilateral S37.511
  contusion S37.529
    bilateral S37.522
    unilateral S37.521
  laceration S37.539
    bilateral S37.532
    unilateral S37.531
  specified type NEC S37.599
    bilateral S37.592
    unilateral S37.591
  unilateral S37.501
    blast injury S37.511
    contusion S37.521
    laceration S37.531
    specified type NEC S37.591
fascia -*see* Injury, muscle
fifth cranial nerve (trigeminal) -*see* Injury,
nerve, trigeminal

Injury --*continued*

finger (nail) S69.9
blood vessel -*see* Injury, blood vessel, finger
contusion -*see* Contusion, finger
dislocation -*see* Dislocation, finger
fracture -*see* Fracture, finger
muscle -*see* Injury, muscle, finger
nerve -*see* Injury, nerve, digital, finger
open -*see* Wound, open, finger
specified NEC S69.8
sprain -*see* Sprain, finger
superficial -*see* Injury, superficial, finger
first cranial nerve (olfactory) -*see* Injury,
nerve, olfactory   flank -*see* Injury, abdomen
foot S99.92
blood vessel -*see* Injury, blood vessel, foot
contusion -*see* Contusion, foot
dislocation -*see* Dislocation, foot
fracture -*see* Fracture, foot
muscle -*see* Injury, muscle, foot
open -*see* Wound, open, foot
specified type NEC S99.82
sprain -*see* Sprain, foot
superficial -*see* Injury, superficial, foot
forceps NOS P15.9
forearm S59.91
blood vessel -*see* Injury, blood vessel,
forearm
contusion -*see* Contusion, forearm
fracture -*see* Fracture, forearm
muscle -*see* Injury, muscle, forearm
nerve -*see* Injury, nerve, forearm
open -*see* Wound, open, forearm
specified NEC S59.81
superficial -*see* Injury, superficial, forearm
forehead S09.90
fourth cranial nerve (trochlear) -*see* Injury,
nerve, trochlear
gallbladder S36.129
contusion S36.122
laceration S36.123
specified NEC S36.128
ganglion
celiac, coeliac -*see* Injury, nerve,
lumbosacral, sympathetic
gasserian -*see* Injury, nerve, trigeminal
stellate -*see* Injury, nerve, thorax,
sympathetic
thoracic sympathetic -*see* Injury, nerve,
thorax, sympathetic
gasserian ganglion -*see* Injury, nerve,
trigeminal
gastric artery -*see* Injury, blood vessel, celiac
artery, branch
gastroduodenal artery -*see* Injury, blood
vessel, celiac artery, branch
gastrointestinal tract -*see* Injury, intra-
abdominal
with open wound into abdominal cavity -*see*
Wound, open, with penetration into
peritoneal cavity
colon -*see* Injury, intestine, large
rectum -*see* Injury, intestine, large, rectum
with open wound into abdominal cavity
S36.61
specified site NEC -*see* Injury, intra-
abdominal, specified, site NEC
stomach -*see* Injury, stomach
small intestine -*see* Injury, intestine, small
genital organ(s)
external S39.94

specified NEC S39.848
internal S37.90
fallopian tube -*see* Injury, fallopian tube
ovary -*see* Injury, ovary
prostate -*see* Injury, prostate
seminal vesicle -*see* Injury, pelvis, organ,
specified site NEC
uterus -*see* Injury, uterus
vas deferens -*see* Injury, pelvis, organ,
specified site NEC
obstetrical trauma O71.9
gland
lacrimal laceration -*see* Injury, eye, specified
site NEC
salivary S09.93
thyroid NEC S19.84
globe (eye) S05.90
specified NEC S05.8X
groin -*see* Injury, abdomen
gum S09.90
hand S69.9
blood vessel -*see* Injury, blood vessel, hand
contusion -*see* Contusion, hand
fracture -*see* Fracture, hand
muscle -*see* Injury, muscle, hand
nerve -*see* Injury, nerve, hand
open -*see* Wound, open, hand
specified NEC S69.8
sprain -*see* Sprain, hand
superficial -*see* Injury, superficial, hand
head S09.90
with loss of consciousness S06.9
specified NEC S09.8
heart S26.90
with hemopericardium S26.00
contusion S26.01
laceration (mild) S26.020
moderate S26.021
major S26.022
specified type NEC S26.09
contusion S26.91
laceration S26.92
specified type NEC S26.99
without hemopericardium S26.10
contusion S26.11
laceration S26.12
specified type NEC S26.19
heel -*see* Injury, foot
hepatic
artery -*see* Injury, blood vessel, celiac artery,
branch
duct -*see* Injury, liver
vein -*see* Injury, vena cava, inferior
hip S79.91
blood vessel -*see* Injury, blood vessel, hip
contusion -*see* Contusion, hip
dislocation -*see* Dislocation, hip
fracture -*see* Fracture, femur, neck
muscle -*see* Injury, muscle, hip
nerve -*see* Injury, nerve, hip
open -*see* Wound, open, hip
sprain -*see* Sprain, hip
superficial -*see* Injury, superficial, hip
specified NEC S79.81
hymen S39.94
hypogastric
blood vessel -*see* Injury, blood vessel, iliac
plexus -*see* Injury, nerve, lumbosacral,
sympathetic
ileum -*see* Injury, intestine, small

iliac region S39.91
instrumental (during surgery) -*see* Laceration,
accidental complicating surgery
birth injury -*see* Birth, injury
nonsurgical -*see* Injury, by site
obstetrical O71.9
bladder O71.5
cervix O71.3
high vaginal O71.4
perineal NOS O70.9
urethra O71.5
uterus O71.5
with rupture or perforation O71.1
internal T14.8
aorta -*see* Injury, aorta
bladder (sphincter) -*see* Injury, bladder
with
ectopic or molar pregnancy O08.6
following ectopic or molar pregnancy
O08.6
obstetrical trauma O71.5
bronchus, bronchi -*see* Injury, intrathoracic,
bronchus
cecum -*see* Injury, intestine, large
cervix (uteri) -*see also* Injury, uterus
with ectopic or molar pregnancy O08.6
following ectopic or molar pregnancy
O08.6
obstetrical trauma O71.3
chest -*see* Injury, intrathoracic
gastrointestinal tract -*see* Injury, intra-
abdominal
heart -*see* Injury, heart
intestine NEC -*see* Injury, intestine
intrauterine -*see* Injury, uterus
mesentery -*see* Injury, intra-abdominal,
specified, site NEC
pelvis, pelvic (organ) S37.90
following ectopic or molar pregnancy
(subsequent episode) O08.6
obstetrical trauma NEC O71.5
rupture or perforation O71.1
specified NEC S39.83
rectum -*see* Injury, intestine, large, rectum
stomach -*see* Injury, stomach
ureter -*see* Injury, ureter
urethra (sphincter) following ectopic or
molar pregnancy O08.6
uterus -*see* Injury, uterus
interscapular area -*see* Injury, thorax -
intestine
large S36.509
ascending (right) S36.500
blast injury (primary) S36.510
secondary S36.590
contusion S36.520
laceration S36.530
specified type NEC S36.590
blast injury (primary) S36.519
ascending (right) S36.510
descending (left) S36.512
rectum S36.61
sigmoid S36.513
specified site NEC S36.518
transverse S36.511
contusion S36.529
ascending (right) S36.520
descending (left) S36.522
rectum S36.62
sigmoid S36.523

Injury --*continued*
    specified site NEC S36.528
    transverse S36.521
   descending (left) S36.502
    blast injury (primary) S36.512
     secondary S36.592
    contusion S36.522
    laceration S36.532
    specified type NEC S36.592
   laceration S36.539
    ascending (right) S36.530
    descending (left) S36.532
    rectum S36.63
    sigmoid S36.533
    specified site NEC S36.538
    transverse S36.531
   rectum S36.60
    blast injury (primary) S36.61
     secondary S36.69
    contusion S36.62
    laceration S36.63
    specified type NEC S36.69
   sigmoid S36.503
    blast injury (primary) S36.513
     secondary S36.593
    contusion S36.523
    laceration S36.533
    specified type NEC S36.593
   specified
    site NEC S36.508
     blast injury (primary) S36.518
      secondary S36.598
     contusion S36.528
     laceration S36.538
     specified type NEC S36.598
    type NEC S36.599
     ascending (right) S36.590
     descending (left) S36.592
     rectum S36.69
     sigmoid S36.593
     specified site NEC S36.598
     transverse S36.591
   transverse S36.501
    blast injury (primary) S36.511
     secondary S36.591
    contusion S36.521
    laceration S36.531
    specified type NEC S36.591
  small S36.409
   blast injury (primary) S36.419
    duodenum S36.410
    secondary S36.499
     duodenum S36.490
     specified site NEC S36.498
    specified site NEC S36.418
   contusion S36.429
    duodenum S36.420
    specified site NEC S36.428
   duodenum S36.400
    blast injury (primary) S36.410
     secondary S36.490
    contusion S36.420
    laceration S36.430
    specified NEC S36.490
   laceration S36.439
    duodenum S36.430
    specified site NEC S36.438
   specified
    type NEC S36.499
     duodenum S36.490
     specified site NEC S36.498

    site NEC S36.408
  intra-abdominal S36.90
   adrenal gland -*see* Injury, adrenal gland
   bladder -*see* Injury, bladder
   colon -*see* Injury, intestine, large
   contusion S36.92
   fallopian tube -*see* Injury, fallopian tube
   gallbladder -*see* Injury, gallbladder
   intestine -*see* Injury, intestine
   laceration S36.93
   liver -*see* Injury, liver
   kidney -*see* Injury, kidney
   ovary -*see* Injury, ovary
   pancreas -*see* Injury, pancreas
   pelvic NOS S37.90
   peritoneum -*see* Injury, intra-abdominal,
    specified, site NEC
   prostate -*see* Injury, prostate
   rectum -*see* Injury, intestine, large, rectum
   retroperitoneum -*see* Injury, intra-
    abdominal, specified, site NEC
   seminal vesicle -*see* Injury, pelvis, organ,
    specified site NEC
   small intestine -*see* Injury, intestine, small
   specified
    site NEC S36.899
     contusion S36.892
     laceration S36.893
     specified type NEC S36.898
    type NEC S36.99
    pelvic S37.90
     specified
      site NEC S37.899
       specified type NEC S37.898
      type NEC S37.99
   spleen -*see* Injury, spleen
   stomach -*see* Injury, stomach
   ureter -*see* Injury, ureter
   urethra -*see* Injury, urethra
   uterus -*see* Injury, uterus
   vas deferens -*see* Injury, pelvis, organ,
    specified site NEC
  intracranial (traumatic) S06.9
   cerebellar hemorrhage, traumatic -*see*
    Injury, intracranial, focal
   cerebral edema, traumatic S06.1X
    diffuse S06.1X
    focal S06.1X
   diffuse (axonal) S06.2X
   epidural hemorrhage (traumatic) S06.4X
   focal brain injury S06.30
    contusion -*see* Contusion, cerebral
    laceration -*see* Laceration, cerebral
    intracerebral hemorrhage, traumatic S06.36
     left side S06.35
     right side S06.34
   subarachnoid hemorrhage, traumatic
    S06.6X
   subdural hemorrhage, traumatic S06.5X
  intraocular -*see* Injury, eyeball, penetrating
  intrathoracic S27.9
   bronchus S27.409
    bilateral S27.402
    blast injury (primary) S27.419
     bilateral S27.412
     secondary -*see* Injury, intrathoracic,
      bronchus, specified type NEC
     unilateral S27.411
    contusion S27.429
     bilateral S27.422

     unilateral S27.421
    laceration S27.439
     bilateral S27.432
     unilateral S27.431
    specified type NEC S27.499
     bilateral S27.492
     unilateral S27.491
    unilateral S27.401
   diaphragm S27.809
    contusion S27.802
    laceration S27.803
    specified type NEC S27.808
   esophagus (thoracic) S27.819
    contusion S27.812
    laceration S27.813
    specified type NEC S27.818
   heart -*see* Injury, heart
   hemopneumothorax S27.2
   hemothorax S27.1
   lung S27.309
    aspiration J69.0
    bilateral S27.302
    blast injury (primary) S27.319
     bilateral S27.312
     secondary -*see* Injury, intrathoracic, lung,
      specified type NEC
     unilateral S27.311
    contusion S27.329
     bilateral S27.322
     unilateral S27.321
    laceration S27.339
     bilateral S27.332
     unilateral S27.331
    specified type NEC S27.399
     bilateral S27.392
     unilateral S27.391
    unilateral S27.301
   pleura S27.60
    laceration S27.63
    specified type NEC S27.69
   pneumothorax S27.0
   specified organ NEC S27.899
    contusion S27.892
    laceration S27.893
    specified type NEC S27.898
   thoracic duct -*see* Injury, intrathoracic,
    specified organ NEC
   thymus gland -*see* Injury, intrathoracic,
    specified organ NEC
   trachea, thoracic S27.50
    blast (primary) S27.51
    contusion S27.52
    laceration S27.53
    specified type NEC S27.59
  iris -*see* Injury, eye, specified site NEC
   penetrating -*see* Injury, eyeball, penetrating
  jaw S09.93
  jejunum -*see* Injury, intestine, small
  joint NOS T14.8
   old or residual -*see* Disorder, joint, specified
    type NEC
  kidney S37.00
   acute (nontraumatic) N17.9
   contusion -*see* Contusion, kidney
   laceration -*see* Laceration, kidney
   specified NEC S37.09
  knee S89.9
   contusion -*see* Contusion, knee
   dislocation -*see* Dislocation, knee

Injury *--continued*

  meniscus (lateral) (medial) *-see* Sprain,
  knee, specified site NEC

    old injury or tear *-see* Derangement, knee,
    meniscus, due to old injury

    open *-see* Wound, open, knee

    specified NEC S89.8

    sprain *-see* Sprain, knee

    superficial *-see* Injury, superficial, knee

  labium (majus) (minus) S39.94

  labyrinth, ear S09.30

  lacrimal apparatus, duct, gland, or sac *-see*
  Injury, eye, specified site NEC

  larynx NEC S19.81

  leg (lower) S89.9

    blood vessel *-see* Injury, blood vessel, leg

    contusion *-see* Contusion, leg

    fracture *-see* Fracture, leg

    muscle *-see* Injury, muscle, leg

    nerve *-see* Injury, nerve, leg

    open *-see* Wound, open, leg

    specified NEC S89.8

    superficial *-see* Injury, superficial, leg

  lens, eye *-see* Injury, eye, specified site NEC

    penetrating *-see* Injury, eyeball, penetrating

  limb NEC T14.8

  lip S09.93

  liver S36.119

    contusion S36.112

    laceration S36.113

      major (stellate) S36.116

      minor S36.114

      moderate S36.115

    specified NEC S36.118

  lower back S39.92

    specified NEC S39.82

  lumbar, lumbosacral (region) S39.92

    plexus *-see* Injury, lumbosacral plexus

  lumbosacral plexus S34.4

  lung *-see also* Injury, intrathoracic, lung

    aspiration J69.0

    transfusion-related (TRALI) J95.84

  lymphatic thoracic duct *-see* Injury,
  intrathoracic, specified organ NEC

  malar region S09.93

  mastoid region S09.90

  maxilla S09.93

  mediastinum *-see* Injury, intrathoracic,
  specified organ NEC

  membrane, brain *-see* Injury, intracranial

  meningeal artery *-see* Injury, intracranial,
  subdural hemorrhage

  meninges (cerebral) *-see* Injury, intracranial

  mesenteric

    artery

      branch S35.299

        laceration (minor) (superficial) S35.291

          major S35.292

        specified NEC S35.298

      inferior S35.239

        laceration (minor) (superficial) S35.231

          major S35.232

        specified NEC S35.238

      superior S35.229

        laceration (minor) (superficial) S35.221

          major S35.222

        specified NEC S35.228

    plexus (inferior) (superior) *-see* Injury,
    nerve, lumbosacral, sympathetic

    vein

      inferior S35.349

Injury *--continued*

    laceration S35.341

    specified NEC S35.348

    superior S35.339

    laceration S35.331

    specified NEC S35.338

  mesentery *-see* Injury, intra-abdominal,
  specified site NEC

  mesosalpinx *-see* Injury, pelvic organ,
  specified site NEC

  middle ear S09.30

  midthoracic region NOS S29.9

  mouth S09.93

  multiple NOS T07

  muscle (and fascia) (and tendon)

    abdomen S39.001

      laceration S39.021

      specified type NEC S39.091

      strain S39.011

    abductor

      thumb, forearm level *-see* Injury, muscle,
      thumb, abductor

    adductor

      thigh S76.20

        laceration S76.22

        specified type NEC S76.29

        strain S76.21

    ankle *-see* Injury, muscle, foot

    anterior muscle group, at leg level (lower)
    S86.20

      laceration S86.22

      specified type NEC S86.29

      strain S86.21

    arm (upper) *-see* Injury, muscle, shoulder

    biceps (parts NEC) S46.20

      laceration S46.22

      long head S46.10

        laceration S46.12

        strain S46.11

        specified type NEC S46.19

      specified type NEC S46.29

      strain S46.21

    extensor

      finger(s) (other than thumb) *-see* Injury,
      muscle, finger by site, extensor

      forearm level, specified NEC *-see* Injury,
      muscle, forearm, extensor

      thumb *-see* Injury, muscle, thumb, extensor

      toe (large) (ankle level) (foot level) *-see*
      Injury, muscle, toe, extensor

    finger

      extensor (forearm level) S56.40

        hand level S66.309

          laceration S66.329

          specified type NEC S66.399

          strain S66.319

        laceration S56.429

        specified type NEC S56.499

        strain S56.419

      flexor (forearm level) S56.10

        hand level S66.109

          laceration S66.129

          specified type NEC S66.199

          strain S66.119

        laceration S56.129

        specified type NEC S56.199

        strain S56.119

      intrinsic S66.509

        laceration S66.529

        specified type NEC S66.599

        strain S66.519

Injury *--continued*

  index

    extensor (forearm level)

      hand level S66.308

        laceration S66.32

        specified type NEC S66.39

        strain S66.31

      specified type NEC S56.492

    flexor (forearm level)

      hand level S66.108

        laceration S66.12

        specified type NEC S66.19

        strain S66.11

      specified type NEC S56.19

      strain S56.11

    intrinsic S66.50

      laceration S66.52

      specified type NEC S66.59

      strain S66.51

  little

    extensor (forearm level)

      hand level S66.30

        laceration S66.32

        specified type NEC S66.39

        strain S66.31

      laceration S56.42

      specified type NEC S56.49

      strain S56.41

    flexor (forearm level)

      hand level S66.10

        laceration S66.12

        specified type NEC S66.19

        strain S66.11

      laceration S56.12

      specified type NEC S56.19

      strain S56.11

    intrinsic S66.50

      laceration S66.52

      specified type NEC S66.59

      strain S66.51

  middle

    extensor (forearm level)

      hand level S66.30

        laceration S66.32

        specified type NEC S66.39

        strain S66.31

      laceration S56.42

      specified type NEC S56.49

      strain S56.41

    flexor (forearm level)

      hand level S66.10

        laceration S66.12

        specified type NEC S66.19

        strain S66.11

      laceration S56.12

      specified type NEC S56.19

      strain S56.11

    intrinsic S66.50

      laceration S66.52

      specified type NEC S66.59

      strain S66.51

  ring

    extensor (forearm level)

      hand level S66.30

        laceration S66.32

        specified type NEC S66.39

        strain S66.31

      laceration S56.42

      specified type NEC S56.49

      strain S56.41

    flexor (forearm level)

Injury --*continued*

    hand level S66.10
      laceration S66.12
      specified type NEC S66.19
      strain S66.11
    laceration S56.12
    specified type NEC S56.19
    strain S56.11
    intrinsic S66.50
      laceration S66.52
      specified type NEC S66.59
      strain S66.51
  flexor
    finger(s) (other than thumb) -*see* Injury, muscle, finger
    forearm level, specified NEC -*see* Injury, muscle, forearm, flexor
    thumb -*see* Injury, muscle, thumb, flexor
    toe (long) (ankle level) (foot level) -*see* Injury, muscle, toe, flexor
  foot S96.90
    intrinsic S96.20
      laceration S96.22
      specified type NEC S96.29
      strain S96.21
    laceration S96.92
    long extensor, toe -*see* Injury, muscle, toe, extensor
    long flexor, toe -*see* Injury, muscle, toe, flexor
    specified
      site NEC S96.80
        laceration S96.82
        specified type NEC S96.89
        strain S96.81
      type NEC S96.99
      strain S96.91
  forearm (level) S56.90
    extensor S56.50
      laceration S56.52
      specified type NEC S56.59
      strain S56.51
    flexor S56.20
      laceration S56.22
      specified type NEC S56.29
      strain S56.21
    laceration S56.92
    specified S56.99
      site NEC S56.80
        laceration S56.82
        strain S56.81
        type NEC S56.89
      strain S56.91
  hand (level) S66.90
    laceration S66.92
    specified
      site NEC S66.80
        laceration S66.82
        specified type NEC S66.89
        strain S66.81
        type NEC S66.99
      strain S66.91
  head S09.10
    laceration S09.12
    specified type NEC S09.19
    strain S09.11
  hip NEC S76.00
    laceration S76.02
    specified type NEC S76.09
    strain S76.01
    intrinsic

  ankle and foot level -*see* Injury, muscle, foot, intrinsic
  finger (other than thumb) -*see* Injury, muscle, finger by site, intrinsic
  foot (level) -*see* Injury, muscle, foot, intrinsic
  thumb -*see* Injury, muscle, thumb, intrinsic
  leg (level) (lower) S86.90
    Achilles tendon -*see* Injury, Achilles tendon
    anterior muscle group -*see* Injury, muscle, anterior muscle group
    laceration S86.92
    peroneal muscle group -*see* Injury, muscle, peroneal muscle group
    posterior muscle group -*see* Injury, muscle, posterior muscle group, leg level
    specified
      site NEC S86.80
        laceration S86.82
        specified type NEC S86.89
        strain S86.81
      type NEC S86.99
    strain S86.91
  long
    extensor toe, at ankle and foot level -*see* Injury, muscle, toe, extensor
    flexor, toe, at ankle and foot level -*see* Injury, muscle, toe, flexor
    head, biceps -*see* Injury, muscle, biceps, long head
  lower back S39.002
    laceration S39.022
    specified type NEC S39.092
    strain S39.012
  neck (level) S16.9
    laceration S16.2
    specified type NEC S16.8
    strain S16.1
  pelvis S39.003
    laceration S39.023
    specified type NEC S39.093
    strain S39.013
  peroneal muscle group, at leg level (lower) S86.30
    laceration S86.32
    specified type NEC S86.39
    strain S86.31
  posterior muscle (group)
    leg level (lower) S86.10
      laceration S86.12
      specified type NEC S86.19
      strain S86.11
    thigh level S76.30
      laceration S76.32
      specified type NEC S76.39
      strain S76.31
  quadriceps (thigh) S76.10
    laceration S76.12
    specified type NEC S76.19
    strain S76.11
  shoulder S46.90
    laceration S46.92
    rotator cuff -*see* Injury, rotator cuff
    specified site NEC S46.80
      laceration S46.82
      strain S46.81
      specified type NEC S46.89
    strain S46.91
    specified type NEC S46.99

  thigh NEC (level) S76.90
    adductor -*see* Injury, muscle, adductor, thigh
    laceration S76.92
    posterior muscle (group) -*see* Injury, muscle, posterior muscle, thigh level
    quadriceps -*see* Injury, muscle, quadriceps
    specified
      site NEC S76.80
        laceration S76.82
        specified type NEC S76.89
        strain S76.81
      type NEC S76.99
    strain S76.91
  thorax (level) S29.009
    back wall S29.002
    front wall S29.001
    laceration S29.029
      back wall S29.022
      front wall S29.021
    specified type NEC S29.099
      back wall S29.092
      front wall S29.091
    strain S29.019
      back wall S29.012
      front wall S29.011
  thumb
    abductor (forearm level) S56.30
      laceration S56.32
      specified type NEC S56.39
      strain S56.31
    extensor (forearm level) S56.30
      hand level S66.20
        laceration S66.22
        specified type NEC S66.29
        strain S66.21
      laceration S56.32
      specified type NEC S56.39
      strain S56.31
    flexor (forearm level) S56.00
      hand level S66.00
        laceration S66.02
        specified type NEC S66.09
        strain S66.01
      laceration S56.02
      specified type NEC S56.09
      strain S56.01
      wrist level -*see* Injury, muscle, thumb, flexor, hand level
    intrinsic S66.40
      laceration S66.42
      specified type NEC S66.49
      strain S66.41
  toe -*see also* Injury, muscle, foot
    extensor, long S96.10
      laceration S96.12
      specified type NEC S96.19
      strain S96.11
    flexor, long S96.00
      laceration S96.02
      specified type NEC S96.09
      strain S96.01
  triceps S46.30
    laceration S46.32
    specified type NEC S46.39
    strain S46.31
  wrist (and hand) level -*see* Injury, muscle, hand
  musculocutaneous nerve -*see* Injury, nerve, musculocutaneous

Injury --*continued*

myocardium -*see* Injury, heart
nape -*see* Injury, neck
nasal (septum) (sinus) S09.92
nasopharynx S09.92
neck S19.9
  specified NEC S19.80
    specified site NEC S19.89
nerve NEC T14.8
  abdomen S34.9
    peripheral S34.6
    specified site NEC S34.8
  abducens S04.4
    contusion S04.4
    laceration S04.4
    specified type NEC S04.4
  abducent -*see* Injury, nerve, abducens
  accessory S04.7
    contusion S04.7
    laceration S04.7
    specified type NEC S04.7
  acoustic S04.6
    contusion S04.6
    laceration S04.6
    specified type NEC S04.6
  ankle S94.9
    cutaneous sensory S94.3
    specified site NEC -*see* subcategory S94.8
  anterior crural, femoral -*see* Injury, nerve, femoral
  arm (upper) S44.9
    axillary -*see* Injury, nerve, axillary
    cutaneous -*see* Injury, nerve, cutaneous, arm
    median -*see* Injury, nerve, median, upper arm
    musculocutaneous -*see* Injury, nerve, musculocutaneous
    radial -*see* Injury, nerve, radial, upper arm
    specified site NEC -*see* subcategory S44.8
    ulnar -*see* Injury, nerve, ulnar, arm
  auditory -*see* Injury, nerve, acoustic
  axillary S44.3
  brachial plexus -*see* Injury, brachial plexus
  cervical sympathetic S14.5
  cranial S04.9
    contusion S04.9
    eighth (acoustic or auditory) -*see* Injury, nerve, acoustic
    eleventh (accessory) -*see* Injury, nerve, accessory
    fifth (trigeminal) -*see* Injury, nerve, trigeminal
    first (olfactory) -*see* Injury, nerve, olfactory
    fourth (trochlear) -*see* Injury, nerve, trochlear
    laceration S04.9
    ninth (glossopharyngeal) -*see* Injury, nerve, glossopharyngeal
    second (optic) -*see* Injury, nerve, optic
    seventh (facial) -*see* Injury, nerve, facial
    sixth (abducent) -*see* Injury, nerve, abducens
    specified
      nerve NEC S04.89
        contusion S04.89
        laceration S04.89
        specified type NEC S04.89
      type NEC S04.9

Injury --*continued*

    tenth (pneumogastric or vagus) -*see* Injury, nerve, vagus
    third (oculomotor) -*see* Injury, nerve, oculomotor
    twelfth (hypoglossal) -*see* Injury, nerve, hypoglossal
  cutaneous sensory
    ankle (level) S94.3
    arm (upper) (level) S44.5
    foot (level) -*see* Injury, nerve, cutaneous sensory, ankle
    forearm (level) S54.3
    hip (level) S74.2
    leg (lower level) S84.2
    shoulder (level) -*see* Injury, nerve, cutaneous sensory, arm
    thigh (level) -*see* Injury, nerve, cutaneous sensory, hip
  deep peroneal -*see* Injury, nerve, peroneal, foot
  digital
    finger S64.4
      index S64.49
      little S64.49
      middle S64.49
      ring S64.49
    thumb S64.3
    toe -*see* Injury, nerve, ankle, specified site NEC
  eighth cranial (acoustic or auditory) -*see* Injury, nerve, acoustic
  eleventh cranial (accessory) -*see* Injury, nerve, accessory
  facial S04.5
    contusion S04.5
    laceration S04.5
    newborn P11.3
    specified type NEC S04.5
  femoral (hip level) (thigh level) S74.1
  fifth cranial (trigeminal) -*see* Injury, nerve, trigeminal
  finger (digital) -*see* Injury, nerve, digital, finger
  first cranial (olfactory) -*see* Injury, nerve, olfactory
  foot S94.9
    cutaneous sensory S94.3
    deep peroneal S94.2
    lateral plantar S94.0
    medial plantar S94.1
    specified site NEC -*see* subcategory S94.8
  forearm (level) S54.9
    cutaneous sensory -*see* Injury, nerve, cutaneous sensory, forearm
    median -*see* Injury, nerve, median
    radial -*see* Injury, nerve, radial
    specified site NEC -*see* subcategory S54.8
    ulnar -*see* Injury, nerve, ulnar
  fourth cranial (trochlear) -*see* Injury, nerve, trochlear
  glossopharyngeal S04.89
    specified type NEC S04.89
  hand S64.9
    median -*see* Injury, nerve, median, hand
    radial -*see* Injury, nerve, radial, hand
    specified NEC -*see* subcategory S64.8
    ulnar -*see* Injury, nerve, ulnar, hand
  hip (level) S74.9
    cutaneous sensory -*see* Injury, nerve, cutaneous sensory, hip

Injury --*continued*

    femoral -*see* Injury, nerve, femoral
    sciatic -*see* Injury, nerve, sciatic
    specified site NEC -*see* subcategory S74.8
  hypoglossal S04.89
    specified type NEC S04.89
  lateral plantar S94.0
  leg (lower) S84.9
    cutaneous sensory -*see* Injury, nerve, cutaneous sensory, leg
    peroneal -*see* Injury, nerve, peroneal
    specified site NEC -*see* subcategory S84.8
    tibial -*see* Injury, nerve, tibial
    upper -*see* Injury, nerve, thigh
  lower
    back -*see* Injury, nerve, abdomen, specified site NEC
      peripheral -*see* Injury, nerve, abdomen, peripheral
    limb -*see* Injury, nerve, leg
  lumbar spinal -*see* Injury, nerve, spinal, lumbar
  lumbar plexus -*see* Injury, nerve, lumbosacral, sympathetic
  lumbosacral
    plexus -*see* Injury, nerve, lumbosacral, sympathetic
    sympathetic S34.5
  medial plantar S94.1
  median (forearm level) S54.1
    hand (level) S64.1
    upper arm (level) S44.1
    wrist (level) -*see* Injury, nerve, median, hand
  musculocutaneous S44.4
  musculospiral (upper arm level) -*see* Injury, nerve, radial, upper arm
  neck S14.9
    peripheral S14.4
    specified site NEC S14.8
    sympathetic S14.5
  ninth cranial (glossopharyngeal) -*see* Injury, nerve, glossopharyngeal
  oculomotor S04.1
    contusion S04.1
    laceration S04.1
    specified type NEC S04.1
  olfactory S04.81
    specified type NEC S04.81
  optic S04.01
    contusion S04.01
    laceration S04.01
    specified type NEC S04.01
  pelvic girdle -*see* Injury, nerve, hip
  pelvis -*see* Injury, nerve, abdomen, specified site NEC
  peripheral -*see* Injury, nerve, abdomen, peripheral
  peripheral NEC T14.8
    abdomen -*see* Injury, nerve, abdomen, peripheral
    lower back -*see* Injury, nerve, abdomen, peripheral
    neck -*see* Injury, nerve, neck, peripheral
    pelvis -*see* Injury, nerve, abdomen, peripheral
    specified NEC T14.8
  peroneal (lower leg level) S84.1
    foot S94.2
  plexus
    brachial -*see* Injury, brachial plexus

Injury *--continued*
- celiac, coeliac *-see* Injury, nerve, lumbosacral, sympathetic
- mesenteric, inferior *-see* Injury, nerve, lumbosacral, sympathetic
- sacral *-see* Injury, lumbosacral plexus
- spinal
  - brachial *-see* Injury, brachial plexus
  - lumbosacral *-see* Injury, lumbosacral plexus
- pneumogastric *-see* Injury, nerve, vagus
- radial (forearm level) S54.2
  - hand (level) S64.2
  - upper arm (level) S44.2
  - wrist (level) *-see* Injury, nerve, radial, hand
- root *-see* Injury, nerve, spinal, root
- sacral plexus *-see* Injury, lumbosacral plexus
- sacral spinal *-see* Injury, nerve, spinal, sacral
- sciatic (hip level) (thigh level) S74.0
- second cranial (optic) *-see* Injury, nerve, optic
- seventh cranial (facial) *-see* Injury, nerve, facial
- shoulder *-see* Injury, nerve, arm
- sixth cranial (abducent) *-see* Injury, nerve, abducens
- spinal
  - plexus *-see* Injury, nerve, plexus, spinal
  - root
    - cervical S14.2
    - dorsal S24.2
    - lumbar S34.21
    - sacral S34.22
    - thoracic *-see* Injury, nerve, spinal, root, dorsal
- splanchnic *-see* Injury, nerve, lumbosacral, sympathetic
- sympathetic NEC *-see* Injury, nerve, lumbosacral, sympathetic
- cervical *-see* Injury, nerve, cervical sympathetic
- tenth cranial (pneumogastric or vagus) *-see* Injury, nerve, vagus
- thigh (level) *-see* Injury, nerve, hip
  - cutaneous sensory *-see* Injury, nerve, cutaneous sensory, hip
  - femoral *-see* Injury, nerve, femoral
  - sciatic *-see* Injury, nerve, sciatic
  - specified NEC *-see* Injury, nerve, hip
- third cranial (oculomotor) *-see* Injury, nerve, oculomotor
- thorax S24.9
  - peripheral S24.3
  - specified site NEC S24.8
  - sympathetic S24.4
- thumb, digital *-see* Injury, nerve, digital, thumb
- tibial (lower leg level) (posterior) S84.0
- toe *-see* Injury, nerve, ankle
- trigeminal S04.3
  - contusion S04.3
  - laceration S04.3
  - specified type NEC S04.3
- trochlear S04.2
  - contusion S04.2
  - laceration S04.2
  - specified type NEC S04.2
- twelfth cranial (hypoglossal) *-see* Injury, nerve, hypoglossal
- ulnar (forearm level) S54.0
  - arm (upper) (level) S44.0

Injury *--continued*
- hand (level) S64.0
  - wrist (level) *-see* Injury, nerve, ulnar, hand
- vagus S04.89
  - specified type NEC S04.89
  - wrist (level) *-see* Injury, nerve, hand
- ninth cranial nerve (glossopharyngeal) *-see* Injury, nerve, glossopharyngeal
- nose (septum) S09.92
- obstetrical O71.9
  - specified NEC O71.89
- occipital (region) (scalp) S09.90
  - lobe *-see* Injury, intracranial
- optic chiasm S04.02
- optic radiation S04.03
- optic tract and pathways S04.03
- orbit, orbital (region) *-see* Injury, eye
  - penetrating (with foreign body) *-see* Injury, eye, orbit, penetrating
  - specified NEC *-see* Injury, eye, specified site NEC
- ovary, ovarian S37.409
  - bilateral S37.402
    - contusion S37.422
    - laceration S37.432
    - specified type NEC S37.492
  - blood vessel *-see* Injury, blood vessel, ovarian
  - contusion S37.429
    - bilateral S37.422
    - unilateral S37.421
  - laceration S37.439
    - bilateral S37.432
    - unilateral S37.431
  - specified type NEC S37.499
    - bilateral S37.492
    - unilateral S37.491
  - unilateral S37.401
    - contusion S37.421
    - laceration S37.431
    - specified type NEC S37.491
- palate (hard) (soft) S09.93
- pancreas S36.209
  - body S36.201
    - contusion S36.221
    - laceration S36.231
      - major S36.261
      - minor S36.241
      - moderate S36.251
    - specified type NEC S36.291
  - contusion S36.229
  - head S36.200
    - contusion S36.220
    - laceration S36.230
      - major S36.260
      - minor S36.240
      - moderate S36.250
    - specified type NEC S36.290
  - laceration S36.239
    - major S36.269
    - minor S36.249
    - moderate S36.259
  - specified type NEC S36.299
  - tail S36.202
    - contusion S36.222
    - laceration S36.232
      - major S36.262
      - minor S36.242
      - moderate S36.252
    - specified type NEC S36.292
- parietal (region) (scalp) S09.90

Injury *--continued*
- lobe *-see* Injury, intracranial
- patellar ligament (tendon) S76.10
  - laceration S76.12
  - specified NEC S76.19
  - strain S76.11
- pelvis, pelvic (floor) S39.93
  - complicating delivery O70.1
  - joint or ligament, complicating delivery O71.6
  - organ S37.90
    - with ectopic or molar pregnancy O08.6
    - complication of abortion *-see* Abortion
    - contusion S37.92
    - following ectopic or molar pregnancy O08.6
    - laceration S37.93
    - obstetrical trauma NEC O71.5
    - specified
      - site NEC S37.899
        - contusion S37.892
        - laceration S37.893
        - specified type NEC S37.898
      - type NEC S37.99
  - specified NEC S39.83
- penis S39.94
- perineum S39.94
- peritoneum S36.81
  - laceration S36.893
- periurethral tissue *-see* Injury, urethra
  - complicating delivery O71.82
- phalanges
  - foot *-see* Injury, foot
  - hand *-see* Injury, hand
- pharynx NEC S19.85
- pleura *-see* Injury, intrathoracic, pleura
- plexus
  - brachial *-see* Injury, brachial plexus
  - cardiac *-see* Injury, nerve, thorax, sympathetic
  - celiac, coeliac *-see* Injury, nerve, lumbosacral, sympathetic
  - esophageal *-see* Injury, nerve, thorax, sympathetic
  - hypogastric *-see* Injury, nerve, lumbosacral, sympathetic
  - lumbar, lumbosacral *-see* Injury, lumbosacral plexus
  - mesenteric *-see* Injury, nerve, lumbosacral, sympathetic
  - pulmonary *-see* Injury, nerve, thorax, sympathetic
- postcardiac surgery (syndrome) I97.0
- prepuce S39.94
- prostate S37.829
  - contusion S37.822
  - laceration S37.823
  - specified type NEC S37.828
- pubic region S39.94
- pudendum S39.94
- pulmonary plexus *-see* Injury, nerve, thorax, sympathetic
- rectovaginal septum NEC S39.83
- rectum *-see* Injury, intestine, large, rectum
- retina *-see* Injury, eye, specified site NEC
  - penetrating *-see* Injury, eyeball, penetrating
- retroperitoneal *-see* Injury, intra-abdominal, specified site NEC
- rotator cuff (muscle(s)) (tendon(s)) S46.00
  - laceration S46.02
  - specified type NEC S46.09

Injury --continued
   strain S46.01
  round ligament -see Injury, pelvic organ,
    specified site NEC
  sacral plexus -see Injury, lumbosacral plexus
  salivary duct or gland S09.93
  scalp S09.90
   newborn (birth injury) P12.9
    due to monitoring (electrode) (sampling
     incision) P12.4
    specified NEC P12.89
     caput succedaneum P12.81
  scapular region -see Injury, shoulder
  sclera -see Injury, eye, specified site NEC
   penetrating -see Injury, eyeball, penetrating
  scrotum S39.94
  second cranial nerve (optic) -see Injury,
   nerve, optic
  seminal vesicle -see Injury, pelvic organ,
   specified site NEC
  seventh cranial nerve (facial) -see Injury,
   nerve, facial
  shoulder S49.9
   blood vessel -see Injury, blood vessel, arm
   contusion -see Contusion, shoulder
   dislocation -see Dislocation, shoulder
   fracture -see Fracture, shoulder
   muscle -see Injury, muscle, shoulder
   nerve -see Injury, nerve, shoulder
   open -see Wound, open, shoulder
   specified type NEC S49.8
   sprain -see Sprain, shoulder girdle
   superficial -see Injury, superficial, shoulder
  sinus
   cavernous -see Injury, intracranial
   nasal S09.92
  sixth cranial nerve (abducent) -see Injury,
   nerve, abducens
  skeleton, birth injury P13.9
   specified part NEC P13.8
  skin NEC T14.8
   surface intact -see Injury, superficial
  skull NEC S09.90
  specified NEC T14.8
  spermatic cord (pelvic region) S37.898
   scrotal region S39.848
  spinal (cord)
   cervical (neck) S14.109
    anterior cord syndrome S14.139
     C1 level S14.131
     C2 level S14.132
     C3 level S14.133
     C4 level S14.134
     C5 level S14.135
     C6 level S14.136
     C7 level S14.137
     C8 level S14.138
    Brown-Séquard syndrome S14.149
     C1 level S14.141
     C2 level S14.142
     C3 level S14.143
     C4 level S14.144
     C5 level S14.145
     C6 level S14.146
     C7 level S14.147
     C8 level S14.148
    C1 level S14.101
    C2 level S14.102
    C3 level S14.103
    C4 level S14.104
    C5 level S14.105

Injury --continued
    C6 level S14.106
    C7 level S14.107
    C8 level S14.108
    central cord syndrome S14.129
     C1 level S14.121
     C2 level S14.122
     C3 level S14.123
     C4 level S14.124
     C5 level S14.125
     C6 level S14.126
     C7 level S14.127
     C8 level S14.128
    complete lesion S14.119
     C1 level S14.111
     C2 level S14.112
     C3 level S14.113
     C4 level S14.114
     C5 level S14.115
     C6 level S14.116
     C7 level S14.117
     C8 level S14.118
    concussion S14.0
    edema S14.0
    incomplete lesion specified NEC S14.159
     C1 level S14.151
     C2 level S14.152
     C3 level S14.153
     C4 level S14.154
     C5 level S14.155
     C6 level S14.156
     C7 level S14.157
     C8 level S14.158
    posterior cord syndrome S14.159
     C1 level S14.151
     C2 level S14.152
     C3 level S14.153
     C4 level S14.154
     C5 level S14.155
     C6 level S14.156
     C7 level S14.157
     C8 level S14.158
   dorsal -see Injury, spinal, thoracic
   lumbar S34.109
    complete lesion S34.119
     L1 level S34.111
     L2 level S34.112
     L3 level S34.113
     L4 level S34.114
     L5 level S34.115
    concussion S34.01
    edema S34.01
    incomplete lesion S34.129
     L1 level S34.121
     L2 level S34.122
     L3 level S34.123
     L4 level S34.124
     L5 level S34.125
     L1 level S34.101
     L2 level S34.102
     L3 level S34.103
     L4 level S34.104
     L5 level S34.105
   nerve root NEC
    cervical -see Injury, nerve, spinal, root,
     cervical
    dorsal -see Injury, nerve, spinal, root,
     dorsal
    lumbar S34.21
    sacral S34.22

Injury --continued
    thoracic -see Injury, nerve, spinal, root,
     dorsal
   plexus
    brachial -see Injury, brachial plexus
    lumbosacral -see Injury, lumbosacral
     plexus
   sacral S34.139
    complete lesion S34.131
    incomplete lesion S34.132
   thoracic S24.109
    anterior cord syndrome S24.139
     T1 level S24.131
     T2 T6 level S24.132
     T7 T10 level S24.133
     T11 T12 level S24.134
    Brown-Séquard syndrome S24.149
     T1 level S24.141
     T2 T6 level S24.142
     T7 T10 level S24.143
     T11 T12 level S24.144
    complete lesion S24.119
     T1 level S24.111
     T2 T6 level S24.112
     T7 T10 level S24.113
     T11 T12 level S24.114
    concussion S24.0
    edema S24.0
    incomplete lesion specified NEC S24.159
     T1 level S24.151
     T2 T6 level S24.152
     T7 T10 level S24.153
     T11 T12 level S24.154
    posterior cord syndrome S24.159
     T1 level S24.151
     T2 T6 level S24.152
     T7 T10 level S24.153
     T11 T12 level S24.154
    T1 level S24.101
    T2 T6 level S24.102
    T7 T10 level S24.103
    T11 T12 level S24.104
  splanchnic nerve -see Injury, nerve,
   lumbosacral, sympathetic
  spleen S36.00
   contusion S36.029
    major S36.021
    minor S36.020
   laceration S36.039
    major (massive) (stellate) S36.032
    moderate S36.031
    superficial (capsular) (minor) S36.030
   specified type NEC S36.09
  splenic artery -see Injury, blood vessel, celiac
   artery, branch
  stellate ganglion -see Injury, nerve, thorax,
   sympathetic
  sternal region S29.9
  stomach S36.30
   contusion S36.32
   laceration S36.33
   specified type NEC S36.39
  subconjunctival -see Injury, eye, conjunctiva
  subcutaneous NEC T14.8
  submaxillary region S09.93
  submental region S09.93
  subungual
   fingers -see Injury, hand
   toes -see Injury, foot
  superficial NEC T14.8
   abdomen, abdominal (wall) S30.92

Injury *--continued*
    abrasion S30.811
    bite S30.871
      insect S30.861
    contusion S30.1
    external constriction S30.841
    foreign body S30.851
  abrasion *-see* Abrasion, by site
  adnexa, eye NEC *-see* Injury, eye, specified
    site NEC
  alveolar process *-see* Injury, superficial, oral
    cavity
  ankle S90.91
    abrasion *-see* Abrasion, ankle
    blister *-see* Blister, ankle
    bite *-see* Bite, ankle
    contusion *-see* Contusion, ankle
    external constriction *-see* Constriction,
    external, ankle
    foreign body *-see* Foreign body,
      superficial, ankle
  anus S30.98
  arm (upper) S40.92
    abrasion *-see* Abrasion, arm
    bite *-see* Bite, superficial, arm
    blister *-see* Blister, arm (upper)
    contusion *-see* Contusion, arm
    external constriction *-see* Constriction,
    external, arm
    foreign body *-see* Foreign body,
      superficial, arm
  auditory canal (external) (meatus) *-see*
    Injury, superficial, ear
  auricle *-see* Injury, superficial, ear
  axilla *-see* Injury, superficial, arm
  back *-see also* Injury, superficial, thorax,
    back
    lower S30.91
      abrasion S30.810
      contusion S30.0
      external constriction S30.840
      superficial
        bite NEC S30.870
          insect S30.860
        foreign body S30.850
  bite NEC *-see* Bite, superficial NEC, by site
  blister *-see* Blister, by site
  breast S20.10
    abrasion *-see* Abrasion, breast
    bite *-see* Bite, superficial, breast
    contusion *-see* Contusion, breast
    external constriction *-see* Constriction,
    external, breast
    foreign body *-see* Foreign body,
      superficial, breast
  brow *-see* Injury, superficial, head, specified
    NEC
  buttock S30.91
  calf *-see* Injury, superficial, leg
  canthus, eye *-see* Injury, superficial,
    periocular area
  cheek (external) *-see* Injury, superficial,
    head, specified NEC
    internal *-see* Injury, superficial, oral cavity
  chest wall *-see* Injury, superficial, thorax
  chin *-see* Injury, superficial, head NEC
  clitoris S30.95
  conjunctiva *-see* Injury, eye, conjunctiva
    with foreign body (in conjunctival sac) *-see*
    Foreign body, conjunctival sac
  contusion *-see* Contusion, by site

Injury *--continued*
  costal region *-see* Injury, superficial, thorax
  digit(s)
    hand *-see* Injury, superficial, finger
  ear (auricle) (canal) (external) S00.40
    abrasion *-see* Abrasion, ear
    bite *-see* Bite, superficial, ear
    contusion *-see* Contusion, ear
    external constriction *-see* Constriction,
    external, ear
    foreign body *-see* Foreign body,
      superficial, ear
  elbow S50.90
    abrasion *-see* Abrasion, elbow
    bite *-see* Bite, superficial, elbow
    blister *-see* Blister, elbow
    contusion *-see* Contusion, elbow
    external constriction *-see* Constriction,
    external, elbow
    foreign body *-see* Foreign body,
      superficial, elbow
  epididymis S30.94
  epigastric region S30.92
  epiglottis *-see* Injury, superficial, throat
  esophagus
    cervical *-see* Injury, superficial, throat
  external constriction *-see* Constriction,
    external, by site
  extremity NEC T14.8
  eyeball NEC *-see* Injury, eye, specified site
    NEC
  eyebrow *-see* Injury, superficial, periocular
    area
  eyelid S00.20
    abrasion *-see* Abrasion, eyelid
    bite *-see* Bite, superficial, eyelid
    contusion *-see* Contusion, eyelid
    external constriction *-see* Constriction,
    external, eyelid
    foreign body *-see* Foreign body,
      superficial, eyelid
  face NEC *-see* Injury, superficial, head,
    specified NEC
  finger(s) S60.949
    abrasion *-see* Abrasion, finger
    bite *-see* Bite, superficial, finger
    blister *-see* Blister, finger
    contusion *-see* Contusion, finger
    external constriction *-see* Constriction,
    external, finger
    foreign body *-see* Foreign body,
      superficial, finger
    insect bite *-see* Bite, by site, superficial,
      insect
    index S60.94
    little S60.94
    middle S60.94
    ring S60.94
  flank S30.92
  foot S90.92
    abrasion *-see* Abrasion, foot
    bite *-see* Bite, foot
    blister *-see* Blister, foot
    contusion *-see* Contusion, foot
    external constriction *-see* Constriction,
    external, foot
    foreign body *-see* Foreign body,
      superficial, foot
  forearm S50.91
    abrasion *-see* Abrasion, forearm
    bite *-see* Bite, forearm, superficial

Injury *--continued*
    blister *-see* Blister, forearm
    contusion *-see* Contusion, forearm
    elbow only *-see* Injury, superficial, elbow
    external constriction *-see* Constriction,
    external, forearm
    foreign body *-see* Foreign body,
      superficial, forearm
  forehead *-see* Injury, superficial, head NEC
  foreign body *-see* Foreign body, superficial
  genital organs, external
    female S30.97
    male S30.96
  globe (eye) *-see* Injury, eye, specified site
    NEC
  groin S30.92
  gum *-see* Injury, superficial, oral cavity
  hand S60.92
    abrasion *-see* Abrasion, hand
    bite *-see* Bite, superficial, hand
    contusion *-see* Contusion, hand
    external constriction *-see* Constriction,
    external, hand
    foreign body *-see* Foreign body,
      superficial, hand
  head S00.90
    ear *-see* Injury, superficial, ear
    eyelid *-see* Injury, superficial, eyelid
    nose S00.30
    oral cavity S00.502
    scalp S00.00
    specified site NEC S00.80
  heel *-see* Injury, superficial, foot
  hip S70.91
    abrasion *-see* Abrasion, hip
    bite *-see* Bite, superficial, hip
    blister *-see* Blister, hip
    contusion *-see* Contusion, hip
    external constriction *-see* Constriction,
    external, hip
    foreign body *-see* Foreign body,
      superficial, hip
  iliac region *-see* Injury, superficial, abdomen
  inguinal region *-see* Injury, superficial,
    abdomen
  insect bite *-see* Bite, by site, superficial,
    insect
  interscapular region *-see* Injury, superficial,
    thorax, back
  jaw *-see* Injury, superficial, head, specified
    NEC
  knee S80.91
    abrasion *-see* Abrasion, knee
    bite *-see* Bite, superficial, knee
    blister *-see* Blister, knee
    contusion *-see* Contusion, knee
    external constriction *-see* Constriction,
    external, knee
    foreign body *-see* Foreign body,
      superficial, knee
  labium (majus) (minus) S30.95
  lacrimal (apparatus) (gland) (sac) *-see*
    Injury, eye, specified site NEC
  larynx *-see* Injury, superficial, throat
  leg (lower) S80.92
    abrasion *-see* Abrasion, leg
    bite *-see* Bite, superficial, leg
    contusion *-see* Contusion, leg
    external constriction *-see* Constriction,
    external, leg

Injury --*continued*

foreign body -*see* Foreign body,
   superficial, leg
knee -*see* Injury, superficial, knee
limb NEC T14.8
lip S00.501
lower back S30.91
lumbar region S30.91
malar region -*see* Injury, superficial, head,
   specified NEC
mammary -*see* Injury, superficial, breast
mastoid region -*see* Injury, superficial, head,
   specified NEC
mouth -*see* Injury, superficial, oral cavity
muscle NEC T14.8
nail NEC T14.8
   finger -*see* Injury, superficial, finger
   toe -*see* Injury, superficial, toe
nasal (septum) -*see* Injury, superficial, nose
neck S10.90
   specified site NEC S10.80
nose (septum) S00.30
occipital region -*see* Injury, superficial,
   scalp
oral cavity S00.502
orbital region -*see* Injury, superficial,
   periocular area
palate -*see* Injury, superficial, oral cavity
palm -*see* Injury, superficial, hand
parietal region -*see* Injury, superficial, scalp
pelvis S30.91
   girdle -*see* Injury, superficial, hip
penis S30.93
perineum
   female S30.95
   male S30.91
periocular area S00.20
   abrasion -*see* Abrasion, eyelid
   bite -*see* Bite, superficial, eyelid
   contusion -*see* Contusion, eyelid
   external constriction -*see* Constriction,
     external, eyelid
   foreign body -*see* Foreign body,
     superficial, eyelid
phalanges
   finger -*see* Injury, superficial, finger
   toe -*see* Injury, superficial, toe
pharynx -*see* Injury, superficial, throat
pinna -*see* Injury, superficial, ear
popliteal space -*see* Injury, superficial, knee
prepuce S30.93
pubic region S30.91
pudendum
   female S30.97
   male S30.96
sacral region S30.91
scalp S00.00
scapular region -*see* Injury, superficial,
   shoulder
sclera -*see* Injury, eye, specified site NEC
scrotum S30.94
shin -*see* Injury, superficial, leg
shoulder S40.91
   abrasion -*see* Abrasion, shoulder
   bite -*see* Bite, superficial, shoulder
   blister -*see* Blister, shoulder
   contusion -*see* Contusion, shoulder
   external constriction -*see* Constriction,
     external, shoulder
   foreign body -*see* Foreign body,
     superficial, shoulder

Injury --*continued*

skin NEC T14.8
sternal region -*see* Injury, superficial,
   thorax, front
subconjunctival -*see* Injury, eye, specified
   site NEC
subcutaneous NEC T14.8
submaxillary region -*see* Injury, superficial,
   head, specified NEC
submental region -*see* Injury, superficial,
   head, specified NEC
subungual
   finger(s) -*see* Injury, superficial, finger
   toe(s) -*see* Injury, superficial, toe
supraclavicular fossa -*see* Injury, superficial,
   neck
supraorbital -*see* Injury, superficial, head,
   specified NEC
temple -*see* Injury, superficial, head,
   specified NEC
temporal region -*see* Injury, superficial,
   head, specified NEC
testis S30.94
thigh S70.92
   abrasion -*see* Abrasion, thigh
   bite -*see* Bite, superficial, thigh
   blister -*see* Blister, thigh
   contusion -*see* Contusion, thigh
   external constriction -*see* Constriction,
     external, thigh
   foreign body -*see* Foreign body,
     superficial, thigh
thorax, thoracic (wall) S20.90
   abrasion -*see* Abrasion, thorax
   back S20.40
   bite -*see* Bite, thorax, superficial
   blister -*see* Blister, thorax
   contusion -*see* Contusion, thorax
   external constriction -*see* Constriction,
     external, thorax
   foreign body -*see* Foreign body,
     superficial, thorax
   front S20.30
throat S10.10
   abrasion S10.11
   bite S10.17
     insect S10.16
   blister S10.12
   contusion S10.0
   external constriction S10.14
   foreign body S10.15
thumb S60.93
   abrasion -*see* Abrasion, thumb
   bite -*see* Bite, superficial, thumb
   blister -*see* Blister, thumb
   contusion -*see* Contusion, thumb
   external constriction -*see* Constriction,
     external, thumb
   foreign body -*see* Foreign body,
     superficial, thumb
   insect bite -*see* Bite, by site, superficial,
     insect
   specified type NEC S60.39
toe(s) S90.93
   abrasion -*see* Abrasion, toe
   bite -*see* Bite, toe
   blister -*see* Blister, toe
   contusion -*see* Contusion, toe
   external constriction -*see* Constriction,
     external, toe

Injury --*continued*

foreign body -*see* Foreign body,
   superficial, toe
   great S90.93
tongue -*see* Injury, superficial, oral cavity
tooth, teeth -*see* Injury, superficial, oral
cavity
trachea S10.10
tunica vaginalis S30.94
tympanum, tympanic membrane -*see* Injury,
   superficial, ear
uvula -*see* Injury, superficial, oral cavity
vagina S30.95
vocal cords -*see* Injury, superficial, throat
vulva S30.95
wrist S60.91
supraclavicular region -*see* Injury, neck
supraorbital S09.93
suprarenal gland (multiple) -*see* Injury,
   adrenal
surgical complication (external or internal
   site) -*see* Laceration, accidental
   complicating surgery   temple S09.90
temporal region S09.90
tendon -*see also* Injury, muscle, by site
   abdomen -*see* Injury, muscle, abdomen
   Achilles -*see* Injury, Achilles tendon
   lower back -*see* Injury, muscle, lower back
   pelvic organs -*see* Injury, muscle, pelvis
tenth cranial nerve (pneumogastric or vagus) -
   see Injury, nerve, vagus
testis S39.94
thigh S79.92
   blood vessel -*see* Injury, blood vessel, hip
   contusion -*see* Contusion, thigh
   fracture -*see* Fracture, femur
   muscle -*see* Injury, muscle, thigh
   nerve -*see* Injury, nerve, thigh
   open -*see* Wound, open, thigh
   specified NEC S79.82
   superficial -*see* Injury, superficial, thigh
third cranial nerve (oculomotor) -*see* Injury,
   nerve, oculomotor
thorax, thoracic S29.9
   blood vessel -*see* Injury, blood vessel,
thorax
   cavity -*see* Injury, intrathoracic
   dislocation -*see* Dislocation, thorax
   external (wall) S29.9
     contusion -*see* Contusion, thorax
     nerve -*see* Injury, nerve, thorax
     open -*see* Wound, open, thorax
     specified NEC S29.8
     sprain -*see* Sprain, thorax
     superficial -*see* Injury, superficial, thorax
   fracture -*see* Fracture, thorax
   internal -*see* Injury, intrathoracic
   intrathoracic organ -*see* Injury, intrathoracic
   sympathetic ganglion -*see* Injury, nerve,
   thorax, sympathetic
throat -*see also* Injury, neck S19.9
thumb S69.9
   blood vessel -*see* Injury, blood vessel,
     thumb
   contusion -*see* Contusion, thumb
   dislocation -*see* Dislocation, thumb
   fracture -*see* Fracture, thumb
   muscle -*see* Injury, muscle, thumb
   nerve -*see* Injury, nerve, digital, thumb
   open -*see* Wound, open, thumb
   specified NEC S69.8

Injury --*continued*
- sprain -*see* Sprain, thumb
- superficial -*see* Injury, superficial, thumb
- thymus (gland) -*see* Injury, intrathoracic, specified organ NEC
- thyroid (gland) NEC S19.84
- toe S99.92
  - contusion -*see* Contusion, toe
  - dislocation -*see* Dislocation, toe
  - fracture -*see* Fracture, toe
  - muscle -*see* Injury, muscle, toe
  - open -*see* Wound, open, toe
  - specified type NEC S99.82
  - sprain -*see* Sprain, toe
  - superficial -*see* Injury, superficial, toe
- tongue S09.93
- tonsil S09.93
- tooth S09.93
- trachea (cervical) NEC S19.82
  - thoracic -*see* Injury, intrathoracic, trachea, thoracic
- transfusion-related acute lung (TRALI) J95.84
- tunica vaginalis S39.94
- twelfth cranial nerve (hypoglossal) -*see* Injury, nerve, hypoglossal
- ureter S37.10
  - contusion S37.12
  - laceration S37.13
  - specified type NEC S37.19
- urethra (sphincter) S37.30
  - at delivery O71.5
  - contusion S37.32
  - laceration S37.33
  - specified type NEC S37.39
- urinary organ S37.90
  - contusion S37.92
  - laceration S37.93
  - specified
    - site NEC S37.899
      - contusion S37.892
      - laceration S37.893
      - specified type NEC S37.898
    - type NEC S37.99
- uterus, uterine S37.60
  - with ectopic or molar pregnancy O08.6
  - blood vessel -*see* Injury, blood vessel, iliac
  - contusion S37.62
  - laceration S37.63
    - cervix at delivery O71.3
  - rupture associated with obstetrics -*see* Rupture, uterus
  - specified type NEC S37.69
- uvula S09.93
- vagina S39.93
  - abrasion S30.814
  - bite S31.45
    - insect S30.864
    - superficial NEC S30.874
  - contusion S30.23
  - crush S38.03
  - during delivery -*see* Laceration, vagina, during delivery
  - external constriction S30.844
  - insect bite S30.864
  - laceration S31.41
    - with foreign body S31.42
  - open wound S31.40
  - puncture S31.43
    - with foreign body S31.44
  - superficial S30.95

Injury --*continued*
- foreign body S30.854
- vas deferens -*see* Injury, pelvic organ, specified site NEC
- vascular NEC T14.8
- vein -*see* Injury, blood vessel
- vena cava (superior) S25.20
  - inferior S35.10
    - laceration (minor) (superficial) S35.11
      - major S35.12
    - specified type NEC S35.19
  - laceration (minor) (superficial) S25.21
    - major S25.22
  - specified type NEC S25.29
- vesical (sphincter) -*see* Injury, bladder
- visual cortex S04.04
- vitreous (humor) S05.90
  - specified NEC S05.8X vocal cord NEC S19.83
- vulva S39.94
  - abrasion S30.814
  - bite S31.45
    - insect S30.864
    - superficial NEC S30.874
  - contusion S30.23
  - crush S38.03
  - during delivery -*see* Laceration, perineum, female, during delivery
  - external constriction S30.844
  - insect bite S30.864
  - laceration S31.41
    - with foreign body S31.42
  - open wound S31.40
  - puncture S31.43
    - with foreign body S31.44
  - superficial S30.95
    - foreign body S30.854
- whiplash (cervical spine) S13.4
- wrist S69.9
  - blood vessel -*see* Injury, blood vessel, hand
  - contusion -*see* Contusion, wrist
  - dislocation -*see* Dislocation, wrist
  - fracture -*see* Fracture, wrist
  - muscle -*see* Injury, muscle, hand
  - nerve -*see* Injury, nerve, hand
  - open -*see* Wound, open, wrist
  - specified NEC S69.8
  - sprain -*see* Sprain, wrist
  - superficial -*see* Injury, superficial, wrist

Inoculation -*see also* Vaccination
- complication or reaction -*see* Complications, vaccination

Insanity, insane -*see also* Psychosis
- adolescent -*see* Schizophrenia
- confusional F28
  - acute or subacute F05
- delusional F22
- senile F03

Insect
- bite -*see* Bite, by site, superficial, insect
- venomous, poisoning NEC (by) -*see* Venom, arthropod

Insensitivity
- adrenocorticotropin hormone (ACTH) E27.49
- androgen E34.50
  - complete E34.51
  - partial E34.52

Insertion
- cord (umbilical) lateral or velamentous O43.12
- intrauterine contraceptive device (encounter for) -*see* Intrauterine contraceptive device

Insolation (sunstroke) T67.0
Insomnia (organic) G47.00
- adjustment F51.02
- adjustment disorder F51.02
- behavioral, of childhood Z73.819
  - combined type Z73.812
  - limit setting type Z73.811
  - sleep-onset association type Z73.810
- childhood Z73.819
- chronic F51.04
  - somatized tension F51.04
- conditioned F51.04
- due to
  - alcohol
    - abuse F10.182
    - dependence F10.282
    - use F10.982
  - amphetamines
    - abuse F15.182
    - dependence F15.282
    - use F15.982
  - anxiety disorder F51.05
  - caffeine
    - abuse F15.182
    - dependence F15.282
    - use F15.982
  - cocaine
    - abuse F14.182
    - dependence F14.282
    - use F14.982
  - depression F51.05
  - drug NEC
    - abuse F19.182
    - dependence F19.282
    - use F19.982
  - medical condition G47.01
  - mental disorder NEC F51.05
  - opioid
    - abuse F11.182
    - dependence F11.282
    - use F11.982
  - psychoactive substance NEC
    - abuse F19.182
    - dependence F19.282
    - use F19.982
  - sedative, hypnotic, or anxiolytic
    - abuse F13.182
    - dependence F13.282
    - use F13.982
  - stimulant NEC
    - abuse F15.182
    - dependence F15.282
    - use F15.982
- fatal familial (FFI) A81.83
- idiopathic F51.01
- learned F51.3
- nonorganic origin F51.01
- not due to a substance or known physiological condition F51.01
  - specified NEC F51.09
- paradoxical F51.03
- primary F51.01
- psychiatric F51.05
- psychophysiologic F51.04
- related to psychopathology F51.05
- short-term F51.02
- specified NEC G47.09
- stress-related F51.02
- transient F51.02
- without objective findings F51.02

Inspiration
food or foreign body -*see* Foreign body, by
site
mucus -*see* Asphyxia, mucus
Inspissated bile syndrome (newborn) P59.1
Instability
emotional (excessive) F60.3
joint (post-traumatic) M25.30
ankle M25.37
due to old ligament injury -*see* Disorder,
ligament
elbow M25.32
flail -*see* Flail, joint
foot M25.37
hand M25.34
hip M25.35
knee M25.36
lumbosacral -*see* subcategory M53.2
prosthesis -*see* Complications, joint
prosthesis, mechanical, displacement, by site
sacroiliac -*see* subcategory M53.2
secondary to
old ligament injury -*see* Disorder, ligament
removal of joint prosthesis M96.89
shoulder (region) M25.31
spine - see subcategory M53.2
wrist M25.33
knee (chronic) M23.5
lumbosacral -*see* subcategory M53.2
nervous F48.8
personality (emotional) F60.3
spine -*see* Instability, joint, spine
vasomotor R55
Institutional syndrome (childhood) F94.2
Institutionalization, affecting child Z62.22
disinhibited attachment F94.2
Insufficiency, insufficient
accommodation, old age H52.4
adrenal (gland) E27.40
primary E27.1
adrenocortical E27.40
drug-induced E27.3
iatrogenic E27.3
primary E27.1
anatomic crown height K08.89
anterior (occlusal) guidance M26.54
anus K62.89
aortic (valve) I35.1
with
mitral (valve) disease I08.0
with tricuspid (valve) disease I08.3
stenosis I35.2
tricuspid (valve) disease I08.2
with mitral (valve) disease I08.3
congenital Q23.1
rheumatic I06.1
with
mitral (valve) disease I08.0
with tricuspid (valve) disease I08.3
stenosis I06.2
with mitral (valve) disease I08.0
with tricuspid (valve) disease I08.3
tricuspid (valve) disease I08.2
with mitral (valve) disease I08.3
specified cause NEC I35.1
syphilitic A52.03
arterial I77.1
basilar G45.0
carotid (hemispheric) G45.1
cerebral I67.81
coronary (acute or subacute) I24.8

Insufficiency, insufficient - *continued*
mesenteric K55.1
peripheral I73.9
precerebral (multiple) (bilateral) G45.2
vertebral G45.0
arteriovenous I99.8
biliary K83.8
cardiac -*see also* Insufficiency, myocardial
due to presence of (cardiac) prosthesis
I97.11
postprocedural I97.11
cardiorenal, hypertensive I13.2
cardiovascular -*see* Disease, cardiovascular
cerebrovascular (acute) I67.81
with transient focal neurological signs and
symptoms G45.8
circulatory NEC I99.8
newborn P29.89
clinical crown length K08.89
convergence H51.11
coronary (acute or subacute) I24.8
chronic or with a stated duration of over 4
weeks I25.89
corticoadrenal E27.40
primary E27.1
dietary E63.9
divergence H51.8
food T73.0
gastroesophageal K22.8
gonadal
ovary E28.39
testis E29.1
heart -*see also* Insufficiency, myocardial
newborn P29.0
valve -*see* Endocarditis
hepatic -*see* Failure, hepatic
idiopathic autonomic G90.09
interocclusal distance of fully erupted teeth
(ridge) M26.36
kidney N28.9
acute N28.9
chronic N18.9
lacrimal (secretion) H04.12
passages -*see* Stenosis, lacrimal
liver -*see* Failure, hepatic
lung -*see* Insufficiency, pulmonary
mental (congenital) -*see* Disability,
intellectual
mesenteric K55.1
mitral (valve) I34.0
with
aortic valve disease I08.0
with tricuspid (valve) disease I08.3
obstruction or stenosis I05.2
with aortic valve disease I08.0
tricuspid (valve) disease I08.1
with aortic (valve) disease I08.3
congenital Q23.3
rheumatic I05.1
with
aortic valve disease I08.0
with tricuspid (valve) disease I08.3
obstruction or stenosis I05.2
with aortic valve disease I08.0
with tricuspid (valve) disease I08.3
tricuspid (valve) disease I08.1
with aortic (valve) disease I08.3
active or acute I01.1
with chorea, rheumatic (Sydenham's)
I02.0
specified cause, except rheumatic I34.0

Insufficiency, insufficient - *continued*
muscle -*see also* Disease, muscle
heart -*see* Insufficiency, myocardial
ocular NEC H50.9
myocardial, myocardium (with
arteriosclerosis) I50.9
with
rheumatic fever (conditions in I00) I09.0
active, acute or subacute I01.2
with chorea I02.0
inactive or quiescent (with chorea) I09.0
congenital Q24.8
hypertensive -*see* Hypertension, heart
newborn P29.0
rheumatic I09.0
active, acute, or subacute I01.2
syphilitic A52.06
nourishment T73.0
pancreatic K86.89
exocrine K86.81
parathyroid (gland) E20.9
peripheral vascular (arterial) I73.9
pituitary E23.0
placental (mother) O36.51
platelets D69.6
prenatal care affecting management of
pregnancy O09.3
progressive pluriglandular E31.0
pulmonary J98.4
acute, following surgery (nonthoracic) J95.2
thoracic J95.1
chronic, following surgery J95.3
following
shock J98.4
trauma J98.4
newborn P28.5
valve I37.1
with stenosis I37.2
congenital Q22.2
rheumatic I09.89
with aortic, mitral or tricuspid (valve)
disease I08.8
pyloric K31.89
renal (acute) N28.9
chronic N18.9
respiratory R06.89
newborn P28.5
rotation -*see* Malrotation
sleep syndrome F51.12
social insurance Z59.7
suprarenal E27.40
primary E27.1
tarso-orbital fascia, congenital Q10.3
testis E29.1
thyroid (gland) (acquired) E03.9
congenital E03.1
tricuspid (valve) (rheumatic) I07.1
with
aortic (valve) disease I08.2
with mitral (valve) disease I08.3
mitral (valve) disease I08.1
with aortic (valve) disease I08.3
obstruction or stenosis I07.2
with aortic (valve) disease I08.2
with mitral (valve) disease I08.3
congenital Q22.8
nonrheumatic I36.1
with stenosis I36.2
urethral sphincter R32
valve, valvular (heart) -*see* Endocarditis
congenital Q24.8

Insufficiency, insufficient - *continued*
vascular I99.8
  intestine K55.9
    acute -*see also* Ischemia, intestine, acute
    K55.059
    mesenteric K55.1
    peripheral I73.9
    renal -*see* Hypertension, kidney
  velopharyngeal
    acquired K13.79
    congenital Q38.8
  venous (chronic) (peripheral) I87.2
  ventricular -*see* Insufficiency, myocardial
  welfare support Z59.7
Insufflation, fallopian Z31.41
Insular -*see* condition **Insulinoma**
  pancreas
    benign D13.7
    malignant C25.4
    uncertain behavior D37.8
  specified site
    benign -*see* Neoplasm, by site, benign
    malignant -*see* Neoplasm, by site, malignant
    uncertain behavior -*see* Neoplasm, by site,
    uncertain behavior
  unspecified site
    benign D13.7
    malignant C25.4
    uncertain behavior D37.8
Insuloma -*see* Insulinoma
Interference
  balancing side M26.56
  non-working side M26.56
Intermenstrual -*see* condition
Intermittent -*see* condition
Internal -*see* condition
Interrogation
  cardiac defibrillator (automatic) (implantable)
  Z45.02
  cardiac pacemaker Z45.018
  cardiac (event) (loop) recorder Z45.09
  infusion pump (implanted) (intrathecal) Z45.1
  neurostimulator Z46.2
Interruption
  aortic arch Q25.21
  bundle of His I44.30
  phase-shift, sleep cycle -*see* Disorder, sleep,
    circadian rhythm
  sleep phase-shift, or 24
  hour sleep-wake cycle -*see* Disorder, sleep,
    circadian rhythm
Interstitial -*see* condition
Intertrigo L30.4
  labialis K13.0
Intervertebral disc -*see* condition
Intestine, intestinal -*see* condition
Intolerance
  carbohydrate K90.49
  disaccharide, hereditary E73.0
  fat NEC K90.49
    pancreatic K90.3
  food K90.49
    dietary counseling and surveillance Z71.3
  fructose E74.10
    hereditary E74.12
  glucose (galactose) E74.39
  gluten K90.41
  lactose E73.9
    specified NEC E73.8
  lysine E72.3
  milk NEC K90.49

Intolerance --*continued*
  lactose E73.9
  protein K90.49
  starch NEC K90.49
  sucrose (isomaltose) E74.31
Intoxicated NEC (without dependence) -*see*
  Alcohol, intoxication
Intoxication
  acid E87.2
  alcoholic (acute) (without dependence) -*see*
    Alcohol, intoxication
  alimentary canal K52.1
  amphetamine (without dependence) -*see*
    Abuse, drug, stimulant, with intoxication
    with dependence -*see* Dependence, drug,
      stimulant, with intoxication
  anxiolytic (acute) (without dependence) -*see*
    Abuse, drug, sedative, with intoxication
    with dependence -*see* Dependence, drug,
      sedative, with intoxication
  caffeine F15.929
    with dependence -*see* Dependence, drug,
      stimulant, with intoxication
  cannabinoids (acute) (without dependence) -
    see Use, cannabis, with intoxication
    with
      abuse -*see* Abuse, drug, cannabis, with
        intoxication
      dependence -*see* Dependence, drug,
        cannabis, with intoxication
  chemical -*see* Table of Drugs and Chemicals
    via placenta or breast milk -*see*
      Absorption, chemical, through placenta
  cocaine (acute) (without dependence) -*see*
    Abuse, drug, cocaine, with intoxication
    with dependence -*see* Dependence, drug,
    cocaine, with intoxication
  drug
    acute (without dependence) -*see* Abuse,
    drug, by type with intoxication
      with dependence -*see* Dependence, drug,
      by type with intoxication
    addictive
      via placenta or breast milk -*see*
      Absorption, drug, addictive, through
      placenta
    newborn P93.8
      gray baby syndrome P93.0
    overdose or wrong substance given or taken
    -*see* Table of Drugs and Chemicals, by drug,
    poisoning
  enteric K52.1
  foodborne A05.9
    bacterial A05.9
    classical (Clostridium botulinum) A05.1
    due to
      Bacillus cereus A05.4
      bacterium A05.9
        specified NEC A05.8
      Clostridium
        botulinum A05.1
        perfringens A05.2
        welchii A05.2
      Salmonella A02.9
        with
          (gastro) enteritis A02.0
          localized infection(s) A02.20
            arthritis A02.23
            meningitis A02.21
            osteomyelitis A02.24
            pneumonia A02.22

Intolerance --*continued*
        pyelonephritis A02.25
        specified NEC A02.29
      sepsis A02.1
      specified manifestation NEC A02.8
      Staphylococcus A05.0
      Vibrio
        parahaemolyticus A05.3
        vulnificus A05.5
    enterotoxin, staphylococcal A05.0
    noxious -*see* Poisoning, food, noxious
  gastrointestinal K52.1
  hallucinogenic (without dependence) -*see*
    Abuse, drug, hallucinogen, with intoxication
    with dependence -*see* Dependence, drug,
      hallucinogen, with intoxication
  hypnotic (acute) (without dependence) -*see*
    Abuse, drug, sedative, with intoxication
    with dependence -*see* Dependence, drug,
      sedative, with intoxication
  inhalant (acute) (without dependence) -*see*
    Abuse, drug, inhalant, with intoxication
    with dependence -*see* Dependence, drug,
      inhalant, with intoxication
  meaning
    inebriation -*see* category F10
    poisoning -*see* Table of Drugs and
    Chemicals
  methyl alcohol (acute) (without dependence) -
    see Alcohol, intoxication
  opioid (acute) (without dependence) -*see*
    Abuse, drug, opioid, with intoxication
    with dependence -*see* Dependence, drug,
      opioid, with intoxication
  pathologic NEC (without dependence) -*see*
    Alcohol, intoxication
  phencyclidine (without dependence) -*see*
    Abuse, drug, hallucinogen, with intoxication
    with dependence -*see* Dependence, drug,
      hallucinogen, with intoxication
  potassium (K) E87.5
  psychoactive substance NEC (without
    dependence) -*see* Abuse, drug, psychoactive
    NEC, with intoxication
    with dependence -*see* Dependence, drug,
      psychoactive NEC, with intoxication
  sedative (acute) (without dependence) -*see*
    Abuse, drug, sedative, with intoxication
    with dependence -*see* Dependence, drug,
      sedative, with intoxication
  serum -*see also* Reaction, serum T80.69
  uremic -*see* Uremia
  volatile solvents (acute) (without dependence)
    -*see* Abuse, drug, inhalant, with intoxication
    with dependence -*see* Dependence, drug,
      inhalant, with intoxication
  water E87.79
Intracranial -*see* condition
Intrahepatic gallbladder Q44.1
Intraligamentous -*see* condition
Intrathoracic -*see also* condition
  kidney Q63.2
Intrauterine contraceptive device
  checking Z30.431
  insertion Z30.430
    immediately following removal Z30.433
  in situ Z97.5
  management Z30.431
  reinsertion Z30.433
  removal Z30.432
  replacement Z30.433
  retention in pregnancy O26.3

Intraventricular -*see* condition
Intrinsic deformity -*see* Deformity
Intubation, difficult or failed T88.4
Intumescence, lens (eye) (cataract) -*see* Cataract
Intussusception (bowel) (colon) (enteric) (ileocecal) (ileocolic) (intestine) (rectum) K56.1
  appendix K38.8
  congenital Q43.8
  ureter (with obstruction) N13.5
Invagination (bowel, colon, intestine or rectum) K56.1
Inversion
  albumin-globulin (A-G) ratio E88.09
  bladder N32.89
  cecum -*see* Intussusception
  cervix N88.8
  chromosome in normal individual Q95.1
  circadian rhythm -*see* Disorder, sleep, circadian rhythm
  nipple N64.59
    congenital Q83.8
    gestational -*see* Retraction, nipple
    puerperal, postpartum -*see* Retraction, nipple
  nyctohemeral rhythm -*see* Disorder, sleep, circadian rhythm
  optic papilla Q14.2
  organ or site, congenital NEC -*see* Anomaly, by site
  sleep rhythm -*see* Disorder, sleep, circadian rhythm
  testis (congenital) Q55.29
  uterus (chronic) (postinfectional) (postpartal, old) N85.5
    postpartum O71.2
  vagina (posthysterectomy) N99.3
  ventricular Q20.5
Investigation -*see also* Examination Z04.9
  clinical research subject (control) (normal comparison) (participant) Z00.6
Involuntary movement, abnormal R25.9
Involution, involutional -*see also* condition
  breast, cystic -*see* Dysplasia, mammary, specified type NEC
  depression (single episode) F32.89
    recurrent episode F33.9
  melancholia (single episode) F32.89
    recurrent episode F33.8
  ovary, senile -*see* Atrophy, ovary
  thymus failure E32.8
I.Q.
  under 20 F73
  20 34 F72
  35 49 F71
  50 69 F70
IRDS (type I) P22.0
  type II P22.1
Irideremia Q13.1
Iridis rubeosis -*see* Disorder, iris, vascular
Iridochoroiditis (panuveitis) -*see* Panuveitis
Iridocyclitis H20.9
  acute H20.0
    hypopyon H20.05
    primary H20.01
    recurrent H20.02
    secondary (noninfectious) H20.04
      infectious H20.03
  chronic H20.1

Iridocyclitis - *continued*
  due to allergy -*see* Iridocyclitis, acute, secondary
  endogenous -*see* Iridocyclitis, acute, primary
  Fuchs' -*see* Cyclitis, Fuchs' heterochromic
  gonococcal A54.32
  granulomatous -*see* Iridocyclitis, chronic
  herpes, herpetic (simplex) B00.51
    zoster B02.32
  hypopyon -*see* Iridocyclitis, acute, hypopyon
  in (due to)
    ankylosing spondylitis M45.9
    gonococcal infection A54.32
    herpes (simplex) virus B00.51
      zoster B02.32
    infectious disease NOS B99
    parasitic disease NOS B89 [*H22*]
    sarcoidosis D86.83
    syphilis A51.43
    tuberculosis A18.54
    zoster B02.32
  lens-induced H20.2
  nongranulomatous -*see* Iridocyclitis, acute
  recurrent -*see* Iridocyclitis, acute, recurrent
  rheumatic -*see* Iridocyclitis, chronic
  subacute -*see* Iridocyclitis, acute
  sympathetic -*see* Uveitis, sympathetic
  syphilitic (secondary) A51.43
  tuberculous (chronic) A18.54
  Vogt-Koyanagi H20.82
Iridocyclochoroiditis (panuveitis) -*see* Panuveitis
Iridodialysis H21.53
Iridodonesis H21.89
Iridoplegia (complete) (partial) (reflex) H57.09
Iridoschisis H21.25
Iris -*see also* condition
  bombé -*see* Membrane, pupillary
Iritis -*see also* Iridocyclitis
  chronic -*see* Iridocyclitis, chronic
  diabetic -*see* E08 E13 with .39
  due to
    herpes simplex B00.51
    leprosy A30.9 [*H22*]
  gonococcal A54.32
  gouty -*see also* Gout, by type M10.9 [*H22*]
  granulomatous -*see* Iridocyclitis, chronic
  lens induced -*see* Iridocyclitis, lens-induced
  papulosa (syphilitic) A52.71
  rheumatic -*see* Iridocyclitis, chronic
  syphilitic (secondary) A51.43
    congenital (early) A50.01
    late A52.71
  tuberculous A18.54
Iron -*see* condition
Iron-miner's lung J63.4
Irradiated enamel (tooth, teeth) K03.89
Irradiation effects, adverse T66
Irreducible, irreducibility -*see* condition
Irregular, irregularity
  action, heart I49.9
  alveolar process K08.89
  bleeding N92.6
  breathing R06.89
  contour of cornea (acquired) -*see* Deformity, cornea
    congenital Q13.4
  contour, reconstructed breast N65.0
  dentin (in pulp) K04.3
  eye movements H55.89

Irregular, irregularity --*continued*
  nystagmus -*see* Nystagmus
    saccadic H55.81
  labor O62.2
  menstruation (cause unknown) N92.6
  periods N92.6
  prostate N42.9
  pupil -*see* Abnormality, pupillary
  reconstructed breast N65.0
  respiratory R06.89
  septum (nasal) J34.2
  shape, organ or site, congenital NEC -*see* Distortion
  sleep-wake pattern (rhythm) G47.23
Irritable, irritability R45.4
  bladder N32.89
  bowel (syndrome) K58.9
    with
      constipation K58.1
      diarrhea K58.0
    mixed K58.2
    psychogenic F45.8
    specified NEC K58.8
  bronchial -*see* Bronchitis
  cerebral, in newborn P91.3
  colon -*see also* Irritable, bowel K58.9
    with diarrhea K58.0
    psychogenic F45.8
  duodenum K59.8
  heart (psychogenic) F45.8
  hip -*see* Derangement, joint, specified type NEC, hip
  ileum K59.8
  infant R68.12
  jejunum K59.8
  rectum K59.8
  stomach K31.89
    psychogenic F45.8
  sympathetic G90.8
  urethra N36.8
Irritation
  anus K62.89
  axillary nerve G54.0
  bladder N32.89
  brachial plexus G54.0
  bronchial -*see* Bronchitis
  cervical plexus G54.2
  cervix -*see* Cervicitis
  choroid, sympathetic -*see* Endophthalmitis
  cranial nerve -*see* Disorder, nerve, cranial
  gastric K31.89
    psychogenic F45.8
  globe, sympathetic -*see* Uveitis, sympathetic
  labyrinth -*see* subcategory H83.2
  lumbosacral plexus G54.1
  meninges (traumatic) -*see* Injury, intracranial
    nontraumatic -*see* Meningismus
  nerve -*see* Disorder, nerve
  nervous R45.0
  penis N48.89
  perineum NEC L29.3
  peripheral autonomic nervous system G90.8
  peritoneum -*see* Peritonitis
  pharynx J39.2
  plantar nerve -*see* Lesion, nerve, plantar
  spinal (cord) (traumatic) -*see also* Injury, spinal cord, by region
    nerve G58.9
      root NEC -*see* Radiculopathy
    nontraumatic -*see* Myelopathy
  stomach K31.89

Irritation - *continued*
  psychogenic F45.8
  sympathetic nerve NEC G90.8
  ulnar nerve -*see* Lesion, nerve, ulnar
  vagina N89.8
Ischemia, ischemic I99.8
  brain -*see* Ischemia, cerebral
  bowel (transient)
    acute -*see also* Ischemia, intestine, acute
      K55.059
    chronic K55.1
    due to mesenteric artery insufficiency K55.1
  cardiac (see Disease, heart, ischemic)
  cardiomyopathy I25.5
  cerebral (chronic) (generalized) I67.82
    arteriosclerotic I67.2
    intermittent G45.9
    newborn P91.0
    recurrent focal G45.8
    transient G45.9
  colon chronic (due to mesenteric artery
    insufficiency) K55.1
  coronary -*see* Disease, heart, ischemic
  demand (coronary) -*see also* Angina I24.8
  heart (chronic or with a stated duration of
    over 4weeks) I25.9
    acute or with a stated duration of 4
  weeks or less I24.9
    subacute I24.9
  infarction, muscle -*see* Infarct, muscle
  intestine (large) (small) (transient) K55.9
    acute K55.059
      diffuse K55.052
      focal K55.051
      large K55.039
        diffuse K55.032
        focal K55.031
      small K55.019
        diffuse K55.012
        focal K55.011
    chronic K55.1
    due to mesenteric artery insufficiency K55.1
  kidney N28.0
  mesenteric, acute -*see also* Ischemia,
    intestine, acute K55.059
  muscle, traumatic T79.6
  myocardium, myocardial (chronic or with a
    stated duration of over 4 weeks) I25.9
    acute, without myocardial infarction I51.3
    silent (asymptomatic) I25.6
    transient of newborn P29.4
  renal N28.0
  retina, retinal -*see* Occlusion, artery, retina
  small bowel
    acute K55.019
      diffuse K55.012
      focal K55.011
    chronic K55.1
    due to mesenteric artery insufficiency K55.1
  spinal cord G95.11
  subendocardial -*see* Insufficiency, coronary
  supply (coronary) -*see also* Angina I25.9
    due to vasospasm I20.1
Ischial spine -*see* condition
Ischialgia -*see* Sciatica
Ischiopagus Q89.4
Ischium, ischial -*see* condition
Ischuria R34
Iselin's disease or osteochondrosis -*see*
  Osteochondrosis, juvenile, metatarsus

Islands of
  parotid tissue in
    lymph nodes Q38.6
    neck structures Q38.6
  submaxillary glands in
    fascia Q38.6
    lymph nodes Q38.6
    neck muscles Q38.6
Islet cell tumor, pancreas D13.7
Isoimmunization NEC -*see also*
  Incompatibility
  affecting management of pregnancy (ABO)
  (with hydrops fetalis) O36.11
    anti-A sensitization O36.11
    anti-B sensitization O36.19
    anti-c sensitization O36.09
    anti-C sensitization O36.09
    anti-e sensitization O36.09
    anti-E sensitization O36.09
    Rh NEC O36.09
      anti-D antibody O36.01
    specified NEC O36.19
  newborn P55.9
    with
      hydrops fetalis P56.0
      kernicterus P57.0
    ABO (blood groups) P55.1
    Rhesus (Rh) factor P55.0
    specified type NEC P55.8
Isolation, isolated
  dwelling Z59.8
  family Z63.79
  social Z60.4
Isoleucinosis E71.19
**Isomerism atrial appendages (with asplenia
  or polysplenia)** Q20.6
Isosporiasis, isosporosis A07.3
Isovaleric acidemia E71.110
Issue of
  medical certificate Z02.79
    for disability determination Z02.71
  repeat prescription (appliance) (glasses)
  (medicinal substance, medicament, medicine)
  Z76.0
    contraception -*see* Contraception
Itch, itching -*see also* Pruritus
  baker's L23.6
  barber's B35.0
  bricklayer's L24.5
  cheese B88.0
  clam digger's B65.3
  coolie B76.9
  copra B88.0
  dew B76.9
  dhobi B35.6
  filarial -*see* Infestation, filarial
  grain B88.0
  grocer's B88.0
  ground B76.9
  harvest B88.0
  jock B35.6
  Malabar B35.5
    beard B35.0
    foot B35.3
    scalp B35.0
  meaning scabies B86
  Norwegian B86
  perianal L29.0
  poultrymen's B88.0
  sarcoptic B86
  scabies B86

Itch, itching --*continued*
  scrub B88.0
  straw B88.0
  swimmer's B65.3
  water B76.9
  winter L29.8
**Ivemark's syndrome (asplenia with
  congenital heart disease)** Q89.01
Ivory bones Q78.2
Ixodiasis NEC B88.8

J

Jaccoud's syndrome -*see* Arthropathy,
  postrheumatic, chronic
Jackson's
  membrane Q43.3
  paralysis or syndrome G83.89
  veil Q43.3
Jacquet's dermatitis (diaper dermatitis) L22
Jadassohn-Pellizari's disease or anetoderma
  L90.2
Jadassohn's
  blue nevus -*see* Nevus
  intraepidermal epithelioma -*see* Neoplasm,
    skin, benign
Jaffe-Lichtenstein (Uehlinger) syndrome -
  see Dysplasia, fibrous, bone NEC
Jakob-Creutzfeldt disease or syndrome -*see*
  Creutzfeldt-Jakob disease or syndrome
Jaksch-Luzet disease D64.89
Jamaican
  neuropathy G92
  paraplegic tropical ataxic-spastic syndrome
    G92
Janet's disease F48.8
Janiceps Q89.4
Jansky Bielschowsky amaurotic idiocy E75.4
Japanese
  B-type encephalitis A83.0
  river fever A75.3
Jaundice (yellow) R17
  acholuric (familial) (splenomegalic) -*see also*
    Spherocytosis
    acquired D59.8
  breast-milk (inhibitor) P59.3
  catarrhal (acute) B15.9
    with hepatic coma B15.0
  cholestatic (benign) R17
  due to or associated with
    delayed conjugation P59.8
      associated with (due to) preterm delivery
        P59.0
    preterm delivery P59.0
  epidemic (catarrhal) B15.9
    with hepatic coma B15.0
    leptospiral A27.0
    spirochetal A27.0
  familial nonhemolytic (congenital) (Gilbert)
    E80.4
    Crigler-Najjar E80.5
  febrile (acute) B15.9
    with hepatic coma B15.0
    leptospiral A27.0
    spirochetal A27.0
  hematogenous D59.9
  hemolytic (acquired) D59.9
    congenital -*see* Spherocytosis
  hemorrhagic (acute) (leptospiral) (spirochetal)
    A27.0
  infectious (acute) (subacute) B15.9

Jaundice (yellow) --*continued*
with hepatic coma B15.0
  leptospiral A27.0
  spirochetal A27.0
leptospiral (hemorrhagic) A27.0
malignant (without coma) K72.90
  with coma K72.91
newborn P59.9
  due to or associated with
    ABO
      antibodies P55.1
      incompatibility, maternal/fetal P55.1
      isoimmunization P55.1
    absence or deficiency of enzyme system
      for bilirubin conjugation (congenital)
      P59.8
    bleeding P58.1
    breast milk inhibitors to conjugation P59.3
      associated with preterm delivery P59.0
    bruising P58.0
    Crigler-Najjar syndrome E80.5
    delayed conjugation P59.8
      associated with preterm delivery P59.0
    drugs or toxins
      given to newborn P58.42
      transmitted from mother P58.41
    excessive hemolysis P58.9
      due to
        bleeding P58.1
        bruising P58.0
        drugs or toxins
          given to newborn P58.42
          transmitted from mother P58.41
        infection P58.2
        polycythemia P58.3
        swallowed maternal blood P58.5
      specified type NEC P58.8
    galactosemia E74.21
    Gilbert syndrome E80.4
    hemolytic disease P55.9
      ABO isoimmunization P55.1
      Rh isoimmunization P55.0
      specified NEC P55.8
    hepatocellular damage P59.20
      specified NEC P59.29
    hereditary hemolytic anemia P58.8
    hypothyroidism, congenital E03.1
    incompatibility, maternal/fetal NOS P55.9
    infection P58.2
    inspissated bile syndrome P59.1
    isoimmunization NOS P55.9
    mucoviscidosis E84.9
    polycythemia P58.3
    preterm delivery P59.0
    Rh
      antibodies P55.0
      incompatibility, maternal/fetal P55.0
      isoimmunization P55.0
    specified cause NEC P59.8
    swallowed maternal blood P58.5
    spherocytosis (congenital) D58.0
neonatal -*see* Jaundice, newborn
nonhemolytic congenital familial (Gilbert)
  E80.4
nuclear, newborn -*see also* Kernicterus of
  newborn P57.9
obstructive -*see also* Obstruction, bile duct
  K83.1
post-immunization -*see* Hepatitis, viral, type,
  B
post-transfusion -*see* Hepatitis, viral, type, B

Jaundice (yellow) --*continued*
regurgitation -*see also* Obstruction, bile duct
  K83.1
serum (homologous) (prophylactic)
  (therapeutic) -*see* Hepatitis, viral, type, B
spirochetal (hemorrhagic) A27.0
symptomatic R17
  newborn P59.9
Jaw -*see* condition
Jaw-winking phenomenon or syndrome
  Q07.8
Jealousy
  alcoholic F10.988
  childhood F93.8
  sibling F93.8
Jejunitis -*see* Enteritis
Jejunostomy status Z93.4
Jejunum, jejunal -*see* condition
Jensen's disease -*see* Inflammation,
  chorioretinal, focal, juxtapapillary
Jerks, myoclonic G25.3
Jervell-Lange-Nielsen syndrome I45.81
Jeune's disease Q77.2
Jigger disease B88.1
Job's syndrome (chronic granulomatous
  disease) D71
Joint -*see also* condition
  mice -*see* Loose, body, joint
  knee M23.4
Jordan's anomaly or syndrome D72.0
Joseph-Diamond-Blackfan anemia
  (congenital hypoplastic) D61.01
Jungle yellow fever A95.0
Jüngling's disease -*see* Sarcoidosis
Juvenile -*see* condition

K

Kahler's disease C90.0
Kakke E51.11
Kala-azar B55.0
Kallmann's syndrome E23.0
Kanner's syndrome (autism) -*see* Psychosis,
  childhood
Kaposi's
  dermatosis (xeroderma pigmentosum) Q82.1
  lichen ruber L44.0
    acuminatus L44.0
  sarcoma
    colon C46.4
    connective tissue C46.1
    gastrointestinal organ C46.4
    lung C46.5
    lymph node (multiple) C46.3
    palate (hard) (soft) C46.2
    rectum C46.4
    skin (multiple sites) C46.0
    specified site NEC C46.7
    stomach C46.4
    unspecified site C46.9
  varicelliform eruption B00.0
  vaccinia T88.1
Kartagener's syndrome or triad (sinusitis,
  bronchiectasis, situs inversus) Q89.3
Karyotype
  with abnormality except iso (Xq) Q96.2
  45,X Q96.0
  46,X
    iso (Xq) Q96.1
  46,XX Q98.3
    with streak gonads Q50.32

Karyotype --*continued*
  hermaphrodite (true) Q99.1
    male Q98.3
  46,XY
    with streak gonads Q56.1
    female Q97.3
    hermaphrodite (true) Q99.1
  47,XXX Q97.0
  47,XXY Q98.0
  47,XYY Q98.5
Kaschin-Beck disease -*see* Disease, Kaschin-
  Beck
Katayama's disease or fever B65.2
Kawasaki's syndrome M30.3
Kayser-Fleischer ring (cornea)
  (pseudosclerosis) H18.04
Kaznelson's syndrome (congenital
  hypoplastic anemia) D61.01
Kearns-Sayre syndrome H49.81
Kedani fever A75.3
Kelis L91.0
Kelly (Patterson) syndrome (sideropenic
  dysphagia) D50.1
Keloid, cheloid L91.0
  acne L73.0
  Addison's L94.0
  cornea -*see* Opacity, cornea
  Hawkin's L91.0
  scar L91.0
Keloma L91.0
Kenya fever A77.1
Keratectasia -*see also* Ectasia, cornea
  congenital Q13.4
Keratinization of alveolar ridge mucosa -
  excessive K13.23
  minimal K13.22
Keratinized residual ridge mucosa -
  excessive K13.23
  minimal K13.22
Keratitis (nodular) (nonulcerative) (simple)
  (zonular) H16.9
  with ulceration (central) (marginal)
    (perforated) (ring) -*see* Ulcer, cornea
  actinic -*see* Photokeratitis
  arborescens (herpes simplex) B00.52
  areolar H16.11
  bullosa H16.8
  deep H16.309
    specified type NEC H16.399
  dendritic (a) (herpes simplex) B00.52
  disciform (is) (herpes simplex) B00.52
    varicella B01.81
  filamentary H16.12
  gonococcal (congenital or prenatal) A54.33
  herpes, herpetic (simplex) B00.52
    zoster B02.33
  in (due to)
    acanthamebiasis B60.13
    adenovirus B30.0
    exanthema -*see also* Exanthem B09
    herpes (simplex) virus B00.52
    measles B05.81
    syphilis A50.31
    tuberculosis A18.52
    zoster B02.33
  interstitial (nonsyphilitic) H16.30
    diffuse H16.32
    herpes, herpetic (simplex) B00.52
      zoster B02.33
    sclerosing H16.33
  specified type NEC H16.39

Keratitis --continued
  syphilitic (congenital) (late) A50.31
  tuberculous A18.52
  macular H16.11
  nummular H16.11
  oyster shuckers' H16.8
  parenchymatous -see Keratitis, interstitial
  petrificans H16.8
  postmeasles B05.81
  punctata
    leprosa A30.9 [H16.14]
    syphilitic (profunda) A50.31
  punctate H16.14
  purulent H16.8
  rosacea L71.8
  sclerosing H16.33
  specified type NEC H16.8
  stellate H16.11
  striate H16.11
  superficial H16.10
    with conjunctivitis -see Keratoconjunctivitis
    due to light -see Photokeratitis
  suppurative H16.8
  syphilitic (congenital) (prenatal) A50.31
  trachomatous A71.1
    sequelae B94.0
  tuberculous A18.52
  vesicular H16.8
  xerotic -see also Keratomalacia H16.8
    vitamin A deficiency E50.4
Keratoacanthoma L85.8
Keratocele -see Descemetocele
Keratoconjunctivitis H16.20
  Acanthamoeba B60.13
  adenoviral B30.0
  epidemic B30.0
  exposure H16.21
  herpes, herpetic (simplex) B00.52
    zoster B02.33
  in exanthema -see also Exanthem B09
  infectious B30.0
  lagophthalmic -see Keratoconjunctivitis,
    specified type NEC
  neurotrophic H16.23
  phlyctenular H16.25
  postmeasles B05.81
  shipyard B30.0
  sicca (Sjogren's) M35.0
    not Sjogren's H16.22
  specified type NEC H16.29
  tuberculous (phlyctenular) A18.52
  vernal H16.26
Keratoconus H18.60
  congenital Q13.4
  stable H18.61
  unstable H18.62
Keratocyst (dental) (odontogenic) -see Cyst,
  calcifying odontogenic
Keratoderma, keratodermia (congenital)
  (palmaris et plantaris) (symmetrical) Q82.8
  acquired L85.1
    in diseases classified elsewhere L86
  climactericum L85.1
  gonococcal A54.89
  gonorrheal A54.89
  punctata L85.2
  Reiter's -see Reiter's disease
Keratodermatocele -see Descemetocele
Keratoglobus H18.79
  congenital Q15.8
    with glaucoma Q15.0

Keratohemia -see Pigmentation, cornea,
  stromal
Keratoiritis -see also Iridocyclitis
  syphilitic A50.39
  tuberculous A18.54
Keratoma L57.0
  palmaris and plantaris hereditarium Q82.8
  senile L57.0
Keratomalacia H18.44
  vitamin A deficiency E50.4
Keratomegaly Q13.4
Keratomycosis B49
  nigrans, nigricans (palmaris) B36.1
Keratopathy H18.9
  band H18.42
  bullous H18.1
  bullous (aphakic), following cataract surgery
    H59.01
Keratoscleritis, tuberculous A18.52
Keratosis L57.0
  actinic L57.0
  arsenical L85.8
  congenital, specified NEC Q80.8
  female genital NEC N94.89
  follicularis Q82.8
    acquired L11.0
    congenita Q82.8
    et parafollicularis in cutem penetrans L87.0
    spinulosa (decalvans) Q82.8
    vitamin A deficiency E50.8
  gonococcal A54.89
  male genital (external) N50.89
  nigricans L83
  obturans, external ear (canal) -see
    Cholesteatoma, external ear
  palmaris et plantaris (inherited) (symmetrical)
    Q82.8
    acquired L85.1
  penile N48.89
  pharynx J39.2
  pilaris, acquired L85.8
  punctata (palmaris et plantaris) L85.2
  scrotal N50.89
  seborrheic L82.1
    inflamed L82.0
  senile L57.0
  solar L57.0
  tonsillaris J35.8
  vagina N89.4
  vegetans Q82.8
  vitamin A deficiency E50.8
  vocal cord J38.3
Kerato-uveitis -see Iridocyclitis
Keraunoparalysis T75.09
Kerion (celsi) B35.0
Kernicterus of newborn (not due to
  isoimmunization) P57.9
  due to isoimmunization (conditions in P55.0
    P55.9) P57.0
  specified type NEC P57.8
Keshan disease E59
Ketoacidosis E87.2
  diabetic -see Diabetes, by type, with
    ketoacidosis
Ketonuria R82.4
Ketosis NEC E88.89
  diabetic -see Diabetes, by type, with
    ketoacidosis
Kew Garden fever A79.1
Kidney -see condition
Kienböck's disease -see also Osteochondrosis,
  juvenile, hand, carpal lunate
  adult M93.1

Kimmelstiel (Wilson) disease -see Diabetes,
  Kimmelstiel (Wilson) disease
Kimura disease D21.9
  specified site (see Neoplasm, connective
    tissue benign)
Kink, kinking
  artery I77.1
  hair (acquired) L67.8
  ileum or intestine -see Obstruction, intestine
  Lane's -see Obstruction, intestine
  organ or site, congenital NEC -see Anomaly,
    by site
  ureter (pelvic junction) N13.5
    with
      hydronephrosis N13.1
        with infection N13.6
      pyelonephritis (chronic) N11.1
    congenital Q62.39
  vein(s) I87.8
    caval I87.1
    peripheral I87.1
Kinnier Wilson's disease (hepatolenticular
  degeneration) E83.01
Kissing spine M48.20
  cervical region M48.22
  cervicothoracic region M48.23
  lumbar region M48.26
  lumbosacral region M48.27
  occipito-atlanto-axial region M48.21
  thoracic region M48.24
  thoracolumbar region M48.25
Klatskin's tumor C24.0
Klauder's disease A26.8
Klebs' disease -see also Glomerulonephritis
  N05.
Klebsiella (K.) pneumoniae, as cause of
  disease classified elsewhere B96.1
Klein (e) Levin syndrome G47.13
Kleptomania F63.2
Klinefelter's syndrome Q98.4
  karyotype 47,XXY Q98.0
  male with more than two X chromosomes
    Q98.1
Klippel-Feil deficiency, disease, or syndrome
  (brevicollis) Q76.1
Klippel's disease I67.2
Klippel-Trenaunay (Weber) syndrome
  Q87.2
Klumpke (Déjerine) palsy, paralysis (birth)
  (newborn) P14.1
Knee -see condition
Knock knee (acquired) M21.06
  congenital Q74.1
Knot(s)
  intestinal, syndrome (volvulus) K56.2
  surfer S89.8
  umbilical cord (true) O69.2
Knotting (of)
  hair L67.8
  intestine K56.2
Knuckle pad (Garrod's) M72.1
Koch's
  infection -see Tuberculosis
  relapsing fever A68.9
Koch-Weeks' conjunctivitis -see
  Conjunctivitis, acute, mucopurulent
Köebner's syndrome Q81.8
Köenig's disease (osteochondritis dissecans) -
  see Osteochondritis, dissecans

Köhler-Pellegrini-Steida disease or
syndrome (calcification, knee joint) -*see*
Bursitis, tibial collateral
Köhler's disease
patellar -*see* Osteochondrosis, juvenile,
patella
tarsal navicular -*see* Osteochondrosis,
juvenile, tarsus
Koilonychia L60.3
congenital Q84.6
Kojevnikov's, epilepsy -*see* Kozhevnikov's
epilepsy
Koplik's spots B05.9
Kopp's asthma E32.8
Korsakoff's (Wernicke) disease, psychosis or
syndrome (alcoholic) F10.96
with dependence F10.26
drug-induced
due to drug abuse -*see* Abuse, drug, by type,
with amnestic disorder
due to drug dependence -*see* Dependence,
drug, by type, with amnestic disorder
nonalcoholic F04
Korsakov's disease, psychosis or syndrome -
see Korsakoff's disease
Korsakow's disease, psychosis or syndrome -
see Korsakoff's disease
Kostmann's disease or syndrome (infantile
genetic agranulocytosis) -*see*
Agranulocytosis
Kozhevnikov's epilepsy G40.109
intractable G40.119
with status epilepticus G40.111
without status epilepticus G40.119
not intractable G40.109
with status epilepticus G40.101
without status epilepticus G40.109
Krabbe's
disease E75.23
syndrome, congenital muscle hypoplasia
Q79.8
Kraepelin-Morel disease -*see* Schizophrenia
Kraft-Weber-Dimitri disease Q85.8
Kraurosis
ani K62.89
penis N48.0
vagina N89.8
vulva N90.4
Kreotoxism A05.9
Krukenberg's
spindle -*see* Pigmentation, cornea, posterior
tumor C79.6
Kufs' disease E75.4
Kugelberg-Welander disease G12.1
Kuhnt-Junius degeneration -*see also*
Degeneration, macula H35.32
Kümmell's disease or spondylitis -*see*
Spondylopathy, traumatic
Kupffer cell sarcoma C22.3
Kuru A81.81
Kussmaul's
disease M30.0
respiration E87.2
in diabetic acidosis -*see* Diabetes, by type,
with ketoacidosis
Kwashiorkor E40
marasmic, marasmus type E42
Kyasanur Forest disease A98.2

Kyphoscoliosis, kyphoscoliotic (acquired) -
see also Scoliosis M41.9
congenital Q67.5
heart (disease) I27.1
sequelae of rickets E64.3
tuberculous A18.01
Kyphosis, kyphotic (acquired) M40.209
cervical region M40.202
cervicothoracic region M40.203
congenital Q76.419
cervical region Q76.412
cervicothoracic region Q76.413
occipito-atlanto-axial region Q76.411
thoracic region Q76.414
thoracolumbar region Q76.415
Morquio-Brailsford type (spinal) -*see also*
subcategory M49.8 E76.219
postlaminectomy M96.3
postradiation therapy M96.2
postural (adolescent) M40.00
cervicothoracic region M40.03
thoracic region M40.04
thoracolumbar region M40.05
secondary NEC M40.10
cervical region M40.12
cervicothoracic region M40.13
thoracic region M40.14
thoracolumbar region M40.15
sequelae of rickets E64.3
specified type NEC M40.299
cervical region M40.292
cervicothoracic region M40.293
thoracic region M40.294
thoracolumbar region M40.295
syphilitic, congenital A50.56
thoracic region M40.204
thoracolumbar region M40.205
tuberculous A18.01
Kyrle disease L87.0

L

Labia, labium -*see* condition
Labile
blood pressure R09.89
vasomotor system I73.9
Labioglossal paralysis G12.29
Labium leporinum -*see* Cleft, lip
Labor -*see* Delivery
Labored breathing -*see* Hyperventilation
Labyrinthitis (circumscribed) (destructive)
(diffuse) (inner ear) (latent) (purulent)
(suppurative) -*see also* subcategory H83.0
syphilitic A52.79
Laceration
with abortion -*see* Abortion, by type,
complicated by laceration of pelvic organs
abdomen, abdominal
wall S31.119
with
foreign body S31.129
penetration into peritoneal cavity S31.619
with foreign body S31.629
epigastric region S31.112
with
foreign body S31.122
penetration into peritoneal cavity
S31.612
with foreign body S31.622
left

Laceration - *continued*
lower quadrant S31.114
with
foreign body S31.124
penetration into peritoneal cavity
S31.614
with foreign body S31.624
upper quadrant S31.111
with
foreign body S31.121
penetration into peritoneal cavity
S31.611
with foreign body S31.621
periumbilic region S31.115
with
foreign body S31.125
penetration into peritoneal cavity
S31.615
with foreign body S31.625
right
lower quadrant S31.113
with
foreign body S31.123
penetration into peritoneal cavity
S31.613
with foreign body S31.623
upper quadrant S31.110
with
foreign body S31.120
penetration into peritoneal cavity
S31.610
with foreign body S31.620
accidental, complicating surgery -*see*
Complications, surgical, accidental puncture
or laceration
Achilles tendon S86.02
adrenal gland S37.813
alveolar (process) -*see* Laceration, oral cavity
ankle S91.01
with
foreign body S91.02
antecubital space -*see* Laceration, elbow
anus (sphincter) S31.831
with
ectopic or molar pregnancy O08.6
foreign body S31.832
complicating delivery -*see* Delivery,
complicated, by, laceration, anus
(sphincter)
following ectopic or molar pregnancy O08.6
nontraumatic, nonpuerperal -*see* Fissure,
anus
arm (upper) S41.11
with foreign body S41.12
lower -*see* Laceration, forearm
auditory canal (external) (meatus) -*see*
Laceration, ear
auricle, ear -*see* Laceration, ear
axilla -*see* Laceration, arm
back -*see also* Laceration, thorax, back
lower S31.010
with
foreign body S31.020
with penetration into retroperitoneal
space S31.021
penetration into retroperitoneal space
S31.011
bile duct S36.13
bladder S37.23
with ectopic or molar pregnancy O08.6
following ectopic or molar pregnancy O08.6

Laceration - *continued*
- obstetrical trauma O71.5
- blood vessel -*see* Injury, blood vessel
- bowel -*see also* Laceration, intestine
  - with ectopic or molar pregnancy O08.6
  - complicating abortion -*see* Abortion, by type, complicated by, specified condition NEC
  - following ectopic or molar pregnancy O08.6
  - obstetrical trauma O71.5
- brain (any part) (cortex) (diffuse) (membrane) -*see also* Injury, intracranial, diffuse
  - during birth P10.8
    - with hemorrhage P10.1
  - focal -*see* Injury, intracranial, focal brain injury   brainstem S06.38
- breast S21.01
  - with foreign body S21.02
- broad ligament S37.893
  - with ectopic or molar pregnancy O08.6
  - following ectopic or molar pregnancy O08.6
  - laceration syndrome N83.8
  - obstetrical trauma O71.6
  - syndrome (laceration) N83.8
- buttock S31.801
  - with foreign body S31.802
  - left S31.821
    - with foreign body S31.822
  - right S31.811
    - with foreign body S31.812
- calf -*see* Laceration, leg
- canaliculus lacrimalis -*see* Laceration, eyelid
- canthus, eye -*see* Laceration, eyelid
- capsule, joint -*see* Sprain
- causing eversion of cervix uteri (old) N86
- central (perineal), complicating delivery O70.9
- cerebellum, traumatic S06.37
- cerebral S06.33
  - left side S06.32
  - during birth P10.8
    - with hemorrhage P10.1
  - right side S06.31
- cervix (uteri)
  - with ectopic or molar pregnancy O08.6
  - following ectopic or molar pregnancy O08.6
  - nonpuerperal, nontraumatic N88.1
  - obstetrical trauma (current) O71.3
  - old (postpartal) N88.1
  - traumatic S37.63
- cheek (external) S01.41
  - with foreign body S01.42
  - internal -*see* Laceration, oral cavity   chest wall -*see* Laceration, thorax
- chin -*see* Laceration, head, specified site NEC
- chordae tendinae NEC I51.1
  - concurrent with acute myocardial infarction -*see* Infarct, myocardium
    - following acute myocardial infarction (current complication) I23.4
- clitoris -*see* Laceration, vulva
- colon -*see* Laceration, intestine, large, colon
- common bile duct S36.13
- cortex (cerebral) -*see* Injury, intracranial, diffuse
- costal region -*see* Laceration, thorax
- cystic duct S36.13
- diaphragm S27.803
- digit(s)
  - hand -*see* Laceration, finger
  - foot -*see* Laceration, toe

Laceration - *continued*
- duodenum S36.430
- ear (canal) (external) S01.31
  - with foreign body S01.32
  - drum S09.2
- elbow S51.01
  - with
    - foreign body S51.02
- epididymis -*see* Laceration, testis
- epigastric region -*see* Laceration, abdomen, wall, epigastric region
- esophagus K22.8
  - traumatic
    - cervical S11.21
      - with foreign body S11.22
    - thoracic S27.813
- eye (ball) S05.3
  - with prolapse or loss of intraocular tissue S05.2
  - penetrating S05.6
- eyebrow -*see* Laceration, eyelid
- eyelid S01.11
  - with foreign body S01.12
- face NEC -*see* Laceration, head, specified site NEC
- fallopian tube S37.539
  - bilateral S37.532
  - unilateral S37.531
- finger(s) S61.219
  - with
    - damage to nail S61.319
      - with
        - foreign body S61.329
    - foreign body S61.229
  - index S61.218
    - with
      - damage to nail S61.318
        - with
          - foreign body S61.328
      - foreign body S61.228
    - left S61.211
      - with
        - damage to nail S61.311
          - with
            - foreign body S61.321
        - foreign body S61.221
    - right S61.210
      - with
        - damage to nail S61.310
          - with
            - foreign body S61.320
        - foreign body S61.220
  - little S61.218
    - with
      - damage to nail S61.318
        - with
          - foreign body S61.328
      - foreign body S61.228
    - left S61.217
      - with
        - damage to nail S61.317
          - with
            - foreign body S61.327
        - foreign body S61.227
    - right S61.216
      - with
        - damage to nail S61.316
          - with
            - foreign body S61.326
        - foreign body S61.226
  - middle S61.218

Laceration - *continued*
- with
  - damage to nail S61.318
    - with
      - foreign body S61.328
  - foreign body S61.228
- left S61.213
  - with
    - damage to nail S61.313
      - with
        - foreign body S61.323
    - foreign body S61.223
- right S61.212
  - with
    - damage to nail S61.312
      - with
        - foreign body S61.322
    - foreign body S61.222
- ring S61.218
  - with
    - damage to nail S61.318
      - with
        - foreign body S61.328
    - foreign body S61.228
  - left S61.215
    - with
      - damage to nail S61.315
        - with
          - foreign body S61.325
      - foreign body S61.225
  - right S61.214
    - with
      - damage to nail S61.314
        - with
          - foreign body S61.324
      - foreign body S61.224
- flank S31.119
  - with foreign body S31.129
- foot (except toe(s) alone) S91.319
  - with foreign body S91.329
  - left S91.312
    - with foreign body S91.322
  - right S91.311
    - with foreign body S91.321
  - toe -*see* Laceration, toe
- forearm S51.819
  - with
    - foreign body S51.829
  - elbow only -*see* Laceration, elbow
  - left S51.812
    - with
      - foreign body S51.822
  - right S51.811
    - with
      - foreign body S51.821
- forehead S01.81
  - with foreign body S01.82
- fourchette O70.0
  - with ectopic or molar pregnancy O08.6
  - complicating delivery O70.0
  - following ectopic or molar pregnancy O08.6
- gallbladder S36.123
- genital organs, external
  - female S31.512
    - with foreign body S31.522
    - vagina -*see* Laceration, vagina
    - vulva -*see* Laceration, vulva
  - male S31.511
    - with foreign body S31.521
    - penis -*see* Laceration, penis
    - scrotum -*see* Laceration, scrotum

Laceration - *continued*

testis *-see* Laceration, testis
groin *-see* Laceration, abdomen, wall
gum *-see* Laceration, oral cavity
hand S61.419
  with
    foreign body S61.429
  finger *-see* Laceration, finger
  left S61.412
    with
      foreign body S61.422
  right S61.411
    with
      foreign body S61.421
  thumb *-see* Laceration, thumb
head S01.91
  with foreign body S01.92
  cheek *-see* Laceration, cheek
  ear *-see* Laceration, ear
  eyelid *-see* Laceration, eyelid
  lip *-see* Laceration, lip
  nose *-see* Laceration, nose
  oral cavity *-see* Laceration, oral cavity
  scalp S01.01
    with foreign body S01.02
  specified site NEC S01.81
    with foreign body S01.82
  temporomandibular area *-see* Laceration, cheek
heart *-see* Injury, heart, laceration
heel *-see* Laceration, foot
hepatic duct S36.13
hip S71.019
  with foreign body S71.029
  left S71.012
    with foreign body S71.022
  right S71.011
    with foreign body S71.021
hymen *-see* Laceration, vagina
hypochondrium *-see* Laceration, abdomen, wall
hypogastric region *-see* Laceration, abdomen, wall
ileum S36.438
inguinal region *-see* Laceration, abdomen, wall
instep *-see* Laceration, foot
internal organ *-see* Injury, by site
interscapular region *-see* Laceration, thorax, back
intestine
  large
    colon S36.539
      ascending S36.530
      descending S36.532
      sigmoid S36.533
      specified site NEC S36.538
    rectum S36.63
    transverse S36.531
  small S36.439
    duodenum S36.430
    specified site NEC S36.438
intra-abdominal organ S36.93
intestine *-see* Laceration, intestine
liver *-see* Laceration, liver
pancreas *-see* Laceration, pancreas
peritoneum S36.81
specified site NEC S36.893
spleen *-see* Laceration, spleen
stomach *-see* Laceration, stomach

Laceration - *continued*

intracranial NEC *-see also* Injury, intracranial, diffuse
  birth injury P10.9
jaw *-see* Laceration, head, specified site NEC
jejunum S36.438
joint capsule *-see* Sprain, by site
kidney S37.03
  major (greater than 3 cm) (massive) (stellate) S37.06
  minor (less than 1 cm) S37.04
  moderate (1 to 3 cm) S37.05
    multiple S37.06
knee S81.01
  with foreign body S81.02
labium (majus) (minus) *-see* Laceration, vulva
lacrimal duct *-see* Laceration, eyelid
large intestine *-see* Laceration, intestine, large
larynx S11.011
  with foreign body S11.012
leg (lower) S81.819
  with foreign body S81.829
  foot *-see* Laceration, foot
  knee *-see* Laceration, knee
  left S81.812
    with foreign body S81.822
  right S81.811
    with foreign body S81.821
  upper *-see* Laceration, thigh
ligament *-see* Sprain
lip S01.511
  with foreign body S01.521
liver S36.113
  major (stellate) S36.116
  minor S36.114
  moderate S36.115
loin *-see* Laceration, abdomen, wall
lower back *-see* Laceration, back, lower
lumbar region *-see* Laceration, back, lower
lung S27.339
  bilateral S27.332
  unilateral S27.331
malar region *-see* Laceration, head, specified site NEC
mammary *-see* Laceration, breast
mastoid region *-see* Laceration, head, specified site NEC
meninges *-see* Injury, intracranial, diffuse
meniscus *-see* Tear, meniscus
mesentery S36.893
mesosalpinx S37.893
mouth *-see* Laceration, oral cavity
muscle *-see* Injury, muscle, by site, laceration
nail
  finger *-see* Laceration, finger, with damage to nail
  toe *-see* Laceration, toe, with damage to nail
nasal (septum) (sinus) *-see* Laceration, nose
nasopharynx *-see* Laceration, head, specified site NEC
neck S11.91
  with foreign body S11.92
  involving
    cervical esophagus S11.21
      with foreign body S11.22
    larynx *-see* Laceration, larynx
    pharynx *-see* Laceration, pharynx
    thyroid gland *-see* Laceration, thyroid gland
    trachea *-see* Laceration, trachea
  specified site NEC S11.81

Laceration - *continued*

  with foreign body S11.82
nerve *-see* Injury, nerve
nose (septum) (sinus) S01.21
  with foreign body S01.22
ocular NOS S05.3
  adnexa NOS S01.11
oral cavity S01.512
  with foreign body S01.522
orbit (eye) *-see* Wound, open, ocular, orbit
ovary S37.439
  bilateral S37.432
  unilateral S37.431
palate *-see* Laceration, oral cavity palm *-see* Laceration, hand
pancreas S36.239
  body S36.231
    major S36.261
    minor S36.241
    moderate S36.251
  head S36.230
    major S36.260
    minor S36.240
    moderate S36.250
  major S36.269
  minor S36.249
  moderate S36.259
  tail S36.232
    major S36.262
    minor S36.242
    moderate S36.252
pelvic S31.010
  with
    foreign body S31.020
      penetration into retroperitoneal cavity S31.021
    penetration into retroperitoneal cavity S31.011
  floor *-see also* Laceration, back, lower
    with ectopic or molar pregnancy O08.6
    complicating delivery O70.1
    following ectopic or molar pregnancy O08.6
    old (postpartal) N81.89
  organ S37.93
    with ectopic or molar pregnancy O08.6
    adrenal gland S37.813
    bladder S37.23
    fallopian tube *-see* Laceration, fallopian tube
    following ectopic or molar pregnancy O08.6
    kidney *-see* Laceration, kidney
    obstetrical trauma O71.5
    ovary *-see* Laceration, ovary
    prostate S37.823
    specified site NEC S37.893
    ureter S37.13
    urethra S37.33
    uterus S37.63
penis S31.21
  with foreign body S31.22
perineum
  female S31.41
    with
      ectopic or molar pregnancy O08.6
      foreign body S31.42
    during delivery O70.9
      first degree O70.0
      fourth degree O70.3
      second degree O70.1

Laceration - *continued*

third degree -*see also* Delivery,
complicated, by, laceration, perineum,
third degree O70.20
old (postpartal) N81.89
postpartal N81.89
secondary (postpartal) O90.1
male S31.119
with foreign body S31.129
periocular area (with or without lacrimal
passages) -*see* Laceration, eyelid
peritoneum S36.893
periumbilic region -*see* Laceration, abdomen,
wall, periumbilic
periurethral tissue -*see* Laceration, urethra
phalanges
finger -*see* Laceration, finger
toe -*see* Laceration, toe
pharynx S11.21
with foreign body S11.22
pinna -*see* Laceration, ear
popliteal space -*see* Laceration, knee
prepuce -*see* Laceration, penis
prostate S37.823
pubic region S31.119
with foreign body S31.129
pudendum -*see* Laceration, genital organs,
external
rectovaginal septum -*see* Laceration, vagina
rectum S36.63
retroperitoneum S36.893
round ligament S37.893
sacral region -*see* Laceration, back, lower
sacroiliac region -*see* Laceration, back, lower
salivary gland -*see* Laceration, oral cavity
scalp S01.01
with foreign body S01.02
scapular region -*see* Laceration, shoulder
scrotum S31.31
with foreign body S31.32
seminal vesicle S37.893
shin -*see* Laceration, leg
shoulder S41.019
with foreign body S41.029
left S41.012
with foreign body S41.022
right S41.011
with foreign body S41.021
small intestine -*see* Laceration, intestine,
small
spermatic cord -*see* Laceration, testis
spinal cord (meninges) -*see also* Injury, spinal
cord, by region
due to injury at birth P11.5
newborn (birth injury) P11.5
spleen S36.039
major (massive) (stellate) S36.032
moderate S36.031
superficial (minor) S36.030
sternal region -*see* Laceration, thorax, front
stomach S36.33
submaxillary region -*see* Laceration, head,
specified site NEC
submental region -*see* Laceration, head,
specified site NEC
subungual
finger(s) -*see* Laceration, finger, with
damage to nail
toe(s) -*see* Laceration, toe, with damage to
nail

Laceration - *continued*

suprarenal gland -*see* Laceration, adrenal
gland
temple, temporal region -*see* Laceration, head,
specified site NEC
temporomandibular area -*see* Laceration,
cheek
tendon -*see* Injury, muscle, by site, laceration
Achilles S86.02
tentorium cerebelli -*see* Injury, intracranial,
diffuse
testis S31.31
with foreign body S31.32
thigh S71.11
with foreign body S71.12
thorax, thoracic (wall) S21.91
with foreign body S21.92
back S21.22
with penetration into thoracic cavity
S21.42
front S21.12
with penetration into thoracic cavity
S21.32
back S21.21
with
foreign body S21.22
with penetration into thoracic cavity
S21.42
penetration into thoracic cavity S21.41
breast -*see* Laceration, breast
front S21.11
with
foreign body S21.12
with penetration into thoracic cavity
S21.32
penetration into thoracic cavity S21.31
thumb S61.019
with
damage to nail S61.119
with
foreign body S61.129
foreign body S61.029
left S61.012
with
damage to nail S61.112
with
foreign body S61.122
foreign body S61.022
right S61.011
with
damage to nail S61.111
with
foreign body S61.121
foreign body S61.021
thyroid gland S11.11
with foreign body S11.12
toe(s) S91.119
with
damage to nail S91.219
with
foreign body S91.229
foreign body S91.129
great S91.113
with
damage to nail S91.213
with
foreign body S91.223
foreign body S91.123
left S91.112
with
damage to nail S91.212

Laceration - *continued*

with
foreign body S91.222
foreign body S91.122
right S91.111
with
damage to nail S91.211
with
foreign body S91.221
foreign body S91.121
lesser S91.116
with
damage to nail S91.216
with
foreign body S91.226
foreign body S91.126
left S91.115
with
damage to nail S91.215
with
foreign body S91.225
foreign body S91.125
right S91.114
with
damage to nail S91.214
with
foreign body S91.224
foreign body S91.124
tongue -*see* Laceration, oral cavity   trachea
S11.021
with foreign body S11.022
tunica vaginalis -*see* Laceration, testis
tympanum, tympanic membrane -*see*
Laceration, ear, drum
umbilical region S31.115
with foreign body S31.125
ureter S37.13
urethra S37.33
with or following ectopic or molar
pregnancy O08.6
obstetrical trauma O71.5
urinary organ NEC S37.893
uterus S37.63
with ectopic or molar pregnancy O08.6
following ectopic or molar pregnancy O08.6
nonpuerperal, nontraumatic N85.8
obstetrical trauma NEC O71.81
old (postpartal) N85.8
uvula -*see* Laceration, oral cavity   vagina
S31.41
with
ectopic or molar pregnancy O08.6
foreign body S31.42
during delivery O71.4
with perineal laceration -*see* Laceration,
perineum, female, during delivery
following ectopic or molar pregnancy O08.6
nonpuerperal, nontraumatic N89.8
old (postpartal) N89.8
vas deferens S37.893
vesical -*see* Laceration, bladder
vocal cords S11.031
with foreign body S11.032
vulva S31.41
with
ectopic or molar pregnancy O08.6
foreign body S31.42
complicating delivery O70.0
following ectopic or molar pregnancy O08.6
nonpuerperal, nontraumatic N90.89
old (postpartal) N90.89

Laceration - *continued*

wrist S61.519
  with
    foreign body S61.529
  left S61.512
    with
      foreign body S61.522
  right S61.511
    with
      foreign body S61.521
Lack of
  achievement in school Z55.3
  adequate
    food Z59.4
    intermaxillary vertical dimension of fully
  erupted teeth M26.36
    sleep Z72.820
  appetite (see Anorexia) R63.0
  awareness R41.9
  care
    in home Z74.2
    of infant (at or after birth) T76.02
      confirmed T74.02
  cognitive functions R41.9
  coordination R27.9
    ataxia R27.0
    specified type NEC R27.8
  development (physiological) R62.50
    failure to thrive (child over 28
days old) R62.51
    adult R62.7
    newborn P92.6
    short stature R62.52
    specified type NEC R62.59
  energy R53.83
  financial resources Z59.6
  food T73.0
  growth R62.52
  heating Z59.1
  housing (permanent) (temporary) Z59.0
    adequate Z59.1
  learning experiences in childhood Z62.898
  leisure time (affecting life-style) Z73.2
  material resources Z59.9
  memory -*see also* Amnesia
    mild, following organic brain damage F06.8
  ovulation N97.0
  parental supervision or control of child Z62.0
  person able to render necessary care Z74.2
  physical exercise Z72.3
  play experience in childhood Z62.898
  posterior occlusal support M26.57
  relaxation (affecting life-style) Z73.2
  sexual
    desire F52.0
    enjoyment F52.1
  shelter Z59.0
  sleep (adequate) Z72.820
  supervision of child by parent Z62.0
  support, posterior occlusal M26.57
  water T73.1
Lacrimal -*see* condition
Lacrimation, abnormal -*see* Epiphora
Lacrimonasal duct -*see* condition
Lactation, lactating (breast) (puerperal, postpartum)
  associated
    cracked nipple O92.13
    retracted nipple O92.03
  defective O92.4

Lactation - disorder NEC O92.79
  excessive O92.6
  failed (complete) O92.3
    partial O92.4
  mastitis NEC -*see* Mastitis, obstetric
  mother (care and/or examination) Z39.1
  nonpuerperal N64.3
Lacticemia, excessive E87.2
Lacunar skull Q75.8
Laennec's cirrhosis K70.30
  with ascites K70.31
  nonalcoholic K74.69
Lafora's disease -*see* Epilepsy, generalized, idiopathic
Lag, lid (nervous) -*see* Retraction, lid
Lagophthalmos (eyelid) (nervous) H02.209
  cicatricial H02.219
    left H02.216
      lower H02.215
      upper H02.214
    right H02.213
      lower H02.212
      upper H02.211
  keratoconjunctivitis -*see* Keratoconjunctivitis
  left H02.206
    lower H02.205
    upper H02.204
  mechanical H02.229
    left H02.226
      lower H02.225
      upper H02.224
    right H02.223
      lower H02.222
      upper H02.221
  paralytic H02.239
    left H02.236
      lower H02.235
      upper H02.234
    right H02.233
      lower H02.232
      upper H02.231
  right H02.203
    lower H02.202
    upper H02.201
Laki-Lorand factor deficiency -*see* Defect, coagulation, specified type NEC
Lalling F80.0
Lambert-Eaton syndrome -*see* Syndrome, Lambert-Eaton
Lambliasis, lambliosis A07.1
Landau-Kleffner syndrome -*see* Epilepsy, specified NEC
Landouzy Déjérine dystrophy or facioscapulohumeral atrophy G71.0
Landouzy's disease (icterohemorrhagic leptospirosis) A27.0
Landry Guillain-Barré, syndrome or paralysis G61.0
Landry's disease or paralysis G61.0
Lane's
  band Q43.3
  kink -*see* Obstruction, intestine
  syndrome K90.2
Langdon Down syndrome -*see* Trisomy, 21
Lapsed immunization schedule status Z28.3
Large
  baby (regardless of gestational age) (4000g to 4499g) P08.1
  ear, congenital Q17.1
  physiological cup Q14.2
  stature R68.89

Large-for-dates NEC (infant) (4000g to 4499g) P08.1
  affecting management of pregnancy O36.6
  exceptionally (4500g or more) P08.0
Larsen-Johansson disease or osteochondrosis -*see* Osteochondrosis, juvenile, patella
Larsen's syndrome (flattened facies and multiple congenital dislocations) Q74.8
Larva migrans
  cutaneous B76.9
    Ancylostoma B76.0
  visceral B83.0
Laryngeal -*see* condition
Laryngismus (stridulus) J38.5
  congenital P28.89
  diphtheritic A36.2
Laryngitis (acute) (edematous) (fibrinous) (infective) (infiltrative) (malignant) (membranous) (phlegmonous) (pneumococcal) (pseudomembranous) (septic) (subglottic) (suppurative) (ulcerative) J04.0
  with
    influenza, flu, or grippe -*see* Influenza, with, laryngitis
    tracheitis (acute) -*see* Laryngotracheitis
  atrophic J37.0
  catarrhal J37.0
  chronic J37.0
    with tracheitis (chronic) J37.1
  diphtheritic A36.2
  due to external agent -*see* Inflammation, respiratory, upper, due to
  Hemophilus influenzae J04.0
  H. influenzae J04.0
  hypertrophic J37.0
  influenzal -*see* Influenza, with, respiratory manifestations NEC
  obstructive J05.0
  sicca J37.0
  spasmodic J05.0
    acute J04.0
  streptococcal J04.0
  stridulous J05.0
  syphilitic (late) A52.73
    congenital A50.59 [*J99*]
      early A50.03 [*J99*]
  tuberculous A15.5
  Vincent's A69.1
Laryngocele (congenital) (ventricular) Q31.3
Laryngofissure J38.7
  congenital Q31.8
Laryngomalacia (congenital) Q31.5
Laryngopharyngitis (acute) J06.0
  chronic J37.0
  due to external agent -*see* Inflammation, respiratory, upper, due to
Laryngoplegia J38.00
  bilateral J38.02
  unilateral J38.01
Laryngoptosis J38.7
Laryngospasm J38.5
Laryngostenosis J38.6
Laryngotracheitis (acute) (Infectional) (infective) (viral) J04.2
  atrophic J37.1
  catarrhal J37.1
  chronic J37.1
  diphtheritic A36.2
  due to external agent -*see* Inflammation, respiratory, upper, due to

Laryngotracheitis - *continued*
  Hemophilus influenzae J04.2
  hypertrophic J37.1
  influenzal -*see* Influenza, with, respiratory
    manifestations NEC
  pachydermic J38.7
  sicca J37.1
  spasmodic J38.5
    acute J05.0
  streptococcal J04.2
  stridulous J38.5
  syphilitic (late) A52.73
    congenital A50.59 [*J99*]
      early A50.03 [*J99*]
  tuberculous A15.5
  Vincent's A69.1
Laryngotracheobronchitis -*see* Bronchitis
Larynx, laryngeal -*see* condition
Lassa fever A96.2
Lassitude -*see* Weakness
Late
  talker R62.0
  walker R62.0
Late effect(s) -*see* Sequelae
Latent -*see* condition
Laterocession -*see* Lateroversion
Lateroflexion -*see* Lateroversion
Lateroversion
  cervix -*see* Lateroversion, uterus
  uterus, uterine (cervix) (postinfectional)
    (postpartal, old) N85.4
    congenital Q51.818
    in pregnancy or childbirth O34.59
Lathyrism -*see* Poisoning, food, noxious, plant
Launois' syndrome (pituitary gigantism)
  E22.0
Launois-Bensaude adenolipomatosis E88.89
Laurence-Moon (Bardet) Biedl syndrome
  Q87.89
Lax, laxity -*see also* Relaxation
  ligament (ous) -*see also* Disorder, ligament
    familial M35.7
    knee -*see* Derangement, knee
  skin (acquired) L57.4
    congenital Q82.8
Laxative habit F55.2
Lazy leukocyte syndrome D70.8
Lead miner's lung J63.6
Leak, leakage
  air NEC J93.82
    postprocedural J95.812
  amniotic fluid -*see* Rupture, membranes,
    premature
  blood (microscopic), fetal, into maternal
    circulation affecting management of
    pregnancy -*see* Pregnancy, complicated by
    cerebrospinal fluid G96.0
    from spinal (lumbar) puncture G97.0
  device, implant or graft -*see also*
    Complications, by site and type, mechanical
    arterial graft NEC -*see* Complication,
      cardiovascular device, mechanical,
      vascular
    breast (implant) T85.43
    catheter NEC T85.638
      urinary T83.038
        cystostomy T83.030
        Hopkins T83.038
        ileostomy T83.038
        indwelling T83.031
        nephrostomy T83.032

Leak, leakage --*continued*
    specified NEC T83.038
    urostomy T83.038
  dialysis (renal) T82.43
    intraperitoneal T85.631
  infusion NEC T82.534
    spinal (epidural) (subdural) T85.630
  gastrointestinal -*see* Complications,
    prosthetic device, mechanical,
    gastrointestinal device
  genital NEC T83.498
    penile prosthesis (cylinder) (implanted)
      (pump) (reservoir) T83.490
    testicular prosthesis T83.491
  heart NEC -*see* Complication,
    cardiovascular device, mechanical
  joint prosthesis -*see* Complications, joint
    prosthesis, mechanical, specified NEC, by
    site
  ocular NEC -*see* Complications, prosthetic
    device, mechanical, ocular device
  orthopedic NEC -*see* Complication,
    orthopedic, device, mechanical
  persistent air J93.82
  specified NEC T85.638
  urinary NEC -*see also* Complication,
    genitourinary, device, urinary, mechanical
    graft T83.23
  vascular NEC -*see* Complication,
    cardiovascular device, mechanical
  ventricular intracranial shunt T85.03
  urine -*see* Incontinence
Leaky heart -*see* Endocarditis
Learning defect (specific) F81.9
Leather bottle stomach C16.9
Leber's
  congenital amaurosis H35.50
  optic atrophy (hereditary) H47.22
Lederer's anemia D59.1
Leeches (external) -*see* Hirudiniasis
Leg -*see* condition
Legg (Calvé) Perthes disease, syndrome or
  osteochondrosis M91.1
Legionellosis A48.1
  nonpneumonic A48.2
Legionnaires'
  disease A48.1
    nonpneumonic A48.2
    pneumonia A48.1
Leigh's disease G31.82
Leiner's disease L21.1
Leiofibromyoma -*see* Leiomyoma
Leiomyoblastoma -*see* Neoplasm, connective
  tissue, benign
Leiomyofibroma -*see also* Neoplasm,
  connective tissue, benign
  uterus (cervix) (corpus) D25.9
Leiomyoma -*see also* Neoplasm, connective
  tissue, benign
  bizarre -*see* Neoplasm, connective tissue,
    benign
  cellular -*see* Neoplasm, connective tissue,
    benign
  epithelioid -*see* Neoplasm, connective tissue,
    benign
  uterus (cervix) (corpus) D25.9
    intramural D25.1
    submucous D25.0
    subserosal D25.2
  vascular -*see* Neoplasm, connective tissue,
    benign

Leiomyoma, leiomyomatosis (intravascular)
  -*see* Neoplasm, connective tissue, uncertain
  behavior
Leiomyosarcoma -*see also* Neoplasm,
  connective tissue, malignant
  epithelioid -*see* Neoplasm, connective tissue,
    malignant
  myxoid -*see* Neoplasm, connective tissue,
    malignant
Leishmaniasis B55.9
  American (mucocutaneous) B55.2
    cutaneous B55.1
  Asian Desert B55.1
  Brazilian B55.2
  cutaneous (any type) B55.1
  dermal -*see also* Leishmaniasis, cutaneous
    post-kala-azar B55.0
  eyelid B55.1
  infantile B55.0
  Mediterranean B55.0
  mucocutaneous (American) (New World)
    B55.2
  naso-oral B55.2
  nasopharyngeal B55.2
  old world B55.1
  tegumentaria diffusa B55.1
  visceral B55.0
Leishmanoid, dermal -*see also* Leishmaniasis,
  cutaneous
  post-kala-azar B55.0
Lenegre's disease I44.2
Lengthening, leg -*see* Deformity, limb,
  unequal length
Lennert's lymphoma -*see* Lymphoma,
  Lennert's
Lennox Gastaut syndrome G40.812
  intractable G40.814
    with status epilepticus G40.813
    without status epilepticus G40.814
  not intractable G40.812
    with status epilepticus G40.811
    without status epilepticus G40.812
Lens -*see* condition
Lenticonus (anterior) (posterior)
  (congenital) Q12.8
Lenticular degeneration, progressive E83.01
Lentiglobus (posterior) (congenital) Q12.8
Lentigo (congenital) L81.4
  maligna -*see also* Melanoma, in situ
    melanoma -*see* Melanoma
Lentivirus, as cause of disease classified
  elsewhere B97.31
Leontiasis
  ossium M85.2
  syphilitic (late) A52.78
    congenital A50.59
Lepothrix A48.8
Lepra -*see* Leprosy
Leprechaunism E34.8
Leprosy A30.
  with muscle disorder A30.9 [*M63.80*]
    ankle A30.9 [*M63.87*]
    foot A30.9 [*M63.87*]
    forearm A30.9 [*M63.83*]
    hand A30.9 [*M63.84*]
    lower leg A30.9 [*M63.86*]
    multiple sites A30.9 [*M63.89*]
    pelvic region A30.9 [*M63.85*]
    shoulder region A30.9 [*M63.81*]
    specified site NEC A30.9 [*M63.88*]
    thigh A30.9 [*M63.85*]

Leprosy --*continued*
upper arm A30.9 [*M63.82*]
anesthetic A30.9
BB A30.3
BL A30.4
borderline (infiltrated) (neuritic) A30.3
lepromatous A30.4
tuberculoid A30.2
BT A30.2
dimorphous (infiltrated) (neuritic) A30.3
I A30.0
indeterminate (macular) (neuritic) A30.0
lepromatous (diffuse) (infiltrated) (macular)
(neuritic) (nodular) A30.5
LL A30.5
macular (early) (neuritic) (simple) A30.9
maculoanesthetic A30.9
mixed A30.3
neural A30.9
nodular A30.5
primary neuritic A30.3
specified type NEC A30.8
TT A30.1
tuberculoid (major) (minor) A30.1
Leptocytosis, hereditary D56.9
Leptomeningitis (chronic) (circumscribed)
(hemorrhagic) (nonsuppurative) -*see*
Meningitis
Leptomeningopathy G96.19
Leptospiral -*see* condition
Leptospirochetal -*see* condition **Leptospirosis**
A27.9
canicola A27.89
due to Leptospira interrogans serovar
icterohaemorrhagiae A27.0
icterohemorrhagica A27.0
pomona A27.89
Weil's disease A27.0
Leptus dermatitis B88.0
Leriche's syndrome (aortic bifurcation
occlusion) I74.09
Leri's pleonosteosis Q78.8
Leri-Weill syndrome Q77.8
Lermoyez' syndrome -*see* Vertigo, peripheral
NEC
Lesch-Nyhan syndrome E79.1
Leser-Trélat disease L82.1
inflamed L82.0
Lesion(s) (nontraumatic)
abducens nerve -*see* Strabismus, paralytic,
sixth nerve
alveolar process K08.9
angiocentric immunoproliferative D47.Z9
anorectal K62.9
aortic (valve) I35.9
auditory nerve - see subcategory H93.3
basal ganglion G25.9
bile duct -*see* Disease, bile duct
biomechanical M99.9
specified type NEC M99.89
abdomen M99.89
acromioclavicular M99.87
cervical region M99.81
cervicothoracic M99.81
costochondral M99.88
costovertebral M99.88
head region M99.80
hip M99.85
lower extremity M99.86
lumbar region M99.83
lumbosacral M99.83

Lesion(s) (nontraumatic) --*continued*
occipitocervical M99.80
pelvic region M99.85
pubic M99.85
rib cage M99.88
sacral region M99.84
sacrococcygeal M99.84
sacroiliac M99.84
specified NEC M99.89
sternochondral M99.88
sternoclavicular M99.87
thoracic region M99.82
thoracolumbar M99.82
upper extremity M99.87
bladder N32.9
bone -*see* Disorder, bone
brachial plexus G54.0
brain G93.9
congenital Q04.9
vascular I67.9
degenerative I67.9
hypertensive I67.4
buccal cavity K13.79
calcified -*see* Calcification
canthus -*see* Disorder, eyelid
carate -*see* Pinta, lesions
cardia K31.9
cardiac -*see also* Disease, heart I51.9
congenital Q24.9
valvular -*see* Endocarditis
cauda equina G83.4
cecum K63.9
cerebral -*see* Lesion, brain
cerebrovascular I67.9
degenerative I67.9
hypertensive I67.4
cervical (nerve) root NEC G54.2
chiasmal -*see* Disorder, optic, chiasm
chorda tympani G51.8
coin, lung R91.1
colon K63.9
combined periodontic
endodontic K05.5
congenital -*see* Anomaly, by site
conjunctiva H11.9
conus medullaris -*see* Injury, conus
medullaris
coronary artery -*see* Ischemia, heart
cranial nerve G52.9
eighth -*see* Disorder, ear
eleventh G52.9
fifth G50.9
first G52.0
fourth -*see* Strabismus, paralytic, fourth
nerve
seventh G51.9
sixth -*see* Strabismus, paralytic, sixth nerve
tenth G52.2
twelfth G52.3
cystic -*see* Cyst
degenerative -*see* Degeneration
duodenum K31.9
edentulous (alveolar) ridge, associated with
trauma, due to traumatic occlusion K06.2
en coup de sabre L94.1
eyelid -*see* Disorder, eyelid
gasserian ganglion G50.8
gastric K31.9
gastroduodenal K31.9
gastrointestinal K63.9
gingiva, associated with trauma K06.2

Lesion(s) (nontraumatic) --*continued*
glomerular
focal and segmental -*see also* N00 N07 with
fourth character .1 N05.1
minimal change -*see also* N00 N07 with
fourth character .0 N05.0
heart (organic) -*see* Disease, heart
hyperchromic, due to pinta (carate) A67.1
hyperkeratotic -*see* Hyperkeratosis
hypothalamic E23.7
ileocecal K63.9
ileum K63.9
iliohypogastric nerve G57.8
inflammatory -*see* Inflammation
intestine K63.9
intracerebral -*see* Lesion, brain
intrachiasmal (optic) -*see* Disorder, optic,
chiasm
intracranial, space-occupying R90.0
joint -*see* Disorder, joint
sacroiliac (old) M53.3
keratotic -*see* Keratosis
kidney -*see* Disease, renal
laryngeal nerve (recurrent) G52.2
lip K13.0
liver K76.9
lumbosacral
plexus G54.1
root (nerve) NEC G54.4
lung (coin) R91.1
maxillary sinus J32.0
mitral I05.9
Morel-Lavallée -*see* Hematoma, by site
motor cortex NEC G93.89
mouth K13.79
nerve G58.9
femoral G57.2
median G56.1
carpal tunnel syndrome -*see* Syndrome,
carpal tunnel
plantar G57.6
popliteal (lateral) G57.3
medial G57.4
radial G56.3
sciatic G57.0
spinal -*see* Injury, nerve, spinal
ulnar G56.2
nervous system, congenital Q07.9
nonallopathic -*see* Lesion, biomechanical
nose (internal) J34.89
obstructive -*see* Obstruction
obturator nerve G57.8
oral mucosa K13.70
organ or site NEC -*see* Disease, by site
osteolytic -*see* Osteolysis
peptic K27.9
periodontal, due to traumatic occlusion K05.5
pharynx J39.2
pigment, pigmented (skin) L81.9
pinta -*see* Pinta, lesions
polypoid -*see* Polyp
prechiasmal (optic) -*see* Disorder, optic,
chiasm
primary -*see also* Syphilis, primary A51.0
carate A67.0
pinta A67.0
yaws A66.0
pulmonary J98.4
valve I37.9
pylorus K31.9
rectosigmoid K63.9

Lesion(s) (nontraumatic) --continued
retina, retinal H35.9
sacroiliac (joint) (old) M53.3
salivary gland K11.9
  benign lymphoepithelial K11.8
saphenous nerve G57.8
sciatic nerve G57.0
secondary -see Syphilis, secondary
shoulder (region) M75.9
  specified NEC M75.8
sigmoid K63.9
sinus (accessory) (nasal) J34.89
skin L98.9
  suppurative L08.0
SLAP S43.43
spinal cord G95.9
  congenital Q06.9
spleen D73.89
stomach K31.9
superior glenoid labrum S43.43
syphilitic -see Syphilis
tertiary -see Syphilis, tertiary
thoracic root (nerve) NEC G54.3
tonsillar fossa J35.9
tooth, teeth K08.9
  white spot
    chewing surface K02.51
    pit and fissure surface K02.51
    smooth surface K02.61
traumatic -see specific type of injury by site
tricuspid (valve) I07.9
  nonrheumatic I36.9
trigeminal nerve G50.9
ulcerated or ulcerative -see Ulcer, skin
uterus N85.9
vagus nerve G52.2
valvular -see Endocarditis
vascular I99.9
  affecting central nervous system I67.9
  following trauma NEC T14.8
  umbilical cord, complicating delivery O69.5
warty -see Verruca
white spot (tooth)
  chewing surface K02.51
  pit and fissure surface K02.51
  smooth surface K02.61
Lethargic -see condition
Lethargy R53.83
Letterer-Siwe's disease C96.0
Leukemia, leukemic C95.9
  acute basophilic C94.8
  acute bilineal C95.0
  acute erythroid C94.0
  acute lymphoblastic C91.0
  acute megakaryoblastic C94.2
  acute megakaryocytic C94.2
  acute mixed lineage C95.0
  acute monoblastic (monoblastic/monocytic)
    C93.0
  acute monocytic (monoblastic/monocytic)
    C93.0
  acute myeloblastic (minimal differentiation)
    (with maturation) C92.0
  acute myeloid
    with
      11q23 abnormality C92.6
      dysplasia of remaining hematopoesis
        and/or myelodysplastic disease in its
        history C92.A-
      multilineage dysplasia C92.A-
      variation of MLL-gene C92.6

Leukemia, leukemic --continued
  M6 (a)(b) C94.0
  M7 C94.2
  acute myelomonocytic C92.5
  acute promyelocytic C92.4
  adult T-cell (HTLV-1 associated) (acute
    variant) (chronic variant) (lymphomatoid
    variant) (smouldering variant) C91.5
  aggressive NK-cell C94.8
  AML (1/ETO) (M0) (M1) (M2) (without a
    FAB classification) C92.0
  AML M3 C92.4
  AML M4 (Eo with inv(16) or t(16;16))
    C92.5
  AML M5 C93.0
  AML M5a C93.0
  AML M5b C93.0
  AML Me with t (15;17) and variants C92.4
  atypical chronic myeloid, BCR/ABL-negative
    C92.2
  biphenotypic acute C95.0
  blast cell C95.0
  Burkitt-type, mature B-cell C91.A-
  chronic lymphocytic, of B-cell type C91.1
  chronic monocytic C93.1
  chronic myelogenous (Philadelphia
    chromosome (Ph1) positive) (t(9;22))
    (q34;q11) (with crisis of blast cells) C92.1
  chronic myeloid, BCR/ABL-positive C92.1
    atypical, BCR/ABL-negative C92.2
  chronic myelomonocytic C93.1
  chronic neutrophilic D47.1
  CMML (1) (2) (with eosinophilia) C93.1
  granulocytic -see also Category C92 C92.9
  hairy cell C91.4
  juvenile myelomonocytic C93.3
  lymphoid C91.9
    specified NEC C91.Z   mast cell C94.3
  mature B-cell, Burkitt-type C91.A-
    monocytic (subacute) C93.9
    specified NEC C93.Z
  myelogenous -see also Category C92 C92.9
  myeloid C92.9
    specified NEC C92.Z   plasma cell C90.1
  plasmacytic C90.1
  prolymphocytic
    of B-cell type C91.3
    of T-cell type C91.6
    specified NEC C94.8
  stem cell, of unclear lineage C95.0
  subacute lymphocytic C91.9
  T-cell large granular lymphocytic C91.Z
  unspecified cell type C95.9
    acute C95.0
    chronic C95.1
Leukemoid reaction -see also Reaction,
  leukemoid D72.823
Leukoaraiosis (hypertensive) I67.81
Leukoariosis -see Leukoaraiosis
Leukocoria -see Disorder, globe, degenerated
  condition, leucocoria
Leukocytopenia D72.819
Leukocytosis D72.829
  eosinophilic D72.1
Leukoderma, leukodermia NEC L81.5
  syphilitic A51.39
    late A52.79
Leukodystrophy E75.29
Leukoedema, oral epithelium K13.29

Leukoencephalitis G04.81
  acute (subacute) hemorrhagic G36.1
    postimmunization or postvaccinal G04.02
  postinfectious G04.01
  subacute sclerosing A81.1
  van Bogaert's (sclerosing) A81.1
Leukoencephalopathy -see also
  Encephalopathy G93.49
  Binswanger's I67.3
  heroin vapor G92
  metachromatic E75.25
  multifocal (progressive) A81.2
  postimmunization and postvaccinal G04.02
  progressive multifocal A81.2
  reversible, posterior G93.6
  van Bogaert's (sclerosing) A81.1
  vascular, progressive I67.3
Leukoerythroblastosis D75.9
Leukokeratosis -see also Leukoplakia
  mouth K13.21
  nicotina palati K13.24
  oral mucosa K13.21
  tongue K13.21
  vocal cord J38.3
Leukokraurosis vulva (e) N90.4
Leukoma (cornea) -see also Opacity, cornea
  adherent H17.0
  interfering with central vision -see Opacity,
    cornea, central
Leukomalacia, cerebral, newborn P91.2
  periventricular P91.2
Leukomelanopathy, hereditary D72.0
Leukonychia (punctata) (striata) L60.8
  congenital Q84.4
Leukopathia unguium L60.8
  congenital Q84.4
Leukopenia D72.819
  basophilic D72.818
  chemotherapy (cancer) induced D70.1
  congenital D70.0
  cyclic D70.0
  drug induced NEC D70.2
    due to cytoreductive cancer chemotherapy
      D70.1
  eosinophilic D72.818
  familial D70.0
  infantile genetic D70.0
  malignant D70.9
  periodic D70.0
  transitory neonatal P61.5
Leukopenic -see condition
Leukoplakia
  anus K62.89
  bladder (postinfectional) N32.89
  buccal K13.21
  cervix (uteri) N88.0
  esophagus K22.8
  gingiva K13.21
  hairy (oral mucosa) (tongue) K13.3
  kidney (pelvis) N28.89
  larynx J38.7
  lip K13.21
  mouth K13.21
  oral epithelium, including tongue (mucosa)
    K13.21
  palate K13.21
  pelvis (kidney) N28.89
  penis (infectional) N48.0
  rectum K62.89
  syphilitic (late) A52.79
  tongue K13.21

Leukoplakia - *continued*
ureter (postinfectional) N28.89
urethra (postinfectional) N36.8
uterus N85.8
vagina N89.4
vocal cord J38.3
vulva N90.4
Leukorrhea N89.8
due to Trichomonas (vaginalis) A59.00
trichomonal A59.00
Leukosarcoma C85.9
Levocardia (isolated) Q24.1
with situs inversus Q89.3
Levotransposition Q20.5
Lev's disease or syndrome (acquired complete heart block) I44.2
Levulosuria *-see* Fructosuria
Levurid L30.2
Lewy body (ies) (dementia) (disease) G31.83
Leyden-Moebius dystrophy G71.0
Leydig cell
carcinoma
specified site *-see* Neoplasm, malignant, by site
unspecified site
female C56.9
male C62.9
tumor
benign
specified site *-see* Neoplasm, benign, by site
unspecified site
female D27.
male D29.2
malignant
specified site *-see* Neoplasm, malignant, by site
unspecified site
female C56.
male C62.9
specified site *-see* Neoplasm, uncertain behavior, by site
unspecified site
female D39.1
male D40.1
Leydig-Sertoli cell tumor
specified site *-see* Neoplasm, benign, by site
unspecified site
female D27.
male D29.2
LGSIL (Low grade squamous intraepithelial lesion on cytologic smear of)
anus R85.612
cervix R87.612
vagina R87.622
Liar, pathologic F60.2
Libido
decreased R68.82
Libman-Sacks disease M32.11
Lice (infestation) B85.2
body (Pediculus corporis) B85.1
crab B85.3
head (Pediculus capitis) B85.0
mixed (classifiable to more than one of the titles B85.0 B85.3) B85.4
pubic (Phthirus pubis) B85.3
Lichen L28.0
albus L90.0
penis N48.0
vulva N90.4
amyloidosis E85.4 [*L99*]

Lichen - *continued*
atrophicus L90.0
penis N48.0
vulva N90.4
congenital Q82.8
myxedematosus L98.5
nitidus L44.1
pilaris Q82.8
acquired L85.8
planopilaris L66.1
planus (chronicus) L43.9
annularis L43.8
bullous L43.1
follicular L66.1
hypertrophic L43.0
moniliformis L44.3
of Wilson L43.9
specified NEC L43.8
subacute (active) L43.3
tropicus L43.3
ruber
acuminatus L44.0
moniliformis L44.3
planus L43.9
sclerosus (et atrophicus) L90.0
penis N48.0
vulva N90.4
scrofulosus (primary) (tuberculous) A18.4
simplex (chronicus) (circumscriptus) L28.0
striatus L44.2
urticatus L28.2
Lichenification L28.0
Lichenoides tuberculosis (primary) A18.4
Lichtheim's disease or syndrome *-see* Degeneration, combined
Lien migrans D73.89
Ligament *-see* condition
Light
for gestational age *-see* Light for dates
headedness R42
Light-for-dates (infant) P05.00
with weight of
499 grams or less P05.01
500 749 grams P05.02
750 999 grams P05.03
1000 1249 grams P05.04
1250 1499 grams P05.05
1500 1749 grams P05.06
1750 1999 grams P05.07
2000 2499 grams P05.08
2500 grams and over P05.09
specified NEC P05.09
and small-for-dates *-see* Small for dates
affecting management of pregnancy O36.59
Lightning (effects) (stroke) (struck by) T75.00
burn *-see* Burn
foot E53.8
shock T75.01
specified effect NEC T75.09
Lightwood-Albright syndrome N25.89
Lightwood's disease or syndrome (renal tubular acidosis) N25.89
Lignac (de Toni) (Fanconi) (Debré) disease or syndrome E72.09
with cystinosis E72.04
Ligneous thyroiditis E06.5
Likoff's syndrome I20.8
Limb *-see* condition
Limbic epilepsy personality syndrome F07.0

Limitation, limited
activities due to disability Z73.6
cardiac reserve *-see* Disease, heart
eye muscle duction, traumatic *-see* Strabismus, mechanical
mandibular range of motion M26.52
Lindau (von Hippel) disease Q85.8
Line(s)
Beau's L60.4
Harris' *-see* Arrest, epiphyseal
Hudson's (cornea) *-see* Pigmentation, cornea, anterior
Stähli's (cornea) *-see* Pigmentation, cornea, anterior
Linea corneae senilis *-see* Change, cornea, senile
Lingua
geographica K14.1
nigra (villosa) K14.3
plicata K14.5
tylosis K13.29
Lingual *-see* condition
Linguatulosis B88.8
Linitis (gastric) plastica C16.9
Lip *-see* condition
Lipedema *-see* Edema
Lipemia *-see also* Hyperlipidemia
retina, retinalis E78.3
Lipidosis E75.6
cerebral (infantile) (juvenile) (late) E75.4
cerebroretinal E75.4
cerebroside E75.22
cholesterol (cerebral) E75.5
glycolipid E75.21
hepatosplenomegalic E78.3
sphingomyelin *-see* Niemann-Pick disease or syndrome
sulfatide E75.29
Lipoadenoma *-see* Neoplasm, benign, by site
Lipoblastoma *-see* Lipoma
Lipoblastomatosis *-see* Lipoma
Lipochondrodystrophy E76.01
Lipodermatosclerosis *-see* Varix, leg, with, inflammation
ulcerated *-see* Varix, leg, with, ulcer, with inflammation by site
Lipochrome histiocytosis (familial) D71
Lipodystrophia progressiva E88.1
Lipodystrophy (progressive) E88.1
insulin E88.1
intestinal K90.81
mesenteric K65.4
Lipofibroma *-see* Lipoma
Lipofuscinosis, neuronal (with ceroidosis) E75.4
Lipogranuloma, sclerosing L92.8
Lipogranulomatosis E78.89
Lipoid *-see also* condition
histiocytosis D76.3
essential E75.29
nephrosis N04.9
proteinosis of Urbach E78.89
Lipoidemia *-see* Hyperlipidemia
Lipoidosis *-see* Lipidosis
Lipoma D17.9
fetal D17.9
fat cell D17.9
infiltrating D17.9
intramuscular D17.9
pleomorphic D17.9
site classification

Lipoma *--continued*
  arms (skin) (subcutaneous) D17.2
  connective tissue D17.30
    intra-abdominal D17.5
    intrathoracic D17.4
    peritoneum D17.79
    retroperitoneum D17.79
    specified site NEC D17.39
    spermatic cord D17.6
  face (skin) (subcutaneous) D17.0
  genitourinary organ NEC D17.72
  head (skin) (subcutaneous) D17.0
  intra-abdominal D17.5
  intrathoracic D17.4
  kidney D17.71
  legs (skin) (subcutaneous) D17.2
  neck (skin) (subcutaneous) D17.0
  peritoneum D17.79
  retroperitoneum D17.79
  skin D17.30
    specified site NEC D17.39
  specified site NEC D17.79
  spermatic cord D17.6
  subcutaneous D17.30
    specified site NEC D17.39
  trunk (skin) (subcutaneous) D17.1
  unspecified D17.9
  spindle cell D17.9
Lipomatosis E88.2
  dolorosa (Dercum) E88.2
  fetal -see Lipoma
  Launois-Bensaude E88.89
Lipomyoma -see Lipoma
Lipomyxoma -see Lipoma
Lipomyxosarcoma -see Neoplasm, connective
  tissue, malignant
Lipoprotein metabolism disorder E78.9
Lipoproteinemia E78.5
  broad-beta E78.2
  floating-beta E78.2
  hyper-pre-beta E78.1
Liposarcoma -see also Neoplasm, connective
  tissue, malignant
  dedifferentiated -see Neoplasm, connective
    tissue, malignant
  differentiated type -see Neoplasm, connective
    tissue, malignant
  embryonal -see Neoplasm, connective tissue,
    malignant
  mixed type -see Neoplasm, connective tissue,
    malignant
  myxoid -see Neoplasm, connective tissue,
    malignant
  pleomorphic -see Neoplasm, connective
    tissue, malignant
  round cell -see Neoplasm, connective tissue,
    malignant
  well differentiated type -see Neoplasm,
    connective tissue, malignant
Liposynovitis prepatellaris E88.89
Lipping, cervix N86
Lipschütz disease or ulcer N76.6
Lipuria R82.0
  schistosomiasis (bilharziasis) B65.0
Lisping F80.0
Lissauer's paralysis A52.17
Lissencephalia, lissencephaly Q04.3
Listeriosis, listerellosis A32.9
  congenital (disseminated) P37.2
  cutaneous A32.0
  neonatal, newborn (disseminated) P37.2
  oculoglandular A32.81
  specified NEC A32.89

Lithemia E79.0
Lithiasis -see Calculus
Lithosis J62.8
Lithuria R82.99
Litigation, anxiety concerning Z65.3
Little leaguer's elbow -see Epicondylitis,
  medial
Little's disease G80.9
Littre's
  gland -see condition
  hernia -see Hernia, abdomen
Littritis -see Urethritis
Livedo (annularis) (racemosa) (reticularis)
  R23.1
Liver -see condition
Living alone (problems with) Z60.2
  with handicapped person Z74.2
Lloyd's syndrome -see Adenomatosis,
  endocrine
Loa Loa, loaiasis, loiasis B74.3
Lobar -see condition
Lobomycosis B48.0
Lobo's disease B48.0
Lobotomy syndrome F07.0
Lobstein (Ekman) disease or syndrome
  Q78.0
Lobster-claw hand Q71.6
Lobulation (congenital) -see also Anomaly,
  by site
  kidney, Q63.1
  liver, abnormal Q44.7
  spleen Q89.09
Lobule, lobular -see condition
Local, localized -see condition
Locked-in state G83.5
Locked twins causing obstructed labor
  O66.1
Locking
  joint -see Derangement, joint, specified type
    NEC
    knee -see Derangement, knee
Lockjaw -see Tetanus
Löffler's
  endocarditis I42.3
  eosinophilia J82
  pneumonia J82
  syndrome (eosinophilic pneumonitis) J82
Loiasis (with conjunctival infestation)
  (eyelid) B74.3
Lone Star fever A77.0
Long
  labor O63.9
    first stage O63.0
    second stage O63.1
  QT syndrome I45.81
Long-term (current) (prophylactic) drug
  therapy (use of)
  agents affecting estrogen receptors and
    estrogen levels NEC Z79.818
  anastrozole (Arimidex) Z79.811
  antibiotics Z79.2
    short-term use - omit code
  anticoagulants Z79.01
  anti-inflammatory, non-steroidal (NSAID)
    Z79.1
  antiplatelet Z79.02
  antithrombotics Z79.02
  aromatase inhibitors Z79.811
  aspirin Z79.82
  birth control pill or patch Z79.3
  bisphosphonates Z79.83

Long-term drug therapy *--continued*
  contraceptive, oral Z79.3
  drug, specified NEC Z79.899
  estrogen receptor downregulators Z79.818
  Evista Z79.810
  exemestane (Aromasin) Z79.811
  Fareston Z79.810
  fulvestrant (Faslodex) Z79.818
  gonadotropin-releasing hormone (GnRH)
    agonist Z79.818
  goserelin acetate (Zoladex) Z79.818
  hormone replacement (postmenopausal)
    Z79.890
  insulin Z79.4
  letrozole (Femara) Z79.811
  leuprolide acetate (leuprorelin) (Lupron)
    Z79.818
  megestrol acetate (Megace) Z79.818
  methadone for pain management Z79.891
  Nolvadex Z79.810
  non-steroidal anti-inflammatories (NSAID)
    Z79.1
  opiate analgesic Z79.891
  oral
    antidiabetic Z79.84
    contraceptive Z79.3
    hypoglycemic Z79.84
  raloxifene (Evista) Z79.810
  selective estrogen receptor modulators
    (SERMs) Z79.810
  steroids
    inhaled Z79.51
    systemic Z79.52
  tamoxifen (Nolvadex) Z79.810
  toremifene (Fareston) Z79.810
Longitudinal stripes or grooves, nails L60.8
  congenital Q84.6
Loop
  intestine -see Volvulus
  vascular on papilla (optic) Q14.2
Loose -see also condition
  body
    joint M24.00
      ankle M24.07
      elbow M24.02
      hand M24.04
      hip M24.05
      knee M23.4
      shoulder (region) M24.01
      specified site NEC M24.08
      vertebra M24.08
      toe M24.07
      wrist M24.03
    knee M23.4
    sheath, tendon -see Disorder, tendon,
      specified type NEC
  cartilage -see Loose, body, joint
  skin and subcutaneous tissue (following
    bariatric surgery weight loss) (following
    dietary weight loss) L98.7
  tooth, teeth K08.89
Loosening
  aseptic
    joint prosthesis -see Complications, joint
      prosthesis, mechanical, loosening, by site
  epiphysis -see Osteochondropathy
  mechanical
    joint prosthesis -see Complications, joint
      prosthesis, mechanical, loosening, by site
Looser-Milkman (Debray) syndrome M83.8
Lop ear (deformity) Q17.3

Lorain (Levi) short stature syndrome E23.0
Lordosis M40.50
  acquired -*see* Lordosis, specified type NEC
  congenital Q76.429
    lumbar region Q76.426
    lumbosacral region Q76.427
    sacral region Q76.428
    sacrococcygeal region Q76.428
    thoracolumbar region Q76.425
  lumbar region M40.56
  lumbosacral region M40.57
  postsurgical M96.4
  postural -*see* Lordosis, specified type NEC
  rachitic (late effect) (sequelae) E64.3
  sequelae of rickets E64.3
  specified type NEC M40.40
    lumbar region M40.46
    lumbosacral region M40.47
    thoracolumbar region M40.45
  thoracolumbar region M40.55
  tuberculous A18.01
Loss (of)
  appetite (see Anorexia) R63.0
    hysterical F50.89
    nonorganic origin F50.89
    psychogenic F50.89
  blood -*see* Hemorrhage
  bone -*see* Loss, substance of, bone
  control, sphincter, rectum R15.9
    nonorganic origin F98.1
  consciousness, transient R55
    traumatic -*see* Injury, intracranial
  elasticity, skin R23.4
  family (member) in childhood Z62.898
  fluid (acute) E86.9
  function of labyrinth -*see* subcategory H83.2
  hair, nonscarring -*see* Alopecia
  hearing -*see also* Deafness
    central NOS H90.5
    conductive H90.2
      bilateral H90.0
      unilateral
        with
          restricted hearing on the contralateral
            side H90.A1
          unrestricted hearing on the contralateral
            side H90.1
    mixed conductive and sensorineural hearing
    loss H90.8
      bilateral H90.6
      unilateral
        with
          restricted hearing on the contralateral
            side H90.A3
          unrestricted hearing on the contralateral
            side H90.7
    neural NOS H90.5
    perceptive NOS H90.5
    sensorineural NOS H90.5
      bilateral H90.3
      unilateral
        with
          restricted hearing on the contralateral
            side H90.A2
          unrestricted hearing on the contralateral
            side H90.4
    sensory NOS H90.5
  height R29.890
  limb or member, traumatic, current -*see*
  Amputation, traumatic
  love relationship in childhood Z62.898

Loss (of) --*continued*
  memory -*see also* Amnesia
    mild, following organic brain damage F06.8
  mind -*see* Psychosis
  occlusal vertical dimension of fully erupted
    teeth M26.37
  organ or part -*see* Absence, by site, acquired
  ossicles, ear (partial) H74.32
  parent in childhood Z63.4
  pregnancy, recurrent N96
    care in current pregnancy O26.2
    without current pregnancy N96
  recurrent pregnancy -*see* Loss, pregnancy,
  recurrent
  self-esteem, in childhood Z62.898
  sense of
    smell -*see* Disturbance, sensation, smell
    taste -*see* Disturbance, sensation, taste
    touch R20.8
  sensory R44.9
    dissociative F44.6
  sexual desire F52.0
  sight (acquired) (complete) (congenital) -*see*
    Blindness
  substance of
    bone -*see* Disorder, bone, density and
    structure, specified NEC
      horizontal alveolar K06.3
    cartilage -*see* Disorder, cartilage, specified
    type NEC
      auricle (ear) -*see* Disorder, pinna, specified
      type NEC
    vitreous (humor) H15.89
  tooth, teeth -*see* Absence, teeth, acquired
  vision, visual H54.7
    both eyes H54.3
    one eye H54.60
      left (normal vision on right) H54.62
      right (normal vision on left) H54.61
    specified as blindness -*see* Blindness
    subjective
      sudden H53.13
      transient H53.12
  vitreous -*see* Prolapse, vitreous
  voice -*see* Aphonia
  weight (abnormal) (cause unknown) R63.4
Louis-Bar syndrome (ataxia-telangiectasia)
  G11.3
Louping ill (encephalitis) A84.8
Louse, lousiness -*see* Lice
Low
  achiever, school Z55.3
  back syndrome M54.5
  basal metabolic rate R94.8
  birthweight (2499 grams or less) P07.10
    with weight of
      1000 1249 grams P07.14
      1250 1499 grams P07.15
      1500 1749 grams P07.16
      1750 1999 grams P07.17
      2000 2499 grams P07.18
    extreme (999 grams or less) P07.00
    with weight of
      499 grams or less P07.01
      500 749 grams P07.02
      750 999 grams P07.03
    for gestational age -*see* Light for dates
  blood pressure -*see also* Hypotension
    reading (incidental) (isolated) (nonspecific)
    R03.1
  cardiac reserve -*see* Disease, heart

Loss (of) --*continued*
  function -*see also* Hypofunction
    kidney N28.9
  hematocrit D64.9
  hemoglobin D64.9
  income Z59.6
  level of literacy Z55.0
  lying
    kidney N28.89
    organ or site, congenital -*see* Malposition,
  congenital
  output syndrome (cardiac) -*see* Failure, heart
  platelets (blood) -*see* Thrombocytopenia
  reserve, kidney N28.89
  salt syndrome E87.1
  self esteem R45.81
  set ears Q17.4
  vision H54.2
    one eye (other eye normal) H54.50
      left (normal vision on right) H54.52
      other eye blind -*see* Blindness
      right (normal vision on left) H54.51
Low-density lipoprotein-type (LDL)
hyperlipoproteinemia E78.00
Lowe's syndrome E72.03
Lown-Ganong-Levine syndrome I45.6
LSD reaction (acute) (without dependence)
  F16.90
  with dependence F16.20
L-shaped kidney Q63.8
Ludwig's angina or disease K12.2
Lues (venerea), luetic -*see* Syphilis
Luetscher's syndrome (dehydration) E86.0
Lumbago, lumbalgia M54.5
  with sciatica M54.4
    due to intervertebral disc disorder M51.17
  due to displacement, intervertebral disc
  M51.27
    with sciatica M51.17
Lumbar -*see* condition
Lumbarization, vertebra, congenital Q76.49
Lumbermen's itch B88.0
Lump -*see* Mass **Lunacy** -*see* Psychosis
Lung -*see* condition
Lupoid (miliary) of Boeck D86.3
Lupus
  anticoagulant D68.62
    with
      hemorrhagic disorder D68.312
      hypercoagulable state D68.62
    finding without diagnosis R76.0
  discoid (local) L93.0
  erythematosus (discoid) (local) L93.0
    disseminated -*see* Lupus, erythematosus,
  systemic
    eyelid H01.129
      left H01.126
        lower H01.125
        upper H01.124
      right H01.123
        lower H01.122
        upper H01.121
  profundus L93.2
  specified NEC L93.2
  subacute cutaneous L93.1
  systemic M32.9
    with organ or system involvement M32.10
      endocarditis M32.11
      lung M32.13
      pericarditis M32.12
      renal (glomerular) M32.14

Lupus - *continued*
    tubulo-interstitial M32.15
        specified organ or system NEC M32.19
    drug-induced M32.0
    inhibitor (presence of) D68.62
        with
            hemorrhagic disorder D68.312
            hypercoagulable state D68.62
            finding without diagnosis R76.0
        specified NEC M32.8
    exedens A18.4
    hydralazine M32.0
        correct substance properly administered -*see* Table of Drugs and Chemicals, by drug, adverse effect
        overdose or wrong substance given or taken -*see* Table of Drugs and Chemicals, by drug, poisoning
    nephritis (chronic) M32.14
    nontuberculous, not disseminated L93.0
    panniculitis L93.2
    pernio (Besnier) D86.3
    systemic -*see* Lupus, erythematosus, systemic
    tuberculous A18.4
        eyelid A18.4
    vulgaris A18.4
        eyelid A18.4
Luteinoma D27.
Lutembacher's disease or syndrome (atrial septal defect with mitral stenosis) Q21.1
Luteoma D27.
Lutz (Splendore-de Almeida) disease -*see* Paracoccidioidomycosis
Luxation -*see also* Dislocation
    eyeball (nontraumatic) -*see* Luxation, globe
        birth injury P15.3
    globe, nontraumatic H44.82
    lacrimal gland -*see* Dislocation, lacrimal gland
    lens (old) (partial) (spontaneous)
        congenital Q12.1
        syphilitic A50.39
Lycanthropy F22
Lyell's syndrome L51.2
    due to drug L51.2
        correct substance properly administered -*see* Table of Drugs and Chemicals, by drug, adverse effect
        overdose or wrong substance given or taken -*see* Table of Drugs and Chemicals, by drug, poisoning
Lyme disease A69.20
Lymph
    gland or node -*see* condition
    scrotum -*see* Infestation, filarial
Lymphadenitis I88.9
    with ectopic or molar pregnancy O08.0
    acute L04.9
        axilla L04.2
        face L04.0
        head L04.0
        hip L04.3
        limb
            lower L04.3
            upper L04.2
        neck L04.0
        shoulder L04.2
        specified site NEC L04.8
        trunk L04.1
    anthracosis (occupational) J60
    any site, except mesenteric I88.9

Lymphadenitis --*continued*
    chronic I88.1
        subacute I88.1
    breast
        gestational -*see* Mastitis, obstetric
        puerperal, postpartum (nonpurulent) O91.22
    chancroidal (congenital) A57
    chronic I88.1
        mesenteric I88.0
    due to
        Brugia (malayi) B74.1
            timori B74.2
        chlamydial lymphogranuloma A55
        diphtheria (toxin) A36.89
        lymphogranuloma venereum A55
        Wuchereria bancrofti B74.0
    following ectopic or molar pregnancy O08.0
    gonorrheal A54.89
    infective -*see* Lymphadenitis, acute
    mesenteric (acute) (chronic) (nonspecific) (subacute) I88.0
        due to Salmonella typhi A01.09
        tuberculous A18.39
    mycobacterial A31.8
    purulent -*see* Lymphadenitis, acute
    pyogenic -*see* Lymphadenitis, acute
    regional, nonbacterial I88.8
    septic -*see* Lymphadenitis, acute
    subacute, unspecified site I88.1
    suppurative -*see* Lymphadenitis, acute
    syphilitic (early) (secondary) A51.49
        late A52.79
    tuberculous -*see* Tuberculosis, lymph gland
    venereal (chlamydial) A55
Lymphadenoid goiter E06.3
Lymphadenopathy (generalized) R59.1
    angioimmunoblastic, with dysproteinemia (AILD) C86.5
    due to toxoplasmosis (acquired) B58.89
        congenital (acute) (subacute) (chronic) P37.1
    localized R59.0
    syphilitic (early) (secondary) A51.49
Lymphadenosis R59.1
Lymphangiectasis I89.0
    conjunctiva H11.89
    postinfectional I89.0
    scrotum I89.0
Lymphangiectatic elephantiasis, nonfilarial I89.0
Lymphangioendothelioma D18.1
    malignant -*see* Neoplasm, connective tissue, malignant
Lymphangioleiomyomatosis J84.81
Lymphangioma D18.1
    capillary D18.1
    cavernous D18.1
    cystic D18.1
    malignant -*see* Neoplasm, connective tissue, malignant
Lymphangiomyoma D18.1
Lymphangiomyomatosis J84.81
Lymphangiosarcoma -*see* Neoplasm, connective tissue, malignant
Lymphangitis I89.1
    with
        abscess
        code by site under Abscess
        cellulitis
        code by site under Cellulitis
        ectopic or molar pregnancy O08.0

Lymphangitis - *continued*
    acute L03.91
    abdominal wall L03.321
    ankle -*see* Lymphangitis, acute, lower limb
    arm -*see* Lymphangitis, acute, upper limb
    auricle (ear) -*see* Lymphangitis, acute, ear
    axilla L03.12
    back (any part) L03.322
    buttock L03.327
    cervical (meaning neck) L03.222
    cheek (external) L03.212
    chest wall L03.323
    digit
        finger -*see* Lymphangitis, acute, finger
        toe -*see* Lymphangitis, acute, toe
    ear (external) H60.1
    external auditory canal -*see* Lymphangitis, acute, ear
    eyelid -*see* Abscess, eyelid
    face NEC L03.212
    finger (intrathecal) (periosteal) (subcutaneous) (subcuticular) L03.02
    foot -*see* Lymphangitis, acute, lower limb
    gluteal (region) L03.327
    groin L03.324
    hand -*see* Lymphangitis, acute, upper limb
    head NEC L03.891
        face (any part, except ear, eye and nose) L03.212
    heel -*see* Lymphangitis, acute, lower limb
    hip -*see* Lymphangitis, acute, lower limb
    jaw (region) L03.212
    knee -*see* Lymphangitis, acute, lower limb
    leg -*see* Lymphangitis, acute, lower limb
    lower limb L03.12
        toe -*see* Lymphangitis, acute, toe
    navel L03.326
    neck (region) L03.222
    orbit, orbital -*see* Cellulitis, orbit
    pectoral (region) L03.323
    perineal, perineum L03.325
    scalp (any part) L03.891
    shoulder -*see* Lymphangitis, acute, upper limb
    specified site NEC L03.898
    thigh -*see* Lymphangitis, acute, lower limb
    thumb (intrathecal) (periosteal) (subcutaneous) (subcuticular) -*see* Lymphangitis, acute, finger
    toe (intrathecal) (periosteal) (subcutaneous) (subcuticular) L03.04
    trunk L03.329
        abdominal wall L03.321
        back (any part) L03.322
        buttock L03.327
        chest wall L03.323
        groin L03.324
        perineal, perineum L03.325
        umbilicus L03.326
    umbilicus L03.326
    upper limb L03.12
        axilla -*see* Lymphangitis, acute, axilla
        finger -*see* Lymphangitis, acute, finger
        thumb -*see* Lymphangitis, acute, finger
        wrist -*see* Lymphangitis, acute, upper limb
    breast
        gestational -*see* Mastitis, obstetric
    chancroidal A57
    chronic (any site) I89.1
    due to
        Brugia (malayi) B74.1

Lymphangitis - *continued*
  timori B74.2
    Wuchereria bancrofti B74.0
  following ectopic or molar pregnancy O08.89
  penis
    acute N48.29
    gonococcal (acute) (chronic) A54.09
  puerperal, postpartum, childbirth O86.89
  strumous, tuberculous A18.2
  subacute (any site) I89.1
  tuberculous -*see* Tuberculosis, lymph gland
Lymphatic (vessel) -*see* condition
Lymphatism E32.8
Lymphectasia I89.0
Lymphedema (acquired) -*see also*
  Elephantiasis
  congenital Q82.0
  hereditary (chronic) (idiopathic) Q82.0
  postmastectomy I97.2
  praecox I89.0
  secondary I89.0
  surgical NEC I97.89
    postmastectomy (syndrome) I97.2
Lymphoblastic -*see* condition
Lymphoblastoma (diffuse) -*see* Lymphoma,
  lymphoblastic (diffuse)
  giant follicular -*see* Lymphoma,
    lymphoblastic (diffuse)
  macrofollicular -*see* Lymphoma,
    lymphoblastic (diffuse)
Lymphocele I89.8
Lymphocytic
  chorioencephalitis (acute) (serous) A87.2
  choriomeningitis (acute) (serous) A87.2
  meningoencephalitis A87.2
Lymphocytoma, benign cutis L98.8
Lymphocytopenia D72.810
Lymphocytosis (symptomatic) D72.820
  infectious (acute) B33.8
Lymphoepithelioma -*see* Neoplasm,
  malignant, by site
Lymphogranuloma (malignant) -*see also*
  Lymphoma, Hodgkin
  chlamydial A55
  inguinale A55
  venereum (any site) (chlamydial) (with
    stricture of rectum) A55
Lymphogranulomatosis (malignant) -*see also*
  Lymphoma, Hodgkin
  benign (Boeck's sarcoid) (Schaumann's)
    D86.1
**Lymphohistiocytosis, hemophagocytic
  (familial)** D76.1
Lymphoid -*see* condition
Lymphoma (of) (malignant) C85.90
  adult T-cell (HTLV-1 associated) (acute
    variant) (chronic variant) (lymphomatoid
    variant) (smouldering variant) C91.5
  anaplastic large cell
    ALK-negative C84.7
    ALK-positive C84.6
    CD30 positive C84.6
    primary cutaneous C86.6
  angioimmunoblastic T-cell C86.5
  BALT C88.4
  B-cell C85.1
  B-precursor C83.5
  blastic NK-cell C86.4
  bronchial-associated lymphoid tissue [BALT-
    lymphoma] C88.4
  Burkitt (atypical) C83.7

Lymphoma - *continued*
  Burkitt-like C83.7
  centrocytic C83.1
  cutaneous follicle center C82.6
  cutaneous T-cell C84.A-
  diffuse follicle center C82.5
  diffuse large cell C83.3
    anaplastic C83.3
    B-cell C83.3
    CD30 positive C83.3
    centroblastic C83.3
    immunoblastic C83.3
    plasmablastic C83.3
    subtype not specified C83.3
    T-cell rich C83.3
  enteropathy type (associated) (intestinal) T-
    cell C86.2
  extranodal NK/T-cell, nasal type C86.0
  extranodal marginal zone B-cell lymphoma of
    mucosa-associated lymphoid tissue [MALT-
    lymphoma] C88.4
  follicular C82.9
    grade
      I C82.0
      II C82.1
      III C82.2
      IIIa C82.3
      IIIb C82.4
    specified NEC C82.8
  hepatosplenic T-cell (alpha-beta) (gamma-
    delta) C86.1
  histiocytic C85.9
    true C96.A
  Hodgkin C81.9
    lymphocyte-rich (classical) C81.4
    lymphocyte depleted (classical) C81.3
    mixed cellularity (classical) C81.2
    nodular sclerosis (classical) C81.1
    specified NEC (classical) C81.7
    lymphocyte-rich classical C81.4
    lymphocyte depleted classical C81.3
    mixed cellularity classical C81.2
    nodular
      lymphocyte predominant C81.0
      sclerosis (classical) C81.1
  intravascular large B-cell C83.8
  Lennert's C84.4
  lymphoblastic B-cell C83.5
  lymphoblastic (diffuse) C83.5
  lymphoblastic T-cell C83.5
  lymphoepithelioid C84.4
  lymphoplasmacytic C83.0
    with IgM-production C88.0
  MALT C88.4
  mantle cell C83.1
  mature T-cell NEC C84.4
  mature T/NK-cell C84.9
    specified NEC C84.Z
  mediastinal (thymic) large B-cell C85.2
  Mediterranean C88.3
  mucosa-associated lymphoid tissue [MALT-
    lymphoma] C88.4
  NK/T cell C84.9
  nodal marginal zone C83.0
  non-follicular (diffuse) C83.9
    specified NEC C83.8
  non-Hodgkin -*see also* Lymphoma, by type
    C85.9
    specified NEC C85.8
  non-leukemic variant of B-CLL C83.0
  peripheral T-cell, not classified C84.4

Lymphoma - *continued*
  primary cutaneous
    anaplastic large cell C86.6
      CD30 positive large T-cell C86.6
  primary effusion B-cell C83.8
  SALT C88.4
  skin-associated lymphoid tissue [SALT-
    lymphoma] C88.4
  small cell B-cell C83.0
  splenic marginal zone C83.0
  subcutaneous panniculitis-like T-cell C86.3
  T-precursor C83.5
  true histiocytic C96.A
Lymphomatosis -*see* Lymphoma
Lymphopathia venereum, veneris A55
Lymphopenia D72.810
Lymphoplasmacytic leukemia -*see* Leukemia,
  chronic lymphocytic, B-cell type
Lymphoproliferation, X linked disease
  D82.3
Lymphoreticulosis, benign (of inoculation)
  A28.1
Lymphorrhea I89.8
Lymphosarcoma (diffuse) -*see also*
  Lymphoma C85.9
Lymphostasis I89.8
Lypemania -*see* Melancholia
**Lysine and hydroxylysine metabolism
  disorder** E72.3
Lyssa -*see* Rabies

M

Macacus ear Q17.3
Maceration, wet feet, tropical (syndrome)
  T69.02
MacLeod's syndrome J43.0
Macrocephalia, macrocephaly Q75.3
Macrocheilia, macrochilia (congenital) Q18.6
Macrocolon -*see also* Megacolon Q43.1
Macrocornea Q15.8
  with glaucoma Q15.0
Macrocytic -*see* condition **Macrocytosis**
  D75.89
**Macrodactylia, macrodactylism (fingers)
  (thumbs)** Q74.0
  toes Q74.2
Macrodontia K00.2
Macrogenia M26.05
**Macrogenitosomia (adrenal) (male)
  (praecox)** E25.9
  congenital E25.0
Macroglobulinemia (idiopathic) (primary)
  C88.0
  monoclonal (essential) D47.2
  Waldenström C88.0
Macroglossia (congenital) Q38.2
  acquired K14.8
**Macrognathia, macrognathism (congenital)
  (mandibular) (maxillary)** M26.09
Macrogyria (congenital) Q04.8
Macrohydrocephalus -*see* Hydrocephalus
Macromastia -*see* Hypertrophy, breast
Macrophthalmos Q11.3
  in congenital glaucoma Q15.0
Macropsia H53.15
Macrosigmoid K59.39
  congenital Q43.2
Macrospondylitis , acromegalic E22.0
Macrostomia (congenital) Q18.4
Macrotia (external ear) (congenital) Q17.1

Macula
cornea, corneal -*see* Opacity, cornea
degeneration (atrophic) (exudative) (senile) -
see also Degeneration, macula
hereditary -*see* Dystrophy, retina
Maculae ceruleae B85.1
Maculopathy, toxic -*see* Degeneration,
macula, toxic
Madarosis (eyelid) H02.729
left H02.726
lower H02.725
upper H02.724
right H02.723
lower H02.722
upper H02.721
Madelung's
deformity (radius) Q74.0
disease
radial deformity Q74.0
symmetrical lipomas, neck E88.89
Madness -*see* Psychosis
Madura
foot B47.9
actinomycotic B47.1
mycotic B47.0
Maduromycosis B47.0
Maffucci's syndrome Q78.4
Magnesium metabolism disorder -*see*
Disorder, metabolism, magnesium
Main en griffe (acquired) -*see also*
Deformity, limb, clawhand
congenital Q74.0
Maintenance (encounter for)
antineoplastic chemotherapy Z51.11
antineoplastic radiation therapy Z51.0
methadone F11.20
Majocchi's
disease L81.7
granuloma B35.8
Major -*see* condition
Malabar itch (any site) B35.5
Malabsorption K90.9
calcium K90.89
carbohydrate K90.49
disaccharide E73.9
fat K90.49
galactose E74.20
glucose (galactose) E74.39
intestinal K90.9
specified NEC K90.89
isomaltose E74.31
lactose E73.9
methionine E72.19
monosaccharide E74.39
postgastrectomy K91.2
postsurgical K91.2
protein K90.49
starch K90.49
sucrose E74.39
syndrome K90.9
postsurgical K91.2
Malacia, bone (adult) M83.9
juvenile -*see* Rickets
Malacoplakia
bladder N32.89
pelvis (kidney) N28.89
ureter N28.89
urethra N36.8
Malacosteon, juvenile -*see* Rickets
Maladaptation -*see* Maladjustment
Maladie de Roger Q21.0

Maladjustment
conjugal Z63.0
involving divorce or estrangement Z63.5
educational Z55.4
family Z63.9
marital Z63.0
involving divorce or estrangement Z63.5
occupational NEC Z56.89
simple, adult -*see* Disorder, adjustment
situational -*see* Disorder, adjustment
social Z60.9
due to
acculturation difficulty Z60.3
discrimination and persecution (perceived)
Z60.5
exclusion and isolation Z60.4
life-cycle (phase of life) transition Z60.0
rejection Z60.4
specified reason NEC Z60.8
Malaise R53.81
Malakoplakia -*see* Malacoplakia
Malaria, malarial (fever) B54
with
blackwater fever B50.8
hemoglobinuric (bilious) B50.8
hemoglobinuria B50.8
accidentally induced (therapeutically)
code by type under Malaria - algid B50.9
cerebral B50.0 *[G94]*
clinically diagnosed (without parasitological
confirmation) B54
congenital NEC P37.4
falciparum P37.3
congestion, congestive B54
continued (fever) B50.9
estivo-autumnal B50.9
falciparum B50.9
with complications NEC B50.8
cerebral B50.0 *[G94]*
severe B50.8
hemorrhagic B54
malariae B52.9
with
complications NEC B52.8
glomerular disorder B52.0
malignant (tertian) -*see* Malaria, falciparum
mixed infections
code to first listed type in B50 B53
ovale B53.0
parasitologically confirmed NEC B53.8
pernicious, acute -*see* Malaria, falciparum
Plasmodium (P.)
falciparum NEC -*see* Malaria, falciparum
malariae NEC B52.9
with Plasmodium
falciparum (and or vivax) -*see* Malaria,
falciparum
vivax -*see also* Malaria, vivax
and falciparum -*see* Malaria, falciparum
ovale B53.0
with Plasmodium malariae -*see also*
Malaria, malariae
and vivax -*see also* Malaria, vivax
and falciparum -*see* Malaria, falciparum
simian B53.1
with Plasmodium malariae -*see also*
Malaria, malariae
and vivax -*see also* Malaria, vivax
and falciparum -*see* Malaria, falciparum
vivax NEC B51.9

Malaria, malarial - *continued*
with Plasmodium falciparum -*see* Malaria,
falciparum
quartan -*see* Malaria, malariae
quotidian -*see* Malaria, falciparum
recurrent B54
remittent B54
specified type NEC (parasitologically
confirmed) B53.8
spleen B54
subtertian (fever) -*see* Malaria, falciparum
tertian (benign) -*see also* Malaria, vivax
malignant B50.9
tropical B50.9
typhoid B54
vivax B51.9
with
complications NEC B51.8
ruptured spleen B51.0
Malassimilation K90.9
Malassez's disease (cystic) N50.89
Mal de los pintos -*see* Pinta
Mal de mer T75.3
Maldescent, testis Q53.9
bilateral Q53.20
abdominal Q53.21
perineal Q53.22
unilateral Q53.10
abdominal Q53.11
perineal Q53.12
Maldevelopment -*see also* Anomaly   brain
Q07.9
colon Q43.9
hip Q74.2
congenital dislocation Q65.2
bilateral Q65.1
unilateral Q65.0
mastoid process Q75.8
middle ear Q16.4
except ossicles Q16.4
ossicles Q16.3
ossicles Q16.3
spine Q76.49
toe Q74.2
Male type pelvis Q74.2
with disproportion (fetopelvic) O33.3
causing obstructed labor O65.3
Malformation (congenital) -*see also* Anomaly
adrenal gland Q89.1
affecting multiple systems with skeletal
changes NEC Q87.5
alimentary tract Q45.9
specified type NEC Q45.8
upper Q40.9
specified type NEC Q40.8
aorta Q25.40
absence Q25.41
aneurysm, congenital Q25.43
aplasia Q25.41
atresia Q25.29
aortic arch Q25.21
coarctation (preductal) (postductal) Q25.1
dilatation, congenital Q25.44
hypoplasia Q25.42
patent ductus arteriosus Q25.0
specified type NEC Q25.49
stenosis Q25.1
supravalvular Q25.3
aortic valve Q23.9
specified NEC Q23.8

MNO

Malformation - *continued*
arteriovenous, aneurysmatic (congenital) Q27.30
  brain Q28.2
  cerebral Q28.2
  peripheral Q27.30
    digestive system Q27.33
    lower limb Q27.32
    other specified site Q27.39
    renal vessel Q27.34
    upper limb Q27.31
  precerebral vessels (nonruptured) Q28.0
auricle
  ear (congenital) Q17.3
    acquired H61.119
      left H61.112
        with right H61.113
      right H61.111
        with left H61.113
bile duct Q44.5
bladder Q64.79
  aplasia Q64.5
  diverticulum Q64.6
  exstrophy -*see* Exstrophy, bladder
  neck obstruction Q64.31
bone Q79.9
  face Q75.9
    specified type NEC Q75.8
  skull Q75.9
    specified type NEC Q75.8
brain (multiple) Q04.9
  arteriovenous Q28.2
  specified type NEC Q04.8
branchial cleft Q18.2
breast Q83.9
  specified type NEC Q83.8
broad ligament Q50.6
bronchus Q32.4
bursa Q79.9
cardiac
  chambers Q20.9
    specified type NEC Q20.8
  septum Q21.9
    specified type NEC Q21.8
cerebral Q04.9
  vessels Q28.3
cervix uteri Q51.9
  specified type NEC Q51.828
Chiari
  Type I G93.5
  Type II Q07.01
choroid (congenital) Q14.3
  plexus Q07.8
circulatory system Q28.9
cochlea Q16.5
cornea Q13.4
coronary vessels Q24.5
corpus callosum (congenital) Q04.0
diaphragm Q79.1
digestive system NEC, specified type NEC Q45.8
dura Q07.9
  brain Q04.9
  spinal Q06.9
ear Q17.9
  causing impairment of hearing Q16.9
  external Q17.9
    accessory auricle Q17.0
    causing impairment of hearing Q16.9
      absence of
        auditory canal Q16.1

Malformation - *continued*
  auricle Q16.0
  macrotia Q17.1
  microtia Q17.2
  misplacement Q17.4
  misshapen NEC Q17.3
  prominence Q17.5
  specified type NEC Q17.8
  inner Q16.5
  middle Q16.4
    absence of eustachian tube Q16.2
    ossicles (fusion) Q16.3
    ossicles Q16.3
    specified type NEC Q17.8
epididymis Q55.4
esophagus Q39.9
  specified type NEC Q39.8
eye Q15.9
  lid Q10.3
  specified NEC Q15.8
fallopian tube Q50.6
genital organ -*see* Anomaly, genitalia
great
  artery Q25.9
    aorta -*see* Malformation, aorta
    pulmonary artery -*see* Malformation, pulmonary, artery
    specified type NEC Q25.8
  vein Q26.9
    anomalous
      portal venous connection Q26.5
      pulmonary venous connection Q26.4
        partial Q26.3
        total Q26.2
    persistent left superior vena cava Q26.1
    portal vein-hepatic artery fistula Q26.6
    specified type NEC Q26.8
    vena cava stenosis, congenital Q26.0
gum Q38.6
hair Q84.2
heart Q24.9
  specified type NEC Q24.8
integument Q84.9
  specified type NEC Q84.8
internal ear Q16.5
intestine Q43.9
  specified type NEC Q43.8
iris Q13.2
joint Q74.9
  ankle Q74.2
  lumbosacral Q76.49
  sacroiliac Q74.2
  specified type NEC Q74.8
kidney Q63.9
  accessory Q63.0
  giant Q63.3
  horseshoe Q63.1
  hydronephrosis Q62.0
  malposition Q63.2
  specified type NEC Q63.8
lacrimal apparatus Q10.6
lip Q38.0
lingual Q38.3
liver Q44.7
lung Q33.9
meninges or membrane (congenital) Q07.9
  cerebral Q04.8
  spinal (cord) Q06.9
middle ear Q16.4
  ossicles Q16.3
mitral valve Q23.9

Malformation - *continued*
  specified NEC Q23.8
Mondini's (congenital) (malformation, cochlea) Q16.5
mouth (congenital) Q38.6
multiple types NEC Q89.7
musculoskeletal system Q79.9
myocardium Q24.8
nail Q84.6
nervous system (central) Q07.9
nose Q30.9
  specified type NEC Q30.8
optic disc Q14.2
orbit Q10.7
ovary Q50.39
palate Q38.5
parathyroid gland Q89.2
pelvic organs or tissues NEC
  in pregnancy or childbirth O34.8
    causing obstructed labor O65.5
penis Q55.69
  aplasia Q55.5
  curvature (lateral) Q55.61
  hypoplasia Q55.62
pericardium Q24.8
peripheral vascular system Q27.9
  specified type NEC Q27.8
pharynx Q38.8
precerebral vessels Q28.1
prostate Q55.4
pulmonary
  arteriovenous Q25.72
  artery Q25.9
    atresia Q25.5
    specified type NEC Q25.79
    stenosis Q25.6
  valve Q22.3
renal artery Q27.2
respiratory system Q34.9
retina Q14.1
scrotum -*see* Malformation, testis and scrotum
seminal vesicles Q55.4
sense organs NEC Q07.9
skin Q82.9
specified NEC Q89.8
spinal
  cord Q06.9
  nerve root Q07.8
spine Q76.49
  kyphosis -*see* Kyphosis, congenital
  lordosis -*see* Lordosis, congenital
spleen Q89.09
stomach Q40.3
  specified type NEC Q40.2
teeth, tooth K00.9
tendon Q79.9
testis and scrotum Q55.20
  aplasia Q55.0
  hypoplasia Q55.1
  polyorchism Q55.21
  retractile testis Q55.22
  scrotal transposition Q55.23
  specified NEC Q55.29
throat Q38.8
thorax, bony Q76.9
thyroid gland Q89.2
tongue (congenital) Q38.3
  hypertrophy Q38.2
  tie Q38.1
trachea Q32.1
tricuspid valve Q22.9

Malformation - *continued*
specified type NEC Q22.8
umbilical cord NEC (complicating delivery) O69.89
umbilicus Q89.9
ureter Q62.8
agenesis Q62.4
duplication Q62.5
malposition -*see* Malposition, congenital, ureter
obstructive defect -*see* Defect, obstructive, ureter
vesico-uretero-renal reflux Q62.7
urethra Q64.79
aplasia Q64.5
duplication Q64.74
posterior valves Q64.2
prolapse Q64.71
stricture Q64.32
urinary system Q64.9
uterus Q51.9
specified type NEC Q51.818
vagina Q52.4
vascular system, peripheral Q27.9
vas deferens Q55.4
atresia Q55.3
venous -*see* Anomaly, vein(s)
vulva Q52.70
Malfunction -*see also* Dysfunction
cardiac electronic device T82.119
electrode T82.110
pulse generator T82.111
specified type NEC T82.118
catheter device NEC T85.618
cystostomy T83.010
dialysis (renal) (vascular) T82.41
intraperitoneal T85.611
infusion NEC T82.514
cranial T85.610
epidural T85.610
intrathecal T85.610
spinal T85.610
subarachnoid T85.610
subdural T85.610
urinary -*see also* Breakdown, device, catheter T83.018
colostomy K94.03
valve K94.03
cystostomy (stoma) N99.512
catheter T83.010
enteric stoma K94.13
enterostomy K94.13
esophagostomy K94.33
gastroenteric K31.89
gastrostomy K94.23
ileostomy K94.13
valve K94.13
intrathecal infusion pump T85.615
jejunostomy K94.13
nervous system device, implant or graft, specified NEC T85.615
pacemaker -*see* Malfunction, cardiac electronic device
prosthetic device, internal -*see* Complications, prosthetic device, by site, mechanical
tracheostomy J95.03
urinary device NEC -*see* Complication, genitourinary, device, urinary, mechanical
valve
colostomy K94.03
heart T82.09

Malfunction - *continued*
ileostomy K94.13
vascular graft or shunt NEC -*see* Complication, cardiovascular device, mechanical, vascular
ventricular (communicating shunt) T85.01
Malherbe's tumor -*see* Neoplasm, skin, benign
Malibu disease L98.8
Malignancy -*see also* Neoplasm, malignant, by site
unspecified site (primary) C80.1
Malignant -*see* condition
Malingerer, malingering Z76.5
Mallet finger (acquired) -*see* Deformity, finger, mallet finger
congenital Q74.0
sequelae of rickets E64.3
Malleus A24.0
Mallory's bodies R89.7
Mallory Weiss syndrome K22.6
Malnutrition E46
degree
first E44.1
mild (protein) E44.1
moderate (protein) E44.0
second E44.0
severe (protein-energy) E43
intermediate form E42
with
kwashiorkor (and marasmus) E42
marasmus E41
third E43
following gastrointestinal surgery K91.2
intrauterine
light-for-dates -*see* Light for dates
small-for-dates -*see* Small for dates
lack of care, or neglect (child) (infant) T76.02
confirmed T74.02
malignant E40
protein E46
calorie E46
mild E44.1
moderate E44.0
severe E43
intermediate form E42
with
kwashiorkor (and marasmus) E42
marasmus E41
energy E46
mild E44.1
moderate E44.0
severe E43
intermediate form E42
with
kwashiorkor (and marasmus) E42
marasmus E41
severe (protein-energy) E43
with
kwashiorkor (and marasmus) E42
marasmus E41
Malocclusion (teeth) M26.4
Angle's M26.219
class I M26.211
class II M26.212
class III M26.213
due to
abnormal swallowing M26.59
mouth breathing M26.59
tongue, lip or finger habits M26.59
temporomandibular (joint) M26.69

Malposition
cervix -*see* Malposition, uterus
congenital
adrenal (gland) Q89.1
alimentary tract Q45.8
lower Q43.8
upper Q40.8
aorta Q25.49
appendix Q43.8
arterial trunk Q20.0
artery (peripheral) Q27.8
coronary Q24.5
digestive system Q27.8
lower limb Q27.8
pulmonary Q25.79
specified site NEC Q27.8
upper limb Q27.8
auditory canal Q17.8
causing impairment of hearing Q16.9
auricle (ear) Q17.4
causing impairment of hearing Q16.9
cervical Q18.2
biliary duct or passage Q44.5
bladder (mucosa) -*see* Exstrophy, bladder
brachial plexus Q07.8
brain tissue Q04.8
breast Q83.8
bronchus Q32.4
cecum Q43.8
clavicle Q74.0
colon Q43.8
digestive organ or tract NEC Q45.8
lower Q43.8
upper Q40.8
ear (auricle) (external) Q17.4
ossicles Q16.3
endocrine (gland) NEC Q89.2
epiglottis Q31.8
eustachian tube Q17.8
eye Q15.8
facial features Q18.8
fallopian tube Q50.6
finger(s) Q68.1
supernumerary Q69.0
foot Q66.9
gallbladder Q44.1
gastrointestinal tract Q45.8
genitalia, genital organ(s) or tract
female Q52.8
external Q52.79
internal NEC Q52.8
male Q55.8
glottis Q31.8
hand Q68.1
heart Q24.8
dextrocardia Q24.0
with complete transposition of viscera Q89.3
hepatic duct Q44.5
hip (joint) Q65.89
intestine (large) (small) Q43.8
with anomalous adhesions, fixation or malrotation Q43.3
joint NEC Q68.8
kidney Q63.2
larynx Q31.8
limb Q68.8
lower Q68.8
upper Q68.8
liver Q44.7
lung (lobe) Q33.8

Malposition - *continued*

nail(s) Q84.6
nerve Q07.8
nervous system NEC Q07.8
nose, nasal (septum) Q30.8
organ or site not listed -*see* Anomaly, by site
ovary Q50.39
pancreas Q45.3
parathyroid (gland) Q89.2
patella Q74.1
peripheral vascular system Q27.8
pituitary (gland) Q89.2
respiratory organ or system NEC Q34.8
rib (cage) Q76.6
  supernumerary in cervical region Q76.5
scapula Q74.0
shoulder Q74.0
spinal cord Q06.8
spleen Q89.09
sternum NEC Q76.7
stomach Q40.2
symphysis pubis Q74.2
thymus (gland) Q89.2
thyroid (gland) (tissue) Q89.2
  cartilage Q31.8
toe(s) Q66.9
  supernumerary Q69.2
tongue Q38.3
trachea Q32.1
ureter Q62.60
  deviation Q62.61
  displacement Q62.62
  ectopia Q62.63
  specified type NEC Q62.69
uterus Q51.818
vein(s) (peripheral) Q27.8
  great Q26.8
vena cava (inferior) (superior) Q26.8
device, implant or graft -*see also*
Complications, by site and type, mechanical
T85.628
  arterial graft NEC -*see* Complication,
cardiovascular device, mechanical, vascular
  breast (implant) T85.42
  catheter NEC T85.628
    cystostomy T83.020
    dialysis (renal) T82.42
      intraperitoneal T85.621
    infusion NEC T82.524
      spinal (epidural) (subdural) T85.620
    urinary -*see also* Displacement, device,
catheter, urinary T83.028
  electronic (electrode) (pulse generator)
(stimulator)
    bone T84.320
    cardiac T82.129
      electrode T82.120
      pulse generator T82.121
      specified type NEC T82.128
    nervous system -*see* Complication,
prosthetic device, mechanical, electronic
nervous system stimulator
    urinary -*see* Complication, genitourinary,
device, urinary, mechanical
  fixation, internal (orthopedic) NEC -*see*
Complication, fixation device, mechanical
  gastrointestinal -*see* Complications,
prosthetic device, mechanical,
gastrointestinal device
  genital NEC T83.428

Malposition - *continued*

intrauterine contraceptive device (string)
T83.32
  penile prosthesis (cylinder) (implanted)
(pump) (reservoir) T83.420
  testicular prosthesis T83.421
  heart NEC -*see* Complication,
cardiovascular device, mechanical
  joint prosthesis -*see* Complication, joint
prosthesis, mechanical
  ocular NEC -*see* Complications, prosthetic
device, mechanical, ocular device
  orthopedic NEC -*see* Complication,
orthopedic, device, mechanical
  specified NEC T85.628
  urinary NEC -*see also* Complication,
genitourinary, device, urinary, mechanical
graft T83.22
  vascular NEC -*see* Complication,
cardiovascular device, mechanical
  ventricular intracranial shunt T85.02
fetus -*see* Pregnancy, complicated by
(management affected by), presentation, fetal
gallbladder K82.8
gastrointestinal tract, congenital Q45.8
heart, congenital NEC Q24.8
joint prosthesis -*see* Complications, joint
prosthesis, mechanical, displacement, by site
stomach K31.89
  congenital Q40.2
tooth, teeth, fully erupted M26.30
uterus (acute) (acquired) (adherent)
(asymptomatic) (postinfectional) (postpartal,
old) N85.4
  anteflexion or anteversion N85.4
    congenital Q51.818
  flexion N85.4
    lateral -*see* Lateroversion, uterus
  inversion N85.5
  lateral (flexion) (version) -*see* Lateroversion,
uterus
    in pregnancy or childbirth -*see* subcategory
O34.5
  retroflexion or retroversion -*see*
Retroversion, uterus

Malposture R29.3

Malrotation

cecum Q43.3
colon Q43.3
intestine Q43.3
kidney Q63.2

Maltreatment

adult
  abandonment
    confirmed T74.01
    suspected T76.01
  confirmed T74.91
  history of Z91.419
  neglect
    confirmed T74.01
    suspected T76.01
  physical abuse
    confirmed T74.11
    suspected T76.11
  psychological abuse
    confirmed T74.31
    suspected T76.31
    history of Z91.411
  sexual abuse
    confirmed T74.21
    suspected T76.21

Maltreatment - *continued*

suspected T76.91
child
  abandonment
    confirmed T74.02
    suspected T76.02
  confirmed T74.92
  history of -*see* History, personal (of), abuse
  neglect
    confirmed T74.02
    history of -*see* History, personal (of), abuse
    suspected T76.02
  physical abuse
    confirmed T74.12
    history of -*see* History, personal (of), abuse
    suspected T76.12
  psychological abuse
    confirmed T74.32
    history of -*see* History, personal (of), abuse
    suspected T76.32
  sexual abuse
    confirmed T74.22
    history of -*see* History, personal (of), abuse
    suspected T76.22
  suspected T76.92
personal history of Z91.89

Malta fever -*see* Brucellosis

Maltworker's lung J67.4

Malunion, fracture -*see* Fracture, by site

Mammillitis N61.0
puerperal, postpartum O91.02

Mammitis -*see* Mastitis

Mammogram (examination) Z12.39
routine Z12.31

Mammoplasia N62

Management (of)
bone conduction hearing device (implanted)
Z45.320
cardiac pacemaker NEC Z45.018
cerebrospinal fluid drainage device Z45.41
cochlear device (implanted) Z45.321
contraceptive Z30.9
  specified NEC Z30.8
implanted device Z45.9
  specified NEC Z45.89
infusion pump Z45.1
procreative Z31.9
  male factor infertility in female Z31.81
  specified NEC Z31.89
prosthesis (external) -*see also* Fitting Z44.9
  implanted Z45.9
    specified NEC Z45.89
renal dialysis catheter Z49.01
vascular access device Z45.2

Mangled -*see* specified injury by site

Mania (monopolar) -*see also* Disorder, mood,
manic episode
with psychotic symptoms F30.2
without psychotic symptoms F30.10
  mild F30.11
  moderate F30.12
  severe F30.13
Bell's F30.8
chronic (recurrent) F31.89
hysterical F44.89
puerperal F30.8
recurrent F31.89

**Manic-depressive insanity, psychosis, or
syndrome** -*see* Disorder, bipolar

Mannosidosis E77.1

Mansonelliasis, mansonellosis B74.4

Manson's
disease B65.1
schistosomiasis B65.1
Manual -*see* condition
Maple-bark-stripper's lung (disease) J67.6
Maple-syrup-urine disease E71.0
Marable's syndrome (celiac artery compression) I77.4
Marasmus E41
due to malnutrition E41
intestinal E41
nutritional E41
senile R54
tuberculous NEC -*see* Tuberculosis **Marble**
bones Q78.2
skin R23.8
Marburg virus disease A98.3
March
fracture -*see* Fracture, traumatic, stress, by site
hemoglobinuria D59.6
Marchesani (Weill) syndrome Q87.0
Marchiafava (Bignami) syndrome or disease G37.1
Marchiafava-Micheli syndrome D59.5
Marcus Gunn's syndrome Q07.8
Marfan's syndrome -*see* Syndrome, Marfan's
Marie-Bamberger disease -*see* Osteoarthropathy, hypertrophic, specified NEC
Marie-Charcot-Tooth neuropathic muscular atrophy G60.0
Marie's
cerebellar ataxia (late-onset) G11.2
disease or syndrome (acromegaly) E22.0
Marie-Strümpell arthritis, disease or spondylitis -*see* Spondylitis, ankylosing
Marion's disease (bladder neck obstruction) N32.0
Marital conflict Z63.0
Mark
port wine Q82.5
raspberry Q82.5
strawberry Q82.5
stretch L90.6
tattoo L81.8
Marker heterochromatin -*see* Extra, marker chromosomes
Maroteaux Lamy syndrome (mild) (severe) E76.29
Marrow (bone)
arrest D61.9
poor function D75.89
Marseilles fever A77.1
Marsh fever -*see* Malaria
Marshall's (hidrotic) ectodermal dysplasia Q82.4
Marsh's disease (exophthalmic goiter) E05.00
with storm E05.01
Masculinization (female) with adrenal hyperplasia E25.9
congenital E25.0
Masculinovoblastoma D27.
Masochism (sexual) F65.51
Mason's lung J62.8
Mass
abdominal R19.00
epigastric R19.06
generalized R19.07
left lower quadrant R19.04

Mass - *continued*
left upper quadrant R19.02
periumbilic R19.05
right lower quadrant R19.03
right upper quadrant R19.01
specified site NEC R19.09
breast N63
chest R22.2
cystic -*see* Cyst
ear H93.8
head R22.0
intra-abdominal (diffuse) (generalized) -*see* Mass, abdominal
kidney N28.89
liver R16.0
localized (skin) R22.9
chest R22.2
head R22.0
limb
lower R22.4
upper R22.3
neck R22.1
trunk R22.2
lung R91.8
malignant -*see* Neoplasm, malignant, by site
neck R22.1
pelvic (diffuse) (generalized) -*see* Mass, abdominal
specified organ NEC -*see* Disease, by site
splenic R16.1
substernal thyroid -*see* Goiter
superficial (localized) R22.9
umbilical (diffuse) (generalized) R19.09
Massive -*see* condition
Mast cell
disease, systemic tissue D47.0
leukemia C94.3
sarcoma C96.2
tumor D47.0
malignant C96.2
Mastalgia N64.4
Masters-Allen syndrome N83.8
Mastitis (acute) (diffuse) (nonpuerperal) (subacute) N61.0
with abscess N61.1
chronic (cystic) -*see* Mastopathy, cystic
cystic (Schimmelbusch's type) -*see* Mastopathy, cystic
fibrocystic -*see* Mastopathy, cystic
infective N61.0
newborn P39.0
interstitial, gestational or puerperal -*see* Mastitis, obstetric
neonatal (noninfective) P83.4
infective P39.0
obstetric (interstitial) (nonpurulent)
associated with
lactation O91.23
pregnancy O91.21
puerperium O91.22
purulent
associated with
lactation O91.13
pregnancy O91.11
puerperium O91.12
periductal -*see* Ectasia, mammary duct
phlegmonous -*see* Mastopathy, cystic
plasma cell -*see* Ectasia, mammary duct
without abscess N61.0
Mastocytoma D47.0
malignant C96.2

Mastocytosis Q82.2
aggressive systemic C96.2
indolent systemic D47.0
malignant C96.2
systemic, associated with clonal hematopoietic non-mast-cell disease (SM-AHNMD) D47.0
Mastodynia N64.4
Mastoid -*see* condition
Mastoidalgia -*see* subcategory H92.0
Mastoiditis (coalescent) (hemorrhagic) (suppurative) H70.9
acute, subacute H70.00
complicated NEC H70.09
subperiosteal H70.01
chronic (necrotic) (recurrent) H70.1
in (due to)
infectious disease NEC B99 [*H75.0*]
parasitic disease NEC B89 [*H75.0*]
tuberculosis A18.03
petrositis -*see* Petrositis
postauricular fistula -*see* Fistula, postauricular
specified NEC H70.89
tuberculous A18.03
Mastopathy, mastopathia N64.9
chronica cystica -*see* Mastopathy, cystic
cystic (chronic) (diffuse) N60.1
with epithelial proliferation N60.3
diffuse cystic -*see* Mastopathy, cystic
estrogenica, oestrogenica N64.89
ovarian origin N64.89
Mastoplasia, mastoplastia N62
Masturbation (excessive) F98.8
Maternal care (for) -*see* Pregnancy (complicated by) (management affected by)
Matheiu's disease (leptospiral jaundice) A27.0
Mauclaire's disease or osteochondrosis -*see* Osteochondrosis, juvenile, hand, metacarpal
Maxcy's disease A75.2
Maxilla, maxillary -*see* condition
May (Hegglin) anomaly or syndrome D72.0
McArdle (Schmid)(Pearson) disease (glycogen storage) E74.04
McCune-Albright syndrome Q78.1
McQuarrie's syndrome (idiopathic familial hypoglycemia) E16.2
Meadow's syndrome Q86.1
Measles (black) (hemorrhagic) (suppressed) B05.9
with
complications NEC B05.89
encephalitis B05.0
intestinal complications B05.4
keratitis (keratoconjunctivitis) B05.81
meningitis B05.1
otitis media B05.3
pneumonia B05.2
French -*see* Rubella
German -*see* Rubella
Liberty -*see* Rubella
Meatitis, urethral -*see* Urethritis
Meatus, meatal -*see* condition
Meat-wrappers' asthma J68.9
Meckel-Gruber syndrome Q61.9
Meckel's diverticulitis, diverticulum (displaced) (hypertrophic) Q43.0
malignant -*see* Table of Neoplasms, small intestine, malignant
Meconium
ileus, newborn P76.0
in cystic fibrosis E84.11

Meconium - *continued*
meaning meconium plug (without cystic fibrosis) P76.0
obstruction, newborn P76.0
due to fecaliths P76.0
in mucoviscidosis E84.11
peritonitis P78.0
plug syndrome (newborn) NEC P76.0
Median -*see also* condition
arcuate ligament syndrome I77.4
bar (prostate) (vesical orifice) -*see* Hyperplasia, prostate
rhomboid glossitis K14.2
Mediastinal shift R93.8
Mediastinitis (acute) (chronic) J98.51
syphilitic A52.73
tuberculous A15.8
Mediastinopericarditis -*see also* Pericarditis
acute I30.9
adhesive I31.0
chronic I31.8
rheumatic I09.2
Mediastinum, mediastinal -*see* condition
Medicine poisoning -*see* Table of Drugs and Chemicals, by drug, poisoning
Mediterranean
fever -*see* Brucellosis
familial M04.1
tick A77.1
kala-azar B55.0
leishmaniasis B55.0
tick fever A77.1
Medulla -*see* condition
Medullary cystic kidney Q61.5
Medullated fibers
optic (nerve) Q14.8
retina Q14.1
Medulloblastoma
desmoplastic C71.6
specified site -*see* Neoplasm, malignant, by site
unspecified site C71.6
Medulloepithelioma -*see also* Neoplasm, malignant, by site
teratoid -*see* Neoplasm, malignant, by site
Medullomyoblastoma
specified site -*see* Neoplasm, malignant, by site
unspecified site C71.6
Meekeren-Ehlers-Danlos syndrome Q79.6
Megacolon (acquired) (functional) (not Hirschsprung's disease) (in) K59.39
Chagas' disease B57.32
congenital, congenitum (aganglionic) Q43.1
Hirschsprung's (disease) Q43.1
toxic NEC K59.31
due to Clostridium difficile A04.7
Megaesophagus (functional) K22.0
congenital Q39.5
in (due to) Chagas' disease B57.31
Megalencephaly Q04.5
Megalerythema (epidemic) B08.3
Megaloappendix Q43.8
Megalocephalous, megalocephaly NEC Q75.3
Megalocornea Q15.8
with glaucoma Q15.0
Megalocytic anemia D53.1
Megalodactylia (fingers) (thumbs) (congenital) Q74.0
toes Q74.2

Megaloduodenum Q43.8
Megaloesophagus (functional) K22.0
congenital Q39.5
Megalogastria (acquired) K31.89
congenital Q40.2
Megalophthalmos Q11.3
Megalopsia H53.15
Megalosplenia -*see* Splenomegaly
Megaloureter N28.82
congenital Q62.2
Megarectum K62.89
Megasigmoid K59.39
congenital Q43.2
Megaureter N28.82
congenital Q62.2
Megavitamin-B6 syndrome E67.2
Megrim -*see* Migraine
Meibomian
cyst, infected -*see* Hordeolum
gland -*see* condition
sty, stye -*see* Hordeolum **Meibomitis** -*see* Hordeolum
Meige-Milroy disease (chronic hereditary edema) Q82.0
Meige's syndrome Q82.0
Melalgia, nutritional E53.8
Melancholia F32.9
climacteric (single episode) F32.89
recurrent episode F33.8
hypochondriac F45.29
intermittent (single episode) F32.89
recurrent episode F33.8
involutional (single episode) F32.89
recurrent episode F33.8
menopausal (single episode) F32.89
recurrent episode F33.8
puerperal F32.89
reactive (emotional stress or trauma) F32.3
recurrent F33.9
senile F03
stuporous (single episode) F32.89
recurrent episode F33.8
Melanemia R79.89
Melanoameloblastoma -*see* Neoplasm, bone, benign
Melanoblastoma -*see* Melanoma
Melanocarcinoma -*see* Melanoma
Melanocytoma, eyeball D31.9
Melanocytosis, neurocutaneous Q82.8
Melanoderma, melanodermia L81.4
Melanodontia, infantile K03.89
Melanodontoclasia K03.89
Melanoepithelioma -*see* Melanoma
(malignant) C43.9
acral lentiginous, malignant -*see* Melanoma, skin, by site
amelanotic -*see* Melanoma, skin, by site
balloon cell -*see* Melanoma, skin, by site
benign -*see* Nevus
desmoplastic, malignant -*see* Melanoma, skin, by site
epithelioid cell -*see* Melanoma, skin, by site
with spindle cell, mixed -*see* Melanoma, skin, by site
in
giant pigmented nevus -*see* Melanoma, skin, by site
Hutchinson's melanotic freckle -*see* Melanoma, skin, by site
junctional nevus -*see* Melanoma, skin, by site

Melanoma (malignant) --*continued*
precancerous melanosis -*see* Melanoma, skin, by site
in situ D03.9
abdominal wall D03.59
ala nasi D03.39
ankle D03.7
anus, anal (margin) (skin) D03.51
arm D03.6
auditory canal D03.2
auricle (ear) D03.2
auricular canal (external) D03.2
axilla, axillary fold D03.59
back D03.59
breast D03.52
brow D03.39
buttock D03.59
canthus (eye) D03.1
cheek (external) D03.39
chest wall D03.59
chin D03.39
choroid D03.8
conjunctiva D03.8
ear (external) D03.2
external meatus (ear) D03.2
eye D03.8
eyebrow D03.39
eyelid (lower) (upper) D03.1
face D03.30
specified NEC D03.39
female genital organ (external) NEC D03.8
finger D03.6
flank D03.59
foot D03.7
forearm D03.6
forehead D03.39
foreskin D03.8
gluteal region D03.59
groin D03.59
hand D03.6
heel D03.7
helix D03.2
hip D03.7
interscapular region D03.59
iris D03.8
jaw D03.39
knee D03.7
labium (majus) (minus) D03.8
lacrimal gland D03.8
leg D03.7
lip (lower) (upper) D03.0
lower limb NEC D03.7
male genital organ (external) NEC D03.8
nail D03.9
finger D03.6
toe D03.7
neck D03.4
nose (external) D03.39
orbit D03.8
penis D03.8
perianal skin D03.51
perineum D03.51
pinna D03.2
popliteal fossa or space D03.7
prepuce D03.8
pudendum D03.8
retina D03.8
retrobulbar D03.8
scalp D03.4
scrotum D03.8
shoulder D03.6

Melanoma (malignant) *--continued*
  specified site NEC D03.8
  submammary fold D03.52
  temple D03.39
  thigh D03.7
  toe D03.7
  trunk NEC D03.59
  umbilicus D03.59
  upper limb NEC D03.6
  vulva D03.8
 juvenile *-see* Nevus
 malignant, of soft parts except skin *-see*
  Neoplasm, connective tissue, malignant
 metastatic
  breast C79.81
  genital organ C79.82
  specified site NEC C79.89
 neurotropic, malignant *-see* Melanoma, skin,
  by site
 nodular *-see* Melanoma, skin, by site
 regressing, malignant *-see* Melanoma, skin,
  by site
 skin C43.9
  abdominal wall C43.59
  ala nasi C43.31
  ankle C43.7
  anus, anal (skin) C43.51
  arm C43.6
  auditory canal (external) C43.2
  auricle (ear) C43.2
  auricular canal (external) C43.2
  axilla, axillary fold C43.59
  back C43.59
  breast (female) (male) C43.52
  brow C43.39
  buttock C43.59
  canthus (eye) C43.1
  cheek (external) C43.39
  chest wall C43.59
  chin C43.39
  ear (external) C43.2
  elbow C43.6
  external meatus (ear) C43.2
  eyebrow C43.39
  eyelid (lower) (upper) C43.1
  face C43.30
   specified NEC C43.39
  female genital organ (external) NEC C51.9
  finger C43.6
  flank C43.59
  foot C43.7
  forearm C43.6
  forehead C43.39
  foreskin C60.0
  glabella C43.39
  gluteal region C43.59
  groin C43.59
  hand C43.6
  heel C43.7
  helix C43.2
  hip C43.7
  interscapular region C43.59
  jaw (external) C43.39
  knee C43.7
  labium C51.9
   majus C51.0
   minus C51.1
  leg C43.7
  lip (lower) (upper) C43.0
  lower limb NEC C43.7
  male genital organ (external) NEC C63.9

Melanoma (malignant) *--continued*
 nail
  finger C43.6
  toe C43.7
 nasolabial groove C43.39
 nates C43.59
 neck C43.4
 nose (external) C43.31
 overlapping site C43.8
 palpebra C43.1
 penis C60.9
 perianal skin C43.51
 perineum C43.51
 pinna C43.2
 popliteal fossa or space C43.7
 prepuce C60.0
 pudendum C51.9
 scalp C43.4
 scrotum C63.2
 shoulder C43.6
 skin NEC C43.9
 submammary fold C43.52
 temple C43.39
 thigh C43.7
 toe C43.7
 trunk NEC C43.59
 umbilicus C43.59
 upper limb NEC C43.6
 vulva C51.9
  overlapping sites C51.8
 spindle cell
  with epithelioid, mixed *-see* Melanoma,
  skin, by site
  type A C69.4
  type B C69.4
 superficial spreading *-see* Melanoma, skin, by
 site
Melanosarcoma *-see also* Melanoma
 epithelioid cell *-see* Melanoma
Melanosis L81.4
 addisonian E27.1
  tuberculous A18.7
 adrenal E27.1
 colon K63.89
 conjunctiva *-see* Pigmentation, conjunctiva
  congenital Q13.89
 cornea (presenile) (senile) *-see also*
 Pigmentation, cornea
  congenital Q13.4
 eye NEC H57.8
  congenital Q15.8
 lenticularis progressiva Q82.1
 liver K76.89
 precancerous *-see also* Melanoma, in situ
  malignant melanoma in *-see* Melanoma
 Riehl's L81.4
 sclera H15.89
  congenital Q13.89
 suprarenal E27.1
 tar L81.4
 toxic L81.4
Melanuria R82.99
MELAS syndrome E88.41
Melasma L81.1
 adrenal (gland) E27.1
 suprarenal (gland) E27.1
Melena K92.1
 with ulcer
 code by site under Ulcer, with hemorrhage
  K27.4
 due to swallowed maternal blood P78.2
 newborn, neonatal P54.1
  due to swallowed maternal blood P78.2

Meleney's
 gangrene (cutaneous) *-see* Ulcer, skin
 ulcer (chronic undermining) *-see* Ulcer, skin
Melioidosis A24.9
 acute A24.1
 chronic A24.2
 fulminating A24.1
 pneumonia A24.1
 pulmonary (chronic) A24.2
  acute A24.1
  subacute A24.2
 sepsis A24.1
 specified NEC A24.3
 subacute A24.2
Melitensis, febris A23.0
Melkersson (Rosenthal) syndrome G51.2
Mellitus, diabetes *-see* Diabetes
Melorheostosis (bone) *-see* Disorder, bone,
 density and structure, specified NEC
Meloschisis Q18.4
Melotia Q17.4
Membrana
 capsularis lentis posterior Q13.89
 epipapillaris Q14.2
Membranacea placenta O43.19
Membranaceous uterus N85.8
Membrane(s), membranous *-see also*
 condition
 cyclitic *-see* Membrane, pupillary
 folds, congenital *-see* Web - Jackson's Q43.3
 over face of newborn P28.9
 premature rupture *-see* Rupture, membranes,
  premature
 pupillary H21.4
  persistent Q13.89
 retained (with hemorrhage) (complicating
 delivery) O72.2
  without hemorrhage O73.1
 secondary cataract *-see* Cataract, secondary
 unruptured (causing asphyxia) *-see* Asphyxia,
  newborn
 vitreous *-see* Opacity, vitreous, membranes
  and strands
Membranitis *-see* Chorioamnionitis
Memory disturbance, lack or loss *-see also*
 Amnesia
 mild, following organic brain damage F06.8
Menadione deficiency E56.1
Menarche
 delayed E30.0
 precocious E30.1
Mendacity, pathologic F60.2
Mendelson's syndrome (due to anesthesia)
 J95.4
 in labor and delivery O74.0
 in pregnancy O29.01
 obstetric O74.0
 postpartum, puerperal O89.01
Ménétrier's disease or syndrome K29.60
 with bleeding K29.61
Ménière's disease, syndrome or vertigo
 H81.0
Meninges, meningeal *-see* condition
Meningioma *-see also* Neoplasm, meninges,
 benign
 angioblastic *-see* Neoplasm, meninges, benign
 angiomatous *-see* Neoplasm, meninges,
  benign
 endotheliomatous *-see* Neoplasm, meninges,
  benign
 fibroblastic *-see* Neoplasm, meninges, benign

Meningioma - *continued*
  fibrous -*see* Neoplasm, meninges, benign
  hemangioblastic -*see* Neoplasm, meninges, benign
  hemangiopericytic -*see* Neoplasm, meninges, benign
  malignant -*see* Neoplasm, meninges, malignant
  meningothelial -*see* Neoplasm, meninges, benign
  meningotheliomatous -*see* Neoplasm, meninges, benign
  mixed -*see* Neoplasm, meninges, benign
  multiple -*see* Neoplasm, meninges, uncertain behavior
  papillary -*see* Neoplasm, meninges, uncertain behavior
  psammomatous -*see* Neoplasm, meninges, benign
  syncytial -*see* Neoplasm, meninges, benign
  transitional -*see* Neoplasm, meninges, benign
Meningiomatosis (diffuse) -*see* Neoplasm, meninges, uncertain behavior
Meningism -*see* Meningismus
Meningismus (infectional) (pneumococcal) R29.1
  due to serum or vaccine R29.1
  influenzal -*see* Influenza, with, manifestations NEC
Meningitis (basal) (basic) (brain) (cerebral) (cervical) (congestive) (diffuse) (hemorrhagic) (infantile) (membranous) (metastatic) (nonspecific) (pontine) (progressive) (simple) (spinal) (subacute) (sympathetic) (toxic) G03.9
  abacterial G03.0
  actinomycotic A42.81
  adenoviral A87.1
  arbovirus A87.8
  aseptic (acute) G03.0
  bacterial G00.9
    Escherichia coli (E. coli) G00.8
    Friedländer (bacillus) G00.8
    gram-negative G00.9
    H. influenzae G00.0
    Klebsiella G00.8
    pneumococcal G00.1
    specified organism NEC G00.8
    staphylococcal G00.3
    streptococcal (acute) G00.2
  benign recurrent (Mollaret) G03.2
  candidal B37.5
  caseous (tuberculous) A17.0
  cerebrospinal A39.0
  chronic NEC G03.1
  clear cerebrospinal fluid NEC G03.0
  coxsackievirus A87.0
  cryptococcal B45.1
  diplococcal (gram positive) A39.0
  echovirus A87.0
  enteroviral A87.0
  eosinophilic B83.2
  epidemic NEC A39.0
  Escherichia coli (E. coli) G00.8
  fibrinopurulent G00.9
    specified organism NEC G00.8
  Friedländer (bacillus) G00.8
  gonococcal A54.81
  gram-negative cocci G00.9
  gram-positive cocci G00.9
  Haemophilus (influenzae) G00.0

Meningitis - *continued*
  H. influenzae G00.0
  in (due to)
    adenovirus A87.1
    African trypanosomiasis B56.9 [*G02*]
    anthrax A22.8
    bacterial disease NEC A48.8 [*G01*]
    Chagas' disease (chronic) B57.41
    chickenpox B01.0
    coccidioidomycosis B38.4
    Diplococcus pneumoniae G00.1
    enterovirus A87.0
    herpes (simplex) virus B00.3
      zoster B02.1
    infectious mononucleosis B27.92
    leptospirosis A27.81
    Listeria monocytogenes A32.11
    Lyme disease A69.21
    measles B05.1
    mumps (virus) B26.1
    neurosyphilis (late) A52.13
    parasitic disease NEC B89 [*G02*]
    poliovirus A80.9 [*G02*]
    preventive immunization, inoculation or vaccination G03.8
    rubella B06.02
    Salmonella infection A02.21
    specified cause NEC G03.8
    Streptococcal pneumoniae G00.1
    typhoid fever A01.01
    varicella B01.0
    viral disease NEC A87.8
    whooping cough A37.90
    zoster B02.1
  infectious G00.9
  influenzal (H. influenzae) G00.0
  Klebsiella G00.8
  leptospiral (aseptic) A27.81
  lymphocytic (acute) (benign) (serous) A87.2
  meningococcal A39.0
  Mima polymorpha G00.8
  Mollaret (benign recurrent) G03.2
  monilial B37.5
  mycotic NEC B49 [*G02*]
  Neisseria A39.0
  nonbacterial G03.0
  nonpyogenic NEC G03.0
  ossificans G96.19
  pneumococcal streptococcus pneumoniae G00.1
  poliovirus A80.9 [*G02*]
  postmeasles B05.1
  purulent G00.9
    specified organism NEC G00.8
  pyogenic G00.9
    specified organism NEC G00.8
  Salmonella (arizonae) (Cholerae-Suis) (enteritidis) (typhimurium) A02.21
  septic G00.9
    specified organism NEC G00.8
  serosa circumscripta NEC G03.0
  serous NEC G93.2
  specified organism NEC G00.8
  sporotrichosis B42.81
  staphylococcal G00.3
  sterile G03.0
  Streptococcal (acute) G00.2
    pneumoniae G00.1
  suppurative G00.9
    specified organism NEC G00.8
  syphilitic (late) (tertiary) A52.13

Meningitis - *continued*
    acute A51.41
    congenital A50.41
    secondary A51.41
  Torula histolytica (cryptococcal) B45.1
  traumatic (complication of injury) T79.8
  tuberculous A17.0
  typhoid A01.01
  viral NEC A87.9
  Yersinia pestis A20.3
Meningocele (spinal) -*see also* Spina bifida
  with hydrocephalus -*see* Spina bifida, by site, with hydrocephalus
  acquired (traumatic) G96.19
  cerebral -*see* Encephalocele
Meningocerebritis -*see* Meningoencephalitis
Meningococcemia A39.4
  acute A39.2
  chronic A39.3
Meningococcus, meningococcal -*see also* condition A39.9
  adrenalitis, hemorrhagic A39.1
  carrier (suspected) of Z22.31
  meningitis (cerebrospinal) A39.0
Meningoencephalitis -*see also* Encephalitis G04.90
  acute NEC -*see also* Encephalitis, viral A86
  bacterial NEC G04.2
  California A83.5
  diphasic A84.1
  eosinophilic B83.2
  epidemic A39.81
  herpesviral, herpetic B00.4
    due to herpesvirus 6 B10.01
    due to herpesvirus 7 B10.09
    specified NEC B10.09
  in (due to)
    blastomycosis NEC B40.81
    diseases classified elsewhere G05.3
    free-living amebae B60.2
    Hemophilus influenzae (H .influenzae) G00.0
    herpes B00.4
      due to herpesvirus 6 B10.01
      due to herpesvirus 7 B10.09
      specified NEC B10.09
    H. influenzae G00.0
    Lyme disease A69.22
    mercury -*see* subcategory T56.1
    mumps B26.2
    Naegleria (amebae) (organisms) (fowleri) B60.2
    Parastrongylus cantonensis B83.2
    toxoplasmosis (acquired) B58.2
      congenital P37.1
  infectious (acute) (viral) A86
  influenzal (H. influenzae) G00.0
  Listeria monocytogenes A32.12
  lymphocytic (serous) A87.2
  mumps B26.2
  parasitic NEC B89 [*G05.3*]
  pneumococcal G04.2
  primary amebic B60.2
  specific (syphilitic) A52.14
  specified organism NEC G04.81
  staphylococcal G04.2
  streptococcal G04.2
  syphilitic A52.14
  toxic NEC G92
    due to mercury -*see* subcategory T56.1
  tuberculous A17.82
  virus NEC A86

Meningoencephalocele -see also
Encephalocele
  syphilitic A52.19
    congenital A50.49
Meningoencephalomyelitis -see also
Meningoencephalitis
  acute NEC (viral) A86
    disseminated G04.00
      postimmunization or postvaccination
        G04.02
      postinfectious G04.01
    due to
      actinomycosis A42.82
      Torula B45.1
      Toxoplasma or toxoplasmosis (acquired)
        B58.2
        congenital P37.1
    postimmunization or postvaccination G04.02
Meningoencephalomyelopathy G96.9
Meningoencephalopathy G96.9
Meningomyelitis -see also
Meningoencephalitis
  bacterial NEC G04.2
  blastomycotic NEC B40.81
  cryptococcal B45.1
  in diseases classified elsewhere G05.4
  meningococcal A39.81
  syphilitic A52.14
  tuberculous A17.82
Meningomyelocele -see also Spina bifida
  syphilitic A52.19
Meningomyeloneuritis -see
Meningoencephalitis
Meningoradiculitis -see Meningitis
Meningovascular -see condition
Menkes' disease or syndrome E83.09
  meaning maple-syrup-urine disease E71.0
Menometrorrhagia N92.1
**Menopause, menopausal (asymptomatic)
(state)** Z78.0
  arthritis (any site) NEC -see Arthritis,
    specified form NEC
  bleeding N92.4
  depression (single episode) F32.89
    agitated (single episode) F32.2
      recurrent episode F33.9
    psychotic (single episode) F32.89
      recurrent episode F33.9
    recurrent episode F33.8
  melancholia (single episode) F32.89
    recurrent episode F33.8
  paranoid state F22
  premature E28.319
    asymptomatic E28.319
      postirradiation E89.40
      postsurgical E89.40
    symptomatic E28.310
      postirradiation E89.41
      postsurgical E89.41
  psychosis NEC F28
  symptomatic N95.1
  toxic polyarthritis NEC -see Arthritis,
    specified form NEC
Menorrhagia (primary) N92.0
  climacteric N92.4
    menopausal N92.4
  menopausal N92.4
  postclimacteric N95.0
  postmenopausal N95.0
  preclimacteric or premenopausal N92.4
  pubertal (menses retained) N92.2

Menostaxis N92.0
Menses, retention N94.89
Menstrual -see Menstruation
  absent -see Amenorrhea
  anovulatory N97.0
  cycle, irregular N92.6
  delayed N91.0
  disorder N93.9
    psychogenic F45.8
  during pregnancy O20.8
  excessive (with regular cycle) N92.0
    with irregular cycle N92.1
    at puberty N92.2
  frequent N92.0
  infrequent -see Oligomenorrhea
  irregular N92.6
    specified NEC N92.5
  latent N92.5
  membranous N92.5
  painful -see also Dysmenorrhea N94.6
    primary N94.4
    psychogenic F45.8
    secondary N94.5
  passage of clots N92.0
  precocious E30.1
  protracted N92.5
  rare -see Oligomenorrhea
  retained N94.89
  retrograde N92.5
  scanty -see Oligomenorrhea
  suppression N94.89
  vicarious (nasal) N94.89
Mental -see also condition
  deficiency -see Disability, intellectual
  deterioration -see Psychosis
  disorder -see Disorder, mental
  exhaustion F48.8
  insufficiency (congenital) -see Disability,
    intellectual
  observation without need for further medical
    care Z03.89
  retardation -see Disability, intellectual
  subnormality -see Disability, intellectual
  upset -see Disorder, mental
Meralgia paresthetica G57.1
Mercurial -see condition
Mercurialism -see subcategory T56.1
**MERRF syndrome (myoclonic epilepsy
  associated with ragged-red fiber)** E88.42
Merkel cell tumor -see Carcinoma, Merkel
  cell
Merocele -see Hernia, femoral
Meromelia
  lower limb -see Defect, reduction, lower limb
    intercalary
      femur -see Defect, reduction, lower limb,
      specified type NEC
        tibiofibular (complete) (incomplete) -see
        Defect, reduction, lower limb
  upper limb -see Defect, reduction, upper limb
    intercalary, humeral, radioulnar -see
    Agenesis, arm, with hand present
Merzbacher-Pelizaeus disease E75.29
Mesaortitis -see Aortitis
Mesarteritis -see Arteritis
Mesencephalitis -see Encephalitis
Mesenchymoma -see also Neoplasm,
  connective tissue, uncertain behavior
  benign -see Neoplasm, connective tissue,
    benign
  malignant -see Neoplasm, connective tissue,
    malignant

Mesenteritis
  retractile K65.4
  sclerosing K65.4
Mesentery, mesenteric -see condition
Mesiodens, mesiodentes K00.1
Mesio-occlusion M26.213
Mesocolon -see condition
Mesonephroma (malignant) -see Neoplasm,
  malignant, by site
  benign -see Neoplasm, benign, by site
Mesophlebitis -see Phlebitis
Mesostromal dysgenesis Q13.89
Mesothelioma (malignant) C45.9
  benign
    mesentery D19.1
    mesocolon D19.1
    omentum D19.1
    peritoneum D19.1
    pleura D19.0
    specified site NEC D19.7
    unspecified site D19.9
  biphasic C45.9
    benign
      mesentery D19.1
      mesocolon D19.1
      omentum D19.1
      peritoneum D19.1
      pleura D19.0
      specified site NEC D19.7
      unspecified site D19.9
  cystic D48.4
  epithelioid C45.9
    benign
      mesentery D19.1
      mesocolon D19.1
      omentum D19.1
      peritoneum D19.1
      pleura D19.0
      specified site NEC D19.7
      unspecified site D19.9
  fibrous C45.9
    benign
      mesentery D19.1
      mesocolon D19.1
      omentum D19.1
      peritoneum D19.1
      pleura D19.0
      specified site NEC D19.7
      unspecified site D19.9
  site classification
    liver C45.7
    lung C45.7
    mediastinum C45.7
    mesentery C45.1
    mesocolon C45.1
    omentum C45.1
    pericardium C45.2
    peritoneum C45.1
    pleura C45.0
      parietal C45.0
    retroperitoneum C45.7
    specified site NEC C45.7
    unspecified C45.9
Metabolic syndrome E88.81
Metagonimiasis B66.8
Metagonimus infestation (intestine) B66.8
Metal
  pigmentation L81.8
  polisher's disease J62.8
Metamorphopsia H53.15

Metaplasia
apocrine (breast) -see Dysplasia, mammary,
specified type NEC
cervix (squamous) -see Dysplasia, cervix
endometrium (squamous) (uterus) N85.8
esophagus K22.7
kidney (pelvis) (squamous) N28.89
myelogenous D73.1
myeloid (agnogenic) (megakaryocytic) D73.1
spleen D73.1
squamous cell, bladder N32.89

Metastasis, metastatic
abscess -see Abscess
calcification E83.59
cancer
from specified site -see Neoplasm,
malignant, by site
to specified site -see Neoplasm, secondary,
by site
deposits (in) -see Neoplasm, secondary, by
site
disease -see also Neoplasm, secondary, by
site C79.9
spread (to) -see Neoplasm, secondary, by site

Metastrongyliasis B83.8

Metatarsalgia M77.4
anterior G57.6
Morton's G57.6

Metatarsus, metatarsal -see also condition
adductus, congenital Q66.22
valgus (abductus), congenital Q66.6
varus (congenital) Q66.22
primus Q66.21

Methadone use -see Use, opioid

Methemoglobinemia D74.9
acquired (with sulfhemoglobinemia) D74.8
congenital D74.0
enzymatic (congenital) D74.0
Hb M disease D74.0
hereditary D74.0
toxic D74.8

Methemoglobinuria -see Hemoglobinuria

Methioninemia E72.19

Methylmalonic acidemia E71.120

**Metritis (catarrhal) (hemorrhagic) (septic)
(suppurative)** -see also Endometritis
cervical -see Cervicitis

Metropathia hemorrhagica N93.8

Metroperitonitis -see Peritonitis, pelvic,
female

Metrorrhagia N92.1
climacteric N92.4
menopausal N92.4
postpartum NEC (atonic) (following delivery
of placenta) O72.1
delayed or secondary O72.2
preclimacteric or premenopausal N92.4
psychogenic F45.8

Metrorrhexis -see Rupture, uterus

Metrosalpingitis N70.91

Metrostaxis N93.8

Metrovaginitis -see Endometritis

Meyer-Schwickerath and Weyers syndrome
Q87.0

Meynert's amentia (nonalcoholic) F04
alcoholic F10.96
with dependence F10.26

Mibelli's disease (porokeratosis) Q82.8

Mice, joint -see Loose, body, joint
knee M23.4

Micrencephalon, micrencephaly Q02

Microalbuminuria R80.9

Microaneurysm, retinal -see also Disorder,
retina, microaneurysms
diabetic -see E08 E13 with .31

Microangiopathy (peripheral) I73.9
thrombotic M31.1

Microcalcifications, breast R92.0

Microcephalus, microcephalic, microcephaly
Q02
due to toxoplasmosis (congenital) P37.1

Microcheilia Q18.7

Microcolon (congenital) Q43.8

Microcornea (congenital) Q13.4

Microcytic -see condition **Microdeletions**
NEC Q93.88

Microdontia K00.2

Microdrepanocytosis D57.40
with crisis (vasoocclusive pain) D57.419
with
acute chest syndrome D57.411
splenic sequestration D57.412

Microembolism
atherothrombotic -see Atheroembolism
retinal -see Occlusion, artery, retina

Microencephalon Q02

Microfilaria streptocerca infestation -see
Onchocerciasis

Microgastria (congenital) Q40.2

Microgenia M26.06

Microgenitalia, congenital
female Q52.8
male Q55.8

Microglioma -see Lymphoma, non-Hodgkin,
specified NEC **Microglossia (congenital)**
Q38.3

**Micrognathia, micrognathism (congenital)
(mandibular) (maxillary)** M26.09

Microgyria (congenital) Q04.3

Microinfarct of heart -see Insufficiency,
coronary

Microlentia (congenital) Q12.8

Microlithiasis, alveolar, pulmonary J84.02

Micromastia N64.82

Micromyelia (congenital) Q06.8

Micropenis Q55.62

Microphakia (congenital) Q12.8

**Microphthalmos, microphthalmia
(congenital)** Q11.2
due to toxoplasmosis P37.1

Micropsia H53.15

Microscopic polyangiitis (polyarteritis)
M31.7

Microsporidiosis B60.8
intestinal A07.8

Microsporon furfur infestation B36.0

Microsporosis -see also Dermatophytosis
nigra B36.1

Microstomia (congenital) Q18.5

Microtia (congenital) (external ear) Q17.2

Microtropia H50.40

**Microvillus inclusion disease (MVD)
(MVID)** Q43.8

Micturition
disorder NEC -see also Difficulty, micturition
R39.198
psychogenic F45.8
frequency R35.0
psychogenic F45.8
hesitancy R39.11
incomplete emptying R39.14
nocturnal R35.1

Micturition - *continued*
painful R30.9
dysuria R30.0
psychogenic F45.8
tenesmus R30.1
poor stream R39.12
position dependent R39.192
split stream R39.13
straining R39.16
urgency R39.15

Mid plane -see condition

Middle
ear -see condition
lobe (right) syndrome J98.19

Miescher's elastoma L87.2

Mietens' syndrome Q87.2

Migraine (idiopathic) G43.909
with refractory migraine G43.919
with status migrainosus G43.911
without status migrainosus G43.919
with aura (acute-onset) (prolonged) (typical)
(without headache) G43.109
with refractory migraine G43.119
with status migrainosus G43.111
without status migrainosus G43.119
intractable G43.119
with status migrainosus G43.111
without status migrainosus G43.119
not intractable G43.109
with status migrainosus G43.101
without status migrainosus G43.109
persistent G43.509
with cerebral infarction G43.609
with refractory migraine G43.619
with status migrainosus G43.611
without status migrainosus G43.619
intractable G43.619
with status migrainosus G43.611
without status migrainosus G43.619
not intractable G43.609
with status migrainosus G43.601
without status migrainosus G43.609
without refractory migraine G43.609
with status migrainosus G43.601
without status migrainosus G43.609
without cerebral infarction G43.509
with refractory migraine G43.519
with status migrainosus G43.511
without status migrainosus G43.519
intractable G43.519
with status migrainosus G43.511
without status migrainosus G43.519
not intractable G43.509
with status migrainosus G43.501
without status migrainosus G43.509
without refractory migraine G43.509
with status migrainosus G43.501
without status migrainosus G43.509
without mention of refractory migraine
G43.109
with status migrainosus G43.101
without status migrainosus G43.109
abdominal G43.D0
with refractory migraine G43.D1
intractable G43.D1
not intractable G43.D0
without refractory migraine G43.D0
basilar -see Migraine, with aura
classical -see Migraine, with aura
common -see Migraine, without aura
complicated G43.109

Migraine --continued
equivalents -see Migraine, with aura
familiar -see Migraine, hemiplegic
hemiplegic G43.409
  with refractory migraine G43.419
    with status migrainosus G43.411
    without status migrainosus G43.419
  intractable G43.419
    with status migrainosus G43.411
    without status migrainosus G43.419
  not intractable G43.409
    with status migrainosus G43.401
    without status migrainosus G43.409
  without refractory migraine G43.409
    with status migrainosus G43.401
    without status migrainosus G43.409
intractable G43.919
  with status migrainosus G43.911
  without status migrainosus G43.919
menstrual G43.829
  with refractory migraine G43.839
    with status migrainosus G43.831
    without status migrainosus G43.839
  intractable G43.839
    with status migrainosus G43.831
    without status migrainosus G43.839
  not intractable 4G43.829
    with status migrainosus G43.821
    without status migrainosus G43.829
  without refractory migraine G43.829
    with status migrainosus G43.821
    without status migrainosus G43.829
menstrually related -see Migraine, menstrual
not intractable G43.909
  with status migrainosus G43.901
  without status migrainosus G43.919
ophthalmoplegic G43.B0
  with refractory migraine G43.B1
  intractable G43.B1
  not intractable G43.B0
  without refractory migraine G43.B0
persistent aura (with, without) cerebral
  infarction -see Migraine, with aura, persistent
preceded or accompanied by transient focal
  neurological phenomena -see Migraine, with
  aura
pre-menstrual -see Migraine, menstrual
pure menstrual -see Migraine, menstrual
retinal -see Migraine, with aura
specified NEC G43.809
  intractable G43.819
    with status migrainosus G43.811
    without status migrainosus G43.819
  not intractable G43.809
    with status migrainosus G43.801
    without status migrainosus G43.809
sporadic -see Migraine, hemiplegic
transformed -see Migraine, without aura,
  chronic
triggered seizures -see Migraine, with aura
without aura G43.009
  with refractory migraine G43.019
    with status migrainosus G43.011
    without status migrainosus G43.019
  chronic G43.709
    with refractory migraine G43.719
      with status migrainosus G43.711
      without status migrainosus G43.719
    intractable
      with status migrainosus G43.711
      without status migrainosus G43.719

Migraine --continued
  not intractable
    with status migrainosus G43.701
    without status migrainosus G43.709
    without refractory migraine G43.709
      with status migrainosus G43.701
      without status migrainosus G43.709
  intractable
    with status migrainosus G43.011
    without status migrainosus G43.019
  not intractable
    with status migrainosus G43.001
    without status migrainosus G43.009
  without mention of refractory migraine
    G43.009
    with status migrainosus G43.001
    without status migrainosus G43.009
  without refractory migraineG43.909
    with status migrainosus G43.901
    without status migrainosus G43.919
Migrant, social Z59.0
Migration, anxiety concerning Z60.3
Migratory, migrating -see also condition
  person Z59.0
  testis Q55.29
Mikity Wilson disease or syndrome P27.0
Mikulicz' disease or syndrome K11.8
Miliaria L74.3
  alba L74.1
  apocrine L75.2
  crystallina L74.1
  profunda L74.2
  rubra L74.0
  tropicalis L74.2
Miliary -see condition **Milium** L72.0
  colloid L57.8
Milk
  crust L21.0
  excessive secretion O92.6
  poisoning -see Poisoning, food, noxious
  retention O92.79
  sickness -see Poisoning, food, noxious
  spots I31.0
Milk-alkali disease or syndrome E83.52
Milk-leg (deep vessels) (nonpuerperal) -see
  Embolism, vein, lower extremity
  complicating pregnancy O22.3
  puerperal, postpartum, childbirth O87.1
Milkman's disease or syndrome M83.8
Milky urine -see Chyluria
Millard-Gubler (Foville) paralysis or
  syndrome G46.3
Millar's asthma J38.5
Miller Fisher syndrome G61.0
Mills' disease -see Hemiplegia
Millstone maker's pneumoconiosis J62.8
Milroy's disease (chronic hereditary edema)
  Q82.0
Minamata disease T56.1
Miners' asthma or lung J60
Minkowski-Chauffard syndrome -see
  Spherocytosis
Minor -see condition
Minor's disease (hematomyelia) G95.19
Minot's disease (hemorrhagic disease),
  newborn P53
Minot-von Willebrand-Jurgens disease or
  syndrome (angiohemophilia) D68.0
Minus (and plus) hand (intrinsic) -see
  Deformity, limb, specified type NEC, forearm
Miosis (pupil) H57.03

Mirizzi's syndrome (hepatic duct stenosis)
  K83.1
Mirror writing F81.0
Misadventure (of) (prophylactic)
  (therapeutic) -see also Complications T88.9
  administration of insulin (by accident) -see
    subcategory T38.3
  infusion -see Complications, infusion
  local applications (of fomentations, plasters,
    etc.) T88.9
    burn or scald -see Burn
    specified NEC T88.8
  medical care (early) (late) T88.9
    adverse effect of drugs or chemicals -see
    Table of Drugs and Chemicals
  medical care (early) (late)
    burn or scald -see Burn
    specified NEC T88.8
    specified NEC T88.8
  surgical procedure (early) (late) -see
    Complications, surgical procedure
  transfusion -see Complications, transfusion
  vaccination or other immunological procedure
    -see Complications, vaccination
Miscarriage O03.9
Misdirection, aqueous H40.83
Misperception, sleep state F51.02
Misplaced, misplacement
  ear Q17.4
  kidney (acquired) N28.89
    congenital Q63.2
  organ or site, congenital NEC -see
    Malposition, congenital
Missed
  abortion O02.1
  delivery O36.4
Missing -see also Absence
  string of intrauterine contraceptive device
    T83.32
Misuse of drugs F19.99
Mitchell's disease (erythromelalgia) I73.81
Mite(s) (infestation) B88.9
  diarrhea B88.0
  grain (itch) B88.0
  hair follicle (itch) B88.0
  in sputum B88.0
Mitral -see condition **Mittelschmerz** N94.0
Mixed -see condition
MMN (multifocal motor neuropathy) G61.82
MNGIE (Mitochondrial
  Neurogastrointestinal Encephalopathy)
  syndrome E88.49
Mobile, mobility
  cecum Q43.3
  excessive -see Hypermobility   gallbladder,
    congenital Q44.1
  kidney N28.89
  organ or site, congenital NEC -see
    Malposition, congenital
Mobitz heart block (atrioventricular) I44.1
Moebius, Möbius
  disease (ophthalmoplegic migraine) -see
    Migraine, ophthalmoplegic
  syndrome Q87.0
    congenital oculofacial paralysis (with other
    anomalies) Q87.0
    ophthalmoplegic migraine -see Migraine,
    ophthalmoplegic
Moeller's glossitis K14.0
Mohr's syndrome (Types I and II) Q87.0
Mola destruens D39.2

Molar pregnancy O02.0
Molarization of premolars K00.2
Molding, head (during birth)
  omit code **Mole (pigmented)** -*see also* Nevus
  blood O02.0
  Breus' O02.0
  cancerous -*see* Melanoma
  carneous O02.0
  destructive D39.2
  fleshy O02.0
  hydatid, hydatidiform (benign) (complicating
  pregnancy) (delivered) (undelivered) O01.9
    classical O01.0
    complete O01.0
    incomplete O01.1
    invasive D39.2
    malignant D39.2
    partial O01.1
  intrauterine O02.0
  invasive (hydatidiform) D39.2
  malignant
    meaning
      malignant hydatidiform mole D39.2
      melanoma -*see* Melanoma
  nonhydatidiform O02.0
  nonpigmented -*see* Nevus
  pregnancy NEC O02.0
  skin -*see* Nevus
  tubal O00.10
    with intrauterine pregnancy O00.11
  vesicular -*see* Mole, hydatidiform
Molimen, molimina (menstrual) N94.3
Molluscum contagiosum (epitheliale) B08.1
Mönckeberg's arteriosclerosis, disease, or
  sclerosis -*see* Arteriosclerosis, extremities
Mondini's malformation (cochlea) Q16.5
Mondor's disease I80.8
Monge's disease T70.29
Monilethrix (congenital) Q84.1
Moniliasis -*see also* Candidiasis B37.9
  neonatal P37.5
Monitoring (encounter for)
  therapeutic drug level Z51.81
Monkey malaria B53.1
Monkeypox B04
Monoarthritis M13.10
  ankle M13.17
  elbow M13.12
  foot joint M13.17
  hand joint M13.14
  hip M13.15
  knee M13.16
  shoulder M13.11
  wrist M13.13
Monoblastic -*see* condition
Monochromat (ism), monochromatopsia
  (acquired) (congenital) H53.51
Monocytic -*see* condition
Monocytopenia D72.818
Monocytosis (symptomatic) D72.821
Monomania -*see* Psychosis **Mononeuritis**
  G58.9
  cranial nerve -*see* Disorder, nerve, cranial
  femoral nerve G57.2
  lateral
    cutaneous nerve of thigh G57.1
    popliteal nerve G57.3
  lower limb G57.9
    specified nerve NEC G57.8
  medial popliteal nerve G57.4
  median nerve G56.1

Monomania - *continued*
  multiplex G58.7
  plantar nerve G57.6
  posterior tibial nerve G57.5
  radial nerve G56.3
  sciatic nerve G57.0
  specified NEC G58.8
  tibial nerve G57.4
  ulnar nerve G56.2
  upper limb G56.9
    specified nerve NEC G56.8
  vestibular -*see* subcategory H93.3
Mononeuropathy G58.9
  carpal tunnel syndrome -*see* Syndrome, carpal
    tunnel
  diabetic NEC -*see* E08 E13with .41
  femoral nerve -*see* Lesion, nerve, femoral
  ilioinguinal nerve G57.8
  in diseases classified elsewhere - see category
    G59
  intercostal G58.0
  lower limb G57.9
    causalgia -*see* Causalgia, lower limb
    femoral nerve -*see* Lesion, nerve, femoral
    meralgia paresthetica G57.1
    plantar nerve -*see* Lesion, nerve, plantar
    popliteal nerve -*see* Lesion, nerve, popliteal
    sciatic nerve -*see* Lesion, nerve, sciatic
    specified NEC G57.8
    tarsal tunnel syndrome -*see* Syndrome, tarsal
    tunnel
  median nerve -*see* Lesion, nerve, median
  multiplex G58.7
  obturator nerve G57.8
  popliteal nerve -*see* Lesion, nerve, popliteal
  radial nerve -*see* Lesion, nerve, radial
  saphenous nerve G57.8
  specified NEC G58.8
  tarsal tunnel syndrome -*see* Syndrome, tarsal
    tunnel
  tuberculous A17.83
  ulnar nerve -*see* Lesion, nerve, ulnar
  upper limb G56.9
    carpal tunnel syndrome -*see* Syndrome,
      carpal tunnel
    causalgia -*see* Causalgia
    median nerve -*see* Lesion, nerve, median
    radial nerve -*see* Lesion, nerve, radial
    specified site NEC G56.8
    ulnar nerve -*see* Lesion, nerve, ulnar
Mononucleosis, infectious B27.90
  with
    complication NEC B27.99
    meningitis B27.92
    polyneuropathy B27.91
  cytomegaloviral B27.10
    with
      complication NEC B27.19
      meningitis B27.12
      polyneuropathy B27.11
  Epstein-Barr (virus) B27.00
    with
      complication NEC B27.09
      meningitis B27.02
      polyneuropathy B27.01
  gammaherpesviral B27.00
    with
      complication NEC B27.09
      meningitis B27.02
      polyneuropathy B27.01
  specified NEC B27.80

Mononucleosis, infectious - *continued*
  with
    complication NEC B27.89
    meningitis B27.82
    polyneuropathy B27.81
Monoplegia G83.3
  congenital (cerebral) G80.8
    spastic G80.1
  embolic (current episode) I63.4
  following
    cerebrovascular disease
      cerebral infarction
        lower limb I69.34
        upper limb I69.33
      intracerebral hemorrhage
        lower limb I69.14
        upper limb I69.13
      lower limb I69.94
      nontraumatic intracranial hemorrhage NEC
        lower limb I69.24
        upper limb I69.23
      specified disease NEC
        lower limb I69.84
        upper limb I69.83
      stroke NOS
        lower limb I69.34
        upper limb I69.33
      subarachnoid hemorrhage
        lower limb I69.04
        upper limb I69.03
        upper limb I69.93
  hysterical (transient) F44.4
  lower limb G83.1
  psychogenic (conversion reaction) F44.4
  thrombotic (current episode) I63.3
  transient R29.818
  upper limb G83.2
Monorchism, monorchidism Q55.0
Monosomy -*see also* Deletion, chromosome
  Q93.9
  specified NEC Q93.89
  whole chromosome
    meiotic nondisjunction Q93.0
    mitotic nondisjunction Q93.1
    mosaicism Q93.1
  X Q96.9
Monster, monstrosity (single) Q89.7
  acephalic Q00.0
  twin Q89.4
Monteggia's fracture (dislocation) S52.27
Mooren's ulcer (cornea) -*see* Ulcer, cornea,
  Mooren's
Moore's syndrome -*see* Epilepsy, specified
  NEC
Mooser-Neill reaction A75.2
Mooser's bodies A75.2
Morbidity not stated or unknown R69
Morbilli -*see* Measles
Morbus -*see also* Disease
  angelicus, anglorum E55.0
  Beigel B36.2
  caducus -*see* Epilepsy
  celiacus K90.0
  comitialis -*see* Epilepsy
  cordis -*see also* Disease, heart I51.9
    valvulorum -*see* Endocarditis
  coxae senilis M16.9
    tuberculous A18.02
  hemorrhagicus neonatorum P53
  maculosus neonatorum P54.5

Morel (Stewart)(Morgagni) syndrome
M85.2
Morel-Kraepelin disease -see Schizophrenia
Morel-Moore syndrome M85.2
Morgagni's
cyst, organ, hydatid, or appendage
female Q50.5
male (epididymal) Q55.4
testicular Q55.29
syndrome M85.2
Morgagni-Stokes-Adams syndrome I45.9
Morgagni-Stewart-Morel syndrome M85.2
Morgagni-Turner (Albright) syndrome
Q96.9
Moria F07.0
Moron (I.Q.50 69) F70
Morphea L94.0
Morphinism (without remission) F11.20
with remission F11.21
Morphinomania (without remission) F11.20
with remission F11.21
**Morquio (Ullrich)(Brailsford) disease or
syndrome** -see Mucopolysaccharidosis
Mortification (dry) (moist) -see Gangrene
**Morton's metatarsalgia
(neuralgia)(neuroma) (syndrome)** G57.6
Morvan's disease or syndrome G60.8
**Mosaicism, mosaic (autosomal)
(chromosomal)**
45,X/other cell lines NEC with abnormal sex
chromosome Q96.4
45,X/46,XX Q96.3
sex chromosome
female Q97.8
lines with various numbers of X
chromosomes Q97.2
male Q98.7
XY Q96.3
Moschowitz' disease M31.1
Mother yaw A66.0
**Motion sickness (from travel, any vehicle)
(from roundabouts or swings)** T75.3
**Mottled, mottling, teeth (enamel) (endemic)
(nonendemic)** K00.3
Mounier-Kuhn syndrome Q32.4
with bronchiectasis J47.9
exacerbation (acute) J47.1
lower respiratory infection J47.0
acquired J98.09
with bronchiectasis J47.9
with
exacerbation (acute) J47.1
lower respiratory infection J47.0
Mountain
sickness T70.29
with polycythemia , acquired (acute) D75.1
tick fever A93.2
Mouse, joint -see Loose, body, joint
knee M23.4
Mouth -see condition **Movable**
coccyx -see subcategory M53.2
kidney N28.89
congenital Q63.8
spleen D73.89
Movements, dystonic R25.8
Moyamoya disease I67.5
**MRSA (Methicillin resistant Staphylococcus
aureus)**
infection A49.02
as the cause of diseases classified elsewhere
B95.62
sepsis A41.02

**MSSA (Methicillin susceptible
Staphylococcus aureus)**
infection A49.01
as the cause of diseases classified elsewhere
B95.61
sepsis A41.01
Mucha-Habermann disease L41.0
**Mucinosis (cutaneous) (focal) (papular)
(reticular erythematous) (skin)** L98.5
oral K13.79
Mucocele
appendix K38.8
buccal cavity K13.79
gallbladder K82.1
lacrimal sac, chronic H04.43
nasal sinus J34.1
nose J34.1
salivary gland (any) K11.6
sinus (accessory) (nasal) J34.1
turbinate (bone) (middle) (nasal) J34.1
uterus N85.8
Mucolipidosis
I E77.1
II, III E77.0
IV E75.11
Mucopolysaccharidosis E76.3
beta-gluduronidase deficiency E76.29
cardiopathy E76.3 [I52]
Hunter's syndrome E76.1
Hurler's syndrome E76.01
Hurler-Scheie syndrome E76.02
Maroteaux Lamy syndrome E76.29
Morquio syndrome E76.219
A E76.210
B E76.211
classic E76.210
Sanfilippo syndrome E76.22
Scheie's syndrome E76.03
specified NEC E76.29
type
I
Hurler's syndrome E76.01
Hurler-Scheie syndrome E76.02
Scheie's syndrome E76.03
II E76.1
III E76.22
IV E76.219
IVA E76.210
IVB E76.211
VI E76.29
VII E76.29
Mucormycosis B46.5
cutaneous B46.3
disseminated B46.4
gastrointestinal B46.2
generalized B46.4
pulmonary B46.0
rhinocerebral B46.1
skin B46.3
subcutaneous B46.3
Mucositis (ulcerative) K12.30
due to drugs NEC K12.32
gastrointestinal K92.81
mouth (oral) (oropharyngeal) K12.30
due to antineoplastic therapy K12.31
due to drugs NEC K12.32
due to radiation K12.33
specified NEC K12.39
viral K12.39
nasal J34.81
oral cavity -see Mucositis, mouth
oral soft tissues -see Mucositis, mouth
vagina and vulva N76.81

Mucositis necroticans agranulocytica -see
Agranulocytosis
Mucous -see also condition
patches (syphilitic) A51.39
congenital A50.07
Mucoviscidosis E84.9
with meconium obstruction E84.11
Mucus
asphyxia or suffocation -see Asphyxia, mucus
in stool R19.5
plug -see Asphyxia, mucus
Muguet B37.0
Mulberry molars (congenital syphilis)
A50.52
Müllerian mixed tumor
specified site -see Neoplasm, malignant, by
site
unspecified site C54.9
Multicystic kidney (development) Q61.4
Multiparity (grand) Z64.1
affecting management of pregnancy, labor
and delivery (supervision only) O09.4
requiring contraceptive management -see
Contraception
Multipartita placenta O43.19
Multiple, multiplex -see also condition
digits (congenital) Q69.9
endocrine neoplasia -see Neoplasia,
endocrine, multiple (MEN)
personality F44.81
Mumps B26.9
arthritis B26.85
complication NEC B26.89
encephalitis B26.2
hepatitis B26.81
meningitis (aseptic) B26.1
meningoencephalitis B26.2
myocarditis B26.82
oophoritis B26.89
orchitis B26.0
pancreatitis B26.3
polyneuropathy B26.84
Mumu -see also Infestation, filarial B74.9
[N51]
Münchhausen's syndrome -see Disorder,
factitious
Münchmeyer's syndrome -see Myositis,
ossificans, progressiva
Mural -see condition
Murmur (cardiac) (heart) (organic) R01.1
abdominal R19.15
aortic (valve) -see Endocarditis, aortic
benign R01.0
diastolic -see Endocarditis
Flint I35.1
functional R01.0
Graham Steell I37.1
innocent R01.0
mitral (valve) -see Insufficiency, mitral
nonorganic R01.0
presystolic, mitral -see Insufficiency, mitral
pulmonic (valve) I37.8
systolic R01.1
tricuspid (valve) I07.9
valvular -see Endocarditis
**Murri's disease (intermittent
hemoglobinuria)** D59.6
Muscle, muscular -see also condition
carnitine (palmitoyltransferase) deficiency
E71.314
Musculoneuralgia -see Neuralgia

Mushroom-workers' (pickers') disease or lung J67.5
Mushrooming hip -see Derangement, joint, specified NEC, hip
Mutation(s)
 factor V Leiden D68.51
 surfactant, of lung J84.83
 prothrombin gene D68.52
Mutism -see also Aphasia
 deaf (acquired) (congenital) NEC H91.3
 elective (adjustment reaction) (childhood) F94.0
 hysterical F44.4
 selective (childhood) F94.0
MVD (microvillus inclusion disease) Q43.8
MVID (microvillus inclusion disease) Q43.8
Myalgia M79.1
 epidemic (cervical) B33.0
 traumatic NEC T14.8
Myasthenia G70.9
 congenital G70.2
 cordis -see Failure, heart
 developmental G70.2
 gravis G70.00
  with exacerbation (acute) G70.01
  in crisis G70.01
 neonatal, transient P94.0
 pseudoparalytica G70.00
  with exacerbation (acute) G70.01
  in crisis G70.01
 stomach, psychogenic F45.8
 syndrome
  in
   diabetes mellitus -see E08 E13 with .44
   neoplastic disease -see also Neoplasm D49.9 [G73.3]
   pernicious anemia D51.0 [G73.3]
   thyrotoxicosis E05.90 [G73.3]
    with thyroid storm E05.91 [G73.3]
Myasthenic M62.81
Mycelium infection B49
Mycetismus -see Poisoning, food, noxious, mushroom
Mycetoma B47.9
 actinomycotic B47.1
 bone (mycotic) B47.9 [M90.80]
 eumycotic B47.0
 foot B47.9
  actinomycotic B47.1
  mycotic B47.0
 madurae NEC B47.9
  mycotic B47.0
 maduromycotic B47.0
 mycotic B47.0
 nocardial B47.1
Mycobacteriosis -see Mycobacterium
Mycobacterium, mycobacterial (infection) A31.9
 anonymous A31.9
 atypical A31.9
  cutaneous A31.1
  pulmonary A31.0
  tuberculous -see Tuberculosis, pulmonary
  specified site NEC A31.8
 avium (intracellulare complex) A31.0
 balnei A31.1
 Battey A31.0
 chelonei A31.8
 cutaneous A31.1
 extrapulmonary systemic A31.8
 fortuitum A31.8

Mycobacterium, mycobacterial - *continued*
 intracellulare (Battey bacillus) A31.0
 kansasii (yellow bacillus) A31.0
 kakaferifu A31.8
 kasongo A31.8
 leprae -see also Leprosy A30.9
 luciflavum A31.1
 marinum (M. balnei) A31.1
 nonspecific -see Mycobacterium, atypical
 pulmonary (atypical) A31.0
  tuberculous -see Tuberculosis, pulmonary
 scrofulaceum A31.8
 simiae A31.8
 systemic, extrapulmonary A31.8
 szulgai A31.8
 terrae A31.8
 triviale A31.8
 tuberculosis (human, bovine) see Tuberculosis
 ulcerans A31.1
 xenopi A31.8
Mycoplasma (M.) pneumoniae, as cause of disease classified elsewhere B96.0
Mycosis, mycotic B49
 cutaneous NEC B36.9
 ear B36.9
  in
   aspergillosis B44.89
   candidiasis B37.84
   moniliasis B37.84
 fungoides (extranodal) (solid organ) C84.0
 mouth B37.0
 nails B35.1
 opportunistic B48.8
 skin NEC B36.9
 specified NEC B48.8
 stomatitis B37.0
 vagina, vaginitis (candidal) B37.3
Mydriasis (pupil) H57.04
Myelatelia Q06.1
Myelinolysis, pontine, central G37.2
Myelitis (acute) (ascending) (childhood) (chronic) (descending) (diffuse) (disseminated) (idiopathic) (pressure) (progressive) (spinal cord) (subacute) -see also Encephalitis G04.91
 herpes simplex B00.82
 herpes zoster B02.24
 in diseases classified elsewhere G05.4
 necrotizing, subacute G37.4
 optic neuritis in G36.0
 post chickenpox B01.12
 postherpetic B02.24
 postimmunization G04.02
 postinfectious NEC G04.89
 postvaccinal G04.02
 specified NEC G04.89
 syphilitic (transverse) A52.14
 toxic G92
 transverse (in demyelinating diseases of central nervous system) G37.3
 tuberculous A17.82
 varicella B01.12
Myeloblastic -see condition
Myeloblastoma
 granular cell -see also Neoplasm, connective tissue
  malignant -see Neoplasm, connective tissue, malignant
  tongue D10.1
Myelocele -see Spina bifida

Myelocystocele -see Spina bifida
Myelocytic -see condition
Myelodysplasia D46.9
 specified NEC D46.Z
 spinal cord (congenital) Q06.1
Myelodysplastic syndrome D46.9
 with
  5q deletion D46.C
  isolated del (5q) chromosomal abnormality D46.C - specified NEC D46.Z
Myeloencephalitis -see Encephalitis
Myelofibrosis D75.81
 with myeloid metaplasia D47.4
 acute C94.4
 idiopathic (chronic) D47.4
 primary D47.1
 secondary D75.81
  in myeloproliferative disease D47.4
Myelogenous -see condition
Myeloid -see condition
Myelokathexis D70.9
Myeloleukodystrophy E75.29
Myelolipoma -see Lipoma
Myeloma (multiple) C90.0
 monostotic C90.3
  plasma cell C90.0
 plasma cell C90.0
 solitary -see also Plasmacytoma, solitary C90.3
Myelomalacia G95.89
Myelomatosis C90.0
Myelomeningitis -see Meningoencephalitis
Myelomeningocele (spinal cord) -see Spina bifida
Myelo-osteo-musculodysplasia hereditaria Q79.8
Myelopathic
 anemia D64.89
 muscle atrophy -see Atrophy, muscle, spinal
 pain syndrome G89.0
Myelopathy (spinal cord) G95.9
 drug-induced G95.89
 in (due to)
  degeneration or displacement, intervertebral disc NEC -see Disorder, disc, with, myelopathy
  infection -see Encephalitis
  intervertebral disc disorder -see also Disorder, disc, with, myelopathy
  mercury -see subcategory T56.1
  neoplastic disease -see also Neoplasm D49.9 [G99.2]
  pernicious anemia D51.0 [G99.2]
  spondylosis -see Spondylosis, with myelopathy NEC
 necrotic (subacute) (vascular) G95.19
 radiation-induced G95.89
 spondylogenic NEC -see Spondylosis, with myelopathy NEC
 toxic G95.89
 transverse, acute G37.3
 vascular G95.19
 vitamin B12 E53.8 [G32.0]
Myelophthisis D61.82
Myeloradiculitis G04.91
Myeloradiculodysplasia (spinal) Q06.1
Myelosarcoma C92.3
Myelosclerosis D75.89
 with myeloid metaplasia D47.4
 disseminated, of nervous system G35
 megakaryocytic D47.4
  with myeloid metaplasia D47.4

Myelosis
  acute C92.0
  aleukemic C92.9
  chronic D47.1
  erythremic (acute) C94.0
  megakaryocytic C94.2
  nonleukemic D72.828
  subacute C92.9
Myiasis (cavernous) B87.9
  aural B87.4
  creeping B87.0
  cutaneous B87.0
  dermal B87.0
  ear (external) (middle) B87.4
  eye B87.2
  genitourinary B87.81
  intestinal B87.82
  laryngeal B87.3
  nasopharyngeal B87.3
  ocular B87.2
  orbit B87.2
  skin B87.0
  specified site NEC B87.89
  traumatic B87.1
  wound B87.1
Myoadenoma, prostate -see Hyperplasia,
  prostate
Myoblastoma
  granular cell -see also Neoplasm, connective
  tissue, benign
    malignant -see Neoplasm, connective tissue,
    malignant
  tongue D10.1
Myocardial -see condition
Myocardiopathy (congestive) (constrictive)
  (familial) (hypertrophic nonobstructive)
  (idiopathic) (infiltrative) (obstructive)
  (primary) (restrictive) (sporadic) -see also
  Cardiomyopathy I42.9
  alcoholic I42.6
  cobalt-beer I42.6
  glycogen storage E74.02 [I43]
  hypertrophic obstructive I42.1
  in (due to)
    beriberi E51.12
    cardiac glycogenosis E74.02 [I43]
    Friedreich's ataxia G11.1 [I43]
    myotonia atrophica G71.11 [I43]
    progressive muscular dystrophy G71.0 [I43]
  obscure (African) I42.8
  secondary I42.9
  thyrotoxic E05.90 [I43]
    with storm E05.91 [I43]
  toxic NEC I42.7
Myocarditis (with
  arteriosclerosis)(chronic)(fibroid)
  (interstitial) (old) (progressive) (senile)
  I51.4
  with
    rheumatic fever (conditions in I00) I09.0
      active -see Myocarditis, acute, rheumatic
      inactive or quiescent (with chorea) I09.0
    active I40.9
      rheumatic I01.2
        with chorea (acute) (rheumatic)
        (Sydenham's) I02.0
    acute or subacute (interstitial) I40.9
      due to
        streptococcus (beta-hemolytic) I01.2
      idiopathic I40.1
      rheumatic I01.2

Myocarditis --continued
  with chorea (acute) (rheumatic)
    (Sydenham's) I02.0
    specified NEC I40.8
  aseptic of newborn B33.22
  bacterial (acute) I40.0
  Coxsackie (virus) B33.22
  diphtheritic A36.81
  eosinophilic I40.1
  epidemic of newborn (Coxsackie) B33.22
  Fiedler's (acute) (isolated) I40.1
  giant cell (acute) (subacute) I40.1
  gonococcal A54.83
  granulomatous (idiopathic) (isolated)
    (nonspecific) I40.1
  hypertensive -see Hypertension, heart
  idiopathic (granulomatous) I40.1
  in (due to)
    diphtheria A36.81
    epidemic louse-borne typhus A75.0 [I41]
    Lyme disease A69.29
    sarcoidosis D86.85
    scarlet fever A38.1
    toxoplasmosis (acquired) B58.81
    typhoid A01.02
    typhus NEC A75.9 [I41]
  infective I40.0
  influenzal -see Influenza, with, myocarditis
  isolated (acute) I40.1
  meningococcal A39.52
  mumps B26.82
  nonrheumatic, active I40.9
  parenchymatous I40.9
  pneumococcal I40.0
  rheumatic (chronic) (inactive) (with chorea)
    I09.0
    active or acute I01.2
      with chorea (acute) (rheumatic)
      (Sydenham's) I02.0
  rheumatoid -see Rheumatoid, carditis
  septic I40.0
  staphylococcal I40.0
  suppurative I40.0
  syphilitic (chronic) A52.06
  toxic I40.8
    rheumatic -see Myocarditis, acute,
    rheumatic
  tuberculous A18.84
  typhoid A01.02
  valvular -see Endocarditis
  virus, viral I40.0
    of newborn (Coxsackie) B33.22
Myocardium, myocardial -see condition
Myocardosis -see Cardiomyopathy
Myoclonus, myoclonic, myoclonia (familial)
  (essential) (multifocal) (simplex) G25.3
  drug-induced G25.3
  epilepsy -see also Epilepsy, generalized,
    specified NEC G40.4
    familial (progressive) G25.3
  epileptica G40.409
    with status epilepticus G40.401
  facial G51.3
  familial progressive G25.3
  Friedreich's G25.3
  jerks G25.3
  massive G25.3
  palatal G25.3
  pharyngeal G25.3
Myocytolysis I51.5
Myodiastasis -see Diastasis, muscle

Myoendocarditis -see Endocarditis
Myoepithelioma -see Neoplasm, benign, by
  site
Myofasciitis (acute) -see Myositis
Myofibroma -see also Neoplasm, connective
  tissue, benign
  uterus (cervix) (corpus) -see Leiomyoma
Myofibromatosis D48.1
  infantile Q89.8
Myofibrosis M62.89
  heart -see Myocarditis
  scapulohumeral -see Lesion, shoulder,
  specified NEC
Myofibrositis M79.7
  scapulohumeral -see Lesion, shoulder,
  specified NEC
Myoglobulinuria, myoglobinuria (primary)
  R82.1
Myokymia, facial G51.4
Myolipoma -see Lipoma
Myoma -see also Neoplasm, connective tissue,
  benign
  malignant -see Neoplasm, connective tissue,
  malignant
  prostate D29.1
  uterus (cervix) (corpus) -see Leiomyoma
Myomalacia M62.89
Myometritis -see Endometritis
Myometrium -see condition
Myonecrosis, clostridial A48.0
Myopathy G72.9
  acute
    necrotizing G72.81
    quadriplegic G72.81
  alcoholic G72.1
  benign congenital G71.2
  central core G71.2
  centronuclear G71.2
  congenital (benign) G71.2
  critical illness G72.81
  distal G71.0
  drug-induced G72.0
  endocrine NEC E34.9 [G73.7]
  extraocular muscles H05.82
  facioscapulohumeral G71.0
  hereditary G71.9
    specified NEC G71.8
  immune NEC G72.49
  in (due to)
    Addison's disease E27.1 [G73.7]
    alcohol G72.1
    amyloidosis E85.0 [G73.7]
    cretinism E00.9 [G73.7]
    Cushing's syndrome E24.9 [G73.7]
    drugs G72.0
    endocrine disease NEC E34.9 [G73.7]
    giant cell arteritis M31.6 [G73.7]
    glycogen storage disease E74.00 [G73.7]
    hyperadrenocorticism E24.9 [G73.7]
    hyperparathyroidism NEC E21.3 [G73.7]
    hypoparathyroidism E20.9 [G73.7]
    hypopituitarism E23.0 [G73.7]
    hypothyroidism E03.9 [G73.7]
    infectious disease NEC B99 [G73.7]
    lipid storage disease E75.6 [G73.7]
    metabolic disease NEC E88.9 [G73.7]
    myxedema E03.9 [G73.7]
    parasitic disease NEC B89 [G73.7]
    polyarteritis nodosa M30.0 [G73.7]
    rheumatoid arthritis -see Rheumatoid,
    myopathy

Myopathy --*continued*
   sarcoidosis D86.87
   scleroderma M34.82
   sicca syndrome M35.03
   Sjögren's syndrome M35.03
   systemic lupus erythematosus M32.19
   thyrotoxicosis (hyperthyroidism) E05.90
     [*G73.7*]
     with thyroid storm E05.91 [*G73.7*]
   toxic agent NEC G72.2
  inflammatory NEC G72.49
  intensive care (ICU) G72.81
  limb-girdle G71.0
  mitochondrial NEC G71.3
  myotonic, proximal (PROMM) G71.11
  myotubular G71.2
  nemaline G71.2
  ocular G71.0
  oculopharyngeal G71.0
  of critical illness G72.81
  primary G71.9
   specified NEC G71.8
  progressive NEC G72.89
  proximal myotonic (PROMM) G71.11
  rod G71.2
  scapulohumeral G71.0
  specified NEC G72.89
  toxic G72.2
Myopericarditis -*see also* Pericarditis
  chronic rheumatic I09.2
Myopia (axial) (congenital) H52.1
  degenerative (malignant) H44.2
  malignant H44.2
  pernicious H44.2
  progressive high (degenerative) H44.2
Myosarcoma -*see* Neoplasm, connective
tissue, malignant
Myosis (pupil) H57.03
  stromal (endolymphatic) D39.0
Myositis M60.9
  clostridial A48.0
  due to posture -*see* Myositis, specified type
   NEC
  epidemic B33.0
  fibrosa or fibrous (chronic), Volkmann's
   T79.6
  foreign body granuloma -*see* Granuloma,
   foreign body
  in (due to)
   bilharziasis B65.9 [*M63.8*]
   cysticercosis B69.81
   leprosy A30.9 [*M63.8*]
   mycosis B49 [*M63.8*]
   sarcoidosis D86.87
   schistosomiasis B65.9 [*M63.8*]
   syphilis
    late A52.78
    secondary A51.49
   toxoplasmosis (acquired) B58.82
   trichinellosis B75 [*M63.8*]
   tuberculosis A18.09
  inclusion body [IBM] G72.41
  infective M60.009
   arm M60.002
    left M60.001
    right M60.000
   leg M60.005
    left M60.004
    right M60.003
   lower limb M60.005
    ankle M60.07

Myositis - *continued*
   foot M60.07
   lower leg M60.06
   thigh M60.05
   toe M60.07
  multiple sites M60.09
  specified site NEC M60.08
  upper limb M60.002
   finger M60.04
   forearm M60.03
   hand M60.04
   shoulder region M60.01
   upper arm M60.02
  interstitial M60.10
   ankle M60.17
   foot M60.17
   forearm M60.13
   hand M60.14
   lower leg M60.16
   multiple sites M60.19
   shoulder region M60.11
   specified site NEC M60.18
   thigh M60.15
   upper arm M60.12
  mycotic B49 [*M63.8*]
  orbital, chronic H05.12
  ossificans or ossifying (circumscripta) -*see*
  also Ossification, muscle, specified NEC
  in (due to)
   burns M61.30
    ankle M61.37
    foot M61.37
    forearm M61.33
    hand M61.34
    lower leg M61.36
    multiple sites M61.39
    pelvic region M61.35
    shoulder region M61.31
    specified site NEC M61.38
    thigh M61.35
    upper arm M61.32
   quadriplegia or paraplegia M61.20
    ankle M61.27
    foot M61.27
    forearm M61.23
    hand M61.24
    lower leg M61.26
    multiple sites M61.29
    pelvic region M61.25
    shoulder region M61.21
    specified site NEC M61.28
    thigh M61.25
    upper arm M61.22
  progressiva M61.10
   ankle M61.17
   finger M61.14
   foot M61.17
   forearm M61.13
   hand M61.14
   lower leg M61.16
   multiple sites M61.19
   pelvic region M61.15
   shoulder region M61.11
   specified site NEC M61.18
   thigh M61.15
   toe M61.17
   upper arm M61.12
  traumatica M61.00
   ankle M61.07
   foot M61.07
   forearm M61.03

Myositis - *continued*
   hand M61.04
   lower leg M61.06
   multiple sites M61.09
   pelvic region M61.05
   shoulder region M61.01
   specified site NEC M61.08
   thigh M61.05
   upper arm M61.02
  purulent -*see* Myositis, infective
  specified type NEC M60.80
   ankle M60.87
   foot M60.87
   forearm M60.83
   hand M60.84
   lower leg M60.86
   multiple sites M60.89
   pelvic region M60.85
   shoulder region M60.81
   specified site NEC M60.88
   thigh M60.85
   upper arm M60.82
  suppurative -*see* Myositis, infective
  traumatic (old) -*see* Myositis, specified type
  NEC
Myospasia impulsiva F95.2
Myotonia (acquisita) (intermittens) M62.89
  atrophica G71.11
  chondrodystrophic G71.13
  congenita (acetazolamide responsive)
   (dominant) (recessive) G71.12
  drug-induced G71.14
  dystrophica G71.11
  fluctuans G71.19
  levior G71.12
  permanens G71.19
  symptomatic G71.19
Myotonic pupil -*see* Anomaly, pupil, function,
  tonic pupil
Myriapodiasis B88.2
Myringitis H73.2
  with otitis media -*see* Otitis, media
  acute H73.00
   bullous H73.01
   specified NEC H73.09
  bullous -*see* Myringitis, acute, bullous
  chronic H73.1
Mysophobia F40.228
Mytilotoxism -*see* Poisoning, fish
Myxadenitis labialis K13.0
Myxedema (adult) (idiocy) (infantile)
  (juvenile) -*see also* Hypothyroidism E03.9
  circumscribed E05.90
   with storm E05.91
  coma E03.5
  congenital E00.1
  cutis L98.5
  localized (pretibial) E05.90
   with storm E05.91
  papular L98.5
Myxochondrosarcoma -*see* Neoplasm,
  cartilage, malignant
Myxofibroma -*see* Neoplasm, connective
tissue, benign
  odontogenic -*see* Cyst, calcifying odontogenic
Myxofibrosarcoma -*see* Neoplasm, connective
tissue, malignant
Myxolipoma D17.9
Myxoliposarcoma -*see* Neoplasm, connective
tissue, malignant

Myxoma -see also Neoplasm, connective
   tissue, benign
   nerve sheath -see Neoplasm, nerve, benign
   odontogenic -see Cyst, calcifying odontogenic
Myxosarcoma -see Neoplasm, connective
   tissue, malignant

N

Naegeli's
   disease Q82.8
   leukemia, monocytic C93.1
Naegleriasis (with meningoencephalitis)
   B60.2
Naffziger's syndrome G54.0
Naga sore -see Ulcer, skin
Nägele's pelvis M95.5
   with disproportion (fetopelvic) O33.0
     causing obstructed labor O65.0
Nail -see also condition
   biting F98.8
   patella syndrome Q87.2
Nanism, nanosomia -see Dwarfism
Nanophyetiasis B66.8
Nanukayami A27.89
Napkin rash L22
Narcolepsy G47.419
   with cataplexy G47.411
   in conditions classified elsewhere G47.429
     with cataplexy G47.421
Narcosis R06.89
Narcotism -see Dependence
NARP (Neuropathy, Ataxia and Retinitis
   pigmentosa) syndrome E88.49
Narrow
   anterior chamber angle H40.03
   gingival width (of periodontal soft tissue)
     K05.5
   pelvis -see Contraction, pelvis
Narrowing -see also Stenosis
   artery I77.1
     auditory, internal I65.8
     basilar -see Occlusion, artery, basilar
     carotid -see Occlusion, artery, carotid
     cerebellar -see Occlusion, artery, cerebellar
     cerebral -see Occlusion, artery, cerebral
     choroidal -see Occlusion, artery, cerebral,
       specified NEC
     communicating posterior -see Occlusion,
       artery, cerebral, specified NEC
     coronary -see also Disease, heart, ischemic,
       atherosclerotic
       congenital Q24.5
         syphilitic A50.54 [I52]
       due to syphilis NEC A52.06
     hypophyseal -see Occlusion, artery, cerebral,
       specified NEC
     pontine -see Occlusion, artery, cerebral,
       specified NEC
     precerebral -see Occlusion, artery,
       precerebral
     vertebral -see Occlusion, artery, vertebral
   auditory canal (external) -see Stenosis,
     external ear canal
   eustachian tube -see Obstruction, eustachian
     tube
   eyelid -see Disorder, eyelid function
   larynx J38.6
   mesenteric artery -see also Ischemia,
     intestine, acute K55.059
   palate M26.89

Narrowing --continued
   palpebral fissure -see Disorder, eyelid
   function
   ureter N13.5
     with infection N13.6
   urethra -see Stricture, urethra
Narrowness, abnormal, eyelid Q10.3
Nasal -see condition
Nasolachrymal, nasolacrimal -see condition
Nasopharyngeal -see also condition
   pituitary gland Q89.2
   torticollis M43.6
Nasopharyngitis (acute) (infective)
(streptococcal) (subacute) J00
   chronic (suppurative) (ulcerative) J31.1
Nasopharynx, nasopharyngeal -see condition
Natal tooth, teeth K00.6
Nausea (without vomiting) R11.0
   with vomiting R11.2
   gravidarum -see Hyperemesis, gravidarum
   marina T75.3
   navalis T75.3
Navel -see condition
Neapolitan fever -see Brucellosis
Near drowning T75.1
Nearsightedness -see Myopia
Near-syncope R55
Nebula, cornea -see Opacity, cornea
Necator americanus infestation B76.1
Necatoriasis B76.1
Neck -see condition **Necrobiosis** R68.89
   lipoidica NEC L92.1
     with diabetes -see E08 E13 with .620
Necrolysis, toxic epidermal L51.2
   due to drug
     correct substance properly administered -see
       Table of Drugs and Chemicals, by drug,
       adverse effect
     overdose or wrong substance given or taken
      -see Table of Drugs and Chemicals, by drug,
      poisoning
Necrophilia F65.89
Necrosis, necrotic (ischemic) -see also
   Gangrene
   adrenal (capsule) (gland) E27.49
   amputation stump (surgical) (late) T87.50
     arm T87.5
     leg T87.5
   antrum J32.0
   aorta (hyaline) -see also Aneurysm, aorta
     cystic medial -see Dissection, aorta
   artery I77.5
   bladder (aseptic) (sphincter) N32.89
   bone -see also Osteonecrosis M87.9
     aseptic or avascular -see Osteonecrosis
       idiopathic M87.00
     ethmoid J32.2
     jaw M27.2
     tuberculous -see Tuberculosis, bone
   brain I67.89
   breast (aseptic) (fat) (segmental) N64.1
   bronchus J98.09
   central nervous system NEC I67.89
   cerebellar I67.89
   cerebral I67.89
   colon -see also Infarct, intestine K55.049
   cornea H18.89
   cortical (acute) (renal) N17.1
   cystic medial (aorta) -see Dissection, aorta
   dental pulp K04.1
   esophagus K22.8

Necrosis, necrotic --continued
   ethmoid (bone) J32.2
   eyelid -see Disorder, eyelid, degenerative
   fat, fatty (generalized) -see also Disorder, soft
   tissue, specified type NEC
     abdominal wall K65.4
     breast (aseptic) (segmental) N64.1
     localized -see Degeneration, by site, fatty
     mesentery K65.4
     omentum K65.4
     pancreas K86.89
     peritoneum K65.4
     skin (subcutaneous), newborn P83.0
     subcutaneous, due to birth injury P15.6
   gallbladder -see Cholecystitis, acute
   heart -see Infarct, myocardium
   hip, aseptic or avascular -see Osteonecrosis,
   by type, femur
   intestine (acute) (hemorrhagic) (massive) -see
   also Infarct, intestine K55.069
   jaw M27.2
   kidney (bilateral) N28.0
     acute N17.9
     cortical (acute) (bilateral) N17.1
       with ectopic or molar pregnancy O08.4
     medullary (bilateral) (in acute renal failure)
       (papillary) N17.2
     papillary (bilateral) (in acute renal failure)
       N17.2
     tubular N17.0
       with ectopic or molar pregnancy O08.4
       complicating
         abortion -see Abortion, by type,
          complicated by, tubular necrosis
         ectopic or molar pregnancy O08.4
         pregnancy -see Pregnancy, complicated
          by, diseases of, specified type or system
          NEC
       following ectopic or molar pregnancy
         O08.4
       traumatic T79.5
   larynx J38.7
   liver (with hepatic failure) (cell) -see Failure,
   hepatic
     hemorrhagic, central K76.2
   lung J85.0
   lymphatic gland -see Lymphadenitis, acute
   mammary gland (fat) (segmental) N64.1
   mastoid (chronic) -see Mastoiditis, chronic
   medullary (acute) (renal) N17.2
   mesentery -see also Infarct, intestine K55.069
     fat K65.4
   mitral valve -see Insufficiency, mitral
   myocardium, myocardial -see Infarct,
     myocardium
   nose J34.0
   omentum (with mesenteric infarction) -see
   also Infarct, intestine K55.069
     fat K65.4
   orbit, orbital -see Osteomyelitis, orbit
   ossicles, ear -see Abnormal, ear ossicles
   ovary N70.92
   pancreas (aseptic) (duct) (fat) K86.89
     acute (infective) -see Pancreatitis, acute
     infective -see Pancreatitis, acute
   papillary (acute) (renal) N17.2
   perineum N90.89
   peritoneum (with mesenteric infarction) -see
   also Infarct, intestine K55.069
     fat K65.4
   pharynx J02.9

Necrosis, necrotic *--continued*
   in granulocytopenia *-see* Neutropenia
     Vincent's A69.1
   phosphorus *-see* subcategory T54.2
   pituitary (gland) E23.0
     postpartum O99.285
     Sheehan O99.285
   pressure *-see* Ulcer, pressure, by site
   pulmonary J85.0
   pulp (dental) K04.1
   radiation *-see* Necrosis, by site
   radium *-see* Necrosis, by site
   renal *-see* Necrosis, kidney   sclera H15.89
   scrotum N50.89
   skin or subcutaneous tissue NEC I96
   spine, spinal (column) *-see also*
    Osteonecrosis, by type, vertebra
     cord G95.19
   spleen D73.5
   stomach K31.89
   stomatitis (ulcerative) A69.0
   subcutaneous fat, newborn P83.8
   subendocardial (acute) I21.4
    chronic I25.89
   suprarenal (capsule) (gland) E27.49
   testis N50.89
   thymus (gland) E32.8
   tonsil J35.8
   trachea J39.8
   tuberculous NEC *-see* Tuberculosis
   tubular (acute) (anoxic) (renal) (toxic) N17.0
    postprocedural N99.0
   vagina N89.8
   vertebra *-see also* Osteonecrosis, by type,
    vertebra
    tuberculous A18.01
   vulva N90.89
   X ray *-see* Necrosis, by site
Necrospermia *-see* Infertility, male
Need (for)
   care provider because (of)
    assistance with personal care Z74.1
    continuous supervision required Z74.3
    impaired mobility Z74.09
    no other household member able to render
    care Z74.2
    specified reason NEC Z74.8
   immunization *-see* Vaccination
   vaccination *-see* Vaccination
Neglect
   adult
    confirmed T74.01
    history of Z91.412
    suspected T76.01
   child (childhood)
    confirmed T74.02
    history of Z62.812
    suspected T76.02
   emotional, in childhood Z62.898
   hemispatial R41.4
   left-sided R41.4
   sensory R41.4
   visuospatial R41.4
Neisserian infection NEC *-see* Gonococcus
Nélaton's syndrome G60.8
Nelson's syndrome E24.1
Nematodiasis (intestinal) B82.0
   Ancylostoma B76.0
Neonatal *-see also* Newborn
   acne L70.4
   bradycardia P29.12

Neonatal - *continued*
   tachycardia P29.11
   screening, abnormal findings on P09
   tooth, teeth K00.6
Neonatorum *-see* condition
Neoplasia
   endocrine, multiple (MEN) E31.20
    type I E31.21
    type IIA E31.22
    type IIB E31.23
   intraepithelial (histologically confirmed)
    anal (AIN) (histologically confirmed)
    K62.82
     grade I K62.82
     grade II K62.82
     severe D01.3
    cervical glandular (histologically confirmed)
    D06.9
    cervix (uteri) (CIN) (histologically
    confirmed) N87.9
     glandular D06.9
     grade I N87.0
     grade II N87.1
     grade III (severe dysplasia) *-see also*
     Carcinoma, cervix uteri, in situ D06.9
    prostate (histologically confirmed) (PIN)
    N42.31
     grade I N42.31
     grade II N42.31
     grade III (severe dysplasia) D07.5
    vagina (histologically confirmed) (VAIN)
    N89.3
     grade I N89.0
     grade II N89.1
     grade III (severe dysplasia) D07.2
    vulva (histologically confirmed) (VIN)
    N90.3
     grade I N90.0
     grade II N90.1
     grade III (severe dysplasia) D07.1
Neoplasm, neoplastic *-see also* Table of
   Neoplasms
   lipomatous, benign *-see* Lipoma
Neovascularization
   ciliary body *-see* Disorder, iris, vascular
   cornea H16.40
    deep H16.44
    ghost vessels *-see* Ghost, vessels
    localized H16.43
    pannus *-see* Pannus
   iris *-see* Disorder, iris, vascular
   retina H35.05
Nephralgia N23
Nephritis, nephritic (albuminuric)
(azotemic) (congenital) (disseminated)
(epithelial) (familial) (focal)
(granulomatous) (hemorrhagic) (infantile)
(nonsuppurative, excretory) (uremic) N05.9
   with
    dense deposit disease N05.6
    diffuse
     crescentic glomerulonephritis N05.7
     endocapillary proliferative
     glomerulonephritis N05.4
     membranous glomerulonephritis N05.2
     mesangial proliferative glomerulonephritis
     N05.3
     mesangiocapillary glomerulonephritis
     N05.5
   edema *-see* Nephrosis

Nephritis, nephritic *--continued*
   focal and segmental glomerular lesions
    N05.1
   foot process disease N04.9
   glomerular lesion
    diffuse sclerosing N05.8
    hypocomplementemic *-see* Nephritis,
     membranoproliferative
    IgA *-see* Nephropathy, IgA
    lobular, lobulonodular *-see* Nephritis,
     membranoproliferative
    nodular *-see* Nephritis,
     membranoproliferative
   lesion of
    glomerulonephritis, proliferative N05.8
    renal necrosis N05.9
   minor glomerular abnormality N05.0
   specified morphological changes NEC
    N05.8
   acute N00.9
   with
    dense deposit disease N00.6
    diffuse
     crescentic glomerulonephritis N00.7
     endocapillary proliferative
     glomerulonephritis N00.4
     membranous glomerulonephritis N00.2
     mesangial proliferative
     glomerulonephritis N00.3
     mesangiocapillary glomerulonephritis
     N00.5
    focal and segmental glomerular lesions
     N00.1
    minor glomerular abnormality N00.0
    specified morphological changes NEC
     N00.8
   amyloid E85.4 [*N08*]
   antiglomerular basement membrane (anti-
    GBM) antibody NEC
    in Goodpasture's syndrome M31.0
   antitubular basement membrane (tubulo-
    interstitial) NEC N12
    toxic *-see* Nephropathy, toxic
   arteriolar *-see* Hypertension, kidney
   arteriosclerotic *-see* Hypertension, kidney
   ascending *-see* Nephritis, tubulo-interstitial
   atrophic N03.9
   Balkan (endemic) N15.0
   calculous, calculus *-see* Calculus, kidney
   cardiac *-see* Hypertension, kidney
   cardiovascular *-see* Hypertension, kidney
   chronic N03.9
   with
    dense deposit disease N03.6
    diffuse
     crescentic glomerulonephritis N03.7
     endocapillary proliferative
     glomerulonephritis N03.4
     membranous glomerulonephritis N03.2
     mesangial proliferative
     glomerulonephritis N03.3
     mesangiocapillary glomerulonephritis
     N03.5
    focal and segmental glomerular lesions
     N03.1
    minor glomerular abnormality N03.0
    specified morphological changes NEC
     N03.8
   arteriosclerotic *-see* Hypertension, kidney
   cirrhotic N26.9
   complicating pregnancy O26.83

Nephritis, nephritic --*continued*
croupous N00.9
degenerative -*see* Nephrosis
diffuse sclerosing N05.8
due to
　diabetes mellitus -*see* E08 E13 with .21
　subacute bacterial endocarditis I33.0
　systemic lupus erythematosus (chronic)
　　M32.14
　typhoid fever A01.09
gonococcal (acute) (chronic) A54.21
hypocomplementemic -*see* Nephritis,
　membranoproliferative
IgA -*see* Nephropathy, IgA
immune complex (circulating) NEC N05.8
infective -*see* Nephritis, tubulo-interstitial
interstitial -*see* Nephritis, tubulo-interstitial
lead N14.3
membranoproliferative (diffuse) (type 1 or 3)
-*see also* N00 N07 with fourth character .5
N05.5
　type 2 -*see also* N00 N07 with fourth
　character .6 N05.6
minimal change N05.0
necrotic, necrotizing NEC -*see also* N00 N07
　with fourth character .8 N05.8
nephrotic -*see* Nephrosis
nodular -*see* Nephritis, membranoproliferative
polycystic Q61.3
　adult type Q61.2
　autosomal
　　dominant Q61.2
　　recessive NEC Q61.19
　childhood type NEC Q61.19
　infantile type NEC Q61.19
poststreptococcal N05.9
　acute N00.9
　chronic N03.9
　rapidly progressive N01.9
proliferative NEC -*see also* N00 N07 with
　fourth character .8 N05.8
purulent -*see* Nephritis, tubulo-interstitial
rapidly progressive N01.9
　with
　　dense deposit disease N01.6
　　diffuse
　　　crescentic glomerulonephritis N01.7
　　　endocapillary proliferative
　　　　glomerulonephritis N01.4
　　　membranous glomerulonephritis N01.2
　　　mesangial proliferative
　　　　glomerulonephritis N01.3
　　　mesangiocapillary glomerulonephritis
　　　　N01.5
　　　focal and segmental glomerular lesions
　　　　N01.1
　　　minor glomerular abnormality N01.0
　　　specified morphological changes NEC
　　　　N01.8
salt losing or wasting NEC N28.89
saturnine N14.3
sclerosing, diffuse N05.8
septic -*see* Nephritis, tubulo-interstitial
specified pathology NEC -*see also* N00 N07
　with fourth character .8 N05.8
subacute N01.9
suppurative -*see* Nephritis, tubulo-interstitial
syphilitic (late) A52.75
　congenital A50.59 [*N08*]
　early (secondary) A51.44
toxic -*see* Nephropathy, toxic

Nephritis, nephritic --*continued*
tubal, tubular -*see* Nephritis, tubulo-interstitial
tuberculous A18.11
tubulo-interstitial (in) N12
　acute (infectious) N10
　chronic (infectious) N11.9
　　nonobstructive N11.8
　　　reflux associated N11.0
　　obstructive N11.1
　　specified NEC N11.8
　due to
　　brucellosis A23.9 [*N16*]
　　cryoglobulinemia D89.1 [*N16*]
　　glycogen storage disease E74.00 [*N16*]
　　Sjögren's syndrome M35.04
　vascular -*see* Hypertension, kidney　war
　N00.9
Nephroblastoma (epithelial) (mesenchymal)
C64
Nephrocalcinosis E83.59 [*N29*]
Nephrocystitis, pustular -*see* Nephritis,
　tubulo-interstitial
Nephrolithiasis (congenital) (pelvis)
　(recurrent) -*see also* Calculus, kidney
Nephroma C64
　mesoblastic D41.0 **Nephronephritis** -*see*
　Nephrosis
Nephronophthisis Q61.5
Nephropathia epidemica A98.5
Nephropathy -*see also* Nephritis N28.9
　with
　　edema -*see* Nephrosis
　　glomerular lesion -*see* Glomerulonephritis
　amyloid, hereditary E85.0
　analgesic N14.0
　　with medullary necrosis, acute N17.2
　Balkan (endemic) N15.0
　chemical -*see* Nephropathy, toxic
　diabetic -*see* E08 E13 with .21
　drug-induced N14.2
　　specified NEC N14.1
　focal and segmental hyalinosis or sclerosis
　　N02.1
　heavy metal-induced N14.3
　hereditary NEC N07.9
　　with
　　　dense deposit disease N07.6
　　　diffuse
　　　　crescentic glomerulonephritis N07.7
　　　　endocapillary proliferative
　　　　　glomerulonephritis N07.4
　　　　membranous glomerulonephritis N07.2
　　　　mesangial proliferative
　　　　　glomerulonephritis N07.3
　　　　mesangiocapillary glomerulonephritis
　　　　　N07.5
　　　focal and segmental glomerular lesions
　　　　N07.1
　　　minor glomerular abnormality N07.0
　　　specified morphological changes NEC
　　　　N07.8
　hypercalcemic N25.89
　hypertensive -*see* Hypertension, kidney
　hypokalemic (vacuolar) N25.89
　IgA N02.8
　　with glomerular lesion N02.9
　　　focal and segmental hyalinosis or sclerosis
　　　　N02.1
　　membranoproliferative (diffuse) N02.5
　　membranous (diffuse) N02.2
　　mesangial proliferative (diffuse) N02.3

Nephropathy --*continued*
　mesangiocapillary (diffuse) N02.5
　proliferative NEC N02.8
　specified pathology NEC N02.8
lead N14.3
membranoproliferative (diffuse) N02.5
membranous (diffuse) N02.2
mesangial (IgA/IgG) -*see* Nephropathy, IgA
　proliferative (diffuse) N02.3
mesangiocapillary (diffuse) N02.5
obstructive N13.8
phenacetin N17.2
phosphate-losing N25.0
potassium depletion N25.89
pregnancy related O26.83
proliferative NEC -*see also* N00 N07 with
　fourth character .8 N05.8
protein-losing N25.89
saturnine N14.3
sickle-cell D57. [*N08*]
toxic NEC N14.4
　due to
　　drugs N14.2
　　　analgesic N14.0
　　　specified NEC N14.1
　　heavy metals N14.3
vasomotor N17.0
water-losing N25.89
Nephroptosis N28.83
Nephropyosis -*see* Abscess, kidney
Nephrorrhagia N28.89
Nephrosclerosis (arteriolar)(arteriosclerotic)
　(chronic) (hyaline) -*see also* Hypertension,
　kidney　hyperplastic -*see* Hypertension,
　kidney　senile N26.9
Nephrosis, nephrotic (Epstein's) (syndrome)
　(congenital) N04.9
　with
　　foot process disease N04.9
　　glomerular lesion N04.1
　　hypocomplementemic N04.5
　acute N04.9
　anoxic -*see* Nephrosis, tubular
　chemical -*see* Nephrosis, tubular
　cholemic K76.7
　diabetic -*see* E08 E13 with .21
　Finnish type (congenital) Q89.8
　hemoglobin N10
　hemoglobinuric -*see* Nephrosis, tubular
　in
　　amyloidosis E85.4 [*N08*]
　　diabetes mellitus -*see* E08 E13 with .21
　　epidemic hemorrhagic fever A98.5
　　malaria (malariae) B52.0
　ischemic -*see* Nephrosis, tubular
　lipoid N04.9
　lower nephron -*see* Nephrosis, tubular
　malarial (malariae) B52.0
　minimal change N04.0
　myoglobin N10
　necrotizing -*see* Nephrosis, tubular
　osmotic (sucrose) N25.89
　radiation N04.9
　syphilitic (late) A52.75
　toxic -*see* Nephrosis, tubular
　tubular (acute) N17.0
　　postprocedural N99.0
　　radiation N04.9
Nephrosonephritis, hemorrhagic (endemic)
A98.5

Nephrostomy
  attention to Z43.6
  status Z93.6
Nerve -*see also* condition
  injury -*see* Injury, nerve, by body site **Nerves**
    R45.0
Nervous -*see also* condition R45.0
  heart F45.8
  stomach F45.8
  tension R45.0
Nervousness R45.0
Nesidioblastoma
  pancreas D13.7
  specified site NEC -*see* Neoplasm, benign, by
    site
  unspecified site D13.7
Nettleship's syndrome Q82.2
Neumann's disease or syndrome L10.1
Neuralgia, neuralgic (acute) M79.2
  accessory (nerve) G52.8
  acoustic (nerve) -*see* subcategory H93.3
  auditory (nerve) -*see* subcategory H93.3
  ciliary G44.009
    intractable G44.001
    not intractable G44.009
  cranial
    nerve -*see also* Disorder, nerve, cranial
      fifth or trigeminal -*see* Neuralgia,
        trigeminal
      postherpetic, postzoster B02.29
  ear -*see* subcategory H92.0
  facialis vera G51.1
  Fothergill's -*see* Neuralgia, trigeminal
  glossopharyngeal (nerve) G52.1
  Horton's G44.099
    intractable G44.091
    not intractable G44.099
  Hunt's B02.21
  hypoglossal (nerve) G52.3
  infraorbital -*see* Neuralgia, trigeminal
  malarial -*see* Malaria
  migrainous G44.009
    intractable G44.001
    not intractable G44.009
  Morton's G57.6
  nerve, cranial -*see* Disorder, nerve, cranial
  nose G52.0
  occipital M54.81
  olfactory G52.0
  penis N48.9
  perineum R10.2
  postherpetic NEC B02.29
    trigeminal B02.22
  pubic region R10.2
  scrotum R10.2
  Sluder's G44.89
  specified nerve NEC G58.8
  spermatic cord R10.2
  sphenopalatine (ganglion) G90.09
  trifacial -*see* Neuralgia, trigeminal
  trigeminal G50.0
    postherpetic, postzoster B02.22
  vagus (nerve) G52.2
  writer's F48.8
    organic G25.89
Neurapraxia -*see* Injury, nerve
Neurasthenia F48.8
  cardiac F45.8
  gastric F45.8
  heart F45.8

Neurilemmoma -*see also* Neoplasm, nerve,
    benign
  acoustic (nerve) D33.3
  malignant -*see also* Neoplasm, nerve,
    malignant
    acoustic (nerve) C72.4
Neurilemmosarcoma -*see* Neoplasm, nerve,
    malignant
Neurinoma -*see* Neoplasm, nerve, benign
Neurinomatosis -*see* Neoplasm, nerve,
    uncertain behavior
Neuritis (rheumatoid) M79.2
  abducens (nerve) -*see* Strabismus, paralytic,
    sixth nerve
  accessory (nerve) G52.8
  acoustic (nerve) -*see also* subcategory H93.3
    in (due to)
      infectious disease NEC B99 [*H94.0*]
      parasitic disease NEC B89 [*H94.0*]
    syphilitic A52.15
  alcoholic G62.1
    with psychosis -*see* Psychosis, alcoholic
  amyloid, any site E85.4 [*G63*]
  auditory (nerve) -*see* subcategory H93.3
  brachial -*see* Radiculopathy
    due to displacement, intervertebral disc -*see*
    Disorder, disc, cervical, with neuritis
  cranial nerve
    due to Lyme disease A69.22
    eighth or acoustic or auditory -*see*
      subcategory H93.3
    eleventh or accessory G52.8
    fifth or trigeminal G51.0
    first or olfactory G52.0
    fourth or trochlear -*see* Strabismus,
      paralytic, fourth nerve
    second or optic -*see* Neuritis, optic
    seventh or facial G51.8
      newborn (birth injury) P11.3
    sixth or abducent -*see* Strabismus, paralytic,
      sixth nerve
    tenth or vagus G52.2
    third or oculomotor -*see* Strabismus,
      paralytic, third nerve
    twelfth or hypoglossal G52.3
  Déjérine-Sottas G60.0
  diabetic (mononeuropathy) -*see* E08 E13 with
    .41
    polyneuropathy -*see* E08 E13 with .42
  due to
    beriberi E51.11
    displacement, prolapse or rupture,
      intervertebral disc -*see* Disorder, disc, with,
      radiculopathy
    herniation, nucleus pulposus M51.9 [*G55*]
  endemic E51.11
  facial G51.8
    newborn (birth injury) P11.3
  general -*see* Polyneuropathy
  geniculate ganglion G51.1
    due to herpes (zoster) B02.21
  gouty -*see also* Gout, by type M10.9 [*G63*]
  hypoglossal (nerve) G52.3
  ilioinguinal (nerve) G57.9
  infectious (multiple) NEC G61.0
  interstitial hypertrophic progressive G60.0
  lumbar M54.16
  lumbosacral M54.17
  multiple -*see also* Polyneuropathy
    endemic E51.11
    infective, acute G61.0

Neuritis - *continued*
  multiplex endemica E51.11
  nerve root -*see* Radiculopathy
  oculomotor (nerve) -*see* Strabismus, paralytic,
    third nerve
  olfactory nerve G52.0
  optic (nerve) (hereditary) (sympathetic) H46.9
    with demyelination G36.0
    in myelitis G36.0
    nutritional H46.2
    papillitis -*see* Papillitis, optic
    retrobulbar H46.1
    specified type NEC H46.8
    toxic H46.3
  peripheral (nerve) G62.9
    multiple -*see* Polyneuropathy
    single -*see* Mononeuritis
  pneumogastric (nerve) G52.2
  postherpetic, postzoster B02.29
  progressive hypertrophic interstitial G60.0
  retrobulbar -*see also* Neuritis, optic,
    retrobulbar
    in (due to)
      late syphilis A52.15
      meningococcal infection A39.82
    meningococcal A39.82
    syphilitic A52.15
  sciatic (nerve) -*see also* Sciatica
    due to displacement of intervertebral disc -
      see Disorder, disc, with, radiculopathy
  serum -*see also* Reaction, serum T80.69
  shoulder-girdle G54.5
  specified nerve NEC G58.8
  spinal (nerve) root -*see* Radiculopathy
  syphilitic A52.15
  thenar (median) G56.1
  thoracic M54.14
  toxic NEC G62.2
  trochlear (nerve) -*see* Strabismus, paralytic,
    fourth nerve
  vagus (nerve) G52.2
Neuroastrocytoma -*see* Neoplasm, uncertain
    behavior, by site
Neuroavitaminosis E56.9 [*G99.8*]
Neuroblastoma - olfactory C30.0
  specified site -*see* Neoplasm, malignant, by
    site
  unspecified site C74.90
Neurochorioretinitis -*see* Chorioretinitis
Neurocirculatory asthenia F45.8
Neurocysticercosis B69.0
Neurocytoma -*see* Neoplasm, benign, by site
Neurodermatitis (circumscribed)
    (circumscripta) (local) L28.0
  atopic L20.81
  diffuse (Brocq) L20.81
  disseminated L20.81
Neuroencephalomyelopathy, optic G36.0
Neuroepithelioma -*see also* Neoplasm,
    malignant, by site
  olfactory C30.0
Neurofibroma -*see also* Neoplasm, nerve,
    benign
  melanotic -*see* Neoplasm, nerve, benign
  multiple -*see* Neurofibromatosis
  plexiform -*see* Neoplasm, nerve, benign

Neurofibromatosis (multiple) (nonmalignant) Q85.00
  acoustic Q85.02
  malignant -see Neoplasm, nerve, malignant
  specified NEC Q85.09
  type 1(von Recklinghausen) Q85.01
  type 2Q85.02
Neurofibrosarcoma -see Neoplasm, nerve, malignant
Neurogenic -see also condition
  bladder -see also Dysfunction, bladder, neuromuscular N31.9
    cauda equina syndrome G83.4
  bowel NEC K59.2
  heart F45.8
Neuroglioma -see Neoplasm, uncertain behavior, by site
Neurolabyrinthitis (of Dix and Hallpike) -see Neuronitis, vestibular
Neurolathyrism -see Poisoning, food, noxious, plant
Neuroleprosy A30.9
Neuroma -see also Neoplasm, nerve, benign
  acoustic (nerve) D33.3
  amputation (stump) (traumatic) (surgical complication) (late) T87.3
    arm T87.3
    leg T87.3
  digital (toe) G57.6
  interdigital G58.8
    lower limb (toe) G57.8
    upper limb G56.8
  intermetatarsal G57.8
  Morton's G57.6
  nonneoplastic
    arm G56.9
    leg G57.9
    lower extremity G57.9
    upper extremity G56.9
  optic (nerve) D33.3
  plantar G57.6
  plexiform -see Neoplasm, nerve, benign
  surgical (nonneoplastic)
    arm G56.9
    leg G57.9
    lower extremity G57.9
    upper extremity G56.9
Neuromyalgia -see Neuralgia
Neuromyasthenia (epidemic) (postinfectious) G93.3
Neuromyelitis G36.9
  ascending G61.0
  optica G36.0
Neuromyopathy G70.9
  paraneoplastic D49.9 [G13.0]
Neuromyotonia (Isaacs) G71.19
Neuronevus -see Nevus
Neuronitis G58.9
  ascending (acute) G57.2
  vestibular H81.2
Neuroparalytic -see condition
Neuropathy, neuropathic G62.9
  acute motor G62.81
  alcoholic G62.1
    with psychosis -see Psychosis, alcoholic
  arm G56.9
  autonomic, peripheral -see Neuropathy, peripheral, autonomic
  axillary G56.9
  bladder N31.9
    atonic (motor) (sensory) N31.2

Neuropathy, neuropathic --continued
  autonomous N31.2
  flaccid N31.2
  nonreflex N31.2
  reflex N31.1
  uninhibited N31.0
  brachial plexus G54.0
  cervical plexus G54.2
  chronic
    progressive segmentally demyelinating G62.89
    relapsing demyelinating G62.89
  Déjérine-Sottas G60.0
  diabetic -see E08 E13 with .40
    mononeuropathy -see E08 E13 with .41
    polyneuropathy -see E08 E13 with .42
  entrapment G58.9
    iliohypogastric nerve G57.8
    ilioinguinal nerve G57.8
    lateral cutaneous nerve of thigh G57.1
    median nerve G56.0
    obturator nerve G57.8
    peroneal nerve G57.3
    posterior tibial nerve G57.5
    saphenous nerve G57.8
    ulnar nerve G56.2
  facial nerve G51.9
  hereditary G60.9
    motor and sensory (types I-IV) G60.0
    sensory G60.8
    specified NEC G60.8
  hypertrophic G60.0
    Charcot-Marie-Tooth G60.0
    Déjérine-Sottas G60.0
    interstitial progressive G60.0
    of infancy G60.0
    Refsum G60.1
  idiopathic G60.9
    progressive G60.3
    specified NEC G60.8
  in association with hereditary ataxia G60.2
  intercostal G58.8
  ischemic -see Disorder, nerve
  Jamaica (ginger) G62.2
  leg NEC G57.9
  lower extremity G57.9
  lumbar plexus G54.1
  median nerve G56.1
  motor and sensory -see also Polyneuropathy
    hereditary (types I-IV) G60.0
  multifocal motor (MMN) G61.82
  multiple (acute) (chronic) -see Polyneuropathy
  optic (nerve) -see also Neuritis, optic
    ischemic H47.01
  paraneoplastic (sensorial) (Denny Brown) D49.9 [G13.0]
  peripheral (nerve) -see also Polyneuropathy G62.9
    autonomic G90.9
      idiopathic G90.09
      in (due to)
        amyloidosis E85.4 [G99.0]
        diabetes mellitus -see E08 E13 with .43
        endocrine disease NEC E34.9 [G99.0]
        gout M10.00 [G99.0]
        hyperthyroidism E05.90 [G99.0]
          with thyroid storm E05.91 [G99.0]
        metabolic disease NEC E88.9 [G99.0]
    idiopathic G60.9
      progressive G60.3

Neuropathy, neuropathic --continued
  in (due to)
    antitetanus serum G62.0
    arsenic G62.2
    drugs NEC G62.0
    lead G62.2
    organophosphate compounds G62.2
    toxic agent NEC G62.2
  plantar nerves G57.6
  progressive
    hypertrophic interstitial G60.0
    inflammatory G62.81
  radicular NEC -see Radiculopathy
  sacral plexus G54.1
  sciatic G57.0
  serum G61.1
  toxic NEC G62.2
  trigeminal sensory G50.8
  ulnar nerve G56.2
  uremic N18.9 [G63]
  vitamin B12 E53.8 [G63]
    with anemia (pernicious) D51.0 [G63]
    due to dietary deficiency D51.3 [G63]
Neurophthisis -see also Disorder, nerve
  peripheral, diabetic -see E08 E13 with .42
Neuroretinitis -see Chorioretinitis
Neuroretinopathy, hereditary optic H47.22
Neurosarcoma -see Neoplasm, nerve, malignant
Neurosclerosis -see Disorder, nerve
Neurosis, neurotic F48.9
  anankastic F42.8
  anxiety (state) F41.1
    panic type F41.0
  asthenic F48.8
  bladder F45.8
  cardiac (reflex) F45.8
  cardiovascular F45.8
  character F60.9
  colon F45.8
  compensation F68.1
  compulsive, compulsion F42.8
  conversion F44.9
  craft F48.8
  cutaneous F45.8
  depersonalization F48.1
  depressive (reaction) (type) F34.1
  environmental F48.8
  excoriation L98.1
  fatigue F48.8
  functional -see Disorder, somatoform
  gastric F45.8
  gastrointestinal F45.8
  heart F45.8
  hypochondriacal F45.21
  hysterical F44.9
  incoordination F45.8
    larynx F45.8
    vocal cord F45.8
  intestine F45.8
  larynx (sensory) F45.8
    hysterical F44.4
  mixed NEC F48.8
  musculoskeletal F45.8
  obsessional F42.8
  obsessive-compulsive F42.8
  occupational F48.8
  ocular NEC F45.8
  organ -see Disorder, somatoform
  pharynx F45.8
  phobic F40.9

Neurosis, neurotic --*continued*
  posttraumatic (situational) F43.10
    acute F43.11
    chronic F43.12
  psychasthenic (type) F48.8
  railroad F48.8
  rectum F45.8
  respiratory F45.8
  rumination F45.8
  sexual F65.9
  situational F48.8
  social F40.10
    generalized F40.11
  specified type NEC F48.8
  state F48.9
    with depersonalization episode F48.1
  stomach F45.8
  traumatic F43.10
    acute F43.11
    chronic F43.12
  vasomotor F45.8
  visceral F45.8
  war F48.8
Neurospongioblastosis diffusa Q85.1
Neurosyphilis (arrested) (early) (gumma) (late) (latent) (recurrent) (relapse) A52.3
  with ataxia (cerebellar) (locomotor) (spastic) (spinal) A52.19
  aneurysm (cerebral) A52.05
  arachnoid (adhesive) A52.13
  arteritis (any artery) (cerebral) A52.04
  asymptomatic A52.2
  congenital A50.40
  dura (mater) A52.13
  general paresis A52.17
  hemorrhagic A52.05
  juvenile (asymptomatic) (meningeal) A50.40
  leptomeninges (aseptic) A52.13
  meningeal, meninges (adhesive) A52.13
  meningitis A52.13
  meningovascular (diffuse) A52.13
  optic atrophy A52.15
  parenchymatous (degenerative) A52.19
  paresis, paretic A52.17
    juvenile A50.45
  remission in (sustained) A52.3
  serological (without symptoms) A52.2
  specified nature or site NEC A52.19
  tabes, tabetic (dorsalis) A52.11
    juvenile A50.45
  taboparesis A52.17
    juvenile A50.45
  thrombosis (cerebral) A52.05
  vascular (cerebral) NEC A52.05
Neurothekeoma -*see* Neoplasm, nerve, benign
Neurotic -*see* Neurosis
Neurotoxemia -*see* Toxemia
Neuroclusion M26.211
Neutropenia, neutropenic (chronic) (genetic) (idiopathic) (immune) (infantile) (malignant) (pernicious) (splenic) D70.9
  congenital (primary) D70.0
  cyclic D70.4
  cytoreductive cancer chemotherapy sequela D70.1
  drug-induced D70.2
    due to cytoreductive cancer chemotherapy D70.1
  due to infection D70.3
  fever D70.9

Neutropenia, neutropenic --*continued*
  neonatal, transitory (isoimmune) (maternal transfer) P61.5
  periodic D70.4
  secondary (cyclic) (periodic) (splenic) D70.4
    drug-induced D70.2
      due to cytoreductive cancer chemotherapy D70.1
  toxic D70.8
Neutrophilia, hereditary giant D72.0
Nevocarcinoma -*see* Melanoma **Nevus** D22.9
  achromic -*see* Neoplasm, skin, benign
  amelanotic -*see* Neoplasm, skin, benign
  angiomatous D18.00
    intra-abdominal D18.03
    intracranial D18.02
    skin D18.01
    specified site NEC D18.09
  araneus I78.1
  balloon cell -*see* Neoplasm, skin, benign
  bathing trunk D48.5
  blue -*see* Neoplasm, skin, benign
    cellular -*see* Neoplasm, skin, benign
    giant -*see* Neoplasm, skin, benign
    Jadassohn's -*see* Neoplasm, skin, benign
    malignant -*see* Melanoma
  capillary D18.00
    intra-abdominal D18.03
    intracranial D18.02
    skin D18.01
    specified site NEC D18.09
  cavernous D18.00
    intra-abdominal D18.03
    intracranial D18.02
    skin D18.01
    specified site NEC D18.09
  cellular -*see* Neoplasm, skin, benign
    blue -*see* Neoplasm, skin, benign
  choroid D31.3
  comedonicus Q82.5
  conjunctiva D31.0
  dermal -*see* Neoplasm, skin, benign
    with epidermal nevus -*see* Neoplasm, skin, benign
  dysplastic -*see* Neoplasm, skin, benign
  eye D31.9
  flammeus Q82.5
  hemangiomatous D18.00
    intra-abdominal D18.03
    intracranial D18.02
    skin D18.01
    specified site NEC D18.09
  iris D31.4
  lacrimal gland D31.5
  lymphatic D18.1
  magnocellular
    specified site -*see* Neoplasm, benign, by site
    unspecified site D31.40
  malignant -*see* Melanoma
  meaning hemangioma D18.00
    intra-abdominal D18.03
    intracranial D18.02
    skin D18.01
    specified site NEC D18.09
  mouth (mucosa) D10.30
    specified site NEC D10.39
    white sponge Q38.6
  multiplex Q85.1
  non-neoplastic I78.1
  oral mucosa D10.30
    specified site NEC D10.39

Nevocarcinoma --*continued*
  white sponge Q38.6
  orbit D31.6
  pigmented
    giant -*see also* Neoplasm, skin, uncertain behavior D48.5
      malignant melanoma in -*see* Melanoma
  portwine Q82.5
  retina D31.2
  retrobulbar D31.6
  sanguineous Q82.5
  senile I78.1
  skin D22.9
    abdominal wall D22.5
    ala nasi D22.39
    ankle D22.7
    anus, anal D22.5
    arm D22.6
    auditory canal (external) D22.2
    auricle (ear) D22.2
    auricular canal (external) D22.2
    axilla, axillary fold D22.5
    back D22.5
    breast D22.5
    brow D22.39
    buttock D22.5
    canthus (eye) D22.1
    cheek (external) D22.39
    chest wall D22.5
    chin D22.39
    ear (external) D22.2
    external meatus (ear) D22.2
    eyebrow D22.39
    eyelid (lower) (upper) D22.1
    face D22.30
      specified NEC D22.39
    female genital organ (external) NEC D28.0
    finger D22.6
    flank D22.5
    foot D22.7
    forearm D22.6
    forehead D22.39
    foreskin D29.0
    genital organ (external) NEC
      female D28.0
      male D29.9
    gluteal region D22.5
    groin D22.5
    hand D22.6
    heel D22.7
    helix D22.2
    hip D22.7
    interscapular region D22.5
    jaw D22.39
    knee D22.7
    labium (majus) (minus) D28.0
    leg D22.7
    lip (lower) (upper) D22.0
    lower limb D22.7
    male genital organ (external) D29.9
    nail D22.9
      finger D22.6
      toe D22.7
    nasolabial groove D22.39
    nates D22.5
    neck D22.4
    nose (external) D22.39
    palpebra D22.1
    penis D29.0
    perianal skin D22.5
    perineum D22.5

Nevocarcinoma --*continued*
  pinna D22.2
  popliteal fossa or space D22.7
  prepuce D29.0
  pudendum D28.0
  scalp D22.4
  scrotum D29.4
  shoulder D22.6
  submammary fold D22.5
  temple D22.39
  thigh D22.7
  toe D22.7
  trunk NEC D22.5
  umbilicus D22.5
  upper limb D22.6
  vulva D28.0
  specified site NEC -*see* Neoplasm, by site,
    benign
  spider I78.1
  stellar I78.1
  strawberry Q82.5
  Sutton's -*see* Neoplasm, skin, benign
  unius lateris Q82.5
  Unna's Q82.5
  vascular Q82.5
  verrucous Q82.5

Newborn (infant) (liveborn) (singleton)
    Z38.2
  acne L70.4
  abstinence syndrome P96.1
  affected by
    abnormalities of membranes P02.9
      specified NEC P02.8
    abruptio placenta P02.1
    amino-acid metabolic disorder, transitory
      P74.8
    amniocentesis (while in utero) P00.6
    amnionitis P02.7
    apparent life threatening event (ALTE)
      R68.13
    bleeding (into)
      cerebral cortex P52.22
      germinal matrix P52.0
      ventricles P52.1
    breech delivery P03.0
    cardiac arrest P29.81
    cardiomyopathy I42.8
      congenital I42.4
    cerebral ischemia P91.0
    Cesarean delivery P03.4
    chemotherapy agents P04.1
    chorioamnionitis P02.7
    cocaine (crack) P04.41
    complications of labor and delivery P03.9
      specified NEC P03.89
    compression of umbilical cord NEC P02.5
    contracted pelvis P03.1
    delivery P03.9
      Cesarean P03.4
      forceps P03.2
      vacuum extractor P03.3
    environmental chemicals P04.6
    entanglement (knot) in umbilical cord P02.5
    fetal (intrauterine)
      growth retardation P05.9
      malnutrition not light or small for
        gestational age P05.2
    forceps delivery P03.2
    heart rate abnormalities
      bradycardia P29.12
      intrauterine P03.819

Newborn - *continued*
    before onset of labor P03.810
    during labor P03.811
  tachycardia P29.11
  hemorrhage (antepartum) P02.1
    cerebellar (nontraumatic) P52.6
    intracerebral (nontraumatic) P52.4
    intracranial (nontraumatic) P52.9
      specified NEC P52.8
    intraventricular (nontraumatic) P52.3
      grade 1 P52.0
      grade 2 P52.1
      grade 3 P52.21
      grade 4 P52.22
    posterior fossa (nontraumatic) P52.6
    subarachnoid (nontraumatic) P52.5
    subependymal P52.0
      with intracerebral extension P52.22
      with intraventricular extension P52.1
        with enlargement of ventricles P52.21
      without intraventricular extension P52.0
  hypoxic ischemic encephalopathy [HIE]
    P91.60
    mild P91.61
    moderate P91.62
    severe P91.63
  induction of labor P03.89
  intestinal perforation P78.0
  intrauterine (fetal) blood loss P50.9
    due to (from)
      cut end of co-twin cord P50.5
      hemorrhage into
        co-twin P50.3
        maternal circulation P50.4
      placenta P50.2
      ruptured cord blood P50.1
      vasa previa P50.0
    specified NEC P50.8
  intrauterine (fetal) hemorrhage P50.9
  intrauterine (in utero) procedure P96.5
  malpresentation (malposition) NEC P03.1
  maternal (complication of) (use of)
    alcohol P04.3
    analgesia (maternal) P04.0
    anesthesia (maternal) P04.0
    blood loss P02.1
    circulatory disease P00.3
    condition P00.9
      specified NEC P00.89
    delivery P03.9
      Cesarean P03.4
      forceps P03.2
      vacuum extractor P03.3
    diabetes mellitus (pre-existing) P70.1
    disorder P00.9
      specified NEC P00.89
    drugs (addictive) (illegal) NEC P04.49
    ectopic pregnancy P01.4
    gestational diabetes P70.0
    hemorrhage P02.1
    hypertensive disorder P00.0
    incompetent cervix P01.0
    infectious disease P00.2
    injury P00.5
    labor and delivery P03.9
    malpresentation before labor P01.7
    maternal death P01.6
    medical procedure P00.7
    medication P04.1
    multiple pregnancy P01.5
    nutritional disorder P00.4

Newborn - *continued*
    oligohydramnios P01.2
    parasitic disease P00.2
    periodontal disease P00.81
    placenta previa P02.0
    polyhydramnios P01.3
    precipitate delivery P03.5
    pregnancy P01.9
      specified P01.8
    premature rupture of membranes P01.1
    renal disease P00.1
    respiratory disease P00.3
    surgical procedure P00.6
    urinary tract disease P00.1
    uterine contraction (abnormal) P03.6
  meconium peritonitis P78.0
  medication (legal) (maternal use)
    (prescribed) P04.1
  membrane abnormalities P02.9
    specified NEC P02.8
  membranitis P02.7
  methamphetamine(s) P04.49
  mixed metabolic and respiratory acidosis
    P84
  neonatal abstinence syndrome P96.1
  noxious substances transmitted via placenta
    or breast milk P04.9
    specified NEC P04.8
  nutritional supplements P04.5
  placenta previa P02.0
  placental
    abnormality (functional) (morphological)
      P02.20
      specified NEC P02.29
    dysfunction P02.29
    infarction P02.29
    insufficiency P02.29
    separation NEC P02.1
    transfusion syndromes P02.3
  placentitis P02.7
  precipitate delivery P03.5
  prolapsed cord P02.4
  respiratory arrest P28.81
  slow intrauterine growth P05.9
  tobacco P04.2
  twin to twin transplacental transfusion P02.3
  umbilical cord (tightly) around neck P02.5
  umbilical cord condition P02.60
    short cord P02.69
    specified NEC P02.69
  uterine contractions (abnormal) P03.6
  vasa previa P02.69
    from intrauterine blood loss P50.0
  apnea P28.4
    primary P28.3
    obstructive P28.4
    sleep (central) (obstructive) (primary) P28.3
  born in hospital Z38.00
    by cesarean Z38.01
  born outside hospital Z38.1
  breast buds P96.89
  breast engorgement P83.4
  check-up -*see* Newborn, examination
  convulsion P90
  dehydration P74.1
  examination
    8 to 28 days old Z00.111
    under 8 days old Z00.110
  fever P81.9
    environmentally induced P81.0
  hyperbilirubinemia P59.9

Newborn - *continued*
  of prematurity P59.0
  hypernatremia P74.2
  hyponatremia P74.2
  infection P39.9
    candidal P37.5
    specified NEC P39.8
    urinary tract P39.3
  jaundice P59.9
    due to
      breast milk inhibitor P59.3
      hepatocellular damage P59.20
        specified NEC P59.29
      preterm delivery P59.0
    of prematurity P59.0
    specified NEC P59.8
  late metabolic acidosis P74.0
  mastitis P39.0
    infective P39.0
    noninfective P83.4
  multiple born NEC Z38.8
    born in hospital Z38.68
      by cesarean Z38.69
    born outside hospital Z38.7
  omphalitis P38.9
    with mild hemorrhage P38.1
    without hemorrhage P38.9
  post-term P08.21
  prolonged gestation (over 42 completed
    weeks) P08.22
  quadruplet Z38.8
    born in hospital Z38.63
      by cesarean Z38.64
    born outside hospital Z38.7
  quintuplet Z38.8
    born in hospital Z38.65
      by cesarean Z38.66
    born outside hospital Z38.7
  seizure P90
  sepsis (congenital) P36.9
    due to
      anaerobes NEC P36.5
      Escherichia coli P36.4
      Staphylococcus P36.30
        aureus P36.2
        specified NEC P36.39
      Streptococcus P36.10
        group B P36.0
        specified NEC P36.19
      specified NEC P36.8
  triplet Z38.8
    born in hospital Z38.61
      by cesarean Z38.62
    born outside hospital Z38.7
  twin Z38.5
    born in hospital Z38.30
      by cesarean Z38.31
    born outside hospital Z38.4
  vomiting P92.09
    bilious P92.01
  weight check Z00.111
Newcastle conjunctivitis or disease B30.8
Nezelof's syndrome (pure alymphocytosis)
  D81.4
Niacin (amide) deficiency E52
Nicolas (Durand) Favre disease A55
Nicotine -*see* Tobacco
Nicotinic acid deficiency E52
Niemann-Pick disease or syndrome E75.249
  specified NEC E75.248
  type

Niemann-Pick disease --*continued*
  A E75.240
  B E75.241
  C E75.242
  D E75.243
Night
  blindness -*see* Blindness, night
  sweats R61
  terrors (child) F51.4
Nightmares (REM sleep type) F51.5
**NIHSS (National Institutes of Health Stroke
  Scale) score** R29.7
Nipple -*see* condition
Nisbet's chancre A57
Nishimoto (Takeuchi) disease I67.5
Nitritoid crisis or reaction -*see* Crisis,
  nitritoid
Nitrosohemoglobinemia D74.8
Njovera A65
Nocardiosis, nocardiasis A43.9
  cutaneous A43.1
  lung A43.0
  pneumonia A43.0
  pulmonary A43.0
  specified site NEC A43.8
Nocturia R35.1
  psychogenic F45.8
Nocturnal -*see* condition
Nodal rhythm I49.8
Node(s) -*see also* Nodule
  Bouchard's (with arthropathy) M15.2
  Haygarth's M15.8
  Heberden's (with arthropathy) M15.1
  larynx J38.7
  lymph -*see* condition
  milker's B08.03
  Osler's I33.0
  Schmorl's -*see* Schmorl's disease
  singer's J38.2
  teacher's J38.2
  tuberculous -*see* Tuberculosis, lymph gland
  vocal cord J38.2
Nodule(s), nodular
  actinomycotic -*see* Actinomycosis
  breast NEC N63
  colloid (cystic), thyroid E04.1
  cutaneous -*see* Swelling, localized
  endometrial (stromal) D26.1
  Haygarth's M15.8
  inflammatory -*see* Inflammation
  juxta-articular
    syphilitic A52.77
    yaws A66.7
  larynx J38.7
  lung, solitary (subsegmental branch of the
    bronchial tree) R91.1
    multiple R91.8
  milker's B08.03
  prostate N40.2
    with lower urinary tract symptoms (LUTS)
      N40.3
    without lower urinary tract symptoms
      (LUTS) N40.2
  pulmonary, solitary (subsegmental branch of
    the bronchial tree) R91.1
  retrocardiac R09.89
  rheumatoid M06.30
    ankle M06.37
    elbow M06.32
    foot joint M06.37
    hand joint M06.34

Nodule(s), nodular - *continued*
  hip M06.35
  knee M06.36
  multiple site M06.39
  shoulder M06.31
  vertebra M06.38
  wrist M06.33
  scrotum (inflammatory) N49.2
  singer's J38.2
  solitary, lung (subsegmental branch of the
    bronchial tree) R91.1
    multiple R91.8
  subcutaneous -*see* Swelling, localized
  teacher's J38.2
  thyroid (cold) (gland) (nontoxic) E04.1
    with thyrotoxicosis E05.20
      with thyroid storm E05.21
    toxic or with hyperthyroidism E05.20
      with thyroid storm E05.21
  vocal cord J38.2
Noma (gangrenous) (hospital) (infective)
  A69.0
  auricle I96
  mouth A69.0
  pudendi N76.89
  vulvae N76.89
Nomad, nomadism Z59.0
**NOMID (neonatal onset multisystemic
  inflammatory disorder)** M04.2
Nonautoimmune hemolytic anemia D59.4
  drug-induced D59.2
Nonclosure -*see also* Imperfect, closure
  ductus arteriosus (Botallo's) Q25.0
  foramen
    botalli Q21.1
    ovale Q21.1
Noncompliance Z91.19
  with
    dietary regimen Z91.11
    dialysis Z91.15
    medical treatment Z91.19
    medication regimen NEC Z91.14
      underdosing -*see also* Table of Drugs and
        Chemicals, categories T36 T50, with final
        character 6 Z91.14
        intentional NEC Z91.128
          due to financial hardship of patient
            Z91.120
        unintentional NEC Z91.138
          due to patient's age related debility
            Z91.130
    renal dialysis Z91.15
Nondescent (congenital) -*see also*
  Malposition, congenital
  cecum Q43.3
  colon Q43.3
  testicle Q53.9
    bilateral Q53.20
      abdominal Q53.21
      perineal Q53.22
    unilateral Q53.10
      abdominal Q53.11
      perineal Q53.12
Nondevelopment
  brain Q02
    part of Q04.3
  heart Q24.8
  organ or site, congenital NEC -*see* Hypoplasia
Nonengagement
  head NEC O32.4
    in labor, causing obstructed labor O64.8

Nonexanthematous tick fever A93.2
Nonexpansion, lung (newborn) P28.0
Nonfunctioning
  cystic duct -*see also* Disease, gallbladder
    K82.8
  gallbladder -*see also* Disease, gallbladder
    K82.8
  kidney N28.9
  labyrinth -*see* subcategory H83.2
Non-Hodgkin lymphoma NEC -*see*
  Lymphoma, non-Hodgkin
Non-working side interference M26.56
Nonimplantation, ovum N97.2
Noninsufflation, fallopian tube N97.1
Non-ketotic hyperglycinemia E72.51
Nonne-Milroy syndrome Q82.0
Nonovulation N97.0
Nonpatent fallopian tube N97.1
Nonpneumatization, lung NEC P28.0
Nonrotation -*see* Malrotation
Nonsecretion, urine -*see* Anuria
Nonunion
  fracture -*see* Fracture, by site
  joint, following fusion or arthrodesis M96.0
  organ or site, congenital NEC -*see* Imperfect,
    closure
  symphysis pubis, congenital Q74.2
Nonvisualization, gallbladder R93.2
Nonvital, nonvitalized tooth K04.99
Noonan's syndrome Q87.1
Normocytic anemia (infectional) due to
  blood loss (chronic) D50.0
  acute D62
Norrie's disease (congenital) Q15.8
North American blastomycosis B40.9
Norwegian itch B86
Nose, nasal -*see* condition
Nosebleed R04.0
Nose-picking F98.8
Nosomania F45.21
Nosophobia F45.22
Nostalgia F43.20
Notch of iris Q13.2
Notching nose, congenital (tip) Q30.2
Nothnagel's
  syndrome -*see* Strabismus, paralytic, third
    nerve
  vasomotor acroparesthesia I73.89
Novy's relapsing fever A68.9
  louse-borne A68.0
  tick-borne A68.1
Noxious
  foodstuffs, poisoning by -*see* Poisoning, food,
    noxious, plant
  substances transmitted through placenta or
    breast milk P04.9
Nucleus pulposus -*see* condition
Numbness R20.0
Nuns' knee -*see* Bursitis, prepatellar
Nursemaid's elbow S53.03
Nutcracker esophagus K22.4
Nutmeg liver K76.1
Nutrient element deficiency E61.9
  specified NEC E61.8
Nutrition deficient or insufficient -*see also*
  Malnutrition E46
  due to
    insufficient food T73.0
    lack of
      care (child) T76.02
        adult T76.01
      food T73.0

Nutritional stunting E45
Nyctalopia (night blindness) -*see* Blindness,
  night
Nycturia R35.1
  psychogenic F45.8
Nymphomania F52.8
Nystagmus H55.00
  benign paroxysmal -*see* Vertigo, benign
    paroxysmal
  central positional H81.4
  congenital H55.01
  dissociated H55.04
  latent H55.02
  miners' H55.09
  positional
    benign paroxysmal H81.4
    central H81.4
  specified form NEC H55.09
  visual deprivation H55.03

O

Obermeyer's relapsing fever (European)
  A68.0
Obesity E66.9
  with alveolar hypoventilation E66.2
  adrenal E27.8
  complicating
    childbirth O99.214
    pregnancy O99.21
    puerperium O99.215
  constitutional E66.8
  dietary counseling and surveillance Z71.3
  drug-induced E66.1
  due to
    drug E66.1
    excess calories E66.09
      morbid E66.01
      severe E66.01
  endocrine E66.8
  endogenous E66.8
  exogenous E66.09
  familial E66.8
  glandular E66.8
  hypothyroid -*see* Hypothyroidism
  hypoventilation syndrome (OHS) E66.2
  morbid E66.01
    with
      alveolar hypoventilation E66.2
      obesity hypoventilation syndrome (OHS)
        E66.2
    due to excess calories E66.01
  nutritional E66.09
  pituitary E23.6
  severe E66.01
  specified type NEC E66.8
Oblique -*see* condition
Obliteration
  appendix (lumen) K38.8
  artery I77.1
  bile duct (noncalculous) K83.1
  common duct (noncalculous) K83.1
  cystic duct -*see* Obstruction, gallbladder
  disease, arteriolar I77.1
  endometrium N85.8
  eye, anterior chamber -*see* Disorder, globe,
    hypotony   fallopian tube N97.1
  lymphatic vessel I89.0
    due to mastectomy I97.2
  organ or site, congenital NEC -*see* Atresia, by
    site

Obliteration - *continued*
  ureter N13.5
    with infection N13.6
  urethra -*see* Stricture, urethra
  vein I87.8
  vestibule (oral) K08.89
Observation (following) (for) (without need
  for further medical care) Z04.9
  accident NEC Z04.3
    at work Z04.2
    transport Z04.1
  adverse effect of drug Z03.6
  alleged rape or sexual assault (victim), ruled
  out
    adult Z04.41
    child Z04.42
  criminal assault Z04.8
  development state
    adolescent Z00.3
    period of rapid growth in childhood Z00.2
    puberty Z00.3
  disease, specified NEC Z03.89
  following work accident Z04.2
  growth and development state -*see*
    Observation, development state
  injuries (accidental) NEC -*see also*
    Observation, accident
  newborn (for)
    suspected condition, related to exposure
      from the mother or birth process -*see*
      Newborn, affected by, maternal
      ruled out Z05.9
        cardiac Z05.0
        connective tissue Z05.73
        gastrointestinal Z05.5
        genetic Z05.41
        genitourinary Z05.6
        immunologic Z05.43
        infectious Z05.1
        metabolic Z05.42
        musculoskeletal Z05.72
        neurological Z05.2
        respiratory Z05.3
        skin and subcutaneous tissue Z05.71
        specified condition NEC Z05.8
  postpartum
    immediately after delivery Z39.0
    routine follow-up Z39.2
  pregnancy (normal) (without complication)
    Z34.9
    high risk O09.9
  suicide attempt, alleged NEC Z03.89
    self-poisoning Z03.6
  suspected, ruled out -*see also* Suspected
  condition, ruled out
    abuse, physical
      adult Z04.71
      child Z04.72
    accident at work Z04.2
    adult battering victim Z04.71
    child battering victim Z04.72
    condition NEC Z03.89
      newborn -*see also* Observation, newborn
      (for), suspected condition, ruled out Z05.9
    drug poisoning or adverse effect Z03.6
    exposure (to)
      anthrax Z03.810
      biological agent NEC Z03.818
    inflicted injury NEC Z04.8
    suicide attempt, alleged Z03.89
      self-poisoning Z03.6

Observation - *continued*
  toxic effects from ingested substance (drug)
    (poison) Z03.6
  toxic effects from ingested substance (drug)
    (poison) Z03.6
Obsession, obsessional state F42.8
  mixed thoughts and acts F42.2
Obsessive-compulsive neurosis or reaction
  F42.8
Obstetric embolism, septic *-see* Embolism,
  obstetric, septic
Obstetrical trauma (complicating delivery)
  O71.9
  with or following ectopic or molar pregnancy
    O08.6
  specified type NEC O71.89
Obstipation *-see* Constipation
Obstruction, obstructed, obstructive
  airway J98.8
    with
      allergic alveolitis J67.9
      asthma J45.909
        with
          exacerbation (acute) J45.901
          status asthmaticus J45.902
      bronchiectasis J47.9
        with
          exacerbation (acute) J47.1
          lower respiratory infection J47.0
      bronchitis (chronic) J44.9
      emphysema J43.9
    chronic J44.9
      with
        allergic alveolitis *-see* Pneumonitis,
          hypersensitivity
        bronchiectasis J47.9
          with
            exacerbation (acute) J47.1
            lower respiratory infection J47.0
    due to
      foreign body *-see* Foreign body, by site,
        causing asphyxia
      inhalation of fumes or vapors J68.9
      laryngospasm J38.5
  ampulla of Vater K83.1
  aortic (heart) (valve) *-see* Stenosis, aortic
  aortoiliac I74.09
  aqueduct of Sylvius G91.1
    congenital Q03.0
      with spina bifida *-see* Spina bifida, by site,
  with hydrocephalus
  Arnold-Chiari *-see* Arnold-Chiari disease
  artery *-see also* Embolism, artery I74.9
    stent *-see* Restenosis, stent
    basilar (complete) (partial) *-see* Occlusion,
      artery, basilar
    carotid (complete) (partial) *-see* Occlusion,
      artery, carotid
    cerebellar *-see* Occlusion, artery, cerebellar
    cerebral (anterior) (middle) (posterior) *-see*
      Occlusion, artery, cerebral
    precerebral *-see* Occlusion, artery,
      precerebral
    renal N28.0
    retinal NEC *-see* Occlusion, artery, retina
    vertebral (complete) (partial) *-see* Occlusion,
      artery, vertebral
  band (intestinal) K56.69
  bile duct or passage (common) (hepatic)
  (noncalculus) K83.1
    with calculus K80.51

Obstruction, obstructed, obstructive --
continued
  congenital (causing jaundice) Q44.3
  biliary (duct) (tract) K83.1
    gallbladder K82.0
  bladder-neck (acquired) N32.0
    congenital Q64.31
    due to hyperplasia (hypertrophy) of prostate
      -see Hyperplasia, prostate
  bowel *-see* Obstruction, intestine
  bronchus J98.09
  canal, ear *-see* Stenosis, external ear canal
  cardia K22.2
  caval veins (inferior) (superior) I87.1
  cecum *-see* Obstruction, intestine
  circulatory I99.8
  colon *-see* Obstruction, intestine
  common duct (noncalculous) K83.1
  coronary (artery) *-see* Occlusion, coronary
  cystic duct *-see also* Obstruction, gallbladder
    with calculus K80.21
  device, implant or graft *-see also*
  Complications, by site and type, mechanical
  T85.698
    arterial graft NEC *-see* Complication,
    cardiovascular device, mechanical, vascular
    catheter NEC T85.628
      cystostomy T83.090
      dialysis (renal) T82.49
        intraperitoneal T85.691
      Hopkins T83.098
      ileostomy T83.098
      infusion NEC T82.594
        spinal (epidural) (subdural) T85.690
      nephrostomy T83.092
      urethral indwelling T83.091
      urinary T83.098
      urostomy T83.098
    due to infection T85.79
    gastrointestinal *-see* Complications,
      prosthetic device, mechanical,
      gastrointestinal device
    genital NEC T83.498
      intrauterine contraceptive device T83.39
      penile prosthesis (cylinder) (implanted)
        (pump) (reservoir) T83.490
      testicular prosthesis T83.491
    heart NEC *-see* Complication,
      cardiovascular device, mechanical
    joint prosthesis *-see* Complications, joint
      prosthesis, mechanical, specified NEC, by
      site
    orthopedic NEC *-see* Complication,
      orthopedic, device, mechanical
    specified NEC T85.628
    urinary NEC *-see also* Complication,
      genitourinary, device, urinary, mechanical
      graft T83.29
    vascular NEC *-see* Complication,
      cardiovascular device, mechanical
    ventricular intracranial shunt T85.09
  due to foreign body accidentally left in
    operative wound T81.529
  duodenum K31.5
  ejaculatory duct N50.89
  esophagus K22.2
  eustachian tube (complete) (partial) H68.10
    cartilaginous (extrinsic) H68.13
      intrinsic H68.12
    osseous H68.11
  fallopian tube (bilateral) N97.1

Obstruction, obstructed, obstructive --
continued
  fecal K56.41
    with hernia *-see* Hernia, by site, with
      obstruction
  foramen of Monro (congenital) Q03.8
    with spina bifida *-see* Spina bifida, by site,
      with hydrocephalus
  foreign body *-see* Foreign body
  gallbladder K82.0
    with calculus, stones K80.21
    congenital Q44.1
  gastric outlet K31.1
  gastrointestinal *-see* Obstruction, intestine
  hepatic K76.89
    duct (noncalculous) K83.1
  hepatobiliary K83.1
  ileum *-see* Obstruction, intestine
  iliofemoral (artery) I74.5
  intestine K56.60
    with
      adhesions (intestinal) (peritoneal) K56.5
    adynamic K56.0
    by gallstone K56.3
    congenital (small) Q41.9
      large Q42.9
        specified part NEC Q42.8
    neurogenic K56.0
      Hirschsprung's disease or megacolon
      Q43.1
    newborn P76.9
      due to
        fecaliths P76.8
        inspissated milk P76.2
        meconium (plug) P76.0
          in mucoviscidosis E84.11
      specified NEC P76.8
    postoperative K91.3
    reflex K56.0
    specified NEC K56.69
    volvulus K56.2
  intracardiac ball valve prosthesis T82.09
  jejunum *-see* Obstruction, intestine
  joint prosthesis *-see* Complications, joint
  prosthesis, mechanical, specified NEC, by site
  kidney (calices) N28.89
  labor *-see* Delivery
  lacrimal (passages) (duct)
    by
      dacryolith *-see* Dacryolith
      stenosis *-see* Stenosis, lacrimal
    congenital Q10.5
    neonatal H04.53
  lacrimonasal duct *-see* Obstruction, lacrimal
  lacteal, with steatorrhea K90.2
  laryngitis *-see* Laryngitis
  larynx NEC J38.6
    congenital Q31.8
  lung J98.4
    disease, chronic J44.9
  lymphatic I89.0
  meconium (plug)
    newborn P76.0
      due to fecaliths P76.0
      in mucoviscidosis E84.11
  mitral *-see* Stenosis, mitral
  nasal J34.89
  nasolacrimal duct *-see also* Obstruction,
  lacrimal
    congenital Q10.5
  nasopharynx J39.2

Obstruction, obstructed, obstructive --
continued
nose J34.89
organ or site, congenital NEC -*see* Atresia, by
site
pancreatic duct K86.89
parotid duct or gland K11.8
pelviureteral junction N13.5
with hydronephrosis N13.0
congenital Q62.39
pharynx J39.2
portal (circulation) (vein) I81
prostate -*see also* Hyperplasia, prostate
valve (urinary) N32.0
pulmonary valve (heart) I37.0
pyelonephritis (chronic) N11.1
pylorus
adult K31.1
congenital or infantile Q40.0
rectosigmoid -*see* Obstruction, intestine
rectum K62.4
renal N28.89
outflow N13.8
pelvis, congenital Q62.39
respiratory J98.8
chronic J44.9
retinal (vessels) H34.9
salivary duct (any) K11.8
with calculus K11.5
sigmoid -*see* Obstruction, intestine
sinus (accessory) (nasal) J34.89
Stensen's duct K11.8
stomach NEC K31.89
acute K31.0
congenital Q40.2
due to pylorospasm K31.3
submandibular duct K11.8
submaxillary gland K11.8
with calculus K11.5
thoracic duct I89.0
thrombotic -*see* Thrombosis
trachea J39.8
tracheostomy airway J95.03
tricuspid (valve) -*see* Stenosis, tricuspid
upper respiratory, congenital Q34.8
ureter (functional) (pelvic junction) NEC
N13.5
with
hydronephrosis N13.1
with infection N13.6
pyelonephritis (chronic) N11.1
congenital Q62.39
due to calculus -*see* Calculus, ureter
urethra NEC N36.8
congenital Q64.39
urinary (moderate) N13.9
due to hyperplasia (hypertrophy) of prostate
-*see* Hyperplasia, prostate
organ or tract (lower) N13.9
prostatic valve N32.0
specified NEC N13.8
uropathy N13.9
uterus N85.8
vagina N89.5
valvular -*see* Endocarditis
vein, venous I87.1
caval (inferior) (superior) I87.1
thrombotic -*see* Thrombosis
vena cava (inferior) (superior) I87.1
vesical NEC N32.0
vesicourethral orifice N32.0

Obstruction, obstructed, obstructive --
continued
congenital Q64.31
vessel NEC I99.8
stent -*see* Restenosis, stent
Obturator -*see* condition
Occlusal wear, teeth K03.0
Occlusio pupillae -*see* Membrane, pupillary
Occlusion, occluded
anus K62.4
congenital Q42.3
with fistula Q42.2
aortoiliac (chronic) I74.09
aqueduct of Sylvius G91.1
congenital Q03.0
with spina bifida -*see* Spina bifida, by site,
with hydrocephalus
artery -*see also* Embolism, artery I74.9
auditory, internal I65.8
basilar I65.1
with
infarction I63.22
due to
embolism I63.12
thrombosis I63.02
brain or cerebral I66.9
with infarction (due to) I63.5
embolism I63.4
thrombosis I63.3
carotid I65.2
with
infarction I63.23
due to
embolism I63.13
thrombosis I63.03
cerebellar (anterior inferior) (posterior
inferior) (superior) I66.3
with infarction I63.54
due to
embolism I63.44
thrombosis I63.34
cerebral I66.9
with infarction I63.50
due to
embolism I63.40
specified NEC I63.49
thrombosis I63.30
specified NEC I63.39
anterior I66.1
with infarction I63.52
due to
embolism I63.42
thrombosis I63.32
middle I66.0
with infarction I63.51
due to
embolism I63.41
thrombosis I63.31
posterior I66.2
with infarction I63.53
due to
embolism I63.43
thrombosis I63.33
specified NEC I66.8
with infarction I63.59
due to
embolism I63.4
thrombosis I63.3
choroidal (anterior) -*see* Occlusion, artery,
precerebral, specified NEC

Occlusion, occluded --*continued*
communicating posterior -*see* Occlusion,
artery, cerebral, specified NEC
complete
coronary I25.82
extremities I70.92
coronary (acute) (thrombotic) (without
myocardial infarction) I24.0
with myocardial infarction -*see* Infarction,
myocardium
chronic total I25.82
complete I25.82
healed or old I25.2
total (chronic) I25.82
hypophyseal -*see* Occlusion, artery,
precerebral, specified NEC
iliac I74.5
lower extremities due to stenosis or stricture
I77.1
mesenteric (embolic) (thrombotic) -*see also*
Infarct, intestine K55.069
perforating -*see* Occlusion, artery, cerebral,
specified NEC
peripheral I77.9
thrombotic or embolic I74.4
pontine -*see* Occlusion, artery, cerebral,
specified NEC
precerebral I65.9
with infarction I63.20
specified NEC I63.29
due to
embolism I63.10
specified NEC I63.19
thrombosis I63.00
specified NEC I63.09
basilar -*see* Occlusion, artery, basilar
carotid -*see* Occlusion, artery, carotid
puerperal O88.23
specified NEC I65.8
with infarction I63.29
due to
embolism I63.19
thrombosis I63.00
vertebral -*see* Occlusion, artery, vertebral
renal N28.0
retinal
central H34.1
partial H34.21
branch H34.23
transient H34.0
spinal -*see* Occlusion, artery, precerebral,
vertebral
total (chronic)
coronary I25.82
extremities I70.92
vertebral I65.0
with
infarction I63.21
due to
embolism I63.11
thrombosis I63.01
basilar artery -*see* Occlusion, artery, basilar
bile duct (common) (hepatic) (noncalculous)
K83.1
bowel -*see* Obstruction, intestine
carotid (artery) (common) (internal) -*see*
Occlusion, artery, carotid
centric (of teeth) M26.59
maximum intercuspation discrepancy
M26.55

Occlusion, occluded --*continued*
cerebellar (artery) -*see* Occlusion, artery, cerebellar
cerebral (artery) -*see* Occlusion, artery, cerebral
cerebrovascular -*see also* Occlusion, artery, cerebral
  with infarction I63.5
cervical canal -*see* Stricture, cervix
cervix (uteri) -*see* Stricture, cervix
choanal Q30.0
choroidal (artery) -*see* Occlusion, artery, precerebral, specified NEC
colon -*see* Obstruction, intestine
communicating posterior artery -*see* Occlusion, artery, precerebral, specified NEC
coronary (artery) (vein) (thrombotic) -*see also* Infarct, myocardium
  chronic total I25.82
  healed or old I25.2
  not resulting in infarction I24.0
  total (chronic) I25.82
cystic duct -*see* Obstruction, gallbladder
embolic -*see* Embolism
fallopian tube N97.1
  congenital Q50.6
gallbladder -*see also* Obstruction, gallbladder
  congenital (causing jaundice) Q44.1
gingiva, traumatic K06.2
hymen N89.6
  congenital Q52.3
hypophyseal (artery) -*see* Occlusion, artery, precerebral, specified NEC
iliac artery I74.5
intestine -*see* Obstruction, intestine
lacrimal passages -*see* Obstruction, lacrimal
lung J98.4
lymph or lymphatic channel I89.0
mammary duct N64.89
mesenteric artery (embolic) (thrombotic) -*see also* Infarct, intestine K55.069
nose J34.89
  congenital Q30.0
organ or site, congenital NEC -*see* Atresia, by site
oviduct N97.1
  congenital Q50.6
peripheral arteries
  due to stricture or stenosis I77.1
  upper extremity I74.2
pontine (artery) -*see* Occlusion, artery, precerebral, specified NEC
posterior lingual, of mandibular teeth M26.29
precerebral artery -*see* Occlusion, artery, precerebral
punctum lacrimale -*see* Obstruction, lacrimal
pupil -*see* Membrane, pupillary
pylorus, adult -*see also* Stricture, pylorus K31.1
renal artery N28.0
retina, retinal
  artery -*see* Occlusion, artery, retinal
  vein (central) H34.81
   engorgement H34.82
   tributary H34.83
  vessels H34.9
spinal artery -*see* Occlusion, artery, precerebral, vertebral
teeth (mandibular) (posterior lingual) M26.29
thoracic duct I89.0

Occlusion, occluded --*continued*
thrombotic -*see* Thrombosis, artery
traumatic
  edentulous (alveolar) ridge K06.2
  gingiva K06.2
  periodontal K05.5
tubal N97.1
ureter (complete) (partial) N13.5
  congenital Q62.10
ureteropelvic junction N13.5
  congenital Q62.11
ureterovesical orifice N13.5
  congenital Q62.12
urethra -*see* Stricture, urethra
uterus N85.8
vagina N89.5
vascular NEC I99.8
vein -*see* Thrombosis
  retinal -*see* Occlusion, retinal, vein
vena cava (inferior) (superior) -*see* Embolism, vena cava
ventricle (brain) NEC G91.1
vertebral (artery) -*see* Occlusion, artery, vertebral
vessel (blood) I99.8
vulva N90.5
Occult
blood in feces (stools) R19.5
Occupational
problems NEC Z56.89
Ochlophobia -*see* Agoraphobia
Ochronosis (endogenous) E70.29
Ocular muscle -*see* condition
Oculogyric crisis or disturbance H51.8
psychogenic F45.8
Oculomotor syndrome H51.9
Oculopathy
syphilitic NEC A52.71
  congenital
   early A50.01
   late A50.30
  early (secondary) A51.43
  late A52.71
Oddi's sphincter spasm K83.4
Odontalgia K08.89
Odontoameloblastoma -*see* Cyst, calcifying odontogenic
Odontoclasia K03.89
Odontodysplasia, regional K00.4
Odontogenesis imperfecta K00.5
Odontoma (ameloblastic) (complex) (compound) (fibroameloblastic) -*see* Cyst, calcifying odontogenic
Odontomyelitis (closed) (open) K04.01
irreversible K04.02
reversible K04.01
Odontorrhagia K08.89
Odontosarcoma, ameloblastic C41.1
upper jaw (bone) C41.0
Oestriasis -*see* Myiasis
Oguchi's disease H53.63
Ohara's disease -*see* Tularemia
OHS (obesity hypoventilation syndrome) E66.2
Oidiomycosis -*see* Candidiasis
Oidium albicans infection -*see* Candidiasis
Old age (without mention of debility) R54
dementia F03
Old (previous) myocardial infarction I25.2
Olfactory -*see* condition
Oligemia -*see* Anemia

Oligoastrocytoma
specified site -*see* Neoplasm, malignant, by site
unspecified site C71.9
Oligocythemia D64.9
Oligodendroblastoma
specified site -*see* Neoplasm, malignant
unspecified site C71.9
Oligodendroglioma
anaplastic type
  specified site -*see* Neoplasm, malignant, by site
  unspecified site C71.9
specified site -*see* Neoplasm, malignant, by site
unspecified site C71.9
Oligodontia -*see* Anodontia
Oligoencephalon Q02
Oligohidrosis L74.4
Oligohydramnios O41.0
Oligohidrosis L74.4
Oligomenorrhea N91.5
primary N91.3
secondary N91.4
Oligophrenia -*see also* Disability, intellectual
phenylpyruvic E70.0
Oligospermia N46.11
due to
  drug therapy N46.121
  efferent duct obstruction N46.123
  infection N46.122
  radiation N46.124
  specified cause NEC N46.129
  systemic disease N46.125
Oligotrichia -*see* Alopecia
Oliguria R34
with, complicating or following ectopic or molar pregnancy O08.4
postprocedural N99.0
Ollier's disease Q78.4
Omentitis -*see* Peritonitis
Omenotocele -*see* Hernia, abdomen, specified site NEC
Omentum, omental -*see* condition
Omphalitis (congenital) (newborn) P38.9
with mild hemorrhage P38.1
without hemorrhage P38.9
not of newborn L08.82
tetanus A33
Omphalocele Q79.2
Omphalomesenteric duct, persistent Q43.0
Omphalorrhagia, newborn P51.9
Omsk hemorrhagic fever A98.1
Onanism (excessive) F98.8
Onchocerciasis, onchocercosis B73.1
with
  eye disease B73.00
   endophthalmitis B73.01
   eyelid B73.09
   glaucoma B73.02
   specified NEC B73.09
  eye NEC B73.00
  eyelid B73.09
Oncocytoma -*see* Neoplasm, benign, by site
Oncovirus, as cause of disease classified elsewhere B97.32
Ondine's curse -*see* Apnea, sleep
Oneirophrenia F23
Onychauxis L60.2
congenital Q84.5

Onychia -see also Cellulitis, digit
  with lymphangitis -see Lymphangitis, acute,
    digit
  candidal B37.2
  dermatophytic B35.1
Onychitis -see also Cellulitis, digit
  with lymphangitis -see Lymphangitis, acute,
    digit
Onychocryptosis L60.0
Onychodystrophy L60.3
  congenital Q84.6
Onychogryphosis, onychogryposis L60.2
Onycholysis L60.1
Onychomadesis L60.8
Onychomalacia L60.3
Onychomycosis (finger) (toe) B35.1
Onycho-osteodysplasia Q87.2
Onychophagia F98.8
Onychophosis L60.8
Onychoptosis L60.8
Onychorrhexis L60.3
  congenital Q84.6
Onychoschizia L60.3
Onyxis (finger) (toe) L60.0
Onyxitis -see also Cellulitis, digit
  with lymphangitis -see Lymphangitis, acute,
    digit
Oophoritis (cystic) (infectional) (interstitial)
  N70.92
  with salpingitis N70.93
  acute N70.02
    with salpingitis N70.03
  chronic N70.12
    with salpingitis N70.13
  complicating abortion -see Abortion, by type,
  complicated by, oophoritis
Oophorocele N83.4
Opacity, opacities - cornea H17.
  central H17.1
  congenital Q13.3
  degenerative -see Degeneration, cornea
  hereditary -see Dystrophy, cornea
  inflammatory -see Keratitis
  minor H17.81
  peripheral H17.82
  sequelae of trachoma (healed) B94.0
  specified NEC H17.89
  enamel (teeth) (fluoride) (nonfluoride) K00.3
  lens -see Cataract
  snowball -see Deposit, crystalline
  vitreous (humor) NEC H43.39
    congenital Q14.0
    membranes and strands H43.31
Opalescent dentin (hereditary) K00.5
Open, opening
  abnormal, organ or site, congenital -see
    Imperfect, closure
  angle with
    borderline
      findings
        high risk H40.02
        low risk H40.01
      intraocular pressure H40.00
    cupping of discs H40.01
    glaucoma (primary) -see Glaucoma, open
    angle
  bite
    anterior M26.220
    posterior M26.221
  false -see Imperfect, closure
  margin on tooth restoration K08.51
  restoration margins of tooth K08.51
  wound -see Wound, open

Operational fatigue F48.8
Operative -see condition
Operculitis -see Periodontitis
Operculum -see Break, retina
Ophiasis L63.2
Ophthalmia -see also Conjunctivitis H10.9
  actinic rays -see Photokeratitis
  allergic (acute) -see Conjunctivitis, acute,
    atopic
  blennorrhagic (gonococcal) (neonatorum)
    A54.31
  diphtheritic A36.86
  Egyptian A71.1
  electrica -see Photokeratitis
  gonococcal (neonatorum) A54.31
  metastatic -see Endophthalmitis, purulent
  migraine -see Migraine, ophthalmoplegic
  neonatorum, newborn P39.1
    gonococcal A54.31
  nodosa H16.24
  purulent -see Conjunctivitis, acute,
    mucopurulent
  spring -see Conjunctivitis, acute, atopic
  sympathetic -see Uveitis, sympathetic
Ophthalmitis -see Ophthalmia
Ophthalmocele (congenital) Q15.8
Ophthalmoneuromyelitis G36.0
Ophthalmoplegia -see also Strabismus,
  paralytic
  anterior internuclear -see Ophthalmoplegia,
    internuclear
  ataxia-areflexia G61.0
  diabetic -see E08 E13 with .39
  exophthalmic E05.00
    with thyroid storm E05.01
  external H49.88
    progressive H49.4
      with pigmentary retinopathy -see Kearns-
        Sayre syndrome
    total H49.3
  internal (complete) (total) H52.51
  internuclear H51.2
  migraine -see Migraine, ophthalmoplegic
  Parinaud's H49.88
  progressive external -see Ophthalmoplegia,
    external, progressive
  supranuclear, progressive G23.1
  total (external) -see Ophthalmoplegia,
    external, total
Opioid(s)
  abuse -see Abuse, drug, opioids
  dependence -see Dependence, drug, opioids
  induced, without use disorder
    anxiety disorder F11.988
    delirium F11.921
    depressive disorder F11.94
    sexual dysfunction F11.981
    sleep disorder F11.982
Opisthognathism M26.09
Opisthorchiasis (felineus) (viverrini) B66.0
Opitz' disease D73.2
Opiumism -see Dependence, drug, opioid
Oppenheim's disease G70.2
Oppenheim-Urbach disease (necrobiosis
  lipoidica diabeticorum) -see E08 E13 with
  .620
Optic nerve -see condition
Orbit -see condition
Orchioblastoma C62.9
Orchitis (gangrenous) (nonspecific) (septic)
  (suppurative) N45.2

Orchitis - continued
  blennorrhagic (gonococcal) (acute) (chronic)
    A54.23
  chlamydial A56.19
  filarial -see also Infestation, filarial B74.9
    [N51]
  gonococcal (acute) (chronic) A54.23
  mumps B26.0
  syphilitic A52.76
  tuberculous A18.15
ORF (virus disease) B08.02
Organic -see also condition
  brain syndrome F09
  heart -see Disease, heart
  mental disorder F09
  psychosis F09
Orgasm
  anejaculatory N53.13
Oriental
  bilharziasis B65.2
  schistosomiasis B65.2
Orifice -see condition
Origin of both great vessels from right
  ventricle Q20.1
Ormond's disease (with ureteral
  obstruction) N13.5
  with infection N13.6
Ornithine metabolism disorder E72.4
Ornithinemia (Type I) (Type II) E72.4
Ornithosis A70
Orotaciduria, oroticaciduria (congenital)
  (hereditary) (pyrimidine deficiency) E79.8
  anemia D53.0
Orthodontics
  adjustment Z46.4
  fitting Z46.4
Orthopnea R06.01
Orthopoxvirus B08.09
  specified NEC B08.09
Os, uterus -see condition
Osgood-Schlatter disease or osteochondrosis
  -see Osteochondrosis, juvenile, tibia
Osler (Weber) Rendu disease I78.0
Osler's nodes I33.0
Osmidrosis L75.0
Osseous -see condition
Ossification
  artery -see Arteriosclerosis
  auricle (ear) -see Disorder, pinna, specified
    type NEC
  bronchial J98.09
  cardiac -see Degeneration, myocardial
  cartilage (senile) -see Disorder, cartilage,
    specified type NEC
  coronary (artery) -see Disease, heart,
    ischemic, atherosclerotic
  diaphragm J98.6
  ear, middle -see Otosclerosis
  falx cerebri G96.19
  fontanel, premature Q75.0
  heart -see also Degeneration, myocardial
    valve -see Endocarditis
  larynx J38.7
  ligament -see Disorder, tendon, specified type
    NEC
    posterior longitudinal -see Spondylopathy,
      specified NEC
  meninges (cerebral) (spinal) G96.19
  multiple, eccentric centers -see Disorder,
    bone, development or growth
  muscle -see also Calcification, muscle

Ossification - *continued*

due to burns *-see* Myositis, ossificans, in, burns

paralytic *-see* Myositis, ossificans, in, quadriplegia

progressive *-see* Myositis, ossificans, progressiva

specified NEC M61.50

ankle M61.57

foot M61.57

forearm M61.53

hand M61.54

lower leg M61.56

multiple sites M61.59

pelvic region M61.55

shoulder region M61.51

specified site NEC M61.58

thigh M61.55

upper arm M61.52

traumatic *-see* Myositis, ossificans, traumatica

myocardium, myocardial *-see* Degeneration, myocardial

penis N48.89

periarticular *-see* Disorder, joint, specified type NEC

pinna *-see* Disorder, pinna, specified type NEC

rider's bone *-see* Ossification, muscle, specified NEC

sclera H15.89

subperiosteal, post-traumatic M89.8X

tendon *-see* Disorder, tendon, specified type NEC

trachea J39.8

tympanic membrane *-see* Disorder, tympanic membrane, specified NEC

vitreous (humor) *-see* Deposit, crystalline

Osteitis - *see also* Osteomyelitis

alveolar M27.3

condensans M85.30

ankle M85.37

foot M85.37

forearm M85.33

hand M85.34

lower leg M85.36

multiple site M85.39

neck M85.38

rib M85.38

shoulder M85.31

skull M85.38

specified site NEC M85.38

thigh M85.35

toe M85.37

upper arm M85.32

vertebra M85.38

deformans M88.9

in (due to)

malignant neoplasm of bone C41.9 [M90.60]

neoplastic disease *-see also* Neoplasm D49.9 [M90.60]

carpus D49.9 [M90.64]

clavicle D49.9 [M90.61]

femur D49.9 [M90.65]

fibula D49.9 [M90.66]

finger D49.9 [M90.64]

humerus D49.9 [M90.62]

ilium D49.9 [M90.65]

ischium D49.9 [M90.65]

metacarpus D49.9 [M90.64]

Osteitis - *continued*

metatarsus D49.9 [M90.67]

multiple sites D49.9 [M90.69]

neck D49.9 [M90.68]

radius D49.9 [M90.63]

rib D49.9 [M90.68]

scapula D49.9 [M90.61]

skull D49.9 [M90.68]

tarsus D49.9 [M90.67]

tibia D49.9 [M90.66]

toe D49.9 [M90.67]

ulna D49.9 [M90.63]

vertebra D49.9 [M90.68]

skull M88.0

specified NEC *-see* Paget's disease, bone, by site

vertebra M88.1

due to yaws A66.6

fibrosa NEC *-see* Cyst, bone, by site

circumscripta *-see* Dysplasia, fibrous, bone NEC

cystica (generalisata) E21.0

disseminata Q78.1

osteoplastica E21.0

fragilitans Q78.0

Garr's (sclerosing) *-see* Osteomyelitis, specified type NEC

jaw (acute) (chronic) (lower) (suppurative) (upper) M27.2

parathyroid E21.0

petrous bone (acute) (chronic) *-see* Petrositis

sclerotic, nonsuppurative *-see* Osteomyelitis, specified type NEC

tuberculosa A18.09

cystica D86.89

multiplex cystoides D86.89

Osteoarthritis M19.90

ankle M19.07

elbow M19.02

foot joint M19.07

generalized M15.9

erosive M15.4

primary M15.0

specified NEC M15.8

hand joint M19.04

first carpometacarpal joint M18.9

hip M16.1

bilateral M16.0

due to hip dysplasia (unilateral) M16.3

bilateral M16.2

interphalangeal

distal (Heberden) M15.1

proximal (Bouchard) M15.2

knee M17.9

bilateral M17.0

shoulder M19.01

spine *-see* Spondylosis

wrist M19.03

post-traumatic NEC M19.92

ankle M19.17

elbow M19.12

foot joint M19.17

hand joint M19.14

first carpometacarpal joint M18.3

bilateral M18.2

hip M16.5

bilateral M16.4

knee M17.3

bilateral M17.2

shoulder M19.11

wrist M19.13

Osteoarthritis - *continued*

primary M19.91

ankle M19.07

elbow M19.02

foot joint M19.07

hand joint M19.04

first carpometacarpal joint M18.1

bilateral M18.0

hip M16.1

bilateral M16.0

knee M17.1

bilateral M17.0

shoulder M19.01

spine *-see* Spondylosis

wrist M19.03

secondary M19.93

ankle M19.27

elbow M19.22

foot joint M19.27

hand joint M19.24

first carpometacarpal joint M18.5

bilateral M18.4

hip M16.7

bilateral M16.6

knee M17.5

bilateral M17.4

multiple M15.3

shoulder M19.21

spine *-see* Spondylosis

wrist M19.23

Osteoarthropathy (hypertrophic) M19.90

ankle *-see* Osteoarthritis, primary, ankle

elbow *-see* Osteoarthritis, primary, elbow

foot joint *-see* Osteoarthritis, primary, foot

hand joint *-see* Osteoarthritis, primary, hand joint

knee joint *-see* Osteoarthritis, primary, knee

multiple site *-see* Osteoarthritis, primary, multiple joint

pulmonary *-see also* Osteoarthropathy, specified type NEC

hypertrophic *-see* Osteoarthropathy, hypertrophic, specified type NEC

secondary hypertrophic *-see* Osteoarthropathy, specified type NEC

shoulder *-see* Osteoarthritis, primary, shoulder

specified joint NEC *-see* Osteoarthritis, primary, specified joint NEC

specified type NEC M89.40

carpus M89.44

clavicle M89.41

femur M89.45

fibula M89.46

finger M89.44

humerus M89.42

ilium M89.459

ischium M89.459

metacarpus M89.44

metatarsus M89.47

multiple sites M89.49

neck M89.48

radius M89.43

rib M89.48

scapula M89.41

skull M89.48

tarsus M89.47

tibia M89.46

toe M89.47

ulna M89.43

vertebra M89.48

Osteoarthropathy
  secondary -see Osteoarthropathy, specified
    type NEC
  spine -see Spondylosis
  wrist -see Osteoarthritis, primary, wrist
Osteoarthrosis (degenerative) (hypertrophic)
(joint) -see also
Osteoarthritis
  deformans alkaptonurica E70.29 [M36.8]
  erosive M15.4
  generalized M15.9
    primary M15.0
  polyarticular M15.9
  spine -see Spondylosis
Osteoblastoma -see Neoplasm, bone, benign
  aggressive -see Neoplasm, bone, uncertain
  behavior
Osteochondroarthrosis deformans endemica
-see Disease, Kaschin-Beck
Osteochondritis -see also Osteochondropathy,
  by site
  Brailsford's -see Osteochondrosis, juvenile,
    radius
  dissecans M93.20
    ankle M93.27
    elbow M93.22
    foot M93.27
    hand M93.24
    hip M93.25
    knee M93.26
    multiple sites M93.29
    shoulder joint M93.21
    specified site NEC M93.28
    wrist M93.23
  juvenile M92.9
    patellar -see Osteochondrosis, juvenile,
    patella
  syphilitic (congenital) (early) A50.02
  [M90.80]
    ankle A50.02 [M90.87]
    elbow A50.02 [M90.82]
    foot A50.02 [M90.87]
    forearm A50.02 [M90.83]
    hand A50.02 [M90.84]
    hip A50.02 [M90.85]
    knee A50.02 [M90.86]
    multiple sites A50.02 [M90.89]
    shoulder joint A50.02 [M90.81]
    specified site NEC A50.02 [M90.88]
Osteochondrodysplasia Q78.9
  with defects of growth of tubular bones and
  spine Q77.9
    specified NEC Q77.8
  specified NEC Q78.8
Osteochondrodystrophy E78.9
Osteochondrolysis -see Osteochondritis,
  dissecans
Osteochondroma -see Neoplasm, bone, benign
Osteochondromatosis D48.0
  syndrome Q78.4
Osteochondromyxosarcoma -see Neoplasm,
  bone, malignant
Osteochondropathy M93.90
  ankle M93.97
  elbow M93.92
  foot M93.97
  hand M93.94
  hip M93.95
  Kienböck's disease of adults M93.1
  knee M93.96
  multiple joints M93.99

Osteochondropathy --continued
  osteochondritis dissecans -see
    Osteochondritis, dissecans
  osteochondrosis -see Osteochondrosis
  shoulder region M93.91
  slipped upper femoral epiphysis -see Slipped,
    epiphysis, upper femoral
  specified joint NEC M93.98
  specified type NEC M93.80
    ankle M93.87
    elbow M93.82
    foot M93.87
    hand M93.84
    hip M93.85
    knee M93.86
    multiple joints M93.89
    shoulder region M93.81
    specified joint NEC M93.88
    wrist M93.83
  syphilitic, congenital
    early A50.02 [M90.80]
    late A50.56 [M90.80]
  wrist M93.93
Osteochondrosarcoma -see Neoplasm, bone,
  malignant
Osteochondrosis -see also Osteochondropathy,
  by site
  acetabulum (juvenile) M91.0
  adult -see Osteochondropathy, specified type
    NEC, by site
  astragalus (juvenile) -see Osteochondrosis,
    juvenile, tarsus
  Blount's -see Osteochondrosis, juvenile, tibia
  Buchanan's M91.0
  Burns' -see Osteochondrosis, juvenile, ulna
  calcaneus (juvenile) -see Osteochondrosis,
    juvenile, tarsus
  capitular epiphysis (femur) (juvenile) -see
    Legg-Calvé Perthes disease
  carpal (juvenile) (lunate) (scaphoid) -see
    Osteochondrosis, juvenile, hand, carpal
    lunate
    adult M93.1
  coxae juvenilis -see Legg-Calvé Perthes
    disease
  deformans juvenilis, coxae -see Legg-Calvé
    Perthes disease
  Diaz's -see Osteochondrosis, juvenile, tarsus
  dissecans (knee) (shoulder) -see
    Osteochondritis, dissecans
  femoral capital epiphysis (juvenile) -see
    Legg-Calvé Perthes disease
  femur (head), juvenile -see Legg-Calvé
    Perthes disease
  fibula (juvenile) -see Osteochondrosis,
    juvenile, fibula
  foot NEC (juvenile) M92.8
  Freiberg's -see Osteochondrosis, juvenile,
    metatarsus
  Haas' (juvenile) -see Osteochondrosis,
    juvenile, humerus
  Haglund's -see Osteochondrosis, juvenile,
    tarsus
  hip (juvenile) -see Legg-Calvé Perthes
    disease
  humerus (capitulum) (head) (juvenile) -see
    Osteochondrosis, juvenile, humerus
  ilium, iliac crest (juvenile) M91.0
  ischiopubic synchondrosis M91.0
  Iselin's -see Osteochondrosis, juvenile,
    metatarsus

Osteochondrosis - continued
  juvenile, juvenilis M92.9
    after congenital dislocation of hip reduction
      -see Osteochondrosis, juvenile, hip,
      specified NEC
    arm -see Osteochondrosis, juvenile, upper
      limb NEC
    capitular epiphysis (femur) -see Legg-Calvé
      Perthes disease
    clavicle, sternal epiphysis -see
      Osteochondrosis, juvenile, upper limb NEC
    coxae -see Legg-Calvé Perthes disease
    deformans M92.9
    fibula M92.5
    foot NEC M92.8
    hand M92.20
      carpal lunate M92.21
      metacarpal head M92.22
      specified site NEC M92.29
    head of femur -see Legg-Calvé Perthes
      disease
    hip and pelvis M91.9
      coxa plana -see Coxa, plana
      femoral head -see Legg-Calvé Perthes
        disease
      pelvis M91.0
      pseudocoxalgia -see Pseudocoxalgia
      specified NEC M91.8
    humerus M92.0
    limb
      lower NEC M92.8
      upper NEC -see Osteochondrosis, juvenile,
      upper limb NEC
    medial cuneiform bone -see
      Osteochondrosis, juvenile, tarsus
    metatarsus M92.7
    patella M92.4
    radius M92.1
    specified site NEC M92.8
    spine M42.00
      cervical region M42.02
      cervicothoracic region M42.03
      lumbar region M42.06
      lumbosacral region M42.07
      multiple sites M42.09
      occipito-atlanto-axial region M42.01
      sacrococcygeal region M42.08
      thoracic region M42.04
      thoracolumbar region M42.05
    tarsus M92.6
    tibia M92.5
    ulna M92.1
    upper limb NEC M92.3
    vertebra (body) (epiphyseal plates) (Calvé's)
      (Scheuermann's) -see Osteochondrosis,
      juvenile, spine
  Kienböck's -see Osteochondrosis, juvenile,
  hand, carpal lunate
    adult M93.1
  Köhler's
    patellar -see Osteochondrosis, juvenile,
  patella
    tarsal navicular -see Osteochondrosis,
    juvenile, tarsus
  Legg-Perthes (Calvé)(Waldenström) -see
    Legg-Calvé Perthes disease
  limb
    lower NEC (juvenile) M92.8
    upper NEC (juvenile) -see Osteochondrosis,
    juvenile, upper limb NEC

Osteochondrosis - *continued*
  lunate bone (carpal) (juvenile) -*see also*
  Osteochondrosis, juvenile, hand, carpal lunate
    adult M93.1
  Mauclaire's -*see* Osteochondrosis, juvenile,
    hand, metacarpal
  metacarpal (head) (juvenile) -*see*
    Osteochondrosis, juvenile, hand, metacarpal
  metatarsus (fifth) (head) (juvenile) (second) -
    see Osteochondrosis, juvenile, metatarsus
  navicular (juvenile) -*see* Osteochondrosis,
    juvenile, tarsus
  os
    calcis (juvenile) -*see* Osteochondrosis,
      juvenile, tarsus
    tibiale externum (juvenile) -*see*
      Osteochondrosis, juvenile, tarsus
  Osgood-Schlatter -*see* Osteochondrosis,
    juvenile, tibia
  Panner's -*see* Osteochondrosis, juvenile,
    humerus
  patellar center (juvenile) (primary)
    (secondary) -*see* Osteochondrosis, juvenile,
    patella
  pelvis (juvenile) M91.0
  Pierson's M91.0
  radius (head) (juvenile) -*see* Osteochondrosis,
    juvenile, radius
  Scheuermann's -*see* Osteochondrosis,
    juvenile, spine
  Sever's -*see* Osteochondrosis, juvenile, tarsus
  Sinding-Larsen -*see* Osteochondrosis,
    juvenile, patella
  spine M42.9
    adult M42.10
      cervical region M42.12
      cervicothoracic region M42.13
      lumbar region M42.16
      lumbosacral region M42.17
      multiple sites M42.19
      occipito-atlanto-axial region M42.11
      sacrococcygeal region M42.18
      thoracic region M42.14
      thoracolumbar region M42.15
    juvenile -*see* Osteochondrosis, juvenile,
  spine
  symphysis pubis (juvenile) M91.0
  syphilitic (congenital) A50.02
  talus (juvenile) -*see* Osteochondrosis,
    juvenile, tarsus
  tarsus (navicular) (juvenile) -*see*
    Osteochondrosis, juvenile, tarsus
  tibia (proximal) (tubercle) (juvenile) -*see*
    Osteochondrosis, juvenile, tibia
  tuberculous -*see* Tuberculosis, bone
  ulna (lower) (juvenile) -*see* Osteochondrosis,
    juvenile, ulna
  van Neck's M91.0
  vertebral -*see* Osteochondrosis, spine
Osteoclastoma D48.0
  malignant -*see* Neoplasm, bone, malignant
Osteodynia -*see* Disorder, bone, specified type
  NEC
Osteodystrophy Q78.9
  azotemic N25.0
  congenital Q78.9
  parathyroid, secondary E21.1
  renal N25.0
Osteofibroma -*see* Neoplasm, bone, benign
Osteofibrosarcoma -*see* Neoplasm, bone,
  malignant

Osteogenesis imperfecta Q78.0
Osteogenic -*see* condition
Osteolysis M89.50
  carpus M89.54
  clavicle M89.51
  femur M89.55
  fibula M89.56
  finger M89.54
  humerus M89.52
  ilium M89.559
  ischium M89.559
  joint prosthesis (periprosthetic) -*see*
    Complications, joint prosthesis, mechanical,
    periprosthetic, osteolysis, by site
  metacarpus M89.54
  metatarsus M89.57
  multiple sites M89.59
  neck M89.58
  periprosthetic -*see* Complications, joint
    prosthesis, mechanical, periprosthetic,
    osteolysis, by site
  radius M89.53
  rib M89.58
  scapula M89.51
  skull M89.58
  tarsus M89.57
  tibia M89.56
  toe M89.57
  ulna M89.53
  vertebra M89.58
Osteoma -*see also* Neoplasm, bone, benign
  osteoid -*see also* Neoplasm, bone, benign
    giant -*see* Neoplasm, bone, benign
Osteomalacia M83.9
  adult M83.9
    drug-induced NEC M83.5
    due to
      malabsorption (postsurgical) M83.2
      malnutrition M83.3
    specified NEC M83.8
  aluminium-induced M83.4
  infantile -*see* Rickets
  juvenile -*see* Rickets
  oncogenic E83.89
  pelvis M83.8
  puerperal M83.0
  senile M83.1
  vitamin-D-resistant in adults E83.31 [*M90.8*]
    carpus E83.31 [*M90.84*]
    clavicle E83.31 [*M90.81*]
    femur E83.31 [*M90.85*]
    fibula E83.31 [*M90.86*]
    finger E83.31 [*M90.84*]
    humerus E83.31 [*M90.82*]
    ilium E83.31 [*M90.859*]
    ischium E83.31 [*M90.859*]
    metacarpus E83.31 [*M90.84*]
    metatarsus E83.31 [*M90.87*]
    multiple sites E83.31 [*M90.89*]
    neck E83.31 [*M90.88*]
    radius E83.31 [*M90.83*]
    rib E83.31 [*M90.88*]
    scapula E83.31 [*M90.819*]
    skull E83.31 [*M90.88*]
    tarsus E83.31 [*M90.879*]
    tibia E83.31 [*M90.869*]
    toe E83.31 [*M90.879*]
    ulna E83.31 [*M90.839*]
    vertebra E83.31 [*M90.88*]

Osteomyelitis (general) (infective) (localized)
(neonatal) (purulent) (septic)
(staphylococcal) (streptococcal)
(suppurative) (with periostitis) M86.9
  acute M86.10
    carpus M86.14
    clavicle M86.11
    femur M86.15
    fibula M86.16
    finger M86.14
    hematogenous M86.00
      carpus M86.04
      clavicle M86.01
      femur M86.05
      fibula M86.06
      finger M86.04
      humerus M86.02
      ilium M86.059
      ischium M86.059
      mandible M27.2
      metacarpus M86.04
      metatarsus M86.07
      multiple sites M86.09
      neck M86.08
      orbit H05.02
      petrous bone -*see* Petrositis
      radius M86.03
      rib M86.08
      scapula M86.01
      skull M86.08
      tarsus M86.07
      tibia M86.06
      toe M86.07
      ulna M86.03
      vertebra -*see* Osteomyelitis, vertebra
    humerus M86.12
    ilium M86.159
    ischium M86.159
    mandible M27.2
    metacarpus M86.14
    metatarsus M86.17
    multiple sites M86.19
    neck M86.18
    orbit H05.02
    petrous bone -*see* Petrositis
    radius M86.13
    rib M86.18
    scapula M86.11
    skull M86.18
    tarsus M86.17
    tibia M86.16
    toe M86.17
    ulna M86.13
    vertebra -*see* Osteomyelitis, vertebra
  chronic (or old) M86.60
    with draining sinus M86.40
      carpus M86.44
      clavicle M86.41
      femur M86.45
      fibula M86.46
      finger M86.44
      humerus M86.42
      ilium M86.459
      ischium M86.459
      mandible M27.2
      metacarpus M86.44
      metatarsus M86.47
      multiple sites M86.49
      neck M86.48
      orbit H05.02
      petrous bone -*see* Petrositis

Osteomyelitis - *continued*
   radius M86.43
   rib M86.48
   scapula M86.41
   skull M86.48
   tarsus M86.47
   tibia M86.46
   toe M86.47
   ulna M86.43
   vertebra *-see* Osteomyelitis, vertebra
   carpus M86.64
   clavicle M86.61
   femur M86.65
   fibula M86.66
   finger M86.64
   hematogenous NEC M86.50
      carpus M86.54
      clavicle M86.51
      femur M86.55
      fibula M86.56
      finger M86.54
      humerus M86.52
      ilium M86.559
      ischium M86.559
      mandible M27.2
      metacarpus M86.54
      metatarsus M86.57
      multifocal M86.30
         carpus M86.34
         clavicle M86.31
         femur M86.35
         fibula M86.36
         finger M86.34
         humerus M86.32
         ilium M86.359
         ischium M86.359
         metacarpus M86.34
         metatarsus M86.37
         multiple sites M86.39
         neck M86.38
         radius M86.33
         rib M86.38
         scapula M86.31
         skull M86.38
         tarsus M86.37
         tibia M86.36
         toe M86.37
         ulna M86.33
         vertebra *-see* Osteomyelitis, vertebra
      multiple sites M86.59
      neck M86.58
      orbit H05.02
      petrous bone *-see* Petrositis
      radius M86.53
      rib M86.58
      scapula M86.51
      skull M86.58
      tarsus M86.57
      tibia M86.56
      toe M86.57
      ulna M86.53
      vertebra *-see* Osteomyelitis, vertebra
   humerus M86.62
   ilium M86.659
   ischium M86.659
   mandible M27.2
   metacarpus M86.64
   metatarsus M86.67
   multifocal *-see* Osteomyelitis, chronic,
      hematogenous, multifocal
   multiple sites M86.69

Osteomyelitis - *continued*
   neck M86.68
   orbit H05.02
   petrous bone *-see* Petrositis
   radius M86.63
   rib M86.68
   scapula M86.61
   skull M86.68
   tarsus M86.67
   tibia M86.66
   toe M86.67
   ulna M86.63
   vertebra *-see* Osteomyelitis, vertebra
   echinococcal B67.2
   Garr's *-see* Osteomyelitis, specified type NEC
   in diabetes mellitus *-see* E08 E13 with .69
   jaw (acute) (chronic) (lower) (neonatal)
      (suppurative) (upper) M27.2
   nonsuppurating *-see* Osteomyelitis, specified
      type NEC
   orbit H05.02
   petrous bone *-see* Petrositis
   Salmonella (arizonae) (cholerae-suis)
      (enteritidis) (typhimurium) A02.24
   sclerosing, nonsuppurative *-see*
      Osteomyelitis, specified type NEC
   specified type NEC *-see also* subcategory
      M86.8X
      mandible M27.2
      orbit H05.02
      petrous bone *-see* Petrositis
      vertebra *-see* Osteomyelitis, vertebra
   subacute M86.20
      carpus M86.24
      clavicle M86.21
      femur M86.25
      fibula M86.26
      finger M86.24
      humerus M86.22
      mandible M27.2
      metacarpus M86.24
      metatarsus M86.27
      multiple sites M86.29
      neck M86.28
      orbit H05.02
      petrous bone *-see* Petrositis
      radius M86.23
      rib M86.28
      scapula M86.21
      skull M86.28
      tarsus M86.27
      tibia M86.26
      toe M86.27
      ulna M86.23
      vertebra *-see* Osteomyelitis, vertebra
   syphilitic A52.77
      congenital (early) A50.02 [*M90.80*]
   tuberculous *-see* Tuberculosis, bone
   typhoid A01.05
   vertebra M46.20
      cervical region M46.22
      cervicothoracic region M46.23
      lumbar region M46.26
      lumbosacral region M46.27
      occipito-atlanto-axial region M46.21
      sacrococcygeal region M46.28
      thoracic region M46.24
      thoracolumbar region M46.25
Osteomyelofibrosis D47.4
Osteomyelosclerosis D75.89

Osteonecrosis M87.9
   due to
      drugs *-see* Osteonecrosis, secondary, due to,
      drugs
      trauma *-see* Osteonecrosis, secondary, due
      to, trauma
   idiopathic aseptic M87.00
      ankle M87.07
      carpus M87.03
      clavicle M87.01
      femur M87.05
      fibula M87.06
      finger M87.04
      humerus M87.02
      ilium M87.050
      ischium M87.050
      metacarpus M87.04
      metatarsus M87.07
      multiple sites M87.09
      neck M87.08
      pelvis M87.050
      radius M87.03
      rib M87.08
      scapula M87.01
      skull M87.08
      tarsus M87.07
      tibia M87.06
      toe M87.07
      ulna M87.03
      vertebra M87.08
   secondary NEC M87.30
      carpus M87.33
      clavicle M87.31
      due to
         drugs M87.10
            carpus M87.13
            clavicle M87.11
            femur M87.15
            fibula M87.16
            finger M87.14
            humerus M87.12
            ilium M87.159
            ischium M87.159
            jaw M87.180
            metacarpus M87.14
            metatarsus M87.17
            multiple sites M87.19
            neck M87.18
            radius M87.13
            rib M87.18
            scapula M87.11
            skull M87.18
            tarsus M87.17
            tibia M87.16
            toe M87.17
            ulna M87.13
            vertebra M87.18
         hemoglobinopathy NEC D58.2 [*M90.50*]
            carpus D58.2 [*M90.54*]
            clavicle D58.2 [*M90.51*]
            femur D58.2 [*M90.55*]
            fibula D58.2 [*M90.56*]
            finger D58.2 [*M90.54*]
            humerus D58.2 [*M90.52*]
            ilium D58.2 [*M90.55*]
            ischium D58.2 [*M90.55*]
            metacarpus D58.2 [*M90.54*]
            metatarsus D58.2 [*M90.57*]
            multiple sites D58.2 [*M90.58*]
            neck D58.2 [*M90.58*]
            radius D58.2 [*M90.53*]

Osteonecrosis - *continued*
rib D58.2 [*M90.58*]
scapula D58.2 [*M90.51*]
skull D58.2 [*M90.58*]
tarsus D58.2 [*M90.57*]
tibia D58.2 [*M90.56*]
toe D58.2 [*M90.57*]
ulna D58.2 [*M90.53*]
vertebra D58.2 [*M90.58*]
trauma (previous) M87.20
carpus M87.23
clavicle M87.21
femur M87.25
fibula M87.26
finger M87.24
humerus M87.22
ilium M87.25
ischium M87.25
metacarpus M87.24
metatarsus M87.27
multiple sites M87.29
neck M87.28
radius M87.23
rib M87.28
scapula M87.21
skull M87.28
tarsus M87.27
tibia M87.26
toe M87.27
ulna M87.23
vertebra M87.28
femur M87.35
fibula M87.36
finger M87.34
humerus M87.32
ilium M87.350
in
caisson disease T70.3 [*M90.50*]
carpus T70.3 [*M90.54*]
clavicle T70.3 [*M90.51*]
femur T70.3 [*M90.55*]
fibula T70.3 [*M90.56*]
finger T70.3 [*M90.54*]
humerus T70.3 [*M90.52*]
ilium T70.3 [*M90.55*]
ischium T70.3 [*M90.55*]
metacarpus T70.3 [*M90.54*]
metatarsus T70.3 [*M90.57*]
multiple sites T70.3 [*M90.59*]
neck T70.3 [*M90.58*]
radius T70.3 [*M90.53*]
rib T70.3 [*M90.58*]
scapula T70.3 [*M90.51*]
skull T70.3 [*M90.58*]
tarsus T70.3 [*M90.57*]
tibia T70.3 [*M90.56*]
toe T70.3 [*M90.57*]
ulna T70.3 [*M90.53*]
vertebra T70.3 [*M90.58*]
ischium M87.350
metacarpus M87.34
metatarsus M87.37
multiple site M87.39
neck M87.38
radius M87.33
rib M87.38
scapula M87.319
skull M87.38
tarsus M87.379
tibia M87.366
toe M87.379

Osteonecrosis - *continued*
ulna M87.33
vertebra M87.38
specified type NEC M87.80
carpus M87.83
clavicle M87.81
femur M87.85
fibula M87.86
finger M87.84
humerus M87.82
ilium M87.85
ischium M87.85
metacarpus M87.84
metatarsus M87.87
multiple sites M87.89
neck M87.88
radius M87.83
rib M87.88
scapula M87.81
skull M87.88
tarsus M87.87
tibia M87.86
toe M87.87
ulna M87.83
vertebra M87.88
Osteo-onycho-arthro-dysplasia Q87.2
Osteo-onychodysplasia, hereditary Q87.2
Osteopathia condensans disseminata Q78.8
Osteopathy -*see also* Osteomyelitis,
Osteonecrosis, Osteoporosis
after poliomyelitis M89.60
carpus M89.64
clavicle M89.61
femur M89.65
fibula M89.66
finger M89.64
humerus M89.62
ilium M89.659
ischium M89.659
metacarpus M89.64
metatarsus M89.67
multiple sites M89.69
neck M89.68
radius M89.63
rib M89.68
scapula M89.61
skull M89.68
tarsus M89.67
tibia M89.66
toe M89.67
ulna M89.63
vertebra M89.68
in (due to)
renal osteodystrophy N25.0
specified diseases classified elsewhere - see
subcategory M90.8
Osteopenia M85.8
borderline M85.8
Osteoperiostitis -*see* Osteomyelitis, specified
type NEC
Osteopetrosis (familial) Q78.2
Osteophyte M25.70
ankle M25.77
elbow M25.72
foot joint M25.77
hand joint M25.74
hip M25.75
knee M25.76
shoulder M25.71
spine M25.78
vertebrae M25.78
wrist M25.73

Osteopoikilosis Q78.8
Osteoporosis (female) (male) M81.0
with current pathological fracture M80.00
age-related M81.0
with current pathologic fracture M80.00
carpus M80.04
clavicle M80.01
fibula M80.06
finger M80.04
humerus M80.02
ilium M80.05
ischium M80.05
metacarpus M80.04
metatarsus M80.07
pelvis M80.05
radius M80.03
scapula M80.01
tarsus M80.07
tibia M80.06
toe M80.07
ulna M80.03
vertebra M80.08
disuse M81.8
with current pathological fracture M80.80
carpus M80.84
clavicle M80.81
fibula M80.86
finger M80.84
humerus M80.82
ilium M80.85
ischium M80.85
metacarpus M80.84
metatarsus M80.87
pelvis M80.85
radius M80.83
scapula M80.81
tarsus M80.87
tibia M80.86
toe M80.87
ulna M80.83
vertebra M80.88
drug-induced -*see* Osteoporosis, specified
type NEC
idiopathic -*see* Osteoporosis, specified type
NEC
involutional -*see* Osteoporosis, age-related
Lequesne M81.6
localized M81.6
postmenopausal M81.0
with pathological fracture M80.00
carpus M80.04
clavicle M80.01
fibula M80.06
finger M80.04
humerus M80.02
ilium M80.05
ischium M80.05
metacarpus M80.04
metatarsus M80.07
pelvis M80.05
radius M80.03
scapula M80.01
tarsus M80.07
tibia M80.06
toe M80.07
ulna M80.03
vertebra M80.08
postoophorectomy -*see* Osteoporosis,
specified type NEC
postsurgical malabsorption -*see* Osteoporosis,
specified type NEC

Osteoporosis - *continued*

post-traumatic -*see* Osteoporosis, specified type NEC

senile -*see* Osteoporosis, age-related

specified type NEC M81.8

with pathological fracture M80.80

carpus M80.84

clavicle M80.81

fibula M80.86

finger M80.84

humerus M80.82

ilium M80.85

ischium M80.85

metacarpus M80.84

metatarsus M80.87

pelvis M80.85

radius M80.83

scapula M80.81

tarsus M80.87

tibia M80.86

toe M80.87

ulna M80.83

vertebra M80.88

Osteopsathyrosis (idiopathica) Q78.0

Osteoradionecrosis, jaw (acute) (chronic) (lower) (suppurative) (upper) M27.2

Osteosarcoma (any form) -*see* Neoplasm, bone, malignant

Osteosclerosis Q78.2

acquired M85.8

congenita Q77.4

fragilitas (generalisata) Q78.2

myelofibrosis D75.81

Osteosclerotic anemia D64.89

Osteosis

cutis L94.2

renal fibrocystic N25.0

Österreicher-Turner syndrome Q87.2

Ostium

atrioventriculare commune Q21.2

primum (arteriosum) (defect) (persistent) Q21.2

secundum (arteriosum) (defect) (patent) (persistent) Q21.1

Ostrum-Furst syndrome Q75.8

Otalgia -*see* subcategory H92.0

Otitis (acute) H66.90

with effusion -*see also* Otitis, media, nonsuppurative

purulent -*see* Otitis, media, suppurative

adhesive - see subcategory H74.1

chronic -*see also* Otitis, media, chronic

with effusion -*see also* Otitis, media, nonsuppurative, chronic

externa H60.9

abscess -*see* Abscess, ear, external

acute (noninfective) H60.50

actinic H60.51

chemical H60.52

contact H60.53

eczematoid H60.54

infective -*see* Otitis, externa, infective

reactive H60.55

specified NEC H60.59

cellulitis -*see* Cellulitis, ear

chronic H60.6

diffuse -*see* Otitis, externa, infective, diffuse

hemorrhagic -*see* Otitis, externa, infective, hemorrhagic

in (due to)

aspergillosis B44.89

Osteoporosis - *continued*

candidiasis B37.84

erysipelas A46 *[H62.40]*

herpes (simplex) virus infection B00.1

zoster B02.8

impetigo L01.00 *[H62.40]*

infectious disease NEC B99 *[H62.4]*

mycosis NEC B36.9 *[H62.40]*

parasitic disease NEC B89 *[H62.40]*

viral disease NEC B34.9 *[H62.40]*

zoster B02.8

infective NEC H60.39

abscess -*see* Abscess, ear, external

cellulitis -*see* Cellulitis, ear

diffuse H60.31

hemorrhagic H60.32

swimmer's ear -*see* Swimmer's, ear

malignant H60.2

mycotic NEC B36.9 *[H62.40]*

in

aspergillosis B44.89

candidiasis B37.84

moniliasis B37.84

necrotizing -*see* Otitis, externa, malignant

Pseudomonas aeruginosa -*see* Otitis, externa, malignant

reactive -*see* Otitis, externa, acute, reactive

specified NEC -*see* subcategory H60.8

tropical NEC B36.9 *[H62.40]*

in

aspergillosis B44.89

candidiasis B37.84

moniliasis B37.84

insidiosa -*see* Otosclerosis

interna -*see* subcategory H83.0

media (hemorrhagic) (staphylococcal) (streptococcal) H66.9

with effusion (nonpurulent) -*see* Otitis, media, nonsuppurative

acute, subacute H66.90

allergic -*see* Otitis, media, nonsuppurative, acute, allergic

exudative -*see* Otitis, media, suppurative, acute

mucoid -*see* Otitis, media, nonsuppurative, acute

necrotizing -*see also* Otitis, media, suppurative, acute

in

measles B05.3

scarlet fever A38.0

nonsuppurative NEC -*see* Otitis, media, nonsuppurative, acute

purulent -*see* Otitis, media, suppurative, acute

sanguinous -*see* Otitis, media, nonsuppurative, acute

secretory -*see* Otitis, media, nonsuppurative, acute, serous

seromucinous -*see* Otitis, media, nonsuppurative, acute

serous -*see* Otitis, media, nonsuppurative, acute, serous

suppurative -*see* Otitis, media, suppurative, acute

allergic -*see* Otitis, media, nonsuppurative

catarrhal -*see* Otitis, media, nonsuppurative

chronic H66.90

with effusion (nonpurulent) -*see* Otitis, media, nonsuppurative, chronic

Osteoporosis - *continued*

allergic -*see* Otitis, media, nonsuppurative, chronic, allergic

benign suppurative -*see* Otitis, media, suppurative, chronic, tubotympanic

catarrhal -*see* Otitis, media, nonsuppurative, chronic, serous

exudative -*see* Otitis, media, nonsuppurative, chronic

mucinous -*see* Otitis, media, nonsuppurative, chronic, mucoid

mucoid -*see* Otitis, media, nonsuppurative, chronic, mucoid

nonsuppurative NEC -*see* Otitis, media, nonsuppurative, chronic

purulent -*see* Otitis, media, suppurative, chronic

secretory -*see* Otitis, media, nonsuppurative, chronic, mucoid

seromucinous -*see* Otitis, media, nonsuppurative, chronic

serous -*see* Otitis, media, nonsuppurative, chronic, serous

suppurative -*see* Otitis, media, suppurative, chronic

transudative -*see* Otitis, media, nonsuppurative, chronic, mucoid

exudative -*see* Otitis, media, suppurative

in (due to) (with)

influenza -*see* Influenza, with, otitis media

measles B05.3

scarlet fever A38.0

tuberculosis A18.6

viral disease NEC B34. *[H67.]*

mucoid -*see* Otitis, media, nonsuppurative

nonsuppurative H65.9

acute or subacute NEC H65.19

allergic H65.11

recurrent H65.11

recurrent H65.19

secretory -*see* Otitis, media, nonsuppurative, serous

serous H65.0

recurrent H65.0

chronic H65.49

allergic H65.41

mucoid H65.3

serous H65.2

postmeasles B05.3

purulent -*see* Otitis, media, suppurative

secretory -*see* Otitis, media, nonsuppurative

seromucinous -*see* Otitis, media, nonsuppurative

serous -*see* Otitis, media, nonsuppurative

suppurative H66.4

acute H66.00

with rupture of ear drum H66.01

recurrent H66.00

with rupture of ear drum H66.01

chronic -*see also* subcategory H66.3

atticoantral H66.2

benign -*see* Otitis, media, suppurative, chronic, tubotympanic

tubotympanic H66.1

transudative -*see* Otitis, media, nonsuppurative

tuberculous A18.6

Otocephaly Q18.2

Otolith syndrome -*see* subcategory H81.8

Otomycosis (diffuse) NEC B36.9 [*H62.40*]
in
  aspergillosis B44.89
  candidiasis B37.84
  moniliasis B37.84
Otoporosis -*see* Otosclerosis
Otorrhagia (nontraumatic) H92.2
  traumatic
  code by Type of injury
Otorrhea H92.1
  cerebrospinal G96.0
Otosclerosis (general) H80.9
  cochlear (endosteal) H80.2
  involving
    otic capsule -*see* Otosclerosis, cochlear
    oval window
      nonobliterative H80.0
      obliterative H80.1
    round window -*see* Otosclerosis, cochlear
  nonobliterative -*see* Otosclerosis, involving,
    oval window, nonobliterative
  obliterative -*see* Otosclerosis, involving, oval
    window, obliterative
  specified NEC H80.8
Otospongiosis -*see* Otosclerosis
Otto's disease or pelvis M24.7
Outcome of delivery Z37.9
  multiple births Z37.9
    all liveborn Z37.50
      quadruplets Z37.52
      quintuplets Z37.53
      sextuplets Z37.54
      specified number NEC Z37.59
      triplets Z37.51
    all stillborn Z37.7
    some liveborn Z37.60
      quadruplets Z37.62
      quintuplets Z37.63
      sextuplets Z37.64
      specified number NEC Z37.69
      triplets Z37.61
  single NEC Z37.9
    liveborn Z37.0
    stillborn Z37.1
  twins NEC Z37.9
    both liveborn Z37.2
    both stillborn Z37.4
    one liveborn, one stillborn Z37.3
Outlet -*see* condition
Ovalocytosis (congenital) (hereditary) -*see*
  Elliptocytosis
Ovarian -*see* Condition
Ovariocele N83.4
Ovaritis (cystic) -*see* Oophoritis
Ovary, ovarian -*see also* condition
  resistant syndrome E28.39
  vein syndrome N13.8
Overactive -*see also* Hyperfunction
  adrenal cortex NEC E27.0
  bladder N32.81
  hypothalamus E23.3
  thyroid -*see* Hyperthyroidism
Overactivity R46.3
  child -*see* Disorder, attention-deficit
  hyperactivity
**Overbite (deep) (excessive) (horizontal)
  (vertical)** M26.29

Overbreathing -*see* Hyperventilation
Overconscientious personality F60.5
Overdevelopment -*see* Hypertrophy
Overdistension -*see* Distension
Overdose, overdosage (drug) -*see* Table of
  Drugs and Chemicals, by drug, poisoning
Overeating R63.2
  nonorganic origin F50.89
  psychogenic F50.89
Overexertion (effects) (exhaustion) T73.3
Overexposure (effects) T73.9
  exhaustion T73.2
Overfeeding -*see* Overeating
  newborn P92.4
Overfill, endodontic M27.52
Overgrowth, bone -*see* Hypertrophy, bone
**Overhanging of dental restorative material
  (unrepairable)** K08.52
Overheated (places) (effects) -*see* Heat
Overjet (excessive horizontal) M26.23
Overlaid, overlying (suffocation) -*see*
  Asphyxia, traumatic, due to mechanical threat
Overlap, excessive horizontal (teeth) M26.23
Overlapping toe (acquired) -*see also*
  Deformity, toe, specified NEC
  congenital (fifth toe) Q66.89
Overload
  circulatory, due to transfusion (blood) (blood
    components) (TACO) E87.71
  fluid E87.70
    due to transfusion (blood) (blood
      components) E87.71
    specified NEC E87.79
  iron, due to repeated red blood cell
    transfusions E83.111
  potassium (K) E87.5
  sodium (Na) E87.0
Overnutrition -*see* Hyperalimentation
Overproduction -*see also* Hypersecretion
  ACTH E27.0
  catecholamine E27.5
  growth hormone E22.0
Overprotection, child by parent Z62.1
Overriding
  aorta Q25.49
  finger (acquired) -*see* Deformity, finger
    congenital Q68.1
  toe (acquired) -*see also* Deformity, toe,
    specified NEC
    congenital Q66.89
Overstrained R53.83
  heart -*see* Hypertrophy, cardiac
Overuse, muscle NEC M70.8
Overweight E66.3
Overworked R53.83
Oviduct -*see* condition
Ovotestis Q56.0
Ovulation (cycle)
  failure or lack of N97.0
  pain N94.0
Ovum -*see* condition
**Owren's disease or syndrome
  (parahemophilia)** D68.2
Ox heart -*see* Hypertrophy, cardiac
Oxalosis E72.53
Oxaluria E72.53
Oxycephaly, oxycephalic Q75.0
  syphilitic, congenital A50.02
Oxyuriasis B80
Oxyuris vermicularis (infestation) B80
Ozena J31.0

P

Pachyderma, pachydermia L85.9
  larynx (verrucosa) J38.7
Pachydermatocele (congenital) Q82.8
Pachydermoperiostosis -*see also*
  Osteoarthropathy, hypertrophic, specified type
  NEC
  clubbed nail M89.40 [*L62*]
Pachygyria Q04.3
**Pachymeningitis (adhesive) (basal) (brain)
  (cervical) (chronic)(circumscribed)
  (external) (fibrous) (hemorrhagic)
  (hypertrophic) (internal) (purulent)
  (spinal) (suppurative)** -*see* Meningitis
Pachyonychia (congenital) Q84.5
Pacinian tumor -*see* Neoplasm, skin, benign
Pad, knuckle or Garrod's M72.1
Paget-Schroetter syndrome I82.890
Paget's disease
  with infiltrating duct carcinoma -*see*
    Neoplasm, breast, malignant
  bone M88.9
    carpus M88.84
    clavicle M88.81
    femur M88.85
    fibula M88.86
    finger M88.84
    humerus M88.82
    ilium M88.85
    in neoplastic disease -*see* Osteitis,
      deformans, in neoplastic disease
    ischium M88.85
    metacarpus M88.84
    metatarsus M88.87
    multiple sites M88.89
    neck M88.88
    radius M88.83
    rib M88.88
    scapula M88.81
    skull M88.0
    tarsus M88.87
    tibia M88.86
    toe M88.87
    ulna M88.83
    vertebra M88.88
  breast (female) C50.01
    male C50.02
  extramammary -*see also* Neoplasm, skin,
  malignant
    anus C21.0
      margin C44.590
      skin C44.590
  intraductal carcinoma -*see* Neoplasm, breast,
  malignant
  malignant -*see* Neoplasm, skin, malignant
    breast (female) C50.01
      male C50.02
    unspecified site (female) C50.01
      male C50.02
  mammary -*see* Paget's disease, breast
  nipple -*see* Paget's disease, breast
  osteitis deformans -*see* Paget's disease, bone
Pain(s) -*see also* Painful R52
  abdominal R10.9
    colic R10.83
    generalized R10.84
      with acute abdomen R10.0
    lower R10.30
      left quadrant R10.32
      pelvic or perineal R10.2

Pain(s) --continued
 periumbilical R10.33
  right quadrant R10.31
 rebound -see Tenderness, abdominal,
 rebound
 severe with abdominal rigidity R10.0
 tenderness -see Tenderness, abdominal
 upper R10.10
  epigastric R10.13
  left quadrant R10.12
  right quadrant R10.11
acute R52
 due to trauma G89.11
 neoplasm related G89.3
 postprocedural NEC G89.18
 post-thoracotomy G89.12
 specified by site
code to Pain, by site
adnexa (uteri) R10.2
anginoid -see Pain, precordial
anus K62.89
arm -see Pain, limb, upper
axillary (axilla) M79.62
back (postural) M54.9
bladder R39.89
 associated with micturition -see Micturition,
 painful
 chronic R39.82
bone -see Disorder, bone, specified type NEC
breast N64.4
broad ligament R10.2
cancer associated (acute) (chronic) G89.3
cecum -see Pain, abdominal
cervicobrachial M53.1
chest (central) R07.9
 anterior wall R07.89
 atypical R07.89
 ischemic I20.9
 musculoskeletal R07.89
 non-cardiac R07.89
 on breathing R07.1
 pleurodynia R07.81
 precordial R07.2
 wall (anterior) R07.89
chronic G89.29
 associated with significant psychosocial
 dysfunction G89.4
 due to trauma G89.21
 neoplasm related G89.3
 postoperative NEC G89.28
 postprocedural NEC G89.28
 post-thoracotomy G89.22
 specified NEC G89.29
coccyx M53.3
colon -see Pain, abdominal
coronary -see Angina
costochondral R07.1
diaphragm R07.1
due to cancer G89.3
due to device, implant or graft -see also
Complications, by site and type, specified
NEC T85.848
 arterial graft NEC T82.848
 breast (implant) T85.848
 catheter NEC T85.848
  dialysis (renal) T82.848
   intraperitoneal T85.848
  infusion NEC T82.848
   spinal (epidural) (subdural) T85.840
  urinary (indwelling) T83.84

Pain(s) --continued
 electronic (electrode) (pulse generator)
 (stimulator)
  bone T84.84
  cardiac T82.847
  nervous system (brain) (peripheral nerve)
   (spinal) T85.840
  urinary T83.84
 fixation, internal (orthopedic) NEC T84.84
 gastrointestinal (bile duct) (esophagus)
  T85.848
 genital NEC T83.84
 heart NEC T82.847
 infusion NEC T85.848
 joint prosthesis T84.84
 ocular (corneal graft) (orbital implant) NEC
  T85.848
 orthopedic NEC T84.84
 specified NEC T85.848
 urinary NEC T83.84
 vascular NEC T82.848
 ventricular intracranial shunt T85.840
due to malignancy (primary) (secondary)
 G89.3
ear -see subcategory H92.0
epigastric, epigastrium R10.13
eye -see Pain, ocular
face, facial R51
 atypical G50.1
female genital organs NEC N94.89
finger -see Pain, limb, upper
flank -see Pain, abdominal
foot -see Pain, limb, lower
gallbladder K82.9
gas (intestinal) R14.1
gastric -see Pain, abdominal
generalized NOS R52
genital organ
 female N94.89
 male N50.89
groin -see Pain, abdominal, lower
hand -see Pain, limb, upper
head -see Headache
heart -see Pain, precordial
infra-orbital -see Neuralgia, trigeminal
intercostal R07.82
intermenstrual N94.0
jaw R68.84
joint M25.50
 ankle M25.57
 elbow M25.52
 finger M25.54
 foot M25.57
 hand M25.54
 hip M25.55
 knee M25.56
 shoulder M25.51
 toe M25.57
 wrist M25.53
kidney N23
laryngeal R07.0
leg -see Pain, limb, lower
limb M79.609
 lower M79.60
  foot M79.67
  lower leg M79.66
  thigh M79.65
  toe M79.67
 upper M79.60
  axilla M79.62
  finger M79.64

Pain(s) --continued
 forearm M79.63
 hand M79.64
 upper arm M79.62
loin M54.5
low back M54.5
lumbar region M54.5
mandibular R68.84
mastoid -see subcategory H92.0
maxilla R68.84
menstrual -see also Dysmenorrhea N94.6
metacarpophalangeal (joint) -see Pain, joint,
 hand
metatarsophalangeal (joint) -see Pain, joint,
 foot
mouth K13.79
muscle -see Myalgia
musculoskeletal -see also Pain, by site M79.1
myofascial M79.1
nasal J34.89
nasopharynx J39.2
neck NEC M54.2
nerve NEC -see Neuralgia
neuromuscular -see Neuralgia
nose J34.89
ocular H57.1
ophthalmic -see Pain, ocular
orbital region -see Pain, ocular
ovary N94.89
over heart -see Pain, precordial
ovulation N94.0
pelvic (female) R10.2
penis N48.89
pericardial -see Pain, precordial
perineal, perineum R10.2
pharynx J39.2
pleura, pleural, pleuritic R07.81
postoperative NOS G89.18
postprocedural NOS G89.18
post-thoracotomy G89.12
precordial (region) R07.2
premenstrual N94.3
psychogenic (persistent) (any site) F45.41
radicular (spinal) -see Radiculopathy
rectum K62.89
respiration R07.1
retrosternal R07.2
rheumatoid, muscular -see Myalgia
rib R07.81
root (spinal) -see Radiculopathy
round ligament (stretch) R10.2
sacroiliac M53.3
sciatic -see Sciatica
scrotum N50.82
seminal vesicle N50.89
shoulder M25.51
spermatic cord N50.89
spinal root -see Radiculopathy
spine M54.9
 cervical M54.2
 low back M54.5
  with sciatica M54.4
 thoracic M54.6
stomach -see Pain, abdominal
substernal R07.2
temporomandibular (joint) M26.62
testis N50.81
thoracic spine M54.6
 with radicular and visceral pain M54.14
throat R07.0
tibia -see Pain, limb, lower

PQR

Pain(s) --*continued*
toe -*see* Pain, limb, lower
tongue K14.6
tooth K08.89
trigeminal -*see* Neuralgia, trigeminal
tumor associated G89.3
ureter N23
urinary (organ) (system) N23
uterus NEC N94.89
vagina R10.2
vertebrogenic (syndrome) M54.89
vesical R39.89
associated with micturition -*see* Micturition, painful
vulva R10.2
Painful -*see also* Pain
coitus
female N94.10
male N53.12
psychogenic F52.6
ejaculation (semen) N53.12
psychogenic F52.6
erection -*see* Priapism
feet syndrome E53.8
joint replacement (hip) (knee) T84.84
menstruation -*see* Dysmenorrhea
psychogenic F45.8
micturition -*see* Micturition, painful
respiration R07.1
scar NEC L90.5
wire sutures T81.89
Painter's colic -*see* subcategory T56.0
Palate -*see* condition
Palatoplegia K13.79
Palatoschisis -*see* Cleft, palate
Palilalia R48.8
Palliative care Z51.5
Pallor R23.1
optic disc, temporal -*see* Atrophy, optic
Palmar -*see also* condition
fascia -*see* condition
Palpable
cecum K63.89
kidney N28.89
ovary N83.8
prostate N42.9
spleen -*see* Splenomegaly
Palpitations (heart) R00.2
psychogenic F45.8
Palsy -*see also* Paralysis G83.9
atrophic diffuse (progressive) G12.22
Bell's -*see also* Palsy, facial
newborn P11.3
brachial plexus NEC G54.0
newborn (birth injury) P14.3
brain -*see* Palsy, cerebral
bulbar (progressive) (chronic) G12.22
of childhood (Fazio-Londe) G12.1
pseudo NEC G12.29
supranuclear (progressive) G23.1
cerebral (congenital) G80.9
ataxic G80.4
athetoid G80.3
choreoathetoid G80.3
diplegic G80.8
spastic G80.1
dyskinetic G80.3
athetoid G80.3
choreoathetoid G80.3
dystonic G80.3
dystonic G80.3

Palsy --*continued*
hemiplegic G80.8
spastic G80.2
mixed G80.8
monoplegic G80.8
spastic G80.1
paraplegic G80.8
spastic G80.1
quadriplegic G80.8
spastic G80.0
spastic G80.1
diplegic G80.1
hemiplegic G80.2
monoplegic G80.1
quadriplegic G80.0
specified NEC G80.1
tetraplegic G80.0
specified NEC G80.8
syphilitic A52.12
congenital A50.49
tetraplegic G80.8
spastic G80.0
cranial nerve -*see also* Disorder, nerve, cranial
multiple G52.7
in
infectious disease B99 [*G53*]
neoplastic disease -*see also* Neoplasm
D49.9 [*G53*]
parasitic disease B89 [*G53*]
sarcoidosis D86.82
creeping G12.22
diver's T70.3
Erb's P14.0
facial G51.0
newborn (birth injury) P11.3
glossopharyngeal G52.1
Klumpke (Déjérine) P14.1
lead -*see* subcategory T56.0
median nerve (tardy) G56.1
nerve G58.9
specified NEC G58.8
peroneal nerve (acute) (tardy) G57.3
progressive supranuclear G23.1
pseudobulbar NEC G12.29
radial nerve (acute) G56.3
seventh nerve -*see also* Palsy, facial
newborn P11.3
shaking -*see* Parkinsonism
spastic (cerebral) (spinal) G80.1
ulnar nerve (tardy) G56.2
wasting G12.29
Paludism -*see* Malaria
Panangiitis M30.0
Panaris, panaritium -*see also* Cellulitis, digit
with lymphangitis -*see* Lymphangitis, acute, digit
Panarteritis nodosa M30.0
brain or cerebral I67.7
Pancake heart R93.1
with cor pulmonale (chronic) I27.81
Pancarditis (acute) (chronic) I51.89
rheumatic I09.89
active or acute I01.8
Pancoast's syndrome or tumor C34.1
Pancolitis, ulcerative (chronic) K51.00
with
complication K51.019
abscess K51.014
fistula K51.013
obstruction K51.012
rectal bleeding K51.011
specified complication NEC K51.018

Pancreas, pancreatic -*see* condition
Pancreatitis (annular) (apoplectic) (calcareous) (edematous) (hemorrhagic) (malignant) (recurrent) (subacute) (suppurative) K85.90
with necrosis (uninfected) K85.91
infected K85.92
acute (without necrosis or infection) K85.90
with necrosis (uninfected) K85.91
infected K85.92
alcohol induced (without necrosis or infection) K85.20
with necrosis (uninfected) K85.21
infected K85.22
biliary (without necrosis or infection) K85.10
with necrosis (uninfected) K85.11
infected K85.12
drug induced (without necrosis or infection) K85.30
with necrosis (uninfected) K85.31
infected K85.32
gallstone (without necrosis or infection) K85.10
with necrosis (uninfected) K85.11
infected K85.12
idiopathic (without necrosis or infection) K85.00
with necrosis (uninfected) K85.01
infected K85.02
specified NEC (without necrosis or infection) K85.80
with necrosis (uninfected) K85.81
infected K85.82
chronic (infectious) K86.1
alcohol-induced K86.0
recurrent K86.1
relapsing K86.1
cystic (chronic) K86.1
cytomegaloviral B25.2
fibrous (chronic) K86.1
gangrenous -*see* Pancreatitis, acute
gallstone (without necrosis or infection) K85.10
with necrosis (uninfected) K85.11
infected K85.12
interstitial (chronic) K86.1
acute -*see also* Pancreatitis, acute K85.80
mumps B26.3
recurrent (chronic) K86.1
relapsing, chronic K86.1
syphilitic A52.74
Pancreatoblastoma -*see* Neoplasm, pancreas, malignant
Pancreolithiasis K86.89
Pancytolysis D75.89
Pancytopenia (acquired) D61.818
with
malformations D61.09
myelodysplastic syndrome -*see* Syndrome, myelodysplastic
antineoplastic chemotherapy induced D61.810
congenital D61.09
drug-induced NEC D61.811
Panencephalitis, subacute, sclerosing A81.1
Panhematopenia D61.9
congenital D61.09
constitutional D61.09
splenic, primary D73.1

Panhemocytopenia D61.9
  congenital D61.09
  constitutional D61.09
Panhypogonadism E29.1
Panhypopituitarism E23.0
  prepubertal E23.0
Panic (attack) (state) F41.0
  reaction to exceptional stress (transient) F43.0
Panmyelopathy, familial, constitutional
  D61.09
Panmyelophthisis D61.82
  congenital D61.09
Panmyelosis (acute) (with myelofibrosis)
  C94.4
Panner's disease -see Osteochondrosis,
  juvenile, humerus
Panneuritis endemica E51.11
Panniculitis (nodular) (nonsuppurative)
  M79.3
  back M54.00
    cervical region M54.02
    cervicothoracic region M54.03
    lumbar region M54.06
    lumbosacral region M54.07
    multiple sites M54.09
    occipito-atlanto-axial region M54.01
    sacrococcygeal region M54.08
    thoracic region M54.04
    thoracolumbar region M54.05
  lupus L93.2
  mesenteric K65.4
  neck M54.02
    cervicothoracic region M54.03
    occipito-atlanto-axial region M54.01
  relapsing M35.6
Panniculus adiposus (abdominal) E65
Pannus (allergic) (cornea) (degenerativus)
  (keratic) H16.42
  abdominal (symptomatic) E65
  trachomatosus, trachomatous (active) A71.1
Panophthalmitis H44.01
Pansinusitis (chronic) (hyperplastic)
  (nonpurulent) (purulent) J32.4
  acute J01.40
    recurrent J01.41
  tuberculous A15.8
Panuveitis (sympathetic) H44.11
Panvalvular disease I08.9
  specified NEC I08.8
PAPA (pyogenic arthritis, pyoderma
  gangrenosum, and acne syndrome) M04.8
Papanicolaou smear, cervix Z12.4
  as part of routine gynecological examination
    Z01.419
    with abnormal findings Z01.411
  for suspected neoplasm Z12.4
  nonspecific abnormal finding R87.619
  routine Z01.419
    with abnormal findings Z01.411
Papilledema (choked disc) H47.10
  associated with
    decreased ocular pressure H47.12
    increased intracranial pressure H47.11
    retinal disorder H47.13
  Foster-Kennedy syndrome H47.14
Papillitis H46.00
  anus K62.89
  chronic lingual K14.4
  necrotizing, kidney N17.2
  optic H46.0
  rectum K62.89
  renal, necrotizing N17.2
  tongue K14.0

Papilloma -see also Neoplasm, benign, by site
  acuminatum (female) (male) (anogenital)
    A63.0
  basal cell L82.1
    inflamed L82.0
  benign pinta (primary) A67.0
  bladder (urinary) (transitional cell) D41.4
  choroid plexus (lateral ventricle) (third
  ventricle) D33.0
    anaplastic C71.5
    fourth ventricle D33.1
    malignant C71.5
  renal pelvis (transitional cell) D41.1
    benign D30.1
  Schneiderian
    specified site -see Neoplasm, benign, by site
    unspecified site D14.0
  serous surface
    borderline malignancy
      specified site -see Neoplasm, uncertain
  behavior, by site
      unspecified site D39.10
    specified site -see Neoplasm, benign, by site
    unspecified site D27.9
  transitional (cell)
    bladder (urinary) D41.4
    inverted type -see Neoplasm, uncertain
      behavior, by site
    renal pelvis D41.1
    ureter D41.2
  ureter (transitional cell) D41.2
    benign D30.2
  urothelial -see Neoplasm, uncertain behavior,
    by site
  villous -see Neoplasm, uncertain behavior, by
    site
    adenocarcinoma in -see Neoplasm,
    malignant, by site
      in situ -see Neoplasm, in situ
  yaws, plantar or palmar A66.1
Papillomata, multiple, of yaws A66.1
Papillomatosis -see also Neoplasm, benign, by
  site
  confluent and reticulated L83
  cystic, breast -see Mastopathy, cystic
  ductal, breast -see Mastopathy, cystic
  intraductal (diffuse) -see Neoplasm, benign,
    by site
  subareolar duct D24
Papillomavirus, as cause of disease classified
  elsewhere B97.7
Papillon-Léage and Psaume syndrome Q87.0
Papule(s) R23.8
  carate (primary) A67.0
  fibrous, of nose D22.39
  Gottron's L94.4
  pinta (primary) A67.0
Papulosis
  lymphomatoid C86.6
  malignant I77.89
Papyraceous fetus O31.0
Para-albuminemia E88.09
Paracephalus Q89.7
Parachute mitral valve Q23.2
Paracoccidioidomycosis B41.9
  disseminated B41.7
  generalized B41.7
  mucocutaneous-lymphangitic B41.8
  pulmonary B41.0
  specified NEC B41.8
  visceral B41.8

Paradentosis K05.4
Paraffinoma T88.8
Paraganglioma D44.7
  adrenal D35.0
    malignant C74.1
  aortic body D44.7
    malignant C75.5
  carotid body D44.6
    malignant C75.4
  chromaffin -see also Neoplasm, benign, by
  site
    malignant -see Neoplasm, malignant, by site
  extra-adrenal D44.7
    malignant C75.5
      specified site -see Neoplasm, malignant, by
        site
      unspecified site C75.5
    specified site -see Neoplasm, uncertain
      behavior, by site
    unspecified site D44.7
  gangliocytic D13.2
    specified site -see Neoplasm, benign, by site
    unspecified site D13.2
  glomus jugulare D44.7
    malignant C75.5
  jugular D44.7
  malignant C75.5
    specified site -see Neoplasm, malignant, by
      site
    unspecified site C75.5
  nonchromaffin D44.7
    malignant C75.5
      specified site -see Neoplasm, malignant, by
        site
      unspecified site C75.5
    specified site -see Neoplasm, uncertain
      behavior, by site
    unspecified site D44.7
  parasympathetic D44.7
    specified site -see Neoplasm, uncertain
      behavior, by site
    unspecified site D44.7
  specified site -see Neoplasm, uncertain
    behavior, by site
  sympathetic D44.7
    specified site -see Neoplasm, uncertain
      behavior, by site
    unspecified site D44.7
  unspecified site D44.7
Parageusia R43.2
  psychogenic F45.8
Paragonimiasis B66.4
Paragranuloma, Hodgkin -see Lymphoma,
  Hodgkin, classical, specified NEC
Parahemophilia -see also Defect, coagulation
  D68.2
Parakeratosis R23.4
  variegata L41.0
Paralysis, paralytic (complete) (incomplete)
  G83.9
  with
    syphilis A52.17
  abducens, abducent (nerve) -see Strabismus,
    paralytic, sixth nerve
  abductor, lower extremity G57.9
  accessory nerve G52.8
  accommodation -see also Paresis, of
    accommodation
    hysterical F44.89
  acoustic nerve (except Deafness) -see
    subcategory H93.3

Paralysis, paralytic --*continued*
 agitans -*see also* Parkinsonism G20
  arteriosclerotic G21.4
 alternating (oculomotor) G83.89
 amyotrophic G12.21
 ankle G57.9
 anus (sphincter) K62.89
 arm -*see* Monoplegia, upper limb
 ascending (spinal), acute G61.0
 association G12.29
 asthenic bulbar G70.00
  with exacerbation (acute) G70.01
  in crisis G70.01
 ataxic (hereditary) G11.9
  general (syphilitic) A52.17
 atrophic G58.9
  infantile, acute -*see* Poliomyelitis, paralytic
  progressive G12.22
  spinal (acute) -*see* Poliomyelitis, paralytic
 axillary G54.0
 Babinski-Nageotte's G83.89
 Bell's G51.0
  newborn P11.3
 Benedikt's G46.3
 birth injury P14.9
  spinal cord P11.5
 bladder (neurogenic) (sphincter) N31.2
 bowel, colon or intestine K56.0
 brachial plexus G54.0
  birth injury P14.3
  newborn (birth injury) P14.3
 brain G83.9
  diplegia G83.0
  triplegia G83.89
 bronchial J98.09
 Brown-Séquard G83.81
 bulbar (chronic) (progressive) G12.22
  infantile -*see* Poliomyelitis, paralytic
  poliomyelitic -*see* Poliomyelitis, paralytic
  pseudo G12.29
 bulbospinal G70.00
  with exacerbation (acute) G70.01
  in crisis G70.01
 cardiac -*see also* Failure, heart I50.9
 cerebrocerebellar, diplegic G80.1
 cervical
  plexus G54.2
  sympathetic G90.09
 Céstan-Chenais G46.3
 Charcot-Marie-Tooth type G60.0
 Clark's G80.9
 colon K56.0
 compressed air T70.3
 compression
  arm G56.9
  leg G57.9
  lower extremity G57.9
  upper extremity G56.9
 congenital (cerebral) -*see* Palsy, cerebral
 conjugate movement (gaze) (of eye) H51.0
  cortical (nuclear) (supranuclear) H51.0
 cordis -*see* Failure, heart
 cranial or cerebral nerve G52.9
 creeping G12.22
 crossed leg G83.89
 crutch -*see* Injury, brachial plexus
 deglutition R13.0
  hysterical F44.4
 dementia A52.17
 descending (spinal) NEC G12.29
 diaphragm (flaccid) J98.6

Paralysis, paralytic --*continued*
 due to accidental dissection of phrenic nerve
  during procedure -*see* Puncture, accidental
  complicating surgery   digestive organs
  NEC K59.8
 diplegic -*see* Diplegia
 divergence (nuclear) H51.8
 diver's T70.3
 Duchenne's
  birth injury P14.0
  due to or associated with
   motor neuron disease G12.22
   muscular dystrophy G71.0
 due to intracranial or spinal birth injury -*see*
  Palsy, cerebral
 embolic (current episode) I63.4
 Erb (Duchenne) (birth) (newborn) P14.0
 Erb's syphilitic spastic spinal A52.17
 esophagus K22.8
 eye muscle (extrinsic) H49.9
  intrinsic -*see also* Paresis, of
  accommodation
 facial (nerve) G51.0
  birth injury P11.3
  congenital P11.3
  following operation NEC -*see* Puncture,
 accidental complicating surgery
  newborn (birth injury) P11.3
 familial (recurrent) (periodic) G72.3
  spastic G11.4
 fauces J39.2
 finger G56.9
 gait R26.1
 gastric nerve (nondiabetic) G52.2
 gaze, conjugate H51.0
 general (progressive) (syphilitic) A52.17
  juvenile A50.45
 glottis J38.00
  bilateral J38.02
  unilateral J38.01
 gluteal G54.1
 Gubler (Millard) G46.3
 hand -*see* Monoplegia, upper limb
 heart -*see* Arrest, cardiac
 hemiplegic -*see* Hemiplegia
 hyperkalemic periodic (familial) G72.3
 hypoglossal (nerve) G52.3
 hypokalemic periodic G72.3
 hysterical F44.4
 ileus K56.0
 infantile -*see also* Poliomyelitis, paralytic
 A80.30
  bulbar -*see* Poliomyelitis, paralytic
  cerebral -*see* Palsy, cerebral
  spastic -*see* Palsy, cerebral, spastic
 infective -*see* Poliomyelitis, paralytic
 inferior nuclear G83.9
 internuclear -*see* Ophthalmoplegia,
 internuclear
 intestine K56.0
 iris H57.09
  due to diphtheria (toxin) A36.89
 ischemic, Volkmann's (complicating trauma)
  T79.6
 Jackson's G83.89
 jake -*see* Poisoning, food, noxious, plant
 Jamaica ginger (jake) G62.2
 juvenile general A50.45
 Klumpke (Déjérine) (birth) (newborn) P14.1
 labioglossal (laryngeal) (pharyngeal) G12.29
 Landry's G61.0

Paralysis, paralytic --*continued*
 laryngeal nerve (recurrent) (superior)
  (unilateral) J38.00
  bilateral J38.02
  unilateral J38.01
 larynx J38.00
  bilateral J38.02
  due to diphtheria (toxin) A36.2
  unilateral J38.01
 lateral G12.21
 lead -*see* subcategory T56.0
 left side -*see* Hemiplegia
 leg G83.1
  both -*see* Paraplegia
  crossed G83.89
  hysterical F44.4
  psychogenic F44.4
  transient or transitory R29.818
   traumatic NEC -*see* Injury, nerve, leg
 levator palpebrae superioris -*see*
  Blepharoptosis, paralytic
 limb -*see* Monoplegia
 lip K13.0
 Lissauer's A52.17
 lower limb -*see* Monoplegia, lower limb
  both -*see* Paraplegia
 lung J98.4
 median nerve G56.1
 medullary (tegmental) G83.89
 mesencephalic NEC G83.89
  tegmental G83.89
 middle alternating G83.89
 Millard-Gubler-Foville G46.3
 monoplegic -*see* Monoplegia
 motor G83.9
 muscle, muscular NEC G72.89
  due to nerve lesion G58.9
  eye (extrinsic) H49.9
   intrinsic -*see* Paresis, of accommodation
   oblique -*see* Strabismus, paralytic, fourth
 nerve
  iris sphincter H21.9
  ischemic (Volkmann's) (complicating
   trauma) T79.6
  progressive G12.21
  pseudohypertrophic G71.0
 musculocutaneous nerve G56.9
 musculospiral G56.9
 nerve -*see also* Disorder, nerve
  abducent -*see* Strabismus, paralytic, sixth
   nerve
  accessory G52.8
  auditory (except Deafness) -*see* subcategory
   H93.3
  birth injury P14.9
  cranial or cerebral G52.9
  facial G51.0
   birth injury P11.3
   congenital P11.3
   newborn (birth injury) P11.3
  fourth or trochlear -*see* Strabismus,
   paralytic, fourth nerve
  newborn (birth injury) P14.9
  oculomotor -*see* Strabismus, paralytic, third
   nerve
  phrenic (birth injury) P14.2
  radial G56.3
  seventh or facial G51.0
   newborn (birth injury) P11.3
  sixth or abducent -*see* Strabismus, paralytic,
 sixth nerve

Paralysis, paralytic --*continued*
  syphilitic A52.15
  third or oculomotor -*see* Strabismus,
    paralytic, third nerve
  trigeminal G50.9
  trochlear -*see* Strabismus, paralytic, fourth
    nerve
  ulnar G56.2
  normokalemic periodic G72.3
  ocular H49.9
    alternating G83.89
  oculofacial, congenital (Moebius) Q87.0
  oculomotor (external bilateral) (nerve) -*see*
    Strabismus, paralytic, third nerve
  palate (soft) K13.79
  paratrigeminal G50.9
  periodic (familial) (hyperkalemic)
    (hypokalemic) (myotonic) (normokalemic)
    (potassium sensitive) (secondary) G72.3
  peripheral autonomic nervous system -*see*
    Neuropathy, peripheral, autonomic
  peroneal (nerve) G57.3
  pharynx J39.2
  phrenic nerve G56.8
  plantar nerve(s) G57.6
  pneumogastric nerve G52.2
  poliomyelitis (current) -*see* Poliomyelitis,
    paralytic
  popliteal nerve G57.3
  postepileptic transitory G83.84
  progressive (atrophic) (bulbar) (spinal)
    G12.22
    general A52.17
    infantile acute -*see* Poliomyelitis, paralytic
    supranuclear G23.1
  pseudobulbar G12.29
  pseudohypertrophic (muscle) G71.0
  psychogenic F44.4
  quadriceps G57.9
  quadriplegic -*see* Tetraplegia
  radial nerve G56.3
  rectus muscle (eye) H49.9
  recurrent isolated sleep G47.53
  respiratory (muscle) (system) (tract) R06.81
    center NEC G93.89
    congenital P28.89
    newborn P28.89
  right side -*see* Hemiplegia
  saturnine - see subcategory T56.0
  sciatic nerve G57.0
  senile G83.9
  shaking -*see* Parkinsonism
  shoulder G56.9
  sleep, recurrent isolated G47.53
  spastic G83.9
    cerebral -*see* Palsy, cerebral, spastic
    congenital (cerebral) -*see* Palsy, cerebral,
      spastic
    familial G11.4
    hereditary G11.4
    quadriplegic G80.0
    syphilitic (spinal) A52.17
  sphincter, bladder -*see* Paralysis, bladder
  spinal (cord) G83.9
    accessory nerve G52.8
    acute -*see* Poliomyelitis, paralytic
    ascending acute G61.0
    atrophic (acute) -*see also* Poliomyelitis,
      paralytic
      spastic, syphilitic A52.17
    congenital NEC -*see* Palsy, cerebral

Paralysis, paralytic --*continued*
  infantile -*see* Poliomyelitis, paralytic
  hereditary G95.89
    progressive G12.21
    sequelae NEC G83.89
  sternomastoid G52.8
  stomach K31.84
    diabetic -*see* Diabetes, by type, with
      gastroparesis
    nerve G52.2
      diabetic -*see* Diabetes, by type, with
      gastroparesis
  stroke -*see* Infarct, brain
  subcapsularis G56.8
  supranuclear (progressive) G23.1
  sympathetic G90.8
    cervical G90.09
    nervous system -*see* Neuropathy, peripheral,
      autonomic
  syndrome G83.9
    specified NEC G83.89
  syphilitic spastic spinal (Erb's) A52.17
  thigh G57.9
  throat J39.2
    diphtheritic A36.0
    muscle J39.2
  thrombotic (current episode) I63.3
  thumb G56.9
  tick -*see* Toxicity, venom, arthropod,
    specified NEC
  Todd's (postepileptic transitory paralysis)
    G83.84
  toe G57.6
  tongue K14.8
  transient R29.5
    arm or leg NEC R29.818
      traumatic NEC -*see* Injury, nerve
  trapezius G52.8
  traumatic, transient NEC -*see* Injury, nerve
  trembling -*see* Parkinsonism
  triceps brachii G56.9
  trigeminal nerve G50.9
  trochlear (nerve) -*see* Strabismus, paralytic,
    fourth nerve
  ulnar nerve G56.2
  upper limb -*see* Monoplegia, upper limb
  uremic N18.9 [*G99.8*]
  uveoparotitic D86.89
  uvula K13.79
    postdiphtheritic A36.0
  vagus nerve G52.2
  vasomotor NEC G90.8
  velum palati K13.79
  vesical -*see* Paralysis, bladder
  vestibular nerve (except Vertigo) -*see*
    subcategory H93.3
  vocal cords J38.00
    bilateral J38.02
    unilateral J38.01
  Volkmann's (complicating trauma) T79.6
  wasting G12.29
  Weber's G46.3
  wrist G56.9
Paramedial urethrovesical orifice Q64.79
Paramenia N92.6
Parametritis -*see also* Disease, pelvis,
  inflammatory N73.2
  acute N73.0
  complicating abortion -*see* Abortion, by type,
    complicated by, parametritis
Parametrium, parametric -*see* condition

Paramnesia -*see* Amnesia
Paramolar K00.1
Paramyloidosis E85.8
Paramyoclonus multiplex G25.3
Paramyotonia (congenita) G71.19
Parangi -*see* Yaws
Paranoia (querulans) F22
  senile F03
Paranoid
  dementia (senile) F03
    praecox -*see* Schizophrenia
  personality F60.0
  psychosis (climacteric) (involutional)
    (menopausal) F22
    psychogenic (acute) F23
    senile F03
  reaction (acute) F23
    chronic F22
  schizophrenia F20.0
  state (climacteric) (involutional)
    (menopausal) (simple) F22
    senile F03
  tendencies F60.0
  traits F60.0
  trends F60.0
  type, psychopathic personality F60.0
Paraparesis -*see* Paraplegia
Paraphasia R47.02
Paraphilia F65.9
Paraphimosis (congenital) N47.2
  chancroidal A57
Paraphrenia, paraphrenic (late) F22
  schizophrenia F20.0
Paraplegia (lower) G82.20
  ataxic -*see* Degeneration, combined, spinal
    cord
  complete G82.21
  congenital (cerebral) G80.8
    spastic G80.1
  familial spastic G11.4
  functional (hysterical) F44.4
  hereditary, spastic G11.4
  hysterical F44.4
  incomplete G82.22
  Pott's A18.01
  psychogenic F44.4
  spastic
    Erb's spinal, syphilitic A52.17
    hereditary G11.4
    tropical G04.1
  syphilitic (spastic) A52.17
  tropical spastic G04.1
Parapoxvirus B08.60
  specified NEC B08.69
Paraproteinemia D89.2
  benign (familial) D89.2
  monoclonal D47.2
  secondary to malignant disease D47.2
Parapsoriasis L41.9
  en plaques L41.4
  guttata L41.1
  large plaque L41.4
  retiform, retiformis L41.5
  small plaque L41.3
  specified NEC L41.8
  varioliformis (acuta) L41.0
Parasitic -*see also* condition
  disease NEC B89
  stomatitis B37.0
  sycosis (beard) (scalp) B35.0
  twin Q89.4

Parasitism B89
  intestinal B82.9
  skin B88.9
  specified -*see* Infestation
Parasitophobia F40.218
Parasomnia G47.50
  due to
    alcohol
      abuse F10.182
      dependence F10.282
      use F10.982
    amphetamines
      abuse F15.182
      dependence F15.282
      use F15.982
    caffeine
      abuse F15.182
      dependence F15.282
      use F15.982
    cocaine
      abuse F14.182
      dependence F14.282
      use F14.982
    drug NEC
      abuse F19.182
      dependence F19.282
      use F19.982
    opioid
      abuse F11.182
      dependence F11.282
      use F11.982
    psychoactive substance NEC
      abuse F19.182
      dependence F19.282
      use F19.982
    sedative, hypnotic, or anxiolytic
      abuse F13.182
      dependence F13.282
      use F13.982
    stimulant NEC
      abuse F15.182
      dependence F15.282
      use F15.982
  in conditions classified elsewhere G47.54
  nonorganic origin F51.8
  organic G47.50
  specified NEC G47.59
Paraspadias Q54.9
Paraspasmus facialis G51.8
Parasuicide (attempt)
  history of (personal) Z91.5
    in family Z81.8
Parathyroid gland -*see* condition
Parathyroid tetany E20.9
Paratrachoma A74.0
Paratyphlitis -*see* Appendicitis
Paratyphoid (fever) -*see* Fever, paratyphoid
Paratyphus -*see* Fever, paratyphoid
Paraurethral duct Q64.79
  nonorganic origin F51.5
Paraurethritis -*see also* Urethritis
  gonococcal (acute) (chronic) (with abscess)
  A54.1
Paravaccinia NEC B08.04
Paravaginitis -*see* Vaginitis
Parencephalitis -*see also* Encephalitis
  sequelae G09
Parent-child conflict -*see* Conflict, parent-
  child - estrangement NEC Z62.890

Paresis -*see also* Paralysis
  accommodation -*see* Paresis, of
    accommodation
  Bernhardt's G57.1
  bladder (sphincter) -*see also* Paralysis,
    bladder
    tabetic A52.17
  bowel, colon or intestine K56.0
  extrinsic muscle, eye H49.9
  general (progressive) (syphilitic) A52.17
    juvenile A50.45
  heart -*see* Failure, heart
  insane (syphilitic) A52.17
  juvenile (general) A50.45
  of accommodation H52.52
  peripheral progressive (idiopathic) G60.3
  pseudohypertrophic G71.0
  senile G83.9
  syphilitic (general) A52.17
    congenital A50.45
  vesical NEC N31.2
Paresthesia -*see also* Disturbance, sensation
  Bernhardt G57.1
Paretic -*see* condition
Parinaud's
  conjunctivitis H10.89
  oculoglandular syndrome H10.89
  ophthalmoplegia H49.88
Parkinsonism (idiopathic) (primary) G20
  with neurogenic orthostatic hypotension
    (symptomatic) G90.3
  arteriosclerotic G21.4
  dementia G31.83 [*F02.80*]
    with behavioral disturbance G31.83
    [*F02.81*]
  due to
    drugs NEC G21.19
      neuroleptic G21.11
  neuroleptic induced G21.11
  postencephalitic G21.3
  secondary G21.9
    due to
      arteriosclerosis G21.4
      drugs NEC G21.19
        neuroleptic G21.11
      encephalitis G21.3
      external agents NEC G21.2
      syphilis A52.19
    specified NEC G21.8
  syphilitic A52.19
  treatment-induced NEC G21.19
  vascular G21.4
Parkinson's disease, syndrome or tremor -
  see Parkinsonism
Parodontitis -*see* Periodontitis
Parodontosis K05.4
Paronychia -*see also* Cellulitis, digit
  with lymphangitis -*see* Lymphangitis, acute,
    digit
  candidal (chronic) B37.2
  tuberculous (primary) A18.4
Parorexia (psychogenic) F50.89
Parosmia R43.1
  psychogenic F45.8
Parotid gland -*see* condition
Parotitis, parotiditis (allergic)(nonspecific
  toxic) (purulent) (septic) (suppurative) -*see*
  also Sialoadenitis
  epidemic -*see* Mumps
  infectious -*see* Mumps
  postoperative K91.89
  surgical K91.89

Parrot fever A70
Parrot's disease (early congenital syphilitic
  pseudoparalysis) A50.02
Parry Romberg syndrome G51.8
Parry's disease or syndrome E05.00
  with thyroid storm E05.01
Pars planitis -*see* Cyclitis
Parsonage (Aldren) Turner syndrome
  G54.5
Parson's disease (exophthalmic goiter)
  E05.00
  with thyroid storm E05.01
Particolored infant Q82.8
Parturition -*see* Delivery **Parulis** K04.7
  with sinus K04.6
Parvovirus, as cause of disease classified
  elsewhere B97.6
Pasini and Pierini's atrophoderma L90.3
Passage
  false, urethra N36.5
  meconium (newborn) during delivery P03.82
  of sounds or bougies -*see* Attention to,
    artificial, opening
Passive -*see* condition
  smoking Z77.22
Pasteurella septica A28.0
Pasteurellosis -*see* Infection, Pasteurella
PAT (paroxysmal atrial tachycardia) I47.1
Patau's syndrome -*see* Trisomy, 13
Patches
  mucous (syphilitic) A51.39
    congenital A50.07
  smokers' (mouth) K13.24
Patellar -*see* condition
Patent -*see also* Imperfect, closure
  canal of Nuck Q52.4
  cervix N88.3
  ductus arteriosus or Botallo's Q25.0
  foramen
    botalli Q21.1
    ovale Q21.1
  interauricular septum Q21.1
  interventricular septum Q21.0
  omphalomesenteric duct Q43.0
  os (uteri) -*see* Patent, cervix
  ostium secundum Q21.1
  urachus Q64.4
  vitelline duct Q43.0
Paterson (Brown)(Kelly) syndrome or web
  D50.1
Pathologic, pathological -*see also* condition
  asphyxia R09.01
  fire-setting F63.1
  gambling F63.0
  ovum O02.0
  resorption, tooth K03.3
  stealing F63.2
Pathology (of) -*see* Disease
  periradicular, associated with previous
    endodontic treatment NEC M27.59
Pattern, sleep-wake, irregular G47.23
Patulous -*see also* Imperfect, closure
  (congenital)
  alimentary tract Q45.8
    lower Q43.8
    upper Q40.8
  eustachian tube H69.0
Pause, sinoatrial I49.5
Paxton's disease B36.2
Pearl(s)
  enamel K00.2
  Epstein's K09.8

Pearl-worker's disease -see Osteomyelitis, specified type NEC
Pectenosis K62.4
Pectoral -see condition
Pectus
  carinatum (congenital) Q67.7
    acquired M95.4
    rachitic sequelae (late effect) E64.3
  excavatum (congenital) Q67.6
    acquired M95.4
    rachitic sequelae (late effect) E64.3
  recurvatum (congenital) Q67.6
Pedatrophia E41
Pederosis F65.4
Pediculosis (infestation) B85.2
  capitis (head-louse) (any site) B85.0
  corporis (body louse) (any site) B85.1
  eyelid B85.0
  mixed (classifiable to more than one of the titles B85.0 B85.3) B85.4
  pubis (pubic louse) (any site) B85.3
  vestimenti B85.1
  vulvae B85.3
Pediculus (infestation) -see Pediculosis
Pedophilia F65.4
Peg-shaped teeth K00.2
Pelade -see Alopecia, areata
Pelger-Huët anomaly or syndrome D72.0
Peliosis (rheumatica) D69.0
  hepatis K76.4
    with toxic liver disease K71.8
Pelizaeus-Merzbacher disease E75.29
Pellagra (alcoholic) (with polyneuropathy) E52
Pellagra-cerebellar-ataxia-renal aminoaciduria syndrome E72.02
Pellegrini (Stieda) disease or syndrome -see Bursitis, tibial collateral
Pellizzi's syndrome E34.8
Pel's crisis A52.11
Pelvic -see also condition
  examination (periodic) (routine) Z01.419
    with abnormal findings Z01.411
  kidney, congenital Q63.2
Pelviolithiasis -see Calculus, kidney
Pelviperitonitis -see also Peritonitis, pelvic
  gonococcal A54.24
  puerperal O85
Pelvis -see condition or type
Pemphigoid L12.9
  benign, mucous membrane L12.1
  bullous L12.0
  cicatricial L12.1
  juvenile L12.2
  ocular L12.1
  specified NEC L12.8
Pemphigus L10.9
  benign familial (chronic) Q82.8
  Brazilian L10.3
  circinatus L13.0
  conjunctiva L12.1
  drug-induced L10.5
  erythematosus L10.4
  foliaceous L10.2
  gangrenous -see Gangrene
  neonatorum L01.03
  ocular L12.1
  paraneoplastic L10.81
  specified NEC L10.89
  syphilitic (congenital) A50.06
  vegetans L10.1
  vulgaris L10.0
  wildfire L10.3

Pendred's syndrome E07.1
Pendulous
  abdomen, in pregnancy -see Pregnancy, complicated by, abnormal, pelvic organs or tissues NEC
  breast N64.89
Penetrating wound -see also Puncture
  with internal injury -see Injury, by site
  eyeball -see Puncture, eyeball
  orbit (with or without foreign body) -see Puncture, orbit
  uterus by instrument with or following ectopic or molar pregnancy O08.6
Penicillosis B48.4
Penis -see condition
Penitis N48.29
Pentalogy of Fallot Q21.8
Pentasomy X syndrome Q97.1
Pentosuria (essential) E74.8
Percreta placenta O43.23
Peregrinating patient -see Disorder, factitious
Perforation, perforated (nontraumatic) (of)
  accidental during procedure (blood vessel) (nerve) (organ) -see Complication, accidental puncture or laceration
  antrum -see Sinusitis, maxillary
  appendix K35.2
    with localized peritonitis K35.3
  atrial septum, multiple Q21.1
  attic, ear -see Perforation, tympanum, attic
  bile duct (common) (hepatic) K83.2
    cystic K82.2
  bladder (urinary)
    with or following ectopic or molar pregnancy O08.6
    obstetrical trauma O71.5
    traumatic S37.29
      at delivery O71.5
  bowel K63.1
    with or following ectopic or molar pregnancy O08.6
    newborn P78.0
    obstetrical trauma O71.5
    traumatic -see Laceration, intestine
  broad ligament N83.8
    with or following ectopic or molar pregnancy O08.6
    obstetrical trauma O71.6
  by
    device, implant or graft -see also Complications, by site and type, mechanical T85.628
      arterial graft NEC -see Complication, cardiovascular device, mechanical, vascular
      breast (implant) T85.49
      catheter NEC T85.698
        cystostomy T83.090
        dialysis (renal) T82.49
          intraperitoneal T85.691
        infusion NEC T82.594
          spinal (epidural) (subdural) T85.690
        urinary -see also Complications, catheter, urinary T83.098
      electronic (electrode) (pulse generator) (stimulator)
        bone T84.390
        cardiac T82.199
          electrode T82.190
          pulse generator T82.191

Peregrinating patient --continued
  specified type NEC T82.198
  nervous system -see Complication, prosthetic device, mechanical, electronic nervous system stimulator
  urinary -see Complication, genitourinary, device, urinary, mechanical
  fixation, internal (orthopedic) NEC -see Complication, fixation device, mechanical
  gastrointestinal -see Complications, prosthetic device, mechanical, gastrointestinal device
  genital NEC T83.498
    intrauterine contraceptive device T83.39
    penile prosthesis T83.490
  heart NEC -see Complication, cardiovascular device, mechanical
  joint prosthesis -see Complications, joint prosthesis, mechanical, specified NEC, by site
  ocular NEC -see Complications, prosthetic device, mechanical, ocular device
  orthopedic NEC -see Complication, orthopedic, device, mechanical
  specified NEC T85.628
  urinary NEC -see also Complication, genitourinary, device, urinary, mechanical
    graft T83.29
  vascular NEC -see Complication, cardiovascular device, mechanical
  ventricular intracranial shunt T85.09
  foreign body left accidentally in operative wound T81.539
  instrument (any) during a procedure, accidental -see Puncture, accidental complicating surgery   cecum K35.2
  with localized peritonitis K35.3
  cervix (uteri) N88.8
    with or following ectopic or molar pregnancy O08.6
    obstetrical trauma O71.3
  colon K63.1
    newborn P78.0
    obstetrical trauma O71.5
    traumatic -see Laceration, intestine, large
  common duct (bile) K83.2
  cornea (due to ulceration) -see Ulcer, cornea, perforated
  cystic duct K82.2
  diverticulum (intestine) K57.80
    with bleeding K57.81
    large intestine K57.20
      with
        bleeding K57.21
        small intestine K57.40
          with bleeding K57.41
    small intestine K57.00
      with
        bleeding K57.01
        large intestine K57.40
          with bleeding K57.41
  ear drum -see Perforation, tympanum
  esophagus K22.3
  ethmoidal sinus -see Sinusitis, ethmoidal
  frontal sinus -see Sinusitis, frontal
  gallbladder K82.2
  heart valve -see Endocarditis
  ileum K63.1
    newborn P78.0
    obstetrical trauma O71.5

Peregrinating patient *--continued*
   traumatic *-see* Laceration, intestine, small
   instrumental, surgical (accidental) (blood
   vessel) (nerve) (organ) *-see* Puncture,
   accidental complicating surgery   intestine
   NEC K63.1
     with ectopic or molar pregnancy O08.6
     newborn P78.0
     obstetrical trauma O71.5
     traumatic *-see* Laceration, intestine
     ulcerative NEC K63.1
      newborn P78.0
   jejunum, jejunal K63.1
     obstetrical trauma O71.5
     traumatic *-see* Laceration, intestine, small
     ulcer *-see* Ulcer, gastrojejunal, with
     perforation
   joint prosthesis *-see* Complications, joint
     prosthesis, mechanical, specified NEC, by
     site
   mastoid (antrum) (cell) *-see* Disorder,
     mastoid, specified NEC
   maxillary sinus *-see* Sinusitis, maxillary
   membrana tympani *-see* Perforation,
     tympanum
   nasal
     septum J34.89
      congenital Q30.3
      syphilitic A52.73
     sinus J34.89
      congenital Q30.8
      due to sinusitis *-see* Sinusitis
   palate *-see also* Cleft, palate Q35.9
     syphilitic A52.79
   palatine vault *-see also* Cleft, palate, hard
     Q35.1
     syphilitic A52.79
      congenital A50.59
   pars flaccida (ear drum) *-see* Perforation,
     tympanum, attic
   pelvic
     floor S31.030
      with
       ectopic or molar pregnancy O08.6
       penetration into retroperitoneal space
        S31.031
       retained foreign body S31.040
        with penetration into retroperitoneal
        space S31.041
      following ectopic or molar pregnancy
       O08.6
      obstetrical trauma O70.1
     organ S37.99
      adrenal gland S37.818
      bladder *-see* Perforation, bladder
      fallopian tube S37.599
       bilateral S37.592
       unilateral S37.591
      kidney S37.09
       obstetrical trauma O71.5
      ovary S37.499
       bilateral S37.492
       unilateral S37.491
      prostate S37.828
      specified organ NEC S37.898
      ureter *-see* Perforation, ureter
      urethra *-see* Perforation, urethra
      uterus *-see* Perforation, uterus
   perineum *-see* Laceration, perineum
   pharynx J39.2
   rectum K63.1

Peregrinating patient *--continued*
   newborn P78.0
     obstetrical trauma O71.5
     traumatic S36.63
   root canal space due to endodontic treatment
     M27.51
   sigmoid K63.1
     newborn P78.0
     obstetrical trauma O71.5
     traumatic S36.533
   sinus (accessory) (chronic) (nasal) J34.89
   sphenoidal sinus *-see* Sinusitis, sphenoidal
   surgical (accidental) (by instrument) (blood
   vessel) (nerve) (organ) *-see* Puncture,
   accidental complicating surgery   traumatic
     external *-see* Puncture
     eye *-see* Puncture, eyeball
     internal organ *-see* Injury, by site
   tympanum, tympanic (membrane) (persistent
   post-traumatic) (postinflammatory) H72.9
     attic H72.1
      multiple *-see* Perforation, tympanum,
     multiple
      total *-see* Perforation, tympanum, total
     central H72.0
      multiple *-see* Perforation, tympanum,
     multiple
      total *-see* Perforation, tympanum, total
     marginal NEC *-see* subcategory H72.2
     multiple H72.81
     pars flaccida *-see* Perforation, tympanum,
     attic
     total H72.82
     traumatic, current episode S09.2
   typhoid, gastrointestinal *-see* Typhoid
   ulcer *-see* Ulcer, by site, with perforation
   ureter N28.89
     traumatic S37.19
   urethra N36.8
     with ectopic or molar pregnancy O08.6
     following ectopic or molar pregnancy O08.6
     obstetrical trauma O71.5
     traumatic S37.39
      at delivery O71.5
   uterus
     with ectopic or molar pregnancy O08.6
     by intrauterine contraceptive device T83.39
     following ectopic or molar pregnancy O08.6
     obstetrical trauma O71.1
     traumatic S37.69
      obstetric O71.1
   uvula K13.79
     syphilitic A52.79
   vagina
     obstetrical trauma O71.4
     other trauma *-see* Puncture, vagina
Periadenitis mucosa necrotica recurrens
   K12.0
Periappendicitis (acute) *-see* Appendicitis
Periarteritis nodosa (disseminated)
   (infectious) (necrotizing) M30.0
Periarthritis (joint) *-see also* Enthesopathy
   Duplay's M75.0
   gonococcal A54.42
   humeroscapularis *-see* Capsulitis, adhesive
   scapulohumeral *-see* Capsulitis, adhesive
   shoulder *-see* Capsulitis, adhesive
   wrist M77.2
Periarthrosis (angioneural) *-see* Enthesopathy
Pericapsulitis, adhesive (shoulder) *-see*
   Capsulitis, adhesive

Pericarditis (with decompensation) (with
   effusion) I31.9
   with rheumatic fever (conditions in I00)
     active *-see* Pericarditis, rheumatic
     inactive or quiescent I09.2
   acute (hemorrhagic) (nonrheumatic) (Sicca)
     I30.9
     with chorea (acute) (rheumatic)
      (Sydenham's) I02.0
     benign I30.8
     nonspecific I30.0
     rheumatic I01.0
      with chorea (acute) (Sydenham's) I02.0
   adhesive or adherent (chronic) (external)
     (internal) I31.0
     acute *-see* Pericarditis, acute
     rheumatic I09.2
   bacterial (acute) (subacute) (with serous or
     seropurulent effusion) I30.1
   calcareous I31.1
   cholesterol (chronic) I31.8
     acute I30.9
   chronic (nonrheumatic) I31.9
     rheumatic I09.2
   constrictive (chronic) I31.1
   coxsackie B33.23
   fibrinocaseous (tuberculous) A18.84
   fibrinopurulent I30.1
   fibrinous I30.8
   fibrous I31.0
   gonococcal A54.83
   idiopathic I30.0
   in systemic lupus erythematosus M32.12
   infective I30.1
   meningococcal A39.53
   neoplastic (chronic) I31.8
     acute I30.9
   obliterans, obliterating I31.0
   plastic I31.0
   pneumococcal I30.1
   postinfarction I24.1
   purulent I30.1
   rheumatic (active) (acute) (with effusion)
     (with pneumonia) I01.0
     with chorea (acute) (rheumatic)
      (Sydenham's) I02.0
     chronic or inactive (with chorea) I09.2
   rheumatoid *-see* Rheumatoid, carditis
   septic I30.1
   serofibrinous I30.8
   staphylococcal I30.1
   streptococcal I30.1
   suppurative I30.1
   syphilitic A52.06
   tuberculous A18.84
   uremic N18.9 *[I32]*
   viral I30.1
Pericardium, pericardial *-see* condition
Pericellulitis *-see* Cellulitis
Pericementitis (chronic) (suppurative) *-see*
   also Periodontitis
   acute K05.20
     generalized *-see* Peridontitis, aggressive,
     generalized
     localized *-see* Peridontitis, aggressive,
     localized
Perichondritis
   auricle *-see* Perichondritis, ear
   bronchus J98.09
   ear (external) H61.00
     acute H61.01

Perichondritis - *continued*
  chronic H61.02
  external auditory canal -*see* Perichondritis, ear
  larynx J38.7
    syphilitic A52.73
    typhoid A01.09
  nose J34.89
  pinna -*see* Perichondritis, ear
  trachea J39.8
Periclasia K05.4
Pericoronitis -*see* Periodontitis
Pericystitis N30.90
  with hematuria N30.91
Peridiverticulitis (intestine) K57.92
  cecum -*see* Diverticulitis, intestine, large
  colon -*see* Diverticulitis, intestine, large
  duodenum -*see* Diverticulitis, intestine, small
  intestine -*see* Diverticulitis, intestine
  jejunum -*see* Diverticulitis, intestine, small
  rectosigmoid -*see* Diverticulitis, intestine,
  large
  rectum -*see* Diverticulitis, intestine, large
  sigmoid -*see* Diverticulitis, intestine, large
Periendocarditis -*see* Endocarditis
Periepididymitis N45.1
Perifolliculitis L01.02
  abscedens, caput, scalp L66.3
  capitis, abscedens (et suffodiens) L66.3
  superficial pustular L01.02
Perihepatitis K65.8
Perilabyrinthitis (acute) -*see* subcategory
  H83.0
Perimeningitis -*see* Meningitis
Perimetritis -*see* Endometritis
Perimetrosalpingitis -*see* Salpingo-oophoritis
Perineocele N81.81
Perinephric, perinephritic -*see* condition
Perinephritis -*see also* Infection, kidney
  purulent -*see* Abscess, kidney
Perineum, perineal -*see* condition
Perineuritis NEC -*see* Neuralgia **Periodic** -*see*
  condition
Periodontitis (chronic) (complex)
  (compound) (local) (simplex) K05.30
  acute K05.20
    generalized K05.229
      moderate K05.222
      severe K05.223
      slight K05.221
    localized K05.219
      moderate K05.212
      severe K05.213
      slight K05.211
  apical K04.5
    acute (pulpal origin) K04.4
  generalized K05.329
    moderate K05.322
    severe K05.323
    slight K05.321
  localized K05.319
    moderate K05.312
    severe K05.313
    slight K05.311
Periodontoclasia K05.4
Periodontosis (juvenile) K05.4
Periods -*see also* Menstruation
  heavy N92.0
  irregular N92.6
  shortened intervals (irregular) N92.1
Perionychia -*see also* Cellulitis, digit
  with lymphangitis -*see* Lymphangitis, acute,
  digit

Perioophoritis -*see* Salpingo-oophoritis
Periorchitis N45.2
Periosteum, periosteal -*see* condition
Periostitis (albuminosa) (circumscribed)
  (diffuse) (infective) (monomelic) -*see also*
  Osteomyelitis
  alveolar M27.3
  alveolodental M27.3
  dental M27.3
  gonorrheal A54.43
  jaw (lower) (upper) M27.2
  orbit H05.03
  syphilitic A52.77
    congenital (early) A50.02 [*M90.80*]
    secondary A51.46
  tuberculous -*see* Tuberculosis, bone
  yaws (hypertrophic) (early) (late) A66.6
  [*M90.80*]
Periostosis (hyperplastic) -*see also* Disorder,
  bone, specified type NEC
  with osteomyelitis -*see* Osteomyelitis,
  specified type NEC
Peripartum
  cardiomyopathy O90.3
Periphlebitis -*see* Phlebitis
Periproctitis K62.89
Periprostatitis -*see* Prostatitis
Perirectal -*see* condition
Perirenal -*see* condition
Perisalpingitis -*see* Salpingo-oophoritis
Perisplenitis (infectional) D73.89
Peristalsis, visible or reversed R19.2
Peritendinitis -*see* Enthesopathy
Peritoneum, peritoneal -*see* condition
Peritonitis (adhesive) (bacterial) (fibrinous)
  (hemorrhagic) (idiopathic) (localized)
  (perforative) (primary) (with adhesions)
  (with effusion) K65.9
  with or following
    abscess K65.1
    appendicitis K35.3
      with perforation or rupture K35.2
      generalized K35.2
      localized K35.3
    diverticular disease (intestine) K57.80
      with bleeding K57.81
      large intestine K57.20
        with
          bleeding K57.21
          small intestine K57.40
            with bleeding K57.41
      small intestine K57.00
        with
          bleeding K57.01
          large intestine K57.40
            with bleeding K57.41
    ectopic or molar pregnancy O08.0
  acute (generalized) K65.0
  aseptic T81.61
  bile, biliary K65.3
  chemical T81.61
  chlamydial A74.81
  complicating abortion -*see* Abortion, by type,
  complicated by, pelvic peritonitis
  congenital P78.1
  chronic proliferative K65.8
  diaphragmatic K65.0
  diffuse K65.0
  diphtheritic A36.89
  disseminated K65.0
  due to

Peritonitis - *continued*
  bile K65.3
  foreign
    body or object accidentally left during a
      procedure (instrument) (sponge) (swab)
      T81.599
    substance accidentally left during a
      procedure (chemical) (powder) (talc)
      T81.61
    talc T81.61
    urine K65.8
  eosinophilic K65.8
    acute K65.0
  fibrocaseous (tuberculous) A18.31
  fibropurulent K65.0
  following ectopic or molar pregnancy O08.0
  general (ized) K65.0
  gonococcal A54.85
  meconium (newborn) P78.0
  neonatal P78.1
    meconium P78.0
  pancreatic K65.0
  paroxysmal, familial E85.0
    benign E85.0
  pelvic
    female N73.5
      acute N73.3
      chronic N73.4
        with adhesions N73.6
    male K65.0
  periodic, familial E85.0
  proliferative, chronic K65.8
  puerperal, postpartum, childbirth O85
  purulent K65.0
  septic K65.0
  specified NEC K65.8
  spontaneous bacterial K65.2
  subdiaphragmatic K65.0
  subphrenic K65.0
  suppurative K65.0
  syphilitic A52.74
    congenital (early) A50.08 [*K67*]
  talc T81.61
  tuberculous A18.31
  urine K65.8
Peritonsillar -*see* condition
Peritonsillitis J36
Perityphlitis K37
Periureteritis N28.89
Periurethral -*see* condition
Periurethritis (gangrenous) -*see* Urethritis
Periuterine -*see* condition
Perivaginitis -*see* Vaginitis
Perivasculitis, retinal H35.06
Perivasitis (chronic) N49.1
Perivesiculitis (seminal) -*see* Vesiculitis
Perlèche NEC K13.0
  due to
    candidiasis B37.83
    moniliasis B37.83
    riboflavin deficiency E53.0
    vitamin B2 (riboflavin) deficiency E53.0
Pernicious -*see* condition
Pernio, perniosis T69.1
Perpetrator (of abuse) -*see* Index to External
  Causes of Injury, Perpetrator
Persecution
  delusion F22
  social Z60.5
Perseveration (tonic) R48.8

Persistence, persistent (congenital)
  anal membrane Q42.3
    with fistula Q42.2
  arteria stapedia Q16.3
  atrioventricular canal Q21.2
  branchial cleft Q18.0
  bulbus cordis in left ventricle Q21.8
  canal of Cloquet Q14.0
  capsule (opaque) Q12.8
  cilioretinal artery or vein Q14.8
  cloaca Q43.7
  communication -see Fistula, congenital
  convolutions
    aortic arch Q25.46
    fallopian tube Q50.6
    oviduct Q50.6
    uterine tube Q50.6
  double aortic arch Q25.45
  ductus arteriosus (Botalli) Q25.0
  fetal
    circulation P29.3
    form of cervix (uteri) Q51.828
    hemoglobin, hereditary (HPFH) D56.4
  foramen
    Botalli Q21.1
    ovale Q21.1
  Gartner's duct Q52.4
  hemoglobin, fetal (hereditary) (HPFH) D56.4
  hyaloid
    artery (generally incomplete) Q14.0
    system Q14.8
  hymen, in pregnancy or childbirth -see
    Pregnancy, complicated by, abnormal, vulva
  lanugo Q84.2
  left
    posterior cardinal vein Q26.8
    root with right arch of aorta Q25.49
    superior vena cava Q26.1
  Meckel's diverticulum Q43.0
    malignant -see Table of Neoplasms, small
      intestine, malignant
  mucosal disease (middle ear) -see Otitis,
    media, suppurative, chronic, tubotympanic
  nail(s), anomalous Q84.6
  omphalomesenteric duct Q43.0
  organ or site not listed -see Anomaly, by site
  ostium
    atrioventriculare commune Q21.2
    primum Q21.2
    secundum Q21.1
  ovarian rests in fallopian tube Q50.6
  pancreatic tissue in intestinal tract Q43.8
  primary (deciduous)
    teeth K00.6
    vitreous hyperplasia Q14.0
  pupillary membrane Q13.89
  right aortic arch Q25.47
  rhesus (Rh) titer -see Complication(s),
    transfusion, incompatibility reaction, Rh
    (factor)
  sinus
    urogenitalis
      female Q52.8
      male Q55.8
    venosus with imperfect incorporation in
      right auricle Q26.8
  thymus (gland) (hyperplasia) E32.0
  thyroglossal duct Q89.2
  thyrolingual duct Q89.2
  truncus arteriosus or communis Q20.0
  tunica vasculosa lentis Q12.2

Persistence, persistent - *continued*
  umbilical sinus Q64.4
  urachus Q64.4
  vitelline duct Q43.0
Person (with)
  admitted for clinical research, as a control
    subject (normal comparison) (participant)
    Z00.6
  awaiting admission to adequate facility
    elsewhere Z75.1
  concern (normal) about sick person in family
    Z63.6
  consulting on behalf of another Z71.0
  feigning illness Z76.5
  living (in)
    alone Z60.2
    boarding school Z59.3
    residential institution Z59.3
    without
      adequate housing (heating) (space) Z59.1
      housing (permanent) (temporary) Z59.0
      person able to render necessary care Z74.2
      shelter Z59.0
  on waiting list Z75.1
  sick or handicapped in family Z63.6
Personality (disorder) F60.9
  accentuation of traits (type A pattern) Z73.1
  affective F34.0
  aggressive F60.3
  amoral F60.2
  anancastic, anankastic F60.5
  antisocial F60.2
  anxious F60.6
  asocial F60.2
  asthenic F60.7
  avoidant F60.6
  borderline F60.3
  change due to organic condition (enduring)
    F07.0
  compulsive F60.5
  cycloid F34.0
  cyclothymic F34.0
  dependent F60.7
  depressive F34.1
  dissocial F60.2
  dual F44.81
  eccentric F60.89
  emotionally unstable F60.3
  expansive paranoid F60.0
  explosive F60.3
  fanatic F60.0
  haltlose type F60.89
  histrionic F60.4
  hyperthymic F34.0
  hypothymic F34.1
  hysterical F60.4
  immature F60.89
  inadequate F60.7
  labile (emotional) F60.3
  mixed (nonspecific) F60.89
  morally defective F60.2
  multiple F44.81
  narcissistic F60.81
  obsessional F60.5
  obsessive (compulsive) F60.5
  organic F07.0
  overconscientious F60.5
  paranoid F60.0
  passive (dependent) F60.7
  passive-aggressive F60.89
  pathologic F60.9

Person (with)
  pattern defect or disturbance F60.9
  pseudopsychopathic (organic) F07.0
  pseudoretarded (organic) F07.0
  psychoinfantile F60.4
  psychoneurotic NEC F60.89
  psychopathic F60.2
  querulant F60.0
  sadistic F60.89
  schizoid F60.1
  self-defeating F60.7
  sensitive paranoid F60.0
  sociopathic (amoral) (antisocial) (asocial)
    (dissocial) F60.2
  specified NEC F60.89
  type A Z73.1
  unstable (emotional) F60.3
Perthes' disease -see Legg-Calvé Perthes
  disease
Pertussis -see also Whooping cough A37.90
Perversion, perverted appetite F50.89
  psychogenic F50.89
  function
    pituitary gland E23.2
    posterior lobe E22.2
  sense of smell and taste R43.8
    psychogenic F45.8
  sexual -see Deviation, sexual
Pervious, congenital -see also Imperfect,
  closure
  ductus arteriosus Q25.0
Pes (congenital) -see also Talipes
  acquired -see also Deformity, limb, foot,
    specified NEC
    planus -see Deformity, limb, flat foot
  adductus Q66.89
  cavus Q66.7
  deformity NEC, acquired -see Deformity,
    limb, foot, specified NEC
  planus (acquired) (any degree) -see also
    Deformity, limb, flat foot
    rachitic sequelae (late effect) E64.3
  valgus Q66.6
Pest, pestis -see Plague
Petechia, petechiae R23.3
  newborn P54.5
Petechial typhus A75.9
Peter's anomaly Q13.4
Petit mal seizure -see Epilepsy, generalized,
  specified NEC
Petit's hernia -see Hernia, abdomen, specified
  site NEC
Petriellidiosis B48.2
Petrositis H70.20
  acute H70.21
  chronic H70.22
Peutz Jeghers disease or syndrome Q85.8
Peyronie's disease N48.6
**PFAPA (periodic fever, aphthous stomatitis,
  pharyngitis, and adenopathy syndrome)**
  M04.8
Pfeiffer's disease -see Mononucleosis,
  infectious
Phagedena (dry) (moist) (sloughing) -see also
  Gangrene
  geometric L88
  penis N48.29
  tropical -see Ulcer, skin
  vulva N76.6
Phagedenic -see condition
Phakoma H35.89

Phakomatosis -see also specific eponymous
   syndromes Q85.9
   Bourneville's Q85.1
   specified NEC Q85.8
Phantom limb syndrome (without pain)
   G54.7
   with pain G54.6
Pharyngeal pouch syndrome D82.1
Pharyngitis (acute) (catarrhal)(gangrenous)
  (infective) (malignant) (membranous)
  (phlegmonous) (pseudomembranous)
  (simple) (subacute) (suppurative)
  (ulcerative) (viral) J02.9
   with influenza, flu, or grippe -see Influenza,
     with, pharyngitis
   aphthous B08.5
   atrophic J31.2
   chlamydial A56.4
   chronic (atrophic) (granular) (hypertrophic)
     J31.2
   coxsackievirus B08.5
   diphtheritic A36.0
   enteroviral vesicular B08.5
   follicular (chronic) J31.2
   fusospirochetal A69.1
   gonococcal A54.5
   granular (chronic) J31.2
   herpesviral B00.2
   hypertrophic J31.2
   infectional, chronic J31.2
   influenzal -see Influenza, with, respiratory
     manifestations NEC
   lymphonodular, acute (enteroviral) B08.8
   pneumococcal J02.8
   purulent J02.9
   putrid J02.9
   septic J02.0
   sicca J31.2
   specified organism NEC J02.8
   staphylococcal J02.8
   streptococcal J02.0
   syphilitic, congenital (early) A50.03
   tuberculous A15.8
   vesicular, enteroviral B08.5
   viral NEC J02.8
Pharyngoconjunctivitis, viral B30.2
Pharyngolaryngitis (acute) J06.0
   chronic J37.0
Pharyngoplegia J39.2
Pharyngotonsillitis, herpesviral B00.2
Pharyngotracheitis, chronic J42
Pharynx, pharyngeal -see condition
Phencyclidine-induced
   anxiety disorder F16.980
   bipolar and related disorder F16.94
   depressive disorder F16.94
   psychotic disorder F16.959
Phenomenon
   Arthus' -see Arthus' phenomenon
   jaw-winking Q07.8
   lupus erythematosus (LE) cell M32.9
   Raynaud's (secondary) I73.00
     with gangrene I73.01
   vasomotor R55
   vasospastic I73.9
   vasovagal R55
   Wenckebach's I44.1
Phenylketonuria E70.1
   classical E70.0
   maternal E70.1

Pheochromoblastoma
   specified site -see Neoplasm, malignant, by
     site
   unspecified site C74.10
Pheochromocytoma - malignant
   specified site -see Neoplasm, malignant, by
     site
   unspecified site C74.10
   specified site -see Neoplasm, benign, by site
   unspecified site D35.00
Phaeohyphomycosis -see Chromomycosis
Pheomycosis -see Chromomycosis
Phimosis (congenital) (due to infection)
   N47.1
   chancroidal A57
Phlebectasia -see also Varix
   congenital Q27.4
Phlebitis (infective) (pyemic) (septic)
  (suppurative) I80.9
   antepartum -see Thrombophlebitis,
     antepartum
   blue -see Phlebitis, leg, deep
   breast, superficial I80.8
   cavernous (venous) sinus -see Phlebitis,
     intracranial (venous) sinus
   cerebral (venous) sinus -see Phlebitis,
     intracranial (venous) sinus
   chest wall, superficial I80.8
   cranial (venous) sinus -see Phlebitis,
     intracranial (venous) sinus
   deep (vessels) -see Phlebitis, leg, deep
   due to implanted device -see Complications,
     by site and type, specified NEC
   during or resulting from a procedure T81.72
   femoral vein (superficial) I80.1
   femoropopliteal vein I80.0
   gestational -see Phlebopathy, gestational
   hepatic veins I80.8
   iliofemoral -see Phlebitis, femoral vein
   intracranial (venous) sinus (any) G08
     nonpyogenic I67.6
   intraspinal venous sinuses and veins G08
     nonpyogenic G95.19
   lateral (venous) sinus -see Phlebitis,
     intracranial (venous) sinus
   leg I80.3
     antepartum -see Thrombophlebitis,
   antepartum
     deep (vessels) NEC I80.20
       iliac I80.21
       popliteal vein I80.22
       specified vessel NEC I80.29
       tibial vein I80.23
     femoral vein (superficial) I80.1
     superficial (vessels) I80.0
   longitudinal sinus -see Phlebitis, intracranial
     (venous) sinus
   lower limb -see Phlebitis, leg
   migrans, migrating (superficial) I82.1
   pelvic
     with ectopic or molar pregnancy O08.0
     following ectopic or molar pregnancy O08.0
     puerperal, postpartum O87.1
   popliteal vein -see Phlebitis, leg, deep,
     popliteal
   portal (vein) K75.1
   postoperative T81.72
   pregnancy -see Thrombophlebitis, antepartum
   puerperal, postpartum, childbirth O87.0
     deep O87.1
     pelvic O87.1

Phlebitis - *continued*
   superficial O87.0
   retina -see Vasculitis, retina
   saphenous (accessory) (great) (long) (small) -
     see Phlebitis, leg, superficial
   sinus (meninges) -see Phlebitis, intracranial
     (venous) sinus
   specified site NEC I80.8
   syphilitic A52.09
   tibial vein -see Phlebitis, leg, deep, tibial
   ulcerative I80.9
     leg -see Phlebitis, leg
   umbilicus I80.8
   uterus (septic) -see Endometritis
   varicose (leg) (lower limb) -see Varix, leg,
     with, inflammation
Phlebofibrosis I87.8
Phleboliths I87.8
Phlebopathy,
   gestational O22.9
   puerperal O87.9
Phlebosclerosis I87.8
Phlebothrombosis -see also Thrombosis
   antepartum -see Thrombophlebitis,
     antepartum
   pregnancy -see Thrombophlebitis, antepartum
   puerperal -see Thrombophlebitis, puerperal
Phlebotomus fever A93.1
Phlegmasia
   alba dolens O87.1
     nonpuerperal -see Phlebitis, femoral vein
   cerulea dolens -see Phlebitis, leg, deep
Phlegmon -see Abscess
Phlegmonous -see condition
Phlyctenulosis (allergic)
  (keratoconjunctivitis) (nontuberculous) -
   see also Keratoconjunctivitis
   cornea -see Keratoconjunctivitis
   tuberculous A18.52
Phobia, phobic F40.9
   animal F40.218
     spiders F40.210
   examination F40.298
   reaction F40.9
   simple F40.298
   social F40.10
     generalized F40.11
   specific (isolated) F40.298
     animal F40.218
       spiders F40.210
     blood F40.230
     injection F40.231
     injury F40.233
     men F40.290
     natural environment F40.228
       thunderstorms F40.220
     situational F40.248
       bridges F40.242
       closed in spaces F40.240
       flying F40.243
       heights F40.241
     specified focus NEC F40.298
     transfusion F40.231
     women F40.291
   specified NEC F40.8
     medical care NEC F40.232
   state F40.9
Phocas' disease -see Mastopathy, cystic
Phocomelia Q73.1
   lower limb -see Agenesis, leg, with foot
     present
   upper limb -see Agenesis, arm, with hand
     present

Phoria H50.50
Phosphate-losing tubular disorder N25.0
Phosphatemia E83.39
Phosphaturia E83.39
Photodermatitis (sun) L56.8
  chronic L57.8
  due to drug L56.8
  light other than sun L59.8
Photokeratitis H16.13
Photophobia H53.14
Photophthalmia -*see* Photokeratitis
Photopsia H53.19
Photoretinitis -*see* Retinopathy, solar
Photosensitivity, photosensitization (sun)
  skin L56.8
  light other than sun L59.8
Phrenitis -*see* Encephalitis
Phrynoderma (vitamin A deficiency) E50.8
Phthiriasis (pubis) B85.3
  with any infestation classifiable to B85.0
  B85.2
  B85.4
Phthirus infestation -*see* Phthiriasis
Phthisis -*see also* Tuberculosis
  bulbi (infectional) -*see* Disorder, globe,
  degenerated condition, atrophy
  eyeball (due to infection) -*see* Disorder,
  globe, degenerated condition, atrophy
Phycomycosis -*see* Zygomycosis
Physalopteriasis B81.8
Physical restraint status Z78.1
Phytobezoar T18.9
  intestine T18.3
  stomach T18.2
Pian -*see* Yaws
Pianoma A66.1
Pica F50.89
  in adults F50.89
  infant or child F98.3
Picking, nose F98.8
Pick-Niemann disease -*see* Niemann-Pick
  disease or syndrome
Pick's
  cerebral atrophy G31.01 [*F02.80*]
    with behavioral disturbance G31.01
    [*F02.81*]
  disease or syndrome (brain) G31.01 [*F02.80*]
    with behavioral disturbance G31.01
    [*F02.81*]
    brain G31.01 [*F02.80*]
     with behavioral disturbance G31.01
     [*F02.81*]
    pericardium (pericardial pseudocirrhosis of
    liver) I31.1
  syndrome
    brain G31.01 [*F02.80*]
     with behavioral disturbance G31.01
     [*F02.81*]
    of heart (pericardial pseudocirrhosis of liver)
    I31.1
Pickwickian syndrome E66.2
Piebaldism E70.39
Piedra (beard) (scalp) B36.8
  black B36.3
  white B36.2
Pierre Robin deformity or syndrome Q87.0
Pierson's disease or osteochondrosis M91.0
Pig-bel A05.2
Pigeon
  breast or chest (acquired) M95.4
    congenital Q67.7

Pigeon - *continued*
  rachitic sequelae (late effect) E64.3
  breeder's disease or lung J67.2
  fancier's disease or lung J67.2
  toe -*see* Deformity, toe, specified NEC
Pigmentation (abnormal) (anomaly) L81.9
  conjunctiva H11.13
  cornea (anterior) H18.01
    posterior H18.05
    stromal H18.06
  diminished melanin formation NEC L81.6
  iron L81.8
  lids, congenital Q82.8
  limbus corneae -*see* Pigmentation, cornea
  metals L81.8
  optic papilla, congenital Q14.2
  retina, congenital (grouped) (nevoid) Q14.1
  scrotum, congenital Q82.8
  tattoo L81.8
Piles -*see also* Hemorrhoids K64.9
Pili
  annulati or torti (congenital) Q84.1
  incarnati L73.1
Pill roller hand (intrinsic) -*see* Parkinsonism
Pilomatrixoma -*see* Neoplasm, skin, benign
  malignant -*see* Neoplasm, skin, malignant
Pilonidal -*see* condition
Pimple R23.8
PIN -*see* Neoplasia, intraepithelial, prostate
Pinched nerve -*see* Neuropathy, entrapment
Pindborg tumor -*see* Cyst, calcifying
  odontogenic
Pineal body or gland -*see* condition
Pinealoblastoma C75.3
Pinealoma D44.5
  malignant C75.3
Pineoblastoma C75.3
Pineocytoma D44.5
Pinguecula H11.15
Pingueculitis H10.81
Pinhole meatus -*see also* Stricture, urethra
  N35.9
Pink
  disease - see subcategory T56.1
  eye -*see* Conjunctivitis, acute, mucopurulent
Pinkus' disease (lichen nitidus) L44.1
Pinpoint
  meatus -*see* Stricture, urethra
  os (uteri) -*see* Stricture, cervix
Pins and needles R20.2
Pinta A67.9
  cardiovascular lesions A67.2
  chancre (primary) A67.0
  erythematous plaques A67.1
  hyperchromic lesions A67.1
  hyperkeratosis A67.1
  lesions A67.9
    cardiovascular A67.2
    hyperchromic A67.1
    intermediate A67.1
    late A67.2
    mixed A67.3
    primary A67.0
  skin (achromic) (cicatricial) (dyschromic)
  A67.2
    hyperchromic A67.1
    mixed (achromic and hyperchromic) A67.3
  papule (primary) A67.0
  skin lesions (achromic) (cicatricial)
  (dyschromic) A67.2
    hyperchromic A67.1
    mixed (achromic and hyperchromic) A67.3
  vitiligo A67.2

Pintids A67.1
Pinworm (disease) (infection) (infestation)
  B80
Piroplasmosis B60.0
Pistol wound -*see* Gunshot wound
Pitchers' elbow -*see* Derangement, joint,
  specified type NEC, elbow
Pithecoid pelvis Q74.2
  with disproportion (fetopelvic) O33.0
    causing obstructed labor O65.0
Pithiatism F48.8
Pitted -*see* Pitting
Pitting -*see also* Edema R60.9
  lip R60.0
  nail L60.8
  teeth K00.4
Pituitary gland -*see* condition
Pituitary snuff-taker's disease J67.8
Pityriasis (capitis) L21.0
  alba L30.5
  circinata (et maculata) L42
  furfuracea L21.0
  Hebra's L26
  lichenoides L41.0
    chronica L41.1
    et varioliformis (acuta) L41.0
  maculata (et circinata) L30.5
  nigra B36.1
  pilaris, Hebra's L44.0
  rosea L42
  rotunda L44.8
  rubra (Hebra) pilaris L44.0
  simplex L30.5
  specified type NEC L30.5
  streptogenes L30.5
  versicolor (scrotal) B36.0
Placenta, placental -*see* Pregnancy,
  complicated by (care of) (management
  affected by), specified condition
Placentitis O41.14
Plagiocephaly Q67.3
Plague A20.9
  abortive A20.8
  ambulatory A20.8
  asymptomatic A20.8
  bubonic A20.0
  cellulocutaneous A20.1
  cutaneobubonic A20.1
  lymphatic gland A20.0
  meningitis A20.3
  pharyngeal A20.8
  pneumonic (primary) (secondary) A20.2
  pulmonary, pulmonic A20.2
  septicemic A20.7
  tonsillar A20.8
    septicemic A20.7
Planning, family
  contraception Z30.9
  procreation Z31.69
Plaque(s)
  artery, arterial -*see* Arteriosclerosis
  calcareous -*see* Calcification
  coronary, lipid rich I25.83
  epicardial I31.8
  erythematous, of pinta A67.1
  Hollenhorst's -*see* Occlusion, artery, retina
  lipid rich, coronary I25.83
  pleural (without asbestos) J92.9
    with asbestos J92.0
  tongue K13.29

Plasmacytoma C90.3
  extramedullary C90.2
  medullary C90.0
  solitary C90.3
Plasmacytopenia D72.818
Plasmacytosis D72.822
Plaster ulcer -*see* Ulcer, pressure, by site
Plateau iris syndrome (post-iridectomy)
  (postprocedural) (without glaucoma)
  H21.82
  with glaucoma H40.22
Platybasia Q75.8
Platyonychia (congenital) Q84.6
  acquired L60.8
Platypelloid pelvis M95.5
  with disproportion (fetopelvic) O33.0
    causing obstructed labor O65.0
  congenital Q74.2
Platyspondylisis Q76.49
Plaut (Vincent) disease -*see also* Vincent's
  A69.1
Plethora R23.2
  newborn P61.1
Pleura, pleural -*see* condition
Pleuralgia R07.81
Pleurisy (acute) (adhesive) (chronic) (costal)
  (diaphragmatic) (double) (dry) (fibrinous)
  (fibrous) (interlobar) (latent) (plastic)
  (primary) (residual) (sicca) (sterile)
  (subacute) (unresolved) R09.1
  with
    adherent pleura J86.0
    effusion J90
      chylous, chyliform J94.0
      tuberculous (non primary) A15.6
        primary (progressive) A15.7
    tuberculosis -*see* Pleurisy, tuberculous (non
      primary)
  encysted -*see* Pleurisy, with effusion
  exudative -*see* Pleurisy, with effusion
  fibrinopurulent, fibropurulent -*see* Pyothorax
  - hemorrhagic -*see* Hemothorax
  pneumococcal J90
  purulent -*see* Pyothorax - septic -*see*
    Pyothorax
  serofibrinous -*see* Pleurisy, with effusion
  seropurulent -*see* Pyothorax
  serous -*see* Pleurisy, with effusion
  staphylococcal J86.9
  streptococcal J90
  suppurative -*see* Pyothorax
  traumatic (post) (current) -*see* Injury,
    intrathoracic, pleura
  tuberculous (with effusion) (non primary)
    A15.6
    primary (progressive) A15.7
Pleuritis sicca -*see* Pleurisy
Pleurobronchopneumonia -*see* Pneumonia,
  broncho-
Pleurodynia R07.81
  epidemic B33.0
  viral B33.0
Pleuropericarditis -*see also* Pericarditis
  acute I30.9
Pleuropneumonia (acute) (bilateral) (double)
  (septic) -*see also* Pneumonia J18.8
  chronic -*see* Fibrosis, lung
Pleuro-pneumonia-like-organism (PPLO), as
  cause of disease classified elsewhere B96.0
Pleurorrhea -*see* Pleurisy, with effusion
Plexitis, brachial G54.0

Plica
  polonica B85.0
  syndrome, knee M67.5
  tonsil J35.8
Plicated tongue K14.5
Plug
  bronchus NEC J98.09
  meconium (newborn) NEC syndrome P76.0
  mucus -*see* Asphyxia, mucus
Plumbism -*see* subcategory T56.0
Plummer's disease E05.20
  with thyroid storm E05.21
Plummer-Vinson syndrome D50.1
Pluricarential syndrome of infancy E40
Plus (and minus) hand (intrinsic) -*see*
  Deformity, limb, specified type NEC, forearm
Pneumathemia -*see* Air, embolism
Pneumatic hammer (drill) syndrome T75.21
Pneumatocele (lung) J98.4
  intracranial G93.89
  tension J44.9
Pneumatosis
  cystoides intestinalis K63.89
  intestinalis K63.89
  peritonei K66.8
Pneumaturia R39.89
Pneumoblastoma -*see* Neoplasm, lung,
  malignant
Pneumocephalus G93.89
Pneumococcemia A40.3
Pneumococcus, pneumococcal -*see* condition
Pneumoconiosis (due to) (inhalation of) J64
  with tuberculosis (any type in A15) J65
  aluminum J63.0
  asbestos J61
  bagasse, bagassosis J67.1
  bauxite J63.1
  beryllium J63.2
  coal miners' (simple) J60
  coalworkers' (simple) J60
  collier's J60
  cotton dust J66.0
  diatomite (diatomaceous earth) J62.8
  dust
    inorganic NEC J63.6
    lime J62.8
    marble J62.8
    organic NEC J66.8
  fumes or vapors (from silo) J68.9
  graphite J63.3
  grinder's J62.8
  kaolin J62.8
  mica J62.8
  millstone maker's J62.8
  mineral fibers NEC J61
  miner's J60
  moldy hay J67.0
  potter's J62.8
  rheumatoid -*see* Rheumatoid, lung
  sandblaster's J62.8
  silica, silicate NEC J62.8
    with carbon J60
  stonemason's J62.8
  talc (dust) J62.0
Pneumocystis carinii pneumonia B59
Pneumocystis jiroveci (pneumonia) B59
Pneumocystosis (with pneumonia) B59
Pneumohemopericardium I31.2
Pneumohemothorax J94.2
  traumatic S27.2
Pneumohydropericardium -*see* Pericarditis

Pneumohydrothorax -*see* Hydrothorax
Pneumomediastinum J98.2
  congenital or perinatal P25.2
Pneumomycosis B49 [*J99*]
Pneumonia (acute) (double) (migratory)
  (purulent) (septic) (unresolved) J18.9
  with
    lung abscess J85.1
      due to specified organism -*see* Pneumonia,
  in (due to)
    influenza -*see* Influenza, with, pneumonia
  adenoviral J12.0
  adynamic J18.2
  alba A50.04
  allergic (eosinophilic) J82
  alveolar -*see* Pneumonia, lobar
  anaerobes J15.8
  anthrax A22.1
  apex, apical -*see* Pneumonia, lobar
  Ascaris B77.81
  aspiration J69.0
    due to
      aspiration of microorganisms
        bacterial J15.9
        viral J12.9
      food (regurgitated) J69.0
      gastric secretions J69.0
      milk (regurgitated) J69.0
      oils, essences J69.1
      solids, liquids NEC J69.8
      vomitus J69.0
    newborn P24.81
      amniotic fluid (clear) P24.11
      blood P24.21
      liquor (amnii) P24.11
      meconium P24.01
      milk P24.31
      mucus P24.11
      food (regurgitated) P24.31
      specified NEC P24.81
      stomach contents P24.31
    postprocedural J95.4
  atypical NEC J18.9
  bacillus J15.9
    specified NEC J15.8
  bacterial J15.9
    specified NEC J15.8
  Bacteroides (fragilis) (oralis)
    (melaninogenicus) J15.8
  basal, basic, basilar -*see* Pneumonia, by type
  bronchiolitis obliterans organized (BOOP)
    J84.89
  broncho-, bronchial (confluent) (croupous)
    (diffuse) (disseminated) (hemorrhagic)
    (involving lobes) (lobar) (terminal) J18.0
    allergic (eosinophilic) J82
    aspiration -*see* Pneumonia, aspiration
    bacterial J15.9
      specified NEC J15.8
    chronic -*see* Fibrosis, lung
    diplococcal J13
    Eaton's agent J15.7
    Escherichia coli (E. coli) J15.5
    Friedländer's bacillus J15.0
    Hemophilus influenzae J14
    hypostatic J18.2
    inhalation -*see also* Pneumonia, aspiration
      due to fumes or vapors (chemical) J68.0
      of oils or essences J69.1
    Klebsiella (pneumoniae) J15.0
    lipid, lipoid J69.1

Pneumonia - *continued*
    endogenous J84.89
    Mycoplasma (pneumoniae) J15.7
    pleuro-pneumonia-like-organisms (PPLO)
      J15.7
    pneumococcal J13
    Proteus J15.6
    Pseudomonas J15.1
    Serratia marcescens J15.6
    specified organism NEC J16.8
    staphylococcal -*see* Pneumonia,
      staphylococcal
    streptococcal NEC J15.4
      group B J15.3
      pneumoniae J13
    viral, virus -*see* Pneumonia, viral
  Butyrivibrio (fibriosolvens) J15.8
  Candida B37.1
  caseous -*see* Tuberculosis, pulmonary
  catarrhal -*see* Pneumonia, broncho
  chlamydial J16.0
    congenital P23.1
  cholesterol J84.89
  cirrhotic (chronic) -*see* Fibrosis, lung
  Clostridium (haemolyticum) (novyi) J15.8
  confluent -*see* Pneumonia, broncho
  congenital (infective) P23.9
    due to
      bacterium NEC P23.6
      Chlamydia P23.1
      Escherichia coli P23.4
      Haemophilus influenzae P23.6
      infective organism NEC P23.8
      Klebsiella pneumoniae P23.6
      Mycoplasma P23.6
      Pseudomonas P23.5
      Staphylococcus P23.2
      Streptococcus (except group B) P23.6
        group B P23.3
      viral agent P23.0
    specified NEC P23.8
  croupous -*see* Pneumonia, lobar
  cryptogenic organizing J84.116
  cytomegalic inclusion B25.0
  cytomegaloviral B25.0
  deglutition -*see* Pneumonia, aspiration
  desquamative interstitial J84.117
  diffuse -*see* Pneumonia, broncho
  diplococcal, diplococcus (broncho-) (lobar)
    J13
  disseminated (focal) -*see* Pneumonia, broncho
  Eaton's agent J15.7
  embolic, embolism -*see* Embolism,
    pulmonary
  Enterobacter J15.6
  eosinophilic J82
  Escherichia coli (E. coli) J15.5
  Eubacterium J15.8
  fibrinous -*see* Pneumonia, lobar
  fibroid, fibrous (chronic) -*see* Fibrosis, lung
  Friedländer's bacillus J15.0
  Fusobacterium (nucleatum) J15.8
  gangrenous J85.0
  giant cell (measles) B05.2
  gonococcal A54.84
  gram-negative bacteria NEC J15.6
    anaerobic J15.8
  Hemophilus influenzae (broncho) (lobar) J14
  human metapneumovirus J12.3
  hypostatic (broncho) (lobar) J18.2
  in (due to)

Pneumonia - *continued*
    actinomycosis A42.0
    adenovirus J12.0
    anthrax A22.1
    ascariasis B77.81
    aspergillosis B44.9
    Bacillus anthracis A22.1
    Bacterium anitratum J15.6
    candidiasis B37.1
    chickenpox B01.2
    Chlamydia J16.0
      neonatal P23.1
    coccidioidomycosis B38.2
      acute B38.0
      chronic B38.1
    cytomegalovirus disease B25.0
    Diplococcus (pneumoniae) J13
    Eaton's agent J15.7
    Enterobacter J15.6
    Escherichia coli (E. coli) J15.5
    Friedländer's bacillus J15.0
    fumes and vapors (chemical) (inhalation)
      J68.0
    gonorrhea A54.84
    Hemophilus influenzae (H. influenzae) J14
    Herellea J15.6
    histoplasmosis B39.2
      acute B39.0
      chronic B39.1
    human metapneumovirus J12.3
    Klebsiella (pneumoniae) J15.0
    measles B05.2
    Mycoplasma (pneumoniae) J15.7
    nocardiosis, nocardiasis A43.0
    ornithosis A70
    parainfluenza virus J12.2
    pleuro-pneumonia-like-organism (PPLO)
      J15.7
    pneumococcus J13
    pneumocystosis (Pneumocystis carinii)
      (Pneumocystis jiroveci) B59
    Proteus J15.6
    Pseudomonas NEC J15.1
      pseudomallei A24.1
    psittacosis A70
    Q fever A78
    respiratory syncytial virus J12.1
    rheumatic fever I00 [*J17*]
    rubella B06.81
    Salmonella (infection) A02.22
      typhi A01.03
    schistosomiasis B65.9 [*J17*]
    Serratia marcescens J15.6
    specified
      bacterium NEC J15.8
      organism NEC J16.8
    spirochetal NEC A69.8
    Staphylococcus J15.20
      aureus (methicillin susceptible) (MSSA)
        J15.211
        methicillin resistant (MRSA) J15.212
      specified NEC J15.29
    Streptococcus J15.4
      group B J15.3
      pneumoniae J13
      specified NEC J15.4
    toxoplasmosis B58.3
    tularemia A21.2
    typhoid (fever) A01.03
    varicella B01.2
    virus -*see* Pneumonia, viral

Pneumonia - *continued*
  whooping cough A37.91
    due to
      Bordetella parapertussis A37.11
      Bordetella pertussis A37.01
      specified NEC A37.81
    Yersinia pestis A20.2
  inhalation of food or vomit -*see* Pneumonia,
    aspiration
  interstitial J84.9
    chronic J84.111
    desquamative J84.117
    due to
      collagen vascular disease J84.17
      known underlying cause J84.17
    idiopathic NOS J84.111
    in disease classified elsewhere J84.17
    lymphocytic (due to collagen vascular
      disease) (in diseases classified elsewhere)
      J84.17
    lymphoid J84.2
    non-specific J84.89
      due to
        collagen vascular disease J84.17
        known underlying cause J84.17
      idiopathic J84.113
      in diseases classified elsewhere J84.17
    plasma cell B59
    pseudomonas J15.1
    usual J84.112
      due to collagen vascular disease J84.17
      idiopathic J84.112
      in diseases classified elsewhere J84.17
  Klebsiella (pneumoniae) J15.0
  lipid, lipoid (exogenous) J69.1
    endogenous J84.89
  lobar (disseminated) (double) (interstitial)
    J18.1
    bacterial J15.9
      specified NEC J15.8
    chronic -*see* Fibrosis, lung
    Escherichia coli (E. coli) J15.5
    Friedländer's bacillus J15.0
    Hemophilus influenzae J14
    hypostatic J18.2
    Klebsiella (pneumoniae) J15.0
    pneumococcal J13
    Proteus J15.6
    Pseudomonas J15.1
    specified organism NEC J16.8
    staphylococcal -*see* Pneumonia,
      staphylococcal
    streptococcal NEC J15.4
    Streptococcus pneumoniae J13
    viral, virus -*see* Pneumonia, viral
  lobular -*see* Pneumonia, broncho
  Löffler's J82
  lymphoid interstitial J84.2
  massive -*see* Pneumonia, lobar
  meconium P24.01
  MRSA (Methicillin resistant Staphylococcus
    aureus) J15.212
  MSSA (methicillin susceptible
    Staphylococcus aureus) J15.211
  multilobar -*see* Pneumonia, by type
  Mycoplasma (pneumoniae) J15.7
  necrotic J85.0
  neonatal P23.9
    aspiration -*see* Aspiration, by substance,
      with pneumonia
  nitrogen dioxide J68.0

Pneumonia - *continued*
organizing J84.89
  due to
    collagen vascular disease J84.17
    known underlying cause J84.17
  in diseases classified elsewhere J84.17
orthostatic J18.2
parainfluenza virus J12.2
parenchymatous -*see* Fibrosis, lung
passive J18.2
patchy -*see* Pneumonia, broncho
Peptococcus J15.8
Peptostreptococcus J15.8
plasma cell (of infants) B59
pleurolobar -*see* Pneumonia, lobar
pleuro-pneumonia-like organism (PPLO)
  J15.7
pneumococcal (broncho) (lobar) J13
Pneumocystis (carinii) (jiroveci) B59
postinfectional NEC B99 [*J17*]
postmeasles B05.2
Proteus J15.6
Pseudomonas J15.1
psittacosis A70
radiation J70.0
respiratory syncytial virus J12.1
resulting from a procedure J95.89
rheumatic I00 [*J17*]
Salmonella (arizonae) (cholerae-suis)
  (enteritidis) (typhimurium) A02.22
  typhi A01.03
  typhoid fever A01.03
SARS-associated coronavirus J12.81
segmented, segmental -*see* Pneumonia,
  broncho- Serratia marcescens J15.6
specified NEC J18.8
  bacterium NEC J15.8
  organism NEC J16.8
  virus NEC J12.89
spirochetal NEC A69.8
staphylococcal (broncho) (lobar) J15.20
  aureus (methicillin susceptible) (MSSA)
    J15.211
    methicillin resistant (MRSA) J15.212
  specified NEC J15.29
static, stasis J18.2
streptococcal NEC (broncho) (lobar) J15.4
  group
    A J15.4
    B J15.3
    specified NEC J15.4
Streptococcus pneumoniae J13
syphilitic, congenital (early) A50.04
traumatic (complication) (early) (secondary)
  T79.8
tuberculous (any) -*see* Tuberculosis,
  pulmonary
tularemic A21.2
varicella B01.2
Veillonella J15.8
ventilator associated J95.851
viral, virus (broncho) (interstitial) (lobar)
  J12.9
  adenoviral J12.0
  congenital P23.0
  human metapneumovirus J12.3
  parainfluenza J12.2
  respiratory syncytial J12.1
  SARS-associated coronavirus J12.81
  specified NEC J12.89
white (congenital) A50.04

Pneumonic -*see* condition
Pneumonitis (acute) (primary) -*see also*
Pneumonia
air-conditioner J67.7
allergic (due to) J67.9
  organic dust NEC J67.8
  red cedar dust J67.8
  sequoiosis J67.8
  wood dust J67.8
aspiration J69.0
  due to
    anesthesia J95.4
      during
        labor and delivery O74.0
        pregnancy O29.01
        puerperium O89.01
    fumes or gases J68.0
  obstetric O74.0
chemical (due to gases, fumes or vapors)
(inhalation) J68.0
  due to anesthesia J95.4
cholesterol J84.89
crack (cocaine) J68.0
chronic -*see* Fibrosis, lung
congenital rubella P35.0
due to
  beryllium J68.0
  cadmium J68.0
  crack (cocaine) J68.0
  detergent J69.8
  fluorocarbon-polymer J68.0
  food, vomit (aspiration) J69.0
  fumes or vapors J68.0
  gases, fumes or vapors (inhalation) J68.0
  inhalation
    blood J69.8
    essences J69.1
    food (regurgitated), milk, vomit J69.0
    oils, essences J69.1
    saliva J69.0
    solids, liquids NEC J69.8
  manganese J68.0
  nitrogen dioxide J68.0
  oils, essences J69.1
  solids, liquids NEC J69.8
  toxoplasmosis (acquired) B58.3
    congenital P37.1
  vanadium J68.0
  ventilator J95.851
eosinophilic J82
hypersensitivity J67.9
  air conditioner lung J67.7
  bagassosis J67.1
  bird fancier's lung J67.2
  farmer's lung J67.0
  maltworker's lung J67.4
  maple bark-stripper's lung J67.6
  mushroom worker's lung J67.5
  specified organic dust NEC J67.8
  suberosis J67.3
interstitial (chronic) J84.89
  acute J84.114
  lymphoid J84.2
  non-specific J84.89
    idiopathic J84.113
lymphoid, interstitial J84.2
meconium P24.01
postanesthetic J95.4
  correct substance properly administered -*see*
  Table of Drugs and Chemicals, by drug,
  adverse effect

Pneumonitis - in labor and delivery O74.0
in pregnancy O29.01
  obstetric O74.0
overdose or wrong substance given or taken
  (by accident) -*see* Table of Drugs and
  Chemicals, by drug, poisoning
postpartum, puerperal O89.01
postoperative J95.4
  obstetric O74.0
radiation J70.0
rubella, congenital P35.0
ventilation (air-conditioning) J67.7
ventilator associated J95.851
wood-dust J67.8
Pneumonoconiosis -*see* Pneumoconiosis
Pneumoparotid K11.8
Pneumopathy NEC J98.4
alveolar J84.09
due to organic dust NEC J66.8
parietoalveolar J84.09
Pneumopericarditis -*see also* Pericarditis
acute I30.9
Pneumopericardium -*see also* Pericarditis
congenital P25.3
newborn P25.3
traumatic (post) -*see* Injury, heart
Pneumophagia (psychogenic) F45.8
Pneumopleurisy, pneumopleuritis -*see also*
Pneumonia J18.8
Pneumopyopericardium I30.1
Pneumopyothorax -*see* Pyopneumothorax -
  with fistula J86.0
Pneumorrhagia -*see also* Hemorrhage, lung
tuberculous -*see* Tuberculosis, pulmonary
Pneumothorax NOS J93.9
acute J93.83
chronic J93.81
congenital P25.1
perinatal period P25.1
postprocedural J95.811
specified NEC J93.83
spontaneous NOS J93.83
  newborn P25.1
  primary J93.11
  secondary J93.12
  tension J93.0
tense valvular, infectional J93.0
tension (spontaneous) J93.0
traumatic S27.0
  with hemothorax S27.2
tuberculous -*see* Tuberculosis, pulmonary
Podagra -*see also* Gout M10.9
Podencephalus Q01.9
Poikilocytosis R71.8
Poikiloderma L81.6
Civatte's L57.3
congenital Q82.8
vasculare atrophicans L94.5
Poikilodermatomyositis M33.10
with
  myopathy M33.12
  respiratory involvement M33.11
  specified organ involvement NEC M33.19
Pointed ear (congenital) Q17.3
Poison ivy, oak, sumac or other plant
dermatitis (allergic) (contact) L23.7
Poisoning (acute) -*see also* Table of Drugs and
Chemicals
algae and toxins T65.82
Bacillus B (aertrycke) (cholerae (suis))
(paratyphosus) (suipestifer) A02.9

Poisoning (acute) --*continued*
  botulinus A05.1
  bacterial toxins A05.9
  berries, noxious -*see* Poisoning, food,
    noxious, berries
  botulism A05.1
  ciguatera fish T61.0
  Clostridium botulinum A05.1
  death-cap (Amanita phalloides) (Amanita
    verna) -*see* Poisoning, food, noxious,
    mushrooms
  drug -*see* Table of Drugs and Chemicals, by
    drug, poisoning
  epidemic, fish (noxious) -*see* Poisoning,
    seafood
    bacterial A05.9
  fava bean D55.0
  fish (noxious) T61.9
    bacterial -*see* Intoxication, foodborne, by
      agent
    ciguatera fish -*see* Poisoning, ciguatera fish
    scombroid fish -*see* Poisoning, scombroid
      fish
    specified type NEC T61.77
  food (acute) (diseased) (infected) (noxious)
    NEC T62.9
    bacterial -*see* Intoxication, foodborne, by
      agent
    due to
      Bacillus (aertrycke) (choleraesuis)
        (paratyphosus) (suipestifer) A02.9
        botulinus A05.1
      Clostridium (perfringens) (Welchii) A05.2
      salmonella (aertrycke) (callinarum)
        (choleraesuis) (enteritidis) (paratyphi)
        (suipestifer) A02.9
        with
          gastroenteritis A02.0
          sepsis A02.1
      staphylococcus A05.0
      Vibrio
        parahaemolyticus A05.3
        vulnificus A05.5
    noxious or naturally toxic T62.9
      berries -*see* subcategory T62.1
      fish -*see* Poisoning, seafood
      mushrooms -*see* subcategory T62.0X
      plants NEC -*see* subcategory T62.2X
      seafood -*see* Poisoning, seafood
      specified NEC -*see* subcategory T62.8X
    ichthyotoxism -*see* Poisoning, seafood
  kreotoxism, food A05.9
  latex T65.81
  lead T56.0
  mushroom -*see* Poisoning, food, noxious,
    mushroom
  mussels -*see also* Poisoning, shellfish
    bacterial -*see* Intoxication, foodborne, by
      agent
  nicotine (tobacco) T65.2
  noxious foodstuffs -*see* Poisoning, food,
    noxious
  plants, noxious -*see* Poisoning, food, noxious,
    plants NEC
  ptomaine -*see* Poisoning, food
  radiation J70.0
  Salmonella (arizonae) (cholerae-suis)
    (enteritidis) (typhimurium) A02.9
  scombroid fish T61.1
  seafood (noxious) T61.9

Poisoning (acute) --*continued*
  bacterial -*see* Intoxication, foodborne, by
    agent
  fish -*see* Poisoning, fish
  shellfish -*see* Poisoning, shellfish
  specified NEC -*see* subcategory T61.8X
  shellfish (amnesic) (azaspiracid) (diarrheic)
    (neurotoxic) (noxious) (paralytic) T61.78
    bacterial -*see* Intoxication, foodborne, by
      agent
    ciguatera mollusk -*see* Poisoning, ciguatera
      fish
  specified substance NEC T65.891
  Staphylococcus, food A05.0
  tobacco (nicotine) T65.2
  water E87.79
Poker spine -*see* Spondylitis, ankylosing
Poland syndrome Q79.8
Polioencephalitis (acute) (bulbar) A80.9
  inferior G12.22
  influenzal -*see* Influenza, with,
    encephalopathy
  superior hemorrhagic (acute) (Wernicke's)
    E51.2
  Wernicke's E51.2
Polioencephalomyelitis (acute) (anterior)
    A80.9
  with beriberi E51.2
Polioencephalopathy, superior hemorrhagic
    E51.2
  with
    beriberi E51.11
    pellagra E52
Poliomeningoencephalitis -*see*
    Meningoencephalitis
Poliomyelitis (acute) (anterior) (epidemic)
    A80.9
  with paralysis (bulbar) -*see* Poliomyelitis,
    paralytic
  abortive A80.4
  ascending (progressive) -*see* Poliomyelitis,
    paralytic
  bulbar (paralytic) -*see* Poliomyelitis, paralytic
  congenital P35.8
  nonepidemic A80.9
  nonparalytic A80.4
  paralytic A80.30
    specified NEC A80.39
    vaccine-associated A80.0
    wild virus
      imported A80.1
      indigenous A80.2
  spinal, acute A80.9
Poliosis (eyebrow) (eyelashes) L67.1
  circumscripta, acquired L67.1
Pollakiuria R35.0
  psychogenic F45.8
Pollinosis J30.1
Pollitzer's disease L73.2
Polyadenitis -*see also* Lymphadenitis
  malignant A20.0
Polyalgia M79.89
Polyangiitis M30.0
  microscopic M31.7
  overlap syndrome M30.8
Polyarteritis
  microscopic M31.7
  nodosa M30.0
    with lung involvement M30.1
    juvenile M30.2
    related condition NEC M30.8

Polyarthralgia -*see* Pain, joint
Polyarthritis, polyarthropathy -*see also*
  Arthritis M13.0
  due to or associated with other specified
    conditions -*see* Arthritis
  epidemic (Australian) (with exanthema)
    B33.1
  infective -*see* Arthritis, pyogenic or pyemic
  inflammatory M06.4
  juvenile (chronic) (seronegative) M08.3
  migratory -*see* Fever, rheumatic
  rheumatic, acute -*see* Fever, rheumatic
Polyarthrosis M15.9
  post-traumatic M15.3
  primary M15.0
  specified NEC M15.8
Polycarential syndrome of infancy E40
Polychondritis (atrophic) (chronic) -*see also*
  Disorder, cartilage, specified type NEC
  relapsing M94.1
Polycoria Q13.2
Polycystic (disease)
  degeneration, kidney Q61.3
    autosomal dominant (adult type) Q61.2
    autosomal recessive (infantile type) NEC
      Q61.19
  kidney Q61.3
    autosomal
      dominant Q61.2
      recessive NEC Q61.19
    autosomal dominant (adult type) Q61.2
    autosomal recessive (childhood type) NEC
      Q61.19
    infantile type NEC Q61.19
  liver Q44.6
  lung J98.4
    congenital Q33.0
  ovary, ovaries E28.2
  spleen Q89.09
Polycythemia (secondary) D75.1
  acquired D75.1
  benign (familial) D75.0
  due to
    donor twin P61.1
    erythropoietin D75.1
    fall in plasma volume D75.1
    high altitude D75.1
    maternal-fetal transfusion P61.1
    stress D75.1
  emotional D75.1
  erythropoietin D75.1
  familial (benign) D75.0
  Gaisböck's (hypertonica) D75.1
  high altitude D75.1
  hypertonica D75.1
  hypoxemic D75.1
  neonatorum P61.1
  nephrogenous D75.1
  relative D75.1
  secondary D75.1
  spurious D75.1
  stress D75.1
  vera D45
Polycytosis cryptogenica D75.1
Polydactylism, polydactyly Q69.9
  toes Q69.2
Polydipsia R63.1
Polydystrophy, pseudo-Hurler E77.0
Polyembryoma -*see* Neoplasm, malignant, by
  site

Polyglandular
  deficiency E31.0
  dyscrasia E31.9
  dysfunction E31.9
  syndrome E31.8
Polyhydramnios O40.
Polymastia Q83.1
Polymenorrhea N92.0
Polymyalgia M35.3
  arteritica, giant cell M31.5
  rheumatica M35.3
    with giant cell arteritis M31.5
Polymyositis (acute) (chronic) (hemorrhagic)
  M33.20
  with
    myopathy M33.22
    respiratory involvement M33.21
    skin involvement -see Dermatopolymyositis
    specified organ involvement NEC M33.29
  ossificans (generalisata) (progressiva) -see
  Myositis, ossificans, progressiva
Polyneuritis, polyneuritic -see also
  Polyneuropathy
  acute (post-) infective G61.0
  alcoholic G62.1
  cranialis G52.7
  demyelinating, chronic inflammatory (CIDP)
    G61.81
  diabetic -see Diabetes, polyneuropathy
  diphtheritic A36.83
  due to lack of vitamin NEC E56.9 [G63]
  endemic E51.11
  erythredema -see subcategory T56.1
  febrile, acute G61.0
  hereditary ataxic G60.1
  idiopathic, acute G61.0
  infective (acute) G61.0
  inflammatory, chronic demyelinating (CIDP)
    G61.81
  nutritional E63.9 [G63]
  postinfective (acute) G61.0
  specified NEC G62.89
Polyneuropathy (peripheral) G62.9
  alcoholic G62.1
  amyloid (Portuguese) E85.1 [G63]
  arsenical G62.2
  critical illness G62.81
  demyelinating, chronic inflammatory (CIDP)
    G61.81
  diabetic -see Diabetes, polyneuropathy
  drug-induced G62.0
  hereditary G60.9
    specified NEC G60.8
  idiopathic G60.9
    progressive G60.3
  in (due to)
    alcohol G62.1
      sequelae G65.2
    amyloidosis, familial (Portuguese) E85.1
      [G63]
    antitetanus serum G61.1
    arsenic G62.2
      sequelae G65.2
    avitaminosis NEC E56.9 [G63]
    beriberi E51.11
    collagen vascular disease NEC M35.9 [G63]
    deficiency (of)
      B (complex) vitamins E53.9 [G63]
      vitamin B6 E53.1 [G63]
    diabetes -see Diabetes, polyneuropathy
    diphtheria A36.83

Polyneuropathy --continued
  drug or medicament G62.0
    correct substance properly administered -
      see Table of Drugs and Chemicals, by
      drug, adverse effect
    overdose or wrong substance given or
  taken -see Table of Drugs and Chemicals, by
  drug, poisoning
    endocrine disease NEC E34.9 [G63]
    herpes zoster B02.23
    hypoglycemia E16.2 [G63]
    infectious
      disease NEC B99 [G63]
      mononucleosis B27.91
    lack of vitamin NEC E56.9 [G63]
    lead G62.2
      sequelae G65.2
    leprosy A30.9 [G63]
    Lyme disease A69.22
    metabolic disease NEC E88.9 [G63]
    microscopic polyangiitis M31.7 [G63]
    mumps B26.84
    neoplastic disease -see also Neoplasm D49.9
      [G63]
    nutritional deficiency NEC E63.9 [G63]
    organophosphate compounds G62.2
      sequelae G65.2
    parasitic disease NEC B89 [G63]
    pellagra E52 [G63]
    polyarteritis nodosa M30.0
    porphyria E80.20 [G63]
    radiation G62.82
    rheumatoid arthritis -see Rheumatoid,
      polyneuropathy
    sarcoidosis D86.89
    serum G61.1
    syphilis (late) A52.15
      congenital A50.43
    systemic
      connective tissue disorder M35.9 [G63]
      lupus erythematosus M32.19
    toxic agent NEC G62.2
      sequelae G65.2
    triorthocresyl phosphate G62.2
      sequelae G65.2
    tuberculosis A17.89
    uremia N18.9 [G63]
    vitamin B12 deficiency E53.8 [G63]
      with anemia (pernicious) D51.0 [G63]
        due to dietary deficiency D51.3 [G63]
    zoster B02.23
  inflammatory G61.9
    chronic demyelinating (CIDP) G61.81
    sequelae G65.1
    specified NEC G61.89
  lead G62.2
    sequelae G65.2
  nutritional NEC E63.9 [G63]
  postherpetic (zoster) B02.23
  progressive G60.3
  radiation-induced G62.82
  sensory (hereditary) (idiopathic) G60.8
  specified NEC G62.89
  syphilitic (late) A52.15
    congenital A50.43
Polyopia H53.8
Polyorchism, polyorchidism Q55.21
Polyosteoarthritis -see also Osteoarthritis,
  generalized M15.9
  post-traumatic M15.3
  specified NEC M15.8

Polyostotic fibrous dysplasia Q78.1
Polyotia Q17.0
Polyp, polypus
  accessory sinus J33.8
  adenocarcinoma in -see Neoplasm, malignant,
    by site
  adenocarcinoma in situ in -see Neoplasm, in
    situ, by site
  adenoid tissue J33.0
  adenomatous -see also Neoplasm, benign, by
    site
    adenocarcinoma in -see Neoplasm,
      malignant, by site
    adenocarcinoma in situ in -see Neoplasm, in
      situ, by site
    carcinoma in -see Neoplasm, malignant, by
      site
    carcinoma in situ in -see Neoplasm, in situ,
      by site
    multiple -see Neoplasm, benign
      adenocarcinoma in -see Neoplasm,
        malignant, by site
      adenocarcinoma in situ in -see Neoplasm,
  in situ, by site
  antrum J33.8
  anus, anal (canal) K62.0
  Bartholin's gland N84.3
  bladder D41.4
  carcinoma in -see Neoplasm, malignant, by
    site
  carcinoma in situ in -see Neoplasm, in situ, by
    site
  cecum D12.0
  cervix (uteri) N84.1
    in pregnancy or childbirth -see Pregnancy,
      complicated by, abnormal, cervix
    mucous N84.1
    nonneoplastic N84.1
  choanal J33.0
  cholesterol K82.4
  clitoris N84.3
  colon K63.5
    adenomatous D12.6
    ascending D12.2
    cecum D12.0
    descending D12.4
    inflammatory K51.40
      with
        abscess K51.414
        complication K51.419
          specified NEC K51.418
        fistula K51.413
        intestinal obstruction K51.412
        rectal bleeding K51.411
    sigmoid D12.5
    transverse D12.3
  corpus uteri N84.0
  dental K04.01
    irreversible K04.02
    reversible K04.01
  duodenum K31.7
  ear (middle) H74.4
  endometrium N84.0
  ethmoidal (sinus) J33.8
  fallopian tube N84.8
  female genital tract N84.9
    specified NEC N84.8
  frontal (sinus) J33.8
  gallbladder K82.4
  gingiva, gum K06.8
  labia, labium (majus) (minus) N84.3

Polyp, polypus - *continued*
  larynx (mucous) J38.1
    adenomatous D14.1
  malignant -*see* Neoplasm, malignant, by site
  maxillary (sinus) J33.8
  middle ear -*see* Polyp, ear (middle)
  myometrium N84.0
  nares
    anterior J33.9
    posterior J33.0
  nasal (mucous) J33.9
    cavity J33.0
    septum J33.0
  nasopharyngeal J33.0
  nose (mucous) J33.9
  oviduct N84.8
  pharynx J39.2
  placenta O90.89
  prostate -*see* Enlargement, enlarged, prostate
  pudenda, pudendum N84.3
  pulpal (dental) K04.01
    irreversible K04.02
    reversible K04.01
  rectum (nonadenomatous) K62.1
    adenomatous -*see* Polyp, adenomatous
  septum (nasal) J33.0
  sinus (accessory) (ethmoidal) (frontal)
    (maxillary) (sphenoidal) J33.8
  sphenoidal (sinus) J33.8
  stomach K31.7
    adenomatous D13.1
  tube, fallopian N84.8
  turbinate, mucous membrane J33.8
  umbilical, newborn P83.6
  ureter N28.89
  urethra N36.2
  uterus (body) (corpus) (mucous) N84.0
    cervix N84.1
    in pregnancy or childbirth -*see* Pregnancy,
      complicated by, tumor, uterus
  vagina N84.2
  vocal cord (mucous) J38.1
  vulva N84.3
Polyphagia R63.2
Polyploidy Q92.7
Polypoid -*see* condition
Polyposis -*see also* Polyp
  coli (adenomatous) D12.6
    adenocarcinoma in C18.9
    adenocarcinoma in situ in -*see* Neoplasm, in
      situ, by site
    carcinoma in C18.9
  colon (adenomatous) D12.6
  familial D12.6
    adenocarcinoma in situ in -*see* Neoplasm, in
      situ, by site
  intestinal (adenomatous) D12.6
  malignant lymphomatous C83.1
  multiple, adenomatous -*see also* Neoplasm,
    benign D36.9
Polyradiculitis -*see* Polyneuropathy
Polyradiculoneuropathy (acute)
  (postinfective) (segmentally demyelinating)
  G61.0
Polyserositis
  due to pericarditis I31.1
  pericardial I31.1
  periodic, familial E85.0
  tuberculous A19.9
    acute A19.1
    chronic A19.8

Polysplenia syndrome Q89.09
Polysyndactyly -*see also* Syndactylism,
  syndactyly Q70.4
Polytrichia L68.3
Polyunguia Q84.6
Polyuria R35.8
  nocturnal R35.1
  psychogenic F45.8
Pompe's disease (glycogen storage) E74.02
Pompholyx L30.1
Poncet's disease (tuberculous rheumatism)
  A18.09
Pond fracture -*see* Fracture, skull
Ponos B55.0
Pons, pontine -*see* condition **Poor**
  aesthetic of existing restoration of tooth
    K08.56
  contractions, labor O62.2
  gingival margin to tooth restoration K08.51
  personal hygiene R46.0
  prenatal care, affecting management of
    pregnancy -*see* Pregnancy, complicated by,
    insufficient, prenatal care
  sucking reflex (newborn) R29.2
  urinary stream R39.12
  vision NEC H54.7
Poradenitis, nostras inguinalis or venerea
  A55
Porencephaly (congenital) (developmental)
  (true) Q04.6
  acquired G93.0
  nondevelopmental G93.0
  traumatic (post) F07.89
Porocephaliasis B88.8
Porokeratosis Q82.8
Poroma, eccrine -*see* Neoplasm, skin, benign
Porphyria (South African) E80.20
  acquired E80.20
  acute intermittent (hepatic) (Swedish) E80.21
  cutanea tarda (hereditary) (symptomatic)
    E80.1
  due to drugs E80.20
    correct substance properly administered -*see*
      Table of Drugs and Chemicals, by drug,
      adverse effect
    overdose or wrong substance given or taken
      -*see* Table of Drugs and Chemicals, by
      drug, poisoning
  erythropoietic (congenital) (hereditary) E80.0
  hepatocutaneous type E80.1
  secondary E80.20
  toxic NEC E80.20
  variegata E80.20
Porphyrinuria -*see* Porphyria
Porphyruria -*see* Porphyria
Portal -*see* condition
Port wine nevus, mark, or stain Q82.5
Posadas-Wernicke disease B38.9
Positive
  culture (nonspecific)
    blood R78.81
    bronchial washings R84.5
    cerebrospinal fluid R83.5
    cervix uteri R87.5
    nasal secretions R84.5
    nipple discharge R89.5
    nose R84.5
      staphylococcus (Methicillin susceptible)
        Z22.321
        Methicillin resistant Z22.322
    peritoneal fluid R85.5

Positive --*continued*
    pleural fluid R84.5
    prostatic secretions R86.5
    saliva R85.5
    seminal fluid R86.5
    sputum R84.5
    synovial fluid R89.5
    throat scrapings R84.5
    urine R82.79
    vagina R87.5
    vulva R87.5
    wound secretions R89.5
  PPD (skin test) R76.11
  serology for syphilis A53.0
    false R76.8
    with signs or symptoms
      code as Syphilis, by site and stage
  skin test, tuberculin (without active
    tuberculosis) R76.11
  test, human immunodeficiency virus (HIV)
    R75
  VDRL A53.0
    with signs or symptoms
      code by site and stage under Syphilis A53.9
  Wassermann reaction A53.0
Postcardiotomy syndrome I97.0
Postcaval ureter Q62.62
Postcholecystectomy syndrome K91.5
Postclimacteric bleeding N95.0
Postcommissurotomy syndrome I97.0
Postconcussional syndrome F07.81
Postcontusional syndrome F07.81
Postcricoid region -*see* condition
Post-dates (40 42
weeks) (pregnancy) (mother) O48.0
  more than 42
weeks gestation O48.1
Postencephalitic syndrome F07.89
Posterior -*see* condition
Posterolateral sclerosis (spinal cord) -*see*
  Degeneration, combined
Postexanthematous -*see* condition
Postfebrile -*see* condition
Postgastrectomy dumping syndrome K91.1
Posthemiplegic chorea -*see* Monoplegia
Posthemorrhagic anemia (chronic) D50.0
  acute D62
  newborn P61.3
Postherpetic neuralgia (zoster) B02.29
  trigeminal B02.22
Posthitis N47.7
Postimmunization complication or reaction -
  see Complications, vaccination
Postinfectious -*see* condition
Postlaminectomy syndrome NEC M96.1
Postleukotomy syndrome F07.0
Postmastectomy lymphedema (syndrome)
  I97.2
Postmaturity, postmature (over 42 weeks)
  maternal (over 42weeks gestation) O48.1
  newborn P08.22
Postmeasles complication NEC -*see also*
  condition B05.89
Postmenopausal
  endometrium (atrophic) N95.8
    suppurative -*see also* Endometritis N71.9
  osteoporosis -*see* Osteoporosis,
  postmenopausal

Postnasal drip R09.82
due to
allergic rhinitis -see Rhinitis, allergic
common cold J00
gastroesophageal reflux -see Reflux,
gastroesophageal
nasopharyngitis -see Nasopharyngitis
other know condition
code to condition
sinusitis -see Sinusitis
Postnatal -see condition
Postoperative (postprocedural) -see
Complication, postoperative
pneumothorax, therapeutic Z98.3
state NEC Z98.890
Postpancreatectomy hyperglycemia E89.1
Postpartum -see Puerperal
Postphlebitic syndrome -see Syndrome,
postthrombotic
Postpoliomyelitic -see also condition
osteopathy -see Osteopathy, after
poliomyelitis
Postpolio (myelitic) syndrome G14
Postprocedural -see also Postoperative
hypoinsulinemia E89.1
Postschizophrenic depression F32.89
Postsurgery status -see also Status (post)
pneumothorax, therapeutic Z98.3
Post-term (40 42
weeks) (pregnancy) (mother) O48.0
infant P08.21
more than 42
weeks gestation (mother) O48.1
Post-traumatic brain syndrome,
nonpsychotic F07.81
Post-typhoid abscess A01.09
Postures, hysterical F44.2
Postvaccinal reaction or complication -see
Complications, vaccination
Postvalvulotomy syndrome I97.0
Potain's
disease (pulmonary edema) -see Edema, lung
syndrome (gastrectasis with dyspepsia) K31.0
Potter's
asthma J62.8
facies Q60.6
lung J62.8
syndrome (with renal agenesis) Q60.6
Pott's
curvature (spinal) A18.01
disease or paraplegia A18.01
spinal curvature A18.01
tumor, puffy -see Osteomyelitis, specified
type NEC
Pouch
bronchus Q32.4
Douglas' -see condition
esophagus, esophageal, congenital Q39.6
acquired K22.5
gastric K31.4
Hartmann's K82.8
pharynx, pharyngeal (congenital) Q38.7
Pouchitis K91.850
Poultrymen's itch B88.0
Poverty NEC Z59.6
extreme Z59.5
Poxvirus NEC B08.8
Prader-Willi syndrome Q87.1
Preauricular appendage or tag Q17.0

Prebetalipoproteinemia (acquired)
(essential) (familial) (hereditary) (primary)
(secondary) E78.1
with chylomicronemia E78.3
Precipitate labor or delivery O62.3
Preclimacteric bleeding (menorrhagia)
N92.4
Precocious
adrenarche E30.1
menarche E30.1
menstruation E30.1
pubarche E30.1
puberty E30.1
central E22.8
sexual development NEC E30.1
thelarche E30.8
Precocity, sexual (constitutional)
(cryptogenic) (female) (idiopathic) (male)
E30.1
with adrenal hyperplasia E25.9
congenital E25.0
Precordial pain R07.2
Predeciduous teeth K00.2
Prediabetes, prediabetic R73.03
complicating
pregnancy -see Pregnancy, complicated by,
diseases of, specified type or system NEC
puerperium O99.89
Predislocation status of hip at birth Q65.6
Pre-eclampsia O14.9
with pre-existing hypertension -see
Hypertension, complicating pregnancy, pre-
existing, with, pre-eclampsia
complicating
childbirth O14.94
puerperium O14.95
mild O14.0
complicating
childbirth O14.04
puerperium O14.05
moderate O14.0
complicating
childbirth O14.04
puerperium O14.05
severe O14.1
with hemolysis, elevated liver enzymes and
low platelet count (HELLP) O14.2
complicating
childbirth O14.24
puerperium O14.25
complicating
childbirth O14.14
puerperium O14.15
Pre-eruptive color change, teeth, tooth K00.8
Pre-excitation atrioventricular conduction
I45.6
Preglaucoma H40.00
Pregnancy (single) (uterine) -see also
Delivery and Puerperal
Note: The Tabular must be reviewed for
assignment of the appropriate character
indicating the trimester of the pregnancy
Note: The Tabular must be reviewed for
assignment of appropriate seventh character
for multiple gestation codes in Chapter 15
abdominal (ectopic) O00.00
with intrauterine pregnancy O00.01
with viable fetus O36.7
ampullar O00.10
with intrauterine pregnancy O00.11
biochemical O02.81

Pregnancy --continued
broad ligament O00.80
with intrauterine pregnancy O00.81
cervical O00.80
with intrauterine pregnancy O00.81
chemical O02.81
complicated NOS O26.9
complicated by (care of) (management
affected by)
abnormal, abnormality
cervix O34.4
causing obstructed labor O65.5
cord (umbilical) O69.9
findings on antenatal screening of mother
O28.9
biochemical O28.1
cytological O28.2
chromosomal O28.5
genetic O28.5
hematological O28.0
radiological O28.4
specified NEC O28.8
ultrasonic O28.3
glucose (tolerance) NEC O99.810
pelvic organs O34.9
specified NEC O34.8
causing obstructed labor O65.5
pelvis (bony) (major) NEC O33.0
perineum O34.7
position
placenta O44.0
with hemorrhage O44.1
uterus O34.59
uterus O34.59
causing obstructed labor O65.5
congenital O34.0
vagina O34.6
causing obstructed labor O65.5
vulva O34.7
causing obstructed labor O65.5
abruptio placentae -see Abruptio placentae
abscess or cellulitis
bladder O23.1
breast O91.11
genital organ or tract O23.9
abuse
physical O9A.31
psychological O9A.51
sexual O9A.41
adverse effect anesthesia O29.9
aspiration pneumonitis O29.01
cardiac arrest O29.11
cardiac complication NEC O29.19
cardiac failure O29.12
central nervous system complication NEC
O29.29
cerebral anoxia O29.21
failed or difficult intubation O29.6
inhalation of stomach contents or
secretions NOS O29.01
local, toxic reaction O29.3X
Mendelson's syndrome O29.01
pressure collapse of lung O29.02
pulmonary complications NEC O29.09
specified NEC O29.8X
spinal and epidural type NEC O29.5X
induced headache O29.4
albuminuria -see also Proteinuria,
gestational O12.1
alcohol use O99.31
amnionitis O41.12

Pregnancy *--continued*

anaphylactoid syndrome of pregnancy O88.01

anemia (conditions in D50 D64) (pre-existing) O99.01

 complicating the puerperium O99.03

antepartum hemorrhage O46.9

 with coagulation defect *-see* Hemorrhage, antepartum, with coagulation defect

 specified NEC O46.8X

appendicitis O99.61

atrophy (yellow) (acute) liver (subacute) O26.61

bariatric surgery status O99.84

bicornis or bicornuate uterus O34.0

biliary tract problems O26.61

breech presentation O32.1

cardiovascular diseases (conditions in I00 I09, I20 I52, I70 I99) O99.41

cerebrovascular disorders (conditions in I60 I69) O99.41

cervical shortening O26.87

cervicitis O23.51

chloasma (gravidarum) O26.89

cholestasis (intrahepatic) O26.61

cholecystitis O99.61

chorioamnionitis O41.12

circulatory system disorder (conditions in I00 I09, I20 I99, O99.41)

compound presentation O32.6

conjoined twins O30.02

connective system disorders (conditions in M00 M99) O99.89

contracted pelvis (general) O33.1

 inlet O33.2

 outlet O33.3

convulsions (eclamptic) (uremic) *-see also* Eclampsia O15.9

cracked nipple O92.11

cystitis O23.1

cystocele O34.8

death of fetus (near term) O36.4

 early pregnancy O02.1

 of one fetus or more in multiple gestation O31.2

deciduitis O41.14

decreased fetal movement O36.81

dental problems O99.61

diabetes (mellitus) O24.91

 gestational (pregnancy induced) *-see* Diabetes, gestational

pre-existing O24.31

 specified NEC O24.81

 type 1 O24.01

 type 2 O24.11

digestive system disorders (conditions in K00 K93) O99.61

diseases of *-see* Pregnancy, complicated by, specified body system disease

 biliary tract O26.61

 blood NEC (conditions in D65 D77) O99.11

 liver O26.61

 specified NEC O99.89

disorders of *-see* Pregnancy, complicated by, specified body system disorder

 amniotic fluid and membranes O41.9

  specified NEC O41.8X

 biliary tract O26.61

 ear and mastoid process (conditions in H60 H95) O99.89

eye and adnexa (conditions in H00 H59) O99.89

 liver O26.61

 skin (conditions in L00 L99) O99.71

 specified NEC O99.89

displacement, uterus NEC O34.59

 causing obstructed labor O65.5

disproportion (due to) O33.9

 fetal (ascites) (hydrops) (meningomyelocele) (sacral teratoma) (tumor) deformities NEC O33.7

 generally contracted pelvis O33.1

 hydrocephalic fetus O33.6

 inlet contraction of pelvis O33.2

 mixed maternal and fetal origin O33.4

 specified NEC O33.8

double uterus O34.0

 causing obstructed labor O65.5

drug use (conditions in F11 F19) O99.32

eclampsia, eclamptic (coma) (convulsions) (delirium) (nephritis) (uremia) *-see also* Eclampsia O15.

ectopic pregnancy *-see* Pregnancy, ectopic

edema O12.0

 with

  gestational hypertension, mild *-see also* Pre-eclampsia O14.0

  proteinuria O12.2

effusion, amniotic fluid *-see* Pregnancy, complicated by, premature rupture of membranes

elderly

 multigravida O09.52

 primigravida O09.51

embolism *-see also* Embolism, obstetric, pregnancy O88.

endocrine diseases NEC O99.28

endometritis O86.12

excessive weight gain O26.0

exhaustion O26.81

 during labor and delivery O75.81

face presentation O32.3

failed induction of labor O61.9

 instrumental O61.1

 mechanical O61.1

 medical O61.0

 specified NEC O61.8

 surgical O61.1

failed or difficult intubation for anesthesia O29.6

false labor (pains) O47.9

 at or after 37 completed weeks of pregnancy O47.1

 before 37 completed weeks of pregnancy O47.0

fatigue O26.81

 during labor and delivery O75.81

fatty metamorphosis of liver O26.61

female genital mutilation O34.8 *[N90.81]*

fetal (maternal care for)

 abnormality or damage O35.9

  acid-base balance O68

  specified type NEC O35.8

 acidemia O68

 acidosis O68

 alkalosis O68

 anemia and thrombocytopenia O36.82

 anencephaly O35.0

 chromosomal abnormality (conditions in Q90 Q99) O35.1

conjoined twins O30.02

damage from

 amniocentesis O35.7

 biopsy procedures O35.7

 drug addiction O35.5

 hematological investigation O35.7

 intrauterine contraceptive device O35.7

 maternal

  alcohol addiction O35.4

  cytomegalovirus infection O35.3

  disease NEC O35.8

  drug addiction O35.5

  listeriosis O35.8

  rubella O35.3

  toxoplasmosis O35.8

  viral infection O35.3

 medical procedure NEC O35.7

 radiation O35.6

death (near term) O36.4

 early pregnancy O02.1

decreased movement O36.81

disproportion due to deformity (fetal) O33.7

excessive growth (large for dates) O36.6

growth retardation O36.59

 light for dates O36.59

 small for dates O36.59

heart rate irregularity (bradycardia) (decelerations) (tachycardia) O76

hereditary disease O35.2

hydrocephalus O35.0

intrauterine death O36.4

poor growth O36.59

 light for dates O36.59

 small for dates O36.59

problem O36.9

 specified NEC O36.89

reduction (elective) O31.3

selective termination O31.3

spina bifida O35.0

thrombocytopenia O36.82

fibroid (tumor) (uterus) O34.1

fissure of nipple O92.11

gallstones O99.61

gastric banding status O99.84

gastric bypass status O99.84

genital herpes (asymptomatic) (history of) (inactive) O98.51

genital tract infection O23.9

glomerular diseases (conditions in N00 N07) O26.83

 with hypertension, pre-existing *-see* Hypertension, complicating, pregnancy, pre-existing, with, renal disease

gonorrhea O98.21

grand multiparity O09.4

habitual aborter *-see* Pregnancy, complicated by, recurrent pregnancy loss

HELLP syndrome (hemolysis, elevated liver enzymes and low platelet count) O14.2

hemorrhage

 antepartum *-see* Hemorrhage, antepartum

 before 20 completed weeks gestation O20.9

  specified NEC O20.8

 due to premature separation, placenta *-see also* Abruptio placentae O45.9

 early O20.9

  specified NEC O20.8

 threatened abortion O20.0

Pregnancy *--continued*
  hemorrhoids O22.4
  hepatitis (viral) O98.41
  herniation of uterus O34.59
  high
    head at term O32.4
    risk *-see* Supervision (of) (for), high-risk
  history of in utero procedure during previous
    pregnancy O09.82
  HIV O98.71
  human immunodeficiency virus (HIV)
    disease O98.71
  hydatidiform mole *-see also* Mole,
    hydatidiform O01.9
  hydramnios O40.
  hydrocephalic fetus (disproportion) O33.6
  hydrops
    amnii O40.
    fetalis O36.2
      associated with isoimmunization *-see*
      also Pregnancy, complicated by,
      isoimmunization O36.11
  hydrorrhea O42.90
  hyperemesis (gravidarum) (mild) *-see also*
    Hyperemesis, gravidarum O21.0
  hypertension *-see* Hypertension,
    complicating pregnancy
  hypertensive
    heart and renal disease, pre-existing *-see*
      Hypertension, complicating, pregnancy,
      pre-existing, with, heart disease, with renal
      disease
    heart disease, pre-existing *-see*
      Hypertension, complicating, pregnancy,
      pre-existing, with, heart disease
    renal disease, pre-existing *-see*
      Hypertension, complicating, pregnancy,
      pre-existing, with, renal disease
  hypotension O26.5
  immune disorders NEC (conditions in D80
    D89) O99.11
  incarceration, uterus O34.51
  incompetent cervix O34.3
  inconclusive fetal viability O36.80
  infection(s) O98.91
    amniotic fluid or sac O41.10
    bladder O23.1
    carrier state NEC O99.830
      streptococcus B O99.820
    genital organ or tract O23.9
      specified NEC O23.59
    genitourinary tract O23.9
    gonorrhea O98.21
    hepatitis (viral) O98.41
    HIV O98.71
    human immunodeficiency virus (HIV)
      O98.71
    kidney O23.0
    nipple O91.01
    parasitic disease O98.91
      specified NEC O98.81
    protozoal disease O98.61
    sexually transmitted NEC O98.31
    specified type NEC O98.81
    syphilis O98.11
    tuberculosis O98.01
    urethra O23.2
    urinary (tract) O23.4
      specified NEC O23.3
    viral disease O98.51

Pregnancy *--continued*
  injury or poisoning (conditions in S00 T88)
    O9A.21
    due to abuse
      physical O9A.31
      psychological O9A.51
      sexual O9A.41
  insufficient
    prenatal care O09.3
    weight gain O26.1
  insulin resistance O26.89
  intrauterine fetal death (near term) O36.4
    early pregnancy O02.1
    multiple gestation (one fetus or more)
      O31.2
  isoimmunization O36.11
    anti-A sensitization O36.11
    anti-B sensitization O36.19
    Rh O36.09
      anti-D antibody O36.01
    specified NEC O36.19
  laceration of uterus NEC O71.81
  malformation
    placenta, placental (vessel) O43.10
      specified NEC O43.19
    uterus (congenital) O34.0
  malnutrition (conditions in E40 E46) O25.1
  maternal hypotension syndrome O26.5
  mental disorders (conditions in F01 F09,
    F20 F99) O99.34
    alcohol use O99.31
    drug use O99.32
    smoking O99.33
  mentum presentation O32.3
  metabolic disorders O99.28
  missed
    abortion O02.1
    delivery O36.4
  multiple gestations O30.9
    conjoined twins O30.02
    specified number of multiples NEC *-see*
      Pregnancy, multiple (gestation), specified
      NEC
    quadruplet *-see* Pregnancy, quadruplet
    specified complication NEC O31.8X
    triplet *-see* Pregnancy, triplet
    twin *-see* Pregnancy, twin
  musculoskeletal condition (conditions is
    M00 M99) O99.89
  necrosis, liver (conditions in K72) O26.61
  neoplasm
    benign
      cervix O34.4
      corpus uteri O34.1
      uterus O34.1
    malignant O9A.11
  nephropathy NEC O26.83
  nervous system condition (conditions in
    G00 G99) O99.35
  nutritional diseases NEC O99.28
  obesity (pre-existing) O99.21
  obesity surgery status O99.84
  oblique lie or presentation O32.2
  older mother *-see* Pregnancy, complicated
    by, elderly
  oligohydramnios O41.0
    with premature rupture of membranes *-see*
      also Pregnancy, complicated by, premature
      rupture of membranes O42.
  onset (spontaneous) of labor after 37
    completed weeks of gestation but before 39
    completed weeks gestation, with delivery by
    (planned) cesarean section O75.82

Pregnancy *--continued*
  oophoritis O23.52
  overdose, drug *-see also* Table of Drugs and
    Chemicals, by drug, poisoning O9A.21
  oversize fetus O33.5
  papyraceous fetus O31.0
  pelvic inflammatory disease O99.89
  periodontal disease O99.61
  peripheral neuritis O26.82
  peritoneal (pelvic) adhesions O99.89
  phlebitis O22.9
  phlebopathy O22.9
  phlebothrombosis (superficial) O22.2
    deep O22.3
  placenta accreta O43.21
  placenta increta O43.22
  placenta percreta O43.23
  placenta previa O44.0
    complete O44.0
      with hemorrhage O44.1
    marginal O44.2
      with hemorrhage O44.3
    partial O44.2
      with hemorrhage O44.3
  placental disorder O43.9
    specified NEC O43.89
  placental dysfunction O43.89
  placental infarction O43.81
  placental insufficiency O36.51
  placental transfusion syndromes
    fetomaternal O43.01
    fetus to fetus O43.02
    maternofetal O43.01
  placentitis O41.14
  pneumonia O99.51
  poisoning *-see also* Table of Drugs and
    Chemicals O9A.21
  polyhydramnios O40
  polymorphic eruption of pregnancy O26.86
  poor obstetric history NEC O09.29
  postmaturity (post-term) (40 to 42 weeks)
    O48.0
    more than 42 completed weeks gestation
      (prolonged) O48.1
  pre-eclampsia O14.9
    mild O14.0
    moderate O14.0
    severe O14.1
      with hemolysis, elevated liver enzymes
      and low platelet count (HELLP) O14.2
  premature labor *-see* Pregnancy,
    complicated by, preterm labor
  premature rupture of membranes O42.90
    full-term, unspecified as to length of time
      between rupture and onset of labor
      O42.92
    with onset of labor
      within 24 hours O42.00
        at or after 37 weeks gestation, onset of
          labor within 24 hours of rupture
          O42.02
        pre-term (before 37 completed weeks of
          gestation) O42.01
      after 24 hours O42.10
        at or after 37 weeks gestation, onset of
          labor more than 24 hours following
          rupture O42.12
        pre-term (before 37 completed weeks of
          gestation) O42.11
    at or after 37 weeks gestation, unspecified
      as to length of time between rupture and
      onset of labor O42.92

Pregnancy --*continued*
    pre-term (before 37 completed weeks of gestation) O42.91
    premature separation of placenta -*see also* Abruptio placentae O45.9
    presentation, fetal
    -*see* Delivery, complicated by, malposition
    preterm delivery O60.10
    preterm labor
      with delivery O60.10
        preterm O60.10
        term O60.20
      second trimester
        with term delivery O60.22
        without delivery O60.02
        with preterm delivery
          second trimester O60.12
          third trimester O60.13
      third trimester
        with term delivery O60.23
        without delivery O60.03
        with third trimester preterm delivery O60.14
      without delivery O60.00
        second trimester O60.02
        third trimester O60.03
    previous history of -*see* Pregnancy,
    supervision of, high-risk
    prolapse, uterus O34.52
    proteinuria (gestational) -*see also*
    Proteinuria, gestational O12.1
      with edema O12.2
    pruritic urticarial papules and plaques of pregnancy (PUPPP) O26.86
    pruritus (neurogenic) O26.89
    psychosis or psychoneurosis (puerperal) F53
    ptyalism O26.89
    PUPPP (pruritic urticarial papules and plaques of pregnancy) O26.86
    pyelitis O23.0
    recurrent pregnancy loss O26.2
    renal disease or failure NEC O26.83
      with secondary hypertension, pre-existing -*see* Hypertension, complicating, pregnancy, pre-existing, secondary
      hypertensive, pre-existing -*see* Hypertension, complicating, pregnancy, pre-existing, with renal disease
    respiratory condition (conditions in J00 J99) O99.51
    retained, retention
      dead ovum O02.0
      intrauterine contraceptive device O26.3
    retroversion, uterus O34.53
    Rh immunization, incompatibility or sensitization NEC O36.09
      anti-D antibody O36.01
    rupture
      amnion (premature) -*see also* Pregnancy, complicated by, premature rupture of membranes O42
      membranes (premature) -*see also* Pregnancy, complicated by, premature rupture of membranes O42
      uterus (during labor) O71.1
        before onset of labor O71.0
    salivation (excessive) O26.89
    salpingitis O23.52
    salpingo-oophoritis O23.52
    sepsis (conditions in A40, A41) O98.81
    size date discrepancy (uterine) O26.84

Pregnancy --*continued*
    skin condition (conditions in L00 L99) O99.71
    smoking (tobacco) O99.33
    social problem O09.7
    specified condition NEC O26.89
    spotting O26.85
    streptococcus group B (GBS) carrier state O99.820
    subluxation of symphysis (pubis) O26.71
    syphilis (conditions in A50 A53) O98.11
    threatened
      abortion O20.0
      labor O47.9
        at or after 37 completed weeks of gestation O47.1
        before 37 completed weeks of gestation O47.0
    thrombophlebitis (superficial) O22.2
    thrombosis O22.9
      cerebral venous O22.5
      cerebrovenous sinus O22.5
      deep O22.3
    tobacco use disorder (smoking) O99.33
    torsion of uterus O34.59
    toxemia O14.9
    transverse lie or presentation O32.2
    tuberculosis (conditions in A15 A19) O98.01
    tumor (benign)
      cervix O34.4
      malignant O9A.11
      uterus O34.1
    unstable lie O32.0
    upper respiratory infection O99.51
    urethritis O23.2
    uterine size date discrepancy O26.84
    vaginitis or vulvitis O23.59
    varicose veins (lower extremities) O22.0
      genitals O22.1
      legs O22.0
      perineal O22.1
      vaginal or vulval O22.1
    venereal disease NEC (conditions in A63.8) O98.31
    venous disorders O22.9
      specified NEC O22.8X
    viral diseases (conditions in A80 B09, B25 B34) O98.51
    very young mother -*see* Pregnancy, complicated by, young mother
    vomiting O21.9
      due to diseases classified elsewhere O21.8
      hyperemesis gravidarum (mild) -*see also* Hyperemesis, gravidarum O21.0
      late (occurring after 20 weeks of gestation) O21.2
    young mother
      multigravida O09.62
      primigravida O09.61
  concealed O09.3
  continuing following
    elective fetal reduction of one or more fetus O31.3
    intrauterine death of one or more fetus O31.2
    spontaneous abortion of one or more fetus O31.1
  cornual O00.80
    with intrauterine pregnancy O00.81
  ectopic (ruptured) O00.90

Pregnancy --*continued*
    with intrauterine pregnancy O00.91
    abdominal O00.00
      with
        intrauterine pregnancy O00.01
        viable fetus O36.7
    cervical O00.80
      with intrauterine pregnancy O00.81
    complicated (by) O08.9
      afibrinogenemia O08.1
      cardiac arrest O08.81
      chemical damage of pelvic organ(s) O08.6
      circulatory collapse O08.3
      defibrination syndrome O08.1
      electrolyte imbalance O08.5
      embolism (amniotic fluid) (blood clot) (pulmonary) (septic) O08.2
      endometritis O08.0
      genital tract and pelvic infection O08.0
      hemorrhage (delayed) (excessive) O08.1
      infection
        genital tract or pelvic O08.0
        kidney O08.83
        urinary tract O08.83
      intravascular coagulation O08.1
      laceration of pelvic organ(s) O08.6
      metabolic disorder O08.5
      oliguria O08.4
      oophoritis O08.0
      parametritis O08.0
      pelvic peritonitis O08.0
      perforation of pelvic organ(s) O08.6
      renal failure or shutdown O08.4
      salpingitis or salpingo-oophoritis O08.0
      sepsis O08.82
      shock O08.83
        septic O08.82
      specified condition NEC O08.89
      tubular necrosis (renal) O08.4
      uremia O08.4
      urinary infection O08.83
      venous complication NEC O08.7
        embolism O08.2
    cornual O00.80
      with intrauterine pregnancy O00.81
    intraligamentous O00.80
      with intrauterine pregnancy O00.81
    mural O00.80
      with intrauterine pregnancy O00.81
    ovarian O00.20
      with intrauterine pregnancy O00.21
    specified site NEC O00.80
      with intrauterine pregnancy O00.81
    tubal (ruptured) O00.10
      with intrauterine pregnancy O00.11
  examination (normal) Z34.9
  high-risk -*see* Pregnancy, supervision of, high-risk
  first Z34.0
  specified Z34.8
  extrauterine -*see* Pregnancy, ectopic
  fallopian O00.10
    with intrauterine pregnancy O00.11
  false F45.8
  gestational carrier Z33.3
  hidden O09.3
  high-risk -*see* Pregnancy, supervision of, high-risk
  incidental finding Z33.1
  interstitial O00.80
    with intrauterine pregnancy O00.81

Pregnancy --*continued*
intraligamentous O00.80
  with intrauterine pregnancy O00.81
intramural O00.80
  with intrauterine pregnancy O00.81
intraperitoneal O00.00
  with intrauterine pregnancy O00.01
isthmian O00.10
  with intrauterine pregnancy O00.11
mesometric (mural) O00.80
  with intrauterine pregnancy O00.81
molar NEC O02.0
  complicated (by) O08.9
    afibrinogenemia O08.1
    cardiac arrest O08.81
    chemical damage of pelvic organ(s) O08.6
    circulatory collapse O08.3
    defibrination syndrome O08.1
    electrolyte imbalance O08.5
    embolism (amniotic fluid) (blood clot)
      (pulmonary) (septic) O08.2
    endometritis O08.0
    genital tract and pelvic infection O08.0
    hemorrhage (delayed) (excessive) O08.1
    infection
      genital tract or pelvic O08.0
      kidney O08.83
      urinary tract O08.83
    intravascular coagulation O08.1
    laceration of pelvic organ(s) O08.6
    metabolic disorder O08.5
    oliguria O08.4
    oophoritis O08.0
    parametritis O08.0
    pelvic peritonitis O08.0
    perforation of pelvic organ(s) O08.6
    renal failure or shutdown O08.4
    salpingitis or salpingo-oophoritis O08.0
    sepsis O08.82
    shock O08.3
      septic O08.82
    specified condition NEC O08.89
    tubular necrosis (renal) O08.4
    uremia O08.4
    urinary infection O08.83
    venous complication NEC O08.7
      embolism O08.2
hydatidiform -*see also* Mole, hydatidiform
  O01.9
multiple (gestation) O30.9
  greater than quadruplets -*see* Pregnancy,
    multiple (gestation), specified NEC
  specified NEC O30.80
    with
      two or more monoamniotic fetuses
        O30.82
      two or more monochorionic fetuses
        O30.81
    two or more monoamniotic fetuses
      O30.82
    two or more monochorionic fetuses
      O30.81
    unable to determine number of placenta
      and number of amniotic sacs O30.89
    unspecified number of placenta and
      unspecified number of amniotic sacs
      O30.80
  mural O00.80
    with intrauterine pregnancy O00.81
  normal (supervision of) Z34.9

Pregnancy --*continued*
high-risk -*see* Pregnancy, supervision of,
  high-risk
  first Z34.0
  specified Z34.8
ovarian O00.20
  with intrauterine pregnancy O00.21
postmature (40 to 42 weeks) O48.0
  more than 42 weeks gestation O48.1
post-term (40 to 42 weeks) O48.0
prenatal care only Z34.9
  high-risk -*see* Pregnancy, supervision of,
    high-risk
  first Z34.0
  specified Z34.8
prolonged (more than 42 weeks gestation)
  O48.1
quadruplet O30.20
  with
    two or more monoamniotic fetuses
      O30.22
    two or more monochorionic fetuses
      O30.21
  two or more monoamniotic fetuses O30.22
  two or more monochorionic fetuses O30.21
  unable to determine number of placenta and
    number of amniotic sacs O30.29
  unspecified number of placenta and
    unspecified number of amniotic sacs
    O30.20
quintuplet -*see* Pregnancy, multiple
  (gestation), specified NEC
sextuplet -*see* Pregnancy, multiple (gestation),
  specified NEC
supervision of
  concealed pregnancy O09.3
  elderly mother
    multigravida O09.52
    primigravida O09.51
  hidden pregnancy O09.3
  high-risk O09.9
    due to (history of)
      ectopic pregnancy O09.1
      elderly -*see* Pregnancy, supervision,
        elderly mother
      grand multiparity O09.4
      infertility O09.0
      insufficient prenatal care O09.3
      in utero procedure during previous
        pregnancy O09.82
      in vitro fertilization O09.81
      molar pregnancy O09.A-
      multiple previous pregnancies O09.4
      older mother -*see* Pregnancy, supervision
        of, elderly mother
      poor reproductive or obstetric history
        NEC O09.29
      pre-term labor O09.21
      previous
        neonatal death O09.29
      social problems O09.7
      specified NEC O09.89
      very young mother -*see* Pregnancy,
        supervision, young mother
    resulting from in vitro fertilization O09.81
  normal Z34.9
    first Z34.0
    specified NEC Z34.8
  young mother
    multigravida O09.62
    primigravida O09.61

Pregnancy --*continued*
triplet O30.10
  with
    two or more monoamniotic fetuses
      O30.12
    two or more monochorionic fetuses
      O30.11
  two or more monoamniotic fetuses O30.12
  two or more monochorionic fetuses O30.11
  unable to determine number of placenta and
    number of amniotic sacs O30.19
  unspecified number of placenta and
    unspecified number of amniotic sacs
    O30.10
tubal (with abortion) (with rupture) O00.10
  with intrauterine pregnancy O00.11
twin O30.00
  conjoined O30.02
  dichorionic/diamniotic (two placenta, two
    amniotic sacs) O30.04
  monochorionic/diamniotic (one placenta,
    two amniotic sacs) O30.03
  monochorionic/monoamniotic (one placenta,
    one amniotic sac) O30.01
  unable to determine number of placenta and
    number of amniotic sacs O30.09
  unspecified number of placenta and
    unspecified number of amniotic sacs
    O30.00
unwanted Z64.0
weeks of gestation
  8 weeks Z3A.08
  9 weeks Z3A.09
  10 weeks Z3A.10
  11 weeks Z3A.11
  12 weeks Z3A.12
  13 weeks Z3A.13
  14 weeks Z3A.14
  15 weeks Z3A.15
  16 weeks Z3A.16
  17 weeks Z3A.17
  18 weeks Z3A.18
  19 weeks Z3A.19
  20 weeks Z3A.20
  21 weeks Z3A.21
  22 weeks Z3A.22
  23 weeks Z3A.23
  24 weeks Z3A.24
  25 weeks Z3A.25
  26 weeks Z3A.26
  27 weeks Z3A.27
  28 weeks Z3A.28
  29 weeks Z3A.29
  30 weeks Z3A.30
  31 weeks Z3A.31
  32 weeks Z3A.32
  33 weeks Z3A.33
  34 weeks Z3A.34
  35 weeks Z3A.35
  36 weeks Z3A.36
  37 weeks Z3A.37
  38 weeks Z3A.38
  39 weeks Z3A.39
  40 weeks Z3A.40
  41 weeks Z3A.41
  42 weeks Z3A.42
  greater than 42 weeks Z3A.49
  less than 8 weeks Z3A.01
  not specified Z3A.00

Preiser's disease -see Osteonecrosis, secondary, due to, trauma, metacarpus
Pre-kwashiorkor -see Malnutrition, severe
Preleukemia (syndrome) D46.9
Preluxation, hip, congenital Q65.6
Premature -see also condition
  adrenarche E27.0
  aging E34.8
  beats I49.40
    atrial I49.1
    auricular I49.1
    supraventricular I49.1
  birth NEC -see Preterm, newborn
  closure, foramen ovale Q21.8
  contraction
    atrial I49.1
    atrioventricular I49.2
    auricular I49.1
    auriculoventricular I49.49
    heart (extrasystole) I49.49
    junctional I49.2
    ventricular I49.3
  delivery -see also Pregnancy, complicated by, preterm labor O60.10
  ejaculation F52.4
  infant NEC -see Preterm, newborn
    light-for-dates -see Light for dates
  labor -see Pregnancy, complicated by, preterm labor
  lungs P28.0
  menopause E28.319
    asymptomatic E28.319
    symptomatic E28.310
  newborn
    extreme (less than 28 completed weeks) -see Immaturity, extreme
    less than 37 completed weeks -see Preterm, newborn
  puberty E30.1
  rupture membranes or amnion -see Pregnancy, complicated by, premature rupture of membranes
  senility E34.8
  thelarche E30.8
  ventricular systole I49.3
Prematurity NEC (less than 37 completed weeks) -see Preterm, newborn
  extreme (less than 28 completed weeks) -see Immaturity, extreme
Premenstrual
  dysphoric disorder (PMDD) F32.81
  tension (syndrome) N94.3
Premolarization, cuspids K00.2
Prenatal
  care, normal pregnancy -see Pregnancy, normal
  screening of mother Z36
  teeth K00.6
Preparatory care for subsequent treatment NEC
  for dialysis Z49.01
    peritoneal Z49.02
Prepartum -see condition
Preponderance, left or right ventricular I51.7
Prepuce -see condition
PRES (posterior reversible encephalopathy syndrome) I67.83
Presbycardia R54
Presbycusis, presbyacusia H91.1
Presbyesophagus K22.8

Presbyophrenia F03
Presbyopia H52.4
Prescription of contraceptives (initial) Z30.019
  barrier Z30.018
  diaphragm Z30.018
  emergency (postcoital) Z30.012
  implantable subdermal Z30.017
  injectable Z30.013
  intrauterine contraceptive device Z30.014
  pills Z30.011
  postcoital (emergency) Z30.012
  repeat Z30.40
    barrier Z30.49
    diaphragm Z30.49
    implantable subdermal Z30.46
    injectable Z30.42
    pills Z30.41
    specified type NEC Z30.49
    transdermal patch hormonal Z30.45
    vaginal ring hormonal Z30.44
  specified type NEC Z30.018
    transdermal patch hormonal Z30.016
    vaginal ring hormonal Z30.015
Presence (of)
  ankle-joint implant (functional) (prosthesis) Z96.66
  aortocoronary (bypass) graft Z95.1
  arterial-venous shunt (dialysis) Z99.2
  artificial
    eye (globe) Z97.0
    heart (fully implantable) (mechanical) Z95.812
      valve Z95.2
    larynx Z96.3
    lens (intraocular) Z96.1
    limb (complete) (partial) Z97.1
      arm Z97.1
        bilateral Z97.15
      leg Z97.1
        bilateral Z97.16
  audiological implant (functional) Z96.29
  bladder implant (functional) Z96.0
  bone
    conduction hearing device Z96.29
    implant (functional) NEC Z96.7
    joint (prosthesis) -see Presence, joint implant
  cardiac
    defibrillator (functional) (with synchronous cardiac pacemaker) Z95.810
    implant or graft Z95.9
      specified type NEC Z95.818
    pacemaker Z95.0
    resynchronization therapy
      defibrillator Z95.810
      pacemaker Z95.0
  cerebrospinal fluid drainage device Z98.2
  cochlear implant (functional) Z96.21
  contact lens (es) Z97.3
  coronary artery graft or prosthesis Z95.5
  CRT-D (cardiac resynchronization therapy defibrillator) Z95.810
  CRT-P (cardiac resynchronization therapy pacemaker) Z95.0
  cardioverter-defibrillator (ICD) Z95.810
  CSF shunt Z98.2
  dental prosthesis device Z97.2
  dentures Z97.2
  device (external) NEC Z97.8
    cardiac NEC Z95.818

Presence (of) --continued
  heart assist Z95.811
  implanted (functional) Z96.9
    specified NEC Z96.89
  prosthetic Z97.8
  ear implant Z96.20
    cochlear implant Z96.21
    myringotomy tube Z96.22
    specified type NEC Z96.29
  elbow-joint implant (functional) (prosthesis) Z96.62
  endocrine implant (functional) NEC Z96.49
  eustachian tube stent or device (functional) Z96.29
  external hearing-aid or device Z97.4
  finger-joint implant (functional) (prosthetic) Z96.69
  functional implant Z96.9
    specified NEC Z96.89
  graft
    cardiac NEC Z95.818
    vascular NEC Z95.828
  hearing-aid or device (external) Z97.4
    implant (bone) (cochlear) (functional) Z96.21
  heart assist device Z95.811
  heart valve implant (functional) Z95.2
    prosthetic Z95.2
    specified type NEC Z95.4
    xenogenic Z95.3
  hip-joint implant (functional) (prosthesis) Z96.64
  ICD (cardioverter-defibrillator) Z95.810
  implanted device (artificial) (functional) (prosthetic) Z96.9
    automatic cardiac defibrillator (with synchronous cardiac pacemaker) Z95.810
    cardiac pacemaker Z95.0
    cochlear Z96.21
    dental Z96.5
    heart Z95.812
    heart valve Z95.2
      prosthetic Z95.2
      specified NEC Z95.4
      xenogenic Z95.3
    insulin pump Z96.41
    intraocular lens Z96.1
    joint Z96.60
      ankle Z96.66
      elbow Z96.62
      finger Z96.69
      hip Z96.64
      knee Z96.65
      shoulder Z96.61
      specified NEC Z96.698
      wrist Z96.63
    larynx Z96.3
    myringotomy tube Z96.22
    otological Z96.20
      cochlear Z96.21
      eustachian stent Z96.29
      myringotomy Z96.22
      specified type NEC Z96.29
      stapes Z96.29
    skin Z96.81
    skull plate Z96.7
    specified NEC Z96.89
    urogenital Z96.0
  insulin pump (functional) Z96.41
  intestinal bypass or anastomosis Z98.0
  intraocular lens (functional) Z96.1

Presence (of) --*continued*
  intrauterine contraceptive device (IUD) Z97.5
  intravascular implant (functional) (prosthetic)
   NEC Z95.9
    coronary artery Z95.5
    defibrillator (with synchronous cardiac
     pacemaker) Z95.810
    peripheral vessel (with angioplasty) Z95.820
  joint implant (prosthetic) (any) Z96.60
   ankle -*see* Presence, ankle joint implant
   elbow -*see* Presence, elbow joint implant
   finger -*see* Presence, finger joint implant
   hip -*see* Presence, hip joint implant
   knee -*see* Presence, knee joint implant
   shoulder -*see* Presence, shoulder joint
  implant
   specified joint NEC Z96.698
   wrist -*see* Presence, wrist joint implant
  knee-joint implant (functional) (prosthesis)
   Z96.65
  laryngeal implant (functional) Z96.3
  mandibular implant (dental) Z96.5
  myringotomy tube(s) Z96.22
  orthopedic-joint implant (prosthetic) (any) -
   see Presence, joint implant
  otological implant (functional) Z96.29
  shoulder-joint implant (functional)
   (prosthesis) Z96.61
  skull-plate implant Z96.7
  spectacles Z97.3
  stapes implant (functional) Z96.29
  systemic lupus erythematosus [SLE] inhibitor
   D68.62
  tendon implant (functional) (graft) Z96.7
  tooth root(s) implant Z96.5
  ureteral stent Z96.0
  urethral stent Z96.0
  urogenital implant (functional) Z96.0
  vascular implant or device Z95.9
   access port device Z95.828
   specified type NEC Z95.828
  wrist-joint implant (functional) (prosthesis)
   Z96.63
Presenile -*see also* condition
  dementia F03
  premature aging E34.8
Presentation, fetal -*see* Delivery , complicated
 by, malposition
Prespondylolisthesis (congenital) Q76.2
Pressure
  area, skin -*see* Ulcer, pressure, by site
  brachial plexus G54.0
  brain G93.5
   injury at birth NEC P11.1
  cerebral -*see* Pressure, brain
  chest R07.89
  cone, tentorial G93.5
  hyposystolic -*see also* Hypotension
   incidental reading, without diagnosis of
   hypotension R03.1
  increased
   intracranial (benign) G93.2
    injury at birth P11.0
   intraocular H40.05
  lumbosacral plexus G54.1
  mediastinum J98.59
  necrosis (chronic) -*see* Ulcer, pressure, by site
  parental, inappropriate (excessive) Z62.6
  sore (chronic) -*see* Ulcer, pressure, by site
  spinal cord G95.20
  ulcer (chronic) -*see* Ulcer, pressure, by site
  venous, increased I87.8

Pre-syncope R55
Preterm
  delivery -*see also* Pregnancy, complicated by,
   preterm labor O60.10
  labor -*see* Pregnancy, complicated by,
   preterm labor
  newborn (infant) P07.30
   gestational age
    28 completed weeks (28 weeks, 0 days
     through 28 weeks, 6 days) P07.31
    29 completed weeks (29 weeks, 0 days
     through 29 weeks, 6 days) P07.32
    30 completed weeks (30 weeks, 0 days
     through 30 weeks, 6 days) P07.33
    31 completed weeks (31 weeks, 0 days
     through 31 weeks, 6 days) P07.34
    32 completed weeks (32 weeks, 0 days
     through 32 weeks, 6 days) P07.35
    33 completed weeks (33 weeks, 0 days
     through 33 weeks, 6 days) P07.36
    34 completed weeks (34 weeks, 0 days
     through 34 weeks, 6 days) P07.37
    35 completed weeks (35 weeks, 0 days
     through 35 weeks, 6 days) P07.38
    36 completed weeks (36 weeks, 0 days
     through 36 weeks, 6 days) P07.39
Previa
  placenta (total) (without hemorrhage) O44.0
   with hemorrhage O44.1
   complete O44.0
    with hemorrhage O44.1
   low -*see also* Delivery, complicated, by,
    placenta, low O44.4
    with hemorrhage O44.5
   marginal O44.2
    with hemorrhage O44.3
   partial O44.2
    with hemorrhage O44.3
  vasa O69.4
Priapism N48.30
  due to
   disease classified elsewhere N48.32
   drug N48.33
   specified cause NEC N48.39
   trauma N48.31
Prickling sensation (skin) R20.2
Prickly heat L74.0
Primary -*see* condition **Primigravida**
  elderly, affecting management of pregnancy,
   labor and delivery (supervision only) -*see*
   Pregnancy, complicated by, elderly,
   primigravida
  older, affecting management of pregnancy,
   labor and delivery (supervision only) -*see*
   Pregnancy, complicated by,
  elderly, primigravida
  very young, affecting management of
   pregnancy, labor and delivery (supervision
   only) -*see* Pregnancy, complicated by,
   young mother, primigravida
Primipara
  elderly, affecting management of pregnancy,
   labor and delivery (supervision only) -*see*
   Pregnancy, complicated by, elderly,
   primigravida
  older, affecting management of pregnancy,
   labor and delivery (supervision only) -*see*
   Pregnancy, complicated by, elderly,
   primigravida
  very young, affecting management of
   pregnancy, labor and delivery (supervision
   only) -*see* Pregnancy, complicated by,
  young mother, primigravida

Primus varus (bilateral) Q66.2
PRIND (Prolonged reversible ischemic
 neurologic deficit) I63.9
Pringle's disease (tuberous sclerosis) Q85.1
Prinzmetal angina I20.1
Prizefighter ear -*see* Cauliflower ear
Problem (with) (related to)
  academic Z55.8
  acculturation Z60.3
  adjustment (to)
   change of job Z56.1
   life-cycle transition Z60.0
   pension Z60.0
   retirement Z60.0
  adopted child Z62.821
  alcoholism in family Z63.72
  atypical parenting situation Z62.9
  bankruptcy Z59.8
  behavioral (adult) F69
   drug seeking Z76.5
  birth of sibling affecting child Z62.898
  care (of)
   provider dependency Z74.9
    specified NEC Z74.8
   sick or handicapped person in family or
   household Z63.6
  child
   abuse (affecting the child) -*see*
    Maltreatment, child
   custody or support proceedings Z65.3
   in welfare custody Z62.21
   in care of non-parental family member
    Z62.21
   in foster care Z62.21
   living in orphanage or group home Z62.22
  child-rearing Z62.9
   specified NEC Z62.898
  communication (developmental) F80.9
  conflict or discord (with)
   boss Z56.4
   classmates Z55.4
   counselor Z64.4
   employer Z56.4
   family Z63.9
    specified NEC Z63.8
   probation officer Z64.4
   social worker Z64.4
   teachers Z55.4
   workmates Z56.4
  conviction in legal proceedings Z65.0
   with imprisonment Z65.1
  counselor Z64.4
  creditors Z59.8
  digestive K92.9
  drug addict in family Z63.72
  ear -*see* Disorder, ear
  economic Z59.9
   affecting care Z59.9
   specified NEC Z59.8
  education Z55.9
   specified NEC Z55.8
  employment Z56.9
   change of job Z56.1
   discord Z56.4
   environment Z56.5
   sexual harassment Z56.81
   specified NEC Z56.89
   stress NEC Z56.6
   stressful schedule Z56.3
   threat of job loss Z56.2
   unemployment Z56.0

Problem (with) (related to) --*continued*
  enuresis, child F98.0
  eye H57.9
  failed examinations (school) Z55.2
  falling Z91.81
  family -*see also* Disruption, family Z63.9
    specified NEC Z63.8
  feeding (elderly) (infant) R63.3
    newborn P92.9
      breast P92.5
      overfeeding P92.4
      slow P92.2
      specified NEC P92.8
      underfeeding P92.3
    nonorganic F50.89
  finance Z59.9
    specified NEC Z59.8
  foreclosure on loan Z59.8
  foster child Z62.822
  frightening experience(s) in childhood
    Z62.898
  genital NEC
    female N94.9
    male N50.9
  health care Z75.9
    specified NEC Z75.8
  hearing -*see* Deafness
  homelessness Z59.0
  housing Z59.9
    inadequate Z59.1
    isolated Z59.8
    specified NEC Z59.8
  identity (of childhood) F93.8
  illegitimate pregnancy (unwanted) Z64.0
  illiteracy Z55.0
  impaired mobility Z74.09
  imprisonment or incarceration Z65.1
  inadequate teaching affecting education Z55.8
  inappropriate (excessive) parental pressure
    Z62.6
  influencing health status NEC Z78.9
  in-law Z63.1
  institutionalization, affecting child Z62.22
  intrafamilial communication Z63.8
  jealousy, child F93.8
  landlord Z59.2
  language (developmental) F80.9
  learning (developmental) F81.9
  legal Z65.3
    conviction without imprisonment Z65.0
    imprisonment Z65.1
    release from prison Z65.2
  life-management Z73.9
    specified NEC Z73.89
  life-style Z72.9
    gambling Z72.6
    high-risk sexual behavior (heterosexual)
      Z72.51
      bisexual Z72.53
      homosexual Z72.52
    inappropriate eating habits Z72.4
    self-damaging behavior NEC Z72.89
    specified NEC Z72.89
    tobacco use Z72.0
  literacy Z55.9
    low level Z55.0
    specified NEC Z55.8
  living alone Z60.2
  lodgers Z59.2
  loss of love relationship in childhood Z62.898
  marital Z63.0

Problem (with) (related to) --*continued*
  involving
    divorce Z63.5
    estrangement Z63.5
    gender identity F66
  mastication K08.89
  medical
    care, within family Z63.6
    facilities Z75.9
      specified NEC Z75.8
  mental F48.9
  multiparity Z64.1
  negative life events in childhood Z62.9
    altered pattern of family relationships
      Z62.898
    frightening experience Z62.898
    loss of
      love relationship Z62.898
      self-esteem Z62.898
    physical abuse (alleged) -*see* Maltreatment,
      child
    removal from home Z62.29
    specified event NEC Z62.898
  neighbor Z59.2
  neurological NEC R29.818
  new step-parent affecting child Z62.898
  none (feared complaint unfounded) Z71.1
  occupational NEC Z56.89
  parent-child -*see* Conflict, parent-child
  personal hygiene Z91.89
  personality F69
  phase-of-life transition, adjustment Z60.0
  presence of sick or disabled person in family
    or household Z63.79
    needing care Z63.6
  primary support group (family) Z63.9
    specified NEC Z63.8
  probation officer Z64.4
  psychiatric F99
  psychosexual (development) F66
  psychosocial Z65.9
    specified NEC Z65.8
  relationship Z63.9
    childhood F93.8
  release from prison Z65.2
  removal from home affecting child Z62.29
  seeking and accepting known hazardous and
    harmful
      behavioral or psychological interventions
        Z65.8
      chemical, nutritional or physical
  interventions Z65.8
  sexual function (nonorganic) F52.9
  sight H54.7
  sleep disorder, child F51.9
  smell -*see* Disturbance, sensation, smell
  social
    environment Z60.9
      specified NEC Z60.8
    exclusion and rejection Z60.4
    worker Z64.4
  speech R47.9
    developmental F80.9
    specified NEC R47.89
  swallowing -*see* Dysphagia
  taste -*see* Disturbance, sensation, taste
  tic, child F95.0
  underachievement in school Z55.3
  unemployment Z56.0
    threatened Z56.2
  unwanted pregnancy Z64.0

Problem (with) (related to) --*continued*
  upbringing Z62.9
    specified NEC Z62.898
  urinary N39.9
  voice production R47.89
  work schedule (stressful) Z56.3
Procedure (surgical)
  converted
    arthroscopic to open Z53.33
    laparoscopic to open Z53.31
    specified procedure NEC to open Z53.39
    thoracoscopic to open Z53.32
  for purpose other than remedying health state
    Z41.9
    specified NEC Z41.8
  not done Z53.9
    because of
      administrative reasons Z53.8
      contraindication Z53.09
        smoking Z53.01
      patient's decision Z53.20
        for reasons of belief or group pressure
          Z53.1
        left against medical advice (AMA)
          Z53.21
      specified reason NEC Z53.29
    specified reason NEC Z53.8
Procidentia (uteri) N81.3
Proctalgia K62.89
  fugax K59.4
  spasmodic K59.4
Proctitis K62.89
  amebic (acute) A06.0
  chlamydial A56.3
  gonococcal A54.6
  granulomatous -*see* Enteritis, regional, large
    intestine
  herpetic A60.1
  radiation K62.7
  tuberculous A18.32
  ulcerative (chronic) K51.20
    with
      complication K51.219
        abscess K51.214
        fistula K51.213
        obstruction K51.212
        rectal bleeding K51.211
        specified NEC K51.218
Proctocele
  female (without uterine prolapse) N81.6
    with uterine prolapse N81.2
      complete N81.3
  male K62.3
Proctocolitis
  food-induced eosinophilic K52.82
  food protein-induced K52.82
  milk protein-induced K52.82
  mucosal -*see* Rectosigmoiditis, ulcerative
Proctoptosis K62.3
Proctorrhagia K62.5
Proctosigmoiditis K63.89
  ulcerative (chronic) -*see* Rectosigmoiditis,
    ulcerative
Proctospasm K59.4
  psychogenic F45.8
Profichet's disease -*see* Disorder, soft tissue,
  specified type NEC
Progeria E34.8
Prognathism (mandibular) (maxillary)
  M26.19

Progonoma (melanotic) -see Neoplasm, benign, by site
Progressive -see condition
Prolactinoma
  specified site -see Neoplasm, benign, by site
  unspecified site D35.2
Prolapse, prolapsed
  anus, anal (canal) (sphincter) K62.2
  arm or hand O32.2
    causing obstructed labor O64.4
  bladder (mucosa) (sphincter) (acquired)
    congenital Q79.4
    female -see Cystocele
    male N32.89
  breast implant (prosthetic) T85.49
  cecostomy K94.09
  cecum K63.4
  cervix, cervical (hypertrophied) N81.2
    anterior lip, obstructing labor O65.5
    congenital Q51.828
    postpartal, old N81.2
    stump N81.85
  ciliary body (traumatic) -see Laceration, eye(ball), with prolapse or loss of interocular tissue
  colon (pedunculated) K63.4
  colostomy K94.09
  disc (intervertebral) -see Displacement, intervertebral disc - eye implant (orbital) T85.398
  lens (ocular) -see Complications, intraocular lens
  fallopian tube N83.4
  gastric (mucosa) K31.89
  genital, female N81.9
    specified NEC N81.89
  globe, nontraumatic -see Luxation, globe
  ileostomy bud K94.19
  intervertebral disc -see Displacement, intervertebral disc
  intestine (small) K63.4
  iris (traumatic) -see Laceration, eye(ball), with prolapse or loss of interocular tissue
    nontraumatic H21.89
  kidney N28.83
    congenital Q63.2
  laryngeal muscles or ventricle J38.7
  liver K76.89
  meatus urinarius N36.8
  mitral (valve) I34.1
  ocular lens implant -see Complications, intraocular lens
  organ or site, congenital NEC -see Malposition, congenital
  ovary N83.4
  pelvic floor, female N81.89
  perineum, female N81.89
  rectum (mucosa) (sphincter) K62.3
    due to trichuris trichuria B79
  spleen D73.89
  stomach K31.89
  umbilical cord
    complicating delivery O69.0
  urachus, congenital Q64.4
  ureter N28.89
    with obstruction N13.5
      with infection N13.6
  ureterovesical orifice N28.89
  urethra (acquired) (infected) (mucosa) N36.8
    congenital Q64.71
  urinary meatus N36.8

Prolapse, prolapsed --continued
  congenital Q64.72
  uterovaginal N81.4
    complete N81.3
    incomplete N81.2
  uterus (with prolapse of vagina) N81.4
    complete N81.3
    congenital Q51.818
    first degree N81.2
    in pregnancy or childbirth -see Pregnancy, complicated by, abnormal, uterus
    incomplete N81.2
    postpartal (old) N81.4
    second degree N81.2
    third degree N81.3
  uveal (traumatic) -see Laceration, eye(ball), with prolapse or loss of interocular tissue
  vagina (anterior) (wall) -see Cystocele
    with prolapse of uterus N81.4
      complete N81.3
      incomplete N81.2
    posterior wall N81.6
    posthysterectomy N99.3
  vitreous (humor) H43.0
    in wound -see Laceration, eye(ball), with prolapse or loss of interocular tissue
  womb -see Prolapse, uterus
Prolapsus, female N81.9
  specified NEC N81.89
Proliferation(s)
  prostate, atypical small acinar N42.32
  primary cutaneous CD30 positive large T-cell C86.6
Proliferative -see condition
Prolonged, prolongation (of)
  bleeding (time) (idiopathic) R79.1
  coagulation (time) R79.1
  gestation (over 42 completed weeks)
    mother O48.1
    newborn P08.22
  interval I44.0
  labor O63.9
    first stage O63.0
    second stage O63.1
  partial thromboplastin time (PTT) R79.1
  pregnancy (more than 42 weeks gestation) O48.1
  prothrombin time R79.1
  QT interval I45.81
  uterine contractions in labor O62.4
Prominence, prominent
  auricle (congenital) (ear) Q17.5
  ischial spine or sacral promontory
    with disproportion (fetopelvic) O33.0
      causing obstructed labor O65.0
  nose (congenital) acquired M95.0
Promiscuity -see High, risk, sexual behavior
Pronation
  ankle -see Deformity, limb, foot, specified NEC
  foot -see also Deformity, limb, foot, specified NEC
    congenital Q74.2
Prophylactic
  administration of
    antibiotics, long-term Z79.2
      short-term use - omit code
    drug -see also Long-term (current) drug therapy (use of) Z79.899
    medication Z79.899

Prophylactic --continued
  organ removal (for neoplasia management) Z40.00
    breast Z40.01
    ovary Z40.02
    specified site NEC Z40.09
  surgery Z40.9
    for risk factors related to malignant neoplasm -see Prophylactic, organ removal
    specified NEC Z40.8
  vaccination Z23
Propionic acidemia E71.121
Proptosis (ocular) -see also Exophthalmos
  thyroid -see Hyperthyroidism, with goiter
Prosecution, anxiety concerning Z65.3
Prosopagnosia R48.3
Prostadynia N42.81
Prostate, prostatic -see condition
Prostatism -see Hyperplasia, prostate
Prostatitis (congestive) (suppurative) (with cystitis) N41.9
  acute N41.0
  cavitary N41.8
  chronic N41.1
  diverticular N41.8
  due to Trichomonas (vaginalis) A59.02
  fibrous N41.1
  gonococcal (acute) (chronic) A54.22
  granulomatous N41.4
  hypertrophic N41.1
  subacute N41.1
  trichomonal A59.02
  tuberculous A18.14
Prostatocystitis N41.3
Prostatorrhea N42.89
Prostatosis N42.82
Prostration R53.83
  heat -see also Heat, exhaustion
    anhydrotic T67.3
    due to
      salt (and water) depletion T67.4
      water depletion T67.3
  nervous F48.8
  senile R54
Protanomaly (anomalous trichromat) H53.54
Protanopia (complete) (incomplete) H53.54
Protection (against) (from) -see Prophylactic
Protein
  deficiency NEC -see Malnutrition
  malnutrition -see Malnutrition
  sickness -see also Reaction, serum T80.69
Proteinemia R77.9
Proteinosis
  alveolar (pulmonary) J84.01
  lipid or lipoid (of Urbach) E78.89
Proteinuria R80.9
  Bence Jones R80.3
  complicating pregnancy -see Proteinuria, gestational
  gestational
    complicating
      childbirth O12.14
      pregnancy O12.1
        with edema O12.2
      puerperium O12.15
  idiopathic R80.0
  isolated R80.0
    with glomerular lesion N06.9
      dense deposit disease N06.6
      diffuse

Proteinuria
  crescentic glomerulonephritis N06.7
  endocapillary proliferative
    glomerulonephritis N06.4
  mesangiocapillary glomerulonephritis
    N06.5
  focal and segmental hyalinosis or sclerosis
    N06.1
  membranous (diffuse) N06.2
  mesangial proliferative (diffuse) N06.3
  minimal change N06.0
  specified pathology NEC N06.8
  orthostatic R80.2
    with glomerular lesion -see Proteinuria,
      isolated, with glomerular lesion
  persistent R80.1
    with glomerular lesion -see Proteinuria,
      isolated, with glomerular lesion
  postural R80.2
    with glomerular lesion -see Proteinuria,
      isolated, with glomerular lesion
  pre-eclamptic -see Pre-eclampsia
  puerperal O12.15
  specified type NEC R80.8
Proteolysis, pathologic D65
**Proteus (mirabilis) (morganii), as cause of
  disease classified elsewhere** B96.4
Prothrombin gene mutation D68.52
Protoporphyria, erythropoietic E80.0
Protozoal -see also condition
  disease B64
  specified NEC B60.8
Protrusion, protrusio - acetabuli M24.7
  acetabulum (into pelvis) M24.7
  device, implant or graft -see also
  Complications, by site and type, mechanical
  T85.698
    arterial graft NEC -see Complication,
      cardiovascular device, mechanical,
      vascular
    breast (implant) T85.49
    catheter NEC T85.698
      cystostomy T83.090
      dialysis (renal) T82.49
        intraperitoneal T85.691
      infusion NEC T82.594
        spinal (epidural) (subdural) T85.690
      urinary -see also Complications, catheter,
  urinary T83.098
    electronic (electrode) (pulse generator)
      (stimulator)
      bone T84.390
      nervous system -see Complication,
        prosthetic device, mechanical, electronic
        nervous system stimulator
    fixation, internal (orthopedic) NEC -see
      Complication, fixation device, mechanical
    gastrointestinal -see Complications,
      prosthetic device, mechanical,
      gastrointestinal device
    genital NEC T83.498
      intrauterine contraceptive device T83.39
      penile prosthesis (cylinder) (implanted)
        (pump) (reservoir) T83.490
      testicular prosthesis T83.491
    heart NEC -see Complication,
      cardiovascular device, mechanical
    joint prosthesis -see Complications, joint
      prosthesis, mechanical, specified NEC, by
      site

Protrusion, protrusio - continued
  ocular NEC -see Complications, prosthetic
    device, mechanical, ocular device
  orthopedic NEC -see Complication,
    orthopedic, device, mechanical
  specified NEC T85.628
  urinary NEC -see also Complication,
    genitourinary, device, urinary, mechanical
    graft T83.29
  vascular NEC -see Complication,
    cardiovascular device, mechanical
  ventricular intracranial shunt T85.09
  intervertebral disc -see Displacement,
    intervertebral disc
  joint prosthesis -see Complications, joint
    prosthesis, mechanical, specified NEC, by
    site
  nucleus pulposus -see Displacement,
    intervertebral disc
Prune belly (syndrome) Q79.4
**Prurigo (ferox) (gravis) (Hebrae) (Hebra's)
  (mitis) (simplex)** L28.2
  Besnier's L20.0
  estivalis L56.4
  nodularis L28.1
  psychogenic F45.8
Pruritus, pruritic (essential) L29.9
  ani, anus L29.0
    psychogenic F45.8
  anogenital L29.3
    psychogenic F45.8
  due to onchocerca volvulus B73.1
  gravidarum -see Pregnancy, complicated by,
    specified pregnancy related condition NEC
  hiemalis L29.8
  neurogenic (any site) F45.8
  perianal L29.0
  psychogenic (any site) F45.8
  scroti, scrotum L29.1
    psychogenic F45.8
  senile, senilis L29.8
  specified NEC L29.8
    psychogenic F45.8
  Trichomonas A59.9
  vulva, vulvae L29.2
    psychogenic F45.8
Pseudarthrosis, pseudoarthrosis (bone) -see
  Nonunion, fracture
  clavicle, congenital Q74.0
  joint, following fusion or arthrodesis M96.0
Pseudoaneurysm -see Aneurysm
Pseudoangioma I81
Pseudoangina (pectoris) -see Angina
Pseudoarteriosus Q28.8
Pseudoarthrosis -see Pseudarthrosis
Pseudobulbar affect (PBA) F48.2
Pseudochromhidrosis L67.8
Pseudocirrhosis, liver, pericardial I31.1
Pseudocowpox B08.03
Pseudocoxalgia M91.3
Pseudocroup J38.5
**Pseudo-Cushing's syndrome, alcohol-
  induced** E24.4
Pseudocyesis F45.8
Pseudocyst
  lung J98.4
  pancreas K86.3
  retina -see Cyst, retina
Pseudoelephantiasis neuroarthritica Q82.0
Pseudoexfoliation, capsule (lens) -see
  Cataract, specified NEC
Pseudofolliculitis barbae L73.1

Pseudoglioma H44.89
**Pseudohemophilia (Bernuth's) (hereditary)
  (type B)** D68.0
  Type A D69.8
  vascular D69.8
Pseudohermaphroditism Q56.3
  adrenal E25.8
  female Q56.2
    with adrenocortical disorder E25.8
    without adrenocortical disorder Q56.2
    adrenal (congenital) E25.0
  male Q56.1
    with
      adrenocortical disorder E25.8
      androgen resistance E34.51
      cleft scrotum Q56.1
      feminizing testis E34.51
      5 alpha-reductase deficiency E29.1
    without gonadal disorder Q56.1
    adrenal E25.8
Pseudo-Hurler's polydystrophy E77.0
Pseudohydrocephalus G93.2
**Pseudohypertrophic muscular dystrophy
  (Erb's)** G71.0
Pseudohypertrophy, muscle G71.0
Pseudohypoparathyroidism E20.1
Pseudoinsomnia F51.03
Pseudoleukemia, infantile D64.89
Pseudomembranous -see condition
Pseudomenses (newborn) P54.6
Pseudomenstruation (newborn) P54.6
**Pseudomeningocele (cerebral) (infective)
  (post-traumatic)** G96.19
  postprocedural (spinal) G97.82
Pseudomonas
  aeruginosa, as cause of disease classified
    elsewhere B96.5
  mallei infection A24.0
    as cause of disease classified elsewhere
      B96.5
  pseudomallei, as cause of disease classified
    elsewhere B96.5
Pseudomyotonia G71.19
Pseudomyxoma peritonei C78.6
**Pseudoneuritis, optic (nerve) (disc) (papilla),
  congenital** Q14.2
**Pseudo-obstruction intestine (acute)
  (chronic) (idiopathic) (intermittent
  secondary) (primary)** K59.8
Pseudopapilledema H47.33
  congenital Q14.2
Pseudoparalysis
  arm or leg R29.818
  atonic, congenital P94.2
Pseudopelade L66.0
Pseudophakia Z96.1
Pseudopolyarthritis, rhizomelic M35.3
Pseudopolycythemia D75.1
Pseudopseudohypoparathyroidism E20.1
Pseudopterygium H11.81
Pseudoptosis (eyelid) -see Blepharochalasis
Pseudopuberty, precocious
  female heterosexual E25.8
  male isosexual E25.8
Pseudorickets (renal) N25.0
Pseudorubella B08.20
Pseudosclerema, newborn P83.8
Pseudosclerosis (brain)
  of Westphal (Strümpell) E83.01
  Jakob's -see Creutzfeldt-Jakob disease or
    syndrome
  spastic -see Creutzfeldt-Jakob disease or
    syndrome

Pseudotetanus -see Convulsions
Pseudotetany R29.0
  hysterical F44.5
Pseudotruncus arteriosus Q25.49
Pseudotuberculosis A28.2
  enterocolitis A04.8
  pasteurella (infection) A28.0
Pseudotumor
  cerebri G93.2
  orbital H05.11
Pseudoxanthoma elasticum Q82.8
Psilosis (sprue) (tropical) K90.1
  nontropical K90.0
Psittacosis A70
Psoitis M60.88
Psoriasis L40.9
  arthropathic L40.50
    arthritis mutilans L40.52
    distal interphalangeal L40.51
    juvenile L40.54
    other specified L40.59
    spondylitis L40.53
  buccal K13.29
  flexural L40.8
  guttate L40.4
  mouth K13.29
  nummular L40.0
  plaque L40.0
  psychogenic F54
  pustular (generalized) L40.1
    palmaris et plantaris L40.3
  specified NEC L40.8
  vulgaris L40.0
Psychasthenia F48.8
Psychiatric disorder or problem F99
Psychogenic -see also condition
  factors associated with physical conditions
    F54
Psychological and behavioral factors
  affecting medical condition F59
Psychoneurosis, psychoneurotic -see also
  Neurosis
  anxiety (state) F41.1
  depersonalization F48.1
  hypochondriacal F45.21
  hysteria F44.9
  neurasthenic F48.8
  personality NEC F60.89
Psychopathy, psychopathic
  affectionless F94.2
  autistic F84.5
  constitution, post-traumatic F07.81
  personality -see Disorder, personality sexual
    -see Deviation, sexual
  state F60.2
Psychosexual identity disorder of childhood
  F64.2
Psychosis, psychotic F29
  acute (transient) F23
    hysterical F44.9
  affective -see Disorder, mood - alcoholic
    F10.959
    with
      abuse F10.159
      anxiety disorder F10.980
        with
          abuse F10.180
          dependence F10.280
      delirium tremens F10.231
      delusions F10.950
        with

Psychosis, psychotic --continued
  abuse F10.150
    dependence F10.250
  dementia F10.97
    with dependence F10.27
  dependence F10.259
  hallucinosis F10.951
    with
      abuse F10.151
      dependence F10.251
  mood disorder F10.94
    with
      abuse F10.14
      dependence F10.24
  paranoia F10.950
    with
      abuse F10.150
      dependence F10.250
  persisting amnesia F10.96
    with dependence F10.26
  amnestic confabulatory F10.96
    with dependence F10.26
  delirium tremens F10.231
  Korsakoff's, Korsakov's, Korsakow's F10.26
  paranoid type F10.950
    with
      abuse F10.150
      dependence F10.250
  anergastic -see Psychosis, organic
  arteriosclerotic (simple type) (uncomplicated)
    F01.50
    with behavioral disturbance F01.51
  childhood F84.0
    atypical F84.8
  climacteric -see Psychosis, involutional
  confusional F29
    acute or subacute F05
    reactive F23
  cycloid F23
  depressive -see Disorder, depressive
  disintegrative (childhood) F84.3
  drug-induced -see F11 F19 with .x59
    paranoid and hallucinatory states -see F11
      F19 with .x50 or .x51
  due to or associated with
    addiction, drug -see F11 F19 with .x59
    dependence
      alcohol F10.259
      drug -see F11 F19 with .x59
    epilepsy F06.8
    Huntington's chorea F06.8
    ischemia, cerebrovascular (generalized)
      F06.8
    multiple sclerosis F06.8
    physical disease F06.8
    presenile dementia F03
    senile dementia F03
    vascular disease (arteriosclerotic) (cerebral)
      F01.50
      with behavioral disturbance F01.51
  epileptic F06.8
  episode F23
    due to or associated with physical condition
      F06.8
  exhaustive F43.0
  hallucinatory, chronic F28
  hypomanic F30.8
  hysterical (acute) F44.9
  induced F24
  infantile F84.0
    atypical F84.8

  infective (acute) (subacute) F05
  involutional F28
    depressive -see Disorder, depressive
    melancholic -see Disorder, depressive
    paranoid (state) F22
  Korsakoff's, Korsakov's, Korsakow's
    (nonalcoholic) F04
    alcoholic F10.96
      in dependence F10.26
    induced by other psychoactive substance -
      see categories F11 F19 with .x5x - mania,
      manic (single episode) F30.2
    recurrent type F31.89
  manic-depressive -see Disorder, bipolar
  menopausal -see Psychosis, involutional
  mixed schizophrenic and affective F25.8
  multi-infarct (cerebrovascular) F01.50
    with behavioral disturbance F01.51
  nonorganic F29
    specified NEC F28
  organic F09
    due to or associated with
      arteriosclerosis (cerebral) -see Psychosis,
        arteriosclerotic
      cerebrovascular disease, arteriosclerotic -
        see Psychosis, arteriosclerotic
      childbirth -see Psychosis, puerperal
      Creutzfeldt-Jakob disease or syndrome -see
        Creutzfeldt-Jakob disease or syndrome
      dependence, alcohol F10.259
      disease
        alcoholic liver F10.259
        brain, arteriosclerotic -see Psychosis,
          arteriosclerotic
        cerebrovascular F01.50
          with behavioral disturbance F01.51
        Creutzfeldt-Jakob -see Creutzfeldt-Jakob
          disease or syndrome
        endocrine or metabolic F06.8
          acute or subacute F05
        liver, alcoholic F10.259
      epilepsy transient (acute) F05
      infection
        brain (intracranial) F06.8
          acute or subacute F05
      intoxication
        alcoholic (acute) F10.259
        drug F19 with .x59 F11
      ischemia, cerebrovascular (generalized) -
        see Psychosis, arteriosclerotic
      puerperium -see Psychosis, puerperal
      trauma, brain (birth) (from electric current)
        (surgical) F06.8
        acute or subacute F05
    infective F06.8
      acute or subacute F05
    post-traumatic F06.8
      acute or subacute F05
  paranoiac F22
  paranoid (climacteric) (involutional)
    (menopausal) F22
    psychogenic (acute) F23
    schizophrenic F20.0
    senile F03
  postpartum F53
  presbyophrenic (type) F03
  presenile F03
  psychogenic (paranoid) F23
    depressive F32.3
  puerperal F53

Psychosis, psychotic --*continued*
  specified type -*see* Psychosis, by type
  reactive (brief) (transient) (emotional stress)
    (psychological trauma) F23
    depressive F32.3
      recurrent F33.3
    excitative type F30.8
  schizoaffective F25.9
    depressive type F25.1
    manic type F25.0
  schizophrenia, schizophrenic -*see*
    Schizophrenia
  schizophrenia-like, in epilepsy F06.2
  schizophreniform F20.81
    affective type F25.9
    brief F23
    confusional type F23
    depressive type F25.1
    manic type F25.0
    mixed type F25.0
  senile NEC F03
    depressed or paranoid type F03
    simple deterioration F03
    specified type - code to condition
  shared F24
  situational (reactive) F23
  symbiotic (childhood) F84.3
  symptomatic F09
Psychosomatic -*see* Disorder, psychosomatic
Psychosyndrome, organic F07.9
Psychotic episode due to or associated with
  physical condition F06.8
Pterygium (eye) H11.00
  amyloid H11.01
  central H11.02
  colli Q18.3
  double H11.03
  peripheral
    progressive H11.05
    stationary H11.04
  recurrent H11.06
Ptilosis (eyelid) -*see* Madarosis
Ptomaine (poisoning) -*see* Poisoning, food
Ptosis -*see also* Blepharoptosis
  adiposa (false) -*see* Blepharoptosis
  breast N64.81
  cecum K63.4
  colon K63.4
  congenital (eyelid) Q10.0
    specified site NEC -*see* Anomaly, by site
  eyelid -*see* Blepharoptosis
    congenital Q10.0
  gastric K31.89
  intestine K63.4
  kidney N28.83
  liver K76.89
  renal N28.83
  splanchnic K63.4
  spleen D73.89
  stomach K31.89
  viscera K63.4
PTP D69.51
Ptyalism (periodic) K11.7
  hysterical F45.8
  pregnancy -*see* Pregnancy, complicated by,
    specified pregnancy related condition NEC
  psychogenic F45.8
Ptyalolithiasis K11.5
Pubarche, precocious E30.1
Pubertas praecox E30.1

Puberty (development state) Z00.3
  bleeding (excessive) N92.2
  delayed E30.0
  precocious (constitutional) (cryptogenic)
    (idiopathic) E30.1
    central E22.8
    due to
      ovarian hyperfunction E28.1
        estrogen E28.0
      testicular hyperfunction E29.0
    premature E30.1
    due to
      adrenal cortical hyperfunction E25.8
      pineal tumor E34.8
      pituitary (anterior) hyperfunction E22.8
Puckering, macula -*see* Degeneration, macula,
  puckering
Pudenda, pudendum -*see* condition
Puente's disease (simple glandular cheilitis)
  K13.0
Puerperal, puerperium (complicated by,
  complications)
  abnormal glucose (tolerance test) O99.815
  abscess
    areola O91.02
      associated with lactation O91.03
    Bartholin's gland O86.19
    breast O91.12
      associated with lactation O91.13
    cervix (uteri) O86.11
    genital organ NEC O86.19
    kidney O86.21
    mammary O91.12
      associated with lactation O91.13
    nipple O91.02
      associated with lactation O91.03
    peritoneum O85
    subareolar O91.12
      associated with lactation O91.13
    urinary tract -*see* Puerperal, infection,
  urinary
    uterus O86.12
    vagina (wall) O86.13
    vaginorectal O86.13
    vulvovaginal gland O86.13
  adnexitis O86.19
  afibrinogenemia, or other coagulation defect
    O72.3
  albuminuria (acute) (subacute) -*see*
    Proteinuria, gestational
  alcohol use O99.315
  anemia O90.81
    pre-existing (pre-pregnancy) O99.03
  anesthetic death O89.8
  apoplexy O99.43
  bariatric surgery status O99.845
  blood disorder NEC O99.13
  blood dyscrasia O72.3
  cardiomyopathy O90.3
  cerebrovascular disorder (conditions in I60
    I69) O99.43
  cervicitis O86.11
  circulatory system disorder O99.43
  coagulopathy (any) O72.3
  complications O90.9
    specified NEC O90.89
  convulsions -*see* Eclampsia
  cystitis O86.22
  cystopyelitis O86.29
  delirium NEC F05
  diabetes O24.93

Puerperal, puerperium - *continued*
  gestational -*see* Puerperal, gestational
    diabetes
    pre-existing O24.33
      specified NEC O24.83
      type 1 O24.03
      type 2 O24.13
  digestive system disorder O99.63
  disease O90.9
    breast NEC O92.29
    cerebrovascular (acute) O99.43
    nonobstetric NEC O99.89
    tubo-ovarian O86.19
    Valsuani's O99.03
  disorder O90.9
    biliary tract O26.63
    lactation O92.70
    liver O26.63
    nonobstetric NEC O99.89
  disruption
    cesarean wound O90.0
    episiotomy wound O90.1
    perineal laceration wound O90.1
  drug use O99.325
  eclampsia (with pre-existing hypertension)
    O15.2
  embolism (pulmonary) (blood clot) -*see*
    Embolism, obstetric, puerperal
  endocrine, nutritional or metabolic disease
    NEC O99.285
  endophlebitis -*see* Puerperal, phlebitis
  endotrachelitis O86.11
  failure
    lactation (complete) O92.3
      partial O92.4
    renal, acute O90.4
  fever (of unknown origin) O86.4
    septic O85
  fissure, nipple O92.12
    associated with lactation O92.13
  fistula
    breast (due to mastitis) O91.12
      associated with lactation O91.13
    nipple O91.02
      associated with lactation O91.03
  galactophoritis O91.22
    associated with lactation O91.23
  galactorrhea O92.6
  gastric banding status O99.845
  gastric bypass status O99.845
  gastrointestinal disease NEC O99.63
  gestational
    diabetes O24.439
      diet controlled O24.430
      insulin (and diet) controlled O24.434
      oral drug controlled (antidiabetic)
        (hypoglycemic) O24.435
    edema O12.05
      with proteinuria O12.25
    proteinuria O12.15
  gonorrhea O98.23
  hematoma, subdural O99.43
  hemiplegia, cerebral O99.355
    due to cerebrovascular disorder O99.43
  hemorrhage O72.1
    brain O99.43
    bulbar O99.43
    cerebellar O99.43
    cerebral O99.43
    cortical O99.43
    delayed or secondary O72.2

Puerperal, puerperium - *continued*
  extradural O99.43
  internal capsule O99.43
  intracranial O99.43
  intrapontine O99.43
  meningeal O99.43
  pontine O99.43
  retained placenta O72.0
  subarachnoid O99.43
  subcortical O99.43
  subdural O99.43
  third stage O72.0
  uterine, delayed O72.2
  ventricular O99.43
  hemorrhoids O87.2
  hepatorenal syndrome O90.4
  hypertension -*see* Hypertension,
    complicating, puerperium
  hypertrophy, breast O92.29
  induration breast (fibrous) O92.29
  infection O86.4
    cervix O86.11
    generalized O85
    genital tract NEC O86.19
      obstetric surgical wound O86.0
    kidney (bacillus coli) O86.21
    maternal O98.93
      carrier state NEC O99.835
      gonorrhea O98.23
      human immunodeficiency virus (HIV)
        O98.73
      protozoal O98.63
      sexually transmitted NEC O98.33
      specified NEC O98.83
      streptococcus group B (GBS) carrier state
        O99.825
      syphilis O98.13
      tuberculosis O98.03
      viral hepatitis O98.43
      viral NEC O98.53
    nipple O91.02
      associated with lactation O91.03
    peritoneum O85
    renal O86.21
    specified NEC O86.89
    urinary (asymptomatic) (tract) NEC O86.20
      bladder O86.22
      kidney O86.21
      specified site NEC O86.29
      urethra O86.22
    vagina O86.13
    vein -*see* Puerperal, phlebitis
  ischemia, cerebral O99.43
  lymphangitis O86.89
    breast O91.22
      associated with lactation O91.23
  malignancy O9A.13
  malnutrition O25.3
  mammillitis O91.02
    associated with lactation O91.03
  mammitis O91.22
    associated with lactation O91.23
  mania F30.8
  mastitis O91.22
    associated with lactation O91.23
    purulent O91.12
      associated with lactation O91.13
  melancholia -*see* Disorder, depressive
  mental disorder NEC O99.345
  metroperitonitis O85
  metrorrhagia -*see* Hemorrhage, postpartum

Puerperal, puerperium - *continued*
  metrosalpingitis O86.19
  metrovaginitis O86.13
  milk leg O87.1
  monoplegia, cerebral O99.43
  mood disturbance O90.6
  necrosis, liver (acute) (subacute) (conditions
    in subcategory K72.0) O26.63
    with renal failure O90.4
  nervous system disorder O99.355
  neuritis O90.89
  obesity (pre-existing prior to pregnancy)
    O99.215
  obesity surgery status O99.845
  occlusion, precerebral artery O99.43
  paralysis
    bladder (sphincter) O90.89
    cerebral O99.43
  paralytic stroke O99.43
  parametritis O85
  paravaginitis O86.13
  pelviperitonitis O85
  perimetritis O86.12
  perimetrosalpingitis O86.19
  perinephritis O86.21
  periphlebitis -*see* Puerperal phlebitis
  peritoneal infection O85
  peritonitis (pelvic) O85
  perivaginitis O86.13
  phlebitis O87.0
    deep O87.1
    pelvic O87.1
    superficial O87.0
  phlebothrombosis, deep O87.1
  phlegmasia alba dolens O87.1
  placental polyp O90.89
  pneumonia, embolic -*see* Embolism, obstetric,
    puerperal
  pre-eclampsia -*see* Pre-eclampsia
  psychosis F53
  pyelitis O86.21
  pyelocystitis O86.29
  pyelonephritis O86.21
  pyelonephrosis O86.21
  pyemia O85
  pyocystitis O86.29
  pyohemia O85
  pyometra O86.12
  pyonephritis O86.21
  pyosalpingitis O86.19
  pyrexia (of unknown origin) O86.4
  renal
    disease NEC O90.89
    failure O90.4
  respiratory disease NEC O99.53
  retention
    decidua -*see* Retention, decidua
    placenta O72.0
    secundines -*see* Retention, secundines
  retracted nipple O92.02
  salpingo-ovaritis O86.19
  salpingoperitonitis O85
  secondary perineal tear O90.1
  sepsis (pelvic) O85
  sepsis O85
  septic thrombophlebitis O86.81
  skin disorder NEC O99.73
  specified condition NEC O99.89
  stroke O99.43
  subinvolution (uterus) O90.89
  subluxation of symphysis (pubis) O26.73

Puerperal, puerperium - *continued*
  suppuration -*see* Puerperal, abscess
  tetanus A34
  thelitis O91.02
    associated with lactation O91.03
  thrombocytopenia O72.3
  thrombophlebitis (superficial) O87.0
    deep O87.1
    pelvic O87.1
    septic O86.81
  thrombosis (venous) -*see* Thrombosis,
    puerperal
  thyroiditis O90.5
  toxemia (eclamptic) (pre-eclamptic) (with
    convulsions) O15.2
  trauma, non-obstetric O9A.23
    caused by abuse (physical) (suspected)
      O9A.33
      confirmed O9A.33
      psychological (suspected) O9A.53
        confirmed O9A.53
      sexual (suspected) O9A.43
        confirmed O9A.43
  uremia (due to renal failure) O90.4
  urethritis O86.22
  vaginitis O86.13
  varicose veins (legs) O87.4
    vulva or perineum O87.8
  venous O87.9
  vulvitis O86.19
  vulvovaginitis O86.13
  white leg O87.1
Puerperium -*see* Puerperal
Pulmolithiasis J98.4
Pulmonary -*see* condition
Pulpitis (acute) (anachoretic) (chronic)
  (hyperplastic) (putrescent) (suppurative)
  (ulcerative) K04.01
  irreversible K04.02
  reversible K04.01
Pulpless tooth K04.99
Pulse
  alternating R00.8
  bigeminal R00.8
  fast R00.0
  feeble, rapid due to shock following injury
    T79.4
  rapid R00.0
  weak R09.89
Pulsus alternans or trigeminus R00.8
Punch drunk F07.81
Punctum lacrimale occlusion -*see*
  Obstruction, lacrimal
Puncture
  abdomen, abdominal
    wall S31.139
      with
        foreign body S31.149
        penetration into peritoneal cavity S31.639
          with foreign body S31.649
      epigastric region S31.132
        with
          foreign body S31.142
          penetration into peritoneal cavity
            S31.632
            with foreign body S31.642
      left
        lower quadrant S31.134
          with
            foreign body S31.144

Puncture --*continued*
    penetration into peritoneal cavity
    S31.634
      with foreign body S31.644
    upper quadrant S31.131
      with
        foreign body S31.141
      penetration into peritoneal cavity
      S31.631
        with foreign body S31.641
   periumbilic region S31.135
    with
      foreign body S31.145
    penetration into peritoneal cavity
    S31.635
      with foreign body S31.645
   right
    lower quadrant S31.133
      with
        foreign body S31.143
      penetration into peritoneal cavity
      S31.633
        with foreign body S31.643
    upper quadrant S31.130
      with
        foreign body S31.140
      penetration into peritoneal cavity
      S31.630
        with foreign body S31.640
accidental, complicating surgery -*see*
Complication, accidental puncture or
laceration
alveolar (process) -*see* Puncture, oral cavity
ankle S91.039
  with
    foreign body S91.049
  left S91.032
    with
      foreign body S91.042
  right S91.031
    with
      foreign body S91.041
anus S31.833
  with foreign body S31.834
arm (upper) S41.139
  with foreign body S41.149
  left S41.132
    with foreign body S41.142
  lower -*see* Puncture, forearm
  right S41.131
    with foreign body S41.141
auditory canal (external) (meatus) -*see*
Puncture, ear
auricle, ear -*see* Puncture, ear
axilla -*see* Puncture, arm
back -*see also* Puncture, thorax, back
  lower S31.030
    with
      foreign body S31.040
        with penetration into retroperitoneal
        space S31.041
      penetration into retroperitoneal space
      S31.031
bladder (traumatic) S37.29
  nontraumatic N32.89
breast S21.039
  with foreign body S21.049
  left S21.032
    with foreign body S21.042
  right S21.031
    with foreign body S21.041

Puncture --*continued*
  buttock S31.803
    with foreign body S31.804
    left S31.823
      with foreign body S31.824
    right S31.813
      with foreign body S31.814
  by
    device, implant or graft -*see* Complications,
    by site and type, mechanical
    foreign body left accidentally in operative
    wound T81.539
    instrument (any) during a procedure,
    accidental -*see* Puncture, accidental
    complicating surgery   calf -*see* Puncture,
    leg
  canaliculus lacrimalis -*see* Puncture, eyelid
  canthus, eye -*see* Puncture, eyelid
  cervical esophagus S11.23
    with foreign body S11.24
  cheek (external) S01.439
    with foreign body S01.449
    left S01.432
      with foreign body S01.442
    right S01.431
      with foreign body S01.441
    internal -*see* Puncture, oral cavity   chest
    wall -*see* Puncture, thorax
  chin -*see* Puncture, head, specified site NEC
  clitoris -*see* Puncture, vulva
  costal region -*see* Puncture, thorax - digit(s)
    hand -*see* Puncture, finger
    foot -*see* Puncture, toe
  ear (canal) (external) S01.339
    with foreign body S01.349
    left S01.332
      with foreign body S01.342
    right S01.331
      with foreign body S01.341
    drum S09.2
  elbow S51.039
    with
      foreign body S51.049
    left S51.032
      with
        foreign body S51.042
    right S51.031
      with
        foreign body S51.041
  epididymis -*see* Puncture, testis
  epigastric region -*see* Puncture, abdomen,
  wall, epigastric
  epiglottis S11.83
    with foreign body S11.84
  esophagus
    cervical S11.23
      with foreign body S11.24
    thoracic S27.818
  eyeball S05.6
    with foreign body S05.5
  eyebrow -*see* Puncture, eyelid
  eyelid S01.13
    with foreign body S01.14
    left S01.132
      with foreign body S01.142
    right S01.131
      with foreign body S01.141
  face NEC -*see* Puncture, head, specified site
  NEC
  finger(s) S61.239
    with

Puncture --*continued*
    damage to nail S61.339
      with
        foreign body S61.349
      foreign body S61.249
    index S61.238
      with
        damage to nail S61.338
          with
            foreign body S61.348
        foreign body S61.248
      left S61.231
        with
          damage to nail S61.331
            with
              foreign body S61.341
          foreign body S61.241
      right S61.230
        with
          damage to nail S61.330
            with
              foreign body S61.340
          foreign body S61.240
    little S61.238
      with
        damage to nail S61.338
          with
            foreign body S61.348
        foreign body S61.248
      left S61.237
        with
          damage to nail S61.337
            with
              foreign body S61.347
          foreign body S61.247
      right S61.236
        with
          damage to nail S61.336
            with
              foreign body S61.346
          foreign body S61.246
    middle S61.238
      with
        damage to nail S61.338
          with
            foreign body S61.348
        foreign body S61.248
      left S61.233
        with
          damage to nail S61.333
            with
              foreign body S61.343
          foreign body S61.243
      right S61.232
        with
          damage to nail S61.332
            with
              foreign body S61.342
          foreign body S61.242
    ring S61.238
      with
        damage to nail S61.338
          with
            foreign body S61.348
        foreign body S61.248
      left S61.235
        with
          damage to nail S61.335
            with
              foreign body S61.345
          foreign body S61.245

Puncture *--continued*
    right S61.234
      with
        damage to nail S61.334
          with
            foreign body S61.344
        foreign body S61.244
    flank S31.139
      with foreign body S31.149
    foot (except toe(s) alone) S91.339
      with foreign body S91.349
      left S91.332
        with foreign body S91.342
      right S91.331
        with foreign body S91.341
      toe *-see* Puncture, toe
    forearm S51.839
      with
        foreign body S51.849
      elbow only *-see* Puncture, elbow
      left S51.832
        with
          foreign body S51.842
      right S51.831
        with
          foreign body S51.841
    forehead *-see* Puncture, head, specified site NEC
    genital organs, external
      female S31.532
        with foreign body S31.542
        vagina *-see* Puncture, vagina
        vulva *-see* Puncture, vulva
      male S31.531
        with foreign body S31.541
        penis *-see* Puncture, penis
        scrotum *-see* Puncture, scrotum
        testis *-see* Puncture, testis
    groin *-see* Puncture, abdomen, wall
    gum *-see* Puncture, oral cavity
    hand S61.439
      with
        foreign body S61.449
      finger *-see* Puncture, finger
      left S61.432
        with
          foreign body S61.442
      right S61.431
        with
          foreign body S61.441
      thumb *-see* Puncture, thumb
    head S01.93
      with foreign body S01.94
      cheek *-see* Puncture, cheek
      ear *-see* Puncture, ear
      eyelid *-see* Puncture, eyelid
      lip *-see* Puncture, oral cavity
      nose *-see* Puncture, nose
      oral cavity *-see* Puncture, oral cavity
      scalp S01.03
        with foreign body S01.04
      specified site NEC S01.83
        with foreign body S01.84
      temporomandibular area *-see* Puncture, cheek
    heart S26.99
      with hemopericardium S26.09
      without hemopericardium S26.19
    heel *-see* Puncture, foot
    hip S71.039
      with foreign body S71.049

Puncture *--continued*
    left S71.032
      with foreign body S71.042
    right S71.031
      with foreign body S71.041
    hymen *-see* Puncture, vagina
    hypochondrium *-see* Puncture, abdomen, wall
    hypogastric region *-see* Puncture, abdomen, wall
    inguinal region *-see* Puncture, abdomen, wall
    instep *-see* Puncture, foot
    internal organs *-see* Injury, by site
    interscapular region *-see* Puncture, thorax, back
    intestine
      large
        colon S36.599
          ascending S36.590
          descending S36.592
          sigmoid S36.593
          specified site NEC S36.598
          transverse S36.591
        rectum S36.69
      small S36.499
        duodenum S36.490
        specified site NEC S36.498
    intra-abdominal organ S36.99
      gallbladder S36.128
      intestine *-see* Puncture, intestine
      liver S36.118
      pancreas *-see* Puncture, pancreas
      peritoneum S36.81
      specified site NEC S36.898
      spleen S36.09
      stomach S36.39
    jaw *-see* Puncture, head, specified site NEC
    knee S81.039
      with foreign body S81.049
      left S81.032
        with foreign body S81.042
      right S81.031
        with foreign body S81.041
    labium (majus) (minus) *-see* Puncture, vulva
    lacrimal duct *-see* Puncture, eyelid
    larynx S11.013
      with foreign body S11.014
    leg (lower) S81.839
      with foreign body S81.849
      foot *-see* Puncture, foot
      knee *-see* Puncture, knee
      left S81.832
        with foreign body S81.842
      right S81.831
        with foreign body S81.841
      upper *-see* Puncture, thigh
    lip S01.531
      with foreign body S01.541
    loin *-see* Puncture, abdomen, wall
    lower back *-see* Puncture, back, lower
    lumbar region *-see* Puncture, back, lower
    malar region *-see* Puncture, head, specified site NEC
    mammary *-see* Puncture, breast
    mastoid region *-see* Puncture, head, specified site NEC
    mouth *-see* Puncture, oral cavity
    nail
      finger *-see* Puncture, finger, with damage to nail
      toe *-see* Puncture, toe, with damage to nail
    nasal (septum) (sinus) *-see* Puncture, nose

Puncture *--continued*
    nasopharynx *-see* Puncture, head, specified site NEC
    neck S11.93
      with foreign body S11.94
      involving
        cervical esophagus *-see* Puncture, cervical esophagus
        larynx *-see* Puncture, larynx
        pharynx *-see* Puncture, pharynx
        thyroid gland *-see* Puncture, thyroid gland
        trachea *-see* Puncture, trachea
      specified site NEC S11.83
        with foreign body S11.84
    nose (septum) (sinus) S01.23
      with foreign body S01.24
    ocular *-see* Puncture, eyeball
    oral cavity S01.532
      with foreign body S01.542
    orbit S05.4
    palate *-see* Puncture, oral cavity   palm *-see* Puncture, hand
    pancreas S36.299
      body S36.291
      head S36.290
      tail S36.292
    pelvis *-see* Puncture, back, lower
    penis S31.23
      with foreign body S31.24
    perineum
      female S31.43
        with foreign body S31.44
      male S31.139
        with foreign body S31.149
    periocular area (with or without lacrimal passages) *-see* Puncture, eyelid
    phalanges
      finger *-see* Puncture, finger
      toe *-see* Puncture, toe
    pharynx S11.23
      with foreign body S11.24
    pinna *-see* Puncture, ear
    popliteal space *-see* Puncture, knee
    prepuce *-see* Puncture, penis
    pubic region S31.139
      with foreign body S31.149
    pudendum *-see* Puncture, genital organs, external
    rectovaginal septum *-see* Puncture, vagina
    sacral region *-see* Puncture, back, lower
    sacroiliac region *-see* Puncture, back, lower
    salivary gland *-see* Puncture, oral cavity
    scalp S01.03
      with foreign body S01.04
    scapular region *-see* Puncture, shoulder
    scrotum S31.33
      with foreign body S31.34
    shin *-see* Puncture, leg
    shoulder S41.039
      with foreign body S41.049
      left S41.032
        with foreign body S41.042
      right S41.031
        with foreign body S41.041
    spermatic cord *-see* Puncture, testis
    sternal region *-see* Puncture, thorax, front
    submaxillary region *-see* Puncture, head, specified site NEC
    submental region *-see* Puncture, head, specified site NEC
    subungual

Puncture --*continued*
  finger(s) -*see* Puncture, finger, with damage
    to nail
  toe -*see* Puncture, toe, with damage to nail
  supraclavicular fossa -*see* Puncture, neck,
    specified site NEC
  temple, temporal region -*see* Puncture, head,
    specified site NEC
  temporomandibular area -*see* Puncture, cheek
  testis S31.33
    with foreign body S31.34
  thigh S71.139
    with foreign body S71.149
    left S71.132
      with foreign body S71.142
    right S71.131
      with foreign body S71.141
  thorax, thoracic (wall) S21.93
    with foreign body S21.94
    back S21.23
      with
        foreign body S21.24
          with penetration S21.44
        penetration S21.43
    breast -*see* Puncture, breast
    front S21.13
      with
        foreign body S21.14
          with penetration S21.34
        penetration S21.33
  throat -*see* Puncture, neck
  thumb S61.039
    with
      damage to nail S61.139
        with
          foreign body S61.149
      foreign body S61.049
    left S61.032
      with
        damage to nail S61.132
          with
            foreign body S61.142
        foreign body S61.042
    right S61.031
      with
        damage to nail S61.131
          with
            foreign body S61.141
        foreign body S61.041
  thyroid gland S11.13
    with foreign body S11.14
  toe(s) S91.139
    with
      damage to nail S91.239
        with
          foreign body S91.249
      foreign body S91.149
    great S91.133
      with
        damage to nail S91.233
          with
            foreign body S91.243
        foreign body S91.143
      left S91.132
        with
          damage to nail S91.232
            with
              foreign body S91.242
          foreign body S91.142
      right S91.131
        with

Puncture --*continued*
      damage to nail S91.231
        with
          foreign body S91.241
      foreign body S91.141
    lesser S91.136
      with
        damage to nail S91.236
          with
            foreign body S91.246
        foreign body S91.146
      left S91.135
        with
          damage to nail S91.235
            with
              foreign body S91.245
          foreign body S91.145
      right S91.134
        with
          damage to nail S91.234
            with
              foreign body S91.244
          foreign body S91.144
  tongue -*see* Puncture, oral cavity   trachea
    S11.023
    with foreign body S11.024
  tunica vaginalis -*see* Puncture, testis
  tympanum, tympanic membrane S09.2
  umbilical region S31.135
    with foreign body S31.145
  uvula -*see* Puncture, oral cavity   vagina
    S31.43
    with foreign body S31.44
  vocal cords S11.033
    with foreign body S11.034
  vulva S31.43
    with foreign body S31.44
  wrist S61.539
    with
      foreign body S61.549
    left S61.532
      with
        foreign body S61.542
    right S61.531
      with
        foreign body S61.541
PUO (pyrexia of unknown origin) R50.9
Pupillary membrane (persistent) Q13.89
Pupillotonia -*see* Anomaly, pupil, function,
  tonic pupil
Purpura D69.2
  abdominal D69.0
  allergic D69.0
  anaphylactoid D69.0
  annularis telangiectodes L81.7
  arthritic D69.0
  autoerythrocyte sensitization D69.2
  autoimmune D69.0
  bacterial D69.0
  Bateman's (senile) D69.2
  capillary fragility (hereditary) (idiopathic)
    D69.8
  cryoglobulinemic D89.1
  Devil's pinches D69.2
  fibrinolytic -*see* Fibrinolysis
  fulminans, fulminous D65
  gangrenous D65
  hemorrhagic, hemorrhagica D69.3
    not due to thrombocytopenia D69.0
  Henoch (Schönlein) (allergic) D69.0

Purpura - *continued*
  hypergammaglobulinemic (benign)
    (Waldenström) D89.0
  idiopathic (thrombocytopenic) D69.3
    nonthrombocytopenic D69.0
  immune thrombocytopenic D69.3
  infectious D69.0
  malignant D69.0
  neonatorum P54.5
  nervosa D69.0
  newborn P54.5
  nonthrombocytopenic D69.2
    hemorrhagic D69.0
    idiopathic D69.0
  nonthrombopenic D69.2
  peliosis rheumatica D69.0
  posttransfusion (post-transfusion) (from
    (fresh) whole blood or blood products)
    D69.51
  primary D69.49
  red cell membrane sensitivity D69.2
  rheumatica D69.0
  Schönlein (Henoch) (allergic) D69.0
  scorbutic E54 [*D77*]
  senile D69.2
  simplex D69.2
  symptomatica D69.0
  telangiectasia annularis L81.7
  thrombocytopenic D69.49
    congenital D69.42
    hemorrhagic D69.3
    hereditary D69.42
    idiopathic D69.3
    immune D69.3
    neonatal, transitory P61.0
    thrombotic M31.1
  thrombohemolytic -*see* Fibrinolysis
  thrombolytic -*see* Fibrinolysis
  thrombopenic D69.49
  thrombotic, thrombocytopenic M31.1
  toxic D69.0
  vascular D69.0
  visceral symptoms D69.0
Purpuric spots R23.3
Purulent -*see* condition
Pus
  in
    stool R19.5
    urine N39.0
  tube (rupture) -*see* Salpingo-oophoritis
Pustular rash L08.0
Pustule (nonmalignant) L08.9
  malignant A22.0
Pustulosis palmaris et plantaris L40.3
Putnam (Dana) disease or syndrome -*see*
  Degeneration, combined
Putrescent pulp (dental) K04.1
Pyarthritis, pyarthrosis -*see* Arthritis,
  pyogenic or pyemic
  tuberculous -*see* Tuberculosis, joint
Pyelectasis -*see* Hydronephrosis
Pyelitis (congenital) (uremic) -*see also*
  Pyelonephritis
  with
    calculus -*see* category N20
      with hydronephrosis N13.2
    contracted kidney N11.9
  acute N10
  chronic N11.9
    with calculus -*see* category N20
      with hydronephrosis N13.2

Pyelitis - *continued*
cystica N28.84
puerperal (postpartum) O86.21
tuberculous A18.11
Pyelocystitis -*see* Pyelonephritis
Pyelonephritis -*see also* Nephritis, tubulo-
interstitial
with
calculus -*see* category N20
with hydronephrosis N13.2
contracted kidney N11.9
acute N10
calculous -*see* category N20
with hydronephrosis N13.2
chronic N11.9
with calculus -*see* category N20
with hydronephrosis N13.2
associated with ureteral obstruction or
stricture N11.1
nonobstructive N11.8
with reflux (vesicoureteral) N11.0
obstructive N11.1
specified NEC N11.8
in (due to)
brucellosis A23.9 [N16]
cryoglobulinemia (mixed) D89.1 [N16]
cystinosis E72.04
diphtheria A36.84
glycogen storage disease E74.09 [N16]
leukemia NEC C95.9 [N16]
lymphoma NEC C85.90 [N16]
multiple myeloma C90.0 [N16]
obstruction N11.1
Salmonella infection A02.25
sarcoidosis D86.84
sepsis A41.9 [N16]
Sjögren's disease M35.04
toxoplasmosis B58.83
transplant rejection T86.91 [N16]
Wilson's disease E83.01 [N16]
nonobstructive N12
with reflux (vesicoureteral) N11.0
chronic N11.8
syphilitic A52.75
Pyelonephrosis (obstructive) N11.1
chronic N11.9
Pyelophlebitis I80.8
Pyeloureteritis cystica N28.85
Pyemia, pyemic (fever) (infection) (purulent)
-*see also* Sepsis
joint -*see* Arthritis, pyogenic or pyemic
liver K75.1
pneumococcal A40.3
portal K75.1
postvaccinal T88.0
puerperal, postpartum, childbirth O85
specified organism NEC A41.89
tuberculous -*see* Tuberculosis, miliary
Pygopagus Q89.4
Pyknoepilepsy (idiopathic) -*see* Pyknolepsy
Pyknolepsy G40.A09
intractable G40.A19
with status epilepticus G40.A11
without status epilepticus G40.A19
not intractable G40.A09
with status epilepticus G40.A01
without status epilepticus G40.A09
Pylephlebitis K75.1
Pyle's syndrome Q78.5
Pylethrombophlebitis K75.1
Pylethrombosis K75.1

Pyloritis K29.90
with bleeding K29.91
Pylorospasm (reflex) NEC K31.3
congenital or infantile Q40.0
newborn Q40.0
neurotic F45.8
psychogenic F45.8
Pylorus, pyloric -*see* condition
Pyoarthrosis -*see* Arthritis, pyogenic or
pyemic
Pyocele
mastoid -*see* Mastoiditis, acute
sinus (accessory) -*see* Sinusitis
turbinate (bone) J32.9
urethra -*see also* Urethritis N34.0
Pyocolpos -*see* Vaginitis
Pyocystitis N30.80
with hematuria N30.81
Pyoderma, pyodermia L08.0
gangrenosum L88
newborn P39.4
phagedenic L88
vegetans L08.81
Pyodermatitis L08.0
vegetans L08.81
Pyogenic -*see* condition
Pyohydronephrosis N13.6
Pyometra, pyometrium, pyometritis -*see*
Endometritis
Pyomyositis (tropical) -*see* Myositis, infective
Pyonephritis N12
Pyonephrosis N13.6
tuberculous A18.11
Pyo-oophoritis -*see* Salpingo-oophoritis
Pyo-ovarium -*see* Salpingo-oophoritis
Pyopericarditis, pyopericardium I30.1
Pyophlebitis -*see* Phlebitis
Pyopneumopericardium I30.1
Pyopneumothorax (infective) J86.9
with fistula J86.0
tuberculous NEC A15.6
Pyosalpinx, pyosalpingitis -*see also* Salpingo-
oophoritis
Pyothorax J86.9
with fistula J86.0
tuberculous NEC A15.6
Pyoureter N28.89
tuberculous A18.11
Pyramidopallidonigral syndrome G20
Pyrexia (of unknown origin) R50.9
atmospheric T67.0
during labor NEC O75.2
heat T67.0
newborn P81.9
environmentally induced P81.0
persistent R50.9
puerperal O86.4
Pyroglobulinemia NEC E88.09
Pyromania F63.1
Pyrosis R12
Pyuria (bacterial) N39.0

Q

Q fever A78
with pneumonia A78
Quadricuspid aortic valve Q23.8
Quadrilateral fever A78
Quadriparesis -*see* Quadriplegia
meaning muscle weakness M62.81

Quadriplegia G82.50
complete
C1 C4 level G82.51
C5 C7 level G82.53
congenital (cerebral) (spinal) G80.8
spastic G80.0
embolic (current episode) I63.4
functional R53.2
incomplete
C1 C4 level G82.52
C5 C7 level G82.54
thrombotic (current episode) I63.3
traumatic - code to injury with seventh
character S
current episode -*see* Injury, spinal (cord),
cervical
Quadruplet, pregnancy -*see* Pregnancy,
quadruplet
Quarrelsomeness F60.3
Queensland fever A77.3
Quervain's disease M65.4
thyroid E06.1
Queyrat's erythroplasia D07.4
penis D07.4
specified site -*see* Neoplasm, skin, in situ
unspecified site D07.4
Quincke's disease or edema T78.3
hereditary D84.1
Quinsy (gangrenous) J36
Quintan fever A79.0
Quintuplet, pregnancy -*see* Pregnancy,
quintuplet

R

Rabbit fever -*see* Tularemia
Rabies A82.9
contact Z20.3
exposure to Z20.3
inoculation reaction -*see* Complications,
vaccination
sylvatic A82.0
urban A82.1
Rachischisis -*see* Spina bifida
Rachitic -*see also* condition
deformities of spine (late effect) (sequelae)
E64.3
pelvis (late effect) (sequelae) E64.3
with disproportion (fetopelvic) O33.0
causing obstructed labor O65.0
Rachitis, rachitism (acute) (tarda) -*see also*
Rickets
renalis N25.0
sequelae E64.3
Radial nerve -*see* condition
Radiation
burn -*see* Burn
effects NOS T66
sickness NOS T66
therapy, encounter for Z51.0
Radiculitis (pressure) (vertebrogenic) -*see*
Radiculopathy
Radiculomyelitis -*see also* Encephalitis
toxic, due to
Clostridium tetani A35
Corynebacterium diphtheriae A36.82
Radiculopathy M54.10
cervical region M54.12
cervicothoracic region M54.13
due to
disc disorder

Radiculopathy
C3 M50.11
C4 M50.11
C5 M50.121
C6 M50.122
C7 M50.123
C8 M50.13
displacement of intervertebral disc -see
Disorder, disc, with, radiculopathy
leg M54.1
lumbar region M54.16
lumbosacral region M54.17
occipito-atlanto-axial region M54.11
postherpetic B02.29
sacrococcygeal region M54.18
syphilitic A52.11
thoracic region (with visceral pain) M54.14
thoracolumbar region M54.15

**Radiodermal burns (acute, chronic, or
occupational)** -see Burn
Radiodermatitis L58.9
acute L58.0
chronic L58.1
Radiotherapy session Z51.0
RAEB (refractory anemia with excess blasts)
D46.2
Rage, meaning rabies -see Rabies
Ragpicker's disease A22.1
Ragsorter's disease A22.1
Raillietiniasis B71.8
Railroad neurosis F48.8
Railway spine F48.8
Raised -see also Elevated
antibody titer R76.0
Rake teeth, tooth M26.39
Rales R09.89
Ramifying renal pelvis Q63.8
Ramsay Hunt disease or syndrome -see also
Hunt's disease B02.21
meaning dyssynergia cerebellaris myoclonica
G11.1
Ranula K11.6
congenital Q38.4
Rape
adult
confirmed T74.21
suspected T76.21
alleged, observation or examination, ruled out
adult Z04.41
child Z04.42
child
confirmed T74.22
suspected T76.22
Rapid
feeble pulse, due to shock, following injury
T79.4
heart (beat) R00.0
psychogenic F45.8
second stage (delivery) O62.3
time-zone change syndrome -see Disorder,
sleep, circadian rhythm, psychogenic
Rarefaction, bone -see Disorder, bone, density
and structure, specified NEC
Rash (toxic) R21
canker A38.9
diaper L22
drug (internal use) L27.0
contact -see also Dermatitis, due to, drugs,
external L25.1
following immunization T88.1
food -see Dermatitis, due to, food

Rash (toxic) --continued
heat L74.0
napkin (psoriasiform) L22
nettle -see Urticaria
pustular L08.0
rose R21
epidemic B06.9
scarlet A38.9
serum -see also Reaction, serum T80.69
wandering tongue K14.1
Rasmussen aneurysm -see Tuberculosis,
pulmonary
Rasmussen encephalitis G04.81
Rat-bite fever A25.9
due to Streptobacillus moniliformis A25.1
spirochetal (morsus muris) A25.0
Rathke's pouch tumor D44.3
Raymond (Céstan) syndrome I65.8
**Raynaud's disease, phenomenon or
syndrome (secondary)** I73.00
with gangrene (symmetric) I73.01
RDS (newborn) (type I) P22.0
type II P22.1
Reaction -see also Disorder
adaptation -see Disorder, adjustment
adjustment (anxiety) (conduct disorder)
(depressiveness) (distress) -see Disorder,
adjustment
with
mutism, elective (child) (adolescent) F94.0
adverse
food (any) (ingested) NEC T78.1
anaphylactic -see Shock, anaphylactic, due
to food
affective -see Disorder, mood
allergic -see Allergy
anaphylactic -see Shock, anaphylactic
anaphylactoid -see Shock, anaphylactic
anesthesia -see Anesthesia, complication
antitoxin (prophylactic) (therapeutic) -see
Complications, vaccination
anxiety F41.1
Arthus -see Arthus' phenomenon
asthenic F48.8
combat and operational stress F43.0
compulsive F42.8
conversion F44.9
crisis, acute F43.0
deoxyribonuclease (DNA) (DNase)
hypersensitivity D69.2
depressive (single episode) F32.9
affective (single episode) F31.4
recurrent episode F33.9
neurotic F34.1
psychoneurotic F34.1
psychotic F32.3
recurrent -see Disorder, depressive,
recurrent
dissociative F44.9
drug NEC T88.7
addictive -see Dependence, drug
transmitted via placenta or breast milk -see
Absorption, drug, addictive, through
placenta
allergic -see Allergy, drug
lichenoid L43.2
newborn P93.8
gray baby syndrome P93.0
overdose or poisoning (by accident) -see
Table of Drugs and Chemicals, by drug,
poisoning

Reaction - continued
photoallergic L56.1
phototoxic L56.0
withdrawal -see Dependence, by drug, with,
withdrawal
infant of dependent mother P96.1
newborn P96.1
wrong substance given or taken (by
accident) -see Table of Drugs and
Chemicals, by drug, poisoning
fear F40.9
child (abnormal) F93.8
febrile nonhemolytic transfusion (FNHTR)
R50.84
fluid loss, cerebrospinal G97.1
foreign
body NEC -see Granuloma, foreign body
in operative wound (inadvertently left) -see
Foreign body, accidentally left during a
procedure
substance accidentally left during a
procedure (chemical) (powder) (talc) T81.60
aseptic peritonitis T81.61
body or object (instrument) (sponge)
(swab) -see Foreign body, accidentally
left during a procedure
specified reaction NEC T81.69
grief -see Disorder, adjustment
Herxheimer's R68.89
hyperkinetic -see Hyperkinesia
hypochondriacal F45.20
hypoglycemic, due to insulin E16.0
with coma (diabetic) -see Diabetes, coma
nondiabetic E15
therapeutic misadventure - see subcategory
T38.3
hypomanic F30.8
hysterical F44.9
immunization -see Complications, vaccination
incompatibility
ABO blood group (infusion) (transfusion) -
see Complication(s), transfusion,
incompatibility reaction, ABO
delayed serologic T80.39
minor blood group (Duffy) (E) (K(ell))
(Kidd) (Lewis) (M) (N) (P) (S) T80.89
Rh (factor) (infusion) (transfusion) -see
Complication(s), transfusion, incompatibility
reaction, Rh (factor)
inflammatory -see Infection
infusion -see Complications, infusion
inoculation (immune serum) -see
Complications, vaccination
insulin T38.3
involutional psychotic -see Disorder,
depressive
leukemoid D72.823
basophilic D72.823
lymphocytic D72.823
monocytic D72.823
myelocytic D72.823
neutrophilic D72.823
LSD (acute)
due to drug abuse -see Abuse, drug,
hallucinogen
due to drug dependence -see Dependence,
drug, hallucinogen
lumbar puncture G97.1
manic-depressive -see Disorder, bipolar
neurasthenic F48.8
neurogenic -see Neurosis

Reaction - *continued*
neurotic F48.9
neurotic-depressive F34.1
nitritoid -*see* Crisis, nitritoid
nonspecific
to
cell mediated immunity measurement of
gamma interferon antigen response
without active tuberculosis R76.12
QuantiFERON-TB test (QFT) without
active tuberculosis R76.12
tuberculin test -*see also* Reaction,
tuberculin skin test R76.11
obsessive-compulsive F42.8
organic, acute or subacute -*see* Delirium
paranoid (acute) F23
chronic F22
senile F03
passive dependency F60.7
phobic F40.9
post-traumatic stress, uncomplicated Z73.3
psychogenic F99
psychoneurotic -*see also* Neurosis
compulsive F42.8
depersonalization F48.1
depressive F34.1
hypochondriacal F45.20
neurasthenic F48.8
obsessive F42.8
psychophysiologic -*see* Disorder, somatoform
psychosomatic -*see* Disorder, somatoform
psychotic -*see* Psychosis
scarlet fever toxin -*see* Complications,
vaccination
schizophrenic F23
acute (brief) (undifferentiated) F23
latent F21
undifferentiated (acute) (brief) F23
serological for syphilis -*see* Serology for
syphilis
serum T80.69
anaphylactic (immediate) -*see also* Shock,
anaphylactic T80.59
specified reaction NEC
due to
administration of blood and blood
products T80.61
immunization T80.62
serum specified NEC T80.69
vaccination T80.62
situational -*see* Disorder, adjustment
somatization -*see* Disorder, somatoform
spinal puncture G97.1
stress (severe) F43.9
acute (agitation) ("daze") (disorientation)
(disturbance of consciousness) (flight
reaction) (fugue) F43.0
specified NEC F43.8
surgical procedure -*see* Complications,
surgical procedure
tetanus antitoxin -*see* Complications,
vaccination
toxic, to local anesthesia T88.59
in labor and delivery O74.4
in pregnancy O29.3X
postpartum, puerperal O89.3
toxin-antitoxin -*see* Complications,
vaccination
transfusion (blood) (bone marrow)
(lymphocytes) (allergic) -*see* Complications,
transfusion

Reaction - *continued*
tuberculin skin test, abnormal R76.11
vaccination (any) -*see* Complications,
vaccination
withdrawing, child or adolescent F93.8
Reactive airway disease -*see* Asthma
Reactive depression -*see* Reaction, depressive
Rearrangement
chromosomal
balanced (in) Q95.9
abnormal individual (autosomal) Q95.2
non-sex (autosomal) chromosomes Q95.2
sex/non-sex chromosomes Q95.3
specified NEC Q95.8
Recalcitrant patient -*see* Noncompliance
Recanalization, thrombus -*see* Thrombosis
Recession, receding
chamber angle (eye) H21.55
chin M26.09
gingival (generalized) (localized)
(postinfective) (postoperative) K06.00
Miller Class I K06.01
Miller Class II K06.02
Miller Class III K06.03
Miller Class IV K06.04
Recklinghausen disease Q85.01
bones E21.0
Reclus' disease (cystic) -*see* Mastopathy,
cystic
Recrudescent typhus (fever) A75.1
Recruitment, auditory H93.21
Rectalgia K62.89
Rectitis K62.89
Rectocele
female (without uterine prolapse) N81.6
with uterine prolapse N81.4
incomplete N81.2
in pregnancy -*see* Pregnancy, complicated by,
abnormal, pelvic organs or tissues NEC
male K62.3
Rectosigmoid junction -*see* condition
Rectosigmoiditis K63.89
ulcerative (chronic) K51.30
with
complication K51.319
abscess K51.314
fistula K51.313
obstruction K51.312
rectal bleeding K51.311
specified NEC K51.318
Rectourethral -*see* condition
Rectovaginal -*see* condition
Rectovesical -*see* condition
Rectum, rectal -*see* condition
Recurrent -*see* condition
pregnancy loss -*see* Loss (of), pregnancy,
recurrent
Red bugs B88.0
Red-cedar lung or pneumonitis J67.8
Red tide -*see also* Table of Drugs and
Chemicals T65.82
Reduced
mobility Z74.09
ventilatory or vital capacity R94.2
Redundant, redundancy
anus (congenital) Q43.8
clitoris N90.89
colon (congenital) Q43.8
foreskin (congenital) N47.8
intestine (congenital) Q43.8
labia N90.69

Redundant, redundancy --*continued*
organ or site, congenital NEC -*see* Accessory
panniculus (abdominal) E65
prepuce (congenital) N47.8
pylorus K31.89
rectum (congenital) Q43.8
scrotum N50.89
sigmoid (congenital) Q43.8
skin L98.7
and subcutaneous tissue L98.7
of face L57.4
eyelids -*see* Blepharochalasis
stomach K31.89
Reduplication -*see* Duplication
Reflex R29.2
hyperactive gag J39.2
pupillary, abnormal -*see* Anomaly, pupil,
function
vasoconstriction I73.9
vasovagal R55
Reflux K21.9
acid K21.9
esophageal K21.9
with esophagitis K21.0
newborn P78.83
gastroesophageal K21.9
with esophagitis K21.0
mitral -*see* Insufficiency, mitral
ureteral -*see* Reflux, vesicoureteral
vesicoureteral (with scarring) N13.70
with
nephropathy N13.729
with hydroureter N13.739
bilateral N13.732
unilateral N13.731
bilateral N13.722
unilateral N13.721
without hydroureter N13.729
bilateral N13.722
unilateral N13.721
pyelonephritis (chronic) N11.0
congenital Q62.7
without nephropathy N13.71
Reforming, artificial openings -*see* Attention
to, artificial, opening
Refractive error -*see* Disorder, refraction
Refsum's disease or syndrome G60.1
Refusal of
food, psychogenic F50.89
treatment (because of) Z53.20
left against medical advice (AMA) Z53.21
patient's decision NEC Z53.29
reasons of belief or group pressure Z53.1
Regional -*see* condition
Regurgitation R11.10
aortic (valve) -*see* Insufficiency, aortic
food -*see also* Vomiting
with reswallowing -*see* Rumination
newborn P92.1
gastric contents -*see* Vomiting
heart -*see* Endocarditis
mitral (valve) -*see* Insufficiency, mitral
congenital Q23.3
myocardial -*see* Endocarditis
pulmonary (valve) (heart) I37.1
congenital Q22.2
syphilitic A52.03
tricuspid -*see* Insufficiency, tricuspid
valve, valvular -*see* Endocarditis
congenital Q24.8
vesicoureteral -*see* Reflux, vesicoureteral

Reifenstein syndrome E34.52
Reinsertion
  implantable subdermal contraceptive Z30.46
  intrauterine contraceptive device Z30.433
Reiter's disease, syndrome, or urethritis
  M02.30
  ankle M02.37
  elbow M02.32
  foot joint M02.37
  hand joint M02.34
  hip M02.35
  knee M02.36
  multiple site M02.39
  shoulder M02.31
  vertebra M02.38
  wrist M02.33
Reichmann's disease or syndrome K31.89
Rejection
  food, psychogenic F50.89
  transplant T86.91
    bone T86.830
      marrow T86.01
    cornea T86.840
    heart T86.21
      with lung(s) T86.31
    intestine T86.850
    kidney T86.11
    liver T86.41
    lung(s) T86.810
      with heart T86.31
    organ (immune or nonimmune cause)
    T86.91
    pancreas T86.890
    skin (allograft) (autograft) T86.820
    specified NEC T86.890
    stem cell (peripheral blood) (umbilical cord)
    T86.5
Relapsing fever A68.9
  Carter's (Asiatic) A68.1
  Dutton's (West African) A68.1
  Koch's A68.9
  louse-borne (epidemic) A68.0
  Novy's (American) A68.1
  Obermeyers's (European) A68.0
  Spirillum A68.9
  tick-borne (endemic) A68.1
Relationship
  occlusal
    open anterior M26.220
    open posterior M26.221
Relaxation
  anus (sphincter) K62.89
    psychogenic F45.8
  arch (foot) -see also Deformity, limb, flat foot
  back ligaments -see Instability, joint, spine
  bladder (sphincter) N31.2
  cardioesophageal K21.9
  cervix -see Incompetency, cervix
  diaphragm J98.6
  joint (capsule) (ligament) (paralytic) -see
    Flail, joint
    congenital NEC Q74.8
  lumbosacral (joint) -see subcategory M53.2
  pelvic floor N81.89
  perineum N81.89
  posture R29.3
  rectum (sphincter) K62.89
  sacroiliac (joint) -see subcategory M53.2
  scrotum N50.89
  urethra (sphincter) N36.44
  vesical N31.2

Release from prison, anxiety concerning
  Z65.2
Remains
  canal of Cloquet Q14.0
  capsule (opaque) Q14.8
Remittent fever (malarial) B54
Remnant
  canal of Cloquet Q14.0
  capsule (opaque) Q14.8
  cervix, cervical stump (acquired)
    (postoperative) N88.8
  cystic duct, postcholecystectomy K91.5
  fingernail L60.8
    congenital Q84.6
  meniscus, knee -see Derangement, knee,
    meniscus, specified NEC
  thyroglossal duct Q89.2
  tonsil J35.8
    infected (chronic) J35.01
  urachus Q64.4
Removal (from) (of)
  artificial
    arm Z44.00
      complete Z44.01
      partial Z44.02
    eye Z44.2
    leg Z44.10
      complete Z44.11
      partial Z44.12
  breast implant Z45.81
  cardiac pulse generator (battery) (end-of-life)
    Z45.010
  catheter (urinary) (indwelling) Z46.6
    from artificial opening -see Attention to,
      artificial, opening
    non-vascular Z46.82
    vascular NEC Z45.2
  drains Z48.03
  device Z46.9
    contraceptive Z30.432
      implantable subdermal Z30.46
    implanted NEC Z45.89
    specified NEC Z46.89
  dressing (nonsurgical) Z48.00
    surgical Z48.01
  external
    fixation device
    code to fracture with seventh character D
  prosthesis, prosthetic device Z44.9
    breast Z44.3
    specified NEC Z44.8
  home in childhood (to foster home or
    institution) Z62.29
  ileostomy Z43.2
  insulin pump Z46.81
  myringotomy device (stent) (tube) Z45.82
  nervous system device NEC Z46.2
    brain neuropacemaker Z46.2
    visual substitution device Z46.2
      implanted Z45.31
  non-vascular catheter Z46.82
  orthodontic device Z46.4
  organ, prophylactic (for neoplasia
    management) -see Prophylactic, organ
    removal
  staples Z48.02
  stent
    ureteral Z46.6
  suture Z48.02
  urinary device Z46.6
  vascular access device or catheter Z45.2

Ren
  arcuatus Q63.1
  mobile, mobilis N28.89
    congenital Q63.8
  unguliformis Q63.1
Renal -see condition
Rendu-Osler-Weber disease or syndrome
  I78.0
Reninoma D41.0
Renon-Delille syndrome E23.3
**Reovirus, as cause of disease classified
  elsewhere** B97.5
Repeated falls NEC R29.6
Replaced chromosome by dicentric ring
  Q93.2
**Replacement by artificial or mechanical
  device or prosthesis of** bladder Z96.0
  blood vessel NEC Z95.828
  bone NEC Z96.7
  cochlea Z96.21
  coronary artery Z95.5
  eustachian tube Z96.29
  eye globe Z97.0
  heart Z95.812
    valve Z95.2
      prosthetic Z95.2
      specified NEC Z95.4
      xenogenic Z95.3
  intestine Z96.89
  joint Z96.60
    hip -see Presence, hip joint implant
    knee -see Presence, knee joint implant
    specified site NEC Z96.698
  larynx Z96.3
  lens Z96.1
  limb(s) -see Presence, artificial, limb
  mandible NEC (for tooth root implant(s))
    Z96.5
  organ NEC Z96.89
  peripheral vessel NEC Z95.828
  stapes Z96.29
  teeth Z97.2
  tendon Z96.7
  tissue NEC Z96.89
  tooth root(s) Z96.5
  vessel NEC Z95.828
    coronary (artery) Z95.5
Request for expert evidence Z04.8
Reserve, decreased or low
  cardiac -see Disease, heart
  kidney N28.89
Residual -see also condition
  ovary syndrome N99.83
  state, schizophrenic F20.5
  urine R39.198
Resistance, resistant (to)
  activated protein C D68.51
  complicating pregnancy O26.89
  insulin E88.81
  organism(s)
    to
      drug Z16.30
        aminoglycosides Z16.29
        amoxicillin Z16.11
        ampicillin Z16.11
        antibiotic(s) Z16.20
          multiple Z16.24
          specified NEC Z16.29
        antifungal Z16.32
        antimicrobial (single) Z16.30
          multiple Z16.35

Resistance, resistant - *continued*
  specified NEC Z16.39
  antimycobacterial (single) Z16.341
    multiple Z16.342
  antiparasitic Z16.31
  antiviral Z16.33
  beta lactam antibiotics Z16.10
    specified NEC Z16.19
  cephalosporins Z16.19
  extended beta lactamase (ESBL) Z16.12
  fluoroquinolones Z16.23
  macrolides Z16.29
  methicillin -*see* MRSA
  multiple drugs (MDRO)
    antibiotics Z16.24
    antimicrobial Z16.35
    antimycobacterials Z16.342
  penicillins Z16.11
  quinine (and related compounds) Z16.31
  quinolones Z16.23
  sulfonamides Z16.29
  tetracyclines Z16.29
  tuberculostatics (single) Z16.341
    multiple Z16.342
  vancomycin Z16.21
  related antibiotics Z16.22
  thyroid hormone E07.89
Resorption
  dental (roots) K03.3
    alveoli M26.79
  teeth (external) (internal) (pathological)
    (roots) K03.3
Respiration
  Cheyne-Stokes R06.3
  decreased due to shock, following injury
    T79.4
  disorder of, psychogenic F45.8
  insufficient, or poor R06.89
    newborn P28.5
  painful R07.1
  sighing, psychogenic F45.8
Respiratory -*see also* condition
  distress syndrome (newborn) (type I) P22.0
    type II P22.1
  syncytial virus, as cause of disease classified
    elsewhere B97.4
Respite care Z75.5
Response (drug)
  photoallergic L56.1
  phototoxic L56.0
Restenosis
  stent
    vascular
      end stent
        adjacent to stent -*see* Arteriosclerosis
        within the stent
          coronary T82.855
          peripheral T82.856
      in stent
        coronary vessel T82.855
        peripheral vessel T82.856
Restless legs (syndrome) G25.81
Restlessness R45.1
Restriction of housing space Z59.1
Restoration (of)
  dental
    aesthetically inadequate or displeasing
      K08.56
    defective K08.50
      specified NEC K08.59
    failure of marginal integrity K08.51

Restoration (of)
  failure of periodontal anatomical integrity
    K08.54
  organ continuity from previous sterilization
    (tuboplasty) (vasoplasty) Z31.0
    aftercare Z31.42
  tooth (existing)
    contours biologically incompatible with oral
      health K08.54
    open margins K08.51
    overhanging K08.52
    poor aesthetic K08.56
    poor gingival margins K08.51
  unsatisfactory, of tooth K08.50
    specified NEC K08.59
Restorative material (dental)
  allergy to K08.55
  fractured K08.539
    with loss of material K08.531
    without loss of material K08.530
  unrepairable overhanging of K08.52
Rests, ovarian, in fallopian tube Q50.6
Restzustand (schizophrenic) F20.5
Retained -*see also* Retention
  cholelithiasis following cholecystectomy
    K91.86
  foreign body fragments (type of) Z18.9
    acrylics Z18.2
    animal quill(s) or spines Z18.31
    cement Z18.83
    concrete Z18.83
    crystalline Z18.83
    depleted isotope Z18.09
    depleted uranium Z18.01
    diethylhexylphthalates Z18.2
    glass Z18.81
    isocyanate Z18.2
    magnetic metal Z18.11
    metal Z18.10
    nonmagnetic metal Z18.12
    nontherapeutic radioactive Z18.09
    organic NEC Z18.39
    plastic Z18.2
    quill(s) (animal) Z18.31
    radioactive (nontherapeutic) NEC Z18.09
    specified NEC Z18.89
    spine(s) (animal) Z18.31
    stone Z18.83
    tooth (teeth) Z18.32
    wood Z18.33
  fragments (type of) Z18.9
    acrylics Z18.2
    animal quill(s) or spines Z18.31
    cement Z18.83
    concrete Z18.83
    crystalline Z18.83
    depleted isotope Z18.09
    depleted uranium Z18.01
    diethylhexylphthalates Z18.2
    glass Z18.81
    isocyanate Z18.2
    magnetic metal Z18.11
    metal Z18.10
    nonmagnetic metal Z18.12
    nontherapeutic radioactive Z18.09
    organic NEC Z18.39
    plastic Z18.2
    quill(s) (animal) Z18.31
    radioactive (nontherapeutic) NEC Z18.09
    specified NEC Z18.89
    spine(s) (animal) Z18.31

Retained --*continued*
  stone Z18.83
  tooth (teeth) Z18.32
  wood Z18.33
  gallstones, following cholecystectomy K91.86
Retardation
  development, developmental, specific -*see*
    Disorder, developmental
  endochondral bone growth -*see* Disorder,
    bone, development or growth
  growth R62.50
    due to malnutrition E45
  mental -*see* Disability, intellectual
  motor function, specific F82
  physical (child) R62.52
    due to malnutrition E45
  reading (specific) F81.0
  spelling (specific) (without reading disorder)
    F81.81
Retching -*see* Vomiting
Retention -*see also* Retained
  bladder -*see* Retention, urine
  carbon dioxide E87.2
  cholelithiasis following cholecystectomy
    K91.86
  cyst -*see* Cyst
  dead
    fetus (at or near term) (mother) O36.4
      early fetal death O02.1
    ovum O02.0
  decidua (fragments) (following delivery)
    (with hemorrhage) O72.2
      without hemorrhage O73.1
  deciduous tooth K00.6
  dental root K08.3
  fecal -*see* Constipation
  fetus
    dead O36.4
      early O02.1
  fluid R60.9
  foreign body -*see also* Foreign body, retained
    current trauma - code as Foreign body, by
    site or type
  gallstones, following cholecystectomy K91.86
  gastric K31.89
  intrauterine contraceptive device, in
    pregnancy -*see* Pregnancy, complicated by,
    retention, intrauterine device
  membranes (complicating delivery) (with
    hemorrhage) O72.2
    with abortion -*see* Abortion, by type
    without hemorrhage O73.1
  meniscus -*see* Derangement, meniscus
  menses N94.89
  milk (puerperal, postpartum) O92.79
  nitrogen, extrarenal R39.2
  ovary syndrome N99.83
  placenta (total) (with hemorrhage) O72.0
    without hemorrhage O73.0
    portions or fragments (with hemorrhage)
      O72.2
      without hemorrhage O73.1
  products of conception
    early pregnancy (dead fetus) O02.1
    following
      delivery (with hemorrhage) O72.2
        without hemorrhage O73.1
  secundines (following delivery) (with
    hemorrhage) O72.0
      without hemorrhage O73.0

Retention - complicating puerperium
  (delayed hemorrhage) O72.2
  partial O72.2
    without hemorrhage O73.1
  smegma, clitoris N90.89
  urine R33.9
    due to hyperplasia (hypertrophy) of prostate
      -see Hyperplasia, prostate
    drug-induced R33.0
    organic R33.8
      drug-induced R33.0
    psychogenic F45.8
    specified NEC R33.8
  water (in tissues) -see Edema
Reticular erythematous mucinosis L98.5
Reticulation, dust -see Pneumoconiosis
Reticulocytosis R70.1
Reticuloendotheliosis
  acute infantile C96.0
  leukemic C91.4
  nonlipid C96.0
Reticulohistiocytoma (giant-cell) D76.3
Reticuloid, actinic L57.1
Reticulosis (skin)
  acute of infancy C96.0
  hemophagocytic, familial D76.1
  histiocytic medullary C96.A
  lipomelanotic I89.8
  malignant (midline) C86.0
  polymorphic C86.0
  Sézary -see Sézary disease
Retina, retinal -see also condition
  dark area D49.81
Retinitis -see also Inflammation, chorioretinal
  albuminurica N18.9 [H32]
  diabetic -see Diabetes, retinitis
  disciformis -see Degeneration, macula
  focal -see Inflammation, chorioretinal, focal
  gravidarum -see Pregnancy, complicated by,
    specified pregnancy related condition NEC
  juxtapapillaris -see Inflammation,
    chorioretinal, focal, juxtapapillary
  luetic -see Retinitis, syphilitic
  pigmentosa H35.52
  proliferans -see Disorder, globe, degenerative,
    specified type NEC
  proliferating -see Disorder, globe,
    degenerative, specified type NEC
  renal N18.9 [H32]
  syphilitic (early) (secondary) A51.43
    central, recurrent A52.71
    congenital (early) A50.01 [H32]
    late A52.71
  tuberculous A18.53
Retinoblastoma C69.2
  differentiated C69.2
  undifferentiated C69.2
Retinochoroiditis -see also Inflammation,
  chorioretinal
  disseminated -see Inflammation,
    chorioretinal, disseminated
    syphilitic A52.71
  focal -see Inflammation, chorioretinal
  juxtapapillaris -see Inflammation,
    chorioretinal, focal, juxtapapillary
Retinopathy (background) H35.00
  arteriosclerotic I70.8 [H35.0]
  atherosclerotic I70.8 [H35.0]
  central serous -see Chorioretinopathy, central
    serous
  Coats H35.02

Retinopathy (background) --continued
  diabetic -see Diabetes, retinopathy
  exudative H35.02
  hypertensive H35.03
  in (due to)
    diabetes -see Diabetes, retinopathy
    sickle-cell disorders D57. [H36]
  of prematurity H35.10
    stage 0 H35.11
    stage 1 H35.12
    stage 2 H35.13
    stage 3 H35.14
    stage 4 H35.15
    stage 5 H35.16
  pigmentary, congenital -see Dystrophy, retina
  proliferative NEC H35.2
    diabetic -see Diabetes, retinopathy,
      proliferative
    sickle-cell D57. [H36]
  solar H31.02
Retinoschisis H33.10
  congenital Q14.1
  specified type NEC H33.19
Retortamoniasis A07.8
Retractile testis Q55.22
Retraction
  cervix -see Retroversion, uterus
  drum (membrane) -see Disorder, tympanic
  membrane, specified NEC
  finger -see Deformity, finger
  lid H02.539
    left H02.536
      lower H02.535
      upper H02.534
    right H02.533
      lower H02.532
      upper H02.531
  lung J98.4
  mediastinum J98.59
  nipple N64.53
    associated with
      lactation O92.03
      pregnancy O92.01
      puerperium O92.02
    congenital Q83.8
  palmar fascia M72.0
  pleura -see Pleurisy
  ring, uterus (Bandl's) (pathological) O62.4
  sternum (congenital) Q76.7
    acquired M95.4
  uterus -see Retroversion, uterus
  valve (heart) -see Endocarditis
Retrobulbar -see condition
Retrocecal -see condition
Retrocession -see Retroversion
Retrodisplacement -see Retroversion
Retroflection, retroflexion -see Retroversion
Retrognathia, retrognathism (mandibular)
  (maxillary) M26.19
Retrograde menstruation N92.5
Retroperineal -see condition
Retroperitoneal -see condition
Retroperitonitis K68.9
Retropharyngeal -see condition
Retroplacental -see condition
Retroposition -see Retroversion
Retroprosthetic membrane T85.398

Retrosternal thyroid (congenital) Q89.2
Retroversion, retroverted
  cervix -see Retroversion, uterus
  female NEC -see Retroversion, uterus
  iris H21.89
  testis (congenital) Q55.29
  uterus (acquired) (acute) (any degree)
    (asymptomatic) (cervix) (postinfectional)
    (postpartal, old) N85.4
    congenital Q51.818
    in pregnancy O34.53
Retrovirus, as cause of disease classified
  elsewhere B97.30
  human
    immunodeficiency, type 2 (HIV 2) B97.35
    T-cell lymphotropic
      type I (HTLV-I) B97.33
      type II (HTLV-II) B97.34
  lentivirus B97.31
  oncovirus B97.32
  specified NEC B97.39
Retrusion, premaxilla (developmental)
  M26.09
Rett's disease or syndrome F84.2
Reverse peristalsis R19.2
Reye's syndrome G93.7
Rh (factor)
  hemolytic disease (newborn) P55.0
  incompatibility, immunization or sensitization
    affecting management of pregnancy NEC
    O36.09
      anti-D antibody O36.01
    newborn P55.0
    transfusion reaction -see Complication(s),
      transfusion, incompatibility reaction, Rh
      (factor)
  negative mother affecting newborn P55.0
  titer elevated -see Complication(s),
    transfusion, incompatibility reaction, Rh
    (factor)
  transfusion reaction -see Complication(s),
    transfusion, incompatibility reaction, Rh
    (factor)
Rhabdomyolysis (idiopathic) NEC M62.82
  traumatic T79.6
Rhabdomyoma -see also Neoplasm,
  connective tissue, benign
  adult -see Neoplasm, connective tissue,
    benign
  fetal -see Neoplasm, connective tissue, benign
  glycogenic -see Neoplasm, connective tissue,
    benign
Rhabdomyosarcoma (any type) -see
  Neoplasm, connective tissue, malignant
Rhabdosarcoma -see Rhabdomyosarcoma
Rhesus (factor) incompatibility -see Rh,
  incompatibility
Rheumatic (acute) (subacute) (chronic)
  adherent pericardium I09.2
  coronary arteritis I01.9
  degeneration, myocardium I09.0
  fever (acute) -see Fever, rheumatic
  heart -see Disease, heart, rheumatic
  myocardial degeneration -see Degeneration,
    myocardium
  myocarditis (chronic) (inactive) (with chorea)
    I09.0
    active or acute I01.2
    with chorea (acute) (rheumatic)
      (Sydenham's) I02.0
  pancarditis, acute I01.8

Rheumatic --*continued*
  with chorea (acute (rheumatic) Sydenham's) I02.0
  pericarditis (active) (acute) (with effusion) (with pneumonia) I01.0
    with chorea (acute) (rheumatic) (Sydenham's) I02.0
  chronic or inactive I09.2
  pneumonia I00 [*J17*]
  torticollis M43.6
  typhoid fever A01.09
Rheumatism (articular) (neuralgic) (nonarticular) M79.0
  gout -*see* Arthritis, rheumatoid
  intercostal, meaning Tietze's disease M94.0
  palindromic (any site) M12.30
    ankle M12.37
    elbow M12.32
    foot joint M12.37
    hand joint M12.34
    hip M12.35
    knee M12.36
    multiple site M12.39
    shoulder M12.31
    specified joint NEC M12.38
    vertebrae M12.38
    wrist M12.33
  sciatic M54.4
Rheumatoid -*see also* condition
  arthritis -*see also* Arthritis, rheumatoid
    with involvement of organs NEC M05.60
      ankle M05.67
      elbow M05.62
      foot joint M05.67
      hand joint M05.64
      hip M05.65
      knee M05.66
      multiple site M05.69
      shoulder M05.61
      vertebra -*see* Spondylitis, ankylosing
      wrist M05.63
    seronegative -*see* Arthritis, rheumatoid, seronegative
    seropositive -*see* Arthritis, rheumatoid, seropositive
  carditis M05.30
    ankle M05.37
    elbow M05.32
    foot joint M05.37
    hand joint M05.34
    hip M05.35
    knee M05.36
    multiple site M05.39
    shoulder M05.31
    vertebra -*see* Spondylitis, ankylosing
    wrist M05.33
  endocarditis -*see* Rheumatoid, carditis
  lung (disease) M05.10
    ankle M05.17
    elbow M05.12
    foot joint M05.17
    hand joint M05.14
    hip M05.15
    knee M05.16
    multiple site M05.19
    shoulder M05.11
    vertebra -*see* Spondylitis, ankylosing
    wrist M05.13
  myocarditis -*see* Rheumatoid, carditis
  myopathy M05.40
    ankle M05.47

Rheumatoid --*continued*
    elbow M05.42
    foot joint M05.47
    hand joint M05.44
    hip M05.45
    knee M05.46
    multiple site M05.49
    shoulder M05.41
    vertebra -*see* Spondylitis, ankylosing
    wrist M05.43
  pericarditis -*see* Rheumatoid, carditis
  polyarthritis -*see* Arthritis, rheumatoid
  polyneuropathy M05.50
    ankle M05.57
    elbow M05.52
    foot joint M05.57
    hand joint M05.54
    hip M05.55
    knee M05.56
    multiple site M05.59
    shoulder M05.51
    vertebra -*see* Spondylitis, ankylosing
    wrist M05.53
  vasculitis M05.20
    ankle M05.27
    elbow M05.22
    foot joint M05.27
    hand joint M05.24
    hip M05.25
    knee M05.26
    multiple site M05.29
    shoulder M05.21
    vertebra -*see* Spondylitis, ankylosing
    wrist M05.23
Rhinitis (atrophic) (catarrhal) (chronic) (croupous) (fibrinous) (granulomatous) (hyperplastic) (hypertrophic) (membranous) (obstructive) (purulent) (suppurative) (ulcerative) J31.0
  with
    sore throat -*see* Nasopharyngitis
  acute J00
  allergic J30.9
    with asthma J45.909
      with
        exacerbation (acute) J45.901
        status asthmaticus J45.902
    due to
      food J30.5
      pollen J30.1
    nonseasonal J30.89
    perennial J30.89
    seasonal NEC J30.2
    specified NEC J30.89
  infective J00
  pneumococcal J00
  syphilitic A52.73
    congenital A50.05 [*J99*]
  tuberculous A15.8
  vasomotor J30.0
Rhinoantritis (chronic) -*see* Sinusitis, maxillary
Rhinodacryolith -*see* Dacryolith
Rhinolith (nasal sinus) J34.89
Rhinomegaly J34.89
Rhinopharyngitis (acute) (subacute) -*see also* Nasopharyngitis
  chronic J31.1
  destructive ulcerating A66.5
  mutilans A66.5
Rhinophyma L71.1

Rhinorrhea J34.89
  cerebrospinal (fluid) G96.0
  paroxysmal -*see* Rhinitis, allergic
  spasmodic -*see* Rhinitis, allergic
Rhinosalpingitis -*see* Salpingitis, eustachian
Rhinoscleroma A48.8
Rhinosporidiosis B48.1
Rhinovirus infection NEC B34.8
Rhizomelic chondrodysplasia punctata E71.540
Rhythm
  atrioventricular nodal I49.8
  disorder I49.9
    coronary sinus I49.8
    ectopic I49.8
    nodal I49.8
  escape I49.9
  heart, abnormal I49.9
  idioventricular I44.2
  nodal I49.8
  sleep, inversion G47.2
    nonorganic origin -*see* Disorder, sleep, circadian rhythm, psychogenic
Rhytidosis facialis L98.8
Rib -*see also* condition
  cervical Q76.5
Riboflavin deficiency E53.0
Rice bodies -*see also* Loose, body, joint
  knee M23.4
Richter syndrome -*see* Leukemia, chronic lymphocytic, B-cell type
Richter's hernia -*see* Hernia, abdomen, with obstruction
Ricinism -*see* Poisoning, food, noxious, plant
Rickets (active) (acute) (adolescent) (chest wall) (congenital) (current) (infantile) (intestinal) E55.0
  adult -*see* Osteomalacia
  celiac K90.0
  hypophosphatemic with nephrotic-glycosuric dwarfism E72.09
  inactive E64.3
  kidney N25.0
  renal N25.0
  sequelae, any E64.3
  vitamin-D-resistant E83.31 [*M90.80*]
Rickettsial disease A79.9
  specified type NEC A79.89
Rickettsialpox (Rickettsia akari) A79.1
Rickettsiosis A79.9
  due to
    Ehrlichia sennetsu A79.81
    Rickettsia akari (rickettsialpox) A79.1
  specified type NEC A79.89
  tick-borne A77.9
  vesicular A79.1
Rider's bone -*see* Ossification, muscle, specified NEC
Ridge, alveolus -*see also* condition
  flabby K06.8
Ridged ear, congenital Q17.3
Riedel's
  lobe, liver Q44.7
  struma, thyroiditis or disease E06.5
Rieger's anomaly or syndrome Q13.81
Riehl's melanosis L81.4
Rietti-Greppi-Micheli anemia D56.9
Rieux's hernia -*see* Hernia, abdomen, specified site NEC
Riga (Fede) disease K14.0
Riggs' disease -*see* Periodontitis

Right aortic arch Q25.47
Right middle lobe syndrome J98.11
Rigid, rigidity -see also condition
   abdominal R19.30
      with severe abdominal pain R10.0
      epigastric R19.36
      generalized R19.37
      left lower quadrant R19.34
      left upper quadrant R19.32
      periumbilic R19.35
      right lower quadrant R19.33
      right upper quadrant R19.31
   articular, multiple, congenital Q68.8
   cervix (uteri) in pregnancy -see Pregnancy,
      complicated by, abnormal, cervix
   hymen (acquired) (congenital) N89.6
   nuchal R29.1
   pelvic floor in pregnancy -see Pregnancy,
      complicated by, abnormal, pelvic organs or
      tissues NEC
   perineum or vulva in pregnancy -see
      Pregnancy, complicated by, abnormal, vulva
   spine -see Dorsopathy, specified NEC
   vagina in pregnancy -see Pregnancy,
      complicated by, abnormal, vagina
Rigors R68.89
   with fever R50.9
Riley Day syndrome G90.1
**RIND (reversible ischemic neurologic
   deficit)** I63.9
Ring(s)
   aorta (vascular) Q25.45
   Bandl's O62.4
   contraction, complicating delivery O62.4
   esophageal, lower (muscular) K22.2
   Fleischer's (cornea) H18.04
   hymenal, tight (acquired) (congenital) N89.6
   Kayser-Fleischer (cornea) H18.04
   retraction, uterus, pathological O62.4
   Schatzki's (esophagus) (lower) K22.2
      congenital Q39.3
   Soemmerring's -see Cataract, secondary
   vascular (congenital) Q25.8
      aorta Q25.45
Ringed hair (congenital) Q84.1
Ringworm B35.9
   beard B35.0
   black dot B35.0
   body B35.4
   Burmese B35.5
   corporeal B35.4
   foot B35.3
   groin B35.6
   hand B35.2
   honeycomb B35.0
   nails B35.1
   perianal (area) B35.6
   scalp B35.0
   specified NEC B35.8
   Tokelau B35.5
Rise, venous pressure I87.8
**Rising, PSA following treatment for
   malignant neoplasm of prostate** R97.21
Risk, suicidal
   meaning personal history of attempted suicide
      Z91.5
   meaning suicidal ideation -see Ideation,
      suicidal
Ritter's disease L00
Rivalry, sibling Z62.891
Rivalta's disease A42.2

River blindness B73.01
Robert's pelvis Q74.2
   with disproportion (fetopelvic) O33.0
      causing obstructed labor O65.0
Robin (Pierre) syndrome Q87.0
Robinow-Silvermann-Smith syndrome Q87.1
**Robinson's (hidrotic) ectodermal dysplasia
   or syndrome** Q82.4
Robles' disease B73.01
Rocky Mountain (spotted) fever A77.0
Roetheln -see Rubella
Roger's disease Q21.0
Rokitansky Aschoff sinuses (gallbladder)
   K82.8
Rolando's fracture (displaced) S62.22
   nondisplaced S62.22
**Romano-Ward (prolonged QT interval)
   syndrome** I45.81
Romberg's disease or syndrome G51.8
Roof, mouth -see condition **Rosacea** L71.9
   acne L71.9
   keratitis L71.8
   specified NEC L71.8
Rosary, rachitic E55.0
Rose
   cold J30.1
   fever J30.1
   rash R21
      epidemic B06.9
Rosenbach's erysipeloid A26.0
Rosenthal's disease or syndrome D68.1
Roseola B09
   infantum B08.20
      due to human herpesvirus 6 B08.21
      due to human herpesvirus 7 B08.22
Rossbach's disease K31.89
   psychogenic F45.8
Ross River disease or fever B33.1
Rostan's asthma (cardiac) -see Failure,
   ventricular, left
Rotation
   anomalous, incomplete or insufficient,
      intestine Q43.3
   cecum (congenital) Q43.3
   colon (congenital) Q43.3
   spine, incomplete or insufficient -see
      Dorsopathy, deforming, specified NEC
   tooth, teeth, fully erupted M26.35
   vertebra, incomplete or insufficient -see
      Dorsopathy, deforming, specified NEC
Rotes Quérol disease or syndrome -see
   Hyperostosis, ankylosing
Roth (Bernhardt) disease or syndrome -see
   Meralgia paraesthetica
Rothmund (Thomson) syndrome Q82.8
Rotor's disease or syndrome E80.6
Round
   back (with wedging of vertebrae) -see
      Kyphosis
   sequelae (late effect) of rickets E64.3
   worms (large) (infestation) NEC B82.0
      Ascariasis -see also Ascariasis B77.9
Roussy Lévy syndrome G60.0
Rubella (German measles) B06.9
   complication NEC B06.09
      neurological B06.00
   congenital P35.0
   contact Z20.4
   exposure to Z20.4
   maternal
      manifest rubella in infant P35.0

Rubella (German measles) --continued
   care for (suspected) damage to fetus O35.3
   suspected damage to fetus affecting
      management of pregnancy O35.3
   specified complications NEC B06.89
Rubeola (meaning measles) -see Measles
   meaning rubella -see Rubella
Rubeosis, iris -see Disorder, iris, vascular
Rubinstein-Taybi syndrome Q87.2
Rudimentary (congenital) -see also Agenesis
   arm -see Defect, reduction, upper limb
   bone Q79.9
   cervix uteri Q51.828
   eye Q11.2
   lobule of ear Q17.3
   patella Q74.1
   respiratory organs in thoracopagus Q89.4
   tracheal bronchus Q32.4
   uterus Q51.818
      in male Q56.1
   vagina Q52.0
Ruled out condition -see Observation,
   suspected
Rumination R11.10
   with nausea R11.2
   disorder of infancy F98.21
   neurotic F42.8
   newborn P92.1
   obsessional F42.8
   psychogenic F42.8
Runeberg's disease D51.0
Runny nose R09.89
Rupia (syphilitic) A51.39
   congenital A50.06
   tertiary A52.79
Rupture, ruptured
   abscess (spontaneous)
      code by site under Abscess
   aneurysm -see Aneurysm
   anus (sphincter) -see Laceration, anus
   aorta, aortic I71.8
      abdominal I71.3
      arch I71.1
      ascending I71.1
      descending I71.8
         abdominal I71.3
         thoracic I71.1
      syphilitic A52.01
      thoracoabdominal I71.5
      thorax, thoracic I71.1
      transverse I71.1
      traumatic -see Injury, aorta, laceration,
         major
      valve or cusp -see also Endocarditis, aortic
         I35.8
   appendix (with peritonitis) K35.2
      with localized peritonitis K35.3
   arteriovenous fistula, brain I60.8
   artery I77.2
   brain -see Hemorrhage, intracranial,
      intracerebral
      coronary -see Infarct, myocardium
      heart -see Infarct, myocardium
      pulmonary I28.8
      traumatic (complication) -see Injury, blood
         vessel
   bile duct (common) (hepatic) K83.2
      cystic K82.2
   bladder (sphincter) (nontraumatic)
      (spontaneous) N32.89
      following ectopic or molar pregnancy O08.6

Rupture, ruptured *--continued*
  obstetrical trauma O71.5
    traumatic S37.29
  blood vessel *-see also* Hemorrhage
    brain *-see* Hemorrhage, intracranial, intracerebral
    heart *-see* Infarct, myocardium
    traumatic (complication) *-see* Injury, blood vessel, laceration, major, by site
  bone *-see* Fracture
  bowel (nontraumatic) K63.1
  brain
    aneurysm (congenital) *-see also* Hemorrhage, intracranial, subarachnoid
      syphilitic A52.05
    hemorrhagic *-see* Hemorrhage, intracranial, intracerebral
  capillaries I78.8
  cardiac (auricle) (ventricle) (wall) I23.3
    with hemopericardium I23.0
    infectional I40.9
    traumatic *-see* Injury, heart
  cartilage (articular) (current) *-see also* Sprain
    knee S83.3
    semilunar *-see* Tear, meniscus
  cecum (with peritonitis) K65.0
    with peritoneal abscess K35.3
    traumatic S36.598
  celiac artery, traumatic *-see* Injury, blood vessel, celiac artery, laceration, major
  cerebral aneurysm (congenital) (see Hemorrhage, intracranial, subarachnoid)
  cervix (uteri)
    with ectopic or molar pregnancy O08.6
    following ectopic or molar pregnancy O08.6
    obstetrical trauma O71.3
    traumatic S37.69
  chordae tendineae NEC I51.1
    concurrent with acute myocardial infarction *-see* Infarct, myocardium
    following acute myocardial infarction (current complication) I23.4
  choroid (direct) (indirect) (traumatic) H31.32
  circle of Willis I60.6
  colon (nontraumatic) K63.1
    traumatic *-see* Injury, intestine, large
  cornea (traumatic) *-see* Injury, eye, laceration
  coronary (artery) (thrombotic) *-see* Infarct, myocardium
  corpus luteum (infected) (ovary) N83.1
  cyst *-see* Cyst
  cystic duct K82.2
  Descemet's membrane *-see* Change, corneal membrane, Descemet's, rupture
    traumatic *-see* Injury, eye, laceration
  diaphragm, traumatic *-see* Injury, intrathoracic, diaphragm
  disc *-see* Rupture, intervertebral disc
  diverticulum (intestine) K57.80
    with bleeding K57.81
    bladder N32.3
    large intestine K57.20
      with
        bleeding K57.21
        small intestine K57.40
          with bleeding K57.41
      small intestine K57.00
        with
          bleeding K57.01
          large intestine K57.40
            with bleeding K57.41

Rupture, ruptured *--continued*
  duodenal stump K31.89
  ear drum (nontraumatic) *-see also* Perforation, tympanum
    traumatic S09.2
      due to blast injury *-see* Injury, blast, ear
  esophagus K22.3
  eye (without prolapse or loss of intraocular tissue) *-see* Injury, eye, laceration
  fallopian tube NEC (nonobstetric) (nontraumatic) N83.8
    due to pregnancy O00.10
      with intrauterine pregnancy O00.11
  fontanel P13.1
  gallbladder K82.2
    traumatic S36.128
  gastric *-see also* Rupture, stomach
    vessel K92.2
  globe (eye) (traumatic) *-see* Injury, eye, laceration
  graafian follicle (hematoma) N83.0
  heart *-see* Rupture, cardiac
  hymen (nontraumatic) (nonintentional) N89.8
  internal organ, traumatic *-see* Injury, by site
  intervertebral disc *-see* Displacement, intervertebral disc
    traumatic *-see* Rupture, traumatic, intervertebral disc
  intestine NEC (nontraumatic) K63.1
    traumatic *-see* Injury, intestine
  iris *-see also* Abnormality, pupillary
    traumatic *-see* Injury, eye, laceration
  joint capsule, traumatic *-see* Sprain
  kidney (traumatic) S37.06
    birth injury P15.8
    nontraumatic N28.89
  lacrimal duct (traumatic) *-see* Injury, eye, specified site NEC
  lens (cataract) (traumatic) *-see* Cataract, traumatic
  ligament, traumatic *-see* Rupture, traumatic, ligament, by site
  liver S36.116
    birth injury P15.0
  lymphatic vessel I89.8
  marginal sinus (placental) (with hemorrhage) *-see* Hemorrhage, antepartum, specified cause NEC
  membrana tympani (nontraumatic) *-see* Perforation, tympanum
  membranes (spontaneous)
    artificial
      delayed delivery following O75.5
    delayed delivery following *-see* Pregnancy, complicated by, premature rupture of membranes
  meningeal artery I60.8
  meniscus (knee) *-see also* Tear, meniscus
    old *-see* Derangement, meniscus
    site other than knee - code as Sprain
  mesenteric artery, traumatic *-see* Injury, mesenteric, artery, laceration, major
  mesentery (nontraumatic) K66.8
    traumatic *-see* Injury, intra-abdominal, specified, site NEC
  mitral (valve) I34.8
  muscle (traumatic) *-see also* Strain
    diastasis *-see* Diastasis, muscle
    nontraumatic M62.10
      ankle M62.17
      foot M62.17

Rupture, ruptured *--continued*
    forearm M62.13
    hand M62.14
    lower leg M62.16
    pelvic region M62.15
    shoulder region M62.11
    specified site NEC M62.18
    thigh M62.15
    upper arm M62.12
    traumatic *-see* Strain, by site
  musculotendinous junction NEC, nontraumatic *-see* Rupture, tendon, spontaneous
  mycotic aneurysm causing cerebral hemorrhage *-see* Hemorrhage, intracranial, subarachnoid
  myocardium, myocardial *-see* Rupture, cardiac
    traumatic *-see* Injury, heart
  nontraumatic, meaning hernia *-see* Hernia
  obstructed *-see* Hernia, by site, obstructed
  operation wound *-see* Disruption, wound, operation
  ovary, ovarian N83.8
    corpus luteum cyst N83.1
    follicle (graafian) N83.0
  oviduct (nonobstetric) (nontraumatic) N83.8
    due to pregnancy O00.10
      with intrauterine pregnancy O00.11
  pancreas (nontraumatic) K86.89
    traumatic S36.299
  papillary muscle NEC I51.2
    following acute myocardial infarction (current complication) I23.5
  pelvic
    floor, complicating delivery O70.1
    organ NEC, obstetrical trauma O71.5
  perineum (nonobstetric) (nontraumatic) N90.89
    complicating delivery *-see* Delivery, complicated, by, laceration, anus (sphincter)
  postoperative wound *-see* Disruption, wound, operation
  prostate (traumatic) S37.828
  pulmonary
    artery I28.8
    valve (heart) I37.8
    vein I28.8
    vessel I28.8
  pus tube *-see* Salpingitis
  pyosalpinx *-see* Salpingitis
  rectum (nontraumatic) K63.1
    traumatic S36.69
  retina, retinal (traumatic) (without detachment) *-see also* Break, retina
    with detachment *-see* Detachment, retina, with retinal, break
  rotator cuff (nontraumatic) M75.10
    complete M75.12
    incomplete M75.11
  sclera *-see* Injury, eye, laceration
  sigmoid (nontraumatic) K63.1
    traumatic S36.593
  spinal cord *-see also* Injury, spinal cord, by region
    due to injury at birth P11.5
    newborn (birth injury) P11.5
  spleen (traumatic) S36.09
    birth injury P15.1
    congenital (birth injury) P15.1
    due to P. vivax malaria B51.0

Rupture, ruptured --*continued*
  nontraumatic D73.5
  spontaneous D73.5
  splenic vein R58
    traumatic -*see* Injury, blood vessel, splenic vein
  stomach (nontraumatic) (spontaneous) K31.89
    traumatic S36.39
  supraspinatus (complete) (incomplete) (nontraumatic) -*see* Tear, rotator cuff
  symphysis pubis
    obstetric O71.6
    traumatic S33.4
  synovium (cyst) M66.10
    ankle M66.17
    elbow M66.12
    finger M66.14
    foot M66.17
    forearm M66.13
    hand M66.14
    pelvic region M66.15
    shoulder region M66.11
    specified site NEC M66.18
    thigh M66.15
    toe M66.17
    upper arm M66.12
    wrist M66.13
  tendon (traumatic) -*see* Strain
    nontraumatic (spontaneous) M66.9
      ankle M66.87
      extensor M66.20
        ankle M66.27
        foot M66.27
        forearm M66.23
        hand M66.24
        lower leg M66.26
        multiple sites M66.29
        pelvic region M66.25
        shoulder region M66.21
        specified site NEC M66.28
        thigh M66.25
        upper arm M66.22
      flexor M66.30
        ankle M66.37
        foot M66.37
        forearm M66.33
        hand M66.34
        lower leg M66.36
        multiple sites M66.39
        pelvic region M66.35
        shoulder region M66.31
        specified site NEC M66.38
        thigh M66.35
        upper arm M66.32
      foot M66.87
      forearm M66.83
      hand M66.84
      lower leg M66.86
      multiple sites M66.89
      pelvic region M66.85
      shoulder region M66.81
      specified
        site NEC M66.88
        tendon M66.80
      thigh M66.85
      upper arm M66.82
  thoracic duct I89.8
  tonsil J35.8
  traumatic
    aorta -*see* Injury, aorta, laceration, major

Rupture, ruptured --*continued*
  diaphragm -*see* Injury, intrathoracic, diaphragm
    external site -*see* Wound, open, by site
    eye -*see* Injury, eye, laceration
    internal organ -*see* Injury, by site
    intervertebral disc
      cervical S13.0
      lumbar S33.0
      thoracic S23.0
    kidney S37.06
    ligament -*see also* Sprain
      ankle -*see* Sprain, ankle
      carpus -*see* Rupture, traumatic, ligament, wrist
      collateral (hand) -*see* Rupture, traumatic, ligament, finger, collateral
      finger (metacarpophalangeal) (interphalangeal) S63.40
        collateral S63.41
          index S63.41
          little S63.41
          middle S63.41
          ring S63.41
        index S63.40
        little S63.40
        middle S63.40
        palmar S63.42
          index S63.42
          little S63.42
          middle S63.42
          ring S63.42
        ring S63.40
        specified site NEC S63.499
          index S63.49
          little S63.49
          middle S63.49
          ring S63.49
        volar plate S63.43
          index S63.43
          little S63.43
          middle S63.43
          ring S63.43
      foot -*see* Sprain, foot
      radial collateral S53.2
      radiocarpal -*see* Rupture, traumatic, ligament, wrist, radiocarpal
      ulnar collateral S53.3
      ulnocarpal -*see* Rupture, traumatic, ligament, wrist, ulnocarpal
      wrist S63.30
        collateral S63.31
        radiocarpal S63.32
        specified site NEC S63.39
        ulnocarpal (palmar) S63.33
    liver S36.116
    membrana tympani -*see* Rupture, ear drum, traumatic
    muscle or tendon -*see* Strain
    myocardium -*see* Injury, heart
    pancreas S36.299
    rectum S36.69
    sigmoid S36.593
    spleen S36.09
    stomach S36.39
    symphysis pubis S33.4
    tympanum, tympanic (membrane) -*see* Rupture, ear drum, traumatic
    ureter S37.19
    uterus S37.69
    vagina -*see* Injury, vagina

Rupture, ruptured --*continued*
  vena cava -*see* Injury, vena cava, laceration, major
  tricuspid (heart) (valve) I07.8
  tube, tubal (nonobstetric) (nontraumatic) N83.8
    abscess -*see* Salpingitis
    due to pregnancy O00.10
      with intrauterine pregnancy O00.11
  tympanum, tympanic (membrane) (nontraumatic) -*see also* Perforation, tympanic membrane H72.9
    traumatic -*see* Rupture, ear drum, traumatic
  umbilical cord, complicating delivery O69.89
  ureter (traumatic) S37.19
    nontraumatic N28.89
  urethra (nontraumatic) N36.8
    with ectopic or molar pregnancy O08.6
    following ectopic or molar pregnancy O08.6
    obstetrical trauma O71.5
    traumatic S37.39
  uterosacral ligament (nonobstetric) (nontraumatic) N83.8
  uterus (traumatic) S37.69
    before labor O71.0
    during or after labor O71.1
    nonpuerperal, nontraumatic N85.8
    pregnant (during labor) O71.1
      before labor O71.0
  vagina -*see* Injury, vagina
  valve, valvular (heart) -*see* Endocarditis
  varicose vein -*see* Varix
  varix -*see* Varix
  vena cava R58
    traumatic -*see* Injury, vena cava, laceration, major
  vesical (urinary) N32.89
  vessel (blood) R58
    pulmonary I28.8
    traumatic -*see* Injury, blood vessel
  viscus R19.8
  vulva complicating delivery O70.0
Russell-Silver syndrome Q87.1
Russian spring-summer type encephalitis A84.0
Rust's disease (tuberculous cervical spondylitis) A18.01
Ruvalcaba-Myhre-Smith syndrome E71.440
Rytand-Lipsitch syndrome I44.2

S

Saber, sabre shin or tibia (syphilitic) A50.56 [*M90.8*]
Sac lacrimal -*see* condition
Saccharomyces infection B37.9
Saccharopinuria E72.3
Saccular -*see* condition **Sacculation**
  aorta (nonsyphilitic) -*see* Aneurysm, aorta
  bladder N32.3
  intralaryngeal (congenital) (ventricular) Q31.3
  larynx (congenital) (ventricular) Q31.3
  organ or site, congenital -*see* Distortion
  pregnant uterus -*see* Pregnancy, complicated by, abnormal, uterus
  ureter N28.89
  urethra N36.1
  vesical N32.3
Sachs' amaurotic familial idiocy or disease E75.02
Sachs-Tay disease E75.02

Sacks-Libman disease M32.11
Sacralgia M53.3
Sacralization Q76.49
Sacrodynia M53.3
Sacroiliac joint -*see* condition
Sacroiliitis NEC M46.1
Sacrum -*see* condition
Saddle
  back -*see* Lordosis
  embolus
    abdominal aorta I74.01
    pulmonary artery I26.92
      with acute cor pulmonale I26.02
  injury   code to condition
  nose M95.0
    due to syphilis A50.57
Sadism (sexual) F65.52
Sadness, postpartal O90.6
Sadomasochism F65.50
Saemisch's ulcer (cornea) -*see* Ulcer, cornea,
  central
Sagging
  skin and subcutaneous tissue (following
  bariatric surgery weight loss) (following
  dietary weight loss) L98.7
Sahib disease B55.0
Sailors' skin L57.8
Saint
  Anthony's fire -*see* Erysipelas
  triad -*see* Hernia, diaphragm
  Vitus' dance -*see* Chorea, Sydenham's
Salaam
  attack(s) -*see* Epilepsy, spasms
  tic R25.8
Salicylism
  abuse F55.8
  overdose or wrong substance given -*see* Table
  of Drugs and Chemicals, by drug, poisoning
Salivary duct or gland -*see* condition
Salivation, excessive K11.7
Salmonella -*see* Infection, Salmonella
Salmonellosis A02.0
Salpingitis (catarrhal) (fallopian tube)
  (nodular) (pseudofollicular) (purulent)
  (septic) N70.91
  with oophoritis N70.93
  acute N70.01
    with oophoritis N70.03
  chlamydial A56.11
  chronic N70.11
    with oophoritis N70.13
  complicating abortion -*see* Abortion, by type,
    complicated by, salpingitis
  ear -*see* Salpingitis, eustachian
  eustachian (tube) H68.00
    acute H68.01
    chronic H68.02
  follicularis N70.11
    with oophoritis N70.13
  gonococcal (acute) (chronic) A54.24
  interstitial, chronic N70.11
    with oophoritis N70.13
  isthmica nodosa N70.11
    with oophoritis N70.13
  specific (gonococcal) (acute) (chronic)
    A54.24
  tuberculous (acute) (chronic) A18.17
  venereal (gonococcal) (acute) (chronic)
    A54.24
Salpingocele N83.4

Salpingo-oophoritis (catarrhal) (purulent)
  (ruptured) (septic) (suppurative) N70.93
  acute N70.03
    with ectopic or molar pregnancy O08.0
    following ectopic or molar pregnancy O08.0
    gonococcal A54.24
  chronic N70.13
  following ectopic or molar pregnancy O08.0
  gonococcal (acute) (chronic) A54.24
  puerperal O86.19
  specific (gonococcal) (acute) (chronic)
    A54.24
  subacute N70.03
  tuberculous (acute) (chronic) A18.17
  venereal (gonococcal) (acute) (chronic)
    A54.24
Salpingo-ovaritis -*see* Salpingo-oophoritis
Salpingoperitonitis -*see* Salpingo-oophoritis
Salzmann's nodular dystrophy -*see*
  Degeneration, cornea, nodular
Sampson's cyst or tumor N80.1
San Joaquin (Valley) fever B38.0
Sandblaster's asthma, lung or
  pneumoconiosis J62.8
Sander's disease (paranoia) F22
Sandfly fever A93.1
Sandhoff's disease E75.01
Sanfilippo (Type B) (Type C) (Type D)
  syndrome E76.22
Sanger-Brown ataxia G11.2
Sao Paulo fever or typhus A77.0
Saponification, mesenteric K65.8
Sarcocele (benign)
  syphilitic A52.76
    congenital A50.59
Sarcocystosis A07.8
Sarcoepiplocele -*see* Hernia
Sarcoepiplomphalocele Q79.2
Sarcoid -*see also* Sarcoidosis
  arthropathy D86.86
  Boeck's D86.9
  Darier-Roussy D86.3
  iridocyclitis D86.83
  meningitis D86.81
  myocarditis D86.85
  myositis D86.87
  pyelonephritis D86.84
  Spiegler-Fendt L08.89
Sarcoidosis D86.9
  with
    cranial nerve palsies D86.82
    hepatic granuloma D86.89
    polyarthritis D86.86
    tubulo-interstitial nephropathy D86.84
  combined sites NEC D86.89
  lung D86.0
    and lymph nodes D86.2
  lymph nodes D86.1
    and lung D86.2
  meninges D86.81
  skin D86.3
  specified type NEC D86.89
Sarcoma (of) -*see also* Neoplasm, connective
  tissue, malignant
  alveolar soft part -*see* Neoplasm, connective
    tissue, malignant
  ameloblastic C41.1
    upper jaw (bone) C41.0
  botryoid -*see* Neoplasm, connective tissue,
    malignant

Sarcoma (of) --*continued*
  botryoides -*see* Neoplasm, connective tissue,
    malignant
  cerebellar C71.6
    circumscribed (arachnoidal) C71.6
  circumscribed (arachnoidal) cerebellar C71.6
  clear cell -*see also* Neoplasm, connective
    tissue, malignant
    kidney C64.
  dendritic cells (accessory cells) C96.4
  embryonal -*see* Neoplasm, connective tissue,
    malignant
  endometrial (stromal) C54.1
    isthmus C54.0
  epithelioid (cell) -*see* Neoplasm, connective
    tissue, malignant
  Ewing's -*see* Neoplasm, bone, malignant
  follicular dendritic cell C96.4
  germinoblastic (diffuse) -*see* Lymphoma,
    diffuse large cell
    follicular -*see* Lymphoma, follicular,
    specified NEC
  giant cell (except of bone) -*see also*
    Neoplasm, connective tissue, malignant
    bone -*see* Neoplasm, bone, malignant
  glomoid -*see* Neoplasm, connective tissue,
    malignant
  granulocytic C92.3
  hemangioendothelial -*see* Neoplasm,
    connective tissue, malignant
  hemorrhagic, multiple -*see* Sarcoma, Kaposi's
  histiocytic C96.A
  Hodgkin -*see* Lymphoma, Hodgkin
  immunoblastic (diffuse) -*see* Lymphoma,
    diffuse large cell
  interdigitating dendritic cell C96.4
  Kaposi's
    colon C46.4
    connective tissue C46.1
    gastrointestinal organ C46.4
    lung C46.5
    lymph node(s) C46.3
    palate (hard) (soft) C46.2
    rectum C46.4
    skin C46.0
    specified site NEC C46.7
    stomach C46.4
    unspecified site C46.9
  Kupffer cell C22.3
  Langerhans cell C96.4
  leptomeningeal -*see* Neoplasm, meninges,
    malignant
  liver NEC C22.4
  lymphangioendothelial -*see* Neoplasm,
    connective tissue, malignant
  lymphoblastic -*see* Lymphoma, lymphoblastic
    (diffuse)
  lymphocytic -*see* Lymphoma, small cell B-
    cell
  mast cell C96.2
  melanotic -*see* Melanoma
  meningeal -*see* Neoplasm, meninges,
    malignant
  meningothelial -*see* Neoplasm, meninges,
    malignant
  mesenchymal -*see also* Neoplasm, connective
    tissue, malignant
    mixed -*see* Neoplasm, connective tissue,
    malignant
  mesothelial -*see* Mesothelioma
  monstrocellular

STUV

Sarcoma (of) --*continued*
  specified site -*see* Neoplasm, malignant, by site
  unspecified site C71.9
  myeloid C92.3
  neurogenic -*see* Neoplasm, nerve, malignant
  odontogenic C41.1
    upper jaw (bone) C41.0
  osteoblastic -*see* Neoplasm, bone, malignant
  osteogenic -*see also* Neoplasm, bone, malignant
    juxtacortical -*see* Neoplasm, bone, malignant
    periosteal -*see* Neoplasm, bone, malignant
  periosteal -*see also* Neoplasm, bone, malignant
    osteogenic -*see* Neoplasm, bone, malignant
  pleomorphic cell -*see* Neoplasm, connective tissue, malignant
  reticulum cell (diffuse) -*see* Lymphoma, diffuse large cell
    nodular -*see* Lymphoma, follicular
    pleomorphic cell type -*see* Lymphoma, diffuse large cell
  rhabdoid -*see* Neoplasm, malignant, by site
  round cell -*see* Neoplasm, connective tissue, malignant
  small cell -*see* Neoplasm, connective tissue, malignant
  soft tissue -*see* Neoplasm, connective tissue, malignant
  spindle cell -*see* Neoplasm, connective tissue, malignant
  stromal (endometrial) C54.1
    isthmus C54.0
  synovial -*see also* Neoplasm, connective tissue, malignant
    biphasic -*see* Neoplasm, connective tissue, malignant
    epithelioid cell -*see* Neoplasm, connective tissue, malignant
    spindle cell -*see* Neoplasm, connective tissue, malignant **Sarcomatosis**
  meningeal -*see* Neoplasm, meninges, malignant
  specified site NEC -*see* Neoplasm, connective tissue, malignant
  unspecified site C80.1
Sarcopenia (age-related) M62.84
Sarcosinemia E72.59
Sarcosporidiosis (intestinal) A07.8
Satiety, early R68.81
Saturnine -*see* condition
Saturnism
  overdose or wrong substance given or taken -*see* Table of Drugs and Chemicals, by drug, poisoning
Satyriasis F52.8
Sauriasis -*see* Ichthyosis
SBE (subacute bacterial endocarditis) I33.0
Scabs R23.4
Scabies (any site) B86
Scaglietti-Dagnini syndrome E22.0
Scald -*see* Burn
Scalenus anticus (anterior) syndrome G54.0
Scales R23.4
Scaling, skin R23.4
Scalp -*see* condition
Scapegoating affecting child Z62.3
Scaphocephaly Q75.0
Scapulalgia M89.8X1

Scapulohumeral myopathy G71.0
Scar, scarring -*see also* Cicatrix L90.5
  adherent L90.5
  atrophic L90.5
  cervix
    in pregnancy or childbirth -*see* Pregnancy, complicated by, abnormal cervix
  cheloid L91.0
  chorioretinal H31.00
    posterior pole macula H31.01
    postsurgical H59.81
    solar retinopathy H31.02
    specified type NEC H31.09
  choroid -*see* Scar, chorioretinal
  conjunctiva H11.24
  cornea H17.9
    xerophthalmic -*see also* Opacity, cornea
      vitamin A deficiency E50.6
  duodenum, obstructive K31.5
  hypertrophic L91.0
  keloid L91.0
  labia N90.89
  lung (base) J98.4
  macula -*see* Scar, chorioretinal, posterior pole
  muscle M62.89
  myocardium, myocardial I25.2
  painful L90.5
  posterior pole (eye) -*see* Scar, chorioretinal, posterior pole
  retina -*see* Scar, chorioretinal
  trachea J39.8
  transmural uterine, in pregnancy O34.29
  uterus N85.8
    in pregnancy O34.29
  vagina N89.8
    postoperative N99.2
  vulva N90.89
Scarabiasis B88.2
Scarlatina (anginosa) (maligna) (ulcerosa) A38.9
  myocarditis (acute) A38.1
    old -*see* Myocarditis
  otitis media A38.0
Scarlet fever (albuminuria) (angina) A38.9
Schamberg's disease (progressive pigmentary dermatosis) L81.7
Schatzki's ring (acquired) (esophagus) (lower) K22.2
  congenital Q39.3
Schaufenster krankheit I20.8
Schaumann's
  benign lymphogranulomatosis D86.1
  disease or syndrome -*see* Sarcoidosis
Scheie's syndrome E76.03
Schenck's disease B42.1
Scheuermann's disease or osteochondrosis - *see* Osteochondrosis, juvenile, spine
Schilder (Flatau) disease G37.0
Schilling-type monocytic leukemia C93.0
Schimmelbusch's disease, cystic mastitis, or hyperplasia -*see* Mastopathy, cystic
Schistosoma infestation -*see* Infestation, Schistosoma
Schistosomiasis B65.9
  with muscle disorder B65.9 [*M63.80*]
    ankle B65.9 [*M63.87*]
    foot B65.9 [*M63.87*]
    forearm B65.9 [*M63.83*]
    hand B65.9 [*M63.84*]
    lower leg B65.9 [*M63.86*]
    multiple sites B65.9 [*M63.89*]

Schistosomiasis - *continued*
    pelvic region B65.9 [*M63.85*]
    shoulder region B65.9 [*M63.81*]
    specified site NEC B65.9 [*M63.88*]
    thigh B65.9 [*M63.85*]
    upper arm B65.9 [*M63.82*]
  Asiatic B65.2
  bladder B65.0
  chestermani B65.8
  colon B65.1
  cutaneous B65.3
  due to
    S. haematobium B65.0
    S. japonicum B65.2
    S. mansoni B65.1
    S. mattheii B65.8
  Eastern B65.2
  genitourinary tract B65.0
  intestinal B65.1
  lung NEC B65.9 [*J99*]
    pneumonia B65.9 [*J17*]
  Manson's (intestinal) B65.1
  oriental B65.2
  pulmonary NEC B65.9 [*J99*]
    pneumonia B65.9
  Schistosoma
    haematobium B65.0
    japonicum B65.2
    mansoni B65.1
  specified type NEC B65.8
  urinary B65.0
  vesical B65.0
Schizencephaly Q04.6
Schizoaffective psychosis F25.9
Schizodontia K00.2
Schizoid personality F60.1
Schizophrenia, schizophrenic F20.9
  acute (brief) (undifferentiated) F23
  atypical (form) F20.3
  borderline F21
  catalepsy F20.2
  catatonic (type) (excited) (withdrawn) F20.2
  cenesthopathic, cenesthesiopathic F20.89
  childhood type F84.5
  chronic undifferentiated F20.5
  cyclic F25.0
  disorganized (type) F20.1
  flexibilitas cerea F20.2
  hebephrenic (type) F20.1
  incipient F21
  latent F21
  negative type F20.5
  paranoid (type) F20.0
  paraphrenic F20.0
  post-psychotic depression F32.89
  prepsychotic F21
  prodromal F21
  pseudoneurotic F21
  pseudopsychopathic F21
  reaction F23
  residual (state) (type) F20.5
  restzustand F20.5
  schizoaffective (type) -*see* Psychosis, schizoaffective
  simple (type) F20.89
  simplex F20.89
  specified type NEC F20.89
  stupor F20.2
  syndrome of childhood F84.5
  undifferentiated (type) F20.3
    chronic F20.5

Schizothymia (persistent) F60.1
Schlatter-Osgood disease or osteochondrosis
-*see* Osteochondrosis, juvenile, tibia
Schlatter's tibia -*see* Osteochondrosis,
juvenile, tibia
Schmidt's syndrome (polyglandular,
autoimmune) E31.0
Schmincke's carcinoma or tumor -*see*
Neoplasm, nasopharynx, malignant
Schmitz (Stutzer) dysentery A03.0
Schmorl's disease or nodes - lumbar region
M51.46
lumbosacral region M51.47
sacrococcygeal region M53.3
thoracic region M51.44
thoracolumbar region M51.45
Schneiderian
papilloma -*see* Neoplasm, nasopharynx,
benign
specified site -*see* Neoplasm, benign, by site
unspecified site D14.0
specified site -*see* Neoplasm, malignant, by
site
unspecified site C30.0
Scholte's syndrome (malignant carcinoid)
E34.0
Scholz (Bielchowsky Henneberg) disease or
syndrome E75.25
Schönlein (Henoch) disease or purpura
(primary) (rheumatic) D69.0
Schottmuller's disease A01.4
Schroeder's syndrome (endocrine
hypertensive) E27.0
Schüller-Christian disease or syndrome
C96.5
Schultze's type acroparesthesia, simple
I73.89
Schultz's disease or syndrome -*see*
Agranulocytosis
Schwalbe-Ziehen-Oppenheim disease G24.1
Schwannoma -*see also* Neoplasm, nerve,
benign
malignant -*see also* Neoplasm, nerve,
malignant
with rhabdomyoblastic differentiation -*see*
Neoplasm, nerve, malignant
melanocytic -*see* Neoplasm, nerve, benign
pigmented -*see* Neoplasm, nerve, benign
Schwannomatosis Q85.03
Schwartz (Jampel) syndrome G71.13
Schwartz Bartter syndrome E22.2
Schweniger-Buzzi anetoderma L90.1
Sciatic -*see* condition
Sciatica (infective)
with lumbago M54.4
due to intervertebral disc disorder -*see*
Disorder, disc, with, radiculopathy
due to displacement of intervertebral disc
(with lumbago) -*see* Disorder, disc, with,
radiculopathy
wallet M54.3
Scimitar syndrome Q26.8
Sclera -*see* condition
Sclerectasia H15.84
Scleredema
adultorum -*see* Sclerosis, systemic
Buschke's -*see* Sclerosis, systemic
newborn P83.0
Sclerema (adiposum) (edematosum)
(neonatorum) (newborn) P83.0
adultorum -*see* Sclerosis, systemic

Scleriasis -*see* Scleroderma
Scleritis H15.00
with corneal involvement H15.04
anterior H15.01
brawny H15.02
in (due to) zoster B02.34
posterior H15.03
specified type NEC H15.09
syphilitic A52.71
tuberculous (nodular) A18.51
Sclerochoroiditis H31.8
Scleroconjunctivitis -*see* Scleritis
Sclerocystic ovary syndrome E28.2
Sclerodactyly, sclerodactylia L94.3
Scleroderma, sclerodermia (acrosclerotic)
(diffuse) (generalized) (progressive)
(pulmonary) -*see also* Sclerosis, systemic
M34.9
circumscribed L94.0
linear L94.1
localized L94.0
newborn P83.8
systemic M34.9
Sclerokeratitis H16.8
tuberculous A18.52
Scleroma nasi A48.8
Scleromalacia (perforans) H15.05
Scleromyxedema L98.5
Sclérose en plaques G35
Sclerosis, sclerotic
adrenal (gland) E27.8
Alzheimer's -*see* Disease, Alzheimer's
amyotrophic (lateral) G12.21
aorta, aortic I70.0
valve -*see* Endocarditis, aortic
artery, arterial, arteriolar, arteriovascular -*see*
Arteriosclerosis
ascending multiple G35
brain (generalized) (lobular) G37.9
artery, arterial I67.2
diffuse G37.0
disseminated G35
insular G35
Krabbe's E75.23
miliary G35
multiple G35
presenile (Alzheimer's) -*see* Disease,
Alzheimer's, early onset
senile (arteriosclerotic) I67.2
stem, multiple G35
tuberous Q85.1
bulbar, multiple G35
bundle of His I44.39
cardiac -*see* Disease, heart, ischemic,
atherosclerotic
cardiorenal -*see* Hypertension, cardiorenal
cardiovascular -*see also* Disease,
cardiovascular
renal -*see* Hypertension, cardiorenal
cerebellar -*see* Sclerosis, brain
cerebral -*see* Sclerosis, brain
cerebrospinal (disseminated) (multiple) G35
cerebrovascular I67.2
choroid -*see* Degeneration, choroid
combined (spinal cord) -*see also*
Degeneration, combined
multiple G35
concentric (Balo) G37.5
cornea -*see* Opacity, cornea
coronary (artery) I25.10
with angina pectoris -*see* Arteriosclerosis,
coronary (artery),   corpus cavernosum

Sclerosis, sclerotic --*continued*
female N90.89
male N48.6
diffuse (brain) (spinal cord) G37.0
disseminated G35
dorsal G35
dorsolateral (spinal cord) -*see* Degeneration,
combined
endometrium N85.5
extrapyramidal G25.9
eye, nuclear (senile) -*see* Cataract, senile,
nuclear
focal and segmental (glomerular) -*see also*
N00 N07 with fourth character .1 N05.1
Friedreich's (spinal cord) G11.1
funicular (spermatic cord) N50.89
general (vascular) -*see* Arteriosclerosis
gland (lymphatic) I89.8
hepatic K74.1
alcoholic K70.2
hereditary
cerebellar G11.9
spinal (Friedreich's ataxia) G11.1
hippocampal G93.81
insular G35
kidney -*see* Sclerosis, renal
larynx J38.7
lateral (amyotrophic) (descending) (primary)
(spinal) G12.21
lens, senile nuclear -*see* Cataract, senile,
nuclear
liver K74.1
with fibrosis K74.2
alcoholic K70.2
alcoholic K70.2
cardiac K76.1
lung -*see* Fibrosis, lung
mastoid -*see* Mastoiditis, chronic
mesial temporal G93.81
mitral I05.8
Mönckeberg's (medial) -*see* Arteriosclerosis,
extremities
multiple (brain stem) (cerebral) (generalized)
(spinal cord) G35
myocardium, myocardial -*see* Disease, heart,
ischemic, atherosclerotic
nuclear (senile), eye -*see* Cataract, senile,
nuclear
ovary N83.8
pancreas K86.89
penis N48.6
peripheral arteries -*see* Arteriosclerosis,
extremities
plaques G35
pluriglandular E31.8
polyglandular E31.8
posterolateral (spinal cord) -*see* Degeneration,
combined
presenile (Alzheimer's) -*see* Disease,
Alzheimer's, early onset
primary, lateral G12.29
progressive, systemic M34.0
pulmonary -*see* Fibrosis, lung
artery I27.0
valve (heart) -*see* Endocarditis, pulmonary
renal N26.9
with
cystine storage disease E72.09

Sclerosis, sclerotic --continued
  hypertensive heart disease (conditions in I11) -see Hypertension, cardiorenal
  arteriolar (hyaline) (hyperplastic) -see Hypertension, kidney
  retina (senile) (vascular) H35.00
  senile (vascular) -see Arteriosclerosis
  spinal (cord) (progressive) G95.89
    ascending G61.0
    combined -see also Degeneration, combined
      multiple G35
      syphilitic A52.11
    disseminated G35
    dorsolateral -see Degeneration, combined
    hereditary (Friedreich's) (mixed form) G11.1
    lateral (amyotrophic) G12.21
    multiple G35
    posterior (syphilitic) A52.11
  stomach K31.89
  subendocardial, congenital I42.4
  systemic M34.9
    with
      lung involvement M34.81
      myopathy M34.82
      polyneuropathy M34.83
    drug-induced M34.2
    due to chemicals NEC M34.2
    progressive M34.0
    specified NEC M34.89
  temporal (mesial) G93.81
  tricuspid (heart) (valve) I07.8
  tuberous (brain) Q85.1
  tympanic membrane -see Disorder, tympanic membrane, specified NEC
  valve, valvular (heart) -see Endocarditis
  vascular -see Arteriosclerosis
  vein I87.8
Scoliosis (acquired) (postural) M41.9
  adolescent (idiopathic) -see Scoliosis, idiopathic, adolescent
  congenital Q67.5
    due to bony malformation Q76.3
    failure of segmentation (hemivertebra) Q76.3
    hemivertebra fusion Q76.3
    postural Q67.5
  idiopathic M41.20
    adolescent M41.129
      cervical region M41.122
      cervicothoracic region M41.123
      lumbar region M41.126
      lumbosacral region M41.127
      thoracic region M41.124
      thoracolumbar region M41.125
    cervical region M41.22
    cervicothoracic region M41.23
    infantile M41.00
      cervical region M41.02
      cervicothoracic region M41.03
      lumbar region M41.06
      lumbosacral region M41.07
      sacrococcygeal region M41.08
      thoracic region M41.04
      thoracolumbar region M41.05
    juvenile M41.119
      cervical region M41.112
      cervicothoracic region M41.113
      lumbar region M41.116
      lumbosacral region M41.117
      thoracic region M41.114
      thoracolumbar region M41.115

Scoliosis - *continued*
  lumbar region M41.26
  lumbosacral region M41.27
  thoracic region M41.24
  thoracolumbar region M41.25
  infantile -see Scoliosis, idiopathic, infantile
  neuromuscular M41.40
    cervical region M41.42
    cervicothoracic region M41.43
    lumbar region M41.46
    lumbosacral region M41.47
    occipito-atlanto-axial region M41.41
    thoracic region M41.44
    thoracolumbar region M41.45
  paralytic -see Scoliosis, neuromuscular
  postradiation therapy M96.5
  rachitic (late effect or sequelae) E64.3 [*M49.80*]
    cervical region E64.3 [*M49.82*]
    cervicothoracic region E64.3 [*M49.83*]
    lumbar region E64.3 [*M49.86*]
    lumbosacral region E64.3 [*M49.87*]
    multiple sites E64.3 [*M49.89*]
    occipito-atlanto-axial region E64.3 [*M49.81*]
    sacrococcygeal region E64.3 [*M49.88*]
    thoracic region E64.3 [*M49.84*]
    thoracolumbar region E64.3 [*M49.85*]
  sciatic M54.4
  secondary (to) NEC M41.50
    cerebral palsy, Friedreich's ataxia, poliomyelitis, neuromuscular disorders -see Scoliosis, neuromuscular
    cervical region M41.52
    cervicothoracic region M41.53
    lumbar region M41.56
    lumbosacral region M41.57
    thoracic region M41.54
    thoracolumbar region M41.55
  specified form NEC M41.80
    cervical region M41.82
    cervicothoracic region M41.83
    lumbar region M41.86
    lumbosacral region M41.87
    thoracic region M41.84
    thoracolumbar region M41.85
  thoracogenic M41.30
    thoracic region M41.34
    thoracolumbar region M41.35
  tuberculous A18.01
Scoliotic pelvis
  with disproportion (fetopelvic) O33.0
    causing obstructed labor O65.0
Scorbutus, scorbutic -see also Scurvy
  anemia D53.2
Score, NIHSS (National Institutes of Health Stroke Scale) R29.7
Scotoma (arcuate) (Bjerrum) (central) (ring) -see also Defect, visual field, localized, scotoma
  scintillating H53.19
Scratch -see Abrasion
Scratchy throat R09.89
Screening (for) Z13.9
  alcoholism Z13.89
  anemia Z13.0
  anomaly, congenital Z13.89
  antenatal, of mother Z36
  arterial hypertension Z13.6
  arthropod-borne viral disease NEC Z11.59
  bacteriuria, asymptomatic Z13.89
  behavioral disorder Z13.89

Screening (for) --continued
  brain injury, traumatic Z13.850
  bronchitis, chronic Z13.83
  brucellosis Z11.2
  cardiovascular disorder Z13.6
  cataract Z13.5
  chlamydial diseases Z11.8
  cholera Z11.0
  chromosomal abnormalities (nonprocreative) NEC Z13.79
  colonoscopy Z12.11
  congenital
    dislocation of hip Z13.89
    eye disorder Z13.5
    malformation or deformation Z13.89
  contamination NEC Z13.88
  cystic fibrosis Z13.228
  dengue fever Z11.59
  dental disorder Z13.84
  depression Z13.89
  developmental handicap Z13.42
    in early childhood Z13.42
    infant Z13.41
  diabetes mellitus Z13.1
  diphtheria Z11.2
  disability, intellectual Z13.42
    infant Z13.41
  disease or disorder Z13.9
    bacterial NEC Z11.2
      intestinal infectious Z11.0
      respiratory tuberculosis Z11.1
    blood or blood-forming organ Z13.0
    cardiovascular Z13.6
    Chagas' Z11.6
    chlamydial Z11.8
    dental Z13.89
    developmental Z13.42
      in child Z13.42
      infant Z13.41
    digestive tract NEC Z13.818
      lower GI Z13.811
      upper GI Z13.810
    ear Z13.5
    endocrine Z13.29
    eye Z13.5
    genitourinary Z13.89
    heart Z13.6
    human immunodeficiency virus (HIV) infection Z11.4
    immunity Z13.0
    infection
      intestinal Z11.0
        specified NEC Z11.6
    infectious Z11.9
    mental Z13.89
    metabolic Z13.228
    neurological Z13.89
    nutritional Z13.21
      metabolic Z13.228
        lipoid disorders Z13.220
    protozoal Z11.6
      intestinal Z11.0
    respiratory Z13.83
    rheumatic Z13.828
    rickettsial Z11.8
    sexually transmitted NEC Z11.3
      human immunodeficiency virus (HIV) Z11.4
    sickle-cell (trait) Z13.0
    skin Z13.89
    specified NEC Z13.89

Screening (for) --continued
- spirochetal Z11.8
- thyroid Z13.29
- vascular Z13.6
- venereal Z11.3
- viral NEC Z11.59
  - human immunodeficiency virus (HIV) Z11.4
  - intestinal Z11.0
- elevated titer Z13.89
- emphysema Z13.83
- encephalitis, viral (mosquito- or tick-borne) Z11.59
- exposure to contaminants (toxic) Z13.88
- fever
  - dengue Z11.59
  - hemorrhagic Z11.59
  - yellow Z11.59
- filariasis Z11.6
- galactosemia Z13.228
- gastrointestinal condition Z13.818
- genetic (nonprocreative)
  - for procreative management -see Testing, genetic, for procreative management
  - disease carrier status (nonprocreative) Z13.71
  - specified NEC (nonprocreative) Z13.79
- genitourinary condition Z13.89
- glaucoma Z13.5
- gonorrhea Z11.3
- gout Z13.89
- helminthiasis (intestinal) Z11.6
- hematopoietic malignancy Z12.89
- hemoglobinopathies NEC Z13.0
- hemorrhagic fever Z11.59
- Hodgkin disease Z12.89
- human immunodeficiency virus (HIV) Z11.4
- human papillomavirus Z11.51
- hypertension Z13.6
- immunity disorders Z13.0
- infection
  - mycotic Z11.8
  - parasitic Z11.8
- ingestion of radioactive substance Z13.88
- intellectual disability Z13.42
  - infant Z13.41
- intestinal
  - helminthiasis Z11.6
  - infectious disease Z11.0
- leishmaniasis Z11.6
- leprosy Z11.2
- leptospirosis Z11.8
- leukemia Z12.89
- lymphoma Z12.89
- malaria Z11.6
- malnutrition Z13.29
  - metabolic Z13.228
  - nutritional Z13.21
- measles Z11.59
- mental disorder Z13.89
- metabolic errors, inborn Z13.228
- multiphasic Z13.89
- musculoskeletal disorder Z13.828
  - osteoporosis Z13.820
- mycoses Z11.8
- myocardial infarction (acute) Z13.6
- neoplasm (malignant) (of) Z12.9
  - bladder Z12.6
  - blood Z12.89
  - breast Z12.39
    - routine mammogram Z12.31

Screening (for) --continued
- cervix Z12.4
- colon Z12.11
- genitourinary organs NEC Z12.79
  - bladder Z12.6
  - cervix Z12.4
  - ovary Z12.73
  - prostate Z12.5
  - testis Z12.71
  - vagina Z12.72
- hematopoietic system Z12.89
- intestinal tract Z12.10
  - colon Z12.11
  - rectum Z12.12
  - small intestine Z12.13
- lung Z12.2
- lymph (glands) Z12.89
- nervous system Z12.82
- oral cavity Z12.81
- prostate Z12.5
- rectum Z12.12
- respiratory organs Z12.2
- skin Z12.83
- small intestine Z12.13
- specified site NEC Z12.89
- stomach Z12.0
- nephropathy Z13.89
- nervous system disorders NEC Z13.858
- neurological condition Z13.89
- osteoporosis Z13.820
- parasitic infestation Z11.9
  - specified NEC Z11.8
- phenylketonuria Z13.228
- plague Z11.2
- poisoning (chemical) (heavy metal) Z13.88
- poliomyelitis Z11.59
- postnatal, chromosomal abnormalities Z13.89
- prenatal, of mother Z36
- protozoal disease Z11.6
  - intestinal Z11.0
- pulmonary tuberculosis Z11.1
- radiation exposure Z13.88
- respiratory condition Z13.83
- respiratory tuberculosis Z11.1
- rheumatoid arthritis Z13.828
- rubella Z11.59
- schistosomiasis Z11.6
- sexually transmitted disease NEC Z11.3
  - human immunodeficiency virus (HIV) Z11.4
- sickle-cell disease or trait Z13.0
- skin condition Z13.89
- sleeping sickness Z11.6
- special Z13.9
  - specified NEC Z13.89
- syphilis Z11.3
- tetanus Z11.2
- trachoma Z11.8
- traumatic brain injury Z13.850
- trypanosomiasis Z11.6
- tuberculosis, respiratory Z11.1
- venereal disease Z11.3
- viral encephalitis (mosquito- or tick-borne) Z11.59
- whooping cough Z11.2
- worms, intestinal Z11.6
- yaws Z11.8
- yellow fever Z11.59

Scrofula, scrofulosis (tuberculosis of cervical lymph glands) A18.2
Scrofulide (primary) (tuberculous) A18.4

Scrofuloderma, scrofulodermia (any site) (primary) A18.4
Scrofulosus lichen (primary) (tuberculous) A18.4
Scrofulous -see condition
Scrotal tongue K14.5
Scrotum -see condition
Scurvy, scorbutic E54
- anemia D53.2
- gum E54
- infantile E54
- rickets E55.0 [M90.80]
Sealpox B08.62
Seasickness T75.3
Seatworm (infection) (infestation) B80
Sebaceous -see also condition
- cyst -see Cyst, sebaceous
Seborrhea, seborrheic L21.9
- capillitii R23.8
- capitis L21.0
- dermatitis L21.9
  - infantile L21.1
- eczema L21.9
  - infantile L21.1
- sicca L21.0
Seckel's syndrome Q87.1
Seclusion, pupil -see Membrane, pupillary
Second hand tobacco smoke exposure (acute) (chronic) Z77.22
- in the perinatal period P96.81
Secondary
- dentin (in pulp) K04.3
- neoplasm, secondaries -see Table of Neoplasms, secondary
Secretion
- antidiuretic hormone, inappropriate E22.2
- catecholamine, by pheochromocytoma E27.5
- hormone
  - antidiuretic, inappropriate (syndrome) E22.2
  - by
    - carcinoid tumor E34.0
    - pheochromocytoma E27.5
  - ectopic NEC E34.2
- urinary
  - excessive R35.8
  - suppression R34
Section
- nerve, traumatic -see Injury, nerve
Sedative, hypnotic, or anxiolytic-induced
- anxiety disorder F13.980
- bipolar and related disorder F13.94
- delirium F13.921
- depressive disorder F13.94
- major neurocognitive disorder F13.97
- mild neurocognitive disorder F13.988
- psychotic disorder F13.959
- sexual dysfunction F13.981
- sleep disorder F13.982
Segmentation, incomplete (congenital) -see also Fusion
- bone NEC Q78.8
- lumbosacral (joint) (vertebra) Q76.49
Seitelberger's syndrome (infantile neuraxonal dystrophy) G31.89
Seizure(s) -see also Convulsions R56.9
- akinetic -see Epilepsy, generalized, specified NEC
- atonic -see Epilepsy, generalized, specified NEC
- autonomic (hysterical) F44.5
- convulsive -see Convulsions

Seizure(s) --*continued*
- cortical (focal) (motor) -*see* Epilepsy, localization-related, symptomatic, with simple partial seizures
- disorder -*see also* Epilepsy G40.909
- due to stroke -*see* Sequelae (of), disease, cerebrovascular, by type, specified NEC
- epileptic -*see* Epilepsy
- febrile (simple) R56.00
  - with status epilepticus G40.901
  - complex (atypical) (complicated) R56.01
    - with status epilepticus G40.901
- grand mal G40.409
  - intractable G40.419
    - with status epilepticus G40.411
    - without status epilepticus G40.419
  - not intractable G40.409
    - with status epilepticus G40.401
    - without status epilepticus G40.409
- heart -*see* Disease, heart
- hysterical F44.5
- intractable G40.919
  - with status epilepticus G40.911
- Jacksonian (focal) (motor type) (sensory type) -*see* Epilepsy, localization-related, symptomatic, with simple partial seizures
- newborn P90
- nonspecific epileptic
  - atonic -*see* Epilepsy, generalized, specified NEC
  - clonic -*see* Epilepsy, generalized, specified NEC
  - myoclonic -*see* Epilepsy, generalized, specified NEC
  - tonic -*see* Epilepsy, generalized, specified NEC
  - tonic-clonic -*see* Epilepsy, generalized, specified NEC
- partial, developing into secondarily generalized seizures
  - complex -*see* Epilepsy, localization-related, symptomatic, with complex partial seizures
  - simple -*see* Epilepsy, localization-related, symptomatic, with simple partial seizures
- petit mal G40.409
  - intractable G40.419
    - with status epilepticus G40.411
    - without status epilepticus G40.419
  - not intractable G40.409
    - with status epilepticus G40.401
    - without status epilepticus G40.409
- post traumatic R56.1
- recurrent G40.909
- specified NEC G40.89
- uncinate -*see* Epilepsy, localization-related, symptomatic, with complex partial seizures

Selenium deficiency, dietary E59
Self-damaging behavior (life-style) Z72.89
Self-harm (attempted)
- history (personal) Z91.5
  - in family Z81.8
Self-mutilation (attempted)
- history (personal) Z91.5
  - in family Z81.8
Self-poisoning
- history (personal) Z91.5
  - in family Z81.8
- observation following (alleged) attempt Z03.6
Semicoma R40.1
Seminal vesiculitis N49.0
Seminoma C62.9
- specified site -*see* Neoplasm, malignant, by site

Senear-Usher disease or syndrome L10.4
Senectus R54
Senescence (without mention of psychosis) R54
Senile, senility -*see also* condition R41.81
- with
  - acute confusional state F05
  - mental changes NOS F03
  - psychosis NEC -*see* Psychosis, senile
- asthenia R54
- cervix (atrophic) N88.8
- debility R54
- endometrium (atrophic) N85.8
- fallopian tube (atrophic) -*see* Atrophy, fallopian tube
- heart (failure) R54
- ovary (atrophic) -*see* Atrophy, ovary
  - premature E34.8
- vagina, vaginitis (atrophic) N95.2
- wart L82.1
Sensation
- burning (skin) R20.8
  - tongue K14.6
- loss of R20.8
- prickling (skin) R20.2
- tingling (skin) R20.2
Sense loss
- smell -*see* Disturbance, sensation, smell
- taste -*see* Disturbance, sensation, taste
- touch R20.8
Sensibility disturbance (cortical) (deep) (vibratory) R20.9
Sensitive, sensitivity -*see also* Allergy
- carotid sinus G90.01
- child (excessive) F93.8
- cold, autoimmune D59.1
- dentin K03.89
- gluten (non-celiac) K90.41
- latex Z91.040
- methemoglobin D74.8
- tuberculin, without clinical or radiological symptoms R76.11
- visual
  - glare H53.71
  - impaired contrast H53.72
Sensitiver Beziehungswahn F22
Sensitization, auto-erythrocytic D69.2
Separation
- anxiety, abnormal (of childhood) F93.0
- apophysis, traumatic
  - code as Fracture, by site
- choroid -*see* Detachment, choroid
- epiphysis, epiphyseal
  - nontraumatic -*see also* Osteochondropathy, specified type NEC
    - upper femoral -*see* Slipped, epiphysis, upper femoral
  - traumatic
    - code as Fracture, by site
- fracture -*see* Fracture
- infundibulum cardiac from right ventricle by a partition Q24.3
- joint (traumatic) (current)
  - code by site under Dislocation
- pubic bone, obstetrical trauma O71.6
- retina, retinal -*see* Detachment, retina
- symphysis pubis, obstetrical trauma O71.6
- tracheal ring, incomplete, congenital Q32.1

Sepsis (generalized) (unspecified organism) A41.9
- with
  - organ dysfunction (acute) (multiple) R65.20
    - with septic shock R65.21
- actinomycotic A42.7
- adrenal hemorrhage syndrome (meningococcal) A39.1
- anaerobic A41.4
- Bacillus anthracis A22.7
- Brucella -*see also* Brucellosis A23.9
- candidal B37.7
- cryptogenic A41.9
- due to device, implant or graft T85.79
  - arterial graft NEC T82.7
  - breast (implant) T85.79
  - catheter NEC T85.79
    - dialysis (renal) T82.7
      - intraperitoneal T85.71
    - infusion NEC T82.7
      - spinal (cranial) (epidural) (intrathecal) (spinal) (subarachnoid) (subdural) T85.735
    - urethral indwelling T83.511
    - urinary T83.518
  - ectopic or molar pregnancy O08.82
  - electronic (electrode) (pulse generator) (stimulator)
    - bone T84.7
    - cardiac T82.7
    - nervous system T85.738
      - brain T85.731
      - neurostimulator generator T85.734
      - peripheral nerve T85.732
      - spinal cord T85.733
    - urinary T83.590
  - fixation, internal (orthopedic) -*see* Complication, fixation device, infection
  - gastrointestinal (bile duct) (esophagus) T85.79
    - neurostimulator electrode (lead) T85.732
  - genital T83.69
  - heart NEC T82.7
    - valve (prosthesis) T82.6
      - graft T82.7
  - joint prosthesis -*see* Complication, joint prosthesis, infection
  - ocular (corneal graft) (orbital implant) T85.79
  - orthopedic NEC T84.7
    - fixation device, internal -*see* Complication, fixation device, infection
  - specified NEC T85.79
  - vascular T82.7
  - ventricular intracranial (communicating) shunt T85.730
- during labor O75.3
- Enterococcus A41.81
- Erysipelothrix (rhusiopathiae) (erysipeloid) A26.7
- Escherichia coli (E. coli) A41.5
- extraintestinal yersiniosis A28.2
- following
  - abortion (subsequent episode) O08.0
    - current episode -*see* Abortion
  - ectopic or molar pregnancy O08.82
  - immunization T88.0
  - infusion, therapeutic injection or transfusion NEC T80.29
- gangrenous A41.9
- gonococcal A54.86

Sepsis --*continued*
  Gram-negative (organism) A41.5
    anaerobic A41.4
  Haemophilus influenzae A41.3
  herpesviral B00.7
  intra-abdominal K65.1
  intraocular -*see* Endophthalmitis, purulent
  Listeria monocytogenes A32.7
  localized - code to specific localized infection
    in operation wound T81.49
    skin -*see* Abscess
  malleus A24.0
  melioidosis A24.1
  meningeal -*see* Meningitis
  meningococcal A39.4
    acute A39.2
    chronic A39.3
  MSSA (Methicillin susceptible
    Staphylococcus aureus) A41.01
  newborn P36.9
    due to
      anaerobes NEC P36.5
      Escherichia coli P36.4
      Staphylococcus P36.30
        aureus P36.2
        specified NEC P36.39
      Streptococcus P36.10
        group B P36.0
        specified NEC P36.19
    specified NEC P36.8
  Pasteurella multocida A28.0
  pelvic, puerperal, postpartum, childbirth O85
  postprocedural T81.49
  pneumococcal A40.3
  puerperal, postpartum, childbirth (pelvic) O85
  Salmonella (arizonae) (cholerae-suis)
    (enteritidis) (typhimurium) A02.1
  severe R65.20
    with septic shock R65.21
  skin, localized -*see* Abscess
  Shigella -*see also* Dysentery, bacillary A03.9
  specified organism NEC A41.89
  Staphylococcus, staphylococcal A41.2
    aureus (methicillin susceptible) (MSSA)
      A41.01
      methicillin resistant (MRSA) A41.02
    coagulase-negative A41.1
    specified NEC A41.1
  Streptococcus, streptococcal A40.9
    agalactiae A40.1
    group
      A A40.0
      B A40.1
      D A41.81
    neonatal P36.10
      group B P36.0
      specified NEC P36.19
    pneumoniae A40.3
    pyogenes A40.0
    specified NEC A40.8
  tracheostomy stoma J95.02
  tularemic A21.7
  umbilical, umbilical cord (newborn) -*see*
    Sepsis, newborn
  Yersinia pestis A20.7
Septate -*see* Septum
Septic -*see* condition
  arm -*see* Cellulitis, upper limb
    with lymphangitis -*see* Lymphangitis, acute,
    upper limb
  embolus -*see* Embolism

Septic --*continued*
  finger -*see* Cellulitis, digit
    with lymphangitis -*see* Lymphangitis, acute,
    digit
  foot -*see* Cellulitis, lower limb
    with lymphangitis -*see* Lymphangitis, acute,
    lower limb
  gallbladder (acute) K81.0
  hand -*see* Cellulitis, upper limb
    with lymphangitis -*see* Lymphangitis, acute,
    upper limb
  joint -*see* Arthritis, pyogenic or pyemic
  leg -*see* Cellulitis, lower limb
    with lymphangitis -*see* Lymphangitis, acute,
    lower limb
  nail -*see also* Cellulitis, digit
    with lymphangitis -*see* Lymphangitis, acute,
    digit
  sore -*see also* Abscess
    throat J02.0
      streptococcal J02.0
  spleen (acute) D73.89
  teeth, tooth (pulpal origin) K04.4
  throat -*see* Pharyngitis
  thrombus -*see* Thrombosis
  toe -*see* Cellulitis, digit
    with lymphangitis -*see* Lymphangitis, acute,
    digit
  tonsils, chronic J35.01
    with adenoiditis J35.03
  uterus -*see* Endometritis
Septicemia A41.9
  meaning sepsis -*see* Sepsis
Septum, septate (congenital) -*see also*
  Anomaly, by site
  anal Q42.3
    with fistula Q42.2
  aqueduct of Sylvius Q03.0
    with spina bifida -*see* Spina bifida, by site,
    with hydrocephalus
  uterus (complete) (partial) Q51.2
  vagina Q52.10
    in pregnancy -*see* Pregnancy, complicated
    by, abnormal vagina
      causing obstructed labor O65.5
    longitudinal Q52.129
      microperforate
        left side Q52.124
        right side Q52.123
      nonobstruction Q52.120
      obstructing Q52.129
        left side Q52.122
        right side Q52.121
    transverse Q52.11
Sequelae (of) -*see also* condition
  abscess, intracranial or intraspinal (conditions
    in G06) G09
  amputation - code to injury with seventh
    character S
  burn and corrosion - code to injury with
    seventh character S
  calcium deficiency E64.8
  cerebrovascular disease -*see* Sequelae,
    disease, cerebrovascular
  childbirth O94
  contusion - code to injury with seventh
    character S
  corrosion -*see* Sequelae, burn and corrosion
  crushing injury - code to injury with seventh
    character S
  disease

Sequelae (of) --*continued*
  cerebrovascular I69.90
    alteration of sensation I69.998
    aphasia I69.920
    apraxia I69.990
    ataxia I69.993
    cognitive deficits I69.91
    disturbance of vision I69.998
    dysarthria I69.922
    dysphagia I69.991
    dysphasia I69.921
    facial droop I69.992
    facial weakness I69.992
    fluency disorder I69.923
    hemiplegia I69.95
    hemorrhage
      intracerebral -*see* Sequelae, hemorrhage,
        intracerebral
      intracranial, nontraumatic NEC -*see*
        Sequelae, hemorrhage, intracranial,
        nontraumatic
      subarachnoid -*see* Sequelae, hemorrhage,
        subarachnoid
    language deficit I69.928
    monoplegia
      lower limb I69.84
      upper limb I69.93
    paralytic syndrome I69.96
    specified effect NEC I69.998
    specified type NEC I69.80
      alteration of sensation I69.898
      aphasia I69.820
      apraxia I69.890
      ataxia I69.893
      cognitive deficits I69.81
      disturbance of vision I69.898
      dysarthria I69.822
      dysphagia I69.891
      dysphasia I69.821
      facial droop I69.892
      facial weakness I69.892
      fluency disorder I69.823
      hemiplegia I69.85
      language deficit I69.828
      monoplegia
        lower limb I69.84
        upper limb I69.83
      paralytic syndrome I69.86
      specified effect NEC I69.898
      speech deficit I69.928
        speech deficit I69.828
      stroke NOS -*see* Sequelae, stroke NOS
  dislocation - code to injury with seventh
    character S
  encephalitis or encephalomyelitis (conditions
    in G04) G09
    in infectious disease NEC B94.8
    viral B94.1
  external cause - code to injury with seventh
    character S
  foreign body entering natural orifice - code to
    injury with seventh character S
  fracture - code to injury with seventh
    character S
  frostbite - code to injury with seventh
    character S
  Hansen's disease B92
  hemorrhage
    intracerebral I69.10
      alteration of sensation I69.198
      aphasia I69.120

Sequelae (of) --*continued*
- apraxia I69.190
- ataxia I69.193
- cognitive deficits I69.11
- disturbance of vision I69.198
- dysarthria I69.122
- dysphagia I69.191
- dysphasia I69.121
- facial droop I69.192
- facial weakness I69.192
- fluency disorder I69.123
- hemiplegia I69.15
- language deficit NEC I69.128
- monoplegia
  - lower limb I69.14
  - upper limb I69.13
- paralytic syndrome I69.16
- specified effect NEC I69.198
- speech deficit NEC I69.128
- intracranial, nontraumatic NEC I69.20
  - alteration of sensation I69.298
  - aphasia I69.220
  - apraxia I69.290
  - ataxia I69.293
  - cognitive deficits I69.21
  - disturbance of vision I69.298
  - dysarthria I69.222
  - dysphagia I69.291
  - dysphasia I69.221
  - facial droop I69.292
  - facial weakness I69.292
  - fluency disorder I69.223
  - hemiplegia I69.25
  - language deficit NEC I69.228
  - monoplegia
    - lower limb I69.24
    - upper limb I69.23
  - paralytic syndrome I69.26
  - specified effect NEC I69.298
  - speech deficit NEC I69.228
  - subarachnoid I69.00
    - alteration of sensation I69.098
    - aphasia I69.020
    - apraxia I69.090
    - ataxia I69.093
    - cognitive deficits -*see* subcategory I69.01
    - disturbance of vision I69.098
    - dysarthria I69.022
    - dysphagia I69.091
    - dysphasia I69.021
    - facial droop I69.092
    - facial weakness I69.092
    - fluency disorder I69.023
    - hemiplegia I69.05
    - language deficit NEC I69.028
    - monoplegia
      - lower limb I69.04
      - upper limb I69.03
    - paralytic syndrome I69.06
    - specified effect NEC I69.098
    - speech deficit NEC I69.028
- hepatitis, viral B94.2
- hyperalimentation E68
- infarction
  - cerebral I69.30
    - alteration of sensation I69.398
    - aphasia I69.320
    - apraxia I69.390
    - ataxia I69.393
    - cognitive deficits I69.31
    - disturbance of vision I69.398

Sequelae (of) --*continued*
- dysarthria I69.322
- dysphagia I69.391
- dysphasia I69.321
- facial droop I69.392
- facial weakness I69.392
- fluency disorder I69.323
- hemiplegia I69.35
- language deficit NEC I69.328
- monoplegia
  - lower limb I69.34
  - upper limb I69.33
- paralytic syndrome I69.36
- specified effect NEC I69.398
- speech deficit NEC I69.328
- infection, pyogenic, intracranial or intraspinal G09
- infectious disease B94.9
  - specified NEC B94.8
- injury - code to injury with seventh character S
- leprosy B92
- meningitis
  - bacterial (conditions in G00) G09
  - other or unspecified cause (conditions in G03) G09
- muscle (and tendon) injury - code to injury with seventh character S
- myelitis -*see* Sequelae, encephalitis
- niacin deficiency E64.8
- nutritional deficiency E64.9
  - specified NEC E64.8
- obstetrical condition O94
- parasitic disease B94.9
- phlebitis or thrombophlebitis of intracranial or intraspinal venous sinuses and veins (conditions in G08) G09
- poisoning - code to poisoning with seventh character S
  - nonmedicinal substance -*see* Sequelae, toxic effect, nonmedicinal substance
- poliomyelitis (acute) B91
- pregnancy O94
- protein-energy malnutrition E64.0
- puerperium O94
- rickets E64.3
- selenium deficiency E64.8
- sprain and strain - code to injury with seventh character S
- stroke NOS I69.30
  - alteration in sensation I69.398
  - aphasia I69.320
  - apraxia I69.390
  - ataxia I69.393
  - cognitive deficits I69.31
  - disturbance of vision I69.398
  - dysarthria I69.322
  - dysphagia I69.391
  - dysphasia I69.321
  - facial droop I69.392
  - facial weakness I69.392
  - hemiplegia I69.35
  - language deficit NEC I69.328
  - monoplegia
    - lower limb I69.34
    - upper limb I69.33
  - paralytic syndrome I69.36
  - specified effect NEC I69.398
  - speech deficit NEC I69.328
- tendon and muscle injury - code to injury with seventh character S

Sequelae (of) --*continued*
- thiamine deficiency E64.8
- trachoma B94.0
- tuberculosis B90.9
  - bones and joints B90.2
  - central nervous system B90.0
  - genitourinary B90.1
  - pulmonary (respiratory) B90.9
  - specified organs NEC B90.8
- viral
  - encephalitis B94.1
  - hepatitis B94.2
- vitamin deficiency NEC E64.8
  - A E64.1
  - B E64.8
  - C E64.2
- wound, open - code to injury with seventh character S

Sequestration -*see also* Sequestrum
- disk -*see* Displacement, intervertebral disk
- lung, congenital Q33.2

Sequestrum
- bone -*see* Osteomyelitis, chronic
- dental M27.2
- jaw bone M27.2
- orbit -*see* Osteomyelitis, orbit
- sinus (accessory) (nasal) -*see* Sinusitis

Sequoiosis lung or pneumonitis J67.8

Serology for syphilis
- doubtful
  - with signs or symptoms
  - code by site and stage under Syphilis
    - follow-up of latent syphilis -*see* Syphilis, latent
- negative, with signs or symptoms
  - code by site and stage under Syphilis
- positive A53.0
  - with signs or symptoms
  - code by site and stage under Syphilis
- reactivated A53.0

Seroma -*see also* Hematoma
- postprocedural -*see* Complication, postprocedural, seroma
- traumatic, secondary and recurrent T79.2

Seropurulent -*see* condition

Serositis, multiple K65.8
- pericardial I31.1
- peritoneal K65.8

Serous -*see* condition

Sertoli cell
- adenoma
  - specified site -*see* Neoplasm, benign, by site
  - unspecified site
    - female D27.9
    - male D29.20
- carcinoma
  - specified site -*see* Neoplasm, malignant, by site
  - unspecified site (male) C62.9
    - female C56.9
- tumor
  - with lipid storage
    - specified site -*see* Neoplasm, benign, by site
    - unspecified site
      - female D27.9
      - male D29.20
  - specified site -*see* Neoplasm, benign, by site
  - unspecified site
    - female D27.9
    - male D29.20

Sertoli-Leydig cell tumor -*see* Neoplasm,
  benign, by site
  specified site -*see* Neoplasm, benign, by site
  unspecified site
    female D27.9
    male D29.20
Serum
  allergy, allergic reaction -*see also* Reaction,
    serum T80.69
    shock -*see also* Shock, anaphylactic T80.59
  arthritis -*see also* Reaction, serum T80.69
  complication or reaction NEC -*see also*
    Reaction, serum T80.69
  disease NEC -*see also* Reaction, serum
    T80.69
  hepatitis -*see also* Hepatitis, viral, type B
    carrier (suspected) of B18.1
  intoxication -*see also* Reaction, serum T80.69
  neuritis -*see also* Reaction, serum T80.69
  neuropathy G61.1
  poisoning NEC -*see also* Reaction, serum
    T80.69
  rash NEC -*see also* Reaction, serum T80.69
  reaction NEC -*see also* Reaction, serum
    T80.69
  sickness NEC -*see also* Reaction, serum
    T80.69
  urticaria -*see also* Reaction, serum T80.69
Sesamoiditis M25.8
Sever's disease or osteochondrosis -*see*
  Osteochondrosis, juvenile, tarsus
Severe sepsis R65.20
  with septic shock R65.21
Sex
  chromosome mosaics Q97.8
    lines with various numbers of X
      chromosomes Q97.2
  education Z70.8
  reassignment surgery status Z87.890
Sextuplet pregnancy -*see* Pregnancy, sextuplet
Sexual
  function, disorder of (psychogenic) F52.9
  immaturity (female) (male) E30.0
  impotence (psychogenic) organic origin NEC
    -*see* Dysfunction, sexual, male
  precocity (constitutional)
    (cryptogenic)(female) (idiopathic) (male)
    E30.1
Sexuality, pathologic -*see* Deviation, sexual
Sézary disease C84.1
Shadow, lung R91.8
Shaking palsy or paralysis -*see* Parkinsonism
Shallowness, acetabulum -*see* Derangement,
  joint, specified type NEC, hip
Shaver's disease J63.1
Sheath (tendon) -*see* condition
Sheathing, retinal vessels H35.01
Shedding
  nail L60.8
  premature, primary (deciduous) teeth K00.6
Sheehan's disease or syndrome E23.0
Shelf, rectal K62.89
Shell teeth K00.5
Shellshock (current) F43.0
  lasting state -*see* Disorder, post-traumatic
    stress
Shield kidney Q63.1
Shift
  auditory threshold (temporary) H93.24
  mediastinal R93.8

**Shifting sleep-work schedule (affecting
  sleep)** G47.26
Shiga (Kruse) dysentery A03.0
Shiga's bacillus A03.0
Shigella (dysentery) -*see* Dysentery, bacillary
Shigellosis A03.9
  Group A A03.0
  Group B A03.1
  Group C A03.2
  Group D A03.3
Shin splints S86.89
Shingles -*see* Herpes, zoster
Shipyard disease or eye B30.0
Shirodkar suture, in pregnancy -*see*
  Pregnancy, complicated by, incompetent
  cervix
Shock R57.9
  with ectopic or molar pregnancy O08.3
  adrenal (cortical) (Addisonian) E27.2
  adverse food reaction (anaphylactic) -*see*
    Shock, anaphylactic, due to food
  allergic -*see* Shock, anaphylactic
  anaphylactic T78.2
    chemical -*see* Table of Drugs and Chemicals
    due to drug or medicinal substance
      correct substance properly administered
        T88.6
      overdose or wrong substance given or
        taken (by accident) -*see* Table of Drugs
        and Chemicals, by drug, poisoning
    due to food (nonpoisonous) T78.00
      additives T78.06
      dairy products T78.07
      eggs T78.08
      fish T78.03
        shellfish T78.02
      fruit T78.04
      milk T78.07
      nuts T78.05
        multiple types T78.05
        peanuts T78.01
      peanuts T78.01
      seeds T78.05
      specified type NEC T78.09
      vegetable T78.04
    following sting(s) -*see* Venom
    immunization T80.52
    serum T80.59
      blood and blood products T80.51
      immunization T80.52
      specified NEC T80.59
      vaccination T80.52
  anaphylactoid -*see* Shock, anaphylactic
  anesthetic
    correct substance properly administered
      T88.2
    overdose or wrong substance given or taken
      -*see* Table of Drugs and Chemicals, by drug,
      poisoning
      specified anesthetic -*see* Table of Drugs
        and Chemicals, by drug, poisoning
  cardiogenic R57.0
  chemical substance -*see* Table of Drugs and
    Chemicals
  complicating ectopic or molar pregnancy
    O08.3
  culture -*see* Disorder, adjustment
  drug
    due to correct substance properly
      administered T88.6

Shock --*continued*
  overdose or wrong substance given or taken
    (by accident) -*see* Table of Drugs and
    Chemicals, by drug, poisoning
  during or after labor and delivery O75.1
  electric T75.4
    (taser) T75.4
  endotoxic R65.21
    postprocedural (resulting from a procedure,
      not elsewhere classified) T81.12
  following
    ectopic or molar pregnancy O08.3
    injury (immediate) (delayed) T79.4
    labor and delivery O75.1
  food (anaphylactic) -*see* Shock, anaphylactic,
    due to food
  from electroshock gun (taser) T75.4
  gram-negative R65.21
    postprocedural (resulting from a procedure,
      not elsewhere classified) T81.12
  hematologic R57.8
  hemorrhagic
    surgery (intraoperative) (postoperative)
      T81.19
    trauma T79.4
  hypovolemic R57.1
    surgical T81.19
    traumatic T79.4
  insulin E15
    therapeutic misadventure - see subcategory
      T38.3
  kidney N17.0
    traumatic (following crushing) T79.5
  liver K72.00
  lightning T75.01
  lung J80
  obstetric O75.1
    with ectopic or molar pregnancy O08.3
    following ectopic or molar pregnancy O08.3
  pleural (surgical) T81.19
    due to trauma T79.4
  postprocedural (postoperative) T81.10
    with ectopic or molar pregnancy O08.3
    cardiogenic T81.11
    endotoxic T81.12
    following ectopic or molar pregnancy O08.3
    gram-negative T81.12
    hypovolemic T81.19
    septic T81.12
    specified type NEC T81.19
  psychic F43.0
  septic (due to severe sepsis) R65.21
  specified NEC R57.8
  surgical T81.10
  taser gun (taser) T75.4
  therapeutic misadventure NEC T81.10
  thyroxin
    overdose or wrong substance given or taken
      -*see* Table of Drugs and Chemicals, by drug,
      poisoning
  toxic, syndrome A48.3
  transfusion -*see* Complications, transfusion
  traumatic (immediate) (delayed) T79.4
Shoemaker's chest M95.4
Short, shortening, shortness
  arm (acquired) -*see also* Deformity, limb,
    unequal length
    congenital Q71.81
    forearm -*see* Deformity, limb, unequal
      length
  bowel syndrome K91.2

Short, shortening, shortness - *continued*
  breath R06.02
  cervical (complicating pregnancy) O26.87
    non-gravid uterus N88.3
  common bile duct, congenital Q44.5
  cord (umbilical), complicating delivery O69.3
  cystic duct, congenital Q44.5
  esophagus (congenital) Q39.8
  femur (acquired) -*see* Deformity, limb,
    unequal length, femur
    congenital -*see* Defect, reduction, lower
    limb, longitudinal, femur
  frenum, frenulum, linguae (congenital) Q38.1
  hip (acquired) -*see also* Deformity, limb,
    unequal length
    congenital Q65.89
  leg (acquired) -*see also* Deformity, limb,
    unequal length
    congenital Q72.81
    lower leg -*see also* Deformity, limb, unequal
    length
  limbed stature, with immunodeficiency D82.2
  lower limb (acquired) -*see also* Deformity,
    limb, unequal length
    congenital Q72.81
  organ or site, congenital NEC -*see* Distortion
  palate, congenital Q38.5
  radius (acquired) -*see also* Deformity, limb,
    unequal length
    congenital -*see* Defect, reduction, upper
    limb, longitudinal, radius
  rib syndrome Q77.2
  stature (child) (hereditary) (idiopathic) NEC
    R62.52
    constitutional E34.3
    due to endocrine disorder E34.3
    Laron-type E34.3
  tendon -*see also* Contraction, tendon
    with contracture of joint -*see* Contraction,
    joint
    Achilles (acquired) M67.0
      congenital Q66.89
    congenital Q79.8
  thigh (acquired) -*see also* Deformity, limb,
    unequal length, femur
    congenital -*see* Defect, reduction, lower
    limb, longitudinal, femur
  tibialis anterior (tendon) -*see* Contraction,
    tendon
  umbilical cord
    complicating delivery O69.3
  upper limb, congenital -*see* Defect, reduction,
    upper limb, specified type NEC
  urethra N36.8
  uvula, congenital Q38.5
  vagina (congenital) Q52.4
Shortsightedness -*see* Myopia
Shoshin (acute fulminating beriberi) E51.11
Shoulder -*see* condition
Shovel-shaped incisors K00.2
Shower, thromboembolic -*see* Embolism
Shunt
  arterial-venous (dialysis) Z99.2
  arteriovenous, pulmonary (acquired) I28.0
    congenital Q25.72
  cerebral ventricle (communicating) in situ
    Z98.2
  surgical, prosthetic, with complications -*see*
    Complications, cardiovascular, device or
    implant
Shutdown, renal N28.9

Shy Drager syndrome G90.3
Sialadenitis, sialadenosis (any gland)
  (chronic) (periodic) (suppurative) -*see*
  Sialoadenitis
Sialectasia K11.8
Sialidosis E77.1
Sialitis, silitis (any gland) (chronic)
  (suppurative) -*see* Sialoadenitis
Sialoadenitis (any gland) (periodic)
  (suppurative) K11.20
  acute K11.21
    recurrent K11.22
  chronic K11.23
Sialadenopathy K11.9
Sialoangitis -*see* Sialoadenitis
Sialodochitis (fibrinosa) -*see* Sialoadenitis
Sialodocholithiasis K11.5
Sialolithiasis K11.5
Sialometaplasia, necrotizing K11.8
Sialorrhea -*see also* Ptyalism
  periodic -*see* Sialoadenitis
Sialosis K11.7
Siamese twin Q89.4
Sibling rivalry Z62.891
Sicard's syndrome G52.7
Sicca syndrome M35.00
  with
    keratoconjunctivitis M35.01
    lung involvement M35.02
    myopathy M35.03
    renal tubulo-interstitial disorders M35.04
  specified organ involvement NEC M35.09
Sick R69
  or handicapped person in family Z63.79
    needing care at home Z63.6
  sinus (syndrome) I49.5
Sick-euthyroid syndrome E07.81
Sickle-cell
  anemia -*see* Disease, sickle-cell
  trait D57.3
Sicklemia -*see also* Disease, sickle-cell
  trait D57.3
Sickness
  air (travel) T75.3
  airplane T75.3
  alpine T70.29
  altitude T70.20
  Andes T70.29
  aviator's T70.29
  balloon T70.29
  car T75.3
  compressed air T70.3
  decompression T70.3
  green D50.8
  milk -*see* Poisoning, food, noxious
  motion T75.3
  mountain T70.29
    acute D75.1
  protein -*see also* Reaction, serum T80.69
  radiation T66
  roundabout (motion) T75.3
  sea T75.3
  serum NEC -*see also* Reaction, serum T80.69
  sleeping (African) B56.9
    by Trypanosoma B56.9
    brucei
      gambiense B56.0
      rhodesiense B56.1
    East African B56.1
    Gambian B56.0

Sickness - *continued*
  Rhodesian B56.1
  West African B56.0
  swing (motion) T75.3
  train (railway) (travel) T75.3
  travel (any vehicle) T75.3
Sideropenia -*see* Anemia, iron deficiency
Siderosilicosis J62.8
Siderosis (lung) J63.4
  eye (globe) -*see* Disorder, globe,
    degenerative, siderosis
Siemens' syndrome (ectodermal dysplasia)
  Q82.8
Sighing R06.89
  psychogenic F45.8
Sigmoid -*see also* condition
  flexure -*see* condition
  kidney Q63.1
Sigmoiditis -*see also* Enteritis K52.9
  infectious A09
  noninfectious K52.9
Silfversköld's syndrome Q78.9
Silicosiderosis J62.8
Silicosis, silicotic (simple) (complicated)
  J62.8
  with tuberculosis J65
Silicotuberculosis J65
Silo-fillers' disease J68.8
  bronchitis J68.0
  pneumonitis J68.0
  pulmonary edema J68.1
Silver's syndrome Q87.1
Simian malaria B53.1
Simmonds' cachexia or disease E23.0
Simons' disease or syndrome (progressive
  lipodystrophy) E88.1
Simple, simplex -*see* condition
Simulation, conscious (of illness) Z76.5
Simultanagnosia (asimultagnosia) R48.3
Sin Nombre virus disease (Hantavirus)
  (cardio) pulmonary syndrome) B33.4
Sinding-Larsen disease or osteochondrosis -
  see Osteochondrosis, juvenile, patella
Singapore hemorrhagic fever A91
Singer's node or nodule J38.2
Single
  atrium Q21.2
  coronary artery Q24.5
  umbilical artery Q27.0
  ventricle Q20.4
Singultus R06.6
  epidemicus B33.0
Sinus -*see also* Fistula
  abdominal K63.89
  arrest I45.5
  arrhythmia I49.8
  bradycardia R00.1
  branchial cleft (internal) (external) Q18.0
  coccygeal -*see* Sinus, pilonidal
  dental K04.6
  dermal (congenital) Q06.8
    with abscess Q06.8
    coccygeal, pilonidal -*see* Sinus, coccygeal
  infected, skin NEC L08.89
  marginal, ruptured or bleeding -*see*
    Hemorrhage, antepartum, specified cause
    NEC
  medial, face and neck Q18.8
  pause I45.5
  pericranii Q01.9
  pilonidal (infected) (rectum) L05.92**S**

Sinus - *continued*
with abscess L05.02
preauricular Q18.1
rectovaginal N82.3
Rokitansky Aschoff (gallbladder) K82.8
sacrococcygeal (dermoid) (infected) -*see*
    Sinus, pilonidal
tachycardia R00.0
    paroxysmal I47.1
tarsi syndrome M25.57
testis N50.89
tract (postinfective) -*see* Fistula
urachus Q64.4
Sinusitis (accessory) (chronic) (hyperplastic) (nasal) (nonpurulent) (purulent) J32.9
acute J01.90
    ethmoidal J01.20
        recurrent J01.21
    frontal J01.10
        recurrent J01.11
    involving more than one sinus, other than
        pansinusitis J01.80
            recurrent J01.81
    maxillary J01.00
        recurrent J01.01
    pansinusitis J01.40
        recurrent J01.41
    recurrent J01.91
    specified NEC J01.80
        recurrent J01.81
    sphenoidal J01.30
        recurrent J01.31
allergic -*see* Rhinitis, allergic
due to high altitude T70.1
ethmoidal J32.2
    acute J01.20
        recurrent J01.21
frontal J32.1
    acute J01.10
        recurrent J01.11
influenzal -*see* Influenza, with, respiratory
    manifestations NEC
involving more than one sinus but not
    pansinusitis J32.8
    acute J01.80
        recurrent J01.81
maxillary J32.0
    acute J01.00
        recurrent J01.01
sphenoidal J32.3
    acute J01.30
        recurrent J01.31
tuberculous, any sinus A15.8
Sinusitis-bronchiectasis-situs inversus (syndrome) (triad) Q89.3
Sipple's syndrome E31.22
Sirenomelia (syndrome) Q87.2
Siriasis T67.0
Sirkari's disease B55.0
Siti A65
Situation, psychiatric F99
Situational
disturbance (transient) -*see* Disorder,
    adjustment
    acute F43.0
maladjustment -*see* Disorder, adjustment
reaction -*see* Disorder, adjustment
    acute F43.0
Situs inversus or transversus (abdominalis) (thoracis) Q89.3

Sixth disease B08.20
due to human herpesvirus 6 B08.21
due to human herpesvirus 7 B08.22
Sjögren-Larsson syndrome Q87.1
Sjögren's syndrome or disease -*see* Sicca
syndrome
Skeletal -*see* condition
Skene's gland -*see* condition
Skenitis -*see* Urethritis
Skerljevo A65
Skevas-Zerfus disease -*see* Toxicity, venom,
marine animal, sea anemone
Skin -*see also* condition
clammy R23.1
donor -*see* Donor, skin
hidebound M35.9
Slate-dressers' or slate-miners' lung J62.8
Sleep
apnea -*see* Apnea, sleep
deprivation Z72.820
disorder or disturbance G47.9
    child F51.9
    nonorganic origin F51.9
    specified NEC G47.8
disturbance G47.9
    nonorganic origin F51.9
drunkenness F51.9
rhythm inversion G47.2
terrors F51.4
walking F51.3
    hysterical F44.89
Sleep hygiene
abuse Z72.821
inadequate Z72.821
poor Z72.821
Sleeping sickness -*see* Sickness, sleeping
Sleeplessness -*see* Insomnia
menopausal N95.1
Sleep-wake schedule disorder G47.20
Slim disease (in HIV infection) B20
Slipped, slipping
epiphysis (traumatic) -*see also*
Osteochondropathy, specified type NEC
    capital femoral (traumatic)
        acute (on chronic) S79.01
    current traumatic
    code as Fracture, by site
        upper femoral (nontraumatic) M93.00
            acute M93.01
                on chronic M93.03
            chronic M93.02
intervertebral disc -*see* Displacement,
intervertebral disc - ligature, umbilical P51.8
patella -*see* Disorder, patella, derangement
NEC
rib M89.8X8
sacroiliac joint -*see* subcategory M53.2
tendon -*see* Disorder, tendon
ulnar nerve, nontraumatic -*see* Lesion, nerve,
    ulnar
vertebra NEC -*see* Spondylolisthesis
Slocumb's syndrome E27.0
Sloughing (multiple) (phagedena) (skin) -*see
also* Gangrene
abscess -*see* Abscess
appendix K38.8
fascia -*see* Disorder, soft tissue, specified type
NEC
scrotum N50.89
tendon -*see* Disorder, tendon
transplanted organ -*see* Rejection, transplant
ulcer -*see* Ulcer, skin

Slow
feeding, newborn P92.2
flow syndrome, coronary I20.8
heart (beat) R00.1
Slowing, urinary stream R39.198
Sluder's neuralgia (syndrome) G44.89
Slurred, slurring speech R47.81
Small (ness)
for gestational age -*see* Small for dates
introitus, vagina N89.6
kidney (unknown cause) N27.9
    bilateral N27.1
    unilateral N27.0
ovary (congenital) Q50.39
pelvis
    with disproportion (fetopelvic) O33.1
        causing obstructed labor O65.1
uterus N85.8
white kidney N03.9
Small-and-light-for-dates -*see* Small for dates
Small-for-dates (infant) P05.10
with weight of
    499 grams or less P05.11
    500 749 grams P05.12
    750 999 grams P05.13
    1000 1249 grams P05.14
    1250 1499 grams P05.15
    1500 1749 grams P05.16
    1750 1999 grams P05.17
    2000 2499 grams P05.18
    2500 grams and over P05.19
specified NEC P05.19
Smallpox B03
Smearing, fecal R15.1
Smith-Lemli-Opitz syndrome E78.72
Smith's fracture S52.54
Smoker -*see* Dependence, drug, nicotine
Smoker's
bronchitis J41.0
cough J41.0
palate K13.24
throat J31.2
tongue K13.24
Smoking
passive Z77.22
Smothering spells R06.81
Snaggle teeth, tooth M26.39
Snapping
finger -*see* Trigger finger
hip -*see* Derangement, joint, specified type
NEC, hip
    involving the iliotibial band M76.3
knee -*see* Derangement, knee
    involving the iliotibial band M76.3
Sneddon-Wilkinson disease or syndrome (sub-corneal pustular dermatosis) L13.1
Sneezing (intractable) R06.7
Sniffing
cocaine
    abuse -*see* Abuse, drug, cocaine
    dependence -*see* Dependence, drug, cocaine
gasoline
    abuse -*see* Abuse, drug, inhalant
    dependence -*see* Dependence, drug, inhalant
glue (airplane)
    abuse -*see* Abuse, drug, inhalant
    drug dependence -*see* Dependence, drug,
    inhalant
Sniffles
newborn P28.89
Snoring R06.83

Snow blindness -see Photokeratitis
Snuffles (non-syphilitic) R06.5
　newborn P28.89
　syphilitic (infant) A50.05 [J99]
Social
　exclusion Z60.4
　　due to discrimination or persecution
　　　(perceived) Z60.5
　migrant Z59.0
　　acculturation difficulty Z60.3
　rejection Z60.4
　　due to discrimination or persecution Z60.5
　role conflict NEC Z73.5
　skills inadequacy NEC Z73.4
　transplantation Z60.3
Sodoku A25.0
Soemmerring's ring -see Cataract, secondary
Soft -see also condition
　nails L60.3
Softening
　bone -see Osteomalacia
　brain (necrotic) (progressive) G93.89
　　congenital Q04.8
　　embolic I63.4
　　hemorrhagic -see Hemorrhage, intracranial,
　　　intracerebral
　　occlusive I63.5
　　thrombotic I63.3
　cartilage M94.2
　　patella M22.4
　cerebellar -see Softening, brain
　cerebral -see Softening, brain
　cerebrospinal -see Softening, brain
　myocardial, heart -see Degeneration,
　　myocardial
　spinal cord G95.89
　stomach K31.89
Soldier's
　heart F45.8
　patches I31.0
Solitary
　cyst, kidney N28.1
　kidney, congenital Q60.0
Solvent abuse -see Abuse, drug, inhalant
　dependence -see Dependence, drug, inhalant
Somatization reaction, somatic reaction -see
　Disorder, somatoform
Somnambulism F51.3
　hysterical F44.89
Somnolence R40.0
　nonorganic origin F51.11
Sonne dysentery A03.3
Soor B37.0
Sore
　bed -see Ulcer, pressure, by site
　chiclero B55.1
　Delhi B55.1
　desert -see Ulcer, skin
　eye H57.1
　Lahore B55.1
　mouth K13.79
　　canker K12.0
　muscle M79.1
　Naga -see Ulcer, skin
　of skin -see Ulcer, skin
　oriental B55.1
　pressure -see Ulcer, pressure, by site
　skin L98.9
　soft A57
　throat (acute) -see also Pharyngitis

Sore --continued
　with influenza, flu, or grippe -see Influenza,
　　with, respiratory manifestations NEC
　chronic J31.2
　coxsackie (virus) B08.5
　diphtheritic A36.0
　herpesviral B00.2
　influenzal -see Influenza, with, respiratory
　　manifestations NEC
　septic J02.0
　streptococcal (ulcerative) J02.0
　viral NEC J02.8
　　coxsackie B08.5
　tropical -see Ulcer, skin
　veldt -see Ulcer, skin
Soto's syndrome (cerebral gigantism) Q87.3
South African cardiomyopathy syndrome
　I42.8
Southeast Asian hemorrhagic fever A91
Spacing
　abnormal, tooth, teeth, fully erupted M26.30
　excessive, tooth, fully erupted M26.32
Spade-like hand (congenital) Q68.1
Spading nail L60.8
　congenital Q84.6
Spanish collar N47.1
Sparganosis B70.1
Spasm(s), spastic, spasticity -see also
　condition R25.2
　accommodation -see Spasm, of
　　accommodation
　ampulla of Vater K83.4
　anus, ani (sphincter) (reflex) K59.4
　　psychogenic F45.8
　artery I73.9
　　cerebral G45.9
　Bell's G51.3
　bladder (sphincter, external or internal)
　　N32.89
　　psychogenic F45.8
　bronchus, bronchiole J98.01
　cardia K22.0
　cardiac I20.1
　carpopedal -see Tetany
　cerebral (arteries) (vascular) G45.9
　cervix, complicating delivery O62.4
　ciliary body (of accommodation) -see Spasm,
　　of accommodation
　colon -see also Irritable, bowel K58.9
　　with diarrhea K58.0
　　psychogenic F45.8
　common duct K83.8
　compulsive -see Tic
　conjugate H51.8
　coronary (artery) I20.1
　diaphragm (reflex) R06.6
　　epidemic B33.0
　　psychogenic F45.8
　duodenum K59.8
　epidemic diaphragmatic (transient) B33.0
　esophagus (diffuse) K22.4
　　psychogenic F45.8
　facial G51.3
　fallopian tube N83.8
　gastrointestinal (tract) K31.89
　　psychogenic F45.8
　glottis J38.5
　　hysterical F44.4
　　psychogenic F45.8
　　　conversion reaction F44.4

Spasm(s), spastic, spasticity --continued
　reflex through recurrent laryngeal nerve
　　J38.5
　habit -see Tic
　heart I20.1
　hemifacial (clonic) G51.3
　hourglass -see Contraction, hourglass
　hysterical F44.4
　infantile -see Epilepsy, spasms
　inferior oblique, eye H51.8
　intestinal -see also Syndrome, irritable bowel
　　K58.9
　　psychogenic F45.8
　larynx, laryngeal J38.5
　　hysterical F44.4
　　psychogenic F45.8
　　　conversion reaction F44.4
　levator palpebrae superioris -see Disorder,
　　eyelid function
　muscle NEC M62.838
　　back M62.830
　nerve, trigeminal G51.0
　nervous F45.8
　nodding F98.4
　occupational F48.8
　oculogyric H51.8
　　psychogenic F45.8
　of accommodation H52.53
　ophthalmic artery -see Occlusion, artery,
　　retina
　perineal, female N94.89
　peroneo-extensor -see also Deformity, limb,
　　flat foot
　pharynx (reflex) J39.2
　　hysterical F45.8
　　psychogenic F45.8
　psychogenic F45.8
　pylorus NEC K31.3
　　adult hypertrophic K31.89
　　congenital or infantile Q40.0
　　psychogenic F45.8
　rectum (sphincter) K59.4
　　psychogenic F45.8
　retinal (artery) -see Occlusion, artery, retina
　sigmoid -see also Syndrome, irritable bowel
　　K58.9
　　psychogenic F45.8
　sphincter of Oddi K83.4
　stomach K31.89
　　neurotic F45.8
　throat J39.2
　　hysterical F45.8
　　psychogenic F45.8
　tic F95.9
　　chronic F95.1
　　transient of childhood F95.0
　tongue K14.8
　torsion (progressive) G24.1
　trigeminal nerve -see Neuralgia, trigeminal
　ureter N13.5
　urethra (sphincter) N35.9
　uterus N85.8
　　complicating labor O62.4
　vagina N94.2
　　psychogenic F52.5
　vascular I73.9
　vasomotor I73.9
　vein NEC I87.8
　viscera -see Pain, abdominal
Spasmodic -see condition
Spasmophilia -see Tetany

Spasmus nutans F98.4
Spastic, spasticity -see also Spasm
  child (cerebral) (congenital) (paralysis) G80.1
Speaker's throat R49.8
Specific, specified -see condition
Speech
  defect, disorder, disturbance, impediment
  R47.9
    psychogenic, in childhood and adolescence
    F98.8
      slurring R47.81
      specified NEC R47.89
Spencer's disease A08.19
Spens' syndrome (syncope with heart block)
  I45.9
Sperm counts (fertility testing) Z31.41
  postvasectomy Z30.8
  reversal Z31.42
Spermatic cord -see condition
Spermatocele N43.40
  congenital Q55.4
  multiple N43.42
  single N43.41
Spermatocystitis N49.0
Spermatocytoma C62.9
  specified site -see Neoplasm, malignant, by
  site
Spermatorrhea N50.89
Sphacelus -see Gangrene
Sphenoidal -see condition
Sphenoiditis (chronic) -see Sinusitis,
  sphenoidal
Sphenopalatine ganglion neuralgia G90.09
Sphericity, increased, lens (congenital) Q12.4
Spherocytosis (congenital) (familial)
  (hereditary) D58.0
  hemoglobin disease D58.0
  sickle-cell (disease) D57.8
Spherophakia Q12.4
Sphincter -see condition
Sphincteritis, sphincter of Oddi -see
  Cholangitis
Sphingolipidosis E75.3
  specified NEC E75.29
Sphingomyelinosis E75.3
Spicule tooth K00.2
Spider
  bite -see Toxicity, venom, spider
  fingers -see Syndrome, Marfan's
  nevus I78.1
  toes -see Syndrome, Marfan's
  vascular I78.1
Spiegler-Fendt
  benign lymphocytoma L98.8
  sarcoid L08.89
Spielmeyer-Vogt disease E75.4
Spina bifida (aperta) Q05.9
  with hydrocephalus NEC Q05.4
  cervical Q05.5
    with hydrocephalus Q05.0
  dorsal Q05.6
    with hydrocephalus Q05.1
  lumbar Q05.7
    with hydrocephalus Q05.2
  lumbosacral Q05.7
    with hydrocephalus Q05.2
  occulta Q76.0
  sacral Q05.8
    with hydrocephalus Q05.3
  thoracic Q05.6
    with hydrocephalus Q05.1
  thoracolumbar Q05.6
    with hydrocephalus Q05.1

Spindle, Krukenberg's -see Pigmentation,
  cornea, posterior
Spine, spinal -see condition
Spiradenoma (eccrine) -see Neoplasm, skin,
  benign
Spirillosis A25.0
Spirillum
  minus A25.0
  obermeieri infection A68.0
Spirochetal -see condition
Spirochetosis A69.9
  arthritic, arthritica A69.9
  bronchopulmonary A69.8
  icterohemorrhagic A27.0
  lung A69.8
Spirometrosis B70.1
Spitting blood -see Hemoptysis
Splanchnoptosis K63.4
Spleen, splenic -see condition
Splenectasis -see Splenomegaly
Splenitis (interstitial) (malignant)
  (nonspecific) D73.89
  malarial -see also Malaria B54 [D77]
  tuberculous A18.85
Splenocele D73.89
Splenomegaly, splenomegalia (Bengal)
  (cryptogenic) (idiopathic) (tropical) R16.1
  with hepatomegaly R16.2
  cirrhotic D73.2
  congenital Q89.09
  congestive, chronic D73.2
  Egyptian B65.1
  Gaucher's E75.22
  malarial -see also Malaria B54 [D77]
  neutropenic D73.81
  Niemann-Pick -see Niemann-Pick disease or
    syndrome
  siderotic D73.2
  syphilitic A52.79
    congenital (early) A50.08 [D77]
Splenopathy D73.9
Splenoptosis D73.89
Splenosis D73.89
Splinter -see Foreign body, superficial, by site
Split, splitting
  foot Q72.7
  hand Q71.6
  heart sounds R01.2
  lip, congenital -see Cleft, lip
  nails L60.3
  urinary stream R39.13
Spondylarthrosis -see Spondylosis
Spondylitis (chronic) -see also
  Spondylopathy, inflammatory
  ankylopoietica -see Spondylitis, ankylosing
  ankylosing (chronic) M45.9
    with lung involvement M45.9 [J99]
    cervical region M45.2
    cervicothoracic region M45.3
    juvenile M08.1
    lumbar region M45.6
    lumbosacral region M45.7
    multiple sites M45.0
    occipito-atlanto-axial region M45.1
    sacrococcygeal region M45.8
    thoracic region M45.4
    thoracolumbar region M45.5
  atrophic (ligamentous) -see Spondylitis,
    ankylosing
  deformans (chronic) -see Spondylosis
  gonococcal A54.41

Spondylitis - continued
  gouty -see also Gout, by type, vertebrae
  M10.08
  in (due to)
    brucellosis A23.9 [M49.80]
      cervical region A23.9 [M49.82]
      cervicothoracic region A23.9 [M49.83]
      lumbar region A23.9 [M49.86]
      lumbosacral region A23.9 [M49.87]
      multiple sites A23.9 [M49.89]
      occipito-atlanto-axial region A23.9
        [M49.81]
      sacrococcygeal region A23.9 [M49.88]
      thoracic region A23.9 [M49.84]
      thoracolumbar region A23.9 [M49.85]
    enterobacteria -see also subcategory M49.8
      A04.9
    tuberculosis A18.01
  infectious NEC -see Spondylopathy, infective
  juvenile ankylosing (chronic) M08.1
  Kümmell's -see Spondylopathy, traumatic
  Marie-Strümpell -see Spondylitis, ankylosing
  muscularis -see Spondylopathy, specified
    NEC
  psoriatic L40.53
  rheumatoid -see Spondylitis, ankylosing
  rhizomelica -see Spondylitis, ankylosing
  sacroiliac NEC M46.1
  senescent, senile -see Spondylosis
  traumatic (chronic) or post-traumatic -see
    Spondylopathy, traumatic
  tuberculous A18.01
  typhosa A01.05
Spondylolisthesis (acquired) (degenerative)
  M43.10
  with disproportion (fetopelvic) O33.0
    causing obstructed labor O65.0
  cervical region M43.12
  cervicothoracic region M43.13
  congenital Q76.2
  lumbar region M43.16
  lumbosacral region M43.17
  multiple sites M43.19
  occipito-atlanto-axial region M43.11
  sacrococcygeal region M43.18
  thoracic region M43.14
  thoracolumbar region M43.15
  traumatic (old) M43.10
    acute
      fifth cervical (displaced) S12.430
        nondisplaced S12.431
        specified type NEC (displaced) S12.450
          nondisplaced S12.451
        type III S12.44
      fourth cervical (displaced) S12.330
        nondisplaced S12.331
        specified type NEC (displaced) S12.350
          nondisplaced S12.351
        type III S12.34
      second cervical (displaced) S12.130
        nondisplaced S12.131
        specified type NEC (displaced) S12.150
          nondisplaced S12.151
        type III S12.14
      seventh cervical (displaced) S12.630
        nondisplaced S12.631
        specified type NEC (displaced) S12.650
          nondisplaced S12.651
        type III S12.64
      sixth cervical (displaced) S12.530
        nondisplaced S12.531

Spondylolisthesis - *continued*
    specified type NEC (displaced) S12.550
      nondisplaced S12.551
      type III S12.54
   third cervical (displaced) S12.230
    nondisplaced S12.231
    specified type NEC (displaced) S12.250
      nondisplaced S12.251
      type III S12.24
Spondylolysis (acquired) M43.00
  cervical region M43.02
  cervicothoracic region M43.03
  congenital Q76.2
  lumbar region M43.06
  lumbosacral region M43.07
   with disproportion (fetopelvic) O33.0
    causing obstructed labor O65.8
  multiple sites M43.09
  occipito-atlanto-axial region M43.01
  sacrococcygeal region M43.08
  thoracic region M43.04
  thoracolumbar region M43.05
Spondylopathy M48.9
  infective NEC M46.50
   cervical region M46.52
   cervicothoracic region M46.53
   lumbar region M46.56
   lumbosacral region M46.57
   multiple sites M46.59
   occipito-atlanto-axial region M46.51
   sacrococcygeal region M46.58
   thoracic region M46.54
   thoracolumbar region M46.55
  inflammatory M46.90
   cervical region M46.92
   cervicothoracic region M46.93
   lumbar region M46.96
   lumbosacral region M46.97
   multiple sites M46.99
   occipito-atlanto-axial region M46.91
   sacrococcygeal region M46.98
  specified type NEC M46.80
   cervical region M46.82
   cervicothoracic region M46.83
   lumbar region M46.86
   lumbosacral region M46.87
   multiple sites M46.89
   occipito-atlanto-axial region M46.81
   sacrococcygeal region M46.88
   thoracic region M46.84
   thoracolumbar region M46.85
  thoracic region M46.94
  thoracolumbar region M46.95
 neuropathic, in
  syringomyelia and syringobulbia G95.0
  tabes dorsalis A52.11
 specified NEC -*see* subcategory M48.8
 traumatic M48.30
  cervical region M48.32
  cervicothoracic region M48.33
  lumbar region M48.36
  lumbosacral region M48.37
  occipito-atlanto-axial region M48.31
  sacrococcygeal region M48.38
  thoracic region M48.34
  thoracolumbar region M48.35
Spondylosis M47.9
 with
  disproportion (fetopelvic) O33.0
   causing obstructed labor O65.0
  myelopathy NEC M47.10

Spondylosis - *continued*
  cervical region M47.12
  cervicothoracic region M47.13
  lumbar region M47.16
  occipito-atlanto-axial region M47.11
  thoracic region M47.14
  thoracolumbar region M47.15
 radiculopathy M47.20
  cervical region M47.22
  cervicothoracic region M47.23
  lumbar region M47.26
  lumbosacral region M47.27
  occipito-atlanto-axial region M47.21
  sacrococcygeal region M47.28
  thoracic region M47.24
  thoracolumbar region M47.25
 specified NEC M47.899
  cervical region M47.892
  cervicothoracic region M47.893
  lumbar region M47.896
  lumbosacral region M47.897
  occipito-atlanto-axial region M47.891
  sacrococcygeal region M47.898
  thoracic region M47.894
  thoracolumbar region M47.895
 traumatic -*see* Spondylopathy, traumatic
 without myelopathy or radiculopathy
  M47.819
  cervical region M47.812
  cervicothoracic region M47.813
  lumbar region M47.816
  lumbosacral region M47.817
  occipito-atlanto-axial region M47.811
  sacrococcygeal region M47.818
  thoracic region M47.814
  thoracolumbar region M47.815
Sponge
 inadvertently left in operation wound -*see*
 Foreign body, accidentally left during a
 procedure
  kidney (medullary) Q61.5
Sponge-diver's disease -*see* Toxicity, venom,
 marine animal, sea anemone
Spongioblastoma (any type) -*see* Neoplasm,
 malignant, by site
 specified site -*see* Neoplasm, malignant, by
 site
 unspecified site C71.9
Spongioneuroblastoma -*see* Neoplasm,
 malignant, by site
Spontaneous -*see also* condition
 fracture (cause unknown) -*see* Fracture,
 pathological **S**
poon nail L60.3
 congenital Q84.6
Sporadic -*see* condition
Sporothrix schenckii infection -*see*
 Sporotrichosis
Sporotrichosis B42.9
 arthritis B42.82
 disseminated B42.7
 generalized B42.7
 lymphocutaneous (fixed) (progressive) B42.1
 pulmonary B42.0
 specified NEC B42.89
Spots, spotting (in) (of)
 Bitot's -*see also* Pigmentation, conjunctiva
  in the young child E50.1
  vitamin A deficiency E50.1
 café, au lait L81.3
 Cayenne pepper I78.1

Spots, spotting --*continued*
 cotton wool, retina -*see* Occlusion, artery,
  retina
 de Morgan's (senile angiomas) I78.1
 Fuchs' black (myopic) H44.2
 intermenstrual (regular) N92.0
  irregular N92.1
 Koplik's B05.9
 liver L81.4
 pregnancy O26.85
 purpuric R23.3
 ruby I78.1
Spotted fever -*see* Fever, spotted N92.3
Sprain (joint) (ligament)
 acromioclavicular joint or ligament S43.5
 ankle S93.40
  calcaneofibular ligament S93.41
  deltoid ligament S93.42
  internal collateral ligament -*see* Sprain,
   ankle, specified ligament NEC
  specified ligament NEC S93.49
  talofibular ligament -*see* Sprain, ankle,
   specified ligament NEC
  tibiofibular ligament S93.43
 anterior longitudinal, cervical S13.4
 atlas, atlanto-axial, atlanto-occipital S13.4
 breast bone -*see* Sprain, sternum
 calcaneofibular -*see* Sprain, ankle
 carpal -*see* Sprain, wrist
 carpometacarpal -*see* Sprain, hand, specified
  site NEC
 cartilage
  costal S23.41
  semilunar (knee) -*see* Sprain, knee, specified
  site NEC
   with current tear -*see* Tear, meniscus
  thyroid region S13.5
  xiphoid -*see* Sprain, sternum
 cervical, cervicodorsal, cervicothoracic S13.4
 chondrosternal S23.421
 coracoclavicular S43.8
 coracohumeral S43.41
 coronary, knee -*see* Sprain, knee, specified
  site NEC
 costal cartilage S23.41
 cricoarytenoid articulation or ligament S13.5
 cricothyroid articulation S13.5
 cruciate, knee -*see* Sprain, knee, cruciate
 deltoid, ankle -*see* Sprain, ankle
 dorsal (spine) S23.3
 elbow S53.40
  radial collateral ligament S53.43
  radiohumeral S53.41
  rupture
   radial collateral ligament -*see* Rupture,
    traumatic, ligament, radial collateral
   ulnar collateral ligament -*see* Rupture,
    traumatic, ligament, ulnar collateral
  specified type NEC S53.49
  ulnar collateral ligament S53.44
  ulnohumeral S53.42
 femur, head -*see* Sprain, hip
 fibular collateral, knee -*see* Sprain, knee,
  collateral
 fibulocalcaneal -*see* Sprain, ankle
 finger(s) S63.61
  index S63.61
  interphalangeal (joint) S63.63
   index S63.63
   little S63.63
   middle S63.63

Sprain - *continued*
- ring S63.63
- little S63.61
- middle S63.61
- ring S63.61
- metacarpophalangeal (joint) S63.65
- specified site NEC S63.69
  - index S63.69
  - little S63.69
  - middle S63.69
  - ring S63.69
- foot S93.60
  - specified ligament NEC S93.69
  - tarsal ligament S93.61
  - tarsometatarsal ligament S93.62
  - toe -*see* Sprain, toe
- hand S63.9
  - finger -*see* Sprain, finger
  - specified site NEC -*see* subcategory S63.8
  - thumb -*see* Sprain, thumb
- head S03.9
- hip S73.10
  - iliofemoral ligament S73.11
  - ischiocapsular (ligament) S73.12
  - specified NEC S73.19
- iliofemoral -*see* Sprain, hip
- innominate
  - acetabulum -*see* Sprain, hip
  - sacral junction S33.6
- internal
  - collateral, ankle -*see* Sprain, ankle
  - semilunar cartilage -*see* Sprain, knee, specified site NEC
- interphalangeal
  - finger -*see* Sprain, finger, interphalangeal (joint)
  - toe -*see* Sprain, toe, interphalangeal joint
- ischiocapsular -*see* Sprain, hip
- ischiofemoral -*see* Sprain, hip
- jaw (articular disc) (cartilage) (meniscus) S03.4
  - old M26.69
- knee S83.9
  - collateral ligament S83.40
    - lateral (fibular) S83.42
    - medial (tibial) S83.41
  - cruciate ligament S83.50
    - anterior S83.51
    - posterior S83.52
  - lateral (fibular) collateral ligament S83.42
  - medial (tibial) collateral ligament S83.41
  - patellar ligament S76.11
  - specified site NEC S83.8X
  - superior tibiofibular joint (ligament) S83.6
- lateral collateral, knee -*see* Sprain, knee, collateral
- lumbar (spine) S33.5
- lumbosacral S33.9
- mandible (articular disc) S03.4
  - old M26.69
- medial collateral, knee -*see* Sprain, knee, collateral
- meniscus
  - jaw S03.4
    - old M26.69
  - knee -*see* Sprain, knee, specified site NEC
    - with current tear -*see* Tear, meniscus
      - old -*see* Derangement, knee, meniscus, due to old tear
  - mandible S03.4
    - old M26.69

Sprain - *continued*
- metacarpal (distal) (proximal) -*see* Sprain, hand, specified site NEC
- metacarpophalangeal -*see* Sprain, finger, metacarpophalangeal (joint)
- metatarsophalangeal -*see* Sprain, toe, metatarsophalangeal joint
- midcarpal -*see* Sprain, hand, specified site NEC
- midtarsal -*see* Sprain, foot, specified site NEC
- neck S13.9
  - anterior longitudinal cervical ligament S13.4
  - atlanto-axial joint S13.4
  - atlanto-occipital joint S13.4
  - cervical spine S13.4
  - cricoarytenoid ligament S13.5
  - cricothyroid ligament S13.5
  - specified site NEC S13.8
  - thyroid region (cartilage) S13.5
- nose S03.8
- orbicular, hip -*see* Sprain, hip
- patella -*see* Sprain, knee, specified site NEC
- patellar ligament S76.11
- pelvis NEC S33.8
- phalanx
  - finger -*see* Sprain, finger
  - toe -*see* Sprain, toe
- pubofemoral -*see* Sprain, hip
- radiocarpal -*see* Sprain, wrist
- radiohumeral -*see* Sprain, elbow
- radius, collateral -*see* Rupture, traumatic, ligament, radial collateral
- rib (cage) S23.41
- rotator cuff (capsule) S43.42
- sacroiliac (region)
  - chronic or old -*see* subcategory M53.2
  - joint S33.6
- scaphoid (hand) -*see* Sprain, hand, specified site NEC
- scapula (r) -*see* Sprain, shoulder girdle, specified site NEC
- semilunar cartilage (knee) -*see* Sprain, knee, specified site NEC
  - with current tear -*see* Tear, meniscus
    - old -*see* Derangement, knee, meniscus, due to old tear
- shoulder joint S43.40
  - acromioclavicular joint (ligament) -*see* Sprain, acromioclavicular joint
  - blade -*see* Sprain, shoulder, girdle, specified site NEC
  - coracoclavicular joint (ligament) -*see* Sprain, coracoclavicular joint
  - coracohumeral ligament -*see* Sprain, coracohumeral joint
  - girdle S43.9
    - specified site NEC S43.8
  - rotator cuff -*see* Sprain, rotator cuff
  - specified site NEC S43.49
  - sternoclavicular joint (ligament) -*see* Sprain, sternoclavicular joint
- spine
  - cervical S13.4
  - lumbar S33.5
  - thoracic S23.3
- sternoclavicular joint S43.6
- sternum S23.429
  - chondrosternal joint S23.421
  - specified site NEC S23.428
  - sternoclavicular (joint) (ligament) S23.420
- symphysis

Sprain - *continued*
- jaw S03.4
  - old M26.69
- mandibular S03.4
  - old M26.69
- talofibular -*see* Sprain, ankle
- tarsal -*see* Sprain, foot, specified site NEC
- tarsometatarsal -*see* Sprain, foot, specified site NEC
- temporomandibular S03.4
  - old M26.69
- thorax S23.9
  - ribs S23.41
  - specified site NEC S23.8
  - spine S23.3
  - sternum -*see* Sprain, sternum
- thumb S63.60
  - interphalangeal (joint) S63.62
  - metacarpophalangeal (joint) S63.64
  - specified site NEC S63.68
- thyroid cartilage or region S13.5
- tibia (proximal end) -*see* Sprain, knee, specified site NEC
- tibial collateral, knee -*see* Sprain, knee, collateral
- tibiofibular
  - distal -*see* Sprain, ankle
  - superior -*see* Sprain, knee, specified site NEC
- toe(s) S93.50
  - great S93.50
  - interphalangeal joint S93.51
    - great S93.51
    - lesser S93.51
  - lesser S93.50
  - metatarsophalangeal joint S93.52
    - great S93.52
    - lesser S93.52
- ulna, collateral -*see* Rupture, traumatic, ligament, ulnar collateral
- ulnohumeral -*see* Sprain, elbow
- wrist S63.50
  - carpal S63.51
  - radiocarpal S63.52
  - specified site NEC S63.59
- xiphoid cartilage -*see* Sprain, sternum

Sprengel's deformity (congenital) Q74.0

Sprue (tropical) K90.1
- celiac K90.0
- idiopathic K90.49
- meaning thrush B37.0
- nontropical K90.0

Spur, bone -*see also* Enthesopathy
- calcaneal M77.3
- iliac crest M76.2
- nose (septum) J34.89

Spurway's syndrome Q78.0

Sputum
- abnormal (amount) (color) (odor) (purulent) R09.3
- blood-stained R04.2
- excessive (cause unknown) R09.3

Squamous -*see also* condition
- epithelium in
  - cervical canal (congenital) Q51.828
  - uterine mucosa (congenital) Q51.818

Squashed nose M95.0
- congenital Q67.4

Squeeze, diver's T70.3

Squint -*see also* Strabismus
- accommodative -*see* Strabismus, convergent concomitant

St. Hubert's disease A82.9
Stab -see also Laceration
  internal organs -see Injury, by site
Stafne's cyst or cavity M27.0
Staggering gait R26.0
  hysterical F44.4
Staghorn calculus -see Calculus, kidney
Stähli's line (cornea) (pigment) -see
  Pigmentation, cornea, anterior
Stain, staining
  meconium (newborn) P96.83
  port wine Q82.5
  tooth, teeth (hard tissues) (extrinsic) K03.6
    due to
      accretions K03.6
      deposits (betel) (black) (green) (materia
        alba) (orange) (soft) (tobacco) K03.6
      metals (copper) (silver) K03.7
      nicotine K03.6
      pulpal bleeding K03.7
      tobacco K03.6
    intrinsic K00.8
Stammering -see also Disorder, fluency
  F80.81
Standstill
  auricular I45.5
  cardiac -see Arrest, cardiac - sinoatrial I45.5
  ventricular -see Arrest, cardiac
Stannosis J63.5
Stanton's disease -see Melioidosis
**Staphylitis (acute) (catarrhal) (chronic)
(gangrenous) (membranous) (suppurative)
(ulcerative)** K12.2
Staphylococcal scalded skin syndrome L00
Staphylococcemia A41.2
Staphylococcus, staphylococcal -see also
  condition
  as cause of disease classified elsewhere B95.8
    aureus (methicillin susceptible) (MSSA)
      B95.61
      methicillin resistant (MRSA) B95.62
    specified NEC, as cause of disease classified
    elsewhere B95.7
Staphyloma (sclera)
  cornea H18.72
  equatorial H15.81
  localized (anterior) H15.82
  posticum H15.83
  ring H15.85
Stargardt's disease -see Dystrophy, retina
Starvation (inanition) (due to lack of food)
  T73.0
  edema -see Malnutrition, severe
Stasis
  bile (noncalculous) K83.1
  bronchus J98.09
    with infection -see Bronchitis
  cardiac -see Failure, heart, congestive
  cecum K59.8
  colon K59.8
  dermatitis I87.2
    with
      varicose ulcer -see Varix, leg, with ulcer,
        with inflammation
      varicose veins -see Varix, leg, with,
        inflammation
    due to postthrombotic syndrome -see
    Syndrome, postthrombotic
  duodenal K31.5
  eczema -see Varix, leg, with, inflammation

Stasis - continued
  edema -see Hypertension, venous (chronic),
    idiopathic
  foot T69.0
  ileocecal coil K59.8
  ileum K59.8
  intestinal K59.8
  jejunum K59.8
  kidney N19
  liver (cirrhotic) K76.1
  lymphatic I89.8
  pneumonia J18.2
  pulmonary -see Edema, lung
  rectal K59.8
  renal N19
    tubular N17.0
  ulcer -see Varix, leg, with, ulcer
    without varicose veins I87.2
  urine -see Retention, urine
  venous I87.8
State (of)
  affective and paranoid, mixed, organic
    psychotic F06.8
  agitated R45.1
    acute reaction to stress F43.0
  anxiety (neurotic) F41.1
  apprehension F41.1
  burn-out Z73.0
  climacteric, female Z78.0
    symptomatic N95.1
  compulsive F42.8
    mixed with obsessional thoughts F42.2
  confusional (psychogenic) F44.89
    acute -see also Delirium
      with
        arteriosclerotic dementia F01.50
          with behavioral disturbance F01.51
        senility or dementia F05
      alcoholic F10.231
      epileptic F05
    reactive (from emotional stress,
      psychological trauma) F44.89
    subacute -see Delirium
  convulsive -see Convulsions
  crisis F43.0
  depressive F32.9
    neurotic F34.1
  dissociative F44.9
  emotional shock (stress) R45.7
  hypercoagulation -see Hypercoagulable
  locked-in G83.5
  menopausal Z78.0
    symptomatic N95.1
  neurotic F48.9
    with depersonalization F48.1
  obsessional F42.8
  oneiroid (schizophrenia-like) F23
  organic
    hallucinatory (nonalcoholic) F06.0
    paranoid (hallucinatory) F06.2
  panic F41.0
  paranoid F22
    climacteric F22
    involutional F22
    menopausal F22
    organic F06.2
    senile F03
    simple F22
  persistent vegetative R40.3
  phobic F40.9
  postleukotomy F07.0

State (of) --continued
  pregnant
    gestational carrier Z33.3
    incidental Z33.1
  psychogenic, twilight F44.89
  psychopathic (constitutional) F60.2
  psychotic, organic -see also Psychosis,
    organic
    mixed paranoid and affective F06.8
    senile or presenile F03
    transient NEC F06.8
      with
        hallucinations F06.0
        depression F06.31
  residual schizophrenic F20.5
  restlessness R45.1
  stress (emotional) R45.7
  tension (mental) F48.9
    specified NEC F48.8
  transient organic psychotic NEC F06.8
    depressive type F06.31
    hallucinatory type F06.0
  twilight
    epileptic F05
    psychogenic F44.89
  vegetative, persistent R40.3
  vital exhaustion Z73.0
  withdrawal, -see Withdrawal, state
Status (post) -see also Presence (of)
  absence, epileptic -see Epilepsy, by type, with
    status epilepticus
  administration of tPA (rtPA) in a different
    facility within the last 24 hours prior to
    admission to current facility Z92.82
  adrenalectomy (unilateral) (bilateral) E89.6
  anastomosis Z98.0
  angioplasty (peripheral) Z98.62
    with implant Z95.820
    coronary artery Z98.61
      with implant Z95.5
  anginosus I20.9
  aortocoronary bypass Z95.1
  arthrodesis Z98.1
  artificial opening (of) Z93.9
    gastrointestinal tract Z93.4
    specified NEC Z93.8
    urinary tract Z93.6
    vagina Z93.8
  asthmaticus -see Asthma, by type, with status
    asthmaticus
  awaiting organ transplant Z76.82
  bariatric surgery Z98.84
  bed confinement Z74.01
  bleb, filtering (vitreous), after glaucoma
    surgery Z98.83
  breast implant Z98.82
    removal Z98.86
  cataract extraction Z98.4
  cholecystectomy Z90.49
  clitorectomy N90.811
    with excision of labia minora N90.812
  colectomy (complete) (partial) Z90.49
  colonization -see Carrier (suspected) of
  colostomy Z93.3
  convulsivus idiopathicus -see Epilepsy, by
    type, with status epilepticus
  coronary artery angioplasty -see Status,
    angioplasty, coronary artery
  cystectomy (urinary bladder) Z90.6
  cystostomy Z93.50
    appendico-vesicostomy Z93.52

Status - *continued*
  cutaneous Z93.51
    specified NEC Z93.59
  delinquent immunization Z28.3
  dental Z98.818
    crown Z98.811
    fillings Z98.811
    restoration Z98.811
    sealant Z98.810
    specified NEC Z98.818
  deployment (current) (military) Z56.82
  dialysis (hemodialysis) (peritoneal) Z99.2
  do not resuscitate (DNR) Z66
  donor -*see* Donor
  embedded fragments -*see* Retained, foreign
    body fragments (type of)
  embedded splinter -*see* Retained, foreign
    body fragments (type of)
  enterostomy Z93.4
  epileptic, epilepticus -*see also* Epilepsy, by
    type, with status epilepticus G40.901
  estrogen receptor
    negative Z17.1
    positive Z17.0
  female genital cutting -*see* Female genital
    mutilation status
  female genital mutilation -*see* Female genital
    mutilation status
  filtering (vitreous) bleb after glaucoma
    surgery Z98.83
  gastrectomy (complete) (partial) Z90.3
  gastric banding Z98.84
  gastric bypass for obesity Z98.84
  gastrostomy Z93.1
  human immunodeficiency virus (HIV)
    infection, asymptomatic Z21
  hysterectomy (complete) (total) Z90.710
    partial (with remaining cervical stump)
      Z90.711
  ileostomy Z93.2
  implant
    breast Z98.82
  infibulation N90.813
  intestinal bypass Z98.0
  jejunostomy Z93.4
  laryngectomy Z90.02
  lapsed immunization schedule Z28.3
  lymphaticus E32.8
  malignancy
    castrate resistant prostate Z19.2
    hormone resistant Z19.2
    hormone sensitive Z19.1
  marmoratus G80.3
  mastectomy (unilateral) (bilateral) Z90.1
  military deployment status (current) Z56.82
    in theater or in support of military war,
      peacekeeping and humanitarian operations
      Z56.82
  nephrectomy (unilateral) (bilateral) Z90.5
  nephrostomy Z93.6
  obesity surgery Z98.84
  oophorectomy
    bilateral Z90.722
    unilateral Z90.721
  organ replacement
    by artificial or mechanical device or
      prosthesis of
      artery Z95.828
      bladder Z96.0
      blood vessel Z95.828
      breast Z97.8

Status - *continued*
  eye globe Z97.0
  heart Z95.812
    valve Z95.2
  intestine Z97.8
  joint Z96.60
    hip -*see* Presence, hip joint implant
    knee -*see* Presence, knee joint implant
    specified site NEC Z96.698
  kidney Z97.8
  larynx Z96.3
  lens Z96.1
  limbs -*see* Presence, artificial, limb
  liver Z97.8
  lung Z97.8
  pancreas Z97.8
  by organ transplant
    (heterologous)(homologous) -*see* Transplant
pacemaker
  brain Z96.89
  cardiac Z95.0
  specified NEC Z96.89
pancreatectomy Z90.410
  complete Z90.410
  partial Z90.411
  total Z90.410
physical restraint Z78.1
pneumonectomy (complete) (partial) Z90.2
pneumothorax, therapeutic Z98.3
postcommotio cerebri F07.81
postoperative (postprocedural) NEC Z98.890
  breast implant Z98.82
  dental Z98.818
    crown Z98.811
    fillings Z98.811
    restoration Z98.811
    sealant Z98.810
    specified NEC Z98.818
  uterine scar Z98.891
  pneumothorax, therapeutic Z98.3
postpartum (routine follow-up) Z39.2
  care immediately after delivery Z39.0
postsurgical (postprocedural) NEC Z98.890
  pneumothorax, therapeutic Z98.3
pregnancy, incidental Z33.1
prosthesis coronary angioplasty Z95.5
pseudophakia Z96.1
renal dialysis (hemodialysis) (peritoneal)
  Z99.2
retained foreign body -*see* Retained, foreign
  body fragments (type of)
reversed jejunal transposition (for bypass)
  Z98.0
salpingo-oophorectomy
  bilateral Z90.722
  unilateral Z90.721
sex reassignment surgery status Z87.890
shunt
  arteriovenous (for dialysis) Z99.2
  cerebrospinal fluid Z98.2
  ventricular (communicating) (for drainage)
    Z98.2
splenectomy Z90.81
thymicolymphaticus E32.8
thymicus E32.8
thymolymphaticus E32.8
thyroidectomy (hypothyroidism) E89.0
tooth (teeth) extraction -*see also* Absence,
  teeth, acquired K08.409

Status - *continued*
  tPA (rtPA) administration in a different
    facility within the last 24 hours prior to
    admission to current facility Z92.82
  tracheostomy Z93.0
  transplant -*see* Transplant
    organ removed Z98.85
  tubal ligation Z98.51
  underimmunization Z28.3
  ureterostomy Z93.6
  urethrostomy Z93.6
  vagina, artificial Z93.8
  vasectomy Z98.52
  wheelchair confinement Z99.3
Stealing
  child problem F91.8
    in company with others Z72.810
  pathological (compulsive) F63.2
Steam burn -*see* Burn
Steatocystoma multiplex L72.2
Steatohepatitis (nonalcoholic) (NASH)
  K75.81
Steatoma L72.3
  eyelid (cystic) -*see* Dermatosis, eyelid
  infected -*see* Hordeolum
Steatorrhea (chronic) K90.9
  with lacteal obstruction K90.2
  idiopathic (adult) (infantile) K90.9
  pancreatic K90.3
  primary K90.0
  tropical K90.1
Steatosis E88.89
  heart -*see* Degeneration, myocardial
  kidney N28.89
  liver NEC K76.0
Steele-Richardson-Olszewski disease or
  syndrome G23.1
Steinbrocker's syndrome G90.8
Steinert's disease G71.11
Stein-Leventhal syndrome E28.2
Stein's syndrome E28.2
STEMI -*see also* - Infarct, myocardium, ST
  elevation I21.3
Stenocardia I20.8
Stenocephaly Q75.8
Stenosis, stenotic (cicatricial) -*see also*
  Stricture
  ampulla of Vater K83.1
  anus, anal (canal) (sphincter) K62.4
    and rectum K62.4
    congenital Q42.3
      with fistula Q42.2
  aorta (ascending) (supraventricular)
    (congenital) Q25.1
    arteriosclerotic I70.0
    calcified I70.0
    supravalvular Q25.3
  aortic (valve) I35.0
    with insufficiency I35.2
    congenital Q23.0
    rheumatic I06.0
      with
        incompetency, insufficiency or
        regurgitation I06.2
          with mitral (valve) disease I08.0
            with tricuspid (valve) disease I08.3
        mitral (valve) disease I08.0
          with tricuspid (valve) disease I08.3
        tricuspid (valve) disease I08.2
          with mitral (valve) disease I08.3
    specified cause NEC I35.0

Stenosis, stenotic --*continued*
  syphilitic A52.03
  aqueduct of Sylvius (congenital) Q03.0
    with spina bifida -*see* Spina bifida, by site,
      with hydrocephalus
    acquired G91.1
  artery NEC -*see also* Arteriosclerosis I77.1
    celiac I77.4
    cerebral -*see* Occlusion, artery, cerebral
    extremities -*see* Arteriosclerosis, extremities
    precerebral -*see* Occlusion, artery,
      precerebral
    pulmonary (congenital) Q25.6
      acquired I28.8
    renal I70.1
    stent
      coronary T82.855
      peripheral T82.856
  bile duct (common) (hepatic) K83.1
    congenital Q44.3
  bladder-neck (acquired) N32.0
    congenital Q64.31
  brain G93.89
  bronchus J98.09
    congenital Q32.3
    syphilitic A52.72
  cardia (stomach) K22.2
    congenital Q39.3
  cardiovascular -*see* Disease, cardiovascular
  caudal M48.08
  cervix, cervical (canal) N88.2
    congenital Q51.828
    in pregnancy or childbirth -*see* Pregnancy,
      complicated by, abnormal cervix
  colon -*see also* Obstruction, intestine
    congenital Q42.9
      specified NEC Q42.8
  colostomy K94.03
  common (bile) duct K83.1
    congenital Q44.3
  coronary (artery) -*see* Disease, heart,
    ischemic, atherosclerotic
  cystic duct -*see* Obstruction, gallbladder
  due to presence of device, implant or graft -
    see also Complications, by site and type,
    specified NEC T85.858
    arterial graft NEC T82.858
    breast (implant) T85.858
    catheter T85.858
      dialysis (renal) T82.858
        intraperitoneal T85.858
      infusion NEC T82.858
        spinal (epidural) (subdural) T85.850
      urinary (indwelling) T83.85
    fixation, internal (orthopedic) NEC T84.85
    gastrointestinal (bile duct) (esophagus)
      T85.858
    genital NEC T83.85
    heart NEC T82.857
    joint prosthesis T84.85
    ocular (corneal graft) (orbital implant) NEC
      T85.858
    orthopedic NEC T84.85
    specified NEC T85.858
    urinary NEC T83.85
    vascular NEC T82.858
    ventricular intracranial shunt T85.850
  duodenum K31.5
    congenital Q41.0
  ejaculatory duct NEC N50.89
  endocervical os -*see* Stenosis, cervix

Stenosis, stenotic --*continued*
  enterostomy K94.13
  esophagus K22.2
    congenital Q39.3
    syphilitic A52.79
      congenital A50.59 [*K23*]
  eustachian tube -*see* Obstruction, eustachian
  tube - external ear canal (acquired) H61.30
    congenital Q16.1
    due to
      inflammation H61.32
      trauma H61.31
    postprocedural H95.81
    specified cause NEC H61.39
  gallbladder -*see* Obstruction, gallbladder
  glottis J38.6
  heart valve (congenital) Q24.8
    aortic Q23.0
    mitral Q23.2
    pulmonary Q22.1
    tricuspid Q22.4
  hepatic duct K83.1
  hymen N89.6
  hypertrophic subaortic (idiopathic) I42.1
  ileum K56.69
    congenital Q41.2
  infundibulum cardia Q24.3
  intervertebral foramina -*see also* Lesion,
  biomechanical, specified NEC
    connective tissue M99.79
      abdomen M99.79
      cervical region M99.71
      cervicothoracic M99.71
      head region M99.70
      lumbar region M99.73
      lumbosacral M99.73
      occipitocervical M99.70
      sacral region M99.74
      sacrococcygeal M99.74
      sacroiliac M99.74
      specified NEC M99.79
      thoracic region M99.72
      thoracolumbar M99.72
    disc M99.79
      abdomen M99.79
      cervical region M99.71
      cervicothoracic M99.71
      head region M99.70
      lower extremity M99.76
      lumbar region M99.73
      lumbosacral M99.73
      occipitocervical M99.70
      pelvic M99.75
      rib cage M99.78
      sacral region M99.74
      sacrococcygeal M99.74
      sacroiliac M99.74
      specified NEC M99.79
      thoracic region M99.72
      thoracolumbar M99.72
      upper extremity M99.77
    osseous M99.69
      abdomen M99.69
      cervical region M99.61
      cervicothoracic M99.61
      head region M99.60
      lower extremity M99.66
      lumbar region M99.63
      lumbosacral M99.63
      occipitocervical M99.60
      pelvic M99.65

Stenosis, stenotic --*continued*
      rib cage M99.68
      sacral region M99.64
      sacrococcygeal M99.64
      sacroiliac M99.64
      specified NEC M99.69
      thoracic region M99.62
      thoracolumbar M99.62
      upper extremity M99.67
    subluxation -*see* Stenosis, intervertebral
      foramina, osseous
  intestine -*see also* Obstruction, intestine
    congenital (small) Q41.9
      large Q42.9
        specified NEC Q42.8
      specified NEC Q41.8
  jejunum K56.69
    congenital Q41.1
  lacrimal (passage)
    canaliculi H04.54
    congenital Q10.5
    duct H04.55
    punctum H04.56
    sac H04.57
  lacrimonasal duct -*see* Stenosis, lacrimal, duct
    congenital Q10.5
  larynx J38.6
    congenital NEC Q31.8
      subglottic Q31.1
    syphilitic A52.73
      congenital A50.59 [*J99*]
  mitral (chronic) (inactive) (valve) I05.0
    with
      aortic valve disease I08.0
      incompetency, insufficiency or
    regurgitation I05.2
    active or acute I01.1
      with rheumatic or Sydenham's chorea I02.0
    congenital Q23.2
    specified cause, except rheumatic I34.2
    syphilitic A52.03
  myocardium, myocardial -*see also*
    Degeneration, myocardial
    hypertrophic subaortic (idiopathic) I42.1
  nares (anterior) (posterior) J34.89
    congenital Q30.0
  nasal duct -*see also* Stenosis, lacrimal, duct
    congenital Q10.5
  nasolacrimal duct -*see also* Stenosis, lacrimal,
  duct
    congenital Q10.5
  neural canal -*see also* Lesion, biomechanical,
  specified NEC
    connective tissue M99.49
      abdomen M99.49
      cervical region M99.41
      cervicothoracic M99.41
      head region M99.40
      lower extremity M99.46
      lumbar region M99.43
      lumbosacral M99.43
      occipitocervical M99.40
      pelvic M99.45
      rib cage M99.48
      sacral region M99.44
      sacrococcygeal M99.44
      sacroiliac M99.44
      specified NEC M99.49
      thoracic region M99.42
      thoracolumbar M99.42
      upper extremity M99.47

Stenosis, stenotic --*continued*
  intervertebral disc M99.59
    abdomen M99.59
    cervical region M99.51
    cervicothoracic M99.51
    head region M99.50
    lower extremity M99.56
    lumbar region M99.53
    lumbosacral M99.53
    occipitocervical M99.50
    pelvic M99.55
    rib cage M99.58
    sacral region M99.54
    sacrococcygeal M99.54
    sacroiliac M99.54
    specified NEC M99.59
    thoracic region M99.52
    thoracolumbar M99.52
    upper extremity M99.57
  osseous M99.39
    abdomen M99.39
    cervical region M99.31
    cervicothoracic M99.31
    head region M99.30
    lower extremity M99.36
    lumbar region M99.33
    lumbosacral M99.33
    pelvic M99.35
    rib cage M99.38
    occipitocervical M99.30
    sacral region M99.34
    sacrococcygeal M99.34
    sacroiliac M99.34
    specified NEC M99.39
    thoracic region M99.32
    thoracolumbar M99.32
    upper extremity M99.37
  subluxation M99.29
    cervical region M99.21
    cervicothoracic M99.21
    head region M99.20
    lower extremity M99.26
    lumbar region M99.23
    lumbosacral M99.23
    occipitocervical M99.20
    pelvic M99.25
    rib cage M99.28
    sacral region M99.24
    sacrococcygeal M99.24
    sacroiliac M99.24
    specified NEC M99.29
    thoracic region M99.22
    thoracolumbar M99.22
    upper extremity M99.27
  organ or site, congenital NEC -*see* Atresia, by site
  papilla of Vater K83.1
  pulmonary (artery) (congenital) Q25.6
    with ventricular septal defect, transposition of aorta, and hypertrophy of right ventricle Q21.3
    acquired I28.8
    in tetralogy of Fallot Q21.3
    infundibular Q24.3
    subvalvular Q24.3
    supravalvular Q25.6
    valve I37.0
      with insufficiency I37.2
      congenital Q22.1
      rheumatic I09.89

Stenosis, stenotic --*continued*
    with aortic, mitral or tricuspid (valve) disease I08.8
    vein, acquired I28.8
    vessel NEC I28.8
  pulmonic (congenital) Q22.1
    infundibular Q24.3
    subvalvular Q24.3
  pylorus (hypertrophic) (acquired) K31.1
    adult K31.1
    congenital Q40.0
    infantile Q40.0
  rectum (sphincter) -*see* Stricture, rectum
  renal artery I70.1
    congenital Q27.1
  salivary duct (any) K11.8
  sphincter of Oddi K83.1
  spinal M48.00
    cervical region M48.02
    cervicothoracic region M48.03
    lumbar region M48.06
    lumbosacral region M48.07
    occipito-atlanto-axial region M48.01
    sacrococcygeal region M48.08
    thoracic region M48.04
    thoracolumbar region M48.05
  stent
    vascular
      end stent
        adjacent to stent -*see* Arteriosclerosis
        within the stent
          coronary T82.855
          peripheral T82.856
      in stent
        coronary vessel T82.855
        peripheral vessel T82.856
  stomach, hourglass K31.2
  subaortic (congenital) Q24.4
    hypertrophic (idiopathic) I42.1
  subglottic J38.6
    congenital Q31.1
    postprocedural J95.5
  trachea J39.8
    congenital Q32.1
    syphilitic A52.73
    tuberculous NEC A15.5
  tracheostomy J95.03
  tricuspid (valve) I07.0
    with
      aortic (valve) disease I08.2
      incompetency, insufficiency or regurgitation I07.2
        with aortic (valve) disease I08.2
          with mitral (valve) disease I08.3
        mitral (valve) disease I08.1
          with aortic (valve) disease I08.3
    congenital Q22.4
    nonrheumatic I36.0
      with insufficiency I36.2
  tubal N97.1
  ureter -*see* Atresia, ureter
  ureteropelvic junction, congenital Q62.11
  ureterovesical orifice, congenital Q62.12
  urethra (valve) -*see also* Stricture, urethra
    congenital Q64.32
  urinary meatus, congenital Q64.33
  vagina N89.5
    congenital Q52.4
    in pregnancy -*see* Pregnancy, complicated by, abnormal vagina
      causing obstructed labor O65.5

Stenosis, stenotic --*continued*
  valve (cardiac) (heart) -*see also* Endocarditis I38
    congenital Q24.8
    aortic Q23.0
    mitral Q23.2
    pulmonary Q22.1
    tricuspid Q22.4
  vena cava (inferior) (superior) I87.1
    congenital Q26.0
  vesicourethral orifice Q64.31
  vulva N90.5
Stent jail T82.897
Stercolith (impaction) K56.41
  appendix K38.1
Stercoraceous, stercoral ulcer K63.3
  anus or rectum K62.6
Stereotypies NEC F98.4
Sterility -*see* Infertility
Sterilization -*see* Encounter (for), sterilization
Sternalgia -*see* Angina
Sternopagus Q89.4
Sternum bifidum Q76.7
Steroid
  effects (adverse) (adrenocortical) (iatrogenic)
    cushingoid E24.2
      correct substance properly administered - *see* Table of Drugs and Chemicals, by drug, adverse effect
      overdose or wrong substance given or taken -*see* Table of Drugs and Chemicals, by drug, poisoning
    diabetes -*see* category E09
      correct substance properly administered - *see* Table of Drugs and Chemicals, by drug, adverse effect
      overdose or wrong substance given or taken -*see* Table of Drugs and Chemicals, by drug, poisoning
    fever R50.2
    insufficiency E27.3
      correct substance properly administered - *see* Table of Drugs and Chemicals, by drug, adverse effect
      overdose or wrong substance given or taken -*see* Table of Drugs and Chemicals, by drug, poisoning
  responder H40.04
Stevens-Johnson disease or syndrome L51.1
  toxic epidermal necrolysis overlap L51.3
Stewart-Morel syndrome M85.2
Sticker's disease B08.3
Sticky eye -*see* Conjunctivitis, acute, mucopurulent
Stieda's disease -*see* Bursitis, tibial collateral
Stiff neck -*see* Torticollis
Stiff-man syndrome G25.82
Stiffness, joint NEC M25.60
  ankle M25.67
  ankylosis -*see* Ankylosis, joint
  contracture -*see* Contraction, joint
  elbow M25.62
  foot M25.67
  hand M25.64
  hip M25.65
  knee M25.66
  shoulder M25.61
  wrist M25.63
Stigmata congenital syphilis A50.59
Stillbirth P95
Still-Felty syndrome -*see* Felty's syndrome

Still's disease or syndrome (juvenile) M08.20
   adult-onset M06.1
   ankle M08.27
   elbow M08.22
   foot joint M08.27
   hand joint M08.24
   hip M08.25
   knee M08.26
   multiple site M08.29
   shoulder M08.21
   vertebra M08.28
   wrist M08.23
Stimulation, ovary E28.1
**Sting (venomous) (with allergic or
   anaphylactic shock)** -see Table of Drugs and
   Chemicals, by animal or substance, poisoning
Stippled epiphyses Q78.8
Stitch
   abscess T81.48
   burst (in operation wound) -see Disruption,
      wound, operation
Stokes-Adams disease or syndrome I45.9
Stokes' disease E05.00
   with thyroid storm E05.01
Stokvis (Talma) disease D74.8
Stoma malfunction
   colostomy K94.03
   enterostomy K94.13
   gastrostomy K94.23
   ileostomy K94.13
   tracheostomy J95.03
Stomach -see condition
Stomatitis (denture) (ulcerative) K12.1
   angular K13.0
      due to dietary or vitamin deficiency E53.0
   aphthous K12.0
   bovine B08.61
   candidal B37.0
   catarrhal K12.1
   diphtheritic A36.89
   due to
      dietary deficiency E53.0
      thrush B37.0
      vitamin deficiency
         B group NEC E53.9
         B2 (riboflavin) E53.0
   epidemic B08.8
   epizootic B08.8
   follicular K12.1
   gangrenous A69.0
   Geotrichum B48.3
   herpesviral, herpetic B00.2
   herpetiformis K12.0
   malignant K12.1
   membranous acute K12.1
   monilial B37.0
   mycotic B37.0
   necrotizing ulcerative A69.0
   parasitic B37.0
   septic K12.1
   spirochetal A69.1
   suppurative (acute) K12.2
   ulceromembranous A69.1
   vesicular K12.1
      with exanthem (enteroviral) B08.4
      virus disease A93.8
   Vincent's A69.1
Stomatocytosis D58.8
Stomatomycosis B37.0
Stomatorrhagia K13.79

Stone(s) -see also Calculus
   bladder (diverticulum) N21.0
   cystine E72.09
   heart syndrome I50.1
   kidney N20.0
   prostate N42.0
   pulpal (dental) K04.2
   renal N20.0
   salivary gland or duct (any) K11.5
   urethra (impacted) N21.1
   urinary (duct) (impacted) (passage) N20.9
      bladder (diverticulum) N21.0
      lower tract N21.9
      specified NEC N21.8
   xanthine E79.8 [N22]
Stonecutter's lung J62.8
**Stonemason's asthma, disease, lung or
   pneumoconiosis** J62.8
Stoppage
   heart -see Arrest, cardiac
   urine -see Retention, urine **Storm, thyroid** -
      see Thyrotoxicosis
Strabismus (congenital) (nonparalytic)
   H50.9
   concomitant H50.40
      convergent -see Strabismus, convergent
         concomitant
      divergent -see Strabismus, divergent
         concomitant
   convergent concomitant H50.00
      accommodative component H50.43
      alternating H50.05
         with
            A pattern H50.06
            specified nonconcomitances NEC H50.08
            V pattern H50.07
      monocular H50.01
         with
            A pattern H50.02
            specified nonconcomitances NEC
               H50.04
            V pattern H50.03
      intermittent H50.31
         alternating H50.32
   cyclotropia H50.41
   divergent concomitant H50.10
      alternating H50.15
         with
            A pattern H50.16
            specified noncomitances NEC H50.18
            V pattern H50.17
      monocular H50.11
         with
            A pattern H50.12
            specified noncomitances NEC H50.14
            V pattern H50.13
         intermittent H50.33
            alternating H50.34
   Duane's syndrome H50.81
   due to adhesions, scars H50.69
   heterophoria H50.50
      alternating H50.55
      cyclophoria H50.54
      esophoria H50.51
      exophoria H50.52
      vertical H50.53
   heterotropia H50.40
      intermittent H50.30
   hypertropia H50.2
   hypotropia -see Hypertropia
   latent H50.50

Strabismus --continued
   mechanical H50.60
      Brown's sheath syndrome H50.61
      specified type NEC H50.69
   monofixation syndrome H50.42
   paralytic H49.9
      abducens nerve H49.2
      fourth nerve H49.1
      Kearns-Sayre syndrome H49.81
      ophthalmoplegia (external)
         progressive H49.4
            with pigmentary retinopathy H49.81
         total H49.3
      sixth nerve H49.2
      specified type NEC H49.88
      third nerve H49.0
      trochlear nerve H49.1
   specified type NEC H50.89
   vertical H50.2
Strain
   back S39.012
   cervical S16.1
   eye NEC -see Disturbance, vision, subjective
   heart -see Disease, heart
   low back S39.012
   mental NOS Z73.3
      work-related Z56.6
   muscle (tendon) -see Injury, muscle, by site,
      strain
   neck S16.1
   postural -see also Disorder, soft tissue, due to
      use
   physical NOS Z73.3
      work-related Z56.6
   psychological NEC Z73.3
   tendon -see Injury, muscle, by site, strain
Straining, on urination R39.16
Strand, vitreous -see Opacity, vitreous,
   membranes and strands
Strangulation, strangulated -see also
   Asphyxia, traumatic
   appendix K38.8
   bladder-neck N32.0
   bowel or colon K56.2
   food or foreign body -see Foreign body, by
      site
   hemorrhoids -see Hemorrhoids, with
      complication
   hernia -see also Hernia, by site, with
      obstruction
      with gangrene -see Hernia, by site, with
         gangrene
   intestine (large) (small) K56.2
      with hernia -see also Hernia, by site, with
         obstruction
         with gangrene -see Hernia, by site, with
            gangrene
   mesentery K56.2
   mucus -see Asphyxia, mucus
   omentum K56.2
   organ or site, congenital NEC -see Atresia, by
      site
   ovary -see Torsion, ovary
   penis N48.89
      foreign body T19.4
   rupture -see Hernia, by site, with obstruction
   stomach due to hernia -see also Hernia, by
      site, with obstruction
      with gangrene -see Hernia, by site, with
         gangrene
   vesicourethral orifice N32.0

Strangury R30.0
Straw itch B88.0
Strawberry
  gallbladder K82.4
  mark Q82.5
  tongue (red) (white) K14.3
Streak(s)
  macula, angioid H35.33
  ovarian Q50.32
Strephosymbolia F81.0
  secondary to organic lesion R48.8
Streptobacillary fever A25.1
Streptobacillosis A25.1
Streptobacillus moniliformis A25.1
Streptococcus, streptococcal -see also
  condition
  as cause of disease classified elsewhere B95.5
  group
    A, as cause of disease classified elsewhere
    B95.0
    B, as cause of disease classified elsewhere
    B95.1
    D, as cause of disease classified elsewhere
    B95.2
  pneumoniae, as cause of disease classified
  elsewhere B95.3
  specified NEC, as cause of disease classified
  elsewhere B95.4
Streptomycosis B47.1
Streptotrichosis A48.8
Stress F43.9
  family -see Disruption, family   fetal P84
  complicating pregnancy O77.9
    due to drug administration O77.1
  mental NEC Z73.3
    work-related Z56.6
  physical NEC Z73.3
    work-related Z56.6
  polycythemia D75.1
  reaction -see also Reaction, stress F43.9
  work schedule Z56.3
Stretching, nerve -see Injury, nerve
**Striae albicantes, atrophicae or distensae
(cutis)** L90.6
Stricture -see also Stenosis
  ampulla of Vater K83.1
  anus (sphincter) K62.4
    congenital Q42.3
      with fistula Q42.2
    infantile Q42.3
      with fistula Q42.2
  aorta (ascending) (congenital) Q25.1
    arteriosclerotic I70.0
    calcified I70.0
    supravalvular, congenital Q25.3
  aortic (valve) -see Stenosis, aortic
  aqueduct of Sylvius (congenital) Q03.0
    with spina bifida -see Spina bifida, by site,
    with hydrocephalus
    acquired G91.1
  artery I77.1
    basilar -see Occlusion, artery, basilar
    carotid -see Occlusion, artery, carotid
    celiac I77.4
    congenital (peripheral) Q27.8
      cerebral Q28.3
      coronary Q24.5
      digestive system Q27.8
      lower limb Q27.8
      retinal Q14.1
      specified site NEC Q27.8

Stricture --continued
      umbilical Q27.0
      upper limb Q27.8
    coronary -see Disease, heart, ischemic,
    atherosclerotic
      congenital Q24.5
    precerebral -see Occlusion, artery,
    precerebral
    pulmonary (congenital) Q25.6
      acquired I28.8
    renal I70.1
    vertebral -see Occlusion, artery, vertebral
  auditory canal (external) (congenital)
    acquired -see Stenosis, external ear canal
  bile duct (common) (hepatic) K83.1
    congenital Q44.3
    postoperative K91.89
  bladder N32.89
    neck N32.0
  bowel -see Obstruction, intestine
  brain G93.89
  bronchus J98.09
    congenital Q32.3
    syphilitic A52.72
  cardia (stomach) K22.2
    congenital Q39.3
  cardiac -see also Disease, heart
    orifice (stomach) K22.2
  cecum -see Obstruction, intestine
  cervix, cervical (canal) N88.2
    congenital Q51.828
    in pregnancy -see Pregnancy, complicated
    by, abnormal cervix
      causing obstructed labor O65.5
  colon -see also Obstruction, intestine
    congenital Q42.9
      specified NEC Q42.8
  colostomy K94.03
  common (bile) duct K83.1
  coronary (artery) -see Disease, heart,
    ischemic, atherosclerotic
  cystic duct -see Obstruction, gallbladder
  digestive organs NEC, congenital Q45.8
  duodenum K31.5
    congenital Q41.0
  ear canal (external) (congenital) Q16.1
    acquired -see Stricture, auditory canal,
    acquired
  ejaculatory duct N50.89
  enterostomy K94.13
  esophagus K22.2
    congenital Q39.3
    syphilitic A52.79
      congenital A50.59 [K23]
  eustachian tube -see also Obstruction,
    eustachian tube
    congenital Q17.8
  fallopian tube N97.1
    gonococcal A54.24
    tuberculous A18.17
  gallbladder -see Obstruction, gallbladder
  glottis J38.6
  heart -see also Disease, heart
    valve -see also Endocarditis I38
      aortic Q23.0
      mitral Q23.4
      pulmonary Q22.1
      tricuspid Q22.4
  hepatic duct K83.1
  hourglass, of stomach K31.2
  hymen N89.6

Stricture --continued
  hypopharynx J39.2
  ileum K56.69
    congenital Q41.2
  intestine -see also Obstruction, intestine
    congenital (small) Q41.9
      large Q42.9
        specified NEC Q42.8
      specified NEC Q41.8
    ischemic K55.1
  jejunum K56.69
    congenital Q41.1
  lacrimal passages -see also Stenosis, lacrimal
    congenital Q10.5
  larynx J38.6
    congenital NEC Q31.8
      subglottic Q31.1
    syphilitic A52.73
      congenital A50.59 [J99]
  meatus
    ear (congenital) Q16.1
      acquired -see Stricture, auditory canal,
      acquired
    osseous (ear) (congenital) Q16.1
      acquired -see Stricture, auditory canal,
      acquired
    urinarius -see also Stricture, urethra
      congenital Q64.33
  mitral (valve) -see Stenosis, mitral
  myocardium, myocardial I51.5
    hypertrophic subaortic (idiopathic) I42.1
  nares (anterior) (posterior) J34.89
    congenital Q30.0
  nasal duct -see also Stenosis, lacrimal, duct
    congenital Q10.5
  nasolacrimal duct -see also Stenosis, lacrimal,
    duct
    congenital Q10.5
  nasopharynx J39.2
    syphilitic A52.73
  nose J34.89
    congenital Q30.0
  nostril (anterior) (posterior) J34.89
    congenital Q30.0
    syphilitic A52.73
      congenital A50.59 [J99]
  organ or site, congenital NEC -see Atresia, by
    site
  os uteri -see Stricture, cervix
  osseous meatus (ear) (congenital) Q16.1
    acquired -see Stricture, auditory canal,
    acquired
  oviduct -see Stricture, fallopian tube
  pelviureteric junction (congenital) Q62.11
    acquired, with hydronephrosis N13.0
  penis, by foreign body T19.4
  pharynx J39.2
  prostate N42.89
  pulmonary, pulmonic
    artery (congenital) Q25.6
      acquired I28.8
      noncongenital I28.8
    infundibulum (congenital) Q24.3
    valve I37.0
      congenital Q22.1
    vein, acquired I28.8
    vessel NEC I28.8
  punctum lacrimale -see also Stenosis,
    lacrimal, punctum
    congenital Q10.5
  pylorus (hypertrophic) K31.1

Stricture --*continued*
  adult K31.1
    congenital Q40.0
    infantile Q40.0
  rectosigmoid K56.69
  rectum (sphincter) K62.4
    congenital Q42.1
      with fistula Q42.0
    due to
      chlamydial lymphogranuloma A55
      irradiation K91.89
      lymphogranuloma venereum A55
    gonococcal A54.6
    inflammatory (chlamydial) A55
    syphilitic A52.74
    tuberculous A18.32
  renal artery I70.1
    congenital Q27.1
  salivary duct or gland (any) K11.8
  sigmoid (flexure) -*see* Obstruction, intestine
  spermatic cord N50.89
  stoma (following) (of)
    colostomy K94.03
    enterostomy K94.13
    gastrostomy K94.23
    ileostomy K94.13
    tracheostomy J95.03
  stomach K31.89
    congenital Q40.2
    hourglass K31.2
  subaortic Q24.4
    hypertrophic (acquired) (idiopathic) I42.1
  subglottic J38.6
  syphilitic NEC A52.79
  trachea J39.8
    congenital Q32.1
    syphilitic A52.73
    tuberculous NEC A15.5
  tracheostomy J95.03
  tricuspid (valve) -*see* Stenosis, tricuspid
  tunica vaginalis N50.89
  ureter (postoperative) N13.5
    with
      hydronephrosis N13.1
        with infection N13.6
      pyelonephritis (chronic) N11.1
    congenital -*see* Atresia, ureter
    tuberculous A18.11
  ureteropelvic junction (congenital) Q62.11
    acquired, with hydronephrosis N13.0
  ureterovesical orifice N13.5
    with infection N13.6
  urethra (organic) (spasmodic) N35.9
    associated with schistosomiasis B65.0 [*N37*]
    congenital Q64.39
      valvular (posterior) Q64.2
    due to
      infection -*see* Stricture, urethra,
        postinfective
      trauma -*see* Stricture, urethra, post-
        traumatic
    gonococcal, gonorrheal A54.01
    infective NEC -*see* Stricture, urethra,
      postinfective
    late effect (sequelae) of injury -*see* Stricture,
      urethra, post-traumatic
    postcatheterization -*see* Stricture, urethra,
      postprocedural
    postinfective NEC
      female N35.12
      male N35.119

Stricture --*continued*
      anterior urethra N35.114
      bulbous urethra N35.112
      meatal N35.111
      membranous urethra N35.113
    postobstetric N35.021
    postoperative -*see* Stricture, urethra,
      postprocedural
    postprocedural
      female N99.12
      male N99.114
        anterior bulbous urethra N99.113
        bulbous urethra N99.111
        fossa navicularis N99.115
        meatal N99.110
        membranous urethra N99.112
    post-traumatic
      female N35.028
        due to childbirth N35.021
      male N35.014
        anterior urethra N35.013
        bulbous urethra N35.011
        meatal N35.010
        membranous urethra N35.012
    sequela (late effect) of
      childbirth N35.021
      injury -*see* Stricture, urethra, post-
        traumatic
    specified cause NEC N35.8
    syphilitic A52.76
    traumatic -*see* Stricture, urethra, post-
      traumatic
    valvular (posterior), congenital Q64.2
  urinary meatus -*see* Stricture, urethra
  uterus, uterine (synechiae) N85.6
    os (external) (internal) -*see* Stricture, cervix
  vagina (outlet) -*see* Stenosis, vagina
  valve (cardiac) (heart) -*see also* Endocarditis
    congenital
      aortic Q23.0
      mitral Q23.2
      pulmonary Q22.1
      tricuspid Q22.4
  vas deferens N50.89
    congenital Q55.4
  vein I87.1
  vena cava (inferior) (superior) NEC I87.1
    congenital Q26.0
  vesicourethral orifice N32.0
    congenital Q64.31
  vulva (acquired) N90.5
Stridor R06.1
  congenital (larynx) P28.89
Stridulous -*see* condition
Stroke (apoplectic) (brain) (embolic)
(ischemic) (paralytic) (thrombotic) I63.9
  epileptic -*see* Epilepsy
  heat T67.0
  in evolution I63.9
  intraoperative
    during cardiac surgery I97.810
    during other surgery I97.811
  lightning -*see* Lightning
  meaning
    cerebral hemorrhage
    code to Hemorrhage, intracranial
    cerebral infarction
    code to Infarction, cerebral
  postprocedural
    following cardiac surgery I97.820
    following other surgery I97.821
  unspecified (NOS) I63.9

Stromatosis, endometrial D39.0
Strongyloidiasis, strongyloidosis B78.9
  cutaneous B78.1
  disseminated B78.7
  intestinal B78.0
Strophulus pruriginosus L28.2
Struck by lightning -*see* Lightning
Struma -*see also* Goiter
  Hashimoto E06.3
  lymphomatosa E06.3
  nodosa (simplex) E04.9
    endemic E01.2
      multinodular E01.1
    multinodular E04.2
      iodine-deficiency related E01.1
    toxic or with hyperthyroidism E05.20
      with thyroid storm E05.21
      multinodular E05.20
        with thyroid storm E05.21
      uninodular E05.10
        with thyroid storm E05.11
    toxicosa E05.20
      with thyroid storm E05.21
      multinodular E05.20
        with thyroid storm E05.21
      uninodular E05.10
        with thyroid storm E05.11
    uninodular E04.1
  ovarii D27.
  Riedel's E06.5
Strumipriva cachexia E03.4
Strümpell-Marie spine -*see* Spondylitis,
  ankylosing
Strümpell-Westphal pseudosclerosis E83.01
Stuart deficiency disease (factor X) D68.2
Stuart-Prower factor deficiency (factor X)
  D68.2
Student's elbow -*see* Bursitis, elbow,
  olecranon
Stump -*see* Amputation
Stunting, nutritional E45
Stupor (catatonic) R40.1
  depressive (single episode) F32.89
    recurrent episode F33.8
  dissociative F44.2
  manic F30.2
  manic-depressive F31.89
  psychogenic (anergic) F44.2
  reaction to exceptional stress (transient) F43.0
Sturge (Weber) (Dimitri) (Kalischer)
  disease or syndrome Q85.8
Stuttering F80.81
  adult onset F98.5
  childhood onset F80.81
  following cerebrovascular disease -*see*
  Disorder, fluency. following cerebrovascular
  disease - in conditions classified elsewhere
  R47.82
Sty, stye (external) (internal) (meibomian)
  (zeisian) -*see* Hordeolum
Subacidity, gastric K31.89
  psychogenic F45.8
Subacute -*see* condition
Subarachnoid -*see* condition
Subcortical -*see* condition
Subcostal syndrome, nerve compression -*see*
  Mononeuropathy, upper limb, specified site
  NEC
Subcutaneous, subcuticular -*see* condition
Subdural -*see* condition
Subendocardium -*see* condition

Subependymoma
  specified site *-see* Neoplasm, uncertain
  behavior, by site
  unspecified site D43.2
Suberosis J67.3
Subglossitis *-see* Glossitis S
Subhemophilia D66
Subinvolution
  breast (postlactational) (postpuerperal)
    N64.89
  puerperal O90.89
  uterus (chronic) (nonpuerperal) N85.3
    puerperal O90.89
Sublingual *-see* condition
Sublinguitis *-see* Sialoadenitis
Subluxatable hip Q65.6
Subluxation *-see also* Dislocation
  acromioclavicular S43.11
  ankle S93.0
  atlantoaxial, recurrent M43.4
    with myelopathy M43.3
  carpometacarpal (joint) NEC S63.05
    thumb S63.04
  complex, vertebral *-see* Complex, subluxation
  congenital *-see also* Malposition, congenital
    hip *-see* Dislocation, hip, congenital, partial
    joint (excluding hip)
      lower limb Q68.8
      shoulder Q68.8
      upper limb Q68.8
  elbow (traumatic) S53.10
    anterior S53.11
    lateral S53.14
    medial S53.13
    posterior S53.12
    specified type NEC S53.19
  finger S63.20
    index S63.20
    interphalangeal S63.22
      distal S63.24
        index S63.24
        little S63.24
        middle S63.24
        ring S63.24
      index S63.22
      little S63.22
      middle S63.22
      proximal S63.23
        index S63.23
        little S63.23
        middle S63.23
        ring S63.23
      ring S63.22
    little S63.20
    metacarpophalangeal S63.21
      index S63.21
      little S63.21
      middle S63.21
      ring S63.21
    middle S63.20
    ring S63.20
  foot S93.30
    specified site NEC S93.33
    tarsal joint S93.31
    tarsometatarsal joint S93.32
    toe *-see* Subluxation, toe
  hip S73.00
    anterior S73.03
      obturator S73.02
    central S73.04
    posterior S73.01

Subluxation - *--continued*
  interphalangeal (joint)
    finger S63.22
      distal joint S63.24
        index S63.24
        little S63.24
        middle S63.24
        ring S63.24
      index S63.22
      little S63.22
      middle S63.22
      proximal joint S63.23
        index S63.23
        little S63.23
        middle S63.23
        ring S63.23
      ring S63.22
    thumb S63.12
      distal joint S63.14
      proximal joint S63.13
    toe S93.13
      great S93.13
      lesser S93.13
  joint prosthesis *-see* Complications, joint
    prosthesis, mechanical, displacement, by site
  knee S83.10
    cap *-see* Subluxation, patella
    patella *-see* Subluxation, patella
    proximal tibia
      anteriorly S83.11
      laterally S83.14
      medially S83.13
      posteriorly S83.12
    specified type NEC S83.19
  lens *-see* Dislocation, lens, partial
  ligament, traumatic *-see* Sprain, by site
  metacarpal (bone)
    proximal end S63.06
  metacarpophalangeal (joint)
    finger S63.21
      index S63.21
      little S63.21
      middle S63.21
      ring S63.21
    thumb S63.11
  metatarsophalangeal joint S93.14
    great toe S93.14
    lesser toe S93.14
  midcarpal (joint) S63.03
  patella S83.00
    lateral S83.01
    recurrent (nontraumatic) *-see* Dislocation,
    patella, recurrent, incomplete
    specified type NEC S83.09
  pathological *-see* Dislocation, pathological
  radial head S53.00
    anterior S53.01
    nursemaid's elbow S53.03
    posterior S53.02
    specified type NEC S53.09
  radiocarpal (joint) S63.02
  radioulnar (joint)
    distal S63.01
    proximal *-see* Subluxation, elbow
  shoulder
    congenital Q68.8
    girdle S43.30
      scapula S43.31
      specified site NEC S43.39
    traumatic S43.00
      anterior S43.01

Subluxation - *--continued*
  inferior S43.03
  posterior S43.02
  specified type NEC S43.08
  sternoclavicular (joint) S43.20
    anterior S43.21
    posterior S43.22
  symphysis (pubis)
  thumb S63.103
    interphalangeal joint *-see* Subluxation,
      interphalangeal (joint), thumb
    metacarpophalangeal joint *-see* Subluxation,
      metacarpophalangeal (joint), thumb
  toe(s) S93.10
    great S93.10
      interphalangeal joint S93.13
      metatarsophalangeal joint S93.14
    interphalangeal joint S93.13
    lesser S93.10
      interphalangeal joint S93.13
      metatarsophalangeal joint S93.14
    metatarsophalangeal joint S93.149
  ulnohumeral joint *-see* Subluxation, elbow
  vertebral
    recurrent NEC *-see* subcategory M43.5
    traumatic
      cervical S13.100
        atlantoaxial joint S13.120
        atlantooccipital joint S13.110
        atloido-occipital joint S13.110
        joint between
          C0 and C1 S13.110
          C1 and C2 S13.120
          C2 and C3 S13.130
          C3 and C4 S13.140
          C4 and C5 S13.150
          C5 and C6 S13.160
          C6 and C7 S13.170
          C7 and T1 S13.180
        occipitoatloid joint S13.110
      lumbar S33.100
        joint between
          L1 and L2 S33.110
          L2 and L3 S33.120
          L3 and L4 S33.130
          L4 and L5 S33.140
      thoracic S23.100
        joint between
          T1 and T2 S23.110
          T2 and T3 S23.120
          T3 and T4 S23.122
          T4 and T5 S23.130
          T5 and T6 S23.132
          T6 and T7 S23.140
          T7 and T8 S23.142
          T8 and T9 S23.150
          T9 and T10 S23.152
          T10 and T11 S23.160
          T11 and T12 S23.162
          T12 and L1 S23.170
  ulna
    distal end S63.07
    proximal end *-see* Subluxation, elbow
  wrist (carpal bone) S63.00
    carpometacarpal joint *-see* Subluxation,
      carpometacarpal (joint)
    distal radioulnar joint *-see* Subluxation,
      radioulnar (joint), distal
    metacarpal bone, proximal *-see* Subluxation,
      metacarpal (bone), proximal end

Subluxation - --*continued*
  midcarpal -*see* Subluxation, midcarpal
    (joint)
  radiocarpal joint -*see* Subluxation,
    radiocarpal (joint)
  recurrent -*see* Dislocation, recurrent, wrist
    specified site NEC S63.09
  ulna -*see* Subluxation, ulna, distal end
Submaxillary -*see* condition
Submersion (fatal) (nonfatal) T75.1
Submucous -*see* condition
Subnormal, subnormality
  accommodation (old age) H52.4
  mental -*see* Disability, intellectual
  temperature (accidental) T68
Subphrenic -*see* condition
Subscapular nerve -*see* condition
Subseptus uterus Q51.2
Subsiding appendicitis K36
Substance (other psychoactive) induced
  anxiety disorder F19.980
  bipolar and related disorder F19.94
  delirium F19.921
  depressive disorder F19.94
  major neurocognitive disorder F19.97
  mild neurocognitive disorder F19.988
  obsessive-compulsive and related disorder
    F19.988
  psychotic disorder F19.959
  sexual dysfunction F19.981
  sleep disorder F19.982
Substernal thyroid E04.9
  congenital Q89.2
Substitution disorder F44.9
Subtentorial -*see* condition
Subthyroidism (acquired) -*see also*
  Hypothyroidism
  congenital E03.1
Succenturiate placenta O43.19
Sucking thumb, child (excessive) F98.8
Sudamen, sudamina L74.1
Sudanese kala-azar B55.0
Sudden
  heart failure -*see* Failure, heart
  hearing loss -*see* Deafness, sudden
Sudeck's atrophy, disease, or syndrome -*see*
  Algoneurodystrophy
Suffocation -*see* Asphyxia, traumatic
Sugar
  blood
    high (transient) R73.9
    low (transient) E16.2
  in urine R81
Suicide, suicidal (attempted) T14.91
  by poisoning -*see* Table of Drugs and
    Chemicals
  history of (personal) Z91.5
    in family Z81.8
  ideation -*see* Ideation, suicidal
  risk
    meaning personal history of attempted
      suicide Z91.5
    meaning suicidal ideation -*see* Ideation,
      suicidal
  tendencies
    meaning personal history of attempted
      suicide Z91.5
    meaning suicidal ideation -*see* Ideation,
      suicidal
  trauma -*see* nature of injury by site
Suipestifer infection -*see* Infection, salmonella

Sulfhemoglobinemia, sulphemoglobinemia
(acquired) (with methemoglobinemia)
  D74.8
Sumatran mite fever A75.3
Summer -*see* condition **Sunburn** L55.9
  due to
    tanning bed (acute) L56.8
      chronic L57.8
    ultraviolet radiation (acute) L56.8
      chronic L57.8
  first degree L55.0
  second degree L55.1
  third degree L55.2
SUNCT (short lasting unilateral
neuralgiform headache with conjunctival
injection and tearing) G44.059
  intractable G44.051
  not intractable G44.059
Sunken acetabulum -*see* Derangement, joint,
  specified type NEC, hip
Sunstroke T67.0
Superfecundation -*see* Pregnancy, multiple
Superfetation -*see* Pregnancy, multiple
Superinvolution (uterus) N85.8
Supernumerary (congenital)
  aortic cusps Q23.8
  auditory ossicles Q16.3
  bone Q79.8
  breast Q83.1
  carpal bones Q74.0
  cusps, heart valve NEC Q24.8
    aortic Q23.8
    mitral Q23.2
    pulmonary Q22.3
  digit(s) Q69.9
  ear (lobule) Q17.0
  fallopian tube Q50.6
  finger Q69.0
  hymen Q52.4
  kidney Q63.0
  lacrimonasal duct Q10.6
  lobule (ear) Q17.0
  mitral cusps Q23.2
  muscle Q79.8
  nipple(s) Q83.3
  organ or site not listed -*see* Accessory
    ossicles, auditory Q16.3
  ovary Q50.31
  oviduct Q50.6
  pulmonary, pulmonic cusps Q22.3
  rib Q76.6
    cervical or first (syndrome) Q76.5
  roots (of teeth) K00.2
  spleen Q89.09
  tarsal bones Q74.2
  teeth K00.1
  testis Q55.29
  thumb Q69.1
  toe Q69.2
  uterus Q51.2
  vagina Q52.1
  vertebra Q76.49
Supervision (of)
  contraceptive -*see* Prescription, contraceptives
  dietary (for) Z71.3
    allergy (food) Z71.3
    colitis Z71.3
    diabetes mellitus Z71.3
    food allergy or intolerance Z71.3
    gastritis Z71.3
    hypercholesterolemia Z71.3

Supervision - *continued*
    hypoglycemia Z71.3
    intolerance (food) Z71.3
    obesity Z71.3
    specified NEC Z71.3
  healthy infant or child Z76.2
    foundling Z76.1
  high-risk pregnancy -*see* Pregnancy,
    complicated by, high, risk
  lactation Z39.1
  pregnancy -*see* Pregnancy, supervision of
Supplemental teeth K00.1
Suppression
  binocular vision H53.34
  lactation O92.5
  menstruation N94.89
  ovarian secretion E28.39
  renal N28.9
  urine, urinary secretion R34
Suppuration, suppurative -*see also* condition
  accessory sinus (chronic) -*see* Sinusitis
  adrenal gland
  antrum (chronic) -*see* Sinusitis, maxillary
  bladder -*see* Cystitis
  brain G06.0
    sequelae G09
  breast N61.1
    puerperal, postpartum or gestational -*see*
      Mastitis, obstetric, purulent
  dental periosteum M27.3
  ear (middle) -*see also* Otitis, media
    external NEC -*see* Otitis, externa, infective
    internal -*see* subcategory H83.0
  ethmoidal (chronic) (sinus) -*see* Sinusitis,
    ethmoidal
  fallopian tube -*see* Salpingo-oophoritis
  frontal (chronic) (sinus) -*see* Sinusitis, frontal
  gallbladder (acute) K81.0
  gum K05.20
    generalized -*see* Peridontitis, aggressive,
      generalized
    localized -*see* Peridontitis, aggressive,
      localized
  intracranial G06.0
  joint -*see* Arthritis, pyogenic or pyemic
  labyrinthine - see subcategory H83.0
  lung -*see* Abscess, lung
  mammary gland N61.1
    puerperal, postpartum O91.12
      associated with lactation O91.13
  maxilla, maxillary M27.2
    sinus (chronic) -*see* Sinusitis, maxillary
  muscle -*see* Myositis, infective
  nasal sinus (chronic) -*see* Sinusitis
  pancreas, acute -*see also* Pancreatitis, acute
    K85.80
  parotid gland -*see* Sialoadenitis
  pelvis, pelvic
    female -*see* Disease, pelvis, inflammatory
    male K65.0
  pericranial -*see* Osteomyelitis
  salivary duct or gland (any) -*see* Sialoadenitis
  sinus (accessory) (chronic) (nasal) -*see*
    Sinusitis
  sphenoidal sinus (chronic) -*see* Sinusitis,
    sphenoidal
  thymus (gland) E32.1
  thyroid (gland) E06.0
  tonsil -*see* Tonsillitis
  uterus -*see* Endometritis
Supraeruption of tooth (teeth) M26.34

Supraglottitis J04.30
  with obstruction J04.31
Suprarenal (gland) -see condition
Suprascapular nerve -see condition
Suprasellar -see condition
Surfer's knots or nodules S89.8
Surgical
  emphysema T81.82
  procedures, complication or misadventure -
    see Complications, surgical procedures
  shock T81.10
Surveillance (of) (for) -see also Observation
  alcohol abuse Z71.41
  contraceptive -see Prescription, contraceptives
  dietary Z71.3
  drug abuse Z71.51
Susceptibility to disease, genetic Z15.89
  malignant neoplasm Z15.09
    breast Z15.01
    endometrium Z15.04
    ovary Z15.02
    prostate Z15.03
    specified NEC Z15.09
  multiple endocrine neoplasia Z15.81
Suspected condition, ruled out -see also
    Observation, suspected
  amniotic cavity and membrane Z03.71
  cervical shortening Z03.75
  fetal anomaly Z03.73
  fetal growth Z03.74
  maternal and fetal conditions NEC Z03.79
  newborn -see also Observation, newborn,
    suspected condition ruled out Z05.9
  oligohydramnios Z03.71
  placental problem Z03.72
  polyhydramnios Z03.71
Suspended uterus
  in pregnancy or childbirth -see Pregnancy,
    complicated by, abnormal uterus
Sutton's nevus D22.9
Suture
  burst (in operation wound) T81.31
    external operation wound T81.31
    internal operation wound T81.32
  inadvertently left in operation wound -see
    Foreign body, accidentally left during a
    procedure
  removal Z48.02
Swab inadvertently left in operation wound -
  see Foreign body, accidentally left during a
    procedure
Swallowed, swallowing
  difficulty -see Dysphagia
  foreign body -see Foreign body, alimentary
    tract
Swan-neck deformity (finger) -see Deformity,
    finger, swan-neck
Swearing, compulsive F42.8
  in Gilles de la Tourette's syndrome F95.2
Sweat, sweats
  fetid L75.0
  night R61
Sweating, excessive R61
Sweeley Klionsky disease E75.21
Sweet's disease or dermatosis L98.2
Swelling (of) R60.9
  abdomen, abdominal (not referable to any
    particular organ) -see Mass, abdominal
  ankle -see Effusion, joint, ankle
  arm M79.89
    forearm M79.89

Swelling --continued
  breast N63
  Calabar B74.3
  cervical gland R59.0
  chest, localized R22.2
  ear H93.8
  extremity (lower) (upper) -see Disorder, soft
    tissue, specified type NEC
  finger M79.89
  foot M79.89
  glands R59.9
    generalized R59.1
    localized R59.0
  hand M79.89
  head (localized) R22.0
  inflammatory -see Inflammation
  intra-abdominal -see Mass, abdominal
  joint -see Effusion, joint
  leg M79.89
    lower M79.89
  limb -see Disorder, soft tissue, specified type
    NEC
  localized (skin) R22.9
    chest R22.2
    head R22.0
    limb
      lower -see Mass, localized, limb, lower
      upper -see Mass, localized, limb, upper
    neck R22.1
    trunk R22.2
  neck (localized) R22.1
  pelvic -see Mass, abdominal
  scrotum N50.89
  splenic -see Splenomegaly   testis N50.89
  toe M79.89
  umbilical R19.09
  wandering, due to Gnathostoma (spinigerum)
    B83.1
  white -see Tuberculosis, arthritis
Swift (Feer) disease
  overdose or wrong substance given or taken -
  see Table of Drugs and Chemicals, by drug,
    poisoning
Swimmer's
  cramp T75.1
  ear H60.33
  itch B65.3
Swimming in the head R42
Swollen -see Swelling
Swyer syndrome Q99.1
Sycosis L73.8
  barbae (not parasitic) L73.8
  contagiosa (mycotic) B35.0
  lupoides L73.8
  mycotic B35.0
  parasitic B35.0
  vulgaris L73.8
Sydenham's chorea -see Chorea, Sydenham's
Sylvatic yellow fever A95.0
Sylvest's disease B33.0
Symblepharon H11.23
  congenital Q10.3
Symond's syndrome G93.2
Sympathetic -see condition
Sympatheticotonia G90.8
Sympathicoblastoma
  specified site -see Neoplasm, malignant, by
    site
  unspecified site C74.90
Sympathogonioma -see Sympathicoblastoma
Symphalangy (fingers) (toes) Q70.9

Symptoms NEC R68.89
  breast NEC N64.59
  development NEC R63.8
  factitious, self-induced -see Disorder,
    factitious
  genital organs, female R10.2
  involving
    abdomen NEC R19.8
    appearance NEC R46.89
    awareness R41.9
      altered mental status R41.82
      amnesia -see Amnesia
      borderline intellectual functioning R41.83
      coma -see Coma
      disorientation R41.0
      neurologic neglect syndrome R41.4
      senile cognitive decline R41.81
      specified symptom NEC R41.89
    behavior NEC R46.89
    cardiovascular system NEC R09.89
    chest NEC R09.89
    circulatory system NEC R09.89
    cognitive functions R41.9
      altered mental status R41.82
      amnesia -see Amnesia
      borderline intellectual functioning R41.83
      coma -see Coma
      disorientation R41.0
      neurologic neglect syndrome R41.4
      senile cognitive decline R41.81
      specified symptom NEC R41.89
    development NEC R62.50
    digestive system NEC R19.8
    emotional state NEC R45.89
      emotional lability R45.86
    food and fluid intake R63.8
    general perceptions and sensations R44.9
      specified NEC R44.8
    musculoskeletal system R29.91
      specified NEC R29.898
    nervous system R29.90
      specified NEC R29.818
    pelvis NEC R19.8
    respiratory system NEC R09.89
    skin and integument R23.9
    urinary system R39.9
  menopausal N95.1
  metabolism NEC R63.8
  neurotic F48.8
  of infancy R68.19
  pelvis NEC, female R10.2
  skin and integument NEC R23.9
  subcutaneous tissue NEC R23.9
Sympus Q74.2
Syncephalus Q89.4
Synchondrosis
  abnormal (congenital) Q78.8
  ischiopubic M91.0
**Synchysis (scintillans) (senile) (vitreous
  body)** H43.89
Syncope (near) (pre-) R55
  anginosa I20.8
  bradycardia R00.1
  cardiac R55
  carotid sinus G90.01
  due to spinal (lumbar) puncture G97.1
  heart R55
  heat T67.1
  laryngeal R05
  psychogenic F48.8
  tussive R05

Syncope --*continued*
  vasoconstriction R55
  vasodepressor R55
  vasomotor R55
  vasovagal R55
Syndactylism, syndactyly Q70.9
  complex (with synostosis)
    fingers Q70.0
    toes Q70.2
  simple (without synostosis)
    fingers Q70.1
    toes Q70.3
Syndrome *-see also* Disease
  5q minus NOS D46.C
  48,XXXX Q97.1
  49,XXXXX Q97.1
  abdominal
    acute R10.0
    muscle deficiency Q79.4
  abnormal innervation H02.519
    left H02.516
      lower H02.515
      upper H02.514
    right H02.513
      lower H02.512
      upper H02.511
  abstinence, neonatal P96.1
  acid pulmonary aspiration, obstetric O74.0
  acquired immunodeficiency *-see* Human,
    immunodeficiency virus (HIV) disease
  acute abdominal R10.0
  acute respiratory distress (adult) (child) J80
    idiopathic J84.114
  Adair-Dighton Q78.0
  Adams-Stokes (Morgagni) I45.9
  adiposogenital E23.6
  adrenal
    hemorrhage (meningococcal) A39.1
    meningococcic A39.1
  adrenocortical *-see* Cushing's, syndrome
  adrenogenital E25.9
    congenital, associated with enzyme
      deficiency E25.0
  afferent loop NEC K91.89
  Alagille's Q44.7
  alcohol withdrawal (without convulsions) *-see*
    Dependence, alcohol, with, withdrawal
  Alder's D72.0
  Aldrich (Wiskott) D82.0
  alien hand R41.4
  Alport Q87.81
  alveolar hypoventilation E66.2
  alveolocapillary block J84.10
  amnesic, amnestic (confabulatory) (due to) -
    see Disorder, amnesic
  amyostatic (Wilson's disease) E83.01
  androgen insensitivity E34.50
    complete E34.51
    partial E34.52
  androgen resistance *-see also* Syndrome,
    androgen insensitivity E34.50
  Angelman Q93.5
  anginal *-see* Angina
  ankyloglossia superior Q38.1
  anterior
    chest wall R07.89
    cord G83.82
    spinal artery G95.19
      compression M47.019
        cervical region M47.012
        cervicothoracic region M47.013

Syndrome *--continued*
        lumbar region M47.016
        occipito-atlanto-axial region M47.011
        thoracic region M47.014
        thoracolumbar region M47.015
    tibial M76.81
  antibody deficiency D80.9
    agammaglobulinemic D80.1
      hereditary D80.0
    congenital D80.0
    hypogammaglobulinemic D80.1
      hereditary D80.0
  anticardiolipin (antibody) D68.61
  antiphospholipid (antibody) D68.61
  aortic
    arch M31.4
    bifurcation I74.09
  aortomesenteric duodenum occlusion K31.5
  apical ballooning (transient left ventricular)
    I51.81
  arcuate ligament I77.4
  argentaffin, argintaffinoma E34.0
  Arnold-Chiari *-see* Arnold-Chiari disease
  Arrillaga-Ayerza I27.0
  arterial tortuosity Q87.82
  arteriovenous steal T82.898
  Asherman's N85.6
  aspiration, of newborn *-see* Aspiration, by
    substance, with pneumonia
    meconium P24.01
  ataxia-telangiectasia G11.3
  auriculotemporal G50.8
  autoerythrocyte sensitization (Gardner-
    Diamond) D69.2
  autoimmune polyglandular E31.0
  autoimmune lymphoproliferative [ALPS]
    D89.82
  autoinflammatory M04.9
    specified type NEC M04.8
  autosomal *-see* Abnormal, autosomes
  Avellis' G46.8
  Ayerza (Arrillaga) I27.0
  Babinski-Nageotte G83.89
  Bakwin-Krida Q78.5
  bare lymphocyte D81.6
  Barré Guillain G61.0
  Barré Liéou M53.0
  Barrett's *-see* Barrett's, esophagus
  Barsony Polgar K22.4
  Barsony Teschendorf K22.4
  Barth E78.71
  Bartter's E26.81
  basal cell nevus Q87.89
  Basedow's E05.00
    with thyroid storm E05.01
  basilar artery G45.0
  Batten-Steinert G71.11
  battered
    baby or child *-see* Maltreatment, child,
      physical abuse
    spouse *-see* Maltreatment, adult, physical
  abuse
  Beals Q87.40
  Beau's I51.5
  Beck's I65.8
  Benedikt's G46.3
  Béquez César (Steinbrinck-Chédiak-Higashi)
    E70.330
  Bernhardt-Roth *-see* Meralgia paresthetica
  Bernheim's I50.9
  big spleen D73.1

Syndrome *--continued*
  bilateral polycystic ovarian E28.2
  Bing-Horton's *-see* Horton's headache
  Birt-Hogg-Dube syndrome Q87.89
  Björck (Thorsen) E34.0
  black
    lung J60
    widow spider bite *-see* Toxicity, venom,
      spider, black widow
  Blackfan-Diamond D61.01
  Blau M04.8
  blind loop K90.2
    congenital Q43.8
    postsurgical K91.2
  blue sclera Q78.0
  blue toe I75.02
  Boder-Sedgewick G11.3
  Boerhaave's K22.3
  Borjeson Forssman Lehmann Q89.8
  Bouillaud's I01.9
  Bourneville (Pringle) Q85.1
  Bouveret (Hoffman) I47.9
  brachial plexus G54.0
  bradycardia-tachycardia I49.5
  brain (nonpsychotic) F09
    with psychosis, psychotic reaction F09
    acute or subacute *-see* Delirium
    congenital *-see* Disability, intellectual
    organic F09
      post-traumatic (nonpsychotic) F07.81
        psychotic F09
    personality change F07.0
    postcontusional F07.81
    post-traumatic, nonpsychotic F07.81
    psycho-organic F09
    psychotic F06.8
  brain stem stroke G46.3
  Brandt's (acrodermatitis enteropathica) E83.2
  broad ligament laceration N83.8
  Brock's J98.11
  bronze baby P83.8
  Brown-Sequard G83.81
  bubbly lung P27.0
  Buchem's M85.2
  Budd-Chiari I82.0
  bulbar (progressive) G12.22
  Bürger-Grütz E78.3
  Burke's K86.89
  Burnett's (milk-alkali) E83.52
  burning feet E53.9
  Bywaters' T79.5
  Call-Fleming I67.841
  carbohydrate-deficient glycoprotein (CDGS)
    E77.8
  carcinogenic thrombophlebitis I82.1
  carcinoid E34.0
  cardiac asthma I50.1
  cardiacos negros I27.0
  cardiofaciocutaneous Q87.89
  cardiopulmonary obesity E66.2
  cardiorenal *-see* Hypertension, cardiorenal
  cardiorespiratory distress (idiopathic),
    newborn P22.0
  cardiovascular renal *-see* Hypertension,
    cardiorenal
  carotid
    artery (hemispheric) (internal) G45.1
    body G90.01
    sinus G90.01
  carpal tunnel G56.0
  Cassidy (Scholte) E34.0

Syndrome --*continued*
  cat cry Q93.4
  cat eye Q92.8
  cauda equina G83.4
  causalgia --*see* Causalgia
  celiac K90.0
    artery compression I77.4
    axis I77.4
  central pain G89.0
  cerebellar
    hereditary G11.9
    stroke G46.4
  cerebellomedullary malformation --*see* Spina
    bifida
  cerebral
    artery
      anterior G46.1
      middle G46.0
      posterior G46.2
    gigantism E22.0
  cervical (root) M53.1
    disc --*see* Disorder, disc, cervical, with
      neuritis
    fusion Q76.1
    posterior, sympathicus M53.0
    rib Q76.5
    sympathetic paralysis G90.2
  cervicobrachial (diffuse) M53.1
  cervicocranial M53.0
  cervicodorsal outlet G54.2
  cervicothoracic outlet G54.0
  Céstan (Raymond) I65.8
  Charcot's (angina cruris) (intermittent
    claudication) I73.9
  Charcot-Weiss-Baker G90.09
  CHARGE Q89.8
  Chédiak-Higashi (Steinbrinck) E70.330
  chest wall R07.1
  Chiari's (hepatic vein thrombosis) I82.0
  Chilaiditi's Q43.3
  child maltreatment --*see* Maltreatment, child
  chondrocostal junction M94.0
  chondroectodermal dysplasia Q77.6
  chromosome 4
short arm deletion Q93.3
  chromosome 5
short arm deletion Q93.4
  chronic
    infantile neurological, cutaneous and
      articular (CINCA) M04.2
    pain G89.4
      personality F68.8
  Clarke-Hadfield K86.89
  Clerambault's automatism G93.89
  Clouston's (hidrotic ectodermal dysplasia)
    Q82.4
  clumsiness, clumsy child F82
  cluster headache G44.009
    intractable G44.001
    not intractable G44.009
  Coffin-Lowry Q89.8
  cold injury (newborn) P80.0
  combined immunity deficiency D81.9
  compartment (deep) (posterior) (traumatic)
    T79.A0
    abdomen T79.A3
    lower extremity (hip, buttock, thigh, leg,
      foot, toes) T79.A2
    nontraumatic
      abdomen M79.A3

Syndrome --*continued*
    lower extremity (hip, buttock, thigh, leg,
      foot, toes) M79.A2
    specified site NEC M79.A9
    upper extremity (shoulder, arm, forearm,
      wrist, hand, fingers) M79.A1
  postprocedural --*see* Syndrome,
    compartment, nontraumatic
  specified site NEC T79.A9
  upper extremity (shoulder, arm, forearm,
    wrist, hand, fingers) T79.A1
  complex regional pain --*see* Syndrome, pain,
  complex regional
  compression T79.5
    anterior spinal --*see* Syndrome, anterior,
      spinal artery, compression
    cauda equina G83.4
    celiac artery I77.4
    vertebral artery M47.029
      occipito-atlanto-axial region M47.021
      cervical region M47.022
  concussion F07.81
  congenital
    affecting multiple systems NEC Q87.89
    central alveolar hypoventilation G47.35
    facial diplegia Q87.0
    muscular hypertrophy cerebral Q87.89
    oculo-auriculovertebral Q87.0
    oculofacial diplegia (Moebius) Q87.0
    rubella (manifest) P35.0
  congestion-fibrosis (pelvic), female N94.89
  congestive dysmenorrhea N94.6
  Conn's E26.01
  connective tissue M35.9
    overlap NEC M35.1
  conus medullaris G95.81
  cord
    anterior G83.82
    posterior G83.83
  coronary
    acute NEC I24.9
    insufficiency or intermediate I20.0
    slow flow I20.8
  Costen's (complex) M26.69
  costochondral junction M94.0
  costoclavicular G54.0
  costovertebral E22.0
  Cowden Q85.8
  craniovertebral M53.0
  Creutzfeldt-Jakob --*see* Creutzfeldt-Jakob
    disease or syndrome
  cri-du-chat Q93.4
  crib death R99
  cricopharyngeal --*see* Dysphagia
  croup J05.0
  CRPS I --*see* Syndrome, pain, complex
    regional I
  crush T79.5
  cubital tunnel --*see* Lesion, nerve, ulnar
  Curschmann (Batten) (Steinert) G71.11
  Cushing's E24.9
    alcohol-induced E24.4
    due to
      alcohol
      drugs E24.2
      ectopic ACTH E24.3
      overproduction of pituitary ACTH E24.0
    drug-induced E24.2
    overdose or wrong substance given or taken
      --*see* Table of Drugs and Chemicals, by drug,
      poisoning

Syndrome --*continued*
  pituitary dependent E24.0
    specified type NEC E24.8
  cryopyrin-associated periodic M04.2
  cryptophthalmos Q87.0
  cystic duct stump K91.5
  Dana-Putnam D51.0
  Danbolt (Cross) (acrodermatitis
    enteropathica) E83.2
  Dandy Walker Q03.1
    with spina bifida Q07.01
  Danlos' Q79.6
  defibrination --*see also* Fibrinolysis
    with
      antepartum hemorrhage --*see* Hemorrhage,
        antepartum, with coagulation defect
      intrapartum hemorrhage --*see* Hemorrhage,
        complicating, delivery
    newborn P60
    postpartum O72.3
  Degos' I77.89
  Déjérine-Roussy G89.0
  delayed sleep phase G47.21
  demyelinating G37.9
  dependence --*see* F10 F19 with fourth
    character .2
  depersonalization (derealization) F48.1
  De Quervain E34.51
  de Toni-Fanconi (Debré) E72.09
    with cystinosis E72.04
  diabetes mellitus-hypertension-nephrosis --*see*
    Diabetes, nephrosis
  diabetes mellitus in newborn infant P70.2
  diabetes-nephrosis --*see* Diabetes, nephrosis
  diabetic amyotrophy --*see* Diabetes,
    amyotrophy
  dialysis associated steal T82.898
  Diamond-Blackfan D61.01
  Diamond-Gardener D69.2
  DIC (diffuse or disseminated intravascular
    coagulopathy) D65
  di George's D82.1
  Dighton's Q78.0
  disequilibrium E87.8
  Döhle body panmyelopathic D72.0
  dorsolateral medullary G46.4
  double athetosis G80.3
  Down --*see also* Down syndrome Q90.9
  Dresbach's (elliptocytosis) D58.1
  Dressler's (postmyocardial infarction) I24.1
    postcardiotomy I97.0
  drug withdrawal, infant of dependent mother
    P96.1
  dry eye H04.12
  due to abnormality
    chromosomal Q99.9
      sex
        female phenotype Q97.9
        male phenotype Q98.9
      specified NEC Q99.8
  dumping (postgastrectomy) K91.1
    nonsurgical K31.89
  Dupré's (meningism) R29.1
  dysmetabolic X E88.81
  dyspraxia, developmental F82
  Eagle-Barrett Q79.4
  Eaton-Lambert --*see* Syndrome, Lambert-
    Eaton
  Ebstein's Q22.5
  ectopic ACTH E24.3
  eczema-thrombocytopenia D82.0

Syndrome --*continued*
  Eddowes' Q78.0
  effort (psychogenic) F45.8
  Eisenmenger's I27.89
  Ehlers-Danlos Q79.6
  Ekman's Q78.0
  electric feet E53.8
  Ellis-van Creveld Q77.6
  empty nest Z60.0
  endocrine-hypertensive E27.0
  entrapment -*see* Neuropathy, entrapment
  eosinophilia-myalgia M35.8
  epileptic -*see also* Epilepsy, by type
    absence G40.A09
      intractable G40.A19
        with status epilepticus G40.A11
        without status epilepticus G40.A19
      not intractable G40.A09
        with status epilepticus G40.A01
        without status epilepticus G40.A09
  Erdheim-Chester (ECD) E88.89
  Erdheim's E22.0
  erythrocyte fragmentation D59.4
  Evans D69.41
  exhaustion F48.8
  extrapyramidal G25.9
    specified NEC G25.89
  eye retraction -*see* Strabismus
  eyelid-malar-mandible Q87.0
  Faber's D50.9
  facial pain, paroxysmal G50.0
  Fallot's Q21.3
  familial cold autoinflammatory M04.2
  familial eczema-thrombocytopenia (Wiskott-Aldrich) D82.0
  Fanconi (de Toni) (Debré) E72.09
    with cystinosis E72.04
  Fanconi's (anemia) (congenital pancytopenia) D61.09
  fatigue
    chronic R53.82
    psychogenic F48.8
  faulty bowel habit K59.39
  Feil-Klippel (brevicollis) Q76.1
  Felty's -*see* Felty's syndrome
  fertile eunuch E23.0
  fetal
    alcohol (dysmorphic) Q86.0
    hydantoin Q86.1
  Fiedler's I40.1
  first arch Q87.0
  fish odor E72.8
  Fisher's G61.0
  Fitzhugh-Curtis
    due to
      Chlamydia trachomatis A74.81
      Neisseria gonorrhorea (gonococcal peritonitis) A54.85
  Fitz's -*see also* Pancreatitis, acute K85.80
  Flajani (Basedow) E05.00
    with thyroid storm E05.01
  flatback -*see* Flatback syndrome - floppy baby P94.2
  iris (intraoperative) (IFIS) H21.81
  mitral valve I34.1
  flush E34.0
  Foix Alajouanine G95.19
  Fong's Q87.2
  food protein-induced enterocolitis K52.21
  foramen magnum G93.5
  Foster-Kennedy H47.14

Syndrome --*continued*
  Foville's (peduncular) G46.3
  fragile X Q99.2
  Franceschetti Q75.4
  Frey's
    auriculotemporal G50.8
    hyperhidrosis L74.52
  Friderichsen-Waterhouse A39.1
  Froin's G95.89
  frontal lobe F07.0
  Fukuhara E88.49
  functional
    bowel K59.9
    prepubertal castrate E29.1
  Gaisböck's D75.1
  ganglion (basal ganglia brain) G25.9
    geniculi G51.1
  Gardner-Diamond D69.2
  gastroesophageal
    junction K22.0
    laceration-hemorrhage K22.6
  gastrojejunal loop obstruction K91.89
  Gee-Herter-Heubner K90.0
  Gelineau's G47.419
    with cataplexy G47.411
  genito-anorectal A55
  Gerstmann-Sträussler-Scheinker (GSS) A81.82
  Gianotti-Crosti L44.4
  giant platelet (Bernard-Soulier) D69.1
  Gilles de la Tourette's F95.2
  goiter-deafness E07.1
  Goldberg Q89.8
  Goldberg-Maxwell E34.51
  Good's D83.8
  Gopalan' (burning feet) E53.8
  Gorlin's Q87.89
  Gougerot-Blum L81.7
  Gouley's I31.1
  Gower's R55
  gray or grey (newborn) P93.0
    platelet D69.1
  Gubler-Millard G46.3
  Guillain-Barré (Strohl) G61.0
  gustatory sweating G50.8
  Hadfield-Clarke K86.89
  hair tourniquet -*see* Constriction, external, by site
  Hamman's J98.19
  hand-foot L27.1
  hand-shoulder G90.8
  hantavirus (cardio) pulmonary (HPS) (HCPS) B33.4
  happy puppet Q93.5
  Harada's H30.81
  Hayem-Faber D50.9
  headache NEC G44.89
    complicated NEC G44.59
  Heberden's I20.8
  Hedinger's E34.0
  Hegglin's D72.0
  HELLP (hemolysis, elevated liver enzymes and low platelet count) O14.2
    complicating
      childbirth O14.24
      puerperium O14.25
  hemolytic-uremic D59.3
  hemophagocytic, infection-associated D76.2
  Henoch-Schönlein D69.0
  hepatic flexure K59.8
  hepatopulmonary K76.81

Syndrome --*continued*
  hepatorenal K76.7
    following delivery O90.4
    postoperative or postprocedural K91.83
    postpartum, puerperal O90.4
  hepatourologic K76.7
  Herter (Gee) (nontropical sprue) K90.0
  Heubner-Herter K90.0
  Heyd's K76.7
  Hilger's G90.09
  histamine-like (fish poisoning) -*see* Poisoning, fish
  histiocytic D76.3
  histiocytosis NEC D76.3
  HIV infection, acute B20
  Hoffmann-Werdnig G12.0
  Hollander-Simons E88.1
  Hoppe-Goldflam G70.00
    with exacerbation (acute) G70.01
    in crisis G70.01
  Horner's G90.2
  hungry bone E83.81
  hunterian glossitis D51.0
  Hutchinson's triad A50.53
  hyperabduction G54.0
  hyperammonemia-hyperornithinemia-homocitrullinemia E72.4
  hypereosinophilic (idiopathic) D72.1
  hyperimmunoglobulin D M04.1
  hyperimmunoglobulin E (IgE) D82.4
  hyperkalemic E87.5
  hyperkinetic -*see* Hyperkinesia
  hypermobility M35.7
  hypernatremia E87.0
  hyperosmolarity E87.0
  hyperperfusion G97.82
  hypersplenic D73.1
  hypertransfusion, newborn P61.1
  hyperventilation F45.8
  hyperviscosity (of serum)
    polycythemic D75.1
    sclerothymic D58.8
  hypoglycemic (familial) (neonatal) E16.2
  hypokalemic E87.6
  hyponatremic E87.1
  hypopituitarism E23.0
  hypoplastic left-heart Q23.4
  hypopotassemia E87.6
  hyposmolality E87.1
  hypotension, maternal O26.5
  hypothenar hammer I73.89
  hypoventilation, obesity (OHS) E66.2
  ICF (intravascular coagulation-fibrinolysis) D65
  idiopathic
    cardiorespiratory distress, newborn P22.0
    nephrotic (infantile) N04.9
  iliotibial band M76.3
  immobility, immobilization (paraplegic) M62.3
  immune reconstitution D89.3
  immune reconstitution inflammatory [IRIS] D89.3
  immunity deficiency, combined D81.9
  immunodeficiency
    acquired -*see* Human, immunodeficiency virus (HIV) disease
    combined D81.9
  impending coronary I20.0
  impingement, shoulder M75.4

Syndrome --*continued*
inappropriate secretion of antidiuretic
    hormone E22.2
infant
    of diabetic mother P70.1
    gestational diabetes P70.0
infantilism (pituitary) E23.0
inferior vena cava I87.1
inspissated bile (newborn) P59.1
institutional (childhood) F94.2
insufficient sleep F51.12
intermediate coronary (artery) I20.0
interspinous ligament -*see* Spondylopathy,
    specified NEC
intestinal
    carcinoid E34.0
    knot K56.2
intravascular coagulation-fibrinolysis (ICF)
    D65
iodine-deficiency, congenital E00.9
    type
        mixed E00.2
        myxedematous E00.1
        neurological E00.0
IRDS (idiopathic respiratory distress,
    newborn) P22.0
irritable
    bowel K58.9
        with
            constipation K58.1
            diarrhea K58.0
        mixed K58.2
        psychogenic F45.8
        specified NEC K58.8
    heart (psychogenic) F45.8
    weakness F48.8
ischemic
    bowel (transient) K55.9
        chronic K55.1
        due to mesenteric artery insufficiency
            K55.1
    steal T82.898
IVC (intravascular coagulopathy) D65
Ivemark's Q89.01
Jaccoud's -*see* Arthropathy, postrheumatic,
    chronic
Jackson's G83.89
Jakob-Creutzfeldt -*see* Creutzfeldt-Jakob
    disease or syndrome
jaw-winking Q07.8
Jervell-Lange-Nielsen I45.81
jet lag G47.25
Job's D71
Joseph-Diamond-Blackfan D61.01
jugular foramen G52.7
Kabuki Q89.8
Kanner's (autism) F84.0
Kartagener's Q89.3
Kelly's D50.1
Kimmelstiel-Wilson -*see* Diabetes, specified
    type, with Kimmelstiel-Wilson disease
Klein (e) Levine G47.13
Klippel-Feil (brevicollis) Q76.1
Köhler-Pellegrini-Steida -*see* Bursitis, tibial
    collateral
Koenig's K59.8
Korsakoff (Wernicke) (nonalcoholic) F04
    alcoholic F10.26
Kostmann's D70.0
Krabbe's congenital muscle hypoplasia Q79.8
labyrinthine - see subcategory H83.2

Syndrome --*continued*
lacunar NEC G46.7
Lambert-Eaton G70.80
    in
        neoplastic disease G73.1
        specified disease NEC G70.81
Landau-Kleffner -*see* Epilepsy, specified
NEC
Larsen's Q74.8
lateral
    cutaneous nerve of thigh G57.1
    medullary G46.4
Launois' E22.0
lazy
    leukocyte D70.8
    posture M62.3
Lemiere I80.8
Lennox Gastaut G40.812
    intractable G40.814
        with status epilepticus G40.813
        without status epilepticus G40.814
    not intractable G40.812
        with status epilepticus G40.811
        without status epilepticus G40.812
lenticular, progressive E83.01
Leopold-Levi's E05.90
Lev's I44.2
Li-Fraumeni Z15.01
Lichtheim's D51.0
Lightwood's N25.89
Lignac (de Toni) (Fanconi) (Debré) E72.09
    with cystinosis E72.04
Likoff's I20.8
limbic epilepsy personality F07.0
liver-kidney K76.7
lobotomy F07.0
Loffler's J82
long arm 18 or 21 deletion Q93.89
long QT I45.81
Louis-Barré G11.3
low
    atmospheric pressure T70.29
    back M54.5
    output (cardiac) I50.9
lower radicular, newborn (birth injury) P14.8
Luetscher's (dehydration) E86.0
Lupus anticoagulant D68.62
Lutembacher's Q21.1
macrophage activation D76.1
    due to infection D76.2
magnesium-deficiency R29.0
Majeed M04.8
Mal de Debarquement R42
malabsorption K90.9
    postsurgical K91.2
malformation, congenital, due to
    alcohol Q86.0
    exogenous cause NEC Q86.8
    hydantoin Q86.1
    warfarin Q86.2
malignant
    carcinoid E34.0
    neuroleptic G21.0
Mallory Weiss K22.6
mandibulofacial dysostosis Q75.4
manic-depressive -*see* Disorder, bipolar
maple-syrup-urine E71.0
Marable's I77.4
Marfan's Q87.40
    with
        cardiovascular manifestations Q87.418

Syndrome --*continued*
    aortic dilation Q87.410
    ocular manifestations Q87.42
    skeletal manifestations Q87.43
Marie's (acromegaly) E22.0
mast cell activation -*see* Activation, mast cell
maternal hypotension -*see* Syndrome,
    hypotension, maternal
May (Hegglin) D72.0
McArdle (Schmidt) (Pearson) E74.04
McQuarrie's E16.2
meconium plug (newborn) P76.0
median arcuate ligament I77.4
Meekeren-Ehlers-Danlos Q79.6
megavitamin-B6 E67.2
Meige G24.4
MELAS E88.41
Mendelson's O74.0
MERRF (myoclonic epilepsy associated with
    ragged-red fibers) E88.42
mesenteric
    artery (superior) K55.1
    vascular insufficiency K55.1
metabolic E88.81
metastatic carcinoid E34.0
micrognathia-glossoptosis Q87.0
midbrain NEC G93.89
middle lobe (lung) J98.19
middle radicular G54.0
migraine -*see also* Migraine G43.909
Mikulicz' K11.8
milk-alkali E83.52
Millard-Gubler G46.3
Miller-Dieker Q93.88
Miller-Fisher G61.0
Minkowski-Chauffard D58.0
Mirizzi's K83.1
MNGIE (Mitochondrial Neurogastrointestinal
    Encephalopathy) E88.49
Möbius, ophthalmoplegic migraine -*see*
    Migraine, ophthalmoplegic
monofixation H50.42
Morel-Moore M85.2
Morel-Morgagni M85.2
Morgagni (Morel) (Stewart) M85.2
Morgagni-Adams-Stokes I45.9
Muckle-Wells M04.2
mucocutaneous lymph node (acute febrile)
    (MCLS) M30.3
multiple endocrine neoplasia (MEN) -*see*
    Neoplasia, endocrine, multiple (MEN)
multiple operations -*see* Disorder, factitious
Mounier-Kuhn Q32.4
    with bronchiectasis J47.9
        with
            exacerbation (acute) J47.1
            lower respiratory infection J47.0
    acquired J98.09
        with bronchiectasis J47.9
            with
                exacerbation (acute) J47.1
                lower respiratory infection J47.0
myasthenic G70.9
    in
        diabetes mellitus -*see* Diabetes,
            amyotrophy
        endocrine disease NEC E34.9 [*G73.3*]
        neoplastic disease -*see also* Neoplasm
            D49.9 [*G73.3*]
        thyrotoxicosis (hyperthyroidism) E05.90
            [*G73.3*]

Syndrome --*continued*

with thyroid storm E05.91 [*G73.3*]
myelodysplastic D46.9
  with
    5q deletion D46.C
    isolated del (5q) chromosomal abnormality D46.C
    lesions, low grade D46.20
    specified NEC D46.Z myelopathic pain G89.0
myeloproliferative (chronic) D47.1
myofascial pain M79.1
Naffziger's G54.0
nail patella Q87.2
NARP (Neuropathy, Ataxia and Retinitis pigmentosa) E88.49
neonatal abstinence P96.1
nephritic -*see also* Nephritis
  with edema -*see* Nephrosis
  acute N00.9
  chronic N03.9
  rapidly progressive N01.9
nephrotic (congenital) -*see also* Nephrosis N04.9
  with
    dense deposit disease N04.6
    diffuse
      crescentic glomerulonephritis N04.7
      endocapillary proliferative glomerulonephritis N04.4
      membranous glomerulonephritis N04.2
      mesangial proliferative glomerulonephritis N04.3
      mesangiocapillary glomerulonephritis N04.5
    focal and segmental glomerular lesions N04.1
    minor glomerular abnormality N04.0
    specified morphological changes NEC N04.8
  diabetic -*see* Diabetes, nephrosis
neurologic neglect R41.4
Nezelof's D81.4
Nonne-Milroy Meige Q82.0
Nothnagel's vasomotor acroparesthesia I73.89
obesity hypoventilation (OHS) E66.2
oculomotor H51.9
ophthalmoplegia-cerebellar ataxia -*see* Strabismus, paralytic, third nerve
oral allergy T78.1
oral-facial-digital Q87.0
organic
  affective F06.30
  amnesic (not alcohol- or drug-induced) F04
  brain F09
  depressive F06.31
  hallucinosis F06.0
  personality F07.0
Ormond's N13.5
oro-facial-digital Q87.0
os trigonum Q68.8
Osler-Weber-Rendu I78.0
osteoporosis-osteomalacia M83.8
Osterreicher-Turner Q87.2
otolith -*see* subcategory H81.8
oto-palatal-digital Q87.0
outlet (thoracic) G54.0
ovary
  polycystic E28.2
  resistant E28.39
  sclerocystic E28.2

Syndrome --*continued*

Owren's D68.2
Paget-Schroetter I82.890
pain -*see also* Pain
  complex regional I G90.50
    lower limb G90.52
    specified site NEC G90.59
    upper limb G90.51
  complex regional II -*see* Causalgia
  painful
    bruising D69.2
    feet E53.8
    prostate N42.81
paralysis agitans -*see* Parkinsonism
paralytic G83.9
  specified NEC G83.89
Parinaud's H51.0
parkinsonian -*see* Parkinsonism
Parkinson's -*see* Parkinsonism
paroxysmal facial pain G50.0
Parry's E05.00
  with thyroid storm E05.01
Parsonage (Aldren) Turner G54.5
patella clunk M25.86
Paterson (Brown) (Kelly) D50.1
pectoral girdle I77.89
pectoralis minor I77.89
Pelger-Huet D72.0
pellagra-cerebellar ataxia-renal aminoaciduria E72.02
pellagroid E52
Pellegrini-Stieda -*see* Bursitis, tibial collateral
pelvic congestion-fibrosis, female N94.89
penta X Q97.1
peptic ulcer -*see* Ulcer, peptic
perabduction I77.89
periodic fever M04.1
periodic fever, aphthous stomatitis, pharyngitis, and adenopathy [PFAPA] M04.8
periodic headache, in adults and children -*see* Headache, periodic syndromes in adults and children
periurethral fibrosis N13.5
phantom limb (without pain) G54.7
  with pain G54.6
pharyngeal pouch D82.1
Pick's -*see* Disease, Pick's
Pickwickian E66.2
PIE (pulmonary infiltration with eosinophilia) J82
pigmentary pallidal degeneration (progressive) G23.0
pineal E34.8
pituitary E22.0
plantar fascia M72.2
placental transfusion -*see* Pregnancy, complicated by, placental transfusion syndromes
plateau iris (post-iridectomy) (postprocedural) H21.82
Plummer-Vinson D50.1
pluricarential of infancy E40
plurideficiency E40
pluriglandular (compensatory) E31.8
  autoimmune E31.0
pneumatic hammer T75.21
polyangiitis overlap M30.8
polycarential of infancy E40
polyglandular E31.8
  autoimmune E31.0

Syndrome --*continued*

polysplenia Q89.09
pontine NEC G93.89
popliteal
  artery entrapment I77.89
  web Q87.89
postcardiac injury
  postcardiotomy I97.0
  postmyocardial infarction I24.1
postcardiotomy I97.0
post chemoembolization
  code to associated conditions
postcholecystectomy K91.5
postcommissurotomy I97.0
postconcussional F07.81
postcontusional F07.81
postencephalitic F07.89
posterior
  cervical sympathetic M53.0
  cord G83.83
  fossa compression G93.5
  reversible encephalopathy (PRES) I67.83
postgastrectomy (dumping) K91.1
postgastric surgery K91.1
postinfarction I24.1
postlaminectomy NEC M96.1
postleukotomy F07.0
postmastectomy lymphedema I97.2
postmyocardial infarction I24.1
postoperative NEC T81.9
  blind loop K90.2
postpartum panhypopituitary (Sheehan) E23.0
postpolio (myelitic) G14
postthrombotic I87.009
  with
    inflammation I87.02
      with ulcer I87.03
    specified complication NEC I87.09
    ulcer I87.01
      with inflammation I87.03
  asymptomatic I87.00
postvagotomy K91.1
postvalvulotomy I97.0
postviral NEC G93.3
  fatigue G93.3
Potain's K31.0
potassium intoxication E87.5
precerebral artery (multiple) (bilateral) G45.2
preinfarction I20.0
preleukemic D46.9
premature senility E34.8
premenstrual dysphoric F32.89
premenstrual tension N94.3
Prinzmetal-Massumi R07.1
prune belly Q79.4
pseudocarpal tunnel (sublimis) -*see* Syndrome, carpal tunnel
pseudoparalytica G70.00
  with exacerbation (acute) G70.01
  in crisis G70.01
pseudo -Turner's Q87.1
psycho-organic (nonpsychotic severity) F07.9
  acute or subacute F05
  depressive type F06.31
  hallucinatory type F06.0
  nonpsychotic severity F07.0
  specified NEC F07.89
pulmonary
  arteriosclerosis I27.0
  dysmaturity (Wilson-Mikity) P27.0
  hypoperfusion (idiopathic) P22.0

Syndrome --*continued*

renal (hemorrhagic) (Goodpasture's) M31.0
pure
  motor lacunar G46.5
  sensory lacunar G46.6
Putnam-Dana D51.0
pyogenic arthritis, pyoderma gangrenosum, and acne [PAPA] M04.8
pyramidopallidonigral G20
pyriformis -*see* Lesion, nerve, sciatic
QT interval prolongation I45.81
radicular NEC -*see* Radiculopathy
  upper limbs, newborn (birth injury) P14.3
rapid time-zone change G47.25
Rasmussen G04.81
Raymond (Céstan) I65.8
Raynaud's I73.00
  with gangrene I73.01
RDS (respiratory distress syndrome, newborn) P22.0
reactive airways dysfunction J68.3
Refsum's G60.1
Reifenstein E34.52
renal glomerulohyalinosis-diabetic -*see* Diabetes, nephrosis
Rendu-Osler-Weber I78.0
residual ovary N99.83
resistant ovary E28.39
respiratory
  distress
    acute J80
      adult J80
      child J80
      idiopathic J84.114
      newborn (idiopathic) (type I) P22.0
      type II P22.1
restless legs G25.81
retinoblastoma (familial) C69.2
retroperitoneal fibrosis N13.5
retroviral seroconversion (acute) Z21
Reye's G93.7
Richter -*see* Leukemia, chronic lymphocytic, B-cell type
Ridley's I50.1
right
  heart, hypoplastic Q22.6
  ventricular obstruction -*see* Failure, heart, congestive
Romano-Ward (prolonged QT interval) I45.81
rotator cuff, shoulder -*see also* Tear, rotator cuff M75.10
Rotes Quérol -*see* Hyperostosis, ankylosing
Roth -*see* Meralgia paresthetica
rubella (congenital) P35.0
Ruvalcaba-Myhre-Smith E71.440
Rytand-Lipsitch I44.2
salt
  depletion E87.1
    due to heat NEC T67.8
      causing heat exhaustion or prostration T67.4
  low E87.1
salt-losing N28.89
Scaglietti-Dagnini E22.0
scalenus anticus (anterior) G54.0
scapulocostal -*see* Mononeuropathy, upper limb, specified site NEC
scapuloperoneal G71.0
schizophrenic, of childhood NEC F84.5

Syndrome --*continued*

Schnitzler D47.2
Scholte's E34.0
Schroeder's E27.0
Schüller-Christian C96.5
Schwachman's -*see* Syndrome, Shwachman's
Schwartz (Jampel) G71.13
Schwartz Bartter E22.2
scimitar Q26.8
sclerocystic ovary E28.2
Seitelberger's G31.89
septicemic adrenal hemorrhage A39.1
seroconversion, retroviral (acute) Z21
serous meningitis G93.2
severe acute respiratory (SARS) J12.81
shaken infant T74.4
shock (traumatic) T79.4
  kidney N17.0
    following crush injury T79.5
  toxic A48.3
shock-lung J80
Shone's
code to specific anomalies
short
  bowel K91.2
  rib Q77.2
shoulder-hand -*see* Algoneurodystrophy
Shwachman's D70.4
sicca -*see* Sicca syndrome
sick
  cell E87.1
  sinus I49.5
sick-euthyroid E07.81
sideropenic D50.1
Siemens' ectodermal dysplasia Q82.4
Silfversköld's Q78.9
Simons' E88.1
sinus tarsi M25.57
sinusitis-bronchiectasis-situs inversus Q89.3
Sipple's E31.22
sirenomelia Q87.2
Slocumb's E27.0
slow flow, coronary I20.8
Sluder's G44.89
Smith-Magenis Q93.88
Sneddon-Wilkinson L13.1
Soto's Q87.3
South African cardiomyopathy I42.8
spasmodic
  upward movement, eyes H51.8
  winking F95.8
Spen's I45.9
splenic
  agenesis Q89.01
  flexure K59.8
  neutropenia D73.81
Spurway's Q78.0
staphylococcal scalded skin L00
steal
  arteriovenous T82.898
  ischemic T82.898
  subclavian G45.8
Stein-Leventhal E28.2
Stein's E28.2
Stevens-Johnson syndrome L51.1
  toxic epidermal necrolysis overlap L51.3
Stewart-Morel M85.2
Stickler Q89.8
stiff baby Q89.8
stiff man G25.82
Still-Felty -*see* Felty's syndrome

Syndrome --*continued*

Stokes (Adams) I45.9
stone heart I50.1
straight back, congenital Q76.49
subclavian steal G45.8
subcoracoid-pectoralis minor G54.0
subcostal nerve compression I77.89
subphrenic interposition Q43.3
superior
  cerebellar artery I63.8
  mesenteric artery K55.1
  semi-circular canal dehiscence H83.8X
  vena cava I87.1
supine hypotensive (maternal) -*see* Syndrome, hypotension, maternal
suprarenal cortical E27.0
supraspinatus -*see also* Tear, rotator cuff M75.10
Susac G93.49
swallowed blood P78.2
sweat retention L74.0
Swyer Q99.1
Symond's G93.2
sympathetic
  cervical paralysis G90.2
  pelvic, female N94.89
systemic inflammatory response (SIRS), of non-infectious origin (without organ dysfunction) R65.10
  with acute organ dysfunction R65.11
tachycardia-bradycardia I49.5
takotsubo I51.81
TAR (thrombocytopenia with absent radius) Q87.2
tarsal tunnel G57.5
teething K00.7
tegmental G93.89
telangiectasic-pigmentation-cataract Q82.8
temporal pyramidal apex -*see* Otitis, media, suppurative, acute
temporomandibular joint-pain-dysfunction M26.62
Terry's H44.2
testicular feminization -*see also* Syndrome, androgen insensitivity E34.51
thalamic pain (hyperesthetic) G89.0
thoracic outlet (compression) G54.0
Thorson-Björck E34.0
thrombocytopenia with absent radius (TAR) Q87.2
thyroid-adrenocortical insufficiency E31.0
tibial
  anterior M76.81
  posterior M76.82
Tietze's M94.0
time-zone (rapid) G47.25
Toni-Fanconi E72.09
  with cystinosis E72.04
Touraine's Q79.8
tourniquet -*see* Constriction, external, by site
toxic shock A48.3
transient left ventricular apical ballooning I51.81
traumatic vasospastic T75.22
Treacher Collins Q75.4
triple X, female Q97.0
trisomy Q92.9
  13 Q91.7
    meiotic nondisjunction Q91.4
    mitotic nondisjunction Q91.5
    mosaicism Q91.5

Syndrome --*continued*
translation Q91.6
18 Q91.3
meiotic nondisjunction Q91.0
mitotic nondisjunction Q91.1
mosaicism Q91.1
translocation Q91.2
20 (q)(p) Q92.8
21 Q90.9
meiotic nondisjunction Q90.0
mitotic nondisjunction Q90.1
mosaicism Q90.1
translocation Q90.2
22 Q92.8
tropical wet feet T69.0
Trousseau's I82.1
tumor lysis (following antineoplastic
chemotherapy) (spontaneous) NEC E88.3
tumor necrosis factor receptor associated
periodic (TRAPS) M04.1
Twiddler's (due to)
automatic implantable defibrillator T82.198
cardiac pacemaker T82.198
Unverricht (Lundborg) -*see* Epilepsy,
generalized, idiopathic
upward gaze H51.8
uremia, chronic -*see also* Disease, kidney,
chronic N18.9
urethral N34.3
urethro-oculo-articular -*see* Reiter's disease
urohepatic K76.7
vago-hypoglossal G52.7
vascular NEC in cerebrovascular disease
G46.8
vasoconstriction, reversible cerebrovascular
I67.841
vasomotor I73.9
vasospastic (traumatic) T75.22
vasovagal R55
van Buchem's M85.2
van der Hoeve's Q78.0
VATER Q87.2
velo-cardio-facial Q93.81
vena cava (inferior) (superior) (obstruction)
I87.1
vertebral
artery G45.0
compression -*see* Syndrome, anterior,
spinal artery, compression
steal G45.0
vertebro-basilar artery G45.0
vertebrogenic (pain) M54.89
vertiginous -*see* Disorder, vestibular function
Vinson-Plummer D50.1
virus B34.9
visceral larva migrans B83.0
visual disorientation H53.8
vitamin B6 deficiency E53.1
vitreal corneal H59.01
vitreous (touch) H59.01
Vogt-Koyanagi H20.82
Volkmann's T79.6
von Schroetter's I82.890
von Willebrand (Jürgen) D68.0
Waldenström-Kjellberg D50.1
Wallenberg's G46.3
water retention E87.79
Waterhouse (Friderichsen) A39.1
Weber-Gubler G46.3
Weber-Leyden G46.3
Weber's G46.3

Syndrome --*continued*
Wegener's M31.30
with
kidney involvement M31.31
lung involvement M31.30
with kidney involvement M31.31
Weingarten's (tropical eosinophilia) J82
Weiss-Baker G90.09
Werdnig-Hoffman G12.0
Wermer's E31.21
Werner's E34.8
Wernicke-Korsakoff (nonalcoholic) F04
alcoholic F10.26
West's -*see* Epilepsy, spasms
Westphal-Strümpell E83.01
wet
feet (maceration) (tropical) T69.0
lung, newborn P22.1
whiplash S13.4
whistling face Q87.0
Wilkie's K55.1
Wilkinson-Sneddon L13.1
Willebrand (Jürgens) D68.0
Wilson's (hepatolenticular degeneration)
E83.01
Wiskott-Aldrich D82.0
withdrawal -*see* Withdrawal, state
drug
infant of dependent mother P96.1
therapeutic use, newborn P96.2
Woakes' (ethmoiditis) J33.1
Wright's (hyperabduction) I77.89
X I20.9
XXXX Q97.1
XXXXX Q97.1
XXXXY Q98.1
XXY Q98.0
yellow nail L60.5
Zahorsky's B08.5
Zellweger syndrome E71.510
Zellweger-like syndrome E71.541
Synechia (anterior) (iris) (posterior) (pupil) -
see also Adhesions, iris
intra-uterine (traumatic) N85.6
Synesthesia R20.8
Syngamiasis, syngamosis B83.3
Synodontia K00.2
Synorchidism, synorchism Q55.1
Synostosis (congenital) Q78.8
astragalo-scaphoid Q74.2
radioulnar Q74.0
Synovial sarcoma -*see* Neoplasm, connective
tissue, malignant
Synovioma (malignant) -*see also* Neoplasm,
connective tissue, malignant
benign -*see* Neoplasm, connective tissue,
benign
Synoviosarcoma -*see* Neoplasm, connective
tissue, malignant
Synovitis -*see also* Tenosynovitis M65.9
crepitant
hand M70.0
wrist M70.03
gonococcal A54.49
gouty -*see* Gout
in (due to)
crystals M65.8
gonorrhea A54.49
syphilis (late) A52.78
use, overuse, pressure -*see* Disorder, soft
tissue, due to use

Synovitis - *continued*
infective NEC -*see* Tenosynovitis, infective
NEC
specified NEC -*see* Tenosynovitis, specified
type NEC
syphilitic A52.78
congenital (early) A50.02
toxic -*see* Synovitis, transient
transient M67.3
ankle M67.37
elbow M67.32
foot joint M67.37
hand joint M67.34
hip M67.35
knee M67.36
multiple site M67.39
pelvic region M67.35
shoulder M67.31
specified joint NEC M67.38
wrist M67.33
traumatic, current -*see* Sprain
tuberculous -*see* Tuberculosis, synovitis
villonodular (pigmented) M12.2
ankle M12.27
elbow M12.22
foot joint M12.27
hand joint M12.24
hip M12.25
knee M12.26
multiple site M12.29
pelvic region M12.25
shoulder M12.21
specified joint NEC M12.28
vertebrae M12.28
wrist M12.23
Syphilid A51.39
congenital A50.06
newborn A50.06
tubercular (late) A52.79
Syphilis, syphilitic (acquired) A53.9
abdomen (late) A52.79
acoustic nerve A52.15
adenopathy (secondary) A51.49
adrenal (gland) (with cortical hypofunction)
A52.79
age under 2
years NOS -*see also* Syphilis, congenital, early
acquired A51.9
alopecia (secondary) A51.32
anemia (late) A52.79 [*D63.8*]
aneurysm (aorta) (ruptured) A52.01
central nervous system A52.05
congenital A50.54 [*I79.0*]
anus (late) A52.74
primary A51.1
secondary A51.39
aorta (arch) (abdominal) (thoracic) A52.02
aneurysm A52.01
aortic (insufficiency) (regurgitation) (stenosis)
A52.03
aneurysm A52.01
arachnoid (adhesive) (cerebral) (spinal)
A52.13
asymptomatic -*see* Syphilis, latent
ataxia (locomotor) A52.11
atrophoderma maculatum A51.39
auricular fibrillation A52.06
bladder (late) A52.76
bone A52.77
secondary A51.46
brain A52.17

Syphilis, syphilitic --*continued*
  breast (late) A52.79
  bronchus (late) A52.72
  bubo (primary) A51.0
  bulbar palsy A52.19
  bursa (late) A52.78
  cardiac decompensation A52.06
  cardiovascular A52.00
  central nervous system (late) (recurrent)
  (relapse) (tertiary) A52.3
    with
      ataxia A52.11
      general paralysis A52.17
        juvenile A50.45
      paresis (general) A52.17
        juvenile A50.45
      tabes (dorsalis) A52.11
        juvenile A50.45
      taboparesis A52.17
        juvenile A50.45
    aneurysm A52.05
    congenital A50.40
      juvenile A50.40
    remission in (sustained) A52.3
    serology doubtful, negative, or positive
      A52.3
    specified nature or site NEC A52.19
    vascular A52.05
  cerebral A52.17
    meningovascular A52.13
    nerves (multiple palsies) A52.15
    sclerosis A52.17
    thrombosis A52.05
  cerebrospinal (tabetic type) A52.12
  cerebrovascular A52.05
  cervix (late) A52.76
  chancre (multiple) A51.0
    extragenital A51.2
    Rollet's A51.0
  Charcot's joint A52.16
  chorioretinitis A51.43
    congenital A50.01
    late A52.71
    prenatal A50.01
  choroiditis -*see* Syphilitic chorioretinitis
  choroidoretinitis -*see* Syphilitic chorioretinitis
  ciliary body (secondary) A51.43
    late A52.71
  colon (late) A52.74
  combined spinal sclerosis A52.11
  condyloma (latum) A51.31
  congenital A50.9
    with
      paresis (general) A50.45
      tabes (dorsalis) A50.45
      taboparesis A50.45
    chorioretinitis, choroiditis A50.01 [*H32*]
    early, or less than 2 years after birth NEC
    A50.2
      with manifestations -*see* Syphilis,
        congenital, early, symptomatic
      latent (without manifestations) A50.1
        negative spinal fluid test A50.1
        serology positive A50.1
      symptomatic A50.09
        cutaneous A50.06
        mucocutaneous A50.07
        oculopathy A50.01
        osteochondropathy A50.02
        pharyngitis A50.03
        pneumonia A50.04

Syphilis, syphilitic --*continued*
    rhinitis A50.05
      visceral A50.08
    interstitial keratitis A50.31
    juvenile neurosyphilis A50.45
    late, or 2 years or more after birth NEC
    A50.7
      chorioretinitis, choroiditis A50.32
      interstitial keratitis A50.31
      juvenile neurosyphilis A50.45
      latent (without manifestations) A50.6
        negative spinal fluid test A50.6
        serology positive A50.6
      symptomatic or with manifestations NEC
      A50.59
        arthropathy A50.55
        cardiovascular A50.54
        Clutton's joints A50.51
        Hutchinson's teeth A50.52
        Hutchinson's triad A50.53
        osteochondropathy A50.56
        saddle nose A50.57
  conjugal A53.9
    tabes A52.11
  conjunctiva (late) A52.71
  contact Z20.2
  cord bladder A52.19
  cornea, late A52.71
  coronary (artery) (sclerosis) A52.06
  coryza, congenital A50.05
  cranial nerve A52.15
    multiple palsies A52.15
  cutaneous -*see* Syphilis, skin
  dacryocystitis (late) A52.71
  degeneration, spinal cord A52.12
  dementia paralytica A52.17
    juvenilis A50.45
  destruction of bone A52.77
  dilatation, aorta A52.01
  due to blood transfusion A53.9
  dura mater A52.13
  ear A52.79
    inner A52.79
      nerve (eighth) A52.15
      neurorecurrence A52.15
  early A51.9
    cardiovascular A52.00
    central nervous system A52.3
    latent (without manifestations) (less than 2
    years after infection) A51.5
      negative spinal fluid test A51.5
      serological relapse after treatment A51.5
      serology positive A51.5
    relapse (treated, untreated) A51.9
    skin A51.39
    symptomatic A51.9
      extragenital chancre A51.2
      primary, except extragenital chancre A51.0
      secondary -*see also* Syphilis, secondary
      A51.39
        relapse (treated, untreated) A51.49
    ulcer A51.39
  eighth nerve (neuritis) A52.15
  endemic A65
  endocarditis A52.03
    aortic A52.03
    pulmonary A52.03
  epididymis (late) A52.76
  epiglottis (late) A52.73
  epiphysitis (congenital) (early) A50.02
  episcleritis (late) A52.71

Syphilis, syphilitic --*continued*
  esophagus A52.79
  eustachian tube A52.73
  exposure to Z20.2
  eye A52.71
  eyelid (late) (with gumma) A52.71
  fallopian tube (late) A52.76
  fracture A52.77
  gallbladder (late) A52.74
  gastric (polyposis) (late) A52.74
  general A53.9
    paralysis A52.17
      juvenile A50.45
  genital (primary) A51.0
  glaucoma A52.71
  gumma NEC A52.79
    cardiovascular system A52.00
    central nervous system A52.3
    congenital A50.59
  heart (block) (decompensation) (disease)
  (failure) A52.06 [*I52*]
    valve NEC A52.03
  hemianesthesia A52.19
  hemianopsia A52.71
  hemiparesis A52.17
  hemiplegia A52.17
  hepatic artery A52.09
  hepatis A52.74
  hepatomegaly, congenital A50.08
  hereditaria tarda -*see* Syphilis, congenital, late
  hereditary -*see* Syphilis, congenital
  Hutchinson's teeth A50.52
  hyalitis A52.71
  inactive -*see* Syphilis, latent
  infantum -*see* Syphilis, congenital
  inherited -*see* Syphilis, congenital
  internal ear A52.79
  intestine (late) A52.74
  iris, iritis (secondary) A51.43
    late A52.71
  joint (late) A52.77
  keratitis (congenital) (interstitial) (late)
    A50.31
  kidney (late) A52.75
  lacrimal passages (late) A52.71
  larynx (late) A52.73
  late A52.9
    cardiovascular A52.00
    central nervous system A52.3
    kidney A52.75
    latent or 2 years or more after infection
    (without manifestations) A52.8
      negative spinal fluid test A52.8
      serology positive A52.8
    paresis A52.17
    specified site NEC A52.79
    symptomatic or with manifestations A52.79
    tabes A52.11
  latent A53.0
    with signs or symptoms
  code by site and stage under Syphilis
    central nervous system A52.2
    date of infection unspecified A53.0
    early, or less than 2 years after infection
    A51.5
    follow-up of latent syphilis A53.0
      date of infection unspecified A53.0
      late, or 2 years or more after infection
      A52.8
    late, or 2 years or more after infection A52.8
    positive serology (only finding) A53.0

Syphilis, syphilitic --*continued*

date of infection unspecified A53.0
early, or less than 2 years after infection
A51.5
late, or 2 years or more after infection
A52.8
lens (late) A52.71
leukoderma A51.39
  late A52.79
lienitis A52.79
lip A51.39
  chancre (primary) A51.2
  late A52.79
Lissauer's paralysis A52.17
liver A52.74
locomotor ataxia A52.11
lung A52.72
lymph gland (early) (secondary) A51.49
  late A52.79
lymphadenitis (secondary) A51.49
macular atrophy of skin A51.39
  striated A52.79
mediastinum (late) A52.73
meninges (adhesive) (brain) (spinal cord)
A52.13
meningitis A52.13
  acute (secondary) A51.41
  congenital A50.41
meningoencephalitis A52.14
meningovascular A52.13
  congenital A50.41
mesarteritis A52.09
  brain A52.04
middle ear A52.77
mitral stenosis A52.03
monoplegia A52.17
mouth (secondary) A51.39
  late A52.79
mucocutaneous (secondary) A51.39
  late A52.79
mucous
  membrane (secondary) A51.39
    late A52.79
  patches A51.39
    congenital A50.07
mulberry molars A50.52
muscle A52.78
myocardium A52.06
nasal sinus (late) A52.73
neonatorum -*see* Syphilis, congenital
nephrotic syndrome (secondary) A51.44
nerve palsy (any cranial nerve) A52.15
  multiple A52.15
nervous system, central A52.3
neuritis A52.15
  acoustic A52.15
neurorecidive of retina A52.19
neuroretinitis A52.19
newborn -*see* Syphilis, congenital
nodular superficial (late) A52.79
nonvenereal A65
nose (late) A52.73
  saddle back deformity A50.57
occlusive arterial disease A52.09
oculopathy A52.71
ophthalmic (late) A52.71
optic nerve (atrophy) (neuritis) (papilla)
A52.15
orbit (late) A52.71
organic A53.9
osseous (late) A52.77

Syphilis, syphilitic --*continued*

osteochondritis (congenital) (early) A50.02
[*M90.80*]
osteoporosis A52.77
ovary (late) A52.76
oviduct (late) A52.76
palate (late) A52.79
pancreas (late) A52.74
paralysis A52.17
  general A52.17
    juvenile A50.45
paresis (general) A52.17
  juvenile A50.45
paresthesia A52.19
Parkinson's disease or syndrome A52.19
paroxysmal tachycardia A52.06
pemphigus (congenital) A50.06
penis (chancre) A51.0
  late A52.76
pericardium A52.06
perichondritis, larynx (late) A52.73
periosteum (late) A52.77
  congenital (early) A50.02 [*M90.80*]
  early (secondary) A51.46
peripheral nerve A52.79
petrous bone (late) A52.77
pharynx (late) A52.73
  secondary A51.39
pituitary (gland) A52.79
pleura (late) A52.73
pneumonia, white A50.04
pontine lesion A52.17
portal vein A52.09
primary A51.0
  anal A51.1
  and secondary -*see* Syphilis, secondary
  central nervous system A52.3
  extragenital chancre NEC A51.2
  fingers A51.2
  genital A51.0
  lip A51.2
  specified site NEC A51.2
  tonsils A51.2
prostate (late) A52.76
ptosis (eyelid) A52.71
pulmonary (late) A52.72
  artery A52.09
pyelonephritis (late) A52.75
recently acquired, symptomatic A51.9
rectum (late) A52.74
respiratory tract (late) A52.73
retina, late A52.71
retrobulbar neuritis A52.15
salpingitis A52.76
sclera (late) A52.71
sclerosis
  cerebral A52.17
  coronary A52.06
  multiple A52.11
scotoma (central) A52.71
scrotum (late) A52.76
secondary (and primary) A51.49
  adenopathy A51.49
  anus A51.39
  bone A51.46
  chorioretinitis, choroiditis A51.43
  hepatitis A51.45
  liver A51.45
  lymphadenitis A51.49
  meningitis (acute) A51.41
  mouth A51.39

Syphilis, syphilitic --*continued*

mucous membranes A51.39
periosteum, periostitis A51.46
pharynx A51.39
relapse (treated, untreated) A51.49
skin A51.39
specified form NEC A51.49
tonsil A51.39
ulcer A51.39
viscera NEC A51.49
vulva A51.39
seminal vesicle (late) A52.76
seronegative with signs or symptoms
code by site and stage under Syphilis
seropositive
  with signs or symptoms
  code by site and stage under Syphilis
  follow-up of latent syphilis -*see* Syphilis,
    latent
  only finding -*see* Syphilis, latent
seventh nerve (paralysis) A52.15
sinus, sinusitis (late) A52.73
skeletal system A52.77
skin (with ulceration) (early) (secondary)
A51.39
  late or tertiary A52.79
small intestine A52.74
spastic spinal paralysis A52.17
spermatic cord (late) A52.76
spinal (cord) A52.12
spleen A52.79
splenomegaly A52.79
spondylitis A52.77
staphyloma A52.71
stigmata (congenital) A50.59
stomach A52.74
synovium A52.78
tabes dorsalis (late) A52.11
  juvenile A50.45
tabetic type A52.11
  juvenile A50.45
taboparesis A52.17
  juvenile A50.45
tachycardia A52.06
tendon (late) A52.78
tertiary A52.9
  with symptoms NEC A52.79
  cardiovascular A52.00
  central nervous system A52.3
  multiple NEC A52.79
  specified site NEC A52.79
testis A52.76
thorax A52.73
throat A52.73
thymus (gland) (late) A52.79
thyroid (late) A52.79
tongue (late) A52.79
tonsil (lingual) (late) A52.73
  primary A51.2
  secondary A51.39
trachea (late) A52.73
tunica vaginalis (late) A52.76
ulcer (any site) (early) (secondary) A51.39
  late A52.79
  perforating A52.79
    foot A52.11
urethra (late) A52.76
urogenital (late) A52.76
uterus (late) A52.76
uveal tract (secondary) A51.43
  late A52.71

Syphilis, syphilitic *--continued*
  uveitis (secondary) A51.43
    late A52.71
  uvula (late) (perforated) A52.79
  vagina A51.0
    late A52.76
  valvulitis NEC A52.03
  vascular A52.00
    brain (cerebral) A52.05
  ventriculi A52.74
  vesicae urinariae (late) A52.76
  viscera (abdominal) (late) A52.74
    secondary A51.49
  vitreous (opacities) (late) A52.71
    hemorrhage A52.71
  vulva A51.0
    late A52.76
    secondary A51.39
Syphiloma A52.79
  cardiovascular system A52.00
  central nervous system A52.3
  circulatory system A52.00
  congenital A50.59
Syphilophobia F45.29
Syringadenoma *-see also* Neoplasm, skin,
  benign
  papillary *-see* Neoplasm, skin, benign
Syringobulbia G95.0
Syringocystadenoma *-see* Neoplasm, skin,
  benign
  papillary *-see* Neoplasm, skin, benign
Syringoma *-see also* Neoplasm, skin, benign
  chondroid *-see* Neoplasm, skin, benign
Syringomyelia G95.0
Syringomyelitis *-see* Encephalitis
Syringomyelocele *-see* Spina bifida
Syringopontia G95.0
System, systemic *-see also* condition
  disease, combined *-see* Degeneration,
    combined
  inflammatory response syndrome (SIRS) of
    non-infectious origin (without organ
    dysfunction) R65.10
    with acute organ dysfunction R65.11
  lupus erythematosus M32.9
    inhibitor present D68.62

T

Tabacism, tabacosis, tabagism *-see also*
  Poisoning, tobacco
  meaning dependence (without remission)
    F17.200
    with
      disorder F17.299
        remission F17.211
        specified disorder NEC F17.298
        withdrawal F17.203
Tabardillo A75.9
  flea-borne A75.2
  louse-borne A75.0
Tabes, tabetic A52.10
  with
    central nervous system syphilis A52.10
    Charcot's joint A52.16
    cord bladder A52.19
    crisis, viscera (any) A52.19
    paralysis, general A52.17
    paresis (general) A52.17
    perforating ulcer (foot) A52.19
  arthropathy (Charcot) A52.16

Tabes, tabetic *--continued*
  bladder A52.19
  bone A52.11
  cerebrospinal A52.12
  congenital A50.45
  conjugal A52.10
  dorsalis A52.11
    juvenile A50.49
  juvenile A50.49
  latent A52.19
  mesenterica A18.39
  paralysis, insane, general A52.17
  spasmodic A52.17
  syphilis (cerebrospinal) A52.12
Taboparalysis A52.17
Taboparesis (remission) A52.17
  juvenile A50.45
TAC (trigeminal autonomic cephalgia) NEC
  G44.099
  intractable G44.091
  not intractable G44.099
Tache noir S60.22
Tachyalimentation K91.2
Tachyarrhythmia, tachyrhythmia *-see*
  Tachycardia
Tachycardia R00.0
  atrial (paroxysmal) I47.1
  auricular I47.1
  AV nodal re-entry (re-entrant) I47.1
  junctional (paroxysmal) I47.1
  newborn P29.11
  nodal (paroxysmal) I47.1
  non-paroxysmal AV nodal I45.89
  paroxysmal (sustained) (nonsustained) I47.9
    with sinus bradycardia I49.5
    atrial (PAT) I47.1
    atrioventricular (AV) (re-entrant) I47.1
      psychogenic F54
    junctional I47.1
      ectopic I47.1
    nodal I47.1
    psychogenic (atrial) (supraventricular)
    (ventricular) F54
    supraventricular (sustained) I47.1
      psychogenic F54
    ventricular I47.2
      psychogenic F54
    psychogenic F45.8
  sick sinus I49.5
  sinoauricular NOS R00.0
    paroxysmal I47.1
  sinus [sinusal] NOS R00.0
    paroxysmal I47.1
  supraventricular I47.1
  ventricular (paroxysmal) (sustained) I47.2
    psychogenic F54
Tachygastria K31.89
Tachypnea R06.82
  hysterical F45.8
  newborn (idiopathic) (transitory) P22.1
  psychogenic F45.8
  transitory, of newborn P22.1
Taenia (infection) (infestation) B68.9
  diminuta B71.0
  echinococcal infestation B67.90
  mediocanellata B68.1
  nana B71.0
  saginata B68.1
  solium (intestinal form) B68.0
    larval form *-see* Cysticercosis
Taeniasis (intestine) *-see* Taenia

TACO (transfusion associated circulatory
  overload) E87.71
Tag (hypertrophied skin) (infected) L91.8
  adenoid J35.8
  anus K64.4
  hemorrhoidal K64.4
  hymen N89.8
  perineal N90.89
  preauricular Q17.0
  sentinel K64.4
  skin L91.8
    accessory (congenital) Q82.8
    anus K64.4
    congenital Q82.8
    preauricular Q17.0
  tonsil J35.8
  urethra, urethral N36.8
  vulva N90.89
Tahyna fever B33.8
Takahara's disease E80.3
Takayasu's disease or syndrome M31.4
Talcosis (pulmonary) J62.0
Talipes (congenital) Q66.89
  acquired, planus *-see* Deformity, limb, flat
    foot
  asymmetric Q66.89
  calcaneovalgus Q66.4
  calcaneovarus Q66.1
  calcaneus Q66.89
  cavus Q66.7
  equinovalgus Q66.6
  equinovarus Q66.0
  equinus Q66.89
  percavus Q66.7
  planovalgus Q66.6
  planus (acquired) (any degree) *-see also*
    Deformity, limb, flat foot
    congenital Q66.5
    due to rickets (sequelae) E64.3
  valgus Q66.6
  varus Q66.3
Tall stature, constitutional E34.4
Talma's disease M62.89
Talon noir S90.3
  hand S60.22
  heel S90.3
  toe S90.1
Tamponade, heart I31.4
Tanapox (virus disease) B08.71
Tangier disease E78.6
Tantrum, child problem F91.8
Tapeworm (infection) (infestation) *-see*
  Infestation, tapeworm
Tapia's syndrome G52.7
TAR (thrombocytopenia with absent radius)
  syndrome Q87.2
Tarral-Besnier disease L44.0
Tarsal tunnel syndrome *-see* Syndrome, tarsal
  tunnel
Tarsalgia *-see* Pain, limb, lower
Tarsitis (eyelid) H01.8
  syphilitic A52.71
  tuberculous A18.4
Tartar (teeth) (dental calculus) K03.6
Tattoo (mark) L81.8
Tauri's disease E74.09
Taurodontism K00.2
Taussig-Bing syndrome Q20.1
Taybi's syndrome Q87.2
Tay Sachs amaurotic familial idiocy or
  disease E75.02

TBI (traumatic brain injury) S06.9
Teacher's node or nodule J38.2
Tear, torn (traumatic) -see also Laceration
  with abortion -see Abortion
  annular fibrosis M51.35
  anus, anal (sphincter) S31.831
    complicating delivery
      with third degree perineal laceration -see
        also Delivery, complicated, by, laceration,
        perineum, third degree O70.20
        with mucosa O70.3
      without third degree perineal laceration
        O70.4
    nontraumatic (healed) (old) K62.81
  articular cartilage, old -see Derangement,
    joint, articular cartilage, by site
  bladder
    with ectopic or molar pregnancy O08.6
    following ectopic or molar pregnancy O08.6
    obstetrical O71.5
    traumatic -see Injury, bladder
  bowel
    with ectopic or molar pregnancy O08.6
    following ectopic or molar pregnancy O08.6
    obstetrical trauma O71.5
  broad ligament
    with ectopic or molar pregnancy O08.6
    following ectopic or molar pregnancy O08.6
    obstetrical trauma O71.6
  bucket handle (knee) (meniscus) -see Tear,
    meniscus
  capsule, joint -see Sprain
  cartilage -see also Sprain
    articular, old -see Derangement, joint,
    articular cartilage, by site
  cervix
    with ectopic or molar pregnancy O08.6
    following ectopic or molar pregnancy O08.6
    obstetrical trauma (current) O71.3
    old N88.1
    traumatic -see Injury, uterus
  dural G97.41
    nontraumatic G96.11
  internal organ -see Injury, by site
  knee cartilage
    articular (current) S83.3
    old -see Derangement, knee, meniscus, due
      to old tear
  ligament -see Sprain
  meniscus (knee) (current injury) S83.209
    bucket-handle S83.20
    lateral
      bucket-handle S83.25
      complex S83.27
      peripheral S83.26
      specified type NEC S83.28
    medial
      bucket-handle S83.21
      complex S83.23
      peripheral S83.22
      specified type NEC S83.24
    old -see Derangement, knee, meniscus, due
      to old tear
    site other than knee - code as Sprain
    specified type NEC S83.20
  muscle -see Strain
  pelvic
    floor, complicating delivery O70.1
    organ NEC, obstetrical trauma O71.5
      with ectopic or molar pregnancy O08.6

Tear, torn - continued
    following ectopic or molar pregnancy
      O08.6
  perineal, secondary O90.1
  periurethral tissue, obstetrical trauma O71.82
    with ectopic or molar pregnancy O08.6
    following ectopic or molar pregnancy O08.6
  rectovaginal septum -see Laceration, vagina
  retina, retinal (without detachment)
    (horseshoe) -see also Break, retina, horseshoe
    with detachment -see Detachment, retina,
      with retinal, break
  rotator cuff (nontraumatic) M75.10
    complete M75.12
    incomplete M75.11
    traumatic S46.01
      capsule S43.42
  semilunar cartilage, knee -see Tear, meniscus
  supraspinatus (complete) (incomplete)
    (nontraumatic) -see also Tear, rotator cuff
    M75.10
  tendon -see Strain
  tentorial, at birth P10.4
  umbilical cord
    complicating delivery O69.89
  urethra
    with ectopic or molar pregnancy O08.6
    following ectopic or molar pregnancy O08.6
    obstetrical trauma O71.5
  uterus -see Injury, uterus
  vagina -see Laceration, vagina
  vessel, from catheter -see Puncture, accidental
  complicating surgery   vulva, complicating
    delivery O70.0
Tear-stone -see Dacryolith
Teeth -see also condition
  grinding
    psychogenic F45.8
    sleep related G47.63
Teething (syndrome) K00.7
Telangiectasia, telangiectasis (verrucous)
  I78.1
  ataxic (cerebellar) (Louis-Bar) G11.3
  familial I78.0
  hemorrhagic, hereditary (congenital) (senile)
    I78.0
  hereditary, hemorrhagic (congenital) (senile)
    I78.0
  juxtafoveal H35.07
  macular H35.07
  parafoveal H35.07
  retinal (idiopathic) (juxtafoveal) (macular)
    (parafoveal) H35.07
  spider I78.1
Telephone scatologia F65.89
Telescoped bowel or intestine K56.1
  congenital Q43.8
Temperature
  body, high (of unknown origin) R50.9
  cold, trauma from T69.9
    newborn P80.0
    specified effect NEC T69.8
Temple -see condition
Temporal -see condition
Temporomandibular joint pain-dysfunction
  syndrome M26.62
Temporosphenoidal -see condition
Tendency
  bleeding -see Defect, coagulation
  suicide

Tendency --continued
    meaning personal history of attempted
      suicide Z91.5
    meaning suicidal ideation -see Ideation,
      suicidal
  to fall R29.6
Tenderness, abdominal R10.819
  epigastric R10.816
  generalized R10.817
  left lower quadrant R10.814
  left upper quadrant R10.812
  periumbilic R10.815
  right lower quadrant R10.813
  right upper quadrant R10.811
  rebound R10.829
    epigastric R10.826
    generalized R10.827
    left lower quadrant R10.824
    left upper quadrant R10.822
    periumbilic R10.825
    right lower quadrant R10.823
    right upper quadrant R10.821
Tendinitis, tendonitis -see also Enthesopathy
  Achilles M76.6
  adhesive -see Tenosynovitis, specified type
    NEC
    shoulder -see Capsulitis, adhesive
  bicipital M75.2
  calcific M65.2
    ankle M65.27
    foot M65.27
    forearm M65.23
    hand M65.24
    lower leg M65.26
    multiple sites M65.29
    pelvic region M65.25
    shoulder M75.3
    specified site NEC M65.28
    thigh M65.25
    upper arm M65.22
  due to use, overuse, pressure -see also
    Disorder, soft tissue, due to use
    specified NEC -see Disorder, soft tissue, due
      to use, specified NEC
  gluteal M76.0
  patellar M76.5
  peroneal M76.7
  psoas M76.1
  tibial (posterior) M76.82
    anterior M76.81
  trochanteric -see Bursitis, hip, trochanteric
Tendon -see condition
Tendosynovitis -see Tenosynovitis
Tenesmus (rectal) R19.8
  vesical R30.1
Tennis elbow -see Epicondylitis, lateral
Tenonitis -see also Tenosynovitis
  eye (capsule) H05.04
Tenontosynovitis -see Tenosynovitis
Tenontothecitis -see Tenosynovitis
Tenophyte -see Disorder, synovium, specified
  type NEC
Tenosynovitis -see also Synovitis M65.9
  adhesive -see Tenosynovitis, specified type
    NEC
    shoulder -see Capsulitis, adhesive
  bicipital (calcifying) -see Tendinitis, bicipital
  gonococcal A54.49
  in (due to)
    crystals M65.8
    gonorrhea A54.49

Tenosynovitis - *continued*
  syphilis (late) A52.78
  use, overuse, pressure -*see also* Disorder,
  soft tissue, due to use
    specified NEC -*see* Disorder, soft tissue,
    due to use, specified NEC
infective NEC M65.1
  ankle M65.17
  foot M65.17
  forearm M65.13
  hand M65.14
  lower leg M65.16
  multiple sites M65.19
  pelvic region M65.15
  shoulder region M65.11
  specified site NEC M65.18
  thigh M65.15
  upper arm M65.12
radial styloid M65.4
shoulder region M65.81
  adhesive -*see* Capsulitis, adhesive
specified type NEC M65.88
  ankle M65.87
  foot M65.87
  forearm M65.83
  hand M65.84
  lower leg M65.86
  multiple sites M65.89
  pelvic region M65.85
  shoulder region M65.81
  specified site NEC M65.88
  thigh M65.85
  upper arm M65.82
tuberculous -*see* Tuberculosis, tenosynovitis
Tenovaginitis -*see* Tenosynovitis
Tension
  arterial, high -*see also* Hypertension
    without diagnosis of hypertension R03.0
  headache G44.209
    intractable G44.201
    not intractable G44.209
  nervous R45.0
  pneumothorax J93.0
  premenstrual N94.3
  state (mental) F48.9
Tentorium -*see* condition
Teratencephalus Q89.8
Teratism Q89.7
Teratoblastoma (malignant) -*see* Neoplasm,
  malignant, by site
Teratocarcinoma -*see also* Neoplasm,
  malignant, by site
  liver C22.7
Teratoma (solid) -*see also* Neoplasm,
  uncertain behavior, by site
  with embryonal carcinoma, mixed -*see*
    Neoplasm, malignant, by site
  with malignant transformation -*see* Neoplasm,
    malignant, by site
  adult (cystic) -*see* Neoplasm, benign, by site
  benign -*see* Neoplasm, benign, by site
  combined with choriocarcinoma -*see*
    Neoplasm, malignant, by site
  cystic (adult) -*see* Neoplasm, benign, by site
  differentiated -*see* Neoplasm, benign, by site
  embryonal -*see also* Neoplasm, malignant, by
    site
    liver C22.7
  immature -*see* Neoplasm, malignant, by site
    liver C22.7

Tenosynovitis - *continued*
  adult, benign, cystic, differentiated type or
  mature D13.4
malignant -*see also* Neoplasm, malignant, by
site
  anaplastic -*see* Neoplasm, malignant, by site
  intermediate -*see* Neoplasm, malignant, by
    site
    specified site -*see* Neoplasm, malignant, by
      site
    unspecified site C62.90
  undifferentiated -*see* Neoplasm, malignant,
    by site
mature -*see* Neoplasm, uncertain behavior, by
site
  malignant -*see* Neoplasm, by site,
    malignant, by site
ovary D27.
  embryonal, immature or malignant C56
solid -*see* Neoplasm, uncertain behavior, by
  site
testis C62.9
  adult, benign, cystic, differentiated type or
    mature D29.2
  scrotal C62.1
  undescended C62.0
Termination
  anomalous -*see also* Malposition, congenital
    right pulmonary vein Q26.3
  pregnancy, elective Z33.2
Ternidens diminutus infestation B81.8
Ternidensiasis B81.8
Terror(s) night (child) F51.4
Terrorism, victim of Z65.4
Terry's syndrome H44.2
Tertiary -*see* condition
Test, tests, testing (for)
  adequacy (for dialysis)
    hemodialysis Z49.31
    peritoneal Z49.32
  blood pressure Z01.30
    abnormal reading -*see* Blood, pressure
  blood-alcohol Z04.8
    positive -*see* Findings, abnormal, in blood -
  blood-drug Z04.8
    positive -*see* Findings, abnormal, in blood -
    blood typing Z01.83
    Rh typing Z01.83
  cardiac pulse generator (battery) Z45.010
  fertility Z31.41
  genetic
    disease carrier status for procreative
    management
      female Z31.430
      male Z31.440
    male partner of patient with recurrent
      pregnancy loss Z31.441
    procreative management NEC
      female Z31.438
      male Z31.448
  hearing Z01.10
    with abnormal findings NEC Z01.118
  HIV (human immunodeficiency virus)
    nonconclusive (in infants) R75
    positive Z21
    seropositive Z21
  immunity status Z01.84
  intelligence NEC Z01.89
  laboratory (as part of a general medical
    examination) Z00.00
    with abnormal finding Z00.01

Test, tests, testing --*continued*
  for medicolegal reason NEC Z04.8
  male partner of patient with recurrent
    pregnancy loss Z31.441
  Mantoux (for tuberculosis) Z11.1
    abnormal result R76.11
  pregnancy, positive first pregnancy -*see*
    Pregnancy, normal, first
  procreative Z31.49
    fertility Z31.41
  skin, diagnostic
    allergy Z01.82
      special screening examination -*see*
    Screening, by name of disease
      Mantoux Z11.1
      tuberculin Z11.1
  specified NEC Z01.89
  tuberculin Z11.1
    abnormal result R76.11
  vision Z01.00
    with abnormal findings Z01.01
  Wassermann Z11.3
    positive -*see* Serology for syphilis, positive
Testicle, testicular, testis -*see also* condition
  feminization syndrome -*see also* Syndrome,
    androgen insensitivity E34.51
  migrans Q55.29
Tetanus, tetanic (cephalic) (convulsions) A35
with
  abortion A34
  ectopic or molar pregnancy O08.0
  following ectopic or molar pregnancy O08.0
  inoculation reaction (due to serum) -*see*
    Complications, vaccination
  neonatorum A33
  obstetrical A34
  puerperal, postpartum, childbirth A34
Tetany (due to) R29.0
  alkalosis E87.3
  associated with rickets E55.0
  convulsions R29.0
    hysterical F44.5
  functional (hysterical) F44.5
  hyperkinetic R29.0
    hysterical F44.5
  hyperpnea R06.4
    hysterical F44.5
    psychogenic F45.8
  hyperventilation -*see also* Hyperventilation
    R06.4
    hysterical F44.5
  neonatal (without calcium or magnesium
    deficiency) P71.3
  parathyroid (gland) E20.9
  parathyroprival E89.2
  post- (para) thyroidectomy E89.2
  postoperative E89.2
  pseudotetany R29.0
  psychogenic (conversion reaction) F44.5
Tetralogy of Fallot Q21.3
Tetraplegia (chronic) -*see also* Quadriplegia
  G82.50
Thailand hemorrhagic fever A91
Thalassanemia -*see* Thalassemia
Thalassemia (anemia) (disease) D56.9
  with other hemoglobinopathy D56.8
  alpha (major) (severe) (triple gene defect)
    D56.0
    minor D56.3
    silent carrier D56.3
    trait D56.3

Thalassemia - *continued*
  beta (severe) D56.1
    homozygous D56.1
    major D56.1
    minor D56.3
    trait D56.3
  delta-beta (homozygous) D56.2
    minor D56.3
    trait D56.3
  dominant D56.8
  hemoglobin
    C D56.8
    E-beta D56.5
  intermedia D56.1
  major D56.1
  minor D56.3
  mixed D56.8
  sickle-cell -*see* Disease, sickle-cell,
    thalassemia
  specified type NEC D56.8
  trait D56.3
  variants D56.8
Thanatophoric dwarfism or short stature
  Q77.1
Thaysen-Gee disease (nontropical sprue)
  K90.0
Thaysen's disease K90.0
Thecoma D27
  luteinized D27
  malignant C56
Thelarche, premature E30.8
Thelaziasis B83.8
Thelitis N61.0
  puerperal, postpartum or gestational -*see*
    Infection, nipple
Therapeutic -*see* condition
Therapy
  drug, long-term (current) (prophylactic)
    agents affecting estrogen receptors and
      estrogen levels NEC Z79.818
    anastrozole (Arimidex) Z79.811
    antibiotics Z79.2
      short-term use - omit code
    anticoagulants Z79.01
    anti-inflammatory Z79.1
    antiplatelet Z79.02
    antithrombotics Z79.02
    aromatase inhibitors Z79.811
    aspirin Z79.82
    birth control pill or patch Z79.3
    bisphosphonates Z79.83
    contraceptive, oral Z79.3
    drug, specified NEC Z79.899
    estrogen receptor downregulators Z79.818
    Evista Z79.810
    exemestane (Aromasin) Z79.811
    Fareston Z79.810
    fulvestrant (Faslodex) Z79.818
    gonadotropin-releasing hormone (GnRH)
      agonist Z79.818
    goserelin acetate (Zoladex) Z79.818
    hormone replacement (postmenopausal)
      Z79.890
    insulin Z79.4
    letrozole (Femara) Z79.811
    leuprolide acetate (leuprorelin) (Lupron)
      Z79.818
    megestrol acetate (Megace) Z79.818
    methadone
      for pain management Z79.891
      maintenance therapy F11.20

Therapy --*continued*
    Nolvadex Z79.810
    opiate analgesic Z79.891
    oral contraceptive Z79.3
    raloxifene (Evista) Z79.810
    selective estrogen receptor modulators
      (SERMs) Z79.810
    short term
  omit code
    steroids
      inhaled Z79.51
      systemic Z79.52
    tamoxifen (Nolvadex) Z79.810
    toremifene (Fareston) Z79.810
Thermic -*see* condition
Thermography (abnormal) -*see also*
  Abnormal, diagnostic imaging R93.8
  breast R92.8
Thermoplegia T67.0
Thesaurismosis, glycogen -*see* Disease,
  glycogen storage
Thiamin deficiency E51.9
  specified NEC E51.8
Thiaminic deficiency with beriberi E51.11
Thibierge-Weissenbach syndrome -*see*
  Sclerosis, systemic
Thickening
  bone -*see* Hypertrophy, bone
  breast N64.59
  endometrium R93.8
  epidermal L85.9
    specified NEC L85.8
  hymen N89.6
  larynx J38.7
  nail L60.2
    congenital Q84.5
  periosteal -*see* Hypertrophy, bone
  pleura J92.9
    with asbestos J92.0
  skin R23.4
  subepiglottic J38.7
  tongue K14.8
  valve, heart -*see* Endocarditis
Thigh -*see* condition
Thinning vertebra -*see* Spondylopathy,
  specified NEC
Thirst, excessive R63.1
  due to deprivation of water T73.1
Thomsen disease G71.12
Thoracic -*see also* condition
  kidney Q63.2
  outlet syndrome G54.0
Thoracogastroschisis (congenital) Q79.8
Thoracopagus Q89.4
Thorax -*see* condition
Thorn's syndrome N28.89
Thorson-Björck syndrome E34.0
Threadworm (infection) (infestation) B80
Threatened
  abortion O20.0
    with subsequent abortion O03.9
  job loss, anxiety concerning Z56.2
  labor (without delivery) O47.9
    at or after 37 completed weeks of gestation
      O47.1
    before 37 completed weeks of gestation
      O47.0
  loss of job, anxiety concerning Z56.2
  miscarriage O20.0
  unemployment, anxiety concerning Z56.2
Three-day fever A93.1

Threshers' lung J67.0
Thrix annulata (congenital) Q84.1
Throat -*see* condition
Thrombasthenia (Glanzmann)
  (hemorrhagic) (hereditary) D69.1
Thromboangiitis I73.1
  obliterans (general) I73.1
    cerebral I67.89
    vessels
      brain I67.89
      spinal cord I67.89
Thromboarteritis -*see* Arteritis
Thromboasthenia (Glanzmann)
  (hemorrhagic) (hereditary) D69.1
Thrombocytasthenia (Glanzmann) D69.1
Thrombocythemia (essential) (hemorrhagic)
  (idiopathic) (primary) D47.3
Thrombocytopathy (dystrophic)
  (granulopenic) D69.1
Thrombocytopenia, thrombocytopenic D69.6
  with absent radius (TAR) Q87.2
  congenital D69.42
  dilutional D69.59
  due to
    drugs D69.59
    extracorporeal circulation of blood D69.59
    (massive) blood transfusion D69.59
    platelet alloimmunization D69.59
  essential D69.3
  heparin induced (HIT) D75.82
  hereditary D69.42
  idiopathic D69.3
  neonatal, transitory P61.0
    due to
      exchange transfusion P61.0
      idiopathic maternal thrombocytopenia
        P61.0
      isoimmunization P61.0
  primary NEC D69.49
    idiopathic D69.3
  puerperal, postpartum O72.3
  secondary D69.59
  transient neonatal P61.0
Thrombocytosis, essential D47.3
  primary D47.3
Thromboembolism -*see* Embolism
Thrombopathy (Bernard-Soulier) D69.1
  constitutional D68.0
  Willebrand-Jurgens D68.0
Thrombopenia -*see* Thrombocytopenia
Thrombophilia D68.59
  primary NEC D68.59
  secondary NEC D68.69
  specified NEC D68.69
Thrombophlebitis I80.9
  antepartum O22.2
    deep O22.3
    superficial O22.2
  cavernous (venous) sinus G08
    complicating pregnancy O22.5
    nonpyogenic I67.6
  cerebral (sinus) (vein) G08
    nonpyogenic I67.6
    sequelae G09
  due to implanted device -*see* Complications,
    by site and type, specified NEC
  during or resulting from a procedure NEC
    T81.72
  femoral vein (superficial) I80.1
  femoropopliteal vein I80.0
  hepatic (vein) I80.8

Thrombophlebitis - continued
idiopathic, recurrent I82.1
iliofemoral I80.1
intracranial venous sinus (any) G08
  nonpyogenic I67.6
  sequelae G09
intraspinal venous sinuses and veins G08
  nonpyogenic G95.19
lateral (venous) sinus G08
  nonpyogenic I67.6
leg I80.299
  superficial I80.0
longitudinal (venous) sinus G08
  nonpyogenic I67.6
lower extremity I80.299
migrans, migrating I82.1
pelvic
  with ectopic or molar pregnancy O08.0
  following ectopic or molar pregnancy O08.0
  puerperal O87.1
popliteal vein -see Phlebitis, leg, deep,
  popliteal
portal (vein) K75.1
postoperative T81.72
pregnancy -see Thrombophlebitis, antepartum
puerperal, postpartum, childbirth O87.0
  deep O87.1
  pelvic O87.1
  septic O86.81
  superficial O87.0
saphenous (greater) (lesser) I80.0
sinus (intracranial) G08
  nonpyogenic I67.6
specified site NEC I80.8
tibial vein I80.23
**Thrombosis, thrombotic (bland) (multiple)
(progressive) (silent) (vessel) I82.90**
anal K64.5
antepartum -see Thrombophlebitis,
  antepartum
aorta, aortic I74.10
  abdominal I74.09
    saddle I74.01
  bifurcation I74.09
  saddle I74.01
  specified site NEC I74.19
  terminal I74.09
  thoracic I74.11
  valve -see Endocarditis, aortic
apoplexy I63.3
artery, arteries (postinfectional) I74.9
  auditory, internal -see Occlusion, artery,
    precerebral, specified NEC
  basilar -see Occlusion, artery, basilar
  carotid (common) (internal) -see Occlusion,
    artery, carotid
  cerebellar (anterior inferior) (posterior
    inferior) (superior) -see Occlusion, artery,
    cerebellar
  cerebral -see Occlusion, artery, cerebral
  choroidal (anterior) -see Occlusion, artery,
    cerebral, specified NEC
  communicating, posterior -see Occlusion,
    artery, cerebral, specified NEC
  coronary -see also Infarct, myocardium
    not resulting in infarction I24.0
  hepatic I74.8
  hypophyseal -see Occlusion, artery, cerebral,
    specified NEC
  iliac I74.5
  limb I74.4

Thrombosis, thrombotic --*continued*
lower I74.3
upper I74.2
meningeal, anterior or posterior -see
  Occlusion, artery, cerebral, specified NEC
mesenteric (with gangrene) -see also Infarct,
  intestine K55.069
ophthalmic -see Occlusion, artery, retina
pontine -see Occlusion, artery, cerebral,
  specified NEC
precerebral -see Occlusion, artery,
  precerebral
pulmonary (iatrogenic) -see Embolism,
  pulmonary
renal N28.0
retinal -see Occlusion, artery, retina
spinal, anterior or posterior G95.11
traumatic NEC T14.8
vertebral -see Occlusion, artery, vertebral
atrium, auricular -see also Infarct,
myocardium
  following acute myocardial infarction
    (current complication) I23.6
  not resulting in infarction I51.3
basilar (artery) -see Occlusion, artery, basilar
brain (artery) (stem) -see also Occlusion,
artery, cerebral
  due to syphilis A52.05
  puerperal O99.43
  sinus -see Thrombosis, intracranial venous
    sinus
capillary I78.8
cardiac -see also Infarct, myocardium
  not resulting in infarction I51.3
  valve -see Endocarditis
carotid (artery) (common) (internal) -see
  Occlusion, artery, carotid
cavernous (venous) sinus -see Thrombosis,
  intracranial venous sinus
cerebellar artery (anterior inferior) (posterior
  inferior) (superior) I66.3
cerebral (artery) -see Occlusion, artery,
  cerebral
cerebrovenous sinus -see also Thrombosis,
  intracranial venous sinus
  puerperium O87.3
chronic I82.91
coronary (artery) (vein) -see also Infarct,
myocardium
  not resulting in infarction I24.0
corpus cavernosum N48.89
cortical I66.9
deep -see Embolism, vein, lower extremity
due to device, implant or graft -see also
  Complications, by site and type, specified
  NEC T85.868
  arterial graft NEC T82.868
  breast (implant) T85.868
  catheter NEC T85.868
    dialysis (renal) T82.868
      intraperitoneal T85.868
    infusion NEC T82.868
      spinal (epidural) (subdural) T85.860
    urinary (indwelling) T83.86
  electronic (electrode) (pulse generator)
  (stimulator)
    bone T84.86
    cardiac T82.867
    nervous system (brain) (peripheral nerve)
    (spinal) T85.860
    urinary T83.86

Thrombosis, thrombotic --*continued*
fixation, internal (orthopedic) NEC T84.86
gastrointestinal (bile duct) (esophagus)
  T85.868
genital NEC T83.86
heart T82.867
joint prosthesis T84.86
ocular (corneal graft) (orbital implant) NEC
  T85.868
orthopedic NEC T84.86
specified NEC T85.868
urinary NEC T83.86
vascular NEC T82.868
ventricular intracranial shunt T85.860
during the puerperium -see Thrombosis,
puerperal
endocardial -see also Infarct, myocardium
  not resulting in infarction I51.3
eye -see Occlusion, retina
genital organ
  female NEC N94.89
    pregnancy -see Thrombophlebitis,
    antepartum
  male N50.1
gestational -see Phlebopathy, gestational
heart (chamber) -see also Infarct, myocardium
  not resulting in infarction I51.3
hepatic (vein) I82.0
  artery I74.8
history (of) Z86.718
intestine (with gangrene) -see also Infarct,
  intestine K55.069
intracardiac NEC (apical) (atrial) (auricular)
  (ventricular) (old) I51.3
intracranial (arterial) I66.9
  venous sinus (any) G08
    nonpyogenic origin I67.6
    puerperium O87.3
intramural -see also Infarct, myocardium
  not resulting in infarction I51.3
intraspinal venous sinuses and veins G08
  nonpyogenic G95.19
kidney (artery) N28.0
lateral (venous) sinus -see Thrombosis,
  intracranial venous sinus
leg -see Thrombosis, vein, lower extremity
  arterial I74.3
liver (venous) I82.0
  artery I74.8
  portal vein I81
longitudinal (venous) sinus -see Thrombosis,
  intracranial venous sinus
lower limb -see Thrombosis, vein, lower
  extremity
lung (iatrogenic) (postoperative) -see
  Embolism, pulmonary
meninges (brain) (arterial) I66.8
mesenteric (artery) (with gangrene) -see also
  Infarct, intestine K55.069
  vein (inferior) (superior) I81
mitral I34.8
mural -see also Infarct, myocardium
  due to syphilis A52.06
  not resulting in infarction I51.3
omentum (with gangrene) -see also Infarct,
  intestine K55.069
ophthalmic -see Occlusion, retina
pampiniform plexus (male) N50.1
parietal -see also Infarct, myocardium
  not resulting in infarction I24.0
penis, superficial vein N48.81

Thrombosis, thrombotic --*continued*
perianal venous K64.5
peripheral arteries I74.4
  upper I74.2
personal history (of) Z86.718
portal I81
  due to syphilis A52.09
precerebral artery -*see* Occlusion, artery,
  precerebral
puerperal, postpartum O87.0
  brain (artery) O99.43
    venous (sinus) O87.3
  cardiac O99.43
  cerebral (artery) O99.43
    venous (sinus) O87.3
  superficial O87.0
pulmonary (artery) (iatrogenic)
  (postoperative) (vein) -*see* Embolism,
  pulmonary
renal (artery) N28.0
  vein I82.3
resulting from presence of device, implant or
  graft -*see* Complications, by site and type,
  specified NEC
retina, retinal -*see* Occlusion, retina
scrotum N50.1
seminal vesicle N50.1
sigmoid (venous) sinus -*see* Thrombosis,
  intracranial venous sinus
sinus, intracranial (any) -*see* Thrombosis,
  intracranial venous sinus
specified site NEC I82.890
  chronic I82.891
spermatic cord N50.1
spinal cord (arterial) G95.11
  due to syphilis A52.09
  pyogenic origin G06.1
spleen, splenic D73.5
  artery I74.8
testis N50.1
tumor -*see* Neoplasm, unspecified behavior,
  by site
traumatic NEC T14.8
tricuspid I07.8
tunica vaginalis N50.1
umbilical cord (vessels), complicating
  delivery O69.5
vas deferens N50.1
vein (acute) I82.90
  antecubital I82.61
    chronic I82.71
  axillary I82.A1
    chronic I82.A2
  basilic I82.61
    chronic I82.71
  brachial I82.62
    chronic I82.72
  brachiocephalic (innominate) I82.290
    chronic I82.291
  cerebral, nonpyogenic I67.6
  cephalic I82.61
    chronic I82.71
  chronic I82.91
  deep (DVT) I82.40
    calf I82.4Z
      chronic I82.5Z
    lower leg I82.4Z
      chronic I82.5Z
    thigh I82.4Y
      chronic I82.5Y
    upper leg I82.4Y

Thrombosis, thrombotic --*continued*
    chronic I82.5y
  femoral I82.41
    chronic I82.51
  iliac (iliofemoral) I82.42
    chronic I82.52
  innominate I82.290
    chronic I82.291
  internal jugular I82.C1
    chronic I82.C2
  lower extremity
    deep I82.40
      chronic I82.50
      specified NEC I82.49
        chronic NEC I82.59
    distal
      deep I82.4Z
    proximal
      deep I82.4Y
        chronic I82.5Y
    superficial I82.81
  perianal K64.5
  popliteal I82.43
    chronic I82.53
  radial I82.62
    chronic I82.72
  renal I82.3
  saphenous (greater) (lesser) I82.81
  specified NEC I82.890
    chronic NEC I82.891
  subclavian I82.B1
    chronic I82.B2
  thoracic NEC I82.290
    chronic I82.291
  tibial I82.44
    chronic I82.54
  ulnar I82.62
    chronic I82.72
  upper extremity I82.60
    chronic I82.70
    deep I82.62
      chronic I82.72
    superficial I82.61
      chronic I82.71
  vena cava
    inferior I82.220
      chronic I82.221
    superior I82.210
      chronic I82.211
  venous, perianal K64.5
  ventricle -*see also* Infarct, myocardium
  following acute myocardial infarction
    (current complication) I23.6
  not resulting in infarction I24.0
Thrombus -*see* Thrombosis
Thrush -*see also* Candidiasis
oral B37.0
newborn P37.5
vaginal B37.3
Thumb -*see also* condition
sucking (child problem) F98.8
Thymitis E32.8
Thymoma (benign) D15.0
malignant C37
Thymus, thymic (gland) -*see* condition
Thyrocele -*see* Goiter
Thyroglossal -*see also* condition
cyst Q89.2
duct, persistent Q89.2
Thyroid (gland) (body) -*see also* condition
hormone resistance E07.89
lingual Q89.2
nodule (cystic) (nontoxic) (single) E04.1

Thyroiditis E06.9
acute (nonsuppurative) (pyogenic)
  (suppurative) E06.0
autoimmune E06.3
chronic (nonspecific) (sclerosing) E06.5
  with thyrotoxicosis, transient E06.2
  fibrous E06.5
  lymphadenoid E06.3
  lymphocytic E06.3
  lymphoid E06.3
de Quervain's E06.1
drug-induced E06.4
fibrous (chronic) E06.5
giant-cell (follicular) E06.1
granulomatous (de Quervain) (subacute)
  E06.1
Hashimoto's (struma lymphomatosa) E06.3
iatrogenic E06.4
ligneous E06.5
lymphocytic (chronic) E06.3
lymphoid E06.3
lymphomatous E06.3
nonsuppurative E06.1
postpartum, puerperal O90.5
pseudotuberculous E06.1
pyogenic E06.0
radiation E06.4
Riedel's E06.5
subacute (granulomatous) E06.1
suppurative E06.0
tuberculous A18.81
viral E06.1
woody E06.5
Thyrolingual duct, persistent Q89.2
Thyromegaly E01.0
Thyrotoxic
crisis -*see* Thyrotoxicosis
heart disease or failure -*see also*
  Thyrotoxicosis E05.90 [143]
  with thyroid storm E05.91 [143]
storm -*see* Thyrotoxicosis
Thyrotoxicosis (recurrent) E05.90
with
  goiter (diffuse) E05.00
    with thyroid storm E05.01
    adenomatous uninodular E05.10
      with thyroid storm E05.11
    multinodular E05.20
      with thyroid storm E05.21
    nodular E05.20
      with thyroid storm E05.21
    uninodular E05.10
      with thyroid storm E05.11
  infiltrative
    dermopathy E05.00
      with thyroid storm E05.01
    ophthalmopathy E05.00
      with thyroid storm E05.01
  single thyroid nodule E05.10
    with thyroid storm E05.11
  thyroid storm E05.91
due to
  ectopic thyroid nodule or tissue E05.30
    with thyroid storm E05.31
  ingestion of (excessive) thyroid material
  E05.40
    with thyroid storm E05.41
  overproduction of thyroid-stimulating
  hormone E05.80
    with thyroid storm E05.81
  specified cause NEC E05.80

Thyrotoxicosis - *continued*
  with thyroid storm E05.81
  factitia E05.40
    with thyroid storm E05.41
  heart E05.90 [*I43*]
    with thyroid storm E05.91 [*I43*]
    failure E05.90 [*I43*]
  neonatal (transient) P72.1
  transient with chronic thyroiditis E06.2
Tibia vara -see Osteochondrosis, juvenile,
    tibia
Tic (disorder) F95.9
  breathing F95.8
  child problem F95.0
  compulsive F95.1
  de la Tourette F95.2
  degenerative (generalized) (localized) G25.69
    facial G25.69
  disorder
    chronic
      motor F95.1
      vocal F95.1
    combined vocal and multiple motor F95.2
    transient F95.0
  douloureux G50.0
    atypical G50.1
    postherpetic, postzoster B02.22
  drug-induced G25.61
  eyelid F95.8
  habit F95.9
    chronic F95.1
    transient of childhood F95.0
  lid, transient of childhood F95.0
  motor-verbal F95.2
  occupational F48.8
  orbicularis F95.8
    transient of childhood F95.0
  organic origin G25.69
  postchoreic G25.69
  provisional F95.0
  psychogenic, compulsive F95.1
  salaam R25.8
  spasm (motor or vocal) F95.9
    chronic F95.1
    transient of childhood F95.0
  specified NEC F95.8
Tick-borne -see condition
Tietze's disease or syndrome M94.0
Tight, tightness
  anus K62.89
  chest R07.89
  fascia (lata) M62.89
  foreskin (congenital) N47.1
  hymen, hymenal ring N89.6
  introitus (acquired) (congenital) N89.6
  rectal sphincter K62.89
  tendon -see Short, tendon
  urethral sphincter N35.9
Tilting vertebra -see Dorsopathy, deforming,
    specified NEC
Timidity, child F93.8
Tin-miner's lung J63.5
Tinea (intersecta) (tarsi) B35.9
  amiantacea L44.8
  asbestina B35.0
  barbae B35.0
  beard B35.0
  black dot B35.0
  blanca B36.2
  capitis B35.0
  corporis B35.4

Tinea - *continued*
  cruris B35.6
  flava B36.0
  foot B35.3
  furfuracea B36.0
  imbricata (Tokelau) B35.5
  kerion B35.0
  manuum B35.2
  microsporic -see Dermatophytosis
  nigra B36.1
  nodosa -see Piedra
  pedis B35.3
  scalp B35.0
  specified site NEC B35.8
  sycosis B35.0
  tonsurans B35.0
  trichophytic -see Dermatophytosis
  unguium B35.1
  versicolor B36.0
Tingling sensation (skin) R20.2
Tinnitus NOS H93.1
  audible H93.1
  aurium H93.1
  pulsatile H93.A-
  subjective H93.1
Tipped tooth (teeth) M26.33
Tipping
  pelvis M95.5
    with disproportion (fetopelvic) O33.0
      causing obstructed labor O65.0
  tooth (teeth), fully erupted M26.33
Tiredness R53.83
Tissue -see condition
Tobacco (nicotine)
  abuse -see Tobacco, use
  dependence -see Dependence, drug, nicotine
  harmful use Z72.0
  heart -see Tobacco, toxic effect
  maternal use, affecting newborn P04.2
  toxic effect -see Table of Drugs and
    Chemicals, by substance, poisoning
    chewing tobacco -see Table of Drugs and
      Chemicals, by substance, poisoning
    cigarettes -see Table of Drugs and
      Chemicals, by substance, poisoning
  use Z72.0
    complicating
      childbirth O99.334
      pregnancy O99.33
      puerperium O99.335
    counseling and surveillance Z71.6
    history Z87.891
  withdrawal state -see also Dependence, drug,
    nicotine F17.203
Tocopherol deficiency E56.0
Todd's
  cirrhosis K74.3
  paralysis (postepileptic) (transitory) G83.84
Toe -see condition
Toilet, artificial opening -see Attention to,
    artificial, opening
Tokelau (ringworm) B35.5
Tollwut -see Rabies
Tommaselli's disease R31.9
  correct substance properly administered -see
    Table of Drugs and Chemicals, by drug,
    adverse effect
  overdose or wrong substance given or taken -
    see Table of Drugs and Chemicals, by drug,
    poisoning
Tongue -see also condition
  tie Q38.1

Tonic pupil -see Anomaly, pupil, function,
    tonic pupil
Toni-Fanconi syndrome (cystinosis) E72.09
  with cystinosis E72.04
Tonsil -see condition
Tonsillitis (acute) (catarrhal) (croupous)
  (follicular) (gangrenous) (infective)
  (lacunar) (lingual) (malignant)
  (membranous) (parenchymatous)
  (phlegmonous) (pseudomembranous)
  (purulent) (septic) (subacute) (suppurative)
  (toxic) (ulcerative) (vesicular) (viral) J03.90
  chronic J35.01
    with adenoiditis J35.03
  diphtheritic A36.0
  hypertrophic J35.01
    with adenoiditis J35.03
  recurrent J03.91
  specified organism NEC J03.80
    recurrent J03.81
  staphylococcal J03.80
    recurrent J03.81
  streptococcal J03.00
    recurrent J03.01
  tuberculous A15.8
  Vincent's A69.1
Tooth, teeth -see condition
Toothache K08.89
Topagnosis R20.8
Tophi -see Gout, chronic
TORCH infection -see Infection, congenital
  without active infection P00.2
Torn -see Tear
Tornwaldt's cyst or disease J39.2
Torsion
  accessory tube -see Torsion, fallopian tube
  adnexa (female) -see Torsion, fallopian tube
  aorta, acquired I77.1
  appendix epididymis N44.04
  appendix testis N44.03
  bile duct (common) (hepatic) K83.8
    congenital Q44.5
  bowel, colon or intestine K56.2
  cervix -see Malposition, uterus
  cystic duct K82.8
  dystonia -see Dystonia, torsion
  epididymis (appendix) N44.04
  fallopian tube N83.52
    with ovary N83.53
  gallbladder K82.8
    congenital Q44.1
  hydatid of Morgagni
    female N83.52
    male N44.03
  kidney (pedicle) (leading to infarction) N28.0
  Meckel's diverticulum (congenital) Q43.0
    malignant -see Table of Neoplasms, small
    intestine, malignant
  mesentery K56.2
  omentum K56.2
  organ or site, congenital NEC -see Anomaly,
    by site
  ovary (pedicle) N83.51
    with fallopian tube N83.53
    congenital Q50.2
  oviduct -see Torsion, fallopian tube - penis
  (acquired) N48.82
    congenital Q55.63
  spasm -see Dystonia, torsion
  spermatic cord N44.02
    extravaginal N44.01

Torsion - *continued*
 intravaginal N44.02
 spleen D73.5
 testis, testicle N44.00
  appendix N44.03
 tibia -*see* Deformity, limb, specified type
  NEC, lower leg
 uterus -*see* Malposition, uterus
Torticollis (intermittent) (spastic) M43.6
 congenital (sternomastoid) Q68.0
 due to birth injury P15.8
 hysterical F44.4
 ocular R29.891
 psychogenic F45.8
  conversion reaction F44.4
 rheumatic M43.6
 rheumatoid M06.88
 spasmodic G24.3
 traumatic, current S13.4
Tortipelvis G24.1
Tortuous
 aortic arch Q25.46
 artery I77.1
 organ or site, congenital NEC -*see* Distortion
 retinal vessel, congenital Q14.1
 ureter N13.8
 urethra N36.8
 vein -*see* Varix
Torture, victim of Z65.4
Torula, torular (histolytica) (infection) -*see*
 Cryptococcosis
Torulosis -*see* Cryptococcosis
Torus (mandibularis) (palatinus) M27.0
 fracture -*see* Fracture, by site, torus
Touraine's syndrome Q79.8
Tourette's syndrome F95.2
Tourniquet syndrome -*see* Constriction,
 external, by site
Tower skull Q75.0
 with exophthalmos Q87.0
Toxemia R68.89
 bacterial -*see* Sepsis
 burn -*see* Burn
 eclamptic (with pre-existing hypertension) -
  see Eclampsia
 erysipelatous -*see* Erysipelas
 fatigue R68.89
 food -*see* Poisoning, food
 gastrointestinal K52.1
 intestinal K52.1
 kidney -*see* Uremia
 malarial -*see* Malaria
 myocardial -*see* Myocarditis, toxic
 of pregnancy -*see* Pre-eclampsia
 pre-eclamptic -*see* Pre-eclampsia
 small intestine K52.1
 staphylococcal, due to food A05.0
 stasis R68.89
 uremic -*see* Uremia
 urinary -*see* Uremia
**Toxemica cerebropathia psychica
 (nonalcoholic)** F04
 alcoholic -*see* Alcohol, amnestic disorder
Toxic (poisoning) -*see also* condition T65.91
 effect -*see* Table of Drugs and Chemicals, by
  substance, poisoning
 shock syndrome A48.3
 thyroid (gland) -*see* Thyrotoxicosis
Toxicemia -*see* Toxemia
Toxicity -*see* Table of Drugs and Chemicals,
 by substance, poisoning

Toxicity --*continued*
 fava bean D55.0
 food, noxious -*see* Poisoning, food
 from drug or nonmedicinal substance -*see*
  Table of Drugs and Chemicals, by drug
Toxicosis -*see also* Toxemia
 capillary, hemorrhagic D69.0
Toxinfection, gastrointestinal K52.1
Toxocariasis B83.0
Toxoplasma, toxoplasmosis (acquired) B58.9
 with
  hepatitis B58.1
  meningoencephalitis B58.2
  ocular involvement B58.00
  other organ involvement B58.89
  pneumonia, pneumonitis B58.3
 congenital (acute) (subacute) (chronic) P37.1
 maternal, manifest toxoplasmosis in infant
  (acute) (subacute) (chronic) P37.1
**tPA (rtPA) administration in a different
 facility within the last 24
 hours prior to admission to current facility**
 Z92.82
Trabeculation, bladder N32.89
Trachea -*see* condition
**Tracheitis (catarrhal) (infantile)
 (membranous) (plastic) (septal)
 (suppurative) (viral)** J04.10
 with
  bronchitis (15 years of age and above) J40
   acute or subacute -*see* Bronchitis, acute
   chronic J42
   tuberculous NEC A15.5
   under 15 years of age J20.9
  laryngitis (acute) J04.2
   chronic J37.1
   tuberculous NEC A15.5
 acute J04.10
  with obstruction J04.11
 chronic J42
  with
   bronchitis (chronic) J42
   laryngitis (chronic) J37.1
 diphtheritic (membranous) A36.89
 due to external agent -*see* Inflammation,
  respiratory, upper, due to
 syphilitic A52.73
 tuberculous A15.5
Trachelitis (nonvenereal) -*see* Cervicitis
Tracheobronchial -*see* condition
**Tracheobronchitis (15
 years of age and above)** -*see also* Bronchitis
 due to
  Bordetella bronchiseptica A37.80
   with pneumonia A37.81
  Francisella tularensis A21.8
Tracheobronchomegaly Q32.4
 with bronchiectasis J47.9
  with
   exacerbation (acute) J47.1
   lower respiratory infection J47.0
 acquired J98.09
  with bronchiectasis J47.9
   with
    exacerbation (acute) J47.1
    lower respiratory infection J47.0
Tracheobronchopneumonitis -*see*
 Pneumonia, broncho-
Tracheocele (external) (internal) J39.8
 congenital Q32.1

Tracheomalacia J39.8
 congenital Q32.0
Tracheopharyngitis (acute) J06.9
 chronic J42
 due to external agent -*see* Inflammation,
  respiratory, upper, due to
Tracheostenosis J39.8
Tracheostomy
 complication -*see* Complication,
  tracheostomy
 status Z93.0
  attention to Z43.0
  malfunctioning J95.03
Trachoma, trachomatous A71.9
 active (stage) A71.1
 contraction of conjunctiva A71.1
 dubium A71.0
 initial (stage) A71.0
 healed or sequelae B94.0
 pannus A71.1
 Türck's J37.0
Traction, vitreomacular H43.82
Train sickness T75.3
Trait(s)
 Hb-S D57.3
 hemoglobin
  abnormal NEC D58.2
   with thalassemia D56.3
  C -*see* Disease, hemoglobin C
  S (Hb-S) D57.3
 Lepore D56.3
 personality, accentuated Z73.1
 sickle-cell D57.3
  with elliptocytosis or spherocytosis D57.3
 type A personality Z73.1
Tramp Z59.0
Trance R41.89
 hysterical F44.89
Transection
 abdomen (partial) S38.3
 aorta (incomplete) -*see also* Injury, aorta
  complete -*see* Injury, aorta, laceration, major
 carotid artery (incomplete) -*see also* Injury,
  blood vessel, carotid, laceration
  complete -*see* Injury, blood vessel, carotid,
  laceration, major
 celiac artery (incomplete) S35.211
  branch (incomplete) S35.291
   complete S35.292
  complete S35.212
 innominate
  artery (incomplete) -*see also* Injury, blood
  vessel, thoracic, innominate, artery,
  laceration
   complete -*see* Injury, blood vessel,
   thoracic, innominate, artery, laceration,
   major
  vein (incomplete) -*see also* Injury, blood
  vessel, thoracic, innominate, vein, laceration
   complete -*see* Injury, blood vessel,
   thoracic, innominate, vein, laceration,
   major
 jugular vein (external) (incomplete) -*see also*
  Injury, blood vessel, jugular vein, laceration
  complete -*see* Injury, blood vessel, jugular
  vein, laceration, major
  internal (incomplete) -*see also* Injury, blood
  vessel, jugular vein, internal, laceration
   complete -*see* Injury, blood vessel, jugular
   vein, internal, laceration, major

Transection - *continued*
mesenteric artery (incomplete) -*see also*
Injury, mesenteric, artery, laceration
   complete -*see* Injury, mesenteric artery,
   laceration, major
pulmonary vessel (incomplete) -*see also*
Injury, blood vessel, thoracic, pulmonary,
laceration
   complete -*see* Injury, blood vessel, thoracic,
   pulmonary, laceration, major
subclavian -*see* Transection, innominate
vena cava (incomplete) -*see also* Injury, vena
cava
   complete -*see* Injury, vena cava, laceration,
   major
vertebral artery (incomplete) -*see also* Injury,
blood vessel, vertebral, laceration
   complete -*see* Injury, blood vessel, vertebral,
   laceration, major

Transaminasemia R74.0

Transfusion
associated (red blood cell) hemochromatosis
  E83.111
blood
  ABO incompatible -*see* Complication(s),
    transfusion, incompatibility reaction, ABO
  minor blood group (Duffy) (E) (K(ell))
    (Kidd) (Lewis) (M) (N) (P) (S) T80.89
  reaction or complication -*see* Complications,
    transfusion
fetomaternal (mother) -*see* Pregnancy,
  complicated by, placenta, transfusion
  syndrome
maternofetal (mother) -*see* Pregnancy,
  complicated by, placenta, transfusion
  syndrome
placental (syndrome) (mother) -*see*
  Pregnancy, complicated by, placenta,
  transfusion syndrome
reaction (adverse) -*see* Complications,
  transfusion
related acute lung injury (TRALI) J95.84
twin-to-twin -*see* Pregnancy, complicated by,
  placenta, transfusion syndrome, fetus to fetus

Transient (meaning homeless) -*see also*
condition Z59.0

Translocation
balanced autosomal Q95.9
  in normal individual Q95.0
chromosomes NEC Q99.8
  balanced and insertion in normal individual
    Q95.0
Down syndrome Q90.2
trisomy
  13 Q91.6
  18 Q91.2
  21 Q90.2

Translucency, iris -*see* Degeneration, iris

**Transmission of chemical substances
through the placenta** -*see* Absorption,
chemical, through placenta

Transparency, lung, unilateral J43.0

Transplant (ed) (status) Z94.9
awaiting organ Z76.82
bone Z94.6
  marrow Z94.81
candidate Z76.82
complication -*see* Complication, transplant
cornea Z94.7
heart Z94.1
  and lung(s) Z94.3

Transplant (ed) (status) --*continued*
valve Z95.2
  prosthetic Z95.2
  specified NEC Z95.4
  xenogenic Z95.3
intestine Z94.82
kidney Z94.0
liver Z94.4
lung(s) Z94.2
  and heart Z94.3
organ (failure) (infection) (rejection) Z94.9
  removal status Z98.85
pancreas Z94.83
skin Z94.5
social Z60.3
specified organ or tissue NEC Z94.89
stem cells Z94.84
tissue Z94.9

Transplants, ovarian, endometrial N80.1

Transposed -*see* Transposition

Transposition (congenital) -*see also*
Malposition, congenital
abdominal viscera Q89.3
aorta (dextra) Q20.3
appendix Q43.8
colon Q43.8
corrected Q20.5
great vessels (complete) (partial) Q20.3
heart Q24.0
  with complete transposition of viscera Q89.3
intestine (large) (small) Q43.8
reversed jejunal (for bypass) (status) Z98.0
scrotum Q55.23
stomach Q40.2
  with general transposition of viscera Q89.3
tooth, teeth, fully erupted M26.30
vessels, great (complete) (partial) Q20.3
viscera (abdominal) (thoracic) Q89.3

Transsexualism F64.0

Transverse -*see also* condition
arrest (deep), in labor O64.0
lie (mother) O32.2
  causing obstructed labor O64.8

Transvestism, transvestitism (dual-role)
F64.1
fetishistic F65.1

Trapped placenta (with hemorrhage) O72.0
without hemorrhage O73.0

**TRAPS (tumor necrosis factor receptor
associated periodic syndrome)** M04.1

Trauma, traumatism -*see also* Injury
acoustic -*see* subcategory H83.3
birth -*see* Birth, injury
complicating ectopic or molar pregnancy
  O08.6
during delivery O71.9
following ectopic or molar pregnancy O08.6
obstetric O71.9
  specified NEC O71.89
occlusal
  primary K08.81
  secondary K08.82

Traumatic -*see also* condition
brain injury S06.9

Treacher Collins syndrome Q75.4

Treitz's hernia -*see* Hernia, abdomen,
specified site NEC

Trematode infestation -*see* Infestation, fluke

Trematodiasis -*see* Infestation, fluke

Trembling paralysis -*see* Parkinsonism

Tremor(s) R25.1
drug induced G25.1
essential (benign) G25.0
familial G25.0
hereditary G25.0
hysterical F44.4
intention G25.2
medication induced postural G25.1
mercurial -*see* subcategory T56.1
Parkinson's -*see* Parkinsonism
psychogenic (conversion reaction) F44.4
senilis R54
specified type NEC G25.2

Trench
fever A79.0
foot -*see* Immersion, foot
mouth A69.1

Treponema pallidum infection -*see* Syphilis

Treponematosis
due to
  T. pallidum -*see* Syphilis
  T. pertenue -*see* Yaws

Triad
Hutchinson's (congenital syphilis) A50.53
Kartagener's Q89.3
Saint's -*see* Hernia, diaphragm

Trichiasis (eyelid) H02.059
with entropion -*see* Entropion
left H02.056
  lower H02.055
  upper H02.054
right H02.053
  lower H02.052
  upper H02.051

Trichinella spiralis (infection) (infestation)
B75

**Trichinellosis, trichiniasis, trichinelliasis,
trichinosis** B75
with muscle disorder B75 [*M63.80*]
  ankle B75 [*M63.87*]
  foot B75 [*M63.87*]
  forearm B75 [*M63.83*]
  hand B75 [*M63.84*]
  lower leg B75 [*M63.86*]
  multiple sites B75 [*M63.89*]
  pelvic region B75 [*M63.85*]
  shoulder region B75 [*M63.81*]
  specified site NEC B75 [*M63.88*]
  thigh B75 [*M63.85*]
  upper arm B75 [*M63.82*]

Trichobezoar T18.9
intestine T18.3
stomach T18.2

Trichocephaliasis, trichocephalosis B79

Trichocephalus infestation B79

Trichoclasis L67.8

Trichoepithelioma -*see also* Neoplasm, skin,
benign
malignant -*see* Neoplasm, skin, malignant

Trichofolliculoma -*see* Neoplasm, skin,
benign

Tricholemmoma -*see* Neoplasm, skin, benign

Trichomoniasis A59.9
bladder A59.03
cervix A59.09
intestinal A07.8
prostate A59.02
seminal vesicles A59.09
specified site NEC A59.8
urethra A59.03
urogenitalis A59.00
vagina A59.01
vulva A59.01

Trichomycosis
  axillaris A48.8
  nodosa, nodularis B36.8
Trichonodosis L67.8
Trichophytid, trichophyton infection -*see*
  Dermatophytosis
Trichophytobezoar T18.9
  intestine T18.3
  stomach T18.2
Trichophytosis -*see* Dermatophytosis
Trichoptilosis L67.8
Trichorrhexis (nodosa) (invaginata) L67.0
Trichosis axillaris A48.8
Trichosporosis nodosa B36.2
Trichostasis spinulosa (congenital) Q84.1
**Trichostrongyliasis, trichostrongylosis (small
  intestine)** B81.2
Trichostrongylus infection B81.2
Trichotillomania F63.3
**Trichromat, trichromatopsia, anomalous
  (congenital)** H53.55
Trichuriasis B79
**Trichuris trichiura (infection) (infestation)
  (any site)** B79
Tricuspid (valve) -*see* condition
Trifid -*see also* Accessory   kidney (pelvis)
  Q63.8
  tongue Q38.3
Trigeminal neuralgia -*see* Neuralgia,
  trigeminal
Trigeminy R00.8
Trigger finger (acquired) M65.30
  congenital Q74.0
  index finger M65.32
  little finger M65.35
  middle finger M65.33
  ring finger M65.34
  thumb M65.31
**Trigonitis (bladder) (chronic)
  (pseudomembranous)** N30.30
  with hematuria N30.31
Trigonocephaly Q75.0
Trilocular heart -*see* Cor triloculare
Trimethylaminuria E72.52
Tripartite placenta O43.19
Triphalangeal thumb Q74.0
Triple -*see also* Accessory
  kidneys Q63.0
  uteri Q51.818
  X, female Q97.0
Triplegia G83.89
  congenital G80.8
Triplet (newborn) -*see also* Newborn, triplet
  complicating pregnancy -*see* Pregnancy,
  triplet
Triplication -*see* Accessory
Triploidy Q92.7
Trismus R25.2
  neonatorum A33
  newborn A33
Trisomy (syndrome) Q92.9
  autosomes Q92.9
  chromosome specified NEC Q92.8
    partial Q92.2
      due to unbalanced translocation Q92.5
    whole (nonsex chromosome)
      meiotic nondisjunction Q92.0
      mitotic nondisjunction Q92.1
      mosaicism Q92.1
  specified NEC Q92.8
  due to

Trisomy (syndrome) --*continued*
  dicentrics -*see* Extra, marker chromosomes
  extra rings -*see* Extra, marker chromosomes
  isochromosomes -*see* Extra, marker
    chromosomes
  specified NEC Q92.8
  whole chromosome Q92.9
    meiotic nondisjunction Q92.0
    mitotic nondisjunction Q92.1
    mosaicism Q92.1
    partial Q92.9
    specified NEC Q92.8
  13 (partial) Q91.7
    meiotic nondisjunction Q91.4
    mitotic nondisjunction Q91.5
    mosaicism Q91.5
    translocation Q91.6
  18 (partial) Q91.3
    meiotic nondisjunction Q91.0
    mitotic nondisjunction Q91.1
    mosaicism Q91.1
    translocation Q91.2
  20 Q92.8
  21 (partial) Q90.9
    meiotic nondisjunction Q90.0
    mitotic nondisjunction Q90.1
    mosaicism Q90.1
    translocation Q90.2
  22 Q92.8
Tritanomaly, tritanopia H53.55
Trombiculosis, trombiculiasis, trombidiosis
  B88.0
Trophedema (congenital) (hereditary) Q82.0
Trophoblastic disease -*see also* Mole,
  hydatidiform O01.9
Tropholymphedema Q82.0
Trophoneurosis NEC G96.8
  disseminated M34.9
Tropical -*see* condition
Trouble -*see also* Disease
  heart -*see* Disease, heart
  kidney -*see* Disease, renal
  nervous R45.0
  sinus -*see* Sinusitis
**Trousseau's syndrome (thrombophlebitis
  migrans)** I82.1
Truancy, childhood
  from school Z72.810
Truncus
  arteriosus (persistent) Q20.0
  communis Q20.0
Trunk -*see* condition
Trypanosomiasis
  African B56.9
    by Trypanosoma brucei
      gambiense B56.0
      rhodesiense B56.1
  American -*see* Chagas' disease
  Brazilian -*see* Chagas' disease - by
    Trypanosoma
      brucei gambiense B56.0
      brucei rhodesiense B56.1
      cruzi -*see* Chagas' disease
  gambiensis, Gambian B56.0
  rhodesiensis, Rhodesian B56.1
  South American -*see* Chagas' disease
  where
    African trypanosomiasis is prevalent B56.9
    Chagas' disease is prevalent B57.2
T-shaped incisors K00.2
Tsutsugamushi (disease) (fever) A75.3

Tube, tubal, tubular -*see* condition
Tubercle -*see also* Tuberculosis
  brain, solitary A17.81
  Darwin's Q17.8
  Ghon, primary infection A15.7
**Tuberculid, tuberculide (indurating,
  subcutaneous) (lichenoid) (miliary)
  (papulonecrotic) (primary) (skin)** A18.4
Tuberculoma -*see also* Tuberculosis
  brain A17.81
  meninges (cerebral) (spinal) A17.1
  spinal cord A17.81
**Tuberculosis, tubercular, tuberculous
  (calcification) (calcified) (caseous)
  (chromogenic acid-fast bacilli)
  (degeneration) (fibrocaseous) (fistula)
  (interstitial) (isolated circumscribed
  lesions) (necrosis) (parenchymatous)
  (ulcerative)** A15.9
  with pneumoconiosis (any condition in J60
    J64) J65
  abdomen (lymph gland) A18.39
  abscess (respiratory) A15.9
    bone A18.03
      hip A18.02
      knee A18.02
      sacrum A18.01
      specified site NEC A18.03
      spinal A18.01
      vertebra A18.01
    brain A17.81
    breast A18.89
    Cowper's gland A18.15
    dura (mater) (cerebral) (spinal) A17.81
    epidural (cerebral) (spinal) A17.81
    female pelvis A18.17
    frontal sinus A15.8
    genital organs NEC A18.10
    genitourinary A18.10
    gland (lymphatic) -*see* Tuberculosis, lymph
      gland
    hip A18.02
    intestine A18.32
    ischiorectal A18.32
    joint NEC A18.02
      hip A18.02
      knee A18.02
      specified NEC A18.02
      vertebral A18.01
    kidney A18.11
    knee A18.02
    latent R76.11
    lumbar (spine) A18.01
    lung -*see* Tuberculosis, pulmonary
    meninges (cerebral) (spinal) A17.0
    muscle A18.09
    perianal (fistula) A18.32
    perinephritic A18.11
    perirectal A18.32
    rectum A18.32
    retropharyngeal A15.8
    sacrum A18.01
    scrofulous A18.2
    scrotum A18.15
    skin (primary) A18.4
    spinal cord A17.81
    spine or vertebra (column) A18.01
    subdiaphragmatic A18.31
    testis A18.15
    urinary A18.13
    uterus A18.17

Tuberculosis, tubercular, tuberculous
--*continued*
accessory sinus -*see* Tuberculosis, sinus
Addison's disease A18.7
adenitis -*see* Tuberculosis, lymph gland
adenoids A15.8
adenopathy -*see* Tuberculosis, lymph gland
adherent pericardium A18.84
adnexa (uteri) A18.17
adrenal (capsule) (gland) A18.7
alimentary canal A18.32
anemia A18.89
ankle (joint) (bone) A18.02
anus A18.32
apex, apical -*see* Tuberculosis, pulmonary
appendicitis, appendix A18.32
arachnoid A17.0
artery, arteritis A18.89
   cerebral A18.89
arthritis (chronic) (synovial) A18.02
   spine or vertebra (column) A18.01
articular -*see* Tuberculosis, joint
ascites A18.31
asthma -*see* Tuberculosis, pulmonary
axilla, axillary (gland) A18.2
bladder A18.12
bone A18.03
   hip A18.02
   knee A18.02
   limb NEC A18.03
   sacrum A18.01
   spine or vertebral column A18.01
bowel (miliary) A18.32
brain A17.81
breast A18.89
broad ligament A18.17
bronchi, bronchial, bronchus A15.5
   ectasia, ectasis (bronchiectasis) -*see*
Tuberculosis, pulmonary
   fistula A15.5
      primary (progressive) A15.7
   gland or node A15.4
      primary (progressive) A15.7
   lymph gland or node A15.4
      primary (progressive) A15.7
bronchiectasis -*see* Tuberculosis, pulmonary
bronchitis A15.5
bronchopleural A15.6
bronchopneumonia, bronchopneumonic -*see*
Tuberculosis, pulmonary
bronchorrhagia A15.5
bronchotracheal A15.5
bronze disease A18.7
buccal cavity A18.83
bulbourethral gland A18.15
bursa A18.09
cachexia A15.9
cardiomyopathy A18.84
caries -*see* Tuberculosis, bone
cartilage A18.02
   intervertebral A18.01
catarrhal -*see* Tuberculosis, respiratory
cecum A18.32
cellulitis (primary) A18.4
cerebellum A17.81
cerebral, cerebrum A17.81
cerebrospinal A17.81
   meninges A17.0
cervical (lymph gland or node) A18.2
cervicitis, cervix (uteri) A18.16

Tuberculosis, tubercular, tuberculous
--*continued*
chest -*see* Tuberculosis, respiratory
   chorioretinitis A18.53
choroid, choroiditis A18.53
ciliary body A18.54
colitis A18.32
collier's J65
colliquativa (primary) A18.4
colon A18.32
complex, primary A15.7
congenital P37.0
conjunctiva A18.59
connective tissue (systemic) A18.89
contact Z20.1
cornea (ulcer) A18.52
Cowper's gland A18.15
coxae A18.02
coxalgia A18.02
cul-de-sac of Douglas A18.17
curvature, spine A18.01
cutis (colliquativa) (primary) A18.4
cyst, ovary A18.18
cystitis A18.12
dactylitis A18.03
diarrhea A18.32
diffuse -*see* Tuberculosis, miliary
digestive tract A18.32
disseminated -*see* Tuberculosis, miliary
duodenum A18.32
dura (mater) (cerebral) (spinal) A17.0
   abscess (cerebral) (spinal) A17.81
dysentery A18.32
ear (inner) (middle) A18.6
   bone A18.03
   external (primary) A18.4
   skin (primary) A18.4
elbow A18.02
emphysema -*see* Tuberculosis, pulmonary
empyema A15.6
encephalitis A17.82
endarteritis A18.89
endocarditis A18.84
   aortic A18.84
   mitral A18.84
   pulmonary A18.84
   tricuspid A18.84
endocrine glands NEC A18.82
endometrium A18.17
enteric, enterica, enteritis A18.32
enterocolitis A18.32
epididymis, epididymitis A18.15
epidural abscess (cerebral) (spinal) A17.81
epiglottis A15.5
episcleritis A18.51
erythema (induratum) (nodosum) (primary)
   A18.4
esophagus A18.83
eustachian tube A18.6
exposure (to) Z20.1
exudative -*see* Tuberculosis, pulmonary
eye A18.50
eyelid (primary) (lupus) A18.4
fallopian tube (acute) (chronic) A18.17
fascia A18.09
fauces A15.8
female pelvic inflammatory disease A18.17
finger A18.03
first infection A15.7
gallbladder A18.83
ganglion A18.09

Tuberculosis, tubercular, tuberculous
--*continued*
gastritis A18.83
gastrocolic fistula A18.32
gastroenteritis A18.32
gastrointestinal tract A18.32
general, generalized -*see* Tuberculosis,
   miliary
genital organs A18.10
genitourinary A18.10
genu A18.02
glandula suprarenalis A18.7
glandular, general A18.2
glottis A15.5
grinder's J65
gum A18.83
hand A18.03
heart A18.84
hematogenous -*see* Tuberculosis, miliary
hemoptysis -*see* Tuberculosis, pulmonary
hemorrhage NEC -*see* Tuberculosis,
   pulmonary
hemothorax A15.6
hepatitis A18.83
hilar lymph nodes A15.4
   primary (progressive) A15.7
hip (joint) (disease) (bone) A18.02
hydropneumothorax A15.6
hydrothorax A15.6
hypoadrenalism A18.7
hypopharynx A15.8
ileocecal (hyperplastic) A18.32
ileocolitis A18.32
ileum A18.32
iliac spine (superior) A18.03
immunological findings only A15.7
indurativa (primary) A18.4
infantile A15.7
infection A15.9
   without clinical manifestations A15.7
infraclavicular gland A18.2
inguinal gland A18.2
inguinalis A18.2
intestine (any part) A18.32
iridocyclitis A18.54
iris, iritis A18.54
ischiorectal A18.32
jaw A18.03
jejunum A18.32
joint A18.02
   vertebral A18.01
keratitis (interstitial) A18.52
keratoconjunctivitis A18.52
kidney A18.11
knee (joint) A18.02
kyphosis, kyphoscoliosis A18.01
laryngitis A15.5
larynx A15.5
latent R76.11
leptomeninges, leptomeningitis (cerebral)
   (spinal) A17.0
lichenoides (primary) A18.4
linguae A18.83
lip A18.83
liver A18.83
lordosis A18.01
lung -*see* Tuberculosis, pulmonary
lupus vulgaris A18.4
lymph gland or node (peripheral) A18.2
   abdomen A18.39
   bronchial A15.4

Tuberculosis, tubercular, tuberculous
--continued
      primary (progressive) A15.7
  cervical A18.2
  hilar A15.4
    primary (progressive) A15.7
  intrathoracic A15.4
    primary (progressive) A15.7
  mediastinal A15.4
    primary (progressive) A15.7
  mesenteric A18.39
  retroperitoneal A18.39
  tracheobronchial A15.4
    primary (progressive) A15.7
  lymphadenitis *-see* Tuberculosis, lymph gland
  lymphangitis *-see* Tuberculosis, lymph gland
  lymphatic (gland) (vessel) *-see* Tuberculosis, lymph gland
  mammary gland A18.89
  marasmus A15.9
  mastoiditis A18.03
  mediastinal lymph gland or node A15.4
    primary (progressive) A15.7
  mediastinitis A15.8
    primary (progressive) A15.7
  mediastinum A15.8
    primary (progressive) A15.7
  medulla A17.81
  melanosis, Addisonian A18.7
  meninges, meningitis (basilar) (cerebral) (cerebrospinal) (spinal) A17.0
  meningoencephalitis A17.82
  mesentery, mesenteric (gland or node) A18.39
  miliary A19.9
    acute A19.2
      multiple sites A19.1
      single specified site A19.0
    chronic A19.8
    specified NEC A19.8
  millstone makers' J65
  miner's J65
  molder's J65
  mouth A18.83
  multiple A19.9
    acute A19.1
    chronic A19.8
  muscle A18.09
  myelitis A17.82
  myocardium, myocarditis A18.84
  nasal (passage) (sinus) A15.8
  nasopharynx A15.8
  neck gland A18.2
  nephritis A18.11
  nerve (mononeuropathy) A17.83
  nervous system A17.9
  nose (septum) A15.8
  ocular A18.50
  omentum A18.31
  oophoritis (acute) (chronic) A18.17
  optic (nerve trunk) (papilla) A18.59
  orbit A18.59
  orchitis A18.15
  organ, specified NEC A18.89
  osseous *-see* Tuberculosis, bone
  osteitis *-see* Tuberculosis, bone
  osteomyelitis *-see* Tuberculosis, bone
  otitis media A18.6
  ovary, ovaritis (acute) (chronic) A18.17
  oviduct (acute) (chronic) A18.17
  pachymeningitis A17.0
  palate (soft) A18.83

Tuberculosis, tubercular, tuberculous
--continued
  pancreas A18.83
  papulonecrotic (a) (primary) A18.4
  parathyroid glands A18.82
  paronychia (primary) A18.4
  parotid gland or region A18.83
  pelvis (bony) A18.03
  penis A18.15
  peribronchitis A15.5
  pericardium, pericarditis A18.84
  perichondritis, larynx A15.5
  periostitis *-see* Tuberculosis, bone
  perirectal fistula A18.32
  peritoneum NEC A18.31
  peritonitis A18.31
  pharynx, pharyngitis A15.8
  phlyctenulosis (keratoconjunctivitis) A18.52
  phthisis NEC *-see* Tuberculosis, pulmonary
  pituitary gland A18.82
  pleura, pleural, pleurisy, pleuritis (fibrinous) (obliterative) (purulent) (simple plastic) (with effusion) A15.6
    primary (progressive) A15.7
  pneumonia, pneumonic *-see* Tuberculosis, pulmonary
  pneumothorax (spontaneous) (tense valvular) *-see* Tuberculosis, pulmonary
  polyneuropathy A17.89
  polyserositis A19.9
    acute A19.1
    chronic A19.8
  potter's J65
  prepuce A18.15
  primary (complex) A15.7
  proctitis A18.32
  prostate, prostatitis A18.14
  pulmonalis *-see* Tuberculosis, pulmonary
  pulmonary (cavitated) (fibrotic) (infiltrative) (nodular) A15.0
    childhood type or first infection A15.7
    primary (complex) A15.7
  pyelitis A18.11
  pyelonephritis A18.11
  pyemia *-see* Tuberculosis, miliary
  pyonephrosis A18.11
  pyopneumothorax A15.6
  pyothorax A15.6
  rectum (fistula) (with abscess) A18.32
  reinfection stage *-see* Tuberculosis, pulmonary
  renal A18.11
  renis A18.11
  respiratory A15.9
    primary A15.7
    specified site NEC A15.8
  retina, retinitis A18.53
  retroperitoneal (lymph gland or node) A18.39
  rheumatism NEC A18.09
  rhinitis A15.8
  sacroiliac (joint) A18.01
  sacrum A18.01
  salivary gland A18.83
  salpingitis (acute) (chronic) A18.17
  sandblaster's J65
  sclera A18.51
  scoliosis A18.01
  scrofulous A18.2
  scrotum A18.15
  seminal tract or vesicle A18.15
  senile A15.9

Tuberculosis, tubercular, tuberculous
--continued
  septic *-see* Tuberculosis, miliary
  shoulder (joint) A18.02
    blade A18.03
  sigmoid A18.32
  sinus (any nasal) A15.8
    bone A18.03
    epididymis A18.15
  skeletal NEC A18.03
  skin (any site) (primary) A18.4
  small intestine A18.32
  soft palate A18.83
  spermatic cord A18.15
  spine, spinal (column) A18.01
    cord A17.81
    medulla A17.81
    membrane A17.0
    meninges A17.0
  spleen, splenitis A18.85
  spondylitis A18.01
  sternoclavicular joint A18.02
  stomach A18.83
  stonemason's J65
  subcutaneous tissue (cellular) (primary) A18.4
  subcutis (primary) A18.4
  subdeltoid bursa A18.83
  submaxillary (region) A18.83
  supraclavicular gland A18.2
  suprarenal (capsule) (gland) A18.7
  swelling, joint (see also category M01) *-see also* Tuberculosis, joint A18.02
  symphysis pubis A18.02
  synovitis A18.09
    articular A18.02
    spine or vertebra A18.01
  systemic *-see* Tuberculosis, miliary
  tarsitis A18.4
  tendon (sheath) *-see* Tuberculosis, tenosynovitis
  tenosynovitis A18.09
    spine or vertebra A18.01
  testis A18.15
  throat A15.8
  thymus gland A18.82
  thyroid gland A18.81
  tongue A18.83
  tonsil, tonsillitis A15.8
  trachea, tracheal A15.5
    lymph gland or node A15.4
      primary (progressive) A15.7
  tracheobronchial A15.5
    lymph gland or node A15.4
      primary (progressive) A15.7
  tubal (acute) (chronic) A18.17
  tunica vaginalis A18.15
  ulcer (skin) (primary) A18.4
    bowel or intestine A18.32
    specified NEC
      code under Tuberculosis, by site
    unspecified site A15.9
  ureter A18.11
  urethra, urethral (gland) A18.13
  urinary organ or tract A18.13
  uterus A18.17
  uveal tract A18.54
  uvula A18.83
  vagina A18.18
  vas deferens A18.15
  verruca, verrucosa (cutis) (primary) A18.4

Tuberculosis, tubercular, tuberculous
--*continued*
  vertebra (column) A18.01
  vesiculitis A18.15
  vulva A18.18
  wrist (joint) A18.02
Tuberculum
  Carabelli -*see* Note at K00.2
  occlusal -*see* Note at K00.2
  paramolare K00.2
Tuberosity, entire maxillary M26.07
Tuberous sclerosis (brain) Q85.1
Tubo-ovarian -*see* condition
Tuboplasty, after previous sterilization
  Z31.0
  aftercare Z31.42
Tubotympanitis, catarrhal (chronic) -*see*
  Otitis, media, nonsuppurative, chronic, serous
Tularemia A21.9
  with
    conjunctivitis A21.1
    pneumonia A21.2
  abdominal A21.3
  bronchopneumonic A21.2
  conjunctivitis A21.1
  cryptogenic A21.3
  enteric A21.3
  gastrointestinal A21.3
  generalized A21.7
  ingestion A21.3
  intestinal A21.3
  oculoglandular A21.1
  ophthalmic A21.1
  pneumonia (any), pneumonic A21.2
  pulmonary A21.2
  sepsis A21.7
  specified NEC A21.8
  typhoidal A21.7
  ulceroglandular A21.0
Tularensis conjunctivitis A21.1
Tumefaction -*see also* Swelling
  liver -*see* Hypertrophy, liver
Tumor -*see also* Neoplasm, unspecified
  behavior, by site
  acinar cell -*see* Neoplasm, uncertain behavior,
    by site
  acinic cell -*see* Neoplasm, uncertain behavior,
    by site
  adenocarcinoid -*see* Neoplasm, malignant, by
    site
  adenomatoid -*see also* Neoplasm, benign, by
  site
    odontogenic -*see* Cyst, calcifying
      odontogenic
  adnexal (skin) -*see* Neoplasm, skin, benign,
    by site
  adrenal
    cortical (benign) D35.0
      malignant C74.0
    rest -*see* Neoplasm, benign, by site
  alpha-cell
    malignant
      pancreas C25.4
      specified site NEC -*see* Neoplasm,
        malignant, by site
      unspecified site C25.4
    pancreas D13.7
    specified site NEC -*see* Neoplasm, benign,
      by site
    unspecified site D13.7
  aneurysmal -*see* Aneurysm

Tumor - *continued*
  aortic body D44.7
    malignant C75.5
  Askin's -*see* Neoplasm, connective tissue,
    malignant
  basal cell -*see also* Neoplasm, skin, uncertain
    behavior D48.5
  Bednar -*see* Neoplasm, skin, malignant
  benign (unclassified) -*see* Neoplasm, benign,
    by site
  beta-cell
    malignant
      pancreas C25.4
      specified site NEC -*see* Neoplasm,
        malignant, by site
      unspecified site C25.4
    pancreas D13.7
    specified site NEC -*see* Neoplasm, benign,
      by site
    unspecified site D13.7
  Brenner D27.9
    borderline malignancy D39.1
    malignant C56
    proliferating D39.1
  bronchial alveolar, intravascular D38.1
  Brooke's -*see* Neoplasm, skin, benign
  brown fat -*see* Lipoma
  Burkitt -*see* Lymphoma, Burkitt
  calcifying epithelial odontogenic -*see* Cyst,
    calcifying odontogenic
  carcinoid
    benign D3A.00
      appendix D3A.020
      ascending colon D3A.022
      bronchus (lung) D3A.090
      cecum D3A.021
      colon D3A.029
      descending colon D3A.024
      duodenum D3A.010
      foregut NOS D3A.094
      hindgut NOS D3A.096
      ileum D3A.012
      jejunum D3A.011
      kidney D3A.093
      large intestine D3A.029
      lung (bronchus) D3A.090
      midgut NOS D3A.095
      rectum D3A.026
      sigmoid colon D3A.025
      small intestine D3A.019
      specified NEC D3A.098
      stomach D3A.092
      thymus D3A.091
      transverse colon D3A.023
    malignant C7A.00
      appendix C7A.020
      ascending colon C7A.022
      bronchus (lung) C7A.090
      cecum C7A.021
      colon C7A.029
      descending colon C7A.024
      duodenum C7A.010
      foregut NOS C7A.094
      hindgut NOS C7A.096
      ileum C7A.012
      jejunum C7A.011
      kidney C7A.093
      large intestine C7A.029
      lung (bronchus) C7A.090
      midgut NOS C7A.095
      rectum C7A.026

Tumor - *continued*
      sigmoid colon C7A.025
      small intestine C7A.019
      specified NEC C7A.098
      stomach C7A.092
      thymus C7A.091
      transverse colon C7A.023
    mesentery metastasis C7B.04
    secondary C7B.00
      bone C7B.03
      distant lymph nodes C7B.01
      liver C7B.02
      peritoneum C7B.04
      specified NEC C7B.09
  carotid body D44.6
    malignant C75.4
  cells -*see also* Neoplasm, unspecified
  behavior, by site
    benign -*see* Neoplasm, benign, by site
    malignant -*see* Neoplasm, malignant, by site
    uncertain whether benign or malignant -*see*
      Neoplasm, uncertain behavior, by site
  cervix, in pregnancy or childbirth -*see*
    Pregnancy, complicated by, tumor, cervix
  chondromatous giant cell -*see* Neoplasm,
    bone, benign
  chromaffin -*see also* Neoplasm, benign, by
  site
    malignant -*see* Neoplasm, malignant, by site
  Cock's peculiar L72.3
  Codman's -*see* Neoplasm, bone, benign
  dentigerous, mixed -*see* Cyst, calcifying
    odontogenic
  dermoid -*see* Neoplasm, benign, by site
    with malignant transformation C56
  desmoid (extra-abdominal) -*see also*
  Neoplasm, connective tissue, uncertain
  behavior
    abdominal -*see* Neoplasm, connective tissue,
      uncertain behavior
  embolus -*see* Neoplasm, secondary, by site
  embryonal (mixed) -*see also* Neoplasm,
  uncertain behavior, by site
    liver C22.7
  endodermal sinus
    specified site -*see* Neoplasm, malignant, by
      site
    unspecified site
      female C56.
      male C62.90
  epithelial
    benign -*see* Neoplasm, benign, by site
    malignant -*see* Neoplasm, malignant, by site
  Ewing's -*see* Neoplasm, bone, malignant, by
    site
  fatty -*see* Lipoma
  fibroid -*see* Leiomyoma
  G cell
    malignant
      pancreas C25.4
      specified site NEC -*see* Neoplasm,
        malignant, by site
      unspecified site C25.4
    specified site -*see* Neoplasm, uncertain
      behavior, by site
    unspecified site D37.8
  germ cell -*see also* Neoplasm, malignant, by
  site
    mixed -*see* Neoplasm, malignant, by site
  ghost cell, odontogenic -*see* Cyst, calcifying
    odontogenic

Tumor - *continued*

giant cell -*see also* Neoplasm, uncertain behavior, by site
  bone D48.0
    malignant -*see* Neoplasm, bone, malignant
    chondromatous -*see* Neoplasm, bone, benign
  malignant -*see* Neoplasm, malignant, by site
  soft parts -*see* Neoplasm, connective tissue, uncertain behavior
    malignant -*see* Neoplasm, connective tissue, malignant
glomus D18.00
  intra-abdominal D18.03
  intracranial D18.02
  jugulare D44.7
    malignant C75.5
  skin D18.01
  specified site NEC D18.09
gonadal stromal -*see* Neoplasm, uncertain behavior, by site
granular cell -*see also* Neoplasm, connective tissue, benign
  malignant -*see* Neoplasm, connective tissue, malignant
granulosa cell D39.1
  juvenile D39.1
  malignant C56
granulosa cell-theca cell D39.1
  malignant C56
Grawitz's C64
hemorrhoidal -*see* Hemorrhoids
hilar cell D27
hilus cell D27
Hürthle cell (benign) D34
  malignant C73
hydatid -*see* Echinococcus
hypernephroid -*see also* Neoplasm, uncertain behavior, by site
interstitial cell -*see also* Neoplasm, uncertain behavior, by site
  benign -*see* Neoplasm, benign, by site
  malignant -*see* Neoplasm, malignant, by site
intravascular bronchial alveolar D38.1
islet cell -*see* Neoplasm, benign, by site
  malignant -*see* Neoplasm, malignant, by site
    pancreas C25.4
    specified site NEC -*see* Neoplasm, malignant, by site
    unspecified site C25.4
  pancreas D13.7
  specified site NEC -*see* Neoplasm, benign, by site
  unspecified site D13.7
juxtaglomerular D41.0
Klatskin's C24.0
Krukenberg's C79.6
Leydig cell -*see* Neoplasm, uncertain behavior, by site
  benign -*see* Neoplasm, benign, by site
    specified site -*see* Neoplasm, benign, by site
    unspecified site
      female D27.9
      male D29.20
  malignant -*see* Neoplasm, malignant, by site
    specified site -*see* Neoplasm, malignant, by site
    unspecified site
      female C56.9
      male C62.90

Tumor - *continued*

  specified site -*see* Neoplasm, uncertain behavior, by site
  unspecified site
    female D39.10
    male D40.10
lipid cell, ovary D27
lipoid cell, ovary D27
malignant -*see also* Neoplasm, malignant, by site C80.1
  fusiform cell (type) C80.1
  giant cell (type) C80.1
  localized, plasma cell -*see* Plasmacytoma, solitary
  mixed NEC C80.1
  small cell (type) C80.1
  spindle cell (type) C80.1
  unclassified C80.1
mast cell D47.0
  malignant C96.2
melanotic, neuroectodermal -*see* Neoplasm, benign, by site
Merkel cell -*see* Carcinoma, Merkel cell
mesenchymal
  malignant -*see* Neoplasm, connective tissue, malignant
  mixed -*see* Neoplasm, connective tissue, uncertain behavior
mesodermal, mixed -*see also* Neoplasm, malignant, by site
  liver C22.4
mesonephric -*see also* Neoplasm, uncertain behavior, by site
  malignant -*see* Neoplasm, malignant, by site
metastatic
  from specified site -*see* Neoplasm, malignant, by site
  of specified site -*see* Neoplasm, malignant, by site
  to specified site -*see* Neoplasm, secondary, by site
mixed NEC -*see also* Neoplasm, benign, by site
  malignant -*see* Neoplasm, malignant, by site
mucinous of low malignant potential
  specified site -*see* Neoplasm, malignant, by site
  unspecified site C56.9
mucocarcinoid
  specified site -*see* Neoplasm, malignant, by site
  unspecified site C18.1
mucoepidermoid -*see* Neoplasm, uncertain behavior, by site
Müllerian, mixed
  specified site -*see* Neoplasm, malignant, by site
  unspecified site C54.9
myoepithelial -*see* Neoplasm, benign, by site
neuroectodermal (peripheral) -*see* Neoplasm, malignant, by site
  primitive
    specified site -*see* Neoplasm, malignant, by site
    unspecified site C71.9
neuroendocrine D3A.8
  malignant poorly differentiated C7A.1
  secondary NEC C7B.8
  specified NEC C7A.8
neurogenic olfactory C30.0
nonencapsulated sclerosing C73

Tumor - *continued*

odontogenic (adenomatoid) (benign) (calcifying epithelial) (keratocystic) (squamous) -*see* Cyst, calcifying odontogenic
  malignant C41.1
    upper jaw (bone) C41.0
ovarian stromal D39.1
ovary, in pregnancy -*see* Pregnancy, complicated by pacinian -*see* Neoplasm, skin, benign
Pancoast's -*see* Pancoast's syndrome -
  papillary -*see also* Papilloma
  cystic D37.9
  mucinous of low malignant potential C56
    specified site -*see* Neoplasm, malignant, by site
    unspecified site C56.9
  serous of low malignant potential
    specified site -*see* Neoplasm, malignant, by site
    unspecified site C56.9
pelvic, in pregnancy or childbirth -*see* Pregnancy, complicated by phantom F45.8
phyllodes D48.6
  benign D24
  malignant -*see* Neoplasm, breast, malignant
Pindborg -*see* Cyst, calcifying odontogenic
placental site trophoblastic D39.2
plasma cell (malignant) (localized) -*see* Plasmacytoma, solitary
polyvesicular vitelline
  specified site -*see* Neoplasm, malignant, by site
  unspecified site
    female C56.9
    male C62.90
Pott's puffy -*see* Osteomyelitis, specified NEC
Rathke's pouch D44.3
retinal anlage -*see* Neoplasm, benign, by site
salivary gland type, mixed -*see* Neoplasm, salivary gland, benign
  malignant -*see* Neoplasm, salivary gland, malignant
Sampson's N80.1
Schmincke's -*see* Neoplasm, nasopharynx, malignant
sclerosing stromal D27
sebaceous -*see* Cyst, sebaceous
secondary -*see* Neoplasm, secondary, by site
  carcinoid C7B.00
    bone C7B.03
    distant lymph nodes C7B.01
    liver C7B.02
    peritoneum C7B.04
    specified NEC C7B.09
  neuroendocrine NEC C7B.8
serous of low malignant potential
  specified site -*see* Neoplasm, malignant, by site
  unspecified site C56.9
Sertoli cell -*see* Neoplasm, benign, by site
  with lipid storage
    specified site -*see* Neoplasm, benign, by site
    unspecified site
      female D27.9
      male D29.20
  specified site -*see* Neoplasm, benign, by site
  unspecified site
    female D27.9

Tumor - *continued*

    male D29.20
Sertoli-Leydig cell *-see* Neoplasm, benign, by site
    specified site *-see* Neoplasm, benign, by site
    unspecified site
        female D27.9
        male D29.20
sex cord (stromal) *-see* Neoplasm, uncertain behavior, by site
    with annular tubules D39.1
skin appendage *-see* Neoplasm, skin, benign
smooth muscle *-see* Neoplasm, connective tissue, uncertain behavior
soft tissue
    benign *-see* Neoplasm, connective tissue, benign
    malignant *-see* Neoplasm, connective tissue, malignant
sternomastoid (congenital) Q68.0
stromal
    endometrial D39.0
    gastric D48.1
        benign D21.4
        malignant C16.9
        uncertain behavior D48.1
    gastrointestinal C49.A-
        benign D21.4
        esophagus C49.A1
        large intestine C49.A4
        malignant C49.A0
            colon C49.A4
            duodenum C49.A3
            esophagus C49.A1
            ileum C49.A3
            jejunum C49.A3
            Meckel diverticulum C49.A3
            large intestine C49.A4
            omentum C49.A9
            peritoneum C49.A9
            rectum C49.A5
            small intestine C49.A3
            specified site NEC C49.A9
            stomach C49.A2
        large intestine C49.A4
        rectum C49.A5
        small intestine C49.A3
        specified site NEC C49.A9
        stomach C49.A2
        uncertain behavior D48.1
    intestine
        benign D21.4
        malignant
            large C49.A4
            small C49.A3
        uncertain behavior D48.1
    ovarian D39.1
    stomach C49.A2
        benign D21.4
        malignant C49.A2
        uncertain behavior D48.1
    testicular D40.10
sweat gland *-see also* Neoplasm, skin, uncertain behavior
    benign *-see* Neoplasm, skin, benign
    malignant *-see* Neoplasm, skin, malignant
syphilitic, brain A52.17
testicular stromal D40.1
theca cell D27
theca cell-granulosa cell D39.1

Tumor - *continued*

Triton, malignant *-see* Neoplasm, nerve, malignant
trophoblastic, placental site D39.2
turban D23.4
uterus (body), in pregnancy or childbirth *-see* Pregnancy, complicated by, tumor, uterus
vagina, in pregnancy or childbirth *-see* Pregnancy, complicated by
varicose *-see* Varix
von Recklinghausen's *-see* Neurofibromatosis
vulva or perineum, in pregnancy or childbirth *-see* Pregnancy, complicated by
    causing obstructed labor O65.5
Warthin's *-see* Neoplasm, salivary gland, benign
Wilms' C64
yolk sac *-see* Neoplasm, malignant, by site
    specified site *-see* Neoplasm, malignant, by site
    unspecified site
        female C56.9
        male C62.90

Tumor lysis syndrome (following antineoplastic chemotherapy) (spontaneous) NEC E88.3
Tumorlet *-see* Neoplasm, uncertain behavior, by site
Tungiasis B88.1
Tunica vasculosa lentis Q12.2
Turban tumor D23.4
Türck's trachoma J37.0
Turner-Kieser syndrome Q87.2
Turner-like syndrome Q87.1
Turner's
    hypoplasia (tooth) K00.4
    syndrome Q96.9
        specified NEC Q96.8
    tooth K00.4
Turner-Ullrich syndrome Q96.9
Tussis convulsiva *-see* Whooping cough
Twiddler's syndrome (due to)
    automatic implantable defibrillator T82.198
    cardiac pacemaker T82.198
Twilight state
    epileptic F05
    psychogenic F44.89
Twin (newborn) *-see also* Newborn, twin
    conjoined Q89.4
    pregnancy *-see* Pregnancy, twin, conjoined
Twinning, teeth K00.2
Twist, twisted
    bowel, colon or intestine K56.2
    hair (congenital) Q84.1
    mesentery K56.2
    omentum K56.2
    organ or site, congenital NEC *-see* Anomaly, by site
    ovarian pedicle *-see* Torsion, ovary
Twitching R25.3
Tylosis (acquired) L84
    buccalis K13.29
    linguae K13.29
    palmaris et plantaris (congenital) (inherited) Q82.8
        acquired L85.1
Tympanism R14.0
Tympanites (abdominal) (intestinal) R14.0
Tympanitis *-see* Myringitis
Tympanosclerosis *-see* subcategory H74.0
Tympanum *-see* condition

Tympany
    abdomen R14.0
    chest R09.89
Type A behavior pattern Z73.1
Typhlitis *-see* Appendicitis
Typhoenteritis *-see* Typhoid
Typhoid (abortive) (ambulant) (any site) (clinical) (fever) (hemorrhagic) (infection) (intermittent) (malignant) (rheumatic) (Widal negative) A01.00
    with pneumonia A01.03
    abdominal A01.09
    arthritis A01.04
    carrier (suspected) of Z22.0
    cholecystitis (current) A01.09
    endocarditis A01.02
    heart involvement A01.02
    inoculation reaction *-see* Complications, vaccination
    meningitis A01.01
    mesenteric lymph nodes A01.09
    myocarditis A01.02
    osteomyelitis A01.05
    perichondritis, larynx A01.09
    pneumonia A01.03
    spine A01.05
    specified NEC A01.09
    ulcer (perforating) A01.09
Typhomalaria (fever) *-see* Malaria
Typhomania A01.00
Typhoperitonitis A01.09
Typhus (fever) A75.9
    abdominal, abdominalis *-see* Typhoid
    African tick A77.1
    amarillic A95.9
    brain A75.9 [*G94*]
    cerebral A75.9 [*G94*]
    classical A75.0
    due to Rickettsia
        prowazekii A75.0
            recrudescent A75.1
        tsutsugamushi A75.3
        typhi A75.2
    endemic (flea-borne) A75.2
    epidemic (louse-borne) A75.0
    exanthematic NEC A75.0
    exanthematicus SAI A75.0
        brillii SAI A75.1
        mexicanus SAI A75.2
        typhus murinus A75.2
    flea-borne A75.2
    India tick A77.1
    Kenya (tick) A77.1
    louse-borne A75.0
    Mexican A75.2
    mite-borne A75.3
    murine A75.2
    North Asian tick-borne A77.2
    petechial A75.9
    Queensland tick A77.3
    rat A75.2
    recrudescent A75.1
    recurrens *-see* Fever, relapsing
    Sao Paulo A77.0
    scrub (China) (India) (Malaysia) (New Guinea) A75.3
    shop (of Malaysia) A75.2
    Siberian tick A77.2
    tick-borne A77.9
    tropical (mite-borne) A75.3

Tyrosinemia E70.21
  newborn, transitory P74.5
Tyrosinosis E70.21
Tyrosinuria E70.29

U

Uhl's anomaly or disease Q24.8
Ulcer, ulcerated, ulcerating, ulceration,
  ulcerative
  alveolar process M27.3
  amebic (intestine) A06.1
    skin A06.7
  anastomotic -see Ulcer, gastrojejunal
  anorectal K62.6
  antral -see Ulcer, stomach
  anus (sphincter) (solitary) K62.6
  aorta -see Aneurysm
  aphthous (oral) (recurrent) K12.0
    genital organ(s)
      female N76.6
      male N50.89
  artery I77.2
  atrophic -see Ulcer, skin
    decubitus -see Ulcer, pressure, by site
  back L98.429
    with
      bone necrosis L98.424
      exposed fat layer L98.422
      muscle necrosis L98.423
      skin breakdown only L98.421
  Barrett's (esophagus) K22.10
    with bleeding K22.11
  bile duct (common) (hepatic) K83.8
  bladder (solitary) (sphincter) NEC N32.89
    bilharzial B65.9 [N33]
    in schistosomiasis (bilharzial) B65.9 [N33]
    submucosal -see Cystitis, interstitial
    tuberculous A18.12
  bleeding K27.4
  bone -see Osteomyelitis, specified type NEC
  bowel -see Ulcer, intestine
  breast N61.1
  bronchus J98.09
  buccal (cavity) (traumatic) K12.1
  Buruli A31.1
  buttock L98.419
    with
      bone necrosis L98.414
      exposed fat layer L98.412
      muscle necrosis L98.413
      skin breakdown only L98.411
  cancerous -see Neoplasm, malignant, by site
  cardia K22.10
    with bleeding K22.11
  cardioesophageal (peptic) K22.10
    with bleeding K22.11
  cecum -see Ulcer, intestine
  cervix (uteri) (decubitus) (trophic) N86
    with cervicitis N72
  chancroidal A57
  chiclero B55.1
  chronic (cause unknown) -see Ulcer, skin
  Cochin-China B55.1
  colon -see Ulcer, intestine
  conjunctiva H10.89
  cornea H16.00
    with hypopyon H16.03
    central H16.01
    dendritic (herpes simplex) B00.52
    marginal H16.04

Ulcer - *continued*
  Mooren's H16.05
  mycotic H16.06
  perforated H16.07
  ring H16.02
  tuberculous (phlyctenular) A18.52
  corpus cavernosum (chronic) N48.5
  crural -see Ulcer, lower limb
  Curling's -see Ulcer, peptic, acute
  Cushing's -see Ulcer, peptic, acute
  cystic duct K82.8
  cystitis (interstitial) -see Cystitis, interstitial
  decubitus -see Ulcer, pressure, by site
  dendritic, cornea (herpes simplex) B00.52
  diabetes, diabetic -see Diabetes, ulcer
  Dieulafoy's K25.0
  due to
    infection NEC -see Ulcer, skin
    radiation NEC L59.8
    trophic disturbance (any region) -see Ulcer,
  skin
    X ray L58.1
  duodenum, duodenal (eroded) (peptic) K26.9
    with
      hemorrhage K26.4
        and perforation K26.6
      perforation K26.5
    acute K26.3
      with
        hemorrhage K26.0
          and perforation K26.2
        perforation K26.1
    chronic K26.7
      with
        hemorrhage K26.4
          and perforation K26.6
        perforation K26.5
  dysenteric A09
  elusive -see Cystitis, interstitial
  endocarditis (acute) (chronic) (subacute) I28.8
  epiglottis J38.7
  esophagus (peptic) K22.10
    with bleeding K22.11
    due to
      aspirin K22.10
        with bleeding K22.11
      gastrointestinal reflux disease K21.0
      ingestion of chemical or medicament
      K22.10
        with bleeding K22.11
    fungal K22.10
      with bleeding K22.11
    infective K22.10
      with bleeding K22.11
    varicose -see Varix, esophagus
  eyelid (region) H01.8
  fauces J39.2
  Fenwick (Hunner) (solitary) -see Cystitis,
  interstitial
  fistulous -see Ulcer, skin
  foot (indolent) (trophic) -see Ulcer, lower
  limb
  frambesial, initial A66.0
  frenum (tongue) K14.0
  gallbladder or duct K82.8
  gangrenous -see Gangrene
  gastric -see Ulcer, stomach
  gastrocolic -see Ulcer, gastrojejunal
  gastroduodenal -see Ulcer, peptic
  gastroesophageal -see Ulcer, stomach
  gastrointestinal -see Ulcer, gastrojejunal

Ulcer - *continued*
  gastrojejunal (peptic) K28.9
    with
      hemorrhage K28.4
        and perforation K28.6
      perforation K28.5
    acute K28.3
      with
        hemorrhage K28.0
          and perforation K28.2
        perforation K28.1
    chronic K28.7
      with
        hemorrhage K28.4
          and perforation K28.6
        perforation K28.5
  gastrojejunocolic -see Ulcer, gastrojejunal
  gingiva K06.8
  gingivitis K05.10
    nonplaque induced K05.11
    plaque induced K05.10
  glottis J38.7
  granuloma of pudenda A58
  gum K06.8
  gumma, due to yaws A66.4
  heel -see Ulcer, lower limb
  hemorrhoid -see also Hemorrhoids, by degree
    K64.8
  Hunner's -see Cystitis, interstitial
  hypopharynx J39.2
  hypopyon (chronic) (subacute) -see Ulcer,
    cornea, with hypopyon
  hypostaticum -see Ulcer, varicose
  ileum -see Ulcer, intestine
  intestine, intestinal K63.3
    with perforation K63.1
    amebic A06.1
    duodenal -see Ulcer, duodenum
    granulocytopenic (with hemorrhage) -see
  Neutropenia
    marginal -see Ulcer, gastrojejunal
    perforating K63.1
      newborn P78.0
    primary, small intestine K63.3
    rectum K62.6
    stercoraceous, stercoral K63.3
    tuberculous A18.32
    typhoid (fever) -see Typhoid
    varicose I86.8
  jejunum, jejunal -see Ulcer, gastrojejunal
  keratitis -see Ulcer, cornea
  knee -see Ulcer, lower limb
  labium (majus) (minus) N76.6
  laryngitis -see Laryngitis
  larynx (aphthous) (contact) J38.7
    diphtheritic A36.2
  leg -see Ulcer, lower limb
  lip K13.0
  Lipschütz's N76.6
  lower limb (atrophic) (chronic) (neurogenic)
  (perforating) (pyogenic) (trophic) (tropical)
  L97.909
    with
      bone necrosis L97.904
      exposed fat layer L97.902
      muscle necrosis L97.903
      skin breakdown only L97.901
    ankle L97.309
      with
        bone necrosis L97.304
        exposed fat layer L97.302

Ulcer - *continued*
  muscle necrosis L97.303
  skin breakdown only L97.301
  left L97.329
    with
      bone necrosis L97.324
      exposed fat layer L97.322
      muscle necrosis L97.323
      skin breakdown only L97.321
  right L97.319
    with
      bone necrosis L97.314
      exposed fat layer L97.312
      muscle necrosis L97.313
      skin breakdown only L97.311
  calf L97.209
    with
      bone necrosis L97.204
      exposed fat layer L97.202
      muscle necrosis L97.203
      skin breakdown only L97.201
    left L97.229
      with
        bone necrosis L97.224
        exposed fat layer L97.222
        muscle necrosis L97.223
        skin breakdown only L97.221
    right L97.219
      with
        bone necrosis L97.214
        exposed fat layer L97.212
        muscle necrosis L97.213
        skin breakdown only L97.211
  decubitus *-see* Ulcer, pressure, by site
  foot specified NEC L97.509
    with
      bone necrosis L97.504
      exposed fat layer L97.502
      muscle necrosis L97.503
      skin breakdown only L97.501
    left L97.529
      with
        bone necrosis L97.524
        exposed fat layer L97.522
        muscle necrosis L97.523
        skin breakdown only L97.521
    right L97.519
      with
        bone necrosis L97.514
        exposed fat layer L97.512
        muscle necrosis L97.513
        skin breakdown only L97.511
  heel L97.409
    with
      bone necrosis L97.404
      exposed fat layer L97.402
      muscle necrosis L97.403
      skin breakdown only L97.401
    left L97.429
      with
        bone necrosis L97.424
        exposed fat layer L97.422
        muscle necrosis L97.423
        skin breakdown only L97.421
    right L97.419
      with
        bone necrosis L97.414
        exposed fat layer L97.412
        muscle necrosis L97.413
        skin breakdown only L97.411
    left L97.929

Ulcer - *continued*
  with
    bone necrosis L97.924
    exposed fat layer L97.922
    muscle necrosis L97.923
    skin breakdown only L97.921
  lower leg NOS L97.909
    with
      bone necrosis L97.904
      exposed fat layer L97.902
      muscle necrosis L97.903
      skin breakdown only L97.901
    left L97.929
      with
        bone necrosis L97.924
        exposed fat layer L97.922
        muscle necrosis L97.923
        skin breakdown only L97.921
    right L97.919
      with
        bone necrosis L97.914
        exposed fat layer L97.912
        muscle necrosis L97.913
        skin breakdown only L97.911
  specified site NEC L97.809
    with
      bone necrosis L97.804
      exposed fat layer L97.802
      muscle necrosis L97.803
      skin breakdown only L97.801
    left L97.829
      with
        bone necrosis L97.824
        exposed fat layer L97.822
        muscle necrosis L97.823
        skin breakdown only L97.821
    right L97.819
      with
        bone necrosis L97.814
        exposed fat layer L97.812
        muscle necrosis L97.813
        skin breakdown only L97.811
  midfoot L97.409
    with
      bone necrosis L97.404
      exposed fat layer L97.402
      muscle necrosis L97.403
      skin breakdown only L97.401
    left L97.429
      with
        bone necrosis L97.424
        exposed fat layer L97.422
        muscle necrosis L97.423
        skin breakdown only L97.421
    right L97.419
      with
        bone necrosis L97.414
        exposed fat layer L97.412
        muscle necrosis L97.413
        skin breakdown only L97.411
  right L97.919
    with
      bone necrosis L97.914
      exposed fat layer L97.912
      muscle necrosis L97.913
      skin breakdown only L97.911
  thigh L97.109
    with
      bone necrosis L97.104
      exposed fat layer L97.102
      muscle necrosis L97.103

Ulcer - *continued*
  skin breakdown only L97.101
  left L97.129
    with
      bone necrosis L97.124
      exposed fat layer L97.122
      muscle necrosis L97.123
      skin breakdown only L97.121
  right L97.119
    with
      bone necrosis L97.114
      exposed fat layer L97.112
      muscle necrosis L97.113
      skin breakdown only L97.111
  toe L97.509
    with
      bone necrosis L97.504
      exposed fat layer L97.502
      muscle necrosis L97.503
      skin breakdown only L97.501
    left L97.529
      with
        bone necrosis L97.524
        exposed fat layer L97.522
        muscle necrosis L97.523
        skin breakdown only L97.521
    right L97.519
      with
        bone necrosis L97.514
        exposed fat layer L97.512
        muscle necrosis L97.513
        skin breakdown only L97.511
  leprous A30.1
  syphilitic A52.19
  varicose *-see* Varix, leg, with, ulcer
  luetic *-see* Ulcer, syphilitic
  lung J98.4
    tuberculous *-see* Tuberculosis, pulmonary
  malignant *-see* Neoplasm, malignant, by site
  marginal NEC *-see* Ulcer, gastrojejunal
  meatus (urinarius) N34.2
  Meckel's diverticulum Q43.0
    malignant *-see* Table of Neoplasms, small
    intestine, malignant
  Meleney's (chronic undermining) *-see* Ulcer,
    skin
  Mooren's (cornea) *-see* Ulcer, cornea,
    Mooren's
  mycobacterial (skin) A31.1
  nasopharynx J39.2
  neck, uterus N86
  neurogenic NEC *-see* Ulcer, skin
  nose, nasal (passage) (infective) (septum)
  J34.0
    skin *-see* Ulcer, skin
    spirochetal A69.8
    varicose (bleeding) I86.8
  oral mucosa (traumatic) K12.1
  palate (soft) K12.1
  penis (chronic) N48.5
  peptic (site unspecified) K27.9
    with
      hemorrhage K27.4
        and perforation K27.6
      perforation K27.5
    acute K27.3
      with
        hemorrhage K27.0
          and perforation K27.2
        perforation K27.1
    chronic K27.7

Ulcer - *continued*

  with
    hemorrhage K27.4
      and perforation K27.6
      perforation K27.5
  esophagus K22.10
    with bleeding K22.11
  newborn P78.82
  perforating K27.5
  skin -*see* Ulcer, skin
  peritonsillar J35.8
  phagedenic (tropical) -*see* Ulcer, skin
  pharynx J39.2
  phlebitis -*see* Phlebitis
  plaster -*see* Ulcer, pressure, by site
  popliteal space -*see* Ulcer, lower limb
  postpyloric -*see* Ulcer, duodenum
  prepuce N47.7
  prepyloric -*see* Ulcer, stomach
  pressure (pressure area) L89.9
    ankle L89.5
    back L89.1
    buttock L89.3
    coccyx L89.15
    contiguous site of back, buttock, hip L89.4
    elbow L89.0
    face L89.81
    head L89.81
    heel L89.6
    hip L89.2
    sacral region (tailbone) L89.15
    specified site NEC L89.89
    stage 1 (healing) (pre-ulcer skin changes limited to persistent focal edema)
      ankle L89.5
      back L89.1
      buttock L89.3
      coccyx L89.15
      contiguous site of back, buttock, hip L89.4
      elbow L89.0
      face L89.81
      head L89.81
      heel L89.6
      hip L89.2
      sacral region (tailbone) L89.15
      specified site NEC L89.89
    stage 2 (healing) (abrasion, blister, partial thickness skin loss involving epidermis and/or dermis)
      ankle L89.5
      back L89.1
      buttock L89.3
      coccyx L89.15
      contiguous site of back, buttock, hip L89.4
      elbow L89.0
      face L89.81
      head L89.81
      heel L89.6
      hip L89.2
      sacral region (tailbone) L89.15
      specified site NEC L89.89
    stage 3 (healing) (full thickness skin loss involving damage or necrosis of subcutaneous tissue)
      ankle L89.5
      back L89.1
      buttock L89.3
      coccyx L89.15

Ulcer - *continued*

      contiguous site of back, buttock, hip L89.4
      elbow L89.0
      face L89.81
      head L89.81
      heel L89.6
      hip L89.2
      sacral region (tailbone) L89.15
      specified site NEC L89.89
    stage 4 (healing) (necrosis of soft tissues through to underlying muscle, tendon, or bone)
      ankle L89.5
      back L89.1
      buttock L89.3
      coccyx L89.15
      contiguous site of back, buttock, hip L89.4
      elbow L89.0
      face L89.81
      head L89.81
      heel L89.6
      hip L89.2
      sacral region (tailbone) L89.15
      specified site NEC L89.89
    unspecified stage
      ankle L89.5
      back L89.1
      buttock L89.3
      coccyx L89.15
      contiguous site of back, buttock, hip L89.4
      elbow L89.0
      face L89.81
      head L89.81
      heel L89.6
      hip L89.2
      sacral region (tailbone) L89.15
      specified site NEC L89.89
    unstageable
      ankle L89.5
      back L89.1
      buttock L89.3
      coccyx L89.15
      contiguous site of back, buttock, hip L89.4
      elbow L89.0
      face L89.81
      head L89.81
      heel L89.6
      hip L89.2
      sacral region (tailbone) L89.15
      specified site NEC L89.89
  primary of intestine K63.3
    with perforation K63.1
  prostate N41.9
  pyloric -*see* Ulcer, stomach
  rectosigmoid K63.3
    with perforation K63.1
  rectum (sphincter) (solitary) K62.6
    stercoraceous, stercoral K62.6
  retina -*see* Inflammation, chorioretinal
  rodent -*see also* Neoplasm, skin, malignant
  sclera -*see* Scleritis
  scrofulous (tuberculous) A18.2
  scrotum N50.89
    tuberculous A18.15
    varicose I86.1
  seminal vesicle N50.89
  sigmoid -*see* Ulcer, intestine

Ulcer - *continued*

  skin (atrophic) (chronic) (neurogenic) (non-healing) (perforating) (pyogenic) (trophic) (tropical) L98.499
    with gangrene -*see* Gangrene
    amebic A06.7
    back -*see* Ulcer, back
    buttock -*see* Ulcer, buttock
    decubitus -*see* Ulcer, pressure
    lower limb -*see* Ulcer, lower limb
    mycobacterial A31.1
    specified site NEC L98.499
      with
        bone necrosis L98.494
        exposed fat layer L98.492
        muscle necrosis L98.493
        skin breakdown only L98.491
    tuberculous (primary) A18.4
    varicose -*see* Ulcer, varicose
  sloughing -*see* Ulcer, skin
  solitary, anus or rectum (sphincter) K62.6
  sore throat J02.9
    streptococcal J02.0
  spermatic cord N50.89
  spine (tuberculous) A18.01
  stasis (venous) -*see* Varix, leg, with, ulcer
    without varicose veins I87.2
  stercoraceous, stercoral K63.3
    with perforation K63.1
    anus or rectum K62.6
  stoma, stomal -*see* Ulcer, gastrojejunal
  stomach (eroded) (peptic) (round) K25.9
    with
      hemorrhage K25.4
        and perforation K25.6
      perforation K25.5
    acute K25.3
      with
        hemorrhage K25.0
          and perforation K25.2
        perforation K25.1
    chronic K25.7
      with
        hemorrhage K25.4
          and perforation K25.6
        perforation K25.5
  stomal -*see* Ulcer, gastrojejunal
  stomatitis K12.1
  stress -*see* Ulcer, peptic
  strumous (tuberculous) A18.2
  submucosal, bladder -*see* Cystitis, interstitial
  syphilitic (any site) (early) (secondary) A51.39
    late A52.79
    perforating A52.79
      foot A52.11
  testis N50.89
  thigh -*see* Ulcer, lower limb
  throat J39.2
    diphtheritic A36.0
  toe -*see* Ulcer, lower limb
  tongue (traumatic) K14.0
  tonsil J35.8
    diphtheritic A36.0
  trachea J39.8
  trophic -*see* Ulcer, skin
  tropical -*see* Ulcer, skin
  tuberculous -*see* Tuberculosis, ulcer
  tunica vaginalis N50.89
  turbinate J34.89
  typhoid (perforating) -*see* Typhoid

Ulcer - *continued*
  unspecified site -*see* Ulcer, skin
  urethra (meatus) -*see* Urethritis
  uterus N85.8
    cervix N86
      with cervicitis N72
    neck N86
      with cervicitis N72
  vagina N76.5
    in Behçet's disease M35.2 [*N77.0*]
    pessary N89.8
  valve, heart I33.0
  varicose (lower limb, any part) -*see also*
  Varix, leg, with, ulcer
    broad ligament I86.2
    esophagus -*see* Varix, esophagus
    inflamed or infected -*see* Varix, leg, with
    ulcer, with inflammation
    nasal septum I86.8
    perineum I86.3
    scrotum I86.1
    specified site NEC I86.8
    sublingual I86.0
    vulva I86.3
  vas deferens N50.89
  vulva (acute) (infectional) N76.6
    in (due to)
      Behçet's disease M35.2 [*N77.0*]
      herpesviral (herpes simplex) infection
        A60.04
      tuberculosis A18.18
  vulvobuccal, recurring N76.6
  X ray L58.1
  yaws A66.4
Ulcerosa scarlatina A38.8
Ulcus -*see also* Ulcer
  cutis tuberculosum A18.4
  duodeni -*see* Ulcer, duodenum
  durum (syphilitic) A51.0
    extragenital A51.2
  gastrojejunale -*see* Ulcer, gastrojejunal
  hypostaticum -*see* Ulcer, varicose
  molle (cutis) (skin) A57
  serpens corneae -*see* Ulcer, cornea, central
  ventriculi -*see* Ulcer, stomach
Ulegyria Q04.8
Ulerythema
  ophryogenes, congenital Q84.2
  sycosiforme L73.8
Ullrich (Bonnevie)(Turner) syndrome -*see
also* Turner's syndrome Q87.1
Ullrich-Feichtiger syndrome Q87.0
Ulnar -*see* condition
Ulorrhagia, ulorrhea K06.8
Umbilicus, umbilical -*see* condition
Unacceptable
  contours of tooth K08.54
  morphology of tooth K08.54
Unavailability (of)
  bed at medical facility Z75.1
  health service-related agencies Z75.4
  medical facilities (at) Z75.3
    due to
      investigation by social service agency
        Z75.2
      lack of services at home Z75.0
      remoteness from facility Z75.3
      waiting list Z75.1
    home Z75.0
    outpatient clinic Z75.3
  schooling Z55.1
  social service agencies Z75.4

Uncinaria americana infestation B76.1
Uncinariasis B76.9
Uncongenial work Z56.5
Unconscious (ness) -*see* Coma
Under observation -*see* Observation
Underachievement in school Z55.3
Underdevelopment -*see also* Undeveloped
  nose Q30.1
  sexual E30.0
Underdosing -*see also* Table of Drugs and
  Chemicals, categories T36 T50, with final
  character 6 Z91.14
  intentional NEC Z91.128
    due to financial hardship of patient Z91.120
  unintentional NEC Z91.138
    due to patient's age related debility Z91.130
Underfeeding, newborn P92.3
Underfill, endodontic M27.53
Underimmunization status Z28.3
Undernourishment -*see* Malnutrition
Undernutrition -*see* Malnutrition
Underweight R63.6
  for gestational age -*see* Light for dates
Underwood's disease P83.0
Undescended -*see also* Malposition, congenital
  cecum Q43.3
  colon Q43.3
  testicle -*see* Cryptorchid
Undeveloped, undevelopment -*see also*
  Hypoplasia
  brain (congenital) Q02
  cerebral (congenital) Q02
  heart Q24.8
  lung Q33.6
  testis E29.1
  uterus E30.0
Undiagnosed (disease) R69
Undulant fever -*see* Brucellosis
Unemployment, anxiety concerning Z56.0
  threatened Z56.2
Unequal length (acquired) (limb) -*see also*
  Deformity, limb, unequal length
  leg -*see also* Deformity, limb, unequal length
    congenital Q72.9
Unextracted dental root K08.3
Unguis incarnatus L60.0
Unhappiness R45.2
Unicornate uterus Q51.4
Unilateral -*see also* condition
  development, breast N64.89
  organ or site, congenital NEC -*see* Agenesis,
    by site
Unilocular heart Q20.8
Union, abnormal -*see also* Fusion
  larynx and trachea Q34.8
Universal mesentery Q43.3
**Unrepairable overhanging of dental
restorative materials** K08.52
Unsatisfactory
  restoration of tooth K08.50
    specified NEC K08.59
  sample of cytologic smear
    anus R85.615
    cervix R87.615
    vagina R87.625
  surroundings Z59.1
  work Z56.5
Unsoundness of mind -*see* Psychosis
Unstable
  back NEC -*see* Instability, joint, spine
  hip (congenital) Q65.6

Unstable --*continued*
  acquired -*see* Derangement, joint, specified
    type NEC, hip
  joint -*see* Instability, joint
    secondary to removal of joint prosthesis
      M96.89
  lie (mother) O32.0
  lumbosacral joint (congenital)
    acquired -*see* subcategory M53.2
  sacroiliac -*see* subcategory M53.2
  spine NEC -*see* Instability, joint, spine
Unsteadiness on feet R26.81
Untruthfulness, child problem F91.8
Unverricht (Lundborg) disease or epilepsy -
see Epilepsy, generalized, idiopathic
Unwanted pregnancy Z64.0
Upbringing, institutional Z62.22
  away from parents NEC Z62.29
  in care of non-parental family member Z62.21
  in foster care Z62.21
  in orphanage or group home Z62.22
  in welfare custody Z62.21
Upper respiratory -*see* condition
Upset
  gastric K30
  gastrointestinal K30
    psychogenic F45.8
  intestinal (large) (small) K59.9
    psychogenic F45.8
  menstruation N93.9
  mental F48.9
  stomach K30
    psychogenic F45.8
Urachus -*see also* condition
  patent or persistent Q64.4
**Urbach-Oppenheim disease (necrobiosis
lipoidica diabeticorum)** -*see* E08 E13 with
.620
Urbach's lipoid proteinosis E78.89
Urbach-Wiethe disease E78.89
Urban yellow fever A95.1
Urea
  blood, high -*see* Uremia
  cycle metabolism disorder -*see* Disorder, urea
  cycle metabolism
Uremia, uremic N19
  with
    ectopic or molar pregnancy O08.4
    polyneuropathy N18.9 [*G63*]
  chronic -*see also* Disease, kidney, chronic
    N18.9
    due to hypertension -*see* Hypertensive,
      kidney complicating
    ectopic or molar pregnancy O08.4
  congenital P96.0
  extrarenal R39.2
  following ectopic or molar pregnancy O08.4
  newborn P96.0
  prenatal R39.2
Ureter, ureteral -*see* condition
Ureteralgia N23
Ureterectasis -*see* Hydroureter
Ureteritis N28.89
  cystica N28.86
  due to calculus N20.1
    with calculus, kidney N20.2
      with hydronephrosis N13.2
  gonococcal (acute) (chronic) A54.21
  nonspecific N28.89
Ureterocele N28.89
  congenital (orthotopic) Q62.31
    ectopic Q62.32

Ureterolith, ureterolithiasis -see Calculus, ureter
Ureterostomy
  attention to Z43.6
  status Z93.6
Urethra, urethral -see condition
Urethralgia R39.89
Urethritis (anterior) (posterior) N34.2
  calculous N21.1
  candidal B37.41
  chlamydial A56.01
  diplococcal (gonococcal) A54.01
   with abscess (accessory gland) (periurethral) A54.1
  gonococcal A54.01
   with abscess (accessory gland) (periurethral) A54.1
  nongonococcal N34.1
   Reiter's -see Reiter's disease
  nonspecific N34.1
  nonvenereal N34.1
  postmenopausal N34.2
  puerperal O86.22
  Reiter's -see Reiter's disease
  specified NEC N34.2
  trichomonal or due to Trichomonas (vaginalis) A59.03
Urethrocele N81.0
  with
   cystocele -see Cystocele
   prolapse of uterus -see Prolapse, uterus
Urethrolithiasis (with colic or infection) N21.1
Urethrorectal -see condition
Urethrorrhagia N36.8
Urethrorrhea R36.9
Urethrostomy
  attention to Z43.6
  status Z93.6
Urethrotrigonitis -see Trigonitis
Urethrovaginal -see condition
Urgency
  fecal R15.2
  hypertensive -see Hypertension
  urinary R39.15
Urhidrosis, uridrosis L74.8
Uric acid in blood (increased) E79.0
Uricacidemia (asymptomatic) E79.0
Uricemia (asymptomatic) E79.0
Uricosuria R82.99
Urinary -see condition
Urination
  frequent R35.0
  painful R30.9
Urine
  blood in -see Hematuria
  discharge, excessive R35.8
  enuresis, nonorganic origin F98.0
  extravasation R39.0
  frequency R35.0
  incontinence R32
   nonorganic origin F98.0
  intermittent stream R39.198
  pus in N39.0
  retention or stasis R33.9
   organic R33.8
    drug-induced R33.0
   psychogenic F45.8
  secretion
   deficient R34
   excessive R35.8

Urine --continued
  frequency R35.0
  stream
   intermittent R39.198
   slowing R39.198
   splitting R39.13
   weak R39.12
Urinemia -see Uremia
Urinoma, urethra N36.8
Uroarthritis, infectious (Reiter's) -see Reiter's disease
Urodialysis R34
Urolithiasis -see Calculus, urinary
Uronephrosis -see Hydronephrosis
Uropathy N39.9
  obstructive N13.9
   specified NEC N13.8
  reflux N13.9
   specified NEC N13.8
  vesicoureteral reflux associated -see Reflux, vesicoureteral
Urosepsis - code to condition
Urticaria L50.9
  with angioneurotic edema T78.3
   hereditary D84.1
  allergic L50.0
  cholinergic L50.5
  chronic L50.8
  cold, familial L50.2
  contact L50.6
  dermatographic L50.3
  due to
   cold or heat L50.2
   drugs L50.0
   food L50.0
   inhalants L50.0
   plants L50.6
   serum -see also Reaction, serum T80.69
  factitial L50.3
  familial cold M04.2
  giant T78.3
   hereditary D84.1
  gigantea T78.3
  idiopathic L50.1
  larynx T78.3
   hereditary D84.1
  neonatorum P83.8
  nonallergic L50.1
  papulosa (Hebra) L28.2
  pigmentosa Q82.2
  recurrent periodic L50.8
  serum -see also Reaction, serum T80.69
  solar L56.3
  specified type NEC L50.8
  thermal (cold) (heat) L50.2
  vibratory L50.4
  xanthelasmoidea Q82.2
Use (of)
  alcohol Z72.89
   with
    intoxication F10.929
    sleep disorder F10.982
   harmful -see Abuse, alcohol
  amphetamines -see Use, stimulant NEC
  caffeine -see Use, stimulant NEC
  cannabis F12.90
   with
    anxiety disorder F12.980
    intoxication F12.929
     with
      delirium F12.921

Use (of) --continued
      perceptual disturbance F12.922
     uncomplicated F12.920
    other specified disorder F12.988
    psychosis F12.959
     delusions F12.950
     hallucinations F12.951
    unspecified disorder F12.99
  cocaine F14.90
   with
    anxiety disorder F14.980
    intoxication F14.929
     with
      delirium F14.921
      perceptual disturbance F14.922
     uncomplicated F14.920
    other specified disorder F14.988
    psychosis F14.959
     delusions F14.950
     hallucinations F14.951
    sexual dysfunction F14.981
    sleep disorder F14.982
    unspecified disorder F14.99
   harmful -see Abuse, drug, cocaine
  drug(s) NEC F19.90
   with sleep disorder F19.982
   harmful -see Abuse, drug, by type
  hallucinogen NEC F16.90
   with
    anxiety disorder F16.980
    intoxication F16.929
     with
      delirium F16.921
     uncomplicated F16.920
    mood disorder F16.94
    other specified disorder F16.988
    perception disorder (flashbacks) F16.983
    psychosis F16.959
     delusions F16.950
     hallucinations F16.951
    unspecified disorder F16.99
   harmful -see Abuse, drug, hallucinogen NEC
  inhalants F18.90
   with
    anxiety disorder F18.980
    intoxication F18.929
     with delirium F18.921
     uncomplicated F18.920
    mood disorder F18.94
    other specified disorder F18.988
    persisting dementia F18.97
    psychosis F18.959
     delusions F18.950
     hallucinations F18.951
    unspecified disorder F18.99
   harmful -see Abuse, drug, inhalant
  methadone -see Use, opioid
  nonprescribed drugs F19.90
   harmful -see Abuse, non-psychoactive substance
  opioid F11.90
   with
    disorder F11.99
     mood F11.94
     sleep F11.982
     specified type NEC F11.988
    intoxication F11.929
     with
      delirium F11.921
      perceptual disturbance F11.922

Use (of) --*continued*
    uncomplicated F11.920
    withdrawal F11.93
  harmful -*see* Abuse, drug, opioid
  patent medicines F19.90
    harmful -*see* Abuse, non-psychoactive
    substance
  psychoactive drug NEC F19.90
    with
      anxiety disorder F19.980
      intoxication F19.929
        with
          delirium F19.921
          perceptual disturbance F19.922
        uncomplicated F19.920
      mood disorder F19.94
      other specified disorder F19.988
      persisting
        amnestic disorder F19.96
        dementia F19.97
      psychosis F19.959
        delusions F19.950
        hallucinations F19.951
      sexual dysfunction F19.981
      sleep disorder F19.982
      unspecified disorder F19.99
      withdrawal F19.939
        with
          delirium F19.931
          perceptual disturbance F19.932
        uncomplicated F19.930
    harmful -*see* Abuse, drug NEC,
    psychoactive NEC
  sedative, hypnotic, or anxiolytic F13.90
    with
      anxiety disorder F13.980
      intoxication F13.929
        with
          delirium F13.921
        uncomplicated F13.920
      other specified disorder F13.988
      persisting
        amnestic disorder F13.96
        dementia F13.97
      psychosis F13.959
        delusions F13.950
        hallucinations F13.951
      sexual dysfunction F13.981
      sleep disorder F13.982
      unspecified disorder F13.99
    harmful -*see* Abuse, drug, sedative,
    hypnotic, or anxiolytic
  stimulant NEC F15.90
    with
      anxiety disorder F15.980
      intoxication F15.929
        with
          delirium F15.921
          perceptual disturbance F15.922
        uncomplicated F15.920
      mood disorder F15.94
      other specified disorder F15.988
      psychosis F15.959
        delusions F15.950
        hallucinations F15.951
      sexual dysfunction F15.981
      sleep disorder F15.982
      unspecified disorder F15.99
      withdrawal F15.93
    harmful -*see* Abuse, drug, stimulant NEC
  tobacco Z72.0

Use (of) --*continued*
    with dependence -*see* Dependence, drug,
    nicotine
  volatile solvents -*see also* Use, inhalant
  F18.90
    harmful -*see* Abuse, drug, inhalant
Usher-Senear disease or syndrome L10.4
Uta B55.1
Uteromegaly N85.2
Uterovaginal -*see* condition
Uterovesical -*see* condition
Uveal -*see* condition
Uveitis (anterior) -*see also* Iridocyclitis
  acute -*see* Iridocyclitis, acute
  chronic -*see* Iridocyclitis, chronic
  due to toxoplasmosis (acquired) B58.09
    congenital P37.1
  granulomatous -*see* Iridocyclitis, chronic
  heterochromic -*see* Cyclitis, Fuchs'
    heterochromic
  lens-induced -*see* Iridocyclitis, lens-induced
  posterior -*see* Chorioretinitis
  sympathetic H44.13
  syphilitic (secondary) A51.43
    congenital (early) A50.01
    late A52.71
  tuberculous A18.54
Uveoencephalitis -*see* Inflammation,
  chorioretinal
Uveokeratitis -*see* Iridocyclitis
Uveoparotitis D86.89
Uvula -*see* condition
**Uvulitis (acute) (catarrhal) (chronic)
(membranous) (suppurative) (ulcerative)**
K12.2

V

Vaccination (prophylactic)
  complication or reaction -*see* Complications,
    vaccination
  delayed Z28.9
  encounter for Z23
  not done -*see* Immunization, not done,
    because (of)
Vaccinia (generalized) (localized) T88.1
  congenital P35.8
  without vaccination B08.011
Vacuum, in sinus (accessory) (nasal) J34.89
Vagabond, vagabondage Z59.0
Vagabond's disease B85.1
Vagina, vaginal -*see* condition
Vaginalitis (tunica) (testis) N49.1
Vaginismus (reflex) N94.2
  functional F52.5
  nonorganic F52.5
  psychogenic F52.5
  secondary N94.2
**Vaginitis (acute) (circumscribed) (diffuse)
(emphysematous) (nonvenereal)
(ulcerative)** N76.0
  with ectopic or molar pregnancy O08.0
  amebic A06.82
  atrophic, postmenopausal N95.2
  bacterial N76.0
  blennorrhagic (gonococcal) A54.02
  candidal B37.3
  chlamydial A56.02
  chronic N76.1
  due to Trichomonas (vaginalis) A59.01
  following ectopic or molar pregnancy O08.0

Vaginitis - *continued*
  gonococcal A54.02
    with abscess (accessory gland) (periurethral)
    A54.1
  granuloma A58
  in (due to)
    candidiasis B37.3
    herpesviral (herpes simplex) infection
    A60.04
    pinworm infection B80 [*N77.1*]
  monilial B37.3
  mycotic (candidal) B37.3
  postmenopausal atrophic N95.2
  puerperal (postpartum) O86.13
  senile (atrophic) N95.2
  subacute or chronic N76.1
  syphilitic (early) A51.0
    late A52.76
  trichomonal A59.01
  tuberculous A18.18
Vaginosis -*see* Vaginitis
Vagotonia G52.2
Vagrancy Z59.0
VAIN -*see* Neoplasia, intraepithelial, vagina
Vallecula -*see* condition
Valley fever B38.0
Valsuani's disease -*see* Anemia, obstetric
Valve, valvular (formation) -*see also*
  condition
  cerebral ventricle (communicating) in situ
    Z98.2
  cervix, internal os Q51.828
  congenital NEC -*see* Atresia, by site
  ureter (pelvic junction) (vesical orifice)
    Q62.39
  urethra (congenital) (posterior) Q64.2
Valvulitis (chronic) -*see* Endocarditis
Valvulopathy -*see* Endocarditis
**Van Bogaert's leukoencephalopathy
(sclerosing) (subacute)** A81.1
**Van Bogaert-Scherer-Epstein disease or
syndrome** E75.5
Van Buchem's syndrome M85.2
Van Creveld-von Gierke disease E74.01
Van der Hoeve (de Kleyn) syndrome Q78.0
Van der Woude's syndrome Q38.0
Van Neck's disease or osteochondrosis
  M91.0
Vanishing lung J44.9
Vapor asphyxia or suffocation T59.9
  specified agent -*see* Table of Drugs and
  Chemicals
Variance, lethal ball, prosthetic heart valve
  T82.09
Variants, thalassemic D56.8
Variations in hair color L67.1
Varicella B01.9
  with
    complications NEC B01.89
    encephalitis B01.11
    encephalomyelitis B01.11
    meningitis B01.0
    myelitis B01.12
    pneumonia B01.2
  congenital P35.8
Varices -*see* Varix
Varicocele (scrotum) (thrombosed) I86.1
  ovary I86.2
  perineum I86.3
  spermatic cord (ulcerated) I86.1

Varicose

aneurysm (ruptured) I77.0
dermatitis -*see* Varix, leg, with, inflammation
eczema -*see* Varix, leg, with, inflammation
phlebitis -*see* Varix, with, inflammation
tumor -*see* Varix
ulcer (lower limb, any part) -*see also* Varix,
  leg, with, ulcer
  anus -*see also* Hemorrhoids K64.8
  esophagus -*see* Varix, esophagus
  inflamed or infected -*see* Varix, leg, with
    ulcer, with inflammation
  nasal septum I86.8
  perineum I86.3
  scrotum I86.1
  specified site NEC I86.8
vein -*see* Varix
vessel -*see* Varix, leg

Varicosis, varicosities, varicosity -*see* Varix
Variola (major) (minor) B03
Varioloid B03
Varix (lower limb) (ruptured) I83.90
with
  edema I83.899
  inflammation I83.10
    with ulcer (venous) I83.209
  pain I83.819
  specified complication NEC I83.899
  stasis dermatitis I83.10
    with ulcer (venous) I83.209
  swelling I83.899
  ulcer I83.009
    with inflammation I83.209
aneurysmal I77.0
asymptomatic I83.9
bladder I86.2
broad ligament I86.2
complicating
  childbirth (lower extremity) O87.4
    anus or rectum O87.2
    genital (vagina, vulva or perineum) O87.8
  pregnancy (lower extremity) O22.0
    anus or rectum O22.4
    genital (vagina, vulva or perineum) O22.1
  puerperium (lower extremity) O87.4
    anus or rectum O87.2
    genital (vagina, vulva, perineum) O87.8
congenital (any site) Q27.8
esophagus (idiopathic) (primary) (ulcerated)
  I85.00
  bleeding I85.01
  congenital Q27.8
  in (due to)
    alcoholic liver disease I85.10
      bleeding I85.11
    cirrhosis of liver I85.10
      bleeding I85.11
    portal hypertension I85.10
      bleeding I85.11
    schistosomiasis I85.10
      bleeding I85.11
    toxic liver disease I85.10
      bleeding I85.11
  secondary I85.10
    bleeding I85.11
gastric I86.4
inflamed or infected I83.10
  ulcerated I83.209
labia (majora) I86.3
leg (asymptomatic) I83.90
  with

Varix - *continued*
edema I83.899
inflammation I83.10
  with ulcer -*see* Varix, leg, with, ulcer,
  with inflammation by site
pain I83.819
specified complication NEC I83.899
swelling I83.899
ulcer I83.009
  with inflammation I83.209
  ankle I83.003
    with inflammation I83.203
  calf I83.002
    with inflammation I83.202
  foot NEC I83.005
    with inflammation I83.205
  heel I83.004
    with inflammation I83.204
  lower leg NEC I83.008
    with inflammation I83.208
  midfoot I83.004
    with inflammation I83.204
  thigh I83.001
    with inflammation I83.201
bilateral (asymptomatic) I83.93
with
  edema I83.893
  pain I83.813
  specified complication NEC I83.893
  swelling I83.893
  ulcer I83.009
    with inflammation I83.209
left (asymptomatic) I83.92
with
  edema I83.892
  pain I83.812
  specified complication NEC I83.892
  swelling I83.892
  inflammation I83.12
    with ulcer -*see* Varix, leg, with, ulcer,
    with inflammation by site
  ulcer I83.029
    with inflammation I83.229
    ankle I83.023
      with inflammation I83.223
    calf I83.022
      with inflammation I83.222
    foot NEC I83.025
      with inflammation I83.225
    heel I83.024
      with inflammation I83.224
    lower leg NEC I83.028
      with inflammation I83.228
    midfoot I83.024
      with inflammation I83.224
    thigh I83.021
      with inflammation I83.221
right (asymptomatic) I83.91
with
  edema I83.891
  pain I83.811
  specified complication NEC I83.891
  swelling I83.891
  inflammation I83.11
    with ulcer -*see* Varix, leg, with, ulcer,
    with inflammation by site
  ulcer I83.019
    with inflammation I83.219
    ankle I83.013
      with inflammation I83.213
    calf I83.012

Varix - *continued*
    with inflammation I83.212
    foot NEC I83.015
      with inflammation I83.215
    heel I83.014
      with inflammation I83.214
    lower leg NEC I83.018
      with inflammation I83.218
    midfoot I83.014
      with inflammation I83.214
    thigh I83.011
      with inflammation I83.211
nasal septum I86.8
orbit I86.8
  congenital Q27.8
ovary I86.2
papillary I78.1
pelvis I86.2
perineum I86.3
pharynx I86.8
placenta O43.89
renal papilla I86.8
retina H35.09
scrotum (ulcerated) I86.1
sigmoid colon I86.8
specified site NEC I86.8
spinal (cord) (vessels) I86.8
spleen, splenic (vein) (with phlebolith) I86.8
stomach I86.4
sublingual I86.0
ulcerated I83.009
  inflamed or infected I83.209
uterine ligament I86.2
vagina I86.8
vocal cord I86.8
vulva I86.3
Vas deferens -*see* condition
Vas deferentitis N49.1
Vasa previa O69.4
hemorrhage from, affecting newborn P50.0
Vascular -*see also* condition
loop on optic papilla Q14.2
spasm I73.9
spider I78.1
Vascularization, cornea -*see*
Neovascularization, cornea
Vasculitis I77.6
allergic D69.0
cryoglobulinemic D89.1
disseminated I77.6
hypocomplementemic M31.8
kidney I77.89
livedoid L95.0
nodular L95.8
retina H35.06
rheumatic -*see* Fever, rheumatic
rheumatoid -*see* Rheumatoid, vasculitis
skin (limited to) L95.9
  specified NEC L95.8
Vasculopathy, necrotizing M31.9
cardiac allograft T86.290
specified NEC M31.8
Vasitis (nodosa) N49.1
tuberculous A18.15
Vasodilation I73.9
Vasomotor -*see* condition
Vasoplasty, after previous sterilization Z31.0
aftercare Z31.42
Vasospasm (vasoconstriction) I73.9
cerebral (cerebrovascular) (artery) I67.848
  reversible I67.841

Vasospasm - *continued*
coronary I20.1
nerve
  arm -*see* Mononeuropathy, upper limb
  brachial plexus G54.0
  cervical plexus G54.2
  leg -*see* Mononeuropathy, lower limb
peripheral NOS I73.9
retina (artery) -*see* Occlusion, artery, retina
Vasospastic -*see* condition
Vasovagal attack (paroxysmal) R55
psychogenic F45.8
VATER syndrome Q87.2
Vater's ampulla -*see* condition
Vegetation, vegetative
adenoid (nasal fossa) J35.8
endocarditis (acute) (any valve) (subacute)
  I33.0
heart (mycotic) (valve) I33.0
Veil
Jackson's Q43.3
Vein, venous -*see* condition
Veldt sore -*see* Ulcer, skin
Velpeau's hernia -*see* Hernia, femoral
Venereal
bubo A55
disease A64
granuloma inguinale A58
lymphogranuloma (Durand-Nicolas-Favre)
  A55
Venofibrosis I87.8
Venom, venomous -*see* Table of Drugs and
Chemicals, by animal or substance, poisoning
Venous -*see* condition
Ventilator lung, newborn P27.8
Ventral -*see* condition
Ventricle, ventricular -*see also* condition
escape I49.3
inversion Q20.5
Ventriculitis (cerebral) -*see also* Encephalitis
G04.90
Ventriculostomy status Z98.2
Vernet's syndrome G52.7
Verneuil's disease (syphilitic bursitis) A52.78
Verruca (due to HPV) (filiformis) (simplex)
(viral) (vulgaris) B07.9
acuminata A63.0
necrogenica (primary) (tuberculosa) A18.4
plana B07.8
plantaris B07.0
seborrheica L82.1
  inflamed L82.0
senile (seborrheic) L82.1
  inflamed L82.0
tuberculosa (primary) A18.4
venereal A63.0
Verrucosities -*see* Verruca
Verruga peruana, peruviana A44.1
Version
with extraction
cervix -*see* Malposition, uterus
uterus (postinfectional) (postpartal, old) -*see*
  Malposition, uterus
Vertebra, vertebral -*see* condition
Vertical talus (congenital) Q66.80
left foot Q66.82
right foot Q66.81
Vertigo R42
auditory -*see* Vertigo, aural
aural H81.31
benign paroxysmal (positional) H81.1

Vertigo - *continued*
central (origin) H81.4
cerebral H81.4
Dix and Hallpike (epidemic) -*see* Neuronitis,
  vestibular
due to infrasound T75.23
epidemic A88.1
  Dix and Hallpike -*see* Neuronitis, vestibular
  Pedersen's -*see* Neuronitis, vestibular
  vestibular neuronitis -*see* Neuronitis,
    vestibular
hysterical F44.89
infrasound T75.23
labyrinthine - see subcategory H81.0
laryngeal R05
malignant positional H81.4
Ménière's -*see* subcategory H81.0
menopausal N95.1
otogenic -*see* Vertigo, aural
paroxysmal positional, benign -*see* Vertigo,
  benign paroxysmal
Pedersen's (epidemic) -*see* Neuronitis,
  vestibular
peripheral NEC H81.39
positional
  benign paroxysmal -*see* Vertigo, benign
  paroxysmal
  malignant H81.4
Very low-density lipoprotein-type (VLDL)
hyperlipoproteinemia E78.1
Vesania -*see* Psychosis
Vesical -*see* condition
Vesicle
cutaneous R23.8
seminal -*see* condition
skin R23.8
Vesicocolic -*see* condition
Vesicoperineal -*see* condition
Vesicorectal -*see* condition
Vesicourethrorectal -*see* condition
Vesicovaginal -*see* condition
Vesicular -*see* condition
Vesiculitis (seminal) N49.0
amebic A06.82
gonorrheal (acute) (chronic) A54.23
trichomonal A59.09
tuberculous A18.15
Vestibulitis (ear) -*see also* subcategory H83.0
nose (external) J34.89
vulvar N94.810
Vestibulopathy , acute peripheral
(recurrent) -*see* Neuronitis, vestibular
Vestige, vestigial -*see also* Persistence
branchial Q18.0
structures in vitreous Q14.0
Vibration
adverse effects T75.20
  pneumatic hammer syndrome T75.21
  specified effect NEC T75.29
  vasospastic syndrome T75.22
  vertigo from infrasound T75.23
exposure (occupational) Z57.7
vertigo T75.23
Vibriosis A28.9
Victim (of)
crime Z65.4
disaster Z65.5
terrorism Z65.4
torture Z65.4
war Z65.5
Vidal's disease L28.0

Villaret's syndrome G52.7
Villous -*see* condition
VIN -*see* Neoplasia, intraepithelial, vulva
Vincent's infection (angina) (gingivitis)
A69.1
stomatitis NEC A69.1
Vinson-Plummer syndrome D50.1
Violence, physical R45.6
Viosterol deficiency -*see* Deficiency, calciferol
Vipoma -*see* Neoplasm, malignant, by site
Viremia B34.9
Virilism (adrenal) E25.9
congenital E25.0
Virilization (female) (suprarenal) E25.9
congenital E25.0
isosexual E28.2
Virulent bubo A57
Virus, viral -*see also* condition
as cause of disease classified elsewhere
  B97.89
cytomegalovirus B25.9
human immunodeficiency (HIV) -*see* Human,
  immunodeficiency virus (HIV) disease
infection -*see* Infection, virus
specified NEC B34.8
swine influenza (viruses that normally cause
  infections in pigs) -*see also* Influenza, due
  to, identified novel influenza A virus J09.X2
West Nile (fever) A92.30
  with
    complications NEC A92.39
    cranial nerve disorders A92.32
    encephalitis A92.31
    encephalomyelitis A92.31
    neurologic manifestation NEC A92.32
    optic neuritis A92.32
    polyradiculitis A92.32
Viscera, visceral -*see* condition
Visceroptosis K63.4
Visible peristalsis R19.2
Vision, visual
binocular, suppression H53.34
blurred, blurring H53.8
  hysterical F44.6
defect, defective NEC H54.7
disorientation (syndrome) H53.8
disturbance H53.9
  hysterical F44.6
double H53.2
examination Z01.00
  with abnormal findings Z01.01
field, limitation (defect) -*see* Defect, visual
  field
hallucinations R44.1
halos H53.19
loss -*see* Loss, vision
  sudden -*see* Disturbance, vision, subjective,
    loss, sudden
low (both eyes) -*see* Low, vision
perception, simultaneous without fusion
  H53.33
Vitality, lack or want of R53.83
newborn P96.89
Vitamin deficiency -*see* Deficiency, vitamin
Vitelline duct, persistent Q43.0
Vitiligo L80
eyelid H02.739
  left H02.736
    lower H02.735
    upper H02.734
  right H02.733

Vitiligo - *continued*
    lower H02.732
    upper H02.731
  pinta A67.2
  vulva N90.89
Vitreal corneal syndrome H59.01
Vitreoretinopathy, proliferative *-see also*
  Retinopathy, proliferative
  with retinal detachment *-see* Detachment,
    retina, traction
Vitreous *-see also* condition
  touch syndrome *-see* Complication,
    postprocedural, following cataract surgery
Vocal cord *-see* condition
Vogt-Koyanagi syndrome H20.82
Vogt's disease or syndrome G80.3
Vogt-Spielmeyer amaurotic idiocy or disease
  E75.4
Voice
  change R49.9
    specified NEC R49.8
  loss *-see* Aphonia
Volhynian fever A79.0
Volkmann's ischemic contracture or
  paralysis (complicating trauma) T79.6
Volvulus (bowel) (colon) (intestine) K56.2
  with perforation K56.2
  congenital Q43.8
  duodenum K31.5
  fallopian tube *-see* Torsion, fallopian tube
  oviduct *-see* Torsion, fallopian tube
  stomach (due to absence of gastrocolic
    ligament) K31.89
Vomiting R11.10
  with nausea R11.2
  asphyxia *-see* Foreign body, by site, causing
    asphyxia, gastric contents
  bilious (cause unknown) R11.14
    in newborn P92.01
    following gastro-intestinal surgery K91.0
  blood *-see* Hematemesis
  causing asphyxia, choking, or suffocation *-see*
    Foreign body, by site
  cyclical G43.A0
    with refractory migraine G43.A1
    intractable G43.A1
    not intractable G43.A0
    psychogenic F50.89
    without refractory migraine G43.A0
  fecal mater R11.13
  following gastrointestinal surgery K91.0
    psychogenic F50.89
  functional K31.89
  hysterical F50.89
  nervous F50.89
  neurotic F50.89
  newborn NEC P92.09
    bilious P92.01
  periodic R11.10
    psychogenic F50.89
  projectile R11.12
  psychogenic F50.89
  uremic *-see* Uremia
  without nausea R11.11
Vomito negro *-see* Fever, yellow
Von Bezold's abscess *-see* Mastoiditis, acute
Von Economo-Cruchet disease A85.8
Von Eulenburg's disease G71.19
Von Gierke's disease E74.01
Von Hippel (Lindau) disease or syndrome
  Q85.8

Von Jaksch's anemia or disease D64.89
Von Recklinghausen
  disease (neurofibromatosis) Q85.01
    bones E21.0
Von Schroetter's syndrome I82.890
Von Willebrand (Jurgens)(Minot) disease
  or syndrome D68.0
Von Zumbusch's disease L40.1
Voyeurism F65.3
Vrolik's disease Q78.0
Vulva *-see* condition
Vulvismus N94.2
Vulvitis (acute) (allergic) (atrophic)
  (hypertrophic) (intertriginous) (senile)
  N76.2
  with ectopic or molar pregnancy O08.0
  adhesive, congenital Q52.79
  blennorrhagic (gonococcal) A54.02
  candidal B37.3
  chlamydial A56.02
  due to Haemophilus ducreyi A57
  following ectopic or molar pregnancy O08.0
  gonococcal A54.02
    with abscess (accessory gland) (periurethral)
    A54.1
  herpesviral A60.04
  leukoplakic N90.4
  monilial B37.3
  puerperal (postpartum) O86.19
  subacute or chronic N76.3
  syphilitic (early) A51.0
    late A52.76
  trichomonal A59.01
  tuberculous A18.18
Vulvodynia N94.819
  specified NEC N94.818
Vulvorectal *-see* condition
Vulvovaginitis (acute) *-see* Vaginitis

W

Waiting list, person on Z75.1
  for organ transplant Z76.82
  undergoing social agency investigation Z75.2
Waldenström-Kjellberg syndrome D50.1
Waldenström
  hypergammaglobulinemia D89.0
  syndrome or macroglobulinemia C88.0
Walking
  difficulty R26.2
    psychogenic F44.4
  sleep F51.3
    hysterical F44.89
Wall, abdominal *-see* condition
Wallenberg's disease or syndrome G46.3
Wallgren's disease I87.8
Wandering
  gallbladder, congenital Q44.1
  in diseases classified elsewhere Z91.83
  kidney, congenital Q63.8
  organ or site, congenital NEC *-see*
    Malposition, congenital, by site
  pacemaker (heart) I49.8
  spleen D73.89
War neurosis F48.8
Wart (due to HPV) (filiform) (infectious)
  (viral) B07.9
  anogenital region (venereal) A63.0
  common B07.8
  external genital organs (venereal) A63.0
  flat B07.8

Wart *--continued*
  Hassal-Henle's (of cornea) H18.49
  Peruvian A44.1
  plantar B07.0
  prosector (tuberculous) A18.4
  seborrheic L82.1
    inflamed L82.0
  senile (seborrheic) L82.1
    inflamed L82.0
  tuberculous A18.4
  venereal A63.0
Warthin's tumor *-see* Neoplasm, salivary
  gland, benign
Wassilieff's disease A27.0
Wasting
  disease R64
    due to malnutrition E41
  extreme (due to malnutrition) E41
  muscle NEC *-see* Atrophy, muscle
Water
  clefts (senile cataract) *-see* Cataract, senile,
    incipient
  deprivation of T73.1
  intoxication E87.79
  itch B76.9
  lack of T73.1
  loading E87.70
  on
    brain *-see* Hydrocephalus
    chest J94.8
  poisoning E87.79
Waterbrash R12
Waterhouse (Friderichsen) syndrome or
  disease (meningococcal) A39.1
Water-losing nephritis N25.89
Watermelon stomach K31.819
  with hemorrhage K31.811
  without hemorrhage K31.819
Watsoniasis B66.8
Wax in ear *-see* Impaction, cerumen
Weak, weakening, weakness (generalized)
  R53.1
  arches (acquired) *-see also* Deformity, limb,
    flat foot
  bladder (sphincter) R32
  facial R29.810
    following
      cerebrovascular disease I69.992
        cerebral infarction I69.392
        intracerebral hemorrhage I69.192
        nontraumatic intracranial hemorrhage
          NEC I69.292
        specified disease NEC I69.892
        stroke I69.392
        subarachnoid hemorrhage I69.092
  foot (double) *-see* Weak, arches
  heart, cardiac *-see* Failure, heart
  mind F70
  muscle M62.81
  myocardium *-see* Failure, heart
  newborn P96.89
  pelvic fundus N81.89
  pubocervical tissue N81.82
  senile R54
  rectovaginal tissue N81.83
  urinary stream R39.12
  valvular *-see* Endocarditis
Wear, worn (with normal or routine use)
  articular bearing surface of internal joint
    prosthesis *-see* Complications, joint
    prosthesis, mechanical, wear of articular
    bearing surfaces, by site

Wear, worn - *continued*
  device, implant or graft -*see* Complications,
    by site, mechanical complication
  tooth, teeth (approximal) (hard tissues)
    (interproximal) (occlusal) K03.0
Weather, weathered
  effects of
    cold T69.9
      specified effect NEC T69.8
    hot -*see* Heat
  skin L57.8
Weaver's syndrome Q87.3
Web, webbed (congenital)
  duodenal Q43.8
  esophagus Q39.4
  fingers Q70.1
  larynx (glottic) (subglottic) Q31.0
  neck (pterygium colli) Q18.3
  Paterson-Kelly D50.1
  popliteal syndrome Q87.89
  toes Q70.3
Weber-Christian disease M35.6
Weber-Cockayne syndrome (epidermolysis bullosa) Q81.8
Weber-Gubler syndrome G46.3
Weber-Leyden syndrome G46.3
Weber-Osler syndrome I78.0
Weber's paralysis or syndrome G46.3
Wedge-shaped or wedging vertebra -*see* Collapse, vertebra NEC
Wegener's granulomatosis or syndrome M31.30
  with
    kidney involvement M31.31
    lung involvement M31.30
      with kidney involvement M31.31
Wegner's disease A50.02
Weight
  1000 2499 grams at birth (low) -*see* Low, birthweight
  999 grams or less at birth (extremely low) - *see* Low, birthweight, extreme
  and length below 10th percentile for gestational age P05.1
  below but length above 10th percentile for gestational age P05.0
  gain (abnormal) (excessive) R63.5
    in pregnancy -*see* Pregnancy, complicated by, excessive weight gain
    low -*see* Pregnancy, complicated by, insufficient, weight gain
  loss (abnormal) (cause unknown) R63.4
Weightlessness (effect of) T75.82
Weil (l) Marchesani syndrome Q87.1
Weil's disease A27.0
Weingarten's syndrome J82
Weir Mitchell's disease I73.81
Weiss-Baker syndrome G90.09
Wells' disease L98.3
Wen -*see* Cyst, sebaceous
Wenckebach's block or phenomenon I44.1
Werdnig-Hoffmann syndrome (muscular atrophy) G12.0
Werlhof's disease D69.3
Wermer's disease or syndrome E31.21
Werner-His disease A79.0
Werner's disease or syndrome E34.8
Wernicke-Korsakoff's syndrome or psychosis (alcoholic) F10.96
  with dependence F10.26
  drug-induced

Wernicke-Korsakoff's syndrome --*continued*
  due to drug abuse -*see* Abuse, drug, by type, with amnestic disorder
  due to drug dependence -*see* Dependence, drug, by type, with amnestic disorder
  nonalcoholic F04
Wernicke-Posadas disease B38.9
Wernicke's
  developmental aphasia F80.2
  disease or syndrome E51.2
  encephalopathy E51.2
  polioencephalitis, superior E51.2
West African fever B50.8
Westphal-Strümpell syndrome E83.01
West's syndrome -*see* Epilepsy, spasms
Wet
  feet, tropical (maceration) (syndrome) -*see* Immersion, foot
  lung (syndrome), newborn P22.1
Wharton's duct -*see* condition
Wheal -*see* Urticaria
Wheezing R06.2
Whiplash injury S13.4
Whipple's disease -*see also* subcategory M14.8 K90.81
Whipworm (disease) (infection) (infestation) B79
Whistling face Q87.0
White -*see also* condition
  kidney, small N03.9
  leg, puerperal, postpartum, childbirth O87.1
  mouth B37.0
  patches of mouth K13.29
  spot lesions, teeth
    chewing surface K02.51
    pit and fissure surface K02.51
    smooth surface K02.61
Whitehead L70.0
Whitlow -*see also* Cellulitis, digit
  with lymphangitis -*see* Lymphangitis, acute, digit
  herpesviral B00.89
Whitmore's disease or fever -*see* Melioidosis
Whooping cough A37.90
  with pneumonia A37.91
  due to Bordetella
    bronchiseptica A37.81
    parapertussis A37.11
    pertussis A37.01
    specified organism NEC A37.81
  due to
    Bordetella
      bronchiseptica A37.80
        with pneumonia A37.81
      parapertussis A37.10
        with pneumonia A37.11
      pertussis A37.00
        with pneumonia A37.01
      specified NEC A37.80
        with pneumonia A37.81
Wichman's asthma J38.5
Wide cranial sutures, newborn P96.3
Widening aorta -*see* Ectasia, aorta
  with aneurysm -*see* Aneurysm, aorta
Wilkie's disease or syndrome K55.1
Wilkinson-Sneddon disease or syndrome L13.1
Willebrand (Jürgens) thrombopathy D68.0
Willige-Hunt disease or syndrome G23.1
Wilms' tumor C64
Wilson-Mikity syndrome P27.0

Wilson's
  disease or syndrome E83.01
  hepatolenticular degeneration E83.01
  lichen ruber L43.9
Window -*see also* Imperfect, closure
  aorticopulmonary Q21.4
Winter -*see* condition
Wiskott-Aldrich syndrome D82.0
Withdrawal state -*see also* Dependence, drug
  by type, with withdrawal
  alcohol
    with perceptual disturbances F10.232
    without perceptual disturbances F10.239
  caffeine F15.93
  cannabis F12.288
  newborn
    correct therapeutic substance properly administered P96.2
    infant of dependent mother P96.1
  therapeutic substance, neonatal P96.2
Witts' anemia D50.8
Witzelsucht F07.0
Woakes' ethmoiditis or syndrome J33.1
Wolff-Hirschorn syndrome Q93.3
Wolff-Parkinson-White syndrome I45.6
Wolhynian fever A79.0
Wolman's disease E75.5
Wood lung or pneumonitis J67.8
Woolly, wooly hair (congenital) (nevus) Q84.1
Woolsorter's disease A22.1
Word
  blindness (congenital) (developmental) F81.0
  deafness (congenital) (developmental) H93.25
Worm(s) (infection) (infestation) -*see also* Infestation, helminth
  guinea B72
  in intestine NEC B82.0
Worm-eaten soles A66.3
Worn out -*see* Exhaustion
  cardiac
    defibrillator (with synchronous cardiac pacemaker) Z45.02
    pacemaker
      battery Z45.010
      lead Z45.018
  device, implant or graft -*see* Complications, by site, mechanical
Worried well Z71.1
Worries R45.82
Wound, open
  abdomen, abdominal
    wall S31.109
      with penetration into peritoneal cavity S31.609
      bite -*see* Bite, abdomen, wall
      epigastric region S31.102
        with penetration into peritoneal cavity S31.602
        bite -*see* Bite, abdomen, wall, epigastric region
        laceration -*see* Laceration, abdomen, wall, epigastric region
        puncture -*see* Puncture, abdomen, wall, epigastric region
      laceration -*see* Laceration, abdomen, wall
    left
      lower quadrant S31.104
        with penetration into peritoneal cavity S31.604

WXYZ

Wound, open - *continued*

bite -*see* Bite, abdomen, wall, left, lower quadrant
laceration -*see* Laceration, abdomen, wall, left, lower quadrant
puncture -*see* Puncture, abdomen, wall, left, lower quadrant
upper quadrant S31.101
with penetration into peritoneal cavity S31.601
bite -*see* Bite, abdomen, wall, left, upper quadrant
laceration -*see* Laceration, abdomen, wall, left, upper quadrant
puncture -*see* Puncture, abdomen, wall, left, upper quadrant
periumbilic region S31.105
with penetration into peritoneal cavity S31.605
bite -*see* Bite, abdomen, wall, periumbilic region
laceration -*see* Laceration, abdomen, wall, periumbilic region
puncture -*see* Puncture, abdomen, wall, periumbilic region
puncture -*see* Puncture, abdomen, wall
right
lower quadrant S31.103
with penetration into peritoneal cavity S31.603
bite -*see* Bite, abdomen, wall, right, lower quadrant
laceration -*see* Laceration, abdomen, wall, right, lower quadrant
puncture -*see* Puncture, abdomen, wall, right, lower quadrant
upper quadrant S31.100
with penetration into peritoneal cavity S31.600
bite -*see* Bite, abdomen, wall, right, upper quadrant
laceration -*see* Laceration, abdomen, wall, right, upper quadrant
puncture -*see* Puncture, abdomen, wall, right, upper quadrant
alveolar (process) -*see* Wound, open, oral cavity
ankle S91.00
bite -*see* Bite, ankle
laceration -*see* Laceration, ankle
puncture -*see* Puncture, ankle
antecubital space -*see* Wound, open, elbow
anterior chamber, eye -*see* Wound, open, ocular
anus S31.839
bite S31.835
laceration -*see* Laceration, anus
puncture -*see* Puncture, anus
arm (upper) S41.10
with amputation -*see* Amputation, traumatic, arm
bite -*see* Bite, arm
forearm -*see* Wound, open, forearm
laceration -*see* Laceration, arm
puncture -*see* Puncture, arm
auditory canal (external) (meatus) -*see* Wound, open, ear
auricle, ear -*see* Wound, open, ear
axilla -*see* Wound, open, arm
back -*see also* Wound, open, thorax, back
lower S31.000

Wound, open - *continued*

with penetration into retroperitoneal space S31.001
bite -*see* Bite, back, lower
laceration -*see* Laceration, back, lower
puncture -*see* Puncture, back, lower
bite -*see* Bite
blood vessel -*see* Injury, blood vessel
breast S21.00
with amputation -*see* Amputation, traumatic, breast
bite -*see* Bite, breast
laceration -*see* Laceration, breast
puncture -*see* Puncture, breast
buttock S31.809
bite -*see* Bite, buttock
laceration -*see* Laceration, buttock
left S31.829
puncture -*see* Puncture, buttock
right S31.819
calf -*see* Wound, open, leg
canaliculus lacrimalis -*see* Wound, open, eyelid
canthus, eye -*see* Wound, open, eyelid
cervical esophagus S11.20
bite S11.25
laceration -*see* Laceration, esophagus, traumatic, cervical
puncture -*see* Puncture, cervical esophagus
cheek (external) S01.40
bite -*see* Bite, cheek
laceration -*see* Laceration, cheek
puncture -*see* Puncture, cheek
internal -*see* Wound, open, oral cavity
chest wall -*see* Wound, open, thorax
chin -*see* Wound, open, head, specified site NEC
choroid -*see* Wound, open, ocular
ciliary body (eye) -*see* Wound, open, ocular
clitoris S31.40
with amputation -*see* Amputation, traumatic, clitoris
bite S31.45
laceration -*see* Laceration, vulva
puncture -*see* Puncture, vulva
conjunctiva -*see* Wound, open, ocular
cornea -*see* Wound, open, ocular
costal region -*see* Wound, open, thorax
Descemet's membrane -*see* Wound, open, ocular
digit(s)
foot -*see* Wound, open, toe
hand -*see* Wound, open, finger
ear (canal) (external) S01.30
with amputation -*see* Amputation, traumatic, ear
bite -*see* Bite, ear
laceration -*see* Laceration, ear
puncture -*see* Puncture, ear
drum S09.2
elbow S51.00
bite -*see* Bite, elbow
laceration -*see* Laceration, elbow
puncture -*see* Puncture, elbow
epididymis -*see* Wound, open, testis
epigastric region S31.102
with penetration into peritoneal cavity S31.602
bite -*see* Bite, abdomen, wall, epigastric region

Wound, open - *continued*

laceration -*see* Laceration, abdomen, wall, epigastric region
puncture -*see* Puncture, abdomen, wall, epigastric region
epiglottis -*see* Wound, open, neck, specified site NEC
esophagus (thoracic) S27.819
cervical -*see* Wound, open, cervical esophagus
laceration S27.813
specified type NEC S27.818
eye -*see* Wound, open, ocular
eyeball -*see* Wound, open, ocular
eyebrow -*see* Wound, open, eyelid
eyelid S01.10
bite -*see* Bite, eyelid
laceration -*see* Laceration, eyelid
puncture -*see* Puncture, eyelid
face NEC -*see* Wound, open, head, specified site NEC
finger(s) S61.209
with
amputation -*see* Amputation, traumatic, finger
damage to nail S61.309
bite -*see* Bite, finger
index S61.208
with
damage to nail S61.308
left S61.201
with
damage to nail S61.301
right S61.200
with
damage to nail S61.300
laceration -*see* Laceration, finger
little S61.208
with
damage to nail S61.308
left S61.207
with damage to nail S61.307
right S61.206
with damage to nail S61.306
middle S61.208
with
damage to nail S61.308
left S61.203
with damage to nail S61.303
right S61.202
with damage to nail S61.302
puncture -*see* Puncture, finger
ring S61.208
with
damage to nail S61.308
left S61.205
with damage to nail S61.305
right S61.204
with damage to nail S61.304
flank -*see* Wound, open, abdomen, wall
foot (except toe(s) alone) S91.30
with amputation -*see* Amputation, traumatic, foot
bite -*see* Bite, foot
laceration -*see* Laceration, foot
puncture -*see* Puncture, foot
toe -*see* Wound, open, toe
forearm S51.80
with
amputation -*see* Amputation, traumatic, forearm

Wound, open - *continued*

bite -*see* Bite, forearm
elbow only -*see* Wound, open, elbow
laceration -*see* Laceration, forearm
puncture -*see* Puncture, forearm
forehead -*see* Wound, open, head, specified
  site NEC
genital organs, external
  with amputation -*see* Amputation, traumatic,
    genital organs
  bite -*see* Bite, genital organ
  female S31.502
    vagina S31.40
    vulva S31.40
  laceration -*see* Laceration, genital organ
  male S31.501
    penis S31.20
    scrotum S31.30
    testes S31.30
  puncture -*see* Puncture, genital organ
globe (eye) -*see* Wound, open, ocular
groin -*see* Wound, open, abdomen, wall
gum -*see* Wound, open, oral cavity
hand S61.40
  with
    amputation -*see* Amputation, traumatic,
      hand
  bite -*see* Bite, hand
  finger(s) -*see* Wound, open, finger
  laceration -*see* Laceration, hand
  puncture -*see* Puncture, hand
  thumb -*see* Wound, open, thumb
head S01.90
  bite -*see* Bite, head
  cheek -*see* Wound, open, cheek
  ear -*see* Wound, open, ear
  eyelid -*see* Wound, open, eyelid
  laceration -*see* Laceration, head
  lip -*see* Wound, open, lip
  nose S01.20
  oral cavity -*see* Wound, open, oral cavity
  puncture -*see* Puncture, head
  scalp -*see* Wound, open, scalp
  specified site NEC S01.80
  temporomandibular area -*see* Wound, open,
    cheek
heel -*see* Wound, open, foot
hip S71.00
  with amputation -*see* Amputation, traumatic,
    hip
  bite -*see* Bite, hip
  laceration -*see* Laceration, hip
  puncture -*see* Puncture, hip
hymen S31.40
  bite -*see* Bite, vulva
  laceration -*see* Laceration, vagina
  puncture -*see* Puncture, vagina
hypochondrium S31.109
  bite -*see* Bite, hypochondrium
  laceration -*see* Laceration, hypochondrium
  puncture -*see* Puncture, hypochondrium
hypogastric region S31.109
  bite -*see* Bite, hypogastric region
  laceration -*see* Laceration, hypogastric
  region
  puncture -*see* Puncture, hypogastric region
iliac (region) -*see* Wound, open, inguinal
  region
inguinal region S31.109
  bite -*see* Bite, abdomen, wall, lower
    quadrant

Wound, open - *continued*

  laceration -*see* Laceration, inguinal region
  puncture -*see* Puncture, inguinal region
instep -*see* Wound, open, foot
interscapular region -*see* Wound, open,
  thorax, back
intraocular -*see* Wound, open, ocular
iris -*see* Wound, open, ocular
jaw -*see* Wound, open, head, specified site
  NEC
knee S81.00
  bite -*see* Bite, knee
  laceration -*see* Laceration, knee
  puncture -*see* Puncture, knee
labium (majus) (minus) -*see* Wound, open,
  vulva
laceration -*see* Laceration, by site
lacrimal duct -*see* Wound, open, eyelid
larynx S11.019
  bite -*see* Bite, larynx
  laceration -*see* Laceration, larynx
  puncture -*see* Puncture, larynx
left
  lower quadrant S31.104
    with penetration into peritoneal cavity
      S31.604
    bite -*see* Bite, abdomen, wall, left, lower
      quadrant
    laceration -*see* Laceration, abdomen, wall,
      left, lower quadrant
    puncture -*see* Puncture, abdomen, wall,
      left, lower quadrant
  upper quadrant S31.101
    with penetration into peritoneal cavity
      S31.601
    bite -*see* Bite, abdomen, wall, left, upper
      quadrant
    laceration -*see* Laceration, abdomen, wall,
      left, upper quadrant
    puncture -*see* Puncture, abdomen, wall,
      left, upper quadrant
leg (lower) S81.80
  with amputation -*see* Amputation, traumatic,
    leg
  ankle -*see* Wound, open, ankle
  bite -*see* Bite, leg
  foot -*see* Wound, open, foot
  knee -*see* Wound, open, knee
  laceration -*see* Laceration, leg
  puncture -*see* Puncture, leg
  toe -*see* Wound, open, toe
  upper -*see* Wound, open, thigh
lip S01.501
  bite -*see* Bite, lip
  laceration -*see* Laceration, lip
  puncture -*see* Puncture, lip
loin S31.109
  bite -*see* Bite, abdomen, wall
  laceration -*see* Laceration, loin
  puncture -*see* Puncture, loin
lower back -*see* Wound, open, back, lower
lumbar region -*see* Wound, open, back, lower
malar region -*see* Wound, open, head,
  specified site NEC
mammary -*see* Wound, open, breast
mastoid region -*see* Wound, open, head,
  specified site NEC
mouth -*see* Wound, open, oral cavity
nail
  finger -*see* Wound, open, finger, with
    damage to nail

Wound, open - *continued*

  toe -*see* Wound, open, toe, with damage to
    nail
nape (neck) -*see* Wound, open, neck
nasal (septum) (sinus) -*see* Wound, open,
  nose
nasopharynx -*see* Wound, open, head,
  specified site NEC
neck S11.90
  bite -*see* Bite, neck
  involving
    cervical esophagus S11.20
    larynx -*see* Wound, open, larynx
    pharynx S11.20
    thyroid S11.10
    trachea (cervical) S11.029
      bite -*see* Bite, trachea
      laceration S11.021
        with foreign body S11.022
      puncture S11.023
        with foreign body S11.024
  laceration -*see* Laceration, neck
  puncture -*see* Puncture, neck
  specified site NEC S11.80
    specified type NEC S11.89
nose (septum) (sinus) S01.20
  with amputation -*see* Amputation, traumatic,
    nose
  bite -*see* Bite, nose
  laceration -*see* Laceration, nose
  puncture -*see* Puncture, nose
ocular S05.90
  avulsion (traumatic enucleation) S05.7
  eyeball S05.6
    with foreign body S05.5
  eyelid -*see* Wound, open, eyelid
  laceration and rupture S05.3
    with prolapse or loss of intraocular tissue
      S05.2
  orbit (penetrating) (with or without foreign
    body) S05.4
  periocular area -*see* Wound, open, eyelid
  specified NEC S05.8X   oral cavity S01.502
  bite S01.552
  laceration -*see* Laceration, oral cavity
  puncture -*see* Puncture, oral cavity
orbit -*see* Wound, open, ocular, orbit
palate -*see* Wound, open, oral cavity   palm -
  see Wound, open, hand
pelvis, pelvic -*see also* Wound, open, back,
  lower
  girdle -*see* Wound, open, hip
penetrating -*see* Puncture, by site
penis S31.20
  with amputation -*see* Amputation, traumatic,
    penis
  bite S31.25
  laceration -*see* Laceration, penis
  puncture -*see* Puncture, penis
perineum
  bite -*see* Bite, perineum
  female S31.502
  laceration -*see* Laceration, perineum
  male S31.501
  puncture -*see* Puncture, perineum
periocular area (with or without lacrimal
  passages) -*see* Wound, open, eyelid
periumbilic region S31.105
  with penetration into peritoneal cavity
    S31.605

Wound, open - *continued*
  bite -*see* Bite, abdomen, wall, periumbilic
    region
  laceration -*see* Laceration, abdomen, wall,
    periumbilic region
  puncture -*see* Puncture, abdomen, wall,
    periumbilic region
  phalanges
    finger -*see* Wound, open, finger
    toe -*see* Wound, open, toe
  pharynx S11.20
  pinna -*see* Wound, open, ear
  popliteal space -*see* Wound, open, knee
  prepuce -*see* Wound, open, penis
  pubic region -*see* Wound, open, back, lower
  pudendum -*see* Wound, open, genital organs,
    external
  puncture wound -*see* Puncture
  rectovaginal septum -*see* Wound, open,
    vagina
  right
    lower quadrant S31.103
      with penetration into peritoneal cavity
        S31.603
      bite -*see* Bite, abdomen, wall, right, lower
        quadrant
      laceration -*see* Laceration, abdomen, wall,
        right, lower quadrant
      puncture -*see* Puncture, abdomen, wall,
        right, lower quadrant
    upper quadrant S31.100
      with penetration into peritoneal cavity
        S31.600
      bite -*see* Bite, abdomen, wall, right, upper
        quadrant
      laceration -*see* Laceration, abdomen, wall,
        right, upper quadrant
      puncture -*see* Puncture, abdomen, wall,
        right, upper quadrant
  sacral region -*see* Wound, open, back, lower
  sacroiliac region -*see* Wound, open, back,
    lower
  salivary gland -*see* Wound, open, oral cavity
  scalp S01.00
    bite S01.05
    laceration -*see* Laceration, scalp
    puncture -*see* Puncture, scalp
  scalpel, newborn (birth injury) P15.8
  scapular region -*see* Wound, open, shoulder
  sclera -*see* Wound, open, ocular
  scrotum S31.30
    with amputation -*see* Amputation, traumatic,
      scrotum
    bite S31.35
    laceration -*see* Laceration, scrotum
    puncture -*see* Puncture, scrotum
  shin -*see* Wound, open, leg
  shoulder S41.00
    with amputation -*see* Amputation, traumatic,
      arm
    bite -*see* Bite, shoulder
    laceration -*see* Laceration, shoulder
    puncture -*see* Puncture, shoulder
  skin NOS T14.8
  spermatic cord -*see* Wound, open, testis
  sternal region -*see* Wound, open, thorax, front
    wall
  submaxillary region -*see* Wound, open, head,
    specified site NEC
  submental region -*see* Wound, open, head,
    specified site NEC

Wound, open - *continued*
  subungual
    finger(s) -*see* Wound, open, finger
    toe(s) -*see* Wound, open, toe
  supraclavicular region -*see* Wound, open,
    neck, specified site NEC
  temple, temporal region -*see* Wound, open,
    head, specified site NEC
  temporomandibular area -*see* Wound, open,
    cheek
  testis S31.30
    with amputation -*see* Amputation, traumatic,
      testes
    bite S31.35
    laceration -*see* Laceration, testis
    puncture -*see* Puncture, testis
  thigh S71.10
    with amputation -*see* Amputation, traumatic,
      hip
    bite -*see* Bite, thigh
    laceration -*see* Laceration, thigh
    puncture -*see* Puncture, thigh
  thorax, thoracic (wall) S21.90
    back S21.20
      with penetration S21.40
    bite -*see* Bite, thorax
    breast -*see* Wound, open, breast
    front S21.10
      with penetration S21.30
    laceration -*see* Laceration, thorax
    puncture -*see* Puncture, thorax
  throat -*see* Wound, open, neck
  thumb S61.009
    with
      amputation -*see* Amputation, traumatic,
        thumb
      damage to nail S61.109
    bite -*see* Bite, thumb
    laceration -*see* Laceration, thumb
    left S61.002
      with
        damage to nail S61.102
    puncture -*see* Puncture, thumb
    right S61.001
      with
        damage to nail S61.101
  thyroid (gland) -*see* Wound, open, neck,
    thyroid
  toe(s) S91.109
    with
      amputation -*see* Amputation, traumatic, toe
      damage to nail S91.209
    bite -*see* Bite, toe
    great S91.103
      with
      damage to nail S91.203
      left S91.102
        with
        damage to nail S91.202
      right S91.101
        with
        damage to nail S91.201
    laceration -*see* Laceration, toe
    lesser S91.106
      with
      damage to nail S91.206
      left S91.105
        with
        damage to nail S91.205
      right S91.104
        with

Wound, open - *continued*
    damage to nail S91.204
    puncture -*see* Puncture, toe
  tongue -*see* Wound, open, oral cavity
  trachea (cervical region) -*see* Wound, open,
    neck, trachea
  tunica vaginalis -*see* Wound, open, testis
  tympanum, tympanic membrane S09.2
    laceration -*see* Laceration, ear, drum
    puncture -*see* Puncture, tympanum
  umbilical region -*see* Wound, open, abdomen,
    wall, periumbilic region
  uvula -*see* Wound, open, oral cavity
  vagina S31.40
    bite S31.45
    laceration -*see* Laceration, vagina
    puncture -*see* Puncture, vagina
  vocal cord S11.039
    bite -*see* Bite, vocal cord
    laceration S11.031
      with foreign body S11.032
    puncture S11.033
      with foreign body S11.034
  vitreous (humor) -*see* Wound, open, ocular
  vulva S31.40
    with amputation -*see* Amputation, traumatic,
      vulva
    bite S31.45
    laceration -*see* Laceration, vulva
    puncture -*see* Puncture, vulva
  wrist S61.50
    bite -*see* Bite, wrist
    laceration -*see* Laceration, wrist
    puncture -*see* Puncture, wrist
Wound, superficial -*see* Injury -*see also*
  specified injury type
Wright's syndrome G54.0
Wrist -*see* condition
Wrong drug (by accident) (given in error) -
  see Table of Drugs and Chemicals, by drug,
  poisoning
Wry neck -*see* Torticollis
Wuchereria (bancrofti) infestation B74.0
Wuchereriasis B74.0
Wuchernde Struma Langhans C73

X

Xanthelasma (eyelid) (palpebrarum) H02.60
  left H02.66
    lower H02.65
    upper H02.64
  right H02.63
    lower H02.62
    upper H02.61
Xanthelasmatosis (essential) E78.2
Xanthinuria, hereditary E79.8
Xanthoastrocytoma
  specified site -*see* Neoplasm, malignant, by
    site
  unspecified site C71.9
Xanthofibroma -*see* Neoplasm, connective
  tissue, benign
Xanthogranuloma D76.3
Xanthoma(s), xanthomatosis (primary)
  (familial) (hereditary) E75.5
  with
    hyperlipoproteinemia
      Type I E78.3
      Type III E78.2
      Type IV E78.1

Xanthoma(s) --*continued*
Type V E78.3
bone (generalisata) C96.5
cerebrotendinous E75.5
cutaneotendinous E75.5
disseminatum (skin) E78.2
eruptive E78.2
hypercholesterinemic E78.00
hypercholesterolemic E78.00
hyperlipidemic E78.5
joint E75.5
multiple (skin) E78.2
tendon (sheath) E75.5
tubo-eruptive E78.2
tuberosum E78.2
tuberous E78.2
verrucous, oral mucosa K13.4
Xanthosis R23.8
Xenophobia F40.10
Xeroderma -*see also* Ichthyosis
acquired L85.0
eyelid H01.149
left H01.146
lower H01.145
upper H01.144
right H01.143
lower H01.142
upper H01.141
pigmentosum Q82.1
vitamin A deficiency E50.8
Xerophthalmia (vitamin A deficiency) E50.7
unrelated to vitamin A deficiency -*see*
Keratoconjunctivitis
Xerosis
conjunctiva H11.14
with Bitot's spots -*see also* Pigmentation,
conjunctiva
vitamin A deficiency E50.1
vitamin A deficiency E50.0
cornea H18.89
with ulceration -*see* Ulcer, cornea
vitamin A deficiency E50.3
vitamin A deficiency E50.2
cutis L85.3
skin L85.3
Xerostomia K11.7
Xiphopagus Q89.4
XO syndrome Q96.9
X ray (of)
abnormal findings -*see* Abnormal, diagnostic
imaging
breast (mammogram) (routine) Z12.31
chest
routine (as part of a general medical
examination) Z00.00
with abnormal findings Z00.01
routine (as part of a general medical
examination) Z00.00
with abnormal findings Z00.01
XXXXY syndrome Q98.1
XXY syndrome Q98.0

Y

Yaba pox (virus disease) B08.72
Yatapoxvirus B08.70
specified NEC B08.79
Yawning R06.89
psychogenic F45.8
Yaws A66.9
bone lesions A66.6

Yaws - *continued*
butter A66.1
chancre A66.0
cutaneous, less than five years after infection
A66.2
early (cutaneous) (macular) (maculopapular)
(micropapular) (papular) A66.2
frambeside A66.2
skin lesions NEC A66.2
eyelid A66.2
ganglion A66.6
gangosis, gangosa A66.5
gumma, gummata A66.4
bone A66.6
gummatous
frambeside A66.4
osteitis A66.6
periostitis A66.6
hydrarthrosis -*see also* subcategory M14.8
A66.6
hyperkeratosis (early) (late) A66.3
initial lesions A66.0
joint lesions -*see also* subcategory M14.8
A66.6
juxta-articular nodules A66.7
late nodular (ulcerated) A66.4
latent (without clinical manifestations) (with
positive serology) A66.8
mother A66.0
mucosal A66.7
multiple papillomata A66.1
nodular, late (ulcerated) A66.4
osteitis A66.6
papilloma, plantar or palmar A66.1
periostitis (hypertrophic) A66.6
specified NEC A66.7
ulcers A66.4
wet crab A66.1
Yeast infection -*see also* Candidiasis B37.9
Yellow
atrophy (liver) -*see* Failure, hepatic
fever -*see* Fever, yellow
jack -*see* Fever, yellow
jaundice -*see* Jaundice
nail syndrome L60.5
Yersiniosis -*see also* Infection, Yersinia
extraintestinal A28.2
intestinal A04.6

Z

Zahorsky's syndrome (herpangina) B08.5
Zellweger's syndrome Q87.89
Zenker's diverticulum (esophagus) K22.5
Ziehen-Oppenheim disease G24.1
Zieve's syndrome K70.0
Zika NOS A92.5
Zinc
deficiency, dietary E60
metabolism disorder E83.2
Zollinger-Ellison syndrome E16.4
Zona -*see* Herpes, zoster
Zoophobia F40.218
Zoster (herpes) -*see* Herpes, zoster
Zygomycosis B46.9
specified NEC B46.8
Zymotic -*see* condition

Neoplasm Table

The list below gives the code numbers for neoplasms by anatomical site. For each site there are six possible code numbers according to whether the neoplasm in question is malignant, benign, in situ, of uncertain behavior, or of unspecified nature. The description of the neoplasm will often indicate which of the six columns is appropriate; e.g., malignant melanoma of skin, benign fibroadenoma of breast, carcinoma in situ of cervix uteri.

Where such descriptors are not present, the remainder of the Index should be consulted where guidance is given to the appropriate column for each morphological (histological) variety listed; e.g., Mesonephroma -see Neoplasm, malignant; Embryoma -see also Neoplasm, uncertain behavior; Disease, Bowen's -see Neoplasm, skin, in situ. However, the guidance in the Index can be overridden if one of the descriptors mentioned above is present; e.g., malignant adenoma of colon is coded to C18.9 and not to D12.6 as the adjective 'malignant' overrides the Index entry 'Adenoma - see also Neoplasm, benign.'

Codes listed with a dash (-) following the code have a required additional character for laterality. The Tabular must be reviewed for the complete code.

	Malignant Primary	Malignant Secondary	Ca in Situ	Benign	Uncertain Behavior	Unspecified Behavior
Neoplasm, neoplastic	C80.1	C79.9	D09.9	D36.9	D48.9	D49.9
- abdomen, abdominal	C76.2	C79.8-	D09.8	D36.7	D48.7	D49.89
- - cavity	C76.2	C79.8-	D09.8	D36.7	D48.7	D49.89
- - organ	C76.2	C79.8-	D09.8	D36.7	D48.7	D49.89
- - viscera	C76.2	C79.8-	D09.8	D36.7	D48.7	D49.89
- - wall—*see also Neoplasm, abdomen, wall, skin*	C44.509	C79.2-	D04.5	D23.5	D48.5	D49.2
- - - connective tissue	C49.4	C79.8-	-	D21.4	D48.1	D49.2
- - - skin	C44.509					
- - - - basal cell carcinoma	C44.519	-	-	-	-	-
- - - - specified type NEC	C44.599	-	-	-	-	-
- - - - squamous cell carcinoma	C44.529	-	-	-	-	-
- abdominopelvic	C76.8	C79.8-		D36.7	D48.7	D49.89
- accessory sinus—*see Neoplasm, sinus*						
- acoustic nerve	C72.4-	C79.49	-	D33.3	D43.3	D49.7
- adenoid (pharynx) (tissue)	C11.1	C79.89	D00.08	D10.6	D37.05	D49.0
- adipose tissue—*see also Neoplasm, connective tissue*	C49.4	C79.89	-	D21.9	D48.1	D49.2
- adnexa (uterine)	C57.4	C79.89	D07.39	D28.7	D39.8	D49.59
- adrenal	C74.9-	C79.7-	D09.3	D35.0-	D44.1-	D49.7
- - capsule	C74.9-	C79.7-	D09.3	D35.0-	D44.1-	D49.7
- - cortex	C74.0-	C79.7-	D09.3	D35.0-	D44.1-	D49.7
- - gland	C74.9-	C79.7-	D09.3	D35.0-	D44.1-	D49.7
- - medulla	C74.1-	C79.7-	D09.3	D35.0-	D44.1-	D49.7
- ala nasi (external)—*see also Neoplasm, skin, nose*	C44.301	C79.2	D04.39	D23.39	D48.5	D49.2
- alimentary canal or tract NEC	C26.9	C78.80	D01.9	D13.9	D37.9	D49.0
- alveolar	C03.9	C79.89	D00.03	D10.39	D37.09	D49.0
- - mucosa	C03.9	C79.89	D00.03	D10.39	D37.09	D49.0
- - - lower	C03.1	C79.89	D00.03	D10.39	D37.09	D49.0
- - - upper	C03.0	C79.89	D00.03	D10.39	D37.09	D49.0
- - ridge or process	C41.1	C79.51	-	D16.5-	D48.0	D49.2
- - - carcinoma	C03.9	C79.8-	-	-	-	-
- - - - lower	C03.1	C79.8-	-	-	-	-
- - - - upper	C03.0	C79.8-	-	-	-	-
- - - lower	C41.1	C79.51	-	D16.5-	D48.0	D49.2
- - - mucosa	C03.9	C79.89	D00.03	D10.39	D37.09	D49.0
- - - - lower	C03.1	C79.89	D00.03	D10.39	D37.09	D49.0
- - - - upper	C03.0	C79.89	D00.03	D10.39	D37.09	D49.0
- - - upper	C41.0	C79.51	-	D16.4-	D48.0	D49.2
- - sulcus	C06.1	C79.89	D00.02	D10.39	D37.09	D49.0
- alveolus	C03.9	C79.89	D00.03	D10.39	D37.09	D49.0
- - lower	C03.1	C79.89	D00.03	D10.39	D37.09	D49.0
- - upper	C03.0	C79.89	D00.03	D10.39	D37.09	D49.0
- ampulla of Vater	C24.1	C78.89	D01.5	D13.5	D37.6	D49.0
- ankle NEC	C76.5-	C79.89	D04.7-	D36.7	D48.7	D49.89
- anorectum, anorectal (junction)	C21.8	C78.5	D01.3	D12.9	D37.8	D49.0
- antecubital fossa or space	C76.4-	C79.89	D04.6-	D36.7	D48.7	D49.89
- antrum (Highmore) (maxillary)	C31.0	C78.39	D02.3	D14.0	D38.5	D49.1
- - pyloric	C16.3	C78.89	D00.2	D13.1	D37.1	D49.0
- - tympanicum	C30.1	C78.39	D02.3	D14.0	D38.5	D49.1

NEOPLASM

	Malignant Primary	Malignant Secondary	Ca in Situ	Benign	Uncertain Behavior	Unspecified Behavior
- anus, anal	C21.0	C78.5	D01.3	D12.9	D37.8	D49.0
- - canal	C21.1	C78.5	D01.3	D12.9	D37.8	D49.0
- - cloacogenic zone	C21.2	C78.5	D01.3	D12.9	D37.8	D49.0
- - margin—see also Neoplasm, anus, skin	C44.500	C79.2	D04.5	D23.5	D48.5	D49.2
- - overlapping lesion with rectosigmoid junction or rectum	C21.8	-	-	-	-	-
- - skin	C44.500	C79.2	D04.5	D23.5	D48.5	D49.2
- - - basal cell carcinoma	C44.510	-	-	-	-	-
- - - specified type NEC	C44.590	-	-	-	-	-
- - - squamous cell carcinoma	C44.520	-	-	-	-	-
- - sphincter	C21.1	C78.5	D01.3	D12.9	D37.8	D49.0
- aorta (thoracic)	C49.3	C79.89	-	D21.3	D48.1	D49.2
- - abdominal	C49.4	C79.89	-	D21.4	D48.1	D49.2
- aortic body	C75.5	C79.89	-	D35.6	D44.7	D49.7
- aponeurosis	C49.9	C79.89	-	D21.9	D48.1	D49.2
- - palmar	C49.1-	C79.89	-	D21.1-	D48.1	D49.2
- - plantar	C49.2-	C79.89	-	D21.2-	D48.1	D49.2
- appendix	C18.1	C78.5	D01.0	D12.1	D37.3	D49.0
- arachnoid	C70.9	C79.49	-	D32.9	D42.9	D49.7
- - cerebral	C70.0	C79.32	-	D32.0	D42.0	D49.7
- - spinal	C70.1	C79.49	-	D32.1	D42.1	D49.7
- areola	C50.0-	C79.81	D05.-	D24.-	D48.6-	D49.3
- arm NEC	C76.4-	C79.89	D04.6-	D36.7	D48.7	D49.89
- artery—see Neoplasm, connective tissue						
- aryepiglottic fold	C13.1	C79.89	D00.08	D10.7	D37.05	D49.0
- - hypopharyngeal aspect	C13.1	C79.89	D00.08	D10.7	D37.05	D49.0
- - laryngeal aspect	C32.1	C78.39	D02.0	D14.1	D38.0	D49.1
- - marginal zone	C13.1	C79.89	D00.08	D10.7	D37.05	D49.0
- arytenoid (cartilage)	C32.3	C78.39	D02.0	D14.1	D38.0	D49.1
- - fold—see Neoplasm, aryepiglottic						
- associated with transplanted organ	C80.2	-	-	-	-	-
- atlas	C41.2	C79.51	-	D16.6	D48.0	D49.2
- atrium, cardiac	C38.0	C79.89	-	D15.1	D48.7	D49.89
- auditory						
- - canal (external) (skin)	C44.20-	C79.2	D04.2-	D23.2-	D48.5	D49.2
- - - internal	C30.1	C78.39	D02.3	D14.0	D38.5	D49.1
- - nerve	C72.4-	C79.49	-	D33.3	D43.3	D49.7
- - tube	C30.1	C78.39	D02.3	D14.0	D38.5	D49.1
- - - opening	C11.2	C79.89	D00.08	D10.6	D37.05	D49.0
- auricle, ear—see also Neoplasm, skin, ear	C44.20-	C79.2	D04.2-	D23.2-	D48.5	D49.2
- auricular canal (external)—see also Neoplasm, skin, ear	C44.20-	C79.2	D04.2-	D23.2-	D48.5	D49.2
- - internal	C30.1	C78.39	D02.3	D14.0	D38.5	D49.2
- autonomic nerve or nervous system NEC (see Neoplasm, nerve, peripheral)						
- axilla, axillary	C76.1	C79.89	D09.8	D36.7	D48.7	D49.89
- - fold—see also Neoplasm, skin, trunk	C44.509	C79.2	D04.5	D23.5	D48.5	D49.2
- back NEC	C76.8	C79.89	D04.5	D36.7	D48.7	D49.89
- Bartholin's gland	C51.0	C79.82	D07.1	D28.0	D39.8	D49.59
- basal ganglia	C71.0	C79.31	-	D33.0	D43.0	D49.6
- basis pedunculi	C71.7	C79.31	-	D33.1	D43.1	D49.6
- bile or biliary (tract)	C24.9	C78.89	D01.5	D13.5	D37.6	D49.0
- - canaliculi (biliferi) (intrahepatic)	C22.1	C78.7	D01.5	D13.4	D37.6	D49.0
- - canals, interlobular	C22.1	C78.89	D01.5	D13.4	D37.6	D49.0
- - duct or passage (common) (cystic) (extrahepatic)	C24.0	C78.89	D01.5	D13.5	D37.6	D49.0
- - - interlobular	C22.1	C78.89	D01.5	D13.4	D37.6	D49.0
- - - intrahepatic	C22.1	C78.7	D01.5	D13.4	D37.6	D49.0
- - - - and extrahepatic	C24.8	C78.89	D01.5	D13.5	D37.6	D49.0
- bladder (urinary)	C67.9	C79.11	D09.0	D30.3	D41.4	D49.4
- - dome	C67.1	C79.11	D09.0	D30.3	D41.4	D49.4
- - neck	C67.5	C79.11	D09.0	D30.3	D41.4	D49.4
- - orifice	C67.9	C79.11	D09.0	D30.3	D41.4	D49.4
- - - ureteric	C67.6	C79.11	D09.0	D30.3	D41.4	D49.4
- - - urethral	C67.5	C79.11	D09.0	D30.3	D41.4	D49.4
- - overlapping lesion	C67.8	-	-	-	-	-
- - sphincter	C67.8	C79.11	D09.0	D30.3	D41.4	D49.4
- - trigone	C67.0	C79.11	D09.0	D30.3	D41.4	D49.4
- - urachus	C67.7	C79.11	D09.0	D30.3	D41.4	D49.4

NEOPLASM TABLE

	Malignant Primary	Malignant Secondary	Ca in Situ	Benign	Uncertain Behavior	Unspecified Behavior
- - wall	C67.9	C79.11	D09.0	D30.3	D41.4	D49.4
- - - anterior	C67.3	C79.11	D09.0	D30.3	D41.4	D49.4
- - - lateral	C67.2	C79.11	D09.0	D30.3	D41.4	D49.4
- - - posterior	C67.4	C79.11	D09.0	D30.3	D41.4	D49.4
- blood vessel—*see Neoplasm, connective tissue*						
- bone (periosteum)	C41.9	C79.51	-	D16.9-	D48.0	D49.2
- - acetabulum	C41.4	C79.51	-	D16.8-	D48.0	D49.2
- - ankle	C40.3-	C79.51	-	D16.3-	-	-
- - arm NEC	C40.0-	C79.51	-	D16.0-	-	-
- - astragalus	C40.3-	C79.51	-	D16.3-	-	-
- - atlas	C41.2	C79.51	-	D16.6-	D48.0	D49.2
- - axis	C41.2	C79.51	-	D16.6-	D48.0	D49.2
- - back NEC	C41.2	C79.51	-	D16.6-	D48.0	D49.2
- - calcaneus	C40.3-	C79.51	-	D16.3-	-	-
- - calvarium	C41.0	C79.51	-	D16.4-	D48.0	D49.2
- - carpus (any)	C40.1-	C79.51	-	D16.1-	-	-
- - cartilage NEC	C41.9	C79.51	-	D16.9-	D48.0	D49.2
- - clavicle	C41.3	C79.51	-	D16.7-	D48.0	D49.2
- - clivus	C41.0	C79.51	-	D16.4-	D48.0	D49.2
- - coccygeal vertebra	C41.4	C79.51	-	D16.8-	D48.0	D49.2
- - coccyx	C41.4	C79.51	-	D16.8-	D48.0	D49.2
- - costal cartilage	C41.3	C79.51	-	D16.7-	D48.0	D49.2
- - costovertebral joint	C41.3	C79.51	-	D16.7-	D48.0	D49.2
- - cranial	C41.0	C79.51	-	D16.4-	D48.0	D49.2
- - cuboid	C40.3-	C79.51	-	D16.3-	-	-
- - cuneiform	C41.9	C79.51	-	D16.9-	D48.0	D49.2
- - elbow	C40.0-	C79.51	-	D16.0-	-	-
- - ethmoid (labyrinth)	C41.0	C79.51	-	D16.4-	D48.0	D49.2
- - face	C41.0	C79.51	-	D16.4-	D48.0	D49.2
- - femur (any part)	C40.2-	C79.51	-	D16.2-	-	-
- - fibula (any part)	C40.2-	C79.51	-	D16.2-	-	-
- - finger (any)	C40.1-	C79.51	-	D16.1-	-	-
- - foot	C40.3-	C79.51	-	D16.3-	-	-
- - forearm	C40.0-	C79.51	-	D16.0-	-	-
- - frontal	C41.0	C79.51	-	D16.4-	D48.0	D49.2
- - hand	C40.1-	C79.51	-	D16.1-	-	-
- - heel	C40.3-	C79.51	-	D16.3-	-	-
- - hip	C41.4	C79.51	-	D16.8-	D48.0	D49.2
- - humerus (any part)	C40.0-	C79.51	-	D16.0-	-	-
- - hyoid	C41.0	C79.51	-	D16.4-	D48.0	D49.2
- - ilium	C41.4	C79.51	-	D16.8-	D48.0	D49.2
- - innominate	C41.4	C79.51	-	D16.8-	D48.0	D49.2
- - intervertebral cartilage or disc	C41.2	C79.51	-	D16.6-	D48.0	D49.2
- - ischium	C41.4	C79.51	-	D16.8-	D48.0	D49.2
- - jaw (lower)	C41.1	C79.51	-	D16.5-	D48.0	D49.2
- - knee	C40.2-	C79.51	-	D16.2-	-	-
- - leg NEC	C40.2-	C79.51	-	D16.2-	-	-
- - limb NEC	C40.9-	C79.51	-	D16.9-	-	-
- - - lower (long bones)	C40.2-	C79.51	-	D16.2-	-	-
- - - - short bones	C40.3-	C79.51	-	D16.3-	-	-
- - - upper (long bones)	C40.0-	C79.51	-	D16.0-	-	-
- - - - short bones	C40.1-	C79.51	-	D16.1-	-	-
- - malar	C41.0	C79.51	-	D16.4-	D48.0	D49.2
- - mandible	C41.1	C79.51	-	D16.5-	D48.0	D49.2
- - marrow NEC (any bone)	C96.9	C79.52	-	-	D47.9	D49.89
- - mastoid	C41.0	C79.51	-	D16.4-	D48.0	D49.2
- - maxilla, maxillary (superior)	C41.0	C79.51	-	D16.4-	D48.0	D49.2
- - - inferior	C41.1	C79.51	-	D16.5-	D48.0	D49.2
- - metacarpus (any)	C40.1-	C79.51	-	D16.1-	-	-
- - metatarsus (any)	C40.3-	C79.51	-	D16.3-	-	-
- - overlapping sites	C40.8-	-	-	-	-	-
- - navicular						
- - - ankle	C40.3-	C79.51	-	-	-	-
- - - hand	C40.1-	C79.51	-	-	-	-
- - nose, nasal	C41.0	C79.51	-	D16.4-	D48.0	D49.2
- - occipital	C41.0	C79.51	-	D16.4-	D48.0	D49.2
- - orbit	C41.0	C79.51	-	D16.4-	D48.0	D49.2
- - parietal	C41.0	C79.51	-	D16.4-	D48.0	D49.2

1573

	Malignant Primary	Malignant Secondary	Ca in Situ	Benign	Uncertain Behavior	Unspecified Behavior
- - patella	C40.2-	C79.51	-	-	-	-
- - pelvic	C41.4	C79.51	-	D16.8	D48.0	D49.2
- - phalanges						
- - - foot	C40.3-	C79.51	-	-	-	-
- - - hand	C40.1-	C79.51	-	-	-	-
- - pubic	C41.4	C79.51	-	D16.8	D48.0	D49.2
- - radius (any part)	C40.0-	C79.51	-	D16.0-		
- - rib	C41.3	C79.51	-	D16.7	D48.0	D49.2
- - sacral vertebra	C41.4	C79.51	-	D16.8	D48.0	D49.2
- - sacrum	C41.4	C79.51	-	D16.8	D48.0	D49.2
- - scaphoid					-	-
- - - of ankle	C40.3-	C79.51	-	-	-	-
- - - of hand	C40.1-	C79.51	-	-	-	-
- - scapula (any part)	C40.0-	C79.51	-	D16.0-	-	-
- - sella turcica	C41.0	C79.51	-	D16.4-	D48.0	D49.2
- - shoulder	C40.0-	C79.51	-	D16.0-	-	-
- - skull	C41.0	C79.51	-	D16.4-	D48.0	D49.2
- - sphenoid	C41.0	C79.51	-	D16.4-	D48.0	D49.2
- - spine, spinal (column)	C41.2	C79.51	-	D16.6	D48.0	D49.2
- - - coccyx	C41.4	C79.51	-	D16.8	D48.0	D49.2
- - - sacrum	C41.4	C79.51	-	D16.8	D48.0	D49.2
- - sternum	C41.3	C79.51	-	D16.7	D48.0	D49.2
- - tarsus (any)	C40.3-	C79.51	-	-	-	-
- - temporal	C41.0	C79.51	-	D16.4-	D48.0	D49.2
- - thumb	C40.1-	C79.51	-	-	-	-
- - tibia (any part)	C40.2-	C79.51	-	-	-	-
- - toe (any)	C40.3-	C79.51	-	-	-	-
- - trapezium	C40.1-	C79.51	-	-	-	-
- - trapezoid	C40.1-	C79.51	-	-	-	-
- - turbinate	C41.0	C79.51	-	D16.4-	D48.0	D49.2
- - ulna (any part)	C40.0-	C79.51	-	D16.0-	-	-
- - unciform	C40.1-	C79.51	-	-	-	-
- - vertebra (column)	C41.2	C79.51	-	D16.6	D48.0	D49.2
- - - coccyx	C41.4	C79.51	-	D16.8	D48.0	D49.2
- - - sacrum	C41.4	C79.51	-	D16.8	D48.0	D49.2
- - vomer	C41.0	C79.51	-	D16.4-	D48.0	D49.2
- - wrist	C40.1-	C79.51	-	-	-	-
- - xiphoid process	C41.3	C79.51	-	D16.7	D48.0	D49.2
- - zygomatic	C41.0	C79.51	-	D16.4-	D48.0	D49.2
- book-leaf (mouth)	C06.89	C79.89	D00.00	D10.39	D37.09	D49.0
- bowel—*see Neoplasm, intestine*						
- brachial plexus	C47.1-	C79.89	-	D36.12	D48.2	D49.2
- brain NEC	C71.9	C79.31	-	D33.2	D43.2	D49.6
- - basal ganglia	C71.0	C79.31	-	D33.0	D43.0	D49.6
- - cerebellopontine angle	C71.6	C79.31	-	D33.1	D43.1	D49.6
- - cerebellum NOS	C71.6	C79.31	-	D33.1	D43.1	D49.6
- - cerebrum	C71.0	C79.31	-	D33.0	D43.0	D49.6
- - choroid plexus	C71.7	C79.31	-	D33.1	D43.1	D49.6
- - corpus callosum	C71.8	C79.31	-	D33.2	D43.2	D49.6
- - corpus striatum	C71.0	C79.31	-	D33.0	D43.0	D49.6
- - cortex (cerebral)	C71.0	C79.31	-	D33.0	D43.0	D49.6
- - frontal lobe	C71.1	C79.31	-	D33.0	D43.0	D49.6
- - globus pallidus	C71.0	C79.31	-	D33.0	D43.0	D49.6
- - hippocampus	C71.2	C79.31	-	D33.0	D43.0	D49.6
- - hypothalamus	C71.0	C79.31	-	D33.0	D43.0	D49.6
- - internal capsule	C71.0	C79.31	-	D33.0	D43.0	D49.6
- - medulla oblongata	C71.7	C79.31	-	D33.1	D43.1	D49.6
- - meninges	C70.0	C79.32	-	D32.0	D42.0	D49.7
- - midbrain	C71.7	C79.31	-	D33.1	D43.1	D49.6
- - occipital lobe	C71.4	C79.31	-	D33.0	D43.0	D49.6
- - overlapping lesion	C71.8	C79.31	-	-	-	-
- - parietal lobe	C71.3	C79.31	-	D33.0	D43.0	D49.6
- - peduncle	C71.7	C79.31	-	D33.1	D43.1	D49.6
- - pons	C71.7	C79.31	-	D33.1	D43.1	D49.6
- - stem	C71.7	C79.31	-	D33.1	D43.1	D49.6
- - tapetum	C71.8	C79.31	-	D33.2	D43.2	D49.6
- - temporal lobe	C71.2	C79.31	-	D33.0	D43.0	D49.6

	Malignant Primary	Malignant Secondary	Ca in Situ	Benign	Uncertain Behavior	Unspecified Behavior
- - thalamus	C71.0	C79.31	-	D33.0	D43.0	D49.6
- - uncus	C71.2	C79.31	-	D33.0	D43.0	D49.6
- - ventricle (floor)	C71.5	C79.31	-	D33.0	D43.0	D49.6
- - - fourth	C71.7	C79.31	-	D33.1	D43.1	D49.6
- branchial (cleft) (cyst) (vestiges)	C10.4	C79.89	D00.08	D10.5	D37.05	D49.0
- breast (connective tissue) (glandular tissue) (soft parts)	C50.9-	C79.81	D05.-	D24.-	D48.6-	D49.3
- - areola	C50.0-	C79.81	D05.-	D24.-	D48.6-	D49.3
- - axillary tail	C50.6-	C79.81	D05.-	D24.-	D48.6-	D49.3
- - central portion	C50.1-	C79.81	D05.-	D24.-	D48.6-	D49.3
- - inner	C50.8-	C79.81	D05.-	D24.-	D48.6-	D49.3
- - lower	C50.8-	C79.81	D05.-	D24.-	D48.6-	D49.3
- - lower-inner quadrant	C50.3-	C79.81	D05.-	D24.-	D48.6-	D49.3
- - lower-outer quadrant	C50.5-	C79.81	D05.-	D24.-	D48.6-	D49.3
- - mastectomy site (skin)—*see also Neoplasm, breast, skin*	C44.501	C79.2	-	-	-	-
- - - specified as breast tissue	C50.8-	C79.81	-	-	-	-
- - midline	C50.8-	C79.81	D05.-	D24.-	D48.6-	D49.3
- - nipple	C50.0-	C79.81	D05.-	D24.-	D48.6-	D49.3
- - outer	C50.8-	C79.81	D05.-	D24.-	D48.6-	D49.3
- - overlapping lesion	C50.8-	-	-	-	-	-
- - skin	C44.501	C79.2	D04.5	D23.5	D48.5	D49.2
- - - basal cell carcinoma	C44.511	-	-	-	-	-
- - - specified type NEC	C44.591	-	-	-	-	-
- - - squamous cell carcinoma	C44.521	-	-	-	-	-
- - tail (axillary)	C50.6-	C79.81	D05.-	D24.-	D48.6-	D49.3
- - upper	C50.8-	C79.81	D05.-	D24.-	D48.6-	D49.3
- - upper-inner quadrant	C50.2-	C79.81	D05.-	D24.-	D48.6-	D49.3
- - upper-outer quadrant	C50.4-	C79.81	D05.-	D24.-	D48.6-	D49.3
- broad ligament	C57.1	C79.82	D07.39	D28.2	D39.8	D49.59
- bronchogenic, bronchogenic (lung)	C34.9-	C78.0-	D02.2-	D14.3-	D38.1	D49.1
- bronchiole	C34.9-	C78.0-	D02.2-	D14.3-	D38.1	D49.1
- bronchus	C34.9-	C78.0-	D02.2-	D14.3-	D38.1	D49.1
- - carina	C34.0-	C78.0-	D02.2-	D14.3-	D38.1	D49.1
- - lower lobe of lung	C34.3-	C78.0-	D02.2-	D14.3-	D38.1	D49.1
- - main	C34.0-	C78.0-	D02.2-	D14.3-	D38.1	D49.1
- - middle lobe of lung	C34.2	C78.0-	D02.21	D14.31	D38.1	D49.1
- - overlapping lesion	C34.8-	-	-	-	-	-
- - upper lobe of lung	C34.1-	C78.0-	D02.2-	D14.3-	D38.1	D49.1
- brow	C44.309	C79.2	D04.39	D23.39	D48.5	D49.2
- - basal cell carcinoma	C44.319	-	-	-	-	-
- - specified type NEC	C44.399	-	-	-	-	-
- - squamous cell carcinoma	C44.329	-	-	-	-	-
- buccal (cavity)	C06.9	C79.89	D00.00	D10.39	D37.09	D49.0
- - commissure	C06.0	C79.89	D00.02	D10.39	D37.09	D49.0
- - groove (lower) (upper)	C06.1	C79.89	D00.02	D10.39	D37.09	D49.0
- - mucosa	C06.0	C79.89	D00.02	D10.39	D37.09	D49.0
- - sulcus (lower) (upper)	C06.1	C79.89	D00.02	D10.39	D37.09	D49.0
- bulbourethral gland	C68.0	C79.19	D09.19	D30.4	D41.3	D49.59
- bursa—*see Neoplasm, connective tissue*						
- buttock NEC	C76.3	C79.89	D04.5	D36.7	D48.7	D49.89
- calf	C76.5-	C79.89	D04.7-	D36.7	D48.7	D49.89
- calvarium	C41.0	C79.51	-	D16.4-	D48.0	D49.2
- calyx, renal	C65.-	C79.0-	D09.19	D30.1-	D41.1-	D49.59
- canal						
- - anal	C21.1	C78.5	D01.3	D12.9	D37.8	D49.0
- - auditory (external)—*see also Neoplasm, skin, ear*	C44.20-	C79.2	D04.2-	D23.2-	D48.5	D49.2
- - auricular (external)—*see also Neoplasm, skin, ear*	C44.20-	C79.2	D04.2-	D23.2-	D48.5	D49.2
- canaliculi, biliary (biliferi) (intrahepatic)	C22.1	C78.7	D01.5	D13.4	D37.6	D49.0
- canthus (eye) (inner) (outer)	C44.10-	C79.2	D04.1-	D23.1-	D48.5	D49.2
- - basal cell carcinoma	C44.11-	-	-	-	-	-
- - specified type NEC	C44.19-	-	-	-	-	-
- - squamous cell carcinoma	C44.12-	-	-	-	-	-
- capillary—*see Neoplasm, connective tissue*						
- caput coli	C18.0	C78.5	D01.0	D12.0	D37.4	D49.0
- carcinoid—*see Tumor, carcinoid*						
- cardia (gastric)	C16.0	C78.89	D00.2	D13.1	D37.1	D49.0
- cardiac orifice (stomach)	C16.0	C78.89	D00.2	D13.1	D37.1	D49.0

	Malignant Primary	Malignant Secondary	Ca in Situ	Benign	Uncertain Behavior	Unspecified Behavior
- cardio-esophageal junction	C16.0	C78.89	D00.2	D13.1	D37.1	D49.0
- cardio-esophagus	C16.0	C78.89	D00.2	D13.1	D37.1	D49.0
- carina (bronchus)	C34.0-	C78.0-	D02.2-	D14.3-	D38.1	D49.1
- carotid (artery)	C49.0	C79.89	-	D21.0	D48.1	D49.2
- - body	C75.4	C79.89	-	D35.5	D44.6	D49.7
- carpus (any bone)	C40.1-	C79.51	-	D16.1-	-	-
- cartilage (articular) (joint)NEC—see also Neoplasm, bone	C41.9	C79.51	-	D16.9-	D48.0	D49.2
- - arytenoid	C32.3	C78.39	D02.0	D14.1	D38.0	D49.1
- - auricular	C49.0	C79.89	-	D21.0	D48.1	D49.2
- - bronchi	C34.0-	C78.39	-	D14.3-	D38.1	D49.1
- - costal	C41.3	C79.51	-	D16.7	D48.0	D49.2
- - cricoid	C32.3	C78.39	D02.0	D14.1	D38.0	D49.1
- - cuneiform	C32.3	C78.39	D02.0	D14.1	D38.0	D49.1
- - ear (external)	C49.0	C79.89	-	D21.0	D48.1	D49.2
- - ensiform	C41.3	C79.51	-	D16.7	D48.0	D49.2
- - epiglottis	C32.1	C78.39	D02.0	D14.1	D38.0	D49.1
- - - anterior surface	C10.1	C79.89	D00.08	D10.5	D37.05	D49.0
- - eyelid	C49.0	C79.89	-	D21.0	D48.1	D49.2
- - intervertebral	C41.2	C79.51	-	D16.6	D48.0	D49.2
- - larynx, laryngeal	C32.3	C78.39	D02.0	D14.1	D38.0	D49.1
- - nose, nasal	C30.0	C78.39	D02.3	D14.0	D38.5	D49.1
- - pinna	C49.0	C79.89	-	D21.0	D48.1	D49.2
- - rib	C41.3	C79.51	-	D16.7	D48.0	D49.2
- - semilunar (knee)	C40.2-	C79.51	-	D16.2-	D48.0	D49.2
- - thyroid	C32.3	C78.39	D02.0	D14.1	D38.0	D49.1
- - trachea	C33	C78.39	D02.1	D14.2	D38.1	D49.1
- cauda equina	C72.1	C79.49	-	D33.4	D43.4	D49.7
- cavity						
- - buccal	C06.9	C79.89	D00.00	D10.30	D37.09	D49.0
- - nasal	C30.0	C78.39	D02.3	D14.0	D38.5	D49.1
- - oral	C06.9	C79.89	D00.00	D10.30	D37.09	D49.0
- - peritoneal	C48.2	C78.6	-	D20.1	D48.4	D49.0
- - tympanic	C30.1	C78.39	D02.3	D14.0	D38.5	D49.1
- cecum	C18.0	C78.5	D01.0	D12.0	D37.4	D49.0
- central nervous system	C72.9	C79.40	-	-	-	-
- cerebellopontine (angle)	C71.6	C79.31	-	D33.1	D43.1	D49.6
- cerebellum, cerebellar	C71.6	C79.31	-	D33.1	D43.1	D49.6
- cerebrum, cerebral (cortex) (hemisphere) (white matter)	C71.0	C79.31	-	D33.0	D43.0	D49.6
- - meninges	C70.0	C79.32	-	D32.0	D42.0	D49.7
- - peduncle	C71.7	C79.31	-	D33.1	D43.1	D49.6
- - ventricle	C71.5	C79.31	-	D33.0	D43.0	D49.6
- - - fourth	C71.7	C79.31	-	D33.1	D43.1	D49.6
- cervical region	C76.0	C79.89	D09.8	D36.7	D48.7	D49.89
- cervix (cervical) (uteri) (uterus)	C53.9	C79.82	D06.9	D26.0	D39.0	D49.59
- - canal	C53.0	C79.82	D06.0	D26.0	D39.0	D49.59
- - endocervix (canal) (gland)	C53.0	C79.82	D06.0	D26.0	D39.0	D49.59
- - exocervix	C53.1	C79.82	D06.1	D26.0	D39.0	D49.59
- - external os	C53.1	C79.82	D06.1	D26.0	D39.0	D49.59
- - internal os	C53.0	C79.82	D06.0	D26.0	D39.0	D49.59
- - nabothian gland	C53.0	C79.82	D06.0	D26.0	D39.0	D49.59
- - overlapping lesion	C53.8	-	-	-	-	-
- - squamocolumnar junction	C53.8	C79.82	D06.7	D26.0	D39.0	D49.59
- - stump	C53.8	C79.82	D06.7	D26.0	D39.0	D49.59
- cheek	C76.0	C79.89	D09.8	D36.7	D48.7	D49.89
- - external	C44.309	C79.2	D04.39	D23.39	D48.5	D49.2
- - - basal cell carcinoma	C44.319	-	-	-	-	-
- - - specified type NEC	C44.399	-	-	-	-	-
- - - squamous cell carcinoma	C44.329	-	-	-	-	-
- - inner aspect	C06.0	C79.89	D00.02	D10.39	D37.09	D49.0
- - internal	C06.0	C79.89	D00.02	D10.39	D37.09	D49.0
- - mucosa	C06.0	C79.89	D00.02	D10.39	D37.09	D49.0
- chest (wall)NEC	C76.1	C79.89	D09.8	D36.7	D48.7	D49.89
- chiasma opticum	C72.3-	C79.49	-	D33.3	D43.3	D49.7
- chin	C44.309	C79.2	D04.39	D23.39	D48.5	D49.2
- - basal cell carcinoma	C44.319	-	-	-	-	-

	Malignant Primary	Malignant Secondary	Ca in Situ	Benign	Uncertain Behavior	Unspecified Behavior
- - specified type NEC	C44.399	-	-	-	-	-
- - squamous cell carcinoma	C44.329	-	-	-	-	-
-choana	C11.3	C79.89	D00.08	D10.6	D37.05	D49.0
- cholangiole	C22.1	C78.89	D01.5	D13.4	D37.6	D49.0
- choledochal duct	C24.0	C78.89	D01.5	D13.5	D37.6	D49.0
- choroid	C69.3-	C79.49	D09.2-	D31.3-	D48.7	D49.81
- - plexus	C71.5	C79.31	-	D33.0	D43.0	D49.6
- ciliary body	C69.4-	C79.49	D09.2-	D31.4-	D48.7	D49.89
- clavicle	C41.3	C79.51	-	D16.7	D48.0	D49.2
- clitoris	C51.2	C79.82	D07.1	D28.0	D39.8	D49.59
- clivus	C41.0	C79.51	-	D16.4-	D48.0	D49.2
- cloacogenic zone	C21.2	C78.5	D01.3	D12.9	D37.8	D49.0
- coccygeal						
- - body or glomus	C49.5	C79.89	-	D21.5	D48.1	D49.2
- - vertebra	C41.4	C79.51	-	D16.8	D48.0	D49.2
- coccyx	C41.4	C79.51	-	D16.8	D48.0	D49.2
- colon—see also Neoplasm, intestine, large	C18.9	C78.5	-	-	-	-
- - with rectum	C19	C78.5	D01.1	D12.7	D37.5	D49.0
- column, spinal—see Neoplasm, spine						
- columnella—see also Neoplasm, skin, face	C44.390	C79.2	D04.39	D23.39	D48.5	D49.2
- commissure						
- - labial, lip	C00.6	C79.89	D00.01	D10.39	D37.01	D49.0
- - laryngeal	C32.0	C78.39	D02.0	D14.1	D38.0	D49.1
- common (bile)duct	C24.0	C78.89	D01.5	D13.5	D37.6	D49.0
- concha—see also Neoplasm, skin, ear	C44.20-	C79.2	D04.2-	D23.2-	D48.5	D49.2
- - nose	C30.0	C78.39	D02.3	D14.0	D38.5	D49.1
- conjunctiva	C69.0-	C79.49	D09.2-	D31.0-	D48.7	D49.89
- connective tissue NEC	C49.9	C79.89	-	D21.9	D48.1	D49.2
Note: For neoplasms of connective tissue (blood vessel, bursa, fascia, ligament, muscle, peripheral nerves, sympathetic and parasympathetic nerves and ganglia, synovia, tendon, etc.) or of morphological types that indicate connective tissue, code according to the list under "Neoplasm, connective tissue". For sites that do not appear in this list, code to neoplasm of that site; e.g., fibrosarcoma, pancreas (C25.9)						
Note: Morphological types that indicate connective tissue appear in their proper place in the alphabetic index with the instruction "see Neoplasm, connective tissue ...."						
- - abdomen	C49.4	C79.89	-	D21.4	D48.1	D49.2
- - abdominal wall	C49.4	C79.89	-	D21.4	D48.1	D49.2
- - ankle	C49.2-	C79.89	-	D21.2-	D48.1	D49.2
- - antecubital fossa or space	C49.1-	C79.89	-	D21.1-	D48.1	D49.2
- - arm	C49.1-	C79.89	-	D21.1-	D48.1	D49.2
- - auricle (ear)	C49.0	C79.89	-	D21.0	D48.1	D49.2
- - axilla	C49.3	C79.89	-	D21.3	D48.1	D49.2
- - back	C49.6	C79.89	-	D21.6	D48.1	D49.2
- - breast—see Neoplasm, breast						
- - buttock	C49.5	C79.89	-	D21.5	D48.1	D49.2
- - calf	C49.2-	C79.89	-	D21.2-	D48.1	D49.2
- - cervical region	C49.0	C79.89	-	D21.0	D48.1	D49.2
- - cheek	C49.0	C79.89	-	D21.0	D48.1	D49.2
- - chest (wall)	C49.3	C79.89	-	D21.3	D48.1	D49.2
- - chin	C49.0	C79.89	-	D21.0	D48.1	D49.2
- - diaphragm	C49.3	C79.89	-	D21.3	D48.1	D49.2
- - ear (external)	C49.0	C79.89	-	D21.0	D48.1	D49.2
- - elbow	C49.1-	C79.89	-	D21.1-	D48.1	D49.2
- - extra rectal	C49.5	C79.89	-	D21.5	D48.1	D49.2
- - extremity	C49.9	C79.89	-	D21.9	D48.1	D49.2
- - - lower	C49.2-	C79.89	-	D21.2-	D48.1	D49.2
- - - upper	C49.1-	C79.89	-	D21.1-	D48.1	D49.2
- - eyelid	C49.0	C79.89	-	D21.0	D48.1	D49.2
- - face	C49.0	C79.89	-	D21.0	D48.1	D49.2
- - finger	C49.1-	C79.89	-	D21.1-	D48.1	D49.2
- - flank	C49.6	C79.89	-	D21.6	D48.1	D49.2
- - foot	C49.2-	C79.89	-	D21.2-	D48.1	D49.2
- - forearm	C49.1-	C79.89	-	D21.1-	D48.1	D49.2

	Malignant Primary	Malignant Secondary	Ca in Situ	Benign	Uncertain Behavior	Unspecified Behavior
- - forehead	C49.0	C79.89	-	D21.0	D48.1	D49.2
- - gastric	C49.4	C79.89	-	D21.4	D48.1	D49.2
- - gastrointestinal	C49.4	C79.89	-	D21.4	D48.1	D49.2
- - gluteal region	C49.5	C79.89	-	D21.5	D48.1	D49.2
- - great vessels NEC	C49.3	C79.89	-	D21.3	D48.1	D49.2
- - groin	C49.5	C79.89	-	D21.5	D48.1	D49.2
- - hand	C49.1-	C79.89	-	D21.1-	D48.1	D49.2
- - head	C49.0	C79.89	-	D21.0	D48.1	D49.2
- - heel	C49.2-	C79.89	-	D21.2-	D48.1	D49.2
- - hip	C49.2-	C79.89	-	D21.2-	D48.1	D49.2
- - hypochondrium	C49.4	C79.89	-	D21.4	D48.1	D49.2
- - iliopsoas muscle	C49.5	C79.89	-	D21.5	D48.1	D49.2
- - infraclavicular region	C49.3	C79.89	-	D21.3	D48.1	D49.2
- - inguinal (canal) (region)	C49.5	C79.89	-	D21.5	D48.1	D49.2
- - intestinal	C49.4	C79.89	-	D21.4	D48.1	D49.2
- - intrathoracic	C49.3	C79.89	-	D21.3	D48.1	D49.2
- - ischiorectal fossa	C49.5	C79.89	-	D21.5	D48.1	D49.2
- - jaw	C03.9	C79.89	D00.03	D10.39	D48.1	D49.0
- - knee	C49.2-	C79.89	-	D21.2-	D48.1	D49.2
- - leg	C49.2-	C79.89	-	D21.2-	D48.1	D49.2
- - limb NEC	C49.9	C79.89	-	D21.9	D48.1	D49.2
- - - lower	C49.2-	C79.89	-	D21.2-	D48.1	D49.2
- - - upper	C49.1-	C79.89	-	D21.1-	D48.1	D49.2
- - nates	C49.5	C79.89	-	D21.5	D48.1	D49.2
- - neck	C49.0	C79.89	-	D21.0	D48.1	D49.2
- - orbit	C69.6-	C79.49	D09.2-	D31.6-	D48.1	D49.89
- - overlapping lesion	C49.8	-	-	-	-	-
- - pararectal	C49.5	C79.89	-	D21.5	D48.1	D49.2
- - para-urethral	C49.5	C79.89	-	D21.5	D48.1	D49.2
- - paravaginal	C49.5	C79.89	-	D21.5	D48.1	D49.2
- - pelvis (floor)	C49.5	C79.89	-	D21.5	D48.1	D49.2
- - pelvo-abdominal	C49.8	C79.89	-	D21.6	D48.1	D49.2
- - perineum	C49.5	C79.89	-	D21.5	D48.1	D49.2
- - perirectal (tissue)	C49.5	C79.89	-	D21.5	D48.1	D49.2
- - periurethral (tissue)	C49.5	C79.89	-	D21.5	D48.1	D49.2
- - popliteal fossa or space	C49.2-	C79.89	-	D21.2-	D48.1	D49.2
- - presacral	C49.5	C79.89	-	D21.5	D48.1	D49.2
- - psoas muscle	C49.4	C79.89	-	D21.4	D48.1	D49.2
- - pterygoid fossa	C49.0	C79.89	-	D21.0	D48.1	D49.2
- - rectovaginal septum or wall	C49.5	C79.89	-	D21.5	D48.1	D49.2
- - rectovesical	C49.5	C79.89	-	D21.5	D48.1	D49.2
- - retroperitoneum	C48.0	C78.6	-	D20.0	D48.3	D49.0
- - sacrococcygeal region	C49.5	C79.89	-	D21.5	D48.1	D49.2
- - scalp	C49.0	C79.89	-	D21.0	D48.1	D49.2
- - scapular region	C49.3	C79.89	-	D21.3	D48.1	D49.2
- - shoulder	C49.1-	C79.89	-	D21.1-	D48.1	D49.2
- - skin (dermis)NEC—see also Neoplasm, skin, by site	C44.90	C79.2	D04.9	D23.9	D48.5	D49.2
- - stomach	C49.4	C79.89	-	D21.4	D48.1	D49.2
- - submental	C49.0	C79.89	-	D21.0	D48.1	D49.2
- - supraclavicular region	C49.0	C79.89	-	D21.0	D48.1	D49.2
- - temple	C49.0	C79.89	-	D21.0	D48.1	D49.2
- - temporal region	C49.0	C79.89	-	D21.0	D48.1	D49.2
- - thigh	C49.2-	C79.89	-	D21.2-	D48.1	D49.2
- - thoracic (duct) (wall)	C49.3	C79.89	-	D21.3	D48.1	D49.2
- - thorax	C49.3	C79.89	-	D21.3	D48.1	D49.2
- - thumb	C49.1-	C79.89	-	D21.1-	D48.1	D49.2
- - toe	C49.2-	C79.89	-	D21.2-	D48.1	D49.2
- - trunk	C49.6	C79.89	-	D21.6	D48.1	D49.2
- - umbilicus	C49.4	C79.89	-	D21.4	D48.1	D49.2
- - vesicorectal	C49.5	C79.89	-	D21.5	D48.1	D49.2
- - wrist	C49.1-	C79.89	-	D21.1-	D48.1	D49.2
- conus medullaris	C72.0	C79.49	-	D33.4	D43.4	D49.7
- cord (true) (vocal)	C32.0	C78.39	D02.0	D14.1	D38.0	D49.1
- - false	C32.1	C78.39	D02.0	D14.1	D38.0	D49.1
- - spermatic	C63.1-	C79.82	D07.69	D29.8	D40.8	D49.59
- - spinal (cervical) (lumbar) (thoracic)	C72.0	C79.49	-	D33.4	D43.4	D49.7

NEOPLASM TABLE

	Malignant Primary	Malignant Secondary	Ca in Situ	Benign	Uncertain Behavior	Unspecified Behavior
- cornea (limbus)	C69.1-	C79.49	D09.2-	D31.1-	D48.7	D49.89
- corpus						
- - albicans	C56.-	C79.6-	D07.39	D27.-	D39.1-	D49.59
- - callosum, brain	C71.0	C79.31	-	D33.2	D43.2	D49.6
- - cavernosum	C60.2	C79.82	D07.4	D29.0	D40.8	D49.59
- - gastric	C16.2	C78.89	D00.2	D13.1	D37.1	D49.0
- - overlapping sites	C54.8	-	-	-	-	-
- - penis	C60.2	C79.82	D07.4	D29.0	D40.8	D49.59
- - striatum, cerebrum	C71.0	C79.31	-	D33.0	D43.0	D49.6
- - uteri	C54.9	C79.82	D07.0	D26.1	D39.0	D49.59
- - - isthmus	C54.0	C79.82	D07.0	D26.1	D39.0	D49.59
- cortex						
- - adrenal	C74.0-	C79.7-	D09.3	D35.0-	D44.1-	D49.7
- - cerebral	C71.0	C79.31	-	D33.0	D43.0	D49.6
- costal cartilage	C41.3	C79.51	-	D16.7	D48.0	D49.2
- costovertebral joint	C41.3	C79.51	-	D16.7	D48.0	D49.2
- Cowper's gland	C68.0	C79.19	D09.19	D30.4	D41.3	D49.59
- cranial (fossa, any)	C71.9	C79.31	-	D33.2	D43.2	D49.6
- - meninges	C70.0	C79.32	-	D32.0	D42.0	D49.7
- - nerve	C72.50	C79.49	-	D33.3	D43.3	D49.7
- - - specified NEC	C72.59	C79.49	-	D33.3	D43.3	D49.7
- craniobuccal pouch	C75.2	C79.89	D09.3	D35.2	D44.3	D49.7
- craniopharyngeal (duct) (pouch)	C75.2	C79.89	D09.3	D35.3	D44.4	D49.7
- cricoid	C13.0	C79.89	D00.08	D10.7	D37.05	D49.0
- - cartilage	C32.3	C79.89	D02.0	D14.1	D38.0	D49.1
- cricopharynx	C13.0	C79.89	D00.08	D10.7	D37.05	D49.0
- crypt of Morgagni	C21.8	C78.5	D01.3	D12.9	D37.8	D49.0
- crystalline lens	C69.4-	C79.49	D09.2-	D31.4-	D48.7	D49.89
- cul-de-sac (Douglas')	C48.1	C78.6	-	D20.1	D48.4	D49.0
- cuneiform cartilage	C32.3	C78.39	D02.0	D14.1	D38.0	D49.1
- cutaneous—*see Neoplasm, skin*						
- cutis—*see Neoplasm, skin*						
- cystic (bile) duct (common)	C24.0	C78.89	D01.5	D13.5	D37.6	D49.0
- dermis—*see Neoplasm, skin*						
- diaphragm	C49.3	C79.89	-	D21.3	D48.1	D49.2
- digestive organs, system, tube, or tract NEC	C26.9	C78.89	D01.9	D13.9	D37.9	D49.0
- disc, intervertebral	C41.2	C79.51	-	D16.6	D48.0	D49.2
- disease, generalized	C80.0	-	-	-	-	-
- disseminated	C80.0	-	-	-	-	-
- Douglas' cul-de-sac or pouch	C48.1	C78.6	-	D20.1	D48.4	D49.0
- duodenojejunal junction	C17.8	C78.4	D01.49	D13.39	D37.2	D49.0
- duodenum	C17.0	C78.4	D01.49	D13.2	D37.2	D49.0
- dura (cranial) (mater)	C70.9	C79.49	-	D32.9	D42.9	D49.7
- - cerebral	C70.0	C79.32	-	D32.0	D42.0	D49.7
- - spinal	C70.1	C79.49	-	D32.1	D42.1	D49.7
- ear (external)—*see also Neoplasm, skin, ear*	C44.20-	C79.2	D04.2-	D23.2-	D48.5	D49.2
- - auricle or auris—*see also Neoplasm, skin, ear*	C44.20-	C79.2	D04.2-	D23.2-	D48.5	D49.2
- - canal, external—*see also Neoplasm, skin, ear*	C44.20-	C79.2	D04.2-	D23.2-	D48.5	D49.2
- - cartilage	C49.0	C79.89	-	D21.0	D48.1	D49.2
- - external meatus—*see also Neoplasm, skin, ear*	C44.20-	C79.2	D04.2-	D23.2-	D48.5	D49.2
- - inner	C30.1	C78.39	D02.3	D14.0	D38.5	D49.1
- - lobule—*see also Neoplasm, skin, ear*	C44.20-	C79.2	D04.2-	D23.2-	D48.5	D49.2
- - middle	C30.1	C78.39	D02.3	D14.0	D38.5	D49.1
- - overlapping lesion with accessory sinuses	C31.8	-	-	-	-	-
- - skin	C44.20-	C79.2	D04.2-	D23.2-	D48.5	D49.2
- - - basal cell carcinoma	C44.21-	-	-	-	-	-
- - - specified type NEC	C44.29-	-	-	-	-	-
- - - squamous cell carcinoma	C44.22-	-	-	-	-	-
- earlobe	C44.20-	C79.2	D04.2-	D23.2-	D48.5	D49.2
- - basal cell carcinoma	C44.21-	-	-	-	-	-
- - specified type NEC	C44.29-	-	-	-	-	-
- - squamous cell carcinoma	C44.22-	-	-	-	-	-
- ejaculatory duct	C63.7	C79.82	D07.69	D29.8	D40.8	D49.59
- elbow NEC	C76.4-	C79.89	D04.6-	D36.7	D48.7	D49.89
- endocardium	C38.0	C79.89	-	D15.1	D48.7	D49.89
- endocervix (canal) (gland)	C53.0	C79.82	D06.0	D26.0	D39.0	D49.59
- endocrine gland NEC	C75.9	C79.89	D09.3	D35.9	D44.9	D49.7
- - pluriglandular	C75.8	C79.89	D09.3	D35.7	D44.9	D49.7

	Malignant Primary	Malignant Secondary	Ca in Situ	Benign	Uncertain Behavior	Unspecified Behavior
- endometrium (gland) (stroma)	C54.1	C79.82	D07.0	D26.1	D39.0	D49.59
- ensiform cartilage	C41.3	C79.51	-	D16.7	D48.0	D49.2
- enteric—*see Neoplasm, intestine*						
- ependyma (brain)	C71.5	C79.31	-	D33.0	D43.0	D49.6
- - fourth ventricle	C71.7	C79.31	-	D33.1	D43.1	D49.6
- epicardium	C38.0	C79.89	-	D15.1	D48.7	D49.89
- epididymis	C63.0-	C79.82	D07.69	D29.3-	D40.8	D49.59
- epidural	C72.9	C79.49	-	D33.9	D43.9	D49.7
- epiglottis	C32.1	C78.39	D02.0	D14.1	D38.0	D49.1
- - anterior aspect or surface	C10.1	C79.89	D00.08	D10.5	D37.05	D49.0
- - cartilage	C32.3	C78.39	D02.0	D14.1	D38.0	D49.1
- - free border (margin)	C10.1	C79.89	D00.08	D10.5	D37.05	D49.0
- - junctional region	C10.8	C79.89	D00.08	D10.5	D37.05	D49.0
- - posterior (laryngeal)surface	C32.1	C78.39	D02.0	D14.1	D38.0	D49.1
- - suprahyoid portion	C32.1	C78.39	D02.0	D14.1	D38.0	D49.1
- esophagogastric junction	C16.0	C78.89	D00.2	D13.1	D37.1	D49.0
- esophagus	C15.9	C78.89	D00.1	D13.0	D37.8	D49.0
- - abdominal	C15.5	C78.89	D00.1	D13.0	D37.8	D49.0
- - cervical	C15.3	C78.89	D00.1	D13.0	D37.8	D49.0
- - distal (third)	C15.5	C78.89	D00.1	D13.0	D37.8	D49.0
- - lower (third)	C15.5	C78.89	D00.1	D13.0	D37.8	D49.0
- - middle (third)	C15.4	C78.89	D00.1	D13.0	D37.8	D49.0
- - overlapping lesion	C15.8	-	-	-	-	-
- - proximal (third)	C15.3	C78.89	D00.1	D13.0	D37.8	D49.0
- - thoracic	C15.4	C78.89	D00.1	D13.0	D37.8	D49.0
- - upper (third)	C15.3	C78.89	D00.1	D13.0	D37.8	D49.0
- ethmoid (sinus)	C31.1	C78.39	D02.3	D14.0	D38.5	D49.1
- - bone or labyrinth	C41.0	C79.51	-	D16.4-	D48.0	D49.2
- eustachian tube	C30.1	C78.39	D02.3	D14.0	D38.5	D49.1
- exocervix	C53.1	C79.82	D06.1	D26.0	D39.0	D49.59
- external						
- - meatus (ear)—*see also Neoplasm, skin, ear*	C44.20-	C79.2	D04.2-	D23.2-	D48.5	D49.2
- - os, cervix uteri	C53.1	C79.82	D06.1	D26.0	D39.0	D49.59
- extradural	C72.9	C79.49	-	D33.9	D43.9	D49.7
- extrahepatic (bile)duct	C24.0	C78.89	D01.5	D13.5	D37.6	D49.0
- - overlapping lesion with gallbladder	C24.8	-	-	-	-	-
- extraocular muscle	C69.6-	C79.49	D09.2-	D31.6-	D48.7	D49.89
- extra rectal	C76.3	C79.89	D09.8	D36.7	D48.7	D49.89
- extremity	C76.8	C79.89	D04.8	D36.7	D48.7	D49.89
- - lower	C76.5-	C79.89	D04.7-	D36.7	D48.7	D49.89
- - upper	C76.4-	C79.89	D04.6-	D36.7	D48.7	D49.89
- eye NEC	C69.9-	C79.49	D09.2	D31.9	D48.7	D49.89
- - overlapping sites	C69.8	-	-	-	-	-
- eyeball	C69.9-	C79.49	D09.2-	D31.9-	D48.7	D49.89
- eyebrow	C44.309	C79.2	D04.39	D23.39	D48.5	D49.2
- - basal cell carcinoma	C44.319	-	-	-	-	-
- - specified type NEC	C44.399	-	-	-	-	-
- - squamous cell carcinoma	C44.329	-	-	-	-	-
- eyelid (lower) (skin) (upper)	C44.10-	-	-	-	-	-
- - basal cell carcinoma	C44.11-	-	-	-	-	-
- - specified type NEC	C44.19-	-	-	-	-	-
- - squamous cell carcinoma	C44.12-	-	-	-	-	-
- - cartilage	C49.0	C79.89	-	D21.0	D48.1	D49.2
- face NEC	C76.0	C79.89	D04.39	D36.7	D48.7	D49.89
- fallopian tube (accessory)	C57.0-	C79.82	D07.39	D28.2	D39.8	D49.59
- falx (cerebella) (cerebri)	C70.0	C79.32	-	D32.0	D42.0	D49.7
- fascia—*see also Neoplasm, connective tissue*						
- - palmar	C49.1-	C79.89	-	D21.1-	D48.1	D49.2
- - plantar	C49.2-	C79.89	-	D21.2-	D48.1	D49.2
- fatty tissue—*see Neoplasm, connective tissue*						
- fauces, faucial NEC	C10.9	C79.89	D00.08	D10.5	D37.05	D49.0
- - pillars	C09.1	C79.89	D00.08	D10.5	D37.05	D49.0
- - tonsil	C09.9	C79.89	D00.08	D10.4	D37.05	D49.0
- femur (any part)	C40.2-	-	-	D16.2-	-	-
- fetal membrane	C58	C79.82	D07.0	D26.7	D39.2	D49.59
- fibrous tissue—*see Neoplasm, connective tissue*						
- fibula (any part)	C40.2-	C79.51	-	D16.2-	-	-

	Malignant Primary	Malignant Secondary	Ca in Situ	Benign	Uncertain Behavior	Unspecified Behavior
- filum terminale	C72.0	C79.49	-	D33.4	D43.4	D49.7
- finger NEC	C76.4-	C79.89	D04.6-	D36.7	D48.7	D49.89
- flank NEC	C76.8	C79.89	D04.5	D36.7	D48.7	D49.89
- follicle, nabothian	C53.0	C79.82	D06.0	D26.0	D39.0	D49.59
- foot NEC	C76.5-	C79.89	D04.7-	D36.7	D48.7	D49.89
- forearm NEC	C76.4-	C79.89	D04.6-	D36.7	D48.7	D49.89
- forehead (skin)	C44.309	C79.2	D04.39	D23.39	D48.5	D49.2
- - basal cell carcinoma	C44.319	-	-	-	-	-
- - specified type NEC	C44.399	-	-	-	-	-
- - squamous cell carcinoma	C44.329	-	-	-	-	-
- foreskin	C60.0	C79.82	D07.4	D29.0	D40.8	D49.59
- fornix						
- - pharyngeal	C11.3	C79.89	D00.08	D10.6	D37.05	D49.0
- - vagina	C52	C79.82	D07.2	D28.1	D39.8	D49.59
- fossa (of)						
- - anterior (cranial)	C71.9	C79.31	-	D33.2	D43.2	D49.6
- - cranial	C71.9	C79.31	-	D33.2	D43.2	D49.6
- - ischiorectal	C76.3	C79.89	D09.8	D36.7	D48.7	D49.89
- - middle (cranial)	C71.9	C79.31	-	D33.2	D43.2	D49.6
- - piriform	C12	C79.89	D00.08	D10.7	D37.05	D49.0
- - pituitary	C75.1	C79.89	D09.3	D35.2	D44.3	D49.7
- - posterior (cranial)	C71.9	C79.31	-	D33.2	D43.2	D49.6
- - pterygoid	C49.0	C79.89	-	D21.0	D48.1	D49.2
- - pyriform	C12	C79.89	D00.08	D10.7	D37.05	D49.0
- - Rosenmüller	C11.2	C79.89	D00.08	D10.6	D37.05	D49.0
- - tonsillar	C09.0	C79.89	D00.08	D10.5	D37.05	D49.0
- fourchette	C51.9	C79.82	D07.1	D28.0	D39.8	D49.59
- frenulum						
- - labii—*see Neoplasm, lip, internal*						
- - linguae	C02.2	C79.89	D00.07	D10.1	D37.02	D49.0
- frontal						
- - bone	C41.0	C79.51	-	D16.4-	D48.0	D49.2
- - lobe, brain	C71.1	C79.31	-	D33.0	D43.0	D49.6
- - pole	C71.1	C79.31	-	D33.0	D43.0	D49.6
- - sinus	C31.2	C78.39	D02.3	D14.0	D38.5	D49.1
- fundus						
- - stomach	C16.1	C78.89	D00.2	D13.1	D37.1	D49.0
- - uterus	C54.3	C79.82	D07.0	D26.1	D39.0	D49.59
- gall duct (extrahepatic)	C24.0	C78.89	D01.5	D13.5	D37.6	D49.0
- - intrahepatic	C22.1	C78.7	D01.5	D13.4	D37.6	D49.0
- gallbladder	C23	C78.89	D01.5	D13.5	D37.6	D49.0
- - overlapping lesion with extrahepatic bile ducts	C24.8	-	-	-	-	-
- ganglia—*see also Neoplasm, nerve, peripheral*	C47.9	C79.89	-	D36.10	D48.2	D49.2
- - basal	C71.0	C79.31	-	D33.0	D43.0	D49.6
- - cranial nerve	C72.50	C79.49	-	D33.3	D43.3	D49.7
- Gartner's duct	C52	C79.82	D07.2	D28.1	D39.8	D49.59
- gastric—*see Neoplasm, stomach*						
- gastrocolic	C26.9	C78.89	D01.9	D13.9	D37.9	D49.0
- gastroesophageal junction	C16.0	C78.89	D00.2	D13.1	D37.1	D49.0
- gastrointestinal (tract)NEC	C26.9	C78.89	D01.9	D13.9	D37.9	D49.0
- generalized	C80.0	-	-	-	-	-
- genital organ or tract						
- - female NEC	C57.9	C79.82	D07.30	D28.9	D39.9	D49.59
- - - overlapping lesion	C57.8	-	-	-	-	-
- - - specified site NEC	C57.7	C79.82	D07.39	D28.7	D39.8	D49.59
- - male NEC	C63.9	C79.82	D07.60	D29.9	D40.9	D49.59
- - - overlapping lesion	C63.8	-	-	-	-	-
- - - specified site NEC	C63.7	C79.82	D07.69	D29.8	D40.8	D49.59
- genitourinary tract						
- - female	C57.9	C79.82	D07.30	D28.9	D39.9	D49.59
- - male	C63.9	C79.82	D07.60	D29.9	D40.9	D49.59
- gingiva (alveolar) (marginal)	C03.9	C79.89	D00.03	D10.39	D37.09	D49.0
- - lower	C03.1	C79.89	D00.03	D10.39	D37.09	D49.0
- - mandibular	C03.1	C79.89	D00.03	D10.39	D37.09	D49.0
- - maxillary	C03.0	C79.89	D00.03	D10.39	D37.09	D49.0
- - upper	C03.0	C79.89	D00.03	D10.39	D37.09	D49.0
- gland, glandular (lymphatic) (system)—*see also Neoplasm, lymph gland*						

	Malignant Primary	Malignant Secondary	Ca in Situ	Benign	Uncertain Behavior	Unspecified Behavior
- - endocrine NEC	C75.9	C79.89	D09.3	D35.9	D44.9	D49.7
- - salivary—*see Neoplasm, salivary gland*						
- glans penis	C60.1	C79.82	D07.4	D29.0	D40.8	D49.59
- globus pallidus	C71.0	C79.31	-	D33.0	D43.0	D49.6
- glomus						
- - coccygeal	C49.5	C79.89	-	D21.5	D48.1	D49.2
- - jugularis	C75.5	C79.89	-	D35.6	D44.7	D49.7
- glosso-epiglottic fold (s)	C10.1	C79.89	D00.08	D10.5	D37.05	D49.0
- glossopalatine fold	C09.1	C79.89	D00.08	D10.5	D37.05	D49.0
- glossopharyngeal sulcus	C09.0	C79.89	D00.08	D10.5	D37.05	D49.0
- glottis	C32.0	C78.39	D02.0	D14.1	D38.0	D49.1
- gluteal region	C76.3	C79.89	D04.5	D36.7	D48.7	D49.89
- great vessels NEC	C49.3	C79.89	-	D21.3	D48.1	D49.2
- groin NEC	C76.3	C79.89	D04.5	D36.7	D48.7	D49.89
- gum	C03.9	C79.89	D00.03	D10.39	D37.09	D49.0
- - lower	C03.1	C79.89	D00.03	D10.39	D37.09	D49.0
- - upper	C03.0	C79.89	D00.03	D10.39	D37.09	D49.0
- hand NEC	C76.4-	C79.89	D04.6-	D36.7	D48.7	D49.89
- head NEC	C76.0	C79.89	D04.4	D36.7	D48.7	D49.89
- heart	C38.0	C79.89	-	D15.1	D48.7	D49.89
- heel NEC	C76.5-	C79.89	D04.7-	D36.7	D48.7	D49.89
- helix—*see also Neoplasm, skin, ear*	C44.20-	C79.2	D04.2-	D23.2-	D48.5	D49.2
- hematopoietic, hemopoietic tissue NEC	C96.9	-	-	-	-	-
- - specified NEC	C96.Z	-	-	-	-	-
- hemisphere, cerebral	C71.0	C79.31	-	D33.0	D43.0	D49.6
- hemorrhoidal zone	C21.1	C78.5	D01.3	D12.9	D37.8	D49.0
- hepatic—*see also Index to disease, by histology*	C22.9	C78.7	D01.5	D13.4	D37.6	D49.0
- - duct (bile)	C24.0	C78.89	D01.5	D13.5	D37.6	D49.0
- - flexure (colon)	C18.3	C78.5	D01.0	D12.3	D37.4	D49.0
- - primary	C22.8	C78.7	D01.5	D13.4	D37.6	D49.0
- hepatobiliary	C24.9	C78.89	D01.5	D13.5	D37.6	D49.0
- hepatoblastoma	C22.2	C78.7	D01.5	D13.4	D37.6	D49.0
- hepatoma	C22.0	C78.7	D01.5	D13.4	D37.6	D49.0
- hilus of lung	C34.0-	C78.0-	D02.2-	D14.3-	D38.1	D49.1
- hip NEC	C76.5-	C79.89	D04.7-	D36.7	D48.7	D49.89
- hippocampus, brain	C71.2	C79.31	-	D33.0	D43.0	D49.6
- humerus (any part)	C40.0-	C79.51	-	D16.0-	-	-
- hymen	C52	C79.82	D07.2	D28.1	D39.8	D49.59
- hypopharynx, hypopharyngeal NEC	C13.9	C79.89	D00.08	D10.7	D37.05	D49.0
- - overlapping lesion	C13.8	-	-	-	-	-
- - postcricoid region	C13.0	C79.89	D00.08	D10.7	D37.05	D49.0
- - posterior wall	C13.2	C79.89	D00.08	D10.7	D37.05	D49.0
- - pyriform fossa (sinus)	C12	C79.89	D00.08	D10.7	D37.05	D49.0
- hypophysis	C75.1	C79.89	D09.3	D35.2	D44.3	D49.7
- hypothalamus	C71.0	C79.31	-	D33.0	D43.0	D49.6
- ileocecum, ileocecal (coil) (junction) (valve)	C18.0	C78.5	D01.0	D12.0	D37.4	D49.0
- ileum	C17.2	C78.4	D01.49	D13.39	D37.2	D49.0
- ilium	C41.4	C79.51	-	D16.8	D48.0	D49.2
- immunoproliferative NEC	C88.9	-	-	-	-	-
- infraclavicular (region)	C76.1	C79.89	D04.5	D36.7	D48.7	D49.89
- inguinal (region)	C76.3	C79.89	D04.5	D36.7	D48.7	D49.89
- insula	C71.0	C79.31	-	D33.0	D43.0	D49.6
- insular tissue (pancreas)	C25.4	C78.89	D01.7	D13.7	D37.8	D49.0
- - brain	C71.0	C79.31	-	D33.0	D43.0	D49.6
- interarytenoid fold	C13.1	C79.89	D00.08	D10.7	D37.05	D49.0
- - hypopharyngeal aspect	C13.1	C79.89	D00.08	D10.7	D37.05	D49.0
- - laryngeal aspect	C32.1	C79.89	D02.0	D14.1	D38.0	D49.1
- - marginal zone	C13.1	C79.89	D00.08	D10.7	D37.05	D49.0
- interdental papillae	C03.9	C79.89	D00.03	D10.39	D37.09	D49.0
- - lower	C03.1	C79.89	D00.03	D10.39	D37.09	D49.0
- - upper	C03.0	C79.89	D00.03	D10.39	D37.09	D49.0
- internal						
- - capsule	C71.0	C79.31	-	D33.0	D43.0	D49.6
- - os (cervix)	C53.0	C79.82	D06.0	D26.0	D39.0	D49.59
- intervertebral cartilage or disc	C41.2	C79.51	-	D16.6	D48.0	D49.2
- intestine, intestinal	C26.0	C78.80	D01.40	D13.9	D37.8	D49.0
- - large	C18.9	C78.5	D01.0	D12.6	D37.4	D49.0

	Malignant Primary	Malignant Secondary	Ca in Situ	Benign	Uncertain Behavior	Unspecified Behavior
- - - appendix	C18.1	C78.5	D01.0	D12.1	D37.3	D49.0
- - - caput coli	C18.0	C78.5	D01.0	D12.0	D37.4	D49.0
- - - cecum	C18.0	C78.5	D01.0	D12.0	D37.4	D49.0
- - - colon	C18.9	C78.5	D01.0	D12.6	D37.4	D49.0
- - - - and rectum	C19	C78.5	D01.1	D12.7	D37.5	D49.0
- - - - ascending	C18.2	C78.5	D01.0	D12.2	D37.4	D49.0
- - - - caput	C18.0	C78.5	D01.0	D12.0	D37.4	D49.0
- - - - descending	C18.6	C78.5	D01.0	D12.4	D37.4	D49.0
- - - - distal	C18.6	C78.5	D01.0	D12.4	D37.4	D49.0
- - - - left	C18.6	C78.5	D01.0	D12.4	D37.4	D49.0
- - - - overlapping lesion	C18.8	-	-	-	-	-
- - - - pelvic	C18.7	C78.5	D01.0	D12.5	D37.4	D49.0
- - - - right	C18.2	C78.5	D01.0	D12.2	D37.4	D49.0
- - - - sigmoid (flexure)	C18.7	C78.5	D01.0	D12.5	D37.4	D49.0
- - - - transverse	C18.4	C78.5	D01.0	D12.3	D37.4	D49.0
- - - hepatic flexure	C18.3	C78.5	D01.0	D12.3	D37.4	D49.0
- - - ileocecum, ileocecal (coil) (valve)	C18.0	C78.5	D01.0	D12.0	D37.4	D49.0
- - - overlapping lesion	C18.8	-	-	-	-	-
- - - sigmoid flexure (lower) (upper)	C18.7	C78.5	D01.0	D12.5	D37.4	D49.0
- - - splenic flexure	C18.5	C78.5	D01.0	D12.3	D37.4	D49.0
- - small	C17.9	C78.4	D01.40	D13.30	D37.2	D49.0
- - - duodenum	C17.0	C78.4	D01.49	D13.2	D37.2	D49.0
- - - ileum	C17.2	C78.4	D01.49	D13.39	D37.2	D49.0
- - - jejunum	C17.1	C78.4	D01.49	D13.39	D37.2	D49.0
- - - overlapping lesion	C17.8	-	-	-	-	-
- - tract NEC	C26.0	C78.89	D01.40	D13.9	D37.8	D49.0
- intra-abdominal	C76.2	C79.89	D09.8	D36.7	D48.7	D49.89
- intracranial NEC	C71.9	C79.31	-	D33.2	D43.2	D49.6
- intrahepatic (bile)duct	C22.1	C78.7	D01.5	D13.4	D37.6	D49.0
- intraocular	C69.9-	C79.49	D09.2-	D31.9-	D48.7	D49.89
- intraorbital	C69.6-	C79.49	D09.2-	D31.6-	D48.7	D49.89
- intrasellar	C75.1	C79.89	D09.3	D35.2	D44.3	D49.7
- intrathoracic (cavity) (organs)	C76.1	C79.89	D09.8	D15.9	D48.7	D49.89
- - specified NEC	C76.1	C79.89	D09.8	D15.7	-	-
- iris	C69.4-	C79.49	D09.2-	D31.4-	D48.7	D49.89
- ischiorectal (fossa)	C76.3	C79.89	D09.8	D36.7	D48.7	D49.89
- ischium	C41.4	C79.51	-	D16.8	D48.0	D49.2
- island of Reil	C71.0	C79.31	-	D33.0	D43.0	D49.6
- islands or islets of Langerhans	C25.4	C78.89	D01.7	D13.7	D37.8	D49.0
- isthmus uteri	C54.0	C79.82	D07.0	D26.1	D39.0	D49.59
- jaw	C76.0	C79.89	D09.8	D36.7	D48.7	D49.89
- - bone	C41.1	C79.51	-	D16.5-	D48.0	D49.2
- - - lower	C41.1	C79.51	-	D16.5-	-	-
- - - upper	C41.0	C79.51	-	D16.4-	-	-
- - carcinoma (any type) (lower) (upper)	C76.0	C79.89	-	-	-	-
- - skin—see also Neoplasm, skin, face	C44.309	C79.2	D04.39	D23.39	D48.5	D49.2
- - soft tissues	C03.9	C79.89	D00.03	D10.39	D37.09	D49.0
- - - lower	C03.1	C79.89	D00.03	D10.39	D37.09	D49.0
- - - upper	C03.0	C79.89	D00.03	D10.39	D37.09	D49.0
- jejunum	C17.1	C78.4	D01.49	D13.39	D37.2	D49.0
- joint NEC—see also Neoplasm, bone	C41.9	C79.51	-	D16.9-	D48.0	D49.2
- - acromioclavicular	C40.0-	C79.51	-	D16.0-	-	-
- - bursa or synovial membrane—see Neoplasm, connective tissue						
- - costovertebral	C41.3	C79.51	-	D16.7	D48.0	D49.2
- - sternocostal	C41.3	C79.51	-	D16.7	D48.0	D49.2
- - temporomandibular	C41.1	C79.51	-	D16.5-	D48.0	D49.2
- junction						
- - anorectal	C21.8	C78.5	D01.3	D12.9	D37.8	D49.0
- - cardioesophageal	C16.0	C78.89	D00.2	D13.1	D37.1	D49.0
- - esophagogastric	C16.0	C78.89	D00.2	D13.1	D37.1	D49.0
- - gastroesophageal	C16.0	C78.89	D00.2	D13.1	D37.1	D49.0
- - hard and soft palate	C05.9	C79.89	D00.00	D10.39	D37.09	D49.0
- - ileocecal	C18.0	C78.5	D01.0	D12.0	D37.4	D49.0
- - pelvirectal	C19	C78.5	D01.1	D12.7	D37.5	D49.0
- - pelviureteric	C65.-	C79.0-	D09.19	D30.1-	D41.1-	D49.59
- - rectosigmoid	C19	C78.5	D01.1	D12.7	D37.5	D49.0
- - squamocolumnar, of cervix	C53.8	C79.82	D06.7	D26.0	D39.0	D49.59

	Malignant Primary	Malignant Secondary	Ca in Situ	Benign	Uncertain Behavior	Unspecified Behavior
- Kaposi's sarcoma—*see Kaposi's, sarcoma*						
- kidney (parenchymal)	C64.-	C79.0-	D09.19	D30.0-	D41.0-	D49.51
- - calyx	C65.-	C79.0-	D09.19	D30.1-	D41.1-	D49.51
- - hilus	C65.-	C79.0-	D09.19	D30.1-	D41.1-	D49.51
- - pelvis	C65.-	C79.0-	D09.19	D30.1-	D41.1-	D49.51
- knee NEC	C76.5-	C79.89	D04.7-	D36.7	D48.7	D49.89
- labia (skin)	C51.9	C79.82	D07.1	D28.0	D39.8	D49.59
- - majora	C51.0	C79.82	D07.1	D28.0	D39.8	D49.59
- - minora	C51.1	C79.82	D07.1	D28.0	D39.8	D49.59
- labial—*see also Neoplasm, lip*	C00.9	C79.89	D00.01	D10.0	D37.01	D49.0
- - sulcus (lower) (upper)	C06.1	C79.89	D00.02	D10.39	D37.09	D49.0
- labium (skin)	C51.9	C79.82	D07.1	D28.0	D39.8	D49.59
- - majus	C51.0	C79.82	D07.1	D28.0	D39.8	D49.59
- - minus	C51.1	C79.82	D07.1	D28.0	D39.8	D49.59
- lacrimal						
- - canaliculi	C69.5-	C79.49	D09.2-	D31.5-	D48.7	D49.89
- - duct (nasal)	C69.5-	C79.49	D09.2-	D31.5-	D48.7	D49.89
- - gland	C69.5-	C79.49	D09.2-	D31.5-	D48.7	D49.89
- - punctum	C69.5-	C79.49	D09.2-	D31.5-	D48.7	D49.89
- - sac	C69.5-	C79.49	D09.2-	D31.5-	D48.7	D49.89
- Langerhans, islands or islets	C25.4	C78.89	D01.7	D13.7	D37.8	D49.0
- laryngopharynx	C13.9	C79.89	D00.08	D10.7	D37.05	D49.0
- larynx, laryngeal NEC	C32.9	C78.39	D02.0	D14.1	D38.0	D49.1
- - aryepiglottic fold	C32.1	C78.39	D02.0	D14.1	D38.0	D49.1
- - cartilage (arytenoid) (cricoid) (cuneiform) (thyroid)	C32.3	C78.39	D02.0	D14.1	D38.0	D49.1
- - commissure (anterior) (posterior)	C32.0	C78.39	D02.0	D14.1	D38.0	D49.1
- - extrinsic NEC	C32.1	C78.39	D02.0	D14.1	D38.0	D49.1
- - - meaning hypopharynx	C13.9	C79.89	D00.08	D10.7	D37.05	D49.0
- - interarytenoid fold	C32.1	C78.39	D02.0	D14.1	D38.0	D49.1
- - intrinsic	C32.0	C78.39	D02.0	D14.1	D38.0	D49.1
- - overlapping lesion	C32.8	-	-	-	-	-
- - ventricular band	C32.1	C78.39	D02.0	D14.1	D38.0	D49.1
- leg NEC	C76.5-	C79.89	D04.7-	D36.7	D48.7	D49.89
- lens, crystalline	C69.4-	C79.49	D09.2-	D31.4-	D48.7	D49.89
- lid (lower) (upper)	C44.10-	C79.2	D04.1-	D23.1-	D48.5	D49.2
- - basal cell carcinoma	C44.11-	-	-	-	-	-
- - specified type NEC	C44.19-	-	-	-	-	-
- - squamous cell carcinoma	C44.12-	-	-	-	-	-
- ligament—*see also Neoplasm, connective tissue*						
- - broad	C57.1	C79.82	D07.39	D28.2	D39.8	D49.59
- - Mackenrodt's	C57.7	C79.82	D07.39	D28.7	D39.8	D49.59
- - non-uterine—*see Neoplasm, connective tissue*						
- - round	C57.2	C79.82	-	D28.2	D39.8	D49.59
- - sacro-uterine	C57.3	C79.82	-	D28.2	D39.8	D49.59
- - uterine	C57.3	C79.82	-	D28.2	D39.8	D49.59
- - utero-ovarian	C57.7	C79.82	D07.39	D28.2	D39.8	D49.59
- - uterosacral	C57.3	C79.82	-	D28.2	D39.8	D49.59
- limb	C76.8	C79.89	D04.8	D36.7	D48.7	D49.89
- - lower	C76.5-	C79.89	D04.7-	D36.7	D48.7	D49.89
- - upper	C76.4-	C79.89	D04.6-	D36.7	D48.7	D49.89
- limbus of cornea	C69.1-	C79.49	D09.2-	D31.1-	D48.7	D49.89
- lingual NEC—*see also Neoplasm, tongue*	C02.9	C79.89	D00.07	D10.1	D37.02	D49.0
- lingula, lung	C34.1-	C78.0-	D02.2-	D14.3-	D38.1	D49.1
- lip	C00.9	C79.89	D00.01	D10.0	D37.01	D49.0
- - buccal aspect—*see Neoplasm, lip, internal*						
- - commissure	C00.6	C79.89	D00.01	D10.0	D37.01	D49.0
- - external	C00.2	C79.89	D00.01	D10.0	D37.01	D49.0
- - - lower	C00.1	C79.89	D00.01	D10.0	D37.01	D49.0
- - - upper	C00.0	C79.89	D00.01	D10.0	D37.01	D49.0
- - frenulum—*see Neoplasm, lip, internal*						
- - inner aspect—*see Neoplasm, lip, internal*						
- - internal	C00.5	C79.89	D00.01	D10.0	D37.01	D49.0
- - - lower	C00.4	C79.89	D00.01	D10.0	D37.01	D49.0
- - - upper	C00.3	C79.89	D00.01	D10.0	D37.01	D49.0
- - lipstick area	C00.2	C79.89	D00.01	D10.0	D37.01	D49.0
- - - lower	C00.1	C79.89	D00.01	D10.0	D37.01	D49.0
- - - upper	C00.0	C79.89	D00.01	D10.0	D37.01	D49.0

	Malignant Primary	Malignant Secondary	Ca in Situ	Benign	Uncertain Behavior	Unspecified Behavior
- - lower	C00.1	C79.89	D00.01	D10.0	D37.01	D49.0
- - - internal	C00.4	C79.89	D00.01	D10.0	D37.01	D49.0
- - mucosa—*see Neoplasm, lip, internal*						
- - oral aspect—*see Neoplasm, lip, internal*						
- - overlapping lesion	C00.8	-	-	-	-	-
- - - with oral cavity or pharynx	C14.8	-	-	-	-	-
- - skin (commissure) (lower) (upper)	C44.00	C79.2	D04.0	D23.0	D48.5	D49.2
- - - basal cell carcinoma	C44.01	-				
- - - specified type NEC	C44.09	-	-	-	-	-
- - - squamous cell carcinoma	C44.02	-	-	-		
- - upper	C00.0	C79.89	D00.01	D10.0	D37.01	D49.0
- - - internal	C00.3	C79.89	D00.01	D10.0	D37.01	D49.0
- - vermilion border	C00.2	C79.89	D00.01	D10.0	D37.01	D49.0
- - - lower	C00.1	C79.89	D00.01	D10.0	D37.01	D49.0
- - - upper	C00.0	C79.89	D00.01	D10.0	D37.01	D49.0
- lipomatous—*see Lipoma, by site*						
- liver—*see also Index to disease, by histology*	C22.9	C78.7	D01.5	D13.4	D37.6	D49.0
- - primary	C22.8	C78.7	D01.5	D13.4	D37.6	D49.0
- lumbosacral plexus	C47.5	C79.89	-	D36.16	D48.2	D49.2
- lung	C34.9-	C78.0-	D02.2-	D14.3-	D38.1	D49.1
- - azygos lobe	C34.1-	C78.0-	D02.2-	D14.3-	D38.1	D49.1
- - carina	C34.0-	C78.0-	D02.2-	D14.3-	D38.1	D49.1
- - hilus	C34.0-	C78.0-	D02.2-	D14.3-	D38.1	D49.1
- - lingula	C34.1-	C78.0-	D02.2-	D14.3-	D38.1	D49.1
- - lobe NEC	C34.9-	C78.0-	D02.2-	D14.3-	D38.1	D49.1
- - lower lobe	C34.3-	C78.0-	D02.2-	D14.3-	D38.1	D49.1
- - main bronchus	C34.0-	C78.0-	D02.2-	D14.3-	D38.1	D49.1
- - mesothelioma—*see Mesothelioma*						
- - middle lobe	C34.2	C78.0-	D02.21	D14.31	D38.1	D49.1
- - overlapping lesion	C34.8-	-	-	-	-	-
- - upper lobe	C34.1-	C78.0-	D02.2-	D14.3-	D38.1	D49.1
- lymph, lymphatic channel NEC	C49.9	C79.89	-	D21.9	D48.1	D49.2
- - gland (secondary)	-	C77.9	-	D36.0	D48.7	D49.89
- - - abdominal	-	C77.2	-	D36.0	D48.7	D49.89
- - - aortic	-	C77.2	-	D36.0	D48.7	D49.89
- - - arm	-	C77.3	-	D36.0	D48.7	D49.89
- - - auricular (anterior) (posterior)	-	C77.0	-	D36.0	D48.7	D49.89
- - - axilla, axillary	-	C77.3	-	D36.0	D48.7	D49.89
- - - brachial	-	C77.3	-	D36.0	D48.7	D49.89
- - - bronchial	-	C77.1	-	D36.0	D48.7	D49.89
- - - bronchopulmonary	-	C77.1	-	D36.0	D48.7	D49.89
- - - celiac	-	C77.2	-	D36.0	D48.7	D49.89
- - - cervical	-	C77.0	-	D36.0	D48.7	D49.89
- - - cervicofacial	-	C77.0	-	D36.0	D48.7	D49.89
- - - Cloquet	-	C77.4	-	D36.0	D48.7	D49.89
- - - colic	-	C77.2	-	D36.0	D48.7	D49.89
- - - common duct	-	C77.2	-	D36.0	D48.7	D49.89
- - - cubital	-	C77.3	-	D36.0	D48.7	D49.89
- - - diaphragmatic	-	C77.1	-	D36.0	D48.7	D49.89
- - - epigastric, inferior	-	C77.1	-	D36.0	D48.7	D49.89
- - - epitrochlear	-	C77.3	-	D36.0	D48.7	D49.89
- - - esophageal	-	C77.1	-	D36.0	D48.7	D49.89
- - - face	-	C77.0	-	D36.0	D48.7	D49.89
- - - femoral	-	C77.4	-	D36.0	D48.7	D49.89
- - - gastric	-	C77.2	-	D36.0	D48.7	D49.89
- - - groin	-	C77.4	-	D36.0	D48.7	D49.89
- - - head	-	C77.0	-	D36.0	D48.7	D49.89
- - - hepatic	-	C77.2	-	D36.0	D48.7	D49.89
- - - hilar (pulmonary)	-	C77.1	-	D36.0	D48.7	D49.89
- - - - splenic	-	C77.2	-	D36.0	D48.7	D49.89
- - - hypogastric	-	C77.5	-	D36.0	D48.7	D49.89
- - - ileocolic	-	C77.2	-	D36.0	D48.7	D49.89
- - - iliac	-	C77.5	-	D36.0	D48.7	D49.89
- - - infraclavicular	-	C77.3	-	D36.0	D48.7	D49.89
- - - inguina, inguinal	-	C77.4	-	D36.0	D48.7	D49.89
- - - innominate	-	C77.1	-	D36.0	D48.7	D49.89
- - - intercostal	-	C77.1	-	D36.0	D48.7	D49.89
- - - intestinal	-	C77.2	-	D36.0	D48.7	D49.89

	Malignant Primary	Malignant Secondary	Ca in Situ	Benign	Uncertain Behavior	Unspecified Behavior
- - - intraabdominal	-	C77.2	-	D36.0	D48.7	D49.89
- - - intrapelvic	-	C77.5	-	D36.0	D48.7	D49.89
- - - intrathoracic	-	C77.1	-	D36.0	D48.7	D49.89
- - - jugular	-	C77.0	-	D36.0	D48.7	D49.89
- - - leg	-	C77.4	-	D36.0	D48.7	D49.89
- - - limb						
- - - - lower	-	C77.4	-	D36.0	D48.7	D49.89
- - - - upper	-	C77.3	-	D36.0	D48.7	D49.89
- - - lower limb	-	C77.4	-	D36.0	D48.7	D49.89
- - - lumbar	-	C77.2	-	D36.0	D48.7	D49.89
- - - mandibular	-	C77.0	-	D36.0	D48.7	D49.89
- - - mediastinal	-	C77.1	-	D36.0	D48.7	D49.89
- - - mesenteric (inferior) (superior)	-	C77.2	-	D36.0	D48.7	D49.89
- - - midcolic	-	C77.2	-	D36.0	D48.7	D49.89
- - - multiple sites in categories C77.0 - C77.5	-	C77.8	-	D36.0	D48.7	D49.89
- - - neck	-	C77.0	-	D36.0	D48.7	D49.89
- - - obturator	-	C77.5	-	D36.0	D48.7	D49.89
- - - occipital	-	C77.0	-	D36.0	D48.7	D49.89
- - - pancreatic	-	C77.2	-	D36.0	D48.7	D49.89
- - - para-aortic	-	C77.2	-	D36.0	D48.7	D49.89
- - - paracervical	-	C77.5	-	D36.0	D48.7	D49.89
- - - parametrial	-	C77.5	-	D36.0	D48.7	D49.89
- - - parasternal	-	C77.1	-	D36.0	D48.7	D49.89
- - - parotid	-	C77.0	-	D36.0	D48.7	D49.89
- - - pectoral	-	C77.3	-	D36.0	D48.7	D49.89
- - - pelvic	-	C77.5	-	D36.0	D48.7	D49.89
- - - peri-aortic	-	C77.2	-	D36.0	D48.7	D49.89
- - - peripancreatic	-	C77.2	-	D36.0	D48.7	D49.89
- - - popliteal	-	C77.4	-	D36.0	D48.7	D49.89
- - - porta hepatis	-	C77.2	-	D36.0	D48.7	D49.89
- - - portal	-	C77.2	-	D36.0	D48.7	D49.89
- - - preauricular	-	C77.0	-	D36.0	D48.7	D49.89
- - - prelaryngeal	-	C77.0	-	D36.0	D48.7	D49.89
- - - presymphysial	-	C77.5	-	D36.0	D48.7	D49.89
- - - pretracheal	-	C77.0	-	D36.0	D48.7	D49.89
- - - primary (any site)NEC	C96.9	-	-	-	-	-
- - - pulmonary (hiler)	-	C77.1	-	D36.0	D48.7	D49.89
- - - pyloric	-	C77.2	-	D36.0	D48.7	D49.89
- - - retroperitoneal	-	C77.2	-	D36.0	D48.7	D49.89
- - - retropharyngeal	-	C77.0	-	D36.0	D48.7	D49.89
- - - Rosenmüller's	-	C77.4	-	D36.0	D48.7	D49.89
- - - sacral	-	C77.5	-	D36.0	D48.7	D49.89
- - - scalene	-	C77.0	-	D36.0	D48.7	D49.89
- - - site NEC	-	C77.9	-	D36.0	D48.7	D49.89
- - - splenic (hilar)	-	C77.2	-	D36.0	D48.7	D49.89
- - - subclavicular	-	C77.3	-	D36.0	D48.7	D49.89
- - - subinguinal	-	C77.4	-	D36.0	D48.7	D49.89
- - - sublingual	-	C77.0	-	D36.0	D48.7	D49.89
- - - submandibular	-	C77.0	-	D36.0	D48.7	D49.89
- - - submaxillary	-	C77.0	-	D36.0	D48.7	D49.89
- - - submental	-	C77.0	-	D36.0	D48.7	D49.89
- - - subscapular	-	C77.3	-	D36.0	D48.7	D49.89
- - - supraclavicular	-	C77.0	-	D36.0	D48.7	D49.89
- - - thoracic	-	C77.1	-	D36.0	D48.7	D49.89
- - - tibial	-	C77.4	-	D36.0	D48.7	D49.89
- - - tracheal	-	C77.1	-	D36.0	D48.7	D49.89
- - - tracheobronchial	-	C77.1	-	D36.0	D48.7	D49.89
- - - upper limb	-	C77.3	-	D36.0	D48.7	D49.89
- - - Virchow's	-	C77.0	-	D36.0	D48.7	D49.89
- - node—*see also Neoplasm, lymph gland*						
- - - primary NEC	C96.9	-	-	-	-	-
- - vessel—*see also Neoplasm, connective tissue*	C49.9	C79.89	-	D21.9	D48.1	D49.2
- Mackenrodt's ligament	C57.7	C79.82	D07.39	D28.7	D39.8	D49.59
- malar	C41.0	C79.51	-	D16.4-	D48.0	D49.2
- - region—*see Neoplasm, cheek*						
- mammary gland—*see Neoplasm, breast*						
- mandible	C41.1	C79.51	-	D16.5-	D48.0	D49.2

	Malignant Primary	Malignant Secondary	Ca in Situ	Benign	Uncertain Behavior	Unspecified Behavior
- - alveolar						
- - - mucosa (carcinoma)	C03.1	C79.89	D00.03	D10.39	D37.09	D49.0
- - - ridge or process	C41.1	C79.51	-	D16.5-	D48.0	D49.2
- marrow (bone)NEC	C96.9	C79.52	-	-	D47.9	D49.89
- mastectomy site (skin)—*see also Neoplasm, breast, skin*	C44.501	C79.2	-	-	-	-
- - specified as breast tissue	C50.8-	C79.81	-	-	-	-
- mastoid (air cells) (antrum) (cavity)	C30.1	C78.39	D02.3	D14.0	D38.5	D49.1
- - bone or process	C41.0	C79.51	-	D16.4-	D48.0	D49.2
- maxilla, maxillary (superior)	C41.0	C79.51	-	D16.4-	D48.0	D49.2
- - alveolar						
- - - mucosa	C03.0	C79.89	D00.03	D10.39	D37.09	D49.0
- - - ridge or process (carcinoma)	C41.0	C79.51	-	D16.4-	D48.0	D49.2
- - antrum	C31.0	C78.39	D02.3	D14.0	D38.5	D49.1
- - carcinoma	C03.0	C79.51	-	-	-	-
- - inferior—*see Neoplasm, mandible*						
- - sinus	C31.0	C78.39	D02.3	D14.0	D38.5	D49.1
- meatus external (ear)—*see also Neoplasm, skin, ear*	C44.20-	C79.2	D04.2-	D23.2-	D48.5	D49.2
- Meckel diverticulum, malignant	C17.3	C78.4	D01.49	D13.39	D37.2	D49.0
- mediastinum, mediastinal	C38.3	C78.1	-	D15.2	D38.3	D49.89
- - anterior	C38.1	C78.1	-	D15.2	D38.3	D49.89
- - posterior	C38.2	C78.1	-	D15.2	D38.3	D49.89
- medulla						
- - adrenal	C74.1-	C79.7-	D09.3	D35.0-	D44.1-	D49.7
- - oblongata	C71.7	C79.31	-	D33.1	D43.1	D49.6
- meibomian gland	C44.10-	C79.2	D04.1-	D23.1-	D48.5	D49.2
- - basal cell carcinoma	C44.11-	-	-	-	-	-
- - specified type NEC	C44.19-	-	-	-	-	-
- - squamous cell carcinoma	C44.12-	-	-	-	-	-
- melanoma—*see Melanoma*						
- meninges	C70.9	C79.49	-	D32.9	D42.9	D49.7
- - brain	C70.0	C79.32	-	D32.0	D42.0	D49.7
- - cerebral	C70.0	C79.32	-	D32.0	D42.0	D49.7
- - cranial	C70.0	C79.32	-	D32.0	D42.0	D49.7
- - intracranial	C70.0	C79.32	-	D32.0	D42.0	D49.7
- - spinal (cord)	C70.1	C79.49	-	D32.1	D42.1	D49.7
- meniscus, knee joint (lateral) (medial)	C40.2-	C79.51	-	D16.2-	D48.0	D49.2
- Merkel cell—*see Carcinoma, Merkel cell*						
- mesentery, mesenteric	C48.1	C78.6	-	D20.1	D48.4	D49.0
- mesoappendix	C48.1	C78.6	-	D20.1	D48.4	D49.0
- mesocolon	C48.1	C78.6	-	D20.1	D48.4	D49.0
- mesopharynx—*see Neoplasm, oropharynx*						
- mesosalpinx	C57.1	C79.82	D07.39	D28.2	D39.8	D49.59
- mesothelial tissue—*see Mesothelioma*						
- mesothelioma—*see Mesothelioma*						
- mesovarium	C57.1	C79.82	D07.39	D28.2	D39.8	D49.59
- metacarpus (any bone)	C40.1-	C79.51	-	D16.1-	-	-
- metastatic NEC—*see also Neoplasm, by site, secondary*	-	C79.9	-	-	-	-
- metatarsus (any bone)	C40.3-	C79.51	-	D16.3-	-	-
- midbrain	C71.7	C79.31	-	D33.1	D43.1	D49.6
- milk duct—*see Neoplasm, breast*						
- mons	C51.9	C79.82	D07.1	D28.0	D39.8	D49.59
- - pubis	C51.9	C79.82	D07.1	D28.0	D39.8	D49.59
- - veneris	C72.9	C79.49	-	D33.9	D43.9	D49.7
- motor tract	C71.9	C79.31	-	D33.2	D43.2	D49.6
- - brain	C72.1	C79.49	-	D33.4	D43.4	D49.7
- - cauda equina	C72.0	C79.49	-	D33.4	D43.4	D49.7
- - spinal	C06.9	C79.89	D00.00	D10.30	D37.09	D49.0
- mouth	C06.89	C79.89	-	-	-	-
- - book-leaf	C04.9	C79.89	D00.06	D10.2	D37.09	D49.0
- - floor	C04.0	C79.89	D00.06	D10.2	D37.09	D49.0
- - - anterior portion	C04.1	C79.89	D00.06	D10.2	D37.09	D49.0
- - - lateral portion	C04.8	-	-	-	-	-
- - - overlapping lesion	C06.80	-	-	-	-	-
- - overlapping NEC	C05.9	C79.89	D00.00	D10.39	D37.09	D49.0
- - - roof	C06.89	C79.89	D00.00	D10.39	D37.09	D49.0
- - specified part NEC						

	Malignant Primary	Malignant Secondary	Ca in Situ	Benign	Uncertain Behavior	Unspecified Behavior
- - vestibule	C06.1	C79.89	D00.00	D10.39	D37.09	D49.0
- mucosa						
- - alveolar (ridge or process)	C03.9	C79.89	D00.03	D10.39	D37.09	D49.0
- - - lower	C03.1	C79.89	D00.03	D10.39	D37.09	D49.0
- - - upper	C03.0	C79.89	D00.03	D10.39	D37.09	D49.0
- - buccal	C06.0	C79.89	D00.02	D10.39	D37.09	D49.0
- - cheek	C06.0	C79.89	D00.02	D10.39	D37.09	D49.0
- - lip—see Neoplasm, lip, internal						
- - nasal	C30.0	C78.39	D02.3	D14.0	D38.5	D49.1
- - oral	C06.0	C79.89	D00.02	D10.39	D37.09	D49.0
- Mullerian duct						
- - female	C57.7	C79.82	D07.39	D28.7	D39.8	D49.59
- - male	C63.7	C79.82	D07.69	D29.8	D40.8	D49.59
- muscle—see also Neoplasm, connective tissue						
- - extraocular	C69.6-	C79.49	D09.2-	D31.6-	D48.7	D49.89
- myocardium	C38.0	C79.89	-	D15.1	D48.7	D49.89
- myometrium	C54.2	C79.82	D07.0	D26.1	D39.0	D49.59
- myopericardium	C38.0	C79.89	-	D15.1	D48.7	D49.89
- nabothian gland (follicle)	C53.0	C79.82	D06.0	D26.0	D39.0	D49.59
- nail—see also Neoplasm, skin, limb	C44.90	C79.2	D04.9	D23.9	D48.5	D49.2
- - finger—see also Neoplasm, skin, limb, upper	C44.60-	C79.2	D04.6-	D23.6-	D48.5	D49.2
- - toe—see also Neoplasm, skin, limb, lower	C44.70-	C79.2	D04.7-	D23.7-	D48.5	D49.2
- nares, naris (anterior) (posterior)	C30.0	C78.39	D02.3	D14.0	D38.5	D49.1
- nasal—see Neoplasm, nose						
- nasolabial groove—see also Neoplasm, skin, face	C44.309	C79.2	D04.39	D23.39	D48.5	D49.2
- nasolacrimal duct	C69.5-	C79.49	D09.2-	D31.5-	D48.7	D49.89
- nasopharynx, nasopharyngeal	C11.9	C79.89	D00.08	D10.6	D37.05	D49.0
- - floor	C11.3	C79.89	D00.08	D10.6	D37.05	D49.0
- - overlapping lesion	C11.8	-	-	-	-	-
- - roof	C11.0	C79.89	D00.08	D10.6	D37.05	D49.0
- - wall	C11.9	C79.89	D00.08	D10.6	D37.05	D49.0
- - - anterior	C11.3	C79.89	D00.08	D10.6	D37.05	D49.0
- - - lateral	C11.2	C79.89	D00.08	D10.6	D37.05	D49.0
- - - posterior	C11.1	C79.89	D00.08	D10.6	D37.05	D49.0
- - - superior	C11.0	C79.89	D00.08	D10.6	D37.05	D49.0
- nates—see also Neoplasm, skin, trunk	C44.509	C79.2	D04.5	D23.5	D48.5	D49.2
- neck NEC	C76.0	C79.89	D09.8	D36.7	D48.7	D49.89
- - skin	C44.40	-	-	-	-	-
- - - basal cell carcinoma	C44.41	-	-	-	-	-
- - - specified type NEC	C44.49	-	-	-	-	-
- - - squamous cell carcinoma	C44.42	-	-	-	-	-
- nerve (ganglion)	C47.9	C79.89	-	D36.10	D48.2	D49.2
- - abducens	C72.59	C79.49	-	D33.3	D43.3	D49.7
- - accessory (spinal)	C72.59	C79.49	-	D33.3	D43.3	D49.7
- - acoustic	C72.4-	C79.49	-	D33.3	D43.3	D49.7
- - auditory	C72.4-	C79.49	-	D33.3	D43.3	D49.7
- - autonomic NEC—see also Neoplasm, nerve, peripheral	C47.9	C79.89	-	D36.10	D48.2	D49.2
- - brachial	C47.1-	C79.89	-	D36.12	D48.2	D49.2
- - cranial	C72.50	C79.49	-	D33.3	D43.3	D49.7
- - - specified NEC	C72.59	C79.49	-	D33.3	D43.3	D49.7
- - facial	C72.59	C79.49	-	D33.3	D43.3	D49.7
- - femoral	C47.2-	C79.89	-	D36.13	D48.2	D49.2
- - ganglion NEC—see also Neoplasm, nerve, peripheral	C47.9	C79.89	-	D36.10	D48.2	D49.2
- - glossopharyngeal	C72.59	C79.49	-	D33.3	D43.3	D49.7
- - hypoglossal	C72.59	C79.49	-	D33.3	D43.3	D49.7
- - intercostal	C47.3	C79.89	-	D36.14	D48.2	D49.2
- - lumbar	C47.6	C79.89	-	D36.17	D48.2	D49.2
- - median	C47.1-	C79.89	-	D36.12	D48.2	D49.2
- - obturator	C47.2-	C79.89	-	D36.13	D48.2	D49.2
- - oculomotor	C72.59	C79.49	-	D33.3	D43.3	D49.7
- - olfactory	C47.2-	C79.49	-	D33.3	D43.3	D49.7
- - optic	C72.3-	C79.49	-	D33.3	D43.3	D49.7
- - parasympathetic NEC	C47.9	C79.89	-	D36.10	D48.2	D49.2
- - peripheral NEC	C47.9	C79.89	-	D36.10	D48.2	D49.2
- - - abdomen	C47.4	C79.89	-	D36.15	D48.2	D49.2

NEOPLASM TABLE

	Malignant Primary	Malignant Secondary	Ca in Situ	Benign	Uncertain Behavior	Unspecified Behavior
- - - abdominal wall	C47.4	C79.89	-	D36.15	D48.2	D49.2
- - - ankle	C47.2-	C79.89	-	D36.13	D48.2	D49.2
- - - antecubital fossa or space	C47.1-	C79.89	-	D36.12	D48.2	D49.2
- - - arm	C47.1-	C79.89	-	D36.12	D48.2	D49.2
- - - auricle (ear)	C47.0	C79.89	-	D36.11	D48.2	D49.2
- - - axilla	C47.3	C79.89	-	D36.12	D48.2	D49.2
- - - back	C47.6	C79.89	-	D36.17	D48.2	D49.2
- - - buttock	C47.5	C79.89	-	D36.16	D48.2	D49.2
- - - calf	C47.2-	C79.89	-	D36.13	D48.2	D49.2
- - - cervical region	C47.0	C79.89	-	D36.11	D48.2	D49.2
- - - cheek	C47.0	C79.89	-	D36.11	D48.2	D49.2
- - - chest (wall)	C47.3	C79.89	-	D36.14	D48.2	D49.2
- - - chin	C47.0	C79.89	-	D36.11	D48.2	D49.2
- - - ear (external)	C47.0	C79.89	-	D36.11	D48.2	D49.2
- - - elbow	C47.1-	C79.89	-	D36.12	D48.2	D49.2
- - - extra rectal	C47.5	C79.89	-	D36.16	D48.2	D49.2
- - - extremity	C47.9	C79.89	-	D36.10	D48.2	D49.2
- - - - lower	C47.2-	C79.89	-	D36.13	D48.2	D49.2
- - - - upper	C47.1-	C79.89	-	D36.12	D48.2	D49.2
- - - eyelid	C47.0	C79.89	-	D36.11	D48.2	D49.2
- - - face	C47.0	C79.89	-	D36.11	D48.2	D49.2
- - - finger	C47.1-	C79.89	-	D36.12	D48.2	D49.2
- - - flank	C47.6	C79.89	-	D36.17	D48.2	D49.2
- - - foot	C47.2-	C79.89	-	D36.13	D48.2	D49.2
- - - forearm	C47.1-	C79.89	-	D36.12	D48.2	D49.2
- - - forehead	C47.0	C79.89	-	D36.11	D48.2	D49.2
- - - gluteal region	C47.5	C79.89	-	D36.16	D48.2	D49.2
- - - groin	C47.5	C79.89	-	D36.16	D48.2	D49.2
- - - hand	C47.1-	C79.89	-	D36.12	D48.2	D49.2
- - - head	C47.0	C79.89	-	D36.11	D48.2	D49.2
- - - heel	C47.2-	C79.89	-	D36.13	D48.2	D49.2
- - - hip	C47.2-	C79.89	-	D36.13	D48.2	D49.2
- - - infraclavicular region	C47.3	C79.89	-	D36.14	D48.2	D49.2
- - - inguinal (canal) (region)	C47.5	C79.89	-	D36.16	D48.2	D49.2
- - - intrathoracic	C47.3	C79.89	-	D36.14	D48.2	D49.2
- - - ischiorectal fossa	C47.5	C79.89	-	D36.16	D48.2	D49.2
- - - knee	C47.2-	C79.89	-	D36.13	D48.2	D49.2
- - - leg	C47.2-	C79.89	-	D36.13	D48.2	D49.2
- - - limb NEC	C47.9	C79.89	-	D36.10	D48.2	D49.2
- - - - lower	C47.2-	C79.89	-	D36.13	D48.2	D49.2
- - - - upper	C47.1-	C79.89	-	D36.12	D48.2	D49.2
- - - nates	C47.5	C79.89	-	D36.16	D48.2	D49.2
- - - neck	C47.0	C79.89	-	D36.11	D48.2	D49.2
- - - orbit	C69.6-	C79.49	-	D31.6-	D48.7	D49.2
- - - pararectal	C47.5	C79.89	-	D36.16	D48.2	D49.2
- - - paraurethral	C47.5	C79.89	-	D36.16	D48.2	D49.2
- - - paravaginal	C47.5	C79.89	-	D36.16	D48.2	D49.2
- - - pelvis (floor)	C47.5	C79.89	-	D36.16	D48.2	D49.2
- - - pelvoabdominal	C47.8	C79.89	-	D36.17	D48.2	D49.2
- - - perineum	C47.5	C79.89	-	D36.16	D48.2	D49.2
- - - perirectal (tissue)	C47.5	C79.89	-	D36.16	D48.2	D49.2
- - - periurethral (tissue)	C47.5	C79.89	-	D36.16	D48.2	D49.2
- - - popliteal fossa or space	C47.2-	C79.89	-	D36.13	D48.2	D49.2
- - - presacral	C47.5	C79.89	-	D36.16	D48.2	D49.2
- - - pterygoid fossa	C47.0	C79.89	-	D36.11	D48.2	D49.2
- - - rectovaginal septum or wall	C47.5	C79.89	-	D36.16	D48.2	D49.2
- - - rectovesical	C47.5	C79.89	-	D36.16	D48.2	D49.2
- - - sacrococcygeal region	C47.5	C79.89	-	D36.16	D48.2	D49.2
- - - scalp	C47.0	C79.89	-	D36.11	D48.2	D49.2
- - - scapular region	C47.3	C79.89	-	D36.14	D48.2	D49.2
- - - shoulder	C47.1-	C79.89	-	D36.12	D48.2	D49.2
- - - submental	C47.0	C79.89	-	D36.11	D48.2	D49.2
- - - supraclavicular region	C47.0	C79.89	-	D36.11	D48.2	D49.2
- - - temple	C47.0	C79.89	-	D36.11	D48.2	D49.2
- - - temporal region	C47.0	C79.89	-	D36.11	D48.2	D49.2
- - - thigh	C47.2-	C79.89	-	D36.13	D48.2	D49.2
- - - thoracic (duct) (wall)	C47.3	C79.89	-	D36.14	D48.2	D49.2
- - - thorax	C47.3	C79.89	-	D36.14	D48.2	D49.2

	Malignant Primary	Malignant Secondary	Ca in Situ	Benign	Uncertain Behavior	Unspecified Behavior
- - - thumb	C47.1-	C79.89	-	D36.12	D48.2	D49.2
- - - toe	C47.2-	C79.89	-	D36.13	D48.2	D49.2
- - - trunk	C47.6	C79.89	-	D36.17	D48.2	D49.2
- - - umbilicus	C47.4	C79.89	-	D36.15	D48.2	D49.2
- - - vesicorectal	C47.5	C79.89	-	D36.16	D48.2	D49.2
- - - wrist	C47.1-	C79.89	-	D36.12	D48.2	D49.2
- - radial	C47.1-	C79.89	-	D36.12	D48.2	D49.2
- - sacral	C47.5	C79.89	-	D36.16	D48.2	D49.2
- - sciatic	C47.2-	C79.89	-	D36.13	D48.2	D49.2
- - spinal NEC	C47.9	C79.89	-	D36.10	D48.2	D49.2
- - - accessory	C72.59	C79.49	-	D33.3	D43.3	D49.7
- - sympathetic NEC—*see also Neoplasm, nerve, peripheral*	C47.9	C79.89	-	D36.10	D48.2	D49.2
- - trigeminal	C72.59	C79.49	-	D33.3	D43.3	D49.7
- - trochlear	C72.59	C79.49	-	D33.3	D43.3	D49.7
- - ulnar	C47.1-	C79.89	-	D36.12	D48.2	D49.2
- - vagus	C72.59	C79.49	-	D33.3	D43.3	D49.7
- nervous system (central)	C72.9	C79.40	-	D33.9	D43.9	D49.7
- - autonomic—*see Neoplasm, nerve, peripheral*						
- - parasympathetic—*see Neoplasm, nerve, peripheral*						
- - specified site NEC	-	C79.49	-	D33.7	D43.8	-
- - sympathetic—*see Neoplasm, nerve, peripheral*						
- nevus—*see Nevus*						
- nipple	C50.0-	C79.81	D05.-	D24.-	-	-
- nose, nasal	C76.0	C79.89	D09.8	D36.7	D48.7	D49.89
- - ala (external) (nasi)—*see also Neoplasm, nose, skin*	C44.301	C79.2	D04.39	D23.39	D48.5	D49.2
- - bone	C41.0	C79.51	-	D16.4-	D48.0	D49.2
- - cartilage	C30.0	C78.39	D02.3	D14.0	D38.5	D49.1
- - cavity	C30.0	C78.39	D02.3	D14.0	D38.5	D49.1
- -choana	C11.3	C79.89	D00.08	D10.6	D37.05	D49.0
- - external (skin)—*see also Neoplasm, nose, skin*	C44.301	C79.2	D04.39	D23.39	D48.5	D49.2
- - fossa	C30.0	C78.39	D02.3	D14.0	D38.5	D49.1
- - internal	C30.0	C78.39	D02.3	D14.0	D38.5	D49.1
- - mucosa	C30.0	C78.39	D02.3	D14.0	D38.5	D49.1
- - septum	C30.0	C78.39	D02.3	D14.0	D38.5	D49.1
- - - posterior margin	C11.3	C79.89	D00.08	D10.6	D37.05	D49.0
- - sinus—*see Neoplasm, sinus*						
- - skin	C44.301	C79.2	D04.39	D23.39	D48.5	D49.2
- - - basal cell carcinoma	C44.311	-	-	-	-	-
- - - specified type NEC	C44.391	-	-	-	-	-
- - - squamous cell carcinoma	C44.321	-	-	-	-	-
- - turbinate (mucosa)	C30.0	C78.39	D02.3	D14.0	D38.5	D49.1
- - - bone	C41.0	C79.51	-	D16.4-	D48.0	D49.2
- - vestibule	C30.0	C78.39	D02.3	D14.0	D38.5	D49.1
- nostril	C30.0	C78.39	D02.3	D14.0	D38.5	D49.1
- nucleus pulposus	C41.2	C79.51	-	D16.6	D48.0	D49.2
- occipital						
- - bone	C41.0	C79.51	-	D16.4-	D48.0	D49.2
- - lobe or pole, brain	C71.4	C79.31	-	D33.0	D43.0	D49.6
- odontogenic—*see Neoplasm, jaw bone*						
- olfactory nerve or bulb	C72.2-	C79.49	-	D33.3	D43.3	D49.7
- olive (brain)	C71.7	C79.31	-	D33.1	D43.1	D49.6
- omentum	C48.1	C78.6	-	D20.1	D48.4	D49.0
- operculum (brain)	C71.0	C79.31	-	D33.0	D43.0	D49.6
- optic nerve, chiasm, or tract	C72.3-	C79.49	-	D33.3	D43.3	D49.7
- oral (cavity)	C06.9	C79.89	D00.00	D10.30	D37.09	D49.0
- - ill-defined	C14.8	C79.89	D00.00	D10.30	D37.09	D49.0
- - mucosa	C06.0	C79.89	D00.02	D10.39	D37.09	D49.0
- orbit	C69.6-	C79.49	D09.2-	D31.6-	D48.7	D49.89
- - autonomic nerve	C69.6-	C79.49	-	D31.6-	D48.7	D49.2
- - bone	C41.0	C79.51	-	D16.4-	D48.0	D49.2
- - eye	C69.6-	C79.49	D09.2-	D31.6-	D48.7	D49.89
- - peripheral nerves	C69.6-	C79.49	-	D31.6-	D48.7	D49.2
- - soft parts	C69.6-	C79.49	D09.2-	D31.6-	D48.7	D49.89
- organ of Zuckerkandl	C75.5	C79.89	-	D35.6	D44.7	D49.7
- oropharynx	C10.9	C79.89	D00.08	D10.5	D37.05	D49.0

	Malignant Primary	Malignant Secondary	Ca in Situ	Benign	Uncertain Behavior	Unspecified Behavior
- - branchial cleft (vestige)	C10.4	C79.89	D00.08	D10.5	D37.05	D49.0
- - junctional region	C10.8	C79.89	D00.08	D10.5	D37.05	D49.0
- - lateral wall	C10.2	C79.89	D00.08	D10.5	D37.05	D49.0
- - overlapping lesion	C10.8	-	-	-	-	-
- - pillars or fauces	C09.1	C79.89	D00.08	D10.5	D37.05	D49.0
- - posterior wall	C10.3	C79.89	D00.08	D10.5	D37.05	D49.0
- - vallecula	C10.0	C79.89	D00.08	D10.5	D37.05	D49.0
- os						
- - external	C53.1	C79.82	D06.1	D26.0	D39.0	D49.59
- - internal	C53.0	C79.82	D06.0	D26.0	D39.0	D49.59
- ovary	C56.-	C79.6-	D07.39	D27.-	D39.1-	D49.59
- oviduct	C57.0-	C79.82	D07.39	D28.2	D39.8	D49.59
- palate	C05.9	C79.89	D00.00	D10.39	D37.09	D49.0
- - hard	C05.0	C79.89	D00.05	D10.39	D37.09	D49.0
- junction of hard and soft palate	C05.9	C79.89	D00.00	D10.39	D37.09	D49.0
- - overlapping lesions	C05.8	-	-	-	-	-
- - soft	C05.1	C79.89	D00.04	D10.39	D37.09	D49.0
- - - nasopharyngeal surface	C11.3	C79.89	D00.08	D10.6	D37.05	D49.0
- - - posterior surface	C11.3	C79.89	D00.08	D10.6	D37.05	D49.0
- - - superior surface	C11.3	C79.89	D00.08	D10.6	D37.05	D49.0
- palatoglossal arch	C09.1	C79.89	D00.00	D10.5	D37.09	D49.0
- palatopharyngeal arch	C09.1	C79.89	D00.00	D10.5	D37.09	D49.0
- pallium	C71.0	C79.31	-	D33.0	D43.0	D49.6
- palpebra	C44.10-	C79.2	D04.1-	D23.1-	D48.5	D49.2
- - basal cell carcinoma	C44.11-	-	-	-	-	-
- - specified type NEC	C44.19-	-	-	-	-	-
- - squamous cell carcinoma	C44.12-	-	-	-	-	-
- pancreas	C25.9	C78.89	D01.7	D13.6	D37.8	D49.0
- - body	C25.1	C78.89	D01.7	D13.6	D37.8	D49.0
- - duct (of Santorini) (of Wirsung)	C25.3	C78.89	D01.7	D13.6	D37.8	D49.0
- - ectopic tissue	C25.7	C78.89	-	D13.6	D37.8	D49.0
- - head	C25.0	C78.89	D01.7	D13.6	D37.8	D49.0
- - islet cells	C25.4	C78.89	D01.7	D13.7	D37.8	D49.0
- - neck	C25.7	C78.89	D01.7	D13.6	D37.8	D49.0
- - overlapping lesion	C25.8	-	-	-	-	-
- - tail	C25.2	C78.89	D01.7	D13.6	D37.8	D49.0
- para-aortic body	C75.5	C79.89	-	D35.6	D44.7	D49.7
- paraganglion NEC	C75.5	C79.89	-	D35.6	D44.7	D49.7
- parametrium	C57.3	C79.82	-	D28.2	D39.8	D49.59
- paranephric	C48.0	C78.6	-	D20.0	D48.3	D49.0
- pararectal	C76.3	C79.89	-	D36.7	D48.7	D49.89
- parasagittal (region)	C76.0	C79.89	D09.8	D36.7	D48.7	D49.89
- parasellar	C72.9	C79.49	-	D33.9	D43.8	D49.7
- parathyroid (gland)	C75.0	C79.89	D09.3	D35.1	D44.2	D49.7
- paraurethral	C76.3	C79.89	-	D36.7	D48.7	D49.89
- - gland	C68.1	C79.19	D09.19	D30.8	D41.8	D49.59
- paravaginal	C76.3	C79.89	-	D36.7	D48.7	D49.89
- parenchyma, kidney	C64.-	C79.0-	D09.19	D30.0-	D41.0-	D49.59
- parietal						
- - bone	C41.0	C79.51	-	D16.4-	D48.0	D49.2
- - lobe, brain	C71.3	C79.31	-	D33.0	D43.0	D49.6
- paroophoron	C57.1	C79.82	D07.39	D28.2	D39.8	D49.59
- parotid (duct) (gland)	C07	C79.89	D00.00	D11.0	D37.030	D49.0
- parovarium	C57.1	C79.82	D07.39	D28.2	D39.8	D49.59
- patella	C40.20	C79.51	-	-	-	-
- peduncle, cerebral	C71.7	C79.31	-	D33.1	D43.1	D49.6
- pelvirectal junction	C19	C78.5	D01.1	D12.7	D37.5	D49.0
- pelvis, pelvic	C76.3	C79.89	D09.8	D36.7	D48.7	D49.89
- - bone	C41.4	C79.51	-	D16.8	D48.0	D49.2
- - floor	C76.3	C79.89	D09.8	D36.7	D48.7	D49.89
- - renal	C65.-	C79.0-	D09.19	D30.1-	D41.1-	D49.59
- - viscera	C76.3	C79.89	D09.8	D36.7	D48.7	D49.89
- - wall	C76.3	C79.89	D09.8	D36.7	D48.7	D49.89
- pelvo-abdominal	C76.8	C79.89	D09.8	D36.7	D48.7	D49.89
- penis	C60.9	C79.82	D07.4	D29.0	D40.8	D49.59
- - body	C60.2	C79.82	D07.4	D29.0	D40.8	D49.59
- - corpus (cavernosum)	C60.2	C79.82	D07.4	D29.0	D40.8	D49.59
- - glans	C60.1	C79.82	D07.4	D29.0	D40.8	D49.59

	Malignant Primary	Malignant Secondary	Ca in Situ	Benign	Uncertain Behavior	Unspecified Behavior
- - overlapping sites	C60.8	-	-	-	-	-
- - skin NEC	C60.9	C79.82	D07.4	D29.0	D40.8	D49.59
- periadrenal (tissue)	C48.0	C78.6	-	D20.0	D48.3	D49.0
- perianal (skin)—*see also Neoplasm, anus, skin*	C44.500	C79.2	D04.5	D23.5	D48.5	D49.2
- pericardium	C38.0	C79.89	-	D15.1	D48.7	D49.89
- perinephric	C48.0	C78.6	-	D20.0	D48.3	D49.0
- perineum	C76.3	C79.89	D09.8	D36.7	D48.7	D49.89
- periodontal tissue NEC	C03.9	C79.89	D00.03	D10.39	D37.09	D49.0
- periosteum—*see Neoplasm, bone*						
- peripancreatic	C48.0	C78.6	-	D20.0	D48.3	D49.0
- peripheral nerve NEC	C47.9	C79.89	-	D36.10	D48.2	D49.2
- perirectal (tissue)	C76.3	C79.89	-	D36.7	D48.7	D49.89
- perirenal (tissue)	C48.0	C78.6	-	D20.0	D48.3	D49.0
- peritoneum, peritoneal (cavity)	C48.2	C78.6	-	D20.1	D48.4	D49.0
- - benign mesothelial tissue—*see Mesothelioma, benign*						
- - overlapping lesion	C48.8	-	-	-	-	-
- - - with digestive organs	C26.9	-	-	-	-	-
- - parietal	C48.1	C78.6	-	D20.1	D48.4	D49.0
- - pelvic	C48.1	C78.6	-	D20.1	D48.4	D49.0
- - specified part NEC	C48.1	C78.6	-	D20.1	D48.4	D49.0
- peritonsillar (tissue)	C76.0	C79.89	D09.8	D36.7	D48.7	D49.89
- periurethral tissue	C76.3	C79.89	-	D36.7	D48.7	D49.89
- phalanges						
- - foot	C40.3-	C79.51	-	D16.3-	-	-
- - hand	C40.1-	C79.51	-	D16.1-	-	-
- pharynx, pharyngeal	C14.0	C79.89	D00.08	D10.9	D37.05	D49.0
- - bursa	C11.1	C79.89	D00.08	D10.6	D37.05	D49.0
- - fornix	C11.3	C79.89	D00.08	D10.6	D37.05	D49.0
- - recess	C11.2	C79.89	D00.08	D10.6	D37.05	D49.0
- - region	C14.0	C79.89	D00.08	D10.9	D37.05	D49.0
- - tonsil	C11.1	C79.89	D00.08	D10.6	D37.05	D49.0
- - wall (lateral) (posterior)	C14.0	C79.89	D00.08	D10.9	D37.05	D49.0
- pia mater	C70.9	C79.40	-	D32.9	D42.9	D49.7
- - cerebral	C70.0	C79.32	-	D32.0	D42.0	D49.7
- - cranial	C70.0	C79.32	-	D32.0	D42.0	D49.7
- - spinal	C70.1	C79.49	-	D32.1	D42.1	D49.7
- pillars of fauces	C09.1	C79.89	D00.08	D10.5	D37.05	D49.0
- pineal (body) (gland)	C75.3	C79.89	D09.3	D35.4	D44.5	D49.7
- pinna (ear)NEC—*see also Neoplasm, skin, ear*	C44.20-	C79.2	D04.2-	D23.2-	D48.5	D49.2
- piriform fossa or sinus	C12	C79.89	D00.08	D10.7	D37.05	D49.0
- pituitary (body) (fossa) (gland) (lobe)	C75.1	C79.89	D09.3	D35.2	D44.3	D49.7
- placenta	C58	C79.82	D07.0	D26.7	D39.2	D49.59
- pleura, pleural (cavity)	C38.4	C78.2	-	D19.0	D38.2	D49.1
- - overlapping lesion with heart or mediastinum	C38.8	-	-	-	-	-
- - parietal	C38.4	C78.2	-	D19.0	D38.2	D49.1
- - visceral	C38.4	C78.2	-	D19.0	D38.2	D49.1
- plexus						
- - brachial	C47.1-	C79.89	-	D36.12	D48.2	D49.2
- - cervical	C47.0	C79.89	-	D36.11	D48.2	D49.2
- - choroid	C71.5	C79.31	-	D33.0	D43.0	D49.6
- - lumbosacral	C47.5	C79.89	-	D36.16	D48.2	D49.2
- - sacral	C47.5	C79.89	-	D36.16	D48.2	D49.2
- pluriendocrine	C75.8	C79.89	D09.3	D35.7	D44.9	D49.7
- pole						
- - frontal	C71.1	C79.31	-	D33.0	D43.0	D49.6
- - occipital	C71.4	C79.31	-	D33.0	D43.0	D49.6
- pons (varolii)	C71.7	C79.31	-	D33.1	D43.1	D49.6
- popliteal fossa or space	C76.5-	C79.89	D04.7-	D36.7	D48.7	D49.89
- postcricoid (region)	C13.0	C79.89	D00.08	D10.7	D37.05	D49.0
- posterior fossa (cranial)	C71.9	C79.31	-	D33.2	D43.2	D49.6
- postnasal space	C11.9	C79.89	D00.08	D10.6	D37.05	D49.0
- prepuce	C60.0	C79.82	D07.4	D29.0	D40.8	D49.59
- prepylorus	C16.4	C78.89	D00.2	D13.1	D37.1	D49.0
- presacral (region)	C76.3	C79.89	-	D36.7	D48.7	D49.89
- prostate (gland)	C61	C79.82	D07.5	D29.1	D40.0	D49.59
- - utricle	C68.0	C79.19	D09.19	D30.4	D41.3	D49.59

NEOPLASM TABLE

	Malignant Primary	Malignant Secondary	Ca in Situ	Benign	Uncertain Behavior	Unspecified Behavior
- pterygoid fossa	C49.0	C79.89	-	D21.0	D48.1	D49.2
- pubic bone	C41.4	C79.51	-	D16.8	D48.0	D49.2
- pudenda, pudendum (female)	C51.9	C79.82	D07.1	D28.0	D39.8	D49.59
- pulmonary—see also Neoplasm, lung	C34.9-	C78.0-	D02.2-	D14.3-	D38.1	D49.1
- putamen	C71.0	C79.31	-	D33.0	D43.0	D49.6
- pyloric						
- - antrum	C16.3	C78.89	D00.2	D13.1	D37.1	D49.0
- - canal	C16.4	C78.89	D00.2	D13.1	D37.1	D49.0
- pylorus	C16.4	C78.89	D00.2	D13.1	D37.1	D49.0
- pyramid (brain)	C71.7	C79.31	-	D33.1	D43.1	D49.6
- pyriform fossa or sinus	C12	C79.89	D00.08	D10.7	D37.05	D49.0
- radius (any part)	C40.0-	C79.51	-	D16.0-	-	D49.7
- Rathke's pouch	C75.1	C79.89	D09.3	D35.2	D44.3	D49.0
- rectosigmoid (junction)	C19	C78.5	D01.1	D12.7	D37.5	D49.0
- - overlapping lesion with anus or rectum	C21.8	-	-	-	-	-
- rectouterine pouch	C48.1	C78.6		D20.1	D48.4	D49.0
- rectovaginal septum or wall	C76.3	C79.89	D09.8	D36.7	D48.7	D49.89
- rectovesical septum	C76.3	C79.89	D09.8	D36.7	D48.7	D49.0
- rectum (ampulla)	C20	C78.5	D01.2	D12.8	D37.5	D49.0
- - and colon	C19	C78.5	D01.1	D12.7	D37.5	-
- - overlapping lesion with anus or rectosigmoid junction	C21.8	-	-	-	-	-
- renal	C64.-	C79.0-	D09.19	D30.0-	D41.0-	D49.51
- - calyx	C65.-	C79.0-	D09.19	D30.1-	D41.1-	D49.51
- - hilus	C65.-	C79.0-	D09.19	D30.1-	D41.1-	D49.51
- - parenchyma	C64.-	C79.0-	D09.19	D30.0-	D41.0-	D49.51
- - pelvis	C65.-	C79.0-	D09.19	D30.1-	D41.1-	D49.51
- respiratory						
- - organs or system NEC	C39.9	C78.30	D02.4	D14.4	D38.6	D49.1
- - tract NEC	C39.9	C78.30	D02.4	D14.4	D38.5	D49.1
- - - upper	C39.0	C78.30	D02.4	D14.4	D38.5	D49.1
- retina	C69.2-	C79.49	D09.2-	D31.2-	D48.7	D49.81
- retrobulbar	C69.6-	C79.49	-	D31.6-	D48.7	D49.89
- retrocecal	C48.0	C78.6	-	D20.0	D48.3	D49.0
- retromolar (area) (triangle) (trigone)	C06.2	C79.89	D00.00	D10.39	D37.09	D49.0
- retro-orbital	C76.0	C79.89	D09.8	D36.7	D48.7	D49.89
- retroperitoneal (space) (tissue)	C48.0	C78.6	-	D20.0	D48.3	D49.0
- retroperitoneum	C48.0	C78.6	-	D20.0	D48.3	D49.0
- retropharyngeal	C14.0	C79.89	D00.08	D10.9	D37.05	D49.0
- retrovesical (septum)	C76.3	C79.89	D09.8	D36.7	D48.7	D49.89
- rhinencephalon	C71.0	C79.31	-	D33.0	D43.0	D49.6
- rib	C41.3	C79.51	-	D16.7	D48.0	D49.2
- Rosenmüller's fossa	C11.2	C79.89	D00.08	D10.6	D37.05	D49.0
- round ligament	C57.2	C79.82	-	D28.2	D39.8	D49.59
- sacrococcyx, sacrococcygeal	C41.4	C79.51		D16.8	D48.0	D49.2
- - region	C76.3	C79.89	D09.8	D36.7	D48.7	D49.89
- sacrouterine ligament	C57.3	C79.82	-	D28.2	D39.8	D49.59
- sacrum, sacral (vertebra)	C41.4	C79.51	-	D16.8	D48.0	D49.2
- salivary gland or duct (major)	C08.9	C79.89	D00.00	D11.9	D37.039	D49.0
- - minor NEC	C06.9	C79.89	D00.00	D10.39	D37.04	D49.0
- - overlapping lesion	C08.9	-	-	-	-	-
- - parotid	C07	C79.89	D00.00	D11.0	D37.030	D49.0
- - pluriglandular	C08.9	C79.89	D00.00	D11.9	D37.039	D49.0
- - sublingual	C08.1	C79.89	D00.00	D11.7	D37.031	D49.0
- - submandibular	C08.0	C79.89	D00.00	D11.7	D37.032	D49.0
- - submaxillary	C08.0	C79.89	D00.00	D11.7	D37.032	D49.0
- salpinx (uterine)	C57.0-	C79.82	D07.39	D28.2	D39.8	D49.59
- Santorini's duct	C25.3	C78.89	D01.7	D13.6	D37.8	D49.0
- scalp	C44.40	C79.2	D04.4	D23.4	D48.5	D49.2
- - basal cell carcinoma	C44.41	-	-	-	-	-
- - specified type NEC	C44.49	-	-	-	-	-
- - squamous cell carcinoma	C44.42	-	-	-	-	-
- scapula (any part)	C40.0-	C79.51	-	D16.0-	-	-
- scapular region	C76.1	C79.89	D09.8	D36.7	D48.7	D49.89
- scar NEC—see also Neoplasm, skin, by site	C44.90	C79.2	D04.9	D23.9	D48.5	D49.2
- sciatic nerve	C47.2-	C79.89	-	D36.13	D48.2	D49.2
- sclera	C69.4-	C79.49	D09.2-	D31.4-	D48.7	D49.89
- scrotum (skin)	C63.2	C79.82	D07.61	D29.4	D40.8	D49.59

	Malignant Primary	Malignant Secondary	Ca in Situ	Benign	Uncertain Behavior	Unspecified Behavior
- sebaceous gland—*see Neoplasm, skin*						
- sella turcica	C75.1	C79.89	D09.3	D35.2	D44.3	D49.7
- - bone	C41.0	C79.51	-	D16.4-	D48.0	D49.2
- semilunar cartilage (knee)	C40.2-	C79.51	-	D16.2-	D48.0	D49.2
- seminal vesicle	C63.7	C79.82	D07.69	D29.8	D40.8	D49.59
- septum						
- - nasal	C30.0	C78.39	D02.3	D14.0	D38.5	D49.1
- - - posterior margin	C11.3	C79.89	D00.08	D10.6	D37.05	D49.0
- - rectovaginal	C76.3	C79.89	D09.8	D36.7	D48.7	D49.89
- - rectovesical	C76.3	C79.89	D09.8	D36.7	D48.7	D49.89
- - urethrovaginal	C57.9	C79.82	D07.30	D28.9	D39.9	D49.59
- - vesicovaginal	C57.9	C79.82	D07.30	D28.9	D39.9	D49.59
- shoulder NEC	C76.4-	C79.89	D04.6-	D36.7	D48.7	D49.89
- sigmoid flexure (lower) (upper)	C18.7	C78.5	D01.0	D12.5	D37.4	D49.0
- sinus (accessory)	C31.9	C78.39	D02.3	D14.0	D38.5	D49.1
- - bone (any)	C41.0	C79.51	-	D16.4-	D48.0	D49.2
- - ethmoidal	C31.1	C78.39	D02.3	D14.0	D38.5	D49.1
- - frontal	C31.2	C78.39	D02.3	D14.0	D38.5	D49.1
- - maxillary	C31.0	C78.39	D02.3	D14.0	D38.5	D49.1
- - nasal, paranasal NEC	C31.9	C78.39	D02.3	D14.0	D38.5	D49.1
- - overlapping lesion	C31.8	-	-	-	-	-
- - pyriform	C12	C79.89	D00.08	D10.7	D37.05	D49.0
- - sphenoid	C31.3	C78.39	D02.3	D14.0	D38.5	D49.1
- skeleton, skeletal NEC	C41.9	C79.51	-	D16.9-	D48.0	D49.2
- Skene's gland	C68.1	C79.19	D09.19	D30.8	D41.8	D49.59
- skin NOS	C44.90	C79.2	D04.9	D23.9	D48.5	D49.2
- - abdominal wall	C44.509	C79.2	D04.5	D23.5	D48.5	D49.2
- - - basal cell carcinoma	C44.519	-	-	-	-	-
- - - specified type NEC	C44.599	-	-	-	-	-
- - - squamous cell carcinoma	C44.529	-	-	-	-	-
- - ala nasi—*see also Neoplasm, nose, skin*	C44.301	C79.2	D04.39	D23.39	D48.5	D49.2
- - ankle—*see also Neoplasm, skin, limb, lower*	C44.70-	C79.2	D04.7-	D23.7-	D48.5	D49.2
- - antecubital space—*see also Neoplasm, skin, limb, upper*	C44.60-	C79.2	D04.6-	D23.6-	D48.5	D49.2
- - anus	C44.500	C79.2	D04.5	D23.5	D48.5	D49.2
- - - basal cell carcinoma	C44.510	-	-	-	-	-
- - - specified type NEC	C44.590	-	-	-	-	-
- - - squamous cell carcinoma	C44.520	-	-	-	-	-
- - arm—*see also Neoplasm, skin, limb, upper*	C44.60-	C79.2	D04.6-	D23.6-	D48.5	D49.2
- - auditory canal (external)—*see also Neoplasm, skin, ear*	C44.20-	C79.2	D04.2-	D23.2-	D48.5	D49.2
- - auricle (ear)—*see also Neoplasm, skin, ear*	C44.20-	C79.2	D04.2-	D23.2-	D48.5	D49.2
- - auricular canal (external)—*see also Neoplasm, skin, ear*	C44.20-	C79.2	D04.2-	D23.2-	D48.5	D49.2
- - axilla, axillary fold—*see also Neoplasm, skin, trunk*	C44.509	C79.2	D04.5	D23.5	D48.5	D49.2
- - back—*see also Neoplasm, skin, trunk*	C44.509	C79.2	D04.5	D23.5	D48.5	D49.2
- - basal cell carcinoma	C44.91					
- - breast	C44.501	C79.2	D04.5	D23.5	D48.5	D49.2
- - - basal cell carcinoma	C44.511	-	-	-	-	-
- - - specified type NEC	C44.591	-	-	-	-	-
- - - squamous cell carcinoma	C44.521	-	-	-	-	-
- - brow—*see also Neoplasm, skin, face*	C44.309	C79.2	D04.39	D23.39	D48.5	D49.2
- - buttock—*see also Neoplasm, skin, trunk*	C44.509	C79.2	D04.5	D23.5	D48.5	D49.2
- - calf—*see also Neoplasm, skin, limb, lower*	C44.70-	C79.2	D04.7-	D23.7-	D48.5	D49.2
- - canthus (eye) (inner) (outer)	C44.10-	C79.2	D04.1-	D23.1-	D48.5	D49.2
- - - basal cell carcinoma	C44.11-	-	-	-	-	-
- - - specified type NEC	C44.19-	-	-	-	-	-
- - - squamous cell carcinoma	C44.12-	-	-	-	-	-
- - cervical region—*see also Neoplasm, skin, neck*	C44.40	C79.2	D04.4	D23.4	D48.5	D49.2
- - cheek (external)—*see also Neoplasm, skin, face*	C44.309	C79.2	D04.39	D23.39	D48.5	D49.2
- - chest (wall)—*see also Neoplasm, skin, trunk*	C44.509	C79.2	D04.5	D23.5	D48.5	D49.2
- - chin—*see also Neoplasm, skin, face*	C44.309	C79.2	D04.39	D23.39	D48.5	D49.2
- - clavicular area—*see also Neoplasm, skin, trunk*	C44.509	C79.2	D04.5	D23.5	D48.5	D49.2
- - clitoris	C51.2	C79.82	D07.1	D28.0	D39.8	D49.59
- - columnella—*see also Neoplasm, skin, face*	C44.309	C79.2	D04.39	D23.39	D48.5	D49.2
- - concha—*see also Neoplasm, skin, ear*	C44.20-	C79.2	D04.2-	D23.2-	D48.5	D49.2

	Malignant Primary	Malignant Secondary	Ca in Situ	Benign	Uncertain Behavior	Unspecified Behavior
- - ear (external)	C44.20-	C79.2	D04.2-	D23.2-	D48.5	D49.2
- - - basal cell carcinoma	C44.21-	-	-	-	-	-
- - - specified type NEC	C44.29-	-	-	-	-	-
- - - squamous cell carcinoma	C44.22-	-	-	-	-	-
- - elbow—*see also Neoplasm, skin, limb, upper*	C44.60-	C79.2	D04.6-	D23.6-	D48.5	D49.2
- - eyebrow—*see also Neoplasm, skin, face*	C44.309	C79.2	D04.39	D23.39	D48.5	D49.2
- - eyelid	C44.10-	C79.2	D04.1-	D23.1-	D48.5	D49.2
- - - basal cell carcinoma	C44.11-	-	-	-	-	-
- - - specified type NEC	C44.19-	-	-	-	-	-
- - - squamous cell carcinoma	C44.12-	-	-	-	-	-
- - face NOS	C44.300	C79.2	D04.30	D23.30	D48.5	D49.2
- - - basal cell carcinoma	C44.310	-	-	-	-	-
- - - specified type NEC	C44.390	-	-	-	-	-
- - - squamous cell carcinoma	C44.320	-	-	-	-	-
- - female genital organs (external)	C51.9	C79.82	D07.1	D28.0	D39.8	D49.59
- - - clitoris	C51.2	C79.82	D07.1	D28.0	D39.8	D49.59
- - - labium NEC	C51.9	C79.82	D07.1	D28.0	D39.8	D49.59
- - - - majus	C51.0	C79.82	D07.1	D28.0	D39.8	D49.59
- - - - minus	C51.1	C79.82	D07.1	D28.0	D39.8	D49.59
- - - pudendum	C51.9	C79.82	D07.1	D28.0	D39.8	D49.59
- - - vulva	C51.9	C79.82	D07.1	D28.0	D39.8	D49.59
- - finger—*see also Neoplasm, skin, limb, upper*	C44.60-	C79.2	D04.6-	D23.6-	D48.5	D49.2
- - flank—*see also Neoplasm, skin, trunk*	C44.509	C79.2	D04.5	D23.5	D48.5	D49.2
- - foot—*see also Neoplasm, skin, limb, lower*	C44.70-	C79.2	D04.7-	D23.7-	D48.5	D49.2
- - forearm—*see also Neoplasm, skin, limb, upper*	C44.60-	C79.2	D04.6-	D23.6-	D48.5	D49.2
- - forehead—*see also Neoplasm, skin, face*	C44.309	C79.2	D04.39	D23.39	D48.5	D49.2
- - glabella—*see also Neoplasm, skin, face*	C44.309	C79.2	D04.39	D23.39	D48.5	D49.2
- - gluteal region—*see also Neoplasm, skin, trunk*	C44.509	C79.2	D04.5	D23.5	D48.5	D49.2
- - groin—*see also Neoplasm, skin, trunk*	C44.509	C79.2	D04.5	D23.5	D48.5	D49.2
- - hand—*see also Neoplasm, skin, limb, upper*	C44.60-	C79.2	D04.6-	D23.6-	D48.5	D49.2
- - head NEC—*see also Neoplasm, skin, scalp*	C44.40	C79.2	D04.4	D23.4	D48.5	D49.2
- - heel—*see also Neoplasm, skin, limb, lower*	C44.70-	C79.2	D04.7-	D23.7-	D48.5	D49.2
- - helix—*see also Neoplasm, skin, ear*	C44.20-	C79.2	D04.2-	D23.2-	D48.5	D49.2
- - hip—*see also Neoplasm, skin, limb, lower*	C44.70-	C79.2	D04.7-	D23.7-	D48.5	D49.2
- - infraclavicular region—*see also Neoplasm, skin, trunk*	C44.509	C79.2	D04.5	D23.5	D48.5	D49.2
- - inguinal region—*see also Neoplasm, skin, trunk*	C44.509	C79.2	D04.5	D23.5	D48.5	D49.2
- - jaw—*see also Neoplasm, skin, face*	C44.309	C79.2	D04.39	D23.39	D48.5	D49.2
- - Kaposi's sarcoma—*see Kaposi's, sarcoma, skin*						
- - knee—*see also Neoplasm, skin, limb, lower*	C44.70-	C79.2	D04.7-	D23.7-	D48.5	D49.2
- - labia						
- - - majora	C51.0	C79.82	D07.1	D28.0	D39.8	D49.59
- - - minora	C51.1	C79.82	D07.1	D28.0	D39.8	D49.59
- - leg—*see also Neoplasm, skin, limb, lower*	C44.70-	C79.2	D04.7-	D23.7-	D48.5	D49.2
- - lid (lower) (upper)	C44.10-	C79.2	D04.1-	D23.1-	D48.5	D49.2
- - - basal cell carcinoma	C44.11-	-	-	-	-	-
- - - specified type NEC	C44.19-	-	-	-	-	-
- - - squamous cell carcinoma	C44.12-	-	-	-	-	-
- - limb NEC	C44.90	C79.2	D04.9	D23.9	D48.5	D49.2
- - - basal cell carcinoma	C44.91					
- - - lower	C44.70-	C79.2	D04.7-	D23.7-	D48.5	D49.2
- - - - basal cell carcinoma	C44.71-	-	-	-	-	-
- - - - specified type NEC	C44.79-	-	-	-	-	-
- - - - squamous cell carcinoma	C44.72-	-	-	-	-	-
- - - upper	C44.60-	C79.2	D04.6-	D23.6-	D48.5	D49.2
- - - - basal cell carcinoma	C44.61-	-	-	-	-	-
- - - - specified type NEC	C44.69-	-	-	-	-	-
- - - - squamous cell carcinoma	C44.62-	-	-	-	-	-
- - lip (lower) (upper)	C44.00	C79.2	D04.0	D23.0	D48.5	D49.2
- - - basal cell carcinoma	C44.01	-	-	-	-	-
- - - specified type NEC	C44.09	-	-	-	-	-
- - - squamous cell carcinoma	C44.02	-	-	-	-	-
- - male genital organs	C63.9	C79.82	D07.60	D29.9	D40.8	D49.59
- - - penis	C60.9	C79.82	D07.4	D29.0	D40.8	D49.59
- - - prepuce	C60.0	C79.82	D07.4	D29.0	D40.8	D49.59
- - - scrotum	C63.2	C79.82	D07.61	D29.4	D40.8	D49.59
- - mastectomy site (skin)—*see also Neoplasm, skin, breast*	C44.501	C79.2	-	-	-	-

	Malignant Primary	Malignant Secondary	Ca in Situ	Benign	Uncertain Behavior	Unspecified Behavior
- - - specified as breast tissue	C50.8-	C79.81	-	-	-	-
- - meatus, acoustic (external)—*see also Neoplasm, skin, ear*	C44.20-	C79.2	D04.2-	D23.2-	D48.5	D49.2
- - melanotic—*see Melanoma*						
- - Merkel cell—*see Carcinoma, Merkel cell*						
- - nates—*see also Neoplasm, skin, trunk*	C44.509	C79.2	D04.5	D23.5	D48.5	D49.2
- - neck	C44.40	C79.2	D04.4	D23.4	D48.5	D49.2
- - - basal cell carcinoma	C44.41	-	-	-	-	-
- - - specified type NEC	C44.49	-	-	-	-	-
- - - squamous cell carcinoma	C44.42	-	-	-	-	-
- - nevus—*see Nevus, skin*						
- - nose (external)—*see also Neoplasm, nose, skin*	C44.301	C79.2	D04.39	D23.39	D48.5	D49.2
- - overlapping lesion	C44.80	-	-	-	-	-
- - - basal cell carcinoma	C44.81	-	-	-	-	-
- - - specified type NEC	C44.89	-	-	-	-	-
- - - squamous cell carcinoma	C44.82	-	-	-	-	-
- - palm—*see also Neoplasm, skin, limb, upper*	C44.60-	C79.2	D04.6-	D23.6-	D48.5	D49.2
- - palpebra	C44.10-	C79.2	D04.1-	D23.1-	D48.5	D49.2
- - - basal cell carcinoma	C44.11-	-	-	-	-	-
- - - specified type NEC	C44.19-	-	-	-	-	-
- - - squamous cell carcinoma	C44.12-	-	-	-	-	-
- - penis NEC	C60.9	C79.82	D07.4	D29.0	D40.8	D49.59
- - perianal—*see also Neoplasm, skin, anus*	C44.500	C79.2	D04.5	D23.5	D48.5	D49.2
- - perineum—*see also Neoplasm, skin, anus*	C44.500	C79.2	D04.5	D23.5	D48.5	D49.2
- - pinna—*see also Neoplasm, skin, ear*	C44.20-	C79.2	D04.2-	D23.2-	D48.5	D49.2
- - plantar—*see also Neoplasm, skin, limb, lower*	C44.70-	C79.2	D04.7-	D23.7-	D48.5	D49.2
- - popliteal fossa or space—*see also Neoplasm, skin, limb, lower*	C44.70-	C79.2	D04.7-	D23.7-	D48.5	D49.2
- - prepuce	C60.0	C79.82	D07.4	D29.0	D40.8	D49.59
- - pubes—*see also Neoplasm, skin, trunk*	C44.509	C79.2	D04.5	D23.5	D48.5	D49.2
- - sacrococcygeal region—*see also Neoplasm, skin, trunk*	C44.509	C79.2	D04.5	D23.5	D48.5	D49.2
- - scalp	C44.40	C79.2	D04.4	D23.4	D48.5	D49.2
- - - basal cell carcinoma	C44.41	-	-	-	-	-
- - - specified type NEC	C44.49	-	-	-	-	-
- - - squamous cell carcinoma	C44.42	-	-	-	-	-
- - scapular region—*see also Neoplasm, skin, trunk*	C44.509	C79.2	D04.5	D23.5	D48.5	D49.2
- - scrotum	C63.2	C79.82	D07.61	D29.4	D40.8	D49.59
- - shoulder—*see also Neoplasm, skin, limb, upper*	C44.60-	C79.2	D04.6-	D23.6-	D48.5	D49.2
- - sole (foot)—*see also Neoplasm, skin, limb, lower*	C44.70-	C79.2	D04.7-	D23.7-	D48.5	D49.2
- - specified sites NEC	C44.80	C79.2	D04.8	D23.9	D48.5	D49.2
- - - basal cell carcinoma	C44.81	-	-	-	-	-
- - - specified type NEC	C44.89	-	-	-	-	-
- - - squamous cell carcinoma	C44.82	-	-	-	-	-
- - specified type NEC	C44.99	-	-	-	-	-
- - squamous cell carcinoma	C44.92	-	-	-	-	-
- - submammary fold—*see also Neoplasm, skin, trunk*	C44.509	C79.2	D04.5	D23.5	D48.5	D49.2
- - supraclavicular region—*see also Neoplasm, skin, neck*	C44.40	C79.2	D04.4	D23.4	D48.5	D49.2
- - temple—*see also Neoplasm, skin, face*	C44.309	C79.2	D04.39	D23.39	D48.5	D49.2
- - thigh—*see also Neoplasm, skin, limb, lower*	C44.70-	C79.2	D04.7-	D23.7-	D48.5	D49.2
- - thoracic wall—*see also Neoplasm, skin, trunk*	C44.509	C79.2	D04.5	D23.5	D48.5	D49.2
- - thumb—*see also Neoplasm, skin, limb, upper*	C44.60-	C79.2	D04.6-	D23.6-	D48.5	D49.2
- - toe—*see also Neoplasm, skin, limb, lower*	C44.70-	C79.2	D04.7-	D23.7-	D48.5	D49.2
- - tragus—*see also Neoplasm, skin, ear*	C44.20-	C79.2	D04.2-	D23.2-	D48.5	D49.2
- - trunk	C44.509	C79.2	D04.5	D23.5	D48.5	D49.2
- - - basal cell carcinoma	C44.519	-	-	-	-	-
- - - specified type NEC	C44.599	-	-	-	-	-
- - - squamous cell carcinoma	C44.529	-	-	-	-	-
- - umbilicus—*see also Neoplasm, skin, trunk*	C44.509	C79.2	D04.5	D23.5	D48.5	D49.2
- - vulva	C51.9	C79.82	D07.1	D28.0	D39.8	D49.59
- - - overlapping lesion	C51.8	-	-	-	-	-
- - wrist—*see also Neoplasm, skin, limb, upper*	C44.60-	C79.2	D04.6-	D23.6-	D48.5	D49.2
- skull	C41.0	C79.51	-	D16.4-	D48.0	D49.2
- soft parts or tissues—*see Neoplasm, connective tissue*						
- specified site NEC	C76.8	C79.89	D09.8	D36.7	D48.7	D49.89
- spermatic cord	C63.1-	C79.82	D07.69	D29.8	D40.8	D49.59

	Malignant Primary	Malignant Secondary	Ca in Situ	Benign	Uncertain Behavior	Unspecified Behavior
- sphenoid	C31.3	C78.39	D02.3	D14.0	D38.5	D49.1
- - bone	C41.0	C79.51	-	D16.4-	D48.0	D49.2
- - sinus	C31.3	C78.39	D02.3	D14.0	D38.5	D49.1
- sphincter						
- - anal	C21.1	C78.5	D01.3	D12.9	D37.8	D49.0
- - of Oddi	C24.0	C78.89	D01.5	D13.5	D37.6	D49.0
- spine, spinal (column)	C41.2	C79.51	-	D16.6	D48.0	D49.2
- - bulb	C71.7	C79.31	-	D33.1	D43.1	D49.6
- - coccyx	C41.4	C79.51	-	D16.8	D48.0	D49.2
- - cord (cervical) (lumbar) (sacral) (thoracic)	C72.0	C79.49	-	D33.4	D43.4	D49.7
- - dura mater	C70.1	C79.49	-	D32.1	D42.1	D49.7
- - lumbosacral	C41.2	C79.51	-	D16.6	D48.0	D49.2
- - marrow NEC	C96.9	C79.52	-	-	D47.9	D49.89
- - membrane	C70.1	C79.49	-	D32.1	D42.1	D49.7
- - meninges	C70.1	C79.49	-	D32.1	D42.1	D49.7
- - nerve (root)	C47.9	C79.89	-	D36.10	D48.2	D49.2
- - pia mater	C70.1	C79.49	-	D32.1	D42.1	D49.7
- - root	C47.9	C79.89	-	D36.10	D48.2	D49.2
- - sacrum	C41.4	C79.51	-	D16.8	D48.0	D49.2
- spleen, splenic NEC	C26.1	C78.89	D01.7	D13.9	D37.8	D49.0
- - flexure (colon)	C18.5	C78.5	D01.0	D12.3	D37.4	D49.0
- stem, brain	C71.7	C79.31	-	D33.1	D43.1	D49.6
- Stensen's duct	C07	C79.89	D00.00	D11.0	D37.030	D49.0
- sternum	C41.3	C79.51	-	D16.7	D48.0	D49.2
- stomach	C16.9	C78.89	D00.2	D13.1	D37.1	D49.0
- - antrum (pyloric)	C16.3	C78.89	D00.2	D13.1	D37.1	D49.0
- - body	C16.2	C78.89	D00.2	D13.1	D37.1	D49.0
- - cardia	C16.0	C78.89	D00.2	D13.1	D37.1	D49.0
- - cardiac orifice	C16.0	C78.89	D00.2	D13.1	D37.1	D49.0
- - corpus	C16.2	C78.89	D00.2	D13.1	D37.1	D49.0
- - fundus	C16.1	C78.89	D00.2	D13.1	D37.1	D49.0
- - greater curvature NEC	C16.6	C78.89	D00.2	D13.1	D37.1	D49.0
- - lesser curvature NEC	C16.5	C78.89	D00.2	D13.1	D37.1	D49.0
- - overlapping lesion	C16.8	-	-	-	-	-
- - prepylorus	C16.4	C78.89	D00.2	D13.1	D37.1	D49.0
- - pylorus	C16.4	C78.89	D00.2	D13.1	D37.1	D49.0
- - wall NEC	C16.9	C78.89	D00.2	D13.1	D37.1	D49.0
- - - anterior NEC	C16.8	C78.89	D00.2	D13.1	D37.1	D49.0
- - - posterior NEC	C16.8	C78.89	D00.2	D13.1	D37.1	D49.0
- stroma, endometrial	C54.1	C79.82	D07.0	D26.1	D39.0	D49.59
- stump, cervical	C53.8	C79.82	D06.7	D26.0	D39.0	D49.59
- subcutaneous (nodule) (tissue)NEC—see Neoplasm, connective tissue						
- subdural	C70.9	C79.32	-	D32.9	D42.9	D49.7
- subglottis, subglottic	C32.2	C78.39	D02.0	D14.1	D38.0	D49.1
- sublingual	C04.9	C79.89	D00.06	D10.2	D37.09	D49.0
- - gland or duct	C08.1	C79.89	D00.00	D11.7	D37.031	D49.0
- submandibular gland	C08.0	C79.89	D00.00	D11.7	D37.032	D49.0
- submaxillary gland or duct	C08.0	C79.89	D00.00	D11.7	D37.032	D49.0
- submental	C76.0	C79.89	D09.8	D36.7	D48.7	D49.89
- subpleural	C34.9-	C78.0-	D02.2-	D14.3-	D38.1	D49.1
- substernal	C38.1	C78.1	-	D15.2	D38.3	D49.89
- sudoriferous, sudoriparous gland, site unspecified	C44.90	C79.2	D04.9	D23.9	D48.5	D49.2
- - specified site—see Neoplasm, skin						
- supraclavicular region	C76.0	C79.89	D09.8	D36.7	D48.7	D49.89
- supraglottis	C32.1	C78.39	D02.0	D14.1	D38.0	D49.1
- suprarenal	C74.9-	C79.7-	D09.3	D35.0-	D44.1-	D49.7
- - capsule	C74.9-	C79.7-	D09.3	D35.0-	D44.1-	D49.7
- - cortex	C74.0-	C79.7-	D09.3	D35.0-	D44.1-	D49.7
- - gland	C74.9-	C79.7-	D09.3	D35.0-	D44.1-	D49.7
- - medulla	C74.1-	C79.7-	D09.3	D35.0-	D44.1-	D49.7
- suprasellar (region)	C71.9	C79.31	-	D33.2	D43.2	D49.6
- supratentorial (brain)NEC	C71.0	C79.31	-	D33.0	D43.0	D49.6
- sweat gland (apocrine) (eccrine), site unspecified	C44.90	C79.2	D04.9	D23.9	D48.5	D49.2
- - specified site—see Neoplasm, skin						
- sympathetic nerve or nervous system NEC	C47.9	C79.89	-	D36.10	D48.2	D49.2
- symphysis pubis	C41.4	C79.51	-	D16.8	D48.0	D49.2
- synovial membrane—see Neoplasm, connective						

	Malignant Primary	Malignant Secondary	Ca in Situ	Benign	Uncertain Behavior	Unspecified Behavior
tissue						
- tapetum, brain	C71.8	C79.31	-	D33.2	D43.2	D49.6
- tarsus (any bone)	C40.3-	C79.51	-	D16.3-	-	-
- temple (skin)—*see also Neoplasm, skin, face*	C44.309	C79.2	D04.39	D23.39	D48.5	D49.2
- temporal						
- - bone	C41.0	C79.51	-	D16.4-	D48.0	D49.2
- - lobe or pole	C71.2	C79.31	-	D33.0	D43.0	D49.6
- - - region	C76.0	C79.89	D09.8	D36.7	D48.7	D49.89
- - - - skin—*see also Neoplasm, skin, face*	C44.309	C79.2	D04.39	D23.39	D48.5	D49.2
- tendon (sheath)—*see Neoplasm, connective tissue*						
- tentorium (cerebelli)	C70.0	C79.32	-	D32.0	D42.0	D49.7
- testis, testes	C62.9-	C79.82	D07.69	D29.2-	D40.1-	D49.59
- - descended	C62.1-	C79.82	D07.69	D29.2-	D40.1-	D49.59
- - ectopic	C62.0-	C79.82	D07.69	D29.2-	D40.1-	D49.59
- - retained	C62.0-	C79.82	D07.69	D29.2-	D40.1-	D49.59
- - scrotal	C62.1-	C79.82	D07.69	D29.2-	D40.1-	D49.59
- - undescended	C62.0-	C79.82	D07.69	D29.2-	D40.1-	D49.59
- - unspecified whether descended or undescended	C62.9-	C79.82	D07.69	D29.2-	D40.1-	D49.59
- thalamus	C71.0	C79.31	-	D33.0	D43.0	D49.6
- thigh NEC	C76.5-	C79.89	D04.7-	D36.7	D48.7	D49.89
- thorax, thoracic (cavity) (organs NEC)	C76.1	C79.89	D09.8	D36.7	D48.7	D49.89
- - duct	C49.3	C79.89	-	D21.3	D48.1	D49.2
- - wall NEC	C76.1	C79.89	D09.8	D36.7	D48.7	D49.89
- throat	C14.0	C79.89	D00.08	D10.9	D37.05	D49.0
- thumb NEC	C76.4-	C79.89	D04.6-	D36.7	D48.7	D49.89
- thymus (gland)	C37	C79.89	D09.3	D15.0	D38.4	D49.89
- thyroglossal duct	C73	C79.89	D09.3	D34	D44.0	D49.7
- thyroid (gland)	C73	C79.89	D09.3	D34	D44.0	D49.7
- - cartilage	C32.3	C78.39	D02.0	D14.1	D38.0	D49.1
- tibia (any part)	C40.2-	C79.51	-	D16.2-	-	-
- toe NEC	C76.5-	C79.89	D04.7-	D36.7	D48.7	D49.89
- tongue	C02.9	C79.89	D00.07	D10.1	D37.02	D49.0
- - anterior (two-thirds)NEC	C02.3	C79.89	D00.07	D10.1	D37.02	D49.0
- - - dorsal surface	C02.0	C79.89	D00.07	D10.1	D37.02	D49.0
- - - ventral surface	C02.2	C79.89	D00.07	D10.1	D37.02	D49.0
- - base (dorsal surface)	C01	C79.89	D00.07	D10.1	D37.02	D49.0
- - border (lateral)	C02.1	C79.89	D00.07	D10.1	D37.02	D49.0
- - dorsal surface NEC	C02.0	C79.89	D00.07	D10.1	D37.02	D49.0
- - fixed part NEC	C01	C79.89	D00.07	D10.1	D37.02	D49.0
- - foramen cecum	C02.0	C79.89	D00.07	D10.1	D37.02	D49.0
- - frenulum linguae	C02.2	C79.89	D00.07	D10.1	D37.02	D49.0
- - junctional zone	C02.8	C79.89	D00.07	D10.1	D37.02	D49.0
- - margin (lateral)	C02.1	C79.89	D00.07	D10.1	D37.02	D49.0
- - midline NEC	C02.0	C79.89	D00.07	D10.1	D37.02	D49.0
- - mobile part NEC	C02.3	C79.89	D00.07	D10.1	D37.02	D49.0
- - overlapping lesion	C02.8	-	-	-	-	-
- - posterior (third)	C01	C79.89	D00.07	D10.1	D37.02	D49.0
- - root	C01	C79.89	D00.07	D10.1	D37.02	D49.0
- - surface (dorsal)	C02.0	C79.89	D00.07	D10.1	D37.02	D49.0
- - - base	C01	C79.89	D00.07	D10.1	D37.02	D49.0
- - - ventral	C02.2	C79.89	D00.07	D10.1	D37.02	D49.0
- - tip	C02.1	C79.89	D00.07	D10.1	D37.02	D49.0
- - tonsil	C02.4	C79.89	D00.07	D10.1	D37.02	D49.0
- tonsil	C09.9	C79.89	D00.08	D10.4	D37.05	D49.0
- - fauces, faucial	C09.9	C79.89	D00.08	D10.4	D37.05	D49.0
- - lingual	C02.4	C79.89	D00.07	D10.1	D37.02	D49.0
- - overlapping sites	C09.8	-	-	-	-	-
- - palatine	C09.9	C79.89	D00.08	D10.4	D37.05	D49.0
- - pharyngeal	C11.1	C79.89	D00.08	D10.6	D37.05	D49.0
- - pillar (anterior) (posterior)	C09.1	C79.89	D00.08	D10.5	D37.05	D49.0
- tonsillar fossa	C09.0	C79.89	D00.08	D10.5	D37.05	D49.0
- tooth socket NEC	C03.9	C79.89	D00.03	D10.39	D37.09	D49.0
- trachea (cartilage) (mucosa)	C33	C78.39	D02.1	D14.2	D38.1	D49.1
- - overlapping lesion with bronchus or lung	C34.8-	-	-	-	-	-
- tracheobronchial	C34.8-	C78.39	D02.1	D14.2	D38.1	D49.1
- - overlapping lesion with lung	C34.8-	-	-	-	-	-
- tragus—*see also Neoplasm, skin, ear*	C44.20-	C79.2	D04.2-	D23.2-	D48.5	D49.2

	Malignant Primary	Malignant Secondary	Ca in Situ	Benign	Uncertain Behavior	Unspecified Behavior
- trunk NEC	C76.8	C79.89	D04.5	D36.7	D48.7	D49.89
- tubo-ovarian	C57.8	C79.82	D07.39	D28.7	D39.8	D49.59
- tunica vaginalis	C63.7	C79.82	D07.69	D29.8	D40.8	D49.59
- turbinate (bone)	C41.0	C79.51	-	D16.4-	D48.0	D49.2
- - nasal	C30.0	C78.39	D02.3	D14.0	D38.5	D49.1
- tympanic cavity	C30.1	C78.39	D02.3	D14.0	D38.5	D49.1
- ulna (any part)	C40.0-	C79.51	-	D16.0-	-	-
- umbilicus, umbilical—see also Neoplasm, skin, trunk	C44.509	C79.2	D04.5	D23.5	D48.5	D49.2
- uncus, brain	C71.2	C79.31	-	D33.0	D43.0	D49.6
- unknown site or unspecified	C80.1	C79.9	D09.9	D36.9	D48.9	D49.9
- urachus	C67.7	C79.11	D09.0	D30.3	D41.4	D49.4
- ureter, ureteral	C66.-	C79.19	D09.19	D30.2-	D41.2-	D49.59
- - orifice (bladder)	C67.6	C79.11	D09.0	D30.3	D41.4	D49.4
- ureter-bladder (junction)	C67.6	C79.11	D09.0	D30.3	D41.4	D49.4
- urethra, urethral (gland)	C68.0	C79.19	D09.19	D30.4	D41.3	D49.59
- - orifice, internal	C67.5	C79.11	D09.0	D30.3	D41.4	D49.4
- urethrovaginal (septum)	C57.9	C79.82	D07.30	D28.9	D39.8	D49.59
- urinary organ or system	C68.9	C79.10	D09.10	D30.9	D41.9	D49.59
- - bladder—see Neoplasm, bladder						
- - overlapping lesion	C68.8	-	-	-	-	-
- - specified sites NEC	C68.8	C79.19	D09.19	D30.8	D41.8	D49.59
- utero-ovarian	C57.8	C79.82	D07.39	D28.7	D39.8	D49.59
- - ligament	C57.1	C79.82	D07.39	D28.2	D39.8	D49.59
- uterosacral ligament	C57.3	C79.82	-	D28.2	D39.8	D49.59
- uterus, uteri, uterine	C55	C79.82	D07.0	D26.9	D39.0	D49.59
- - adnexa NEC	C57.4	C79.82	D07.39	D28.7	D39.8	D49.59
- - body	C54.9	C79.82	D07.0	D26.1	D39.0	D49.59
- - cervix	C53.9	C79.82	D06.9	D26.0	D39.0	D49.59
- - cornu	C54.9	C79.82	D07.0	D26.1	D39.0	D49.59
- - corpus	C54.9	C79.82	D07.0	D26.1	D39.0	D49.59
- - endocervix (canal) (gland)	C53.0	C79.82	D06.0	D26.0	D39.0	D49.59
- - endometrium	C54.1	C79.82	D07.0	D26.1	D39.0	D49.59
- - exocervix	C53.1	C79.82	D06.1	D26.0	D39.0	D49.59
- - external os	C53.1	C79.82	D06.1	D26.0	D39.0	D49.59
- - fundus	C54.3	C79.82	D07.0	D26.1	D39.0	D49.59
- - internal os	C53.0	C79.82	D06.0	D26.0	D39.0	D49.59
- - isthmus	C54.0	C79.82	D07.0	D26.1	D39.0	D49.59
- - ligament	C57.3	C79.82	-	D28.2	D39.8	D49.59
- - - broad	C57.1	C79.82	D07.39	D28.2	D39.8	D49.59
- - - round	C57.2	C79.82	-	D28.2	D39.8	D49.59
- - lower segment	C54.0	C79.82	D07.0	D26.1	D39.0	D49.59
- - myometrium	C54.2	C79.82	D07.0	D26.1	D39.0	D49.59
- - overlapping sites	C54.8	-	-	-	-	-
- - squamocolumnar junction	C53.8	C79.82	D06.7	D26.0	D39.0	D49.59
- - tube	C57.0-	C79.82	D07.39	D28.2	D39.8	D49.59
- utricle, prostatic	C68.0	C79.19	D09.19	D30.4	D41.3	D49.59
- uveal tract	C69.4-	C79.49	D09.2-	D31.4-	D48.7	D49.89
- uvula	C05.2	C79.89	D00.04	D10.39	D37.09	D49.0
- vagina, vaginal (fornix) (vault) (wall)	C52	C79.82	D07.2	D28.1	D39.8	D49.59
- vaginovesical	C57.9	C79.82	D07.30	D28.9	D39.9	D49.59
- - septum	C57.9	C79.82	D07.30	D28.9	D39.9	D49.59
- vallecula (epiglottis)	C10.0	C79.89	D00.08	D10.5	D37.05	D49.0
- vas deferens	C63.1-	C79.82	D07.69	D29.8	D40.8	D49.59
- vascular—see Neoplasm, connective tissue						
- Vater's ampulla	C24.1	C78.89	D01.5	D13.5	D37.6	D49.0
- vein, venous—see Neoplasm, connective tissue						
- vena cava (abdominal) (inferior)	C49.4	C79.89	-	D21.4	D48.1	D49.2
- - superior	C49.3	C79.89	-	D21.3	D48.1	D49.2
- ventricle (cerebral) (floor) (lateral) (third)	C71.5	C79.31	-	D33.0	D43.0	D49.6
- - cardiac (left) (right)	C38.0	C79.89	-	D15.1	D48.7	D49.89
- - fourth	C71.7	C79.31	-	D33.1	D43.1	D49.6
- ventricular band of larynx	C32.1	C78.39	D02.0	D14.1	D38.0	D49.1
- ventriculus—see Neoplasm, stomach						
- vermillion border—see Neoplasm, lip						
- vermis, cerebellum	C71.6	C79.31	-	D33.1	D43.1	D49.6
- vertebra (column)	C41.2	C79.51	-	D16.6	D48.0	D49.2
- - coccyx	C41.4	C79.51	-	D16.8-	D48.0	D49.2

	Malignant Primary	Malignant Secondary	Ca in Situ	Benign	Uncertain Behavior	Unspecified Behavior
- - marrow NEC	C96.9	C79.52	-	-	D47.9	D49.89
- - sacrum	C41.4	C79.51	-	D16.8-	D48.0	D49.2
- vesical—*see Neoplasm, bladder*						
- vesicle, seminal	C63.7	C79.82	D07.69	D29.8	D40.8	D49.59
- vesicocervical tissue	C57.9	C79.82	D07.30	D28.9	D39.9	D49.59
- vesicorectal	C76.3	C79.82	D09.8	D36.7	D48.7	D49.89
- vesicovaginal	C57.9	C79.82	D07.30	D28.9	D39.9	D49.59
- - septum	C57.9	C79.82	D07.30	D28.9	D39.8	D49.59
- vessel (blood)—*see Neoplasm, connective tissue*						
- vestibular gland, greater	C51.0	C79.82	D07.1	D28.0	D39.8	D49.59
- vestibule						
- - mouth	C06.1	C79.89	D00.00	D10.39	D37.09	D49.0
- - nose	C30.0	C78.39	D02.3	D14.0	D38.5	D49.1
- Virchow's gland	C77.0	C77.0	-	D36.0	D48.7	D49.89
- viscera NEC	C76.8	C79.89	D09.8	D36.7	D48.7	D49.89
- vocal cords (true)	C32.0	C78.39	D02.0	D14.1	D38.0	D49.1
- - false	C32.1	C78.39	D02.0	D14.1	D38.0	D49.1
- vomer	C41.0	C79.51	-	D16.4-	D48.0	D49.2
- vulva	C51.9	C79.82	D07.1	D28.0	D39.8	D49.59
- vulvovaginal gland	C51.0	C79.82	D07.1	D28.0	D39.8	D49.59
- Waldeyer's ring	C14.2	C79.89	D00.08	D10.9	D37.05	D49.0
- Wharton's duct	C08.0	C79.89	D00.00	D11.7	D37.032	D49.0
- white matter (central) (cerebral)	C71.0	C79.31	-	D33.0	D43.0	D49.6
- windpipe	C33	C78.39	D02.1	D14.2	D38.1	D49.1
- Wirsung's duct	C25.3	C78.89	D01.7	D13.6	D37.8	D49.0
- wolffian (body) (duct)						
- - female	C57.7	C79.82	D07.39	D28.7	D39.8	D49.59
- - male	C63.7	C79.82	D07.69	D29.8	D40.8	D49.59
- womb—*see Neoplasm, uterus*						
- wrist NEC	C76.4-	C79.89	D04.6-	D36.7	D48.7	D49.89
- xiphoid process	C41.3	C79.51	-	D16.7	D48.0	D49.2
- Zuckerkandl organ	C75.5	C79.89	-	D35.6	D44.7	D49.7

Table Of Drugs And Chemicals

Substance	Poisoning, Accidental (unintentional)	Poisoning, Intentional Self-harm	Poisoning, Assault	Poisoning, Undetermined	Adverse effect	Underdosing
1-propanol	T51.3X1	T51.3X2	T51.3X3	T51.3X4	--	--
2-propanol	T51.2X1	T51.2X2	T51.2X3	T51.2X4	--	--
2,4-D (dichlorophen-oxyacetic acid)	T60.3X1	T60.3X2	T60.3X3	T60.3X4	--	--
2,4-toluene diisocyanate	T65.0X1	T65.0X2	T65.0X3	T65.0X4	--	--
2,4,5-T (trichloro-phenoxyacetic acid)	T60.1X1	T60.1X2	T60.1X3	T60.1X4	--	--
14-hydroxydihydro-morphinone	T40.2X1	T40.2X2	T40.2X3	T40.2X4	T40.2X5	T40.2X6
ABOB	T37.5X1	T37.5X2	T37.5X3	T37.5X4	T37.5X5	T37.5X6
Abrine	T62.2X1	T62.2X2	T62.2X3	T62.2X4	--	--
Abrus (seed)	T62.2X1	T62.2X2	T62.2X3	T62.2X4	--	--
Absinthe	T51.0X1	T51.0X2	T51.0X3	T51.0X4	--	--
beverage	T51.0X1	T51.0X2	T51.0X3	T51.0X4	--	--
Acaricide	T60.8X1	T60.8X2	T60.8X3	T60.8X4	--	--
Acebutolol	T44.7X1	T44.7X2	T44.7X3	T44.7X4	T44.7X5	T44.7X6
Acecarbromal	T42.6X1	T42.6X2	T42.6X3	T42.6X4	T42.6X5	T42.6X6
Aceclidine	T44.1X1	T44.1X2	T44.1X3	T44.1X4	T44.1X5	T44.1X6
Acedapsone	T37.0X1	T37.0X2	T37.0X3	T37.0X4	T37.0X5	T37.0X6
Acefylline piperazine	T48.6X1	T48.6X2	T48.6X3	T48.6X4	T48.6X5	T48.6X6
Acemorphan	T40.2X1	T40.2X2	T40.2X3	T40.2X4	T40.2X5	T40.2X6
Acenocoumarin	T45.511	T45.512	T45.513	T45.514	T45.515	T45.516
Acenocoumarol	T45.511	T45.512	T45.513	T45.514	T45.515	T45.516
Acepifylline	T48.6X1	T48.6X2	T48.6X3	T48.6X4	T48.6X5	T48.6X6
Acepromazine	T43.3X1	T43.3X2	T43.3X3	T43.3X4	T43.3X5	T43.3X6
Acesulfamethoxypyridazine	T37.0X1	T37.0X2	T37.0X3	T37.0X4	T37.0X5	T37.0X6
Acetal	T52.8X1	T52.8X2	T52.8X3	T52.8X4	--	--
Acetaldehyde (vapor)	T52.8X1	T52.8X2	T52.8X3	T52.8X4	--	--
liquid	T65.891	T65.892	T65.893	T65.894	--	--
P-Acetamidophenol	T39.1X1	T39.1X2	T39.1X3	T39.1X4	T39.1X5	T39.1X6
Acetaminophen	T39.1X1	T39.1X2	T39.1X3	T39.1X4	T39.1X5	T39.1X6
Acetaminosalol	T39.1X1	T39.1X2	T39.1X3	T39.1X4	T39.1X5	T39.1X6
Acetanilide	T39.1X1	T39.1X2	T39.1X3	T39.1X4	T39.1X5	T39.1X6
Acetarsol	T37.3X1	T37.3X2	T37.3X3	T37.3X4	T37.3X5	T37.3X6
Acetazolamide	T50.2X1	T50.2X2	T50.2X3	T50.2X4	T50.2X5	T50.2X6
Acetiamine	T45.2X1	T45.2X2	T45.2X3	T45.2X4	T45.2X5	T45.2X6
Acetic						
acid	T54.2X1	T54.2X2	T54.2X3	T54.2X4	--	--
with sodium acetate (ointment)	T49.3X1	T49.3X2	T49.3X3	T49.3X4	T49.3X5	T49.3X6
ester (solvent) (vapor)	T52.8X1	T52.8X2	T52.8X3	T52.8X4	--	--
irrigating solution	T50.3X1	T50.3X2	T50.3X3	T50.3X4	T50.3X5	T50.3X6
medicinal (lotion)	T49.2X1	T49.2X2	T49.2X3	T49.2X4	T49.2X5	T49.2X6
anhydride	T65.891	T65.892	T65.893	T65.894	--	--
ether (vapor)	T52.8X1	T52.8X2	T52.8X3	T52.8X4	--	--
Acetohexamide	T38.3X1	T38.3X2	T38.3X3	T38.3X4	T38.3X5	T38.3X6
Acetohydroxamic acid	T50.991	T50.992	T50.993	T50.994	T50.995	T50.996
Acetomenaphthone	T45.7X1	T45.7X2	T45.7X3	T45.7X4	T45.7X5	T45.7X6
Acetomorphine	T40.1X1	T40.1X2	T40.1X3	T40.1X4	T40.1X5	--
Acetone (oils)	T52.4X1	T52.4X2	T52.4X3	T52.4X4	--	--
chlorinated	T52.4X1	T52.4X2	T52.4X3	T52.4X4	--	--
vapor	T52.4X1	T52.4X2	T52.4X3	T52.4X4	--	--
Acetonitrile	T52.8X1	T52.8X2	T52.8X3	T52.8X4	--	--
Acetophenazine	T43.3X1	T43.3X2	T43.3X3	T43.3X4	T43.3X5	T43.3X6
Acetophenetedin	T39.1X1	T39.1X2	T39.1X3	T39.1X4	T39.1X5	T39.1X6
Acetophenone	T52.4X1	T52.4X2	T52.4X3	T52.4X4	--	--
Acetorphine	T40.2X1	T40.2X2	T40.2X3	T40.2X4	--	--
Acetosulfone (sodium)	T37.1X1	T37.1X2	T37.1X3	T37.1X4	T37.1X5	T37.1X6
Acetrizoate (sodium)	T50.8X1	T50.8X2	T50.8X3	T50.8X4	T50.8X5	T50.8X6
Acetrizoic acid	T50.8X1	T50.8X2	T50.8X3	T50.8X4	T50.8X5	T50.8X6
Acetyl						
bromide	T53.6X1	T53.6X2	T53.6X3	T53.6X4	--	--
chloride	T53.6X1	T53.6X2	T53.6X3	T53.6X4	--	--
Acetylcarbromal	T42.6X1	T42.6X2	T42.6X3	T42.6X4	T42.6X5	T42.6X6
Acetylcholine						
chloride	T44.1X1	T44.1X2	T44.1X3	T44.1X4	T44.1X5	T44.1X6
derivative	T44.1X1	T44.1X2	T44.1X3	T44.1X4	T44.1X5	T44.1X6
Acetylcysteine	T48.4X1	T48.4X2	T48.4X3	T48.4X4	T48.4X5	T48.4X6

Substance	Poisoning, Accidental (unintentional)	Poisoning, Intentional Self-harm	Poisoning, Assault	Poisoning, Undetermined	Adverse effect	Underdosing
Acetyldigitoxin	T46.0X1	T46.0X2	T46.0X3	T46.0X4	T46.0X5	T46.0X6
Acetyldigoxin	T46.0X1	T46.0X2	T46.0X3	T46.0X4	T46.0X5	T46.0X6
Acetyldihydrocodeine	T40.2X1	T40.2X2	T40.2X3	T40.2X4	--	--
Acetyldihydrocodeinone	T40.2X1	T40.2X2	T40.2X3	T40.2X4	--	--
Acetylene (gas)	T59.891	T59.892	T59.893	T59.894	--	--
dichloride	T53.6X1	T53.6X2	T53.6X3	T53.6X4	--	--
incomplete combustion of	T58.11	T58.12	T58.13	T58.14	--	--
industrial	T59.891	T59.892	T59.893	T59.894	--	--
tetrachloride	T53.6X1	T53.6X2	T53.6X3	T53.6X4	--	--
vapor	T53.6X1	T53.6X2	T53.6X3	T53.6X4	--	--
Acetylpheneturide	T42.6X1	T42.6X2	T42.6X3	T42.6X4	T42.6X5	T42.6X6
Acetylphenylhydrazine	T39.8X1	T39.8X2	T39.8X3	T39.8X4	T39.8X5	T39.8X6
Acetylsalicylic acid (salts)	T39.011	T39.012	T39.013	T39.014	T39.015	T39.016
enteric coated	T39.011	T39.012	T39.013	T39.014	T39.015	T39.016
Acetylsulfamethoxypyridazine	T37.0X1	T37.0X2	T37.0X3	T37.0X4	T37.0X5	T37.0X6
Achromycin	T36.4X1	T36.4X2	T36.4X3	T36.4X4	T36.4X5	T36.4X6
ophthalmic preparation	T49.5X1	T49.5X2	T49.5X3	T49.5X4	T49.5X5	T49.5X6
topical NEC	T49.0X1	T49.0X2	T49.0X3	T49.0X4	T49.0X5	T49.0X6
Aciclovir	T37.5X1	T37.5X2	T37.5X3	T37.5X4	T37.5X5	T37.5X6
Acid (corrosive) NEC	T54.2X1	T54.2X2	T54.2X3	T54.2X4	--	--
Acidifying agent NEC	T50.901	T50.902	T50.903	T50.904	T50.905	T50.906
Acipimox	T46.6X1	T46.6X2	T46.6X3	T46.6X4	T46.6X5	T46.6X6
Acitretin	T50.991	T50.992	T50.993	T50.994	T50.995	T50.996
Aclarubicin	T45.1X1	T45.1X2	T45.1X3	T45.1X4	T45.1X5	T45.1X6
Aclatonium napadisilate	T48.1X1	T48.1X2	T48.1X3	T48.1X4	T48.1X5	T48.1X6
Aconite (wild)	T46.991	T46.992	T46.993	T46.994	T46.995	T46.996
Aconitine	T46.991	T46.992	T46.993	T46.994	T46.995	T46.996
Aconitum ferox	T46.991	T46.992	T46.993	T46.994	T46.995	T46.996
Acridine	T65.6X1	T65.6X2	T65.6X3	T65.6X4	--	--
vapor	T59.891	T59.892	T59.893	T59.894	--	--
Acriflavine	T37.91	T37.92	T37.93	T37.94	T37.95	T37.96
Acriflavinium chloride	T49.0X1	T49.0X2	T49.0X3	T49.0X4	T49.0X5	T49.0X6
Acrinol	T49.0X1	T49.0X2	T49.0X3	T49.0X4	T49.0X5	T49.0X6
Acrisorcin	T49.0X1	T49.0X2	T49.0X3	T49.0X4	T49.0X5	T49.0X6
Acrivastine	T45.0X1	T45.0X2	T45.0X3	T45.0X4	T45.0X5	T45.0X6
Acrolein (gas)	T59.891	T59.892	T59.893	T59.894	--	--
liquid	T54.1X1	T54.1X2	T54.1X3	T54.1X4	--	--
Acrylamide	T65.891	T65.892	T65.893	T65.894	--	--
Acrylic resin	T49.3X1	T49.3X2	T49.3X3	T49.3X4	T49.3X5	T49.3X6
Acrylonitrile	T65.891	T65.892	T65.893	T65.894	--	--
Actaea spicata	T62.2X1	T62.2X2	T62.2X3	T62.2X4	--	--
berry	T62.1X1	T62.1X2	T62.1X3	T62.1X4	--	--
Acterol	T37.3X1	T37.3X2	T37.3X3	T37.3X4	T37.3X5	T37.3X6
ACTH	T38.811	T38.812	T38.813	T38.814	T38.815	T38.816
Actinomycin C	T45.1X1	T45.1X2	T45.1X3	T45.1X4	T45.1X5	T45.1X6
Actinomycin D	T45.1X1	T45.1X2	T45.1X3	T45.1X4	T45.1X5	T45.1X6
Activated charcoal—*see also Charcoal, medicinal*	T47.6X1	T47.6X2	T47.6X3	T47.6X4	T47.6X5	T47.6X6
Acyclovir	T37.5X1	T37.5X2	T37.5X3	T37.5X4	T37.5X5	T37.5X6
Adenine	T45.2X1	T45.2X2	T45.2X3	T45.2X4	T45.2X5	T45.2X6
arabinoside	T37.5X1	T37.5X2	T37.5X3	T37.5X4	T37.5X5	T37.5X6
Adenosine (phosphate)	T46.2X1	T46.2X2	T46.2X3	T46.2X4	T46.2X5	T46.2X6
ADH	T38.891	T38.892	T38.893	T38.894	T38.895	T38.896
Adhesive NEC	T65.891	T65.892	T65.893	T65.894	--	--
Adicillin	T36.0X1	T36.0X2	T36.0X3	T36.0X4	T36.0X5	T36.0X6
Adiphenine	T44.3X1	T44.3X2	T44.3X3	T44.3X4	T44.3X5	T44.3X6
Adipiodone	T50.8X1	T50.8X2	T50.8X3	T50.8X4	T50.8X5	T50.8X6
Adjunct, pharmaceutical	T50.901	T50.902	T50.903	T50.904	T50.905	T50.906
Adrenal (extract, cortex or medulla) (glucocorticoids)(hormones)(mineralocorticoids)	T38.0X1	T38.0X2	T38.0X3	T38.0X4	T38.0X5	T38.0X6
ENT agent	T49.6X1	T49.6X2	T49.6X3	T49.6X4	T49.6X5	T49.6X6
ophthalmic preparation	T49.5X1	T49.5X2	T49.5X3	T49.5X4	T49.5X5	T49.5X6
topical NEC	T49.0X1	T49.0X2	T49.0X3	T49.0X4	T49.0X5	T49.0X6
Adrenaline	T44.5X1	T44.5X2	T44.5X3	T44.5X4	T44.5X5	T44.5X6
Adrenalin—see Adrenaline						

Substance	Poisoning, Accidental (unintentional)	Poisoning, Intentional Self-harm	Poisoning, Assault	Poisoning, Undetermined	Adverse effect	Underdosing
Adrenergic NEC	T44.901	T44.902	T44.903	T44.904	T44.905	T44.906
blocking agent NEC	T44.8X1	T44.8X2	T44.8X3	T44.8X4	T44.8X5	T44.8X6
beta, heart	T44.7X1	T44.7X2	T44.7X3	T44.7X4	T44.7X5	T44.7X6
specified NEC	T44.991	T44.992	T44.993	T44.994	T44.995	T44.996
Adrenochrome						
(mono) semicarbazone	T46.991	T46.992	T46.993	T46.994	T46.995	T46.996
derivative	T46.991	T46.992	T46.993	T46.994	T46.995	T46.996
Adrenocorticotrophic hormone	T38.811	T38.812	T38.813	T38.814	T38.815	T38.816
Adrenocorticotrophin	T38.811	T38.812	T38.813	T38.814	T38.815	T38.816
Adriamycin	T45.1X1	T45.1X2	T45.1X3	T45.1X4	T45.1X5	T45.1X6
Aerosol spray NEC	T65.91	T65.92	T65.93	T65.94	--	--
Aerosporin	T36.8X1	T36.8X2	T36.8X3	T36.8X4	T36.8X5	T36.8X6
ENT agent	T49.6X1	T49.6X2	T49.6X3	T49.6X4	T49.6X5	T49.6X6
ophthalmic preparation	T49.5X1	T49.5X2	T49.5X3	T49.5X4	T49.5X5	T49.5X6
topical NEC	T49.0X1	T49.0X2	T49.0X3	T49.0X4	T49.0X5	T49.0X6
Aethusa cynapium	T62.2X1	T62.2X2	T62.2X3	T62.2X4	--	--
Afghanistan black	T40.7X1	T40.7X2	T40.7X3	T40.7X4	T40.7X5	T40.7X6
Aflatoxin	T64.01	T64.02	T64.03	T64.04	--	--
Afloqualone	T42.8X1	T42.8X2	T42.8X3	T42.8X4	T42.8X5	T42.8X6
African boxwood	T62.2X1	T62.2X2	T62.2X3	T62.2X4	--	--
Agar	T47.4X1	T47.4X2	T47.4X3	T47.4X4	T47.4X5	T47.4X6
Agonist						
predominantly						
alpha-adrenoreceptor	T44.4X1	T44.4X2	T44.4X3	T44.4X4	T44.4X5	T44.4X6
beta-adrenoreceptor	T44.5X1	T44.5X2	T44.5X3	T44.5X4	T44.5X5	T44.5X6
Agricultural agent NEC	T65.91	T65.92	T65.93	T65.94	--	--
Agrypnal	T42.3X1	T42.3X2	T42.3X3	T42.3X4	T42.3X5	T42.3X6
AHLG	T50.Z11	T50.Z12	T50.Z13	T50.Z14	T50.Z15	T50.Z16
Air contaminant (s) , source/type NOS	T65.91	T65.92	T65.93	T65.94	--	--
Ajmaline	T46.2X1	T46.2X2	T46.2X3	T46.2X4	T46.2X5	T46.2X6
Akee	T62.1X1	T62.1X2	T62.1X3	T62.1X4	--	--
Akrinol	T49.0X1	T49.0X2	T49.0X3	T49.0X4	T49.0X5	T49.0X6
Akritoin	T37.8X1	T37.8X2	T37.8X3	T37.8X4	T37.8X5	T37.8X6
Alacepril	T46.4X1	T46.4X2	T46.4X3	T46.4X4	T46.4X5	T46.4X6
Alantolactone	T37.4X1	T37.4X2	T37.4X3	T37.4X4	T37.4X5	T37.4X6
Albamycin	T36.8X1	T36.8X2	T36.8X3	T36.8X4	T36.8X5	T36.8X6
Albendazole	T37.4X1	T37.4X2	T37.4X3	T37.4X4	T37.4X5	T37.4X6
Albumin						
bovine	T45.8X1	T45.8X2	T45.8X3	T45.8X4	T45.8X5	T45.8X6
human serum	T45.8X1	T45.8X2	T45.8X3	T45.8X4	T45.8X5	T45.8X6
salt-poor	T45.8X1	T45.8X2	T45.8X3	T45.8X4	T45.8X5	T45.8X6
normal human serum	T45.8X1	T45.8X2	T45.8X3	T45.8X4	T45.8X5	T45.8X6
Albuterol	T48.6X1	T48.6X2	T48.6X3	T48.6X4	T48.6X5	T48.6X6
Albutoin	T42.0X1	T42.0X2	T42.0X3	T42.0X4	T42.0X5	T42.0X6
Alclometasone	T49.0X1	T49.0X2	T49.0X3	T49.0X4	T49.0X5	T49.0X6
Alcohol	T51.91	T51.92	T51.93	T51.94	--	--
absolute	T51.0X1	T51.0X2	T51.0X3	T51.0X4	--	--
beverage	T51.0X1	T51.0X2	T51.0X3	T51.0X4	--	--
allyl	T51.8X1	T51.8X2	T51.8X3	T51.8X4	--	--
amyl	T51.3X1	T51.3X2	T51.3X3	T51.3X4	--	--
antifreeze	T51.1X1	T51.1X2	T51.1X3	T51.1X4	--	--
beverage	T51.0X1	T51.0X2	T51.0X3	T51.0X4	--	--
butyl	T51.3X1	T51.3X2	T51.3X3	T51.3X4	--	--
dehydrated	T51.0X1	T51.0X2	T51.0X3	T51.0X4	--	--
beverage	T51.0X1	T51.0X2	T51.0X3	T51.0X4	--	--
denatured	T51.0X1	T51.0X2	T51.0X3	T51.0X4	--	--
deterrent NEC	T50.6X1	T50.6X2	T50.6X3	T50.6X4	T50.6X5	T50.6X6
diagnostic (gastric function)	T50.8X1	T50.8X2	T50.8X3	T50.8X4	T50.8X5	T50.8X6
ethyl	T51.0X1	T51.0X2	T51.0X3	T51.0X4	--	--
beverage	T51.0X1	T51.0X2	T51.0X3	T51.0X4	--	--
grain	T51.0X1	T51.0X2	T51.0X3	T51.0X4	--	--
beverage	T51.0X1	T51.0X2	T51.0X3	T51.0X4	--	--
industrial	T51.2X1	T51.2X2	T51.2X3	T51.2X4	--	--
isopropyl						

Substance	Poisoning, Accidental (unintentional)	Poisoning, Intentional Self-harm	Poisoning, Assault	Poisoning, Undetermined	Adverse effect	Underdosing
methyl	T51.1X1	T51.1X2	T51.1X3	T51.1X4	--	--
preparation for consumption	T51.0X1	T51.0X2	T51.0X3	T51.0X4	--	--
propyl	T51.3X1	T51.3X2	T51.3X3	T51.3X4	--	--
secondary	T51.2X1	T51.2X2	T51.2X3	T51.2X4	--	--
radiator	T51.1X1	T51.1X2	T51.1X3	T51.1X4	--	--
rubbing	T51.2X1	T51.2X2	T51.2X3	T51.2X4	--	--
specified type NEC	T51.8X1	T51.8X2	T51.8X3	T51.8X4	--	--
surgical	T51.0X1	T51.0X2	T51.0X3	T51.0X4	--	--
vapor (from any type of Alcohol)	T59.891	T59.892	T59.893	T59.894	--	--
wood	T51.1X1	T51.1X2	T51.1X3	T51.1X4	--	--
Alcuronium (chloride)	T48.1X1	T48.1X2	T48.1X3	T48.1X4	T48.1X5	T48.1X6
Aldactone	T50.0X1	T50.0X2	T50.0X3	T50.0X4	T50.0X5	T50.0X6
Aldesulfone sodium	T37.1X1	T37.1X2	T37.1X3	T37.1X4	T37.1X5	T37.1X6
Aldicarb	T60.0X1	T60.0X2	T60.0X3	T60.0X4	--	--
Aldomet	T46.5X1	T46.5X2	T46.5X3	T46.5X4	T46.5X5	T46.5X6
Aldosterone	T50.0X1	T50.0X2	T50.0X3	T50.0X4	T50.0X5	T50.0X6
Aldrin (dust)	T60.1X1	T60.1X2	T60.1X3	T60.1X4	--	--
Aleve—see Naproxen						
Alexitol sodium	T47.1X1	T47.1X2	T47.1X3	T47.1X4	T47.1X5	T47.1X6
Alfacalcidol	T45.2X1	T45.2X2	T45.2X3	T45.2X4	T45.2X5	T45.2X6
Alfadolone	T41.1X1	T41.1X2	T41.1X3	T41.1X4	T41.1X5	T41.1X6
Alfaxalone	T41.1X1	T41.1X2	T41.1X3	T41.1X4	T41.1X5	T41.1X6
Alfentanil	T40.4X1	T40.4X2	T40.4X3	T40.4X4	T40.4X5	T40.4X6
Alfuzosin (hydrochloride)	T44.8X1	T44.8X2	T44.8X3	T44.8X4	T44.8X5	T44.8X6
Algae (harmful) (toxin)	T65.821	T65.822	T65.823	T65.824	--	--
Algeldrate	T47.1X1	T47.1X2	T47.1X3	T47.1X4	T47.1X5	T47.1X6
Algin	T47.8X1	T47.8X2	T47.8X3	T47.8X4	T47.8X5	T47.8X6
Alglucerase	T45.3X1	T45.3X2	T45.3X3	T45.3X4	T45.3X5	T45.3X6
Alidase	T45.3X1	T45.3X2	T45.3X3	T45.3X4	T45.3X5	T45.3X6
Alimemazine	T43.3X1	T43.3X2	T43.3X3	T43.3X4	T43.3X5	T43.3X6
Aliphatic thiocyanates	T65.0X1	T65.0X2	T65.0X3	T65.0X4	--	--
Alizapride	T45.0X1	T45.0X2	T45.0X3	T45.0X4	T45.0X5	T45.0X6
Alkali (caustic)	T54.3X1	T54.3X2	T54.3X3	T54.3X4	--	--
Alkaline antiseptic solution (aromatic)	T49.6X1	T49.6X2	T49.6X3	T49.6X4	T49.6X5	T49.6X6
Alkalinizing agents (medicinal)	T50.901	T50.902	T50.903	T50.904	T50.905	T50.906
Alkalizing agent NEC	T50.901	T50.902	T50.903	T50.904	T50.905	T50.906
Alka-seltzer	T39.011	T39.012	T39.013	T39.014	T39.015	T39.016
Alkavervir	T46.5X1	T46.5X2	T46.5X3	T46.5X4	T46.5X5	T46.5X6
Alkonium (bromide)	T49.0X1	T49.0X2	T49.0X3	T49.0X4	T49.0X5	T49.0X6
Alkylating drug NEC	T45.1X1	T45.1X2	T45.1X3	T45.1X4	T45.1X5	T45.1X6
antimyeloproliferative	T45.1X1	T45.1X2	T45.1X3	T45.1X4	T45.1X5	T45.1X6
lymphatic	T45.1X1	T45.1X2	T45.1X3	T45.1X4	T45.1X5	T45.1X6
Alkylisocyanate	T65.0X1	T65.0X2	T65.0X3	T65.0X4	--	--
Allantoin	T49.4X1	T49.4X2	T49.4X3	T49.4X4	T49.4X5	T49.4X6
Allegron	T43.011	T43.012	T43.013	T43.014	T43.015	T43.016
Allethrin	T49.0X1	T49.0X2	T49.0X3	T49.0X4	T49.0X5	T49.0X6
Allobarbital	T42.3X1	T42.3X2	T42.3X3	T42.3X4	T42.3X5	T42.3X6
Allopurinol	T50.4X1	T50.4X2	T50.4X3	T50.4X4	T50.4X5	T50.4X6
Allyl						
Alcohol	T51.8X1	T51.8X2	T51.8X3	T51.8X4	--	--
disulfide	T46.6X1	T46.6X2	T46.6X3	T46.6X4	T46.6X5	T46.6X6
Allylestrenol	T38.5X1	T38.5X2	T38.5X3	T38.5X4	T38.5X5	T38.5X6
Allylisopropylacetylurea	T42.6X1	T42.6X2	T42.6X3	T42.6X4	T42.6X5	T42.6X6
Allylisopropylmalonylurea	T42.3X1	T42.3X2	T42.3X3	T42.3X4	T42.3X5	T42.3X6
Allylthiourea	T49.3X1	T49.3X2	T49.3X3	T49.3X4	T49.3X5	T49.3X6
Allyltribromide	T42.6X1	T42.6X2	T42.6X3	T42.6X4	T42.6X5	T42.6X6
Allypropymal	T42.3X1	T42.3X2	T42.3X3	T42.3X4	T42.3X5	T42.3X6
Almagate	T47.1X1	T47.1X2	T47.1X3	T47.1X4	T47.1X5	T47.1X6
Almasilate	T47.1X1	T47.1X2	T47.1X3	T47.1X4	T47.1X5	T47.1X6
Almitrine	T50.7X1	T50.7X2	T50.7X3	T50.7X4	T50.7X5	T50.7X6
Aloes	T47.2X1	T47.2X2	T47.2X3	T47.2X4	T47.2X5	T47.2X6
Aloglutamol	T47.1X1	T47.1X2	T47.1X3	T47.1X4	T47.1X5	T47.1X6
Aloin	T47.2X1	T47.2X2	T47.2X3	T47.2X4	T47.2X5	T47.2X6
Aloxidone	T42.2X1	T42.2X2	T42.2X3	T42.2X4	T42.2X5	T42.2X6
Alpha						

TABLE OF DRUGS AND CHEMICALS

Substance	Poisoning, Accidental (unintentional)	Poisoning, Intentional Self-harm	Poisoning, Assault	Poisoning, Undetermined	Adverse effect	Underdosing
acetyldigoxin	T46.0X1	T46.0X2	T46.0X3	T46.0X4	T46.0X5	T46.0X6
adrenergic blocking drug	T44.6X1	T44.6X2	T44.6X3	T44.6X4	T44.6X5	T44.6X6
amylase	T45.3X1	T45.3X2	T45.3X3	T45.3X4	T45.3X5	T45.3X6
tocoferol (acetate)	T45.2X1	T45.2X2	T45.2X3	T45.2X4	T45.2X5	T45.2X6
tocopherol	T45.2X1	T45.2X2	T45.2X3	T45.2X4	T45.2X5	T45.2X6
Alphadolone	T41.1X1	T41.1X2	T41.1X3	T41.1X4	T41.1X5	T41.1X6
Alphaprodine	T40.4X1	T40.4X2	T40.4X3	T40.4X4	T40.4X5	T40.4X6
Alphaxalone	T41.1X1	T41.1X2	T41.1X3	T41.1X4	T41.1X5	T41.1X6
Alprazolam	T42.4X1	T42.4X2	T42.4X3	T42.4X4	T42.4X5	T42.4X6
Alprenolol	T44.7X1	T44.7X2	T44.7X3	T44.7X4	T44.7X5	T44.7X6
Alprostadil	T46.7X1	T46.7X2	T46.7X3	T46.7X4	T46.7X5	T46.7X6
Alsactide	T38.811	T38.812	T38.813	T38.814	T38.815	T38.816
Alseroxylon	T46.5X1	T46.5X2	T46.5X3	T46.5X4	T46.5X5	T46.5X6
Alteplase	T45.611	T45.612	T45.613	T45.614	T45.615	T45.616
Altizide	T50.2X1	T50.2X2	T50.2X3	T50.2X4	T50.2X5	T50.2X6
Altretamine	T45.1X1	T45.1X2	T45.1X3	T45.1X4	T45.1X5	T45.1X6
Alum (medicinal)	T49.4X1	T49.4X2	T49.4X3	T49.4X4	T49.4X5	T49.4X6
nonmedicinal (ammonium) (potassium)	T56.891	T56.892	T56.893	T56.894	--	--
Aluminium, aluminum						
acetate	T49.2X1	T49.2X2	T49.2X3	T49.2X4	T49.2X5	T49.2X6
solution	T49.0X1	T49.0X2	T49.0X3	T49.0X4	T49.0X5	T49.0X6
aspirin	T39.011	T39.012	T39.013	T39.014	T39.015	T39.016
bis (acetylsalicylate)	T39.011	T39.012	T39.013	T39.014	T39.015	T39.016
carbonate (gel, basic)	T47.1X1	T47.1X2	T47.1X3	T47.1X4	T47.1X5	T47.1X6
chlorhydroxide-complex	T47.1X1	T47.1X2	T47.1X3	T47.1X4	T47.1X5	T47.1X6
chloride	T49.2X1	T49.2X2	T49.2X3	T49.2X4	T49.2X5	T49.2X6
clofibrate	T46.6X1	T46.6X2	T46.6X3	T46.6X4	T46.6X5	T46.6X6
diacetate	T49.2X1	T49.2X2	T49.2X3	T49.2X4	T49.2X5	T49.2X6
glycinate	T47.1X1	T47.1X2	T47.1X3	T47.1X4	T47.1X5	T47.1X6
hydroxide (gel)	T47.1X1	T47.1X2	T47.1X3	T47.1X4	T47.1X5	T47.1X6
hydroxide-magnesium carb. gel	T47.1X1	T47.1X2	T47.1X3	T47.1X4	T47.1X5	T47.1X6
magnesium silicate	T47.1X1	T47.1X2	T47.1X3	T47.1X4	T47.1X5	T47.1X6
nicotinate	T46.7X1	T46.7X2	T46.7X3	T46.7X4	T46.7X5	T46.7X6
ointment (surgical) (topical)	T49.3X1	T49.3X2	T49.3X3	T49.3X4	T49.3X5	T49.3X6
phosphate	T47.1X1	T47.1X2	T47.1X3	T47.1X4	T47.1X5	T47.1X6
salicylate	T39.091	T39.092	T39.093	T39.094	T39.095	T39.096
silicate	T47.1X1	T47.1X2	T47.1X3	T47.1X4	T47.1X5	T47.1X6
sodium silicate	T47.1X1	T47.1X2	T47.1X3	T47.1X4	T47.1X5	T47.1X6
subacetate	T49.2X1	T49.2X2	T49.2X3	T49.2X4	T49.2X5	T49.2X6
sulfate	T49.0X1	T49.0X2	T49.0X3	T49.0X4	T49.0X5	T49.0X6
tannate	T47.6X1	T47.6X2	T47.6X3	T47.6X4	T47.6X5	T47.6X6
topical NEC	T49.3X1	T49.3X2	T49.3X3	T49.3X4	T49.3X5	T49.3X6
Alurate	T42.3X1	T42.3X2	T42.3X3	T42.3X4	T42.3X5	T42.3X6
Alverine	T44.3X1	T44.3X2	T44.3X3	T44.3X4	T44.3X5	T44.3X6
Alvodine	T40.2X1	T40.2X2	T40.2X3	T40.2X4	T40.2X5	T40.2X6
Amanita phalloides	T62.0X1	T62.0X2	T62.0X3	T62.0X4	--	--
Amanitine	T62.0X1	T62.0X2	T62.0X3	T62.0X4	--	--
Amantadine	T42.8X1	T42.8X2	T42.8X3	T42.8X4	T42.8X5	T42.8X6
Ambazone	T49.6X1	T49.6X2	T49.6X3	T49.6X4	T49.6X5	T49.6X6
Ambenonium (chloride)	T44.0X1	T44.0X2	T44.0X3	T44.0X4	T44.0X5	T44.0X6
Ambroxol	T48.4X1	T48.4X2	T48.4X3	T48.4X4	T48.4X5	T48.4X6
Ambuphylline	T48.6X1	T48.6X2	T48.6X3	T48.6X4	T48.6X5	T48.6X6
Ambutonium bromide	T44.3X1	T44.3X2	T44.3X3	T44.3X4	T44.3X5	T44.3X6
Amcinonide	T49.0X1	T49.0X2	T49.0X3	T49.0X4	T49.0X5	T49.0X6
Amdinocilline	T36.0X1	T36.0X2	T36.0X3	T36.0X4	T36.0X5	T36.0X6
Ametazole	T50.8X1	T50.8X2	T50.8X3	T50.8X4	T50.8X5	T50.8X6
Amethocaine	T41.3X1	T41.3X2	T41.3X3	T41.3X4	T41.3X5	T41.3X6
regional	T41.3X1	T41.3X2	T41.3X3	T41.3X4	T41.3X5	T41.3X6
spinal	T41.3X1	T41.3X2	T41.3X3	T41.3X4	T41.3X5	T41.3X6
Amethopterin	T45.1X1	T45.1X2	T45.1X3	T45.1X4	T45.1X5	T45.1X6
Amezinium metilsulfate	T44.991	T44.992	T44.993	T44.994	T44.995	T44.996
Amfebutamone	T43.291	T43.292	T43.293	T43.294	T43.295	T43.296
Amfepramone	T50.5X1	T50.5X2	T50.5X3	T50.5X4	T50.5X5	T50.5X6
Amfetamine	T43.621	T43.622	T43.623	T43.624	T43.625	T43.626

TABLE OF DRUGS AND CHEMICALS

Substance	Poisoning, Accidental (unintentional)	Poisoning, Intentional Self-harm	Poisoning, Assault	Poisoning, Undetermined	Adverse effect	Underdosing
Amfetaminil	T43.621	T43.622	T43.623	T43.624	T43.625	T43.626
Amfomycin	T36.8X1	T36.8X2	T36.8X3	T36.8X4	T36.8X5	T36.8X6
Amidefrine mesilate	T48.5X1	T48.5X2	T48.5X3	T48.5X4	T48.5X5	T48.5X6
Amidone	T40.3X1	T40.3X2	T40.3X3	T40.3X4	T40.3X5	T40.3X6
Amidopyrine	T39.2X1	T39.2X2	T39.2X3	T39.2X4	T39.2X5	T39.2X6
Amidotrizoate	T50.8X1	T50.8X2	T50.8X3	T50.8X4	T50.8X5	T50.8X6
Amiflamine	T43.1X1	T43.1X2	T43.1X3	T43.1X4	T43.1X5	T43.1X6
Amikacin	T36.5X1	T36.5X2	T36.5X3	T36.5X4	T36.5X5	T36.5X6
Amikhelline	T46.3X1	T46.3X2	T46.3X3	T46.3X4	T46.3X5	T46.3X6
Amiloride	T50.2X1	T50.2X2	T50.2X3	T50.2X4	T50.2X5	T50.2X6
Aminacrine	T49.0X1	T49.0X2	T49.0X3	T49.0X4	T49.0X5	T49.0X6
Amineptine	T43.011	T43.012	T43.013	T43.014	T43.015	T43.016
Aminitrozole	T37.3X1	T37.3X2	T37.3X3	T37.3X4	T37.3X5	T37.3X6
Amino acids	T50.3X1	T50.3X2	T50.3X3	T50.3X4	T50.3X5	T50.3X6
Aminoacetic acid (derivatives)	T50.3X1	T50.3X2	T50.3X3	T50.3X4	T50.3X5	T50.3X6
Aminoacridine	T49.0X1	T49.0X2	T49.0X3	T49.0X4	T49.0X5	T49.0X6
Aminobenzoic acid (-p)	T49.3X1	T49.3X2	T49.3X3	T49.3X4	T49.3X5	T49.3X6
4-Aminobutyric acid	T43.8X1	T43.8X2	T43.8X3	T43.8X4	T43.8X5	T43.8X6
Aminocaproic acid	T45.621	T45.622	T45.623	T45.624	T45.625	T45.626
Aminoethylisothiourium	T45.8X1	T45.8X2	T45.8X3	T45.8X4	T45.8X5	T45.8X6
Aminofenazone	T39.2X1	T39.2X2	T39.2X3	T39.2X4	T39.2X5	T39.2X6
Aminoglutethimide	T45.1X1	T45.1X2	T45.1X3	T45.1X4	T45.1X5	T45.1X6
Aminohippuric acid	T50.8X1	T50.8X2	T50.8X3	T50.8X4	T50.8X5	T50.8X6
Aminomethylbenzoic acid	T45.691	T45.692	T45.693	T45.694	T45.695	T45.696
Aminometradine	T50.2X1	T50.2X2	T50.2X3	T50.2X4	T50.2X5	T50.2X6
Aminopentamide	T44.3X1	T44.3X2	T44.3X3	T44.3X4	T44.3X5	T44.3X6
Aminophenazone	T39.2X1	T39.2X2	T39.2X3	T39.2X4	T39.2X5	T39.2X6
Aminophenol	T54.0X1	T54.0X2	T54.0X3	T54.0X4	--	--
4-Aminophenol derivatives	T39.1X1	T39.1X2	T39.1X3	T39.1X4	T39.1X5	T39.1X6
Aminophenylpyridone	T43.591	T43.592	T43.593	T43.594	T43.595	T43.596
Aminophylline	T48.6X1	T48.6X2	T48.6X3	T48.6X4	T48.6X5	T48.6X6
Aminopterin sodium	T45.1X1	T45.1X2	T45.1X3	T45.1X4	T45.1X5	T45.1X6
Aminopyrine	T39.2X1	T39.2X2	T39.2X3	T39.2X4	T39.2X5	T39.2X6
8-Aminoquinoline drugs	T37.2X1	T37.2X2	T37.2X3	T37.2X4	T37.2X5	T37.2X6
Aminorex	T50.5X1	T50.5X2	T50.5X3	T50.5X4	T50.5X5	T50.5X6
Aminosalicylic acid	T37.1X1	T37.1X2	T37.1X3	T37.1X4	T37.1X5	T37.1X6
Aminosalylum	T37.1X1	T37.1X2	T37.1X3	T37.1X4	T37.1X5	T37.1X6
Amiodarone	T46.2X1	T46.2X2	T46.2X3	T46.2X4	T46.2X5	T46.2X6
Amiphenazole	T50.7X1	T50.7X2	T50.7X3	T50.7X4	T50.7X5	T50.7X6
Amiquinsin	T46.5X1	T46.5X2	T46.5X3	T46.5X4	T46.5X5	T46.5X6
Amisometradine	T50.2X1	T50.2X2	T50.2X3	T50.2X4	T50.2X5	T50.2X6
Amisulpride	T43.591	T43.592	T43.593	T43.594	T43.595	T43.596
Amitriptyline	T43.011	T43.012	T43.013	T43.014	T43.015	T43.016
Amitriptylinoxide	T43.011	T43.012	T43.013	T43.014	T43.015	T43.016
Amlexanox	T48.6X1	T48.6X2	T48.6X3	T48.6X4	T48.6X5	T48.6X6
Ammonia (fumes) (gas) (vapor)	T59.891	T59.892	T59.893	T59.894	--	--
aromatic spirit	T48.991	T48.992	T48.993	T48.994	T48.995	T48.996
liquid (household)	T54.3X1	T54.3X2	T54.3X3	T54.3X4	--	--
Ammoniated mercury	T49.0X1	T49.0X2	T49.0X3	T49.0X4	T49.0X5	T49.0X6
Ammonium						
acid tartrate	T49.5X1	T49.5X2	T49.5X3	T49.5X4	T49.5X5	T49.5X6
bromide	T42.6X1	T42.6X2	T42.6X3	T42.6X4	T42.6X5	T42.6X6
carbonate	T54.3X1	T54.3X2	T54.3X3	T54.3X4	--	--
chloride	T50.991	T50.992	T50.993	T50.994	T50.995	T50.996
expectorant	T48.4X1	T48.4X2	T48.4X3	T48.4X4	T48.4X5	T48.4X6
compounds (household) NEC	T54.3X1	T54.3X2	T54.3X3	T54.3X4	--	--
fumes (any usage)	T59.891	T59.892	T59.893	T59.894	--	--
industrial	T54.3X1	T54.3X2	T54.3X3	T54.3X4	--	--
ichthyosulronate	T49.4X1	T49.4X2	T49.4X3	T49.4X4	T49.4X5	T49.4X6
mandelate	T37.91	T37.92	T37.93	T37.94	T37.95	T37.96
sulfamate	T60.3X1	T60.3X2	T60.3X3	T60.3X4	--	--
sulfonate resin	T47.8X1	T47.8X2	T47.8X3	T47.8X4	T47.8X5	T47.8X6
Amobarbital (sodium)	T42.3X1	T42.3X2	T42.3X3	T42.3X4	T42.3X5	T42.3X6
Amodiaquine	T37.2X1	T37.2X2	T37.2X3	T37.2X4	T37.2X5	T37.2X6
Amopyroquin (e)	T37.2X1	T37.2X2	T37.2X3	T37.2X4	T37.2X5	T37.2X6

Substance	Poisoning, Accidental (unintentional)	Poisoning, Intentional Self-harm	Poisoning, Assault	Poisoning, Undetermined	Adverse effect	Underdosing
Amoxapine	T43.011	T43.012	T43.013	T43.014	T43.015	T43.016
Amoxicillin	T36.0X1	T36.0X2	T36.0X3	T36.0X4	T36.0X5	T36.0X6
Amperozide	T43.591	T43.592	T43.593	T43.594	T43.595	T43.596
Amphenidone	T43.591	T43.592	T43.593	T43.594	T43.595	T43.596
Amphetamine NEC	T43.621	T43.622	T43.623	T43.624	T43.625	T43.626
Amphomycin	T36.8X1	T36.8X2	T36.8X3	T36.8X4	T36.8X5	T36.8X6
Amphotalide	T37.4X1	T37.4X2	T37.4X3	T37.4X4	T37.4X5	T37.4X6
Amphotericin B	T36.7X1	T36.7X2	T36.7X3	T36.7X4	T36.7X5	T36.7X6
topical	T49.0X1	T49.0X2	T49.0X3	T49.0X4	T49.0X5	T49.0X6
Ampicillin	T36.0X1	T36.0X2	T36.0X3	T36.0X4	T36.0X5	T36.0X6
Amprotropine	T44.3X1	T44.3X2	T44.3X3	T44.3X4	T44.3X5	T44.3X6
Amsacrine	T45.1X1	T45.1X2	T45.1X3	T45.1X4	T45.1X5	T45.1X6
Amygdaline	T62.2X1	T62.2X2	T62.2X3	T62.2X4	--	--
Amyl						
acetate	T52.8X1	T52.8X2	T52.8X3	T52.8X4	--	--
vapor	T59.891	T59.892	T59.893	T59.894	--	--
alcohol	T51.3X1	T51.3X2	T51.3X3	T51.3X4	--	--
chloride	T53.6X1	T53.6X2	T53.6X3	T53.6X4	--	--
formate	T52.8X1	T52.8X2	T52.8X3	T52.8X4	--	--
nitrite	T46.3X1	T46.3X2	T46.3X3	T46.3X4	T46.3X5	T46.3X6
propionate	T65.891	T65.892	T65.893	T65.894	--	--
Amylase	T47.5X1	T47.5X2	T47.5X3	T47.5X4	T47.5X5	T47.5X6
Amyleine, regional	T41.3X1	T41.3X2	T41.3X3	T41.3X4	T41.3X5	T41.3X6
Amylene						
dichloride	T53.6X1	T53.6X2	T53.6X3	T53.6X4	--	--
hydrate	T51.3X1	T51.3X2	T51.3X3	T51.3X4	--	--
Amylmetacresol	T49.6X1	T49.6X2	T49.6X3	T49.6X4	T49.6X5	T49.6X6
Amylobarbitone	T42.3X1	T42.3X2	T42.3X3	T42.3X4	T42.3X5	T42.3X6
Amylocaine, regional	T41.3X1	T41.3X2	T41.3X3	T41.3X4	T41.3X5	T41.3X6
infiltration (subcutaneous)	T41.3X1	T41.3X2	T41.3X3	T41.3X4	T41.3X5	T41.3X6
nerve block (peripheral) (plexus)	T41.3X1	T41.3X2	T41.3X3	T41.3X4	T41.3X5	T41.3X6
spinal	T41.3X1	T41.3X2	T41.3X3	T41.3X4	T41.3X5	T41.3X6
topical (surface)	T41.3X1	T41.3X2	T41.3X3	T41.3X4	T41.3X5	T41.3X6
Amylopectin	T47.6X1	T47.6X2	T47.6X3	T47.6X4	T47.6X5	T47.6X6
Amytal (sodium)	T42.3X1	T42.3X2	T42.3X3	T42.3X4	T42.3X5	T42.3X6
Anabolic steroid	T38.7X1	T38.7X2	T38.7X3	T38.7X4	T38.7X5	T38.7X6
Analeptic NEC	T50.7X1	T50.7X2	T50.7X3	T50.7X4	T50.7X5	T50.7X6
Analgesic	T39.91	T39.92	T39.93	T39.94	T39.95	T39.96
anti-inflammatory NEC	T39.91	T39.92	T39.93	T39.94	T39.95	T39.96
propionic acid derivative	T39.311	T39.312	T39.313	T39.314	T39.315	T39.316
antirheumatic NEC	T39.4X1	T39.4X2	T39.4X3	T39.4X4	T39.4X5	T39.4X6
aromatic NEC	T39.1X1	T39.1X2	T39.1X3	T39.1X4	T39.1X5	T39.1X6
narcotic NEC	T40.601	T40.602	T40.603	T40.604	T40.605	T40.606
combination	T40.601	T40.602	T40.603	T40.604	T40.605	T40.606
obstetric	T40.601	T40.602	T40.603	T40.604	T40.605	T40.606
non-narcotic NEC	T39.91	T39.92	T39.93	T39.94	T39.95	T39.96
combination	T39.91	T39.92	T39.93	T39.94	T39.95	T39.96
pyrazole	T39.2X1	T39.2X2	T39.2X3	T39.2X4	T39.2X5	T39.2X6
specified NEC	T39.8X1	T39.8X2	T39.8X3	T39.8X4	T39.8X5	T39.8X6
Analgin	T39.2X1	T39.2X2	T39.2X3	T39.2X4	T39.2X5	T39.2X6
Anamirta cocculus	T62.1X1	T62.1X2	T62.1X3	T62.1X4	--	--
Ancillin	T36.0X1	T36.0X2	T36.0X3	T36.0X4	T36.0X5	T36.0X6
Ancrod	T45.691	T45.692	T45.693	T45.694	T45.695	T45.696
Androgen	T38.7X1	T38.7X2	T38.7X3	T38.7X4	T38.7X5	T38.7X6
Androgen-estrogen mixture	T38.7X1	T38.7X2	T38.7X3	T38.7X4	T38.7X5	T38.7X6
Androstalone	T38.7X1	T38.7X2	T38.7X3	T38.7X4	T38.7X5	T38.7X6
Androstanolone	T38.7X1	T38.7X2	T38.7X3	T38.7X4	T38.7X5	T38.7X6
Androsterone	T38.7X1	T38.7X2	T38.7X3	T38.7X4	T38.7X5	T38.7X6
Anemone pulsatilla	T62.2X1	T62.2X2	T62.2X3	T62.2X4	--	--
Anesthesia						
caudal	T41.3X1	T41.3X2	T41.3X3	T41.3X4	T41.3X5	T41.3X6
endotracheal	T41.0X1	T41.0X2	T41.0X3	T41.0X4	T41.0X5	T41.0X6
epidural	T41.3X1	T41.3X2	T41.3X3	T41.3X4	T41.3X5	T41.3X6
inhalation	T41.0X1	T41.0X2	T41.0X3	T41.0X4	T41.0X5	T41.0X6

Substance	Poisoning, Accidental (unintentional)	Poisoning, Intentional Self-harm	Poisoning, Assault	Poisoning, Undetermined	Adverse effect	Underdosing
local	T41.3X1	T41.3X2	T41.3X3	T41.3X4	T41.3X5	T41.3X6
mucosal	T41.3X1	T41.3X2	T41.3X3	T41.3X4	T41.3X5	T41.3X6
muscle relaxation	T48.1X1	T48.1X2	T48.1X3	T48.1X4	T48.1X5	T48.1X6
nerve blocking	T41.3X1	T41.3X2	T41.3X3	T41.3X4	T41.3X5	T41.3X6
plexus blocking	T41.3X1	T41.3X2	T41.3X3	T41.3X4	T41.3X5	T41.3X6
potentiated	T41.201	T41.202	T41.203	T41.204	T41.205	T41.206
rectal	T41.201	T41.202	T41.203	T41.204	T41.205	T41.206
general	T41.201	T41.202	T41.203	T41.204	T41.205	T41.206
local	T41.3X1	T41.3X2	T41.3X3	T41.3X4	T41.3X5	T41.3X6
regional	T41.3X1	T41.3X2	T41.3X3	T41.3X4	T41.3X5	T41.3X6
surface	T41.3X1	T41.3X2	T41.3X3	T41.3X4	T41.3X5	T41.3X6
Anesthetic NEC—see also Anesthesia	T41.41	T41.42	T41.43	T41.44	T41.45	T41.46
with muscle relaxant	T41.201	T41.202	T41.203	T41.204	T41.205	T41.206
general	T41.201	T41.202	T41.203	T41.204	T41.205	T41.206
local	T41.3X1	T41.3X2	T41.3X3	T41.3X4	T41.3X5	T41.3X6
gaseous NEC	T41.0X1	T41.0X2	T41.0X3	T41.0X4	T41.0X5	T41.0X6
general NEC	T41.201	T41.202	T41.203	T41.204	T41.205	T41.206
halogenated hydrocarbon derivatives NEC	T41.0X1	T41.0X2	T41.0X3	T41.0X4	T41.0X5	T41.0X6
infiltration NEC	T41.3X1	T41.3X2	T41.3X3	T41.3X4	T41.3X5	T41.3X6
intravenous NEC	T41.1X1	T41.1X2	T41.1X3	T41.1X4	T41.1X5	T41.1X6
local NEC	T41.3X1	T41.3X2	T41.3X3	T41.3X4	T41.3X5	T41.3X6
rectal	T41.201	T41.202	T41.203	T41.204	T41.205	T41.206
general	T41.201	T41.202	T41.203	T41.204	T41.205	T41.206
local	T41.3X1	T41.3X2	T41.3X3	T41.3X4	T41.3X5	T41.3X6
regional NEC	T41.3X1	T41.3X2	T41.3X3	T41.3X4	T41.3X5	T41.3X6
spinal NEC	T41.3X1	T41.3X2	T41.3X3	T41.3X4	T41.3X5	T41.3X6
thiobarbiturate	T41.1X1	T41.1X2	T41.1X3	T41.1X4	T41.1X5	T41.1X6
topical	T41.3X1	T41.3X2	T41.3X3	T41.3X4	T41.3X5	T41.3X6
Aneurine	T45.2X1	T45.2X2	T45.2X3	T45.2X4	T45.2X5	T45.2X6
Angio-Conray	T50.8X1	T50.8X2	T50.8X3	T50.8X4	T50.8X5	T50.8X6
Angiotensin	T44.5X1	T44.5X2	T44.5X3	T44.5X4	T44.5X5	T44.5X6
Angiotensinamide	T44.991	T44.992	T44.993	T44.994	T44.995	T44.996
Anhydrohydroxy-progesterone	T38.5X1	T38.5X2	T38.5X3	T38.5X4	T38.5X5	T38.5X6
Anhydron	T50.2X1	T50.2X2	T50.2X3	T50.2X4	T50.2X5	T50.2X6
Anileridine	T40.4X1	T40.4X2	T40.4X3	T40.4X4	T40.4X5	T40.4X6
Aniline (dye) (liquid)	T65.3X1	T65.3X2	T65.3X3	T65.3X4	--	--
analgesic	T39.1X1	T39.1X2	T39.1X3	T39.1X4	T39.1X5	T39.1X6
derivatives, therapeutic NEC	T39.1X1	T39.1X2	T39.1X3	T39.1X4	T39.1X5	T39.1X6
vapor	T65.3X1	T65.3X2	T65.3X3	T65.3X4	--	--
Aniscoropine	T44.3X1	T44.3X2	T44.3X3	T44.3X4	T44.3X5	T44.3X6
Anise oil	T47.5X1	T47.5X2	T47.5X3	T47.5X4	T47.5X5	T47.5X6
Anisidine	T65.3X1	T65.3X2	T65.3X3	T65.3X4	--	--
Anisindione	T45.511	T45.512	T45.513	T45.514	T45.515	T45.516
Anisotropine methyl-bromide	T44.3X1	T44.3X2	T44.3X3	T44.3X4	T44.3X5	T44.3X6
Anistreplase	T45.611	T45.612	T45.613	T45.614	T45.615	T45.616
Anorexiant (central)	T50.5X1	T50.5X2	T50.5X3	T50.5X4	T50.5X5	T50.5X6
Anorexic agents	T50.5X1	T50.5X2	T50.5X3	T50.5X4	T50.5X5	T50.5X6
Ansamycin	T36.6X1	T36.6X2	T36.6X3	T36.6X4	T36.6X5	T36.6X6
Ant (bite) (sting)	T63.421	T63.422	T63.423	T63.424	--	--
Ant poison—see Insecticide						
Antabuse	T50.6X1	T50.6X2	T50.6X3	T50.6X4	T50.6X5	T50.6X6
Antacid NEC	T47.1X1	T47.1X2	T47.1X3	T47.1X4	T47.1X5	T47.1X6
Antagonist						
Aldosterone	T50.0X1	T50.0X2	T50.0X3	T50.0X4	T50.0X5	T50.0X6
alpha-adrenoreceptor	T44.6X1	T44.6X2	T44.6X3	T44.6X4	T44.6X5	T44.6X6
anticoagulant	T45.7X1	T45.7X2	T45.7X3	T45.7X4	T45.7X5	T45.7X6
beta-adrenoreceptor	T44.7X1	T44.7X2	T44.7X3	T44.7X4	T44.7X5	T44.7X6
extrapyramidal NEC	T44.3X1	T44.3X2	T44.3X3	T44.3X4	T44.3X5	T44.3X6
folic acid	T45.1X1	T45.1X2	T45.1X3	T45.1X4	T45.1X5	T45.1X6
H2 receptor	T47.0X1	T47.0X2	T47.0X3	T47.0X4	T47.0X5	T47.0X6
heavy metal	T45.8X1	T45.8X2	T45.8X3	T45.8X4	T45.8X5	T45.8X6
narcotic analgesic	T50.7X1	T50.7X2	T50.7X3	T50.7X4	T50.7X5	T50.7X6
opiate	T50.7X1	T50.7X2	T50.7X3	T50.7X4	T50.7X5	T50.7X6
pyrimidine	T45.1X1	T45.1X2	T45.1X3	T45.1X4	T45.1X5	T45.1X6
serotonin	T46.5X1	T46.5X2	T46.5X3	T46.5X4	T46.5X5	T46.5X6

Substance	Poisoning, Accidental (unintentional)	Poisoning, Intentional Self-harm	Poisoning, Assault	Poisoning, Undetermined	Adverse effect	Underdosing
Antazolin (e)	T45.0X1	T45.0X2	T45.0X3	T45.0X4	T45.0X5	T45.0X6
Anterior pituitary hormone NEC	T38.811	T38.812	T38.813	T38.814	T38.815	T38.816
Anthelmintic NEC	T37.4X1	T37.4X2	T37.4X3	T37.4X4	T37.4X5	T37.4X6
Anthiolimine	T37.4X1	T37.4X2	T37.4X3	T37.4X4	T37.4X5	T37.4X6
Anthralin	T49.4X1	T49.4X2	T49.4X3	T49.4X4	T49.4X5	T49.4X6
Anthramycin	T45.1X1	T45.1X2	T45.1X3	T45.1X4	T45.1X5	T45.1X6
Antiadrenergic NEC	T44.8X1	T44.8X2	T44.8X3	T44.8X4	T44.8X5	T44.8X6
Antiallergic NEC	T45.0X1	T45.0X2	T45.0X3	T45.0X4	T45.0X5	T45.0X6
Anti-anemic (drug) (preparation)	T45.8X1	T45.8X2	T45.8X3	T45.8X4	T45.8X5	T45.8X6
Antiandrogen NEC	T38.6X1	T38.6X2	T38.6X3	T38.6X4	T38.6X5	T38.6X6
Antianxiety drug NEC	T43.501	T43.502	T43.503	T43.504	T43.505	T43.506
Antiaris toxicaria	T65.891	T65.892	†65.893	T65.894	--	--
Antiarteriosclerotic drug	T46.6X1	T46.6X2	T46.6X3	T46.6X4	T46.6X5	T46.6X6
Antiasthmatic drug NEC	T48.6X1	T48.6X2	T48.6X3	T48.6X4	T48.6X5	T48.6X6
Antibiotic NEC	T36.91	T36.92	T36.93	T36.94	T36.95	T36.96
aminoglycoside	T36.5X1	T36.5X2	T36.5X3	T36.5X4	T36.5X5	T36.5X6
anticancer	T45.1X1	T45.1X2	T45.1X3	T45.1X4	T45.1X5	T45.1X6
antifungal	T36.7X1	T36.7X2	T36.7X3	T36.7X4	T36.7X5	T36.7X6
antimycobacterial	T36.5X1	T36.5X2	T36.5X3	T36.5X4	T36.5X5	T36.5X6
antineoplastic	T45.1X1	T45.1X2	T45.1X3	T45.1X4	T45.1X5	T45.1X6
cephalosporin (group)	T36.1X1	T36.1X2	T36.1X3	T36.1X4	T36.1X5	T36.1X6
chloramphenicol (group)	T36.2X1	T36.2X2	T36.2X3	T36.2X4	T36.2X5	T36.2X6
ENT	T49.6X1	T49.6X2	T49.6X3	T49.6X4	T49.6X5	T49.6X6
eye	T49.5X1	T49.5X2	T49.5X3	T49.5X4	T49.5X5	T49.5X6
fungicidal (local)	T49.0X1	T49.0X2	T49.0X3	T49.0X4	T49.0X5	T49.0X6
intestinal	T36.8X1	T36.8X2	T36.8X3	T36.8X4	T36.8X5	T36.8X6
b-lactam NEC	T36.1X1	T36.1X2	T36.1X3	T36.1X4	T36.1X5	T36.1X6
local	T49.0X1	T49.0X2	T49.0X3	T49.0X4	T49.0X5	T49.0X6
macrolides	T36.3X1	T36.3X2	T36.3X3	T36.3X4	T36.3X5	T36.3X6
polypeptide	T36.8X1	T36.8X2	T36.8X3	T36.8X4	T36.8X5	T36.8X6
specified NEC	T36.8X1	T36.8X2	T36.8X3	T36.8X4	T36.8X5	T36.8X6
tetracycline (group)	T36.4X1	T36.4X2	T36.4X3	T36.4X4	T36.4X5	T36.4X6
throat	T49.6X1	T49.6X2	T49.6X3	T49.6X4	T49.6X5	T49.6X6
Anticancer agents NEC	T45.1X1	T45.1X2	T45.1X3	T45.1X4	T45.1X5	T45.1X6
Anticholesterolemic drug NEC	T46.6X1	T46.6X2	T46.6X3	T46.6X4	T46.6X5	T46.6X6
Anticholinergic NEC	T44.3X1	T44.3X2	T44.3X3	T44.3X4	T44.3X5	T44.3X6
Anticholinesterase	T44.0X1	T44.0X2	T44.0X3	T44.0X4	T44.0X5	T44.0X6
organophosphorus	T44.0X1	T44.0X2	T44.0X3	T44.0X4	T44.0X5	T44.0X6
insecticide	T60.0X1	T60.0X2	T60.0X3	T60.0X4	--	--
nerve gas	T59.891	T59.892	T59.893	T59.894	--	--
reversible	T44.0X1	T44.0X2	T44.0X3	T44.0X4	T44.0X5	T44.0X6
ophthalmological	T49.5X1	T49.5X2	T49.5X3	T49.5X4	T49.5X5	T49.5X6
Anticoagulant NEC	T45.511	T45.512	T45.513	T45.514	T45.515	T45.516
Antagonist	T45.7X1	T45.7X2	T45.7X3	T45.7X4	T45.7X5	T45.7X6
Anti-common-cold drug NEC	T48.5X1	T48.5X2	T48.5X3	T48.5X4	T48.5X5	T48.5X6
Anticonvulsant	T42.71	T42.72	T42.73	T42.74	T42.75	T42.76
barbiturate	T42.3X1	T42.3X2	T42.3X3	T42.3X4	T42.3X5	T42.3X6
combination (with barbiturate)	T42.3X1	T42.3X2	T42.3X3	T42.3X4	T42.3X5	T42.3X6
hydantoin	T42.0X1	T42.0X2	T42.0X3	T42.0X4	T42.0X5	T42.0X6
hypnotic NEC	T42.6X1	T42.6X2	T42.6X3	T42.6X4	T42.6X5	T42.6X6
oxazolidinedione	T42.2X1	T42.2X2	T42.2X3	T42.2X4	T42.2X5	T42.2X6
pyrimidinedione	T42.6X1	T42.6X2	T42.6X3	T42.6X4	T42.6X5	T42.6X6
specified NEC	T42.6X1	T42.6X2	T42.6X3	T42.6X4	T42.6X5	T42.6X6
succinimide	T42.2X1	T42.2X2	T42.2X3	T42.2X4	T42.2X5	T42.2X6
Anti-D immunoglobulin (human)	T50.Z11	T50.Z12	T50.Z13	T50.Z14	T50.Z15	T50.Z16
Antidepressant	T43.201	T43.202	T43.203	T43.204	T43.205	T43.206
monoamine oxidase inhibitor	T43.1X1	T43.1X2	T43.1X3	T43.1X4	T43.1X5	T43.1X6
selective serotonin norepinephrine reuptake inhibitor	T43.211	T43.212	T43.213	T43.214	T43.215	T43.216
selective serotonin reuptake inhibitor	T43.221	T43.222	T43.223	T43.224	T43.225	T43.226
specified NEC	T43.291	T43.292	T43.293	T43.294	T43.295	T43.296
tetracyclic	T43.021	T43.022	T43.023	T43.024	T43.025	T43.026
triazolopyridine	T43.211	T43.212	T43.213	T43.214	T43.215	T43.216
tricyclic	T43.011	T43.012	T43.013	T43.014	T43.015	T43.016

Substance	Poisoning, Accidental (unintentional)	Poisoning, Intentional Self-harm	Poisoning, Assault	Poisoning, Undetermined	Adverse effect	Underdosing
Antidiabetic NEC	T38.3X1	T38.3X2	T38.3X3	T38.3X4	T38.3X5	T38.3X6
biguanide	T38.3X1	T38.3X2	T38.3X3	T38.3X4	T38.3X5	T38.3X6
and sulfonyl combined	T38.3X1	T38.3X2	T38.3X3	T38.3X4	T38.3X5	T38.3X6
combined	T38.3X1	T38.3X2	T38.3X3	T38.3X4	T38.3X5	T38.3X6
sulfonylurea	T38.3X1	T38.3X2	T38.3X3	T38.3X4	T38.3X5	T38.3X6
Antidiarrheal drug NEC	T47.6X1	T47.6X2	T47.6X3	T47.6X4	T47.6X5	T47.6X6
absorbent	T47.6X1	T47.6X2	T47.6X3	T47.6X4	T47.6X5	T47.6X6
Antidiphtheria serum	T50.Z11	T50.Z12	T50.Z13	T50.Z14	T50.Z15	T50.Z16
Antidiuretic hormone	T38.891	T38.892	T38.893	T38.894	T38.895	T38.896
Antidote NEC	T50.6X1	T50.6X2	T50.6X3	T50.6X4	T50.6X5	T50.6X6
heavy metal	T45.8X1	T45.8X2	T45.8X3	T45.8X4	T45.8X5	T45.8X6
Antidysrhythmic NEC	T46.2X1	T46.2X2	T46.2X3	T46.2X4	T46.2X5	T46.2X6
Antiemetic drug	T45.0X1	T45.0X2	T45.0X3	T45.0X4	T45.0X5	T45.0X6
Antiepilepsy agent	T42.71	T42.72	T42.73	T42.74	T42.75	T42.76
combination	T42.5X1	T42.5X2	T42.5X3	T42.5X4	T42.5X5	T42.5X6
mixed	T42.5X1	T42.5X2	T42.5X3	T42.5X4	T42.5X5	T42.5X6
specified, NEC	T42.6X1	T42.6X2	T42.6X3	T42.6X4	T42.6X5	T42.6X6
Antiestrogen NEC	T38.6X1	T38.6X2	T38.6X3	T38.6X4	T38.6X5	T38.6X6
Antifertility pill	T38.4X1	T38.4X2	T38.4X3	T38.4X4	T38.4X5	T38.4X6
Antifibrinolytic drug	T45.621	T45.622	T45.623	T45.624	T45.625	T45.626
Antifilarial drug	T37.4X1	T37.4X2	T37.4X3	T37.4X4	T37.4X5	T37.4X6
Antiflatulent	T47.5X1	T47.5X2	T47.5X3	T47.5X4	T47.5X5	T47.5X6
Antifreeze	T65.91	T65.92	T65.93	T65.94	--	--
alcohol	T51.1X1	T51.1X2	T51.1X3	T51.1X4	--	--
ethylene glycol	T51.8X1	T51.8X2	T51.8X3	T51.8X4	--	--
Antifungal						
antibiotic (systemic)	T36.7X1	T36.7X2	T36.7X3	T36.7X4	T36.7X5	T36.7X6
anti-infective NEC	T37.91	T37.92	T37.93	T37.94	T37.95	T37.96
disinfectant, local	T49.0X1	T49.0X2	T49.0X3	T49.0X4	T49.0X5	T49.0X6
nonmedicinal (spray)	T60.3X1	T60.3X2	T60.3X3	T60.3X4	--	--
topical	T49.0X1	T49.0X2	T49.0X3	T49.0X4	T49.0X5	T49.0X6
Anti-gastric-secretion drug NEC	T47.1X1	T47.1X2	T47.1X3	T47.1X4	T47.1X5	T47.1X6
Antigonadotrophin NEC	T38.6X1	T38.6X2	T38.6X3	T38.6X4	T38.6X5	T38.6X6
Antihallucinogen	T43.501	T43.502	T43.503	T43.504	T43.505	T43.506
Antihelmintics	T37.4X1	T37.4X2	T37.4X3	T37.4X4	T37.4X5	T37.4X6
Antihemophilic						
factor	T45.8X1	T45.8X2	T45.8X3	T45.8X4	T45.8X5	T45.8X6
fraction	T45.8X1	T45.8X2	T45.8X3	T45.8X4	T45.8X5	T45.8X6
globulin concentrate	T45.7X1	T45.7X2	T45.7X3	T45.7X4	T45.7X5	T45.7X6
human plasma	T45.8X1	T45.8X2	T45.8X3	T45.8X4	T45.8X5	T45.8X6
plasma, dried	T45.7X1	T45.7X2	T45.7X3	T45.7X4	T45.7X5	T45.7X6
Antihemorrhoidal preparation	T49.2X1	T49.2X2	T49.2X3	T49.2X4	T49.2X5	T49.2X6
Antiheparin drug	T45.7X1	T45.7X2	T45.7X3	T45.7X4	T45.7X5	T45.7X6
Antihistamine	T45.0X1	T45.0X2	T45.0X3	T45.0X4	T45.0X5	T45.0X6
Antihookworm drug	T37.4X1	T37.4X2	T37.4X3	T37.4X4	T37.4X5	T37.4X6
Anti-human lymphocytic globulin	T50.Z11	T50.Z12	T50.Z13	T50.Z14	T50.Z15	T50.Z16
Antihyperlipidemic drug	T46.6X1	T46.6X2	T46.6X3	T46.6X4	T46.6X5	T46.6X6
Antihypertensive drug NEC	T46.5X1	T46.5X2	T46.5X3	T46.5X4	T46.5X5	T46.5X6
Anti-infective NEC	T37.91	T37.92	T37.93	T37.94	T37.95	T37.96
anthelmintic	T37.4X1	T37.4X2	T37.4X3	T37.4X4	T37.4X5	T37.4X6
antibiotics	T36.91	T36.92	T36.93	T36.94	T36.95	T36.96
specified NEC	T36.8X1	T36.8X2	T36.8X3	T36.8X4	T36.8X5	T36.8X6
antimalarial	T37.2X1	T37.2X2	T37.2X3	T37.2X4	T37.2X5	T37.2X6
antimycobacterial NEC	T37.1X1	T37.1X2	T37.1X3	T37.1X4	T37.1X5	T37.1X6
antibiotics	T36.5X1	T36.5X2	T36.5X3	T36.5X4	T36.5X5	T36.5X6
antiprotozoal NEC	T37.3X1	T37.3X2	T37.3X3	T37.3X4	T37.3X5	T37.3X6
blood	T37.2X1	T37.2X2	T37.2X3	T37.2X4	T37.2X5	T37.2X6
antiviral	T37.5X1	T37.5X2	T37.5X3	T37.5X4	T37.5X5	T37.5X6
arsenical	T37.8X1	T37.8X2	T37.8X3	T37.8X4	T37.8X5	T37.8X6
bismuth, local	T49.0X1	T49.0X2	T49.0X3	T49.0X4	T49.0X5	T49.0X6
ENT	T49.6X1	T49.6X2	T49.6X3	T49.6X4	T49.6X5	T49.6X6
eye NEC	T49.5X1	T49.5X2	T49.5X3	T49.5X4	T49.5X5	T49.5X6
heavy metals NEC	T37.8X1	T37.8X2	T37.8X3	T37.8X4	T37.8X5	T37.8X6
local NEC	T49.0X1	T49.0X2	T49.0X3	T49.0X4	T49.0X5	T49.0X6
specified NEC	T49.0X1	T49.0X2	T49.0X3	T49.0X4	T49.0X5	T49.0X6

TABLE OF DRUGS AND CHEMICALS

Substance	Poisoning, Accidental (unintentional)	Poisoning, Intentional Self-harm	Poisoning, Assault	Poisoning, Undetermined	Adverse effect	Underdosing
mixed	T37.91	T37.92	T37.93	T37.94	T37.95	T37.96
ophthalmic preparation	T49.5X1	T49.5X2	T49.5X3	T49.5X4	T49.5X5	T49.5X6
topical NEC	T49.0X1	T49.0X2	T49.0X3	T49.0X4	T49.0X5	T49.0X6
Anti-inflammatory drug NEC	T39.391	T39.392	T39.393	T39.394	T39.395	T39.396
local	T49.0X1	T49.0X2	T49.0X3	T49.0X4	T49.0X5	T49.0X6
nonsteroidal NEC	T39.391	T39.392	T39.393	T39.394	T39.395	T39.396
propionic acid derivative	T39.311	T39.312	T39.313	T39.314	T39.315	T39.316
specified NEC	T39.391	T39.392	T39.393	T39.394	T39.395	T39.396
Antikaluretic	T50.3X1	T50.3X2	T50.3X3	T50.3X4	T50.3X5	T50.3X6
Antiknock (tetraethyl lead)	T56.0X1	T56.0X2	T56.0X3	T56.0X4	--	--
Antilipemic drug NEC	T46.6X1	T46.6X2	T46.6X3	T46.6X4	T46.6X5	T46.6X6
Antimalarial	T37.2X1	T37.2X2	T37.2X3	T37.2X4	T37.2X5	T37.2X6
prophylactic NEC	T37.2X1	T37.2X2	T37.2X3	T37.2X4	T37.2X5	T37.2X6
pyrimidine derivative	T37.2X1	T37.2X2	T37.2X3	T37.2X4	T37.2X5	T37.2X6
Antimetabolite	T45.1X1	T45.1X2	T45.1X3	T45.1X4	T45.1X5	T45.1X6
Antimitotic agent	T45.1X1	T45.1X2	T45.1X3	T45.1X4	T45.1X5	T45.1X6
Antimony (compounds) (vapor) NEC	T56.891	T56.892	T56.893	T56.894	--	--
anti-infectives	T37.8X1	T37.8X2	T37.8X3	T37.8X4	T37.8X5	T37.8X6
dimercaptosuccinate	T37.3X1	T37.3X2	T37.3X3	T37.3X4	T37.3X5	T37.3X6
hydride	T56.891	T56.892	T56.893	T56.894	--	--
pesticide (vapor)	T60.8X1	T60.8X2	T60.8X3	T60.8X4	--	--
potassium (sodium) tartrate	T37.8X1	T37.8X2	T37.8X3	T37.8X4	T37.8X5	T37.8X6
sodium dimercaptosuccinate	T37.3X1	T37.3X2	T37.3X3	T37.3X4	T37.3X5	T37.3X6
tartrated	T37.8X1	T37.8X2	T37.8X3	T37.8X4	T37.8X5	T37.8X6
Antimuscarinic NEC	T44.3X1	T44.3X2	T44.3X3	T44.3X4	T44.3X5	T44.3X6
Antimycobacterial drug NEC	T37.1X1	T37.1X2	T37.1X3	T37.1X4	T37.1X5	T37.1X6
antibiotics	T36.5X1	T36.5X2	T36.5X3	T36.5X4	T36.5X5	T36.5X6
combination	T37.1X1	T37.1X2	T37.1X3	T37.1X4	T37.1X5	T37.1X6
Antinausea drug	T45.0X1	T45.0X2	T45.0X3	T45.0X4	T45.0X5	T45.0X6
Antinematode drug	T37.4X1	T37.4X2	T37.4X3	T37.4X4	T37.4X5	T37.4X6
Antineoplastic NEC	T45.1X1	T45.1X2	T45.1X3	T45.1X4	T45.1X5	T45.1X6
alkaloidal	T45.1X1	T45.1X2	T45.1X3	T45.1X4	T45.1X5	T45.1X6
antibiotics	T45.1X1	T45.1X2	T45.1X3	T45.1X4	T45.1X5	T45.1X6
combination	T45.1X1	T45.1X2	T45.1X3	T45.1X4	T45.1X5	T45.1X6
estrogen	T38.5X1	T38.5X2	T38.5X3	T38.5X4	T38.5X5	T38.5X6
steroid	T38.7X1	T38.7X2	T38.7X3	T38.7X4	T38.7X5	T38.7X6
Antiparasitic drug (systemic)	T37.91	T37.92	T37.93	T37.94	T37.95	T37.96
local	T49.0X1	T49.0X2	T49.0X3	T49.0X4	T49.0X5	T49.0X6
specified NEC	T37.8X1	T37.8X2	T37.8X3	T37.8X4	T37.8X5	T37.8X6
Antiparkinsonism drug NEC	T42.8X1	T42.8X2	T42.8X3	T42.8X4	T42.8X5	T42.8X6
Antiperspirant NEC	T49.2X1	T49.2X2	T49.2X3	T49.2X4	T49.2X5	T49.2X6
Antiphlogistic NEC	T39.4X1	T39.4X2	T39.4X3	T39.4X4	T39.4X5	T39.4X6
Antiplatyhelmintic drug	T37.4X1	T37.4X2	T37.4X3	T37.4X4	T37.4X5	T37.4X6
Antiprotozoal drug NEC	T37.3X1	T37.3X2	T37.3X3	T37.3X4	T37.3X5	T37.3X6
blood	T37.2X1	T37.2X2	T37.2X3	T37.2X4	T37.2X5	T37.2X6
local	T49.0X1	T49.0X2	T49.0X3	T49.0X4	T49.0X5	T49.0X6
Antipruritic drug NEC	T49.1X1	T49.1X2	T49.1X3	T49.1X4	T49.1X5	T49.1X6
Antipsychotic drug	T43.501	T43.502	T43.503	T43.504	T43.505	T43.506
specified NEC	T43.591	T43.592	T43.593	T43.594	T43.595	T43.596
Antipyretic	T39.91	T39.92	T39.93	T39.94	T39.95	T39.96
specified NEC	T39.8X1	T39.8X2	T39.8X3	T39.8X4	T39.8X5	T39.8X6
Antipyrine	T39.2X1	T39.2X2	T39.2X3	T39.2X4	T39.2X5	T39.2X6
Antirabies hyperimmune serum	T50.Z11	T50.Z12	T50.Z13	T50.Z14	T50.Z15	T50.Z16
Antirheumatic NEC	T39.4X1	T39.4X2	T39.4X3	T39.4X4	T39.4X5	T39.4X6
Antirigidity drug NEC	T42.8X1	T42.8X2	T42.8X3	T42.8X4	T42.8X5	T42.8X6
Antischistosomal drug	T37.4X1	T37.4X2	T37.4X3	T37.4X4	T37.4X5	T37.4X6
Antiscorpion sera	T50.Z11	T50.Z12	T50.Z13	T50.Z14	T50.Z15	T50.Z16
Antiseborrheics	T49.4X1	T49.4X2	T49.4X3	T49.4X4	T49.4X5	T49.4X6
Antiseptics (external) (medicinal)	T49.0X1	T49.0X2	T49.0X3	T49.0X4	T49.0X5	T49.0X6
Antistine	T45.0X1	T45.0X2	T45.0X3	T45.0X4	T45.0X5	T45.0X6
Antitapeworm drug	T37.4X1	T37.4X2	T37.4X3	T37.4X4	T37.4X5	T37.4X6
Antitetanus immunoglobulin	T50.Z11	T50.Z12	T50.Z13	T50.Z14	T50.Z15	T50.Z16
Antithyroid drug NEC	T38.2X1	T38.2X2	T38.2X3	T38.2X4	T38.2X5	T38.2X6
Antitoxin	T50.Z11	T50.Z12	T50.Z13	T50.Z14	T50.Z15	T50.Z16

TABLE OF DRUGS AND CHEMICALS

Substance	Poisoning, Accidental (unintentional)	Poisoning, Intentional Self-harm	Poisoning, Assault	Poisoning, Undetermined	Adverse effect	Underdosing
diphtheria	T50.Z11	T50.Z12	T50.Z13	T50.Z14	T50.Z15	T50.Z16
gas gangrene	T50.Z11	T50.Z12	T50.Z13	T50.Z14	T50.Z15	T50.Z16
tetanus	T50.Z11	T50.Z12	T50.Z13	T50.Z14	T50.Z15	T50.Z16
Antitrichomonal drug	T37.3X1	T37.3X2	T37.3X3	T37.3X4	T37.3X5	T37.3X6
Antituberculars	T37.1X1	T37.1X2	T37.1X3	T37.1X4	T37.1X5	T37.1X6
antibiotics	T36.5X1	T36.5X2	T36.5X3	T36.5X4	T36.5X5	T36.5X6
Antitussive NEC	T48.3X1	T48.3X2	T48.3X3	T48.3X4	T48.3X5	T48.3X6
codeine mixture	T40.2X1	T40.2X2	T40.2X3	T40.2X4	T40.2X5	T40.2X6
opiate	T40.2X1	T40.2X2	T40.2X3	T40.2X4	T40.2X5	T40.2X6
Antivaricose drug	T46.8X1	T46.8X2	T46.8X3	T46.8X4	T46.8X5	T46.8X6
Antivenin, antivenom (sera)	T50.Z11	T50.Z12	T50.Z13	T50.Z14	T50.Z15	T50.Z16
crotaline	T50.Z11	T50.Z12	T50.Z13	T50.Z14	T50.Z15	T50.Z16
spider bite	T50.Z11	T50.Z12	T50.Z13	T50.Z14	T50.Z15	T50.Z16
Antivertigo drug	T45.0X1	T45.0X2	T45.0X3	T45.0X4	T45.0X5	T45.0X6
Antiviral drug NEC	T37.5X1	T37.5X2	T37.5X3	T37.5X4	T37.5X5	T37.5X6
eye	T49.5X1	T49.5X2	T49.5X3	T49.5X4	T49.5X5	T49.5X6
Antiwhipworm drug	T37.4X1	T37.4X2	T37.4X3	T37.4X4	T37.4X5	T37.4X6
Antrol—see also by specific chemical	T60.91	T60.92	T60.93	T60.94	--	--substance
fungicide	T60.91	T60.92	T60.93	T60.94	--	--
ANTU (alpha naphthylthiourea)	T60.4X1	T60.4X2	T60.4X3	T60.4X4	--	--
Apalcillin	T36.0X1	T36.0X2	T36.0X3	T36.0X4	T36.0X5	T36.0X6
APC	T48.5X1	T48.5X2	T48.5X3	T48.5X4	T48.5X5	T48.5X6
Aplonidine	T44.4X1	T44.4X2	T44.4X3	T44.4X4	T44.4X5	T44.4X6
Apomorphine	T47.7X1	T47.7X2	T47.7X3	T47.7X4	T47.7X5	T47.7X6
Appetite depressants, central	T50.5X1	T50.5X2	T50.5X3	T50.5X4	T50.5X5	T50.5X6
Apraclonidine (hydrochloride)	T44.4X1	T44.4X2	T44.4X3	T44.4X4	T44.4X5	T44.4X6
Apresoline	T46.5X1	T46.5X2	T46.5X3	T46.5X4	T46.5X5	T46.5X6
Aprindine	T46.2X1	T46.2X2	T46.2X3	T46.2X4	T46.2X5	T46.2X6
Aprobarbital	T42.3X1	T42.3X2	T42.3X3	T42.3X4	T42.3X5	T42.3X6
Apronalide	T42.6X1	T42.6X2	T42.6X3	T42.6X4	T42.6X5	T42.6X6
Aprotinin	T45.621	T45.622	T45.623	T45.624	T45.625	T45.626
Aptocaine	T41.3X1	T41.3X2	T41.3X3	T41.3X4	T41.3X5	T41.3X6
Aqua fortis	T54.2X1	T54.2X2	T54.2X3	T54.2X4	--	--
Ara-A	T37.5X1	T37.5X2	T37.5X3	T37.5X4	T37.5X5	T37.5X6
Ara-C	T45.1X1	T45.1X2	T45.1X3	T45.1X4	T45.1X5	T45.1X6
Arachis oil	T49.3X1	T49.3X2	T49.3X3	T49.3X4	T49.3X5	T49.3X6
cathartic	T47.4X1	T47.4X2	T47.4X3	T47.4X4	T47.4X5	T47.4X6
Aralen	T37.2X1	T37.2X2	T37.2X3	T37.2X4	T37.2X5	T37.2X6
Arecoline	T44.1X1	T44.1X2	T44.1X3	T44.1X4	T44.1X5	T44.1X6
Arginine	T50.991	T50.992	T50.993	T50.994	T50.995	T50.996
glutamate	T50.991	T50.992	T50.993	T50.994	T50.995	T50.996
Argyrol	T49.0X1	T49.0X2	T49.0X3	T49.0X4	T49.0X5	T49.0X6
EN	T agent	T49.6X1	T49.6X2	T49.6X3	T49.6X4	T49.6X5
T49.6X6						
ophthalmic preparation	T49.5X1	T49.5X2	T49.5X3	T49.5X4	T49.5X5	T49.5X6
Aristocort	T38.0X1	T38.0X2	T38.0X3	T38.0X4	T38.0X5	T38.0X6
ENT agent	T49.6X1	T49.6X2	T49.6X3	T49.6X4	T49.6X5	T49.6X6
ophthalmic preparation	T49.5X1	T49.5X2	T49.5X3	T49.5X4	T49.5X5	T49.5X6
topical NEC	T49.0X1	T49.0X2	T49.0X3	T49.0X4	T49.0X5	T49.0X6
Aromatics, corrosive	T54.1X1	T54.1X2	T54.1X3	T54.1X4	--	--
disinfectants	T54.1X1	T54.1X2	T54.1X3	T54.1X4	--	--
Arsenate of lead	T57.0X1	T57.0X2	T57.0X3	T57.0X4	--	--
herbicide	T57.0X1	T57.0X2	T57.0X3	T57.0X4	--	--
Arsenic, arsenicals (compounds) (dust) (vapor) NEC	T57.0X1	T57.0X2	T57.0X3	T57.0X4	--	--
anti-infectives	T37.8X1	T37.8X2	T37.8X3	T37.8X4	T37.8X5	T37.8X6
pesticide (dust) (fumes)	T57.0X1	T57.0X2	T57.0X3	T57.0X4	--	--
Arsine (gas)	T57.0X1	T57.0X2	T57.0X3	T57.0X4	--	--
Arsphenamine (silver)	T37.8X1	T37.8X2	T37.8X3	T37.8X4	T37.8X5	T37.8X6
Arsthinol	T37.3X1	T37.3X2	T37.3X3	T37.3X4	T37.3X5	T37.3X6
Artane	T44.3X1	T44.3X2	T44.3X3	T44.3X4	T44.3X5	T44.3X6
Arthropod (venomous) NEC	T63.481	T63.482	T63.483	T63.484	--	--
Articaine	T41.3X1	T41.3X2	T41.3X3	T41.3X4	T41.3X5	T41.3X6
Asbestos	T57.8X1	T57.8X2	T57.8X3	T57.8X4	--	--
Ascaridole	T37.4X1	T37.4X2	T37.4X3	T37.4X4	T37.4X5	T37.4X6

TABLE OF DRUGS AND CHEMICALS

Substance	Poisoning, Accidental (unintentional)	Poisoning, Intentional Self-harm	Poisoning, Assault	Poisoning, Undetermined	Adverse effect	Underdosing
Ascorbic acid	T45.2X1	T45.2X2	T45.2X3	T45.2X4	T45.2X5	T45.2X6
Asiaticoside	T49.0X1	T49.0X2	T49.0X3	T49.0X4	T49.0X5	T49.0X6
Asparaginase	T45.1X1	T45.1X2	T45.1X3	T45.1X4	T45.1X5	T45.1X6
Aspidium (oleoresin)	T37.4X1	T37.4X2	T37.4X3	T37.4X4	T37.4X5	T37.4X6
Aspirin (aluminum) (soluble)	T39.011	T39.012	T39.013	T39.014	T39.015	T39.016
Aspoxicillin	T36.0X1	T36.0X2	T36.0X3	T36.0X4	T36.0X5	T36.0X6
Astemizole	T45.0X1	T45.0X2	T45.0X3	T45.0X4	T45.0X5	T45.0X6
Astringent (local)	T49.2X1	T49.2X2	T49.2X3	T49.2X4	T49.2X5	T49.2X6
specified NEC	T49.2X1	T49.2X2	T49.2X3	T49.2X4	T49.2X5	T49.2X6
Astromicin	T36.5X1	T36.5X2	T36.5X3	T36.5X4	T36.5X5	T36.5X6
Ataractic drug NEC	T43.501	T43.502	T43.503	T43.504	T43.505	T43.506
Atenolol	T44.7X1	T44.7X2	T44.7X3	T44.7X4	T44.7X5	T44.7X6
Atonia drug, intestinal	T47.4X1	T47.4X2	T47.4X3	T47.4X4	T47.4X5	T47.4X6
Atophan	T50.4X1	T50.4X2	T50.4X3	T50.4X4	T50.4X5	T50.4X6
Atracurium besilate	T48.1X1	T48.1X2	T48.1X3	T48.1X4	T48.1X5	T48.1X6
Atropine	T44.3X1	T44.3X2	T44.3X3	T44.3X4	T44.3X5	T44.3X6
derivative	T44.3X1	T44.3X2	T44.3X3	T44.3X4	T44.3X5	T44.3X6
methonitrate	T44.3X1	T44.3X2	T44.3X3	T44.3X4	T44.3X5	T44.3X6
Attapulgite	T47.6X1	T47.6X2	T47.6X3	T47.6X4	T47.6X5	T47.6X6
Auramine	T65.891	T65.892	T65.893	T65.894	--	--
dye	T65.6X1	T65.6X2	T65.6X3	T65.6X4	--	--
fungicide	T60.3X1	T60.3X2	T60.3X3	T60.3X4	--	--
Auranofin	T39.4X1	T39.4X2	T39.4X3	T39.4X4	T39.4X5	T39.4X6
Aurantiin	T46.991	T46.992	T46.993	T46.994	T46.995	T46.996
Aureomycin	T36.4X1	T36.4X2	T36.4X3	T36.4X4	T36.4X5	T36.4X6
ophthalmic preparation	T49.5X1	T49.5X2	T49.5X3	T49.5X4	T49.5X5	T49.5X6
topical NEC	T49.0X1	T49.0X2	T49.0X3	T49.0X4	T49.0X5	T49.0X6
Aurothioglucose	T39.4X1	T39.4X2	T39.4X3	T39.4X4	T39.4X5	T39.4X6
Aurothioglycanide	T39.4X1	T39.4X2	T39.4X3	T39.4X4	T39.4X5	T39.4X6
Aurothiomalate sodium	T39.4X1	T39.4X2	T39.4X3	T39.4X4	T39.4X5	T39.4X6
Aurotioprol	T39.4X1	T39.4X2	T39.4X3	T39.4X4	T39.4X5	T39.4X6
Automobile fuel	T52.0X1	T52.0X2	T52.0X3	T52.0X4	--	--
Autonomic nervous system agent NEC	T44.901	T44.902	T44.903	T44.904	T44.905	T44.906
Avlosulfon	T37.1X1	T37.1X2	T37.1X3	T37.1X4	T37.1X5	T37.1X6
Avomine	T42.6X1	T42.6X2	T42.6X3	T42.6X4	T42.6X5	T42.6X6
Axerophthol	T45.2X1	T45.2X2	T45.2X3	T45.2X4	T45.2X5	T45.2X6
Azacitidine	T45.1X1	T45.1X2	T45.1X3	T45.1X4	T45.1X5	T45.1X6
Azacyclonol	T43.591	T43.592	T43.593	T43.594	T43.595	T43.596
Azadirachta	T60.2X1	T60.2X2	T60.2X3	T60.2X4	--	--
Azanidazole	T37.3X1	T37.3X2	T37.3X3	T37.3X4	T37.3X5	T37.3X6
Azapetine	T46.7X1	T46.7X2	T46.7X3	T46.7X4	T46.7X5	T46.7X6
Azapropazone	T39.2X1	T39.2X2	T39.2X3	T39.2X4	T39.2X5	T39.2X6
Azaribine	T45.1X1	T45.1X2	T45.1X3	T45.1X4	T45.1X5	T45.1X6
Azaserine	T45.1X1	T45.1X2	T45.1X3	T45.1X4	T45.1X5	T45.1X6
Azatadine	T45.0X1	T45.0X2	T45.0X3	T45.0X4	T45.0X5	T45.0X6
Azatepa	T45.1X1	T45.1X2	T45.1X3	T45.1X4	T45.1X5	T45.1X6
Azathioprine	T45.1X1	T45.1X2	T45.1X3	T45.1X4	T45.1X5	T45.1X6
Azelaic acid	T49.0X1	T49.0X2	T49.0X3	T49.0X4	T49.0X5	T49.0X6
Azelastine	T45.0X1	T45.0X2	T45.0X3	T45.0X4	T45.0X5	T45.0X6
Azidocillin	T36.0X1	T36.0X2	T36.0X3	T36.0X4	T36.0X5	T36.0X6
Azidothymidine	T37.5X1	T37.5X2	T37.5X3	T37.5X4	T37.5X5	T37.5X6
Azinphos (ethyl) (methyl)	T60.0X1	T60.0X2	T60.0X3	T60.0X4	--	--
Aziridine (chelating)	T54.1X1	T54.1X2	T54.1X3	T54.1X4	--	--
Azithromycin	T36.3X1	T36.3X2	T36.3X3	T36.3X4	T36.3X5	T36.3X6
Azlocillin	T36.0X1	T36.0X2	T36.0X3	T36.0X4	T36.0X5	T36.0X6
Azobenzene smoke	T65.3X1	T65.3X2	T65.3X3	T65.3X4	--	--
acaricide	T60.8X1	T60.8X2	T60.8X3	T60.8X4	--	--
Azosulfamide	T37.0X1	T37.0X2	T37.0X3	T37.0X4	T37.0X5	T37.0X6
AZT	T37.5X1	T37.5X2	T37.5X3	T37.5X4	T37.5X5	T37.5X6
Aztreonam	T36.1X1	T36.1X2	T36.1X3	T36.1X4	T36.1X5	T36.1X6
Azulfidine	T37.0X1	T37.0X2	T37.0X3	T37.0X4	T37.0X5	T37.0X6
Azuresin	T50.8X1	T50.8X2	T50.8X3	T50.8X4	T50.8X5	T50.8X6
Bacampicillin	T36.0X1	T36.0X2	T36.0X3	T36.0X4	T36.0X5	T36.0X6
Bacillus						

Substance	Poisoning, Accidental (unintentional)	Poisoning, Intentional Self-harm	Poisoning, Assault	Poisoning, Undetermined	Adverse effect	Underdosing
lactobacillus	T47.8X1	T47.8X2	T47.8X3	T47.8X4	T47.8X5	T47.8X6
subtilis	T47.6X1	T47.6X2	T47.6X3	T47.6X4	T47.6X5	T47.6X6
Bacimycin	T49.0X1	T49.0X2	T49.0X3	T49.0X4	T49.0X5	T49.0X6
ophthalmic preparation	T49.5X1	T49.5X2	T49.5X3	T49.5X4	T49.5X5	T49.5X6
Bacitracin zinc	T49.0X1	T49.0X2	T49.0X3	T49.0X4	T49.0X5	T49.0X6
with neomycin	T49.0X1	T49.0X2	T49.0X3	T49.0X4	T49.0X5	T49.0X6
ENT agent	T49.6X1	T49.6X2	T49.6X3	T49.6X4	T49.6X5	T49.6X6
ophthalmic preparation	T49.5X1	T49.5X2	T49.5X3	T49.5X4	T49.5X5	T49.5X6
topical NEC	T49.0X1	T49.0X2	T49.0X3	T49.0X4	T49.0X5	T49.0X6
Baclofen	T42.8X1	T42.8X2	T42.8X3	T42.8X4	T42.8X5	T42.8X6
Baking soda	T50.991	T50.992	T50.993	T50.994	T50.995	T50.996
BAL	T45.8X1	T45.8X2	T45.8X3	T45.8X4	T45.8X5	T45.8X6
Bambuterol	T48.6X1	T48.6X2	T48.6X3	T48.6X4	T48.6X5	T48.6X6
Bamethan (sulfate)	T46.7X1	T46.7X2	T46.7X3	T46.7X4	T46.7X5	T46.7X6
Bamifylline	T48.6X1	T48.6X2	T48.6X3	T48.6X4	T48.6X5	T48.6X6
Bamipine	T45.0X1	T45.0X2	T45.0X3	T45.0X4	T45.0X5	T45.0X6
Baneberry—see Actaea spicata						
Banewort—see Belladonna						
Barbenyl	T42.3X1	T42.3X2	T42.3X3	T42.3X4	T42.3X5	T42.3X6
Barbexaclone	T42.6X1	T42.6X2	T42.6X3	T42.6X4	T42.6X5	T42.6X6
Barbital	T42.3X1	T42.3X2	T42.3X3	T42.3X4	T42.3X5	T42.3X6
sodium	T42.3X1	T42.3X2	T42.3X3	T42.3X4	T42.3X5	T42.3X6
Barbitone	T42.3X1	T42.3X2	T42.3X3	T42.3X4	T42.3X5	T42.3X6
Barbiturate NEC	T42.3X1	T42.3X2	T42.3X3	T42.3X4	T42.3X5	T42.3X6
with tranquilizer	T42.3X1	T42.3X2	T42.3X3	T42.3X4	T42.3X5	T42.3X6
anesthetic (intravenous)	T41.1X1	T41.1X2	T41.1X3	T41.1X4	T41.1X5	T41.1X6
Barium (carbonate) (chloride) (sulfite)	T57.8X1	T57.8X2	T57.8X3	T57.8X4	--	--
diagnostic agent	T50.8X1	T50.8X2	T50.8X3	T50.8X4	T50.8X5	T50.8X6
pesticide	T60.4X1	T60.4X2	T60.4X3	T60.4X4	--	--
rodenticide	T60.4X1	T60.4X2	T60.4X3	T60.4X4	--	--
sulfate (medicinal)	T50.8X1	T50.8X2	T50.8X3	T50.8X4	T50.8X5	T50.8X6
Barrier cream	T49.3X1	T49.3X2	T49.3X3	T49.3X4	T49.3X5	T49.3X6
Basic fuchsin	T49.0X1	T49.0X2	T49.0X3	T49.0X4	T49.0X5	T49.0X6
Battery acid or fluid	T54.2X1	T54.2X2	T54.2X3	T54.2X4	--	--
Bay rum	T51.8X1	T51.8X2	T51.8X3	T51.8X4	--	--
BCG (vaccine)	T50.A91	T50.A92	T50.A93	T50.A94	T50.A95	T50.A96
BCNU	T45.1X1	T45.1X2	T45.1X3	T45.1X4	T45.1X5	T45.1X6
Bearsfoot	T62.2X1	T62.2X2	T62.2X3	T62.2X4	--	--
Beclamide	T42.6X1	T42.6X2	T42.6X3	T42.6X4	T42.6X5	T42.6X6
Beclomethasone	T44.5X1	T44.5X2	T44.5X3	T44.5X4	T44.5X5	T44.5X6
Bee (sting) (venom)	T63.441	T63.442	T63.443	T63.444	--	--
Befunolol	T49.5X1	T49.5X2	T49.5X3	T49.5X4	T49.5X5	T49.5X6
Bekanamycin	T36.5X1	T36.5X2	T36.5X3	T36.5X4	T36.5X5	T36.5X6
Belladonna—see also Nightshade						
alkaloids	T44.3X1	T44.3X2	T44.3X3	T44.3X4	T44.3X5	T44.3X6
extract	T44.3X1	T44.3X2	T44.3X3	T44.3X4	T44.3X5	T44.3X6
herb	T44.3X1	T44.3X2	T44.3X3	T44.3X4	T44.3X5	T44.3X6
Bemegride	T50.7X1	T50.7X2	T50.7X3	T50.7X4	T50.7X5	T50.7X6
Benactyzine	T44.3X1	T44.3X2	T44.3X3	T44.3X4	T44.3X5	T44.3X6
Benadryl	T45.0X1	T45.0X2	T45.0X3	T45.0X4	T45.0X5	T45.0X6
Benaprizine	T44.3X1	T44.3X2	T44.3X3	T44.3X4	T44.3X5	T44.3X6
Benazepril	T46.4X1	T46.4X2	T46.4X3	T46.4X4	T46.4X5	T46.4X6
Bencyclane	T46.7X1	T46.7X2	T46.7X3	T46.7X4	T46.7X5	T46.7X6
Bendazol	T46.3X1	T46.3X2	T46.3X3	T46.3X4	T46.3X5	T46.3X6
Bendrofluazide	T50.2X1	T50.2X2	T50.2X3	T50.2X4	T50.2X5	T50.2X6
Bendroflumethiazide	T50.2X1	T50.2X2	T50.2X3	T50.2X4	T50.2X5	T50.2X6
Benemid	T50.4X1	T50.4X2	T50.4X3	T50.4X4	T50.4X5	T50.4X6
Benethamine penicillin	T36.0X1	T36.0X2	T36.0X3	T36.0X4	T36.0X5	T36.0X6
Benexate	T47.1X1	T47.1X2	T47.1X3	T47.1X4	T47.1X5	T47.1X6
Benfluorex	T46.6X1	T46.6X2	T46.6X3	T46.6X4	T46.6X5	T46.6X6
Benfotiamine	T45.2X1	T45.2X2	T45.2X3	T45.2X4	T45.2X5	T45.2X6
Benisone	T49.0X1	T49.0X2	T49.0X3	T49.0X4	T49.0X5	T49.0X6
Benomyl	T60.0X1	T60.0X2	T60.0X3	T60.0X4	--	--
Benoquin	T49.8X1	T49.8X2	T49.8X3	T49.8X4	T49.8X5	T49.8X6
Benoxinate	T41.3X1	T41.3X2	T41.3X3	T41.3X4	T41.3X5	T41.3X6

Substance	Poisoning, Accidental (unintentional)	Poisoning, Intentional Self-harm	Poisoning, Assault	Poisoning, Undetermined	Adverse effect	Underdosing
Benperidol	T43.4X1	T43.4X2	T43.4X3	T43.4X4	T43.4X5	T43.4X6
Benproperine	T48.3X1	T48.3X2	T48.3X3	T48.3X4	T48.3X5	T48.3X6
Benserazide	T42.8X1	T42.8X2	T42.8X3	T42.8X4	T42.8X5	T42.8X6
Bentazepam	T42.4X1	T42.4X2	T42.4X3	T42.4X4	T42.4X5	T42.4X6
Bentiromide	T50.8X1	T50.8X2	T50.8X3	T50.8X4	T50.8X5	T50.8X6
Bentonite	T49.3X1	T49.3X2	T49.3X3	T49.3X4	T49.3X5	T49.3X6
Benzalbutyramide	T46.6X1	T46.6X2	T46.6X3	T46.6X4	T46.6X5	T46.6X6
Benzalkonium (chloride)	T49.0X1	T49.0X2	T49.0X3	T49.0X4	T49.0X5	T49.0X6
ophthalmic preparation	T49.5X1	T49.5X2	T49.5X3	T49.5X4	T49.5X5	T49.5X6
Benzamidosalicylate (calcium)	T37.1X1	T37.1X2	T37.1X3	T37.1X4	T37.1X5	T37.1X6
Benzamine	T41.3X1	T41.3X2	T41.3X3	T41.3X4	T41.3X5	T41.3X6
lactate	T49.1X1	T49.1X2	T49.1X3	T49.1X4	T49.1X5	T49.1X6
Benzamphetamine	T50.5X1	T50.5X2	T50.5X3	T50.5X4	T50.5X5	T50.5X6
Benzapril hydrochloride	T46.5X1	T46.5X2	T46.5X3	T46.5X4	T46.5X5	T46.5X6
Benzathine benzylpenicillin	T36.0X1	T36.0X2	T36.0X3	T36.0X4	T36.0X5	T36.0X6
Benzathine penicillin	T36.0X1	T36.0X2	T36.0X3	T36.0X4	T36.0X5	T36.0X6
Benzatropine	T42.8X1	T42.8X2	T42.8X3	T42.8X4	T42.8X5	T42.8X6
Benzbromarone	T50.4X1	T50.4X2	T50.4X3	T50.4X4	T50.4X5	T50.4X6
Benzcarbimine	T45.1X1	T45.1X2	T45.1X3	T45.1X4	T45.1X5	T45.1X6
Benzedrex	T44.991	T44.992	T44.993	T44.994	T44.995	T44.996
Benzedrine (amphetamine)	T43.621	T43.622	T43.623	T43.624	T43.625	T43.626
Benzenamine	T65.3X1	T65.3X2	T65.3X3	T65.3X4	--	--
Benzene	T52.1X1	T52.1X2	T52.1X3	T52.1X4	--	--
homologues (acetyl) (dimethyl) (methyl) (solvent)	T52.2X1	T52.2X2	T52.2X3	T52.2X4	--	--
Benzethonium (chloride)	T49.0X1	T49.0X2	T49.0X3	T49.0X4	T49.0X5	T49.0X6
Benzfetamine	T50.5X1	T50.5X2	T50.5X3	T50.5X4	T50.5X5	T50.5X6
Benzhexol	T44.3X1	T44.3X2	T44.3X3	T44.3X4	T44.3X5	T44.3X6
Benzhydramine (chloride)	T45.0X1	T45.0X2	T45.0X3	T45.0X4	T45.0X5	T45.0X6
Benzidine	T65.891	T65.892	T65.893	T65.894	--	--
Benzilonium bromide	T44.3X1	T44.3X2	T44.3X3	T44.3X4	T44.3X5	T44.3X6
Benzimidazole	T60.3X1	T60.3X2	T60.3X3	T60.3X4	--	--
Benzin (e) —see Ligroin						
Benziodarone	T46.3X1	T46.3X2	T46.3X3	T46.3X4	T46.3X5	T46.3X6
Benznidazole	T37.3X1	T37.3X2	T37.3X3	T37.3X4	T37.3X5	T37.3X6
Benzocaine	T41.3X1	T41.3X2	T41.3X3	T41.3X4	T41.3X5	T41.3X6
Benzodiapin	T42.4X1	T42.4X2	T42.4X3	T42.4X4	T42.4X5	T42.4X6
Benzodiazepine NEC	T42.4X1	T42.4X2	T42.4X3	T42.4X4	T42.4X5	T42.4X6
Benzoic acid	T49.0X1	T49.0X2	T49.0X3	T49.0X4	T49.0X5	T49.0X6
with salicylic acid	T49.0X1	T49.0X2	T49.0X3	T49.0X4	T49.0X5	T49.0X6
Benzoin (tincture)	T48.5X1	T48.5X2	T48.5X3	T48.5X4	T48.5X5	T48.5X6
Benzol (benzene)	T52.1X1	T52.1X2	T52.1X3	T52.1X4	--	--
vapor	T52.0X1	T52.0X2	T52.0X3	T52.0X4	--	--
Benzomorphan	T40.2X1	T40.2X2	T40.2X3	T40.2X4	T40.2X5	T40.2X6
Benzonatate	T48.3X1	T48.3X2	T48.3X3	T48.3X4	T48.3X5	T48.3X6
Benzophenones	T49.3X1	T49.3X2	T49.3X3	T49.3X4	T49.3X5	T49.3X6
Benzopyrone	T46.991	T46.992	T46.993	T46.994	T46.995	T46.996
Benzothiadiazides	T50.2X1	T50.2X2	T50.2X3	T50.2X4	T50.2X5	T50.2X6
Benzoxonium chloride	T49.0X1	T49.0X2	T49.0X3	T49.0X4	T49.0X5	T49.0X6
Benzoyl peroxide	T49.0X1	T49.0X2	T49.0X3	T49.0X4	T49.0X5	T49.0X6
Benzoylpas calcium	T37.1X1	T37.1X2	T37.1X3	T37.1X4	T37.1X5	T37.1X6
Benzperidin	T43.591	T43.592	T43.593	T43.594	T43.595	T43.596
Benzperidol	T43.591	T43.592	T43.593	T43.594	T43.595	T43.596
Benzphetamine	T50.5X1	T50.5X2	T50.5X3	T50.5X4	T50.5X5	T50.5X6
Benzpyrinium bromide	T44.1X1	T44.1X2	T44.1X3	T44.1X4	T44.1X5	T44.1X6
Benzquinamide	T45.0X1	T45.0X2	T45.0X3	T45.0X4	T45.0X5	T45.0X6
Benzthiazide	T50.2X1	T50.2X2	T50.2X3	T50.2X4	T50.2X5	T50.2X6
Benztropine						
anticholinergic	T44.3X1	T44.3X2	T44.3X3	T44.3X4	T44.3X5	T44.3X6
antiparkinson	T42.8X1	T42.8X2	T42.8X3	T42.8X4	T42.8X5	T42.8X6
Benzydamine	T49.0X1	T49.0X2	T49.0X3	T49.0X4	T49.0X5	T49.0X6
Benzyl						
acetate	T52.8X1	T52.8X2	T52.8X3	T52.8X4	--	--
alcohol	T49.0X1	T49.0X2	T49.0X3	T49.0X4	T49.0X5	T49.0X6

Substance	Poisoning, Accidental (unintentional)	Poisoning, Intentional Self-harm	Poisoning, Assault	Poisoning, Undetermined	Adverse effect	Underdosing
benzoate	T49.0X1	T49.0X2	T49.0X3	T49.0X4	T49.0X5	T49.0X6
Benzoic acid	T49.0X1	T49.0X2	T49.0X3	T49.0X4	T49.0X5	T49.0X6
morphine	T40.2X1	T40.2X2	T40.2X3	T40.2X4	--	--
nicotinate	T46.6X1	T46.6X2	T46.6X3	T46.6X4	T46.6X5	T46.6X6
penicillin	T36.0X1	T36.0X2	T36.0X3	T36.0X4	T36.0X5	T36.0X6
Benzylhydrochlorthia-zide	T50.2X1	T50.2X2	T50.2X3	T50.2X4	T50.2X5	T50.2X6
Benzylpenicillin	T36.0X1	T36.0X2	T36.0X3	T36.0X4	T36.0X5	T36.0X6
Benzylthiouracil	T38.2X1	T38.2X2	T38.2X3	T38.2X4	T38.2X5	T38.2X6
Bephenium hydroxy-naphthoate	T37.4X1	T37.4X2	T37.4X3	T37.4X4	T37.4X5	T37.4X6
Bepridil	T46.1X1	T46.1X2	T46.1X3	T46.1X4	T46.1X5	T46.1X6
Bergamot oil	T65.891	T65.892	T65.893	T65.894	--	--
Bergapten	T50.991	T50.992	T50.993	T50.994	T50.995	T50.996
Berries, poisonous	T62.1X1	T62.1X2	T62.1X3	T62.1X4	--	--
Beryllium (compounds)	T56.7X1	T56.7X2	T56.7X3	T56.7X4	--	--
b-acetyldigoxin	T46.0X1	T46.0X2	T46.0X3	T46.0X4	T46.0X5	T46.0X6
beta adrenergic blocking agent, heart	T44.7X1	T44.7X2	T44.7X3	T44.7X4	T44.7X5	T44.7X6
b-benzalbutyramide	T46.6X1	T46.6X2	T46.6X3	T46.6X4	T46.6X5	T46.6X6
Betacarotene	T45.2X1	T45.2X2	T45.2X3	T45.2X4	T45.2X5	T45.2X6
b-eucaine	T49.1X1	T49.1X2	T49.1X3	T49.1X4	T49.1X5	T49.1X6
Beta-Chlor	T42.6X1	T42.6X2	T42.6X3	T42.6X4	T42.6X5	T42.6X6
b-galactosidase	T47.5X1	T47.5X2	T47.5X3	T47.5X4	T47.5X5	T47.5X6
Betahistine	T46.7X1	T46.7X2	T46.7X3	T46.7X4	T46.7X5	T46.7X6
Betaine	T47.5X1	T47.5X2	T47.5X3	T47.5X4	T47.5X5	T47.5X6
Betamethasone	T49.0X1	T49.0X2	T49.0X3	T49.0X4	T49.0X5	T49.0X6
topical	T49.0X1	T49.0X2	T49.0X3	T49.0X4	T49.0X5	T49.0X6
Betamicin	T36.8X1	T36.8X2	T36.8X3	T36.8X4	T36.8X5	T36.8X6
Betanidine	T46.5X1	T46.5X2	T46.5X3	T46.5X4	T46.5X5	T46.5X6
b-sitosterol (s)	T46.6X1	T46.6X2	T46.6X3	T46.6X4	T46.6X5	T46.6X6
Betaxolol	T44.7X1	T44.7X2	T44.7X3	T44.7X4	T44.7X5	T44.7X6
Betazole	T50.8X1	T50.8X2	T50.8X3	T50.8X4	T50.8X5	T50.8X6
Bethanechol	T44.1X1	T44.1X2	T44.1X3	T44.1X4	T44.1X5	T44.1X6
chloride	T44.1X1	T44.1X2	T44.1X3	T44.1X4	T44.1X5	T44.1X6
Bethanidine	T46.5X1	T46.5X2	T46.5X3	T46.5X4	T46.5X5	T46.5X6
Betoxycaine	T41.3X1	T41.3X2	T41.3X3	T41.3X4	T41.3X5	T41.3X6
Betula oil	T49.3X1	T49.3X2	T49.3X3	T49.3X4	T49.3X5	T49.3X6
Bevantolol	T44.7X1	T44.7X2	T44.7X3	T44.7X4	T44.7X5	T44.7X6
Bevonium metilsulfate	T44.3X1	T44.3X2	T44.3X3	T44.3X4	T44.3X5	T44.3X6
Bezafibrate	T46.6X1	T46.6X2	T46.6X3	T46.6X4	T46.6X5	T46.6X6
Bezitramide	T40.4X1	T40.4X2	T40.4X3	T40.4X4	T40.4X5	T40.4X6
BHA	T50.991	T50.992	T50.993	T50.994	T50.995	T50.996
Bhang	T40.7X1	T40.7X2	T40.7X3	T40.7X4	T40.7X5	T40.7X6
BHC (medicinal)	T49.0X1	T49.0X2	T49.0X3	T49.0X4	T49.0X5	T49.0X6
nonmedicinal (vapor)	T53.6X1	T53.6X2	T53.6X3	T53.6X4	--	--
Bialamicol	T37.3X1	T37.3X2	T37.3X3	T37.3X4	T37.3X5	T37.3X6
Bibenzonium bromide	T48.3X1	T48.3X2	T48.3X3	T48.3X4	T48.3X5	T48.3X6
Bibrocathol	T49.5X1	T49.5X2	T49.5X3	T49.5X4	T49.5X5	T49.5X6
Bichloride of mercury—see Mercury, chloride						
Bichromates (calcium) (potassium) (sodium)	T57.8X1	T57.8X2	T57.8X3	T57.8X4	--	- (crystals)
fumes	T56.2X1	T56.2X2	T56.2X3	T56.2X4	--	--
Biclotymol	T49.6X1	T49.6X2	T49.6X3	T49.6X4	T49.6X5	T49.6X6
Bicucculine	T50.7X1	T50.7X2	T50.7X3	T50.7X4	T50.7X5	T50.7X6
Bifemelane	T43.291	T43.292	T43.293	T43.294	T43.295	T43.296
Biguanide derivatives, oral	T38.3X1	T38.3X2	T38.3X3	T38.3X4	T38.3X5	T38.3X6
Bile salts	T47.5X1	T47.5X2	T47.5X3	T47.5X4	T47.5X5	T47.5X6
Biligrafin	T50.8X1	T50.8X2	T50.8X3	T50.8X4	T50.8X5	T50.8X6
Bilopaque	T50.8X1	T50.8X2	T50.8X3	T50.8X4	T50.8X5	T50.8X6
Binifibrate	T46.6X1	T46.6X2	T46.6X3	T46.6X4	T46.6X5	T46.6X6
Binitrobenzol	T65.3X1	T65.3X2	T65.3X3	T65.3X4	--	--
Bioflavonoid (s)	T46.991	T46.992	T46.993	T46.994	T46.995	T46.996
Biological substance NEC	T50.901	T50.902	T50.903	T50.904	T50.905	T50.906
Biotin	T45.2X1	T45.2X2	T45.2X3	T45.2X4	T45.2X5	T45.2X6
Biperiden	T44.3X1	T44.3X2	T44.3X3	T44.3X4	T44.3X5	T44.3X6
Bisacodyl	T47.2X1	T47.2X2	T47.2X3	T47.2X4	T47.2X5	T47.2X6
Bisbentiamine	T45.2X1	T45.2X2	T45.2X3	T45.2X4	T45.2X5	T45.2X6
Bisbutiamine	T45.2X1	T45.2X2	T45.2X3	T45.2X4	T45.2X5	T45.2X6

Substance	Poisoning, Accidental (unintentional)	Poisoning, Intentional Self-harm	Poisoning, Assault	Poisoning, Undetermined	Adverse effect	Underdosing
Bisdequalinium (salts) (diacetate)	T49.6X1	T49.6X2	T49.6X3	T49.6X4	T49.6X5	T49.6X6
Bishydroxycoumarin	T45.511	T45.512	T45.513	T45.514	T45.515	T45.516
Bismarsen	T37.8X1	T37.8X2	T37.8X3	T37.8X4	T37.8X5	T37.8X6
Bismuth salts	T47.6X1	T47.6X2	T47.6X3	T47.6X4	T47.6X5	T47.6X6
aluminate	T47.1X1	T47.1X2	T47.1X3	T47.1X4	T47.1X5	T47.1X6
anti-infectives	T37.8X1	T37.8X2	T37.8X3	T37.8X4	T37.8X5	T37.8X6
formic iodide	T49.0X1	T49.0X2	T49.0X3	T49.0X4	T49.0X5	T49.0X6
glycolylarsenate	T49.0X1	T49.0X2	T49.0X3	T49.0X4	T49.0X5	T49.0X6
nonmedicinal (compounds) NEC	T65.91	T65.92	T65.93	T65.94	--	--
subcarbonate	T47.6X1	T47.6X2	T47.6X3	T47.6X4	T47.6X5	T47.6X6
subsalicylate	T37.8X1	T37.8X2	T37.8X3	T37.8X4	T37.8X5	T37.8X6
sulfarsphenamine	T37.8X1	T37.8X2	T37.8X3	T37.8X4	T37.8X5	T37.8X6
Bisoprolol	T44.7X1	T44.7X2	T44.7X3	T44.7X4	T44.7X5	T44.7X6
Bisoxatin	T47.2X1	T47.2X2	T47.2X3	T47.2X4	T47.2X5	T47.2X6
Bisulepin (hydrochloride)	T45.0X1	T45.0X2	T45.0X3	T45.0X4	T45.0X5	T45.0X6
Bithionol	T37.8X1	T37.8X2	T37.8X3	T37.8X4	T37.8X5	T37.8X6
anthelminthic	T37.4X1	T37.4X2	T37.4X3	T37.4X4	T37.4X5	T37.4X6
Bitolterol	T48.6X1	T48.6X2	T48.6X3	T48.6X4	T48.6X5	T48.6X6
Bitoscanate	T37.4X1	T37.4X2	T37.4X3	T37.4X4	T37.4X5	T37.4X6
Bitter almond oil	T62.8X1	T62.8X2	T62.8X3	T62.8X4	--	--
Bittersweet	T62.2X1	T62.2X2	T62.2X3	T62.2X4	--	--
Black						
flag	T60.91	T60.92	T60.93	T60.94	--	--
henbane	T62.2X1	T62.2X2	T62.2X3	T62.2X4	--	--
leaf (40)	T60.91	T60.92	T60.93	T60.94	--	--
widow spider (bite)	T63.311	T63.312	T63.313	T63.314	--	--
antivenin	T50.Z11	T50.Z12	T50.Z13	T50.Z14	T50.Z15	T50.Z16
Blast furnace gas (carbon monoxide from)	T58.8X1	T58.8X2	T58.8X3	T58.8X4	--	--
Bleach	T54.91	T54.92	T54.93	T54.94	--	--
Bleaching agent (medicinal)	T49.4X1	T49.4X2	T49.4X3	T49.4X4	T49.4X5	T49.4X6
Bleomycin	T45.1X1	T45.1X2	T45.1X3	T45.1X4	T45.1X5	T45.1X6
Blockain	T41.3X1	T41.3X2	T41.3X3	T41.3X4	T41.3X5	T41.3X6
infiltration (subcutaneous)	T41.3X1	T41.3X2	T41.3X3	T41.3X4	T41.3X5	T41.3X6
nerve block (peripheral) (plexus)	T41.3X1	T41.3X2	T41.3X3	T41.3X4	T41.3X5	T41.3X6
topical (surface)	T41.3X1	T41.3X2	T41.3X3	T41.3X4	T41.3X5	T41.3X6
Blockers, calcium channel	T46.1X1	T46.1X2	T46.1X3	T46.1X4	T46.1X5	T46.1X6
Blood (derivatives) (natural) (plasma) (whole)	T45.8X1	T45.8X2	T45.8X3	T45.8X4	T45.8X5	T45.8X6
dried	T45.8X1	T45.8X2	T45.8X3	T45.8X4	T45.8X5	T45.8X6
drug affecting NEC	T45.91	T45.92	T45.93	T45.94	T45.95	T45.96
expander NEC	T45.8X1	T45.8X2	T45.8X3	T45.8X4	T45.8X5	T45.8X6
fraction NEC	T45.8X1	T45.8X2	T45.8X3	T45.8X4	T45.8X5	T45.8X6
substitute (macromolecular)	T45.8X1	T45.8X2	T45.8X3	T45.8X4	T45.8X5	T45.8X6
Blue velvet	T40.2X1	T40.2X2	T40.2X3	T40.2X4	--	--
Bone meal	T62.8X1	T62.8X2	T62.8X3	T62.8X4	--	--
Bonine	T45.0X1	T45.0X2	T45.0X3	T45.0X4	T45.0X5	T45.0X6
Bopindolol	T44.7X1	T44.7X2	T44.7X3	T44.7X4	T44.7X5	T44.7X6
Boracic acid	T49.0X1	T49.0X2	T49.0X3	T49.0X4	T49.0X5	T49.0X6
ENT agent	T49.6X1	T49.6X2	T49.6X3	T49.6X4	T49.6X5	T49.6X6
ophthalmic preparation	T49.5X1	T49.5X2	T49.5X3	T49.5X4	T49.5X5	T49.5X6
Borane complex	T57.8X1	T57.8X2	T57.8X3	T57.8X4	--	--
Borate (s)	T57.8X1	T57.8X2	T57.8X3	T57.8X4	--	--
buffer	T50.991	T50.992	T50.993	T50.994	T50.995	T50.996
cleanser	T54.91	T54.92	T54.93	T54.94	--	--
sodium	T57.8X1	T57.8X2	T57.8X3	T57.8X4	--	--
Borax (cleanser)	T54.91	T54.92	T54.93	T54.94	--	--
Bordeaux mixture	T60.3X1	T60.3X2	T60.3X3	T60.3X4	--	--
Boric acid	T49.0X1	T49.0X2	T49.0X3	T49.0X4	T49.0X5	T49.0X6
ENT agent	T49.6X1	T49.6X2	T49.6X3	T49.6X4	T49.6X5	T49.6X6
ophthalmic preparation	T49.5X1	T49.5X2	T49.5X3	T49.5X4	T49.5X5	T49.5X6
Bornaprine	T44.3X1	T44.3X2	T44.3X3	T44.3X4	T44.3X5	T44.3X6
Boron	T57.8X1	T57.8X2	T57.8X3	T57.8X4	--	--
hydride NEC	T57.8X1	T57.8X2	T57.8X3	T57.8X4	--	--
fumes or gas	T57.8X1	T57.8X2	T57.8X3	T57.8X4	--	--
trifluoride	T59.891	T59.892	T59.893	T59.894	--	--

Substance	Poisoning, Accidental (unintentional)	Poisoning, Intentional Self-harm	Poisoning, Assault	Poisoning, Undetermined	Adverse effect	Underdosing
Botox	T48.291	T48.292	T48.293	T48.294	T48.295	T48.296
Botulinus anti-toxin (type A, B)	T50.Z11	T50.Z12	T50.Z13	T50.Z14	T50.Z15	T50.Z16
Brake fluid vapor	T59.891	T59.892	T59.893	T59.894	--	--
Brallobarbital	T42.3X1	T42.3X2	T42.3X3	T42.3X4	T42.3X5	T42.3X6
Bran (wheat)	T47.4X1	T47.4X2	T47.4X3	T47.4X4	T47.4X5	T47.4X6
Brass (fumes)	T56.891	T56.892	T56.893	T56.894	--	--
Brasso	T52.0X1	T52.0X2	T52.0X3	T52.0X4	--	--
Bretylium tosilate	T46.2X1	T46.2X2	T46.2X3	T46.2X4	T46.2X5	T46.2X6
Brevital (sodium)	T41.1X1	T41.1X2	T41.1X3	T41.1X4	T41.1X5	T41.1X6
Brinase	T45.3X1	T45.3X2	T45.3X3	T45.3X4	T45.3X5	T45.3X6
British antilewisite	T45.8X1	T45.8X2	T45.8X3	T45.8X4	T45.8X5	T45.8X6
Brodifacoum	T60.4X1	T60.4X2	T60.4X3	T60.4X4	--	--
Bromal (hydrate)	T42.6X1	T42.6X2	T42.6X3	T42.6X4	T42.6X5	T42.6X6
Bromazepam	T42.4X1	T42.4X2	T42.4X3	T42.4X4	T42.4X5	T42.4X6
Bromazine	T45.0X1	T45.0X2	T45.0X3	T45.0X4	T45.0X5	T45.0X6
Brombenzylcyanide	T59.3X1	T59.3X2	T59.3X3	T59.3X4	--	--
Bromelains	T45.3X1	T45.3X2	T45.3X3	T45.3X4	T45.3X5	T45.3X6
Bromethalin	T60.4X1	T60.4X2	T60.4X3	T60.4X4	--	--
Bromhexine	T48.4X1	T48.4X2	T48.4X3	T48.4X4	T48.4X5	T48.4X6
Bromide salts	T42.6X1	T42.6X2	T42.6X3	T42.6X4	T42.6X5	T42.6X6
Bromindione	T45.511	T45.512	T45.513	T45.514	T45.515	T45.516
Bromine						
compounds (medicinal)	T42.6X1	T42.6X2	T42.6X3	T42.6X4	T42.6X5	T42.6X6
sedative	T42.6X1	T42.6X2	T42.6X3	T42.6X4	T42.6X5	T42.6X6
vapor	T59.891	T59.892	T59.893	T59.894	--	--
Bromisoval	T42.6X1	T42.6X2	T42.6X3	T42.6X4	T42.6X5	T42.6X6
Bromisovalum	T42.6X1	T42.6X2	T42.6X3	T42.6X4	T42.6X5	T42.6X6
Bromobenzylcyanide	T59.3X1	T59.3X2	T59.3X3	T59.3X4	--	--
Bromochlorosalicylani-lide	T49.0X1	T49.0X2	T49.0X3	T49.0X4	T49.0X5	T49.0X6
Bromocriptine	T42.8X1	T42.8X2	T42.8X3	T42.8X4	T42.8X5	T42.8X6
Bromodiphenhydramine	T45.0X1	T45.0X2	T45.0X3	T45.0X4	T45.0X5	T45.0X6
Bromoform	T42.6X1	T42.6X2	T42.6X3	T42.6X4	T42.6X5	T42.6X6
Bromophenol blue reagent	T50.991	T50.992	T50.993	T50.994	T50.995	T50.996
Bromopride	T47.8X1	T47.8X2	T47.8X3	T47.8X4	T47.8X5	T47.8X6
Bromosalicylchloranitide	T49.0X1	T49.0X2	T49.0X3	T49.0X4	T49.0X5	T49.0X6
Bromosalicylhydroxamic acid	T37.1X1	T37.1X2	T37.1X3	T37.1X4	T37.1X5	T37.1X6
Bromo-seltzer	T39.1X1	T39.1X2	T39.1X3	T39.1X4	T39.1X5	T39.1X6
Bromoxynil	T60.3X1	T60.3X2	T60.3X3	T60.3X4	--	--
Bromperidol	T43.4X1	T43.4X2	T43.4X3	T43.4X4	T43.4X5	T43.4X6
Brompheniramine	T45.0X1	T45.0X2	T45.0X3	T45.0X4	T45.0X5	T45.0X6
Bromsulfophthalein	T50.8X1	T50.8X2	T50.8X3	T50.8X4	T50.8X5	T50.8X6
Bromural	T42.6X1	T42.6X2	T42.6X3	T42.6X4	T42.6X5	T42.6X6
Bromvaletone	T42.6X1	T42.6X2	T42.6X3	T42.6X4	T42.6X5	T42.6X6
Bronchodilator NEC	T48.6X1	T48.6X2	T48.6X3	T48.6X4	T48.6X5	T48.6X6
Brotizolam	T42.4X1	T42.4X2	T42.4X3	T42.4X4	T42.4X5	T42.4X6
Brovincamine	T46.7X1	T46.7X2	T46.7X3	T46.7X4	T46.7X5	T46.7X6
Brown recluse spider (bite) (venom)	T63.331	T63.332	T63.333	T63.334	--	--
Brown spider (bite) (venom)	T63.391	T63.392	T63.393	T63.394	--	--
Broxaterol	T48.6X1	T48.6X2	T48.6X3	T48.6X4	T48.6X5	T48.6X6
Broxuridine	T45.1X1	T45.1X2	T45.1X3	T45.1X4	T45.1X5	T45.1X6
Broxyquinoline	T37.8X1	T37.8X2	T37.8X3	T37.8X4	T37.8X5	T37.8X6
Bruceine	T48.291	T48.292	T48.293	T48.294	T48.295	T48.296
Brucia	T62.2X1	T62.2X2	T62.2X3	T62.2X4	--	--
Brucine	T65.1X1	T65.1X2	T65.1X3	T65.1X4	--	--
Brunswick green—see Copper						
Bruten—see Ibuprofen						
Bryonia	T47.2X1	T47.2X2	T47.2X3	T47.2X4	T47.2X5	T47.2X6
Buclizine	T45.0X1	T45.0X2	T45.0X3	T45.0X4	T45.0X5	T45.0X6
Buclosamide	T49.0X1	T49.0X2	T49.0X3	T49.0X4	T49.0X5	T49.0X6
Budesonide	T44.5X1	T44.5X2	T44.5X3	T44.5X4	T44.5X5	T44.5X6
Budralazine	T46.5X1	T46.5X2	T46.5X3	T46.5X4	T46.5X5	T46.5X6
Bufferin	T39.011	T39.012	T39.013	T39.014	T39.015	T39.016
Buflomedil	T46.7X1	T46.7X2	T46.7X3	T46.7X4	T46.7X5	T46.7X6
Buformin	T38.3X1	T38.3X2	T38.3X3	T38.3X4	T38.3X5	T38.3X6
Bufotenine	T40.991	T40.992	T40.993	T40.994	--	--

Substance	Poisoning, Accidental (unintentional)	Poisoning, Intentional Self-harm	Poisoning, Assault	Poisoning, Undetermined	Adverse effect	Underdosing
Bufrolin	T48.6X1	T48.6X2	T48.6X3	T48.6X4	T48.6X5	T48.6X6
Bufylline	T48.6X1	T48.6X2	T48.6X3	T48.6X4	T48.6X5	T48.6X6
Bulk filler	T50.5X1	T50.5X2	T50.5X3	T50.5X4	T50.5X5	T50.5X6
cathartic	T47.4X1	T47.4X2	T47.4X3	T47.4X4	T47.4X5	T47.4X6
Bumetanide	T50.1X1	T50.1X2	T50.1X3	T50.1X4	T50.1X5	T50.1X6
Bunaftine	T46.2X1	T46.2X2	T46.2X3	T46.2X4	T46.2X5	T46.2X6
Bunamiodyl	T50.8X1	T50.8X2	T50.8X3	T50.8X4	T50.8X5	T50.8X6
Bunazosin	T44.6X1	T44.6X2	T44.6X3	T44.6X4	T44.6X5	T44.6X6
Bunitrolol	T44.7X1	T44.7X2	T44.7X3	T44.7X4	T44.7X5	T44.7X6
Buphenine	T46.7X1	T46.7X2	T46.7X3	T46.7X4	T46.7X5	T46.7X6
Bupivacaine	T41.3X1	T41.3X2	T41.3X3	T41.3X4	T41.3X5	T41.3X6
infiltration (subcutaneous)	T41.3X1	T41.3X2	T41.3X3	T41.3X4	T41.3X5	T41.3X6
nerve block (peripheral) (plexus)	T41.3X1	T41.3X2	T41.3X3	T41.3X4	T41.3X5	T41.3X6
spinal	T41.3X1	T41.3X2	T41.3X3	T41.3X4	T41.3X5	T41.3X6
Bupranolol	T44.7X1	T44.7X2	T44.7X3	T44.7X4	T44.7X5	T44.7X6
Buprenorphine	T40.4X1	T40.4X2	T40.4X3	T40.4X4	T40.4X5	T40.4X6
Bupropion	T43.291	T43.292	T43.293	T43.294	T43.295	T43.296
Burimamide	T47.1X1	T47.1X2	T47.1X3	T47.1X4	T47.1X5	T47.1X6
Buserelin	T38.891	T38.892	T38.893	T38.894	T38.895	T38.896
Buspirone	T43.591	T43.592	T43.593	T43.594	T43.595	T43.596
Busulfan, busulphan	T45.1X1	T45.1X2	T45.1X3	T45.1X4	T45.1X5	T45.1X6
Butabarbital (sodium)	T42.3X1	T42.3X2	T42.3X3	T42.3X4	T42.3X5	T42.3X6
Butabarbitone	T42.3X1	T42.3X2	T42.3X3	T42.3X4	T42.3X5	T42.3X6
Butabarpal	T42.3X1	T42.3X2	T42.3X3	T42.3X4	T42.3X5	T42.3X6
Butacaine	T41.3X1	T41.3X2	T41.3X3	T41.3X4	T41.3X5	T41.3X6
Butalamine	T46.7X1	T46.7X2	T46.7X3	T46.7X4	T46.7X5	T46.7X6
Butalbital	T42.3X1	T42.3X2	T42.3X3	T42.3X4	T42.3X5	T42.3X6
Butallylonal	T42.3X1	T42.3X2	T42.3X3	T42.3X4	T42.3X5	T42.3X6
Butamben	T41.3X1	T41.3X2	T41.3X3	T41.3X4	T41.3X5	T41.3X6
Butamirate	T48.3X1	T48.3X2	T48.3X3	T48.3X4	T48.3X5	T48.3X6
Butane (distributed in mobile container)	T59.891	T59.892	T59.893	T59.894	--	--
distributed through pipes	T59.891	T59.892	T59.893	T59.894	--	--
incomplete combustion	T58.11	T58.12	T58.13	T58.14	--	--
Butanilicaine	T41.3X1	T41.3X2	T41.3X3	T41.3X4	T41.3X5	T41.3X6
Butanol	T51.3X1	T51.3X2	T51.3X3	T51.3X4	--	--
Butanone, 2-butanone	T52.4X1	T52.4X2	T52.4X3	T52.4X4	--	--
Butantrone	T49.4X1	T49.4X2	T49.4X3	T49.4X4	T49.4X5	T49.4X6
Butaperazine	T43.3X1	T43.3X2	T43.3X3	T43.3X4	T43.3X5	T43.3X6
Butazolidin	T39.2X1	T39.2X2	T39.2X3	T39.2X4	T39.2X5	T39.2X6
Butetamate	T48.6X1	T48.6X2	T48.6X3	T48.6X4	T48.6X5	T48.6X6
Butethal	T42.3X1	T42.3X2	T42.3X3	T42.3X4	T42.3X5	T42.3X6
Butethamate	T44.3X1	T44.3X2	T44.3X3	T44.3X4	T44.3X5	T44.3X6
Buthalitone (sodium)	T41.1X1	T41.1X2	T41.1X3	T41.1X4	T41.1X5	T41.1X6
Butisol (sodium)	T42.3X1	T42.3X2	T42.3X3	T42.3X4	T42.3X5	T42.3X6
Butizide	T50.2X1	T50.2X2	T50.2X3	T50.2X4	T50.2X5	T50.2X6
Butobarbital	T42.3X1	T42.3X2	T42.3X3	T42.3X4	T42.3X5	T42.3X6
sodium	T42.3X1	T42.3X2	T42.3X3	T42.3X4	T42.3X5	T42.3X6
Butobarbitone	T42.3X1	T42.3X2	T42.3X3	T42.3X4	T42.3X5	T42.3X6
Butoconazole (nitrate)	T49.0X1	T49.0X2	T49.0X3	T49.0X4	T49.0X5	T49.0X6
Butorphanol	T40.4X1	T40.4X2	T40.4X3	T40.4X4	T40.4X5	T40.4X6
Butriptyline	T43.011	T43.012	T43.013	T43.014	T43.015	T43.016
Butropium bromide	T44.3X1	T44.3X2	T44.3X3	T44.3X4	T44.3X5	T44.3X6
Butter of antimony—see Antimony						
Buttercups	T62.2X1	T62.2X2	T62.2X3	T62.2X4	--	--
Butyl						
acetate (secondary)	T52.8X1	T52.8X2	T52.8X3	T52.8X4	--	--
alcohol	T51.3X1	T51.3X2	T51.3X3	T51.3X4	--	--
aminobenzoate	T41.3X1	T41.3X2	T41.3X3	T41.3X4	T41.3X5	T41.3X6
butyrate	T52.8X1	T52.8X2	T52.8X3	T52.8X4	--	--
carbinol	T51.3X1	T51.3X2	T51.3X3	T51.3X4	--	--
carbitol	T52.3X1	T52.3X2	T52.3X3	T52.3X4	--	--
cellosolve	T52.3X1	T52.3X2	T52.3X3	T52.3X4	--	--
chloral (hydrate)	T42.6X1	T42.6X2	T42.6X3	T42.6X4	T42.6X5	T42.6X6
formate	T52.8X1	T52.8X2	T52.8X3	T52.8X4	--	--

Substance	Poisoning, Accidental (unintentional)	Poisoning, Intentional Self-harm	Poisoning, Assault	Poisoning, Undetermined	Adverse effect	Underdosing
lactate	T52.8X1	T52.8X2	T52.8X3	T52.8X4	--	--
propionate	T52.8X1	T52.8X1	T52.8X3	T52.8X4	--	--
scopolamine bromide	T44.3X1	T44.3X2	T44.3X3	T44.3X4	T44.3X5	T44.3X6
thiobarbital sodium	T41.1X1	T41.1X2	T41.1X3	T41.1X4	T41.1X5	T41.1X6
Butylated hydroxy-anisole	T50.991	T50.992	T50.993	T50.994	T50.995	T50.996
Butylchloral hydrate	T42.6X1	T42.6X2	T42.6X3	T42.6X4	T42.6X5	T42.6X6
Butyltoluene	T52.2X1	T52.2X2	T52.2X3	T52.2X4	--	--
Butyn	T41.3X1	T41.3X2	T41.3X3	T41.3X4	T41.3X5	T41.3X6
Butyrophenone (-based tranquilizers)	T43.4X1	T43.4X2	T43.4X3	T43.4X4	T43.4X5	T43.4X6
Cabergoline	T42.8X1	T42.8X2	T42.8X3	T42.8X4	T42.8X5	T42.8X6
Cacodyl, cacodylic acid	T57.0X1	T57.0X2	T57.0X3	T57.0X4	--	--
Cactinomycin	T45.1X1	T45.1X2	T45.1X3	T45.1X4	T45.1X5	T45.1X6
Cade oil	T49.4X1	T49.4X2	T49.4X3	T49.4X4	T49.4X5	T49.4X6
Cadexomer iodine	T49.0X1	T49.0X2	T49.0X3	T49.0X4	T49.0X5	T49.0X6
Cadmium (chloride) (fumes) (oxide)	T56.3X1	T56.3X2	T56.3X3	T56.3X4	--	--
sulfide (medicinal) NEC	T49.4X1	T49.4X2	T49.4X3	T49.4X4	T49.4X5	T49.4X6
Cadralazine	T46.5X1	T46.5X2	T46.5X3	T46.5X4	T46.5X5	T46.5X6
Caffeine	T43.611	T43.612	T43.613	T43.614	T43.615	T43.616
Calabar bean	T62.2X1	T62.2X2	T62.2X3	T62.2X4	--	--
Caladium seguinum	T62.2X1	T62.2X2	T62.2X3	T62.2X4	--	--
Calamine (lotion)	T49.3X1	T49.3X2	T49.3X3	T49.3X4	T49.3X5	T49.3X6
Calcifediol	T45.2X1	T45.2X2	T45.2X3	T45.2X4	T45.2X5	T45.2X6
Calciferol	T45.2X1	T45.2X2	T45.2X3	T45.2X4	T45.2X5	T45.2X6
Calcitonin	T50.991	T50.992	T50.993	T50.994	T50.995	T50.996
Calcitriol	T45.2X1	T45.2X2	T45.2X3	T45.2X4	T45.2X5	T45.2X6
Calcium	T50.3X1	T50.3X2	T50.3X3	T50.3X4	T50.3X5	T50.3X6
actylsalicylate	T39.011	T39.012	T39.013	T39.014	T39.015	T39.016
benzamidosalicylate	T37.1X1	T37.1X2	T37.1X3	T37.1X4	T37.1X5	T37.1X6
bromide	T42.6X1	T42.6X2	T42.6X3	T42.6X4	T42.6X5	T42.6X6
bromolactobionate	T42.6X1	T42.6X2	T42.6X3	T42.6X4	T42.6X5	T42.6X6
carbaspirin	T39.011	T39.012	T39.013	T39.014	T39.015	T39.016
carbimide	T50.6X1	T50.6X2	T50.6X3	T50.6X4	T50.6X5	T50.6X6
carbonate	T47.1X1	T47.1X2	T47.1X3	T47.1X4	T47.1X5	T47.1X6
chloride	T50.991	T50.992	T50.993	T50.994	T50.995	T50.996
anhydrous	T50.991	T50.992	T50.993	T50.994	T50.995	T50.996
cyanide	T57.8X1	T57.8X2	T57.8X3	T57.8X4	--	--
dioctyl sulfosuccinate	T47.4X1	T47.4X2	T47.4X3	T47.4X4	T47.4X5	T47.4X6
disodium edathamil	T45.8X1	T45.8X2	T45.8X3	T45.8X4	T45.8X5	T45.8X6
disodium edetate	T45.8X1	T45.8X2	T45.8X3	T45.8X4	T45.8X5	T45.8X6
dobesilate	T46.991	T46.992	T46.993	T46.994	T46.995	T46.996
EDTA	T45.8X1	T45.8X2	T45.8X3	T45.8X4	T45.8X5	T45.8X6
ferrous citrate	T45.4X1	T45.4X2	T45.4X3	T45.4X4	T45.4X5	T45.4X6
folinate	T45.8X1	T45.8X2	T45.8X3	T45.8X4	T45.8X5	T45.8X6
glubionate	T50.3X1	T50.3X2	T50.3X3	T50.3X4	T50.3X5	T50.3X6
gluconate	T50.3X1	T50.3X2	T50.3X3	T50.3X4	T50.3X5	T50.3X6
gluconogalactogluc-onate	T50.3X1	T50.3X2	T50.3X3	T50.3X4	T50.3X5	T50.3X6
hydrate, hydroxide	T54.3X1	T54.3X2	T54.3X3	T54.3X4	--	--
hypochlorite	T54.3X1	T54.3X2	T54.3X3	T54.3X4	--	--
iodide	T48.4X1	T48.4X2	T48.4X3	T48.4X4	T48.4X5	T48.4X6
ipodate	T50.8X1	T50.8X2	T50.8X3	T50.8X4	T50.8X5	T50.8X6
lactate	T50.3X1	T50.3X2	T50.3X3	T50.3X4	T50.3X5	T50.3X6
leucovorin	T45.8X1	T45.8X2	T45.8X3	T45.8X4	T45.8X5	T45.8X6
mandelate	T37.91	T37.92	T37.93	T37.94	T37.95	T37.96
oxide	T54.3X1	T54.3X2	T54.3X3	T54.3X4	--	--
pantothenate	T45.2X1	T45.2X2	T45.2X3	T45.2X4	T45.2X5	T45.2X6
phosphate	T50.3X1	T50.3X2	T50.3X3	T50.3X4	T50.3X5	T50.3X6
salicylate	T39.091	T39.092	T39.093	T39.094	T39.095	T39.096
salts	T50.3X1	T50.3X2	T50.3X3	T50.3X4	T50.3X5	T50.3X6
Calculus-dissolving drug	T50.991	T50.992	T50.993	T50.994	T50.995	T50.996
Calomel	T49.0X1	T49.0X2	T49.0X3	T49.0X4	T49.0X5	T49.0X6
Caloric agent	T50.3X1	T50.3X2	T50.3X3	T50.3X4	T50.3X5	T50.3X6
Calusterone	T38.7X1	T38.7X2	T38.7X3	T38.7X4	T38.7X5	T38.7X6
Camazepam	T42.4X1	T42.4X2	T42.4X3	T42.4X4	T42.4X5	T42.4X6
Camomile	T49.0X1	T49.0X2	T49.0X3	T49.0X4	T49.0X5	T49.0X6
Camoquin	T37.2X1	T37.2X2	T37.2X3	T37.2X4	T37.2X5	T37.2X6

Substance	Poisoning, Accidental (unintentional)	Poisoning, Intentional Self-harm	Poisoning, Assault	Poisoning, Undetermined	Adverse effect	Underdosing
Camphor						
insecticide	T60.2X1	T60.2X2	T60.2X3	T60.2X4	--	--
medicinal	T49.8X1	T49.8X2	T49.8X3	T49.8X4	T49.8X5	T49.8X6
Camylofin	T44.3X1	T44.3X2	T44.3X3	T44.3X4	T44.3X5	T44.3X6
Cancer chemotherapy drug regimen	T45.1X1	T45.1X2	T45.1X3	T45.1X4	T45.1X5	T45.1X6
Candeptin	T49.0X1	T49.0X2	T49.0X3	T49.0X4	T49.0X5	T49.0X6
Candicidin	T49.0X1	T49.0X2	T49.0X3	T49.0X4	T49.0X5	T49.0X6
Cannabinol	T40.7X1	T40.7X2	T40.7X3	T40.7X4	T40.7X5	T40.7X6
Cannabis (derivatives)	T40.7X1	T40.7X2	T40.7X3	T40.7X4	T40.7X5	T40.7X6
Canned heat	T51.1X1	T51.1X2	T51.1X3	T51.1X4	--	--
Canrenoic acid	T50.0X1	T50.0X2	T50.0X3	T50.0X4	T50.0X5	T50.0X6
Canrenone	T50.0X1	T50.0X2	T50.0X3	T50.0X4	T50.0X5	T50.0X6
Cantharides, cantharidin, cantharis	T49.8X1	T49.8X2	T49.8X3	T49.8X4	T49.8X5	T49.8X6
Canthaxanthin	T50.991	T50.992	T50.993	T50.994	T50.995	T50.996
Capillary-active drug NEC	T46.901	T46.902	T46.903	T46.904	T46.905	T46.906
Capreomycin	T36.8X1	T36.8X2	T36.8X3	T36.8X4	T36.8X5	T36.8X6
Capsicum	T49.4X1	T49.4X2	T49.4X3	T49.4X4	T49.4X5	T49.4X6
Captafol	T60.3X1	T60.3X2	T60.3X3	T60.3X4	--	--
Captan	T60.3X1	T60.3X2	T60.3X3	T60.3X4	--	--
Captodiame, captodiamine	T43.591	T43.592	T43.593	T43.594	T43.595	T43.596
Captopril	T46.4X1	T46.4X2	T46.4X3	T46.4X4	T46.4X5	T46.4X6
Caramiphen	T44.3X1	T44.3X2	T44.3X3	T44.3X4	T44.3X5	T44.3X6
Carazolol	T44.7X1	T44.7X2	T44.7X3	T44.7X4	T44.7X5	T44.7X6
Carbachol	T44.1X1	T44.1X2	T44.1X3	T44.1X4	T44.1X5	T44.1X6
Carbacrylamine (resin)	T50.3X1	T50.3X2	T50.3X3	T50.3X4	T50.3X5	T50.3X6
Carbamate (insecticide)	T60.0X1	T60.0X2	T60.0X3	T60.0X4	--	--
Carbamate (sedative)	T42.6X1	T42.6X2	T42.6X3	T42.6X4	T42.6X5	T42.6X6
herbicide	T60.0X1	T60.0X2	T60.0X3	T60.0X4	--	--
insecticide	T60.0X1	T60.0X2	T60.0X3	T60.0X4	--	--
Carbamazepine	T42.1X1	T42.1X2	T42.1X3	T42.1X4	T42.1X5	T42.1X6
Carbamide	T47.3X1	T47.3X2	T47.3X3	T47.3X4	T47.3X5	T47.3X6
peroxide	T49.0X1	T49.0X2	T49.0X3	T49.0X4	T49.0X5	T49.0X6
topical	T49.8X1	T49.8X2	T49.8X3	T49.8X4	T49.8X5	T49.8X6
Carbamylcholine chloride	T44.1X1	T44.1X2	T44.1X3	T44.1X4	T44.1X5	T44.1X6
Carbaril	T60.0X1	T60.0X2	T60.0X3	T60.0X4	--	--
Carbarsone	T37.3X1	T37.3X2	T37.3X3	T37.3X4	T37.3X5	T37.3X6
Carbaryl	T60.0X1	T60.0X2	T60.0X3	T60.0X4	--	--
Carbaspirin	T39.011	T39.012	T39.013	T39.014	T39.015	T39.016
Carbazochrome (salicylate) (sodium sulfonate)	T49.4X1	T49.4X2	T49.4X3	T49.4X4	T49.4X5	T49.4X6
Carbenicillin	T36.0X1	T36.0X2	T36.0X3	T36.0X4	T36.0X5	T36.0X6
Carbenoxolone	T47.1X1	T47.1X2	T47.1X3	T47.1X4	T47.1X5	T47.1X6
Carbetapentane	T48.3X1	T48.3X2	T48.3X3	T48.3X4	T48.3X5	T48.3X6
Carbethyl salicylate	T39.091	T39.092	T39.093	T39.094	T39.095	T39.096
Carbidopa (with levodopa)	T42.8X1	T42.8X2	T42.8X3	T42.8X4	T42.8X5	T42.8X6
Carbimazole	T38.2X1	T38.2X2	T38.2X3	T38.2X4	T38.2X5	T38.2X6
Carbinol	T51.1X1	T51.1X2	T51.1X3	T51.1X4	--	--
Carbinoxamine	T45.0X1	T45.0X2	T45.0X3	T45.0X4	T45.0X5	T45.0X6
Carbiphene	T39.8X1	T39.8X2	T39.8X3	T39.8X4	T39.8X5	T39.8X6
Carbitol	T52.3X1	T52.3X2	T52.3X3	T52.3X4	--	--
Carbo medicinalis	T47.6X1	T47.6X2	T47.6X3	T47.6X4	T47.6X5	T47.6X6
Carbocaine	T41.3X1	T41.3X2	T41.3X3	T41.3X4	T41.3X5	T41.3X6
infiltration (subcutaneous)	T41.3X1	T41.3X2	T41.3X3	T41.3X4	T41.3X5	T41.3X6
nerve block (peripheral) (plexus)	T41.3X1	T41.3X2	T41.3X3	T41.3X4	T41.3X5	T41.3X6
topical (surface)	T41.3X1	T41.3X2	T41.3X3	T41.3X4	T41.3X5	T41.3X6
Carbocisteine	T48.4X1	T48.4X2	T48.4X3	T48.4X4	T48.4X5	T48.4X6
Carbocromen	T46.3X1	T46.3X2	T46.3X3	T46.3X4	T46.3X5	T46.3X6
Carbol fuchsin	T49.0X1	T49.0X2	T49.0X3	T49.0X4	T49.0X5	T49.0X6
Carbolic acid—see also Phenol	T54.0X1	T54.0X2	T54.0X3	T54.0X4	--	--
Carbolonium (bromide)	T48.1X1	T48.1X2	T48.1X3	T48.1X4	T48.1X5	T48.1X6
Carbomycin	T36.8X1	T36.8X2	T36.8X3	T36.8X4	T36.8X5	T36.8X6
bisulfide (liquid)	T65.4X1	T65.4X2	T65.4X3	T65.4X4	--	--
vapor	T65.4X1	T65.4X2	T65.4X3	T65.4X4	--	--
dioxide (gas)	T59.7X1	T59.7X2	T59.7X3	T59.7X4	--	--
medicinal	T41.5X1	T41.5X2	T41.5X3	T41.5X4	T41.5X5	T41.5X6

Substance	Poisoning, Accidental (unintentional)	Poisoning, Intentional Self-harm	Poisoning, Assault	Poisoning, Undetermined	Adverse effect	Underdosing
nonmedicinal	T59.7X1	T59.7X2	T59.7X3	T59.7X4	--	--
snow	T49.4X1	T49.4X2	T49.4X3	T49.4X4	T49.4X5	T49.4X6
disulfide (liquid)	T65.4X1	T65.4X2	T65.4X3	T65.4X4	--	--
vapor	T65.4X1	T65.4X2	T65.4X3	T65.4X4	--	--
monoxide (from incomplete combustion)	T58.91	T58.92	T58.93	T58.94	--	--
blast furnace gas	T58.8X1	T58.8X2	T58.8X3	T58.8X4	--	--
butane (distributed in mobile container)	T58.11	T58.12	T58.13	T58.14	--	--
distributed through pipes	T58.11	T58.12	T58.13	T58.14	--	--
charcoal fumes	T58.2X1	T58.2X2	T58.2X3	T58.2X4	--	--
coal	T58.2X1	T58.2X2	T58.2X3	T58.2X4	--	--
coke (in domestic stoves, fireplaces)	T58.2X1	T58.2X2	T58.2X3	T58.2X4	--	--
gas (piped)	T58.11	T58.12	T58.13	T58.14	--	--
solid (in domestic stoves, fireplaces)	T58.2X1	T58.2X2	T58.2X3	T58.2X4	--	--
exhaust gas (motor) not in transit	T58.01	T58.02	T58.03	T58.04	--	--
combustion engine, any not in watercraft	T58.01	T58.02	T58.03	T58.04	--	--
farm tractor, not in transit	T58.01	T58.02	T58.03	T58.04	--	--
gas engine	T58.01	T58.02	T58.03	T58.04	--	--
motor pump	T58.01	T58.02	T58.03	T58.04	--	--
motor vehicle, not in transit	T58.01	T58.02	T58.03	T58.04	--	--
fuel (in domestic use)	T58.2X1	T58.2X2	T58.2X3	T58.2X4	--	--
gas (piped)	T58.11	T58.12	T58.13	T58.14	--	--
in mobile container	T58.11	T58.12	T58.13	T58.14	--	--
piped (natural)	T58.11	T58.12	T58.13	T58.14	--	--
utility	T58.11	T58.12	T58.13	T58.14	--	--
in mobile container	T58.11	T58.12	T58.13	T58.14	--	--
illuminating gas	T58.11	T58.12	T58.13	T58.14	--	--
industrial fuels or gases, any	T58.8X1	T58.8X2	T58.8X3	T58.8X4	--	--
kerosene (in domestic stoves, fireplaces)	T58.2X1	T58.2X2	T58.2X3	T58.2X4	--	--
kiln gas or vapor	T58.8X1	T58.8X2	T58.8X3	T58.8X4	--	--
motor exhaust gas, not in transit	T58.01	T58.02	T58.03	T58.04	--	--
piped gas (manufactured) (natural)	T58.11	T58.12	T58.13	T58.14	--	--
producer gas	T58.8X1	T58.8X2	T58.8X3	T58.8X4	--	--
propane (distributed in mobile container)	T58.11	T58.12	T58.13	T58.14	--	--
distributed through pipes	T58.11	T58.12	T58.13	T58.14	--	--
specified source NEC	T58.8X1	T58.8X2	T58.8X3	T58.8X4	--	--
stove gas	T58.11	T58.12	T58.13	T58.14	--	--
piped	T58.11	T58.12	T58.13	T58.14	--	--
utility gas	T58.11	T58.12	T58.13	T58.14	--	--
piped	T58.11	T58.12	T58.13	T58.14	--	--
water gas	T58.11	T58.12	T58.13	T58.14	--	--
wood (in domestic stoves, fireplaces)	T58.2X1	T58.2X2	T58.2X3	T58.2X4	--	--
tetrachloride (vapor) NEC	T53.0X1	T53.0X2	T53.0X3	T53.0X4	--	--
liquid (cleansing agent) NEC	T53.0X1	T53.0X2	T53.0X3	T53.0X4	--	--
solvent	T53.0X1	T53.0X2	T53.0X3	T53.0X4	--	--
Carbonic acid gas	T59.7X1	T59.7X2	T59.7X3	T59.7X4	--	--
anhydrase inhibitor NEC	T50.2X1	T50.2X2	T50.2X3	T50.2X4	T50.2X5	T50.2X6
Carbophenothion	T60.0X1	T60.0X2	T60.0X3	T60.0X4	--	--
Carboplatin	T45.1X1	T45.1X2	T45.1X3	T45.1X4	T45.1X5	T45.1X6
Carboprost	T48.0X1	T48.0X2	T48.0X3	T48.0X4	T48.0X5	T48.0X6
Carboquone	T45.1X1	T45.1X2	T45.1X3	T45.1X4	T45.1X5	T45.1X6
Carbowax	T49.3X1	T49.3X2	T49.3X3	T49.3X4	T49.3X5	T49.3X6
Carboxymethyl-cellulose	T47.4X1	T47.4X2	T47.4X3	T47.4X4	T47.4X5	T47.4X6
S-Carboxymethyl-cysteine	T48.4X1	T48.4X2	T48.4X3	T48.4X4	T48.4X5	T48.4X6
Carbrital	T42.3X1	T42.3X2	T42.3X3	T42.3X4	T42.3X5	T42.3X6
Carbromal	T42.6X1	T42.6X2	T42.6X3	T42.6X4	T42.6X5	T42.6X6
Carbutamide	T38.3X1	T38.3X2	T38.3X3	T38.3X4	T38.3X5	T38.3X6
Carbuterol	T48.6X1	T48.6X2	T48.6X3	T48.6X4	T48.6X5	T48.6X6
Cardiac						
depressants	T46.2X1	T46.2X2	T46.2X3	T46.2X4	T46.2X5	T46.2X6
rhythm regulator	T46.2X1	T46.2X2	T46.2X3	T46.2X4	T46.2X5	T46.2X6
specified NEC	T46.2X1	T46.2X2	T46.2X3	T46.2X4	T46.2X5	T46.2X6
Cardiografin	T50.8X1	T50.8X2	T50.8X3	T50.8X4	T50.8X5	T50.8X6
Cardio-green	T50.8X1	T50.8X2	T50.8X3	T50.8X4	T50.8X5	T50.8X6
Cardiotonic (glycoside) NEC	T46.0X1	T46.0X2	T46.0X3	T46.0X4	T46.0X5	T46.0X6
Cardiovascular drug NEC	T46.901	T46.902	T46.903	T46.904	T46.905	T46.906

Substance	Poisoning, Accidental (unintentional)	Poisoning, Intentional Self-harm	Poisoning, Assault	Poisoning, Undetermined	Adverse effect	Underdosing
Cardrase	T50.2X1	T50.2X2	T50.2X3	T50.2X4	T50.2X5	T50.2X6
Carfecillin	T36.0X1	T36.0X2	T36.0X3	T36.0X4	T36.0X5	T36.0X6
Carfenazine	T43.3X1	T43.3X2	T43.3X3	T43.3X4	T43.3X5	T43.3X6
Carfusin	T49.0X1	T49.0X2	T49.0X3	T49.0X4	T49.0X5	T49.0X6
Carindacillin	T36.0X1	T36.0X2	T36.0X3	T36.0X4	T36.0X5	T36.0X6
Carisoprodol	T42.8X1	T42.8X2	T42.8X3	T42.8X4	T42.8X5	T42.8X6
Carmellose	T47.4X1	T47.4X2	T47.4X3	T47.4X4	T47.4X5	T47.4X6
Carminative	T47.5X1	T47.5X2	T47.5X3	T47.5X4	T47.5X5	T47.5X6
Carmofur	T45.1X1	T45.1X2	T45.1X3	T45.1X4	T45.1X5	T45.1X6
Carmustine	T45.1X1	T45.1X2	T45.1X3	T45.1X4	T45.1X5	T45.1X6
Carotene	T45.2X1	T45.2X2	T45.2X3	T45.2X4	T45.2X5	T45.2X6
Carphenazine	T43.3X1	T43.3X2	T43.3X3	T43.3X4	T43.3X5	T43.3X6
Carpipramine	T42.4X1	T42.4X2	T42.4X3	T42.4X4	T42.4X5	T42.4X6
Carprofen	T39.311	T39.312	T39.313	T39.314	T39.315	T39.316
Carpronium chloride	T44.3X1	T44.3X2	T44.3X3	T44.3X4	T44.3X5	T44.3X6
Carrageenan	T47.8X1	T47.8X2	T47.8X3	T47.8X4	T47.8X5	T47.8X6
Carteolol	T44.7X1	T44.7X2	T44.7X3	T44.7X4	T44.7X5	T44.7X6
Carter's Little Pills	T47.2X1	T47.2X2	T47.2X3	T47.2X4	T47.2X5	T47.2X6
Cascara (sagrada)	T47.2X1	T47.2X2	T47.2X3	T47.2X4	T47.2X5	T47.2X6
Cassava	T62.2X1	T62.2X2	T62.2X3	T62.2X4	--	--
Castellani's paint	T49.0X1	T49.0X2	T49.0X3	T49.0X4	T49.0X5	T49.0X6
Castor						
bean	T62.2X1	T62.2X2	T62.2X3	T62.2X4	--	--
oil	T47.2X1	T47.2X2	T47.2X3	T47.2X4	T47.2X5	T47.2X6
Catalase	T45.3X1	T45.3X2	T45.3X3	T45.3X4	T45.3X5	T45.3X6
Caterpillar (sting)	T63.431	T63.432	T63.433	T63.434	--	--
Catha (edulis) (tea)	T43.691	T43.692	T43.693	T43.694	--	--
Cathartic NEC	T47.4X1	T47.4X2	T47.4X3	T47.4X4	T47.4X5	T47.4X6
anthacene derivative	T47.2X1	T47.2X2	T47.2X3	T47.2X4	T47.2X5	T47.2X6
bulk	T47.4X1	T47.4X2	T47.4X3	T47.4X4	T47.4X5	T47.4X6
contact	T47.2X1	T47.2X2	T47.2X3	T47.2X4	T47.2X5	T47.2X6
emollient NEC	T47.4X1	T47.4X2	T47.4X3	T47.4X4	T47.4X5	T47.4X6
irritant NEC	T47.2X1	T47.2X2	T47.2X3	T47.2X4	T47.2X5	T47.2X6
mucilage	T47.4X1	T47.4X2	T47.4X3	T47.4X4	T47.4X5	T47.4X6
saline	T47.3X1	T47.3X2	T47.3X3	T47.3X4	T47.3X5	T47.3X6
vegetable	T47.2X1	T47.2X2	T47.2X3	T47.2X4	T47.2X5	T47.2X6
Cathine	T50.5X1	T50.5X2	T50.5X3	T50.5X4	T50.5X5	T50.5X6
Cathomycin	T36.8X1	T36.8X2	T36.8X3	T36.8X4	T36.8X5	T36.8X6
Cation exchange resin	T50.3X1	T50.3X2	T50.3X3	T50.3X4	T50.3X5	T50.3X6
Caustic (s) NEC	T54.91	T54.92	T54.93	T54.94	--	--
alkali	T54.3X1	T54.3X2	T54.3X3	T54.3X4	--	--
hydroxide	T54.3X1	T54.3X2	T54.3X3	T54.3X4	--	--
potash	T54.3X1	T54.3X2	T54.3X3	T54.3X4	--	--
soda	T54.3X1	T54.3X2	T54.3X3	T54.3X4	--	--
specified NEC	T54.91	T54.92	T54.93	T54.94	--	--
Ceepryn	T49.0X1	T49.0X2	T49.0X3	T49.0X4	T49.0X5	T49.0X6
ENT agent	T49.6X1	T49.6X2	T49.6X3	T49.6X4	T49.6X5	T49.6X6
lozenges	T49.6X1	T49.6X2	T49.6X3	T49.6X4	T49.6X5	T49.6X6
Cefacetrile	T36.1X1	T36.1X2	T36.1X3	T36.1X4	T36.1X5	T36.1X6
Cefaclor	T36.1X1	T36.1X2	T36.1X3	T36.1X4	T36.1X5	T36.1X6
Cefadroxil	T36.1X1	T36.1X2	T36.1X3	T36.1X4	T36.1X5	T36.1X6
Cefalexin	T36.1X1	T36.1X2	T36.1X3	T36.1X4	T36.1X5	T36.1X6
Cefaloglycin	T36.1X1	T36.1X2	T36.1X3	T36.1X4	T36.1X5	T36.1X6
Cefaloridine	T36.1X1	T36.1X2	T36.1X3	T36.1X4	T36.1X5	T36.1X6
Cefalosporins	T36.1X1	T36.1X2	T36.1X3	T36.1X4	T36.1X5	T36.1X6
Cefalotin	T36.1X1	T36.1X2	T36.1X3	T36.1X4	T36.1X5	T36.1X6
Cefamandole	T36.1X1	T36.1X2	T36.1X3	T36.1X4	T36.1X5	T36.1X6
Cefamycin antibiotic	T36.1X1	T36.1X2	T36.1X3	T36.1X4	T36.1X5	T36.1X6
Cefapirin	T36.1X1	T36.1X2	T36.1X3	T36.1X4	T36.1X5	T36.1X6
Cefatrizine	T36.1X1	T36.1X2	T36.1X3	T36.1X4	T36.1X5	T36.1X6
Cefazedone	T36.1X1	T36.1X2	T36.1X3	T36.1X4	T36.1X5	T36.1X6
Cefazolin	T36.1X1	T36.1X2	T36.1X3	T36.1X4	T36.1X5	T36.1X6
Cefbuperazone	T36.1X1	T36.1X2	T36.1X3	T36.1X4	T36.1X5	T36.1X6
Cefetamet	T36.1X1	T36.1X2	T36.1X3	T36.1X4	T36.1X5	T36.1X6

Substance	Poisoning, Accidental (unintentional)	Poisoning, Intentional Self-harm	Poisoning, Assault	Poisoning, Undetermined	Adverse effect	Underdosing
Cefixime	T36.1X1	T36.1X2	T36.1X3	T36.1X4	T36.1X5	T36.1X6
Cefmenoxime	T36.1X1	T36.1X2	T36.1X3	T36.1X4	T36.1X5	T36.1X6
Cefmetazole	T36.1X1	T36.1X2	T36.1X3	T36.1X4	T36.1X5	T36.1X6
Cefminox	T36.1X1	T36.1X2	T36.1X3	T36.1X4	T36.1X5	T36.1X6
Cefonicid	T36.1X1	T36.1X2	T36.1X3	T36.1X4	T36.1X5	T36.1X6
Cefoperazone	T36.1X1	T36.1X2	T36.1X3	T36.1X4	T36.1X5	T36.1X6
Ceforanide	T36.1X1	T36.1X2	T36.1X3	T36.1X4	T36.1X5	T36.1X6
Cefotaxime	T36.1X1	T36.1X2	T36.1X3	T36.1X4	T36.1X5	T36.1X6
Cefotetan	T36.1X1	T36.1X2	T36.1X3	T36.1X4	T36.1X5	T36.1X6
Cefotiam	T36.1X1	T36.1X2	T36.1X3	T36.1X4	T36.1X5	T36.1X6
Cefoxitin	T36.1X1	T36.1X2	T36.1X3	T36.1X4	T36.1X5	T36.1X6
Cefpimizole	T36.1X1	T36.1X2	T36.1X3	T36.1X4	T36.1X5	T36.1X6
Cefpiramide	T36.1X1	T36.1X2	T36.1X3	T36.1X4	T36.1X5	T36.1X6
Cefradine	T36.1X1	T36.1X2	T36.1X3	T36.1X4	T36.1X5	T36.1X6
Cefroxadine	T36.1X1	T36.1X2	T36.1X3	T36.1X4	T36.1X5	T36.1X6
Cefsulodin	T36.1X1	T36.1X2	T36.1X3	T36.1X4	T36.1X5	T36.1X6
Ceftazidime	T36.1X1	T36.1X2	T36.1X3	T36.1X4	T36.1X5	T36.1X6
Cefteram	T36.1X1	T36.1X2	T36.1X3	T36.1X4	T36.1X5	T36.1X6
Ceftezole	T36.1X1	T36.1X2	T36.1X3	T36.1X4	T36.1X5	T36.1X6
Ceftizoxime	T36.1X1	T36.1X2	T36.1X3	T36.1X4	T36.1X5	T36.1X6
Ceftriaxone	T36.1X1	T36.1X2	T36.1X3	T36.1X4	T36.1X5	T36.1X6
Cefuroxime	T36.1X1	T36.1X2	T36.1X3	T36.1X4	T36.1X5	T36.1X6
Cefuzonam	T36.1X1	T36.1X2	T36.1X3	T36.1X4	T36.1X5	T36.1X6
Celestone	T38.0X1	T38.0X2	T38.0X3	T38.0X4	T38.0X5	T38.0X6
topical	T49.0X1	T49.0X2	T49.0X3	T49.0X4	T49.0X5	T49.0X6
Celiprolol	T44.7X1	T44.7X2	T44.7X3	T44.7X4	T44.7X5	T44.7X6
Cell stimulants and proliferants	T49.8X1	T49.8X2	T49.8X3	T49.8X4	T49.8X5	T49.8X6
Cellosolve	T52.91	T52.92	T52.93	T52.94	--	--
Cellulose						
cathartic	T47.4X1	T47.4X2	T47.4X3	T47.4X4	T47.4X5	T47.4X6
hydroxyethyl	T47.4X1	T47.4X2	T47.4X3	T47.4X4	T47.4X5	T47.4X6
nitrates (topical)	T49.3X1	T49.3X2	T49.3X3	T49.3X4	T49.3X5	T49.3X6
oxidized	T49.4X1	T49.4X2	T49.4X3	T49.4X4	T49.4X5	T49.4X6
Centipede (bite)	T63.411	T63.412	T63.413	T63.414	--	--
Central nervous system						
depressants	T42.71	T42.72	T42.73	T42.74	T42.75	T42.76
anesthetic (general) NEC	T41.201	T41.202	T41.203	T41.204	T41.205	T41.206
gases NEC	T41.0X1	T41.0X2	T41.0X3	T41.0X4	T41.0X5	T41.0X6
intravenous	T41.1X1	T41.1X2	T41.1X3	T41.1X4	T41.1X5	T41.1X6
barbiturates	T42.3X1	T42.3X2	T42.3X3	T42.3X4	T42.3X5	T42.3X6
benzodiazepines	T42.4X1	T42.4X2	T42.4X3	T42.4X4	T42.4X5	T42.4X6
bromides	T42.6X1	T42.6X2	T42.6X3	T42.6X4	T42.6X5	T42.6X6
cannabis sativa	T40.7X1	T40.7X2	T40.7X3	T40.7X4	T40.7X5	T40.7X6
chloral hydrate	T42.6X1	T42.6X2	T42.6X3	T42.6X4	T42.6X5	T42.6X6
ethanol	T51.0X1	T51.0X2	T51.0X3	T51.0X4	--	--
hallucinogenics	T40.901	T40.902	T40.903	T40.904	T40.905	T40.906
hypnotics	T42.71	T42.72	T42.73	T42.74	T42.75	T42.76
specified NEC	T42.6X1	T42.6X2	T42.6X3	T42.6X4	T42.6X5	T42.6X6
muscle relaxants	T42.8X1	T42.8X2	T42.8X3	T42.8X4	T42.8X5	T42.8X6
paraldehyde	T42.6X1	T42.6X2	T42.6X3	T42.6X4	T42.6X5	T42.6X6
sedatives; sedative-hypnotics	T42.71	T42.72	T42.73	T42.74	T42.75	T42.76
mixed NEC	T42.6X1	T42.6X2	T42.6X3	T42.6X4	T42.6X5	T42.6X6
specified NEC	T42.6X1	T42.6X2	T42.6X3	T42.6X4	T42.6X5	T42.6X6
muscle-tone depressants	T42.8X1	T42.8X2	T42.8X3	T42.8X4	T42.8X5	T42.8X6
stimulants	T43.601	T43.602	T43.603	T43.604	T43.605	T43.606
amphetamines	T43.621	T43.622	T43.623	T43.624	T43.625	T43.626
analeptics	T50.7X1	T50.7X2	T50.7X3	T50.7X4	T50.7X5	T50.7X6
antidepressants	T43.201	T43.202	T43.203	T43.204	T43.205	T43.206
opiate antagonists	T50.7X1	T50.7X2	T50.7X3	T50.7X4	T50.7X5	T50.7X6
specified NEC	T43.691	T43.692	T43.693	T43.694	T43.695	T43.696
Cephalexin	T36.1X1	T36.1X2	T36.1X3	T36.1X4	T36.1X5	T36.1X6
Cephaloglycin	T36.1X1	T36.1X2	T36.1X3	T36.1X4	T36.1X5	T36.1X6
Cephaloridine	T36.1X1	T36.1X2	T36.1X3	T36.1X4	T36.1X5	T36.1X6
Cephalosporins	T36.1X1	T36.1X2	T36.1X3	T36.1X4	T36.1X5	T36.1X6
N (adicillin)	T36.0X1	T36.0X2	T36.0X3	T36.0X4	T36.0X5	T36.0X6

Substance	Poisoning, Accidental (unintentional)	Poisoning, Intentional Self-harm	Poisoning, Assault	Poisoning, Undetermined	Adverse effect	Underdosing
Cephalothin	T36.1X1	T36.1X2	T36.1X3	T36.1X4	T36.1X5	T36.1X6
Cephalotin	T36.1X1	T36.1X2	T36.1X3	T36.1X4	T36.1X5	T36.1X6
Cephradine	T36.1X1	T36.1X2	T36.1X3	T36.1X4	T36.1X5	T36.1X6
Cerbera (odallam)	T62.2X1	T62.2X2	T62.2X3	T62.2X4	--	--
Cerberin	T46.0X1	T46.0X2	T46.0X3	T46.0X4	T46.0X5	T46.0X6
Cerebral stimulants	T43.601	T43.602	T43.603	T43.604	T43.605	T43.606
psychotherapeutic	T43.601	T43.602	T43.603	T43.604	T43.605	T43.606
specified NEC	T43.691	T43.692	T43.693	T43.694	T43.695	T43.696
Cerium oxalate	T45.0X1	T45.0X2	T45.0X3	T45.0X4	T45.0X5	T45.0X6
Cerous oxalate	T45.0X1	T45.0X2	T45.0X3	T45.0X4	T45.0X5	T45.0X6
Ceruletide	T50.8X1	T50.8X2	T50.8X3	T50.8X4	T50.8X5	T50.8X6
Cetalkonium (chloride)	T49.0X1	T49.0X2	T49.0X3	T49.0X4	T49.0X5	T49.0X6
Cethexonium chloride	T49.0X1	T49.0X2	T49.0X3	T49.0X4	T49.0X5	T49.0X6
Cetiedil	T46.7X1	T46.7X2	T46.7X3	T46.7X4	T46.7X5	T46.7X6
Cetirizine	T45.0X1	T45.0X2	T45.0X3	T45.0X4	T45.0X5	T45.0X6
Cetomacrogol	T50.991	T50.992	T50.993	T50.994	T50.995	T50.996
Cetotiamine	T45.2X1	T45.2X2	T45.2X3	T45.2X4	T45.2X5	T45.2X6
Cetoxime	T45.0X1	T45.0X2	T45.0X3	T45.0X4	T45.0X5	T45.0X6
Cetraxate	T47.1X1	T47.1X2	T47.1X3	T47.1X4	T47.1X5	T47.1X6
Cetrimide	T49.0X1	T49.0X2	T49.0X3	T49.0X4	T49.0X5	T49.0X6
Cetrimonium (bromide)	T49.0X1	T49.0X2	T49.0X3	T49.0X4	T49.0X5	T49.0X6
Cetylpyridinium chloride	T49.0X1	T49.0X2	T49.0X3	T49.0X4	T49.0X5	T49.0X6
ENT agent	T49.6X1	T49.6X2	T49.6X3	T49.6X4	T49.6X5	T49.6X6
lozenges	T49.6X1	T49.6X2	T49.6X3	T49.6X4	T49.6X5	T49.6X6
Cevadilla—see Sabadilla						
Cevitamic acid	T45.2X1	T45.2X2	T45.2X3	T45.2X4	T45.2X5	T45.2X6
Chalk, precipitated	T47.1X1	T47.1X2	T47.1X3	T47.1X4	T47.1X5	T47.1X6
Chamomile	T49.0X1	T49.0X2	T49.0X3	T49.0X4	T49.0X5	T49.0X6
Ch'an su	T46.0X1	T46.0X2	T46.0X3	T46.0X4	T46.0X5	T46.0X6
Charcoal	T47.6X1	T47.6X2	T47.6X3	T47.6X4	T47.6X5	T47.6X6
activated—see also Charcoal, medicinal	T47.6X1	T47.6X2	T47.6X3	T47.6X4	T47.6X5	T47.6X6
fumes (Carbon monoxide)	T58.2X1	T58.2X2	T58.2X3	T58.2X4	--	--
industrial	T58.8X1	T58.8X2	T58.8X3	T58.8X4	--	--
medicinal (activated)	T47.6X1	T47.6X2	T47.6X3	T47.6X4	T47.6X5	T47.6X6
antidiarrheal	T47.6X1	T47.6X2	T47.6X3	T47.6X4	T47.6X5	T47.6X6
poison control	T47.8X1	T47.8X2	T47.8X3	T47.8X4	T47.8X5	T47.8X6
specified use other than for diarrhea	T47.8X1	T47.8X2	T47.8X3	T47.8X4	T47.8X5	T47.8X6
topical	T49.8X1	T49.8X2	T49.8X3	T49.8X4	T49.8X5	T49.8X6
Chaulmosulfone	T37.1X1	T37.1X2	T37.1X3	T37.1X4	T37.1X5	T37.1X6
Chelating agent NEC	T50.6X1	T50.6X2	T50.6X3	T50.6X4	T50.6X5	T50.6X6
Chelidonium majus	T62.2X1	T62.2X2	T62.2X3	T62.2X4	--	--
Chemical substance NEC	T65.91	T65.92	T65.93	T65.94	--	--
Chenodeoxycholic acid	T47.5X1	T47.5X2	T47.5X3	T47.5X4	T47.5X5	T47.5X6
Chenodiol	T47.5X1	T47.5X2	T47.5X3	T47.5X4	T47.5X5	T47.5X6
Chenopodium	T37.4X1	T37.4X2	T37.4X3	T37.4X4	T37.4X5	T37.4X6
Cherry laurel	T62.2X1	T62.2X2	T62.2X3	T62.2X4	--	--
Chinidin (e)	T46.2X1	T46.2X2	T46.2X3	T46.2X4	T46.2X5	T46.2X6
Chiniofon	T37.8X1	T37.8X2	T37.8X3	T37.8X4	T37.8X5	T37.8X6
Chlophedianol	T48.3X1	T48.3X2	T48.3X3	T48.3X4	T48.3X5	T48.3X6
Chloral	T42.6X1	T42.6X2	T42.6X3	T42.6X4	T42.6X5	T42.6X6
derivative	T42.6X1	T42.6X2	T42.6X3	T42.6X4	T42.6X5	T42.6X6
hydrate	T42.6X1	T42.6X2	T42.6X3	T42.6X4	T42.6X5	T42.6X6
Chloralamide	T42.6X1	T42.6X2	T42.6X3	T42.6X4	T42.6X5	T42.6X6
Chloralodol	T42.6X1	T42.6X2	T42.6X3	T42.6X4	T42.6X5	T42.6X6
Chloralose	T60.4X1	T60.4X2	T60.4X3	T60.4X4	--	--
Chlorambucil	T45.1X1	T45.1X2	T45.1X3	T45.1X4	T45.1X5	T45.1X6
Chloramine	T57.8X1	T57.8X2	T57.8X3	T57.8X4	--	--
T	T49.0X1	T49.0X2	T49.0X3	T49.0X4	T49.0X5	T49.0X6
topical	T49.0X1	T49.0X2	T49.0X3	T49.0X4	T49.0X5	T49.0X6
Chloramphenicol	T36.2X1	T36.2X2	T36.2X3	T36.2X4	T36.2X5	T36.2X6
ENT agent	T49.6X1	T49.6X2	T49.6X3	T49.6X4	T49.6X5	T49.6X6
ophthalmic preparation	T49.5X1	T49.5X2	T49.5X3	T49.5X4	T49.5X5	T49.5X6
topical NEC	T49.0X1	T49.0X2	T49.0X3	T49.0X4	T49.0X5	T49.0X6
Chlorate (potassium) (sodium) NEC	T60.3X1	T60.3X2	T60.3X3	T60.3X4	--	--

Substance	Poisoning, Accidental (unintentional)	Poisoning, Intentional Self-harm	Poisoning, Assault	Poisoning, Undetermined	Adverse effect	Underdosing
herbicide	T60.3X1	T60.3X2	T60.3X3	T60.3X4	--	--
Chlorazanil	T50.2X1	T50.2X2	T50.2X3	T50.2X4	T50.2X5	T50.2X6
Chlorbenzene, chlorbenzol	T53.7X1	T53.7X2	T53.7X3	T53.7X4	--	--
Chlorbenzoxamine	T44.3X1	T44.3X2	T44.3X3	T44.3X4	T44.3X5	T44.3X6
Chlorbutol	T42.6X1	T42.6X2	T42.6X3	T42.6X4	T42.6X5	T42.6X6
Chlorcyclizine	T45.0X1	T45.0X2	T45.0X3	T45.0X4	T45.0X5	T45.0X6
Chlordan (e) (dust)	T60.1X1	T60.1X2	T60.1X3	T60.1X4	--	--
Chlordantoin	T49.0X1	T49.0X2	T49.0X3	T49.0X4	T49.0X5	T49.0X6
Chlordiazepoxide	T42.4X1	T42.4X2	T42.4X3	T42.4X4	T42.4X5	T42.4X6
Chlordiethyl benzamide	T49.3X1	T49.3X2	T49.3X3	T49.3X4	T49.3X5	T49.3X6
Chloresium	T49.8X1	T49.8X2	T49.8X3	T49.8X4	T49.8X5	T49.8X6
Chlorethiazol	T42.6X1	T42.6X2	T42.6X3	T42.6X4	T42.6X5	T42.6X6
Chlorethyl—see Ethyl chloride						
Chloretone	T42.6X1	T42.6X2	T42.6X3	T42.6X4	T42.6X5	T42.6X6
Chlorex	T53.6X1	T53.6X2	T53.6X3	T53.6X4	--	--
insecticide	T60.1X1	T60.1X2	T60.1X3	T60.1X4	--	--
Chlorfenvinphos	T60.0X1	T60.0X2	T60.0X3	T60.0X4	--	--
Chlorhexadol	T42.6X1	T42.6X2	T42.6X3	T42.6X4	T42.6X5	T42.6X6
Chlorhexamide	T45.1X1	T45.1X2	T45.1X3	T45.1X4	T45.1X5	T45.1X6
Chlorhexidine	T49.0X1	T49.0X2	T49.0X3	T49.0X4	T49.0X5	T49.0X6
Chlorhydroxyquinolin	T49.0X1	T49.0X2	T49.0X3	T49.0X4	T49.0X5	T49.0X6
Chloride of lime (bleach)	T54.3X1	T54.3X2	T54.3X3	T54.3X4	--	--
Chlorimipramine	T43.011	T43.012	T43.013	T43.014	T43.015	T43.016
Chlorinated						
camphene	T53.6X1	T53.6X2	T53.6X3	T53.6X4	--	--
diphenyl	T53.7X1	T53.7X2	T53.7X3	T53.7X4	--	--
hydrocarbons NEC	T53.91	T53.92	T53.93	T53.94	--	--
solvents	T53.91	T53.92	T53.93	T53.94	--	--
lime (bleach)	T54.3X1	T54.3X2	T54.3X3	T54.3X4	--	--
and boric acid solution	T49.0X1	T49.0X2	T49.0X3	T49.0X4	T49.0X5	T49.0X6
naphthalene (insecticide)	T60.1X1	T60.1X2	T60.1X3	T60.1X4	--	--
industrial (non-pesticide)	T53.7X1	T53.7X2	T53.7X3	T53.7X4	--	--
pesticide NEC	T60.8X1	T60.8X2	T60.8X3	T60.8X4	--	--
soda—see also sodium hypochlorite						
solution	T49.0X1	T49.0X2	T49.0X3	T49.0X4	T49.0X5	T49.0X6
Chlorine (fumes) (gas)	T59.4X1	T59.4X2	T59.4X3	T59.4X4	--	--
bleach	T54.3X1	T54.3X2	T54.3X3	T54.3X4	--	--
compound gas NEC	T59.4X1	T59.4X2	T59.4X3	T59.4X4	--	--
disinfectant	T59.4X1	T59.4X2	T59.4X3	T59.4X4	--	--
releasing agents NEC	T59.4X1	T59.4X2	T59.4X3	T59.4X4	--	--
Chlorisondamine chloride	T46.991	T46.992	T46.993	T46.994	T46.995	T46.996
Chlormadinone	T38.5X1	T38.5X2	T38.5X3	T38.5X4	T38.5X5	T38.5X6
Chlormephos	T60.0X1	T60.0X2	T60.0X3	T60.0X4	--	--
Chlormerodrin	T50.2X1	T50.2X2	T50.2X3	T50.2X4	T50.2X5	T50.2X6
Chlormethiazole	T42.6X1	T42.6X2	T42.6X3	T42.6X4	T42.6X5	T42.6X6
Chlormethine	T45.1X1	T45.1X2	T45.1X3	T45.1X4	T45.1X5	T45.1X6
Chlormethylenecycline	T36.4X1	T36.4X2	T36.4X3	T36.4X4	T36.4X5	T36.4X6
Chlormezanone	T42.6X1	T42.6X2	T42.6X3	T42.6X4	T42.6X5	T42.6X6
Chloroacetic acid	T60.3X1	T60.3X2	T60.3X3	T60.3X4	--	--
Chloroacetone	T59.3X1	T59.3X2	T59.3X3	T59.3X4	--	--
Chloroacetophenone	T59.3X1	T59.3X2	T59.3X3	T59.3X4	--	--
Chloroaniline	T53.7X1	T53.7X2	T53.7X3	T53.7X4	--	--
Chlorobenzene, chlorobenzol	T53.7X1	T53.7X2	T53.7X3	T53.7X4	--	--
Chlorobromomethane (fire extinguisher)	T53.6X1	T53.6X2	T53.6X3	T53.6X4	--	--
Chlorobutanol	T49.0X1	T49.0X2	T49.0X3	T49.0X4	T49.0X5	T49.0X6
Chlorocresol	T49.0X1	T49.0X2	T49.0X3	T49.0X4	T49.0X5	T49.0X6
Chlorodehydro-methyltestosterone	T38.7X1	T38.7X2	T38.7X3	T38.7X4	T38.7X5	T38.7X6
Chlorodinitrobenzene	T53.7X1	T53.7X2	T53.7X3	T53.7X4	--	--
dust or vapor	T53.7X1	T53.7X2	T53.7X3	T53.7X4	--	--
Chlorodiphenyl	T53.7X1	T53.7X2	T53.7X3	T53.7X4	--	--
Chloroethane—see Ethyl chloride						
Chloroethylene	T53.6X1	T53.6X2	T53.6X3	T53.6X4	--	--
Chlorofluorocarbons	T53.5X1	T53.5X2	T53.5X3	T53.5X4	--	--
Chloroform (fumes) (vapor)	T53.1X1	T53.1X2	T53.1X3	T53.1X4	--	--
anesthetic	T41.0X1	T41.0X2	T41.0X3	T41.0X4	T41.0X5	T41.0X6

Substance	Poisoning, Accidental (unintentional)	Poisoning, Intentional Self-harm	Poisoning, Assault	Poisoning, Undetermined	Adverse effect	Underdosing
solvent	T53.1X1	T53.1X2	T53.1X3	T53.1X4	--	--
water, concentrated	T41.0X1	T41.0X2	T41.0X3	T41.0X4	T41.0X5	T41.0X6
Chloroguanide	T37.2X1	T37.2X2	T37.2X3	T37.2X4	T37.2X5	T37.2X6
Chloromycetin	T36.2X1	T36.2X2	T36.2X3	T36.2X4	T36.2X5	T36.2X6
ENT agent	T49.6X1	T49.6X2	T49.6X3	T49.6X4	T49.6X5	T49.6X6
ophthalmic preparation	T49.5X1	T49.5X2	T49.5X3	T49.5X4	T49.5X5	T49.5X6
otic solution	T49.6X1	T49.6X2	T49.6X3	T49.6X4	T49.6X5	T49.6X6
topical NEC	T49.0X1	T49.0X2	T49.0X3	T49.0X4	T49.0X5	T49.0X6
Chloronitrobenzene	T53.7X1	T53.7X2	T53.7X3	T53.7X4	--	--
dust or vapor	T53.7X1	T53.7X2	T53.7X3	T53.7X4	--	--
Chlorophacinone	T60.4X1	T60.4X2	T60.4X3	T60.4X4	--	--
Chlorophenol	T53.7X1	T53.7X2	T53.7X3	T53.7X4	--	--
Chlorophenothane	T60.1X1	T60.1X2	T60.1X3	T60.1X4	--	--
Chlorophyll	T50.991	T50.992	T50.993	T50.994	T50.995	T50.996
Chloropicrin (fumes)	T53.6X1	T53.6X2	T53.6X3	T53.6X4	--	--
fumigant	T60.8X1	T60.8X2	T60.8X3	T60.8X4	--	--
fungicide	T60.3X1	T60.3X2	T60.3X3	T60.3X4	--	--
pesticide	T60.8X1	T60.8X2	T60.8X3	T60.8X4	--	--
Chloroprocaine	T41.3X1	T41.3X2	T41.3X3	T41.3X4	T41.3X5	T41.3X6
infiltration (subcutaneous)	T41.3X1	T41.3X2	T41.3X3	T41.3X4	T41.3X5	T41.3X6
nerve block (peripheral) (plexus)	T41.3X1	T41.3X2	T41.3X3	T41.3X4	T41.3X5	T41.3X6
spinal	T41.3X1	T41.3X2	T41.3X3	T41.3X4	T41.3X5	T41.3X6
Chloroptic	T49.5X1	T49.5X2	T49.5X3	T49.5X4	T49.5X5	T49.5X6
Chloropurine	T45.1X1	T45.1X2	T45.1X3	T45.1X4	T45.1X5	T45.1X6
Chloropyramine	T45.0X1	T45.0X2	T45.0X3	T45.0X4	T45.0X5	T45.0X6
Chloropyrifos	T60.0X1	T60.0X2	T60.0X3	T60.0X4	--	--
Chloropyrilene	T45.0X1	T45.0X2	T45.0X3	T45.0X4	T45.0X5	T45.0X6
Chloroquine	T37.2X1	T37.2X2	T37.2X3	T37.2X4	T37.2X5	T37.2X6
Chlorothalonil	T60.3X1	T60.3X2	T60.3X3	T60.3X4	--	--
Chlorothen	T45.0X1	T45.0X2	T45.0X3	T45.0X4	T45.0X5	T45.0X6
Chlorothiazide	T50.2X1	T50.2X2	T50.2X3	T50.2X4	T50.2X5	T50.2X6
Chlorothymol	T49.4X1	T49.4X2	T49.4X3	T49.4X4	T49.4X5	T49.4X6
Chlorotrianisene	T38.5X1	T38.5X2	T38.5X3	T38.5X4	T38.5X5	T38.5X6
Chlorovinyldichloro-arsine, not in war	T57.0X1	T57.0X2	T57.0X3	T57.0X4	--	--
Chloroxine	T49.4X1	T49.4X2	T49.4X3	T49.4X4	T49.4X5	T49.4X6
Chloroxylenol	T49.0X1	T49.0X2	T49.0X3	T49.0X4	T49.0X5	T49.0X6
Chlorphenamine	T45.0X1	T45.0X2	T45.0X3	T45.0X4	T45.0X5	T45.0X6
Chlorphenesin	T42.8X1	T42.8X2	T42.8X3	T42.8X4	T42.8X5	T42.8X6
topical (antifungal)	T49.0X1	T49.0X2	T49.0X3	T49.0X4	T49.0X5	T49.0X6
Chlorpheniramine	T45.0X1	T45.0X2	T45.0X3	T45.0X4	T45.0X5	T45.0X6
Chlorphenoxamine	T45.0X1	T45.0X2	T45.0X3	T45.0X4	T45.0X5	T45.0X6
Chlorphentermine	T50.5X1	T50.5X2	T50.5X3	T50.5X4	T50.5X5	T50.5X6
Chlorprocaine—see Chloroprocaine						
Chlorproguanil	T37.2X1	T37.2X2	T37.2X3	T37.2X4	T37.2X5	T37.2X6
Chlorpromazine	T43.3X1	T43.3X2	T43.3X3	T43.3X4	T43.3X5	T43.3X6
Chlorpropamide	T38.3X1	T38.3X2	T38.3X3	T38.3X4	T38.3X5	T38.3X6
Chlorprothixene	T43.4X1	T43.4X2	T43.4X3	T43.4X4	T43.4X5	T43.4X6
Chlorquinaldol	T49.0X1	T49.0X2	T49.0X3	T49.0X4	T49.0X5	T49.0X6
Chlorquinol	T49.0X1	T49.0X2	T49.0X3	T49.0X4	T49.0X5	T49.0X6
Chlortalidone	T50.2X1	T50.2X2	T50.2X3	T50.2X4	T50.2X5	T50.2X6
Chlortetracycline	T36.4X1	T36.4X2	T36.4X3	T36.4X4	T36.4X5	T36.4X6
Chlorthalidone	T50.2X1	T50.2X2	T50.2X3	T50.2X4	T50.2X5	T50.2X6
Chlorthiophos	T60.0X1	T60.0X2	T60.0X3	T60.0X4	--	--
Chlortrianisene	T38.5X1	T38.5X2	T38.5X3	T38.5X4	T38.5X5	T38.5X6
Chlor-Trimeton	T45.0X1	T45.0X2	T45.0X3	T45.0X4	T45.0X5	T45.0X6
Chlorthion	T60.0X1	T60.0X2	T60.0X3	T60.0X4	--	--
Chlorzoxazone	T42.8X1	T42.8X2	T42.8X3	T42.8X4	T42.8X5	T42.8X6
Choke damp	T59.7X1	T59.7X2	T59.7X3	T59.7X4	--	--
Cholagogues	T47.5X1	T47.5X2	T47.5X3	T47.5X4	T47.5X5	T47.5X6
Cholebrine	T50.8X1	T50.8X2	T50.8X3	T50.8X4	T50.8X5	T50.8X6
Cholecalciferol	T45.2X1	T45.2X2	T45.2X3	T45.2X4	T45.2X5	T45.2X6
Cholecystokinin	T50.8X1	T50.8X2	T50.8X3	T50.8X4	T50.8X5	T50.8X6
Cholera vaccine	T50.A91	T50.A92	T50.A93	T50.A94	T50.A95	T50.A96
Choleretic	T47.5X1	T47.5X2	T47.5X3	T47.5X4	T47.5X5	T47.5X6

Substance	Poisoning, Accidental (unintentional)	Poisoning, Intentional Self-harm	Poisoning, Assault	Poisoning, Undetermined	Adverse effect	Underdosing
Cholesterol-lowering agents	T46.6X1	T46.6X2	T46.6X3	T46.6X4	T46.6X5	T46.6X6
Cholestyramine (resin)	T46.6X1	T46.6X2	T46.6X3	T46.6X4	T46.6X5	T46.6X6
Cholic acid	T47.5X1	T47.5X2	T47.5X3	T47.5X4	T47.5X5	T47.5X6
Choline	T48.6X1	T48.6X2	T48.6X3	T48.6X4	T48.6X5	T48.6X6
chloride	T50.991	T50.992	T50.993	T50.994	T50.995	T50.996
dihydrogen citrate	T50.991	T50.992	T50.993	T50.994	T50.995	T50.996
salicylate	T39.091	T39.092	T39.093	T39.094	T39.095	T39.096
theophyllinate	T48.6X1	T48.6X2	T48.6X3	T48.6X4	T48.6X5	T48.6X6
Cholinergic (drug) NEC	T44.1X1	T44.1X2	T44.1X3	T44.1X4	T44.1X5	T44.1X6
muscle tone enhancer	T44.1X1	T44.1X2	T44.1X3	T44.1X4	T44.1X5	T44.1X6
organophosphorus	T44.0X1	T44.0X2	T44.0X3	T44.0X4	T44.0X5	T44.0X6
insecticide	T60.0X1	T60.0X2	T60.0X3	T60.0X4	--	--
nerve gas	T59.891	T59.892	T59.893	T59.894	--	--
trimethyl ammonium propanediol	T44.1X1	T44.1X2	T44.1X3	T44.1X4	T44.1X5	T44.1X6
Cholinesterase reactivator	T50.6X1	T50.6X2	T50.6X3	T50.6X4	T50.6X5	T50.6X6
Cholografin	T50.8X1	T50.8X2	T50.8X3	T50.8X4	T50.8X5	T50.8X6
Chorionic gonadotropin	T38.891	T38.892	T38.893	T38.894	T38.895	T38.896
Chromate	T56.2X1	T56.2X2	T56.2X3	T56.2X4	--	--
dust or mist	T56.2X1	T56.2X2	T56.2X3	T56.2X4	--	--
lead—see also lead	T56.0X1	T56.0X2	T56.0X3	T56.0X4	--	--
paint	T56.0X1	T56.0X2	T56.0X3	T56.0X4	--	--
Chromic						
acid	T56.2X1	T56.2X2	T56.2X3	T56.2X4	--	--
dust or mist	T56.2X1	T56.2X2	T56.2X3	T56.2X4	--	--
phosphate 32P	T45.1X1	T45.1X2	T45.1X3	T45.1X4	T45.1X5	T45.1X6
Chromium	T56.2X1	T56.2X2	T56.2X3	T56.2X4	--	--
compounds—see Chromate						
sesquioxide	T50.8X1	T50.8X2	T50.8X3	T50.8X4	T50.8X5	T50.8X6
Chromomycin A3	T45.1X1	T45.1X2	T45.1X3	T45.1X4	T45.1X5	T45.1X6
Chromonar	T46.3X1	T46.3X2	T46.3X3	T46.3X4	T46.3X5	T46.3X6
Chromyl chloride	T56.2X1	T56.2X2	T56.2X3	T56.2X4	--	--
Chrysarobin	T49.4X1	T49.4X2	T49.4X3	T49.4X4	T49.4X5	T49.4X6
Chrysazin	T47.2X1	T47.2X2	T47.2X3	T47.2X4	T47.2X5	T47.2X6
Chymar	T45.3X1	T45.3X2	T45.3X3	T45.3X4	T45.3X5	T45.3X6
ophthalmic preparation	T49.5X1	T49.5X2	T49.5X3	T49.5X4	T49.5X5	T49.5X6
Chymopapain	T45.3X1	T45.3X2	T45.3X3	T45.3X4	T45.3X5	T45.3X6
Chymotrypsin	T45.3X1	T45.3X2	T45.3X3	T45.3X4	T45.3X5	T45.3X6
ophthalmic preparation	T49.5X1	T49.5X2	T49.5X3	T49.5X4	T49.5X5	T49.5X6
Cianidanol	T50.991	T50.992	T50.993	T50.994	T50.995	T50.996
Cianopramine	T43.011	T43.012	T43.013	T43.014	T43.015	T43.016
Cibenzoline	T46.2X1	T46.2X2	T46.2X3	T46.2X4	T46.2X5	T46.2X6
Ciclacillin	T36.0X1	T36.0X2	T36.0X3	T36.0X4	T36.0X5	T36.0X6
Ciclobarbital—see Hexobarbital						
Ciclonicate	T46.7X1	T46.7X2	T46.7X3	T46.7X4	T46.7X5	T46.7X6
Ciclopirox (olamine)	T49.0X1	T49.0X2	T49.0X3	T49.0X4	T49.0X5	T49.0X6
Ciclosporin	T45.1X1	T45.1X2	T45.1X3	T45.1X4	T45.1X5	T45.1X6
Cicuta maculata or virosa	T62.2X1	T62.2X2	T62.2X3	T62.2X4	--	--
Cicutoxin	T62.2X1	T62.2X2	T62.2X3	T62.2X4	--	--
Cigarette lighter fluid	T52.0X1	T52.0X2	T52.0X3	T52.0X4	--	--
Cigarettes (tobacco)	T65.221	T65.222	T65.223	T65.224	--	--
Ciguatoxin	T61.01	T61.02	T61.03	T61.04	--	--
Cilazapril	T46.4X1	T46.4X2	T46.4X3	T46.4X4	T46.4X5	T46.4X6
Cimetidine	T47.0X1	T47.0X2	T47.0X3	T47.0X4	T47.0X5	T47.0X6
Cimetropium bromide	T44.3X1	T44.3X2	T44.3X3	T44.3X4	T44.3X5	T44.3X6
Cinchocaine	T41.3X1	T41.3X2	T41.3X3	T41.3X4	T41.3X5	T41.3X6
topical (surface)	T41.3X1	T41.3X2	T41.3X3	T41.3X4	T41.3X5	T41.3X6
Cinchona	T37.2X1	T37.2X2	T37.2X3	T37.2X4	T37.2X5	T37.2X6
Cinchonine alkaloids	T37.2X1	T37.2X2	T37.2X3	T37.2X4	T37.2X5	T37.2X6
Cinchophen	T50.4X1	T50.4X2	T50.4X3	T50.4X4	T50.4X5	T50.4X6
Cinepazide	T46.7X1	T46.7X2	T46.7X3	T46.7X4	T46.7X5	T46.7X6
Cinnamedrine	T48.5X1	T48.5X2	T48.5X3	T48.5X4	T48.5X5	T48.5X6
Cinnarizine	T45.0X1	T45.0X2	T45.0X3	T45.0X4	T45.0X5	T45.0X6
Cinoxacin	T37.8X1	T37.8X2	T37.8X3	T37.8X4	T37.8X5	T37.8X6
Ciprofibrate	T46.6X1	T46.6X2	T46.6X3	T46.6X4	T46.6X5	T46.6X6
Ciprofloxacin	T36.8X1	T36.8X2	T36.8X3	T36.8X4	T36.8X5	T36.8X6

TABLE OF DRUGS AND CHEMICALS

Substance	Poisoning, Accidental (unintentional)	Poisoning, Intentional Self-harm	Poisoning, Assault	Poisoning, Undetermined	Adverse effect	Underdosing
Cisapride	T47.8X1	T47.8X2	T47.8X3	T47.8X4	T47.8X5	T47.8X6
Cisplatin	T45.1X1	T45.1X2	T45.1X3	T45.1X4	T45.1X5	T45.1X6
Citalopram	T43.221	T43.222	T43.223	T43.224	T43.225	T43.226
Citanest	T41.3X1	T41.3X2	T41.3X3	T41.3X4	T41.3X5	T41.3X6
infiltration (subcutaneous)	T41.3X1	T41.3X2	T41.3X3	T41.3X4	T41.3X5	T41.3X6
nerve block (peripheral) (plexus)	T41.3X1	T41.3X2	T41.3X3	T41.3X4	T41.3X5	T41.3X6
Citric acid	T47.5X1	T47.5X2	T47.5X3	T47.5X4	T47.5X5	T47.5X6
Citrovorum (factor)	T45.8X1	T45.8X2	T45.8X3	T45.8X4	T45.8X5	T45.8X6
Claviceps purpurea	T62.2X1	T62.2X2	T62.2X3	T62.2X4	--	--
Clavulanic acid	T36.1X1	T36.1X2	T36.1X3	T36.1X4	T36.1X5	T36.1X6
Cleaner, cleansing agent, type not specified	T65.891	T65.892	T65.893	T65.894	--	--
of paint or varnish	T52.91	T52.92	T52.93	T52.94	--	--
specified type NEC	T65.891	T65.892	T65.893	T65.894	--	--
Clebopride	T47.8X1	T47.8X2	T47.8X3	T47.8X4	T47.8X5	T47.8X6
Clefamide	T37.3X1	T37.3X2	T37.3X3	T37.3X4	T37.3X5	T37.3X6
Clemastine	T45.0X1	T45.0X2	T45.0X3	T45.0X4	T45.0X5	T45.0X6
Clematis vitalba	T62.2X1	T62.2X2	T62.2X3	T62.2X4	--	--
Clemizole	T45.0X1	T45.0X2	T45.0X3	T45.0X4	T45.0X5	T45.0X6
penicillin	T36.0X1	T36.0X2	T36.0X3	T36.0X4	T36.0X5	T36.0X6
Clenbuterol	T48.6X1	T48.6X2	T48.6X3	T48.6X4	T48.6X5	T48.6X6
Clidinium bromide	T44.3X1	T44.3X2	T44.3X3	T44.3X4	T44.3X5	T44.3X6
Clindamycin	T36.8X1	T36.8X2	T36.8X3	T36.8X4	T36.8X5	T36.8X6
Clinofibrate	T46.6X1	T46.6X2	T46.6X3	T46.6X4	T46.6X5	T46.6X6
Clioquinol	T37.8X1	T37.8X2	T37.8X3	T37.8X4	T37.8X5	T37.8X6
Cliradon	T40.2X1	T40.2X2	T40.2X3	T40.2X4	--	--
Clobazam	T42.4X1	T42.4X2	T42.4X3	T42.4X4	T42.4X5	T42.4X6
Clobenzorex	T50.5X1	T50.5X2	T50.5X3	T50.5X4	T50.5X5	T50.5X6
Clobetasol	T49.0X1	T49.0X2	T49.0X3	T49.0X4	T49.0X5	T49.0X6
Clobetasone	T49.0X1	T49.0X2	T49.0X3	T49.0X4	T49.0X5	T49.0X6
Clobutinol	T48.3X1	T48.3X2	T48.3X3	T48.3X4	T48.3X5	T48.3X6
Clocortolone	T38.0X1	T38.0X2	T38.0X3	T38.0X4	T38.0X5	T38.0X6
Clodantoin	T49.0X1	T49.0X2	T49.0X3	T49.0X4	T49.0X5	T49.0X6
Clodronic acid	T50.991	T50.992	T50.993	T50.994	T50.995	T50.996
Clofazimine	T37.1X1	T37.1X2	T37.1X3	T37.1X4	T37.1X5	T37.1X6
Clofedanol	T48.3X1	T48.3X2	T48.3X3	T48.3X4	T48.3X5	T48.3X6
Clofenamide	T50.2X1	T50.2X2	T50.2X3	T50.2X4	T50.2X5	T50.2X6
Clofenotane	T49.0X1	T49.0X2	T49.0X3	T49.0X4	T49.0X5	T49.0X6
Clofezone	T39.2X1	T39.2X2	T39.2X3	T39.2X4	T39.2X5	T39.2X6
Clofibrate	T46.6X1	T46.6X2	T46.6X3	T46.6X4	T46.6X5	T46.6X6
Clofibride	T46.6X1	T46.6X2	T46.6X3	T46.6X4	T46.6X5	T46.6X6
Cloforex	T50.5X1	T50.5X2	T50.5X3	T50.5X4	T50.5X5	T50.5X6
Clomethiazole	T42.6X1	T42.6X2	T42.6X3	T42.6X4	T42.6X5	T42.6X6
Clometocillin	T36.0X1	T36.0X2	T36.0X3	T36.0X4	T36.0X5	T36.0X6
Clomifene	T38.5X1	T38.5X2	T38.5X3	T38.5X4	T38.5X5	T38.5X6
Clomiphene	T38.5X1	T38.5X2	T38.5X3	T38.5X4	T38.5X5	T38.5X6
Clomipramine	T43.011	T43.012	T43.013	T43.014	T43.015	T43.016
Clomocycline	T36.4X1	T36.4X2	T36.4X3	T36.4X4	T36.4X5	T36.4X6
Clonazepam	T42.4X1	T42.4X2	T42.4X3	T42.4X4	T42.4X5	T42.4X6
Clonidine	T46.5X1	T46.5X2	T46.5X3	T46.5X4	T46.5X5	T46.5X6
Clonixin	T39.8X1	T39.8X2	T39.8X3	T39.8X4	T39.8X5	T39.8X6
Clopamide	T50.2X1	T50.2X2	T50.2X3	T50.2X4	T50.2X5	T50.2X6
Clopenthixol	T43.4X1	T43.4X2	T43.4X3	T43.4X4	T43.4X5	T43.4X6
Cloperastine	T48.3X1	T48.3X2	T48.3X3	T48.3X4	T48.3X5	T48.3X6
Clophedianol	T48.3X1	T48.3X2	T48.3X3	T48.3X4	T48.3X5	T48.3X6
Cloponone	T36.2X1	T36.2X2	T36.2X3	T36.2X4	T36.2X5	T36.2X6
Cloprednol	T38.0X1	T38.0X2	T38.0X3	T38.0X4	T38.0X5	T38.0X6
Cloral betaine	T42.6X1	T42.6X2	T42.6X3	T42.6X4	T42.6X5	T42.6X6
Cloramfenicol	T36.2X1	T36.2X2	T36.2X3	T36.2X4	T36.2X5	T36.2X6
Clorazepate (dipotassium)	T42.4X1	T42.4X2	T42.4X3	T42.4X4	T42.4X5	T42.4X6
Clorexolone	T50.2X1	T50.2X2	T50.2X3	T50.2X4	T50.2X5	T50.2X6
Clorfenamine	T45.0X1	T45.0X2	T45.0X3	T45.0X4	T45.0X5	T45.0X6
Clorgiline	T43.1X1	T43.1X2	T43.1X3	T43.1X4	T43.1X5	T43.1X6
Clorotepine	T44.3X1	T44.3X2	T44.3X3	T44.3X4	T44.3X5	T44.3X6
Clorox (bleach)	T54.91	T54.92	T54.93	T54.94	--	--

Substance	Poisoning, Accidental (unintentional)	Poisoning, Intentional Self-harm	Poisoning, Assault	Poisoning, Undetermined	Adverse effect	Underdosing
Clorprenaline	T48.6X1	T48.6X2	T48.6X3	T48.6X4	T48.6X5	T48.6X6
Clortermine	T50.5X1	T50.5X2	T50.5X3	T50.5X4	T50.5X5	T50.5X6
Clotiapine	T43.591	T43.592	T43.593	T43.594	T43.595	T43.596
Clotiazepam	T42.4X1	T42.4X2	T42.4X3	T42.4X4	T42.4X5	T42.4X6
Clotibric acid	T46.6X1	T46.6X2	T46.6X3	T46.6X4	T46.6X5	T46.6X6
Clotrimazole	T49.0X1	T49.0X2	T49.0X3	T49.0X4	T49.0X5	T49.0X6
Cloxacillin	T36.0X1	T36.0X2	T36.0X3	T36.0X4	T36.0X5	T36.0X6
Cloxazolam	T42.4X1	T42.4X2	T42.4X3	T42.4X4	T42.4X5	T42.4X6
Cloxiquine	T49.0X1	T49.0X2	T49.0X3	T49.0X4	T49.0X5	T49.0X6
Clozapine	T42.4X1	T42.4X2	T42.4X3	T42.4X4	T42.4X5	T42.4X6
Coagulant NEC	T45.7X1	T45.7X2	T45.7X3	T45.7X4	T45.7X5	T45.7X6
Coal (carbon monoxide from) —see also Carbon, monoxide, coal	T58.2X1	T58.2X2	T58.2X3	T58.2X4	--	--
oil—see Kerosene						
tar	T49.1X1	T49.1X2	T49.1X3	T49.1X4	T49.1X5	T49.1X6
fumes	T59.891	T59.892	T59.893	T59.894	--	--
medicinal (ointment)	T49.4X1	T49.4X2	T49.4X3	T49.4X4	T49.4X5	T49.4X6
analgesics NEC	T39.2X1	T39.2X2	T39.2X3	T39.2X4	T39.2X5	T39.2X6
naphtha (solvent)	T52.0X1	T52.0X2	T52.0X3	T52.0X4	--	--
Cobalamine	T45.2X1	T45.2X2	T45.2X3	T45.2X4	T45.2X5	T45.2X6
Cobalt (nonmedicinal) (fumes) (industrial)	T56.891	T56.892	T56.893	T56.894	--	--
medicinal (trace) (chloride)	T45.8X1	T45.8X2	T45.8X3	T45.8X4	T45.8X5	T45.8X6
Cobra (venom)	T63.041	T63.042	T63.043	T63.044	--	--
Coca (leaf)	T40.5X1	T40.5X2	T40.5X3	T40.5X4	T40.5X5	T40.5X6
Cocaine	T40.5X1	T40.5X2	T40.5X3	T40.5X4	T40.5X5	T40.5X6
topical anesthetic	T41.3X1	T41.3X2	T41.3X3	T41.3X4	T41.3X5	T41.3X6
Cocarboxylase	T45.3X1	T45.3X2	T45.3X3	T45.3X4	T45.3X5	T45.3X6
Coccidioidin	T50.8X1	T50.8X2	T50.8X3	T50.8X4	T50.8X5	T50.8X6
Cocculus indicus	T62.1X1	T62.1X2	T62.1X3	T62.1X4	--	--
Cochineal	T65.6X1	T65.6X2	T65.6X3	T65.6X4	--	--
medicinal products	T50.991	T50.992	T50.993	T50.994	T50.995	T50.996
Codeine	T40.2X1	T40.2X2	T40.2X3	T40.2X4	T40.2X5	T40.2X6
Cod-liver oil	T45.2X1	T45.2X2	T45.2X3	T45.2X4	T45.2X5	T45.2X6
Coenzyme A	T50.991	T50.992	T50.993	T50.994	T50.995	T50.996
Coffee	T62.8X1	T62.8X2	T62.8X3	T62.8X4	--	--
Cogalactoiso-merase	T50.991	T50.992	T50.993	T50.994	T50.995	T50.996
Cogentin	T44.3X1	T44.3X2	T44.3X3	T44.3X4	T44.3X5	T44.3X6
Coke fumes or gas (carbon monoxide)	T58.2X1	T58.2X2	T58.2X3	T58.2X4	--	--
industrial use	T58.8X1	T58.8X2	T58.8X3	T58.8X4	--	--
Colace	T47.4X1	T47.4X2	T47.4X3	T47.4X4	T47.4X5	T47.4X6
Colaspase	T45.1X1	T45.1X2	T45.1X3	T45.1X4	T45.1X5	T45.1X6
Colchicine	T50.4X1	T50.4X2	T50.4X3	T50.4X4	T50.4X5	T50.4X6
Colchicum	T62.2X1	T62.2X2	T62.2X3	T62.2X4	--	--
Cold cream	T49.3X1	T49.3X2	T49.3X3	T49.3X4	T49.3X5	T49.3X6
Colecalciferol	T45.2X1	T45.2X2	T45.2X3	T45.2X4	T45.2X5	T45.2X6
Colestipol	T46.6X1	T46.6X2	T46.6X3	T46.6X4	T46.6X5	T46.6X6
Colestyramine	T46.6X1	T46.6X2	T46.6X3	T46.6X4	T46.6X5	T46.6X6
Colimycin	T36.8X1	T36.8X2	T36.8X3	T36.8X4	T36.8X5	T36.8X6
Colistimethate	T36.8X1	T36.8X2	T36.8X3	T36.8X4	T36.8X5	T36.8X6
Colistin	T36.8X1	T36.8X2	T36.8X3	T36.8X4	T36.8X5	T36.8X6
sulfate (eye preparation)	T49.5X1	T49.5X2	T49.5X3	T49.5X4	T49.5X5	T49.5X6
Collagen	T50.991	T50.992	T50.993	T50.994	T50.995	T50.996
Collagenase	T49.4X1	T49.4X2	T49.4X3	T49.4X4	T49.4X5	T49.4X6
Collodion	T49.3X1	T49.3X2	T49.3X3	T49.3X4	T49.3X5	T49.3X6
Colocynth	T47.2X1	T47.2X2	T47.2X3	T47.2X4	T47.2X5	T47.2X6
Colophony adhesive	T49.3X1	T49.3X2	T49.3X3	T49.3X4	T49.3X5	T49.3X6
Colorant—see also Dye	T50.991	T50.992	T50.993	T50.994	T50.995	T50.996
Coloring matter—see Dye (s)						
Combustion gas (after combustion) —see Carbon, monoxide						
prior to combustion	T59.891	T59.892	T59.893	T59.894	--	--
Compazine	T43.3X1	T43.3X2	T43.3X3	T43.3X4	T43.3X5	T43.3X6
Compound						
42 (warfarin)	T60.4X1	T60.4X2	T60.4X3	T60.4X4	--	--
269 (endrin)	T60.1X1	T60.1X2	T60.1X3	T60.1X4	--	--

TABLE OF DRUGS AND CHEMICALS

Substance	Poisoning, Accidental (unintentional)	Poisoning, Intentional Self-harm	Poisoning, Assault	Poisoning, Undetermined	Adverse effect	Underdosing
497 (dieldrin)	T60.1X1	T60.1X2	T60.1X3	T60.1X4	--	--
1080 (sodium fluoroacetate)	T60.4X1	T60.4X2	T60.4X3	T60.4X4	--	--
3422 (parathion)	T60.0X1	T60.0X2	T60.0X3	T60.0X4	--	--
3911 (phorate)	T60.0X1	T60.0X2	T60.0X3	T60.0X4	--	--
3956 (toxaphene)	T60.1X1	T60.1X2	T60.1X3	T60.1X4	--	--
4049 (malathion)	T60.0X1	T60.0X2	T60.0X3	T60.0X4	--	--
4069 (malathion)	T60.0X1	T60.0X2	T60.0X3	T60.0X4	--	--
4124 (dicapthon)	T60.0X1	T60.0X2	T60.0X3	T60.0X4	--	--
E (cortisone)	T38.0X1	T38.0X2	T38.0X3	T38.0X4	T38.0X5	T38.0X6
F (hydrocortisone)	T38.0X1	T38.0X2	T38.0X3	T38.0X4	T38.0X5	T38.0X6
Congener, anabolic	T38.7X1	T38.7X2	T38.7X3	T38.7X4	T38.7X5	T38.7X6
Congo red	T50.8X1	T50.8X2	T50.8X3	T50.8X4	T50.8X5	T50.8X6
Coniine, conine	T62.2X1	T62.2X2	T62.2X3	T62.2X4	--	--
Conium (maculatum)	T62.2X1	T62.2X2	T62.2X3	T62.2X4	--	--
Conjugated estrogenic substances	T38.5X1	T38.5X2	T38.5X3	T38.5X4	T38.5X5	T38.5X6
Contac	T48.5X1	T48.5X2	T48.5X3	T48.5X4	T48.5X5	T48.5X6
Contact lens solution	T49.5X1	T49.5X2	T49.5X3	T49.5X4	T49.5X5	T49.5X6
Contraceptive (oral)	T38.4X1	T38.4X2	T38.4X3	T38.4X4	T38.4X5	T38.4X6
vaginal	T49.8X1	T49.8X2	T49.8X3	T49.8X4	T49.8X5	T49.8X6
Contrast medium, radiography	T50.8X1	T50.8X2	T50.8X3	T50.8X4	T50.8X5	T50.8X6
Convallaria glycosides	T46.0X1	T46.0X2	T46.0X3	T46.0X4	T46.0X5	T46.0X6
Convallaria majalis	T62.2X1	T62.2X2	T62.2X3	T62.2X4	--	--
berry	T62.1X1	T62.1X2	T62.1X3	T62.1X4	--	--
Copper (dust) (fumes) (nonmedicinal) NEC	T56.4X1	T56.4X2	T56.4X3	T56.4X4	--	--
arsenate, arsenite	T57.0X1	T57.0X2	T57.0X3	T57.0X4	--	--
insecticide	T60.2X1	T60.2X2	T60.2X3	T60.2X4	--	--
emetic	T47.7X1	T47.7X2	T47.7X3	T47.7X4	T47.7X5	T47.7X6
fungicide	T60.3X1	T60.3X2	T60.3X3	T60.3X4	--	--
gluconate	T49.0X1	T49.0X2	T49.0X3	T49.0X4	T49.0X5	T49.0X6
insecticide	T60.2X1	T60.2X2	T60.2X3	T60.2X4	--	--
medicinal (trace)	T45.8X1	T45.8X2	T45.8X3	T45.8X4	T45.8X5	T45.8X6
oleate	T49.0X1	T49.0X2	T49.0X3	T49.0X4	T49.0X5	T49.0X6
sulfate	T56.4X1	T56.4X2	T56.4X3	T56.4X4	--	--
cupric	T56.4X1	T56.4X2	T56.4X3	T56.4X4	--	--
fungicide	T60.3X1	T60.3X2	T60.3X3	T60.3X4	--	--
medicinal						
ear	T49.6X1	T49.6X2	T49.6X3	T49.6X4	T49.6X5	T49.6X6
emetic	T47.7X1	T47.7X2	T47.7X3	T47.7X4	T47.7X5	T47.7X6
eye	T49.5X1	T49.5X2	T49.5X3	T49.5X4	T49.5X5	T49.5X6
cuprous	T56.4X1	T56.4X2	T56.4X3	T56.4X4	--	--
fungicide	T60.3X1	T60.3X2	T60.3X3	T60.3X4	--	--
medicinal						
ear	T49.6X1	T49.6X2	T49.6X3	T49.6X4	T49.6X5	T49.6X6
emetic	T47.7X1	T47.7X2	T47.7X3	T47.7X4	T47.7X5	T47.7X6
eye	T49.5X1	T49.5X2	T49.5X3	T49.5X4	T49.5X5	T49.5X6
Copperhead snake (bite) (venom)	T63.061	T63.062	T63.063	T63.064	--	--
Coral (sting)	T63.691	T63.692	T63.693	T63.694	--	--
snake (bite) (venom)	T63.021	T63.022	T63.023	T63.024	--	--
Corbadrine	T49.6X1	T49.6X2	T49.6X3	T49.6X4	T49.6X5	T49.6X6
Cordite	T65.891	T65.892	T65.893	T65.894	--	--
vapor	T59.891	T59.892	T59.893	T59.894	--	--
Cordran	T49.0X1	T49.0X2	T49.0X3	T49.0X4	T49.0X5	T49.0X6
Corn cures	T49.4X1	T49.4X2	T49.4X3	T49.4X4	T49.4X5	T49.4X6
Corn starch	T49.3X1	T49.3X2	T49.3X3	T49.3X4	T49.3X5	T49.3X6
Cornhusker's lotion	T49.3X1	T49.3X2	T49.3X3	T49.3X4	T49.3X5	T49.3X6
Coronary vasodilator NEC	T46.3X1	T46.3X2	T46.3X3	T46.3X4	T46.3X5	T46.3X6
Corrosive NEC	T54.91	T54.92	T54.93	T54.94	--	--
acid NEC	T54.2X1	T54.2X2	T54.2X3	T54.2X4	--	--
aromatics	T54.1X1	T54.1X2	T54.1X3	T54.1X4	--	--
disinfectant	T54.1X1	T54.1X2	T54.1X3	T54.1X4	--	--
fumes NEC	T54.91	T54.92	T54.93	T54.94	--	--
specified NEC	T54.91	T54.92	T54.93	T54.94	--	--
sublimate	T56.1X1	T56.1X2	T56.1X3	T56.1X4	--	--
Cortate	T38.0X1	T38.0X2	T38.0X3	T38.0X4	T38.0X5	T38.0X6

Substance	Poisoning, Accidental (unintentional)	Poisoning, Intentional Self-harm	Poisoning, Assault	Poisoning, Undetermined	Adverse effect	Underdosing
Cort-Dome	T38.0X1	T38.0X2	T38.0X3	T38.0X4	T38.0X5	T38.0X6
ENT agent	T49.6X1	T49.6X2	T49.6X3	T49.6X4	T49.6X5	T49.6X6
ophthalmic preparation	T49.5X1	T49.5X2	T49.5X3	T49.5X4	T49.5X5	T49.5X6
topical NEC	T49.0X1	T49.0X2	T49.0X3	T49.0X4	T49.0X5	T49.0X6
Cortef	T38.0X1	T38.0X2	T38.0X3	T38.0X4	T38.0X5	T38.0X6
ENT agent	T49.6X1	T49.6X2	T49.6X3	T49.6X4	T49.6X5	T49.6X6
ophthalmic preparation	T49.5X1	T49.5X2	T49.5X3	T49.5X4	T49.5X5	T49.5X6
topical NEC	T49.0X1	T49.0X2	T49.0X3	T49.0X4	T49.0X5	T49.0X6
Corticosteroid	T38.0X1	T38.0X2	T38.0X3	T38.0X4	T38.0X5	T38.0X6
ENT agent	T49.6X1	T49.6X2	T49.6X3	T49.6X4	T49.6X5	T49.6X6
mineral	T50.0X1	T50.0X2	T50.0X3	T50.0X4	T50.0X5	T50.0X6
ophthalmic	T49.5X1	T49.5X2	T49.5X3	T49.5X4	T49.5X5	T49.5X6
topical NEC	T49.0X1	T49.0X2	T49.0X3	T49.0X4	T49.0X5	T49.0X6
Corticotropin	T38.811	T38.812	T38.813	T38.814	T38.815	T38.816
Cortisol	T49.0X1	T49.0X2	T49.0X3	T49.0X4	T49.0X5	T49.0X6
ENT agent	T49.6X1	T49.6X2	T49.6X3	T49.6X4	T49.6X5	T49.6X6
ophthalmic preparation	T49.5X1	T49.5X2	T49.5X3	T49.5X4	T49.5X5	T49.5X6
topical NEC	T49.0X1	T49.0X2	T49.0X3	T49.0X4	T49.0X5	T49.0X6
Cortisone (acetate)	T38.0X1	T38.0X2	T38.0X3	T38.0X4	T38.0X5	T38.0X6
ENT agent	T49.6X1	T49.6X2	T49.6X3	T49.6X4	T49.6X5	T49.6X6
ophthalmic preparation	T49.5X1	T49.5X2	T49.5X3	T49.5X4	T49.5X5	T49.5X6
topical NEC	T49.0X1	T49.0X2	T49.0X3	T49.0X4	T49.0X5	T49.0X6
Cortivazol	T38.0X1	T38.0X2	T38.0X3	T38.0X4	T38.0X5	T38.0X6
Cortogen	T38.0X1	T38.0X2	T38.0X3	T38.0X4	T38.0X5	T38.0X6
ENT agent	T49.6X1	T49.6X2	T49.6X3	T49.6X4	T49.6X5	T49.6X6
ophthalmic preparation	T49.5X1	T49.5X2	T49.5X3	T49.5X4	T49.5X5	T49.5X6
Cortone	T38.0X1	T38.0X2	T38.0X3	T38.0X4	T38.0X5	T38.0X6
ENT agent	T49.6X1	T49.6X2	T49.6X3	T49.6X4	T49.6X5	T49.6X6
ophthalmic preparation	T49.5X1	T49.5X2	T49.5X3	T49.5X4	T49.5X5	T49.5X6
Cortril	T38.0X1	T38.0X2	T38.0X3	T38.0X4	T38.0X5	T38.0X6
ENT agent	T49.6X1	T49.6X2	T49.6X3	T49.6X4	T49.6X5	T49.6X6
ophthalmic preparation	T49.5X1	T49.5X2	T49.5X3	T49.5X4	T49.5X5	T49.5X6
topical NEC	T49.0X1	T49.0X2	T49.0X3	T49.0X4	T49.0X5	T49.0X6
Corynebacterium parvum	T45.1X1	T45.1X2	T45.1X3	T45.1X4	T45.1X5	T45.1X6
Cosmetic preparation	T49.8X1	T49.8X2	T49.8X3	T49.8X4	T49.8X5	T49.8X6
Cosmetics	T49.8X1	T49.8X2	T49.8X3	T49.8X4	T49.8X5	T49.8X6
Cosyntropin	T38.811	T38.812	T38.813	T38.814	T38.815	T38.816
Cotarnine	T45.7X1	T45.7X2	T45.7X3	T45.7X4	T45.7X5	T45.7X6
Co-trimoxazole	T36.8X1	T36.8X2	T36.8X3	T36.8X4	T36.8X5	T36.8X6
Cottonseed oil	T49.3X1	T49.3X2	T49.3X3	T49.3X4	T49.3X5	T49.3X6
Cough mixture (syrup)	T48.4X1	T48.4X2	T48.4X3	T48.4X4	T48.4X5	T48.4X6
containing opiates	T40.2X1	T40.2X2	T40.2X3	T40.2X4	T40.2X5	T40.2X6
expectorants	T48.4X1	T48.4X2	T48.4X3	T48.4X4	T48.4X5	T48.4X6
Coumadin	T45.511	T45.512	T45.513	T45.514	T45.515	T45.516
rodenticide	T60.4X1	T60.4X2	T60.4X3	T60.4X4	--	--
Coumaphos	T60.0X1	T60.0X2	T60.0X3	T60.0X4	--	--
Coumarin	T45.511	T45.512	T45.513	T45.514	T45.515	T45.516
Coumetarol	T45.511	T45.512	T45.513	T45.514	T45.515	T45.516
Cowbane	T62.2X1	T62.2X2	T62.2X3	T62.2X4	--	--
Cozyme	T45.2X1	T45.2X2	T45.2X3	T45.2X4	T45.2X5	T45.2X6
Crack	T40.5X1	T40.5X2	T40.5X3	T40.5X4	--	--
Crataegus extract	T46.0X1	T46.0X2	T46.0X3	T46.0X4	T46.0X5	T46.0X6
Creolin	T54.1X1	T54.1X2	T54.1X3	T54.1X4	--	--
disinfectant	T54.1X1	T54.1X2	T54.1X3	T54.1X4	--	--
Creosol (compound)	T49.0X1	T49.0X2	T49.0X3	T49.0X4	T49.0X5	T49.0X6
Creosote (coal tar) (beechwood)	T49.0X1	T49.0X2	T49.0X3	T49.0X4	T49.0X5	T49.0X6
medicinal (expectorant)	T48.4X1	T48.4X2	T48.4X3	T48.4X4	T48.4X5	T48.4X6
syrup	T48.4X1	T48.4X2	T48.4X3	T48.4X4	T48.4X5	T48.4X6
Cresol (s)	T49.0X1	T49.0X2	T49.0X3	T49.0X4	T49.0X5	T49.0X6
and soap solution	T49.0X1	T49.0X2	T49.0X3	T49.0X4	T49.0X5	T49.0X6
Cresyl acetate	T49.0X1	T49.0X2	T49.0X3	T49.0X4	T49.0X5	T49.0X6
Cresylic acid	T49.0X1	T49.0X2	T49.0X3	T49.0X4	T49.0X5	T49.0X6
Crimidine	T60.4X1	T60.4X2	T60.4X3	T60.4X4	--	--
Croconazole	T37.8X1	T37.8X2	T37.8X3	T37.8X4	T37.8X5	T37.8X6
Cromoglicic acid	T48.6X1	T48.6X2	T48.6X3	T48.6X4	T48.6X5	T48.6X6

Substance	Poisoning, Accidental (unintentional)	Poisoning, Intentional Self-harm	Poisoning, Assault	Poisoning, Undetermined	Adverse effect	Underdosing
Cromolyn	T48.6X1	T48.6X2	T48.6X3	T48.6X4	T48.6X5	T48.6X6
Cromonar	T46.3X1	T46.3X2	T46.3X3	T46.3X4	T46.3X5	T46.3X6
Cropropamide	T39.8X1	T39.8X2	T39.8X3	T39.8X4	T39.8X5	T39.8X6
with crotethamide	T50.7X1	T50.7X2	T50.7X3	T50.7X4	T50.7X5	T50.7X6
Crotamiton	T49.0X1	T49.0X2	T49.0X3	T49.0X4	T49.0X5	T49.0X6
Crotethamide	T39.8X1	T39.8X2	T39.8X3	T39.8X4	T39.8X5	T39.8X6
with cropropamide	T50.7X1	T50.7X2	T50.7X3	T50.7X4	T50.7X5	T50.7X6
Croton (oil)	T47.2X1	T47.2X2	T47.2X3	T47.2X4	T47.2X5	T47.2X6
chloral	T42.6X1	T42.6X2	T42.6X3	T42.6X4	T42.6X5	T42.6X6
Crude oil	T52.0X1	T52.0X2	T52.0X3	T52.0X4	--	--
Cryogenine	T39.8X1	T39.8X2	T39.8X3	T39.8X4	T39.8X5	T39.8X6
Cryolite (vapor)	T60.1X1	T60.1X2	T60.1X3	T60.1X4	--	--
insecticide	T60.1X1	T60.1X2	T60.1X3	T60.1X4	--	--
Cryptenamine (tannates)	T46.5X1	T46.5X2	T46.5X3	T46.5X4	T46.5X5	T46.5X6
Crystal violet	T49.0X1	T49.0X2	T49.0X3	T49.0X4	T49.0X5	T49.0X6
Cuckoopint	T62.2X1	T62.2X2	T62.2X3	T62.2X4	--	--
Cumetharol	T45.511	T45.512	T45.513	T45.514	T45.515	T45.516
Cupric						
acetate	T60.3X1	T60.3X2	T60.3X3	T60.3X4	--	--
acetoarsenite	T57.0X1	T57.0X2	T57.0X3	T57.0X4	--	--
arsenate	T57.0X1	T57.0X2	T57.0X3	T57.0X4	--	--
gluconate	T49.0X1	T49.0X2	T49.0X3	T49.0X4	T49.0X5	T49.0X6
oleate	T49.0X1	T49.0X2	T49.0X3	T49.0X4	T49.0X5	T49.0X6
sulfate	T56.4X1	T56.4X2	T56.4X3	T56.4X4	--	--
Cuprous sulfate—see also Copper sulfate	T56.4X1	T56.4X2	T56.4X3	T56.4X4	--	--
Curare, curarine	T48.1X1	T48.1X2	T48.1X3	T48.1X4	T48.1X5	T48.1X6
Cyamemazine	T43.3X1	T43.3X2	T43.3X3	T43.3X4	T43.3X5	T43.3X6
Cyamopsis tetragono-loba	T46.6X1	T46.6X2	T46.6X3	T46.6X4	T46.6X5	T46.6X6
Cyanacetyl hydrazide	T37.1X1	T37.1X2	T37.1X3	T37.1X4	T37.1X5	T37.1X6
Cyanic acid (gas)	T59.891	T59.892	T59.893	T59.894	--	--
Cyanide (s) (compounds) (potassium) (sodium) NEC	T65.0X1	T65.0X2	T65.0X3	T65.0X4	--	--
dust or gas (inhalation) NEC	T57.3X1	T57.3X2	T57.3X3	T57.3X4	--	--
fumigant	T65.0X1	T65.0X2	T65.0X3	T65.0X4	--	--
hydrogen	T57.3X1	T57.3X2	T57.3X3	T57.3X4	--	--
mercuric—see Mercury						
pesticide (dust) (fumes)	T65.0X1	T65.0X2	T65.0X3	T65.0X4	--	--
Cyanoacrylate adhesive	T49.3X1	T49.3X2	T49.3X3	T49.3X4	T49.3X5	T49.3X6
Cyanocobalamin	T45.8X1	T45.8X2	T45.8X3	T45.8X4	T45.8X5	T45.8X6
Cyanogen (chloride) (gas) NEC	T59.891	T59.892	T59.893	T59.894	--	--
Cyclacillin	T36.0X1	T36.0X2	T36.0X3	T36.0X4	T36.0X5	T36.0X6
Cyclaine	T41.3X1	T41.3X2	T41.3X3	T41.3X4	T41.3X5	T41.3X6
Cyclamate	T50.991	T50.992	T50.993	T50.994	T50.995	T50.996
Cyclamen europaeum	T62.2X1	T62.2X2	T62.2X3	T62.2X4	--	--
Cyclandelate	T46.7X1	T46.7X2	T46.7X3	T46.7X4	T46.7X5	T46.7X6
Cyclazocine	T50.7X1	T50.7X2	T50.7X3	T50.7X4	T50.7X5	T50.7X6
Cyclizine	T45.0X1	T45.0X2	T45.0X3	T45.0X4	T45.0X5	T45.0X6
Cyclobarbital	T42.3X1	T42.3X2	T42.3X3	T42.3X4	T42.3X5	T42.3X6
Cyclobarbitone	T42.3X1	T42.3X2	T42.3X3	T42.3X4	T42.3X5	T42.3X6
Cyclobenzaprine	T48.1X1	T48.1X2	T48.1X3	T48.1X4	T48.1X5	T48.1X6
Cyclodrine	T44.3X1	T44.3X2	T44.3X3	T44.3X4	T44.3X5	T44.3X6
Cycloguanil embonate	T37.2X1	T37.2X2	T37.2X3	T37.2X4	T37.2X5	T37.2X6
Cyclohexane	T52.8X1	T52.8X2	T52.8X3	T52.8X4	--	--
Cyclohexanol	T51.8X1	T51.8X2	T51.8X3	T51.8X4	--	--
Cyclohexanone	T52.4X1	T52.4X2	T52.4X3	T52.4X4	--	--
Cycloheximide	T60.3X1	T60.3X2	T60.3X3	T60.3X4	--	--
Cyclohexyl acetate	T52.8X1	T52.8X2	T52.8X3	T52.8X4	--	--
Cycloleucin	T45.1X1	T45.1X2	T45.1X3	T45.1X4	T45.1X5	T45.1X6
Cyclomethycaine	T41.3X1	T41.3X2	T41.3X3	T41.3X4	T41.3X5	T41.3X6
Cyclopentamine	T44.4X1	T44.4X2	T44.4X3	T44.4X4	T44.4X5	T44.4X6
Cyclopenthiazide	T50.2X1	T50.2X2	T50.2X3	T50.2X4	T50.2X5	T50.2X6
Cyclopentolate	T44.3X1	T44.3X2	T44.3X3	T44.3X4	T44.3X5	T44.3X6
Cyclophosphamide	T45.1X1	T45.1X2	T45.1X3	T45.1X4	T45.1X5	T45.1X6
Cycloplegic drug	T49.5X1	T49.5X2	T49.5X3	T49.5X4	T49.5X5	T49.5X6

Substance	Poisoning, Accidental (unintentional)	Poisoning, Intentional Self-harm	Poisoning, Assault	Poisoning, Undetermined	Adverse effect	Underdosing
Cyclopropane	T41.291	T41.292	T41.293	T41.294	T41.295	T41.296
Cyclopyrabital	T39.8X1	T39.8X2	T39.8X3	T39.8X4	T39.8X5	T39.8X6
Cycloserine	T37.1X1	T37.1X2	T37.1X3	T37.1X4	T37.1X5	T37.1X6
Cyclosporin	T45.1X1	T45.1X2	T45.1X3	T45.1X4	T45.1X5	T45.1X6
Cyclothiazide	T50.2X1	T50.2X2	T50.2X3	T50.2X4	T50.2X5	T50.2X6
Cycrimine	T44.3X1	T44.3X2	T44.3X3	T44.3X4	T44.3X5	T44.3X6
Cyhalothrin	T60.1X1	T60.1X2	T60.1X3	T60.1X4	--	--
Cymarin	T46.0X1	T46.0X2	T46.0X3	T46.0X4	T46.0X5	T46.0X6
Cypermethrin	T60.1X1	T60.1X2	T60.1X3	T60.1X4	--	--
Cyphenothrin	T60.2X1	T60.2X2	T60.2X3	T60.2X4	--	--
Cyproheptadine	T45.0X1	T45.0X2	T45.0X3	T45.0X4	T45.0X5	T45.0X6
Cyproterone	T38.6X1	T38.6X2	T38.6X3	T38.6X4	T38.6X5	T38.6X6
Cysteamine	T50.6X1	T50.6X2	T50.6X3	T50.6X4	T50.6X5	T50.6X6
Cytarabine	T45.1X1	T45.1X2	T45.1X3	T45.1X4	T45.1X5	T45.1X6
Cytisus						
laburnum	T62.2X1	T62.2X2	T62.2X3	T62.2X4	--	--
scoparius	T62.2X1	T62.2X2	T62.2X3	T62.2X4	--	--
Cytochrome C	T47.5X1	T47.5X2	T47.5X3	T47.5X4	T47.5X5	T47.5X6
Cytomel	T38.1X1	T38.1X2	T38.1X3	T38.1X4	T38.1X5	T38.1X6
Cytosine arabinoside	T45.1X1	T45.1X2	T45.1X3	T45.1X4	T45.1X5	T45.1X6
Cytoxan	T45.1X1	T45.1X2	T45.1X3	T45.1X4	T45.1X5	T45.1X6
Cytozyme	T45.7X1	T45.7X2	T45.7X3	T45.7X4	T45.7X5	T45.7X6
2,4-D	T60.3X1	T60.3X2	T60.3X3	T60.3X4	--	--
Dacarbazine	T45.1X1	T45.1X2	T45.1X3	T45.1X4	T45.1X5	T45.1X6
Dactinomycin	T45.1X1	T45.1X2	T45.1X3	T45.1X4	T45.1X5	T45.1X6
DADPS	T37.1X1	T37.1X2	T37.1X3	T37.1X4	T37.1X5	T37.1X6
Dakin's solution	T49.0X1	T49.0X2	T49.0X3	T49.0X4	T49.0X5	T49.0X6
Dalapon (sodium)	T60.3X1	T60.3X2	T60.3X3	T60.3X4	--	--
Dalmane	T42.4X1	T42.4X2	T42.4X3	T42.4X4	T42.4X5	T42.4X6
Danazol	T38.6X1	T38.6X2	T38.6X3	T38.6X4	T38.6X5	T38.6X6
Danilone	T45.511	T45.512	T45.513	T45.514	T45.515	T45.516
Danthron	T47.2X1	T47.2X2	T47.2X3	T47.2X4	T47.2X5	T47.2X6
Dantrolene	T42.8X1	T42.8X2	T42.8X3	T42.8X4	T42.8X5	T42.8X6
Dantron	T47.2X1	T47.2X2	T47.2X3	T47.2X4	T47.2X5	T47.2X6
Daphne (gnidium) (mezereum)	T62.2X1	T62.2X2	T62.2X3	T62.2X4	--	--
berry	T62.1X1	T62.1X2	T62.1X3	T62.1X4	--	--
Dapsone	T37.1X1	T37.1X2	T37.1X3	T37.1X4	T37.1X5	T37.1X6
Daraprim	T37.2X1	T37.2X2	T37.2X3	T37.2X4	T37.2X5	T37.2X6
Darnel	T62.2X1	T62.2X2	T62.2X3	T62.2X4	--	--
Darvon	T39.8X1	T39.8X2	T39.8X3	T39.8X4	T39.8X5	T39.8X6
Daunomycin	T45.1X1	T45.1X2	T45.1X3	T45.1X4	T45.1X5	T45.1X6
Daunorubicin	T45.1X1	T45.1X2	T45.1X3	T45.1X4	T45.1X5	T45.1X6
DBI	T38.3X1	T38.3X2	T38.3X3	T38.3X4	T38.3X5	T38.3X6
D-Con	T60.91	T60.92	T60.93	T60.94	--	--
insecticide	T60.2X1	T60.2X2	T60.2X3	T60.2X4	--	--
rodenticide	T60.4X1	T60.4X2	T60.4X3	T60.4X4	--	--
DDAVP	T38.891	T38.892	T38.893	T38.894	T38.895	T38.896
DDE (bis (chlorophenyl) -dichloroethylene)	T60.2X1	T60.2X2	T60.2X3	T60.2X4	--	--
DDS	T37.1X1	T37.1X2	T37.1X3	T37.1X4	T37.1X5	T37.1X6
DDT (dust)	T60.1X1	T60.1X2	T60.1X3	T60.1X4	--	--
Deadly nightshade—see also Belladonna	T62.2X1	T62.2X2	T62.2X3	T62.2X4	--	--
berry	T62.1X1	T62.1X2	T62.1X3	T62.1X4	--	--
Deamino-D-arginine vasopressin	T38.891	T38.892	T38.893	T38.894	T38.895	T38.896
Deanol (aceglumate)	T50.991	T50.992	T50.993	T50.994	T50.995	T50.996
Debrisoquine	T46.5X1	T46.5X2	T46.5X3	T46.5X4	T46.5X5	T46.5X6
Decaborane	T57.8X1	T57.8X2	T57.8X3	T57.8X4	--	--
fumes	T59.891	T59.892	T59.893	T59.894	--	--
Decadron	T38.0X1	T38.0X2	T38.0X3	T38.0X4	T38.0X5	T38.0X6
ENT agent	T49.6X1	T49.6X2	T49.6X3	T49.6X4	T49.6X5	T49.6X6
ophthalmic preparation	T49.5X1	T49.5X2	T49.5X3	T49.5X4	T49.5X5	T49.5X6
topical NEC	T49.0X1	T49.0X2	T49.0X3	T49.0X4	T49.0X5	T49.0X6
Decahydronaphthalene	T52.8X1	T52.8X2	T52.8X3	T52.8X4	--	--
Decalin	T52.8X1	T52.8X2	T52.8X3	T52.8X4	--	--
Decamethonium (bromide)	T48.1X1	T48.1X2	T48.1X3	T48.1X4	T48.1X5	T48.1X6
Decholin	T47.5X1	T47.5X2	T47.5X3	T47.5X4	T47.5X5	T47.5X6

Substance	Poisoning, Accidental (unintentional)	Poisoning, Intentional Self-harm	Poisoning, Assault	Poisoning, Undetermined	Adverse effect	Underdosing
Declomycin	T36.4X1	T36.4X2	T36.4X3	T36.4X4	T36.4X5	T36.4X6
Decongestant, nasal (mucosa)	T48.5X1	T48.5X2	T48.5X3	T48.5X4	T48.5X5	T48.5X6
combination	T48.5X1	T48.5X2	T48.5X3	T48.5X4	T48.5X5	T48.5X6
Deet	T60.8X1	T60.8X2	T60.8X3	T60.8X4	--	--
Deferoxamine	T45.8X1	T45.8X2	T45.8X3	T45.8X4	T45.8X5	T45.8X6
Deflazacort	T38.0X1	T38.0X2	T38.0X3	T38.0X4	T38.0X5	T38.0X6
Deglycyrrhizinized extract of licorice	T48.4X1	T48.4X2	T48.4X3	T48.4X4	T48.4X5	T48.4X6
Dehydrocholic acid	T47.5X1	T47.5X2	T47.5X3	T47.5X4	T47.5X5	T47.5X6
Dehydroemetine	T37.3X1	T37.3X2	T37.3X3	T37.3X4	T37.3X5	T37.3X6
Dekalin	T52.8X1	T52.8X2	T52.8X3	T52.8X4	--	--
Delalutin	T38.5X1	T38.5X2	T38.5X3	T38.5X4	T38.5X5	T38.5X6
Delorazepam	T42.4X1	T42.4X2	T42.4X3	T42.4X4	T42.4X5	T42.4X6
Delphinium	T62.2X1	T62.2X2	T62.2X3	T62.2X4	--	--
Deltamethrin	T60.1X1	T60.1X2	T60.1X3	T60.1X4	--	--
Deltasone	T38.0X1	T38.0X2	T38.0X3	T38.0X4	T38.0X5	T38.0X6
Deltra	T38.0X1	T38.0X2	T38.0X3	T38.0X4	T38.0X5	T38.0X6
Delvinal	T42.3X1	T42.3X2	T42.3X3	T42.3X4	T42.3X5	T42.3X6
Demecarium (bromide)	T49.5X1	T49.5X2	T49.5X3	T49.5X4	T49.5X5	T49.5X6
Demeclocycline	T36.4X1	T36.4X2	T36.4X3	T36.4X4	T36.4X5	T36.4X6
Demecolcine	T45.1X1	T45.1X2	T45.1X3	T45.1X4	T45.1X5	T45.1X6
Demegestone	T38.5X1	T38.5X2	T38.5X3	T38.5X4	T38.5X5	T38.5X6
Demelanizing agents	T49.8X1	T49.8X2	T49.8X3	T49.8X4	T49.8X5	T49.8X6
Demephion -O and -S	T60.0X1	T60.0X2	T60.0X3	T60.0X4	--	--
Demerol	T40.2X1	T40.2X2	T40.2X3	T40.2X4	T40.2X5	T40.2X6
Demethylchlortetracycline	T36.4X1	T36.4X2	T36.4X3	T36.4X4	T36.4X5	T36.4X6
Demethyltetracycline	T36.4X1	T36.4X2	T36.4X3	T36.4X4	T36.4X5	T36.4X6
Demeton -O and -S	T60.0X1	T60.0X2	T60.0X3	T60.0X4	--	--
Demulcent (external)	T49.3X1	T49.3X2	T49.3X3	T49.3X4	T49.3X5	T49.3X6
specified NEC	T49.3X1	T49.3X2	T49.3X3	T49.3X4	T49.3X5	T49.3X6
Demulen	T38.4X1	T38.4X2	T38.4X3	T38.4X4	T38.4X5	T38.4X6
Denatured alcohol	T51.0X1	T51.0X2	T51.0X3	T51.0X4	--	--
Dendrid	T49.5X1	T49.5X2	T49.5X3	T49.5X4	T49.5X5	T49.5X6
Dental drug, topical application NEC	T49.7X1	T49.7X2	T49.7X3	T49.7X4	T49.7X5	T49.7X6
Dentifrice	T49.7X1	T49.7X2	T49.7X3	T49.7X4	T49.7X5	T49.7X6
Deodorant spray (feminine hygiene)	T49.8X1	T49.8X2	T49.8X3	T49.8X4	T49.8X5	T49.8X6
Deoxycortone	T50.0X1	T50.0X2	T50.0X3	T50.0X4	T50.0X5	T50.0X6
2-Deoxy-5-fluorouridine	T45.1X1	T45.1X2	T45.1X3	T45.1X4	T45.1X5	T45.1X6
5-Deoxy-5-fluorouridine	T45.1X1	T45.1X2	T45.1X3	T45.1X4	T45.1X5	T45.1X6
Deoxyribonuclease (pancreatic)	T45.3X1	T45.3X2	T45.3X3	T45.3X4	T45.3X5	T45.3X6
Depilatory	T49.4X1	T49.4X2	T49.4X3	T49.4X4	T49.4X5	T49.4X6
Deprenalin	T42.8X1	T42.8X2	T42.8X3	T42.8X4	T42.8X5	T42.8X6
Deprenyl	T42.8X1	T42.8X2	T42.8X3	T42.8X4	T42.8X5	T42.8X6
Depressant, appetite	T50.5X1	T50.5X2	T50.5X3	T50.5X4	T50.5X5	T50.5X6
Depressant						
appetite (central)	T50.5X1	T50.5X2	T50.5X3	T50.5X4	T50.5X5	T50.5X6
cardiac	T46.2X1	T46.2X2	T46.2X3	T46.2X4	T46.2X5	T46.2X6
central nervous system (anesthetic) —see also Central nervous system, depressants	T42.71	T42.72	T42.73	T42.74	T42.75	T42.76
general anesthetic	T41.201	T41.202	T41.203	T41.204	T41.205	T41.206
muscle tone	T42.8X1	T42.8X2	T42.8X3	T42.8X4	T42.8X5	T42.8X6
muscle tone, central	T42.8X1	T42.8X2	T42.8X3	T42.8X4	T42.8X5	T42.8X6
psychotherapeutic	T43.501	T43.502	T43.503	T43.504	T43.505	T43.506
Deptropine	T45.0X1	T45.0X2	T45.0X3	T45.0X4	T45.0X5	T45.0X6
Dequalinium (chloride)	T49.0X1	T49.0X2	T49.0X3	T49.0X4	T49.0X5	T49.0X6
Derris root	T60.2X1	T60.2X2	T60.2X3	T60.2X4	--	--
Deserpidine	T46.5X1	T46.5X2	T46.5X3	T46.5X4	T46.5X5	T46.5X6
Desferrioxamine	T45.8X1	T45.8X2	T45.8X3	T45.8X4	T45.8X5	T45.8X6
Desipramine	T43.011	T43.012	T43.013	T43.014	T43.015	T43.016
Deslanoside	T46.0X1	T46.0X2	T46.0X3	T46.0X4	T46.0X5	T46.0X6
Desloughing agent	T49.4X1	T49.4X2	T49.4X3	T49.4X4	T49.4X5	T49.4X6
Desmethylimipramine	T43.011	T43.012	T43.013	T43.014	T43.015	T43.016
Desmopressin	T38.891	T38.892	T38.893	T38.894	T38.895	T38.896
Desocodeine	T40.2X1	T40.2X2	T40.2X3	T40.2X4	T40.2X5	T40.2X6

Substance	Poisoning, Accidental (unintentional)	Poisoning, Intentional Self-harm	Poisoning, Assault	Poisoning, Undetermined	Adverse effect	Underdosing
Desogestrel	T38.5X1	T38.5X2	T38.5X3	T38.5X4	T38.5X5	T38.5X6
Desomorphine	T40.2X1	T40.2X2	T40.2X3	T40.2X4	--	--
Desonide	T49.0X1	T49.0X2	T49.0X3	T49.0X4	T49.0X5	T49.0X6
Desoximetasone	T49.0X1	T49.0X2	T49.0X3	T49.0X4	T49.0X5	T49.0X6
Desoxycorticosteroid	T50.0X1	T50.0X2	T50.0X3	T50.0X4	T50.0X5	T50.0X6
Desoxycortone	T50.0X1	T50.0X2	T50.0X3	T50.0X4	T50.0X5	T50.0X6
Desoxyephedrine	T43.621	T43.622	T43.623	T43.624	T43.625	T43.626
Detaxtran	T46.6X1	T46.6X2	T46.6X3	T46.6X4	T46.6X5	T46.6X6
Detergent	T49.2X1	T49.2X2	T49.2X3	T49.2X4	T49.2X5	T49.2X6
external medication	T49.2X1	T49.2X2	T49.2X3	T49.2X4	T49.2X5	T49.2X6
local	T49.2X1	T49.2X2	T49.2X3	T49.2X4	T49.2X5	T49.2X6
medicinal	T49.2X1	T49.2X2	T49.2X3	T49.2X4	T49.2X5	T49.2X6
nonmedicinal	T55.1X1	T55.1X2	T55.1X3	T55.1X4	--	--
specified NEC	T55.1X1	T55.1X2	T55.1X3	T55.1X4	--	--
Deterrent, alcohol	T50.6X1	T50.6X2	T50.6X3	T50.6X4	T50.6X5	T50.6X6
Detoxifying agent	T50.6X1	T50.6X2	T50.6X3	T50.6X4	T50.6X5	T50.6X6
Detrothyronine	T38.1X1	T38.1X2	T38.1X3	T38.1X4	T38.1X5	T38.1X6
Dettol (external medication)	T49.0X1	T49.0X2	T49.0X3	T49.0X4	T49.0X5	T49.0X6
Dexamethasone	T38.0X1	T38.0X2	T38.0X3	T38.0X4	T38.0X5	T38.0X6
ENT agent	T49.6X1	T49.6X2	T49.6X3	T49.6X4	T49.6X5	T49.6X6
ophthalmic preparation	T49.5X1	T49.5X2	T49.5X3	T49.5X4	T49.5X5	T49.5X6
topical NEC	T49.0X1	T49.0X2	T49.0X3	T49.0X4	T49.0X5	T49.0X6
Dexamfetamine	T43.621	T43.622	T43.623	T43.624	T43.625	T43.626
Dexamphetamine	T43.621	T43.622	T43.623	T43.624	T43.625	T43.626
Dexbrompheniramine	T45.0X1	T45.0X2	T45.0X3	T45.0X4	T45.0X5	T45.0X6
Dexchlorpheniramine	T45.0X1	T45.0X2	T45.0X3	T45.0X4	T45.0X5	T45.0X6
Dexedrine	T43.621	T43.622	T43.623	T43.624	T43.625	T43.626
Dexetimide	T44.3X1	T44.3X2	T44.3X3	T44.3X4	T44.3X5	T44.3X6
Dexfenfluramine	T50.5X1	T50.5X2	T50.5X3	T50.5X4	T50.5X5	T50.5X6
Dexpanthenol	T45.2X1	T45.2X2	T45.2X3	T45.2X4	T45.2X5	T45.2X6
Dextran (40) (70) (150)	T45.8X1	T45.8X2	T45.8X3	T45.8X4	T45.8X5	T45.8X6
Dextriferron	T45.4X1	T45.4X2	T45.4X3	T45.4X4	T45.4X5	T45.4X6
Dextro calcium pantothenate	T45.2X1	T45.2X2	T45.2X3	T45.2X4	T45.2X5	T45.2X6
Dextro pantothenyl alcohol	T45.2X1	T45.2X2	T45.2X3	T45.2X4	T45.2X5	T45.2X6
Dextroamphetamine	T43.621	T43.622	T43.623	T43.624	T43.625	T43.626
Dextromethorphan	T48.3X1	T48.3X2	T48.3X3	T48.3X4	T48.3X5	T48.3X6
Dextromoramide	T40.4X1	T40.4X2	T40.4X3	T40.4X4	--	--
topical	T49.8X1	T49.8X2	T49.8X3	T49.8X4	T49.8X5	T49.8X6
Dextropropoxyphene	T40.4X1	T40.4X2	T40.4X3	T40.4X4	T40.4X5	T40.4X6
Dextrorphan	T40.2X1	T40.2X2	T40.2X3	T40.2X4	T40.2X5	T40.2X6
Dextrose	T50.3X1	T50.3X2	T50.3X3	T50.3X4	T50.3X5	T50.3X6
concentrated solution, intravenous	T46.8X1	T46.8X2	T46.8X3	T46.8X4	T46.8X5	T46.8X6
Dextrothyroxin	T38.1X1	T38.1X2	T38.1X3	T38.1X4	T38.1X5	T38.1X6
Dextrothyroxine sodium	T38.1X1	T38.1X2	T38.1X3	T38.1X4	T38.1X5	T38.1X6
DFP	T44.0X1	T44.0X2	T44.0X3	T44.0X4	T44.0X5	T44.0X6
DHE	T37.3X1	T37.3X2	T37.3X3	T37.3X4	T37.3X5	T37.3X6
45	T46.5X1	T46.5X2	T46.5X3	T46.5X4	T46.5X5	T46.5X6
Diabinese	T38.3X1	T38.3X2	T38.3X3	T38.3X4	T38.3X5	T38.3X6
Diacetone alcohol	T52.4X1	T52.4X2	T52.4X3	T52.4X4	--	--
Diacetyl monoxime	T50.991	T50.992	T50.993	T50.994	--	--
Diacetylmorphine	T40.1X1	T40.1X2	T40.1X3	T40.1X4	T40.1X5	--
Diachylon plaster	T49.4X1	T49.4X2	T49.4X3	T49.4X4	T49.4X5	T49.4X6
Diaethylstilboestrolum	T38.5X1	T38.5X2	T38.5X3	T38.5X4	T38.5X5	T38.5X6
Diagnostic agent NEC	T50.8X1	T50.8X2	T50.8X3	T50.8X4	T50.8X5	T50.8X6
Dial (soap)	T49.2X1	T49.2X2	T49.2X3	T49.2X4	T49.2X5	T49.2X6
sedative	T42.3X1	T42.3X2	T42.3X3	T42.3X4	T42.3X5	T42.3X6
Dialkyl carbonate	T52.91	T52.92	T52.93	T52.94	--	--
Diallylbarbituric acid	T42.3X1	T42.3X2	T42.3X3	T42.3X4	T42.3X5	T42.3X6
Diallymal	T42.3X1	T42.3X2	T42.3X3	T42.3X4	T42.3X5	T42.3X6
Dialysis solution (intraperitoneal)	T50.3X1	T50.3X2	T50.3X3	T50.3X4	T50.3X5	T50.3X6
Diaminodiphenylsulfone	T37.1X1	T37.1X2	T37.1X3	T37.1X4	T37.1X5	T37.1X6
Diamorphine	T40.1X1	T40.1X2	T40.1X3	T40.1X4	T40.1X5	--
Diamox	T50.2X1	T50.2X2	T50.2X3	T50.2X4	T50.2X5	T50.2X6
Diamthazole	T49.0X1	T49.0X2	T49.0X3	T49.0X4	T49.0X5	T49.0X6
Dianthone	T47.2X1	T47.2X2	T47.2X3	T47.2X4	T47.2X5	T47.2X6

TABLE OF DRUGS AND CHEMICALS

Substance	Poisoning, Accidental (unintentional)	Poisoning, Intentional Self-harm	Poisoning, Assault	Poisoning, Undetermined	Adverse effect	Underdosing
Diaphenylsulfone	T37.0X1	T37.0X2	T37.0X3	T37.0X4	T37.0X5	T37.0X6
Diasone (sodium)	T37.1X1	T37.1X2	T37.1X3	T37.1X4	T37.1X5	T37.1X6
Diastase	T47.5X1	T47.5X2	T47.5X3	T47.5X4	T47.5X5	T47.5X6
Diatrizoate	T50.8X1	T50.8X2	T50.8X3	T50.8X4	T50.8X5	T50.8X6
Diazepam	T42.4X1	T42.4X2	T42.4X3	T42.4X4	T42.4X5	T42.4X6
Diazinon	T60.0X1	T60.0X2	T60.0X3	T60.0X4	--	--
Diazomethane (gas)	T59.891	T59.892	T59.893	T59.894	--	--
Diazoxide	T46.5X1	T46.5X2	T46.5X3	T46.5X4	T46.5X5	T46.5X6
Dibekacin	T36.5X1	T36.5X2	T36.5X3	T36.5X4	T36.5X5	T36.5X6
Dibenamine	T44.6X1	T44.6X2	T44.6X3	T44.6X4	T44.6X5	T44.6X6
Dibenzepin	T43.011	T43.012	T43.013	T43.014	T43.015	T43.016
Dibenzheptropine	T45.0X1	T45.0X2	T45.0X3	T45.0X4	T45.0X5	T45.0X6
Dibenzyline	T44.6X1	T44.6X2	T44.6X3	T44.6X4	T44.6X5	T44.6X6
Diborane (gas)	T59.891	T59.892	T59.893	T59.894	--	--
Dibromochloropropane	T60.8X1	T60.8X2	T60.8X3	T60.8X4	--	--
Dibromodulcitol	T45.1X1	T45.1X2	T45.1X3	T45.1X4	T45.1X5	T45.1X6
Dibromoethane	T53.6X1	T53.6X2	T53.6X3	T53.6X4	--	--
Dibromomannitol	T45.1X1	T45.1X2	T45.1X3	T45.1X4	T45.1X5	T45.1X6
Dibromopropamidine isethionate	T49.0X1	T49.0X2	T49.0X3	T49.0X4	T49.0X5	T49.0X6
Dibrompropamidine	T49.0X1	T49.0X2	T49.0X3	T49.0X4	T49.0X5	T49.0X6
Dibucaine	T41.3X1	T41.3X2	T41.3X3	T41.3X4	T41.3X5	T41.3X6
topical (surface)	T41.3X1	T41.3X2	T41.3X3	T41.3X4	T41.3X5	T41.3X6
Dibunate sodium	T48.3X1	T48.3X2	T48.3X3	T48.3X4	T48.3X5	T48.3X6
Dibutoline sulfate	T44.3X1	T44.3X2	T44.3X3	T44.3X4	T44.3X5	T44.3X6
Dicamba	T60.3X1	T60.3X2	T60.3X3	T60.3X4	--	--
Dicapthon	T60.0X1	T60.0X2	T60.0X3	T60.0X4	--	--
Dichlobenil	T60.3X1	T60.3X2	T60.3X3	T60.3X4	--	--
Dichlone	T60.3X1	T60.3X2	T60.3X3	T60.3X4	--	--
Dichloralphenozone	T42.6X1	T42.6X2	T42.6X3	T42.6X4	T42.6X5	T42.6X6
Dichlorbenzidine	T65.3X1	T65.3X2	T65.3X3	T65.3X4	--	--
Dichlorhydrin	T52.8X1	T52.8X2	T52.8X3	T52.8X4	--	--
Dichlorhydroxyquinoline	T37.8X1	T37.8X2	T37.8X3	T37.8X4	T37.8X5	T37.8X6
Dichlorobenzene	T53.7X1	T53.7X2	T53.7X3	T53.7X4	--	--
Dichlorobenzyl alcohol	T49.6X1	T49.6X2	T49.6X3	T49.6X4	T49.6X5	T49.6X6
Dichlorodifluoromethane	T53.5X1	T53.5X2	T53.5X3	T53.5X4	--	--
Dichloroethane	T52.8X1	T52.8X2	T52.8X3	T52.8X4	--	--
Sym-Dichloroethyl ether	T53.6X1	T53.6X2	T53.6X3	T53.6X4	--	--
Dichloroethyl sulfide, not in war	T59.891	T59.892	T59.893	T59.894	--	--
Dichloroethylene	T53.6X1	T53.6X2	T53.6X3	T53.6X4	--	--
Dichloroformoxine, not in war	T59.891	T59.892	T59.893	T59.894	--	--
Dichlorohydrin, alpha-dichlorohydrin	T52.8X1	T52.8X2	T52.8X3	T52.8X4	--	--
Dichloromethane (solvent)	T53.4X1	T53.4X2	T53.4X3	T53.4X4	--	--
vapor	T53.4X1	T53.4X2	T53.4X3	T53.4X4	--	--
Dichloronaphthoquinone	T60.3X1	T60.3X2	T60.3X3	T60.3X4	--	--
Dichlorophen	T37.4X1	T37.4X2	T37.4X3	T37.4X4	T37.4X5	T37.4X6
2,4-Dichlorophenoxyacetic acid	T60.3X1	T60.3X2	T60.3X3	T60.3X4	--	--
Dichloropropene	T60.3X1	T60.3X2	T60.3X3	T60.3X4	--	--
Dichloropropionic acid	T60.3X1	T60.3X2	T60.3X3	T60.3X4	--	--
Dichlorphenamide	T50.2X1	T50.2X2	T50.2X3	T50.2X4	T50.2X5	T50.2X6
Dichlorvos	T60.0X1	T60.0X2	T60.0X3	T60.0X4	--	--
Diclofenac	T39.391	T39.392	T39.393	T39.394	T39.395	T39.396
Diclofenamide	T50.2X1	T50.2X2	T50.2X3	T50.2X4	T50.2X5	T50.2X6
Diclofensine	T43.291	T43.292	T43.293	T43.294	T43.295	T43.296
Diclonixine	T39.8X1	T39.8X2	T39.8X3	T39.8X4	T39.8X5	T39.8X6
Dicloxacillin	T36.0X1	T36.0X2	T36.0X3	T36.0X4	T36.0X5	T36.0X6
Dicophane	T49.0X1	T49.0X2	T49.0X3	T49.0X4	T49.0X5	T49.0X6
Dicoumarol, dicoumarin, dicumarol	T45.511	T45.512	T45.513	T45.514	T45.515	T45.516
Dicrotophos	T60.0X1	T60.0X2	T60.0X3	T60.0X4	--	--
Dicyanogen (gas)	T65.0X1	T65.0X2	T65.0X3	T65.0X4	--	--
Dicyclomine	T44.3X1	T44.3X2	T44.3X3	T44.3X4	T44.3X5	T44.3X6
Dicycloverine	T44.3X1	T44.3X2	T44.3X3	T44.3X4	T44.3X5	T44.3X6
Dideoxycytidine	T37.5X1	T37.5X2	T37.5X3	T37.5X4	T37.5X5	T37.5X6
Dideoxyinosine	T37.5X1	T37.5X2	T37.5X3	T37.5X4	T37.5X5	T37.5X6

TABLE OF DRUGS AND CHEMICALS

Substance	Poisoning, Accidental (unintentional)	Poisoning, Intentional Self-harm	Poisoning, Assault	Poisoning, Undetermined	Adverse effect	Underdosing
Dieldrin (vapor)	T60.1X1	T60.1X2	T60.1X3	T60.1X4	--	--
Diemal	T42.3X1	T42.3X2	T42.3X3	T42.3X4	T42.3X5	T42.3X6
Dienestrol	T38.5X1	T38.5X2	T38.5X3	T38.5X4	T38.5X5	T38.5X6
Dienoestrol	T38.5X1	T38.5X2	T38.5X3	T38.5X4	T38.5X5	T38.5X6
Dietetic drug NEC	T50.901	T50.902	T50.903	T50.904	T50.905	T50.906
Diethazine	T42.8X1	T42.8X2	T42.8X3	T42.8X4	T42.8X5	T42.8X6
Diethyl						
barbituric acid	T42.3X1	T42.3X2	T42.3X3	T42.3X4	T42.3X5	T42.3X6
carbamazine	T37.4X1	T37.4X2	T37.4X3	T37.4X4	T37.4X5	T37.4X6
carbinol	T51.3X1	T51.3X2	T51.3X3	T51.3X4	--	--
carbonate	T52.8X1	T52.8X2	T52.8X3	T52.8X4	--	--
ether (vapor) —see also ether	T41.0X1	T41.0X2	T41.0X3	T41.0X4	T41.0X5	T41.0X6
oxide	T52.8X1	T52.8X2	T52.8X3	T52.8X4	--	--
propion	T50.5X1	T50.5X2	T50.5X3	T50.5X4	T50.5X5	T50.5X6
stilbestrol	T38.5X1	T38.5X2	T38.5X3	T38.5X4	T38.5X5	T38.5X6
toluamide (nonmedicinal)	T60.8X1	T60.8X2	T60.8X3	T60.8X4	--	--
medicinal	T49.3X1	T49.3X2	T49.3X3	T49.3X4	T49.3X5	T49.3X6
Diethylcarbamazine	T37.4X1	T37.4X2	T37.4X3	T37.4X4	T37.4X5	T37.4X6
Diethylene						
dioxide	T52.8X1	T52.8X2	T52.8X3	T52.8X4	--	--
glycol (monoacetate) (monobutyl ether) (monoethyl ether)	T52.3X1	T52.3X2	T52.3X3	T52.3X4	--	--
Diethylhexylphthalate	T65.891	T65.892	T65.893	T65.894	--	--
Diethylpropion	T50.5X1	T50.5X2	T50.5X3	T50.5X4	T50.5X5	T50.5X6
Diethylstilbestrol	T38.5X1	T38.5X2	T38.5X3	T38.5X4	T38.5X5	T38.5X6
Diethylstilboestrol	T38.5X1	T38.5X2	T38.5X3	T38.5X4	T38.5X5	T38.5X6
Diethylsulfone-diethylmethane	T42.6X1	T42.6X2	T42.6X3	T42.6X4	T42.6X5	T42.6X6
Diethyltoluamide	T49.0X1	T49.0X2	T49.0X3	T49.0X4	T49.0X5	T49.0X6
Diethyltryptamine (DET)	T40.991	T40.992	T40.993	T40.994	--	--
Difebarbamate	T42.3X1	T42.3X2	T42.3X3	T42.3X4	T42.3X5	T42.3X6
Difencloxazine	T40.2X1	T40.2X2	T40.2X3	T40.2X4	T40.2X5	T40.2X6
Difenidol	T45.0X1	T45.0X2	T45.0X3	T45.0X4	T45.0X5	T45.0X6
Difenoxin	T47.6X1	T47.6X2	T47.6X3	T47.6X4	T47.6X5	T47.6X6
Difetarsone	T37.3X1	T37.3X2	T37.3X3	T37.3X4	T37.3X5	T37.3X6
Diffusin	T45.3X1	T45.3X2	T45.3X3	T45.3X4	T45.3X5	T45.3X6
Diflorasone	T49.0X1	T49.0X2	T49.0X3	T49.0X4	T49.0X5	T49.0X6
Diflos	T44.0X1	T44.0X2	T44.0X3	T44.0X4	T44.0X5	T44.0X6
Diflubenzuron	T60.1X1	T60.1X2	T60.1X3	T60.1X4	--	--
Diflucortolone	T49.0X1	T49.0X2	T49.0X3	T49.0X4	T49.0X5	T49.0X6
Diflunisal	T39.091	T39.092	T39.093	T39.094	T39.095	T39.096
Difluoromethyldopa	T42.8X1	T42.8X2	T42.8X3	T42.8X4	T42.8X5	T42.8X6
Difluorophate	T44.0X1	T44.0X2	T44.0X3	T44.0X4	T44.0X5	T44.0X6
Digestant NEC	T47.5X1	T47.5X2	T47.5X3	T47.5X4	T47.5X5	T47.5X6
Digitalin (e)	T46.0X1	T46.0X2	T46.0X3	T46.0X4	T46.0X5	T46.0X6
Digitalis (leaf) (glycoside)	T46.0X1	T46.0X2	T46.0X3	T46.0X4	T46.0X5	T46.0X6
lanata	T46.0X1	T46.0X2	T46.0X3	T46.0X4	T46.0X5	T46.0X6
purpurea	T46.0X1	T46.0X2	T46.0X3	T46.0X4	T46.0X5	T46.0X6
Digitoxin	T46.0X1	T46.0X2	T46.0X3	T46.0X4	T46.0X5	T46.0X6
Digitoxose	T46.0X1	T46.0X2	T46.0X3	T46.0X4	T46.0X5	T46.0X6
Digoxin	T46.0X1	T46.0X2	T46.0X3	T46.0X4	T46.0X5	T46.0X6
Digoxine	T46.0X1	T46.0X2	T46.0X3	T46.0X4	T46.0X5	T46.0X6
Dihydralazine	T46.5X1	T46.5X2	T46.5X3	T46.5X4	T46.5X5	T46.5X6
Dihydrazine	T46.5X1	T46.5X2	T46.5X3	T46.5X4	T46.5X5	T46.5X6
Dihydrocodeine	T40.2X1	T40.2X2	T40.2X3	T40.2X4	T40.2X5	T40.2X6
Dihydrocodeinone	T40.2X1	T40.2X2	T40.2X3	T40.2X4	T40.2X5	T40.2X6
Dihydroergocornine	T46.7X1	T46.7X2	T46.7X3	T46.7X4	T46.7X5	T46.7X6
Dihydroergocristine (mesilate)	T46.7X1	T46.7X2	T46.7X3	T46.7X4	T46.7X5	T46.7X6
Dihydroergokryptine	T46.7X1	T46.7X2	T46.7X3	T46.7X4	T46.7X5	T46.7X6
Dihydroergotamine	T46.5X1	T46.5X2	T46.5X3	T46.5X4	T46.5X5	T46.5X6
Dihydroergotoxine	T46.7X1	T46.7X2	T46.7X3	T46.7X4	T46.7X5	T46.7X6
mesilate	T46.7X1	T46.7X2	T46.7X3	T46.7X4	T46.7X5	T46.7X6
Dihydrohydroxycodeinone	T40.2X1	T40.2X2	T40.2X3	T40.2X4	T40.2X5	T40.2X6
Dihydrohydroxymorphinone	T40.2X1	T40.2X2	T40.2X3	T40.2X4	T40.2X5	T40.2X6
Dihydroisocodeine	T40.2X1	T40.2X2	T40.2X3	T40.2X4	T40.2X5	T40.2X6
Dihydromorphine	T40.2X1	T40.2X2	T40.2X3	T40.2X4	--	--

1638

Substance	Poisoning, Accidental (unintentional)	Poisoning, Intentional Self-harm	Poisoning, Assault	Poisoning, Undetermined	Adverse effect	Underdosing
Dihydromorphinone	T40.2X1	T40.2X2	T40.2X3	T40.2X4	T40.2X5	T40.2X6
Dihydrostreptomycin	T36.5X1	T36.5X2	T36.5X3	T36.5X4	T36.5X5	T36.5X6
Dihydrotachysterol	T45.2X1	T45.2X2	T45.2X3	T45.2X4	T45.2X5	T45.2X6
Dihydroxyaluminum aminoacetate	T47.1X1	T47.1X2	T47.1X3	T47.1X4	T47.1X5	T47.1X6
Dihydroxyaluminum sodium carbonate	T47.1X1	T47.1X2	T47.1X3	T47.1X4	T47.1X5	T47.1X6
Dihydroxyanthraquinone	T47.2X1	T47.2X2	T47.2X3	T47.2X4	T47.2X5	T47.2X6
Dihydroxycodeinone	T40.2X1	T40.2X2	T40.2X3	T40.2X4	T40.2X5	T40.2X6
Dihydroxypropyl theophylline	T50.2X1	T50.2X2	T50.2X3	T50.2X4	T50.2X5	T50.2X6
Diiodohydroxyquin	T37.8X1	T37.8X2	T37.8X3	T37.8X4	T37.8X5	T37.8X6
topical	T49.0X1	T49.0X2	T49.0X3	T49.0X4	T49.0X5	T49.0X6
Diiodohydroxyquinoline	T37.8X1	T37.8X2	T37.8X3	T37.8X4	T37.8X5	T37.8X6
Diiodotyrosine	T38.2X1	T38.2X2	T38.2X3	T38.2X4	T38.2X5	T38.2X6
Diisopromine	T44.3X1	T44.3X2	T44.3X3	T44.3X4	T44.3X5	T44.3X6
Diisopropylamine	T46.3X1	T46.3X2	T46.3X3	T46.3X4	T46.3X5	T46.3X6
Diisopropylfluorophos-phonate	T44.0X1	T44.0X2	T44.0X3	T44.0X4	T44.0X5	T44.0X6
Dilantin	T42.0X1	T42.0X2	T42.0X3	T42.0X4	T42.0X5	T42.0X6
Dilaudid	T40.2X1	T40.2X2	T40.2X3	T40.2X4	T40.2X5	T40.2X6
Dilazep	T46.3X1	T46.3X2	T46.3X3	T46.3X4	T46.3X5	T46.3X6
Dill	T47.5X1	T47.5X2	T47.5X3	T47.5X4	T47.5X5	T47.5X6
Diloxanide	T37.3X1	T37.3X2	T37.3X3	T37.3X4	T37.3X5	T37.3X6
Diltiazem	T46.1X1	T46.1X2	T46.1X3	T46.1X4	T46.1X5	T46.1X6
Dimazole	T49.0X1	T49.0X2	T49.0X3	T49.0X4	T49.0X5	T49.0X6
Dimefline	T50.7X1	T50.7X2	T50.7X3	T50.7X4	T50.7X5	T50.7X6
Dimefox	T60.0X1	T60.0X2	T60.0X3	T60.0X4	--	--
Dimemorfan	T48.3X1	T48.3X2	T48.3X3	T48.3X4	T48.3X5	T48.3X6
Dimenhydrinate	T45.0X1	T45.0X2	T45.0X3	T45.0X4	T45.0X5	T45.0X6
Dimercaprol (British anti-lewisite)	T45.8X1	T45.8X2	T45.8X3	T45.8X4	T45.8X5	T45.8X6
Dimercaptopropanol	T45.8X1	T45.8X2	T45.8X3	T45.8X4	T45.8X5	T45.8X6
Dimestrol	T38.5X1	T38.5X2	T38.5X3	T38.5X4	T38.5X5	T38.5X6
Dimetane	T45.0X1	T45.0X2	T45.0X3	T45.0X4	T45.0X5	T45.0X6
Dimethicone	T47.1X1	T47.1X2	T47.1X3	T47.1X4	T47.1X5	T47.1X6
Dimethindene	T45.0X1	T45.0X2	T45.0X3	T45.0X4	T45.0X5	T45.0X6
Dimethisoquin	T49.1X1	T49.1X2	T49.1X3	T49.1X4	T49.1X5	T49.1X6
Dimethisterone	T38.5X1	T38.5X2	T38.5X3	T38.5X4	T38.5X5	T38.5X6
Dimethoate	T60.0X1	T60.0X2	T60.0X3	T60.0X4	--	--
Dimethocaine	T41.3X1	T41.3X2	T41.3X3	T41.3X4	T41.3X5	T41.3X6
Dimethoxanate	T48.3X1	T48.3X2	T48.3X3	T48.3X4	T48.3X5	T48.3X6
Dimethyl						
arsine, arsinic acid	T57.0X1	T57.0X2	T57.0X3	T57.0X4	--	--
carbinol	T51.2X1	T51.2X2	T51.2X3	T51.2X4	--	--
carbonate	T52.8X1	T52.8X2	T52.8X3	T52.8X4	--	--
diguanide	T38.3X1	T38.3X2	T38.3X3	T38.3X4	T38.3X5	T38.3X6
ketone	T52.4X1	T52.4X2	T52.4X3	T52.4X4	--	--
vapor	T52.4X1	T52.4X2	T52.4X3	T52.4X4	--	--
meperidine	T40.2X1	T40.2X2	T40.2X3	T40.2X4	T40.2X5	T40.2X6
parathion	T60.0X1	T60.0X2	T60.0X3	T60.0X4	--	--
phthlate	T49.3X1	T49.3X2	T49.3X3	T49.3X4	T49.3X5	T49.3X6
polysiloxane	T47.8X1	T47.8X2	T47.8X3	T47.8X4	T47.8X5	T47.8X6
sulfate (fumes)	T59.891	T59.892	T59.893	T59.894	--	--
liquid	T65.891	T65.892	T65.893	T65.894	--	--
sulfoxide (nonmedicinal)	T52.8X1	T52.8X2	T52.8X3	T52.8X4	--	--
medicinal	T49.4X1	T49.4X2	T49.4X3	T49.4X4	T49.4X5	T49.4X6
tryptamine	T40.991	T40.992	T40.993	T40.994	--	--
tubocurarine	T48.1X1	T48.1X2	T48.1X3	T48.1X4	T48.1X5	T48.1X6
Dimethylamine sulfate	T49.4X1	T49.4X2	T49.4X3	T49.4X4	T49.4X5	T49.4X6
Dimethylformamide	T52.8X1	T52.8X2	T52.8X3	T52.8X4	--	--
Dimethyltubocurarinium chloride	T48.1X1	T48.1X2	T48.1X3	T48.1X4	T48.1X5	T48.1X6
Dimeticone	T47.1X1	T47.1X2	T47.1X3	T47.1X4	T47.1X5	T47.1X6
Dimetilan	T60.0X1	T60.0X2	T60.0X3	T60.0X4	--	--
Dimetindene	T45.0X1	T45.0X2	T45.0X3	T45.0X4	T45.0X5	T45.0X6
Dimetotiazine	T43.3X1	T43.3X2	T43.3X3	T43.3X4	T43.3X5	T43.3X6
Dimorpholamine	T50.7X1	T50.7X2	T50.7X3	T50.7X4	T50.7X5	T50.7X6
Dimoxyline	T46.3X1	T46.3X2	T46.3X3	T46.3X4	T46.3X5	T46.3X6
Dinitrobenzene	T65.3X1	T65.3X2	T65.3X3	T65.3X4	--	--

Substance	Poisoning, Accidental (unintentional)	Poisoning, Intentional Self-harm	Poisoning, Assault	Poisoning, Undetermined	Adverse effect	Underdosing
vapor	T59.891	T59.892	T59.893	T59.894	--	--
Dinitrobenzol	T65.3X1	T65.3X2	T65.3X3	T65.3X4	--	--
vapor	T59.891	T59.892	T59.893	T59.894	--	--
Dinitrobutylphenol	T65.3X1	T65.3X2	T65.3X3	T65.3X4	--	--
Dinitro (-ortho-) cresol (pesticide) (spray)	T65.3X1	T65.3X2	T65.3X3	T65.3X4	--	--
Dinitrocyclohexylphenol	T65.3X1	T65.3X2	T65.3X3	T65.3X4	--	--
Dinitrophenol	T65.3X1	T65.3X2	T65.3X3	T65.3X4	--	--
Dinoprost	T48.0X1	T48.0X2	T48.0X3	T48.0X4	T48.0X5	T48.0X6
Dinoprostone	T48.0X1	T48.0X2	T48.0X3	T48.0X4	T48.0X5	T48.0X6
Dinoseb	T60.3X1	T60.3X2	T60.3X3	T60.3X4	--	--
Dioctyl sulfosuccinate (calcium) (sodium)	T47.4X1	T47.4X2	T47.4X3	T47.4X4	T47.4X5	T47.4X6
Diodone	T50.8X1	T50.8X2	T50.8X3	T50.8X4	T50.8X5	T50.8X6
Diodoquin	T37.8X1	T37.8X2	T37.8X3	T37.8X4	T37.8X5	T37.8X6
Dionin	T40.2X1	T40.2X2	T40.2X3	T40.2X4	T40.2X5	T40.2X6
Diosmin	T46.991	T46.992	T46.993	T46.994	T46.995	T46.996
Dioxane	T52.8X1	T52.8X2	T52.8X3	T52.8X4	--	--
Dioxathion	T60.0X1	T60.0X2	T60.0X3	T60.0X4	--	--
Dioxin	T53.7X1	T53.7X2	T53.7X3	T53.7X4	--	--
Dioxopromethazine	T43.3X1	T43.3X2	T43.3X3	T43.3X4	T43.3X5	T43.3X6
Dioxyline	T46.3X1	T46.3X2	T46.3X3	T46.3X4	T46.3X5	T46.3X6
Dipentene	T52.8X1	T52.8X2	T52.8X3	T52.8X4	--	--
Diperodon	T41.3X1	T41.3X2	T41.3X3	T41.3X4	T41.3X5	T41.3X6
Diphacinone	T60.4X1	T60.4X2	T60.4X3	T60.4X4	--	--
Diphemanil	T44.3X1	T44.3X2	T44.3X3	T44.3X4	T44.3X5	T44.3X6
metilsulfate	T44.3X1	T44.3X2	T44.3X3	T44.3X4	T44.3X5	T44.3X6
Diphenadione	T45.511	T45.512	T45.513	T45.514	T45.515	T45.516
rodenticide	T60.4X1	T60.4X2	T60.4X3	T60.4X4	--	--
Diphenhydramine	T45.0X1	T45.0X2	T45.0X3	T45.0X4	T45.0X5	T45.0X6
Diphenidol	T45.0X1	T45.0X2	T45.0X3	T45.0X4	T45.0X5	T45.0X6
Diphenoxylate	T47.6X1	T47.6X2	T47.6X3	T47.6X4	T47.6X5	T47.6X6
Diphenylamine	T65.3X1	T65.3X2	T65.3X3	T65.3X4	--	--
Diphenylbutazone	T39.2X1	T39.2X2	T39.2X3	T39.2X4	T39.2X5	T39.2X6
Diphenylchloroarsine, not in war	T57.0X1	T57.0X2	T57.0X3	T57.0X4	--	--
Diphenylhydantoin	T42.0X1	T42.0X2	T42.0X3	T42.0X4	T42.0X5	T42.0X6
Diphenylmethane dye	T52.1X1	T52.1X2	T52.1X3	T52.1X4	--	--
Diphenylpyraline	T45.0X1	T45.0X2	T45.0X3	T45.0X4	T45.0X5	T45.0X6
Diphtheria						
antitoxin	T50.Z11	T50.Z12	T50.Z13	T50.Z14	T50.Z15	T50.Z16
toxoid	T50.A91	T50.A92	T50.A93	T50.A94	T50.A95	T50.A96
with tetanus toxoid	T50.A21	T50.A22	T50.A23	T50.A24	T50.A25	T50.A26
with pertussis component	T50.A11	T50.A12	T50.A13	T50.A14	T50.A15	T50.A16
vaccine	T50.A91	T50.A92	T50.A93	T50.A94	T50.A95	T50.A96
combination						
including pertussis	T50.A11	T50.A12	T50.A13	T50.A14	T50.A15	T50.A16
without pertussis	T50.A21	T50.A22	T50.A23	T50.A24	T50.A25	T50.A26
Diphylline	T50.2X1	T50.2X2	T50.2X3	T50.2X4	T50.2X5	T50.2X6
Dipipanone	T40.4X1	T40.4X2	T40.4X3	T40.4X4	--	--
Dipivefrine	T49.5X1	T49.5X2	T49.5X3	T49.5X4	T49.5X5	T49.5X6
Diplovax	T50.B91	T50.B92	T50.B93	T50.B94	T50.B95	T50.B96
Diprophylline	T50.2X1	T50.2X2	T50.2X3	T50.2X4	T50.2X5	T50.2X6
Dipropyline	T48.291	T48.292	T48.293	T48.294	T48.295	T48.296
Dipyridamole	T46.3X1	T46.3X2	T46.3X3	T46.3X4	T46.3X5	T46.3X6
Dipyrone	T39.2X1	T39.2X2	T39.2X3	T39.2X4	T39.2X5	T39.2X6
Diquat (dibromide)	T60.3X1	T60.3X2	T60.3X3	T60.3X4	--	--
Disinfectant	T65.891	T65.892	T65.893	T65.894	--	--
alkaline	T54.3X1	T54.3X2	T54.3X3	T54.3X4	--	--
aromatic	T54.1X1	T54.1X2	T54.1X3	T54.1X4	--	--
intestinal	T37.8X1	T37.8X2	T37.8X3	T37.8X4	T37.8X5	T37.8X6
Disipal	T42.8X1	T42.8X2	T42.8X3	T42.8X4	T42.8X5	T42.8X6
Disodium edetate	T50.6X1	T50.6X2	T50.6X3	T50.6X4	T50.6X5	T50.6X6
Disoprofol	T41.291	T41.292	T41.293	T41.294	T41.295	T41.296
Disopyramide	T46.2X1	T46.2X2	T46.2X3	T46.2X4	T46.2X5	T46.2X6
Distigmine (bromide)	T44.0X1	T44.0X2	T44.0X3	T44.0X4	T44.0X5	T44.0X6
Disulfamide	T50.2X1	T50.2X2	T50.2X3	T50.2X4	T50.2X5	T50.2X6
Disulfanilamide	T37.0X1	T37.0X2	T37.0X3	T37.0X4	T37.0X5	T37.0X6

Substance	Poisoning, Accidental (unintentional)	Poisoning, Intentional Self-harm	Poisoning, Assault	Poisoning, Undetermined	Adverse effect	Underdosing
Disulfiram	T50.6X1	T50.6X2	T50.6X3	T50.6X4	T50.6X5	T50.6X6
Disulfoton	T60.0X1	T60.0X2	T60.0X3	T60.0X4	--	--
Dithiazanine iodide	T37.4X1	T37.4X2	T37.4X3	T37.4X4	T37.4X5	T37.4X6
Dithiocarbamate	T60.0X1	T60.0X2	T60.0X3	T60.0X4	--	--
Dithranol	T49.4X1	T49.4X2	T49.4X3	T49.4X4	T49.4X5	T49.4X6
Diucardin	T50.2X1	T50.2X2	T50.2X3	T50.2X4	T50.2X5	T50.2X6
Diupres	T50.2X1	T50.2X2	T50.2X3	T50.2X4	T50.2X5	T50.2X6
Diuretic NEC	T50.2X1	T50.2X2	T50.2X3	T50.2X4	T50.2X5	T50.2X6
benzothiadiazine	T50.2X1	T50.2X2	T50.2X3	T50.2X4	T50.2X5	T50.2X6
carbonic acid anhydrase inhibitors	T50.2X1	T50.2X2	T50.2X3	T50.2X4	T50.2X5	T50.2X6
furfuryl NEC	T50.2X1	T50.2X2	T50.2X3	T50.2X4	T50.2X5	T50.2X6
loop (high-ceiling)	T50.1X1	T50.1X2	T50.1X3	T50.1X4	T50.1X5	T50.1X6
mercurial NEC	T50.2X1	T50.2X2	T50.2X3	T50.2X4	T50.2X5	T50.2X6
osmotic	T50.2X1	T50.2X2	T50.2X3	T50.2X4	T50.2X5	T50.2X6
purine NEC	T50.2X1	T50.2X2	T50.2X3	T50.2X4	T50.2X5	T50.2X6
saluretic NEC	T50.2X1	T50.2X2	T50.2X3	T50.2X4	T50.2X5	T50.2X6
sulfonamide	T50.2X1	T50.2X2	T50.2X3	T50.2X4	T50.2X5	T50.2X6
thiazide NEC	T50.2X1	T50.2X2	T50.2X3	T50.2X4	T50.2X5	T50.2X6
xanthine	T50.2X1	T50.2X2	T50.2X3	T50.2X4	T50.2X5	T50.2X6
Diurgin	T50.2X1	T50.2X2	T50.2X3	T50.2X4	T50.2X5	T50.2X6
Diuril	T50.2X1	T50.2X2	T50.2X3	T50.2X4	T50.2X5	T50.2X6
Diuron	T60.3X1	T60.3X2	T60.3X3	T60.3X4	--	--
Divalproex	T42.6X1	T42.6X2	T42.6X3	T42.6X4	T42.6X5	T42.6X6
Divinyl ether	T41.0X1	T41.0X2	T41.0X3	T41.0X4	T41.0X5	T41.0X6
Dixanthogen	T49.0X1	T49.0X2	T49.0X3	T49.0X4	T49.0X5	T49.0X6
Dixyrazine	T43.3X1	T43.3X2	T43.3X3	T43.3X4	T43.3X5	T43.3X6
D-lysergic acid diethylamide	T40.8X1	T40.8X2	T40.8X3	T40.8X4	T40.8X5	--
DMCT	T36.4X1	T36.4X2	T36.4X3	T36.4X4	T36.4X5	T36.4X6
DMSO—see Dimethyl sulfoxide						
DNBP	T60.3X1	T60.3X2	T60.3X3	T60.3X4	--	--
DNOC	T65.3X1	T65.3X2	T65.3X3	T65.3X4	--	--
Dobutamine	T44.5X1	T44.5X2	T44.5X3	T44.5X4	T44.5X5	T44.5X6
DOCA	T38.0X1	T38.0X2	T38.0X3	T38.0X4	T38.0X5	T38.0X6
Docusate sodium	T47.4X1	T47.4X2	T47.4X3	T47.4X4	T47.4X5	T47.4X6
Dodicin	T49.0X1	T49.0X2	T49.0X3	T49.0X4	T49.0X5	T49.0X6
Dofamium chloride	T49.0X1	T49.0X2	T49.0X3	T49.0X4	T49.0X5	T49.0X6
Dolophine	T40.3X1	T40.3X2	T40.3X3	T40.3X4	T40.3X5	T40.3X6
Doloxene	T39.8X1	T39.8X2	T39.8X3	T39.8X4	T39.8X5	T39.8X6
Domestic gas (after combustion) —see Gas, utility						
prior to combustion	T59.891	T59.892	T59.893	T59.894	--	--
Domiodol	T48.4X1	T48.4X2	T48.4X3	T48.4X4	T48.4X5	T48.4X6
Domiphen (bromide)	T49.0X1	T49.0X2	T49.0X3	T49.0X4	T49.0X5	T49.0X6
Domperidone	T45.0X1	T45.0X2	T45.0X3	T45.0X4	T45.0X5	T45.0X6
Dopa	T42.8X1	T42.8X2	T42.8X3	T42.8X4	T42.8X5	T42.8X6
Dopamine	T44.991	T44.992	T44.993	T44.994	T44.995	T44.996
Doriden	T42.6X1	T42.6X2	T42.6X3	T42.6X4	T42.6X5	T42.6X6
Dormiral	T42.3X1	T42.3X2	T42.3X3	T42.3X4	T42.3X5	T42.3X6
Dormison	T42.6X1	T42.6X2	T42.6X3	T42.6X4	T42.6X5	T42.6X6
Dornase	T48.4X1	T48.4X2	T48.4X3	T48.4X4	T48.4X5	T48.4X6
Dorsacaine	T41.3X1	T41.3X2	T41.3X3	T41.3X4	T41.3X5	T41.3X6
Dosulepin	T43.011	T43.012	T43.013	T43.014	T43.015	T43.016
Dothiepin	T43.011	T43.012	T43.013	T43.014	T43.015	T43.016
Doxantrazole	T48.6X1	T48.6X2	T48.6X3	T48.6X4	T48.6X5	T48.6X6
Doxapram	T50.7X1	T50.7X2	T50.7X3	T50.7X4	T50.7X5	T50.7X6
Doxazosin	T44.6X1	T44.6X2	T44.6X3	T44.6X4	T44.6X5	T44.6X6
Doxepin	T43.011	T43.012	T43.013	T43.014	T43.015	T43.016
Doxifluridine	T45.1X1	T45.1X2	T45.1X3	T45.1X4	T45.1X5	T45.1X6
Doxorubicin	T45.1X1	T45.1X2	T45.1X3	T45.1X4	T45.1X5	T45.1X6
Doxycycline	T36.4X1	T36.4X2	T36.4X3	T36.4X4	T36.4X5	T36.4X6
Doxylamine	T45.0X1	T45.0X2	T45.0X3	T45.0X4	T45.0X5	T45.0X6
Dramamine	T45.0X1	T45.0X2	T45.0X3	T45.0X4	T45.0X5	T45.0X6
Drano (drain cleaner)	T54.3X1	T54.3X2	T54.3X3	T54.3X4	--	--
Dressing, live pulp	T49.7X1	T49.7X2	T49.7X3	T49.7X4	T49.7X5	T49.7X6

TABLE OF DRUGS AND CHEMICALS

Substance	Poisoning, Accidental (unintentional)	Poisoning, Intentional Self-harm	Poisoning, Assault	Poisoning, Undetermined	Adverse effect	Underdosing
Drocode	T40.2X1	T40.2X2	T40.2X3	T40.2X4	T40.2X5	T40.2X6
Dromoran	T40.2X1	T40.2X2	T40.2X3	T40.2X4	T40.2X5	T40.2X6
Dromostanolone	T38.7X1	T38.7X2	T38.7X3	T38.7X4	T38.7X5	T38.7X6
Dronabinol	T40.7X1	T40.7X2	T40.7X3	T40.7X4	T40.7X5	T40.7X6
Droperidol	T43.591	T43.592	T43.593	T43.594	T43.595	T43.596
Dropropizine	T48.3X1	T48.3X2	T48.3X3	T48.3X4	T48.3X5	T48.3X6
Drostanolone	T38.7X1	T38.7X2	T38.7X3	T38.7X4	T38.7X5	T38.7X6
Drotaverine	T44.3X1	T44.3X2	T44.3X3	T44.3X4	T44.3X5	T44.3X6
Drotrecogin alfa	T45.511	T45.512	T45.513	T45.514	T45.515	T45.516
Drug NEC	T50.901	T50.902	T50.903	T50.904	T50.905	T50.906
specified NEC	T50.991	T50.992	T50.993	T50.994	T50.995	T50.996
DTIC	T45.1X1	T45.1X2	T45.1X3	T45.1X4	T45.1X5	T45.1X6
Duboisine	T44.3X1	T44.3X2	T44.3X3	T44.3X4	T44.3X5	T44.3X6
Dulcolax	T47.2X1	T47.2X2	T47.2X3	T47.2X4	T47.2X5	T47.2X6
Duponol (C) (EP)	T49.2X1	T49.2X2	T49.2X3	T49.2X4	T49.2X5	T49.2X6
Durabolin	T38.7X1	T38.7X2	T38.7X3	T38.7X4	T38.7X5	T38.7X6
Dyclone	T41.3X1	T41.3X2	T41.3X3	T41.3X4	T41.3X5	T41.3X6
Dyclonine	T41.3X1	T41.3X2	T41.3X3	T41.3X4	T41.3X5	T41.3X6
Dydrogesterone	T38.5X1	T38.5X2	T38.5X3	T38.5X4	T38.5X5	T38.5X6
Dye NEC	T65.6X1	T65.6X2	T65.6X3	T65.6X4	--	--
antiseptic	T49.0X1	T49.0X2	T49.0X3	T49.0X4	T49.0X5	T49.0X6
diagnostic agents	T50.8X1	T50.8X2	T50.8X3	T50.8X4	T50.8X5	T50.8X6
pharmaceutical NEC	T50.901	T50.902	T50.903	T50.904	T50.905	T50.906
Dyflos	T44.0X1	T44.0X2	T44.0X3	T44.0X4	T44.0X5	T44.0X6
Dymelor	T38.3X1	T38.3X2	T38.3X3	T38.3X4	T38.3X5	T38.3X6
Dynamite	T65.3X1	T65.3X2	T65.3X3	T65.3X4	--	--
fumes	T59.891	T59.892	T59.893	T59.894	--	--
Dyphylline	T44.3X1	T44.3X2	T44.3X3	T44.3X4	T44.3X5	T44.3X6
Ear drug NEC	T49.6X1	T49.6X2	T49.6X3	T49.6X4	T49.6X5	T49.6X6
Ear preparations	T49.6X1	T49.6X2	T49.6X3	T49.6X4	T49.6X5	T49.6X6
Echothiophate, echothiopate, ecothiopate	T49.5X1	T49.5X2	T49.5X3	T49.5X4	T49.5X5	T49.5X6
Econazole	T49.0X1	T49.0X2	T49.0X3	T49.0X4	T49.0X5	T49.0X6
Ecothiopate iodide	T49.5X1	T49.5X2	T49.5X3	T49.5X4	T49.5X5	T49.5X6
Ecstasy	T43.621	T43.622	T43.623	T43.624	T43.625	T43.626
Ectylurea	T42.6X1	T42.6X2	T42.6X3	T42.6X4	T42.6X5	T42.6X6
Edathamil disodium	T45.8X1	T45.8X2	T45.8X3	T45.8X4	T45.8X5	T45.8X6
Edecrin	T50.1X1	T50.1X2	T50.1X3	T50.1X4	T50.1X5	T50.1X6
Edetate, disodium (calcium)	T45.8X1	T45.8X2	T45.8X3	T45.8X4	T45.8X5	T45.8X6
Edoxudine	T49.5X1	T49.5X2	T49.5X3	T49.5X4	T49.5X5	T49.5X6
Edrophonium	T44.0X1	T44.0X2	T44.0X3	T44.0X4	T44.0X5	T44.0X6
chloride	T44.0X1	T44.0X2	T44.0X3	T44.0X4	T44.0X5	T44.0X6
EDTA	T50.6X1	T50.6X2	T50.6X3	T50.6X4	T50.6X5	T50.6X6
Eflornithine	T37.2X1	T37.2X2	T37.2X3	T37.2X4	T37.2X5	T37.2X6
Efloxate	T46.3X1	T46.3X2	T46.3X3	T46.3X4	T46.3X5	T46.3X6
Elase	T49.8X1	T49.8X2	T49.8X3	T49.8X4	T49.8X5	T49.8X6
Elastase	T47.5X1	T47.5X2	T47.5X3	T47.5X4	T47.5X5	T47.5X6
Elaterium	T47.2X1	T47.2X2	T47.2X3	T47.2X4	T47.2X5	T47.2X6
Elcatonin	T50.991	T50.992	T50.993	T50.994	T50.995	T50.996
Elder	T62.2X1	T62.2X2	T62.2X3	T62.2X4	--	--
berry, (unripe)	T62.1X1	T62.1X2	T62.1X3	T62.1X4	--	--
Electrolyte balance drug	T50.3X1	T50.3X2	T50.3X3	T50.3X4	T50.3X5	T50.3X6
Electrolytes NEC	T50.3X1	T50.3X2	T50.3X3	T50.3X4	T50.3X5	T50.3X6
Electrolytic agent NEC	T50.3X1	T50.3X2	T50.3X3	T50.3X4	T50.3X5	T50.3X6
Elemental diet	T50.901	T50.902	T50.903	T50.904	T50.905	T50.906
Elliptinium acetate	T45.1X1	T45.1X2	T45.1X3	T45.1X4	T45.1X5	T45.1X6
Embramine	T45.0X1	T45.0X2	T45.0X3	T45.0X4	T45.0X5	T45.0X6
Emepronium (salts)	T44.3X1	T44.3X2	T44.3X3	T44.3X4	T44.3X5	T44.3X6
bromide	T44.3X1	T44.3X2	T44.3X3	T44.3X4	T44.3X5	T44.3X6
Emetic NEC	T47.7X1	T47.7X2	T47.7X3	T47.7X4	T47.7X5	T47.7X6
Emetine	T37.3X1	T37.3X2	T37.3X3	T37.3X4	T37.3X5	T37.3X6
Emollient NEC	T49.3X1	T49.3X2	T49.3X3	T49.3X4	T49.3X5	T49.3X6
Emorfazone	T39.8X1	T39.8X2	T39.8X3	T39.8X4	T39.8X5	T39.8X6
Emylcamate	T43.591	T43.592	T43.593	T43.594	T43.595	T43.596
Enalapril	T46.4X1	T46.4X2	T46.4X3	T46.4X4	T46.4X5	T46.4X6
Enalaprilat	T46.4X1	T46.4X2	T46.4X3	T46.4X4	T46.4X5	T46.4X6

Substance	Poisoning, Accidental (unintentional)	Poisoning, Intentional Self-harm	Poisoning, Assault	Poisoning, Undetermined	Adverse effect	Underdosing
Encainide	T46.2X1	T46.2X2	T46.2X3	T46.2X4	T46.2X5	T46.2X6
Endocaine	T41.3X1	T41.3X2	T41.3X3	T41.3X4	T41.3X5	T41.3X6
Endosulfan	T60.2X1	T60.2X2	T60.2X3	T60.2X4	--	--
Endothall	T60.3X1	T60.3X2	T60.3X3	T60.3X4	--	--
Endralazine	T46.5X1	T46.5X2	T46.5X3	T46.5X4	T46.5X5	T46.5X6
Endrin	T60.1X1	T60.1X2	T60.1X3	T60.1X4	--	--
Enflurane	T41.0X1	T41.0X2	T41.0X3	T41.0X4	T41.0X5	T41.0X6
Enhexymal	T42.3X1	T42.3X2	T42.3X3	T42.3X4	T42.3X5	T42.3X6
Enocitabine	T45.1X1	T45.1X2	T45.1X3	T45.1X4	T45.1X5	T45.1X6
Enovid	T38.4X1	T38.4X2	T38.4X3	T38.4X4	T38.4X5	T38.4X6
Enoxacin	T36.8X1	T36.8X2	T36.8X3	T36.8X4	T36.8X5	T36.8X6
Enoxaparin (sodium)	T45.511	T45.512	T45.513	T45.514	T45.515	T45.516
Enpiprazole	T43.591	T43.592	T43.593	T43.594	T43.595	T43.596
Enprofylline	T48.6X1	T48.6X2	T48.6X3	T48.6X4	T48.6X5	T48.6X6
Enprostil	T47.1X1	T47.1X2	T47.1X3	T47.1X4	T47.1X5	T47.1X6
ENT preparations (anti-infectives)	T49.6X1	T49.6X2	T49.6X3	T49.6X4	T49.6X5	T49.6X6
Enterogastrone	T38.891	T38.892	T38.893	T38.894	T38.895	T38.896
Enviomycin	T36.8X1	T36.8X2	T36.8X3	T36.8X4	T36.8X5	T36.8X6
Enzodase	T45.3X1	T45.3X2	T45.3X3	T45.3X4	T45.3X5	T45.3X6
Enzyme NEC	T45.3X1	T45.3X2	T45.3X3	T45.3X4	T45.3X5	T45.3X6
depolymerizing	T49.8X1	T49.8X2	T49.8X3	T49.8X4	T49.8X5	T49.8X6
fibrolytic	T45.3X1	T45.3X2	T45.3X3	T45.3X4	T45.3X5	T45.3X6
gastric	T47.5X1	T47.5X2	T47.5X3	T47.5X4	T47.5X5	T47.5X6
intestinal	T47.5X1	T47.5X2	T47.5X3	T47.5X4	T47.5X5	T47.5X6
local action	T49.4X1	T49.4X2	T49.4X3	T49.4X4	T49.4X5	T49.4X6
proteolytic	T49.4X1	T49.4X2	T49.4X3	T49.4X4	T49.4X5	T49.4X6
thrombolytic	T45.3X1	T45.3X2	T45.3X3	T45.3X4	T45.3X5	T45.3X6
EPAB	T41.3X1	T41.3X2	T41.3X3	T41.3X4	T41.3X5	T41.3X6
Epanutin	T42.0X1	T42.0X2	T42.0X3	T42.0X4	T42.0X5	T42.0X6
Ephedra	T44.991	T44.992	T44.993	T44.994	T44.995	T44.996
Ephedrine	T44.991	T44.992	T44.993	T44.994	T44.995	T44.996
Epichlorhydrin, epichlorohydrin	T52.8X1	T52.8X2	T52.8X3	T52.8X4	--	--
Epicillin	T36.0X1	T36.0X2	T36.0X3	T36.0X4	T36.0X5	T36.0X6
Epiestriol	T38.5X1	T38.5X2	T38.5X3	T38.5X4	T38.5X5	T38.5X6
Epilim—see Sodium valproate						
Epimestrol	T38.5X1	T38.5X2	T38.5X3	T38.5X4	T38.5X5	T38.5X6
Epinephrine	T44.5X1	T44.5X2	T44.5X3	T44.5X4	T44.5X5	T44.5X6
Epirubicin	T45.1X1	T45.1X2	T45.1X3	T45.1X4	T45.1X5	T45.1X6
Epitiostanol	T38.7X1	T38.7X2	T38.7X3	T38.7X4	T38.7X5	T38.7X6
Epitizide	T50.2X1	T50.2X2	T50.2X3	T50.2X4	T50.2X5	T50.2X6
EPN	T60.0X1	T60.0X2	T60.0X3	T60.0X4	--	--
EPO	T45.8X1	T45.8X2	T45.8X3	T45.8X4	T45.8X5	T45.8X6
Epoetin alpha	T45.8X1	T45.8X2	T45.8X3	T45.8X4	T45.8X5	T45.8X6
Epomediol	T50.991	T50.992	T50.993	T50.994	T50.995	T50.996
Epoprostenol	T45.521	T45.522	T45.523	T45.524	T45.525	T45.526
Epoxy resin	T65.891	T65.892	T65.893	T65.894	--	--
Eprazinone	T48.4X1	T48.4X2	T48.4X3	T48.4X4	T48.4X5	T48.4X6
Epsilon amino-caproic acid	T45.621	T45.622	T45.623	T45.624	T45.625	T45.626
Epsom salt	T47.3X1	T47.3X2	T47.3X3	T47.3X4	T47.3X5	T47.3X6
Eptazocine	T40.4X1	T40.4X2	T40.4X3	T40.4X4	T40.4X5	T40.4X6
Equanil	T43.591	T43.592	T43.593	T43.594	T43.595	T43.596
Equisetum	T62.2X1	T62.2X2	T62.2X3	T62.2X4	--	--
diuretic	T50.2X1	T50.2X2	T50.2X3	T50.2X4	T50.2X5	T50.2X6
Ergobasine	T48.0X1	T48.0X2	T48.0X3	T48.0X4	T48.0X5	T48.0X6
Ergocalciferol	T45.2X1	T45.2X2	T45.2X3	T45.2X4	T45.2X5	T45.2X6
Ergoloid mesylates	T46.7X1	T46.7X2	T46.7X3	T46.7X4	T46.7X5	T46.7X6
Ergometrine	T48.0X1	T48.0X2	T48.0X3	T48.0X4	T48.0X5	T48.0X6
Ergonovine	T48.0X1	T48.0X2	T48.0X3	T48.0X4	T48.0X5	T48.0X6
Ergot NEC	T64.81	T64.82	T64.83	T64.84	--	--
derivative	T48.0X1	T48.0X2	T48.0X3	T48.0X4	T48.0X5	T48.0X6
medicinal (alkaloids)	T48.0X1	T48.0X2	T48.0X3	T48.0X4	T48.0X5	T48.0X6
prepared	T48.0X1	T48.0X2	T48.0X3	T48.0X4	T48.0X5	T48.0X6
Ergotamine	T46.5X1	T46.5X2	T46.5X3	T46.5X4	T46.5X5	T46.5X6
Ergotocine	T48.0X1	T48.0X2	T48.0X3	T48.0X4	T48.0X5	T48.0X6

Substance	Poisoning, Accidental (unintentional)	Poisoning, Intentional Self-harm	Poisoning, Assault	Poisoning, Undetermined	Adverse effect	Underdosing
Ergotrate	T48.0X1	T48.0X2	T48.0X3	T48.0X4	T48.0X5	T48.0X6
Eritrityl tetranitrate	T46.3X1	T46.3X2	T46.3X3	T46.3X4	T46.3X5	T46.3X6
Erythrityl tetranitrate	T46.3X1	T46.3X2	T46.3X3	T46.3X4	T46.3X5	T46.3X6
Erythrol tetranitrate	T46.3X1	T46.3X2	T46.3X3	T46.3X4	T46.3X5	T46.3X6
Erythromycin (salts)	T36.3X1	T36.3X2	T36.3X3	T36.3X4	T36.3X5	T36.3X6
ophthalmic preparation	T49.5X1	T49.5X2	T49.5X3	T49.5X4	T49.5X5	T49.5X6
topical NEC	T49.0X1	T49.0X2	T49.0X3	T49.0X4	T49.0X5	T49.0X6
Erythropoietin	T45.8X1	T45.8X2	T45.8X3	T45.8X4	T45.8X5	T45.8X6
human	T45.8X1	T45.8X2	T45.8X3	T45.8X4	T45.8X5	T45.8X6
Escin	T46.991	T46.992	T46.993	T46.994	T46.995	T46.996
Esculin	T45.2X1	T45.2X2	T45.2X3	T45.2X4	T45.2X5	T45.2X6
Esculoside	T45.2X1	T45.2X2	T45.2X3	T45.2X4	T45.2X5	T45.2X6
ESDT (ether-soluble tar distillate)	T49.1X1	T49.1X2	T49.1X3	T49.1X4	T49.1X5	T49.1X6
Eserine	T49.5X1	T49.5X2	T49.5X3	T49.5X4	T49.5X5	T49.5X6
Esflurbiprofen	T39.311	T39.312	T39.313	T39.314	T39.315	T39.316
Eskabarb	T42.3X1	T42.3X2	T42.3X3	T42.3X4	T42.3X5	T42.3X6
Eskalith	T43.8X1	T43.8X2	T43.8X3	T43.8X4	T43.8X5	T43.8X6
Esmolol	T44.7X1	T44.7X2	T44.7X3	T44.7X4	T44.7X5	T44.7X6
Estanozolol	T38.7X1	T38.7X2	T38.7X3	T38.7X4	T38.7X5	T38.7X6
Estazolam	T42.4X1	T42.4X2	T42.4X3	T42.4X4	T42.4X5	T42.4X6
Estradiol	T38.5X1	T38.5X2	T38.5X3	T38.5X4	T38.5X5	T38.5X6
with testosterone	T38.7X1	T38.7X2	T38.7X3	T38.7X4	T38.7X5	T38.7X6
benzoate	T38.5X1	T38.5X2	T38.5X3	T38.5X4	T38.5X5	T38.5X6
Estramustine	T45.1X1	T45.1X2	T45.1X3	T45.1X4	T45.1X5	T45.1X6
Estriol	T38.5X1	T38.5X2	T38.5X3	T38.5X4	T38.5X5	T38.5X6
Estrogen	T38.5X1	T38.5X2	T38.5X3	T38.5X4	T38.5X5	T38.5X6
with progesterone	T38.5X1	T38.5X2	T38.5X3	T38.5X4	T38.5X5	T38.5X6
conjugated	T38.5X1	T38.5X2	T38.5X3	T38.5X4	T38.5X5	T38.5X6
Estrone	T38.5X1	T38.5X2	T38.5X3	T38.5X4	T38.5X5	T38.5X6
Estropipate	T38.5X1	T38.5X2	T38.5X3	T38.5X4	T38.5X5	T38.5X6
Etacrynate sodium	T50.1X1	T50.1X2	T50.1X3	T50.1X4	T50.1X5	T50.1X6
Etacrynic acid	T50.1X1	T50.1X2	T50.1X3	T50.1X4	T50.1X5	T50.1X6
Etafedrine	T48.6X1	T48.6X2	T48.6X3	T48.6X4	T48.6X5	T48.6X6
Etafenone	T46.3X1	T46.3X2	T46.3X3	T46.3X4	T46.3X5	T46.3X6
Etambutol	T37.1X1	T37.1X2	T37.1X3	T37.1X4	T37.1X5	T37.1X6
Etamiphyllin	T48.6X1	T48.6X2	T48.6X3	T48.6X4	T48.6X5	T48.6X6
Etamivan	T50.7X1	T50.7X2	T50.7X3	T50.7X4	T50.7X5	T50.7X6
Etamsylate	T45.7X1	T45.7X2	T45.7X3	T45.7X4	T45.7X5	T45.7X6
Etebenecid	T50.4X1	T50.4X2	T50.4X3	T50.4X4	T50.4X5	T50.4X6
Ethacridine	T49.0X1	T49.0X2	T49.0X3	T49.0X4	T49.0X5	T49.0X6
Ethacrynic acid	T50.1X1	T50.1X2	T50.1X3	T50.1X4	T50.1X5	T50.1X6
Ethadione	T42.2X1	T42.2X2	T42.2X3	T42.2X4	T42.2X5	T42.2X6
Ethambutol	T37.1X1	T37.1X2	T37.1X3	T37.1X4	T37.1X5	T37.1X6
Ethamide	T50.2X1	T50.2X2	T50.2X3	T50.2X4	T50.2X5	T50.2X6
Ethamivan	T50.7X1	T50.7X2	T50.7X3	T50.7X4	T50.7X5	T50.7X6
Ethamsylate	T45.7X1	T45.7X2	T45.7X3	T45.7X4	T45.7X5	T45.7X6
Ethanol	T51.0X1	T51.0X2	T51.0X3	T51.0X4	--	--
beverage	T51.0X1	T51.0X2	T51.0X3	T51.0X4	--	--
Ethanolamine oleate	T46.8X1	T46.8X2	T46.8X3	T46.8X4	T46.8X5	T46.8X6
Ethaverine	T44.3X1	T44.3X2	T44.3X3	T44.3X4	T44.3X5	T44.3X6
Ethchlorvynol	T42.6X1	T42.6X2	T42.6X3	T42.6X4	T42.6X5	T42.6X6
Ethebenecid	T50.4X1	T50.4X2	T50.4X3	T50.4X4	T50.4X5	T50.4X6
Ether (vapor)	T41.0X1	T41.0X2	T41.0X3	T41.0X4	T41.0X5	T41.0X6
anesthetic	T41.0X1	T41.0X2	T41.0X3	T41.0X4	T41.0X5	T41.0X6
divinyl	T41.0X1	T41.0X2	T41.0X3	T41.0X4	T41.0X5	T41.0X6
ethyl (medicinal)	T41.0X1	T41.0X2	T41.0X3	T41.0X4	T41.0X5	T41.0X6
nonmedicinal	T52.8X1	T52.8X2	T52.8X3	T52.8X4	--	--
petroleum—see Ligroin						
solvent	T52.8X1	T52.8X2	T52.8X3	T52.8X4	--	--
Ethiazide	T50.2X1	T50.2X2	T50.2X3	T50.2X4	T50.2X5	T50.2X6
Ethidium chloride (vapor)	T59.891	T59.892	T59.893	T59.894	--	--
Ethinamate	T42.6X1	T42.6X2	T42.6X3	T42.6X4	T42.6X5	T42.6X6
Ethinylestradiol, ethinyloestradiol	T38.5X1	T38.5X2	T38.5X3	T38.5X4	T38.5X5	T38.5X6
with						
levonorgestrel	T38.4X1	T38.4X2	T38.4X3	T38.4X4	T38.4X5	T38.4X6

Substance	Poisoning, Accidental (unintentional)	Poisoning, Intentional Self-harm	Poisoning, Assault	Poisoning, Undetermined	Adverse effect	Underdosing
norethisterone	T38.4X1	T38.4X2	T38.4X3	T38.4X4	T38.4X5	T38.4X6
Ethiodized oil (131 I)	T50.8X1	T50.8X2	T50.8X3	T50.8X4	T50.8X5	T50.8X6
Ethion	T60.0X1	T60.0X2	T60.0X3	T60.0X4	--	--
Ethionamide	T37.1X1	T37.1X2	T37.1X3	T37.1X4	T37.1X5	T37.1X6
Ethioniamide	T37.1X1	T37.1X2	T37.1X3	T37.1X4	T37.1X5	T37.1X6
Ethisterone	T38.5X1	T38.5X2	T38.5X3	T38.5X4	T38.5X5	T38.5X6
Ethobral	T42.3X1	T42.3X2	T42.3X3	T42.3X4	T42.3X5	T42.3X6
Ethocaine (infiltration) (topical)	T41.3X1	T41.3X2	T41.3X3	T41.3X4	T41.3X5	T41.3X6
nerve block (peripheral) (plexus)	T41.3X1	T41.3X2	T41.3X3	T41.3X4	T41.3X5	T41.3X6
spinal	T41.3X1	T41.3X2	T41.3X3	T41.3X4	T41.3X5	T41.3X6
Ethoheptazine	T40.4X1	T40.4X2	T40.4X3	T40.4X4	T40.4X5	T40.4X6
Ethopropazine	T44.3X1	T44.3X2	T44.3X3	T44.3X4	T44.3X5	T44.3X6
Ethosuximide	T42.2X1	T42.2X2	T42.2X3	T42.2X4	T42.2X5	T42.2X6
Ethotoin	T42.0X1	T42.0X2	T42.0X3	T42.0X4	T42.0X5	T42.0X6
Ethoxazene	T37.91	T37.92	T37.93	T37.94	T37.95	T37.96
Ethoxazorutoside	T46.991	T46.992	T46.993	T46.994	T46.995	T46.996
2-Ethoxyethanol	T52.3X1	T52.3X2	T52.3X3	T52.3X4	--	--
Ethoxzolamide	T50.2X1	T50.2X2	T50.2X3	T50.2X4	T50.2X5	T50.2X6
Ethyl						
acetate	T52.8X1	T52.8X2	T52.8X3	T52.8X4	--	--
alcohol	T51.0X1	T51.0X2	T51.0X3	T51.0X4	--	--
beverage	T51.0X1	T51.0X2	T51.0X3	T51.0X4	--	--
aldehyde (vapor)	T59.891	T59.892	T59.893	T59.894	--	--
liquid	T52.8X1	T52.8X2	T52.8X3	T52.8X4	--	--
aminobenzoate	T41.3X1	T41.3X2	T41.3X3	T41.3X4	T41.3X5	T41.3X6
aminophenothiazine	T43.3X1	T43.3X2	T43.3X3	T43.3X4	T43.3X5	T43.3X6
benzoate	T52.8X1	T52.8X2	T52.8X3	T52.8X4	--	--
biscoumacetate	T45.511	T45.512	T45.513	T45.514	T45.515	T45.516
bromide (anesthetic)	T41.0X1	T41.0X2	T41.0X3	T41.0X4	T41.0X5	T41.0X6
carbamate	T45.1X1	T45.1X2	T45.1X3	T45.1X4	T45.1X5	T45.1X6
carbinol	T51.3X1	T51.3X2	T51.3X3	T51.3X4	--	--
carbonate	T52.8X1	T52.8X2	T52.8X3	T52.8X4	--	--
chaulmoograte	T37.1X1	T37.1X2	T37.1X3	T37.1X4	T37.1X5	T37.1X6
chloride (anesthetic)	T41.0X1	T41.0X2	T41.0X3	T41.0X4	T41.0X5	T41.0X6
anesthetic (local)	T41.3X1	T41.3X2	T41.3X3	T41.3X4	T41.3X5	T41.3X6
inhaled	T41.0X1	T41.0X2	T41.0X3	T41.0X4	T41.0X5	T41.0X6
local	T49.4X1	T49.4X2	T49.4X3	T49.4X4	T49.4X5	T49.4X6
solvent	T53.6X1	T53.6X2	T53.6X3	T53.6X4	--	--
dibunate	T48.3X1	T48.3X2	T48.3X3	T48.3X4	T48.3X5	T48.3X6
dichloroarsine (vapor)	T57.0X1	T57.0X2	T57.0X3	T57.0X4	--	--
estranol	T38.7X1	T38.7X2	T38.7X3	T38.7X4	T38.7X5	T38.7X6
ether—see also ether	T52.8X1	T52.8X2	T52.8X3	T52.8X4	--	--
formate NEC (solvent)	T52.0X1	T52.0X2	T52.0X3	T52.0X4	--	--
fumarate	T49.4X1	T49.4X2	T49.4X3	T49.4X4	T49.4X5	T49.4X6
hydroxyisobutyrate NEC (solvent)	T52.8X1	T52.8X2	T52.8X3	T52.8X4	--	--
iodoacetate	T59.3X1	T59.3X2	T59.3X3	T59.3X4	--	--
lactate NEC (solvent)	T52.8X1	T52.8X2	T52.8X3	T52.8X4	--	--
loflazepate	T42.4X1	T42.4X2	T42.4X3	T42.4X4	T42.4X5	T42.4X6
mercuric chloride	T56.1X1	T56.1X2	T56.1X3	T56.1X4	--	--
methylcarbinol	T51.8X1	T51.8X2	T51.8X3	T51.8X4	--	--
morphine	T40.2X1	T40.2X2	T40.2X3	T40.2X4	T40.2X5	T40.2X6
noradrenaline	T48.6X1	T48.6X2	T48.6X3	T48.6X4	T48.6X5	T48.6X6
oxybutyrate NEC (solvent)	T52.8X1	T52.8X2	T52.8X3	T52.8X4	--	--
Ethylene (gas)	T59.891	T59.892	T59.893	T59.894	--	--
anesthetic (general)	T41.0X1	T41.0X2	T41.0X3	T41.0X4	T41.0X5	T41.0X6
chlorohydrin	T52.8X1	T52.8X2	T52.8X3	T52.8X4	--	--
vapor	T53.6X1	T53.6X2	T53.6X3	T53.6X4	--	--
dichloride	T52.8X1	T52.8X2	T52.8X3	T52.8X4	--	--
vapor	T53.6X1	T53.6X2	T53.6X3	T53.6X4	--	--
dinitrate	T52.3X1	T52.3X2	T52.3X3	T52.3X4	--	--
glycol (s)	T52.8X1	T52.8X2	T52.8X3	T52.8X4	--	--
dinitrate	T52.3X1	T52.3X2	T52.3X3	T52.3X4	--	--
monobutyl ether	T52.3X1	T52.3X2	T52.3X3	T52.3X4	--	--
imine	T54.1X1	T54.1X2	T54.1X3	T54.1X4	--	--

Substance	Poisoning, Accidental (unintentional)	Poisoning, Intentional Self-harm	Poisoning, Assault	Poisoning, Undetermined	Adverse effect	Underdosing
oxide (fumigant) (nonmedicinal)	T59.891	T59.892	T59.893	T59.894	--	--
medicinal	T49.0X1	T49.0X2	T49.0X3	T49.0X4	T49.0X5	T49.0X6
Ethylenediamine theophylline	T48.6X1	T48.6X2	T48.6X3	T48.6X4	T48.6X5	T48.6X6
Ethylenediaminetetra-acetic acid	T50.6X1	T50.6X2	T50.6X3	T50.6X4	T50.6X5	T50.6X6
Ethylenedinitrilotetra-acetate	T50.6X1	T50.6X2	T50.6X3	T50.6X4	T50.6X5	T50.6X6
Ethylestrenol	T38.7X1	T38.7X2	T38.7X3	T38.7X4	T38.7X5	T38.7X6
Ethylhydroxycellulose	T47.4X1	T47.4X2	T47.4X3	T47.4X4	T47.4X5	T47.4X6
Ethylidene						
chloride NEC	T53.6X1	T53.6X2	T53.6X3	T53.6X4	--	--
diacetate	T60.3X1	T60.3X2	T60.3X3	T60.3X4	--	--
dicoumarin	T45.511	T45.512	T45.513	T45.514	T45.515	T45.516
dicoumarol	T45.511	T45.512	T45.513	T45.514	T45.515	T45.516
diethyl ether	T52.0X1	T52.0X2	T52.0X3	T52.0X4	--	--
Ethylmorphine	T40.2X1	T40.2X2	T40.2X3	T40.2X4	T40.2X5	T40.2X6
Ethylnorepinephrine	T48.6X1	T48.6X2	T48.6X3	T48.6X4	T48.6X5	T48.6X6
Ethylparachlorophen-oxyisobutyrate	T46.6X1	T46.6X2	T46.6X3	T46.6X4	T46.6X5	T46.6X6
Ethynodiol	T38.4X1	T38.4X2	T38.4X3	T38.4X4	T38.4X5	T38.4X6
with mestranol diacetate	T38.4X1	T38.4X2	T38.4X3	T38.4X4	T38.4X5	T38.4X6
Etidocaine	T41.3X1	T41.3X2	T41.3X3	T41.3X4	T41.3X5	T41.3X6
infiltration (subcutaneous)	T41.3X1	T41.3X2	T41.3X3	T41.3X4	T41.3X5	T41.3X6
nerve (peripheral) (plexus)	T41.3X1	T41.3X2	T41.3X3	T41.3X4	T41.3X5	T41.3X6
Etidronate	T50.991	T50.992	T50.993	T50.994	T50.995	T50.996
Etidronic acid (disodium salt)	T50.991	T50.992	T50.993	T50.994	T50.995	T50.996
Etifoxine	T42.6X1	T42.6X2	T42.6X3	T42.6X4	T42.6X5	T42.6X6
Etilefrine	T44.4X1	T44.4X2	T44.4X3	T44.4X4	T44.4X5	T44.4X6
Etilfen	T42.3X1	T42.3X2	T42.3X3	T42.3X4	T42.3X5	T42.3X6
Etinodiol	T38.4X1	T38.4X2	T38.4X3	T38.4X4	T38.4X5	T38.4X6
Etiroxate	T46.6X1	T46.6X2	T46.6X3	T46.6X4	T46.6X5	T46.6X6
Etizolam	T42.4X1	T42.4X2	T42.4X3	T42.4X4	T42.4X5	T42.4X6
Etodolac	T39.391	T39.392	T39.393	T39.394	T39.395	T39.396
Etofamide	T37.3X1	T37.3X2	T37.3X3	T37.3X4	T37.3X5	T37.3X6
Etofibrate	T46.6X1	T46.6X2	T46.6X3	T46.6X4	T46.6X5	T46.6X6
Etofylline	T46.7X1	T46.7X2	T46.7X3	T46.7X4	T46.7X5	T46.7X6
clofibrate	T46.6X1	T46.6X2	T46.6X3	T46.6X4	T46.6X5	T46.6X6
Etoglucid	T45.1X1	T45.1X2	T45.1X3	T45.1X4	T45.1X5	T45.1X6
Etomidate	T41.1X1	T41.1X2	T41.1X3	T41.1X4	T41.1X5	T41.1X6
Etomide	T39.8X1	T39.8X2	T39.8X3	T39.8X4	T39.8X5	T39.8X6
Etomidoline	T44.3X1	T44.3X2	T44.3X3	T44.3X4	T44.3X5	T44.3X6
Etoposide	T45.1X1	T45.1X2	T45.1X3	T45.1X4	T45.1X5	T45.1X6
Etorphine	T40.2X1	T40.2X2	T40.2X3	T40.2X4	T40.2X5	T40.2X6
Etoval	T42.3X1	T42.3X2	T42.3X3	T42.3X4	T42.3X5	T42.3X6
Etozolin	T50.1X1	T50.1X2	T50.1X3	T50.1X4	T50.1X5	T50.1X6
Etretinate	T50.991	T50.992	T50.993	T50.994	T50.995	T50.996
Etryptamine	T43.691	T43.692	T43.693	T43.694	T43.695	T43.696
Etybenzatropine	T44.3X1	T44.3X2	T44.3X3	T44.3X4	T44.3X5	T44.3X6
Etynodiol	T38.4X1	T38.4X2	T38.4X3	T38.4X4	T38.4X5	T38.4X6
Eucaine	T41.3X1	T41.3X2	T41.3X3	T41.3X4	T41.3X5	T41.3X6
Eucalyptus oil	T49.7X1	T49.7X2	T49.7X3	T49.7X4	T49.7X5	T49.7X6
Eucatropine	T49.5X1	T49.5X2	T49.5X3	T49.5X4	T49.5X5	T49.5X6
Eucodal	T40.2X1	T40.2X2	T40.2X3	T40.2X4	T40.2X5	T40.2X6
Euneryl	T42.3X1	T42.3X2	T42.3X3	T42.3X4	T42.3X5	T42.3X6
Euphthalmine	T44.3X1	T44.3X2	T44.3X3	T44.3X4	T44.3X5	T44.3X6
Eurax	T49.0X1	T49.0X2	T49.0X3	T49.0X4	T49.0X5	T49.0X6
Euresol	T49.4X1	T49.4X2	T49.4X3	T49.4X4	T49.4X5	T49.4X6
Euthroid	T38.1X1	T38.1X2	T38.1X3	T38.1X4	T38.1X5	T38.1X6
Evans blue	T50.8X1	T50.8X2	T50.8X3	T50.8X4	T50.8X5	T50.8X6
Evipal	T42.3X1	T42.3X2	T42.3X3	T42.3X4	T42.3X5	T42.3X6
sodium	T41.1X1	T41.1X2	T41.1X3	T41.1X4	T41.1X5	T41.1X6
Evipan	T42.3X1	T42.3X2	T42.3X3	T42.3X4	T42.3X5	T42.3X6
sodium	T41.1X1	T41.1X2	T41.1X3	T41.1X4	T41.1X5	T41.1X6
Exalamide	T49.0X1	T49.0X2	T49.0X3	T49.0X4	T49.0X5	T49.0X6
Exalgin	T39.1X1	T39.1X2	T39.1X3	T39.1X4	T39.1X5	T39.1X6
Excipients, pharmaceutical	T50.901	T50.902	T50.903	T50.904	T50.905	T50.906
Exhaust gas (engine) (motor vehicle)	T58.01	T58.02	T58.03	T58.04	--	--
Ex-Lax (phenolphthalein)	T47.2X1	T47.2X2	T47.2X3	T47.2X4	T47.2X5	T47.2X6

Substance	Poisoning, Accidental (unintentional)	Poisoning, Intentional Self-harm	Poisoning, Assault	Poisoning, Undetermined	Adverse effect	Underdosing
Expectorant NEC	T48.4X1	T48.4X2	T48.4X3	T48.4X4	T48.4X5	T48.4X6
Extended insulin zinc suspension	T38.3X1	T38.3X2	T38.3X3	T38.3X4	T38.3X5	T38.3X6
External medications (skin) (mucous membrane)	T49.91	T49.92	T49.93	T49.94	T49.95	T49.96
dental agent	T49.7X1	T49.7X2	T49.7X3	T49.7X4	T49.7X5	T49.7X6
ENT agent	T49.6X1	T49.6X2	T49.6X3	T49.6X4	T49.6X5	T49.6X6
ophthalmic preparation	T49.5X1	T49.5X2	T49.5X3	T49.5X4	T49.5X5	T49.5X6
specified NEC	T49.8X1	T49.8X2	T49.8X3	T49.8X4	T49.8X5	T49.8X6
Extrapyramidal antagonist NEC	T44.3X1	T44.3X2	T44.3X3	T44.3X4	T44.3X5	T44.3X6
Eye agents (anti-infective)	T49.5X1	T49.5X2	T49.5X3	T49.5X4	T49.5X5	T49.5X6
Eye drug NEC	T49.5X1	T49.5X2	T49.5X3	T49.5X4	T49.5X5	T49.5X6
FAC (fluorouracil + doxorubicin + cyclophosphamide)	T45.1X1	T45.1X2	T45.1X3	T45.1X4	T45.1X5	T45.1X6
Factor						
I (fibrinogen)	T45.8X1	T45.8X2	T45.8X3	T45.8X4	T45.8X5	T45.8X6
III (thromboplastin)	T45.8X1	T45.8X2	T45.8X3	T45.8X4	T45.8X5	T45.8X6
VIII (antihemophilic Factor) (concentrate)	T45.8X1	T45.8X2	T45.8X3	T45.8X4	T45.8X5	T45.8X6
IX complex	T45.7X1	T45.7X2	T45.7X3	T45.7X4	T45.7X5	T45.7X6
human	T45.8X1	T45.8X2	T45.8X3	T45.8X4	T45.8X5	T45.8X6
Famotidine	T47.0X1	T47.0X2	T47.0X3	T47.0X4	T47.0X5	T47.0X6
Fat suspension, intravenous	T50.991	T50.992	T50.993	T50.994	T50.995	T50.996
Fazadinium bromide	T48.1X1	T48.1X2	T48.1X3	T48.1X4	T48.1X5	T48.1X6
Febarbamate	T42.3X1	T42.3X2	T42.3X3	T42.3X4	T42.3X5	T42.3X6
Fecal softener	T47.4X1	T47.4X2	T47.4X3	T47.4X4	T47.4X5	T47.4X6
Fedrilate	T48.3X1	T48.3X2	T48.3X3	T48.3X4	T48.3X5	T48.3X6
Felodipine	T46.1X1	T46.1X2	T46.1X3	T46.1X4	T46.1X5	T46.1X6
Felypressin	T38.891	T38.892	T38.893	T38.894	T38.895	T38.896
Femoxetine	T43.221	T43.222	T43.223	T43.224	T43.225	T43.226
Fenalcomine	T46.3X1	T46.3X2	T46.3X3	T46.3X4	T46.3X5	T46.3X6
Fenamisal	T37.1X1	T37.1X2	T37.1X3	T37.1X4	T37.1X5	T37.1X6
Fenazone	T39.2X1	T39.2X2	T39.2X3	T39.2X4	T39.2X5	T39.2X6
Fenbendazole	T37.4X1	T37.4X2	T37.4X3	T37.4X4	T37.4X5	T37.4X6
Fenbutrazate	T50.5X1	T50.5X2	T50.5X3	T50.5X4	T50.5X5	T50.5X6
Fencamfamine	T43.691	T43.692	T43.693	T43.694	T43.695	T43.696
Fendiline	T46.1X1	T46.1X2	T46.1X3	T46.1X4	T46.1X5	T46.1X6
Fenetylline	T43.691	T43.692	T43.693	T43.694	T43.695	T43.696
Fenflumizole	T39.391	T39.392	T39.393	T39.394	T39.395	T39.396
Fenfluramine	T50.5X1	T50.5X2	T50.5X3	T50.5X4	T50.5X5	T50.5X6
Fenobarbital	T42.3X1	T42.3X2	T42.3X3	T42.3X4	T42.3X5	T42.3X6
Fenofibrate	T46.6X1	T46.6X2	T46.6X3	T46.6X4	T46.6X5	T46.6X6
Fenoprofen	T39.311	T39.312	T39.313	T39.314	T39.315	T39.316
Fenoterol	T48.6X1	T48.6X2	T48.6X3	T48.6X4	T48.6X5	T48.6X6
Fenoverine	T44.3X1	T44.3X2	T44.3X3	T44.3X4	T44.3X5	T44.3X6
Fenoxazoline	T48.5X1	T48.5X2	T48.5X3	T48.5X4	T48.5X5	T48.5X6
Fenproporex	T50.5X1	T50.5X2	T50.5X3	T50.5X4	T50.5X5	T50.5X6
Fenquizone	T50.2X1	T50.2X2	T50.2X3	T50.2X4	T50.2X5	T50.2X6
Fentanyl	T40.4X1	T40.4X2	T40.4X3	T40.4X4	T40.4X5	T40.4X6
Fentazin	T43.3X1	T43.3X2	T43.3X3	T43.3X4	T43.3X5	T43.3X6
Fenthion	T60.0X1	T60.0X2	T60.0X3	T60.0X4	--	--
Fenticlor	T49.0X1	T49.0X2	T49.0X3	T49.0X4	T49.0X5	T49.0X6
Fenylbutazone	T39.2X1	T39.2X2	T39.2X3	T39.2X4	T39.2X5	T39.2X6
Feprazone	T39.2X1	T39.2X2	T39.2X3	T39.2X4	T39.2X5	T39.2X6
Fer de lance (bite) (venom)	T63.061	T63.062	T63.063	T63.064	--	--
Ferric—see also Iron						
chloride	T45.4X1	T45.4X2	T45.4X3	T45.4X4	T45.4X5	T45.4X6
citrate	T45.4X1	T45.4X2	T45.4X3	T45.4X4	T45.4X5	T45.4X6
hydroxide						
colloidal	T45.4X1	T45.4X2	T45.4X3	T45.4X4	T45.4X5	T45.4X6
polymaltose	T45.4X1	T45.4X2	T45.4X3	T45.4X4	T45.4X5	T45.4X6
pyrophosphate	T45.4X1	T45.4X2	T45.4X3	T45.4X4	T45.4X5	T45.4X6
Ferritin	T45.4X1	T45.4X2	T45.4X3	T45.4X4	T45.4X5	T45.4X6
Ferrocholinate	T45.4X1	T45.4X2	T45.4X3	T45.4X4	T45.4X5	T45.4X6
Ferrodextrane	T45.4X1	T45.4X2	T45.4X3	T45.4X4	T45.4X5	T45.4X6
Ferropolimaler	T45.4X1	T45.4X2	T45.4X3	T45.4X4	T45.4X5	T45.4X6

Substance	Poisoning, Accidental (unintentional)	Poisoning, Intentional Self-harm	Poisoning, Assault	Poisoning, Undetermined	Adverse effect	Underdosing
Ferrous—see also Iron						
phosphate	T45.4X1	T45.4X2	T45.4X3	T45.4X4	T45.4X5	T45.4X6
salt	T45.4X1	T45.4X2	T45.4X3	T45.4X4	T45.4X5	T45.4X6
with folic acid	T45.4X1	T45.4X2	T45.4X3	T45.4X4	T45.4X5	T45.4X6
Ferrous fumerate, gluconate, lactate, salt NEC, sulfate (medicinal)	T45.4X1	T45.4X2	T45.4X3	T45.4X4	T45.4X5	T45.4X6
Ferrovanadium (fumes)	T59.891	T59.892	T59.893	T59.894	--	--
Ferrum—see Iron						
Fertilizers NEC	T65.891	T65.892	T65.893	T65.894	--	--
with herbicide mixture	T60.3X1	T60.3X2	T60.3X3	T60.3X4	--	--
Fetoxilate	T47.6X1	T47.6X2	T47.6X3	T47.6X4	T47.6X5	T47.6X6
Fiber, dietary	T47.4X1	T47.4X2	T47.4X3	T47.4X4	T47.4X5	T47.4X6
Fiberglass	T65.831	T65.832	T65.833	T65.834	--	--
Fibrinogen (human)	T45.8X1	T45.8X2	T45.8X3	T45.8X4	T45.8X5	T45.8X6
Fibrinolysin (human)	T45.691	T45.692	T45.693	T45.694	T45.695	T45.696
Fibrinolysis						
affecting drug	T45.601	T45.602	T45.603	T45.604	T45.605	T45.606
inhibitor NEC	T45.621	T45.622	T45.623	T45.624	T45.625	T45.626
Fibrinolytic drug	T45.611	T45.612	T45.613	T45.614	T45.615	T45.616
Filix mas	T37.4X1	T37.4X2	T37.4X3	T37.4X4	T37.4X5	T37.4X6
Filtering cream	T49.3X1	T49.3X2	T49.3X3	T49.3X4	T49.3X5	T49.3X6
Fiorinal	T39.011	T39.012	T39.013	T39.014	T39.015	T39.016
Firedamp	T59.891	T59.892	T59.893	T59.894	--	--
Fish, noxious, nonbacterial	T61.91	T61.92	T61.93	T61.94	--	--
ciguatera	T61.01	T61.02	T61.03	T61.04	--	--
scombroid	T61.11	T61.12	T61.13	T61.14	--	--
shell	T61.781	T61.782	T61.783	T61.784	--	--
specified NEC	T61.771	T61.772	T61.773	T61.774	--	--
Flagyl	T37.3X1	T37.3X2	T37.3X3	T37.3X4	T37.3X5	T37.3X6
Flavine adenine dinucleotide	T45.2X1	T45.2X2	T45.2X3	T45.2X4	T45.2X5	T45.2X6
Flavodic acid	T46.991	T46.992	T46.993	T46.994	T46.995	T46.996
Flavoxate	T44.3X1	T44.3X2	T44.3X3	T44.3X4	T44.3X5	T44.3X6
Flaxedil	T48.1X1	T48.1X2	T48.1X3	T48.1X4	T48.1X5	T48.1X6
Flaxseed (medicinal)	T49.3X1	T49.3X2	T49.3X3	T49.3X4	T49.3X5	T49.3X6
Flecainide	T46.2X1	T46.2X2	T46.2X3	T46.2X4	T46.2X5	T46.2X6
Fleroxacin	T36.8X1	T36.8X2	T36.8X3	T36.8X4	T36.8X5	T36.8X6
Floctafenine	T39.8X1	T39.8X2	T39.8X3	T39.8X4	T39.8X5	T39.8X6
Flomax	T44.6X1	T44.6X2	T44.6X3	T44.6X4	T44.6X5	T44.6X6
Flomoxef	T36.1X1	T36.1X2	T36.1X3	T36.1X4	T36.1X5	T36.1X6
Flopropione	T44.3X1	T44.3X2	T44.3X3	T44.3X4	T44.3X5	T44.3X6
Florantyrone	T47.5X1	T47.5X2	T47.5X3	T47.5X4	T47.5X5	T47.5X6
Floraquin	T37.8X1	T37.8X2	T37.8X3	T37.8X4	T37.8X5	T37.8X6
Florinef	T38.0X1	T38.0X2	T38.0X3	T38.0X4	T38.0X5	T38.0X6
ENT agent	T49.6X1	T49.6X2	T49.6X3	T49.6X4	T49.6X5	T49.6X6
ophthalmic preparation	T49.5X1	T49.5X2	T49.5X3	T49.5X4	T49.5X5	T49.5X6
topical NEC	T49.0X1	T49.0X2	T49.0X3	T49.0X4	T49.0X5	T49.0X6
Flowers of sulfur	T49.4X1	T49.4X2	T49.4X3	T49.4X4	T49.4X5	T49.4X6
Floxuridine	T45.1X1	T45.1X2	T45.1X3	T45.1X4	T45.1X5	T45.1X6
Fluanisone	T43.4X1	T43.4X2	T43.4X3	T43.4X4	T43.4X5	T43.4X6
Flubendazole	T37.4X1	T37.4X2	T37.4X3	T37.4X4	T37.4X5	T37.4X6
Fluclorolone acetonide	T49.0X1	T49.0X2	T49.0X3	T49.0X4	T49.0X5	T49.0X6
Flucloxacillin	T36.0X1	T36.0X2	T36.0X3	T36.0X4	T36.0X5	T36.0X6
Fluconazole	T37.8X1	T37.8X2	T37.8X3	T37.8X4	T37.8X5	T37.8X6
Flucytosine	T37.8X1	T37.8X2	T37.8X3	T37.8X4	T37.8X5	T37.8X6
Fludeoxyglucose (18F)	T50.8X1	T50.8X2	T50.8X3	T50.8X4	T50.8X5	T50.8X6
Fludiazepam	T42.4X1	T42.4X2	T42.4X3	T42.4X4	T42.4X5	T42.4X6
Fludrocortisone	T50.0X1	T50.0X2	T50.0X3	T50.0X4	T50.0X5	T50.0X6
ENT agent	T49.6X1	T49.6X2	T49.6X3	T49.6X4	T49.6X5	T49.6X6
ophthalmic preparation	T49.5X1	T49.5X2	T49.5X3	T49.5X4	T49.5X5	T49.5X6
topical NEC	T49.0X1	T49.0X2	T49.0X3	T49.0X4	T49.0X5	T49.0X6
Fludroxycortide	T49.0X1	T49.0X2	T49.0X3	T49.0X4	T49.0X5	T49.0X6
Flufenamic acid	T39.391	T39.392	T39.393	T39.394	T39.395	T39.396
Fluindione	T45.511	T45.512	T45.513	T45.514	T45.515	T45.516
Flumequine	T37.8X1	T37.8X2	T37.8X3	T37.8X4	T37.8X5	T37.8X6
Flumethasone	T49.0X1	T49.0X2	T49.0X3	T49.0X4	T49.0X5	T49.0X6

Substance	Poisoning, Accidental (unintentional)	Poisoning, Intentional Self-harm	Poisoning, Assault	Poisoning, Undetermined	Adverse effect	Underdosing
Flumethiazide	T50.2X1	T50.2X2	T50.2X3	T50.2X4	T50.2X5	T50.2X6
Flumidin	T37.5X1	T37.5X2	T37.5X3	T37.5X4	T37.5X5	T37.5X6
Flunarizine	T46.7X1	T46.7X2	T46.7X3	T46.7X4	T46.7X5	T46.7X6
Flunidazole	T37.8X1	T37.8X2	T37.8X3	T37.8X4	T37.8X5	T37.8X6
Flunisolide	T48.6X1	T48.6X2	T48.6X3	T48.6X4	T48.6X5	T48.6X6
Flunitrazepam	T42.4X1	T42.4X2	T42.4X3	T42.4X4	T42.4X5	T42.4X6
Fluocinolone (acetonide)	T49.0X1	T49.0X2	T49.0X3	T49.0X4	T49.0X5	T49.0X6
Fluocinonide	T49.0X1	T49.0X2	T49.0X3	T49.0X4	T49.0X5	T49.0X6
Fluocortin (butyl)	T49.0X1	T49.0X2	T49.0X3	T49.0X4	T49.0X5	T49.0X6
Fluocortolone	T49.0X1	T49.0X2	T49.0X3	T49.0X4	T49.0X5	T49.0X6
Fluohydrocortisone	T38.0X1	T38.0X2	T38.0X3	T38.0X4	T38.0X5	T38.0X6
ENT agent	T49.6X1	T49.6X2	T49.6X3	T49.6X4	T49.6X5	T49.6X6
ophthalmic preparation	T49.5X1	T49.5X2	T49.5X3	T49.5X4	T49.5X5	T49.5X6
topical NEC	T49.0X1	T49.0X2	T49.0X3	T49.0X4	T49.0X5	T49.0X6
Fluonid	T49.0X1	T49.0X2	T49.0X3	T49.0X4	T49.0X5	T49.0X6
Fluopromazine	T43.3X1	T43.3X2	T43.3X3	T43.3X4	T43.3X5	T43.3X6
Fluoracetate	T60.8X1	T60.8X2	T60.8X3	T60.8X4	--	--
Fluorescein	T50.8X1	T50.8X2	T50.8X3	T50.8X4	T50.8X5	T50.8X6
Fluorhydrocortisone	T50.0X1	T50.0X2	T50.0X3	T50.0X4	T50.0X5	T50.0X6
Fluoride (nonmedicinal) (pesticide) (sodium) NEC	T60.8X1	T60.8X2	T60.8X3	T60.8X4	--	--
hydrogen—see Hydrofluoric acid						
medicinal NEC	T50.991	T50.992	T50.993	T50.994	T50.995	T50.996
dental use	T49.7X1	T49.7X2	T49.7X3	T49.7X4	T49.7X5	T49.7X6
not pesticide NEC	T54.91	T54.92	T54.93	T54.94	--	--
stannous	T49.7X1	T49.7X2	T49.7X3	T49.7X4	T49.7X5	T49.7X6
Fluorinated corticosteroids	T38.0X1	T38.0X2	T38.0X3	T38.0X4	T38.0X5	T38.0X6
Fluorine (gas)	T59.5X1	T59.5X2	T59.5X3	T59.5X4	--	--
salt—see Fluoride (s)						
Fluoristan	T49.7X1	T49.7X2	T49.7X3	T49.7X4	T49.7X5	T49.7X6
Fluormetholone	T49.0X1	T49.0X2	T49.0X3	T49.0X4	T49.0X5	T49.0X6
Fluoroacetate	T60.8X1	T60.8X2	T60.8X3	T60.8X4	--	--
Fluorocarbon monomer	T53.6X1	T53.6X2	T53.6X3	T53.6X4	--	--
Fluorocytosine	T37.8X1	T37.8X2	T37.8X3	T37.8X4	T37.8X5	T37.8X6
Fluorodeoxyuridine	T45.1X1	T45.1X2	T45.1X3	T45.1X4	T45.1X5	T45.1X6
Fluorometholone	T49.0X1	T49.0X2	T49.0X3	T49.0X4	T49.0X5	T49.0X6
Fluorophosphate insecticide	T60.0X1	T60.0X2	T60.0X3	T60.0X4	--	--
Fluorosol	T46.3X1	T46.3X2	T46.3X3	T46.3X4	T46.3X5	T46.3X6
Fluorouracil	T45.1X1	T45.1X2	T45.1X3	T45.1X4	T45.1X5	T45.1X6
Fluorphenylalanine	T49.5X1	T49.5X2	T49.5X3	T49.5X4	T49.5X5	T49.5X6
Fluothane	T41.0X1	T41.0X2	T41.0X3	T41.0X4	T41.0X5	T41.0X6
Fluoxetine	T43.221	T43.222	T43.223	T43.224	T43.225	T43.226
Fluoxymesterone	T38.7X1	T38.7X2	T38.7X3	T38.7X4	T38.7X5	T38.7X6
Flupenthixol	T43.4X1	T43.4X2	T43.4X3	T43.4X4	T43.4X5	T43.4X6
Flupentixol	T43.4X1	T43.4X2	T43.4X3	T43.4X4	T43.4X5	T43.4X6
Fluphenazine	T43.3X1	T43.3X2	T43.3X3	T43.3X4	T43.3X5	T43.3X6
Fluprednidene	T49.0X1	T49.0X2	T49.0X3	T49.0X4	T49.0X5	T49.0X6
Fluprednisolone	T38.0X1	T38.0X2	T38.0X3	T38.0X4	T38.0X5	T38.0X6
Fluradoline	T39.8X1	T39.8X2	T39.8X3	T39.8X4	T39.8X5	T39.8X6
Flurandrenolide	T49.0X1	T49.0X2	T49.0X3	T49.0X4	T49.0X5	T49.0X6
Flurandrenolone	T49.0X1	T49.0X2	T49.0X3	T49.0X4	T49.0X5	T49.0X6
Flurazepam	T42.4X1	T42.4X2	T42.4X3	T42.4X4	T42.4X5	T42.4X6
Flurbiprofen	T39.311	T39.312	T39.313	T39.314	T39.315	T39.316
Flurobate	T49.0X1	T49.0X2	T49.0X3	T49.0X4	T49.0X5	T49.0X6
Fluroxene	T41.0X1	T41.0X2	T41.0X3	T41.0X4	T41.0X5	T41.0X6
Fluspirilene	T43.591	T43.592	T43.593	T43.594	T43.595	T43.596
Flutamide	T38.6X1	T38.6X2	T38.6X3	T38.6X4	T38.6X5	T38.6X6
Flutazolam	T42.4X1	T42.4X2	T42.4X3	T42.4X4	T42.4X5	T42.4X6
Fluticasone propionate	T49.1X1	T49.1X2	T49.1X3	T49.1X4	T49.1X5	T49.1X6
Flutoprazepam	T42.4X1	T42.4X2	T42.4X3	T42.4X4	T42.4X5	T42.4X6
Flutropium bromide	T48.6X1	T48.6X2	T48.6X3	T48.6X4	T48.6X5	T48.6X6
Fluvoxamine	T43.221	T43.222	T43.223	T43.224	T43.225	T43.226
Folacin	T45.8X1	T45.8X2	T45.8X3	T45.8X4	T45.8X5	T45.8X6
Folic acid	T45.8X1	T45.8X2	T45.8X3	T45.8X4	T45.8X5	T45.8X6

TABLE OF DRUGS AND CHEMICALS

Substance	Poisoning, Accidental (unintentional)	Poisoning, Intentional Self-harm	Poisoning, Assault	Poisoning, Undetermined	Adverse effect	Underdosing
with ferrous salt	T45.2X1	T45.2X2	T45.2X3	T45.2X4	T45.2X5	T45.2X6
antagonist	T45.1X1	T45.1X2	T45.1X3	T45.1X4	T45.1X5	T45.1X6
Folinic acid	T45.8X1	T45.8X2	T45.8X3	T45.8X4	T45.8X5	T45.8X6
Folium stramoniae	T48.6X1	T48.6X2	T48.6X3	T48.6X4	T48.6X5	T48.6X6
Follicle-stimulating hormone, human	T38.811	T38.812	T38.813	T38.814	T38.815	T38.816
Folpet	T60.3X1	T60.3X2	T60.3X3	T60.3X4	--	--
Fominoben	T48.3X1	T48.3X2	T48.3X3	T48.3X4	T48.3X5	T48.3X6
Food, foodstuffs, noxious, nonbacterial, NEC	T62.91	T62.92	T62.93	T62.94	--	--
berries	T62.1X1	T62.1X2	T62.1X3	T62.1X4	--	--
fish—see also Fish	T61.91	T61.92	T61.93	T61.94	--	--
mushrooms	T62.0X1	T62.0X2	T62.0X3	T62.0X4	--	--
plants	T62.2X1	T62.2X2	T62.2X3	T62.2X4	--	--
seafood	T61.91	T61.92	T61.93	T61.94	--	--
specified NEC	T61.8X1	T61.8X2	T61.8X3	T61.8X4	--	--
seeds	T62.2X1	T62.2X2	T62.2X3	T62.2X4	--	--
shellfish	T61.781	T61.782	T61.783	T61.784	--	--
specified NEC	T62.8X1	T62.8X2	T62.8X3	T62.8X4	--	--
Fool's parsley	T62.2X1	T62.2X2	T62.2X3	T62.2X4	--	--
Formaldehyde (solution), gas or vapor	T59.2X1	T59.2X2	T59.2X3	T59.2X4	--	--
fungicide	T60.3X1	T60.3X2	T60.3X3	T60.3X4	--	--
Formalin	T59.2X1	T59.2X2	T59.2X3	T59.2X4	--	--
fungicide	T60.3X1	T60.3X2	T60.3X3	T60.3X4	--	--
vapor	T59.2X1	T59.2X2	T59.2X3	T59.2X4	--	--
Formic acid	T54.2X1	T54.2X2	T54.2X3	T54.2X4	--	--
vapor	T59.891	T59.892	T59.893	T59.894	--	--
Foscarnet sodium	T37.5X1	T37.5X2	T37.5X3	T37.5X4	T37.5X5	T37.5X6
Fosfestrol	T38.5X1	T38.5X2	T38.5X3	T38.5X4	T38.5X5	T38.5X6
Fosfomycin	T36.8X1	T36.8X2	T36.8X3	T36.8X4	T36.8X5	T36.8X6
Fosfonet sodium	T37.5X1	T37.5X2	T37.5X3	T37.5X4	T37.5X5	T37.5X6
Fosinopril	T46.4X1	T46.4X2	T46.4X3	T46.4X4	T46.4X5	T46.4X6
sodium	T46.4X1	T46.4X2	T46.4X3	T46.4X4	T46.4X5	T46.4X6
Fowler's solution	T57.0X1	T57.0X2	T57.0X3	T57.0X4	--	--
Foxglove	T62.2X1	T62.2X2	T62.2X3	T62.2X4	--	--
Framycetin	T36.5X1	T36.5X2	T36.5X3	T36.5X4	T36.5X5	T36.5X6
Frangula	T47.2X1	T47.2X2	T47.2X3	T47.2X4	T47.2X5	T47.2X6
extract	T47.2X1	T47.2X2	T47.2X3	T47.2X4	T47.2X5	T47.2X6
Frei antigen	T50.8X1	T50.8X2	T50.8X3	T50.8X4	T50.8X5	T50.8X6
Freon	T53.5X1	T53.5X2	T53.5X3	T53.5X4	--	--
Fructose	T50.3X1	T50.3X2	T50.3X3	T50.3X4	T50.3X5	T50.3X6
Frusemide	T50.1X1	T50.1X2	T50.1X3	T50.1X4	T50.1X5	T50.1X6
FSH	T38.811	T38.812	T38.813	T38.814	T38.815	T38.816
Ftorafur	T45.1X1	T45.1X2	T45.1X3	T45.1X4	T45.1X5	T45.1X6
Fuel						
automobile	T52.0X1	T52.0X2	T52.0X3	T52.0X4	--	--
exhaust gas, not in transit	T58.01	T58.02	T58.03	T58.04	--	--
vapor NEC	T52.0X1	T52.0X2	T52.0X3	T52.0X4	--	--
gas (domestic use) —see also Carbon, monoxide, fuel, utility	T59.891	T59.892	T59.893	T59.894	--	--
utility	T59.891	T59.892	T59.893	T59.894	--	--
in mobile container	T59.891	T59.892	T59.893	T59.894	--	--
incomplete combustion of—see Carbon, monoxide, fuel, utility						
piped (natural)	T59.891	T59.892	T59.893	T59.894	--	--
industrial, incomplete combustion	T58.8X1	T58.8X2	T58.8X3	T58.8X4	--	--
Fugillin	T36.8X1	T36.8X2	T36.8X3	T36.8X4	T36.8X5	T36.8X6
Fulminate of mercury	T56.1X1	T56.1X2	T56.1X3	T56.1X4	--	--
Fulvicin	T36.7X1	T36.7X2	T36.7X3	T36.7X4	T36.7X5	T36.7X6
Fumadil	T36.8X1	T36.8X2	T36.8X3	T36.8X4	T36.8X5	T36.8X6
Fumagillin	T36.8X1	T36.8X2	T36.8X3	T36.8X4	T36.8X5	T36.8X6
Fumaric acid	T49.4X1	T49.4X2	T49.4X3	T49.4X4	T49.4X5	T49.4X6
Fumes (from)	T59.91	T59.92	T59.93	T59.94	--	--
carbon monoxide—see Carbon, monoxide						
charcoal (domestic use) —see Charcoal, fumes						
chloroform—see Chloroform						
coke (in domestic stoves, fireplaces) —see Coke						

Substance	Poisoning, Accidental (unintentional)	Poisoning, Intentional Self-harm	Poisoning, Assault	Poisoning, Undetermined	Adverse effect	Underdosing
fumes						
corrosive NEC	T54.91	T54.92	T54.93	T54.94	--	--
ether—see ether						
freons	T53.5X1	T53.5X2	T53.5X3	T53.5X4	--	--
hydrocarbons	T59.891	T59.892	T59.893	T59.894	--	--
petroleum (liquefied)	T59.891	T59.892	T59.893	T59.894	--	--
distributed through pipes (pure or mixed with air)	T59.891	T59.892	T59.893	T59.894	--	--
lead—see lead						
metal—see Metals, or the specified metal						
nitrogen dioxide	T59.0X1	T59.0X2	T59.0X3	T59.0X4	--	--
pesticides—see Pesticides						
petroleum (liquefied)	T59.891	T59.892	T59.893	T59.894	--	--
distributed through pipes (pure or mixed with air)	T59.891	T59.892	T59.893	T59.894	--	--
polyester	T59.891	T59.892	T59.893	T59.894	--	--
specified source NEC—see also substance specified	T59.891	T59.892	T59.893	T59.894	--	--
sulfur dioxide	T59.1X1	T59.1X2	T59.1X3	T59.1X4	--	--
Fumigant NEC	T60.91	T60.92	T60.93	T60.94	--	--
Fungi, noxious, used as food	T62.0X1	T62.0X2	T62.0X3	T62.0X4	--	--
Fungicide NEC (nonmedicinal)	T60.3X1	T60.3X2	T60.3X3	T60.3X4	--	--
Fungizone	T36.7X1	T36.7X2	T36.7X3	T36.7X4	T36.7X5	T36.7X6
topical	T49.0X1	T49.0X2	T49.0X3	T49.0X4	T49.0X5	T49.0X6
Furacin	T49.0X1	T49.0X2	T49.0X3	T49.0X4	T49.0X5	T49.0X6
Furadantin	T37.91	T37.92	T37.93	T37.94	T37.95	T37.96
Furazolidone	T37.8X1	T37.8X2	T37.8X3	T37.8X4	T37.8X5	T37.8X6
Furazolium chloride	T49.0X1	T49.0X2	T49.0X3	T49.0X4	T49.0X5	T49.0X6
Furfural	T52.8X1	T52.8X2	T52.8X3	T52.8X4	--	--
Furnace (coal burning) (domestic) , gas from	T58.2X1	T58.2X2	T58.2X3	T58.2X4	--	--
industrial	T58.8X1	T58.8X2	T58.8X3	T58.8X4	--	--
Furniture polish	T65.891	T65.892	T65.893	T65.894	--	--
Furosemide	T50.1X1	T50.1X2	T50.1X3	T50.1X4	T50.1X5	T50.1X6
Furoxone	T37.91	T37.92	T37.93	T37.94	T37.95	T37.96
Fursultiamine	T45.2X1	T45.2X2	T45.2X3	T45.2X4	T45.2X5	T45.2X6
Fusafungine	T36.8X1	T36.8X2	T36.8X3	T36.8X4	T36.8X5	T36.8X6
Fusel oil (any) (amyl) (butyl) (propyl) , vapor	T51.3X1	T51.3X2	T51.3X3	T51.3X4	--	--
Fusidate (ethanolamine) (sodium)	T36.8X1	T36.8X2	T36.8X3	T36.8X4	T36.8X5	T36.8X6
Fusidic acid	T36.8X1	T36.8X2	T36.8X3	T36.8X4	T36.8X5	T36.8X6
Fytic acid, nonasodium	T50.6X1	T50.6X2	T50.6X3	T50.6X4	T50.6X5	T50.6X6
GABA	T43.8X1	T43.8X2	T43.8X3	T43.8X4	T43.8X5	T43.8X6
Gadopentetic acid	T50.8X1	T50.8X2	T50.8X3	T50.8X4	T50.8X5	T50.8X6
Galactose	T50.3X1	T50.3X2	T50.3X3	T50.3X4	T50.3X5	T50.3X6
b-Galactosidase	T47.5X1	T47.5X2	T47.5X3	T47.5X4	T47.5X5	T47.5X6
Galantamine	T44.0X1	T44.0X2	T44.0X3	T44.0X4	T44.0X5	T44.0X6
Gallamine (triethiodide)	T48.1X1	T48.1X2	T48.1X3	T48.1X4	T48.1X5	T48.1X6
Gallium citrate	T50.991	T50.992	T50.993	T50.994	T50.995	T50.996
Gallopamil	T46.1X1	T46.1X2	T46.1X3	T46.1X4	T46.1X5	T46.1X6
Gamboge	T47.2X1	T47.2X2	T47.2X3	T47.2X4	T47.2X5	T47.2X6
Gamimune	T50.Z11	T50.Z12	T50.Z13	T50.Z14	T50.Z15	T50.Z16
Gamma globulin	T50.Z11	T50.Z12	T50.Z13	T50.Z14	T50.Z15	T50.Z16
Gamma-aminobutyric acid	T43.8X1	T43.8X2	T43.8X3	T43.8X4	T43.8X5	T43.8X6
Gamma-benzene hexachloride (medicinal)	T49.0X1	T49.0X2	T49.0X3	T49.0X4	T49.0X5	T49.0X6
nonmedicinal, vapor	T53.6X1	T53.6X2	T53.6X3	T53.6X4	--	--
Gamma-BHC (medicinal) —see also Gamma benzene hexachloride	T49.0X1	T49.0X2	T49.0X3	T49.0X4	T49.0X5	T49.0X6
Gamulin	T50.Z11	T50.Z12	T50.Z13	T50.Z14	T50.Z15	T50.Z16
Ganciclovir (sodium)	T37.5X1	T37.5X2	T37.5X3	T37.5X4	T37.5X5	T37.5X6
Ganglionic blocking drug NEC	T44.2X1	T44.2X2	T44.2X3	T44.2X4	T44.2X5	T44.2X6
specified NEC	T44.2X1	T44.2X2	T44.2X3	T44.2X4	T44.2X5	T44.2X6
Ganja	T40.7X1	T40.7X2	T40.7X3	T40.7X4	T40.7X5	T40.7X6
Garamycin	T36.5X1	T36.5X2	T36.5X3	T36.5X4	T36.5X5	T36.5X6
ophthalmic preparation	T49.5X1	T49.5X2	T49.5X3	T49.5X4	T49.5X5	T49.5X6
topical NEC	T49.0X1	T49.0X2	T49.0X3	T49.0X4	T49.0X5	T49.0X6

Substance	Poisoning, Accidental (unintentional)	Poisoning, Intentional Self-harm	Poisoning, Assault	Poisoning, Undetermined	Adverse effect	Underdosing
Gardenal	T42.3X1	T42.3X2	T42.3X3	T42.3X4	T42.3X5	T42.3X6
Gardepanyl	T42.3X1	T42.3X2	T42.3X3	T42.3X4	T42.3X5	T42.3X6
Gas	T59.91	T59.92	T59.93	T59.94	--	--
acetylene	T59.891	T59.892	T59.893	T59.894	--	--
incomplete combustion of	T58.11	T58.12	T58.13	T58.14	--	--
air contaminants, source or type not specified	T59.91	T59.92	T59.93	T59.94	--	--
anesthetic	T41.0X1	T41.0X2	T41.0X3	T41.0X4	T41.0X5	T41.0X6
blast furnace	T58.8X1	T58.8X2	T58.8X3	T58.8X4	--	--
butane—see butane						
carbon monoxide—see Carbon, monoxide						
chlorine	T59.4X1	T59.4X2	T59.4X3	T59.4X4		
coal	T58.2X1	T58.2X2	T58.2X3	T58.2X4	--	--
cyanide	T57.3X1	T57.3X2	T57.3X3	T57.3X4	--	--
dicyanogen	T65.0X1	T65.0X2	T65.0X3	T65.0X4	--	--
domestic—see Domestic gas						
exhaust	T58.01	T58.02	T58.03	T58.04	--	--
from utility (for cooking, heating, or lighting) (after combustion) —see Carbon, monoxide, fuel, utility						
prior to combustion	T59.891	T59.892	T59.893	T59.894	--	--
from wood or coal-burning stove or fireplace	T58.2X1	T58.2X2	T58.2X3	T58.2X4	--	--
fuel (domestic use) (after combustion) —see also Carbon, monoxide, fuel						
industrial use	T58.8X1	T58.8X2	T58.8X3	T58.8X4	--	--
prior to combustion	T59.891	T59.892	T59.893	T59.894	--	--
utility	T59.891	T59.892	T59.893	T59.894	--	--
in mobile container	T59.891	T59.892	T59.893	T59.894	--	--
incomplete combustion of—see Carbon, monoxide, fuel, utility						
piped (natural)	T59.891	T59.892	T59.893	T59.894	--	--
garage	T58.01	T58.02	T58.03	T58.04	--	--
hydrocarbon NEC	T59.891	T59.892	T59.893	T59.894	--	--
incomplete combustion of—see Carbon, monoxide, fuel, utility						
liquefied—see butane						
piped	T59.891	T59.892	T59.893	T59.894	--	--
hydrocyanic acid	T65.0X1	T65.0X2	T65.0X3	T65.0X4	--	--
illuminating (after combustion)	T58.11	T58.12	T58.13	T58.14	--	--
prior to combustion	T59.891	T59.892	T59.893	T59.894	--	--
incomplete combustion, any—see Carbon, monoxide						
kiln	T58.8X1	T58.8X2	T58.8X3	T58.8X4	--	--
lacrimogenic	T59.3X1	T59.3X2	T59.3X3	T59.3X4	--	--
liquefied petroleum—see butane						
marsh	T59.891	T59.892	T59.893	T59.894	--	--
motor exhaust, not in transit	T58.01	T58.02	T58.03	T58.04	--	--
mustard, not in war	T59.891	T59.892	T59.893	T59.894	--	--
natural	T59.891	T59.892	T59.893	T59.894	--	--
nerve, not in war	T59.91	T59.92	T59.93	T59.94	--	--
oil	T52.0X1	T52.0X2	T52.0X3	T52.0X4	--	--
petroleum (liquefied) (distributed in mobile containers)	T59.891	T59.892	T59.893	T59.894	--	--
piped (pure or mixed with air)	T59.891	T59.892	T59.893	T59.894	--	--
piped (manufactured) (natural) NEC	T59.891	T59.892	T59.893	T59.894	--	--
producer	T58.8X1	T58.8X2	T58.8X3	T58.8X4	--	--
propane—see propane						
refrigerant (chlorofluoro-carbon)	T53.5X1	T53.5X2	T53.5X3	T53.5X4	--	--
not chlorofluoro-carbon	T59.891	T59.892	T59.893	T59.894	--	--
sewer	T59.91	T59.92	T59.93	T59.94	--	--
specified source NEC	T59.91	T59.92	T59.93	T59.94	--	--
stove (after combustion)	T58.11	T58.12	T58.13	T58.14	--	--
prior to combustion	T59.891	T59.892	T59.893	T59.894	--	--
tear	T59.3X1	T59.3X2	T59.3X3	T59.3X4	--	--
therapeutic	T41.5X1	T41.5X2	T41.5X3	T41.5X4	T41.5X5	T41.5X6
utility (for cooking, heating, or lighting) (piped)	T59.891	T59.892	T59.893	T59.894	--	--

Substance	Poisoning, Accidental (unintentional)	Poisoning, Intentional Self-harm	Poisoning, Assault	Poisoning, Undetermined	Adverse effect	Underdosing
NEC						
in mobile container	T59.891	T59.892	T59.893	T59.894	--	--
incomplete combustion of—see Carbon, monoxide, fuel, utilty						
piped (natural)	T59.891	T59.892	T59.893	T59.894	--	--
water	T58.11	T58.12	T58.13	T58.14	--	--
incomplete combustion of—see Carbon, monoxide, fuel, utility						
Gaseous substance—see Gas						
Gasoline	T52.0X1	T52.0X2	T52.0X3	T52.0X4	--	--
vapor	T52.0X1	T52.0X2	T52.0X3	T52.0X4	--	--
Gastric enzymes	T47.5X1	T47.5X2	T47.5X3	T47.5X4	T47.5X5	T47.5X6
Gastrografin	T50.8X1	T50.8X2	T50.8X3	T50.8X4	T50.8X5	T50.8X6
Gastrointestinal drug	T47.91	T47.92	T47.93	T47.94	T47.95	T47.96
biological	T47.8X1	T47.8X2	T47.8X3	T47.8X4	T47.8X5	T47.8X6
specified NEC	T47.8X1	T47.8X2	T47.8X3	T47.8X4	T47.8X5	T47.8X6
Gaultheria procumbens	T62.2X1	T62.2X2	T62.2X3	T62.2X4	--	--
Gefarnate	T44.3X1	T44.3X2	T44.3X3	T44.3X4	T44.3X5	T44.3X6
Gelatin (intravenous)	T45.8X1	T45.8X2	T45.8X3	T45.8X4	T45.8X5	T45.8X6
absorbable (sponge)	T45.7X1	T45.7X2	T45.7X3	T45.7X4	T45.7X5	T45.7X6
Gelfilm	T49.8X1	T49.8X2	T49.8X3	T49.8X4	T49.8X5	T49.8X6
Gelfoam	T45.7X1	T45.7X2	T45.7X3	T45.7X4	T45.7X5	T45.7X6
Gelsemine	T50.991	T50.992	T50.993	T50.994	T50.995	T50.996
Gelsemium (sempervirens)	T62.2X1	T62.2X2	T62.2X3	T62.2X4	--	--
Gemeprost	T48.0X1	T48.0X2	T48.0X3	T48.0X4	T48.0X5	T48.0X6
Gemfibrozil	T46.6X1	T46.6X2	T46.6X3	T46.6X4	T46.6X5	T46.6X6
Gemonil	T42.3X1	T42.3X2	T42.3X3	T42.3X4	T42.3X5	T42.3X6
Gentamicin	T36.5X1	T36.5X2	T36.5X3	T36.5X4	T36.5X5	T36.5X6
ophthalmic preparation	T49.5X1	T49.5X2	T49.5X3	T49.5X4	T49.5X5	T49.5X6
topical NEC	T49.0X1	T49.0X2	T49.0X3	T49.0X4	T49.0X5	T49.0X6
Gentian	T47.5X1	T47.5X2	T47.5X3	T47.5X4	T47.5X5	T47.5X6
violet	T49.0X1	T49.0X2	T49.0X3	T49.0X4	T49.0X5	T49.0X6
Gepefrine	T44.4X1	T44.4X2	T44.4X3	T44.4X4	T44.4X5	T44.4X6
Gestonorone caproate	T38.5X1	T38.5X2	T38.5X3	T38.5X4	T38.5X5	T38.5X6
Gexane	T49.0X1	T49.0X2	T49.0X3	T49.0X4	T49.0X5	T49.0X6
Gila monster (venom)	T63.111	T63.112	T63.113	T63.114	--	--
Ginger	T47.5X1	T47.5X2	T47.5X3	T47.5X4	T47.5X5	T47.5X6
Jamaica—see Jamaica, ginger						
Gitalin	T46.0X1	T46.0X2	T46.0X3	T46.0X4	T46.0X5	T46.0X6
amorphous	T46.0X1	T46.0X2	T46.0X3	T46.0X4	T46.0X5	T46.0X6
Gitaloxin	T46.0X1	T46.0X2	T46.0X3	T46.0X4	T46.0X5	T46.0X6
Gitoxin	T46.0X1	T46.0X2	T46.0X3	T46.0X4	T46.0X5	T46.0X6
Glafenine	T39.8X1	T39.8X2	T39.8X3	T39.8X4	T39.8X5	T39.8X6
Glandular extract (medicinal) NEC	T50.Z91	T50.Z92	T50.Z93	T50.Z94	T50.Z95	T50.Z96
Glaucarubin	T37.3X1	T37.3X2	T37.3X3	T37.3X4	T37.3X5	T37.3X6
Glibenclamide	T38.3X1	T38.3X2	T38.3X3	T38.3X4	T38.3X5	T38.3X6
Glibornuride	T38.3X1	T38.3X2	T38.3X3	T38.3X4	T38.3X5	T38.3X6
Gliclazide	T38.3X1	T38.3X2	T38.3X3	T38.3X4	T38.3X5	T38.3X6
Glimidine	T38.3X1	T38.3X2	T38.3X3	T38.3X4	T38.3X5	T38.3X6
Glipizide	T38.3X1	T38.3X2	T38.3X3	T38.3X4	T38.3X5	T38.3X6
Gliquidone	T38.3X1	T38.3X2	T38.3X3	T38.3X4	T38.3X5	T38.3X6
Glisolamide	T38.3X1	T38.3X2	T38.3X3	T38.3X4	T38.3X5	T38.3X6
Glisoxepide	T38.3X1	T38.3X2	T38.3X3	T38.3X4	T38.3X5	T38.3X6
Globin zinc insulin	T38.3X1	T38.3X2	T38.3X3	T38.3X4		
Globulin						
antilymphocytic	T50.Z11	T50.Z12	T50.Z13	T50.Z14	T50.Z15	T50.Z16
antirhesus	T50.Z11	T50.Z12	T50.Z13	T50.Z14	T50.Z15	T50.Z16
antivenin	T50.Z11	T50.Z12	T50.Z13	T50.Z14	T50.Z15	T50.Z16
antiviral	T50.Z11	T50.Z12	T50.Z13	T50.Z14	T50.Z15	T50.Z16
Glucagon	T38.3X1	T38.3X2	T38.3X3	T38.3X4	T38.3X5	T38.3X6
Glucocorticoids	T38.0X1	T38.0X2	T38.0X3	T38.0X4	T38.0X5	T38.0X6
Glucocorticosteroid	T38.0X1	T38.0X2	T38.0X3	T38.0X4	T38.0X5	T38.0X6
Gluconic acid	T50.991	T50.992	T50.993	T50.994	T50.995	T50.996
Glucosamine sulfate	T39.4X1	T39.4X2	T39.4X3	T39.4X4	T39.4X5	T39.4X6

Substance	Poisoning, Accidental (unintentional)	Poisoning, Intentional Self-harm	Poisoning, Assault	Poisoning, Undetermined	Adverse effect	Underdosing
Glucose	T50.3X1	T50.3X2	T50.3X3	T50.3X4	T50.3X5	T50.3X6
with sodium chloride	T50.3X1	T50.3X2	T50.3X3	T50.3X4	T50.3X5	T50.3X6
Glucosulfone sodium	T37.1X1	T37.1X2	T37.1X3	T37.1X4	T37.1X5	T37.1X6
Glucurolactone	T47.8X1	T47.8X2	T47.8X3	T47.8X4	T47.8X5	T47.8X6
Glue NEC	T52.8X1	T52.8X2	T52.8X3	T52.8X4	--	--
Glutamic acid	T47.5X1	T47.5X2	T47.5X3	T47.5X4	T47.5X5	T47.5X6
Glutaral (medicinal)	T49.0X1	T49.0X2	T49.0X3	T49.0X4	T49.0X5	T49.0X6
nonmedicinal	T65.891	T65.892	T65.893	T65.894	--	--
Glutaraldehyde (nonmedicinal)	T65.891	T65.892	T65.893	T65.894	--	--
medicinal	T49.0X1	T49.0X2	T49.0X3	T49.0X4	T49.0X5	T49.0X6
Glutathione	T50.6X1	T50.6X2	T50.6X3	T50.6X4	T50.6X5	T50.6X6
Glutethimide	T42.6X1	T42.6X2	T42.6X3	T42.6X4	T42.6X5	T42.6X6
Glyburide	T38.3X1	T38.3X2	T38.3X3	T38.3X4	T38.3X5	T38.3X6
Glycerin	T47.4X1	T47.4X2	T47.4X3	T47.4X4	T47.4X5	T47.4X6
Glycerol	T47.4X1	T47.4X2	T47.4X3	T47.4X4	T47.4X5	T47.4X6
borax	T49.6X1	T49.6X2	T49.6X3	T49.6X4	T49.6X5	T49.6X6
intravenous	T50.3X1	T50.3X2	T50.3X3	T50.3X4	T50.3X5	T50.3X6
iodinated	T48.4X1	T48.4X2	T48.4X3	T48.4X4	T48.4X5	T48.4X6
Glycerophosphate	T50.991	T50.992	T50.993	T50.994	T50.995	T50.996
Glyceryl						
gualacolate	T48.4X1	T48.4X2	T48.4X3	T48.4X4	T48.4X5	T48.4X6
nitrate	T46.3X1	T46.3X2	T46.3X3	T46.3X4	T46.3X5	T46.3X6
triacetate (topical)	T49.0X1	T49.0X2	T49.0X3	T49.0X4	T49.0X5	T49.0X6
trinitrate	T46.3X1	T46.3X2	T46.3X3	T46.3X4	T46.3X5	T46.3X6
Glycine	T50.3X1	T50.3X2	T50.3X3	T50.3X4	T50.3X5	T50.3X6
Glyclopyramide	T38.3X1	T38.3X2	T38.3X3	T38.3X4	T38.3X5	T38.3X6
Glycobiarsol	T37.3X1	T37.3X2	T37.3X3	T37.3X4	T37.3X5	T37.3X6
Glycols (ether)	T52.3X1	T52.3X2	T52.3X3	T52.3X4	--	--
Glyconiazide	T37.1X1	T37.1X2	T37.1X3	T37.1X4	T37.1X5	T37.1X6
Glycopyrrolate	T44.3X1	T44.3X2	T44.3X3	T44.3X4	T44.3X5	T44.3X6
Glycopyrronium	T44.3X1	T44.3X2	T44.3X3	T44.3X4	T44.3X5	T44.3X6
bromide	T44.3X1	T44.3X2	T44.3X3	T44.3X4	T44.3X5	T44.3X6
Glycoside, cardiac (stimulant)	T46.0X1	T46.0X2	T46.0X3	T46.0X4	T46.0X5	T46.0X6
Glycyclamide	T38.3X1	T38.3X2	T38.3X3	T38.3X4	T38.3X5	T38.3X6
Glycyrrhiza extract	T48.4X1	T48.4X2	T48.4X3	T48.4X4	T48.4X5	T48.4X6
Glycyrrhizic acid	T48.4X1	T48.4X2	T48.4X3	T48.4X4	T48.4X5	T48.4X6
Glycyrrhizinate potassium	T48.4X1	T48.4X2	T48.4X3	T48.4X4	T48.4X5	T48.4X6
Glymidine sodium	T38.3X1	T38.3X2	T38.3X3	T38.3X4	T38.3X5	T38.3X6
Glyphosate	T60.3X1	T60.3X2	T60.3X3	T60.3X4	--	--
Glyphylline	T48.6X1	T48.6X2	T48.6X3	T48.6X4	T48.6X5	T48.6X6
Gold						
colloidal (l98Au)	T45.1X1	T45.1X2	T45.1X3	T45.1X4	T45.1X5	T45.1X6
salts	T39.4X1	T39.4X2	T39.4X3	T39.4X4	T39.4X5	T39.4X6
Golden sulfide of antimony	T56.891	T56.892	T56.893	T56.894	--	--
Goldylocks	T62.2X1	T62.2X2	T62.2X3	T62.2X4	--	--
Gonadal tissue extract	T38.901	T38.902	T38.903	T38.904	T38.905	T38.906
female	T38.5X1	T38.5X2	T38.5X3	T38.5X4	T38.5X5	T38.5X6
male	T38.7X1	T38.7X2	T38.7X3	T38.7X4	T38.7X5	T38.7X6
Gonadorelin	T38.891	T38.892	T38.893	T38.894	T38.895	T38.896
Gonadotropin	T38.891	T38.892	T38.893	T38.894	T38.895	T38.896
chorionic	T38.891	T38.892	T38.893	T38.894	T38.895	T38.896
pituitary	T38.811	T38.812	T38.813	T38.814	T38.815	T38.816
Goserelin	T45.1X1	T45.1X2	T45.1X3	T45.1X4	T45.1X5	T45.1X6
Grain alcohol	T51.0X1	T51.0X2	T51.0X3	T51.0X4	--	--
Gramicidin	T49.0X1	T49.0X2	T49.0X3	T49.0X4	T49.0X5	T49.0X6
Granisetron	T45.0X1	T45.0X2	T45.0X3	T45.0X4	T45.0X5	T45.0X6
Gratiola officinalis	T62.2X1	T62.2X2	T62.2X3	T62.2X4	--	--
Grease	T65.891	T65.892	T65.893	T65.894	--	--
Green hellebore	T62.2X1	T62.2X2	T62.2X3	T62.2X4	--	--
Green soap	T49.2X1	T49.2X2	T49.2X3	T49.2X4	T49.2X5	T49.2X6
Grifulvin	T36.7X1	T36.7X2	T36.7X3	T36.7X4	T36.7X5	T36.7X6
Griseofulvin	T36.7X1	T36.7X2	T36.7X3	T36.7X4	T36.7X5	T36.7X6
Growth hormone	T38.811	T38.812	T38.813	T38.814	T38.815	T38.816
Guaiac reagent	T50.991	T50.992	T50.993	T50.994	T50.995	T50.996
Guaiacol derivatives	T48.4X1	T48.4X2	T48.4X3	T48.4X4	T48.4X5	T48.4X6

Substance	Poisoning, Accidental (unintentional)	Poisoning, Intentional Self-harm	Poisoning, Assault	Poisoning, Undetermined	Adverse effect	Underdosing
Guaifenesin	T48.4X1	T48.4X2	T48.4X3	T48.4X4	T48.4X5	T48.4X6
Guaimesal	T48.4X1	T48.4X2	T48.4X3	T48.4X4	T48.4X5	T48.4X6
Guaiphenesin	T48.4X1	T48.4X2	T48.4X3	T48.4X4	T48.4X5	T48.4X6
Guamecycline	T36.4X1	T36.4X2	T36.4X3	T36.4X4	T36.4X5	T36.4X6
Guanabenz	T46.5X1	T46.5X2	T46.5X3	T46.5X4	T46.5X5	T46.5X6
Guanacline	T46.5X1	T46.5X2	T46.5X3	T46.5X4	T46.5X5	T46.5X6
Guanadrel	T46.5X1	T46.5X2	T46.5X3	T46.5X4	T46.5X5	T46.5X6
Guanatol	T37.2X1	T37.2X2	T37.2X3	T37.2X4	T37.2X5	T37.2X6
Guanethidine	T46.5X1	T46.5X2	T46.5X3	T46.5X4	T46.5X5	T46.5X6
Guanfacine	T46.5X1	T46.5X2	T46.5X3	T46.5X4	T46.5X5	T46.5X6
Guano	T65.891	T65.892	T65.893	T65.894	--	--
Guanochlor	T46.5X1	T46.5X2	T46.5X3	T46.5X4	T46.5X5	T46.5X6
Guanoclor	T46.5X1	T46.5X2	T46.5X3	T46.5X4	T46.5X5	T46.5X6
Guanoctine	T46.5X1	T46.5X2	T46.5X3	T46.5X4	T46.5X5	T46.5X6
Guanoxabenz	T46.5X1	T46.5X2	T46.5X3	T46.5X4	T46.5X5	T46.5X6
Guanoxan	T46.5X1	T46.5X2	T46.5X3	T46.5X4	T46.5X5	T46.5X6
Guar gum (medicinal)	T46.6X1	T46.6X2	T46.6X3	T46.6X4	T46.6X5	T46.6X6
Hachimycin	T36.7X1	T36.7X2	T36.7X3	T36.7X4	T36.7X5	T36.7X6
Hair						
dye	T49.4X1	T49.4X2	T49.4X3	T49.4X4	T49.4X5	T49.4X6
preparation NEC	T49.4X1	T49.4X2	T49.4X3	T49.4X4	T49.4X5	T49.4X6
Halazepam	T42.4X1	T42.4X2	T42.4X3	T42.4X4	T42.4X5	T42.4X6
Halcinolone	T49.0X1	T49.0X2	T49.0X3	T49.0X4	T49.0X5	T49.0X6
Halcinonide	T49.0X1	T49.0X2	T49.0X3	T49.0X4	T49.0X5	T49.0X6
Halethazole	T49.0X1	T49.0X2	T49.0X3	T49.0X4	T49.0X5	T49.0X6
Hallucinogen NEC	T40.901	T40.902	T40.903	T40.904	T40.905	T40.906
Halofantrine	T37.2X1	T37.2X2	T37.2X3	T37.2X4	T37.2X5	T37.2X6
Halofenate	T46.6X1	T46.6X2	T46.6X3	T46.6X4	T46.6X5	T46.6X6
Halometasone	T49.0X1	T49.0X2	T49.0X3	T49.0X4	T49.0X5	T49.0X6
Haloperidol	T43.4X1	T43.4X2	T43.4X3	T43.4X4	T43.4X5	T43.4X6
Haloprogin	T49.0X1	T49.0X2	T49.0X3	T49.0X4	T49.0X5	T49.0X6
Halotex	T49.0X1	T49.0X2	T49.0X3	T49.0X4	T49.0X5	T49.0X6
Halothane	T41.0X1	T41.0X2	T41.0X3	T41.0X4	T41.0X5	T41.0X6
Haloxazolam	T42.4X1	T42.4X2	T42.4X3	T42.4X4	T42.4X5	T42.4X6
Halquinols	T49.0X1	T49.0X2	T49.0X3	T49.0X4	T49.0X5	T49.0X6
Hamamelis	T49.2X1	T49.2X2	T49.2X3	T49.2X4	T49.2X5	T49.2X6
Haptendextran	T45.8X1	T45.8X2	T45.8X3	T45.8X4	T45.8X5	T45.8X6
Harmonyl	T46.5X1	T46.5X2	T46.5X3	T46.5X4	T46.5X5	T46.5X6
Hartmann's solution	T50.3X1	T50.3X2	T50.3X3	T50.3X4	T50.3X5	T50.3X6
Hashish	T40.7X1	T40.7X2	T40.7X3	T40.7X4	T40.7X5	T40.7X6
Hawaiian Woodrose seeds	T40.991	T40.992	T40.993	T40.994	--	--
HCB	T60.3X1	T60.3X2	T60.3X3	T60.3X4	--	--
HCH	T53.6X1	T53.6X2	T53.6X3	T53.6X4	--	--
medicinal	T49.0X1	T49.0X2	T49.0X3	T49.0X4	T49.0X5	T49.0X6
HCN	T57.3X1	T57.3X2	T57.3X3	T57.3X4	--	--
Headache cures, drugs, powders NEC	T50.901	T50.902	T50.903	T50.904	T50.905	T50.906
Heavenly Blue (morning glory)	T40.991	T40.992	T40.993	T40.994	--	--
Heavy metal antidote	T45.8X1	T45.8X2	T45.8X3	T45.8X4	T45.8X5	T45.8X6
Hedaquinium	T49.0X1	T49.0X2	T49.0X3	T49.0X4	T49.0X5	T49.0X6
Hedge hyssop	T62.2X1	T62.2X2	T62.2X3	T62.2X4	--	--
Heet	T49.8X1	T49.8X2	T49.8X3	T49.8X4	T49.8X5	T49.8X6
Helenin	T37.4X1	T37.4X2	T37.4X3	T37.4X4	T37.4X5	T37.4X6
Helium (nonmedicinal) NEC	T59.891	T59.892	T59.893	T59.894	--	--
medicinal	T48.991	T48.992	T48.993	T48.994	T48.995	T48.996
Hellebore (black) (green) (white)	T62.2X1	T62.2X2	T62.2X3	T62.2X4	--	--
Hematin	T45.8X1	T45.8X2	T45.8X3	T45.8X4	T45.8X5	T45.8X6
Hematinic preparation	T45.8X1	T45.8X2	T45.8X3	T45.8X4	T45.8X5	T45.8X6
Hematological agent	T45.91	T45.92	T45.93	T45.94	T45.95	T45.96
specified NEC	T45.8X1	T45.8X2	T45.8X3	T45.8X4	T45.8X5	T45.8X6
Hemlock	T62.2X1	T62.2X2	T62.2X3	T62.2X4	--	--
Hemostatic	T45.621	T45.622	T45.623	T45.624	T45.625	T45.626
drug, systemic	T45.621	T45.622	T45.623	T45.624	T45.625	T45.626
Hemostyptic	T49.4X1	T49.4X2	T49.4X3	T49.4X4	T49.4X5	T49.4X6
Henbane	T62.2X1	T62.2X2	T62.2X3	T62.2X4	--	--

Substance	Poisoning, Accidental (unintentional)	Poisoning, Intentional Self-harm	Poisoning, Assault	Poisoning, Undetermined	Adverse effect	Underdosing
Heparin (sodium)	T45.511	T45.512	T45.513	T45.514	T45.515	T45.516
action reverser	T45.7X1	T45.7X2	T45.7X3	T45.7X4	T45.7X5	T45.7X6
Heparin-fraction	T45.511	T45.512	T45.513	T45.514	T45.515	T45.516
Heparinoid (systemic)	T45.511	T45.512	T45.513	T45.514	T45.515	T45.516
Hepatic secretion stimulant	T47.8X1	T47.8X2	T47.8X3	T47.8X4	T47.8X5	T47.8X6
Hepatitis B						
immune globulin	T50.Z11	T50.Z12	T50.Z13	T50.Z14	T50.Z15	T50.Z16
vaccine	T50.B91	T50.B92	T50.B93	T50.B94	T50.B95	T50.B96
Hepronicate	T46.7X1	T46.7X2	T46.7X3	T46.7X4	T46.7X5	T46.7X6
Heptabarb	T42.3X1	T42.3X2	T42.3X3	T42.3X4	T42.3X5	T42.3X6
Heptabarbital	T42.3X1	T42.3X2	T42.3X3	T42.3X4	T42.3X5	T42.3X6
Heptabarbitone	T42.3X1	T42.3X2	T42.3X3	T42.3X4	T42.3X5	T42.3X6
Heptachlor	T60.1X1	T60.1X2	T60.1X3	T60.1X4	--	--
Heptalgin	T40.2X1	T40.2X2	T40.2X3	T40.2X4	T40.2X5	T40.2X6
Heptaminol	T46.3X1	T46.3X2	T46.3X3	T46.3X4	T46.3X5	T46.3X6
Herbicide NEC	T60.3X1	T60.3X2	T60.3X3	T60.3X4	--	--
Heroin	T40.1X1	T40.1X2	T40.1X3	T40.1X4	T40.1X5	--
Herplex	T49.5X1	T49.5X2	T49.5X3	T49.5X4	T49.5X5	T49.5X6
HES	T45.8X1	T45.8X2	T45.8X3	T45.8X4	T45.8X5	T45.8X6
Hesperidin	T46.991	T46.992	T46.993	T46.994	T46.995	T46.996
Hetacillin	T36.0X1	T36.0X2	T36.0X3	T36.0X4	T36.0X5	T36.0X6
Hetastarch	T45.8X1	T45.8X2	T45.8X3	T45.8X4	T45.8X5	T45.8X6
HETP	T60.0X1	T60.0X2	T60.0X3	T60.0X4	--	--
Hexachlorobenzene (vapor)	T60.3X1	T60.3X2	T60.3X3	T60.3X4	--	--
Hexachlorocyclohexane	T53.6X1	T53.6X2	T53.6X3	T53.6X4	--	--
Hexachlorophene	T49.0X1	T49.0X2	T49.0X3	T49.0X4	T49.0X5	T49.0X6
Hexadiline	T46.3X1	T46.3X2	T46.3X3	T46.3X4	T46.3X5	T46.3X6
Hexadimethrine (bromide)	T45.7X1	T45.7X2	T45.7X3	T45.7X4	T45.7X5	T45.7X6
Hexadylamine	T46.3X1	T46.3X2	T46.3X3	T46.3X4	T46.3X5	T46.3X6
Hexaethyl tetraphos-phate	T60.0X1	T60.0X2	T60.0X3	T60.0X4	--	--
Hexafluorenium bromide	T48.1X1	T48.1X2	T48.1X3	T48.1X4	T48.1X5	T48.1X6
Hexafluronium (bromide)	T48.1X1	T48.1X2	T48.1X3	T48.1X4	T48.1X5	T48.1X6
Hexa-germ	T49.2X1	T49.2X2	T49.2X3	T49.2X4	T49.2X5	T49.2X6
Hexahydrobenzol	T52.8X1	T52.8X2	T52.8X3	T52.8X4	--	--
Hexahydrocresol (s)	T51.8X1	T51.8X2	T51.8X3	T51.8X4	--	--
arsenide	T57.0X1	T57.0X2	T57.0X3	T57.0X4	--	--
arseniurated	T57.0X1	T57.0X2	T57.0X3	T57.0X4	--	--
cyanide	T57.3X1	T57.3X2	T57.3X3	T57.3X4	--	--
gas	T59.891	T59.892	T59.893	T59.894	--	--
Fluoride (liquid)	T57.8X1	T57.8X2	T57.8X3	T57.8X4	--	--
vapor	T59.891	T59.892	T59.893	T59.894	--	--
phophorated	T60.0X1	T60.0X2	T60.0X3	T60.0X4	--	--
sulfate	T57.8X1	T57.8X2	T57.8X3	T57.8X4	--	--
sulfide (gas)	T59.6X1	T59.6X2	T59.6X3	T59.6X4	--	--
arseniurated	T57.0X1	T57.0X2	T57.0X3	T57.0X4	--	--
sulfurated	T57.8X1	T57.8X2	T57.8X3	T57.8X4	--	--
Hexahydrophenol	T51.8X1	T51.8X2	T51.8X3	T51.8X4	--	--
Hexalen	T51.8X1	T51.8X2	T51.8X3	T51.8X4	--	--
Hexamethonium bromide	T44.2X1	T44.2X2	T44.2X3	T44.2X4	T44.2X5	T44.2X6
Hexamethylene	T52.8X1	T52.8X2	T52.8X3	T52.8X4	--	--
Hexamethylmelamine	T45.1X1	T45.1X2	T45.1X3	T45.1X4	T45.1X5	T45.1X6
Hexamidine	T49.0X1	T49.0X2	T49.0X3	T49.0X4	T49.0X5	T49.0X6
Hexamine (mandelate)	T37.8X1	T37.8X2	T37.8X3	T37.8X4	T37.8X5	T37.8X6
Hexanone, 2-hexanone	T52.4X1	T52.4X2	T52.4X3	T52.4X4	--	--
Hexanuorenium	T48.1X1	T48.1X2	T48.1X3	T48.1X4	T48.1X5	T48.1X6
Hexapropymate	T42.6X1	T42.6X2	T42.6X3	T42.6X4	T42.6X5	T42.6X6
Hexasonium iodide	T44.3X1	T44.3X2	T44.3X3	T44.3X4	T44.3X5	T44.3X6
Hexcarbacholine bromide	T48.1X1	T48.1X2	T48.1X3	T48.1X4	T48.1X5	T48.1X6
Hexemal	T42.3X1	T42.3X2	T42.3X3	T42.3X4	T42.3X5	T42.3X6
Hexestrol	T38.5X1	T38.5X2	T38.5X3	T38.5X4	T38.5X5	T38.5X6
Hexethal (sodium)	T42.3X1	T42.3X2	T42.3X3	T42.3X4	T42.3X5	T42.3X6
Hexetidine	T37.8X1	T37.8X2	T37.8X3	T37.8X4	T37.8X5	T37.8X6
Hexobarbital	T42.3X1	T42.3X2	T42.3X3	T42.3X4	T42.3X5	T42.3X6
rectal	T41.291	T41.292	T41.293	T41.294	T41.295	T41.296
sodium	T41.1X1	T41.1X2	T41.1X3	T41.1X4	T41.1X5	T41.1X6

Substance	Poisoning, Accidental (unintentional)	Poisoning, Intentional Self-harm	Poisoning, Assault	Poisoning, Undetermined	Adverse effect	Underdosing
Hexobendine	T46.3X1	T46.3X2	T46.3X3	T46.3X4	T46.3X5	T46.3X6
Hexocyclium	T44.3X1	T44.3X2	T44.3X3	T44.3X4	T44.3X5	T44.3X6
metilsulfate	T44.3X1	T44.3X2	T44.3X3	T44.3X4	T44.3X5	T44.3X6
Hexoestrol	T38.5X1	T38.5X2	T38.5X3	T38.5X4	T38.5X5	T38.5X6
Hexone	T52.4X1	T52.4X2	T52.4X3	T52.4X4	--	--
Hexoprenaline	T48.6X1	T48.6X2	T48.6X3	T48.6X4	T48.6X5	T48.6X6
Hexylcaine	T41.3X1	T41.3X2	T41.3X3	T41.3X4	T41.3X5	T41.3X6
Hexylresorcinol	T52.2X1	T52.2X2	T52.2X3	T52.2X4	--	--
HGH (human growth hormone)	T38.811	T38.812	T38.813	T38.814	T38.815	T38.816
Hinkle's pills	T47.2X1	T47.2X2	T47.2X3	T47.2X4	T47.2X5	T47.2X6
Histalog	T50.8X1	T50.8X2	T50.8X3	T50.8X4	T50.8X5	T50.8X6
Histamine (phosphate)	T50.8X1	T50.8X2	T50.8X3	T50.8X4	T50.8X5	T50.8X6
Histoplasmin	T50.8X1	T50.8X2	T50.8X3	T50.8X4	T50.8X5	T50.8X6
Holly berries	T62.2X1	T62.2X2	T62.2X3	T62.2X4	--	--
Homatropine	T44.3X1	T44.3X2	T44.3X3	T44.3X4	T44.3X5	T44.3X6
methylbromide	T44.3X1	T44.3X2	T44.3X3	T44.3X4	T44.3X5	T44.3X6
Homochlorcyclizine	T45.0X1	T45.0X2	T45.0X3	T45.0X4	T45.0X5	T45.0X6
Homosalate	T49.3X1	T49.3X2	T49.3X3	T49.3X4	T49.3X5	T49.3X6
Homo-tet	T50.Z11	T50.Z12	T50.Z13	T50.Z14	T50.Z15	T50.Z16
Hormone	T38.801	T38.802	T38.803	T38.804	T38.805	T38.806
adrenal cortical steroids	T38.0X1	T38.0X2	T38.0X3	T38.0X4	T38.0X5	T38.0X6
androgenic	T38.7X1	T38.7X2	T38.7X3	T38.7X4	T38.7X5	T38.7X6
anterior pituitary NEC	T38.811	T38.812	T38.813	T38.814	T38.815	T38.816
antidiabetic agents	T38.3X1	T38.3X2	T38.3X3	T38.3X4	T38.3X5	T38.3X6
antidiuretic	T38.891	T38.892	T38.893	T38.894	T38.895	T38.896
cancer therapy	T45.1X1	T45.1X2	T45.1X3	T45.1X4	T45.1X5	T45.1X6
follicle stimulating	T38.811	T38.812	T38.813	T38.814	T38.815	T38.816
gonadotropic	T38.891	T38.892	T38.893	T38.894	T38.895	T38.896
pituitary	T38.811	T38.812	T38.813	T38.814	T38.815	T38.816
growth	T38.811	T38.812	T38.813	T38.814	T38.815	T38.816
luteinizing	T38.811	T38.812	T38.813	T38.814	T38.815	T38.816
ovarian	T38.5X1	T38.5X2	T38.5X3	T38.5X4	T38.5X5	T38.5X6
oxytocic	T48.0X1	T48.0X2	T48.0X3	T48.0X4	T48.0X5	T48.0X6
parathyroid (derivatives)	T50.991	T50.992	T50.993	T50.994	T50.995	T50.996
pituitary (posterior) NEC	T38.891	T38.892	T38.893	T38.894	T38.895	T38.896
anterior	T38.811	T38.812	T38.813	T38.814	T38.815	T38.816
specified, NEC	T38.891	T38.892	T38.893	T38.894	T38.895	T38.896
thyroid	T38.1X1	T38.1X2	T38.1X3	T38.1X4	T38.1X5	T38.1X6
Hornet (sting)	T63.451	T63.452	T63.453	T63.454	--	--
Horse anti-human lymphocytic serum	T50.Z11	T50.Z12	T50.Z13	T50.Z14	T50.Z15	T50.Z16
Horticulture agent NEC	T65.91	T65.92	T65.93	T65.94	--	--
with pesticide	T60.91	T60.92	T60.93	T60.94	--	--
Human						
albumin	T45.8X1	T45.8X2	T45.8X3	T45.8X4	T45.8X5	T45.8X6
growth hormone (HGH)	T38.811	T38.812	T38.813	T38.814	T38.815	T38.816
immune serum	T50.Z11	T50.Z12	T50.Z13	T50.Z14	T50.Z15	T50.Z16
Hyaluronidase	T45.3X1	T45.3X2	T45.3X3	T45.3X4	T45.3X5	T45.3X6
Hyazyme	T45.3X1	T45.3X2	T45.3X3	T45.3X4	T45.3X5	T45.3X6
Hycodan	T40.2X1	T40.2X2	T40.2X3	T40.2X4	T40.2X5	T40.2X6
Hydantoin derivative NEC	T42.0X1	T42.0X2	T42.0X3	T42.0X4	T42.0X5	T42.0X6
Hydeltra	T38.0X1	T38.0X2	T38.0X3	T38.0X4	T38.0X5	T38.0X6
Hydergine	T44.6X1	T44.6X2	T44.6X3	T44.6X4	T44.6X5	T44.6X6
Hydrabamine penicillin	T36.0X1	T36.0X2	T36.0X3	T36.0X4	T36.0X5	T36.0X6
Hydralazine	T46.5X1	T46.5X2	T46.5X3	T46.5X4	T46.5X5	T46.5X6
Hydrargaphen	T49.0X1	T49.0X2	T49.0X3	T49.0X4	T49.0X5	T49.0X6
Hydrargyri amino-chloridum	T49.0X1	T49.0X2	T49.0X3	T49.0X4	T49.0X5	T49.0X6
Hydrastine	T48.291	T48.292	T48.293	T48.294	T48.295	T48.296
Hydrazine	T54.1X1	T54.1X2	T54.1X3	T54.1X4	--	--
monoamine oxidase inhibitors	T43.1X1	T43.1X2	T43.1X3	T43.1X4	T43.1X5	T43.1X6
Hydrazoic acid, azides	T54.2X1	T54.2X2	T54.2X3	T54.2X4	--	--
Hydriodic acid	T48.4X1	T48.4X2	T48.4X3	T48.4X4	T48.4X5	T48.4X6
Hydrocarbon gas	T59.891	T59.892	T59.893	T59.894	--	--
incomplete combustion of—see Carbon, monoxide, fuel, utility						

Substance	Poisoning, Accidental (unintentional)	Poisoning, Intentional Self-harm	Poisoning, Assault	Poisoning, Undetermined	Adverse effect	Underdosing
liquefied (mobile container)	T59.891	T59.892	T59.893	T59.894	--	--
piped (natural)	T59.891	T59.892	T59.893	T59.894	--	--
Hydrochloric acid (liquid)	T54.2X1	T54.2X2	T54.2X3	T54.2X4	--	--
medicinal (digestant)	T47.5X1	T47.5X2	T47.5X3	T47.5X4	T47.5X5	T47.5X6
vapor	T59.891	T59.892	T59.893	T59.894	--	--
Hydrochlorothiazide	T50.2X1	T50.2X2	T50.2X3	T50.2X4	T50.2X5	T50.2X6
Hydrocodone	T40.2X1	T40.2X2	T40.2X3	T40.2X4	T40.2X5	T40.2X6
Hydrocortisone (derivatives)	T38.0X1	T38.0X2	T38.0X3	T38.0X4	T38.0X5	T38.0X6
aceponate	T49.0X1	T49.0X2	T49.0X3	T49.0X4	T49.0X5	T49.0X6
ENT agent	T49.6X1	T49.6X2	T49.6X3	T49.6X4	T49.6X5	T49.6X6
ophthalmic preparation	T49.5X1	T49.5X2	T49.5X3	T49.5X4	T49.5X5	T49.5X6
topical NEC	T49.0X1	T49.0X2	T49.0X3	T49.0X4	T49.0X5	T49.0X6
Hydrocortone	T38.0X1	T38.0X2	T38.0X3	T38.0X4	T38.0X5	T38.0X6
ENT agent	T49.6X1	T49.6X2	T49.6X3	T49.6X4	T49.6X5	T49.6X6
ophthalmic preparation	T49.5X1	T49.5X2	T49.5X3	T49.5X4	T49.5X5	T49.5X6
topical NEC	T49.0X1	T49.0X2	T49.0X3	T49.0X4	T49.0X5	T49.0X6
Hydrocyanic acid (liquid)	T57.3X1	T57.3X2	T57.3X3	T57.3X4	--	--
gas	T65.0X1	T65.0X2	T65.0X3	T65.0X4	--	--
Hydroflumethiazide	T50.2X1	T50.2X2	T50.2X3	T50.2X4	T50.2X5	T50.2X6
Hydrofluoric acid (liquid)	T54.2X1	T54.2X2	T54.2X3	T54.2X4	--	--
vapor	T59.891	T59.892	T59.893	T59.894	--	--
Hydrogen	T59.891	T59.892	T59.893	T59.894	--	--
arsenide	T57.0X1	T57.0X2	T57.0X3	T57.0X4	--	--
arseniureted	T57.0X1	T57.0X2	T57.0X3	T57.0X4	--	--
chloride	T57.8X1	T57.8X2	T57.8X3	T57.8X4	--	--
cyanide (salts)	T57.3X1	T57.3X2	T57.3X3	T57.3X4	--	--
gas	T57.3X1	T57.3X2	T57.3X3	T57.3X4	--	--
Fluoride	T59.5X1	T59.5X2	T59.5X3	T59.5X4	--	--
vapor	T59.5X1	T59.5X2	T59.5X3	T59.5X4	--	--
peroxide	T49.0X1	T49.0X2	T49.0X3	T49.0X4	T49.0X5	T49.0X6
phosphureted	T57.1X1	T57.1X2	T57.1X3	T57.1X4	--	--
sulfide	T59.6X1	T59.6X2	T59.6X3	T59.6X4	--	--
arseniureted	T57.0X1	T57.0X2	T57.0X3	T57.0X4	--	--
sulfureted	T59.6X1	T59.6X2	T59.6X3	T59.6X4	--	--
Hydromethylpyridine	T46.7X1	T46.7X2	T46.7X3	T46.7X4	T46.7X5	T46.7X6
Hydromorphinol	T40.2X1	T40.2X2	T40.2X3	T40.2X4	--	--
Hydromorphinone	T40.2X1	T40.2X2	T40.2X3	T40.2X4	T40.2X5	T40.2X6
Hydromorphone	T40.2X1	T40.2X2	T40.2X3	T40.2X4	T40.2X5	T40.2X6
Hydromox	T50.2X1	T50.2X2	T50.2X3	T50.2X4	T50.2X5	T50.2X6
Hydrophilic lotion	T49.3X1	T49.3X2	T49.3X3	T49.3X4	T49.3X5	T49.3X6
Hydroquinidine	T46.2X1	T46.2X2	T46.2X3	T46.2X4	T46.2X5	T46.2X6
Hydroquinone	T52.2X1	T52.2X2	T52.2X3	T52.2X4	--	--
vapor	T59.891	T59.892	T59.893	T59.894	--	--
Hydrosulfuric acid (gas)	T59.6X1	T59.6X2	T59.6X3	T59.6X4	--	--
Hydrotalcite	T47.1X1	T47.1X2	T47.1X3	T47.1X4	T47.1X5	T47.1X6
Hydrous wool fat	T49.3X1	T49.3X2	T49.3X3	T49.3X4	T49.3X5	T49.3X6
Hydroxide, caustic	T54.3X1	T54.3X2	T54.3X3	T54.3X4	--	--
Hydroxocobalamin	T45.8X1	T45.8X2	T45.8X3	T45.8X4	T45.8X5	T45.8X6
Hydroxyamphetamine	T49.5X1	T49.5X2	T49.5X3	T49.5X4	T49.5X5	T49.5X6
Hydroxycarbamide	T45.1X1	T45.1X2	T45.1X3	T45.1X4	T45.1X5	T45.1X6
Hydroxychloroquine	T37.8X1	T37.8X2	T37.8X3	T37.8X4	T37.8X5	T37.8X6
Hydroxydihydrocodeinone	T40.2X1	T40.2X2	T40.2X3	T40.2X4	T40.2X5	T40.2X6
Hydroxyestrone	T38.5X1	T38.5X2	T38.5X3	T38.5X4	T38.5X5	T38.5X6
Hydroxyethyl starch	T45.8X1	T45.8X2	T45.8X3	T45.8X4	T45.8X5	T45.8X6
Hydroxymethylpenta-none	T52.4X1	T52.4X2	T52.4X3	T52.4X4	--	--
Hydroxyphenamate	T43.591	T43.592	T43.593	T43.594	T43.595	T43.596
Hydroxyphenylbutazone	T39.2X1	T39.2X2	T39.2X3	T39.2X4	T39.2X5	T39.2X6
Hydroxyprogesterone	T38.5X1	T38.5X2	T38.5X3	T38.5X4	T38.5X5	T38.5X6
caproate	T38.5X1	T38.5X2	T38.5X3	T38.5X4	T38.5X5	T38.5X6
Hydroxyquinoline (derivatives) NEC	T37.8X1	T37.8X2	T37.8X3	T37.8X4	T37.8X5	T37.8X6
Hydroxystilbamidine	T37.3X1	T37.3X2	T37.3X3	T37.3X4	T37.3X5	T37.3X6
Hydroxytoluene (nonmedicinal)	T54.0X1	T54.0X2	T54.0X3	T54.0X4	--	--
medicinal	T49.0X1	T49.0X2	T49.0X3	T49.0X4	T49.0X5	T49.0X6
Hydroxyurea	T45.1X1	T45.1X2	T45.1X3	T45.1X4	T45.1X5	T45.1X6
Hydroxyzine	T43.591	T43.592	T43.593	T43.594	T43.595	T43.596

Substance	Poisoning, Accidental (unintentional)	Poisoning, Intentional Self-harm	Poisoning, Assault	Poisoning, Undetermined	Adverse effect	Underdosing
Hyoscine	T44.3X1	T44.3X2	T44.3X3	T44.3X4	T44.3X5	T44.3X6
Hyoscyamine	T44.3X1	T44.3X2	T44.3X3	T44.3X4	T44.3X5	T44.3X6
Hyoscyamus	T44.3X1	T44.3X2	T44.3X3	T44.3X4	T44.3X5	T44.3X6
dry extract	T44.3X1	T44.3X2	T44.3X3	T44.3X4	T44.3X5	T44.3X6
Hypaque	T50.8X1	T50.8X2	T50.8X3	T50.8X4	T50.8X5	T50.8X6
Hypertussis	T50.Z11	T50.Z12	T50.Z13	T50.Z14	T50.Z15	T50.Z16
Hypnotic	T42.71	T42.72	T42.73	T42.74	T42.75	T42.76
anticonvulsant	T42.71	T42.72	T42.73	T42.74	T42.75	T42.76
specified NEC	T42.6X1	T42.6X2	T42.6X3	T42.6X4	T42.6X5	T42.6X6
Hypochlorite	T49.0X1	T49.0X2	T49.0X3	T49.0X4	T49.0X5	T49.0X6
Hypophysis, posterior	T38.891	T38.892	T38.893	T38.894	T38.895	T38.896
Hypotensive NEC	T46.5X1	T46.5X2	T46.5X3	T46.5X4	T46.5X5	T46.5X6
Hypromellose	T49.5X1	T49.5X2	T49.5X3	T49.5X4	T49.5X5	T49.5X6
Ibacitabine	T37.5X1	T37.5X2	T37.5X3	T37.5X4	T37.5X5	T37.5X6
Ibopamine	T44.991	T44.992	T44.993	T44.994	T44.995	T44.996
Ibufenac	T39.311	T39.312	T39.313	T39.314	T39.315	T39.316
Ibuprofen	T39.311	T39.312	T39.313	T39.314	T39.315	T39.316
Ibuproxam	T39.311	T39.312	T39.313	T39.314	T39.315	T39.316
Ibuterol	T48.6X1	T48.6X2	T48.6X3	T48.6X4	T48.6X5	T48.6X6
Ichthammol	T49.0X1	T49.0X2	T49.0X3	T49.0X4	T49.0X5	T49.0X6
Ichthyol	T49.4X1	T49.4X2	T49.4X3	T49.4X4	T49.4X5	T49.4X6
Idarubicin	T45.1X1	T45.1X2	T45.1X3	T45.1X4	T45.1X5	T45.1X6
Idrocilamide	T42.8X1	T42.8X2	T42.8X3	T42.8X4	T42.8X5	T42.8X6
Ifenprodil	T46.7X1	T46.7X2	T46.7X3	T46.7X4	T46.7X5	T46.7X6
Ifosfamide	T45.1X1	T45.1X2	T45.1X3	T45.1X4	T45.1X5	T45.1X6
Iletin	T38.3X1	T38.3X2	T38.3X3	T38.3X4	T38.3X5	T38.3X6
Ilex	T62.2X1	T62.2X2	T62.2X3	T62.2X4	--	--
Illuminating gas (after combustion)	T58.11	T58.12	T58.13	T58.14	--	--
prior to combustion	T59.891	T59.892	T59.893	T59.894	--	--
Ilopan	T45.2X1	T45.2X2	T45.2X3	T45.2X4	T45.2X5	T45.2X6
Iloprost	T46.7X1	T46.7X2	T46.7X3	T46.7X4	T46.7X5	T46.7X6
Ilotycin	T36.3X1	T36.3X2	T36.3X3	T36.3X4	T36.3X5	T36.3X6
ophthalmic preparation	T49.5X1	T49.5X2	T49.5X3	T49.5X4	T49.5X5	T49.5X6
topical NEC	T49.0X1	T49.0X2	T49.0X3	T49.0X4	T49.0X5	T49.0X6
Imidazole-4-carboxamide	T45.1X1	T45.1X2	T45.1X3	T45.1X4	T45.1X5	T45.1X6
Imipenem	T36.0X1	T36.0X2	T36.0X3	T36.0X4	T36.0X5	T36.0X6
Imipramine	T43.011	T43.012	T43.013	T43.014	T43.015	T43.016
Iminostilbene	T42.1X1	T42.1X2	T42.1X3	T42.1X4	T42.1X5	T42.1X6
Immu-G	T50.Z11	T50.Z12	T50.Z13	T50.Z14	T50.Z15	T50.Z16
Immuglobin	T50.Z11	T50.Z12	T50.Z13	T50.Z14	T50.Z15	T50.Z16
Immune						
globulin	T50.Z11	T50.Z12	T50.Z13	T50.Z14	T50.Z15	T50.Z16
serum globulin	T50.Z11	T50.Z12	T50.Z13	T50.Z14	T50.Z15	T50.Z16
Immunoglobin human (intravenous) (normal)	T50.Z11	T50.Z12	T50.Z13	T50.Z14	T50.Z15	T50.Z16
unmodified	T50.Z11	T50.Z12	T50.Z13	T50.Z14	T50.Z15	T50.Z16
Immunosuppressive drug	T45.1X1	T45.1X2	T45.1X3	T45.1X4	T45.1X5	T45.1X6
Immu-tetanus	T50.Z11	T50.Z12	T50.Z13	T50.Z14	T50.Z15	T50.Z16
Indalpine	T43.221	T43.222	T43.223	T43.224	T43.225	T43.226
Indanazoline	T48.5X1	T48.5X2	T48.5X3	T48.5X4	T48.5X5	T48.5X6
Indandione (derivatives)	T45.511	T45.512	T45.513	T45.514	T45.515	T45.516
Indapamide	T46.5X1	T46.5X2	T46.5X3	T46.5X4	T46.5X5	T46.5X6
Indendione (derivatives)	T45.511	T45.512	T45.513	T45.514	T45.515	T45.516
Indenolol	T44.7X1	T44.7X2	T44.7X3	T44.7X4	T44.7X5	T44.7X6
Inderal	T44.7X1	T44.7X2	T44.7X3	T44.7X4	T44.7X5	T44.7X6
Indian						
hemp	T40.7X1	T40.7X2	T40.7X3	T40.7X4	T40.7X5	T40.7X6
tobacco	T62.2X1	T62.2X2	T62.2X3	T62.2X4	--	--
Indigo carmine	T50.8X1	T50.8X2	T50.8X3	T50.8X4	T50.8X5	T50.8X6
Indobufen	T45.521	T45.522	T45.523	T45.524	T45.525	T45.526
Indocin	T39.2X1	T39.2X2	T39.2X3	T39.2X4	T39.2X5	T39.2X6
Indocyanine green	T50.8X1	T50.8X2	T50.8X3	T50.8X4	T50.8X5	T50.8X6
Indometacin	T39.391	T39.392	T39.393	T39.394	T39.395	T39.396
Indomethacin	T39.391	T39.392	T39.393	T39.394	T39.395	T39.396
farnesil	T39.4X1	T39.4X2	T39.4X3	T39.4X4	T39.4X5	T39.4X6

Substance	Poisoning, Accidental (unintentional)	Poisoning, Intentional Self-harm	Poisoning, Assault	Poisoning, Undetermined	Adverse effect	Underdosing
Indoramin	T44.6X1	T44.6X2	T44.6X3	T44.6X4	T44.6X5	T44.6X6
Industrial						
alcohol	T51.0X1	T51.0X2	T51.0X3	T51.0X4	--	--
fumes	T59.891	T59.892	T59.893	T59.894	--	--
solvents (fumes) (vapors)	T52.91	T52.92	T52.93	T52.94	--	--
Influenza vaccine	T50.B91	T50.B92	T50.B93	T50.B94	T50.B95	T50.B96
Ingested substance NEC	T65.91	T65.92	T65.93	T65.94	--	--
INH	T37.1X1	T37.1X2	T37.1X3	T37.1X4	T37.1X5	T37.1X6
Inhalation, gas (noxious) —see Gas Inhibitor						
angiotensin-converting enzyme	T46.4X1	T46.4X2	T46.4X3	T46.4X4	T46.4X5	T46.4X6
carbonic anhydrase	T50.2X1	T50.2X2	T50.2X3	T50.2X4	T50.2X5	T50.2X6
fibrinolysis	T45.621	T45.622	T45.623	T45.624	T45.625	T45.626
monoamine oxidase NEC	T43.1X1	T43.1X2	T43.1X3	T43.1X4	T43.1X5	T43.1X6
hydrazine	T43.1X1	T43.1X2	T43.1X3	T43.1X4	T43.1X5	T43.1X6
postsynaptic	T43.8X1	T43.8X2	T43.8X3	T43.8X4	T43.8X5	T43.8X6
prothrombin synthesis	T45.511	T45.512	T45.513	T45.514	T45.515	T45.516
Ink	T65.891	T65.892	T65.893	T65.894	--	--
Inorganic substance NEC	T57.91	T57.92	T57.93	T57.94	--	--
Inosine pranobex	T37.5X1	T37.5X2	T37.5X3	T37.5X4	T37.5X5	T37.5X6
Inositol	T50.991	T50.992	T50.993	T50.994	T50.995	T50.996
nicotinate	T46.7X1	T46.7X2	T46.7X3	T46.7X4	T46.7X5	T46.7X6
Inproquone	T45.1X1	T45.1X2	T45.1X3	T45.1X4	T45.1X5	T45.1X6
Insect (sting) , venomous	T63.481	T63.482	T63.483	T63.484	--	--
ant	T63.421	T63.422	T63.423	T63.424	--	--
bee	T63.441	T63.442	T63.443	T63.444	--	--
caterpillar	T63.431	T63.432	T63.433	T63.434	--	--
hornet	T63.451	T63.452	T63.453	T63.454	--	--
wasp	T63.461	T63.462	T63.463	T63.464	--	--
Insecticide NEC	T60.91	T60.92	T60.93	T60.94	--	--
carbamate	T60.0X1	T60.0X2	T60.0X3	T60.0X4	--	--
chlorinated	T60.1X1	T60.1X2	T60.1X3	T60.1X4	--	--
mixed	T60.91	T60.92	T60.93	T60.94	--	--
organochlorine	T60.1X1	T60.1X2	T60.1X3	T60.1X4	--	--
organophosphorus	T60.0X1	T60.0X2	T60.0X3	T60.0X4	--	--
Insular tissue extract	T38.3X1	T38.3X2	T38.3X3	T38.3X4	T38.3X5	T38.3X6
Insulin (amorphous) (globin) (isophane) (Lente) (NPH) (Semilente) (Ultralente)	T38.3X1	T38.3X2	T38.3X3	T38.3X4	T38.3X5	T38.3X6
defalan	T38.3X1	T38.3X2	T38.3X3	T38.3X4	T38.3X5	T38.3X6
human	T38.3X1	T38.3X2	T38.3X3	T38.3X4	T38.3X5	T38.3X6
injection, soluble	T38.3X1	T38.3X2	T38.3X3	T38.3X4	T38.3X5	T38.3X6
biphasic	T38.3X1	T38.3X2	T38.3X3	T38.3X4	T38.3X5	T38.3X6
intermediate acting	T38.3X1	T38.3X2	T38.3X3	T38.3X4	T38.3X5	T38.3X6
protamine zinc	T38.3X1	T38.3X2	T38.3X3	T38.3X4	T38.3X5	T38.3X6
slow acting	T38.3X1	T38.3X2	T38.3X3	T38.3X4	T38.3X5	T38.3X6
zinc						
protamine injection	T38.3X1	T38.3X2	T38.3X3	T38.3X4	T38.3X5	T38.3X6
suspension (amorphous) (crystalline)	T38.3X1	T38.3X2	T38.3X3	T38.3X4	T38.3X5	T38.3X6
Interferon (alpha) (beta) (gamma)	T37.5X1	T37.5X2	T37.5X3	T37.5X4	T37.5X5	T37.5X6
Intestinal motility control drug	T47.6X1	T47.6X2	T47.6X3	T47.6X4	T47.6X5	T47.6X6
biological	T47.8X1	T47.8X2	T47.8X3	T47.8X4	T47.8X5	T47.8X6
Intranarcon	T41.1X1	T41.1X2	T41.1X3	T41.1X4	T41.1X5	T41.1X6
Intravenous						
amino acids	T50.991	T50.992	T50.993	T50.994	T50.995	T50.996
fat suspension	T50.991	T50.992	T50.993	T50.994	T50.995	T50.996
Inulin	T50.8X1	T50.8X2	T50.8X3	T50.8X4	T50.8X5	T50.8X6
Invert sugar	T50.3X1	T50.3X2	T50.3X3	T50.3X4	T50.3X5	T50.3X6
Inza—see Naproxen						
Iobenzamic acid	T50.8X1	T50.8X2	T50.8X3	T50.8X4	T50.8X5	T50.8X6
Iocarmic acid	T50.8X1	T50.8X2	T50.8X3	T50.8X4	T50.8X5	T50.8X6
Iocetamic acid	T50.8X1	T50.8X2	T50.8X3	T50.8X4	T50.8X5	T50.8X6
Iodamide	T50.8X1	T50.8X2	T50.8X3	T50.8X4	T50.8X5	T50.8X6
Iodide NEC—see also Iodine	T49.0X1	T49.0X2	T49.0X3	T49.0X4	T49.0X5	T49.0X6
mercury (ointment)	T49.0X1	T49.0X2	T49.0X3	T49.0X4	T49.0X5	T49.0X6
methylate	T49.0X1	T49.0X2	T49.0X3	T49.0X4	T49.0X5	T49.0X6
potassium (expectorant) NEC	T48.4X1	T48.4X2	T48.4X3	T48.4X4	T48.4X5	T48.4X6

Substance	Poisoning, Accidental (unintentional)	Poisoning, Intentional Self-harm	Poisoning, Assault	Poisoning, Undetermined	Adverse effect	Underdosing
Iodinated						
contrast medium	T50.8X1	T50.8X2	T50.8X3	T50.8X4	T50.8X5	T50.8X6
glycerol	T48.4X1	T48.4X2	T48.4X3	T48.4X4	T48.4X5	T48.4X6
human serum albumin (131I)	T50.8X1	T50.8X2	T50.8X3	T50.8X4	T50.8X5	T50.8X6
Iodine (antiseptic, external) (tincture) NEC	T49.0X1	T49.0X2	T49.0X3	T49.0X4	T49.0X5	T49.0X6
125—see also Radiation sickness, and Exposure to radioactivce isotopes	T50.8X1	T50.8X2	T50.8X3	T50.8X4	T50.8X5	T50.8X6
therapeutic	T50.991	T50.992	T50.993	T50.994	T50.995	T50.996
131—see also Radiation sickness, and Exposure to radioactivce isotopes	T50.8X1	T50.8X2	T50.8X3	T50.8X4	T50.8X5	T50.8X6
therapeutic	T38.2X1	T38.2X2	T38.2X3	T38.2X4	T38.2X5	T38.2X6
diagnostic	T50.8X1	T50.8X2	T50.8X3	T50.8X4	T50.8X5	T50.8X6
for thyroid conditions (antithyroid)	T38.2X1	T38.2X2	T38.2X3	T38.2X4	T38.2X5	T38.2X6
solution	T49.0X1	T49.0X2	T49.0X3	T49.0X4	T49.0X5	T49.0X6
vapor	T59.891	T59.892	T59.893	T59.894	--	--
Iodipamide	T50.8X1	T50.8X2	T50.8X3	T50.8X4	T50.8X5	T50.8X6
Iodized (poppy seed) oil	T50.8X1	T50.8X2	T50.8X3	T50.8X4	T50.8X5	T50.8X6
Iodobismitol	T37.8X1	T37.8X2	T37.8X3	T37.8X4	T37.8X5	T37.8X6
Iodochlorhydroxyquin	T37.8X1	T37.8X2	T37.8X3	T37.8X4	T37.8X5	T37.8X6
topical	T49.0X1	T49.0X2	T49.0X3	T49.0X4	T49.0X5	T49.0X6
Iodochlorhydroxyquinoline	T37.8X1	T37.8X2	T37.8X3	T37.8X4	T37.8X5	T37.8X6
Iodocholesterol (131I)	T50.8X1	T50.8X2	T50.8X3	T50.8X4	T50.8X5	T50.8X6
Iodoform	T49.0X1	T49.0X2	T49.0X3	T49.0X4	T49.0X5	T49.0X6
Iodohippuric acid	T50.8X1	T50.8X2	T50.8X3	T50.8X4	T50.8X5	T50.8X6
Iodopanoic acid	T50.8X1	T50.8X2	T50.8X3	T50.8X4	T50.8X5	T50.8X6
Iodophthalein (sodium)	T50.8X1	T50.8X2	T50.8X3	T50.8X4	T50.8X5	T50.8X6
Iodopyracet	T50.8X1	T50.8X2	T50.8X3	T50.8X4	T50.8X5	T50.8X6
Iodoquinol	T37.8X1	T37.8X2	T37.8X3	T37.8X4	T37.8X5	T37.8X6
Iodoxamic acid	T50.8X1	T50.8X2	T50.8X3	T50.8X4	T50.8X5	T50.8X6
Iofendylate	T50.8X1	T50.8X2	T50.8X3	T50.8X4	T50.8X5	T50.8X6
Ioglycamic acid	T50.8X1	T50.8X2	T50.8X3	T50.8X4	T50.8X5	T50.8X6
Iohexol	T50.8X1	T50.8X2	T50.8X3	T50.8X4	T50.8X5	T50.8X6
Ion exchange resin						
anion	T47.8X1	T47.8X2	T47.8X3	T47.8X4	T47.8X5	T47.8X6
cation	T50.3X1	T50.3X2	T50.3X3	T50.3X4	T50.3X5	T50.3X6
cholestyramine	T46.6X1	T46.6X2	T46.6X3	T46.6X4	T46.6X5	T46.6X6
intestinal	T47.8X1	T47.8X2	T47.8X3	T47.8X4	T47.8X5	T47.8X6
Iopamidol	T50.8X1	T50.8X2	T50.8X3	T50.8X4	T50.8X5	T50.8X6
Iopanoic acid	T50.8X1	T50.8X2	T50.8X3	T50.8X4	T50.8X5	T50.8X6
Iophenoic acid	T50.8X1	T50.8X2	T50.8X3	T50.8X4	T50.8X5	T50.8X6
Iopodate, sodium	T50.8X1	T50.8X2	T50.8X3	T50.8X4	T50.8X5	T50.8X6
Iopodic acid	T50.8X1	T50.8X2	T50.8X3	T50.8X4	T50.8X5	T50.8X6
Iopromide	T50.8X1	T50.8X2	T50.8X3	T50.8X4	T50.8X5	T50.8X6
Iopydol	T50.8X1	T50.8X2	T50.8X3	T50.8X4	T50.8X5	T50.8X6
Iotalamic acid	T50.8X1	T50.8X2	T50.8X3	T50.8X4	T50.8X5	T50.8X6
Iothalamate	T38.2X1	T38.2X2	T38.2X3	T38.2X4	T38.2X5	T38.2X6
Iothiouracil	T50.8X1	T50.8X2	T50.8X3	T50.8X4	T50.8X5	T50.8X6
Iotrol	T50.8X1	T50.8X2	T50.8X3	T50.8X4	T50.8X5	T50.8X6
Iotrolan	T50.8X1	T50.8X2	T50.8X3	T50.8X4	T50.8X5	T50.8X6
Iotroxate	T50.8X1	T50.8X2	T50.8X3	T50.8X4	T50.8X5	T50.8X6
Iotroxic acid	T50.8X1	T50.8X2	T50.8X3	T50.8X4	T50.8X5	T50.8X6
Ioversol	T50.8X1	T50.8X2	T50.8X3	T50.8X4	T50.8X5	T50.8X6
Ioxaglate	T50.8X1	T50.8X2	T50.8X3	T50.8X4	T50.8X5	T50.8X6
Ioxaglic acid	T50.8X1	T50.8X2	T50.8X3	T50.8X4	T50.8X5	T50.8X6
Ioxitalamic acid	T47.7X1	T47.7X2	T47.7X3	T47.7X4	T47.7X5	T47.7X6
Ipecac	T48.4X1	T48.4X2	T48.4X3	T48.4X4	T48.4X5	T48.4X6
Ipecacuanha	T50.8X1	T50.8X2	T50.8X3	T50.8X4	T50.8X5	T50.8X6
Ipodate, calcium	T42.3X1	T42.3X2	T42.3X3	T42.3X4	T42.3X5	T42.3X6
Ipral	T48.6X1	T48.6X2	T48.6X3	T48.6X4	T48.6X5	T48.6X6
Ipratropium (bromide)	T46.3X1	T46.3X2	T46.3X3	T46.3X4	T46.3X5	T46.3X6
Ipriflavone	T43.011	T43.012	T43.013	T43.014	T43.015	T43.016
Iprindole	T43.1X1	T43.1X2	T43.1X3	T43.1X4	T43.1X5	T43.1X6
Iproclozide	T50.8X1	T50.8X2	T50.8X3	T50.8X4	T50.8X5	T50.8X6
Iprofenin						

Substance	Poisoning, Accidental (unintentional)	Poisoning, Intentional Self-harm	Poisoning, Assault	Poisoning, Undetermined	Adverse effect	Underdosing
Iproheptine	T49.2X1	T49.2X2	T49.2X3	T49.2X4	T49.2X5	T49.2X6
Iproniazid	T43.1X1	T43.1X2	T43.1X3	T43.1X4	T43.1X5	T43.1X6
Iproplatin	T45.1X1	T45.1X2	T45.1X3	T45.1X4	T45.1X5	T45.1X6
Iproveratril	T46.1X1	T46.1X2	T46.1X3	T46.1X4	T46.1X5	T46.1X6
Iron (compounds) (medicinal) NEC	T45.4X1	T45.4X2	T45.4X3	T45.4X4	T45.4X5	T45.4X6
ammonium	T45.4X1	T45.4X2	T45.4X3	T45.4X4	T45.4X5	T45.4X6
dextran injection	T45.4X1	T45.4X2	T45.4X3	T45.4X4	T45.4X5	T45.4X6
nonmedicinal	T56.891	T56.892	T56.893	T56.894	--	--
salts	T45.4X1	T45.4X2	T45.4X3	T45.4X4	T45.4X5	T45.4X6
sorbitex	T45.4X1	T45.4X2	T45.4X3	T45.4X4	T45.4X5	T45.4X6
sorbitol citric acid complex	T45.4X1	T45.4X2	T45.4X3	T45.4X4	T45.4X5	T45.4X6
Irrigating fluid (vaginal)	T49.8X1	T49.8X2	T49.8X3	T49.8X4	T49.8X5	T49.8X6
eye	T49.5X1	T49.5X2	T49.5X3	T49.5X4	T49.5X5	T49.5X6
Isepamicin	T36.5X1	T36.5X2	T36.5X3	T36.5X4	T36.5X5	T36.5X6
Isoaminile (citrate)	T48.3X1	T48.3X2	T48.3X3	T48.3X4	T48.3X5	T48.3X6
Isoamyl nitrite	T46.3X1	T46.3X2	T46.3X3	T46.3X4	T46.3X5	T46.3X6
Isobenzan	T60.1X1	T60.1X2	T60.1X3	T60.1X4	--	--
Isobutyl acetate	T52.8X1	T52.8X2	T52.8X3	T52.8X4	--	--
Isocarboxazid	T43.1X1	T43.1X2	T43.1X3	T43.1X4	T43.1X5	T43.1X6
Isoconazole	T49.0X1	T49.0X2	T49.0X3	T49.0X4	T49.0X5	T49.0X6
Isocyanate	T65.0X1	T65.0X2	T65.0X3	T65.0X4	--	--
Isoephedrine	T44.991	T44.992	T44.993	T44.994	T44.995	T44.996
Isoetarine	T48.6X1	T48.6X2	T48.6X3	T48.6X4	T48.6X5	T48.6X6
Isoethadione	T42.2X1	T42.2X2	T42.2X3	T42.2X4	T42.2X5	T42.2X6
Isoetharine	T44.5X1	T44.5X2	T44.5X3	T44.5X4	T44.5X5	T44.5X6
Isoflurane	T41.0X1	T41.0X2	T41.0X3	T41.0X4	T41.0X5	T41.0X6
Isoflurophate	T44.0X1	T44.0X2	T44.0X3	T44.0X4	T44.0X5	T44.0X6
Isomaltose, ferric complex	T45.4X1	T45.4X2	T45.4X3	T45.4X4	T45.4X5	T45.4X6
Isometheptene	T44.3X1	T44.3X2	T44.3X3	T44.3X4	T44.3X5	T44.3X6
Isoniazid	T37.1X1	T37.1X2	T37.1X3	T37.1X4	T37.1X5	T37.1X6
with						
rifampicin	T36.6X1	T36.6X2	T36.6X3	T36.6X4	T36.6X5	T36.6X6
thioacetazone	T37.1X1	T37.1X2	T37.1X3	T37.1X4	T37.1X5	T37.1X6
Isonicotinic acid hydrazide	T37.1X1	T37.1X2	T37.1X3	T37.1X4	T37.1X5	T37.1X6
Isonipecaine	T40.4X1	T40.4X2	T40.4X3	T40.4X4	T40.4X5	T40.4X6
Isopentaquine	T37.2X1	T37.2X2	T37.2X3	T37.2X4	T37.2X5	T37.2X6
Isophane insulin	T38.3X1	T38.3X2	T38.3X3	T38.3X4	T38.3X5	T38.3X6
Isophorone	T65.891	T65.892	T65.893	T65.894	--	--
Isophosphamide	T45.1X1	T45.1X2	T45.1X3	T45.1X4	T45.1X5	T45.1X6
Isopregnenone	T38.5X1	T38.5X2	T38.5X3	T38.5X4	T38.5X5	T38.5X6
Isoprenaline	T48.6X1	T48.6X2	T48.6X3	T48.6X4	T48.6X5	T48.6X6
Isopromethazine	T43.3X1	T43.3X2	T43.3X3	T43.3X4	T43.3X5	T43.3X6
Isopropamide	T44.3X1	T44.3X2	T44.3X3	T44.3X4	T44.3X5	T44.3X6
iodide	T44.3X1	T44.3X2	T44.3X3	T44.3X4	T44.3X5	T44.3X6
Isopropanol	T51.2X1	T51.2X2	T51.2X3	T51.2X4	--	--
Isopropyl						
acetate	T52.8X1	T52.8X2	T52.8X3	T52.8X4	--	--
alcohol	T51.2X1	T51.2X2	T51.2X3	T51.2X4	--	--
medicinal	T49.4X1	T49.4X2	T49.4X3	T49.4X4	T49.4X5	T49.4X6
ether	T52.8X1	T52.8X2	T52.8X3	T52.8X4	--	--
Isopropylaminophenazone	T39.2X1	T39.2X2	T39.2X3	T39.2X4	T39.2X5	T39.2X6
Isoproterenol	T48.6X1	T48.6X2	T48.6X3	T48.6X4	T48.6X5	T48.6X6
Isosorbide dinitrate	T46.3X1	T46.3X2	T46.3X3	T46.3X4	T46.3X5	T46.3X6
Isothipendyl	T45.0X1	T45.0X2	T45.0X3	T45.0X4	T45.0X5	T45.0X6
Isotretinoin	T50.991	T50.992	T50.993	T50.994	T50.995	T50.996
Isoxazolyl penicillin	T36.0X1	T36.0X2	T36.0X3	T36.0X4	T36.0X5	T36.0X6
Isoxicam	T39.391	T39.392	T39.393	T39.394	T39.395	T39.396
Isoxsuprine	T46.7X1	T46.7X2	T46.7X3	T46.7X4	T46.7X5	T46.7X6
Ispagula	T47.4X1	T47.4X2	T47.4X3	T47.4X4	T47.4X5	T47.4X6
husk	T47.4X1	T47.4X2	T47.4X3	T47.4X4	T47.4X5	T47.4X6
Isradipine	T46.1X1	T46.1X2	T46.1X3	T46.1X4	T46.1X5	T46.1X6
I-thyroxine sodium	T38.1X1	T38.1X2	T38.1X3	T38.1X4	T38.1X5	T38.1X6
Itraconazole	T37.8X1	T37.8X2	T37.8X3	T37.8X4	T37.8X5	T37.8X6
Itramin tosilate	T46.3X1	T46.3X2	T46.3X3	T46.3X4	T46.3X5	T46.3X6
Ivermectin	T37.4X1	T37.4X2	T37.4X3	T37.4X4	T37.4X5	T37.4X6

Substance	Poisoning, Accidental (unintentional)	Poisoning, Intentional Self-harm	Poisoning, Assault	Poisoning, Undetermined	Adverse effect	Underdosing
Izoniazid	T37.1X1	T37.1X2	T37.1X3	T37.1X4	T37.1X5	T37.1X6
with thioacetazone	T37.1X1	T37.1X2	T37.1X3	T37.1X4	T37.1X5	T37.1X6
Jalap	T47.2X1	T47.2X2	T47.2X3	T47.2X4	T47.2X5	T47.2X6
Jamaica						
dogwood (bark)	T39.8X1	T39.8X2	T39.8X3	T39.8X4	T39.8X5	T39.8X6
ginger	T65.891	T65.892	T65.893	T65.894	--	--
root	T62.2X1	T62.2X2	T62.2X3	T62.2X4	--	--
Jatropha	T62.2X1	T62.2X2	T62.2X3	T62.2X4	--	--
curcas	T62.2X1	T62.2X2	T62.2X3	T62.2X4	--	--
Jectofer	T45.4X1	T45.4X2	T45.4X3	T45.4X4	T45.4X5	T45.4X6
Jellyfish (sting)	T63.621	T63.622	T63.623	T63.624	--	--
Jequirity (bean)	T62.2X1	T62.2X2	T62.2X3	T62.2X4	--	--
Jimson weed (stramonium)	T62.2X1	T62.2X2	T62.2X3	T62.2X4	--	--
seeds	T62.2X1	T62.2X2	T62.2X3	T62.2X4	--	
Josamycin	T36.3X1	T36.3X2	T36.3X3	T36.3X4	T36.3X5	T36.3X6
Juniper tar	T49.1X1	T49.1X2	T49.1X3	T49.1X4	T49.1X5	T49.1X6
Kallidinogenase	T46.7X1	T46.7X2	T46.7X3	T46.7X4	T46.7X5	T46.7X6
Kallikrein	T46.7X1	T46.7X2	T46.7X3	T46.7X4	T46.7X5	T46.7X6
Kanamycin	T36.5X1	T36.5X2	T36.5X3	T36.5X4	T36.5X5	T36.5X6
Kantrex	T36.5X1	T36.5X2	T36.5X3	T36.5X4	T36.5X5	T36.5X6
Kaolin	T47.6X1	T47.6X2	T47.6X3	T47.6X4	T47.6X5	T47.6X6
light	T47.6X1	T47.6X2	T47.6X3	T47.6X4	T47.6X5	T47.6X6
Karaya (gum)	T47.4X1	T47.4X2	T47.4X3	T47.4X4	T47.4X5	T47.4X6
Kebuzone	T39.2X1	T39.2X2	T39.2X3	T39.2X4	T39.2X5	T39.2X6
Kelevan	T60.1X1	T60.1X2	T60.1X3	T60.1X4	--	--
Kemithal	T41.1X1	T41.1X2	T41.1X3	T41.1X4	T41.1X5	T41.1X6
Kenacort	T38.0X1	T38.0X2	T38.0X3	T38.0X4	T38.0X5	T38.0X6
Keratolytic drug NEC	T49.4X1	T49.4X2	T49.4X3	T49.4X4	T49.4X5	T49.4X6
anthracene	T49.4X1	T49.4X2	T49.4X3	T49.4X4	T49.4X5	T49.4X6
Keratoplastic NEC	T49.4X1	T49.4X2	T49.4X3	T49.4X4	T49.4X5	T49.4X6
Kerosene, kerosine (fuel) (solvent) NEC	T52.0X1	T52.0X2	T52.0X3	T52.0X4	--	--
insecticide	T52.0X1	T52.0X2	T52.0X3	T52.0X4	--	--
vapor	T52.0X1	T52.0X2	T52.0X3	T52.0X4	--	--
Ketamine	T41.291	T41.292	T41.293	T41.294	T41.295	T41.296
Ketazolam	T42.4X1	T42.4X2	T42.4X3	T42.4X4	T42.4X5	T42.4X6
Ketazon	T39.2X1	T39.2X2	T39.2X3	T39.2X4	T39.2X5	T39.2X6
Ketobemidone	T40.4X1	T40.4X2	T40.4X3	T40.4X4	--	--
Ketoconazole	T49.0X1	T49.0X2	T49.0X3	T49.0X4	T49.0X5	T49.0X6
Ketols	T52.4X1	T52.4X2	T52.4X3	T52.4X4	--	--
Ketone oils	T52.4X1	T52.4X2	T52.4X3	T52.4X4	--	--
Ketoprofen	T39.311	T39.312	T39.313	T39.314	T39.315	T39.316
Ketorolac	T39.8X1	T39.8X2	T39.8X3	T39.8X4	T39.8X5	T39.8X6
Ketotifen	T45.0X1	T45.0X2	T45.0X3	T45.0X4	T45.0X5	T45.0X6
Khat	T43.691	T43.692	T43.693	T43.694	--	--
Khellin	T46.3X1	T46.3X2	T46.3X3	T46.3X4	T46.3X5	T46.3X6
Khelloside	T46.3X1	T46.3X2	T46.3X3	T46.3X4	T46.3X5	T46.3X6
Kiln gas or vapor (carbon monoxide)	T58.8X1	T58.8X2	T58.8X3	T58.8X4	--	--
Kitasamycin	T36.3X1	T36.3X2	T36.3X3	T36.3X4	T36.3X5	T36.3X6
Konsyl	T47.4X1	T47.4X2	T47.4X3	T47.4X4	T47.4X5	T47.4X6
Kosam seed	T62.2X1	T62.2X2	T62.2X3	T62.2X4	--	--
Krait (venom)	T63.091	T63.092	T63.093	T63.094	--	--
Kwell (insecticide)	T60.1X1	T60.1X2	T60.1X3	T60.1X4	--	--
anti-infective (topical)	T49.0X1	T49.0X2	T49.0X3	T49.0X4	T49.0X5	T49.0X6
Labetalol	T44.8X1	T44.8X2	T44.8X3	T44.8X4	T44.8X5	T44.8X6
Laburnum (seeds)	T62.2X1	T62.2X2	T62.2X3	T62.2X4	--	--
leaves	T62.2X1	T62.2X2	T62.2X3	T62.2X4	--	--
Lachesine	T49.5X1	T49.5X2	T49.5X3	T49.5X4	T49.5X5	T49.5X6
Lacidipine	T46.5X1	T46.5X2	T46.5X3	T46.5X4	T46.5X5	T46.5X6
Lacquer	T65.6X1	T65.6X2	T65.6X3	T65.6X4	--	--
Lacrimogenic gas	T59.3X1	T59.3X2	T59.3X3	T59.3X4	--	--
Lactated potassic saline	T50.3X1	T50.3X2	T50.3X3	T50.3X4	T50.3X5	T50.3X6
Lactic acid	T49.8X1	T49.8X2	T49.8X3	T49.8X4	T49.8X5	T49.8X6
Lactobacillus						
acidophilus	T47.6X1	T47.6X2	T47.6X3	T47.6X4	T47.6X5	T47.6X6

Substance	Poisoning, Accidental (unintentional)	Poisoning, Intentional Self-harm	Poisoning, Assault	Poisoning, Undetermined	Adverse effect	Underdosing
compound	T47.6X1	T47.6X2	T47.6X3	T47.6X4	T47.6X5	T47.6X6
bifidus, lyophilized	T47.6X1	T47.6X2	T47.6X3	T47.6X4	T47.6X5	T47.6X6
bulgaricus	T47.6X1	T47.6X2	T47.6X3	T47.6X4	T47.6X5	T47.6X6
sporogenes	T47.6X1	T47.6X2	T47.6X3	T47.6X4	T47.6X5	T47.6X6
Lactoflavin	T45.2X1	T45.2X2	T45.2X3	T45.2X4	T45.2X5	T45.2X6
Lactose (as excipient)	T50.901	T50.902	T50.903	T50.904	T50.905	T50.906
Lactuca (virosa) (extract)	T42.6X1	T42.6X2	T42.6X3	T42.6X4	T42.6X5	T42.6X6
Lactucarium	T42.6X1	T42.6X2	T42.6X3	T42.6X4	T42.6X5	T42.6X6
Lactulose	T47.3X1	T47.3X2	T47.3X3	T47.3X4	T47.3X5	T47.3X6
Laevo—see Levo-						
Lanatosides	T46.0X1	T46.0X2	T46.0X3	T46.0X4	T46.0X5	T46.0X6
Lanolin	T49.3X1	T49.3X2	T49.3X3	T49.3X4	T49.3X5	T49.3X6
Largactil	T43.3X1	T43.3X2	T43.3X3	T43.3X4	T43.3X5	T43.3X6
Larkspur	T62.2X1	T62.2X2	T62.2X3	T62.2X4	--	--
Laroxyl	T43.011	T43.012	T43.013	T43.014	T43.015	T43.016
Lasix	T50.1X1	T50.1X2	T50.1X3	T50.1X4	T50.1X5	T50.1X6
Lassar's paste	T49.4X1	T49.4X2	T49.4X3	T49.4X4	T49.4X5	T49.4X6
Latamoxef	T36.1X1	T36.1X2	T36.1X3	T36.1X4	T36.1X5	T36.1X6
Latex	T65.811	T65.812	T65.813	T65.814	--	--
Lathyrus (seed)	T62.2X1	T62.2X2	T62.2X3	T62.2X4	--	--
Laudanum	T40.0X1	T40.0X2	T40.0X3	T40.0X4	T40.0X5	T40.0X6
Laudexium	T48.1X1	T48.1X2	T48.1X3	T48.1X4	T48.1X5	T48.1X6
Laughing gas	T41.0X1	T41.0X2	T41.0X3	T41.0X4	T41.0X5	T41.0X6
Laurel, black or cherry	T62.2X1	T62.2X2	T62.2X3	T62.2X4	--	--
Laurolinium	T49.0X1	T49.0X2	T49.0X3	T49.0X4	T49.0X5	T49.0X6
Lauryl sulfoacetate	T49.2X1	T49.2X2	T49.2X3	T49.2X4	T49.2X5	T49.2X6
Laxative NEC	T47.4X1	T47.4X2	T47.4X3	T47.4X4	T47.4X5	T47.4X6
osmotic	T47.3X1	T47.3X2	T47.3X3	T47.3X4	T47.3X5	T47.3X6
saline	T47.3X1	T47.3X2	T47.3X3	T47.3X4	T47.3X5	T47.3X6
stimulant	T47.2X1	T47.2X2	T47.2X3	T47.2X4	T47.2X5	T47.2X6
L-dopa	T42.8X1	T42.8X2	T42.8X3	T42.8X4	T42.8X5	T42.8X6
Lead (dust) (fumes) (vapor) NEC	T56.0X1	T56.0X2	T56.0X3	T56.0X4	--	--
acetate	T49.2X1	T49.2X2	T49.2X3	T49.2X4	T49.2X5	T49.2X6
alkyl (fuel additive)	T56.0X1	T56.0X2	T56.0X3	T56.0X4	--	--
anti-infectives	T37.8X1	T37.8X2	T37.8X3	T37.8X4	T37.8X5	T37.8X6
antiknock compound (tetraethyl)	T56.0X1	T56.0X2	T56.0X3	T56.0X4	--	--
arsenate, arsenite (dust) (herbicide) (insecticide) (vapor)	T57.0X1	T57.0X2	T57.0X3	T57.0X4	--	--
carbonate	T56.0X1	T56.0X2	T56.0X3	T56.0X4	--	--
paint	T56.0X1	T56.0X2	T56.0X3	T56.0X4	--	--
chromate	T56.0X1	T56.0X2	T56.0X3	T56.0X4	--	--
paint	T56.0X1	T56.0X2	T56.0X3	T56.0X4	--	--
dioxide	T56.0X1	T56.0X2	T56.0X3	T56.0X4	--	--
inorganic	T56.0X1	T56.0X2	T56.0X3	T56.0X4	--	--
iodide	T56.0X1	T56.0X2	T56.0X3	T56.0X4	--	--
pigment (paint)	T56.0X1	T56.0X2	T56.0X3	T56.0X4	--	--
monoxide (dust)	T56.0X1	T56.0X2	T56.0X3	T56.0X4	--	--
paint	T56.0X1	T56.0X2	T56.0X3	T56.0X4	--	--
organic	T56.0X1	T56.0X2	T56.0X3	T56.0X4	--	--
oxide	T56.0X1	T56.0X2	T56.0X3	T56.0X4	--	--
paint	T56.0X1	T56.0X2	T56.0X3	T56.0X4	--	--
paint	T56.0X1	T56.0X2	T56.0X3	T56.0X4	--	--
salts	T56.0X1	T56.0X2	T56.0X3	T56.0X4	--	--
specified compound NEC	T56.0X1	T56.0X2	T56.0X3	T56.0X4	--	--
tetra-ethyl	T56.0X1	T56.0X2	T56.0X3	T56.0X4	--	--
Lebanese red	T40.7X1	T40.7X2	T40.7X3	T40.7X4	T40.7X5	T40.7X6
Lefetamine	T39.8X1	T39.8X2	T39.8X3	T39.8X4	T39.8X5	T39.8X6
Lenperone	T43.4X1	T43.4X2	T43.4X3	T43.4X4	T43.4X5	T43.4X6
Lente lietin (insulin)	T38.3X1	T38.3X2	T38.3X3	T38.3X4	T38.3X5	T38.3X6
Leptazol	T50.7X1	T50.7X2	T50.7X3	T50.7X4	T50.7X5	T50.7X6
Leptophos	T60.0X1	T60.0X2	T60.0X3	T60.0X4	--	--
Leritine	T40.2X1	T40.2X2	T40.2X3	T40.2X4	T40.2X5	T40.2X6
Letosteine	T48.4X1	T48.4X2	T48.4X3	T48.4X4	T48.4X5	T48.4X6
Letter	T38.1X1	T38.1X2	T38.1X3	T38.1X4	T38.1X5	T38.1X6
Lettuce opium	T42.6X1	T42.6X2	T42.6X3	T42.6X4	T42.6X5	T42.6X6

Substance	Poisoning, Accidental (unintentional)	Poisoning, Intentional Self-harm	Poisoning, Assault	Poisoning, Undetermined	Adverse effect	Underdosing
Leucinocaine	T41.3X1	T41.3X2	T41.3X3	T41.3X4	T41.3X5	T41.3X6
Leucocianidol	T46.991	T46.992	T46.993	T46.994	T46.995	T46.996
Leucovorin (factor)	T45.8X1	T45.8X2	T45.8X3	T45.8X4	T45.8X5	T45.8X6
Leukeran	T45.1X1	T45.1X2	T45.1X3	T45.1X4	T45.1X5	T45.1X6
Leuprolide	T38.891	T38.892	T38.893	T38.894	T38.895	T38.896
Levalbuterol	T48.6X1	T48.6X2	T48.6X3	T48.6X4	T48.6X5	T48.6X6
Levallorphan	T50.7X1	T50.7X2	T50.7X3	T50.7X4	T50.7X5	T50.7X6
Levamisole	T37.4X1	T37.4X2	T37.4X3	T37.4X4	T37.4X5	T37.4X6
Levanil	T42.6X1	T42.6X2	T42.6X3	T42.6X4	T42.6X5	T42.6X6
Levarterenol	T44.4X1	T44.4X2	T44.4X3	T44.4X4	T44.4X5	T44.4X6
Levdropropizine	T48.3X1	T48.3X2	T48.3X3	T48.3X4	T48.3X5	T48.3X6
Levobunolol	T49.5X1	T49.5X2	T49.5X3	T49.5X4	T49.5X5	T49.5X6
Levocabastine (hydrochloride)	T45.0X1	T45.0X2	T45.0X3	T45.0X4	T45.0X5	T45.0X6
Levocarnitine	T50.991	T50.992	T50.993	T50.994	T50.995	T50.996
Levodopa	T42.8X1	T42.8X2	T42.8X3	T42.8X4	T42.8X5	T42.8X6
with carbidopa	T42.8X1	T42.8X2	T42.8X3	T42.8X4	T42.8X5	T42.8X6
Levo-dromoran	T40.2X1	T40.2X2	T40.2X3	T40.2X4	T40.2X5	T40.2X6
Levoglutamide	T50.991	T50.992	T50.993	T50.994	T50.995	T50.996
Levoid	T38.1X1	T38.1X2	T38.1X3	T38.1X4	T38.1X5	T38.1X6
Levo-iso-methadone	T40.3X1	T40.3X2	T40.3X3	T40.3X4	T40.3X5	T40.3X6
Levomepromazine	T43.3X1	T43.3X2	T43.3X3	T43.3X4	T43.3X5	T43.3X6
Levonordefrin	T49.6X1	T49.6X2	T49.6X3	T49.6X4	T49.6X5	T49.6X6
Levonorgestrel	T38.4X1	T38.4X2	T38.4X3	T38.4X4	T38.4X5	T38.4X6
with ethinylestradiol	T38.5X1	T38.5X2	T38.5X3	T38.5X4	T38.5X5	T38.5X6
Levopromazine	T43.3X1	T43.3X2	T43.3X3	T43.3X4	T43.3X5	T43.3X6
Levoprome	T42.6X1	T42.6X2	T42.6X3	T42.6X4	T42.6X5	T42.6X6
Levopropoxyphene	T40.4X1	T40.4X2	T40.4X3	T40.4X4	T40.4X5	T40.4X6
Levopropylhexedrine	T50.5X1	T50.5X2	T50.5X3	T50.5X4	T50.5X5	T50.5X6
Levoproxyphylline	T48.6X1	T48.6X2	T48.6X3	T48.6X4	T48.6X5	T48.6X6
Levorphanol	T40.4X1	T40.4X2	T40.4X3	T40.4X4	T40.4X5	T40.4X6
Levothyroxine	T38.1X1	T38.1X2	T38.1X3	T38.1X4	T38.1X5	T38.1X6
sodium	T38.1X1	T38.1X2	T38.1X3	T38.1X4	T38.1X5	T38.1X6
Levsin	T44.3X1	T44.3X2	T44.3X3	T44.3X4	T44.3X5	T44.3X6
Levulose	T50.3X1	T50.3X2	T50.3X3	T50.3X4	T50.3X5	T50.3X6
Lewisite (gas) , not in war	T57.0X1	T57.0X2	T57.0X3	T57.0X4	--	--
Librium	T42.4X1	T42.4X2	T42.4X3	T42.4X4	T42.4X5	T42.4X6
Lidex	T49.0X1	T49.0X2	T49.0X3	T49.0X4	T49.0X5	T49.0X6
Lidocaine	T41.3X1	T41.3X2	T41.3X3	T41.3X4	T41.3X5	T41.3X6
regional	T41.3X1	T41.3X2	T41.3X3	T41.3X4	T41.3X5	T41.3X6
spinal	T41.3X1	T41.3X2	T41.3X3	T41.3X4	T41.3X5	T41.3X6
Lidofenin	T50.8X1	T50.8X2	T50.8X3	T50.8X4	T50.8X5	T50.8X6
Lidoflazine	T46.1X1	T46.1X2	T46.1X3	T46.1X4	T46.1X5	T46.1X6
Lighter fluid	T52.0X1	T52.0X2	T52.0X3	T52.0X4	--	--
Lignin hemicellulose	T47.6X1	T47.6X2	T47.6X3	T47.6X4	T47.6X5	T47.6X6
Lignocaine	T41.3X1	T41.3X2	T41.3X3	T41.3X4	T41.3X5	T41.3X6
regional	T41.3X1	T41.3X2	T41.3X3	T41.3X4	T41.3X5	T41.3X6
spinal	T41.3X1	T41.3X2	T41.3X3	T41.3X4	T41.3X5	T41.3X6
Ligroin (e) (solvent)	T52.0X1	T52.0X2	T52.0X3	T52.0X4	--	--
vapor	T59.891	T59.892	T59.893	T59.894	--	--
Ligustrum vulgare	T62.2X1	T62.2X2	T62.2X3	T62.2X4	--	--
Lily of the valley	T62.2X1	T62.2X2	T62.2X3	T62.2X4	--	--
Lime (chloride)	T54.3X1	T54.3X2	T54.3X3	T54.3X4	--	--
Limonene	T52.8X1	T52.8X2	T52.8X3	T52.8X4	--	--
Lincomycin	T36.8X1	T36.8X2	T36.8X3	T36.8X4	T36.8X5	T36.8X6
Lindane (insecticide) (nonmedicinal) (vapor)	T53.6X1	T53.6X2	T53.6X3	T53.6X4	--	--
medicinal	T49.0X1	T49.0X2	T49.0X3	T49.0X4	T49.0X5	T49.0X6
Liniments NEC	T49.91	T49.92	T49.93	T49.94	T49.95	T49.96
Linoleic acid	T46.6X1	T46.6X2	T46.6X3	T46.6X4	T46.6X5	T46.6X6
Linolenic acid	T46.6X1	T46.6X2	T46.6X3	T46.6X4	T46.6X5	T46.6X6
Linseed	T47.4X1	T47.4X2	T47.4X3	T47.4X4	T47.4X5	T47.4X6
Liothyronine	T38.1X1	T38.1X2	T38.1X3	T38.1X4	T38.1X5	T38.1X6
Liotrix	T38.1X1	T38.1X2	T38.1X3	T38.1X4	T38.1X5	T38.1X6
Lipancreatin	T47.5X1	T47.5X2	T47.5X3	T47.5X4	T47.5X5	T47.5X6
Lipo-alprostadil	T46.7X1	T46.7X2	T46.7X3	T46.7X4	T46.7X5	T46.7X6

Substance	Poisoning, Accidental (unintentional)	Poisoning, Intentional Self-harm	Poisoning, Assault	Poisoning, Undetermined	Adverse effect	Underdosing
Lipo-Lutin	T38.5X1	T38.5X2	T38.5X3	T38.5X4	T38.5X5	T38.5X6
Lipotropic drug NEC	T50.901	T50.902	T50.903	T50.904	T50.905	T50.906
Liquefied petroleum gases	T59.891	T59.892	T59.893	T59.894	--	--
piped (pure or mixed with air)	T59.891	T59.892	T59.893	T59.894	--	--
Liquid						
paraffin	T47.4X1	T47.4X2	T47.4X3	T47.4X4	T47.4X5	T47.4X6
petrolatum	T47.4X1	T47.4X2	T47.4X3	T47.4X4	T47.4X5	T47.4X6
topical	T49.3X1	T49.3X2	T49.3X3	T49.3X4	T49.3X5	T49.3X6
specified NEC	T65.891	T65.892	T65.893	T65.894	--	--
substance	T65.91	T65.92	T65.93	T65.94	--	--
Liquor creosolis compositus	T65.891	T65.892	T65.893	T65.894	--	--
Liquorice	T48.4X1	T48.4X2	T48.4X3	T48.4X4	T48.4X5	T48.4X6
extract	T47.8X1	T47.8X2	T47.8X3	T47.8X4	T47.8X5	T47.8X6
Lisinopril	T46.4X1	T46.4X2	T46.4X3	T46.4X4	T46.4X5	T46.4X6
Lisuride	T42.8X1	T42.8X2	T42.8X3	T42.8X4	T42.8X5	T42.8X6
Lithane	T43.8X1	T43.8X2	T43.8X3	T43.8X4	T43.8X5	T43.8X6
Lithium	T56.891	T56.892	T56.893	T56.894	--	--
gluconate	T43.591	T43.592	T43.593	T43.594	T43.595	T43.596
salts (carbonate)	T43.591	T43.592	T43.593	T43.594	T43.595	T43.596
Lithonate	T43.8X1	T43.8X2	T43.8X3	T43.8X4	T43.8X5	T43.8X6
Liver						
extract	T45.8X1	T45.8X2	T45.8X3	T45.8X4	T45.8X5	T45.8X6
for parenteral use	T45.8X1	T45.8X2	T45.8X3	T45.8X4	T45.8X5	T45.8X6
fraction 1	T45.8X1	T45.8X2	T45.8X3	T45.8X4	T45.8X5	T45.8X6
hydrolysate	T45.8X1	T45.8X2	T45.8X3	T45.8X4	T45.8X5	T45.8X6
Lizard (bite) (venom)	T63.121	T63.122	T63.123	T63.124	--	--
LMD	T45.8X1	T45.8X2	T45.8X3	T45.8X4	T45.8X5	T45.8X6
Lobelia	T62.2X1	T62.2X2	T62.2X3	T62.2X4	--	--
Lobeline	T50.7X1	T50.7X2	T50.7X3	T50.7X4	T50.7X5	T50.7X6
Local action drug NEC	T49.8X1	T49.8X2	T49.8X3	T49.8X4	T49.8X5	T49.8X6
Locorten	T49.0X1	T49.0X2	T49.0X3	T49.0X4	T49.0X5	T49.0X6
Lofepramine	T43.011	T43.012	T43.014	T43.015	T43.016	
Lolium temulentum	T62.2X1	T62.2X2	T62.2X3	T62.2X4	--	--
Lomotil	T47.6X1	T47.6X2	T47.6X3	T47.6X4	T47.6X5	T47.6X6
Lomustine	T45.1X1	T45.1X2	T45.1X3	T45.1X4	T45.1X5	T45.1X6
Lonidamine	T45.1X1	T45.1X2	T45.1X3	T45.1X4	T45.1X5	T45.1X6
Loperamide	T47.6X1	T47.6X2	T47.6X3	T47.6X4	T47.6X5	T47.6X6
Loprazolam	T42.4X1	T42.4X2	T42.4X3	T42.4X4	T42.4X5	T42.4X6
Lorajmine	T46.2X1	T46.2X2	T46.2X3	T46.2X4	T46.2X5	T46.2X6
Loratidine	T45.0X1	T45.0X2	T45.0X3	T45.0X4	T45.0X5	T45.0X6
Lorazepam	T42.4X1	T42.4X2	T42.4X3	T42.4X4	T42.4X5	T42.4X6
Lorcainide	T46.2X1	T46.2X2	T46.2X3	T46.2X4	T46.2X5	T46.2X6
Lormetazepam	T42.4X1	T42.4X2	T42.4X3	T42.4X4	T42.4X5	T42.4X6
Lotions NEC	T49.91	T49.92	T49.93	T49.94	T49.95	T49.96
Lotusate	T42.3X1	T42.3X2	T42.3X3	T42.3X4	T42.3X5	T42.3X6
Lovastatin	T46.6X1	T46.6X2	T46.6X3	T46.6X4	T46.6X5	T46.6X6
Lowila	T49.2X1	T49.2X2	T49.2X3	T49.2X4	T49.2X5	T49.2X6
Loxapine	T43.591	T43.592	T43.593	T43.594	T43.595	T43.596
Lozenges (throat)	T49.6X1	T49.6X2	T49.6X3	T49.6X4	T49.6X5	T49.6X6
LSD	T40.8X1	T40.8X2	T40.8X3	T40.8X4	T40.8X5	--
L-Tryptophan—see amino acid						
Lubricant, eye	T49.5X1	T49.5X2	T49.5X3	T49.5X4	T49.5X5	T49.5X6
Lubricating oil NEC	T52.0X1	T52.0X2	T52.0X3	T52.0X4	--	--
Lucanthone	T37.4X1	T37.4X2	T37.4X3	T37.4X4	T37.4X5	T37.4X6
Luminal	T42.3X1	T42.3X2	T42.3X3	T42.3X4	T42.3X5	T42.3X6
Lung irritant (gas) NEC	T59.91	T59.92	T59.93	T59.94	--	--
Luteinizing hormone	T38.811	T38.812	T38.813	T38.814	T38.815	T38.816
Lutocylol	T38.5X1	T38.5X2	T38.5X3	T38.5X4	T38.5X5	T38.5X6
Lutromone	T38.5X1	T38.5X2	T38.5X3	T38.5X4	T38.5X5	T38.5X6
Lututrin	T48.291	T48.292	T48.293	T48.294	T48.295	T48.296
Lye (concentrated)	T54.3X1	T54.3X2	T54.3X3	T54.3X4	--	--
Lygranum (skin test)	T50.8X1	T50.8X2	T50.8X3	T50.8X4	T50.8X5	T50.8X6
Lymecycline	T36.4X1	T36.4X2	T36.4X3	T36.4X4	T36.4X5	T36.4X6
Lymphogranuloma venereum antigen	T50.8X1	T50.8X2	T50.8X3	T50.8X4	T50.8X5	T50.8X6
Lynestrenol	T38.4X1	T38.4X2	T38.4X3	T38.4X4	T38.4X5	T38.4X6

Substance	Poisoning, Accidental (unintentional)	Poisoning, Intentional Self-harm	Poisoning, Assault	Poisoning, Undetermined	Adverse effect	Underdosing
Lyovac Sodium Edecrin	T50.1X1	T50.1X2	T50.1X3	T50.1X4	T50.1X5	T50.1X6
Lypressin	T38.891	T38.892	T38.893	T38.894	T38.895	T38.896
Lysergic acid diethylamide	T40.8X1	T40.8X2	T40.8X3	T40.8X4	T40.8X5	--
Lysergide	T40.8X1	T40.8X2	T40.8X3	T40.8X4	T40.8X5	--
Lysine vasopressin	T38.891	T38.892	T38.893	T38.894	T38.895	T38.896
Lysol	T54.1X1	T54.1X2	T54.1X3	T54.1X4	--	--
Lysozyme	T49.0X1	T49.0X2	T49.0X3	T49.0X4	T49.0X5	T49.0X6
Lytta (vitatta)	T49.8X1	T49.8X2	T49.8X3	T49.8X4	T49.8X5	T49.8X6
Mace	T59.3X1	T59.3X2	T59.3X3	T59.3X4	--	--
Macrogol	T50.991	T50.992	T50.993	T50.994	T50.995	T50.996
Macrolide						
anabolic drug	T38.7X1	T38.7X2	T38.7X3	T38.7X4	T38.7X5	T38.7X6
antibiotic	T36.3X1	T36.3X2	T36.3X3	T36.3X4	T36.3X5	T36.3X6
Mafenide	T49.0X1	T49.0X2	T49.0X3	T49.0X4	T49.0X5	T49.0X6
Magaldrate	T47.1X1	T47.1X2	T47.1X3	T47.1X4	T47.1X5	T47.1X6
Magic mushroom	T40.991	T40.992	T40.993	T40.994	--	--
Magnamycin	T36.8X1	T36.8X2	T36.8X3	T36.8X4	T36.8X5	T36.8X6
Magnesia magma	T47.1X1	T47.1X2	T47.1X3	T47.1X4	T47.1X5	T47.1X6
Magnesium NEC	T56.891	T56.892	T56.893	T56.894	--	--
carbonate	T47.1X1	T47.1X2	T47.1X3	T47.1X4	T47.1X5	T47.1X6
citrate	T47.4X1	T47.4X2	T47.4X3	T47.4X4	T47.4X5	T47.4X6
hydroxide	T47.1X1	T47.1X2	T47.1X3	T47.1X4	T47.1X5	T47.1X6
oxide	T47.1X1	T47.1X2	T47.1X3	T47.1X4	T47.1X5	T47.1X6
peroxide	T49.0X1	T49.0X2	T49.0X3	T49.0X4	T49.0X5	T49.0X6
salicylate	T39.091	T39.092	T39.093	T39.094	T39.095	T39.096
silicofluoride	T50.3X1	T50.3X2	T50.3X3	T50.3X4	T50.3X5	T50.3X6
sulfate	T47.4X1	T47.4X2	T47.4X3	T47.4X4	T47.4X5	T47.4X6
thiosulfate	T45.0X1	T45.0X2	T45.0X3	T45.0X4	T45.0X5	T45.0X6
trisilicate	T47.1X1	T47.1X2	T47.1X3	T47.1X4	T47.1X5	T47.1X6
Malathion (medicinal)	T49.0X1	T49.0X2	T49.0X3	T49.0X4	T49.0X5	T49.0X6
insecticide	T60.0X1	T60.0X2	T60.0X3	T60.0X4	--	--
Male fern extract	T37.4X1	T37.4X2	T37.4X3	T37.4X4	T37.4X5	T37.4X6
M-AMSA	T45.1X1	T45.1X2	T45.1X3	T45.1X4	T45.1X5	T45.1X6
Mandelic acid	T37.8X1	T37.8X2	T37.8X3	T37.8X4	T37.8X5	T37.8X6
Manganese (dioxide) (salts)	T57.2X1	T57.2X2	T57.2X3	T57.2X4	--	--
medicinal	T50.991	T50.992	T50.993	T50.994	T50.995	T50.996
Mannitol	T47.3X1	T47.3X2	T47.3X3	T47.3X4	T47.3X5	T47.3X6
hexanitrate	T46.3X1	T46.3X2	T46.3X3	T46.3X4	T46.3X5	T46.3X6
Mannomustine	T45.1X1	T45.1X2	T45.1X3	T45.1X4	T45.1X5	T45.1X6
MAO inhibitors	T43.1X1	T43.1X2	T43.1X3	T43.1X4	T43.1X5	T43.1X6
Mapharsen	T37.8X1	T37.8X2	T37.8X3	T37.8X4	T37.8X5	T37.8X6
Maphenide	T49.0X1	T49.0X2	T49.0X3	T49.0X4	T49.0X5	T49.0X6
Maprotiline	T43.021	T43.022	T43.023	T43.024	T43.025	T43.026
Marcaine	T41.3X1	T41.3X2	T41.3X3	T41.3X4	T41.3X5	T41.3X6
infiltration (subcutaneous)	T41.3X1	T41.3X2	T41.3X3	T41.3X4	T41.3X5	T41.3X6
nerve block (peripheral) (plexus)	T41.3X1	T41.3X2	T41.3X3	T41.3X4	T41.3X5	T41.3X6
Marezine	T45.0X1	T45.0X2	T45.0X3	T45.0X4	T45.0X5	T45.0X6
Marihuana	T40.7X1	T40.7X2	T40.7X3	T40.7X4	T40.7X5	T40.7X6
Marijuana	T40.7X1	T40.7X2	T40.7X3	T40.7X4	T40.7X5	T40.7X6
Marine (sting)	T63.691	T63.692	T63.693	T63.694	--	--
animals (sting)	T63.691	T63.692	T63.693	T63.694	--	--
plants (sting)	T63.711	T63.712	T63.713	T63.714	--	--
Marplan	T43.1X1	T43.1X2	T43.1X3	T43.1X4	T43.1X5	T43.1X6
Marsh gas	T59.891	T59.892	T59.893	T59.894	--	--
Marsilid	T43.1X1	T43.1X2	T43.1X3	T43.1X4	T43.1X5	T43.1X6
Matulane	T45.1X1	T45.1X2	T45.1X3	T45.1X4	T45.1X5	T45.1X6
Mazindol	T50.5X1	T50.5X2	T50.5X3	T50.5X4	T50.5X5	T50.5X6
MCPA	T60.3X1	T60.3X2	T60.3X3	T60.3X4	--	--
MDMA	T43.621	T43.622	T43.623	T43.624	T43.625	T43.626
Meadow saffron	T62.2X1	T62.2X2	T62.2X3	T62.2X4	--	--
Measles virus vaccine (attenuated)	T50.B91	T50.B92	T50.B93	T50.B94	T50.B95	T50.B96
Meat, noxious	T62.8X1	T62.8X2	T62.8X3	T62.8X4	--	--
Meballymal	T42.3X1	T42.3X2	T42.3X3	T42.3X4	T42.3X5	T42.3X6
Mebanazine	T43.1X1	T43.1X2	T43.1X3	T43.1X4	T43.1X5	T43.1X6

TABLE OF DRUGS AND CHEMICALS

Substance	Poisoning, Accidental (unintentional)	Poisoning, Intentional Self-harm	Poisoning, Assault	Poisoning, Undetermined	Adverse effect	Underdosing
Mebaral	T42.3X1	T42.3X2	T42.3X3	T42.3X4	T42.3X5	T42.3X6
Mebendazole	T37.4X1	T37.4X2	T37.4X3	T37.4X4	T37.4X5	T37.4X6
Mebeverine	T44.3X1	T44.3X2	T44.3X3	T44.3X4	T44.3X5	T44.3X6
Mebhydrolin	T45.0X1	T45.0X2	T45.0X3	T45.0X4	T45.0X5	T45.0X6
Mebumal	T42.3X1	T42.3X2	T42.3X3	T42.3X4	T42.3X5	T42.3X6
Mebutamate	T43.591	T43.592	T43.593	T43.594	T43.595	T43.596
Mecamylamine	T44.2X1	T44.2X2	T44.2X3	T44.2X4	T44.2X5	T44.2X6
Mechlorethamine	T45.1X1	T45.1X2	T45.1X3	T45.1X4	T45.1X5	T45.1X6
Mecillinam	T36.0X1	T36.0X2	T36.0X3	T36.0X4	T36.0X5	T36.0X6
Meclizine (hydrochloride)	T45.0X1	T45.0X2	T45.0X3	T45.0X4	T45.0X5	T45.0X6
Meclocycline	T36.4X1	T36.4X2	T36.4X3	T36.4X4	T36.4X5	T36.4X6
Meclofenamate	T39.391	T39.392	T39.393	T39.394	T39.395	T39.396
Meclofenamic acid	T39.391	T39.392	T39.393	T39.394	T39.395	T39.396
Meclofenoxate	T43.691	T43.692	T43.693	T43.694	T43.695	T43.696
Meclozine	T45.0X1	T45.0X2	T45.0X3	T45.0X4	T45.0X5	T45.0X6
Mecobalamin	T45.8X1	T45.8X2	T45.8X3	T45.8X4	T45.8X5	T45.8X6
Mecoprop	T60.3X1	T60.3X2	T60.3X3	T60.3X4	--	--
Mecrilate	T49.3X1	T49.3X2	T49.3X3	T49.3X4	T49.3X5	T49.3X6
Mecysteine	T48.4X1	T48.4X2	T48.4X3	T48.4X4	T48.4X5	T48.4X6
Medazepam	T42.4X1	T42.4X2	T42.4X3	T42.4X4	T42.4X5	T42.4X6
Medicament NEC	T50.901	T50.902	T50.903	T50.904	T50.905	T50.906
Medinal	T42.3X1	T42.3X2	T42.3X3	T42.3X4	T42.3X5	T42.3X6
Medomin	T42.3X1	T42.3X2	T42.3X3	T42.3X4	T42.3X5	T42.3X6
Medrogestone	T38.5X1	T38.5X2	T38.5X3	T38.5X4	T38.5X5	T38.5X6
Medroxalol	T44.8X1	T44.8X2	T44.8X3	T44.8X4	T44.8X5	T44.8X6
Medroxyprogesterone acetate (depot)	T38.5X1	T38.5X2	T38.5X3	T38.5X4	T38.5X5	T38.5X6
Medrysone	T49.0X1	T49.0X2	T49.0X3	T49.0X4	T49.0X5	T49.0X6
Mefenamic acid	T39.391	T39.392	T39.393	T39.394	T39.395	T39.396
Mefenorex	T50.5X1	T50.5X2	T50.5X3	T50.5X4	T50.5X5	T50.5X6
Mefloquine	T37.2X1	T37.2X2	T37.2X3	T37.2X4	T37.2X5	T37.2X6
Mefruside	T50.2X1	T50.2X2	T50.2X3	T50.2X4	T50.2X5	T50.2X6
Megahallucinogen	T40.901	T40.902	T40.903	T40.904	T40.905	T40.906
Megestrol	T38.5X1	T38.5X2	T38.5X3	T38.5X4	T38.5X5	T38.5X6
Meglumine						
antimoniate	T37.8X1	T37.8X2	T37.8X3	T37.8X4	T37.8X5	T37.8X6
diatrizoate	T50.8X1	T50.8X2	T50.8X3	T50.8X4	T50.8X5	T50.8X6
iodipamide	T50.8X1	T50.8X2	T50.8X3	T50.8X4	T50.8X5	T50.8X6
iotroxate	T50.8X1	T50.8X2	T50.8X3	T50.8X4	T50.8X5	T50.8X6
MEK (methyl ethyl ketone)	T52.4X1	T52.4X2	T52.4X3	T52.4X4	--	--
Meladinin	T49.3X1	T49.3X2	T49.3X3	T49.3X4	T49.3X5	T49.3X6
Meladrazine	T44.3X1	T44.3X2	T44.3X3	T44.3X4	T44.3X5	T44.3X6
Melaleuca alternifolia oil	T49.0X1	T49.0X2	T49.0X3	T49.0X4	T49.0X5	T49.0X6
Melanizing agents	T49.3X1	T49.3X2	T49.3X3	T49.3X4	T49.3X5	T49.3X6
Melanocyte-stimulating hormone	T38.891	T38.892	T38.893	T38.894	T38.895	T38.896
Melarsonyl potassium	T37.3X1	T37.3X2	T37.3X3	T37.3X4	T37.3X5	T37.3X6
Melarsoprol	T37.3X1	T37.3X2	T37.3X3	T37.3X4	T37.3X5	T37.3X6
Melia azedarach	T62.2X1	T62.2X2	T62.2X3	T62.2X4	--	--
Melitracen	T43.011	T43.012	T43.013	T43.014	T43.015	T43.016
Mellaril	T43.3X1	T43.3X2	T43.3X3	T43.3X4	T43.3X5	T43.3X6
Meloxine	T49.3X1	T49.3X2	T49.3X3	T49.3X4	T49.3X5	T49.3X6
Melperone	T43.4X1	T43.4X2	T43.4X3	T43.4X4	T43.4X5	T43.4X6
Melphalan	T45.1X1	T45.1X2	T45.1X3	T45.1X4	T45.1X5	T45.1X6
Memantine	T43.8X1	T43.8X2	T43.8X3	T43.8X4	T43.8X5	T43.8X6
Menadiol	T45.7X1	T45.7X2	T45.7X3	T45.7X4	T45.7X5	T45.7X6
sodium sulfate	T45.7X1	T45.7X2	T45.7X3	T45.7X4	T45.7X5	T45.7X6
Menadione	T45.7X1	T45.7X2	T45.7X3	T45.7X4	T45.7X5	T45.7X6
sodium bisulfite	T45.7X1	T45.7X2	T45.7X3	T45.7X4	T45.7X5	T45.7X6
Menaphthone	T45.7X1	T45.7X2	T45.7X3	T45.7X4	T45.7X5	T45.7X6
Menaquinone	T45.7X1	T45.7X2	T45.7X3	T45.7X4	T45.7X5	T45.7X6
Menatetrenone	T45.7X1	T45.7X2	T45.7X3	T45.7X4	T45.7X5	T45.7X6
Meningococcal vaccine	T50.A91	T50.A92	T50.A93	T50.A94	T50.A95	T50.A96
Menningovax (-AC) (-C)	T50.A91	T50.A92	T50.A93	T50.A94	T50.A95	T50.A96
Menotropins	T38.811	T38.812	T38.813	T38.814	T38.815	T38.816
Menthol	T48.5X1	T48.5X2	T48.5X3	T48.5X4	T48.5X5	T48.5X6
Mepacrine	T37.2X1	T37.2X2	T37.2X3	T37.2X4	T37.2X5	T37.2X6

Substance	Poisoning, Accidental (unintentional)	Poisoning, Intentional Self-harm	Poisoning, Assault	Poisoning, Undetermined	Adverse effect	Underdosing
Meparfynol	T42.6X1	T42.6X2	T42.6X3	T42.6X4	T42.6X5	T42.6X6
Mepartricin	T36.7X1	T36.7X2	T36.7X3	T36.7X4	T36.7X5	T36.7X6
Mepazine	T43.3X1	T43.3X2	T43.3X3	T43.3X4	T43.3X5	T43.3X6
Mepenzolate	T44.3X1	T44.3X2	T44.3X3	T44.3X4	T44.3X5	T44.3X6
bromide	T44.3X1	T44.3X2	T44.3X3	T44.3X4	T44.3X5	T44.3X6
Meperidine	T40.4X1	T40.4X2	T40.4X3	T40.4X4	T40.4X5	T40.4X6
Mephebarbital	T42.3X1	T42.3X2	T42.3X3	T42.3X4	T42.3X5	T42.3X6
Mephenamin (e)	T42.8X1	T42.8X2	T42.8X3	T42.8X4	T42.8X5	T42.8X6
Mephenesin	T42.8X1	T42.8X2	T42.8X3	T42.8X4	T42.8X5	T42.8X6
Mephenhydramine	T45.0X1	T45.0X2	T45.0X3	T45.0X4	T45.0X5	T45.0X6
Mephenoxalone	T42.8X1	T42.8X2	T42.8X3	T42.8X4	T42.8X5	T42.8X6
Mephentermine	T44.991	T44.992	T44.993	T44.994	T44.995	T44.996
Mephenytoin	T42.0X1	T42.0X2	T42.0X3	T42.0X4	T42.0X5	T42.0X6
with phenobarbital	T42.3X1	T42.3X2	T42.3X3	T42.3X4	T42.3X5	T42.3X6
Mephobarbital	T42.3X1	T42.3X2	T42.3X3	T42.3X4	T42.3X5	T42.3X6
Mephosfolan	T60.0X1	T60.0X2	T60.0X3	T60.0X4	--	--
Mepindolol	T44.7X1	T44.7X2	T44.7X3	T44.7X4	T44.7X5	T44.7X6
Mepiperphenidol	T44.3X1	T44.3X2	T44.3X3	T44.3X4	T44.3X5	T44.3X6
Mepitiostane	T38.7X1	T38.7X2	T38.7X3	T38.7X4	T38.7X5	T38.7X6
Mepivacaine	T41.3X1	T41.3X2	T41.3X3	T41.3X4	T41.3X5	T41.3X6
epidural	T41.3X1	T41.3X2	T41.3X3	T41.3X4	T41.3X5	T41.3X6
Meprednisone	T38.0X1	T38.0X2	T38.0X3	T38.0X4	T38.0X5	T38.0X6
Meprobam	T43.591	T43.592	T43.593	T43.594	T43.595	T43.596
Meprobamate	T43.591	T43.592	T43.593	T43.594	T43.595	T43.596
Meproscillarin	T46.0X1	T46.0X2	T46.0X3	T46.0X4	T46.0X5	T46.0X6
Meprylcaine	T41.3X1	T41.3X2	T41.3X3	T41.3X4	T41.3X5	T41.3X6
Meptazinol	T39.8X1	T39.8X2	T39.8X3	T39.8X4	T39.8X5	T39.8X6
Mepyramine	T45.0X1	T45.0X2	T45.0X3	T45.0X4	T45.0X5	T45.0X6
Mequitazine	T43.3X1	T43.3X2	T43.3X3	T43.3X4	T43.3X5	T43.3X6
Meralluride	T50.2X1	T50.2X2	T50.2X3	T50.2X4	T50.2X5	T50.2X6
Merbaphen	T50.2X1	T50.2X2	T50.2X3	T50.2X4	T50.2X5	T50.2X6
Merbromin	T49.0X1	T49.0X2	T49.0X3	T49.0X4	T49.0X5	T49.0X6
Mercaptobenzothiazole salts	T49.0X1	T49.0X2	T49.0X3	T49.0X4	T49.0X5	T49.0X6
Mercaptomerin	T50.2X1	T50.2X2	T50.2X3	T50.2X4	T50.2X5	T50.2X6
Mercaptopurine	T45.1X1	T45.1X2	T45.1X3	T45.1X4	T45.1X5	T45.1X6
Mercumatilin	T50.2X1	T50.2X2	T50.2X3	T50.2X4	T50.2X5	T50.2X6
Mercuramide	T50.2X1	T50.2X2	T50.2X3	T50.2X4	T50.2X5	T50.2X6
Mercurochrome	T49.0X1	T49.0X2	T49.0X3	T49.0X4	T49.0X5	T49.0X6
Mercurophylline	T50.2X1	T50.2X2	T50.2X3	T50.2X4	T50.2X5	T50.2X6
Mercury, mercurial, mercuric, mercurous (compounds) (cyanide) (fumes) (nonmedicinal) (vapor) NEC	T56.1X1	T56.1X2	T56.1X3	T56.1X4	--	--
ammoniated	T49.0X1	T49.0X2	T49.0X3	T49.0X4	T49.0X5	T49.0X6
anti-infective						
local	T49.0X1	T49.0X2	T49.0X3	T49.0X4	T49.0X5	T49.0X6
systemic	T37.8X1	T37.8X2	T37.8X3	T37.8X4	T37.8X5	T37.8X6
topical	T49.0X1	T49.0X2	T49.0X3	T49.0X4	T49.0X5	T49.0X6
chloride (ammoniated)	T49.0X1	T49.0X2	T49.0X3	T49.0X4	T49.0X5	T49.0X6
fungicide	T56.1X1	T56.1X2	T56.1X3	T56.1X4	--	--
diuretic NEC	T50.2X1	T50.2X2	T50.2X3	T50.2X4	T50.2X5	T50.2X6
fungicide	T56.1X1	T56.1X2	T56.1X3	T56.1X4	--	--
organic (fungicide)	T56.1X1	T56.1X2	T56.1X3	T56.1X4	--	--
oxide, yellow	T49.0X1	T49.0X2	T49.0X3	T49.0X4	T49.0X5	T49.0X6
Mersalyl	T50.2X1	T50.2X2	T50.2X3	T50.2X4	T50.2X5	T50.2X6
Merthiolate	T49.0X1	T49.0X2	T49.0X3	T49.0X4	T49.0X5	T49.0X6
ophthalmic preparation	T49.5X1	T49.5X2	T49.5X3	T49.5X4	T49.5X5	T49.5X6
Meruvax	T50.B91	T50.B92	T50.B93	T50.B94	T50.B95	T50.B96
Mesalazine	T47.8X1	T47.8X2	T47.8X3	T47.8X4	T47.8X5	T47.8X6
Mescal buttons	T40.991	T40.992	T40.993	T40.994	--	--
Mescaline	T40.991	T40.992	T40.993	T40.994	--	--
Mesna	T48.4X1	T48.4X2	T48.4X3	T48.4X4	T48.4X5	T48.4X6
Mesoglycan	T46.6X1	T46.6X2	T46.6X3	T46.6X4	T46.6X5	T46.6X6
Mesoridazine	T43.3X1	T43.3X2	T43.3X3	T43.3X4	T43.3X5	T43.3X6
Mestanolone	T38.7X1	T38.7X2	T38.7X3	T38.7X4	T38.7X5	T38.7X6

TABLE OF DRUGS AND CHEMICALS

Substance	Poisoning, Accidental (unintentional)	Poisoning, Intentional Self-harm	Poisoning, Assault	Poisoning, Undetermined	Adverse effect	Underdosing
Mesterolone	T38.7X1	T38.7X2	T38.7X3	T38.7X4	T38.7X5	T38.7X6
Mestranol	T38.5X1	T38.5X2	T38.5X3	T38.5X4	T38.5X5	T38.5X6
Mesulergine	T42.8X1	T42.8X2	T42.8X3	T42.8X4	T42.8X5	T42.8X6
Mesulfen	T49.0X1	T49.0X2	T49.0X3	T49.0X4	T49.0X5	T49.0X6
Mesuximide	T42.2X1	T42.2X2	T42.2X3	T42.2X4	T42.2X5	T42.2X6
Metabutethamine	T41.3X1	T41.3X2	T41.3X3	T41.3X4	T41.3X5	T41.3X6
Metactesylacetate	T49.0X1	T49.0X2	T49.0X3	T49.0X4	T49.0X5	T49.0X6
Metacycline	T36.4X1	T36.4X2	T36.4X3	T36.4X4	T36.4X5	T36.4X6
Metaldehyde (snail killer) NEC	T60.8X1	T60.8X2	T60.8X3	T60.8X4	--	--
Metals (heavy) (nonmedicinal)	T56.91	T56.92	T56.93	T56.94	--	--
dust, fumes, or vapor NEC	T56.91	T56.92	T56.93	T56.94	--	--
light NEC	T56.91	T56.92	T56.93	T56.94	--	--
dust, fumes, or vapor NEC	T56.91	T56.92	T56.93	T56.94	--	--
specified NEC	T56.891	T56.892	T56.893	T56.894	--	--
thallium	T56.811	T56.812	T56.813	T56.814	--	--
Metamfetamine	T43.621	T43.622	T43.623	T43.624	T43.625	T43.626
Metamizole sodium	T39.2X1	T39.2X2	T39.2X3	T39.2X4	T39.2X5	T39.2X6
Metampicillin	T36.0X1	T36.0X2	T36.0X3	T36.0X4	T36.0X5	T36.0X6
Metamucil	T47.4X1	T47.4X2	T47.4X3	T47.4X4	T47.4X5	T47.4X6
Metandienone	T38.7X1	T38.7X2	T38.7X3	T38.7X4	T38.7X5	T38.7X6
Metandrostenolone	T38.7X1	T38.7X2	T38.7X3	T38.7X4	T38.7X5	T38.7X6
Metaphen	T49.0X1	T49.0X2	T49.0X3	T49.0X4	T49.0X5	T49.0X6
Metaphos	T60.0X1	T60.0X2	T60.0X3	T60.0X4	--	--
Metapramine	T43.011	T43.012	T43.013	T43.014	T43.015	T43.016
Metaproterenol	T48.291	T48.292	T48.293	T48.294	T48.295	T48.296
Metaraminol	T44.4X1	T44.4X2	T44.4X3	T44.4X4	T44.4X5	T44.4X6
Metaxalone	T42.8X1	T42.8X2	T42.8X3	T42.8X4	T42.8X5	T42.8X6
Metenolone	T38.7X1	T38.7X2	T38.7X3	T38.7X4	T38.7X5	T38.7X6
Metergoline	T42.8X1	T42.8X2	T42.8X3	T42.8X4	T42.8X5	T42.8X6
Metescufylline	T46.991	T46.992	T46.993	T46.994	T46.995	T46.996
Metetoin	T42.0X1	T42.0X2	T42.0X3	T42.0X4	T42.0X5	T42.0X6
Metformin	T38.3X1	T38.3X2	T38.3X3	T38.3X4	T38.3X5	T38.3X6
Methacholine	T44.1X1	T44.1X2	T44.1X3	T44.1X4	T44.1X5	T44.1X6
Methacycline	T36.4X1	T36.4X2	T36.4X3	T36.4X4	T36.4X5	T36.4X6
Methadone	T40.3X1	T40.3X2	T40.3X3	T40.3X4	T40.3X5	T40.3X6
Methallenestril	T38.5X1	T38.5X2	T38.5X3	T38.5X4	T38.5X5	T38.5X6
Methallenoestril	T38.5X1	T38.5X2	T38.5X3	T38.5X4	T38.5X5	T38.5X6
Methamphetamine	T43.621	T43.622	T43.623	T43.624	T43.625	T43.626
Methampyrone	T39.2X1	T39.2X2	T39.2X3	T39.2X4	T39.2X5	T39.2X6
Methandienone	T38.7X1	T38.7X2	T38.7X3	T38.7X4	T38.7X5	T38.7X6
Methandriol	T38.7X1	T38.7X2	T38.7X3	T38.7X4	T38.7X5	T38.7X6
Methandrostenolone	T38.7X1	T38.7X2	T38.7X3	T38.7X4	T38.7X5	T38.7X6
Methane	T59.891	T59.892	T59.893	T59.894	--	--
Methanethiol	T59.891	T59.892	T59.893	T59.894	--	--
Methaniazide	T37.1X1	T37.1X2	T37.1X3	T37.1X4	T37.1X5	T37.1X6
Methanol (vapor)	T51.1X1	T51.1X2	T51.1X3	T51.1X4	--	--
Methantheline	T44.3X1	T44.3X2	T44.3X3	T44.3X4	T44.3X5	T44.3X6
Methanthelinium bromide	T44.3X1	T44.3X2	T44.3X3	T44.3X4	T44.3X5	T44.3X6
Methaphenilene	T45.0X1	T45.0X2	T45.0X3	T45.0X4	T45.0X5	T45.0X6
Methapyrilene	T45.0X1	T45.0X2	T45.0X3	T45.0X4	T45.0X5	T45.0X6
Methaqualone (compound)	T42.6X1	T42.6X2	T42.6X3	T42.6X4	T42.6X5	T42.6X6
Metharbital	T42.3X1	T42.3X2	T42.3X3	T42.3X4	T42.3X5	T42.3X6
Methazolamide	T50.2X1	T50.2X2	T50.2X3	T50.2X4	T50.2X5	T50.2X6
Methdilazine	T43.3X1	T43.3X2	T43.3X3	T43.3X4	T43.3X5	T43.3X6
Methedrine	T43.621	T43.622	T43.623	T43.624	T43.625	T43.626
Methenamine (mandelate)	T37.8X1	T37.8X2	T37.8X3	T37.8X4	T37.8X5	T37.8X6
Methenolone	T38.7X1	T38.7X2	T38.7X3	T38.7X4	T38.7X5	T38.7X6
Methergine	T48.0X1	T48.0X2	T48.0X3	T48.0X4	T48.0X5	T48.0X6
Methetoin	T42.0X1	T42.0X2	T42.0X3	T42.0X4	T42.0X5	T42.0X6
Methiacil	T38.2X1	T38.2X2	T38.2X3	T38.2X4	T38.2X5	T38.2X6
Methicillin	T36.0X1	T36.0X2	T36.0X3	T36.0X4	T36.0X5	T36.0X6
Methimazole	T38.2X1	T38.2X2	T38.2X3	T38.2X4	T38.2X5	T38.2X6
Methiodal sodium	T50.8X1	T50.8X2	T50.8X3	T50.8X4	T50.8X5	T50.8X6
Methionine	T50.991	T50.992	T50.993	T50.994	T50.995	T50.996
Methisazone	T37.5X1	T37.5X2	T37.5X3	T37.5X4	T37.5X5	T37.5X6

Substance	Poisoning, Accidental (unintentional)	Poisoning, Intentional Self-harm	Poisoning, Assault	Poisoning, Undetermined	Adverse effect	Underdosing
Methisoprinol	T37.5X1	T37.5X2	T37.5X3	T37.5X4	T37.5X5	T37.5X6
Methitural	T42.3X1	T42.3X2	T42.3X3	T42.3X4	T42.3X5	T42.3X6
Methixene	T44.3X1	T44.3X2	T44.3X3	T44.3X4	T44.3X5	T44.3X6
Methobarbital, methobarbitone	T42.3X1	T42.3X2	T42.3X3	T42.3X4	T42.3X5	T42.3X6
Methocarbamol	T42.8X1	T42.8X2	T42.8X3	T42.8X4	T42.8X5	T42.8X6
skeletal muscle relaxant	T48.1X1	T48.1X2	T48.1X3	T48.1X4	T48.1X5	T48.1X6
Methohexital	T41.1X1	T41.1X2	T41.1X3	T41.1X4	T41.1X5	T41.1X6
Methohexitone	T41.1X1	T41.1X2	T41.1X3	T41.1X4	T41.1X5	T41.1X6
Methoin	T42.0X1	T42.0X2	T42.0X3	T42.0X4	T42.0X5	T42.0X6
Methopholine	T39.8X1	T39.8X2	T39.8X3	T39.8X4	T39.8X5	T39.8X6
Methopromazine	T43.3X1	T43.3X2	T43.3X3	T43.3X4	T43.3X5	T43.3X6
Methorate	T48.3X1	T48.3X2	T48.3X3	T48.3X4	T48.3X5	T48.3X6
Methoserpidine	T46.5X1	T46.5X2	T46.5X3	T46.5X4	T46.5X5	T46.5X6
Methotrexate	T45.1X1	T45.1X2	T45.1X3	T45.1X4	T45.1X5	T45.1X6
Methotrimeprazine	T43.3X1	T43.3X2	T43.3X3	T43.3X4	T43.3X5	T43.3X6
Methoxa-Dome	T49.3X1	T49.3X2	T49.3X3	T49.3X4	T49.3X5	T49.3X6
Methoxamine	T44.4X1	T44.4X2	T44.4X3	T44.4X4	T44.4X5	T44.4X6
Methoxsalen	T50.991	T50.992	T50.993	T50.994	T50.995	T50.996
Methoxyaniline	T65.3X1	T65.3X2	T65.3X3	T65.3X4	--	--
Methoxybenzyl penicillin	T36.0X1	T36.0X2	T36.0X3	T36.0X4	T36.0X5	T36.0X6
Methoxychlor	T53.7X1	T53.7X2	T53.7X3	T53.7X4	--	--
Methoxy-DDT	T53.7X1	T53.7X2	T53.7X3	T53.7X4	--	--
2-Methoxyethanol	T52.3X1	T52.3X2	T52.3X3	T52.3X4	--	--
Methoxyflurane	T41.0X1	T41.0X2	T41.0X3	T41.0X4	T41.0X5	T41.0X6
Methoxyphenamine	T48.6X1	T48.6X2	T48.6X3	T48.6X4	T48.6X5	T48.6X6
Methoxypromazine	T43.3X1	T43.3X2	T43.3X3	T43.3X4	T43.3X5	T43.3X6
5-Methoxypsoralen (5-MOP)	T50.991	T50.992	T50.993	T50.994	T50.995	T50.996
8-Methoxypsoralen (8-MOP)	T50.991	T50.992	T50.993	T50.994	T50.995	T50.996
Methscopolamine bromide	T44.3X1	T44.3X2	T44.3X3	T44.3X4	T44.3X5	T44.3X6
Methsuximide	T42.2X1	T42.2X2	T42.2X3	T42.2X4	T42.2X5	T42.2X6
Methyclothiazide	T50.2X1	T50.2X2	T50.2X3	T50.2X4	T50.2X5	T50.2X6
Methyl						
acetate	T52.4X1	T52.4X2	T52.4X3	T52.4X4	--	--
acetone	T52.4X1	T52.4X2	T52.4X3	T52.4X4	--	--
acrylate	T65.891	T65.892	T65.893	T65.894	--	--
alcohol	T51.1X1	T51.1X2	T51.1X3	T51.1X4	--	--
aminophenol	T65.3X1	T65.3X2	T65.3X3	T65.3X4	--	--
amphetamine	T43.621	T43.622	T43.623	T43.624	T43.625	T43.626
androstanolone	T38.7X1	T38.7X2	T38.7X3	T38.7X4	T38.7X5	T38.7X6
atropine	T44.3X1	T44.3X2	T44.3X3	T44.3X4	T44.3X5	T44.3X6
benzene	T52.2X1	T52.2X2	T52.2X3	T52.2X4	--	--
benzoate	T52.8X1	T52.8X2	T52.8X3	T52.8X4	--	--
benzol	T52.2X1	T52.2X2	T52.2X3	T52.2X4	--	--
bromide (gas)	T59.891	T59.892	T59.893	T59.894	--	--
fumigant	T60.8X1	T60.8X2	T60.8X3	T60.8X4	--	--
butanol	T51.3X1	T51.3X2	T51.3X3	T51.3X4	--	--
carbinol	T51.1X1	T51.1X2	T51.1X3	T51.1X4	--	--
carbonate	T52.8X1	T52.8X2	T52.8X3	T52.8X4	--	--
CCNU	T45.1X1	T45.1X2	T45.1X3	T45.1X4	T45.1X5	T45.1X6
cellosolve	T52.91	T52.92	T52.93	T52.94	--	--
cellulose	T47.4X1	T47.4X2	T47.4X3	T47.4X4	T47.4X5	T47.4X6
chloride (gas)	T59.891	T59.892	T59.893	T59.894	--	--
chloroformate	T59.3X1	T59.3X2	T59.3X3	T59.3X4	--	--
cyclohexane	T52.8X1	T52.8X2	T52.8X3	T52.8X4	--	--
cyclohexanol	T51.8X1	T51.8X2	T51.8X3	T51.8X4	--	--
cyclohexanone	T52.8X1	T52.8X2	T52.8X3	T52.8X4	--	--
cyclohexyl acetate	T52.8X1	T52.8X2	T52.8X3	T52.8X4	--	--
demeton	T60.0X1	T60.0X2	T60.0X3	T60.0X4	--	--
dihydromorphinone	T40.2X1	T40.2X2	T40.2X3	T40.2X4	T40.2X5	T40.2X6
ergometrine	T48.0X1	T48.0X2	T48.0X3	T48.0X4	T48.0X5	T48.0X6
ergonovine	T48.0X1	T48.0X2	T48.0X3	T48.0X4	T48.0X5	T48.0X6
ethyl ketone	T52.4X1	T52.4X2	T52.4X3	T52.4X4	--	--
glucamine antimonate	T37.8X1	T37.8X2	T37.8X3	T37.8X4	T37.8X5	T37.8X6
hydrazine	T65.891	T65.892	T65.893	T65.894	--	--

TABLE OF DRUGS AND CHEMICALS

Substance	Poisoning, Accidental (unintentional)	Poisoning, Intentional Self-harm	Poisoning, Assault	Poisoning, Undetermined	Adverse effect	Underdosing
iodide	T65.891	T65.892	T65.893	T65.894	--	--
isobutyl ketone	T52.4X1	T52.4X2	T52.4X3	T52.4X4	--	--
isothiocyanate	T60.3X1	T60.3X2	T60.3X3	T60.3X4	--	--
mercaptan	T59.891	T59.892	T59.893	T59.894	--	--
morphine NEC	T40.2X1	T40.2X2	T40.2X3	T40.2X4	T40.2X5	T40.2X6
nicotinate	T49.4X1	T49.4X2	T49.4X3	T49.4X4	T49.4X5	T49.4X6
paraben	T49.0X1	T49.0X2	T49.0X3	T49.0X4	T49.0X5	T49.0X6
parafynol	T42.6X1	T42.6X2	T42.6X3	T42.6X4	T42.6X5	T42.6X6
parathion	T60.0X1	T60.0X2	T60.0X3	T60.0X4	--	--
peridol	T43.4X1	T43.4X2	T43.4X3	T43.4X4	T43.4X5	T43.4X6
phenidate	T43.631	T43.632	T43.633	T43.634	T43.635	T43.636
prednisolone	T38.0X1	T38.0X2	T38.0X3	T38.0X4	T38.0X5	T38.0X6
ENT agent	T49.6X1	T49.6X2	T49.6X3	T49.6X4	T49.6X5	T49.6X6
ophthalmic preparation	T49.5X1	T49.5X2	T49.5X3	T49.5X4	T49.5X5	T49.5X6
topical NEC	T49.0X1	T49.0X2	T49.0X3	T49.0X4	T49.0X5	T49.0X6
propylcarbinol	T51.3X1	T51.3X2	T51.3X3	T51.3X4	--	--
rosaniline NEC	T49.0X1	T49.0X2	T49.0X3	T49.0X4	T49.0X5	T49.0X6
salicylate	T49.2X1	T49.2X2	T49.2X3	T49.2X4	T49.2X5	T49.2X6
sulfate (fumes)	T59.891	T59.892	T59.893	T59.894	--	--
liquid	T52.8X1	T52.8X2	T52.8X3	T52.8X4	--	--
sulfonal	T42.6X1	T42.6X2	T42.6X3	T42.6X4	T42.6X5	T42.6X6
testosterone	T38.7X1	T38.7X2	T38.7X3	T38.7X4	T38.7X5	T38.7X6
thiouracil	T38.2X1	T38.2X2	T38.2X3	T38.2X4	T38.2X5	T38.2X6
Methylamphetamine	T43.621	T43.622	T43.623	T43.624	T43.625	T43.626
Methylated spirit	T51.1X1	T51.1X2	T51.1X3	T51.1X4	--	--
Methylatropine nitrate	T44.3X1	T44.3X2	T44.3X3	T44.3X4	T44.3X5	T44.3X6
Methylbenactyzium bromide	T44.3X1	T44.3X2	T44.3X3	T44.3X4	T44.3X5	T44.3X6
Methylbenzethonium chloride	T49.0X1	T49.0X2	T49.0X3	T49.0X4	T49.0X5	T49.0X6
Methylcellulose	T47.4X1	T47.4X2	T47.4X3	T47.4X4	T47.4X5	T47.4X6
laxative	T47.4X1	T47.4X2	T47.4X3	T47.4X4	T47.4X5	T47.4X6
Methylchlorophenoxy-acetic acid	T60.3X1	T60.3X2	T60.3X3	T60.3X4	--	--
Methyldopa	T46.5X1	T46.5X2	T46.5X3	T46.5X4	T46.5X5	T46.5X6
Methyldopate	T46.5X1	T46.5X2	T46.5X3	T46.5X4	T46.5X5	T46.5X6
Methylene						
blue	T50.6X1	T50.6X2	T50.6X3	T50.6X4	T50.6X5	T50.6X6
chloride or dichloride (solvent) NEC	T53.4X1	T53.4X2	T53.4X3	T53.4X4	--	--
Methylenedioxyamphetamine	T43.621	T43.622	T43.623	T43.624	T43.625	T43.626
Methylenedioxymethamphetamine	T43.621	T43.622	T43.623	T43.624	T43.625	T43.626
Methylergometrine	T48.0X1	T48.0X2	T48.0X3	T48.0X4	T48.0X5	T48.0X6
Methylergonovine	T48.0X1	T48.0X2	T48.0X3	T48.0X4	T48.0X5	T48.0X6
Methylestrenolone	T38.5X1	T38.5X2	T38.5X3	T38.5X4	T38.5X5	T38.5X6
Methylethyl cellulose	T50.991	T50.992	T50.993	T50.994	T50.995	T50.996
Methylhexabital	T42.3X1	T42.3X2	T42.3X3	T42.3X4	T42.3X5	T42.3X6
Methylmorphine	T40.2X1	T40.2X2	T40.2X3	T40.2X4	T40.2X5	T40.2X6
Methylparaben (ophthalmic)	T49.5X1	T49.5X2	T49.5X3	T49.5X4	T49.5X5	T49.5X6
Methylparafynol	T42.6X1	T42.6X2	T42.6X3	T42.6X4	T42.6X5	T42.6X6
Methylpentynol, methylpenthynol	T42.6X1	T42.6X2	T42.6X3	T42.6X4	T42.6X5	T42.6X6
Methylphenidate	T43.631	T43.632	T43.633	T43.634	T43.635	T43.636
Methylphenobarbital	T42.3X1	T42.3X2	T42.3X3	T42.3X4	T42.3X5	T42.3X6
Methylpolysiloxane	T47.1X1	T47.1X2	T47.1X3	T47.1X4	T47.1X5	T47.1X6
Methylprednisolone—see Methyl, prednisolone						
Methylrosaniline	T49.0X1	T49.0X2	T49.0X3	T49.0X4	T49.0X5	T49.0X6
Methylrosanilinium chloride	T49.0X1	T49.0X2	T49.0X3	T49.0X4	T49.0X5	T49.0X6
Methyltestosterone	T38.7X1	T38.7X2	T38.7X3	T38.7X4	T38.7X5	T38.7X6
Methylthionine chloride	T50.6X1	T50.6X2	T50.6X3	T50.6X4	T50.6X5	T50.6X6
Methylthioninium chloride	T50.6X1	T50.6X2	T50.6X3	T50.6X4	T50.6X5	T50.6X6
Methylthiouracil	T38.2X1	T38.2X2	T38.2X3	T38.2X4	T38.2X5	T38.2X6
Methyprylon	T42.6X1	T42.6X2	T42.6X3	T42.6X4	T42.6X5	T42.6X6
Methysergide	T46.5X1	T46.5X2	T46.5X3	T46.5X4	T46.5X5	T46.5X6
Metiamide	T47.1X1	T47.1X2	T47.1X3	T47.1X4	T47.1X5	T47.1X6
Meticillin	T36.0X1	T36.0X2	T36.0X3	T36.0X4	T36.0X5	T36.0X6
Meticrane	T50.2X1	T50.2X2	T50.2X3	T50.2X4	T50.2X5	T50.2X6
Metildigoxin	T46.0X1	T46.0X2	T46.0X3	T46.0X4	T46.0X5	T46.0X6
Metipranolol	T49.5X1	T49.5X2	T49.5X3	T49.5X4	T49.5X5	T49.5X6
Metirosine	T46.5X1	T46.5X2	T46.5X3	T46.5X4	T46.5X5	T46.5X6

Substance	Poisoning, Accidental (unintentional)	Poisoning, Intentional Self-harm	Poisoning, Assault	Poisoning, Undetermined	Adverse effect	Underdosing
Metisazone	T37.5X1	T37.5X2	T37.5X3	T37.5X4	T37.5X5	T37.5X6
Metixene	T44.3X1	T44.3X2	T44.3X3	T44.3X4	T44.3X5	T44.3X6
Metizoline	T48.5X1	T48.5X2	T48.5X3	T48.5X4	T48.5X5	T48.5X6
Metoclopramide	T45.0X1	T45.0X2	T45.0X3	T45.0X4	T45.0X5	T45.0X6
Metofenazate	T43.3X1	T43.3X2	T43.3X3	T43.3X4	T43.3X5	T43.3X6
Metofoline	T39.8X1	T39.8X2	T39.8X3	T39.8X4	T39.8X5	T39.8X6
Metolazone	T50.2X1	T50.2X2	T50.2X3	T50.2X4	T50.2X5	T50.2X6
Metopon	T40.2X1	T40.2X2	T40.2X3	T40.2X4	T40.2X5	T40.2X6
Metoprine	T45.1X1	T45.1X2	T45.1X3	T45.1X4	T45.1X5	T45.1X6
Metoprolol	T44.7X1	T44.7X2	T44.7X3	T44.7X4	T44.7X5	T44.7X6
Metrifonate	T60.0X1	T60.0X2	T60.0X3	T60.0X4	--	--
Metrizamide	T50.8X1	T50.8X2	T50.8X3	T50.8X4	T50.8X5	T50.8X6
Metrizoic acid	T50.8X1	T50.8X2	T50.8X3	T50.8X4	T50.8X5	T50.8X6
Metronidazole	T37.8X1	T37.8X2	T37.8X3	T37.8X4	T37.8X5	T37.8X6
Metycaine	T41.3X1	T41.3X2	T41.3X3	T41.3X4	T41.3X5	T41.3X6
infiltration (subcutaneous)	T41.3X1	T41.3X2	T41.3X3	T41.3X4	T41.3X5	T41.3X6
nerve block (peripheral) (plexus)	T41.3X1	T41.3X2	T41.3X3	T41.3X4	T41.3X5	T41.3X6
topical (surface)	T41.3X1	T41.3X2	T41.3X3	T41.3X4	T41.3X5	T41.3X6
Metyrapone	T50.8X1	T50.8X2	T50.8X3	T50.8X4	T50.8X5	T50.8X6
Mevinphos	T60.0X1	T60.0X2	T60.0X3	T60.0X4	--	--
Mexazolam	T42.4X1	T42.4X2	T42.4X3	T42.4X4	T42.4X5	T42.4X6
Mexenone	T49.3X1	T49.3X2	T49.3X3	T49.3X4	T49.3X5	T49.3X6
Mexiletine	T46.2X1	T46.2X2	T46.2X3	T46.2X4	T46.2X5	T46.2X6
Mezereon	T62.2X1	T62.2X2	T62.2X3	T62.2X4	--	--
berries	T62.1X1	T62.1X2	T62.1X3	T62.1X4	--	--
Mezlocillin	T36.0X1	T36.0X2	T36.0X3	T36.0X4	T36.0X5	T36.0X6
Mianserin	T43.021	T43.022	T43.023	T43.024	T43.025	T43.026
Micatin	T49.0X1	T49.0X2	T49.0X3	T49.0X4	T49.0X5	T49.0X6
Miconazole	T49.0X1	T49.0X2	T49.0X3	T49.0X4	T49.0X5	T49.0X6
Micronomicin	T36.5X1	T36.5X2	T36.5X3	T36.5X4	T36.5X5	T36.5X6
Midazolam	T42.4X1	T42.4X2	T42.4X3	T42.4X4	T42.4X5	T42.4X6
Midecamycin	T36.3X1	T36.3X2	T36.3X3	T36.3X4	T36.3X5	T36.3X6
Mifepristone	T38.6X1	T38.6X2	T38.6X3	T38.6X4	T38.6X5	T38.6X6
Milk of magnesia	T47.1X1	T47.1X2	T47.1X3	T47.1X4	T47.1X5	T47.1X6
Millipede (tropical) (venomous)	T63.411	T63.412	T63.413	T63.414	--	--
Miltown	T43.591	T43.592	T43.593	T43.594	T43.595	T43.596
Milverine	T44.3X1	T44.3X2	T44.3X3	T44.3X4	T44.3X5	T44.3X6
Minaprine	T43.291	T43.292	T43.293	T43.294	T43.295	T43.296
Minaxolone	T41.291	T41.292	T41.293	T41.294	T41.295	T41.296
Mineral						
acids	T54.2X1	T54.2X2	T54.2X3	T54.2X4	--	--
oil (laxative) (medicinal)	T47.4X1	T47.4X2	T47.4X3	T47.4X4	T47.4X5	T47.4X6
emulsion	T47.2X1	T47.2X2	T47.2X3	T47.2X4	T47.2X5	T47.2X6
nonmedicinal	T52.0X1	T52.0X2	T52.0X3	T52.0X4	--	--
topical	T49.3X1	T49.3X2	T49.3X3	T49.3X4	T49.3X5	T49.3X6
salt NEC	T50.3X1	T50.3X2	T50.3X3	T50.3X4	T50.3X5	T50.3X6
spirits	T52.0X1	T52.0X2	T52.0X3	T52.0X4	--	--
Mineralocorticosteroid	T50.0X1	T50.0X2	T50.0X3	T50.0X4	T50.0X5	T50.0X6
Minocycline	T36.4X1	T36.4X2	T36.4X3	T36.4X4	T36.4X5	T36.4X6
Minoxidil	T46.7X1	T46.7X2	T46.7X3	T46.7X4	T46.7X5	T46.7X6
Miokamycin	T36.3X1	T36.3X2	T36.3X3	T36.3X4	T36.3X5	T36.3X6
Miotic drug	T49.5X1	T49.5X2	T49.5X3	T49.5X4	T49.5X5	T49.5X6
Mipafox	T60.0X1	T60.0X2	T60.0X3	T60.0X4	--	--
Mirex	T60.1X1	T60.1X2	T60.1X3	T60.1X4	--	--
Mirtazapine	T43.021	T43.022	T43.023	T43.024	T43.025	T43.026
Misonidazole	T37.3X1	T37.3X2	T37.3X3	T37.3X4	T37.3X5	T37.3X6
Misoprostol	T47.1X1	T47.1X2	T47.1X3	T47.1X4	T47.1X5	T47.1X6
Mithramycin	T45.1X1	T45.1X2	T45.1X3	T45.1X4	T45.1X5	T45.1X6
Mitobronitol	T45.1X1	T45.1X2	T45.1X3	T45.1X4	T45.1X5	T45.1X6
Mitoguazone	T45.1X1	T45.1X2	T45.1X3	T45.1X4	T45.1X5	T45.1X6
Mitolactol	T45.1X1	T45.1X2	T45.1X3	T45.1X4	T45.1X5	T45.1X6
Mitomycin	T45.1X1	T45.1X2	T45.1X3	T45.1X4	T45.1X5	T45.1X6
Mitopodozide	T45.1X1	T45.1X2	T45.1X3	T45.1X4	T45.1X5	T45.1X6
Mitotane	T45.1X1	T45.1X2	T45.1X3	T45.1X4	T45.1X5	T45.1X6

TABLE OF DRUGS AND CHEMICALS

Substance	Poisoning, Accidental (unintentional)	Poisoning, Intentional Self-harm	Poisoning, Assault	Poisoning, Undetermined	Adverse effect	Underdosing
Mitoxantrone	T45.1X1	T45.1X2	T45.1X3	T45.1X4	T45.1X5	T45.1X6
Mivacurium chloride	T48.1X1	T48.1X2	T48.1X3	T48.1X4	T48.1X5	T48.1X6
Miyari bacteria	T47.6X1	T47.6X2	T47.6X3	T47.6X4	T47.6X5	T47.6X6
Moclobemide	T43.1X1	T43.1X2	T43.1X3	T43.1X4	T43.1X5	T43.1X6
Moderil	T46.5X1	T46.5X2	T46.5X3	T46.5X4	T46.5X5	T46.5X6
Mofebutazone	T39.2X1	T39.2X2	T39.2X3	T39.2X4	T39.2X5	T39.2X6
Mogadon—see Nitrazepam						
Molindone	T43.591	T43.592	T43.593	T43.594	T43.595	T43.596
Molsidomine	T46.3X1	T46.3X2	T46.3X3	T46.3X4	T46.3X5	T46.3X6
Mometasone	T49.0X1	T49.0X2	T49.0X3	T49.0X4	T49.0X5	T49.0X6
Monistat	T49.0X1	T49.0X2	T49.0X3	T49.0X4	T49.0X5	T49.0X6
Monkshood	T62.2X1	T62.2X2	T62.2X3	T62.2X4	--	--
Monoamine oxidase inhibitor NEC	T43.1X1	T43.1X2	T43.1X3	T43.1X4	T43.1X5	T43.1X6
hydrazine	T43.1X1	T43.1X2	T43.1X3	T43.1X4	T43.1X5	T43.1X6
Monobenzone	T49.4X1	T49.4X2	T49.4X3	T49.4X4	T49.4X5	T49.4X6
Monochloroacetic acid	T60.3X1	T60.3X2	T60.3X3	T60.3X4	--	--
Monochlorobenzene	T53.7X1	T53.7X2	T53.7X3	T53.7X4	--	--
Monoethanolamine	T46.8X1	T46.8X2	T46.8X3	T46.8X4	T46.8X5	T46.8X6
oleate	T46.8X1	T46.8X2	T46.8X3	T46.8X4	T46.8X5	T46.8X6
Monooctanoin	T50.991	T50.992	T50.993	T50.994	T50.995	T50.996
Monophenylbutazone	T39.2X1	T39.2X2	T39.2X3	T39.2X4	T39.2X5	T39.2X6
Monosodium glutamate	T65.891	T65.892	T65.893	T65.894	--	--
Monosulfiram	T49.0X1	T49.0X2	T49.0X3	T49.0X4	T49.0X5	T49.0X6
Monoxide, carbon—see Carbon, monoxide						
Monoxidine hydrochloride	T46.1X1	T46.1X2	T46.1X3	T46.1X4	T46.1X5	T46.1X6
Monuron	T60.3X1	T60.3X2	T60.3X3	T60.3X4	--	--
Moperone	T43.4X1	T43.4X2	T43.4X3	T43.4X4	T43.4X5	T43.4X6
Mopidamol	T45.1X1	T45.1X2	T45.1X3	T45.1X4	T45.1X5	T45.1X6
MOPP (mechloreth-amine + vincristine + prednisone + procarba-zine)	T45.1X1	T45.1X2	T45.1X3	T45.1X4	T45.1X5	T45.1X6
Morfin	T40.2X1	T40.2X2	T40.2X3	T40.2X4	T40.2X5	T40.2X6
Morinamide	T37.1X1	T37.1X2	T37.1X3	T37.1X4	T37.1X5	T37.1X6
Morning glory seeds	T40.991	T40.992	T40.993	T40.994	--	--
Moroxydine	T37.5X1	T37.5X2	T37.5X3	T37.5X4	T37.5X5	T37.5X6
Morphazinamide	T37.1X1	T37.1X2	T37.1X3	T37.1X4	T37.1X5	T37.1X6
Morphine	T40.2X1	T40.2X2	T40.2X3	T40.2X4	T40.2X5	T40.2X6
antagonist	T50.7X1	T50.7X2	T50.7X3	T50.7X4	T50.7X5	T50.7X6
Morpholinylethylmorphine	T40.2X1	T40.2X2	T40.2X3	T40.2X4	--	--
Morsuximide	T42.2X1	T42.2X2	T42.2X3	T42.2X4	T42.2X5	T42.2X6
Mosapramine	T43.591	T43.592	T43.593	T43.594	T43.595	T43.596
Moth balls—see also Pesticides	T60.2X1	T60.2X2	T60.2X3	T60.2X4	--	--
naphthalene	T60.2X1	T60.2X2	T60.2X3	T60.2X4	--	--
paradichlorobenzene	T60.1X1	T60.1X2	T60.1X3	T60.1X4	--	--
Motor exhaust gas	T58.01	T58.02	T58.03	T58.04	--	--
Mouthwash (antiseptic) (zinc chloride)	T49.6X1	T49.6X2	T49.6X3	T49.6X4	T49.6X5	T49.6X6
Moxastine	T45.0X1	T45.0X2	T45.0X3	T45.0X4	T45.0X5	T45.0X6
Moxaverine	T44.3X1	T44.3X2	T44.3X3	T44.3X4	T44.3X5	T44.3X6
Moxisylyte	T46.7X1	T46.7X2	T46.7X3	T46.7X4	T46.7X5	T46.7X6
Mucilage, plant	T47.4X1	T47.4X2	T47.4X3	T47.4X4	T47.4X5	T47.4X6
Mucolytic drug	T48.4X1	T48.4X2	T48.4X3	T48.4X4	T48.4X5	T48.4X6
Mucomyst	T48.4X1	T48.4X2	T48.4X3	T48.4X4	T48.4X5	T48.4X6
Mucous membrane agents (external)	T49.91	T49.92	T49.93	T49.94	T49.95	T49.96
specified NEC	T49.8X1	T49.8X2	T49.8X3	T49.8X4	T49.8X5	T49.8X6
Mumps						
immune globulin (human)	T50.Z11	T50.Z12	T50.Z13	T50.Z14	T50.Z15	T50.Z16
skin test antigen	T50.8X1	T50.8X2	T50.8X3	T50.8X4	T50.8X5	T50.8X6
vaccine	T50.B91	T50.B92	T50.B93	T50.B94	T50.B95	T50.B96
Mumpsvax	T50.B91	T50.B92	T50.B93	T50.B94	T50.B95	T50.B96
Mupirocin	T49.0X1	T49.0X2	T49.0X3	T49.0X4	T49.0X5	T49.0X6
Muriatic acid—see Hydrochloric acid						
Muromonab-CD3	T45.1X1	T45.1X2	T45.1X3	T45.1X4	T45.1X5	T45.1X6
Muscle-action drug NEC	T48.201	T48.202	T48.203	T48.204	T48.205	T48.206
Muscle affecting agents NEC	T48.201	T48.202	T48.203	T48.204	T48.205	T48.206
oxytocic	T48.0X1	T48.0X2	T48.0X3	T48.0X4	T48.0X5	T48.0X6
relaxants	T48.201	T48.202	T48.203	T48.204	T48.205	T48.206

Substance	Poisoning, Accidental (unintentional)	Poisoning, Intentional Self-harm	Poisoning, Assault	Poisoning, Undetermined	Adverse effect	Underdosing
central nervous system	T42.8X1	T42.8X2	T42.8X3	T42.8X4	T42.8X5	T42.8X6
skeletal	T48.1X1	T48.1X2	T48.1X3	T48.1X4	T48.1X5	T48.1X6
smooth	T44.3X1	T44.3X2	T44.3X3	T44.3X4	T44.3X5	T44.3X6
Muscle relaxant—see Relaxant, muscle						
Muscle-tone depressant, central NEC	T42.8X1	T42.8X2	T42.8X3	T42.8X4	T42.8X5	T42.8X6
specified NEC	T42.8X1	T42.8X2	T42.8X3	T42.8X4	T42.8X5	T42.8X6
Mushroom, noxious	T62.0X1	T62.0X2	T62.0X3	T62.0X4	--	--
Mussel, noxious	T61.781	T61.782	T61.783	T61.784	--	--
Mustard (emetic)	T47.7X1	T47.7X2	T47.7X3	T47.7X4	T47.7X5	T47.7X6
black	T47.7X1	T47.7X2	T47.7X3	T47.7X4	T47.7X5	T47.7X6
gas, not in war	T59.91	T59.92	T59.93	T59.94	--	--
nitrogen	T45.1X1	T45.1X2	T45.1X3	T45.1X4	T45.1X5	T45.1X6
Mustine	T45.1X1	T45.1X2	T45.1X3	T45.1X4	T45.1X5	T45.1X6
M-vac	T45.1X1	T45.1X2	T45.1X3	T45.1X4	T45.1X5	T45.1X6
Mycifradin	T36.5X1	T36.5X2	T36.5X3	T36.5X4	T36.5X5	T36.5X6
topical	T49.0X1	T49.0X2	T49.0X3	T49.0X4	T49.0X5	T49.0X6
Mycitracin	T36.8X1	T36.8X2	T36.8X3	T36.8X4	T36.8X5	T36.8X6
ophthalmic preparation	T49.5X1	T49.5X2	T49.5X3	T49.5X4	T49.5X5	T49.5X6
Mycostatin	T36.7X1	T36.7X2	T36.7X3	T36.7X4	T36.7X5	T36.7X6
topical	T49.0X1	T49.0X2	T49.0X3	T49.0X4	T49.0X5	T49.0X6
Mycotoxins	T64.81	T64.82	T64.83	T64.84	--	--
aflatoxin	T64.01	T64.02	T64.03	T64.04	--	--
specified NEC	T64.81	T64.82	T64.83	T64.84	--	--
Mydriacyl	T44.3X1	T44.3X2	T44.3X3	T44.3X4	T44.3X5	T44.3X6
Mydriatic drug	T49.5X1	T49.5X2	T49.5X3	T49.5X4	T49.5X5	T49.5X6
Myelobromal	T45.1X1	T45.1X2	T45.1X3	T45.1X4	T45.1X5	T45.1X6
Myleran	T45.1X1	T45.1X2	T45.1X3	T45.1X4	T45.1X5	T45.1X6
Myochrysin (e)	T39.2X1	T39.2X2	T39.2X3	T39.2X4	T39.2X5	T39.2X6
Myoneural blocking agents	T48.1X1	T48.1X2	T48.1X3	T48.1X4	T48.1X5	T48.1X6
Myralact	T49.0X1	T49.0X2	T49.0X3	T49.0X4	T49.0X5	T49.0X6
Myristica fragrans	T62.2X1	T62.2X2	T62.2X3	T62.2X4	--	--
Myristicin	T65.891	T65.892	T65.893	T65.894	--	--
Mysoline	T42.3X1	T42.3X2	T42.3X3	T42.3X4	T42.3X5	T42.3X6
Nabilone	T40.7X1	T40.7X2	T40.7X3	T40.7X4	T40.7X5	T40.7X6
Nabumetone	T39.391	T39.392	T39.393	T39.394	T39.395	T39.396
Nadolol	T44.7X1	T44.7X2	T44.7X3	T44.7X4	T44.7X5	T44.7X6
Nafcillin	T36.0X1	T36.0X2	T36.0X3	T36.0X4	T36.0X5	T36.0X6
Nafoxidine	T38.6X1	T38.6X2	T38.6X3	T38.6X4	T38.6X5	T38.6X6
Naftazone	T46.991	T46.992	T46.993	T46.994	T46.995	T46.996
Naftidrofuryl (oxalate)	T46.7X1	T46.7X2	T46.7X3	T46.7X4	T46.7X5	T46.7X6
Naftifine	T49.0X1	T49.0X2	T49.0X3	T49.0X4	T49.0X5	T49.0X6
Nail polish remover	T52.91	T52.92	T52.93	T52.94	--	--
Nalbuphine	T40.4X1	T40.4X2	T40.4X3	T40.4X4	T40.4X5	T40.4X6
Naled	T60.0X1	T60.0X2	T60.0X3	T60.0X4	--	--
Nalidixic acid	T37.8X1	T37.8X2	T37.8X3	T37.8X4	T37.8X5	T37.8X6
Nalorphine	T50.7X1	T50.7X2	T50.7X3	T50.7X4	T50.7X5	T50.7X6
Naloxone	T50.7X1	T50.7X2	T50.7X3	T50.7X4	T50.7X5	T50.7X6
Naltrexone	T50.7X1	T50.7X2	T50.7X3	T50.7X4	T50.7X5	T50.7X6
Namenda	T43.8X1	T43.8X2	T43.8X3	T43.8X4	T43.8X5	T43.8X6
Nandrolone	T38.7X1	T38.7X2	T38.7X3	T38.7X4	T38.7X5	T38.7X6
Naphazoline	T48.5X1	T48.5X2	T48.5X3	T48.5X4	T48.5X5	T48.5X6
Naphtha (painters') (petroleum)	T52.0X1	T52.0X2	T52.0X3	T52.0X4	--	--
solvent	T52.0X1	T52.0X2	T52.0X3	T52.0X4	--	--
vapor	T52.0X1	T52.0X2	T52.0X3	T52.0X4	--	--
Naphthalene (non-chlorinated)	T60.2X1	T60.2X2	T60.2X3	T60.2X4	--	--
chlorinated	T60.1X1	T60.1X2	T60.1X3	T60.1X4	--	--
vapor	T60.1X1	T60.1X2	T60.1X3	T60.1X4	--	--
insecticide or moth repellent	T60.2X1	T60.2X2	T60.2X3	T60.2X4	--	--
chlorinated	T60.1X1	T60.1X2	T60.1X3	T60.1X4	--	--
vapor	T60.2X1	T60.2X2	T60.2X3	T60.2X4	--	--
chlorinated	T60.1X1	T60.1X2	T60.1X3	T60.1X4	--	--
Naphthol	T65.891	T65.892	T65.893	T65.894	--	--
Naphthylamine	T65.891	T65.892	T65.893	T65.894	--	--
Naphthylthiourea (ANTU)	T60.4X1	T60.4X2	T60.4X3	T60.4X4	--	--

Substance	Poisoning, Accidental (unintentional)	Poisoning, Intentional Self-harm	Poisoning, Assault	Poisoning, Undetermined	Adverse effect	Underdosing
Naprosyn—see Naproxen						
Naproxen	T39.311	T39.312	T39.313	T39.314	T39.315	T39.316
Narcotic (drug)	T40.601	T40.602	T40.603	T40.604	T40.605	T40.606
analgesic NEC	T40.601	T40.602	T40.603	T40.604	T40.605	T40.606
antagonist	T50.7X1	T50.7X2	T50.7X3	T50.7X4	T50.7X5	T50.7X6
specified NEC	T40.691	T40.692	T40.693	T40.694	T40.695	T40.696
synthetic	T40.4X1	T40.4X2	T40.4X3	T40.4X4	T40.4X5	T40.4X6
Narcotine	T48.3X1	T48.3X2	T48.3X3	T48.3X4	T48.3X5	T48.3X6
Nardil	T43.1X1	T43.1X2	T43.1X3	T43.1X4	T43.1X5	T43.1X6
Nasal drug NEC	T49.6X1	T49.6X2	T49.6X3	T49.6X4	T49.6X5	T49.6X6
Natamycin	T49.0X1	T49.0X2	T49.0X3	T49.0X4	T49.0X5	T49.0X6
Natrium cyanide—see Cyanide (s)						
Natural						
blood (product)	T45.8X1	T45.8X2	T45.8X3	T45.8X4	T45.8X5	T45.8X6
gas (piped)	T59.891	T59.892	T59.893	T59.894	--	--
incomplete combustion	T58.11	T58.12	T58.13	T58.14	--	--
Nealbarbital	T42.3X1	T42.3X2	T42.3X3	T42.3X4	T42.3X5	T42.3X6
Nectadon	T48.3X1	T48.3X2	T48.3X3	T48.3X4	T48.3X5	T48.3X6
Nedocromil	T48.6X1	T48.6X2	T48.6X3	T48.6X4	T48.6X5	T48.6X6
Nefopam	T39.8X1	T39.8X2	T39.8X3	T39.8X4	T39.8X5	T39.8X6
Nematocyst (sting)	T63.691	T63.692	T63.693	T63.694	--	--
Nembutal	T42.3X1	T42.3X2	T42.3X3	T42.3X4	T42.3X5	T42.3X6
Nemonapride	T43.591	T43.592	T43.593	T43.594	T43.595	T43.596
Neoarsphenamine	T37.8X1	T37.8X2	T37.8X3	T37.8X4	T37.8X5	T37.8X6
Neocinchophen	T50.4X1	T50.4X2	T50.4X3	T50.4X4	T50.4X5	T50.4X6
Neomycin (derivatives)	T36.5X1	T36.5X2	T36.5X3	T36.5X4	T36.5X5	T36.5X6
with						
bacitracin	T49.0X1	T49.0X2	T49.0X3	T49.0X4	T49.0X5	T49.0X6
neostigmine	T44.0X1	T44.0X2	T44.0X3	T44.0X4	T44.0X5	T44.0X6
ENT agent	T49.6X1	T49.6X2	T49.6X3	T49.6X4	T49.6X5	T49.6X6
ophthalmic preparation	T49.5X1	T49.5X2	T49.5X3	T49.5X4	T49.5X5	T49.5X6
topical NEC	T49.0X1	T49.0X2	T49.0X3	T49.0X4	T49.0X5	T49.0X6
Neonal	T42.3X1	T42.3X2	T42.3X3	T42.3X4	T42.3X5	T42.3X6
Neoprontosil	T37.0X1	T37.0X2	T37.0X3	T37.0X4	T37.0X5	T37.0X6
Neosalvarsan	T37.8X1	T37.8X2	T37.8X3	T37.8X4	T37.8X5	T37.8X6
Neosilversalvarsan	T37.8X1	T37.8X2	T37.8X3	T37.8X4	T37.8X5	T37.8X6
Neosporin	T36.8X1	T36.8X2	T36.8X3	T36.8X4	T36.8X5	T36.8X6
ENT agent	T49.6X1	T49.6X2	T49.6X3	T49.6X4	T49.6X5	T49.6X6
opthalmic preparation	T49.5X1	T49.5X2	T49.5X3	T49.5X4	T49.5X5	T49.5X6
topical NEC	T49.0X1	T49.0X2	T49.0X3	T49.0X4	T49.0X5	T49.0X6
Neostigmine bromide	T44.0X1	T44.0X2	T44.0X3	T44.0X4	T44.0X5	T44.0X6
Neraval	T42.3X1	T42.3X2	T42.3X3	T42.3X4	T42.3X5	T42.3X6
Neravan	T42.3X1	T42.3X2	T42.3X3	T42.3X4	T42.3X5	T42.3X6
Nerium oleander	T62.2X1	T62.2X2	T62.2X3	T62.2X4	--	--
Nerve gas, not in war	T59.91	T59.92	T59.93	T59.94	--	--
Nesacaine	T41.3X1	T41.3X2	T41.3X3	T41.3X4	T41.3X5	T41.3X6
infiltration (subcutaneous)	T41.3X1	T41.3X2	T41.3X3	T41.3X4	T41.3X5	T41.3X6
nerve block (peripheral) (plexus)	T41.3X1	T41.3X2	T41.3X3	T41.3X4	T41.3X5	T41.3X6
Netilmicin	T36.5X1	T36.5X2	T36.5X3	T36.5X4	T36.5X5	T36.5X6
Neurobarb	T42.3X1	T42.3X2	T42.3X3	T42.3X4	T42.3X5	T42.3X6
Neuroleptic drug NEC	T43.501	T43.502	T43.503	T43.504	T43.505	T43.506
Neuromuscular blocking drug	T48.1X1	T48.1X2	T48.1X3	T48.1X4	T48.1X5	T48.1X6
Neutral insulin injection	T38.3X1	T38.3X2	T38.3X3	T38.3X4	T38.3X5	T38.3X6
Neutral spirits	T51.0X1	T51.0X2	T51.0X3	T51.0X4	--	--
beverage	T51.0X1	T51.0X2	T51.0X3	T51.0X4	--	--
Niacin	T46.7X1	T46.7X2	T46.7X3	T46.7X4	T46.7X5	T46.7X6
Niacinamide	T45.2X1	T45.2X2	T45.2X3	T45.2X4	T45.2X5	T45.2X6
Nialamide	T43.1X1	T43.1X2	T43.1X3	T43.1X4	T43.1X5	T43.1X6
Niaprazine	T42.6X1	T42.6X2	T42.6X3	T42.6X4	T42.6X5	T42.6X6
Nicametate	T46.7X1	T46.7X2	T46.7X3	T46.7X4	T46.7X5	T46.7X6
Nicardipine	T46.1X1	T46.1X2	T46.1X3	T46.1X4	T46.1X5	T46.1X6
Nicergoline	T46.7X1	T46.7X2	T46.7X3	T46.7X4	T46.7X5	T46.7X6
Nickel (carbonyl) (tetra-carbonyl) (fumes) (vapor)	T56.891	T56.892	T56.893	T56.894	--	--
Nickelocene	T56.891	T56.892	T56.893	T56.894	--	--

Substance	Poisoning, Accidental (unintentional)	Poisoning, Intentional Self-harm	Poisoning, Assault	Poisoning, Undetermined	Adverse effect	Underdosing
Niclosamide	T37.4X1	T37.4X2	T37.4X3	T37.4X4	T37.4X5	T37.4X6
Nicofuranose	T46.7X1	T46.7X2	T46.7X3	T46.7X4	T46.7X5	T46.7X6
Nicomorphine	T40.2X1	T40.2X2	T40.2X3	T40.2X4	--	--
Nicorandil	T46.3X1	T46.3X2	T46.3X3	T46.3X4	T46.3X5	T46.3X6
Nicotiana (plant)	T62.2X1	T62.2X2	T62.2X3	T62.2X4	--	--
Nicotinamide	T45.2X1	T45.2X2	T45.2X3	T45.2X4	T45.2X5	T45.2X6
Nicotine (insecticide) (spray) (sulfate) NEC	T60.2X1	T60.2X2	T60.2X3	T60.2X4	--	--
from tobacco	T65.291	T65.292	T65.293	T65.294	--	--
cigarettes	T65.221	T65.222	T65.223	T65.224	--	--
not insecticide	T65.291	T65.292	T65.293	T65.294	--	--
Nicotinic acid	T46.7X1	T46.7X2	T46.7X3	T46.7X4	T46.7X5	T46.7X6
Nicotinyl alcohol	T46.7X1	T46.7X2	T46.7X3	T46.7X4	T46.7X5	T46.7X6
Nicoumalone	T45.511	T45.512	T45.513	T45.514	T45.515	T45.516
Nifedipine	T46.1X1	T46.1X2	T46.1X3	T46.1X4	T46.1X5	T46.1X6
Nifenazone	T39.2X1	T39.2X2	T39.2X3	T39.2X4	T39.2X5	T39.2X6
Nifuraldezone	T37.91	T37.92	T37.93	T37.94	T37.95	T37.96
Nifuratel	T37.8X1	T37.8X2	T37.8X3	T37.8X4	T37.8X5	T37.8X6
Nifurtimox	T37.3X1	T37.3X2	T37.3X3	T37.3X4	T37.3X5	T37.3X6
Nifurtoinol	T37.8X1	T37.8X2	T37.8X3	T37.8X4	T37.8X5	T37.8X6
Nightshade, deadly (solanum) —see also Belladonna	T62.2X1	T62.2X2	T62.2X3	T62.2X4	--	--
berry	T62.1X1	T62.1X2	T62.1X3	T62.1X4	--	--
Nikethamide	T50.7X1	T50.7X2	T50.7X3	T50.7X4	T50.7X5	T50.7X6
Nilstat	T36.7X1	T36.7X2	T36.7X3	T36.7X4	T36.7X5	T36.7X6
topical	T49.0X1	T49.0X2	T49.0X3	T49.0X4	T49.0X5	T49.0X6
Nilutamide	T38.6X1	T38.6X2	T38.6X3	T38.6X4	T38.6X5	T38.6X6
Nimesulide	T39.391	T39.392	T39.393	T39.394	T39.395	T39.396
Nimetazepam	T42.4X1	T42.4X2	T42.4X3	T42.4X4	T42.4X5	T42.4X6
Nimodipine	T46.1X1	T46.1X2	T46.1X3	T46.1X4	T46.1X5	T46.1X6
Nimorazole	T37.3X1	T37.3X2	T37.3X3	T37.3X4	T37.3X5	T37.3X6
Nimustine	T45.1X1	T45.1X2	T45.1X3	T45.1X4	T45.1X5	T45.1X6
Niridazole	T37.4X1	T37.4X2	T37.4X3	T37.4X4	T37.4X5	T37.4X6
Nisentil	T40.2X1	T40.2X2	T40.2X3	T40.2X4	T40.2X5	T40.2X6
Nisoldipine	T46.1X1	T46.1X2	T46.1X3	T46.1X4	T46.1X5	T46.1X6
Nitramine	T65.3X1	T65.3X2	T65.3X3	T65.3X4	--	--
Nitrate, organic	T46.3X1	T46.3X2	T46.3X3	T46.3X4	T46.3X5	T46.3X6
Nitrazepam	T42.4X1	T42.4X2	T42.4X3	T42.4X4	T42.4X5	T42.4X6
Nitrefazole	T50.6X1	T50.6X2	T50.6X3	T50.6X4	T50.6X5	T50.6X6
Nitrendipine	T46.1X1	T46.1X2	T46.1X3	T46.1X4	T46.1X5	T46.1X6
Nitric						
acid (liquid)	T54.2X1	T54.2X2	T54.2X3	T54.2X4	--	--
vapor	T59.891	T59.892	T59.893	T59.894	--	--
oxide (gas)	T59.0X1	T59.0X2	T59.0X3	T59.0X4	--	--
Nitrimidazine	T37.3X1	T37.3X2	T37.3X3	T37.3X4	T37.3X5	T37.3X6
Nitrite, amyl (medicinal) (vapor)	T46.3X1	T46.3X2	T46.3X3	T46.3X4	T46.3X5	T46.3X6
Nitroaniline	T65.3X1	T65.3X2	T65.3X3	T65.3X4	--	--
vapor	T59.891	T59.892	T59.893	T59.894	--	--
Nitrobenzene, nitrobenzol	T65.3X1	T65.3X2	T65.3X3	T65.3X4	--	--
vapor	T65.3X1	T65.3X2	T65.3X3	T65.3X4	--	--
Nitrocellulose	T65.891	T65.892	T65.893	T65.894	--	--
lacquer	T65.891	T65.892	T65.893	T65.894	--	--
Nitrodiphenyl	T65.3X1	T65.3X2	T65.3X3	T65.3X4	--	--
Nitrofural	T49.0X1	T49.0X2	T49.0X3	T49.0X4	T49.0X5	T49.0X6
Nitrofurantoin	T37.8X1	T37.8X2	T37.8X3	T37.8X4	T37.8X5	T37.8X6
Nitrofurazone	T49.0X1	T49.0X2	T49.0X3	T49.0X4	T49.0X5	T49.0X6
Nitrogen	T59.0X1	T59.0X2	T59.0X3	T59.0X4	--	--
mustard	T45.1X1	T45.1X2	T45.1X3	T45.1X4	T45.1X5	T45.1X6
Nitroglycerin, nitro-glycerol (medicinal)	T46.3X1	T46.3X2	T46.3X3	T46.3X4	T46.3X5	T46.3X6
nonmedicinal	T65.5X1	T65.5X2	T65.5X3	T65.5X4	--	--
fumes	T65.5X1	T65.5X2	T65.5X3	T65.5X4	--	--
Nitroglycol	T52.3X1	T52.3X2	T52.3X3	T52.3X4	--	--
Nitrohydrochloric acid	T54.2X1	T54.2X2	T54.2X3	T54.2X4	--	--
Nitromersol	T49.0X1	T49.0X2	T49.0X3	T49.0X4	T49.0X5	T49.0X6
Nitronaphthalene	T65.891	T65.892	T65.893	T65.894	--	--

Substance	Poisoning, Accidental (unintentional)	Poisoning, Intentional Self-harm	Poisoning, Assault	Poisoning, Undetermined	Adverse effect	Underdosing
Nitrophenol	T54.0X1	T54.0X2	T54.0X3	T54.0X4	--	--
Nitropropane	T52.8X1	T52.8X2	T52.8X3	T52.8X4	--	--
Nitroprusside	T46.5X1	T46.5X2	T46.5X4	T46.5X4	T46.5X5	T46.5X6
Nitrosodimethylamine	T65.3X1	T65.3X2	T65.3X3	T65.3X4	--	--
Nitrothiazol	T37.4X1	T37.4X2	T37.4X3	T37.4X4	T37.4X5	T37.4X6
Nitrotoluene, nitrotoluol	T65.3X1	T65.3X2	T65.3X3	T65.3X4	--	--
vapor	T65.3X1	T65.3X2	T65.3X3	T65.3X4	--	--
Nitrous						
acid (liquid)	T54.2X1	T54.2X2	T54.2X3	T54.2X4	--	--
fumes	T59.891	T59.892	T59.893	T59.894	--	--
ether spirit	T46.3X1	T46.3X2	T46.3X4	T46.3X4	T46.3X5	T46.3X6
oxide	T41.0X1	T41.0X2	T41.0X3	T41.0X4	T41.0X5	T41.0X6
Nitroxoline	T37.8X1	T37.8X2	T37.8X3	T37.8X4	T37.8X5	T37.8X6
Nitrozone	T49.0X1	T49.0X2	T49.0X3	T49.0X4	T49.0X5	T49.0X6
Nizatidine	T47.0X1	T47.0X2	T47.0X3	T47.0X4	T47.0X5	T47.0X6
Nizofenone	T43.8X1	T43.8X2	T43.8X3	T43.8X4	T43.8X5	T43.8X6
Noctec	T42.6X1	T42.6X2	T42.6X3	T42.6X4	T42.6X5	T42.6X6
Noludar	T42.6X1	T42.6X2	T42.6X3	T42.6X4	T42.6X5	T42.6X6
Nomegestrol	T38.5X1	T38.5X2	T38.5X3	T38.5X4	T38.5X5	T38.5X6
Nomifensine	T43.291	T43.292	T43.293	T43.294	T43.295	T43.296
Nonoxinol	T49.8X1	T49.8X2	T49.8X3	T49.8X4	T49.8X5	T49.8X6
Nonylphenoxy (polyethoxy-ethanol)	T49.8X1	T49.8X2	T49.8X3	T49.8X4	T49.8X5	T49.8X6
Noptil	T42.3X1	T42.3X2	T42.3X3	T42.3X4	T42.3X5	T42.3X6
Noradrenaline	T44.4X1	T44.4X2	T44.4X3	T44.4X4	T44.4X5	T44.4X6
Noramidopyrine	T39.2X1	T39.2X2	T39.2X3	T39.2X4	T39.2X5	T39.2X6
methanesulfonate sodium	T39.2X1	T39.2X2	T39.2X3	T39.2X4	T39.2X5	T39.2X6
Norbormide	T60.4X1	T60.4X2	T60.4X3	T60.4X4	--	--
Nordazepam	T42.4X1	T42.4X2	T42.4X3	T42.4X4	T42.4X5	T42.4X6
Norepinephrine	T44.4X1	T44.4X2	T44.4X3	T44.4X4	T44.4X5	T44.4X6
Norethandrolone	T38.7X1	T38.7X2	T38.7X3	T38.7X4	T38.7X5	T38.7X6
Norethindrone	T38.4X1	T38.4X2	T38.4X3	T38.4X4	T38.4X5	T38.4X6
Norethisterone (acetate) (enantate)	T38.4X1	T38.4X2	T38.4X3	T38.4X4	T38.4X5	T38.4X6
with ethinylestradiol	T38.5X1	T38.5X2	T38.5X3	T38.5X4	T38.5X5	T38.5X6
Noretynodrel	T38.5X1	T38.5X2	T38.5X3	T38.5X4	T38.5X5	T38.5X6
Norfenefrine	T44.4X1	T44.4X2	T44.4X3	T44.4X4	T44.4X5	T44.4X6
Norfloxacin	T36.8X1	T36.8X2	T36.8X3	T36.8X4	T36.8X5	T36.8X6
Norgestrel	T38.4X1	T38.4X2	T38.4X3	T38.4X4	T38.4X5	T38.4X6
Norgestrienone	T38.4X1	T38.4X2	T38.4X3	T38.4X4	T38.4X5	T38.4X6
Norlestrin	T38.4X1	T38.4X2	T38.4X3	T38.4X4	T38.4X5	T38.4X6
Norlutin	T38.4X1	T38.4X2	T38.4X3	T38.4X4	T38.4X5	T38.4X6
Normal serum albumin (human), salt-poor	T45.8X1	T45.8X2	T45.8X3	T45.8X4	T45.8X5	T45.8X6
Normethandrone	T38.5X1	T38.5X2	T38.5X3	T38.5X4	T38.5X5	T38.5X6
Normison—see Benzodiazepines						
Normorphine	T40.2X1	T40.2X2	T40.2X3	T40.2X4	--	--
Norpseudoephedrine	T50.5X1	T50.5X2	T50.5X3	T50.5X4	T50.5X5	T50.5X6
Nortestosterone (furanpropionate)	T38.7X1	T38.7X2	T38.7X3	T38.7X4	T38.7X5	T38.7X6
Nortriptyline	T43.011	T43.012	T43.013	T43.014	T43.015	T43.016
Noscapine	T48.3X1	T48.3X2	T48.3X3	T48.3X4	T48.3X5	T48.3X6
Nose preparations	T49.6X1	T49.6X2	T49.6X3	T49.6X4	T49.6X5	T49.6X6
Novobiocin	T36.5X1	T36.5X2	T36.5X3	T36.5X4	T36.5X5	T36.5X6
Novocain (infiltration) (topical)	T41.3X1	T41.3X2	T41.3X3	T41.3X4	T41.3X5	T41.3X6
nerve block (peripheral) (plexus)	T41.3X1	T41.3X2	T41.3X3	T41.3X4	T41.3X5	T41.3X6
spinal	T41.3X1	T41.3X2	T41.3X3	T41.3X4	T41.3X5	T41.3X6
Noxious foodstuff	T62.91	T62.92	T62.93	T62.94	--	--
specified NEC	T62.8X1	T62.8X2	T62.8X3	T62.8X4	--	--
Noxiptiline	T43.011	T43.012	T43.013	T43.014	T43.015	T43.016
Noxytiolin	T49.0X1	T49.0X2	T49.0X3	T49.0X4	T49.0X5	T49.0X6
NPH lletin (insulin)	T38.3X1	T38.3X2	T38.3X3	T38.3X4	T38.3X5	T38.3X6
Numorphan	T40.2X1	T40.2X2	T40.2X3	T40.2X4	T40.2X5	T40.2X6
Nunol	T42.3X1	T42.3X2	T42.3X3	T42.3X4	T42.3X5	T42.3X6
Nupercaine (spinal anesthetic)	T41.3X1	T41.3X2	T41.3X3	T41.3X4	T41.3X5	T41.3X6
topical (surface)	T41.3X1	T41.3X2	T41.3X3	T41.3X4	T41.3X5	T41.3X6
Nutmeg oil (liniment)	T49.3X1	T49.3X2	T49.3X3	T49.3X4	T49.3X5	T49.3X6
Nutritional supplement	T50.901	T50.902	T50.903	T50.904	T50.905	T50.906
Nux vomica	T65.1X1	T65.1X2	T65.1X3	T65.1X4	--	--

Substance	Poisoning, Accidental (unintentional)	Poisoning, Intentional Self-harm	Poisoning, Assault	Poisoning, Undetermined	Adverse effect	Underdosing
Nydrazid	T37.1X1	T37.1X2	T37.1X3	T37.1X4	T37.1X5	T37.1X6
Nylidrin	T46.7X1	T46.7X2	T46.7X3	T46.7X4	T46.7X5	T46.7X6
Nystatin	T36.7X1	T36.7X2	T36.7X3	T36.7X4	T36.7X5	T36.7X6
topical	T49.0X1	T49.0X2	T49.0X3	T49.0X4	T49.0X5	T49.0X6
Nytol	T45.0X1	T45.0X2	T45.0X3	T45.0X4	T45.0X5	T45.0X6
Obidoxime chloride	T50.6X1	T50.6X2	T50.6X3	T50.6X4	T50.6X5	T50.6X6
Octafonium (chloride)	T49.3X1	T49.3X2	T49.3X3	T49.3X4	T49.3X5	T49.3X6
Octamethyl pyrophos-phoramide	T60.0X1	T60.0X2	T60.0X3	T60.0X4	--	--
Octanoin	T50.991	T50.992	T50.993	T50.994	T50.995	T50.996
Octatropine methyl-bromide	T44.3X1	T44.3X2	T44.3X3	T44.3X4	T44.3X5	T44.3X6
Octotiamine	T45.2X1	T45.2X2	T45.2X3	T45.2X4	T45.2X5	T45.2X6
Octoxinol (9)	T49.8X1	T49.8X2	T49.8X3	T49.8X4	T49.8X5	T49.8X6
Octreotide	T38.991	T38.992	T38.993	T38.994	T38.995	T38.996
Octyl nitrite	T46.3X1	T46.3X2	T46.3X3	T46.3X4	T46.3X5	T46.3X6
Oestradiol	T38.5X1	T38.5X2	T38.5X3	T38.5X4	T38.5X5	T38.5X6
Oestriol	T38.5X1	T38.5X2	T38.5X3	T38.5X4	T38.5X5	T38.5X6
Oestrogen	T38.5X1	T38.5X2	T38.5X3	T38.5X4	T38.5X5	T38.5X6
Oestrone	T38.5X1	T38.5X2	T38.5X3	T38.5X4	T38.5X5	T38.5X6
Ofloxacin	T36.8X1	T36.8X2	T36.8X3	T36.8X4	T36.8X5	T36.8X6
Oil (of)	T65.891	T65.892	T65.893	T65.894	--	--
bitter almond	T62.8X1	T62.8X2	T62.8X3	T62.8X4	--	--
cloves	T49.7X1	T49.7X2	T49.7X3	T49.7X4	T49.7X5	T49.7X6
colors	T65.6X1	T65.6X2	T65.6X3	T65.6X4	--	--
fumes	T59.891	T59.892	T59.893	T59.894	--	--
lubricating	T52.0X1	T52.0X2	T52.0X3	T52.0X4	--	--
Niobe	T52.8X1	T52.8X2	T52.8X3	T52.8X4	--	--
vitriol (liquid)	T54.2X1	T54.2X2	T54.2X3	T54.2X4	--	--
fumes	T54.2X1	T54.2X2	T54.2X3	T54.2X4	--	--
wintergreen (bitter) NEC	T49.3X1	T49.3X2	T49.3X3	T49.3X4	T49.3X5	T49.3X6
Oily preparation (for skin)	T49.3X1	T49.3X2	T49.3X3	T49.3X4	T49.3X5	T49.3X6
Ointment NEC	T49.3X1	T49.3X2	T49.3X3	T49.3X4	T49.3X5	T49.3X6
Olanzapine	T43.591	T43.592	T43.593	T43.594	T43.595	T43.596
Oleander	T62.2X1	T62.2X2	T62.2X3	T62.2X4	--	--
Oleandomycin	T36.3X1	T36.3X2	T36.3X3	T36.3X4	T36.3X5	T36.3X6
Oleandrin	T46.0X1	T46.0X2	T46.0X3	T46.0X4	T46.0X5	T46.0X6
Oleic acid	T46.6X1	T46.6X2	T46.6X3	T46.6X4	T46.6X5	T46.6X6
Oleovitamin A	T45.2X1	T45.2X2	T45.2X3	T45.2X4	T45.2X5	T45.2X6
Oleum ricini	T47.2X1	T47.2X2	T47.2X3	T47.2X4	T47.2X5	T47.2X6
Olive oil (medicinal) NEC	T47.4X1	T47.4X2	T47.4X3	T47.4X4	T47.4X5	T47.4X6
Olivomycin	T45.1X1	T45.1X2	T45.1X3	T45.1X4	T45.1X5	T45.1X6
Olsalazine	T47.8X1	T47.8X2	T47.8X3	T47.8X4	T47.8X5	T47.8X6
Omeprazole	T47.1X1	T47.1X2	T47.1X3	T47.1X4	T47.1X5	T47.1X6
OMPA	T60.0X1	T60.0X2	T60.0X3	T60.0X4	--	--
Oncovin	T45.1X1	T45.1X2	T45.1X3	T45.1X4	T45.1X5	T45.1X6
Ondansetron	T45.0X1	T45.0X2	T45.0X3	T45.0X4	T45.0X5	T45.0X6
Ophthaine	T41.3X1	T41.3X2	T41.3X3	T41.3X4	T41.3X5	T41.3X6
Ophthetic	T41.3X1	T41.3X2	T41.3X3	T41.3X4	T41.3X5	T41.3X6
Opiate NEC	T40.601	T40.602	T40.603	T40.604	T40.605	T40.606
antagonists	T50.7X1	T50.7X2	T50.7X3	T50.7X4	T50.7X5	T50.7X6
Opioid NEC	T40.2X1	T40.2X2	T40.2X3	T40.2X4	T40.2X5	T40.2X6
Opipramol	T43.011	T43.012	T43.013	T43.014	T43.015	T43.016
Opium alkaloids (total)	T40.0X1	T40.0X2	T40.0X3	T40.0X4	T40.0X5	T40.0X6
standardized powdered	T40.0X1	T40.0X2	T40.0X3	T40.0X4	T40.0X5	T40.0X6
tincture (camphorated)	T40.0X1	T40.0X2	T40.0X3	T40.0X4	T40.0X5	T40.0X6
Oracon	T38.4X1	T38.4X2	T38.4X3	T38.4X4	T38.4X5	T38.4X6
Oragrafin	T50.8X1	T50.8X2	T50.8X3	T50.8X4	T50.8X5	T50.8X6
Oral contraceptives	T38.4X1	T38.4X2	T38.4X3	T38.4X4	T38.4X5	T38.4X6
Oral rehydration salts	T50.3X1	T50.3X2	T50.3X3	T50.3X4	T50.3X5	T50.3X6
Orazamide	T50.991	T50.992	T50.993	T50.994	T50.995	T50.996
Orciprenaline	T48.291	T48.292	T48.293	T48.294	T48.295	T48.296
Organidin	T48.4X1	T48.4X2	T48.4X3	T48.4X4	T48.4X5	T48.4X6
Organonitrate NEC	T46.3X1	T46.3X2	T46.3X3	T46.3X4	T46.3X5	T46.3X6
Organophosphates	T60.0X1	T60.0X2	T60.0X3	T60.0X4	--	--
Orimune	T50.B91	T50.B92	T50.B93	T50.B94	T50.B95	T50.B96

Substance	Poisoning, Accidental (unintentional)	Poisoning, Intentional Self-harm	Poisoning, Assault	Poisoning, Undetermined	Adverse effect	Underdosing
Orinase	T38.3X1	T38.3X2	T38.3X3	T38.3X4	T38.3X5	T38.3X6
Ormeloxifene	T38.6X1	T38.6X2	T38.6X3	T38.6X4	T38.6X5	T38.6X6
Ornidazole	T37.3X1	T37.3X2	T37.3X3	T37.3X4	T37.3X5	T37.3X6
Ornithine aspartate	T50.991	T50.992	T50.993	T50.994	T50.995	T50.996
Ornoprostil	T47.1X1	T47.1X2	T47.1X3	T47.1X4	T47.1X5	T47.1X6
Orphenadrine (hydrochloride)	T42.8X1	T42.8X2	T42.8X3	T42.8X4	T42.8X5	T42.8X6
Ortal (sodium)	T42.3X1	T42.3X2	T42.3X3	T42.3X4	T42.3X5	T42.3X6
Orthoboric acid	T49.0X1	T49.0X2	T49.0X3	T49.0X4	T49.0X5	T49.0X6
ENT agent	T49.6X1	T49.6X2	T49.6X3	T49.6X4	T49.6X5	T49.6X6
ophthalmic preparation	T49.5X1	T49.5X2	T49.5X3	T49.5X4	T49.5X5	T49.5X6
Orthocaine	T41.3X1	T41.3X2	T41.3X3	T41.3X4	T41.3X5	T41.3X6
Orthodichlorobenzene	T53.7X1	T53.7X2	T53.7X3	T53.7X4	--	--
Ortho-Novum	T38.4X1	T38.4X2	T38.4X3	T38.4X4	T38.4X5	T38.4X6
Orthotolidine (reagent)	T54.2X1	T54.2X2	T54.2X3	T54.2X4	--	--
Osmic acid (liquid)	T54.2X1	T54.2X2	T54.2X3	T54.2X4	--	--
fumes	T54.2X1	T54.2X2	T54.2X3	T54.2X4	--	--
Osmotic diuretics	T50.2X1	T50.2X2	T50.2X3	T50.2X4	T50.2X5	T50.2X6
Otilonium bromide	T44.3X1	T44.3X2	T44.3X3	T44.3X4	T44.3X5	T44.3X6
Otorhinolaryngological drug NEC	T49.6X1	T49.6X2	T49.6X3	T49.6X4	T49.6X5	T49.6X6
Ouabain (e)	T46.0X1	T46.0X2	T46.0X3	T46.0X4	T46.0X5	T46.0X6
Ovarian						
hormone	T38.5X1	T38.5X2	T38.5X3	T38.5X4	T38.5X5	T38.5X6
stimulant	T38.5X1	T38.5X2	T38.5X3	T38.5X4	T38.5X5	T38.5X6
Ovral	T38.4X1	T38.4X2	T38.4X3	T38.4X4	T38.4X5	T38.4X6
Ovulen	T38.4X1	T38.4X2	T38.4X3	T38.4X4	T38.4X5	T38.4X6
Oxacillin	T36.0X1	T36.0X2	T36.0X3	T36.0X4	T36.0X5	T36.0X6
Oxalic acid	T54.2X1	T54.2X2	T54.2X3	T54.2X4	--	--
ammonium salt	T50.991	T50.992	T50.993	T50.994	T50.995	T50.996
Oxamniquine	T37.4X1	T37.4X2	T37.4X3	T37.4X4	T37.4X5	T37.4X6
Oxanamide	T43.591	T43.592	T43.593	T43.594	T43.595	T43.596
Oxandrolone	T38.7X1	T38.7X2	T38.7X3	T38.7X4	T38.7X5	T38.7X6
Oxantel	T37.4X1	T37.4X2	T37.4X3	T37.4X4	T37.4X5	T37.4X6
Oxapium iodide	T44.3X1	T44.3X2	T44.3X3	T44.3X4	T44.3X5	T44.3X6
Oxaprotiline	T43.021	T43.022	T43.023	T43.024	T43.025	T43.026
Oxaprozin	T39.311	T39.312	T39.313	T39.314	T39.315	T39.316
Oxatomide	T45.0X1	T45.0X2	T45.0X3	T45.0X4	T45.0X5	T45.0X6
Oxazepam	T42.4X1	T42.4X2	T42.4X3	T42.4X4	T42.4X5	T42.4X6
Oxazimedrine	T50.5X1	T50.5X2	T50.5X3	T50.5X4	T50.5X5	T50.5X6
Oxazolam	T42.4X1	T42.4X2	T42.4X3	T42.4X4	T42.4X5	T42.4X6
Oxazolidine derivatives	T42.2X1	T42.2X2	T42.2X3	T42.2X4	T42.2X5	T42.2X6
Oxazolidinedione (derivative)	T42.2X1	T42.2X2	T42.2X3	T42.2X4	T42.2X5	T42.2X6
Ox bile extract	T47.5X1	T47.5X2	T47.5X3	T47.5X4	T47.5X5	T47.5X6
Oxcarbazepine	T42.1X1	T42.1X2	T42.1X3	T42.1X4	T42.1X5	T42.1X6
Oxedrine	T44.4X1	T44.4X2	T44.4X3	T44.4X4	T44.4X5	T44.4X6
Oxeladin (citrate)	T48.3X1	T48.3X2	T48.3X3	T48.3X4	T48.3X5	T48.3X6
Oxendolone	T38.5X1	T38.5X2	T38.5X3	T38.5X4	T38.5X5	T38.5X6
Oxetacaine	T41.3X1	T41.3X2	T41.3X3	T41.3X4	T41.3X5	T41.3X6
Oxethazine	T41.3X1	T41.3X2	T41.3X3	T41.3X4	T41.3X5	T41.3X6
Oxetorone	T39.8X1	T39.8X2	T39.8X3	T39.8X4	T39.8X5	T39.8X6
Oxiconazole	T49.0X1	T49.0X2	T49.0X3	T49.0X4	T49.0X5	T49.0X6
Oxidizing agent NEC	T54.91	T54.92	T54.93	T54.94	--	--
Oxipurinol	T50.4X1	T50.4X2	T50.4X3	T50.4X4	T50.4X5	T50.4X6
Oxitriptan	T43.291	T43.292	T43.293	T43.294	T43.295	T43.296
Oxitropium bromide	T48.6X1	T48.6X2	T48.6X3	T48.6X4	T48.6X5	T48.6X6
Oxodipine	T46.1X1	T46.1X2	T46.1X3	T46.1X4	T46.1X5	T46.1X6
Oxolamine	T48.3X1	T48.3X2	T48.3X3	T48.3X4	T48.3X5	T48.3X6
Oxolinic acid	T37.8X1	T37.8X2	T37.8X3	T37.8X4	T37.8X5	T37.8X6
Oxomemazine	T43.3X1	T43.3X2	T43.3X3	T43.3X4	T43.3X5	T43.3X6
Oxophenarsine	T37.3X1	T37.3X2	T37.3X3	T37.3X4	T37.3X5	T37.3X6
Oxprenolol	T44.7X1	T44.7X2	T44.7X3	T44.7X4	T44.7X5	T44.7X6
Oxsoralen	T49.3X1	T49.3X2	T49.3X3	T49.3X4	T49.3X5	T49.3X6
Oxtriphylline	T48.6X1	T48.6X2	T48.6X3	T48.6X4	T48.6X5	T48.6X6
Oxybate sodium	T41.291	T41.292	T41.293	T41.294	T41.295	T41.296
Oxybuprocaine	T41.3X1	T41.3X2	T41.3X3	T41.3X4	T41.3X5	T41.3X6
Oxybutynin	T44.3X1	T44.3X2	T44.3X3	T44.3X4	T44.3X5	T44.3X6

Substance	Poisoning, Accidental (unintentional)	Poisoning, Intentional Self-harm	Poisoning, Assault	Poisoning, Undetermined	Adverse effect	Underdosing
Oxychlorosene	T49.0X1	T49.0X2	T49.0X3	T49.0X4	T49.0X5	T49.0X6
Oxycodone	T40.2X1	T40.2X2	T40.2X3	T40.2X4	T40.2X5	T40.2X6
Oxyfedrine	T46.3X1	T46.3X2	T46.3X3	T46.3X4	T46.3X5	T46.3X6
Oxygen	T41.5X1	T41.5X2	T41.5X3	T41.5X4	T41.5X5	T41.5X6
Oxylone	T49.0X1	T49.0X2	T49.0X3	T49.0X4	T49.0X5	T49.0X6
ophthalmic preparation	T49.5X1	T49.5X2	T49.5X3	T49.5X4	T49.5X5	T49.5X6
Oxymesterone	T38.7X1	T38.7X2	T38.7X3	T38.7X4	T38.7X5	T38.7X6
Oxymetazoline	T48.5X1	T48.5X2	T48.5X3	T48.5X4	T48.5X5	T48.5X6
Oxymetholone	T38.7X1	T38.7X2	T38.7X3	T38.7X4	T38.7X5	T38.7X6
Oxymorphone	T40.2X1	T40.2X2	T40.2X3	T40.2X4	T40.2X5	T40.2X6
Oxypertine	T43.591	T43.592	T43.593	T43.594	T43.595	T43.596
Oxyphenbutazone	T39.2X1	T39.2X2	T39.2X3	T39.2X4	T39.2X5	T39.2X6
Oxyphencyclimine	T44.3X1	T44.3X2	T44.3X3	T44.3X4	T44.3X5	T44.3X6
Oxyphenisatine	T47.2X1	T47.2X2	T47.2X3	T47.2X4	T47.2X5	T47.2X6
Oxyphenonium bromide	T44.3X1	T44.3X2	T44.3X3	T44.3X4	T44.3X5	T44.3X6
Oxypolygelatin	T45.8X1	T45.8X2	T45.8X3	T45.8X4	T45.8X5	T45.8X6
Oxyquinoline (derivatives)	T37.8X1	T37.8X2	T37.8X3	T37.8X4	T37.8X5	T37.8X6
Oxytetracycline	T36.4X1	T36.4X2	T36.4X3	T36.4X4	T36.4X5	T36.4X6
Oxytocic drug NEC	T48.0X1	T48.0X2	T48.0X3	T48.0X4	T48.0X5	T48.0X6
Oxytocin (synthetic)	T48.0X1	T48.0X2	T48.0X3	T48.0X4	T48.0X5	T48.0X6
Ozone	T59.891	T59.892	T59.893	T59.894	--	--
PABA	T49.3X1	T49.3X2	T49.3X3	T49.3X4	T49.3X5	T49.3X6
Packed red cells	T45.8X1	T45.8X2	T45.8X3	T45.8X4	T45.8X5	T45.8X6
Padimate	T49.3X1	T49.3X2	T49.3X3	T49.3X4	T49.3X5	T49.3X6
Paint NEC	T65.6X1	T65.6X2	T65.6X3	T65.6X4	--	--
cleaner	T52.91	T52.92	T52.93	T52.94	--	--
fumes NEC	T59.891	T59.892	T59.893	T59.894	--	--
lead (fumes)	T56.0X1	T56.0X2	T56.0X3	T56.0X4	--	--
solvent NEC	T52.8X1	T52.8X2	T52.8X3	T52.8X4	--	--
stripper	T52.8X1	T52.8X2	T52.8X3	T52.8X4	--	--
Palfium	T40.2X1	T40.2X2	T40.2X3	T40.2X4	--	--
Palm kernel oil	T50.991	T50.992	T50.993	T50.994	T50.995	T50.996
Paludrine	T37.2X1	T37.2X2	T37.2X3	T37.2X4	T37.2X5	T37.2X6
PAM (pralidoxime)	T50.6X1	T50.6X2	T50.6X3	T50.6X4	T50.6X5	T50.6X6
Pamaquine (naphthoute)	T37.2X1	T37.2X2	T37.2X3	T37.2X4	T37.2X5	T37.2X6
Panadol	T39.1X1	T39.1X2	T39.1X3	T39.1X4	T39.1X5	T39.1X6
Pancreatic						
digestive secretion stimulant	T47.8X1	T47.8X2	T47.8X3	T47.8X4	T47.8X5	T47.8X6
dornase	T45.3X1	T45.3X2	T45.3X3	T45.3X4	T45.3X5	T45.3X6
Pancreatin	T47.5X1	T47.5X2	T47.5X3	T47.5X4	T47.5X5	T47.5X6
Pancrelipase	T47.5X1	T47.5X2	T47.5X3	T47.5X4	T47.5X5	T47.5X6
Pancuronium (bromide)	T48.1X1	T48.1X2	T48.1X3	T48.1X4	T48.1X5	T48.1X6
Pangamic acid	T45.2X1	T45.2X2	T45.2X3	T45.2X4	T45.2X5	T45.2X6
Panthenol	T45.2X1	T45.2X2	T45.2X3	T45.2X4	T45.2X5	T45.2X6
topical	T49.8X1	T49.8X2	T49.8X3	T49.8X4	T49.8X5	T49.8X6
Pantopon	T40.0X1	T40.0X2	T40.0X3	T40.0X4	T40.0X5	T40.0X6
Pantothenic acid	T45.2X1	T45.2X2	T45.2X3	T45.2X4	T45.2X5	T45.2X6
Panwarfin	T45.511	T45.512	T45.513	T45.514	T45.515	T45.516
Papain	T47.5X1	T47.5X2	T47.5X3	T47.5X4	T47.5X5	T47.5X6
digestant	T47.5X1	T47.5X2	T47.5X3	T47.5X4	T47.5X5	T47.5X6
Papaveretum	T40.0X1	T40.0X2	T40.0X3	T40.0X4	T40.0X5	T40.0X6
Papaverine	T44.3X1	T44.3X2	T44.3X3	T44.3X4	T44.3X5	T44.3X6
Para-acetamidophenol	T39.1X1	T39.1X2	T39.1X3	T39.1X4	T39.1X5	T39.1X6
Para-aminobenzoic acid	T49.3X1	T49.3X2	T49.3X3	T49.3X4	T49.3X5	T49.3X6
Para-aminophenol derivatives	T39.1X1	T39.1X2	T39.1X3	T39.1X4	T39.1X5	T39.1X6
Para-aminosalicylic acid	T37.1X1	T37.1X2	T37.1X3	T37.1X4	T37.1X5	T37.1X6
Paracetaldehyde	T42.6X1	T42.6X2	T42.6X3	T42.6X4	T42.6X5	T42.6X6
Paracetamol	T39.1X1	T39.1X2	T39.1X3	T39.1X4	T39.1X5	T39.1X6
Parachlorophenol (camphorated)	T49.0X1	T49.0X2	T49.0X3	T49.0X4	T49.0X5	T49.0X6
Paracodin	T40.2X1	T40.2X2	T40.2X3	T40.2X4	T40.2X5	T40.2X6
Paradione	T42.2X1	T42.2X2	T42.2X3	T42.2X4	T42.2X5	T42.2X6
Paraffin (s) (wax)	T52.0X1	T52.0X2	T52.0X3	T52.0X4	--	--
liquid (medicinal)	T47.4X1	T47.4X2	T47.4X3	T47.4X4	T47.4X5	T47.4X6
nonmedicinal	T52.0X1	T52.0X2	T52.0X3	T52.0X4	--	--

Substance	Poisoning, Accidental (unintentional)	Poisoning, Intentional Self-harm	Poisoning, Assault	Poisoning, Undetermined	Adverse effect	Underdosing
Paraformaldehyde	T60.3X1	T60.3X2	T60.3X3	T60.3X4	--	--
Paraldehyde	T42.6X1	T42.6X2	T42.6X3	T42.6X4	T42.6X5	T42.6X6
Paramethadione	T42.2X1	T42.2X2	T42.2X3	T42.2X4	T42.2X5	T42.2X6
Paramethasone	T38.0X1	T38.0X2	T38.0X3	T38.0X4	T38.0X5	T38.0X6
acetate	T49.0X1	T49.0X2	T49.0X3	T49.0X4	T49.0X5	T49.0X6
Paraoxon	T60.0X1	T60.0X2	T60.0X3	T60.0X4	--	--
Paraquat	T60.3X1	T60.3X2	T60.3X3	T60.3X4	--	--
Parasympatholytic NEC	T44.3X1	T44.3X2	T44.3X3	T44.3X4	T44.3X5	T44.3X6
Parasympathomimetic drug NEC	T44.1X1	T44.1X2	T44.1X3	T44.1X4	T44.1X5	T44.1X6
Parathion	T60.0X1	T60.0X2	T60.0X3	T60.0X4	--	--
Parathormone	T50.991	T50.992	T50.993	T50.994	T50.995	T50.996
Parathyroid extract	T50.991	T50.992	T50.993	T50.994	T50.995	T50.996
Paratyphoid vaccine	T50.A91	T50.A92	T50.A93	T50.A94	T50.A95	T50.A96
Paredrine	T44.4X1	T44.4X2	T44.4X3	T44.4X4	T44.4X5	T44.4X6
Paregoric	T40.0X1	T40.0X2	T40.0X3	T40.0X4	T40.0X5	T40.0X6
Pargyline	T46.5X1	T46.5X2	T46.5X3	T46.5X4	T46.5X5	T46.5X6
Paris green	T57.0X1	T57.0X2	T57.0X3	T57.0X4	--	--
insecticide	T57.0X1	T57.0X2	T57.0X3	T57.0X4	--	--
Parnate	T43.1X1	T43.1X2	T43.1X3	T43.1X4	T43.1X5	T43.1X6
Paromomycin	T36.5X1	T36.5X2	T36.5X3	T36.5X4	T36.5X5	T36.5X6
Paroxypropione	T45.1X1	T45.1X2	T45.1X3	T45.1X4	T45.1X5	T45.1X6
Parzone	T40.2X1	T40.2X2	T40.2X3	T40.2X4	T40.2X5	T40.2X6
PAS	T37.1X1	T37.1X2	T37.1X3	T37.1X4	T37.1X5	T37.1X6
Pasiniazid	T37.1X1	T37.1X2	T37.1X3	T37.1X4	T37.1X5	T37.1X6
PBB (polybrominated biphenyls)	T65.891	T65.892	T65.893	T65.894	--	--
PCB	T65.891	T65.892	T65.893	T65.894	--	--
PCP						
meaning pentachlorophenol	T60.1X1	T60.1X2	T60.1X3	T60.1X4	--	--
fungicide	T60.3X1	T60.3X2	T60.3X3	T60.3X4	--	--
herbicide	T60.3X1	T60.3X2	T60.3X3	T60.3X4	--	--
insecticide	T60.1X1	T60.1X2	T60.1X3	T60.1X4	--	--
meaning phencyclidine	T40.991	T40.992	T40.993	T40.994	--	--
Peach kernel oil (emulsion)	T47.4X1	T47.4X2	T47.4X3	T47.4X4	T47.4X5	T47.4X6
Peanut oil (emulsion) NEC	T47.4X1	T47.4X2	T47.4X3	T47.4X4	T47.4X5	T47.4X6
topical	T49.3X1	T49.3X2	T49.3X3	T49.3X4	T49.3X5	T49.3X6
Pearly Gates (morning glory seeds)	T40.991	T40.992	T40.993	T40.994	--	--
Pecazine	T43.3X1	T43.3X2	T43.3X3	T43.3X4	T43.3X5	T43.3X6
Pectin	T47.6X1	T47.6X2	T47.6X3	T47.6X4	T47.6X5	T47.6X6
Pefloxacin	T37.8X1	T37.8X2	T37.8X3	T37.8X4	T37.8X5	T37.8X6
Pegademase, bovine	T50.Z91	T50.Z92	T50.Z93	T50.Z94	T50.Z95	T50.Z96
Pelletierine tannate	T37.4X1	T37.4X2	T37.4X3	T37.4X4	T37.4X5	T37.4X6
Pemirolast (potassium)	T48.6X1	T48.6X2	T48.6X3	T48.6X4	T48.6X5	T48.6X6
Pemoline	T50.7X1	T50.7X2	T50.7X3	T50.7X4	T50.7X5	T50.7X6
Pempidine	T44.2X1	T44.2X2	T44.2X3	T44.2X4	T44.2X5	T44.2X6
Penamecillin	T36.0X1	T36.0X2	T36.0X3	T36.0X4	T36.0X5	T36.0X6
Penbutolol	T44.7X1	T44.7X2	T44.7X3	T44.7X4	T44.7X5	T44.7X6
Penethamate	T36.0X1	T36.0X2	T36.0X3	T36.0X4	T36.0X5	T36.0X6
Penfluridol	T43.591	T43.592	T43.593	T43.594	T43.595	T43.596
Penflutizide	T50.2X1	T50.2X2	T50.2X3	T50.2X4	T50.2X5	T50.2X6
Pengitoxin	T46.0X1	T46.0X2	T46.0X3	T46.0X4	T46.0X5	T46.0X6
Penicillamine	T50.6X1	T50.6X2	T50.6X3	T50.6X4	T50.6X5	T50.6X6
Penicillin (any)	T36.0X1	T36.0X2	T36.0X3	T36.0X4	T36.0X5	T36.0X6
Penicillinase	T45.3X1	T45.3X2	T45.3X3	T45.3X4	T45.3X5	T45.3X6
Penicilloyl polylysine	T50.8X1	T50.8X2	T50.8X3	T50.8X4	T50.8X5	T50.8X6
Penimepicycline	T36.4X1	T36.4X2	T36.4X3	T36.4X4	T36.4X5	T36.4X6
Pentachloroethane	T53.6X1	T53.6X2	T53.6X3	T53.6X4	--	--
Pentachloronaphthalene	T53.7X1	T53.7X2	T53.7X3	T53.7X4	--	--
Pentachlorophenol (pesticide)	T60.1X1	T60.1X2	T60.1X3	T60.1X4	--	--
fungicide	T60.3X1	T60.3X2	T60.3X3	T60.3X4	--	--
herbicide	T60.3X1	T60.3X2	T60.3X3	T60.3X4	--	--
insecticide	T60.1X1	T60.1X2	T60.1X3	T60.1X4	--	--
Pentaerythritol	T46.3X1	T46.3X2	T46.3X3	T46.3X4	T46.3X5	T46.3X6
chloral	T42.6X1	T42.6X2	T42.6X3	T42.6X4	T42.6X5	T42.6X6
tetranitrate NEC	T46.3X1	T46.3X2	T46.3X3	T46.3X4	T46.3X5	T46.3X6
Pentaerythrityl tetranitrate	T46.3X1	T46.3X2	T46.3X3	T46.3X4	T46.3X5	T46.3X6

Substance	Poisoning, Accidental (unintentional)	Poisoning, Intentional Self-harm	Poisoning, Assault	Poisoning, Undetermined	Adverse effect	Underdosing
Pentagastrin	T50.8X1	T50.8X2	T50.8X3	T50.8X4	T50.8X5	T50.8X6
Pentalin	T53.6X1	T53.6X2	T53.6X3	T53.6X4	--	--
Pentamethonium bromide	T44.2X1	T44.2X2	T44.2X3	T44.2X4	T44.2X5	T44.2X6
Pentamidine	T37.3X1	T37.3X2	T37.3X3	T37.3X4	T37.3X5	T37.3X6
Pentanol	T51.3X1	T51.3X2	T51.3X3	T51.3X4	--	--
Pentapyrrolinium (bitartrate)	T44.2X1	T44.2X2	T44.2X3	T44.2X4	T44.2X5	T44.2X6
Pentaquine	T37.2X1	T37.2X2	T37.2X3	T37.2X4	T37.2X5	T37.2X6
Pentazocine	T40.4X1	T40.4X2	T40.4X3	T40.4X4	T40.4X5	T40.4X6
Pentetrazole	T50.7X1	T50.7X2	T50.7X3	T50.7X4	T50.7X5	T50.7X6
Penthienate bromide	T44.3X1	T44.3X2	T44.3X3	T44.3X4	T44.3X5	T44.3X6
Pentifylline	T46.7X1	T46.7X2	T46.7X3	T46.7X4	T46.7X5	T46.7X6
Pentobarbital	T42.3X1	T42.3X2	T42.3X3	T42.3X4	T42.3X5	T42.3X6
sodium	T42.3X1	T42.3X2	T42.3X3	T42.3X4	T42.3X5	T42.3X6
Pentobarbitone	T42.3X1	T42.3X2	T42.3X3	T42.3X4	T42.3X5	T42.3X6
Pentolonium tartrate	T44.2X1	T44.2X2	T44.2X3	T44.2X4	T44.2X5	T44.2X6
Pentosan polysulfate (sodium)	T39.8X1	T39.8X2	T39.8X3	T39.8X4	T39.8X5	T39.8X6
Pentostatin	T45.1X1	T45.1X2	T45.1X3	T45.1X4	T45.1X5	T45.1X6
Pentothal	T41.1X1	T41.1X2	T41.1X3	T41.1X4	T41.1X5	T41.1X6
Pentoxifylline	T46.7X1	T46.7X2	T46.7X3	T46.7X4	T46.7X5	T46.7X6
Pentoxyverine	T48.3X1	T48.3X2	T48.3X3	T48.3X4	T48.3X5	T48.3X6
Pentrinat	T46.3X1	T46.3X2	T46.3X3	T46.3X4	T46.3X5	T46.3X6
Pentylenetetrazole	T50.7X1	T50.7X2	T50.7X3	T50.7X4	T50.7X5	T50.7X6
Pentylsalicylamide	T37.1X1	T37.1X2	T37.1X3	T37.1X4	T37.1X5	T37.1X6
Pentymal	T42.3X1	T42.3X2	T42.3X3	T42.3X4	T42.3X5	T42.3X6
Peplomycin	T45.1X1	T45.1X2	T45.1X3	T45.1X4	T45.1X5	T45.1X6
Peppermint (oil)	T47.5X1	T47.5X2	T47.5X3	T47.5X4	T47.5X5	T47.5X6
Pepsin	T47.5X1	T47.5X2	T47.5X3	T47.5X4	T47.5X5	T47.5X6
digestant	T47.5X1	T47.5X2	T47.5X3	T47.5X4	T47.5X5	T47.5X6
Pepstatin	T47.1X1	T47.1X2	T47.1X3	T47.1X4	T47.1X5	T47.1X6
Peptavlon	T50.8X1	T50.8X2	T50.8X3	T50.8X4	T50.8X5	T50.8X6
Perazine	T43.3X1	T43.3X2	T43.3X3	T43.3X4	T43.3X5	T43.3X6
Percaine (spinal)	T41.3X1	T41.3X2	T41.3X3	T41.3X4	T41.3X5	T41.3X6
topical (surface)	T41.3X1	T41.3X2	T41.3X3	T41.3X4	T41.3X5	T41.3X6
Perchloroethylene	T53.3X1	T53.3X2	T53.3X3	T53.3X4	--	--
medicinal	T37.4X1	T37.4X2	T37.4X3	T37.4X4	T37.4X5	T37.4X6
vapor	T53.3X1	T53.3X2	T53.3X3	T53.3X4	--	--
Percodan	T40.2X1	T40.2X2	T40.2X3	T40.2X4	T40.2X5	T40.2X6
Percogesic—see also acetaminophen	T45.0X1	T45.0X2	T45.0X3	T45.0X4	T45.0X5	T45.0X6
Percorten	T38.0X1	T38.0X2	T38.0X3	T38.0X4	T38.0X5	T38.0X6
Pergolide	T42.8X1	T42.8X2	T42.8X3	T42.8X4	T42.8X5	T42.8X6
Pergonal	T38.811	T38.812	T38.813	T38.814	T38.815	T38.816
Perhexilene	T46.3X1	T46.3X2	T46.3X3	T46.3X4	T46.3X5	T46.3X6
Perhexiline (maleate)	T46.3X1	T46.3X2	T46.3X3	T46.3X4	T46.3X5	T46.3X6
Periactin	T45.0X1	T45.0X2	T45.0X3	T45.0X4	T45.0X5	T45.0X6
Periciazine	T43.3X1	T43.3X2	T43.3X3	T43.3X4	T43.3X5	T43.3X6
Periclor	T42.6X1	T42.6X2	T42.6X3	T42.6X4	T42.6X5	T42.6X6
Perindopril	T46.4X1	T46.4X2	T46.4X3	T46.4X4	T46.4X5	T46.4X6
Perisoxal	T39.8X1	T39.8X2	T39.8X3	T39.8X4	T39.8X5	T39.8X6
Peritoneal dialysis solution	T50.3X1	T50.3X2	T50.3X3	T50.3X4	T50.3X5	T50.3X6
Peritrate	T46.3X1	T46.3X2	T46.3X3	T46.3X4	T46.3X5	T46.3X6
Perlapine	T42.4X1	T42.4X2	T42.4X3	T42.4X4	T42.4X5	T42.4X6
Permanganate	T65.891	T65.892	T65.893	T65.894	--	--
Permethrin	T60.1X1	T60.1X2	T60.1X3	T60.1X4	--	--
Pernocton	T42.3X1	T42.3X2	T42.3X3	T42.3X4	T42.3X5	T42.3X6
Pernoston	T42.3X1	T42.3X2	T42.3X3	T42.3X4	T42.3X5	T42.3X6
Peronine	T40.2X1	T40.2X2	T40.2X3	T40.2X4	--	--
Perphenazine	T43.3X1	T43.3X2	T43.3X3	T43.3X4	T43.3X5	T43.3X6
Pertofrane	T43.011	T43.012	T43.013	T43.014	T43.015	T43.016
Pertussis						
immune serum (human)	T50.Z11	T50.Z12	T50.Z13	T50.Z14	T50.Z15	T50.Z16
vaccine (with diphtheria toxoid) (with tetanus toxoid)	T50.A11	T50.A12	T50.A13	T50.A14	T50.A15	T50.A16
Peruvian balsam	T49.0X1	T49.0X2	T49.0X3	T49.0X4	T49.0X5	T49.0X6
Peruvoside	T46.0X1	T46.0X2	T46.0X3	T46.0X4	T46.0X5	T46.0X6

Substance	Poisoning, Accidental (unintentional)	Poisoning, Intentional Self-harm	Poisoning, Assault	Poisoning, Undetermined	Adverse effect	Underdosing
Pesticide (dust) (fumes) (vapor) NEC	T60.91	T60.92	T60.93	T60.94	--	--
arsenic	T57.0X1	T57.0X2	T57.0X3	T57.0X4	--	--
chlorinated	T60.1X1	T60.1X2	T60.1X3	T60.1X4	--	--
cyanide	T65.0X1	T65.0X2	T65.0X3	T65.0X4	--	--
kerosene	T52.0X1	T52.0X2	T52.0X3	T52.0X4	--	--
mixture (of compounds)	T60.91	T60.92	T60.93	T60.94	--	--
naphthalene	T60.2X1	T60.2X2	T60.2X3	T60.2X4	--	--
organochlorine (compounds)	T60.1X1	T60.1X2	T60.1X3	T60.1X4	--	--
petroleum (distillate) (products) NEC	T60.8X1	T60.8X2	T60.8X3	T60.8X4	--	--
specified ingredient NEC	T60.8X1	T60.8X2	T60.8X3	T60.8X4	--	--
strychnine	T65.1X1	T65.1X2	T65.1X3	T65.1X4	--	--
thallium	T60.4X1	T60.4X2	T60.4X3	T60.4X4	--	--
Pethidine	T40.4X1	T40.4X2	T40.4X3	T40.4X4	T40.4X5	T40.4X6
Petrichloral	T42.6X1	T42.6X2	T42.6X3	T42.6X4	T42.6X5	T42.6X6
Petrol	T52.0X1	T52.0X2	T52.0X3	T52.0X4	--	--
vapor	T52.0X1	T52.0X2	T52.0X3	T52.0X4	--	--
Petrolatum	T49.3X1	T49.3X2	T49.3X3	T49.3X4	T49.3X5	T49.3X6
hydrophilic	T49.3X1	T49.3X2	T49.3X3	T49.3X4	T49.3X5	T49.3X6
liquid	T47.4X1	T47.4X2	T47.4X3	T47.4X4	T47.4X5	T47.4X6
topical	T49.3X1	T49.3X2	T49.3X3	T49.3X4	T49.3X5	T49.3X6
nonmedicinal	T52.0X1	T52.0X2	T52.0X3	T52.0X4	--	--
red veterinary	T49.3X1	T49.3X2	T49.3X3	T49.3X4	T49.3X5	T49.3X6
white	T49.3X1	T49.3X2	T49.3X3	T49.3X4	T49.3X5	T49.3X6
Petroleum (products) NEC	T52.0X1	T52.0X2	T52.0X3	T52.0X4	--	--
benzine (s) —see Ligroin						
ether—see Ligroin						
jelly—see Petrolatum						
naphtha—see Ligroin						
pesticide	T60.8X1	T60.8X2	T60.8X3	T60.8X4	--	--
solids	T52.0X1	T52.0X2	T52.0X3	T52.0X4	--	--
solvents	T52.0X1	T52.0X2	T52.0X3	T52.0X4	--	--
vapor	T52.0X1	T52.0X2	T52.0X3	T52.0X4	--	--
Peyote	T40.991	T40.992	T40.993	T40.994	--	--
Phanodorm, phanodorn	T42.3X1	T42.3X2	T42.3X3	T42.3X4	T42.3X5	T42.3X6
Phanquinone	T37.3X1	T37.3X2	T37.3X3	T37.3X4	T37.3X5	T37.3X6
Phanquone	T37.3X1	T37.3X2	T37.3X3	T37.3X4	T37.3X5	T37.3X6
Pharmaceutical						
adjunct NEC	T50.901	T50.902	T50.903	T50.904	T50.905	T50.906
excipient NEC	T50.901	T50.902	T50.903	T50.904	T50.905	T50.906
sweetener	T50.901	T50.902	T50.903	T50.904	T50.905	T50.906
viscous agent	T50.901	T50.902	T50.903	T50.904	T50.905	T50.906
Phemitone	T42.3X1	T42.3X2	T42.3X3	T42.3X4	T42.3X5	T42.3X6
Phenacaine	T41.3X1	T41.3X2	T41.3X3	T41.3X4	T41.3X5	T41.3X6
Phenacemide	T42.6X1	T42.6X2	T42.6X3	T42.6X4	T42.6X5	T42.6X6
Phenacetin	T39.1X1	T39.1X2	T39.1X3	T39.1X4	T39.1X5	T39.1X6
Phenadoxone	T40.2X1	T40.2X2	T40.2X3	T40.2X4	--	--
Phenaglycodol	T43.591	T43.592	T43.593	T43.594	T43.595	T43.596
Phenantoin	T42.0X1	T42.0X2	T42.0X3	T42.0X4	T42.0X5	T42.0X6
Phenaphthazine reagent	T50.991	T50.992	T50.993	T50.994	T50.995	T50.996
Phenazocine	T40.4X1	T40.4X2	T40.4X3	T40.4X4	T40.4X5	T40.4X6
Phenazone	T39.2X1	T39.2X2	T39.2X3	T39.2X4	T39.2X5	T39.2X6
Phenazopyridine	T39.8X1	T39.8X2	T39.8X3	T39.8X4	T39.8X5	T39.8X6
Phenbenicillin	T36.0X1	T36.0X2	T36.0X3	T36.0X4	T36.0X5	T36.0X6
Phenbutrazate	T50.5X1	T50.5X2	T50.5X3	T50.5X4	T50.5X5	T50.5X6
Phencyclidine	T40.991	T40.992	T40.993	T40.994	T40.995	T40.996
Phendimetrazine	T50.5X1	T50.5X2	T50.5X3	T50.5X4	T50.5X5	T50.5X6
Phenelzine	T43.1X1	T43.1X2	T43.1X3	T43.1X4	T43.1X5	T43.1X6
Phenemal	T42.3X1	T42.3X2	T42.3X3	T42.3X4	T42.3X5	T42.3X6
Phenergan	T42.6X1	T42.6X2	T42.6X3	T42.6X4	T42.6X5	T42.6X6
Pheneticillin	T36.0X1	T36.0X2	T36.0X3	T36.0X4	T36.0X5	T36.0X6
Pheneturide	T42.6X1	T42.6X2	T42.6X3	T42.6X4	T42.6X5	T42.6X6
Phenformin	T38.3X1	T38.3X2	T38.3X3	T38.3X4	T38.3X5	T38.3X6
Phenglutarimide	T44.3X1	T44.3X2	T44.3X3	T44.3X4	T44.3X5	T44.3X6
Phenicarbazide	T39.8X1	T39.8X2	T39.8X3	T39.8X4	T39.8X5	T39.8X6
Phenindamine	T45.0X1	T45.0X2	T45.0X3	T45.0X4	T45.0X5	T45.0X6

Substance	Poisoning, Accidental (unintentional)	Poisoning, Intentional Self-harm	Poisoning, Assault	Poisoning, Undetermined	Adverse effect	Underdosing
Phenindione	T45.511	T45.512	T45.513	T45.514	T45.515	T45.516
Pheniprazine	T43.1X1	T43.1X2	T43.1X3	T43.1X4	T43.1X5	T43.1X6
Pheniramine	T45.0X1	T45.0X2	T45.0X3	T45.0X4	T45.0X5	T45.0X6
Phenisatin	T47.2X1	T47.2X2	T47.2X3	T47.2X4	T47.2X5	T47.2X6
Phenmetrazine	T50.5X1	T50.5X2	T50.5X3	T50.5X4	T50.5X5	T50.5X6
Phenobal	T42.3X1	T42.3X2	T42.3X3	T42.3X4	T42.3X5	T42.3X6
Phenobarbital	T42.3X1	T42.3X2	T42.3X3	T42.3X4	T42.3X5	T42.3X6
with						
mephenytoin	T42.3X1	T42.3X2	T42.3X3	T42.3X4	T42.3X5	T42.3X6
phenytoin	T42.3X1	T42.3X2	T42.3X3	T42.3X4	T42.3X5	T42.3X6
sodium	T42.3X1	T42.3X2	T42.3X3	T42.3X4	T42.3X5	T42.3X6
Phenobarbitone	T42.3X1	T42.3X2	T42.3X3	T42.3X4	T42.3X5	T42.3X6
Phenobutiodil	T50.8X1	T50.8X2	T50.8X3	T50.8X4	T50.8X5	T50.8X6
Phenoctide	T49.0X1	T49.0X2	T49.0X3	T49.0X4	T49.0X5	T49.0X6
Phenol	T49.0X1	T49.0X2	T49.0X3	T49.0X4	T49.0X5	T49.0X6
disinfectant	T54.0X1	T54.0X2	T54.0X3	T54.0X4	--	--
in oil injection	T46.8X1	T46.8X2	T46.8X3	T46.8X4	T46.8X5	T46.8X6
medicinal	T49.1X1	T49.1X2	T49.1X3	T49.1X4	T49.1X5	T49.1X6
nonmedicinal NEC	T54.0X1	T54.0X2	T54.0X3	T54.0X4	--	--
pesticide	T60.8X1	T60.8X2	T60.8X3	T60.8X4	--	--
red	T50.8X1	T50.8X2	T50.8X3	T50.8X4	T50.8X5	T50.8X6
Phenolic preparation	T49.1X1	T49.1X2	T49.1X3	T49.1X4	T49.1X5	T49.1X6
Phenolphthalein	T47.2X1	T47.2X2	T47.2X3	T47.2X4	T47.2X5	T47.2X6
Phenolsulfonphthalein	T50.8X1	T50.8X2	T50.8X3	T50.8X4	T50.8X5	T50.8X6
Phenomorphan	T40.2X1	T40.2X2	T40.2X3	T40.2X4	--	--
Phenonyl	T42.3X1	T42.3X2	T42.3X3	T42.3X4	T42.3X5	T42.3X6
Phenoperidine	T40.4X1	T40.4X2	T40.4X3	T40.4X4	--	--
Phenopyrazone	T46.991	T46.992	T46.993	T46.994	T46.995	T46.996
Phenoquin	T50.4X1	T50.4X2	T50.4X3	T50.4X4	T50.4X5	T50.4X6
Phenothiazine (psychotropic) NEC	T43.3X1	T43.3X2	T43.3X3	T43.3X4	T43.3X5	T43.3X6
insecticide	T60.2X1	T60.2X2	T60.2X3	T60.2X4	--	--
Phenothrin	T49.0X1	T49.0X2	T49.0X3	T49.0X4	T49.0X5	T49.0X6
Phenoxybenzamine	T46.7X1	T46.7X2	T46.7X3	T46.7X4	T46.7X5	T46.7X6
Phenoxyethanol	T49.0X1	T49.0X2	T49.0X3	T49.0X4	T49.0X5	T49.0X6
Phenoxymethyl penicillin	T36.0X1	T36.0X2	T36.0X3	T36.0X4	T36.0X5	T36.0X6
Phenprobamate	T42.8X1	T42.8X2	T42.8X3	T42.8X4	T42.8X5	T42.8X6
Phenprocoumon	T45.511	T45.512	T45.513	T45.514	T45.515	T45.516
Phensuximide	T42.2X1	T42.2X2	T42.2X3	T42.2X4	T42.2X5	T42.2X6
Phentermine	T50.5X1	T50.5X2	T50.5X3	T50.5X4	T50.5X5	T50.5X6
Phenthicillin	T36.0X1	T36.0X2	T36.0X3	T36.0X4	T36.0X5	T36.0X6
Phentolamine	T46.7X1	T46.7X2	T46.7X3	T46.7X4	T46.7X5	T46.7X6
Phenyl						
butazone	T39.2X1	T39.2X2	T39.2X3	T39.2X4	T39.2X5	T39.2X6
enediamine	T65.3X1	T65.3X2	T65.3X3	T65.3X4	--	--
hydrazine	T65.3X1	T65.3X2	T65.3X3	T65.3X4	--	--
antineoplastic	T45.1X1	T45.1X2	T45.1X3	T45.1X4	T45.1X5	T45.1X6
mercuric compounds—see Mercury						
salicylate	T49.3X1	T49.3X2	T49.3X3	T49.3X4	T49.3X5	T49.3X6
Phenylalanine mustard	T45.1X1	T45.1X2	T45.1X3	T45.1X4	T45.1X5	T45.1X6
Phenylbutazone	T39.2X1	T39.2X2	T39.2X3	T39.2X4	T39.2X5	T39.2X6
Phenylenediamine	T65.3X1	T65.3X2	T65.3X3	T65.3X4	--	--
Phenylephrine	T44.4X1	T44.4X2	T44.4X3	T44.4X4	T44.4X5	T44.4X6
Phenylethylbiguanide	T38.3X1	T38.3X2	T38.3X3	T38.3X4	T38.3X5	T38.3X6
Phenylmercuric						
acetate	T49.0X1	T49.0X2	T49.0X3	T49.0X4	T49.0X5	T49.0X6
borate	T49.0X1	T49.0X2	T49.0X3	T49.0X4	T49.0X5	T49.0X6
nitrate	T49.0X1	T49.0X2	T49.0X3	T49.0X4	T49.0X5	T49.0X6
Phenylmethylbarbitone	T42.3X1	T42.3X2	T42.3X3	T42.3X4	T42.3X5	T42.3X6
Phenylpropanol	T47.5X1	T47.5X2	T47.5X3	T47.5X4	T47.5X5	T47.5X6
Phenylpropanolamine	T44.991	T44.992	T44.993	T44.994	T44.995	T44.996
Phenylsulfthion	T60.0X1	T60.0X2	T60.0X3	T60.0X4	--	--
Phenyltoloxamine	T45.0X1	T45.0X2	T45.0X3	T45.0X4	T45.0X5	T45.0X6
Phenyramidol, phenyramidon	T39.8X1	T39.8X2	T39.8X3	T39.8X4	T39.8X5	T39.8X6
Phenytoin	T42.0X1	T42.0X2	T42.0X3	T42.0X4	T42.0X5	T42.0X6

TABLE OF DRUGS AND CHEMICALS

Substance	Poisoning, Accidental (unintentional)	Poisoning, Intentional Self-harm	Poisoning, Assault	Poisoning, Undetermined	Adverse effect	Underdosing
with Phenobarbital	T42.3X1	T42.3X2	T42.3X3	T42.3X4	T42.3X5	T42.3X6
pHisoHex	T49.2X1	T49.2X2	T49.2X3	T49.2X4	T49.2X5	T49.2X6
Pholcodine	T48.3X1	T48.3X2	T48.3X3	T48.3X4	T48.3X5	T48.3X6
Pholedrine	T46.991	T46.992	T46.993	T46.994	T46.995	T46.996
Phorate	T60.0X1	T60.0X2	T60.0X3	T60.0X4	--	--
Phosdrin	T60.0X1	T60.0X2	T60.0X3	T60.0X4	--	--
Phosfolan	T60.0X1	T60.0X2	T60.0X3	T60.0X4	--	--
Phosgene (gas)	T59.891	T59.892	T59.893	T59.894	--	--
Phosphamidon	T60.0X1	T60.0X2	T60.0X3	T60.0X4	--	--
Phosphate	T65.891	T65.892	T65.893	T65.894	--	--
laxative	T47.4X1	T47.4X2	T47.4X3	T47.4X4	T47.4X5	T47.4X6
organic	T60.0X1	T60.0X2	T60.0X3	T60.0X4	--	--
solvent	T52.91	T52.92	T52.93	T52.94	--	--
tricresyl	T65.891	T65.892	T65.893	T65.894	--	--
Phosphine	T57.1X1	T57.1X2	T57.1X3	T57.1X4	--	--
fumigant	T57.1X1	T57.1X2	T57.1X3	T57.1X4	--	--
Phospholine	T49.5X1	T49.5X2	T49.5X3	T49.5X4	T49.5X5	T49.5X6
Phosphoric acid	T54.2X1	T54.2X2	T54.2X3	T54.2X4	--	--
Phosphorus (compound) NEC	T57.1X1	T57.1X2	T57.1X3	T57.1X4	--	--
pesticide	T60.0X1	T60.0X2	T60.0X3	T60.0X4	--	--
Phthalates	T65.891	T65.892	T65.893	T65.894	--	--
Phthalic anhydride	T65.891	T65.892	T65.893	T65.894	--	--
Phthalimidoglutarimide	T42.6X1	T42.6X2	T42.6X3	T42.6X4	T42.6X5	T42.6X6
Phthalylsulfathiazole	T37.0X1	T37.0X2	T37.0X3	T37.0X4	T37.0X5	T37.0X6
Phylloquinone	T45.7X1	T45.7X2	T45.7X3	T45.7X4	T45.7X5	T45.7X6
Physeptone	T40.3X1	T40.3X2	T40.3X3	T40.3X4	T40.3X5	T40.3X6
Physostigma venenosum	T62.2X1	T62.2X2	T62.2X3	T62.2X4	--	--
Physostigmine	T49.5X1	T49.5X2	T49.5X3	T49.5X4	T49.5X5	T49.5X6
Phytolacca decandra	T62.2X1	T62.2X2	T62.2X3	T62.2X4	--	--
berries	T62.1X1	T62.1X2	T62.1X3	T62.1X4	--	--
Phytomenadione	T45.7X1	T45.7X2	T45.7X3	T45.7X4	T45.7X5	T45.7X6
Phytonadione	T45.7X1	T45.7X2	T45.7X3	T45.7X4	T45.7X5	T45.7X6
Picoperine	T48.3X1	T48.3X2	T48.3X3	T48.3X4	T48.3X5	T48.3X6
Picosulfate (sodium)	T47.2X1	T47.2X2	T47.2X3	T47.2X4	T47.2X5	T47.2X6
Picric (acid)	T54.2X1	T54.2X2	T54.2X3	T54.2X4	--	--
Picrotoxin	T50.7X1	T50.7X2	T50.7X3	T50.7X4	T50.7X5	T50.7X6
Piketoprofen	T49.0X1	T49.0X2	T49.0X3	T49.0X4	T49.0X5	T49.0X6
Pilocarpine	T44.1X1	T44.1X2	T44.1X3	T44.1X4	T44.1X5	T44.1X6
Pilocarpus (jaborandi) extract	T44.1X1	T44.1X2	T44.1X3	T44.1X4	T44.1X5	T44.1X6
Pilsicainide (hydrochloride)	T46.2X1	T46.2X2	T46.2X3	T46.2X4	T46.2X5	T46.2X6
Pimaricin	T36.7X1	T36.7X2	T36.7X3	T36.7X4	T36.7X5	T36.7X6
Pimeclone	T50.7X1	T50.7X2	T50.7X3	T50.7X4	T50.7X5	T50.7X6
Pimelic ketone	T52.8X1	T52.8X2	T52.8X3	T52.8X4	--	--
Pimethixene	T45.0X1	T45.0X2	T45.0X3	T45.0X4	T45.0X5	T45.0X6
Piminodine	T40.2X1	T40.2X2	T40.2X3	T40.2X4	T40.2X5	T40.2X6
Pimozide	T43.591	T43.592	T43.593	T43.594	T43.595	T43.596
Pinacidil	T46.5X1	T46.5X2	T46.5X3	T46.5X4	T46.5X5	T46.5X6
Pinaverium bromide	T44.3X1	T44.3X2	T44.3X3	T44.3X4	T44.3X5	T44.3X6
Pinazepam	T42.4X1	T42.4X2	T42.4X3	T42.4X4	T42.4X5	T42.4X6
Pindolol	T44.7X1	T44.7X2	T44.7X3	T44.7X4	T44.7X5	T44.7X6
Pindone	T60.4X1	T60.4X2	T60.4X3	T60.4X4	--	--
Pine oil (disinfectant)	T65.891	T65.892	T65.893	T65.894	--	--
Pinkroot	T37.4X1	T37.4X2	T37.4X3	T37.4X4	T37.4X5	T37.4X6
Pipadone	T40.2X1	T40.2X2	T40.2X3	T40.2X4	--	--
Pipamazine	T45.0X1	T45.0X2	T45.0X3	T45.0X4	T45.0X5	T45.0X6
Pipamperone	T43.4X1	T43.4X2	T43.4X3	T43.4X4	T43.4X5	T43.4X6
Pipazetate	T48.3X1	T48.3X2	T48.3X3	T48.3X4	T48.3X5	T48.3X6
Pipemidic acid	T37.8X1	T37.8X2	T37.8X3	T37.8X4	T37.8X5	T37.8X6
Pipenzolate bromide	T44.3X1	T44.3X2	T44.3X3	T44.3X4	T44.3X5	T44.3X6
Piperacetazine	T43.3X1	T43.3X2	T43.3X3	T43.3X4	T43.3X5	T43.3X6
Piperacillin	T36.0X1	T36.0X2	T36.0X3	T36.0X4	T36.0X5	T36.0X6
Piperazine	T37.4X1	T37.4X2	T37.4X3	T37.4X4	T37.4X5	T37.4X6
estrone sulfate	T38.5X1	T38.5X2	T38.5X3	T38.5X4	T38.5X5	T38.5X6
Piper cubeba	T62.2X1	T62.2X2	T62.2X3	T62.2X4	--	--
Piperidione	T48.3X1	T48.3X2	T48.3X3	T48.3X4	T48.3X5	T48.3X6

Substance	Poisoning, Accidental (unintentional)	Poisoning, Intentional Self-harm	Poisoning, Assault	Poisoning, Undetermined	Adverse effect	Underdosing
Piperidolate	T44.3X1	T44.3X2	T44.3X3	T44.3X4	T44.3X5	T44.3X6
Piperocaine	T41.3X1	T41.3X2	T41.3X3	T41.3X4	T41.3X5	T41.3X6
infiltration (subcutaneous)	T41.3X1	T41.3X2	T41.3X3	T41.3X4	T41.3X5	T41.3X6
nerve block (peripheral) (plexus)	T41.3X1	T41.3X2	T41.3X3	T41.3X4	T41.3X5	T41.3X6
topical (surface)	T41.3X1	T41.3X2	T41.3X3	T41.3X4	T41.3X5	T41.3X6
Piperonyl butoxide	T60.8X1	T60.8X2	T60.8X3	T60.8X4	--	--
Pipethanate	T44.3X1	T44.3X2	T44.3X3	T44.3X4	T44.3X5	T44.3X6
Pipobroman	T45.1X1	T45.1X2	T45.1X3	T45.1X4	T45.1X5	T45.1X6
Pipotiazine	T43.3X1	T43.3X2	T43.3X3	T43.3X4	T43.3X5	T43.3X6
Pipoxizine	T45.0X1	T45.0X2	T45.0X3	T45.0X4	T45.0X5	T45.0X6
Pipradrol	T43.691	T43.692	T43.693	T43.694	T43.695	T43.696
Piprinhydrinate	T45.0X1	T45.0X2	T45.0X3	T45.0X4	T45.0X5	T45.0X6
Pirarubicin	T45.1X1	T45.1X2	T45.1X3	T45.1X4	T45.1X5	T45.1X6
Pirazinamide	T37.1X1	T37.1X2	T37.1X3	T37.1X4	T37.1X5	T37.1X6
Pirbuterol	T48.6X1	T48.6X2	T48.6X3	T48.6X4	T48.6X5	T48.6X6
Pirenzepine	T47.1X1	T47.1X2	T47.1X3	T47.1X4	T47.1X5	T47.1X6
Piretanide	T50.1X1	T50.1X2	T50.1X3	T50.1X4	T50.1X5	T50.1X6
Piribedil	T42.8X1	T42.8X2	T42.8X3	T42.8X4	T42.8X5	T42.8X6
Piridoxilate	T46.3X1	T46.3X2	T46.3X3	T46.3X4	T46.3X5	T46.3X6
Piritramide	T40.4X1	T40.4X2	T40.4X3	T40.4X4	--	--
Piromidic acid	T37.8X1	T37.8X2	T37.8X3	T37.8X4	T37.8X5	T37.8X6
Piroxicam	T39.391	T39.392	T39.393	T39.394	T39.395	T39.396
beta-cyclodextrin complex	T39.8X1	T39.8X2	T39.8X3	T39.8X4	T39.8X5	T39.8X6
Pirozadil	T46.6X1	T46.6X2	T46.6X3	T46.6X4	T46.6X5	T46.6X6
Piscidia (bark) (erythrina)	T39.8X1	T39.8X2	T39.8X3	T39.8X4	T39.8X5	T39.8X6
Pitch	T65.891	T65.892	T65.893	T65.894	--	--
Pitkin's solution	T41.3X1	T41.3X2	T41.3X3	T41.3X4	T41.3X5	T41.3X6
Pitocin	T48.0X1	T48.0X2	T48.0X3	T48.0X4	T48.0X5	T48.0X6
Pitressin (tannate)	T38.891	T38.892	T38.893	T38.894	T38.895	T38.896
Pituitary extracts (posterior)	T38.891	T38.892	T38.893	T38.894	T38.895	T38.896
anterior	T38.811	T38.812	T38.813	T38.814	T38.815	T38.816
Pituitrin	T38.891	T38.892	T38.893	T38.894	T38.895	T38.896
Pivampicillin	T36.0X1	T36.0X2	T36.0X3	T36.0X4	T36.0X5	T36.0X6
Pivmecillinam	T36.0X1	T36.0X2	T36.0X3	T36.0X4	T36.0X5	T36.0X6
Placental hormone	T38.891	T38.892	T38.893	T38.894	T38.895	T38.896
Placidyl	T42.6X1	T42.6X2	T42.6X3	T42.6X4	T42.6X5	T42.6X6
Plague vaccine	T50.A91	T50.A92	T50.A93	T50.A94	T50.A95	T50.A96
Plant						
food or fertilizer NEC	T65.891	T65.892	T65.893	T65.894	--	--
containing herbicide	T60.3X1	T60.3X2	T60.3X3	T60.3X4	--	--
noxious, used as food	T62.2X1	T62.2X2	T62.2X3	T62.2X4	--	--
berries	T62.1X1	T62.1X2	T62.1X3	T62.1X4	--	--
seeds	T62.2X1	T62.2X2	T62.2X3	T62.2X4	--	--
specified type NEC	T62.2X1	T62.2X2	T62.2X3	T62.2X4	--	--
Plasma	T45.8X1	T45.8X2	T45.8X3	T45.8X4	T45.8X5	T45.8X6
expander NEC	T45.8X1	T45.8X2	T45.8X3	T45.8X4	T45.8X5	T45.8X6
protein fraction (human)	T45.8X1	T45.8X2	T45.8X3	T45.8X4	T45.8X5	T45.8X6
Plasmanate	T45.8X1	T45.8X2	T45.8X3	T45.8X4	T45.8X5	T45.8X6
Plasminogen (tissue) activator	T45.611	T45.612	T45.613	T45.614	T45.615	T45.616
Plaster dressing	T49.3X1	T49.3X2	T49.3X3	T49.3X4	T49.3X5	T49.3X6
Plastic dressing	T49.3X1	T49.3X2	T49.3X3	T49.3X4	T49.3X5	T49.3X6
Plegicil	T43.3X1	T43.3X2	T43.3X3	T43.3X4	T43.3X5	T43.3X6
Plicamycin	T45.1X1	T45.1X2	T45.1X3	T45.1X4	T45.1X5	T45.1X6
Podophyllotoxin	T49.8X1	T49.8X2	T49.8X3	T49.8X4	T49.8X5	T49.8X6
Podophyllum (resin)	T49.4X1	T49.4X2	T49.4X3	T49.4X4	T49.4X5	T49.4X6
Poison NEC	T65.91	T65.92	T65.93	T65.94	--	--
Poisonous berries	T62.1X1	T62.1X2	T62.1X3	T62.1X4	--	--
Pokeweed (any part)	T62.2X1	T62.2X2	T62.2X3	T62.2X4	--	--
Poldine metilsulfate	T44.3X1	T44.3X2	T44.3X3	T44.3X4	T44.3X5	T44.3X6
Polidexide (sulfate)	T46.6X1	T46.6X2	T46.6X3	T46.6X4	T46.6X5	T46.6X6
Polidocanol	T46.8X1	T46.8X2	T46.8X3	T46.8X4	T46.8X5	T46.8X6
Poliomyelitis vaccine	T50.B91	T50.B92	T50.B93	T50.B94	T50.B95	T50.B96
Polish (car) (floor) (furni-ture) (metal) (porcelain) (silver)	T65.891	T65.892	T65.893	T65.894	--	--

Substance	Poisoning, Accidental (unintentional)	Poisoning, Intentional Self-harm	Poisoning, Assault	Poisoning, Undetermined	Adverse effect	Underdosing
abrasive	T65.891	T65.892	T65.893	T65.894	--	--
porcelain	T65.891	T65.892	T65.893	T65.894	--	--
Poloxalkol	T47.4X1	T47.4X2	T47.4X3	T47.4X4	T47.4X5	T47.4X6
Poloxamer	T47.4X1	T47.4X2	T47.4X3	T47.4X4	T47.4X5	T47.4X6
Polyaminostyrene resins	T50.3X1	T50.3X2	T50.3X3	T50.3X4	T50.3X5	T50.3X6
Polycarbophil	T47.4X1	T47.4X2	T47.4X3	T47.4X4	T47.4X5	T47.4X6
Polychlorinated biphenyl	T65.891	T65.892	T65.893	T65.894	--	--
Polycycline	T36.4X1	T36.4X2	T36.4X3	T36.4X4	T36.4X5	T36.4X6
Polyester fumes	T59.891	T59.892	T59.893	T59.894	--	--
Polyester resin hardener	T52.91	T52.92	T52.93	T52.94	--	--
fumes	T59.891	T59.892	T59.893	T59.894	--	--
Polyestradiol phosphate	T38.5X1	T38.5X2	T38.5X3	T38.5X4	T38.5X5	T38.5X6
Polyethanolamine alkyl sulfate	T49.2X1	T49.2X2	T49.2X3	T49.2X4	T49.2X5	T49.2X6
Polyethylene adhesive	T49.3X1	T49.3X2	T49.3X3	T49.3X4	T49.3X5	T49.3X6
Polyferose	T45.4X1	T45.4X2	T45.4X3	T45.4X4	T45.4X5	T45.4X6
Polygeline	T45.8X1	T45.8X2	T45.8X3	T45.8X4	T45.8X5	T45.8X6
Polymyxin	T36.8X1	T36.8X2	T36.8X3	T36.8X4	T36.8X5	T36.8X6
B	T36.8X1	T36.8X2	T36.8X3	T36.8X4	T36.8X5	T36.8X6
ENT agent	T49.6X1	T49.6X2	T49.6X3	T49.6X4	T49.6X5	T49.6X6
topical NEC	T49.0X1	T49.0X2	T49.0X3	T49.0X4	T49.0X5	T49.0X6
E sulfate (eye preparation)	T49.5X1	T49.5X2	T49.5X3	T49.5X4	T49.5X5	T49.5X6
Polynoxylin	T49.0X1	T49.0X2	T49.0X3	T49.0X4	T49.0X5	T49.0X6
Polyoestradiol phosphate	T38.5X1	T38.5X2	T38.5X3	T38.5X4	T38.5X5	T38.5X6
Polyoxymethyleneurea	T49.0X1	T49.0X2	T49.0X3	T49.0X4	T49.0X5	T49.0X6
Polysilane	T47.8X1	T47.8X2	T47.8X3	T47.8X4	T47.8X5	T47.8X6
Polytetrafluoroethylene (inhaled)	T59.891	T59.892	T59.893	T59.894	--	--
Polythiazide	T50.2X1	T50.2X2	T50.2X3	T50.2X4	T50.2X5	T50.2X6
Polyvidone	T45.8X1	T45.8X2	T45.8X3	T45.8X4	T45.8X5	T45.8X6
Polyvinylpyrrolidone	T45.8X1	T45.8X2	T45.8X3	T45.8X4	T45.8X5	T45.8X6
Pontocaine (hydrochloride) (infiltration) (topical)	T41.3X1	T41.3X2	T41.3X3	T41.3X4	T41.3X5	T41.3X6
nerve block (peripheral) (plexus)	T41.3X1	T41.3X2	T41.3X3	T41.3X4	T41.3X5	T41.3X6
spinal	T41.3X1	T41.3X2	T41.3X3	T41.3X4	T41.3X5	T41.3X6
Porfiromycin	T45.1X1	T45.1X2	T45.1X3	T45.1X4	T45.1X5	T45.1X6
Posterior pituitary hormone NEC	T38.891	T38.892	T38.893	T38.894	T38.895	T38.896
Pot	T40.7X1	T40.7X2	T40.7X3	T40.7X4	T40.7X5	T40.7X6
Potash (caustic)	T54.3X1	T54.3X2	T54.3X3	T54.3X4	--	--
Potassic saline injection (lactated)	T50.3X1	T50.3X2	T50.3X3	T50.3X4	T50.3X5	T50.3X6
Potassium (salts) NEC	T50.3X1	T50.3X2	T50.3X3	T50.3X4	T50.3X5	T50.3X6
aminobenzoate	T45.8X1	T45.8X2	T45.8X3	T45.8X4	T45.8X5	T45.8X6
aminosalicylate	T37.1X1	T37.1X2	T37.1X3	T37.1X4	T37.1X5	T37.1X6
antimony ' tartrate'	T37.8X1	T37.8X2	T37.8X3	T37.8X4	T37.8X5	T37.8X6
arsenite (solution)	T57.0X1	T57.0X2	T57.0X3	T57.0X4	--	--
bichromate	T56.2X1	T56.2X2	T56.2X3	T56.2X4	--	--
bisulfate	T47.3X1	T47.3X2	T47.3X3	T47.3X4	T47.3X5	T47.3X6
bromide	T42.6X1	T42.6X2	T42.6X3	T42.6X4	T42.6X5	T42.6X6
canrenoate	T50.0X1	T50.0X2	T50.0X3	T50.0X4	T50.0X5	T50.0X6
carbonate	T54.3X1	T54.3X2	T54.3X3	T54.3X4	--	--
chlorate NEC	T65.891	T65.892	T65.893	T65.894	--	--
chloride	T50.3X1	T50.3X2	T50.3X3	T50.3X4	T50.3X5	T50.3X6
citrate	T50.991	T50.992	T50.993	T50.994	T50.995	T50.996
cyanide	T65.0X1	T65.0X2	T65.0X3	T65.0X4	--	--
ferric hexacyanoferrate (medicinal)	T50.6X1	T50.6X2	T50.6X3	T50.6X4	T50.6X5	T50.6X6
nonmedicinal	T65.891	T65.892	T65.893	T65.894	--	--
Fluoride	T57.8X1	T57.8X2	T57.8X3	T57.8X4	--	--
glucaldrate	T47.1X1	T47.1X2	T47.1X3	T47.1X4	T47.1X5	T47.1X6
hydroxide	T54.3X1	T54.3X2	T54.3X3	T54.3X4	--	--
iodate	T49.0X1	T49.0X2	T49.0X3	T49.0X4	T49.0X5	T49.0X6
iodide	T48.4X1	T48.4X2	T48.4X3	T48.4X4	T48.4X5	T48.4X6
nitrate	T57.8X1	T57.8X2	T57.8X3	T57.8X4	--	--
oxalate	T65.891	T65.892	T65.893	T65.894	--	--
perchlorate (nonmedicinal) NEC	T65.891	T65.892	T65.893	T65.894	--	--
antithyroid	T38.2X1	T38.2X2	T38.2X3	T38.2X4	T38.2X5	T38.2X6
medicinal	T38.2X1	T38.2X2	T38.2X3	T38.2X4	T38.2X5	T38.2X6
Permanganate (nonmedicinal)	T65.891	T65.892	T65.893	T65.894	--	--

Substance	Poisoning, Accidental (unintentional)	Poisoning, Intentional Self-harm	Poisoning, Assault	Poisoning, Undetermined	Adverse effect	Underdosing
medicinal	T49.0X1	T49.0X2	T49.0X3	T49.0X4	T49.0X5	T49.0X6
sulfate	T47.2X1	T47.2X2	T47.2X3	T47.2X4	T47.2X5	T47.2X6
Potassium-removing resin	T50.3X1	T50.3X2	T50.3X3	T50.3X4	T50.3X5	T50.3X6
Potassium-retaining drug	T50.3X1	T50.3X2	T50.3X3	T50.3X4	T50.3X5	T50.3X6
Povidone	T45.8X1	T45.8X2	T45.8X3	T45.8X4	T45.8X5	T45.8X6
iodine	T49.0X1	T49.0X2	T49.0X3	T49.0X4	T49.0X5	T49.0X6
Practolol	T44.7X1	T44.7X2	T44.7X3	T44.7X4	T44.7X5	T44.7X6
Prajmalium bitartrate	T46.2X1	T46.2X2	T46.2X3	T46.2X4	T46.2X5	T46.2X6
Pralidoxime (iodide)	T50.6X1	T50.6X2	T50.6X3	T50.6X4	T50.6X5	T50.6X6
chloride	T50.6X1	T50.6X2	T50.6X3	T50.6X4	T50.6X5	T50.6X6
Pramiverine	T44.3X1	T44.3X2	T44.3X3	T44.3X4	T44.3X5	T44.3X6
Pramocaine	T49.1X1	T49.1X2	T49.1X3	T49.1X4	T49.1X5	T49.1X6
Pramoxine	T49.1X1	T49.1X2	T49.1X3	T49.1X4	T49.1X5	T49.1X6
Prasterone	T38.7X1	T38.7X2	T38.7X3	T38.7X4	T38.7X5	T38.7X6
Pravastatin	T46.6X1	T46.6X2	T46.6X3	T46.6X4	T46.6X5	T46.6X6
Prazepam	T42.4X1	T42.4X2	T42.4X3	T42.4X4	T42.4X5	T42.4X6
Praziquantel	T37.4X1	T37.4X2	T37.4X3	T37.4X4	T37.4X5	T37.4X6
Prazitone	T43.291	T43.292	T43.293	T43.294	T43.295	T43.296
Prazosin	T44.6X1	T44.6X2	T44.6X3	T44.6X4	T44.6X5	T44.6X6
Prednicarbate	T49.0X1	T49.0X2	T49.0X3	T49.0X4	T49.0X5	T49.0X6
Prednimustine	T45.1X1	T45.1X2	T45.1X3	T45.1X4	T45.1X5	T45.1X6
Prednisolone	T38.0X1	T38.0X2	T38.0X3	T38.0X4	T38.0X5	T38.0X6
ENT agent	T49.6X1	T49.6X2	T49.6X3	T49.6X4	T49.6X5	T49.6X6
ophthalmic preparation	T49.5X1	T49.5X2	T49.5X3	T49.5X4	T49.5X5	T49.5X6
steaglate	T49.0X1	T49.0X2	T49.0X3	T49.0X4	T49.0X5	T49.0X6
topical NEC	T49.0X1	T49.0X2	T49.0X3	T49.0X4	T49.0X5	T49.0X6
Prednisone	T38.0X1	T38.0X2	T38.0X3	T38.0X4	T38.0X5	T38.0X6
Prednylidene	T38.0X1	T38.0X2	T38.0X3	T38.0X4	T38.0X5	T38.0X6
Pregnandiol	T38.5X1	T38.5X2	T38.5X3	T38.5X4	T38.5X5	T38.5X6
Pregneninolone	T38.5X1	T38.5X2	T38.5X3	T38.5X4	T38.5X5	T38.5X6
Preludin	T43.691	T43.692	T43.693	T43.694	T43.695	T43.696
Premarin	T38.5X1	T38.5X2	T38.5X3	T38.5X4	T38.5X5	T38.5X6
Premedication anesthetic	T41.201	T41.202	T41.203	T41.204	T41.205	T41.206
Prenalterol	T44.5X1	T44.5X2	T44.5X3	T44.5X4	T44.5X5	T44.5X6
Prenoxdiazine	T48.3X1	T48.3X2	T48.3X3	T48.3X4	T48.3X5	T48.3X6
Prenylamine	T46.3X1	T46.3X2	T46.3X3	T46.3X4	T46.3X5	T46.3X6
Preparation H	T49.8X1	T49.8X2	T49.8X3	T49.8X4	T49.8X5	T49.8X6
Preparation, local	T49.4X1	T49.4X2	T49.4X3	T49.4X4	T49.4X5	T49.4X6
Preservative (nonmedicinal)	T65.891	T65.892	T65.893	T65.894	--	--
medicinal	T50.901	T50.902	T50.903	T50.904	T50.905	T50.906
wood	T60.91	T60.92	T60.93	T60.94	--	--
Prethcamide	T50.7X1	T50.7X2	T50.7X3	T50.7X4	T50.7X5	T50.7X6
Pride of China	T62.2X1	T62.2X2	T62.2X3	T62.2X4	--	--
Pridinol	T44.3X1	T44.3X2	T44.3X3	T44.3X4	T44.3X5	T44.3X6
Prifinium bromide	T44.3X1	T44.3X2	T44.3X3	T44.3X4	T44.3X5	T44.3X6
Prilocaine	T41.3X1	T41.3X2	T41.3X3	T41.3X4	T41.3X5	T41.3X6
infiltration (subcutaneous)	T41.3X1	T41.3X2	T41.3X3	T41.3X4	T41.3X5	T41.3X6
nerve block peripheral (plexus)	T41.3X1	T41.3X2	T41.3X3	T41.3X4	T41.3X5	T41.3X6
regional	T41.3X1	T41.3X2	T41.3X3	T41.3X4	T41.3X5	T41.3X6
Primaquine	T37.2X1	T37.2X2	T37.2X3	T37.2X4	T37.2X5	T37.2X6
Primidone	T42.6X1	T42.6X2	T42.6X3	T42.6X4	T42.6X5	T42.6X6
Primula (veris)	T62.2X1	T62.2X2	T62.2X3	T62.2X4	--	--
Prinadol	T40.2X1	T40.2X2	T40.2X3	T40.2X4	T40.2X5	T40.2X6
Priscol, Priscoline	T44.6X1	T44.6X2	T44.6X3	T44.6X4	T44.6X5	T44.6X6
Pristinamycin	T36.3X1	T36.3X2	T36.3X3	T36.3X4	T36.3X5	T36.3X6
Privet	T62.2X1	T62.2X2	T62.2X3	T62.2X4	--	--
berries	T62.1X1	T62.1X2	T62.1X3	T62.1X4	--	--
Privine	T44.4X1	T44.4X2	T44.4X3	T44.4X4	T44.4X5	T44.4X6
Pro-Banthine	T44.3X1	T44.3X2	T44.3X3	T44.3X4	T44.3X5	T44.3X6
Probarbital	T42.3X1	T42.3X2	T42.3X3	T42.3X4	T42.3X5	T42.3X6
Probenecid	T50.4X1	T50.4X2	T50.4X3	T50.4X4	T50.4X5	T50.4X6
Probucol	T46.6X1	T46.6X2	T46.6X3	T46.6X4	T46.6X5	T46.6X6
Procainamide	T46.2X1	T46.2X2	T46.2X3	T46.2X4	T46.2X5	T46.2X6
Procaine	T41.3X1	T41.3X2	T41.3X3	T41.3X4	T41.3X5	T41.3X6

Substance	Poisoning, Accidental (unintentional)	Poisoning, Intentional Self-harm	Poisoning, Assault	Poisoning, Undetermined	Adverse effect	Underdosing
benzylpenicillin	T36.0X1	T36.0X2	T36.0X3	T36.0X4	T36.0X5	T36.0X6
nerve block (periphreal) (plexus)	T41.3X1	T41.3X2	T41.3X3	T41.3X4	T41.3X5	T41.3X6
penicillin G	T36.0X1	T36.0X2	T36.0X3	T36.0X4	T36.0X5	T36.0X6
regional	T41.3X1	T41.3X2	T41.3X3	T41.3X4	T41.3X5	T41.3X6
spinal	T41.3X1	T41.3X2	T41.3X3	T41.3X4	T41.3X5	T41.3X6
Procalmidol	T43.591	T43.592	T43.593	T43.594	T43.595	T43.596
Procarbazine	T45.1X1	T45.1X2	T45.1X3	T45.1X4	T45.1X5	T45.1X6
Procaterol	T44.5X1	T44.5X2	T44.5X3	T44.5X4	T44.5X5	T44.5X6
Prochlorperazine	T43.3X1	T43.3X2	T43.3X3	T43.3X4	T43.3X5	T43.3X6
Procyclidine	T44.3X1	T44.3X2	T44.3X3	T44.3X4	T44.3X5	T44.3X6
Producer gas	T58.8X1	T58.8X2	T58.8X3	T58.8X4	--	--
Profadol	T40.4X1	T40.4X2	T40.4X3	T40.4X4	T40.4X5	T40.4X6
Profenamine	T44.3X1	T44.3X2	T44.3X3	T44.3X4	T44.3X5	T44.3X6
Profenil	T44.3X1	T44.3X2	T44.3X3	T44.3X4	T44.3X5	T44.3X6
Proflavine	T49.0X1	T49.0X2	T49.0X3	T49.0X4	T49.0X5	T49.0X6
Progabide	T42.6X1	T42.6X2	T42.6X3	T42.6X4	T42.6X5	T42.6X6
Progesterone	T38.5X1	T38.5X2	T38.5X3	T38.5X4	T38.5X5	T38.5X6
Progestin	T38.5X1	T38.5X2	T38.5X3	T38.5X4	T38.5X5	T38.5X6
oral contraceptive	T38.4X1	T38.4X2	T38.4X3	T38.4X4	T38.4X5	T38.4X6
Progestogen NEC	T38.5X1	T38.5X2	T38.5X3	T38.5X4	T38.5X5	T38.5X6
Progestone	T38.5X1	T38.5X2	T38.5X3	T38.5X4	T38.5X5	T38.5X6
Proglumide	T47.1X1	T47.1X2	T47.1X3	T47.1X4	T47.1X5	T47.1X6
Proguanil	T37.2X1	T37.2X2	T37.2X3	T37.2X4	T37.2X5	T37.2X6
Prolactin	T38.811	T38.812	T38.813	T38.814	T38.815	T38.816
Prolintane	T43.691	T43.692	T43.693	T43.694	T43.695	T43.696
Proloid	T38.1X1	T38.1X2	T38.1X3	T38.1X4	T38.1X5	T38.1X6
Proluton	T38.5X1	T38.5X2	T38.5X3	T38.5X4	T38.5X5	T38.5X6
Promacetin	T37.1X1	T37.1X2	T37.1X3	T37.1X4	T37.1X5	T37.1X6
Promazine	T43.3X1	T43.3X2	T43.3X3	T43.3X4	T43.3X5	T43.3X6
Promedol	T40.2X1	T40.2X2	T40.2X3	T40.2X4	--	--
Promegestone	T38.5X1	T38.5X2	T38.5X3	T38.5X4	T38.5X5	T38.5X6
Promethazine (teoclate)	T43.3X1	T43.3X2	T43.3X3	T43.3X4	T43.3X5	T43.3X6
Promin	T37.1X1	T37.1X2	T37.1X3	T37.1X4	T37.1X5	T37.1X6
Pronase	T45.3X1	T45.3X2	T45.3X3	T45.3X4	T45.3X5	T45.3X6
Pronestyl (hydrochloride)	T46.2X1	T46.2X2	T46.2X3	T46.2X4	T46.2X5	T46.2X6
Pronetalol	T44.7X1	T44.7X2	T44.7X3	T44.7X4	T44.7X5	T44.7X6
Prontosil	T37.0X1	T37.0X2	T37.0X3	T37.0X4	T37.0X5	T37.0X6
Propachlor	T60.3X1	T60.3X2	T60.3X3	T60.3X4	--	--
Propafenone	T46.2X1	T46.2X2	T46.2X3	T46.2X4	T46.2X5	T46.2X6
Propallylonal	T42.3X1	T42.3X2	T42.3X3	T42.3X4	T42.3X5	T42.3X6
Propamidine	T49.0X1	T49.0X2	T49.0X3	T49.0X4	T49.0X5	T49.0X6
Propane (distributed in mobile container)	T59.891	T59.892	T59.893	T59.894	--	--
distributed through pipes	T59.891	T59.892	T59.893	T59.894	--	--
incomplete combustion	T58.11	T58.12	T58.13	T58.14	--	--
Propanidid	T41.291	T41.292	T41.293	T41.294	T41.295	T41.296
Propanil	T60.3X1	T60.3X2	T60.3X3	T60.3X4	--	--
1-Propanol	T51.3X1	T51.3X2	T51.3X3	T51.3X4	--	--
2-Propanol	T51.2X1	T51.2X2	T51.2X3	T51.2X4	--	--
Propantheline	T44.3X1	T44.3X2	T44.3X3	T44.3X4	T44.3X5	T44.3X6
bromide	T44.3X1	T44.3X2	T44.3X3	T44.3X4	T44.3X5	T44.3X6
Proparacaine	T41.3X1	T41.3X2	T41.3X3	T41.3X4	T41.3X5	T41.3X6
Propatylnitrate	T46.3X1	T46.3X2	T46.3X3	T46.3X4	T46.3X5	T46.3X6
Propicillin	T36.0X1	T36.0X2	T36.0X3	T36.0X4	T36.0X5	T36.0X6
Propiolactone	T49.0X1	T49.0X2	T49.0X3	T49.0X4	T49.0X5	T49.0X6
Propiomazine	T45.0X1	T45.0X2	T45.0X3	T45.0X4	T45.0X5	T45.0X6
Propionaldehyde (medicinal)	T42.6X1	T42.6X2	T42.6X3	T42.6X4	T42.6X5	T42.6X6
Propionate (calcium) (sodium)	T49.0X1	T49.0X2	T49.0X3	T49.0X4	T49.0X5	T49.0X6
Propion gel	T49.0X1	T49.0X2	T49.0X3	T49.0X4	T49.0X5	T49.0X6
Propitocaine	T41.3X1	T41.3X2	T41.3X3	T41.3X4	T41.3X5	T41.3X6
infiltration (subcutaneous)	T41.3X1	T41.3X2	T41.3X3	T41.3X4	T41.3X5	T41.3X6
nerve block (peripheral) (plexus)	T41.3X1	T41.3X2	T41.3X3	T41.3X4	T41.3X5	T41.3X6
Propofol	T41.291	T41.292	T41.293	T41.294	T41.295	T41.296
Propoxur	T60.0X1	T60.0X2	T60.0X3	T60.0X4	--	--
Propoxycaine	T41.3X1	T41.3X2	T41.3X3	T41.3X4	T41.3X5	T41.3X6
infiltration (subcutaneous)	T41.3X1	T41.3X2	T41.3X3	T41.3X4	T41.3X5	T41.3X6

Substance	Poisoning, Accidental (unintentional)	Poisoning, Intentional Self-harm	Poisoning, Assault	Poisoning, Undetermined	Adverse effect	Underdosing
nerve block (peripheral) (plexus)	T41.3X1	T41.3X2	T41.3X3	T41.3X4	T41.3X5	T41.3X6
topical (surface)	T41.3X1	T41.3X2	T41.3X3	T41.3X4	T41.3X5	T41.3X6
Propoxyphene	T40.4X1	T40.4X2	T40.4X3	T40.4X4	T40.4X5	T40.4X6
Propranolol	T44.7X1	T44.7X2	T44.7X3	T44.7X4	T44.7X5	T44.7X6
Propyl						
alcohol	T51.3X1	T51.3X2	T51.3X3	T51.3X4	--	--
carbinol	T51.3X1	T51.3X2	T51.3X3	T51.3X4	--	--
hexadrine	T44.4X1	T44.4X2	T44.4X3	T44.4X4	T44.4X5	T44.4X6
iodone	T50.8X1	T50.8X2	T50.8X3	T50.8X4	T50.8X5	T50.8X6
thiouracil	T38.2X1	T38.2X2	T38.2X3	T38.2X4	T38.2X5	T38.2X6
Propylaminopheno-thiazine	T43.3X1	T43.3X2	T43.3X3	T43.3X4	T43.3X5	T43.3X6
Propylene	T59.891	T59.892	T59.893	T59.894	--	--
Propylhexedrine	T48.5X1	T48.5X2	T48.5X3	T48.5X4	T48.5X5	T48.5X6
Propyliodone	T50.8X1	T50.8X2	T50.8X3	T50.8X4	T50.8X5	T50.8X6
Propylparaben (ophthalmic)	T49.5X1	T49.5X2	T49.5X3	T49.5X4	T49.5X5	T49.5X6
Propylthiouracil	T38.2X1	T38.2X2	T38.2X3	T38.2X4	T38.2X5	T38.2X6
Propyphenazone	T39.2X1	T39.2X2	T39.2X3	T39.2X4	T39.2X5	T39.2X6
Proquazone	T39.391	T39.392	T39.393	T39.394	T39.395	T39.396
Proscillaridin	T46.0X1	T46.0X2	T46.0X3	T46.0X4	T46.0X5	T46.0X6
Prostacyclin	T45.521	T45.522	T45.523	T45.524	T45.525	T45.526
Prostaglandin (I2)	T45.521	T45.522	T45.523	T45.524	T45.525	T45.526
E1	T46.7X1	T46.7X2	T46.7X3	T46.7X4	T46.7X5	T46.7X6
E2	T48.0X1	T48.0X2	T48.0X3	T48.0X4	T48.0X5	T48.0X6
F2 alpha	T48.0X1	T48.0X2	T48.0X3	T48.0X4	T48.0X5	T48.0X6
Prostigmin	T44.0X1	T44.0X2	T44.0X3	T44.0X4	T44.0X5	T44.0X6
Prosultiamine	T45.2X1	T45.2X2	T45.2X3	T45.2X4	T45.2X5	T45.2X6
Protamine sulfate	T45.7X1	T45.7X2	T45.7X3	T45.7X4	T45.7X5	T45.7X6
zinc insulin	T38.3X1	T38.3X2	T38.3X3	T38.3X4	T38.3X5	T38.3X6
Protease	T47.5X1	T47.5X2	T47.5X3	T47.5X4	T47.5X5	T47.5X6
Protectant, skin NEC	T49.3X1	T49.3X2	T49.3X3	T49.3X4	T49.3X5	T49.3X6
Protein hydrolysate	T50.991	T50.992	T50.993	T50.994	T50.995	T50.996
Prothiaden—see Dothiepin hydrochloride						
Prothionamide	T37.1X1	T37.1X2	T37.1X3	T37.1X4	T37.1X5	T37.1X6
Prothipendyl	T43.591	T43.592	T43.593	T43.594	T43.595	T43.596
Prothoate	T60.0X1	T60.0X2	T60.0X3	T60.0X4	--	--
Prothrombin						
activator	T45.7X1	T45.7X2	T45.7X3	T45.7X4	T45.7X5	T45.7X6
synthesis inhibitor	T45.511	T45.512	T45.513	T45.514	T45.515	T45.516
Protionamide	T37.1X1	T37.1X2	T37.1X3	T37.1X4	T37.1X5	T37.1X6
Protirelin	T38.891	T38.892	T38.893	T38.894	T38.895	T38.896
Protokylol	T48.6X1	T48.6X2	T48.6X3	T48.6X4	T48.6X5	T48.6X6
Protopam	T50.6X1	T50.6X2	T50.6X3	T50.6X4	T50.6X5	T50.6X6
Protoveratrine (s) (A) (B)	T46.5X1	T46.5X2	T46.5X3	T46.5X4	T46.5X5	T46.5X6
Protriptyline	T43.011	T43.012	T43.013	T43.014	T43.015	T43.016
Provera	T38.5X1	T38.5X2	T38.5X3	T38.5X4	T38.5X5	T38.5X6
Provitamin A	T45.2X1	T45.2X2	T45.2X3	T45.2X4	T45.2X5	T45.2X6
Proxibarbal	T42.3X1	T42.3X2	T42.3X3	T42.3X4	T42.3X5	T42.3X6
Proxymetacaine	T41.3X1	T41.3X2	T41.3X3	T41.3X4	T41.3X5	T41.3X6
Proxyphylline	T48.6X1	T48.6X2	T48.6X3	T48.6X4	T48.6X5	T48.6X6
Prozac—see Fluoxetine hydrochloride						
Prunus						
laurocerasus	T62.2X1	T62.2X2	T62.2X3	T62.2X4	--	--
virginiana	T62.2X1	T62.2X2	T62.2X3	T62.2X4	--	--
Prussian blue						
commercial	T65.891	T65.892	T65.893	T65.894	--	--
therapeutic	T50.6X1	T50.6X2	T50.6X3	T50.6X4	T50.6X5	T50.6X6
Prussic acid	T65.0X1	T65.0X2	T65.0X3	T65.0X4	--	--
vapor	T57.3X1	T57.3X2	T57.3X3	T57.3X4	--	--
Pseudoephedrine	T44.991	T44.992	T44.993	T44.994	T44.995	T44.996
Psilocin	T40.991	T40.992	T40.993	T40.994	--	--
Psilocybin	T40.991	T40.992	T40.993	T40.994	--	--
Psilocybine	T40.991	T40.992	T40.993	T40.994	--	--
Psoralene (nonmedicinal)	T65.891	T65.892	T65.893	T65.894	--	--
Psoralens (medicinal)	T50.991	T50.992	T50.993	T50.994	T50.995	T50.996

Substance	Poisoning, Accidental (unintentional)	Poisoning, Intentional Self-harm	Poisoning, Assault	Poisoning, Undetermined	Adverse effect	Underdosing
PSP (phenolsulfonphthalein)	T50.8X1	T50.8X2	T50.8X3	T50.8X4	T50.8X5	T50.8X6
Psychodysleptic drug NEC	T40.901	T40.902	T40.903	T40.904	T40.905	T40.906
Psychostimulant	T43.601	T43.602	T43.603	T43.604	T43.605	T43.606
amphetamine	T43.621	T43.622	T43.623	T43.624	T43.625	T43.626
caffeine	T43.611	T43.612	T43.613	T43.614	T43.615	T43.616
methylphenidate	T43.631	T43.632	T43.633	T43.634	T43.635	T43.636
specified NEC	T43.691	T43.692	T43.693	T43.694	T43.695	T43.696
Psychotherapeutic drug NEC	T43.91	T43.92	T43.93	T43.94	T43.95	T43.96
antidepressants—see also Antidepressant	T43.201	T43.202	T43.203	T43.204	T43.205	T43.206
specified NEC	T43.8X1	T43.8X2	T43.8X3	T43.8X4	T43.8X5	T43.8X6
tranquilizers NEC	T43.501	T43.502	T43.503	T43.504	T43.505	T43.506
Psychotomimetic agents	T40.901	T40.902	T40.903	T40.904	T40.905	T40.906
Psychotropic drug NEC	T43.91	T43.92	T43.93	T43.94	T43.95	T43.96
specified NEC	T43.8X1	T43.8X2	T43.8X3	T43.8X4	T43.8X5	T43.8X6
Psyllium hydrophilic mucilloid	T47.4X1	T47.4X2	T47.4X3	T47.4X4	T47.4X5	T47.4X6
Pteroylglutamic acid	T45.8X1	T45.8X2	T45.8X3	T45.8X4	T45.8X5	T45.8X6
Pteroyltriglutamate	T45.1X1	T45.1X2	T45.1X3	T45.1X4	T45.1X5	T45.1X6
PTFE—see Polytetrafluoroethylene						
Pulp						
devitalizing paste	T49.7X1	T49.7X2	T49.7X3	T49.7X4	T49.7X5	T49.7X6
dressing	T49.7X1	T49.7X2	T49.7X3	T49.7X4	T49.7X5	T49.7X6
Pulsatilla	T62.2X1	T62.2X2	T62.2X3	T62.2X4	--	--
Pumpkin seed extract	T37.4X1	T37.4X2	T37.4X3	T37.4X4	T37.4X5	T37.4X6
Purex (bleach)	T54.91	T54.92	T54.93	T54.94	--	--
Purgative NEC—see also Cathartic	T47.4X1	T47.4X2	T47.4X3	T47.4X4	T47.4X5	T47.4X6
Purine analogue (antineoplastic)	T45.1X1	T45.1X2	T45.1X3	T45.1X4	T45.1X5	T45.1X6
Purine diuretics	T50.2X1	T50.2X2	T50.2X3	T50.2X4	T50.2X5	T50.2X6
Purinethol	T45.1X1	T45.1X2	T45.1X3	T45.1X4	T45.1X5	T45.1X6
PVP	T45.8X1	T45.8X2	T45.8X3	T45.8X4	T45.8X5	T45.8X6
Pyrabital	T39.8X1	T39.8X2	T39.8X3	T39.8X4	T39.8X5	T39.8X6
Pyramidon	T39.2X1	T39.2X2	T39.2X3	T39.2X4	T39.2X5	T39.2X6
Pyrantel	T37.4X1	T37.4X2	T37.4X3	T37.4X4	T37.4X5	T37.4X6
Pyrathiazine	T45.0X1	T45.0X2	T45.0X3	T45.0X4	T45.0X5	T45.0X6
Pyrazinamide	T37.1X1	T37.1X2	T37.1X3	T37.1X4	T37.1X5	T37.1X6
Pyrazinoic acid (amide)	T37.1X1	T37.1X2	T37.1X3	T37.1X4	T37.1X5	T37.1X6
Pyrazole (derivatives)	T39.2X1	T39.2X2	T39.2X3	T39.2X4	T39.2X5	T39.2X6
Pyrazolone analgesic NEC	T39.2X1	T39.2X2	T39.2X3	T39.2X4	T39.2X5	T39.2X6
Pyrethrin, pyrethrum (nonmedicinal)	T60.2X1	T60.2X2	T60.2X3	T60.2X4	--	--
Pyrethrum extract	T49.0X1	T49.0X2	T49.0X3	T49.0X4	T49.0X5	T49.0X6
Pyribenzamine	T45.0X1	T45.0X2	T45.0X3	T45.0X4	T45.0X5	T45.0X6
Pyridine	T52.8X1	T52.8X2	T52.8X3	T52.8X4	--	--
aldoxime methiodide	T50.6X1	T50.6X2	T50.6X3	T50.6X4	T50.6X5	T50.6X6
aldoxime methyl chloride	T50.6X1	T50.6X2	T50.6X3	T50.6X4	T50.6X5	T50.6X6
vapor	T59.891	T59.892	T59.893	T59.894	--	--
Pyridium	T39.8X1	T39.8X2	T39.8X3	T39.8X4	T39.8X5	T39.8X6
Pyridostigmine bromide	T44.0X1	T44.0X2	T44.0X3	T44.0X4	T44.0X5	T44.0X6
Pyridoxal phosphate	T45.2X1	T45.2X2	T45.2X3	T45.2X4	T45.2X5	T45.2X6
Pyridoxine	T45.2X1	T45.2X2	T45.2X3	T45.2X4	T45.2X5	T45.2X6
Pyrilamine	T45.0X1	T45.0X2	T45.0X3	T45.0X4	T45.0X5	T45.0X6
Pyrimethamine	T37.2X1	T37.2X2	T37.2X3	T37.2X4	T37.2X5	T37.2X6
with sulfadoxine	T37.2X1	T37.2X2	T37.2X3	T37.2X4	T37.2X5	T37.2X6
Pyrimidine antagonist	T45.1X1	T45.1X2	T45.1X3	T45.1X4	T45.1X5	T45.1X6
Pyriminil	T60.4X1	T60.4X2	T60.4X3	T60.4X4	--	--
Pyrithione zinc	T49.4X1	T49.4X2	T49.4X3	T49.4X4	T49.4X5	T49.4X6
Pyrithyldione	T42.6X1	T42.6X2	T42.6X3	T42.6X4	T42.6X5	T42.6X6
Pyrogallic acid	T49.0X1	T49.0X2	T49.0X3	T49.0X4	T49.0X5	T49.0X6
Pyrogallol	T49.0X1	T49.0X2	T49.0X3	T49.0X4	T49.0X5	T49.0X6
Pyroxylin	T49.3X1	T49.3X2	T49.3X3	T49.3X4	T49.3X5	T49.3X6
Pyrrobutamine	T45.0X1	T45.0X2	T45.0X3	T45.0X4	T45.0X5	T45.0X6
Pyrrolizidine alkaloids	T62.8X1	T62.8X2	T62.8X3	T62.8X4	--	--
Pyrvinium chloride	T37.4X1	T37.4X2	T37.4X3	T37.4X4	T37.4X5	T37.4X6
PZI	T38.3X1	T38.3X2	T38.3X3	T38.3X4	T38.3X5	T38.3X6
Quaalude	T42.6X1	T42.6X2	T42.6X3	T42.6X4	T42.6X5	T42.6X6
Quarternary ammonium						
anti-infective	T49.0X1	T49.0X2	T49.0X3	T49.0X4	T49.0X5	T49.0X6

Substance	Poisoning, Accidental (unintentional)	Poisoning, Intentional Self-harm	Poisoning, Assault	Poisoning, Undetermined	Adverse effect	Underdosing
ganglion blocking	T44.2X1	T44.2X2	T44.2X3	T44.2X4	T44.2X5	T44.2X6
parasympatholytic	T44.3X1	T44.3X2	T44.3X3	T44.3X4	T44.3X5	T44.3X6
Quazepam	T42.4X1	T42.4X2	T42.4X3	T42.4X4	T42.4X5	T42.4X6
Quicklime	T54.3X1	T54.3X2	T54.3X3	T54.3X4	--	--
Quillaja extract	T48.4X1	T48.4X2	T48.4X3	T48.4X4	T48.4X5	T48.4X6
Quinacrine	T37.2X1	T37.2X2	T37.2X3	T37.2X4	T37.2X5	T37.2X6
Quinaglute	T46.2X1	T46.2X2	T46.2X3	T46.2X4	T46.2X5	T46.2X6
Quinalbarbital	T42.3X1	T42.3X2	T42.3X3	T42.3X4	T42.3X5	T42.3X6
Quinalbarbitone sodium	T42.3X1	T42.3X2	T42.3X3	T42.3X4	T42.3X5	T42.3X6
Quinalphos	T60.0X1	T60.0X2	T60.0X3	T60.0X4	--	--
Quinapril	T46.4X1	T46.4X2	T46.4X3	T46.4X4	T46.4X5	T46.4X6
Quinestradiol	T38.5X1	T38.5X2	T38.5X3	T38.5X4	T38.5X5	T38.5X6
Quinestradol	T38.5X1	T38.5X2	T38.5X3	T38.5X4	T38.5X5	T38.5X6
Quinestrol	T38.5X1	T38.5X2	T38.5X3	T38.5X4	T38.5X5	T38.5X6
Quinethazone	T50.2X1	T50.2X2	T50.2X3	T50.2X4	T50.2X5	T50.2X6
Quingestanol	T38.4X1	T38.4X2	T38.4X3	T38.4X4	T38.4X5	T38.4X6
Quinidine	T46.2X1	T46.2X2	T46.2X3	T46.2X4	T46.2X5	T46.2X6
Quinine	T37.2X1	T37.2X2	T37.2X3	T37.2X4	T37.2X5	T37.2X6
Quiniobine	T37.8X1	T37.8X2	T37.8X3	T37.8X4	T37.8X5	T37.8X6
Quinisocaine	T49.1X1	T49.1X2	T49.1X3	T49.1X4	T49.1X5	T49.1X6
Quinocide	T37.2X1	T37.2X2	T37.2X3	T37.2X4	T37.2X5	T37.2X6
Quinoline (derivatives) NEC	T37.8X1	T37.8X2	T37.8X3	T37.8X4	T37.8X5	T37.8X6
Quinupramine	T43.011	T43.012	T43.013	T43.014	T43.015	T43.016
Quotane	T41.3X1	T41.3X2	T41.3X3	T41.3X4	T41.3X5	T41.3X6
Rabies						
immune globulin (human)	T50.Z11	T50.Z12	T50.Z13	T50.Z14	T50.Z15	T50.Z16
vaccine	T50.B91	T50.B92	T50.B93	T50.B94	T50.B95	T50.B96
Racemoramide	T40.2X1	T40.2X2	T40.2X3	T40.2X4	--	--
Racemorphan	T40.2X1	T40.2X2	T40.2X3	T40.2X4	T40.2X5	T40.2X6
Racepinefrin	T44.5X1	T44.5X2	T44.5X3	T44.5X4	T44.5X5	T44.5X6
Raclopride	T43.591	T43.592	T43.593	T43.594	T43.595	T43.596
Radiator alcohol	T51.1X1	T51.1X2	T51.1X3	T51.1X4	--	--
Radioactive drug NEC	T50.8X1	T50.8X2	T50.8X3	T50.8X4	T50.8X5	T50.8X6
Radio-opaque (drugs) (materials)	T50.8X1	T50.8X2	T50.8X3	T50.8X4	T50.8X5	T50.8X6
Ramifenazone	T39.2X1	T39.2X2	T39.2X3	T39.2X4	T39.2X5	T39.2X6
Ramipril	T46.4X1	T46.4X2	T46.4X3	T46.4X4	T46.4X5	T46.4X6
Ranitidine	T47.0X1	T47.0X2	T47.0X3	T47.0X4	T47.0X5	T47.0X6
Ranunculus	T62.2X1	T62.2X2	T62.2X3	T62.2X4	--	--
Rat poison NEC	T60.4X1	T60.4X2	T60.4X3	T60.4X4	--	--
Rattlesnake (venom)	T63.011		T63.013	T63.014	--	--
Raubasine	T46.7X1	T46.7X2	T46.7X3	T46.7X4	T46.7X5	T46.7X6
Raudixin	T46.5X1	T46.5X2	T46.5X3	T46.5X4	T46.5X5	T46.5X6
Rautensin	T46.5X1	T46.5X2	T46.5X3	T46.5X4	T46.5X5	T46.5X6
Rautina	T46.5X1	T46.5X2	T46.5X3	T46.5X4	T46.5X5	T46.5X6
Rautotal	T46.5X1	T46.5X2	T46.5X3	T46.5X4	T46.5X5	T46.5X6
Rauwiloid	T46.5X1	T46.5X2	T46.5X3	T46.5X4	T46.5X5	T46.5X6
Rauwoldin	T46.5X1	T46.5X2	T46.5X3	T46.5X4	T46.5X5	T46.5X6
Rauwolfia (alkaloids)	T46.5X1	T46.5X2	T46.5X3	T46.5X4	T46.5X5	T46.5X6
Razoxane	T45.1X1	T45.1X2	T45.1X3	T45.1X4	T45.1X5	T45.1X6
Realgar	T57.0X1	T57.0X2	T57.0X3	T57.0X4	--	--
Recombinant (R) —see specific protein						
Red blood cells, packed	T45.8X1	T45.8X2	T45.8X3	T45.8X4	T45.8X5	T45.8X6
Red squill (scilliroside)	T60.4X1	T60.4X2	T60.4X3	T60.4X4	--	--
Reducing agent, industrial NEC	T65.891	T65.892	T65.893	T65.894	--	--
Refrigerant gas (chlorofluoro-carbon)	T53.5X1	T53.5X2	T53.5X3	T53.5X4	--	--
not chlorofluoro-carbon	T59.891	T59.892	T59.893	T59.894	--	--
Regroton	T50.2X1	T50.2X2	T50.2X3	T50.2X4	T50.2X5	T50.2X6
Rehydration salts (oral)	T50.3X1	T50.3X2	T50.3X3	T50.3X4	T50.3X5	T50.3X6
Rela	T42.8X1	T42.8X2	T42.8X3	T42.8X4	T42.8X5	T42.8X6
Relaxant, muscle						
anesthetic	T48.1X1	T48.1X2	T48.1X3	T48.1X4	T48.1X5	T48.1X6
central nervous system	T42.8X1	T42.8X2	T42.8X3	T42.8X4	T42.8X5	T42.8X6
skeletal NEC	T48.1X1	T48.1X2	T48.1X3	T48.1X4	T48.1X5	T48.1X6
smooth NEC	T44.3X1	T44.3X2	T44.3X3	T44.3X4	T44.3X5	T44.3X6

Substance	Poisoning, Accidental (unintentional)	Poisoning, Intentional Self-harm	Poisoning, Assault	Poisoning, Undetermined	Adverse effect	Underdosing
Remoxipride	T43.591	T43.592	T43.593	T43.594	T43.595	T43.596
Renese	T50.2X1	T50.2X2	T50.2X3	T50.2X4	T50.2X5	T50.2X6
Renografin	T50.8X1	T50.8X2	T50.8X3	T50.8X4	T50.8X5	T50.8X6
Replacement solution	T50.3X1	T50.3X2	T50.3X3	T50.3X4	T50.3X5	T50.3X6
Reproterol	T48.6X1	T48.6X2	T48.6X3	T48.6X4	T48.6X5	T48.6X6
Rescinnamine	T46.5X1	T46.5X2	T46.5X3	T46.5X4	T46.5X5	T46.5X6
Reserpin (e)	T46.5X1	T46.5X2	T46.5X3	T46.5X4	T46.5X5	T46.5X6
Resorcin, resorcinol (nonmedicinal)	T65.891	T65.892	T65.893	T65.894	--	--
medicinal	T49.4X1	T49.4X2	T49.4X3	T49.4X4	T49.4X5	T49.4X6
Respaire	T48.4X1	T48.4X2	T48.4X3	T48.4X4	T48.4X5	T48.4X6
Respiratory drug NEC	T48.901	T48.902	T48.903	T48.904	T48.905	T48.906
antiasthmatic NEC	T48.6X1	T48.6X2	T48.6X3	T48.6X4	T48.6X5	T48.6X6
anti-common-cold NEC	T48.5X1	T48.5X2	T48.5X3	T48.5X4	T48.5X5	T48.5X6
expectorant NEC	T48.4X1	T48.4X2	T48.4X3	T48.4X4	T48.4X5	T48.4X6
stimulant	T48.901	T48.902	T48.903	T48.904	T48.905	T48.906
Retinoic acid	T49.0X1	T49.0X2	T49.0X3	T49.0X4	T49.0X5	T49.0X6
Retinol	T45.2X1	T45.2X2	T45.2X3	T45.2X4	T45.2X5	T45.2X6
Rh (D) immune globulin (human)	T50.Z11	T50.Z12	T50.Z13	T50.Z14	T50.Z15	T50.Z16
Rhodine	T39.011	T39.012	T39.013	T39.014	T39.015	T39.016
RhoGAM	T50.Z11	T50.Z12	T50.Z13	T50.Z14	T50.Z15	T50.Z16
Rhubarb						
dry extract	T47.2X1	T47.2X2	T47.2X3	T47.2X4	T47.2X5	T47.2X6
tincture, compound	T47.2X1	T47.2X2	T47.2X3	T47.2X4	T47.2X5	T47.2X6
Ribavirin	T37.5X1	T37.5X2	T37.5X3	T37.5X4	T37.5X5	T37.5X6
Riboflavin	T45.2X1	T45.2X2	T45.2X3	T45.2X4	T45.2X5	T45.2X6
Ribostamycin	T36.5X1	T36.5X2	T36.5X3	T36.5X4	T36.5X5	T36.5X6
Ricin	T62.2X1	T62.2X2	T62.2X3	T62.2X4	--	--
Ricinus communis	T62.2X1	T62.2X2	T62.2X3	T62.2X4	--	--
Rickettsial vaccine NEC	T50.A91	T50.A92	T50.A93	T50.A94	T50.A95	T50.A96
Rifabutin	T36.6X1	T36.6X2	T36.6X3	T36.6X4	T36.6X5	T36.6X6
Rifamide	T36.6X1	T36.6X2	T36.6X3	T36.6X4	T36.6X5	T36.6X6
Rifampicin	T36.6X1	T36.6X2	T36.6X3	T36.6X4	T36.6X5	T36.6X6
with isoniazid	T37.1X1	T37.1X2	T37.1X3	T37.1X4	T37.1X5	T37.1X6
Rifampin	T36.6X1	T36.6X2	T36.6X3	T36.6X4	T36.6X5	T36.6X6
Rifamycin	T36.6X1	T36.6X2	T36.6X3	T36.6X4	T36.6X5	T36.6X6
Rifaximin	T36.6X1	T36.6X2	T36.6X3	T36.6X4	T36.6X5	T36.6X6
Rimantadine	T37.5X1	T37.5X2	T37.5X3	T37.5X4	T37.5X5	T37.5X6
Rimazolium metilsulfate	T39.8X1	T39.8X2	T39.8X3	T39.8X4	T39.8X5	T39.8X6
Rimifon	T37.1X1	T37.1X2	T37.1X3	T37.1X4	T37.1X5	T37.1X6
Rimiterol	T48.6X1	T48.6X2	T48.6X3	T48.6X4	T48.6X5	T48.6X6
Ringer (lactate) solution	T50.3X1	T50.3X2	T50.3X3	T50.3X4	T50.3X5	T50.3X6
Ristocetin	T36.8X1	T36.8X2	T36.8X3	T36.8X4	T36.8X5	T36.8X6
Ritalin	T43.631	T43.632	T43.633	T43.634	T43.635	T43.636
Ritodrine	T44.5X1	T44.5X2	T44.5X3	T44.5X4	T44.5X5	T44.5X6
Roach killer—see Insecticide						
Rociverine	T44.3X1	T44.3X2	T44.3X3	T44.3X4	T44.3X5	T44.3X6
Rocky Mountain spotted fever vaccine	T50.A91	T50.A92	T50.A93	T50.A94	T50.A95	T50.A96
Rodenticide NEC	T60.4X1	T60.4X2	T60.4X3	T60.4X4	--	--
Rohypnol	T42.4X1	T42.4X2	T42.4X3	T42.4X4	T42.4X5	T42.4X6
Rokitamycin	T36.3X1	T36.3X2	T36.3X3	T36.3X4	T36.3X5	T36.3X6
Rolaids	T47.1X1	T47.1X2	T47.1X3	T47.1X4	T47.1X5	T47.1X6
Rolitetracycline	T36.4X1	T36.4X2	T36.4X3	T36.4X4	T36.4X5	T36.4X6
Romilar	T48.3X1	T48.3X2	T48.3X3	T48.3X4	T48.3X5	T48.3X6
Ronifibrate	T46.6X1	T46.6X2	T46.6X3	T46.6X4	T46.6X5	T46.6X6
Rosaprostol	T47.1X1	T47.1X2	T47.1X3	T47.1X4	T47.1X5	T47.1X6
Rose bengal sodium (131I)	T50.8X1	T50.8X2	T50.8X3	T50.8X4	T50.8X5	T50.8X6
Rose water ointment	T49.3X1	T49.3X2	T49.3X3	T49.3X4	T49.3X5	T49.3X6
Rosoxacin	T37.8X1	T37.8X2	T37.8X3	T37.8X4	T37.8X5	T37.8X6
Rotenone	T60.2X1	T60.2X2	T60.2X3	T60.2X4	--	--
Rotoxamine	T45.0X1	T45.0X2	T45.0X3	T45.0X4	T45.0X5	T45.0X6
Rough-on-rats	T60.4X1	T60.4X2	T60.4X3	T60.4X4	--	--
Roxatidine	T47.0X1	T47.0X2	T47.0X3	T47.0X4	T47.0X5	T47.0X6
Roxithromycin	T36.3X1	T36.3X2	T36.3X3	T36.3X4	T36.3X5	T36.3X6
Rt-PA	T45.611	T45.612	T45.613	T45.614	T45.615	T45.616
Rubbing alcohol	T51.2X1	T51.2X2	T51.2X3	T51.2X4	--	--

Substance	Poisoning, Accidental (unintentional)	Poisoning, Intentional Self-harm	Poisoning, Assault	Poisoning, Undetermined	Adverse effect	Underdosing
Rubefacient	T49.4X1	T49.4X2	T49.4X3	T49.4X4	T49.4X5	T49.4X6
Rubella vaccine	T50.B91	T50.B92	T50.B93	T50.B94	T50.B95	T50.B96
Rubeola vaccine	T50.B91	T50.B92	T50.B93	T50.B94	T50.B95	T50.B96
Rubidium chloride Rb82	T50.8X1	T50.8X2	T50.8X3	T50.8X4	T50.8X5	T50.8X6
Rubidomycin	T45.1X1	T45.1X2	T45.1X3	T45.1X4	T45.1X5	T45.1X6
Rue	T62.2X1	T62.2X2	T62.2X3	T62.2X4	--	--
Rufocromomycin	T45.1X1	T45.1X2	T45.1X3	T45.1X4	T45.1X5	T45.1X6
Russel's viper venin	T45.7X1	T45.7X2	T45.7X3	T45.7X4	T45.7X5	T45.7X6
Ruta (graveolens)	T62.2X1	T62.2X2	T62.2X3	T62.2X4	--	--
Rutinum	T46.991	T46.992	T46.993	T46.994	T46.995	T46.996
Rutoside	T46.991	T46.992	T46.993	T46.994	T46.995	T46.996
Sabadilla (plant)	T62.2X1	T62.2X2	T62.2X3	T62.2X4	--	--
pesticide	T60.2X1	T60.2X2	T60.2X3	T60.2X4	--	--
Saccharated iron oxide	T45.8X1	T45.8X2	T45.8X3	T45.8X4	T45.8X5	T45.8X6
Saccharin	T50.901	T50.902	T50.903	T50.904	T50.905	T50.906
Saccharomyces boulardii	T47.6X1	T47.6X2	T47.6X3	T47.6X4	T47.6X5	T47.6X6
Safflower oil	T46.6X1	T46.6X2	T46.6X3	T46.6X4	T46.6X5	T46.6X6
Safrazine	T43.1X1	T43.1X2	T43.1X3	T43.1X4	T43.1X5	T43.1X6
Salazosulfapyridine	T37.0X1	T37.0X2	T37.0X3	T37.0X4	T37.0X5	T37.0X6
Salbutamol	T48.6X1	T48.6X2	T48.6X3	T48.6X4	T48.6X5	T48.6X6
Salicylamide	T39.091	T39.092	T39.093	T39.094	T39.095	T39.096
Salicylate NEC	T39.091	T39.092	T39.093	T39.094	T39.095	T39.096
methyl	T49.3X1	T49.3X2	T49.3X3	T49.3X4	T49.3X5	T49.3X6
theobromine calcium	T50.2X1	T50.2X2	T50.2X3	T50.2X4	T50.2X5	T50.2X6
Salicylazosulfapyridine	T37.0X1	T37.0X2	T37.0X3	T37.0X4	T37.0X5	T37.0X6
Salicylhydroxamic acid	T49.0X1	T49.0X2	T49.0X3	T49.0X4	T49.0X5	T49.0X6
Salicylic acid	T49.4X1	T49.4X2	T49.4X3	T49.4X4	T49.4X5	T49.4X6
with benzoic acid	T49.4X1	T49.4X2	T49.4X3	T49.4X4	T49.4X5	T49.4X6
congeners	T39.091	T39.092	T39.093	T39.094	T39.095	T39.096
derivative	T39.091	T39.092	T39.093	T39.094	T39.095	T39.096
salts	T39.091	T39.092	T39.093	T39.094	T39.095	T39.096
Salinazid	T37.1X1	T37.1X2	T37.1X3	T37.1X4	T37.1X5	T37.1X6
Salmeterol	T48.6X1	T48.6X2	T48.6X3	T48.6X4	T48.6X5	T48.6X6
Salol	T49.3X1	T49.3X2	T49.3X3	T49.3X4	T49.3X5	T49.3X6
Salsalate	T39.091	T39.092	T39.093	T39.094	T39.095	T39.096
Salt substitute	T50.901	T50.902	T50.903	T50.904	T50.905	T50.906
Salt-replacing drug	T50.901	T50.902	T50.903	T50.904	T50.905	T50.906
Salt-retaining mineralocorticoid	T50.0X1	T50.0X2	T50.0X3	T50.0X4	T50.0X5	T50.0X6
Saluretic NEC	T50.2X1	T50.2X2	T50.2X3	T50.2X4	T50.2X5	T50.2X6
Saluron	T50.2X1	T50.2X2	T50.2X3	T50.2X4	T50.2X5	T50.2X6
Salvarsan 606 (neosilver) (silver)	T37.8X1	T37.8X2	T37.8X3	T37.8X4	T37.8X5	T37.8X6
Sambucus canadensis	T62.2X1	T62.2X2	T62.2X3	T62.2X4	--	--
berry	T62.1X1	T62.1X2	T62.1X3	T62.1X4	--	--
Sandril	T46.5X1	T46.5X2	T46.5X3	T46.5X4	T46.5X5	T46.5X6
Sanguinaria canadensis	T62.2X1	T62.2X2	T62.2X3	T62.2X4	--	--
Saniflush (cleaner)	T54.2X1	T54.2X2	T54.2X3	T54.2X4	--	--
Santonin	T37.4X1	T37.4X2	T37.4X3	T37.4X4	T37.4X5	T37.4X6
Santyl	T49.8X1	T49.8X2	T49.8X3	T49.8X4	T49.8X5	T49.8X6
Saralasin	T46.5X1	T46.5X2	T46.5X3	T46.5X4	T46.5X5	T46.5X6
Sarcolysin	T45.1X1	T45.1X2	T45.1X3	T45.1X4	T45.1X5	T45.1X6
Sarkomycin	T45.1X1	T45.1X2	T45.1X3	T45.1X4	T45.1X5	T45.1X6
Saroten	T43.011	T43.012	T43.013	T43.014	T43.015	T43.016
Saturnine—see Lead						
Savin (oil)	T49.4X1	T49.4X2	T49.4X3	T49.4X4	T49.4X5	T49.4X6
Scammony	T47.2X1	T47.2X2	T47.2X3	T47.2X4	T47.2X5	T47.2X6
Scarlet red	T49.8X1	T49.8X2	T49.8X3	T49.8X4	T49.8X5	T49.8X6
Scheele's green	T57.0X1	T57.0X2	T57.0X3	T57.0X4	--	--
insecticide	T57.0X1	T57.0X2	T57.0X3	T57.0X4	--	--
Schizontozide (blood) (tissue)	T37.2X1	T37.2X2	T37.2X3	T37.2X4	T37.2X5	T37.2X6
Schradan	T60.0X1	T60.0X2	T60.0X3	T60.0X4	--	--
Schweinfurth green	T57.0X1	T57.0X2	T57.0X3	T57.0X4	--	--
insecticide	T57.0X1	T57.0X2	T57.0X3	T57.0X4	--	--
Scilla, rat poison	T60.4X1	T60.4X2	T60.4X3	T60.4X4	--	--
Scillaren	T60.4X1	T60.4X2	T60.4X3	T60.4X4	--	--

Substance	Poisoning, Accidental (unintentional)	Poisoning, Intentional Self-harm	Poisoning, Assault	Poisoning, Undetermined	Adverse effect	Underdosing
Sclerosing agent	T46.8X1	T46.8X2	T46.8X3	T46.8X4	T46.8X5	T46.8X6
Scombrotoxin	T61.11	T61.12	T61.13	T61.14	--	--
Scopolamine	T44.3X1	T44.3X2	T44.3X3	T44.3X4	T44.3X5	T44.3X6
Scopolia extract	T44.3X1	T44.3X2	T44.3X3	T44.3X4	T44.3X5	T44.3X6
Scouring powder	T65.891	T65.892	T65.893	T65.894	--	--
Sea						
anemone (sting)	T63.631	T63.632	T63.633	T63.634	--	--
cucumber (sting)	T63.691	T63.692	T63.693	T63.694	--	--
snake (bite) (venom)	T63.091	T63.092	T63.093	T63.094	--	--
urchin spine (puncture)	T63.691	T63.692	T63.693	T63.694	--	--
Seafood	T61.91	T61.92	T61.93	T61.94	--	--
specified NEC	T61.8X1	T61.8X2	T61.8X3	T61.8X4	--	--
Secbutabarbital	T42.3X1	T42.3X2	T42.3X3	T42.3X4	T42.3X5	T42.3X6
Secbutabarbitone	T42.3X1	T42.3X2	T42.3X3	T42.3X4	T42.3X5	T42.3X6
Secnidazole	T37.3X1	T37.3X2	T37.3X3	T37.3X4	T37.3X5	T37.3X6
Secobarbital	T42.3X1	T42.3X2	T42.3X3	T42.3X4	T42.3X5	T42.3X6
Seconal	T42.3X1	T42.3X2	T42.3X3	T42.3X4	T42.3X5	T42.3X6
Secretin	T50.8X1	T50.8X2	T50.8X3	T50.8X4	T50.8X5	T50.8X6
Sedative NEC	T42.71	T42.72	T42.73	T42.74	T42.75	T42.76
mixed NEC	T42.6X1	T42.6X2	T42.6X3	T42.6X4	T42.6X5	T42.6X6
Sedormid	T42.6X1	T42.6X2	T42.6X3	T42.6X4	T42.6X5	T42.6X6
Seed disinfectant or dressing	T60.8X1	T60.8X2	T60.8X3	T60.8X4	--	--
Seeds (poisonous)	T62.2X1	T62.2X2	T62.2X3	T62.2X4	--	--
Selegiline	T42.8X1	T42.8X2	T42.8X3	T42.8X4	T42.8X5	T42.8X6
Selenium NEC	T56.891	T56.892	T56.893	T56.894	--	--
disulfide or sulfide	T49.4X1	T49.4X2	T49.4X3	T49.4X4	T49.4X5	T49.4X6
fumes	T59.891	T59.892	T59.893	T59.894	--	--
sulfide	T49.4X1	T49.4X2	T49.4X3	T49.4X4	T49.4X5	T49.4X6
Selenomethionine (75Se)	T50.8X1	T50.8X2	T50.8X3	T50.8X4	T50.8X5	T50.8X6
Selsun	T49.4X1	T49.4X2	T49.4X3	T49.4X4	T49.4X5	T49.4X6
Semustine	T45.1X1	T45.1X2	T45.1X3	T45.1X4	T45.1X5	T45.1X6
Senega syrup	T48.4X1	T48.4X2	T48.4X3	T48.4X4	T48.4X5	T48.4X6
Senna	T47.2X1	T47.2X2	T47.2X3	T47.2X4	T47.2X5	T47.2X6
Sennoside A+B	T47.2X1	T47.2X2	T47.2X3	T47.2X4	T47.2X5	T47.2X6
Septisol	T49.2X1	T49.2X2	T49.2X3	T49.2X4	T49.2X5	T49.2X6
Seractide	T38.811	T38.812	T38.813	T38.814	T38.815	T38.816
Serax	T42.4X1	T42.4X2	T42.4X3	T42.4X4	T42.4X5	T42.4X6
Serenesil	T42.6X1	T42.6X2	T42.6X3	T42.6X4	T42.6X5	T42.6X6
Serenium (hydrochloride)	T37.91	T37.92	T37.93	T37.94	T37.95	T37.96
Serepax—see Oxazepam						
Sermorelin	T38.891	T38.892	T38.893	T38.894	T38.895	T38.896
Sernyl	T41.1X1	T41.1X2	T41.1X3	T41.1X4	T41.1X5	T41.1X6
Serotonin	T50.991	T50.992	T50.993	T50.994	T50.995	T50.996
Serpasil	T46.5X1	T46.5X2	T46.5X3	T46.5X4	T46.5X5	T46.5X6
Serrapeptase	T45.3X1	T45.3X2	T45.3X3	T45.3X4	T45.3X5	T45.3X6
Serum						
antibotulinus	T50.Z11	T50.Z12	T50.Z13	T50.Z14	T50.Z15	T50.Z16
anticytotoxic	T50.Z11	T50.Z12	T50.Z13	T50.Z14	T50.Z15	T50.Z16
antidiphtheria	T50.Z11	T50.Z12	T50.Z13	T50.Z14	T50.Z15	T50.Z16
antimeningococcus	T50.Z11	T50.Z12	T50.Z13	T50.Z14	T50.Z15	T50.Z16
anti-Rh	T50.Z11	T50.Z12	T50.Z13	T50.Z14	T50.Z15	T50.Z16
anti-snake-bite	T50.Z11	T50.Z12	T50.Z13	T50.Z14	T50.Z15	T50.Z16
antitetanic	T50.Z11	T50.Z12	T50.Z13	T50.Z14	T50.Z15	T50.Z16
antitoxic	T50.Z11	T50.Z12	T50.Z13	T50.Z14	T50.Z15	T50.Z16
complement (inhibitor)	T45.8X1	T45.8X2	T45.8X3	T45.8X4	T45.8X5	T45.8X6
convalescent	T50.Z11	T50.Z12	T50.Z13	T50.Z14	T50.Z15	T50.Z16
hemolytic complement	T45.8X1	T45.8X2	T45.8X3	T45.8X4	T45.8X5	T45.8X6
immune (human)	T50.Z11	T50.Z12	T50.Z13	T50.Z14	T50.Z15	T50.Z16
protective NEC	T50.Z11	T50.Z12	T50.Z13	T50.Z14	T50.Z15	T50.Z16
Setastine	T45.0X1	T45.0X2	T45.0X3	T45.0X4	T45.0X5	T45.0X6
Setoperone	T43.591	T43.592	T43.593	T43.594	T43.595	T43.596
Sewer gas	T59.91	T59.92	T59.93	T59.94	--	--
Shampoo	T55.0X1	T55.0X2	T55.0X3	T55.0X4	--	--
Shellfish, noxious, nonbacterial	T61.781	T61.782	T61.783	T61.784	--	--
Sildenafil	T46.7X1	T46.7X2	T46.7X3	T46.7X4	T46.7X5	T46.7X6

Substance	Poisoning, Accidental (unintentional)	Poisoning, Intentional Self-harm	Poisoning, Assault	Poisoning, Undetermined	Adverse effect	Underdosing
Silibinin	T50.991	T50.992	T50.993	T50.994	T50.995	T50.996
Silicone NEC	T65.891	T65.892	T65.893	T65.894	--	--
medicinal	T49.3X1	T49.3X2	T49.3X3	T49.3X4	T49.3X5	T49.3X6
Silvadene	T49.0X1	T49.0X2	T49.0X3	T49.0X4	T49.0X5	T49.0X6
Silver	T49.0X1	T49.0X2	T49.0X3	T49.0X4	T49.0X5	T49.0X6
anti-infectives	T49.0X1	T49.0X2	T49.0X3	T49.0X4	T49.0X5	T49.0X6
arsphenamine	T37.8X1	T37.8X2	T37.8X3	T37.8X4	T37.8X5	T37.8X6
colloidal	T49.0X1	T49.0X2	T49.0X3	T49.0X4	T49.0X5	T49.0X6
nitrate	T49.0X1	T49.0X2	T49.0X3	T49.0X4	T49.0X5	T49.0X6
ophthalmic preparation	T49.5X1	T49.5X2	T49.5X3	T49.5X4	T49.5X5	T49.5X6
toughened (keratolytic)	T49.4X1	T49.4X2	T49.4X3	T49.4X4	T49.4X5	T49.4X6
nonmedicinal (dust)	T56.891	T56.892	T56.893	T56.894	--	--
protein	T49.5X1	T49.5X2	T49.5X3	T49.5X4	T49.5X5	T49.5X6
salvarsan	T37.8X1	T37.8X2	T37.8X3	T37.8X4	T37.8X5	T37.8X6
sulfadiazine	T49.4X1	T49.4X2	T49.4X3	T49.4X4	T49.4X5	T49.4X6
Silymarin	T50.991	T50.992	T50.993	T50.994	T50.995	T50.996
Simaldrate	T47.1X1	T47.1X1	T47.1X3	T47.1X4	T47.1X5	T47.1X6
Simazine	T60.3X1	T60.3X2	T60.3X3	T60.3X4	--	--
Simethicone	T47.1X1	T47.1X2	T47.1X3	T47.1X4	T47.1X5	T47.1X6
Simfibrate	T46.6X1	T46.6X2	T46.6X3	T46.6X4	T46.6X5	T46.6X6
Simvastatin	T46.6X1	T46.6X2	T46.6X3	T46.6X4	T46.6X5	T46.6X6
Sincalide	T50.8X1	T50.8X2	T50.8X3	T50.8X4	T50.8X5	T50.8X6
Sinequan	T43.011	T43.012	T43.013	T43.014	T43.015	T43.016
Singoserp	T46.5X1	T46.5X2	T46.5X3	T46.5X4	T46.5X5	T46.5X6
Sintrom	T45.511	T45.512	T45.513	T45.514	T45.515	T45.516
Sisomicin	T36.5X1	T36.5X2	T36.5X3	T36.5X4	T36.5X5	T36.5X6
Sitosterols	T46.6X1	T46.6X2	T46.6X3	T46.6X4	T46.6X5	T46.6X6
Skeletal muscle relaxants	T48.1X1	T48.1X2	T48.1X3	T48.1X4	T48.1X5	T48.1X6
Skin						
agents (external)	T49.91	T49.92	T49.93	T49.94	T49.95	T49.96
specified NEC	T49.8X1	T49.8X2	T49.8X3	T49.8X4	T49.8X5	T49.8X6
test antigen	T50.8X1	T50.8X2	T50.8X3	T50.8X4	T50.8X5	T50.8X6
Sleep-eze	T45.0X1	T45.0X2	T45.0X3	T45.0X4	T45.0X5	T45.0X6
Sleeping draught, pill	T42.71	T42.72	T42.73	T42.74	T42.75	T42.76
Smallpox vaccine	T50.B11	T50.B12	T50.B13	T50.B14	T50.B15	T50.B16
Smelter fumes NEC	T56.91	T56.92	T56.93	T56.94	--	--
Smog	T59.1X1	T59.1X2	T59.1X3	T59.1X4	--	--
Smoke NEC	T59.811	T59.812	T59.813	T59.814	--	--
Smooth muscle relaxant	T44.3X1	T44.3X2	T44.3X3	T44.3X4	T44.3X5	T44.3X6
Snail killer NEC	T60.8X1	T60.8X2	T60.8X3	T60.8X4	--	--
Snake venom or bite	T63.001	T63.002	T63.003	T63.004	--	--
hemocoagulase	T45.7X1	T45.7X2	T45.7X3	T45.7X4	T45.7X5	T45.7X6
Snuff	T65.211	T65.212	T65.213	T65.214	--	--
Soap (powder) (product)	T55.0X1	T55.0X2	T55.0X3	T55.0X4	--	--
enema	T47.4X1	T47.4X2	T47.4X3	T47.4X4	T47.4X5	T47.4X6
medicinal, soft	T49.2X1	T49.2X2	T49.2X3	T49.2X4	T49.2X5	T49.2X6
superfatted	T49.2X1	T49.2X2	T49.2X3	T49.2X4	T49.2X5	T49.2X6
Sobrerol	T48.4X1	T48.4X2	T48.4X3	T48.4X4	T48.4X5	T48.4X6
Soda (caustic)	T54.3X1	T54.3X2	T54.3X3	T54.3X4	--	--
bicarb	T47.1X1	T47.1X2	T47.1X3	T47.1X4	T47.1X5	T47.1X6
chlorinated—see Sodium, hypochlorite						
Sodium						
acetosulfone	T37.1X1	T37.1X2	T37.1X3	T37.1X4	T37.1X5	T37.1X6
acetrizoate	T50.8X1	T50.8X2	T50.8X3	T50.8X4	T50.8X5	T50.8X6
acid phosphate	T50.3X1	T50.3X2	T50.3X3	T50.3X4	T50.3X5	T50.3X6
alginate	T47.8X1	T47.8X2	T47.8X3	T47.8X4	T47.8X5	T47.8X6
amidotrizoate	T50.8X1	T50.8X2	T50.8X3	T50.8X4	T50.8X5	T50.8X6
aminopterin	T45.1X1	T45.1X2	T45.1X3	T45.1X4	T45.1X5	T45.1X6
amylosulfate	T47.8X1	T47.8X2	T47.8X3	T47.8X4	T47.8X5	T47.8X6
amytal	T42.3X1	T42.3X2	T42.3X3	T42.3X4	T42.3X5	T42.3X6
antimony gluconate	T37.3X1	T37.3X2	T37.3X3	T37.3X4	T37.3X5	T37.3X6
arsenate	T57.0X1	T57.0X2	T57.0X3	T57.0X4	--	--
aurothiomalate	T39.4X1	T39.4X2	T39.4X3	T39.4X4	T39.4X5	T39.4X6
aurothiosulfate	T39.4X1	T39.4X2	T39.4X3	T39.4X4	T39.4X5	T39.4X6

TABLE OF DRUGS AND CHEMICALS

Substance	Poisoning, Accidental (unintentional)	Poisoning, Intentional Self-harm	Poisoning, Assault	Poisoning, Undetermined	Adverse effect	Underdosing
barbiturate	T42.3X1	T42.3X2	T42.3X3	T42.3X4	T42.3X5	T42.3X6
basic phosphate	T47.4X1	T47.4X2	T47.4X3	T47.4X4	T47.4X5	T47.4X6
bicarbonate	T47.1X1	T47.1X2	T47.1X3	T47.1X4	T47.1X5	T47.1X6
bichromate	T57.8X1	T57.8X2	T57.8X3	T57.8X4	--	--
biphosphate	T50.3X1	T50.3X2	T50.3X3	T50.3X4	T50.3X5	T50.3X6
bisulfate	T65.891	T65.892	T65.893	T65.894	--	--
borate						
cleanser	T57.8X1	T57.8X2	T57.8X3	T57.8X4	--	--
eye	T49.5X1	T49.5X2	T49.5X3	T49.5X4	T49.5X5	T49.5X6
therapeutic	T49.8X1	T49.8X2	T49.8X3	T49.8X4	T49.8X5	T49.8X6
bromide	T42.6X1	T42.6X2	T42.6X3	T42.6X4	T42.6X5	T42.6X6
cacodylate (nonmedicinal) NEC	T50.8X1	T50.8X2	T50.8X3	T50.8X4	T50.8X5	T50.8X6
anti-infective	T37.8X1	T37.8X2	T37.8X3	T37.8X4	T37.8X5	T37.8X6
herbicide	T60.3X1	T60.3X2	T60.3X3	T60.3X4	--	--
calcium edetate	T45.8X1	T45.8X2	T45.8X3	T45.8X4	T45.8X5	T45.8X6
carbonate NEC	T54.3X1	T54.3X2	T54.3X3	T54.3X4	--	--
chlorate NEC	T65.891	T65.892	T65.893	T65.894	--	--
herbicide	T54.91	T54.92	T54.93	T54.94	--	--
chloride	T50.3X1	T50.3X2	T50.3X3	T50.3X4	T50.3X5	T50.3X6
with glucose	T50.3X1	T50.3X2	T50.3X3	T50.3X4	T50.3X5	T50.3X6
chromate	T65.891	T65.892	T65.893	T65.894	--	--
citrate	T50.991	T50.992	T50.993	T50.994	T50.995	T50.996
cromoglicate	T48.6X1	T48.6X2	T48.6X3	T48.6X4	T48.6X5	T48.6X6
cyanide	T65.0X1	T65.0X2	T65.0X3	T65.0X4	--	--
cyclamate	T50.3X1	T50.3X2	T50.3X3	T50.3X4	T50.3X5	T50.3X6
dehydrocholate	T45.8X1	T45.8X2	T45.8X3	T45.8X4	T45.8X5	T45.8X6
diatrizoate	T50.8X1	T50.8X2	T50.8X3	T50.8X4	T50.8X5	T50.8X6
dibunate	T48.4X1	T48.4X2	T48.4X3	T48.4X4	T48.4X5	T48.4X6
dioctyl sulfosuccinate	T47.4X1	T47.4X2	T47.4X3	T47.4X4	T47.4X5	T47.4X6
dipantoyl ferrate	T45.8X1	T45.8X2	T45.8X3	T45.8X4	T45.8X5	T45.8X6
edetate	T45.8X1	T45.8X2	T45.8X3	T45.8X4	T45.8X5	T45.8X6
ethacrynate	T50.1X1	T50.1X2	T50.1X3	T50.1X4	T50.1X5	T50.1X6
feredetate	T45.8X1	T45.8X2	T45.8X3	T45.8X4	T45.8X5	T45.8X6
Fluoride—see Fluoride						
fluoroacetate (dust) (pesticide)	T60.4X1	T60.4X2	T60.4X3	T60.4X4	--	--
free salt	T50.3X1	T50.3X2	T50.3X3	T50.3X4	T50.3X5	T50.3X6
fusidate	T36.8X1	T36.8X2	T36.8X3	T36.8X4	T36.8X5	T36.8X6
glucaldrate	T47.1X1	T47.1X2	T47.1X3	T47.1X4	T47.1X5	T47.1X6
glucosulfone	T37.1X1	T37.1X2	T37.1X3	T37.1X4	T37.1X5	T37.1X6
glutamate	T45.8X1	T45.8X2	T45.8X3	T45.8X4	T45.8X5	T45.8X6
hydrogen carbonate	T50.3X1	T50.3X2	T50.3X3	T50.3X4	T50.3X5	T50.3X6
hydroxide	T54.3X1	T54.3X2	T54.3X3	T54.3X4	--	--
hypochlorite (bleach) NEC	T54.3X1	T54.3X2	T54.3X3	T54.3X4	--	--
disinfectant	T54.3X1	T54.3X2	T54.3X3	T54.3X4	--	--
medicinal (anti-infective) (external)	T49.0X1	T49.0X2	T49.0X3	T49.0X4	T49.0X5	T49.0X6
vapor	T54.3X1	T54.3X2	T54.3X3	T54.3X4	--	--
hyposulfite	T49.0X1	T49.0X2	T49.0X3	T49.0X4	T49.0X5	T49.0X6
indigotin disulfonate	T50.8X1	T50.8X2	T50.8X3	T50.8X4	T50.8X5	T50.8X6
iodide	T50.991	T50.992	T50.993	T50.994	T50.995	T50.996
I-131	T50.8X1	T50.8X2	T50.8X3	T50.8X4	T50.8X5	T50.8X6
therapeutic	T38.2X1	T38.2X2	T38.2X3	T38.2X4	T38.2X5	T38.2X6
iodohippurate (131I)	T50.8X1	T50.8X2	T50.8X3	T50.8X4	T50.8X5	T50.8X6
iopodate	T50.8X1	T50.8X2	T50.8X3	T50.8X4	T50.8X5	T50.8X6
iothalamate	T50.8X1	T50.8X2	T50.8X3	T50.8X4	T50.8X5	T50.8X6
iron edetate	T45.4X1	T45.4X2	T45.4X3	T45.4X4	T45.4X5	T45.4X6
lactate (compound solution)	T45.8X1	T45.8X2	T45.8X3	T45.8X4	T45.8X5	T45.8X6
lauryl (sulfate)	T49.2X1	T49.2X2	T49.2X3	T49.2X4	T49.2X5	T49.2X6
L-triiodothyronine	T38.1X1	T38.1X2	T38.1X3	T38.1X4	T38.1X5	T38.1X6
magnesium citrate	T50.991	T50.992	T50.993	T50.994	T50.995	T50.996
mersalate	T50.2X1	T50.2X2	T50.2X3	T50.2X4	T50.2X5	T50.2X6
metasilicate	T65.891	T65.892	T65.893	T65.894	--	--
metrizoate	T50.8X1	T50.8X2	T50.8X3	T50.8X4	T50.8X5	T50.8X6
monofluoroacetate (pesticide)	T60.1X1	T60.1X2	T60.1X3	T60.1X4	--	--
morrhuate	T46.8X1	T46.8X2	T46.8X3	T46.8X4	T46.8X5	T46.8X6
nafcillin	T36.0X1	T36.0X2	T36.0X3	T36.0X4	T36.0X5	T36.0X6

Substance	Poisoning, Accidental (unintentional)	Poisoning, Intentional Self-harm	Poisoning, Assault	Poisoning, Undetermined	Adverse effect	Underdosing
nitrate (oxidizing agent)	T65.891	T65.892	T65.893	T65.894	--	--
nitrite	T50.6X1	T50.6X2	T50.6X3	T50.6X4	T50.6X5	T50.6X6
nitroferricyanide	T46.5X1	T46.5X2	T46.5X3	T46.5X4	T46.5X5	T46.5X6
nitroprusside	T46.5X1	T46.5X2	T46.5X3	T46.5X4	T46.5X5	T46.5X6
oxalate	T65.891	T65.892	T65.893	T65.894	--	--
oxide/peroxide	T65.891	T65.892	T65.893	T65.894	--	--
oxybate	T41.291	T41.292	T41.293	T41.294	T41.295	T41.296
para-aminohippurate	T50.8X1	T50.8X2	T50.8X3	T50.8X4	T50.8X5	T50.8X6
perborate (nonmedicinal) NEC	T65.891	T65.892	T65.893	T65.894	--	--
medicinal	T49.0X1	T49.0X2	T49.0X3	T49.0X4	T49.0X5	T49.0X6
soap	T55.0X1	T55.0X2	T55.0X3	T55.0X4	--	--
percarbonate—see Sodium, perborate						
pertechnetate Tc99m	T50.8X1	T50.8X2	T50.8X3	T50.8X4	T50.8X5	T50.8X6
phosphate						
cellulose	T45.8X1	T45.8X2	T45.8X3	T45.8X4	T45.8X5	T45.8X6
dibasic	T47.2X1	T47.2X2	T47.2X3	T47.2X4	T47.2X5	T47.2X6
monobasic	T47.2X1	T47.2X2	T47.2X3	T47.2X4	T47.2X5	T47.2X6
phytate	T50.6X1	T50.6X2	T50.6X3	T50.6X4	T50.6X5	T50.6X6
picosulfate	T47.2X1	T47.2X2	T47.2X3	T47.2X4	T47.2X5	T47.2X6
polyhydroxyaluminium monocarbonate	T47.1X1	T47.1X2	T47.1X3	T47.1X4	T47.1X5	T47.1X6
polystyrene sulfonate	T50.3X1	T50.3X2	T50.3X3	T50.3X4	T50.3X5	T50.3X6
propionate	T49.0X1	T49.0X2	T49.0X3	T49.0X4	T49.0X5	T49.0X6
propyl hydroxybenzoate	T50.991	T50.992	T50.993	T50.994	T50.995	T50.996
psylliate	T46.8X1	T46.8X2	T46.8X3	T46.8X4	T46.8X5	T46.8X6
removing resins	T50.3X1	T50.3X2	T50.3X3	T50.3X4	T50.3X5	T50.3X6
salicylate	T39.091	T39.092	T39.093	T39.094	T39.095	T39.096
salt NEC	T50.3X1	T50.3X2	T50.3X3	T50.3X4	T50.3X5	T50.3X6
selenate	T60.2X1	T60.2X2	T60.2X3	T60.2X4	--	--
stibogluconate	T37.3X1	T37.3X2	T37.3X3	T37.3X4	T37.3X5	T37.3X6
sulfate	T47.4X1	T47.4X2	T47.4X3	T47.4X4	T47.4X5	T47.4X6
sulfoxone	T37.1X1	T37.1X2	T37.1X3	T37.1X4	T37.1X5	T37.1X6
tetradecyl sulfate	T46.8X1	T46.8X2	T46.8X3	T46.8X4	T46.8X5	T46.8X6
thiopental	T41.1X1	T41.1X2	T41.1X3	T41.1X4	T41.1X5	T41.1X6
thiosalicylate	T39.091	T39.092	T39.093	T39.094	T39.095	T39.096
thiosulfate	T50.6X1	T50.6X2	T50.6X3	T50.6X4	T50.6X5	T50.6X6
tolbutamide	T38.3X1	T38.3X2	T38.3X3	T38.3X4	T38.3X5	T38.3X6
(L) -triiodothyronine	T38.1X1	T38.1X2	T38.1X3	T38.1X4	T38.1X5	T38.1X6
tyropanoate	T50.8X1	T50.8X2	T50.8X3	T50.8X4	T50.8X5	T50.8X6
valproate	T42.6X1	T42.6X2	T42.6X3	T42.6X4	T42.6X5	T42.6X6
versenate	T50.6X1	T50.6X2	T50.6X3	T50.6X4	T50.6X5	T50.6X6
Sodium-free salt	T50.901	T50.902	T50.903	T50.904	T50.905	T50.906
Sodium-removing resin	T50.3X1	T50.3X2	T50.3X3	T50.3X4	T50.3X5	T50.3X6
Soft soap	T55.0X1	T55.0X2	T55.0X3	T55.0X4	--	--
Solanine	T62.2X1	T62.2X2	T62.2X3	T62.2X4	--	--
berries	T62.1X1	T62.1X2	T62.1X3	T62.1X4	--	--
Solanum dulcamara	T62.2X1	T62.2X2	T62.2X3	T62.2X4	--	--
berries	T62.1X1	T62.1X2	T62.1X3	T62.1X4	--	--
Solapsone	T37.1X1	T37.1X2	T37.1X3	T37.1X4	T37.1X5	T37.1X6
Solar lotion	T49.3X1	T49.3X2	T49.3X3	T49.3X4	T49.3X5	T49.3X6
Solasulfone	T37.1X1	T37.1X2	T37.1X3	T37.1X4	T37.1X5	T37.1X6
Soldering fluid	T65.891	T65.892	T65.893	T65.894	--	--
Solid substance	T65.91	T65.92	T65.93	T65.94	--	--
specified NEC	T65.891	T65.892	T65.893	T65.894	--	--
Solvent, industrial NEC	T52.91	T52.92	T52.93	T52.94	--	--
naphtha	T52.0X1	T52.0X2	T52.0X3	T52.0X4	--	--
petroleum	T52.0X1	T52.0X2	T52.0X3	T52.0X4	--	--
specified NEC	T52.8X1	T52.8X2	T52.8X3	T52.8X4	--	--
Soma	T42.8X1	T42.8X2	T42.8X3	T42.8X4	T42.8X5	T42.8X6
Somatorelin	T38.891	T38.892	T38.893	T38.894	T38.895	T38.896
Somatostatin	T38.991	T38.992	T38.993	T38.994	T38.995	T38.996
Somatotropin	T38.811	T38.812	T38.813	T38.814	T38.815	T38.816
Somatrem	T38.811	T38.812	T38.813	T38.814	T38.815	T38.816
Somatropin	T38.811	T38.812	T38.813	T38.814	T38.815	T38.816
Sominex	T45.0X1	T45.0X2	T45.0X3	T45.0X4	T45.0X5	T45.0X6

Substance	Poisoning, Accidental (unintentional)	Poisoning, Intentional Self-harm	Poisoning, Assault	Poisoning, Undetermined	Adverse effect	Underdosing
Somnos	T42.6X1	T42.6X2	T42.6X3	T42.6X4	T42.6X5	T42.6X6
Somonal	T42.3X1	T42.3X2	T42.3X3	T42.3X4	T42.3X5	T42.3X6
Soneryl	T42.3X1	T42.3X2	T42.3X3	T42.3X4	T42.3X5	T42.3X6
Soothing syrup	T50.901	T50.902	T50.903	T50.904	T50.905	T50.906
Sopor	T42.6X1	T42.6X2	T42.6X3	T42.6X4	T42.6X5	T42.6X6
Soporific	T42.71	T42.72	T42.73	T42.74	T42.75	T42.76
Soporific drug	T42.71	T42.72	T42.73	T42.74	T42.75	T42.76
specified type NEC	T42.6X1	T42.6X2	T42.6X3	T42.6X4	T42.6X5	T42.6X6
Sorbide nitrate	T46.3X1	T46.3X2	T46.3X3	T46.3X4	T46.3X5	T46.3X6
Sorbitol	T47.4X1	T47.4X2	T47.4X3	T47.4X4	T47.4X5	T47.4X6
Sotalol	T44.7X1	T44.7X2	T44.7X3	T44.7X4	T44.7X5	T44.7X6
Sotradecol	T46.8X1	T46.8X2	T46.8X3	T46.8X4	T46.8X5	T46.8X6
Soysterol	T46.6X1	T46.6X2	T46.6X3	T46.6X4	T46.6X5	T46.6X6
Spacoline	T44.3X1	T44.3X2	T44.3X3	T44.3X4	T44.3X5	T44.3X6
Spanish fly	T49.8X1	T49.8X2	T49.8X3	T49.8X4	T49.8X5	T49.8X6
Sparine	T43.3X1	T43.3X2	T43.3X3	T43.3X4	T43.3X5	T43.3X6
Sparteine	T48.0X1	T48.0X2	T48.0X3	T48.0X4	T48.0X5	T48.0X6
Spasmolytic						
anticholinergics	T44.3X1	T44.3X2	T44.3X3	T44.3X4	T44.3X5	T44.3X6
autonomic	T44.3X1	T44.3X2	T44.3X3	T44.3X4	T44.3X5	T44.3X6
bronchial NEC	T48.6X1	T48.6X2	T48.6X3	T48.6X4	T48.6X5	T48.6X6
quaternary ammonium	T44.3X1	T44.3X2	T44.3X3	T44.3X4	T44.3X5	T44.3X6
skeletal muscle NEC	T48.1X1	T48.1X2	T48.1X3	T48.1X4	T48.1X5	T48.1X6
Spectinomycin	T36.5X1	T36.5X2	T36.5X3	T36.5X4	T36.5X5	T36.5X6
Speed	T43.621	T43.622	T43.623	T43.624	T43.625	T43.626
Spermicide	T49.8X1	T49.8X2	T49.8X3	T49.8X4	T49.8X5	T49.8X6
Spider (bite) (venom)	T63.391	T63.392	T63.393	T63.394	--	--
antivenin	T50.Z11	T50.Z12	T50.Z13	T50.Z14	T50.Z15	T50.Z16
Spigelia (root)	T37.4X1	T37.4X2	T37.4X3	T37.4X4	T37.4X5	T37.4X6
Spindle inactivator	T50.4X1	T50.4X2	T50.4X3	T50.4X4	T50.4X5	T50.4X6
Spiperone	T43.4X1	T43.4X2	T43.4X3	T43.4X4	T43.4X5	T43.4X6
Spiramycin	T36.3X1	T36.3X2	T36.3X3	T36.3X4	T36.3X5	T36.3X6
Spirapril	T46.4X1	T46.4X2	T46.4X3	T46.4X4	T46.4X5	T46.4X6
Spirilene	T43.591	T43.592	T43.593	T43.594	T43.595	T43.596
Spirit (s) (neutral) NEC	T51.0X1	T51.0X2	T51.0X3	T51.0X4	--	--
beverage	T51.0X1	T51.0X2	T51.0X3	T51.0X4	--	--
industrial	T51.0X1	T51.0X2	T51.0X3	T51.0X4	--	--
mineral	T52.0X1	T52.0X2	T52.0X3	T52.0X4	--	--
of salt—see Hydrochloric acid						
surgical	T51.0X1	T51.0X2	T51.0X3	T51.0X4	--	--
Spironolactone	T50.0X1	T50.0X2	T50.0X3	T50.0X4	T50.0X5	T50.0X6
Spiroperidol	T43.4X1	T43.4X2	T43.4X3	T43.4X4	T43.4X5	T43.4X6
Sponge, absorbable (gelatin)	T45.7X1	T45.7X2	T45.7X3	T45.7X4	T45.7X5	T45.7X6
Sporostacin	T49.0X1	T49.0X2	T49.0X3	T49.0X4	T49.0X5	T49.0X6
Spray (aerosol)	T65.91	T65.92	T65.93	T65.94	--	--
cosmetic	T65.891	T65.892	T65.893	T65.894	--	--
medicinal NEC	T50.901	T50.902	T50.903	T50.904	T50.905	T50.906
pesticides—see Pesticides						
specified content—see specific substance						
Spurge flax	T62.2X1	T62.2X2	T62.2X3	T62.2X4	--	--
Spurges	T62.2X1	T62.2X2	T62.2X3	T62.2X4	--	--
Sputum viscosity-lowering drug	T48.4X1	T48.4X2	T48.4X3	T48.4X4	T48.4X5	T48.4X6
Squill	T46.0X1	T46.0X2	T46.0X3	T46.0X4	T46.0X5	T46.0X6
rat poison	T60.4X1	T60.4X2	T60.4X3	T60.4X4	--	--
Squirting cucumber (cathartic)	T47.2X1	T47.2X2	T47.2X3	T47.2X4	T47.2X5	T47.2X6
Stains	T65.6X1	T65.6X2	T65.6X3	T65.6X4	--	--
Stannous fluoride	T49.7X1	T49.7X2	T49.7X3	T49.7X4	T49.7X5	T49.7X6
Stanolone	T38.7X1	T38.7X2	T38.7X3	T38.7X4	T38.7X5	T38.7X6
Stanozolol	T38.7X1	T38.7X2	T38.7X3	T38.7X4	T38.7X5	T38.7X6
Staphisagria or stavesacre (pediculicide)	T49.0X1	T49.0X2	T49.0X3	T49.0X4	T49.0X5	T49.0X6
Starch	T50.901	T50.902	T50.903	T50.904	T50.905	T50.906
Stelazine	T43.3X1	T43.3X2	T43.3X3	T43.3X4	T43.3X5	T43.3X6
Stemetil	T43.3X1	T43.3X2	T43.3X3	T43.3X4	T43.3X5	T43.3X6
Stepronin	T48.4X1	T48.4X2	T48.4X3	T48.4X4	T48.4X5	T48.4X6
Sterculia	T47.4X1	T47.4X2	T47.4X3	T47.4X4	T47.4X5	T47.4X6

Substance	Poisoning, Accidental (unintentional)	Poisoning, Intentional Self-harm	Poisoning, Assault	Poisoning, Undetermined	Adverse effect	Underdosing
Sternutator gas	T59.891	T59.892	T59.893	T59.894	--	--
Steroid	T38.0X1	T38.0X2	T38.0X3	T38.0X4	T38.0X5	T38.0X6
anabolic	T38.7X1	T38.7X2	T38.7X3	T38.7X4	T38.7X5	T38.7X6
androgenic	T38.7X1	T38.7X2	T38.7X3	T38.7X4	T38.7X5	T38.7X6
antineoplastic, hormone	T38.7X1	T38.7X2	T38.7X3	T38.7X4	T38.7X5	T38.7X6
estrogen	T38.5X1	T38.5X2	T38.5X3	T38.5X4	T38.5X5	T38.5X6
ENT agent	T49.6X1	T49.6X2	T49.6X3	T49.6X4	T49.6X5	T49.6X6
ophthalmic preparation	T49.5X1	T49.5X2	T49.5X3	T49.5X4	T49.5X5	T49.5X6
topical NEC	T49.0X1	T49.0X2	T49.0X3	T49.0X4	T49.0X5	T49.0X6
Stibine	T56.891	T56.892	T56.893	T56.894	--	--
Stibogluconate	T37.3X1	T37.3X2	T37.3X3	T37.3X4	T37.3X5	T37.3X6
Stibophen	T37.4X1	T37.4X2	T37.4X3	T37.4X4	T37.4X5	T37.4X6
Stilbamidine (isetionate)	T37.3X1	T37.3X2	T37.3X3	T37.3X4	T37.3X5	T37.3X6
Stilbestrol	T38.5X1	T38.5X2	T38.5X3	T38.5X4	T38.5X5	T38.5X6
Stilboestrol	T38.5X1	T38.5X2	T38.5X3	T38.5X4	T38.5X5	T38.5X6
Stimulant						
central nervous system—see also Psychostimulant	T43.601	T43.602	T43.603	T43.604	T43.605	T43.606
analeptics	T50.7X1	T50.7X2	T50.7X3	T50.7X4	T50.7X5	T50.7X6
opiate antagonist	T50.7X1	T50.7X2	T50.7X3	T50.7X4	T50.7X5	T50.7X6
psychotherapeutic NEC—see also Psychotherapeutic drug	T43.601	T43.602	T43.603	T43.604	T43.605	T43.606
specified NEC	T43.691	T43.692	T43.693	T43.694	T43.695	T43.696
respiratory	T48.901	T48.902	T48.903	T48.904	T48.905	T48.906
Stone-dissolving drug	T50.901	T50.902	T50.903	T50.904	T50.905	T50.906
Storage battery (cells) (acid)	T54.2X1	T54.2X2	T54.2X3	T54.2X4	--	--
Stovaine	T41.3X1	T41.3X2	T41.3X3	T41.3X4	T41.3X5	T41.3X6
infiltration (subcutaneous)	T41.3X1	T41.3X2	T41.3X3	T41.3X4	T41.3X5	T41.3X6
nerve block (peripheral) (plexus)	T41.3X1	T41.3X2	T41.3X3	T41.3X4	T41.3X5	T41.3X6
spinal	T41.3X1	T41.3X2	T41.3X3	T41.3X4	T41.3X5	T41.3X6
topical (surface)	T41.3X1	T41.3X2	T41.3X3	T41.3X4	T41.3X5	T41.3X6
Stovarsal	T37.8X1	T37.8X2	T37.8X3	T37.8X4	T37.8X5	T37.8X6
Stove gas—see Gas, stove						
Stoxil	T49.5X1	T49.5X2	T49.5X3	T49.5X4	T49.5X5	T49.5X6
Stramonium	T48.6X1	T48.6X2	T48.6X3	T48.6X4	T48.6X5	T48.6X6
natural state	T62.2X1	T62.2X2	T62.2X3	T62.2X4	--	--
Streptodornase	T45.3X1	T45.3X2	T45.3X3	T45.3X4	T45.3X5	T45.3X6
Streptoduocin	T36.5X1	T36.5X2	T36.5X3	T36.5X4	T36.5X5	T36.5X6
Streptokinase	T45.611	T45.612	T45.613	T45.614	T45.615	T45.616
Streptomycin (derivative)	T36.5X1	T36.5X2	T36.5X3	T36.5X4	T36.5X5	T36.5X6
Streptonivicin	T36.5X1	T36.5X2	T36.5X3	T36.5X4	T36.5X5	T36.5X6
Streptovarycin	T36.5X1	T36.5X2	T36.5X3	T36.5X4	T36.5X5	T36.5X6
Streptozocin	T45.1X1	T45.1X2	T45.1X3	T45.1X4	T45.1X5	T45.1X6
Streptozotocin	T45.1X1	T45.1X2	T45.1X3	T45.1X4	T45.1X5	T45.1X6
Stripper (paint) (solvent)	T52.8X1	T52.8X2	T52.8X3	T52.8X4	--	--
Strobane	T60.1X1	T60.1X2	T60.1X3	T60.1X4	--	--
Strofantina	T46.0X1	T46.0X2	T46.0X3	T46.0X4	T46.0X5	T46.0X6
Strophanthin (g) (k)	T46.0X1	T46.0X2	T46.0X3	T46.0X4	T46.0X5	T46.0X6
Strophanthus	T46.0X1	T46.0X2	T46.0X3	T46.0X4	T46.0X5	T46.0X6
Strophantin	T46.0X1	T46.0X2	T46.0X3	T46.0X4	T46.0X5	T46.0X6
Strophantin-g	T46.0X1	T46.0X2	T46.0X3	T46.0X4	T46.0X5	T46.0X6
Strychnine (nonmedicinal) (pesticide) (salts)	T65.1X1	T65.1X2	T65.1X3	T65.1X4	--	--
medicinal	T48.291	T48.292	T48.293	T48.294	T48.295	T48.296
Strychnos (ignatii)—see Strychnine						
Styramate	T42.8X1	T42.8X2	T42.8X3	T42.8X4	T42.8X5	T42.8X6
Styrene	T65.891	T65.892	T65.893	T65.894	--	--
Succinimide, antiepileptic or anticonvulsant	T42.2X1	T42.2X2	T42.2X3	T42.2X4	T42.2X5	T42.2X6
mercuric—see Mercury						
Succinylcholine	T48.1X1	T48.1X2	T48.1X3	T48.1X4	T48.1X5	T48.1X6
Succinylsulfathiazole	T37.0X1	T37.0X2	T37.0X3	T37.0X4	T37.0X5	T37.0X6
Sucralfate	T47.1X1	T47.1X2	T47.1X3	T47.1X4	T47.1X5	T47.1X6
Sucrose	T50.3X1	T50.3X2	T50.3X3	T50.3X4	T50.3X5	T50.3X6
Sufentanil	T40.4X1	T40.4X2	T40.4X3	T40.4X4	T40.4X5	T40.4X6
Sulbactam	T36.0X1	T36.0X2	T36.0X3	T36.0X4	T36.0X5	T36.0X6

Substance	Poisoning, Accidental (unintentional)	Poisoning, Intentional Self-harm	Poisoning, Assault	Poisoning, Undetermined	Adverse effect	Underdosing
Sulbenicillin	T36.0X1	T36.0X2	T36.0X3	T36.0X4	T36.0X5	T36.0X6
Sulbentine	T49.0X1	T49.0X2	T49.0X3	T49.0X4	T49.0X5	T49.0X6
Sulfacetamide	T49.0X1	T49.0X2	T49.0X3	T49.0X4	T49.0X5	T49.0X6
ophthalmic preparation	T49.5X1	T49.5X2	T49.5X3	T49.5X4	T49.5X5	T49.5X6
Sulfachlorpyridazine	T37.0X1	T37.0X2	T37.0X3	T37.0X4	T37.0X5	T37.0X6
Sulfacitine	T37.0X1	T37.0X2	T37.0X3	T37.0X4	T37.0X5	T37.0X6
Sulfadiasulfone sodium	T37.0X1	T37.0X2	T37.0X3	T37.0X4	T37.0X5	T37.0X6
Sulfadiazine	T37.0X1	T37.0X2	T37.0X3	T37.0X4	T37.0X5	T37.0X6
silver (topical)	T49.0X1	T49.0X2	T49.0X3	T49.0X4	T49.0X5	T49.0X6
Sulfadimethoxine	T37.0X1	T37.0X2	T37.0X3	T37.0X4	T37.0X5	T37.0X6
Sulfadimidine	T37.0X1	T37.0X2	T37.0X3	T37.0X4	T37.0X5	T37.0X6
Sulfadoxine	T37.0X1	T37.0X2	T37.0X3	T37.0X4	T37.0X5	T37.0X6
with pyrimethamine	T37.2X1	T37.2X2	T37.2X3	T37.2X4	T37.2X5	T37.2X6
Sulfaethidole	T37.0X1	T37.0X2	T37.0X3	T37.0X4	T37.0X5	T37.0X6
Sulfafurazole	T37.0X1	T37.0X2	T37.0X3	T37.0X4	T37.0X5	T37.0X6
Sulfaguanidine	T37.0X1	T37.0X2	T37.0X3	T37.0X4	T37.0X5	T37.0X6
Sulfalene	T37.0X1	T37.0X2	T37.0X3	T37.0X4	T37.0X5	T37.0X6
Sulfaloxate	T37.0X1	T37.0X2	T37.0X3	T37.0X4	T37.0X5	T37.0X6
Sulfaloxic acid	T37.0X1	T37.0X2	T37.0X3	T37.0X4	T37.0X5	T37.0X6
Sulfamazone	T39.2X1	T39.2X2	T39.2X3	T39.2X4	T39.2X5	T39.2X6
Sulfamerazine	T37.0X1	T37.0X2	T37.0X3	T37.0X4	T37.0X5	T37.0X6
Sulfameter	T37.0X1	T37.0X2	T37.0X3	T37.0X4	T37.0X5	T37.0X6
Sulfamethazine	T37.0X1	T37.0X2	T37.0X3	T37.0X4	T37.0X5	T37.0X6
Sulfamethizole	T37.0X1	T37.0X2	T37.0X3	T37.0X4	T37.0X5	T37.0X6
Sulfamethoxazole	T37.0X1	T37.0X2	T37.0X3	T37.0X4	T37.0X5	T37.0X6
with trimethoprim	T36.8X1	T36.8X2	T36.8X3	T36.8X4	T36.8X5	T36.8X6
Sulfamethoxydiazine	T37.0X1	T37.0X2	T37.0X3	T37.0X4	T37.0X5	T37.0X6
Sulfamethoxypyridazine	T37.0X1	T37.0X2	T37.0X3	T37.0X4	T37.0X5	T37.0X6
Sulfamethylthiazole	T37.0X1	T37.0X2	T37.0X3	T37.0X4	T37.0X5	T37.0X6
Sulfametoxydiazine	T37.0X1	T37.0X2	T37.0X3	T37.0X4	T37.0X5	T37.0X6
Sulfamidopyrine	T39.2X1	T39.2X2	T39.2X3	T39.2X4	T39.2X5	T39.2X6
Sulfamonomethoxine	T37.0X1	T37.0X2	T37.0X3	T37.0X4	T37.0X5	T37.0X6
Sulfamoxole	T37.0X1	T37.0X2	T37.0X3	T37.0X4	T37.0X5	T37.0X6
Sulfamylon	T49.0X1	T49.0X2	T49.0X3	T49.0X4	T49.0X5	T49.0X6
Sulfan blue (diagnostic dye)	T50.8X1	T50.8X2	T50.8X3	T50.8X4	T50.8X5	T50.8X6
Sulfanilamide	T37.0X1	T37.0X2	T37.0X3	T37.0X4	T37.0X5	T37.0X6
Sulfanilylguanidine	T37.0X1	T37.0X2	T37.0X3	T37.0X4	T37.0X5	T37.0X6
Sulfaperin	T37.0X1	T37.0X2	T37.0X3	T37.0X4	T37.0X5	T37.0X6
Sulfaphenazole	T37.0X1	T37.0X2	T37.0X3	T37.0X4	T37.0X5	T37.0X6
Sulfaphenylthiazole	T37.0X1	T37.0X2	T37.0X3	T37.0X4	T37.0X5	T37.0X6
Sulfaproxyline	T37.0X1	T37.0X2	T37.0X3	T37.0X4	T37.0X5	T37.0X6
Sulfapyridine	T37.0X1	T37.0X2	T37.0X3	T37.0X4	T37.0X5	T37.0X6
Sulfapyrimidine	T37.0X1	T37.0X2	T37.0X3	T37.0X4	T37.0X5	T37.0X6
Sulfarsphenamine	T37.8X1	T37.8X2	T37.8X3	T37.8X4	T37.8X5	T37.8X6
Sulfasalazine	T37.0X1	T37.0X2	T37.0X3	T37.0X4	T37.0X5	T37.0X6
Sulfasuxidine	T37.0X1	T37.0X2	T37.0X3	T37.0X4	T37.0X5	T37.0X6
Sulfasymazine	T37.0X1	T37.0X2	T37.0X3	T37.0X4	T37.0X5	T37.0X6
Sulfated amylopectin	T47.8X1	T47.8X2	T47.8X3	T47.8X4	T47.8X5	T47.8X6
Sulfathiazole	T37.0X1	T37.0X2	T37.0X3	T37.0X4	T37.0X5	T37.0X6
Sulfatostearate	T49.2X1	T49.2X2	T49.2X3	T49.2X4	T49.2X5	T49.2X6
Sulfinpyrazone	T50.4X1	T50.4X2	T50.4X3	T50.4X4	T50.4X5	T50.4X6
Sulfiram	T49.0X1	T49.0X2	T49.0X3	T49.0X4	T49.0X5	T49.0X6
Sulfisomidine	T37.0X1	T37.0X2	T37.0X3	T37.0X4	T37.0X5	T37.0X6
Sulfisoxazole	T37.0X1	T37.0X2	T37.0X3	T37.0X4	T37.0X5	T37.0X6
ophthalmic preparation	T49.5X1	T49.5X2	T49.5X3	T49.5X4	T49.5X5	T49.5X6
Sulfobromophthalein (sodium)	T50.8X1	T50.8X2	T50.8X3	T50.8X4	T50.8X5	T50.8X6
Sulfobromphthalein	T50.8X1	T50.8X2	T50.8X3	T50.8X4	T50.8X5	T50.8X6
Sulfogaiacol	T48.4X1	T48.4X2	T48.4X3	T48.4X4	T48.4X5	T48.4X6
Sulfomyxin	T36.8X1	T36.8X2	T36.8X3	T36.8X4	T36.8X5	T36.8X6
Sulfonal	T42.6X1	T42.6X2	T42.6X3	T42.6X4	T42.6X5	T42.6X6
Sulfonamide NEC	T37.0X1	T37.0X2	T37.0X3	T37.0X4	T37.0X5	T37.0X6
eye	T49.5X1	T49.5X2	T49.5X3	T49.5X4	T49.5X5	T49.5X6
Sulfonazide	T37.1X1	T37.1X2	T37.1X3	T37.1X4	T37.1X5	T37.1X6
Sulfones	T37.1X1	T37.1X2	T37.1X3	T37.1X4	T37.1X5	T37.1X6
Sulfonethylmethane	T42.6X1	T42.6X2	T42.6X3	T42.6X4	T42.6X5	T42.6X6

Substance	Poisoning, Accidental (unintentional)	Poisoning, Intentional Self-harm	Poisoning, Assault	Poisoning, Undetermined	Adverse effect	Underdosing
Sulfonmethane	T42.6X1	T42.6X2	T42.6X3	T42.6X4	T42.6X5	T42.6X6
Sulfonphthal, sulfonphthol	T50.8X1	T50.8X2	T50.8X3	T50.8X4	T50.8X5	T50.8X6
Sulfonylurea derivatives, oral	T38.3X1	T38.3X2	T38.3X3	T38.3X4	T38.3X5	T38.3X6
Sulforidazine	T43.3X1	T43.3X2	T43.3X3	T43.3X4	T43.3X5	T43.3X6
Sulfoxone	T37.1X1	T37.1X2	T37.1X3	T37.1X4	T37.1X5	T37.1X6
Sulfur, sulfurated, sulfuric, sulfurous, sulfuryl (compounds NEC) (medicinal)	T49.4X1	T49.4X2	T49.4X3	T49.4X4	T49.4X5	T49.4X6
acid	T54.2X1	T54.2X2	T54.2X3	T54.2X4	--	--
dioxide (gas)	T59.1X1	T59.1X2	T59.1X3	T59.1X4	--	--
ether—see Ether (s)						
hydrogen	T59.6X1	T59.6X2	T59.6X3	T59.6X4	--	--
medicinal (keratolytic) (ointment) NEC	T49.4X1	T49.4X2	T49.4X3	T49.4X4	T49.4X5	T49.4X6
ointment	T49.0X1	T49.0X2	T49.0X3	T49.0X4	T49.0X5	T49.0X6
pesticide (vapor)	T60.91	T60.92	T60.93	T60.94	--	--
vapor NEC	T59.891	T59.892	T59.893	T59.894	--	--
Sulfuric acid	T54.2X1	T54.2X2	T54.2X3	T54.2X4	--	--
Sulglicotide	T47.1X1	T47.1X2	T47.1X3	T47.1X4	T47.1X5	T47.1X6
Sulindac	T39.391	T39.392	T39.393	T39.394	T39.395	T39.396
Sulisatin	T47.2X1	T47.2X2	T47.2X3	T47.2X4	T47.2X5	T47.2X6
Sulisobenzone	T49.3X1	T49.3X2	T49.3X3	T49.3X4	T49.3X5	T49.3X6
Sulkowitch's reagent	T50.8X1	T50.8X2	T50.8X3	T50.8X4	T50.8X5	T50.8X6
Sulmetozine	T44.3X1	T44.3X2	T44.3X3	T44.3X4	T44.3X5	T44.3X6
Suloctidil	T46.7X1	T46.7X2	T46.7X3	T46.7X4	T46.7X5	T46.7X6
Sulph—see also Sulf-						
Sulphadiazine	T37.0X1	T37.0X2	T37.0X3	T37.0X4	T37.0X5	T37.0X6
Sulphadimethoxine	T37.0X1	T37.0X2	T37.0X3	T37.0X4	T37.0X5	T37.0X6
Sulphadimidine	T37.0X1	T37.0X2	T37.0X3	T37.0X4	T37.0X5	T37.0X6
Sulphadione	T37.1X1	T37.1X2	T37.1X3	T37.1X4	T37.1X5	T37.1X6
Sulphafurazole	T37.0X1	T37.0X2	T37.0X3	T37.0X4	T37.0X5	T37.0X6
Sulphamethizole	T37.0X1	T37.0X2	T37.0X3	T37.0X4	T37.0X5	T37.0X6
Sulphamethoxazole	T37.0X1	T37.0X2	T37.0X3	T37.0X4	T37.0X5	T37.0X6
Sulphan blue	T50.8X1	T50.8X2	T50.8X3	T50.8X4	T50.8X5	T50.8X6
Sulphaphenazole	T37.0X1	T37.0X2	T37.0X3	T37.0X4	T37.0X5	T37.0X6
Sulphapyridine	T37.0X1	T37.0X2	T37.0X3	T37.0X4	T37.0X5	T37.0X6
Sulphasalazine	T37.0X1	T37.0X2	T37.0X3	T37.0X4	T37.0X5	T37.0X6
Sulphinpyrazone	T50.4X1	T50.4X2	T50.4X3	T50.4X4	T50.4X5	T50.4X6
Sulpiride	T43.591	T43.592	T43.593	T43.594	T43.595	T43.596
Sulprostone	T48.0X1	T48.0X2	T48.0X3	T48.0X4	T48.0X5	T48.0X6
Sulpyrine	T39.2X1	T39.2X2	T39.2X3	T39.2X4	T39.2X5	T39.2X6
Sultamicillin	T36.0X1	T36.0X2	T36.0X3	T36.0X4	T36.0X5	T36.0X6
Sulthiame	T42.6X1	T42.6X2	T42.6X3	T42.6X4	T42.6X5	T42.6X6
Sultiame	T42.6X1	T42.6X2	T42.6X3	T42.6X4	T42.6X5	T42.6X6
Sultopride	T43.591	T43.592	T43.593	T43.594	T43.595	T43.596
Sumatriptan	T39.8X1	T39.8X2	T39.8X3	T39.8X4	T39.8X5	T39.8X6
Sunflower seed oil	T46.6X1	T46.6X2	T46.6X3	T46.6X4	T46.6X5	T46.6X6
Superinone	T48.4X1	T48.4X2	T48.4X3	T48.4X4	T48.4X5	T48.4X6
Suprofen	T39.311	T39.312	T39.313	T39.314	T39.315	T39.316
Suramin (sodium)	T37.4X1	T37.4X2	T37.4X3	T37.4X4	T37.4X5	T37.4X6
Surfacaine	T41.3X1	T41.3X2	T41.3X3	T41.3X4	T41.3X5	T41.3X6
Surital	T41.1X1	T41.1X2	T41.1X3	T41.1X4	T41.1X5	T41.1X6
Sutilains	T45.3X1	T45.3X2	T45.3X3	T45.3X4	T45.3X5	T45.3X6
Suxamethonium (chloride)	T48.1X1	T48.1X2	T48.1X3	T48.1X4	T48.1X5	T48.1X6
Suxethonium (chloride)	T48.1X1	T48.1X2	T48.1X3	T48.1X4	T48.1X5	T48.1X6
Suxibuzone	T39.2X1	T39.2X2	T39.2X3	T39.2X4	T39.2X5	T39.2X6
Sweet niter spirit	T46.3X1	T46.3X2	T46.3X3	T46.3X4	T46.3X5	T46.3X6
Sweet oil (birch)	T49.3X1	T49.3X2	T49.3X3	T49.3X4	T49.3X5	T49.3X6
Sweetener	T50.901	T50.902	T50.903	T50.904	T50.905	T50.906
Sym-dichloroethyl ether	T53.6X1	T53.6X2	T53.6X3	T53.6X4	--	--
Sympatholytic NEC	T44.8X1	T44.8X2	T44.8X3	T44.8X4	T44.8X5	T44.8X6
haloalkylamine	T44.8X1	T44.8X2	T44.8X3	T44.8X4	T44.8X5	T44.8X6
Sympathomimetic NEC	T44.901	T44.902	T44.903	T44.904	T44.905	T44.906
anti-common-cold	T48.5X1	T48.5X2	T48.5X3	T48.5X4	T48.5X5	T48.5X6
bronchodilator	T48.6X1	T48.6X2	T48.6X3	T48.6X4	T48.6X5	T48.6X6
specified NEC	T44.991	T44.992	T44.993	T44.994	T44.995	T44.996

Substance	Poisoning, Accidental (unintentional)	Poisoning, Intentional Self-harm	Poisoning, Assault	Poisoning, Undetermined	Adverse effect	Underdosing
Synagis	T50.B91	T50.B92	T50.B93	T50.B94	T50.B95	T50.B96
Synalar	T49.0X1	T49.0X2	T49.0X3	T49.0X4	T49.0X5	T49.0X6
Synthroid	T38.1X1	T38.1X2	T38.1X3	T38.1X4	T38.1X5	T38.1X6
Syntocinon	T48.0X1	T48.0X2	T48.0X3	T48.0X4	T48.0X5	T48.0X6
Syrosingopine	T46.5X1	T46.5X2	T46.5X3	T46.5X4	T46.5X5	T46.5X6
Systemic drug	T45.91	T45.92	T45.93	T45.94	T45.95	T45.96
specified NEC	T45.8X1	T45.8X2	T45.8X3	T45.8X4	T45.8X5	T45.8X6
2,4,5-T	T60.3X1	T60.3X2	T60.3X3	T60.3X4	--	--
Tablets—see also specified substance	T50.901	T50.902	T50.903	T50.904	T50.905	T50.906
Tace	T38.5X1	T38.5X2	T38.5X3	T38.5X4	T38.5X5	T38.5X6
Tacrine	T44.0X1	T44.0X2	T44.0X3	T44.0X4	T44.0X5	T44.0X6
Tadalafil	T46.7X1	T46.7X2	T46.7X3	T46.7X4	T46.7X5	T46.7X6
Talampicillin	T36.0X1	T36.0X2	T36.0X3	T36.0X4	T36.0X5	T36.0X6
Talbutal	T42.3X1	T42.3X2	T42.3X3	T42.3X4	T42.3X5	T42.3X6
Talc powder	T49.3X1	T49.3X2	T49.3X3	T49.3X4	T49.3X5	T49.3X6
Talcum	T49.3X1	T49.3X2	T49.3X3	T49.3X4	T49.3X5	T49.3X6
Taleranol	T38.6X1	T38.6X2	T38.6X3	T38.6X4	T38.6X5	T38.6X6
Tamoxifen	T38.6X1	T38.6X2	T38.6X3	T38.6X4	T38.6X5	T38.6X6
Tamsulosin	T44.6X1	T44.6X2	T44.6X3	T44.6X4	T44.6X5	T44.6X6
Tandearil, tanderil	T39.2X1	T39.2X2	T39.2X3	T39.2X4	T39.2X5	T39.2X6
Tannic acid	T49.2X1	T49.2X2	T49.2X3	T49.2X4	T49.2X5	T49.2X6
medicinal (astringent)	T49.2X1	T49.2X2	T49.2X3	T49.2X4	T49.2X5	T49.2X6
Tannin—see Tannic acid						
Tansy	T62.2X1	T62.2X2	T62.2X3	T62.2X4	--	--
TAO	T36.3X1	T36.3X2	T36.3X3	T36.3X4	T36.3X5	T36.3X6
Tapazole	T38.2X1	T38.2X2	T38.2X3	T38.2X4	T38.2X5	T38.2X6
Tar NEC	T52.0X1	T52.0X2	T52.0X3	T52.0X4	--	--
camphor	T60.1X1	T60.1X2	T60.1X3	T60.1X4	--	--
distillate	T49.1X1	T49.1X2	T49.1X3	T49.1X4	T49.1X5	T49.1X6
fumes	T59.891	T59.892	T59.893	T59.894	--	--
medicinal	T49.1X1	T49.1X2	T49.1X3	T49.1X4	T49.1X5	T49.1X6
ointment	T49.1X1	T49.1X2	T49.1X3	T49.1X4	T49.1X5	T49.1X6
Taractan	T43.591	T43.592	T43.593	T43.594	T43.595	T43.596
Tarantula (venomous)	T63.321	T63.322	T63.323	T63.324	--	--
Tartar emetic	T37.8X1	T37.8X2	T37.8X3	T37.8X4	T37.8X5	T37.8X6
Tartaric acid	T65.891	T65.892	T65.893	T65.894	--	--
Tartrate, laxative	T47.4X1	T47.4X2	T47.4X3	T47.4X4	T47.4X5	T47.4X6
Tartrated antimony (anti-infective)	T37.8X1	T37.8X2	T37.8X3	T37.8X4	T37.8X5	T37.8X6
Tauromustine	T45.1X1	T45.1X2	T45.1X3	T45.1X4	T45.1X5	T45.1X6
TCA—see Trichloroacetic acid						
TCDD	T53.7X1	T53.7X2	T53.7X3	T53.7X4	--	--
TDI (vapor)	T65.0X1	T65.0X2	T65.0X3	T65.0X4	--	--
Tear						
gas	T59.3X1	T59.3X2	T59.3X3	T59.3X4	--	--
solution	T49.5X1	T49.5X2	T49.5X3	T49.5X4	T49.5X5	T49.5X6
Teclothiazide	T50.2X1	T50.2X2	T50.2X3	T50.2X4	T50.2X5	T50.2X6
Teclozan	T37.3X1	T37.3X2	T37.3X3	T37.3X4	T37.3X5	T37.3X6
Tegafur	T45.1X1	T45.1X2	T45.1X3	T45.1X4	T45.1X5	T45.1X6
Tegretol	T42.1X1	T42.1X2	T42.1X3	T42.1X4	T42.1X5	T42.1X6
Teicoplanin	T36.8X1	T36.8X2	T36.8X3	T36.8X4	T36.8X5	T36.8X6
Telepaque	T50.8X1	T50.8X2	T50.8X3	T50.8X4	T50.8X5	T50.8X6
Tellurium	T56.891	T56.892	T56.893	T56.894	--	--
fumes	T56.891	T56.892	T56.893	T56.894	--	--
TEM	T45.1X1	T45.1X2	T45.1X3	T45.1X4	T45.1X5	T45.1X6
Temazepam	T42.4X1	T42.4X2	T42.4X3	T42.4X4	T42.4X5	T42.4X6
Temocillin	T36.0X1	T36.0X2	T36.0X3	T36.0X4	T36.0X5	T36.0X6
Tenamfetamine	T43.621	T43.622	T43.623	T43.624	T43.625	T43.626
Teniposide	T45.1X1	T45.1X2	T45.1X3	T45.1X4	T45.1X5	T45.1X6
Tenitramine	T46.3X1	T46.3X2	T46.3X3	T46.3X4	T46.3X5	T46.3X6
Tenoglicin	T48.4X1	T48.4X2	T48.4X3	T48.4X4	T48.4X5	T48.4X6
Tenonitrozole	T37.3X1	T37.3X2	T37.3X3	T37.3X4	T37.3X5	T37.3X6
Tenoxicam	T39.391	T39.392	T39.393	T39.394	T39.395	T39.396
TEPA	T45.1X1	T45.1X2	T45.1X3	T45.1X4	T45.1X5	T45.1X6
TEPP	T60.0X1	T60.0X2	T60.0X3	T60.0X4	--	--
Teprotide	T46.5X1	T46.5X2	T46.5X3	T46.5X4	T46.5X5	T46.5X6

Substance	Poisoning, Accidental (unintentional)	Poisoning, Intentional Self-harm	Poisoning, Assault	Poisoning, Undetermined	Adverse effect	Underdosing
Terazosin	T44.6X1	T44.6X2	T44.6X3	T44.6X4	T44.6X5	T44.6X6
Terbufos	T60.0X1	T60.0X2	T60.0X3	T60.0X4	--	--
Terbutaline	T48.6X1	T48.6X2	T48.6X3	T48.6X4	T48.6X5	T48.6X6
Terconazole	T49.0X1	T49.0X2	T49.0X3	T49.0X4	T49.0X5	T49.0X6
Terfenadine	T45.0X1	T45.0X2	T45.0X3	T45.0X4	T45.0X5	T45.0X6
Teriparatide (acetate)	T50.991	T50.992	T50.993	T50.994	T50.995	T50.996
Terizidone	T37.1X1	T37.1X2	T37.1X3	T37.1X4	T37.1X5	T37.1X6
Terlipressin	T38.891	T38.892	T38.893	T38.894	T38.895	T38.896
Terodiline	T46.3X1	T46.3X2	T46.3X3	T46.3X4	T46.3X5	T46.3X6
Teroxalene	T37.4X1	T37.4X2	T37.4X3	T37.4X4	T37.4X5	T37.4X6
Terpin (cis) hydrate	T48.4X1	T48.4X2	T48.4X3	T48.4X4	T48.4X5	T48.4X6
Terramycin	T36.4X1	T36.4X2	T36.4X3	T36.4X4	T36.4X5	T36.4X6
Tertatolol	T44.7X1	T44.7X2	T44.7X3	T44.7X4	T44.7X5	T44.7X6
Tessalon	T48.3X1	T48.3X2	T48.3X3	T48.3X4	T48.3X5	T48.3X6
Testolactone	T38.7X1	T38.7X2	T38.7X3	T38.7X4	T38.7X5	T38.7X6
Testosterone	T38.7X1	T38.7X2	T38.7X3	T38.7X4	T38.7X5	T38.7X6
Tetanus toxoid or vaccine	T50.A91	T50.A92	T50.A93	T50.A94	T50.A95	T50.A96
antitoxin	T50.Z11	T50.Z12	T50.Z13	T50.Z14	T50.Z15	T50.Z16
immune globulin (human)	T50.Z11	T50.Z12	T50.Z13	T50.Z14	T50.Z15	T50.Z16
toxoid	T50.A91	T50.A92	T50.A93	T50.A94	T50.A95	T50.A96
with diphtheria toxoid	T50.A21	T50.A22	T50.A23	T50.A24	T50.A25	T50.A26
with pertussis	T50.A11	T50.A12	T50.A13	T50.A14	T50.A15	T50.A16
Tetrabenazine	T43.591	T43.592	T43.593	T43.594	T43.595	T43.596
Tetracaine	T41.3X1	T41.3X2	T41.3X3	T41.3X4	T41.3X5	T41.3X6
nerve block (peripheral) (plexus)	T41.3X1	T41.3X2	T41.3X3	T41.3X4	T41.3X5	T41.3X6
regional	T41.3X1	T41.3X2	T41.3X3	T41.3X4	T41.3X5	T41.3X6
spinal	T41.3X1	T41.3X2	T41.3X3	T41.3X4	T41.3X5	T41.3X6
Tetrachlorethylene—see Tetrachloroethylene						
Tetrachlormethiazide	T50.2X1	T50.2X2	T50.2X3	T50.2X4	T50.2X5	T50.2X6
2,3,7,8-Tetrachlorodibenzo-p-dioxin	T53.7X1	T53.7X2	T53.7X3	T53.7X4	--	--
Tetrachloroethane	T53.6X1	T53.6X2	T53.6X3	T53.6X4	--	--
vapor	T53.6X1	T53.6X2	T53.6X3	T53.6X4	--	--
paint or varnish	T53.6X1	T53.6X2	T53.6X3	T53.6X4	--	--
Tetrachloroethylene (liquid)	T53.3X1	T53.3X2	T53.3X3	T53.3X4	--	--
medicinal	T37.4X1	T37.4X2	T37.4X3	T37.4X4	T37.4X5	T37.4X6
vapor	T53.3X1	T53.3X2	T53.3X3	T53.3X4	--	--
Tetrachloromethane—see Carbon tetrachloride						
Tetracosactide	T38.811	T38.812	T38.813	T38.814	T38.815	T38.816
Tetracosactrin	T38.811	T38.812	T38.813	T38.814	T38.815	T38.816
Tetracycline	T36.4X1	T36.4X2	T36.4X3	T36.4X4	T36.4X5	T36.4X6
ophthalmic preparation	T49.5X1	T49.5X2	T49.5X3	T49.5X4	T49.5X5	T49.5X6
topical NEC	T49.0X1	T49.0X2	T49.0X3	T49.0X4	T49.0X5	T49.0X6
Tetradifon	T60.8X1	T60.8X2	T60.8X3	T60.8X4	--	--
Tetradotoxin	T61.771	T61.772	T61.773	T61.774	--	--
Tetraethyl						
lead	T56.0X1	T56.0X2	T56.0X3	T56.0X4	--	--
pyrophosphate	T60.0X1	T60.0X2	T60.0X3	T60.0X4	--	--
Tetraethylammonium chloride	T44.2X1	T44.2X2	T44.2X3	T44.2X4	T44.2X5	T44.2X6
Tetraethylthiuram disulfide	T50.6X1	T50.6X2	T50.6X3	T50.6X4	T50.6X5	T50.6X6
Tetrahydroaminoacridine	T44.0X1	T44.0X2	T44.0X3	T44.0X4	T44.0X5	T44.0X6
Tetrahydrocannabinol	T40.7X1	T40.7X2	T40.7X3	T40.7X4	T40.7X5	T40.7X6
Tetrahydrofuran	T52.8X1	T52.8X2	T52.8X3	T52.8X4	--	--
Tetrahydronaphthalene	T52.8X1	T52.8X2	T52.8X3	T52.8X4	--	--
Tetrahydrozoline	T49.5X1	T49.5X2	T49.5X3	T49.5X4	T49.5X5	T49.5X6
Tetralin	T52.8X1	T52.8X2	T52.8X3	T52.8X4	--	--
Tetramethrin	T60.2X1	T60.2X2	T60.2X3	T60.2X4	--	--
Tetramethylthiuram (disulfide) NEC	T60.3X1	T60.3X2	T60.3X3	T60.3X4	--	--
medicinal	T49.0X1	T49.0X2	T49.0X3	T49.0X4	T49.0X5	T49.0X6
Tetramisole	T37.4X1	T37.4X2	T37.4X3	T37.4X4	T37.4X5	T37.4X6
Tetranicotinoyl fructose	T46.7X1	T46.7X2	T46.7X3	T46.7X4	T46.7X5	T46.7X6
Tetrazepam	T42.4X1	T42.4X2	T42.4X3	T42.4X4	T42.4X5	T42.4X6
Tetronal	T42.6X1	T42.6X2	T42.6X3	T42.6X4	T42.6X5	T42.6X6
Tetryl	T65.3X1	T65.3X2	T65.3X3	T65.3X4	--	--
Tetrylammonium chloride	T44.2X1	T44.2X2	T44.2X3	T44.2X4	T44.2X5	T44.2X6

Substance	Poisoning, Accidental (unintentional)	Poisoning, Intentional Self-harm	Poisoning, Assault	Poisoning, Undetermined	Adverse effect	Underdosing
Tetryzoline	T49.5X1	T49.5X2	T49.5X3	T49.5X4	T49.5X5	T49.5X6
Thalidomide	T45.1X1	T45.1X2	T45.1X3	T45.1X4	T45.1X5	T45.1X6
Thallium (compounds) (dust) NEC	T56.811	T56.812	T56.813	T56.814	--	--
pesticide	T60.4X1	T60.4X2	T60.4X3	T60.4X4	--	--
THC	T40.7X1	T40.7X2	T40.7X3	T40.7X4	T40.7X5	T40.7X6
Thebacon	T48.3X1	T48.3X2	T48.3X3	T48.3X4	T48.3X5	T48.3X6
Thebaine	T40.2X1	T40.2X2	T40.2X3	T40.2X4	T40.2X5	T40.2X6
Thenoic acid	T49.6X1	T49.6X2	T49.6X3	T49.6X4	T49.6X5	T49.6X6
Thenyldiamine	T45.0X1	T45.0X2	T45.0X3	T45.0X4	T45.0X5	T45.0X6
Theobromine (calcium salicylate)	T48.6X1	T48.6X2	T48.6X3	T48.6X4	T48.6X5	T48.6X6
sodium salicylate	T48.6X1	T48.6X2	T48.6X3	T48.6X4	T48.6X5	T48.6X6
Theophyllamine	T48.6X1	T48.6X2	T48.6X3	T48.6X4	T48.6X5	T48.6X6
Theophylline	T48.6X1	T48.6X2	T48.6X3	T48.6X4	T48.6X5	T48.6X6
aminobenzoic acid	T48.6X1	T48.6X2	T48.6X3	T48.6X4	T48.6X5	T48.6X6
ethylenediamine	T48.6X1	T48.6X2	T48.6X3	T48.6X4	T48.6X5	T48.6X6
piperazine p-amino-benzoate	T48.6X1	T48.6X2	T48.6X3	T48.6X4	T48.6X5	T48.6X6
Thiabendazole	T37.4X1	T37.4X2	T37.4X3	T37.4X4	T37.4X5	T37.4X6
Thialbarbital	T41.1X1	T41.1X2	T41.1X3	T41.1X4	T41.1X5	T41.1X6
Thiamazole	T38.2X1	T38.2X2	T38.2X3	T38.2X4	T38.2X5	T38.2X6
Thiambutosine	T37.1X1	T37.1X2	T37.1X3	T37.1X4	T37.1X5	T37.1X6
Thiamine	T45.2X1	T45.2X2	T45.2X3	T45.2X4	T45.2X5	T45.2X6
Thiamphenicol	T36.2X1	T36.2X2	T36.2X3	T36.2X4	T36.2X5	T36.2X6
Thiamylal	T41.1X1	T41.1X2	T41.1X3	T41.1X4	T41.1X5	T41.1X6
sodium	T41.1X1	T41.1X1	T41.1X3	T41.1X4	T41.1X5	T41.1X6
Thiazesim	T43.291	T43.292	T43.293	T43.294	T43.295	T43.296
Thiazides (diuretics)	T50.2X1	T50.2X2	T50.2X3	T50.2X4	T50.2X5	T50.2X6
Thiazinamium metilsulfate	T43.3X1	T43.3X2	T43.3X3	T43.3X4	T43.3X5	T43.3X6
Thiethylperazine	T43.3X1	T43.3X2	T43.3X3	T43.3X4	T43.3X5	T43.3X6
Thimerosal	T49.0X1	T49.0X2	T49.0X3	T49.0X4	T49.0X5	T49.0X6
ophthalmic preparation	T49.5X1	T49.5X2	T49.5X3	T49.5X4	T49.5X5	T49.5X6
Thioacetazone	T37.1X1	T37.1X2	T37.1X3	T37.1X4	T37.1X5	T37.1X6
with isoniazid	T37.1X1	T37.1X2	T37.1X3	T37.1X4	T37.1X5	T37.1X6
Thiobarbital sodium	T41.1X1	T41.1X2	T41.1X3	T41.1X4	T41.1X5	T41.1X6
Thiobarbiturate anesthetic	T41.1X1	T41.1X2	T41.1X3	T41.1X4	T41.1X5	T41.1X6
Thiobismol	T37.8X1	T37.8X2	T37.8X3	T37.8X4	T37.8X5	T37.8X6
Thiobutabarbital sodium	T41.1X1	T41.1X2	T41.1X3	T41.1X4	T41.1X5	T41.1X6
Thiocarbamate (insecticide)	T60.0X1	T60.0X2	T60.0X3	T60.0X4	--	--
Thiocarbamide	T38.2X1	T38.2X2	T38.2X3	T38.2X4	T38.2X5	T38.2X6
Thiocarbarsone	T37.8X1	T37.8X2	T37.8X3	T37.8X4	T37.8X5	T37.8X6
Thiocarlide	T37.1X1	T37.1X2	T37.1X3	T37.1X4	T37.1X5	T37.1X6
Thioctamide	T50.991	T50.992	T50.993	T50.994	T50.995	T50.996
Thioctic acid	T50.991	T50.992	T50.993	T50.994	T50.995	T50.996
Thiofos	T60.0X1	T60.0X2	T60.0X3	T60.0X4	--	--
Thioglycolate	T49.4X1	T49.4X2	T49.4X3	T49.4X4	T49.4X5	T49.4X6
Thioglycolic acid	T65.891	T65.892	T65.893	T65.894	--	--
Thioguanine	T45.1X1	T45.1X2	T45.1X3	T45.1X4	T45.1X5	T45.1X6
Thiomercaptomerin	T50.2X1	T50.2X2	T50.2X3	T50.2X4	T50.2X5	T50.2X6
Thiomerin	T50.2X1	T50.2X2	T50.2X3	T50.2X4	T50.2X5	T50.2X6
Thiomersal	T49.0X1	T49.0X2	T49.0X3	T49.0X4	T49.0X5	T49.0X6
Thionazin	T60.0X1	T60.0X2	T60.0X3	T60.0X4	--	--
Thiopental (sodium)	T41.1X1	T41.1X2	T41.1X3	T41.1X4	T41.1X5	T41.1X6
Thiopentone (sodium)	T41.1X1	T41.1X2	T41.1X3	T41.1X4	T41.1X5	T41.1X6
Thiopropazate	T43.3X1	T43.3X2	T43.3X3	T43.3X4	T43.3X5	T43.3X6
Thioproperazine	T43.3X1	T43.3X2	T43.3X3	T43.3X4	T43.3X5	T43.3X6
Thioridazine	T43.3X1	T43.3X2	T43.3X3	T43.3X4	T43.3X5	T43.3X6
Thiosinamine	T49.3X1	T49.3X2	T49.3X3	T49.3X4	T49.3X5	T49.3X6
Thiotepa	T45.1X1	T45.1X2	T45.1X3	T45.1X4	T45.1X5	T45.1X6
Thiothixene	T43.4X1	T43.4X2	T43.4X3	T43.4X4	T43.4X5	T43.4X6
Thiouracil (benzyl) (methyl) (propyl)	T38.2X1	T38.2X2	T38.2X3	T38.2X4	T38.2X5	T38.2X6
Thiourea	T38.2X1	T38.2X2	T38.2X3	T38.2X4	T38.2X5	T38.2X6
Thiphenamil	T44.3X1	T44.3X2	T44.3X3	T44.3X4	T44.3X5	T44.3X6
Thiram	T60.3X1	T60.3X2	T60.3X3	T60.3X4	--	--
medicinal	T49.2X1	T49.2X2	T49.2X3	T49.2X4	T49.2X5	T49.2X6
Thonzylamine (systemic)	T45.0X1	T45.0X2	T45.0X3	T45.0X4	T45.0X5	T45.0X6
mucosal decongestant	T48.5X1	T48.5X2	T48.5X3	T48.5X4	T48.5X5	T48.5X6

Substance	Poisoning, Accidental (unintentional)	Poisoning, Intentional Self-harm	Poisoning, Assault	Poisoning, Undetermined	Adverse effect	Underdosing
Thorazine	T43.3X1	T43.3X2	T43.3X3	T43.3X4	T43.3X5	T43.3X6
Thorium dioxide suspension	T50.8X1	T50.8X2	T50.8X3	T50.8X4	T50.8X5	T50.8X6
Thornapple	T62.2X1	T62.2X2	T62.2X3	T62.2X4	--	--
Throat drug NEC	T49.6X1	T49.6X2	T49.6X3	T49.6X4	T49.6X5	T49.6X6
Thrombin	T45.7X1	T45.7X2	T45.7X3	T45.7X4	T45.7X5	T45.7X6
Thrombolysin	T45.611	T45.612	T45.613	T45.614	T45.615	T45.616
Thromboplastin	T45.7X1	T45.7X2	T45.7X3	T45.7X4	T45.7X5	T45.7X6
Thurfyl nicotinate	T46.7X1	T46.7X2	T46.7X3	T46.7X4	T46.7X5	T46.7X6
Thymol	T49.0X1	T49.0X2	T49.0X3	T49.0X4	T49.0X5	T49.0X6
Thymopentin	T37.5X1	T37.5X2	T37.5X3	T37.5X4	T37.5X5	T37.5X6
Thymoxamine	T46.7X1	T46.7X2	T46.7X3	T46.7X4	T46.7X5	T46.7X6
Thymus extract	T38.891	T38.892	T38.893	T38.894	T38.895	T38.896
Thyreotrophic hormone	T38.811	T38.812	T38.813	T38.814	T38.815	T38.816
Thyroglobulin	T38.1X1	T38.1X2	T38.1X3	T38.1X4	T38.1X5	T38.1X6
Thyroid (hormone)	T38.1X1	T38.1X2	T38.1X3	T38.1X4	T38.1X5	T38.1X6
Thyrolar	T38.1X1	T38.1X2	T38.1X3	T38.1X4	T38.1X5	T38.1X6
Thyrotrophin	T38.811	T38.812	T38.813	T38.814	T38.815	T38.816
Thyrotropic hormone	T38.811	T38.812	T38.813	T38.814	T38.815	T38.816
Thyroxine	T38.1X1	T38.1X2	T38.1X3	T38.1X4	T38.1X5	T38.1X6
Tiabendazole	T37.4X1	T37.4X2	T37.4X3	T37.4X4	T37.4X5	T37.4X6
Tiamizide	T50.2X1	T50.2X2	T50.2X3	T50.2X4	T50.2X5	T50.2X6
Tianeptine	T43.291	T43.292	T43.293	T43.294	T43.295	T43.296
Tiapamil	T46.1X1	T46.1X2	T46.1X3	T46.1X4	T46.1X5	T46.1X6
Tiapride	T43.591	T43.592	T43.593	T43.594	T43.595	T43.596
Tiaprofenic acid	T39.311	T39.312	T39.313	T39.314	T39.315	T39.316
Tiaramide	T39.8X1	T39.8X2	T39.8X3	T39.8X4	T39.8X5	T39.8X6
Ticarcillin	T36.0X1	T36.0X2	T36.0X3	T36.0X4	T36.0X5	T36.0X6
Ticlatone	T49.0X1	T49.0X2	T49.0X3	T49.0X4	T49.0X5	T49.0X6
Ticlopidine	T45.521	T45.522	T45.523	T45.524	T45.525	T45.526
Ticrynafen	T50.1X1	T50.1X2	T50.1X3	T50.1X4	T50.1X5	T50.1X6
Tidiacic	T50.991	T50.992	T50.993	T50.994	T50.995	T50.996
Tiemonium	T44.3X1	T44.3X2	T44.3X3	T44.3X4	T44.3X5	T44.3X6
iodide	T44.3X1	T44.3X2	T44.3X3	T44.3X4	T44.3X5	T44.3X6
Tienilic acid	T50.1X1	T50.1X2	T50.1X3	T50.1X4	T50.1X5	T50.1X6
Tifenamil	T44.3X1	T44.3X2	T44.3X3	T44.3X4	T44.3X5	T44.3X6
Tigan	T45.0X1	T45.0X2	T45.0X3	T45.0X4	T45.0X5	T45.0X6
Tigloidine	T44.3X1	T44.3X2	T44.3X3	T44.3X4	T44.3X5	T44.3X6
Tilactase	T47.5X1	T47.5X2	T47.5X3	T47.5X4	T47.5X5	T47.5X6
Tiletamine	T41.291	T41.292	T41.293	T41.294	T41.295	T41.296
Tilidine	T40.4X1	T40.4X2	T40.4X3	T40.4X4	--	--
Timepidium bromide	T44.3X1	T44.3X2	T44.3X3	T44.3X4	T44.3X5	T44.3X6
Timiperone	T43.4X1	T43.4X2	T43.4X3	T43.4X4	T43.4X5	T43.4X6
Timolol	T44.7X1	T44.7X2	T44.7X3	T44.7X4	T44.7X5	T44.7X6
Tin (chloride) (dust) (oxide) NEC	T56.6X1	T56.6X2	T56.6X3	T56.6X4	--	--
anti-infectives	T37.8X1	T37.8X2	T37.8X3	T37.8X4	T37.8X5	T37.8X6
Tincture, iodine—see Iodine						
Tindal	T43.3X1	T43.3X2	T43.3X3	T43.3X4	T43.3X5	T43.3X6
Tinidazole	T37.3X1	T37.3X2	T37.3X3	T37.3X4	T37.3X5	T37.3X6
Tinoridine	T39.8X1	T39.8X2	T39.8X3	T39.8X4	T39.8X5	T39.8X6
Tiocarlide	T37.1X1	T37.1X2	T37.1X3	T37.1X4	T37.1X5	T37.1X6
Tioclomarol	T45.511	T45.512	T45.513	T45.514	T45.515	T45.516
Tioconazole	T49.0X1	T49.0X2	T49.0X3	T49.0X4	T49.0X5	T49.0X6
Tioguanine	T45.1X1	T45.1X2	T45.1X3	T45.1X4	T45.1X5	T45.1X6
Tiopronin	T50.991	T50.992	T50.993	T50.994	T50.995	T50.996
Tiotixene	T43.4X1	T43.4X2	T43.4X3	T43.4X4	T43.4X5	T43.4X6
Tioxolone	T49.4X1	T49.4X2	T49.4X3	T49.4X4	T49.4X5	T49.4X6
Tipepidine	T48.3X1	T48.3X2	T48.3X3	T48.3X4	T48.3X5	T48.3X6
Tiquizium bromide	T44.3X1	T44.3X2	T44.3X3	T44.3X4	T44.3X5	T44.3X6
Tiratricol	T38.1X1	T38.1X2	T38.1X3	T38.1X4	T38.1X5	T38.1X6
Tisopurine	T50.4X1	T50.4X2	T50.4X3	T50.4X4	T50.4X5	T50.4X6
Titanium (compounds) (vapor)	T56.891	T56.892	T56.893	T56.894	--	--
dioxide	T49.3X1	T49.3X2	T49.3X3	T49.3X4	T49.3X5	T49.3X6
ointment	T49.3X1	T49.3X2	T49.3X3	T49.3X4	T49.3X5	T49.3X6
oxide	T49.3X1	T49.3X2	T49.3X3	T49.3X4	T49.3X5	T49.3X6

Substance	Poisoning, Accidental (unintentional)	Poisoning, Intentional Self-harm	Poisoning, Assault	Poisoning, Undetermined	Adverse effect	Underdosing
tetrachloride	T56.891	T56.892	T56.893	T56.894	--	--
Titanocene	T56.891	T56.892	T56.893	T56.894	--	--
Titroid	T38.1X1	T38.1X2	T38.1X3	T38.1X4	T38.1X5	T38.1X6
Tizanidine	T42.8X1	T42.8X2	T42.8X3	T42.8X4	T42.8X5	T42.8X6
TMTD	T60.3X1	T60.3X2	T60.3X3	T60.3X4	--	--
TNT (fumes)	T65.3X1	T65.3X2	T65.3X3	T65.3X4	--	--
Toadstool	T62.0X1	T62.0X2	T62.0X3	T62.0X4	--	--
Tobacco NEC	T65.291	T65.292	T65.293	T65.294	--	--
cigarettes	T65.221	T65.222	T65.223	T65.224	--	--
Indian	T62.2X1	T62.2X2	T62.2X3	T62.2X4	--	--
smoke, second-hand	T65.221	T65.222	T65.223	T65.224	--	--
Tobramycin	T36.5X1	T36.5X2	T36.5X3	T36.5X4	T36.5X5	T36.5X6
Tocainide	T46.2X1	T46.2X2	T46.2X3	T46.2X4	T46.2X5	T46.2X6
Tocoferol	T45.2X1	T45.2X2	T45.2X3	T45.2X4	T45.2X5	T45.2X6
Tocopherol	T45.2X1	T45.2X2	T45.2X3	T45.2X4	T45.2X5	T45.2X6
acetate	T45.2X1	T45.2X2	T45.2X3	T45.2X4	T45.2X5	T45.2X6
Tocosamine	T48.0X1	T48.0X2	T48.0X3	T48.0X4	T48.0X5	T48.0X6
Todralazine	T46.5X1	T46.5X2	T46.5X3	T46.5X4	T46.5X5	T46.5X6
Tofisopam	T42.4X1	T42.4X2	T42.4X3	T42.4X4	T42.4X5	T42.4X6
Tofranil	T43.011	T43.012	T43.013	T43.014	T43.015	T43.016
Toilet deodorizer	T65.891	T65.892	T65.893	T65.894	--	--
Tolamolol	T44.7X1	T44.7X2	T44.7X3	T44.7X4	T44.7X5	T44.7X6
Tolazamide	T38.3X1	T38.3X2	T38.3X3	T38.3X4	T38.3X5	T38.3X6
Tolazoline	T46.7X1	T46.7X2	T46.7X3	T46.7X4	T46.7X5	T46.7X6
Tolbutamide (sodium)	T38.3X1	T38.3X2	T38.3X3	T38.3X4	T38.3X5	T38.3X6
Tolciclate	T49.0X1	T49.0X2	T49.0X3	T49.0X4	T49.0X5	T49.0X6
Tolmetin	T39.391	T39.392	T39.393	T39.394	T39.395	T39.396
Tolnaftate	T49.0X1	T49.0X2	T49.0X3	T49.0X4	T49.0X5	T49.0X6
Tolonidine	T46.5X1	T46.5X2	T46.5X3	T46.5X4	T46.5X5	T46.5X6
Toloxatone	T42.6X1	T42.6X2	T42.6X3	T42.6X4	T42.6X5	T42.6X6
Tolperisone	T44.3X1	T44.3X2	T44.3X3	T44.3X4	T44.3X5	T44.3X6
Tolserol	T42.8X1	T42.8X2	T42.8X3	T42.8X4	T42.8X5	T42.8X6
Toluene (liquid)	T52.2X1	T52.2X2	T52.2X3	T52.2X4	--	--
diisocyanate	T65.0X1	T65.0X2	T65.0X3	T65.0X4	--	--
Toluidine	T65.891	T65.892	T65.893	T65.894	--	--
vapor	T59.891	T59.892	T59.893	T59.894	--	--
Toluol (liquid)	T52.2X1	T52.2X2	T52.2X3	T52.2X4	--	--
vapor	T52.2X1	T52.2X2	T52.2X3	T52.2X4	--	--
Toluylenediamine	T65.3X1	T65.3X2	T65.3X3	T65.3X4	--	--
Tolylene-2,4-diisocyanate	T65.0X1	T65.0X2	T65.0X3	T65.0X4	--	--
Tonic NEC	T50.901	T50.902	T50.903	T50.904	T50.905	T50.906
Topical action drug NEC	T49.91	T49.92	T49.93	T49.94	T49.95	T49.96
ear, nose or throat	T49.6X1	T49.6X2	T49.6X3	T49.6X4	T49.6X5	T49.6X6
eye	T49.5X1	T49.5X2	T49.5X3	T49.5X4	T49.5X5	T49.5X6
skin	T49.91	T49.92	T49.93	T49.94	T49.95	T49.96
specified NEC	T49.8X1	T49.8X2	T49.8X3	T49.8X4	T49.8X5	T49.8X6
Toquizine	T44.3X1	T44.3X2	T44.3X3	T44.3X4	T44.3X5	T44.3X6
Toremifene	T38.6X1	T38.6X2	T38.6X3	T38.6X4	T38.6X5	T38.6X6
Tosylchloramide sodium	T49.8X1	T49.8X2	T49.8X3	T49.8X4	T49.8X5	T49.8X6
Toxaphene (dust) (spray)	T60.1X1	T60.1X2	T60.1X3	T60.1X4	--	--
Toxin, diphtheria (Schick Test)	T50.8X1	T50.8X2	T50.8X3	T50.8X4	T50.8X5	T50.8X6
Toxoid						
combined	T50.A21	T50.A22	T50.A23	T50.A24	T50.A25	T50.A26
diphtheria	T50.A91	T50.A92	T50.A93	T50.A94	T50.A95	T50.A96
tetanus	T50.A91	T50.A92	T50.A93	T50.A94	T50.A95	T50.A96
Trace element NEC	T45.8X1	T45.8X2	T45.8X3	T45.8X4	T45.8X5	T45.8X6
Tractor fuel NEC	T52.0X1	T52.0X2	T52.0X3	T52.0X4	--	--
Tragacanth	T50.991	T50.992	T50.993	T50.994	T50.995	T50.996
Tramadol	T40.4X1	T40.4X2	T40.4X3	T40.4X4	T40.4X5	T40.4X6
Tramazoline	T48.5X1	T48.5X2	T48.5X3	T48.5X4	T48.5X5	T48.5X6
Tranexamic acid	T45.621	T45.622	T45.623	T45.624	T45.625	T45.626
Tranilast	T45.0X1	T45.0X2	T45.0X3	T45.0X4	T45.0X5	T45.0X6
Tranquilizer NEC	T43.501	T43.502	T43.503	T43.504	T43.505	T43.506
with hypnotic or sedative	T42.6X1	T42.6X2	T42.6X3	T42.6X4	T42.6X5	T42.6X6
benzodiazepine NEC	T42.4X1	T42.4X2	T42.4X3	T42.4X4	T42.4X5	T42.4X6

Substance	Poisoning, Accidental (unintentional)	Poisoning, Intentional Self-harm	Poisoning, Assault	Poisoning, Undetermined	Adverse effect	Underdosing
butyrophenone NEC	T43.4X1	T43.4X2	T43.4X3	T43.4X4	T43.4X5	T43.4X6
carbamate	T43.591	T43.592	T43.593	T43.594	T43.595	T43.596
dimethylamine	T43.3X1	T43.3X2	T43.3X3	T43.3X4	T43.3X5	T43.3X6
ethylamine	T43.3X1	T43.3X2	T43.3X3	T43.3X4	T43.3X5	T43.3X6
hydroxyzine	T43.591	T43.592	T43.593	T43.594	T43.595	T43.596
major NEC	T43.501	T43.502	T43.503	T43.504	T43.505	T43.506
penothiazine NEC	T43.3X1	T43.3X2	T43.3X3	T43.3X4	T43.3X5	T43.3X6
phenothiazine-based	T43.3X1	T43.3X2	T43.3X3	T43.3X4	T43.3X5	T43.3X6
piperazine NEC	T43.3X1	T43.3X2	T43.3X3	T43.3X4	T43.3X5	T43.3X6
piperidine	T43.3X1	T43.3X2	T43.3X3	T43.3X4	T43.3X5	T43.3X6
propylamine	T43.3X1	T43.3X2	T43.3X3	T43.3X4	T43.3X5	T43.3X6
specified NEC	T43.591	T43.592	T43.593	T43.594	T43.595	T43.596
thioxanthene NEC	T43.591	T43.592	T43.593	T43.594	T43.595	T43.596
Tranxene	T42.4X1	T42.4X2	T42.4X3	T42.4X4	T42.4X5	T42.4X6
Tranylcypromine	T43.1X1	T43.1X2	T43.1X3	T43.1X4	T43.1X5	T43.1X6
Trapidil	T46.3X1	T46.3X2	T46.3X3	T46.3X4	T46.3X5	T46.3X6
Trasentine	T44.3X1	T44.3X2	T44.3X3	T44.3X4	T44.3X5	T44.3X6
Travert	T50.3X1	T50.3X2	T50.3X3	T50.3X4	T50.3X5	T50.3X6
Trazodone	T43.211	T43.212	T43.213	T43.214	T43.215	T43.216
Trecator	T37.1X1	T37.1X2	T37.1X3	T37.1X4	T37.1X5	T37.1X6
Treosulfan	T45.1X1	T45.1X2	T45.1X3	T45.1X4	T45.1X5	T45.1X6
Tretamine	T45.1X1	T45.1X2	T45.1X3	T45.1X4	T45.1X5	T45.1X6
Tretinoin	T49.0X1	T49.0X2	T49.0X3	T49.0X4	T49.0X5	T49.0X6
Tretoquinol	T48.6X1	T48.6X2	T48.6X3	T48.6X4	T48.6X5	T48.6X6
Triacetin	T49.0X1	T49.0X2	T49.0X3	T49.0X4	T49.0X5	T49.0X6
Triacetoxyanthracene	T49.4X1	T49.4X2	T49.4X3	T49.4X4	T49.4X5	T49.4X6
Triacetyloleandomycin	T36.3X1	T36.3X2	T36.3X3	T36.3X4	T36.3X5	T36.3X6
Triamcinolone	T49.0X1	T49.0X2	T49.0X3	T49.0X4	T49.0X5	T49.0X6
ENT agent	T49.6X1	T49.6X2	T49.6X3	T49.6X4	T49.6X5	T49.6X6
hexacetonide	T49.0X1	T49.0X2	T49.0X3	T49.0X4	T49.0X5	T49.0X6
ophthalmic preparation	T49.5X1	T49.5X2	T49.5X3	T49.5X4	T49.5X5	T49.5X6
topical NEC	T49.0X1	T49.0X2	T49.0X3	T49.0X4	T49.0X5	T49.0X6
Triampyzine	T44.3X1	T44.3X2	T44.3X3	T44.3X4	T44.3X5	T44.3X6
Triamterene	T50.2X1	T50.2X2	T50.2X3	T50.2X4	T50.2X5	T50.2X6
Triazine (herbicide)	T60.3X1	T60.3X2	T60.3X3	T60.3X4	--	--
Triaziquone	T45.1X1	T45.1X2	T45.1X3	T45.1X4	T45.1X5	T45.1X6
Triazolam	T42.4X1	T42.4X2	T42.4X3	T42.4X4	T42.4X5	T42.4X6
Triazole (herbicide)	T60.3X1	T60.3X2	T60.3X3	T60.3X4	--	--
Tribenoside	T46.991	T46.992	T46.993	T46.994	T46.995	T46.996
Tribromacetaldehyde	T42.6X1	T42.6X2	T42.6X3	T42.6X4	T42.6X5	T42.6X6
Tribromoethanol, rectal	T41.291	T41.292	T41.293	T41.294	T41.295	T41.296
Tribromomethane	T42.6X1	T42.6X2	T42.6X3	T42.6X4	T42.6X5	T42.6X6
Trichlorethane	T53.2X1	T53.2X2	T53.2X3	T53.2X4	--	--
Trichlorethylene	T53.2X1	T53.2X2	T53.2X3	T53.2X4	--	--
Trichlorfon	T60.0X1	T60.0X2	T60.0X3	T60.0X4	--	--
Trichlormethiazide	T50.2X1	T50.2X2	T50.2X3	T50.2X4	T50.2X5	T50.2X6
Trichlormethine	T45.1X1	T45.1X2	T45.1X3	T45.1X4	T45.1X5	T45.1X6
Trichloroacetic acid, Trichloracetic acid	T54.2X1	T54.2X2	T54.2X3	T54.2X4	--	--
medicinal	T49.4X1	T49.4X2	T49.4X3	T49.4X4	T49.4X5	T49.4X6
Trichloroethane	T53.2X1	T53.2X2	T53.2X3	T53.2X4	--	--
Trichloroethanol	T42.6X1	T42.6X2	T42.6X3	T42.6X4	T42.6X5	T42.6X6
Trichloroethyl phosphate	T42.6X1	T42.6X2	T42.6X3	T42.6X4	T42.6X5	T42.6X6
Trichloroethylene (liquid) (vapor)	T53.2X1	T53.2X2	T53.2X3	T53.2X4	--	--
anesthetic (gas)	T41.0X1	T41.0X2	T41.0X3	T41.0X4	T41.0X5	T41.0X6
vapor NEC	T53.2X1	T53.2X2	T53.2X3	T53.2X4	--	--
Trichlorofluoromethane NEC	T53.5X1	T53.5X2	T53.5X3	T53.5X4	--	--
Trichloronate	T60.0X1	T60.0X2	T60.0X3	T60.0X4	--	--
2,4,5-Trichlorophen-oxyacetic acid	T60.3X1	T60.3X2	T60.3X3	T60.3X4	--	--
Trichloropropane	T53.6X1	T53.6X2	T53.6X3	T53.6X4	--	--
Trichlorotriethylamine	T45.1X1	T45.1X2	T45.1X3	T45.1X4	T45.1X5	T45.1X6
Trichomonacides NEC	T37.3X1	T37.3X2	T37.3X3	T37.3X4	T37.3X5	T37.3X6
Trichomycin	T36.7X1	T36.7X2	T36.7X3	T36.7X4	T36.7X5	T36.7X6
Triclobisonium chloride	T49.0X1	T49.0X2	T49.0X3	T49.0X4	T49.0X5	T49.0X6
Triclocarban	T49.0X1	T49.0X2	T49.0X3	T49.0X4	T49.0X5	T49.0X6

Substance	Poisoning, Accidental (unintentional)	Poisoning, Intentional Self-harm	Poisoning, Assault	Poisoning, Undetermined	Adverse effect	Underdosing
Triclofos	T42.6X1	T42.6X2	T42.6X3	T42.6X4	T42.6X5	T42.6X6
Triclosan	T49.0X1	T49.0X2	T49.0X3	T49.0X4	T49.0X5	T49.0X6
Tricresyl phosphate	T65.891	T65.892	T65.893	T65.894	--	--
solvent	T52.91	T52.92	T52.93	T52.94	--	--
Tricyclamol chloride	T44.3X1	T44.3X2	T44.3X3	T44.3X4	T44.3X5	T44.3X6
Tridesilon	T49.0X1	T49.0X2	T49.0X3	T49.0X4	T49.0X5	T49.0X6
Tridihexethyl iodide	T44.3X1	T44.3X2	T44.3X3	T44.3X4	T44.3X5	T44.3X6
Tridione	T42.2X1	T42.2X2	T42.2X3	T42.2X4	T42.2X5	T42.2X6
Trientine	T45.8X1	T45.8X2	T45.8X3	T45.8X4	T45.8X5	T45.8X6
Triethanolamine NEC	T54.3X1	T54.3X2	T54.3X3	T54.3X4	--	--
detergent	T54.3X1	T54.3X2	T54.3X3	T54.3X4	--	--
trinitrate (biphosphate)	T46.3X1	T46.3X2	T46.3X3	T46.3X4	T46.3X5	T46.3X6
Triethanomelamine	T45.1X1	T45.1X2	T45.1X3	T45.1X4	T45.1X5	T45.1X6
Triethylenemelamine	T45.1X1	T45.1X2	T45.1X3	T45.1X4	T45.1X5	T45.1X6
Triethylenephosphoramide	T45.1X1	T45.1X2	T45.1X3	T45.1X4	T45.1X5	T45.1X6
Triethylenethiophosphoramide	T45.1X1	T45.1X2	T45.1X3	T45.1X4	T45.1X5	T45.1X6
Trifluoperazine	T43.3X1	T43.3X2	T43.3X3	T43.3X4	T43.3X5	T43.3X6
Trifluoroethyl vinyl ether	T41.0X1	T41.0X2	T41.0X3	T41.0X4	T41.0X5	T41.0X6
Trifluperidol	T43.4X1	T43.4X2	T43.4X3	T43.4X4	T43.4X5	T43.4X6
Triflupromazine	T43.3X1	T43.3X2	T43.3X3	T43.3X4	T43.3X5	T43.3X6
Trifluridine	T37.5X1	T37.5X2	T37.5X3	T37.5X4	T37.5X5	T37.5X6
Triflusal	T45.521	T45.522	T45.523	T45.524	T45.525	T45.526
Trihexyphenidyl	T44.3X1	T44.3X2	T44.3X3	T44.3X4	T44.3X5	T44.3X6
Triiodothyronine	T38.1X1	T38.1X2	T38.1X3	T38.1X4	T38.1X5	T38.1X6
Trilene	T41.0X1	T41.0X2	T41.0X3	T41.0X4	T41.0X5	T41.0X6
Trilostane	T38.991	T38.992	T38.993	T38.994	T38.995	T38.996
Trimebutine	T44.3X1	T44.3X2	T44.3X3	T44.3X4	T44.3X5	T44.3X6
Trimecaine	T41.3X1	T41.3X2	T41.3X3	T41.3X4	T41.3X5	T41.3X6
Trimeprazine (tartrate)	T44.3X1	T44.3X2	T44.3X3	T44.3X4	T44.3X5	T44.3X6
Trimetaphan camsilate	T44.2X1	T44.2X2	T44.2X3	T44.2X4	T44.2X5	T44.2X6
Trimetazidine	T46.7X1	T46.7X2	T46.7X3	T46.7X4	T46.7X5	T46.7X6
Trimethadione	T42.2X1	T42.2X2	T42.2X3	T42.2X4	T42.2X5	T42.2X6
Trimethaphan	T44.2X1	T44.2X2	T44.2X3	T44.2X4	T44.2X5	T44.2X6
Trimethidinium	T44.2X1	T44.2X2	T44.2X3	T44.2X4	T44.2X5	T44.2X6
Trimethobenzamide	T45.0X1	T45.0X2	T45.0X3	T45.0X4	T45.0X5	T45.0X6
Trimethoprim	T37.8X1	T37.8X2	T37.8X3	T37.8X4	T37.8X5	T37.8X6
with sulfamethoxazole	T36.8X1	T36.8X2	T36.8X3	T36.8X4	T36.8X5	T36.8X6
Trimethylcarbinol	T51.3X1	T51.3X2	T51.3X3	T51.3X4	--	--
Trimethylpsoralen	T49.3X1	T49.3X2	T49.3X3	T49.3X4	T49.3X5	T49.3X6
Trimeton	T45.0X1	T45.0X2	T45.0X3	T45.0X4	T45.0X5	T45.0X6
Trimetrexate	T45.1X1	T45.1X2	T45.1X3	T45.1X4	T45.1X5	T45.1X6
Trimipramine	T43.011	T43.012	T43.013	T43.014	T43.015	T43.016
Trimustine	T45.1X1	T45.1X2	T45.1X3	T45.1X4	T45.1X5	T45.1X6
Trinitrine	T46.3X1	T46.3X2	T46.3X3	T46.3X4	T46.3X5	T46.3X6
Trinitrobenzol	T65.3X1	T65.3X2	T65.3X3	T65.3X4	--	--
Trinitrophenol	T65.3X1	T65.3X2	T65.3X3	T65.3X4	--	--
Trinitrotoluene (fumes)	T65.3X1	T65.3X2	T65.3X3	T65.3X4	--	--
Trional	T42.6X1	T42.6X2	T42.6X3	T42.6X4	T42.6X5	T42.6X6
Triorthocresyl phosphate	T65.891	T65.892	T65.893	T65.894	--	--
Trioxide of arsenic	T57.0X1	T57.0X2	T57.0X3	T57.0X4	--	--
Trioxysalen	T49.4X1	T49.4X2	T49.4X3	T49.4X4	T49.4X5	T49.4X6
Tripamide	T50.2X1	T50.2X2	T50.2X3	T50.2X4	T50.2X5	T50.2X6
Triparanol	T46.6X1	T46.6X2	T46.6X3	T46.6X4	T46.6X5	T46.6X6
Tripelennamine	T45.0X1	T45.0X2	T45.0X3	T45.0X4	T45.0X5	T45.0X6
Triperiden	T44.3X1	T44.3X2	T44.3X3	T44.3X4	T44.3X5	T44.3X6
Triperidol	T43.4X1	T43.4X2	T43.4X3	T43.4X4	T43.4X5	T43.4X6
Triphenylphosphate	T65.891	T65.892	T65.893	T65.894	--	--
Triple						
bromides	T42.6X1	T42.6X2	T42.6X3	T42.6X4	T42.6X5	T42.6X6
carbonate	T47.1X1	T47.1X2	T47.1X3	T47.1X4	T47.1X5	T47.1X6
vaccine						
DPT	T50.A11	T50.A12	T50.A13	T50.A14	T50.A15	T50.A16
including pertussis	T50.A11	T50.A12	T50.A13	T50.A14	T50.A15	T50.A16
MMR	T50.B91	T50.B92	T50.B93	T50.B94	T50.B95	T50.B96
Triprolidine	T45.0X1	T45.0X2	T45.0X3	T45.0X4	T45.0X5	T45.0X6

Substance	Poisoning, Accidental (unintentional)	Poisoning, Intentional Self-harm	Poisoning, Assault	Poisoning, Undetermined	Adverse effect	Underdosing
Trisodium hydrogen edetate	T50.6X1	T50.6X2	T50.6X3	T50.6X4	T50.6X5	T50.6X6
Trisoralen	T49.3X1	T49.3X2	T49.3X3	T49.3X4	T49.3X5	T49.3X6
Trisulfapyrimidines	T37.0X1	T37.0X2	T37.0X3	T37.0X4	T37.0X5	T37.0X6
Trithiozine	T44.3X1	T44.3X2	T44.3X3	T44.3X4	T44.3X5	T44.3X6
Tritiozine	T44.3X1	T44.3X2	T44.3X3	T44.3X4	T44.3X5	T44.3X6
Tritoqualine	T45.0X1	T45.0X2	T45.0X3	T45.0X4	T45.0X5	T45.0X6
Trofosfamide	T45.1X1	T45.1X2	T45.1X3	T45.1X4	T45.1X5	T45.1X6
Troleandomycin	T36.3X1	T36.3X2	T36.3X3	T36.3X4	T36.3X5	T36.3X6
Trolnitrate (phosphate)	T46.3X1	T46.3X2	T46.3X3	T46.3X4	T46.3X5	T46.3X6
Tromantadine	T37.5X1	T37.5X2	T37.5X3	T37.5X4	T37.5X5	T37.5X6
Trometamol	T50.2X1	T50.2X2	T50.2X3	T50.2X4	T50.2X5	T50.2X6
Tromethamine	T50.2X1	T50.2X2	T50.2X3	T50.2X4	T50.2X5	T50.2X6
Tronothane	T41.3X1	T41.3X2	T41.3X3	T41.3X4	T41.3X5	T41.3X6
Tropacine	T44.3X1	T44.3X2	T44.3X3	T44.3X4	T44.3X5	T44.3X6
Tropatepine	T44.3X1	T44.3X2	T44.3X3	T44.3X4	T44.3X5	T44.3X6
Tropicamide	T44.3X1	T44.3X2	T44.3X3	T44.3X4	T44.3X5	T44.3X6
Trospium chloride	T44.3X1	T44.3X2	T44.3X3	T44.3X4	T44.3X5	T44.3X6
Troxerutin	T46.991	T46.992	T46.993	T46.994	T46.995	T46.996
Troxidone	T42.2X1	T42.2X2	T42.2X3	T42.2X4	T42.2X5	T42.2X6
Tryparsamide	T37.3X1	T37.3X2	T37.3X3	T37.3X4	T37.3X5	T37.3X6
Trypsin	T45.3X1	T45.3X2	T45.3X3	T45.3X4	T45.3X5	T45.3X6
Tryptizol	T43.011	T43.012	T43.013	T43.014	T43.015	T43.016
TSH	T38.811	T38.812	T38.813	T38.814	T38.815	T38.816
Tuaminoheptane	T48.5X1	T48.5X2	T48.5X3	T48.5X4	T48.5X5	T48.5X6
Tuberculin, purified protein derivative (PPD)	T50.8X1	T50.8X2	T50.8X3	T50.8X4	T50.8X5	T50.8X6
Tubocurare	T48.1X1	T48.1X2	T48.1X3	T48.1X4	T48.1X5	T48.1X6
Tubocurarine (chloride)	T48.1X1	T48.1X2	T48.1X3	T48.1X4	T48.1X5	T48.1X6
Tulobuterol	T48.6X1	T48.6X2	T48.6X3	T48.6X4	T48.6X5	T48.6X6
Turpentine (spirits of)	T52.8X1	T52.8X2	T52.8X3	T52.8X4	--	--
vapor	T52.8X1	T52.8X2	T52.8X3	T52.8X4	--	--
Tybamate	T43.591	T43.592	T43.593	T43.594	T43.595	T43.596
Tyloxapol	T48.4X1	T48.4X2	T48.4X3	T48.4X4	T48.4X5	T48.4X6
Tymazoline	T48.5X1	T48.5X2	T48.5X3	T48.5X4	T48.5X5	T48.5X6
Typhoid-paratyphoid vaccine	T50.A91	T50.A92	T50.A93	T50.A94	T50.A95	T50.A96
Typhus vaccine	T50.A91	T50.A92	T50.A93	T50.A94	T50.A95	T50.A96
Tyropanoate	T50.8X1	T50.8X2	T50.8X3	T50.8X4	T50.8X5	T50.8X6
Tyrothricin	T49.6X1	T49.6X2	T49.6X3	T49.6X4	T49.6X5	T49.6X6
ENT agent	T49.6X1	T49.6X2	T49.6X3	T49.6X4	T49.6X5	T49.6X6
ophthalmic preparation	T49.5X1	T49.5X2	T49.5X3	T49.5X4	T49.5X5	T49.5X6
Ufenamate	T39.391	T39.392	T39.393	T39.394	T39.395	T39.396
Ultraviolet light protectant	T49.3X1	T49.3X2	T49.3X3	T49.3X4	T49.3X5	T49.3X6
Undecenoic acid	T49.0X1	T49.0X2	T49.0X3	T49.0X4	T49.0X5	T49.0X6
Undecoylium	T49.0X1	T49.0X2	T49.0X3	T49.0X4	T49.0X5	T49.0X6
Undecylenic acid (derivatives)	T49.0X1	T49.0X2	T49.0X3	T49.0X4	T49.0X5	T49.0X6
Unna's boot	T49.3X1	T49.3X2	T49.3X3	T49.3X4	T49.3X5	T49.3X6
Unsaturated fatty acid	T46.6X1	T46.6X2	T46.6X3	T46.6X4	T46.6X5	T46.6X6
Uracil mustard	T45.1X1	T45.1X2	T45.1X3	T45.1X4	T45.1X5	T45.1X6
Uramustine	T45.1X1	T45.1X2	T45.1X3	T45.1X4	T45.1X5	T45.1X6
Urapidil	T46.5X1	T46.5X2	T46.5X3	T46.5X4	T46.5X5	T46.5X6
Urari	T48.1X1	T48.1X2	T48.1X3	T48.1X4	T48.1X5	T48.1X6
Urate oxidase	T50.4X1	T50.4X2	T50.4X3	T50.4X4	T50.4X5	T50.4X6
Urea	T47.3X1	T47.3X2	T47.3X3	T47.3X4	T47.3X5	T47.3X6
peroxide	T49.0X1	T49.0X2	T49.0X3	T49.0X4	T49.0X5	T49.0X6
stibamine	T37.4X1	T37.4X2	T37.4X3	T37.4X4	T37.4X5	T37.4X6
topical	T49.8X1	T49.8X2	T49.8X3	T49.8X4	T49.8X5	T49.8X6
Urethane	T45.1X1	T45.1X2	T45.1X3	T45.1X4	T45.1X5	T45.1X6
Urginea (maritima) (scilla) —see Squill						
Uric acid metabolism drug NEC	T50.4X1	T50.4X2	T50.4X3	T50.4X4	T50.4X5	T50.4X6
Uricosuric agent	T50.4X1	T50.4X2	T50.4X3	T50.4X4	T50.4X5	T50.4X6
Urinary anti-infective	T37.8X1	T37.8X2	T37.8X3	T37.8X4	T37.8X5	T37.8X6
Urofollitropin	T38.811	T38.812	T38.813	T38.814	T38.815	T38.816
Urokinase	T45.611	T45.612	T45.613	T45.614	T45.615	T45.616
Urokon	T50.8X1	T50.8X2	T50.8X3	T50.8X4	T50.8X5	T50.8X6
Ursodeoxycholic acid	T50.991	T50.992	T50.993	T50.994	T50.995	T50.996

Substance	Poisoning, Accidental (unintentional)	Poisoning, Intentional Self-harm	Poisoning, Assault	Poisoning, Undetermined	Adverse effect	Underdosing
Ursodiol	T50.991	T50.992	T50.993	T50.994	T50.995	T50.996
Urtica	T62.2X1	T62.2X2	T62.2X3	T62.2X4	--	--
Utility gas—see Gas, utility						
Vaccine NEC	T50.Z91	T50.Z92	T50.Z93	T50.Z94	T50.Z95	T50.Z96
antineoplastic	T50.Z91	T50.Z92	T50.Z93	T50.Z94	T50.Z95	T50.Z96
bacterial NEC	T50.A91	T50.A92	T50.A93	T50.A94	T50.A95	T50.A96
with						
other bacterial component	T50.A21	T50.A22	T50.A23	T50.A24	T50.A25	T50.A26
pertussis component	T50.A11	T50.A12	T50.A13	T50.A14	T50.A15	T50.A16
viral-rickettsial component	T50.A21	T50.A22	T50.A23	T50.A24	T50.A25	T50.A26
mixed NEC	T50.A21	T50.A22	T50.A23	T50.A24	T50.A25	T50.A26
BCG	T50.A91	T50.A92	T50.A93	T50.A94	T50.A95	T50.A96
cholera	T50.A91	T50.A92	T50.A93	T50.A94	T50.A95	T50.A96
diphtheria	T50.A91	T50.A92	T50.A93	T50.A94	T50.A95	T50.A96
with tetanus	T50.A21	T50.A22	T50.A23	T50.A24	T50.A25	T50.A26
and pertussis	T50.A11	T50.A12	T50.A13	T50.A14	T50.A15	T50.A16
influenza	T50.B91	T50.B92	T50.B93	T50.B94	T50.B95	T50.B96
measles	T50.B91	T50.B92	T50.B93	T50.B94	T50.B95	T50.B96
with mumps and rubella	T50.B91	T50.B92	T50.B93	T50.B94	T50.B95	T50.B96
meningococcal	T50.A91	T50.A92	T50.A93	T50.A94	T50.A95	T50.A96
mumps	T50.B91	T50.B92	T50.B93	T50.B94	T50.B95	T50.B96
paratyphoid	T50.A91	T50.A92	T50.A93	T50.A94	T50.A95	T50.A96
pertussis	T50.A11	T50.A12	T50.A13	T50.A14	T50.A15	T50.A16
with diphtheria	T50.A11	T50.A12	T50.A13	T50.A14	T50.A15	T50.A16
and tetanus	T50.A11	T50.A12	T50.A13	T50.A14	T50.A15	T50.A16
with other component	T50.A11	T50.A12	T50.A13	T50.A14	T50.A15	T50.A16
plague	T50.A91	T50.A92	T50.A93	T50.A94	T50.A95	T50.A96
poliomyelitis	T50.B91	T50.B92	T50.B93	T50.B94	T50.B95	T50.B96
poliovirus	T50.B91	T50.B92	T50.B93	T50.B94	T50.B95	T50.B96
rabies	T50.B91	T50.B92	T50.B93	T50.B94	T50.B95	T50.B96
respiratory syncytial virus	T50.B91	T50.B92	T50.B93	T50.B94	T50.B95	T50.B96
rickettsial NEC	T50.A91	T50.A92	T50.A93	T50.A94	T50.A95	T50.A96
with						
bacterial component	T50.A21	T50.A22	T50.A23	T50.A24	T50.A25	T50.A26
Rocky Mountain spotted fever	T50.A91	T50.A92	T50.A93	T50.A94	T50.A95	T50.A96
rubella	T50.B91	T50.B92	T50.B93	T50.B94	T50.B95	T50.B96
sabin oral	T50.B91	T50.B92	T50.B93	T50.B94	T50.B95	T50.B96
smallpox	T50.B11	T50.B12	T50.B13	T50.B14	T50.B15	T50.B16
TAB	T50.A91	T50.A92	T50.A93	T50.A94	T50.A95	T50.A96
tetanus	T50.A91	T50.A92	T50.A93	T50.A94	T50.A95	T50.A96
typhoid	T50.A91	T50.A92	T50.A93	T50.A94	T50.A95	T50.A96
typhus	T50.A91	T50.A92	T50.A93	T50.A94	T50.A95	T50.A96
viral NEC	T50.B91	T50.B92	T50.B93	T50.B94	T50.B95	T50.B96
yellow fever	T50.B91	T50.B92	T50.B93	T50.B94	T50.B95	T50.B96
Vaccinia immune globulin	T50.Z11	T50.Z12	T50.Z13	T50.Z14	T50.Z15	T50.Z16
Vaginal contraceptives	T49.8X1	T49.8X2	T49.8X3	T49.8X4	T49.8X5	T49.8X6
Valerian						
root	T42.6X1	T42.6X2	T42.6X3	T42.6X4	T42.6X5	T42.6X6
tincture	T42.6X1	T42.6X2	T42.6X3	T42.6X4	T42.6X5	T42.6X6
Valethamate bromide	T44.3X1	T44.3X2	T44.3X3	T44.3X4	T44.3X5	T44.3X6
Valisone	T49.0X1	T49.0X2	T49.0X3	T49.0X4	T49.0X5	T49.0X6
Valium	T42.4X1	T42.4X2	T42.4X3	T42.4X4	T42.4X5	T42.4X6
Valmid	T42.6X1	T42.6X2	T42.6X3	T42.6X4	T42.6X5	T42.6X6
Valnoctamide	T42.6X1	T42.6X2	T42.6X3	T42.6X4	T42.6X5	T42.6X6
Valproate (sodium)	T42.6X1	T42.6X2	T42.6X3	T42.6X4	T42.6X5	T42.6X6
Valproic acid	T42.6X1	T42.6X2	T42.6X3	T42.6X4	T42.6X5	T42.6X6
Valpromide	T42.6X1	T42.6X2	T42.6X3	T42.6X4	T42.6X5	T42.6X6
Vanadium	T56.891	T56.892	T56.893	T56.894	--	--
Vancomycin	T36.8X1	T36.8X2	T36.8X3	T36.8X4	T36.8X5	T36.8X6
Vapor—see also Gas	T59.91	T59.92	T59.93	T59.94	--	--
kiln (carbon monoxide)	T58.8X1	T58.8X2	T58.8X3	T58.8X4	--	--
lead—see lead						
specified source NEC	T59.891	T59.892	T59.893	T59.894	--	--
Vardenafil	T46.7X1	T46.7X2	T46.7X3	T46.7X4	T46.7X5	T46.7X6
Varicose reduction drug	T46.8X1	T46.8X2	T46.8X3	T46.8X4	T46.8X5	T46.8X6

Substance	Poisoning, Accidental (unintentional)	Poisoning, Intentional Self-harm	Poisoning, Assault	Poisoning, Undetermined	Adverse effect	Underdosing
Varnish	T65.4X1	T65.4X2	T65.4X3	T65.4X4	--	--
cleaner	T52.91	T52.92	T52.93	T52.94	--	--
Vaseline	T49.3X1	T49.3X2	T49.3X3	T49.3X4	T49.3X5	T49.3X6
Vasodilan	T46.7X1	T46.7X2	T46.7X3	T46.7X4	T46.7X5	T46.7X6
Vasodilator						
coronary NEC	T46.3X1	T46.3X2	T46.3X3	T46.3X4	T46.3X5	T46.3X6
peripheral NEC	T46.7X1	T46.7X2	T46.7X3	T46.7X4	T46.7X5	T46.7X6
Vasopressin	T38.891	T38.892	T38.893	T38.894	T38.895	T38.896
Vasopressor drugs	T38.891	T38.892	T38.893	T38.894	T38.895	T38.896
Vecuronium bromide	T48.1X1	T48.1X2	T48.1X3	T48.1X4	T48.1X5	T48.1X6
Vegetable extract, astringent	T49.2X1	T49.2X2	T49.2X3	T49.2X4	T49.2X5	T49.2X6
Venlafaxine	T43.211	T43.212	T43.213	T43.214	T43.215	T43.216
Venom, venomous (bite) (sting)	T63.91	T63.92	T63.93	T63.94	--	--
amphibian NEC	T63.831	T63.832	T63.833	T63.834	--	--
animal NEC	T63.891	T63.892	T63.893	T63.894	--	--
ant	T63.421	T63.422	T63.423	T63.424	--	--
arthropod NEC	T63.481	T63.482	T63.483	T63.484	--	--
bee	T63.441	T63.442	T63.443	T63.444	--	--
centipede	T63.411	T63.412	T63.413	T63.414	--	--
fish	T63.591	T63.592	T63.593	T63.594	--	--
frog	T63.811	T63.812	T63.813	T63.814	--	--
hornet	T63.451	T63.452	T63.453	T63.454	--	--
insect NEC	T63.481	T63.482	T63.483	T63.484	--	--
lizard	T63.121	T63.122	T63.123	T63.124	--	--
marine						
animals	T63.691	T63.692	T63.693	T63.694	--	--
bluebottle	T63.611	T63.612	T63.613	T63.614	--	--
jellyfish NEC	T63.621	T63.622	T63.623	T63.624	--	--
Portugese Man-o-war	T63.611	T63.612	T63.613	T63.614	--	--
sea anemone	T63.631	T63.632	T63.633	T63.634	--	--
specified NEC	T63.691	T63.692	T63.693	T63.694	--	--
fish	T63.591	T63.592	T63.593	T63.594	--	--
plants	T63.711	T63.712	T63.713	T63.714	--	--
sting ray	T63.511	T63.512	T63.513	T63.514	--	--
millipede (tropical)	T63.411	T63.412	T63.413	T63.414	--	--
plant NEC	T63.791	T63.792	T63.793	T63.794	--	--
marine	T63.711	T63.712	T63.713	T63.714	--	--
reptile	T63.191	T63.192	T63.193	T63.194	--	--
gila monster	T63.111	T63.112	T63.113	T63.114	--	--
lizard NEC	T63.121	T63.122	T63.123	T63.124	--	--
scorpion	T63.2X1	T63.2X2	T63.2X3	T63.2X4	--	--
snake	T63.001	T63.002	T63.003	T63.004	--	--
African NEC	T63.081	T63.082	T63.083	T63.084	--	--
American (North) (South) NEC	T63.061	T63.062	T63.063	T63.064	--	--
Asian	T63.081	T63.082	T63.083	T63.084	--	--
Australian	T63.071	T63.072	T63.073	T63.074	--	--
cobra	T63.041	T63.042	T63.043	T63.044	--	--
coral snake	T63.021	T63.022	T63.023	T63.024	--	--
rattlesnake	T63.011	T63.012	T63.013	T63.014	--	--
specified NEC	T63.091	T63.092	T63.093	T63.094	--	--
taipan	T63.031	T63.032	T63.033	T63.034	--	--
specified NEC	T63.891	T63.892	T63.893	T63.894	--	--
spider	T63.301	T63.302	T63.303	T63.304	--	--
black widow	T63.311	T63.312	T63.313	T63.314	--	--
brown recluse	T63.331	T63.332	T63.333	T63.334	--	--
specified NEC	T63.391	T63.392	T63.393	T63.394	--	--
tarantula	T63.321	T63.322	T63.323	T63.324	--	--
sting ray	T63.511	T63.512	T63.513	T63.514	--	--
toad	T63.821	T63.822	T63.823	T63.824	--	--
wasp	T63.461	T63.462	T63.463	T63.464	--	--
Venous sclerosing drug NEC	T46.8X1	T46.8X2	T46.8X3	T46.8X4	T46.8X5	T46.8X6
Ventolin—see Albuterol						
Veramon	T42.3X1	T42.3X2	T42.3X3	T42.3X4	T42.3X5	T42.3X6
Verapamil	T46.1X1	T46.1X2	T46.1X3	T46.1X4	T46.1X5	T46.1X6

TABLE OF DRUGS AND CHEMICALS

Substance	Poisoning, Accidental (unintentional)	Poisoning, Intentional Self-harm	Poisoning, Assault	Poisoning, Undetermined	Adverse effect	Underdosing
Veratrine	T46.5X1	T46.5X2	T46.5X3	T46.5X4	T46.5X5	T46.5X6
Veratrum						
album	T62.2X1	T62.2X2	T62.2X3	T62.2X4	--	--
alkaloids	T46.5X1	T46.5X2	T46.5X3	T46.5X4	T46.5X5	T46.5X6
viride	T62.2X1	T62.2X2	T62.2X3	T62.2X4	--	--
Verdigris	T60.3X1	T60.3X2	T60.3X3	T60.3X4	--	--
Veronal	T42.3X1	T42.3X2	T42.3X3	T42.3X4	T42.3X5	T42.3X6
Veroxil	T37.4X1	T37.4X2	T37.4X3	T37.4X4	T37.4X5	T37.4X6
Versenate	T50.6X1	T50.6X2	T50.6X3	T50.6X4	T50.6X5	T50.6X6
Versidyne	T39.8X1	T39.8X2	T39.8X3	T39.8X4	T39.8X5	T39.8X6
Vetrabutine	T48.0X1	T48.0X2	T48.0X3	T48.0X4	T48.0X5	T48.0X6
Vidarabine	T37.5X1	T37.5X2	T37.5X3	T37.5X4	T37.5X5	T37.5X6
Vienna						
green	T57.0X1	T57.0X2	T57.0X3	T57.0X4	--	--
insecticide	T60.2X1	T60.2X2	T60.2X3	T60.2X4	--	--
red	T57.0X1	T57.0X2	T57.0X3	T57.0X4	--	--
pharmaceutical dye	T50.991	T50.992	T50.993	T50.994	T50.995	T50.996
Vigabatrin	T42.6X1	T42.6X2	T42.6X3	T42.6X4	T42.6X5	T42.6X6
Viloxazine	T43.291	T43.292	T43.293	T43.294	T43.295	T43.296
Viminol	T39.8X1	T39.8X2	T39.8X3	T39.8X4	T39.8X5	T39.8X6
Vinbarbital, vinbarbitone	T42.3X1	T42.3X2	T42.3X3	T42.3X4	T42.3X5	T42.3X6
Vinblastine	T45.1X1	T45.1X2	T45.1X3	T45.1X4	T45.1X5	T45.1X6
Vinburnine	T46.7X1	T46.7X2	T46.7X3	T46.7X4	T46.7X5	T46.7X6
Vincamine	T45.1X1	T45.1X2	T45.1X3	T45.1X4	T45.1X5	T45.1X6
Vincristine	T45.1X1	T45.1X2	T45.1X3	T45.1X4	T45.1X5	T45.1X6
Vindesine	T45.1X1	T45.1X2	T45.1X3	T45.1X4	T45.1X5	T45.1X6
Vinesthene, vinethene	T41.0X1	T41.0X2	T41.0X3	T41.0X4	T41.0X5	T41.0X6
Vinorelbine tartrate	T45.1X1	T45.1X2	T45.1X3	T45.1X4	T45.1X5	T45.1X6
Vinpocetine	T46.7X1	T46.7X2	T46.7X3	T46.7X4	T46.7X5	T46.7X6
Vinyl						
acetate	T65.891	T65.892	T65.893	T65.894	--	--
bital	T42.3X1	T42.3X2	T42.3X3	T42.3X4	T42.3X5	T42.3X6
bromide	T65.891	T65.892	T65.893	T65.894	--	--
chloride	T59.891	T59.892	T59.893	T59.894	--	--
ether	T41.0X1	T41.0X2	T41.0X3	T41.0X4	T41.0X5	T41.0X6
Vinylbital	T42.3X1	T42.3X2	T42.3X3	T42.3X4	T42.3X5	T42.3X6
Vinylidene chloride	T65.891	T65.892	T65.893	T65.894	--	--
Vioform	T37.8X1	T37.8X2	T37.8X3	T37.8X4	T37.8X5	T37.8X6
topical	T49.0X1	T49.0X2	T49.0X3	T49.0X4	T49.0X5	T49.0X6
Viomycin	T36.8X1	T36.8X2	T36.8X3	T36.8X4	T36.8X5	T36.8X6
Viosterol	T45.2X1	T45.2X2	T45.2X3	T45.2X4	T45.2X5	T45.2X6
Viper (venom)	T63.091	T63.092	T63.093	T63.094	--	--
Viprynium	T37.4X1	T37.4X2	T37.4X3	T37.4X4	T37.4X5	T37.4X6
Viquidil	T46.7X1	T46.7X2	T46.7X3	T46.7X4	T46.7X5	T46.7X6
Viral vaccine NEC	T50.B91	T50.B92	T50.B93	T50.B94	T50.B95	T50.B96
Virginiamycin	T36.8X1	T36.8X2	T36.8X3	T36.8X4	T36.8X5	T36.8X6
Virugon	T37.5X1	T37.5X2	T37.5X3	T37.5X4	T37.5X5	T37.5X6
Viscous agent	T50.901	T50.902	T50.903	T50.904	T50.905	T50.906
Visine	T49.5X1	T49.5X2	T49.5X3	T49.5X4	T49.5X5	T49.5X6
Visnadine	T46.3X1	T46.3X2	T46.3X3	T46.3X4	T46.3X5	T46.3X6
Vitamin NEC	T45.2X1	T45.2X2	T45.2X3	T45.2X4	T45.2X5	T45.2X6
A	T45.2X1	T45.2X2	T45.2X3	T45.2X4	T45.2X5	T45.2X6
B NEC	T45.2X1	T45.2X2	T45.2X3	T45.2X4	T45.2X5	T45.2X6
nicotinic acid	T46.7X1	T46.7X2	T46.7X3	T46.7X4	T46.7X5	T46.7X6
B1	T45.2X1	T45.2X2	T45.2X3	T45.2X4	T45.2X5	T45.2X6
B2	T45.2X1	T45.2X2	T45.2X3	T45.2X4	T45.2X5	T45.2X6
B6	T45.2X1	T45.2X2	T45.2X3	T45.2X4	T45.2X5	T45.2X6
B12	T45.2X1	T45.2X2	T45.2X3	T45.2X4	T45.2X5	T45.2X6
B15	T45.2X1	T45.2X2	T45.2X3	T45.2X4	T45.2X5	T45.2X6
C	T45.2X1	T45.2X2	T45.2X3	T45.2X4	T45.2X5	T45.2X6
D	T45.2X1	T45.2X2	T45.2X3	T45.2X4	T45.2X5	T45.2X6
D2	T45.2X1	T45.2X2	T45.2X3	T45.2X4	T45.2X5	T45.2X6
D3	T45.2X1	T45.2X2	T45.2X3	T45.2X4	T45.2X5	T45.2X6
E	T45.2X1	T45.2X2	T45.2X3	T45.2X4	T45.2X5	T45.2X6
E acetate	T45.2X1	T45.2X2	T45.2X3	T45.2X4	T45.2X5	T45.2X6

Substance	Poisoning, Accidental (unintentional)	Poisoning, Intentional Self-harm	Poisoning, Assault	Poisoning, Undetermined	Adverse effect	Underdosing
hematopoietic	T45.8X1	T45.8X2	T45.8X3	T45.8X4	T45.8X5	T45.8X6
K NEC	T45.7X1	T45.7X2	T45.7X3	T45.7X4	T45.7X5	T45.7X6
K1	T45.7X1	T45.7X2	T45.7X3	T45.7X4	T45.7X5	T45.7X6
K2	T45.7X1	T45.7X2	T45.7X3	T45.7X4	T45.7X5	T45.7X6
PP	T45.2X1	T45.2X2	T45.2X3	T45.2X4	T45.2X5	T45.2X6
ulceroprotectant	T47.1X1	T47.1X2	T47.1X3	T47.1X4	T47.1X5	T47.1X6
Vleminckx's solution	T49.4X1	T49.4X2	T49.4X3	T49.4X4	T49.4X5	T49.4X6
Voltaren—see Diclofenac sodium						
Warfarin	T45.511	T45.512	T45.513	T45.514	T45.515	T45.516
rodenticide	T60.4X1	T60.4X2	T60.4X3	T60.4X4	--	--
sodium	T60.4X1	T60.4X2	T60.4X3	T60.4X4	--	--
Wasp (sting)	T63.461	T63.462	T63.463	T63.464	--	--
Water						
balance drug	T50.3X1	T50.3X2	T50.3X3	T50.3X4	T50.3X5	T50.3X6
distilled	T50.3X1	T50.3X2	T50.3X3	T50.3X4	T50.3X5	T50.3X6
gas—see Gas, water						
incomplete combustion of—see Carbon, monoxide, fuel, utility						
hemlock	T62.2X1	T62.2X2	T62.2X3	T62.2X4	--	--
moccasin (venom)	T63.061	T63.062	T63.063	T63.064	--	--
purified	T50.3X1	T50.3X2	T50.3X3	T50.3X4	T50.3X5	T50.3X6
Wax (paraffin) (petroleum)	T52.0X1	T52.0X2	T52.0X3	T52.0X4	--	--
automobile	T65.891	T65.892	T65.893	T65.894	--	--
floor	T52.0X1	T52.0X2	T52.0X3	T52.0X4	--	--
Weed killers NEC	T60.3X1	T60.3X2	T60.3X3	T60.3X4	--	--
Welldorm	T42.6X1	T42.6X2	T42.6X3	T42.6X4	T42.6X5	T42.6X6
White						
arsenic	T57.0X1	T57.0X2	T57.0X3	T57.0X4	--	--
hellebore	T62.2X1	T62.2X2	T62.2X3	T62.2X4	--	--
lotion (keratolytic)	T49.4X1	T49.4X2	T49.4X3	T49.4X4	T49.4X5	T49.4X6
spirit	T52.0X1	T52.0X2	T52.0X3	T52.0X4	--	--
Whitewash	T65.891	T65.892	T65.893	T65.894	--	--
Whole blood (human)	T45.8X1	T45.8X2	T45.8X3	T45.8X4	T45.8X5	T45.8X6
Wild						
black cherry	T62.2X1	T62.2X2	T62.2X3	T62.2X4	--	--
poisonous plants NEC	T62.2X1	T62.2X2	T62.2X3	T62.2X4	--	--
Window cleaning fluid	T65.891	T65.892	T65.893	T65.894	--	--
Wintergreen (oil)	T49.3X1	T49.3X2	T49.3X3	T49.3X4	T49.3X5	T49.3X6
Wisterine	T62.2X1	T62.2X2	T62.2X3	T62.2X4	--	--
Witch hazel	T49.2X1	T49.2X2	T49.2X3	T49.2X4	T49.2X5	T49.2X6
Wood alcohol or spirit	T51.1X1	T51.1X2	T51.1X3	T51.1X4	--	--
Wool fat (hydrous)	T49.3X1	T49.3X2	T49.3X3	T49.3X4	T49.3X5	T49.3X6
Woorali	T48.1X1	T48.1X2	T48.1X3	T48.1X4	T48.1X5	T48.1X6
Wormseed, American	T37.4X1	T37.4X2	T37.4X3	T37.4X4	T37.4X5	T37.4X6
Xamoterol	T44.5X1	T44.5X2	T44.5X3	T44.5X4	T44.5X5	T44.5X6
Xanthine diuretics	T50.2X1	T50.2X2	T50.2X3	T50.2X4	T50.2X5	T50.2X6
Xanthinol nicotinate	T46.7X1	T46.7X2	T46.7X3	T46.7X4	T46.7X5	T46.7X6
Xanthotoxin	T49.3X1	T49.3X2	T49.3X3	T49.3X4	T49.3X5	T49.3X6
Xantinol nicotinate	T46.7X1	T46.7X2	T46.7X3	T46.7X4	T46.7X5	T46.7X6
Xantocillin	T36.0X1	T36.0X2	T36.0X3	T36.0X4	T36.0X5	T36.0X6
Xenon (127Xe) (133Xe)	T50.8X1	T50.8X2	T50.8X3	T50.8X4	T50.8X5	T50.8X6
Xenysalate	T49.4X1	T49.4X2	T49.4X3	T49.4X4	T49.4X5	T49.4X6
Xibornol	T37.8X1	T37.8X2	T37.8X3	T37.8X4	T37.8X5	T37.8X6
Xigris	T45.511	T45.512	T45.513	T45.514	T45.515	T45.516
Xipamide	T50.2X1	T50.2X2	T50.2X3	T50.2X4	T50.2X5	T50.2X6
Xylene (vapor)	T52.2X1	T52.2X2	T52.2X3	T52.2X4	--	--
Xylocaine (infiltration) (topical)	T41.3X1	T41.3X2	T41.3X3	T41.3X4	T41.3X5	T41.3X6
nerve block (peripheral) (plexus)	T41.3X1	T41.3X2	T41.3X3	T41.3X4	T41.3X5	T41.3X6
spinal	T41.3X1	T41.3X2	T41.3X3	T41.3X4	T41.3X5	T41.3X6
Xylol (vapor)	T52.2X1	T52.2X2	T52.2X3	T52.2X4	--	--
Xylometazoline	T48.5X1	T48.5X2	T48.5X3	T48.5X4	T48.5X5	T48.5X6
Yeast	T45.2X1	T45.2X2	T45.2X3	T45.2X4	T45.2X5	T45.2X6
dried	T45.2X1	T45.2X2	T45.2X3	T45.2X4	T45.2X5	T45.2X6
Yellow						

Substance	Poisoning, Accidental (unintentional)	Poisoning, Intentional Self-harm	Poisoning, Assault	Poisoning, Undetermined	Adverse effect	Underdosing
fever vaccine	T50.B91	T50.B92	T50.B93	T50.B94	T50.B95	T50.B96
jasmine	T62.2X1	T62.2X2	T62.2X3	T62.2X4	--	--
phenolphthalein	T47.2X1	T47.2X2	T47.2X3	T47.2X4	T47.2X5	T47.2X6
Yew	T62.2X1	T62.2X2	T62.2X3	T62.2X4	--	--
Yohimbic acid	T40.991	T40.992	T40.993	T40.994	T40.995	T40.996
Zactane	T39.8X1	T39.8X2	T39.8X3	T39.8X4	T39.8X5	T39.8X6
Zalcitabine	T37.5X1	T37.5X2	T37.5X3	T37.5X4	T37.5X5	T37.5X6
Zaroxolyn	T50.2X1	T50.2X2	T50.2X3	T50.2X4	T50.2X5	T50.2X6
Zephiran (topical)	T49.0X1	T49.0X2	T49.0X3	T49.0X4	T49.0X5	T49.0X6
ophthalmic preparation	T49.5X1	T49.5X2	T49.5X3	T49.5X4	T49.5X5	T49.5X6
Zeranol	T38.7X1	T38.7X2	T38.7X3	T38.7X4	T38.7X5	T38.7X6
Zerone	T51.1X1	T51.1X2	T51.1X3	T51.1X4	--	--
Zidovudine	T37.5X1	T37.5X2	T37.5X3	T37.5X4	T37.5X5	T37.5X6
Zimeldine	T43.221	T43.222	T43.223	T43.224	T43.225	T43.226
Zinc (compounds) (fumes) (vapor) NEC	T56.5X1	T56.5X2	T56.5X3	T56.5X4	--	--
anti-infectives	T49.0X1	T49.0X2	T49.0X3	T49.0X4	T49.0X5	T49.0X6
antivaricose	T46.8X1	T46.8X2	T46.8X3	T46.8X4	T46.8X5	T46.8X6
bacitracin	T49.0X1	T49.0X2	T49.0X3	T49.0X4	T49.0X5	T49.0X6
chloride (mouthwash)	T49.6X1	T49.6X2	T49.6X3	T49.6X4	T49.6X5	T49.6X6
chromate	T56.5X1	T56.5X2	T56.5X3	T56.5X4	--	--
gelatin	T49.3X1	T49.3X2	T49.3X3	T49.3X4	T49.3X5	T49.3X6
oxide	T49.3X1	T49.3X2	T49.3X3	T49.3X4	T49.3X5	T49.3X6
plaster	T49.3X1	T49.3X2	T49.3X3	T49.3X4	T49.3X5	T49.3X6
peroxide	T49.0X1	T49.0X2	T49.0X3	T49.0X4	T49.0X5	T49.0X6
pesticides	T56.5X1	T56.5X2	T56.5X3	T56.5X4	--	--
phosphide	T60.4X1	T60.4X2	T60.4X3	T60.4X4	--	--
pyrithionate	T49.4X1	T49.4X2	T49.4X3	T49.4X4	T49.4X5	T49.4X6
stearate	T49.3X1	T49.3X2	T49.3X3	T49.3X4	T49.3X5	T49.3X6
sulfate	T49.5X1	T49.5X2	T49.5X3	T49.5X4	T49.5X5	T49.5X6
ENT agent	T49.6X1	T49.6X2	T49.6X3	T49.6X4	T49.6X5	T49.6X6
ophthalmic solution	T49.5X1	T49.5X2	T49.5X3	T49.5X4	T49.5X5	T49.5X6
topical NEC	T49.0X1	T49.0X2	T49.0X3	T49.0X4	T49.0X5	T49.0X6
undecylenate	T49.0X1	T49.0X2	T49.0X3	T49.0X4	T49.0X5	T49.0X6
Zineb	T60.0X1	T60.0X2	T60.0X3	T60.0X4	--	--
Zinostatin	T45.1X1	T45.1X2	T45.1X3	T45.1X4	T45.1X5	T45.1X6
Zipeprol	T48.3X1	T48.3X2	T48.3X3	T48.3X4	T48.3X5	T48.3X6
Zofenopril	T46.4X1	T46.4X2	T46.4X3	T46.4X4	T46.4X5	T46.4X6
Zolpidem	T42.6X1	T42.6X2	T42.6X3	T42.6X4	T42.6X5	T42.6X6
Zomepirac	T39.391	T39.392	T39.393	T39.394	T39.395	T39.396
Zopiclone	T42.6X1	T42.6X2	T42.6X3	T42.6X4	T42.6X5	T42.6X6
Zorubicin	T45.1X1	T45.1X2	T45.1X3	T45.1X4	T45.1X5	T45.1X6
Zotepine	T43.591	T43.592	T43.593	T43.594	T43.595	T43.596
Zovant	T45.511	T45.512	T45.513	T45.514	T45.515	T45.516
Zoxazolamine	T42.8X1	T42.8X2	T42.8X3	T42.8X4	T42.8X5	T42.8X6
Zuclopenthixol	T43.4X1	T43.4X2	T43.4X3	T43.4X4	T43.4X5	T43.4X6
Zygadenus (venenosus)	T62.2X1	T62.2X2	T62.2X3	T62.2X4	--	--
Zyprexa	T43.591	T43.592	T43.593	T43.594	T43.595	T43.596

Accident -- *continued*

streetcar (traffic) V76.9
  nontraffic V76.3
    while boarding or alighting V76.4
three wheeled motor vehicle (traffic)
  V72.9
  nontraffic V72.3
    while boarding or alighting V72.4
truck (traffic) V74.9
  nontraffic V74.3
    while boarding or alighting V74.4
two wheeled motor vehicle (traffic)
  V72.9
  nontraffic V72.3
    while boarding or alighting V72.4
van (traffic) V73.9
  nontraffic V73.3
    while boarding or alighting V73.4
driver
  collision (with)
    animal (traffic) V70.5
      being ridden (traffic) V76.5
        nontraffic V76.0
      nontraffic V70.0
    animal-drawn vehicle (traffic) V76.5
      nontraffic V76.0
    bus (traffic) V74.5
      nontraffic V74.0
    car (traffic) V73.5
      nontraffic V73.0
    motor vehicle NOS (traffic) V79.40
      nontraffic V79.00
        specified type NEC (traffic) V79.49
          nontraffic V79.09
    pedal cycle (traffic) V71.5
      nontraffic V71.0
    pickup truck (traffic) V73.5
      nontraffic V73.0
    railway vehicle (traffic) V75.5
      nontraffic V75.0
    specified vehicle NEC (traffic) V76.5
      nontraffic V76.0
    stationary object (traffic) V77.5
      nontraffic V77.0
    streetcar (traffic) V76.5
      nontraffic V76.0
    three wheeled motor vehicle (traffic)
      V72.5
      nontraffic V72.0
    truck (traffic) V74.5
      nontraffic V74.0
    two wheeled motor vehicle (traffic)
      V72.5
      nontraffic V72.0
    van (traffic) V73.5
      nontraffic V73.0
  noncollision accident (traffic) V78.5
    nontraffic V78.0
  noncollision accident (traffic) V78.9
    nontraffic V78.3
      while boarding or alighting V78.4
  nontraffic V79.3
hanger-on
  collision (with)
    animal (traffic) V70.7
      being ridden (traffic) V76.7
        nontraffic V76.2
      nontraffic V70.2
    animal-drawn vehicle (traffic) V76.7
      nontraffic V76.2
    bus (traffic) V74.7

Accident -- *continued*

      nontraffic V74.2
    car (traffic) V73.7
      nontraffic V73.2
    pedal cycle (traffic) V71.7
      nontraffic V71.2
    pickup truck (traffic) V73.7
      nontraffic V73.2
    railway vehicle (traffic) V75.7
      nontraffic V75.2
    specified vehicle NEC (traffic) V76.7
      nontraffic V76.2
    stationary object (traffic) V77.7
      nontraffic V77.2
    streetcar (traffic) V76.7
      nontraffic V76.2
    three wheeled motor vehicle (traffic)
      V72.7
      nontraffic V72.2
    truck (traffic) V74.7
      nontraffic V74.2
    two wheeled motor vehicle (traffic)
      V72.7
      nontraffic V72.2
    van (traffic) V73.7
      nontraffic V73.2
  noncollision accident (traffic) V78.7
    nontraffic V78.2
passenger
  collision (with)
    animal (traffic) V70.6
      being ridden (traffic) V76.6
        nontraffic V76.1
      nontraffic V70.1
    animal-drawn vehicle (traffic) V76.6
      nontraffic V76.1
    bus (traffic) V74.6
      nontraffic V74.1
    car (traffic) V73.6
      nontraffic V73.1
    motor vehicle NOS (traffic) V79.50
      nontraffic V79.10
        specified type NEC (traffic) V79.59
          nontraffic V79.19
    pedal cycle (traffic) V71.6
      nontraffic V71.1
    pickup truck (traffic) V73.6
      nontraffic V73.1
    railway vehicle (traffic) V75.6
      nontraffic V75.1
    specified vehicle NEC (traffic) V76.6
      nontraffic V76.1
    stationary object (traffic) V77.6
      nontraffic V77.1
    streetcar (traffic) V76.6
      nontraffic V76.1
    three wheeled motor vehicle (traffic)
      V72.6
      nontraffic V72.1
    truck (traffic) V74.6
      nontraffic V74.1
    two wheeled motor vehicle (traffic)
      V72.6
      nontraffic V72.1
    van (traffic) V73.6
      nontraffic V73.1
  noncollision accident (traffic) V78.6
    nontraffic V78.1
  specified type NEC V79.88
    military vehicle V79.81
cable car, not on rails V98.0

Accident -- *continued*

on rails -*see* Accident, transport, streetcar
  occupant
car occupant V49.9
  ambulance occupant -*see* Accident,
  transport, ambulance occupant
  collision (with)
    animal (traffic) V40.9
      being ridden (traffic) V46.9
        nontraffic V46.3
        while boarding or alighting V46.4
      nontraffic V40.3
        while boarding or alighting V40.4
    animal-drawn vehicle (traffic) V46.9
      nontraffic V46.3
        while boarding or alighting V46.4
    bus (traffic) V44.9
      nontraffic V44.3
        while boarding or alighting V44.4
    car (traffic) V43.92
      nontraffic V43.32
        while boarding or alighting V43.42
    motor vehicle NOS (traffic) V49.60
      nontraffic V49.20
        specified type NEC (traffic) V49.69
          nontraffic V49.29
    pedal cycle (traffic) V41.9
      nontraffic V41.3
        while boarding or alighting V41.4
    pickup truck (traffic) V43.93
      nontraffic V43.33
        while boarding or alighting V43.43
    railway vehicle (traffic) V45.9
      nontraffic V45.3
        while boarding or alighting V45.4
    specified vehicle NEC (traffic) V46.9
      nontraffic V46.3
        while boarding or alighting V46.4
    sport utility vehicle (traffic) V43.91
      nontraffic V43.31
        while boarding or alighting V43.41
    stationary object (traffic) V47.92
      nontraffic V47.32
        while boarding or alighting V47.4
    streetcar (traffic) V46.9
      nontraffic V46.3
        while boarding or alighting V46.4
    three wheeled motor vehicle (traffic)
      V42.9
      nontraffic V42.3
        while boarding or alighting V42.4
    truck (traffic) V44.9
      nontraffic V44.3
        while boarding or alighting V44.4
    two wheeled motor vehicle (traffic)
      V42.9
      nontraffic V42.3
        while boarding or alighting V42.4
    van (traffic) V43.94
      nontraffic V43.34
        while boarding or alighting V43.44
  driver
    collision (with)
      animal (traffic) V40.5
        being ridden (traffic) V46.5
          nontraffic V46.0
        nontraffic V40.0
      animal-drawn vehicle (traffic) V46.5
        nontraffic V46.0
      bus (traffic) V44.5
        nontraffic V44.0

Accident -- *continued*
  specified vehicle NEC (traffic) V26.9
    nontraffic V26.2
    while boarding or alighting V26.3
  stationary object (traffic) V27.9
    nontraffic V27.2
    while boarding or alighting V27.3
  streetcar (traffic) V26.9
    nontraffic V26.2
    while boarding or alighting V26.3
  three wheeled motor vehicle (traffic)
      V22.9
    nontraffic V22.2
    while boarding or alighting V22.3
  truck (traffic) V24.9
    nontraffic V24.2
    while boarding or alighting V24.3
  two wheeled motor vehicle (traffic)
      V22.9
    nontraffic V22.2
    while boarding or alighting V22.3
  van (traffic) V23.9
    nontraffic V23.2
    while boarding or alighting V23.3
driver
  collision (with)
    animal (traffic) V20.4
      being ridden (traffic) V26.4
        nontraffic V26.0
      nontraffic V20.0
    animal-drawn vehicle (traffic) V26.4
      nontraffic V26.0
    bus (traffic) V24.4
      nontraffic V24.0
    car (traffic) V23.4
      nontraffic V23.0
    motor vehicle NOS (traffic) V29.40
      nontraffic V29.00
      specified type NEC (traffic) V29.49
        nontraffic V29.09
    pedal cycle (traffic) V21.4
      nontraffic V21.0
    pickup truck (traffic) V23.4
      nontraffic V23.0
    railway vehicle (traffic) V25.4
      nontraffic V25.0
    specified vehicle NEC (traffic) V26.4
      nontraffic V26.0
    stationary object (traffic) V27.4
      nontraffic V27.0
    streetcar (traffic) V26.4
      nontraffic V26.0
    three wheeled motor vehicle (traffic)
        V22.4
      nontraffic V22.0
    truck (traffic) V24.4
      nontraffic V24.0
    two wheeled motor vehicle (traffic)
        V22.4
      nontraffic V22.0
    van (traffic) V23.4
      nontraffic V23.0
  noncollision accident (traffic) V28.4
    nontraffic V28.0
  noncollision accident (traffic) V28.9
    nontraffic V28.2
    while boarding or alighting V28.3
  nontraffic V29.3
passenger
  collision (with)
    animal (traffic) V20.5

Accident -- *continued*
  being ridden (traffic) V26.5
    nontraffic V26.1
    nontraffic V20.1
  animal-drawn vehicle (traffic) V26.5
    nontraffic V26.1
  bus (traffic) V24.5
    nontraffic V24.1
  car (traffic) V23.5
    nontraffic V23.1
  motor vehicle NOS (traffic) V29.50
    nontraffic V29.10
    specified type NEC (traffic) V29.59
      nontraffic V29.19
  pedal cycle (traffic) V21.5
    nontraffic V21.1
  pickup truck (traffic) V23.5
    nontraffic V23.1
  railway vehicle (traffic) V25.5
    nontraffic V25.1
  specified vehicle NEC (traffic) V26.5
    nontraffic V26.1
  stationary object (traffic) V27.5
    nontraffic V27.1
  streetcar (traffic) V26.5
    nontraffic V26.1
  three wheeled motor vehicle (traffic)
      V22.5
    nontraffic V22.1
  truck (traffic) V24.5
    nontraffic V24.1
  two wheeled motor vehicle (traffic)
      V22.5
    nontraffic V22.1
  van (traffic) V23.5
    nontraffic V23.1
noncollision accident (traffic) V28.5
  nontraffic V28.1
specified type NEC V29.88
  military vehicle V29.81
motor vehicle NEC occupant (traffic)
    V89.2
occupant (of)
  aircraft (powered) V95.9
    fixed wing
      commercial -*see* Accident, transport,
    aircraft, occupant, powered, fixed wing,
    commercial
      private -*see* Accident, transport,
    aircraft, occupant, powered, fixed wing,
    private
      nonpowered V96.9
      specified NEC V95.8
  airport battery-powered vehicle -*see*
  Accident, transport, industrial vehicle
  occupant
  all-terrain vehicle (ATV) -*see* Accident,
  transport, all-terrain vehicle occupant
  animal-drawn vehicle -*see* Accident,
  transport, animal-drawn vehicle occupant
  automobile -*see* Accident, transport, car
  occupant
  balloon V96.00
  battery-powered vehicle -*see* Accident,
  transport, industrial vehicle occupant
  bicycle -*see* Accident, transport, pedal
  cyclist
    motorized -*see* Accident, transport,
    motorcycle rider
  boat NEC -*see* Accident, watercraft

Accident -- *continued*
  bulldozer -*see* Accident, transport,
  construction vehicle occupant
  bus -*see* Accident, transport, bus
  occupant
  cable car (on rails) -*see also* Accident,
  transport, streetcar occupant
    not on rails V98.0
  car -*see also* Accident, transport, car
  occupant
    cable (on rails) -*see also* Accident,
    transport, streetcar occupant
      not on rails V98.0
    coach -*see* Accident, transport, bus
    occupant
    coal-car -*see* Accident, transport,
    industrial vehicle occupant
    digger -*see* Accident, transport,
    construction vehicle occupant
    dump truck -*see* Accident, transport,
    construction vehicle occupant
    earth-leveler -*see* Accident, transport,
    construction vehicle occupant
    farm machinery (self-propelled) -*see*
    Accident, transport, agricultural
    vehicle occupant
    forklift -*see* Accident, transport,
    industrial vehicle occupant
    glider (unpowered) V96.20
      hang V96.10
      powered (microlight) (ultralight) -*see*
      Accident, transport, aircraft, occupant,
      powered, glider
    glider (unpowered) NEC V96.20
    hang-glider V96.10
    harvester -*see* Accident, transport,
    agricultural vehicle occupant
    heavy (transport) vehicle -*see* Accident,
    transport, truck occupant
    helicopter -*see* Accident, transport,
    aircraft, occupant, helicopter
    ice-yacht V98.2
    kite (carrying person) V96.8
    land-yacht V98.1
    logging car -*see* Accident, transport,
    industrial vehicle occupant
    mechanical shovel -*see* Accident,
    transport, construction vehicle
    occupant
    microlight -*see* Accident, transport,
    aircraft, occupant, powered, glider
    minibus -*see* Accident, transport, pickup
    truck occupant
    minivan -*see* Accident, transport, pickup
    truck occupant
    moped -*see* Accident, transport,
    motorcycle
    motor scooter -*see* Accident, transport,
    motorcycle
    motorcycle (with sidecar) -*see* Accident,
    transport, motorcycle
    pedal cycle -*see also* Accident, transport,
    pedal cyclist
    pick-up (truck) -*see* Accident, transport,
    pickup truck occupant
    railway (train) (vehicle) (subterranean)
    (elevated) -*see* Accident, transport,
    railway vehicle occupant
    rickshaw -*see* Accident, transport, pedal
    cycle

Accident -- *continued*

motorized -*see* Accident, transport, three-wheeled motor vehicle

    pedal driven -*see* Accident, transport, pedal cyclist

road-roller -*see* Accident, transport, construction vehicle occupant

ship NOS V94.9

ski-lift (chair) (gondola) V98.3

snowmobile -*see* Accident, transport, snowmobile occupant

spacecraft, spaceship -*see* Accident, transport, aircraft, occupant, spacecraft

sport utility vehicle -*see* Accident, transport, pickup truck occupant

streetcar (interurban) (operating on public street or highway) -*see* Accident, transport, streetcar occupant

SUV -*see* Accident, transport, pickup truck occupant

téléférique V98.0

three-wheeled vehicle (motorized) -*see also* Accident, transport, three-wheeled motor vehicle occupant

    nonmotorized -*see* Accident, transport, pedal cycle

tractor (farm) (and trailer) -*see* Accident, transport, agricultural vehicle occupant

train -*see* Accident, transport, railway vehicle occupant

tram -*see* Accident, transport, streetcar occupant

    in mine or quarry -*see* Accident, transport, industrial vehicle occupant

tricycle -*see* Accident, transport, pedal cycle

    motorized -*see* Accident, transport, three-wheeled motor vehicle

trolley -*see* Accident, transport, streetcar occupant

    in mine or quarry -*see* Accident, transport, industrial vehicle occupant

tub, in mine or quarry -*see* Accident, transport, industrial vehicle occupant

ultralight -*see* Accident, transport, aircraft, occupant, powered, glider

van -*see* Accident, transport, van occupant

vehicle NEC V89.9

    heavy transport -*see* Accident, transport, truck occupant

    motor (traffic) NEC V89.2

      nontraffic NEC V89.0

watercraft NOS V94.9

    causing drowning -*see* Drowning, resulting from accident to boat

parachutist V97.29

    after accident to aircraft -*see* Accident, transport, aircraft

    entangled in object V97.21

    injured on landing V97.22

pedal cyclist V19.9

    collision (with)

      animal (traffic) V10.9

        being ridden (traffic) V16.9

          nontraffic V16.2

          while boarding or alighting V16.3

        nontraffic V10.2

        while boarding or alighting V10.3

      animal-drawn vehicle (traffic) V16.9

        nontraffic V16.2

Accident -- *continued*

        while boarding or alighting V16.3

      bus (traffic) V14.9

        nontraffic V14.2

        while boarding or alighting V14.3

      car (traffic) V13.9

        nontraffic V13.2

        while boarding or alighting V13.3

      motor vehicle NOS (traffic) V19.60

        nontraffic V19.20

        specified type NEC (traffic) V19.69

          nontraffic V19.29

      pedal cycle (traffic) V11.9

        nontraffic V11.2

        while boarding or alighting V11.3

      pickup truck (traffic) V13.9

        nontraffic V13.2

        while boarding or alighting V13.3

      railway vehicle (traffic) V15.9

        nontraffic V15.2

        while boarding or alighting V15.3

      specified vehicle NEC (traffic) V16.9

        nontraffic V16.2

        while boarding or alighting V16.3

      stationary object (traffic) V17.9

        nontraffic V17.2

        while boarding or alighting V17.3

      streetcar (traffic) V16.9

        nontraffic V16.2

        while boarding or alighting V16.3

      three wheeled motor vehicle (traffic) V12.9

        nontraffic V12.2

        while boarding or alighting V12.3

      truck (traffic) V14.9

        nontraffic V14.2

        while boarding or alighting V14.3

      two wheeled motor vehicle (traffic) V12.9

        nontraffic V12.2

        while boarding or alighting V12.3

      van (traffic) V13.9

        nontraffic V13.2

        while boarding or alighting V13.3

    driver

      collision (with)

        animal (traffic) V10.4

          being ridden (traffic) V16.4

            nontraffic V16.0

          nontraffic V10.0

        animal-drawn vehicle (traffic) V16.4

          nontraffic V16.0

        bus (traffic) V14.4

          nontraffic V14.0

        car (traffic) V13.4

          nontraffic V13.0

        motor vehicle NOS (traffic) V19.40

          nontraffic V19.00

          specified type NEC (traffic) V19.49

            nontraffic V19.09

        pedal cycle (traffic) V11.4

          nontraffic V11.0

        pickup truck (traffic) V13.4

          nontraffic V13.0

        railway vehicle (traffic) V15.4

          nontraffic V15.0

        specified vehicle NEC (traffic) V16.4

          nontraffic V16.0

        stationary object (traffic) V17.4

          nontraffic V17.0

        streetcar (traffic) V16.4

Accident -- *continued*

          nontraffic V16.0

        three wheeled motor vehicle (traffic) V12.4

          nontraffic V12.0

        truck (traffic) V14.4

          nontraffic V14.0

        two wheeled motor vehicle (traffic) V12.4

          nontraffic V12.0

        van (traffic) V13.4

          nontraffic V13.0

      noncollision accident (traffic) V18.4

        nontraffic V18.0

    noncollision accident (traffic) V18.9

      nontraffic V18.2

      while boarding or alighting V18.3

    nontraffic V19.3

    passenger

      collision (with)

        animal (traffic) V10.5

          being ridden (traffic) V16.5

            nontraffic V16.1

          nontraffic V10.1

        animal-drawn vehicle (traffic) V16.5

          nontraffic V16.1

        bus (traffic) V14.5

          nontraffic V14.1

        car (traffic) V13.5

          nontraffic V13.1

        motor vehicle NOS (traffic) V19.50

          nontraffic V19.10

          specified type NEC (traffic) V19.59

            nontraffic V19.19

        pedal cycle (traffic) V11.5

          nontraffic V11.1

        pickup truck (traffic) V13.5

          nontraffic V13.1

        railway vehicle (traffic) V15.5

          nontraffic V15.1

        specified vehicle NEC (traffic) V16.5

          nontraffic V16.1

        stationary object (traffic) V17.5

          nontraffic V17.1

        streetcar (traffic) V16.5

          nontraffic V16.1

        three wheeled motor vehicle (traffic) V12.5

          nontraffic V12.1

        truck (traffic) V14.5

          nontraffic V14.1

        two wheeled motor vehicle (traffic) V12.5

          nontraffic V12.1

        van (traffic) V13.5

          nontraffic V13.1

      noncollision accident (traffic) V18.5

        nontraffic V18.1

    specified type NEC V19.88

      military vehicle V19.81

    pedestrian

      conveyance (occupant) V09.9

      babystroller V00.828

        collision (with) V09.9

          animal being ridden or animal drawn vehicle V06.99

            nontraffic V06.09

            traffic V06.19

          bus or heavy transport V04.99

            nontraffic V04.09

            traffic V04.19

Accident -- *continued*
traffic V05.11
streetcar V06.91
nontraffic V06.01
traffic V06.11
stationary object V00.122
two- or three-wheeled motor vehicle
V02.91
nontraffic V02.01
traffic V02.11
vehicle V09.9
animal-drawn V06.91
nontraffic V06.01
traffic V06.11
motor
nontraffic V09.00
traffic V09.20
fall V00.121
in-line V00.118
collision- -*see also* Accident,
transport, pedestrian, conveyance
occupant, roller skates, collision
with stationary object V00.112
fall V00.111
nontraffic V09.1
involving motor vehicle NEC
V09.00
traffic V09.3
involving motor vehicle NEC
V09.20
rolling shoes V00.158
colliding with stationary object
V00.152
fall V00.151
rolling type NEC V00.188
collision (with) V09.9
animal being ridden or animal drawn
vehicle V06.99
nontraffic V06.09
traffic V06.19
bus or heavy transport V04.99
nontraffic V04.09
traffic V04.19
car V03.99
nontraffic V03.09
traffic V03.19
pedal cycle V01.99
nontraffic V01.09
traffic V01.19
pick-up truck or van V03.99
nontraffic V03.09
traffic V03.19
railway (train) (vehicle) V05.99
nontraffic V05.09
traffic V05.19
stationary object V00.182
streetcar V06.99
nontraffic V06.09
traffic V06.19
two- or three-wheeled motor vehicle
V02.99
nontraffic V02.09
traffic V02.19
vehicle V09.9
animal-drawn V06.99
nontraffic V06.09
traffic V06.19
motor
nontraffic V09.00
traffic V09.20
fall V00.181

in-line roller skate -*see* Accident,
transport, pedestrian, conveyance,
roller skate, in-line
nontraffic V09.1
involving motor vehicle NEC
V09.00
roller skate -*see* Accident, transport,
pedestrian, conveyance, roller skate
scooter (non-motorized) -*see*
Accident, transport, pedestrian,
conveyance, scooter
skateboard -*see* Accident, transport,
pedestrian, conveyance, skateboard
traffic V09.3
involving motor vehicle NEC
V09.20
scooter (non-motorized) V00.148
collision (with) V09.9
animal being ridden or animal drawn
vehicle V06.99
nontraffic V06.09
traffic V06.19
bus or heavy transport V04.99
nontraffic V04.09
traffic V04.19
car V03.99
nontraffic V03.09
traffic V03.19
pedal cycle V01.99
nontraffic V01.09
traffic V01.19
pick-up truck or van V03.99
nontraffic V03.09
traffic V03.19
railway (train) (vehicle) V05.99
nontraffic V05.09
traffic V05.19
streetcar V06.99
nontraffic V06.09
traffic V06.19
stationary object V00.142
two- or three-wheeled motor vehicle
V02.99
nontraffic V02.09
traffic V02.19
vehicle V09.9
animal-drawn V06.99
nontraffic V06.09
traffic V06.19
motor
nontraffic V09.00
traffic V09.20
fall V00.141
nontraffic V09.1
involving motor vehicle NEC
V09.00
traffic V09.3
involving motor vehicle NEC
V09.20
skate board V00.138
collision (with) V09.9
animal being ridden or animal drawn
vehicle V06.92
nontraffic V06.02
traffic V06.12
bus or heavy transport V04.92
nontraffic V04.02
traffic V04.12
car V03.92
nontraffic V03.02

Accident -- *continued*
traffic V03.12
pedal cycle V01.92
nontraffic V01.02
traffic V01.12
pick-up truck or van V03.92
nontraffic V03.02
traffic V03.12
railway (train) (vehicle) V05.92
nontraffic V05.02
traffic V05.12
streetcar V06.92
nontraffic V06.02
traffic V06.12
stationary object V00.132
two- or three-wheeled motor vehicle
V02.92
nontraffic V02.02
traffic V02.12
vehicle V09.9
animal-drawn V06.92
nontraffic V06.02
traffic V06.12
motor
nontraffic V09.00
traffic V09.20
fall V00.131
nontraffic V09.1
involving motor vehicle NEC
V09.00
traffic V09.3
involving motor vehicle NEC
V09.20
sled V00.228
collision (with) V09.9
animal being ridden or animal drawn
vehicle V06.99
nontraffic V06.09
traffic V06.19
bus or heavy transport V04.99
nontraffic V04.09
traffic V04.19
car V03.99
nontraffic V03.09
traffic V03.19
pedal cycle V01.99
nontraffic V01.09
traffic V01.19
pick-up truck or van V03.99
nontraffic V03.09
traffic V03.19
railway (train) (vehicle) V05.99
nontraffic V05.09
traffic V05.19
streetcar V06.99
nontraffic V06.09
traffic V06.19
stationary object V00.222
two- or three-wheeled motor vehicle
V02.99
nontraffic V02.09
traffic V02.19
vehicle V09.9
animal-drawn V06.99
nontraffic V06.09
traffic V06.19
motor
nontraffic V09.00
traffic V09.20
fall V00.221
nontraffic V09.1

Accident -- *continued*

    involving motor vehicle NEC
      V09.00
    traffic V09.3
    involving motor vehicle NEC
      V09.20
  skis (snow) V00.328
    collision (with) V09.9
    animal being ridden or animal drawn
      vehicle V06.99
      nontraffic V06.09
      traffic V06.19
    bus or heavy transport V04.99
      nontraffic V04.09
      traffic V04.19
    car V03.99
      nontraffic V03.09
      traffic V03.19
    pedal cycle V01.99
      nontraffic V01.09
      traffic V01.19
    pick-up truck or van V03.99
      nontraffic V03.09
      traffic V03.19
    railway (train) (vehicle) V05.99
      nontraffic V05.09
      traffic V05.19
    streetcar V06.99
      nontraffic V06.09
      traffic V06.19
    stationary object V00.322
    two- or three-wheeled motor vehicle
      V02.99
      nontraffic V02.09
      traffic V02.19
    vehicle V09.9
      animal-drawn V06.99
      nontraffic V06.09
      traffic V06.19
      motor
      nontraffic V09.00
      traffic V09.20
    fall V00.321
    nontraffic V09.1
    involving motor vehicle NEC
      V09.00
    traffic V09.3
    involving motor vehicle NEC
      V09.20
  snow board V00.318
    collision (with) V09.9
    animal being ridden or animal drawn
      vehicle V06.99
      nontraffic V06.09
      traffic V06.19
    bus or heavy transport V04.99
      nontraffic V04.09
      traffic V04.19
    car V03.99
      nontraffic V03.09
      traffic V03.19
    pedal cycle V01.99
      nontraffic V01.09
      traffic V01.19
    pick-up truck or van V03.99
      nontraffic V03.09
      traffic V03.19
    railway (train) (vehicle) V05.99
      nontraffic V05.09
      traffic V05.19
    streetcar V06.99

-- continued

    nontraffic V06.09
    traffic V06.19
    stationary object V00.312
    two- or three-wheeled motor vehicle
      V02.99
      nontraffic V02.09
      traffic V02.19
    vehicle V09.9
      animal-drawn V06.99
      nontraffic V06.09
      traffic V06.19
      motor
      nontraffic V09.00
      traffic V09.20
    fall V00.311
    nontraffic V09.1
    involving motor vehicle NEC
      V09.00
    traffic V09.3
    involving motor vehicle NEC
      V09.20
  specified type NEC V00.898
    collision (with) V09.9
    animal being ridden or animal drawn
      vehicle V06.99
      nontraffic V06.09
      traffic V06.19
    bus or heavy transport V04.99
      nontraffic V04.09
      traffic V04.19
    car V03.99
      nontraffic V03.09
      traffic V03.19
    pedal cycle V01.99
      nontraffic V01.09
      traffic V01.19
    pick-up truck or van V03.99
      nontraffic V03.09
      traffic V03.19
    railway (train) (vehicle) V05.99
      nontraffic V05.09
      traffic V05.19
    streetcar V06.99
      nontraffic V06.09
      traffic V06.19
    stationary object V00.892
    two- or three-wheeled motor vehicle
      V02.99
      nontraffic V02.09
      traffic V02.19
    vehicle V09.9
      animal-drawn V06.99
      nontraffic V06.09
      traffic V06.19
      motor
      nontraffic V09.00
      traffic V09.20
    fall V00.891
    nontraffic V09.1
    involving motor vehicle NEC
      V09.00
    traffic V09.3
    involving motor vehicle NEC
      V09.20
  traffic V09.3
    involving motor vehicle V09.20
    military V09.21
    specified type NEC V09.29
  wheelchair (powered) V00.818
    collision (with) V09.9

-- continued

  animal being ridden or animal drawn
    vehicle V06.99
    nontraffic V06.09
    traffic V06.19
  bus or heavy transport V04.99
    nontraffic V04.09
    traffic V04.19
  car V03.99
    nontraffic V03.09
    traffic V03.19
  pedal cycle V01.99
    nontraffic V01.09
    traffic V01.19
  pick-up truck or van V03.99
    nontraffic V03.09
    traffic V03.19
  railway (train) (vehicle) V05.99
    nontraffic V05.09
    traffic V05.19
  streetcar V06.99
    nontraffic V06.09
    traffic V06.19
  stationary object V00.812
  two- or three-wheeled motor vehicle
    V02.99
    nontraffic V02.09
    traffic V02.19
  vehicle V09.9
    animal-drawn V06.99
    nontraffic V06.09
    traffic V06.19
    motor
    nontraffic V09.00
    traffic V09.20
  fall V00.811
  nontraffic V09.1
    involving motor vehicle NEC
      V09.00
  traffic V09.3
    involving motor vehicle NEC
      V09.20
  wheeled shoe V00.158
    colliding with stationary object
      V00.152
    fall V00.151
  on foot -*see also* Accident, pedestrian
    collision (with)
    animal being ridden or animal drawn
      vehicle V06.90
      nontraffic V06.00
      traffic V06.10
    bus or heavy transport V04.90
      nontraffic V04.00
      traffic V04.10
    car V03.90
      nontraffic V03.00
      traffic V03.10
    pedal cycle V01.90
      nontraffic V01.00
      traffic V01.10
    pick-up truck or van V03.90
      nontraffic V03.00
      traffic V03.10
    railway (train) (vehicle) V05.90
      nontraffic V05.00
      traffic V05.10
    streetcar V06.90
      nontraffic V06.00
      traffic V06.10

Accident -- *continued*

nontraffic V33.2
noncollision accident (traffic) V38.7
  nontraffic V38.2
passenger
  collision (with)
    animal (traffic) V30.6
      being ridden (traffic) V36.6
        nontraffic V36.1
      nontraffic V30.1
    animal-drawn vehicle (traffic) V36.6
      nontraffic V36.1
    bus (traffic) V34.6
      nontraffic V34.1
    car (traffic) V33.6
      nontraffic V33.1
    motor vehicle NOS (traffic) V39.50
      nontraffic V39.10
      specified type NEC (traffic) V39.59
        nontraffic V39.19
    pedal cycle (traffic) V31.6
      nontraffic V31.1
    pickup truck (traffic) V33.6
      nontraffic V33.1
    railway vehicle (traffic) V35.6
      nontraffic V35.1
    specified vehicle NEC (traffic) V36.6
      nontraffic V36.1
    stationary object (traffic) V37.6
      nontraffic V37.1
    streetcar (traffic) V36.6
      nontraffic V36.1
    three wheeled motor vehicle (traffic)
      V32.6
      nontraffic V32.1
    truck (traffic) V34.6
      nontraffic V34.1
    two wheeled motor vehicle (traffic)
      V32.6
      nontraffic V32.1
    van (traffic) V33.6
      nontraffic V33.1
  noncollision accident (traffic) V38.6
    nontraffic V38.1
specified type NEC V39.89
  military vehicle V39.81
tractor (farm) (and trailer) -*see* Accident,
transport, agricultural vehicle occupant
tram -*see* Accident, transport, streetcar
  in mine or quarry -*see* Accident,
transport, industrial vehicle occupant
trolley -*see* Accident, transport, streetcar
  in mine or quarry -*see* Accident,
transport, industrial vehicle occupant
truck (heavy) occupant V69.9
  collision (with)
    animal (traffic) V60.9
      being ridden (traffic) V66.9
        nontraffic V66.3
        while boarding or alighting V66.4
      nontraffic V60.3
      while boarding or alighting V60.4
    animal-drawn vehicle (traffic) V66.9
      nontraffic V66.3
      while boarding or alighting V66.4
    bus (traffic) V64.9
      nontraffic V64.3
      while boarding or alighting V64.4
    car (traffic) V63.9
      nontraffic V63.3
      while boarding or alighting V63.4

Accident -- *continued*

motor vehicle NOS (traffic) V69.60
  nontraffic V69.20
  specified type NEC (traffic) V69.69
    nontraffic V69.29
pedal cycle (traffic) V61.9
  nontraffic V61.3
  while boarding or alighting V61.4
pickup truck (traffic) V63.9
  nontraffic V63.3
  while boarding or alighting V63.4
railway vehicle (traffic) V65.9
  nontraffic V65.3
  while boarding or alighting V65.4
specified vehicle NEC (traffic) V66.9
  nontraffic V66.3
  while boarding or alighting V66.4
stationary object (traffic) V67.9
  nontraffic V67.3
  while boarding or alighting V67.4
streetcar (traffic) V66.9
  nontraffic V66.3
  while boarding or alighting V66.4
three wheeled motor vehicle (traffic)
  V62.9
  nontraffic V62.3
  while boarding or alighting V62.4
truck (traffic) V64.9
  nontraffic V64.3
  while boarding or alighting V64.4
two wheeled motor vehicle (traffic)
  V62.9
  nontraffic V62.3
  while boarding or alighting V62.4
van (traffic) V63.9
  nontraffic V63.3
  while boarding or alighting V63.4
driver
  collision (with)
    animal (traffic) V60.5
      being ridden (traffic) V66.5
        nontraffic V66.0
      nontraffic V60.0
    animal-drawn vehicle (traffic) V66.5
      nontraffic V66.0
    bus (traffic) V64.5
      nontraffic V64.0
    car (traffic) V63.5
      nontraffic V63.0
    motor vehicle NOS (traffic) V69.40
      nontraffic V69.00
      specified type NEC (traffic) V69.49
        nontraffic V69.09
    pedal cycle (traffic) V61.5
      nontraffic V61.0
    pickup truck (traffic) V63.5
      nontraffic V63.0
    railway vehicle (traffic) V65.5
      nontraffic V65.0
    specified vehicle NEC (traffic) V66.5
      nontraffic V66.0
    stationary object (traffic) V67.5
      nontraffic V67.0
    streetcar (traffic) V66.5
      nontraffic V66.0
    three wheeled motor vehicle (traffic)
      V62.5
      nontraffic V62.0
    truck (traffic) V64.5
      nontraffic V64.0

Accident -- *continued*

two wheeled motor vehicle (traffic)
  V62.5
  nontraffic V62.0
  van (traffic) V63.5
  nontraffic V63.0
noncollision accident (traffic) V68.5
  nontraffic V68.0
dump -*see* Accident, transport,
construction vehicle occupant
hanger-on
  collision (with)
    animal (traffic) V60.7
      being ridden (traffic) V66.7
        nontraffic V66.2
      nontraffic V60.2
    animal-drawn vehicle (traffic) V66.7
      nontraffic V66.2
    bus (traffic) V64.7
      nontraffic V64.2
    car (traffic) V63.7
      nontraffic V63.2
    pedal cycle (traffic) V61.7
      nontraffic V61.2
    pickup truck (traffic) V63.7
      nontraffic V63.2
    railway vehicle (traffic) V65.7
      nontraffic V65.2
    specified vehicle NEC (traffic) V66.7
      nontraffic V66.2
    stationary object (traffic) V67.7
      nontraffic V67.2
    streetcar (traffic) V66.7
      nontraffic V66.2
    three wheeled motor vehicle (traffic)
      V62.7
      nontraffic V62.2
    truck (traffic) V64.7
      nontraffic V64.2
    two wheeled motor vehicle (traffic)
      V62.7
      nontraffic V62.2
    van (traffic) V63.7
      nontraffic V63.2
  noncollision accident (traffic) V68.7
    nontraffic V68.2
noncollision accident (traffic) V68.9
  nontraffic V68.3
  while boarding or alighting V68.4
nontraffic V69.3
passenger
  collision (with)
    animal (traffic) V60.6
      being ridden (traffic) V66.6
        nontraffic V66.1
      nontraffic V60.1
    animal-drawn vehicle (traffic) V66.6
      nontraffic V66.1
    bus (traffic) V64.6
      nontraffic V64.1
    car (traffic) V63.6
      nontraffic V63.1
    motor vehicle NOS (traffic) V69.50
      nontraffic V69.10
      specified type NEC (traffic) V69.59
        nontraffic V69.19
    pedal cycle (traffic) V61.6
      nontraffic V61.1
    pickup truck (traffic) V63.6
      nontraffic V63.1
    railway vehicle (traffic) V65.6

Accident -- *continued*
   nontraffic V65.1
      specified vehicle NEC (traffic) V66.6
         nontraffic V66.1
      stationary object (traffic) V67.6
         nontraffic V67.1
      streetcar (traffic) V66.6
         nontraffic V66.1
      three wheeled motor vehicle (traffic)
         V62.6
         nontraffic V62.1
      truck (traffic) V64.6
         nontraffic V64.1
      two wheeled motor vehicle (traffic)
         V62.6
         nontraffic V62.1
      van (traffic) V63.6
         nontraffic V63.1
   noncollision accident (traffic) V68.6
      nontraffic V68.1
   pickup -*see* Accident, transport, pickup
   truck occupant
      specified type NEC V69.88
      military vehicle V69.81
   van occupant V59.9
      collision (with)
         animal (traffic) V50.9
            being ridden (traffic) V56.9
               nontraffic V56.3
               while boarding or alighting V56.4
            nontraffic V50.3
            while boarding or alighting V50.4
         animal-drawn vehicle (traffic) V56.9
            nontraffic V56.3
            while boarding or alighting V56.4
         bus (traffic) V54.9
            nontraffic V54.3
            while boarding or alighting V54.4
         car (traffic) V53.9
            nontraffic V53.3
            while boarding or alighting V53.4
         motor vehicle NOS (traffic) V59.60
            nontraffic V59.20
            specified type NEC (traffic) V59.69
               nontraffic V59.29
         pedal cycle (traffic) V51.9
            nontraffic V51.3
            while boarding or alighting V51.4
         pickup truck (traffic) V53.9
            nontraffic V53.3
            while boarding or alighting V53.4
         railway vehicle (traffic) V55.9
            nontraffic V55.3
            while boarding or alighting V55.4
         specified vehicle NEC (traffic) V56.9
            nontraffic V56.3
            while boarding or alighting V56.4
         stationary object (traffic) V57.9
            nontraffic V57.3
            while boarding or alighting V57.4
         streetcar (traffic) V56.9
            nontraffic V56.3
            while boarding or alighting V56.4
         three wheeled motor vehicle (traffic)
            V52.9
            nontraffic V52.3
            while boarding or alighting V52.4
         truck (traffic) V54.9
            nontraffic V54.3
            while boarding or alighting V54.4

Accident -- *continued*
      two wheeled motor vehicle (traffic)
         V52.9
         nontraffic V52.3
         while boarding or alighting V52.4
      van (traffic) V53.9
         nontraffic V53.3
         while boarding or alighting V53.4
   driver
      collision (with)
         animal (traffic) V50.5
            being ridden (traffic) V56.5
               nontraffic V56.0
            nontraffic V50.0
         animal-drawn vehicle (traffic) V56.5
            nontraffic V56.0
         bus (traffic) V54.5
            nontraffic V54.0
         car (traffic) V53.5
            nontraffic V53.0
         motor vehicle NOS (traffic) V59.40
            nontraffic V59.00
            specified type NEC (traffic) V59.49
               nontraffic V59.09
         pedal cycle (traffic) V51.5
            nontraffic V51.0
         pickup truck (traffic) V53.5
            nontraffic V53.0
         railway vehicle (traffic) V55.5
            nontraffic V55.0
         specified vehicle NEC (traffic) V56.5
            nontraffic V56.0
         stationary object (traffic) V57.5
            nontraffic V57.0
         streetcar (traffic) V56.5
            nontraffic V56.0
         three wheeled motor vehicle (traffic)
            V52.5
            nontraffic V52.0
         truck (traffic) V54.5
            nontraffic V54.0
         two wheeled motor vehicle (traffic)
            V52.5
            nontraffic V52.0
         van (traffic) V53.5
            nontraffic V53.0
      noncollision accident (traffic) V58.5
         nontraffic V58.0
   noncollision accident (traffic) V58.9
      nontraffic V58.3
      while boarding or alighting V58.4
   nontraffic V59.3
   hanger-on
      collision (with)
         animal (traffic) V50.7
            being ridden (traffic) V56.7
               nontraffic V56.2
            nontraffic V50.2
         animal-drawn vehicle (traffic) V56.7
            nontraffic V56.2
         bus (traffic) V54.7
            nontraffic V54.2
         car (traffic) V53.7
            nontraffic V53.2
         pedal cycle (traffic) V51.7
            nontraffic V51.2
         pickup truck (traffic) V53.7
            nontraffic V53.2
         railway vehicle (traffic) V55.7
            nontraffic V55.2
         specified vehicle NEC (traffic) V56.7

Accident -- *continued*
            nontraffic V56.2
         stationary object (traffic) V57.7
            nontraffic V57.2
         streetcar (traffic) V56.7
            nontraffic V56.2
         three wheeled motor vehicle (traffic)
            V52.7
            nontraffic V52.2
         truck (traffic) V54.7
            nontraffic V54.2
         two wheeled motor vehicle (traffic)
            V52.7
            nontraffic V52.2
         van (traffic) V53.7
            nontraffic V53.2
      noncollision accident (traffic) V58.7
         nontraffic V58.2
   passenger
      collision (with)
         animal (traffic) V50.6
            being ridden (traffic) V56.6
               nontraffic V56.1
            nontraffic V50.1
         animal-drawn vehicle (traffic) V56.6
            nontraffic V56.1
         bus (traffic) V54.6
            nontraffic V54.1
         car (traffic) V53.6
            nontraffic V53.1
         motor vehicle NOS (traffic) V59.50
            nontraffic V59.10
            specified type NEC (traffic) V59.59
               nontraffic V59.19
         pedal cycle (traffic) V51.6
            nontraffic V51.1
         pickup truck (traffic) V53.6
            nontraffic V53.1
         railway vehicle (traffic) V55.6
            nontraffic V55.1
         specified vehicle NEC (traffic) V56.6
            nontraffic V56.1
         stationary object (traffic) V57.6
            nontraffic V57.1
         streetcar (traffic) V56.6
            nontraffic V56.1
         three wheeled motor vehicle (traffic)
            V52.6
            nontraffic V52.1
         truck (traffic) V54.6
            nontraffic V54.1
         two wheeled motor vehicle (traffic)
            V52.6
            nontraffic V52.1
         van (traffic) V53.6
            nontraffic V53.1
      noncollision accident (traffic) V58.6
         nontraffic V58.1
      specified type NEC V59.88
         military vehicle V59.81
   watercraft occupant -*see* Accident,
      watercraft
   vehicle NEC V89.9
   animal-drawn NEC -*see* Accident,
      transport, animal-drawn vehicle occupant
   special
      agricultural -*see* Accident, transport,
         agricultural vehicle occupant
      construction -*see* Accident, transport,
         construction vehicle occupant
      industrial -*see* Accident, transport,
         industrial vehicle occupant

Accident -- *continued*
  three-wheeled NEC (motorized) -*see*
    Accident, transport, three-wheeled
    motor vehicle occupant
  watercraft V94.9
  causing
    drowning -*see* Drowning, due to, accident
      to, watercraft
    injury NEC V91.89
      crushed between craft and object
        V91.19
        powered craft V91.13
          ferry boat V91.11
          fishing boat V91.12
          jet skis V91.13
          liner V91.11
          merchant ship V91.10
          passenger ship V91.11
        unpowered craft V91.18
          canoe V91.15
          inflatable V91.16
          kayak V91.15
          sailboat V91.14
          surf-board V91.18
          windsurfer V91.18
      fall on board V91.29
        powered craft V91.23
          ferry boat V91.21
          fishing boat V91.22
          jet skis V91.23
          liner V91.21
          merchant ship V91.20
          passenger ship V91.21
        unpowered craft
          canoe V91.25
          inflatable V91.26
          kayak V91.25
          sailboat V91.24
      fire on board causing burn V91.09
        powered craft V91.03
          ferry boat V91.01
          fishing boat V91.02
          jet skis V91.03
          liner V91.01
          merchant ship V91.00
          passenger ship V91.01
        unpowered craft V91.08
          canoe V91.05
          inflatable V91.06
          kayak V91.05
          sailboat V91.04
          surf-board V91.08
          water skis V91.07
          windsurfer V91.08
      hit by falling object V91.39
        powered craft V91.33
          ferry boat V91.31
          fishing boat V91.32
          jet skis V91.33
          liner V91.31
          merchant ship V91.30
          passenger ship V91.31
        unpowered craft V91.38
          canoe V91.35
          inflatable V91.36
          kayak V91.35
          sailboat V91.34
          surf-board V91.38
          water skis V91.37
          windsurfer V91.38
      specified type NEC V91.89

Accident -- *continued*
      powered craft V91.83
        ferry boat V91.81
        fishing boat V91.82
        jet skis V91.83
        liner V91.81
        merchant ship V91.80
        passenger ship V91.81
      unpowered craft V91.88
        canoe V91.85
        inflatable V91.86
        kayak V91.85
        sailboat V91.84
        surf-board V91.88
        water skis V91.87
        windsurfer V91.88
    due to, caused by cataclysm -*see* Forces of
      nature, by type
    military NEC V94.818
      with civilian watercraft V94.810
      civilian in water injured by V94.811
    nonpowered, struck by
      nonpowered vessel V94.22
      powered vessel V94.21
    specified type NEC V94.89
    striking swimmer
      powered V94.11
      unpowered V94.12

Acid throwing (assault) Y08.89
**Activity (involving) (of victim at time of
event)** Y93.9
  aerobic and step exercise (class) Y93.A3
  alpine skiing Y93.23
  animal care NEC Y93.K9
  arts and handcrafts NEC Y93.D9
  athletics NEC Y93.79
  athletics played as a team or group NEC
    Y93.69
  athletics played individually NEC Y93.59
  baking Y93.G3
  ballet Y93.41
  barbells Y93.B3
  BASE (Building, Antenna, Span, Earth)
    jumping Y93.33
  baseball Y93.64
  basketball Y93.67
  bathing (personal) Y93.E1
  beach volleyball Y93.68
  bike riding Y93.55
  blackout game Y93.85
  boogie boarding Y93.18
  bowling Y93.54
  boxing Y93.71
  brass instrument playing Y93.J4
  building construction Y93.H3
  bungee jumping Y93.34
  calisthenics Y93.A2
  canoeing (in calm and turbulent water)
    Y93.16
  capture the flag Y93.6A
  cardiorespiratory exercise NEC Y93.A9
  caregiving (providing) NEC Y93.F9
    bathing Y93.F1
    lifting Y93.F2
  cellular
    communication device Y93.C2
    telephone Y93.C2
  challenge course Y93.A5
  cheerleading Y93.45
  choking game Y93.85
  circuit training Y93.A4

Activity -- *continued*
  cleaning
    floor Y93.E5
  climbing NEC Y93.39
    mountain Y93.31
    rock Y93.31
    wall Y93.31
  clothing care and maintenance NEC Y93.E9
  combatives Y93.75
  computer
    keyboarding Y93.C1
    technology NEC Y93.C9
  confidence course Y93.A5
  construction (building) Y93.H3
  cooking and baking Y93.G3
  cool down exercises Y93.A2
  cricket Y93.69
  crocheting Y93.D1
  cross country skiing Y93.24
  dancing (all types) Y93.41
  digging
    dirt Y93.H1
  dirt digging Y93.H1
  dishwashing Y93.G1
  diving (platform) (springboard) Y93.12
    underwater Y93.15
  dodge ball Y93.6A
  downhill skiing Y93.23
  drum playing Y93.J2
  dumbbells Y93.B3
  electronic
    devices NEC Y93.C9
      hand held interactive Y93.C2
    game playing (using) (with)
      interactive device Y93.C2
      keyboard or other stationary device
        Y93.C1
  elliptical machine Y93.A1
  exercise(s)
    machines ((primarily) for)
      cardiorespiratory conditioning Y93.A1
      muscle strengthening Y93.B1
    muscle strengthening (non-machine) NEC
      Y93.B9
  external motion NEC Y93.I9
    rollercoaster Y93.I1
  fainting game Y93.85
  field hockey Y93.65
  figure skating (pairs) (singles) Y93.21
  flag football Y93.62
  floor mopping and cleaning Y93.E5
  food preparation and clean up Y93.G1
  football (American) NOS Y93.61
    flag Y93.62
    tackle Y93.61
    touch Y93.62
  four square Y93.6A
  free weights Y93.B3
  frisbee (ultimate) Y93.74
  furniture
    building Y93.D3
    finishing Y93.D3
    repair Y93.D3
  game playing (electronic)
    using keyboard or other stationary device
      Y93.C1
    using interactive device Y93.C2
  gardening Y93.H2
  golf Y93.53
  grass drills Y93.A6
  grilling and smoking food Y93.G2

Activity -- *continued*
grooming and shearing an animal Y93.K3
guerilla drills Y93.A6
gymnastics (rhythmic) Y93.43
handball Y93.73
handcrafts NEC Y93.D9
hand held interactive electronic device Y93.C2
hang gliding Y93.35
hiking (on level or elevated terrain) Y93.01
hockey (ice) Y93.22
  field Y93.65
horseback riding Y93.52
household (interior) maintenance NEC Y93.E9
ice NEC Y93.29
  dancing Y93.21
  hockey Y93.22
  skating Y93.21
inline roller skating Y93.51
ironing Y93.E4
judo Y93.75
jumping (off) NEC Y93.39
  BASE (Building, Antenna, Span, Earth) Y93.33
  bungee Y93.34
  jacks Y93.A2
  rope Y93.56
jumping jacks Y93.A2
jumping rope Y93.56
karate Y93.75
kayaking (in calm and turbulent water) Y93.16
keyboarding (computer) Y93.C1
kickball Y93.6A
knitting Y93.D1
lacrosse Y93.65
land maintenance NEC Y93.H9
landscaping Y93.H2
laundry Y93.E2
machines (exercise)
  primarily for cardiorespiratory conditioning Y93.A1
  primarily for muscle strengthening Y93.B1
maintenance
  exterior building NEC Y93.H9
  household (interior) NEC Y93.E9
  land Y93.H9
  property Y93.H9
marching (on level or elevated terrain) Y93.01
martial arts Y93.75
microwave oven Y93.G3
milking an animal Y93.K2
mopping (floor) Y93.E5
mountain climbing Y93.31
muscle strengthening
  exercises (non-machine) NEC Y93.B9
  machines Y93.B1
musical keyboard (electronic) playing Y93.J1
Nordic skiing Y93.24
obstacle course Y93.A5
oven (microwave) Y93.G3
packing up and unpacking in moving to a new residence Y93.E6
parasailing Y93.19
pass out game Y93.85
percussion instrument playing NEC Y93.J2
personal
  bathing and showering Y93.E1

Activity -- *continued*
  hygiene NEC Y93.E8
  showering Y93.E1
physical games generally associated with school recess, summer camp and children Y93.6A
physical training NEC Y93.A9
piano playing Y93.J1
pilates Y93.B4
platform diving Y93.12
playing musical instrument
  brass instrument Y93.J4
  drum Y93.J2
  musical keyboard (electronic) Y93.J1
  percussion instrument NEC Y93.J2
  piano Y93.J1
  string instrument Y93.J3
  winds instrument Y93.J4
property maintenance
  exterior NEC Y93.H9
  interior NEC Y93.E9
pruning (garden and lawn) Y93.H2
pull-ups Y93.B2
push-ups Y93.B2
racquetball Y93.73
rafting (in calm and turbulent water) Y93.16
raking (leaves) Y93.H1
rappelling Y93.32
refereeing a sports activity Y93.81
residential relocation Y93.E6
rhythmic gymnastics Y93.43
rhythmic movement NEC Y93.49
riding
  horseback Y93.52
  rollercoaster Y93.I1
rock climbing Y93.31
rollercoaster riding Y93.I1
roller skating (inline) Y93.51
rough housing and horseplay Y93.83
rowing (in calm and turbulent water) Y93.16
rugby Y93.63
running Y93.02
SCUBA diving Y93.15
sewing Y93.D2
shoveling Y93.H1
  dirt Y93.H1
  snow Y93.H1
showering (personal) Y93.E1
sit-ups Y93.B2
skateboarding Y93.51
skating (ice) Y93.21
  roller Y93.51
skiing (alpine) (downhill) Y93.23
  cross country Y93.24
  Nordic Y93.24
  water Y93.17
sledding (snow) Y93.23
sleeping (sleep) Y93.84
smoking and grilling food Y93.G2
snorkeling Y93.15
snow NEC Y93.29
  boarding Y93.23
  shoveling Y93.H1
  sledding Y93.23
  tubing Y93.23
soccer Y93.66
softball Y93.64
specified NEC Y93.89
spectator at an event Y93.82
sports NEC Y93.79

Activity -- *continued*
sports played as a team or group NEC Y93.69
sports played individually NEC Y93.59
springboard diving Y93.12
squash Y93.73
stationary bike Y93.A1
step (stepping) exercise (class) Y93.A3
stepper machine Y93.A1
stove Y93.G3
string instrument playing Y93.J3
surfing Y93.18
  wind Y93.18
swimming Y93.11
tackle football Y93.61
tap dancing Y93.41
tennis Y93.73
tobogganing Y93.23
touch football Y93.62
track and field events (non-running) Y93.57
  running Y93.02
trampoline Y93.44
treadmill Y93.A1
trimming shrubs Y93.H2
tubing (in calm and turbulent water) Y93.16
  snow Y93.23
ultimate frisbee Y93.74
underwater diving Y93.15
unpacking in moving to a new residence Y93.E6
use of stove, oven and microwave oven Y93.G3
vacuuming Y93.E3
volleyball (beach) (court) Y93.68
wake boarding Y93.17
walking an animal Y93.K1
walking (on level or elevated terrain) Y93.01
  an animal Y93.K1
wall climbing Y93.31
warm up and cool down exercises Y93.A2
water NEC Y93.19
  aerobics Y93.14
  craft NEC Y93.19
  exercise Y93.14
  polo Y93.13
  skiing Y93.17
  sliding Y93.18
  survival training and testing Y93.19
weeding (garden and lawn) Y93.H2
wind instrument playing Y93.J4
windsurfing Y93.18
wrestling Y93.72
yoga Y93.42
Adverse effect of drugs -*see* Table of Drugs and Chemicals
Aerosinusitis
-*see* Air, pressure
After-effect, late -*see* Sequelae
Air
blast in war operations -*see* War operations, air blast
pressure
  change, rapid
    during
      ascent W94.29
        while (in) (surfacing from)
          aircraft W94.23
          deep water diving W94.21
          underground W94.22
      descent W94.39

Air -- *continued*
  in
    aircraft W94.31
    water W94.32
  high, prolonged W94.0
  low, prolonged W94.12
    due to residence or long visit at high
      altitude W94.11
Alpine sickness W94.11
Altitude sickness W94.11
Anaphylactic shock, anaphylaxis -*see* Table
  of Drugs and Chemicals
Andes disease W94.11
Arachnidism, arachnoidism X58
Arson (with intent to injure or kill) X97
Asphyxia, asphyxiation
  by
    food (bone) (seed) -*see* categories T17 and
      T18
    gas -*see also* Table of Drugs and
      Chemicals
      legal
        execution -*see* Legal, intervention, gas
        intervention -*see* Legal, intervention,
      gas
  from
    fire -*see also* Exposure, fire
      in war operations -*see* War operations,
      fire
    ignition -*see* Ignition
    vomitus T17.81
  in war operations -*see* War operations,
    restriction of airway
Aspiration
  food (any type) (into respiratory tract) (with
    asphyxia, obstruction respiratory tract,
    suffocation) -*see* categories T17 and T18
  foreign body -*see* Foreign body, aspiration
  vomitus (with asphyxia, obstruction
    respiratory tract, suffocation) T17.81
Assassination (attempt) -*see* Assault
Assault (homicidal) (by) (in) Y09
  arson X97
  bite (of human being) Y04.1
  bodily force Y04.8
    bite Y04.1
    bumping into Y04.2
    sexual -*see* subcategories T74.0, T76.0
    unarmed fight Y04.0
  bomb X96.9
    antipersonnel X96.0
    fertilizer X96.3
    gasoline X96.1
    letter X96.2
    petrol X96.1
    pipe X96.3
    specified NEC X96.8
  brawl (hand) (fists) (foot) (unarmed) Y04.0
  burning, burns (by fire) NEC X97
    acid Y08.89
    caustic, corrosive substance Y08.89
    chemical from swallowing caustic,
      corrosive substance -*see* Table of Drugs
      and Chemicals
    cigarette(s) X97
    hot object X98.9
      fluid NEC X98.2
      household appliance X98.3
      specified NEC X98.8
      steam X98.0
      tap water X98.1

Assault (homicidal) -- *continued*
    vapors X98.0
    scalding -*see* Assault, burning
    steam X98.0
    vitriol Y08.89
  caustic, corrosive substance (gas) Y08.89
  crashing of
    aircraft Y08.81
    motor vehicle Y03.8
      pushed in front of Y02.0
      run over Y03.0
      specified NEC Y03.8
  cutting or piercing instrument X99.9
    dagger X99.2
    glass X99.0
    knife X99.1
    specified NEC X99.8
    sword X99.2
  dagger X99.2
  drowning (in) X92.9
    bathtub X92.0
    natural water X92.3
    specified NEC X92.8
    swimming pool X92.1
      following fall X92.2
  dynamite X96.8
  explosive(s) (material) X96.9
  fight (hand) (fists) (foot) (unarmed) Y04.0
    with weapon -*see* Assault, by type of
      weapon
  fire X97
  firearm X95.9
    airgun X95.01
    handgun X93
    hunting rifle X94.1
    larger X94.9
      specified NEC X94.8
    machine gun X94.2
    shotgun X94.0
    specified NEC X95.8
  gunshot (wound) NEC -*see* Assault, firearm,
    by type
  incendiary device X97
  injury Y09
    to child due to criminal abortion attempt
      NEC Y08.89
  knife X99.1
  late effect of -*see* X92 Y08 with 7th
    character S
  placing before moving object NEC Y02.8
    motor vehicle Y02.0
  poisoning -*see* categories T36 T65 with 7th
    character S
  puncture, any part of body -*see* Assault,
    cutting or piercing instrument
  pushing
    before moving object NEC Y02.8
    motor vehicle Y02.0
    subway train Y02.1
    train Y02.1
  from high place Y01
  rape T74.2
  scalding -*see* Assault, burning
  sequelae of -*see* X92 Y08 with 7th character
    S
  sexual (by bodily force) T74.2
  shooting -*see* Assault, firearm
  specified means NEC Y08.89
  stab, any part of body -*see* Assault, cutting
    or piercing instrument
  steam X98.0

Assault (homicidal) -- *continued*
  striking against
    other person Y04.2
    sports equipment Y08.09
      baseball bat Y08.02
      hockey stick Y08.01
  struck by
    sports equipment Y08.09
      baseball bat Y08.02
      hockey stick Y08.01
  submersion -*see* Assault, drowning
  violence Y09
  weapon Y09
    blunt Y00
    cutting or piercing -*see* Assault, cutting or
      piercing instrument
    firearm -*see* Assault, firearm
  wound Y09
    cutting or piercing -*see* Assault, cutting or
      instrument
    gunshot -*see* Assault, firearm
    knife X99.1
    piercing -*see* Assault, cutting or piercing
      instrument
    puncture -*see* Assault, cutting or piercing
      instrument
    stab -*see* Assault, cutting or piercing
      instrument **Attack by mammals NEC**
      W55.89
Avalanche -*see* Landslide
Aviator's disease
  -*see* Air, pressure

B

Barotitis, barodontalgia, barosinusitis,
  barotrauma (otitic) (sinus)   -*see* Air,
  pressure
Battered (baby) (child) (person)
  (syndrome) X58
Bayonet wound W26.1
  in
    legal intervention -*see* Legal, intervention,
      sharp object, bayonet
    war operations -*see* War operations,
      combat
  stated as undetermined whether accidental
    or intentional Y28.8
  suicide (attempt) X78.2
Bean in nose -*see* categories T17 and T18
Bed set on fire NEC -*see* Exposure, fire,
  uncontrolled, building, bed
Beheading (by guillotine)
  homicide X99.9
  legal execution -*see* Legal, intervention
Bending, injury in (prolonged) (static)
  X50.1
Bends
  -*see* Air, pressure, change
Bite, bitten by
  alligator W58.01
  arthropod (nonvenomous) NEC W57
  bull W55.21
  cat W55.01
  cow W55.21
  crocodile W58.11
  dog W54.0
  goat W55.31
  hoof stock NEC W55.31
  horse W55.11
  human being (accidentally) W50.3

Bite, bitten by -- *continued*
with intent to injure or kill Y04.1
as, or caused by, a crowd or human
stampede (with fall) W52
assault Y04.1
homicide (attempt) Y04.1
in
fight Y04.1
insect (nonvenomous) W57
lizard (nonvenomous) W59.01
mammal NEC W55.81
marine W56.31
marine animal (nonvenomous) W56.81
millipede W57
moray eel W56.51
mouse W53.01
person(s) (accidentally) W50.3
with intent to injure or kill Y04.1
as, or caused by, a crowd or human
stampede (with fall) W52
assault Y04.1
homicide (attempt) Y04.1
in
fight Y04.1
pig W55.41
raccoon W55.51
rat W53.11
reptile W59.81
lizard W59.01
snake W59.11
turtle W59.21
terrestrial W59.81
rodent W53.81
mouse W53.01
rat W53.11
specified NEC W53.81
squirrel W53.21
shark W56.41
sheep W55.31
snake (nonvenomous) W59.11
spider (nonvenomous) W57
squirrel W53.21
Blast (air) in war operations -*see* War
operations, blast
Blizzard X37.2
Blood alcohol level Y90.9
less than 20mg/100ml Y90.0
presence in blood, level not specified Y90.9
20 39mg/100ml Y90.1
40 59mg/100ml Y90.2
60 79mg/100ml Y90.3
80 99mg/100ml Y90.4
100 119mg/100ml Y90.5
120 199mg/100ml Y90.6
200 239mg/100ml Y90.7
Blow X58
by law-enforcing agent, police (on duty) -
see Legal, intervention, manhandling
blunt object -*see* Legal, intervention, blunt
object
Blowing up -*see* Explosion
Brawl (hand) (fists) (foot) Y04.0
Breakage (accidental) (part of) ladder
(causing fall) W11
scaffolding (causing fall) W12
Broken
glass, contact with -*see* Contact, with, glass
power line (causing electric shock) W85

Bumping against, into (accidentally)
object NEC W22.8
with fall -*see* Fall, due to, bumping against,
object
caused by crowd or human stampede (with
fall) W52
sports equipment W21.9
person(s) W51
with fall W03
due to ice or snow W00.0
assault Y04.2
caused by, a crowd or human stampede
(with fall) W52
homicide (attempt) Y04.2
sports equipment W21.9
Burn, burned, burning (accidental) (by)
(from) (on)
acid NEC -*see* Table of Drugs and
Chemicals
bed linen -*see* Exposure, fire, uncontrolled,
in building, bed
blowtorch X08.8
with ignition of clothing NEC X06.2
nightwear X05
bonfire, campfire (controlled) -*see also*
Exposure, fire, controlled, not in building
uncontrolled -*see* Exposure, fire,
uncontrolled, not in building
candle X08.8
with ignition of clothing NEC X06.2
nightwear X05
caustic liquid, substance (external) (internal)
NEC -*see* Table of Drugs and Chemicals
chemical (external) (internal) -*see also*
Table of Drugs and Chemicals
in war operations -*see* War operations. fire
cigar(s) or cigarette(s) X08.8
with ignition of clothing NEC X06.2
nightwear X05
clothes, clothing NEC (from controlled fire)
X06.2
with conflagration -*see* Exposure, fire,
uncontrolled, building
not in building or structure -*see*
Exposure, fire, uncontrolled, not in
building
cooker (hot) X15.8
stated as undetermined whether accidental
or intentional Y27.3
suicide (attempt) X77.3
electric blanket X16
engine (hot) X17
fire, flames -*see* Exposure, fire
flare, Very pistol -*see* Discharge, firearm
NEC
heat
from appliance (electrical) (household)
X15.8
cooker X15.8
hotplate X15.2
kettle X15.8
light bulb X15.8
saucepan X15.3
skillet X15.3
stove X15.0
stated as undetermined whether
accidental or intentional Y27.3
suicide (attempt) X77.3
toaster X15.1
in local application or packing during
medical or surgical procedure Y63.5

Burn, burned, burning -- *continued*
heating
appliance, radiator or pipe X16
homicide (attempt) -*see* Assault, burning
hot
air X14.1
cooker X15.8
drink X10.0
engine X17
fat X10.2
fluid NEC X12
food X10.1
gases X14.1
heating appliance X16
household appliance NEC X15.8
kettle X15.8
liquid NEC X12
machinery X17
metal (molten) (liquid) NEC X18
object (not producing fire or flames) NEC
X19
oil (cooking) X10.2
pipe(s) X16
radiator X16
saucepan (glass) (metal) X15.3
stove (kitchen) X15.0
substance NEC X19
caustic or corrosive NEC -*see* Table of
Drugs and Chemicals
toaster X15.1
tool X17
vapor X13.1
water (tap) -*see* Contact, with, hot, tap
water
hotplate X15.2
suicide (attempt) X77.3
ignition -*see* Ignition
in war operations -*see* War operations, fire
inflicted by other person X97
by hot objects, hot vapor, and steam -*see*
Assault, burning, hot object
internal, from swallowed caustic, corrosive
liquid, substance -*see* Table of Drugs and
Chemicals
iron (hot) X15.8
stated as undetermined whether accidental
or intentional Y27.3
suicide (attempt) X77.3
kettle (hot) X15.8
stated as undetermined whether accidental
or intentional Y27.3
suicide (attempt) X77.3
lamp (flame) X08.8
with ignition of clothing NEC X06.2
nightwear X05
lighter (cigar) (cigarette) X08.8
with ignition of clothing NEC X06.2
nightwear X05
lightning -see subcategory T75.0
causing fire -*see* Exposure, fire
liquid (boiling) (hot) NEC X12
stated as undetermined whether accidental
or intentional Y27.2
suicide (attempt) X77.2
local application of externally applied
substance in medical or surgical care
Y63.5
on board watercraft
due to
accident to watercraft V91.09
powered craft V91.03

Burn, burned, burning -- *continued*
 ferry boat V91.01
 fishing boat V91.02
 jet skis V91.03
 liner V91.01
 merchant ship V91.00
 passenger ship V91.01
 unpowered craft V91.08
  canoe V91.05
  inflatable V91.06
  kayak V91.05
  sailboat V91.04
  surf-board V91.08
  water skis V91.07
  windsurfer V91.08
 fire on board V93.09
  ferry boat V93.01
  fishing boat V93.02
  jet skis V93.03
  liner V93.01
  merchant ship V93.00
  passenger ship V93.01
  powered craft NEC V93.03
  sailboat V93.04
  specified heat source NEC on board
   V93.19
  ferry boat V93.11
  fishing boat V93.12
  jet skis V93.13
  liner V93.11
  merchant ship V93.10
  passenger ship V93.11
  powered craft NEC V93.13
  sailboat V93.14
machinery (hot) X17
matches X08.8
 with ignition of clothing NEC X06.2
  nightwear X05
mattress -*see* Exposure, fire, uncontrolled,
  building, bed
medicament, externally applied Y63.5
metal (hot) (liquid) (molten) NEC X18
nightwear (nightclothes, nightdress, gown,
  pajamas, robe) X05
object (hot) NEC X19
pipe (hot) X16
 smoking X08.8
  with ignition of clothing NEC X06.2
   nightwear X05
powder -*see* Powder burn
radiator (hot) X16
saucepan (hot) (glass) (metal) X15.3
 stated as undetermined whether accidental
  or intentional Y27.3
 suicide (attempt) X77.3
self-inflicted X76
 stated as undetermined whether accidental
  or intentional Y26
steam X13.1
 pipe X16
  stated as undetermined whether
   accidental or intentional Y27.8
 stated as undetermined whether accidental
  or intentional Y27.0
 suicide (attempt) X77.0
stove (hot) (kitchen) X15.0
 stated as undetermined whether accidental
  or intentional Y27.3
 suicide (attempt) X77.3
substance (hot) NEC X19
 boiling X12

Burn, burned, burning -- *continued*
 stated as undetermined whether
  accidental or intentional Y27.2
  suicide (attempt) X77.2
 molten (metal) X18
 suicide (attempt) NEC X76
  hot
   household appliance X77.3
   object X77.9
 stated as undetermined whether accidental
  or intentional Y27.0
 therapeutic misadventure
  heat in local application or packing during
   medical or surgical procedure Y63.5
  overdose of radiation Y63.2
 toaster (hot) X15.1
  stated as undetermined whether accidental
   or intentional Y27.3
  suicide (attempt) X77.3
 tool (hot) X17
 torch, welding X08.8
  with ignition of clothing NEC X06.2
   nightwear X05
 trash fire (controlled) -*see* Exposure, fire,
  controlled, not in building
  uncontrolled -*see* Exposure, fire,
   uncontrolled, not in building
 vapor (hot) X13.1
  stated as undetermined whether accidental
   or intentional Y27.0
  suicide (attempt) X77.0
 Very pistol -*see* Discharge, firearm NEC
Butted by animal W55.82
 bull W55.22
 cow W55.22
 goat W55.32
 horse W55.12
 pig W55.42
 sheep W55.32

C

Caisson disease
 -*see* Air, pressure, change
Campfire (exposure to) (controlled) -*see*
  also Exposure, fire, controlled, not in
  building
 uncontrolled -*see* Exposure, fire,
  uncontrolled, not in building
Capital punishment (any means) -*see* Legal,
  intervention
Car sickness T75.3
Casualty (not due to war) NEC X58
 war -*see* War operations
Cat
 bite W55.01
 scratch W55.03
Cataclysm, cataclysmic (any injury) NEC -
  see Forces of nature
Catching fire -*see* Exposure, fire
Caught
 between
  folding object W23.0
  objects (moving) (stationary and moving)
   W23.0
  and machinery -*see* Contact, with, by
   type of machine
   stationary W23.1
  sliding door and door frame W23.0
 by, in

Caught -- *continued*
 machinery (moving parts of) -*see* Contact,
  with, by type of machine
 washing-machine wringer W23.0
 under packing crate (due to losing grip)
  W23.1
**Cave-in caused by cataclysmic earth
 surface movement or eruption** -*see*
 Landslide
Change(s) in air pressure
 -*see* Air, pressure, change
**Choked, choking (on) (any object except
 food or vomitus)** food (bone) (seed) -
 see categories T17 and T18
 vomitus T17.81
Civil insurrection -*see* War operations
Cloudburst (any injury) X37.8
**Cold, exposure to (accidental) (excessive)
 (extreme) (natural) (place) NEC** -*see*
 Exposure, cold
Collapse
 building W20.1
  burning (uncontrolled fire) X00.2
 dam or man-made structure (causing earth
  movement) X36.0
 machinery -*see* Contact, with, by type of
  machine
 structure W20.1
  burning (uncontrolled fire) X00.2
Collision (accidental) NEC -*see also*
  Accident, transport V89.9
 pedestrian W51
  with fall W03
   due to ice or snow W00.0
   involving pedestrian conveyance -*see*
    Accident, transport, pedestrian,
    conveyance
  and
   crowd or human stampede (with fall)
    W52
   object W22.8
    with fall -*see* Fall, due to, bumping
     against, object
 person(s) -*see* Collision, pedestrian
 transport vehicle NEC V89.9
  and
   avalanche, fallen or not moving -*see*
    Accident, transport
    falling or moving -*see* Landslide
   landslide, fallen or not moving -*see*
    Accident, transport
    falling or moving -*see* Landslide
  due to cataclysm -*see* Forces of nature, by
   type
  intentional, purposeful suicide (attempt) -
   see Suicide, collision
Combustion, spontaneous -*see* Ignition
**Complication (delayed) of or following
 (medical or surgical procedure)** Y84.9
 with misadventure -*see* Misadventure
 amputation of limb(s) Y83.5
 anastomosis (arteriovenous) (blood vessel)
  (gastrojejunal) (tendon) (natural or
  artificial material) Y83.2
 aspiration (of fluid) Y84.4
  tissue Y84.8
 biopsy Y84.8
 blood
  sampling Y84.7
  transfusion
   procedure Y84.8

Complication -- *continued*
  bypass Y83.2
  catheterization (urinary) Y84.6
    cardiac Y84.0
  colostomy Y83.3
  cystostomy Y83.3
  dialysis (kidney) Y84.1
  drug -*see* Table of Drugs and Chemicals
  due to misadventure -*see* Misadventure
  duodenostomy Y83.3
  electroshock therapy Y84.3
  external stoma, creation of Y83.3
  formation of external stoma Y83.3
  gastrostomy Y83.3
  graft Y83.2
  hypothermia (medically-induced) Y84.8
  implant, implantation (of)
    artificial
      internal device (cardiac pacemaker)
        (electrodes in brain) (heart valve
        prosthesis) (orthopedic) Y83.1
      material or tissue (for anastomosis or
        bypass) Y83.2
        with creation of external stoma Y83.3
    natural tissues (for anastomosis or bypass)
      Y83.2
      with creation of external stoma Y83.3
  infusion
    procedure Y84.8
  injection -*see* Table of Drugs and Chemicals
    procedure Y84.8
  insertion of gastric or duodenal sound Y84.5
  insulin-shock therapy Y84.3
  paracentesis (abdominal) (thoracic)
    (aspirative) Y84.4
  procedures other than surgical operation -*see*
    Complication of or following, by type of
    procedure
  radiological procedure or therapy Y84.2
  removal of organ (partial) (total) NEC
    Y83.6
  sampling
    blood Y84.7
    fluid NEC Y84.4
    tissue Y84.8
  shock therapy Y84.3
  surgical operation NEC -*see also*
    Complication of or following, by type of
    operation Y83.9
    reconstructive NEC Y83.4
      with
        anastomosis, bypass or graft Y83.2
        formation of external stoma Y83.3
      specified NEC Y83.8
  transfusion -*see also* Table of Drugs and
    Chemicals
    procedure Y84.8
  transplant, transplantation (heart) (kidney)
    (liver) (whole organ, any) Y83.0
    partial organ Y83.4
  ureterostomy Y83.3
  vaccination -*see also* Table of Drugs and
    Chemicals
    procedure Y84.8
Compression
  divers' squeeze
  -*see* Air, pressure, change
  trachea by
    food (lodged in esophagus) -*see* categories
      T17 and T18
    vomitus (lodged in esophagus) T17.81

Conflagration -*see* Exposure, fire,
  uncontrolled
Constriction (external)
  hair W49.01
  jewelry W49.04
  ring W49.04
  rubber band W49.03
  specified item NEC W49.09
  string W49.02
  thread W49.02
Contact (accidental) with
  abrasive wheel (metalworking) W31.1
  alligator W58.09
    bite W58.01
    crushing W58.03
    strike W58.02
  amphibian W62.9
    frog W62.0
    toad W62.1
  animal (nonvenomous) NEC W64
    marine W56.89
      bite W56.81
      dolphin -*see* Contact, with, dolphin
      fish NEC -*see* Contact, with, fish
      mammal -*see* Contact, with, mammal,
    marine
      orca -*see* Contact, with, orca
      sea lion -*see* Contact, with, sea lion
      shark -*see* Contact, with, shark
      strike W56.82
  animate mechanical force NEC W64
  arrow W21.89
    not thrown, projected or falling W45.8
  arthropods (nonvenomous) W57
  axe W27.0
  band-saw (industrial) W31.2
  bayonet -*see* Bayonet wound
  bee(s) X58
  bench-saw (industrial) W31.2
  bird W61.99
    bite W61.91
    chicken -*see* Contact, with, chicken
    duck -*see* Contact, with, duck
    goose -*see* Contact, with, goose
    macaw -*see* Contact, with, macaw
    parrot -*see* Contact, with, parrot
    psittacine -*see* Contact, with, psittacine
    strike W61.92
    turkey -*see* Contact, with, turkey
  blender W29.0
  boiling water X12
    stated as undetermined whether
      accidental or intentional Y27.2
    suicide (attempt) X77.2
  bore, earth-drilling or mining (land)
    (seabed) W31.0
  buffalo -*see* Contact, with, hoof stock NEC
  bull W55.29
    bite W55.21
    gored W55.22
    strike W55.22
  bumper cars W31.81
  camel -*see* Contact, with, hoof stock NEC
  can
    lid W26.8
    opener W27.4
      powered W29.0
  cat W55.09
    bite W55.01
    scratch W55.03
  caterpillar (venomous) X58

Contact (accidental) -- *continued*
  centipede (venomous) X58
  chain
    hoist W24.0
      agricultural operations W30.89
    saw W29.3
  chicken W61.39
    peck W61.33
    strike W61.32
  chisel W27.0
  circular saw W31.2
  cobra X58
  combine (harvester) W30.0
  conveyer belt W24.1
  cooker (hot) X15.8
    stated as undetermined whether
      accidental or intentional Y27.3
    suicide (attempt) X77.3
  coral X58
  cotton gin W31.82
  cow W55.29
    bite W55.21
    strike W55.22
  crane W24.0
    agricultural operations W30.89
  crocodile W58.19
    bite W58.11
    crushing W58.13
    strike W58.12
  dagger W26.1
    stated as undetermined whether
      accidental or intentional Y28.2
    suicide (attempt) X78.2
  dairy equipment W31.82
  dart W21.89
    not thrown, projected or falling W45.8
  deer -*see* Contact, with, hoof stock NEC
  derrick W24.0
    agricultural operations W30.89
    hay W30.2
  dog W54.8
    bite W54.0
    strike W54.1
  dolphin W56.09
    bite W56.01
    strike W56.02
  donkey -*see* Contact, with, hoof stock NEC
  drill (powered) W29.8
    earth (land) (seabed) W31.0
    nonpowered W27.8
  drive belt W24.0
    agricultural operations W30.89
  dry ice -*see* Exposure, cold, man-made
  dryer (clothes) (powered) (spin) W29.2
  duck W61.69
    bite W61.61
    strike W61.62
  earth ( )
    drilling machine (industrial) W31.0
    scraping machine in stationary use
      W31.83
  edge of stiff paper W26.2
  electric
    beater W29.0
    blanket X16
    fan W29.2
      commercial W31.82
    knife W29.1
    mixer W29.0
  elevator (building) W24.0
    agricultural operations W30.89

Contact (accidental) -- *continued*
- molding W31.2
- overhead plane W31.2
- power press, metal W31.1
- prime mover W31.3
- printing W31.89
- radial saw W31.2
- recreational W31.81
- roller-coaster W31.81
- rolling mill, metal W31.1
- sander W31.2
- seabed drill W31.0
- shaft
  - hoist W31.0
  - lift W31.0
- specified NEC W31.89
- spinning W31.89
- steam engine W31.3
- transmission W24.1
- undercutter W31.0
- water driven turbine W31.3
- weaving W31.89
- woodworking or forming (industrial) W31.2
- mammal (feces) (urine) W55.89
  - bull -*see* Contact, with, bull
  - cat -*see* Contact, with, cat
  - cow -*see* Contact, with, cow
  - goat -*see* Contact, with, goat
  - hoof stock -*see* Contact, with, hoof stock
  - horse -*see* Contact, with, horse
  - marine W56.39
    - dolphin -*see* Contact, with, dolphin
    - orca -*see* Contact, with, orca
    - sea lion -*see* Contact, with, sea lion
    - specified NEC W56.39
      - bite W56.31
      - strike W56.32
  - pig -*see* Contact, with, pig
  - raccoon -*see* Contact, with, raccoon
  - rodent -*see* Contact, with, rodent
  - sheep -*see* Contact, with, sheep
  - specified NEC W55.89
    - bite W55.81
    - strike W55.82
- marine
  - animal W56.89
    - bite W56.81
    - dolphin -*see* Contact, with, dolphin
    - fish NEC -*see* Contact, with, fish
    - mammal -*see* Contact, with, mammal, marine
    - orca -*see* Contact, with, orca
    - sea lion -*see* Contact, with, sea lion
    - shark -*see* Contact, with, shark
    - strike W56.82
- meat
  - grinder (domestic) W29.0
    - industrial W31.82
    - nonpowered W27.4
  - slicer (domestic) W29.0
    - industrial W31.82
- merry go round W31.81
- metal, hot (liquid) (molten) NEC X18
- millipede W57
- nail W45.0
  - gun W29.4
- needle (sewing) W27.3
  - hypodermic W46.0
    - contaminated W46.1
- object (blunt) NEC

Contact (accidental) -- *continued*
- hot NEC X19
- legal intervention -*see* Legal, intervention, blunt object
- sharp NEC W45.8
  - inflicted by other person NEC W45.8
    - stated as
      - intentional homicide (attempt) -*see* Assault, cutting or piercing instrument
    - legal intervention -*see* Legal, intervention, sharp object
    - self-inflicted X78.9
- orca W56.29
  - bite W56.21
  - strike W56.22
- overhead plane W31.2
- paper (as sharp object) W26.2
- paper-cutter W27.5
- parrot W61.09
  - bite W61.01
  - strike W61.02
- pig W55.49
  - bite W55.41
  - strike W55.42
- pipe, hot X16
- pitchfork W27.1
- plane (metal) (wood) W27.0
  - overhead W31.2
- plant thorns, spines, sharp leaves or other mechanisms W60
- powered
  - garden cultivator W29.3
  - household appliance, implement, or machine W29.8
  - saw (industrial) W31.2
    - hand W29.8
- printing machine W31.89
- psittacine bird W61.29
  - bite W61.21
  - macaw -*see* Contact, with, macaw
  - parrot -*see* Contact, with, parrot
  - strike W61.22
- pulley (block) (transmission) W24.0
  - agricultural operations W30.89
- raccoon W55.59
  - bite W55.51
  - strike W55.52
- radial-saw (industrial) W31.2
- radiator (hot) X16
- rake W27.1
- rattlesnake X58
- reaper W30.0
- reptile W59.89
  - lizard -*see* Contact, with, lizard
  - snake -*see* Contact, with, snake
  - specified NEC W59.89
    - bite W59.81
    - crushing W59.83
    - strike W59.82
  - turtle -*see* Contact, with, turtle
- rivet gun (powered) W29.4
- road scraper -*see* Accident, transport, construction vehicle
- rodent (feces) (urine) W53.89
  - bite W53.81
  - mouse W53.09
    - bite W53.01
  - rat W53.19
    - bite W53.11
  - specified NEC W53.89
    - bite W53.81

Contact (accidental) -- *continued*
- squirrel W53.29
  - bite W53.21
- roller coaster W31.81
- rope NEC W24.0
  - agricultural operations W30.89
- saliva -*see* Contact, with, by type of animal
- sander W29.8
  - industrial W31.2
- saucepan (hot) (glass) (metal) X15.3
- saw W27.0
  - band (industrial) W31.2
  - bench (industrial) W31.2
  - chain W29.3
  - hand W27.0
- sawing machine, metal W31.1
- scissors W27.2
- scorpion X58
- screwdriver W27.0
  - powered W29.8
- sea
  - anemone, cucumber or urchin (spine) X58
  - lion W56.19
    - bite W56.11
    - strike W56.12
- serpent -*see* Contact, with, snake, by type
- sewing-machine (electric) (powered) W29.2
  - not powered W27.8
- shaft (hoist) (lift) (transmission) NEC W24.0
  - agricultural W30.89
- shark W56.49
  - bite W56.41
  - strike W56.42
- sharp object(s) W26.9
  - specified NEC W26.8
- shears (hand) W27.2
  - powered (industrial) W31.1
    - domestic W29.2
- sheep W55.39
  - bite W55.31
  - strike W55.32
- shovel W27.8
  - steam -*see* Accident, transport, construction vehicle
- snake (nonvenomous) W59.19
  - bite W59.11
  - crushing W59.13
  - strike W59.12
- spade W27.1
- spider (venomous) X58
- spin-drier W29.2
- spinning machine W31.89
- splinter W45.8
- sports equipment W21.9
- staple gun (powered) W29.8
- steam X13.1
  - engine W31.3
  - inhalation X13.0
  - pipe X16
  - shovel W31.89
- stove (hot) (kitchen) X15.0
- substance, hot NEC X19
  - molten (metal) X18
- sword W26.1
  - assault X99.2
  - stated as undetermined whether accidental or intentional Y28.2
  - suicide (attempt) X78.2
- tarantula X58
- thresher W30.0

Contact (accidental) -- *continued*
  tin can lid W26.8
  toad W62.1
  toaster (hot) X15.1
  tool W27.8
    hand (not powered) W27.8
      auger W27.0
      axe W27.0
      can opener W27.4
      chisel W27.0
      fork W27.4
      garden W27.1
      handsaw W27.0
      hoe W27.1
      ice-pick W27.4
      kitchen utensil W27.4
      manual
        lawn mower W27.1
        sewing machine W27.8
      meat grinder W27.4
      needle (sewing) W27.3
        hypodermic W46.0
          contaminated W46.1
      paper cutter W27.5
      pitchfork W27.1
      rake W27.1
      scissors W27.2
      screwdriver W27.0
      specified NEC W27.8
      workbench W27.0
    hot X17
    powered W29.8
      blender W29.0
        commercial W31.82
      can opener W29.0
        commercial W31.82
      chainsaw W29.3
      clothes dryer W29.2
        commercial W31.82
      dishwasher W29.2
        commercial W31.82
      edger W29.3
      electric fan W29.2
        commercial W31.82
      electric knife W29.1
      food processor W29.0
        commercial W31.82
      garbage disposal W29.0
        commercial W31.82
      garden tool W29.3
      hedge trimmer W29.3
      ice maker W29.0
        commercial W31.82
      kitchen appliance W29.0
        commercial W31.82
      lawn mower W28
      meat grinder W29.0
        commercial W31.82
      mixer W29.0
        commercial W31.82
      rototiller W29.3
      sewing machine W29.2
        commercial W31.82
      washing machine W29.2
        commercial W31.82
  transmission device (belt, cable, chain, gear, pinion, shaft) W24.1
    agricultural operations W30.89
  turbine (gas) (water-driven) W31.3
  turkey W61.49
    peck W61.43

Contact (accidental) -- *continued*
  strike W61.42
  turtle (nonvenomous) W59.29
    bite W59.21
    strike W59.22
    terrestrial W59.89
      bite W59.81
      crushing W59.83
      strike W59.82
  under-cutter W31.0
  urine -*see* Contact, with, by type of animal
  vehicle
    agricultural use (transport) -*see* Accident, transport, agricultural vehicle
      not on public highway W30.81
    industrial use (transport) -*see* Accident, transport, industrial vehicle
      not on public highway W31.83
    off-road use (transport) -*see* Accident, transport, all-terrain or off-road vehicle
      not on public highway W31.83
    special construction use (transport) -*see* Accident, transport, construction vehicle
      not on public highway W31.83
  venomous
    animal X58
    arthropods X58
    lizard X58
    marine animal NEC X58
    marine plant NEC X58
    millipedes (tropical) X58
    plant(s) X58
    snake X58
    spider X58
    viper X58
  washing-machine (powered) W29.2
  wasp X58
  weaving-machine W31.89
  winch W24.0
    agricultural operations W30.89
  wire NEC W24.0
    agricultural operations W30.89
  wood slivers W45.8
  yellow jacket X58
  zebra -*see* Contact, with, hoof stock NEC
  pressure X50.9
  stress X50.9
Coup de soleil X32
Crash
  aircraft (in transit) (powered) V95.9
    balloon V96.01
    fixed wing NEC (private) V95.21
      commercial V95.31
    glider V96.21
      hang V96.11
      powered V95.11
    helicopter V95.01
    in war operations -*see* War operations, destruction of aircraft
    microlight V95.11
    nonpowered V96.9
      specified NEC V96.8
    powered NEC V95.8
    stated as
      homicide (attempt) Y08.81
      suicide (attempt) X83.0
    ultralight V95.11
  spacecraft V95.41
  transport vehicle NEC -*see also* Accident, transport V89.9
    homicide (attempt) Y03.8
    motor NEC (traffic) V89.2

Crash -- *continued*
    homicide (attempt) Y03.8
    suicide (attempt) -*see* Suicide, collision
Cruelty (mental) (physical) (sexual) X58
Crushed (accidentally) X58
  between objects (moving) (stationary and moving) W23.0
    stationary W23.1
  by
    alligator W58.03
    avalanche NEC -*see* Landslide
    cave-in W20.0
      caused by cataclysmic earth surface movement -*see* Landslide
    crocodile W58.13
    crowd or human stampede W52
    falling
      aircraft V97.39
        in war operations -*see* War operations, destruction of aircraft
      earth, material W20.0
        caused by cataclysmic earth surface movement -*see* Landslide
      object NEC W20.8
    landslide NEC -*see* Landslide
    lizard (nonvenomous) W59.09
    machinery -*see* Contact, with, by type of machine
    reptile NEC W59.89
    snake (nonvenomous) W59.13
  in
    machinery -*see* Contact, with, by type of machine
Cut, cutting (any part of body) (accidental) -*see also* Contact, with, by object or machine
  during medical or surgical treatment as misadventure -*see* Index to Diseases and Injuries, Complications
  homicide (attempt) -*see* Assault, cutting or piercing instrument
  inflicted by other person -*see* Assault, cutting or piercing instrument
  legal
    execution -*see* Legal, intervention
    intervention -*see* Legal, intervention, sharp object
  machine NEC -*see also* Contact, with, by type of machine W31.9
  self-inflicted -*see* Suicide, cutting or piercing instrument
  suicide (attempt) -*see* Suicide, cutting or piercing instrument
Cyclone (any injury) X37.1

D

Decapitation (accidental circumstances) NEC X58
  homicide X99.9
  legal execution -*see* Legal, intervention
Dehydration from lack of water X58
Deprivation X58
Derailment (accidental)
  railway (rolling stock) (train) (vehicle) (without antecedent collision) V81.7
    with antecedent collision -*see* Accident, transport, railway vehicle occupant
  streetcar (without antecedent collision) V82.7
    with antecedent collision -*see* Accident, transport, streetcar occupant

Descent
parachute (voluntary) (without accident to aircraft) V97.29
due to accident to aircraft -*see* Accident, transport, aircraft
Desertion X58
Destitution X58
Disability, late effect or sequela of injury - *see* Sequelae
Discharge (accidental)
airgun W34.010
assault X95.01
homicide (attempt) X95.01
stated as undetermined whether accidental or intentional Y24.0
suicide (attempt) X74.01
BB gun -*see* Discharge, airgun
firearm (accidental) W34.00
assault X95.9
handgun (pistol) (revolver) W32.0
assault X93
homicide (attempt) X93
legal intervention -*see* Legal, intervention, firearm, handgun
stated as undetermined whether accidental or intentional Y22
suicide (attempt) X72
homicide (attempt) X95.9
hunting rifle W33.02
assault X94.1
homicide (attempt) X94.1
legal intervention
injuring
bystander Y35.032
law enforcement personnel Y35.031
suspect Y35.033
stated as undetermined whether accidental or intentional Y23.1
suicide (attempt) X73.1
larger W33.00
assault X94.9
homicide (attempt) X94.9
hunting rifle -*see* Discharge, firearm, hunting rifle
legal intervention -*see* Legal, intervention, firearm by type of firearm
machine gun -*see* Discharge, firearm, machine gun
shotgun -*see* Discharge, firearm, shotgun
specified NEC W33.09
assault X94.8
homicide (attempt) X94.8
legal intervention
injuring
bystander Y35.092
law enforcement personnel Y35.091
suspect Y35.093
stated as undetermined whether accidental or intentional Y23.8
suicide (attempt) X73.8
stated as undetermined whether accidental or intentional Y23.9
suicide (attempt) X73.9
legal intervention
injuring
bystander Y35.002
law enforcement personnel Y35.001
suspect Y35.03
using rubber bullet
injuring
bystander Y35.042

Discharge (accidental) -- *continued*
law enforcement personnel Y35.041
suspect Y35.043
machine gun W33.03
assault X94.2
homicide (attempt) X94.2
legal intervention -*see* Legal, intervention, firearm, machine gun
stated as undetermined whether accidental or intentional Y23.3
suicide (attempt) X73.2
pellet gun -*see* Discharge, airgun
shotgun W33.01
assault X94.0
homicide (attempt) X94.0
legal intervention -*see* Legal, intervention, firearm, specified NEC
stated as undetermined whether accidental or intentional Y23.0
suicide (attempt) X73.0
specified NEC W34.09
assault X95.8
homicide (attempt) X95.8
legal intervention -*see* Legal, intervention, firearm, specified NEC
stated as undetermined whether accidental or intentional Y24.8
suicide (attempt) X74.8
stated as undetermined whether accidental or intentional Y24.9
suicide (attempt) X74.9
Very pistol W34.09
assault X95.8
homicide (attempt) X95.8
stated as undetermined whether accidental or intentional Y24.8
suicide (attempt) X74.8
firework(s) W39
stated as undetermined whether accidental or intentional Y25
gas-operated gun NEC W34.018
airgun -*see* Discharge, airgun
assault X95.09
homicide (attempt) X95.09
paintball gun -*see* Discharge, paintball gun
stated as undetermined whether accidental or intentional Y24.8
suicide (attempt) X74.09
gun NEC -*see also* Discharge, firearm NEC
air -*see* Discharge, airgun
BB -*see* Discharge, airgun
for single hand use -*see* Discharge, firearm, handgun
hand -*see* Discharge, firearm, handgun
machine -*see* Discharge, firearm, machine gun
other specified -*see* Discharge, firearm NEC
paintball -*see* Discharge, paintball gun
pellet -*see* Discharge, airgun
handgun -*see* Discharge, firearm, handgun
machine gun -*see* Discharge, firearm, machine gun
paintball gun W34.011
assault X95.02
homicide (attempt) X95.02
stated as undetermined whether accidental or intentional Y24.8
suicide (attempt) X74.02
pistol -*see* Discharge, firearm, handgun
flare -*see* Discharge, firearm, Very pistol

Discharge (accidental) -- *continued*
pellet -*see* Discharge, airgun
Very -*see* Discharge, firearm, Very pistol
revolver -*see* Discharge, firearm, handgun
rifle (hunting) -*see* Discharge, firearm, hunting rifle
shotgun -*see* Discharge, firearm, shotgun
spring-operated gun NEC W34.018
assault X95.09
homicide (attempt) X95.09
stated as undetermined whether accidental or intentional Y24.8
suicide (attempt) X74.09
Disease
Andes W94.11
aviator's
-*see* Air, pressure
range W94.11
Diver's disease, palsy, paralysis, squeeze -*see* Air, pressure
Diving (into water) -*see* Accident, diving
Dog bite W54.0
Dragged by transport vehicle NEC -*see also* Accident, transport V09.9
Drinking poison (accidental) -*see* Table of Drugs and Chemicals
Dropped (accidentally) while being carried or supported by other person W04
Drowning (accidental) W74
assault X92.9
due to
accident (to)
machinery -*see* Contact, with, by type of machine
watercraft V90.89
burning V90.29
powered V90.23
merchant ship V90.20
passenger ship V90.21
fishing boat V90.22
jet skis V90.23
unpowered V90.28
canoe V90.25
inflatable V90.26
kayak V90.25
sailboat V90.24
water skis V90.27
crushed V90.39
powered V90.33
merchant ship V90.30
passenger ship V90.31
fishing boat V90.32
jet skis V90.33
unpowered V90.38
canoe V90.35
inflatable V90.36
kayak V90.35
sailboat V90.34
water skis V90.37
overturning V90.09
powered V90.03
merchant ship V90.00
passenger ship V90.01
fishing boat V90.02
jet skis V90.03
unpowered V90.08
canoe V90.05
inflatable V90.06
kayak V90.05
sailboat V90.04
sinking V90.19

Drowning (accidental) -- *continued*
   powered V90.13
    merchant ship V90.10
    passenger ship V90.11
    fishing boat V90.12
    jet skis V90.13
   unpowered V90.18
    canoe V90.15
    inflatable V90.16
    kayak V90.15
    sailboat V90.14
   specified type NEC V90.89
   powered V90.83
    merchant ship V90.80
    passenger ship V90.81
    fishing boat V90.82
    jet skis V90.83
   unpowered V90.88
    canoe V90.85
    inflatable V90.86
    kayak V90.85
    sailboat V90.84
    water skis V90.87
 avalanche -*see* Landslide
 cataclysmic
   earth surface movement NEC -*see* Forces of nature, earth movement
   storm -*see* Forces of nature, cataclysmic storm
 cloudburst X37.8
 cyclone X37.1
 fall overboard (from) V92.09
   powered craft V92.03
    ferry boat V92.01
    liner V92.01
    merchant ship V92.00
    passenger ship V92.01
    fishing boat V92.02
    jet skis V92.03
   unpowered craft V92.08
    canoe V92.05
    inflatable V92.06
    kayak V92.05
    sailboat V92.04
    surf-board V92.08
    water skis V92.07
    windsurfer V92.08
 resulting from
   accident to watercraft -*see* Drowning, due to, accident to, watercraft
   being washed overboard (from) V92.29
    powered craft V92.23
     ferry boat V92.21
     liner V92.21
     merchant ship V92.20
     passenger ship V92.21
     fishing boat V92.22
     jet skis V92.23
    unpowered craft V92.28
     canoe V92.25
     inflatable V92.26
     kayak V92.25
     sailboat V92.24
     surf-board V92.28
     water skis V92.27
     windsurfer V92.28
   motion of watercraft V92.19
    powered craft V92.13
     ferry boat V92.11
     liner V92.11
     merchant ship V92.10

Drowning (accidental) -- *continued*
     passenger ship V92.11
     fishing boat V92.12
     jet skis V92.13
    unpowered craft
     canoe V92.15
     inflatable V92.16
     kayak V92.15
     sailboat V92.14
 hurricane X37.0
 jumping into water from watercraft (involved in accident) -*see also* Drowning, due to, accident to, watercraft without accident to or on watercraft W16.711
 tidal wave NEC -*see* Forces of nature, tidal wave
 torrential rain X37.8
 following
   fall
    into
     bathtub W16.211
     bucket W16.221
     fountain -*see* Drowning, following, fall, into, water, specified NEC
     quarry -*see* Drowning, following, fall, into, water, specified NEC
     reservoir -*see* Drowning, following, fall, into, water, specified NEC
     swimming-pool W16.011
      striking
       bottom W16.021
       wall W16.031
      stated as undetermined whether accidental or intentional Y21.3
      suicide (attempt) X71.2
     water NOS W16.41
     natural (lake) (open sea) (river) (stream) (pond) W16.111
      striking
       bottom W16.121
       side W16.131
     specified NEC W16.311
      striking
       bottom W16.321
       wall W16.331
   overboard NEC -*see* Drowning, due to, fall overboard
   jump or dive
    from boat W16.711
     striking bottom W16.721
    into
     fountain -*see* Drowning, following, jump or dive, into, water, specified NEC
     quarry -*see* Drowning, following, jump or dive, into, water, specified NEC
     reservoir -*see* Drowning, following, jump or dive, into, water, specified NEC
     swimming-pool W16.511
      striking
       bottom W16.521
       wall W16.531
      suicide (attempt) X71.2
     water NOS W16.91
     natural (lake) (open sea) (river) (stream) (pond) W16.611
     specified NEC W16.811
      striking
       bottom W16.821
       wall W16.831
     striking bottom W16.621

Drowning (accidental) -- *continued*
 homicide (attempt) X92.9
 in
   bathtub (accidental) W65
    assault X92.0
    following fall W16.211
     stated as undetermined whether accidental or intentional Y21.1
    stated as undetermined whether accidental or intentional Y21.0
    suicide (attempt) X71.0
   lake -*see* Drowning, in, natural water
   natural water (lake) (open sea) (river) (stream) (pond) W69
    assault X92.3
    following
     dive or jump W16.611
      striking bottom W16.621
     fall W16.111
      striking
       bottom W16.121
       side W16.131
    stated as undetermined whether accidental or intentional Y21.4
    suicide (attempt) X71.3
   quarry -*see* Drowning, in, specified place NEC
   quenching tank -*see* Drowning, in, specified place NEC
   reservoir -*see* Drowning, in, specified place NEC
   river -*see* Drowning, in, natural water
   sea -*see* Drowning, in, natural water
   specified place NEC W73
    assault X92.8
    following
     dive or jump W16.811
      striking
       bottom W16.821
       wall W16.831
     fall W16.311
      striking
       bottom W16.321
       wall W16.331
    stated as undetermined whether accidental or intentional Y21.8
    suicide (attempt) X71.8
   stream -*see* Drowning, in, natural water
   swimming-pool W67
    assault X92.1
     following fall X92.2
    following
     dive or jump W16.511
      striking
       bottom W16.521
       wall W16.531
     fall W16.011
      striking
       bottom W16.021
       wall W16.031
    stated as undetermined whether accidental or intentional Y21.2
     following fall Y21.3
    suicide (attempt) X71.1
     following fall X71.2
   war operations -*see* War operations, restriction of airway
 resulting from accident to watercraft see Drowning, due to, accident, watercraft
 self-inflicted X71.9
 stated as undetermined whether accidental or intentional Y21.9
 suicide (attempt) X71.9

E

Earth (surface) movement NEC -*see* Forces of nature, earth movement
Earth falling (on) W20.0
  caused by cataclysmic earth surface movement or eruption -*see* Landslide
Earthquake (any injury) X34
Effect(s) (adverse) of
  air pressure (any) -*see* Air, pressure
  cold, excessive (exposure to) -*see* Exposure, cold
  heat (excessive) -*see* Heat
  hot place (weather) -*see* Heat
  insolation X30
  late -*see* Sequelae
  motion -*see* Motion
  nuclear explosion or weapon in war operations -*see* War operations, nuclear weapon
  radiation -*see* Radiation
  travel -*see* Travel
Electric shock (accidental) (by) (in) -*see* Exposure, electric current
Electrocution (accidental) -*see* Exposure, electric current
Endotracheal tube wrongly placed during anesthetic procedure
Entanglement
  in
    bed linen, causing suffocation -*see* category T71
    wheel of pedal cycle V19.88
Entry of foreign body or material -*see* Foreign body
Environmental pollution related condition-see Z57
Execution, legal (any method) -*see* Legal, intervention
Exhaustion
  cold -*see* Exposure, cold
  due to excessive exertion -*see also* Overexertion X50.9
  heat -*see* Heat
Explosion (accidental) (of) (with secondary fire) W40.9
  acetylene W40.1
  aerosol can W36.1
  air tank (compressed) (in machinery) W36.2
  aircraft (in transit) (powered) NEC V95.9
    balloon V96.05
    fixed wing NEC (private) V95.25
      commercial V95.35
    glider V96.25
      hang V96.15
      powered V95.15
    helicopter V95.05
    in war operations -*see* War operations, destruction of aircraft
    microlight V95.15
    nonpowered V96.9
      specified NEC V96.8
    powered NEC V95.8
    stated as
      homicide (attempt) Y03.8
      suicide (attempt) X83.0
    ultralight V95.15
  anesthetic gas in operating room W40.1
  antipersonnel bomb W40.8
    assault X96.0
    homicide (attempt) X96.0

Explosion (accidental) -- *continued*
  suicide (attempt) X75
  assault X96.9
  bicycle tire W37.0
  blasting (cap) (materials) W40.0
  boiler (machinery), not on transport vehicle W35
  on watercraft -*see* Explosion, in, watercraft
  butane W40.1
  caused by other person X96.9
  coal gas W40.1
  detonator W40.0
  dump (munitions) W40.8
  dynamite W40.0
    in
      assault X96.8
      homicide (attempt) X96.8
      legal intervention
        injuring
          bystander Y35.112
          law enforcement personnel Y35.111
          suspect Y35.113
      suicide (attempt) X75
  explosive (material) W40.9
  gas W40.1
  in blasting operation W40.0
  specified NEC W40.8
    in
      assault X96.8
      homicide (attempt) X96.8
      legal intervention
        injuring
          bystander Y35.192
          law enforcement personnel Y35.191
          suspect Y35.193
      suicide (attempt) X75
  factory (munitions) W40.8
  fertilizer bomb W40.8
    assault X96.3
    homicide (attempt) X96.3
    suicide (attempt) X75
  firearm (parts) NEC W34.19
    airgun W34.110
    BB gun W34.110
    gas, air or spring-operated gun NEC W34.118
    handgun W32.1
    hunting rifle W33.12
    larger firearm W33.10
      specified NEC W33.19
    machine gun W33.13
    paintball gun W34.111
    pellet gun W34.110
    shotgun W33.11
    Very pistol [flare] W34.19
  fire-damp W40.1
  fireworks W39
  gas (coal) (explosive) W40.1
    cylinder W36.9
      aerosol can W36.1
      air tank W36.2
      pressurized W36.3
      specified NEC W36.8
  gasoline (fumes) (tank) not in moving motor vehicle W40.1
    bomb W40.8
      assault X96.1
      homicide (attempt) X96.1
      suicide (attempt) X75
    in motor vehicle -*see* Accident, transport, by type of vehicle

Explosion (accidental) -- *continued*
  grain store W40.8
  grenade W40.8
    in
      assault X96.8
      homicide (attempt) X96.8
      legal intervention
        injuring
          bystander Y35.192
          law enforcement personnel Y35.191
          suspect Y35.193
      suicide (attempt) X75
  handgun (parts) -*see* Explosion, firearm, handgun (parts) homicide (attempt) X96.9
  antipersonnel bomb -*see* Explosion, antipersonnel bomb
  fertilizer bomb -*see* Explosion, fertilizer bomb
  gasoline bomb -*see* Explosion, gasoline bomb
  letter bomb -*see* Explosion, letter bomb
  pipe bomb -*see* Explosion, pipe bomb
  specified NEC X96.8
  hose, pressurized W37.8
  hot water heater, tank (in machinery) W35
  on watercraft -*see* Explosion, in, watercraft
  in, on
    dump W40.8
    factory W40.8
    mine (of explosive gases) NEC W40.1
    watercraft V93.59
      powered craft V93.53
        ferry boat V93.51
        fishing boat V93.52
        jet skis V93.53
        liner V93.51
        merchant ship V93.50
        passenger ship V93.51
        sailboat V93.54
  letter bomb W40.8
    assault X96.2
    homicide (attempt) X96.2
    suicide (attempt) X75
  machinery -*see also* Contact, with, by type of machine
    on board watercraft -*see* Explosion, in, watercraft
    pressure vessel -*see* Explosion, by type of vessel
  methane W40.1
  mine W40.1
  missile NEC W40.8
  mortar bomb W40.8
    in
      assault X96.8
      homicide (attempt) X96.8
      legal intervention
        injuring
          bystander Y35.192
          law enforcement personnel Y35.191
          suspect Y35.193
      suicide (attempt) X75
  munitions (dump) (factory) W40.8
  pipe, pressurized W37.8
    bomb W40.8
      assault X96.4
      homicide (attempt) X96.4
      suicide (attempt) X75
  pressure, pressurized
    cooker W38

Explosion (accidental) -- *continued*
    gas tank (in machinery) W36.3
    hose W37.8
    pipe W37.8
    specified device NEC W38
    tire W37.8
      bicycle W37.0
    vessel (in machinery) W38
    propane W40.1
    self-inflicted X75
    shell (artillery) NEC W40.8
      during war operations -*see* War operations,
        explosion
      in
        legal intervention
          injuring
            bystander Y35.122
            law enforcement personnel Y35.121
            suspect Y35.123
      war -*see* War operations, explosion
    spacecraft V95.45
    steam or water lines (in machinery) W37.8
    stove W40.9
    stated as undetermined whether accidental
      or intentional Y25
    suicide (attempt) X75
    tire, pressurized W37.8
      bicycle W37.0
    undetermined whether accidental or
      intentional Y25
    vehicle tire NEC W37.8
      bicycle W37.0
    war operations -*see* War operations,
      explosion

Exposure (to) X58
    air pressure change -*see* Air, pressure
    cold (accidental) (excessive) (extreme)
      (natural) (place) X31
      assault Y08.89
      due to
        man-made conditions W93.8
          dry ice (contact) W93.01
            inhalation W93.02
          liquid air (contact) (hydrogen)
            (nitrogen) W93.11
            inhalation W93.12
          refrigeration unit (deep freeze) W93.2
      suicide (attempt) X83.2
      weather (conditions) X31
      homicide (attempt) Y08.89
      self-inflicted X83.2
    due to abandonment or neglect X58
    electric current W86.8
      appliance (faulty) W86.8
        domestic W86.0
      caused by other person Y08.89
      conductor (faulty) W86.1
      control apparatus (faulty) W86.1
      electric power generating plant,
        distribution station W86.1
      electroshock gun -*see* Exposure, electric
        current, taser
      high-voltage cable W85
      homicide (attempt) Y08.89
      legal execution -*see* Legal, intervention,
        specified means NEC
      lightning -*see* subcategory T75.0
      live rail W86.8
      misadventure in medical or surgical
        procedure in electroshock therapy Y63.4
      motor (electric) (faulty) W86.8

Exposure (to) -- *continued*
      domestic W86.0
      self-inflicted X83.1
      specified NEC W86.8
        domestic W86.0
      stun gun -*see* Exposure, electric current,
        taser
      suicide (attempt) X83.1
      taser W86.8
        assault Y08.89
        legal intervention -*see* category Y35
        self-harm (intentional) X83.8
        undetermined intent Y33
      third rail W86.8
      transformer (faulty) W86.1
      transmission lines W85
    environmental tobacco smoke X58
    excessive
      cold -*see* Exposure, cold
      heat (natural) NEC X30
        man-made W92
    factor(s) NOS X58
      environmental NEC X58
        man-made NEC W99
      natural NEC -*see* Forces of nature
      specified NEC X58
    fire, flames (accidental) X08.8
      assault X97
      campfire -*see* Exposure, fire, controlled,
        not in building
      controlled (in)
        with ignition (of) clothing -*see also*
        Ignition, clothes X06.2
          nightwear X05
      bonfire -*see* Exposure, fire, controlled,
      not in building
      brazier (in building or structure) -*see also*
      Exposure, fire, controlled, building
        not in building or structure -*see*
      Exposure, fire, controlled, not in building
      building or structure X02.0
        with
          fall from building X02.3
          injury due to building collapse X02.2
          from building X02.5
          smoke inhalation X02.1
        hit by object from building X02.4
        specified mode of injury NEC X02.8
      fireplace, furnace or stove -*see* Exposure,
      fire, controlled, building
      not in building or structure X03.0
        with
          fall X03.3
          smoke inhalation X03.1
        hit by object X03.4
        specified mode of injury NEC X03.8
      trash -*see* Exposure, fire, controlled, not
      in building
      fireplace -*see* Exposure, fire, controlled,
      building
      fittings or furniture (in building or
      structure) (uncontrolled) -*see* Exposure,
      fire, uncontrolled, building
      forest (uncontrolled) -*see* Exposure, fire,
      uncontrolled, not in building
      grass (uncontrolled) -*see* Exposure, fire,
      uncontrolled, not in building
      hay (uncontrolled) -*see* Exposure, fire,
      uncontrolled, not in building
      homicide (attempt) X97
      ignition of highly flammable material X04

Exposure (to) -- *continued*
    in, of, on, starting in
      machinery -*see* Contact, with, by type of
      machine
      motor vehicle (in motion) -*see also*
      Accident, transport, occupant by type of
      vehicle V87.8
        with collision -*see* Collision
      railway rolling stock, train, vehicle
      V81.81
        with collision -*see* Accident, transport,
        railway vehicle occupant
      street car (in motion) V82.8
        with collision -*see* Accident, transport,
        streetcar occupant
      transport vehicle NEC -*see also*
      Accident, transport
        with collision -*see* Collision
      war operations -*see also* War operations,
      fire
        from nuclear explosion -*see* War
      operations, nuclear weapons
      watercraft (in transit) (not in transit)
      V91.09
        localized -*see* Burn, on board
      watercraft, due to, fire on board
        powered craft V91.03
          ferry boat V91.01
          fishing boat V91.02
          jet skis V91.03
          liner V91.01
          merchant ship V91.00
          passenger ship V91.01
        unpowered craft V91.08
          canoe V91.05
          inflatable V91.06
          kayak V91.05
          sailboat V91.04
          surf-board V91.08
          waterskis V91.07
          windsurfer V91.08
      lumber (uncontrolled) -*see* Exposure, fire,
      uncontrolled, not in building
      mine (uncontrolled) -*see* Exposure, fire,
      uncontrolled, not in building
      prairie (uncontrolled) -*see* Exposure, fire,
      uncontrolled, not in building
      resulting from
        explosion -*see* Explosion
        lightning X08.8
      self-inflicted X76
      specified NEC X08.8
      started by other person X97
      stove -*see* Exposure, fire, controlled,
      building
      stated as undetermined whether accidental
      or intentional Y26
      suicide (attempt) X76
      tunnel (uncontrolled) -*see* Exposure, fire,
      uncontrolled, not in building
      uncontrolled
        in building or structure X00.0
          with
            fall from building X00.3
            injury due to building collapse X00.2
            jump from building X00.5
            smoke inhalation X00.1
          bed X08.00
            due to
              cigarette X08.01
              specified material NEC X08.09

Exposure (to) -- *continued*
    furniture NEC X08.20
      due to
        cigarette X08.21
        specified material NEC X08.29
    hit by object from building X00.4
    sofa X08.10
      due to
        cigarette X08.11
        specified material NEC X08.19
    specified mode of injury NEC X00.8
    not in building or structure (any) X01.0
      with
        fall X01.3
        smoke inhalation X01.1
      hit by object X01.4
      specified mode of injury NEC X01.8
    undetermined whether accidental or
      intentional Y26
    forces of nature NEC -*see* Forces of nature
    G-forces (abnormal) W49.9
    gravitational forces (abnormal) W49.9
    heat (natural) NEC -*see* Heat
    high-pressure jet (hydraulic) (pneumatic)
      W49.9
    hydraulic jet W49.9
    inanimate mechanical force W49.9
    jet, high-pressure (hydraulic) (pneumatic)
      W49.9
    lightning -*see* subcategory T75.0
      causing fire -*see* Exposure, fire
    mechanical forces NEC W49.9
      animate NEC W64
      inanimate NEC W49.9
    noise W42.9
      supersonic W42.0
    noxious substance -*see* Table of Drugs and
      Chemicals
    pneumatic jet W49.9
    prolonged in deep-freeze unit or refrigerator
      W93.2
    radiation -*see* Radiation
    smoke -*see also* Exposure, fire
      tobacco, second hand Z77.22
    specified factors NEC X58
    sunlight X32
      man-made (sun lamp) W89.8
        tanning bed W89.1
    supersonic waves W42.0
    transmission line(s), electric W85
    vibration W49.9
    waves
      infrasound W49.9
      sound W42.9
      supersonic W42.0
    weather NEC -*see* Forces of nature
External cause status Y99.9
    child assisting in compensated work for
      family Y99.8
    civilian activity done for financial or other
      compensation Y99.0
    civilian activity done for income or pay
      Y99.0
    family member assisting in compensated
      work for other family member Y99.8
    hobby not done for income Y99.8
    leisure activity Y99.8
    military activity Y99.1
    off-duty activity of military personnel Y99.8
    recreation or sport not for income or while a
      student Y99.8

External cause status -- *continued*
    specified NEC Y99.8
    student activity Y99.8
    volunteer activity Y99.2

F

Factors, supplemental
    alcohol
      blood level
        less than 20mg/100ml Y90.0
        presence in blood, level not specified
          Y90.9
        20 39mg/100ml Y90.1
        40 59mg/100ml Y90.2
        60 79mg/100ml Y90.3
        80 99mg/100ml Y90.4
        100 119mg/100ml Y90.5
        120 199mg/100ml Y90.6
        200 239mg/100ml Y90.7
        240mg/100ml or more Y90.8
      presence in blood, but level not specified
        Y90.9
    environmental-pollution-related condition-
      see Z57
    nosocomial condition Y95
    work-related condition Y99.0
Failure
    in suture or ligature during surgical
      procedure Y65.2
    mechanical, of instrument or apparatus (any)
      (during any medical or surgical
      procedure) Y65.8
    sterile precautions (during medical and
      surgical care) -*see* Misadventure, failure,
      sterile precautions, by type of procedure
    to
      introduce tube or instrument Y65.4
        endotracheal tube during anesthesia
          Y65.3
      make curve (transport vehicle) NEC -*see*
        Accident, transport
      remove tube or instrument Y65.4
Fall, falling (accidental) W19
    building W20.1
      burning (uncontrolled fire) X00.3
    down
      embankment W17.81
      escalator W10.0
      hill W17.81
      ladder W11
      ramp W10.2
      stairs, steps W10.9
    due to
      bumping against
        object W18.00
          sharp glass W18.02
          specified NEC W18.09
          sports equipment W18.01
        person W03
          due to ice or snow W00.0
          on pedestrian conveyance -*see*
          Accident, transport, pedestrian,
          conveyance
      collision with another person W03
        due to ice or snow W00.0
        involving pedestrian conveyance -*see*
        Accident, transport, pedestrian,
        conveyance
      grocery cart tipping over W17.82
      ice or snow W00.9

Fall, falling (accidental) -- *continued*
    from one level to another W00.2
      on stairs or steps W00.1
      involving pedestrian conveyance -*see*
      Accident, transport, pedestrian,
      conveyance
      on same level W00.0
    slipping (on moving sidewalk) W01.0
      with subsequent striking against object
        W01.10
        furniture W01.190
        sharp object W01.119
          glass W01.110
          power tool or machine W01.111
          specified NEC W01.118
        specified NEC W01.198
    striking against
      object W18.00
        sharp glass W18.02
        specified NEC W18.09
        sports equipment W18.01
      person W03
        due to ice or snow W00.0
        on pedestrian conveyance -*see*
        Accident, transport, pedestrian,
        conveyance
    earth (with asphyxia or suffocation (by
      pressure)) -*see* Earth, falling
    from, off, out of
    aircraft NEC (with accident to aircraft
      NEC) V97.0
      while boarding or alighting V97.1
    balcony W13.0
    bed W06
    boat, ship, watercraft NEC (with drowning
      or submersion) -*see* Drowning, due to,
      fall overboard
      with hitting bottom or object V94.0
    bridge W13.1
    building W13.9
      burning (uncontrolled fire) X00.3
    cavity W17.2
    chair W07
    cherry picker W17.89
    cliff W15
    dock W17.4
    embankment W17.81
    escalator W10.0
    flagpole W13.8
    furniture NEC W08
    grocery cart W17.82
    haystack W17.89
    high place NEC W17.89
      stated as undetermined whether
      accidental or intentional Y30
    hole W17.2
    incline W10.2
    ladder W11
    lifting device W17.89
    machine, machinery -*see also* Contact,
      with, by type of machine
      not in operation W17.89
    manhole W17.1
    mobile elevated work platform [MEWP]
      W17.89
    motorized mobility scooter W05.2
    one level to another NEC W17.89
      intentional, purposeful, suicide (attempt)
      X80
      stated as undetermined whether
      accidental or intentional Y30

Fall, falling (accidental) -- *continued*
  pit W17.2
  playground equipment W09.8
    jungle gym W09.2
    slide W09.0
    swing W09.1
  quarry W17.89
  railing W13.9
  ramp W10.2
  roof W13.2
  scaffolding W12
  scooter (nonmotorized) W05.1
    motorized mobility W05.2
  sky lift W17.89
  stairs, steps W10.9
    curb W10.1
    due to ice or snow W00.1
    escalator W10.0
    incline W10.2
    ramp W10.2
    sidewalk curb W10.1
    specified NEC W10.8
  stepladder W11
  storm drain W17.1
  streetcar NEC V82.6
    with antecedent collision -*see* Accident,
    transport, streetcar occupant
    while boarding or alighting V82.4
  structure NEC W13.8
    burning (uncontrolled fire) X00.3
  table W08
  toilet W18.11
    with subsequent striking against object
    W18.12
  train NEC V81.6
    during derailment (without antecedent
    collision) V81.7
      with antecedent collision -*see* Accident,
    transport, railway vehicle occupant
    while boarding or alighting V81.4
  transport vehicle after collision -*see*
    Accident, transport, by type of vehicle,
    collision
  tree W14
  vehicle (in motion) NEC -*see also*
    Accident, transport V89.9
    motor NEC -*see also* Accident, transport,
    occupant, by type of vehicle V87.8
    stationary W17.89
      while boarding or alighting -*see*
    Accident, transport, by type of vehicle,
    while boarding or alighting
  viaduct W13.8
  wall W13.8
  watercraft -*see also* Drowning, due to, fall
    overboard
    with hitting bottom or object V94.0
  well W17.0
  wheelchair, non-moving W05.0
    powered -*see* Accident, transport,
    pedestrian, conveyance occupant,
    specified type NEC
  window W13.4
  in, on
    aircraft NEC V97.0
      with accident to aircraft V97.0
      while boarding or alighting V97.1
    bathtub (empty) W18.2
      filled W16.212
        causing drowning W16.211
    escalator W10.0

Fall, falling (accidental) -- *continued*
  incline W10.2
  ladder W11
  machine, machinery -*see* Contact, with, by
    type of machine
  object, edged, pointed or sharp (with cut) -
    see Fall, by type
  playground equipment W09.8
    jungle gym W09.2
    slide W09.0
    swing W09.1
  ramp W10.2
  scaffolding W12
  shower W18.2
    causing drowning W16.211
  staircase, stairs, steps W10.9
    curb W10.1
    due to ice or snow W00.1
    escalator W10.0
    incline W10.2
    specified NEC W10.8
  streetcar (without antecedent collision)
    V82.5
    with antecedent collision -*see* Accident,
    transport, streetcar occupant
    while boarding or alighting V82.4
  train (without antecedent collision) V81.5
    with antecedent collision -*see* Accident,
    transport, railway vehicle occupant
    during derailment (without antecedent
    collision) V81.7
      with antecedent collision -*see* Accident,
    transport, railway vehicle occupant
    while boarding or alighting V81.4
  transport vehicle after collision -*see*
    Accident, transport, by type of vehicle,
    collision
  watercraft V93.39
    due to
      accident to craft V91.29
        powered craft V91.23
          ferry boat V91.21
          fishing boat V91.22
          jet skis V91.23
          liner V91.21
          merchant ship V91.20
          passenger ship V91.21
        unpowered craft
          canoe V91.25
          inflatable V91.26
          kayak V91.25
          sailboat V91.24
      powered craft V93.33
        ferry boat V93.31
        fishing boat V93.32
        jet skis V93.33
        liner V93.31
        merchant ship V93.30
        passenger ship V93.31
      unpowered craft V93.38
        canoe V93.35
        inflatable V93.36
        kayak V93.35
        sailboat V93.34
        surf-board V93.38
        windsurfer V93.38
  into
    cavity W17.2
    dock W17.4
    fire -*see* Exposure, fire, by type
    haystack W17.89

Fall, falling (accidental) -- *continued*
    hole W17.2
    lake -*see* Fall, into, water
    manhole W17.1
    moving part of machinery -*see* Contact,
      with, by type of machine
    ocean -*see* Fall, into, water
    opening in surface NEC W17.89
    pit W17.2
    pond -*see* Fall, into, water
    quarry W17.89
    river -*see* Fall, into, water
    shaft W17.89
    storm drain W17.1
    stream -*see* Fall, into, water
    swimming pool -*see also* Fall, into, water,
      in, swimming pool
      empty W17.3
    tank W17.89
    water W16.42
      causing drowning W16.41
      from watercraft -*see* Drowning, due to,
      fall overboard
      hitting diving board W21.4
      in
        bathtub W16.212
          causing drowning W16.211
        bucket W16.222
          causing drowning W16.221
        natural body of water W16.112
          causing drowning W16.111
          striking
            bottom W16.122
              causing drowning W16.121
            side W16.132
              causing drowning W16.131
        specified water NEC W16.312
          causing drowning W16.311
          striking
            bottom W16.322
              causing drowning W16.321
            wall W16.332
              causing drowning W16.331
        swimming pool W16.012
          causing drowning W16.011
          striking
            bottom W16.022
              causing drowning W16.021
            wall W16.032
              causing drowning W16.031
        utility bucket W16.222
          causing drowning W16.221
    well W17.0
  involving
    bed W06
    chair W07
    furniture NEC W08
    glass -*see* Fall, by type
    playground equipment W09.8
      jungle gym W09.2
      slide W09.0
      swing W09.1
    roller blades -*see* Accident, transport,
      pedestrian, conveyance
    skateboard(s) -*see* Accident, transport,
      pedestrian, conveyance
    skates (ice) (in line) (roller) -*see* Accident,
      transport, pedestrian, conveyance
    skis -*see* Accident, transport, pedestrian,
      conveyance
    table W08

Fall, falling (accidental) -- *continued*
  wheelchair, non-moving W05.0
    powered -*see* Accident, transport,
      pedestrian, conveyance, specified type
      NEC
  object -*see* Struck by, object, falling
  off
    toilet W18.11
      with subsequent striking against object
        W18.12
    on same level W18.30
    due to
      specified NEC W18.39
      stepping on an object W18.31
    out of
      bed W06
      building NEC W13.8
      chair W07
      furniture NEC W08
      wheelchair, non-moving W05.0
        powered -*see* Accident, transport,
          pedestrian, conveyance, specified type
          NEC
    window W13.4
  over
    animal W01.0
    cliff W15
    embankment W17.81
    small object W01.0
  rock W20.8
  same level W18.30
    from
      being crushed, pushed, or stepped on by a
        crowd or human stampede W52
      collision, pushing, shoving, by or with
        other person W03
      slipping, stumbling, tripping W01.0
    involving ice or snow W00.0
      involving skates (ice) (roller), skateboard,
        skis -*see* Accident, transport, pedestrian,
        conveyance
  snowslide (avalanche) -*see* Landslide
  stone W20.8
  structure W20.1
    burning (uncontrolled fire) X00.3
  through
    bridge W13.1
    floor W13.3
    roof W13.2
    wall W13.8
    window W13.4
  timber W20.8
  tree (caused by lightning) W20.8
  while being carried or supported by other
    person(s) W04
Fallen on by
  animal (not being ridden) NEC W55.89
Felo-de-se -*see* Suicide
Fight (hand) (fists) (foot) -*see* Assault, fight
Fire (accidental) -*see* Exposure, fire
Firearm discharge -*see* Discharge, firearm
Fireball effects from nuclear explosion in
  war operations -*see* War operations,
  nuclear weapons
Fireworks (explosion) W39
Flash burns from explosion -*see* Explosion
Flood (any injury) (caused by) X38
  collapse of man-made structure causing
    earth movement X36.0
  tidal wave -*see* Forces of nature, tidal wave

Food (any type) in
  air passages (with asphyxia, obstruction, or
    suffocation) -*see* categories T17 and T18
  alimentary tract causing asphyxia (due to
    compression of trachea) -*see* categories
    T17 and T18
Forces of nature X39.8
  avalanche X36.1
    causing transport accident -*see* Accident,
      transport, by type of vehicle
  blizzard X37.2
  cataclysmic storm X37.9
    with flood X38
    blizzard X37.2
    cloudburst X37.8
    cyclone X37.1
    dust storm X37.3
    hurricane X37.0
    specified storm NEC X37.8
    storm surge X37.0
    tornado X37.1
    twister X37.1
    typhoon X37.0
  cloudburst X37.8
  cold (natural) X31
  cyclone X37.1
  dam collapse causing earth movement
    X36.0
  dust storm X37.3
  earth movement X36.1
    earthquake X34
    caused by dam or structure collapse X36.0
  earthquake X34
  flood (caused by) X38
    dam collapse X36.0
    tidal wave -*see* Forces of nature, tidal wave
  heat (natural) X30
  hurricane X37.0
  landslide X36.1
    causing transport accident -*see* Accident,
      transport, by type of vehicle
  lightning -see subcategory T75.0
    causing fire -*see* Exposure, fire
  mudslide X36.1
    causing transport accident -*see* Accident,
      transport, by type of vehicle
  radiation (natural) X39.08
    radon X39.01
  radon X39.01
  specified force NEC X39.8
  storm surge X37.0
  structure collapse causing earth movement
    X36.0
  sunlight X32
  tidal wave X37.41
    due to
      earthquake X37.41
      landslide X37.43
      storm X37.42
      volcanic eruption X37.41
  tornado X37.1
  tsunami X37.41
  twister X37.1
  typhoon X37.0
  volcanic eruption X35
Foreign body
  aspiration -*see* Index to Diseases and
    Injuries, Foreign body, respiratory tract
  embedded in skin W45
  entering through skin W45.8
    can lid W26.8

Foreign body -- *continued*
  nail W45.0
  paper W26.2
  specified NEC W45.8
  splinter W45.8
Forest fire (exposure to) -*see* Exposure, fire,
  uncontrolled, not in building
Found injured X58
  from exposure (to) -*see* Exposure
  on
    highway, road (way), street V89.9
    railway right of way V81.9
Fracture (circumstances unknown or
  unspecified) X58
  due to specified cause NEC X58
Freezing -*see* Exposure, cold **Frostbite** X31
  due to man-made conditions -*see* Exposure,
    cold, man-made **Frozen** -*see* Exposure,
    cold

G

Gored by bull W55.22
Gunshot wound W34.00

H

Hailstones, injured by X39.8
Hanged herself or himself -*see* Hanging,
  self-inflicted
Hanging (accidental) -*see also* category T71
  legal execution -*see* Legal, intervention,
    specified means NEC
Heat (effects of) (excessive) X30
  due to
    man-made conditions W92
      on board watercraft V93.29
        fishing boat V93.22
        merchant ship V93.20
        passenger ship V93.21
        sailboat V93.24
        specified powered craft NEC V93.23
      weather (conditions) X30
  from
    electric heating apparatus causing burning
      X16
    nuclear explosion in war operations -*see*
      War operations, nuclear weapons
  inappropriate in local application or packing
    in medical or surgical procedure Y63.5
Hemorrhage
  delayed following medical or surgical
    treatment without mention of
    misadventure -*see* Index to Diseases and
    Injuries, Complication(s)
  during medical or surgical treatment as
    misadventure -*see* Index to Diseases and
    Injuries, Complication(s)
High
  altitude (effects)   -*see* Air, pressure, low
  level of radioactivity, effects -*see* Radiation
  pressure (effects)   -*see* Air, pressure, high
  temperature, effects -*see* Heat
Hit, hitting (accidental) by -*see* Struck by
Hitting against -*see* Striking against
Homicide (attempt) (justifiable) -*see*
  Assault
Hot
  place, effects -*see also* Heat
  weather, effects X30

House fire (uncontrolled) -see Exposure, fire, uncontrolled, building
Humidity, causing problem X39.8
Hunger X58
Hurricane (any injury) X37.0
Hypobarism, hypobaropathy -see Air, pressure, low

I

Ictus
caloris -see also Heat
solaris X30
Ignition (accidental) -see also Exposure, fire X08.8
anesthetic gas in operating room W40.1
apparel X06.2
from highly flammable material X04
nightwear X05
bed linen (sheets) (spreads) (pillows) (mattress) -see Exposure, fire, uncontrolled, building, bed
benzine X04
clothes, clothing NEC (from controlled fire) X06.2
from
highly flammable material X04
ether X04
in operating room W40.1
explosive material -see Explosion
gasoline X04
jewelry (plastic) (any) X06.0
kerosene X04
material
explosive -see Explosion
highly flammable with secondary explosion X04
nightwear X05
paraffin X04
petrol X04
Immersion (accidental) -see also Drowning
hand or foot due to cold (excessive) X31
Implantation of quills of porcupine W55.89
Inanition (from) (hunger) X58
thirst X58
Inappropriate operation performed
correct operation on wrong side or body part (wrong side) (wrong site) Y65.53
operation intended for another patient done on wrong patient Y65.52
wrong operation performed on correct patient Y65.51
Inattention after, at birth (homicidal intent) (infanticidal intent) X58
Incident, adverse
device
anesthesiology Y70.8
accessory Y70.2
diagnostic Y70.0
miscellaneous Y70.8
monitoring Y70.0
prosthetic Y70.2
rehabilitative Y70.1
surgical Y70.3
therapeutic Y70.1
cardiovascular Y71.8
accessory Y71.2
diagnostic Y71.0
miscellaneous Y71.8
monitoring Y71.0
prosthetic Y71.2
rehabilitative Y71.1

Incident, adverse -- *continued*
surgical Y71.3
therapeutic Y71.1
gastroenterology Y73.8
accessory Y73.2
diagnostic Y73.0
miscellaneous Y73.8
monitoring Y73.0
prosthetic Y73.2
rehabilitative Y73.1
surgical Y73.3
therapeutic Y73.1
general
hospital Y74.8
accessory Y74.2
diagnostic Y74.0
miscellaneous Y74.8
monitoring Y74.0
prosthetic Y74.2
rehabilitative Y74.1
surgical Y74.3
therapeutic Y74.1
surgical Y81.8
accessory Y81.2
diagnostic Y81.0
miscellaneous Y81.8
monitoring Y81.0
prosthetic Y81.2
rehabilitative Y81.1
surgical Y81.3
therapeutic Y81.1
gynecological Y76.8
accessory Y76.2
diagnostic Y76.0
miscellaneous Y76.8
monitoring Y76.0
prosthetic Y76.2
rehabilitative Y76.1
surgical Y76.3
therapeutic Y76.1
medical Y82.9
specified type NEC Y82.8
neurological Y75.8
accessory Y75.2
diagnostic Y75.0
miscellaneous Y75.8
monitoring Y75.0
prosthetic Y75.2
rehabilitative Y75.1
surgical Y75.3
therapeutic Y75.1
obstetrical Y76.8
accessory Y76.2
diagnostic Y76.0
miscellaneous Y76.8
monitoring Y76.0
prosthetic Y76.2
rehabilitative Y76.1
surgical Y76.3
therapeutic Y76.1
ophthalmic Y77.8
accessory Y77.2
diagnostic Y77.0
miscellaneous Y77.8
monitoring Y77.0
prosthetic Y77.2
rehabilitative Y77.1
surgical Y77.3
therapeutic Y77.1
orthopedic Y79.8
accessory Y79.2
diagnostic Y79.0
miscellaneous Y79.8

Incident, adverse -- *continued*
monitoring Y79.0
prosthetic Y79.2
rehabilitative Y79.1
surgical Y79.3
therapeutic Y79.1
otorhinolaryngological Y72.8
accessory Y72.2
diagnostic Y72.0
miscellaneous Y72.8
monitoring Y72.0
prosthetic Y72.2
rehabilitative Y72.1
surgical Y72.3
therapeutic Y72.1
personal use Y74.8
accessory Y74.2
diagnostic Y74.0
miscellaneous Y74.8
monitoring Y74.0
prosthetic Y74.2
rehabilitative Y74.1
surgical Y74.3
therapeutic Y74.1
physical medicine Y80.8
accessory Y80.2
diagnostic Y80.0
miscellaneous Y80.8
monitoring Y80.0
prosthetic Y80.2
rehabilitative Y80.1
surgical Y80.3
therapeutic Y80.1
plastic surgical Y81.8
accessory Y81.2
diagnostic Y81.0
miscellaneous Y81.8
monitoring Y81.0
prosthetic Y81.2
rehabilitative Y81.1
surgical Y81.3
therapeutic Y81.1
radiological Y78.8
accessory Y78.2
diagnostic Y78.0
miscellaneous Y78.8
monitoring Y78.0
prosthetic Y78.2
rehabilitative Y78.1
surgical Y78.3
therapeutic Y78.1
urology Y73.8
accessory Y73.2
diagnostic Y73.0
miscellaneous Y73.8
monitoring Y73.0
prosthetic Y73.2
rehabilitative Y73.1
surgical Y73.3
therapeutic Y73.1
Incineration (accidental) -see Exposure, fire
Infanticide -see Assault
Infrasound waves (causing injury) W49.9
Ingestion
foreign body (causing injury) (with obstruction) -see Foreign body, alimentary canal
poisonous
plant(s) X58
substance NEC -see Table of Drugs and Chemicals

Inhalation

excessively cold substance, man-made -see
Exposure, cold, man-made
food (any type) (into respiratory tract) (with
asphyxia, obstruction respiratory tract,
suffocation) -see categories T17 and T18
foreign body -see Foreign body, aspiration
gastric contents (with asphyxia, obstruction
respiratory passage, suffocation) T17.81
hot air or gases X14.0
liquid air, hydrogen, nitrogen W93.12
suicide (attempt) X83.2
steam X13.0
assault X98.0
stated as undetermined whether accidental
or intentional Y27.0
suicide (attempt) X77.0
toxic gas -see Table of Drugs and Chemicals
vomitus (with asphyxia, obstruction
respiratory passage, suffocation) T17.81

Injury, injured (accidental(ly)) NOS X58
by, caused by, from
assault -see Assault
law-enforcing agent, police, in course of
legal intervention -see Legal intervention
suicide (attempt) X83.8
due to, in
civil insurrection -see War operations
fight -see also Assault, fight Y04.0
war operations -see War operations
homicide -see also Assault Y09
inflicted (by)
in course of arrest (attempted), suppression
of disturbance, maintenance of order, by
law-enforcing agents -see Legal
intervention
other person
stated as
accidental X58
intentional, homicide (attempt) -see
Assault
undetermined whether accidental or
intentional Y33
purposely (inflicted) by other person(s) -see
Assault
self-inflicted X83.8
stated as accidental X58
specified cause NEC X58
undetermined whether accidental or
intentional Y33

Insolation, effects X30

Insufficient nourishment X58

Interruption of respiration (by)
food (lodged in esophagus) -see categories
T17 and T18
vomitus (lodged in esophagus) T17.81

Intervention, legal -see Legal intervention

Intoxication
drug -see Table of Drugs and Chemicals
poison -see Table of Drugs and Chemicals

J

Jammed (accidentally)
between objects (moving) (stationary and
moving) W23.0
stationary W23.1

Jumped, jumping
before moving object NEC X81.8
motor vehicle X81.0
subway train X81.1
train X81.1

Jumped, jumping -- continued
undetermined whether accidental or
intentional Y31
from
boat (into water) voluntarily, without
accident (to or on boat) W16.712
with
accident to or on boat -see Accident,
watercraft
drowning or submersion W16.711
suicide (attempt) X71.3
striking bottom W16.722
causing drowning W16.721
building -see also Jumped, from, high
place W13.9
burning (uncontrolled fire) X00.5
high place NEC W17.89
suicide (attempt) X80
undetermined whether accidental or
intentional Y30
structure -see also Jumped, from, high
place W13.9
burning (uncontrolled fire) X00.5
into water W16.92
causing drowning W16.91
from, off watercraft -see Jumped, from,
boat
in
natural body W16.612
causing drowning W16.611
striking bottom W16.622
causing drowning W16.621
specified place NEC W16.812
causing drowning W16.811
striking
bottom W16.822
causing drowning W16.821
wall W16.832
causing drowning W16.831
swimming pool W16.512
causing drowning W16.511
striking
bottom W16.522
causing drowning W16.521
wall W16.532
causing drowning W16.531
suicide (attempt) X71.3

K

Kicked by
animal NEC W55.82
person(s) (accidentally) W50.1
with intent to injure or kill Y04.0
as, or caused by, a crowd or human
stampede (with fall) W52
assault Y04.0
homicide (attempt) Y04.0
in
fight Y04.0
legal intervention
injuring
bystander Y35.812
law enforcement personnel Y35.811
suspect Y35.813

Kicking
against
object W22.8
sports equipment W21.9
stationary W22.09
sports equipment W21.89

Kicking -- continued
person -see Striking against, person
sports equipment W21.9
carpet stretcher with knee X50.3

Killed, killing (accidentally) NOS -see also
Injury X58
in
action -see War operations
brawl, fight (hand) (fists) (foot) Y04.0
by weapon -see also Assault
cutting, piercing -see Assault, cutting or
piercing instrument
firearm -see Discharge, firearm, by
type, homicide
self
stated as
accident NOS X58
suicide -see Suicide
undetermined whether accidental or
intentional Y33

Kneeling (prolonged) (static) X50.1

Knocked down (accidentally) (by) NOS
X58
animal (not being ridden) NEC -see also
Struck by, by type of animal
crowd or human stampede W52
person W51
in brawl, fight Y04.0
transport vehicle NEC -see also Accident,
transport V09.9

L

Laceration NEC -see Injury

Lack of
care (helpless person) (infant) (newborn)
X58
food except as result of abandonment or
neglect X58
due to abandonment or neglect X58
water except as result of transport accident
X58
due to transport accident -see Accident,
transport, by type
helpless person, infant, newborn X58

Landslide (falling on transport vehicle)
X36.1
caused by collapse of man-made structure
X36.0

Late effect -see Sequelae

Legal
execution (any method) -see Legal,
intervention
intervention (by)
baton -see Legal, intervention, blunt
object, baton
bayonet -see Legal, intervention, sharp
object, bayonet
blow -see Legal, intervention,
manhandling
blunt object
baton
injuring
bystander Y35.312
law enforcement personnel Y35.311
suspect Y35.313
injuring
bystander Y35.302
law enforcement personnel Y35.301
suspect Y35.303
specified NEC
injuring
bystander Y35.392

Legal -- *continued*

law enforcement personnel Y35.391
  suspect Y35.393
stave
  injuring
    bystander Y35.392
  law enforcement personnel Y35.391
  suspect Y35.393
bomb -*see* Legal, intervention, explosive
cutting or piercing instrument -*see* Legal,
  intervention, sharp object
dynamite -*see* Legal, intervention,
  explosive, dynamite
explosive(s)   dynamite
  injuring
    bystander Y35.112
  law enforcement personnel Y35.111
  suspect Y35.113
grenade
  injuring
    bystander Y35.192
  law enforcement personnel Y35.191
  suspect Y35.193
injuring
  bystander Y35.102
  law enforcement personnel Y35.101
  suspect Y35.103
mortar bomb
  injuring
    bystander Y35.192
  law enforcement personnel Y35.191
  suspect Y35.193
shell
  injuring
    bystander Y35.122
  law enforcement personnel Y35.121
  suspect Y35.123
specified NEC
  injuring
    bystander Y35.192
  law enforcement personnel Y35.191
  suspect Y35.193
firearm(s) (discharge)   handgun
  injuring
    bystander Y35.022
  law enforcement personnel Y35.021
  suspect Y35.023
injuring
  bystander Y35.002
  law enforcement personnel Y35.001
  suspect Y35.003
machine gun
  injuring
    bystander Y35.012
  law enforcement personnel Y35.011
  suspect Y35.013
rifle pellet
  injuring
    bystander Y35.032
  law enforcement personnel Y35.031
  suspect Y35.033
rubber bullet
  injuring
    bystander Y35.042
  law enforcement personnel Y35.041
  suspect Y35.043
shotgun -*see* Legal, intervention, firearm,
  specified NEC
specified NEC
  injuring
    bystander Y35.092

Legal -- *continued*

law enforcement personnel Y35.091
  suspect Y35.093
gas (asphyxiation) (poisoning)   injuring
  bystander Y35.202
  law enforcement personnel Y35.201
  suspect Y35.203
specified NEC
  injuring
    bystander Y35.292
  law enforcement personnel Y35.291
  suspect Y35.293
tear gas
  injuring
    bystander Y35.212
  law enforcement personnel Y35.211
  suspect Y35.213
grenade -*see* Legal, intervention,
  explosive, grenade
injuring
  bystander Y35.92
  law enforcement personnel Y35.91
  suspect Y35.93
late effect (of) -*see* with 7th character S
  Y35
manhandling
  injuring
    bystander Y35.812
  law enforcement personnel Y35.811
  suspect Y35.813
sequelae (of) -*see* with 7th character S Y35
sharp objects
  bayonet
    injuring
      bystander Y35.412
    law enforcement personnel Y35.411
    suspect Y35.413
  injuring
    bystander Y35.402
  law enforcement personnel Y35.401
  suspect Y35.403
  specified NEC
    injuring
      bystander Y35.492
    law enforcement personnel Y35.491
    suspect Y35.493
specified means NEC
  injuring
    bystander Y35.892
  law enforcement personnel Y35.891
  suspect Y35.893
stabbing -*see* Legal, intervention, sharp
  object
stave -*see* Legal, intervention, blunt object,
  stave
tear gas -*see* Legal, intervention, gas, tear
  gas
truncheon -*see* Legal, intervention, blunt
  object, stave
Lifting -*see also* Overexertion
  heavy objects X50.0
  weights X50.0
Lightning (shock) (stroke) (struck by) -*see*
  subcategory T75.0
  causing fire -*see* Exposure, fire
Loss of control (transport vehicle) NEC -
  see Accident, transport
Lost at sea NOS -*see* Drowning, due to, fall
  overboard

Low

pressure (effects) -*see* Air, pressure, low
temperature (effects) -*see* Exposure, cold
Lying before train, vehicle or other moving
  object X81.8
subway train X81.1
train X81.1
undetermined whether accidental or
  intentional Y31
Lynching -*see* Assault

M

Malfunction (mechanism or component)
  (of)   firearm W34.10
airgun W34.110
BB gun W34.110
gas, air or spring-operated gun NEC
  W34.118
handgun W32.1
hunting rifle W33.12
larger firearm W33.10
  specified NEC W33.19
machine gun W33.13
paintball gun W34.111
pellet gun W34.110
shotgun W33.11
specified NEC W34.19
Very pistol [flare] W34.19
handgun -*see* Malfunction, firearm, handgun
Maltreatment -*see* Perpetrator
Mangled (accidentally) NOS X58
Manhandling (in brawl, fight) Y04.0
legal intervention -*see* Legal, intervention,
  manhandling
Manslaughter (nonaccidental) -*see* Assault
Mauled by animal NEC W55.89
Medical procedure, complication of
  (delayed or as an abnormal reaction
  without mention of misadventure) -*see*
  Complication of or following, by
  specified type of procedure
due to or as a result of misadventure -*see*
  Misadventure
Melting (due to fire) -*see also* Exposure, fire
apparel NEC X06.3
clothes, clothing NEC X06.3
  nightwear X05
fittings or furniture (burning building)
  (uncontrolled fire) X00.8
nightwear X05
plastic jewelry X06.1
Mental cruelty X58
Military operations (injuries to military
  and civilians occurring during
  peacetime on military property and
  during routine military exercises and
  operations) (by) (from) (involving)
  Y37.90
air blast Y37.20
aircraft
  destruction -*see* Military operations,
  destruction of aircraft
airway restriction -*see* Military operations,
  restriction of airways
asphyxiation -*see* Military operations,
  restriction of airways
biological weapons Y37.6X-
blast Y37.20
blast fragments Y37.20
blast wave Y37.20

Military operations -- *continued*
blast wind Y37.20
bomb Y37.20
  dirty Y37.50
  gasoline Y37.31
  incendiary Y37.31
  petrol Y37.31
bullet Y37.43
  incendiary Y37.32
  rubber Y37.41
chemical weapons Y37.7X-
combat
  hand to hand (unarmed) combat Y37.44
  using blunt or piercing object Y37.45
conflagration -*see* Military operations, fire
conventional warfare NEC Y37.49
depth-charge Y37.01
destruction of aircraft Y37.10
  due to
    air to air missile Y37.11
    collision with other aircraft Y37.12
    detonation (accidental) of onboard
      munitions and explosives Y37.14
    enemy fire or explosives Y37.11
    explosive placed on aircraft Y37.11
    onboard fire Y37.13
    rocket propelled grenade [RPG] Y37.11
    small arms fire Y37.11
    surface to air missile Y37.11
    specified NEC Y37.19
detonation (accidental) of
  onboard marine weapons Y37.05
  own munitions or munitions launch device
    Y37.24
dirty bomb Y37.50
explosion (of) Y37.20
  aerial bomb Y37.21
  bomb NOS -*see also* Military operations,
    bomb(s) Y37.20
  own munitions or munitions launch device
    (accidental) Y37.24
  fragments Y37.20
  grenade Y37.29
  guided missile Y37.22
  improvised explosive device [IED]
    (person-borne) (roadside) (vehicle-borne)
    Y37.23
  land mine Y37.29
  marine mine (at sea) (in harbor) Y37.02
  marine weapon Y37.00
    specified NEC Y37.09
  sea-based artillery shell Y37.03
  specified NEC Y37.29
  torpedo Y37.04
fire Y37.30
  specified NEC Y37.39
firearms
  discharge Y37.43
  pellets Y37.42
flamethrower Y37.33
fragments (from) (of)
  improvised explosive device [IED]
    (person-borne) (roadside) (vehicle-borne)
    Y37.26
  munitions Y37.25
  specified NEC Y37.29
  weapons Y37.27
friendly fire Y37.92
hand to hand (unarmed) combat Y37.44
hot substances -*see* Military operations, fire
incendiary bullet Y37.32

Military operations -- *continued*
nuclear weapon (effects of) Y37.50
  acute radiation exposure Y37.54
  blast pressure Y37.51
  direct blast Y37.51
  direct heat Y37.53
  fallout exposure Y37.54
  fireball Y37.53
  indirect blast (struck or crushed by blast
    debris) (being thrown by blast) Y37.52
  ionizing radiation (immediate exposure)
    Y37.54
  nuclear radiation Y37.54
  radiation
    ionizing (immediate exposure) Y37.54
    nuclear Y37.54
    thermal Y37.53
  specified NEC Y37.59
  secondary effects Y37.54
  thermal radiation Y37.53
restriction of air (airway) - - intentional
  Y37.46
  unintentional Y37.47
rubber bullets Y37.41
shrapnel NOS Y37.29
suffocation -*see* Military operations,
  restriction of airways
unconventional warfare NEC Y37.7X-
underwater blast NOS Y37.00
warfare
  conventional NEC Y37.49
  unconventional NEC Y37.7X-
weapons
  biological weapons Y37.6X
  chemical Y37.7X-
  nuclear (effects of) Y37.50
    acute radiation exposure Y37.54
    blast pressure Y37.51
    direct blast Y37.51
    direct heat Y37.53
    fallout exposure Y37.54
    fireball Y37.53
    indirect blast (struck or crushed by blast
      debris) (being thrown by blast) Y37.52
    radiation
      ionizing (immediate exposure) Y37.54
      nuclear Y37.54
      thermal Y37.53
    secondary effects Y37.54
    specified NEC Y37.59
  of mass destruction [WMD] Y37.91
  weapon of mass destruction [WMD]
    Y37.91

**Misadventure(s) to patient(s) during
  surgical or medical care** Y69
contaminated medical or biological
  substance (blood, drug, fluid) Y64.9
  administered (by) NEC Y64.9
    immunization Y64.1
    infusion Y64.0
    injection Y64.1
    specified means NEC Y64.8
    transfusion Y64.0
    vaccination Y64.1
excessive amount of blood or other fluid
  during transfusion or infusion Y63.0
failure
  in dosage Y63.9
    electroshock therapy Y63.4
    inappropriate temperature (too hot or too
      cold) in local application and packing
      Y63.5

Misadventure(s) to patient(s) -- *continued*
infusion
  excessive amount of fluid Y63.0
  incorrect dilution of fluid Y63.1
insulin-shock therapy Y63.4
nonadministration of necessary drug or
  biological substance Y63.6
overdose -*see* Table of Drugs and
  Chemicals
  radiation, in therapy Y63.2
radiation
  overdose Y63.2
specified procedure NEC Y63.8
transfusion
  excessive amount of blood Y63.0
mechanical, of instrument or apparatus
  (any) (during any procedure) Y65.8
sterile precautions (during procedure)
  Y62.9
  aspiration of fluid or tissue (by puncture
    or catheterization, except heart) Y62.6
  biopsy (except needle aspiration) Y62.8
    needle (aspirating) Y62.6
  blood sampling Y62.6
  catheterization Y62.6
    heart Y62.5
  dialysis (kidney) Y62.2
  endoscopic examination Y62.4
  enema Y62.8
  immunization Y62.3
  infusion Y62.1
  injection Y62.3
  needle biopsy Y62.6
  paracentesis (abdominal) (thoracic)
    Y62.6
  perfusion Y62.2
  puncture (lumbar) Y62.6
  removal of catheter or packing Y62.8
  specified procedure NEC Y62.8
  surgical operation Y62.0
  transfusion Y62.1
  vaccination Y62.3
suture or ligature during surgical procedure
  Y65.2
to introduce or to remove tube or
  instrument -*see* Failure, to
hemorrhage -*see* Index to Diseases and
  Injuries, Complication(s)
inadvertent exposure of patient to radiation
  Y63.3
inappropriate
  operation performed -*see* Inappropriate
    operation performed
  temperature (too hot or too cold) in local
    application or packing Y63.5
infusion -*see also* Misadventure, by type,
  infusion Y69
  excessive amount of fluid Y63.0
  incorrect dilution of fluid Y63.1
  wrong fluid Y65.1
mismatched blood in transfusion Y65.0
nonadministration of necessary drug or
  biological substance Y63.6
overdose -*see* Table of Drugs and Chemicals
  radiation (in therapy) Y63.2
perforation -*see* Index to Diseases and
  Injuries, Complication(s)
performance of inappropriate operation -*see*
  Inappropriate operation performed
puncture -*see* Index to Diseases and Injuries,
  Complication(s)

Misadventure(s) to patient(s) -- *continued*
  specified type NEC Y65.8
    failure
      suture or ligature during surgical
        operation Y65.2
      to introduce or to remove tube or
        instrument -*see* Failure, to
    infusion of wrong fluid Y65.1
    performance of inappropriate operation -
      see Inappropriate operation performed
    transfusion of mismatched blood Y65.0
    wrong
      fluid in infusion Y65.1
      placement of endotracheal tube during
        anesthetic procedure Y65.3
    transfusion -*see* Misadventure, by type,
      transfusion
      excessive amount of blood Y63.0
      mismatched blood Y65.0
    wrong
      drug given in error -*see* Table of Drugs and
        Chemicals
      fluid in infusion Y65.1
      placement of endotracheal tube during
        anesthetic procedure Y65.3
Mismatched blood in transfusion Y65.0
Motion sickness T75.3
Mountain sickness W94.11
Mudslide (of cataclysmic nature) -*see*
  Landslide
Murder (attempt) -*see* Assault

N

Nail
  contact with W45.0
    gun W29.4
  embedded in skin W45.0
Neglect (criminal) (homicidal intent) X58
Noise (causing injury) (pollution) W42.9
  supersonic W42.0
Nonadministration (of)
  drug or biological substance (necessary)
    Y63.6
  surgical and medical care Y66
Nosocomial condition Y95

O

Object
  falling
    from, in, on, hitting
      machinery -*see* Contact, with, by type of
        machine
  set in motion by
    accidental explosion or rupture of pressure
      vessel W38
    firearm -*see* Discharge, firearm, by type
    machine (ry) -*see* Contact, with, by type of
      machine
Overdose (drug) -*see* Table of Drugs and
  Chemicals
  radiation Y63.2
Overexertion X50.9
  from
    prolonged static or awkward postures
      X50.1
    repetitive movements X50.3
    specified strenuous movements or postures
      NEC X50.9
    strenuous movement or load X50.0

Overexposure (accidental) (to)
  cold -*see also* Exposure, cold X31
    due to man-made conditions -*see*
      Exposure, cold, man-made
  heat -*see also* Heat X30
  radiation -*see* Radiation
  radioactivity W88.0
  sun (sunburn) X32
  weather NEC -*see* Forces of nature
  wind NEC -*see* Forces of nature
Overheated -*see* Heat
Overturning (accidental)
  machinery -*see* Contact, with, by type of
    machine
  transport vehicle NEC -*see also* Accident,
    transport V89.9
  watercraft (causing drowning, submersion) -
    see also Drowning, due to, accident to,
    watercraft, overturning
    causing injury except drowning or
      submersion -*see* Accident, watercraft,
      causing, injury NEC

P

Parachute descent (voluntary) (without
  accident to aircraft) V97.29
  due to accident to aircraft -*see* Accident,
    transport, aircraft
Pecked by bird W61.99
Perforation during medical or surgical
  treatment as misadventure -*see* Index to
  Diseases and Injuries, Complication(s)
Perpetrator, perpetration, of assault,
  maltreatment and neglect (by) Y07.9
  boyfriend Y07.03
  brother Y07.410
    stepbrother Y07.435
  coach Y07.53
  cousin
    female Y07.491
    male Y07.490
  daycare provider Y07.519
    at-home
      adult care Y07.512
      childcare Y07.510
    care center
      adult care Y07.513
      childcare Y07.511
  family member NEC Y07.499
  father Y07.11
    adoptive Y07.13
    foster Y07.420
    stepfather Y07.430
  foster father Y07.420
  foster mother Y07.421
  girl friend Y07.04
  healthcare provider Y07.529
    mental health Y07.521
    specified NEC Y07.528
  husband Y07.01
  instructor Y07.53
  mother Y07.12
    adoptive Y07.14
    foster Y07.421
    stepmother Y07.433
  nonfamily member Y07.50
    specified NEC Y07.59
  nurse Y07.528
  occupational therapist Y07.528
  partner of parent

Perpetrator, perpetration -- *continued*
    female Y07.434
    male Y07.432
  physical therapist Y07.528
  sister Y07.411
  speech therapist Y07.528
  stepbrother Y07.435
  stepfather Y07.430
  stepmother Y07.433
  stepsister Y07.436
  teacher Y07.53
  wife Y07.02
Piercing -*see* Contact, with, by type of object
  or machine
Pinched
  between objects (moving) (stationary and
    moving) W23.0
  stationary W23.1
Pinned under machine (ry) -*see* Contact,
  with, by type of machine
Place of occurrence Y92.9
  abandoned house Y92.89
  airplane Y92.813
  airport Y92.520
  ambulatory health services establishment
    NEC Y92.538
  ambulatory surgery center Y92.530
  amusement park Y92.831
  apartment (co-op) -*see* Place of occurrence,
    residence, apartment
  assembly hall Y92.29
  bank Y92.510
  barn Y92.71
  baseball field Y92.320
  basketball court Y92.310
  beach Y92.832
  boarding house -*see* Place of occurrence,
    residence, boarding house
  boat Y92.814
  bowling alley Y92.39
  bridge Y92.89
  building under construction Y92.61
  bus Y92.811
    station Y92.521
  cafe Y92.511
  campsite Y92.833
  campus -*see* Place of occurrence, school
  canal Y92.89
  car Y92.810
  casino Y92.59
  children's home -*see* Place of occurrence,
    residence, institutional, orphanage
  church Y92.22
  cinema Y92.26
  clubhouse Y92.29
  coal pit Y92.64
  college (community) Y92.214
  condominium -*see* Place of occurrence,
    residence, apartment
  construction area -*see* Place of occurrence,
    industrial and construction area
  convalescent home -*see* Place of occurrence,
    residence, institutional, nursing home
  court-house Y92.240
  cricket ground Y92.328
  cultural building Y92.258
    art gallery Y92.250
    museum Y92.251
    music hall Y92.252
    opera house Y92.253
    specified NEC Y92.258

Place of occurrence -- *continued*
- driveway Y92.113
- garage Y92.114
- garden Y92.116
- kitchen Y92.110
- specified NEC Y92.118
- swimming pool Y92.115
- yard Y92.116
- prison Y92.149
  - bathroom Y92.142
  - cell Y92.143
  - courtyard Y92.147
  - dining room Y92.141
  - kitchen Y92.140
  - specified NEC Y92.148
  - swimming pool Y92.146
- reform school Y92.159
  - bathroom Y92.152
  - bedroom Y92.153
  - dining room Y92.151
  - driveway Y92.154
  - garage Y92.155
  - garden Y92.157
  - kitchen Y92.150
  - specified NEC Y92.158
  - swimming pool Y92.156
  - yard Y92.157
- school dormitory Y92.169
  - bathroom Y92.162
  - bedroom Y92.163
  - dining room Y92.161
  - kitchen Y92.160
  - specified NEC Y92.168
- specified NEC Y92.199
  - bathroom Y92.192
  - bedroom Y92.193
  - dining room Y92.191
  - driveway Y92.194
  - garage Y92.195
  - garden Y92.197
  - kitchen Y92.190
  - specified NEC Y92.198
  - swimming pool Y92.196
  - yard Y92.197
- kitchen Y92.000
- mobile home Y92.029
  - bathroom Y92.022
  - bedroom Y92.023
  - dining room Y92.021
  - driveway Y92.024
  - garage Y92.025
  - garden Y92.027
  - kitchen Y92.020
  - specified NEC Y92.028
  - swimming pool Y92.026
  - yard Y92.027
- specified place in residence NEC Y92.008
- specified residence type NEC Y92.099
  - bathroom Y92.091
  - bedroom Y92.092
  - driveway Y92.093
  - garage Y92.094
  - garden Y92.096
  - kitchen Y92.090
  - specified NEC Y92.098
  - swimming pool Y92.095
  - yard Y92.096
- restaurant Y92.511
- riding school Y92.39
- river Y92.828
- road Y92.488

Place of occurrence -- *continued*
- rodeo ring Y92.39
- rugby field Y92.328
- same day surgery center Y92.530
- sand pit Y92.64
- school (private) (public) (state) Y92.219
  - college Y92.214
  - daycare center Y92.210
  - elementary school Y92.211
  - high school Y92.213
  - kindergarten Y92.211
  - middle school Y92.212
  - specified NEC Y92.218
  - trace school Y92.215
  - university Y92.214
  - vocational school Y92.215
- sea (shore) Y92.832
- senior citizen center Y92.29
- service area
  - airport Y92.520
  - bus station Y92.521
  - gas station Y92.524
  - highway rest stop Y92.523
  - railway station Y92.522
- shipyard Y92.62
- shop (commercial) Y92.513
- sidewalk Y92.480
- silo Y92.79
- skating rink (roller) Y92.331
  - ice Y92.330
- slaughter house Y92.86
- soccer field Y92.322
- specified place NEC Y92.89
- sports area Y92.39
  - athletic
    - court Y92.318
      - basketball Y92.310
      - specified NEC Y92.318
      - squash Y92.311
      - tennis Y92.312
    - field Y92.328
      - baseball Y92.320
      - cricket ground Y92.328
      - football Y92.321
      - hockey Y92.328
      - soccer Y92.322
      - specified NEC Y92.328
  - golf course Y92.39
  - gymnasium Y92.39
  - riding school Y92.39
  - skating rink (roller) Y92.331
    - ice Y92.330
  - stadium Y92.39
  - swimming pool Y92.34
- squash court Y92.311
- stadium Y92.39
- steeplechasing course Y92.39
- store Y92.512
- stream Y92.828
- street and highway Y92.410
  - bike path Y92.482
  - freeway Y92.411
  - highway ramp Y92.415
  - interstate highway Y92.411
  - local residential or business street Y92.414
  - motorway Y92.411
  - parkway Y92.412
  - parking lot Y92.481
  - sidewalk Y92.480
  - specified NEC Y92.488
- state road Y92.413

Place of occurrence -- *continued*
- subway car Y92.816
- supermarket Y92.512
- swamp Y92.828
- swimming pool (public) Y92.34
  - private (at) Y92.095
    - boarding house Y92.045
    - military base Y92.136
    - mobile home Y92.026
    - nursing home Y92.125
    - orphanage Y92.115
    - prison Y92.146
    - reform school Y92.156
    - single family residence Y92.016
- synagogue Y92.22
- television station Y92.59
- tennis court Y92.312
- theater Y92.254
- trade area Y92.59
  - bank Y92.510
  - cafe Y92.511
  - casino Y92.59
  - garage Y92.59
  - hotel Y92.59
  - market Y92.512
  - office building Y92.59
  - radio station Y92.59
  - restaurant Y92.511
  - shop Y92.513
  - shopping mall Y92.59
  - store Y92.512
  - supermarket Y92.512
  - television station Y92.59
  - warehouse Y92.59
- trailer park, residential -*see* Place of occurrence, residence, mobile home
- trailer site NOS Y92.89
- train Y92.815
  - station Y92.522
- truck Y92.812
- tunnel under construction Y92.69
- urgent (health) care center Y92.532
- university Y92.214
- vehicle (transport) Y92.818
  - airplane Y92.813
  - boat Y92.814
  - bus Y92.811
  - car Y92.810
  - specified NEC Y92.818
  - subway car Y92.816
  - train Y92.815
  - truck Y92.812
- warehouse Y92.59
- water reservoir Y92.89
- wilderness area Y92.828
  - desert Y92.820
  - forest Y92.821
  - marsh Y92.828
  - mountain Y92.828
  - prairie Y92.828
  - specified NEC Y92.828
  - swamp Y92.828
- workshop Y92.69
- yard, private Y92.096
  - boarding house Y92.046
  - single family house Y92.017
  - mobile home Y92.027
- youth center Y92.29
- zoo (zoological garden) Y92.834

Plumbism -*see* Table of Drugs and Chemicals, lead

Poisoning (accidental) (by) *-see also* Table
of Drugs and Chemicals
by plant, thorns, spines, sharp leaves or
other mechanisms NEC X58
carbon monoxide
generated by
motor vehicle *-see* Accident, transport
watercraft (in transit) (not in transit)
V93.89
ferry boat V93.81
fishing boat V93.82
jet skis V93.83
liner V93.81
merchant ship V93.80
passenger ship V93.81
powered craft NEC V93.83
caused by injection of poisons into skin by
plant thorns, spines, sharp leaves X58
marine or sea plants (venomous) X58
exhaust gas
generated by
motor vehicle *-see* Accident, transport
watercraft (in transit) (not in transit)
V93.89
ferry boat V93.81
fishing boat V93.82
jet skis V93.83
liner V93.81
merchant ship V93.80
passenger ship V93.81
powered craft NEC V93.83
fumes or smoke due to
explosion *-see also* Explosion W40.9
fire *-see* Exposure, fire
ignition *-see* Ignition
gas
in legal intervention *-see* Legal,
intervention, gas
legal execution *-see* Legal, intervention,
gas
in war operations *-see* War operations
legal
execution *-see* Legal, intervention, gas
intervention
by gas *-see* Legal, intervention, gas
other specified means *-see* Legal,
intervention, specified means NEC
Powder burn (by) (from)
airgun W34.110
BB gun W34.110
firearm NEC W34.19
gas, air or spring-operated gun NEC
W34.118
handgun W32.1
hunting rifle W33.12
larger firearm W33.10
specified NEC W33.19
machine gun W33.13
paintball gun W34.111
pellet gun W34.110
shotgun W33.11
Very pistol [flare] W34.19
**Premature cessation (of) surgical and
medical care** Y66
Privation (food) (water) X58
Procedure (operation)
correct, on wrong side or body part (wrong
side) (wrong site) Y65.53
intended for another patient done on wrong
patient Y65.52

Procedure (operation) *-- continued*
performed on patient not scheduled for
surgery Y65.52
performed on wrong patient Y65.52
wrong, performed on correct patient Y65.51
Prolonged
sitting in transport vehicle *-see* Travel, by
type of vehicle
stay in
high altitude as cause of anoxia,
barodontalgia, barotitis or hypoxia
W94.11
weightless environment X52
Pulling, excessive *-see also* Overexertion
X50.9
Puncture, puncturing *-see also* Contact,
with, by type of object or machine
by
plant thorns, spines, sharp leaves or other
mechanisms NEC W60
during medical or surgical treatment as
misadventure *-see* Index to Diseases and
Injuries, Complication(s)
Pushed, pushing (accidental) (injury in)
by other person(s) (accidental) W51
with fall W03
due to ice or snow W00.0
as, or caused by, a crowd or human
stampede (with fall) W52
before moving object NEC Y02.8
motor vehicle Y02.0
subway train Y02.1
train Y02.1
from
high place NEC
in accidental circumstances W17.89
stated as
intentional, homicide (attempt) Y01
undetermined whether accidental or
intentional Y30
transport vehicle NEC *-see also*
Accident, transport V89.9
stated as
intentional, homicide (attempt) Y08.89
overexertion X50.9

R

Radiation (exposure to) arc lamps W89.0
atomic power plant (malfunction) NEC
W88.1
complication of or abnormal reaction to
medical radiotherapy Y84.2
electromagnetic, ionizing W88.0
gamma rays W88.1
in
war operations (from or following nuclear
explosion) *-see* War operations
inadvertent exposure of patient (receiving
test or therapy) Y63.3
infrared (heaters and lamps) W90.1
excessive heat from W92
ionized, ionizing (particles, artificially
accelerated) radioisotopes W88.1
specified NEC W88.8
x-rays W88.0
isotopes, radioactive *-see* Radiation,
radioactive isotopes
laser(s) W90.2
in war operations *-see* War operations
misadventure in medical care Y63.2

Radiation (exposure to) *-- continued*
light sources (man-made visible and
ultraviolet) W89.9
natural X32
specified NEC W89.8
tanning bed W89.1
welding light W89.0
man-made visible light W89.9
specified NEC W89.8
tanning bed W89.1
welding light W89.0
microwave W90.8
misadventure in medical or surgical
procedure Y63.2
natural NEC X39.08
radon X39.01
overdose (in medical or surgical procedure)
Y63.2
radar W90.0
radioactive isotopes (any) W88.1
atomic power plant malfunction W88.1
misadventure in medical or surgical
treatment Y63.2
radiofrequency W90.0
radium NEC W88.1
sun X32
ultraviolet (light) (man-made) W89.9
natural X32
specified NEC W89.8
tanning bed W89.1
welding light W89.0
welding arc, torch, or light W89.0
excessive heat from W92
x-rays (hard) (soft) W88.0
Range disease W94.11
Rape (attempted) T74.2
Rat bite W53.11
Reaching (prolonged) (static) X50.1
Reaction, abnormal to medical procedure -
see also Complication of or following, by
type of procedure Y84.9
with misadventure *-see* Misadventure
biologicals *-see* Table of Drugs and
Chemicals
drugs *-see* Table of Drugs and Chemicals
vaccine *-see* Table of Drugs and Chemicals
Recoil
airgun W34.110
BB gun W34.110
firearm NEC W34.19
gas, air or spring-operated gun NEC
W34.118
handgun W32.1
hunting rifle W33.12
larger firearm W33.10
specified NEC W33.19
machine gun W33.13
paintball gun W34.111
pellet W34.110
shotgun W33.11
Very pistol [flare] W34.19
Reduction in
atmospheric pressure
-see Air, pressure, change
**Rock falling on or hitting (accidentally)
(person)** W20.8
in cave-in W20.0
Run over (accidentally) (by)
animal (not being ridden) NEC W55.89
machinery *-see* Contact, with, by specified
type of machine

Run over (accidentally) -- continued
  transport vehicle NEC -see also Accident,
    transport V09.9
    intentional homicide (attempt) Y03.0
    motor NEC V09.20
      intentional homicide (attempt) Y03.0
Running
  before moving object X81.8
  motor vehicle X81.0
Running off, away
  animal (being ridden) -see also Accident,
    transport V80.918
    not being ridden W55.89
  animal-drawn vehicle NEC -see also
    Accident, transport V80.928
  highway, road (way), street
    transport vehicle NEC -see also Accident,
      transport V89.9
Rupture pressurized devices -see Explosion,
  by type of device

S

Saturnism -see Table of Drugs and
  Chemicals, lead
Scald, scalding (accidental) (by) (from) (in)
  X19
  air (hot) X14.1
  gases (hot) X14.1
  homicide (attempt) -see Assault, burning,
    hot object
  inflicted by other person
    stated as intentional, homicide (attempt) -
      see Assault, burning, hot object
  liquid (boiling) (hot) NEC X12
    stated as undetermined whether accidental
      or intentional Y27.2
    suicide (attempt) X77.2
  local application of externally applied
    substance in medical or surgical care
    Y63.5
  metal (molten) (liquid) (hot) NEC X18
  self-inflicted X77.9
  stated as undetermined whether accidental
    or intentional Y27.8
  steam X13.1
    assault X98.0
    stated as undetermined whether accidental
      or intentional Y27.0
    suicide (attempt) X77.0
  vapor (hot) X13.1
    assault X98.0
    stated as undetermined whether accidental
      or intentional Y27.0
    suicide (attempt) X77.0
Scratched by
  cat W55.03
  person(s) (accidentally) W50.4
    with intent to injure or kill Y04.0
    as, or caused by, a crowd or human
      stampede (with fall) W52
    assault Y04.0
    homicide (attempt) Y04.0
    in
      fight Y04.0
      legal intervention
        injuring
          bystander Y35.892
          law enforcement personnel Y35.891
          suspect Y35.893

Seasickness T75.3
Self-harm NEC -see also External cause by
  type, undetermined whether accidental or
  intentional
  intentional -see Suicide
  poisoning NEC -see Table of drugs and
    biologicals, accident
Self-inflicted (injury) NEC -see also
  External cause by type, undetermined
  whether accidental or intentional
  intentional -see Suicide
  poisoning NEC -see Table of drugs and
    biologicals, accident
Sequelae (of)
  accident NEC -see W00 X58 with 7th
    character S
  assault (homicidal) (any means) -see X92
    Y08 with 7th character S
  homicide, attempt (any means) -see X92
    Y08 with 7th character S
  injury undetermined whether accidentally or
    purposely inflicted -see Y21 Y33 with 7th
    character S
  intentional self-harm (classifiable to X71
    X83) -see X71 X83 with 7th character S
  legal intervention -see with 7th character S
    Y35
  motor vehicle accident -see V00 V99 with
    7th character S
  suicide, attempt (any means) -see X71 X83
    with 7th character S
  transport accident -see V00 V99 with 7th
    character S
  war operations -see War operations **Shock**
  electric -see Exposure, electric current
  from electric appliance (any) (faulty) W86.8
    domestic W86.0
  suicide (attempt) X83.1
Shooting, shot (accidental(ly)) -see also
  Discharge, firearm, by type
  herself or himself -see Discharge, firearm by
    type, self-inflicted
  homicide (attempt) -see Discharge, firearm
    by type, homicide
  in war operations -see War operations
  inflicted by other person -see Discharge,
    firearm by type, homicide
    accidental -see Discharge, firearm, by type
    of firearm
  legal
    execution -see Legal, intervention, firearm
    intervention -see Legal, intervention,
      firearm
  self-inflicted -see Discharge, firearm by
    type, suicide
    accidental -see Discharge, firearm, by type
    of firearm
  suicide (attempt) -see Discharge, firearm by
    type, suicide
Shoving (accidentally) by other person -see
  Pushed, by other person
Sickness
  alpine W94.11
  motion -see Motion
  mountain W94.11
Sinking (accidental)
  watercraft (causing drowning, submersion) -
    see also Drowning, due to, accident to,
    watercraft, sinking
  causing injury except drowning or
    submersion -see Accident, watercraft,
    causing, injury NEC

Siriasis X32
Sitting (prolonged) (static) X50.1
Slashed wrists -see Cut, self-inflicted
Slipping (accidental) (on same level) (with
  fall) W01.0
  on
    ice W00.0
      with skates -see Accident, transport,
        pedestrian, conveyance
    mud W01.0
    oil W01.0
    snow W00.0
      with skis -see Accident, transport,
        pedestrian, conveyance
    surface (slippery) (wet) NEC W01.0
  without fall W18.40
    due to
      specified NEC W18.49
      stepping from one level to another
        W18.43
      stepping into hole or opening W18.42
      stepping on object W18.41
Sliver, wood, contact with W45.8
Smoldering (due to fire) -see Exposure, fire
Sodomy (attempted) by force T74.2
Sound waves (causing injury) W42.9
  supersonic W42.0
Splinter, contact with W45.8
Stab, stabbing -see Cut
Standing (prolonged) (static) X50.1
Starvation X58
Status of external cause Y99.9
  child assisting in compensated work for
    family Y99.8
  civilian activity done for financial or other
    compensation Y99.0
  civilian activity done for income or pay
    Y99.0
  family member assisting in compensated
    work for other family member Y99.8
  hobby not done for income Y99.8
  leisure activity Y99.8
  military activity Y99.1
  off-duty activity of military personnel Y99.8
  recreation or sport not for income or while a
    student Y99.8
  specified NEC Y99.8
  student activity Y99.8
  volunteer activity Y99.2
Stepped on
  by
    animal (not being ridden) NEC W55.89
    crowd or human stampede W52
    person W50.0
Stepping on
  object W22.8
    with fall W18.31
    sports equipment W21.9
    stationary W22.09
      sports equipment W21.89
  person W51
    by crowd or human stampede W52
  sports equipment W21.9
Sting
  arthropod, nonvenomous W57
  insect, nonvenomous W57
Storm (cataclysmic) -see Forces of nature,
  cataclysmic storm
Straining, excessive -see also Overexertion
  X50.9
Strangling -see Strangulation

Struck (accidentally) -- *continued*
  in sports W21.9
    assault Y08.09
    ball W21.00
      baseball W21.03
      basketball W21.05
      football W21.01
      golf ball W21.04
      soccer W21.02
      soft ball W21.07
      specified NEC W21.09
      volleyball W21.06
    bat or racquet
      baseball bat W21.11
        assault Y08.02
      golf club W21.13
        assault Y08.09
      specified NEC W21.19
        assault Y08.09
      tennis racquet W21.12
        assault Y08.09
    hockey (ice)
      field
        puck W21.221
        stick W21.211
      puck W21.220
      stick W21.210
        assault Y08.01
    specified NEC W21.89
  other person(s) W50.0
    with
      blunt object W22.8
        intentional, homicide (attempt) Y00
      sports equipment W21.9
      undetermined whether accidental or
        intentional Y29
    fall W03
      due to ice or snow W00.0
  as, or caused by, a crowd or human
    stampede (with fall) W52
    assault Y04.2
    homicide (attempt) Y04.2
  in legal intervention
    injuring
      bystander Y35.812
      law enforcement personnel Y35.811
      suspect Y35.813
    sports equipment W21.9
  police (on duty) -*see* Legal, intervention,
    manhandling
    with blunt object -*see* Legal, intervention,
      blunt object
  sports equipment W21.9
    assault Y08.09
    ball W21.00
      baseball W21.03
      basketball W21.05
      football W21.01
      golf ball W21.04
      soccer W21.02
      soft ball W21.07
      specified NEC W21.09
      volleyball W21.06
    bat or racquet
      baseball bat W21.11
        assault Y08.02
      golf club W21.13
        assault Y08.09
      specified NEC W21.19
      tennis racquet W21.12
        assault Y08.09

Struck (accidentally) -- *continued*
  cleats (shoe) W21.31
  foot wear NEC W21.39
  football helmet W21.81
  hockey (ice)
    field
      puck W21.221
      stick W21.211
    puck W21.220
    stick W21.210
      assault Y08.01
  skate blades W21.32
  specified NEC W21.89
    assault Y08.09
  thunderbolt -*see* subcategory T75.0
  causing fire -*see* Exposure, fire
  transport vehicle NEC -*see also* Accident,
    transport V09.9
  intentional, homicide (attempt) Y03.0
  motor NEC -*see also* Accident, transport
    V09.20
  homicide Y03.0
  vehicle (transport) NEC -*see* Accident,
    transport, by type of vehicle
  stationary (falling from jack, hydraulic lift,
    ramp) W20.8
Stumbling
  over
    animal NEC W01.0
      with fall W18.09
    carpet, rug or (small) object W22.8
      with fall W18.09
    person W51
      with fall W03
        due to ice or snow W00.0
  without fall W18.40
    due to
      specified NEC W18.49
      stepping from one level to another
        W18.43
      stepping into hole or opening W18.42
      stepping on object W18.41
Submersion (accidental) -*see* Drowning
**Suffocation (accidental) (by external
    means) (by pressure) (mechanical)** -*see
    also* category T71
  due to, by
    avalanche -*see* Landslide
    explosion -*see* Explosion
    fire -*see* Exposure, fire
    food, any type (aspiration) (ingestion)
      (inhalation) -*see* categories T17 and T18
    ignition -*see* Ignition
    landslide -*see* Landslide
    machine (ry) -*see* Contact, with, by type of
      machine
    vomitus (aspiration) (inhalation) T17.81
  in
    burning building X00.8
Suicide, suicidal (attempted) (by) X83.8
  blunt object X79
  burning, burns X76
    hot object X77.9
      fluid NEC X77.2
      household appliance X77.3
      specified NEC X77.8
      steam X77.0
      tap water X77.1
      vapors X77.0
  caustic substance -*see* Table of Drugs and
    Chemicals

Suicide, suicidal -- *continued*
  cold, extreme X83.2
  collision of motor vehicle with
    motor vehicle X82.0
    specified NEC X82.8
    train X82.1
    tree X82.2
  crashing of aircraft X83.0
  cut (any part of body) X78.9
  cutting or piercing instrument X78.9
    dagger X78.2
    glass X78.0
    knife X78.1
    specified NEC X78.8
    sword X78.2
  drowning (in) X71.9
    bathtub X71.0
    natural water X71.3
    specified NEC X71.8
    swimming pool X71.1
      following fall X71.2
  electrocution X83.1
  explosive(s) (material) X75
  fire, flames X76
  firearm X74.9
    airgun X74.01
    handgun X72
    hunting rifle X73.1
    larger X73.9
      specified NEC X73.8
    machine gun X73.2
    shotgun X73.0
    specified NEC X74.8
  hanging X83.8
  hot object -*see* Suicide, burning, hot object
  jumping
    before moving object X81.8
      motor vehicle X81.0
      subway train X81.1
      train X81.1
    from high place X80
  late effect of attempt -*see* X71 X83 with 7th
    character S
  lying before moving object, train, vehicle
    X81.8
  poisoning -*see* Table of Drugs and
    Chemicals
  puncture (any part of body) -*see* Suicide,
    cutting or piercing instrument
  scald -*see* Suicide, burning, hot object
  sequelae of attempt -*see* X71 X83 with 7th
    character S
  sharp object (any) -*see* Suicide, cutting or
    piercing instrument
  shooting -*see* Suicide, firearm
  specified means NEC X83.8
  stab (any part of body) -*see* Suicide, cutting
    or piercing instrument
  steam, hot vapors X77.0
  strangulation X83.8
  submersion -*see* Suicide, drowning
  suffocation X83.8
  wound NEC X83.8
Sunstroke X32
Supersonic waves (causing injury) W42.0
**Surgical procedure, complication of
    (delayed or as an abnormal reaction
    without mention of misadventure)** -*see
    also* Complication of or following, by
    type of procedure
  due to or as a result of misadventure -*see*
    Misadventure

Swallowed, swallowing
  foreign body *-see* Foreign body, alimentary
    canal
  poison *-see* Table of Drugs and Chemicals
  substance
    caustic or corrosive *-see* Table of Drugs
      and Chemicals
    poisonous *-see* Table of Drugs and
      Chemicals

T

Tackle in sport W03
Terrorism (involving) Y38.80
  biological weapons Y38.6X-
  chemical weapons Y38.7X-
  conflagration Y38.3X-
  drowning and submersion Y38.89
  explosion Y38.2X-
    destruction of aircraft Y38.1X
    marine weapons Y38.0X-
  fire Y38.3X-
  firearms Y38.4X-
  hot substances Y38.3X-
  lasers Y38.89
  nuclear weapons Y38.5X-
  piercing or stabbing instruments Y38.89
  secondary effects Y38.9X-
  specified method NEC Y38.89
  suicide bomber Y38.81
Thirst X58
Threat to breathing
  aspiration *-see* Aspiration
  due to cave-in, falling earth or substance
    NEC -see category T71
Thrown (accidentally)
  against part (any) of or object in transport
    vehicle (in motion) NEC *-see also*
    Accident, transport
  from
    high place, homicide (attempt) Y01
    machinery *-see* Contact, with, by type of
      machine
    transport vehicle NEC *-see also* Accident,
      transport V89.9
  off *-see* Thrown, from
Thunderbolt -see subcategory T75.0
  causing fire *-see* Exposure, fire
Tidal wave (any injury) NEC *-see* Forces of
    nature, tidal wave
Took
  overdose (drug) *-see* Table of Drugs and
    Chemicals
  poison *-see* Table of Drugs and Chemicals
Tornado (any injury) X37.1
Torrential rain (any injury) X37.8
Torture X58
Trampled by animal NEC W55.89
Trapped (accidentally)
  between objects (moving) (stationary and
    moving) *-see* Caught
  by part (any) of
    motorcycle V29.88
    pedal cycle V19.88
    transport vehicle NEC *-see also* Accident,
      transport V89.9
Travel (effects) (sickness) T75.3

Tree falling on or hitting (accidentally)
  (person) W20.8
Tripping
  over
    animal W01.0
      with fall W01.0
    carpet, rug or (small) object W22.8
      with fall W18.09
    person W51
      with fall W03
        due to ice or snow W00.0
    without fall W18.40
      due to
        specified NEC W18.49
        stepping from one level to another
          W18.43
        stepping into hole or opening W18.42
        stepping on object W18.41
Twisted by person(s) (accidentally) W50.2
  with intent to injure or kill Y04.0
  as, or caused by, a crowd or human
    stampede (with fall) W52
  assault Y04.0
  homicide (attempt) Y04.0
  in
    fight Y04.0
    legal intervention *-see* Legal, intervention,
      manhandling
Twisting (prolonged) (static) X50.1

U

Underdosing of necessary drugs,
  medicaments or biological substances
  Y63.6
Undetermined intent (contact) (exposure)
  automobile collision Y32
  blunt object Y29
  drowning (submersion) (in) Y21.9
    bathtub Y21.0
      after fall Y21.1
    natural water (lake) (ocean) (pond) (river)
      (stream) Y21.4
    specified place NEC Y21.8
    swimming pool Y21.2
      after fall Y21.3
  explosive material Y25
  fall, jump or push from high place Y30
  falling, lying or running before moving
    object Y31
  fire Y26
  firearm discharge Y24.9
    airgun (BB) (pellet) Y24.0
    handgun (pistol) (revolver) Y22
    hunting rifle Y23.1
    larger Y23.9
      hunting rifle Y23.1
      machine gun Y23.3
      military Y23.2
      shotgun Y23.0
      specified type NEC Y23.8
    machine gun Y23.3
    military Y23.2
    shotgun Y23.0
    specified type NEC Y24.8
    Very pistol Y24.8
  hot object Y27.9
    fluid NEC Y27.2
    household appliance Y27.3
    specified object NEC Y27.8

Undetermined intent -- *continued*
    steam Y27.0
    tap water Y27.1
    vapor Y27.0
  jump, fall or push from high place Y30
  lying, falling or running before moving
    object Y31
  motor vehicle crash Y32
  push, fall or jump from high place Y30
  running, falling or lying before moving
    object Y31
  sharp object Y28.9
    dagger Y28.2
    glass Y28.0
    knife Y28.1
    specified object NEC Y28.8
    sword Y28.2
  smoke Y26
  specified event NEC Y33
Use of hand as hammer X50.3

V

Vibration (causing injury) W49.9
Victim (of)
  avalanche *-see* Landslide
  earth movements NEC *-see* Forces of nature,
    earth movement
  earthquake X34
  flood *-see* Flood
  landslide *-see* Landslide
  lightning -see subcategory T75.0
    causing fire *-see* Exposure, fire
  storm (cataclysmic) NEC *-see* Forces of
    nature, cataclysmic storm
  volcanic eruption X35
Volcanic eruption (any injury) X35
Vomitus, gastric contents in air passages
  (with asphyxia, obstruction or
  suffocation) T17.81

W

Walked into stationary object (any)
  W22.09
  furniture W22.03
  lamppost W22.02
  wall W22.01
War operations (injuries to military
  personnel and civilians during war,
  civil insurrection and peacekeeping
  missions) (by) (from) (involving)
  Y36.90
  after cessation of hostilities Y36.89
    explosion (of)
      bomb placed during war operations
        Y36.82
      mine placed during war operations
        Y36.81
      specified NEC Y36.88
    air blast Y36.20
    aircraft
      destruction *-see* War operations,
        destruction of aircraft
      airway restriction *-see* War operations,
        restriction of airways
      asphyxiation *-see* War operations, restriction
        of airways
    biological weapons Y36.6X-
    blast Y36.20

War operations -- *continued*

blast fragments Y36.20
blast wave Y36.20
blast wind Y36.20
bomb Y36.20
  dirty Y36.50
  gasoline Y36.31
  incendiary Y36.31
  petrol Y36.31
bullet Y36.43
  incendiary Y36.32
  rubber Y36.41
chemical weapons Y36.7X-
combat
  hand to hand (unarmed) combat Y36.44
  using blunt or piercing object Y36.45
conflagration -*see* War operations, fire
conventional warfare NEC Y36.49
depth-charge Y36.01
destruction of aircraft Y36.10
  due to
    air to air missile Y36.11
    collision with other aircraft Y36.12
    detonation (accidental) of onboard
    munitions and explosives Y36.14
    enemy fire or explosives Y36.11
    explosive placed on aircraft Y36.11
    onboard fire Y36.13
    rocket propelled grenade [RPG] Y36.11
    small arms fire Y36.11
    surface to air missile Y36.11
  specified NEC Y36.19
detonation (accidental) of
  onboard marine weapons Y36.05
  own munitions or munitions launch device
    Y36.24
dirty bomb Y36.50
explosion (of) Y36.20
  after cessation of hostilities
    bomb placed during war operations
    Y36.82
    mine placed during war operations
    Y36.81
  aerial bomb Y36.21
  bomb NOS -*see also* War operations,
    bomb(s) Y36.20
  own munitions or munitions launch device
    (accidental) Y36.24
  fragments Y36.20
  grenade Y36.29
  guided missile Y36.22
  improvised explosive device [IED]
    (person-borne) (roadside) (vehicle-borne)
    Y36.23
  land mine Y36.29
  marine mine (at sea) (in harbor) Y36.02
  marine weapon Y36.00
    specified NEC Y36.09
  sea-based artillery shell Y36.03
  specified NEC Y36.29
  torpedo Y36.04
fire Y36.30
  specified NEC Y36.39
firearms
  discharge Y36.43
  pellets Y36.42
flamethrower Y36.33
fragments (from) (of)
  improvised explosive device [IED]
    (person-borne) (roadside) (vehicle-borne)
    Y36.26

War operations -- *continued*

  munitions Y36.25
  specified NEC Y36.29
  weapons Y36.27
friendly fire Y36.92
hand to hand (unarmed) combat Y36.44
hot substances -*see* War operations, fire
incendiary bullet Y36.32
nuclear weapon (effects of) Y36.50
  acute radiation exposure Y36.54
  blast pressure Y36.51
  direct blast Y36.51
  direct heat Y36.53
  fallout exposure Y36.54
  fireball Y36.53
  indirect blast (struck or crushed by blast
    debris) (being thrown by blast) Y36.52
  ionizing radiation (immediate exposure)
    Y36.54
  nuclear radiation Y36.54
  radiation
    ionizing (immediate exposure) Y36.54
    nuclear Y36.54
    thermal Y36.53
  specified NEC Y36.59
  secondary effects Y36.54
  thermal radiation Y36.53
restriction of air (airway)   intentional
    Y36.46
  unintentional Y36.47
rubber bullets Y36.41
shrapnel NOS Y36.29
suffocation -*see* War operations, restriction
  of airways
unconventional warfare NEC Y36.7X-
underwater blast NOS Y36.00
warfare
  conventional NEC Y36.49
  unconventional NEC Y36.7X-
weapons
  biological weapons Y36.6X-
  chemical Y36.7X-
  nuclear (effects of) Y36.50
    acute radiation exposure Y36.54
    blast pressure Y36.51
    direct blast Y36.51
    direct heat Y36.53
    fallout exposure Y36.54
    fireball Y36.53
    indirect blast (struck or crushed by blast
    debris) (being thrown by blast) Y36.52
    radiation
      ionizing (immediate exposure) Y36.54
      nuclear Y36.54
      thermal Y36.53
    secondary effects Y36.54
    specified NEC Y36.59
  of mass destruction [WMD] Y36.91
  weapon of mass destruction [WMD] Y36.91

Washed
  away by flood -*see* Flood
  off road by storm (transport vehicle) -*see*
    Forces of nature, cataclysmic storm
Weather exposure NEC -*see* Forces of
  nature
Weightlessness (causing injury) (effects of)
  (in spacecraft, real or simulated) X52
Work related condition Y99.0
Wound (accidental) NEC -*see also* Injury
  X58
  battle -*see also* War operations Y36.90
  gunshot -*see* Discharge, firearm by type

Wreck transport vehicle NEC -*see also*
  Accident, transport V89.9
Wrong
  device implanted into correct surgical site
    Y65.51
  fluid in infusion Y65.1
  procedure (operation) on correct patient
    Y65.51
  patient, procedure performed on Y65.52

List Of Three Digit Categories

CHAPTER 1: CERTAIN INFECTIOUS AND PARASITIC DISEASES (A00-B99)

A00 Cholera

A01 Typhoid and paratyphoid fevers

A02 Other salmonella infections

A03 Shigellosis

A04 Other bacterial intestinal infections

A05 Other bacterial foodborne intoxications, not elsewhere classified

A06 Amebiasis

A07 Other protozoal intestinal diseases

A08 Viral and other specified intestinal infections

A09 Infectious gastroenteritis and colitis unspecified

A15 Respiratory tuberculosis

A17 Tuberculosis of nervous system

A18 Tuberculosis of other organs

A19 Miliary tuberculosis

A20 Plague

A21 Tularemia

A22 Anthrax

A23 Brucellosis

A24 Glanders and melioidosis

A25 Rat-bite fever

A26 Erysipeloid

A27 Leptospirosis

A28 Other zoonotic bacterial diseases, not elsewhere classified

A30 Leprosy (Hansen's disease)

A31 Infection due to other mycobacteria

A32 Listeriosis

A33 Tetanus neonatorum

A34 Obstetrical tetanus

A35 Other tetanus

A36 Diphtheria

A37 Whooping cough

A38 Scarlet fever

A39 Meningococcal infection

A40 Streptococcal sepsis

A41 Other sepsis

A42 Actinomycosis

A43 Nocardiosis

A44 Bartonellosis

A46 Erysipelas

A48 Other bacterial diseases, not elsewhere classified

A49 Staphylococcal infection of unspecified site

A50 Congenital syphilis

A51 Early syphilis

A52 Late syphilis

A53 Other and unspecified syphilis

A54 Gonococcal infection

A55 Chlamydial lymphogranuloma (venereum)

A56 Other sexually transmitted chlamydial diseases

A57 Chancroid

A58 Granuloma inguinale

A59 Trichomoniasis

A60 Anogenital herpesviral [herpes simplex] infections

A63 Other predominantly sexually transmitted diseases, not elsewhere classified

A64 Unspecified sexually transmitted disease

A65 Nonvenereal syphilis

A66 Yaws

A67 Pinta [carate]

A68 Relapsing fevers

A69 Other spirochetal infections

A70 Chlamydia psittaci infections

A71 Trachoma

A74 Other diseases caused by chlamydiae

A75 Typhus fever

A77 Spotted fever [tick-borne rickettsioses]

A78 Q fever

A79 Other rickettsioses

A80 Acute poliomyelitis

A81 Atypical virus infections of central nervous system

A82 Rabies

A83 Mosquito-borne viral encephalitis

A84 Tick-borne viral encephalitis

A85 Other viral encephalitis, not elsewhere classified

A86 Unspecified viral encephalitis

A87 Viral meningitis

A88 Other viral infections of central nervous system, not elsewhere classified

A89 Unspecified viral infection of central nervous system

A90 Dengue fever [classical dengue]

A91 Dengue hemorrhagic fever

A92 Other mosquito-borne viral fevers

A93 Other arthropod-borne viral fevers, not elsewhere classified

A94 Unspecified arthropod-borne viral fever

A95 Yellow fever

A96 Arenaviral hemorrhagic fever

A98 Other viral hemorrhagic fevers, not elsewhere classified

A99 Unspecified viral hemorrhagic fever

B00 Herpesviral [herpes simplex] infections

B01 Varicella [chickenpox]

B02 Zoster [herpes zoster]

B03 Smallpox

B04 Monkeypox

B05 Measles

B06 Rubella [German measles]

B07 Viral warts

B08 Cowpox

B09 Other human herpesviruses

B10 Other human herpesviruses

B15 Acute hepatitis A

B16 Acute hepatitis B

B17 Other acute viral hepatitis

B18 Chronic viral hepatitis

B19 Unspecified viral hepatitis

B20 Human immunodeficiency virus [HIV] disease

B25 Cytomegaloviral disease

B26 Mumps

B27 Infectious mononucleosis

B30 Viral conjunctivitis

B33 Other viral diseases, not elsewhere classified

B34 Viral infection of unspecified site

B35 Dermatophytosis

B36 Other superficial mycoses

B37 Candidiasis

B38 Coccidioidomycosis

B39 Histoplasmosis

B40 Blastomycosis

B41 Paracoccidioidomycosis

B42 Sporotrichosis

B43 Chromomycosis and pheomycotic abscess

B44 Aspergillosis

B45 Cryptococcosis

B46 Zygomycosis

B47 Mycetoma

B48 Other mycoses, not elsewhere classified

B49 Unspecified mycosis

B50 Plasmodium falciparum malaria

B51 Plasmodium vivax malaria

B52 Plasmodium malariae malaria

B53 Other specified malaria

B54 Unspecified malaria

B55 Leishmaniasis

B56 African trypanosomiasis

B57 Chagas' disease

B58 Toxoplasmosis

B59 Pneumocystosis

B60 Other protozoal diseases, not elsewhere classified

B64 Unspecified protozoal disease

B65 Schistosomiasis [bilharziasis]

B66 Other fluke infections

B67 Echinococcosis

B68 Taeniasis

B69	Cysticercosis	**C14**	Malignant neoplasm of other and ill-defined sites in the lip, oral cavity and pharynx	**C57**	Malignant neoplasm of other and unspecified female genital organs
B70	Diphyllobothriasis and sparganosis			**C58**	Malignant neoplasm of placenta
B71	Other cestode infections	**C15**	Malignant neoplasm of esophagus	**C60**	Malignant neoplasm of penis
B72	Dracunculiasis	**C16**	Malignant neoplasm of stomach	**C61**	Malignant neoplasm of prostate
B73	Onchocerciasis	**C17**	Malignant neoplasm of small intestine	**C62**	Malignant neoplasm of testis
B74	Filariasis	**C18**	Malignant neoplasm of colon	**C63**	Malignant neoplasm of other and unspecified male genital organs
B75	Trichinellosis	**C19**	Malignant neoplasm of rectosigmoid junction		
B76	Hookworm diseases			**C64**	Malignant neoplasm of kidney, except renal pelvis
B77	Ascariasis	**C20**	Malignant neoplasm of rectum		
B78	Strongyloidiasis	**C21**	Malignant neoplasm of anus and anal canal	**C65**	Malignant neoplasm of renal pelvis
B79	Trichuriasis			**C66**	Malignant neoplasm of ureter
B80	Enterobiasis	**C22**	Malignant neoplasm of liver and intrahepatic bile ducts	**C67**	Malignant neoplasm of bladder
B81	Other intestinal helminthiases, not elsewhere classified			**C68**	Malignant neoplasm of other and unspecified urinary organs
		C23	Malignant neoplasm of gallbladder		
B82	Unspecified intestinal parasitism	**C24**	Malignant neoplasm of other and unspecified parts of biliary tract	**C69**	Malignant neoplasm of eye and adnexa
B83	Other helminthiases			**C70**	Malignant neoplasm of meninges
B85	Pediculosis and phthiriasis	**C25**	Malignant neoplasm of pancreas	**C71**	Malignant neoplasm of brain
B86	Scabies	**C26**	Malignant neoplasm of other and ill-defined digestive organs	**C72**	Malignant neoplasm of spinal cord, cranial nerves and other parts of central nervous system
B87	Myiasis				
B88	Other infestations	**C30**	Malignant neoplasm of nasal cavity and middle ear		
B89	Unspecified parasitic disease			**C73**	Malignant neoplasm of thyroid gland
B90	Sequelae of tuberculosis	**C31**	Malignant neoplasm of accessory sinuses	**C74**	Malignant neoplasm of adrenal gland
B91	Sequelae of poliomyelitis			**C75**	Malignant neoplasm of other endocrine glands and related structures
B92	Sequelae of leprosy	**C32**	Malignant neoplasm of larynx		
B94	Sequelae of other and unspecified infectious and parasitic diseases	**C33**	Malignant neoplasm of trachea	**C76**	Malignant neoplasm of other and ill-defined sites
		C34	Malignant neoplasm of bronchus and lung		
B95	Streptococcus, Staphylococcus, and Enterococcus as the cause of diseases classified elsewhere	**C37**	Malignant neoplasm of thymus	**C77**	Secondary and unspecified malignant neoplasm of lymph nodes
		C38	Malignant neoplasm of heart, mediastinum and pleura	**C78**	Secondary malignant neoplasm of respiratory and digestive organs
B96	Other bacterial agents as the cause of diseases classified elsewhere	**C39**	Malignant neoplasm of other and ill-defined sites in the respiratory system and intrathoracic organs	**C79**	Secondary malignant neoplasm of other and unspecified sites
B97	Viral agents as the cause of diseases classified elsewhere			**C7A**	Malignant neuroendocrine tumors
		C40	Malignant neoplasm of bone and articular cartilage of limbs	**C7B**	Secondary neuroendocrine tumors
B99	Other and unspecified infectious diseases			**C80**	Malignant neoplasm without specification of site
		C41	Malignant neoplasm of bone and articular cartilage of other and unspecified sites		
				C81	Hodgkin lymphoma
CHAPTER 2: NEOPLASMS (C00-D49)				**C82**	Follicular lymphoma
		C43	Malignant melanoma of skin	**C83**	Non-follicular lymphoma
C00	Malignant neoplasm of lip	**C44**	Other and unspecified malignant neoplasm of skin	**C84**	Mature T/NK-cell lymphomas
C01	Malignant neoplasm of base of tongue			**C85**	Other specified and unspecified types of non-Hodgkin lymphoma
C02	Malignant neoplasm of other and unspecified parts of tongue	**C45**	Mesothelioma		
		C46	Kaposi's sarcoma	**C86**	Other specified types of T/NK-cell lymphoma
C03	Malignant neoplasm of gum	**C47**	Malignant neoplasm of peripheral nerves and autonomic nervous system		
C04	Malignant neoplasm of floor of mouth			**C88**	Malignant immunoproliferative diseases and certain other B-cell lymphomas
C05	Malignant neoplasm of palate	**C48**	Malignant neoplasm of retroperitoneum and peritoneum		
C06	Malignant neoplasm of other and unspecified parts of mouth			**C90**	Multiple myeloma and malignant plasma cell neoplasms
		C49	Malignant neoplasm of other connective and soft tissue		
C07	Malignant neoplasm of parotid gland			**C91**	Lymphoid leukemia
C08	Malignant neoplasm of other and unspecified major salivary glands	**C4A**	Merkel cell carcinoma	**C92**	Myeloid leukemia
		C50	Malignant neoplasm of breast	**C93**	Monocytic leukemia
C09	Malignant neoplasm of tonsil	**C52**	Malignant neoplasm of vagina	**C94**	Other leukemias of specified cell type
C10	Malignant neoplasm of oropharynx	**C53**	Malignant neoplasm of cervix uteri	**C95**	Leukemia of unspecified cell type
C11	Malignant neoplasm of nasopharynx	**C54**	Malignant neoplasm of corpus uteri	**C96**	Other and unspecified malignant neoplasms of lymphoid, hematopoietic and related tissue
C12	Malignant neoplasm of pyriform sinus	**C55**	Malignant neoplasm of uterus, part unspecified		
C13	Malignant neoplasm of hypopharynx	**C56**	Malignant neoplasm of ovary		

D00 Carcinoma in situ of oral cavity, esophagus and stomach

D01 Carcinoma in situ of other and unspecified digestive organs

D02 Carcinoma in situ of middle ear and respiratory system

D03 Melanoma in situ

D04 Carcinoma in situ of skin

D05 Carcinoma in situ of breast

D06 Carcinoma in situ of cervix uteri

D07 Carcinoma in situ of other and unspecified genital organs

D09 Carcinoma in situ of other and unspecified sites

D10 Benign neoplasm of mouth and pharynx

D11 Benign neoplasm of major salivary glands

D12 Benign neoplasm of colon, rectum, anus and anal canal

D13 Benign neoplasm of other and ill-defined parts of digestive system

D14 Benign neoplasm of middle ear and respiratory system

D15 Benign neoplasm of other and unspecified intrathoracic organs

D16 Benign neoplasm of bone and articular cartilage

D17 Benign lipomatous neoplasm

D18 Hemangioma and lymphangioma, any site

D19 Benign neoplasm of mesothelial tissue

D20 Benign neoplasm of soft tissue of retroperitoneum and peritoneum

D21 Other benign neoplasms of connective and other soft tissue

D22 Melanocytic nevi

D23 Other benign neoplasms of skin

D24 Benign neoplasm of breast

D25 Leiomyoma of uterus

D26 Other benign neoplasms of uterus

D27 Benign neoplasm of ovary

D28 Benign neoplasm of other and unspecified female genital organs

D29 Benign neoplasm of male genital organs

D30 Benign neoplasm of urinary organs

D31 Benign neoplasm of eye and adnexa

D32 Benign neoplasm of meninges

D33 Benign neoplasm of brain and other parts of central nervous system

D34 Benign neoplasm of thyroid gland

D35 Benign neoplasm of other and unspecified endocrine glands

D36 Benign neoplasm of other and unspecified sites

D37 Neoplasm of uncertain behavior of oral cavity and digestive organs

D38 Neoplasm of uncertain behavior of middle ear and respiratory and intrathoracic organs

D39 Neoplasm of uncertain behavior of female genital organs

D3A Benign carcinoid tumor of unspecified site

D40 Neoplasm of uncertain behavior of male genital organs

D41 Neoplasm of uncertain behavior of urinary organs

D42 Neoplasm of uncertain behavior of meninges

D43 Neoplasm of uncertain behavior of brain and central nervous system

D44 Neoplasm of uncertain behavior of endocrine glands

D45 Polycythemia vera

D46 Myelodysplastic syndromes

D47 Other neoplasms of uncertain behavior of lymphoid, hematopoietic and related tissue

D48 Neoplasm of uncertain behavior of other and unspecified sites

D49 Neoplasms of unspecified behavior

CHAPTER 3: DISEASES OF THE BLOOD AND BLOOD-FORMING ORGANS AND CERTAIN DISORDERS INVOLVING THE IMMUNE MECHANISM (D50-D89)

D50 Iron deficiency anemia

D51 Vitamin B12 deficiency anemia

D52 Folate deficiency anemia

D53 Other nutritional anemias

D55 Anemia due to enzyme disorders

D56 Thalassemia

D57 Sickle-cell disorders

D58 Other hereditary hemolytic anemias

D59 Acquired hemolytic anemia

D60 Acquired pure red cell aplasia [erythroblastopenia]

D61 Other aplastic anemias and other bone marrow failure syndromes

D62 Acute posthemorrhagic anemia

D63 Anemia in chronic diseases classified elsewhere

D64 Other anemias

D65 Disseminated intravascular coagulation [defibrination syndrome]

D66 Hereditary factor VIII deficiency

D67 Hereditary factor IX deficiency

D68 Other coagulation defects

D69 Purpura and other hemorrhagic conditions

D70 Neutropenia

D71 Functional disorders of polymorphonuclear neutrophils

D72 Other disorders of white blood cells

D73 Diseases of spleen

D74 Methemoglobinemia

D75 Other and unspecified diseases of blood and blood-forming organs

D76 Other specified diseases with participation of lymphoreticular and reticulohistiocytic tissue

D77 Other disorders of blood and blood-forming organs in diseases classified elsewhere

D78 Intraoperative and postprocedural complications of the spleen

D80 Immunodeficiency with predominantly antibody defects

D81 Combined immunodeficiencies

D82 Immunodeficiency associated with other major defects

D83 Common variable immunodeficiency

D84 Other immunodeficiencies

D86 Sarcoidosis

D89 Other disorders involving the immune mechanism, not elsewhere classified

CHAPTER 4: ENDOCRINE, NUTRITIONAL AND METABOLIC DISEASES (E00-E89)

E00 Congenital iodine-deficiency syndrome

E01 Iodine-deficiency related thyroid disorders and allied conditions

E02 Subclinical iodine-deficiency hypothyroidism

E03 Other hypothyroidism

E04 Other nontoxic goiter

E05 Thyrotoxicosis [hyperthyroidism]

E06 Thyroiditis

E07 Other disorders of thyroid

E08 Diabetes mellitus due to underlying condition

E09 Drug or chemical induced diabetes mellitus

E10 Type 1 diabetes mellitus

E11 Type 2 diabetes mellitus

E13 Other specified diabetes mellitus

E15 Nondiabetic hypoglycemic coma

E16 Other disorders of pancreatic internal secretion

E20 Hypoparathyroidism

E21 Hyperparathyroidism and other disorders of parathyroid gland

E22 Hyperfunction of pituitary gland

E23 Hypofunction and other disorders of the pituitary gland

E24 Cushing's syndrome

E25 Adrenogenital disorders

E26 Hyperaldosteronism

E27 Other disorders of adrenal gland

E28 Ovarian dysfunction

E29 Testicular dysfunction

E30 Disorders of puberty, not elsewhere classified

E31 Polyglandular dysfunction

E32 Diseases of thymus

E34 Other endocrine disorders

E35 Disorders of endocrine glands in diseases classified elsewhere

E36 Intraoperative complications of endocrine system

E40 Kwashiorkor

E41 Nutritional marasmus

E42 Marasmic kwashiorkor

E43 Unspecified severe protein-calorie malnutrition

E44 Protein-calorie malnutrition of moderate and mild degree

E45 Retarded development following protein-calorie malnutrition

E46 Unspecified protein-calorie malnutrition

E50 Vitamin A deficiency

E51 Thiamine deficiency

E52 Niacin deficiency [pellagra]

E53 Deficiency of other B group vitamins

E54 Ascorbic acid deficiency

E55 Vitamin D deficiency

E56 Other vitamin deficiencies

E58 Dietary calcium deficiency

E59 Dietary selenium deficiency

E60 Dietary zinc deficiency

E61 Deficiency of other nutrient elements

E63 Other nutritional deficiencies

E64 Sequelae of malnutrition and other nutritional deficiencies

E65 Localized adiposity

E66 Overweight and obesity

E67 Other hyperalimentation

E68 Sequelae of hyperalimentation

E70 Disorders of aromatic amino-acid metabolism

E71 Disorders of branched-chain amino-acid metabolism and fatty-acid metabolism

E72 Other disorders of amino-acid metabolism

E73 Lactose intolerance

E74 Other disorders of carbohydrate metabolism

E75 Disorders of sphingolipid metabolism and other lipid storage disorders

E76 Disorders of glycosaminoglycan metabolism

E77 Disorders of glycoprotein metabolism

E78 Disorders of lipoprotein metabolism and other lipidemias

E79 Disorders of purine and pyrimidine metabolism

E80 Disorders of porphyrin and bilirubin metabolism

E83 Disorders of mineral metabolism

E84 Cystic fibrosis

E85 Amyloidosis

E86 Volume depletion

E87 Other disorders of fluid, electrolyte and acid-base balance

E88 Other and unspecified metabolic disorders

E89 Postprocedural endocrine and metabolic complications and disorders, not elsewhere classified

CHAPTER 5: MENTAL, BEHAVIORAL AND NEURODEVELOPMENTAL DISORDERS (F01-F99)

F01 Vascular dementia

F02 Dementia in other diseases classified elsewhere

F03 Unspecified dementia

F04 Amnestic disorder due to known physiological condition

F05 Delirium due to known physiological condition

F06 Unspecified dementia

F07 Other mental disorders due to known physiological condition

F09 Personality and behavioral disorders due to known physiological condition

F10 Alcohol related disorders

F11 Opioid related disorders

F12 Cannabis related disorders

F13 Sedative, hypnotic, or anxiolytic related disorders

F14 Cocaine related disorders

F15 Other stimulant related disorders

F16 Hallucinogen related disorders

F17 Nicotine dependence

F18 Inhalant related disorders

F19 Other psychoactive substance related disorders

F21 Schizotypal disorder

F22 Delusional disorders

F23 Brief psychotic disorder

F24 Shared psychotic disorder

F25 Schizoaffective disorders

F28 Other psychotic disorder not due to a substance or known physiological condition

F29 Unspecified psychosis not due to a substance or known physiological condition

F30 Manic episode

F31 Bipolar disorder

F32 Major depressive disorder, single episode

F33 Major depressive disorder, recurrent

F34 Persistent mood [affective] disorders

F39 Unspecified mood [affective] disorder

F40 Phobic anxiety disorders

F41 Other anxiety disorders

F42 Obsessive-compulsive disorder

F43 Reaction to severe stress, and adjustment disorders

F44 Dissociative and conversion disorders

F45 Somatoform disorders

F48 Other nonpsychotic mental disorders

F50 Eating disorders

F51 Sleep disorders not due to a substance or known physiological condition

F52 Sexual dysfunction not due to a substance or known physiological condition

F53 Puerperal psychosis

F54 Psychological and behavioral factors associated with disorders or diseases classified elsewhere

F55 Abuse of non-psychoactive substances

F59 Unspecified behavioral syndromes associated with physiological disturbances and physical factors

F60 Specific personality disorders

F63 Impulse disorders

F64 Gender identity disorders

F65 Paraphilias

F66 Other sexual disorders

F68 Other disorders of adult personality and behavior

F69 Unspecified disorder of adult personality and behavior

F70 Mild intellectual disabilities

F71 Moderate mental retardation

F72 Severe intellectual disabilities

F73 Profound intellectual disabilities

F78 Other intellectual disabilities

F79 Unspecified intellectual disabilities

F80 Specific developmental disorders of speech and language

F81 Specific developmental disorders of scholastic skills

F82 Specific developmental disorder of motor function

F84 Pervasive developmental disorders

F88 Other disorders of psychological development

F89 Unspecified disorder of psychological development

F90 Attention-deficit hyperactivity disorders

F91 Conduct disorders

F93 Emotional disorders with onset specific to childhood

F94 Disorders of social functioning with onset specific to childhood and adolescence

F95 Tic disorder

F98 Other behavioral and emotional disorders with onset usually occurring in childhood and adolescence

F99 Mental disorder not otherwise specified

CHAPTER 6: DISEASES OF THE NERVOUS SYSTEM (G00-G99)

G00 Bacterial meningitis, not elsewhere classified

G01 Meningitis in bacterial diseases classified elsewhere

G02 Meningitis in other infectious and parasitic diseases classified elsewhere

G03 Meningitis due to other and unspecified causes

G04 Encephalitis, myelitis and encephalomyelitis

G05 Encephalitis, myelitis and encephalomyelitis in diseases classified elsewhere

G06 Intracranial and intraspinal abscess and granuloma

G07 Intracranial and intraspinal abscess and granuloma in diseases classified elsewhere

G08 Intracranial and intraspinal phlebitis and thrombophlebitis

G09 Sequelae of inflammatory diseases of central nervous system

G10 Huntington's disease

G11 Hereditary ataxia

G12 Spinal muscular atrophy and related syndromes

G13 Systemic atrophies primarily affecting central nervous system in diseases classified elsewhere

G14 Postpolio syndrome

G20 Parkinson's disease

G21 Secondary parkinsonism

G23 Other degenerative diseases of basal ganglia

G24 Dystonia

G25 Other extrapyramidal and movement disorders

G26 Extrapyramidal and movement disorders in diseases classified elsewhere

G30 Alzheimer's disease

G31 Other degenerative diseases of nervous system, not elsewhere classified

G32 Other degenerative disorders of nervous system in diseases classified elsewhere

G35 Multiple sclerosis

G36 Other acute disseminated demyelination

G37 Other demyelinating diseases of central nervous system

G40 Epilepsy and recurrent seizures

G43 Migraine

G44 Other headache syndromes

G45 Transient cerebral ischemic attacks and related syndromes

G46 Vascular syndromes of brain in cerebrovascular diseases

G47 Sleep disorders

G50 Disorders of trigeminal nerve

G51 Facial nerve disorders

G52 Disorders of other cranial nerves

G53 Cranial nerve disorders in diseases classified elsewhere

G54 Nerve root and plexus disorders

G55 Mononeuropathies of upper limb

G56 Mononeuropathies of lower limb

G57 Mononeuropathy in diseases classified elsewhere

G58 Other mononeuropathies

G59 Hereditary and idiopathic neuropathy

G60 Disorders of trigeminal nerve

G61 Inflammatory polyneuropathy

G62 Other and unspecified polyneuropathies

G63 Polyneuropathy in diseases classified elsewhere

G64 Other disorders of peripheral nervous system

G65 Sequelae of inflammatory and toxic polyneuropathies

G70 Myasthenia gravis and other myoneural disorders

G71 Primary disorders of muscles

G72 Other and unspecified myopathies

G73 Malignant neoplasm of thyroid gland

G80 Cerebral palsy

G81 Hemiplegia and hemiparesis

G82 Paraplegia (paraparesis) and quadriplegia (quadriparesis)

G83 Other paralytic syndromes

G89 Pain, not elsewhere classified

G90 Disorders of autonomic nervous system

G91 Hydrocephalus

G92 Toxic encephalopathy

G93 Other disorders of brain

G94 Other disorders of brain in diseases classified elsewhere

G95 Other and unspecified diseases of spinal cord

G96 Other disorders of central nervous system

G97 Intraoperative and postprocedural complications and disorders of nervous system, not elsewhere classified

G98 Other disorders of nervous system not elsewhere classified

G99 Other disorders of nervous system in diseases classified elsewhere

CHAPTER 7: DISEASES OF THE EYE AND ADNEXA (H00-H59)

H00 Hordeolum and chalazion

H01 Other inflammation of eyelid

H02 Other disorders of eyelid

H04 Disorders of lacrimal system

H05 Disorders of orbit

H10 Conjunctivitis

H11 Other disorders of conjunctiva

H15 Disorders of sclera

H16 Keratitis

H17 Corneal scars and opacities

H18 Other disorders of cornea

H20 Iridocyclitis

H21 Other disorders of iris and ciliary body

H22 Disorders of iris and ciliary body in diseases classified elsewhere

H25 Age-related cataract

H26 Other cataract

H27 Other disorders of lens

H28 Cataract in diseases classified elsewhere

H30 Chorioretinal inflammation

H31 Other disorders of choroid

H32 Chorioretinal disorders in diseases classified elsewhere

H33 Retinal detachments and breaks

H34 Retinal vascular occlusions

H35 Other retinal disorders

H36 Retinal disorders in diseases classified elsewhere

H40 Glaucoma

H42 Glaucoma in diseases classified elsewhere

H43 Disorders of vitreous body

H44 Disorders of globe

H46 Optic neuritis

H47 Other disorders of optic [2nd] nerve and visual pathways

H49 Paralytic strabismus

H50 Other strabismus

H51 Other disorders of binocular movement

H52 Disorders of refraction and accommodation

H53 Visual disturbances

H54 Blindness and low vision

H55 Nystagmus and other irregular eye movements

H57 Other disorders of eye and adnexa

H59 Intraoperative and postprocedural complications and disorders of eye and adnexa, not elsewhere classified

CHAPTER 8: DISEASES OF THE EAR AND MASTOID PROCESS (H60-H95)

H60 Otitis externa

H61 Other disorders of external ear

H62 Disorders of external ear in diseases classified elsewhere

H65 Nonsuppurative otitis media

H66 Suppurative and unspecified otitis media

H67 Otitis media in diseases classified elsewhere

H68 Eustachian salpingitis and obstruction

H69 Other and unspecified disorders of Eustachian tube

H70 Mastoiditis and related conditions

H71 Cholesteatoma of middle ear

H72 Perforation of tympanic membrane

H73 Other disorders of tympanic membrane

H74 Other disorders of middle ear mastoid

H75 Other disorders of middle ear and mastoid in diseases classified elsewhere

H80 Otosclerosis

H81 Disorders of vestibular function

H82 Vertiginous syndromes in diseases classified elsewhere

H83 Other diseases of inner ear

H90 Conductive and sensorineural hearing loss

H91 Other and unspecified hearing loss

H92 Otalgia and effusion of ear

H93 Other disorders of ear, not elsewhere classified

H94 Other disorders of ear in diseases classified elsewhere

H95 Intraoperative and postprocedural complications and disorders of ear and mastoid process, not elsewhere classified

CHAPTER 9: DISEASES OF THE CIRCULATORY SYSTEM (I00-I99)

I00 Rheumatic fever without heart involvement

I01 Rheumatic fever with heart involvement

I02 Rheumatic chorea

I05 Rheumatic mitral valve diseases

I06 Rheumatic aortic valve diseases

I07 Rheumatic tricuspid valve diseases

I08 Multiple valve diseases

I09 Other rheumatic heart diseases

I10 Essential (primary) hypertension

I11 Hypertensive heart disease

I12 Hypertensive chronic kidney disease

I13 Hypertensive heart and chronic kidney disease

I15 Secondary hypertension

I16 Hypertensive crisis

I20 Angina pectoris

I21 ST elevation (STEMI) and non-ST elevation (NSTEMI) myocardial infarction

I22 Subsequent ST elevation (STEMI) and non-ST elevation (NSTEMI) myocardial infarction

I23 Certain current complications following ST elevation (STEMI) and non-ST

elevation (NSTEMI) myocardial infarction (within the 28 day period)

I24 Other acute ischemic heart diseases

I25 Chronic ischemic heart disease

I26 Pulmonary embolism

I27 Other pulmonary heart diseases

I28 Other diseases of pulmonary vessels

I30 Acute pericarditis

I31 Other diseases of pericardium

I32 Pericarditis in diseases classified elsewhere

I33 Acute and subacute endocarditis

I34 Nonrheumatic mitral valve disorders

I35 Nonrheumatic aortic valve disorders

I36 Nonrheumatic tricuspid valve disorders

I37 Nonrheumatic pulmonary valve disorders

I38 Endocarditis, valve unspecified

I39 Endocarditis and heart valve disorders in diseases classified elsewhere

I40 Acute myocarditis

I41 Myocarditis in diseases classified elsewhere

I42 Cardiomyopathy

I43 Cardiomyopathy in diseases classified elsewhere

I44 Atrioventricular and left bundle-branch block

I45 Other conduction disorders

I46 Cardiac arrest

I47 Paroxysmal tachycardia

I48 Atrial fibrillation and flutter

I49 Other cardiac arrhythmias

I50 Heart failure

I51 Complications and ill-defined descriptions of heart disease

I52 Other heart disorders in diseases classified elsewhere

I60 Nontraumatic subarachnoid hemorrhage

I61 Nontraumatic intracerebral hemorrhage

I62 Other and unspecified nontraumatic intracranial hemorrhage

I63 Cerebral infarction

I65 Occlusion and stenosis of precerebral arteries, not resulting in cerebral infarction

I66 Occlusion and stenosis of cerebral arteries, not resulting in cerebral infarction

I67 Other cerebrovascular diseases

I68 Cerebrovascular disorders in diseases classified elsewhere

I69 Sequelae of cerebrovascular disease

I70 Atherosclerosis

I71 Aortic aneurysm and dissection

I72 Other aneurysm

I73 Other peripheral vascular diseases

I74 Arterial embolism and thrombosis

I75 Atheroembolism

I76 Other disorders of arteries and arterioles

I77 Diseases of capillaries

I78 Disorders of arteries, arterioles and capillaries in diseases classified elsewhere

I79 Disorders of arteries, arterioles and capillaries in diseases classified elsewhere

I80 Phlebitis and thrombophlebitis

I81 Portal vein thrombosis

I82 Other venous embolism and thrombosis

I83 Varicose veins of lower extremities

I84 Unspecified thrombosed hemorrhoids

I85 Esophageal varices

I86 Varicose veins of other sites

I87 Other disorders of veins

I88 Nonspecific lymphadenitis

I89 Other noninfective disorders of lymphatic vessels and lymph nodes

I95 Hypotension

I96 Gangrene, not elsewhere classified

I97 Intraoperative and postprocedural complications and disorders of circulatory system, not elsewhere classified

I99 Other and unspecified disorders of circulatory system

CHAPTER 10: DISEASES OF THE RESPIRATORY SYSTEM (J00-J99)

J00 Acute nasopharyngitis [common cold]

J01 Acute sinusitis

J02 Acute nasopharyngitis [common cold]

J03 Acute tonsillitis

J04 Acute laryngitis and tracheitis

J05 Acute obstructive laryngitis [croup] and epiglottitis

J06 Acute upper respiratory infections of multiple and unspecified sites

J09 Influenza due to certain identified influenza viruses

J10 Influenza due to other identified influenza virus

J12 Viral pneumonia, not elsewhere classified

J13 Pneumonia due to Streptococcus pneumoniae

J14 Pneumonia due to Hemophilus influenzae

J15 Bacterial pneumonia, not elsewhere classified

J16 Pneumonia due to other infectious organisms, not elsewhere classified

J17 Pneumonia in diseases classified elsewhere

J18 Pneumonia, unspecified organism

J20	Acute bronchitis
J21	Acute bronchiolitis
J22	Unspecified acute lower respiratory infection
J30	Vasomotor and allergic rhinitis
J31	Chronic rhinitis, nasopharyngitis and pharyngitis
J32	Chronic sinusitis
J33	Nasal polyp
J34	Other and unspecified disorders of nose and nasal sinuses
J35	Chronic diseases of tonsils and adenoids
J36	Peritonsillar abscess
J37	Chronic laryngitis and laryngotracheitis
J38	Diseases of vocal cords and larynx, not elsewhere classified
J39	Other diseases of upper respiratory tract
J40	Bronchitis, not specified as acute or chronic
J41	Simple and mucopurulent chronic bronchitis
J42	Unspecified chronic bronchitis
J43	Emphysema
J44	Other chronic obstructive pulmonary disease
J45	Asthma
J47	Bronchiectasis
J60	Coalworker's pneumoconiosis
J61	Pneumoconiosis due to asbestos and other mineral fibers
J62	Pneumoconiosis due to dust containing silica
J63	Pneumoconiosis due to other inorganic dusts
J64	Unspecified pneumoconiosis
J65	Pneumoconiosis associated with tuberculosis
J66	Airway disease due to specific organic dust
J67	Hypersensitivity pneumonitis due to organic dust
J68	Respiratory conditions due to inhalation of chemicals, gases, fumes and vapors
J69	Pneumonitis due to solids and liquids
J70	Respiratory conditions due to other external agents
J80	Acute respiratory distress syndrome
J81	Pulmonary edema
J82	Pulmonary eosinophilia, not elsewhere classified
J84	Other interstitial pulmonary diseases
J85	Abscess of lung and mediastinum
J86	Pyothorax
J90	Pleural effusion, not elsewhere classified
J91	Pleural effusion in conditions classified elsewhere
J92	Pleural plaque

J93	Pneumothorax and air leak
J94	Other pleural conditions
J95	Intraoperative and postprocedural complications and disorders of respiratory system, not elsewhere classified
J96	Respiratory failure, not elsewhere classified
J98	Other respiratory disorders
J99	Respiratory disorders in diseases classified elsewhere

CHAPTER 11: DISEASES OF THE DIGESTIVE SYSTEM (K00-K95)

K00	Disorders of tooth development and eruption
K01	Embedded and impacted teeth
K02	Dental caries
K03	Other diseases of hard tissues of teeth
K04	Diseases of pulp and periapical tissues
K05	Gingivitis and periodontal diseases
K06	Other disorders of gingiva and edentulous alveolar ridge
K08	Other disorders of teeth and supporting structures
K09	Cysts of oral region, not elsewhere classified
K11	Diseases of salivary glands
K12	Stomatitis and related lesions
K13	Other diseases of lip and oral mucosa
K14	Diseases of tongue
K20	Esophagitis
K21	Gastro-esophageal reflux disease
K22	Other diseases of esophagus
K23	Disorders of esophagus in diseases classified elsewhere
K25	Gastric ulcer
K26	Duodenal ulcer
K27	Peptic ulcer, site unspecified
K28	Gastrojejunal ulcer
K29	Gastritis and duodenitis
K30	Functional dyspepsia
K31	Other diseases of stomach and duodenum
K35	Acute appendicitis
K36	Other appendicitis
K37	Unspecified appendicitis
K38	Other diseases of appendix
K40	Inguinal hernia
K41	Femoral hernia
K42	Umbilical hernia
K43	Ventral hernia
K44	Diaphragmatic hernia
K45	Other abdominal hernia
K46	Unspecified abdominal hernia

K50	Crohn's disease [regional enteritis]
K51	Ulcerative colitis
K52	Other and unspecified noninfective gastroenteritis and colitis
K55	Vascular disorders of intestine
K56	Paralytic ileus and intestinal obstruction without hernia
K57	Diverticular disease of intestine
K58	Irritable bowel syndrome
K59	Fissure and fistula of anal and rectal regions
K60	Abscess of anal and rectal regions
K61	Other diseases of anus and rectum
K62	Other diseases of intestine
K63	Hemorrhoids and perianal venous thrombosis
K65	Peritonitis
K66	Other disorders of peritoneum
K67	Disorders of peritoneum in infectious diseases classified elsewhere
K68	Disorders of retroperitoneum
K70	Alcoholic liver disease
K71	Toxic liver disease
K72	Hepatic failure, not elsewhere classified
K73	Chronic hepatitis, not elsewhere classified
K74	Fibrosis and cirrhosis of liver
K75	Other inflammatory liver diseases
K76	Other diseases of liver
K77	Liver disorders in diseases classified elsewhere
K80	Cholelithiasis
K81	Cholecystitis
K82	Other diseases of gallbladder
K83	Other diseases of biliary tract
K85	Acute pancreatitis
K86	Other diseases of pancreas
K87	Disorders of gallbladder biliary tract and pancreas in diseases classified elsewhere
K90	Intestinal malabsorption
K91	Intraoperative and postprocedural complications and disorders of digestive system, not elsewhere classified
K92	Other diseases of digestive system
K94	Complications of artificial openings of the digestive system
K95	Complications of bariatric procedures

CHAPTER 12: DISEASES OF THE SKIN AND SUBCUTANEOUS TISSUE (L00-L99)

L00	Staphylococcal scalded skin syndrome
L01	Impetigo
L02	Cutaneous abscess, furuncle and carbuncle
L03	Cellulitis and acute lymphangitis
L04	Acute lymphadenitis

L05 Pilonidal cyst and sinus

L08 Other local infections of skin and subcutaneous tissue

L08 Other specified local infections of the skin and subcutaneous tissue

L10 Pemphigus

L11 Other acantholytic disorders

L12 Pemphigoid

L13 Other bullous disorders

L14 Bullous disorders in diseases classified elsewhere

L20 Atopic dermatitis

L21 Seborrheic dermatitis

L22 Diaper dermatitis

L23 Allergic contact dermatitis

L24 Irritant contact dermatitis

L25 Unspecified contact dermatitis

L26 Exfoliative dermatitis

L27 Dermatitis due to substances taken internally

L28 Lichen simplex chronicus and prurigo

L29 Pruritus

L30 Other and unspecified dermatitis

L40 Psoriasis

L41 Parapsoriasis

L42 Pityriasis rosea

L43 Lichen planus

L44 Other papulosquamous disorders

L45 Papulosquamous disorders in diseases classified elsewhere

L49 Exfoliation due to erythematous conditions according to extent of body surface involved

L50 Urticaria

L51 Erythema multiforme

L52 Erythema nodosum

L53 Other erythematous conditions

L54 Erythema in diseases classified elsewhere

L55 Sunburn

L56 Other acute skin changes due to ultraviolet radiation

L57 Skin changes due to chronic exposure to nonionizing radiation

L58 Radiodermatitis

L59 Other disorders of skin and subcutaneous tissue related to radiation

L60 Nail disorders

L62 Nail disorders in diseases classified elsewhere

L63 Alopecia areata

L64 Androgenic alopecia

L65 Other nonscarring hair loss

L66 Cicatricial alopecia [scarring hair loss]

L67 Hair color and hair shaft abnormalities

L68 Hypertrichosis

L70 Acne

L71 Rosacea

L72 Follicular cysts of skin and subcutaneous tissue

L73 Other follicular disorders

L74 Eccrine sweat disorders

L75 Apocrine sweat disorders

L76 Intraoperative and postprocedural complications of skin and subcutaneous tissue

L80 Vitiligo

L81 Other disorders of pigmentation

L82 Seborrheic keratosis

L83 Acanthosis nigricans

L84 Corns and callosities

L85 Other epidermal thickening

L86 Keratoderma in diseases classified elsewhere

L87 Transepidermal elimination disorders

L88 Pyoderma gangrenosum

L89 Pressure ulcer

L90 Atrophic disorders of skin

L91 Hypertrophic disorders of skin

L92 Granulomatous disorders of skin and subcutaneous tissue

L93 Lupus erythematosus

L94 Other localized connective tissue disorders

L95 Vasculitis limited to skin, not elsewhere classified

L97 Non-pressure chronic ulcer of lower limb, not elsewhere classified

L98 Other disorders of skin and subcutaneous tissue, not elsewhere classified

L99 Other disorders of skin and subcutaneous tissue in diseases classified elsewhere

CHAPTER 13: DISEASES OF THE MUSCULOSKELETAL SYSTEM AND CONNECTIVE TISSUE (M00-M99)

M00 Pyogenic arthritis

M01 Direct infections of joint in infectious and parasitic diseases classified elsewhere

M02 Postinfective and reactive arthropathies

M04 Autoinflammatory syndromes

M05 Rheumatoid arthritis with rheumatoid factor

M06 Other rheumatoid arthritis

M07 Enteropathic arthropathies

M08 Juvenile arthritis

M10 Idiopathic gout unspecified site

M11 Other crystal arthropathies

M12 Other and unspecified arthropathy

M13 Other arthritis

M14 Arthropathies in other diseases classified elsewhere

M15 Polyosteoarthritis

M16 Osteoarthritis of hip

M17 Osteoarthritis of knee

M18 Osteoarthritis of first carpometacarpal joint

M19 Other and unspecified osteoarthritis

M1A Idiopathic chronic gout unspecified site without tophus (tophi)

M20 Acquired deformities of fingers and toes

M21 Other acquired deformities of limbs

M22 Disorder of patella

M23 Internal derangement of knee

M24 Other specific joint derangements

M25 Other joint disorder, not elsewhere classified

M26 Dentofacial anomalies [including malocclusion]

M27 Other diseases of jaws

M30 Polyarteritis nodosa and related conditions

M31 Other necrotizing vasculopathies

M32 Systemic lupus erythematosus (SLE)

M33 Dermatopolymyositis

M34 Systemic sclerosis [scleroderma]

M35 Other systemic involvement of connective tissue

M36 Systemic disorders of connective tissue in diseases classified elsewhere

M40 Kyphosis and lordosis

M41 Scoliosis

M42 Spinal osteochondrosis

M43 Other deforming dorsopathies

M45 Ankylosing spondylitis

M46 Other inflammatory spondylopathies

M47 Spondylosis

M48 Other spondylopathies

M49 Spondylopathies in diseases classified elsewhere

M50 Cervical disc disorders

M51 Thoracic, thoracolumbar, and lumbosacral intervertebral disc disorders

M53 Other and unspecified dorsopathies, not elsewhere classified

M54 Dorsalgia

M60 Myositis

M61 Calcification and ossification of muscle

M62 Other disorders of muscle

M63 Disorders of muscle in diseases classified elsewhere

M65 Synovitis and tenosynovitis

M66 Spontaneous rupture of synovium and tendon

M67 Other disorders of synovium and tendon

M70 Soft tissue disorders related to use, overuse and pressure

M71 Other bursopathies

M72 Fibroblastic disorders

M75 Shoulder lesions

M76 Enthesopathies, lower limb, excluding foot

M77 Other enthesopathies

M79 Other and unspecified soft tissue disorders, not elsewhere classified

M80 Osteoporosis with current pathological fracture

M81 Osteoporosis without current pathological fracture

M83 Puerperal osteomalacia

M84 Disorder of continuity of bone

M85 Other disorders of bone density and structure

M86 Osteomyelitis

M87 Osteonecrosis

M88 Osteitis deformans [Paget's disease of bone]

M89 Other disorders of bone

M90 Osteopathies in diseases classified elsewhere

M91 Juvenile osteochondrosis of hip and pelvis

M92 Other juvenile osteochondrosis

M93 Other osteochondropathies

M94 Other disorders of cartilage

M95 Other acquired deformities of musculoskeletal system and connective tissue

M96 Intraoperative and postprocedural complications and disorders of musculoskeletal system, not elsewhere classified

M97 Periprosthetic fracture around internal prosthetic joint

M99 Biomechanical lesions, not elsewhere classified

CHAPTER 14: DISEASES OF THE GENITOURINARY SYSTEM (N00-N99)

N00 Acute nephritic syndrome

N01 Rapidly progressive nephritic syndrome

N02 Recurrent and persistent hematuria

N03 Chronic nephritic syndrome

N04 Nephrotic syndrome

N05 Unspecified nephritic syndrome

N06 Isolated proteinuria with specified morphological lesion

N07 Hereditary nephropathy, not elsewhere classified

N08 Glomerular disorders in diseases classified elsewhere

N10 Acute tubulointerstitial nephritis

N11 Chronic tubulointerstitial nephritis

N12 Tubulo-interstitial nephritis not specified as acute or chronic

N13 Obstructive and reflux uropathy

N14 Drug- and heavy-metal-induced tubulointerstitial and tubular conditions

N15 Other renal tubulointerstitial diseases

N16 Renal tubulointerstitial disorders in diseases classified elsewhere

N17 Acute kidney failure

N18 Chronic kidney disease (CKD)

N19 Unspecified kidney failure

N20 Calculus of kidney and ureter

N21 Calculus of lower urinary tract

N22 Calculus of urinary tract in diseases classified elsewhere

N23 Unspecified renal colic

N25 Disorders resulting from impaired renal tubular function

N26 Unspecified contracted kidney

N27 Small kidney of unknown cause

N28 Other disorders of kidney and ureter, not elsewhere classified

N29 Other disorders of kidney and ureter in diseases classified elsewhere

N30 Cystitis

N31 Neuromuscular dysfunction of bladder, not elsewhere classified

N32 Other disorders of bladder

N34 Urethritis and urethral syndrome

N35 Urethral stricture

N36 Other disorders of urethra

N37 Urethral disorders in diseases classified elsewhere

N39 Other disorders of urinary system

N40 Enlarged prostate

N41 Inflammatory diseases of prostate

N42 Other and unspecified disorders of prostate

N43 Hydrocele and spermatocele

N44 Noninflammatory disorders of testis

N45 Orchitis and epididymitis

N46 Male infertility

N47 Disorders of prepuce

N48 Other disorders of penis

N49 Inflammatory disorders of male genital organs, not elsewhere classified

N50 Other and unspecified disorders of male genital organs

N51 Disorders of male genital organs in diseases classified elsewhere

N52 Male erectile dysfunction

N53 Other male sexual dysfunction

N60 Benign mammary dysplasia

N61 Inflammatory disorders of breast

N62 Hypertrophy of breast

N63 Unspecified lump in breast

N64 Other disorders of breast

N65 Deformity and disproportion of reconstructed breast

N70 Salpingitis and oophoritis

N71 Acute inflammatory disease of uterus

N72 Inflammatory disease of cervix uteri

N73 Other female pelvic inflammatory diseases

N74 Female pelvic inflammatory disorders in diseases classified elsewhere

N75 Diseases of Bartholin's gland

N76 Other inflammation of vagina and vulva

N77 Vulvovaginal ulceration and inflammation in diseases classified elsewhere

N80 Endometriosis

N81 Female genital prolapse

N82 Fistulae involving female genital tract

N83 Noninflammatory disorders of ovary, fallopian tube and broad ligament

N84 Polyp of female genital tract

N85 Other noninflammatory disorders of uterus, except cervix

N86 Erosion and ectropion of cervix uteri

N87 Dysplasia of cervix uteri

N88 Other noninflammatory disorders of cervix uteri

N89 Other noninflammatory disorders of vagina

N90 Other noninflammatory disorders of vulva and perineum

N91 Absent, scanty and rare menstruation

N92 Excessive, frequent and irregular menstruation

N93 Other abnormal uterine and vaginal bleeding

N94 Pain and other conditions associated with female genital organs and menstrual cycle

N95 Menopausal and other perimenopausal disorders

N96 Recurrent pregnancy loss

N97 Female infertility

N98 Complications associated with artificial fertilization

N99 Intraoperative and postprocedural complications and disorders of genitourinary system, not elsewhere classified

CHAPTER 15: PREGNANCY, CHILDBIRTH AND THE PUERPERIUM (O00-O9A)

O00 Ectopic pregnancy

O00 Anencephaly and similar malformations

O01 Hydatidiform mole

O02 Other abnormal products of conception

O03 Spontaneous abortion

O04	Complications following (induced) termination of pregnancy
O07	Failed attempted termination of pregnancy
O07	Other congenital malformations of nervous system
O08	Complications following ectopic and molar pregnancy
O09	Supervision of high risk pregnancy
O10	Pre-existing hypertension complicating pregnancy, childbirth and the puerperium
O11	Pre-existing hypertension with pre-eclampsia
O12	Gestational [pregnancy-induced] edema and proteinuria without hypertension
O13	Gestational [pregnancy-induced] hypertension without significant proteinuria
O14	Pre-eclampsia
O15	Eclampsia
O16	Unspecified maternal hypertension
O20	Hemorrhage in early pregnancy
O21	Excessive vomiting in pregnancy
O22	Venous complications and hemorrhoids in pregnancy
O23	Infections of genitourinary tract in pregnancy
O24	Diabetes mellitus in pregnancy, childbirth, and the puerperium
O25	Malnutrition in pregnancy, childbirth and the puerperium
O26	Maternal care for other conditions predominantly related to pregnancy
O28	Abnormal findings on antenatal screening of mother
O29	Complications of anesthesia during pregnancy
O30	Multiple gestation
O31	Complications specific to multiple gestation
O32	Maternal care for malpresentation of fetus
O33	Maternal care for disproportion
O34	Maternal care for abnormality of pelvic organs
O35	Maternal care for known or suspected fetal abnormality and damage
O36	Maternal care for other fetal problems
O40	Polyhydramnios
O41	Other disorders of amniotic fluid and membranes
O42	Premature rupture of membranes
O43	Placental disorders
O44	Placenta previa
O45	Premature separation of placenta [abruptio placentae]
O46	Antepartum hemorrhage, not elsewhere classified
O47	False labor

O48	Late pregnancy
O60	Preterm labor
O61	Failed induction of labor
O62	Abnormalities of forces of labor
O63	Long labor
O64	Obstructed labor due to malposition and malpresentation of fetus
O65	Obstructed labor due to maternal pelvic abnormality
O66	Other obstructed labor
O67	Labor and delivery complicated by intrapartum hemorrhage, not elsewhere classified
O68	Labor and delivery complicated by abnormality of fetal acid-base balance
O69	Labor and delivery complicated by umbilical cord complications
O70	Perineal laceration during delivery
O71	Other obstetric trauma
O72	Postpartum hemorrhage
O73	Retained placenta and membranes, without hemorrhage
O74	Complications of anesthesia during labor and delivery
O75	Other complications of labor and delivery, not elsewhere classified
O76	Abnormality in fetal heart rate and rhythm complicating labor and delivery
O77	Other fetal stress complicating labor and delivery
O80	Encounter for full-term uncomplicated delivery
O82	Encounter for cesarean delivery without indication
O85	Puerperal sepsis
O86	Other puerperal infections
O87	Venous complications and hemorrhoids in the puerperium
O88	Obstetric embolism
O89	Complications of anesthesia during the puerperium
O90	Complications of the puerperium, not elsewhere classified
O91	Infections of breast associated with pregnancy, the puerperium and lactation
O92	Other disorders of breast and disorders of lactation associated with pregnancy and the puerperium
O94	Sequelae of complication of pregnancy, childbirth, and the puerperium
O98	Maternal infectious and parasitic diseases classifiable elsewhere but complicating pregnancy, childbirth and the puerperium
O99	Other maternal diseases classifiable elsewhere but complicating pregnancy, childbirth and the puerperium
O9A	Maternal malignant neoplasms, traumatic injuries and abuse classifiable elsewhere but complicating pregnancy, childbirth and the puerperium

CHAPTER 16: CERTAIN CONDITIONS ORIGINATING IN THE PERINATAL PERIOD (P00-P96)

P00	Newborn (suspected to be) affected by maternal conditions that may be unrelated to present pregnancy
P01	Newborn (suspected to be) affected by maternal complications of pregnancy
P02	Newborn (suspected to be) affected by complications of placenta, cord and membranes
P03	Newborn (suspected to be) affected by other complications of labor and delivery
P04	Newborn (suspected to be) affected by noxious substances transmitted via placenta or breast milk
P05	Disorders of newborn related to slow fetal growth and fetal malnutrition
P07	Disorders of newborn related to short gestation and low birth weight, not elsewhere classified
P08	Disorders of newborn related to long gestation and high birth weight
P09	Abnormal findings on neonatal screening
P10	Intracranial laceration and hemorrhage due to birth injury
P11	Other birth injuries to central nervous system
P12	Birth injury to scalp
P13	Birth injury to skeleton
P14	Birth injury to peripheral nervous system
P15	Other birth injuries
P19	Metabolic acidemia in newborn
P22	Respiratory distress of newborn
P23	Congenital pneumonia
P24	Neonatal aspiration
P25	Interstitial emphysema and related conditions originating in the perinatal period
P26	Pulmonary hemorrhage originating in the perinatal period
P27	Chronic respiratory disease originating in the perinatal period
P28	Other respiratory conditions originating in the perinatal period
P29	Cardiovascular disorders originating in the perinatal period
P35	Congenital viral diseases
P36	Bacterial sepsis of newborn
P37	Other congenital infectious and parasitic diseases
P38	Omphalitis of newborn
P39	Other infections specific to the perinatal period
P50	Newborn affected by intrauterine (fetal) blood loss
P51	Umbilical hemorrhage of newborn

P52	Intracranial nontraumatic hemorrhage of newborn
P53	Hemorrhagic disease of newborn
P54	Other neonatal hemorrhages
P55	Hemolytic disease of newborn
P56	Hydrops fetalis due to hemolytic disease
P57	Kernicterus
P58	Neonatal jaundice due to other excessive hemolysis
P59	Neonatal jaundice from other and unspecified causes
P60	Disseminated intravascular coagulation of newborn
P61	Other perinatal hematological disorders
P70	Transitory disorders of carbohydrate metabolism specific to newborn
P71	Transitory neonatal disorders of calcium and magnesium metabolism
P72	Other transitory neonatal endocrine disorders
P74	Other transitory neonatal electrolyte and metabolic disturbances
P76	Other intestinal obstruction of newborn
P77	Necrotizing enterocolitis of newborn
P78	Other perinatal digestive system disorders
P80	Hypothermia of newborn
P81	Other disturbances of temperature regulation of newborn
P83	Other conditions of integument specific to newborn
P84	Other problems with newborn
P90	Convulsions of newborn
P91	Other disturbances of cerebral status of newborn
P92	Feeding problems of newborn
P93	Reactions and intoxications due to drugs administered to newborn
P94	Disorders of muscle tone of newborn
P95	Stillbirth
P96	Other conditions originating in the perinatal period

CHAPTER 17: CONGENITAL MALFORMATIONS, DEFORMATIONS AND CHROMOSOMAL ABNORMALITIES (Q00-Q99)

Q01	Encephalocele
Q02	Microcephaly
Q03	Congenital hydrocephalus
Q04	Other congenital malformations of brain
Q05	Spina bifida
Q06	Other congenital malformations of spinal cord
Q10	Congenital malformations of eyelid, lacrimal apparatus and orbit

Q11	Anophthalmos, microphthalmos and macrophthalmos
Q12	Congenital lens malformations
Q13	Congenital malformations of anterior segment of eye
Q14	Congenital malformations of posterior segment of eye
Q15	Other congenital malformations of eye
Q16	Congenital malformations of ear causing impairment of hearing
Q17	Other congenital malformations of ear
Q18	Other congenital malformations of face and neck
Q20	Congenital malformations of cardiac chambers and connections
Q21	Congenital malformations of cardiac septa
Q22	Congenital malformations of pulmonary and tricuspid valves
Q23	Congenital malformations of aortic and mitral valves
Q24	Other congenital malformations of heart
Q25	Congenital malformations of great arteries
Q26	Congenital malformations of great veins
Q27	Other congenital malformations of peripheral vascular system
Q28	Other congenital malformations of circulatory system
Q30	Congenital malformations of nose
Q31	Congenital malformations of larynx
Q32	Congenital malformations of trachea and bronchus
Q33	Congenital malformations of lung
Q34	Other congenital malformations of respiratory system
Q35	Cleft palate
Q36	Cleft lip
Q37	Cleft palate with cleft lip
Q38	Other congenital malformations of tongue, mouth and pharynx
Q39	Congenital malformations of esophagus
Q40	Other congenital malformations of upper alimentary tract
Q41	Congenital absence, atresia and stenosis of small intestine
Q42	Congenital absence, atresia and stenosis of large intestine
Q43	Other congenital malformations of intestine
Q44	Congenital malformations of gallbladder, bile ducts and liver
Q45	Other congenital malformations of digestive system
Q50	Congenital malformations of ovaries, fallopian tubes and broad ligaments
Q51	Congenital malformations of uterus and cervix

Q52	Other congenital malformations of female genitalia
Q53	Undescended and ectopic testicle
Q54	Hypospadias
Q55	Other congenital malformations of male genital organs
Q56	Indeterminate sex and pseudohermaphroditism
Q60	Renal agenesis and other reduction defects of kidney
Q61	Cystic kidney disease
Q62	Congenital obstructive defects of renal pelvis and congenital malformations of ureter
Q63	Other congenital malformations of kidney
Q64	Other congenital malformations of urinary system
Q65	Congenital deformities of hip
Q66	Congenital deformities of feet
Q67	Congenital musculoskeletal deformities of head, face, spine and chest
Q68	Other congenital musculoskeletal deformities
Q69	Polydactyly
Q70	Syndactyly
Q71	Reduction defects of upper limb
Q72	Reduction defects of lower limb
Q73	Reduction defects of unspecified limb
Q74	Other congenital malformations of limb(s)
Q75	Other congenital malformations of skull and face bones
Q76	Congenital malformations of spine and bony thorax
Q77	Osteochondrodysplasia with defects of growth of tubular bones and spine
Q78	Other osteochondrodysplasias
Q79	Congenital malformations of musculoskeletal system, not elsewhere classified
Q80	Congenital ichthyosis
Q81	Epidermolysis bullosa
Q82	Other congenital malformations of skin
Q83	Congenital malformations of breast
Q84	Other congenital malformations of integument
Q85	Phakomatoses, not elsewhere classified
Q86	Congenital malformation syndromes due to known exogenous causes, not elsewhere classified
Q87	Other specified congenital malformation syndromes affecting multiple systems
Q89	Other congenital malformations, not elsewhere classified
Q90	Down syndrome
Q91	Trisomy 18 and Trisomy 13
Q92	Other trisomies and partial trisomies of the autosomes, not elsewhere classified

Q93	Monosomies and deletions from the autosomes, not elsewhere classified	R36	Urethral discharge	R82	Other and unspecified abnormal findings in urine
Q95	Balanced rearrangements and structural markers, not elsewhere classified	R37	Sexual dysfunction, unspecified	R83	Abnormal findings in cerebrospinal fluid
Q96	Turner's syndrome	R39	Other and unspecified symptoms and signs involving the genitourinary system	R84	Abnormal findings in specimens from respiratory organs and thorax
Q97	Other sex chromosome abnormalities, female phenotype, not elsewhere classified	R40	Somnolence, stupor and coma	R85	Abnormal findings in specimens from digestive organs and abdominal cavity
Q98	Other sex chromosome abnormalities, male phenotype, not elsewhere classified	R41	Other symptoms and signs involving cognitive functions and awareness	R86	Abnormal findings in specimens from male genital organs

R00 — R99, etc.

CHAPTER 18: SYMPTOMS, SIGNS AND ABNORMAL CLINICAL AND LABORATORY FINDINGS, NOT ELSEWHERE CLASSIFIED (R00-R99)

R42 Dizziness and giddiness

R43 Disturbances of smell and taste

R87 Abnormal findings in specimens from female genital organs

R88 Abnormal findings in other body fluids and substances

R00 Abnormalities of heart beat

R44 Other symptoms and signs involving general sensations and perceptions

R89 Abnormal findings in specimens from other organs, systems and tissues

R01 Cardiac murmurs and other cardiac sounds

R45 Symptoms and signs involving emotional state

R90 Abnormal findings on diagnostic imaging of central nervous system

R03 Abnormal blood-pressure reading, without diagnosis

R46 Symptoms and signs involving appearance and behavior

R91 Abnormal findings on diagnostic imaging of lung

R04 Hemorrhage from respiratory passages

R47 Speech disturbances, not elsewhere classified

R92 Abnormal and inconclusive findings on diagnostic imaging of breast

R05 Cough

R48 Dyslexia and other symbolic dysfunctions, not elsewhere classified

R93 Abnormal findings on diagnostic imaging of other body structures

R06 Abnormalities of breathing

R49 Voice and resonance disorders

R94 Abnormal results of function studies

R07 Pain in throat and chest

R50 Fever of other and unknown origin

R97 Abnormal tumor markers

R09 Other symptoms and signs involving the circulatory and respiratory system

R51 Headache

R99 Ill-defined and unknown cause of mortality

R10 Abdominal and pelvic pain

R52 Pain, unspecified

R11 Nausea and vomiting

R53 Malaise and fatigue

R12 Heartburn

R54 Age-related physical debility

CHAPTER 19: INJURY, POISONING AND CERTAIN OTHER CONSEQUENCES OF EXTERNAL CAUSES (S00-T88)

R13 Aphagia and dysphagia

R55 Syncope and collapse

R14 Flatulence and related conditions

R56 Convulsions, not elsewhere classified

R15 Fecal incontinence

R57 Shock, not elsewhere classified

S00 Superficial injury of head

R16 Hepatomegaly and splenomegaly, not elsewhere classified

R58 Hemorrhage not elsewhere classified

S00 Insect bite (nonvenomous) of scalp, initial encounter

R17 Unspecified jaundice

R59 Enlarged lymph nodes

S01 Open wound of head

R18 Ascites

R60 Edema, not elsewhere classified

S02 Fracture of skull and facial bones

R19 Other symptoms and signs involving the digestive system and abdomen

R61 Generalized hyperhidrosis

S03 Dislocation and sprain of joints and ligaments of head

R20 Disturbances of skin sensation

R62 Lack of expected normal physiological development in childhood and adults

S04 Injury of cranial nerve

R21 Rash and other nonspecific skin eruption

R63 Symptoms and signs concerning food and fluid intake

S05 Injury of eye and orbit

R22 Localized swelling, mass and lump of skin and subcutaneous tissue

R64 Cachexia

S06 Intracranial injury

R23 Other skin changes

R65 Symptoms and signs specifically associated with systemic inflammation and infection

S07 Crushing injury of head

R25 Abnormal involuntary movements

S08 Avulsion and traumatic amputation of part of head

R26 Abnormalities of gait and mobility

R68 Other general symptoms and signs

S09 Other and unspecified injuries of head

R27 Other lack of coordination

R70 Elevated erythrocyte sedimentation rate and abnormality of plasma viscosity

S10 Superficial injury of neck

R29 Other symptoms and signs involving the nervous and musculoskeletal systems

R71 Abnormality of red blood cells

S10 Abrasion of unspecified part of neck, initial encounter

R30 Pain associated with micturition

R73 Elevated blood glucose level

S11 Open wound of neck

R31 Hematuria

R74 Abnormal serum enzyme levels

S12 Fracture of cervical vertebra and other parts of neck

R32 Unspecified urinary incontinence

R75 Inconclusive laboratory evidence of human immunodeficiency virus [HIV]

S13 Dislocation and sprain of joints and ligaments at neck level

R33 Retention of urine

R76 Other abnormal immunological findings in serum

S14 Injury of nerves and spinal cord at neck level

R34 Polyuria

R77 Other abnormalities of plasma proteins

S15 Injury of blood vessels at neck level

R35 Polyuria

R78 Findings of drugs and other substances, not normally found in blood

S16 Injury of muscle, fascia and tendon at neck level

R79 Other abnormal findings of blood chemistry

R80 Proteinuria

R81 Glycosuria

S17	Crushing injury of neck	**S49**	Other and unspecified injuries of shoulder and upper arm	**S89**	Other and unspecified injuries of lower leg
S19	Other specified and unspecified injuries of neck	**S50**	Superficial injury of elbow and forearm	**S90**	Superficial injury of ankle, foot and toes
S20	Superficial injury of thorax	**S51**	Open wound of elbow and forearm	**S91**	Open wound of ankle, foot and toes
S20	Abrasion of unspecified parts of thorax, initial encounter	**S52**	Fracture of forearm	**S92**	Fracture of foot and toe, except ankle
S21	Open wound of thorax	**S53**	Dislocation and sprain of joints and ligaments of elbow	**S93**	Dislocation and sprain of joints and ligaments at ankle, foot and toe level
S22	Fracture of rib(s), sternum and thoracic spine	**S54**	Injury of nerves at forearm level	**S93**	Dislocation and sprain of joints and ligaments at ankle, foot and toe
S23	Dislocation and sprain of joints and ligaments of thorax	**S55**	Injury of blood vessels at forearm level	**S94**	Injury of nerves at ankle and foot level
S24	Injury of nerves and spinal cord at thorax level	**S56**	Injury of muscle, fascia and tendon at forearm level	**S95**	Injury of blood vessels at ankle and foot level
S25	Injury of blood vessels of thorax	**S57**	Crushing injury of elbow and forearm	**S96**	Injury of muscle and tendon at ankle and foot level
S26	Injury of heart	**S58**	Traumatic amputation of elbow and forearm	**S97**	Crushing injury of ankle and foot
S27	Injury of other and unspecified intrathoracic organs	**S59**	Other and unspecified injuries of elbow and forearm	**S98**	Traumatic amputation of ankle and foot
S28	Crushing injury of thorax, and traumatic amputation of part of thorax	**S60**	Superficial injury of wrist, hand and fingers	**S99**	Other and unspecified injuries of ankle and foot
S29	Other and unspecified injuries of thorax	**S61**	Open wound of wrist, hand and fingers	**T07**	Unspecified multiple injuries
S30	Superficial injury of abdomen, lower back, pelvis and external genitals	**S62**	Fracture at wrist and hand level	**T14**	Injury of unspecified body region
				T15	Foreign body on external eye
S30	Blister (nonthermal) of lower back and pelvis, initial encounter	**S63**	Dislocation and sprain of joints and ligaments at wrist and hand level	**T16**	Foreign body in ear
S31	Open wound of abdomen, lower back, pelvis and external genitals	**S64**	Injury of nerves at wrist and hand level	**T17**	Foreign body in respiratory tract
				T18	Foreign body in alimentary tract
S32	Fracture of lumbar spine and pelvis	**S65**	Injury of blood vessels at wrist and hand level	**T19**	Foreign body in genitourinary tract
S33	Dislocation and sprain of joints and ligaments of lumbar spine and pelvis	**S66**	Injury of muscle, fascia and tendon at wrist and hand level	**T20**	Burn and corrosion of head, face, and neck
S34	Injury of lumbar and sacral spinal cord and nerves at abdomen, lower back and pelvis level	**S67**	Crushing injury of wrist, hand and fingers	**T21**	Burn and corrosion of trunk
		S68	Traumatic amputation of wrist, hand and fingers	**T22**	Burn and corrosion of shoulder and upper limb, except wrist and hand
S35	Injury of blood vessels at abdomen, lower back and pelvis level	**S69**	Other and unspecified injuries of wrist, hand and finger(s)	**T23**	Burn and corrosion of wrist and hand
S36	Injury of intra-abdominal organs	**S70**	Superficial injury of hip and thigh	**T24**	Burn and corrosion of lower limb, except ankle and foot
S36	Injury of intra-abdominal organs	**S71**	Open wound of hip and thigh	**T25**	Burn and corrosion of ankle and foot
S37	Injury of urinary and pelvic organs	**S72**	Fracture of femur	**T26**	Burn and corrosion confined to eye and adnexa
S38	Crushing injury and traumatic amputation of abdomen, lower back, pelvis and external genitals	**S73**	Dislocation and sprain of joint and ligaments of hip	**T27**	Burn and corrosion of respiratory tract
		S74	Injury of nerves at hip and thigh level	**T28**	Burn and corrosion of other internal organs
S39	Other and unspecified injuries of abdomen, lower back, pelvis and external genitals	**S75**	Injury of blood vessels at hip and thigh level	**T30**	Burn and corrosion, body region unspecified
		S76	Injury of muscle, fascia and tendon at hip and thigh level	**T31**	Burns classified according to extent of body surface involved
S40	Superficial injury of shoulder and upper arm	**S77**	Crushing injury of hip and thigh	**T32**	Corrosions classified according to extent of body surface involved
S41	Open wound of shoulder and upper arm	**S78**	Traumatic amputation of hip and thigh	**T33**	Superficial frostbite
S42	Fracture of shoulder and upper arm	**S79**	Other and unspecified injuries of hip and thigh	**T34**	Frostbite with tissue necrosis
S43	Dislocation and sprain of joints and ligaments of shoulder girdle	**S80**	Superficial injury of knee and lower leg	**T36**	Poisoning by, adverse effect of and underdosing of systemic antibiotics
S44	Injury of nerves at shoulder and upper arm level	**S81**	Open wound of knee and lower leg	**T37**	Poisoning by, adverse effect of and underdosing of other systemic anti-infectives and antiparasitics
S45	Injury of blood vessels at shoulder and upper arm level	**S82**	Fracture of lower leg, including ankle		
		S83	Dislocation and sprain of joints and ligaments of knee	**T38**	Poisoning by, adverse effect of and underdosing of hormones and their synthetic substitutes and antagonists, not elsewhere classified
S46	Injury of muscle, fascia and tendon at shoulder and upper arm level	**S84**	Injury of nerves at lower leg level		
S47	Crushing injury of shoulder and upper arm	**S85**	Injury of blood vessels at lower leg level		
S48	Traumatic amputation of shoulder and upper arm	**S86**	Injury of muscle, fascia and tendon at lower leg level	**T39**	Poisoning by, adverse effect of and underdosing of nonopioid analgesics, antipyretics and antirheumatics
		S87	Crushing injury of lower leg		
		S88	Traumatic amputation of lower leg		

T40 Poisoning by, adverse effect of and underdosing of narcotics and psychodysleptics [hallucinogens]

T41 Poisoning by, adverse effect of and underdosing of anesthetics and therapeutic gases

T42 Poisoning by, adverse effect of and underdosing of antiepileptic, sedative-hypnotic and antiparkinsonism drugs

T43 Poisoning by, adverse effect of and underdosing of psychotropic drugs, not elsewhere classified

T44 Poisoning by, adverse effect of and underdosing of drugs primarily affecting the autonomic nervous system

T45 Poisoning by, adverse effect of and underdosing of primarily systemic and hematological agents, not elsewhere classified

T46 Poisoning by, adverse effect of and underdosing of agents primarily affecting the cardiovascular system

T47 Poisoning by, adverse effect of and underdosing of agents primarily affecting the gastrointestinal system

T48 Poisoning by, adverse effect of and underdosing of agents primarily acting on smooth and skeletal muscles and the respiratory system

T49 Poisoning by, adverse effect of and underdosing of topical agents primarily affecting skin and mucous membrane and by ophthalmological, otorhinolaryngological and dental drugs

T50 Poisoning by, adverse effect of and underdosing of diuretics and other and unspecified drugs, medicaments and biological substances

T51 Toxic effect of alcohol

T52 Toxic effect of organic solvents

T53 Toxic effect of halogen derivatives of aliphatic and aromatic hydrocarbons

T54 Toxic effect of corrosive substances

T55 Toxic effect of soaps and detergents

T56 Toxic effect of metals

T57 Toxic effect of other inorganic substances

T58 Toxic effect of carbon monoxide

T59 Toxic effect of other gases, fumes and vapors

T60 Toxic effect of pesticides

T61 Toxic effect of noxious substances eaten as seafood

T62 Toxic effect of other noxious substances eaten as food

T63 Toxic effect of contact with venomous animals and plants

T64 Toxic effect of aflatoxin and other mycotoxin food contaminants

T65 Toxic effect of other and unspecified substances

T66 Radiation sickness, unspecified

T67 Effects of heat and light

T68 Hypothermia

T69 Other effects of reduced temperature

T70 Effects of air pressure and water pressure

T71 Asphyxiation

T73 Effects of other deprivation

T74 Adult and child abuse, neglect and other maltreatment, confirmed

T75 Other and unspecified effects of other external causes

T76 Adult and child abuse, neglect and other maltreatment, suspected

T78 Adverse effects, not elsewhere classified

T79 Certain early complications of trauma, not elsewhere classified

T80 Complications following infusion, transfusion and therapeutic injection

T81 Complications of procedures, not elsewhere classified

T82 Complications of cardiac and vascular prosthetic devices, implants and grafts

T83 Complications of genitourinary prosthetic devices, implants and grafts

T84 Complications of internal orthopedic prosthetic devices, implants and grafts

T85 Complications of other internal prosthetic devices, implants and grafts

T86 Complications of transplanted organs and tissue

T87 Complications peculiar to reattachment and amputation

T88 Other complications of surgical and medical care, not elsewhere classified

CHAPTER 20: EXTERNAL CAUSES OF MORBIDITY (V00-Y99)

V00 Pedestrian conveyance accident

V01 Pedestrian injured in collision with pedal cycle

V03 Pedestrian injured in collision with car, pick-up truck or van

V05 Pedestrian injured in collision with railway train or railway vehicle

V06 Pedestrian injured in collision with other nonmotor vehicle

V09 Pedestrian injured in other and unspecified transport accidents

V10 Pedal cycle rider injured in collision with pedestrian or animal

V13 Pedal cycle rider injured in collision with car, pick-up truck or van

V15 Pedal cycle rider injured in collision with railway train or railway vehicle

V17 Pedal cycle rider injured in collision with fixed or stationary object

V18 Pedal cycle rider injured in noncollision transport accident

V19 Pedal cycle rider injured in other and unspecified transport accidents

V20 Motorcycle rider injured in collision with pedestrian or animal

V21 Motorcycle rider injured in collision with pedal cycle

V23 Motorcycle rider injured in collision with car, pick-up truck or van

V25 Motorcycle rider injured in collision with railway train or railway vehicle

V26 Motorcycle rider injured in collision with other nonmotor vehicle

V27 Motorcycle rider injured in collision with fixed or stationary object

V28 Motorcycle rider injured in noncollision transport accident

V29 Motorcycle rider injured in other and unspecified transport accidents

V40 Car occupant injured in collision with pedestrian or animal

V43 Car occupant injured in collision with car, pick-up truck or van

V45 Car occupant injured in collision with railway train or railway vehicle

V46 Car occupant injured in collision with other nonmotor vehicle

V47 Car occupant injured in collision with fixed or stationary object

V48 Car occupant injured in noncollision transport accident

V49 Car occupant injured in other and unspecified transport accidents

V57 Occupant of pick-up truck or van injured in collision with fixed or stationary object

V58 Occupant of pick-up truck or van injured in noncollision transport accident

V59 Occupant of pick-up truck or van injured in other and unspecified transport accidents

V69 Occupant of heavy transport vehicle injured in other and unspecified transport accidents

V78 Bus occupant injured in noncollision transport accident

V80 Animal-rider or occupant of animal-drawn vehicle injured in transport accident

V81 Occupant of railway train or railway vehicle injured in transport accident

V82 Occupant of powered streetcar injured in transport accident

V83 Occupant of special vehicle mainly used on industrial premises injured in transport accident

V86 Occupant of special all-terrain or other off-road motor vehicle, injured in transport accident

V87 Traffic accident of specified type but victim's mode of transport unknown

V88 Nontraffic accident of specified type but victim's mode of transport unknown

V89	Motor- or nonmotor-vehicle accident, type of vehicle unspecified
V90	Drowning and submersion due to accident to watercraft
V91	Other injury due to accident to watercraft
V92	Drowning and submersion due to accident on board watercraft, without accident to watercraft
V93	Other injury due to accident on board watercraft, without accident to watercraft
V94	Other and unspecified water transport accidents
V95	Accident to powered aircraft causing injury to occupant
V96	Accident to nonpowered aircraft causing injury to occupant
V97	Other specified air transport accidents
V98	Other specified transport accidents
V99	Unspecified transport accident
W01	Fall on same level from slipping, tripping and stumbling
W03	Other fall on same level due to collision with another person
W05	Fall from non-moving wheelchair, nonmotorized scooter and motorized mobility scooter
W06	Fall from bed
W07	Fall from chair
W08	Fall from other furniture
W09	Fall on and from playground equipment
W10	Fall on and from stairs and steps
W11	Fall on and from ladder
W12	Fall on and from scaffolding
W13	Fall from, out of or through building or structure
W14	Fall from tree
W15	Fall from cliff
W16	Fall, jump or diving into water
W17	Other fall from one level to another
W18	Other slipping, tripping and stumbling and falls
W19	Unspecified fall
W20	Struck by thrown, projected or falling object
W21	Striking against or struck by sports equipment
W22	Striking against or struck by other objects
W23	Caught, crushed, jammed or pinched in or between objects
W24	Contact with lifting and transmission devices, not elsewhere classified
W26	Contact with knife, sword or dagger
W27	Contact with nonpowered hand tool
W28	Contact with powered lawn mower
W29	Contact with other powered hand tools and household machinery

W30	Contact with agricultural machinery
W31	Contact with other and unspecified machinery
W32	Accidental handgun discharge and malfunction
W33	Accidental rifle, shotgun and larger firearm discharge and malfunction
W34	Accidental discharge and malfunction from other and unspecified firearms and guns
W35	Explosion and rupture of boiler
W36	Explosion and rupture of gas cylinder
W38	Explosion and rupture of other specified pressurized devices
W39	Discharge of firework
W40	Explosion of other materials
W42	Exposure to noise
W45	Foreign body or object entering through skin
W46	Contact with hypodermic needle
W49	Exposure to other inanimate mechanical forces
W50	Accidental hit, strike, kick, twist, bite or scratch by another person
W51	Accidental striking against or bumped into by another person
W52	Crushed, pushed or stepped on by crowd or human stampede
W53	Contact with rodent
W54	Contact with dog
W55	Contact with other mammals
W57	Bitten or stung by nonvenomous insect and other nonvenomous arthropods
W59	Contact with other nonvenomous reptiles
W64	Exposure to other animate mechanical forces
W65	Accidental drowning and submersion while in bath-tub
W67	Accidental drowning and submersion while in swimming-pool
W69	Accidental drowning and submersion while in natural water
W74	Unspecified cause of accidental drowning and submersion
W85	Exposure to electric transmission lines
W86	Exposure to other specified electric current
W88	Exposure to ionizing radiation
W89	Exposure to man-made visible and ultraviolet light
W90	Exposure to other nonionizing radiation
W92	Exposure to excessive heat of man-made origin
W93	Exposure to excessive cold of man-made origin
W94	Exposure to high and low air pressure and changes in air pressure

W99	Exposure to other man-made environmental factors
X00	Exposure to uncontrolled fire in building or structure
X01	Exposure to uncontrolled fire, not in building or structure
X02	Exposure to controlled fire in building or structure
X03	Exposure to controlled fire, not in building or structure
X04	Exposure to ignition of highly flammable material
X05	Exposure to ignition or melting of nightwear
X06	Exposure to ignition or melting of other clothing and apparel
X08	Exposure to other specified smoke, fire and flames
X11	Contact with hot tap-water
X12	Contact with other hot fluids
X19	Contact with other heat and hot substances
X30	Exposure to excessive natural heat
X31	Exposure to excessive natural cold
X34	Earthquake
X35	Volcanic eruption
X36	Avalanche, landslide and other earth movements
X37	Cataclysmic storm
X38	Flood
X39	Exposure to other forces of nature
X50	Overexertion and strenuous or repetitive movements
X52	Prolonged stay in weightless environment
X58	Exposure to other specified factors
X71	Intentional self-harm by drowning and submersion
X72	Intentional self-harm by handgun discharge
X73	Intentional self-harm by rifle, shotgun and larger firearm discharge
X74	Intentional self-harm by other and unspecified firearm and gun discharge
X75	Intentional self-harm by explosive material
X76	Intentional self-harm by smoke, fire and flames
X77	Intentional self-harm by steam, hot vapors and hot objects
X78	Intentional self-harm by sharp object
X80	Intentional self-harm by jumping from a high place
X81	Intentional self-harm by jumping or lying in front of moving object
X82	Intentional self-harm by crashing of motor vehicle
X83	Intentional self-harm by other specified means

X92 Assault by drowning and submersion

X93 Assault by handgun discharge

X94 Assault by rifle, shotgun and larger firearm discharge

X95 Assault by other and unspecified firearm and gun discharge

X96 Assault by explosive material

X97 Assault by smoke, fire and flames

X98 Assault by steam, hot vapors and hot objects

X99 Assault by sharp object

Y00 Assault by blunt object

Y01 Assault by pushing from high place

Y02 Assault by pushing or placing victim in front of moving object

Y03 Assault by crashing of motor vehicle

Y04 Assault by bodily force

Y07 Perpetrator of assault, maltreatment and neglect

Y08 Assault by other specified means

Y09 Assault by unspecified means

Y22 Handgun discharge, undetermined intent

Y23 Rifle, shotgun and larger firearm discharge, undetermined intent

Y24 Other and unspecified firearm discharge, undetermined intent

Y25 Contact with explosive material, undetermined intent

Y26 Exposure to smoke, fire and flames, undetermined intent

Y27 Contact with steam, hot vapors and hot objects, undetermined intent

Y28 Contact with sharp object, undetermined intent

Y30 Falling, jumping or pushed from a high place, undetermined intent

Y31 Falling, lying or running before or into moving object, undetermined intent

Y32 Crashing of motor vehicle, undetermined intent

Y33 Other specified events, undetermined intent

Y35 Legal intervention

Y36 Operations of war

Y38 Terrorism

Y62 Failure of sterile precautions during surgical and medical care

Y63 Failure in dosage during surgical and medical care

Y64 Contaminated medical or biological substances

Y65 Other misadventures during surgical and medical care

Y69 Unspecified misadventure during surgical and medical care

Y83 Surgical operation and other surgical procedures as the cause of abnormal reaction of the patient, or of later

Y84 Other medical procedures as the cause of abnormal reaction of the patient, or of later complication, without

Y92 Place of occurrence of the external cause

Y93 Activity codes

Y99 External cause status

CHAPTER 21: FACTORS INFLUENCING HEALTH STATUS AND CONTACT WITH HEALTH SERVICES (Z00-Z99)

Z00 Encounter for general examination without complaint, suspected or reported diagnosis

Z01 Encounter for other special examination without complaint, suspected or reported diagnosis

Z02 Encounter for administrative examination

Z03 Encounter for medical observation for suspected diseases and conditions ruled out

Z04 Encounter for examination and observation for other reasons

Z05 Encounter for observation and evaluation of newborn for suspected diseases and conditions ruled out

Z08 Encounter for follow-up examination after completed treatment for malignant neoplasm

Z09 Encounter for follow-up examination after completed treatment for conditions other than malignant neoplasm

Z11 Encounter for screening for infectious and parasitic diseases

Z12 Encounter for screening for malignant neoplasms

Z13 Encounter for screening for other diseases and disorders

Z14 Genetic carrier

Z15 Genetic susceptibility to disease

Z16 Resistance to antimicrobial drugs

Z17 Estrogen receptor status

Z18 Retained foreign body fragments

Z19 Hormone sensitivity malignancy status

Z20 Contact with and (suspected) exposure to communicable diseases

Z21 Asymptomatic human immunodeficiency virus [HIV] infection status

Z22 Carrier of infectious disease

Z23 Encounter for immunization

Z28 Immunization not carried out and underimmunization status

Z29 Encounter for other prophylactic measures

Z30 Encounter for contraceptive management

Z31 Encounter for procreative management

Z32 Encounter for pregnancy test and childbirth and childcare instruction

Z33 Pregnant state

Z34 Encounter for supervision of normal pregnancy

Z36 Encounter for antenatal screening of mother

Z37 Outcome of delivery

Z38 Liveborn infants according to place of birth and type of delivery

Z39 Encounter for maternal postpartum care and examination

Z3A Weeks of gestation

Z40 Encounter for prophylactic surgery

Z41 Encounter for procedures for purposes other than remedying health state

Z42 Encounter for plastic and reconstructive surgery following medical procedure

Z43 Encounter for attention to artificial openings

Z44 Encounter for fitting and adjustment of external prosthetic device

Z45 Encounter for adjustment and management of implanted device

Z46 Encounter for fitting and adjustment of other devices

Z47 Orthopedic aftercare

Z48 Encounter for other postprocedural aftercare

Z49 Encounter for attention to artificial openings

Z51 Encounter for other aftercare and medical care

Z52 Donors of organs and tissues

Z53 Persons encountering health services for specific procedures and treatment, not carried out

Z55 Problems related to education and literacy

Z56 Problems related to employment and unemployment

Z57 Occupational exposure to risk factors

Z59 Problems related to housing and economic circumstances

Z60 Problems related to social environment

Z62 Problems related to upbringing

Z63 Other problems related to primary support group, including family circumstances

Z64 Problems related to certain psychosocial circumstances

Z65 Problems related to other psychosocial services

Z65 Problems related to other psychosocial circumstances

Z68 Body mass index [BMI]

Z69 Encounter for mental health services for victim and perpetrator of abuse

Z70 Counseling related to sexual attitude, behavior and orientation

Z71 Persons encountering health services for other counseling and medical advice, not elsewhere classified

Z72 Problems related to lifestyle

Z73 Problems related to life management difficulty

Z74 Problems related to care provider dependency

Z75 Problems related to medical facilities and other health care

Z76 Persons encountering health services in other circumstances

Z77 Other contact with and (suspected) exposures hazardous to health

Z78 Other specified health status

Z79 Long term (current) drug therapy

Z80 Family history of primary malignant neoplasm

Z81 Family history of mental and behavioral disorders

Z82 Family history of certain disabilities and chronic diseases (leading to disablement)

Z83 Family history of other specific disorders

Z84 Family history of other conditions

Z85 Personal history of malignant neoplasm

Z86 Personal history of certain other diseases

Z87 Personal history of other diseases and conditions

Z88 Allergy status to drugs, medicaments and biological substances

Z89 Acquired absence of limb

Z90 Acquired absence of organs, not elsewhere classified

Z91 Personal risk factors, not elsewhere classified

Z92 Personal history of medical treatment

Z93 Artificial opening status

Z94 Transplanted organ and tissue status

Z95 Presence of cardiac and vascular implants and grafts

Z96 Presence of other functional implants

Z97 Presence of other devices

Z98 Other postprocedural states

Z99 Dependence on enabling machines and devices, not elsewhere classified